DeLisa's

Physical Medicine and Rehabilitation

PRINCIPLES AND PRACTICE

SIXTH EDITION

DeLisa's

Physical Medicine and Rehabilitation

PRINCIPLES AND PRACTICE

SIXTH EDITION

EDITOR-IN-CHIEF

Walter R. Frontera, MD, PhD, MA (Hon.), FRCP (Lond.)
Professor
Department of Physical Medicine, Rehabilitation, and Sports Medicine
Department of Physiology and Biophysics
University of Puerto Rico School of Medicine
San Juan, Puerto Rico

EDITOR EMERITUS

Joel A. DeLisa, MD, MS
Emeritus Professor
Department of Physical Medicine & Rehabilitation
Rutgers New Jersey Medical School
Newark, New Jersey
Clinical Professor
Department of Neurosurgery and Physical Medicine and Rehabilitation
University of New Mexico School of Medicine
Albuquerque, New Mexico
Clinical Professor
Department of Medical Education & Clinical Sciences
Elson S. College of Medicine
Washington State University
Spokane, Washington

EDITORS

Jeffrey R. Basford, MD, PhD
Professor
Department of Physical Medicine and Rehabilitation
Mayo Clinic
Rochester, Minnesota

William L. Bockenek, MD
Professor
Department of Physical Medicine and Rehabilitation
Carolinas Medical Center/Atrium Health
Chair of PMR, Chief Medical Officer
Carolinas Rehabilitation
Charlotte, North Carolina

John Chae, MD
Professor and Chair
Physical Medicine & Rehabilitation
Case Western Reserve University
Vice President, Research and Sponsored Programs
MetroHealth Research Institute
MetroHealth System
Cleveland, Ohio

Lawrence R. Robinson, MD
Professor and Chief, PM&R
Department of Medicine
University of Toronto
Chief, Rehabilitation
St. John's Rehab
Sunnybrook Health Sciences Centre
Toronto, Ontario, Canada

ASSOCIATE EDITORS

Michael L. Boninger, MD
Joanne Borg-Stein, MD
Gregory T. Carter, MD, MS

Leighton Chan, MD, MPH
Gerard E. Francisco, MD
Helen Hoenig, MD, MPH

Alan M. Jette, PhD, PT
Heidi Prather, DO

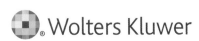

Philadelphia • Baltimore • New York • London
Buenos Aires • Hong Kong • Sydney • Tokyo

Acquisitions Editor: Robin Najar
Development Editor: Ashley Fischer
Editorial Coordinator: Emily Buccieri
Production Project Manager: David Saltzberg
Design Coordinator: Joan Wendt, Joseph Clark
Manufacturing Coordinator: Beth Welsh
Prepress Vendor: SPi Global

6th edition

Copyright © 2020 Wolters Kluwer

Library of Congress Cataloging-in-Publication Data

Names: Frontera, Walter R., 1955- editor.
Title: DeLisa's physical medicine and rehabilitation : principles and practice / editor-in-chief, Walter R. Frontera ; editor emeritus, Joel A. DeLisa ; editors, Jeffrey Basford, William Bockenek, John Chae, Lawrence R. Robinson ; associate editors, Michael Boninger, Joanne Borg-Stein, Gregory T. Carter, Leighton Chan, Gerard Francisco, Helen Hoenig, Alan Jette, Heidi Prather.
Other titles: DeLisa's Physical medicine and rehabilitation | Physical medicine & rehabilitation | Physical medicine and rehabilitation
Description: Sixth edition. | Philadelphia : Wolters Kluwer, [2020] | Includes bibliographical references and index.
Identifiers: LCCN 2019003514 | ISBN 9781496374967
Subjects: | MESH: Physical and Rehabilitation Medicine—methods | Rehabilitation
Classification: LCC RM930 | NLM WB 320 | DDC 615.8/2—dc23 LC record available at https://lccn.loc.gov/2019003514

To Our Patients
*who inspire us to continually strive to improve their health,
function, and quality of life*

To Our Teachers
*who encouraged us to develop a scientific approach to medicine
and instilled in us the need for continuous learning*

To Our Students
*who challenge and stimulate us to stay at the cutting edge;
they are our hope for the future*

To Our Colleagues
*who have gone before us, who are with us
and who will follow us*

To Our Families
who provided the support and patience necessary

CONTENTS

PART V

Major Conditions: General Rehabilitation

PART VI

Secondary Conditions and Complications

PART VII

Special Populations

PART VIII

Management Methods

PART IX

Scientific Advances

Sally B. Alcott, MD
Senior Associate Consultant
Department of Physical Medicine & Rehabilitation
Mayo Clinic
Scottsdale/Phoenix, Arizona
Medical Director
Inpatient Rehabilitation Facility
Mayo Clinic
Phoenix, Arizona
Medical Director
Geriatric Residency, Physical Therapy Residency
   Program
Mayo Clinic
School of Health Sciences
Scottsdale/Phoenix, Arizona

Marcalee S. Alexander, MD
Clinical Professor of PM&R
Department of Physical Medicine and
   Rehabilitation
School of Medicine
University of Alabama
Birmingham, Alabama

Shruti Amin, MD
Resident Physician
Texas Tech University Health Sciences Center
El Paso, Texas

Prin Amorapanth, MD, PhD
Assistant Professor
Department of Rehabilitation Medicine
NYU Langone Physical Medicine and
   Rehabilitation Associates
New York, New York

Karen L. Andrews, MD
Associate Professor of Physical Medicine and
   Rehabilitation
College of Medicine and Science
Mayo Clinic
Director, Amputee Rehabilitation Services
Director, Vascular Ulcer/Wound Healing Center
Physical Medicine and Rehabilitation Gonda
   Vascular Center
Mayo Clinic
Rochester, Minnesota

Thiru M. Annaswamy, MD, MA
Professor
Physical Medicine and Rehabilitation
University of Texas Southwestern Medical Center
Staff Physician and Section Chief
VA North Texas Health Care System/Dallas VA
   Medical Center
Dallas, Texas

John R. Bach, MD
Professor of PM&R
Department of Physical Medicine & Rehabilitation
Professor of Neurology
Department of Neurology
Rutgers University New Jersey Medical School
Director
Center for Ventilatory Management Alternatives
   and Pulmonary Rehabilitation
University Hospital
Newark, New Jersey

Patrick J. Bachoura, MD
Physician Intern
Pediatric Medicine
LAC-USC
Los Angeles, California
Resident Physician
Family Medicine
Presbyterian Intercommunity Hospital
Whittier, California

Luis Baerga-Varela, MD
Assistant Professor
Department of Physical Medicine and
   Rehabilitation
University of Puerto Rico Medical School
San Juan, Puerto Rico

Christopher H. Bailey, MD
Fellow, Pain Medicine
Department of Anesthesiology
Mayo Clinic Arizona
Phoenix, Arizona

Matthew T. Santa Barbara, MD
Resident Physician
Physical Medicine & Rehabilitation
University of Pittsburgh Medical Center
Pittsburgh, Pennsylvania

Matthew N. Bartels, MD, MPH
Professor and Chairman
Department of Rehabilitation Medicine
Albert Einstein College of Medicine
Attending and Chairman
Montefiore Health System
Bronx, New York

Jeffrey R. Basford, MD, PhD
Professor
Department of Physical Medicine and
   Rehabilitation
Mayo Clinic
Rochester, Minnesota

Carolyn M. Baum, PhD, OTR/L, FAOTA
Elias Michael Director and Professor of
   Occupational Therapy, Neurology and Social
   Work
Program in Occupational Therapy
School of Medicine
Washington University
St. Louis, Missouri

**G. David Baxter, TD, BSc (Hons), DPhil,
MBA**
Professor
Centre for Health, Activity, and Rehabilitation
   Research
University of Otago
Dunedin, Otago, New Zealand

Bruce E. Becker, MD, MS
Clinical Professor
Department of Rehabilitation Medicine
University of Washington School of Medicine
Seattle, Washington

Abrahm J. Behnam, MD, MS
Resident Physician
Department of Anesthesiology and Perioperative
   Medicine
Penn State College of Medicine
Penn State Health Milton S. Hershey Medical
   Center
Hershey, Pennsylvania

Jessica B. Berry, MD
Assistant Professor
Physical Medicine and Rehabilitation
University of Pittsburgh
Medical Director of Stroke Rehabilitation
UPMC Mercy
Pittsburgh, Pennsylvania

Francois A. Bethoux, MD
Professor of Medicine
Cleveland Clinic Lerner College of Medicine of
   Case Western Reserve University
Associate Staff
Neurological Institute/Mellen Center
   for MS
Cleveland Clinic
Cleveland, Ohio

Jerome Bickenbach, LLB, PhD
Professor
Health Science & Health Policy
Lucerne University
Lucerne, Switzerland
Head
Disability Policy Group
Swiss Paraplegic Research
Nottwil, Switzerland

Cheri A. Blauwet, MD
Assistant Professor
Department of Physical Medicine and
   Rehabilitation
Harvard Medical School
Charlestown, Massachusetts
Chair, Medical Committee
International Paralympic Committee
Bonn, Germany

Cathy Bodine, PhD, CCC-SLP
Associate Professor
Bioengineering, Orthopedics, Pediatrics and
   Physical Medicine and Rehabilitation
University of Colorado
Denver, Colorado

Michael L. Boninger, MD
UPMC Endow Professor and Vice Chair for
   Research
Physical Medicine & Rehabilitation
University of Pittsburgh
Physician Researcher
Human Engineer Research Laboratory
VA Pittsburgh Health Care System
Pittsburgh, Pennsylvania

Joanne Borg-Stein, MD
Associate Professor and Associate Chair
Chief, Division of Sports and Musculoskeletal
    Rehabilitation
Associate Director, Harvard/Spaulding Sports
    Medicine Fellowship
Department of Physical Medicine and Rehabilitation
Harvard Medical School
Wellesley, Massachusetts

Steven W. Brose, DO
Chief, Spinal Cord Injury and Disorders Service
Physical Rehabilitation
Syracuse VA Medical Center
Syracuse, New York

Morgan Brubaker, DO
Assistant Clinical Professor
Physical Medicine & Rehabilitation
University of Colorado School of Medicine
Office of the Dean
Aurora, Colorado
Attending Physician
Craig Hospital
Englewood, Colorado

Luis R. Burgos-Anaya, MD, DABR
Musculoskeletal Radiologist
Department of Diagnostic Radiology
Hospital Pavia Santurce
San Juan, Puerto Rico

**Ian D. Cameron, MBBS, PhD (Med),
FAFRM (RACP)**
Professor of Rehabilitation Medicine
John Walsh Centre for Rehabilitation Research
Kolling Institute
Faculty of Medicine and Health
University of Sydney
St Leonards, New South Wales, Australia
Senior Staff Specialist
Division of Rehabilitation and Aged Care
Hornsby Ku-ring-gai Health Service and
    Southern NSW Local Health District
Hornsby, New South Wales, Australia

Gregory T. Carter, MD, MS
Chief Medical Officer
St. Lukes Rehabilitation Institute
Clinical Professor
Elson S Floyd College of Medicine
Washington State University RiverPoint Campus
Spokane, Washington

Sara E. Cartwright, MD
Fellow
Physical Medicine & Rehabilitation
University of Cincinnati
Cincinnati Children's Hospital
Cincinnati, Ohio

John Chae, MD
Professor and Chair
Physical Medicine & Rehabilitation
Case Western Reserve University
Vice President, Research and Sponsored Programs
MetroHealth Research Institute
MetroHealth System
Cleveland, Ohio

Lauren A. Chambers, DO
Resident
Department of Physical Medicine and Rehabilitation
Carolinas Rehabilitation
Charlotte, North Carolina

Leighton Chan, MD, MPH
Chief
Rehabilitation Medicine Department
National Institutes of Health
Bethesda, Maryland

Shuo-Hsiu (James) Chang, PT, PhD
Assistant Professor
Department of Physical Medicine and
    Rehabilitation
McGovern Medical School
The University of Texas Health Science Center
    at Houston
Administrative Director of The NeuroRecovery
    Research Center
TIRR Memorial Hermann
Houston, Texas

Eric T. Chen, MD
Resident Physician
Department of Rehabilitation Medicine
University of Washington
Seattle, Washington

Yi-Pin Chiang, MD, PhD
Assistant Professor
Department of Medicine
Mackay Medical College
New Taipei City, Taiwan
Director
Department of Rehabilitation Medicine
MacKay Memorial Hospital
Taipei City, Taiwan

David A. DeLambo, RhD
Professor
Department of Rehabilitation and Counseling
University of Wisconsin–Stout
Menomonie, Wisconsin

Armen G. Derian, MD
Interventional Pain Fellow
Division of Pain Medicine
Department of Anesthesiology
Mayo Clinic Arizona
Phoenix, Arizona

Harmeet S. Dhani, MD, MSc
Resident Physician
Department of Surgery
The George Washington University
Washington, District of Columbia

Sabrina Donzelli, MD
Expert Clinician and Researcher
ISICO (Italian Scientific Spine Institute)
Milan, Italy

Alberto Esquenazi, MD
Chair and Professor of PM&R
Director, Gait & Motion Analysis Laboratory
MossRehab and Einstein Healthcare Network
Elkins Park, Pennsylvania

Marlís González Fernández, MD, PhD
Associate Professor, Vice Chair, Clinical Affairs
Department of Physical Medicine and
    Rehabilitation
Johns Hopkins University School of Medicine
Managing Director of Outpatient Rehabilitation
    Services
Johns Hopkins Rehabilitation Network
Johns Hopkins Medicine
Baltimore, Maryland

Nicholas P. Fey, PhD
Assistant Professor
Department of Bioengineering
The University of Texas at Dallas
Richardson, Texas
Department of Physical Medicine and Rehabilitation
UT Southwestern Medical Center
Dallas, Texas

Steve R. Fisher, PT, PhD, GCS
Associate Professor
Department of Physical Therapy
School of Health Professions
University of Texas Medical Branch
Galveston, Texas

Steven R. Flanagan, MD
Professor and Chair
Department of Rehabilitation Medicine
New York University School of Medicine
Medical Director of Rusk Rehabilitation
New York University Langone Health
New York, New York

Gerard E. Francisco, MD
Professor and Chair
Physical Medicine and Rehabilitation
McGovern Medical School
The University of Texas Health Science Center
Chief Medical Officer and Director of
    The NeuroRecovery Research Center
TIRR Memorial Hermann
Houston, Texas

John A. Freeman, MD
Assistant Professor of Anesthesiology and
    Physical Medicine & Rehabilitation
Department of Anesthesiology
Consultant and Chair
Division of Pain Medicine
Mayo Clinic Arizona
Phoenix, Arizona

**Walter R. Frontera, MD, PhD, MA (Hon.),
FRCP**
Professor
Department of Physical Medicine,
    Rehabilitation, and Sports Medicine
Department of Physiology and Biophysics
University of Puerto Rico School of Medicine
San Juan, Puerto Rico

Adrielle L. Fry, MD
Evergreen Sport and Spine Care
EvergreenHealth
Kirkland, Washington

Andrea Dompieri Furlan, MD, PhD
Assistant Professor
Department of Medicine
University of Toronto
Senior Scientist
Toronto Rehabilitation Institute
University Health Network
Toronto, Ontario, Canada

Heidi N. Fusco, MD
Assistant Professor
Department of Rehabilitation Medicine
Rusk Rehabilitation Hospital and NYU Langone
    Medical Center
Medical Director
Brain Injury Unit
Queens Nassau Nursing and Rehabilitation Center
New York, New York

Chan Gao, MD, PhD
Resident Physician
Department of Physical Medicine and
    Rehabilitation
Vanderbilt University Medical Center
Nashville, Tennessee

Russell Gelfman, MD
Assistant Professor of Physical Medicine and
    Rehabilitation
College of Medicine and Science
Mayo Clinic
Consultant
Mayo Clinic
Rochester, Minnesota

Lynn H. Gerber, MD
University Professor
Health Administration and Policy
George Mason University
Fairfax, Virginia
Director for Research, Medicine
Fairfax Medical Campus, Inova Health
Falls Church, Virginia

Francesca Gimigliano, MD, PhD
Associate Professor
Department of Mental and Physical Health and
    Preventive Medicine
University of Campania "Luigi Vanvitelli"
Napoli, Italy

Mario Giraldo-Prieto, MD
Researcher
Departamento de Medicina Física y
    Rehabilitación
University of Antioquia
Medellín, Antioquia, Colombia

James E. Graham, PhD, DC
Professor
Department of Occupational Therapy
Colorado State University
Fort Collins, Colorado

Stephen P. Gulley, PhD, MSW
Lecturer
Heller School, Health, Science, Society and
    Policy Program
Brandeis University
Waltham, Massachusetts
Research Associate
Rehabilitation Medicine Department
National Institutes of Health, Mark O. Hatfield
    Clinical Research Center
Bethesda, Maryland

Janet F. Haas, MD
Physician
Department of Medicine
Pennsylvania Hospital
Philadelphia, Pennsylvania

Andrew J. Haig, MD
Professor Emeritus
Physical Medicine & Rehabilitation
University of Michigan
Williston, Vermont

Jay J. Han, MD
Professor and Vice Chair
Department of Physical Medicine &
    Rehabilitation
School of Medicine
University of California, Irvine
Orange, California

Thida Han, PsyD, LP
Psychologist
Courage Kenny Psychological Associates
Courage Kenny Rehabilitation Institute at
    United Hospital
Saint Paul, Minnesota

Kathryn Ann Hansen, MSN, ANP-BC
Director of Clinical Operations
Osher Center for Integrative Medicine at Vanderbilt
Department of Physical Medicine and
    Rehabilitation
Vanderbilt University School of Nursing
Nashville, Tennessee

Pamela Hansen, MD
Associate Professor
Physical Medicine & Rehabilitation
University of Utah, Health
Salt Lake City, Utah

Amanda L. Harrington, MD
Assistant Professor
Physical Medicine and Rehabilitation
University of Pittsburgh
Director of Spinal Cord Injury Services
UPMC Mercy
Pittsburgh, Pennsylvania

Anne L. Hart, PT, PhD
Associate Professor
Department of Physical Therapy and Athlete
    Training
Northern Arizona University
Flagstaff, Arizona
Chair, Classification Committee
International Paralympic Committee
Bonn, Germany

Allen W. Heinemann, PhD
Professor
Department of Physical Medicine and
    Rehabilitation
Northwestern University
Director
Center for Rehabilitation Outcomes Research
Shirley Ryan AbilityLab
Chicago, Illinois

Marni G. Hillinger, MD
Integrative Physiatrist
Scripps Center for Integrative Medicine
Scripps Health
La Jolla, California

Mark A. Hirsch, PhD
Director of Residency Research Education
Department of PM&R
Carolinas Medical Center
Senior Scientist
Carolinas Rehabilitation
Charlotte, North Carolina

Helen Hoenig, MD, MPH
Professor, Division of Geriatrics
Department of Medicine
Duke University Medical Center
Chief
Physical Medicine & Rehabilitation Service
Durham VA Health Care System
Durham, North Carolina

Debra B. Homa, PhD
Professor
Department of Rehabilitation and Counseling
University of Wisconsin–Stout
Menomonie, Wisconsin

Matthew T. Houdek, MD
Assistant Professor, Senior Associate Consultant
Orthopedic Surgery
Mayo Clinic
Rochester, Minnesota

Ileana Michelle Howard, MD
Clinical Associate Professor
Rehabilitation Medicine
University of Washington
Outpatient Medical Director
Rehabilitation Care Services
VA Puget Sound Healthcare System
Seattle, Washington

Lisa Huynh, MD
Clinical Assistant Professor
Physical Medicine and Rehabilitation Section
Department of Orthopaedics
Stanford University
Redwood City, California

Brian S. Im, MD
Assistant Professor
Physical Medicine & Rehabilitation
New York University
Director of Brain Injury Rehabilitation
New York University Langone Medical Center
New York, New York

Didem Inanoglu, MD
Associate Professor
Department of Physical Medicine and
    Rehabilitation
University of Texas Southwestern Medical
    Center
Director, Fellowship Program
Pediatric Rehabilitation Medicine
Children's Health System of Texas
Dallas, Texas

Nitin B. Jain, MD, MSPH
Associate Professor
Department of Physical Medicine and
    Rehabilitation
Vanderbilt University School of Medicine
Nashville, Tennessee

Alan M. Jette, PhD, PT
Professor of Interprofessional Studies
Rehabilitation Sciences Program
Department of Physical Therapy
MGH Institute of Health Professions
Boston, Massachusetts

Galen O. Joe, MD
Deputy Chief/Chief of Consultation Services
Rehabilitation Medicine Department
Clinical Research Center
National Institutes of Health
Bethesda, Maryland

Stephen C. Johnson, MD, MS
Clinical Assistant Professor
Department of Rehabilitation Medicine
University of Washington
Attending Physician
Harborview Medical Center
Seattle, Washington

Nanette C. Joyce, DO, MAS
Associate Clinical Professor
Physical Medicine and Rehabilitation
Davis School of Medicine
University of California
Sacramento, California

Zahra Kadivar, PT, PhD, NCS
Manager of Outpatient Rehabilitation
  Services
Brain Injury Program
TIRR Memorial Hermann
Houston, Texas

David J. Kennedy, MD
Professor and Chair
Physical Medicine and Rehabilitation
Vanderbilt University Medical Center
Stallworth Rehabilitation Hospital at Vanderbilt
  University Medical Center
Nashville, Tennessee

Steven Craig Kirshblum, MD
Professor and Chair
Department of Physical Medicine &
  Rehabilitation
Rutgers New Jersey Medical School
Newark, New Jersey
Senior Medical Officer and Director of SCI
  Services
Kessler Institute for Rehabilitation
West Orange, New Jersey

Sasha E. Knowlton, MD
Instructor
Department of Physical Medicine and
  Rehabilitation
Harvard Medical School
Boston, Massachusetts
Assistant Director of Cancer Rehabilitation
Spaulding Rehabilitation Hospital
Charlestown, Massachusetts

Jayme S. Knutson, PhD
Associate Professor
Physical Medicine and Rehabilitation
Case Western Reserve University
Director of Research
MetroHealth Rehabilitation Institute
MetroHealth System
Cleveland, Ohio

Patrick Kortebein, MD
Clinical Professor
Physical Medicine & Rehabilitation
University of California–Davis
Sacramento, California
Assistant Chief of Service
Physical Medicine & Rehabilitation Service
VA Mather
Mather, California

Michael A. Kryger, MD, MS
Assistant Professor
Department of Physical Medicine and
  Rehabilitation
Penn State University
Director of Spinal Cord Injury Medicine
Penn State Health Rehabilitation Hospital
Hershey, Pennsylvania

**Dinesh Kumbhare, MD, PhD, FRCPC,
FAAPMR**
Associate Professor
Division of Physical Medicine and
  Rehabilitation
Department of Medicine
University of Toronto
Toronto, Ontario, Canada

Susan Kurrle, MBBS, PhD, DipGerMed
Curran Professor in Health Care of
  Older People
Faculty of Medicine and Health
University of Sydney
Sydney, New South Wales, Australia
Senior Staff Specialist Geriatrician
Division of Rehabilitation and Aged Care
Hornsby Ku-ring-gai Health Service
Hornsby, New South Wales, Australia

Byron W. Lai, PhD
Postdoctoral Research Associate
University of Alabama at Birmingham
Birmingham, Alabama

Jorge Laíns, MD
Invited Professor
Medical Dentistry School
Catholic University
Viseu, Portugal
Head of PRM Outpatient Department and
  Continuum Care Unit
Deputy of the Medical Director and Chair of the
  Medical Education Department
Rehabilitation Centre for the Central Region of
  Portugal–Rovisco
Tocha, Portugal

Alicia H. Lazeski, MD
Staff Physician
Physical Medicine & Rehabilitation
OrthoCarolina
Charlotte, North Carolina

Danbi Lee, PhD, OTD
Assistant Professor
Division of Occupational Therapy
Department of Rehabilitation Medicine
University of Washington
Seattle, Washington

Henry L. Lew, MD, PhD
Tenured Professor and Chair
Communication Sciences and Disorders
School of Medicine
University of Hawaii
Consulting Physician of Orthopedics
Queen's Hospital
Honolulu, Hawaii

Jan Lexell, MD, PhD, DPhil h.c.
Professor of Rehabilitation Medicine
Department of Neuroscience, Rehabilitation
  Medicine
Uppsala University
Senior Consultant in Neurological Rehabilitation
Department of Rehabilitation Medicine
Uppsala University Hospital
Uppsala, Sweden
Member, Medical Committee
International Paralympic Committee
Bonn, Germany

Leonard S.W. Li, MD
Honorary Clinical Professor
Division of Rehabilitation
Department of Medicine
Queen Mary Hospital
LKS Faculty of Medicine
University of Hong Kong
Hong Kong Island, Hong Kong SAR, China
Director of Neurological Rehabilitation Centre
Virtus Medical Tower
Central, Hong Kong SAR, China

Jesse A. Lieberman, MD, MSPH
Associate Professor
Department of Physical Medicine and Rehabilitation
Carolinas Rehabilitation
Charlotte, North Carolina

Frank E. Lorch, MD
Professor of PMR
Physical Medicine and Rehabilitation
Carolinas Rehabilitation/Carolinas Medical
  Center/Atrium Health
Charlotte, North Carolina

Melinda S. Loveless, MD
Clinical Assistant Professor
Department of Rehabilitation Medicine
University of Washington
Attending Physician
Harborview Medical Center
Seattle, Washington

**Angela Mailis-Gagnon, MD, MSc,
FRCPC (PhysMed)**
Clinical Adjunct Professor
Department of Medicine
University of Toronto
Toronto, Ontario, Canada
Director, Pain and Wellness Center
Vaughan, Ontario, Canada

Gerard A. Malanga, MD
Clinical Professor of PM&R
Rutgers School of Medicine–New Jersey Medical
  School
Newark, New Jersey

Michael Masi, DPT
Physical Therapist
Carolinas Rehabilitation
Atrium Health
Charlotte, North Carolina

Mary E. Matsumoto, MD
Assistant Professor
Department of Rehabilitation Medicine
University of Minnesota
Staff Physician
Physical Medicine and Rehabilitation
Minneapolis VA Health Care System
Minneapolis, Minnesota

Zachary L. McCormick, MD
Assistant Professor, Director of Clinical Spine
  Research
Physical Medicine and Rehabilitation
School of Medicine
University of Utah
Salt Lake City, Utah

Lindsey C. McKernan, PhD
Assistant Professor
Psychiatry & Behavioral Sciences
Physical Medicine & Rehabilitation
Vanderbilt University Medical Center
Nashville, Tennessee

Amie Brown (Jackson) McLain, MD
Chair and Professor
Department of Physical Medicine and
  Rehabilitation
School of Medicine
University of Alabama at Birmingham
University of Alabama at Birmingham Health
  System
Birmingham, Alabama

Jose R. Medina-Inojosa, MD, MSc
Research Associate
Division of Preventive Cardiology
Department of Cardiovascular Medicine
Mayo Clinic
Rochester, Minnesota

John L. Melvin, MD, MMSc
Emeritus Professor and Chair
Department of Rehabilitation Medicine
Thomas Jefferson University and Hospital
Philadelphia, Pennsylvania

William Micheo, MD
Professor and Chair
Department of Physical Medicine,
    Rehabilitation, and Sports Medicine
School of Medicine
University of Puerto Rico
San Juan, Puerto Rico

Gerardo Miranda-Comas, MD
Assistant Professor
Rehabilitation and Human Performance
Icahn School of Medicine
New York, New York

Nimish Mittal, MBBS, MD
Assistant Professor
Physical Medicine and Rehabilitation
University of Toronto
Active Staff of PM&R
Toronto Rehabilitation Institute
Toronto, Ontario, Canada

Diana M. Molinares, MD
Cancer Rehabilitation Fellow
Palliative, Rehabilitation & Integrative Medicine
MD Anderson Cancer Center
Houston, Texas

Rachel W. Mulheren, PhD
Assistant Professor
Department of Psychological Sciences,
    Communication Sciences Program
Case Western Reserve University
Cleveland, Ohio

Alessandra Negrini, PT
Assistant Technical Director
ISICO (Italian Scientific Spine Institute)
Milano, Italy

Stefano Negrini, MD
Associate Professor
Clinical and Experimental Sciences
University of Brescia
Brescia, Italy
Scientific Director
IRCCS Fondazione Don Carlo Gnocchi
Milan, Italy

Edgar Colón Negron, MD, FACR
Professor
Department of Radiological Sciences
School of Medicine
University of Puerto Rico
San Juan, Puerto Rico

Melissa J. Neisen, MD
Assistant Professor
Department of Radiology
Mayo Clinic Alix School of Medicine
Vascular Interventional Radiologist
Mayo Clinic
Rochester, Minnesota

Vu Q. C. Nguyen, MD, MBA
Professor and Vice Chair of Academics
Residency Program Director
Department of PM&R
Carolinas Medical Center
Vice President of the Medical Staff
Medical Director of Stroke Rehabilitation
Medical Director of Specialty Clinics
Carolinas Rehabilitation
Charlotte, North Carolina

Randolph J. Nudo, PhD, FAHA, FASNR
University Distinguished Professor, Vice Chair
    of Research
Department of Rehabilitation Medicine
University of Kansas Medical Center
Kansas City, Kansas

Marcia K. O'Malley, PhD
Stanley C. Moore Professor
Department of Mechanical Engineering
Rice University
Director of Rehabilitation Engineering
TIRR Memorial Hermann
Houston, Texas

Kenneth J. Ottenbacher, PhD, OTR
Professor and Director
Division of Rehabilitation Sciences
School of Health Professions
University of Texas Medical Branch
Galveston, Texas

Sabrina Paganoni, MD, PhD
Assistant Professor
Department of Physical Medicine and
    Rehabilitation
Harvard Medical School
Physiatrist
Spaulding Rehabilitation Hospital
Boston, Massachusetts

Kelly L. D. Pham, MD
Acting Assistant Professor
Physical Medicine & Rehabilitation
    Department
University of Washington
Pediatric Physiatrist
Department of Pediatric Rehabilitation
    Medicine
Seattle Children's Hospital
Seattle, Washington

Joseph P. Pillion, PhD
Assistant Professor
Department of Physical Medicine and
    Rehabilitation
Johns Hopkins University School of Medicine
Director of Audiology
Kennedy Krieger Institute
Baltimore, Maryland

Ela B. Plow, PhD, PT
Assistant Professor of Neurology
Cleveland Clinic Lerner College of Medicine
Assistant Staff
Biomedical Engineering
Lerner Research Institute
Physical Medicine & Rehabilitation
Center for Neurological Restoration
Neurological Institute
Cleveland Clinic Foundation
Cleveland, Ohio

Heidi Prather, DO
Professor
Division of Physical Medicine and
    Rehabilitation
Washington University School of Medicine
St. Louis, Missouri

Vishwa S. Raj, MD
Associate Professor
PM&R
Carolinas Medical Center at Atrium Health
Director of Oncology Rehabilitation
Carolinas Rehabilitation
Charlotte, North Carolina

Stephanie Rand, DO
Assistant Professor, PM&R
Rehabilitation Medicine
Albert Einstein College of Medicine
Associate Program Director, PM&R
Montefiore Medical Center
Bronx, New York

Elizabeth K. Rasch, PT, PhD
Staff Scientist and Chief
Epidemiology and Biostatistics Section
Rehabilitation Medicine Department
NIH Clinical Center
Bethesda, Maryland

Gargi D. Raval, MD
Assistant Professor
Physical Medicine and Rehabilitation
UT Southwestern Medical Center
Staff Physician
VA North Texas Healthcare System/Dallas VA
    Medical Center
Dallas, Texas

Ramona Raya, MD
Associate Professor
Department of Medicine
Virginia Commonwealth University
Inpatient Rheumatologist
Inova Fairfax Hospital
Falls Church, Virginia

Ronald K. Reeves, MD
Associate Professor
Department of PM&R
Mayo Clinic College of Medicine
Rochester, Minnesota

Brian Richardson, PT, MS, SCS, CSCS
Physical Therapist
Vanderbilt Orthopaedic Institute-Rehabilitation
    Services
Vanderbilt University Medical Center
Nashville, Tennessee

Stephanie K. Rigot, DPT
Graduate Student Researcher
Department of Biomedical Engineering
University of Pittsburgh
Pittsburgh, Pennsylvania

James H. Rimmer, PhD
Lakeshore Foundation Endowed Chair in Health
    Promotion and Rehabilitation Sciences
Director of Research
Lakeshore Foundation
University of Alabama at Birmingham
Birmingham, Alabama

Melinda R. Ring, MD, FACP, ABOIM
Executive Director
Osher Center for Integrative Medicine at
    Northwestern University
Drs. Pat and Carl Greer Distinguished Physician
    in Integrative Medicine
Clinical Associate Professor of Medicine and
    Medical Social Sciences
Northwestern University Feinberg School of
    Medicine
Chicago, Illinois

Sonya Rissmiller, MD
Faculty MD
Sports Medicine and Injury Care
Carolinas Rehabilitation
Charlotte, North Carolina

Lawrence R. Robinson, MD
Professor and Chief, PM&R
Department of Medicine
University of Toronto
Chief, Rehabilitation
St. John's Rehab
Sunnybrook Health Sciences Centre
Toronto, Ontario, Canada

Daniel E. Rohe, PhD, ABPP (Rp)
Consultant in Psychology
Physical Medicine and Rehabilitation
Mayo Clinic College of Medicine
Rochester, Minnesota

Michele Romano, PT
Chief
Department of Rehabilitation
ISICO (Italian Scientific Spine Institute)
Milano, Italy

Nicole F. Rup, MD
Faculty Physician
Physical Medicine and Rehabilitation
Carolinas Rehabilitation
Charlotte, North Carolina

Lisa Marie Ruppert, MD
Assistant Professor
Rehabilitation Medicine
Weill Cornell Medical College
Assistant Attending
Neurology–Rehabilitation Medicine Service
Memorial Sloan Kettering Cancer Center
New York, New York

Nourma Sajid, MD
Physician of Internal Medicine, PGY-1
Internal Medicine Department
Nassau University Medical Center
East Meadow, New York

Jeffrey C. Schneider, MD
Associate Professor
Physical Medicine & Rehabilitation
Harvard Medical School
Medical Director, Trauma & Burn Rehabilitation
Spaulding Rehabilitation Hospital
Boston, Massachusetts

Rajani Sebastian, PhD, CCC-SLP
Assistant Professor
Department of Physical Medicine and
    Rehabilitation
Johns Hopkins University School of Medicine
Baltimore, Maryland

Melissa Selb, MS
ICF Research Branch Coordinator and
    Project Scientist
Swiss Paraplegic Research
Nottwil, Switzerland

Vivan P. Shah, MD
Resident Physician
Department of Physical Medicine and
    Rehabilitation
Beaumont Health
Taylor, Michigan
Medical Scribe
Rutgers New Jersey Medical School
Newark, New Jersey

Julie K. Silver, MD
Associate Professor and Associate Chair
Department of Physical Medicine and
    Rehabilitation
Harvard Medical School
Boston, Massachusetts
Associate Chair and Director of Cancer
    Rehabilitation
Spaulding Rehabilitation Hospital
Charlestown, Massachusetts

Mary D. Slavin, PT, PhD
Director, Education and Training Health
    Outcomes Unit
Department of Health Law, Policy &
    Management
Boston University School of Public Health
Boston, Massachusetts

Gwendolyn Sowa, MD, PhD
Professor and Chair
Department of Physical Medicine and
    Rehabilitation
University of Pittsburgh
Director
UPMC Rehabilitation Institute
Pittsburgh, Pennsylvania

Joel Stein, MD
Simon Baruch Professor and Chair
Rehabilitation and Regenerative Medicine
Vagelos College of Physicians and Surgeons of
    Columbia University
Professor and Chair
Department of Rehabilitation Medicine
Weill Cornell Medical College
Physiatrist-in-Chief
Rehabilitation Medicine
New York–Presbyterian Hospital
New York, New York

Todd P. Stitik, MD, RMSK
Professor
Department of Physical Medicine &
    Rehabilitation
Rutgers New Jersey Medical School
Director, Occupational/Musculoskeletal
    Medicine
University Hospital
Newark, New Jersey

**Lee Stoner, PhD, MPH, FRSPH, SFHEA,
FACSM, ACSM-EIM, ACSM-CEP**
Assistant Professor
Exercise and Sport Science
University of North Carolina at Chapel Hill
Chapel Hill, North Carolina

Gerold Stucki, MD, MS
Professor and Chair
Department of Health Sciences and Health Policy
University of Lucerne
Lucerne, Switzerland
Director
Swiss Paraplegic Research (SPF)
Nottwil, Switzerland

Jennifer L. Sullivan, MASc
Research Engineer
Department of Mechanical Engineering
Rice University
Houston, Texas

Megan M. Sweeney, BS, MPHc
Medical Student Research Associate
Family Medicine & Public Health
UC San Diego School of Medicine
Clinical Research Specialist
Integrative Medicine Research
Scripps Center for Integrative Medicine
La Jolla, California

Samuel Talisman, OTD, OTR/L
Occupational Therapy Neurologic Fellow
Department of Occupational Therapy
Trinity Washington University
MedStar National Rehabilitation Hospital
Washington, District of Columbia

Carmen M. Terzic, MD, PhD
Professor of Physical Medicine and Rehabilitation
Mayo Clinic College of Medicine
Chair and Consultant
Mayo Clinic
Rochester, Minnesota

Mark A. Thomas, MD
Associate Professor, PM&R
Rehabilitation Medicine
Albert Einstein College of Medicine
Program Director, PM&R
Montefiore Medical Center
Bronx, New York

Donna C. Tippett, MPH, MA, CCC-SLP
Associate Professor
Departments of Neurology, Otolaryngology—
    Head and Neck Surgery, and Physical
    Medicine & Rehabilitation
Johns Hopkins University School of Medicine
Baltimore, Maryland

Dorothy Weiss Tolchin, MD, EdM
Instructor (Part-time)
Physical Medicine and Rehabilitation
Harvard Medical School
Boston, Massachusetts
Research Staff
Spaulding Rehabilitation Hospital
Charlestown, Massachusetts

Carlo Trevisan, MD
Adjunct Professor
Scuola di Specializzazione in Ortopedia e
    Traumatologia
Università degli Studi Milano Bicocca
Milano, Italia
Chief of Department
UOC Ortopedia e Traumatologia
Ospedale Bolognini Seriate–ASST Bergamo Est
Seriate, Italia

Erika L. Trovato, DO, BS
Associate Professor
Rehabilitation Medicine
Albert Einstein School of Medicine
Bronx, New York
Brain Injury Attending Physician
Burke Rehabilitation Hospital
White Plains, New York

Tobias J. Tsai, MD
Clinical Assistant Professor
Department of Physical Medicine &
    Rehabilitation
Carolinas Rehabilitation
Medical Director, Pediatric Rehabilitation
Atrium Health Levine Children's
    Hospital
Charlotte, North Carolina

Wen-Chung Tsai, MD, PhD
Professor
School of Medicine
Chang Gung University
Vice-superintendent
Department of Physical Medicine and
    Rehabilitation
Chang Gung Memorial Hospital, Taoyuan
Taoyuan City, Taiwan

Yetsa A. Tuakli-Wosornu, MD, MPH
Assistant Clinical Professor
Department of Chronic Disease Epidemiology
Yale School of Public Health
New Haven, Connecticut
Member, Medical Committee
International Blind Sports Federation
Bonn, Germany

Heikki Uustal, MD
Associate Professor
Physical Medicine and Rehabilitation
Rutgers Robert Wood Johnson Medical School
Piscataway, New Jersey
Attending Physiatrist and Medical Director,
    Prosthetic/Orthotic Team
Rehabilitation Medicine
JFK Johnson Rehabilitation Institute
Edison, New Jersey

Josh Verson, MD
Resident Physician
Department of Emergency Medicine
The University of Arizona Health Sciences
    College of Medicine
Tucson, Arizona

Tyng-Guey Wang, MD
Professor
Department of Physical Medicine of Rehabilitation
School Medicine
National Taiwan University
Attending Physician
National Taiwan University Hospital
Taipei, Taiwan

Katie Weatherhogg, MD
Medical Practice Lead
Physical Medicine & Rehabilitation
University of Colorado
Medical Center of the Rockies
Loveland, Colorado

Mary Alissa Willis, MD
Staff Neurologist, Associate Program Director,
    Neurology Residency
Neurological Institute/Mellen Center for
    Multiple Sclerosis
Cleveland Clinic
Cleveland, Ohio

Richard D. Wilson, MD
Associate Professor
Department of Physical Medicine and Rehabilitation
Case Western Reserve University
Director
Division of Neurologic Rehabilitation
MetroHealth Rehabilitation Institute
The MetroHealth System
Cleveland, Ohio

Timothy J. Wolf, OTD, PhD, OTR/L, FAOTA
Associate Professor and Chair
Department of Occupational Therapy
University of Missouri
Columbia, Missouri

Lynn A. Worobey, PhD, DPT, ATP
Research Assistant Professor
Physical Medicine & Rehabilitation
University of Pittsburgh
Pittsburgh, Pennsylvania

Fabio Zaina, MD
Consultant
ISICO (Italian Scientific Spine Institute)
Milan, Italy

Rebecca Wilson Zingg, DO
Assistant Professor
Physical Medicine & Rehabilitation
University of Utah, Health
Salt Lake City, Utah

The field of *Physical Medicine and Rehabilitation* focuses on the restoration of health and function and reintegration of the patient into the community. The goal of *DeLisa's Physical Medicine and Rehabilitation: Principles and Practice* is to organize, summarize, discuss, and make available knowledge in the field to assist the developing or established practitioner in these endeavors. This sixth edition responds to the dramatic increase in information and knowledge in the field of physical medicine and rehabilitation since the publication of the fifth edition. This edition also introduces a major reorganization of chapters and a classification of the chapters in new sections.

The content of this book has been extensively revised and expanded. There are 5 new chapters and over 20 major revisions in this edition. Our goal is to provide a comprehensive, thorough, evidence-based, and multidisciplinary discussion covering the depth and breadth of the science of physical medicine and rehabilitation and the evidence that supports current best practice. Chapters cover the scientific fundamentals of our field as well as the state-of-the-art clinical interventions used in the treatment and rehabilitation of patients with a wide variety of diseases and disabilities. Authors for each chapter were chosen for their experience and expertise in their given topic. This text reflects the efforts of over two hundred contributing authors representing all parts of the world.

The editorial board for this edition has changed. Walter R. Frontera, MD, PhD, continues his role as the Editor-in-Chief and Joel A. DeLisa, MD, as Editor Emeritus. In addition, a wonderful group of four editors and eight associate editors have worked diligently to make this sixth edition a world class treatise.

The editors of this edition would like to express their appreciation to each of the editors and authors of previous editions. Their work has contributed in a special way to this current version. We also would like to acknowledge the hard work of the authors of this current edition; they have helped create an excellent source of knowledge for those interested in physical medicine and rehabilitation. Their commitment and dedication have made this an exciting and productive effort.

We hope this sixth edition of *DeLisa's Physical Medicine and Rehabilitation: Principles and Practice* contributes significantly to the advancement of the field. As an essential resource for the training and continuing education of medical rehabilitation professionals, this text will help ensure that the care they provide to people with disabling conditions is of the highest quality, resulting in improvement in their health, function, and quality of life.

Walter R. Frontera
Joel A. DeLisa
Jeffrey Basford
William Bockenek
John Chae
Lawrence R. Robinson
Michael L. Boninger
Joanne Borg-Stein
Gregory T. Carter
Leighton Chan
Gerard E. Francisco
Helen Hoenig
Alan M. Jette
Heidi Prather

PART I Principles of Assessment and Evaluation

CHAPTER 1

John A. Freeman
Sally B. Alcott

Armen G. Derian
Christopher H. Bailey

Clinical Evaluation

OVERVIEW

Physical medicine and rehabilitation focuses on the restoration of function and the subsequent reintegration of the patient into the community. As with other branches of medicine, the cornerstone of physical medicine and rehabilitation is a meticulous and thorough clinical evaluation of the patient through history taking and physical examination. Therapeutic intervention by physiatrists must be based on proper assessment of the patient. Impaired function cannot be isolated from preexisting and concurrent medical problems or from the social circumstances of the individual patient.

Evaluation of Function

Medical diagnosis focuses on the historical clues and physical findings that lead the examiner to the correct identification of disease. After a medical diagnosis is established, the physiatrist must ascertain functional consequences of the disease. Appropriate clinical evaluation requires the examiner to have a clear understanding of the distinctions among the disease, body functions, activity limitations, and participation restrictions.

If a disease cannot be eliminated or its severity cannot be reduced through medical or surgical means, measures are used to minimize its impact on functioning. For example, a weak muscle can be strengthened or a hearing impairment can be minimized with the use of an electronic aid. For successful rehabilitation, the physiatrist must not only address the consequences of impaired functioning directly but also identify intact functional capabilities. When intact capabilities and their use are augmented and adapted to new uses, functional independence can be enhanced.

Case 1

AW had gained much enjoyment and self-esteem as a competitive runner before a spinal cord injury that left him with paraplegia. During and after inpatient rehabilitation, he vigorously pursued a cardiovascular and upper extremity conditioning program. He obtained an ultra-lightweight sport wheelchair and resumed competitive athletics as a wheelchair racer, winning several regional races.

Comment: AW's intact capabilities included normal arm strength, a competitive spirit, and self-discipline. Through augmentation of upper body fitness and adaptation with the use of an appropriate wheelchair, he regained enjoyment and self-esteem in his athletic endeavors.

Sometimes it is not possible to ascertain the specific disease responsible for a patient's constellation of historical, physical, and laboratory findings. Medical management must then address the symptoms of the patient. Although diagnosis is highly desirable, it is not a prerequisite to the identification and subsequent management of functional loss. To determine the expectations of future activity in relation to past activity, the physiatrist should attempt to characterize the temporal nature of the disease process over time.

Case 2

FZ, a 62-year-old woman, had difficulty climbing stairs. When questioned, she revealed that she and her husband had been in the habit of taking a 30-minute evening walk for many years. However, 2 years earlier, fatigue began to limit her walk to no more than a few blocks. During the previous year, she had had difficulty rising from low seating and reluctantly quit taking walks. Most recently she finds stair climbing a challenge and requires assistance with tub bathing.

FZ reported no sensory deficits. Physical examination showed hypotonic muscle stretch reflexes and predominantly proximal muscle weakness. Electrodiagnostic studies and muscle biopsy demonstrated a noninflammatory myopathy; however, further extensive evaluation failed to determine a cause. FZ was provided with a bath bench, a toilet seat riser, a lightweight folding wheelchair for long-distance mobility, and a rolling walker for short distances. She was instructed in safe ambulation with the assistive device, operation of the wheelchair, energy conservation techniques, and the proper placement of bathroom safety bars. Safe automobile operation was documented, and she was provided with documentation to obtain a handicapped parking permit. The functional impact of potentially progressive muscle weakness was discussed with her, and she was given supportive counseling.

When FZ returned for a follow-up examination 1 month later, muscle testing showed only a slight progression of her weakness, and her functional capabilities were unchanged. Another follow-up examination was scheduled for 6 weeks later.

Comment: Although a specific diagnosis was not established, rehabilitation intervention addressed the patient's specific functional losses. Serial evaluations at regular follow-up intervals allowed the physiatrist to identify functional loss and maximize functional independence.

Comprehensiveness of Evaluation
The scope of physical medicine and rehabilitation encompasses more than a single organ system. Attention to the whole person is paramount. The objective of the physiatrist is to eliminate disability and restore functioning. The goal is to empower the individual to attain the fullest possible physical, mental, social, and economic independence by maximizing activity and participation. Consequently, the evaluation must assess not only the disease but also the way the disease affects and is affected by the person's family and social environment, vocational responsibilities and economic state, avocational interests, hopes, and dreams.

Cases 3 and 4
CC, a 63-year-old piano tuner, had a left cerebral infarction manifested only as minimal dysfunction of the dominant right hand. Despite demonstrating discrete function of the digits of the involved hand on physical examination, he was psychologically devastated to find that he could no longer accomplish the fine and precise motor patterns necessary to continue in his profession.

BD, a 63-year-old corporate attorney, had a left cerebral infarction resulting in severe spastic weakness of his nondominant upper extremity. He completed some paperwork every day during his inpatient rehabilitation and returned to full-time employment shortly after finishing treatment.

Comment: For each person, the degree of functional impairment is uniquely and disproportionately related to the extent of resultant limitations in activity and restrictions in participation.

Interdisciplinary Nature of Evaluation
Although most of this chapter addresses the patient history and physical examination as related to the rehabilitation evaluation, these are only part of the comprehensive rehabilitation assessment. This statement is not meant to diminish the usefulness of these traditional tools for the physician. Both are of critical importance and serve as the basis for further evaluation; yet, by their very nature, they are also limited. Speech and language disorders can inhibit communication. Subjective interpretation of the facts by the patient and the family can cloud the objective assessment of function. Performance cannot be optimally assessed by interview and physical examination alone.

For example, asking the patient about ambulation skills during the interview may identify a potential problem, but such skills can only be assessed objectively and reliably by having the physician and physical therapist observe the patient's ambulation in various situations. Likewise, the occupational therapist must assess the performance of activities of daily living, and the rehabilitation nurse must assess the safety and judgment of the hospitalized patient. The speech therapist furnishes a measured assessment of language function and, through special communication skills, may obtain information from the patient that was missed during the interview. The rehabilitation psychologist provides a quantified and standardized assessment of cognitive and perceptual function and a skilled assessment of the patient's current psychological state. Through interaction with the patient's family and employer, the social worker can provide useful information that is otherwise unavailable regarding the patient's social support system and economic resources. The concept of the physical medicine and rehabilitation team applies not only to evaluation of the patient but also to ongoing management of the rehabilitation process in the outpatient as well as the inpatient practice setting.

SETTING AND PURPOSE

Because of the expanding scope of physical medicine and rehabilitation, the evaluation setting can be diverse. A necessary corollary to the setting is the purpose of the evaluation. Both the setting and the purpose will affect the format and extent of the evaluation. Traditionally, the inpatient rehabilitation unit or the outpatient physiatry clinic has been the optimal setting for a comprehensive evaluation by the entire rehabilitation team. However, in these days of increasing medical costs and intervention by the government and other third-party payers, creative approaches may be required to accomplish comprehensive rehabilitation evaluations in the clinic and elsewhere in the community (**Table 1-1**).

PATIENT HISTORY

Ordinarily, the patient history is obtained in an interview of the patient by the physiatrist. If communication disorders and cognitive deficits are encountered during the evaluation, additional corroborative information must be obtained from significant others accompanying the patient. The spouse and family members can be valuable resources. The physiatrist may also find it necessary to interview other caregivers, such as paid attendants, public health nurses, and home health agency aides.

The major components of the patient history are the chief report of symptoms, the history of the present illness, the functional history, the past medical history, a review of systems, the patient profile, and the family history.

Chief Report of Symptoms
The goal in assessing the chief report of symptoms is to document the patient's primary concern in his or her own words. Patients often report an impairment in the form of a symptom that may suggest a certain disease or group of diseases. A report of "chest pain when I walk up a flight of stairs" suggests cardiac disease, whereas a report that "my hands ache and go numb when I drive" hints at carpal tunnel syndrome.

TABLE 1-1	The Physical Medicine and Rehabilitation Evaluation: Setting and Purpose
Setting	**Purpose**
Hospital	
Inpatient rehabilitation unit	Comprehensive evaluation by the rehabilitation team
Off-service consultation	Assessment by physiatrist of potential for rehabilitation benefit
Clinic	
General physiatry clinic	Comprehensive evaluation by the team
	Assessment by physiatrist of potential for rehabilitation benefit
	Thorough evaluation of musculoskeletal or spine disorder
Special clinic	Thorough evaluation of specific disease group (e.g., muscular dystrophy or sports injury)
Day rehabilitation program	Comprehensive evaluation by rehabilitation team
Impairment or disability clinic	Evaluation determined by requirement of referring agency (e.g., workers' compensation or Social Security Administration)
Community nursing home	Comprehensive evaluation by rehabilitation team
	Limited assessment by selected members of rehabilitation team
	Assessment by physiatrist of potential for rehabilitation benefit
School	Limited evaluation of functioning
	Limited evaluation for participation in sports
Transitional living facilities	Comprehensive evaluation by rehabilitation team
	Limited assessment of specific problem

Of equal importance is the recognition that a chief report of impaired function may also be the first implication of activity limitation or participation restriction. A homemaker's report that "my balance has been getting worse and I've fallen several times" may be related to disease involving the vestibular system and to disability created by unsafe ambulation. Similarly, a farmer's declaration that "I can no longer climb up onto my tractor" not only suggests a neuromuscular or orthopedic disease but also conveys that the disorder has resulted in disability because the patient is not able to fulfill vocational expectations.

History of Present Illness

The history of the present illness is obtained when the patient relates the development of the present illness. When necessary, patients should be asked to define the specific words they use. Specific questions relating to a particular symptom can also help focus the interview. Using these techniques, the physician can gently guide the patient to follow a chronologic sequence and to fully describe the symptoms and their consequences. Above all, the patient should be allowed to tell the story. More than one symptom may be elicited during the interview, and the physician should document each problem in an orderly fashion (**Table 1-2**) (1).

TABLE 1-2	Analysis of Symptoms

1. Date of onset
2. Character and severity
3. Location and extension
4. Time relationships
5. Associated symptoms
6. Aggravating and alleviating factors
7. Previous treatment and effects
8. Progress, noting remission and exacerbations

From Mayo Clinic Department of Neurology. *Mayo Clinic Examinations in Neurology.* 7th ed. St. Louis, MO: Mosby; 1998. Used with permission of Mayo Foundation for Medical Education and Research.

A complete list of the patient's current medications should be obtained. Polypharmacy is commonly encountered in people with chronic disease, at times with striking adverse effects. Side effects of medications can further impede cognition, psychological state, vascular reflexes, balance, bowel and bladder control, muscle tone, and coordination already impaired by the present illness or injury.

The history of the present illness should include a record of handedness, which is important in many areas of rehabilitation.

Functional History

The physiatric evaluation of a patient with chronic disease often reveals impaired function. The functional history enables the physiatrist to characterize the disabilities that have resulted from disease and to identify remaining functional capabilities. Some physicians consider the functional history to be part of the history of the present illness, whereas others view it as a separate segment of the patient interview. The examiner must know not only the functional status associated with the present illness but also the premorbid level of function.

Although the specific organization of the activities of daily living varies somewhat, the following elements of personal independence are constant: communication, eating, grooming, bathing, toileting, dressing, bed activities, transfers, and mobility.

When obtaining the functional history, the physician may record in a descriptive paragraph the patient's level of independence in each activity. However, functional stability is best communicated, followed over time, and made accessible for study when the physician uses a standard functional assessment scale, as discussed in Chapter 7,8, and 15.

Communication

Because a major component of physical medicine and rehabilitation practice is patient education, effective communication is essential. The interviewer must assess the patient's communication options. In the clinical situation, this aspect of the evaluation blurs the distinction between history and physical examination. It is difficult to interact with the patient in a meaningful way without coincidentally examining his or her ability to communicate; significant speech and language deficiencies become obvious. However, for purposes of discussion, certain facets of the assessment relate more specifically to the history and will be discussed here. Additional facets are presented below in the section on the physical examination.

Speech and language pathology has provided clinicians with numerous classification systems for speech and language disorders (see Chapter 13). From a functional view, the elements of communication hinge on four abilities related to speech and language (2):

1. Listening
2. Reading
3. Speaking
4. Writing

By assessing these factors as well as comprehension and memory, the examiner can determine a patient's communication abilities. Representative questions include the following:

1. Do you have difficulty hearing?
2. Do you use a hearing aid?
3. Do you have difficulty reading?
4. Do you need glasses to read?
5. Do others find it hard to understand what you say?
6. Do you have problems putting your thoughts into words?
7. Do you have difficulty finding words?
8. Can you write?
9. Can you type?
10. Do you use any communication aids?

Eating

The abilities to place solid food and liquids to the mouth, to chew, and to swallow are basic skills taken for granted by able-bodied people. However, in patients with neurologic, orthopedic, or oncologic disorders, these tasks can be formidable. Dysfunctional eating is associated with far-reaching consequences, such as malnutrition, aspiration pneumonitis, and depression. As in the assessment of other skills for activities of daily living, eating function should be assessed specifically and methodically.

Representative questions include the following:

1. Can you eat without help?
2. Do you have difficulty opening containers or pouring liquids?
3. Can you cut meat?
4. Do you have difficulty handling a fork, knife, or spoon?
5. Do you have problems bringing food or beverages to your mouth?
6. Do you have problems chewing?
7. Do you have difficulty swallowing solids or liquids?
8. Do you ever cough or choke while eating?
9. Do you regurgitate food or liquids through your nose?

Patients with nasogastric or gastrostomy tubes should be asked who helps them prepare and administer their feedings. The type, quantity, and schedule of feedings should be recorded.

Grooming

Grooming may not be considered as important as feeding. However, impaired functioning that leads to deficits in grooming can have deleterious effects on hygiene as well as on body image and self-esteem. Consequently, grooming skills should be of real concern to the rehabilitation team.

Representative questions include the following:

1. Can you brush your teeth without help?
2. Can you remove and replace your dentures without help?
3. Do you have problems fixing or combing your hair?
4. Can you apply your makeup independently?
5. Do you have problems shaving?
6. Can you apply deodorant without assistance?

Bathing

The ability to maintain cleanliness also has far-reaching physical and psychosocial implications. Deficits in cleaning can result in skin maceration and ulceration, skin and systemic infections, and the spread of disease to others. Patients should be questioned about their ability to bath independently.

Representative questions include the following:

1. Can you take a tub bath or shower without assistance?
2. Do you feel safe in the tub or shower?
3. Do you use a bath bench or shower chair?
4. Can you accomplish a sponge bath without help?
5. Are there parts of your body that you cannot reach?

For patients with sensory deficits, bathing is also a convenient time for skin inspection, and inquiry about the patient's inspection habits should be made. For patients using a wheelchair, walker, or other mobility device, architectural barriers to bathroom entry should be determined.

Toileting

To the cognitively intact person, incontinence of stool or urine can be a psychologically devastating deficit of personal independence. Ineffective bowel or bladder control has an adverse impact on self-esteem, body image, and sexuality, and it can lead to participation restriction. The soiling of skin and clothing can result in ulceration, infection, and urologic complications. The physiatrist should be thorough yet sensitive as they pursue questioning about toileting dependency.

Representative questions include the following:

1. Can you use the toilet without assistance?
2. Do you need help with clothing before or after using the toilet?
3. Do you need help with cleaning after a bowel movement?

For patients with indwelling urinary catheters, the usual management of the catheter and leg bag should be examined. If bladder emptying is accomplished by intermittent catheterization, the examiner should determine who performs the catheterization and should have a clear understanding of his or her technique. For patients who have had ostomies for urine or feces, the examiner should determine who cares for the ostomy and should ask the patient to describe the technique.

Feminine hygiene is generally performed while on or near the toilet, so at this point in the interview, it may be appropriate to ask about problems with the use of sanitary napkins or tampons.

Dressing

We dress to go out into the world to be employed in the workplace, to dine in restaurants, to be entertained in public places, and to visit friends. Even at home, convention dictates that we dress to entertain anyone except close friends and family. We dress for protection, warmth, self-esteem, and pleasure.

Dependency in dressing can result in a severe limitation to personal independence and should be investigated thoroughly during the rehabilitation interview.

Representative questions include the following:
1. Do you dress daily?
2. What articles of clothing do you regularly wear?
3. Do you require assistance putting on or taking off your underwear, shirt, slacks, skirt, dress, coat, stockings, panty hose, shoes, tie, or coat?
4. Do you need help with buttons, zippers, hooks, snaps, or shoelaces?
5. Do you use clothing modifications?

Bed Activities

The most basic stage of functional mobility is independence in bed activities. The importance of this functional level should not be underestimated. Persons who cannot turn from side to side to redistribute pressure and periodically expose their skin to the air are at high risk for development of pressure sores over bony prominences and skin maceration from heat and occlusion. For the person who cannot stand upright to dress, bridging (lifting the hips off the bed in the supine position) will allow the donning of underwear and slacks. Independence is likewise enhanced by an ability to move between a recumbent position and a sitting position. Sitting balance is required to accomplish many other activities of daily living, including transfers.

Representative questions include the following:
1. When lying down, can you turn onto your front, back, and sides without assistance?
2. Can you lift your hips off the bed when lying on your back?
3. Do you need help to sit or lie down?
4. Do you have difficulty maintaining a seated position?
5. Can you operate the bed controls on an electric hospital bed?

Transfers

The second stage of functional mobility is independence in transfers. Being able to move between a wheelchair and the bed, toilet, bath bench, shower chair, standard seating, or car seat often serves as a precursor to independence in other areas. Although a male patient can use a urinal to void without having to transfer, a female patient cannot be independent in bladder care without the ability to transfer to the toilet and will probably require an indwelling catheter. Travel by airplane or train is difficult without the ability to transfer from the wheelchair to other seating. Bathing or showering is not independent without the ability to move to the bath bench or shower chair. The inability to transfer to a car seat precludes the use of a motor vehicle with standard seats. Also included in this category is the ability to rise from a seated position to a standing position. Low seats without arm supports present a much greater problem than straight-backed chairs with arm supports.

Representative questions include the following:
1. Can you move to and from the wheelchair to the bed, toilet, bath bench, shower chair, standard seating, or car seat without assistance?
2. Can you get out of bed without difficulty?
3. Do you require assistance to rise to a standing position from either a low or a high seat?
4. Can you get on and off the toilet without help?

Mobility

Wheelchair Mobility

Although wheelchair independence is more likely than walking to be inhibited by architectural barriers, it provides excellent mobility for the person who is not able to walk. With efficiently engineered, lightweight manual wheelchairs, the energy expenditure required to wheel on flat ground is only slightly greater than that of walking. With the addition of a motorized drive, battery power, and controls for speed and direction, a wheelchair can be propelled even by a person who lacks the upper extremity strength necessary to propel a manual wheelchair, and it can thus help maintain independence in mobility.

Quantification of manual wheelchair skills can be accomplished in several ways. Patients may report in feet, yards, meters, or city blocks the distance that they are able to traverse before resting. Alternatively, the number of minutes they can continuously propel the chair can be specified, or the environment in which they are able to use the chair can be described (e.g., within a single room, around the house, or throughout the community).

Representative questions include the following:
1. Do you propel your wheelchair yourself?
2. Do you need help to lock the wheelchair brakes before transfers?
3. Do you require assistance to cross high-pile carpets, rough ground, or inclines in your wheelchair?
4. How far or how many minutes can you wheel before you must rest?
5. Can you move independently about your living room, bedroom, and kitchen?
6. Do you go out to stores, to restaurants, and to friends' homes?

With any of these functional levels of wheelchair mobility, patients should be asked what keeps them from going farther afield and whether they need help lifting the wheelchair into and out of an automobile.

Ambulation

The final level of mobility is ambulation. In the narrowest sense of the word, ambulation is walking, and we have used this definition to simplify the following discussion. However, within the sphere of rehabilitation, ambulation may be any useful means of movement from one place to another. In the view of many rehabilitation professionals, the person with a bilateral above-knee amputation ambulates with a manual wheelchair, the patient with C4 tetraplegia ambulates with a motorized wheelchair, and the survivor of polio in an underdeveloped country might ambulate by crawling. Driving a motor vehicle may also be considered a form of ambulation. Ambulation ability can be quantified the same way wheelchair mobility is quantified. Persons may report the distance they are able to walk, how long they can walk before they require a rest period, and the scope of the environment within which they walk.

Representative questions include the following:
1. Do you walk unaided?
2. Do you use a cane, crutches, or a walker to walk?
3. How far or how many minutes can you walk before you must rest?
4. What stops you from going farther?

5. Do you feel unsteady or do you fall?
6. Can you go upstairs and downstairs unassisted?
7. Do you go out to stores, to restaurants, and to friends' homes?
8. Can you use public transportation (e.g., the bus or subway) without assistance?

Operation of a Motor Vehicle

In the perception of many patients, full independence in mobility is not attained without the ability to operate a motor vehicle on one's own. Although driving skills are by no means necessary for urban dwellers with readily available public transportation, they may be essential to persons living in a suburban or rural environment. Driving skills should always be assessed in patients of driving age.

Representative questions include the following:
1. Do you have a valid driver's license?
2. Do you own a car?
3. Do you drive your car to stores, to restaurants, and to friends' homes?
4. Do you drive in heavy traffic or over long distances?
5. Do you drive in low light or after sunset?
6. Do you use hand controls or other automobile modifications?
7. Have you been involved in any motor vehicle accidents or received any citations for improper operation of a motor vehicle since your illness or injury?

Past Medical History

The past medical history is a record of any major illness, trauma, or health maintenance since the patient's birth. The effects of certain past conditions will continue to affect the present level of function. Identifying these conditions affords an opportunity to better characterize the patient's baseline level of function before the present disorder. The examiner must take special care to decipher whether the patient's diagnostic terms accurately represent the true diagnoses. Although many past conditions associated with extensive immobilization, deconditioning, and disability are themselves amenable to rehabilitation measures, such conditions tend to affect the goals for future rehabilitation efforts.

Case 5

PB, a 66-year-old woman, was referred for rehabilitation after an above-knee amputation of her right leg because of vascular disease. Her past history was notable for a right cerebral infarction 7 years earlier. Despite comprehensive rehabilitation after the stroke, PB was able to walk only one block with a quadruped cane and an ankle-foot orthosis because of spastic left hemiparesis.

Comment: After prosthetic fitting and training, most people in this age group with an above-knee amputation regain ambulation skills, albeit with a cane or other gait aid. However, because PB had a preexisting ambulation disability due to the left hemiparesis that had occurred before amputation, her rehabilitation goals included a wheelchair prescription, with consideration of a hemichair if she could not wheel with her left arm, and training in wheelchair activities. Although ambulation beyond a few yards was not feasible, a preparatory prosthesis with a manual knee lock was provided on a trial basis to determine whether it aided in transfers. For PB, ambulation

disability was dictated more by her previous impairments than by impairments associated with her present illness.

All elements of the standard past medical history should be completed; however, a history of neurologic, cardiopulmonary, or musculoskeletal disease should alert the physiatrist to special needs of the patient. Psychiatric disorders are also of special interest to the physiatrist and are discussed below in the section on the psychological and psychiatric history.

Neurologic Disorders

Most frequently encountered in older populations but possibly present in any age group, a past history of neurologic disease can have a tremendous impact on the rehabilitation outcome of an unrelated current illness. Whether congenital or acquired, preexisting cognitive impairment places restrictions on educationally oriented rehabilitation intervention. Disorders with sensory manifestations such as loss of touch, pain, or joint position or afflictions that are characterized by perceptual dysfunction can retard the patient's ability to monitor performance during the acquisition of new functional skills. These maladies also render patients more likely to be unresponsive to soft tissue injury from prolonged or excessive skin surface pressures during long periods of immobility. When these conditions are coupled with preexisting visual or auditory impairment, the function is further encumbered. Likewise, new motor learning can be inhibited by a residual motor deficit that results in spasticity, weakness, or decreased endurance. A diligent search for antecedent neurologic disease should be a fundamental part of the rehabilitation evaluation.

Cardiopulmonary Disorders

For patients with motor disabilities, the activities of daily living require more than the normal expenditure of energy. When preexisting cardiopulmonary disorders limit the patient's capacity to tolerate the greater energy expenditures imposed by motor impairment, they can result in additional functional deficits. This is also the case with many forms of hematologic, renal, and hepatic dysfunction. The physician should gather as much cardiopulmonary data as needed to estimate cardiac reserve accurately. Only when disease of the cardiopulmonary system is identified and addressed can medical intervention be initiated and rehabilitation tailored to maximize cardiac reserve.

Musculoskeletal Disorders

Weakness, joint ankylosis, or instability from previous trauma or arthritis, amputation, and other musculoskeletal dysfunctions can all affect functional capacity deleteriously. A search for such disorders is a necessary prerequisite to a complete physiatric evaluation.

Review of Systems

The systems should be thoroughly reviewed to screen for clues to disease not otherwise identified in the history of the present illness or in the past medical history. Many diseases have the potential to cause adverse effects on rehabilitation outcomes. However, as described previously, certain disorders are of special interest to the physiatrist. This part of the evaluation considers constitutional, head and neck, respiratory, cardiovascular, gastrointestinal, genitourinary, musculoskeletal, neurologic, psychiatric, endocrine, and dermatologic symptoms.

Constitutional Symptoms

Of particular interest to the examiner are suggestions of infection and nutritional deficiency. Fatigue can be a prominent symptom in patients with neurologic and neuromuscular conditions such as stroke, multiple sclerosis, amyotrophic lateral sclerosis, or poliomyelitis sequelae, or with other conditions such as obstructive sleep apnea or chronic pain syndromes.

Head and Neck Symptoms

Vision, hearing, and swallowing deficits must be identified.

Respiratory Symptoms

Any pulmonary condition that inhibits delivery of oxygen to the tissues will adversely affect endurance. Symptoms such as dyspnea, cough, sputum, hemoptysis, wheezing, and pleuritic chest pain should be identified.

Cardiovascular Symptoms

The manifestations of heart disease restrict cardiac reserve and endurance. When identified, many cardiovascular conditions can be ameliorated through medical management. Identifying arrhythmias may help prevent recurrent strokes of embolic cause. The presence of chest pain, dyspnea, orthopnea, palpitations, or light-headedness should be determined.

Peripheral vascular disease is the leading cause of amputation. The potential for ulceration and gangrene caused by bed rest, orthoses, pressure garments, and other rehabilitation equipment can be minimized if peripheral disease is recognized. The patient should be asked about claudication, foot ulcers, and varicosities.

Gastrointestinal Symptoms

Almost any form of gastrointestinal tract disease can result in nutritional deficiency, a particularly insidious condition that limits rehabilitation efforts more frequently than previously realized (3). Bowel control is of special interest for patients with neurologic disorders. These patients should be asked about incontinence, bowel care techniques, and use of laxatives.

Genitourinary Symptoms

Manifestations of neurogenic bladder must be sought. Questions should be asked about specific fluid intake, voiding schedules, specific bladder-emptying techniques, urgency, frequency, incontinence, retention and incomplete emptying, sensation of fullness and voiding, dysuria, pyuria, infections, flank pain, hematuria, and renal stones.

For female patients, a menstrual and pregnancy history should be obtained, and inquiries should focus on dyspareunia, vaginal and clitoral sensation, and orgasm. Male patients should be asked about erection, ejaculation, progeny, and pain during intercourse.

Musculoskeletal Symptoms

The musculoskeletal system review must be thorough because of the likelihood of musculoskeletal dysfunction in patients in a rehabilitation program. The examiner should ask about muscle pain, weakness, fasciculation, atrophy, hypertrophy, skeletal deformities and fractures, limited joint motion, joint stiffness, joint pain, and swelling of soft tissues and joints.

Neurologic Symptoms

Because of the increased prevalence of neurologic disorders in patients in a rehabilitation program, a methodical neurologic review should always be performed. The following areas should be addressed: sense of smell, diplopia, blurred vision, visual field cuts, imbalance, vertigo, tinnitus, weakness, tremors, involuntary movements, convulsions, depressed consciousness, ataxia, loss of touch, pain, temperature, dysesthesia, hyperpathia, and changes in memory and thinking.

Chewing, swallowing, hearing, reading, and speaking may be addressed in either the functional history or the review of systems.

Psychiatric Symptoms

Psychological and psychiatric issues can be discussed during the review of symptoms. However, we prefer to explore this area while obtaining the psychosocial history for the patient profile.

Endocrine Symptoms

Screening questions should be presented to address intolerance to hot or cold, excessive sweating, increase in urine, increase in thirst, and changes in skin, hair distribution, and voice.

Dermatologic Symptoms

Rash, itching, pigmentation, moisture or dryness, texture, changes in hair growth, and nail changes should be questioned.

Patient Profile

The patient profile provides the interviewer with information about the patient's present and past psychological state, social milieu, and vocational background.

Personal History

Psychological and Psychiatric History

Any present illness accompanied by functional loss can be psychologically challenging. A quiescent major psychiatric disturbance may resurface during such stressful times and may hinder or halt rehabilitation efforts. When the examiner is able to identify a history of psychiatric dysfunction, the necessary support systems to lessen the likelihood of recrudescence can be applied prophylactically during rehabilitation. The examiner should seek a history of previous psychiatric hospitalization, psychotropic pharmacologic intervention, or psychotherapy. The patient should be screened for past or current anxiety, depression and other mood changes, sleep disturbances, delusions, hallucinations, obsessive and phobic ideas, and past major and minor psychiatric illnesses. A review of the patient's prior and current responses to stress often helps the rehabilitation team to better understand and modify behavioral responses to catastrophic illness or trauma. Therefore, it is important to know the patient's emotional responses to previous illness and family troubles and to know how the stress of the current illness is being addressed. If initial screening suggests any abnormality, a clinical psychologist can conduct tests to clarify psychological symptoms or to identify a personality disturbance.

Lifestyle

Leisure activities can promote both physical health and emotional health. The patient's leisure habits should be reviewed to identify special rehabilitation measures that might return independence in these activities. Examples of questions to consider include the following (4):

What sorts of interests do you have?

1. Do you enjoy physical endeavors, sports, the outdoors, and mechanical avocations (i.e., motor oriented) more than sedentary activities?
2. Are you more interested in intellectual pursuits (i.e., symbol oriented) than physical endeavors?
3. Do you derive the most pleasure from social interactions, organizations, and group functions (i.e., interpersonally oriented)?
4. Have you been actively pursuing any of these interests?

The work-oriented person without avocational interests before the present illness will need recreational counseling during rehabilitation.

Diet

Inadequate nutrition may inhibit rehabilitation efforts. In addition, even after initial myocardial and cerebrovascular events due to atherosclerosis, some secondary prevention can be accomplished through dietary intervention. The examiner should determine the patient's ability to prepare meals and snacks, as well as the patient's usual dietary habits and special diets.

Alcohol and Drugs

Drug, alcohol, and nicotine use must be assessed. Patients with cognitive, perceptual, and motor deficits can be further impaired to a dangerous degree through substance abuse. The use of alcohol or drugs is frequently a factor in head and spinal cord injuries. Identifying abuse and dependency provides an opportunity to help the patient modify future behavior through counseling. The CAGE questionnaire is a brief but useful screening vehicle for assessing alcohol abuse and dependency (**Table 1-3**); a single affirmative answer should initiate further investigation (5).

Social History

Family

Catastrophic illness in a family member places enormous stress on the rest of the family. When the family is already facing other problems with interaction, health, or substance abuse, the potential is greater for disintegration of the family unit. This tendency is unfortunate because the availability of a sturdy support system of family and friends can be as predictive of disposition as it is of functional outcome. The examiner should determine the patient's marriage history and marital status and should obtain the names and ages of other family members who live in the home. The established roles of each member should be understood clearly (e.g., who handles the finances, the cooking, the cleaning, or the discipline). The

examiner should also determine whether other family members live nearby. To ascertain the availability of all potential assistants, the examiner should inquire about their willingness and ability to participate in the care of the patient and about their work or school schedule.

Home

The patient's home design should be reviewed to identify architectural barriers. The examiner should determine whether the patient owns or rents the home, the location of the home (e.g., urban, suburban, or rural), the distance between the home and rehabilitation services, the number of steps into the home, the presence of (or room for) entry ramps, and the accessibility of the kitchen, bath, bedroom, and living room.

Vocational History

Education and Training

Although education does not predict intellectual function, the educational level achieved by the patient may suggest intellectual skills upon which the rehabilitation team can draw during the patient's convalescence. In addition, when coupled with the assessment of physical function, the educational background will dictate future educational and training needs. After determining the years of education completed by the patient and whether high school, undergraduate, or graduate degrees were obtained, the examiner should review the patient's performance. The acquisition of special skills, licenses, and certifications should be noted. Future vocational goals are always important to address but are of particular concern with adolescent patients. A discussion of these goals should indicate the need for and the type of interest, aptitude, and skills testing and any appropriate vocational counseling.

Work History

An understanding of the patient's work experience can help determine the need for further education and training. It also provides an idea of the patient's motivation, reliability, and self-discipline. The duration and type of previous jobs and the reason for job changes should be recorded. Not only titles but also actual job descriptions must be obtained, and the patient should be asked about architectural barriers within the workplace. These principles also apply to the patient who works at home. In addition, the examiner should define the specific expectations related to meal preparation, shopping, home maintenance, cleaning, child rearing, and discipline. Finally, the examiner should ask where clothes are washed and whether architectural barriers prevent the patient from reaching appliances or areas in the home and yard.

Finances

The physical medicine and rehabilitation team, in particular the social worker or case manager, should have a basic understanding of the patient's income, investment, and insurance resources, disability classifications, and debts. This financial information is important in determining the services and assistance to which an individual patient may be entitled.

Family History

The family history can be used to identify hereditary disease in the family and to assess the health of people in the patient's home support system. Knowledge of the health and fitness of the spouse and other family members can aid dismissal planning.

TABLE 1-3   **The CAGE Questionnaire**

1. Have you ever felt you ought to **C**ut down on your drinking?
2. Have people **A**nnoyed you by criticizing your drinking?
3. Have you ever felt bad or **G**uilty about your drinking?
4. Have you ever had a drink first thing in the morning to steady your nerves or get rid of a hangover (**E**ye-opener)?

PHYSICAL EXAMINATION

The physical examination performed by the physiatrist has much in common with the general medical examination. Of necessity, it is a well-practiced art. Through perceptions gleaned from observation, palpation, percussion, and auscultation, the examining physician seeks physical findings to support and formulate the diagnosis and to screen for other conditions not suggested by the patient history.

The physical examination also differs from the general medical examination. After investigating the physical findings that help to establish the medical diagnosis, the physiatrist still has two principal tasks:

1. To scrutinize the patient for physical findings that can help define the functional impairments emanating from the disease
2. To identify the patient's remaining physical, psychological, and intellectual strengths that can serve as the base for reestablishing functioning

Physical medicine and rehabilitation emphasizes the orthopedic and neurologic examinations and makes assessment of function an integral part of the overall physical examination.

Severe motor, cognitive, and communication impairments make it difficult or impossible for some patients to follow the directions of the physician, and these impairments limit certain traditional physical examination maneuvers. Thus, creativity is often required to accomplish the examination. Expert examination skills are particularly necessary in such situations.

We assume that the reader is competent in the performance of the general medical examination (6). The following discussion places priority on the aspects of the physical examination that have special relevance to physical medicine and rehabilitation. The major segments of the physical examination are vital signs and general appearance, integument and lymphatics, head, eyes, ears, nose, mouth and throat, neck, chest, heart and peripheral vascular system, abdomen, genitourinary system and rectum, musculoskeletal system, neurologic examination, and functional examination.

Vital Signs and General Appearance

The recording of blood pressure, pulse, temperature, weight, and general observations is important. The identification of hypertension may be meaningful to the secondary prevention of stroke and myocardial infarction. Supine, sitting, and standing blood pressures should be obtained to rule out orthostasis in any patient who has had unexplained falls, light-headedness, or dizziness. Tachycardia can be the initial manifestation of sepsis in a patient with high-level tetraplegia, or it can suggest pulmonary embolism in an immobilized patient. Initial weight recordings are invaluable to identify and follow up malnutrition, obesity, and fluid and electrolyte disorders common after various forms of brain injury. A notation should be made if patients act hostile, tense, or agitated or if their behavior is uncooperative, inappropriate, or preoccupied.

Integument and Lymphatics

Skin disorders are frequently encountered in patients undergoing physical rehabilitation. Prolonged pressure in patients with peripheral vascular disease, sensory disorders, immobility, and altered consciousness often results in damage to skin and underlying tissues. Many diseases common to disabled persons, and their treatments, render the skin more prone to trauma and infection. Skin problems that are only somewhat bothersome to able-bodied people can be devastating to persons with disabilities when they interfere with the use of prostheses, orthoses, and other devices.

The patient's skin should be inspected in appropriate lighting. By considering the skin as each separate body region is examined, the physiatrist can study the entire body surface without total exposure of the patient. In particular, the skin over bony prominences and in contact with prosthetic and orthotic devices should be examined for lichenification, erythema, or breakdown. Intertriginous areas should be inspected for maceration and ulceration; the distal lower extremities in patients with vascular disease should be examined for pigmentation, hair loss, and breakdown; and the hands and feet in insensate patients should be observed for unrecognized trauma. All common lymph node sites should be palpated for enlargement and tenderness, and areas of edema should be palpated for pitting.

Head

The head should be inspected for signs of past or present trauma. Gentle palpation should be performed for evidence of previous trauma or neurosurgical procedures, shunt pumps, and other craniofacial abnormalities. Auscultation for bruits should be done when considering vascular malformations.

Eyes

Unrecognized acuity errors can hamper rehabilitation efforts, especially in patients needing adequate eyesight to compensate for disorders of other sensory systems. With the patient's usual eyewear in place, far and near vision should be tested with the use of standard charts. If charts are not available, the patient's vision can be compared with the examiner's vision by object identification and description for far vision and by reading materials of several print sizes for near vision. Findings can be substantiated with refraction when circumstances permit. An ophthalmoscopic examination should be performed; if dilatory agents are necessary, one with a short duration can be used; notation should be made in the patient's chart of the time of administration and the name of the preparation. Evidence of erythema and inflammation of the globe or conjunctiva should be sought; aphasic patients and those with altered consciousness may not adequately express the pain of acute glaucoma or the discomfort of conjunctivitis. The eyes of comatose patients should be inspected for inadequate lid closure; deficient lubrication should be compensated for to prevent corneal ulcerations.

Ears

Unrecognized hearing impairment can limit rehabilitation efforts. Hearing acuity can be checked with the "watch test" or by having the patient listen to and repeat words that are whispered. If a unilateral hearing deficit is identified, the Weber test and the Rinne test can be used to determine whether it is a nerve or conductive loss. Findings can be substantiated with an audiogram. An otoscopic examination should be performed. If otorrhea is present in a head-injured patient, Benedict's solution can be used to assess the presence of sugar, which indicates cerebrospinal fluid.

Nose

A routine examination of the nose, including olfactory function, is generally sufficient. Clear or blood-tinged drainage in a head-injured patient may indicate the presence of cerebrospinal fluid.

Mouth and Throat

The oral and pharyngeal mucosa should be inspected for poor hygiene and infections (e.g., candidiasis in patients taking corticosteroids or broad-spectrum antibiotics), the teeth for disrepair, and the gums for gingivitis or hypertrophy. Dentures should be checked for fit and maintenance. In patients with arthritis or trauma, the temporomandibular joints should be inspected and palpated for crepitation, tenderness, swelling, or limited motion. Any of these problems can impair food and fluid intake, resulting in poor nutrition.

Neck

A routine examination of the neck is generally sufficient. The examiner should listen for carotid bruits in patients with atherosclerosis and cerebrovascular disorders. In patients with musculoskeletal disorders, range of motion (ROM) should be assessed. However, neck motion need not be checked in patients with recent trauma or chronic polyarthritis until radiographic studies have ruled out fracture or instability.

Chest

Tolerance to exercise is considerably affected by pulmonary function. For patients whose exercise tolerance is already compromised by neurologic or musculoskeletal disease, the examiner must search rigorously for pulmonary dysfunction to minimize the deficit. The standard medical maneuvers are usually sufficient; however, certain aspects of the chest examination merit mention.

The chest wall should be inspected to note the rate, amplitude, and rhythm of breathing. The presence of cough, hiccups, labored breathing, accessory muscle activity, and chest wall deformities should be noted. Respiration may be restricted by rheumatologic disorders such as advanced spondyloarthropathies and scleroderma. Likewise, restrictive pulmonary disease with hypoventilation is common in muscular dystrophy and other neuromuscular diseases, severe kyphoscoliosis, and chronic spinal cord injuries. Tachypnea and tachycardia may be the only readily apparent manifestations of pulmonary embolism, pneumonia, or sepsis after a high-level spinal cord injury. The finding of a barrel chest may lead the examiner to identify obstructive pulmonary disease so that medical management can minimize its effect on functioning.

The patient should be instructed to cough, and the force and efficiency of this action should be noted. If the cough is weak, the patient can be assisted by exerting manual pressure over the abdomen coincidentally with the cough to observe the effect. The chest wall should be palpated for tenderness, deformity, and transmitted sounds. During the acute care of a head-injured patient, rib fractures may be missed. Percussion should be performed to document diaphragmatic level and excursion. Auscultation should be performed to characterize breath sounds and to identify wheezes, rubs, rhonchi, and rales. Pneumonitis can be especially insidious in the immunosuppressed patient.

When pulmonary disease is suspected, further investigation with pulmonary function tests and a determination of blood gas levels may need to be undertaken. If the patient has a tracheostomy, the skin around the opening should be examined, the type of apparatus recorded, and cuff leaks noted. Screening for breast malignancy may be necessary in women and men alike.

Heart and Peripheral Vascular System

As with pulmonary disease, cardiovascular dysfunction can adversely affect exercise tolerance already encumbered by neurologic or musculoskeletal disease. When cardiovascular disorders are identified, intervention can relieve or reduce deleterious effects on exercise tolerance and general health. Implementation of appropriate secondary prevention measures for embolic stroke is contingent upon the identification of arrhythmias, valvular disease, and congenital anomalies.

In the clinical situation, peripheral circulation is usually assessed during examination of the patient's limbs. When bracing is being considered, the examiner should search for the pallor and cool dystrophic skin of arterial occlusive disease; inappropriate devices may lead to edema and subsequent skin breakdown. Deep venous thrombosis is a major risk to immobilized patients, who should be examined for varicose and incompetent veins. Bedside Doppler studies should be used as necessary to help delineate arterial or venous concerns such as Raynaud phenomenon.

Abdomen

In many patients, the general medical examination of the abdomen is the only necessary screen to identify abnormality and to assess gastrointestinal tract symptoms. In patients with widespread spasticity (e.g., due to multiple sclerosis or myelopathy), inspection and auscultation should precede palpation and percussion. Manipulation of the abdominal wall often results in a wave of increased tone that will temporarily impede the rest of the abdominal examination. Vigorous abdominal palpation in patients with disordered peristalsis from certain central nervous system diseases may initiate regurgitation of stomach contents. Such patients should be examined gently when they are in a partially reclined position.

Genitourinary System and Rectum

During any comprehensive evaluation, the genitalia should be examined. A thorough evaluation of the male and female genitalia is particularly necessary for patients with disorders of continence, micturition, and sexual function. Incontinence in patients of either sex and in male patients using an external collecting device such as the condom catheter can result in maceration and ulceration. Thus, the penile skin in male patients, the periurethral mucosa in female patients, and all intertriginous perineal areas should be examined. The scrotal contents should be palpated for orchitis and epididymitis in male patients with indwelling catheters. Incontinence from neurogenic causes is common in patients undergoing rehabilitation; however, the examiner should check for a cystocele or other structural cause of incontinence that can be remediated. Patients with long-term use of indwelling catheters should be checked for external urethral meatal ulceration, and male patients should be checked for penile fistulas. If urinary retention is suspected, the physical examination should be followed by an in-and-out catheterization to measure residual urine.

The rehabilitation assessment is not complete without digital examination of the rectum and anus to check anal tone and perineal sensation. In any patient with suspected central nervous system, autonomic, or pelvic disease, the bulbocavernosus reflex should be evaluated to monitor sphincter tone by firmly compressing the glans of the penis or clitoris with one hand while inserting the index finger of the other hand into the anus. Sphincter tone is increased with many upper motor neuron lesions, whereas it is decreased or absent with lesions peripheral to the sacral cord (S2-4).

Musculoskeletal System

Disorders of the musculoskeletal system are a major portion of the pathologic conditions addressed by the rehabilitation physician. The examiner must possess expert skills in the evaluation of all musculoskeletal components and should systematically assess the bone, joint, cartilage, ligament, tendon, and muscle in each body region. Accomplishing this task requires full familiarity with surface landmarks and underlying anatomical features.

The assignment of many examination components to the neurologic or musculoskeletal examination is arbitrary because the neuromusculoskeletal function is so integrated. Examination of the musculoskeletal system is divided into inspection, palpation, ROM assessment, joint stability assessment, and muscle strength testing.

Inspection

Musculoskeletal inspection should be performed for scoliosis, abnormal kyphosis, and lordosis; joint deformity, amputation, and absence and asymmetry of body parts (leg-length discrepancy); soft tissue swelling, mass, scar, and defect; and muscle fasciculations, atrophy, hypertrophy, and rupture. At times, the dysfunction may be subtle and decipherable only through careful observation. While proceeding with the examination, the physician should note any wary and tentative movements of the patient indicative of pain, any exaggerated and inconsistent conduct indicative of malingering, and any bizarre behavior indicative of conversion reaction.

Palpation

Localized abnormalities (e.g., areas of tenderness or deformity) identified through inspection and any body regions of concern to the patient should be palpated to ascertain their structural origins. For an abnormality, it is important to first determine whether its basic consistency is that of soft tissue or bone and whether it is of normal anatomical structure. An attempt should be made to further identify soft tissue abnormalities as pitting or nonpitting edema, synovitis, or mass lesions.

All skeletal elements near areas of hemorrhage and ecchymosis in patients with altered consciousness should be palpated. The elderly patient with traumatic subdural hematoma may have an extremity fracture associated with a fall. During the critical care of a motorcyclist with a head injury, an incidental fracture may have been missed. Likewise, any in-hospital fall by a confused patient warrants a search for occult bony trauma.

ROM Assessment

Human joint motion is measured during clinical evaluation by many health care professionals for various reasons, including initial evaluation, evaluation of treatment procedure, feedback to the patient, assessment of work capacity, or research studies. When identifying a starting point for measuring the ROM of a joint, we prefer to regard the anatomical position as the baseline (zero starting point). If rotation is being measured, the midway point between the normal rotation range should be the zero starting point (7).

Considerable variation exists among the ROM measurements of individuals. Factors such as age, sex, conditioning, obesity, and genetics can influence the normal ROM. The American Academy of Orthopaedic Surgeons has reported the average ROM measurements for joints in the human body (8).

When the patient does not assist the examiner during an assessment, the measurement is a passive ROM. If the patient performs the ROM maneuver without assistance, then the range is an active ROM. If comparisons are made between active and passive ROMs, the starting position, stabilization, goniometer, alignment, and type of goniometer should be the same.

Different methods are available for recording the results of ROM measurements. Graphic recordings are often helpful for providing feedback to the patient or a third party. Sometimes the difference between the patient's ROM and a normal ROM is of special interest to the examiner, such as when the surgeon wants to evaluate finger motion periodically as a guide to recovery after a hand operation.

The goniometer position, starting position, and average ROM of the more commonly measured joints are shown in **Figures 1-1** through **1-26**.

(Text continues on page 18)

FIGURE 1-1. Shoulder flexion. (Courtesy of J.F. Lehmann, MD.)

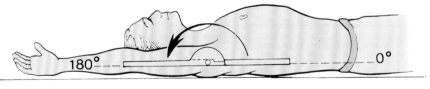

Starting position	Measurement

Supine
Arm at side with
  hand pronated
	Sagittal plane
	Substitution to avoid:
	  Arching back
	  Rotating trunk
	Goniometer:
	  Axis lateral to joint and
	    just below acromion
	  Shaft parallel to
	    midaxillary line of trunk
	  Shaft parallel to midline of
	    humerus

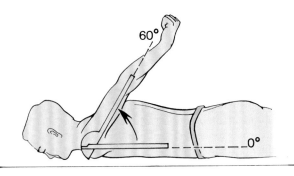

Starting position

Prone
Arm at side with hand
  pronated

Measurement

Sagittal plane
Substitution to avoid:
  Lifting shoulder from table
  Rotating trunk
Goniometer: same as in
  Figure 1-1

FIGURE 1-2. Shoulder hyperextension. (Courtesy of J.F. Lehmann, MD.)

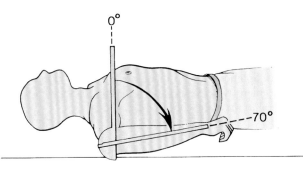

Starting position

Supine
Arm abducted to 90°
  and elbow off table
Elbow flexed to 90°
  and hand pronated
Forearm perpendicular
  to floor

Measurement

Transverse plane
Substitution to avoid:
  Protracting shoulder
  Rotating trunk
  Changing angle at shoulder or
    elbow
Goniometer:
  Axis through longitudinal axis
    of humerus
  Shaft perpendicular to floor
  Shaft parallel to midline or
    forearm

FIGURE 1-4. Shoulder internal rotation. (Courtesy of J.F. Lehmann, MD.)

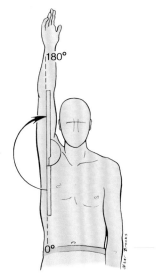

Starting position

Supine
Arm at side

Measurement

Frontal plane (must externally rotate
  shoulder to obtain maximum)
Substitution to avoid:
  Lateral motion of trunk
  Rotating trunk
Goniometer:
  Axis anterior to joint and in line with
    acromion
  Shaft parallel to midline of trunk
  Shaft parallel to midline of humerus

FIGURE 1-3. Shoulder abduction. (Courtesy of J.F. Lehmann, MD.)

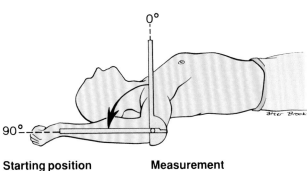

Starting position

Same as in Figure
  1-2

Measurement

Transverse plane
Substitution to avoid:
  Arching back
  Rotating trunk
  Changing angle at shoulder or
    elbow
Goniometer: same as in Figure
  1-4

FIGURE 1-5. Shoulder external rotation. (Courtesy of J.F. Lehmann, MD.)

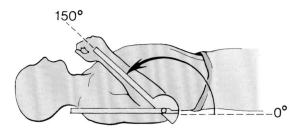

Starting position

Supine
Arm at side with elbow
    straight
Hand supinated

Measurement

Sagittal plane
Goniometer:
    Axis lateral to joint and
        through epicondyles of
        humerus
    Shaft parallel to midline of
        humerus
    Shaft parallel to midline of
        forearm

FIGURE 1-6.   Elbow flexion. (Courtesy of J.F. Lehmann, MD.)

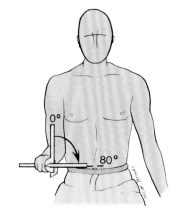

Starting position

Sitting (or standing)
Arm at side with elbow
    held close to trunk
Elbow bent to 90°
Forearm in neutral
    position between
    pronation and
    supination
Wrist in neutral position
Pencil held securely in
    midpalmar crease

Measurement

Transverse plane
Substitution to avoid:
    Rotating trunk
    Moving arm
    Changing angle at elbow
    Angulating wrist
Goniometer:
    Axis through longitudinal
        axis of forearm
    Shaft parallel to midline of
        humerus
    Shaft parallel to pencil (on
        thumb side)

FIGURE 1-8.   Forearm pronation. (Courtesy of J.F. Lehmann, MD.)

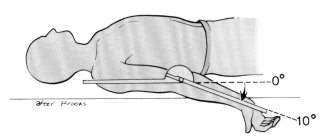

FIGURE 1-7.   Elbow hyperextension. Demonstration of the method of measuring excessive mobility past the normal starting position. (Courtesy of J.F. Lehmann, MD.)

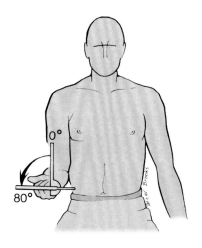

Starting position

Same as in Figure 1-8

Measurement

Same as in Figure 1-8

FIGURE 1-9.   Forearm supination. (Courtesy of J.F. Lehmann, MD.)

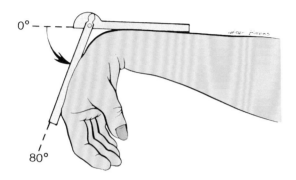

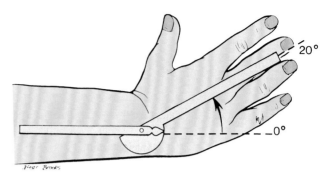

Starting position

Elbow bent
Forearm and wrist
  in neutral
  position

Measurement

Sagittal plane
Goniometer:
  Axis over dorsum of wrist (in line
    with third metacarpal bone)
  Shaft on mid-dorsum of forearm
  Shaft on mid-dorsum of hand

FIGURE 1-10.   Wrist flexion. (Courtesy of J.F. Lehmann, MD.)

Starting position

Forearm pronated
Wrist in neutral position

Measurement

Frontal plane
Goniometer:
  Axis over dorsum of wrist
    centered at midcarpal bone
  Shaft on mid-dorsum of
    forearm
  Shaft on shaft of third
    metacarpal bone

FIGURE 1-12.   Wrist radial deviation. (Courtesy of J.F. Lehmann, MD.)

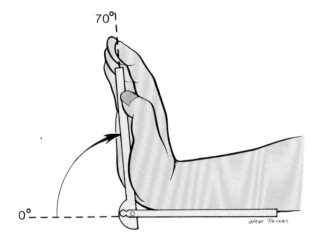

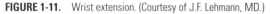

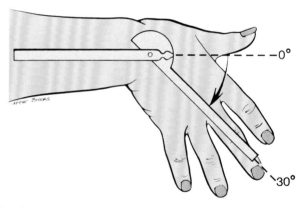

Starting position

Same as in Figure 1-12

Measurement

Same as in Figure 1-12

FIGURE 1-13.   Wrist ulnar deviation. (Courtesy of J.F. Lehmann, MD.)

Starting position

Same as in Figure 1-10

Measurement

Sagittal plane
Goniometer:
  Axis on ventral surface of
    wrist (in line with third
    metacarpal bone)
  Shaft on midventral surface
    of forearm
  Shaft on midpalmar surface
    of hand

FIGURE 1-11.   Wrist extension. (Courtesy of J.F. Lehmann, MD.)

FIGURE 1-14. First metacarpophalangeal flexion. (Courtesy of J.F. Lehmann, MD.)

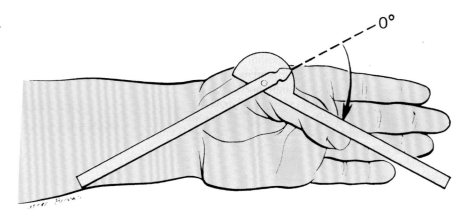

Starting position

Elbow slightly flexed
Hand supinated
Fingers and thumb extended

Measurement

Frontal plane
Goniometer:
    Axis on lateral aspect of
      metacarpophalangeal joint
    Shaft parallel to midline of
      first metacarpal bone
    Shaft parallel to midline of
      proximal phalanx

FIGURE 1-15. Second, third, and fourth metacarpophalangeal flexion. (Courtesy of J.F. Lehmann, MD.)

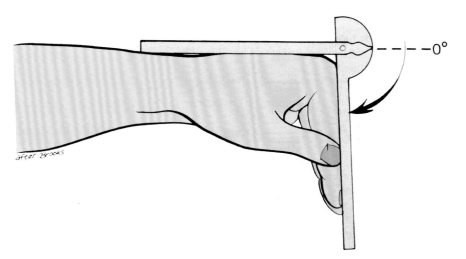

Starting position

Elbow flexed
Hand pronated
Wrist in neutral position

Measurement

Sagittal plane
Goniometer:
    Axis on mid-dorsum of joint
    Shaft on mid-dorsum of
      metacarpal bone
    Shaft on mid-dorsum of
      proximal phalanx

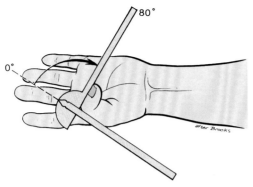

Starting position

Elbow flexed
Forearm supinated
Interphalangeal joint
    extended

Measurement

Frontal plane
Goniometer:
    Axis on lateral aspect of
        interphalangeal joint
    Shaft parallel to midline of
        proximal phalanx
    Shaft parallel to midline of
        distal phalanx

FIGURE 1-16.   First interphalangeal flexion. (Courtesy of J.F. Lehmann, MD.)

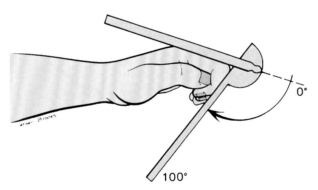

Starting position

Elbow flexed
Forearm pronated
Interphalangeal joint extended

Measurement

Sagittal plane
Goniometer:
    Axis over dorsal aspect of joint
    Shaft over mid-dorsum of
        proximal phalanx
    Shaft over mid-dorsum of more
        distal phalanx

FIGURE 1-17.   Second, third, and fourth interphalangeal flexion. (Courtesy of J.F. Lehmann, MD.)

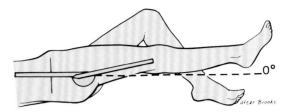

FIGURE 1-18.   Hip extension. See Figure 1-19. (Courtesy of J.F. Lehmann, MD.)

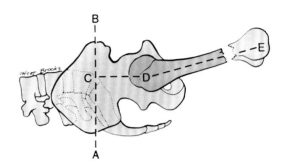

Starting position

Lying on side (or supine)
Lower leg bent for support

Measurement

Sagittal plane
Draw line from anterosuperior to
    posterosuperior iliac spines (*B–A*)
Drop a perpendicular to the greater
    trochanter (*C–D*)
Center axis of goniometer at greater
    trochanter (*D*)
Shaft along perpendicular (*C–D*)
Shaft along shaft of femur (*D–E*)

FIGURE 1-19.   Hip extension. (Courtesy of J.F. Lehmann, MD.)

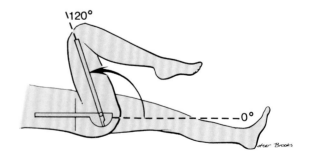

Starting position

Lying on side or supine (may
    flex lower knee slightly for
    support)

Measurement

Sagittal plane
Relocate greater trochanter and
    redraw C–D, as described in
    Figure 1-19
Goniometer placement is the
    same as in Figure 1-19

FIGURE 1-20.   Hip flexion. (Courtesy of J.F. Lehmann, MD.)

FIGURE 1-21.   Hip abduction. (Courtesy of J.F. Lehmann, MD.)

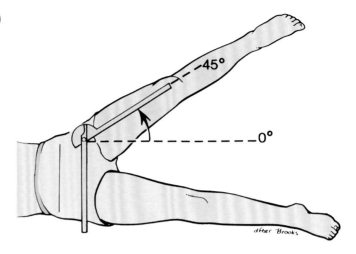

FIGURE 1-22.   Hip adduction. (Courtesy of J.F. Lehmann, MD.)

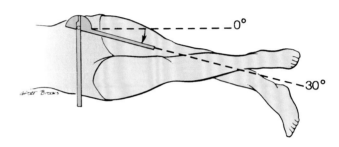

Starting position

Supine
Leg extended and in neutral
    position

Measurement

Frontal plane
Mark both anterosuperior iliac
    spines, and draw a line
    between them
Goniometer:
    Axis over hip joint
    Shaft parallel to line between
        spines of ilium
    Shaft along shaft of femur

FIGURE 1-23.   Hip internal rotation **(left)** and hip external rotation **(right)**. (Courtesy of J.F. Lehmann, MD.)

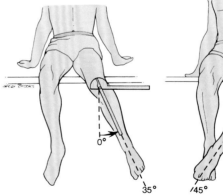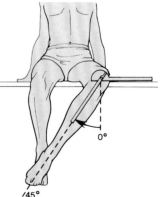

Starting position

Prone, sitting, or supine
    (indicate position on
    record)
Knee flexed to 90°

Measurement

Transverse plane
Substitution to avoid:
    Rotating trunk
    Lifting thigh from table
Goniometer:
    Axis through longitudinal
        axis of femur
    Shaft parallel to table
    Shaft parallel to lower part
        of leg

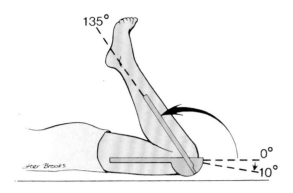

Starting position

Prone (or supine with hip flexed if rectus femoris limits motion)

Measurement

Sagittal plane
Goniometer:
   Axis through knee joint
   Shaft along midthigh
   Shaft along fibula

FIGURE 1-24.   Knee flexion. (Courtesy of J.F. Lehmann, MD.)

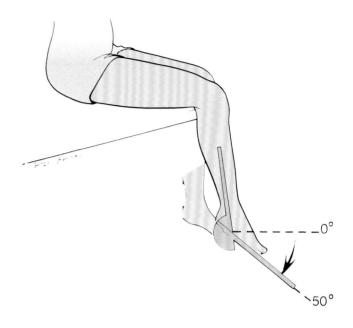

Starting position

Same as in Figure 1-25

Measurement

Same as in Figure 1-25

FIGURE 1-26.   Ankle plantar flexion. (Courtesy of J.F. Lehmann, MD.)

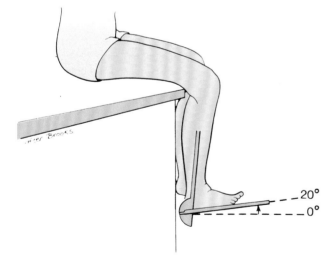

Starting position

Sitting
Knee flexed to 90°
Foot at 90° angle to leg

Measurement

Sagittal plane
Goniometer:
   Axis on sole of foot
   Shaft along fibula
   Shaft along fifth metatarsal
     bone

FIGURE 1-25.   Ankle dorsiflexion. (Courtesy of J.F. Lehmann, MD.)

Joint Stability Assessment

Joint stability is the capacity of the structural elements of a joint to resist the forces of an inappropriate vector. It is determined by the degree of bony congruity, cartilaginous and capsular integrity, and ligament and muscle strength and by the forces applied to the joint. For example, the ball-and-socket arrangement of the hip joint is inherently stable because of bony congruity, whereas the glenohumeral joint must rely on musculoligamentous support because of the incongruity of the spherical humeral head in relation to the shallow curve of the glenoid fossa.

Joint stability is often compromised by disorders commonly treated by physical medicine and rehabilitation staff. For example, inflammatory synovitis associated with polyarthritis weakens the joint capsule and surrounding ligaments, and the resulting pain inhibits muscle contraction. This inhibition renders the involved joint susceptible to trauma from normal and abnormal forces and leads to joint instability. Similarly, traumatic and neurogenic conditions may commonly result in instability of peripheral and axial joints.

Excessive joint motion is often identified during the ROM assessment. However, several specialized physical examination maneuvers (e.g., the Larson test, the Lachman test, or the pivot shift test) can be used to assess individual joint integrity. Although a discussion of these tests is beyond the scope of this chapter, excellent texts are available on them (6,9,10).

The stability of each joint should be assessed in an orderly fashion. A routine series of individual joint maneuvers should be used as part of the general examination, and additional tests should be performed as necessary to identify more subtle instability when indicated by the history or general examination.

If joint instability is recognized or suspected during the physical examination, subsequent radiographic studies can often be helpful for quantifying the extent of instability. At times, flexion-extension views of the spine and stressed joint views of extremity joints can be informative; however, these should not be considered until the physical examination and nonstressed films have determined that such maneuvers are safe.

Muscle Strength Testing

Manual muscle testing provides an important means of assessing strength but also can be used to assess weakness. The examiner should keep in mind many factors that can affect patient effort during testing. These factors include age, sex, pain, fatigue, low motivation, fear, misunderstanding of the test, and the presence of lower or upper motor neuron disease.

Lower motor neuron disease results in patterns of motor loss that depend on the location of the disease. For example, peripheral neuropathy results in a pattern of weakness in the muscles supplied by the affected nerve, whereas poliomyelitis results in residual weakness that is often scattered. The flaccid characteristic of a paretic muscle or muscle group in lower motor neuron disease allows the testing procedure to be uncomplicated by the spasticity or rigidity of upper motor neuron disease. Knowledge of the appearance of the muscle surface when a muscle undergoes atrophy from lower motor neuron disease also can be helpful to the clinician. If the joint crossed by the muscle being tested is unstable because of a chronic flaccid state, the grade of weakness may be difficult to estimate.

Upper motor neuron disease frequently results in spastic muscles that make manual testing challenging. For example, the antagonist muscle may be spastic and resist the action of the muscle being tested, or contractures may have developed that complicate the testing by limiting the available ROM.

Detailed discussions of the technique of manual muscle testing can be found in the publications of Kendall et al. (11) and Hislop and Montgomery (12). The anatomical basis for manual muscle testing of the major groups of muscles is discussed below (1).

ANATOMICAL INFORMATION REQUIRED TO TEST INDIVIDUAL MUSCLE STRENGTH

In the description of each test below, which is based on the format used in *Mayo Clinic Examinations in Neurology* (1), the name of each muscle is followed by the corresponding peripheral nerve and spinal segmental supply. Different authorities give considerable variability in segmental supply, particularly for certain muscles. Anatomical variation also exists both in the plexus and in the peripheral nerves. Therefore, the segments listed here cannot be regarded as absolute. The "action" sections identify only the principal and important secondary or accessory functions that are useful in testing. The positions and the movements in each test refer first to the patient. When the movement is adequately indicated by the action of

the muscle, it has been omitted here. Unless otherwise stated, "resistance" refers to pressure applied by the examiner in the opposite direction of the patient's movement. For brevity and uniformity, we have given methods of testing that involve the patient initiating action against the resistance of the examiner, except when the other method is distinctly more applicable, but we do not mean to imply a preference for this method. We have often given the location of the belly of the muscle and its tendon so as to stress the importance of observation and palpation in identifying the muscle's function. We have listed only those participating muscles with a definite action in the movement being tested that may substitute in part or in whole for the muscle being reviewed.

The following text has been adapted with permission from the Mayo Foundation for Medical Education and Research (1).

Trapezius (Fig. 1-27)
Spinal accessory nerve (**Fig.** 1-29).

Action
Elevation, retraction (adduction), and rotation (lateral angle upward) of the scapula, providing fixation of the scapula during movement of the arm.

Test
1. Elevation (shrugging) of the shoulder against resistance tests the upper portion, which is readily visible.
2. Bracing the shoulder (backward movement and adduction of the scapula) primarily tests the middle portion.
3. Abduction of the arm against resistance intensifies the winging of the scapula that may be present in paresis of the trapezius muscle (as in spinal accessory neuropathy).

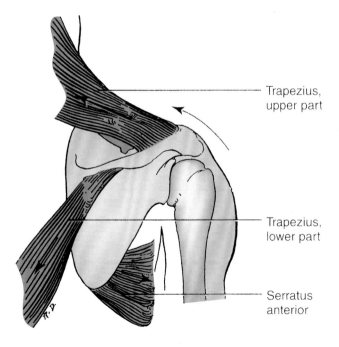

FIGURE 1-27. Upward rotators of the scapula. (From Jenkins DB. *Hollinshead's Functional Anatomy of the Limbs and Back.* 8th ed. Philadelphia, PA: WB Saunders; 2002:99. Used with permission of Mayo Foundation for Medical Education and Research.)

In isolated trapezius palsy with the shoulder girdle at rest, the scapula is displaced downward laterally and rotated so that the superior angle is farther from the spine than the inferior angle. The lateral displacement is due in part to the unopposed action of the serratus anterior. The vertebral border, particularly at the inferior angle, is flared. These changes are accentuated when the arm is abducted from the side against resistance. On flexion (forward elevation) of the arm, however, this flaring of the inferior angle virtually disappears. These features are important in distinguishing paresis of the trapezius from that of the serratus anterior, because both conditions produce winging of the scapula.

Participating Muscles

1. Elevation: levator scapulae (third and fourth cervical nerves and dorsal scapular nerve, C3-5)
2. Retraction: rhomboids
3. Upward rotation: serratus anterior

Rhomboids (Fig. 1-28)

Dorsal scapular nerve from the anterior ramus, C4, C5 (**Fig. 1-29**).

Action

Retraction (adduction) of the scapula and elevation of its vertebral border.

Test

The hand is on the hip; the arm is held backward and rotated medially. The examiner attempts to force the patient's elbow laterally and forward while observing and palpating the muscle bellies medial to the scapula.

Participating Muscles

Trapezius; levator scapulae with elevation of the medial border of the scapula.

Serratus Anterior (See Fig. 1-27)

Long thoracic nerve from the anterior rami, C5-7 (see **Fig. 1-29**). See Appendix A.

Action

1. Protraction (lateral and forward movement) of the scapula while it is kept close to the thorax
2. Assistance in the upward rotation of the scapula

Test

The patient's outstretched arm is thrust forward against a wall or against resistance provided by the examiner.

Isolated palsy results in comparatively little change in the appearance of the shoulder girdle at rest. However, there is slight winging of the inferior angle of the scapula and a slight shift medially toward the spine. When the outstretched arm is thrust forward, the entire scapula, particularly its inferior angle, shifts backward away from the thorax, producing the characteristic wing effect. Abduction of the arm laterally, however, produces comparatively little winging, compared with the manifestations of paralysis of the trapezius.

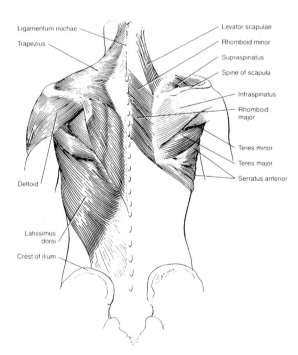

FIGURE 1-28. Musculature of the shoulder, posterior view. (From Jenkins DB. *Hollinshead's Functional Anatomy of the Limbs and Back.* 8th ed. Philadelphia, PA: WB Saunders; 2002:89. Used with permission of Mayo Foundation for Medical Education and Research.)

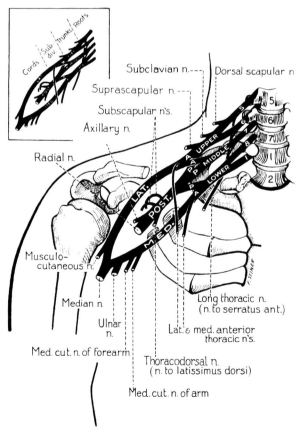

FIGURE 1-29. Brachial plexus. (Reprinted with permisison from Premkumar K. *Anatomy and Physiology: The Massage Connection.* 3rd ed. Baltimore, MD: Lippincott Williams & Wilkins; 2011:139.)

Supraspinatus (Fig. 1-30)

Suprascapular nerve from the upper trunk of the brachial plexus, C5, C6 (see **Fig. 1-29**). See Appendix B.

Action

Initiation of abduction of the arm from the side of the body.

Test

The above action is tested against resistance.

Atrophy may be detected just above the spine of the scapula, but the trapezius overlies the supraspinatus, and atrophy of either muscle will produce a depression in this area. Scapular fixation is important in this test.

Participating Muscle

Deltoid.

Infraspinatus (Fig. 1-31)

Suprascapular nerve from the upper trunk of the brachial plexus, C5, C6 (see **Fig. 1-29**). See Appendix B.

Action

Lateral (external) rotation of the arm at the shoulder.

Test

The elbow is at the side and flexed 90 degrees. The patient resists the examiner's attempt to push the hand medially toward the abdomen.

The muscle is palpable, and atrophy may be visible below the spine of the scapula.

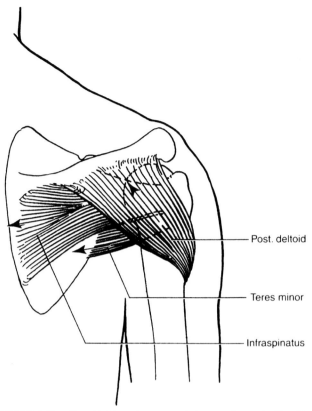

FIGURE 1-31. The chief lateral rotators of the arm. (From Jenkins DB. *Hollinshead's Functional Anatomy of the Limbs and Back.* 8th ed. Philadelphia, PA: WB Saunders; 2002:106. Used with permission of Mayo Foundation for Medical Education and Research.)

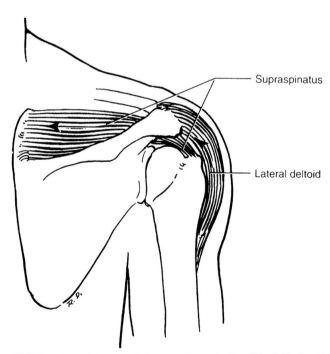

FIGURE 1-30. Abductors of the arm. (From Jenkins DB. *Hollinshead's Functional Anatomy of the Limbs and Back.* 8th ed. Philadelphia, PA: WB Saunders; 2002:103. Used with permission of Mayo Foundation for Medical Education and Research.)

Participating Muscles

Teres minor (axillary nerve); deltoid (posterior fibers).

Pectoralis Major (Fig. 1-32)

See **Figure 1-29** and Appendix A.
   1. Clavicular portion (lateral pectoral nerve from the lateral cord of the plexus, C5-7).
   2. Sternal portion (medial pectoral nerve from the medial cord of the plexus, lateral pectoral nerve, C6-8, T1).

Action

   1. Adduction and medial rotation of the arm.
   2. Clavicular portion: assistance in flexion of the arm.

Test

   1. The arm is in front of the body. The patient resists the examiner's attempt to force it laterally.
   2. The two portions of the muscle are visible and palpable.

Latissimus Dorsi (Fig. 1-33)

Thoracodorsal nerve from the posterior cord of the plexus, C6-8 (see **Fig. 1-29**). See Appendix C.

Action

Adduction, extension, and medial rotation of the arm.

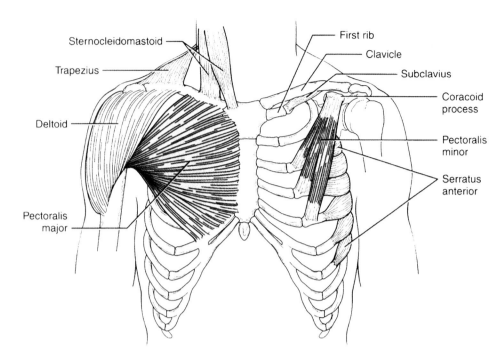

FIGURE 1-32. The pectoral (*shaded*) and related muscles. (From Jenkins DB. *Hollinshead's Functional Anatomy of the Limbs and Back.* 8th ed. Philadelphia, PA: WB Saunders; 2002:85. Used with permission of Mayo Foundation for Medical Education and Research.)

Test

The arm is in abduction to the horizontal position. Downward and backward movement against resistance is applied under the elbow.

The muscle should be observed and palpated in and below the posterior axillary fold. When the patient coughs, a brisk contraction of the normal latissimus dorsi can be felt at the inferior angle of the scapula.

Teres Major (Fig. 1-33A)

Lower subscapular nerve from the posterior cord of the plexus, C5-7 (see **Fig. 1-29**). See Appendix C.

Action

Same as for the latissimus dorsi.

Test

Same as for the latissimus dorsi. The muscle is visible and palpable at the lower lateral border of the scapula.

Deltoid (Fig. 1-33C; See Fig. 1-32)

Axillary nerve from the posterior cord of the plexus, C5, C6 (see **Fig. 1-29**). See Appendix D.

Action

1. Abduction of the arm.
2. Flexion (forward movement) and medial rotation of the arm: anterior fibers.
3. Extension (backward movement) and lateral rotation of the arm: posterior fibers.

Test

1. The arm is almost horizontal in abduction. The patient resists the examiner's efforts to depress the elbow. Paralysis of the deltoid leads to conspicuous atrophy and serious disability, because the other muscles that

participate in abduction of the arm (the supraspinatus, trapezius, and serratus anterior—the last two by rotating the scapula) cannot compensate for the deltoid's lack of function.

2. Flexion and extension of the arm are tested against resistance.

Participating Muscles

1. Abduction: given above.
2. Flexion: pectoralis major (clavicular portion); biceps.
3. Extension: latissimus dorsi; teres major.

Subscapularis (Fig. 1-33B)

Upper and lower subscapular nerves from the posterior cord of the plexus, C5-7 (see **Fig. 1-29**). See Appendix G.

Action

Medial (internal) rotation of the arm at the shoulder.

Test

The patient's elbow is at the side and flexed 90 degrees. The patient resists the examiner's attempt to pull the hand laterally.

Because this muscle is not accessible to observation or palpation, it is necessary to gauge the activity of other muscles that produce this movement. The pectoralis major is the most powerful medial rotator of the arm; hence, paralysis of the subscapularis alone results in relatively little weakness of this movement.

Participating Muscles

Pectoralis major; deltoid (anterior fibers); teres major; latissimus dorsi.

Biceps; Brachialis (Fig. 1-34)

Musculocutaneous nerve from the lateral cord of the plexus, C5, C6 (see **Fig. 1-29**).

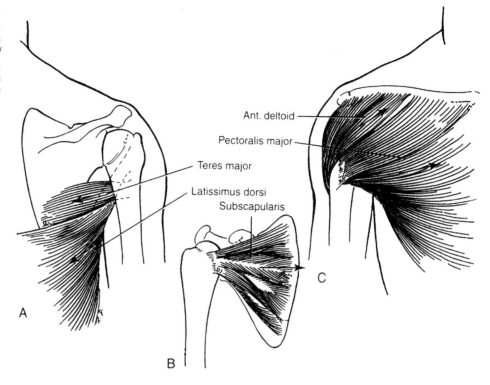

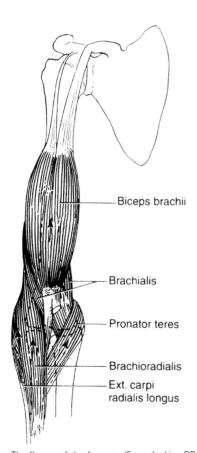

FIGURE 1-34. The flexors of the forearm. (From Jenkins DB. *Hollinshead's Functional Anatomy of the Limbs and Back.* 8th ed. Philadelphia, PA: WB Saunders; 2002:129. Used with permission of Mayo Foundation for Medical Education and Research.)

Action

1. Biceps: flexion and supination of the forearm and assistance in flexion of the arm at the shoulder.
2. Brachialis: flexion of the forearm at the elbow.

Test

Flexion of the forearm is tested against resistance. The forearm should be in supination to decrease participation of the brachioradialis.

Triceps (Fig. 1-35)

Radial nerve, which is a continuation of the posterior cord of the plexus, C6-8 (see **Fig. 1-29**). See Appendix A.

Action

Extension of the forearm at the elbow.

Test

The forearm is in mid flexion. The patient resists the examiner's effort to flex the forearm farther. Slight weakness is more easily detected when starting with the forearm almost completely flexed.

Brachioradialis (Fig. 1-36)

Radial nerve, C5, C6 (see **Fig. 1-29**). See Appendix E.

Action

Flexion of the forearm at the elbow.

Test

Flexion of the forearm is tested against resistance, with the forearm midway between pronation and supination. The belly of the muscle stands out prominently on the upper surface of

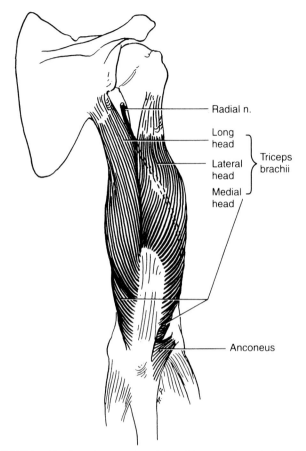

FIGURE 1-35. Posterior muscles of the right arm. (From Jenkins DB. *Hollinshead's Functional Anatomy of the Limbs and Back*. 8th ed. Philadelphia, PA: WB Saunders; 2002:122. Used with permission of Mayo Foundation for Medical Education and Research.)

the forearm, tending to bridge the angle between the forearm and the arm.

Participating Muscles
Biceps; brachialis.

Supinator (See Fig. 1-36)
Posterior interosseous nerve from the radial nerve, C5, C6 (see **Fig. 1-29**). See Appendix A.

Action
Supination of the forearm.

Test
The forearm is in full extension and supination. The patient tries to maintain supination while the examiner attempts to pronate the forearm and palpate the biceps.

Resistance to pronation by the intact supinator can usually be felt before there is appreciable contraction of the biceps.

Extensor Carpi Radialis Longus (Fig. 1-37)
Radial nerve, C6, C7 (see **Fig. 1-29**). See Appendix A.

Action
Extension (dorsiflexion) and radial abduction of the hand at the wrist.

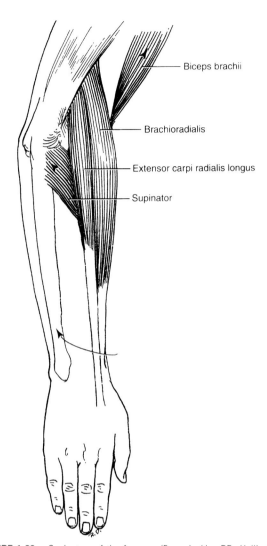

FIGURE 1-36. Supinators of the forearm. (From Jenkins DB. *Hollinshead's Functional Anatomy of the Limbs and Back*. 8th ed. Philadelphia, PA: WB Saunders; 2002:173. Used with permission of Mayo Foundation for Medical Education and Research.)

Test
The forearm is in almost complete pronation. Dorsiflexion of the wrist is tested against resistance applied to the dorsum of the hand downward and toward the ulnar side.

The tendon is palpable just above its insertion into the base of the second metacarpal bone. To minimize participation of the extensors of the digits, the patient should relax the fingers and thumb but flex them somewhat.

Extensor Carpi Radialis Brevis (See Fig. 1-37)
Posterior interosseous nerve from the radial nerve, C6, C7 (see **Fig. 1-29**). See Appendix A.

Action
Extension (dorsiflexion) of the hand at the wrist.

Test
The forearm is in complete pronation. Dorsiflexion of the wrist is tested against resistance applied straight downward to the dorsum of the hand.

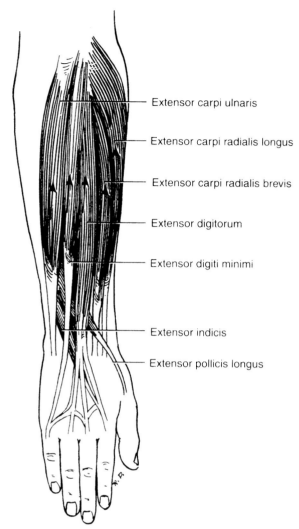

FIGURE 1-37. Extensors at the wrist. (From Jenkins DB. *Hollinshead's Functional Anatomy of the Limbs and Back.* 8th ed. Philadelphia, PA: WB Saunders; 2002:174. Used with permission of Mayo Foundation for Medical Education and Research.)

The tendon is palpable just proximal to the base of the third metacarpal bone. To minimize participation of the extensors of the digits, the patient should relax the fingers and thumb but flex them somewhat.

Extensor Carpi Ulnaris (See Fig. 1-37)

Posterior interosseous nerve from the radial nerve, C7, C8 (see **Fig. 1-29**). See Appendix A.

Action

Extension (dorsiflexion) and ulnar deviation of the hand at the wrist.

Test

The forearm is in pronation. Dorsiflexion and ulnar deviation of the wrist are tested against resistance applied to the dorsum of the hand downward and toward the radial side.

The tendon is palpable just below or above the distal end of the ulna. To minimize participation of the extensors of the digits, the patient should relax the fingers but flex them somewhat.

Extensor Digitorum Communis (See Fig. 1-37)

Posterior interosseous nerve from the radial nerve, C7, C8 (see **Fig. 1-29**). See Appendix A.

Action

1. Extension of the fingers, principally at the metacarpophalangeal joints.
2. Assistance in extension (dorsiflexion) of the wrist.

Test

The forearm is in pronation. The wrist is stabilized in a straight position. Extension of the fingers at the metacarpophalangeal joints is tested against resistance applied to the proximal phalanges.

The distal portions of the fingers may be somewhat relaxed but slightly flexed. The tendons are visible and palpable over the dorsum of the hand.

Extension at the interphalangeal joints is a function primarily of the interossei (ulnar nerve) and the lumbricals (median and ulnar nerves).

To minimize the action of the common extensor, the physiatrist can individually test the extensor digiti quinti and extensor indicis (posterior interosseous nerve, C7, C8), which are proper extensors of the little finger and the index finger, respectively, while the other fingers are flexed. In a thin person's hand, these tendons can usually be identified.

Abductor Pollicis Longus (See Fig. 1-39)

Posterior interosseous nerve from the radial nerve, C7, C8. See Appendix A.

Action

1. Radial abduction of the thumb (in the same plane as that of the palm, in contradistinction to palmar abduction, which is movement perpendicular to the plane of the palm).
2. Assistance in radial abduction and flexion of the hand at the wrist.

Test

1. The hand is on the edge (the forearm is midway between pronation and supination).
2. Radial abduction of the thumb is tested against resistance applied to the metacarpal.

The tendon, which forms the anterior (volar) boundary of the "anatomic snuffbox," is palpable just above its insertion into the base of the metacarpal bone.

Participating Muscle

Extensor pollicis brevis.

Extensor Pollicis Brevis

Posterior interosseous nerve from the radial nerve, C7, C8. See Appendix A.

Action

1. Extension of the proximal phalanx of the thumb.
2. Assistance in radial abduction and extension of the metacarpal of the thumb.

Test

The hand is on the edge. The wrist and the metacarpal of the thumb are stabilized by the examiner. Extension of the proximal phalanx is tested against resistance applied to that phalanx, while the distal phalanx is in flexion to minimize the action of the extensor pollicis longus.

At the wrist, the tendon lies just posterior (dorsal) to the tendon of the abductor pollicis longus.

Participating Muscle

Extensor pollicis longus.

Extensor Pollicis Longus (See Fig. 1-37)

Posterior interosseous nerve from the radial nerve, C7, C8. See Appendix A.

Action

1. Extension of all parts of the thumb but specifically extension of the distal phalanx.
2. Assistance in adduction of the thumb.

Test

The hand is on the edge. The wrist and the metacarpal and proximal phalanx of the thumb are stabilized by the examiner, with the thumb close to the palm at its radial border. Extension of the distal phalanx is tested against resistance.

If the patient is permitted to flex the wrist or abduct the thumb away from the palm, some extension of the phalanges results simply from lengthening the path of the extensor tendon. At the wrist, the tendon forms the posterior (dorsal) boundary of the anatomic snuffbox.

The characteristic result of radial nerve palsy is wrist-drop. Extension of the fingers at the interphalangeal joints is still possible by virtue of the action of the interossei and lumbricals, but extension of the thumb is lost.

Pronator Teres (Fig. 1-38)

Median nerve, C6, C7 (see **Fig. 1-29**). See Appendix B.

Action

Pronation of the forearm.

Test

The elbow is at the side of the trunk, the forearm is in flexion to the right angle, and the arm is in lateral rotation at the shoulder to eliminate the effect of gravity, which favors pronation in most positions. Pronation of the forearm is tested against resistance, starting from a position of moderate supination.

Participating Muscle

Pronator quadratus (anterior interosseous branch of the median nerve, C7, C8, T1).

Flexor Carpi Radialis (Figs. 1-38 and 1-39)

Median nerve, C6, C7 (see **Fig. 1-29**). See Appendix B.

Action

1. Flexion (palmar flexion) of the hand at the wrist.
2. Assistance in radial abduction of the hand.

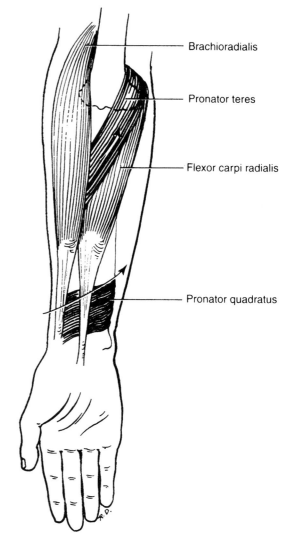

FIGURE 1-38. Pronators of the forearm. (From Jenkins DB. *Hollinshead's Functional Anatomy of the Limbs and Back.* 8th ed. Philadelphia, PA: WB Saunders; 2002:172. Used with permission of Mayo Foundation for Medical Education and Research.)

Test

1. Flexion of the hand is tested against resistance applied to the palm.
2. The fingers should be relaxed to minimize participation of their flexors. The tendon is the more lateral (radial) of the two conspicuous tendons on the volar aspect of the wrist.

In complete median nerve palsy, flexion of the wrist is considerably weakened but can still be performed by the flexor carpi ulnaris (ulnar nerve), assisted to some extent by the abductor pollicis longus (radial nerve). In this event, ulnar deviation of the hand usually accompanies flexion.

Palmaris Longus (See Fig. 1-39)

Median nerve, C7, C8, T1 (see **Fig. 1-29**). See Appendix B.

Action

Flexion of the hand at the wrist.

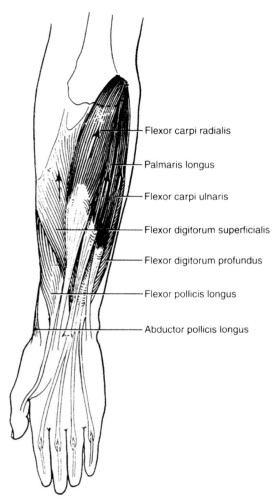

FIGURE 1-39. Flexors at the wrist. (From Jenkins DB. *Hollinshead's Functional Anatomy of the Limbs and Back.* 8th ed. Philadelphia, PA: WB Saunders; 2002:174. Used with permission of Mayo Foundation for Medical Education and Research.)

Test
Same as that for flexor carpi radialis. The tendon is palpable at the ulnar side of the tendon of the flexor carpi radialis.

Flexor Carpi Ulnaris (See Fig. 1-39)
Ulnar nerve, C7, C8, T1 (see **Fig. 1-29**). See Appendix C.

Action
1. Flexion and ulnar deviation of the hand at the wrist.
2. Fixation of the pisiform bone during contraction of the abductor digiti quinti.

Test
Flexion and ulnar deviation of the hand are tested against resistance applied to the ulnar side of the palm in the direction of extension and radial abduction. The fingers should be relaxed. The tendon is palpable proximal to the pisiform bone.

Flexor Digitorum Superficialis (See Fig. 1-39)
Median nerve, C7, C8 (see **Fig. 1-29**). See Appendix B.

Action
1. Flexion primarily of the middle phalanges of the fingers at the first interphalangeal joints; flexion secondarily of the proximal phalanges at the metacarpophalangeal joints.
2. Assistance in flexion of the hand at the wrist.

Test
The wrist is in a neutral position; the proximal phalanges are stabilized. Flexion of the middle phalanx of each finger is tested against resistance applied to that phalanx, with the distal phalanx relaxed.

Flexor Digitorum Profundus
See **Figure 1-39** and Appendices B and C.
1. Radial portion: usually to digits II and III (median nerve and its anterior interosseous branch C7, C8, T1).
2. Ulnar portion: usually to digits IV and V (ulnar nerve, C7, C8, T1).

Action
1. Flexion primarily of the distal phalanges of the fingers; flexion secondarily of other phalanges.
2. Assistance in flexion of the hand at the wrist.

Test
1. Flexion of the distal phalanges is tested against resistance, with the proximal and middle phalanges stabilized in extension.
2. With the middle and distal phalanges folded over the edge of the examiner's hand, the patient resists the examiner's attempt to extend the distal phalanges.

Flexor Pollicis Longus (See Fig. 1-39)
Anterior interosseous branch of the median nerve, C7, C8, T1. See Appendix A.

Action
1. Flexion of the thumb, particularly the distal phalanx.
2. Assistance in ulnar adduction of the thumb.

Test
Flexion of the distal phalanx is tested against resistance, with the thumb in the position of palmar adduction and with stabilization of the metacarpal and the proximal phalanx.

Abductor Pollicis Brevis (Fig. 1-40)
Median nerve, C8, T1 (see **Fig. 1-29**). See Appendix A.

Action
1. Palmar abduction of the thumb (perpendicular to the plane of the palm).
2. Assistance in opposition and in flexion of the proximal phalanx of the thumb.

Test
Palmar abduction of the thumb is tested against resistance applied at the metacarpophalangeal joint.

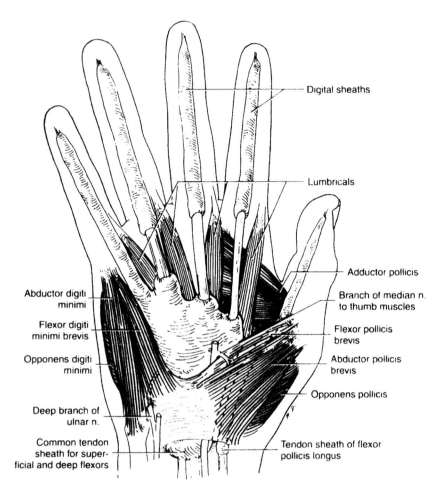

Digital sheaths

Lumbricals

Abductor digiti minimi

Flexor digiti minimi brevis

Opponens digiti minimi

Deep branch of ulnar n.

Common tendon sheath for superficial and deep flexors

Adductor pollicis

Branch of median n. to thumb muscles

Flexor pollicis brevis

Abductor pollicis brevis

Opponens pollicis

Tendon sheath of flexor pollicis longus

FIGURE 1-40. Short muscles of the thumb and little finger (*dark shading*), and flexor tendon sheaths of the hand (*light shading*). (From Jenkins DB. *Hollinshead's Functional Anatomy of the Limbs and Back.* 8th ed. Philadelphia, PA: WB Saunders; 2002:187. Used with permission of Mayo Foundation for Medical Education and Research.)

The muscle is readily visible and palpable in the thenar eminence.

Participating Muscle
Flexor pollicis brevis (superficial head).

Opponens Pollicis (See Fig. 1-40)
Median nerve, C8, T1 (see **Fig. 1-29**). See Appendix B.

Action
Movement of the first metacarpal across the palm, rotating it into opposition.

Test
The thumb is in opposition. The examiner attempts to rotate and draw the thumb back to its usual position.

Participating Muscles
Abductor pollicis brevis; flexor pollicis brevis.

Flexor Pollicis Brevis (Fig. 1-40)
Superficial head (median nerve, C8, T1); deep head (ulnar nerve, C8, T1) (see **Fig. 1-29**). See Appendix B.

Action
1. Flexion of the proximal phalanx of the thumb.
2. Assistance in opposition, ulnar adduction (entire muscle), and palmar abduction (superficial head) of the thumb.

Test
1. The thumb is in the position of palmar adduction, with stabilization of the metacarpal.
2. Flexion of the proximal phalanx is tested against resistance applied to that phalanx, while the distal phalanx is as relaxed as possible.

Participating Muscles
Flexor pollicis longus; abductor pollicis brevis; adductor pollicis.

Severe median nerve palsy produces the "simian" hand, wherein the thumb tends to lie in the same plane as the palm, with the volar surface facing more anteriorly than normal. Atrophy of the muscles of the thenar eminence is usually conspicuous.

Three muscles supplied, at least in part, by the ulnar nerve have already been described: the flexor carpi ulnaris, the flexor digitorum profundus, and the flexor pollicis brevis. The remaining muscles supplied by this nerve are described below.

Hypothenar Muscles (See Fig. 1-40)
Ulnar nerve, C8, T1 (see **Fig. 1-29**). See Appendix C.

Action
1. Abductor digiti minimi and flexor digiti minimi: abduction and flexion (proximal phalanx) of the little finger.
2. Opponens digiti minimi: opposition of the little finger toward the thumb.
3. All three muscles: palmar elevation of the head of the fifth metacarpal, helping to cup the palm.

Test
The action usually tested is abduction of the little finger (against resistance).

The abductor digiti minimi is readily observed and palpated at the ulnar border of the palm. Opposition of the thumb and the little finger can be tested together by gauging the force required to separate the tips of the two digits when opposed or by attempting to withdraw a piece of paper clasped between the tips of the digits.

Interossei (Fig. 1-41)
Ulnar nerve, C8, T1 (see **Fig. 1-29**). See Appendix C and Figure 1-42.

Action
1. Dorsal: abduction of the index, middle, and ring fingers from the middle line of the middle finger (double action on the middle finger: both radial and ulnar abduction; radial abduction of the index finger; ulnar abduction of the ring finger).
2. First dorsal: adduction (especially palmar adduction) of the thumb.
3. Palmar: adduction of the index, ring, and little fingers toward the middle finger.
4. Both sets: flexion of metacarpophalangeal joints and simultaneous extension of the interphalangeal joints.

Test
1. Abduction and adduction of the individual fingers are tested against resistance, with the fingers extended. Adduction can be tested by retention of a slip of paper between the fingers and between the thumb and the index finger, as the examiner attempts to withdraw it.
2. Ability of the patient to flex the proximal phalanges and simultaneously extend the distal phalanges.
3. Extension of the middle phalanges of the fingers against resistance while the examiner stabilizes the proximal phalanges in hyperextension.

The long extensors of the fingers (radial nerve) and the lumbrical muscles (median and ulnar nerves) assist in extension of the middle and distal phalanges. The first dorsal interosseous is readily observed and palpated in the space between the index finger and the thumb.

Adductor Pollicis (see Fig. 1-42)
Ulnar nerve, C8, T1 (see **Fig. 1-29**). See Appendix C.

Action
Adduction of the thumb in both the ulnar and the palmar directions (in the plane of the palm and perpendicular to the palm, respectively). Assistance in flexion of the proximal phalanx.

Test
Adduction in each plane is tested against resistance by retention of a slip of paper between the thumb and the radial border of the hand and between the thumb and the palm, without flexion of the distal phalanx.

It is often possible to palpate the edge of the adductor pollicis just volar to the proximal part of the first dorsal interosseous.

Participating Muscles
1. Ulnar adduction: first dorsal interosseous; flexor pollicis longus; extensor pollicis longus; flexor pollicis brevis.
2. Palmar adduction: first dorsal interosseous, in particular; extensor pollicis longus.

Flexors of the Neck
Cervical nerves, C1-6.

Test
Sitting or supine: flexion of the neck, with the chin on the chest, is tested against resistance applied to the forehead.

Extensors of the Neck (Fig. 1-43)
Cervical nerves, C1-T1.

Test
Sitting or prone: extension of the neck is tested against resistance applied to the occiput.

Diaphragm
Phrenic nerves, C3-5.

Action
Abdominal respiration (inspiration) is distinguished from thoracic respiration (inspiration), which is produced principally by the intercostal muscles.

Test
1. The patient is observed for protrusion of the upper portion of the abdomen during deep inspiration when the thoracic cage is splinted.
2. The patient is observed for ability to sniff.
3. Litten phenomenon (successive retraction of the lower intercostal spaces during inspiration) may be observed if the patient's body habitus permits, such as in thin individuals.
4. Diaphragmatic movements are observed fluoroscopically. Unilateral phrenic nerve palsy leads to diaphragmatic movement on one side but not the other (Litten sign).

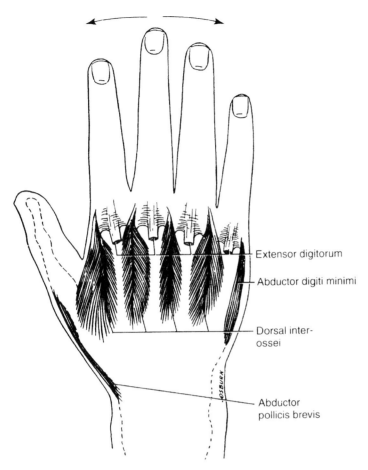

Extensor digitorum

Abductor digiti minimi

Dorsal inter-ossei

Abductor pollicis brevis

FIGURE 1-41. Dorsal view of the chief abductors of the digits. (From Jenkins DB. *Hollinshead's Functional Anatomy of the Limbs and Back.* 8th ed. Philadelphia, PA: WB Saunders; 2002:212. Used with permission of Mayo Foundation for Medical Education and Research.)

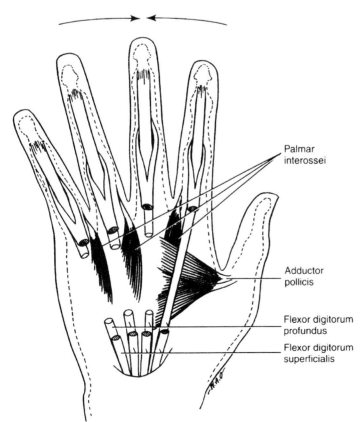

Palmar interossei

Adductor pollicis

Flexor digitorum profundus

Flexor digitorum superficialis

FIGURE 1-42. The chief adductors of the digits. (From Jenkins DB. *Hollinshead's Functional Anatomy of the Limbs and Back.* 8th ed. Philadelphia, PA: WB Saunders; 2002:213. Used with permission of Mayo Foundation for Medical Education and Research.)

Weakness of the diaphragm should be suspected in disease of the spinal cord when the deltoid or biceps is paralyzed, because these muscles are supplied by neurons situated close to those that innervate the diaphragm.

Intercostal Muscles

Intercostal nerves, T1-11.

Action

Expansion of the thorax anteroposteriorly and transversely, producing thoracic inspiration.

Test

1. Observation and palpation of the expansion of the thoracic cage during deep inspiration while maintaining pressure against the thorax.
2. Observation for asymmetric movement of the thorax, particularly during deep inspiration.
3. Other more general tests of function of the respiratory muscles are as follows:
   a. Observation of the patient for rapid shallow respiration, flaring of ala nasi, and the use of accessory muscles of respiration.
   b. Ability of the patient to repeat three or four numbers without pausing for breath.
   c. Ability of the patient to hold his or her breath for 15 seconds.

Anterior Abdominal Muscles

Upper (T6-9); lower (T10-L1).

Test

1. Supine: flexion of the neck is tested against resistance applied to the forehead by the examiner. Contraction of the abdominal muscles can be observed and palpated. Upward movement of the umbilicus is associated with weakness of the lower abdominal muscles (Beevor sign).
2. Supine: hands on the occiput. Flexion of the trunk by anterior abdominal muscles is followed by flexion of the pelvis on the thighs by the hip flexors (chiefly iliopsoas) to reach a sitting position. The examiner holds down the patient's legs.

Completion of this test can exclude significant weakness of either the abdominal muscles or the flexors of the hips. Weak abdominal muscles, in the presence of strong hip flexors, result in hyperextension of the lumbar spine during attempts to elevate the legs or to rise to a sitting position.

Extensors of the Back

See **Figure 1-43**.

Test

Prone: with the hands clasped over the buttocks, the patient elevates his or her head and shoulders off the table while the examiner holds down the patient's legs.

The gluteal and hamstring muscles fix the pelvis on the thigh.

Iliopsoas (Fig. 1-44)

Psoas major (lumbar plexus, L2-4); iliacus (femoral nerve, L2-4). See Appendix H.

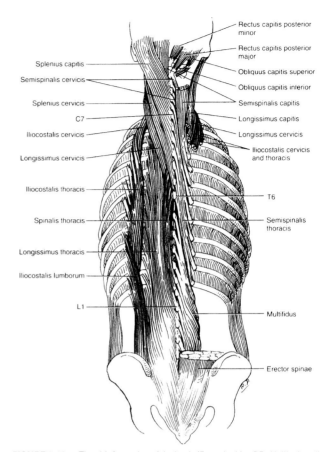

FIGURE 1-43. The chief muscles of the back. (From Jenkins DB. *Hollinshead's Functional Anatomy of the Limbs and Back.* 8th ed. Philadelphia, PA: WB Saunders; 2002:236. Used with permission of Mayo Foundation for Medical Education and Research.)

Action

Flexion of the thigh at the hip.

Test

1. Sitting: flexion of the thigh is tested by raising a knee against resistance by the examiner.
2. Supine: flexion of the thigh is tested by raising an extended leg off the table and maintaining it against downward pressure applied by the examiner just above the knee.

Participating Muscles

Rectus femoris and sartorius (both: femoral nerve, L2-4); tensor fasciae latae (superior gluteal nerve, L4, L5).

Adductor Magnus, Longus, Brevis (See Fig. 1-44)

Obturator nerve, L2-4; part of adductor magnus is supplied by sciatic nerve, L5, and functions with hamstrings. See Appendix I.

Action

Adduction of the thigh principally.

Test

Sitting or supine: the knees are held together while the examiner attempts to separate them.

The legs also can be tested separately and the muscles palpated.

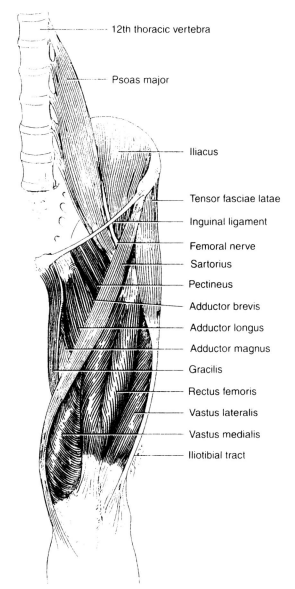

FIGURE 1-44. The superficial muscles of the anterior aspect of the thigh. (From Jenkins DB. *Hollinshead's Functional Anatomy of the Limbs and Back.* 8th ed. Philadelphia, PA: WB Saunders; 2002:281. Used with permission of Mayo Foundation for Medical Education and Research.)

Participating Muscles
Gluteus maximus; gracilis (obturator nerve, L2-4).

Abductors of the Thigh (Fig. 1-45)
Superior gluteal nerve, L4, L5, S1.
1. Gluteus medius and gluteus minimus principally.
2. Tensor fasciae latae to a lesser extent.

Action
1. Abduction and medial rotation of the thigh.
2. Tensor fasciae latae assists in flexion of the thigh at the hip.

Test
1. Sitting: the knees are approximated against resistance by the examiner. In this position, the gluteus maximus and some of the other lateral rotators of the thigh

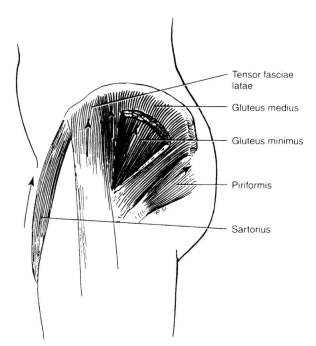

FIGURE 1-45. The abductors of the thigh. (From Jenkins DB. *Hollinshead's Functional Anatomy of the Limbs and Back.* 8th ed. Philadelphia, PA: WB Saunders; 2002:315. Used with permission of Mayo Foundation for Medical Education and Research.)

function as abductors, hence diminishing the accuracy of the test.
2. Supine: same test as for abductors, above, but more exact.
3. Lying on opposite side: the hip is abducted (moved upward) while the examiner presses downward on the lower leg and stabilizes the pelvis.

The tensor fasciae latae and, to a lesser extent, the gluteus medius can be palpated.

Medial Rotators of the Thigh (See Fig. 1-45)
Same as abductors; superior gluteal nerve, L4, L5, S1.

Test
Sitting or supine: the knee is flexed to 90 degrees. Medial rotation of the thigh is tested against resistance applied by the examiner at the knee and the ankle in an attempt to rotate the thigh laterally.

Lateral Rotators of the Thigh (Fig. 1-46)
L4, L5, S1, S2.
1. Gluteus maximus (inferior gluteal nerve, L5, S1, S2) chiefly.
2. Obturator internus and gemellus superior (nerve to obturator internus, L5, S1, S2).
3. Quadratus femoris and gemellus inferior (nerve to quadratus femoris, L4, L5, S1).

Test
Sitting or supine: the knee is flexed to 90 degrees. Lateral rotation of the thigh is tested against an attempt by the examiner to rotate the thigh medially.

The gluteus maximus is the muscle principally tested, and it can be observed and palpated in the prone position.

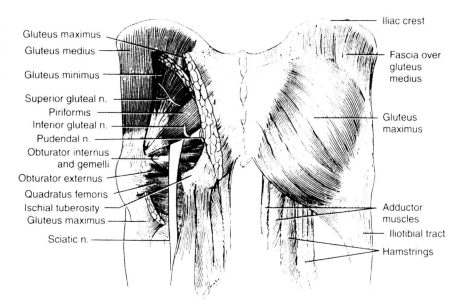

FIGURE 1-46. The musculature of the gluteal region. (From Jenkins DB. *Hollinshead's Functional Anatomy of the Limbs and Back.* 8th ed. Philadelphia, PA: WB Saunders; 2002:300. Used with permission of Mayo Foundation for Medical Education and Research.)

Gluteus Maximus (See Fig. 1-46)

Inferior gluteal nerve, L5, S1, S2.

Action

1. Extension of the thigh at the hip.
2. Lateral rotation of the thigh.
3. Assistance in adduction of the thigh.

Test

1. Sitting or supine: starting with the thigh slightly raised, extension (downward movement) of the thigh is tested against resistance applied by the examiner under the distal part of the thigh. In this rather crude test, the muscle cannot be observed or readily palpated.
2. Prone: the knee is well flexed to minimize the participation of the hamstrings. Extension of the thigh is tested by raising the knee from the table against downward pressure applied by the examiner to the distal part of the thigh. The muscle is accessible to observation and palpation in this position.

Quadriceps Femoris (Fig. 1-47)

Femoral nerve, L2-4. See Appendix H.

Action

1. Extension of the leg at the knee.
2. Rectus femoris assists in flexion of the thigh at the hip.

Test

1. Sitting or supine: the lower leg is in moderate extension.
2. Maintenance of extension is tested against effort by the examiner to flex the patient's leg at the knee.

Atrophy is easily noted.

Hamstrings (Fig. 1-48)

Sciatic nerve, L4, L5, S1, S2. See Appendix J. Biceps femoris: external hamstring (L5, S1, S2). Semitendinosus and semimembranosus: internal hamstrings (L4, L5, S1, S2).

Action

1. Flexion of the leg at the knee.
2. All but the short head of the biceps femoris assist in extension of the thigh at the hip.

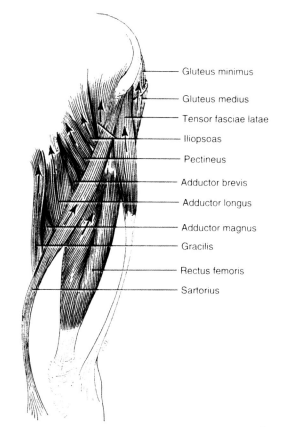

FIGURE 1-47. Flexors of the thigh. (From Jenkins DB. *Hollinshead's Functional Anatomy of the Limbs and Back.* 8th ed. Philadelphia, PA: WB Saunders; 2002:317. Used with permission of Mayo Foundation for Medical Education and Research.)

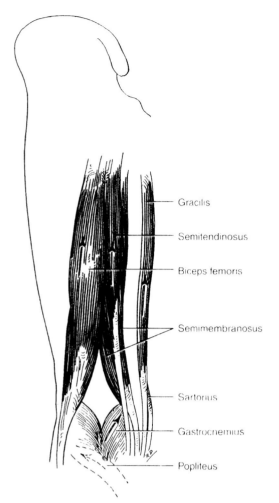

FIGURE 1-48. The flexors of the leg. (From Jenkins DB. *Hollinshead's Functional Anatomy of the Limbs and Back.* 8th ed. Philadelphia, PA: WB Saunders; 2002:320. Used with permission of Mayo Foundation for Medical Education and Research.)

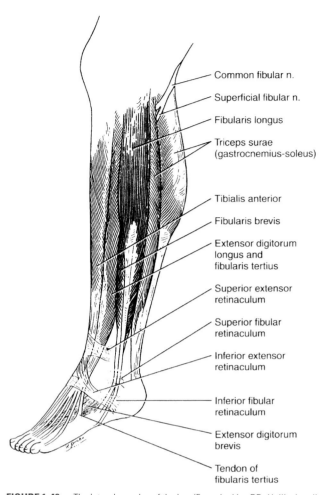

FIGURE 1-49. The lateral muscles of the leg. (From Jenkins DB. *Hollinshead's Functional Anatomy of the Limbs and Back.* 8th ed. Philadelphia, PA: WB Saunders; 2002:338. Used with permission of Mayo Foundation for Medical Education and Research.)

Test
1. Sitting: flexion of the lower leg is tested against resistance.
2. Prone: the knee is partly flexed. Further flexion is tested against resistance.

Observation and palpation of the muscles and the tendons are important for proper interpretation.

Anterior Tibialis (Fig. 1-49)
Deep peroneal nerve, L4, L5, S1. See Appendix K and **Figure 1-50**.

Action
Dorsiflexion and inversion (particularly in the dorsiflexed position) of the foot.

Test
Dorsiflexion of the foot is tested against resistance applied to the dorsum of the foot downward and toward eversion.

The belly of the muscle just lateral to the shin and the tendon medially on the dorsal aspect of the ankle should be

observed and palpated to be certain that dorsiflexion is not being accomplished by the extensor digitorum longus without contraction of the anterior tibialis. Atrophy is conspicuous.

Participating Muscles
1. Dorsiflexion: extensor hallucis longus; extensor digitorum longus.
2. Inversion: posterior tibialis.

Extensor Hallucis Longus (See Figs. 1-49 and 1-50)
Deep peroneal nerve, L5, S1. See Appendix K.

Action
Extension of the great toe and dorsiflexion of the foot.

Test
Extension of the great toe is tested against resistance, while the foot is stabilized in a neutral position.

The tendon is palpable between the tendons of the anterior tibialis and the extensor digitorum longus.

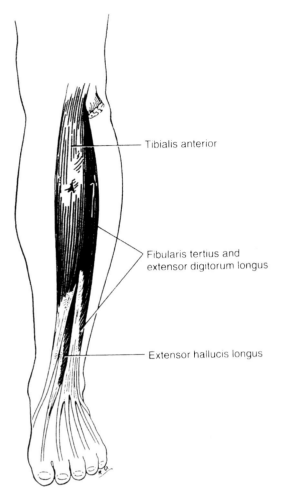

FIGURE 1-50. The dorsiflexors of the foot. (From Jenkins DB. *Hollinshead's Functional Anatomy of the Limbs and Back.* 8th ed. Philadelphia, PA: WB Saunders; 2002:345. Used with permission of Mayo Foundation for Medical Education and Research.)

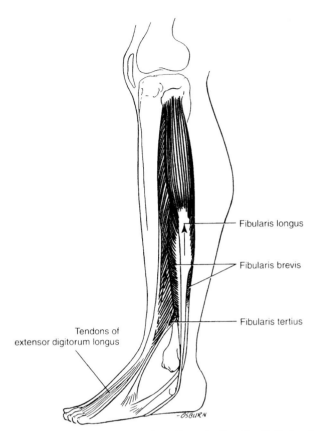

FIGURE 1-51. Evertors of the foot. (From Jenkins DB. *Hollinshead's Functional Anatomy of the Limbs and Back.* 8th ed. Philadelphia, PA: WB Saunders; 2002:346. Used with permission of Mayo Foundation for Medical Education and Research.)

Extensor Digitorum Longus (See Figs. 1-49 and 1-50)

Deep peroneal nerve, L4, L5, S1. See Appendix K.

Action

Extension of the lateral four toes and dorsiflexion of the foot.

Test

Extension of the lateral four toes and dorsiflexion of the foot are tested against resistance.

The tendons are visible and palpable on the dorsal aspect of the ankle and the foot lateral to the tendon of the extensor hallucis longus.

Extensor Digitorum Brevis (See Fig. 1-49)

Deep peroneal nerve, L4, L5, S1. See Appendix K.

Action

Assists in the extension of all the toes except the little toe.

Test

The belly of the muscle is observed and palpated on the lateral aspect of the dorsum of the foot during toe extension.

Peroneus Longus, Brevis (Fibularis Longus, Brevis) (Fig. 1-51)

Superficial peroneal nerve, L5, S1. See Appendix L.

Action

1. Eversion of the foot.
2. Assistance in plantar flexion of the foot.

Test

The foot is in plantar flexion. Eversion is tested against resistance applied by the examiner to the lateral border of the foot.

The tendons are palpable just above and behind the external malleolus. Atrophy may be visible over the anterolateral aspect of the lower extremity.

Gastrocnemius; Soleus (Fig. 1-52)

Tibial nerve, L5, S1, S2. See Appendix J.

Action

1. Plantar flexion of the foot.
2. The gastrocnemius also flexes the knee and cannot act effectively to plantar flex the foot when the knee is well flexed.

Test

1. The knee is extended to test both muscles. The knee is flexed principally to test the soleus.
2. Plantar flexion of the foot is tested against resistance.

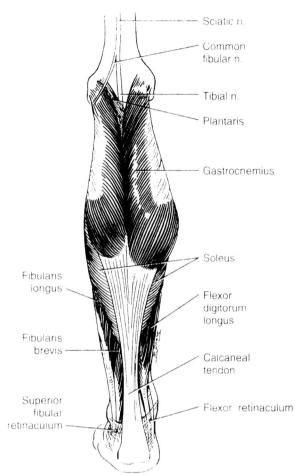

FIGURE 1-52. Musculature of the calf of the leg. (From Jenkins DB. *Hollinshead's Functional Anatomy of the Limbs and Back.* 8th ed. Philadelphia, PA: WB Saunders; 2002:333. Used with permission of Mayo Foundation for Medical Education and Research.)

The muscles and tendon should be observed and palpated. Atrophy is readily visible. The gastrocnemius and soleus are strong muscles, and leverage in testing favors the patient rather than the examiner. For this reason, slight weakness is difficult to detect by resisting flexion of the ankle or by pressing against the flexed foot in the direction of extension. Consequently, the strength of these muscles should be tested against the weight of the patient's body. The patient should stand on one foot and plantar flex the foot to lift himself or herself directly and fully upward. It may be necessary for the examiner to hold the patient steady while this test is performed.

Participating Muscles
Long flexors of the toes; posterior tibialis, fibularis longus, and fibularis brevis (particularly near the extreme plantar flexion).

Posterior Tibialis (Fig. 1-53)
Posterior tibial nerve, L5, S1. See Appendix J.

Action
1. Inversion of the foot.
2. Assistance in plantar flexion of the foot.

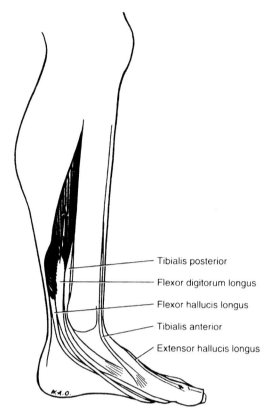

FIGURE 1-53. Invertors of the foot. (From Jenkins DB. *Hollinshead's Functional Anatomy of the Limbs and Back.* 8th ed. Philadelphia, PA: WB Saunders; 2002:345. Used with permission of Mayo Foundation for Medical Education and Research.)

Test
The foot is in complete plantar flexion. Inversion is tested against resistance applied to the medial border of the foot and directed toward eversion and slightly toward dorsiflexion.

This maneuver virtually eliminates participation of the anterior tibialis in inversion. The toes should be relaxed to prevent participation of the long flexors of the toes.

Long Flexors of the Toes (See Fig. 1-53)
Posterior tibial nerve, L5, S1. See Appendix J.
1. Flexor digitorum longus.
2. Flexor hallucis longus.

Action
1. Plantar flexion of the toes, especially at the distal interphalangeal joints.
2. Assistance in plantar flexion and inversion of the foot.

Test
1. The foot is stabilized in a neutral position. Plantar flexion of the toes is tested against resistance applied to the distal phalanges.
2. Weakness of the long toe flexors results in inability to curl the tips of the toes under the foot against resistance. (See intrinsic foot muscle testing below.)

Intrinsic Muscles of the Foot

Virtually all muscles except the extensor digitorum brevis (medial and lateral plantar nerves from the posterior tibial nerve, L5, S1, S2).

Action

The flexion of the proximal phalanges during extension of the distal phalanges is an action comparable to that of the intrinsic muscles of the hand.

Test

The patient's foot is stabilized in a neutral position, and plantar flexion of the toes is tested against resistance applied to the distal phalanges. (Same maneuver as that in the test of the long toe flexors.)

Neurologic Examination

With the exception of the musculoskeletal examination, no other component of the standard physical examination is more important to the physical medicine and rehabilitation assessment than the neurologic examination. Although often conducted to identify disease, the neurologic examination provides the physiatrist with an opportunity to identify both the neurologic impairments to be addressed and the residual abilities to be used in maximizing the functional outcome for the patient.

Although it is customary to record the results of the neurologic examination in a separate portion of the examination report, the neurologic examination is rarely performed all at one time. The examiner often finds it convenient to integrate the appropriate portions of the neurologic examination into the assessment of a specific region of the body. For example, cranial nerve assessment often is performed with other components of the head and neck examination, because the patient is positioned appropriately for both. For purposes of discussion, the neurologic examination is addressed separately and is divided into assessments of mental status, speech and language function, cranial nerves, reflexes, central motor integration, sensation, and perception. Muscle strength is discussed in the section on examination of the musculoskeletal system. The assessment of complex motor activities is discussed in the section "Functional Examination." The reader is referred to *Mayo Clinic Examinations in Neurology* for a comprehensive discussion of the neurologic evaluation (1).

Mental Status

Level of Consciousness

Before performing a formal mental status examination, the examiner should determine the patient's level of consciousness. Qualitative terms such as "drowsy," "lethargic," and "stuporous" are useful in a descriptive sense, but they suffer from a lack of precise definition. "Stuporous" to one examiner may mean "lethargic" to another. A definitive classification of mental status requires a standardized approach (13–15). In the Glasgow Coma Scale, the examiner classifies the patient's eye, motor, and verbal responses to verbal and physical stimuli according to a numerical scale that is quantifiable and reproducible **(Table 1-4)** (16). Such a standardized scale is necessary to assess changes over time and to facilitate communication among physicians, nurses, therapists, and family members. In

TABLE 1-4	Glasgow Coma Scale*[a]
Response	**Score**
Eye-opening, E	
Spontaneous	E 4
To speech	E 3
To pain	E 2
Nil	E 1
Best motor response, M	
Obeys	M 6
Localizes	M 5
Withdraws	M 4
Abnormal flexion	M 3
Extensor response	M 2
Nil	M 1
Verbal response, V	
Orientated	V 5
Confused conversation	V 4
Inappropriate words	V 3
Incomprehensible sounds	V 2
Nil	V 1

[a]Coma score (E + M + V) = 3 to 15.
Reprinted from Teasdale G, Jennett B. Assessment of coma and impaired consciousness. A practical scale. *Lancet.* 1974;304(7872):81–84. Copyright © 1974 Elsevier. With permission.

patients with traumatic brain injury, other aspects of the neurologic assessment, such as pupillary responses, ocular movements, and respiration, will provide information about the cause of altered consciousness but do not quantifiably relate in a statistical sense to eventual outcome.

Cognitive Evaluation

With the conscious patient, assessment of mental status begins when the physician enters the room and continues throughout the examination. However, as with the assessment of the level of consciousness, a formal approach to the mental status examination can help the examiner to identify and quantify specific impairments and residual capacity, to recognize subtle temporal changes, and to facilitate communication among caregivers. A commonly used clinical tool for evaluating the patient's mental status is the Folstein Mini-Mental Status Examination (13). Excellent systems have been developed to assess intellectual performance in specific populations (10,16). Although systems may or may not include perceptual testing, speech and language assessment, or an inventory of thought processing, certain components of the evaluation remain constant.

Orientation

The patient is asked to report his or her name, address, and telephone number and the building (e.g., hospital or clinic), city, state, year, month, and day.

Attention

Attention is assessed with digit repetition; the patient is asked to repeat a series of random numbers. Two numbers are used initially (e.g., 4 and 9); if the patient answers correctly, the sequence is increased by one more digit with each additional repetition until the patient either repeats seven digits correctly or makes a mistake. The number of digits repeated correctly should be noted.

Recall

Three numbers or three objects are listed, and the patient is asked to remember them for repetition later. In 5 minutes, the patient is asked to recall the list, and the number of correct responses is recorded. If all responses are correct, recall responses are obtained again at 10 minutes and at 15 minutes.

General Fund of Information

Questions are asked appropriate to the patient's age, cultural interests, and educational background. For example, the names of the past five US presidents or leaders of other countries, the current US vice president, and the governor of the patient's home state can be requested, or inquiries can be made for information about current events and other nearly universal subjects (e.g., world wars and basic scientific principles).

Calculations

The patient is asked to count by sevens, and the last correct response is recorded. Arithmetic calculations of increasing difficulty are presented.

Proverbs

An explanation of three common proverbs is requested. The patient is assessed as to whether he or she can abstract the principle from the adage and explain it in concrete terms.

Similarities

The patient is asked to describe what is common to an orange and an apple, to a desk and a bookcase, and to a cup and a fork. The number of correct responses is recorded.

Judgment

The patient is presented with three problems (e.g., smelling smoke in a movie theater, finding a stamped and addressed envelope on the sidewalk, and locating a friend in an unfamiliar city) and asked how to handle each situation.

Speech and Language Function

As with the assessment of mental status, the analysis of communicative function occurs throughout the entire examination. The patient should be evaluated for the presence and extent of aphasia, apraxia, and dysarthria and for any residual communicative skills (17,18). At times, effort is required to discriminate among the disorders of aphasia, apraxia of speech, and language dysfunction associated with a more generalized cognitive deficit. Expert assessment of speech production and language processing can be valuable for diagnosis of neurologic disease (see Chapter 13). However, as described in the preceding section, assessment of the four basic elements of communication (i.e., listening, reading, speaking, and writing) provides a practical framework for functional evaluation.

Listening

After first determining that the patient does not have a significant hearing loss, had been able to speak the examiner's language before the onset of disease, and has the requisite motor and visual skills, the physician should test the patient's auditory comprehension, noting the extent of his or her ability to follow specific directions without gestures from the examiner. Often, it is useful to characterize the degree of impairment with stepped commands. First, the patient's ability to follow one-step commands is assessed by asking him or her to perform three different single motor activities, such as "take off

your glasses," "touch your nose," and "open the book." Each command should be given separately, and a prolonged pause should be allowed to observe the response. These responses are rated and notation is made of whether the patient requires pantomime of the activity before performing the task. If two of the three responses are correct, an assessment should be made of the patient's skill at following two-step commands, such as "touch your nose, then take off your glasses," "point to the window, then close the book," and "touch my hand, then touch your knee." If the patient can follow two-step commands, then an assessment of his or her ability to follow three-step commands is conducted in a similar fashion. A simple object such as a toothbrush is held up, and the patient is asked to demonstrate its use. This request is repeated at least two more times with different objects. If speech is functional, the patient is asked to repeat a short phrase that is spoken. The response should be observed for perseveration and jargon.

Reading

It is important to verify that the patient had reading skills before the onset of the neurologic disorder. The patient should be asked to read a short written command and perform the activity; the patient also can be asked to follow written two-step and three-step commands. If writing is otherwise functional, the patient should be asked to read aloud what he or she has written.

Speaking

If auditory comprehension is adequate, language production can be tested in several ways. An object is indicated, and the patient is asked to name it and state its function; at least three objects are used. The patient is asked to report his or her name, hometown, telephone number, or another simple verifiable fact. A picture can be shown and the patient asked to describe it. Tests for phonation and resonance deficits are performed by asking the patient to say a prolonged "aaah" and by observing for force and steadiness of pitch and tone. The patient should be asked to say "pa-pa-pa" to test lip closure, "ta-ta-ta" to test tongue function, and "ka-ka-ka" to test speed, regulatory, and posterior pharyngeal function. If reading is otherwise functional, articulation can be further assessed by having the patient read aloud a short passage containing various vowels and consonants.

Writing

The patient should be asked to write his or her name, address, telephone number, and a brief paragraph.

Cranial Nerves

Cranial Nerve I (Olfactory)

Olfactory function should be evaluated routinely. Deficits are common after head trauma.

Cranial Nerve II (Optic)

Visual field testing of each eye should be performed, with a temporary patch over the contralateral eye. It is best to test each quadrant diagonally to identify any quadrantanopia. Although visual double simultaneous stimulation may be more correctly classified under cortical sensation, it is convenient to assess for extinction during visual field testing, after full fields have been verified. Visual acuity is discussed in the section on "Eye Examination."

Cranial Nerves III (Oculomotor), IV (Trochlear), and VI (Abducens)

Visual pathways are assessed by evaluating the pupil size, pupillary reactions, and extraocular movements. Strabismus is evaluated by testing corneal light reflections.

Cranial Nerve V (Trigeminal)

The muscles of mastication and facial sensation should be tested.

Cranial Nerve VIII (Vestibulocochlear)

The patient should be examined for nystagmus. Auditory function is discussed in the section on "Ear Examination."

Cranial Nerves VII (Facial), IX (Glossopharyngeal), X (Vagus), and XII (Hypoglossal)

Isolating individual cranial nerve function emanating from the lower part of the brainstem is difficult. Cranial nerves are often grouped by function. Evaluation should be conducted of taste (nerves VII, IX, and X), muscles of facial expression (nerve VII) and articulation (nerves VII, IX, X, and XII), and swallowing function (nerves IX, X, and XII).

Cranial Nerve XI (Accessory)

The function of sternocleidomastoid and trapezius is frequently assessed during manual muscle testing.

Brainstem- and visual-evoked responses, electromyography and other forms of electrodiagnostic testing, and swallowing videofluoroscopy are often necessary for better delineation of dysfunction of cranial nerves and their brainstem interactions.

Reflexes

Muscle Stretch Reflexes

Muscle stretch reflexes should be tested when the patient is relaxed. The commonly tested muscles are the biceps (C5, C6), triceps (C6-8), brachioradialis (C5, C6), quadriceps (L2-4), and gastrocnemius-soleus (L5, S1, S2). The reflexes of the masseter (cranial nerve V), internal hamstring (L4, L5, S1, S2), and external hamstring (L5, S1, S2) are tested in select cases. The patient should be observed for clonus.

Superficial Reflexes

Segmental reflexes are often helpful for localizing the lesion. These include the corneal (cranial nerves V and VII), gag (cranial nerves IX and X), anal (S3-5), and plantar (L5, S1, S2) reflexes. At times, it is useful to include the epigastric (T6-9), midabdominal (T9-11), hypogastric (T11, T12, L1), and cremasteric (L1, L2) reflexes.

Pathologic Reflexes

Elicitation of the Babinski reflex should be attempted. In questionable cases, the confirmatory Chaddock, Oppenheim, and Stransky reflexes should be tested.

Central Motor Integration

Muscle Tone

Spasticity, rigidity, and hypotonicity can be assessed by evaluating the patient's resistance to passive movement, pendulousness, and ability to posturally fixate.

Coordination

Coordination in the upper extremities can be assessed with the finger-nose, finger-nose-finger, and knee-pat tests. Coordination in the lower extremities can be evaluated with the toe-finger and heel-knee-shin test.

Alternate Motion Rate

The tongue-wiggle, finger-wiggle, and foot-pat tests can be used to identify subtle spasticity, rigidity, and incoordination.

Involuntary Movements

The patient should be observed for tremors, chorea, athetosis, ballismus, dystonia, myoclonus, asterixis, and tics. If present, these should be described in the neurologic report.

Apraxia

Apraxia is the failure of motor planning and execution without deficits in strength, coordination, or sensation; however, deficits of strength, coordination, and sensation are often also present because of the extent of the lesion. Automatic motor activities can be observed while the patient manipulates a pen or pencil, handles clothing, and moves about the examination room; then, the patient's ability to perform some of the same maneuvers on command can be assessed. The patient should be asked to touch his or her nose, drink from a glass, put a pencil in the glass, and use scissors. The patient should then be asked to perform these activities without the objects with each hand. Inefficient or fumbling movements or inability to accomplish the task should be noted. Dressing apraxia can be assessed by asking the patient to put on a coat. To assess for more subtle deficits, the examiner should first turn one sleeve of the coat inside out. Constructional apraxia can be evaluated by asking the patient to copy a geometric design or draw the face of a clock.

Sensation

Superficial Sensation

Light touch can be tested with a wisp of cotton, superficial pain with a single-use pin, and temperature with two test tubes, one with hot tap water and the other with cold tap water. Abnormal findings should be recorded on a drawing of the human figure and compared with standard charts of spinal dermatomes and peripheral nerves (1).

Deep Sensation

The evaluation of joint position sense begins with the distal joints of the hand and foot and moves proximally until normal sensation is identified. Testing for deep pain in the upper extremities can be done by hyperextension of small finger joints and in the lower extremities by firm compression of the calf muscles or Achilles tendon. Vibration sense is often evaluated, but its isolated absence does not result in functional deficit.

Cortical Sensation

If superficial and deep sensations are intact, two-point discrimination, graphesthesia, stereognosis, and double simultaneous stimulation can be evaluated.

Perception

Disorders of perception are most common with lesions of the nondominant parietal lobe but also can occur with lesions on the dominant side.

Agnosia

Agnosia is the failure to recognize familiar objects despite intact vision, hearing, sensation, and language function (although language is also often deficient because of the extent of the lesion). Pictures of common objects or the objects themselves are shown, and the patient is asked to identify them and describe their components. Agnosia of body parts can be assessed by asking the patient to identify his or her (or the examiner's) arm, finger, or eye. Unilateral environmental neglect can be assessed by observing ambulation or wheelchair operation for difficulty clearing corners and doorjambs, extinction on double simultaneous stimulation, and failure to scan the complete page width when asked to read a passage or cross out all the occurrences of the letter E. Body scheme agnosias can be evaluated by searching for denial of obvious physical impairments when the patient is asked to describe them.

Right-Left Disorientation

If agnosia of body parts is not present, the patient should be asked to indicate various body parts on the right and the left sides.

Other Perceptual Tests

If perceptual deficits are identified with the maneuvers described above, the examiner should test for additional deficits, such as impaired geographic and spatial orientation and figure-ground relationships. Comprehensive, formal, and quantitative testing of perception by a psychologist and an occupational therapist is warranted if any deficits are found during the physical examination.

Functional Examination

After impairments have been identified, the consequences of each impairment for the function of the patient must be appraised. Prediction of functional status should not be attempted from the history and physical examination; instead, function should be examined. For a comprehensive assessment, the patient must be evaluated by individual physical medicine and rehabilitation team members in settings where the activities are actually performed. Bathing skills should be observed by the occupational therapist or the rehabilitation nurse in the bathroom while the patient attempts to bathe; eating skills should be analyzed by the occupational therapist while the patient eats a meal; and car transfer skills should be assessed by the physical therapist with the use of the patient's car. Each team member will use unique skills to contribute to a comprehensive determination of functional status. Many functional evaluative processes cannot be accomplished at a single point. Safety and judgment can be assessed only by observing the patient in varying situations within both the rehabilitation environment and the community.

However, in many instances, the physiatrist must glean a basic view of the functional status at the time of the initial evaluation. For instance, in the clinic, the physician may be consulted to determine a patient's need for rehabilitation services. It is unlikely that the physician will be able to observe the patient during a meal, in the bathroom, or in the process of transferring to and from a car. In such cases, the physician must use creativity to place the patient in situations similar to those of daily life. Examples are given below. Components of the communication assessment were discussed in the sections "History and Physical Examination" and will not be repeated here.

Eating

The patient should be asked to use examining equipment in place of feeding utensils to demonstrate proficiency in bringing food to the mouth. If aspiration has not already been identified, the patient should be provided with a glass of water and asked to drink.

Grooming

The patient should be asked to comb his or her hair and to mimic the activities of brushing teeth or putting on makeup.

Bathing

The patient should be asked to mimic the activities of bathing. It is important to note if any body parts cannot be reached by the patient, particularly the back, the scalp, and the axilla and arm contralateral to hemiparesis.

Toileting

The patient must have adequate unsupported sitting balance, must have the requisite wrist and hand motion to reach the perineum adequately, must be able to handle toilet paper, and must be able to rise from low seating.

Dressing

The patient should be observed during undressing before the examination and dressing after completion of the examination. The examiner should explain the purpose of the observation and should be accompanied by a nurse or aide.

Bed Activities

During the physical examination, the examiner should note whether the patient has difficulty moving between the seated and the supine positions. It should also be determined whether the patient can roll from front to back and back to front and whether the patient can raise the pelvis off the examining table while supine.

Transfers

The patient should be observed rising from seating with and without armrests and moving between the bed and a chair.

Wheelchair Mobility

The patient should be asked to demonstrate wheeling straight ahead and turning, on both carpeted and noncarpeted floors, if available; locking the brakes; and manipulating the leg rests.

Ambulation

To adequately recognize disturbances of gait, the examiner must be able to view body parts. If the examining room is secluded, the assessment can be performed with the patient wearing only the underwear. If privacy is not possible, the patient should have access to washable or disposable shorts. If the examiner does not already have knowledge of the patient's ambulation skills, the patient should be provided with a safety belt before gait is assessed. To discern specific gait abnormalities, the examiner must study both the individual components and the composite activity. The patient should be observed from the front, back, and each side. If the patient experiences pain during ambulation, its temporal relationship to the gait cycle should be noted. This analysis must be approached in an orderly fashion. One routine for gait analysis is outlined in **Table 1-5** (4,19). See Chapter 4 for a comprehensive discussion of gait.

Operation of a Motor Vehicle

Driving ability can be assessed best in an automobile. However, the examiner can gain some information about the patient's motor abilities for driving by asking the patient to demonstrate the motions of operating the pedals and hand controls.

TABLE 1-5	Gait Analysis

Standing balance
   Observe for steadiness of position; push the patient off balance and note the patient's attempts to regain balanced posture
Individual body part movements during walking
   Observe for fixed or abnormal posture and inadequate, excessive, or asymmetrical movement of body parts
   Head and trunk: listing or tilting, shoulder dipping, elevation, depression, protraction, and retraction
   Arm swing: protecting positioning or posturing
   Pelvis and hip: hip hiking, dropping (Trendelenburg), or lateral thrust
   Knee: genu valgum, varum, or recurvatum
   Foot and ankle: excessive inversion or eversion
Gait cycle factors
   Cadence: rate, symmetry, fluidity, and consistency
   Stride width: narrow or broad based; knee and ankle clearance
   Stride length: shortened, lengthened, or asymmetrical
   Stance phase: initial contact, loading response, toe off; knee stability during all components of stance; coordination of knee and ankle movements
   Swing phase: adequate and synchronized knee flexion and ankle dorsiflexion during swing, abduction, or circumduction

Quantitation of Function

Several scales can be used to document and quantify functional status in activities of daily living. These are extremely useful in assessing a patient's rehabilitation progress (see Chapter 7). When validated and standardized, these scales are essential tools for analysis of rehabilitation outcome for a series of patients participating in a specific intervention program. When they are used by multiple rehabilitation centers to share data, relevant information can be obtained to advance the field and to assess the cost versus the benefit of rehabilitation. Physicians should develop expertise in the use of these valuable tools.

However, the data collection for most validated functional scales requires additional time because they require interdisciplinary input; therefore, the initial documentation of functional status by the physician must be practical and complete. One such system is shown in **Figure 1-54**. Findings from both the history and the physical examination should be used to define functional status.

FIGURE 1-54. Sample of a functional status record.

FUNCTIONAL STATUS

NAME *John Doe*
      3-418-448   L Hemiparesis

ACTIVITY	Independent	Independent with aids	Requires Assistance	Dependent
Listening		aid - L ear		
Reading			verbal cues to scan L	
Speaking	dysarthria			
Writing	✓			
Eating			set up meal; needs rocker knife; scoop plate	
Grooming			verbal cues for L body shave L face	
Bathing			verbal cues for L body wash R trunk	
Toileting		bladder with urinal	1 person assist for transfer to commode	
Dressing			1 person assist lower body; fasteners	
Bed Activities		hospital bed with bed rails		
Transfers			verbal cues; lock brakes protect L arm & judgement	
Wheel Chair			verbal cues to scan L unlock wc brakes	
Ambulation				✓
Driving				✓

If the activity is Independent or Dependent, mark with a check
If the activity is Independent with Aids, list the aids needed
If the activity Requires Assistance, describe the assistance and list the aids needed

TABLE 1-6   **Example of Summary, Problem List, and Plan**

Summary

A 55-year-old male carpenter with a left hearing deficit and poorly treated hypertension presents 4 days after sudden moderate left-side spastic hemiparesis with moderate sensory deficits, left neglect, nocturnal bladder incontinence, and dysarthria. He is alert, oriented, and normotensive; motor function in his left hip and knee is returning; and he has an elevated serum cholesterol level. He is divorced, lives alone, and has no close family. Computed tomography of the head shows moderate right subcortical infarction. Evidence of ischemia is not shown in the electrocardiogram.

Medical problems and plans

1. Right hemisphere infarction with motor, sensory, perceptual, and speech deficits: monitor neuromuscular function, maintain ROM, control spasticity (air splint, positioning, possible medications), provide motor reeducation, and provide patient education and risk factor
2. Hypertension: monitor systolic/diastolic blood pressure and treat with antihypertensive agents as appropriate
3. Dyslipidemia: low-fat diet, patient education about diet and food preparation, and lipid-lowering agents
4. Urinary incontinence: check residual urine volume and culture specimens; treat urosepsis. If residual volume is low, offer urinal frequently, with or without nocturnal condom catheterization. If residual volume is high, begin 1,800-mL fluid intake schedule with catheterization every 6 hours, urodynamics, and bladder retraining

Rehabilitation problems and plans

1. Communication deficits: speech pathologist for evaluation and therapy
2. Left neglect: OT for perceptual testing, retraining, and compensation; verbal clues to scan left; RN and PT to reinforce OT
3. Left sensory deficits: monitor skin; offer patient education on care of insensate skin
4. Self-care deficits: OT for upper extremity ROM, reeducation about strengthening, ADL retraining, adaptive aids
5. Safety and judgment deficits: four bed rails, RN monitoring at night, verbal clues, physical spotting
6. Transfer deficits: PT for retraining, left wheelchair brake extension
7. Mobility deficits: PT for lower extremity ROM, reeducation about strengthening, gait retraining, gait aids
8. Driving dependency: retesting and retraining with improvement
9. Community reentry and poor support system: assess home for architectural barriers, assess home health services, identify additional social support
10. Reactive depression: refer for psychological support
11. Vocational issues: consider prevocational counseling and testing

ADL, activities of daily living; OT, occupational therapy; PT, physical therapy; RN, registered nurse; ROM, range of motion.

SUMMARY AND PROBLEM LIST

After obtaining the history, performing the physical examination, and recording the results, the physiatrist should summarize the findings, construct a problem list, and formulate a plan.

A summary of findings can be a useful component of the written record. In a few sentences, a summary can provide a succinct description of relevant findings in the history and examination.

For the management of chronic diseases, physiatrists must commonly address myriad physical, psychological, social, and vocational problems. Weed's (20) problem-oriented medical record has been applied to the management of patients undergoing rehabilitation (21–24). Although the use of the problem list itself is the essential factor, a consensus as to the organization and the use of the entire system in the rehabilitation setting has proved challenging. The recommendation of Grabois (23) that medical and rehabilitation problems be separately listed is beneficial. In addition, it may be helpful to delineate individual plans for each problem at the conclusion of the workup (**Table 1-6**).

REFERENCES

1. Mayo Clinic Department of Neurology. *Mayo Clinic Examinations in Neurology.* 7th ed. St. Louis, MO: Mosby; 1998.
2. Darley FL. Treatment of acquired aphasia. *Adv Neurol.* 1975;7:111–145.
3. Newmark SR, Sublett D, Black J, et al. Nutritional assessment in a rehabilitation unit. *Arch Phys Med Rehabil.* 1981;62:279–282.
4. Stolov WC, Hays RM. Evaluation of the patient. In: Kottke JF, Lehmann JF, eds. *Krusen's Handbook of Physical Medicine and Rehabilitation.* 4th ed. Philadelphia, PA: WB Saunders; 1990:1–19.
5. Ewing JA. Detecting alcoholism: the CAGE questionnaire. *JAMA.* 1984;252:1905–1907.
6. LeBlond RF, DeGowin RL, Brown DD, eds. *DeGowin's Diagnostic Examination.* 8th ed. New York: McGraw-Hill Medical Publishing Division; 2004.
7. Norkin CC, White DJ, eds. *Measurement of Joint Motion: A Guide to Goniometry.* 2nd ed. Philadelphia, PA: FA Davis; 1995.
8. American Academy of Orthopaedic Surgeons, ed. *Joint Motion: Method of Measuring and Recording.* Edinburgh, UK: Churchill Livingstone; 1988.
9. D'Ambrosia RD. *Musculoskeletal Disorders: Regional Examination and Differential Diagnosis.* 2nd ed. Philadelphia, PA: Lippincott; 1986.
10. Hoppenfeld S, ed. *Physical Examination of the Spine and Extremities.* New York, NY: Appleton-Century-Crofts; 1976.
11. Kendall FP, McCreary EK, Provance PG, eds. *Muscles, Testing and Function.* 4th ed. Philadelphia, PA: Lippincott Williams & Wilkins; 1999.
12. Hislop HJ, Montgomery J, eds. *Daniels and Worthingham's Muscle Testing: Techniques of Manual Examination.* 7th ed. Philadelphia, PA: WB Saunders; 2002.
13. Folstein MF, Folstein SE, McHugh PR. "Mini-mental state": a practical method for grading the cognitive state of patients for the clinician. *J Psychiatr Res.* 1975;12:189–198.
14. Levin HS, O'Donnell VM, Grossman RG. The Galveston orientation and amnesia test: a practical scale to assess cognition after head injury. *J Nerv Ment Dis.* 1979;167:675–684.
15. Strub RL, Black FW, eds. *The Mental Status Examination in Neurology.* 4th ed. Philadelphia, PA: FA Davis; 2000.
16. Jennett B, Teasdale G, eds. *Management of Head Injuries.* Philadelphia, PA: FA Davis; 1981.
17. Hegde MN. *A Coursebook on Aphasia and Other Neurogenic Language Disorders.* 2nd ed. San Diego, CA: Singular Publishing Group; 1998.
18. Robey RR. A meta-analysis of clinical outcomes in the treatment of aphasia. *J Speech Lang Hear Res.* 1998;41:172–187.
19. Lehmann JF, de Lateur BJ. Gait analysis: diagnosis and management. In: Kottke FJ, Lehmann JF, eds. *Krusen's Handbook of Physical Medicine and Rehabilitation.* 4th ed. Philadelphia, PA: WB Saunders; 1990:108–125.
20. Weed LL, ed. *Medical Records, Medical Education, and Patient Care: The Problem-Oriented Record as a Basic Tool.* Cleveland, OH: The Press of Case Western Reserve University; 1971.
21. Dinsdale SM, Gent M, Kline G, et al. Problem oriented medical records: their impact on staff communication, attitudes and decision making. *Arch Phys Med Rehabil.* 1975;56:269–274.
22. Dinsdale SM, Mossman PL, Gullickson G Jr, et al. The problem-oriented medical record in rehabilitation. *Arch Phys Med Rehabil.* 1970;51:488–492.
23. Grabois M. The problem-oriented medical record: modification and simplification for rehabilitation medicine. *South Med J.* 1977;70:1383–1385.
24. Milhous RL. The problem-oriented medical record in rehabilitation management and training. *Arch Phys Med Rehabil.* 1972;53:182–185.

APPENDICES

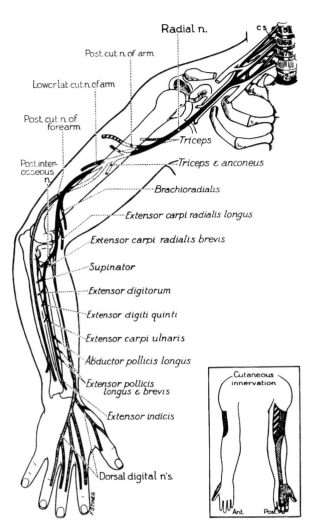

Radial n.

Post. cut. n. of arm

Lower lat. cut. n. of arm

Post. cut. n. of forearm

Post. inter-osseous n.

Triceps

Triceps & anconeus

Brachioradialis

Extensor carpi radialis longus

Extensor carpi radialis brevis

Supinator

Extensor digitorum

Extensor digiti quinti

Extensor carpi ulnaris

Abductor pollicis longus

Extensor pollicis longus & brevis

Extensor indicis

Dorsal digital n's.

Cutaneous innervation

Ant.   Post.

APPENDIX A. Long thoracic nerve; thoracic anterior nerve. (Reprinted from Haymaker W, Woodhall B, eds. *Peripheral Nerve Injuries: Principles of Diagnosis.* 2nd ed. Philadelphia, PA: WB Saunders Company; 1953:223. Copyright © 1953 Elsevier. With permission.)

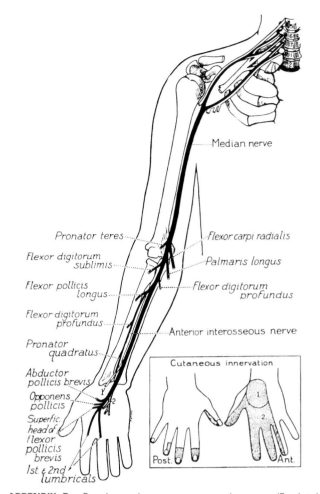

Median nerve

Pronator teres

Flexor digitorum sublimis

Flexor pollicis longus

Flexor digitorum profundus

Pronator quadratus

Abductor pollicis brevis

Opponens pollicis

Superfic. head of flexor pollicis brevis

1st & 2nd lumbricals

Flexor carpi radialis

Palmaris longus

Flexor digitorum profundus

Anterior interosseous nerve

Cutaneous innervation

Post.   Ant.

APPENDIX B. Dorsal scapular nerve; suprascapular nerve. (Reprinted from Haymaker W, Woodhall B, eds. *Peripheral Nerve Injuries: Principles of Diagnosis.* 2nd ed. Philadelphia, PA: WB Saunders Company; 1953:229. Copyright © 1953 Elsevier. With permission.)

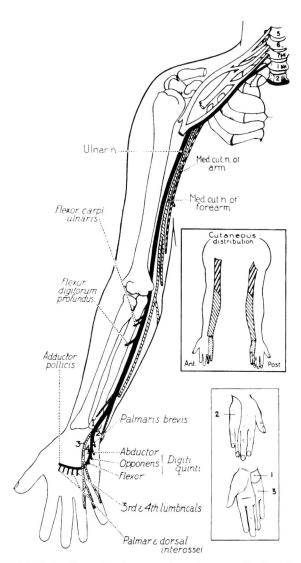

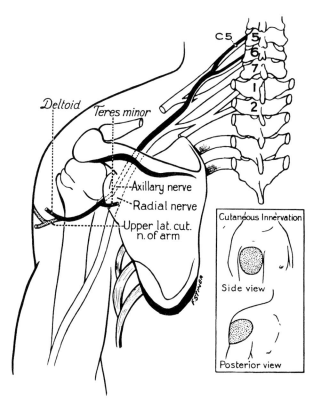

APPENDIX D. Axillary nerve. (Reprinted from Haymaker W, Woodhall B, eds. *Peripheral Nerve Injuries: Principles of Diagnosis.* 2nd ed. Philadelphia, PA: WB Saunders Company; 1953:235. Copyright © 1953 Elsevier. With permission.)

APPENDIX C. Thoracodorsal nerve; subscapular nerve. (Reprinted from Haymaker W, Woodhall B, eds. *Peripheral Nerve Injuries: Principles of Diagnosis.* 2nd ed. Philadelphia, PA: WB Saunders Company; 1953:233. Copyright © 1953 Elsevier. With permission.)

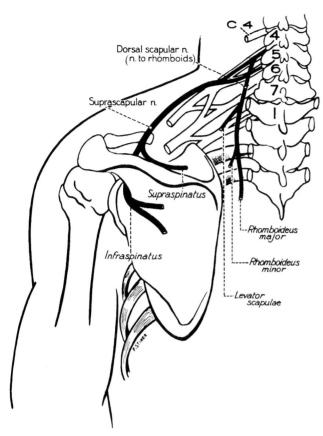

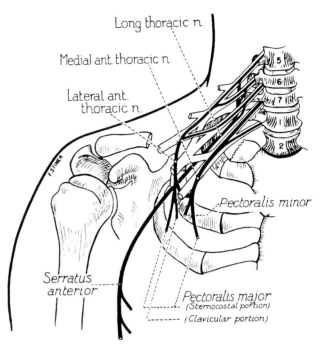

APPENDIX F. Median nerve. (Reprinted from Haymaker W, Woodhall B, eds. *Peripheral Nerve Injuries: Principles of Diagnosis*. 2nd ed. Philadelphia, PA: WB Saunders Company; 1953:242. Copyright © 1953 Elsevier. With permission.)

APPENDIX E. Radial nerve. (Reprinted from Haymaker W, Woodhall B, eds. *Peripheral Nerve Injuries: Principles of Diagnosis*. 2nd ed. Philadelphia, PA: WB Saunders Company; 1953:265. Copyright © 1953 Elsevier. With permission.)

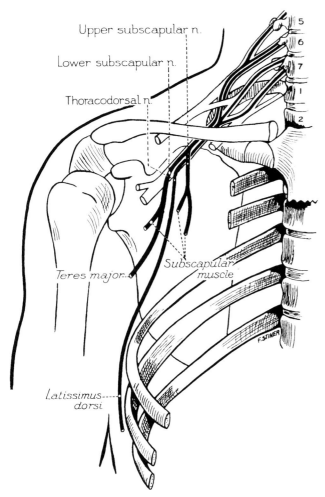

APPENDIX G. Ulnar nerve. (Reprinted from Haymaker W, Woodhall B, eds. *Peripheral Nerve Injuries: Principles of Diagnosis.* 2nd ed. Philadelphia, PA: WB Saunders Company; 1953:252. Copyright © 1953 Elsevier. With permission.)

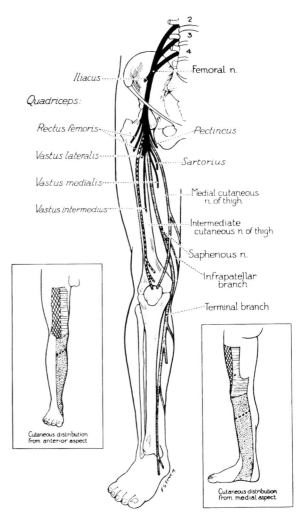

APPENDIX H. Femoral nerve. (Reprinted from Haymaker W, Woodhall B, eds. *Peripheral Nerve Injuries: Principles of Diagnosis.* 2nd ed. Philadelphia, PA: WB Saunders Company; 1953:282. Copyright © 1953 Elsevier. With permission.)

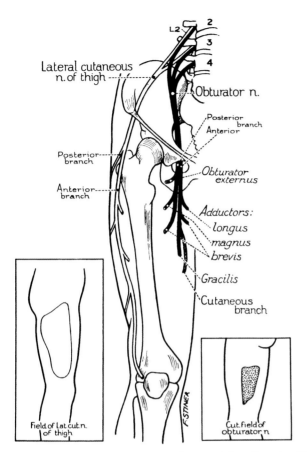

APPENDIX I. Lateral cutaneous nerve. (Reprinted from Haymaker W, Woodhall B, eds. *Peripheral Nerve Injuries: Principles of Diagnosis.* 2nd ed. Philadelphia, PA: WB Saunders Company; 1953:279. Copyright © 1953 Elsevier. With permission.)

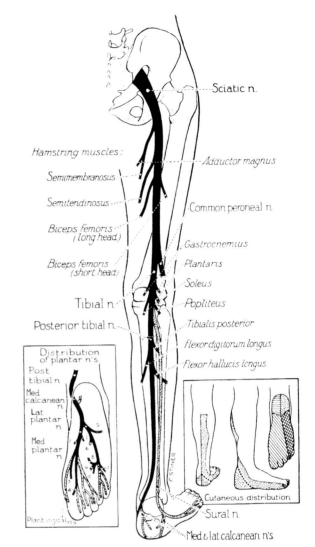

APPENDIX J. Sciatic nerve; tibial nerve; posterior tibial nerve. (Reprinted from Haymaker W, Woodhall B, eds. *Peripheral Nerve Injuries: Principles of Diagnosis.* 2nd ed. Philadelphia, PA: WB Saunders Company; 1953:290. Copyright © 1953 Elsevier. With permission.)

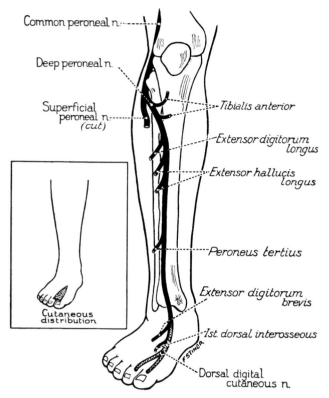

APPENDIX K.   Deep peroneal nerve. (Reprinted from Haymaker W, Woodhall B, eds. *Peripheral Nerve Injuries: Principles of Diagnosis.* 2nd ed. Philadelphia, PA: WB Saunders Company; 1953:293. Copyright © 1953 Elsevier. With permission.)

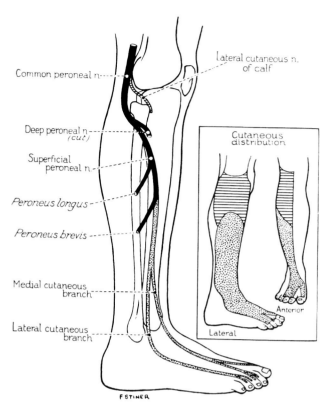

APPENDIX L.   Superficial peroneal nerve. (Reprinted from Haymaker W, Woodhall B, eds. *Peripheral Nerve Injuries: Principles of Diagnosis.* 2nd ed. Philadelphia, PA: WB Saunders Company; 1953:292. Copyright © 1953 Elsevier. With permission.)

CHAPTER 2

Assessment of Human Muscle Function

To move is all mankind can do, and for such the sole executant is muscle.

Sir Charles Sherrington, Edinburgh, 1937–1938

The relevance of skeletal muscle to the performance of all types of physical activities (i.e., therapeutic, recreational, occupational, athletic, and others) and the successful participation in daily life and societal obligations should be well appreciated by all those who work in rehabilitation. Skeletal muscle plays an important role, primary and/or secondary, in the pathophysiology of many diseases, and skeletal muscle function is the key to defining the nature and extent of impairments and activity limitations. Thus, understanding how skeletal muscle works, how to measure skeletal muscle function, and how to interpret the results of various physiologic and functional tests is a necessary component of the education of all physiatrists and rehabilitation professionals. It is worth noting that this understanding is of special value to the advancement of research in the rehabilitation sciences because many biologic and functional outcome variables used in scientific studies are directly associated with the function and structure of skeletal muscle. Finally, this chapter discusses this topic in the context of what is known about human skeletal muscle in health and disease. We will not review the extensive literature on muscle function based on studies in various animal models. With very few exceptions, the references will be those from human studies.

WHY MUSCLE?

The main function of the approximately 600 muscles in the human body is to convert chemical energy (i.e., fat and carbohydrates) into mechanical energy and thereby generate force. This force is transmitted from the active muscle fibers to the tendons with the help of the sarcolemma, special extracellular protein complexes, and connective tissue elements. The action of the tendons on bony structures results in the conversion of the force into joint and limb stability and movement and displacement of individual body parts or the body as a unit. In principle, force generation can occur during brief moments, resulting in what is generally referred to as *muscle strength*, or force generation can be maintained over a period of time referred to as *muscle endurance*. In the clinical setting, the failure to generate force during a brief moment is what we generally call *muscle weakness*, as opposed to the inability to maintain force, which we refer to as *muscle fatigue*.

Skeletal muscle comprises 40% to 45% of the total body mass (1–3), and 55% of total muscle mass is distributed in the lower limbs. Muscle contains approximately 50% to 75% of the total body protein (4,5), and protein turnover in muscle represents 30% to 50% of the total body protein turnover (3,6). More than half of the protein in muscle is found in the thick (myosin) and thin (actin) contractile filaments that generate and regulate force production (5,7). Actin and myosin account for more than 80% of the protein in the myofibrillar complex. In addition to force generation, skeletal muscles contribute to basal metabolism; produce heat to maintain core temperature; regulate blood glucose; serve as storage for carbohydrates, lipids, and amino acids; contribute to energy production during exercise; and protect internal organs (8).

During illness, nitrogen must be mobilized from muscle to provide amino acids to the immune system, liver, and other organs. Thus, if sufficient nitrogen is not available due to muscle wasting associated with aging, immobilization, or severe illness, the body's capacity to withstand an acute insult declines. The relationship between muscle function, illness, morbidity, and mortality is more obvious if one considers that morbidity becomes demonstrable at a 5% loss of lean mass and that the loss of 40% of lean body mass (LBM) is fatal (9). Finally, the extensive and considerable plasticity demonstrated by skeletal muscle under various conditions and in response to environmental influences such as bed rest, exercise training, and electrical stimulation makes it an ideal target for therapeutic and rehabilitative interventions.

From a functional point of view, skeletal muscle strength has been associated with comfortable and maximal walking speed (10,11), the incidence and prevalence of disability (12–14), balance (13), time to rise from a chair (15,16), ability to climb stairs (17), incidence of falls (18), and survival rate (19,20). Muscle power, a related but distinct property of skeletal muscle, also shows a positive and significant association with functional status (21). This evidence provides strong support to the conclusion that enhancing and maintaining muscle strength and muscle endurance throughout the life span, whether it is through prevention or rehabilitation, may reduce the prevalence of limitations in recreational, household, daily, and personal care activities, both in health and disease (22).

MUSCLE ACTIONS AND UNITS OF MEASUREMENT

The need to use consistent terminology, definitions, and measurement units across research studies, in educational programs, and in clinical rehabilitation is of great importance. Furthermore, measuring devices must be reliable and valid indicators of muscle function. Muscle function and structure can be quantified using the International System of Units, a refinement of the metric system (23–25) (**Table 2-1**).

TABLE 2-1	**Examples of Units for Assessing Muscle Structure and Function**
Mass	Kilograms (kg)
Distance	Meter (m)
Time	Second (s)
Force (mass × acceleration)	Newton (N)
Work (force × distance)	Joule (J)
Power (force × velocity)	Watt (W)
Velocity	Meters per second (m/s)
Torque	Newton-meter (Nm)
Angle	Radian (rad)
Angular velocity	Radians per second (rad/s)
Volume	Liter (L)

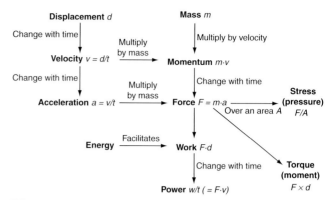

FIGURE 2-1. Physical and biomechanical concepts relevant to the assessment of human skeletal muscle function. Note the relevance of time on several variables, such as displacement, velocity, and work. Also, note the sequence of formulas leading from mass to power. (From Siff MC. Biomechanical foundations of strength and power training. In: Zatsiorsky V, ed. *Biomechanics in Sport*. 1st ed. Oxford: Blackwell Science; 2000:103–139. Copyright © 2000 International Olympic Committee. Reprinted by permission of John Wiley & Sons, Inc.)

All types of muscle actions result in the production of force or torque (tendency of a force to produce rotation about an axis). When the force is applied against an immovable object and there is no joint angular movement, the action is called *static* (isometric). Work is defined as the product of force × distance and power as the ratio of work over time. Therefore, by definition, because during a static muscle action the distance is zero, no work is performed and no power is produced.

When the muscle action results in the displacement of a given mass or body part at the same time that the origin and insertion of a muscle move *closer together*, the action is called *dynamic* (isotonic) *concentric* or *shortening* action. When the action results in the displacement of a given mass, and the origin and insertion of a muscle move *further apart*, the action is called *dynamic eccentric* or *lengthening* action. Both concentric and eccentric muscle actions result in work (force × distance), by convention called positive in the first case and negative in the latter. During many natural activities such as walking and running, concentric muscle actions occur in immediate combination with eccentric actions and are referred to as the *stretch-shortening cycle* (26,27).

In these activities such as jumping and running upstairs, the rate at which force is developed is more important than generating maximal force. Thus, power ([work/time] or [force × velocity]) and not strength becomes the limiting factor. Some of the most important physical and biomechanical concepts in the study and measurement of muscle function are illustrated in **Figure 2-1** (28).

Isokinetic muscle actions are dynamic and could be concentric or eccentric. This kind of muscle action is characterized by a combination of constant angular velocity and variable resistance. The resistance generated by the isokinetic device varies throughout the range of motion in order to match the torque generated by the muscle at each angle of the range of motion. It should be recognized that isokinetic actions represent an artificial situation that does not usually occur in nature outside of a laboratory. Many devices have been developed to measure muscle torque, work, power, and endurance based on the isokinetic concept. Isokinetic dynamometers, although expensive, are found in many research laboratories as well as in rehabilitation clinics (**Fig. 2-2**). Advantages of these devices include the objective quantification of muscle function, the immediate availability of reports, the provision of feedback to the patient, their high reproducibility, and the opportunity to standardize sequential testing for follow-up purposes during

the rehabilitation process. Disadvantages include the cost, lack of portability, and limited specificity in relation to muscle actions typical of daily activities.

The terms *open kinetic chain* and *closed kinetic chain* are used to describe two forms of muscle contractions and movements. The kinetic chain is a concept that describes a body segment as a series of mobile segments and linkages (29–31). In the case of the lower extremities, this chain allows forward propulsion during gait. When the foot is in contact with the ground, the kinetic chain is considered to be closed. When the

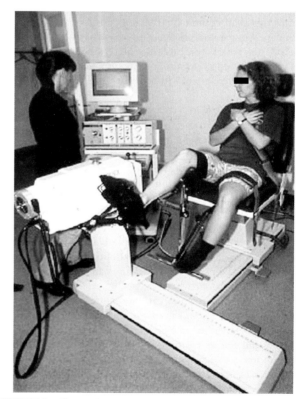

FIGURE 2-2. Picture of an isokinetic dynamometer. Here, the torque of the ankle dorsiflexor muscles is measured.

foot is off the ground, the chain is said to be open. Examples of open kinetic chain exercises used in rehabilitation programs are leg extension, leg curls, arm curls, and bench press exercises. Exercises such as leg press, squats, and push-ups are examples of closed kinetic chain exercises. Closed kinetic chain exercises tend to activate agonist and antagonist muscle groups simultaneously (e.g., the knee extensors and flexors during squat exercises) and tend to be more functional (32). Both types of exercises could result in significant functional improvements after reconstruction of the anterior cruciate ligament (31).

Energetics of Muscle Actions

The energy needed for the muscle to perform its mechanical functions is supplied by three different energy-producing biochemical pathways (**Fig. 2-3**). The relative contribution of each pathway is determined by the duration and intensity of the muscle actions (also, see Chapter 49). Performance of a particular task is determined not only by the integrity and capacity of the sarcomeric proteins but also by the ability of these pathways to supply adenosine triphosphate (ATP). Thus, the results of the functional tests discussed later could be used as indicators of the status of the biochemical pathways. The low strength and/or endurance performance scores in patients with various neuromuscular diseases may relate to abnormalities in these pathways.

In general, short-duration tasks lasting up to 10 seconds depend on existing stores of ATP and creatine phosphate (CP) (33,34). These two stores are readily available and therefore could be used instantaneously. However, from a quantitative point of view, these ATP and CP stores are very small and have a limited ability to sustain muscle performance over time. Activities lasting between 10 seconds and 2 minutes are driven by the process of anaerobic glycolysis fueled by the transport of glucose into the muscle cell or the breakdown (glycogenolysis) of intramuscular carbohydrates (35–39). Finally, the energy for activities lasting more than 2 minutes is supplied mainly by

the oxidative pathways in the mitochondria. The fuel for these pathways can be derived from the end product of anaerobic glycolysis, circulating fatty acids, or intramuscular lipid stores (40,41).

In real life, these biochemical processes combine in various proportions to provide ATP during physical activity and exercise. Activities can be classified as "predominantly" dependent on a particular pathway, since very few activities can be considered purely dependent on any given pathway. In other words, a given activity may require a combination of all three processes, depending on fluctuations in the intensity of the exercise. For example, when a person is walking on a level at a comfortable speed, ATP supply may depend predominantly on oxidative pathways. Confronted with an incline or hill, the contribution of the glycolytic pathways increases. Another example in a different type of activity is the sprint at the end of a marathon race requiring the activation of the glycolytic pathway in a predominantly oxidative event.

Functional Characteristics of Skeletal Muscle

Muscle Strength

Muscle strength can be defined as the maximal force (or torque) generated by a muscle or muscle group at a specified velocity. Because strength depends on force production, it is generally measured in Newtons (N) or Newton-meters (Nm) in the case of torque. When reporting measurements of muscle strength, the type of muscle action must be stated (25). In other words, strength can be static (at different joint angles), dynamic (concentric or eccentric), or isokinetic (at different angular velocities).

It should be clear that there is no single strength measurement and that different kinds of strength can be expressed. Furthermore, under static conditions, force is influenced by fiber (and sarcomere) length (42) and mechanical leverage. Moreover, under dynamic conditions, the level of force is

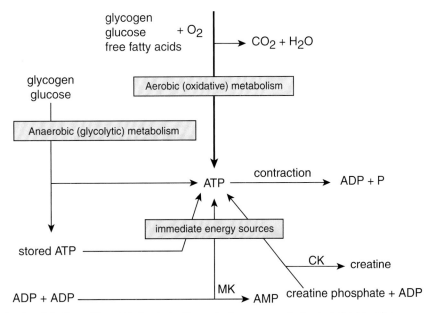

FIGURE 2-3. Schematic drawing of the three different biochemical pathways for the energy production in skeletal muscles.

influenced by the velocity of the movement (42). These relationships are two of the most fundamental biologic properties of skeletal muscle and must be understood to appreciate the meaning of the results of functional tests. For example, the patient's performance during a manual muscle test will not be reliable unless the test is always done at the same joint angle.

The force-length relationship illustrates how the sarcomere length, which defines the degree of overlap between actin and myosin and the formation of crossbridges, determines force (**Fig. 2-4**). The optimal sarcomere length varies with the type of activity. For example, the optimal sarcomere length has been reported to be in the region around the plateau for ankle bending (43), walking (44), and jumping (45) activities and in the descending limb for slow pedaling (46). On the other hand, the force-velocity curve demonstrates a gradient of strength that ranges from the highest level during fast eccentric actions to the lowest level during fast concentric actions (**Fig. 2-5**). Static actions generate more than dynamic concentric actions but less force than dynamic eccentric actions, independent of the velocity.

Testing of Muscle Strength

Various methods and devices are used to measure the different types of muscle strength (47). These methods used in clinical practice and research require a maximal voluntary action on the part of the patient or volunteer. This is dependent on the ability of higher central nervous centers to recruit and modulate the frequency of discharge of the appropriate spinal motoneuron pool. The implication is that all those factors that influence the activation of the neuromuscular system such as age, various disorders in the central and peripheral

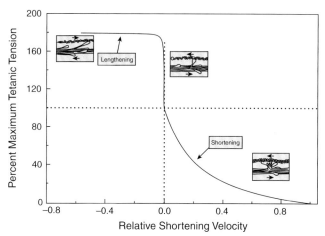

FIGURE 2-5.   Force-velocity relationship of skeletal muscle. *Insets* show schematic representations of actin-myosin crossbridges. Static (isometric) strength (relative shortening velocity = 0) is higher than force at any given velocity of movement during concentric (shortening) muscle actions. On the other hand, eccentric (lengthening) muscle actions at any given velocity generate higher forces than static actions. (Reprinted with permission from Lieber RL. *Skeletal Muscle Structure and Function: Implications for Rehabilitation and Sports Medicine.* 1st ed. Baltimore, MD: Williams & Wilkins; 1992.)

nervous system, presence of pain, joint swelling, medications, fear and anxiety over the test, lack of motivation, time of the day, and environmental conditions such as noise may have a significant effect on strength measurements and should be controlled for or factored into the analysis of the results (48–50). Needless to say, testing conditions must be standardized as much as possible, the same device and/or method and testing protocol must be used when repeated measurements are required, the subject must be encouraged to make a maximal effort during the test, and the presence of symptoms such as pain should be considered when interpreting the measurements. Furthermore, for comparisons among groups, it may be necessary to adjust for differences in muscle/body size using statistical techniques (51). Even under optimal conditions, a valid and reliable level may require that the strength test be repeated more than once (52). Over the last decade, there has been a growing interest in, and a gradual development of, the statistical methods for the analysis of reliability. Today, there is a general agreement that a comprehensive set of several statistical methods are required to fully address the reliability of a measurement method (53).

Manual Muscle Testing

The method of muscle strength measurement used most frequently in the busy clinical setting is manual muscle testing. This technique uses a subjective scale (**Table 2-2**) that ranges from zero (complete paralysis) to normal strength (erroneously called *normal muscle power* by some authors) and is generally known as the "Classification of the Medical Research Council of Great Britain" (54,55). The tester's perception of the strength of a given muscle is influenced by the duration of the tester's effort and the force applied during the test (56). The manual muscle testing scale is characterized by a fairly high level of intra- and interrater variability that limits its usefulness for research studies and clinical follow-up (57). To distinguish

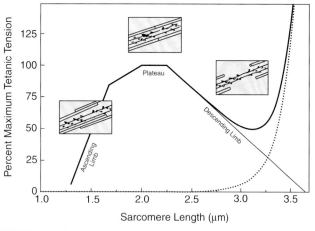

FIGURE 2-4.   Force-length relationship of skeletal muscle. *Insets* show schematic representations of crossbridges. An optimal length results in the largest number of actin-myosin crossbridges (plateau). When the muscle (or sarcomere) has been stretched too much (descending limb; sarcomere length > 3.0 µm), no active force is produced by the actin-myosin crossbridges. However, a level of force can be recorded as a result of the contribution of the passive elastic elements, including cytoskeletal proteins such as titin and nebulin and components of the sarcolemma. During the ascending limb (sarcomere length < 1.75 µm), overlap of myofilaments interferes with actin-myosin crossbridge formation. (Reprinted with permission from Lieber RL. *Skeletal Muscle Structure and Function: Implications for Rehabilitation and Sports Medicine.* 1st ed. Baltimore, MD: Williams & Wilkins; 1992.)

TABLE 2-2	Scale for Manual Muscle Testing			
Numeric Scale	**Descriptor**	**Original Scale**		**Comments**
0	Zero	No contraction		Complete paralysis
1	Trace	Flicker or trace of contraction		No palpable muscle action
2	Poor	Active movement with gravity eliminated		Some authors require full range of movement
3	Fair	Active movement against gravity		Some authors require full range of movement; no resistance
4	Good	Active movement against gravity and resistance		Examiner can overcome
5	Normal	Normal strength		Examiner cannot overcome

among the various degrees of muscle strength within a given level, this scale has been modified with the addition of intermediate levels (e.g., 4+ and 4–). Although clinically useful, there is no evidence that this modification increases the validity or the reliability of the method. It should be understood that this method represents an estimate of static strength at the tested joint angle. Extrapolation of the results to other joint angles and especially to dynamic actions must be done with great caution. In addition, manual muscle testing may not be valid for persons with central nervous system lesions with only synergistic muscle activation.

Static (Isometric) Maximal Voluntary Contraction

A static maximal voluntary contraction (MVC) refers to a condition in which a person attempts to recruit as many muscle fibers in a muscle as possible for the purpose of developing force (25). Although the need for a maximal voluntary effort applies to all forms of strength testing, the term *maximal voluntary contraction* is frequently associated with static strength testing (58). Devices such as handheld dynamometers, cable tensiometers, force transducers, and isokinetic (angular velocity set at zero) dynamometers can be used to measure static muscle strength. Several studies (59–61) have shown good intra- and interrater reliability for the handheld dynamometer in various patient populations. The simplicity and portability of these devices make it an attractive clinical instrument.

The validity of the strength measurement depends on the activation level of the nervous system. Merton (62) introduced the use of electrical stimulation superimposed on a static maximal effort in an attempt to activate directly those motor units and muscle fibers not stimulated by the voluntary effort of the subject. The stimulus is applied to the motor nerve during the MVC, and if the force increases, it indicates a suboptimal activation of motor units by the central nervous system. This is often referred to as *central activation failure* (CAF) (63). In many studies, single impulse stimulation has been used to detect CAF. It has been shown that high-frequency maximal train stimulation may improve the detection of CAF during static (isometric) knee extensions (58,63). This may be important in the clinical assessment of weakness, as it may distinguish weakness caused by CAF from that due to muscle wasting. This, in turn, could have very important implications for the design and evaluation of effective muscle-strengthening exercise therapy. The simultaneous assessment of CAF and muscle mass is advantageous and will facilitate the identification of the mechanism underlying muscle weakness in a particular patient. It is generally considered that healthy men and women, even above the age of 70, have the ability to fully activate their muscles during an MVC (64,65).

Repetition Maximum

During the course of physical rehabilitation and research studies involving exercise training, muscle strength is frequently measured using the one repetition maximum (1 RM) method. In the case of the extensors of the knee, DeLorme (66) defined the 1 RM as the maximum weight that can be lifted with one repetition with the knee going into complete extension. The proper unit of strength measurement is the Newton (N), but in this test, strength is commonly expressed as the mass in kilograms (kg) of the lifted load. This is a simple, valid, and reliable method that uses relatively inexpensive equipment and has been shown to be safe even in the elderly population (67). One drawback is that, by definition, it requires full active range of motion, a condition that some patients with joint pain, swelling, or contractures may be unable to satisfy. Also, if the test is not properly performed and too many repetitions are used to determine the 1 RM, muscle fatigue may interfere with the subject's ability to generate maximal force.

The concept of a continuum of repetition is frequently used when designing strength-conditioning programs (68). The RM refers to the exact resistance that allows a specific number of repetitions to be performed. **Figure 2-6** shows the relationship between RM, number of repetitions, and muscle physiologic characteristic affected by training at a specific level.

Isokinetic Strength

A number of isokinetic devices have been used to measure muscle strength in research laboratories and rehabilitation clinics (see **Fig. 2-2**). Although several muscle groups have been studied with these devices, most of the information concerns the knee, ankle (**Fig. 2-7**), and shoulder muscle groups. The lever arm is aligned with the axis of rotation of the joint to be tested, and proximal and distal segments are stabilized using Velcro straps limiting the contribution of agonists. The tester

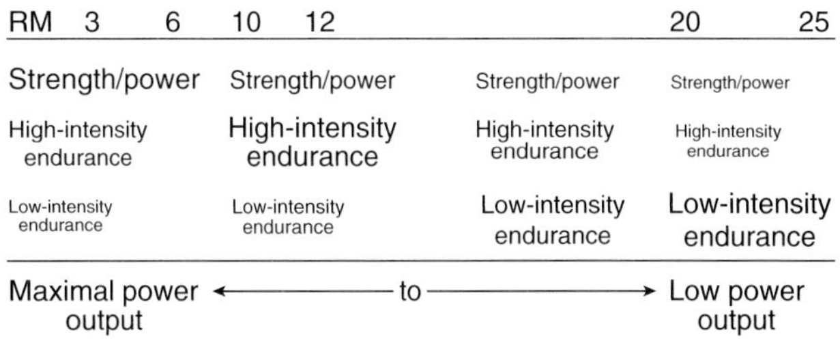

FIGURE 2-6. Theoretical repetition maximum (RM) continuum. Note the relationship between the number of repetitions and the specific muscle physiologic characteristic affected by training at the specific level. (Reprinted with permission from Fleck SJ, Kraemer WJ. Designing Resistance Training Programs. 3rd ed. Champaign, IL: Human Kinetics; 2004:167.)

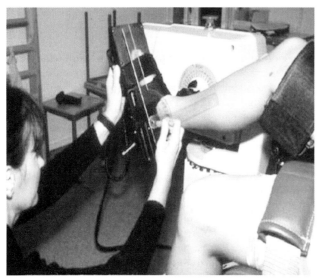

FIGURE 2-7. A handheld goniometer is used to define 0 degrees of the ankle joint (i.e., the tibia being perpendicular to the sole of the foot) before the assessment of isokinetic torque in the ankle dorsiflexor muscles.

sets the angular velocity (available range 0 to 450 degrees per second or 0 to 7.9 rad per second), and the research subjects or patients are usually asked to complete three to five maximal repetitions, with the maximal torque used as a measurement of strength.

Individual brands of isokinetic dynamometers have been shown to be reliable (49,50,52,69–71), including measurements of isokinetic eccentric strength (50,70) and strength in patients with Duchenne or Becker muscular dystrophies (72) or stroke (73,74). Reliability is usually best at low angular velocities and gradually decreases with increased angular velocity. At very high velocities (e.g., above 180 degrees per second), reliability is often considered poor. The comparison of strength values among the different brands of isokinetic dynamometers appears to be less valid. The spectrum of indicators of muscle function provided includes measurements of muscle work (integrated area under the curve), endurance (see later), agonists/antagonists ratios, and differences between sides that can be used to assess for muscle imbalances and asymmetries and for making clinical decisions such as when to decide that an athlete is ready to return to competitive sports (75) (also, see Chapter 41). On the other hand, the devices are expensive, the isokinetic nature of the muscle action does not allow for direct comparisons with daily activities, and the range of angular velocities does not extend to the speed of many sports and daily actions. Finally, measurements of isokinetic strength at various angular velocities have been used to study, *in vivo*, the whole muscle torque-velocity curve and the effects of strength training on muscle contractile behavior (76–78). These studies require the use of torque at multiple given joint angles rather than peak torque over the continuum of available angles in order to control for the effect of muscle length on force development.

Muscle Power

Leg extensor power could be a very important measurement in sports as well as in rehabilitation because power is more relevant for time-dependent/time-critical activities than strength.

Power has been shown to correlate with gait speed, time to rise from a chair, stair-climb time, and self-reported disability (79,80). In addition, power declines with aging at a faster rate than strength (81). The maximum leg extension power output produced by both legs and each leg separately can be estimated using a power rig bench or resistance training machines. The power rig bench measures force and velocity of leg movement, whereas the test using resistance training machines is based on the performance of one repetition at a percentage of the 1 RM. Peak power has been reported to occur usually at 70% of the 1 RM using the resistance training machines (21). Several test trials are usually performed with a 45- to 60-second rest between trials and the maximum value recorded. The coefficient of variation of this method is 6% (82).

Other investigators have designed power tests that combine an eccentric muscle action followed by a concentric action of the same muscle group with a very brief static action in between (83). This is a test of the stretch-shortening cycle (84). A mat or platform that is connected to a timer is used to measure flight time (time spent off the ground) during a vertical jump from which jump height can be calculated. The jump is preceded by a countermovement or semisquat position. The output is fed into a computer for analysis and calculation of muscle power.

Muscle Endurance (and Fatigue)

The definitions of *endurance* and *fatigue* vary with the source. For the purpose of this chapter, *endurance* will be defined as the "time limit of a person's ability to maintain either a static force or a power level involving combinations of concentric and/or eccentric muscular actions" (25). Endurance can be measured in seconds. Fatigue, on the other hand, is the inability to maintain a given level of force output (85). Alternatively, *neuromuscular fatigue* can be defined as "any reduction in the force-generating capacity of the total neuromuscular system" and can be due to factors that affect muscle fibers, the neuromuscular junction, and/or the nervous system (86). In humans, fatigue results in the loss of voluntary force and power production (87), a reduction in electrically stimulated maximal force and the maximum rate of force development (88), altered recruitment pattern of muscles (89), impaired neuromuscular performance in activities such as jumping (90), and even a reduction in sensory function such as the acuity of the joint movement sense (91). Methods used to measure these effects could be good indicators of the presence and degree of fatigue in younger and older populations (92).

In the context of the study of muscle performance, endurance could be divided into central (cardiovascular) and peripheral (local muscular) types. Several physiologic systems are involved in the expression of endurance and the avoidance of fatigue, including the nervous (central and peripheral), cardiovascular, hormonal, and metabolic systems. It is likely that the contribution of each system to endurance and fatigue depends on factors such as the type of activity, environmental conditions, nutritional status, and fitness level. Measurements of muscle endurance represent an integrated evaluation of several of these systems.

The basic mechanisms underlying muscle fatigue have not been precisely defined, although our understanding of this phenomenon has been substantially enhanced by recent research. Several excellent reviews summarize the available literature and discuss the contribution to fatigue of many of the components of the neuromuscular system (93–95). Clearly, each and every step along the chain of transmission of the electrical and chemical signals from the brain to the actin-myosin crossbridges and the biochemical pathways that supply fuel for muscle action is a potential site of failure. The development of fatigue is significantly influenced by the fiber type composition of skeletal muscle as the effector organ (96). Other relevant factors include central and peripheral mechanisms (97), such as changes in the excitability of the motor cortex or inadequate neural drive upstream of the motor cortex (98,99). This type of fatigue is of particular significance in neurologic rehabilitation, as it is considered prevalent in various nervous system disorders such as multiple sclerosis and stroke (100).

At the cellular level, the role of changes in the ADP/ATP ratio and the concentration of inorganic phosphate have received strong support (101,102) challenging the traditional view that accumulation of lactic acid and hydrogen ions is the main biochemical correlate of muscle fatigue. Others have highlighted the importance of cation pumps such as the Na^+/K^+ ATPase (103) and the Ca^+ ATPase (104) in maintaining muscle excitability and preventing muscle fatigue. Cellular factors may also play a role in muscle fatigue in disorders of the central nervous system such as multiple sclerosis and amyotrophic lateral sclerosis (105,106). A recent review summarizes the various molecular and cellular mechanisms that interact under various conditions, resulting in the clinical phenomenon called muscle fatigue (107).

Absolute and Relative Endurance

One simple test of dynamic endurance is to count the number of repetitions that a subject/patient can do with a given load. Similarly, a test of static endurance could measure the length of time that a given level of force can be maintained. Since both tests use an absolute load or level of force, stronger subjects/patients will be tested at a relatively lower percentage of their strength than weaker subjects. For example, a dynamic test conducted using a 40-kg load represents 40% and 80% of the strength of individuals with a 1 RM test of 100 and 50 kg, respectively. Tested at a lower percentage of his or her strength, the stronger individual will demonstrate better endurance.

To control for the effects of muscle and body size, a similar testing paradigm can be used, but based on a percentage of the individual's strength. This relative endurance test requires the performance of as many repetitions as possible using, for example, 50% of the dynamic strength of the individual. It can also be done by asking the individual to maintain a relative level of static force for as long as possible. The relative endurance test limits the influence of body or muscle size on the measurement and may allow for a better way to compare different groups of patients.

Fatigue Indices

Isokinetic devices have been used to quantify muscle fatigue and endurance by measuring relative losses in peak torque and/or work during a standardized test. For example, the ratio between peak torque or work performed during the first and last three or five repetitions of a series of repetitions, usually 25 to 100, depending on the muscle group under study, has been used as an index of muscle fatigue. Since the calculation of work performed is based on the integration of the area under the curve, it is important to make sure that, during the test, the joint moves through the entire predetermined range of motion. Studies that have measured both fatigue and strength reproducibility using isokinetic dynamometers have found that isokinetic fatigue tests are less reliable than isokinetic strength tests (108–110). In a study of the reliability of an isokinetic fatigue test for concentric ankle dorsiflexion, it was shown that fatigue indices using decreases in peak torque were more reliable than an index based on relative decreases in work, but that all indices showed acceptable to good reliability (111).

A similar approach has been used by other investigators, but during static muscle actions. A combination of the percent reduction in force over a given period of time and the average augmentation with electrical stimulation superimposed during contractions has been proposed as a clinically useful method of quantifying muscle fatigue (112).

Spectral Analysis of the Surface Electromyographic Signal

Spectral analysis of the surface electromyographic signal is based on the idea that, during the performance of static muscle actions, a reduction of the median frequency correlates with the drop in force and therefore is an indirect indicator of muscle fatigue (109). The median frequency reflects muscle fiber conduction velocity and motor unit recruitment and therefore is influenced by the fiber type composition of the muscle. Some authors have proposed that a shift in the mean power frequency of the electromyography (EMG) is actually a selective indicator of fatigue of the fast-twitch motor units (113) and that subjects with higher concentrations of fibers expressing type II myosin heavy chain (MHC) isoform displayed greater reductions in median frequency of EMG and muscle fiber conduction velocity during exercise (114).

Another approach based on the study of changes in the EMG signal during voluntary contractions has been proposed by Merletti and Roy (115). They studied the rate of spectral compression of the surface EMG signal during the early phases of static voluntary muscle actions of the tibialis anterior. The slope of the median frequency during the first 30 seconds correlated with endurance time. The authors proposed the use of this technique in the clinical setting in part because the test does not require the use of muscle actions to failure.

Nuclear Magnetic Resonance

Nuclear magnetic resonance (NMR) is used to study the metabolic correlates of muscle fatigue at rest and during exercise (**Fig. 2-8**). Changes in intracellular pH, concentrations of inorganic phosphate, phosphocreatine (PCr), ADP, and ATP resulting from the metabolic demands imposed on active muscles can be monitored in real time at rest, during exercise and fatiguing conditions, and during the recovery period (116). The speed at which a muscle recovers from these metabolic alterations is a good indicator of the fitness level of the muscle and the individual. An interesting point is that the accumulation of these metabolites alters the conduction of the action potential and explains the changes in the spectral content of the EMG signal mentioned earlier. This technique has the advantage of being noninvasive. However, it is expensive and not readily available in many clinical facilities.

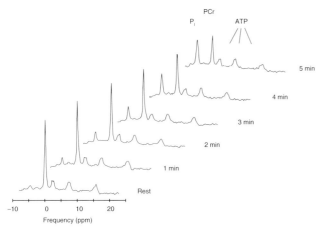

FIGURE 2-8. NMR spectra from the calf muscles of a sprint athlete at rest and during 5 minutes of progressive exercise. Note the reduction in phosphocreatine (PCr) and the accumulation of inorganic phosphate (Pi) with progression of exercise. Also, note the relative conservation of adenosine triphosphate (ATP), which protects the muscle cell from permanent damage. (Reprinted with permission from McCully KK, Vandenborne K, Demeirleir K, et al. Muscle metabolism in track athletes, using 31P magnetic resonance spectroscopy. *Can J Physiol Pharmacol.* 1992;70(10):1353–1359.)

Other Tests of Muscle Properties Related to Fatigue and Endurance

Near-Infrared Spectroscopy and Microdialysis

Near-infrared spectroscopy (NIRS) is a noninvasive research technique to measure oxygen (O_2) through tissues up to 10 cm in depth (117). NIRS can be used to investigate the delivery and utilization of oxygen in response to exercise and in the clinical setting to assess circulatory and metabolic abnormalities (118). Quantitative measures of blood flow are also possible using NIRS.

Microdialysis is an invasive research technique that has allowed mechanistic investigations to be performed in human skeletal muscle. The microdialysis catheter has been equated to an artificial blood vessel, which is introduced into the tissue. By means of this "vessel," the concentrations of compounds in the interstitial space of skeletal muscle (as well as other tissues) can be monitored. A number of important observations on the *in vivo* regulation of lipolysis, carbohydrate metabolism, and blood flow in human skeletal muscle and adipose tissue have been made using microdialysis (119).

STRUCTURAL CHARACTERISTICS OF SKELETAL MUSCLE

The Relationship Between Function and Structure

The relationship between the structure and the function of biologic systems has received significant scientific attention. Ewald Weibel, the great Swiss morphologist, concluded in his book on the structure and function of the mammalian respiratory system that, "I have become convinced not only that structure determines function, but that functional demand also determines structural design, be it through evolution or by modulation of design features" (120). The importance of function as a determinant of form has also been emphasized by

Russell et al. (121). In their review, they demonstrated how the functional demands imposed on muscle cells result in adaptations in muscle cell shape, size, and functions such as force production.

Based on the previous paragraph, a discussion about muscle function cannot be comprehensive unless some of the structural and architectural features of skeletal muscle are analyzed. The level of force and power generated by an active muscle is influenced by several factors including muscle size, fiber angle of insertion, and sarcomere length (122,123). Muscle length contributes to shortening velocity, and muscle fiber type composition is an important determinant of speed and endurance. We will now discuss some of the measurements of muscle structure that are used in rehabilitation clinics and research laboratories.

Body Composition: Estimating and Measuring Muscle Mass in Humans

The human body is composed of various types of tissues (including skeletal muscle) with different chemical consistency. The study of body composition allows a determination of the amount and anatomic quality of these components (124). Body composition is associated with health status and functional capacity, among other outcomes. The study of body composition can be accomplished using different compartment models (**Fig. 2-9**) (125). Skeletal muscle and its constituents, although sometimes measured indirectly, are important components in each of these models. The chemical composition of muscle has been described as approximately 75% water and 20% protein, with the remaining 5% made up of inorganic salts and other substances that include high-energy phosphates, urea, lactic acid, calcium, magnesium, phosphorus, enzymes, potassium, sodium, chloride, amino acids, fats, and carbohydrates (4,126).

The traditional gold standard in the study of human body composition, hydrodensitometry or underwater weighing, and the more recent air displacement (plethysmography) is based

Five Level Model

N, Ca, P, K, Na, Cl	Lipid	Adipocytes	Adipose Tissue
H	Water	Cells	
C			Skeletal Muscle
		Extracellular Fluid	Visceral Organs & Residual
O	Proteins		
	Glycogen		
		Extracellular Solids	
	Minerals		Skeleton
Atomic	*Molecular*	*Cellular*	*Tissue-System*

FIGURE 2-9. Multiple compartment models for the study of human body composition. Note the relative contribution of skeletal muscle and its atomic, molecular, and cellular components in each of the models. (From Wang ZM, Pierson RN Jr, Heymsfield SB. The five-level model: a new approach to organizing body-composition research. *Am J Clin Nutr.* 1992;56(1):19–28. Reproduced by permission of Oxford University Press.)

on a two-compartment model. This model divides the body into fat mass (FM) and fat-free mass (FFM). In this context, the use of the term *fat-free mass* is thought not to be very accurate, since the nonfat component includes a small percentage of essential fat stores within the central nervous system, bone marrow, and internal organs. Thus, LBM is a more appropriate designation. LBM includes essential fat, muscle, and bone. Hydrodensitometry estimates body density (127), which is then used to calculate FM with the Siri equation, assuming a constant density for FM and LBM (128):

$$\text{Percent body fat} = \frac{495}{\text{density}} - 450$$

where density = mass (in air)/loss of mass in water (or mass in air, mass in water). Accurate determination of density requires correction for water temperature. Finally, LBM is obtained by subtracting FM from the total body mass.

Elements at the atomic level can be quantified using neutron activation techniques (129,130). This is relevant to our topic of discussion because, as mentioned earlier, muscle is an important source of nitrogen. In addition, most of the potassium present in the body is intracellular, and a large amount is present in myofibers. The use of whole-body counters, special instruments capable of detecting radiation from the decay of the naturally occurring radioactive isotope of potassium, allows quantification of cell body mass and, indirectly, lean body and muscle mass (129,130).

Techniques such as dual-energy x-ray absorptiometry (DEXA) are used to quantify bone, fat (both subcutaneous and visceral) mass, and skeletal muscle mass (131,132). Total body and appendicular estimates can be obtained (131) at a lower cost and radiation exposure than with computerized tomography (CT). The most accurate *in vivo* methods of measuring muscle size, muscle mass, and segmental body composition are imaging techniques such as CT and magnetic resonance imaging (MRI) (see later).

Muscle Size

A reasonable, but not always accurate, estimate of muscle size at a given limb level can be obtained in the clinic by measuring limb circumference with a metric tape. However, these measurements include fat, bone, and other noncontractile tissues. Furthermore, such measurements cannot be corrected for changes in limb circumference related to fluid shifts or tissue edema. In pathologic conditions where muscle is replaced by connective tissue and/or fat, such as in certain myopathic conditions, measurements of limb circumference can be very misleading.

Reliable estimates of muscle cross-sectional area can be obtained with modern techniques such as ultrasound (133,134), CT (135), or MRI (135–137). Ultrasound has been used extensively because of its simplicity, its low cost, and the fact that it does not involve exposure to radiation. However, it does not provide an optimal distinction of the borders between the various tissues. Another application for ultrasound techniques has been the *in vivo* study of the architecture of the muscle tendon complex (138). Measurements of tendon length, muscle fascicle length, pennation angle of muscle fibers, tendon elongation during muscle contraction, tendon strain, and related properties have been done *in vivo* in

humans. These measurements can help us understand muscle function. For example, because muscle fibers consist of sarcomeres in series, the muscle fiber length indicates the velocity potential of a muscle during contraction. The longer fascicles in the vastus lateralis muscle result in faster velocity than that occurs with the medial gastrocnemius. However, the tendon of the medial gastrocnemius has a higher compliance and therefore a greater potential to store elastic energy (139).

Both CT and MRI have been widely used to obtain valid (using cadaver measurements as the standard) and reliable measurements of total thigh, muscle, subcutaneous fat, and bone cross-sectional areas in health and disease (135,140). In both CT- and MRI-based methodologies, anatomic cross-sectional area refers to the area measured from a single cross section of the muscle. The measurement is made perpendicular to the long axis of the muscle. Because in pennate muscles, like the quadriceps femoris, fibers do not run parallel to the longitudinal axis of the muscle, these measurements underestimate the true muscle area (141; **Fig. 2-10**). On the other hand, if measurements of muscle volume obtained by MRI are combined with estimates of muscle fiber length from cadavers, physiologic cross-sectional area can be calculated with reasonable accuracy (142,143).

Both CT and MRI have been shown to provide valid estimates of muscle cross-sectional area (135). The higher-definition MRI provides better area estimates than CT images. The latter tends to systematically overestimate anatomic cross-sectional area by 10% to 20% (144). Both MRI and CT have been shown to have high intrarater and interrater reliability and are capable of detecting exercise training–induced adaptations in

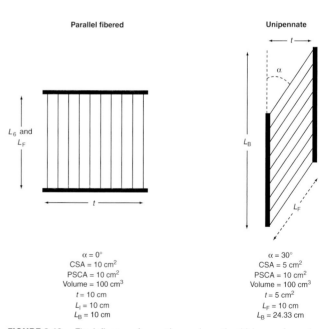

FIGURE 2-10. The influence of pennation angle on the thickness of muscle and estimations of muscle size. CSA, anatomic cross-sectional area; PCSA, physiologic cross-sectional area. These two muscles have the same number of fibers of the same thickness. By increasing the pennation angle α, thickness of the muscle (CSA) belly decreases. The pennation angle allows more of the muscle mass to be closer to the joint, reducing the resistance to movement. (From Fukunaga T, Roy RR, Shellock FG, et al. Physiological cross-sectional area of human leg muscles based on magnetic resonance imaging. *J Orthop Res.* 1992;10:926–934.)

skeletal muscle (77,145,146). T1-weighed MRI allows muscle tissue and noncontractile tissue components (connective tissue, subcutaneous and interstitial adipose tissue) to be separated (135,145). Cross-sectional images of the human thigh and leg obtained using MRI are presented in **Figure 2-11** (137). Computer-based image analysis systems can be used to quantify the composition of muscle, fat, and connective tissue by assigning different density values to the different tissue components. Muscle attenuation, a function of tissue density and chemical composition, has been shown to relate to its lipid content (146). Furthermore, since disease and exercise training may alter both the contractile and noncontractile components of the limb, it is very useful to be able to quantify changes in these two compartments (145,147).

MRI has also been used to assess the level of activation of different muscles or parts of muscles during volitional exercise and neuromuscular electrical stimulation (148,149). MRI can provide a noninvasive way to quantitatively evaluate and localize muscle activity. The underlying mechanism that explains this phenomenon is the accumulation of osmolites (phosphate, lactate, sodium) in the cytoplasm during exercise, resulting in the influx of fluid and an increase in muscle T2 relaxation. A practical application of this technique is the use of the T2 relaxation times to evaluate muscle activation during specific exercises. (For a detailed discussion of radiologic techniques, see Chapter 5.) For example, a recent study demonstrated that both the "empty can" and the "full can" exercises activate the

supraspinatus muscle to a larger extent than the horizontal abduction exercise (150). This information could be used to design the optimal combination of exercises for strengthening rehabilitation programs. Thus, only those exercises that activate a large proportion of the injured or weak muscles are included in the rehabilitation program.

When comparing different patient populations, subjects with different levels of physical fitness, or measurements done before and after exercise training, we must take into account the fact that force varies with size (**Fig. 2-12**) and that larger individuals will be stronger if absolute strength is used as an outcome. These comparisons should only be made after strength is adjusted for differences in muscle physiologic cross-sectional area or volume or for the amount of noncontractile tissue components. The ratio between force generated and measurements of muscle area is known as specific force and has been used as an index of "muscle quality" (143,151–153). A simple ratio, however, may not be the best way of adjusting muscle strength, and more sophisticated statistical treatment may be needed (154–157).

Muscle Biopsy Techniques

Despite recent advances in noninvasive muscle-imaging techniques, analysis of small samples of human skeletal muscle is still the only way to determine various changes in the fiber population as a result of an intervention or to investigate the underlying pathophysiologic mechanisms of muscle

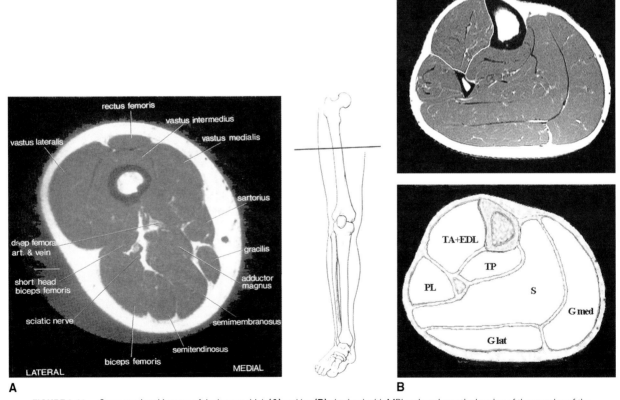

A   B

FIGURE 2-11.   Cross-sectional images of the human thigh **(A)** and leg **(B)** obtained with MRI and a schematic drawing of the muscles of the leg. Note the clear difference in density of the muscle (contractile) and fat and connective (noncontractile) tissues. (Reprinted with permission from Berquist TH. *MRI of the Musculoskeletal System.* 3rd ed. Philadelphia, PA: Lippincott Williams & Wilkins; 1996.)

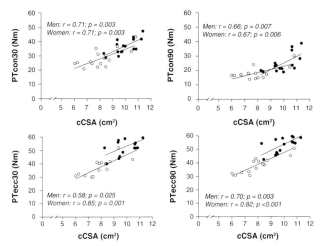

FIGURE 2-12. Relationship between muscle strength and size in humans. Note that the correlation is not 1, suggesting that factors other than muscle size (e.g., motor unit activation, fiber type distribution, muscle fiber quality) explain a significant percentage of the variability in muscle strength among subjects or patients.

dysfunction. Muscle biopsies for various morphologic and biochemical studies can be obtained with the open and percutaneous (needle or semiopen conchotome) biopsy techniques (**Fig. 2-13**). The needle biopsy technique was introduced by Duchenne in 1868 (158) and has been successfully adapted or modified by others (159–163) for the study of neuromuscular

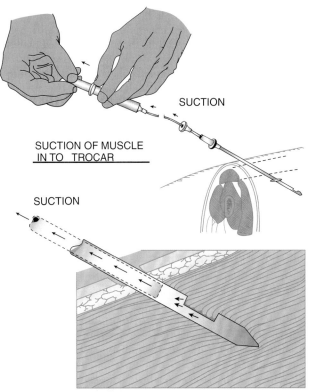

FIGURE 2-13. The needle muscle biopsy technique. This technique can be used to obtain muscle samples for research studies and for clinical diagnosis. The application of suction enhances the amount of tissue obtained for analysis. (Reprinted with permission from Mubarak SJ, Chambers HG, Wenger DR. Percutaneous muscle biopsy in the diagnosis of neuromuscular disease. *J Pediatr Orthop.* 1992;12(2):191–196.)

and systemic diseases affecting skeletal muscle (164–166), adaptations to exercise training (167–169), and aging (170). An alternative technique is the semiopen conchotome technique (171,172), which usually yields larger samples than the needle technique. With either technique, the procedure is done under local anesthesia and is usually well tolerated by research subjects and patients. Ultrasound (172,173) and MRI (174) have been used to guide the placement of the biopsy needle to the area of interest in the muscle under study. The skeletal muscles most frequently biopsied are the vastus lateralis, lateral gastrocnemius, triceps surae, tibialis anterior, and biceps brachii.

It must be noted that a biopsy sample represents a very small fraction of all the fibers in a large muscle such as the vastus lateralis. A biopsy sample from this muscle may contain several hundred to a few thousand fibers, compared with hundreds of thousands in the whole muscle. Thus, because there is significant intramuscular variability in the distribution of fiber types, more than one sample may be needed to obtain a good estimate of the fiber type proportion (175). The determination of fiber size and capillarity, however, appears to be less problematic. It has been suggested that one biopsy sample may suffice (174–178), although several small samples are advantageous when muscle fiber areas are determined (179).

Muscle Fiber Size and Type Distribution

Muscle is a heterogeneous tissue composed of fibers of different sizes and types (180). Histologic and histochemical techniques have been used for more than half a century to study muscle cross sections under light microscopy (181,182). Over the last decades, immunocytochemical techniques have been introduced. These techniques use chemical reagents (stains) that react with components of the muscle fiber, allowing the visualization and assessment of various structural and functional muscle characteristics such as fiber size and shape, fiber type distribution, capillary supply, enzyme activity, nuclei distribution, satellite cells, intracellular carbohydrates and lipid stores, amount of intercellular connective tissue, degree of fat infiltration, presence of intracellular structures such as inclusion bodies, and others.

Table 2-3 summarizes the most common staining procedures of human muscle biopsies. Many of these techniques are used as part of the clinical investigation of muscle biopsies (e.g., to diagnose a specific neuromuscular disorder). Other procedures are used to investigate pathologic changes in general, and yet others are only used for research.

Muscle biopsy cross sections can be stained with hematoxylin and eosin for the evaluation of the general morphology of muscle fibers, including its size, shape, and location of nuclei. The identification of capillaries in the muscle biopsy cross section can be accomplished with the periodic acid–Schiff amylase stain or immunocytochemical procedures with antibodies against laminin or *Ulex europaeus* agglutinin I (UEA) lectin (183). This is an important property of skeletal muscle, given the fact that capillarity changes significantly with exercise training, disease (e.g., peripheral vascular disease), and immobilization. A qualitative assessment of various oxidative and glycolytic enzymes can be done with specific enzymatic stains such as succinate dehydrogenase (SDH), NADH tetrazolium reductase (NADH-TR), α-glycerophosphate dehydrogenase (GPDH), cytochrome C oxidase (COX), and phosphofructokinase

TABLE 2-3   Examples of Staining Procedures of Human Muscle Biopsies

Histologic stains

Hematoxylin and eosin (H&E)	Stains nuclei and cytoplasm, used to assess general structure, location of nuclei, inflammation, regeneration
Periodic acid–Schiff (PAS)	Glycogen, shows abnormal accumulations of glycogen and related metabolic disorders
Oil red O or Sudan Black	Lipid droplets
Modified Gomori trichrome	Stains mitochondria, nuclei, used to visualize ragged red fibers with excess mitochondria

Histochemical stains

Myosin ATPase at pH 4.3, 4.6, and 9.4	Used to visualize and differentiate muscle fiber types
Oxidative enzymes	
NADH	Stains intermyofibrillar material such as mitochondria, sarcoplasmic reticulum, T tubules, target fibers
SDH	Stains mitochondria (complex II, encoded entirely in nuclear DNA), visualizes subsarcolemmal and intermyofibrillar distribution, indicates excess mitochondrial activity
COX	Stains mitochondria (complex IV), used to detect mitochondrial myopathies that lack the enzyme
Other enzymes	
PFK	This enzyme is active in the glycolysis and absent in type VII glycogenosis
Myophosphorylase	Indicates excess of glycolytic activity or absence, as in McArdle's disease (type V glycogenosis)

Immunocytochemical stains

UEA	Stains capillaries
Dystrophin	Duchenne and Becker muscular dystrophy
Desmin and vimentin	Cytoskeletal proteins, used to visualize congenital myopathies and myopathies with cytoplasmic bodies
Lymphocyte markers	Used to visualize mononuclear inflammatory cells
N-CAM	Used to visualize regenerating and denervated fibers

(PFK). Finally, qualitative and quantitative estimates of lipid and carbohydrate content are possible via histochemical and biochemical methods. The glycogen depletion technique has been used for several decades to identify the pattern of activation of motor units in various types of exercises; the reader is referred to other publications on this subject for more details (184).

The mATPase stain is one of the most widely used to visualize the fiber population and evaluate changes in the size and proportion of the different fiber types following an intervention such as detraining (**Fig. 2-14**). Based on the mATPase activity, the human muscle fiber population is commonly classified into types I, IIA, IIB, and IIC (185). This original mATPase-based semiqualitative classification of muscle fibers

has been expanded, and seven different human muscle fiber types are now being identified: I, IC, IIC, IIAC, IIA, IIAB, and IIB (186,187). Perrie and Bumford (188) refined the electrophoretic techniques and separated the human MHCs into three isoforms: I, IIa, and IIx, which have been shown to correlate with the three major mATPase-based fiber types (189–191). It is now known that the mATPase-based type IIB fibers correspond to MHC IIx identified by gel electrophoresis (192,193). Studies of single muscle fibers have also shown that fibers can contain a mixture of MHC isoforms. The mATPase types IC, IIC, and IIAC coexpress the MHC I and IIa to a varying degree, whereas type IIAB fibers coexpress MHC IIa and IIx (187). As the enzyme histochemical and electrophoretic techniques can yield different information, it is recommended that both techniques are used when the muscle fiber type population is quantified (194).

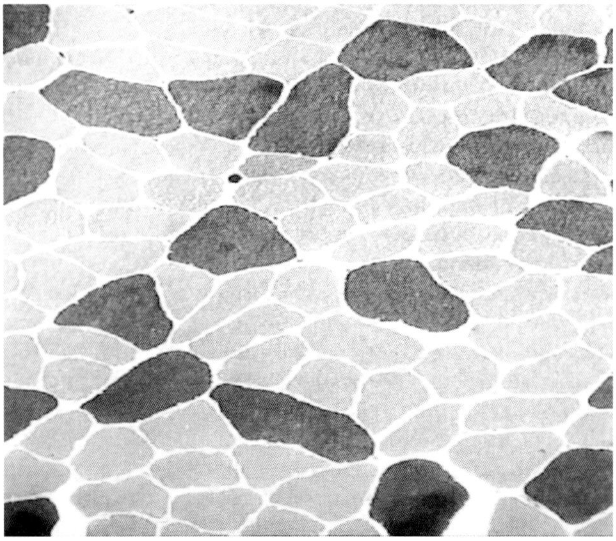

STUDIES OF SINGLE MUSCLE FIBERS

The percutaneous biopsy technique has been used to obtain muscle fiber segments for the study of the morphologic, contractile, and biochemical properties of single human skeletal muscle fibers (195,196). These single fibers are permeabilized with high glycerol concentrations and a detergent solution, resulting in breaks in the sarcolemma and the sarcoplasmic reticulum. The absence of these barriers permits the rapid diffusion of calcium into the cell and its interaction with troponin C, triggering the cascade of events that lead to force generation. Before these experiments are done, the fibers are attached to a force transducer that measures force generation during activation and a servomotor that controls the sarcomere length (**Fig. 2-15**). An image analysis system is used to measure sarcomere length, muscle fiber length, diameter, and depth; the latter two are used to calculate fiber cross-sectional area.

FIGURE 2-14. Microscopic image of a muscle biopsy from the human tibialis anterior muscle visualizing type I (lightly stained) and type II (heavily stained) fibers.

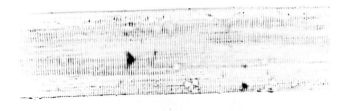

100 µm

FIGURE 2-15.   Light microscopy image of a human single muscle fiber. The fiber is attached to a force transducer and a lever system to control its length. Notice the well-preserved striation pattern.

Measurements of maximal static force, peak power, and shortening velocity are obtained by activating the fiber with calcium (156,157,197). Using a different experimental protocol, the force-velocity and force-power relationships of the single fibers can also be studied. When contractility studies are completed, the fiber segment is submitted to protein gel electrophoresis to determine the expression of MHC isoforms and thereby the fiber type (**Fig. 2-16**). This electrophoretic technique has the advantage over the ATPase stain of allowing the identification of hybrid fibers, fibers expressing simultaneously two or more MHC isoforms.

The single muscle fiber method complements the techniques used to measure *in vivo* muscle function by making it possible to study the contractile behavior of single fibers in the absence of confounding variables such as the influence of the nervous system, the presence of intercellular connective tissue,

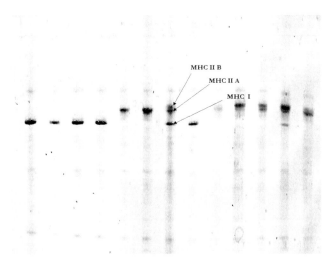

MHC II B
MHC II A
MHC I

FIGURE 2-16.   Protein gel electrophoresis (SDS-PAGE) of human skeletal muscle single fibers for fiber type identification. One muscle fiber per lane. Most fibers express one myosin heavy chain isoform (bands). Notice also the hybrid fibers simultaneously expressing more than one myosin heavy chain isoform (i.e., third lane from right).

the heterogeneity of muscle fiber type distribution, and the connectivity to the tendon-bone interface. Adjusting measurements of contractility for differences in muscle fiber size has been used as an index of muscle fiber quality.

FUNCTIONAL TESTS OF MUSCLE PERFORMANCE

In a clinical setting, it is sometimes not practical or efficient to evaluate muscle function with expensive devices and time-consuming laboratory-based tests. Furthermore, in research and patient care, there is a need to measure performance in tasks that are more similar to activities of daily living (ADLs) and instrumental activities of daily living (IADLs) than many sophisticated laboratory tests. These two considerations have resulted in the development of simple, inexpensive, and easy-to-administer tests of neuromuscular function or performance. These measurements do not represent direct evaluations of skeletal muscle or any other isolated physiologic characteristic but rather an integrated response of the human body to the demands of a particular task. However, muscle strength and power correlate well with test performance scores. These tests are described in various publications together with normative data (20,21,198,199), and some of them will be described later.

Chair Stand Time
In general, the chair stand time test (198,199) requires a chair with arms and a seat placed against a wall for support and safety. Subjects should sit all the way back in the chair with their back against the back of the chair. The feet should be placed so that the knee is in a 90-degree angle. The patient or research subject is instructed to stand up and sit back down as fast as possible for five or ten repetitions with the arms crossed at the chest. Time is measured with a stopwatch to the nearest 0.01 second and stopped after the last stand. The subjects should come to a complete stand each time and completely sit down with their backs against the back of the chair each time. This test can be considered an indirect index of knee extensor function, since this muscle group produces 72% of the power needed to rise from a chair (15).

Stair-Climbing Power
A standard stair flight with handrails on each side is used for the stair-climbing test (200). Subjects are instructed to ascend stairs as quickly as possible using the handrail and/or an assistive device if necessary. The test is started with both of the subject's feet on the bottom step. The subject is instructed to climb up the steps as quickly as possible. A stopwatch is used and stopped when both feet are planted at the top step. Time is recorded to the nearest 0.01 second, and the best of two trials (separated by a 2-minute rest period) is taken. Power, in watts, is calculated using the following equation:

$$\frac{\text{body weight } (\text{kg}) \times \text{vertical distance } (\text{m})}{\text{time } (\text{s}) \div 60} \div 6.12$$

(Note that 6.12 kg-m/min = 1 watt.)

Habitual and Maximal Walking Speed

Walking speed correlates with strength of the ankle dorsi-flexors and knee extensors (10,201–203) and leg extension power (203). This relationship has been shown to be nonlinear (10). In other words, the decline in gait time with increases in strength is curvilinear, and there is a threshold value below which the relationship is lost. In longitudinal studies, baseline strength of the knee extensors has been shown to be a good predictor of 2- and 4-year decline in walking velocity (201). Walking speed is also correlated with isokinetic knee extensor and flexor torque in chronic stroke patients; strength for the paretic limb explains up to 50% of the variance in gait performance (204).

Walking speed can be measured to the nearest 0.01 second as the mean of two trials using a stopwatch and a set distance or a gait speed monitor. The subject or patient will start the test with feet parallel and both heels and toes on the floor. For the habitual walking speed test, patients or subjects are instructed to walk at their normal or comfortable speed. During the maximal walking speed test, they are required to walk as quickly as possible. Speed is recorded after subjects walked a given distance to control for individual differences in acceleration. Measurements of walking speed have been shown to be highly reliable in a number of patient groups (205).

The 6-Minute Walk Test

The 6-minute walk test requires that subjects walk for 6 minutes covering as much ground as possible at a pace that would allow them to talk without becoming short of breath (206). The test may be conducted in a circular track or on a level course. The subject is allowed to rest but instructed to continue walking if possible. The tester times the walk with a stopwatch. After 6 minutes, the distance walked is measured.

Although sometimes considered a test of aerobic capacity, endurance, and survival in patients with heart disease (207), it has been shown that performance in the 6-minute walk test correlates with lower extremity muscle strength and power (204,208). Performance in this test depends on multiple physiologic, psychological, and health factors (209). Muscle strength, balance, medication use, and age explain the largest proportion of the variance in the performance of this test.

MUSCLE FUNCTION, EXERCISE TRAINING, AND FUNCTIONAL PERFORMANCE

In this chapter, we have emphasized that muscle function is related to performance. In rehabilitation, improvements of physiologic capacity are only relevant if these improvements have functional consequences, reduce disability, and increase participation. However, the association between muscle function and functional performance is not necessarily linear (210) (Fig. 2-17). In the presence of disease and with a high degree of muscle function, exercise could serve as a means of preventing the deleterious consequences of disease progression and inactivity. When chronic illness has resulted in severe functional losses, exercise training may be used as a form of recreation. In the steep part of the curve, a relatively small loss of muscle function could result in disproportionate reduction in performance. Thus, even minor adaptations to exercise training could preserve functional capacity and independence. The

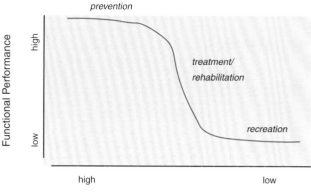

FIGURE 2-17. The nonlinear relationship between muscle function (e.g., muscle strength) and functional performance (e.g., walking ability) and the differential effects of exercise on functional performance, depending on the degree of disease progression. (Reprinted with permission from Lexell J. Muscle structure and function in chronic neurological disorders. The potential of exercise to improve activities of daily living. *Exerc Sports Sci Rev.* 2000;28(2):80–84.)

minimal level of muscle function needed to achieve this goal remains to be determined.

CONCLUSION

Understanding the role of skeletal muscle in health and disease is of paramount importance for those interested in rehabilitation medicine. A wide range of techniques and methods have been developed to assess muscle function and structure. Becoming proficient in their applicability and use is relevant to patient care, education, and research in physical medicine and rehabilitation.

REFERENCES

1. Clarys JP, Martin AD, Drinkwater DT. Gross tissue weights in the human body by cadaver dissection. *Hum Biol.* 1984;56:459–473.
2. Rooyackers OE, Nair KS. Hormonal regulation of human muscle protein metabolism. *Annu Rev Nutr.* 1997;17:457–485.
3. Houston ME. Gaining weight: the scientific basis of increasing skeletal muscle mass. *Can J Appl Physiol.* 1999;24:305–316.
4. Frontera WR, Ochala J. Skeletal muscle: a brief review of structure and function. *Calcif Tissue Int.* 2015;96:183–195.
5. Balagopal P, Ford GC, Ebenstein DB. Mass spectrometric method for determination of [^{13}C] leucine enrichment in human muscle protein. *Anal Biochem.* 1996;239:77–85.
6. Balagopal P, Ljungqvist O, Nair SK. Skeletal muscle myosin heavy-chain synthesis rate in healthy humans. *Am J Physiol.* 1997;272:E45–E50.
7. Perry SV. *Molecular Mechanisms in Striated Muscle.* Cambridge, MA: Cambridge University Press; 1996.
8. Wilmore JH, Costill DL. *Physiology of Exercise.* 2nd ed. Champaign, IL: Human Kinetics; 1999.
9. Roubenoff R, Castaieda C. Sarcopenia—understanding the dynamics of aging muscle. *JAMA.* 2001;286:1230–1231.
10. Buchner DM, Larson EB, Wagner EH, et al. Evidence for a non-linear relationship between leg strength and gait speed. *Age Ageing.* 1996;25:386–391.
11. Rantanen T, Guralnik JM, Izmirlian G, et al. Association of muscle strength with maximum walking speed in disabled older women. *Am J Phys Med Rehabil.* 1998;77:299–305.
12. Rantanen T, Guralnik JM, Leveille S, et al. Racial differences in muscle strength in disabled older women. *J Gerontol Biol Sci.* 1998;53A:B355–B361.
13. Rantanen T, Guralnik JM, Ferrucci L, et al. Coimpairments: strength and balance as predictors of severe walking disability. *J Gerontol Med Sci.* 1999;54A:M172–M176.
14. Rantanen T, Guralnik JM, Sakari-Rantala R, et al. Disability, physical activity, and muscle strength in older women: the women's health and aging study. *Arch Phys Med Rehabil.* 1999;80:130–135.
15. Millington PJ, Myklebust BM, Shambers GM. Biomechanical analysis of the sit-to-stand motion in elderly persons. *Arch Phys Med Rehabil.* 1992;73:609–617.

16. Wretenberg P, Arborelius UP. Power and work produced in different leg muscle groups when rising from a chair. *Eur J Appl Physiol.* 1994;68:413–417.

17. Schroll M, Avlund K, Davidsen M. Predictors of five-year functional ability in a longitudinal survey of men and women aged 75 to 80. The 1914-population in Glostrup, Denmark. *Aging Clin Exp Res.* 1997;9:143–152.

18. Lipsitz LA, Nakajima I, Gagnon M, et al. Muscle strength and fall rates among residents of Japanese and American nursing homes: an international cross-cultural study. *J Am Geriatr Soc.* 1994;42:953–959.

19. Laukkanen P, Heikkinen E, Kauppinen M. Muscle strength and mobility as predictors of survival in 75–84-year-old people. *Age Ageing.* 1995;24:468–473.

20. Katzmarzyk PT, Craig CL. Musculoskeletal fitness and risk of mortality. *Med Sci Sports Exerc.* 2002;34:740–744.

21. Bean JF, Kiely DK, Herman S, et al. The relationship between leg power and physical performance in mobility-limited older people. *J Am Geriatr Soc.* 2002;50:461–467.

22. Brill PA, Macera CA, Davis DR, et al. Muscular strength and physical function. *Med Sci Sports Exerc.* 2000;32:412–416.

23. Knuttgen HG. Force, work, power, and exercise. *Med Sci Sports.* 1978;10:227–228.

24. Knuttgen HG. Quantifying exercise performance with SI units. *Physician Sports Med.* 1986;14:157–161.

25. Knuttgen HG, Kraemer WJ. Terminology and measurement in exercise performance. *J Strength Cond Res.* 1987;1:1–10.

26. Komi PV. Physiological and biomechanical correlates of muscle function: effects of muscle structure and stretch-shortening cycle on force and speed. *Exerc Sports Sci Rev.* 1984;12:81–121.

27. Svantesson U. *Eccentric-Concentric Plantar Flexion Muscle Action. Studies of Muscle Strength and Fatigue in Normal Subjects and in Patients After Stroke [thesis].* Sweden: Göteborg University; 1997.

28. Siff MC. Biomechanical foundations of strength and power training. In: Zatsiorsky V, ed. *Biomechanics in Sport.* Oxford, UK: Blackwell Science; 2000:103–139.

29. Macintyre J, Lloyd-Smith R. Overuse running injuries. In: Renstrom PAFH, ed. *Sports Injuries.* Oxford, UK: Blackwell Science; 1993:139–160.

30. Beynnon BD, Johnson RJ, Fleming BC, et al. The strain behavior of the anterior cruciate ligament during squatting and active flexion-extension. A comparison of an open and a closed kinetic chain exercise. *Am J Sports Med.* 1997;25:823–829.

31. Hooper DM, Morrissey MC, Drechsler W, et al. Open and closed kinetic chain exercises in the early period after anterior cruciate ligament reconstruction. Improvements in level walking, stair ascent, and stair descent. *Am J Sports Med.* 2001;29:167–174.

32. Kvist J, Gillquist J. Sagittal plane knee translation and electromyographic activity during closed and open kinetic chain exercises in anterior cruciate ligament-deficient patients and control subjects. *Am J Sports Med.* 2001;29:72–82.

33. Blei ML, Conley KE, Kushmerick MJ. Separate measures of ATP utilization and recovery in human skeletal muscle. *J Physiol.* 1993;465:203–222.

34. Walter G, Vandenborne K, McCully KK, et al. Noninvasive measurement of phosphocreatine recovery kinetics in single human muscles. *Am J Physiol Cell Physiol.* 1997;272:C525–C534.

35. Spriet LL. Anaerobic metabolism in human skeletal muscle during short-term, intense activity. *Can J Physiol Pharmacol.* 1992;70:157–165.

36. Bogdanis GC, Nevill ME, Boobis LH, et al. Contribution of phosphocreatine and aerobic metabolism to energy supply during repeated sprint exercise. *J Appl Physiol.* 1996;80:876–884.

37. Conley KE, Blei ML, Richards TL, et al. Activation of glycolysis in human muscle in vivo. *Am J Physiol Cell Physiol.* 1997;273:C306–C315.

38. Conley KE, Kushmerick MJ, Jubrias SA. Glycolysis is independent of oxygenation state in stimulated human skeletal muscle in vivo. *J Physiol.* 1998;511:935–945.

39. Bogdanis GC, Nevill ME, Lakomy HKA, et al. Power output and muscle metabolism during and following recovery from 10 and 20 s of maximal sprint exercise in humans. *Acta Physiol Scand.* 1998;163:261–272.

40. Romlin JA, Coyle EF, Sidossis LS, et al. Regulation of endogenous fat and carbohydrate metabolism in relation to exercise intensity and duration. *Am J Physiol Endocrinol Metab.* 1993;265:E380–E391.

41. Van Loon LJC, Greenhaff PL, Constantin-Teodosiu D, et al. The effects of increasing exercise intensity on muscle fuel utilisation in humans. *J Physiol.* 2001;536: 295–304.

42. Lieber RL. *Skeletal Muscle Structure and Function: Implications for Rehabilitation and Sports Medicine.* Baltimore, MD: Williams & Wilkins; 1992.

43. Kubo K, Kanehisa H, Takeshita D, et al. In vivo dynamics of human medial gastrocnemius muscle-tendon complex during stretch-shortening cycle exercise. *Acta Physiol Scand.* 2000;170:127–135.

44. Fukunaga T, Kubo K, Kawakami Y, et al. In vivo behavior of human muscle tendon during walking. *Proc Biol Sci.* 2001;268:229–233.

45. Kurokawa S, Fukunaga T, Fukashiro S. Behavior of fascicles and tendinous structures of human gastrocnemius during vertical jumping. *J Appl Physiol.* 2001;90:1349–1358.

46. Muraoka T, Kawakami Y, Tachi M, et al. Muscle fiber and tendon length changes in the human vastus lateralis during slow pedaling. *J Appl Physiol.* 2001;91:2035–2040.

47. McDougall JD, Wenger HA, Green HJ. *Physiological Testing of the High-Performance Athlete.* Champaign, IL: Human Kinetics; 1991.

48. Martin A, Carpenter A, Guissard N. Effect of time of day in force variation in a human muscle. *Muscle Nerve.* 1999;22:1380–1387.

49. Holmback AM, Porter MM, Downham D, et al. Reliability of isokinetic ankle dorsiflexor strength measurements in healthy young men and women. *Scand J Rehabil Med.* 1999;31:229–239.

50. Holmback AM, Porter MM, Downham D, et al. Ankle dorsiflexor muscle performance in healthy young men and women: reliability of eccentric peak torque and work measurements. *Scand J Rehabil Med.* 2000;32:1–7.

51. Jaric S. Muscle strength testing. Use of normalization for body size. *Sports Med.* 2002;32:615–631.

52. Frontera WR, Hughes VA, Dallal GE, et al. Reliability of isokinetic muscle strength testing in 45- to 78-year-old men and women. *Arch Phys Med Rehabil.* 1993;74:1181–1185.

53. Lexell J, Downham D. Analysis of reliability of measurements in rehabilitation research and clinical practice. *Am J Phys Med Rehabil.* 2005;84:719–723.

54. Medical Research Council. *Aids to the Investigation of Peripheral Nerve Injuries: War Memorandum No. 7.* Revised 2nd ed. London, UK: Her Majesty's Stationery Office; 1943.

55. McPeak LA. The psychiatric history and physical examination. In: Braddom RL, Buschbacher R, Dumitru D, et al., eds. *Physical Medicine and Rehabilitation.* Philadelphia, PA: WB Saunders; 1996:3–42.

56. Nicholas JA, Sapega A, Kraus H, et al. Factors influencing manual muscle tests in physical therapy. *J Bone Joint Surg.* 1978;60A:186–190.

57. Escobar DM, Henricson EK, Mayhew J, et al. Clinical evaluator reliability for quantitative and manual muscle testing measures of strength in children. *Muscle Nerve.* 2001;24:787–793.

58. Miller M, Downham D, Lexell J. Superimposed single impulse and pulse train electrical stimulation: a quantitative assessment during submaximal isometric knee extension in young, healthy men. *Muscle Nerve.* 1999;22:1038–1046.

59. Kilmer DD, McCrory MA, Wright NC, et al. Hand-held dynamometry reliability in persons with neuropathic weakness. *Arch Phys Med Rehabil.* 1997;78:1364–1368.

60. Beenakker EA, van der Hoeven JH, Fock JM, et al. Reference values of maximum isometric muscle force obtained in 270 children aged 4–16 years by hand-held dynamometry. *Neuromuscul Disord.* 2001;11:441–446.

61. Phillips BA, Lo SK, Mastaglia FL. Muscle force measured using break testing with a hand-held myometer in normal subjects aged 20 to 69 years. *Arch Phys Med Rehabil.* 2000;81:653–661.

62. Merton PA. Voluntary strength and fatigue. *J Physiol (Lond).* 1954;123:553–564.

63. Kent-Braun J, Le Blanc R. Quantitation of central activation failure during maximal voluntary contractions in humans. *Muscle Nerve.* 1996;19:861–869.

64. Miller M, Downham DY, Lexell J. Voluntary activation and central activation failure in the knee extensors of young and old individuals. *Am J Phys Med Rehabil.* 2006;85:945–950.

65. Miller M, Downham DY, Lexell J. Voluntary activation and central activation failure in the knee extensors of young men and women. *Scand J Med Sci Sports.* 2006;16:274–281.

66. DeLorme TL. Restoration of muscle power by heavy resistance exercise. *J Bone Joint Surg.* 1945;27:645–667.

67. Shaw CE, McCully KK, Posner JD. Injuries during the one repetition maximum assessment in the elderly. *J Cardiopulm Rehabil.* 1999;15:283–287.

68. Fleck SJ, Kraemer WJ. *Designing Resistance Training Programs.* 2nd ed. Champaign, IL: Human Kinetics; 1997.

69. Feiring DC, Ellenbecker TS, Derscheid GL. Test-retest reliability of the Biodex isokinetic dynamometer. *J Occup Sports Phys Ther.* 1990;11:298–300.

70. Kramer JF. Reliability of knee extensor and flexor torques during continuous concentric–eccentric cycles. *Arch Phys Med Rehabil.* 1990;71:460–464.

71. Snow CJ, Blacklin K. Reliability of knee flexor peak torque measurements from a standardized test protocol on a Kin/Com dynamometer. *Arch Phys Med Rehabil.* 1992;73:15–21.

72. Barr AE, Diamond BE, Wade CK, et al. Reliability of testing measures in Duchenne or Becker muscular dystrophy. *Arch Phys Med Rehabil.* 1991;72:315–319.

73. Flansbjer U-B, Holmbäck AM, Downham D, et al. What change in isokinetic knee muscle strength can be detected in men and women with hemiparesis after stroke? *Clin Rehabil.* 2005;19:514–522.

74. Kristensen OH, Stenager E, Dalgas U. Muscle strength and poststroke hemiplegia: a systematic review of muscle strength assessment and muscle strength impairment. *Arch Phys Med Rehabil.* 2017;98:368–380.

75. Kyritsis P, Bahr R, Landreau P, et al. Likelihood of ACL graft rupture: not meeting six clinical discharge criteria before return to sport is associated with a four times greater risk of rupture. *Br J Sports Med.* 2016;50:946–951.

76. Caiozzo VJ, Perrine JJ, Edgerton VR. Training-induced alterations of the in vivo force-velocity relationship of human muscle. *J Appl Physiol.* 1981;51:750–754.

77. Frontera WR, Meredith CN, O'Reilly KP, et al. Strength conditioning in older men: skeletal muscle hypertrophy and improved function. *J Appl Physiol.* 1988;64:1038–1044.

78. Harries UJ, Bassey EJ. Torque-velocity relationships for the knee extensors in women in their 3rd and 7th decades. *Eur J Appl Physiol.* 1990;60:187–190.

79. Bassey EJ, Fiatarone MA, O'Neill EF, et al. Leg extensor power and functional performance in very old men and women. *Clin Sci.* 1992;82:321–327.

80. Foldavari M, Clark M, Laviolette MJA, et al. Association of muscle power with functional status in community dwelling elderly women. *Med Sci Sports Exerc.* 1999;31:S378.

81. Metter EJ, Conwit R, Tobin J, et al. Age associated loss of power and strength in the upper extremities in men and women. *J Gerontol Biol Sci.* 1997;52A:B267–B276.

82. Bassey EJ, Short AH. A new method for measuring power output in a single leg extension: feasibility, reliability, and validity. *Eur J Appl Physiol.* 1990;60:385–390.

83. Bosco C, Luhtanen P, Komi PV. A simple method for measurement of mechanical power in jumping. *Eur J Appl Physiol.* 1983;50:273–282.

84. Komi PV, Nicol C. Stretch-shortening cycle of muscle function. In: Zatsiorsky V, ed. *Biomechanics in Sport*. Oxford, UK: Blackwell Science; 2000:87–102.

85. Edwards RHT. Human muscle function and fatigue: physiological mechanisms. In: *CIBA Foundation Symposium No. 82*. London, UK: Pitman Medical; 1981:1–18.

86. Bigland-Ritchie B, Woods JJ. Changes in muscle contractile properties and neural control during human muscular fatigue. *Muscle Nerve*. 1984;7:691–699.

87. James C, Sacco P, Jones DA. Loss of power during fatigue of human leg muscles. *J Physiol*. 1995;484:237–246.

88. Beelen A, Sargeant AJ, Jones DA, et al. Fatigue and recovery of voluntary and electrically elicited dynamic force in humans. *J Physiol*. 1995;484:227–235.

89. Akima H, Foley JM, Prior BM, et al. Vastus lateralis fatigue alters recruitment of musculus quadriceps femoris in humans. *J Appl Physiol*. 2002;92:679–684.

90. Nicol C, Komi PV, Marconnet P. Fatigue effects of marathon running on neuromuscular performance. I. Changes in muscle force and stiffness characteristics. *Scand J Med Sci Sports*. 1991;1:10–17.

91. Pedersen J, Lonn J, Hellström F, et al. Localized muscle fatigue decreases the acuity of the movement sense in the human shoulder. *Med Sci Sports Exerc*. 1999;31:1047–1052.

92. Allman BL, Rice CL. Neuromuscular fatigue and aging: central and peripheral factors. *Muscle Nerve*. 2002;25:785–796.

93. Fitts RH. Cellular mechanisms of muscle fatigue. *Physiol Rev*. 1994;74:49–94.

94. Allen DG, Lannergren J, Westerblad H. Muscle cell function during prolonged activity: cellular mechanisms of fatigue. *Exp Physiol*. 1995;80:497–527.

95. Sejersted OM, Bahr R, Hallen J, et al. Muscle performance—fatigue, recovery, and trainability. *Acta Physiol Scand*. 1998;162:181–182.

96. Stephenson DG, Lamb GD, Stephenson GMM. Events off the excitation-contraction-relaxation (E-C-R) cycle in fast- and slow-twitch mammalian muscle fibres relevant to muscle fatigue. *Acta Physiol Scand*. 1998;162:229–245.

97. Kent-Braun JA. Central and peripheral contributions to muscle fatigue in humans during sustained maximal effort. *Eur J Appl Physiol*. 1999;80:57–63.

98. Taylor JL, Butler JE, Allen GM, et al. Changes in motor cortex excitability during human muscle fatigue. *J Physiol*. 1996;490:519–528.

99. Gandevia SC, Allen GM, Butler JE, et al. Supraspinal factors in human muscle fatigue: evidence for suboptimal output from the motor cortex. *J Physiol*. 1996;490:529–536.

100. Sheean GL, Murray NMF, Rothwell JC, et al. An electrophysiological study of the mechanism of fatigue in multiple sclerosis. *Brain*. 1997;120:299–315.

101. Westerblad H, Allen DG, Bruton JD, et al. Mechanisms underlying the reduction of isometric tension in skeletal muscle fatigue. *Acta Physiol Scand*. 1998;162:253–260.

102. Westerblad H, Allen DG, Lannnergren J. Muscle fatigue: lactic acid or inorganic phosphate the major cause? *News Physiol Sci*. 2002;17:17–21.

103. Clausen T, Nielsen OB, Harrison AP, et al. The Na⁺, K⁺ pump and muscle excitability. *Acta Physiol Scand*. 1998;162:183–190.

104. Green HJ. Cation pumps in skeletal muscle: potential role in muscle fatigue. *Acta Physiol Scand*. 1998;162:201–213.

105. Sharma KR, Kent-Braun J, Mynhier MA, et al. Evidence of an abnormal intramuscular component of fatigue in multiple sclerosis. *Muscle Nerve*. 1995;18:1403–1411.

106. Sharma KR, Miller RG. Electrical and mechanical properties of skeletal muscle underlying increased fatigue in patients with amyotrophic lateral sclerosis. *Muscle Nerve*. 1996;19:1391–1400.

107. Wan J-J, Qin Z, Wang P-Y, et al. Muscle fatigue: general understanding and treatment. *Exp Mol Med*. 2017;49:e384.

108. Gleeson NP, Mercer TH. The utility of isokinetic dynamometry in the assessment of human muscle fatigue. *Sports Med*. 1996;21:18–34.

109. Pincivero DM, Lephart SM, Karunakara RG. Effects of intrasession rest interval on strength recovery and reliability during high intensity exercise. *J Strength Cond Res*. 1997;12:152–156.

110. Burdett RG, Van Swearingen J. Reliability of isokinetic muscle endurance tests. *J Orthop Sports Phys Ther*. 1987;8:484–488.

111. Porter MM, Holmback AM, Lexell J. Reliability of concentric ankle dorsiflexion fatigue testing. *Can J Appl Physiol*. 2002;27:116–127.

112. Robinson LR, Mustovic EH, Lieber PS, et al. A technique for quantifying and determining the site of isometric muscle fatigue in the clinical setting. *Arch Phys Med Rehabil*. 1990;71:901–904.

113. Gerdle B, Fugl-Meyer AR. Is the mean power frequency shift of the EMG a selective indicator of fatigue of the fast twitch motor units? *Acta Physiol Scand*. 1992;145:129–138.

114. Taylor AD, Bronks R, Smith P, et al. Myoelectric evidence of peripheral muscle fatigue during exercise in severe hypoxia: some references to m. vastus lateralis myosin heavy chain composition. *Eur J Appl Physiol*. 1997;75:151–159.

115. Merletti R, Roy S. Myoelectric and mechanical manifestations of muscle fatigue in voluntary contractions. *J Occup Sports Phys Ther*. 1996;24:342–353.

116. McCully KK, Vandenborne K, Demeirleir K, et al. Muscle metabolism in track athletes, using ³¹P magnetic resonance spectroscopy. *Can J Physiol Pharmacol*. 1992;70:1353–1359.

117. Irwin MS, Thorniley MS, Dore CJ, et al. Near infra-red spectroscopy: a noninvasive monitor of perfusion and oxygenation within the microcirculation of limbs and flaps. *Br J Plast Surg*. 1995;48:14–22.

118. Boushel R, Langberg H, Olesen J, et al. Monitoring tissue oxygen availability with near infra-red spectroscopy (NIRS) in health and disease. *Scand J Med Sci Sports*. 2001;11:213–222.

119. Henriksson J. Microdialysis of skeletal muscle at rest. *Proc Nutr Soc*. 1999;58:919–923.

120. Weibel E. *The Pathway for Oxygen. Structure and Function in the Mammalian Respiratory System*. Cambridge, MA: Harvard University Press; 1984.

121. Russell B, Motlagh D, Ashley WW. Form follows function: how muscle shape is regulated by work. *J Appl Physiol*. 2000;88:1127–1132.

122. Fukunaga T, Ichinose Y, Ito M, et al. Determination of fascicle length and pennation in a contracting human muscle in vivo. *J Appl Physiol*. 1997;82:354–358.

123. Kumagai K, Abe T, Brechue WF, et al. Sprint performance is related to muscle fascicle length in male 100-m sprinters. *J Appl Physiol*. 2000;88:811–816.

124. Tosato M, Marzetti E, Cesari M, et al. Measurement of muscle mass in sarcopenia: from imaging to biochemical markers. *Aging Clin Exp Res*. 2017;29:19-27.

125. Wang ZM, Pierson RN Jr, Heymsfield SB. The five-level model: a new approach to organizing body-composition research. *Am J Clin Nutr*. 1992;56:19–28.

126. McArdle WD, Katch FI, Katch VI. *Exercise Physiology: Energy, Nutrition, and Human Performance*. 4th ed. Baltimore, MD: Williams & Wilkins; 1996:316.

127. Visser M, Gallagher D, Deurenberg P, et al. Density of fat-free body mass: relationship with race, age, and level of body fatness. *Am J Physiol Endocrinol Metab*. 1997;272:E781–E787.

128. Siri WE. Gross composition of the body. In: Lawrence JH, Tobias CA, eds. *Advances in Biological and Medical Physics*. Vol. 4. New York: Academic Press; 1956.

129. Cohn SH, Vartsky D, Yasumura S. Compartmental body composition based on total-body nitrogen, potassium, and calcium. *Am J Physiol*. 1980;239:E524–E530.

130. Nelson ME, Fiatarone MA, Layne JE, et al. Analysis of body-composition techniques and models for detecting change in soft tissue with strength training. *Am J Clin Nutr*. 1996;63:678–686.

131. Wang W, Wang Z, Faith M, et al. Regional skeletal muscle measurement: evaluation of new dual-energy X-ray absorptiometry model. *J Appl Physiol*. 1999;87:1163–1171.

132. Shih R, Wang Z, Heo M, et al. Lower limb skeletal muscle mass: development of a dual-energy X-ray absorptiometry prediction model. *J Appl Physiol*. 2000;89:1380–1386.

133. Sipila S, Suominen H. Muscle ultrasonography and computed tomography in elderly trained and untrained women. *Muscle Nerve*. 1993;16:294–300.

134. Kanehisa H, Ikegawa S, Fukunaga T. Comparison of muscle cross-sectional area and strength between untrained women and men. *Eur J Appl Physiol*. 1994;68:148–154.

135. Mitsiopoulos N, Baumgartner RN, Heymsfield SB, et al. Cadaver validation of skeletal muscle measurement by magnetic resonance imaging and computerized tomography. *J Appl Physiol*. 1998;85:115–122.

136. Fukunaga T, Roy RR, Shellock FG, et al. Physiological cross-sectional area of human leg muscles based on magnetic resonance imaging. *J Orthop Res*. 1992;10:926–934.

137. Berquist TH. *MRI of the Musculoskeletal System*. Philadelphia, PA: Lippincott-Raven; 1996.

138. Fukunaga T, Kawakami Y, Kubo K, et al. Muscle and tendon interaction during human movements. *Exerc Sport Sci Rev*. 2002;30:106–110.

139. Muramatsu T, Muraoka M, Takeshita D, et al. Mechanical properties of tendon and aponeurosis of human gastrocnemius muscle in vivo. *J Appl Physiol*. 2001;90:1671–1678.

140. Phoenix J, Betal D, Roberts N, et al. Objective quantification of muscle and fat in human dystrophic muscle by magnetic resonance image analysis. *Muscle Nerve*. 1996;19:302–310.

141. Challis JH. Muscle-tendon architecture and athletic performance. In: Zatsiorsky V, ed. *Biomechanics in Sport*. Oxford, UK: Blackwell Science; 2000:33–55.

142. Narici MV, Landoni L, Minetti AE. Assessment of human knee extensor muscle stress from in vivo physiological cross-sectional area and strength measurements. *Eur J Appl Physiol*. 1992;65:438–444.

143. Fukunaga T, Roy RR, Shellock FG, et al. Specific tension of human plantar flexors and dorsiflexors. *J Appl Physiol*. 1996;80:158–165.

144. Engstrom CM, Loeb GE, Reid JG, et al. Morphometry of the human thigh muscles. A comparison between anatomical sections and computed tomographic and magnetic resonance images. *J Physiol*. 1991;176:139–156.

145. Holmbäck AM, Askaner K, Holtas S, et al. Assessment of contractile and non-contractile components in human skeletal muscle by magnetic resonance imaging. *Muscle Nerve*. 2002;25:251–258.

146. Goodpaster BH, Kelley DE, Thaete FL, et al. Skeletal muscle attenuation determined by computed tomography is associated with skeletal muscle lipid content. *J Appl Physiol*. 2000;89:104–110.

147. Rozenberg D, Martelli V, Vieira L, et al. Utilization of non-invasive imaging tools for assessment of peripheral skeletal muscle size and composition in chronic lung disease: a systematic review. *Respir Med*. 2017;131:125–134.

148. Meyer RA, Prior BM. Functional magnetic resonance imaging of muscle. *Exerc Sport Sci Rev*. 2000;28:89–92.

149. Ogino M, Shiba N, Maeda T, et al. MRI quantification of muscle activity after volitional exercise and neuromuscular electrical stimulation. *Am J Phys Med Rehabil*. 2002;81:446–451.

150. Takeda Y, Kashiwaguchi S, Endo K, et al. The most effective exercise for strengthening the supraspinatus muscle: evaluation by magnetic resonance imaging. *Am J Sports Med*. 2002;30:374–381.

151. Maganaris CN, Baltzopoulos V, Ball D, et al. In vivo specific tension of human skeletal muscle. *J Appl Physiol*. 2001;90:865–872.

152. Klein CS, Rice CL, Marsh GD. Normalized force activation, and coactivation in the arm muscles of young and old men. *J Appl Physiol*. 2001;91:1341–1349.

153. Bamman MM, Newcomer BR, Larson-Meyer DE, et al. Evaluation of the strength–size relationship *in vivo* using various muscle size indices. *Med Sci Sports Exerc*. 2000;32:1307–1313.

154. Dowling JJ, Cardone N. Relative cross-sectional areas of upper and lower extremity muscles and implications for force prediction. *Int J Sports Med.* 1994;15:453–459.

155. Bruce SA, Phillips SK, Woledge RC. Interpreting the relationship between force and cross-sectional area in human muscle. *Med Sci Sports Exerc.* 1997;29:677–683.

156. Frontera WR, Suh D, Krivickas L, et al. Skeletal muscle fiber quality in older men and women. *Am J Physiol Cell Physiol.* 2000;279:C611–C618.

157. Krivickas LS, Dorer DJ, Ochala J, et al. Relationship between force and size in human single muscle fibres. *Exp Physiol.* 2011;96:539–547.

158. Duchenne GB. Recherches sur la paralysie musculaire pseudohypertrophique ou paralysie myo-sclérosique. I. Symptomatologie. Marche, durée, terminaison. *Arch Gen Med.* 1868;11:179.

159. Bergstrom J. Muscle electrolytes in man. *Scand J Clin Lab Med.* 1962;14:511–513.

160. Edwards RHT. Percutaneous needle-biopsy of skeletal muscle in diagnosis and research. *Lancet.* 1971;2:593–595.

161. Evans WJ, Phinney SD, Young VR. Suction applied to a muscle biopsy maximizes sample size. *Med Sci Sports Exerc.* 1982;14:101–102.

162. Dietrichson P, Coakley J, Smith PEM. Conchotome and needle percutaneous biopsy of skeletal muscle. *J Neurol Neurosurg Psychiatry.* 1987;50:1461–1467.

163. Hennesey JV, Chromiak JA, Dellaventura S, et al. Increase in percutaneous muscle biopsy yield with a suction-enhancement technique. *J Appl Physiol.* 1997;82:1739–1742.

164. Mubarak SJ, Chambers HG, Wenger DR. Percutaneous muscle biopsy in the diagnosis of neuromuscular disease. *J Pediatr Orthop.* 1992;12:191–196.

165. Magistris MR, Kohler A, Pizzolato G. Needle muscle biopsy in the investigation of neuromuscular disorders. *Muscle Nerve.* 1998;21:194–200.

166. Edwards RHT, Round JM, Jones DA. Needle biopsy of skeletal muscle: a review of 10 years experience. *Muscle Nerve.* 1983;6:676–683.

167. Staron RS, Hikida RS, Murray TF. Assessment of skeletal muscle damage in successive biopsies from strength-trained and untrained men and women. *Eur J Appl Physiol.* 1992;65:258–264.

168. Viru A. Contemporary state and further perspectives on using muscle biopsies for metabolism studies in sportsmen. *Med Sport (Roma).* 1994;47:371–376.

169. Jansson E. Methodology and actual perspectives of the evaluation of muscular enzymes in skeletal muscle by biopsy during rest, exercise, and detraining. *Med Sport (Roma).* 1994;47:377–383.

170. Coggan A. Muscle biopsy as a tool in the study of aging. *J Gerontol.* 1995;50A(special issue):30–34.

171. Henriksson KG. "Semi-open" muscle biopsy technique. A simple outpatient procedure. *Acta Neurol Scand.* 1979;59:317–323.

172. Heckmatt JZ, Dubowitz V. Diagnostic advantage of needle muscle biopsy and ultrasound imaging in the detection of focal pathology in a girl with limb girdle dystrophy. *Muscle Nerve.* 1985;8:705–709.

173. Shalabi A, Eriksson K, Jansson E, et al. Ultrasound-guided percutaneous biopsies of the semitendinosus muscle following ACL reconstruction—a methodological description. *Int J Sports Med.* 2002;23:202–206.

174. Nurenberg P, Giddings CJ, Stray-Gundersen J, et al. MR imaging-guided muscle biopsy for correlation of increased signal intensity with ultrastructural change and delayed-onset muscle soreness after exercise. *Radiology.* 1992;184:865–869.

175. Lexell J, Taylor C, Sjostrom M. Analysis of sampling errors in biopsy techniques using data from whole muscle cross sections. *J Appl Physiol.* 1985;59:1228–1236.

176. Blomstrand E, Celsing F, Friden J, et al. How to calculate human muscle fibre areas in biopsy samples-methodological considerations. *Acta Physiol Scand.* 1984;122:545–551.

177. McCall GE, Byrnes WC, Dickinson AL, et al. Sample size required for the accurate determination of fiber area and capillarity of human skeletal muscle. *Can J Appl Physiol.* 1998;23:594–599.

178. Porter MM, Coolage CW, Lexell J. Biopsy sampling requirements for the estimation of muscle capillarization. *Muscle Nerve.* 2002;26:546–548.

179. Lexell J, Taylor CC. Variability in muscle fibre areas in whole human quadriceps muscle: how to reduce sampling errors in biopsy techniques. *Clin Physiol.* 1989;9:333–342.

180. Greising SM, Gransee HM, Mantilla CB, et al. Systems biology of skeletal muscle: fiber type as an organizing principle. *Wiley Interdiscip Rev Syst Biol Med.* 2012;4:457–473.

181. Dubowitz V, Brooke MH. *Muscle Biopsy: A Modern Approach.* Philadelphia, PA: WB Saunders; 1973.

182. Brumback RA, Leech RW. *Color Atlas of Muscle Histochemistry.* Littleton, MA: PSG Publishing; 1984.

183. Lexell J. Muscle capillarization: morphological and morphometrical analysis of biopsy samples. *Muscle Nerve.* 1997;5(suppl):S110–S112.

184. Henriksson J, Hickner RC. Training-induced adaptations in skeletal muscle. In: Harries M, Williams C, Stanish WD, et al., eds. *Oxford Textbook of Sports Medicine.* Oxford, UK: Oxford University Press; 1994:27–45.

185. Brooke MH, Kaiser KK. Muscle fibre types: how many and what kind? *Arch Neurol.* 1970;23:369–379.

186. Staron RS, Johnson P. Myosin polymorphism and differential expression in adult human skeletal muscle. *Comp Biochem Physiol B.* 1993;106:463–475.

187. Staron RS. Human skeletal muscle fiber types: delineation, development, and distribution. *Can J Appl Physiol.* 1997;22:307–327.

188. Perrie WT, Bumford SJ. Electrophoretic separation of myosin isoenzymes. Implications for the histochemical demonstration of fibre types in biopsy specimens of human skeletal muscles. *J Neurol Sci.* 1986;73:89–96.

189. Adams GR, Hather BM, Baldwin KM, et al. Skeletal muscle myosin heavy chain composition and resistance training. *J Appl Physiol.* 1993;74:911–915.

190. Staron RS. Correlation between myofibrillar ATPase activity and myosin heavy chain composition in single human muscle fibers. *Histochemistry.* 1991;96:21–24.

191. Staron RS, Hikida RS. Histochemical, biochemical, and ultrastructural analyses of single human muscle fibers, with special reference to the C-fiber population. *J Histochem Cytochem.* 1992;40:563–568.

192. Ennion S, Santana Pereira JAA, Sargeant AJ, et al. Characterization of human skeletal muscle fibres according to the myosin heavy chain they express. *J Muscle Res Cell Motil.* 1995;16:35–43.

193. Smerdu V, Karsch-Mizrachi I, Campione M, et al. Type IIx myosin heavy chain transcripts are expressed in type IIb fibers of human skeletal muscle. *Am J Physiol.* 1994;267:C1723–C1728.

194. Fry AC, Allemeir CA, Staron RS. Correlation between percentage fibre type area and myosin heavy chain content in human skeletal muscle. *Eur J Appl Physiol.* 1994;68:246–251.

195. Larsson L, Salviati G. A technique for studies of the contractile apparatus in single human muscle fibre segments obtained by percutaneous biopsy. *Acta Physiol Scand.* 1992;146:485–495.

196. Larsson L, Moss RL. Maximum velocity of shortening in relation to myosin isoform composition in single fibres from human skeletal muscles. *J Physiol.* 1993;472:595–614.

197. Krivickas L, Suh D, Wilkins J, et al. Age- and gender-related differences in maximum shortening velocity of skeletal muscle fibers. *Am J Physical Med Rehabil.* 2001;80:447–455.

198. Guralnik JM, Simonsick EM, Ferucci L, et al. A short physical performance battery assessing lower extremity function: association with self-reported disability and prediction of mortality and nursing home admission. *J Gerontol Med Sci.* 1994;49:M85–M94.

199. Guralnik JM, Ferruci L, Simonsick EM, et al. Lower extremity function in persons over the age of 70 years as a predictor of subsequent disability. *N Engl J Med.* 1995;332:556–561.

200. Margaria R, Aghemo P, Rovelli E. Measurement of muscular power (anaerobic) in man. *J Appl Physiol.* 1966;21:1662–1664.

201. Gibbs J, Hughes S, Dunlop J. Predictors of change in walking velocity in older adults. *J Am Geriatr Soc.* 1996;44:126–132.

202. Kwon IS, Oldaker S, Schrager M, et al. Relationship between muscle strength and the time taken to complete a standardized walk-turn-walk test. *J Gerontol Biol Sci.* 2001;56A:B398–B404.

203. Rantanen T, Avela J. Leg extension power and walking speed in very old people living independently. *J Gerontol Med Sci.* 1997;52A:M225–M231.

204. Flansbjer U-B, Downham D, Lexell J. Knee muscle strength, gait performance and participation after stroke. *Arch Phys Med Rehabil.* 2006;87:974–980.

205. Flansbjer U-B, Holmbäck AM, Downham D, et al. Reliability of gait performance tests in men and women with hemiparesis after stroke. *J Rehabil Med.* 2005;37:75–82.

206. Harada N, Chiu V, Stewart AL. Mobility-related function in older adults: assessment with a 6-minute walk test. *Arch Phys Med Rehabil.* 1999;80:837–841.

207. Cahalin LP, Mathier MA, Semigram MJ, et al. The six-minute walk test predicts peak oxygen uptake and survival in patients with advanced heart failure. *Chest.* 1996;110:325–332.

208. Bean JF, Kiely DK, Leveille SG, et al. The six-minute walk test in mobility limited elders: what is being measured? *J Gerontol Biol Sci.* 2002;57:M751–M756.

209. Lord SR, Menz HB. Physiologic, psychologic, and health predictors of 6-minute walk performance in older people. *Arch Phys Med Rehabil.* 2002;83:907–911.

210. Lexell J. Muscle structure and function in chronic neurological disorders. The potential of exercise to improve activities of daily living. *Exerc Sports Sci Rev.* 2000;28:80–84.

Electrodiagnostic Evaluation of the Peripheral Nervous System

The ability to perform high-quality electrodiagnostic studies is a critical skill for the practicing physiatrist. Electrodiagnosis is an important extension of the physical examination as it can detect minor abnormalities when physical examination cannot. Moreover, the electrodiagnostic examination can:

- Localize the site of nerve impairment
- Provide insight into the pathophysiology of a nerve lesion
- Quantify the degree of axon loss
- Estimate prognosis for recovery
- Quantitatively track disease processes over time

PREPARING FOR THE ELECTRODIAGNOSTIC EXAMINATION

There are several key steps to prepare for the electrodiagnostic examination, including review of referral materials, eliciting the patient's history, performing a directed physical examination, developing a differential diagnosis, and putting together a plan for the electrodiagnostic evaluation.

Review of referral materials: The electrodiagnostic consultant should start by reviewing the question from the referring physician so that one knows what is being asked for. Without reviewing this information first, it is easy to be misled into another diagnostic pathway and never answer the referring physician's question. If there is any uncertainty about what is being asked, or if the question does not seem to make sense, it is often helpful to talk to the referring physician. If it is not possible to address the question being asked, one should have that discussion with the referring physician before starting the electrodiagnostic study.

Patient history: A focused patient history allows one to establish a differential diagnosis before performing the physical examination and then the electrodiagnostic evaluation. The history should start off with the chief complaint, but should also include exacerbating or relieving factors and past medical history. It is often useful to ask what medications the patient is taking so that one is not later surprised by a risk factor polyneuropathy (e.g., diabetes), for example. Parts of the past medical history may be especially contributory to the differential diagnosis such as diabetes, history of cancer, or toxic exposures. When one starts to consider diseases that may be hereditary, it is always wise to ask about any family history of neuromuscular problems.

Physical examination: The examination needs to be focused and adapted to the individual presentation of the patient. Typically, it is useful to assess muscle strength not only in the involved body part but in bilateral upper and lower limbs. One should get a good sense of the distribution of sensory loss. Two techniques are particularly helpful in this regard. First, in mild sensory loss, it is often helpful to compare with an area of intact sensation and ask, "If this is 100 (testing intact area), how much is this (testing abnormal area)?" Generally, losses of small percentages are not meaningful. Second, if an area of abnormal or absent sensation is clearly established, it is useful to map this out, putting small pen marks where sensation changes from abnormal to intact.

Muscle stretch reflexes are one of the few objective indicators of nerve or muscle disease. Hyperreflexia usually suggests an upper motor neuron etiology, while diminished reflexes or areflexia is more consistent with a peripheral nerve or lower motor neuron (LMN) process.

Provocative signs can be somewhat helpful but have limited diagnostic accuracy. One may consider Spurling's sign for cervical radiculopathy, straight leg raise sign for lumbar radiculopathy, Tinel's, Phalen's, or flick sign for carpal tunnel syndrome (CTS), and other maneuvers. Generally, these provocative signs have a limited specificity (1).

After completing the clinical assessment above, one should establish and write down a differential diagnosis. One can consider the differential diagnosis starting from most likely to least likely or starting centrally in the nervous system and work peripherally so that important possibilities are not overlooked. It is generally wise to include the diagnosis the referring physician has suggested on your list, since you want to be able to answer his or her question in your final report.

One should then establish a plan for diagnostic testing based upon the differential diagnoses and what elements of electrodiagnostic study are needed to assess for those possible diagnoses. One may elect to modify this plan as initial information is attained, and in fact, this is often an iterative process. However, without going through the rigor of developing (and writing down) a plan based on the differential diagnosis, one will miss important findings (**Fig. 3-1**).

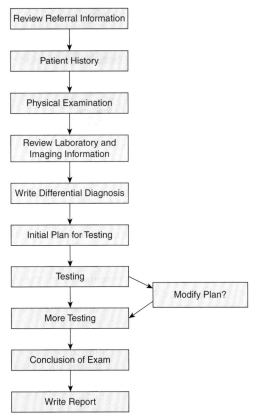

FIGURE 3-1. The process used for electrodiagnostic evaluation.

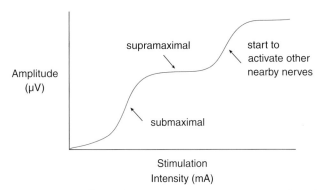

FIGURE 3-2. Amplitude of a motor or sensory response as currently used for stimulation is increased. Note the plateau at supramaximal stimulation. Increasing past this point will eventually activate other nearby nerves and the amplitude can go up again as a result.

TYPES OF ELECTRODIAGNOSTIC TESTING

This chapter will cover frequently used electrodiagnostic techniques including nerve action potentials (sensory and mixed), motor nerve conduction studies, late responses (F waves, H waves, and A waves), needle electromyography (EMG), and repetitive stimulation.

Sensory Nerve Action Potentials and Compound Nerve Action Potentials

Sensory nerve action potentials (SNAPs) and compound nerve action potentials (CNAPs) both involve electrical stimulation of nerves and recording of the synchronized discharge of axons within the nerve at some distance from the point of stimulation. SNAPs are responses that only involve sensory axons, whereas CNAPs may involve sensory axons, motor axons, or a mixture of both.

To standardize stimulation levels, the nerve is stimulated supramaximally, meaning that all the axons are electrically activated. In practice, this means that stimulator intensity (in milliamperes or mA) is gradually increased while monitoring the size of the nerve response. When the response from the nerve gets no larger as the intensity continues to increase, this indicates that all the available axons have been activated and further increases in stimulation will activate no more axons. Increasing the stimulator substantially above this level will sometimes activate other nearby nerves, and responses from these other nerves can be recorded from the same recording electrodes (**Fig. 3-2**) through volume conduction; this is to be avoided.

One records from the same nerve at a specified or measured distance away from the stimulation and records the synchronized discharge of all the axons that have been activated (**Fig. 3-3**).

Several items are then measured from the nerve action potential. Most commonly, these include the latency and amplitude of the response. The latency is measured from the time of stimulation to the onset or the peak of the response. The advantage of measuring to the onset is that this represents the fastest conducted fibers. The advantage of measuring latency to the peak is that the peak is more reliably determined

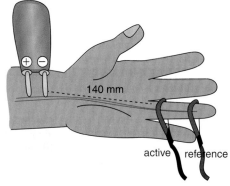

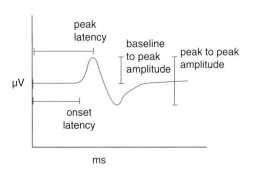

FIGURE 3-3. Sensory nerve action potential (SNAP) recorded from digital nerves. Latency reflects the speed of conduction and amplitude is a measure of the number of functioning sensory axons. Conduction velocity can be calculated by dividing the distance by the onset latency.

and less influenced by the sensitivity of the display or the amplifier. In either case, one should have reference (normal) data, which have been derived using the same technique. The amplitude or size of the response can be measured from baseline to peak or from peak to peak, again depending upon how the reference data were collected. Conduction velocity is in units of distance over time, in this case meters per second (m/s), which is the same as millimeters per millisecond (mm/ms). In the case of nerve action potentials, one can measure the distance between stimulation and recording and divide that by onset latency to obtain the velocity in m/s.

The latency can be prolonged and velocity slowed by a number of both physiologic and pathologic processes:

- *Cold* prolongs latency, by about 0.2 ms/°C. Slowing of nerve conduction velocity (NCV) is generally in the range of about 5%/°C.
- *Age* influences latency and conduction velocity. Initially, children are born with conduction velocities about half of that of adults. As their nerves become better myelinated, these values approach adult values around age 3. Later, in the fifth and sixth decades, velocities start to slow again but not to the degree of that seen in infancy. For this reason, reference values are often adjusted for age.
- *Loss of myelin* will cause slowing of conduction velocity and increase in latencies. When demyelination becomes severe enough, however, conduction block will occur.

The amplitude of the response is affected by several factors.

- *Cold* tends to increase the amplitude of the response if the recording electrodes are over a cold area of the limb. Cold slows the opening and, to a greater extent, the closing of sodium channels. As a result, more charge is exchanged across the axon plasma membrane and a greater size axon potential is elicited.
- Amplitude is also dependent upon the *distance of the electrodes from the generator source*. The electrical potential amplitude falls off rapidly with distance as one moves further from the nerve. Thus, nerve conduction studies in which the generator is close to the skin (such as recording from the fingers) usually generate a bigger amplitude response than when one is recording from proximal areas of the limb (where the nerves are located deeper).
- If one *loses axons*, the amplitude falls roughly in proportion to the degree of axon loss. A reduction in amplitude can result from axon loss occurring between the stimulating and recording electrodes, in which case changes in the potentials would be seen immediately. However, SNAP amplitudes will also be reduced if sensory axons are affected anywhere from their cell bodies (which are located in the dorsal root ganglion or DRG) distally. In such cases, the axons undergo degeneration, and by 10 days after a proximal loss of sensory neurons or axons, the distal response will disappear due to axonal degeneration. If lesions are proximal to the DRG (i.e., most radiculopathies), then the distal axons will remain connected to their cell bodies in the DRG and will conduct normally, even if the patient has complete anesthesia in the relevant area.

Sensory nerve conduction studies can be most useful in diagnosis of nerve injuries that are distal to the DRG, including plexopathies, entrapment neuropathies, and polyneuropathies.

Sensory nerve conduction studies should usually be normal in the setting of radiculopathies (when injury is typically proximal to the DRG), central nervous system disorders, neuromuscular junction (NMJ) diseases, and myopathies (the latter two because recordings are obtained from nerve, and not muscle).

There are several potential limitations in utilizing SNAP or CNAP studies. First, these can be technically challenging to obtain when responses are small, such as in people with polyneuropathies, people with thick or calloused skin, or older individuals. It can be challenging as well in unusual nerves that are not commonly studied. Hence, in less frequently studied nerves, one should interpret the absence of a response with caution and consider studying the contralateral limb as well as other sensory nerves. Electronic averaging of responses can be useful to elicit small-amplitude responses that would otherwise be unnoticeable in the baseline electronic noise.

As mentioned above, temperature will have significant impact on sensory nerve conduction studies. One should consider that the limb might be cold if latencies are prolonged but amplitudes are large. In contrast, in disease states, latencies would be prolonged but amplitudes would usually be small. If one is unsure about whether temperature is having an influential effect, it is best to warm the limb. This author puts the limb into a plastic bag and then submerges it in a bucket or sink filled with warm water for 5 minutes. There are many other techniques, including warm air (e.g., from a hair dryer), infrared lamps, and other methods.

Compound Muscle Action Potentials and Motor Nerve Conduction Studies

Compound muscle action potentials (CMAPs) involve electrical stimulation of nerves and recording of the synchronized discharge of muscle fibers in the muscle supplied by the stimulated nerve.

As above for sensory nerves, the nerve is stimulated supramaximally. But, as opposed to the SNAP or CNAP, one now records not from axons but from muscle fibers at a specified or measured distance away from the stimulation and records the synchronized discharge of all the muscle fibers that have been activated (**Fig. 3-4**).

As with SNAPs, several measurements are taken from the CMAP. The amplitude or size of the response is usually measured from baseline to peak. The latency is measured to the onset of the response. Conduction velocity is more complicated to calculate than for SNAPs. Because the latency includes not only conduction time along the nerve but also time for NMJ transmission (about 1 ms), one cannot simply divide the distance between stimulation and recording by the distal latency. Instead, we stimulate at two points along the nerve and take the difference in distance divided by the difference in latency to derive a conduction velocity (see **Fig. 3-4**).

Latency can be affected by the same factors as for SNAPs: cold, age, and loss of myelin. Because we are recording from muscle instead of nerve, CMAP amplitude is dependent upon different factors than SNAPs. These include

- Number of motor axons
- Integrity of the NMJ
- Number of muscle fibers

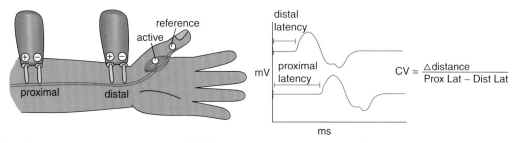

FIGURE 3-4. Compound muscle action potential (CMAP) recorded from a thenar muscle. Stimulation at the wrist and elbow is demonstrated. Nerve conduction velocity (NCV) cannot be calculated from one point of stimulation, as the latency reflects not only nerve conduction time but also neuromuscular transmission time and muscle fiber conduction time. Consequently, NCV is calculated from two points of stimulation, by dividing the distance between the two points by the latency difference.

The CMAP will fall roughly in proportion to the degree of motor axon loss (or, in the case of myopathies, muscle fiber loss). As opposed to the SNAP (where lesions anywhere from the DRG distally cause an amplitude reduction), a reduction in CMAP amplitude can result from lesions from the anterior horn cell (the motor neuron cell body) distally. By 7 days after a proximal loss of motor cell bodies or axons, the distal response will disappear due to axonal degeneration; this occurs earlier than for the SNAP due to earlier failure of the NMJ (2).

Conduction block is the observation that stimulation of nerves proximally produces a significantly smaller response than distal stimulation does. This can be seen in CMAPs when there is demyelination. In this case, the axons are excitable and intact distally and so produce a normal response when stimulation is distal to the injury site. However, when demyelination is severe enough, proximal stimulation does propagate across the injury site, and a smaller or absent response is seen. One can usually "inch" along the nerve and find a focal site of block. Pure axonal injuries will not typically produce conduction block; in those cases, the injured axons undergo wallerian degeneration distally and are excitable neither above nor below the site of pathology.

Temporal dispersion results from the asynchronous arrival of impulses at the recording electrode. One will typically observe a prolonged duration CMAP and/or a more complex waveform with multiple turns or phases. This usually results from patchy demyelination that affects some fibers more than others and is only seen in acquired (not hereditary) demyelination. In these cases, the demyelination causes slowing but is not severe enough to cause conduction block.

Motor nerve conduction studies can be most useful in diagnosis of lesions that affect the LMN or surrounding myelin. This includes significant spinal root lesions, plexopathies, entrapment neuropathies, and polyneuropathies.

Late Responses

While the typical motor and sensory conduction studies mentioned above rely on conduction proceeding distally in the limbs, there are several responses, known as late responses, that depend upon conduction proceeding proximally in the peripheral nervous system, and thus these occur with longer latency.

The F wave was so named because it was originally discovered in the foot (3). Physiologically, F waves depend upon conduction proximally to the motor neuron cell body. Since axons conduct in both directions, when motor axons are activated distally in the limb, they conduct both proximally and distally.

For most axons, the impulse travels proximally, past the axon hillock, into the motor neuron and ends. But for a small number (about 3% to 5%), the depolarization traverses through the dendritic tree and comes back through the axon hillock after it is no longer refractory (about 1 ms). As a result, a small late response will be recorded from the muscle after enough time for a round trip from the stimulus site, back to the spinal cord, and then back to muscle (**Fig. 3-5**). The reference (normal) values in humans are about 32 ms in the upper limbs and 55 ms in the lower limbs (4).

The technique is similar to motor conduction studies but has several important differences (5). The sweep speed needs to be slow enough to capture the F waves (50 ms in the upper limb and 100 ms in the lower limb). Since F waves are smaller than CMAPs, sensitivity needs to be sufficient to observe these responses (200 to 500 μV/div); most EMG instruments have split screens with the first part of the sweep (e.g., first 20 ms) at 2 to 5 mV/div to observe the CMAP and the latter part of the sweep at 200 to 500 μV/div. Conventional teaching is that the cathode should be placed proximally along the nerve with the anode distally to avoid proximal anodal block, but this probably makes little or no difference (6) as long as the cathode is placed at the same location. Conventional teaching is also that the stimulation should be supramaximal, but latencies are similar even with submaximal stimulation (7).

Since F waves are typically derived from different populations of motor neurons for each response, the latency and appearance vary with each stimulation. Thus, measuring latency is more complicated than for a CMAP or SNAP, where the latency is the same with each stimulation. Because of this variability, one must acquire multiple F waves (typically 10 to 20) and take measurements that account for this inherent variability. Most commonly, one obtains either the minimal latency (the shortest latency of multiple responses) or the mean latency (the average latency). The minimal latency is easiest to measure and is most commonly used. However, the minimal latency will depend upon the number of responses obtained. As more responses are recorded, the chances of finding a shorter latency response increase and the minimal latency will drop. The mean latency, on the other hand, is more time-consuming to measure since one must mark all the F-wave responses obtained. But mean values are less dependent upon sample size and the measure will be more stable, making it a more reliable parameter.

There are other latency measures that are also sometimes used. Maximal latency reflects the speed of conduction of the slower motor axons. Chronodispersion is measured as the

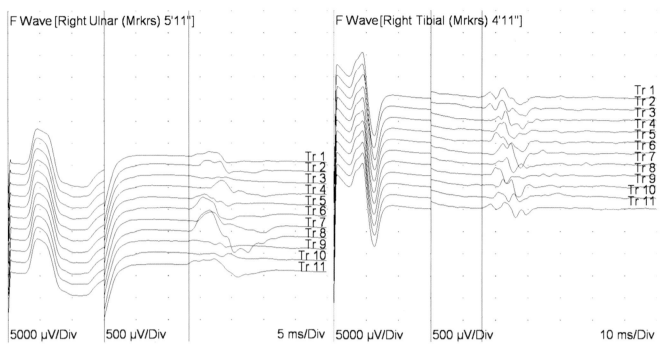

F Wave [Right Ulnar (Mrkrs) 5'11"]

F Wave [Right Tibial (Mrkrs) 4'11"]

Tr 1
Tr 2
Tr 3
Tr 4
Tr 5
Tr 6
Tr 7
Tr 8
Tr 9
Tr 10
Tr 11

Tr 1
Tr 2
Tr 3
Tr 4
Tr 5
Tr 6
Tr 7
Tr 8
Tr 9
Tr 10
Tr 11

5000 µV/Div 500 µV/Div 5 ms/Div 5000 µV/Div 500 µV/Div 10 ms/Div

FIGURE 3-5. Ulnar **(left)** and tibial **(right)** F waves. Note the variability in waveforms with each stimulation.

difference between the shortest and longest F-wave latencies. Greater chronodispersion may indicate selective slowing of some motor axons more than others and can be expected in acquired demyelinating neuropathies (3).

Not every motor nerve stimulation results in an F wave. Persistence or penetrance is measured as the percentage of stimulations that produce an F wave. Persistence is altered by many factors (including activity level), and generally low persistence is not considered a diagnostic finding (8). Absence of F waves, however, is considered abnormal in tibial or median nerves, but may be of uncertain significance in other nerves.

Amplitude of the F wave can be measured, usually as a percentage of the corresponding CMAP. This, however, is also variable and is usually not typically used as a diagnostic finding.

As above, there are many measures one can obtain from F waves. A problem is that each measure has a false-positive rate, which, if the reference (normal) values were analyzed optimally, is about 2.5%. As one performs more comparisons with reference (normal) data, each comparison roughly adds 2.5% to the false-positive rate. Thus, if one were to analyze minimal latency, mean latency, chronodispersion (the difference between shortest and longest latency F waves), persistence, and amplitude, there is roughly a 12.5% chance that at least one of these five measures would be "abnormal" in the healthy population.

Consequently, it is this author's preference to only measure the mean or minimal latency, or indicate if the response is absent.

Although F waves will be abnormal in many clinical settings, they provide *unique* information in relatively few diagnoses. Probably the most useful setting for F waves is when evaluating for acquired demyelinating polyneuropathies, such as acute inflammatory demyelinating polyradiculoneuropathy (AIDP or Guillain-Barré syndrome) (9). In these disorders, the

most proximal and distal ends of the peripheral nervous system (i.e., roots and distal axons) are affected first. As a result, one of the earliest findings on nerve conduction studies is absence of F waves or prolongation of F-wave latencies, presumably reflecting slowing or conduction block at the root level. This may be the only finding early in the disease process.

F waves also provide unique information regarding proximal conduction in early traumatic nerve lesions and will demonstrate changes before distal axon wallerian degeneration occurs and before changes appear on needle EMG. There is some evidence that F waves may change after walking in lumbar spinal stenosis (10), though it is unclear how F waves should contribute to the diagnosis of lumbar spinal stenosis (11).

There are a number of limitations with F waves. First, since they involve only a few of the total pool of motor axons, lesions affecting only some of the axons can be missed. For instance, F waves are generally not helpful for detecting radiculopathies (12), although some authors have reported more frequent abnormalities (13). Since most muscles have more than one root supplying them, normal F waves can be obtained via the other root supply, thereby bypassing slowing via the involved root. Another limitation is that F waves measure conduction over a long distance. This limits their ability to detect focal pathology that causes only focal slowing across a short segment of nerve, which is then diluted by much longer segments of normal nerve conduction. In addition to the above, F waves are generally recorded from only distal limb muscles. In proximal muscles, the F-wave latency is so short (it does not have far to go to the spinal cord and back) that the F wave is buried in the CMAP response.

H waves (named after Dr. P. Hoffman who described it in 1918) utilize a pathway similar to a muscle stretch reflex (3). In a muscle stretch reflex, the receptors in the muscle spindle are activated by sudden stretch of the muscle. This sends a wave of depolarization proximally up the large diameter Ia sensory fibers, to the spinal cord. At the spinal cord, there is a monosynaptic reflex to the α-motor neuron and the descending motor axons are activated. H waves use a similar pathway, but the wave of depolarization starts upstream at the Ia afferent fiber instead of at the muscle spindle (14).

In healthy adults, H waves are easily elicited primarily in the soleus and the flexor carpi radialis muscles. Young children have H waves in many more muscles (before descending inhibitory motor pathways are fully developed). Patients with upper motor neuron lesions will also have easily elicited H waves in many other muscles (15).

When recording H waves, the sweep speed needs to be slow enough to capture the response (50 ms analysis times in the upper limb and 100 ms in the lower limb). Sensitivity needs to be sufficient to observe these responses although H waves are typically larger than F waves. Similar to F waves, conventional teaching is that the cathode should be placed proximally along the nerve with the anode distally. However, one often uses less current if one stimulates through the knee, with a small 1-cm disk electrode over the tibial nerve (midway between the hamstring tendons at the popliteal fossa) and a 3-cm electrode (the type usually used as a ground electrode) anteriorly over the patella (16). Stimulation is best accomplished with long-duration pulses (0.5 to 1.0 ms), since these preferentially activate the large Ia afferent nerve fibers that initiate the reflex arc (17). Stimulation should be at a level that produces the largest H wave, which is usually submaximal for the M wave (**Fig. 3-6**). Higher levels of stimulation are thought to inhibit H waves at the spinal level (3).

Latency is measured to the onset of the response—that is, the first departure from the baseline. Since the perceived onset will depend upon the display sensitivity (18), it's usually preferable to use a consistent display gain for measurement—ideally the same one used as for one's reference values (e.g., 500 µV per division). Latencies will depend upon height or leg length, and most reference values take this into account. Side-to-side latency differences are more sensitive for detecting abnormalities than comparing a measured latency to reference values. A side-to-side latency difference exceeding 1.2 ms is likely abnormal for the tibial H wave (19). Amplitude of the H wave is variable and is also best compared to the other side. When the smaller response is less than 40% of the larger response, this is likely abnormal (19).

Although H waves will be abnormal in many clinical settings, they provide unique information in relatively few diagnoses. The most useful setting for H waves is when evaluating for S1 radiculopathies. H waves are likely more sensitive for detecting S1 radiculopathies than is needle EMG (20). It is postulated that H waves can detect demyelination or sensory axon loss, while needle EMG only detects motor axon loss. H waves, however, provide less information about acuity or chronicity than needle EMG; they usually disappear early (or immediately) after onset of a radiculopathy and often never return. Obtaining and measuring H waves in the upper limbs is more challenging. They are somewhat more difficult to elicit than in the lower limb and the onset is often obscured by the preceding M wave.

The A wave is another response that is sometimes noted during studies in which one is trying to record late responses. The

FIGURE 3-6. H wave recorded from the soleus with tibial nerve stimulation at the popliteal fossa. The top trace represents the optimal response (labeled Tr 7). The traces going from Tr 1 to Tr 22 represent recordings with increasing current. Note that the H wave appears with lower stimulation levels. As stimulation is increased, the M wave appears and the H wave is attenuated.

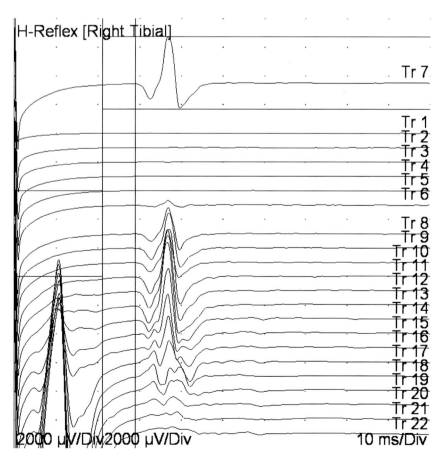

H-Reflex [Right Tibial]

Tr 7

Tr 1
Tr 2
Tr 3
Tr 4
Tr 5
Tr 6

Tr 8
Tr 9
Tr 10
Tr 11
Tr 12
Tr 13
Tr 14
Tr 15
Tr 16
Tr 17
Tr 18
Tr 19
Tr 20
Tr 21
Tr 22

2000 µV/Div 2000 µV/Div   10 ms/Div

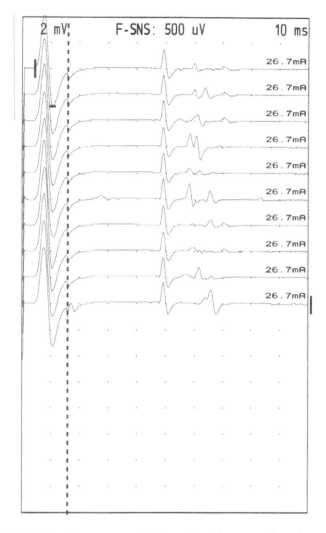

FIGURE 3-7. A waves are noted in this tracing during attempted recording of F waves in the tibial nerve. A constant A wave is noted at about 50 ms, in the middle of the sweep. The constant nature of the waveform distinguishes it from the later F wave, which is variable.

A wave is a stable, small response that is the same with every stimulation (**Fig. 3-7**). These can appear with either submaximal or supramaximal stimulation. The proposed physiology is activation of motor axons due to either axon branching (usually seen with submaximal stimulation) or ephaptic transmission (seen with supramaximal stimulation) (**Fig. 3-8**). These are usually considered abnormal though relatively nonspecific, and they are sometimes seen in the tibial nerve of healthy individuals (21). When seen with only submaximal stimulation, they may represent chronic nerve lesions with subsequent reinnervation and axon branching (22). A waves elicited with supramaximal stimulation are likely due to ephaptic transmission. These are sometimes seen in acute demyelinating polyneuropathies (e.g., AIDP) since demyelination creates an ideal setting for ephaptic transmission (see **Fig. 3-8**).

Needle Electromyography

Needle EMG is a very sensitive and useful technique for detecting pathology in the LMN, NMJ, and muscle. Key to an understanding of needle EMG is a familiarity with the concept of the motor unit (**Fig. 3-9**). The motor unit consists of the motor neuron cell body (which, for the limbs, resides in the anterior horns of the spinal cord), the axon, and all the muscle fibers the axon supplies. The number of muscle fibers innervated per axon varies widely. For small muscles that control very fine movements (e.g., extraocular muscles or laryngeal muscles), there may be only 4 to 6 muscle fibers per axon. In large muscles for which force is more important than fine control, such as the quadriceps, there are over 1,000 muscle fibers per axon (23).

In healthy individuals, if one leaves a recording needle in a muscle at rest, it is usually electrically quiet. When the individual gives a small voluntary contraction and activates the motor unit, a motor unit action potential (MUAP) can be recorded from the muscle (see **Fig. 3-9**). The MUAP represents the synchronous discharge of all the muscle fibers supplied by the axon. As more force is produced, these MUAPs fire more rapidly, and additional motor units are recruited until there are many MUAPs firing rapidly and none can be individually distinguished.

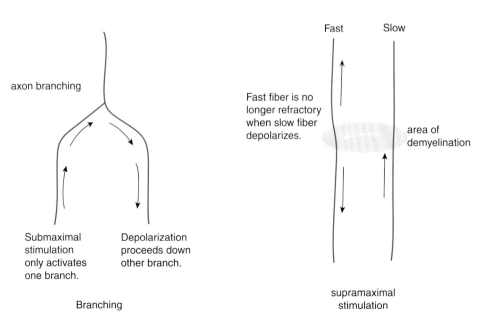

FIGURE 3-8. Physiologic mechanism for A waves. There are two purported mechanisms for A-wave production. Some nerves may have branching either due to prior injury or anatomic variants. In that case, depolarization can proceed up one branch and then down the other (**left**). In other cases (**right**), there may be an area of demyelination, which allows ephaptic transmission from one axon to another. In this case, the faster fiber has already depolarized at the site of demyelination, so collision due to refractory period does not prevent conduction distally to the muscle.

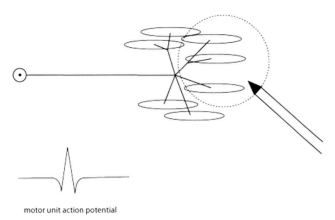

motor unit action potential

FIGURE 3-9. A representation of a motor unit—composed of a single motor neuron cell body, a single axon, and all the muscle fibers supplied by the axon. The motor unit action potential (MUAP) represents the synchronous discharge of all the muscle fibers in the motor unit.

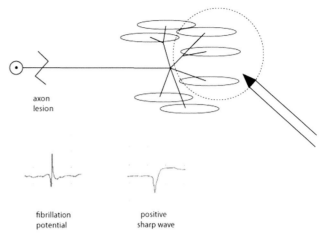

axon lesion

fibrillation potential   positive sharp wave

FIGURE 3-10. After denervation, single muscle fibers fire spontaneously, creating fibrillation potentials or positive sharp waves.

There are a number of potentials that can be recorded at rest (spontaneous potentials), some in healthy individuals, but most representing disease processes. When moving the needle electrode through the muscle, there is normally a brief electrical discharge from the muscle, known as insertional activity. This is usually high frequency and brief, usually lasting less than 300 ms (depending to some extent on examiner technique). Insertional activity can be prolonged, with discharges persisting longer after needle movement than normal. Prolonged or increased insertional activity can be seen in early denervation, in some myopathies, and in some inherited syndromes (24), but is usually not considered diagnostic when seen in isolation. Reduced insertional activity is measured along a different dimension than increased insertional activity (which is measured in time). Reduced insertional activity refers to reduced amplitude or absence of the burst of muscle fiber discharges when moving the needle through muscle. Reduced insertional activity is seen when there are no resting muscle membrane potentials in the area of study, such as muscle fibrosis (long-term denervation), muscle necrosis (e.g., compartment syndrome (25)), or if is not in muscle (but, for instance, in adipose tissue).

In healthy individuals, one can easily enter the motor point of the muscle where there are abundant NMJs. When this occurs, one records endplate noise and endplate spikes. Endplate noise consists of small irregular potentials that sound (when played over a loudspeaker) like the sound of a seashell held up to one's ear. They result from spontaneously released vesicles of acetylcholine (miniature endplate potentials or MEPPs). Endplate spikes are very brief (<5 ms duration) spikes with initially negative (upward) deflections, and they create a sputtering irregular sound similar to fat in a frying pan. They result from MEPPs summating to form localized endplate potentials (EPPs). These are normal findings, but one should pull back the needle electrode slightly and move to a different area for two reasons. These are typically painful areas to explore and the endplate spikes, when viewed from a distance, can take on an initial positivity and look like fibrillation potentials.

Fibrillation potentials and positive sharp waves represent abnormal spontaneous single muscle fiber discharges and are frequently seen in impairment of the LMN, NMJ, or muscle (26). They both represent single muscle fiber discharges and are seen in mostly the same disorders. Fibrillation potentials (**Fig. 3-10**) are short-duration (1 to 5 ms), regularly firing spikes with an initial positivity (downward deflection). They are likely recorded by the needle electrode from outside the muscle fiber. Positive sharp waves (see **Fig. 3-10**) have a sharp initially positive (downward) deflection but have a duration of 10 to 30 ms, and they fire regularly. It is suspected that positive sharp waves are recorded from pierced or injured muscle fibers (27–29).

Both fibrillation potentials and positive sharp waves are seen in a variety of disorders and neither is specific to denervation (hence, one should not use the term denervation potentials). They are commonly seen in disorders of motor neurons, motor axons, the NMJ (presynaptic more commonly than postsynaptic), and muscle (inflammatory myopathies and dystrophies more commonly). Upper motor neuron injury (e.g., spinal cord injury, stroke, and traumatic brain injury) can also produce fibrillation potentials and positive sharp waves in weak muscles, though less commonly than LMN impairments do.

When fibrillation potentials and positive sharp waves are recorded, one usually grades them on a 1+ to 4+ scale (**Box 3-1**). This is an ordinal scale but not a ratio or interval scale. Thus, we know that a grading of 2+ represents more axon loss than 1+, but not necessarily twice as much. Moreover, a finding of 4+ fibrillations does not mean that all axons have been lost—this can be seen in partial axon loss (30). Some authors have reported that positive sharp waves and fibrillations can be

BOX 3-1

Fibrillation and Positive Sharp Wave

Grading	Grade Characteristics
0	None
1+	Persistent single runs >1 s in two areas
2+	Moderate runs >1 s in three or more areas
3+	Many discharges in most muscle regions
4+	Continuous discharges in all areas of the muscle, baseline often obscured

seen in normal paraspinal and foot muscles (31–33), but other authors have not found this to be common (34).

Complex repetitive discharges (CRDs) can be seen in a variety of chronic neuropathic and myopathic conditions. It is believed that CRDs result from abnormal muscle membranes that allow ephaptic transmission (i.e., a depolarizing muscle fiber activates an adjacent muscle fiber via local currents, not via any synapse). A pacer muscle cell fires regularly, thereby activating adjacent muscle fibers, which then fire in a sustained rhythmic pattern. CRDs are constant iterative discharges that appear and disappear suddenly without variation in firing rate or amplitude. They sound like steadily operating machinery. They are not usually considered normal findings, but suggest chronic axon or muscle fiber loss. CRDs are most commonly seen in chronic neuropathic and myopathic conditions but are not specific to either one. Some authors report that they can be found normally in select muscles such as the iliopsoas (35). If they are found in a myotomal distribution, they can be considered diagnostic of radiculopathy (12).

Fasciculation potentials represent spontaneous discharges of an entire motor unit or a large part of a motor unit. They often originate in the anterior horn cell but can also originate distally along the axon or a branch of the axon (36). Fasciculation potentials are recognized by their appearance and rhythm of firing. Individually, they look like a single motor unit, because that is what is firing. However, they can be distinguished from a voluntary motor unit by their random discharge pattern. These discharges are spontaneous and not under voluntary control. To observe fasciculation potentials, one must often wait with the needle quietly in the muscles without moving the needle for a minute or more. Altering the sweep speed to a lower slower sweep (e.g., 100 ms per division) is often helpful.

Fasciculation potentials can be seen in a variety of disorders. Benign fasciculations are common. When asked, approximately 50% of people report fasciculations in their calves, worse with activity and sometimes increased with the use of caffeine (37). Fasciculation potentials are also seen in thyrotoxicosis and exposure to anticholinesterase medications. They can be seen in radiculopathies and chronic neuropathies as well. Perhaps the most worrisome disease in which fasciculations can be seen is motor neuron disease. Amyotrophic lateral sclerosis (ALS) and other variants of motor neuron disease can present with fasciculation potentials. The primary method by which benign fasciculations can be distinguished from those associated with disease is by the "company they keep." In motor neuron and other progressive disease processes, one will often see fibrillation potentials, positive sharp waves, and large-amplitude long-duration motor unit potentials, along with the fasciculation potentials. Benign fasciculations do not present with these other findings. Fasciculations associated with motor neuron disease tend to be less frequent in firing rate, and they tend to be larger in amplitude, polyphasic, and longer duration (reflecting the concurrent ongoing reinnervation), but these differences are not usually sufficient to be diagnostic.

Myokymia is often thought of as a grouped fasciculation. Myokymic discharges represent groups of motor units firing in a burst pattern, usually with a regular burst rate (38). These discharges, when played over the EMG instrument's loudspeaker, are often described as sounding like marching soldiers. However, the bursts can be quite different in both their duration and discharge rate, making recognition sometimes difficult. Myokymia is distinguished from CRDs because of the bursting nature rather than a single on and off with constant firing as seen in CRDs. Myokymic discharges are also distinguished from myotonic discharges because the former do not change in firing frequency or amplitude.

Myokymia can be seen in a variety of conditions. Facial myokymia can be seen in multiple sclerosis, pontine gliomas, and other brainstem disorders. Limb myokymia can occur in the presence of radiation plexopathy (39). When patients have had radiation for breast cancer, Hodgkin's lymphoma, or other malignant tumors, some will present with a later-onset plexopathy. The diagnostic question is whether the plexopathy represents tumor invasion or delayed onset radiation plexopathy. Tumor invasion in the brachial plexus tends to present with painful lower trunk lesions and a Horner's syndrome. Radiation plexitis presents with upper trunk lesions, paresthesias, and myokymia. Thus, myokymia argues for a diagnosis of radiation plexopathy in these cases. Limb myokymia can be seen in some chronic radiculopathies and entrapment neuropathies.

Myotonia is a discharge that originates in single muscle fibers. It is believed to be due to abnormal chloride conductance across the muscle cell membrane. These discharges are noted by their unique waxing and waning quality, both in frequency and in amplitude. Because the firing frequency changes, the pitch produced over the loudspeakers changes as well, and one hears sounds often described as a "dive bomber" or "revving motorcycle." The amplitude of the response also changes over time making the sound louder and softer during the discharge pattern. This can be distinguished from CRD because of its changing nature (CRDs are noticeably constant in firing frequency and amplitude).

Myotonia can be seen in a variety of muscle disorders including myotonic dystrophy, myotonia congenita, paramyotonia, and other disorders (40). Myotonic dystrophy is an unusual myopathy in that distal muscles are affected more than proximal muscles, and the same is true for where one might record these discharges. Distal hand muscles are often most affected. Since myotonia originates from muscle, it is not expected in patients with neuropathic disease.

A possible variant of myotonia is the syndrome of diffusely abnormal increased insertional activity, also known as "EMG disease." This disorder is an autosomally dominant inherited syndrome and presents with increased insertional activity and persistent positive sharp waves in essentially all muscles tested in the body (24). One can tell, however, that the patient does not have a true neuropathic disease because there are no fibrillation potentials, motor unit potentials are normal in morphology and size, and recruitment is normal. Because of the diffuse positive sharp waves, these patients can often be erroneously diagnosed with motor neuron disease or other serious disorders. It is difficult to know whether this syndrome produces symptoms or not, since those coming to the EMG laboratory are usually selected for some symptoms to start with. However, relatives of the patient with this disorder are often asymptomatic.

Motor Unit Analysis

Examination of MUAPs yields important information about the integrity of the motor unit and whether there are changes in axons, muscle fibers, or the NMJ. The MUAP, as mentioned earlier, represents the synchronous discharge of all the muscle fibers supplied by a single motor neuron. Duration of the

MUAP is largely influenced by the size of the motor unit territory; that is, the number of muscle fibers supplied by the single axon that are within the recording area of the needle electrode. Duration of the MUAP is not markedly affected by proximity of the depolarizing muscle fibers to the needle electrode.

Amplitude of the MUAP is also related to motor unit territory but is more influenced by the proximity of the discharging muscle fibers to the recording electrode. When the needle is close to the depolarizing muscle fibers, the amplitude is much larger than when it is some distance away. Thus, motor unit duration is a more reliable indication indicator of motor unit territory than is amplitude. There are reference values established for concentric electrodes for most of the major muscles in the body (41). These vary according to muscle and age. More proximal muscles, and especially bulbar muscles, have shorter-duration MUAPs. MUAP duration tends to increase with age.

MUAPs are polyphasic when there are more than five phases. A phase represents a change in direction that crosses the baseline. Thus, one can calculate the number of phases as the number of baseline crossings plus one. Changes in direction that do not extend across the baseline are not counted as a phase (these are better referred to as "turns"). The presence of polyphasic MUAPs alone is usually not diagnostic, since most normal muscles have a small percentage (approximately 20%) of polyphasic MUAPs. However, polyphasic, long-duration, large-amplitude MUAPs are usually seen in neuropathies, and polyphasic, short-duration, small-amplitude MUAPs are typically seen in myopathic conditions or disorders of the NMJ.

In neuropathic conditions, two types of reinnervation may be noted that change the MUAP morphology. When nerve injuries are incomplete, some axons are spared and others undergo wallerian degeneration. In this case, the remaining intact axons send distal sprouts to reinnervate the denervated muscle fibers. These sprouts are initially poorly myelinated and immature, which results in less synchronous discharge of muscle fibers than when seen normally. Consequently, one will observe polyphasic long-duration large-amplitude MUAPs (**Fig. 3-11**). As these new sprouts mature and become better myelinated, the MUAPs are less polyphasic because the muscle

fibers fire synchronously again. Thus, late after reinnervation by axon sprouting, the examiner will see large-amplitude long-duration but not polyphasic MUAPs.

In cases of complete axon loss, the picture is different. In these cases, there is no distal axonal sprouting because there are no viable distal axons. Rather, one is dependent upon axons regrowing from the site of nerve injury down to the muscle. When these new axons first reach the denervated muscle, they innervate just a few muscle fibers. These new MUAPs (which used to be called nascent potentials) are typically short in duration, polyphasic, and small in amplitude because the axons have supplied only a few muscle fibers. As these axons continue to sprout, they become larger and longer duration and stay polyphasic until the new sprouts mature several months after reinnervation.

Whether reinnervation occurs by distal axon sprouting or axon regrowth from the site of injury, recruitment will be reduced and fast firing. Because there are fewer MUAPs, the existing motor units will fire more rapidly than normal, and there will be fewer MUAPs firing even with maximum contraction.

The model for myopathic changes in MUAPs can be thought of as random loss of muscle fibers within the motor unit (**Fig. 3-12**). Since there are reduced numbers of muscle fibers, the MUAP duration and amplitude will be reduced. These MUAPs are polyphasic possibly due to less muscle fibers in the motor unit or possibly due to temporal dispersion along muscle fibers that conduct at different speeds in the setting of muscle disease. In either case, in myopathies, one sees small-amplitude short-duration polyphasic MUAPs. These MUAPs are recruited early with many MUAPs appearing on the EMG screen during even small levels of force generation. It is difficult to isolate a single MUAP in patients with the most severe myopathies.

NMJ disease can result in MUAPs that appear, in many ways, just like those seen in a myopathy. Because not all the NMJs are able to activate their muscle fibers, there are less functional muscle fibers per motor unit, and the duration and amplitude of the MUAPs are reduced. A feature commonly found in NMJ disease that is not seen in myopathy, however, is that of motor unit instability. Since the NMJs will fire variably and unreliably, the entire MUAP will vary in its size

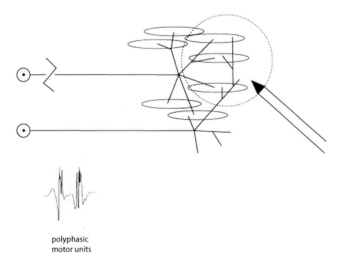

polyphasic
motor units

FIGURE 3-11. After reinnervation, one observes long-duration, large-amplitude, polyphasic motor unit action potentials (MUAPs). Over time, new sprouts and neuromuscular junctions mature and ultimately MUAPs become large amplitude and long duration.

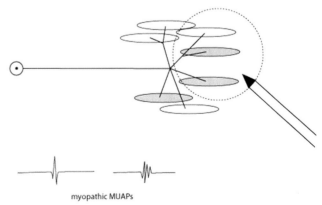

myopathic MUAPs

FIGURE 3-12. In myopathies, one can model motor units as having fewer functioning muscle fibers. Consequently, motor unit action potentials are smaller in amplitude and shorter in duration. They are also frequently polyphasic.

and morphology as muscle fibers either fire or do not fire with each successive MUAP discharge. This motor unit instability can be seen in NMJ disease as well as in recent reinnervation, since in the latter case the NMJs are also not mature and reliable. To observe motor unit instability, it is most helpful to look at MUAPs with a trigger and delay line so that the MUAP fires repetitively at the same location on the screen.

After MUAPs are assessed, one should then evaluate motor unit recruitment. Healthy individuals applying a small force will recruit a single motor unit firing slowly, typically at about 5 Hz. As more force is exerted, this motor unit will speed up to 10 to 12 Hz and produce greater levels of force. However, as the firing rate reaches about 12 to 15 Hz (depending on the muscle), a second motor unit is then recruited to allow additional force production. In this way, muscle forces are generated both by increasing rates of motor unit firing and by increasing the number of motor units firing. Normally, at full contraction, there are many motor units firing rapidly and the baseline cannot be distinguished.

There are generally three types of abnormalities of recruitment. Sometimes patients have insufficient central drive from the upper motor neurons to generate high levels of motor unit firing. This could be due to pain, poor voluntary effort, or upper motor neuron impairments. In these cases, one sees less than the full number of MUAPs, but the ones that are present fire slowly due to reduced upper motor neuron drive. This is often termed *central recruitment*.

In other cases, there is sufficient upper motor neuron drive, but there are reduced numbers of motor units available to participate in force production due to motor neuron or axon loss. In these cases, the initial motor units fire more rapidly before a second motor unit is recruited because there are fewer motor units available to recruit. In extreme cases, there may be only one or two motor units firing very rapidly (up to 30 to 40 Hz) without any additional motor units firing. This is typically termed *reduced recruitment* (or in cases where there are only very few motor units, discrete recruitment). It is distinguished from central recruitment in that the motor unit firing rate is quite fast.

A third abnormality one can see in motor unit recruitment is *early recruitment*. This is typically seen in myopathies or NMJ defects. With early recruitment, since each motor unit in a myopathy produces less force than normal, more motor units are recruited sooner or earlier than normal for a given level of force generation. The examiner asks the patient to produce a small amount of force but notes many MUAPs firing, more than expected for that level of force. In many cases of early recruitment, it is difficult to have a patient fire just one MUAP; it's usually either many or none. Thus, early recruitment represents many MUAPs firing for a low level of force production. Assessing early recruitment requires both measurement of force (whether qualitative or quantitative) and observation of MUAP firing patterns.

Repetitive Stimulation Studies

Repetitive stimulation studies are primarily useful for detection of NMJ abnormalities. To understand the underlying reasoning of how one performs NMJ studies, one needs to first briefly review the physiology of NMJ function, which is well reviewed elsewhere (42).

Normally, when a motor axon is depolarized, the wave of polarization travels toward the axon terminal as a result of the propagation of opening and closing of sodium channels. When it reaches the terminal end of the motor axon near the endplate, voltage-gated calcium channels are activated. The opening of these channels allows an influx of calcium ions (Ca^{2+}) into the presynaptic terminal. The opening of the voltage-gated and voltage-dependent calcium channels and the resulting Ca^{2+} influx result in an increase of intracellular Ca^{2+} at the presynaptic terminal for about 100 to 200 ms before it is pumped out and the intra-axonal Ca^{2+} is returned to the resting state. This influx of calcium allows acetylcholine vesicles to fuse with the presynaptic membrane and release quanta of acetylcholine into the extracellular space at the synapse.

In healthy individuals, the presynaptic terminal releases three to five times as much acetylcholine as is required to activate the postsynaptic membrane of the corresponding muscle fiber. This extra amount of acetylcholine release is known as the safety factor. While there is normally a large safety factor for the first discharge of a motor neuron, the amount of acetylcholine released drops with successive discharges when the nerve is activated at 2 to 3 Hz. However, because the safety factor is so large, there is still more than enough acetylcholine to activate the muscle fiber (**Fig. 3-13**).

Once acetylcholine is released into the synaptic cleft, it encounters acetylcholinesterase, the enzyme so named because it hydrolyzes acetylcholine molecules. This enzyme does not

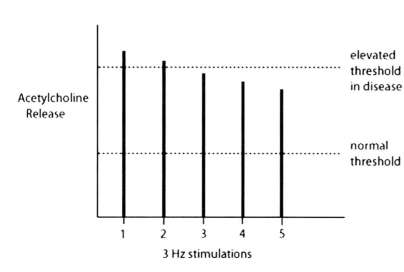

FIGURE 3-13. Normally, the quantity of acetylcholine (Ach) released by the presynaptic neuron drops with successive stimulations at 3 Hz. Because of the normal safety factor, all releases are still higher than the threshold for muscle fiber activation. In postsynaptic diseases, the threshold is higher and the quantity of Ach released falls below threshold.

"know" whether the acetylcholine it is digesting has just come from the presynaptic terminal or has already been used to activate the postsynaptic receptors. It digests the acetylcholine it encounters either way. Due to this enzymatic activity, it is estimated that only about half of the acetylcholine released from the presynaptic terminal makes it to the postsynaptic receptors. Once the acetylcholine reaches the postsynaptic receptors, it creates localized areas of membrane depolarization known as EPPs. These EPPs then summate temporally and spatially to create a muscle membrane depolarization and the muscle fiber discharges.

Exercise also has significant influences on NMJ physiology. Immediately after exercise, one sees postexercise potentiation or facilitation. In part, this is due to the fact that motor units fire at rates approaching 30 Hz with tetanic voluntary contraction. At 30 Hz rates, there is roughly 33 ms between each axon depolarization, which is less than the time needed for the Ca^{2+} to be pumped out of the presynaptic terminal. Thus, with exercise, Ca^{2+} builds up in the presynaptic terminal, and this further facilitates release of acetylcholine. When the safety factor is intact, this is not noticed because there is already more than enough acetylcholine to fully depolarize the muscle fiber. However, when the safety factor is reduced in disease states, postexercise potentiation will improve NMJ function compared to preexercise. This is termed postexercise facilitation.

There is also a phenomenon of postexercise exhaustion, which occurs 2 to 4 minutes after sustained exercise. In this period of postexercise exhaustion, there is less acetylcholine released than in the preexercise condition. Again, in healthy individuals, this would not be noticed because of the large safety factor. However, in individuals with marginal or reduced safety factors, some NMJs will not fire, and the CMAP will be reduced in amplitude.

There are several steps of the electrodiagnostic examination to keep in mind when evaluating an individual with possible NMJ disease (43). First, one should perform a standard motor nerve conduction study of the muscle and nerve to be studied with repetitive stimulation. This is to both assess the resting amplitude of the response and to be sure that the nerve under study does not have a prior or subclinical injury that could alter the results of NMJ testing.

The second step is to record the distal CMAP at rest and then again *immediately* after 10 seconds of maximum voluntary isometric exercise (**Table 3-1**). This procedure is used to look for any postexercise facilitation. If presynaptic diseases of the NMJ are present, the initial resting CMAP will be low in amplitude but will increase markedly after 10 seconds of exercise since Ca^{2+} buildup within the presynaptic terminal occurs and acetylcholine release is greatly facilitated.

The third step is to perform repetitive stimulation at slow rates of 2 or 3 Hz (**Table 3-1**). Generally, trains of five stimulations are sufficient. When stimulating at 3 Hz, there are 333 ms between each stimulation. This allows for essentially a full return of baseline or resting state of Ca^{2+} concentration, and there is no significant facilitation of acetylcholine release. As discussed above, there is depletion of the immediately available stores of acetylcholine vesicles and resultant diminution of acetylcholine release with each successive stimulation. In healthy individuals, while the acetylcholine release is reduced with each successive stimulation, the CMAP remains stable and unchanged because of the large safety factor. Most laboratories consider amplitude decrements of less than 10% between the first stimulation and the fourth or fifth to be acceptable. However, in the setting of NMJ diseases, when the safety factor is diminished, a reduction in CMAP with progressive stimulations will exceed the reference range. To be considered abnormal, the reduction should be more than 10% decrement compared to the baseline value.

There are several technical points to be aware of when performing repetitive stimulation studies. First, temperature is critical. When the temperature is below 34°C, enzymatic activity of acetylcholine esterase is reduced. As a result, cold causes an increase in acetylcholine levels within the NMJ, which compensates for any pathologic reduction of the safety factor. This reduces the likelihood of detecting decrements that might be present otherwise. Second, a stable recording baseline is important. The movement of the limb has to be minimized so it does not create signal artifacts in the recordings. Many laboratories will attempt to immobilize the part of the limb being studied, although this is more difficult with proximal or bulbar muscles. The choice of the nerve muscle pair is also crucial. NMJ diseases, especially myasthenia gravis (MG), tend

TABLE 3-1	**Expected Findings with Single and Repetitive Stimulation in Healthy Individuals, Compared to Myasthenia Gravis (Postsynaptic Defect) and Lambert-Eaton Myasthenic Syndrome (LEMS)**		
	Normal	**Myasthenia Gravis**	**LEMS**
Single CMAP at rest	Norm	Norm	Small
Compare single CMAP immediately after 10-s exercise	No Δ	No Δ	↑↑ >100% increase
Preexercise 3-Hz stimulation compare first to fifth	No Δ	Decrement >10%	Decrement >10% all responses are very small
Postexercise potentiation 3-Hz stimulation compare first to fifth immediately after 30-s exercise	No Δ	Less decrement than pre-exercise	Decrement >10% but all responses are bigger than pre-exercise
Postexercise exhaustion 3-Hz stimulation compare first to fifth 2–4 min after 30-s exercise	No Δ	Decrement >10% more pronounced than pre-exercise	Decrement >10% with all responses small as pre-exercise
High-frequency stimulation or exercise 30–50-Hz stimulation comparing last to first (10 s of exercise has similar effects)	↑ ≤40% increase	↑ ≤40% increase	↑↑ >100% increase

to affect proximal muscles more than distal muscles. However, the proximal studies are technically more difficult than the more distal limb nerve muscle pairs. Thus, many laboratories will start with the ulnar nerve recording from the abductor digiti minimi (ADM). If this is normal, then most laboratories will proceed to a proximal limb muscle such as the trapezius (stimulate spinal accessory nerve) or the deltoid (stimulate at Erb's point). Finally, if these two studies are normal, then the study of the facial nerve recording from nasalis can yield important information. While the latter technique is more sensitive, it is also more vulnerable to movement artifact.

After the initial series of five stimulations at 3 Hz, one should then repeat studies both immediately after exercise (to look for postexercise potentiation) and several minutes after exercise (to look for postexercise exhaustion). After the preexercise testing, one asks the patient to maximally contract the muscle for 30 or 60 seconds. Immediately postexercise, one then gives another series of five stimulations as before the exercise. This series is repeated again at 1-minute intervals until 4 minutes postexercise. By performing this procedure, one assesses for postexercise facilitation (or potentiation) immediately after exercise and for postexercise exhaustion, which typically occurs at 2 to 4 minutes postexercise.

In some cases, high-frequency repetitive stimulation is used. This is particularly helpful when the patient is not able to voluntarily exercise and when one is looking for a presynaptic disease such as Lambert-Eaton myasthenic syndrome (LEMS) or botulism. Stimulation rates are set in the 30- to 50-Hz range, which means there are only 20 to 33 ms between each successive stimulation. At these rates, the subsequent stimuli occur too frequently for the presynaptic nerve terminal to pump out the extra influx of Ca^{2+}. Thus, calcium concentration builds up in the presynaptic terminal, and consequently, acetylcholine release is markedly increased. High-frequency repetitive stimulation is primarily used to look for postexercise facilitation and is mostly useful in presynaptic defects. Healthy patients have a moderate increase in CMAP size with these rates of stimulation, known as pseudofacilitation. The phenomenon is not likely due to mechanical artifact. While some have postulated that hypersynchronization of the muscle fiber action potentials is the cause, a more convincing explanation, for which there is now experimental evidence, is that the muscle fibers undergo hyperpolarization, due to the intramuscular release of norepinephrine and consequent stimulation of the electrogenic Na^+/K^+ pump (44).

One generally groups NMJ defects into presynaptic and postsynaptic types. MG is the most common postsynaptic NMJ disease. The pathophysiology has been postulated to result from acetylcholine receptor antibodies likely generated from an autoimmune process. These antibodies act as antagonists against the acetylcholine receptors at the postsynaptic cleft of the NMJ. In addition, there are marked distortions of the NMJ with a widened cleft and fewer infoldings postsynaptically well visualized on morphologic studies by electron microscopy (45,46). This is helpful for electromyographers to keep in mind since the widened cleft means that there is a greater chance that acetylcholinesterase will digest the acetylcholine before it reaches the postsynaptic cleft. Moreover, for the acetylcholine molecules that do reach the postsynaptic membrane, there are fewer available receptors to activate; hence, there is a much reduced safety factor.

In MG, one usually sees relatively normal CMAPs at rest and little change immediately after exercise. However, with slow repetitive stimulation (2 to 3 Hz), one will often observe a reduction in the CMAP maximal at the fourth or fifth stimulation in the series. As mentioned above, the decrement needs to be greater than 10% to be considered normal. Repetitive stimulation in these patients should also display a repair of the decrement immediately after exercise due to postexercise potentiation. At 2 to 4 minutes after exercise, when postexercise exhaustion occurs, a more marked decrement is seen than in the preexercise phase. At times, patients with more subtle disease will demonstrate no decrement preexercise but will demonstrate a significant decrement 2 to 4 minutes postexercise. Thus, when evaluating for potential MG, one should always complete the series of postexercise runs of repetitive stimulation as described above. With high-frequency repetitive stimulation, patients with MG show only small increments as do normal individuals due to pseudofacilitation (described above).

LEMS is due to an abnormality in the voltage-gated calcium channels located in the presynaptic terminal (47). It is most commonly associated with small cell lung cancer but can also be seen in other cancers and some autoimmune disorders, and it is rarely idiopathic.

Patients with LEMS demonstrate very small CMAPs at rest (48). However, immediately after 10 seconds of exercise, the CMAP increases in size dramatically due to the enhanced release of acetylcholine precipitated by brief periods of exercise and consequent increase in calcium ion concentration within the presynaptic terminal. The results are quite striking and few other diseases cause CMAP amplitude to increase so impressively. To be diagnostic, the increase in CMAP amplitude needs to be at least 100%, that is, a doubling of the initial CMAP. The CMAP does not increase in size above normal values but simply goes from a very small initial amplitude to one that is closer to the healthy range.

With repetitive stimulation at slow rates, patients with LEMS will demonstrate a decrement between the first and fourth potential that is not unlike that seen in MG. This is related to the abnormal safety factor that is seen in LEMS as well as MG. However, what will be noted is that in the series of five stimulations immediately postexercise, all of the CMAPs will be much larger than they were in the pre-exercise condition. At 2 to 4 minutes postexercise, the CMAPs fall to their baseline levels and the results become similar to what was seen at rest.

It is in the setting of LEMS that high-frequency repetitive stimulation is most useful. With stimulation rates of 30 Hz or more, there is a buildup of Ca^{2+} in the presynaptic terminal, which tends to overcome the initial defect. As a result, the CMAP becomes more than double its resting amplitude, often approaching a near-normal amplitude.

Botulism is another example of presynaptic NMJ disease. In this case, it is not the voltage-gated Ca^{2+} channels that are impaired but rather the ability of the presynaptic vesicle membrane to fuse with axon terminal plasma membrane and release acetylcholine (49). The effect of botulism on electrodiagnostic findings is conceptually similar to that seen in LEMS. However, in the real word, the presentation of botulism tends to be more variable, and not all cases will have marked increments with fast repetitive stimulation or marked postexercise facilitation.

There are a number of limitations in NMJ testing. First, the sensitivity of repetitive stimulation studies is probably only about 60% to 70% in cases of MG even with technically well-performed studies utilizing exercise (50,51); specificity, however, is very good. The reasons for only moderate sensitivity are likely multifold and are beyond the scope of discussion here. Single fiber EMG, which is not being reviewed in this chapter, has a greater sensitivity than repetitive stimulation. Similarly, repetitive stimulation is not as sensitive for presynaptic impairments as is single fiber EMG. Cold can have a significant influence on these studies and cause false-negative results. Patients who are on anticholinesterase medication such as pyridostigmine will not demonstrate the same degree of abnormalities as those who are without the medication. Finally, good examiners always keep in mind the technical aspects, with the most concerning one being errors introduced by limb movement. With repetitive stimulation, there is often considerable limb movement unless one is vigilant. Limb movement alters the position of the recording, the stimulating electrodes, and their contact to the skin. In this way, movement can bring the stimulation to less than supramaximal, which could mimic a decrement.

DISEASE PROCESSES

Entrapment Neuropathies

There are a variety of entrapment neuropathies that commonly present to the electrodiagnostic laboratory for evaluation. The most common ones, which will be discussed here, include median neuropathy at the wrist (CTS), ulnar neuropathy at the elbow (UNE), radial neuropathy at the spiral groove, fibular neuropathy at the fibular head, and tarsal tunnel syndrome.

There are a few general concepts regarding entrapment neuropathies to keep in mind as one evaluates these various neuropathies. First, entrapment of a nerve typically first produces demyelination and conduction slowing in more mild cases. As demyelination progresses, the electrophysiologic changes progress from slowing to conduction block. With more severe entrapments, axon loss can then occur. There is some variation in this general principle across nerves since some nerves, such as tibial nerve at the ankle or ulnar nerve at the elbow, are more prone to axon loss than others such as the median nerve at the wrist or the fibula nerve at the knee.

In entrapment neuropathies, the largest diameter fibers are usually affected first. This means that large diameter sensory fibers will first demonstrate slowing and conduction block, and only with more progressive lesions will the slightly smaller diameter motor fibers be affected.

Not all fascicles are affected equally by a nerve entrapment. For example, UNE often spares fascicles supplying the two ulnar-innervated forearm muscles, flexor carpi ulnaris and flexor digitorum profundus (52). Similarly, in the median nerve at the wrist, the fascicles supplying the ring finger and long finger are more commonly affected than those supplying the index finger (53). In fibular neuropathy, it is more common to have deep fibular nerve involvement than it is to have changes in the distribution of the superficial fibular nerve. These variations in fascicular vulnerability need to be considered in interpretation. For instance, one should not assume that if there is evidence of denervation in ulnar-innervated hand muscles, but forearm muscles are normal, the lesion is distal to the elbow or at the wrist.

Perhaps the most important principle to remember is that one should think about one's approach carefully before starting the evaluation. Clinicians can run into a common pitfall by doing some initial testing and, if findings are normal, then proceeding with additional testing. Since each test performed carries a 2.5% false-positive rate, more tests will introduce a higher rate of false-positive error if not analyzed appropriately. This false-positive rate can quickly add up to unacceptable levels as multiple independent tests are performed.

Median Neuropathy at the Wrist

Median neuropathy at the wrist, which is usually responsible for CTS, is the most common entrapment neuropathy to be referred to electrodiagnostic laboratories in the United States (54). Symptoms commonly include hand numbness and weakness (55). The patient often does not localize the numbness to simply the median distribution but rather indicates that the whole hand becomes numb (56). A complaint of dropping things is frequent. Symptoms are usually worse at night and patients may occasionally report they "flick" their wrist to relieve symptoms.

On examination, one may find weakness of the thenar muscles and possibly some mildly reduced sensation. There are a number of physical signs such as Tinel's sign, Phalen's sign, and the flick sign that are suggestive of CTS. However, the sensitivity and specificity of these tests are not high (1) and they should not be used to make or rule out a diagnosis.

There are a number of risk factors for CTS, which have been well documented in the literature (57). In polyneuropathies, nerves are more susceptible to superimposed entrapment such as in the case of diabetes. Diseases in which there is more synovial tissue at the wrist such as rheumatoid arthritis also increase the risk of CTS by about threefold. Individuals who have work that involves high repetition and high force involving hand muscles are at significantly increased risk of CTS (58). Obesity is also a risk factor (59).

Since detection of slowing of median nerve conduction across the wrist is the most useful way to localize the entrapment neuropathy, this should be the focus of one's electrodiagnostic assessment. There have been many approaches described for diagnosing CTS with nerve conduction studies. For more in-depth coverage, readers are encouraged to review other articles (60,61). One's general approach should be to measure sensory and motor conduction across the wrist and to compare latencies with nearby nerves in the hand such as the radial or ulnar nerve that do not traverse the carpal tunnel. This helps to exclude the effects of temperature, age, and other factors such as polyneuropathy that may influence nerve conduction. As with most entrapment neuropathies, sensory fibers are usually affected first. Rarely, motor axons are preferentially affected possibly because of focal compression of the recurrent branch of the median nerve or selective effects on fascicles within the median nerve at the wrist (62).

There are many approaches for evaluating median sensory conductions across the wrist, and it is critical to think through these alternative approaches before testing the patient. In particular, as mentioned above, one should not adopt the methodology of performing one test and, upon finding a normal result, performing another test until one finds an abnormality. Although this might seem tempting intuitively, it is risky since each additional test performed carries a 2.5% false-positive rate. These rates are roughly additive as each new test is performed.

When selecting sensory nerve conduction studies, one should select studies that are (in descending order of importance):

- Specific (few false positives)
- Sensitive (few false negatives)

- Reliable (obtain the same results today and tomorrow)
- Least influenced by covariates such as temperature and age

There are three sensory conduction studies that have been shown to be reasonably good in terms of the criteria mentioned above (63). These are demonstrated in **Figure 3-14**. Comparison of median and ulnar conduction to the ring finger allows the detection of median nerve slowing in comparison to the ulnar nerve, which does not traverse the carpal tunnel. A median-ulnar difference exceeding 0.4 ms is likely abnormal. Similarly, comparison of the median and radial nerve to the thumb has similar advantages. Here, a difference exceeding 0.5 ms

is probably abnormal. The third test, which has good evidence from the literature, is the median and ulnar comparison across the palm over an 8-cm distance. This study should demonstrate no more than a 0.3-ms difference in healthy individuals.

This author has also published extensively on a method to summarize these three tests into one result known as the combined sensory index or CSI (since the television show Crime Scene Investigation has become popular, this is now being called the Robinson Index). To calculate the CSI, one performs all three of the studies mentioned above and adds the latency differences (median minus ulnar or median minus radial) together (when these are negative, i.e., the median is faster,

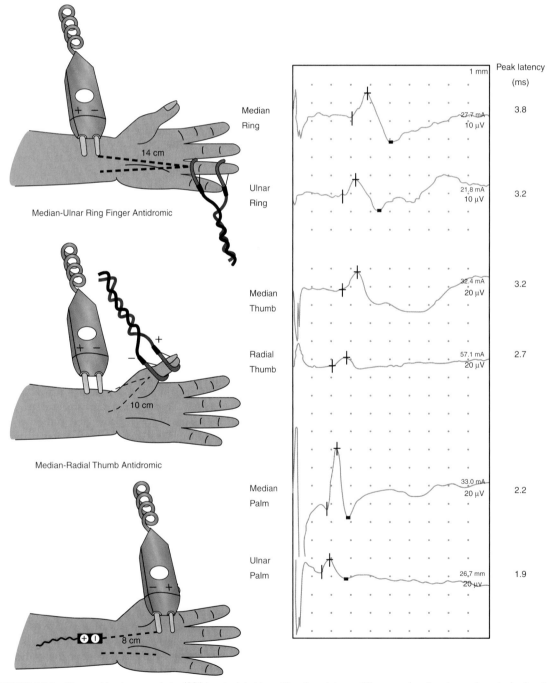

FIGURE 3-14.   The combined sensory index (CSI) is calculated by adding three latency differences: (median ring – ulnar ring) + (median thumb – radial thumb) + (median palm – ulnar palm). Normally, this sum is less than 1 ms. In this case it is 0.6 + 0.5 + 0.3 = 1.4 ms.

a negative number is used). The CSI, because it summarizes three different tests, has been shown to be highly specific and more sensitive than the individual tests (64). It is also more reliable than single tests when one studies the same patient on two different occasions (65). A CSI of 1.0 ms or more is considered abnormal (64).

Motor nerve conduction studies are also, as mentioned above, an essential component of the electrodiagnostic evaluation of CTS. These should be performed even if sensory conduction studies are normal. Most commonly, studies are performed with stimulation of the median nerve at the wrist and recording over the abductor pollicis brevis (APB). Generally, latencies exceeding 4.5 ms are considered abnormal. It is not useful to compare one median nerve with the other side because of the frequency of bilateral CTS. However, some electromyographers compare the median motor latency with the ulnar motor latency; a difference exceeding 1.5 ms is considered abnormal. While some authors do advocate stimulating both at the wrist and at the palm (66), it is difficult to stimulate only the median nerve in the palm, and one can be easily misled into a false diagnosis if the ulnar nerve is stimulated in the palm (67).

Needle EMG is sometimes useful in evaluating patients with CTS (68). There is not a consensus about when thenar muscle EMG should be performed. It is this author's practice to perform needle EMG of the thenar muscles in three settings:

- Patients in whom the motor response is abnormal (this group has a higher yield)
- Patients with a history of trauma (in which axon loss is more likely)
- Patients with a clinical presentation that suggests another possible diagnosis (such as radiculopathy or plexopathy)

Ulnar Neuropathy at the Elbow

Ulnar neuropathy at the elbow (UNE) is another common entrapment neuropathy presenting to the electrodiagnostic medical consultant. The etiology of UNE varies but can be due to acute injury, entrapment in the cubital tunnel (under the aponeurosis between the two heads of the flexor carpi ulnaris), or prolonged stretching of the nerve in the ulnar groove when the elbow is held in the flexed position (69). Tardy ulnar palsy is a result of prior elbow injury causing an elbow deformity and slowly progressive injury to the ulnar nerve.

Symptoms of ulnar neuropathy typically include numbness over the small finger and the ulnar half of the ring finger. Generally, an UNE also affects sensation over the dorsum of the hand on the ulnar side, an area supplied by the dorsal ulnar cutaneous nerve, which branches from the ulnar nerve proximal to the wrist. In contrast, ulnar nerve lesions at the wrist spare the dorsal ulnar cutaneous territory because they occur distal to this branch point. UNE should spare sensation over the medial forearm. This area is supplied by the medial antebrachial cutaneous nerve originating from the medial cord of the brachial plexus and should be spared in UNE.

Patients often also present with weakness of ulnar hand muscles complaining that they have difficulty holding small objects and difficulty with grip strength. They may sometimes notice atrophy of the first dorsal interosseous (FDI) muscle.

On physical examination, one will often note weakness of interosseous muscles, atrophy of the FDI, and reduced sensation in the ulnar nerve territory in the hand. One may also find a Froment's sign indicating weakness of the adductor pollicis and the FDI (70). A Tinel's sign can often be noted at the elbow, but this is nonspecific and can be seen in a number of normal healthy individuals.

Because sensory conduction is difficult to reliably record across the elbow, most electromyographers will rely upon motor conduction studies of the ulnar nerve (61). There are a number of technical elements to keep in mind when performing these studies. First, it is advisable to record from both the ADM and the FDI at the same time utilizing two channels of the EMG instrument. Although each muscle has similar sensitivity for detecting UNE, there is not a complete overlap and sometimes one muscle will demonstrate conduction block when the other one does not (71). Stimulation usually is at the wrist, below the elbow, and above the elbow. When stimulating across the elbow, one should have the elbow in a flexed position with a roughly 70 to 90 degree angle. This is important because it stretches the nerve through the ulnar groove. If the elbow is not bent, the nerve is still long enough to accommodate elbow flexion, but is redundant upon itself; therefore, surface measurement across the skin will underestimate the true distance and the calculated conduction velocity will be too slow.

There has been considerable discussion in the literature about the appropriate distances to use between the above and below elbow stimulation sites. Earlier literature suggested that in general, one should have at least 10 cm of distance between stimulation sites (72). However, this was based upon measurements of error in the 1970s when measuring latencies on equipment using much older technology. Similar studies have now been repeated utilizing modern digital equipment (73), and this has demonstrated that a 6-cm distance should usually be sufficient and would have error similar to the 10-cm distance 30 years ago.

When performing ulnar motor conduction studies, one must be aware of the potential of Martin-Gruber anastomosis. This anastomosis is said to be present in 15% to 20% of individuals and typically involves fibers crossing from the median nerve to the ulnar nerve in the proximal forearm (74). At times, the fibers can originate from the anterior interosseous nerve rather than the main branch of the median nerve. In the presence of Martin-Gruber anastomosis, one will record a normal large-amplitude response from the ADM and FDI when stimulating the ulnar nerve at the wrist. However, while stimulating the ulnar nerve at or below the elbow, one will note a decreased amplitude response because one is stimulating only the ulnar nerve fibers and not those that cross in the proximal forearm. To the inexperienced electromyographer, this can masquerade as conduction block in the proximal forearm and can result in an erroneous diagnosis. The hint of a Martin-Gruber anastomosis rather than ulnar neuropathy in the forearm or elbow is that this drop in amplitude occurs between the wrist and below the elbow and not across the elbow. The presence of this anomalous innervation can be proven by stimulating the median nerve at the elbow and recording from the ADM and FDI muscles; when a crossover exists, a sizable response can be recorded from these usually ulnar-innervated muscles (75).

There are two ways to decide if the across elbow velocity is acceptable. Some authors advocate comparing ulnar conduction across the elbow to that recorded in the forearm. However, this comparison is flawed in that it assumes that ulnar conduction in the forearm is unaffected by a neuropathy proximally at the elbow (71). Unfortunately, this is not the case since with axon loss, there is distal slowing due to preferential loss of the faster-conducting fibers. As a result, comparison between the two segments is not valid. The other method for determining whether the conduction is normal is to compare the velocity to reference values. This has been shown to be preferable in terms of sensitivity and specificity (71). Our laboratory uses a reference value of 48 m/s as a lower limit of normal.

When there is concern for UNE, it is frequently useful to perform ulnar "inching" studies. These studies involve stimulation of the ulnar nerve at 2-cm increments across the elbow looking for any focal slowing or conduction block. Latency differences exceeding 0.7 ms or amplitude differences exceeding 10% are suggestive of a focal lesion (76). It is preferable to see both latency and amplitude changes as well as changes in morphology to be certain of a focal lesion. Because the distances are small, and the error in measurement is large as a percentage, one should not consider the conduction velocity of inching studies in m/s but rather look at the established reference values (≤0.7 ms) for latency differences across 2 cm.

Ulnar sensory conduction studies can be useful at times. When stimulating at the wrist and recording at the small finger, responses are usually small in amplitude or absent. It is difficult to reliably and consistently record ulnar sensory conduction across the elbow recording at the small finger. The response from the dorsal ulnar cutaneous nerve can be helpful. In UNE, it should be affected to a similar degree as the ulnar sensory response to the small finger, whereas it should be spared in ulnar neuropathy at the wrist.

Needle EMG should generally be performed in patients referred for UNE including the ADM, FDI, and the flexor digitorum profundus. However, the FDP is often spared in UNE to its fascicles residing a relatively protected position within the nerve. When there are abnormalities in the ulnar-innervated hand muscles, it is helpful to check non–ulnar-innervated C8/T1 muscles (e.g., APB or extensor indicis [EI]) to look for root or plexus lesions that might mimic an ulnar neuropathy.

Radial Nerve at the Humerus

In the absence of trauma, radial nerve entrapments are much less common than entrapments of the median or ulnar nerves in the upper limb. This is in contrast to traumatic neuropathies where radial nerve injuries are more common due to the proximity of the nerve to the humerus as it traverses along the spiral groove. The radial nerve is most typically affected along the spiral groove of the humerus, after the nerve has given branches to the triceps and the anconeus muscles but before it gives branches to the brachioradialis and the finger and wrist extensors. The site of the lesion is also proximal to the division of the nerve into superficial and deep branches (77).

Patients typically present with symptoms of weakness when opening their hand and extending their wrist. They also report weak grip strength since grip is weaker with the wrist in flexion than it is with an extension. Patients will also report numbness in the radial distribution on the dorsum of the hand with a proximal radial neuropathy.

On physical examination, the primary finding on strength testing will be weakness of wrist and finger extension (78). There are several special points that can help improve accuracy when examining the patient with possible radial neuropathy. First, it is difficult to isolate the brachioradialis muscle, which is the first muscle supplied after the spiral groove, on manual muscle testing. It is best to test this muscle with the forearm in the neutral position and to flex the elbow while palpating and observing the brachioradialis muscle visually. Although the biceps and other elbow flexors are strong enough to substitute for the brachioradialis, one can usually palpate or visually appreciate a side-to-side difference when this muscle is weak. Another point to keep in mind is that the extensor digitorum and other finger extensors supplied by the radial nerve primarily produce extension at the MCP (metacarpal phalangeal) joints. It is the ulnar-innervated lumbricals and interossei that contribute to extension at the interphalangeal (IP) joints. As a result, extension of the fingers at the proximal interphalangeal joint (PIP) and distal interphalangeal joint (DIP) joints may be intact even with a complete radial neuropathy. Finally, one should be aware that when a patient has a radial neuropathy and weak finger extension, testing finger abduction (i.e., the interosseous muscles) will produce apparent weakness. This is not because of true muscle weakness but rather because testing finger abduction while the MCP joints are in a flexed position produces much less force than when they are fully extended. For this reason, it is helpful to have the patient lay his or her hand on a table or a book to complete testing of interosseous muscle function.

Physical examination will also usually show reduced sensation in the radial distribution of the hand and an absent brachioradialis muscle stretch reflex. Since the injury is commonly distal to the branch supplying the triceps, the reflex at the triceps is typically intact.

In cases of radial neuropathy, needle EMG is often more useful than motor nerve conduction studies. Both recording and stimulation of the radial motor nerve can be problematic. Recording of the radial motor response is typically achieved with surface electrodes placed over the EI muscle. This is sometimes satisfactory but does suffer from the problem that other forearm muscles in the posterior compartment also contribute to this response via volume conduction. Probably the most useful setting for motor conduction studies in the assessment of radial neuropathy is to evaluate the surface amplitude for the EI with stimulation of the nerve in the distal forearm. This distally evoked amplitude gives an indication of how many axons are viable and has been shown to correlate with the prognosis in radial neuropathy (79). Radial sensory responses are useful to evaluate for evidence of sensory axon loss and to evaluate whether the lesion is proximal to the branching of the radial nerve into superficial and deep branches.

Needle EMG is usually the most useful electrodiagnostic assessment. One should generally consider studying the triceps muscle to look for evidence of denervation. If there is denervation in this muscle, then it is usually wise to proceed proximally to the deltoid muscle, which is also innervated by the posterior cord of the brachial plexus. If this is abnormal as well, then a broader evaluation of the limb is clearly indicated.

Distally, it is useful to study the brachioradialis muscle since this is the first muscle to be innervated after the spiral groove (the anconeus muscle is innervated by the same branch as supplies the medial head of the triceps). The other muscles in the forearm that are useful to study include the extensor carpi radialis, extensor digitorum, and the extensor indicis. It has been demonstrated that two of the more useful prognostic signs in radial neuropathy are presence or absence of a radial motor response to the EI and the degree of recruitment noted in the brachioradialis muscle (79).

Fibular Neuropathy

The fibular nerve (the preferred name for the nerve formerly known as peroneal) (77) is the most commonly affected nerve in the lower limb. It is particularly vulnerable to pressure as it crosses just behind the fibular head near the knee. It can also be affected by prolonged knee flexion or squatting and hence can be seen in prolonged labor and in those with occupations requiring prolonged squatting, such as strawberry pickers (80). This is the most common lower limb nerve injury in athletes (81). Sometimes athletes can also have intraneural fibular nerve cysts, which are thought to develop from synovial fluid tracking along the intra-articular branch of the small branches innervating the knee joint.

The most common symptom of fibular neuropathy is weakness of dorsiflexion, presenting with foot slap or dragging of the foot when walking (82). Patients also have sensory loss over the dorsum of the foot, but rarely is this a prominent or presenting complaint.

Electrodiagnostic assessment generally includes motor and sensory conduction studies as well as needle EMG in the lower limb (83). Motor nerve conduction studies are often performed with recording over the extensor digitorum brevis (EDB) muscle. The EDB muscle is useful when studying the fibular nerve in the leg region, and it provides a conduction velocity between the fibular head and the ankle. On the other hand, the EDB is not a functionally useful muscle, and in moderately severe fibular neuropathies, or in polyneuropathies, the response may be absent. Thus, it is wise to record from both the EDB and the tibialis anterior (TA) muscles at the same time. The TA has the advantage of being a functionally more important muscle and it may at times be present when the EDB is absent (84). Recently, it has been shown that hip and knee position have an influence on measured NCVs; hip flexion stretches the fibular nerve and increases measured velocity by an average of 2.5 m/s (85).

Sensory responses can be recorded from the superficial fibular nerve. This is helpful to distinguish between a proximal L5 root lesion (in which sensory conduction should be normal) and a more distal fibular nerve lesion. However, it is usually not otherwise helpful for localization. This response can also at times be misleading since a selective deep fibular nerve lesion will spare the superficial fibular sensory response.

Needle EMG can be very helpful in localization of fibular nerve lesions. It is usually helpful to study the TA and fibularis longus (formerly peroneus longus) muscles to evaluate both the deep and superficial branches. In order to exclude a more proximal lesion, one studies the short head of the biceps femoris since this muscle is supplied by the fibular division of the sciatic nerve proximal to fibular head. If this muscle is abnormal, then a wider examination of the lower limb is indicated.

The EDB muscle can be studied with needle EMG but has a high frequency of false-positive results (33). It is also often useful to study tibial-innervated muscles in the leg to exclude a more proximal sciatic lesion or a proximal root lesion.

Prognosis of fibular nerve lesions in large part is determined by both the amplitude of the motor responses and by the degree of motor unit recruitment in the TA muscle (84). Those with good recruitment in TA and present CMAP responses in TA and EDB generally do quite well.

Tibial Nerve

Neuropathy affecting the tibial nerve is relatively rare compared to the other nerve lesions discussed above. This is likely related to the relatively protected position of the tibial nerve within the leg and foot. Moreover, the fascicular anatomy of the tibial nerve is such that it has many small fascicles, which are resistant to injury (86). In comparison, the fibular nerve is made up of a few larger fascicles, which are more susceptible to entrapment and trauma as well as stretching (86). The tibial nerve can occasionally be injured at the ankle such as with posttraumatic tibial neuropathy at the ankle after calcaneal fractures, or other foot injuries.

Patients with tibial neuropathy at the ankle can present with numbness or paresthesias in the sole of the foot (87). They may have predominant symptoms in either the lateral or medial plantar nerve distribution or occasionally in the calcaneal nerve distribution. As noted above, this can occur after trauma to the ankle or foot but may also be occasionally seen without history of injury. The etiology of nontraumatic tarsal tunnel syndrome is unclear. Some studies have shown that varicose veins, accessory muscles, or other space-occupying lesions within the tarsal tunnel may be noted in these patients based on MRI or ultrasound examinations (88,89). Other investigators hypothesize that the hyperpronated foot, especially in runners, can predispose one to tarsal tunnel syndrome, but this is more controversial.

There are several nerve conduction studies that can be performed to evaluate for possible tarsal tunnel syndrome (87,90). Motor conduction studies can be performed to muscles supplied by the medial and the lateral plantar nerves. One stimulates the tibial nerve at the ankle and records from the abductor hallucis and the abductor digiti quinti pedis at the same time. There are reference values for these two muscles in the literature, but one must be especially careful about temperature control since cold feet will markedly prolong the distal latencies. These motor studies are reported to be less sensitive than CNAP studies in the diagnosis of tarsal tunnel syndrome (91).

One can also perform CNAPs of the medial and lateral plantar nerves in the foot (92). This involves stimulation of the medial and lateral plantar nerves on the sole of the foot while recording proximally just above the medial malleolus. This is a CNAP rather than a SNAP since one is in part activating motor axons antidromically in addition to the orthodromic sensory potentials. Reportedly, these studies are more sensitive to demonstrate abnormalities than motor nerve conduction studies. However, these CNAP responses are usually quite small and often difficult to obtain. Thus, absence of a response is not diagnostic by itself. An asymmetrically delayed latency is more suggestive of a diagnosis of tarsal tunnel syndrome.

Needle EMG of intrinsic foot muscles can also be useful to assess for tibial neuropathy at the ankle. Some authors believe that tarsal tunnel syndrome can be a primarily axonal injury and thus EMG may be more useful at detecting this axon loss than the nerve conduction studies (93). This point, however, is not universally accepted. Needle EMG is usually performed on a medial plantar–innervated muscle such as the abductor hallucis and a lateral plantar–innervated muscle such as one of the interossei. The FDI muscle can be used, but there is a high incidence of this muscle being jointly innervated by the deep fibular nerve (94). Thus, it is preferable to study the fourth dorsal interosseous muscle, between the fourth and fifth metatarsal bones. One must be cautious in interpreting findings on needle EMG in the intrinsic foot muscles since some studies have demonstrated a high incidence of false-positive results in otherwise healthy individuals (33). The abductor hallucis and interosseous muscles are less likely to show abnormalities than the EDB. However, one should still be cautious in interpreting mild or subtle changes.

Traumatic Neuropathies

Traumatic injury to peripheral nerves results in considerable disability across the world. In peacetime, peripheral nerve injuries commonly result from trauma due to motor vehicle accidents and less commonly from penetrating trauma, falls, and industrial accidents. Of all patients admitted to level I trauma centers, it is estimated that roughly 2% to 3% have peripheral nerve injuries (95,96). If plexus and root injuries are also included, the incidence is about 5% (95).

In the upper limb, the radial nerve is most commonly injured, followed by ulnar and median nerves (95,96). Lower limb peripheral nerve injuries are less common, with the sciatic most frequently injured, followed by fibular and rarely tibial or femoral nerves.

Seddon has used the terms "neurapraxia," "axonotmesis," and "neurotmesis" to describe peripheral nerve injuries (97). Neurapraxia is a comparatively mild injury with motor and sensory loss but no evidence of wallerian degeneration. The nerve conducts normally distally. Focal demyelination and ischemia are thought to be the etiologies of conduction block. Recovery may occur within hours, days, weeks, or up to a few months. Axonotmesis is commonly seen in crush injuries, nerve stretch injuries (such as from motor vehicle accidents and falls), or percussion injuries (such as from blast wounds). The axons and their myelin sheaths are broken, yet the surrounding stroma (i.e., the Schwann tubes, endoneurium, and perineurium) is at least partially intact. Degeneration occurs, but subsequent axonal regrowth may proceed along endoneurial tubes if they are sufficiently preserved. Recovery ultimately depends upon the degree of internal disorganization in the nerve as well as the distance to the end organ.

Neurotmesis describes a nerve that has been either completely severed or is so markedly disorganized by scar tissue that axonal regrowth is impossible. Examples are sharp injury, some traction injuries, and percussion injuries, or injection of noxious drugs. Prognosis for spontaneous recovery is quite poor without surgical intervention.

Optimal timing of electrodiagnostic studies will vary according to clinical circumstances. For circumstances in which it is important to define an injury very early, initial studies at 7 to 10 days may be useful at localization and separating conduction block from axonotmesis. On the other hand, when clinical circumstances permit waiting, studies at 3 to 4 weeks

postinjury will provide much more diagnostic information, because fibrillations will be apparent on needle EMG. Finally, in cases where a nerve injury is surgically confirmed and needle EMG is used only to document recovery, initial studies at a few months postinjury may be most useful.

Changes may be seen in the CMAP, late responses (F and H waves), SNAP, and needle EMG. Each of these studies has a somewhat different time course; they will also vary according to the severity of nerve injury.

In purely neurapraxic injuries, the CMAP will change immediately after injury, assuming one can stimulate both above and below the site of the nerve injury (**Fig. 3-15**). When recording from distal muscles and stimulating distal to the site of the injury, the CMAP should be normal because no axonal loss and no wallerian degeneration has occurred. Moving the site of stimulation proximal to the injury will produce a smaller or absent CMAP, as conduction in some or all fibers is blocked. In addition to conduction block, partial injuries also often demonstrate concomitant slowing across the injury site. This slowing may be due to either loss of faster-conducting fibers or demyelination of surviving fibers.

Electrodiagnostically, complete axonotmesis and complete neurotmesis cannot be differentiated, because the difference between these types of injuries is in the integrity of the supporting structures, which have no electrophysiologic function. Thus, these injuries can be grouped together as axonotmesis for the purpose of this discussion. Immediately after axonotmesis and for a "few days" thereafter, the CMAP and motor conduction studies look the same as those seen in a neurapraxic lesion. Nerve segments distal to the injury remain excitable and demonstrate normal conduction, whereas proximal stimulation results in an absent or small response from distal muscles. Early on, this picture looks the same as conduction block and can be confused with neurapraxia. Hence, neurapraxia and axonotmesis cannot be distinguished until sufficient time for wallerian degeneration in all motor fibers has occurred, typically about 9 days postinjury (98).

After enough time has passed for wallerian degeneration to occur, the amplitude of the CMAP elicited with distal stimulation will fall. This starts at about day 3 and is complete by about day 9 (98). Thus, in complete axonotmesis at day 9, one has a very different picture from neurapraxia. There are absent responses both above and below the injury. Partial axon loss injuries will produce small-amplitude motor responses, with the amplitude of the CMAP roughly proportional to the number of surviving axons.

F waves may change immediately after the onset of a neurapraxic injury. In complete conduction block, responses will be absent. However, in partial injuries, changes can be more subtle, because F waves are dependent upon only 3% to 5% of the axon population to elicit a response (3). Thus, partial injuries may have normal minimal F-wave latencies and mean latencies, with reduced or possibly normal penetrance. Although F waves are conceptually appealing for detecting proximal injuries (e.g., brachial plexopathies), only in a few instances do they truly provide useful additional or unique information. They are sometimes useful in very early proximal injuries when conventional studies are normal because stimulation does not occur proximal to the lesion.

The SNAP and CNAP show changes similar to the CMAP after focal nerve injury. With neurapraxia, there is focal

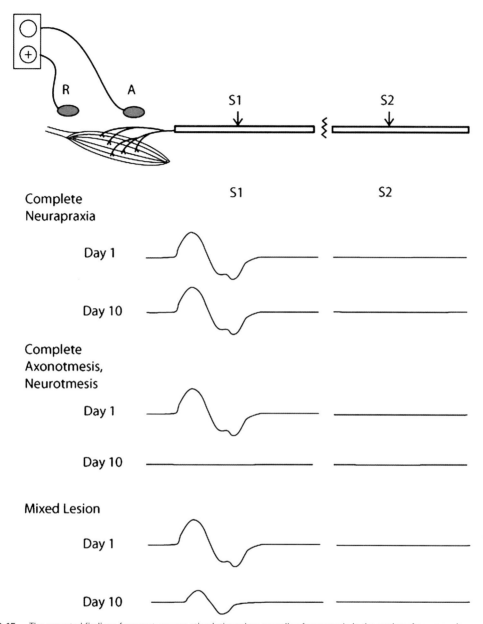

FIGURE 3-15. The expected findings from motor nerve stimulation when recording from muscle in the setting of neurapraxia, axonotmesis, and neurotmesis. Note that one cannot resolve the differences at day 1. It is only after axonal degeneration has proceeded that the distal compound muscle action potential drops in amplitude.

conduction block at the site of the lesion, with preserved distal amplitude. Immediately after axonotmesis and for a few days thereafter, the SNAP looks the same, as with a neurapraxic lesion. Nerve segments distal to the injury remain excitable and demonstrate normal conduction, whereas proximal stimulation results in an absent or small response. It takes slightly longer for sensory nerve studies to demonstrate loss of amplitude than for motor studies, that is, 11 days versus 9 days, due to the earlier failure of NMJ transmission compared with nerve conduction.

On needle EMG, in neurapraxic injuries, the most apparent changes will be in recruitment. These occur immediately after injury. In complete injuries (i.e., complete conduction block), there will be no MUAPs. In incomplete neurapraxic injuries, there will be reduced numbers of MUAPs firing more rapidly than normal (i.e., reduced or discrete recruitment). Because no axon loss occurs in neurapraxic injuries, there will be no axonal sprouting and no changes in MUAP morphology (e.g., duration, amplitude, or phasicity) at any time after injury.

With axonotmesis, needle EMG will demonstrate fibrillation potentials and positive sharp waves a number of days after injury. The time between injury and onset of fibrillation potentials will be dependent in part upon the length of the distal nerve stump. When the distal nerve stump is short, it takes only 10 to 14 days for fibrillations to develop. With a longer distal nerve stump (e.g., ulnar-innervated hand muscles in a brachial plexopathy), 21 to 30 days is required for full development of fibrillation potentials and positive sharp waves (99). Thus, the electrodiagnostic medicine consultant needs to be aware of the time since injury so that severity is not underestimated when a study is performed early after injury and so that development of increased fibrillation potentials over time is not misinterpreted as a worsening of the injury.

Fibrillation potential size decreases over time since injury. Kraft (100) has demonstrated that fibrillations initially are several hundred microvolts in the first few months after injury. However, when injuries are more than 1 year old, they are unlikely to be more than 100 µV in size.

Fibrillations may also occur after direct muscle injury as well as nerve injury. Partanen and Danner (101) have demonstrated that patients after muscle biopsy have persistent fibrillation potentials starting after 6 to 7 days and extending for up to 11 months. In patients who have undergone multiple trauma, coexisting direct muscle injury is common and can be potentially misleading when trying to localize a lesion.

When there are surviving axons after an incomplete axonal injury, remaining MUAPs are initially normal in morphology but demonstrate reduced or discrete recruitment. Axonal sprouting will be manifested by changes in morphology of existing motor units. Amplitude will increase, duration will become prolonged, and the percentage of polyphasic MUAPs will increase as motor unit territory increases (102,103). In complete injuries, the only possible mechanism of recovery is axonal regrowth from the injury site. The earliest needle EMG finding in this case is the presence of small, polyphasic, often unstable MUAPs previously referred to as "nascent potentials." (This term is now discouraged because it implies an etiology; it is preferred to simply describe the size, duration, and phasicity of the MUAP.) Observation of these potentials is dependent upon establishing axon regrowth as well as new NMJs, and this observation represents the earliest evidence of reinnervation, usually preceding the onset of clinically evident voluntary movement (102). When performing the examination looking for new MUAPs, one must be sure to accept only "crisp," nearby MUAPs with a short rise time, because distant potentials recorded from other muscles can be deceptive.

Determining the pathophysiology of a peripheral nerve traumatic injury can help with estimating prognosis. Those injuries that are completely or largely neurapraxic have a good prognosis for recovery within a few months (usually up to 3 months postinjury). Resolution of ischemia and remyelination should be complete by this time.

In axonotmesis, recovery will depend upon axonal sprouting and regeneration. Hence, there will be some early recovery followed possibly by a later recovery if or when regenerating axons reach their end organs. The amplitude of the CMAP provides some guide to prognosis. In facial nerve lesions, it has been demonstrated that patients with CMAP amplitudes 30% or more of the other side have an excellent outcome, those with 10% to 30% have good but not always complete recovery, and those with less than 10% have a poor outcome (104). There is some evidence, however, that outcomes are better in peripheral nerves than in the facial nerve (79,84).

Complete axonotmesis and neurotmesis have the worst prognosis. Recovery depends solely upon axonal regeneration, which may or may not occur, depending upon the degree of injury to the nerve. In many cases of complete axon loss, it is not possible to know the degree of nerve injury except by surgical exploration with or without intraoperative recording or looking for evidence of early reinnervation after the injury. As a consequence, it is often recommended to wait 2 to

4 months and look for evidence of reinnervation in previously completely denervated muscles near the site of the injury (105,106). Those injuries that have some spontaneous recovery are usually treated conservatively, because operative repair is unlikely to improve upon natural recovery. Those with no evidence of axonal regrowth often have operative exploration with possible grafting.

Radiculopathy

Radiculopathy is another common reason for electrodiagnostic assessment. The electrodiagnostic evaluation can be useful to assess for the presence of active radiculopathy, for identifying which root(s) are involved, and exploring other possible diagnoses that may be confused with root disease (12).

The typical clinical presentation of radiculopathy is well covered in other chapters. Most commonly, it involves pain starting from the neck or the back and extending into the upper or lower limb. It is often accompanied by sensory symptoms and sometimes by weakness. Physical examination may show weakness, depressed reflexes, and positive relevant provocative signs (such as straight leg raise test or Spurling's sign). Although sensory loss is often found, this is not as predominant or as well circumscribed as it might be in peripheral nerve lesions.

The etiology of radiculopathy can be multifactorial (107). There are certain structural injuries such as disk protrusions and bony lesions that can press upon the root. However, the electrodiagnostic medical consultant should keep in mind that there are other causes of radiculopathy as well. Neoplasms either at the root or spinal cord level can look like a radiculopathy. There are metabolic or inflammatory processes such as diabetes or vasculitis, which can produce a radiculopathy without significant structural changes apparent on imaging studies. There are also infectious causes such as herpes zoster that can affect the roots. Thus, not all radiculopathies are caused by disk or bony impingement.

In general, the most useful electrodiagnostic assessment in radiculopathy is needle EMG. There have been studies suggesting how many muscles should be studied in a limb when assessing for possibly radiculopathy (108,109). It is generally preferable to examine at least six muscles in the lower limb and six muscles in the upper limb (including paraspinal muscles) to reach a high degree of sensitivity on needle EMG. When the paraspinal muscles are not available, such as after surgical intervention, then one should increase the number of limb muscles to eight to achieve a similar degree of sensitivity.

The selection of muscles should be tailored to each patient depending on which root level is in question. For example, if the patient's symptoms are more in the C6 distribution, one should include more C6 level muscles and perhaps fewer muscles at the C8 or T1 levels. When symptoms are nonspecific, then one should design an electrodiagnostic evaluation that includes multiple roots and multiple peripheral nerves within the limb. Examples of commonly used screens are in **Box 3-2**.

The key to diagnosing radiculopathy is to find evidence of denervation in at least two muscles within a single myotome (the distribution of muscles supplied by a single root) but supplied by different peripheral nerves (12). For example, evidence of denervation in the TA and fibularis longus muscles would

BOX 3-2

Sample Radiculopathy Screens for Needle EMG

Upper Limb Radiculopathy Screen	Lower Limb Radiculopathy Screen
Deltoid	Vastus medialis
Biceps	Tensor fascia lata
Pronator teres	Tibialis anterior
Triceps	Medial gastrocnemius
First dorsal interosseous	Biceps femoris long head
Cervical paraspinal muscles	Lumbar paraspinal muscles

not be sufficient to diagnose an L5 radiculopathy because both muscles are within the common fibular nerve distribution. However, the same changes in the TA and tensor fascia lata would be much more suggestive of a root lesion.

It's useful to consider which findings are diagnostic when found in a myotomal distribution. Most electromyographers would agree that evidence of the following potentials in a myotomal distribution would be diagnostic:

- Fibrillation potentials
- Positive sharp waves
- Complex repetitive discharges
- Fasciculation potentials

It is more controversial as to which MUAP changes should be considered diagnostic. If there are very large-amplitude, long-duration, polyphasic MUAPs in a myotomal distribution, then one might interpret the study as suggestive of chronic radiculopathy with reinnervation. However, one should not diagnose a radiculopathy based solely upon increased numbers of polyphasic MUAPs, since these are often found in otherwise healthy individuals in many muscles (12).

The paraspinal muscles can be useful to localize an injury to the root level, since these muscles are supplied by the posterior primary ramus of the root. Evidence of denervation in these muscles, combined with the limb muscles, is suggestive of root pathology. At the same time, one should be cautious in interpreting paraspinal findings. Some authors have reported the presence of fibrillation potentials and positive sharp waves in otherwise healthy individuals in the lumbar and cervical paraspinal muscles, with an increasing frequency with age (32,110), but not all investigators have corroborated these findings (34). Moreover, there are other causes for fibrillation potentials in the paraspinal muscles besides radiculopathy. For instance, myopathies, prior spine surgery, recent prior needle intervention, metastatic muscle lesions, and diabetes can all cause paraspinal abnormalities without significant radiculopathy. Moreover, the paraspinal muscles are not localizing since most of the muscles are multisegmentally innervated (111). Localization is primarily achieved through analysis of limb muscle findings.

In addition to needle EMG, H waves can be useful in diagnosing S1 radiculopathies. The primary advantage of H waves in the assessment of radiculopathy is that they will detect sensory axon loss, conduction block, and demyelination in the root, whereas needle EMG only detects loss of motor axons (20). Side-to-side differences in H-wave latency exceeding 1.2 to 1.5 ms are likely abnormal. A limitation is that any injury along the pathway (from the soleus muscle to the S1 root) can cause abnormalities in this response. Moreover, H-wave abnormalities

do not indicate chronicity, and these responses can be abnormal in very acute or very chronic or old root lesions.

Sensory responses should usually be normal in root pathology since here the injury is proximal to the DRG. F waves are generally of little use in evaluation of radiculopathy. It is believed that since muscles are supplied by more than one root, the responses traverse more than one root proximally, and a single intact root can produce normal F-wave latencies.

The electrodiagnostic medical consultant is often asked about the sensitivity of needle EMG and comparison to imaging studies. Generally, the EMG is considered to have a sensitivity for radiculopathy in the range of 70% to 80% compared to clinical presentation (108,112,113). This is in contrast to imaging studies, which are often reported with sensitivities exceeding 90%.

Sensitivity, however, is not the only figure of merit. One should be equally or even more concerned about specificity, that is, the ability to detect absence of disease and to avoid false-positive findings (64). Specificity of needle EMG, using the approach discussed above, is excellent, likely exceeding 95%. If one were to make a diagnosis based solely upon paraspinal findings or a few polyphasic motor units, the specificity would be less. In contrast, the specificity of imaging is much lower. Many studies have reported imaging specificities in the 60% to 70% range, with a false-positive rate of 30% to 40% (114). Thus, a primary advantage of needle EMG is the high specificity it offers in comparison to imaging studies.

Plexopathy

The assessment of brachial and lumbosacral plexopathy is aided considerably by the electrodiagnostic examination (115). The etiologies of brachial plexopathy are varied. Most common in adults are motorcycle crashes, motor vehicle crashes, falls, and industrial injuries, which account for the great majority of brachial plexus lesions. It is estimated that 2% to 3% of patients coming to level 1 trauma centers have a brachial plexus injury (95). There are other causes of brachial plexus lesions such as neuralgic amyotrophy, radiation plexitis, tumor invasion, true neurogenic thoracic outlet syndrome, and others.

Lumbosacral plexopathies are much less common. Traumatic lumbosacral plexopathies occur in less than 1% of patients with pelvic fractures (116). The placement of the lumbosacral plexus within the pelvis offers a great deal of protection compared to the relatively vulnerable brachial plexus in the upper limb and shoulder. The lumbosacral plexus nevertheless can be affected by trauma, radiation plexitis, tumor, diabetes, and neuralgic amyotrophy, all of which are rare.

Patients with plexopathy can present variably. Typically, there is pain in the limb (but not the spine) and there are sensory symptoms in the limb. Occasionally, patients present with a plexopathy after breast cancer and subsequent radiation; those with radiation plexitis typically have upper trunk distribution paresthesias, whereas those with tumor invasion present with lower trunk painful lesions (39). Physical examination is usually remarkable for weakness, significant sensory loss outside of a single peripheral nerve distribution, and reduced reflexes.

Sensory nerve conduction studies can be very useful to differentiate plexus injuries from more proximal root pathology. As has been discussed above, root injuries will have normal SNAPs, whereas plexus injuries (distal to the DRG) will have abnormal or absent sensory responses. This fact can be used to screen the brachial plexus. For example, one can evaluate the upper trunk through the use of median and radial nerve sensory testing to the thumb (C6). The middle trunk can be evaluated by stimulating the median nerve and recording from the long finger (C7), and the lower trunk can be evaluated by testing the ulnar sensory potential to the small finger (C8) (117). If these are all intact, it would argue strongly against a brachial plexus injury affecting the upper, middle, or lower trunks. Similarly, one can use SNAPs in the lower limb to evaluate for peripheral nerve or plexus injuries versus root pathology.

The reader should be aware of a rather unique setting in which the presence of normal sensory potentials is a very poor prognostic sign. When a patient is evaluated for traumatic brachial plexopathy, at times they will have complete root injuries such as root avulsion rather than a more distal brachial plexus lesion. When the roots have been avulsed from the spinal cord, this is a very poor prognosis and there is essentially no likelihood of recovery. In this setting, the SNAPs will be normal because the dorsal root ganglia have been avulsed along with the plexus and there is no subsequent degeneration of sensory axons. However, needle EMG will be consistent with complete denervation and no motor responses will be obtainable. In this case, presence of normal sensory potentials generally suggests root avulsion and a very poor prognosis for recovery, though these findings do not always agree with imaging studies (118).

Motor nerve conduction studies are also useful in the assessment of brachial plexopathy, particularly for prognosis. One can determine the degree of axon loss by recording from an affected muscle and stimulating the nerve distal to the lesion. For example, in the case of an upper trunk plexus lesion, one might stimulate the musculocutaneous nerve and record from biceps. A large-amplitude response here, assuming enough time has occurred for wallerian degeneration, would indicate a rather good prognosis since there is unlikely to be severe axon loss.

Needle EMG can also be helpful in diagnosing and localizing brachial plexopathy. These are usually very extensive evaluations. This author generally finds it helpful to draw out the plexus in question and can make sure that a muscle supplied by each of the significant branches off the plexus is tested on needle EMG. Paraspinal muscles are also useful as abnormalities there will suggest a more proximal root injury.

F-wave responses can be helpful early on in a possible brachial plexus lesion, before motor or sensory conduction studies have changed and before needle EMG shows abnormalities. Absence of F waves may indicate a proximal injury particularly if distal conduction is intact. However, it should be remembered that an abnormality anywhere along the course of the F wave will produce an abnormal response. In the setting of more chronic pathology, it is rare that the F wave will show a unique abnormality that is not apparent on other nerve conduction studies or needle EMG.

Polyneuropathies

The goal of electrodiagnostic evaluation in assessing peripheral polyneuropathies is to both detect abnormalities and classify the neuropathy into one of six broad groups. One should also determine whether there are other lesions (such as spinal stenosis) that can produce similar clinical presentations.

It's useful to consider six categories in which one can place peripheral polyneuropathies. These are well covered in other references (119). The six categories will be discussed briefly below.

Uniform Demyelinating Neuropathies

Uniform demyelinating neuropathies are inherited neuropathies in which myelin is abnormal throughout the peripheral nervous system. Examples include Charcot-Marie-Tooth disease (type 1), Refsum's disease, Dejerine-Sottas disease, and others. Because of the diffuse abnormality of myelin, one sees uniform nonsegmental changes. In these uniform demyelinating neuropathies, one sees diffuse slowing of NCVs (without patchiness), prolonged distal latencies, and prolonged or absent F-wave responses. There is generally no conduction block or temporal dispersion. Generally, motor fibers are more affected than sensory fibers. Needle EMG can reveal mild evidence of distal denervation, but this is not as marked as the slowing that is apparent on nerve conduction studies.

Segmental Demyelinating Neuropathies

Segmental demyelinating neuropathies are acquired neuropathies (not inherited) that present with patchy demyelination along the peripheral nervous system. Examples include acute inflammatory demyelinating polyradiculoneuropathy and chronic inflammatory demyelinating polyradiculoneuropathy (AIDP and CIDP), monoclonal gammopathies of undetermined significance, multiple myeloma, and others. The hallmark of this category is patchiness of abnormalities. Generally, there are five findings seen on nerve conduction studies in this group including

1. Prolonged distal latencies
2. Prolonged or absent F-wave responses
3. Patchy slowing (faster in some areas, slower in other areas of the same nerve)
4. Conduction block
5. Temporal dispersion

This can generally be differentiated from the inherited neuropathies mentioned above by the presence of patchy slowing, conduction block, and temporal dispersion. Needle EMG will often show patchy denervation in more severe cases. Motor findings are more prominent than sensory findings in these patients. Many of these patients will have sparing of sural SNAPs but relatively greater abnormalities noted in the upper limb sensory responses. Prognosis in these cases has been shown to correlate best with the distal CMAP amplitudes (120). When amplitudes are larger than 10% of the lower limit of normal, prognosis is generally good.

Sensory Neuropathy or Neuronopathy

Sensory neurons can be selectively affected at their cell bodies (neuronopathy) or axons (neuropathy). There are a variety of processes that predominantly affect sensory nerves. At the cell body level, there is an entity that is known as dorsal root ganglionitis or sensory neuronopathy. This represents death of the cell body within the DRG and subsequent loss of sensory axons. Most commonly, this is seen as a paraneoplastic presentation, but occasionally autoimmune diseases can present with the same findings (121,122). Selective loss of sensory axons distally can be seen in a variety of toxins such as B6 toxicity, cis-platinum exposure, and others.

The hallmark of this category is the absence of SNAPs or reduction in their amplitudes. When these presentations are severe, one will be unable to obtain a sensory response anywhere in the limbs. In general, motor nerve conduction and needle EMG are normal as expected with selective involvement of sensory nerves.

Motor Greater than Sensory Axon Loss

Motor greater than sensory neuropathies are rare. In evaluating these patients, one should be wary of other diseases that can present with similar findings such as motor neuron disease, NMJ disease, or myopathy. Selective motor neuropathies can be seen in acute porphyria, heavy metal exposure, and exposure to vinca alkaloids (123), among other conditions. Occasionally, inherited neuropathies (e.g., Charcot-Marie-Tooth disease type 2) also present this way (124).

The primary abnormality in this category is reduced amplitude or absent motor responses with relatively normal SNAPs. Needle EMG usually shows length-dependent evidence of denervation in the limb muscles with more distal muscles showing greater abnormalities than proximal limb muscles. There is usually not significant slowing of nerve conduction studies in this group, although mild slowing could be present due to loss of faster-conducting fibers.

Motor and Sensory Axon Loss

This is the most common presentation of polyneuropathy and has the greatest number of etiologies among all the categories. This group includes the majority of toxic exposures, paraneoplastic conditions, infectious diseases (such as HIV), and other etiologies. One sees reduced amplitude sensory and motor potential on nerve conduction studies with relatively little slowing. Needle EMG also shows length-dependent evidence of denervation worse in the distal muscles of the limb. In many cases, the exact etiology of these polyneuropathies remains undetermined even after extensive investigation. Only about 60% of these patients will ultimately have an etiologic diagnosis. Guidelines can help direct the laboratory workup of these patients (125,126).

Motor and Sensory Axon Loss and Demyelination

There are two common diseases that present with motor and sensory axon loss and demyelination: diabetes and uremia. These two diseases present with a mixture of reduction of SNAP amplitudes, reduced amplitude CMAPs, mild-to-moderate slowing of conduction, and evidence of denervation worse distally in the limbs.

Approach to Polyneuropathies

When evaluating possible polyneuropathy, it's reasonable to start by performing motor and sensory conduction studies and F waves in one upper limb and one lower limb. This author's approach is generally to perform the following nerve conductions: sural sensory, fibular motor, fibular F wave, ulnar sensory, ulnar motor, and ulnar F wave (the advantage of ulnar nerve studies is that it avoids possible misinterpretation resulting from median neuropathy at the wrist). If the symptoms are primarily in the lower limb and the lower limb nerve conduction studies are normal, it may not be necessary to study the upper limb.

Needle EMG should be performed routinely because it is more sensitive at detecting motor axon loss than nerve conduction studies. The TA and soleus muscles are useful muscles, and occasionally one may study an interosseous muscle in the foot. When there are abnormalities seen in the lower limb, other muscles should be studied in the lower limb as well as some upper limb muscles to determine whether this represents a distal greater than proximal gradient.

The electromyographer needs to be aware of the effects of temperature upon nerve conduction studies. If the limb is excessively cold, less than 32°C, it is generally preferable to warm up the limb with a hairdryer, warm water, or other methodology. The use of correction factors, particularly for correction across many degrees of temperature, is discouraged.

In writing the report, it is usually not possible to definitively indicate the cause of the polyneuropathy in the patient being studied. However, one can indicate the category as discussed above and include a differential diagnosis, which fits with the clinical presentation.

Myopathy

EMG is useful in the assessment of patients with possible muscle disease.

Generally, patients presenting with a possible myopathy will primarily report symptoms of proximal weakness. They often report difficulty climbing stairs, difficulty brushing their hair or teeth, and at times difficulty with breathing or coughing. Some patients will have muscle pain or tenderness. If there are any sensory symptoms, then an alternative diagnosis should be considered. On examination, one will generally note proximal greater than distal weakness. Trendelenburg's sign is often present and may be either compensated or uncompensated. Reflexes are usually preserved until late in the progression of the disease.

The diagnosis of a specific myopathy depends upon multiple evaluations. First, the clinical presentation needs to be consistent with myopathy. In addition, laboratory values should usually show elevated muscle enzymes such as creatine kinase. Muscle biopsy is often important to arrive at a more definitive diagnosis in terms of what type of myopathy is present. Finally, EMG can demonstrate abnormalities that can help in determining the presence and activity and sometimes help with diagnosis of the myopathy (127,128).

In general, one should approach the patient with myopathy by studying only one side of the patient (right or left). This is important because many patients will have a subsequent muscle biopsy and it is preferable to avoid histologic examination of muscles that have had a recent needle EMG examination. Muscle trauma from the EMG needle can sometimes mimic changes from inflammation.

It is often helpful to study both proximal and distal muscles in the limb to look for a proximal greater than distal gradient since proximal muscles should be affected considerably more than distal muscles. One major exception to this rule is myotonic dystrophy, which presents with distal findings greater than proximal (129). Even though they are not easily biopsied, the EMG evaluation should usually include paraspinal muscles as they are very sensitive. It is also wise to include muscles that can be biopsied on the contralateral side such as quadriceps, biceps, or deltoid.

On needle EMG, many acquired myopathies and inherited dystrophies will be associated with fibrillations and positive sharp waves, especially when there is inflammation. It is hypothesized that inflammation induces segmental necrosis. As a result of this focal necrosis, distal portions of the muscle fibers are functionally denervated and fibrillate. When there is no inflammation, such as with chronic steroid myopathy (which produces selective type II fiber atrophy), needle EMG will be relatively normal at rest. In inflammatory myopathies, the presence of fibrillation potentials and positive sharp waves is suggestive of more active disease, whereas muscles studied in those with treated disease will often have no significant spontaneous activity (130,131). CRDs are commonly seen in myopathies, especially in chronic inflammatory myopathies, though they are not specific for muscle disease. At times, one will see needle EMG potentials in muscles that will help refine the diagnosis further. For instance, the presence of myotonic discharges will indicate that the patient may have a myotonic syndrome such as myotonic dystrophy, myotonia congenita, acid maltase deficiency, or other rare diseases.

As mentioned earlier, MUAPs in myopathies are generally small in amplitude, brief in duration, and sometimes polyphasic. They are recruited in an "early" pattern with many MUAPs firing despite small amounts of force.

On nerve conduction studies, SNAPs should generally be normal without any significant slowing or changes in amplitude. On the other hand, CMAPs may be reduced in size, proportional to the degree of muscle fiber loss. Conduction velocity is usually preserved.

After the needle EMG has been completed, it is often helpful for the electromyographer to suggest some potential contralateral muscles for subsequent muscle biopsy. Generally, it is good to select a muscle with moderate disease. If one selects a muscle with very severe electrodiagnostic changes, often the muscle biopsy will be read as end-stage muscle disease and will offer little specificity as to the etiology.

At times, the EMG is especially useful in inflammatory myopathies treated with steroids. In those patients with polymyositis who have initial recovery but later weakness, there is often a question as to whether this represents recurrence of the inflammatory disease or new steroid myopathy. In disease recurrence, one sees increased spontaneous activity such as fibrillation potentials and positive sharp waves (132). However, if a patient has steroid myopathy, which does not cause segmental necrosis or muscle fiber loss, one will see a relatively normal needle EMG both in terms of spontaneous activity and initially recruited MUAPs (133).

Critical illness myopathy is probably the most common myopathy seen in patients admitted to the hospital (134). This commonly coexists with critical illness polyneuropathy, but the former has a better prognosis (135). Findings are not always pronounced, but usually demonstrate small-amplitude CMAPs, normal SNAPs (unless there is coexisting polyneuropathy), and proximal greater than distal needle EMG abnormalities. It is often difficult to examine MUAPs since these patients are often not alert enough to produce a muscle contraction. There are recently described techniques for direct muscle stimulation, which have suggested that much of the weakness noted in the ICU is due to critical illness myopathy (136).

Motor Neuron Disease

Motor neuron disease can have multiple presentations, which are well covered in other chapters in this textbook, the most common of which is ALS. ALS is characterized by both upper UMN and LMN loss as well as involvement of both bulbar and limb muscles. ALS usually starts off with focal weakness without any sensory loss and with little or no pain. The weakness can be in the distal upper or lower limb or, especially in the older individuals, in the bulbar musculature. Fasciculations are often noted by the patient and reported to the physician.

There are several symptoms and/or signs that make the diagnosis of ALS unlikely including presence of sensory symptoms such as numbness or tingling, presence of urinary incontinence, or deficits in extraocular muscles.

There are other variants of motor neuron disease in addition to ALS (137). Primary lateral sclerosis (PLS) presents with selective involvement of the corticospinal tracks in the brain and spinal cord. These patients have upper motor neuron syndromes without significant atrophy or evidence of LMN loss. They have a somewhat better prognosis than ALS, but some eventually progress into full-blown ALS. Progressive bulbar palsy (PBP) starts off with weakness primarily in the bulbar muscles. Most commonly, patients present with slurring of speech or difficulty swallowing. This often quickly evolves into full-blown ALS and has a worse prognosis than if the onset were in the limbs instead. Spinal muscular atrophy (SMA) is a predominantly LMN loss, which has a slower disease progression and somewhat better prognosis than does ALS. It does not have prominent upper motor neuron features. Monomelic amyotrophy looks like ALS clinically but is confined to one limb and has a much better prognosis. It usually has both upper and LMN features in one limb without any sensory changes.

With respect to ALS, physical examination usually shows weakness in either one limb or, as the disease becomes advanced, more diffusely. There is often dysphagia and slurring of speech, which are worrisome signs. There should be no significant sensory loss unless there is a coexisting lesion such as sensory polyneuropathy. Reflexes are typically brisk, consistent with the upper motor neuron involvement. However, at the same time, there is usually muscle atrophy, which suggests LMN loss.

When evaluating a patient with possible motor neuron disease, it is best for the patient if the electromyographer can identify some other (treatable) cause of the patient's symptoms. At times, myopathies, NMJ diseases, cervical spinal stenosis, and multifocal motor neuropathy with conduction block (138) can all mimic ALS. In contrast to ALS, these are treatable diseases without rapid progression to death.

Nerve conduction studies are first performed to evaluate for polyneuropathy or to look for multifocal motor neuropathy with conduction block. It is generally useful to study one motor and one sensory nerve in an upper and lower limb, with multiple sites of stimulation, in addition to F waves. In ALS, these are usually normal except for potentially reduced amplitudes of the CMAPs. If there is conduction block, then other diagnoses should be considered.

Needle EMG is often performed according to the diagnostic requirements of the El Escorial criteria (139), though the more recent Awaji criteria allow for earlier diagnosis (140). These criteria divide the body into four regions: bulbar, cervical, thoracic, and lumbosacral. The electromyographer should

TABLE 3-2	**Awaji Criteria Summary**
Definite	Clinical or neurophysiologic evidence of UMN and LMN dysfunction in the bulbar region and at least two spinal regions, or three spinal regions
Probable	Clinical or neurophysiologic evidence of UMN and LMN dysfunction in at least two spinal regions with some UMN signs rostral to the LMN signs
Possible	Clinical or neurophysiologic evidence of UMN and LMN dysfunction in one region, or UMN signs evident in two regions, or LMN dysfunction evident rostral to UMN signs

The definition of LMN dysfunction using the Awaji criteria is (a) presence of fibrillation potentials and positive sharp waves or fasciculation potentials, (b) evidence of reinnervation (large-amplitude, long-duration polyphasic motor unit action potentials), and (c) reduced interference on full contraction with increased firing motor unit rate upon voluntary contraction. In order for a region to be classified as affected, the neurophysiologic changes have to be evident in a minimum of two muscles innervated by different nerve roots and nerves for spinal and lumbosacral regions and a minimum of one muscle in the bulbar/thoracic regions. The assessment of upper motor neuron dysfunction remains clinically based.

study muscles from each of these regions to look for evidence of denervation, fasciculation potentials, or reinnervation. The Awaji criteria are summarized in **Table 3-2** (141).

The thoracic paraspinal muscles are especially important to study because they are commonly affected in motor neuron disease (142). Moreover, when abnormal, they help to exclude the presence of combined cervical and lumbar spinal stenosis, which could result in abnormalities in both the upper and lower limbs. Likewise, the bulbar muscles are very important because when abnormal, they help to exclude spine disease as the cause of the patient's presentation.

The primary finding on needle EMG is that of acute denervation, with positive sharp waves and fibrillations. Although fasciculation potentials are not required for a definitive diagnosis, their presence is much more suggestive of motor neuron disease than when they are absent. The presence of large-amplitude polyphasic long-duration MUAPs is suggestive of chronic reinnervation and should be seen in the limbs as well as evidence of denervation. Often, reduced recruitment with rapid firing of MUAPs is one of the first findings in ALS. Since progressive motor neuron loss can often be compensated by distal sprouting, there may not be prominent fibrillation potentials early in the disease.

Generally, when evaluating the patient with motor neuron disease, it is preferable not to discuss the findings or even the differential diagnosis with the patient or in front of the patient unless he or she has already been discussing this with a referring physician. Getting into a discussion during the study often prompts questions, which the electromyographer is not prepared to answer.

REPORT WRITING

After the electrodiagnostic examination has been completed, one then writes the electrodiagnostic report. This usually includes several elements such as:

- Identifying information (name, medical record number, date of birth, name of referring physician, name of examining physician, and date of study).

- Brief history and physical (enough to support your differential diagnosis, but not so long as to repeat extensive notes from the medial record).
- *Electrodiagnostic data* should be presented in tabular form with pertinent findings listed in the tables. Most recent electrodiagnostic instruments can automatically prepare these reports in a word processing document, but the electromyographer should use caution when employing this feature. Because the instruments will automatically place cursors on all waveforms, at times the automated reports will give cursor information when no response is in fact present. The electromyographer should review these tables to make sure that they are accurate and that responses are listed as absent when they are unobtainable.
- Summary of findings (how you interpret the findings— e.g., "there is evidence of acute denervation in the C7 myotome" or "there is slowing of median motor and sensory conduction across the wrist"). The physician should not repeat what's in the data tables in this section.
- The *impression or conclusion* should be succinct and should clearly address the referring physician's question. It should include whether the study was normal or abnormal, which diagnoses were ruled in, important diagnoses that were ruled out, pathophysiology, and prognosis when appropriate. This section should be able to stand alone, since some referring physicians will only read this part of the report. It should also give the side (right or left) and the pathophysiology (e.g., axon loss or demyelination). At times, the electromyographer will not have a final diagnosis but will have a differential diagnosis, and this should be clearly stated in the impression (it is better to give a differential diagnosis than to simply guess what it might be).
- At times, the study will be normal. In these cases, the electrodiagnostic medical consultant will want to report, "There is no electrodiagnostic evidence of...." Other times, the electromyographer will have a different diagnosis than the referring diagnosis. In these cases, one should comment on the referring diagnosis as well as the diagnosis found during the study.

Guidelines for what should go in the report are also available on the website of the American Association of Electrodiagnostic and Neuromuscular Medicine (http://www.aanem.org/practiceissues/practiceguidelines/practiceguidelines.cfm).

In most cases, one should assume that the patient may read the medical record and take care in the use of wording that might be offensive or might be interpreted as derogatory (e.g., obese or argumentative).

SUMMARY

In summary, the electrodiagnostic evaluation is critical to the understanding of nerve and muscle disease, to the management of peripheral nervous system disease, and to assessing prognosis for a variety of lesions that the physiatrist will encounter. It is an important tool that extends the clinical skills of the physiatrist in assessing and treating patients with diseases or injuries to the peripheral nervous system.

REFERENCES

1. Hansen PA, Micklesen P, Robinson LR. Clinical utility of the flick maneuver in diagnosing carpal tunnel syndrome. *Am J Phys Med Rehabil.* 2004;83:363–367.
2. Robinson LR. Traumatic injury to peripheral nerves. *Muscle Nerve.* 2000;23:863–873.
3. Fisher MA. AAEM minimonograph #13: H reflexes and F waves: physiology and clinical indications. *Muscle Nerve.* 1992;15:1223–1233.
4. Mesrati F, Vecchierini MF. F-waves: neurophysiology and clinical value. *Neurophysiol Clin.* 2004;34:217–243.
5. Panayiotopoulos CP, Chroni E. F-waves in clinical neurophysiology: a review, methodological issues and overall value in peripheral neuropathies. *Electroencephalogr Clin Neurophysiol.* 1996;101:365–374.
6. Dreyer SJ, Dumitru D, King JC. Anodal block V anodal stimulation. Fact or fiction. *Am J Phys Med Rehabil.* 1993;72:10–18.
7. DiBenedetto M, Gale SD, Adarmes D, et al. F-wave acquisition using low-current stimulation. *Muscle Nerve.* 2003;28:82–86.
8. Taniguchi S, Kimura J, Yanagisawa T, et al. Rest-induced suppression of anterior horn cell excitability as measured by F waves: comparison between volitionally inactivated and control muscles. *Muscle Nerve.* 2008;37:343–349.
9. Vucic S, Cairns KD, Black KR, et al. Neurophysiologic findings in early acute inflammatory demyelinating polyradiculoneuropathy. *Clin Neurophysiol.* 2004;115:2329–2335.
10. Wallbom AS, Geisser ME, Haig AJ, et al. Alterations of F wave parameters after exercise in symptomatic lumbar spinal stenosis. *Am J Phys Med Rehabil.* 2008;87:270–274.
11. Bal S, Celiker R, Palaoglu S, et al. F wave studies of neurogenic intermittent claudication in lumbar spinal stenosis. *Am J Phys Med Rehabil.* 2006;85:135–140.
12. Wilbourn AJ, Aminoff MJ. AAEE minimonograph #32: the electrophysiologic examination in patients with radiculopathies. *Muscle Nerve.* 1988;11:1099–1114.
13. Toyokura M, Furukawa T. F wave duration in mild S1 radiculopathy: comparison between the affected and unaffected sides. *Clin Neurophysiol.* 2002;113:1231–1235.
14. Misiaszek JE. The H-reflex as a tool in neurophysiology: its limitations and uses in understanding nervous system function. *Muscle Nerve.* 2003;28:144–160.
15. Raynor EM, Shefner JM. Recurrent inhibition is decreased in patients with amyotrophic lateral sclerosis. *Neurology.* 1994;44:2148–2153.
16. Little JW, Hayward LF, Halar E. Monopolar recording of H reflexes at various sites. *Electromyogr Clin Neurophysiol.* 1989;29:213–219.
17. Panizza M, Nilsson J, Hallett M. Optimal stimulus duration for the H reflex. *Muscle Nerve.* 1989;12:576–579.
18. Gitter AJ, Stolov WC. AAEM minimonograph #16: instrumentation and measurement in electrodiagnostic medicine—Part II. *Muscle Nerve.* 1995;18:812–824.
19. Jankus WR, Robinson LR, Little JW. Normal limits of side-to-side H-reflex amplitude variability. *Arch Phys Med Rehabil.* 1994;75:3–7.
20. Braddom RI, Johnson EW. Standardization of H reflex and diagnostic use in SI radiculopathy. *Arch Phys Med Rehabil.* 1974;55:161–166.
21. Rowin J, Meriggioli MN. Electrodiagnostic significance of supramaximally stimulated A-waves. *Muscle Nerve.* 2000;23:1117–1120.
22. Fullerton PM, Gilliatt RW. Axon reflexes in human motor nerve fibres. *J Neurol Neurosurg Psychiatry.* 1965;28:1–11.
23. Floeter MK. Structure and Function of Muscle Fibers and Motor Units. Cambridge, UK: Cambridge University Press; 2010.
24. Wright KC, Ramsey-Goldman R, Nielsen VK, et al. Syndrome of diffuse abnormal insertional activity: case report and family study. *Arch Phys Med Rehabil.* 1988;69:534–536.
25. Ceyssens C, Van de Walle JP, Bruyninckx F, et al. The anterior compartment syndrome in the lower leg. Review and role of the EMG examination. *Acta Belg Med Phys.* 1990;13:195–199.
26. Daube JR. AAEM minimonograph #11: needle examination in clinical electromyography. *Muscle Nerve.* 1991;14:685–700.
27. Dumitru D. Single muscle fiber discharges (insertional activity, end-plate potentials, positive sharp waves, and fibrillation potentials): a unifying proposal. *Muscle Nerve.* 1996;19:221–226; discussion 7–30.
28. Dumitru D, Martinez CT. Propagated insertional activity: a model of positive sharp wave generation. *Muscle Nerve.* 2006;34:457–462.
29. Dumitru D, Santa Maria DL. Positive sharp wave origin: evidence supporting the electrode initiation hypothesis. *Muscle Nerve.* 2007;36:349–356.
30. Herbison GJ, Jaweed MM, Ditunno JF Jr. Acetylcholine sensitivity and fibrillation potentials in electrically stimulated crush-denervated rat skeletal muscle. *Arch Phys Med Rehabil.* 1983;64:217–220.
31. Date ES, Mar EY, Bugola MR, et al. The prevalence of lumbar paraspinal spontaneous activity in asymptomatic subjects. *Muscle Nerve.* 1996;19:350–354.
32. Date ES, Kim BJ, Yoon JS, et al. Cervical paraspinal spontaneous activity in asymptomatic subjects. *Muscle Nerve.* 2006;34:361–364.
33. Gatens PF, Saeed MA. Electromyographic findings in the intrinsic muscles of normal feet. *Arch Phys Med Rehabil.* 1982;63:317–318.
34. Dumitru D, Diaz CA, King JC. Prevalence of denervation in paraspinal and foot intrinsic musculature. *Am J Phys Med Rehabil.* 2001;80:482–490.
35. Kimura J. *Electrodiagnosis in Diseases of Nerve and Muscle: Principles and Practice.* 3rd ed. Oxford, UK/New York: Oxford University Press; 2001.
36. Layzer RB. The origin of muscle fasciculations and cramps. *Muscle Nerve.* 1994;17:1243–1249.
37. Jansen PH, van Dijck JA, Verbeek AL, et al. Estimation of the frequency of the muscular pain-fasciculation syndrome and the muscular cramp-fasciculation syndrome in the adult population. *Eur Arch Psychiatry Clin Neurosci.* 1991;241:102–104.
38. Gutmann L. AAEM minimonograph #37: facial and limb myokymia. *Muscle Nerve.* 1991;14:1043–1049.
39. Lederman RJ, Wilbourn AJ. Brachial plexopathy: recurrent cancer or radiation? *Neurology.* 1984;34:1331–1335.
40. Miller TM. Differential diagnosis of myotonic disorders. *Muscle Nerve.* 2008;37:293–299.
41. Sacco G, Buchthal F, Rosenfalck P. Motor unit potentials at different ages. *Arch Neurol.* 1962;6:366–373.
42. Rich MM. The control of neuromuscular transmission in health and disease. *Neuroscientist.* 2006;12:134–142.
43. Chiou-Tan FY. Electromyographic approach to neuromuscular junction disorders repetitive nerve stimulation and single-fiber electromyography. *Phys Med Rehabil Clin N Am.* 2003;14:387–401.
44. McComas AJ, Galea V, Einhorn RW. Pseudofacilitation: a misleading term. *Muscle Nerve.* 1994;17:599–607.
45. Kalamida D, Poulas K, Avramopoulou V, et al. Muscle and neuronal nicotinic acetylcholine receptors. Structure, function and pathogenicity. *FEBS J.* 2007;274:3799–3845.
46. Massey JM. Acquired myasthenia gravis. *Neurol Clin.* 1997;15:577–595.
47. Adams PJ, Snutch TP. Calcium channelopathies: voltage-gated calcium channels. *Subcell Biochem.* 2007;45:215–251.
48. Sanders DB. Electrophysiologic tests of neuromuscular transmission. *Suppl Clin Neurophysiol.* 2004;57:167–169.
49. Shukla HD, Sharma SK. Clostridium botulinum: a bug with beauty and weapon. *Crit Rev Microbiol.* 2005;31:11–18.
50. Zinman LH, O'Connor PW, Dadson KE, et al. Sensitivity of repetitive facial-nerve stimulation in patients with myasthenia gravis. *Muscle Nerve.* 2006;33:694–696.
51. Niks EH, Badrising UA, Verschuuren JJ, et al. Decremental response of the nasalis and hypothenar muscles in myasthenia gravis. *Muscle Nerve.* 2003;28:236–238.
52. Campbell WW, Pridgeon RM, Riaz G, et al. Sparing of the flexor carpi ulnaris in ulnar neuropathy at the elbow. *Muscle Nerve.* 1989;12:965–967.
53. Terzis S, Paschalis C, Metallinos IC, et al. Early diagnosis of carpal tunnel syndrome: comparison of sensory conduction studies of four fingers. *Muscle Nerve.* 1998;21:1543–1545.
54. Mondelli M, Giannini F, Giacchi M. Carpal tunnel syndrome incidence in a general population. *Neurology.* 2002;58:289–294.
55. D'Arcy CA, McGee S. The rational clinical examination. Does this patient have carpal tunnel syndrome? *JAMA.* 2000;283:3110–3117.
56. Stevens JC, Smith BE, Weaver AL, et al. Symptoms of 100 patients with electromyographically verified carpal tunnel syndrome. *Muscle Nerve.* 1999;22:1448–1456.
57. Stevens JC, Beard CM, O'Fallon WM, et al. Conditions associated with carpal tunnel syndrome. *Mayo Clin Proc.* 1992;67:541–548.
58. Kozak A, Schedlbauer G, Wirth T, et al. Association between work-related biomechanical risk factors and the occurrence of carpal tunnel syndrome: an overview of systematic reviews and a meta-analysis of current research. *BMC Musculoskelet Disord.* 2015;16:231.
59. Werner RA, Albers JW, Franzblau A, et al. The relationship between body mass index and the diagnosis of carpal tunnel syndrome. *Muscle Nerve.* 1994;17:632–636.
60. Robinson LR. Electrodiagnosis of carpal tunnel syndrome. *Phys Med Rehabil Clin N Am.* 2007;18:733–746, vi.
61. Campbell WW. Guidelines in electrodiagnostic medicine. Practice parameter for electrodiagnostic studies in ulnar neuropathy at the elbow. *Muscle Nerve Suppl.* 1999;8:S171–S205.
62. Cosgrove JL, Chase PM, Mast NJ. Thenar motor syndrome: median mononeuropathy of the hand. *Am J Phys Med Rehabil.* 2002;81:421–423.
63. Jackson DA, Clifford JC. Electrodiagnosis of mild carpal tunnel syndrome. *Arch Phys Med Rehabil.* 1989;70:199–204.
64. Robinson LR, Micklesen PJ, Wang L. Strategies for analyzing nerve conduction data: superiority of a summary index over single tests. *Muscle Nerve.* 1998;21:1166–1171.
65. Lew HL, Wang L, Robinson LR. Test-retest reliability of combined sensory index: implications for diagnosing carpal tunnel syndrome. *Muscle Nerve.* 2000;23:1261–1264.
66. Lesser EA, Venkatesh S, Preston DC, et al. Stimulation distal to the lesion in patients with carpal tunnel syndrome. *Muscle Nerve.* 1995;18:503–507.
67. Park TA, Welshofer JA, Dzwierzynski WW, et al. Median "pseudoneurapraxia" at the wrist: reassessment of palmar stimulation of the recurrent median nerve. *Arch Phys Med Rehabil.* 2001;82:190–197.
68. Wee AS. Needle electromyography in carpal tunnel syndrome. *Electromyogr Clin Neurophysiol.* 2002;42:253–256.
69. Kincaid JC. AAEE minimonograph #31: the electrodiagnosis of ulnar neuropathy at the elbow. *Muscle Nerve.* 1988;11:1005–1015.
70. Froment J. Prehension and the sign of the thumb in paralysis of the ulnar nerve. *Bull Hosp Joint Dis.* 1972;33:193–196.
71. Shakir A, Micklesen PJ, Robinson LR. Which motor nerve conduction study is best in ulnar neuropathy at the elbow? *Muscle Nerve.* 2004;29:585–590.
72. Maynard FM, Stolov WC. Experimental error in determination of nerve conduction velocity. *Arch Phys Med Rehabil.* 1972;53:362–372.

73. Landau ME, Diaz MI, Barner KC, et al. Optimal distance for segmental nerve conduction studies revisited. *Muscle Nerve*. 2003;27:367–369.

74. Gutmann L. AAEM minimonograph #2: important anomalous innervations of the extremities. *Muscle Nerve*. 1993;16:339–347.

75. Robinson LR. Pseudo-ulnar neuropathy. *Am J Phys Med Rehabil*. 2005;84:481.

76. Kanakamedala RV, Simons DG, Porter RW, et al. Ulnar nerve entrapment at the elbow localized by short segment stimulation. *Arch Phys Med Rehabil*. 1988;69:959–963.

77. Federative Committee on Anatomical Terminology. *Terminologia Anatomica: International Anatomical Terminology*. Stuttgart, Germany/New York, NY: Thieme; 1998.

78. Carlson N, Logigian EL. Radial neuropathy. *Neurol Clin*. 1999;17:499–523, vi.

79. Malikowski T, Micklesen PJ, Robinson LR. Prognostic values of electrodiagnostic studies in traumatic radial neuropathy. *Muscle Nerve*. 2007;36:364–367.

80. Seppalainen AM, Aho K, Uusitupa M. Strawberry pickers' foot drop. *Br Med J*. 1977;2:767.

81. Krivickas LS, Wilbourn AJ. Peripheral nerve injuries in athletes: a case series of over 200 injuries. *Semin Neurol*. 2000;20:225–232.

82. Katirji B. Peroneal neuropathy. *Neurol Clin*. 1999;17:567–591, vii.

83. Marciniak C, Armon C, Wilson J, et al. Practice parameter: utility of electrodiagnostic techniques in evaluating patients with suspected peroneal neuropathy: an evidence-based review. *Muscle Nerve*. 2005;31:520–527.

84. Derr JJ, Micklesen P, Robinson LR. Predicting recovery after fibular nerve injury: which electrodiagnostic features are most useful? *Am J Phys Med Rehabil*. 2009;88(7):547–553.

85. Broadhurst PK, Robinson LR. Effect of hip and knee position on nerve conduction in the common fibular nerve. *Muscle Nerve*. 2017;56(3):519–521.

86. Sunderland S. *Nerves and Nerve Injuries*. 2nd ed. Edinburgh, UK/New York, NY: Churchill Livingstone; distributed by Longman; 1978.

87. Oh SJ, Meyer RD. Entrapment neuropathies of the tibial (posterior tibial) nerve. *Neurol Clin*. 1999;17:593–615, vii.

88. Kerr R, Frey C. MR imaging in tarsal tunnel syndrome. *J Comput Assist Tomogr*. 1991;15:280–286.

89. Finkel JE. Tarsal tunnel syndrome. *Magn Reson Imaging Clin N Am*. 1994;2:67–78.

90. Patel AT, Gaines K, Malamut R, et al. Usefulness of electrodiagnostic techniques in the evaluation of suspected tarsal tunnel syndrome: an evidence-based review. *Muscle Nerve*. 2005;32:236–240.

91. Galardi G, Amadio S, Maderna L, et al. Electrophysiologic studies in tarsal tunnel syndrome. Diagnostic reliability of motor distal latency, mixed nerve and sensory nerve conduction studies. *Am J Phys Med Rehabil*. 1994;73:193–198.

92. DeLisa JA, Saeed MA. The tarsal tunnel syndrome. *Muscle Nerve*. 1983;6:664–670.

93. Kraft GH. Tarsal tunnel syndrome: a case report and review of the literature. *Orthopedics*. 1986;9:32.

94. Akita K, Niiro N, Murakami G, et al. First dorsal interosseous muscle of the foot and its innervation. *Clin Anat*. 1999;12:12–15.

95. Noble J, Munro CA, Prasad VS, et al. Analysis of upper and lower extremity peripheral nerve injuries in a population of patients with multiple injuries. *J Trauma*. 1998;45:116–122.

96. Selecki BR, Ring IT, Simpson DA, et al. Trauma to the central and peripheral nervous systems. Part II: a statistical profile of surgical treatment in New South Wales. *Aust N Z J Surg*. 1982;52:111–116.

97. Seddon HJ. *Surgical Disorders of the Peripheral Nerves*. 2nd ed. New York, NY: Churchill Livingstone; 1975:21–23.

98. Chaudhry V, Glass JD, Griffin JW. Wallerian degeneration in peripheral nerve disease. *Neurol Clin*. 1992;10:613–627.

99. Thesleff S. Trophic functions of the neuron. II. Denervation and regulation of muscle. Physiological effects of denervation of muscle. *Ann N Y Acad Sci*. 1974;228:89–104.

100. Kraft GH. Fibrillation potential amplitude and muscle atrophy following peripheral nerve injury. *Muscle Nerve*. 1990;13:814–821.

101. Partanen JV, Danner R. Fibrillation potentials after muscle injury in humans. *Muscle Nerve*. 1982;5:S70–S73.

102. Dorfman LJ. Quantitative clinical electrophysiology in the evaluation of nerve injury and regeneration. *Muscle Nerve*. 1990;13:822–828.

103. Erminio F, Buchthal F, Rosenfalck P. Motor unit territory and muscle fiber concentration in paresis due to peripheral nerve injury and anterior horn cell involvement. *Neurology*. 1959;9:657–671.

104. Sillman JS, Niparko JK, Lee SS, et al. Prognostic value of evoked and standard electromyography in acute facial paralysis. *Otolaryngol Head Neck Surg*. 1992;107:377–381.

105. Kline DG. Surgical repair of peripheral nerve injury. *Muscle Nerve*. 1990;13:843–852.

106. Wood MB. *Surgical Approach to Peripheral Nerve System Trauma 1998 AAEM Course C: Electrodiagnosis in Traumatic Conditions*. Rochester, NY: American Association of Electrodiagnostic Medicine; 1998:27–36.

107. Lipetz JS. Pathophysiology of inflammatory, degenerative, and compressive radiculopathies. *Phys Med Rehabil Clin N Am*. 2002;13:439–449.

108. Dillingham TR, Lauder TD, Andary M, et al. Identifying lumbosacral radiculopathies: an optimal electromyographic screen. *Am J Phys Med Rehabil*. 2000;79:496–503.

109. Dillingham TR, Lauder TD, Andary M, et al. Identification of cervical radiculopathies: optimizing the electromyographic screen. *Am J Phys Med Rehabil*. 2001;80:84–91.

110. Nardin RA, Raynor EM, Rutkove SB. Fibrillations in lumbosacral paraspinal muscles of normal subjects. *Muscle Nerve*. 1998;21:1347–1349.

111. Haig AJ. Lumbar paraspinal muscles. *Arch Phys Med Rehabil*. 1994;75:491.

112. Nardin RA, Patel MR, Gudas TF, et al. Electromyography and magnetic resonance imaging in the evaluation of radiculopathy. *Muscle Nerve*. 1999;22:151–155.

113. Weber F, Albert U. Electrodiagnostic examination of lumbosacral radiculopathies. *Electromyogr Clin Neurophysiol*. 2000;40:231–236.

114. Jensen MC, Brant-Zawadzki MN, Obuchowski N, et al. Magnetic resonance imaging of the lumbar spine in people without back pain. *N Engl J Med*. 1994;331:69–73.

115. Ferrante MA, Wilbourn AJ. Electrodiagnostic approach to the patient with suspected brachial plexopathy. *Neurol Clin*. 2002;20:423–450.

116. Kutsy RL, Robinson LR, Routt ML Jr. Lumbosacral plexopathy in pelvic trauma. *Muscle Nerve*. 2000;23:1757–1760.

117. Ferrante MA, Wilbourn AJ. The utility of various sensory nerve conduction responses in assessing brachial plexopathies. *Muscle Nerve*. 1995;18:879–889.

118. Trojaborg W. Clinical, electrophysiological, and myelographic studies of 9 patients with cervical spinal root avulsions: discrepancies between EMG and X-ray findings. *Muscle Nerve*. 1994;17:913–922.

119. Donofrio PD, Albers JW. AAEM minimonograph #34: polyneuropathy: classification by nerve conduction studies and electromyography. *Muscle Nerve*. 1990;13:889–903.

120. Miller RG, Peterson GW, Daube JR, et al. Prognostic value of electrodiagnosis in Guillain-Barre syndrome. *Muscle Nerve*. 1988;11:769–774.

121. Kuntzer T, Antoine JC, Steck AJ. Clinical features and pathophysiological basis of sensory neuronopathies (ganglionopathies). *Muscle Nerve*. 2004;30:255–268.

122. Gwathmey KG. Sensory neuronopathies. *Muscle Nerve*. 2016;53:8–19.

123. Carozzi VA, Canta A, Chiorazzi A. Chemotherapy-induced peripheral neuropathy: what do we know about mechanisms? *Neurosci Lett*. 2015;596:90–107.

124. Bird TD. Charcot-Marie-Tooth neuropathy type 2. In: Pagon RA, Adam MP, Ardinger HH, et al., eds. *GeneReviews(R)*. Seattle, WA: University of Washington, Seattle University of Washington, Seattle. GeneReviews is a registered trademark of the University of Washington, Seattle. All rights reserved; 1993.

125. England JD, Gronseth GS, Franklin G, et al. Evaluation of distal symmetric polyneuropathy: the role of autonomic testing, nerve biopsy, and skin biopsy (an evidence-based review). *Muscle Nerve*. 2009;39:106–115.

126. England JD, Gronseth GS, Franklin G, et al. Evaluation of distal symmetric polyneuropathy: the role of laboratory and genetic testing (an evidence-based review). *Muscle Nerve*. 2009;39:116–125.

127. Bromberg MB. The role of electrodiagnostic studies in the diagnosis and management of polymyositis. *Compr Ther*. 1992;18:17–22.

128. Robinson LR. AAEM case report #22: polymyositis. *Muscle Nerve*. 1991;14:310–315.

129. Morgenlander JC, Massey JM. Myotonic dystrophy. *Semin Neurol*. 1991;11:236–243.

130. Dinsdale SM, Cole TM, Zaki FG, et al. Measurements of disease activity in dermatomyositis. *Arch Phys Med Rehabil*. 1971;52:201–206 passim.

131. Streib EW, Wilbourn AJ, Mitsumoto H. Spontaneous electrical muscle fiber activity in polymyositis and dermatomyositis. *Muscle Nerve*. 1979;2:14–18.

132. Blijham PJ, Hengstman GJ, Hama-Amin AD, et al. Needle electromyographic findings in 98 patients with myositis. *Eur Neurol*. 2006;55:183–188.

133. Pearson CM, Bohan A. The spectrum of polymyositis and dermatomyositis. *Med Clin North Am*. 1977;61:439–457.

134. Jolley SE, Bunnell AE, Hough CL. ICU-acquired weakness. *Chest*. 2016;150:1129–1140.

135. Bird SJ, Rich MM. Critical illness myopathy and polyneuropathy. *Curr Neurol Neurosci Rep*. 2002;2:527–533.

136. Lefaucheur JP, Nordine T, Rodriguez P, et al. Origin of ICU acquired paresis determined by direct muscle stimulation. *J Neurol Neurosurg Psychiatry*. 2006;77:500–506.

137. Krivickas LS. Amyotrophic lateral sclerosis and other motor neuron diseases. *Phys Med Rehabil Clin N Am*. 2003;14:327–345.

138. Van Asseldonk JT, Franssen H, Van den Berg-Vos RM, et al. Multifocal motor neuropathy. *Lancet Neurol*. 2005;4:309–319.

139. Brooks BR. El Escorial World Federation of Neurology criteria for the diagnosis of amyotrophic lateral sclerosis. Subcommittee on Motor Neuron Diseases/Amyotrophic Lateral Sclerosis of the World Federation of Neurology Research Group on Neuromuscular Diseases and the El Escorial "Clinical limits of amyotrophic lateral sclerosis" workshop contributors. *J Neurol Sci*. 1994;124(suppl): 96–107.

140. Costa J, Swash M, de Carvalho M. Awaji criteria for the diagnosis of amyotrophic lateral sclerosis: a systematic review. *Arch Neurol*. 2012;69:1410–1416.

141. Geevasinga N, Loy CT, Menon P, et al. Awaji criteria improves the diagnostic sensitivity in amyotrophic lateral sclerosis: a systematic review using individual patient data. *Clin Neurophysiol*. 2016;127:2684–2691.

142. Kuncl RW, Cornblath DR, Griffin JW. Assessment of thoracic paraspinal muscles in the diagnosis of ALS. *Muscle Nerve*. 1988;11:484–492.

CHAPTER 4

Thiru M. Annaswamy   Didem Inanoglu
Nicholas P. Fey   Gargi D. Raval

Human Walking

Walking is one of the most basic and essential forms of human movement. It is one of human's most highly valued movements as it serves the purpose of locomotion. Disorder of walking is a very common reason why a patient visits her doctor. Understanding human walking or gait will help the physician evaluate his patient's complaints of walking difficulty and gather information that might clarify the problem, leading to more optimal management. Although related, the associated biomechanical and clinical aspects of arising from sitting and starting and stopping walking will not be addressed in this chapter.

NORMAL HUMAN GAIT

The human gait pattern is normally a fluid and continuous movement forward. The basic unit of walking is the *gait cycle*, which is typically recorded from the time one foot strikes the ground until that same foot strikes the ground again and starts the next cycle. During one gait cycle, the distance traversed is defined as one *stride* (**Table 4-1**). Each stride is made up of two steps that are normally symmetrical in length, one *step* by each foot. The frequency of stepping is known as the *cadence* (steps/min). The speed of walking is calculated as the cadence times the step length. In practice, walking speed is often computed by recording the time needed to traverse a measured distance (e.g., 50-ft walking speed) (1).

Gait Cycle Definitions

The gait cycle is divided into segments (**Fig. 4-1**) that serve specific functions, each for a limited time during the gait cycle. There are two phases of gait. Each lower limb supports the body on the ground during its *stance* phase and then propels it forward during its *swing* phase. The basic function of walking involves each foot in turn either advancing forward (limb advancement task) as a step or supporting the body weight (weight acceptance task) and balancing (single-limb support task) during the advancement of the contralateral lower limb. A period of double-limb support (DLS) occurs that makes up 10% of the gait cycle for each step. During DLS, the weight is transferred from one foot to the other in a complex coordinated pattern known as weight acceptance (or loading) and weight release (preswing) for each of the respective limbs (see **Fig. 4-1**). During each gait cycle, limb muscles produce a carefully timed pattern of activity that causes limb acceleration and deceleration. This muscle activity pattern must overcome gravity, as represented by the vertical component of the ground reaction force (GRF), and provide forward propulsion

(**Figs. 4-2** and **4-3**). For purposes of discussion, the detailed descriptions below are given with the focus on the right lower limb.

Gait Cycle Tasks and Activities

The stance phase of gait begins with the task of weight acceptance. Weight acceptance, also called loading, is a decelerating portion of the gait cycle where the foot must stop after traveling at about 4 m/s during the end of swing phase. This sudden stop requires controlled braking involving simultaneous action of the ankle, knee, and hip. At the same time, the left leg is involved in the equally complex task of liftoff to initiate its swing phase, thereby, putting both feet in a DLS period. At initial contact, the right ankle is in a few degrees of dorsiflexion at heel strike and then rapidly plantar flexes under the control of an eccentric (lengthening) contraction of the ankle dorsiflexors (primarily anterior tibialis), until the foot is flat on the ground. Simultaneously, the right knee begins to flex under the eccentric control of the quadriceps (loading response period), and the trunk reaches its lowest point during the cycle. The right hip, which was flexed approximately 40 degrees at heel strike, begins to extend on the pelvis as the trunk smoothly continues forward. The forward momentum of the trunk is slowed by contraction of the hip extensors, the gluteus maximus, and the long hamstrings, resulting in controlled hip extension. The hip and pelvis rotate opposite to one another at the same time, the right hip internally rotating on the pelvis. The stance limb's hip extension and internal rotation have a critical role on forward propulsion compared to ankle power, which is considered less important (2).

As the left foot leaves the ground, the right hip continues to rotate internally as that limb enters the single-limb support portion of stance phase. The right ankle begins to passively dorsiflex as the tibia tilts forward and the pelvis lowers on the left. The pelvis is also moving laterally to the right so that the center of mass (COM) of the body is aligned over the right foot for optimal balance. During this period, the pelvis and COM of the body are rising. To achieve this, some of the kinetic energy of forward motion is converted into potential energy as the trunk rises against the force of gravity (3).

In the middle of single-limb stance (SLS) phase, the ankle reaches maximum dorsiflexion and the heel begins to rise. This heel rise signals a major shift in the right leg's function in the gait cycle as it ends its decelerating role and begins to serve as the acceleration for its swing phase. The foot now rocks over to the forefoot as the knee extends, and the pelvis (not the hip) maximally rotates externally, and the right hip maximally

TABLE 4-1	Sample Temporal Gait Parameters During Comfortable Walking on Level Surfaces in an Unimpaired Adult and in a Patient with Left Hemiplegia		
Temporal Gait Parameter	Unimpaired Adult	Left Hemiplegia	
		Left	Right
Velocity (m/s)	1.33	0.77	0.79
Cadence (steps/min)	113	98.4	98.4
Stride length (m)	1.41	0.94	0.97
Stance (% gait cycle)	62	62.3	63.9
Swing (% gait cycle)	38	37.7	36.1
Double support (% gait cycle)	24	32	28
Opposite foot off (%)		13.1	9.84
Opposite foot contact (%)		49.2	50.8
Single support (s)		0.44	0.50
Step length (m)		0.45	0.49
Step time (s)		0.62	0.60
Stride time (s)		1.22	1.22

Reprinted from Balaban B, Tok F. *Gait disturbances in patients with stroke.* PM&R. 2014;6(7):635–642. Copyright © 2014 American Academy of Physical Medicine and Rehabilitation. With permission.

extends in preparation for opposite heel strike. The left lower limb is fully stretched out for its heel strike so that the pelvis is supported and the drop of the COM of the body is minimized.

The right leg must now shift weight support to the left lower limb while accelerating the right leg into its swing phase. During this DLS period during which weight transfer occurs, the ankle is actively plantar flexed by concentric action of the gastrocnemius, soleus, posterior tibialis, and lesser plantar flexors. These forces contribute primarily to the vertical components of the GRF. At the same time, right hip flexion is being produced by the iliacus, psoas, and tensor fascia lata muscles, and the left hip internal rotators are causing forward rotation of the right pelvis. These left hip muscles contribute much to the horizontal forces or forward propulsion of the right lower limb. As toe-off occurs because of this combined push and pull on the right lower limb, its stance phase concludes and swing phase is initiated.

At the beginning of swing phase, the right leg continues to accelerate as hip flexion, knee flexion, and ankle dorsiflexion

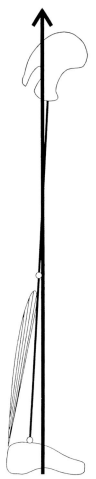

FIGURE 4-2. Quiet standing. The GRF, represented by the *solid line* with an *arrow*, is located anterior to the knee and ankle and posterior to the hip. The soleus muscle is active to stabilize the lower limb. (Courtesy of D. Casey Kerrigan, MD, with permission.)

combine to cause the toe to pass over the ground cleanly. Typically, the toe reaches a minimum height of less than 2.5 cm at the middle of the swing phase. This minimal elevation conserves energy by minimizing the amount of work done against gravity. This closeness to the ground can be a safety problem, causing stumbles on uneven ground, but the gains of energy efficiency caused by reducing the step height are

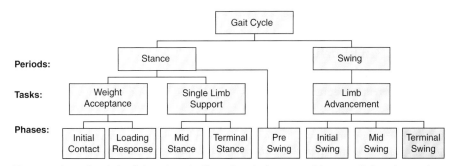

FIGURE 4-1. Phases, tasks, and periods of the gait cycle. The gait cycle is separated into two distinct phases of stance and swing. Functional tasks include weight acceptance and single-limb support during stance and limb advancement during swing. The stance phase of the gait cycle includes the periods of initial contact, loading response, midstance, terminal stance, and preswing. The swing phase includes initial swing, midswing, and terminal swing.

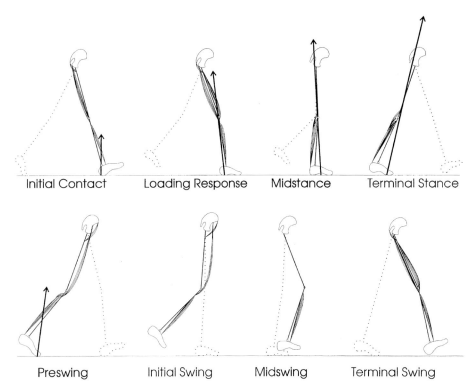

Initial Contact   Loading Response   Midstance   Terminal Stance

Preswing   Initial Swing   Midswing   Terminal Swing

FIGURE 4-3. The eight phases of the gait cycle include initial contact, loading response, midstance, terminal stance, preswing, initial swing, midswing, and terminal swing. The GRF vector is represented by a *solid line* with an *arrow*. The active muscles (**top row,** *left to right,* knee flexors and ankle dorsiflexors, knee flexors and ankle dorsiflexors, ankle plantar flexors, ankle plantar flexors; **bottom row,** *left to right,* knee extensors and ankle plantar flexors, knee extensors and ankle dorsiflexors, ankle dorsiflexors, knee extensors, and ankle dorsiflexors) are shown during each phase of the gait cycle. The uninvolved limb is shown as a *dotted line.* (Courtesy of D. Casey Kerrigan, MD, with permission.)

important enough for this safety risk. The energy-conserving nature of the gait cycle, in part attributable to these mechanics and its highly repetitive and symmetrical nature, will be discussed in more detail, but most of us have experienced the rapid fatigue caused by high stepping (steppage gait) when traversing deep snow or the lack of repetitive steps when walking on very uneven ground.

The second half of the swing phase returns the right leg into a role of decelerating as the forward motion is slowed in preparation for heel strike. The ankle is held in dorsiflexion while the hip flexes and the knee extends. This combination, along with the forward rotation of the right pelvis and external rotation of the right hip, results in maximal length of the step. Any injury or dysfunction of a joint or muscle-tendon unit that reduces the step length will have a major impact on the efficiency of walking. At the end of swing, the hip extensors serve to brake the forward flexion of the hip; and, at faster gait speeds, the hamstrings slow and control the knee extension. The speed of the leg and foot must be controlled to prevent slipping at heel strike.

DETERMINANTS OF GAIT AND ENERGY CONSERVATION

Energy is consumed in three different categories during walking (4). First, there is the work of moving the body's mass through the required distance in a period of time. Second, there is the work done to accomplish the up-and-down motion of the trunk for each step as the pelvis rises to a position above a single supporting leg during midstance and is lowered during double support when it lies between the two lower limbs supporting it at opposite angles. Third, energy is being consumed by the body for general, or basal, metabolism. Because work

requires energy and faster walking involves more work, there is an energy cost. However, since the constant basal metabolic rate continues, as well as some muscular energy consumption for standing, the total energy consumed per unit distance traveled is seen to decrease initially as speed increases from a very slow walking speed. As an optimal speed is reached that is traditionally called comfortable walking, the combined metabolic rate is most efficient for traveling over the ground (**Fig. 4-4**). The higher energy requirements of faster walking and running require greater work output by the muscles (5,6).

The vertical displacement of the body is minimized by a number of factors that are known as the *determinants of gait* (7). These determinants operate independently but simultaneously to produce a smooth sinusoidal vertical and horizontal path, which has one vertical peak and trough for each step. There is also one lateral sinusoid, or curve, for each stride as the body moves toward the supporting foot during each cycle. To illustrate the effects of the determinants of gait, they are removed and replaced in models of the gait cycle. This "compass gait" analysis was restudied by Della Croce et al. (8) with the inclusion of data recorded in a gait lab, largely reaffirming the model. However, we would like to note that subsequent studies have shown that sinusoidal vertical and horizontal paths of the COM of the body are not purely accomplished by passive dynamical exchange of potential and kinetic energies (6,9–11). Rather, both active (i.e., muscles) and passive (i.e., gravity) mechanisms contribute to human gait, which have been highlighted extensively in forward dynamics modeling and simulation studies (9,10,12,13). In addition, the human legs have significant mass, and thus mechanisms to both support and propel the legs in addition to the upper body are important when examining human gait and identification of gait deficits.

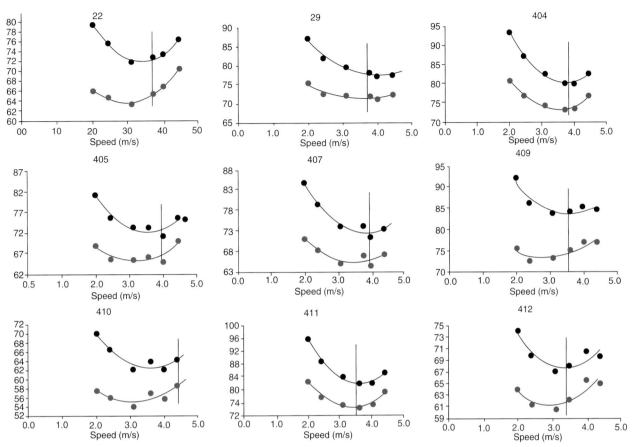

FIGURE 4-4. Graphs demonstrating energy cost of walking and running at preferred speed are optimal compared to slower or higher speeds. (From Rathkey JK, Wall-Scheffler CM. People choose to run at their optimal speed. *Am J Phys Anthropol.* 2017;163(1):85–93. Copyright © 2014 Wiley Periodicals, Inc. Reprinted by permission of John Wiley & Sons, Inc.)

With regard to the determinants of gait, the first is the rotation of the pelvis. During each step, the pelvis rotates forward on the side of the swinging limb. The axis of this rotation is the hip joint of the stance leg, which undergoes internal rotation. As the pelvis forms a bridge between the two hips, it reduces the angle of intersection of the thighs to reduce the vertical descent of the trunk.

The pelvic Trendelenburg motion, or pelvic list, is another determinant. The pelvis drops a few degrees so that the hip of the leg in swing phase is lower than the hip of the stance limb. This reduces the vertical rise of the COM of the trunk and reduces the work of lifting this mass. The cost of this pelvic list is to reduce the space for toe clearance, but this is an affordable cost. Pelvic list, as well as rotation, has been shown to decrease at slower speeds (14). This fact, and the data that reveal that these motions are less important modifiers of the vertical movement of the COM (8), suggests that these movements are important to the control of the momentum during forward propulsion.

Knee flexion in stance phase is an important determinant of gait for two reasons. First, it provides a shock-absorbing mechanism at the beginning of the stance phase. The reduction of the shock of foot impact on the floor helps to maintain momentum and thereby reduces energy loss of stopping and restarting the gait cycle. Also, the knee flexion in stance reduces

the height of the hip joint in midstance. This additional height reduction prevents energy loss from lifting the body but at the cost of quadriceps muscle work.

Lateral displacement of the pelvis also occurs during each step. The pelvis and trunk must move to the stance side to balance the COM of the trunk above the stance foot. This also aligns the tibia into the vertical position during stance. This determinant of gait is a net loss of energy since it causes upward movement of the body, but it is necessary for balance in bipedal gait.

The trunk and shoulder rotate during normal gait in a direction opposite to the pelvic rotation. This 180-degree phase shift of total trunk movement balances the angular acceleration so that balance and forward momentum are maintained. Smooth, coordinated movement here is an energy advantage.

The obliquity of the subtalar joint provides a unique relationship between the motion of the foot and that of the shank. Dorsiflexion of the foot causes lateral movement of the forefoot and vice versa. During stance, the passive dorsiflexion of the ankle, therefore, causes internal rotation of the tibia to partially match that similar movement in the hip. This combined rotation is then reversed during the end of stance or weight release.

Sagittal plane foot and ankle movement is referred to as the three "rockers." The three components are at heel strike, during foot flat, and during toe-off. Each of these has work- and energy-saving factors. For the first rocker, the dorsiflexion of the foot causes the heel to stick out and produce a net lengthening of leg length to maximize the length of the step. This extra length is quickly lost during weight acceptance, when it is no longer needed. Also during this time, the resisting ankle dorsiflexion muscles provide a shock-absorbing descent of the forefoot. During the second rocker, dorsiflexion of the foot occurs during midstance. This serves to reduce the length of the leg until the pelvis passes in front of the ankle. As the heel rises after midstance, the third rocker occurs. The elevation of the heel increases the leg length during push-off and so limits the amount of drop that is experienced by the pelvis. The rockers of the heel, midfoot and forefoot, are therefore useful in minimizing the vertical work of the body movement. The second utility of the rockers is to provide a rolling-like mechanism of foot during stance so that momentum is preserved. Della Croce's work suggests that heel rise and forefoot support may be the most important determinants of gait (8).

QUANTITATIVE GAIT ANALYSIS

Kinetics and Kinematics

A complete understanding of gait requires knowledge of the kinetics of movement in addition to the kinematics of motion discussed in the preceding sections. Kinetics is the science of forces and moments acting on bodies to cause motion. Gait kinetics explains the global and local causes of the motions of gait.

The basic principles of kinetics are Newton's three laws of motion. The first is that a body (of mass m) will change velocity (accelerate (a) or decelerate) only if a force is applied to it. Also, this change in velocity (v) per unit time (t) is proportional to the force ($F = ma$ and $a = \Delta v/\Delta t$). The second law states that the rate of change of momentum of a body is directly proportional to the force applied, and this change in momentum takes place in the direction of the applied force. Newton's third law, the law of action and reaction, is very important for the study of gait and other aspects of biomechanics. This law relates the forces interacting between the foot and the floor as always being equal and opposite. One can therefore measure the forces of ground reaction on the foot with a force plate and begin to understand the net forces acting on the lower limb and on the body as a whole.

The GRF is represented by three directions perpendicular to each other: horizontal (fore/aft), side to side, and vertical. One can also measure the twisting or rotational load on the force plate as the rotating limb is constrained from moving by friction. The force plate also allows the direct calculation of the center of pressure on the foot. During stance phase, the center of pressure starts at the medial heel. As foot flat occurs and the limb progresses to single stance, the center of pressure typically moves laterally as it progresses forward. Then, after heel rise and into weight release, the center is in the forefoot, progressing to the medial side again.

From the center of pressure, the net vector of the three GRFs can be located at each instant during gait (see **Fig. 4-3**). This force vector (i.e., a force that has magnitude and direction) acts on each of the limb segments as well as each joint. The perpendicular distance between the GRF and each joint defines an external moment arm, or leverage, that when multiplied by the force creates a moment of rotation, or torque, about the joint's axis.

Through the process known as inverse dynamics, these forces and moments can be calculated sequentially and distally from the ground and foot to joints between proximal body segments such as the pelvis and trunk. It is important to note that joint moments calculated via inverse dynamics can only be produced by muscles and joint structures (e.g., bony structures and ligaments) that span a given joint. Thus, biarticular muscles can contribute to the joint moment of two joints through their differing muscle moment arms at each joint.

Changes in vertical position of the trunk COM result in changes in the potential energy, and forces causing changes in velocity of limb segments will affect the kinetic energy. Only small amounts of energy change are seen in the transverse and frontal planes, and so studies of gait usually focus on only the energy changes in the sagittal plane relating to forward progression and vertical support.

Power is defined as work per unit time and is usually calculated at each joint as the product of joint moment and angular velocity. The net power of each joint is shown in **Figure 4-5**. Keep in mind that this net power is not the same as the individual muscle power or the metabolic power representing those changes in energy levels. It is only the balanced result of those interactions with the GRF. This net power at each joint can represent generation of energy (+) or absorption of energy (−). For example, study the knee power in **Figure 4-5**. The power is initially negative (decelerating) as the extensor torque produced by the quadriceps is overcome by the flexion moment of the ground reaction. As the trunk progresses forward, the GRF vector angles forward and reduces the flexion moment as the knee stabilizes. Later, the extensor muscles and GRF produce extension together, and the net power is positive (accelerating). A final important note pertaining to interpretations of joint power is that unlike joint moments, musculature spanning any joint in the body can contribute to power of a given joint through dynamic coupling (13,15). As all body segments are linked together, musculature has the potential to accelerate any joint (i.e., contributing to its velocity and thus power) due to the propagation of intersegmental forces within each segment. Thus, interpretations of muscle contributions to joint power are not as straightforward as their contributions to joint moments.

Electromyography in Gait Analysis

Actively contracting muscles under neural control produce electromyographic (EMG) activity. This EMG signal is easily recorded and amplified so that the muscle activity can be correlated with the kinematics and kinetics of gait. In carefully controlled experiments of isometric contraction, a linear relationship exists between the EMG signal and the muscle force. However, this relationship is greatly disrupted by the movement of the muscles during gait, so EMG does not give accurate information about muscle forces (16). For example, EMG analysis of the rectus femoris' role as a hip flexor in early swing phase demonstrates that higher-amplitude EMG signals are produced at faster walking speeds (17). The muscle must exert greater force to flex the hip more rapidly, but the relationship

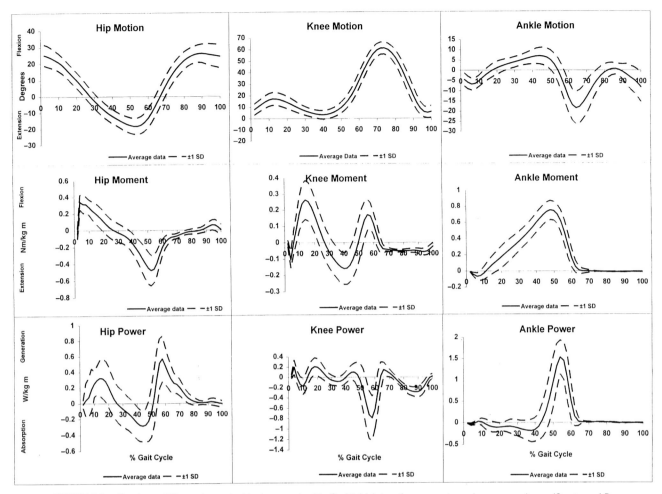

FIGURE 4-5. Kinetics and kinematics at the hip, knee, and ankle. Sagittal joint motion, moments, and power are shown. (Courtesy of D. Casey Kerrigan, MD, with permission.)

is nonlinear and complex, and one is still unable to make quantitative conclusions about muscle force from EMG signals alone. For example, muscle fibers can be arranged linearly along a muscle such as the biceps or in a multipennate fashion such as the deltoid. These muscle architecture differences as well as differences in lever arm lengths (distance between the tendon and the axis of movement) may also influence force production, but these influences are not represented in corresponding EMG signal changes.

Multichannel amplifiers are used in gait laboratories to record from several muscles simultaneous to the recording of kinematic motion (**Fig. 4-6**). The electrodes used for this recording may be either surface electrodes or flexible intramuscular (IM) wire electrodes (16). Surface electrodes are noninvasive and record a larger volume of the target muscle. They are unable to record signals from deep muscles and may record unwanted signals from muscles that are adjacent to the target muscle. Wire electrodes can be located to record more precisely from any muscle, including those that are deep. However, in addition to being more painful, the wire electrodes may dislodge or break during activity. EMG also allows the measurement of muscle fatigue during sustained activity. As lactic acid accumulates in a muscle with exercise, the membrane propagation of the action potential (AP) is

slowed. This slowing of velocity is seen as a reduction in the frequency of the recorded EMG signals (16).

DEVELOPMENT OF MATURE GAIT

Normal adults perform the task of walking without significant active thought or effort. It is a process that is learned and eventually mastered in childhood. Normal gait development is a complex process. Pathologic gait is even more complex, and walking is considered to be a sensitive measure of neuromuscular development (18). Understanding the development of gait is critical to any physician examining and treating children with neuromuscular conditions. To appreciate subtle normal variations, to identify pathologic findings, and to ensure optimal interventions, a physician must have a thorough knowledge of normal development, understand its relationship to gait, and use a systematic approach (19).

The first few years of life are characterized by the most rapid growth in the human life span (20). During this period of maturation of the central and peripheral nervous systems, and musculoskeletal growth, the development of gait emerges according to a typical pattern of motor development: rostral to caudal, proximal to distal, and mass movement to specific action (20,21). Although there is variation in the development

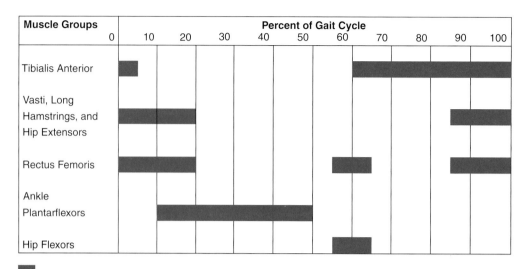

FIGURE 4-6. General muscle group activity as a percentage of the gait cycle in normals. (Courtesy of D. Casey Kerrigan, MD, with permission.)

of each child, achievement of certain motor skills like head control, rolling, sitting, and pulling to stand is needed before a child can master supported or independent walking. Balance and support are two major skills a child practices before progressing to supported walking (walking while holding onto objects) at age 8 to 10 months (22).

With a child's supported walking, there are some features that are in contrast to those of adults: increased hip flexion and ankle dorsiflexion, decreased knee extension, slower walking speed, increased variability, and decreased smoothness. Around the age of 12 months, children progress to independent walking. This immature and inconsistent gait of "toddler" shows wide-based support, increased hip flexion, and lack of reciprocal arm swing (23). According to Sutherland et al., when a child begins to walk, he or she uses a high guard position with the shoulders abducted and the elbows flexed. The hip usually remains externally rotated, the knees are in relative extension, and there is toe strike at initial contact with increased ankle plantar flexion during stance. There is circumduction to clear the externally rotated and extended lower extremities (24). By the time the child reaches 2 years of age, arm swing becomes reciprocal and there is heel-first initial contact similar to adult gait. During swing, dorsiflexion allows for limb clearance, and during stance, there is greater stability due to increased duration of SLS. By age 3, most of the adult kinematic patterns are present; however, maturation continues until about age 7 when the adult gait pattern is developed (25).

In studying human walking, Sutherland et al. proposed five important determinants of mature gait: duration of SLS, walking velocity, cadence, step length, and the ratio of pelvic span to ankle spread (25,26). The gait of a toddler demonstrates significant changes in each of these determinants as he or she approaches gait maturity. The duration of SLS increases steadily from 32% of the gait cycle at 1 year to 38% at age 7 years (25,26). The most rapid changes were observed in children before 2½ years of age. Walking speed increases as a child progresses from supported to independent walking; however, children are inconsistent in their ability to

manage their walking speed (27). Average speed in independent walkers is found to be 64 cm/s, in contrast to 39 cm/s for supported walkers (28). Furthermore, increased cadence seems to be the main reason for the noticeable increase in walking velocity in the toddler. Sutherland (26) reported that walking velocity increases with age in a linear manner from 1 to 3 years, at a rate of 11 cm/s/y, and from 4 to 7 years, the rate of change diminishes to 4.5 cm/s/y with a continued linear relationship. As independent walking matures, there is a decrease in cadence with an increase in stride length with a net result of faster walking speed (23,26). The primary reduction in cadence occurs between the ages of 1 and 2 years, with a gradual decrease thereafter. The cadence at 7 years is noted to be 26% greater than in a normal adult (26). As one would expect, the stride length increases with height, and this leads to faster walking for taller children (and adults). Todd et al. have developed a mathematical equation that defines this nonlinear relationship for children during development without regard to age (29). Sutherland et al. defined the ratio of pelvic span to ankle spread, their fifth determinant of mature gait, as the ratio of body width at the anterior superior iliac spine and distance between ankle centers during double support (26). They found that the ratio increased in a linear fashion from ages 1 to 3 years and then remained constant.

The trend of muscle timing during the toddler years is to shorten the duration of muscle action during the gait cycle and establish normal phasing by reducing unnecessary muscle activity (23). Quadriceps and hamstring activities are prolonged in a toddler but approach normal timing by 2 years (26). No change was seen in the gluteus medius EMG activity with increasing age; however, there was shortening of the time that the gluteus maximus was active during stance phase. Medial and lateral hamstring activities were primarily prolonged, during stance phase, in the immature gait of 12- to 18-month children, with mature patterns emerging around the age of 2 years. Similar findings were also observed for the tibialis anterior and gastrocnemius-soleus muscle complex when referring to the late swing phase and premature stance phase activities seen in these muscles (26). Despite age-related differences, the fundamental components of gait develop at a very early age. As a result, any deviation from normal or step-to-step variability may be an indication of gait pathology both in children and adults. Different investigators described fundamental gait tasks differently (30). Perry developed the notion of three functional gait tasks: weight acceptance, single-limb support, and swing limb advancement. Winter described three elements of walking: support control to prevent collapse against gravity; balance control of head, arms, and trunk (HAT) acting as inverted pendulum; and coordinated lower limb movement during swing. Finally, Gage identified five prerequisites of normal gait: stability during stance, clearance during swing, prepositioning of swing foot before IC, adequate step length, and energy conservation (31). While functional subclassification of the gait cycle differed among investigators, their work collectively lead to better clinical application of gait analysis in children.

GAIT DISORDERS

Pediatric Gait Disorders

When assessing children with gait pathology, it is important to differentiate primary injury from secondary abnormalities and compensatory strategies. A systemic assessment starts with observational gait analysis, includes detailed clinical examination, and establishes a review of each joint, in each plane, and for each phase of gait (32). Joint range of motion, muscle strength and tone, fixed contractures, and rotational deformities of long bones (transverse plane) need to be noted. Functional assessment measures may be used. Patient's gait is assessed from the side (sagittal plane) and front and back (coronal plane). Then if needed, patients may be referred to instrumented gait analysis (IGA) for dynamic measures. IGA may help identify specific impairments, monitor progression of neuromuscular disease, plan surgical and nonsurgical interventions, evaluate postoperative outcomes, and assess the effects of orthoses and prostheses.

Gait in Cerebral Palsy

The development of gait in children with cerebral palsy (CP) is substantially different from their able-bodied peers due to the primary neurologic injury and the secondary musculoskeletal complications. In general, their gait development relates to the topographical type of CP and the gross motor function classification system (GMFCS) levels. For example, children with mild spastic diplegia (GMFCS I or II) typically achieve independent walking between the ages of 2 and 4 years.

Gait abnormalities in CP often include deviations at multiple joints and in multiple planes of motion. Trunk sway, Trendelenburg gait, scissoring, and circumduction occur at trunk and hip level. Knee abnormalities include stiff knee, flexed knee, and recurvatum. At the ankle level, foot drop or equinus gaits are common. Multiple segment involvement may result in in-toeing or out-toeing. Over the past few decades, the use of IGA has improved the evaluation of children with developmental disabilities, particularly CP and myelomeningocele. With the use of IGA, the classification of gait function at both the joint level and in relation to the patterns of movement across multiple joints is possible. Gait in CP is now classified based on combination of specific kinematic and kinetic patterns that result from abnormal muscle tone, loss of strength,

balance, and selective motor control and joint contractures. This allows treatment decisions to be made based on function and impact at joint level. IGA has also shown that there is a measurable deterioration in gait parameters in CP without intervention (33). Some of the changes seen include decreased walking speed, increased duration of double support, decreased range of motion in the sagittal plane with increasing stiffness at the hip and knee, and a gradual shift from equinus through neutral to calcaneus at the ankle.

Among the various types of CP, the spastic form is the most prevalent. For ambulatory diplegic or hemiplegic children, common gait deviations have been described: scissoring, jump, crouch, stiff-knee gait, and equinus (34,35). Stiff-knee gait with decreased knee flexion throughout the gait cycle due to overactive rectus femoris is commonly observed in children with hemiplegia. In jump gait, there is excessive hip and knee flexion with ankle equinus and is the most common diplegic gait pattern in young children. In crouch gait, hip and knee flexion occurs together with ankle dorsiflexion and is seen in older diplegic children. It may be iatrogenic due to overlengthening of muscles and is commonly progressive leading to decline in function. Excessive lower extremity adduction with internal rotation, scissoring, may coexist with crouch and jump gait. While planning interventions for abnormal gait in children with CP, it is important to identify and address specific impairments. Common approach in treatment includes reducing spasticity, correcting the lever arm dysfunction or bone malalignment resulting from fixed contractures, and addressing muscle insufficiency. The data from IGA in CP have resulted in changes in surgical recommendations (36,37), postop care (34), and development of orthotics and new surgical techniques. Although one might assume that the spasticity evident on static examination is the main culprit responsible for the abnormal movement patterns, IGA has revealed abnormal dynamic muscle activation patterns, including excessive cocontraction of agonists and antagonists, with resultant increased joint stiffness and weakening of agonist force production as playing a more central role (31). Hamstring spasticity has been proposed as being primarily responsible for the crouch position, but IGA has additionally identified hip or knee flexion contractures, ankle plantar flexion contractures, and ankle plantar-flexor weakness as being contributory (31,38,39). More recently, in a large group of CP patients including children with both unilateral and bilateral involvement, functioning in GMFCS levels I to IV, the authors found the likelihood of having equinus and in-toeing decreased, while crouch and out-toeing increased with age and higher GMFCS level and when prior surgery had been done (40). With better understanding of the changes that take place naturally with age, clinicians can avoid iatrogenic problems and unnecessary treatments.

Adult Gait Disorders

An abnormal gait pattern is usually apparent from the patient's history and observational gait analysis. When presented with a patient with abnormal gait, it is important to determine during initial evaluation whether the abnormal movement patterns (a) have been adapted as compensatory strategies, which are functionally beneficial; (b) pose potentially detrimental functional consequences, such as increased fall risk, excessive energy expenditure, or adverse joint stresses that may predispose to degenerative changes; or (c) bear cosmetic significance to the patient and/or family. Quantitative kinematic and kinetic data from gait analysis can then be used to differentiate the primary gait deviations from those that are secondary (or compensatory) (41,42).

Initial observational evaluation should assess the symmetry and smoothness of movements, including trunk movement, arm swing, stride length, width of gait base, balance, and degree of effort. The examiner should note the portion of the gait cycle during which a particular deviation occurs. Subsequently, if safe and feasible, the patient can be asked to walk faster and slower, with and without use of any handheld gait aid or orthosis and up and down an incline and stairs. This enhanced observational evaluation can elicit important information that may better guide the examiner. Then, a more systematic and methodical evaluation should be performed, focusing on specific segments and joints and including quantitative gait analysis when available and appropriate.

When interventions are planned to improve a patient's gait, the patient's ambulatory goals need to be determined and agreed upon with the clinician at the outset. In addition to addressing the primary gait abnormality, contributing factors that may affect the patient's ambulatory potential should also be addressed. When reversible muscular weakness is a contributor, strengthening exercises may be appropriate. Irreversible or long-standing weakness can be addressed with appropriate orthoses and handheld gait aids along with a manual wheelchair or powered mobility device as indicated. If spasticity is present that may not be functionally beneficial (43), spasticity-reducing interventions that may be considered include physical therapy; oral, injectable, and intrathecal pharmacologic agents; tendon surgery; or implants. For patients with gait abnormalities who wear a lower limb prosthesis or orthosis, adjusting or replacing prosthetic or orthotic components may be necessary in addition.

The sections below describe in detail the characteristics of specific neurologic and/or physical conditions that result in gait abnormalities as well as specific named gait disorders, which can be applied more broadly to numerous conditions.

Spastic Gait

Injury to the central nervous system, such as hemiplegic stroke, is a very common cause of gait disorder, particularly spastic gait. Spasticity is broadly defined as a passive resistance to stretch, while hypertonicity refers to abnormal activation of the muscle. Both factors are prevalent in individuals with neurologic injury; however, the gait of these individuals is usually described as spastic. Characteristic kinematic features of gait following stroke are lower gait speed and marked asymmetry of stepping (44,45). Other well-noted kinematic deviations from normal gait are reduced percentage of the gait cycle in single-limb support on the paretic limb, prolonged period of weight release for the hemiparetic limb during DLS, and prolonged paretic swing time (44–46).

See **Table 4-1** for spatiotemporal gait data in an illustrative case example of a patient with left hemiplegia.

Typical kinetic abnormalities include greater GRF moment after initial contact and at push-off in the unaffected leg compared to the affected leg, positive extensor moment at the affected knee throughout the gait cycle (normal gait features a flexor moment in early stance), and reduced power bursts compared to normal gait (44). As a result of these abnormal gait characteristics, the overall energy expenditure of walking is about 50% to 67% higher in patients with hemiplegic gait compared to healthy controls (44).

Transfemoral (Above-Knee) Amputation Gait

Another example of a condition that results in numerous gait disorders is a patient who has undergone a transfemoral (TF) amputation. We will assume that this patient has a midthigh level of amputation, no significant hip flexion contracture, use of an ischial containment socket, and an optimal prosthetic suspension. The shorter the residual limb is, the shorter the lever available to control the prosthesis, resulting in the hip abductors on the prosthetic side becoming less effective in stabilizing the pelvis (38). The ischial containment or narrow medial-lateral socket is usually preferred to the older quadrilateral socket design, because of advantages in both comfort and biomechanics (47). Finally, suboptimal suspension results in a functionally long prosthetic limb, with resultant difficulty clearing the foot during mid-swing phase unless compensatory motions (e.g., hip hiking or an abducted gait on the prosthetic side or vaulting on the intact side) are performed. Prosthetic knee stability is of paramount importance to the TF amputee, whose remaining quadriceps can no longer serve the function of controlling knee flexion during loading. During the initial weight acceptance portion of stance phase, the prosthetic knee unit will be more stable when the GRF line passes anterior to the knee. For a TF amputee with a longer, stable residual limb and normal strength, the prosthetist may elect to place the axis of rotation of the knee unit anterior to the trochanter-knee-ankle (TKA) line—the line drawn during static alignment that passes through the greater trochanter, knee, and ankle joint centers in the sagittal plane—to provide "voluntary control" over prosthetic knee stability (38). Although this situation requires greater voluntary activation of the hip extensors beginning at the moment of heel strike, which via closed-chain kinetics effects accelerates the knee into extension, the advantage is easier knee flexion during terminal stance and preswing, since the GRF line is more readily positioned posterior to the knee joint axis (48,49). On the other hand, for a TF amputee with a weakened residual limb, the prosthetic knee joint axis would be placed posterior to the TKA line to afford greater knee stability but with the disadvantage of greater difficulty achieving knee flexion during late stance. Current prosthetic technology provides greater knee stability during early stance and more readily achieved knee flexion during late stance with mechanical polycentric knees, simple fluid or pneumatic-controlled knees, and the increasingly popular microprocessor-controlled knee units (50). With regard to the prosthetic foot and ankle, the more rapidly the prosthetic foot advances from heel strike to foot flat, the more rapidly the GRF line progresses to a position anterior to the knee joint axis, with a resultant extension moment at the knee. Any restriction in ankle plantar flexion, such as may result from an excessively stiff plantar flexion bumper in a single-axis prosthetic foot, would serve to destabilize the prosthetic knee during early stance. Given that there is an ankle dorsiflexion moment from midstance to terminal stance, unchecked dorsiflexion, such as can result from a worn dorsiflexion bumper in a single-axis prosthetic foot, would predispose to late-stance phase buckling of the pros- thetic knee because of unrestricted forward motion of the prosthetic shank (38).

Transtibial Amputee Gait

We will now consider a patient who has undergone a transtib- ial amputation. For purposes of this example, we will assume an average length of residual limb and absence of significant knee or hip flexion contractures. We will assume PTB socket with adequate suspension and a single-axis foot. Though pros- thetic advances continue to work toward mimicking normal joint motion and gait, there are still some notable differences in gait in the transtibial amputee. In general, unilateral trans- tibial amputees will have shorter stance phase, longer swing phase, and less push-off force on the prosthetic side compared to sound limb (9,51). Some of the differences in transtibial amputee gait can be attributed to the absence of the ankle plantar flexor muscles. Ankle plantar flexors play a pivotal role in providing trunk support and forward propulsion and initiating swing in normal gait (9). In the absence of ankle musculature, unilateral transtibial amputees develop some compensatory patterns to achieve functional gait (52–54). At the beginning of stance phase at heel strike, there is energy transfer to the prosthetic foot and tibia. The heel rocker then rotates the foot and tibia forward. In transtibial prosthetic gait, the tibial shank only rotates forward at half the normal rate, and heel-only support is longer in duration than in normal gait (55). Since the foot is in dorsiflexed position longer, it leads to knee flexion moment and there is greater instability (56). The more rapidly the prosthetic proceeds to foot flat and the GRF passes anterior to the knee, there is more stability. Another dif- ference is that in transtibial amputee gait, knee flexion range is less than in normal gait after heel strike. In the transtibial amputee, knee flexion range is approximately 6 to 10 degrees compared to approximately 18 degrees in a normal gait (57– 59). The quadriceps muscles contract to control the rate of knee flexion during weight acceptance (59,60). In the trans- tibial amputee, the quadriceps fire with more intensity than in normal gait correlated with increase in EMG activity (58). The shorter arc of knee flexion during loading response and also the fixed relationship between the shank of the prosthesis and the forefoot create more demand on the quadriceps muscle. The hamstrings and semimembranosus also fire with increased intensity than in normal gait, which may help to control hip motion (54,58).

At the hip, motion is similar to that in normal gait, but there is an increase of about 10 degrees in hip flexion dur- ing loading response (57,59,61). The gluteus maximus fires with more intensity and duration during weight acceptance leading to trunk leaning slightly forward. This forward lean reduces the flexion moment at the knee and therefore reduces the force on quadriceps to stabilize the knee (56,57). Another important consideration in transtibial amputee is the impact on the sound limb (62). During transfer of support to the sound limb, a foot component such as SACH foot increases loading force on the opposite limb (60,63,64). As dorsiflex- ion is more limited in this foot design, there is early heel rise resulting in body elevation as the foot rolls forward, creating a drop on the sound side. Though the exact mechanism is still unknown, other studies have implicated abnormal fron- tal- and transverse-plane knee loading characteristics across

changing gait speeds as well as the duration of prosthesis use (62) in higher incidence of knee osteoarthritis in older trans- tibial amputees who are long-time users (65,66). Newer foot designs that are designed to store and release energy passively or with active power do not impart as large a loading force on the opposite limb (60,67). Recent studies have shown that foot/ankle stiffness is an important independent device property, which can be used to guide prosthetic selection and prescription (68). Foot/ankle stiffness was shown to have widespread influences on bilateral GRFs, kinematics, kinetics, and electromyography of the legs (68,69).

Aged Gait

Many of the gait changes seen in elderly individuals may be attributed to their reduced walking speed (70,71). However, differences that persist when healthy elderly individuals walk both at comfortable walking speeds and at speeds comparable to those of young adults include reduced peak hip extension, increased anterior pelvic tilt, and reduced ankle plantar flexion and power generation, possibly caused by ankle plantar-flexor muscle weakness (70). Reduced gait velocity, resulting from reductions in both stride length and cadence, has been shown to correlate with lower limb muscle strength in older persons, but the muscle group that is primarily responsible has been variably suggested to be the ankle dorsiflexors (72), ankle plan- tar flexors (73), knee extensors and hip flexors (74), and hip extensors (75).

Falls in the elderly may be due to a variety of factors impacting one or more of several organ systems related to bal- ance, such as disturbances of the visual, vestibular, cognitive, sensory, and other systems (76). However, falls occur in elderly individuals without evident predisposing factors. Although kinematic gait studies have not revealed significant differences between fallers and nonfallers, kinetic gait studies have shown increased peak hip flexion moment in stance, reduced peak hip extension moment, reduced knee flexion moment in preswing, and reduced knee power absorption in preswing phase (77). Further, the abnormalities in both energetics and fall risks associated with aging gait may be attributed to the identified "organizational shift" of elderly individuals to rely on proximal musculature as opposed to distal musculature when negotiat- ing increased demands of gait, such as walking over increasing incline grades (78).

Foot Drop or Equinus Gait

A foot drop or ankle equinus condition may be due to weak- ness of the anterior compartment (dorsiflexor) muscles of the leg, ankle plantar flexor spasticity, or an ankle plantar flexion contracture. In the case of dorsiflexor weakness, a foot slap may occur immediately following heel strike in mild weakness, or, if severe, the forefoot makes initial contact in stance phase (79). Gait analysis with EMG can determine if there is inap- propriate plantar flexor activity during swing. All three causes of ankle equinus, depending on severity, may increase the risk of tripping and rate of falls and increase the need for com- pensatory ipsilateral knee and hip flexion (steppage gait) or contralateral pelvic tilting and hip vaulting during gait. These compensatory motions can reduce toe drag and improve foot clearance during swing but also increase overall energy expen- diture by increasing the vertical displacement of COM and visually have poor cosmesis.

With the exception of the ankle plantar flexor contracture, an ankle-foot orthosis (AFO) is typically used to compensate for foot drop (80). Spastic ankle plantar flexors usually necessitate a rigid, solid (nonarticulated, to reduce activation of the plantar flexors' stretch reflex) AFO designed to maintain a 90-degree (neutral) position of ankle dorsiflexion (if achievable). In the absence of significant spasticity, however, spring-assisted dorsiflexion is often used. This type of component can be incorporated into both plastic and double metal upright AFO designs and allows partial ankle motion—from neutral to up to full ankle dorsiflexion—with less adverse effect during stance phase compared with a solid plastic AFO or fixed-ankle metal AFO. Either an AFO with assisted dorsiflexion or an AFO that allows no ankle motion will usually prevent ankle plantar flexion beyond neutral (via a 90-degree plantar flexion stop), resulting in little difference between the two from initial contact through loading response. The inability of the ankle in an AFO to plantar flex beyond neutral keeps the GRF line posterior to the knee, resulting in a knee flexion moment from initial contact through midstance. However, from midstance to terminal stance, a solid AFO does not allow the tibia to move progressively forward via dorsiflexion, which interferes with the second of the "three rockers" described earlier, and instead necessitates early heel rise from knee flexion. Neither AFO design allows ankle plantar flexion to occur as would normally take place from terminal stance through preswing. Maintaining foot clearance in a narrow range is critical during initial and midswing phases, and both AFO designs prevent toe drag by restricting plantar flexion. A recent systematic review revealed that AFOs have beneficial effects on ankle kinematics, stance phase knee kinematics as well as ankle and foot forces, and overall energy cost of walking (81).

Weak Calf Gait

In contrast to ankle dorsiflexor weakness, which affects the entire swing phase and the first half of stance phase, weakness of the ankle plantar flexors results in deviations involving the second half of stance phase. In normal gait, the ankle plantar flexors contract eccentrically to control the rate at which the tibia advances forward over the supporting foot. Weakness of this muscle group, as may result from such conditions as Achilles tendon injury, tibial nerve injury, S1 radiculopathy, or lower lumbar myelomeningocele, results in excessive and untimely forward progression of the tibia during the midstance to late-stance phase (2). This excessive passive ankle dorsiflexion during terminal stance prevents normal heel rise, which functionally shortens the stance limb and reduces the effect of the toe (or third) rocker. This leads to premature contralateral initial foot contact that decreases stride length (79). It is the shortened step, not deficient "push-off," that impairs forward progression in the presence of calf weakness (2). The failure of vertical support from the calf also causes ipsilateral pelvic drop, which lowers the body COM (8). The excessive drop in the body COM results in marked energy loss, since the pelvis must rise again to a normal height during the stance phase of the sound limb.

Gluteus Medius (Waddling or Trendelenburg) Gait

The gluteus medius is the primary hip abductor; the gluteus minimus and tensor fascia lata are secondary hip abductors; and all three share the same spinal root and peripheral nerve supplies. With open-chain kinetics (when the foot is unrestrained), activation of the hip abductors results in hip abduction. However, with "closed-chain" kinetics (when the foot is in contact with a surface such as the floor), activation of the hip abductors does not result in lower limb movement, because of friction between the foot and the supporting surface. Rather, the angle between the femur and the pelvis is increased by pelvic tilting (assuming the pelvis is unrestrained). During normal gait, the hip abductors—chiefly the gluteus medius—are active during SLS to limit the degree to which the contralateral pelvis lists (or dips) downward. Normally, this is limited to 5 degrees of pelvic list (Inman's second major determinant of gait) (82). Excessive pelvic tilt, or instability of the pelvis in the coronal plane due to hip abductor weakness, may present as difficulty with foot clearance during midswing phase on the opposite side. A gluteus medius–type gait, classically described as Trendelenburg gait (83), may be due to hip abductor weakness, hip joint pain, or both. The excessive energy demands of an uncompensated gluteus medius gait—characterized by excessive pelvic list, lateral protrusion of the pelvis on the affected side during stance phase, and an obligatory steppage gait on the contralateral side, thereby creating the appearance of a pronounced waddle—are somewhat lessened by a compensated gluteus medius gait in which the person employs excessive trunk leaning over the affected limb with an associated medial pelvic deviation during stance phase (79). This effectively reduces the large hip adductor moment that results from unloading the contralateral limb and that is normally controlled by fully functioning hip abductors. A lesser demand for a forceful contraction of the hip abductors results in a lesser axial, or compressive, load on the hip joint surfaces. In addition to ipsilateral trunk lean during stance phase, further reduction in hip joint loading may be achieved using a cane in the opposite hand. Finally, the gluteus medius gait, in contrast to most other gait deviations, becomes *less* evident with *faster* walking, since the shorter duration of stance phase means that there is a shorter time period over which the weakened hip abductors must act to try to stabilize the pelvis.

Stiff-Knee Gait

Reduced knee flexion during the swing phase of gait results in an appearance of a "stiff leg" or "stiff knee," which is the reason behind the moniker-stiff-knee gait. Some characteristics of stiff-knee gait include a large moment of inertia, compensatory maneuvers such as ipsilateral hip circumduction or hip hiking, contralateral hip vaulting, and excessive pelvic motion. If these compensatory mechanisms are inadequate, one might observe ipsilateral toe drag as well. The net effect is higher vertical displacement of the body's COM, resulting in energy inefficiency and poor cosmesis. The most commonly implicated muscle spasticity in stiff-knee gait is spasticity of the knee extensors, especially the quadriceps muscles. Other causes may include weak hip flexors and poor ankle mechanics. Dynamic EMG analysis will reveal inappropriate knee extensor activity during preswing or initial swing when quadriceps spasticity is the cause and overactivity of the ankle plantar flexors in preswing when plantar flexor spasticity is the cause (44). IGA can also identify abnormalities in hip, knee, or ankle power, when those are the primary causes of stiff-knee gait.

Knee Recurvatum Gait

Dynamic knee recurvatum, back-kneeing, or hyperextension of the knee during stance can be a particularly painful gait disorder. It may predispose the knee to injury from overstretch of ligament and posterior capsular structures as the (external) GRF and the (internal) muscle force combine to create a knee extension moment (84). Other characteristics of knee recurvatum gait include increased ipsilateral hip flexion (due to increased hip flexion moment) during stance and increased lumbar lordosis (to compensate for the large hip flexion moment). This gait is highly energy inefficient and painful and can predispose the knee to further injury. The commonly implicated cause of knee recurvatum gait is ankle plantar flexor spasticity, particularly early in the stance phase, which drives the GRF moment anterior to the knee, thereby driving it into hyperextension (79). Other causes may include ankle plantar flexion contracture, weak ankle plantar flexors, or knee extensors. Dynamic EMG or IGA can identify the primary causative factors by revealing inappropriate muscle activity or abnormal joint forces or moments (44).

Crouched Gait

Crouched gait is described by its striking feature of excessive knee flexion during stance. This places higher demand on the knee extensors, which can fatigue quickly, and can also increase the risk of falling due to fatigue, pain, and instability. The common causative factors for this gait disorder include spasticity of the hamstring muscles, or hip flexors, or contracture of the hamstrings or hip flexors. IGA and dynamic EMG can determine if there is elevated hip flexion or knee flexion moment in early stance, which will help identify the source of the problem.

Foot Varus Gait

This gait disorder is characterized by excessive inversion of the foot during swing. The adverse consequences of this gait deviation include increased risk of tripping and falls and higher likelihood of injury to the lateral ligamentous structures of the foot and ankle. Anterior or posterior tibialis spasticity is the most commonly implicated cause, which can be easily identified by inappropriate activity during the swing phase of gait. Weak ankle evertors can be a potential factor as well.

Scissoring Gait

Excessive hip adduction during swing and in stance can result in the appearance of scissoring, thereby causing scissoring gait. Spasticity in the hip adductors is the most commonly implicated cause of this gait disorder. In addition to poor cosmetic appearance of this gait, other consequences are higher risk of falling due to tripping and stumbling. In addition, if the hip adductor spasticity is severe, it can interfere with toileting, dressing, and personal hygiene as well. Other factors that may cause scissoring gait include hip adductor contracture and the rare occurrence of (contralateral) hip abductor spasticity.

Reduced Hip Extension Gait

Reduced hip extension moment during terminal stance may shorten the contralateral leg's step length, increase pelvic motion and/or knee flexion, and result in the appearance of a stiff hip gait or reduced hip extension gait. This energy-inefficient gait pattern is typically caused by spastic ipsilateral hip flexors. Other causes included hip flexion contracture or decreased ipsilateral step length due to other causes. The cause can be identified using dynamic EMG and evaluating hip and ankle kinetics by IGA.

GAIT INTERVENTIONS TO DELIVER LOCAL ASSISTANCE

Several techniques have been applied to influence "local" mechanics of individuals during gait. Surgical procedures such as rectus femoris release have been used to eliminate the detrimental effect of abnormal rectus femoris activity, with resultant enhanced initial swing phase knee flexion in patients with CP and hemiplegic stroke patients (85–91). Motor nerve block of the rectus femoris has been shown to improve maximal swing phase knee flexion, the slope of the knee motion curve at toe-off, and gait speed in patients with spastic stiff-legged gait who also had sufficient hip flexor strength and no abnormal EMG activity of the vastus muscles during the initial swing phase (92). Alcohol neurolysis of the sciatic nerve to reduce hamstring spasticity in hemiplegic stroke patients has produced beneficial effects lasting 6 months (93). Selective dorsal rhizotomy in CP patients has been shown to normalize cocontraction during knee extension but was without benefit to cocontraction during ankle plantar flexion in the majority of the time (94).

Electrical stimulation of nerves and muscles has a long history in attempts to improve the functional walking in persons with upper motor neuron injury and spastic paralysis (95–97). Liberson, as early as in the 1960s, envisioned an electrical replacement for the ankle-foot orthoses (97). Later work expanded this concept into complex systems that use multiple sites of stimulation with implanted wires to produce more complex movements (98–100). Further development of this technology has redirected attention on Liberson's concept of a device that is simple and safe enough for home use as an exercise and training device (98,101,102). In persons with hemiplegia after stroke and incomplete spinal cord injury (SCI), these electrical stimulators activate the fibular nerve during swing phase to produce walking patterns that are faster, farther, and more efficient and with improved toe clearance (99,100,102). The improved toe clearance comes with the finding that fibular nerve stimulation improves knee flexion as well as ankle dorsiflexion (95,99). In addition, the evidence makes it clear that this method of treatment has a training effect and results in sustained improvement in walking when the stimulator is inactive (99,102,103). These devices are increasingly being used in clinical practice (98) and are theorized to have a training effect that represents central nervous system reorganization rather than just peripheral improvements in muscle tone, range of motion, and muscle strength (103).

Another advance in the local management of gait disorders associated with spasticity and dystonia has been the application of botulinum toxin (BTX) types A and B. BTX is available in the United States and many other countries for therapeutic use. When compared to other muscle tone–reducing options, these toxins have the advantage of producing selective, graded weakness in individual muscles with a predictable recovery over several weeks. However, large muscles may not respond adequately to the recommended maximum cumulative dose of 400 units of BTX-A, gait analysis may identify a muscle or muscles that reduce the efficiency of gait (104), and BTX can reduce the contractile force of the selected muscle. The analysis might be a simple, clinical observation of gait as part of a neurologic exam, or it might be a sophisticated, multichannel EMG recording of muscle activity during the gait cycle. At the time of injection, needle electromyography may confirm motor unit activity at rest, or electrical muscle stimulation may be used to direct the injection into the muscle identified by the exam during walking.

An example of this type of treatment includes treatment of ankle inversion by BTX injection of the tibialis posterior muscle (in some cases with additional dosing of the tibialis anterior) (43). During the ensuing weeks, the weakened muscles will require orthotic support so that stable walking can be practiced (105); however, the treatment can reduce pressure at the lateral malleolus and other areas so that pain and pressure ulcers are improved. The result can include improved walking speed and step length (106,107). Adductor muscle scissoring of the thighs can also be improved with BTX treatment. A risk to be considered is the potential loss of extensor tone in the lower limbs upon which the patient has been relying for standing and walking. While the rehab team may be able to teach a compensation for this weakness, in many cases, the patient will need to wait for the BTX to wear off so that the useful tone returns to the legs. Dosing information for BTXs A and B are available for both adults and children (108,109). Typically, injections are repeated at 3- to 4-month intervals if the offending muscle tone reoccurs (110). Side effects, in addition to muscle weakness or fatigue, include nausea or "flulike symptoms" and symptoms associated with anticholinergics such as dry mouth. BTX treatment has eliminated the use of tendon transfer surgery for many patients (109). It needs to be noted, however, that BTXs have not yet been approved for this use by the U.S. Food and Drug Administration and that serious complications, including some deaths, have been reported. However, numerous authorities have produced practice guidelines for this therapy (108–111) and most US health care plans pay for the treatment.

Treatment with BTX is an adjunct to other physical and pharmacologic treatment of specific conditions resulting in disordered muscle tone, covered in more detail in other chapters of this text. Oral and intrathecal baclofen therapies have been shown to improve walking velocity in appropriately selected patients with upper motor neuron disorders, for example (106,110). However, it should always be remembered that the primary treatment of abnormal tone is a consistent stretching exercise program (with active exercise as is practical for the individual) that improves the health of the muscles (108,109).

Finally, wearable assistive devices (prostheses and orthoses) have shown considerable advancement over the last decade from devices that are mechanically passive such as hinges, springs, and dampers to devices that have self-contained motors and active actuation systems to provide net energy to the user (112–116). A few of these research advancements seek to deliver not only localized joint assistance in specific modes of gait (117), but they seek to interpret user intent to allow for seamless and intuitive switching between varying modes such as level ground, stairs, and ramps, with impressive initial research findings (118).

GAIT INTERVENTIONS TO PROMOTE MOTOR ADAPTATION

We conclude this chapter with a brief discussion of training interventions that seek to engage plasticity of the nervous system to facilitate neuromotor recovery. One widely used intervention is body weight–supported treadmill training (BWSTT), a more recently developed approach to gait rehabilitation being utilized with increasing frequency for patients with diminished or absent supraspinal control. Although this technique was initially developed and then used with varying degrees of success following SCI (119–121), BWSTT has since been a component of locomotor rehabilitation for patients with stroke, traumatic brain injury (TBI), Parkinson's disease, and lumbar stenosis (122–128), among other conditions. In addition, improvement in cardiovascular fitness from BWSTT has been documented in patients after a stroke or TBI (129,130).

Most commonly, BWSTT employs upright walking on a motorized treadmill while the patient wears a suspension harness to reduce GRF by a specified percentage. In other scenarios, systems such as ZeroG (Aretech, Inc.) or FLOAT (Lutz Medical Engineering, Inc.) can be used to dynamically and precisely control specific levels of body weight support and allow individual to freely ambulate overground (131). In either scenario, typically two therapists (and sometimes a third to facilitate upright posture) manually position and guide each lower limb to achieve repetitive, rhythmic stepping motions. To reduce therapist effort and improve the repeatability of locomotor training, commercially available robotic devices have been developed to increase the volume of stepping practice (132–134). Another proposed technologic refinement in the setting of hemiparetic gait has been a computer-controlled, dynamic system to precisely regulate the magnitude and timing—with respect to gait cycle events—of body weight support provided to the user.

In addition to BWSTT, other training paradigms have been proposed and studied in the literature, both in normal gait scenarios and in destabilizing and challenging locomotor scenarios, to assess if individuals can learn to manage neurologic and physical constraints of their condition in a beneficial way. Approaches seeking to engage motor learning for improved function such as treadmill-delivered perturbation-based training for fall prevention of transtibial individuals (135), variable speed split-belt treadmill paradigms to improve step symmetry of individuals post stroke (136), and "high-intensity stepping training" physical therapy to improve locomotion of individuals post stroke (137) have demonstrated promising results to date in this area of translational study. Most of these paradigms have been used to see if short-term acute shaping of task performance can be facilitated, whereas long-term retention as well as generalization to other gait tasks may be viewed as the ultimate goal. However, currently, there is limited scientific evidence that locomotor training such as BWSTT is superior to conventional physical therapy–guided exercise program (138) although another review article suggested that electromechanical-assisted gait training with and without partial body weight support such as end-effector devices may be superior to exoskeleton device walkers in achieving optimal gait outcomes after stroke (139).

ACKNOWLEDGMENTS

Vivek Kadyan, MD, was our coauthor in this chapter as it appeared in the predecessor edition of this textbook. Some of his previous phrasing and other contributions are retained.

D. Casey Kerrigan, MD, created some figures for a previous edition that she authored and that have been retained.

REFERENCES

1. Ditunno JF Jr, Barbeau H, Dobkin BH, et al. Validity of the walking scale for spinal cord injury and other domains of function in a multicenter clinical trial. *Neurorehabil Neural Repair.* 2007;21(6):539–550.
2. Sadeghi H, Sadeghi S, Allard P, et al. Lower limb muscle power relationships in bilateral able-bodied gait. *Am J Phys Med Rehabil.* 2001;80(11):821–830.
3. Aissaoui R, Allard P, Junqua A, et al. Internal work estimation in three-dimensional gait analysis. *Med Biol Eng Comput.* 1996;34(6):467–471.
4. Rose J, Morgan D, Gamble J. Energetics of walking. In: Rose J, Gamble J, eds. *Human Walking.* 3rd ed. Baltimore, MD: Lippincott Williams & Wilkins; 2005:77–102.
5. Rathkey JK, Wall-Scheffler CM. People choose to run at their optimal speed. *Am J Phys Anthropol.* 2017;163(1):85–93.
6. Umberger BR. Stance and swing phase costs in human walking. *J R Soc Interface.* 2010;7(50):1329–1340.
7. Inman VT, Ralston H, Todd FN. Human locomotion. In: Rose J, Gamble J, eds. *Human Walking.* 3rd ed. Baltimore, MD: Lippincott Williams & Wilkins; 2005:1–22.
8. Della Croce U, Riley PO, Lelas JL, et al. A refined view of the determinants of gait. *Gait Posture.* 2001;14(2):79–84.
9. Neptune RR, Kautz SA, Zajac FE. Contributions of the individual ankle plantar flexors to support, forward progression and swing initiation during walking. *J Biomech.* 2001;34(11):1387–1398.
10. Neptune RR, Zajac FE, Kautz SA. Muscle force redistributes segmental power for body progression during walking. *Gait Posture.* 2004;19(2):194–205.
11. Neptune RR, Zajac FE, Kautz SA. Muscle mechanical work requirements during normal walking: the energetic cost of raising the body's center-of-mass is significant. *J Biomech.* 2004;37(5):817–825.
12. Neptune RR, Sasaki K, Kautz SA. The effect of walking speed on muscle function and mechanical energetics. *Gait Posture.* 2008;28(1):135–143.
13. Zajac FE, Neptune RR, Kautz SA. Biomechanics and muscle coordination of human walking: part II: lessons from dynamical simulations and clinical implications. *Gait Posture.* 2003;17(1):1–17.
14. Taylor NF, Goldie PA, Evans OM. Angular movements of the pelvis and lumbar spine during self-selected and slow walking speeds. *Gait Posture.* 1999;9(2):88–94.
15. Zajac FE, Neptune RR, Kautz SA. Biomechanics and muscle coordination of human walking. Part I: introduction to concepts, power transfer, dynamics and simulations. *Gait Posture.* 2002;16(3):215–232.
16. Basmajian J, DeLuca C. *Muscles Alive: Their Functions Revealed by Electromyography.* Baltimore, MD: Lippincott Williams & Wilkins; 1985.
17. Nene A, Mayagoitia R, Veltink P. Assessment of rectus femoris function during initial swing phase. *Gait Posture.* 1999;9(1):1–9.
18. Rose SA, Ounpuu S, DeLuca PA. Strategies for the assessment of pediatric gait in the clinical setting. *Phys Ther.* 1991;71(12):961–980.
19. Chambers HG, Sutherland DH. A practical guide to gait analysis. *J Am Acad Orthop Surg.* 2002;10(3):222–231.
20. Carpenter D, Batley R, Johnson E. Developmental evaluation of infants and children. *Phys Med Rehabil Clin N Am.* 1996;7:561–582.
21. Dunn BH. Musculoskeletal assessment: gait assessment. *Orthop Nurs.* 1982;1(3):33–37.
22. Johnson EW, Spiegel MH. Ambulation problems in very young children. *JAMA.* 1961;175:858–863.
23. Kermoian R, Johanson M, Butler E, et al. Development of gait. In: Rose J, Gamble J, eds. *Human Walking.* 3rd ed. Baltimore, MD: Lippincott Williams & Wilkins; 2005:119–130.
24. Chambers HG. Pediatric gait analysis. In: Perry J, Burnfield J, eds. *Gait Analysis: Normal and Pathological Function.* 2nd ed. Thorofare, NJ: Slack; 2010:341–363.
25. Sutherland DH, Olshen R, Cooper L, et al. The development of mature gait. *J Bone Joint Surg Am.* 1980;62(3):336–353.
26. Sutherland D. The development of mature walking. *Clin Dev Med.* 1988;104/105:1–227.
27. Grieve D, Gear R. The relationships between length of stride, step frequency, time of swing and speed of walking for children and adults. *Ergonomics.* 1996;9:379–399.
28. Statham L, Murray MP. Early walking patterns of normal children. *Clin Orthop Relat Res.* 1971;79:8–24.
29. Todd FN, Lamoreux LW, Skinner SR, et al. Variations in the gait of normal children. A graph applicable to the documentation of abnormalities. *J Bone Joint Surg Am.* 1989;71(2):196–204.
30. Carollo J, Matthews D. Quantitative assessment of gait: a systemic approach. In: Alexander M, Matthews D, eds. *Pediatric Rehabilitation Principles and Practice.* 5th ed. New York: Demos Medical; 2015:78–112.
31. Gage JR. Gait analysis. An essential tool in the treatment of cerebral palsy. *Clin Orthop Relat Res.* 1993;(288):126–134.
32. Feng J, Wick J, Bompiani E, et al. Application of gait analysis in pediatric orthopaedics. *Curr Orthop Pract.* 2016;27:455–464.
33. Bell KJ, Ounpuu S, DeLuca PA, et al. Natural progression of gait in children with cerebral palsy. *J Pediatr Orthop.* 2002;22(5):677–682.
34. Kay RM, Dennis S, Rethlefsen S, et al. Impact of postoperative gait analysis on orthopaedic care. *Clin Orthop Relat Res.* 2000;(374):259–264.
35. Novachek T. Orthopedic treatment of muscle contractures. In: Gage JR, Schwartz MH, Koop SE, et al., eds. *The Identification and Treatment of Gait Problems in Cerebral Palsy.* 2nd ed. London, UK: Mac Keith Press; 2009:445–472.
36. DeLuca PA, Davis RB III, Ounpuu S, et al. Alterations in surgical decision making in patients with cerebral palsy based on three-dimensional gait analysis. *J Pediatr Orthop.* 1997;17(5):608–614.
37. Kay RM, Dennis S, Rethlefsen S, et al. The effect of preoperative gait analysis on orthopaedic decision making. *Clin Orthop Relat Res.* 2000;(372):217–222.
38. Michael J. Lower limb prosthetics: implications and applications. In: Rose J, Gamble J, eds. *Human Walking.* Baltimore, MD: Lippincott Williams & Wilkins; 2005:185–192.
39. Sutherland DH, Cooper L. The pathomechanics of progressive crouch gait in spastic diplegia. *Orthop Clin North Am.* 1978;9(1):143–154.
40. Rethlefsen SA, Blumstein G, Kay RM, et al. Prevalence of specific gait abnormalities in children with cerebral palsy revisited: influence of age, prior surgery, and Gross Motor Function Classification System level. *Dev Med Child Neurol.* 2017;59(1):79–88.
41. Kerrigan DC, Glenn MB. An illustration of clinical gait laboratory use to improve rehabilitation management. *Am J Phys Med Rehabil.* 1994;73(6):421–427.
42. Saleh M, Murdoch G. In defence of gait analysis. Observation and measurement in gait assessment. *J Bone Joint Surg Br.* 1985;67(2):237–241.
43. Cioni M, Esquenazi A, Hirai B. Effects of botulinum toxin-A on gait velocity, step length, and base of support of patients with dynamic equinovarus foot. *Am J Phys Med Rehabil.* 2006;85(7):600–606.
44. Balaban B, Tok F. Gait disturbances in patients with stroke. *PM R.* 2014;6(7):635–642.
45. Goldie PA, Matyas TA, Evans OM. Gait after stroke: initial deficit and changes in temporal patterns for each gait phase. *Arch Phys Med Rehabil.* 2001;82(8):1057–1065.
46. De Quervain IA, Simon SR, Leurgans S, et al. Gait pattern in the early recovery period after stroke. *J Bone Joint Surg Am.* 1996;78(10):1506–1514.
47. Czerniecki JM. Rehabilitation in limb deficiency. 1. Gait and motion analysis. *Arch Phys Med Rehabil.* 1996;77(3 suppl):S3–S8.
48. Murray MP, Mollinger LA, Sepic SB, et al. Gait patterns in above-knee amputee patients: hydraulic swing control vs constant-friction knee components. *Arch Phys Med Rehabil.* 1983;64(8):339–345.
49. Murray MP, Sepic SB, Gardner GM, et al. Gait patterns of above-knee amputees using constant-friction knee components. *Bull Prosthet Res.* 1980;10-34:35–45.
50. Huang ME, Levy CE, Webster JB. Acquired limb deficiencies. 3. Prosthetic components, prescriptions, and indications. *Arch Phys Med Rehabil.* 2001;82(3 suppl 1):S17–S24.
51. Mattes SJ, Martin PE, Royer TD. Walking symmetry and energy cost in persons with unilateral transtibial amputations: matching prosthetic and intact limb inertial properties. *Arch Phys Med Rehabil.* 2000;81(5):561–568.
52. Silverman AK, Fey NP, Portillo A, et al. Compensatory mechanisms in below-knee amputee gait in response to increasing steady-state walking speeds. *Gait Posture.* 2008;28(4):602–609.
53. Winter DA, Sienko SE. Biomechanics of below-knee amputee gait. *J Biomech.* 1988;21(5):361–367.
54. Fey NP, Silverman AK, Neptune RR. The influence of increasing steady-state walking speed on muscle activity in below-knee amputees. *J Electromyogr Kinesiol.* 2010;20(1):155–161.
55. Van Jaarsveld HW, Grootenboer HJ, De Vries J. Accelerations due to impact at heel strike using below-knee prosthesis. *Prosthet Orthot Int.* 1990;14(2):63–66.
56. Perry J. Amputee gait. In: Smith DG, Michael J, Bowker JH, eds. *Atlas of Amputations and Limb Deficiencies: Surgical, Prosthetic and Rehabilitation Principles.* 3rd ed. Rosemont, IL: American Academy of Orthopaedic Surgeons; 2005.
57. Gitter A, Czerniecki JM, DeGroot DM. Biomechanical analysis of the influence of prosthetic feet on below-knee amputee walking. *Am J Phys Med Rehabil.* 1991;70(3):142–148.
58. Powers CM, Rao S, Perry J. Knee kinetics in trans-tibial amputee gait. *Gait Posture.* 1998;8(1):1–7.
59. Torburn L, Perry J, Ayyappa E, et al. Below-knee amputee gait with dynamic elastic response prosthetic feet: a pilot study. *J Rehabil Res Dev.* 1990;27(4):369–384.
60. Barth D, Schumacher L, Sienko-Thomas S. Gait analysis and energy cost of below knee amputees wearing six different prosthetic feet. *J Prosthet Orthot.* 1992;4:63–75.
61. Barr AE, Siegel KL, Danoff JV, et al. Biomechanical comparison of the energy-storing capabilities of SACH and Carbon Copy II prosthetic feet during the stance phase of gait in a person with below-knee amputation. *Phys Ther.* 1992;72(5):344–354.

62. Fey NP, Neptune RR. 3D intersegmental knee loading in below-knee amputees across steady-state walking speeds. *Clin Biomech (Bristol, Avon)*. 2012;27(4):409–414.

63. Perry J, Shanfield S. Efficiency of dynamic elastic response prosthetic feet. *J Rehabil Res Dev*. 1993;30(1):137–143.

64. Powers CM, Torburn L, Perry J, et al. Influence of prosthetic foot design on sound limb loading in adults with unilateral below-knee amputations. *Arch Phys Med Rehabil*. 1994;75(7):825–829.

65. Gailey R, Allen K, Castles J, et al. Review of secondary physical conditions associated with lower-limb amputation and long-term prosthesis use. *J Rehabil Res Dev*. 2008;45(1):15–29.

66. Lemaire ED, Fisher FR. Osteoarthritis and elderly amputee gait. *Arch Phys Med Rehabil*. 1994;75(10):1094–1099.

67. Fey NP, Klute GK, Neptune RR. Optimization of prosthetic foot stiffness to reduce metabolic cost and intact knee loading during below-knee amputee walking: a theoretical study. *J Biomech Eng*. 2012;134(11):111005.

68. Fey NP, Klute GK, Neptune RR. The influence of energy storage and return foot stiffness on walking mechanics and muscle activity in below-knee amputees. *Clin Biomech (Bristol, Avon)*. 2011;26(10):1025–1032.

69. Fey NP, Klute GK, Neptune RR. Altering prosthetic foot stiffness influences foot and muscle function during below-knee amputee walking: a modeling and simulation analysis. *J Biomech*. 2013;46(4):637–644.

70. Kerrigan DC, Todd MK, Della Croce U, et al. Biomechanical gait alterations independent of speed in the healthy elderly: evidence for specific limiting impairments. *Arch Phys Med Rehabil*. 1998;79(3):317–322.

71. Murray MP, Kory RC, Clarkson BH. Walking patterns in healthy old men. *J Gerontol*. 1969;24(2):169–178.

72. Judge J, Smyers D, Wolfson L. Muscle strength gait measures in older adults. *J Am Geriatr Soc*. 1992;40:SA27.

73. Bendall MJ, Bassey EJ, Pearson MB. Factors affecting walking speed of elderly people. *Age Ageing*. 1989;18(5):327–332.

74. Chang RW, Dunlop D, Gibbs J, et al. The determinants of walking velocity in the elderly. An evaluation using regression trees. *Arthritis Rheum*. 1995;38(3):343–350.

75. Burnfield JM, Josephson KR, Powers CM, et al. The influence of lower extremity joint torque on gait characteristics in elderly men. *Arch Phys Med Rehabil*. 2000;81(9):1153–1157.

76. McMillan GJ, Hubbard RE. Frailty in older inpatients: what physicians need to know. *QJM*. 2012;105(11):1059–1065.

77. Kerrigan DC, Lee LW, Nieto TJ, et al. Kinetic alterations independent of walking speed in elderly fallers. *Arch Phys Med Rehabil*. 2000;81(6):730–735.

78. DeVita P, Hortobagyi T. Age causes a redistribution of joint torques and powers during gait. *J Appl Physiol*. 2000;88(5):1804–1811.

79. Adams J, Perry J. Gait analysis: clinical decision making. In: Rose J, Gamble J, eds. *Human Walking*. Baltimore, MD: Lippincott Williams & Wilkins; 2005:165–184.

80. Lehmann JF. Biomechanics of ankle-foot orthoses: prescription and design. *Arch Phys Med Rehabil*. 1979;60(5):200–207.

81. Tyson SF, Sadeghi-Demneh E, Nester CJ. A systematic review and meta-analysis of the effect of an ankle-foot orthosis on gait biomechanics after stroke. *Clin Rehabil*. 2013;27(10):879–891.

82. Saunders JB, Inman VT, Eberhart HD. The major determinants in normal and pathological gait. *J Bone Joint Surg Am*. 1953;35-a(3):543–558.

83. Cassidy L, Bandela S, Wooten C, et al. Friedrich Trendelenburg: historical background and significant medical contributions. *Clin Anat*. 2014;27(6):815–820.

84. Kerrigan DC, Deming LC, Holden MK. Knee recurvatum in gait: a study of associated knee biomechanics. *Arch Phys Med Rehabil*. 1996;77(7):645–650.

85. Chambers H, Lauer A, Kaufman K, et al. Prediction of outcome after rectus femoris surgery in cerebral palsy: the role of cocontraction of the rectus femoris and vastus lateralis. *J Pediatr Orthop*. 1998;18(6):703–711.

86. Gage JR, Perry J, Hicks RR, et al. Rectus femoris transfer to improve knee function of children with cerebral palsy. *Dev Med Child Neurol*. 1987;29(2):159–166.

87. Hadley N, Chambers C, Scarborough N, et al. Knee motion following multiple soft-tissue releases in ambulatory patients with cerebral palsy. *J Pediatr Orthop*. 1992;12(3):324–328.

88. Ounpuu S, Muik E, Davis RB III, et al. Rectus femoris surgery in children with cerebral palsy. Part I: the effect of rectus femoris transfer location on knee motion. *J Pediatr Orthop*. 1993;13(3):325–330.

89. Perry J. Distal rectus femoris transfer. *Dev Med Child Neurol*. 1987;29(2):153–158.

90. Sutherland DH, Larsen LJ, Mann R. Rectus femoris release in selected patients with cerebral palsy: a preliminary report. *Dev Med Child Neurol*. 1975;17(1):26–34.

91. Waters RL, Garland DE, Perry J, et al. Stiff-legged gait in hemiplegia: surgical correction. *J Bone Joint Surg Am*. 1979;61(6a):927–933.

92. Sung DH, Bang HJ. Motor branch block of the rectus femoris: its effectiveness in stiff-legged gait in spastic paresis. *Arch Phys Med Rehabil*. 2000;81(7):910–915.

93. Chua KS, Kong KH. Alcohol neurolysis of the sciatic nerve in the treatment of hemiplegic knee flexor spasticity: clinical outcomes. *Arch Phys Med Rehabil*. 2000;81(10):1432–1435.

94. Buckon CE, Thomas SS, Harris GE, et al. Objective measurement of muscle strength in children with spastic diplegia after selective dorsal rhizotomy. *Arch Phys Med Rehabil*. 2002;83(4):454–460.

95. Cozean CD, Pease WS, Hubbell SL. Biofeedback and functional electric stimulation in stroke rehabilitation. *Arch Phys Med Rehabil*. 1988;69(6):401–405.

96. Granat MH, Maxwell DJ, Ferguson AC, et al. Peroneal stimulator; evaluation for the correction of spastic drop foot in hemiplegia. *Arch Phys Med Rehabil*. 1996;77(1):19–24.

97. Liberson WT, Holmquest HJ, Scot D, et al. Functional electrotherapy: stimulation of the peroneal nerve synchronized with the swing phase of the gait of hemiplegic patients. *Arch Phys Med Rehabil*. 1961;42:101–105.

98. Bethoux F, Rogers HL, Nolan KJ, et al. The effects of peroneal nerve functional electrical stimulation versus ankle-foot orthosis in patients with chronic stroke: a randomized controlled trial. *Neurorehabil Neural Repair*. 2014;28(7):688–697.

99. Daly JJ, Roenigk K, Holcomb J, et al. A randomized controlled trial of functional neuromuscular stimulation in chronic stroke subjects. *Stroke*. 2006;37(1):172–178.

100. Kobetic R, Triolo RJ, Marsolais EB. Muscle selection and walking performance of multichannel FES systems for ambulation in paraplegia. *IEEE Trans Rehabil Eng*. 1997;5(1):23–29.

101. Kim CM, Eng JJ, Whittaker MW. Effects of a simple functional electric system and/or a hinged ankle-foot orthosis on walking in persons with incomplete spinal cord injury. *Arch Phys Med Rehabil*. 2004;85(10):1718–1723.

102. Stein RB, Chong S, Everaert DG, et al. A multicenter trial of a footdrop stimulator controlled by a tilt sensor. *Neurorehabil Neural Repair*. 2006;20(3):371–379.

103. Ladouceur M, Barbeau H. Functional electrical stimulation-assisted walking for persons with incomplete spinal injuries: longitudinal changes in maximal overground walking speed. *Scand J Rehabil Med*. 2000;32(1):28–36.

104. Galli M, Cimolin V, Valente EM, et al. Computerized gait analysis of botulinum toxin treatment in children with cerebral palsy. *Disabil Rehabil*. 2007;29(8):659–664.

105. Desloovere K, Molenaers G, De Cat J, et al. Motor function following multilevel botulinum toxin type A treatment in children with cerebral palsy. *Dev Med Child Neurol*. 2007;49(1):56–61.

106. Francisco GE, Boake C. Improvement in walking speed in poststroke spastic hemiplegia after intrathecal baclofen therapy: a preliminary study. *Arch Phys Med Rehabil*. 2003;84(8):1194–1199.

107. Wong AM, Chen CL, Chen CP, et al. Clinical effects of botulinum toxin A and phenol block on gait in children with cerebral palsy. *Am J Phys Med Rehabil*. 2004;83(4):284–291.

108. Brin MF. Dosing, administration, and a treatment algorithm for use of botulinum toxin A for adult-onset spasticity. Spasticity Study Group. *Muscle Nerve Suppl*. 1997;6:S208–S220.

109. Russman BS, Tilton A, Gormley ME Jr. Cerebral palsy: a rational approach to a treatment protocol, and the role of botulinum toxin in treatment. *Muscle Nerve Suppl*. 1997;6:S181–S193.

110. Graham HK, Aoki KR, Autti-Ramo I, et al. Recommendations for the use of botulinum toxin type A in the management of cerebral palsy. *Gait Posture*. 2000;11(1):67–79.

111. Assessment: the clinical usefulness of botulinum toxin-A in treating neurologic disorders. Report of the Therapeutics and Technology Assessment Subcommittee of the American Academy of Neurology. *Neurology*. 1990;40(9):1332–1336.

112. Au S, Berniker M, Herr H. Powered ankle-foot prosthesis to assist level-ground and stair-descent gaits. *Neural Netw*. 2008;21(4):654–666.

113. Sup F, Bohara A, Goldfarb M. Design and control of a powered transfemoral prosthesis. *Int J Robot Res*. 2008;27(2):263–273.

114. Banala SK, Kim SH, Agrawal SK, et al. Robot assisted gait training with active leg exoskeleton (ALEX). *IEEE Trans Neural Syst Rehabil Eng*. 2009;17(1):2–8.

115. Veneman JF, Kruidhof R, Hekman EE, et al. Design and evaluation of the LOPES exoskeleton robot for interactive gait rehabilitation. *IEEE Trans Neural Syst Rehabil Eng*. 2007;15(3):379–386.

116. Zoss AB, Kazerooni H, Chu A. Biomechanical design of the Berkeley lower extremity exoskeleton (BLEEX). *IEEE/ASME Trans Mechatr*. 2006;11(2):128–138.

117. Fey NP, Simon AM, Young AJ, et al. Controlling knee swing initiation and ankle plantarflexion with an active prosthesis on level and inclined surfaces at variable walking speeds. *IEEE J Transl Eng Health Med*. 2014;2:1–12.

118. Hargrove LJ, Young AJ, Simon AM, et al. Intuitive control of a powered prosthetic leg during ambulation: a randomized clinical trial. *JAMA*. 2015;313(22):2244–2252.

119. Barbeau H, Fung J. The role of rehabilitation in the recovery of walking in the neurological population. *Curr Opin Neurol*. 2001;14(6):735–740.

120. Dobkin B, Barbeau H, Deforge D, et al. The evolution of walking-related outcomes over the first 12 weeks of rehabilitation for incomplete traumatic spinal cord injury: the multicenter randomized Spinal Cord Injury Locomotor Trial. *Neurorehabil Neural Repair*. 2007;21(1):25–35.

121. Protas EJ, Holmes SA, Qureshy H, et al. Supported treadmill ambulation training after spinal cord injury: a pilot study. *Arch Phys Med Rehabil*. 2001;82(6):825–831.

122. Miyai I, Fujimoto Y, Ueda Y, et al. Treadmill training with body weight support: its effect on Parkinson's disease. *Arch Phys Med Rehabil*. 2000;81(7):849–852.

123. Peurala SH, Tarkka IM, Pitkanen K, et al. The effectiveness of body weight-supported gait training and floor walking in patients with chronic stroke. *Arch Phys Med Rehabil*. 2005;86(8):1557–1564.

124. Sullivan KJ, Knowlton BJ, Dobkin BH. Step training with body weight support: effect of treadmill speed and practice paradigms on poststroke locomotor recovery. *Arch Phys Med Rehabil*. 2002;83(5):683–691.

125. Toole T, Maitland CG, Warren E, et al. The effects of loading and unloading treadmill walking on balance, gait, fall risk, and daily function in Parkinsonism. *NeuroRehabilitation*. 2005;20(4):307–322.

126. Visintin M, Barbeau H, Korner-Bitensky N, et al. A new approach to retrain gait in stroke patients through body weight support and treadmill stimulation. *Stroke*. 1998;29(6):1122–1128.

127. Vo AN, Kamen LB, Shih VC, et al. Rehabilitation of orthopedic and rheumatologic disorders. 5. Lumbar spinal stenosis. *Arch Phys Med Rehabil*. 2005;86(3 suppl 1):S69–S76.

128. Werner C, Bardeleben A, Mauritz KH, et al. Treadmill training with partial body weight support and physiotherapy in stroke patients: a preliminary comparison. *Eur J Neurol.* 2002;9(6):639–644.

129. Hesse S, Werner C, Paul T, et al. Influence of walking speed on lower limb muscle activity and energy consumption during treadmill walking of hemiparetic patients. *Arch Phys Med Rehabil.* 2001;82(11):1547–1550.

130. Mossberg KA, Orlander EE, Norcross JL. Cardiorespiratory capacity after weight-supported treadmill training in patients with traumatic brain injury. *Phys Ther.* 2008;88(1):77–87.

131. Hidler JM, Stienen AHA, Vallery H. Robotic devices for overground gait and balance training. In: Reinkensmeyer D, Dietz V, eds. *Neurorehabilitation Technology.* 2nd ed. Switzerland, AG: Springer International; 2016:483–492.

132. Colombo G, Joerg M, Schreier R, et al. Treadmill training of paraplegic patients using a robotic orthosis. *J Rehabil Res Dev.* 2000;37(6):693–700.

133. Winchester P, Querry R. Robotic orthoses for body weight-supported treadmill training. *Phys Med Rehabil Clin N Am.* 2006;17(1):159–172.

134. Wirz M, Zemon DH, Rupp R, et al. Effectiveness of automated locomotor training in patients with chronic incomplete spinal cord injury: a multicenter trial. *Arch Phys Med Rehabil.* 2005;86(4):672–680.

135. Kaufman KR, Wyatt MP, Sessoms PH, et al. Task-specific fall prevention training is effective for warfighters with transtibial amputations. *Clin Orthop Relat Res.* 2014;472(10):3076–3084.

136. Reisman DS, Wityk R, Silver K, et al. Locomotor adaptation on a split-belt treadmill can improve walking symmetry post-stroke. *Brain.* 2007;130(7):1861–1872.

137. Holleran CL, Straube DD, Kinnaird CR, et al. Feasibility and potential efficacy of high-intensity stepping training in variable contexts in subacute and chronic stroke. *Neurorehabil Neural Repair.* 2014;28(7):643–651.

138. Duncan PW, Sullivan KJ, Behrman AL, et al. Body-weight-supported treadmill rehabilitation after stroke. *N Engl J Med.* 2011;364(21):2026–2036.

139. Mehrholz J, Pohl M. Electromechanical-assisted gait training after stroke: a systematic review comparing end-effector and exoskeleton devices. *J Rehabil Med.* 2012;44(3):193–199.

CHAPTER 5

Edgar Colón Negron
Luis R. Burgos-Anaya

Imaging Techniques

A brief presentation of imaging techniques of interest to the physiatrist must necessarily be selective. Because the diagnosis and initial treatment of fractures are primarily the responsibility of the orthopedic surgeon, with the rehabilitation professional typically involved only later in the course, a full discussion of fractures is not presented in this chapter. Only those fractures that bring patients under the long-term care of the physiatrist are included (e.g., vertebral fractures with the potential to damage the spinal cord). Similarly, tumors and infectious processes are deemphasized. Rather, emphasis is placed on imaging degenerative musculoskeletal processes, spine and head trauma, stroke, and degenerative central nervous system (CNS) diseases commonly seen by the physiatrist. We will also cover imaging in sport medicine as this is a rapidly changing area in radiology and review the current applications of diagnostic ultrasound in the evaluation of musculoskeletal disorders.

MUSCULOSKELETAL IMAGING

The important role played by radiology in the diagnosis of diseases has come at the expense of increased radiation exposure to the general population. With the advent of new technology, such as positron emission tomography (PET) studies and multidetector computed tomography (MDCT) technology, there has been a sharp increase in the number of radiographic examinations performed and as a consequence an increase in the cumulative radiation dose to the individual patient. Overall, there has been a sevenfold increase in radiation exposure to the population of the United States from medical radiation since the early 1980s. An expected outcome of the increase in radiation exposure is a higher incidence of malignancy. Therefore, increased awareness is needed in issues concerning radiation safety. Ionizing radiation, especially at high doses, is known to increase the risk of developing cancer. It is estimated that medical exposure might be responsible for 1% of cancer diagnoses in the United States. This rate is expected to increase in the coming years due to the increased number of examinations performed today.

The scientific measurement for the effective dose of radiation is the millisievert (mSv). The background radiation dose for the average person in the United States is about 3 mSv per year. This is secondary to cosmic radiation and naturally occurring radioactive materials. By comparison, the effective radiation dose for a spinal CT is equivalent to 6 mSv or 2 years of natural background radiation. Radiation exposure is particularly important in pregnant women and pediatric patients due to the cumulative life effect of radiation exposure

at a younger age. In nuclear medicine examinations, special precautions are needed. Some of the radiopharmaceuticals used in nuclear medicine can pass into the milk of lactating women (1).

The relative radiation level (RRL) is a radiation measurement used to calculate effective dose. This is the dose used to estimate population total radiation risk associated with an imaging procedure. This takes into account the sensitivity of different body organs and tissues. This estimate cannot assess the specific risk of an individual patient.

The advent of the MDCT scanner has increased the applicability of CT imaging technique for the assessment of the musculoskeletal system. This technology allows for the acquisition of large data set in the axial plane that can be reconstructed in multiple planes of imaging with the use of multiplanar reconstruction (MPR) algorithms. Any anatomical part in the human body can now be scanned in the axial plane, and the anatomical information can later be reconstructed in the sagittal, coronal, or any orthogonal plane desired in order to better assess complex anatomical structures (2). CT provides poor contrast resolution to evaluate the soft tissues since the soft tissue radiodensity of the cartilage, tendons, and muscle is similar. Thus, we cannot resolve adequate soft tissue differences between these structures. For example, the articular cartilage can only be assessed with CT after contrast is introduced in the joint space, such as is the case with CT arthrography. CT, however, provides superb spatial resolution that allows for the accurate evaluation of structures including bone density and trabecular pattern.

CT images may be displayed with various windows suitable to resolve different structures. Bone window images provide the highest resolution of compact and cancellous bone. Soft tissue window offers moderate resolution of muscle, tendon, ligament, fat, cartilage, and neural structures.

The good resolution and enhanced contrast of MRI for soft tissue structures, together with its direct multiplanar imaging capability, make it a superb modality for evaluating all the principal constituents of the musculoskeletal system. Although a technical discussion of the physics of MRI is beyond the scope of this chapter, the physiatrist should know the normal and abnormal MRI appearance of various tissues to be able to look at an MR image with confidence and explain the findings to a patient.

The MRI signal intensity of any tissue primarily reflects its proton density, its T1 relaxation time, and its T2 relaxation time. Various techniques, including manipulating the repetition time (TR) between the application of radiofrequency pulses or the echo time (TE) between the radiofrequency pulse and the recording of a signal (i.e., echo) produced by the tissue, can emphasize the proton density, T1 relaxation time, or T2 relaxation time features of any tissue (3). The TR and TE are expressed in milliseconds. The most commonly used technique is spin echo, in which short TR and TE will emphasize the T1 relaxation time of a tissue, the so-called T1-weighted image. In general, an image is said to be T1 weighted if TR is less than 1,000 milliseconds (ms) and TE is less than 30 ms (e.g., TR = 500 ms, TE = 20 ms). A T2-weighted image generally is accomplished with a TR longer than 1,500 ms and a TE greater than 60 ms (e.g., TR = 2,000 ms, TE = 85 ms). Proton density images are obtained with a long TR and a short TE (e.g., TR = 2,000 ms, TE = 20 ms).

Compact bone, fibrocartilage, ligaments, and tendons produce very low signal intensity due to their low proton density and appear hypointense (black) both on T1- and T2-weighted sequences (**Fig. 5-1**). The Muscle demonstrates moderately

low signal intensity and appears relatively hypointense (dark gray) both on T1- and T2-weighted sequences. Peripheral nerves demonstrate slightly higher signal intensity than the muscle because of the fat content of their myelinated fibers. Hyaline cartilage produces moderate signal intensity on T2-weighted sequences and appears light gray. Fat produces very high signal intensity and appears bright on T1- and T2-weighted sequences. Because fat is frequently situated adjacent to ligaments and tendons, it can provide a high-contrast interface for evaluating the integrity of these structures. Adult bone marrow also shows high signal intensity in the appendicular skeleton because of its high fat content and intermediate-to-high signal intensity in the axial skeleton due to the presence of red marrow. The signal changes with time in response to the normal conversion of hematopoietic to nonhematopoietic marrow that occurs normally related to the aging process. Most normal body fluids that are not flowing show

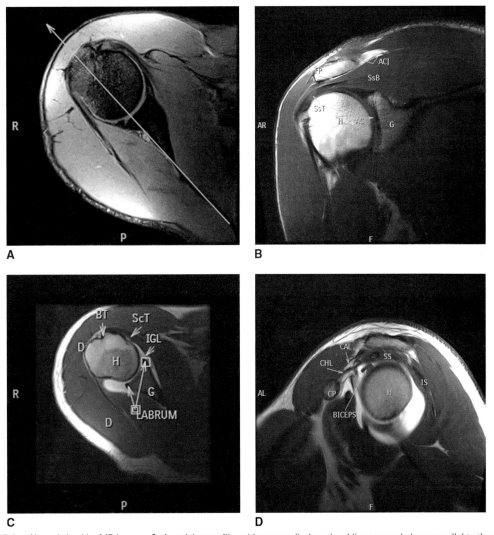

FIGURE 5-1. Normal shoulder MR images. **A:** An axial scout film with cursors displays the oblique coronal planes parallel to the plane of the scapula (long arrow perpendicular to the glenohumeral joint), which allow optimal visualization of the supraspinatus. **B:** An oblique coronal image demonstrates the supraspinatus muscle belly (*SsB*), supraspinatus tendon (*SsT*), subacromial-subdeltoid fat plane (*FP*), acromioclavicular joint (*ACJ*), deltoid muscle (*D*), articular cartilage of humeral head and glenoid (*AC*), glenoid (*G*), and humeral head (*H*). **C:** An axial image displays the humeral head (*H*), glenoid (*G*), glenoid labrum (*L*), inferior glenohumeral ligament (*IGL*), deltoid muscle (*D*), subscapularis tendon (*ScT*), and biceps tendon (*BT*). **D:** A sagittal section demonstrates good resolution of the coracoacromial ligament (*CAL*) extending from the coracoid process (*CP*) to the acromion; CP, supraspinatus (*SS*), and infraspinatus (*IS*).

low signal intensity on T1-weighted images and high signal intensity on T2-weighted images.

Pathologic processes such as tumor, infection, and abnormal fluids (e.g., edema, joint effusion) show intermediate signal intensity on T1-weighted images and become very hyperintense on T2-weighted images. Pathologic calcifications demonstrate very low signal intensity on both T1- and T2-weighted images.

The direct multiplanar imaging capability of MRI is particularly useful in evaluating obliquely oriented musculoskeletal structures such as the supraspinatus tendon, the cruciate ligaments, and the lateral collateral ligaments of the ankle among others.

MRI has proved useful in evaluating traumatic, degenerative, inflammatory, and neoplastic pathology of the limbs and spine. It is useful in detecting acute or chronic traumatic injuries and degenerative conditions involving bones, muscles, tendons, ligaments, fibrocartilage, and nerves. Bone pathology, particularly well detected by MRI, includes contusions, osteochondral injuries, stress fractures, marrow replacement by neoplastic cells, and ischemic necrosis. Muscle lesions that MRI is especially sensitive at identifying include strain or contusion, complete rupture, compartment syndrome, myopathies, and atrophy (4). Tendon conditions well depicted by MRI include partial and complete tear, tendinopathy, and tenosynovitis. MRI is also very sensitive for detecting partial or complete ligament tears. Fibrocartilaginous injuries or diseases well delineated by MRI include pathology of the menisci, the glenoid labrum, the triangular fibrocartilage of the wrist, and the intervertebral discs. Nerve entrapments well visualized by MRI include spinal nerve encroachment by disc disease or spinal stenosis and carpal tunnel syndrome (CTS) or other entrapment syndromes. Enhanced imaging of normal and injured peripheral nerves can be obtained using a short-tau inversion recovery (STIR) excitation-emission sequence due to the increased sensitivity to free water content associated with tissue edema using this MR recording protocol. This pulse sequences suppress the signal from fat and increased the signal from areas of high water content including edema in the musculoskeletal system. This is the most popular sequence for the evaluation of trauma and inflammatory reactions in the bones, joints, and soft tissues. The increased signal generated by injured nerves using STIR pulse sequences probably reflects an increase in free water content of the nerve due to altered axoplasmic flow, axonal and/or myelin degeneration, and endoneurial or perineurial edema due to a breakdown in the blood-nerve barrier (5). MRI imaging of acutely denervated skeletal muscle shows increased MR signal using the STIR sequence, due to intramuscular edema, when there is significant muscular weakness and well-defined changes indicating muscle denervation on needle electromyography (6).

Osteomyelitis causes a reduction in bone marrow signal intensity on T1-weighted images because of the replacement of normal fatty marrow by inflammatory exudate. In T2-weighted images, these areas of active infection become hyperintense.

MRI has particular value in evaluating both bone and soft tissue neoplasms. Most of them demonstrate moderately low signal intensity on T1-weighted images and very high signal intensity on T2-weighted images.

Every effort should be made to order the examination, which is best indicated to address the clinical concerns of the patient. To aid in this regard, the American College of Radiology (acr.org) has established guidelines for the appropriate use of imaging to answer specific clinical questions. The appropriateness criteria can be of help when deciding which imaging study to order.

Shoulder

Plain film radiographic evaluation of the shoulder should include frontal examinations with internal and external humeral rotation. If there is a question of instability or dislocation, axillary view, a scapular Y view, or both should be obtained. There have been several reports that recommend the use of a 30-degree caudad-angled radiograph or a suprascapular outlet view for the assessment of the anterior acromion in cases of suspected shoulder impingement. Since these are special views, they must be requested, as routine shoulder radiographs do not include axillary or suprascapular outlet views. The RRL for plain film radiographic examinations of the shoulder is less than 0.1 mSv, which is considered minimal.

MRI has become important in evaluating many shoulder abnormalities very familiar to the physiatrist. These include impingement syndrome, other rotator cuff abnormalities, instability syndrome, and bicipital tendon abnormalities. It is also useful in demonstrating arthritic changes, occult fractures, ischemic necrosis, and intra-articular bodies. MRI with intra-articular contrast is now considered the modality of choice for the evaluation of labral and capsular pathology. The use of MRI for shoulder evaluation avoids radiation exposure to the nearby thyroid gland, which can occur with CT examinations. The excellent visualization of the bone marrow by MRI permits early diagnosis of ischemic necrosis, infection, and primary or metastatic tumors.

Because of the oblique orientation of the scapula on the chest wall and the consequent anterolateral facing direction of the glenoid, the direct multiplanar imaging capability of MRI provides optimal visualization of all the important shoulder structures. An oblique coronal image parallel to the plane of the scapula provide full-length views of the rotator cuff musculature, especially the supraspinatus, and is the best plane for the evaluation of injuries to the biceps-labral complex (BLC) (**Fig. 5-1A** and **B**). Coronal oblique images can also provide information about the presence of impingement upon the supraspinatus by the acromion and osteophytes in the presence of acromioclavicular joint osteoarthritis. Oblique sagittal imaging planes parallel to the glenoid provide cross-sectional views of the rotator cuff apparatus and evaluate the anatomical configuration of the coracoacromial arch and the presence of impingement (**Fig. 5-1D**). Axial imaging planes provide good visualization of the anterior and posterior capsular apparatus, glenoid labrum, bony glenoid rim, and humeral head (**Fig. 5-1C**).

SHOULDER IMPINGEMENT SYNDROME AND SUPRASPINATUS INJURY

The MRI findings of shoulder impingement syndrome and its associated supraspinatus injury are best seen on oblique coronal MR images that visualize the full length of the supraspinatus muscle belly and tendon (**Fig. 5-1B**). The normal muscle belly displays moderately low signal intensity. The tendon is visualized as an intermediate–signal-intensity structure that blends with the low signal intensity of the superior capsule as it courses to its insertion on the greater tubercle of the humerus. The tendon demonstrates smooth tapering from medial to lateral into its insertion in the greater tuberosity. The inferior aspect of the tendon is delimited below by the moderate signal intensity of the hyaline cartilage on the superior aspect of the humeral head. The superior aspects of both the muscle belly and tendon are delimited by a high–signal-intensity subacromial and subdeltoid fat plane. The normal subacromial-subdeltoid bursa is not specifically visualized because its walls are separated only by monomolecular layers of a synovial-type fluid, but it is situated between the supraspinatus tendon and the fat plane. Above the fat plane, the clavicle, acromioclavicular joint, acromion, and deltoid muscle are demonstrated on different oblique coronal sections.

Although rotator cuff impingement is a clinical diagnosis, MRI can provide direct visualization of the constituents to the coracoacromial arch and their relationship to the supraspinatus (**Fig. 5-2A** and **B**). Downward slanting of the acromion in the coronal or the sagittal plane, a thickened coracoacromial ligament or inferior osteophytes within the acromioclavicular joint can exert mass effect upon the supraspinatus. This has been implied as being in part responsible for chronic tears of the supraspinatus (7).

Neer stated that 95% of rotator cuff tears are associated with chronic impingement syndrome (7) and described three stages in the progression of rotator cuff injury based on this extrinsic model. These can be visualized by MRI (7–9). Stage 1 is characterized by edema and hemorrhage within the supraspinatus tendon characteristic of an early tendinitis. On MRI, there is focal tendon thickening and diffuse moderate increase in signal intensity within the tendon (**Fig. 5-3A–C**). In stage 2, Neer described both inflammation and fibrosis within the tendon. MRI shows this as thinning and irregularity of the tendon. Stage 3 is a frank tear of the supraspinatus tendon. On MRI, complete tears are noted by a discontinuity of the tendon with a well-defined focus of high signal intensity on

T2-weighted images (**Fig. 5-4**). The most susceptible area is the critical zone of hypovascularity, located about 1 cm from the insertion (10). With small or partial tears, there is no retraction of the muscle-tendon junction, the subacromial-subdeltoid fat plane is commonly obliterated, and fluid may accumulate in the subacromial-subdeltoid bursa, which becomes hyperintense on T2-weighted images. There also may be effusion of the shoulder joint, which may extend inferiorly along the tendon sheath about the long head of the biceps. With a complete supraspinatus tendon tear, the muscle belly may retract medially, and atrophy may occur as the tear becomes chronic (**Fig. 5-5A** and **B**). Muscle atrophy appears as areas of high signal intensity because of fatty replacement within the muscle belly and decreased muscle mass. Finally, the acromiohumeral interval narrows as the humeral head migrates superiorly, because of the loss of supraspinatus restraint to the deltoid tendency to sublux the humerus superiorly during abduction.

SHOULDER INSTABILITY AND DISRUPTION OF THE ANTERIOR CAPSULAR MECHANISM

For the assessment of shoulder instability and labral tears, it is imperative that intra-articular contrast medium be injected in order to be able to evaluate the entire articular labrum, glenoid fossa, and capsular mechanism (11). Axial MR images provide the best visualization of the anterior and posterior glenoid labrum, capsule, and lower rotator cuff muscles (see **Fig. 5-1**). Anteriorly, the moderate–signal-intensity subscapularis muscle belly and its low–signal-intensity tendon are visualized. The tendon fuses with the low–signal-intensity anterior capsule as it courses to its insertion on the lesser tubercle. The fibrocartilaginous anterior and posterior labrum appear as low–signal-intensity triangular or rounded areas attached to the glenoid rim. The higher–signal-intensity intra-articular contrast opposed the hyaline cartilage surfaces of the glenoid and humeral head. The posterior capsule is visualized as a low-intensity area blending with the deep surface of infraspinatus

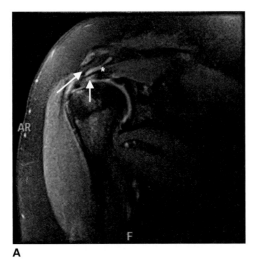 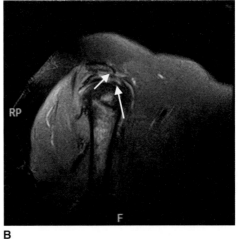

FIGURE 5-2. **A:** Coronal oblique T2-weighted pulse sequence with fat suppression demonstrates downward slanting to the acromion (*long arrow*), which is against the supraspinatus tendon (*asterisk*). Note focal area of increased signal at the myotendinous junction of the SsT (*short arrow*). **B:** Sagittal oblique T2WI with fat suppression demonstrates to a better advantage the inferior slanting to the acromion against the SsT (*short arrow*). Note focal tendinosis (*long arrow*).

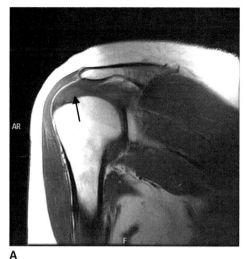

A

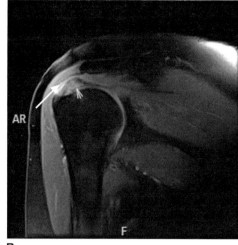

B

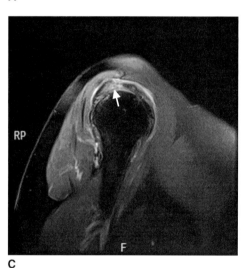

C

FIGURE 5-3. **A:** T1-weighted MRI of focal supraspinatus tendinosis demonstrating focal thickening and slight increase of signal intensity to the tendon (*arrow*). **B:** Coronal oblique T2-weighted fat suppressed sequence with increased signal intensity within the area of tendinosis (*arrowhead*). There is fluid within the adjacent subdeltoid bursa (*long arrow*). **C:** Sagittal oblique T2-weighted fat suppressed image demonstrates the area of increased signal to be within the anterior-superior portion of the rotator cuff representing fibers of the supraspinatus tendon (*short arrow*).

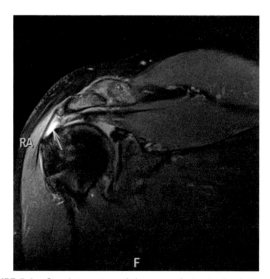

FIGURE 5-4. Complete rupture of the supraspinatus tendon is seen in a T2-weighted MRI. There is fluid filling the gap (*arrow*), and there is retraction to the tendon fibers underneath the acromion.

and teres minor muscles as they extend to their insertions on the greater tubercle of the humerus. The long tendon of the biceps is demonstrated as a round, low–signal-intensity area within the bicipital groove.

Shoulder instability and the associated disruption of the anterior capsular mechanism can cause chronic shoulder pain and disability. The instability may be caused by an acute traumatic episode or can occur with no history of a traumatic event. Both recurrent traumatic subluxation and nontraumatic instability are typically associated with disruption of the anterior capsular mechanism. Anteriorly, where most instability occurs, this mechanism includes the subscapularis muscle and tendon, the anterior joint capsule, three underlying glenohumeral ligaments, the synovial lining, and the anterior labrum. With instability, the labrum shows tears, separation from the glenoid rim, or degeneration. Also, frequently present are medial stripping of the capsule from its normal attachment to the labrum and glenoid rim, an enlarged fluid-filled subscapular bursa secondary to joint effusion, attenuation of the glenohumeral ligaments, and injury or laxity of the subscapularis muscle or tendon.

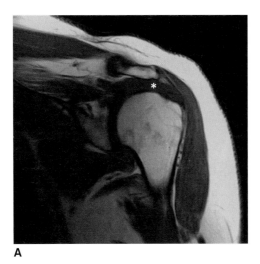
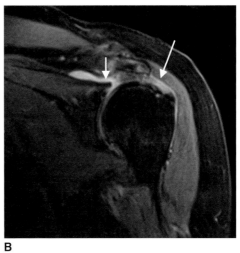

FIGURE 5-5. Complete rotator cuff tear. **A:** Coronal oblique T1-weighted image. There is intermediate signal intensity (*asterisk*) from the inflammatory reaction replacing the normal low signal to the SS tendon. **B:** The edge (*short arrow*) to the retracted tendon is at the level of the superior labrum. There is increased signal intensity filling the gap of the retracted tendon (*long arrow*).

In an MRI, labral tears may be visualized as discrete linear areas of increased signal intensity within the normal signal void of the labrum (**Figs. 5-6** and **5-7**). These areas show moderate intensity on T1-weighted images and high intensity on T2-weighted images. With recurrent dislocation or subluxation, the labrum can become fragmented or attenuated.

Capsular detachment from the scapula (i.e., stripping) is visualized by T2-weighted MRI as an area of high–signal-intensity fluid dissecting medially from the glenoid rim. With trauma to the subscapularis tendon, there can be medial retraction of the muscle-tendon junction when the tendon is completely ruptured. Chronic atrophy of the subscapularis muscle belly is identified by high–signal-intensity fatty replacement. The glenoid marrow underlying a labral detachment may show pathologically decreased signal intensity even before the plain film radiograph shows an osseous Bankart lesion. MRI and CT can be used to visualize Bankart fractures of the anterior glenoid and the Hill-Sachs compression deformity of the

posterolateral humeral head (12,13) and are both useful in the assessment of the extent of a Hill-Sachs defect in patients with engaging lesions. Patients with the rarer posterior instability show similar posterior labral, capsular, and muscular defects.

TENDINOPATHY OR TEARS OF OTHER ROTATOR CUFF MUSCLES

Tendinopathy and tears can involve the subscapularis, infraspinatus, teres minor, or biceps tendons, although far less commonly than the supraspinatus. Early tendinopathy can be seen as increased or decreased thickness to the tendon with an area of increased signal intensity on T2-weighted sequences. This can progress to frank rupture of the tendon with a high–signal-intensity area at the site of the tear on T2-weighted images and may be associated with joint effusion or fluid in the subdeltoid bursa. A complete tear will eventually cause muscle retraction and atrophy.

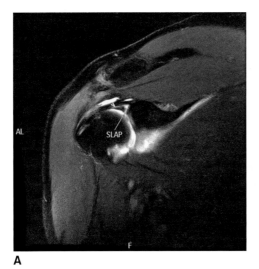
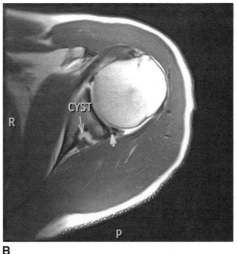

FIGURE 5-6. SLAP lesion and posterior labral tear in a patient with history of posterior instability. **A:** Coronal oblique T1-weighted fat suppressed MR arthrogram demonstrates increased signal intensity within the BLC extending on the biceps tendon (*arrowhead*) characteristic of a type IV SLAP lesion. **B:** Axial T1-weighted MR arthrogram demonstrates increased signal within the posterior labrum (*arrowhead*). There is a cyst within the posterior aspect of the spinoglenoid notch with high–signal-intensity contrast extending into the cyst.

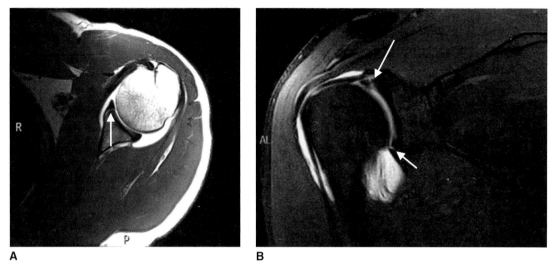

FIGURE 5-7. Bankart lesion. **A:** Axial T1-weighted images of a left shoulder MR arthrogram demonstrate the fibrocartilaginous Bankart lesion of the anterior glenoid labrum (*arrow*). **B:** Coronal T1-weighted fat suppression demonstrates the inferior (*short arrow*) and the superior (*long arrow*) extensions of the labral tears.

Calcific tendinopathy (**Fig. 5-8**) of the rotator cuff tendons is a common clinical entity most commonly affecting the supraspinatus in middle age persons. It is slightly more common in females and can affect multiple tendons in the body. It is, however, far more frequent in the supraspinatus and other rotator cuff tendons. Although the exact etiology is unknown, it is felt to be secondary to chronic ischemia of the tendon fibers.

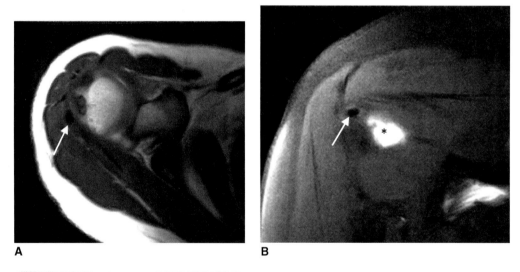

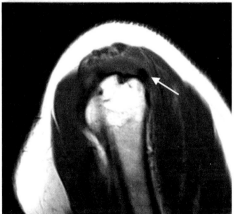

FIGURE 5-8. Calcific tendinosis of the infraspinatus tendon. Axial T1WI (**A**) and coronal oblique T2WI (**B**) with fat suppression demonstrating a focal area of decreased signal within the fibers of the distal infraspinatus (*arrow*). Note high–signal-intensity fluid within the posterior joint (*asterisk*). **C:** Sagittal oblique T1WI shows the calcification within the posterior fibers of the infraspinatus (*arrow*).

Fluid within the bicipital groove surrounding the long head of the biceps tendon can be produced by either biceps tenosynovitis or a shoulder joint effusion because the tendon sheath normally communicates with the shoulder joint. Minimal fluid could be a normal variant and not necessarily relates to the presence of rotator cuff pathology. Rupture of the biceps tendon is demonstrated by the absence of the biceps tendon within the intertubercular sulcus and by distal retraction of the muscle, which is seen on imaging the arm (14). Dislocation of the biceps tendon is identified by medial displacement of the biceps tendon out of the intertubercular sulcus.

ISCHEMIC NECROSIS OF THE HUMERAL HEAD

As in other joints, ischemic necrosis of the humeral head is depicted as an area of decreased signal intensity within the subarticular bone marrow in T1-weighted images. On T2-weighted images, curvilinear bright bands surrounding areas of decreased signal intensity, the so-called tram track sign, represent reactive marrow surrounding the core of a dead bone (15). Ischemic necrosis is more fully described with the hip, where its incidence is higher.

ELBOW

Plain film radiographic examination of the elbows should be the initial evaluation for patients with chronic elbow pain. Radiographs can be useful for the assessment of calcium within the joint compartment or periarticular soft tissues. Standard frontal and lateral radiographs are used for the routine evaluation of the elbow joint. Radiographic examination of the elbow has a minimal RRL.

MRI has not been applied to the evaluation of elbow pathology as extensively as it has been to other large joints (16). However, improving imaging techniques and the use of surface coils permit superb visualization of the bony, ligamentous, muscular, and neurovascular structures around the elbow. Common elbow injuries evaluated with MRI are usually related to sports (weightlifting, throwing, and racquet sports) or compartmental nerve entrapment.

Axial MRI views of the elbow region permit good visualization of the biceps, brachialis, triceps, and all the extensor and flexor muscles of the forearm (**Fig. 5-9A**). High–signal-intensity fat planes and low–signal-intensity intermuscular septa permit clear delineation of each muscle and their tendon insertion or origin. Axial images clearly depict brachial, ulnar, and radial

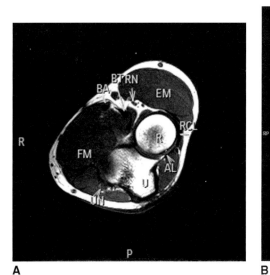

A

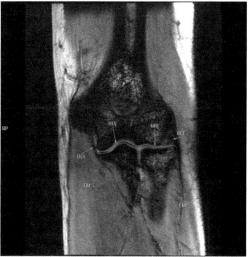

B

FIGURE 5-9. Normal elbow as seen on T1-weighted MR images. **A:** The axial MRI displays the ulna (*U*), radius (*R*), annular ligament (*AL*), radial collateral ligament (*RCL*), brachial artery (*BA*), biceps tendon (*BT*), forearm flexor muscles (*FM*), forearm extensor muscles (*EM*), ulnar nerve (*UN*), and radial nerve (*RN*). **B:** The coronal MRI displays the humeroulnar joint (*HUJ*), humeroradial joint (*HRJ*), radial collateral ligament (*RCL*), ulnar collateral ligament (*UCL*), forearm flexor muscles (*FM*), and forearm extensor muscles (*EM*). **C:** The sagittal MRI through the humeroulnar joint demonstrates the biceps tendon (*BT*), brachialis (*Br*), and triceps (*T*).

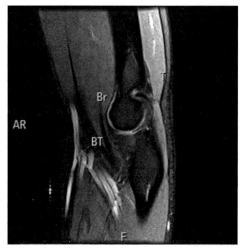

C

arteries and all the subcutaneous and deep veins. They also allow identification of the ulnar nerve within the cubital tunnel and the radial nerve in the brachioradialis-brachialis interval and under the supinator muscle arcade of Frohse, where it is commonly entrapped. The median nerve is visualized at its common elbow entrapment sites, including under the bicipital aponeurosis, between the heads of the pronator teres, and under the fibrous arch of the flexor digitorum superficialis.

The humeroulnar, humeroradial, and proximal radioulnar joint spaces and articular cartilages are well visualized on both coronal and sagittal MR images (**Fig. 5-9B** and **C**). The low–signal-intensity ulnar collateral, radial collateral, and annular ligaments are depicted on both axial and coronal MR images. Sagittal images delineate the anterior and posterior subsynovial fat pads.

MRI has the capability of directly visualizing degenerative or traumatic abnormalities of the annular and the radial and ulnar collateral ligamentous complexes. A sprain appears in MRI as thickened or thinned ligament with surrounding high T2 signal intensity. The collateral ligaments may show degeneration in association with adjacent epicondylosis. The affected ligament commonly shows thickening and intermediate signal intensity. Full-thickness ligament tears or avulsions appear as discontinuities and irregularity of the normal low–signal-intensity ligament. The T2-weighted images disclose hyperintense edema and hemorrhage between the torn ends of the ligament extending into the joint interval and adjacent soft tissues. A partial-thickness tear appears as high T2 fluid signal intensity within an uninterrupted ligament (**Fig. 5-10**).

MRI also provides good visualization of the sites of muscle injury and denervation about the elbow (17) (**Fig. 5-11A** and **B**). Acute muscle denervation is demonstrated by increased T2-weighted signal intensity within the specific muscle group supplied by the injured or the affected nerve. Increased

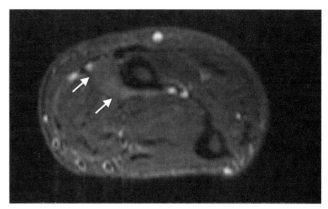

FIGURE 5-11. Impingement to the anterior interosseous branch of the median nerve, Kiloh-Nevin syndrome. Axial STIR (short-tau inversion recovery) sequence at the level of the distal forearm. On this fat suppressed sequence, there is increased signal intensity to the fibers of the flexor pollicis longus muscle as can be appreciated with acute (stage I) or subacute (stage II) impingement (*arrow*). (Courtesy of Zehava Rosenberg, NY.)

intramuscular T2-weighted signal intensity is due to muscle edema. Chronic muscle denervation is demonstrated by increased intramuscular T1-weighted signal intensity, related to muscle atrophy and fatty infiltration. Acute muscle injuries present with intramuscular edema and hemorrhage. Increased thickening, increased signal intensity, and discontinuity of tendon fibers are the findings commonly observed in tendon tears (**Fig. 5-12A** and **B**).

MRI has the ability to demonstrate tendinopathy involving the common extensor and flexor tendon origins from the lateral and medial aspects of the humerus with findings similar to those described in tendinopathy about the shoulder. It also can display abnormalities of the radial and ulnar collateral ligament complexes.

Wrist

Plain film radiography and CT provide good visualization of the osseous structures of the wrist. Most physicians agree that the imaging evaluation of a painful hand and wrist should begin with radiographs. This inexpensive study may establish a specific diagnosis in arthritis, injury, infection, and wrist instability. Standard anteroposterior (AP) and lateral radiographs of the wrist are enough for most clinical problems (18). Additional views can be ordered to assess specific clinical problems, such as scaphoid views in patients with trauma and pain in the snuffbox. In the specific setting of wrist trauma, further imaging studies should be considered in the presence of negative radiographic examinations due to the high incidence of missed occult fractures. The relative radiation dose for radiographic examinations of the wrist is low. The ability of MRI to visualize soft tissue pathology already has been shown to be of great value in assessing CTS and may prove useful in imaging cases of unexplained wrist pain (19–21). MR arthrography provides detailed information about ligamentous disorders in and about the wrist.

Axial MR images through the wrist from the distal radioulnar joint to the metacarpals provide excellent visualization of all the bones, joints, ligaments, muscles, tendons, nerves, and vessels in the wrist area (**Fig. 5-13A–D**). They also clearly display all the boundaries and contents of the carpal tunnel and Guyon's canal.

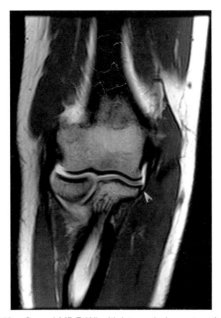

FIGURE 5-10. Coronal MR T1WI with intra-articular contrast in a 22-year-old baseball player with medial elbow pain. There is a partial tear (*arrowhead*) at the insertion of the ulnar collateral ligament into the coronoid process of the ulna. Note the minimal amount of contrast extending between the bone cortex and the distal ligament attachment.

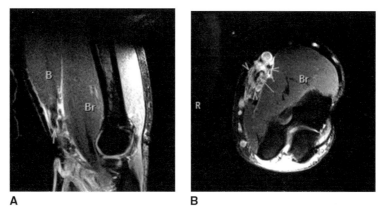

FIGURE 5-12. Sagittal **(A)** and axial **(B)** FSE T2-weighted fat suppressed images of the distal arm in a patient with a complete biceps tear. **A:** The tendon free margin is retracted (*long arrow* in **A**). **B:** There is significant edema (*arrowheads*) surrounding the retracted tendon (*long arrow*). B, biceps muscle; Br, brachialis muscle.

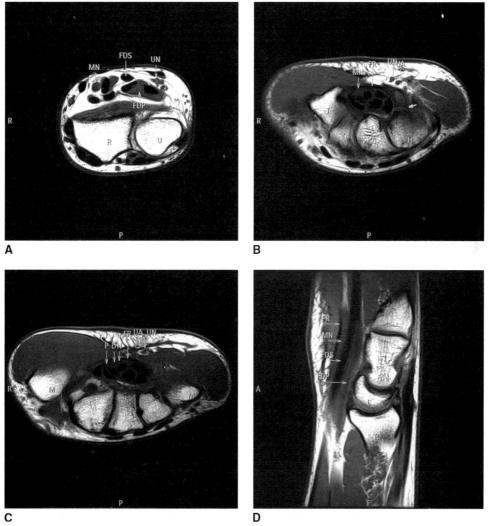

FIGURE 5-13. Normal wrist anatomy as seen on T1-weighted MR images. Axial MR images are at the levels of the distal radioulnar joint **(A)**, the proximal **(B)**, and the distal carpal tunnel **(C)**. **D:** Longitudinal MRI through the median nerve within the carpal tunnel. C, capitate; FDP, flexor digitorum profundus; FDS, flexor digitorum superficialis; FR, flexor retinaculum; H, hamate; L, lunate; MN, median nerve; PDN, palmar digital branches of the median nerve; R, radius; T, trapezium; U, ulna; UA, ulnar artery; UN, ulnar nerve. Note fracture through the base of the hook of the hamate (*arrow* in **B**).

CARPAL TUNNEL SYNDROME

MRI can serve as an adjunct diagnostic tool for CTS when the clinical or neurophysiologic findings are equivocal. The carpal tunnel is a fibro-osseous space with little fat that contains the flexor tendons and the median nerve. The flexor retinaculum composes the volar aspect of the tunnel and normally shows slight palmar bowing. The median nerve courses through the tunnel within its volar and radial aspect, and it can be differentiated from the adjacent tendons because it shows relative higher signal intensity. The carpal tunnel and its contents are best evaluated in the axial plane and should be scrutinized at three standard locations: distal radioulnar joint before the median nerves enter the tunnel, proximal tunnel, at the level of the pisiform and the distal tunnel, and at the level of the hook of the hamate.

There are four universal findings of CTS visible by MRI regardless of etiology (20):

1. Swelling of the median nerve (i.e., pseudoganglion) in the proximal part of the carpal tunnel at the level of the pisiform. This is best evaluated by comparing the size of the median nerve at the level of the distal radioulnar joint with its size at the proximal tunnel.
2. Increased signal intensity of the edematous median nerve on T2-weighted images.

3. Palmar bowing of the flexor retinaculum, determined by a bowing ratio of more than 15%. The bowing ratio is calculated by drawing a line from the trapezium to the hook of the hamate on the axial plane. The distance from this line to the flexor retinaculum is divided by the previously calculated length.
4. Flattening of the median nerve in the distal carpal tunnel at the level of the hamate (**Fig. 5-14A–D**).

MRI also has the potential to establish the cause of CTS. Some of the etiologies visualized by MRI include traumatic tenosynovitis, rheumatoid tenosynovitis, a ganglion cyst of a carpal joint, excessive fat within the carpal tunnel, a hypertrophied adductor pollicis muscle in the floor of the carpal tunnel, and a persistent median artery (22).

MRI also provides a means of postoperative evaluation of those patients in whom the symptoms persist, to ensure that the flexor retinaculum has been completely incised and that there are no other complicating postoperative factors producing continuing discomfort. When the flexor retinaculum has been completely incised, the incision site is well documented by MRI, and the contents of the carpal tunnel are typically displaced forward (**Fig. 5-15A**). If the distal part of the flexor retinaculum has been incompletely incised, this can be demonstrated by MRI, and the preoperative MRI findings of CTS will persist (**Fig. 5-15B and C**).

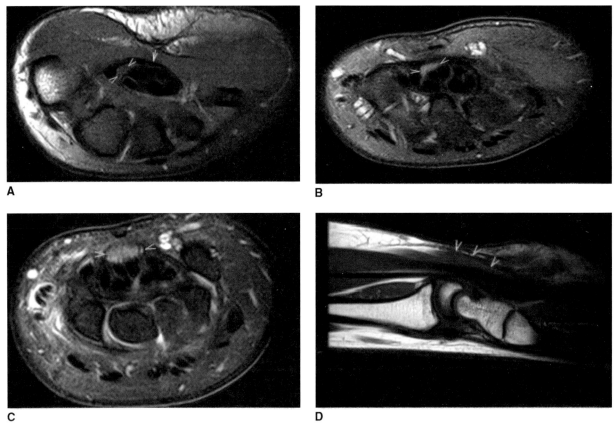

A B

C D

FIGURE 5-14.   Axial FSE T2-weighted fat suppressed images (**A–C**) and sagittal T1-weighted image in a patient with carpal tunnel syndrome. **A and B:** There is a normal size to the nerve within the tunnel (*arrowheads*). **C:** There is thickening, increased girth, and increased signal intensity proximal to the flexor retinaculum (*arrowheads*). **D:** Note tapering to the nerve as it approaches the carpal tunnel in the sagittal view (*arrowheads*).

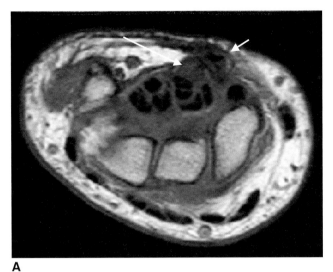

A

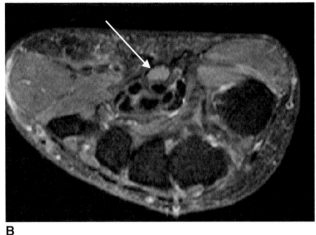

B

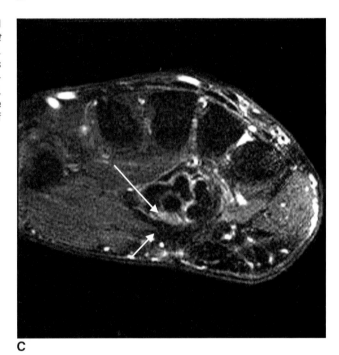

C

FIGURE 5-15. Postoperative MR of carpal tunnel syndrome. **A:** Axial T1-weighted image. There has been release to the flexor retinaculum (*short arrow*). The median nerve (*long arrow*) insinuates through the surgical defect. **B:** Axial T2-weighted fat suppressed image. The median nerve (*arrow*) has intermediate signal and is better delineated. **C:** Patient with failed carpal tunnel release. There is a linear area of decreased signal intensity (*short arrow*), which was found to represent a fibrous band at surgery. The median nerve (*long arrow*) is flattened underneath the fibrous band. (**A and B:** Courtesy of Zehava Rosenberg, NY. **C:** Courtesy of Mark Kransdorf, FL.)

OTHER WRIST ABNORMALITIES

MRI can also visualize postincisional neuromas as lobulated masses in the typical location of the palmar cutaneous branches of the median nerve. Other peripheral nerve tumors such as schwannomas (**Fig. 5-16**) and neurofibromas can be well recognized as well. It can also demonstrate tenosynovitis involving any of the tendons crossing the wrist. MRI also displays marrow abnormalities such as ischemic necrosis of the proximal fragment of a scaphoid fracture and avascular necrosis of the lunate, where the marrow shows reduced signal intensity (23). MRI has the ability to evaluate the integrity of the intrinsic/extrinsic ligaments of the wrist and the triangular fibrocartilage complex (TFCC) (24). The TFCC, scapholunate, and lunotriquetral ligaments are best evaluated with MR arthrography (**Fig. 5-17**).

Hip

In order to fully evaluate patients who present with hip pain, the following radiographic views can be considered: an AP view of the pelvis, a cross-table lateral view, a 45- or 90-degree Dunn view, a frog leg lateral view, and a false profile view. Frontal and frog leg views are the standard radiographs performed for the assessment of hip joint abnormalities; however, they are not optimal when assessing for hip dysplasia and femoroacetabular impingement (25). The presence of osteoarthritis, bone tumors, and soft tissue calcifications can be assessed with plain films.

MRI of the hip is usually performed without contrast and includes standard axial, coronal, and sagittal planes. Intra-articular contrast should be considered when evaluating the integrity of the articular cartilage and the articular labrum. The normal marrow of the femoral head epiphysis and the greater trochanter displays very high signal intensity both on the T1- and on the T2-weighted sequences and is surrounded by a thin layer of compact bone that appears as a signal void. However, in children and young adults, the marrow of the femoral neck and shaft normally shows lower signal intensity, because it contains some residual hematopoietic marrow. The acetabulum has imaging characteristics similar to those of the femoral neck.

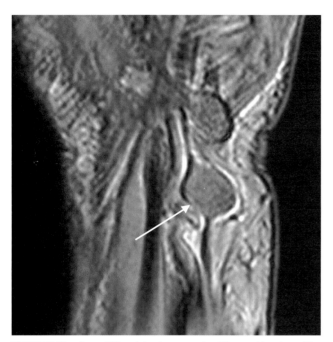

FIGURE 5-16. Coronal T2-weighted sequence in a 72-year-old patient with a palpable hypothenar mass. There is a rounded soft tissue mass (*arrow*) within the ulnar nerve proximal to the retinaculum representing a schwannoma of the ulnar nerve. (Courtesy of Dr. Mark Kransdorf, Jacksonville, FL.)

The periphery of the hip joint interval displays the moderate signal intensity of the apposed hyaline cartilage surfaces of the femoral head and acetabulum, whereas the centrally situated acetabular notch contains high–signal-intensity fat. The thick, very-low–signal-intensity, hip joint capsule blends with the acetabular labrum proximally and the cortex of the femoral neck distally. The labrum demonstrates uniform decreased signal intensity in all pulse sequences. All the muscles, nerves, and blood vessels crossing the hip are well visualized.

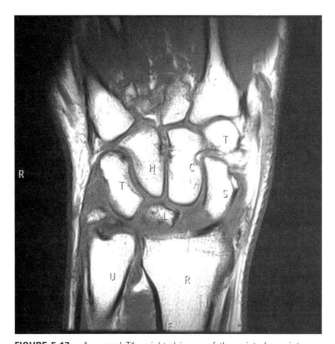

FIGURE 5-17. A coronal T1-weighted image of the wrist shows intermediate signal intensity and increased distance to the scapholunate interval (*arrow*), representing a scapholunate ligament tear.

ISCHEMIC NECROSIS

One of the common indications for MRI of the hip is to determine the presence of ischemic necrosis. This is bone death produced by a compromised blood supply. It also has been called *avascular necrosis, osteonecrosis,* or *aseptic necrosis.* Predisposing factors that should raise the physician's index of suspicion include corticosteroid therapy, alcoholism, known hip trauma, chronic pancreatitis, Gaucher's disease, sickle cell disease, exposure to hypobaric conditions, subcapital fractures, childhood septic arthritis or osteomyelitis of the hip, and congenital hip dislocation (15,26). If not detected early, the disease can progress and finally undergo irreversible collapse of the femoral head. MRI has been demonstrated to be even more sensitive and specific than bone scintigraphy for the early diagnosis of ischemic necrosis of the femoral head (27–30).

On T1-weighted MRI, the foci of ischemic necrosis of the femoral head appear as homogeneous or heterogeneous well-delimited or diffuse areas of decreased signal intensity in the shape of rings, bands, wedges, or crescents or in an irregular configuration (**Fig. 5-18A–C**) (31,32). The low signal intensity is caused by the death of marrow fat and replacement of the marrow by a fibrous connective tissue. Some cases show a lower signal band surrounding the lesion, and this has been attributed to healing sclerotic bone at the interface between normal and necrotic bone. On T2-weighted images, many cases show a double-line sign with a high–signal-intensity zone just inside of a low–signal-intensity margin. This is thought to be produced by granulation tissue surrounded by sclerotic bone (30–32).

FEMOROACETABULAR IMPINGEMENT

Femoroacetabular impingement is another cause of hip pain that may initially have a nonspecific clinical presentation. Pain can be elicited on physical exam by passive movement of the thigh into full flexion, adduction, and internal rotation (33). Radiographs often help to identify anatomical variations such as dysplasia of the femoral neck (**Fig. 5-19**), sphericity of the femoral head, or acetabular overcoverage. MR arthrography (**Fig. 5-20**) can be helpful for the assessment of early chondral loss or labral tears.

OTHER HIP ABNORMALITIES

Primary bone marrow edema syndrome refers to abnormal signal to the femoral head and neck with decreased signal intensity on T1-weighted images and hyperintense signal on the T2-weighted sequences in a heterogeneous geographic pattern. It can affect any bone but is more frequent at the femoral head and neck, the knee, and bones of the lower extremities. Patients affected with this condition typically do not have predisposing conditions. MRI also has been found to be very useful for identifying stress or occult fractures. These appear as low–signal-intensity areas containing an oblique or wavy line of still lower signal intensity, representing the actual fracture site. On T2-weighted, fat suppressed images, the marrow demonstrates increased signal intensity due to the associated marrow edema. MRI also can identify many types of soft tissue abnormalities about the hip, including synovial cysts, periarticular bursitis, and soft tissue masses and articular abnormalities such as synovial chondromatosis.

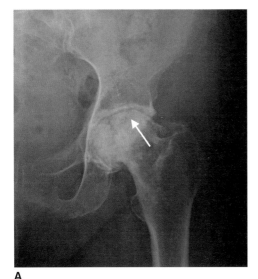

A

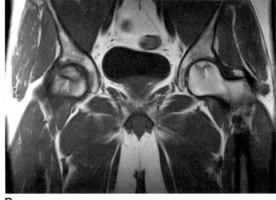

B

FIGURE 5-18. **A:** Frontal radiograph on patient with advanced left hip AVN. There is sclerosis to the femoral head and collapse (*arrow*) to the articular surface. Bilateral ischemic necrosis of the femoral head in a different patient. **B:** Bilateral ischemic necrosis of the femoral head in a different patient. Coronal T1-weighted, serpiginous areas of decreased signal intensity are well demarcated within the subchondral marrow (*arrowheads*). **C:** Coronal T2-weighted fat suppressed images. There is edema within the right femoral head (*arrowheads*). The left femoral heads demonstrate a serpiginous area of increased signal intensity. These findings are characteristic of AVN.

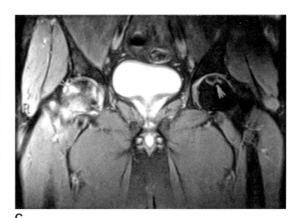

C

Knee

Patients complaining of traumatic or nontraumatic knee pain should undergo plain film radiographic examination with AP and lateral (Lat) knee radiographs. Axial views of the patella (Merchant or sunrise) are important in patients with anterior knee pain. When evaluating for radiographic evidence of early osteoarthritis, standing views of the knees should be ordered. Standing views with the knee slightly flexed can better predict the degree of cartilaginous loss within the posterior-medial and lateral knee compartments (34,35).

When a patient has persistent knee pain and normal radiographs or when there are symptoms of internal derangement, an MRI of the knee is the next evaluation of choice. MRI of the knee is the most commonly performed nonneurologic MRI study (36).

MENISCAL INJURIES

MRI provides excellent assessment of the menisci. Sagittal MR images provide good views of the anterior and posterior horns and a fair view of the body of both menisci. In more central sections, both horns of the menisci appear as wedge-shaped signal voids contrasted on their superior and inferior surfaces by the moderate signal intensity of the hyaline cartilage on the

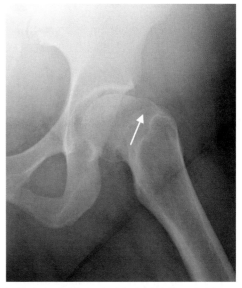

FIGURE 5-19. Lateral radiograph of the left hip. There is a bump along the superior margin of the left femoral head-neck junction (*arrow*) that makes for an aspherical configuration of the femoral head. This is characteristic of Cam-type femoroacetabular impingement.

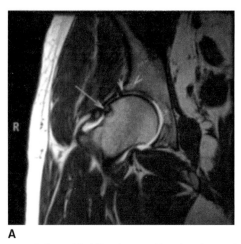 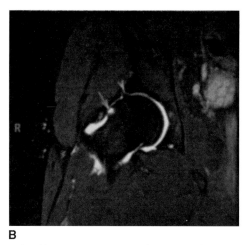

A **B**

FIGURE 5-20. **A:** Coronal T1 MR arthrogram. There is an intermediate–signal-intensity subcortical cyst (herniation pit) related to pressure erosion from the incongruent joint (*large arrow*). A labral tear (*short arrow*) and remodeling to the superior acetabulum (*arrowhead*) are well appreciated. **B:** Coronal PD fat suppressed with intra-articular contrast. The subcortical cyst is hyperintense (*large arrow*). The labral tear is better delineated (*arrowhead*).

articular surfaces of the femur and tibia. In more peripheral sections through the body, where the images are tangential to the circumference of the meniscus, they appear bow tie shaped (**Fig. 5-21**). Coronal MR images provide the best visualization of the bodies of the menisci, where they appear as wedge-shaped structures.

There are three types of meniscal findings visualized by MRI in the presence of tears or degeneration (15,37,38). One is the presence of small globular or irregular high–signal-intensity foci confined to the interior of the meniscus. This is considered to be an early type of mucoid degeneration. A second type of meniscal finding is the presence of a linear region of increased signal intensity within the meniscus that does not extend to either the femoral or tibial articular surface of the meniscus but may extend to the meniscocapsular junction. Histologically, this represents fragmentation and separation of

the fibrocartilage and is considered by many to be an intrameniscal tear. The significance of the globular or linear signals that do not extend to either articular surface of the meniscus is unclear (39). Frank meniscal tears are demonstrated by MRI as linear or irregular areas of signal intensity that extend to one or both articular surfaces of the meniscus, or to the meniscal free edge, seen in two consecutive MR images (**Fig. 5-22**). The high signal intensity is produced by synovial fluid in the crevices within the meniscus. These meniscal tears can be classified as horizontal, longitudinal, and radial meniscal root tears or complex tears. Horizontal tears are more common in older patients in the presence of degenerative joint disease (DJD). They run parallel to the tibial plateau and may extend to the superior or inferior articular surfaces or the inner free edge of the meniscus. They are associated to parameniscal cysts if the tear extends to the periphery of the meniscus. Vertical longitudinal tears are more common in younger patients after knee trauma and extend perpendicular to the tibial plateau to the superior and/or inferior articular surfaces in the long axis of the meniscus. Bucket-handle tears are longitudinal tears where the inner meniscal fragment is displaced toward the intercondylar notch (**Fig. 5-22C and D**). Radial tears extend from the inner free margin perpendicular to the longitudinal fibers of the meniscus, causing a loss of meniscal hoop strength and possible meniscal extrusion, allowing more stress to the femoral and tibial articular surfaces, leading to chondromalacia and osteoarthritis. Meniscal root tears are typically radial tears through the meniscal roots, also leading to loss of meniscal hoop strength and meniscal extrusion. Meniscal root tears are better visualized in coronal fluid–sensitive sequences. Complex tears result from a combination of longitudinal, horizontal, or radial tears. At times, menisci are macerated due to repeated trauma or chronic degeneration that may cause a gross distortion of meniscal shape, and the meniscus may then appear to have a truncated apex or to be grossly small with a free fragment.

Other meniscal abnormalities well visualized by MRI include discoid meniscus, meniscal/parameniscal cysts, and abnormalities involving the postoperative meniscus. In discoid meniscus, typically involving the lateral meniscus, there is a continuous bridge of meniscal tissue between the anterior

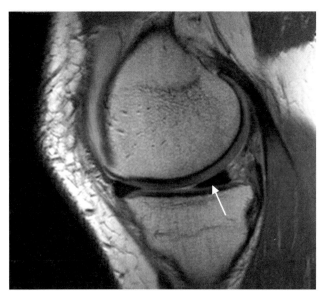

FIGURE 5-21. Sagittal MR images through a normal peripheral meniscus. The anterior and the posterior (*arrow*) horns appear wedge (triangular) in shape.

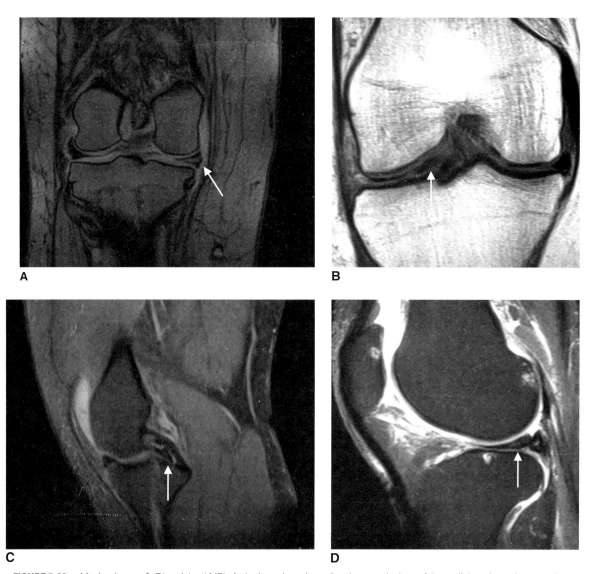

FIGURE 5-22. Meniscal tears. **A:** T1-weighted MRI of a horizontal tear (*arrow*) at the posterior horn of the medial meniscus that extends to its tibial articular surface. **B:** Coronal PD-weighted image of a bucket-handle tear. There is a displaced fragment from the lateral meniscus into the intercondylar fossa (*arrow*). **C:** Sagittal FSE-PD fat suppressed sequence of a double "PCL sign." The displaced fragment from a bucket-handle tear (*arrow*) projects anterior to the PCL. **D:** Sagittal PD fat suppressed sequence through the lateral tibiofemoral joint demonstrates the double delta sign. The displaced anterior horn from a large flap injury is projecting anterior to the posterior horn (*arrow*).

and the posterior horns in the central part of the joint. A discoid meniscus can be diagnosed when the meniscal body in the coronal plane measures 15 mm or more or when three or more bow tie shapes are seen in the sagittal images through the meniscal body, in 4-mm-thick sagittal slices (normally, there are up to two bow ties in the sagittal plane through the meniscal body). Parameniscal cysts are usually associated with underlying horizontal meniscal tears through which synovial fluid collects at the meniscocapsular junction (40). They show high signal intensity on T2-weighted images. MRI also can be used to evaluate the postmeniscectomy patient with continuing or recurrent symptomatology (37). It can detect an incompletely excised meniscal tear, retained meniscal fragments, or a tear developing within the residual part of the meniscus. MR arthrography with gadolinium can be helpful to distinguish between retears and old healed tears that might still show increased signal intensity on T2-weighted images (41).

CRUCIATE LIGAMENT INJURIES

The cruciate ligaments are best visualized by sagittal or oblique sagittal MR images that display the full length of the ligaments (**Fig. 5-23A**). On straight sagittal images, the slender nature of the anterior cruciate ligament and its oblique course cause a volume-averaging effect that averages fat signal intensity about the ligaments with the normal low signal intensity of the ligament so that the anterior cruciate ligament frequently does not appear as a complete signal void. Furthermore, straight sagittal images typically fail to demonstrate the anterior cruciate ligament femoral attachment because of its oblique orientation in both sagittal and coronal planes. Oblique sagittal images that parallel the ligament show the full thickness and length of the anterior cruciate ligament without subjecting it to partial volume averaging (42). In the extended position of the knee, which is typically used for MR images, the anterior cruciate

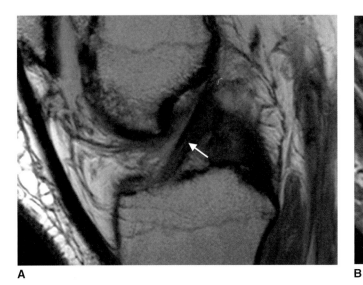

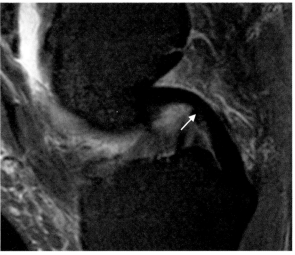

FIGURE 5-23. Normal cruciate ligaments. **A:** An oblique sagittal MRI parallel to the anterior cruciate ligament demonstrates excellent visualization of all borders and attachments of the anterior cruciate ligament (*arrow*). **B:** A T2-weighted MRI of the posterior cruciate ligament (*arrow*), which is normally posteriorly bowed when the knee is extended.

ligament is normally taut. The posterior cruciate ligament is a thicker ligament and is therefore well visualized on straight sagittal MR images (**Fig. 5-23B**). It can be visualized as a signal void structure from its attachment to the posterior tibial intercondylar area to its attachment on the medial femoral condyle. With the knee extended, the posterior cruciate ligament is visualized as thick and posteriorly bowed. It straightens with knee flexion. Axial images can be very helpful to evaluate the femoral insertion of the anterior and the posterior cruciate ligaments.

The MRI appearance of an anterior cruciate ligament injury depends on the site and degree of disruption, as well

as the age of the tear. A complete tear may be visualized as a discontinuity of the ligament (**Fig. 5-24A–D**). In the acute complete tear, the interval between the torn ends of the ligament is often occupied by a mass of intermediate signal intensity on T1-weighted images that appears hyperintense on T2-weighted images (43). At other times, the torn ligament may present as a fusiform or irregular soft tissue mass of intermediate signal intensity on T1-weighted images that appears hyperintense on T2-weighted images. These fluid masses are usually a combination of edema and hemorrhage, and there may be an associated joint effusion. If the ligament tears from

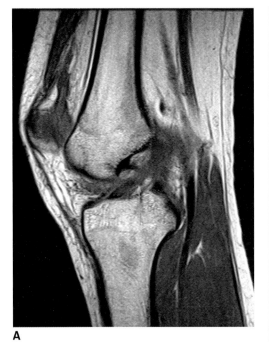

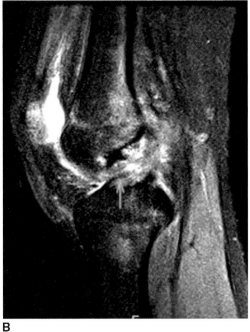

FIGURE 5-24. Acute ACL injury, spectrum of findings. Sagittal PD **(A)** and sagittal PD **(B)** fat suppressed sequences. The *arrow* demonstrates the torn ACL resting against the tibial spine. There is diffuse marrow edema with increased signal intensity on the T2-weighted sequence.

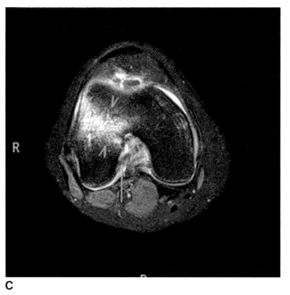
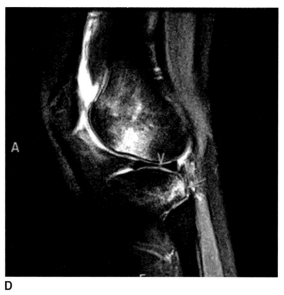

C   **D**

FIGURE 5-24. (*Continued*) **C:** Axial T2-weighted fat suppressed sequence. The *long arrow* is pointing to the ACL fibers. There is edema anterior to the ACL. The *arrowheads* demarcate an area of marrow edema within the lateral femoral condyle. **D:** There is bone marrow edema within the posterior tibial plateau (*long arrow*) and the anterior femoral condyle (*arrowhead* over the femoral condyle). There is a small radial tear to the free inner margin of the lateral meniscus (*arrowhead*).

its femoral attachment, the axial images will show fluid signal between the lateral femoral condyle and the expected ligament insertion. In partial tears, there is no complete discontinuity, but a ligament that appears intact on a T1-weighted image may show a hyperintense signal on T2-weighted images, or the ligament may display an interrupted or concave anterior or posterior margin when the knee is extended (40). In chronic anterior cruciate ligament deficiency, there may be a complete absence of the ligament, or there may be only remnants remaining in its usual location. Some secondary signs of anterior cruciate ligament injury may be present. These include a forward shift of the tibia, uncovering of the inferior surface

of the posterior horn to the lateral meniscus by the posterior lateral tibial plateau, and anterior bowing or buckling of the posterior cruciate ligament caused by the position of the knee within the coil, which duplicates the knee position of an anterior drawer or Lachman test (37).

On T1-weighted MR images, partial tears of the posterior cruciate ligament typically appear as foci of increased signal intensity within the normal black signal void of the ligament. These appear hyperintense on T2-weighted images. With complete tears, a frank discontinuity is visualized with an intervening fluid mass that becomes hyperintense on T2-weighted images (**Fig. 5-25**). The gap between the ends of a completely torn posterior cruciate ligament can be exaggerated by imaging the knee in flexion, which tenses the posterior cruciate ligament.

COLLATERAL LIGAMENT INJURIES

The collateral ligaments are best visualized by coronal MR images (**Fig. 5-26**). The medial collateral ligament appears as a narrow low–signal-intensity band extending from the medial epicondyle of the femur to an attachment on the anteromedial aspect of the tibia 5 to 6 cm below the joint line. It is overlaid at its tibial attachment by the tendons of the pes anserinus, which are separated from it by an intervening anserine bursa that is not visualized unless it is inflamed. Deep to the tibial collateral ligament, the medial capsular ligament, sometimes called the deep portion of the tibial collateral ligament, has femoral and tibial attachments close to the joint interval and deep attachments to the medial meniscus, referred to as the meniscofemoral and meniscotibial or coronary ligaments. Valgus and rotatory stresses can injure the medial capsular ligament or the tibial collateral ligament, usually in that order (37). In a complete rupture (i.e., grade III injury), MRI can show discontinuity, serpentine ligamentous borders, and edema within adjacent connective tissues. In a partial tear

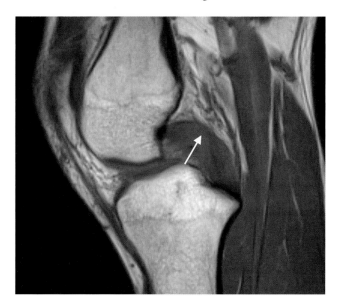

FIGURE 5-25. Sagittal T1-weighted image of a chronic PCL tear. The *arrow* points to the thickened posterior cruciate ligament. Intermediate signal intensity is replacing the normal hypointensity of the ligament.

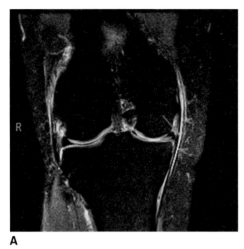 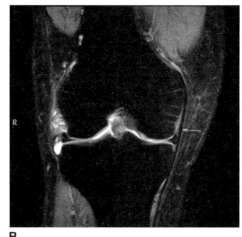

A   **B**

FIGURE 5-26. Tibial collateral ligament tear (MCL). **A:** Coronal T2-weighted fat suppressed sequences of grade I injury. There is edema (*arrowheads*) overlying the intact fibers of the MCL (*long arrow*). **B:** Normal MCL (*arrow*).

(i.e., grade II injury) or in the case of microtears confined to the ligament substance (i.e., grade I injury), the ligament may show no discontinuity, but the overlying subcutaneous fat typically demonstrates edema and hemorrhage, which is indicated by moderate signal intensity on T1-weighted images and high signal intensity on T2-weighted images. Injury to the tibial collateral ligament is commonly associated with injuries to the anterior cruciate ligament and medial meniscus.

The lateral collateral complex commonly refers to the lateral supporting structures of the knee, whose main components are the iliotibial tract, the lateral collateral ligament, the long head of the biceps femoris, the arcuate ligament and the popliteofibular ligament. These structures are best seen on axial and coronal MR images as a low–signal-intensity band extending somewhat obliquely from the lateral femoral epicondyle to the fibular head. The lateral collateral ligament is usually injured by varus and rotatory stresses to the knee, although its frequency of injury is less than that of the tibial collateral ligament. The MRI findings of the injured fibular collateral ligament are similar to those for the tibial collateral ligament.

OTHER KNEE ABNORMALITIES

Patellar tendinitis (jumper's knee) is demonstrated by MRI as an area of edema within the patellar ligament (i.e., tendon) at its patellar (**Fig. 5-27**) or tibial tuberosity attachment. There is also associated edema in the adjacent subcutaneous fat or the infrapatellar fat pad.

Ischemic necrosis about the knee most commonly involves the weight-bearing surface of the medial femoral condyle, and its MRI findings are as described for the hip. Osteochondral injuries, previously known as osteochondritis dissecans, occur mainly in adolescents and involve a partial or total separation of a segment of articular cartilage and subchondral bone from the underlying bone (37). It commonly involves the intercondylar portion of the medial femoral condyle articular surface. It is visualized on T1-weighted MR images as a low–signal-intensity region in the subchondral bone with or without disruption of the overlying articular cartilage (**Fig. 5-28A** and **B**). If the involved osteochondral segment becomes completely

separated from the underlying bone, it becomes an intra-articular loose body. The role of MRI in osteochondritis dissecans is mainly to determine the stability of the fragment, because the treatment hinges on this issue.

Chondromalacia patella can be diagnosed and graded noninvasively by MRI (38). In stage I, the posterior patellar articular cartilage demonstrates local areas of cartilage swelling with decreased signal intensity on both T1- and T2-weighted images. Stage II is characterized by irregularity of the patellar articular cartilage with areas of thinning. Stage III demonstrates complete absence of the articular cartilage with synovial fluid extending through this cartilaginous ulcer to the subchondral bone (**Fig. 5-29**).

Popliteal (i.e., Baker's) cysts and other synovial cysts about the knee appear hyperintense on T2-weighted images

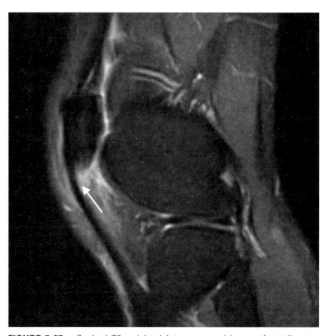

FIGURE 5-27. Sagittal T2-weighted fat suppressed image of patellar tendinitis. The *arrow* points to the increased signal intensity within the proximal tendon fibers and the adjacent infrapatellar fat pad.

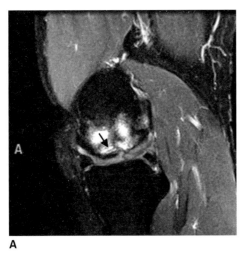
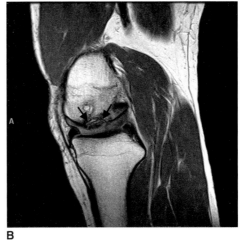

A **B**

FIGURE 5-28. Osteochondral lesion (previously osteochondritis dissecans). T2-weighted fat suppressed **(A)** and PD **(B)** sequences. **A:** There is a hyperintense T2 signal at the interface of the OC lesion and the adjacent cortex compatible with an unstable fragment (*arrow*). **B:** The lesion is well demarcated by a hypointense rim (*short arrows*).

(**Fig. 5-30A–D**). They can be visualized on axial, sagittal, or coronal images. Popliteal cysts are usually an enlargement of the semimembranosus-gastrocnemius bursa, which is located between the tendon of insertion of the semimembranosus and the tendon of origin of the medial head of the gastrocnemius. Popliteal cysts may communicate with the knee joint and therefore may be caused by chronic knee joint pathology that produces effusion. A previously undescribed bursa is now known to be consistently present between the tibial collateral ligament and a major slip of the semimembranosus tendon that extends beneath it and may serve to clarify many cases of previously unexplained medial knee pain (44). Inflammation of this bursa is well demonstrated by MRI (**Fig. 5-31A and B**).

Ankle

Patients that complain of ankle pain of greater than 6-month duration should undergo radiographic examination of the

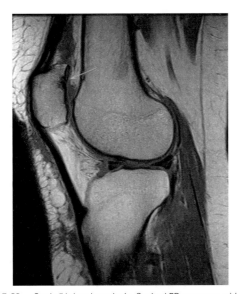

FIGURE 5-29. Grade IV chondromalacia. Sagittal PD sequence with grade IV chondromalacia. There is a full-thickness defect (*arrow*) with subchondral bone sclerosis and early subchondral cyst formation within the proximal patella.

ankle joint including AP, lateral, and mortise views. Patients with acute ankle injuries that meet Ottawa rules-inclusion criteria should also undergo radiographic examinations first (45). These criteria include inability to bear weight immediately after the injury and bone tenderness at the posterior edge and tip of either malleolus. MRI is valuable as a screening modality for assessing a variety of painful chronic ankle disorders (46–49).

LIGAMENT INJURIES

MRI provides a noninvasive means of directly imaging all the ligaments in the vicinity of the ankle as well as all the other osseous and soft tissues. Axial MR images provide good visualization of the tibiofibular ligaments and the tibiofibular mortise. The anterior talofibular ligament is the most commonly injured ligament at the ankle joint. On MRI, the ligament appears as a low–signal-intensity band extending anteromedially from the lateral malleolus to gain attachment to the talus just anterior to its fibular articular surface (**Fig. 5-32A**) (48). The calcaneofibular ligament is visualized as a low–signal-intensity structure extending from the lateral malleolus to the calcaneus, with the peroneus longus and brevis tendons situated superficial to its fibular end (**Fig. 5-32B**). The posterior talofibular ligament is visualized as a wide, low–signal-intensity structure extending from the deep surface of the lateral malleolus to a broad attachment on the talus from its fibular articular surface to its posterior process (**Fig. 5-32C**).

MRI of ankle ligament injuries offers accurate and noninvasive evaluation of the site and severity of both acute ankle ligament injuries and chronic ankle instability (45,49).

The mechanism of injury of the lateral collateral ligaments typically involves plantar flexion and inversion, and they are usually injured in a predictable sequence from anterior to posterior. The anterior talofibular ligament is the most commonly injured, followed by injury to the calcaneofibular and posterior talofibular ligaments. The major MRI finding in a complete rupture (i.e., grade III sprain) of the anterior talofibular ligament is a complete discontinuity of the ligament

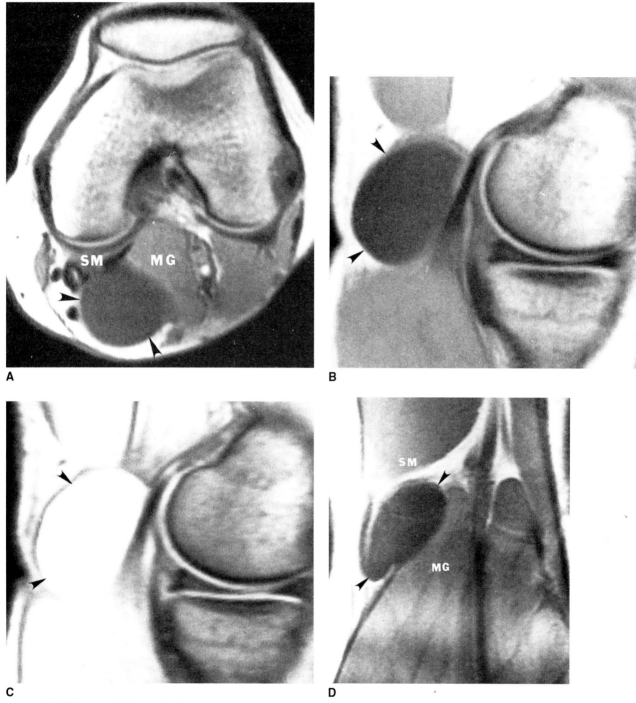

FIGURE 5-30.   Baker's cyst. **A:** A T1-weighted axial MRI demonstrates a hypointense Baker's cyst (*arrowheads*) in the interval between the semimembranosus (*SM*) and the medial head of the gastrocnemius (*MG*). T1-weighted **(B)** and T2-weighted **(C)** sagittal MR images through Baker's cyst (*arrowheads*). Note that the hypointense fluid in the cyst in the T1-weighted image becomes hyperintense on the T2-weighted image. **D:** A coronal T1-weighted image locates the cyst between the SM and the MG (*arrowheads*).

visualized at all imaging levels (**Fig. 5-33A and B**). This is accompanied by periarticular edema or hemorrhage and joint effusion. The edema and effusion are visualized with moderate signal intensity on T1-weighted MR images and hyperintensity on T2-weighted images. A partial tear (i.e., grade II sprain) of the anterior talofibular ligament is visualized on MRI as a discontinuity of the upper part of the ligament, with the lower

portion remaining intact. Again, there is periarticular edema, hemorrhage, and joint effusion. Grade II sprains of the calcaneofibular ligament may appear as a longitudinal splitting or waviness of the ligament with fluid accumulation within the tendon sheath of the overlying peroneal tendons (**Fig. 5-34**).

In contrast to the three discrete lateral collateral ligaments, the medial collateral or deltoid ligament is a continuous

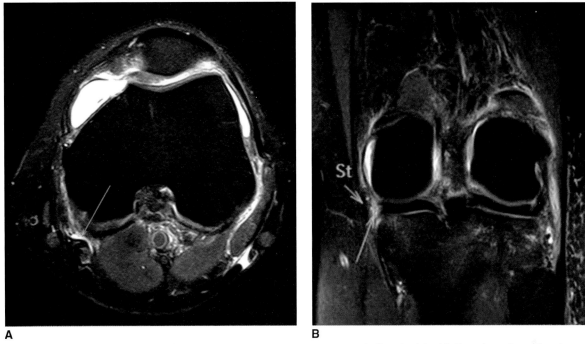

A   **B**

FIGURE 5-31.   Axial **(A)** and coronal **(B)** T2-weighted PD fat suppressed sequences. **A:** There is minimal fluid anterior to the semimembranosus (*long arrow*). **B:** The fluid is deep to the semitendinosus (*St*) and superficial to the meniscocapsular junction of the medial meniscus (*long arrow* in **B**).

ligamentous sheet with the apex attached to the tibial malleolus and distal broad base attachments in the navicular bone, talar neck, spring ligament, sustentaculum tali of the calcaneus, and posterior talus. The posterior tibiotalar part of the deltoid ligament is its thickest and strongest (50). The deltoid ligament can be visualized by either axial or coronal MRI. Axial images allow simultaneous visualization of all parts of the deltoid ligament, the overlying flexor retinaculum, and the walls and contents of the tarsal tunnel (**Fig. 5-35A**). The contents of the four compartments under the flexor retinaculum include, from anterior to posterior, the tibialis posterior tendon, flexor digitorum longus tendon, posterior tibial artery, tibial nerve, and flexor hallucis longus tendon. Coronal MR images through the deltoid ligament display the proximal and distal attachments of each part of the deltoid ligament (**Fig. 5-35B**).

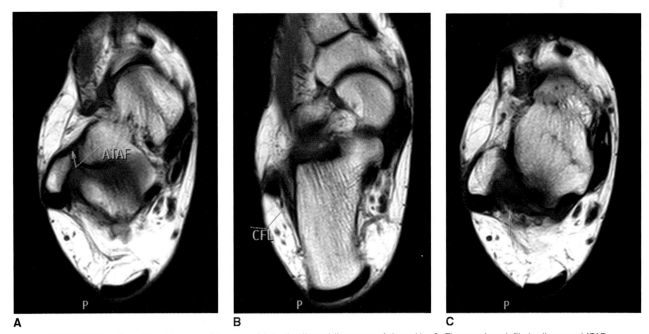

A   **B**   **C**

FIGURE 5-32.   T1-weighted images of the normal lateral collateral ligaments of the ankle. **A:** The anterior talofibular ligament (*ATAF*) extends from the fibular malleolus to the neck of the talus. **B:** The calcaneofibular ligament (*CFL*) attaches to the calcaneus and is deep to the peroneus tendons. **C:** The strong talofibular ligament (between *arrows*).

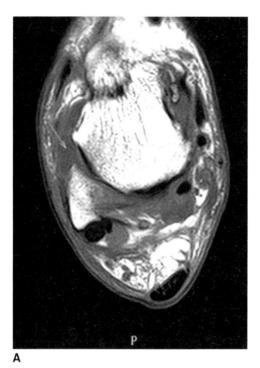
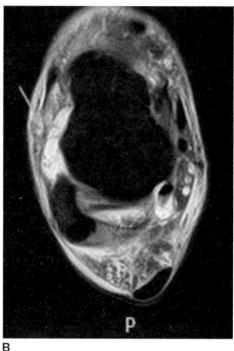

A   **B**

FIGURE 5-33.   Complete rupture of the anterior talofibular ligament. Axial T1-weighted **(A)** and T2-weighted fat suppressed sequences **(B)**. There is discontinuity to the ligament fibers (*arrows*) and associated soft tissue swelling.

MRI has the potential to visualize even grade I sprains, which are microtears confined to the interior of the ligament. The minute foci of edema and hemorrhage accompanying such tears become hyperintense on T2-weighted images. Findings compatible with such grade I tears have been identified in the posterior tibiotalar portion of the deltoid ligament. They are frequently accompanied by fluid within the tendon sheath of the overlying tibialis posterior.

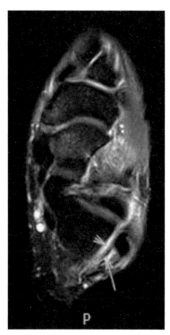

FIGURE 5-34.   Partial tear to the calcaneofibular ligament. There is thickening and increased signal within the ligament fibers (*long arrow*) and edema within the soft tissues between the ligament and the calcaneus (*arrowhead*).

In chronic ankle instability, MR images show thinned, lengthened, wavy ligaments in some locations and thickened, scarred ligaments in others.

OTHER ANKLE ABNORMALITIES

Technetium-99 scintigraphy has been valuable for detecting stress fractures of metatarsal and tarsal bones. CT, as well as MR, is highly accurate for the detection of osteochondral fractures. In foot pain of undetermined etiology, MRI is an excellent screening modality because it permits direct evaluation of all osseous and soft tissue structures.

MRI is superior to any other modality in displaying tendon pathology (45,46). In tenosynovitis, MRI detects fluid within the tendon sheath as having moderate signal intensity on T1-weighted images and as hyperintense on T2-weighted images. Tendinosis is commonly observed in the Achilles, tibialis posterior, flexor hallucis longus, tibialis anterior, and peroneal tendons (**Fig. 5-36**). Tendinosis is visualized as a focal or diffuse thickening of the tendon that may show areas of increased signal intensity on T2-weighted images. Plantar fasciitis shows similar changes within the plantar aponeurosis (**Fig. 5-37**). With a complete tendon rupture, axial MR images show absence of the tendon replaced by high–signal-intensity fluid or edema. Sagittal and coronal MR images display the site of discontinuity, with edema occupying the gap and surrounding the torn ends of the tendon.

Stress fractures of the tarsal or metatarsal bones appear on MRI as linear areas of decreased marrow signal intensity. There are adjacent areas of marrow edema that are hypointense relative to marrow fat on T1-weighted images and hyperintense on T2-weighted images (46). By MRI, osteochondral fractures (e.g., of the talar dome) have an appearance similar to

FIGURE 5-35. Normal tibial collateral ligament (i.e., deltoid ligament) and contents of the tarsal tunnel. **A:** Axial T1-weighted image demonstrates the deltoid ligament (*DL*), flexor retinacula (*FR*), tibialis posterior (*TP*), flexor digitorum longus (*FDL*), posterior tibialis artery and vein (*PTA/V*), posterior tibialis nerve (*PTN*), and the flexor hallucis longus (*FHL*). **B:** Coronal T2-weighted fat suppressed image demonstrating the superficial (*arrowhead*) and the deep (*arrows*) fibers of the deltoid ligament.

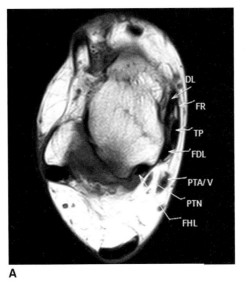
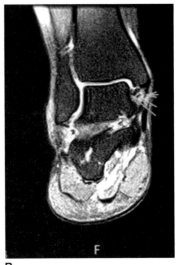

A

B

that of osteochondritis dissecans of the knee. The primary task of MRI is to determine the stability of the fragment by demonstrating the integrity of the articular cartilage and the absence of fluid between the osteochondral fragment and the parent bone. Synovial cysts of intertarsal joint origin demonstrate moderate signal intensity on T1-weighted images and high signal intensity on T2-weighted images.

Osteoarthritis

Osteoarthritis or DJD is an asymmetric, usually bilateral, mechanical degenerative process that involves joints significantly involved in weight bearing, such as the hip, knee, and spine, and those involved in frequent repetitive mechanical trauma, such as the distal interphalangeal joints of the fingers, trapezium-first metacarpal joint, trapezium-scaphoid joint, and metatarsophalangeal joint of the great toe. It is the most common arthritis, and it is estimated that 80% of the population of more than 50 years of age will show radiographic evidence of osteoarthritis. The most common radiographic findings include the following:

- Nonuniform loss of joint space caused by cartilage degeneration in high load areas (e.g., the superior aspect of the hip and medial knee)
- Sclerosis of the subchondral bone
- Osteophyte formation at the margins of the articular surface

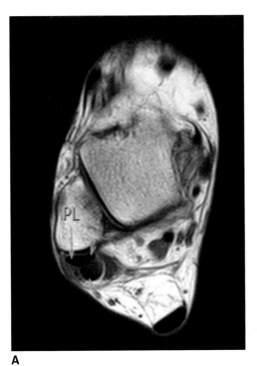
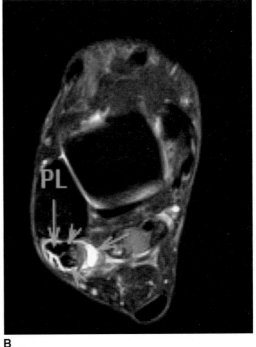

A

B

FIGURE 5-36. **A:** Axial T1-weighted image at the level of the talar dome. There is thickening and splitting to the fibers of the peroneus brevis (*short arrows*). Note normal signal and configuration to the peroneus longus (PL). **B:** Axial PD fat suppressed sequence. The split fibers of the peroneus brevis are better depicted (*arrowheads*). There is an effusion within the tendon sheath (*short arrow*).

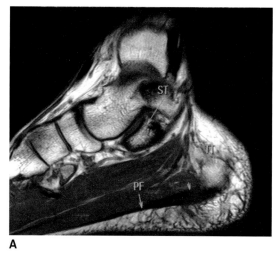
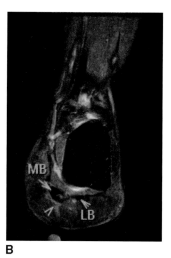

A   **B**

FIGURE 5-37.   A: Sagittal T1-weighted image of the hindfoot. There is thickening and increased signal (*short arrow*) within the proximal fibers of the plantar fascia (*PF*). TT, tarsal tunnel; ST, sustentaculum talus. **B:** Coronal T2-weighted fat suppressed sequence. There is asymmetric thickening and increased signal to the medial bundle of the plantar fascia (*MB*). Edema extends into the adjacent fat (*arrowhead*). Note normal thickness and signal to the lateral bundle (*LB*).

- Cyst-like rarefactions in the subchondral bone that may collapse to produce marked joint deformities
- Adjacent soft tissue swelling (e.g., that which occurs with Heberden's nodes of the distal interphalangeal joints of the fingers) (**Fig. 5-38**) (51)

Rheumatoid Arthritis

Rheumatoid arthritis is a connective tissue disorder that can affect any synovial joint in the body. It is a bilateral and symmetric inflammatory degenerative disease that involves the following joints in the order of decreasing frequency: small joints of the hands and feet, with the exception of the distal interphalangeal joints, knees, hips, cervical spine shoulders, and elbows.

The major radiographic findings include the following:
- Symmetric periarticular *soft tissue swelling*
- Juxta-articular *osteoporosis* proceeding to diffuse osteoporosis

- *Erosions* of the intracapsular portions of the articulating bones not covered by cartilage, which can proceed to severe subchondral bone erosion
- Uniform joint space narrowing
- Synovial cysts (e.g., Baker's cysts behind the knee)
- Subluxations (e.g., boutonniere or swan-neck deformities of the fingers and palmar and ulnar subluxation of the proximal phalanges on the metacarpal heads) (**Fig. 5-39A and B**) (52)

Seronegative Spondyloarthropathies

These disorders are all linked to the human leukocyte antigen (HLA)-B27 histocompatibility antigen. These groups of diseases include ankylosing spondylitis, inflammatory bowel disease, psoriatic arthritis, and reactive arthritis. They are characterized by osseous ankylosis, proliferative new bone

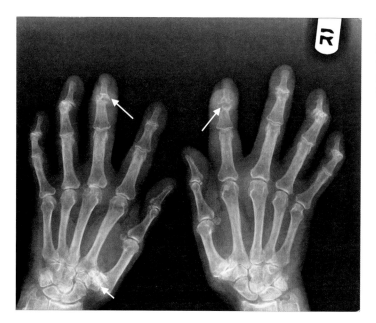

FIGURE 5-38.   Frontal projection of both hands demonstrates joint space narrowing, marginal osteophytosis, subchondral bone sclerosis involving the distal interphalangeal joints and the triscaphae joints (*short arrow*) of the hands and wrist. In this patient, there are erosions on the right second DIP and left third DIP joints (*long arrow*) that suggest erosive OA.

FIGURE 5-39. Frontal projections of both hands. There is extensive erosive disease within the wrist joints bilaterally; ulnar subluxations to the second MCP, to the third MCP, and to the fourth PIP; and radial subluxation to the fifth PIP on the left.

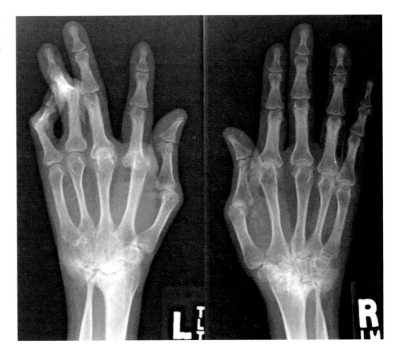

formation (syndesmophytes), and predominantly axial (spinal and sacroiliac) involvement.

Gout

Gout is a metabolic disorder that most commonly involves the feet, especially the first metatarsophalangeal joint, as well as the ankles, knees, hands, and elbows in asymmetric fashion. It is produced by a deposition of monosodium urate crystals in tissues with a poor blood supply, such as cartilage, tendon sheaths, and bursae. The radiographic features of gout typically do not appear until after 4 to 6 years of episodic arthritis. Radiographic features characteristic of gout include the following:

- Tophi or periarticular soft tissue nodules/masses created by the deposition of urate crystals that may contain calcium
- Tophi-induced periarticular or intra-articular bone erosion
- Prominent cortical edges overhanging the tophi and well-defined bone erosions (with sclerotic margins) (**Fig. 5-40**) (52)
- Random distribution, without marked osteoporosis

Calcium Pyrophosphate Dihydrate Deposition Disease

It is also known as *pseudogout* and has the classic triad of pain, cartilage calcification, and joint destruction. Chondrocalcinosis at the knee, wrist, or symphysis pubis is virtually diagnostic of calcium pyrophosphate dihydrate (CPPD) deposition disease (**Fig. 5-41**).

Diffuse Idiopathic Skeletal Hyperostosis

Diffuse idiopathic skeletal hyperostosis (DISH) is not really an arthropathy because it spares synovium, articular cartilage, and articular osseous surfaces. It is a fairly common ossification process involving ligamentous and tendinous attachments to bones and occurs in 12% of the elderly (53). It most commonly

affects the thoracic spine but also may involve the pelvis, foot, knee, and elbow. It can involve ossification of all the ligaments surrounding the vertebral bodies, particularly the anterior longitudinal ligament. Ossification of the posterior longitudinal ligament (OPLL) can also be seen. This is reported to be more common in individuals of Asian descent and can be responsible for significant spinal canal stenosis. By definition, DISH must involve a flowing ossification of at least four contiguous vertebral bodies (**Fig. 5-42A** and **B**). There must be normal disc spaces and facet joints, without joint sclerosis.

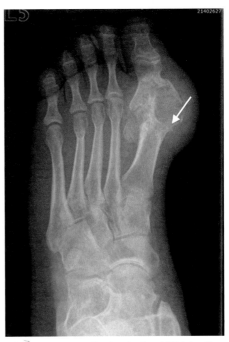

FIGURE 5-40. Gout arthritis affecting the first MTP joint. There are large periarticular bone erosions with overhanging edges (*arrow*) and significant soft tissue swelling.

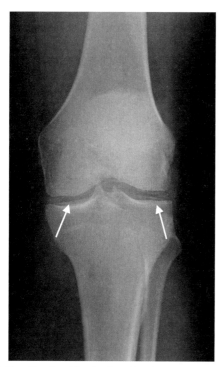

FIGURE 5-41. Chondrocalcinosis. Frontal radiograph of the right knee. Calcifications (*arrows*) are present within the medial and lateral tibiofemoral joint along the expected location of the meniscus.

SPINE AND SPINAL CORD IMAGING

It is clear, after multiple research studies to assess the usefulness of imaging in low back pain, that uncomplicated acute low back pain is a benign, self-limited condition that does not warrant any imaging studies. The vast majority of patients are back to their usual activities within 30 days. Radiographic evaluation of the lumbar spine includes frontal and lateral radiographs. These are indicated in the evaluation of back pain and weight loss, after mild trauma in patients older than 50 years old and in patients with unexplained fever, immunosuppression, history of cancer, prolonged use of steroids, and focal neurologic or disabling symptoms. Oblique views are useful for the assessment of defects to the pars interarticularis when suspecting spondylolysis, for the evaluation of the nerve root foramina and to better assess the facet joints. The relative radiation dose level for a routine radiographic examination of the lumbar spine is between 1 and 10 mSv (54). Although plain radiographs remain valuable for detecting many types of spine fractures and degenerative changes, the high resolution of osseous and soft tissue structures provided by CT and MRI has made these modalities invaluable for the diagnosis of degenerative, traumatic, neoplastic, and infectious diseases of the spinal column and spinal cord.

Degenerative Spine Disorders

CT and MRI provide complementary information about degenerative diseases of the spine. MRI is often the modality of choice in assessing degenerative changes within the spine due to its superior soft tissue contrast and lack of radiation exposure. CT has superior spatial resolution and provides better conspicuity of osseous and calcified structures. The advent of MDCT technology allows for superb reconstruction in the sagittal and the coronal planes that allows for better depiction of pathologic processes and hardware evaluation in the postoperative spine (55). MRI permits noninvasive visualization of the spinal cord and subarachnoid space within the spinal canal and the nerve roots within the neural foramina. Discrimination of these structures by CT requires injection of intrathecal contrast agents. MRI has a superior ability to

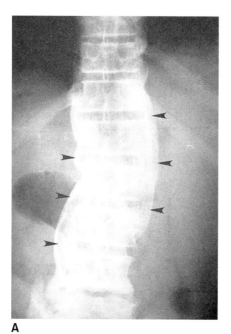

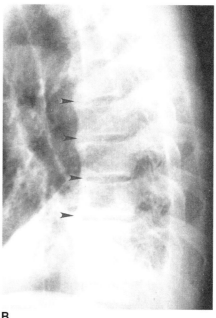

A   **B**

FIGURE 5-42. Diffuse idiopathic skeletal hyperostosis. Frontal **(A)** and lateral **(B)** radiographs of the lower thoracic spine. There are flowing ossifications (*arrowheads*) of the paraspinal ligaments bridging more than four segments of the spine. Note relative preservation of the intervertebral disc spaces.

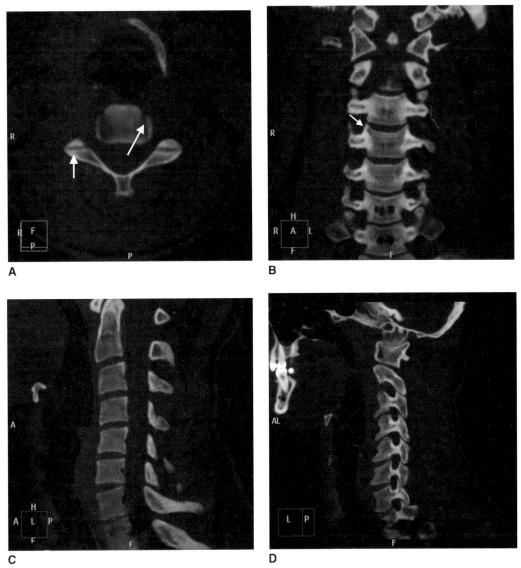

FIGURE 5-43. MDCT of the normal cervical spine. **A:** Bone window CT of the cervical spine in the axial plane at the level of C5-6 displays normal facet joints (*short arrow*) and Luschka joints (*long arrow*). **B:** Coronal multiplanar reformatted images (MPR) through the level of the uncovertebral joints (*arrow*). **C:** Midplane sagittal reconstructed images of the cervical spine shows mild reverse of the normal lordosis that could be secondary to spasm or associated to positioning. Note adequate alignment and no intersegmental subluxations. **D:** Sagittal oblique MPR demonstrates the nerve root foramina, uncovertebral joints, and facet joints.

evaluate intramedullary abnormalities. It also offers direct multiplanar imaging capabilities.

Axial CT images of the normal cervical and lumbar spine (**Figs. 5-43** and **5-44**) provide good visualization of all osseous elements, including the facet joints. In the cervical spine, the uncovertebral joints (i.e., Luschka) are well depicted with coronal reformatted and sagittal oblique images. Sagittal oblique images through the lumbar spine provide excellent anatomical reconstruction of the pars interarticularis for the assessment of spondylolysis. Soft tissue windows typically permit visualization of the moderate radiodensity of the soft tissue structures, such as the intervertebral disc, ligamentum flavum, and thecal sac. Sagittal images provide assessment of anatomical alignment and intersegmental instability and allows for adequate evaluation of foraminal stenosis. The epidural fat contains the internal vertebral venous plexus, which can be enhanced by a circulating bolus of contrast material to improve visualization

of soft tissue encroachments into the spinal canal, such as herniated discs. Introduction of contrast material into the subarachnoid space (i.e., CT myelography) delimits the contained spinal cord and the nerve roots (**Fig. 5-45**).

The introduction of MDCT technology allows for the acquisitions of multiple thin cut images in the axial plane that can be reconstructed in the sagittal and the coronal planes. The high spatial resolution of the acquired data allows for near-perfect isometric reconstruction in different planes. In addition, computer-generated volume rendering images provide superb 3D images of the spine (**Fig. 5-46A–C**).

Sagittal T1-weighted MR images of the cervical, thoracic, or lumbar spine provide excellent noninvasive survey to evaluate patients with suspected regional spinal pathology. Midsagittal T1-weighted images display the high–signal-intensity marrow of the vertebrae bordered by low–signal-intensity cortical bone. Structures displaying very low signal intensity include

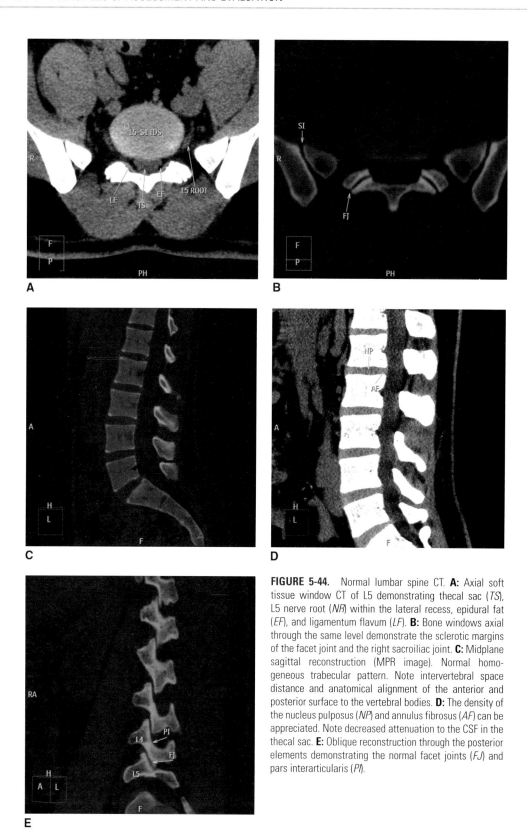

FIGURE 5-44. Normal lumbar spine CT. **A:** Axial soft tissue window CT of L5 demonstrating thecal sac (*TS*), L5 nerve root (*NR*) within the lateral recess, epidural fat (*EF*), and ligamentum flavum (*LF*). **B:** Bone windows axial through the same level demonstrate the sclerotic margins of the facet joint and the right sacroiliac joint. **C:** Midplane sagittal reconstruction (MPR image). Normal homogeneous trabecular pattern. Note intervertebral space distance and anatomical alignment of the anterior and posterior surface to the vertebral bodies. **D:** The density of the nucleus pulposus (*NP*) and annulus fibrosus (*AF*) can be appreciated. Note decreased attenuation to the CSF in the thecal sac. **E:** Oblique reconstruction through the posterior elements demonstrating the normal facet joints (*FJ*) and pars interarticularis (*PI*).

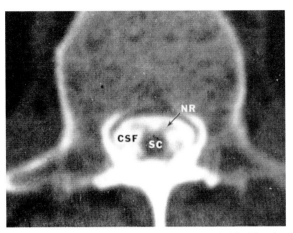

FIGURE 5-45. Metrizamide CT myelogram at L1 level delimiting the spinal cord (*SC*), the nerve roots (*NR*) arising from the cord, and the contrast-enhanced CSF.

the peripheral part of the annulus fibrosis of the intervertebral disc, all ligaments, the dura, and the cerebrospinal fluid (CSF), and these are usually indistinguishable from each other (**Fig. 5-47A–C**). The nucleus pulposus and the inner portion of the annulus fibrosis show moderate signal intensity. The spinal cord and the nerve roots display moderate signal intensity, which is well contrasted against the low–signal-intensity CSF. Collections of epidural fat, which are largest at lumbar levels, produce high signal intensity on T1- and T2-weighted images. On T2-weighted MR images, CSF and the normal well-hydrated nucleus pulposus assume high signal intensity.

Degenerative Disc Disease

The intervertebral disc space is a cartilaginous joint with a central nucleus pulposus surrounded by an annulus fibrosis. Degenerative change in the nucleus pulposus is termed intervertebral osteochondrosis (**Fig. 5-48A** and **B**). Early signs of disc disease may include loss of fluid signal within the

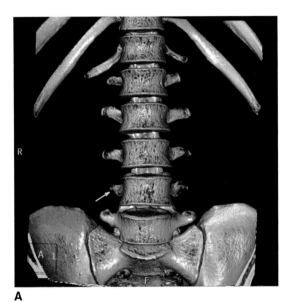

A

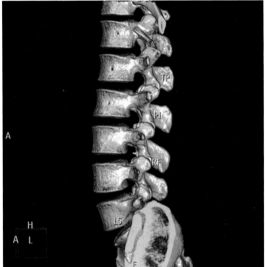

B

FIGURE 5-46. Volume rendering images of the normal lumbar spine. **A:** Coronal (frontal) projection. *Arrow* points to a hypoplastic right transverse process, a normal anatomical variant. **B:** Sagittal (lateral) view, note relationship of pars interarticularis (*PI*) to the facet joint (*FJ*) and root foramina (*RF*). **C:** Midplane sagittal view through the central canal. Facet joint (*FJ*), pars interarticularis (*PI*), and pedicle (*P*).

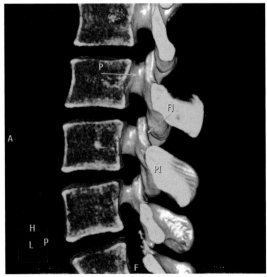

C

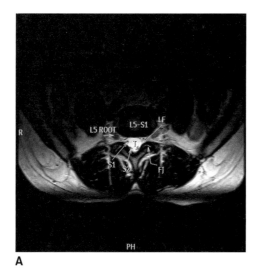

A

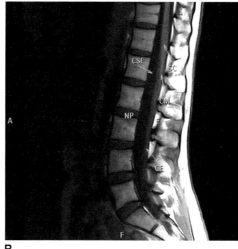

B

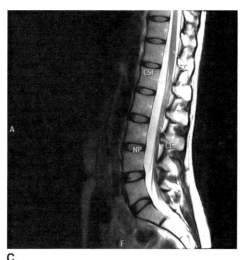

C

FIGURE 5-47. MRI of the normal spine and spinal cord. **A:** A T2-weighted axial MRI at the L5-S1 disk level shows the thecal sac (*T*) as an area of high signal intensity, the nerve roots (*S1, S2*) within the posterior thecal sac are of low signal intensity. Note the ligamentum flavum (*LF*) and fluid within the facet joints (*FJ*) with high–signal-intensity fluid. **B:** T1-weighted midsagittal MRI of the lumbosacral spine displays the nucleus pulposus (*NP*) of the intervertebral discs, spinal cord (*SC*), conus medullaris (*CM*), and nerve roots of the cauda equina (*CE*) as areas of moderate signal intensity. Cerebrospinal fluid (*CSF*) is of low signal intensity, and epidural fat (*E*) is hyperintense. **C:** T2-weighted midsagittal MRI of the lumbosacral spine demonstrates the increased intensity of the nucleus pulposus (*NP*) and CSF.

nucleus pulposus (dehydration), which results in decreased signal within the central portion of the disc on T2-weighted images, and blurring of the transition between the nucleus pulposus and the annulus fibrosis. This is followed later by narrowing of the intervertebral disc and irregularity to the endplates. Endplate changes including the signal abnormalities appreciated within the marrow of the subchondral bone are referred to as *Modic changes* (56). Modic type I changes are characterized by signal of edema that is decreased signal on T1-weighted images and increased signal on T2-weighted images. Type II changes (**Fig. 5-49A** and **B**) follow the signal characteristic of fat, with intermediate to increased signal on T1-weighted images and increased signal on T2-weighted images. This is the most common type of reactive endplate changes appreciated on degenerative osteochondrosis. Type III changes represent osseous sclerosis, characterized by decreased signal on both the T1- and the T2-weighted images.

When the disc becomes degenerated, it may undergo tearing of the annulus fibrosis collagen bundles, which is often a precursor to herniation of the nucleus pulposus, particularly at the posterolateral aspect of the disc. Protrusion is herniation of the nucleus pulposus that is contained by the annulus. In the axial plane, it usually demonstrates a base broader than

the height against the parent disc (57). Extrusion is defined as a herniation of the nucleus pulposus beyond the fibers of the peripheral annulus. In the axial plane, it can demonstrate a narrower base in relationship to the height of the herniation. A sequestered or free fragment is an extruded disc without contiguity to the parent disc. The majority of disc herniation are central or paracentral (subarticular) in location. The loss of the load-diffusing function of the normal disc also causes facet joint osteoarthrosis and marginal osteophytosis of the vertebral body ends (spondylosis deformans) by virtue of the increased loads these joints must bear.

Cervical Disc Herniation

Disc herniation is typically preceded by degenerative changes in the mucopolysaccharides of the nucleus pulposus, which produce fibrillation of the collagen (58). This eventually causes dehydration and loss of disc volume. As a result, the nucleus pulposus no longer serves as a normal load-dispersing mechanism, and excessive stress is borne by the annulus fibrosis. This produces annular fissuring and tears that can culminate in herniation of the nucleus. The loss of the load-diffusing function of the normal disc also causes facet joint degeneration and marginal osteophytosis of the vertebral body ends by virtue of the increased loads these joints must bear.

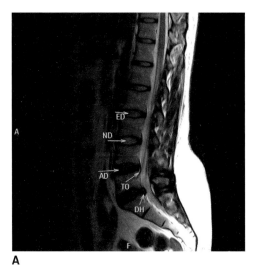
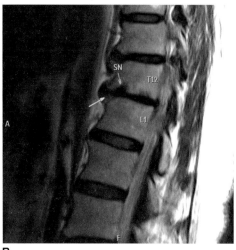

A **B**

FIGURE 5-48. **A:** Sagittal T2WI of the lumbar spine demonstrating different stages of intervertebral osteochondrosis. Normal disk (*ND*) demonstrates increased signal to the nucleus pulposus and normal height. With early degeneration (*ED*), the nucleus pulposus loses signal in part related to the decreased water content of the intervertebral disc but preserves the intervertebral height. With advanced degeneration (*AD*), there is near complete loss to the normal signal of the intervertebral disk and early traction osteophyte formation (*TO*). Note herniated disk (*DH*) at the L5-S1 segment. **B:** Advanced degenerative osteochondrosis on a different patient. There is loss of the intervertebral disk height, Schmorl's node formation (*SN*) representing endplate herniation, and moderate traction osteophyte formation (*arrow*).

Cervical disc herniation occurs with less frequency than lumbar disc herniation. About 90% of cervical disc herniations occur, in order of decreasing frequency, at C5-6, C6-7, and C4-5 levels (59,60). On CT examination, a herniated cervical disc appears as a dense soft tissue mass protruding from the disc space centrally or paracentrally into the spinal canal or posterolaterally into the neural foramen (**Fig. 5-50**).

On T1-weighted MR images, the herniated cervical disc appears as a posterior extension of the moderate signal intensity of the disc into the low–signal-intensity region of the thecal sac (**Fig. 5-51A and B**). Because the spinal cord appears as a relatively high–signal-intensity structure outlined by the low–signal-intensity CSF, the relationship of the herniated disc to the spinal cord can be visualized directly by MRI. On

T2-weighted MR images, the degenerated disc appears as a narrowed disc interval. The disc herniation appears as a moderate– to low–signal-intensity impingement on the now high–signal-intensity CSF. The posterior margin of the herniated disc may have a very-low–signal-intensity margin interfacing with the CSF. This may be a posterior longitudinal ligament elevated by the herniated disc, or it may be fragments of the posterior part of the annulus fibrosis (59). T2-weighted images also permit evaluation of the relationship of the herniated disc to the spinal cord to determine its probability of causing a patient's myelopathic findings (**Fig. 5-52A and B**). It is sometimes difficult to differentiate lateral herniations of the disc into the neural foramen from osteophytic encroachments by MRI because they may both demonstrate low signal intensity.

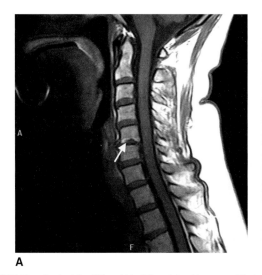
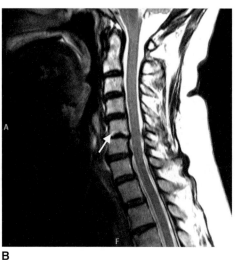

A **B**

FIGURE 5-49. Sagittal T1- **(A)** and T2- **(B)** weighted images with degenerative osteochondrosis of the cervical spine. There is decreased T2 signal to most intervertebral discs, decreased disc height throughout, annular bulge, and traction osteophytosis. Note increased signal to the inferior endplate of C5 both on the T1- and T2-weighted images (*arrows*) characteristic of Modic type II changes.

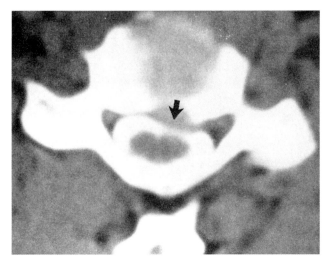

FIGURE 5-50. CT evaluation of a herniated C5-6 nucleus pulposus. An axial CT myelogram shows a radiodense protrusion of the C5-6 disc (*arrow*) that distorts the left anterior aspect of both the thecal sac and the spinal cord.

In these circumstances, CT provides good differentiation between bone and soft tissue density.

Cervical Spinal Stenosis and Foraminal Stenosis

Cervical spinal stenosis can be congenital or acquired. In the less common congenital stenosis, a small spinal canal is produced by short pedicles and thick laminae (60). It commonly remains asymptomatic until degenerative changes are superimposed on the congenital stenosis later in life. Acquired stenosis can be produced by a host of hypertrophic degenerative changes often collectively referred to as cervical spondylosis. These include osteophytic lipping of the posterior margins of the vertebral body ends bordering the disc, hypertrophic degenerative changes involving Luschka's joints or the facet joints, buckling or hypertrophy of the ligamenta flava, and OPLL. All these structures border the spinal canal; therefore,

hypertrophic degenerative changes can produce spinal canal stenosis. Because Luschka's joints, the facet joints, and the ligamenta flava also border the neural foramen, their involvement by degenerative processes can produce foraminal stenosis.

Although hypertrophic degenerative changes of any of the structures bordering the spinal canal or neural foramen can occur in isolation, they are commonly precipitated by intervertebral disc degeneration. As the disc degenerates and loses its normal load-dispersing ability, loads tend to become concentrated on the vertebral body margin toward which the spine is bent. This excessive loading can produce marginal osteophytes around the entire circumference of the vertebral body endplates. Those osteophytes developing on the posterior margin can encroach on the spinal canal to produce spinal stenosis (**Fig. 5-53A** and **B**). Luschka (i.e., uncovertebral) joints are situated between the uncinate processes that protrude from the lateral or posterolateral margins of the upper surface of the vertebral bodies and a reciprocal convexity on the lateral aspect of the inferior surface of the next higher vertebral body. Recent evidence indicates that they are not true joints. Rather, they are degenerative clefts within the lateral part of the intervertebral disc that begin in the second decade of life (61). The increased loading of Luschka joints produced by these degenerative changes produces bony spurs that can extend posteriorly into the lateral part of the spinal canal or posterolaterally into the neural foramen (**Fig. 5-54A–C**).

Disc degeneration is accompanied by dehydration and loss of disc height, with decreased space between vertebral bodies resulting in increased facet joint loads. The resultant facet joint degeneration involves cartilage erosion with joint space narrowing, subchondral bone sclerosis, and osteophyte formation. The osteophytes may encroach on the spinal canal or the neural foramen. Loss of disc height results in decrease of the laminae interspace, which causes the ligamentum flavum to buckle and bulge into the spinal canal, contributing to the spinal stenosis. Because the ligamentum flavum continues laterally into the facet joint capsule, buckling of this part of the ligamentum flavum can cause foraminal stenosis. OPLL occurs more commonly at cervical than at other vertebral levels. It is best

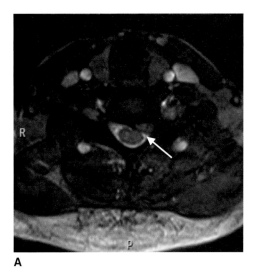

A

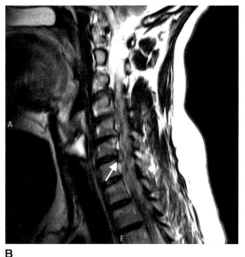

B

FIGURE 5-51. **A:** T2*-weighted axial MRI of the cervical spine shows a left posterolateral C5-6 nucleus pulposus (*arrow*) indenting the thecal sac and extending into the ostium of the ipsilateral nerve root foramina. **B:** A T2-weighted left parasagittal MRI shows the disc fragment (*arrow*) impinging upon the intermediate–signal-intensity thecal sac and low–signal-intensity posterior longitudinal ligament.

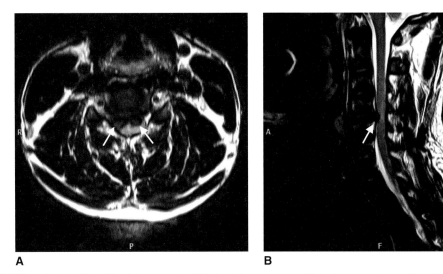

FIGURE 5-52. **A:** Axial T2-weighted image at the C4-5 level demonstrates a bilobed protrusion (*arrows*) contained in the midline by the posterior longitudinal ligament. Note complete obliteration of the normal CSF signal anterior to the cord, posterior displacement, and compression of the cord. **B:** The herniated disc (*arrow*) elevates the posterior longitudinal ligament, compresses the cervical cord, which demonstrates increased signal intensity as a sign of myelopathy.

visualized via CT, where it appears as an ossification extending over several vertebral levels, separated from the posterior margin of the vertebral bodies by a thin radiolucent interval (**Fig. 5-55A** and **B**).

When any of these potential causes of cervical stenosis sufficiently narrow the spinal canal, cord compression can produce myelopathic signs and symptoms. Spinal stenosis most frequently narrows the AP dimension of the spinal canal. Although the cross-sectional area of the spinal canal is smallest at the C4 and C7 levels, the smallest AP diameter is usually at the C3 through C5 levels (60). It has been stated that all spinal stenosis that reduces the AP dimension to less than 10 mm could produce quadriplegia (62).

Although the uppermost cervical cord segments are nearly round, at most cervical levels, the cord has an elliptical outline with its major axis transversely oriented. With encroachment of the cord by spinal stenosis, it is usually first flattened anteriorly by an encroaching osteophyte. With progression, the anterior median fissure becomes indented and widened until the cord assumes a kidney bean shape (**Fig. 5-56**) (45). The lateral funiculi may become tapered anterolaterally because of tension on the denticulate ligaments. The cord may become notched dorsally because of posterior white column atrophy. It has been estimated that a 30% reduction in cord cross-sectional area may be required to produce signs of ascending and descending tract degeneration (63).

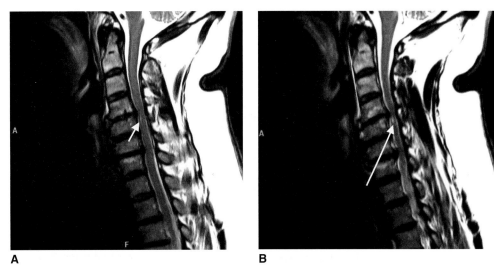

FIGURE 5-53. Midplane sagittal **(A)** and right parasagittal **(B)** T2-weighted images in a patient with congenital stenosis and superimposed degenerative spondylosis with central canal narrowing and cord compression. There is increased AP dimension to the C4, C5, and C6 vertebral bodies. Annular bulge and hypertrophy to the supporting ligamentous structures are responsible for compression of the cord. There is linear increased signal to the cord on the T2-weighted image (*arrow*) compatible with early myelopathy.

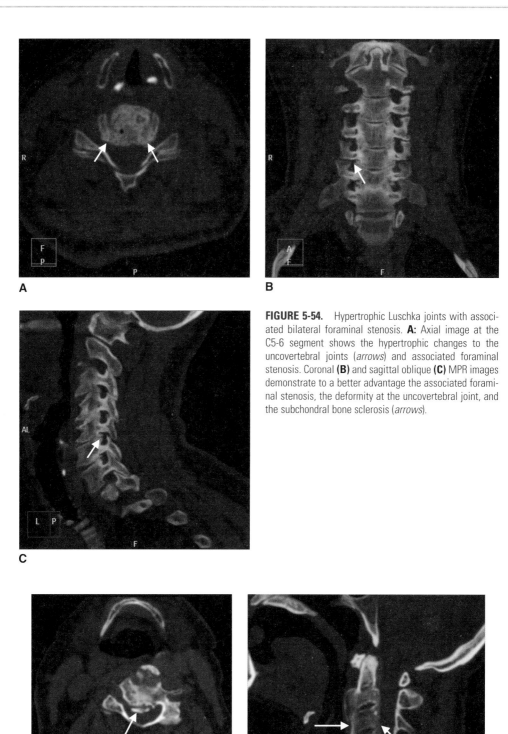

FIGURE 5-54.   Hypertrophic Luschka joints with associated bilateral foraminal stenosis. **A:** Axial image at the C5-6 segment shows the hypertrophic changes to the uncovertebral joints (*arrows*) and associated foraminal stenosis. Coronal **(B)** and sagittal oblique **(C)** MPR images demonstrate to a better advantage the associated foraminal stenosis, the deformity at the uncovertebral joint, and the subchondral bone sclerosis (*arrows*).

FIGURE 5-55.   Ossification of the posterior longitudinal ligament (OPLL). **A:** Axial CT at the level of C3 demonstrates the calcification to the fibers of the posterior longitudinal ligament (*arrow*). There is narrowing to the central canal by the mass effect exerted by the enlarged calcified ligament. **B:** Sagittal multiplanar reformatted image. There are flowing calcifications within the anterior longitudinal ligament (*short arrows*). The calcification extends from C2 up to C7. The OPLL (*long arrow*) extends from C2 up to the proximal border of C5.

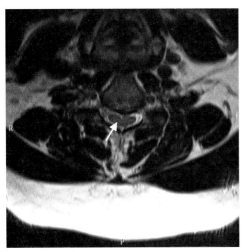

FIGURE 5-56. Axial T2-weighted images in the same patient as in **Figure 5-54**. Note deformity to the cord that has assumed a bean shape in the transaxial plane. There is compression and increased signal intensity to the cord compatible with myelopathy (*arrow*).

Thoracic Spine Abnormalities

Both thoracic disc herniation and thoracic spinal stenosis are rare compared with cervical and lumbar level disease. When thoracic disc herniation does occur, it most frequently involves discs below T8 (64). The CT findings are similar to those of cervical levels, except that calcification of the disc protrusion is more common at thoracic levels. The causes as well as CT and MRI findings of thoracic spinal stenosis are similar to those at cervical levels.

Lumbar Disc Herniation

The correlation of lumbar disc herniation with a patient's complaints of low back pain or sciatica is not always clearly established. It has been estimated that as many as 20% of patients

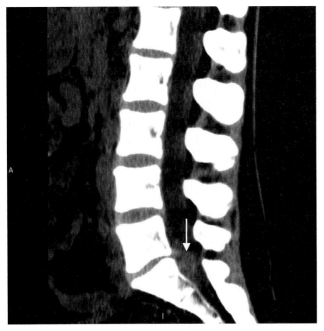

FIGURE 5-57. Sagittal reconstructed image of an MDCT acquisition of the lumbar spine demonstrates a large disc protrusion (*arrow*).

with radiologic findings of disc herniation are asymptomatic (65). Furthermore, when disc herniation occurs in symptomatic patients, other findings are often present that also could explain the clinical findings. Lumbar disc herniations occur most frequently posterolaterally because the annulus is thinnest in the posterior quadrants and reinforced in the midline by the posterior longitudinal ligament. Also, flexion is the most prevalent lumbar spine motion, which places greatest stress on the posterior part of the disc. When the disc herniates to the posterolateral direction, it frequently does not impinge on the spinal nerve roots emerging from the neural foramen to which the disc is related, because the nerve roots occupy the upper portion of the foramen, whereas the disc is situated in the anterior wall of the lower part of the foramen. Therefore, when the L5-S1 disc herniates posterolaterally, it frequently spares the L5 nerve roots, exiting through the upper portion of the L5-S1 neural foramen. Instead, it more commonly involves the S1 nerve roots that descend across the posterolateral aspect of the L5-S1 disc before their exit from the S1 sacral foramina. Less common lumbar disc herniations are placed centrally or far laterally. Central herniations can involve any or all of the rootlets of the cauda equina. The infrequent far lateral herniations occur outside of the neural foramina. When present, they usually impinge on the ventral ramus that has just emerged from that foramen.

Noncontrast CT has been described as being accurate in diagnosing disc herniations. On CT examination, the herniated disc appears as a focal protrusion of the disc that displaces the epidural fat (**Fig. 5-57**). The herniated disc material is typically slightly hyperdense relative to the non–contrast-enhanced dural sac and its adjacent nerve roots. The dural sac or adjacent nerve roots may be seen to be indented, displaced, or compressed. In more lateral herniations, the soft tissue material of the disc can encroach on the neural foramen or the extraforaminal soft tissues, where it also displaces fat, and here, it may encroach on the dorsal root ganglion, the spinal nerve, or its ventral ramus. Herniated lumbar discs may calcify or contain gas. Extruded disc fragments can become separated from the disc and are thus able to migrate superiorly, inferiorly, or laterally. A herniated disc should be distinguished from a bulging annulus. A bulging annulus is produced by dehydration and volume loss within the nucleus pulposus. In contrast to the focal protrusion of a herniated disc, the bulging annulus typically has a symmetrical smooth contour, bulging beyond all margins of the vertebral body.

On T1-weighted sagittal and axial MR images, the herniated lumbar disc appears as a moderate–signal-intensity intrusion into the high–signal-intensity epidural fat or on the moderate– to low–signal-intensity thecal sac or the lumbar nerve roots within their dural sleeves (**Fig. 5-58A and B**). Similarly, disc herniation into the neural foramen is visualized by a moderate–signal-intensity mass displacing the foraminal fat and encroaching on the dorsal root ganglion or nerve roots.

On T2-weighted sagittal MR images, the low signal intensity of a degenerated disc contrasts sharply with the high signal intensity of the nucleus pulposus of adjacent well-hydrated discs (**Fig. 5-59**). Any intrusion of the low–signal-intensity disc herniation on the thecal sac is well seen because of the high–signal-intensity myelographic effect of the CSF on T2-weighted images.

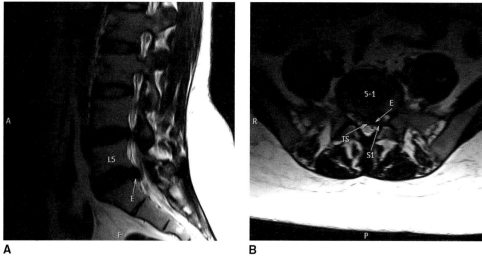

FIGURE 5-58. **A:** Left parasagittal T2WI of the lumbar spine with an extruded disk at the L5-S1 segment. **B:** Axial T2WI demonstrates elevation of the thecal sac (*TS*) by the extrusion (*E*). There is mass effect and posterior displacement of the first sacral root (*S1*).

Discography remains a controversial diagnostic imaging modality. It appears that its major diagnostic value lies in the reproduction of the patient's specific pain on contrast injection of a given disc, with controls demonstrating that injection of adjacent discs produces either no pain or referred pain (66). Discography, especially when combined with CT, may provide information about degeneration and the extent of fissures and rupture.

Lumbar Spinal Stenosis and Foraminal Stenosis

Like cervical stenosis, lumbar spinal stenosis is frequently precipitated by disc degeneration with subsequent marginal osteophytosis of the vertebral body ends, hypertrophic degeneration of the facet joints, and bulging of the ligamenta flava. Lumbar stenosis may be lateral, central, or combined. The lower lumbar vertebrae normally have shorter pedicles that cause the superior articular processes to intrude into the spinal canal to cut off narrow lateral recesses (**Fig. 5-60A–E**). The lateral recesses are bordered by the pedicles laterally, the vertebral body anteriorly, and, most important, the superior articular processes posteriorly. The lateral recesses are occupied by the nerve roots of the next spinal nerve to exit as they descend within their dural sleeve. Osteophytes that develop on the anteromedial margin of the superior articular processes of the next lower vertebra are most likely to encroach on the lateral recess to produce lateral stenosis. Because the inferior articular processes of the next higher vertebra are situated posterior-medial to the superior articular processes, osteophytes developing on their anterior margin are more likely to produce central stenosis. In central stenosis, any or all of the rootlets of the cauda equina can be encroached on. Vertebral body margin osteophytes and buckling of the ligamentum flavum can contribute to lumbar spinal stenosis.

Hypertrophic degenerative changes involving the facet joints can also encroach on the posterior aspect of the neural foramen and produce foraminal stenosis with compression of the nerve roots exiting that foramen. Therefore, hypertrophic degenerative changes involving a single superior articular process can involve the roots of two closely adjacent nerves, with the possibility of producing both foraminal and lateral spinal stenosis. With disc degeneration and loss of disc height, the neural foramen can be further compromised by the upward and forward displacement of the superior articular process into the upper part of the neural foramen, where the nerve roots are situated. In addition, because of the obliquity of the facet joint, the accompanying downward displacement of the inferior articular process of the next higher vertebra can produce retrolisthesis (i.e., backward displacement) of its vertebral body into the upper portion of the neural foramen. By standard myelography, the protruding disc anteriorly and the bulging ligamenta flava posteriorly can produce an hourglass appearance of the thecal sac (**Fig. 5-61**). By CT, all osteophytes are clearly visualized, and measurements of the AP dimension of lateral recesses that are less than 3 mm are strongly suggestive of lateral stenosis (67). The hypertrophic changes producing central and foraminal stenosis are also well visualized. Sagittal reformations are especially helpful in evaluating foraminal stenosis.

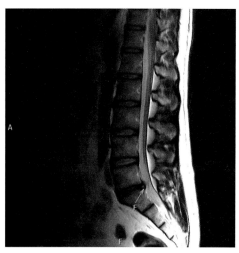

FIGURE 5-59. Small central extrusion (*E*) at the L5-S1 segment. Note decreased signal to the intervertebral disk when compared to the remaining intervertebral segments, a sign of degeneration.

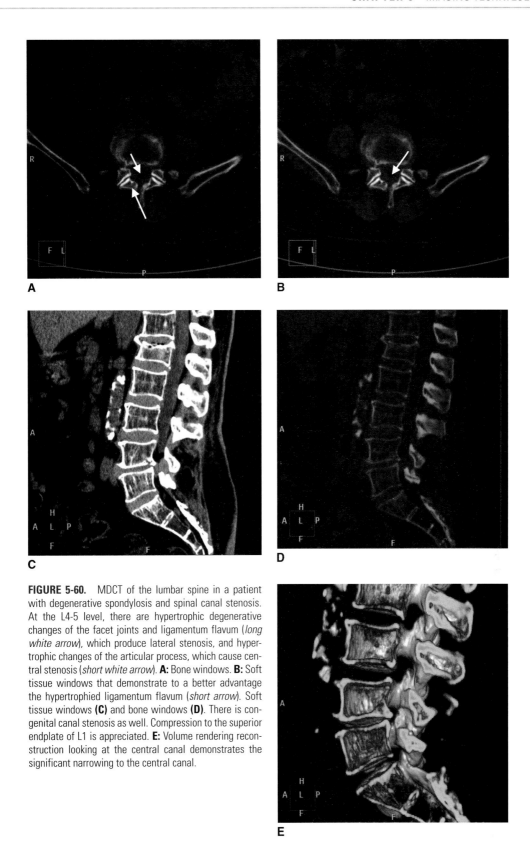

FIGURE 5-60. MDCT of the lumbar spine in a patient with degenerative spondylosis and spinal canal stenosis. At the L4-5 level, there are hypertrophic degenerative changes of the facet joints and ligamentum flavum (*long white arrow*), which produce lateral stenosis, and hypertrophic changes of the articular process, which cause central stenosis (*short white arrow*). **A:** Bone windows. **B:** Soft tissue windows that demonstrate to a better advantage the hypertrophied ligamentum flavum (*short arrow*). Soft tissue windows **(C)** and bone windows **(D)**. There is congenital canal stenosis as well. Compression to the superior endplate of L1 is appreciated. **E:** Volume rendering reconstruction looking at the central canal demonstrates the significant narrowing to the central canal.

Facet anatomy is well seen by MRI, with subchondral bone appearing as a signal void. On T1-weighted images, articular cartilage is visualized as a moderate–signal-intensity interval between the subchondral bones of the two articular processes. This becomes more signal intense on T2-weighted images. Facet joint degeneration appears as an irregularity or reduction in the thickness of the articular cartilage. Osteophytes are usually displayed as signal voids encroaching into the foramen, lateral recess, or spinal canal. Occasionally, osteophytes show high–signal-intensity interior, indicating the presence of marrow.

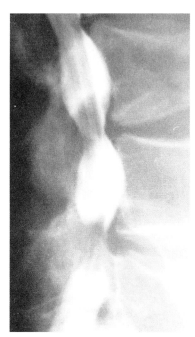

FIGURE 5-61. Lumbar spinal stenosis caused by both protruding discs and bulging ligamentum flavum. Lateral myelogram showing the hourglass appearance of the thecal sac.

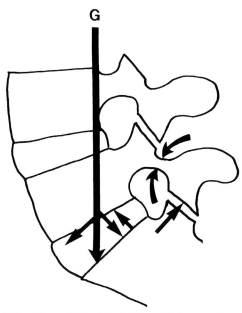

FIGURE 5-62. The gravitational load (*G*) is applied across the lumbosacral junction. The equal and opposite forces acting on the inferior aspect of the L5 body and the anterior aspect of the inferior articular process of L5 cause shearing stresses to be concentrated on the pars interarticularis of L5 (*curved arrows*). This produces the stress fracture of spondylolysis.

Spondylolysis and Spondylolisthesis

Spondylolysis is a defect in the pars interarticularis, commonly involving the L5 and occasionally the L4 vertebrae. Most spondylolysis is thought to be produced by repetitive stress. The gravitational and muscular loads acting across the steep incline of the upper surface of the sacrum can be resolved into a shearing component, which tends to displace the L5 vertebral body forward on S1, and a compressive component at right angles to the superior surface of S1 (**Fig. 5-62**). In accordance with Newton's third law, S1 will exert an equal and opposite force against the inferior aspect of the L5 vertebral body. The tendency of L5 to be displaced forward on S1 is primarily resisted by the impaction of the inferior articular processes of L5 on the superior articular processes of S1. Again, Newton's third law dictates that there will be an equal and opposite force exerted against the inferior articular process of L5. The upward and forward force of the sacral body on the L5 body and the upward and backward force of the superior articular process of the sacrum on the inferior articular process of L5 cause shearing stresses to be concentrated on the pars interarticularis, and this can produce a stress fracture.

Spondylolisthesis is an anterior subluxation of one vertebral body on another. It can occur at any vertebral level, but the mechanics of the lumbosacral junction cause a higher incidence at this level. The most common cause at this level is spondylolysis, where the impaction of the inferior articular process of L5 or L4 will no longer be able to resist forward displacement of the vertebral body. Whether or not a spondylolisthesis follows a spondylolysis is largely determined by the resistance of the other supporting structures of the lumbosacral junction, which include the intervertebral disc, the anterior longitudinal ligament, and the iliolumbar ligaments. When they fail, the lysis becomes a listhesis. Other causes of spondylolisthesis include degenerative changes in the facet joints and

disc that produce joint instability, fractures, dysplasia of the upper sacrum or the neural arch of L5, generalized pathology such as Paget's disease, or iatrogenically induced laminectomy or facetectomy (67).

On oblique plain films, spondylolysis is visualized as a break in the neck of the "Scotty dog" outline, which is produced by the ipsilateral transverse process forming a nose; the ipsilateral pedicle, an eye; the pars interarticularis, a neck; the ipsilateral inferior articular process, a forelimb; the lamina, a body; the contralateral inferior articular process, a hind limb; and the spinous process, a tail (**Fig. 5-63**). When spondylolysis

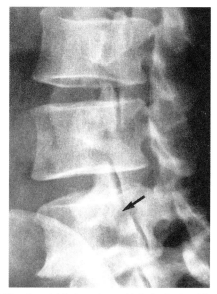

FIGURE 5-63. Spondylolysis and spondylolisthesis. An oblique radiograph demonstrates a spondylolytic defect in the pars interarticularis of L4 (*arrow*). Note the intact neck in the "Scotty dog" outline in the L3 vertebra.

is suspected clinically or on plain film studies, a volumetric CT with sagittal reconstruction, MR, or plain film examination with nuclear medicine scintigraphy can be useful for diagnosis (**Fig. 5-64A** and **B**) (68).

Spondylolisthesis is graded by the amount of subluxation, with grade I being a forward displacement of less than 25%; grade II, a forward displacement of 25% to 50%; grade III, a displacement of 50% to 75%; and grade IV, a displacement of greater than 75%. Grading the spondylolisthesis is usually accomplished by lateral plain films or sagittal reconstructed images in CT (**Fig. 5-64C** and **D**).

On CT, the defect of spondylolysis is differentiated from the facet joint interval by its location at the axial level of the pedicles rather than at the level of the neural foramen, as well as by the defect irregular margins and adjacent sclerosis. By MRI, the defect in the pars is visualized as a low–signal-intensity zone within the high–signal-intensity marrow of the pars.

Spinal Trauma

Although much spinal trauma is well visualized on plain films, CT has a number of advantages over this modality. These include the demonstration of fractures not seen in plain films, an accurate determination of the amount of spinal canal encroachment by fracture fragments (**Fig. 5-65A** and **B**), the identification of neural foramen impingement by fractures involving its boundaries, and a more precise evaluation of facet disruption.

MR can display impingement on the dural sac or the spinal cord by bone fragments, as well as any resultant cord contusion (**Fig. 5-65C**). It can demonstrate acute cord enlargement as a sign of cord edema or hemorrhage and cord atrophy. CT myelography can be used to diagnose posttraumatic cystic myelopathy because the cyst will take up the contrast and be displayed as a well-marginated, homogeneous, high-density region within the cord. When MRI is not available or contra-indicated, CT myelography can be used to assess the degree of

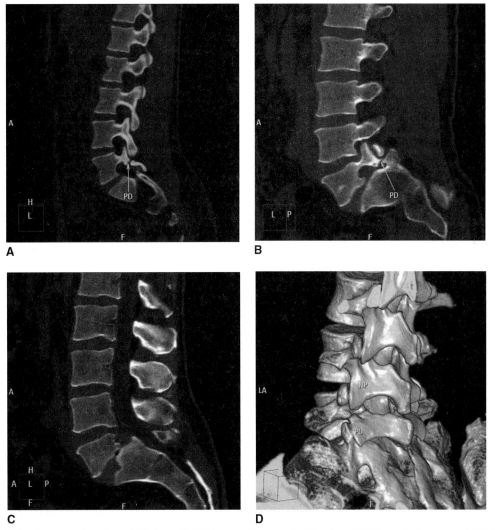

FIGURE 5-64. Spondylolysis and spondylolisthesis. **A:** Right parasagittal reconstruction of an MDCT demonstrates a spondylolytic defect in the pars interarticularis of L5 (PD *arrow*). **B:** Parasagittal reconstructed image forms a volumetric CT demonstrating the pars defect in a patient with stage II spondylolisthesis (PD *arrow*). **C:** Midplane sagittal reconstruction demonstrates grade II spondylolisthesis. **D:** Volume rendering, oblique posterior view demonstrating the pars defect (*PD*) and a normal pars (*NP*) above.

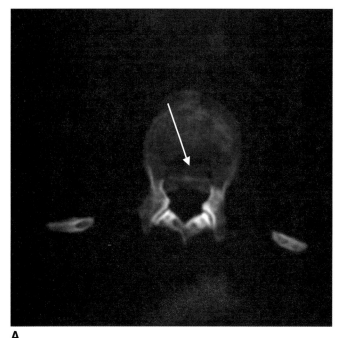

A

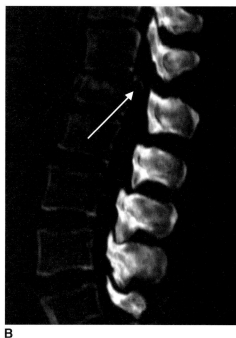

B

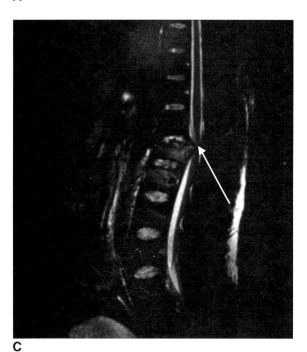

C

FIGURE 5-65. MDCT visualization of spinal trauma. **A:** CT of a burst fracture of L1 shows displacement of a fracture fragment into the spinal canal (*arrow*). There is significant comminution to the superior articular surface of the vertebral body. **B:** Sagittal MPR reconstruction demonstrates the large fragment (*arrow*) extending into the spinal canal. There is mild compression of the superior endplate of L2. **C:** Sagittal T2-weighted MR image demonstrates increased signal intensity to the bone marrow of the L1 and L2 vertebral bodies due to the presence of edema and hemorrhage. There is posterior displacement of the conus and proximal cauda equina in the spinal canal. Increased signal to the conus (*arrow*) is compatible with a cord contusion.

spinal canal stenosis and cord compression. CT also can better demonstrate the signs of vertebral instability seen on plain radiographs (**Fig. 5-66A–C**) (69). These signs include the following:

- Vertebral displacements involving the whole vertebra or fracture fragments
- Widening of the interspinous interval, which implies injury to the posterior spinal ligaments secondary to hyperflexion injury
- Increased dimensions of the vertebral canal in the sagittal or coronal plane often evaluated by an increased interpedicular distance, which implies a complete disruption of the vertebral body in the sagittal plane

- Widening of the facet joint interval, which implies ligamentous disruption
- Disruption of the alignment of the posterior aspect of the vertebral bodies, such as occurs in burst fractures or lap-seat belt fractures (**Fig. 5-67**)

T1-weighted sagittal and axial MR images provide the best evaluation of vertebral alignment and the bony and ligamentous boundaries of the spinal canal. They also allow the best delineation of the low signal intensity of a traumatic syringomyelia against the higher signal intensity of the surrounding spinal cord. T2-weighted sagittal MR images that produce a high–signal-intensity CSF provide the best estimate of the

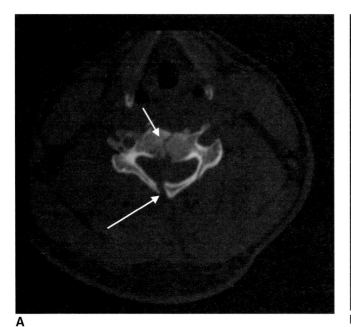

A

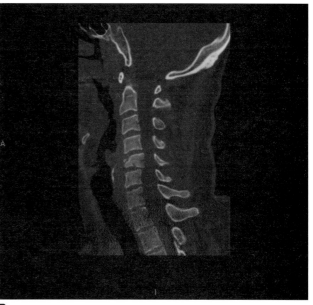

B

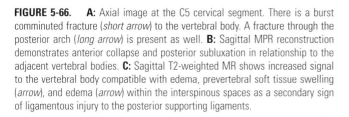

FIGURE 5-66. **A:** Axial image at the C5 cervical segment. There is a burst comminuted fracture (*short arrow*) to the vertebral body. A fracture through the posterior arch (*long arrow*) is present as well. **B:** Sagittal MPR reconstruction demonstrates anterior collapse and posterior subluxation in relationship to the adjacent vertebral bodies. **C:** Sagittal T2-weighted MR shows increased signal to the vertebral body compatible with edema, prevertebral soft tissue swelling (*arrow*), and edema (*arrow*) within the interspinous spaces as a secondary sign of ligamentous injury to the posterior supporting ligaments.

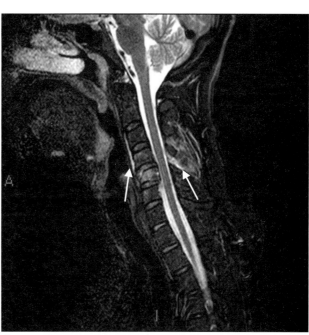

C

degree of encroachment of a bony fragment on the thecal sac or the spinal cord.

MRI has a number of advantages over other modalities for imaging spinal trauma. First, it permits evaluation of vertebral alignment at the cervicothoracic junction of the spine, which is relatively inaccessible by other modalities. Second, it provides a means to evaluate adjacent soft tissue damage. For example, hemorrhage in the prevertebral space that can occur with hyperextension injuries is identified on T2-weighted images as a high–signal-intensity area. MRI also identifies high–signal-intensity hemorrhage in the posterior paravertebral muscles that can occur secondary to hyperflexion injuries. In addition, MRI is the most sensitive modality for the assessment of ligamentous injuries as it detects edema within

the supporting ligaments, a finding not assessed by any other imaging modality (see **Figs. 5-65** and **5-66C**). Of importance is the fact that MRI provides a noninvasive means of evaluating the relationship of retropulsed vertebral body fragments or anteriorly displaced neural arch fragments to the spinal cord (see **Fig. 5-65C**). In most centers, MRI has replaced myelography as the procedure of choice for evaluating the effects of vertebral trauma on the spinal cord. Most importantly, MRI can evaluate the extent and type of spinal cord injury (69,70).

An acutely injured spinal cord tends to enlarge, thereby filling the spinal canal and displacing the epidural fat. This can be visualized by both CT and MRI. MRI is valuable in the early stages of spinal cord injury in determining the type of spinal cord injury and the prognosis for recovery. It can identify the

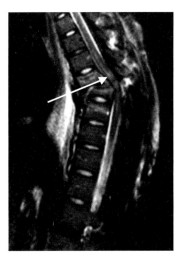

FIGURE 5-67. Sagittal T2-weighted image of the thoracic spine. There is a fracture dislocation (Chance fracture) at the C7-T1 interspace. There is bone marrow edema of the C7, T1, and T2 vertebral bodies and extensive prevertebral soft tissue swelling. Edema is also appreciated within the posterior supporting structures. There is compression and edema (*white arrow*) to the cord extending from C6 up to the T2 segment.

level and completeness of cord transection by direct visualization of the transection site. In the nontransected cord, it can discriminate cord hemorrhage from cord contusion with edema. Spinal cord contusion with edema causes high signal intensity on T2-weighted images within the first 24 hours of injury. Acute hemorrhage of less than 24 hours' duration appears as a low–signal-intensity area on T2-weighted images. Within a few days of the trauma, the subacute hemorrhage site becomes hyperintense on T2-weighted images as a result of the accumulation of paramagnetic methemoglobin (**Fig. 5-68**). Khurana et al. found that the type of injury visualized by MRI correlated with the patient's recovery of neurologic function (70,71). Those patients with cord contusion and edema exhibited significant functional recovery, whereas those with hemorrhage made little functional progress. Therefore, the MRI

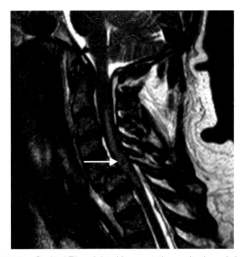

FIGURE 5-68. Sagittal T2-weighted image at the cervicothoracic junction in a patient with fracture dislocation at the C5-6 segment. There is compression and swelling of the cord. A focal area of decreased signal within the cord secondary to methemoglobin deposition associated with the acute bleed (*arrow*).

characteristics of the injury may provide the clinician with important prognostic data.

MRI is also invaluable for identifying late sequelae of spinal cord trauma, including myelomalacia and posttraumatic spinal cord cysts or syringomyelia. Myelomalacia is thought to develop within an injured segment of the spinal cord as a result of ischemia or the release of enzymes from damaged spinal cord tissues, or both (72). The myelomalacic area is made up of the products of neuronal degeneration, scar tissue, and microcysts. It is thought that the myelomalacic areas become larger intramedullary cysts because the scar tissue about the injured cord tethers the cord to the dura so that the episodic changes in CSF pressure that occur during daily activities tend to be concentrated on the injured cord segment as stretching forces. It is hypothesized that these stresses cause coalescence of the myelomalacic microcysts into a progressively enlarging gross cyst. CSF is theorized to enter the cysts along enlarged perivascular Virchow-Robin spaces that connect the subarachnoid space to the cyst (70).

On T1-weighted images, myelomalacia appears within the segment of the spinal cord near the area of injury as a region of lower signal intensity than the spinal cord but higher signal intensity than the CSF. It has indistinct margins with the surrounding spinal cord. In contrast, intramedullary cysts have signal intensity approximating that of CSF and sharply marginated borders with the surrounding spinal cord or an adjacent area of myelomalacia. The development of an intramedullary cyst in a spinal cord of a patient whose clinical picture had previously stabilized may cause the patient to develop progressive sensory and motor deficits. Although myelomalacia has no definitive treatment mode, a spinal cord cyst can be surgically decompressed with a shunt to achieve improvement or at least an arrest of the patient's neurologic deterioration. Therefore, the MRI distinction between cysts and myelomalacia is important. MRI can also be used in postoperative follow-up to ensure that the cyst has been fully decompressed and that the catheter is continuing to function to prevent reaccumulation of fluid within the cyst.

Atlantoaxial Instability

Spine instability is the loss of the spine motion segment integrity, where force produces greater displacement than normal, causing deformity and pain. Atlantoaxial instability can be produced by softening, laxity, or rupture of the transverse atlantal, alar, and apical ligaments of the dens (i.e., odontoid). These ligaments hold the odontoid in its proper position against the anterior arch of the atlas and below the level of the foramen magnum. Such ligamentous changes can be produced by rheumatoid arthritis, Down's syndrome, or traumatic rupture. Rheumatoid changes that destroy the articular cartilage and bone of the atlantoaxial joints can further increase the instability. Atlantoaxial instability also can be caused by odontoid abnormalities, such as an unfused apical portion of the odontoid (i.e., os odontoideum), or by odontoid fractures.

Normally, the cartilaginous radiolucent interval between the anterior arch of the atlas and the dens does not exceed 3 mm in the adult. With ligamentous abnormalities, lateral radiographs of the flexed cervical spine may show a posterior subluxation of the odontoid into the spinal canal that increases the atlas-dens interval to more than 3 mm. When posterior subluxation of the odontoid exceeds 9 mm, it is likely to compromise the spinal cord and produce neurologic abnormalities (73). There also can be a superior subluxation of the odontoid above the level of the foramen magnum that can cause death by impingement on the medulla or the vertebral arteries. These subluxations are well visualized by CT and MRI. MRI also can directly evaluate the ligaments. CT myelography and MR images in the axial or sagittal planes can assess the involvement of the spinal cord or medulla by the subluxation.

BRAIN IMAGING

The following section will be dedicated to brain imaging relevant to rehabilitation. Emphasis is placed on the imaging of ischemic and hemorrhagic strokes, head trauma, and common degenerative diseases. The imaging of brain neoplasms and infections will not be covered in this section, as it is beyond the scope of this text.

Stroke

The term *stroke* refers to both transient and permanent neurologic signs and symptoms of a nontraumatic vascular etiology (see Chapter 18). Imaging of acute stroke should help (a) exclude intracranial hemorrhage; (b) differentiate between irreversibly affected brain tissue and reversibly impaired tissue ("tissue at risk"), which can benefit from early treatment; and (c) identify arterial stenosis or occlusion. Tissue at risk, or *penumbra*, refers to an area of reduced perfusion and loss of function, yet whose neurons are still viable. Therefore, once hemorrhage has been ruled out, timely reperfusion of this tissue with thrombolytics may prevent neuronal cell death and help re-establish normal function (74). CT continues to be the initial imaging modality for most acute stroke patients for three reasons. First, CT detects intracerebral hemorrhage with great specificity and sensitivity because freshly extravasated blood is more radiodense than either gray or white matter. Second, MRI is unable to detect the oxyhemoglobin that predominates in the hemorrhage in the early hours after a stroke because it is a nonparamagnetic substance. Third, the uncooperativeness of many acute stroke patients during the long MRI scan times and the incompatibility of monitoring equipment with strong magnetic fields often preclude early MRI examination. Current stroke diagnostic protocols follow a multimodal approach that can include non–contrast-enhanced CT, CT perfusion, CT angiography (CTA), conventional MRI, MR angiography (MRA), and diffusion- and perfusion-weighted MR imaging techniques, in order to establish early diagnosis and subsequently select appropriate therapy.

ISCHEMIC STROKE

Cerebral ischemia can be produced by thrombosis of large extracranial or small intracerebral vessels, emboli originating from atherosclerotic plaques or thrombi within more proximal vessels or the heart. In addition, decreased perfusion of systemic origin, such as shock, decreased cardiac output, or respiratory failure can also cause cerebral ischemia with or without infarction.

Cerebral ischemia can be completely or partially reversible or irreversible leading to neuronal cell death, commonly known as *infarction*. Once blood flow to the brain is decreased or interrupted for a sufficient period of time, the chemical pumps within the neuronal cell membranes cease to function adequately, disturbing normal electrolyte homeostasis. Extracellular water subsequently rushes into the affected neuronal cells. This cascade of events initially causes neurons to halt cellular function in an attempt to survive. This "stunned" cell population is potentially salvageable with prompt reperfusion. If adequate reperfusion does not occur in a timely fashion, irreversible neuronal cell death will occur.

Edema related to infarction involves both gray and white matter and has certain CT and MRI findings. Nonenhanced CT is the initial study of choice in patients with suspected stroke, as it is readily available, can be performed quickly, and is highly sensitive in the detection of cerebral hemorrhage. On nonenhanced CT, edema related to a cerebral infarction appears as a hypodense or low attenuation area, which means that it appears darker than expected. Early nonenhanced CT signs of ischemic cerebral infarction in the middle cerebral artery (MCA) territory are as follows: (a) obscuration of the lentiform nucleus, sometimes referred to as the *disappearing basal ganglia sign*, which can be seen as early as 2 hours after symptom onset (75) (**Fig. 5-69**); (b) insular ribbon sign, which refers to hypoattenuation of the insular cortex (**Fig. 5-70**); and (c) hyperdense MCA sign, which refers to a fresh thrombus within the artery and can be seen as soon as 90 minutes after the event (**Fig. 5-71**). It is important to note that this sign implicates occlusion and not necessarily infarction. Nevertheless, nonenhanced CT is usually negative during the first few hours after an ischemic infarct, and it is only later that areas of hypoattenuation can be identified with associated effacement of the adjacent cortical sulci (**Fig. 5-72**).

Edema reaches its peak at 3 to 5 days, and by this time, non–contrast-enhanced CT typically demonstrates a well-defined hypodense area that usually corresponds to the vascular territory of one of the cerebral arteries or its branches.

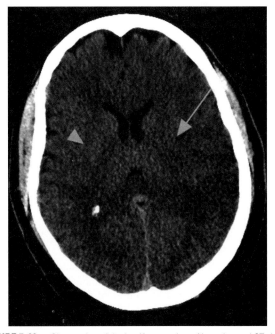

FIGURE 5-69. Obscuration of the lentiform nucleus. Nonenhanced CT shows effacement of the left lentiform nucleus (*arrow*). Compare with normal lentiform nucleus on the right (*arrowhead*).

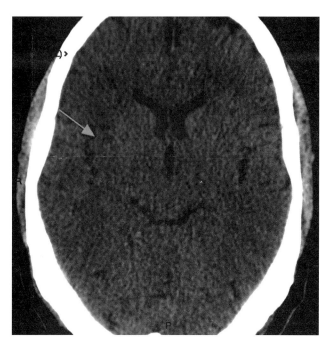

FIGURE 5-70. Insular ribbon sign. CT changes of slight hypodensity, loss of normal gray-white matter differentiation, and effacement of overlying cortical sulci in the region of the right insula (*arrow*).

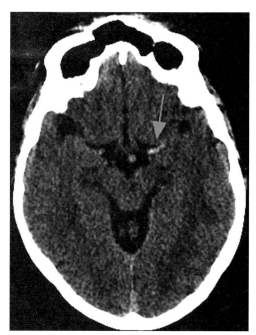

FIGURE 5-71. MCA hyperdense sign. Tubular hyperdensity at location of the left middle cerebral artery (*arrow*), compatible with intraluminal thrombus.

With large infarctions, brain swelling can eventually lead to brain herniation or obstructive hydrocephalus (**Fig. 5-73A** and **B**). With subsequent degeneration and phagocytosis of the infarcted brain tissue, there is volume loss that causes an increase in size of the overlying cortical sulci and underlying ventricles (76). When the infarction is caused by a systemically induced general reduction in brain perfusion, the infarcted areas correspond to the border zones between the territories of the major cerebral arteries because perfusion is most tenuous here (**Fig. 5-74**). Emboli can at times be directly visualized by noncontrast CT as increased attenuation within the lumen of the arteries. It is important to note that hemorrhage can not only occur de novo related to a hemorrhagic infarct, but that it can also occur within an ischemic infarct, as a consequence of reperfusion injury due to blood-brain barrier breakdown. When the latter occurs, it appears as a hyperdense mass within the hypodense edema of the infarct (**Fig. 5-75**).

Injection of intravenous (IV) contrast provides no brain enhancement in the 1st day or 2 after a stroke. Contrast enhancement must await sufficient damage to the blood-brain barrier. It reaches its peak at 1 to 2 weeks and usually ceases to occur after 2 or 3 months (77). The greatest vascular damage to intact vessels is at the periphery of the infarct. Therefore, contrast-enhanced CT frequently visualizes a contrast-enhanced ring about the infarcted area or in the immediately adjacent cortical gyri, a phenomenon known as *luxury perfusion* (**Fig. 5-76A** and **B**) (76).

Conventional MRI is more sensitive and specific than CT for the detection of acute ischemic brain infarcts, within the first few hours after the onset of symptoms. On MRI, the edema of an early infarct is of low signal intensity on T1-weighted images with corresponding high signal intensity on FLAIR (fluid-attenuated inversion recovery) and T2-weighted images (**Fig. 5-77A** and **B**). In addition, there is loss of gray-white matter differentiation, sulcal effacement,

and mass effect analogous to CT imaging findings. With the administration of IV gadolinium-diethylenetriaminepentaacetic acid (DTPA), a damaged blood-brain barrier can often be visualized as a hyperintense area on T1-weighted images. MRI is more sensitive than CT at detecting lacunar infarcts, which are small infarcts of less than 1.5 cm (76) typically located in the basal ganglia and periventricular areas and at the brainstem (**Fig. 5-78A** and **B**). Lacunar infarcts are most commonly caused by hypertension or diabetes-induced arteriolar occlusive disease of the deeply penetrating arteries, such as the

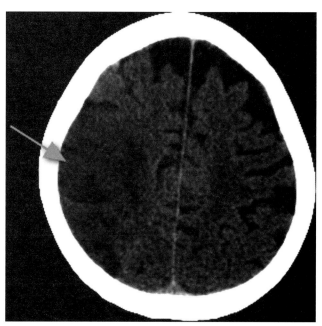

FIGURE 5-72. Postinjury edema has peaked, and the infarcted area is shown as a distinct hypodensity conforming to the territory of the right middle cerebral artery (*arrow*).

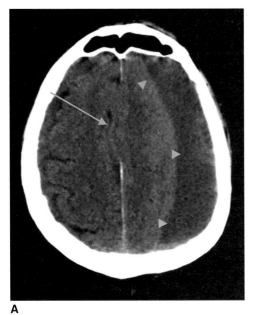
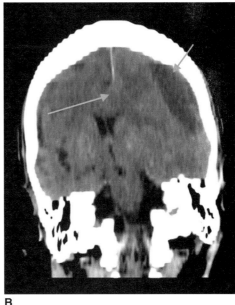

A   **B**

FIGURE 5-73. **A:** Axial CT scan examination with large left subdural hematoma (*arrowheads*) and early subfalcine herniation (*long arrow*). **B:** Coronal multiplanar reformatted image (MPR) demonstrates to a better advantage the mass effect and the subfalcine herniation (*long arrow*). The subdural hematoma has a lentiform shape (*short arrow*).

lenticulostriate branches of the middle cerebral arteries. MRI is also superior to CT in detecting ischemic infarcts of the posterior cranial fossa, because MR images are not degraded by osseous structures as is the case with CT. Another powerful imaging sequence is diffusion-weighted MR imaging (DWI). Water molecules normally move within tissues in a random fashion known as *Brownian motion*. As was discussed earlier, acute stroke produces an electrolyte imbalance, which causes water molecules to rush into the intracellular compartment, where free random motion is no longer possible and therefore falling into a state of restricted diffusion. DW images reflect restricted diffusion as a signal increase, which corresponds with a signal drop in its accompanying sequence, the apparent diffusion coefficient (ADC) map. The combination of increased

signal in the DW images and decreased signal in the ADC map is compatible with an infarct in the appropriate clinical setting, as other entities such as viscous abscesses and dense masses such as lymphomas can have a similar restricted diffusion pattern (**Fig. 5-79A** and **B**). One of the key features of DWI of acute cerebral ischemia is that it becomes positive as soon as 30 minutes after the insult and can remain positive for 5 days or more (78).

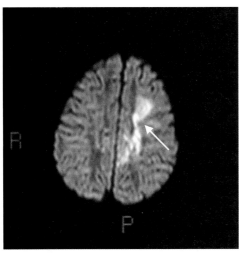

FIGURE 5-74. Axial diffusion-weighted images (DWI) of an acute watershed infarct at the left superior frontal lobe. Increase signal intensity (*arrow*) represents restricted diffusion.

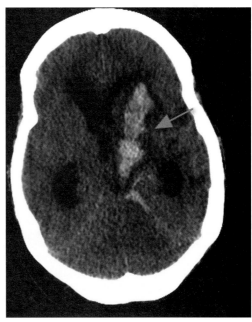

FIGURE 5-75. There is a hyperdense region at the left basal ganglia and thalamus surrounded by hypodense rim of edema, compatible with hemorrhagic transformation of an ischemic stroke (*arrow*). The patient had suffered an ischemic stroke 12 days earlier.

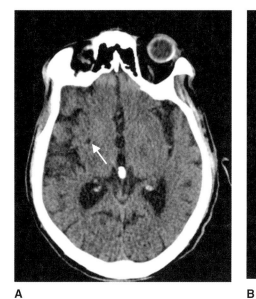

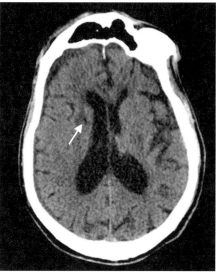

A   **B**

FIGURE 5-76. Axial CT images of the brain of a patient with small focal areas of low attenuation representing lacunar infarcts within the right inferior basal ganglia (*arrow*) **(A)** and within the caudate nucleus (*arrow*) **(B)**.

Nonenhanced CT is highly sensitive in detecting intracranial bleeds, which, in the setting of an ischemic stroke, represents hemorrhagic transformation. In MR imaging, T2*-weighted gradient-echo sequences depict areas of hemorrhage as focal regions of low signal intensity, secondary to a phenomenon known as *blooming* (**Fig. 5-80**).

As was stated before, cerebral ischemia can be reversible. A tissue that is potentially salvageable with prompt recanalization is referred to as *penumbra*. The goal of stroke imaging is to document an infarct, to exclude hemorrhage, and to differentiate infarcted from salvageable tissue (penumbra) in an effort to guide thrombolytic therapy and save as much

brain tissue as possible. CT and MR imaging techniques that are currently being used with this purpose in mind will be briefly discussed. CT perfusion is a technique in which a bolus of contrast is injected into the patient with simultaneous imaging of a slice of tissue, usually chosen at the level of the basal ganglia, because it represents the three major vascular territories: anterior, middle, and posterior cerebral arteries. The three main parameters obtained and compared throughout the slice are cerebral blood volume (CBV), cerebral blood flow (CBF), and mean transit time (MTT). In general terms, a mismatch between these parameters usually represents tissue suffering reversible ischemia or penumbra. MR perfusion is a

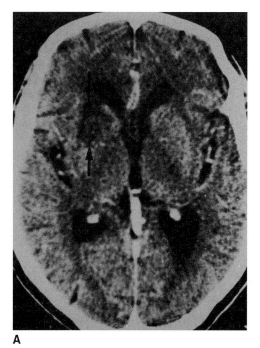

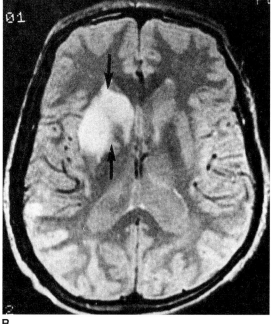

A   **B**

FIGURE 5-77.   Subacute ischemic infarct. **A:** Axial CT image demonstrates an area of decreased attenuation (*arrow*) within the head of the caudate nucleus. **B:** Axial proton density (PD) sequence. There is increased signal intensity (*arrow*) due to restricted diffusion characteristic of an infarct.

FIGURE 5-78. Lacunar infarcts. **A:** CT shows multiple bilateral lacunar infarcts as small hypodense areas (*arrows*). **B:** By MRI, these infarcts are shown as multiple hyperintense areas (*arrows*).

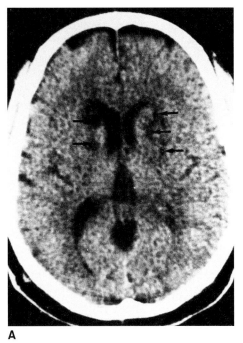
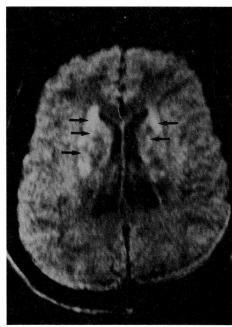

A   B

contrast-dependent technique also utilized to determine the amount, if any, of salvageable brain tissue. In general terms, when a perfusion defect matches a diffusion defect, irreversible infarction has occurred. On the other hand, a perfusion-diffusion mismatch represents an area of reversible ischemia or penumbra, where infarction can possibly be avoided with timely thrombolytic treatment.

CTA is a technique that uses IV contrast to image extra-cranial and intracranial blood vessels. Different methods are utilized to reconstruct the arterial system, in an attempt to identify the cause of the patient's symptoms, usually an obstructing thrombus or embolus, which is seen as a cutoff in one or various vessels. CTA information is commonly used to guide intra-arterial or mechanical thrombolysis in stroke centers. Just as in CTA, MRA can also be performed following injection of IV contrast. Nevertheless, MRI has the added

bonus of being able to perform angiograms without having to inject contrast material based on the MR properties of flowing blood; a useful proposition in patients with renal insufficiency. Contrast-enhanced MRA findings are analogous to CTA findings; nevertheless, in non–contrast-enhanced (time-of-flight) MRAs, normal vessels are depicted as a flow void, and intra-arterial thrombus is seen as an area of increased signal intensity (**Fig. 5-81**).

Cerebral venous thrombosis is caused by aseptic or septic etiologies and can lead to infarction in a nonarterial distribution. This rare cause of infarction has characteristic imaging features. Whether the thrombosis involves a deep cerebral vein or a dural venous sinus, the thrombus can be detected on a noncontrast CT as a hyperdensity within the vein (79). The hyperdensity may have a hypodense center, implying a residual lumen. In a contrast-enhanced CT, a thrombus appears as a

FIGURE 5-79. Ischemic infarct. Restricted diffusion is shown as increased signal intensity in the diffusion-weighted image **(A)** with corresponding signal drop in the ADC map **(B)** (*large arrows*).

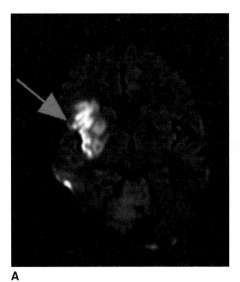
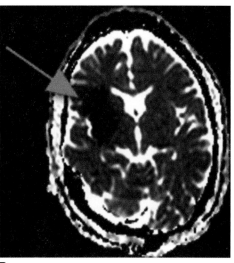

A   B

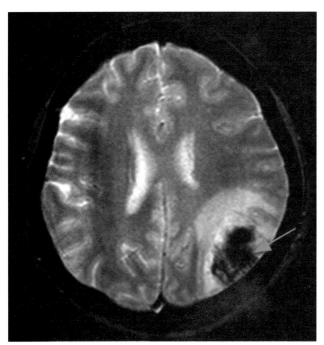

FIGURE 5-80. Axial gradient echo T2* image shows an irregular area of signal drop with surrounding high–signal-intensity edema at the left superior parietal lobe (*arrow*), compatible with a hemorrhagic stroke.

filling defect, with tortuous dilated collateral venous channels occasionally demonstrated around the thrombosed vein. By MRI, while the thrombus is still in the oxyhemoglobin stage, which is isodense to brain tissue, it can be suspected by the absence of the normal flow void in that vessel. In the deoxy-hemoglobin stage, the thrombus is hypointense on T1, and

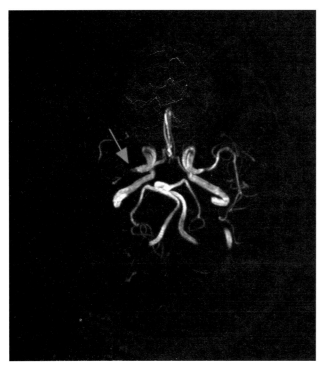

FIGURE 5-81. Right middle cerebral artery thrombosis by MRA. *Arrow* points to vessel cutoff.

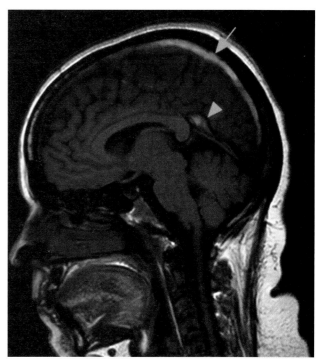

FIGURE 5-82. Deep venous thrombosis. Sagittal noncontrast T1-weighted image. *Arrow* points to a thrombus-filled hyperintense superior sagittal sinus. *Arrowhead* points to a thrombus-filled hyperintense straight sinus.

in the later methemoglobin stage, it becomes hyperintense on T1-weighted images. The venous thrombus typically does not proceed to the hemosiderin phase because it usually lyses spontaneously and flow is reestablished. Contrast and non–contrast-enhanced MR venography techniques can also be utilized to diagnose venous thrombosis (**Fig. 5-82**).

A stroke-like clinical presentation frequently encountered in the ER is a transient ischemic attack (TIA). A TIA is a functional neurologic disturbance usually lasting a few minutes, which clears completely within 24 hours. TIAs typically produce no CT or MRI findings, yet one third of these patients eventually will suffer a cerebral infarction, 20% of them within the 1st month after the episode. Some stroke centers perform an MRI to all patients who suffered a TIA, as occasionally small acute infarcts are found.

HEMORRHAGIC STROKE

A stroke is considered hemorrhagic if blood is found within the first 24 hours after initial symptoms. When blood is noted after this time, it is usually hemorrhagic transformation of an ischemic stroke, which is due to reperfusion injury. Hypertension is the most common cause of intraparenchymal hemorrhage, which can also be caused by ruptured aneurysm, by arteriovenous malformation, and, more rarely, by infarction, neoplasms, blood coagulation defects, and cerebral arteritis (79). Common hemorrhage sites include the putamen and the thalamus, which receive their major blood supply from the lenticulostriate and the thalamogeniculate arteries, respectively.

Because freshly extravasated blood is more radiodense than gray or white matter, an acute hemorrhagic stroke is well visualized by CT as a hyperdense region usually conforming to an arterial distribution (**Fig. 5-83A** and **B**). The radiodensity

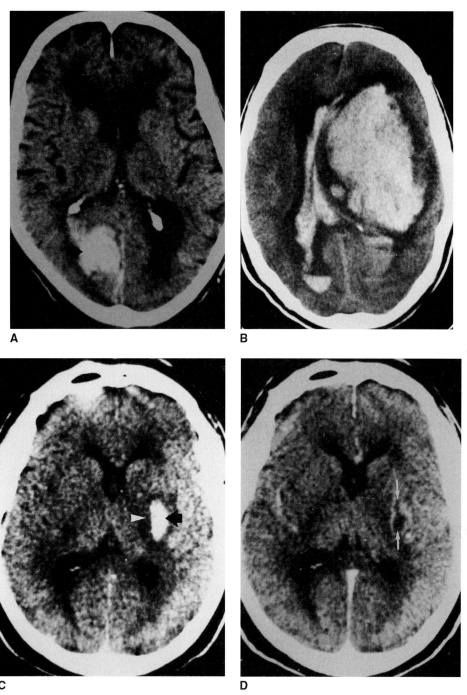

FIGURE 5-83. CT evaluation of early and evolving hemorrhagic strokes. **A:** Recent hemorrhagic stroke has occurred in the distribution of the right posterior cerebral artery, which appears hyperdense (*arrows*). **B:** A massive hypertensive hemorrhage involving most of the interior of the left cerebral hemisphere with intraventricular hemorrhage, midline shift to the right, and herniation of the left hemisphere under the falx cerebri. **C:** A 5-day-old hemorrhagic stroke involving the lenticular nucleus shows a hyperdense hemorrhagic center (*arrow*) and a hypodense edematous rim (*arrowhead*). **D:** The same stroke patient displays replacement of the hyperdense hemorrhage with a narrow hypodense interval (*arrows*) several months later.

of the blood clot increases over 3 days because of clot retraction, serum extrusion, and hemoglobin concentration. The extruded serum may form a hypodense rim around the hyperdense clot (**Fig. 5-83C**). As edema develops over 3 to 5 days, the hypodense rim may increase. Eventually, the hyperdensity of the clot gradually fades and usually disappears by 2 months, leaving only a narrow hypodense slit to mark the site where hemorrhage took place (**Fig. 5-83D**).

The appearance of hemorrhage by MRI depends on the state of the hemoglobin in the hemorrhage (79). The oxyhemoglobin present in a fresh hemorrhage is nonparamagnetic; therefore, very early hemorrhage is not detected by MRI. Within a few hours, the oxyhemoglobin will be converted to deoxyhemoglobin, which is a paramagnetic substance. Intracellular deoxyhemoglobin will cause acute hemorrhage to appear very hypointense on T2-weighted images and

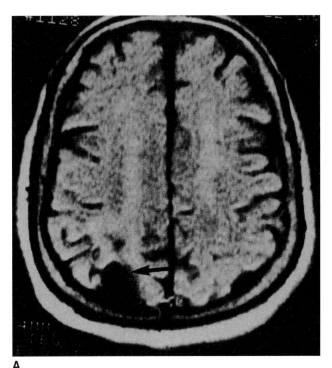
A

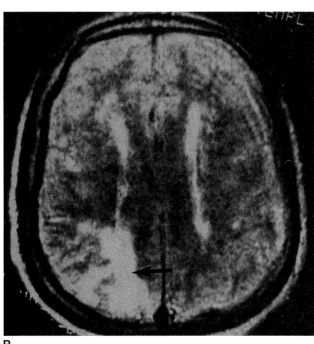
B

FIGURE 5-84. MRI evaluation of hemorrhagic stroke. **A:** An acute hemorrhagic stroke involving the occipital lobe appears hypointense (*arrow*). **B:** In the subacute phase, the same area appears hyperintense (*arrow*).

slightly hypointense or isointense on T1-weighted images (**Fig. 5-84A**). By 3 to 7 days, intracellular deoxyhemoglobin is oxidized to methemoglobin as the clot enters the subacute phase. Although a subacute hemorrhage has several subphases in which the signal intensity of methemoglobin varies, in general, methemoglobin appears hyperintense on both T1- and T2-weighted images (**Fig. 5-84B**). Because the conversion to methemoglobin begins at the periphery of the clot, early in the subacute phase, a hemorrhage can have a hyperintense margin and a central hypointense region still containing deoxyhemoglobin. Eventually, the entire region of subacute hemorrhage becomes hyperintense. Over several months, the methemoglobin is gradually resorbed, and the clot develops a rim of hemosiderin-containing macrophages. Hemosiderin is hypointense on both T1- and T2-weighted images. Therefore, a chronic hemorrhage of several months' duration often has a hyperintense methemoglobin center and a hypointense hemosiderin rim. Because the hemosiderin deposits remain indefinitely, an old hemorrhage of several years' duration shows up as a totally hypointense area. Gradient-echo sequences have recently been added to many brain MRI protocols, as they are very sensitive in the detection of degrading blood products, which appear as areas of hypointensity. As can be seen, CT provides the very earliest information about cerebral hemorrhage, whereas MRI is the better technique for determining hemorrhage age.

SUBARACHNOID AND INTRAVENTRICULAR HEMORRHAGE

Subarachnoid and intraventricular hemorrhage can be spontaneous, as in the case of a bleeding aneurysm or arteriovenous malformation, or secondary to trauma. CT is the imaging modality of choice for evaluating these types of hemorrhages because hemorrhage appears hyperdense from its onset. However, subarachnoid hemorrhage is not as radiodense as epidural or subdural hemorrhage because the blood will be diluted by CSF. Unless blood replaces at least 70% of the CSF, the subarachnoid hemorrhage remains isodense to adjacent gray matter (80). When the volume of blood is sufficient to make the hemorrhage hyperdense, it accumulates in the extensions and expansions of the subarachnoid space. Subarachnoid hemorrhage appears as linear radiodensities within the sulci or fissures or as larger aggregations in the basal cisterns (**Fig. 5-85**). MRI will not visualize a very early hemorrhage when oxyhemoglobin, a nonparamagnetic substance, is the

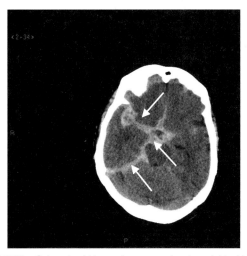

FIGURE 5-85. Subarachnoid hemorrhage secondary to a right middle cerebral artery aneurysm. CT shows this condition as hemorrhagic radiodensities within sulci and cisterns (*arrows*).

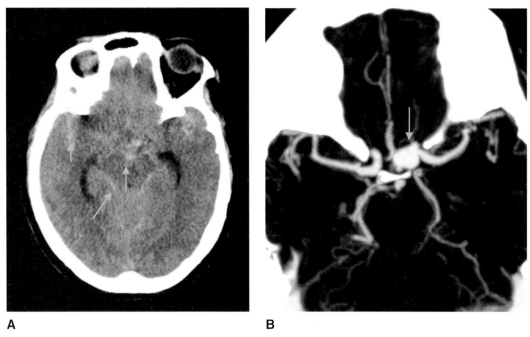

A **B**

FIGURE 5-86. **A:** CT of an anterior cerebral artery aneurysm (*arrows*) that produced a subarachnoid hemorrhage with secondary hydrocephalus. **B:** Axial collapse image of a time-of-flight (TOF) MR angiogram in a different patient. The *arrow* points to a large aneurysm arising from the left anterior communicating artery.

primary constituent, and thus, CT is the study of choice in the very early stages. Subarachnoid and intraventricular hemorrhage can cause communicating hydrocephalus by virtue of red blood cells blocking the arachnoid granulations, the CSF resorption sites.

Aneurysms and arteriovenous malformations can be detected directly by contrast-enhanced CT and MRI or by their flow void characteristics on non–contrast-enhanced MR images (**Fig. 5-86A** and **B**).

TRAUMATIC BRAIN INJURIES

Head injury can be produced by direct contact or impact loading, where impacts either set a resting head in motion or stop a moving head, or can be produced by impulse or inertial loading, where the head is suddenly placed in motion or suddenly stopped without impact (81) (see Chapter 19). Impulse or inertial loading is commonly referred to in the literature as *acceleration-deceleration mechanism*, which commonly produces tissue shearing injuries. Fractures and epidural hematomas are produced only by impact loading, but other types of head injury can be produced by either type of loading. Head injury is typically categorized as focal or diffuse. Focal injuries include extracerebral hemorrhages such as epidural or subdural hematomas, intraparenchymal hematomas, cerebral contusion or laceration, and fractures. Diffuse brain injuries include diffuse axonal injury, diffuse cerebral swelling, and edema. Furthermore, traumatic head injuries can be classified as primary or secondary, where primary injuries are a direct result of trauma, such as contusions and diffuse axonal injury, and secondary injuries are an indirect sequelae of trauma such as edema, infarctions, or herniation.

CT is typically the initial imaging modality of choice for patients suffering head trauma, because it is very accurate at detecting the depressed fractures and acute hematomas that require emergency surgery. Its other advantages include rapid scanning with continuation of close monitoring of critically injured patients. MRI has the disadvantages of longer scans, high susceptibility to motion artifacts by uncooperative patients, inability to detect very recent hemorrhage, and difficulty evaluating fractures because of the signal void characteristics of cortical bone.

EPIDURAL HEMATOMA

Epidural hematoma is caused by tears of the middle meningeal artery or vein or of a dural venous sinus. The blood accumulates in the interval between the inner table of the calvarium and the dura by gradually stripping the dura from its bony attachment. CT visualizes the epidural hematoma as a well-localized biconvex radiodense mass (81) (**Fig. 5-87**). It is commonly, though not invariably, associated with a skull fracture. It causes mass effect upon the adjacent brain parenchyma with effacement of the underlying sulci, compression of the brain and ventricles, and possible contralateral midline shift. It is important to note that midline shift can be responsible for a secondary injury caused by subfalcine herniation, which is herniation of the cingulate gyrus under the falx cerebri, and can eventually lead to ipsilateral anterior cerebral artery infarction. When there is a question about whether the mass might be intraparenchymal, contrast injection enhances the dura, establishing the epidural position of the clot. As the clot lyses over the next few weeks, it shrinks and changes to isodense and then hypodense relative to the brain. The inner aspect of the clot vascularizes, and this may produce a thicker rim of enhancement on late contrast studies. The overlying dura may calcify. Epidural hematoma may be associated with subdural, subarachnoid, or intraparenchymal hemorrhages.

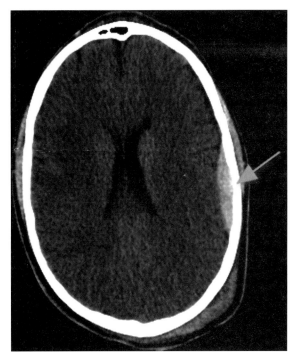

FIGURE 5-87.   Epidural hematoma. Nonenhanced CT scan of the head shows a left parietal biconvex extra-axial hyperdensity (*arrow*).

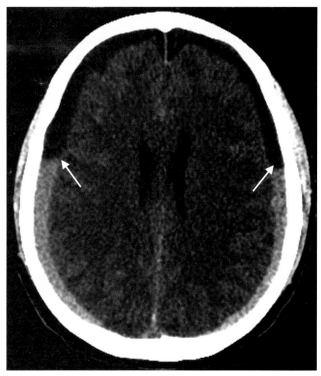

FIGURE 5-88.   Bilateral panhemispheric chronic subdural hematomas with superimposed acute bleed and hematocrit levels (*arrows*).

SUBDURAL HEMATOMA

Subdural hematoma is most commonly caused by acceleration-deceleration shearing stresses that rupture the bridging veins that extend from the cerebrum to the fixed dural venous sinuses. The blood accumulates in the subdural space. Because the subdural space is a potential space surrounding all external surfaces of the brain, subdural hemorrhage tends to spread extensively over the brain.

On CT examination, the typical acute subdural hematoma appears as a diffuse crescent-shaped radiodensity that may extend onto many surfaces of the brain, including the cerebral convexity, skull base, interhemispheric fissure, upper or lower surface of the tentorium, and areas around the brain stem (**Fig. 5-88**). One way to differentiate subdural from epidural hematomas is that subdural hematomas cross suture lines yet do not cross midline, whereas epidural hematomas do not cross suture lines yet can cross the midline.

There are two ways of classifying subdural hematomas based on their changing radiographic appearance over time (81). One scheme divides them into acute (i.e., more radiodense than adjacent gray matter), subacute (i.e., isodense to gray matter), and chronic (i.e., hypodense to gray matter). Another scheme simply lumps the subacute and chronic into the chronic category. The subdural hematoma typically effaces the adjacent gyri, produces inward displacement of the gray-white matter junction, and may compress the ventricle or cause brain herniation under the falx or through the tentorium.

As the subdural hematoma ages, the hemoglobin protein producing its radiodensity is broken down and removed, and a vascular granulation tissue develops along its inner surface. Over a few weeks, the subdural hematoma usually becomes isodense or hypodense to gray matter (82). Because of volume loss, the chronic subdural hematoma may lose its concave inner border and become more focal, even occasionally assuming a biconvex outline. Isodense subdural hematomas are more difficult to discriminate. Their presence can be implied indirectly by their mass effects on the underlying brain. An injection of contrast material will enhance both the vascular membrane and the displaced cortical vessels, allowing discrimination of the hematoma from the adjacent cortex.

Patients who present first with a chronic subdural hematoma may have no recollection of any antecedent trauma because the traumatic episode may have been so slight that it was forgotten. Chronic hematomas commonly involve the elderly, where loss of cerebral volume puts the bridging veins under increased stress and makes them more susceptible to rupture by minor trauma.

MRI has valuable unique imaging properties that make it very sensitive to the detection of some extracerebral hemorrhages. First, the high signal intensity that subacute hematomas display on T1- and T2-weighted images makes MRI more sensitive than CT for detecting hematomas that are isodense by CT (81). Even chronic subdural hematomas remain hyperintense to CSF and gray matter for several months, which is long after they have become isodense or hypodense on CT. Also, the ability of MRI to discern the displaced signal voids of cortical or dural vessels facilitates the identification of small extracerebral hemorrhages. In addition, when the hematoma collects around the obliquely placed tentorium, axial CT images may average it into adjacent tissues. In these cases, the multiplanar imaging properties of MRI can be very valuable. Also, small hematomas next to the calvarium can be better seen by MRI because they are contrasted against the osseous signal void.

CONTUSIONS AND INTRAPARENCHYMAL HEMORRHAGE

Focal parenchymal injuries such as contusions and intraparenchymal hemorrhage usually develop as a result of contact of the brain with the osseous walls of the cranial cavity. The coup-type injuries occur at the point of contact, and the contrecoup injuries occur on the opposite side of the brain. Contusions often occur in areas where the walls of the cranial cavity are irregular, such as the anterior and middle cranial fossae. Therefore, frontal and temporal lobe contusions are common as the brain glides along these irregular surfaces (83) (**Fig. 5-89A** and **B**).

Cerebral contusions are heterogeneous lesions containing edema, hemorrhage, and necrosis, with any element predominating. When blood makes a major contribution, the contusion appears on CT as a poorly delimited irregular area of hyperdensity. A contusion with mostly edema or necrosis may not be detectable immediately, but after a few days, it appears as a hypodense region. Where there is a general admixture of elements, contusions may have a heterogeneous density. Old contusions appear as hypodense areas. By MRI, the edematous and necrotic areas have low signal intensity on T1-weighted images and high signal intensity on T2-weighted images, and thus, MRI is more sensitive than CT in identifying these nonhemorrhagic contusions. The areas of hemorrhage in a contusion older than a few days will be hyperintense on both T1- and T2-weighted images. Intraparenchymal hemorrhage differs from contusions by having better demarcated areas of more homogeneous hemorrhage. The CT and MRI characteristics of acute and evolving intraparenchymal hemorrhage are the same as for hemorrhagic stroke.

DIFFUSE BRAIN INJURIES

Diffuse brain injuries include diffuse axonal injury, diffuse cerebral swelling, and edema. Diffuse axonal injury is produced by high shearing stresses that occur at different parts of the brain, including the gray matter-white matter interface. These shearing stresses cause axonal stretching commonly involving the corpus callosum, anterior commissure, and upper brain stem. Blood vessels may or may not be disrupted. When vessels are uninterrupted, the scattered small areas of edema are best demonstrated by T1-weighted MR images as slightly hypointense or isointense regions that become hyperintense on T2-weighted images. When vessel disruption produces hemorrhages, they appear early on CT as multiple sites of hyperdensity (**Fig. 5-90**).

Diffuse cerebral swelling occurs with many types of head injury. It is thought to be produced by a rapidly increased volume of circulating blood. By MRI and CT, the general brain enlargement is visualized by an obliteration or encroachment of the normal CSF spaces: the cortical sulci, the perimesencephalic and basal cisterns, and the ventricles (83). By CT, the enlarged brain may show slightly increased density.

In generalized cerebral edema, the enlarged brain also encroaches on the CSF spaces, but by CT, the edema produces a generalized hypodensity that usually takes longer to develop than diffuse cerebral swelling (**Fig. 5-91**). The edema may obscure gray matter-white matter boundaries.

Both diffuse brain swelling and generalized cerebral edema are emergencies, because if not treated promptly they may lead to brain herniation sometimes with fatal outcomes.

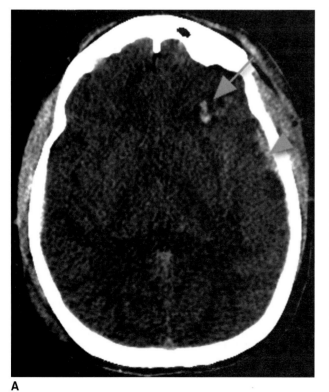

A

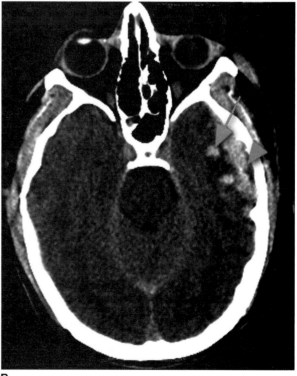

B

FIGURE 5-89. **A:** Nonenhanced CT scan shows a small left frontal hyperdense hemorrhagic foci (*arrow*). Acute extra-axial bleed is also noted (*arrowhead*). **B:** Left temporal posttraumatic hemorrhagic contusions (*arrow*). Overlying acute extra-axial bleed is noted (*arrowhead*).

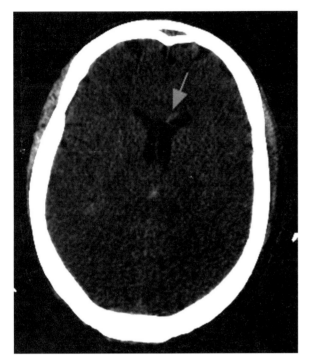

FIGURE 5-90. Diffuse axonal injury. Nonenhanced CT scan shows hemorrhagic foci at the genu of the corpus callosum (*arrow*).

PENETRATING TRAUMA

Bullets and other types of penetrating objects will cause brain laceration by both the penetrating objects and the fragments of subcutaneous tissues, bone, and dura driven into the brain. The imbedded fragments of the foreign object and bone are well visualized by CT, as are the accompanying cerebral edema and various types of intracerebral or extracerebral hemorrhage.

COMPLICATIONS OF BRAIN INJURY

Brain injuries may be accompanied by a number of late or long-term complications. These secondary brain injuries include cerebral herniations, which may occur under the falx cerebri or through the tentorium. Herniations can cause compression of adjacent brain substance or vessels, with the production of secondary signs and symptoms (**Fig. 5-92**). Penetrating injuries or fractures can injure nearby large or small vessels, producing thrombosis, embolism, traumatic aneurysm formation, or internal carotid-cavernous sinus fistula. Basal skull fractures involving the dura and arachnoid can cause CSF leaks that show up as CSF rhinorrhea or otorrhea. Local or diffuse brain swelling can compress the cerebral aqueduct or fourth ventricle, producing obstructive hydrocephalus. Subarachnoid hemorrhage may obstruct CSF resorption and cause a late-developing communicating hydrocephalus. Focal cerebral atrophy can occur at sites of infarction, hemorrhage, or trauma. Generalized atrophy can follow diffuse injuries and can be demonstrated by an increased size of sulci, fissures, cisterns, and ventricles.

Degenerative Diseases of the CNS

Degenerative diseases of the CNS include the wide spectrum of gray and white matter diseases, general degenerative changes of aging, and the dementias.

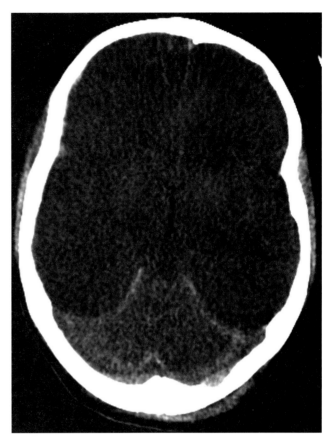

FIGURE 5-91. Diffuse brain edema. Nonenhanced CT scan shows diffuse hypodensity with sulci effacement and loss of gray/white matter differentiation. Mass effect is causing almost complete obliteration of the ventricular system. Compare low parenchymal attenuation with normal cerebellar density.

WHITE MATTER DISEASES

White matter diseases can be divided into demyelinating diseases, in which the white matter is normally formed and then pathologically destroyed, and dysmyelinating diseases, in which there is usually a genetically determined enzymatic disorder that interferes with the normal production or maintenance of myelin (84). The enzymatic disturbances are relatively rare; therefore, their imaging characteristics will not be described.

The most common of the demyelinating disorders is multiple sclerosis (MS). The demyelinating plaques of MS are better visualized by MRI than by CT. In fact, MRI has become the primary complementary test to confirm a clinical diagnosis of MS. It also provides a quantitative means of evaluating the present state of a patient's disease and a mode of following its progress (85). Although the T1-weighted MR images are usually normal, the FLAIR and T2-weighted images demonstrate MS plaques as high–signal-intensity areas. These are most frequently seen in the periventricular white matter, especially around the atrium and the tips of the anterior and posterior horns of the lateral ventricles (**Fig. 5-93A and B**). The high–signal-intensity plaques also can be seen in other white matter areas of the cerebral hemispheres, the brainstem, and even the upper spinal cord. When these lesions are seen in patients younger than 40 years of age, they tend to be relatively specific for MS (84). In patients more than 50 years of age,

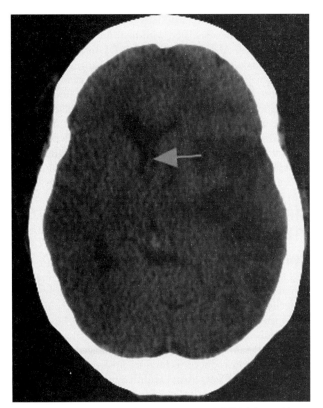

FIGURE 5-92. Nonenhanced CT scan shows a left MCA infarct with mass effect causing contralateral midline shift (*arrow*) corresponding to subfalcine herniation.

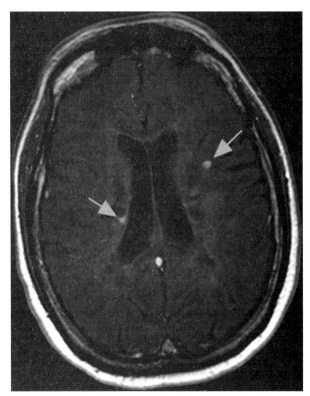

FIGURE 5-94. Active MS. T1 gadolinium-enhanced MR image shows periventricular enhancing MS plaques (*arrows*).

the MRI findings of MS are similar to findings in some aging brains, and correlation with the clinical findings helps establish the diagnosis. Recent MS plaques that involve damage to the blood-brain barrier frequently enhance with the use of IV gadolinium-DTPA (**Fig. 5-94**).

CT demonstrates MS plaques with less reliability than does MRI. On CT, these plaques appear as areas of hypodensity. Recent plaques in the acute phase of an exacerbation of the disease will have damage to the blood-brain barrier, and IV contrast will then enhance the periphery of the lesion. In the chronic plaque, no contrast enhancement occurs on CT or

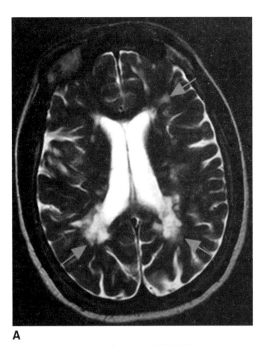

A

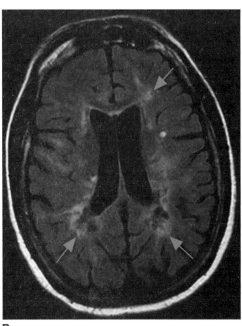

B

FIGURE 5-93. T2-weighted **(A)** and FLAIR **(B)** MRI demonstrates the periventricular demyelinating plaques of MS as hyperintense areas (*arrows*) adjacent to the anterior horns and atria of the lateral ventricles.

MRI. Other demyelinating diseases, although numerous, are of relatively low incidence and therefore are not described.

GRAY MATTER DISEASES

At present, MRI is being used clinically to discriminate a number of movement disorders that are characterized by changes in the size or iron content of a number of deep gray matter nuclei (86). Normal nuclei that contain high iron levels, such as the globus pallidus, reticular part of the substantia nigra, red nucleus, and dentate nucleus of the cerebellum, appear hypointense on T2-weighted images. In Parkinson's disease, T2-weighted MRI shows a hypointensity in the putamen that may exceed the normal hypointensity of the globus pallidus. In Huntington's chorea, MRI consistently shows atrophy of the head of the caudate with associated dilation of the adjacent frontal horn of the lateral ventricle. Some patients with Huntington's chorea also show a hypointensity of the caudate or putamen on T2-weighted images and atrophy predominating in the frontal lobe. Some forms of secondary dystonia show increased signal intensity of the putamen and caudate in T2-weighted images.

Age-Related Changes and Dementing Disorders

The aging brain is characterized on CT or MRI as demonstrating volume increases in both cortical sulci and ventricles (**Fig. 5-95**). T2-weighted MR images also frequently display small areas of hyperintense signal along the anterolateral margins of the anterior horns of the lateral ventricles. These changes may or may not be associated with neurologic findings.

Patients with Alzheimer's disease (AD) and other dementing disorders consistently show these age changes, but because many normal elderly do also, these changes cannot be used to diagnose AD. However, the absence of these findings typically excludes AD. Findings more specifically related to AD are those involving the temporal lobe. The earliest findings in AD involve atrophy of the temporal lobe with dilation of the temporal horn of the lateral ventricle, as well as dilation of the choroidal and hippocampal fissures caused by atrophy of the hippocampus, subiculum, and parahippocampal gyrus (87).

EMERGING IMAGING TECHNOLOGIES OF INTEREST TO THE PHYSIATRIST

Advanced MR Imaging Techniques

Since the advent of medical imaging using nuclear magnetic resonance (NMR), there has been a continuous advance in this technology with improvements in spatial resolution, as well as the introduction of new methods that allow for the rapid acquisition of images and the ability to image different aspects of dynamic function within the imaged tissues. Most of the initially introduced techniques involved the imaging of static structural characteristics at different points in parenchymal tissue. Proton density imaging basically reflects the concentration of water and the electrochemical environment of the water-based protons in the tissues. When water-based protons are actively in motion during the standard MRI imaging sequence, a "flow artifact" is created. However, if one is actually interested in the imaging of proton movement, then the flow artifact becomes a flow signal to be recorded. This is the basis for both MRA, which is actually the imaging of proton flow within the vascular spaces, and for diffusion-weighted imaging (DWI) and diffusion-tensor MR imaging (DTI), which are the imaging of the molecular diffusion of water molecules through tissue. When techniques are employed to image the diffusion of specific molecular species related to tissue metabolism, one can develop MR-based imaging techniques that allow one to image the active perfusion of tissues as well as their metabolic activity. This is the basis for perfusion-weighted and functional MRI (fMRI). Functional changes in the brain occur at relatively rapid rates during performance, and in order to image these changes, images must be acquired at a very rapid rate. Echo planar imaging (EPI) is a method for MR image acquisition that optimizes the image acquisition algorithm so that an entire image is acquired within a single TR period. EPI permits the acquisition of tomographic images at "video" rates of 15 to 30 images a second or down to as low as 20 ms per image, depending on the pulse sequence employed. EPI has been particularly important for the advancement of fMRI of the brain but is also used in DWI to reduce motion artifact.

MAGNETIC RESONANCE ANGIOGRAPHY

Conventional angiography uses x-ray methods that involve introduction of an iodine-based radio-opaque dye into the vascular space through an intravascular catheter, followed by imaging of the distribution of the dye within different vascular compartments. This technique involves the invasive

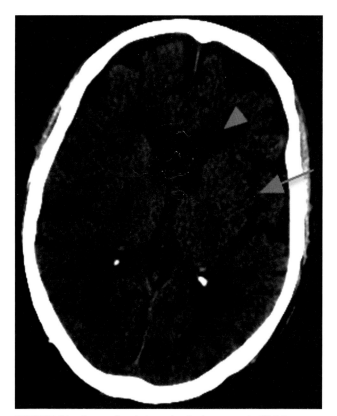

FIGURE 5-95. A case of cortical atrophy of aging as seen by CT. Enlargement of cortical sulci and sylvian fissures (*arrow*) with ex vacuo ventricular dilation (*arrowhead*).

introduction of the dye via intra-arterial catheterization and potential problems resulting from the physical introduction and threading of the catheter, as well as allergic reactions to the dye. The technique can be used to produce a structural image of a vascular tree but does not provide direct information regarding the relative flow of the blood within the tree. MRA, on the other hand, involves no introduction of dye, except in the contrast-enhanced technique described later, and no need for invasive catheter introduction. The technique takes advantage of the principle of signal-intensity attenuation from a region in which the imaged protons are actively in motion, producing a dark-signal "flow void" that marks a vascular structure containing moving blood seen on a standard T1-weighted image. MRA produces images of dynamically flowing blood, with the intensity of the image signal being proportional to the actual blood flow velocity. MRA, therefore, provides a dynamic image of circulatory flow rather than a static image of a vascular structure as is obtained with conventional x-ray angiography. Generally, there are three different methods used to produce MRA images: time of flight, phase-contrast angiography, and contrast-enhanced angiography.

As was described above, time-of-flight imaging involves utilizing the normal loss of signal produced by moving intravascular protons, seen as a signal drop or "void," to create images of the vascular tree. Phase-contrast angiography involves the application of a bipolar magnetic field gradient pulse. Two imaging sequences are performed in which the first has a positive bipolar gradient pulse and the second has a negative bipolar gradient pulse and the raw data from the two images are then subtracted. The signals emitted by stationary spin sources cancel out, whereas the signals emitted from flowing sources will add up. The net effect is to produce an image of proton spins that are flowing. In contrast-enhanced MRA, the imaging of the vessels relies on the difference between the T1 relaxation time of the blood and that of the surrounding tissues after a paramagnetic contrast agent has been injected into the blood. The agent reduces the T1 relaxation time in the blood relative to the surrounding tissues. This technique generally provides a higher-quality imaging of structural vascular anomalies comparable to that obtained with x-ray angiography. In addition, MRA techniques are normally obtained in conjunction with conventional MRI sequences, and therefore, information regarding surrounding brain parenchyma also becomes available. An example of a normal contrast-enhanced MRA is shown in **Figure 5-96A** and **B**.

The disadvantages of MRA over conventional x-ray angiography are that the images are not quite as clear using MRA, the time for acquisition of the study is significantly longer with MRA, and the study involves an extended period of time in the scanner which may not be tolerated by claustrophobic patients. An example of an MRA study of the head demonstrating occlusion of the left internal carotid artery is shown in **Figure 5-97**.

FLUID-ATTENUATED INVERSION RECOVERY IMAGING

Another MR imaging pulse sequence that has been usefully applied is the so-called FLAIR imaging method. In this imaging technique, T2 is heavily weighted with a short TE (e.g., 160 ms) and a very long TR (e.g., 10,000 ms) with the selection of an inversion interval, TI, so as to null out any mass fluid-containing spaces such as the cerebral ventricles or the subarachnoid space overlying the cortical surface. This creates a significant contrast between CSF and parenchymal brain

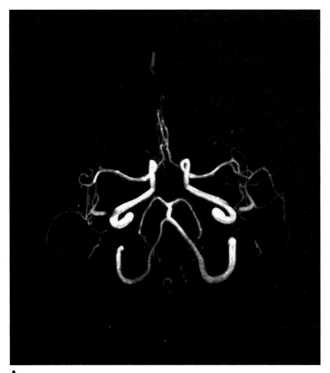

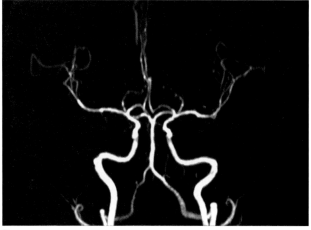

A   B

FIGURE 5-96.   **A and B:** Normal magnetic resonance angiogram (MRA).

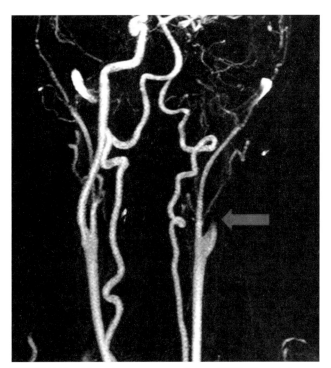

FIGURE 5-97. Magnetic resonance angiogram (MRA). The left internal carotid artery is occluded (*arrow*). The right internal carotid artery is normal.

tissue that enhances the identification of edema, periventricular white matter lesions, as well as cortical and gray-white matter junction lesions. It has been shown to be useful in conditions involving the subcortical white matter such as MS (88). Studies using FLAIR MR sequences to evaluate white matter lesions in severe traumatic brain injury (TBI) suggest that the white matter lesion "load" associated with diffuse axonal injury, as detected by this sequence, correlates with the severity of the clinical presentation and the eventual clinical outcome (89–91). FLAIR images are generally more sensitive in the identification of white matter lesions than conventional T2-weighted images or T2–fast spin echo techniques. However, the technique is also subject to CSF pulsation artifact and to vascular flow artifact, which can limit its utility in certain situations. A FLAIR image of a left MCA territory stroke is shown in **Figure 5-98** and compared to a corresponding T2-weighted image (**Fig. 5-99**).

DIFFUSION-WEIGHTED IMAGING

Diffusion is a physical property of molecules whereby they move randomly via Brownian motion and spread out through a medium in accordance with their thermal energy. The rate of diffusion for a particular molecule in a particular environment is measured by the diffusion coefficient. Molecular diffusion is influenced by concentration (i.e., chemical) gradients, as well as by mechanical tissue structure that can confer a directional ("anisotropic") component. For example, in the muscle or in cerebral white matter, anisotropic tissue structure creates a preferred pathway for water diffusion parallel to muscle or nerve fibers, and the direction of diffusion is largely uniform across each imaged voxel. Diffusion of polarized molecules may also be influenced by an electrical potential gradient. Diffusion imaging is performed in the same general manner

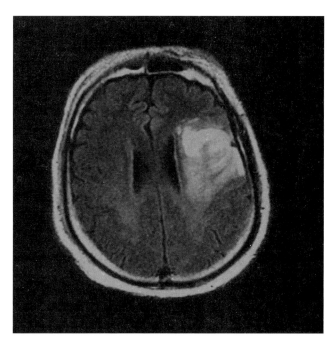

FIGURE 5-98. MR FLAIR image of an acute left middle cerebral artery stroke.

as phase-contrast angiography, described earlier, except that the amplitudes of the bipolar magnetic field gradients are increased greatly so as to be able to image the relatively small distances and slower velocities associated with molecular diffusion as opposed to blood flow. Rapid image acquisition techniques such as echoplanar imaging are used to limit the influence of motion artifact. The direct MR signal cannot differentiate between diffusion-related motion in extracellular

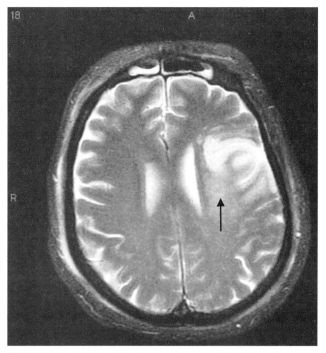

FIGURE 5-99. MR T2-weighted image of an acute left middle cerebral artery stroke. Note increased signal to the subcortical white matter of the left temporal lobe and frontal lobe operculum and decreased gray-white matter differentiation due to parenchymal swelling and edema (*arrow*).

fluid, blood flow, perfusion, and tissue pulsation–related motion. Thus, what is being imaged is not actually a true tissue diffusion coefficient, but rather an ADC. Since diffusion-weighted images are strongly T2-weighted because of the long probe times of the magnetic field gradients, a calculation can be performed to separate T2 relaxation effects from diffusion-related changes in the signal and derive the ADC. A map of ADCs can then be calculated for specific regions of interest from the diffusion-weighted image.

DWI is most usefully applied to the problem of early detection of brain infarction. The diffusion coefficient of ischemic brain tissue rapidly *decreases* within minutes of onset of tissue ischemia (92). While a standard T2-weighted MRI examination can detect brain ischemia/infarction as early as 3 hours after onset (see **Fig. 5-99**), DWI can detect ischemia within minutes (**Fig. 5-100**). One possible explanation for this rapid change is that cytotoxic ischemia causes a movement of water from extracellular to intracellular spaces as the cells rapidly swell due to a failure of the sodium ATP-dependent pump. This membrane-based pump, which appears exquisitely sensitive to ATP availability, normally maintains water equilibrium across cell membranes and thereby regulates cell volume by controlling intracellular and extracellular cation concentrations. The resulting decrease in average diffusion of water-dependent protons in the ischemic region is detected as an area of increased signal intensity on the diffusion-weighted MR image. Signal intensity rapidly rises with tissue ischemia with the diffusion coefficient for water reduced by as much as 50% within minutes after onset of ischemia. With the emergence of new early interventions for acute cerebrovascular thrombosis, improved patient selection and triage at a very early point in the evolution of cerebral ischemia could be achieved with DWI. Furthermore, the changes noted during acute ischemia on DWI, particularly when compared with MR perfusion images described earlier, may indicate reversible tissue dysfunction and may be very helpful in selecting patients for early thrombolytic intervention for acute cerebrovascular thrombosis (93,94).

Additional applications of DWI involve the assessment of *restricted* diffusion due to the anisotropic structure of surrounding tissue such as the myelinated fiber tracts in cerebral white matter and in the spinal cord. The assessment of restricted diffusion involves computing an ADC for each of six different directions for each voxel in the image and using this to derive a diffusion *tensor*. This technique has been called *diffusion tensor imaging* (DTI). Using geometric methods to determine the degree of loss of anisotropic diffusion in subcortical white matter, it is possible to document white matter disruption such as focal dislocation, tearing, swelling, and infiltration. It is also possible to map out the structure and direction of major subcortical white matter tracts using a technique called *diffusion tensor tractography* (95). DWI and fMRI have been used together to map out altered white matter anatomy and to identify eloquent cortical regions for movement and language generation in process of planning brain tumor excisions. Imaging information can be used so that displaced but intact fiber tracts can be preserved and critical cortical regions can be left unharmed. There is now also ongoing active research to evaluate the application of DWI to the assessment and recovery from diffuse axonal injury due to TBI (96,97). Recent studies with limited numbers of patients suggest that DWI may be a helpful technique for detecting the presence and localizing the zones of damage in TBI due to diffuse axonal injury when standard imaging methods show no abnormality (98–100). This is clearly an evolving area with some currently used imaging applications and important future research.

IN VIVO MAGNETIC RESONANCE SPECTROSCOPY IMAGING

Although most of the MR signal that is typically examined in clinical imaging comes from water-based protons, it is possible to study specific resonances from other sources in order to image other metabolically important molecules in the tissue. Although it is relatively easy to obtain a detailed NMR spectrum from a bulk sample as is typically done in NMR-based analytical chemistry, it is much more difficult to obtain the full spectrum from a spatially restricted volume of tissue. A number of different approaches have been taken to develop spectroscopic imaging techniques that would permit the recording of the NMR spectrum for each voxel in an image. However, because the concentration of most metabolic molecular species of interest (e.g., lactic acid) is typically several orders of magnitude less than that of water or fat in different tissues, the proton-NMR signals from water and fat must be suppressed when performing proton spectroscopy of metabolites, and large magnetic fields are also required to permit improved signal-to-noise ratio so that these much smaller spectral peaks can be registered clearly. At present, *in vivo* MR spectroscopy imaging is being used in a wide range of clinical as well as research applications.

PERFUSION-WEIGHTED IMAGING AND FMRI

Perfusion-weighted imaging (PWI) of the brain is obtained by rapidly injecting a paramagnetic dye (e.g., gadolinium) intravenously and imaging the appearance of the dye in perfused brain tissue. Its utility in stroke imaging, particularly when used in conjunction with DWI, was discussed earlier in the section on ischemic stroke. fMRI depends on the coupling of neuronal firing to local changes in metabolic rate that are, in turn, linked to changes in local perfusion of normal brain tissue. In a locally active region of brain tissue, there is an increase in oxygen

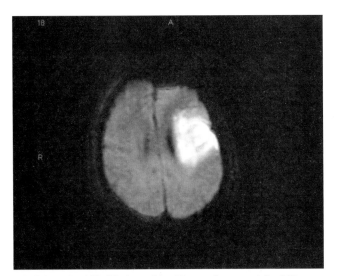

FIGURE 5-100. MR diffusion-weighted image of an acute left middle cerebral artery stroke.

extraction to support the increased metabolic rate of the tissue. However, there is also an increase in local CBF to support the active region, which increases oxygen delivery to the area to the point where it exceeds that which is actually required. There is therefore a relative *decrease* in the local concentration of deoxyhemoglobin at the postcapillary level in activated tissue. Deoxyhemoglobin contains iron and is paramagnetic, thus diminishing signal intensity on a T2-weighted image. Since deoxyhemoglobin is decreased in activated tissue, there is a net increase in signal intensity in this region on the T2-weighted image. This is a small signal but can be recovered from the background by averaging together several images obtained by rapid-acquisition EPI methods. The images are obtained while the subject is engaged in performing a specific continuous activating task such as repetitively moving the fingers of one hand or performing an extended cognitive task. This fMRI technique is referred to as *blood-oxygen-level–dependent imaging*, or BOLD. A number of other techniques have also been developed for use in fMRI applications (101). **Table 5-1** provides a brief description of the various MR imaging techniques that have been touched on in this chapter and provides a synopsis of their different applications and limitations.

TABLE 5-1	A Comparison of MR Imaging Methods			
MR Method	**Excitation-Emission Sequence**	**What Is Imaged?**	**Applications**	**Limitations**
T1-weighted	TR: short (<1,000 ms) TE: short (<30 ms) Spin echo technique	T1 contrast. Fluid is dark. Fat is white. Brain parenchyma is gray. Tumor and edema are gray or dark. Ligament and tendon are dark. Methemoglobin (hemoglobin breakdown product >7 d) has high signal intensity	Best spatial resolution for connective tissue anatomy and bone marrow and trabecular anatomy Myelin distribution and mucoid degeneration of tendons/menisci. Used for all post-contrast imaging—e.g., with gadolinium Identify subacute to chronic hemorrhage	Poor tissue edema contrast resolution. Poor sensitivity to pathologic lesions since most lesions involve increased tissue or edema fluid and T1 is not sensitive to the appearance of tissue fluid associated with acute inflammatory reaction or pathologic tissue changes
T2-weighted	TR: long (>1,500 ms) TE: long (>60 ms) E.g., FSE technique	T2 contrast. Fluid is white. Fat is variable. Brain parenchyma is gray. Tumor and edema are white (hyperintense). Ligament and tendon are dark	Regions with high free water content have high signal intensity—e.g., CSF, edema, nucleus pulposus, synovial fluid, abscess, and hyperacute hemorrhage (<1 d). Sensitive to pathologic appearance of fluid in parenchymal tissue	Difficult-to-see high-intensity lesions adjacent to CSF or other free fluid regions—CSF has high signal intensity, as do T2 lesions; therefore, tissue lesions at CSF interface are obscured
STIR	TR: long (>4,000 ms) TE: short (<50 ms) TI: short values to null out fatty tissue	Very sensitive to tissue edema Water content in soft tissue (e.g., nerve and muscle) produces a high signal intensity. Fat is suppressed	MR neurography Muscle pathology imaging Pathologic fracture, bone edema, ligamentous or tendinous injury imaging	Poor spatial resolution but suitable to large body parts such as the limbs and trunk or pelvis
FLAIR	TR: long (e.g., 9,000 ms) TE: long (e.g., 130 ms) Heavily T2-weighted TI adjusted to null out free fluid signal (e.g., 2,200 ms)	Heavily T2-weighted with bulk water suppression, but without extracellular fluid/tissue edema suppression	White matter T2 lesions seen more clearly than with T2-weighted Applied to MS, DAI/TBI, Lyme, HIV, brain infarction/ischemia	CSF pulsation artifact Blood flow artifact Requires careful adjustment of TI, especially when CSF is abnormal
MRA	Phase-contrast imaging; bipolar MFG	Flowing spins	Blood flow; angiography. Noninvasive screening for cerebrovascular anomalies (e.g., cerebral aneurysms)	Longer study time Lower spatial resolution compared with x-ray angiography
DWI	EPIA TR: long (e.g., 10,000 ms) Heavily T2-weighted Phase-contrast imaging with large-amplitude bipolar MFGs Spin echo	Diffusing spins. To look at "restricted" or "anisotropic" diffusion, a diffusion "tensor" of directionally specific diffusion rates is computed for each voxel. DTI can be used to compute pathways of white fiber tracts (i.e., diffusion tensor tractography) and focal white matter disruption	Ischemia; acute stroke; TBI; DAI Held to be exquisitely and nearly immediately sensitive to the effects of ischemia on the brain tissue due to focal reduction in diffusion of extracellular water in the ischemic region. H_2O moves into intracellular space due to metabolic failure of ATP-dependent membrane-based Na-K pump Tissue perfusion assessment	Motion artifact; MR measurement cannot differentiate diffusion from local blood flow or tissue pulsation; T2-weighted due to long probe time. Can correct for effect of T2 weighting by calculating map of ADC values

Continued

TABLE 5-1	A Comparison of MR Imaging Methods *(Continued)*			
MR Method	**Excitation-Emission Sequence**	**What Is Imaged?**	**Applications**	**Limitations**
PWI	TR: short TE: short Images taken while contrast medium (e.g., gadolinium) is power-injected intravenously at a fixed rate	Appearance of blood-conducted paramagnetic contrast medium in different brain regions		Involves dye injection using specialized equipment to control rate of infusion
fMRI-BOLD	EPIA; T2-weighted; multiple image averaging to extract deoxyhemoglobin signal	Spatially localized tissue decrease in deoxyhemoglobin in regions of functionally related metabolic activation	Local tissue activation in functional brain activation/physiologic studies	Must average images to extract small deoxyhemoglobin signal Limited temporal resolution Subject must be cooperative and able to continuously perform the activation task

Note: The exact choices of parameter settings for TR, TE, and TI will vary according to the size of the static external magnetic field and various design details of the MR instrument.

ADC, apparent diffusion coefficient; DTI, diffusion tensor imaging; DWI, diffusion-weighted imaging; EPIA, echo planar image acquisition; FLAIR, fluid-attenuated inversion recovery; fMRI-BOLD, functional magnetic resonance imaging-blood-oxygen-level–dependent technique; FSE, fast spin echo; MFG, magnetic field gradient; MRA, magnetic resonance angiography; PWI, perfusion-weighted imaging; STIR, short-tau inversion recovery; T1, longitudinal relaxation time (aka "spin-lattice relaxation time"—magnetization relaxation parallel to the static external magnetic field); T2, transverse relaxation time (aka "spin-spin relaxation time," magnetization relaxation perpendicular to static external magnetic field, "precession"); TE, echo record time between RF pulse and signal recording window; TI, inversion recovery time; TR, repetition time between each new excitation-emission sequence.

Susceptibility-Weighted Imaging

Susceptibility-weighted imaging (SWI) is a 3D gradient-echo sequence, which provides high-resolution images based on local tissue magnetic susceptibility and on BOLD effects (102,103). Magnetic susceptibility is related to loss of signal in voxels with magnetic field nonuniformities, due to greater $T2^*$ decay. SWI was originally intended for submillimeter cerebral vein imaging without the use of contrast agents, based on the fact that deoxygenated venous blood produces more magnetic field inhomogeneities than oxygenized arterial blood. Nevertheless, it was soon realized that the sensitivity of SWI of deoxygenated blood, as well as its sensitivity in detecting subtle susceptibility differences, allowed for many more imaging applications (104). In addition, with the new 3T scanners, SWI of the entire brain can be performed in less than 4 minutes (103). At present, most of the applications of SWI are in the field of neuroradiology, among which are TBI, hemorrhagic disorders, vascular malformations, cerebral infarctions, tumors, and neurodegenerative disorders associated with intracranial calcifications or iron deposition. When adding SWI sequences, in addition to diffusion-weighted and perfusion-weighted sequences, to the standard MR protocol, a more complete understanding of the disease process in question is accomplished, particularly when dealing with neurovascular and neurodegenerative disorders (103).

Ultrasound Imaging of the Muscle, Nerve, Connective Tissues, and Joints

Ultrasound imaging (USI) involves the creation of visual images from the reflection of high-frequency mechanical waves back from different interfaces within the imaged tissues (see Chapter 6). Medical USI uses the ability of high-frequency sound to penetrate through multiple layers of tissue so that images can be constructed of the structures lying under the skin. Surfaces at which sound conductance changes generate

an echo back to the transducer, depending on how much the sound conductance changes at the interface. Various different probes are available for USI. A transverse linear array probe is able to image from relatively flat surfaces and can be used to study soft tissues of the limbs or trunk. High-frequency transducers offer the best-quality imaging of anatomic details for soft tissue neuromusculoskeletal examination (see **Fig. 5-100**).

USI OF THE MUSCLE

The appearance of a muscle with USI is determined by the complex interweaving of fibrous tissue and myocytes in the stromal architecture of the muscle. Reflections arise at interfaces between relatively dense fibrous tissue and relatively soft muscle tissue, where fibrous tissue wraps around individual muscle fascicles. In sagittal section, these fascicular interfaces form longitudinal striations along the length of the muscle. With an axial section of the muscle, the end-on view of the fascicular structure produces a stippled cellular mosaic pattern (**Fig. 5-101**). The echogenicity of the muscle depends on the relative density of the fibrous matrix. In the presence of disuse atrophy, the echogenicity of the muscle increases as a result of volume loss in the myocytes and increased fibrofatty tissue content of the muscle.

Muscle injuries account for up to one third of all sports-related injuries in elite sports. Muscle injuries result from either direct trauma or indirect trauma following eccentric muscle contraction. The most common mechanism of injury of muscles in elite athletes is related to indirect muscle injury (muscle strain), usually at the myotendinous junction. Blunt trauma is the most common mechanism of direct muscle injury in sports that may involve collisions. Multiple classification and grading systems have been proposed, with categorical grading systems based on sonographic findings still in use. Grade 1 muscle strains may show a normal appearance of the muscle fibers but sometimes may present as focal or diffuse

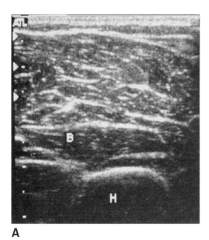
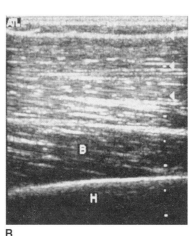

A   **B**

FIGURE 5-101. Normal biceps muscle on USI. The biceps muscle is labeled *B* and the humerus underneath it is labeled *H*. **A:** The axial image of the muscle. **B:** The sagittal image of the muscle. Note the normal striatal structure in the two views.

ill-defined hyperechoic areas within the muscle at the site of injury. Grade 2 muscle strain manifests as partial disruption of the muscle fibers, sometimes associated with an intramuscular hematoma. Grade 3 muscle strains demonstrate complete disruption (100% of the cross-sectional area) of the muscle with retraction of the proximal fibers. An intramuscular hematoma may also be seen in grade 3 injuries. Perifascial edema may be present and can be seen with any grade of muscle injury. The normal cortical bone surfaces are smooth and echogenic with posterior acoustic shadowing. The subcortical bone and underlying marrow cannot be evaluated with ultrasound, a disadvantage when compared to MRI. Tendons tend to be intermediate between cortical bone and muscle in terms of echogenicity and have a dense nonpulsatile fibrillar pattern that helps to separate their appearance from vessels and nerves (105). Furthermore, they can be readily recognized by having the subject contract the muscle connected to the visualized tendon so that its active movement can be directly observed. This highlights one of the very unique and valuable features of USI: its ability to generate real-time images of structures that are dynamically active. The ultrasound image is constantly being updated on the screen at video rates to produce a "live-action" dynamic imaging of the tissue structure. Thus, it is possible to evaluate the relative motility of different structures and the "slide" that occurs at tissue interfaces as active and passive movements are elicited during imaging. When a normal contracting muscle is imaged, the muscle can be seen to enlarge in cross section with irregular jerky motions seen within the muscle bulk. These appear to be contractions of individual fascicles during voluntary contraction of motor units. Fasciculations can be readily identified on real-time USI as a sudden isolated limited contraction within the muscle. USI allows for specific indications as to the intramuscular location of the motor unit generating the fasciculation. Also, dynamic USI can evaluate intrafascial or interfascial muscle herniation.

USI OF PERIPHERAL NERVE

USI can also be applied to the imaging of peripheral nerves. Nerves can have either an echogenic cross section when surrounded by relatively hypoechoic tissues or a relatively hypoechoic appearance in surrounding tissues that are relatively hyperechoic. With high-resolution USI, a stippled transverse cross-sectional appearance can be seen reflecting the

fascicular internal structure of the nerve. Nerves can be differentiated from the three other major tubular structures: tendons/ligaments, arteries, and veins. Tendons/ligaments have well-defined anatomic locations, are densely hyperechoic, and can be made to move in a specific manner with appropriate patient movements. Arteries tend to pulsate regularly and veins collapse when compressed.

The median nerve can be readily identified in a transverse cross section of the wrist just proximal to the transverse carpal ligament. It lies just above the tendons of the flexor sublimis and deep to the palmaris tendon at this point and has a flattened oval appearance. In sagittal section, it is seen as a relatively hypoechoic structure with tendons above and below it. When the fingers are flexed, the flexor digitorum sublimis tendons can be seen moving back and forth under the static image of the nerve. In the axial transverse image, the nerve is not fixed and changes its shape readily with wrist and finger motion. With full flexion of the fingers into the palm of the hand, the median nerve initially rises and then dives down into a deep pocket formed by the first sublimis tendon above, the flexor pollicis longus tendon medially, and the first profundus tendon below. When the nerve becomes pathologically enlarged, some of this dynamic motion of the nerve is lost. It is also possible to generate images of the ulnar nerve as it passes around the elbow (**Fig. 5-102**).

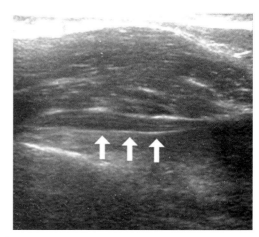

FIGURE 5-102. Longitudinal image of the ulnar nerve (*arrows*) proximal to the medial epicondyle. Note the striated appearance and homogeneous echotexture. High echogenic fat delineates the nerve.

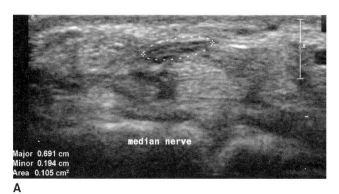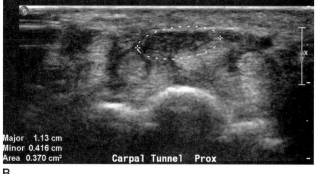

A **B**

FIGURE 5-103. Cross-sectional sonographic images at the level of the carpal tunnel. **A:** Normal median nerve. **B:** There is diffuse enlargement to the median nerve with an area of 0.370 cm³, well above the upper limits of normal (0.15 cm³). (Image courtesy of Dr. Rogelio Muñoz, Puerto Rico.)

In patients presenting with CTS, some changes are consistently noted on USI. Some "doming" of the flexor retinaculum may be present, reflecting a generalized enlargement of the contents of the tunnel. There may be some observable compression of the nerve, usually at the distal edge of the flexor retinaculum. The nerve appears less deformable with compression and movement and may have increased blood flows associated with it, which can be detected with Doppler ultrasound. Finally, the nerve often is noted to be significantly enlarged (**Fig. 5-103**). The reason for this enlargement may be a combination of local edema, increased intrafascicular fibrous tissue development within the nerve (related to chronic inflammation), or a backup of axoplasmic fluid flow caused by compression. Furthermore, the nerve appears to be less mobile within the carpal segment, particularly with rapid repetitive motions of the wrist and fingers. USI can therefore provide some useful qualitative information about anatomic changes in the median nerve associated with CTS (**Fig. 5-104**). Imaging of the contents of the carpal tunnel can also detect other problems that could be contributing to CTS symptoms, such as nerve and ganglion cysts, synovial cysts, and osteophytes (106). USI has also been applied to the study of enlarged nerves in the hereditary motor and sensory neuropathies, to studies of ulnar nerve entrapment in the cubital tunnel, and to evaluation of the brachial plexus.

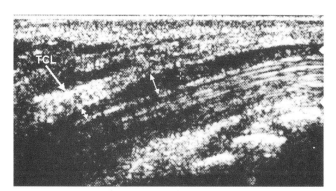

FIGURE 5-104. A sagittal section of the median nerve in which there is evidence of compression of the nerve under the transverse carpal ligament (TCL). Note the swelling of the nerve proximal to where it goes deep to the TCL. *White double headed arrows* demonstrate the compression of the nerve with reduction in nerve diameter under the TCL and the enlargement of the nerve proximal to the TCL.

USI OF JOINTS

Ultrasound is currently used for the evaluation of joint internal derangement. The shoulder, elbow, wrist, hip, knee, and ankle articulations are routinely evaluated with ultrasound for ligament, tendon, cartilage, and fibrocartilage abnormalities. Current ultrasound technology allows imaging of structures not only during rest but also in real time during controlled limb movements, so that movement-dependent changes in anatomic relationship (e.g., shoulder impingement and snapping syndromes) can be visualized and evaluated. Different USI findings can be seen in muscle tear and rupture, tendon tear, tendonitis, ligament tears, and various soft tissue overuse syndromes. Evaluation with USI, in the hands of a well-trained individual who understands the underlying anatomy and pathophysiology, as well as the advantages and limitations of ultrasound technology, can be very helpful in the differential diagnosis of musculoskeletal complaints and the assessment of extent and severity of a musculoskeletal injury or condition. A detailed review of the application of musculoskeletal ultrasound is beyond the scope of this chapter, but interested readers are referred to available sources (107,108).

REFERENCES

1. Amis ES. Butler PR. ACR white paper on radiation dose in medicine: three years later. *J Am Coll Radiol.* 2010;7:865–870.
2. Pretorius S, Fishman EK. Volume-rendered three-dimensional spiral CT: musculoskeletal applications. *Radiographics.* 1999;19:1143–1160.
3. Seeger LL, Lufkin RB. Physical principles of MRI. In: Bassett LW, Gold RH, Seeger LL, eds. *MRI Atlas of the Musculoskeletal System.* London, UK: Martin Dunitz; 1989:11–24.
4. Deutsch AL, Mink JH. Magnetic resonance imaging of musculoskeletal injuries. *Radiol Clin North Am.* 1989;27:983–1002.
5. Filler AG, Howe FA, Hayes CE, et al. Application of magnetic resonance neurography in the evaluation of patients with peripheral nerve pathology. *J Neurosurg.* 1996;85:299–309.
6. West GA, Haynor DR, Goodkin R, et al. Magnetic resonance imaging signal changes in denervated muscle after peripheral nerve injury. *Neurosurgery.* 1994;35:1077–1086.
7. Neer CS. Impingement lesions. *Clin Orthop.* 1983;173:70–77.
8. Morag Y, Jacobson J, et al. MR imaging of rotator cuff injury: what the clinician needs to know. *Radiographics.* 2006;26:1045–1065.
9. Murray PJ, Shaffer BS. Clinical update: MR imaging of the shoulder. *Sports Med Arthrosc Rev.* 2009;17(1):40–48.
10. Berquist TH. Shoulder and arm. In: Berquist TH, ed. *MRI of the Musculoskeletal System.* Philadelphia, PA: Lippincott-Raven; 1996:517–607.
11. Waldt S, Bukart AJ, Imhoff AB, et al. Anterior shoulder instability: accuracy of MR arthrography in the classification of anteroinferior labroligamentous injuries. *Radiology.* 2005;237:578–583.
12. Workman TL, Burkhard TK, Resnick D. Hill Sachs lesion, comparison of detection with MR imaging, radiography and arthroscopy. *Radiology.* 1992;185:847–852.

13. Bencardino JT, Gyftopoulos S, Palmer W. Imaging in anterior glenohumeral instability. *Radiology.* 2013;269(2):232–337.

14. Motamedi D, Everist B, et al. Pitfalls in shoulder MRI: Part 2. Biceps tendon, bursae and cysts, incidental and postsurgical findings, and artifacts. *AJR Am J Roentgenol.* 2014;203:508–515.

15. Murphey MD, Foreman KL, et al. From the radiologic pathologic archives; imaging of osteonecrosis: radiologic pathologic correlation. *Radiographics.* 2014;34:1003–1028.

16. Crosby NE, Greenberg JA. Radiographic evaluation of the elbow. *J Hand Surg [Am].* 2014;39(7):1408–1414.

17. Bencardino JT, Rosenberg ZS. Entrapment neuropathies of the upper extremity. In: Stoller DW, ed. *Magnetic Resonance Imaging in Orthopedics and Sports Medicine.* 3rd ed. Philadelphia, PA: Lippincott Williams & Wilkins; 2006:1933–1976.

18. Mann F, Wilson A, Gilula L. Radiographic evaluation of the wrist: what does the hand surgeon wants to know? *Radiology.* 1992;184:15–24.

19. Mesgarzadeh M, Schneck CD, Bonakdarpour A. Carpal tunnel: MR imaging. Part I. Normal anatomy. *Radiology.* 1989;171:743–749.

20. Mesgarzadeh M, Schneck CD, Bonakdarpour A, et al. Carpal tunnel: MR imaging. Part II. Carpal tunnel syndrome. *Radiology.* 1989;171: 749–754.

21. Mesgarzadeh M, Schneck CD, Bonakdarpour A. The wrist and hand. In: Bassett LW, Gold RH, Seeger LL, eds. *MRI Atlas of the Musculoskeletal System.* London, UK: Martin Dunitz; 1989:139–174.

22. Mesgarzadeh M, Triola J, Schneck CD. Carpal tunnel syndrome: MR imaging diagnosis. *Magn Reson Imaging Clin N Am.* 1995;3:249–264.

23. Quinn SF, Belsole RJ, Greene TL, et al. Advanced imaging of the wrist. *Radiographics.* 1988;9:229–246.

24. Schoenberg N, Rosenberg ZS. Magnetic resonance imaging of the elbow, wrist and hand. In: Beltran J, ed. *Current Review of MRI.* Philadelphia, PA: Current Medicine; 1995:215–228.

25. Clohisy JC, Carlisle JC, Beaulé PE, et al. A systematic approach to the plain film evaluation of the young adult hip. *J Bone Joint Surg Am.* 2008;90(suppl 4):47–66.

26. Ficat RP, Arlet J. Bone necrosis of known etiology. In: Hungerford D, ed. *Ischemia and Necrosis of Bone.* Baltimore, MD: Williams & Wilkins; 1980:111–130.

27. McGlade CT, Bassett LH. The hip. In: Bassett LW, Gold RH, Seeger LL, eds. *MRI Atlas of the Musculoskeletal System.* London, UK: Martin Dunitz; 1989: 175–214.

28. Coleman BG, Kressel HY, Dalinka MK, et al. Radiographically negative avascular necrosis: detection with MR imaging. *Radiology.* 1988;168:525–528.

29. Tervonen O, Mueller DM, Matterson EL, et al. Clinically occult avascular necrosis of the hip: prevalence in an asymptomatic population at risk. *Radiology.* 1992;182:845–847.

30. Resnick D, Sweet DE, Madowell JE. Osteonecrosis and osteochondrosis. In: Resnick D, ed. *Bone and Joint Imaging.* Philadelphia, PA: WB Saunders; 1996:941–977.

31. Totty WG, Murphy WA, Ganz WI, et al. Magnetic resonance imaging of the normal and ischemic femoral head. *AJR Am J Roentgenol.* 1984;143:1273–1280.

32. Mitchell DG, Rao VM, Dalinka MK, et al. Femoral head avascular necrosis: correlation of MR imaging, radiographic staging, radionuclide imaging and clinical findings. *Radiology.* 1987;162:709–715.

33. Ganz R, Parvazi J, Beck M, et al. Femoroacetabular impingement: a cause for osteoarthritis of the hip. *Clin Orthop Relat Res.* 2003;417:112–220.

34. Hayes CW, Conway WF. Evaluation of articular cartilage: radiographic and cross sectional imaging techniques. *Radiographics.* 1992;12(3):409–428.

35. Brandt KD, Fife RS, Braunstein EM, et al. Radiographic grading of the severity of knee osteoarthritis; relation of the Kellgren and Lawrence grade to a grade based on joint space narrowing and correlation with arthroscopic evidence of articular degeneration. *Arthritis Rheum.* 1991;34(11):1381–1386.

36. Vincken PW, ter Braak AP, van Erkel AR, et al. MR imaging: effectiveness and costs at triage of patients with nonacute knee symptoms. *Radiology.* 2007;242(1):85–93

37. Langer JE, Meyer SJF, Dalinka MK. Imaging of the knee. *Radiol Clin North Am.* 1990;28:975–990.

38. Hartzman S, Gold RH. The knee. In: Bassett LW, Gold RH, Seeger LL, eds. *MRI Atlas of the Musculoskeletal System.* London, UK: Martin Dunitz; 1989:215–265.

39. Dillon EH, Pope CF, Jokl P, et al. Follow-up of grade 2 meniscal abnormalities in the stable knee. *Radiology.* 1991;181:849–852.

40. Burk DL, Mitchell DG, Rifkin MD, et al. Recent advances in magnetic imaging of the knee. *Radiol Clin North Am.* 1990;28:379–393.

41. Fox MG, Graham JA, et al. Prospective evaluation of agreement and accuracy in the diagnosis of meniscal tears: MR arthrography a short time after injection versus CT arthrography after a moderate delay. *AJR Am J Roentgenol.* 2016;207:142–149.

42. Mesgarzadeh M, Schneck CD, Bonakdarpour A. Magnetic resonance imaging of the knee: correlation with normal anatomy. *Radiographics.* 1988;8:707–733.

43. Vahey TN, Broome DR, Kayes KJ, et al. Acute and chronic tears of the anterior cruciate ligament: differential features of MR imaging. *Radiology.* 1991;181:251–253.

44. Hennigan SP, Schneck CD, Mesgarzadeh M, et al. The semimembranosus–tibial collateral ligament bursa. *J Bone Joint Surg Am.* 1994;76:1322–1327.

45. Anis AH, Stiell IG, Stewart DG, et al. Cost-effectiveness analysis of the Ottawa Ankle Rules. *Ann Emerg Med.* 1995;26(4):422–428.

46. Kier R, McCarthy S, Dietz MJ, et al. MR appearance of painful conditions of the ankle. *Radiographics.* 1991;11:401–414.

47. Perrich KD, Goodwin DW, et al. Ankle ligaments on MRI: appearance of normal and injured ligaments. *AJR Am J Roentgenol.* 2009;193;687–695.

48. Schneck CD, Mesgarzadeh M, Bonakdarpour A, et al. MR imaging of the most commonly injured ankle ligaments. Part I. Normal anatomy. *Radiology.* 1992;184:499–506.

49. Schneck CD, Mesgarzadeh M, Bonakdarpour A. MR imaging of the most commonly injured ankle ligaments. Part II. Ligament injuries. *Radiology.* 1992;184:507–512.

50. Siegler S, Block J, Schneck C. The mechanical characteristics of the collateral ligaments of the human ankle joint. *Foot Ankle.* 1988;8:234–242.

51. Brower AC. *Arthritis in Black and White.* Philadelphia, PA: WB Saunders; 1988:213–230.

52. Schumacher EH. *Primer on the Rheumatic Diseases.* Atlanta, GA: Arthritis Foundation; 1988:60–76.

53. Brower AC. *Arthritis in Black and White.* Philadelphia, PA: WB Saunders; 1988: 243–256.

54. Davis PC, Wippold FJ, Brunberg JA, et al. ACR appropriateness criteria on low back pain. *J Am Coll Radiol.* 2009;6(6):401–407.

55. Williams AL, Gornet MF, Burkis JK. CT evaluation of lumbar interbody fusion: current concepts. *AJNR Am J Neuroradiol.* 2005;26:2057–2066.

56. Modic MT, Herfkens RJ. Intervertebral disk: normal age-related changes in MR signal intensity. *Radiology.* 1990;177:332–334.

57. Fardon DF, Milette PC. Nomenclature and classification of lumbar disc pathology (Recommendations of the Combined Task Forces of the North American Spine Society, American Society of Spine Radiology and American Society of Neuroradiology). *Spine.* 2001;26:E93–E113.

58. Inoue N, Espinosa Orias A. Biomechanics of intervertebral disc degeneration. *Orthop Clin North Am.* 2011;42(4):487–499.

59. Jahnke RW, Hart BL. Cervical stenosis, spondylosis and herniated disc disease. *Radiol Clin North Am.* 1991;29:777–791.

60. Yi JS, Cha JG, et al. Imaging of herniated discs of the cervical spine: inter-modality differences between 64-slice multidetector CT and 1.5 T MRI. *Korean J Radiol.* 2015; 16(4):881–888.

61. Sherk HH, Lapinski AS. Developmental anatomy of the cervical spine. In: Benzel EC, ed. *The Cervical Spine.* 5th ed. Philadelphia, PA: Wolters Klugwer/Lippincott Williams and Wilkins. 2012:34–42.

62. Hartman J. Anatomy and clinical significance of the uncinated process and uncovertebral joint: a comprehensive review. *Clin Anat.* 2014;27(3):431–440.

63. Penning L, Wilmink JT, Van Worden HH, et al. CT myelographic findings in degenerative disorders of the cervical spine: clinical significance. *AJR Am J Roentgenol.* 1986; 146:793–801.

64. McAllister VL, Sage MR. The radiology of thoracic disc protrusion. *Clin Radiol.* 1976;27:291–299.

65. Brinjikji W, Luetmer PH, et al. Systematic literature review of imaging features of spinal degeneration in asymptomatic populations. *AJNR Am J Neuroradiol.* 2015; 36(4):811–816.

66. Bogduk N, Aprill C, Derby R. Discography. In: White AH, Schofferman JA, eds. *Spine Care.* St. Louis, MO: CV Mosby; 1995:219–238.

67. Ciric L, Mikhael MA, Tarkington JA, et al. The lateral recess syndrome: a variant of spinal stenosis. *J Neurosurg.* 1980;53:433–443.

68. Campbell RSD, Grainger AJ, Hide IG, et al. Juvenile spondylolysis: a comparative analysis of CT, SPECT and MRI. *Skeletal Radiol.* 2005;34:63–76.

69. Parizel PR, van der Zijden T, et al. Trauma of the spine and spinal cord: imaging strategies. *Eur Spine J.* 2010;19(suppl 1):8–17.

70. Khurana B, Sheehan SE, et al. Traumatic thoracolumbar spine injuries: what the spine surgeon wants to know. *Radiographics.* 2013;33:2031–2046.

71. MiYanji F, Furlan JC, et al. Acute cervical traumatic spinal cord injury: MR imaging findings correlated with neurological outcome-prospective study with 100 consecutive patients. *Radiology.* 2007;243(3):820–827.

72. Quencer RM. Post-traumatic spinal cord cysts: characterization with CT, MRI and sonography. In: Latchaw RE, ed. *MR and CT Imaging of the Head, Neck and Spine.* St. Louis, MO: Mosby-Year Book; 1991:1257–1267.

73. Weissman BNW, Aliabadi P, Weinfeld MS, et al. Prognostic features of atlanto-axial subluxation in rheumatoid arthritis patients. *Radiology.* 1982;144:745–751.

74. Tomandl BF, Klotz E, Handschu R, et al. Comprehensive imaging of ischemic stroke with multisection CT. *Radiographics.* 2003;23:565–592.

75. Saenz RC. The disappearing basal ganglia sign. *Radiology.* 2005;234:242–243.

76. Hecht ST, Eelkema EA, Latchaw RE. Cerebral ischemia and infarction. In: Latchaw RE, ed. *MR and CT Imaging of the Head, Neck and Spine.* St. Louis, MO: Mosby-Year Book; 1991:145–169.

77. Inoue Y, Takemoto K, Miyamoto T, et al. Sequential computed tomography scans in acute cerebral infarction. *Radiology.* 1980;135:655–662.

78. Srinivasan A, Goyal M, Al Azrib F, et al. State-of-the-art imaging of acute stroke. *Radiographics.* 2006;26:S75–S95.

79. Heit JJ, Iv M, Wintermark M. Imaging of intracranial hemorrhage. *J Stroke.* 2017;19(1):11–27.

80. Verma RK, Kottke R, et al. Detecting subarachnoid hemorrhage: comparison of combined FLAIR/SWI versus CT. *Eur J Radiol.* 2013;82(9):1539–1545.

81. Hijaz TA, Cento EA, et al. Imaging of head trauma. *Radiol Clin North Am.* 2011;49: 81–103.

82. Bergstrom M, Ericson K, Levander B, et al. Variations with time of the attenuation values of intracranial hematomas. *J Comput Assist Tomogr.* 1977;1:57–63.

83. Pussaint TY, Moeller KK. Imaging of pediatric head trauma. *Neuroimaging Clin N Am.* 2002;12:271–292.

84. Sarbu N, Shih R, et al. White matter diseases with radiologic-pathologic correlation. *Radiographics.* 2016;36:1426–1447.

85. Gebarski SS. The passionate man plays his part: neuroimaging and multiple sclerosis. *Radiology.* 1988;169:275–276.

86. Drayer BP. Brain iron and movement disorders. In: Latchaw RE, ed. *MR and CT Imaging of the Head, Neck and Spine.* St. Louis, MO: Mosby-Year Book; 1991:399–412.

87. Murray AD. Imaging approaches for dementia. *AJNR Am J Neuroradiol.* 2012; 33(10):1836–1844.

88. Bakshi R, Ariyaratana S, Benedict RHB, et al. Fluid-attenuated inversion recovery magnetic resonance imaging detects cortical and juxtacortical multiple sclerosis lesions. *Arch Neurol.* 2001;58:742–748.

89. Pierallini A, Pantano P, Fantozzi LM, et al. Correlation between MRI findings and long-term outcome in patients with severe brain trauma. *Neuroradiology.* 2000;42:860–867.

90. Ashikaga R, Araki Y, Ishida O. MRI of head injury using FLAIR. *Neuroradiology.* 1997;39:239–342.

91. Takaoka M, Tabuse H, Kumura E, et al. Semiquantitative analysis of corpus callosum injury using magnetic resonance imaging indicates clinical severity in patients with diffuse axonal injury. *J Neurol Neurosurg Psychiatry.* 2002;73:289–293.

92. Moseley ME, Cohen Y, Kucharczyk J, et al. Diffusion-weighted MR imaging of anisotropic water diffusion in cat central nervous system. *Radiology.* 1990;176:439–445.

93. Romero JM, Schaefer PW, Grant PE, et al. Diffusion MR imaging of acute ischemic stroke. *Neuroimaging Clin N Am.* 2002;12:35–53.

94. Warach S. New imaging strategies for patient selection for thrombolytic and neuroprotective therapies. *Neurology.* 2001;57(5 suppl 2):S48–S52.

95. Basser PJ, Pajevic S, Pierpaoli C, et al. In vivo fiber tractography using DT–MRI data. *Magn Reson Med.* 2000;44:625–632.

96. Pierpaoli C, Barnett A, Pajevic S, et al. Water diffusion changes in Wallerian degeneration and their dependence on white matter architecture. *Neuroimage.* 2001;13:1174–1185.

97. Alsop DC, Murai H, Detre JA, et al. Detection of acute pathologic changes following experimental traumatic brain injury using diffusion-weighted magnetic resonance imaging. *J Trauma.* 1996;13:151–521.

98. Arfanakis K, Haughton VM, Carew JD, et al. Diffusion tensor MR imaging in diffuse axonal injury. *AJNR Am J Neuroradiol.* 2002;23:794–802.

99. Nakahara M, Ericson K, Bellander BM. Diffusion-weighted MR and apparent diffusion coefficient in the evaluation of severe brain injury. *Acta Radiol.* 2001;42:365–369.

100. Liu AY, Maldjian JA, Bagley LJ, et al. Traumatic brain injury: diffusion-weighted MR imaging findings. *AJNR Am J Neuroradiol.* 1999;20:1636–1641.

101. Buxton RB. *Introduction to Functional Magnetic Resonance Imaging: Principles and Techniques.* Cambridge, UK: Cambridge University Press; 2001.

102. Haacke EM, Mittal S, Wu Z, et al. Susceptibility–weighted imaging: technical aspects and clinical applications. Part I. *AJNR Am J Neuroradiol.* 2009;30:19–30.

103. Mittal S, Wu Z, Neelavalli J, et al. Susceptibility-weighted imaging: technical aspects and clinical applications. Part II. *AJNR Am J Neuroradiol.* 2009;30:232–252.

104. Deistung A, Rauscher A, Sedlacik J, et al. GUIBOLD: a graphical user interface for image reconstruction and data analysis in susceptibility-weighted MR imaging. *Radiographics.* 2008;28:639–651.

105. McNally E, eds. *Practical Musculoskeltal Utrasound.* 2nd Ed. Churchill Livingston Elsevier; 2014.

106. Van Holsbeeck MT, Joseph HI. Sonography of the elbow, wrist and hand. In: Van Holsbeeck MT, Joseph HI, eds. *Musculoskeletal Ultrasound.* 2nd ed. St. Louis, MO: Mosby; 2001:517–572.

107. Van Holsbeeck MT, Joseph HI, eds. *Musculoskeletal Ultrasound.* 2nd ed. St. Louis, MO: Mosby; 2001.

108. Jacobson JA, eds. *Fundamentals of Musculoskeletal Ultrasound.* 3rd ed. Elsevier; 2018.

CHAPTER 6

Yi-Pin Chiang Tyng-Guey Wang
Wen-Chung Tsai Henry L. Lew

Diagnostic Ultrasound

INTRODUCTION

With recent advances in computer technology, equipment miniaturization, reduced cost, and ease of use, the clinical applications of diagnostic ultrasound (U/S) have spread across various medical specialties, including musculoskeletal medicine. In this chapter, we review several common pathologies of the shoulder, the elbow, and the knee to demonstrate the utility of diagnostic U/S in musculoskeletal medicine. Detailed procedures for examining the upper and lower extremities have been described in two recent publications (1,2) and are only briefly mentioned in this chapter.

Two major imaging modalities for detection of soft tissue injuries are magnetic resonance imaging (MRI) and U/S (see Chapter 5 on Imaging Techniques). Musculoskeletal U/S is, by no means, a replacement of MRI. Instead, it should be viewed as an extension of our physical examination. Typically, MRI can reveal static features of muscles, tendons, nerves, and bones with excellent resolution. However, when compared with U/S, the disadvantages of MRI are (a) its limited accessibility in the clinic, (b) longer examination time, and (c) higher cost. On the other hand, modern musculoskeletal U/S can provide high-resolution and real-time imaging of the nerves, tendons, muscles, and joint recesses, provided that the structures are not too deep or obscured by hyperechoic body parts (3).

Musculoskeletal U/S plays a role not only in the assessment of soft tissue pathologies but also as an adjunct to a number of common interventional procedures. When used appropriately, U/S guidance improves the accuracy of steroid injection into joint cavities, bursa, and tendon sheaths, thus improving its therapeutic efficacy (4,5) and thereby reducing the risk of iatrogenic complications. By the same token, the application of U/S for regional nerve blocks is also gaining popularity (6,7). In a recent study, ultrasonography has been successfully used to locate the sacral hiatus for caudal epidural injections (8). Moreover, U/S-guided sacroiliac joint injection, facet joint injection, and medial branch block have been advocated as viable options over fluoroscopy- and computed tomography–guided techniques (9–11).

U/S images vary with the reflection of the U/S waves, the amount of which defines the echogenicity. Thus, common terms used to describe the anatomic structures in the areas of interest include "hyperechoic (means the echogenicity is brighter than it should be)," "isoechoic," "hypoechoic (means darker)," and "anechoic (nothing to be seen in area of interest)." In ultrasonography reports, the images are also described in terms of the plane within which the scanning was performed, either longitudinal or transverse. Typically, a linear array probe is used in musculoskeletal examination, as its wider view and higher near-field resolution provide good images of superficial structures. **Figure 6-1** shows an example of a U/S machine and the transducer probes. The degree of U/S penetration also depends on its frequency. Probes with higher frequency ranges (7 to 12 MHz) are commonly used to assess very superficial structures. Probes with lower frequency ranges (5 to 7.5 MHz) are often used to assess structures that are deeper, since they allow greater tissue penetration (3). In addition, power Doppler, a technique that takes into account the velocity of red blood cells being scanned, can be used to indirectly demonstrate blood flow within the scanned area. In the three sections below, we review the imaging of several common musculoskeletal pathologies, (a) the shoulder, (b) the elbow, and (c) the knee.

EXAMPLES OF SHOULDER PATHOLOGY

Supraspinatus Tendon Tear

Supraspinatus tendon tears are commonly seen in individuals participating in sports such as baseball, tennis, or swimming. Pain on resisted shoulder abduction suggests pathology of the supraspinatus tendon. On long-axis scan, a normal supraspinatus tendon should appear as a beak-shaped, echogenic fibrillar structure extending under the acromion, between the humeral head and the subacromial/subdeltoid bursa. On short-axis scan, the tendon appears as a band of medium-level echogenic structures, deep to the subdeltoid bursa and superficial to the hypoechoic hyaline cartilage on the humeral head. A partial-thickness tear is demonstrated as a focal anechoic lesion (**Fig. 6-2A**) or as a mixed "hyperechoic and hypoechoic" focus in the poorly vascularized critical zone of the supraspinatus tendon. The main sonographic features of a full-thickness tear include focal nonvisualization (or anechoic defect) through the width of the tendon, as demonstrated on both of the long- and short-axis views (**Fig. 6-2B and C**) (12).

There is inherent interobserver variability in the detection and characterization of supraspinatus tendon tears (12,13). However, with standardized diagnostic criteria, high-quality scanning equipment, and well-trained sonographers, several studies have reported sensitivities and specificities exceeding 90% in the detection of full-thickness tears of supraspinatus tendon (14–16). Even though the detection of partial-thickness tears and differentiation from focal tendinopathy is often challenging, a meta-analysis reported that the pooled sensitivities and specificities to detect partial-thickness tears exceeded 80% (17). Furthermore, quantitative ultrasound may facilitate the detection of rotator cuff pathology (18).

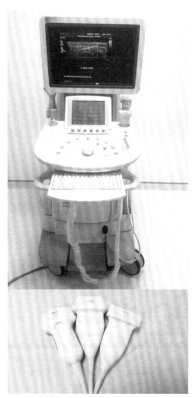

FIGURE 6-1. Basic instrumentation. An example of a diagnostic U/S machine (*upper*) and the transducer probes (*lower*). U/S images are generated when pulses of U/S from the transducer produce echoes at tissue or organ boundaries. Between pulse transmissions, the transducer serves as a detector of echoes, which are processed to form an anatomic image.

Calcific Tendinopathy of the Rotator Cuff

Calcific tendinopathy of the shoulder is a common disorder, characterized by the deposition of calcium, predominately hydroxyapatite within the rotator cuff tendons. The deposition is most often at the insertion of the supraspinatus tendon on the greater tuberosity followed by the infraspinatus and the subscapularis (19). The diagnosis of calcific tendinopathy is mainly based on standard radiographs which can demonstrate the size and location of the calcific deposition. Ultrasound can define the tendon involved and guide therapeutic procedures. In ultrasonography, rotator cuff calcifications appear as echogenic focus with or without acoustic shadowing (**Fig. 6-3A** and **B**). The shape of the calcification focus can be curvilinear, granular, or nodular (19). Furthermore, the calcifications in tendons can be either symptomatic or asymptomatic. For symptomatic rotator cuff calcification, conservative therapeutic options include oral nonsteroidal anti-inflammatory drug, local steroid injection, and shockwave therapy. Ultrasound can not only localize the lesion but also guide steroid injection precisely to the calcified areas. Furthermore, ultrasound-guided percutaneous needle aspiration and lavage is claimed to be effective to treat calcific tendinopathy (20).

Subacromial-Subdeltoid Bursitis

Subacromial-subdeltoid bursitis is often associated with repeated trauma; in middle-aged or older individuals, it tends to be linked with overuse or degenerative changes in the rotator cuff (21). A normal bursa should appear on U/S as a thin hypoechoic stripe, covered by a narrow layer of echogenic peribursal fat, located between the underlying supraspinatus tendon and the overlying deltoid muscle. Typically, it is less than 2 mm in thickness, even counting the hypoechoic layer of fluid located between the two sides of the bursa (22).

Fluid accumulation within the subacromial/subdeltoid bursa is often noted in patients with infectious or inflammatory bursitis (**Fig. 6-4**). However, it can also be observed in patients with full-thickness tear of rotator cuff tendon or in individuals with shoulder impingement syndrome (23). If a needle intervention is deemed necessary, U/S can be utilized to guide bursal fluid aspiration or steroid injection (4).

Bicipital Tenosynovitis

Bicipital tenosynovitis is an inflammation of the long head of the biceps where the tendon passes through the bicipital groove. When the biceps tendon is inflamed, local tenderness in the bicipital groove and an increasing painful arc (painful sensation when the shoulder is flexed from 30 to 120 degrees) are often present. When a clinician is uncertain about the accuracy of the Yergason's supination test or Speed's test (24,25), he or she may consider the use of U/S to improve its diagnosis and treatment.

The long head of the biceps brachii originates at the supraglenoid tubercle, and glenoid labrum in the most superior portion of the glenoid. It lies in the bony groove between the greater tuberosity and the lesser tuberosity of the humeral head. The transverse bicipital ligament keeps the tendon confined within the groove. On short-axis scan, with the arm in neutral position, the long head of biceps tendon of a normal subject is visualized as an oval-shaped, echogenic structure within the bicipital groove. In ultrasonography, the tendon is typically seen as an array of echogenic fibrillar lines, emerging from beneath the acromion and traversing distally to the musculoskeletal junction, where it becomes indistinguishable from the muscle belly.

In biceps tendinopathy, effusion in the tendon sheath is associated with focal tenderness and often with heterogeneity of the tendon. It was demonstrated that the power Doppler signal was more frequently observed medial to the biceps tendon in shoulders with clinically diagnosed biceps disorder (**Fig. 6-5A and B**) (26). Fluid accumulation in bicipital tendon sheath may indicate intra-articular pathology rather than biceps tendon pathology *per se* because of the connection of the sheath with the glenohumeral joint (27). Bicipital sheath effusion may also be seen in supraspinatus tendon tear (28).

EXAMPLES OF ELBOW PATHOLOGY

Lateral Epicondylitis

Lateral epicondylitis is usually caused by repetitive traction of the common extensor tendon (CET) at its osteotendinous attachment to the lateral humeral epicondyle (29). Diagnosis is usually made clinically, without any need for imaging. U/S provides direct visualization of the CET for both the patient and the clinician and can provide confirmatory signs in the evaluation process (30,31). In the longitudinal view via U/S examination, the CET should appear as an echogenic beak-shaped structure (**Fig. 6-6A**). Main U/S features of a "tennis elbow" may include swelling of the tendon, partial tear,

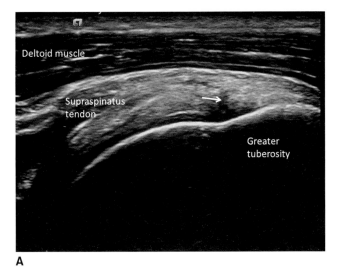

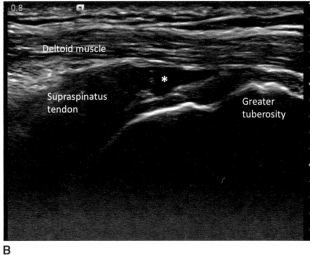

A   **B**

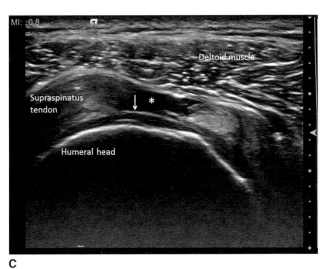

C

FIGURE 6-2. Tear of supraspinatus tendon. **A:** A long-axis scan of supraspinatus tendon with a partial-thickness tear reveals a hypoechoic defect (*white arrow*) on the articular side of the tendon. **B:** A long-axis scan of supraspinatus tendon with a full-thickness tear reveals an irregular anechoic defect (*white asterisk*) throughout the width of the tendon. **C:** A short-axis scan of supraspinatus tendon with a full-thickness tear reveals an anechoic defect (*white asterisk*) inside the tendon and a hyperechoic line (*white arrow*) between the defect and the hypoechoic cartilage of the humeral head (cartilage interface sign).

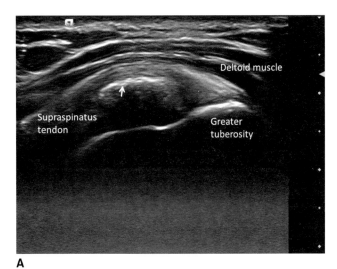

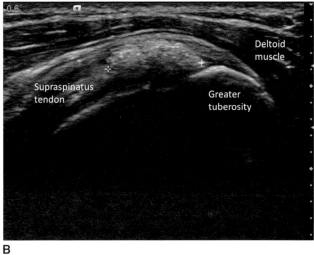

A   **B**

FIGURE 6-3. Calcific tendinopathy of supraspinatus tendon. **A:** A long-axis scan of supraspinatus tendon reveals a curvilinear hyperechoic focus (*arrow*) with faint posterior acoustic shadowing within the tendon. **B:** A long-axis scan of supraspinatus tendon reveals an intratendinous hyperechoic soft-tissue structure ("+" indicates the edges of the calcification structure).

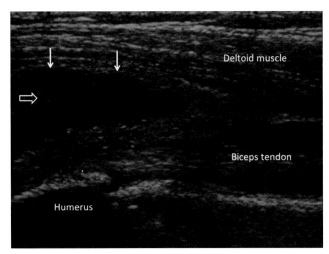

FIGURE 6-4. Subacromial-subdeltoid bursitis. Scanning parallel to the axis of the biceps tendon reveals distension of the bursa (*white arrows*), with irregular synovial thickening (*white void arrow*).

calcification, and hyperemia. In **Figure 6-6B**, the diffuse, thickened hypoechoic area with loss of normal fibrillar pattern is compatible with tendinopathy. A focal anechoic area on ultrasonography indicates a complete or partial rupture of the CET, which may require surgical intervention. As expected, calcification of the tendon can be seen as echogenic foci within the CET with or without acoustic shadow beneath the lesion (**Fig. 6-6C**). Cystic lesions can occasionally be seen around the CET. With Doppler imaging, hypervascularity of the CET (**Fig. 6-6D**) is suggestive of focal hyperemia and active inflammation.

Ulnar Collateral Ligament Rupture

An ulnar collateral ligament (UCL) tear may result from either acute or chronic valgus stress to the elbow. Repeated overhead throwing or pitching is a common cause of UCL injury (32,33). Traditionally, MRI has been widely used for assessment of UCL injury. However, U/S not only can visualize the

UCL in a static view (**Fig. 6-7A** and **B**) but also can evaluate the related structures during motion. A dynamic U/S study can assess joint laxity by comparing the degree of joint widening of both arms during valgus stress. Both U/S and MRI have been used to assess UCL injury, and their diagnostic accuracies are quite comparable (34). In another study, 26 asymptomatic major league professional baseball pitchers were assessed by U/S. When compared to the nonpitching arms, the pitching arms were found to have thicker UCL anterior bands and wider joint spaces (35).

EXAMPLES OF KNEE PATHOLOGY

Knee Effusion

For U/S detection of knee effusion, it is best to place the patient in a supine position, with a pillow below the knee, and the knee either extended or slightly bent. The transducer is placed longitudinally along the axis of quadriceps tendon (**Fig. 6-8A**). The suprapatellar recess is located between the quadriceps tendon and the prefemoral fat (**Fig. 6-8B**). The normal suprapatellar recess is slit-like, with the thickness no more than 2 mm (36). Knee effusion is demonstrated as a distended suprapatellar recess with anechoic space (**Fig. 6-8C**), which is easily compressed, and without vascularity on power Doppler imaging. In repeated injuries or inflammatory arthritis such as rheumatoid arthritis, synovium hypertrophy can occur within the suprapatellar recess. The enlarged synovium often appears as a hyperechoic mass, either attached to the wall of the suprapatellar recess or floating within it (**Fig. 6-8D**). As in other scenarios, increased synovial vascularity indicates active inflammation. If a large amount of effusion is noted after an injury, one should suspect internal knee derangement, which may be better diagnosed with MRI and arthroscopy (37).

Patellar Tendinopathy

Patients with patellar tendinopathy (also known as "jumper knee") may complain of anterior knee pain while jumping or going downstairs. Local tenderness over the patellar tendon is

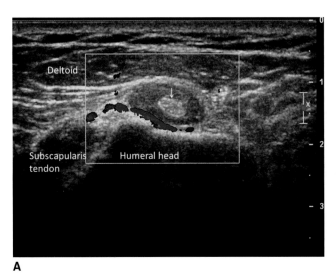

A

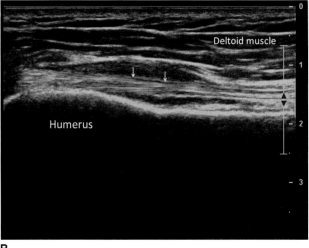

B

FIGURE 6-5. Bicipital tenosynovitis. **A:** A short-axis scan at the level of the bicipital groove shows anechoic fluid accumulation surrounding a tender, thickened biceps tendon (so called "target sign") (*white arrow*) in a patient with biceps tenosynovitis. **B:** On long-axis scan, fluid accumulation around the tendon (*white arrows*) is noted.

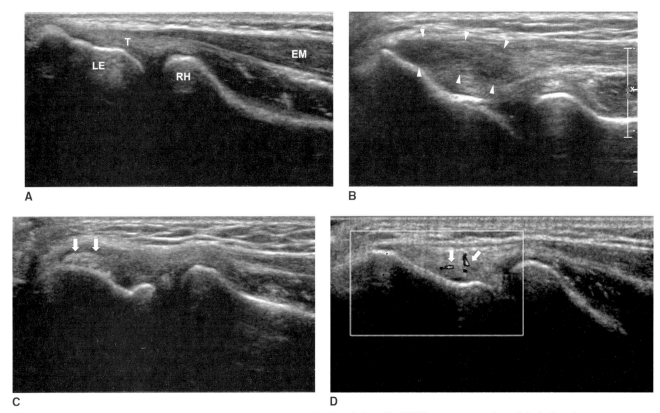

FIGURE 6-6. Lateral epicondylitis. **A:** Normal sonographic image of the lateral elbow. The CET (*T*) presents as an echogenic beak-shaped structure, while the extensor muscle (*EM*) is relatively hypoechoic. LE, lateral epicondyle; RH, radial head. **B:** Swelling of the tendon is seen as hypoechoic thickening with loss of normal fibrillar pattern (between the *arrowheads*) near its insertion. **C:** Calcification (*arrows*) deposit is seen inside the tendon. **D:** Doppler image indicates a hypervascular status inside the tendon (*arrows*). This is frequently seen in an actively inflamed tendon.

a common manifestation. When scanning the patellar tendon, the patient should be placed in supine position, with the patellar tendon tightened by flexing the knee to 60 to 80 degrees (**Fig. 6-9A**). The normal longitudinal patellar tendon should appear as parallel, fibrillar, echogenic structures (**Fig. 6-9B**). Commonly observed sonographic findings of patellar tendinopathy include loss of fibrillar pattern, reduced echogenicity, and tendon hypertrophy in comparison with the contralateral knee (38). This is demonstrated in **Figure 6-8C**. Increased vascularity on power Doppler examination (**Fig. 6-9D**) suggests an acute inflammatory process. Studies have also shown that the presence of abnormal sonographic findings in the patellar tendon, even in the absence of subjective symptomatology,

is associated with the higher risk of future patellar tendon injury (39).

Muscular Injury

Muscular injury is quite common in athletes. It may result from direct trauma or may sometimes be caused by overstretching, especially with insufficient warm-up. On U/S, normal muscle should appear as feather-like, longitudinal fibrils. Muscle tear will manifest as a disruption of muscular fibrils. An anechoic area within an injured muscle suggests hematoma or effusion (**Fig. 6-10A**). On U/S, the severity of muscle injury can be divided into three grades. In grade I injury, no obvious muscular fibril rupture is observed, indicating a minor injury.

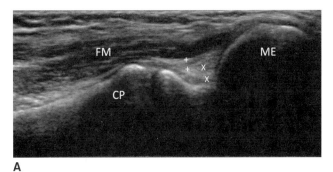

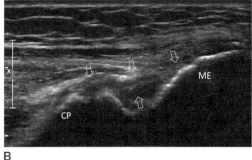

FIGURE 6-7. Elbow UCL rupture. **A:** Normal UCL. The anterior band of UCL is seen on U/S as having two components, the superficial component (between "++") and the deep component (between "xx"). **B:** Ruptured UCL showed swelling and blurring of the ligament (*open arrows*). ME, medial epicondyle of humerus; CP, coronoid process of ulnar bone; FM, flexor muscle.

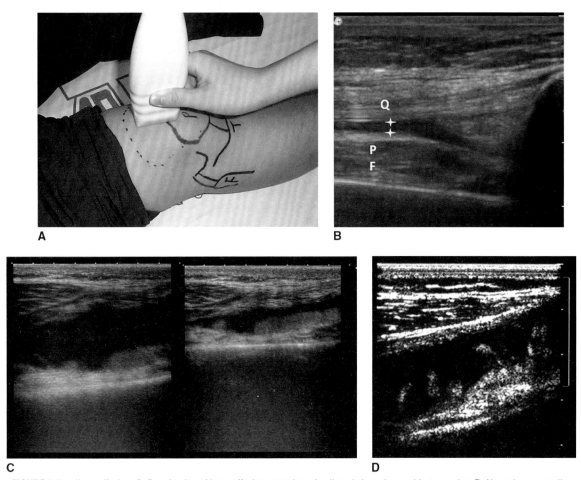

FIGURE 6-8. Knee effusion. **A:** Examination of knee effusion: transducer is aligned along the quadriceps tendon. **B:** Normal suprapatellar recess (between markers) is slit-like, located between the quadriceps (*Q*) tendon and prefemoral fat (*PF*). **C:** Effusion of knee demonstrates itself as a distended anechoic mass, which is easily compressed. **D:** Hyperechoic villus is seen floating within the suprapatellar recess.

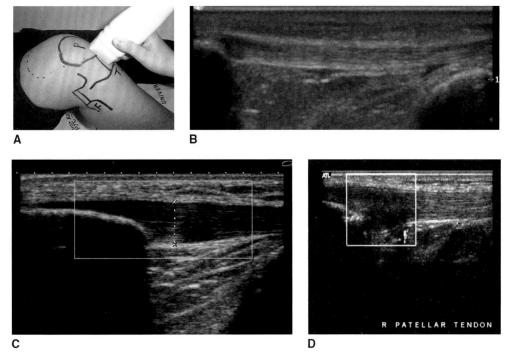

FIGURE 6-9. Patellar tendinopathy. **A:** Examination of patellar tendon: the knee is flexed to 60 to 80 degrees to stretch the patellar tendon. **B:** Normal sonogram of patellar tendon shows the typical hyperechoic fibrillar pattern. **C:** Sonogram of patellar tendon tendinopathy reveals reduced echogenicity and increased thickness. **D:** Increased vascularity of patellar tendon is revealed, indicating active inflammation of the patellar tendon.

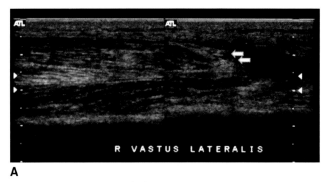
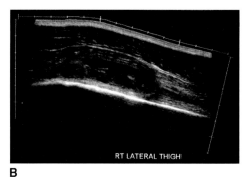

A   **B**

FIGURE 6-10.   Muscle tear. **A:** Anechoic gap is seen within the quadriceps tendon, representing a tear. The round end of the ruptured muscle is well defined on sonogram (*arrows*). **B:** A wider view of the ruptured quadriceps muscle reveals the extent of the injury.

Echogenicity of the injured muscle may be reduced due to swelling or bleeding. In grade II injury, fibrillar tear can be observed, with disruption of the normal muscular texture. An anechoic area due to either local hematoma or effusion is often apparent. Sometimes, the ruptured end of muscular fibril floats within the local effusion and is referred to as the "bell clapper sign." In grade III injury, the muscle tear is unfortunately complete. The round end of the ruptured "stump" can be seen, and the muscle gap will widen during stretching. An example of a complete quadriceps tear is seen in **Figure 6-10B**.

Posterior Cruciate Ligament Injury

Unlike the anterior cruciate ligament, the posterior cruciate ligament (PCL) can be clearly visualized on U/S examination (40). When scanning the PCL, the patient should be placed in prone position, with the knee extended. The transducer is located between the lateral margin of the medial femoral condyle and the midportion of the tibial intercondylar region (**Fig. 6-11A**). The normal PCL should appear as a hypoechoic, fan-shaped structure (**Fig. 6-11B**). Rupture is suspected when the thickness of PCL at the tibial spine is greater than 10 mm and with a waxy posterior margin (41) (**Fig. 6-11C and D**).

The above-mentioned examples present a limited selection of common musculoskeletal pathologies encountered by practicing physiatrists. Together they serve as a brief introduction to the clinical applications of musculoskeletal U/S. There are numerous other conditions that U/S can be used for diagnostic, therapeutic, and research purposes, such as for evaluation of the median nerve in carpal tunnel syndrome (42). The integrity of ankle ligaments and tendons can also be evaluated with U/S (43). Moreover, U/S characteristics of plantar fasciitis have been well established (44), and injection of steroid under U/S guidance had been shown to be effective (45). There are many other applications of U/S that are beyond the scope of this chapter. Readers are encouraged to refer to musculoskeletal U/S textbooks for more thorough descriptions (46).

CONCLUSION

The ability to perform dynamic examinations with real-time visualization and rapid side-to-side comparisons makes U/S eminently suitable for the diagnosis of musculoskeletal pathologies. In addition to assisting with initial diagnosis, U/S images can also be used in guiding needle injections and in assessing the recovery process. While helpful, musculoskeletal U/S is, by no means, a replacement for other diagnostic methods such as MRI and arthroscopy. Instead, it should be viewed as an extension of our physical examination. Limitations of

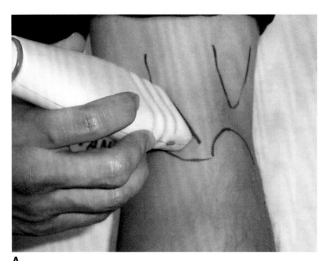
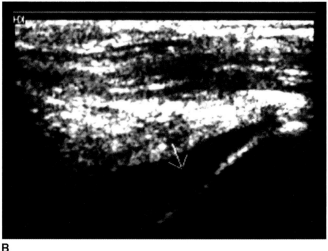

A   **B**

FIGURE 6-11.   PCL injury. **A:** The patient is in prone position, with knee extended. The transducer is aligned between the lateral margin of the medial condyle and the intercondylar region of the femur. **B:** The PCL reveals itself as fan-like hypoechoic band due to anisotropy (*arrow*).

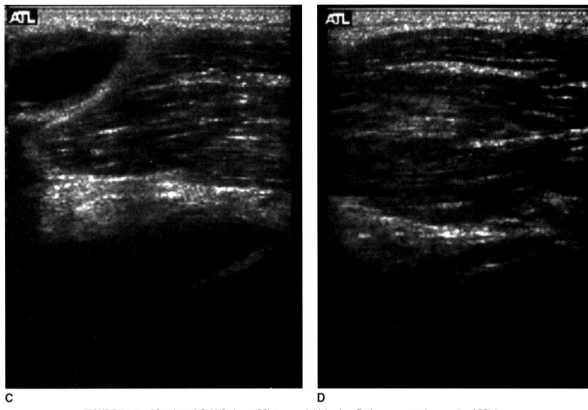

C   **D**

FIGURE 6-11. (*Continued*) **C:** U/S shows PCL tear and thickening. **D:** A waxy posterior margin of PCL is seen.

U/S include its dependence on the experience of the operator and a relatively long learning curve. Adequate training and supervision may minimize these limitations; however, training opportunities and certification for musculoskeletal U/S are currently not standardized. Despite these limitations, U/S, when used appropriately, provides an important adjunct to physical examination to aid in the diagnosis and thus in the treatment of common musculoskeletal pathologies.

REFERENCES

1. Lew HL, Chen CP, Wang TG, et al. Diagnostic ultrasound in musculoskeletal medicine. Part 1: introduction and examination of the upper limb. *Am J Phys Med Rehabil*. 2007;86(4):310–321.
2. Chew K, Stevens K, Wang TG, et al. Introduction to diagnostic musculoskeletal ultrasound. Part 2: examination of the lower limb. *Am J Phys Med Rehabil*. 2008;87(3):238–248.
3. Fornage BD. *Ultrasound of the Extremities*. Paris: Vigot; 1991.
4. Chen MJL, Lew HL, Hsu TZ, et al. Ultrasound-guided shoulder injections in the treatment of subacromial bursitis. *Am J Phys Med Rehabil*. 2006;85:31–35.
5. Tsai WC, Hsu TZ, Chen CPC, et al. Plantar fasciitis treated with local steroid injection: comparison between sonographic and palpation guidance. *J Clin Ultrasound*. 2006;34:12–16.
6. Marhofer P, Schrogendorfer K, Koinig H, et al. Ultrasonographic guidance improves sensory block and onset time of three-in-one blocks. *Anesth Analg*. 1997;85:854–857.
7. Marhofer P, Schrogendorfer K, Wallner T, et al. Ultrasonographic guidance reduces the amount of local anesthetic for 3-in-1 blocks. *Reg Anesth Pain Med*. 1998;23:584–588.
8. Chen CPC, Tang SFT, Hsu TZ, et al. Ultrasound guidance in caudal epidural needle placement. *Anesthesiology*. 2004;101:181–184.
9. Pekkafalı MZ, Kıralp MZ, Başekim CÇ, et al. Sacroiliac joint injections: performed with sonographic guidance. *J Ultrasound Med*. 2003;22:553–559.
10. Greher M, Scharbert G, Kamolz LP, et al. Ultrasound-guided lumbar facet nerve block: a sonoanatomic study of a new methodologic approach. *Anesthesiology*. 2004;100:1242–1248.
11. Galiano K, Obwegeser AA, Bodner G, et al. Ultrasound guidance for facet joint injections in the lumbar spine: a computed tomography-controlled feasibility study. *Anesth Analg*. 2005;101:579–583.
12. van Holsbeeck MT, Kolowich PA, Eyler WR, et al. US depiction of partial-thickness tear of the rotator cuff. *Radiology*. 1995;197(2):443–446.
13. Naredo E, Moller I, Moragues C, et al. Interobserver reliability in musculoskeletal ultrasonography: results from a "Teach the Teachers" rheumatologist course. *Ann Rheum Dis*. 2006;65(1):14–19.
14. Middleton WD, Teefey SA, Yamaguchi K. Sonography of the rotator cuff: analysis of interobserver variability. *AJR Am J Roentgenol*. 2004;183(5):1465–1468.
15. Teefey SA, Hasan SA, Middleton WD, et al. Ultrasonography of the rotator cuff. A comparison of ultrasonographic and arthroscopic findings in one hundred consecutive cases. *J Bone Joint Surg Am*. 2000;82(4):498–504.
16. Teefey SA, Rubin DA, Middleton WD, et al. Detection and quantification of rotator cuff tears. Comparison of ultrasonographic, magnetic resonance imaging, and arthroscopic findings in seventy-one consecutive cases. *J Bone Joint Surg Am*. 2004;86-A(4):708–716.
17. Smith TO, Back T, Toms AP, et al. Diagnostic accuracy of ultrasound for rotator cuff tears in adults: a systematic review and meta-analysis. *Clin Radiol*. 2011;66(11):1036–1048.
18. Chang KV, Chen WS, Wang TG, et al. Quantitative ultrasound facilitates the exploration of morphological association of the long head biceps tendon with supraspinatus tendon full thickness tear. *PLoS One*. 2014;9(11):e113803.
19. Sansone V, Consonni O, Maiorano E, et al. Calcific tendinopathy of the rotator cuff: the correlation between pain and imaging features in symptomatic and asymptomatic female shoulders. *Skeletal Radiol*. 2016;45(1):49–55.
20. Serafini G, Sconfienza LM, Lacelli F, et al. Rotator cuff calcific tendonitis: short-term and 10-year outcomes after two-needle us-guided percutaneous treatment—nonrandomized controlled trial. *Radiology*. 2009;252(1):157–164.
21. Reid DC. *Sports Injury Assessment and Rehabilitation*. New York: Churchill Livingstone; 1992.
22. van Holsbeeck M, Introcaso J. Sonography of the postoperative shoulder. *AJR Am J Roentgenol*. 1989;152(1):202.
23. van Holsbeeck M, Strouse PJ. Sonography of the shoulder: evaluation of the sub-acromial-subdeltoid bursa. *AJR Am J Roentgenol*. 1993;160(3):561–564.
24. Holtby R, Razmjou H. Accuracy of the Speed's and Yergason's tests in detecting biceps pathology and SLAP lesions: comparison with arthroscopic findings. *Arthroscopy*. 2004;20(3):231–236.
25. Naredo E, Aguado P, De Miguel E, et al. Painful shoulder: comparison of physical examination and ultrasonographic findings. *Ann Rheum Dis*. 2002;61(2):132–136.
26. Chang KV, Wu SH, Lin SH, et al. Power Doppler presentation of shoulders with biceps disorder. *Arch Phys Med Rehabil*. 2010;91(4):624–631.
27. McNally E. *Practical Musculoskeletal Ultrasound*. Philadelphia, PA: Elsevier Churchill Livingstone; 2005.
28. Dondelinger RF. *Peripheral Musculoskeletal Ultrasound Atlas*. Stuttgart, Germany; New York: G. Thieme Verlag; Thieme Medical Publishers; 1996.

29. Regan W, Wold LE, Coonrad R, et al. Microscopic histopathology of chronic refractory lateral epicondylitis. *Am J Sports Med*. 1992;20:746–749.

30. Chiang YP, Hsieh SF, Lew HL. The role of ultrasonography in the differential diagnosis and treatment of tennis elbow. *Am J Phys Med Rehabil*. 2012;91: 94–95.

31. Wang YC, Lew RJ, Lee CW, et al. Adding a transverse scan in the ultrasound diagnosis of extensor tendinopathy. *Am J Phys Med Rehabil*. 2017;96(5):e93–e94.

32. Azar FM, Andrews JR, Wilk KE, et al. Operative treatment of ulnar collateral ligament injuries of the elbow in athletes. *Am J Sports Med*. 2000;28:16–23.

33. Hyman J, Breazeale NM, Altchek DW. Valgus instability of the elbow in athletes. *Clin Sports Med*. 2001;20:25–45, viii.

34. De Smet AA, Winter TC, Best TM, et al. Dynamic sonography with valgus stress to assess elbow ulnar collateral ligament injury in baseball pitchers. *Skeletal Radiol*. 2002;31:671–676.

35. Nazarian LN, McShane JM, Ciccotti MG, et al. Dynamic US of the anterior band of the ulnar collateral ligament of the elbow in asymptomatic major league baseball pitchers. *Radiology*. 2003;227:149–154.

36. Delaunoy I, Feipel V, Appelboom T, et al. Sonography detection threshold for knee effusion. *Clin Rheumatol*. 2003;22(6):391–392.

37. Wang CY, Wang HK, Hsu CY, et al. Role of sonographic examination in traumatic knee internal derangement. *Arch Phys Med Rehabil*. 2007;88(8):984–987.

38. Na YC, Wang C-L, Shieh JY, et al. Ultrasonographic examination of patellar tendinitis. *Formos J Med*. 1999;3(1):20–25.

39. Malliaras P, Cook J. Patellar tendons with normal imaging and pain: change in imaging and pain status over a volleyball season. *Clin J Sport Med*. 2006;16(5):388–391.

40. Wang TG, Wang CL, Hsu TC, et al. Sonographic evaluation of the posterior cruciate ligament in amputated specimens and normal subjects. *J Ultrasound Med*. 1999;18(9):647–653.

41. Chew K, Stevens K, Wang TG, et al. Introduction to musculoskeletal diagnostic ultrasound, part II: examination of the lower limb. *Am J Phys Med Rehabil*. 2008;87(3):238–248.

42. Sernik RA, et al. Ultrasound features of carpal tunnel syndrome: a prospective case-control study. *Skeletal Radiol*. 2008;37(1):49–53.

43. Khoury V, et al. Ultrasound of ankle and foot: overuse and sports injuries. *Semin Musculoskelet Radiol*. 2007;11(2):149–161.

44. Wu CH, Chen WS, Wang TG. Plantar fascia softening in plantar fasciitis with normal B-mode sonography. *Skeletal Radiol*. 2015;44:1603–1607.

45. Tsai WC, et al. Treatment of proximal plantar fasciitis with ultrasound-guided steroid injection. *Arch Phys Med Rehabil*. 2000;81(10):1416–1421.

46. Batmaz İ, Malas FU, Özçakar L. Ultrasound Evaluation of the knee. In: Özçakar L, ed. *Musculoskeletal Ultrasound in Physical and Rehabilitation Medicine*. Milan, Italy: Edi-Ermes; 2014:99–110.

CHAPTER 7

Carolyn M. Baum
Timothy J. Wolf
Samuel Talisman

Functional Evaluation and Management of Self-Care and Other Activities of Daily Living

DEFINING ACTIVITIES OF DAILY LIFE

As we address the Functional Evaluation and Management of Self-Care and Other Activities of Daily Living, it is necessary for us to give context to the changes that Activities of Daily Living have undergone since it was first conceptualized as a record of achievement (1) and in the 1940s as the physical demands of daily life. In the 1950s, Rehabilitation Medicine used the term functional therapy to address the activities of daily life. Dr. Coulter (2) described functional therapy as "prescribed activities planned to assist in the restoration of articular and muscular function" (p. 452); Bennett (3) described the specific use of physical, occupational, and recreational therapy to assist the patient to "pass" the test items representing the common obstacles encountered in daily living in a normal environment (p. 351). Buchwald (4) described functional training as the physical reconditioning of the patient through a carefully devised exercise and activity program to make him (or her) able to handle his (or her) body in the most efficient way, so as to be as independent as possible.

There have been some major advances in our understanding and the importance of activities of daily living since these early times in rehabilitation. Science has expanded our understanding of how motor, cognitive, sensory, psychological, and physiologic issues contribute to function and performance in daily life. In addition to the advances in science, the rehabilitation community has been highly influenced by the changes in policy initiated by the disability community in an effort to demedicalize the issues faced by individuals who live with challenges that result in problems that are not fully addressed by medical recovery. These individuals require an inclusive environment to be independent. A major international initiative has influenced the delivery of rehabilitation services. The International Classification of Functioning, Disability, and Health, known more commonly as ICF (a classification of function and health), was developed by consumers and rehabilitation professionals and was adopted by the WHO member states in 1991 (5). The ICF requires the rehabilitation community to address the activities, participation, and environmental needs that will enable them to overcome the barriers that limit their performance, as they return to their communities to live their lives and manage their health.

Rehabilitation has traditionally relied on a measure of functional independence (FIM) to report the patient's capacity for activities of daily learning (ADL). As rehabilitation is asked to focus on participation and community integration, the FIM does not indicate the person's capacity to perform Instrumental Activities of Daily Living (IADL), which includes not only caring for self but also caring for others, maintaining a household, and using community resources. This chapter addresses this expanded approach that rehabilitation professionals must assess and address to manage the issues that an impairment can have on the daily lives of the people that they will serve in their rehabilitation programs.

Figure 7-1 demonstrates FIM scores for 911 persons 6 month following discharge from a major U.S. hospital for stroke. With few exceptions, people who had FIM scores even from 108 to 126 had not fully reintegrated into their communities as measured by the Reintegration to Normal Living (**Fig. 7-1**). These data support the importance for rehabilitation professionals to introduce community integration to address the residual IADL problems that are faced when home and trying to get back to family, work, and community activities demanded by their roles.

Given the complexity of addressing the issues that underlie the assessment and intervention of activities of daily living, it is helpful to use the Person-Environment-Occupational-Performance model (6) to organize this chapter to prepare rehabilitation professionals to address the needs of our patients in an interdisciplinary and continuum of care model.

THE PERSON-ENVIRONMENT-OCCUPATIONAL-PERFORMANCE MODEL

The Person-Environment-Occupation-Performance (PEOP) model (6) is a conceptual representation of a system or process and the relationships among its components. All aspects of the model must be addressed in rehabilitation interventions to prepare the patients to reengage in their lives after an illness or disability has either temporarily or permanently altered their ability to carry out the activities and participate in their daily lives.

PEOP has drawn on theories that provide a developmental context and support our understanding of what people do.

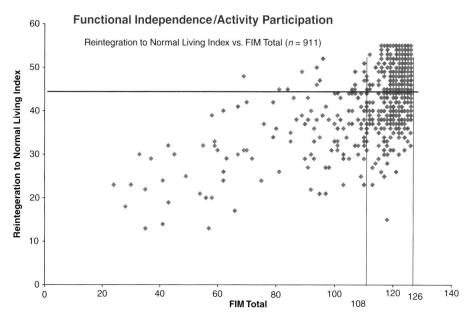

FIGURE 7-1.   A typically used measure to record activities of daily living in the United States and in some international rehabilitation facilities is the functional independence measure (FIM) x. It gives a picture in time of the level of independence of a person across the basic level of physical and cognitive functions. The score indicates the level of assistance the person needs. A score of 6, or modified independence (a total score of 108), reports that the person may use a device but needs no physical assistance.

PEOP has adopted principles that recognize the value and characteristics of daily activities within a developmental perspective including (a) the drive for engagement; (b) the complex and multidimensional nature of body systems and body function factors; (c) the importance of the environmental context; and (d) influence of daily activities on health and well-being of the individual (6). **Figure 7-2** produces an overview of the model.

Rehabilitation professionals can never know the whole story of the person-environment-occupation-performance for an individual. However, effective services require the incorporation of the patient's perspective as much as possible in evaluations, interventions, and outcome measures. A *narrative* provides "important background information from the client in a story format that describes the perception of the current situation and is used to establish goals" (7). In a personal narrative, rehabilitation professionals learn about the patient's perceptions and meanings, choices and responsibilities, and attitudes and motivations.

Person factors are "factors intrinsic to individual(s) that include psychological, cognitive, sensory, motor, physiological, and meaning/sense-making/spiritual characteristics that support or limit occupational performance" (7). *Psychological factors* include motivation, self-concept, self-esteem, sense of identity, self-efficacy, metacognition, self-awareness, emotional state, and narrative. *Cognition* includes memory, thought organization, attention, awareness, reasoning, decision-making, and executive function. *Sensory factors* (somatosensory, olfactory, gustatory, visual, auditory, proprioceptive, and tactile senses) and *motor factors* (motor learning, motor planning [praxis], postural control, motor learning) are associated with the neurobehavioral systems. *Physiologic* factors

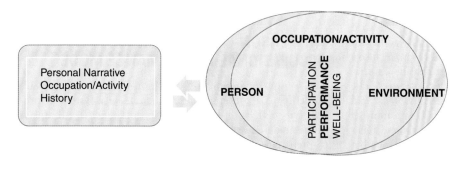

PEOP Model: Enabling Everyday Living

Occupational performance (doing) enables participation (engagement) in everyday life That contributes to the well-being (health and quality of life) of individuals. Adapted from the PEOP MODEL (Baum, Christiansen & Bass, 2015)

FIGURE 7-2.   Person-environment-occupation-performance (PEOP) model. (Adapted from Christiansen CH, Baum CM, Bass JD. *Occupational Therapy: Performance, Participation, and Well-Being.* 4th ed. Thorofare, NJ: Slack Incorporated; 2014. Reprinted with permission from SLACK Incorporated.)

TABLE 7-1	**Occupational/Activity Assessments**		
Occupational/Activity Assessments History	**Self-Report/ Performance**	**Description**	**Where It Can Be Obtained**
Canadian Occupational Performance Measure (COPM)		A measure of client's perceived occupational performance in self-care, productivity, and leisure. The client rates each occupation according to importance, performance, and satisfaction on a 10-pt scale.	Canadian Association of Occupational Therapists: www.caot.ca or www.thecopm.ca
Activity Card Sort (ACS)	Self-report	An instrument to help clients describe their engagement in social, instrumental, and leisure activities before and after a medical event.	American Occupational Therapy Association: www.aota.org
Occupational Performance History Interview (OPHI-II)	Self-report	A subjective measure that uses semistructured interview, rating scale, and life history narrative to identify themes of occupational adaptation including occupational identity, occupational competence, and the impact of occupational behavior settings.	American Occupational Therapy Association: www.aota.org
Activity Measure for Post–Acute Care (AM-PAC)	Performance	An item bank of functional activities likely to be encountered by most adults during daily routines within the context of either an inpatient episode of care or outpatient postacute services (8).	Boston University Activity Measure for Post–Acute Care: am-pac.com

include strength, endurance, flexibility, activity levels, stress, sleep patterns, nutrition, and general health.

Environment factors are "factors extrinsic to individual(s) that include culture, social, physical and natural, policy, and technology characteristics that support or limit occupational performance" (7). *Cultural factors* include values, beliefs, customs, rituals, and time use. *Social factors* address social determinants of health, social support, and social capital. *Physical factors* include the physical and natural environment with features such as accessibility, usability, geography, terrain, climate, and air quality along with the technology characteristics of tools and assistive devices. *Policy factors* include all the characteristics that govern or influence access to resources. *Technology* includes an array of general and specific supports for performance in mobility, communication, and occupations requiring sensory, cognitive, or manipulation function. All of these factors contribute to a person's capacity to perform his or her activities of daily living, and collectively, the rehabilitation team must understand how to recognize the problems that must be addressed in rehabilitation and working with the patient and family to prepare for discharge.

OVERVIEW OF THE ISSUES THAT IMPACT FUNCTION

Each rehabilitation discipline will contribute to the functional assessment of the patient to understand how the capabilities of the person and the barriers they will face must be considered in their recovery and community reintegration phases after rehabilitation. This is not intended to be a comprehensive review or list of measures but rather an overview of commonly employed measures used in clinical practice. The decision as to which tools to use depends on the client's condition, the client's goals, the point in recovery at which the assessment is being used, the therapist's training, as well as any restrictions/preferences from the facility where the assessment is taking place.

Occupation/activity or the things people do every day include the activities, tasks, and roles that individuals want and need to do as they execute tasks and are engaged and involved

in the situations that contribute to their well-being and quality of life (7). **Table 7-1** identifies measures to determine what a patient has done before a rehabilitation admission.

Factors That Support Activities of Daily Life

Each of the factors in the PEOP model will be introduced in the context of how they impact daily life and why they must be addressed by physicians, therapists, and nurses when they provide the critical rehabilitation services. Measures that relate to each factor are included in the tables. **Table 7-2** identifies traditional ADL measures that record basic activities of daily living.

Cognition

A typical adult needs cognitive functions to participate in everyday life. These functions include attention, memory, social awareness, communication, executive functions, and awareness (9). Disabilities often cause disruptions in cognitive processes, making it harder to engage in daily activities. A majority of patients with cognitive impairments have associated deficits in activities of daily living, occupational engagement, and rehabilitative success (10,11). There is often a relationship between cognitive impact and depression, which contributes to impairments in social skills, work, and role functioning (12,13).

Cognition may be impaired in unpredictable and various ways. A number of cognitive functions must be screened for memory, attention, processing speed, executive functioning, language, and visuospatial abilities (14,15) as they often go unnoticed especially if the impacts are not obvious. This means rehabilitation patients may not know that they are living with cognitive impairment, leaving these consequences untreated, even though daily activities may be affected (16).

The higher-level cognitive impairments associated with neurologic and metabolic conditions are complicated when there are concurrent mental health issues. Executive functioning includes higher-level cognitive processes, like controlling actions, judgment, and decision-making, which are important to performance in all occupations (17). Executive functioning issues are prevalent in the rehabilitation population and are also common in people with depression (10,18,19). People

TABLE 7-2	Activity of Daily Living Assessments		
Activities of Daily Living Assessments	**Self-Report/ Performance**	**Description**	**Where It Can Be Obtained**
Functional Independence Measure (FIM)	Performance	An objective measure of disability according to the level of assistance required to perform self-care, communication, and cognitive activities.	Uniform Data System for Medical Rehabilitation: www.udsmr.org
Barthel Index (BI)	Performance	An assessment of functional independence in personal care and mobility for hospitalized patients with neuromuscular or musculoskeletal disorders.	Internet Stroke Center: www.stroke-center.org
Arnadottir OT-ADL Neurobehavioral Evaluation (A-ONE)	Performance	An assessment used to identify neurobehavioral dysfunctions and how they relate to functional performance deficits. The client performs a series of ADL tasks that are scored according to a Functional Independence Scale (FIS) and a Neurobehavioral Impairment Scale (NIS).	Cote R, Hachinski V, Shurvell B, et al. The Canadian Neurological Scale: a preliminary study in acute stroke. *Stroke*. 1986;17(4):731–737.

with depression score lower on executive function tasks and have limited ability to inhibit irrelevant information when working on a task, an important executive feature to completing tasks efficiently (18). In addition, people with depression are slower to complete executive functioning tasks, consistent with findings that processing speed is severely impacted by depression (12,20). Executive functioning is an indicator of functional status, predicting recovery from disability participation in rehabilitation, and functional independence (14,15,21). Limitations in executive dysfunction are predictive of poor functional outcomes (19).

The rehabilitation team must identify the cognitive issues the patient is experiencing. If patients require repeated instruction, additional cueing, or reminders to stay focused, a neuropsychological examination and a functional cognition assessment is warranted and treatment must help patients employ strategies to manage the tasks that will support their accomplishment of goals.

Table 7-3 identifies measures to assess cognitive performance in IADL.

Table 7-4 identifies common assessments to identify cognitive issues faced by patients.

Psychological

The mental health issues occurring with many individuals receiving rehabilitation include loss of sense of self, uncertainty about the future, stress over the loss of social relationships, and feelings of guilt; all may lead to depression and anxiety (22). Furthermore, frustration, sadness, and distress may come from the limitations of imposing feelings of overwhelming life changes (22). There is a cyclical relationship that may follow mental health issues, wherein distress prevents engagement in social activities, leading to further distress. These depressive and anxious thought pathways are the same that cause impairments in other areas. For example, apathy and loss of pleasure in activities, which are symptoms of depression, may lead to lower effort during demanding tasks, leading to lower performance (17).

Mental health problems that impact psychological functioning also affect engagement in everyday life. Lowered self-efficacy relates to a lack of confidence in one's own performance, which is associated with lower independence in daily activities (23). Changes in personality, which can take various unpredictable forms, can alter a person's perceived identity (24). Lowered self-esteem and emotional regulation issues may limit a person's emotional adjustment to new circumstances

TABLE 7-3	Instrumental Activities of Daily Living Assessments		
Instrumental Activities of Daily Living Assessments	**Self-Report/ Performance**	**Description**	**Where It Can Be Obtained**
Performance Assessment of Self-Care Skills (PASS)	Performance	A measure of the client's ability to live independently and safely in the community based on 26 ADL/IADL tasks. Performance components of each task include independence, adequacy, and safety.	The assessment can be obtained by contacting: PASS@shrs.pitt.edu
Assessment of Motor and Process Skills (AMPS)	Performance	An assessment of motor and process skills observed in ADL/IADL tasks. Quality of performance is assessed in terms of effort, efficiency, safety, and independence in 16 motor and 20 process skill items.	The AMPS manual and software can be purchased online at www.ampsintl.com
Lawton Instrumental Activities of Daily Living Scale (IADLS)	Self and proxy-report	An interview of a person's ability to perform 8 IADL tasks, including telephone use, shopping, meal prep, housekeeping, laundry, transportation, medication management, and finances.	Graf C. The Lawton Instrumental Activities of Daily Living Scale. *Am J Nurs*. 2008;108(4):52–62.
Fitness to Drive Screening (FTDS)	Proxy-report	A computerized screening tool that assesses driving habits and skills in order to identify at-risk older drivers. Completed by family members and/or caregivers.	www.fitnesstodrivescreening.com

TABLE 7-4	Cognitive Assessments		
Cognition Assessments	**Self-Report/Performance**	**Description**	**Where It Can Be Obtained**
Montreal Cognitive Assessment (MoCA)	Performance	A rapid screen of global cognitive abilities designed to detect mild cognitive impairment.	http://www.mocatest.org/
Executive Function Performance Test (EFPT)	Performance	An assessment of executive functioning in task performance in simple cooking, telephone use, medication management, and bill payment. Performance components of each task include initiation, organization, sequencing, judgment and safety, and completion.	Program in Occupational Therapy, Washington University School of Medicine: www.ot.wustl.edu/about/resources/assessment
Behavioral Inattention Test (BIT)	Performance	A performance-based assessment designed to provide information about the interference of visual inattention and unilateral spatial neglect in daily activities.	Pearson: www.pearsonclinical.com
Self-Awareness of Deficits Interview (SADI)	Self-report	Assesses intellectual awareness via semistructured interviews. Specifically measures awareness of deficits, awareness of functional consequences of deficits, and ability to set realistic goals for the future.	Contact the author, Jennifer Flemming, PhD: j.flemming@uq.edu.au
Complex Task Performance Assessment (CTPA)	Performance	A performance-based, work-oriented assessment of executive function.	Program in Occupational Therapy, Washington University School of Medicine: www.ot.wustl.edu/about/resources/assessment

(25). Finally, apathy can impact motivation to participate in daily life and recovery (26).

Because these mental health issues will affect a person's ability to sustain motivation for rehabilitation and daily life activities, planning for managing these psychosocial issues must be included in the case plan.

Table 7-5 lists psychological assessments to identify patients who may need psychological services.

Physiologic

The bodily responses that change in people receiving rehabilitation are as remarkable as the changes in the brain. Sleep and appetite disturbances are common (27). Psychological stress is shown to activate the sympathetic nervous system, which causes a physiologic increase in blood pressure and atherosclerosis (28). The acute fatigue caused by lower physical fitness impairs long-term physical health and is also associated with lower health-related quality of life and thoughts about suicide (29–31). Complications such as depression and apathy decrease desire to participate in exercise rehabilitation activities, which would otherwise lead to improved fitness (32,33).

Patients with higher pain levels are more likely to have depression than those without pain and are more likely to have suicidal thoughts (34). Psychological stressors, such as decreased social participation, can cause activation of physical pain as well as emotional pain (35).

Problems with sexual responses in persons with neurologic, mental, and physical health issues relate to an altered experience of sexuality and sexual activity. Personality changes from acquiring a disability can cause a person to appear less sexually desirable, especially considering changes such as irritability are not compatible with a sexual mood (36). People with depression report negative feelings from unresolved sexual problems such as "anger, abandonment, helplessness, or aversion," further decreasing the likelihood of sexual activity due to this negative association (36).

Issues of sleep, pain, and sexuality must be addressed as part of the rehabilitation plan as they are central to how a person will manage his or her daily life activities as the person returns to roles and responsibilities after discharge.

Table 7-6 identifies physiologic measures to help in case of planning.

TABLE 7-5	Psychological Assessments		
Psychological Assessments	**Self-Report/Performance**	**Description**	**Where It Can Be Obtained**
Center for Epidemiologic Studies Depression Scale (CES-D)	Self-report	A self-report measure that assesses the severity of symptoms of depression.	Radloff LS. The CES-D Scale: a self-reported depression scale for research in the general population. *Appl Psychol Meas.* 1997;1:385–401.
State-Trait Anxiety Inventory (STAI)	Self-report	A self-report measure that assesses the presence and severity of symptoms of anxiety in terms of current feelings (state) and long-term anxiety.	Mind Garden Inc.: http://www.mindgarden.com
Beck Depression Scale	Self-report	A screening tool that quantifies severity of depression.	Pearson: www.pearsonclinical.com

TABLE 7-6	Physiologic Assessments		
Physiologic Assessments	**Self-Report/Performance**	**Description**	**Where It Can Be Obtained**
Berg Balance Scale	Performance	A 14-item assessment of fall risk in adult populations.	Internet Stroke Center: www.strokecenter.org
6-Minute Walk Test	Performance	An assessment of aerobic capacity/endurance as determined by distance walked over 6 minutes.	Rehab Measures: www.rehabmeasures.org
Epworth Sleepiness Scale (ESS)	Self-report	A subjective measure of a client's tendency to feel sleepy in daily occupations.	www.epworthsleepinessscale.com
Pain Intensity Scale: Numerical Rating Scale (NRS) and Visual Analog Scale (VAS)	Self-report	A scale that prompts the patient to quantify pain according to intensity of the experience. Rating scale may be numeric (0 = no pain, 10 = worst pain imaginable) or visual (facial expressions of discomfort).	Universally available

Motor

Most rehabilitation patients have changes in movement as well, compromising a person's capacity for complicated movements essential to daily tasks. The movements of both upper and lower extremities may be impacted. While physical activity can help with the recovery from deficits, patients with diminished mental health are overall less active and participate less than other people (32,37). Motivation, which is impacted by issues such as depression, may limit desire to engage in activity and motor recovery (33,38).

Limited motor recovery may cause long-term problems with activities of daily living (39). Plateaus in motor recovery may cause frustration and sadness, contributing to greater mental health issues (33). Depression lowers the ability to use sensory feedback to facilitate motor recovery and motor learning (40). Motivation, which is impacted by issues such as depression, also influences motor recovery (33,38). Decreased desire to participate in exercise activities limits the benefits of rehabilitation (32,33). The mental health effects on motor recovery show a cycle between decreased motor functioning and decreased mental health.

Decreased mobility is related to declines in mental health, which is also linked to reduction in activity and participation that may otherwise facilitate balance recovery (41,42). Reduced self-efficacy in balance and in falls are both linked to worse balance, motor and physical functioning, and perceived

health status (41). Balance and falls self-efficacy is also related to less activity and participation, more so than physical problems (41). Self-efficacy problems complete a cycle of fear of falling, where decreased participation in activities leads to decreased balance and strength, leading to further fear of falling and avoidance of activities (43).

Rehabilitation traditionally focuses on motor problems. The related problems of depression and poor motivation must be addressed to help people and their families realize the impact on balance, fall risk decreased activities.

Table 7-7 identifies common motor tests.

Sensory

A sense of hope and continued effort in rehabilitation are important to recovery (44). Therefore, the feelings of hopelessness and decreased motivation typified by depression and other mental health issues may hinder sensory recovery, similar to motor recovery (33). The sensory changes that occur in rehabilitation patients are difficult to predict as are the impacts of sensory changes on daily life (45). Hearing impairments such as sound recognition and localization are associated with severe functional limitation and less safety during daily activities (45,46). Changes in olfaction and gustatory functioning are associated with performance and participation changes, such as difficulties preparing and eating food and increased social isolation (47). Poor olfactory functioning also impacts

TABLE 7-7	Motor Assessments		
Motor Assessments	**Self-Report/Performance**	**Description**	**Where It Can Be Obtained**
Wolf Motor Function Test	Performance	Quantitative assessment of upper extremity motor deficits as observed through functional tasks.	http://stroke.ahajournals.org/content/strokeaha/32/7/1635.full.pdf
Block and Box	Performance	An objective measure of unilateral gross manual dexterity.	Kit available for purchase from Patterson Medical: www.pattersonmedical.com
Action Research Arm Test	Performance	A quantitative measure of upper extremity functioning as observed through grasp, grip, pinch, and gross movements.	Internet Stroke Center: www.strokecenter.org
Functional Reach	Performance	An assessment of dynamic functional reach by measuring the maximum distance one can reach forward while maintaining balance in a fixed standing position. The modified version conducts the assessment from a fixed sitting position.	Rehab Measures: www.rehabmeasures.org

mental health through depression and mood changes (47,48). Mental health factors such as personality changes and social changes may impact vestibular perception (33,49). In return, the vestibular system may affect mental factors such as self-consciousness, mood, and depression (49).

Somatosensation, that is, information regarding the body surface and its interaction with the environment, is important to motor performance of daily life skills and use of limbs in daily activities (50–52). Somatosensation impairments limit motor recovery, as the deficits may lead to ignorance of impaired limbs, preventing their use in activities (50). When attempting to recover from such impairments, emotions such as frustration, despair, and self-worthlessness, and changes in self-confidence and personal identity, may arise from somatosensory function loss (52). Patients must be taught to pay increased attention to affected limbs to facilitate somatosensory function, but mental stress may decrease the person's attentional capacity (53,54).

Visual deficits may damage participation and performance in a breadth of daily activities, including reading, outdoor mobility, driving, leisure, and shopping (51,55). The limitations in daily activities following vision impairment may contribute to low self-esteem and self-efficacy, which then further limit daily participation and performance (33).

Sensory issues and their resolution relate to a person's sense of meaning throughout his or her rehabilitation. The rehabilitation team must recognize the sensory issues of vision, auditory, gustatory, and olfactory in addition to the somatosensory and vestibular issues as they all support the daily life activities associated with nutrition, safety, and pleasure in daily life activities.

Table 7-8 identifies common sensory tests to use in planning care.

Social Support

Social support involves the person having supportive resources including emotional support, tougher support, informational support, and companionship (56). From our medical training, we have long understood the environment at the cellular level. As we work with people who receive our care to recover and adjust to a new self, we must understand how the environment gives context and support to their recovery and adaptation.

Developing social support improves depression, functional ability, and health-related quality of life (57,58). However, more disability is associated with overall lower levels of social support, and this association is intensified in people with mental health issues (59,60). Additionally, people with higher levels of functional impairment or depression may benefit less from increased social support than others (60). The poor social support rehabilitation patients receive is associated with depression and worse treatment outcomes, further damaging their recovery and their mental health, and increasing the need for health care services (61,62).

The type of social support received may explain how the support impacts a person's abilities and mental health. Perceived social support is associated with depression and depressive symptoms, while actual social support is not consistently reported to be (61). This perceived functional support is also related to integrating into the community, as well as personal optimism, subjective well-being, and meaning in life (63,64).

Most social support is provided by informal caregivers, who are not paid and are often family. They are central to managing patients' physical, emotional, and physical and safety needs (65). Community integration requires maintaining social support. The patient may have physical and cognitive issues, which increase the dependency on others to perform activities, complicated by a lack of transport, which may contribute to decreases in socially related activities (61). Fear of falling, anxiety over walking, and self-consciousness also prevent engagement in social activities, as patients may choose not to go out in order to protect their self-esteem (61,66).

All of these issues require that caregivers and friends understand the importance of social support in supporting people's activities as they make the transition to home. The rehabilitation team should look for ways to bring friends and family into rehabilitation facilities to help the patient engage in activities and conversation to encourage social support.

Culture

A person's race, ethnicity, age, religion, or language is often how people are culturally classified (67). However, this ignores the complicated interactions between these elements, as well as how the person experiences them. Understanding the unique

TABLE 7-8	Sensory Assessments			
Sensory Assessments	**Self-Report/Performance**	**Description**		**Where It Can Be Obtained**
Semmes-Weinstein monofilaments	Performance	A quantitative test of light touch detection and deep touch.		Commercially available through: www.amazon.com; www.pattersonmedical.com; www.alimed.com
Wrist Position Test	Performance	A quantitative test of limb positioning sense at the wrist.		SENSe Manual can be purchased through: www.florey.edu.au/stroke
Light House Near Acuity	Performance	A criterion-referenced, objective measure of near visual acuity with use of a lettered visual acuity card.		Optelec: www.shoplowvision.com
Whisper Test	Performance	An assessment of hearing loss in adult populations.		No purchase necessary
Odor Identification Test	Performance	An assessment of odor identification through presentation of familiar smells which the client identifies by choosing from a set of possible names or pictures.		www.nihtoolbox.org

cultural perspective of each patient and the people involved in their care is important to properly understanding how to treat and communicate with them (68,69).

While individual cultural experiences are essential to identify in each patient, acknowledging the differences in the prevalence of health issues and access to health care services among cultural groups is necessary to understand. Using race and ethnicity as examples, people who are black, are American Indian and Alaska Natives, or have multiple races have higher than average prevalence of stroke in the United States (70,71). People who are black have higher rates of depression than the rest of the population (72). People who are African-American, Hispanic-American, and Asian-American are all at higher risk for mental health issues due to discrimination and racism (73). However, they are significantly less likely than Caucasian-Americans to utilize mental health services due to factors such as social stigma, lack of sufficient insurance coverage, and mistrust of medical systems (73). Knowing how people experience specific cultural phenomena can impact treatment.

Another cultural consideration to recognize is a person's adjustment to disability. A person may feel shameful about his or her disability and avoid social participation, think that disability is a fate with no solution, or feel solely responsible for his or her recovery (74). These viewpoints can be limiting and damaging to a person's willingness to seek help in dealing with a disability and may shape views of recovery.

The narrative conducted by a member of the rehabilitation team should explore the cultural aspects of the person including what they think has happened to them and why. Such information will help in planning client-centered care.

Physical Environment

Physical obstacles may be especially hard to remove, preventing the accomplishment of desired tasks and reach individual goals for recovery. Unfortunately, if a person has trouble navigating the physical environment, it may be difficult to get help or report the issue to have it resolved (75). It also involves intricate planning to figure out if the physical environment will cause problems in a future activity, especially if it is in the community, which may decrease motivation to participate in desired occupations (75).

Discharge location must be considered in the quality of a patient's recovery. Being in the hospital can contribute to low motivation due to low levels of activity and feelings of disempowerment present in the role of being a patient (76). Physical activity levels remain low in inpatient rehabilitation settings (77). Patients get more steps and expend higher amounts of energy at home, possibly due to increased personal responsibility for rehabilitation (78).

People who live near more green space are less affected by stressful life events and have better perceived mental health (79). Those with less green space near their living environment report loneliness and a perceived shortage of social support (59,80). Noise is another characteristic of the physical environment that limits activity and participation (81). Air pollution is positively correlated with poststroke mortality, indicating potential health complications for those living in polluted areas (82). The features of the physical environment determine how that setting will help or hinder recovery.

In some locations, physical and structural barriers cause the largest problems with activity and participation (83). Such barriers may make certain activities inaccessible. Within the home, residential buildings may not be designed well enough to support performance in activities, requiring design modifications (84). In the community, the construction of buildings may not support completion of tasks for people with disabilities (84). Barriers in the physical environment can influence depression, while an accessible physical environment can moderate depressive symptoms (85).

Rehabilitation professionals are placing more emphasis on the physical environment including home visits and consultation with families on safe and accessible environments. Emphasis on sharing resources of accessible community facilities including fitness, restaurants, and community centers should be routine to discharge. Such information will support community reentry.

ASSISTIVE TECHNOLOGY

Providing people with assistive technology (AT) helps them perform their necessary occupations (86). Technology can come in several varieties, including seating and mobility, computers and computer access technology, and cognitive technologies, and tools to support special interests (86).

Overall, the use of assistive devices for self-care and mobility limitations is positively related to well-being (87). If used correctly, AT can improve one's participation in activity to closer resemble one's participation before one's disability and align a person's self-image (88). Poor mental health can prevent proper AT use, however. Limitations in self-care and mobility are negatively associated with well-being, and AT may be seen as a solution to such problems (87,89). However, improper use of AT devices may cause patients to feel unwanted attention, threatening their desires to blend in (88). This identity confusion that can occur during recovery may cause patients to disregard AT because they feel it sets them apart from others (22,88,89). They also need training to use and integrate AT successfully into their daily activities. The relationship between a patient and AT will only remain positive if equipment is matched to the client's personal goals, preferences, and environment (89).

AT has become central to supporting people's daily life. Rehabilitation professionals should be careful to help the person choose what he or she wants to learn to use; if not, it may sit unused.

OVERVIEW OF INTERVENTION APPROACHES

An overview of the major categories of rehabilitation interventions is briefly described in the following sections. A basic understanding of intervention approaches is necessary for all health care professionals to know. This knowledge will facilitate assessment and decisions to refer clients for services needed to support to engagement in everyday life activity. Determination of the most appropriate treatment approach requires collaboration among the client, caregiver, and health care team; however, the approach is targeted at helping the client achieve the highest level of independence possible. The therapeutic approach that is the best match intervention considers the client's needs, desires, and expectations as well as capacity for learning, the prognosis for the impairments, the time available for intervention, and the anticipated discharge environment.

Remediation

Remediation is the reduction of functional or structural impairments or the acquisition/reacquisition of skills in the area of skilled movement, cognition, or social function. In this approach, one expects that lost skill or ability will be regained. Rehabilitation approaches are used to establish or reestablish the client's skills, habits, and routines. Consequently, the use of this approach implies an active learning process whereby patients must adapt to functional and environmental limitations as they affect the demands of everyday life. The initial acquisition of skills by those who are developmentally or congenitally disabled at birth is a markedly different learning process from the reacquisition of daily living skills by those who have been independent at such tasks before experiencing a disabling condition. When the goals of remediation are to develop skills in a person with a congenital condition, the training process is described as rehabilitative. When the goal is to achieve previous functional levels for a person with an acquired disability, the training process is described as restorative.

The best candidates for remediation or restoration of skills are often based on the clients' specific condition and prognosis. Clients with neurodegenerative diseases for example are often not good candidates for remediation-based approaches; however, clients with orthopedic injuries typically are good candidates. To participate in remediation-based approaches, patients have to be able to monitor their own errors and often use appropriate strategies to minimize deficits. In this case, the treatment session is used to develop a practice strategy and the client practices self-care at each opportunity whether or not the therapist is present. Problems occurring between treatments are discussed, and possible solutions can be practiced during the next treatment session. Implied in the process of remediation is the ability to learn; however, the process by which one is able to learn is guided by one's cognitive capacity (see Learning Strategies below).

Compensation

Compensation is the use of techniques, devices, or any other form of external support to help clients complete activities in spite of nonmodifiable impairments. These compensations may include the use of caregivers and/or personal care assistants, environmental modifications, the use of AT, the use of mobility devices, etc. The therapist's role is determining when these compensations are necessary, identifying potential compensatory strategies that can help maximize independence in the client's chosen activity, and providing training the client and/or the client's caregiver in the correct use of the compensatory method. Compensation techniques are very often used in conjunction with remediation-based approaches to help clients maintain their highest level of independence with activity while they are working to regain function. A clear example of when compensatory strategies are often used is with individuals with spinal cord injuries by helping to train attendants or families to help them complete ADL and IADL. As is the case with remediation-based approaches,

implied in this approach is the ability to learn and methods for training are often guided by the client's cognitive capacity to learn new skills.

Learning Strategies

As research has unveiled the importance of specific learning strategies in both acquisition and reacquisition of functional skills, rehabilitation professionals have incorporated these strategies into training. There are a variety of classification schemes for describing these learning strategies. In practice, four stages of learning described by Bertoti are helpful in differentiating between the initial stages of learning (e.g., acquisition) and the long-term stages of learning that may include maintenance, fluency or proficiency, and generalization (90).

Optimal learning in the initial stages requires different strategies from those for retention or long-term learning, but most of the teaching strategies are used at both the initial and long-term learning strategies, albeit in different ways. Some of those strategies for learning are highlighted in **Table 7-9**. Research also indicates that learning is enhanced when the learner engages in a naturally occurring task versus use of progressive resistive exercise and by using real objects in a natural context (91–94).

The strategies employed by the therapist are guided by the client's cognitive capacity to learn and ability to employ strategies to complete a task. The therapist's role is to promote the highest level of independence possible, which in essence means providing the least guidance and cueing necessary to complete the task. The overall goal of rehabilitation is to be able to generalize knowledge gained to novel environments and different tasks. To achieve this, general knowledge and strategies are taught since general knowledge transfers better than task specific knowledge (95). The subtlety in the underlying effect of these general strategies lies in how they are taught to the client. Currently most rehabilitation is provided using direct instruction, which means the therapist is in essence telling the client what to do (96). By instructing in this way, even if the therapist is teaching strategies, the problem-solving component of learning is minimized and therefore the patient is not trained in a way that will be available for use when direct instruction is not available. The contrast to direct instruction is guided discovery where the therapist uses guided questions and prompts to allow the client to discover strategies on his or her own, thereby providing support to the client to problem solve on his or her own (97). Using guided discovery with a general strategy to help clients learn their own task-specific strategies has been demonstrated to be an effective way to not only improve ADL/IADL performance but also to transfer and generalize outside the clinic (98). In order to use this approach, clients must have a high level of awareness as they need to be aware of their deficits and recognize when they are making errors (99). For those clients without the ability to do this, direct instruction/behavioral training focused on task performance instead of strategy training would be necessary to help them learn new activities.

Instruction

Instruction prior to initiation of any task is crucial for motivation and for clarification about the task and can take the forms of verbal, demonstration, and modeling. Verbal instructions help to focus the client's attention on important aspects of the task.

TABLE 7-9	Resources for Families		
Purpose	**Resource**	**Description**	**Where to Find**
Caregiving	Caregiver Action Network	This network connects caregivers of people with a variety of conditions.	http://caregiveraction.org/
Computer Skills and Typing	Infogrip	This assistive technology retailer provides alternative computer equipment, including mice and keyboards, to accommodate people with disabilities.	http://www.infogrip.com/
Mental Health	National Alliance of Mental Illness (NAMI)	This organization includes free information and referrals for mental health and related services.	http://www.nami.org/
Exercise	YMCA	This association has exercise facilities and classes across the United States.	www.ymca.net
Parenting	Through the Looking Glass (TLG)	This organization offers education and support for parents with disabilities.	http://www.lookingglass.org/
Sexuality and Intimacy	American Association of Sexuality Educators, Counselors, and Therapists	This association includes a "locate a professional" option to find local sexuality educators, counselors, and therapists.	https://www.aasect.org/
Work	Job Accommodation Network	This network offers free guidance on workplace accommodations and employment issues for people with disabilities.	http://askjan.org/
Transportation	National Aging and Disability Transportation Center	The NADTC provides education on transportation choices available in the community and how to access them. It offers one-on-one assistance, and includes a "Looking for a ride?" button, which helps find local transportation services.	http://www.nadtc.org/
Finances	Foundation for Health Coverage Education	The foundation offers simplified insurance eligibility information to assist with access to coverage.	https://coverageforall.org/
General	RESNA (Rehab Engineering and Assistive Technology Society of North America)	RESNA provides technical assistance to people with disabilities, including awareness, access, acquisition, and advocacy. The Web site includes a database for financial aid for state technology assistance programs.	http://www.resna.org/

The therapist may choose to break down verbal instruction into one or two essential elements. Verbal instructions that are both brief and clear are the most helpful to clients. In addition, a therapist may use demonstration or modeling of the task to either replace or enhance the verbal instructions. Demonstrating how the client is to achieve the task has clearly been demonstrated to promote learning; however, this type of learning is often not expected to transfer. Therefore, direct instruction should be reserved for two primary purposes: (a) to clarify task expectations for the client and (b) for clients who are unable to recognize when they are making errors consistently and require direct instruction to complete a task accurately and safely. This type of learning is often referred to as behavioral learning, behavioral training, and/or task training (100). Cueing, feedback, reinforcement, and many of behavioral training techniques can be used to accomplish this type of learning (100).

Self-Management

Management of the chronic symptoms from stroke is essential for healthy living and to reduce chances of a secondary stroke (101,102). Most rehabilitation efforts are focused on restoring function with little effort given to living with longer-term impairments, which are common with many conditions we serve, for example, individuals with stroke; however, while not often used as part of rehabilitation practice, chronic disease management approaches like self-management education have been used widely and are effective to fill this need.

Self-management programs are designed to help individuals learn to manage their health conditions. Self-management has

many definitions but is most often described as an individual's ability to manage the symptoms, treatment, physical and psychosocial consequences, and lifestyle changes inherent with living with a chronic disease (103). With conditions such as asthma and diabetes, the concept of self-management has been widely evaluated and proven effective (103). A common program often cited in the literature is the chronic disease self-management program (CDSMP). The CDSMP was created to address symptom management across multiple diagnoses such as diabetes, arthritis, MS, and heart disease. The CDSMP is a 6-week program that helps participants develop strategies and techniques to address emotions, pain, appropriate exercises, medication, effective communication, nutrition, decision-making, and treatment evaluation (104). The CDSMP has been widely researched with individuals with a variety of health conditions including stroke and been found to improve establishment of personalized strategies to manage symptoms and impairments (104). While programs like the CDSMP exist, individuals with chronic neurologic conditions like stroke are rarely provided any self-management education. This may be in part due to the unique and complex deficits individuals with neurologic conditions experience, which would require self-management programs to include additional content. This content may include supporting self-management of more social roles and managing emotional well-being and new medical tasks they may need (105). Specific again to individuals with stroke, the Improving Participation after Stroke Self-Management Program (IPASS) was created to address this need for a more robust self-management program that further addressed participation in everyday activity (106). The IPASS follows the structure of the CDSMP; however, it also includes an additional seven sessions focused on improving self-efficacy to manage participation in the home, community, and work activities (106,107). The PEOP model of practice from occupational therapy guides the efficacy building process of the seven sessions by helping participants problem solve to identify how their occupations are impacted by person-centered factors and environmental factors (106). Participants then problem solve to identify strategies to change the person, activity, or environment to increase participation in activities (106). Research on the IPASS with individuals with stroke found an increase in self-efficacy in managing chronic health conditions and an increase in participation in the home, community, and work activities (106); however, even in light of the work with the IPASS, the development and use of self-management programs with individuals/groups commonly seen in rehabilitation settings is an ongoing need.

Resources

Providing clients with resources that they can choose to use in the future allows them to seek further help for such problems. Resources can be given to clients so they can follow up with issues that may not be addressed in their formal rehabilitation or for follow-up on issues that arise after discharge from rehabilitation. Once a client is discharged, it may become more difficult for him or her to reach assistance if needed. Issues such as lack of knowledge or financial resources create barriers in the event that unforeseen problems arise that limit their ability to further their recovery and reintegration into society. Community resources can serve to address such needs. Community resources should be tailored to each client based on cost, location, and area of need addressed.

Resources to Help Patients Transition to Daily Life in Community

Table 7-9 identifies resources that can be reviewed with the patient and family as they make plans for the next stages in the patient's return to activities that are important and meaningful for them to do.

OVERALL GOALS OF THE REHABILITATION TEAM'S EFFORTS TO SUPPORT DAILY LIFE FUNCTION

The overall goal of rehabilitation is to enable a person to do the things that are necessary and important for them to do. Rehabilitation cannot focus on the person caring for themselves (ADL) and anticipate that they can do anything. People have roles and responsibilities that are central to their family, work, and community lives. Rehabilitation certainly begins their recovery and adaptation, but the process takes weeks, months, and in some cases years. By focusing on the skills that support activities that are important to the patient, the team can address the patient's medical and health needs in addition to the communication, movement, and performance issues that will prepare the patient and his/her family to continue the rehabilitation with home health, home safety, self-management, and long-term health and fitness that will allow the person to be who they want to be and do what they want to do.

Rehabilitation is a team approach and the patient and family are on the team.

REFERENCES

1. Sheldon MP. A physical achievement record for use with crippled children. *J Health Phys Educ.* 1935;6(5):30–31, 60.
2. Coulter JS. Occupational therapy in a private general hospital. *Journal of the American Medical Association*, 1944;126(6):360–367.
3. Bennett RL. Rehabilitation in poliomyelitis. In: Kessler HH, ed. *The Principles and Practice of Rehabilitation.* Philadelphia, PA: Lea & Febiger; 1950:324–360.
4. Buchwald E. *Physical Rehabilitation for Daily Living.* New York: McGraw-Hill; 1952.
5. WHO. *International Classification of Functioning, Disability and Health.* Geneva: The World Health Organization; 2001.
6. Baum CM, Christiansen CH, Bass JD. The person-environment-occupation-performance model. In: Christiansen CH, Baum CM, Bass JD, eds. *Occupational Therapy: Performance, Participation and Well-Being.* Thorafare, NJ: Slack Inc.; 2015:49–56.
7. Bass JD, Baum CM, Christiansen CH, Interventions and outcomes: the person-environment-occupation-performance (PEOP) occupational therapy process. In: Christiansen CH, Baum CM, Bass JD, eds. *Occupational Therapy: Performance, Participation and Well-Being.* Thorafare, NJ: Slack Inc.; 2015:57–80.
8. Jette AM. et al. Beyond function: predicting participation in a rehabilitation cohort. *Arch Phys Med Rehabil.* 2005;86(11):2087–2094.
9. Maeir A, Rotenberg-Shpigelman S. Person factors: cognition. In: Christiansen CH, Baum CM, eds. *Occupational Therapy: Performance, Participation and Well-Being.* Thorofare, NJ: Slack Inc.; 2015:233–247.
10. Arauz A, et al. Vascular cognitive disorders and depression after first-ever stroke: the fogarty-Mexico stroke cohort. *Cerebrovasc Dis.* 2014;38(4):284–289.
11. Taylor GH, Broomfield NM. Cognitive assessment and rehabilitation pathway for stroke (CARPS). *Top Stroke Rehabil.* 2013;20(3):270–282.
12. Bora E, et al. Cognitive impairment in euthymic major depressive disorder: a meta-analysis. *Psychol Med.* 2013;43(10):2017–2026.
13. Woo YS, et al. Cognitive deficits as a mediator of poor occupational function in remitted major depressive disorder patients. *Clin Psychopharmacol Neurosci.* 2016;14(1):1–16.
14. Park YH, et al. Executive function as a strong predictor of recovery from disability in patients with acute stroke: a preliminary study. *J Stroke Cerebrovasc Dis.* 2015;24(3):554–561.
15. Muir RT, et al. Trail making test elucidates neural substrates of specific poststroke executive dysfunctions. *Stroke.* 2015;46(10):2755–2761.
16. Knopman DS, et al. Association of prior stroke with cognitive function and cognitive impairment: a population-based study. *Arch Neurol.* 2009;66(5):614–619.
17. Porter RJ, Bourke C, Gallagher P. Neuropsychological impairment in major depression: its nature, origin and clinical significance. *Aust N Z J Psychiatry.* 2007;41(2):115–128.
18. Gohier B, et al. Cognitive inhibition and working memory in unipolar depression. *J Affect Disord.* 2009;116(1):100–105.
19. Roussel M, et al. The behavioral and cognitive executive disorders of stroke: the GREFEX Study. *PLoS One.* 2016;11(1):e0147602.
20. Mahurin RK, et al. Trail making test errors and executive function in schizophrenia and depression. *Clin Neuropsychol.* 2006;20(2):271–288.
21. Royall DR, et al. Declining executive control in normal aging predicts change in functional status: the Freedom House Study. *J Am Geriatr Soc.* 2004;52(3):346–352.
22. DeJean D, et al. Patient experiences of depression and anxiety with chronic disease: a systematic review and qualitative meta-synthesis. *Ont Health Technol Assess Ser.* 2013;13(16):1–33.
23. Frost Y, et al. Self-care self-efficacy correlates with independence in basic activities of daily living in individuals with chronic stroke. *J Stroke Cerebrovasc Dis.* 2015;24(7):1649–1655.
24. Ferro JM, Caeiro L, Santos C. Poststroke emotional and behavior impairment: a narrative review. *Cerebrovasc Dis.* 2009;27(suppl 1):197–203.
25. Vickery CD, et al. Multilevel modeling of self-esteem change during acute inpatient stroke rehabilitation. *Rehabil Psychol.* 2009;54(4):372.
26. Hackett ML, et al. Neuropsychiatric outcomes of stroke. *Lancet Neurol.* 2014;13(5):525–534.
27. Nakase T, et al. Outstanding symptoms of poststroke depression during the acute phase of stroke. *PLoS One.* 2016;11(10):e0163038.
28. Truelsen T, et al. Self-reported stress and risk of stroke the Copenhagen City heart study. *Stroke.* 2003;34(4):856–862.
29. Lerdal A, Gay CL. Fatigue in the acute phase after first stroke predicts poorer physical health 18 months later. *Neurology.* 2013;81(18):1581–1587.
30. Tang W-K, et al. Is fatigue associated with suicidality in stroke? *Arch Phys Med Rehabil.* 2011;92(8):1336–1338.
31. Tang WK, et al. Is fatigue associated with short-term health-related quality of life in stroke? *Arch Phys Med Rehabil.* 2010;91(10):1511–1515.
32. Kramer S, et al. Energy expenditure and cost during walking after stroke: a systematic review. *Arch Phys Med Rehabil.* 2016;97(4):619–632.
33. Gillen G. *Psychological Aspects of Stroke Rehabilitation: A Function-Based Approach.* 4th ed. St. Louis, MO: Elsevier; 2011.
34. Tang WK, et al. Is pain associated with suicidality in stroke? *Arch Phys Med Rehabil.* 2013;94(5):863–866.

35. Kross E, et al. Social rejection shares somatosensory representations with physical pain. *Proc Natl Acad Sci.* 2011;108(15):6270–6275.

36. Hattjar B. *Sexuality and Occupational Therapy: Strategies for Persons with Disabilities.* Bethesda, MD: American Occupational Therapy Association, Inc./AOTA Press; 2012.

37. English C, et al. Physical activity and sedentary behaviors in people with stroke living in the community: a systematic review. *Phys Ther.* 2014;94(2):185.

38. Subramanian SK, et al. Arm motor recovery using a virtual reality intervention in chronic stroke: randomized control trial. *Neurorehabil Neural Repair.* 2013;27(1):13–23.

39. Cirstea M, Levin M. Improvement of arm movement patterns and endpoint control depends on type of feedback during practice in stroke survivors. *Neurorehabil Neural Repair.* 2007;21(5):398–411.

40. Subramanian SK, et al. Depressive symptoms influence use of feedback for motor learning and recovery in chronic stroke. *Restor Neurol Neurosci.* 2015;33(5):727–740.

41. Schmid AA, et al. Balance and balance self-efficacy are associated with activity and participation after stroke: a cross-sectional study in people with chronic stroke. *Arch Phys Med Rehabil.* 2012;93(6):1101–1107.

42. Schmid AA, et al. Balance is associated with quality of life in chronic stroke. *Top Stroke Rehabil.* 2013;20(4):340–346.

43. Delbaere K, et al. Fear-related avoidance of activities, falls and physical frailty: a prospective community-based cohort study. *Age Ageing.* 2004;33(4):368–373.

44. Barker RN, Brauer SG. Upper limb recovery after stroke: the stroke survivors' perspective. *Disabil Rehabil.* 2005;27(20):1213–1223.

45. Carey L. Person factors: sensory. In: Christiansen CH, Baum CM, eds. *Occupational Therapy: Performance, Participation and Well-Being.* Thorofare, NJ: Slack; 2015:249–265.

46. Bamiou D-E, et al. Patient-reported auditory functions after stroke of the central auditory pathway. *Stroke.* 2012;43(5):1285–1289.

47. Wehling E, et al. Olfactory dysfunction in chronic stroke patients. *BMC Neurol.* 2015;15(1):199.

48. Croy I, Nordin S, Hummel T. Olfactory disorders and quality of life—an updated review. *Chem Senses.* 2014;39(3):185–194.

49. Lopez C. The vestibular system: balancing more than just the body. *Curr Opin Neurol.* 2016;29(1):74–83.

50. Carey LM. Touch and body sensation. In: Carey LM, ed. *Stroke Rehabilitation: Insights from Neuroscience and Imaging.* New York: Oxford University Press; 2012.

51. Carey LM. et al. Same intervention–different reorganization: the impact of lesion location on training-facilitated somatosensory recovery after stroke. *Neurorehabil Neural Repair.* 2016;30(10):988–1000.

52. Doyle SD, Bennett S, Dudgeon B. Upper limb post-stroke sensory impairments: the survivor's experience. *Disabil Rehabil.* 2014;36(12):993–1000.

53. Bannister LC, et al. Improvement in touch sensation after stroke is associated with resting functional connectivity changes. *Front Neurol.* 2015;6:165.

54. Stawski RS, Sliwinski MJ, Smyth JM. Stress-related cognitive interference predicts cognitive function in old age. *Psychol Aging.* 2006;21(3):535.

55. Rowe F, et al. Visual impairment following stroke: do stroke patients require vision assessment? *Age Ageing.* 2009;38(2):188–193.

56. Friedland, J., & McColl, M. Social support and psychosocial dysfunction after stroke: buffering effects in a community sample. *Arch Phys Med Rehabil.* 1987;68(8):475–480.

57. Huang CY, et al. Mediating roles of social support on poststroke depression and quality of life in patients with ischemic stroke. *J Clin Nurs.* 2010;19(19–20):2752–2762.

58. Kruithof WJ, et al. Associations between social support and stroke survivors' health-related quality of life—a systematic review. *Patient Educ Couns.* 2013;93(2):169–176.

59. Kamenov K, et al. Factors related to social support in neurological and mental disorders. *PLoS One.* 2016;11(2):e0149356.

60. Van Orden KA, et al. The association between higher social support and lower depressive symptoms among aging services clients is attenuated at higher levels of functional impairment. *Int J Geriatr Psychiatry.* 2015;30(10):1085–1092.

61. Northcott S, et al. A systematic review of the impact of stroke on social support and social networks: associated factors and patterns of change. *Clin Rehabil.* 2016;30(8):811–831.

62. ten Have M, et al. Combined effect of mental disorder and low social support on care service use for mental health problems in the Dutch general population. *Psychol Med.* 2002;32(2):311.

63. Beckley MN. The influence of the quality and quantity of social support in the promotion of community participation following stroke. *Aust Occup Ther J.* 2007;54(3):215–220.

64. Shao J, et al. Well-being of elderly stroke survivors in Chinese communities: mediating effects of meaning in life. *Aging Ment Health.* 2014;18(4):435–443.

65. Bugge C, Alexander H, Hagen S. Stroke patients' informal caregivers. *Stroke.* 1999;30(8):1517–1523.

66. Northcott S, Hilari K. Why do people lose their friends after a stroke? *Int J Lang Commun Disord.* 2011;46(5):524–534.

67. Padilla R. Environment factors: culture. In: Christiansen CH, Baum CM, Bass JD, eds. *Occupational Therapy: Performance, Participation and Well-Being.* Thorofare, NJ: Slack Inc.; 2015:335–358.

68. Iwama MK. Revisiting culture in occupational therapy: a meaningful endeavor. *OTJR (Thorofare N J)* 2004;24(1):2–3.

69. Perkinson MA, et al. Therapeutic partnerships: occupational therapy and home-based care. In: Christiansen CH, Matuska KM, eds. *Ways of Living: Adaptive Strategies for Special Needs.* Bethesda, MD: AOTA Press; 2011:519–532.

70. Benjamin EJ, et al. Heart disease and stroke statistics—2017 update: a report from the American Heart Association. *Circulation.* 2017;135(10):e146–e603.

71. Centers for Disease Control and Prevention. Prevalence of stroke—United States, 2006–2010. *MMWR Morb Mortal Wkly Rep.* 2012;61(20):379.

72. Pratt LA, Brody DJ. Depression in the United States household population, 2005–2006. *NCHS Data Brief.* 2008:1–8.

73. Agency for Healthcare Research and Quality. *2010 National Healthcare Disparities Report.* 2010. Available from: https://archive.ahrq.gov/research/findings/nhqrdr/nhdr10/Chap2b.html

74. Ripat J, Woodgate R. The intersection of culture, disability and assistive technology. *Disabil Rehabil Assist Technol.* 2011;6(2):87–96.

75. Hammel J, et al. Environmental barriers and supports to everyday participation: a qualitative insider perspective from people with disabilities. *Arch Phys Med Rehabil.* 2015;96(4):578–588.

76. Holmqvist LW, von Koch L. Environmental factors in stroke rehabilitation. *BMJ.* 2001;322(7301):1501–1502.

77. Åstrand A, et al. Poststroke physical activity levels no higher in rehabilitation than in the acute hospital. *J Stroke Cerebrovasc Dis.* 2016;25(4):938–945.

78. Vanroy C, et al. Physical activity in chronic home-living and sub-acute hospitalized stroke patients using objective and self-reported measures. *Top Stroke Rehabil.* 2016;23(2):98–105.

79. Van den Berg AE, et al. Green space as a buffer between stressful life events and health. *Soc Sci Med.* 2010;70(8):1203–1210.

80. Maas J, et al. Social contacts as a possible mechanism behind the relation between green space and health. *Health Place.* 2009;15(2):586–595.

81. Snogren M, Sunnerhagen KS. Description of functional disability among younger stroke patients: exploration of activity and participation and environmental factors. *Int J Rehabil Res.* 2009;32(2):124–31.

82. Wilker EH, et al. Residential proximity to high-traffic roadways and poststroke mortality. *J Stroke Cerebrovasc Dis.* 2013;22(8):e366–e372.

83. Zhang L, et al. Barriers to activity and participation for stroke survivors in rural China. *Arch Phys Med Rehabil.* 2015;96(7):1222–1228.

84. Randström KB, Asplund K, Svedlund M. Impact of environmental factors in home rehabilitation—a qualitative study from the perspective of older persons using the International Classification of Functioning, Disability and Health to describe facilitators and barriers. *Disabil Rehabil.* 2012;34(9):779–787.

85. Zhang L. A study in persons later after stroke of the relationships between social participation, environmental factors and depression. *Clin Rehabil.* 2017;31(3):394–402.

86. Polgar JM. Environmental factors: technology. In: Christiansen CH, Baum CM, Bass JD, eds. *Occupational Therapy: Performance, Participation, and Well-Being.* Thorofare, NJ: Slack; 2015:441–464.

87. Lin I-F, Wu H-S. Activity limitations, use of assistive devices or personal help, and well-being: variation by education. *J Gerontol B Psychol Sci Soc Sci.* 2014;69(suppl 1):S16–S25.

88. Pape TL-B, Kim J, Weiner B. The shaping of individual meanings assigned to assistive technology: a review of personal factors. *Disabil Rehabil.* 2002;24(1–3):5–20.

89. Scherer MJ, Glueckauf R. Assessing the benefits of assistive technologies for activities and participation. *Rehabil Psychol.* 2005;50(2):132–141.

90. Bertoti DB. *Functional Neurorehabilitation Through the Life Span.* Philadelphia, PA: F. A. Davis; 2004.

91. Trombly CA, Wu C. Effect of rehabilitation tasks on organization of movement after stroke. *Am J Occup Ther.* 1999;53(4):333–344.

92. Trombly CA, Ma H. A synthesis of the effects of occupational therapy for persons with stroke. Part 1: restoration of roles, tasks, and activities. *Am J Occup Ther.* 2002;56:250–259.

93. Wu C, Trombley CA, Lin K, et al. Effects of object affordances on reaching performance in persons with and without cerebrovascular accident. *Am J Occup Ther.* 1998;52(6):447–456.

94. Wu C, Trombly CA, Lin K, et al. A kinematic study of contextual effects on reaching performance in persons with and without stroke: influences of object availability. *Arch Phys Med Rehabil.* 2000;81(1):95–101.

95. Geusgens CA, et al. Occurrence and measurement of transfer in cognitive rehabilitation: a critical review. *J Rehabil Med.* 2007;39(6):425–439.

96. Skidmore ER. Training to optimize learning after traumatic brain injury. *Curr Phys Med Rehabil Rep.* 2015;3(2):99–105.

97. Polatajko HJ, Mandich AD, McEwen S. Cognitive orientation to daily occupational performance (CO-OP): a cognitive-based intervention for children and adults. In: Katz N, ed. *Cognition, Occupation and Participation Across the Life Span.* Bethesda, MD: AOTA Press; 2012:299–321.

98. McEwen S, et al. Combined cognitive-strategy and task-specific training improve transfer to untrained activities in subacute stroke: an exploratory randomized controlled trial. *Neurorehabil Neural Repair.* 2015;29(6):526–536.

99. Haskins E. *Cognitive Rehabilitation Manual: Translating Evidence-Based Recommendations into Practice.* Vol 1. Reston, VA: American Congress of Rehabilitation Medicine; 2012.

100. Giles GM. Cognitive versus functional approaches to rehabilitation after traumatic brain injury: commentary on a randomized controlled trial. *Am J Occup Ther.* 2010;64(1):182–185.

101. Center for Disease Control. *Know the Facts About Stroke.* 2013. Available from: https://www.cdc.gov/stroke/materials_for_patients.htm

102. Howard VG, et al. An approach to coordinate efforts to reduce the public health burden of stroke: the Delta States Stroke Consortium. *Prev Chronic Dis.* 2004;1(4):1–7.

103. Lennon S, McKenna S, Jones F. Self-management programmes for people post stroke: a systematic review. *Clin Rehabil.* 2013;27(10):867–878.

104. Lorig KR, et al. Chronic disease self-management program: 2-year health status and health care utilization outcomes. *Med Care.* 2001;39(11):1217–1223.

105. Parke HL, et al. Self-management support interventions for stroke survivors: a systematic meta-review. *PLoS One.* 2015;10(7):e0131448.

106. Wolf TJ, et al. The development of the improving participation after stroke self-management program (IPASS): an exploratory randomized clinical study. *Top Stroke Rehabil.* 2016;23(4):284–292.

107. Bandura A. Self-efficacy mechanism in human agency. *Am Psychol.* 1982;37(2):122.

Disability Determination in Relation to Work

Including a chapter on disability determination in a medical textbook, as it relates to an individual's work or ability to work, might suggest that this aspect of disability can be reliably determined and that a validated method for health care providers to perform this determination is available. However, these issues often serve as robust topics for debate among those who understand and have an interest in the methods and processes utilized. In spite of this debate, many stakeholders have a need for an assessment of a person's "disability" and frequently ask physician and nonphysician medical providers to perform this task. For those who may be asked, this chapter provides an introduction to the concepts involved in the medical determination of disability in this context. Included are common conceptual models of disability, work disability terminology, functional assessments of disability, major disability systems in the United States, and the independent medical examination (IME).

MODELS OF DISABLEMENT

Since the beginning of the specialty, the evaluation and treatment of physical impairments and associated disabilities have fallen within the clinical scope of practice of physical medicine and rehabilitation (1). However, physicians from many specialties, as well as nonphysicians, are commonly involved in the process of determining disability.

To a major degree, the definition of disability depends upon the context to which it is being applied and who is asking. Health care providers are frequently asked to provide determinations of the disability of their patients for various reasons. However, while standardized guidelines for the purpose of impairment evaluation can be applied during a medical encounter, an adequate evaluation of disability requires a deeper understanding of the health condition of the individual, the contextual factors of the environment in which the individual interacts, and various personal factors (2,3). Therefore, let us begin with an overview of models of disablement in order to provide a common framework for understanding.

One of the earlier attempts to conceptualize the disablement process was proposed by Nagi (4,5). His work was later used as the basis for the Institute of Medicine (IOM; now known as the National Academy of Medicine) model to help define the criteria for Social Security Disability Insurance (SSDI) and Supplemental Security Income (SSI). In this model, disability can be described as an *expression of a physical or mental limitation in a social context* (6). However, an alternative model,

the International Classification of Impairments, Disabilities and Handicaps (ICIDH), was developed by the World Health Organization (WHO) to classify the consequences of diseases, injuries, and other disorders on the lives of individuals (7). This model distinguishes impairment, disability, and handicap resulting from diseases. *The American Medical Association (AMA) Guides to the Evaluation of Permanent Impairment*, Fifth Edition, includes concepts from this model of disablement into the impairment rating process (8). This classification system enjoyed widespread acceptance but was criticized because it did not clarify the role of the social and physical environment, giving an impression of encouraging the medicalization of disablement. Further revision and input from stakeholders eventually resulted in the *International Classification of Functioning, Disability and Health (ICF)* (9). The ICF provides a standard language and framework for the classification of health and health-related domains (see Chapter 9). These domains help to describe changes in body function and structure, what an individual with a health condition can do (level of capacity), and what they actually do in their usual environment (level of performance). In ICF, *functioning* refers to all body functions and body structures, activities, and participation, while *disability* refers to impairments, activity limitations, and participation restrictions that may occur with a health condition. ICF also lists *contextual factors* (environmental and personal factors) that interact with all these components. *The AMA Guides to the Evaluation of Permanent Impairment*, Sixth Edition, initiated the inclusion of this model of disablement into the impairment rating process (10). However, the use of the AMA Guides for the unintended purpose of evaluating work disability has been controversial (10–13). Furthermore, for disability compensation, the ICF model of disability has been contrasted with the one initially proposed by the IOM (14,15). As noted above, the IOM model draws from the experiences common to disability systems, such as those within Social Security, which are designed to compensate individuals who meet certain entitlement criteria and who demonstrate losses in key domains (**Fig. 8-1**). The IOM model includes the concepts of impairment, functional limitation, and disability as well as mediating factors (e.g., lifestyle and behavioral, biologic, and environmental), but also addresses the effects of disablement on quality of life. In addition to its use for Social Security, this model is felt to be preferable for use in the Veterans Administration. The Committee on Medical Evaluation of Veterans for Disability Compensation felt that

FIGURE 8-1. The enabling-disabling process. (Republished with permission of National Academies Press from Committee on Assessing Rehabilitation Science and Engineering, Institute of Medicine, Brandt EN, Pope AM, eds. *Enabling America: Assessing the Role of Rehabilitation Science and Engineering.* Washington, DC: National Academy Press, 1997; permission conveyed through Copyright Clearance Center, Inc.)

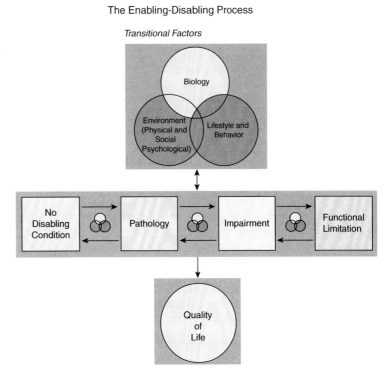

the IOM definition was not inconsistent with the ICF (16). The concepts from this model are operationalized to determine the amount of cash benefits provided by veterans' disability programs, as well as workers' compensation (**Fig. 8-2**). However, concern has been expressed as to the relative weight placed upon each of the domains by the various disability systems and a generally poor understanding by the medical community regarding the metrics used to define and measure some of the domains (17). Until these differences in defining disability are reconciled and the procedures used to determine it are proven to be reliable and valid, the model concepts one applies for disability determinations will likely continue to evolve.

WORK DISABILITY TERMINOLOGY

Regardless of the issues with interpreting the models of disablement, obtaining detailed information and assessing the contextual factors affecting disability should always be part of the care of patients who are unable to work, even if the disabling condition is temporary. For instance, when a treating physician and patient are engaged with the patient's employer in the return-to-work process following an injury or illness, there is the potential for the successful cooperation of all parties in a less adversarial and more effective process. Under these circumstances, disability can be understood as the decreased

FIGURE 8-2. The consequences of an injury or disease. (Republished with permission of National Academies Press from Committee on Medical Evaluation of Veterans for Disability Compensation, McGeary M, Ford MA, McCutchen SR, Barnes DK, eds. *A 21st Century System for Evaluating Veterans for Disability Benefits.* Washington, DC: National Academy Press, 2007; permission conveyed through Copyright Clearance Center, Inc.)

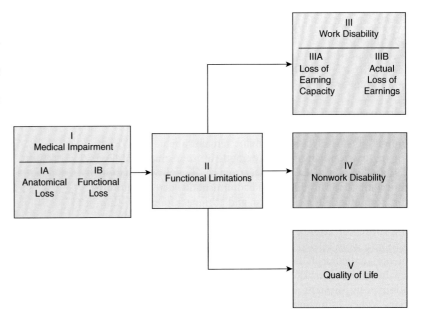

ability to perform certain *essential job functions* or the *substantial and material duties of an occupation.*

In addition to treating the underlying medical condition, the physician's role is to evaluate the nature of the impairment and outline the accommodations required to function in the workplace without further injury as outlined in a work ability report. This process can be facilitated by specifying temporary *work restrictions* that, if accommodated, will allow an employee to work on modified *duty*. This individual will then be considered to have a *temporary partial disability*. If the necessary accommodations are not feasible, then the individual will be off work. If the individual needs to be off work, it is considered a *temporary total disability*. If the medical condition is one that results in permanent impairment, the physician can assist the individual to remain at work or to find suitable alternative work by providing an assessment of permanent restrictions and work capacity to allow for the possibility of accommodation within the context of the Americans with Disabilities Act (ADA) (18) and the ADA Amendments Act (ADAAA) (19). This individual will then have a *permanent partial disability (PPD)*. If the medical condition is so severe that competitive employment is not feasible, there is a *permanent total disability*. The dynamics of this process should be understood and embraced by physicians as part of the care of patients with major medical illnesses affecting their ability to work or as a specific knowledge base for the efficient treatment of work-related injuries.

In addition to providing a work-ability form for the purpose of accommodation, there are times when an individual seeks compensation as a result of a functional limitation. In these situations, the definition of disability is often narrowed to specify the functional effects of an injury (such as the effects from pain and suffering for tort claims) or the inability to earn a living as a result of an illness or injury for workers' compensation, Social Security, and private disability insurance. In the absence of objective anatomic impairment, it is often challenging for a patient's physician to objectively determine that an individual *cannot* continue to work. This often leads to questioning of the motivation of the individual by physicians, insurers, or government agencies involved in providing the compensation. The term *motivation* can be construed as intentional for secondary gain or malingering, but it is often unintentional, occurring as a result of pain intolerance, pain-related fear, depression, catastrophizing, posttraumatic stress disorder, job factors, perceived injustice, or illness behavior. In fact, researchers have identified over 100 different determinants affecting the process of returning to work after illness or injury (20).

FUNCTIONAL ASSESSMENTS OF DISABILITY

How to objectively assess disability remains a major challenge for the medical community. Methods of measuring disability common to survey research differ from the disability evaluation procedures used in judicial and administrative determinations for accommodation, benefits, and compensation (21–23). Since there are often considerable differences when comparing self-report, clinical examination, and functional testing for assessing work-related limitations, clinicians should be aware of the subtleties of the various options (24). Administrative disability determinations tend to rely on the medical evaluation of impairment and variably on an assessment of function, either estimated, particularly for temporary medical

conditions, or often in the form of a functional capacity evaluation (FCE) for permanent conditions. However, FCEs have other uses, including preemployment screening and planning treatment following a work injury, in addition to determining physical disability and work capacity for administrative case closure. This later situation of the forensic application of the FCE grew out of the use of therapists as vocational expert witnesses for individuals with work limitations (25).

An FCE performed by an occupational or physical therapist may consist of several components, including record review, self-administered questionnaire, interview, physical measures, physiologic measures, functional measures, and a comparison of testing results to job requirements (26). The intention is to evaluate an individual's capacity to perform physical work activities. Physical measures may include range of motion, strength, and coordination. Physiologic measures may include heart rate and endurance. Functional measures may include lifting, carrying, pushing, pulling, sitting, standing, walking, reaching, stooping, crouching, balancing, climbing, and dexterity. These measures are quantified and expressed in terms of weight and/or frequency as appropriate. Frequency can be categorized as *rare*, up to 5% of the workday; *occasional*, 6% to 33% of the workday; *frequent*, 34% to 66% of the workday; and *constant*, 67% or more of the workday. Strength requirements required for specific occupations can be categorized as described in **Table 8-1**.

There are many different FCEs commonly used by therapists. An incomplete listing would include Blankenship, Ergos Work Simulator and Ergo-Kit variation, Isernhagen Work System (WorkWell), BTE (Hanoun Medical), Physical Work Performance Evaluation (ErgoScience), Key, Ergos, ARCON, and AssessAbility (27). While often advertised as "objective" methods to measure work abilities, there is no single standardized FCE, and the observations required for many FCE procedures rely on the expert assessment of therapists. For most methods, there is insufficient research to document reliability, validity, and potential examiner bias (28–30). As opposed to being thought of as an "objective" test, FCEs should be considered complementary behavioral tests influenced by multiple factors, including physical ability, beliefs, and perceptions

TABLE 8-1	**Strength Requirements Classification**	
Degree of Strength	**Amount of Lifting/ Carrying**	**Posture; Other Activities**
Sedentary work	Occasional: ≤10#	Primarily sitting; walking and standing at most occasionally
Light work	≤20#, ≤10# frequently	Significant walking/standing *or* primarily sitting but requiring pushing and pulling of arm and/or leg controls
Medium work	≤50#, ≤20# frequently	Unspecified
Heavy work	≤100#, ≤50# frequently	Unspecified
Very heavy work	>100#, ≥50# frequently	Unspecified

Reproduced from Chio A, Mora G, Lauria G. Pain in amyotrophic lateral sclerosis. *Lancet Neurol.* 2017;16(2):144–157. Copyright © 2016 Elsevier. With permission.

(31,32). Another particularly challenging aspect of the FCE is that there is no scientifically validated method of measuring sincerity of effort (33). However, it is possible to detect sub-maximal physical capacity in certain conditions (34).

Research on the reliability of medical evaluations of work disability indicates a high variation in medical judgments (35). It has also been shown that in the context of musculoskeletal disability assessments, physicians will often change their opinion regarding the physical work ability of claimants when FCE information is provided, despite the limitations of FCEs (36). Therefore, standardizing the evaluation process, along with the development and testing of instruments to improve reliability in evaluation of disability, is clearly needed (35).

As for now, the literature suggests that both performance-based and self-report measures of disability should be used in an effort to obtain a comprehensive picture of an individual's disability (37). For the assessment of functional limitations in workers applying for disability benefit, a combination of questionnaires, performance tests, or interviews together with professional clinical judgment is recommended (38). In relation to returning to work, an FCE may be useful to determine if an employee is capable of performing in a specific job, but the FCE cannot predict whether or not reinjury will occur (39).

MAJOR DISABILITY SYSTEMS IN THE UNITED STATES

The terms impairment and disability are frequently misinterpreted and often used somewhat interchangeably and incorrectly because of similarities in the administrative processes. For example, physicians may be asked to use the AMA Guides to provide an impairment rating following a work-related injury (e.g., Iowa), which will be used to calculate disability benefits to which an injured worker is entitled. A worker with the same injury in another state may need to have an impairment rating (e.g., Minnesota) or a disability rating (e.g., Wisconsin) from a state-specified schedule. The process for Social Security disability is entirely different, as will be reviewed later. This situation results from the fact that different systems and jurisdictions rate and provide compensation for physical impairments and disability differently.

Tort Liability

Although not a disability system *per se*, impairment evaluations may be performed in the context of tort liability. A *tort* is defined in common law as a civil wrong that results in loss or harm to a person resulting in legal liability for the person committing the wrongful act. Prior to workers' compensation legislation, tort claims could arise from work injuries. However, common law proved to be an insufficient mechanism for addressing the needs of injured workers and their families. Therefore, tort claims requiring disability determinations tend to arise in the context of personal injury cases, such as accidents or medical malpractice (40). In these situations, the AMA Guides may be used as a proxy to assess the severity of impairments. In addition to this use for some legal claims, several major U.S. disability systems utilize disability determinations, including workers' compensation, Social Security, private disability insurance, and various federal disability programs. These systems are briefly introduced in the following sections.

Workers' Compensation

Prior to the early 20th century, the civil courts, using the common law of torts, were the only option for the redress of disputes involving employment-related injuries, illnesses, and deaths. In the United States, workers' compensation, often referred to as the *grand bargain* between employers (capital) and workers (labor), developed around the beginning of the 20th century as a result of the fact that the legal tort system was an unpredictable and unfair method of compensating injured workers. Under tort law, it was difficult for the worker to establish negligence on the part of the employer, who could utilize three defenses under common law (41)

1. *Assumption of risk—the worker knew the risks of the job and accepted those risks by accepting the job.*
2. *Fellow-servant—the injury was caused by a coworker and not the employer's negligence.*
3. *Contributory negligence—the worker's actions or failure to exercise due care resulted in the injury.*

Workers' compensation is a no-fault system that provides medical and wage replacement benefits to the injured worker for injuries, illnesses, and death that occur on the job and financial benefits to dependents of workers killed on the job without regard to negligence. In exchange for these benefits, workers give up their rights to sue their employer (41).

Before workers' compensation, many employers would purchase liability policies to insure against losses from work injury claims. These insurance policies were essentially mandated following passage of workers' compensation laws, with some exceptions based upon number of employees or self-insurance. Most workers in the United States are covered by workers' compensation, and in most cases it is regulated by the states through various insurance arrangements (**Table 8-2**) (42). While all 50 states and the District of Columbia have workers' compensation, there is no federal requirement or standards for state systems, which contributes to the lack of standardization when it comes to disability determination for workers' compensation purposes as alluded to earlier. In addition, in the early 1970s there was concern about benefit inequity among the states, which led to a National Commission on State Workmen's Compensation Laws. This commission outlined five major objectives for a comprehensive program to serve as a model (43–45):

1. *Broad coverage of employees and of work-related injuries and diseases by extending protection to as many workers as feasible, and to all work-related injuries and diseases*
2. *Substantial protection against interruption of income by replacing a high proportion of a disabled worker's lost earnings by workers' compensation benefits*
3. *Provision of sufficient medical care and rehabilitation services to promptly restore the injured worker's physical condition and earning capacity*
4. *Encouragement of safety to reduce the number of work-related injuries and diseases though economic incentives*
5. *An effective system for delivery of the benefits and services to achieve the first four basic objectives*

States were never legally required to follow these recommendations, and unfortunately, there have been recent concerns that state workers' compensation benefits have been reduced over time. These reductions, due to state legislative policy changes, may be shifting some of the costs associated

TABLE 8-2	State Workers' Compensation Insurance Arrangements, 2013	
Exclusive State Fund	**Competitive State Fund**	**Private Insurance**
Ohio	California	Alabama
North Dakota	Colorado	Alaska
Washington	Hawaii	Arizona
Wyoming	Idaho	Arkansas
	Kentucky	Connecticut
	Louisiana	Delaware
	Maryland	District of Columbia
	Missouri	Florida
	Montana	Georgia
	New Mexico	Illinois
	New York	Indiana
	Oklahoma	Iowa
	Oregon	Kansas
	Pennsylvania	Maine
	Rhode Island	Massachusetts
	South Carolina	Michigan
	Texas	Minnesota
	Utah	Mississippi
		Nebraska
		Nevada
		New Hampshire
		New Jersey
		North Carolina
		South Dakota
		Tennessee
		Vermont
		Virginia
		West Virginia
		Wisconsin

Data from Sengupta I, Baldwin ML. *Workers' Compensation: Benefits, Coverage, and Costs, 2013.* National Academy of Social Insurance; 2015:22–23. Available from: https://www.nasi.org/sites/default/files/research/NASI_Work_Comp_Year_2015.pdf

with injuries, illnesses, and deaths in the workplace to the employee or social programs, such as SSDI and Medicare (41).

Social Security

The Old-Age, Survivors, and Disability Insurance program of the Social Security Administration (SSA), referred to by the acronym "OASDI," began in 1935 (46). There were no provisions for disability insurance until the disability program was implemented in the 1956 Amendments to the Social Security Act, which established the SSDI program for workers who became totally and permanently disabled. A separate SSA disability program, Supplemental Security Income (SSI), began in 1974 to assist financially indigent people who were disabled, blind, or aged 65 or older.

The SSA is headed by a Commissioner and has a central office located in Maryland; however, individual claims services are provided by local Social Security offices. Disability Determination Services (DDS), which has agencies in each state, makes the decision on work disability. An evaluation team within the agency obtains and reviews medical evidence from treatment sources in order to make the determination. If an individual has submitted a claim for disability and does not agree with the decisions made on the claim, appeals can be filed (47).

For the purposes of SSDI, one is considered "disabled" if he/she cannot engage in any *substantial gainful activity* because of physical or mental impairment. This means any type of work considering age, education, and work experience, not only previous work. It does not matter whether the work exists in the immediate area, whether a job is available, or whether the individual is hirable. The impairment(s) must be determined medically by a doctor, result from objective anatomical, physiologic, or psychological abnormalities and be expected to either result in death or last for at least 12 consecutive months (47).

SSDI disability determinations are *not* based upon a rating schedule. One is either disabled or not disabled. There is no *percentage of disability* caused by a given impairment, even though patients may often request this from their physicians. Furthermore, the medical evidence needs to document that the level of impairment is severe. A severe impairment *significantly* limits "physical or mental ability to perform basic work activities, such as: sitting, standing, walking, lifting, carrying, handling, reaching, pushing, pulling, climbing, stooping, crouching, seeing, hearing, speaking; understanding, carrying out and remembering simple instructions; using judgment; responding appropriately to supervision, coworkers, and usual work situations; and dealing with changes in a routine work setting" (47). For physical conditions, these limitations are documented on a physical Residual Functional Capacity (RFC) form[1]. Psychological conditions have their own form. An RFC form completed by a treating medical provider can greatly improve a disabled individual's chance of securing Social Security disability benefits. Medical evidence alone may establish disability if the evidence shows the presence of an impairment included in the Listing of Impairments (48), or the evidence shows an impairing condition that is medically the same as a listed impairment, and the person is not engaged in any substantial gainful activity. DDS, at their expense, may require a consultative examination from a treating provider or independent consultant to "(a) gather more evidence because the evidence obtained is not enough to make a disability decision; (b) obtain more detailed medical findings about the impairment(s); (c) obtain technical or specialized medical information; (d) resolve conflicts or differences in medical findings; or (e) resolve the issue of the ability to engage in substantial gainful activity" (47).

Private Disability Insurance

There are two main types of personal disability insurance: (a) short-term, which replaces a portion of your salary, usually 60% to 70%, for a specified period that is often less than 6 months but can last up to a year after an illness, injury, or childbirth; and (b) long-term, which replaces your salary, usually 40% to 60%, until the disability ends. However, benefits may end after a specified time or at retirement age, depending upon the policy. Disability policies vary in their definition of *disabled*, with some paying only if you cannot work any job for which you are qualified and others paying if you cannot perform your own occupation. Only 33% of the private sector workforce has long-term disability insurance (49).

---

[1]A copy of the RFC form is accessible at: https://secure.ssa.gov/apps10/poms/images/SSA4/G-SSA-4734-U8-1.pdf

Federal Employees' Compensation Act

In 1916, the Federal Employees' Compensation Act (FECA) extended workers' compensation principles that were developing in the states to nearly all federal employees (41). The law applies to all federal civilian employees in the executive, legislative, and judicial branches of government. It also includes federal jurors, state and local law enforcement officers operating in a federal capacity, employees of the U.S. Postal Service, and Peace Corps and the Civil Air Patrol. It is a no-fault system, so that federal employees cannot sue the federal government (50).

Longshore and Harbor Workers' Compensation Act

The Longshore and Harbor Workers' Compensation Act (LHWCA), enacted in 1927, provides workers' compensation benefits for private-sector workers engaged in the loading, unloading, building, or breaking of vessels that operate on the navigable waters of the United States (41). It also covers other groups of private-sector workers including (a) employees of the District of Columbia; (b) overseas military and public works contractors; (c) civilian employees of nonappropriated fund instrumentalities of the Armed Forces, such as service clubs and post exchanges; and (d) employees working on the Outer Continental Shelf in the exploration and the development of natural resources, such as workers on offshore oil platforms (41). It is a no-fault system administered by the U.S. Department of Labor (50).

Federal Employers Liability Act and Jones Act

The Federal Employers Liability Act (FELA) was passed by congress in the late 19th century and early 20th century in response to deaths associated with work on the railroads. Under FELA, railroad workers can sue for damages for a work-related railroad injury, including wage loss, loss of benefits, medical expenses, rehabilitation costs, as well as pain and suffering. Unlike workers' compensation, FELA requires the injured worker to prove that the railroad was negligent (40).

The Jones Act covers civilian sailors for permanent disability suffered while in the service of a ship on navigable waters. Similar to FELA, the injured worker must file suit against the ship's owner or master. Suits are often settled out of court (40).

Federal Black Lung Program

This workers' compensation program provides financial and medical benefits to coal miners with black lung disease and to dependents of miners who die from the disease. Diagnosis is ascertained through specific chest x-ray findings using the International Labour Organization (ILO) classification system. The x-rays must be read by "B-readers" certified by the National Institute for Occupational Health and Safety (NIOSH). Disability claims are referenced against standards published by the U.S. Department of Labor for spirometric and arterial blood gas values (40).

Energy Employees Occupational Illness Compensation Program Act

The Energy Employees Occupational Illness Compensation Program Act (EEOICPA) was enacted in 2000 and provides financial and medical benefits to workers who were involved in the development, research, and testing of atomic weapons (41). EEOICPA provides lump-sum cash benefits and medical benefits to "(a) Department of Energy (DOE) employees or contractors and atomic weapons industry workers with specified types of cancer likely caused by exposure to radiation or chronic silicosis likely caused by the mining of tunnels for atomic weapons testing; (b) beryllium workers with chronic beryllium disease; and (c) uranium miners, millers, and ore transporters provided benefits under the Radiation Exposure Compensation Act (RECA)" (41). It is also a program that provides workers' compensation benefits based upon "degree of disability and impairment and medical benefits to former DOE contractor employees with illnesses or deaths caused by occupational exposure to any toxic substance" (41).

Department of Veterans Affairs Disability Compensation

Veterans Affairs (VA) eligibility is based upon an honorable and general discharge from active military service. Disability compensation is a monthly benefit paid to veterans with injuries or diseases that were incurred in or aggravated during active duty, active duty for training, or inactive duty training who are at least 10% disabled. The benefit amount is adjusted according to the degree of disability, on a scale from 10% to 100%, in increments of 10%. In order to be eligible, the veteran must have medical evidence of a current physical or mental disability *and* evidence of a relationship between the disability and an injury, disease, or event in military service (*service connected*). This relationship must be established by medical records or medical opinions. There are certain conditions where the cause of the disability is presumed to be from service, including "former prisoners of war; veterans who have certain chronic or tropical diseases that become evident within a specific period of time after discharge from service; veterans who were exposed to ionizing radiation, mustard gas, or Lewisite while in service; veterans who were exposed to certain herbicides, such as by serving in Vietnam; and veterans who served in Southwest Asia during the Gulf War" (51). The process of application for benefits, examination, worksheets utilized, and the schedule for rating are unique to the VA system and can be reviewed elsewhere (52).

OVERVIEW OF THE INDEPENDENT MEDICAL EXAMINATION

The IME is a specialized evaluation performed by a health provider to provide information for a third party. Health providers, such as physicians, dentists, or chiropractors are asked to make formal assessments within their own specialty. The third party is often an insurer, employer, attorney, or a disability case manager. The purposes may include confirmation or contradiction of diagnoses; determining if further testing or treatment is necessary; commenting on functional limitations or work restrictions; evaluating impairment, prognosis, causality; and whether or not maximum medical improvement (MMI) has been reached (53). In workers' compensation, IME examiners are typically given specific questions to answer because the requesting party has doubts about some aspect of the validity of the affected individual or the medical treatment they are receiving. In particular, a common reason for the evaluation is to answer the question as to why the claimant is not getting better (*severity of the medical problem*) or if there is a need for continuing work disability (*degree of impairment*).

Ethics

The ethical issues surrounding the IME are important topics. While it is easy to understand that any physician performing an IME should remain impartial, in practice, impartiality is challenging because of the many potential conflicts of interest. Self-interest should never be a consideration even though the reimbursement for the evaluation is coming from a third party and future referrals may be dependent upon the favorability of the opinions. There is no standard approach to address this conflict, but it has been suggested that total time spent or total income derived from IMEs may warrant specialty board review or potential intervention of state medical boards in cases of abuse in order to encourage examiner adherence to ethical guidelines when performing IMEs (54). Conversely, many patients expect a physician-patient relationship whenever they interact with a physician, and they expect the physician to be supportive and to provide advice. This conflict is addressed by informing the examinee, prior to any assessment, that they are being evaluated as a claimant and that there is no physician-patient relationship (see section on Medicolegal Issues) (55). The absence of a formal physician-patient relationship does not reduce the obligation to treat the person being evaluated in an ethical and professional manner even though the purpose of the IME is to prepare and present an expert opinion to the requesting party. For this to occur, it is necessary to go beyond advocacy for the individual and consider the interests of the individual and society as a whole, where it is recognized that free medical care and/or wage replacement, as specified for many of these social programs, has potential inherent disincentives to recovery that may promote disability. Furthermore, physician actions, regardless of their intent, that result in excessive or inappropriate diagnostic and therapeutic efforts, or passive approaches that result in prolongation of claims, may help to inappropriately prolong disability. Such treatment approaches may contribute to a failure to achieve the greatest possible functional outcome for an individual.

Evaluating and Reporting Requirements

The evaluation should include a review of the medical records, a complete history of the current condition from the individual, a past history of any diagnostic tests for similar conditions, a work history, summary of the diagnostic studies available at the time of evaluation, prior treatment, and a comprehensive examination. During the examination, the examiner should observe for any nonphysiologic findings, such as those described by Waddell for low back pain (56). Lastly, any surveillance information, such as video taken of the examinee prior to arriving for the evaluation, should be reviewed. Based upon the information gathered, the examiner should then be prepared to provide opinions on the issues outlined in the following sections and respond to any other specific interrogatories put forth by the party requesting the evaluation.

Diagnosis: Impairment, Disability, and Prognosis

The medical diagnosis can be straightforward when the history, physical examination findings, and diagnostic studies are all correlated with a specific medical condition, such as a lumbar radiculopathy. However, at times, the symptoms do not correlate with the exam findings or diagnostic studies. A common dilemma is how to assess functionally limiting musculoskeletal pain in the absence of any objective findings or in the setting of diagnostic tests reflecting changes that can occur as a result of normal aging. There are no easy answers, but it is often helpful to take into account the demeanor and behavior of the individual during the evaluation to assist with the decision. A person who has had no prior similar injuries, a good work history, and a consistent examination but no neurologic deficits or obvious structural abnormalities on imaging may have experienced a sprain/strain that has become chronic. One should also be prepared to comment on comorbidities, such as depression, that can contribute to persistent pain (57). Formal psychological testing can often clarify the nonstructural determinants of disability (58). For those individuals with more well-defined medical conditions, one should be able to comment on the likelihood of further improvement and possibility of having residual impairments.

Causality and Apportionment

The question of *causality* will often arise in the situation of a work-related injury or illness, since the condition must be related to a work activity or exposure in order to be eligible for coverage through workers' compensation. Causality refers to a cause and effect relationship where the incident or exposure caused the condition, often stated to *within a reasonable degree of medical probability* to satisfy legal standards. *Medically probable* is an opinion that something is more likely than not (likelihood of causation >50%), as opposed to *medically possible* (likelihood of causation ≤50%). Ideally, the workplace incident or exposure should be the "proximate cause" (59). This implies that the condition arose from a specific event and without that event, the condition would not have occurred. For acute injuries, a thorough history, taking into account details of the onset of the condition and any previous similar conditions, can often assist with this determination. For gradually developing illnesses due to workplace exposures, including conditions felt secondary to cumulative trauma, forceful or repetitive occupational activities, in the absence of a history of similar avocational activities, such as woodworking, sewing, sports, or other repetitive activities may be regarded as work related.

If more than one condition is present, or there is a history of prior similar conditions requiring treatment and having residual or preexisting impairment, it is necessary to consider *apportionment* to assign a percentage to each condition. In addition, preexisting age-related or degenerative conditions need to be taken into account. However, in many workers' compensation jurisdictions, the workplace event or exposure only needs to be sufficient to contribute to aggravation or progression of the condition beyond the normally occurring progression to be considered work related.

Necessity and Appropriateness of Diagnostic Testing and Treatments Rendered

The examiner should ensure that a sufficient and thorough diagnostic workup and treatment period have been provided. Excessive testing or prolonged passive treatments may not be medically necessary. Otherwise, the examining clinician should confirm that the diagnostic testing and treatment were "reasonably necessary" to address the work-related condition or personal injury.

Additional Diagnostic Testing and Treatments Needed

The examiner is encouraged to recommend additional tests and treatments if they are reasonably necessary to diagnose the condition or to improve or accelerate the eventual outcome. However, recommending excessive diagnostic tests and additional symptomatic care, particularly in the setting of chronic pain, can be counterproductive. If a true chronic pain syndrome is present, recommending multidisciplinary, cognitive-behavioral approaches should be considered to achieve improved functioning despite pain.

Maximum Medical Improvement

Maximum medical improvement (MMI) is the point when further medical intervention or treatment is reasonably unlikely to improve the underlying impairment (60). The sixth edition of the *Guides* no longer specifies the duration of sufficient healing, but a "sufficient healing period" has occurred when the medical condition has resolved, or when there is no reasonable evidence of ongoing or anticipated progress toward resolution of the condition. This is also often referred to as reaching a *healing plateau*. MMI determination should be based primarily on lack of demonstrable progress toward reducing impairment or achieving measurable functional gains, and should not be confused with persistent symptoms, which may or may not resolve with time.

Sometimes an individual has a condition that has improved to the point of stability, but which may be expected to worsen in the future. This person would meet criteria for MMI, but it would be appropriate either to comment that additional treatment will likely be needed in the future to provide a medical basis for reopening a claim in the future or to estimate the likely future needs to maintain or minimize the progression of impairment.

Impairment Rating and Apportionment

Permanent impairment should not be rated until the individual has reached MMI, unless otherwise statutorily mandated. For example, in Minnesota, the insurer is expected to pay PPD benefits as soon as permanency is apparent and payable, such as for an amputation, even though the healing period may not have ended yet. They must pay the current minimum rating, referred to as the minimum ascertainable PPD, now and then pay any remaining PPD that is due when a final rating is appropriate. Otherwise, if using the AMA *Guides*, the permanent total or partial impairment associated with the condition should be determined according to methods and procedures outlined in the book (60). For situations where there has been a previous rating of an organ system, any new permanent impairment should be apportioned taking into account prior ratings.

Work Ability

The ability to return to work, particularly when there is a concern about the speed of recovery, is a frequent question posed to the IME physician. Many job descriptions provided by employers do not have detailed physical requirements to perform the job. In these cases, having a formal job analysis and the results of a FCE can assist in the determination of work ability (see prior section on functional assessments).

Medicolegal Issues

While there is no legal consensus, courts have tended to favor the view that the IME creates at least a limited physician-patient relationship, sufficient to allow for certain malpractice claims. IME physicians are felt to have the following legal duties to their patients (61): (a) the duty not to cause injury during the examination, (b) the duty to diagnose significant medical conditions accurately, (c) the duty to disclose significant findings in a reasonable manner, and (d) the duty to maintain confidentiality. It has been recommended that prior to conducting an IME, physicians should inform claimants who will receive medical information or findings arising from the evaluation, and obtain written authorization for such disclosures before conducting the IME, using a HIPAA (Health Insurance Portability and Accountability Act) compliant authorization form (61).

The IME physician should expect to be deposed or offer courtroom testimony in the future regarding the findings and opinions rendered following a disability determination. This could occur months or even years from the time of the IME, so the report should be carried out in a thorough, systematic, and detailed manner. At times, it is not possible to remember details from the encounter except as documented in the report.

MEDICAL IMPAIRMENT RATING

Purpose and Derivation of the AMA *Guides*

The AMA *Guides to the Evaluation of Permanent Impairment* (henceforth the *Guides*) was originally published as a series of articles in JAMA starting in 1958 and then subsequently compiled into a single volume in 1971 (13). It has been developed and refined through several editions to standardize the method of evaluating and reporting medical impairment of any human organ system (60). The *Guides* serve as a tool to convert medically assessed permanent impairment into numerical values or *ratings*, which are expressed as a percentage of loss of function for whichever organ system is involved. Reportedly, as of July 2016, 32 states require physicians to use some edition of the *Guides* in making their assessments of permanent impairment for injured workers and 15 more allow the use of the *Guides*, making them an important reference standard for medical disability claims evaluations (62). The sixth edition is the current edition; however, prior editions are still mandated in some jurisdictions. The fifth edition needed revision to address a number of shortcomings (13). The major criticisms were that "(a) the *Guides* failed to provide a comprehensive, valid, reliable, unbiased, and evidence-based rating system; (b) impairment ratings did not adequately or accurately reflect perceived and actual loss of function; and (c) numerical ratings were more the representation of legal fiction than medical reality" (11). The goals for the sixth edition were to address the criticisms by enhancing the validity and reliability of ratings with an emphasis on a diagnosis-based approach, improving internal consistency with the adoption of an ICF-based template for five functionally based impairment classes across all organ systems, and applying standardized activities of daily living (ADL) assessment methods to the impairment ratings (63). The consequent effect on the ratings shows a significant difference between average whole person impairment ratings when comparing the sixth edition with the fifth edition, but not when comparing the sixth edition with the fourth edition, suggesting that average ratings from the fifth edition had increased from the fourth edition without any clear or intended scientific rationale (64).

Limitations of the AMA *Guides*

The *Guides* provides a disclaimer that it is not to be used for direct estimates of work disability (60). However, as already discussed, impairment percentages derived according to the AMA *Guides* are used by many states to determine disability percentages for workers' compensation purposes. One of the criticisms of the *Guides* is that they are designed to measure the severity of impairment as opposed to disability. While impairment refers to the loss of function of a body part, disability implies the loss of ability to participate in major life activities, including the ability to work, and consequently the ability to earn a living. With workers' compensation, financial losses resulting from work disability provide the basis for indemnity benefits. It has been shown, at least for the fifth edition, that impairment ratings are accurate predictors of disability severity on average (65). However, there are differences across body regions between impairment ratings and loss of earnings, with spine impairments, for example, being associated with 22% higher earning losses in comparison to similar knee impairments, suggesting that work disability varies across body regions differently than impairment ratings and suggesting that someone with a similar spine impairment rating relative to someone with a knee injury would be underpaid for the economic loss (65).

Another concern regarding impairment versus disability arises with chronic pain (66). Impairment is assessed according to predetermined measurable criteria. The subjectivity inherent in the assessment of pain can be measured using only subjective criteria. So, even though pain can result in disability, the *Guides* typically accounts for this at the organ system level as a contributing modifier of ADLs for diagnosis-based impairment ratings (63). In the rare situation where persistent pain cannot be attributed to an organ system and diagnosis-based source, a "pain rating" can be applied, but it is capped at 3% (60). In general, the physician examiner can frequently expect to encounter elements of symptom magnification, particularly in the presence of chronicity and pain. Exaggerated displays of pain behavior and related inconsistencies should not significantly influence the impairment rating, which is based on other objective criteria.

SUMMARY

Many social systems exist to provide a means for fair and equitable compensation for those individuals with disabilities that impact their ability to earn a living. Physicians are required for the processes to function properly. Since this chapter only provides a brief introduction to the concepts involved in the medical determination of work disability, including common conceptual models of disability, terminology, functional assessments, major disability systems in the United States, and the IME, the interested learner is encouraged to pursue further education and training in this subject area.

REFERENCES

1. Kottke FJ, Knapp ME. The development of physiatry before 1950. *Arch Phys Med Rehabil.* 1988;69(Spec No):4–14.
2. Martins AC. Using the International Classification of Functioning, Disability and Health (ICF) to address facilitators and barriers to participation at work. *Work.* 2015;50(4):585–593.
3. Keratar R, et al. Work disabilities and unmet needs for health care and rehabilitation among jobseekers: a community-level investigation using multidimensional work ability assessments. *Scand J Prim Health Care.* 2016;34(4):343–351.
4. Nagi SZ. A study in the evaluation of disability and rehabilitation potential: concepts, methods, and procedures. *Am J Public Health Nations Health.* 1964;54:1568–1579.
5. Nagi SZ, ed. *Disability and Rehabilitation: Legal, Clinical, and Self-Concepts and Measurement.* Columbus, OH: Ohio State University Press; 1969.
6. Masala C, Petretto DR. From disablement to enablement: conceptual models of disability in the 20th century. *Disabil Rehabil.* 2008;30(17):1233–1244.
7. WHO. *International Classification of Impairments, Disabilities and Handicaps: A Manual of Classification Relating to the Consequences of Disease.* Geneva, Switzerland: World Health Organization; 1980.
8. Cocchiarella L, Lord SJ; American Medical Association. *Master the AMA Guides Fifth: A Medical and Legal Transition to the Guides to the Evaluation of Permanent Impairment.* 5th ed. Chicago, IL: AMA Press; 2001:ix, 401.
9. WHO. *International Classification of Functioning, Disability and Health.* Geneva, Switzerland: World Health Organization; 2001.
10. Rondinelli RD, Genovese E, Brigham CR, eds. *Guides to the Evaluation of Permanent Impairment.* 6th ed. Chicago, IL: American Medical Association; 2008.
11. Spieler EA, et al. Recommendations to guide revision of the Guides to the Evaluation of Permanent Impairment. *JAMA.* 2000;283(4):519–523.
12. Causey J, McFarren T. In search of a method: permanent disability assessment revisited. *New Solut.* 2000;10(3):207–215.
13. Rondinelli RD, Katz RT. Merits and shortcomings of the American Medical Association Guides to the Evaluation of Permanent Impairment, 5th edition. A physiatric perspective. *Phys Med Rehabil Clin N Am.* 2002;13(2):355–370, x.
14. Pope AM, Tarlov AR, eds. *Disability in America: A National Agenda for Prevention.* Washington, DC: Institute of Medicine, National Academy Press; 1991.
15. Pope AM, Brandt EN Jr. *Enabling America: Assessing the Role of Rehabilitation Science and Engineering.* Washington, DC: National Academies Press; 1997.
16. McGeary M, Ford M, McCutchen S; IOM Committee on Medical Evaluation of Veterans for Disability Compensation. *A 21st Century System for Evaluating Veterans for Disability Benefits. The Rating Schedule.* Washington, DC: National Academies Press; 2007.
17. Rondinelli RD. Changes for the new AMA Guides to impairment ratings: implications and applications for physician disability evaluations. *PM R.* 2009;1(7):643–656.
18. West J. *The Americans with Disabilities Act: From Policy to Practice.* New York: Milbank Memorial Fund; 1991.
19. Long AB. *Introducing the New and Improved Americans with Disabilities Act: Assessing the ADA Amendments Act of 2008.* Nw. U. L. Rev. Colloquy; 2008.
20. Krause N, et al. Determinants of duration of disability and return-to-work after work-related injury and illness: challenges for future research. *Am J Ind Med.* 2001;40(4):464–484.
21. Gelfman R, et al. Correlates of upper extremity disability in medical transcriptionists. *J Occup Rehabil.* 2010;20(3):340–348.
22. Nagi SZ. *Disability and Rehabilitation: Legal, Clinical, and Self-concepts and Measurements.* Columbus, OH: Ohio State University Press; 1970.
23. Yelin E, Nevitt M, Epstein W. Toward an epidemiology of work disability. *Milbank Mem Fund Q Health Soc.* 1980;58(3):386–415.
24. Brouwer S, et al. Comparing self-report, clinical examination and functional testing in the assessment of work-related limitations in patients with chronic low back pain. *Disabil Rehabil.* 2005;27(17):999–1005.
25. Smith SL. The forensic model of occupational therapy. *Occup Ther Health Care.* 1984;1(1):17–22.
26. King PM, Tuckwell N, Barrett TE. A critical review of functional capacity evaluations. *Phys Ther.* 1998;78(8):852–866.
27. Chen JJ. Functional capacity evaluation & disability. *Iowa Orthop J.* 2007;27:121–127.
28. Tramposh AK. The functional capacity evaluation: measuring maximal work abilities. *Occup Med.* 1992;7(1):113–124.
29. Innes E, Straker L. A clinician's guide to work-related assessments: 3—administration and interpretation problems. *Work.* 1998;11(2):207–219.
30. Gouttebarge V, et al. Reliability and validity of Functional Capacity Evaluation methods: a systematic review with reference to Blankenship system, Ergos work simulator, Ergo-Kit and Isernhagen work system. *Int Arch Occup Environ Health.* 2004;77(8):527–537.
31. Gross DP, Battie MC. Factors influencing results of functional capacity evaluations in workers' compensation claimants with low back pain. *Phys Ther.* 2005;85(4):315–322.
32. Rudy TE, Lieber SJ, Boston JR. Functional capacity assessment: influence of behavioral and environmental factors. *J Back Musculoskelet Rehabil.* 1996;6(3):277–288.
33. Lechner DE, Bradbury SF, Bradley LA. Detecting sincerity of effort: a summary of methods and approaches. *Phys Ther.* 1998;78(8):867–888.
34. van der Meer S, et al. Which instruments can detect submaximal physical and functional capacity in patients with chronic nonspecific back pain? A systematic review. *Spine (Phila Pa 1976).* 2013;38(25):E1608–E1615.
35. Barth J, et al. Inter-rater agreement in evaluation of disability: systematic review of reproducibility studies. *BMJ.* 2017;356:j14.
36. Wind H, et al. Effect of Functional Capacity Evaluation information on the judgment of physicians about physical work ability in the context of disability claims. *Int Arch Occup Environ Health.* 2009;82(9):1087–1096.

37. Reneman MF, et al. Concurrent validity of questionnaire and performance-based disability measurements in patients with chronic nonspecific low back pain. *J Occup Rehabil*. 2002;12(3):119–129.

38. Spanjer J, Groothoff JW, Brouwer S. Instruments used to assess functional limitations in workers applying for disability benefit: a systematic review. *Disabil Rehabil*. 2011;33(23–24):2143–2150.

39. Johns REJ, Colledge AL, Holmes EB. Introduction to fitness for duty. In: Andersson GBJ, Demeter SL, Smith GM, eds. *Disability Evaluation*. 2nd ed. St. Louis, MO: Mosby/AMAp; 2003:709–738.

40. Rondinelli RD, Katz RT. *Impairment Rating and Disability Evaluation*. Philadelphia, PA: WB Saunders Company; 2000.

41. Szymendera SD. *Workers' Compensation: Overview and Issues*. Washington, DC: Congressional Research Service; 2017.

42. Sengupta I, Baldwin ML. *Workers' Compensation: Benefits, Coverage, and Costs, 2013*. Washington, DC: National Academy of Social Insurance; 2015.

43. Burton JF, Jr. The National Commission on State Workmen's Compensation Laws: a year later. *Arch Environ Health*. 1974;29(1):34–38.

44. Hellmuth GA. Medical recommendations and the National Commission on State Workmen's Compensation Laws. *IMS Ind Med Surg*. 1972;41(7):20–24.

45. Howe HF. Developments subsequent to report of National Commission on State Workmen's Compensation Laws. *J Occup Med*. 1973;15(8):657–658.

46. Kearney JR. Social Security and the "D" in OASDI: the history of a Federal Program insuring earners against disability. *Soc Secur Bull*. 2006;66(3):1–27.

47. https://www.ssa.gov/disability/professionals/bluebook/general-info.htm

48. https://www.ssa.gov/disability/professionals/bluebook/AdultListings.htm

49. https://www.ssa.gov/news/press/factsheets/basicfact-alt.pdf

50. Ranavaya MI, Rondinelli RD. The major U.S. disability and compensation systems: origins and historical overview. In: Katz RT, Rondinelli RD, eds. *Impairment Rating and Disability Evaluation*. Philadelphia, PA: WB Saunders; 2000:3–16.

51. http://www.benefits.va.gov/COMPENSATION/types-disability.asp

52. Oboler S. Disability evaluation under the department of veterans affairs. In: Katz RT, Rondinelli RD, eds. *Impairment Rating and Disability Evaluation*. Philadelphia, PA: W.W. Saunders Company; 2000:187–217.

53. Kraus J. The independent medical examination and the functional capacity evaluation. *Occup Med*. 1997;12(3):525–556.

54. Spencer RF. Are independent medical examiners truly independent? *Pain Physician*. 2010;13(1):92–93; author reply 93–94.

55. Ameis A, Zasler ND. The independent medical examination. *Phys Med Rehabil Clin N Am*. 2002;13(2):259–286, ix.

56. Waddell G, et al. Nonorganic physical signs in low-back pain. *Spine (Phila Pa 1976)*. 1980;5(2):117–125.

57. Velly AM, Mohit S. Epidemiology of pain and relation to psychiatric disorders. *Prog Neuropsychopharmacol Biol Psychiatry*. 2017;87(Pt B):159–167.

58. Committee on Psychological Testing, Including Validity Testing, for Social Security Administration Disability Determinations; Board on the Health of Select Populations; Institute of Medicine. *Psychological Testing in the Service of Disability Determination*. Washington, DC: National Academies Press (US); 2015.

59. Foye PM, et al. Industrial medicine and acute musculoskeletal rehabilitation. 5. Effective medical management of industrial injuries: from causality to case closure. *Arch Phys Med Rehabil*. 2002;83(3 suppl 1):S19–S24, S33–S39.

60. Rondinelli RD, Genovese E, Brigham CR. *Guides to the Evaluation of Permanent Impairment*. 6th ed. Chicago, IL: American Medical Association; 2008.

61. Baum K. Independent medical examinations: an expanding source of physician liability. *Ann Intern Med*. 2005;142(12 Pt 1):974–978.

62. https://www.lexisnexis.com/legalnewsroom/workers-compensation/b/recent-cases-news-trends-developments/archive/2016/07/21/latest-developments-in-state-handling-of-ama-guidelines.aspx?Redirected=true

63. Rondinelli RD. Changes for the new AMA Guides to impairment ratings, 6th edition: implications and applications for physician disability evaluations. *PM R*. 2009;1(7):643–656.

64. Brigham C, Uejo C, McEntire A, et al. Comparative analysis of AMA Guides ratings by the fourth, fifth, and sixth editions. *AMA Guides Newsl*. 2010;81.

65. Seabury SA, Neuhauser F, Nuckols T. American Medical Association impairment ratings and earnings losses due to disability. *J Occup Environ Med*. 2013;55(3):286–291.

66. Robinson JP, Turk DC, Loeser JD. Pain, impairment, and disability in the AMA guides. *J Law Med Ethics*. 2004;32(2):315–326, 191.

CHAPTER 9

Gerold Stucki   Melissa Selb
Jerome Bickenbach   John L. Melvin

The International Classification of Functioning, Disability, and Health

The health of an individual, and by extension of a population, can best be understood in terms of the actual experience of living with a health condition—whether it is a congenital disorder, an injury, an acute or chronic health condition, or the natural process of ageing. Since the myriad of ways in which health can be compromised are unavoidable, and ageing is an inevitable process of the accumulating molecular and cellular damage (1), living with a health condition is a universal human experience. The lived experience of health, moreover, can be operationalized as **functioning**—understood both biomedically, in terms of the functions and structures of the body and the resulting intrinsic capacity of a person to perform simple or complex activities, as well as the actual performance of those activities in interaction with features of the person's physical, human-built, and social environment (2).

The notion of functioning is at the core of the World Health Organization's (WHO) *International Classification of Functioning, Disability and Health* (ICF) endorsed by the 54th World Health Assembly in 2001 (3). Since then, the ICF has proven to be a robust and widely applicable conceptual framework for documenting functioning information (4), and, more generally, the international common language of functioning and disability (5). Functioning is also the key concept that animates rehabilitation theory and practice (6). Conceptually, rehabilitation can be characterized as the health strategy that aims at the optimization of a person's functioning in interaction with the environment (7,8). In light of population ageing and the increase in prevalence of chronic noncommunicable diseases, the focus of health care will increasingly turn to the need to optimize functioning in addition to preventing premature death. Given these trends, rehabilitation will become the key health strategy of the 21st century (9).

The objective of this chapter is to introduce the reader to the ICF and in particular to the central notion of functioning, explaining how functioning relates to rehabilitation practice within the health system. In the first two sections, we present how functioning provides an operationalization of health and how, as a consequence, it constitutes—after mortality and morbidity—the third health indicator that defines the outcome of interest of rehabilitation in particular and health care in general. In the third section, we place functioning more broadly into the context of the health sciences and rehabilitation research, and in the final four sections, we review considerations relevant to the documentation of functioning

information for clinical decision-making and, more broadly, as the key precondition for a learning health system.

ICF: WHO'S OPERATIONALIZATION OF HEALTH

Since its foundation in 1948, the WHO has officially defined health as the "state of complete physical, mental and social well-being and not merely the absence of disease or infirmity" (10). Over the years, this aspirational definition has been criticized for its unrealistic expectation of "complete health" (11) and the confusion created by equating health with well-being, especially social well-being (12,13). Whether it is useful to try to define health or not (14), it is clear that the health sciences and health care practice requires an *operationalization of health* to work with. An operationalization makes it possible to describe states of health in a universal and comparable manner, setting the stage both for evaluation of health care interventions and the measurement of health for the health sciences and for rehabilitation and health systems research in general (6,15).

Unlike a purely theoretical definition of health, an operationalization must not only meet scientific measurement criteria but also accord with our basic intuitions about why our health matters to us. It must be useful in the explanation as to why we have made such an enormous societal investment in the institutions of health care provision. And indeed, it is here where the notion of functioning becomes relevant: health matters to us because health problems interfere with our lives and what we want to do. If we find it difficult to climb stairs, walk as far as we used to, clean or dress ourselves as quickly as we need to, read a book, make and keep friends, do all the housework we have to, or perform our job—when these limitations are associated with diseases, injuries, and other health conditions, then they are inextricably linked to how our bodies and minds function. Problems in health are problems in functioning. Health matters to us, in other words, because of our lived experience of health and its impact on our daily functioning.

Arguably, this approach to understanding health preserves the spirit of WHO's original 1948 "aspirational" definition of health (10). The 1948 definition insisted that health is not the same as the absence of pathologies or diseases but that it implicitly acknowledges the importance of a person's environment and its impact on the lived experience of health (10).

This is the functioning approach. While commonsense may demand that we abandon the utopian notion that health is "complete well-being," keeping the insight that health has far more to do with living our lives and achieving our life goals preserves the aspirational value of the WHO definition (16).

WHO's ICF was developed in order to provide a new perspective for describing and understanding a person's lived experience of health in terms of the notion of functioning. WHO's *International Classification of Diseases* (ICD) (17) had been developed as an international language of diagnosis to collect data relevant to morbidity and mortality. What was missing was a classification for information about living with a health condition in order to be able to collect data relevant to functioning. This was a paradigm-shifting change in focus (16). In this chapter, the dimensions of this paradigm shift will be described in detail in the context of rehabilitation, and primarily as it affects the information documentation requirements for rehabilitation practice and management.

The ICF serves as a conceptual framework and practical lens for describing the lived experience of health in a meaningful and useful manner for rehabilitation practitioners aiming to optimize functioning, for policy-makers to shape health systems to effectively respond to the functioning needs of the population, and finally, for researchers who seek to explain functioning and its determinants and thereby to understand not only rehabilitation as a health strategy but health itself (16).

Conceptual Framework and Structure

As a model of functioning and problems with functioning, the ICF represents the culmination in conceptual developments that resulted in a model in which states of functioning and disability are outcomes of interactions between intrinsic health features of the person and the full context in which the person lives and acts, in terms of environmental and personal factors (3). The debate between the "medical model" and the "social model" of disability that waged during the 1970s and 80s resolved itself into a broader consensus by the time the ICF was being developed at the end of the 1990s (18). This consensus recognized that when people experience problems with functioning, the underlying determinants of this involve both the person's health state, and specifically the negative impact on the person's functioning that the health condition produces, as well as the many factors associated with the overall environmental and personal context in which the person lives and acts. This interactive, person and environment, construct, although novel in some areas of medicine, was well known in the domain of rehabilitation practice (19).

This so-called interactional model of functioning and disability is called the "biopsychosocial" model in the ICF. The ICF model is interactional in the sense that it identifies the two primary classes of determinants of functioning and disability—namely, Health Conditions and Contextual Factors. Health Conditions are broadly characterized as diseases (acute or chronic), disorders, injuries, trauma, or any other "natural" circumstance such as pregnancy, ageing, stress, congenital anomaly, or genetic predisposition. These are to be coded using the ICD (17). The 11th revision of the ICD (ICD-11) is currently being finalized and is anticipated to include a list of "functioning properties" directly associated with specific health conditions, thereby increasing the usefulness of joint application of the two WHO international classifications (20,21).

As a classification, ICF is structured in a manner that mirrors its underlying conceptual framework. As displayed in **Figure 9-1**, there are two basic parts of the ICF as a classification: part 1 classifies functioning and disability in terms of two components: (a) Body Functions and Structures and (b)

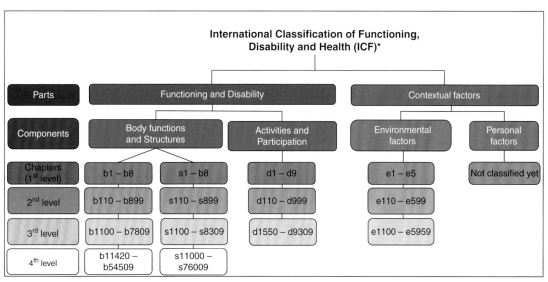

Example for different levels:

First or chapter level	b2	Sensory functions and pain
Second level	b280	Sensation of pain
Third level	b2801	Pain in body part
Fourth level	b28013	Pain in back

*Personal Factors, a component within the Contextual Factors, are not classified yet and Body Functions and Body Structures, a component within Functioning and Disability, is the only component with 4th level categories.

FIGURE 9-1. The structure of the ICF classifications. (Adapted from Prodinger B, Tennant A, Stucki G, et al. Harmonizing routinely collected health information for strengthening quality management in health systems: requirements and practice. *J Health Serv Res Policy.* 2016;21(4):223–228. Copyright © 2016 SAGE Publications.)

Activities and Participation. Part 2 comprises the Contextual Factors, namely the components of Environmental Factors and Personal Factors. Although the Personal Factor component is not developed in the ICF, work has been done to provide guidance in the use of a subset of these factors, for example psychological personal factors (22). In the first part, ICF consists of a classification of Body Functions (physiologic functions of body systems, including psychological functions) and a parallel classification of Body Structures (anatomical parts of the body such as organs, limbs, and their components). Both classifications are arranged by body systems and together provide an international common language and coding scheme for information about body-level functioning. Problems at this level are termed "impairments." Secondly, there is a classification of Activities and Participation that provides an international language and coding scheme for information about all of the activities, tasks, and behaviors that human beings engage in, from the very simple (e.g., d110 Watching) to the more complex (e.g., d510 Washing oneself), as well as the more socially constructed and complex interpersonal and social engagements with others across the major life activities (e.g., d710 Basic interpersonal interactions, d830 Higher education, d850 Remunerative employment; d950 Political life and citizenship). The ICF divides this classification into Activities ("execution of a task or action by an individual") and Participation ("involvement in a life situation"). Although the classification conceptually represents a single, unbroken continuum from simple to complex tasks and actions, in clinical practice and research it may be helpful to make an informal distinction between those actions that are "close" to the person (Activities) and those that are more "distant" and socially constructed (Participation).

In Part 2, there is the essential component of the ICF model of functioning, namely Environmental Factors. These factors range from climate and other physical conditions, to the human-built environment and products, human relationships, attitudes, and complex services, systems, and policies across several basic societal domains (e.g., housing, communications, transportation, media, economic, social security, health, education, labor and political). The Environmental Factors classification is fundamental to the underlying conceptual framework of the ICF in which functioning, and problems with functioning, or disability, are understood as outcomes of the interaction between the health conditions a person experiences and the person's overall environmental context. This classification allows for the collection of information about the person's actual, real-world context, and in particular whether, and the extent to which, that environment facilitates or hinders the performance of actions.

Taking all of the classifications together, the ICF contains a total of 1,495 meaningful, discrete, and mutually exclusive elements of information called categories. These categories are cumulatively exhaustive and cover the entire spectrum of human functioning and the environment. The categories are organized by means of a standard hierarchically nested structure with, depending on the classification, up to four levels as shown in **Figure 9-1**. The ICF categories are denoted by unique alphanumeric codes (the letters b, s, d, and e followed by one to five digits) for collecting information both at the individual or clinical level, or the group level for programming development and evaluation, and at the overall population level for health systems and policy research, development, and implementation.

In order to denote the level of functioning or positive or negative environmental impact for any category, the ICF suggests using qualifiers that form part of the coding scheme. In the case of Environmental Factors, the qualifier indicates whether, and the degree to which, the factor is a facilitator or barrier, positively or negatively impacting the individual's functioning. Body Functions and Body Structures rely on a single severity qualifier and several more specific qualifiers of position and location. Activities and Participation identify severity in terms of capacity and performance qualifiers (described below). All of the severity qualifiers use the same generic five-point scale ("0" = no problem, "1" = mild problem, "2" = moderate problem, "3" = severe problem, "4" = complete problem) (3). There are also other scales, including interval scales to indicate functioning level, such as the numeric rating scale used in the case example described below.

Biologic Health and Lived Health

The ICF provides an international standard language of functioning terminology as well as a classification for the consistent documentation and reporting of information about both bodily health and the lived experience of health. What has in the rehabilitation literature been variously labeled as "functional loss," "functional limitation," or "functional incapacity," is in the ICF consistently and systematically defined (23).

Each category of functioning in the ICF—whether Body Functions and Structure, or Activity and Participation—is a distinct and meaningful component of the overall lived experience of a health condition. This entails, firstly, that the ICF is only applicable in the context of a health condition. There are, for complex domains such as employment, different reasons why a person may not perform optimally, but the ICF is only concerned with capturing information of functioning of persons experiencing a health condition of any sort and any degree of severity. Secondly, each functioning category represents a component that can be experienced at any point along a continuum from total absence of functioning (or in the case of Body Structures, absence, deviation, discontinuity of a body part) to full functioning. This range is reflected in the generic five-point scale for the severity qualifiers. In the ICF, functioning is a matter of more or less rather than present or not present.

The continuous nature of functioning categories is an essential conceptual feature of the ICF and reflects the reality of the lived experience of health. The continuity of each functioning category entails that there is no predetermined threshold point on the continuum in which the level of functioning becomes a problem or disability. For example, for a category in Body Functions—say b2100 Visual Acuity functions—the ICF does not predetermine where on the continuum of visual acuity a person will experience an impairment of visual acuity. Total absence of visual acuity is obviously impairment (blindness) and total presence is obviously not, but where on the continuum impairment begins is not predetermined by the ICF. This threshold or cut-off point is left to research and standardization, possibly in terms of population norms. For this reason, the ICF does not identify who has impairment or a disability and who does not. For a similar reason, the ICF does not purport to identify two distinct groups of people in a population, those with disabilities and those without. That is not the function of the ICF. For social reasons—for example, eligibility for social supports or services—thresholds will be administratively created and applied. Optimally these should be based on the insights of clinical practice and research in the form of transparent and stable standardization. In short, although the ICF is perfectly well suited for disability assessment and eligibility determination for social services and supports, the ICF does not determine who is eligible and who is not (24).

The ICF is WHO's paradigm-shifting instrument for describing the lived experience of health in terms of functioning that can serve as the operationalization of health, suitable for measurement purposes (25). At the heart of the ICF conceptual framework is a fundamental distinction that transforms the intuitive interactional or "person-environment" model of functioning into a powerful scientific tool. This is the distinction captured by the notions of *capacity* and *performance*. This distinction is represented by the two severity qualifiers found in the Activities and Participation classification, but its significance goes far beyond this technical application.

The ICF notion of *capacity* is a theoretical construct (statistically, a latent trait) that in practice is essentially a clinical inference based on information about the underlying health conditions and observations of what people do given their impairments. Capacity constitutes the intrinsic health state of a person, independent of the environment. Capacity is composed of all physiologic and psychological functions and anatomical structures of the body, and, by virtue of these functions in various combinations, results in the "capacity" of the person to perform all human activities, from the very simple to the very complex. A person's capacity should be understood to be independent of the external, environmental determinants that may facilitate or hinder the actual execution of these activities.

Performance, on the other hand, presumes a person's capacity but goes beyond it to describe the extent to which the person actually performs or executes activities, simple or complex, fully in the context of, and in interaction with, all aspects of that person's environment. Performance is not a theoretical construct, but a full factual description of what actually takes place. Hence, the performance of human action always depends on features of the person's environment (physical, human-built, social, political, and cultural), as these shape all of what people do and, by extension, what complex social roles they perform (spouse, father, student, employee, and so on). Environmental factors may make it harder to perform activities (e.g., poor air quality, inaccessible and nonaccommodating physical environments, or stigma and discrimination, and social exclusion), or make it easier to perform activities (e.g., assistive technology, accessible buildings, supportive attitudes, and social arrangements).

The lived experience of health is therefore determined by both the intrinsic health state of a person and the overall physical and social environment in which that person lives. Information about relatively simple activities such like grasping, standing, or even walking can be gathered by simple observation. Although information about the level of performance of complex activities, such as making friends, going to school, or participating in cultural activities, is far more intricate and socially constructed, it is nearly always possible to adequately describe the level of a person's performance taking

into account both a person's biologic health and his or her actual environment.

This suggests that a distinction needs to be made within the lived experience of health between **biologic health** and **lived health** (26). Capacity identifies the domain of biologic health, while performance captures the complementary experience of lived health. All of this information, it should be noted, is "etiologically neutral" in the sense that it does not explicitly refer to any particular underlying cause, be it disease, injury, or natural process such as ageing. It is a basic clinical observation that people with very different diseases can experience the same kinds of problem in functioning, while people with the same diseases can experience very different functioning problems, especially if they live in very different environments (2).

The ICF in effect characterizes in general terms the goal or objective of any intervention, health and social, that is designed to respond to functioning needs: an intervention should be designed to optimize intrinsic health capacity as much as possible and to translate that capacity into performance in interaction with environment. This translation of biologic health into lived health is characteristic of health interventions and is fundamental to rehabilitation interventions (9,16,26).

ICF for Physical Medicine and Rehabilitation

The distinction between biologic and lived health has several powerful applications in rehabilitation practice and health systems research. First of all, as described in detail in the sections on documenting functioning below, the distinction—operationalized in terms of the ICF constructs of capacity and performance—makes it possible to document functioning and analyze these data in a standardized and internationally comparable manner across the continuum of care. Furthermore, as described later in this chapter, ICF functioning data can inform clinical decision-making and, at the programming and systems level, makes it possible to create and maintain a "learning health system" for continuous clinical quality management in rehabilitation and evidence-informed policy.

The ICF also provides a representation of how Physical Medicine and Rehabilitation (PMR) professionals organize rehabilitation. The conceptual framework of the ICF includes components familiar to PMR specialists, although perhaps not by the terms the ICF uses. PMR encounters with patients are generally precipitated by patient-perceived restrictions in the performance in important life experiences, such as work, recreation, moving from place to place, and independence in self-care. Presented with these patient complaints, PMR specialists seek to determine the impairments that contribute to these restrictions in a patient's lived experience of health, seeking information regarding physiologic, pathophysiologic, and psychological body functions and anatomic structures, and their impact on the ability of the patient to perform life activities.

Usually, the PMR specialist focuses first on the capacity to perform these activities in a neutral environment, such as exists in rehabilitation treatment centers or other clinical settings. Of course, the PMR specialist, such as a physician, will also collect information regarding the health condition associated with these limitations in terms of capacity and performance. PMR specialists are also well aware that environmental factors, such as physical barriers, both natural and person-made; social attitudes; and other social restrictions, seriously impact the successful performance of life activities of all people, but particularly those with limitations in functioning. They also recognize that personal factors, such as life experiences, age, and overall approach to life may influence the extent of a person's recovery of functioning. In short, the PMR specialist takes into account all of the ICF components when developing, usually with the patient and other rehabilitation professionals, the treatment plan designed to optimize patient functioning and enhancing their performance of activities in fundamental life experiences.

To fully appreciate how the ICF contributes to our understanding of rehabilitation, as one of the basic health strategies (7,8), it is necessary to describe how functioning is the third health indicator after mortality and morbidity (26).

FUNCTIONING: THIRD AND KEY HEALTH INDICATOR FOR REHABILITATION

Traditionally, epidemiology is characterized as the study of how often diseases and other health conditions occur in different population groups and why, including studies that identify patterns, causes, and effects of health conditions on the population (27). Accordingly, the health indicators traditionally employed in epidemiologic research are mortality—the indicator of a population's length of life and the survival of individuals with health conditions—and morbidity—the indicator for number, distribution, and duration of health conditions in the population (28). The data for these two indicators can be coded with ICD. Yet, these two indicators, although essential indicators for population health, are of limited value in understanding people's lived experience of health in light of their health conditions, and in interaction with their environment.

For this reason, WHO has suggested a more comprehensive sense of epidemiology as "the study of the distribution and determinants of health-related states or events (including disease), and the application of this study to the control of diseases and other health problems" (28). There is a strong case to be made that comprehensive epidemiology works with three health indicators, mortality, morbidity, and functioning (16). The functioning indicator can supplement the epidemiology

of morbidity and mortality by including information about a population's lived experience of health condition, as well as being a measure of the outcome of clinical interventions (26).

Moreover, by analytically distinguishing biologic health (captured by information about the person's intrinsic capacity) and lived health (captured by information about performance) health scientists can use functioning as a health indicator to elucidate approaches to the primary objective of a health system: to achieve and maintain population health. Since 1978 and the Declaration of Alma Ata (29) four health strategies have been recognized: promotive, preventive, curative, and rehabilitative. More recently, the palliative strategy has been added (30). In practice, these strategies are combined to effectively address the individual's health needs. Still, given the goals of each strategy, the most relevant health indicator and information coding standard are different for each strategy (26). **Table 9-1** displays these differences and presents the main use cases for which health information is applicable.

The primary goal of the health strategy of prevention is to prevent the occurrence of health conditions and premature mortality in the population. Prevention targets risk factors that are characterized in the ICF as Environmental and Personal Factors. In prevention, morbidity and mortality are the relevant indicators; functioning can be used to report on the level of biologic health preserved thanks to the nonoccurrence of health conditions. Health promotion also targets known risk factors and aims to improve people's intrinsic health capacity. Thus, the key indicator for health promotion is functioning, from the perspective of biologic health. Since the curative strategy aims at the restoration of full health (or if that is not an option, then remission and disease control), its key indicator is mortality. At the same time, cure is a matter of optimal management of a health condition, and minimization of complications and comorbidities, so information about morbidity is also relevant. Although the curative strategy seeks to improve biologic health, it is indifferent to the rest of the lived experience of health, since this is affected by Environmental Factors and these factors are outside the scope of the curative strategy. Finally, the goal of the palliative strategy is to optimize wellbeing during the dying process, which is more a matter of a person's appraisal of his or her lived experience.

TABLE 9-1	The Main Health Strategies of the Health System, their Goals, and Indicators		
Strategy	**Health Goal**	**Health Indicator**	
Preventive	Prevent the occurrence of health conditions	Morbidity	ICD
	Prevent mortality related to the occurrence of health conditions	Mortality	ICD
	Prevent the loss of functioning related to the occurrence of health conditions	Biologic health (intrinsic health capacity)	ICF ICD
Promotive	Optimal health	Biologic health (intrinsic health capacity)	ICF
Curative	Cure (full recovery)	Mortality	ICD
	Remission	Mobility	ICD-11
	Disease control	Functioning (intrinsic health capacity)	ICD-11
Rehabilitative	**Optimal functioning**	**Functioning**	**ICF**
Palliative	Optimize wellbeing	Appraised functioning (quality of life)	ICF

Adapted with permission from Salomon J, Mathers C, Chatterji S, et al. Quantifying individual levels of health: definitions, concepts, and measurement issues. In: Murray CJL, Evans CJL, eds. *Health Systems Performance Assessment: Debates, Methods and Empiricism.* WHO: Geneva, 2003:301–318.

Key Indicator for Rehabilitation

The point of this review of the health strategies is to highlight the significance of functioning for the rehabilitative strategy. Functioning is clearly the key indicator for rehabilitation (7,13,14). It was the adoption of the ICF that made it possible to rethink the conceptual foundations of rehabilitation as a health strategy by professional organizations and researchers. Accordingly, the goal of rehabilitation was identified as that of enabling people with health conditions experiencing or likely to experience disability to achieve and maintain optimal functioning in interaction with the environment (5,7). A modified version of this characterization of rehabilitation was used by WHO in its *World Report on Disability* in 2011 (31) and in the same year, the International Society for Physical and Rehabilitation Medicine (ISPRM) developed its conceptual definition of rehabilitation (7), which was further modified for PMR explicitly and endorsed by ISPRM in 2011 (8).

Throughout these developments, the underlying consensus was that the focus of rehabilitation is on living with a health condition, whether acute, chronic, or progressively debilitating, to optimize functioning and the lived experience of health. Rehabilitation aims to optimize a person's functioning by improving both biologic health and lived health in concert. Rehabilitation achieves this through the provision of the best treatment for health conditions to optimize the person's intrinsic health capacity, by strengthening a person's psychological resources and assets, facilitating the person's immediate environment, and finally and most importantly, by translating the potential from these improvements into better lived health (26).

Future of Rehabilitation and Functioning Information

We now have strong evidence of fundamental demographic and epidemiologic trends—rapidly increasing population ageing and the transition to a higher incidence and prevalence of chronic, noncommunicable diseases—coupled with improved access to emergency, trauma, and curative medical care, which has led to a profound shift in emphasis in future health care (18). Longer life expectancies, increasing survival rates, and rising prevalence of chronic diseases means that there will be a global increase in the health burden associated with limitations in functioning (32). Added to this is the rise of multimorbidity associated with ageing, leading to more older adults experiencing difficulties in functioning, which in turn means more years of life lived with one or several problems of functioning (33). If populations continue to experience more and more limitations in functioning and live longer with these limitations, then, given that the aim of rehabilitation is to optimize functioning, the global need for rehabilitation should increase. Rehabilitation may well become the key health strategy of the 21st century (9).

In its recent *Rehabilitation 2030: A Call for Action*, WHO has made an urgent call to scale up rehabilitation, primarily in low- and medium-resource countries, and to strengthen rehabilitation services within the health system across the globe (34). This call follows on from WHO's global disability action plan 2014 to 2021, which listed actions that needed to be taken by WHO, Member States, and partners in order to strengthen and extend rehabilitation services across the world (35). In background documents to the Call for Action, WHO has cited the evidence for population ageing and other epidemiologic trends and estimates, in terms of the Global Burden of Disease data, the overall population of people with health conditions for which rehabilitation is likely beneficial. These documents conclude that as rehabilitation needs will be increasing dramatically, the worldwide unmet need for rehabilitation will also increase, given the inadequacy of the current workforce of physicians, nurses, and skilled rehabilitation professionals in most countries, especially in the African, Eastern Mediterranean, and Southeast Asian regions (34).

In the Call for Action, rehabilitation is characterized as "a set of interventions designed to optimize functioning and reduce disability in individuals with health conditions in interaction with their environment" (36). Rehabilitation is not restricted to individuals with severe disabilities, but may be needed by anyone with a health condition who experiences some form and severity of limitation in functioning in some domain—mobility, vision, or cognition. Moreover, rehabilitation "is a highly person-centered health strategy; treatment caters to the underlying health condition(s) as well as goals and preferences of the user." Key to rehabilitation is that it addresses functioning, both in terms of biologic health and lived health, in order to optimize the capacity of a person with a health condition and, by interventions involving personal and environmental factors, to optimize the performance of the person. Because of the essential role that functioning plays in rehabilitation, WHO also recognizes that the task of strengthening rehabilitation services requires functioning information. The Call for Action, therefore, specifically includes the call "for stakeholders to enhance HIS [health information system] by including system level rehabilitation data and information on functioning, utilizing the ICF" (37).

Mainstreaming Functioning Information in Health Information Systems

As argued above, functioning information—information about what matters most to people about their health—is required for the description of the intervention outcomes of all health strategies, but especially for rehabilitation, given its goal of optimizing functioning in persons with health conditions (2). More specifically, PMR practice depends on the availability of functioning information for assessment, selection of interventions, and evaluation of outcomes (see section on clinical decision-making) (38). Finally, a case can also be made that functioning information is an essential input into all six of WHO's basic components of a health system, not merely in the health information system but also in service delivery, the workforce, information systems, essential medicines, financing, and leadership and governance (39–41).

In short, from the perspective of the overall health system, but especially in light of the increasing importance of the rehabilitation health strategy, a strong case can be made for ensuring the availability of functioning information for a variety of purposes. However, this presumes that the health system has a sufficiently robust health information system to secure access to functioning information for rehabilitation and across the health system as a whole. A health information system collects, standardizes, codes, and manages information relevant to indicators of health status, determinants of health, and health systems (42).

Particularly, information on functioning needs to be sustainably mainstreamed within the health information since it is essential to decision-making in rehabilitation at all levels. For clinicians, functioning information guides goal-setting and outcome evaluation across the continuum of rehabilitation care as well as across the continuum and phases of treatment (acute care, post–acute care, and long-term care). At the facility or programming level, functioning information that is aggregated from clinical settings can be used to monitor clinical outcomes and improve service planning and quality assurance. Finally, at the policy level, aggregated functioning information gives policy-makers a source of evidence for developing rehabilitation policies and programs and monitoring their impact. Functioning information is the prerequisite for continuous quality improvement of a learning health system at all three levels (38).

A social, political and financial commitment to mainstreaming the full range of functioning information is arguably justifiable because of the immense value and practical usefulness at all levels of the health system from clinical interventions to programming evaluation and policy development. But this is not to ignore or downplay the considerable practical hurdles that need to be overcome to routinely collect, standardize, and mainstream functioning data into the health information system. In the sections that follow on functioning in the health sciences and approaches for documenting functioning data using the ICF in rehabilitation and along the continuum of care, we will explore how these hurdles can be overcome.

FUNCTIONING IN THE HEALTH SCIENCES

To appreciate the broad scope of the scientific application of the ICF and the value of the notion of functioning, and to situate human functioning and rehabilitation research within the health sciences, it is worth pausing and describing how the ICF can provide a conceptualization of the health sciences (43).

Research across the health sciences has expanded astonishingly over the last century in response to the long-standing, social objective of maintaining and improving the health of individuals and populations and limiting the impact of disability. This research has achieved its current status and complexity because of the contribution of a variety of scientific disciplines from different intellectual traditions, including the humanities and social sciences, the natural sciences, and engineering. At the most abstract level, health systems reflect an equally complex interaction between people's health states, and responding health needs, and the organized response to those needs and requirement by society through its health and health-impacting social systems. As this is a broader interpretation of the basic person-environment interaction upon which ICF—and rehabilitation practice itself—is built, this suggests that the ICF offers a conceptual framework for understanding both the aims and objectives of health systems, and their overall structure.

Recalling ICF's operationalization of health in terms of the lived experience of health, the importance of the concept of functioning, and the resulting conceptual distinction between biologic health and lived health, a proposed conceptual definition of the health sciences is as follows:

> …the study of a person's functioning in interaction with the environment, in light of health conditions and given his or her psychological resources, and of the response by society to the individual's and the overall population's health needs through its health system and related social systems including labor, social affairs and education. (43)

This conceptualization can be further developed as a matrix for capturing the full range of scientific fields of study involved in the modern health sciences (those addressing the person as well as the social response) as well as shared methodologic approaches.

Concepts for Human Functioning and Rehabilitation Research

It has been recognized for some time that rehabilitation research, given its focus on functioning and its complex interdisciplinary structure, would profit from an organizing framework (44). It is clear that the conception of the health sciences applies to interdisciplinary rehabilitation practice and research, which suggests that the notion of functioning can provide the necessary framework. We can understand human functioning sciences as a multidisciplinary approach to the understanding of the full scope of the lived experience of health—from the biomedical through to all aspects of the societal response to functioning needs ("from cell to society"), and rehabilitation research, both applied and clinical, as a multidisciplinary approach to understanding the comprehensive assessment and interventions used clinically to optimize functioning.

DOCUMENTING FUNCTIONING WITH THE ICF

Four Steps

In order to realize the full potential of functioning information, especially for rehabilitation clinical services, service management, evidence-informed policy, and, more generally, scientific inquiry, the standardized documentation of functioning information is a prerequisite. As a general matter, when documenting scientific information it is essential to distinguish "what to measure" from "how to measure" (45,46). In terms of using the ICF as an information standard for functioning information, a four-step approach has evolved (4) that addresses four essential issues: (a) what ICF categories to document; (b) what perspective—capacity or performance—to adopt; (c) what data collection tools to apply; and (d) what measurement approach to use for reporting. An overview of these four steps is presented in **Table 9-2**.

Step 1

The first step, deciding what ICF categories to document, is a daunting challenge since there are more than 1,400 ICF categories available for documentation. This is not only far more than are required in practical contexts, but far too many to be feasibly included in a health information system. A practical solution is to rely on the results of the multiyear ICF Core Set project carried out by the ICF Research Branch, a cooperation partner within the WHO Collaborating Centre in Germany (DIMDI) and hosted by Swiss Paraplegic Research

TABLE 9-2	Overview of the Four Steps to Document Functioning with the ICF	
Steps	**Considerations**	**Example: Swiss Spinal Cord Injury Cohort Study (SwiSCI)**
1. ICF categories	Two points are important to consider in selecting ICF categories. The identified categories • are representative for all relevant aspects of functioning • which entails that as many categories are provided as needed but as few as possible to minimize burden in data management while maximizing comprehensiveness	*ICF Generic Set (ICF Generic-7) and ICF Rehabilitation Set (ICF Generic-30)* to make it possible to compare across health conditions *ICF Core Sets for Spinal Cord Injury in the early postacute and long-term context* to capture the relevant aspects of functioning of people with spinal cord injury (SCI) along the continuum of care
2. Perspective	Three perspectives on health can be identified: • Biologic health • Lived health • Appraised health	Primarily *lived health* since the main objective of SwiSCI is to describe the lived experience of people living with SCI in Switzerland
3. Data collection tools	In selecting appropriate tools, the principles of comparability, efficiency, nonredundancy, reliability, validity, and feasibility have to be taken into account. Two complementary approaches are available: 1. Existing data collection tools linked to the ICF 2. ICF-based data collection tools	*Existing data collection tools* have been used and linked to the ICF • since their psychometric properties have long been established • to ensure comparability with the tools commonly used in SCI research and practice
4. Approach for reporting	Preference for interval-scale-based scorings	For SwiSCI, two approaches for creating interval-scale-based metrics were applied: 1. creation of an ICF-based metric based on items from existing instruments linked to relevant ICF categories, e.g., all items linked to ICF categories within the ICF chapter d4 Mobility were cocalibrated into a metric for d4 Mobility 2. interval-scale-based scoring for each data collection tool, e.g., Spinal Cord Independence Measure—Self-Report (SCIM-SR), Utrecht Scale for Evaluation of Rehabilitation-Participation (USER-P), or instruments measuring psychological-personal factors such as feelings, beliefs, motives, and patterns of experience and behavior

Adapted from Stucki G, Prodinger B, Bickenbach J. Four steps to follow when documenting functioning with the International Classification of Functioning, Disability and Health. *Eur J Phys Rehabil Med.* 2017;53:144–149.

(www.ICF-research-branch.org), together with WHO, ISPRM and several partner organizations, institutions, and clinicians and scientists. A manual available in several languages (Chinese, English, French, German, Italian, Japanese, Korean, and Spanish) provides background on the development of core sets and practical information on how to select and apply them (47).

An ICF Core Set is a minimal data set that is based on the perspective of people who share the lived experience of the same health condition (e.g., multiple sclerosis, breast cancer, depression), condition groups (e.g., cardiopulmonary, neurologic condition, or context—such as acute and postacute, vocational rehabilitation), joined with the perspective of health service providers along the continuum of care and the life span. The idea is to identify a selection of categories from the complete ICF classification that provides a tool for describing functioning. In clinical practice, for example, the purpose of an ICF Core Set is to present the most relevant ICF categories for a specific health condition or context in order to support an interdisciplinary and comprehensive description of functioning relevant to the patient's lived experience (48). Currently, there are 37 ICF Core Sets for specific conditions and settings, including the ten most burdensome chronic health conditions.

The ICF Core Sets were each developed by means of a rigorous, multimethod scientific procedure: evidence was first gathered from four preparatory studies—an empirical multicenter study, a systematic literature review, a qualitative study, and an expert survey. These results serve as the starting point for a structured decision-making and consensus process at an international conference, during which participating health professionals and other experts decide on the ICF categories to be included in the first version of the ICF Core Set. Ideally, this first version of the ICF Core Set is validated and modified as necessary (49).

Another set of ICF categories are the ICF Generic Sets. These can be used alone or in combination with ICF Core Sets. The ICF Generic-7 Set is particularly useful for health statistics and public health purposes. It can be used to compare functioning across health conditions, settings, contexts, countries, and population groups in terms of only 7 ICF categories that are key indicators of health and functioning. The ICF Generic-7 is also valuable for clinical use as it depicts the very core of functioning, and provides at a glance, initial insight into a patient's level of functioning that is clear and understandable to any health or health-related professional involved. Most importantly, the ICF Generic-7 ensures comparability across health conditions (50). The ICF Generic-7 is included in a larger set called ICF Generic-30 (also referred to as the Rehabilitation Set) (51) that has particular relevance to rehabilitation and for documenting functioning in a clinical context across health conditions and along the continuum of care.

Unlike condition-specific and context-specific ICF Core Sets, the ICF Generic Sets were developed psychometrically. The ICF Generic-7 is composed of seven second level ICF categories from Body Functions and Activities and Participation that have been statistically determined to be generally applicable across health conditions and contexts. The ICF Generic-30 was similarly developed. This ensures that these two ICF Generic Sets identify ICF categories useful for brief documentation of functioning across conditions, settings, and countries (50,51).

It is important to note that ICF Generic Sets and ICF Core Sets can be used in combination as they rely on the same ICF categories. Most importantly, it is generally preferable not only to use a context-specific or health-condition specific ICF Core Set but also to use it in combination with an ICF Generic Set. Depending on one's purposes, one may prefer to combine Core Sets with either the ICF Generic-7 Set or the ICF-Generic-30 Set. An example is the specification of ICF Sets for clinical quality management (52).

Step 2

The second of the four steps requires a determination of the perspective of functioning. The question here is whether the aim is to document biologic health—that is, a person's intrinsic health capacity, independent of environmental facilitator or barrier—or lived health—the person's actual performance of an activity, fully taking into account the interaction between capacity and the person's environment. It is also possible to step outside the realm of the ICF, restricted to the description of functioning, and use the same ICF categories for an entirely different perspective, namely, the person's satisfaction with, or appraisal of, his or her capacity or performance in an area of functioning. This, for example, would be the kind of information that is needed for a quality of life or subjective well-being data collection exercise.

Step 3

The third step is the most difficult and complex to perform, but is key to the entire documentation process—namely identifying the data collection tools that are best suited to collect data on the selected ICF categories and taking into account the selected perspective. There are many existing clinical tests, self-administered questionnaires, or patient-reported outcomes (or PROs) and other data collection tools that are already linked to the ICF and ICF Core Sets (53). The Functional Independence Measure and the Barthel Index, widely used in rehabilitation, have been cocalibrated by means of the ICF using Rasch measurement theory (54). Existing tools can be linked to the ICF using the available linking protocols that have been developed for this purpose (55,56). However, care must be taken since some tools do not clearly distinguish the two perspectives—capacity and performance. Many of the available functional capacity evaluations use the capacity perspective, while self-administered questionnaires, especially activities of daily living (ADL) and instrumental ADL tools, often presume the performance perspective (4).

There have been some recent developments in response to the need for ICF-based clinical tools and PROs. The ASAS Health Index is an example of a ICF Core Set based

PRO developed for outcome evaluation in ankylosing spondylitis (57). Another example is the Work Rehabilitation Questionnaire (WORQ). Based on the ICF Core Set for vocational rehabilitation, WORQ was developed for assessing and evaluating functioning in vocational rehabilitation settings (58,59). Under development for the system-wide implementation of the ICF in health care is also an expert-administered, ICF Clinical Tool using simplified descriptions of ICF categories and a numerical rating scale (60).

Step 4

Finally, as the fourth step, it is important for standardized documentation of functioning information to use a statistically rigorous approach to measurement when answering the "how to measure" question. Sound measurement is best achieved through an interval scale metric, which can be achieved through statistical transformations using both qualitative linking to cocalibrate instruments with different response options (55,56) and quantitative mapping (61–63) to create the interval scale metric. Such a scale makes it possible for subsequent parametric analysis as well as ensuring the comparability of information along the continuum of care and over time, which is essential, for example, for cohort studies.

Standardized Documentation of Functioning Along the Continuum of Care

Information about functioning, whether biomedical information about body functions and structures, or information about an individual's performance of activities, is of considerable importance to both patients and their clinicians, wherever they are in the continuum of health care (2). To access this information at the clinical level, from acute care to rehabilitation care and community care, there needs to be a standardized system of documenting functioning. When aggregated, these data from clinical professional-patient interactions are also important for evaluating services and developing policies and programs (39). As we saw, the ICF provides such a standardized reference system for functioning information. The ICF not only addresses the issue of what to document but also, by means of qualitative linking and quantitative mapping (60–62), addresses the issue of which of the wide range of currently used data collection tools, including clinical tests and outcome assessment instruments, are most suitable to use for documentation (4).

Standardized Systems of Documenting Functioning: National Examples

The effective use of functioning information at multiple levels within national health systems requires that this information be fully integrated into national health information systems (2). At the systems level, functioning information is essential for the provision, evaluation and planning of rehabilitation services. It is also an important indicator of the effectiveness of the health strategies other than rehabilitation: preventive, promotive, curative, and palliative. At the service level, functioning information provides an indicator of quality performance, and the potential basis for benchmarking of services. At the clinical level, functioning information is important not only to PMR but also to most clinical disciplines, particularly primary care and geriatrics.

For functioning information to describe the sequential status of patients at the clinical level, its documentation must occur at different time points during the course of rehabilitation services. This is necessary for the monitoring of functioning outcomes and the periodic updating of clinical interventions (42). For these applications to be successful, there must be common data items from each clinical visit to permit comparisons from one time point to another. Although specific categories of functioning for individual patients can be followed for clinical purposes, tracking patient functioning generally requires sequential scores that are conceptually coherent and metrically sound (26,64).

The successful implementation of functioning-based health information systems at these three levels presents unique challenges, since it depends upon developing links among health care practice, science, and health systems governance (65). The Physical and Rehabilitation Medicine Section and Board of the Union of Medical Specialists in Europe (UEMS-PRM) has discussed these challenges and has operationalized approaches and developed plans to address them concretely through an implementation action plan.

The International Society of Physical and Rehabilitation Medicine (ISPRM), as part of its collaborative work plan with the WHO, has also addressed these issues, including in particular the implementation of system-wide functioning information systems at the national level. Initiatives in line with WHO's own efforts towards system-wide implementation of functioning information documentation have been lanched at the regional and country levels, specifically in Europe (65–68), China (60,66), Japan (69), and Switzerland (70). What is currently missing is a country-wide demonstration project involving the implementation of a clinical quality management system for the continuous improvement of rehabilitation, both at the level of clinical care for individual patients and at the level of rehabilitation service provision. Currently this gap is being filled by important developments in Malaysia.

The Malaysian Experience

In Malaysia, the Department of Rehabilitation Medicine at the University Malaya Medical Centre (UMMC) has initiated a project to develop a Malaysian-wide clinical quality management system for the continuous improvement of rehabilitation, both at the level of clinical care for individual patients and at the level of provision of rehabilitation services (CQM-R Malaysia) (52). This project is unique and will serve as a model for others wishing to implement a clinical quality management system for rehabilitation that relies on the documentation of functioning along the continuum of care.

The Malaysian project began with a situation analysis to understand the provision of rehabilitation services in the country along the continuum of care and from the perspectives of the three mentioned ministries that provide these services. The situation analysis involved expert consultations and site visits that gathered information about the services available from each participating institution. This led to a comprehensive description of rehabilitation services in Malaysia, guided by the International Classification of Services Organization in Rehabilitation (ICSO-R) (71,72).

The project's steering group identified and provided descriptions for seven types of rehabilitation services across the continuum of care: rehabilitation in acute care, general postacute

rehabilitation, specialized postacute rehabilitation, general outpatient rehabilitation, specialized outpatient rehabilitation, rehabilitation in primary care, and vocational rehabilitation. For each of the rehabilitation service types, the steering group proposed clinical assessment schedules (CLASs) (67). Each CLAS consists of a list of ICF categories, the assessment tools used to collect the relevant information, the patient group targeted, and the time points for documentation. The ICF categories used for the CLASs relied on existing ICF sets: the ICF Generic-6, Generic-7, Generic-30, as well as a collection of ICF Core Sets. (See **Table 9-3**.)

The steering group felt that the ICF Generic-7 Set (50) should be the minimum standard for documentation of functioning information by all rehabilitation services from acute and postacute care to the community. For documentation of functioning in general as well as for specialized rehabilitation services, the steering group recommended the ICF Generic-30 Set as the minimum standard (51). With 21 Activity and Participation categories and 9 Body Function categories, the ICF-Generic-30 allows rehabilitation professionals to track a patient's functioning across a wide range of health conditions requiring rehabilitation along the continuum of care. For specialized postacute rehabilitation facilities, the steering group recommended the ICF Generic-30 Set and the ICF Core Sets for postacute care (76,80). To address comorbidities for general and specialized rehabilitation services, the group recommended that clinicians use the ICF Generic-30 Set and relevant ICF Core Set(s) for various chronic conditions. To track patient functioning over time, sequential scores for each of the categories of the relevant ICF sets will be calculated and interpreted using scoring algorithms and corresponding transformation tables (64).

🛜 eFigure 9-1 sets out the ICF categories of the ICF Generic-6 Set, the ICF Generic-7 Set, and the ICF Generic-30 Set. As an example of the options available for more complete functioning documentation for specialized rehabilitation, 🛜 eFigure 9-1 shows the ICF categories of the ICF Core Set for spinal cord injury (SCI), alone and combined with the ICF Generic-30 Set. The ICF Core Set for vocational rehabilitation is also shown for use when the rehabilitation goals include vocational rehabilitation.

The Malaysian experience provides a number of insights that are useful for the development of national clinical quality management systems for rehabilitation and documenting functioning along the continuum of care:

1. National health systems need to describe the configuration of rehabilitation services that exist in their countries, using a structured classification system.
2. Stakeholder input and acceptance is critical to success.
3. Different rehabilitation services along the continuum of care may require more and more specific information documentation than do other services.
4. For patient tracking, there must be sets of comparable data collected at sequential points during the rehabilitation process, preferably along the entire continuum of care.

Documenting Functioning at the Population Level: WHO's Model Disability Survey

As the United Nations specialty agency for health, WHO has a responsibility to provide technical support to countries to assist in standardized collection of internationally comparable health

TABLE 9-3	Framework for the Specification of Clinical Assessment Schedules (CLASs)[a]		
Rehabilitation Services	**Patient Group Receiving Specific Rehabilitation Services**	**Selected Default ICF Set(s)**	**Selected Optional ICF Set(s)**
Rehabilitation in Acute Care Assessment and interventions are performed by therapists in the acute wards of a hospital. The primary physicians are usually not physical and rehabilitation medicine (PRM) specialists; the non-PRM physician can directly refer patients to the relevant therapists. PRM physicians may consult on complex cases. The PRM specialist assesses and decides if individual patients should participate in a postacute rehabilitation program.	Hospitalized patients across a range of health conditions	ICF Generic-6 Set (50) *ICF Generic-6 Score*	ICF Acute Core Sets • Neurological (73) • Cardiopulmonary (74) • Musculoskeletal (75)
General Postacute Rehabilitation Rehabilitation assessment and interventions are performed by a multidisciplinary team led and coordinated by a PRM specialist. Depending on the availability of a rehabilitation ward or beds dedicated for rehabilitation patients, patients may receive the rehabilitation care in a rehabilitation or acute ward.	Hospitalized patients across a range of health conditions. Patients usually come from an acute ward of a hospital and need further rehabilitation treatment in the rehabilitation ward, but this does not require specialized rehabilitation.	ICF Generic-30 Set (51) *ICF Generic-30 Score*	ICF Postacute Core Sets (76) • Neurological (77) • Cardiopulmonary (78) • Musculoskeletal (79) • Geriatric (80)
Specialized Postacute Rehabilitation Rehabilitation assessment and interventions are performed by a specialized multidisciplinary team led and coordinated by PRM specialist. The multidisciplinary team is generally more comprehensive than available for general postacute rehabilitation. Patients with specific and complex health conditions and functioning limitations are assigned to the rehabilitation ward. Pediatric patients are assigned to the pediatric ward. Each specialized rehabilitation service has its own dedicated multidisciplinary team. Occasionally, patients will have short periods of discharge home to facilitate integration into the community.	Hospitalized patients with a specific health condition or geriatric patients	ICF Generic-30 Set *ICF Generic-30 Score* + Relevant ICF Core Set (4) (e.g., for SCI [81–83], for TBI [84]) *Relevant ICF Core Set Score*	*Documentation of Comorbidity.* ICF Postacute Core Sets • Neurologic • Cardiopulmonary • Musculoskeletal • Geriatric

[a]**Using the Malaysian experience as a case example.** For each rehabilitation services a proposal for a default or minimum ICF set and a proposal for optional ICF sets are shown.

and disability information. More recently, that obligation has focused on the United Nations' *Convention on the Rights of Persons with Disabilities* (CRPD) (85) and in particular Article 33 that requires countries to collect appropriate information to "promote, protect and monitor implementation of the present Convention." WHO has responded by developing and piloting a Model Disability Survey (MDS) (86). The primary objective of the MDS is to collect population-level data on people with disability in order to understand the lived experience of health in a manner that disentangles the impact of the health state from that of barriers and facilitators in the person's physical, human-built, attitudinal, and social environments.

As a general population survey, the MDS will provide detailed and nuanced information on the lives of people with disability. It will allow direct comparison between groups with differing levels and profiles of disability, including comparison to people without disability. Unlike other standardized approaches to disability data collection, the MDS does not view disability as an attribute of the person due to impairments or specific health conditions. Furthermore, disability is understood as a continuum, ranging from none or very low to very high levels of disability. Disability is therefore a matter of degree, making the experience of disability varying and diverse. This continuum can be partitioned using specific thresholds to estimate the prevalence of severe, moderate, and mild disability in a country.

For disability measurement purposes, the two key ICF concepts of capacity and performance are used to structure the questions in the MDS. Capacity-oriented questions capture the intrinsic physical and mental capacities of a person, determined by the person's health state. Performance questions target the respondents' lived experience of health in their real-life environment. Disability measurement made possible by the MDS takes into account environmental barriers that can have a strong disabling effect.

Realizing the need for brief tools for the sound and valid collection of disability data, and suitable for incorporation in existing national surveys, WHO has responded by developing a brief version of the MDS. A first technical expert consultation was organized in late 2015 to identify appropriate questions of the MDS for a brief version. This was followed by a series of expert consultations and application of statistical methods to ensure robustness and reliability. In August 2016, the brief version of the MDS—including brief sets of questions targeting capacity, performance, and environmental factors—was created. The brief MDS is an important milestone in disability measurement as it provides countries and interested agencies with a brief but powerful tool to assess disability in other surveys and data collection platforms. This brief MDS is already being implemented in several countries (86).

ICF IN CLINICAL DECISION-MAKING

Clinical decision-making and rehabilitation management are critically dependent on functioning information (2). To achieve the objective of rehabilitation, that is, to optimize functioning, rehabilitation management requires functioning information to (a) describe the status of those receiving rehabilitation; (b) identify the categories of functioning in need of improvement; (c) describe the goals of intervention programs; (d) match the assignment of treating professionals to the areas of their expertise; and (e) evaluate the results of the interventions. Specifically, PMR as the medical specialty of functioning requires functioning information to achieve its goals (8).

As mentioned above, functioning information can be analyzed in terms of biologic health, a person's intrinsic health capacity in terms of physiologic and psychological processes and anatomical structures of the body and capacity limitations, and lived health, namely the person's actual performance of activities across the domains of activities and participation in interaction with the person's environments (2,87). To accomplish this, several requirements must be met so that this information can be included as an integral component of health information systems:

- The language of functioning must be *uniform and consistent*. This is necessary for visit-to-visit comparative purposes, for communication among treating rehabilitation professionals, for consistent identification of needed interventions, for consistent matching of assignments to treating professionals, and for the assessment of the achievement of goals.
- Functioning information needs to be *comprehensive* and identify all needed interventions, including those directed at body functions and structures, capacity and performance, and environmental factors. Comprehensive functioning information is needed to describe in sufficient detail the functioning status of persons receiving rehabilitation, the goals of rehabilitation programs, and the outcomes of these programs.
- Functioning information needs to be *relevant*, that is, it needs to include categories of functioning that reflect what is important to patients as well as categories required to identify needed interventions.
- Functioning information needs to be *documented without undue burden*. The acceptance by professionals of the need to document functioning information will depend on their belief that the benefits of doing so exceed the disadvantages.

It is widely recognized by rehabilitation professionals and researchers worldwide that the ICF provides a framework for the documentation of functioning information that meets all of these requirements. The ICF provides a uniform and consistent language of functioning for communication among stakeholders in rehabilitation and for the description of functioning that can be modified to enhance understanding in specific cultural contexts (31,60,66). ICF categories are key elements of CLASs (67) that provide information for patient assignments to appropriate rehabilitation services, for matching the needs of patients to the competencies of various rehabilitation professionals and for monitoring functioning outcomes. The burden of documentation can be lessened by relying on ICF Core Sets and generic sets, which greatly reduce the number of categories that need to be taken into account.

Rehabilitation Management

Effective rehabilitation requires the application of specific management approaches based upon the standardized documentation of functioning. These include CLASs, rehabilitation plans, and Rehab-Cycles (38). As mentioned above, CLASs include ICF categories, identification of the assessment tools used to collect the information, the patient group targeted, and the time points for documentation (67). The rehabilitation plan describes the interventions along the continuum of care that are targeted to address a person's functioning needs. The need for a plan may be triggered by an acute health event (such as a stroke) causing limitations in functioning or by the functioning needs of a person with a chronic condition living in the community (38). Rehabilitation plans include more than interventions to improve functioning; they may also include strategies to provide for environmental support, for example home care, supported living services, and access to financial programs.

Finally, the Rehab-Cycle can be used for rehabilitation clinical decision-making to monitor progress and adjust interventions through the continuum of care. It includes four phases: assessment, assignment, intervention, and evaluation (48,88–90). Assessment is the identification of problems, needs, and shared goals and identification of the functioning targets for interventions. Assignment includes assigning appropriate rehabilitation professionals to provide the needed interventions. After the intervention, evaluation determines whether the goals for each intervention target were met by comparing the status of the person during the initial assessment with the status after the interventions. Information from the evaluation phase informs the next Rehab-Cycle assessment phase or discharge planning. The Rehab-Cycles are iterative and provide the framework for sequential rehabilitation interventions and monitoring functioning. **Table 9-4** shows the relationship between rehabilitation management, standardized documentation, and clinical decision-making in sequential rehabilitation cycles (19,38,48,89,90–93).

How to Apply Functioning Information in the Rehab-Cycle

The ICF is useful in providing the functioning framework utilized in all four phases of the Rehab-Cycle. It guides the structured and practical approach of the Rehab-Cycle in identifying and documenting patient problems and the information from technical and clinical examinations. It facilitates communication among rehabilitation team members with respect to problems, shared goals, types of interventions, and the specific interventions themselves, as well as between the rehabilitation team and the patient. Used consistently, the ICF provides an opportunity to improve the understanding that stakeholders in other clinical settings, insurers, and case managers have of the functioning status of rehabilitation patients and of the rehabilitation process (48,89,90).

For each phase of the Rehab-Cycle, an ICF documentation tool is available: the ICF Assessment Sheet and the ICF Categorical Profile for the assessment phase, the ICF Intervention Table for the assignment and intervention phases and the ICF Evaluation Display for the evaluation phase.

TABLE 9-4	Rehabilitation Management: Patient Assigned to Consecutive Rehabilitation Services

Goals	Actions
• **Standardized Documentation** Documenting a person's functioning as specified in clinical assessment schedules for consecutive rehabilitation services • **Individual Rehabilitation Plan** Devising and adjusting an individual rehabilitation plan in partnership with the patient or his/her proxy	• **Clinical decision-making in sequential Rehab-Cycles** • Assessment of functioning and specification of functioning goals for the long-term (expected functioning level of a person returning to or living in the community); mid-term (expected functioning level at the end of the stay at a consecutive rehabilitation service); and short-term (expected functioning upon completion of the next Rehab-Cycle). • Assignment of rehabilitation professionals to clinical interventions aimed at functioning targets related to the short-term functioning goals. • Evaluation of short-, mid-, and long-term functioning goal achievement against a predicted functioning trajectory (calculated with cumulative data of patients with similar health conditions, functioning and personal characteristics). • Reassessment and planning of the next Rehab-Cycle in light of mid-term and long-term goals as specified in the rehabilitation plan.

Adapted from Stucki G, Bickenbach J. Functioning information in the learning health system. *Eur J Phys Rehabil Med.* 2017;53:139–143.

These tools facilitate the documentation, planning, and implementation of rehabilitation management. Their use results in transparent documentation and open communication among rehabilitation team members throughout each Rehab-Cycle and during subsequent Rehab-Cycles (45,48,90). **Figure 9-2** lists the tools and shows their relationships to the four phases of the Rehab-Cycle (94).

How to Apply the Four Steps of the Rehab-Cycle

The framework of the Rehab-Cycle combined with its documentation tools provides a practical approach to the management of patients receiving rehabilitation services. To demonstrate their use in actual clinical practice, the Swiss Paraplegic Research and the Swiss Paraplegic Center (an acute and specialized rehabilitation center for SCI and spinal cord diseases) prepared a series of case studies that described their existing rehabilitation processes utilizing the Rehab-Cycle and corresponding ICF-based documentation tools (89,94–97). The case studies involved persons living with SCI of different ages and gender, and whose SCI varied by etiology and levels of severity. Each case study highlights a specific theme, such as community reintegration, SCI in older persons, and SCI and chronic pain management. Cases involving other health conditions such as low back pain and traumatic brain injury also

demonstrate how these ICF-based documentation tools can be used within the Rehab-Cycle framework (92,98).

The application of the ICF documentation tools to each phase of the Rehab-Cycle involves significant detail in order to accurately reflect the steps of the rehabilitation management of actual patients. The discussion and tables explaining their utilizations are based on the following case example (99).

L sustained a SCI injury classified as complete paraplegia as the result of a climbing accident. She lacked complete motor and sensory function below the 8th thoracic vertebrae. After 4 months of initial rehabilitation at a specialized postacute rehabilitation facility for SCI, L regained a degree of independence in self-care and was able to transfer to and from her wheelchair. At this time point, she began a new Rehab-Cycle that, among other things, addressed her physical fitness and expressed wish to participate in sports again—both of which were expected to contribute to community reintegration and independent living. She is about to enter her second Rehab-Cycle.

Assessment

During the assessment phase, the multidisciplinary rehabilitation team, together with the patient, documents a comprehensive picture of the patient's functioning. This includes problems in functioning and the contextual factors that might influence them. The information for the assessment is gathered from all of the available sources, including the patient's case history, various clinical and diagnostic tests, patient-reported questionnaires, patient interviews, and other observations (47). To further patient-oriented rehabilitation management, the rehabilitation team documents this information from both the perspectives of the rehabilitation professionals and the patient and organizes it by the ICF components (93,100).

The clinical documentation tool associated with the assessment phase of the Rehab-Cycle is the ICF Assessment Sheet, which documents the patient's problems and strengths. There are separate sections for entries from the patient's perspective and the health professional perspective. The sheet also distinguishes entries for body functions and structures, and activities and participation. In addition, there are sections for the entry of environmental and personal factors that may facilitate functioning or provide barriers to it. 📶 **eTable 9-1** shows the entries in the ICF Assessment Sheet related to the case example.

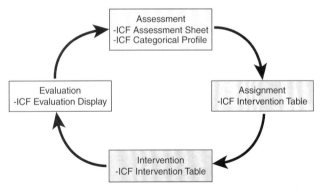

FIGURE 9-2. Rehab-Cycle and corresponding ICF-based documentation tools. (Adapted from Prodinger B, Tennant A, Stucki G, et al. Harmonizing routinely collected health information for strengthening quality management in health systems: requirements and practice. *J Health Serv Res Policy.* 2016;21(4):223–228. Copyright © 2016 SAGE Publications.)

The information from the assessment forms the basis for the patient's functioning profile, long-term and short-term goals, and intervention targets, that is, those areas of functioning for which a goal is identified and interventions proposed (48,88,90). To prepare the profile, the rehabilitation team first identifies the appropriate ICF set or combination of sets in light of the patient's underlying health condition, including comorbidities or secondary health conditions. The ICF Core Set Manual for Clinical Practice (47) is available in English, French, German, Spanish, Italian, Chinese, Japanese, and Korean, and is a good source of information for selecting the appropriate set(s). At the level of service provision along the continuum of care ICF information can be shared as described in the discussion of the Malaysian experience above. Once the rehabilitation team has identified the ICF set(s) to use, they then rate the extent to which the patient is having problems in functioning areas represented by the categories of selected ICF set(s). The ICF categories and their ratings form the functioning profile of the patient. To ensure that the goals are patient oriented, the team together with the patient use the assessment information to establish goals for the rehabilitation interventions.

The clinical documentation tool for profiling and goal setting is the ICF Categorical Profile. The rehabilitation team and the patient establish global goals, the highest-level goal they are aiming for, and the desired outcome after successful completion of rehabilitation. In L's case, the global goal was "community reintegration." A service-program goal is an intermediate goal a patient aims to achieve as an endpoint of a specific Rehab-Cycle. In L's case, this was "independence in daily living." There are also more specific goals called "cycle goals," which are short-term goals or "stepping stones" toward achieving the service-program goal. In L's case, she and the rehabilitation team defined "independence in self-care," "improvement in mobility," and "increased participation in recreation and leisure" (specifically in sports activities) as the cycle goals to address with specific interventions (99).

The ICF Categorical Profile also shows the ICF categories the team has selected as important when profiling the patient's functioning, the extent to which the patient is having problems in each ICF category at the time of assessment, and the expected improvement at the end of the Rehab-Cycle. 🛜 **eFigure 9-2** shows the ICF Categorical Profile that describes the goals and functioning profile of L (99).

In L's ICF Categorical Profile, the extent of her problems is expressed using a scale of 0 to 10 from "no problem" to "complete problem" for body functions, body structures and activities, and participation. A plus sign (+) after the rating designates a positive impact of environmental and personal factors on functioning. Other approaches have used different scales, in particular the 0 to 4 scoring for the severity qualifier that is provided in the ICF itself. The results of the assessment phase and the content of the ICF Categorical Profile provide information for the assignment phase.

Assignment

In the assignment phase, intervention decisions are made to address the intervention targets identified in the assessment phase, and rehabilitation professionals responsible for providing these interventions are assigned (48,90). The clinical documentation tool for the assignment phase is the ICF Intervention Table, which supports the coordination of responsibilities and resources, avoiding unnecessary redundancy of resources or gaps in services through miscommunication. 🛜 **eFigure 9-3** shows the ICF Intervention Table displaying the intervention targets, interventions, and health professional assignments for L's rehabilitation program (30).

While the intervention targets specified in the ICF Intervention Table are ICF coded, the interventions themselves can be coded using the International Classification of Health Interventions (ICHI). The ICHI is a system of classifying health interventions that is under development by the WHO (101,102). The intervention codes of the ICHI can be linked to the ICF codes, matching interventions to the targets to which the interventions are directed. The current absence of a generally accepted international classification for health interventions has resulted in multiple national classifications that often are limited in scope and make international comparisons difficult (103).

Intervention (Management)

During the intervention phase, the rehabilitation team conducts and regularly monitors the interventions implemented to address the intervention targets (48,85). The ICF Intervention Table is also used as the documentation tool for this phase. It shows the functioning level observed at the initial assessment, the goal value expected after the interventions, and the actual value after the interventions. This table only displays the ICF categories selected as intervention targets from those originally assessed (99).

Evaluation

During the evaluation phase, a determination is made whether the goals set for each intervention target during the assessment phase have been achieved. This involves comparing the patient's functioning status after completing interventions with the status before the intervention phase. The outcome of the assessment during the evaluation phase contributes to further rehabilitation planning for a subsequent Rehab-Cycle (48,90). The documentation tool associated with the evaluation phase is the ICF Evaluation Display. See 🛜 **eFigure 9-4** (90).

The ICF Evaluation Display is an extended version of the ICF Categorical Profile, providing a visualization showing at a glance whether goals were achieved. It displays the results of the original assessment and the assessment completed during the evaluation phase. The results are represented by the ICF categories selected as intervention targets during the assessment phase and are visualized as bar graphs—one graph depicting the original assessment and the other depicting the evaluation phase assessment. Each bar in the respective graph reflects the rating given for each intervention target. The ICF Evaluation Display also shows the goal achievement of each intervention target.

It is important to note that this "before-after" picture of change in functioning status between the two time points does not necessarily signify that the change is due to the intervention itself or whether the intervention has been effective or not. Although some rehabilitation professionals employ goal attainment itself as an outcome measure or a measure to demonstrate effectiveness of services in rehabilitation practice (104), appropriate measurement standards should be adhered to, and this requires using interval-scale metrics for determining goal achievement (64,105). As mentioned above, determining a measurement standard is the final step in the process of documenting ICF functioning information (4).

In short, functioning information is critically important for both rehabilitation clinical decision-making and the process of rehabilitation management that builds on these clinical judgments. One of the important uses of functioning information is to make periodic adjustments to rehabilitation interventions that are guided by sequential assessments. Functioning information developed through patient-oriented clinical activities lends itself, when aggregated, to evaluating rehabilitation services and development of policy. This sets the stage for using the ICF, and functioning information, to improve the entire health system into which rehabilitation, as one of the prominent health strategies, fits. Functioning information allows health systems to "learn."

ICF IN THE LEARNING HEALTH SYSTEM

To evaluate the performance of any system, especially one as complex as a national health system, it is important to be clear about the resource input and the service or product outcome in order to determine whether expected results have been achieved (106). In the case of rehabilitation services located within the health system, the designed results are the following: at the clinical level, improvements in functioning for patients; at the meso-level, sustainable rehabilitation services and continuity of services care across settings; and at the macro level, suitable rehabilitation policies to guide comprehensive rehabilitation programming to meet population requirements. These information requirements that make these system performance evaluations possible presume a coordinated data collection at each level (65). Routine collection of functioning information provides the essential data precondition for what has been termed the "learning health system" in which research, clinical practice, programming, and policies are aligned in terms of what the U.S. Institute of Medicine (now National Academy of Medicine) described in 2007 as the "cyclical dynamics" of continuous improvement at all levels (107).

Health systems "learn" when they can continuously identify issues, create responses, implement changes, observe the consequences, respond to the results of the implementation, and revise and reshape the response accordingly. Health systems learn, in short, from success and failure. But a health system can only learn if it has the capacity to identify and understand systematic weaknesses and constraints, successes and innovations, and craft and implement interventions that avoid or mitigate the effects of what does not work and enhance synergies that encourage what does work (108).

At the micro-level, standardized documentation of a person's functioning is essential for clinical decision-making along the continuum of care, and can be used to devise a rehabilitation plan that incorporates the Rehab-Cycle from assessment to evaluation (48,88,90). In terms of the ICF model, the gap between the level of a person's capacity to perform an activity and his or her performance identifies the positive or negative impact of the person's environment on performance. With standardized information about functioning, it is possible at the clinical level to compare actual functioning improvements against expected or desired functioning outcomes. These results, for reference classes of patients, can create trajectories

from which the health system can use to "learn" to assure quality management.

The management of rehabilitation service provision—the meso-level of the health system—tracks service use inputs and processes (such as human resources, service infrastructures as well as delivery mechanism) against service outcomes. Again, functioning information, routinely collected, helps the system to learn by systematically comparing outcomes with inputs and processes, to detect whether, for example, there are subpopulations that are not achieving expected outcomes or exhibiting predicted trajectories. Failure to achieve desired functioning outcomes can then be addressed by health service managers and revisions made to inputs or processes (65).

Finally, at the macro-level of policy and programming, routinely collecting functioning information makes it possible to assess whether, and the degree to which, the rehabilitation system as a whole is producing the desired impact at the population level. At this level, functioning data are used to monitor the impact on the population as a whole to signal potential health system failures and suggest ways to improve results through modifications to service management and programming. Standard, population-based functioning data are derived from censuses, health surveys, household surveys, or population-based disability surveys, although these rarely contain sufficient and comparable functioning data that can be used to evaluate overall rehabilitation system impact.

The previously mentioned WHO innovative survey, the MDS, would be particularly useful at the macro-level as it collects functioning information at the population level, and distinguishes the impact of health limitations in capacity from performance limitations that result from the impact of environmental factors. Another example of a source of population data for macro-level analysis is a health condition–specific survey that does provide detailed functioning information for that subpopulation. An example of this is the ICF-based Swiss survey for people living with spinal cord injury (SCI) (SwiSCI) (109,110) and the International SCI Survey (InSCI) (111). For population information to accurately assess the impact of rehabilitation programming on the population, these data need to be reconciled with data collected by service providers at the facility level. (One limitation to this process is the fact that facility level data are geographically limited and may not be fully representative of the population as a whole (112).) **Table 9-5** shows the continuous improvement of the health system's response to population and individual functioning needs at the macro-, meso-, and micro levels.

In the context of rehabilitation services, therefore, there are two important learning "cycles": the first involves the macro- and meso-levels in which information about rehabilitation programming cycle to the policy level so that rehabilitation policy reflects the successes and failures at the meso-level of management. This can be called the "functioning-informed policy learning cycle." The second is concerned with clinical quality management and links the micro-level of clinical practice to the meso-level of programming so that successes and failures at the clinical levels are used to improve programming that sustains successes and avoids failures. This can be called the "continuous clinical quality management cycle."

The ISPRM initiative to standardize functioning information documentation in the the national health systems of China,

TABLE 9-5 Continuous Improvement of the Health System's Response to Population and Individual Functioning Needs: Macro-, Meso-, and Micro Levels

Health System Level	Goal	Process of Continuous Improvement of the Health System's Response to Population and Individual Functioning Needs
Macro-level Rehabilitation policies guiding rehabilitation programming	Rehabilitation policy Development of rehabilitation policies addressing a country's population functioning needs	• Monitoring country functioning needs with general population and subpopulation surveys; • Evaluation of rehabilitation policies against the backdrop of how a population's functioning needs are met; • Analysis and potential modification of rehabilitation policies in light of evaluation results.
	Rehabilitation programming Specification of a comprehensive set of rehabilitation service programs addressing the functioning needs of specific subpopulations along the continuum of care in a defined geographical area	• Monitoring functioning outcomes achieved across realized rehabilitation service programs; • Improvement of rehabilitation programming in light of monitoring results, results reported by other countries, and scientific evidence from quasi-experimental studies comparing rehabilitation programming across geographical areas and over time.
Meso-level Realizing rehabilitation service programs through provision of individual rehabilitation services	Rehabilitation service program Optimizing the operational management of a rehabilitation service program through provision of a set of individual rehabilitation services	• Benchmarking functioning outcomes across individual rehabilitation services (adjusted for case-mix); • Identification of modifiable inputs associated with favorable functioning outcomes (e.g., physical infrastructure and organization of the rehabilitation service; work force; use of information, products, and procedure inputs); • Anonymous feedback to individual rehabilitation services.
	Rehabilitation service Optimizing rehabilitation service provision	• Monitoring functioning outcomes over time; • Stepwise revision of rehabilitation service provision in light of anonymous feedback from benchmarking and new scientific evidence on best rehabilitation service provision (sequential quasi-experiments).
Micro-level Rehabilitation management for an individual patient assigned to consecutive rehabilitation services	Standardized documentation Documenting a person's functioning as specified in clinical assessment schedules for consecutive rehabilitation services	• Functioning-informed clinical decision-making during consecutive rehabilitation services (i.e., assignment of the patient to consecutive rehabilitation services; assignment of clinical interventions provided by rehabilitation professionals; monitoring of functioning outcomes)
	Rehabilitation plan Devising and adjusting an individual rehabilitation plan in partnership with the patient or his/her proxy	Clinical decision-making in sequential rehabilitation cycles: • Assessment of functioning and specification of functioning goals for the long-term (expected functioning level of a person returning to or living in the community); mid-term (expected functioning level at the end of the stay at a consecutive rehabilitation service); and short-term (expected functioning upon completion of the next rehabilitation cycle); • Assignment of rehabilitation professionals to clinical interventions aimed at functioning targets related to the short-term functioning goals; • Evaluation of short-, mid-, and long-term functioning goal achievement against a predicted functioning trajectory (calculated with cumulative data of patients with similar health conditions, functioning, and personal characteristics); • Reassessment and planning of the next rehabilitation cycle in light of mid-term and long-term goals as specified in the rehabilitation plan.

Adapted from Stucki G, Bickenbach J. Functioning information in the learning health system. *Eur J Phys Rehabil Med.* 2017;53:139–143.

Japan, and Switzerland as described above are examples of experiments in implementing learning health systems for rehabiltation.

In the United States, the importance of routinely collecting functioning information, and aggregating and reporting it for quality improvement, has been recognized since 1987 with the Uniform Data System for Medical Rehabilitation. Although not ICF based, this system has provided detailed summaries to subscribing rehabilitation hospitals and units, long-term care hospitals, skilled nursing facilities, and pediatric and outpatient facilities of the data submitted by these facilities. These detailed summaries compare data collected from these facilities to regional and national benchmarks, which they use for quality management and compliance with the standards of accrediting organizations (113). More recently, the US Centers for Medicare and Medicaid Services (CMS), in compliance with legislative mandates, has expanded the information it requires rehabilitation facilities to record and submit for each discharged patient (114). Self-care outcome items based on the Continuity Assessment Record and Evaluation (CARE) Tool (115) are among those added. CMS plans to use these self-care outcome data to initiate a publically reported benchmarking quality measure (116). These US initiatives provide opportunities for the development of future

ICF-based clinical quality management programs through the established method of converting scores of functioning measurement tools into ICF standardized reports through scoring algorithms and related transformation tables (61).

Strategies to Overcome the Challenges of ICF Implementation

Despite the widespread acceptance of ICF use in rehabilitation practice (65,117), we recognize that there are challenges to implementing the ICF in routine clinical practice (66). Often, these challenges are due to misconceptions about the ICF and how it can be used. Here are three of these misconceptions:

Challenge A: There is No Need to Implement the ICF, Since it is Just Another Outcome Measure

The ICF is not an outcome measure; it is a classification that can be used as the starting point for tool development, and many other applications. ICF-based tools have been developed, and these would enhance clinical decision-making and outcome evaluation by providing additional evidence (16,118).

Challenge B: ICF is too Complex for Use in Daily Clinical Routine (65)

Rehabilitation professionals may perceive the ICF as complex. Usually, this is the result of unfamiliarity, which can be addressed by providing ICF training, ideally as part of the academic curriculum (119–123). To make ICF use in daily routine easier, ICF-based tools, such as those described in the section *Documenting functioning with the ICF: Four Steps* (e.g., ICF Core Sets, ASAS Health Index), have been developed. The section *How to apply functioning information in the Rehab-Cycle* also outlines a simple approach for using ICF-based tools in routine rehabilitation management.

Challenge C: ICF Would Add an Additional Burden to an Already Full Routine of Daily Service Provision

Clinicians are free to use the tools they already know. The results of these tools can be converted to functioning scores (at an overall level, domain level, or individual level) and represented by ICF standardized reporting. There is, therefore, no additional burden. In addition, to reduce the time for using ICF-based tools, these tools could be integrated into the existing health information system. This is how clinicians who wish a more comprehensive and standardized way to document and report the functioning of patients can proceed.

Alternatively, one can use an ICF-based tool where available. It has been shown in the implementation of an ICF-based tool in neurorehabilitation assessments (120) that the more often it was used, the easier and less time consuming it became. The ICF tool also had the advantage of making multidisciplinary patient progress meetings more efficient.

As one can see, there are strategies to overcome the challenges of ICF implementation in routine rehabilitation practice.

SUMMARY

The World Health Organization's *ICF* constitutes a paradigm shift in our understanding of health, the operation of health systems, and the nature and value of rehabilitation as a health strategy. At the core of the ICF is the notion of "functioning" that captures a person's lived experience of their health and structures the information needed by all participants in health—practitioners whose objective is to optimize functioning in their patients, policy-makers who shape the health system to respond to people's functioning needs, and researchers who aim to explain and influence functioning (16). The ICF not only provides the operationalization of health but also is a conceptual framework and structure for describing functioning and disability, as well as a classification that provides an international information reference for functioning information.

In this chapter, recent work in the application of the ICF, and in particular the notion of functioning, has been surveyed at all levels of the health system, particularly from the perspective of rehabilitation and PRM practice. Functioning is not only the third health indicator along with mortality and morbidity, it also identifies the goal of rehabilitation. Thus the goal of rehabilitation is that of enabling people with health conditions experiencing or likely to experience disability to achieve and maintain optimal functioning in interaction with the environment.

This chapter expands on the role and value of functioning information across the health system and especially for rehabilitation. Functioning information is an essential component of the health information system of a robust and effective health system. More broadly, functioning information helps to comprehend and organize the health systems in general. The chapter explains recent developments toward standardized documentation of functioning information along the continuum of care, and provides national examples of such standardized systems under development. At the clinical level, the role of functioning information in clinical decisions is described and applied to rehabilitation practice and management.

Bringing these components together, the chapter ends by making the case for the role of functioning information, based on the ICF, in creating health systems that "learn" and progressively improve services by aligning research, clinical practice, programming, and policies to achieve continuous improvement at all levels. Continuous quality management and continuous evidence-based policy development are essential features of the health systems of the future, and will be achievable through the understanding gained from the ICF and functioning information.

ACKNOWLEDGMENT

The authors would like to thank Cristiana Baffone and Susanne Stucki for their help in the preparation of the manuscript.

REFERENCES

1. World Health Organization. *World Report on Ageing and Health*. Geneva, Switzerland: WHO; 2015.
2. Stucki G, Bickenbach J, Melvin J. Strengthening rehabilitation in health systems worldwide by integrating information on functioning in national health information systems. *Am J Phys Med Rehabil*. 2017;96:677–681.
3. World Health Organization. *The International Classification of Functioning, Disability and Health (ICF)*. Geneva, Switzerland: WHO; 2001.
4. Stucki G, Prodinger B, Bickenbach J. Four steps to follow when documenting functioning with the International Classification of Functioning, Disability and Health. *Eur J Phys Rehabil Med*. 2017;53:144–149.
5. Stucki G, Cieza A, Melvin J. The International Classification of Functioning, Disability and Health (ICF): a unifying model for the conceptual description of the rehabilitation strategy. *J Rehabil Med*. 2007;39:279–285.
6. Grimby G, Melvin J, Stucki G, eds. The ICF: a unifying model for the conceptualization, organization and development of human functioning and rehabilitation research. *J Rehabil Med*. 2007;39:273–344.
7. Meyer T, Gutenbrunner C, Bickenbach J, et al. Towards a conceptual description of rehabilitation as a health strategy. *J Rehabil Med*. 2011;43:765–769.
8. Gutenbrunner C, Meyer T, Melvin J, et al. Towards a conceptual description of physical and rehabilitation medicine. *J Rehabil Med*. 2011;43:760–764.

9. Stucki G, Bickenbach J, Gutenbrunner C, et al. Rehabilitation: the health strategy of the 21st century. *J Rehabil Med.* 2018;50:309–316.

10. World Health Organization. *The Constitution of the World Health Organization. [Internet].* Available from: http://www.who.int/governance/eb/who_constitution_en.pdf

11. Callahan D. The WHO definition of 'health'. *Hastings Cent Stud.* 1973;1:77–87.

12. Larson JS. The conceptualization of health. *Med Care Res Rev.* 1999;56:123–136.

13. Saracci R. The World Health Organisation needs to reconsider its definition of health. *Br Med J.* 1997;314:1409–1410.

14. Jadad AR, O'Grady L. How should health be defined? *Br Med J.* 2008;337:a2900.

15. Stucki G, Reinhardt JD, Grimby G, et al. Developing "human functioning and rehabilitation research" from the comprehensive perspective. *J Rehabil Med.* 2007;39:665–671.

16. Stucki G. Olle Höök Lectureship 2015: the World Health Organization's paradigm shift and implementation of the International Classification of Functioning, Disability and Health in Rehabilitation. *J Rehabil Med.* 2016;48:486–493.

17. World Health Organization. *The International Classification of Diseases.* 4th ed. Geneva, Switzerland: WHO; 2010. Available from: http://www.who.int/classifications/icd/en/

18. Bickenbach JE, Chatterji S, Badley EM, et al. Models of disablement, universalism and the ICIDH. *Soc Sci Med.* 1999;48:1173–1187.

19. Stucki G. International Classification of Functioning, Disability, and Health (ICF): a promising framework and classification for rehabilitation medicine. *Am J Phys Med Rehabil.* 2005;84:733–740.

20. Selb M, Kohler F, Robinson Nicol MM, et al. ICD-11: a comprehensive picture of health, an update on the ICD-ICF joint use initiative. *J Rehabil Med.* 2015;47:2–8.

21. Escorpizo R, Kostanjsek N, Kennedy C, et al. Harmonizing WHO's International Classification of Diseases (ICD) and International Classification of Functioning, Disability and Health (ICF): importance and methods to link disease and functioning. *BMC Public Health.* 2013;13:742.

22. Geyh S, Muller R, Peter C, et al. Capturing the psychologic-personal perspective in spinal cord injury. *Am J Phys Med Rehabil.* 2011;90(suppl):S79–S96.

23. Stucki G, Boonen A, Tugwell P, et al. The World Health Organisation International Classification of Functioning, Disability and Health: a conceptual model and interface for the OMERACT process. *J Rheumatol.* 2007;34:600–606.

24. Bickenbach J, Posarac A, Cieza A, et al. *Assessing Disability in Working Age Population: A Paradigm Shift: From Impairment and Functional Limitation to the Disability Approach. Report No: ACS14124.* Washington, DC: The World Bank; 2015.

25. Salomon J, Mathers C, Chatterji S, et al. Quantifying individual levels of health: definitions, concepts, and measurement issues. In: Murray CJL, Evans CJL, eds. *Health Systems Performance Assessment: Debates, Methods and Empiricism.* Geneva, Switzerland: WHO; 2003:301–318.

26. Stucki G, Bickenbach J. Functioning: the third health indicator in the health system and the key indicator for rehabilitation. *Eur J Phys Rehabil Med.* 2017;53:134–138.

27. BMJ. *What is Epidemiology? [Internet]*; 2016. Available from: http://www.bmj.com/about-bmj/resources-readers/publications/epidemiology-uninitiated/1-what-epidemiology [cited March 24, 2017].

28. World Health Organization. *Epidemiology. [Internet]*; 2016. Available from: http://www.who.int/topics/epidemiology/en/ [cited March 24, 2017].

29. World Health Organization. Declaration of Alma-Ata. International Conference on Primary Health Care, Alma-Ata, USSR, September 6–12, 1978 [Internet]; 1978. Available from: http://www.who.int/publications/almaata_declaration_en.pdf?ua=1 [cited March 24, 2017].

30. World Health Organization. *Universal Health Coverage. [Internet].* Available from: http://www.who.int/mediacentre/factsheets/fs395/en/ [cited March 24, 2017].

31. World Health Organization; World Bank. *World Report on Disability.* Geneva, Switzerland: WHO; 2011.

32. Murray CJL, Barber RM, Foreman KJ, et al. Global, regional, and national disability-adjusted life years (DALYs) for 306 diseases and injuries and healthy life expectancy (HALE) for 188 countries, 1990–2013: quantifying the epidemiological transition. *Lancet.* 2015;386:2145–2191.

33. Chatterji S, Byles J, Cutler D, et al. Health, functioning, and disability in older adults—present status and future implications. *Lancet.* 2015;385:563–575.

34. World Health Organization. *Rehabilitation 2030: A Call for Action. [Internet]*; 2017. Available from: http://www.who.int/disabilities/care/rehab-2030/en/ [cited March 24, 2017].

35. World Health Organization. *Global Disability Action Plan 2014–2021: Better Health for All People with Disability.* Geneva, Switzerland: WHO; 2014.

36. World Health Organization. Rehabilitation: key for health in the 21st century. In: *Rehabilitation 2030: A Call for Action. [Internet]*; 2017. Available from: http://www.who.int/disabilities/care/rehab-2030/en/ [cited March 24, 2017].

37. World Health Organization. Health information systems and rehabilitation. In: *Rehabilitation 2030: A Call for Action. [Internet]*; 2017. Available from: http://www.who.int/disabilities/care/rehab-2030/en/ [cited March 24, 2017].

38. Stucki G, Bickenbach J. Functioning information in the learning health system. *Eur J Phys Rehabil Med.* 2017;53:139–143.

39. World Health Organization. *Everybody's Business: Strengthening Health Systems to Improve Health Outcomes. WHO's Framework for Action.* Geneva, Switzerland: WHO; 2007.

40. World Health Organization. *Systems Thinking for Health Systems Strengthening.* Geneva, Switzerland: Alliance for Health Policy and Systems Research and WHO; 2009.

41. World Health Organization. *Monitoring the Building Blocks of Health Systems: A Handbook of Indicators and their Measurement Strategies.* Geneva, Switzerland: WHO; 2010.

42. World Health Organization. *Framework and Standards for Country Health Information Systems.* 2nd ed. Geneva, Switzerland: WHO; 2012.

43. Stucki G, Rubinelli S, Reinhardt JD. Towards a common understanding of the health sciences. *Gesundheitswesen.* 2016;78:e78–e82.

44. Grimby G, Melvin J, Stucki G. The ICF: a unifying model for the conceptualization, organization and development of human functioning and rehabilitation research. Foreword. *J Rehabil Med.* 2007;39:277–278.

45. Cieza A, Boldt C, Ballert CS, et al. Setting up a cohort study on functioning: deciding what to measure. *Am J Phys Med Rehabil.* 2011;90:S17–S28.

46. Fekete C, Boldt C, Post M, et al. How to measure what matters: development and application of guiding principles to select measurement instruments in an epidemiologic study on functioning. *Am J Phys Med Rehabil.* 2011;90:S29–S38.

47. Bickenbach J, Cieza A, Rauch A, et al., eds. *ICF Core Sets: Manual for Clinical Practice for the ICF.* Cambridge, MA: Hogrefe; 2012.

48. Avellanet M, Selb M, Stucki G, et al. Utility of using the ICF Core Sets in clinical practice. *Rehabilitación.* 2015;49:197–201.

49. Selb M, Escorpizo R, Kostanjsek N, et al. A guide on how to develop an International Classification of Functioning, Disability and Health Core Set. *Eur J Phys Rehabil Med.* 2015;51:105–117.

50. Cieza A, Oberhauser C, Bickenbach J, et al. Towards a minimal generic set of domains of functioning and health. *BMC Public Health.* 2014;14:218.

51. Prodinger B, Cieza A, Oberhauser C, et al. Toward the International Classification of Functioning, Disability and Health (ICF) rehabilitation set: a minimal generic set of domains for rehabilitation as a health strategy. *Arch Phys Med Rehabil.* 2016;97:875–884.

52. Engkasan JP, Stucki G, Ali S, et al. Implementation of clinical quality management for rehabilitation in Malaysia. *J Rehabil Med.* 2018;50(4):346–357.

53. Cieza A, Brockow T, Ewert T, et al. Linking health-status measurements to the international classification of functioning, disability and health. *J Rehabil Med.* 2002;34:205–210.

54. Prodinger B, O'Connor RJ, Stucki G, et al. Establishing score equivalence of the Functional Independence Measure (FIM™) motor scale and the Barthel Index, utilising the International Classification of Functioning, Disability and Health (ICF) and Rasch Measurement Theory. *J Rehabil Med.* 2017;49(5):416–422.

55. Cieza A, Geyh S, Chatterji S, et al. ICF linking rules: an update based on lessons learned. *J Rehabil Med.* 2005;37:212–218.

56. Cieza A, Fayed N, Bickenbach J, et al. Refinements of the ICF Linking Rules to strengthen their potential for establishing comparability of health information. *Disabil Rehabil.* 2016:1–10.

57. Kiltz U, van der Heijde D, Boonen A, et al. Development of a health index in patients with ankylosing spondylitis (ASAS HI): final result of a global initiative based on the ICF guided by ASAS. *Ann Rheum Dis.* 2015;74:830–835.

58. Escorpizo R, Ekholm J, Gmunder HP, et al. Developing a Core Set to describe functioning in vocational rehabilitation using the international classification of functioning, disability, and health (ICF). *J Rehabil Med.* 2010;20:502–511.

59. Finger M, Escorpizo R, Bostan C, et al. Work rehabilitation questionnaire (WORQ): development and preliminary psychometric evidence of an ICF-based questionnaire for vocational rehabilitation. *J Occup Rehabil.* 2014;24:498–510.

60. Li J, Prodinger B, Reinhardt JD, et al. Towards the system-wide implementation of the International Classification of Functioning, Disability and Health in routine practice: lessons from a pilot study in China. *J Rehabil Med.* 2016;48:502–507.

61. Prodinger B, Tennant A, Stucki G. Standardized reporting of functioning information on ICF-based common metrics. *Eur J Phys Rehabil Med.* 2018;54(1):110–117.

62. Prodinger B, Tennant A, Stucki G, et al. Harmonizing routinely collected health information for strengthening quality management in health systems: requirements and practice. *J Health Serv Res Policy.* 2016;21:223–228.

63. La Porta F, Franceschini M, Caselli S, et al. Unified Balance Scale: an activity-based, bed to community, and aetiology-independent measure of balance calibrated with Rasch analysis. *J Rehabil Med.* 2011;43:435–444.

64. Prodinger B, Ballert CS, Brach M, et al. Toward standardized reporting for a cohort study on functioning: the Swiss Spinal Cord Injury Cohort Study. *J Rehabil Med.* 2016;48:189–196.

65. Stucki G, Zampolini M, Juocevicius A, et al. Practice, science and governance in interaction: European effort for the system-wide implementation of the International Classification of Functioning, Disability and Health (ICF) in Physical and Rehabilitation Medicine. *Eur J Phys Rehabil Med.* 2017;53:299–307.

66. Prodinger B, Reinhardt JD, Selb M, et al. Towards system-wide implementation of the International Classification of Functioning, Disability and Health (ICF) in routine practice: developing simple, intuitive descriptions of ICF categories in the ICF Generic and Rehabilitation Set. *J Rehabil Med.* 2016;48:508–514.

67. Prodinger B, Scheel-Sailer A, Escorpizo R, et al. European initiative for the application of the International Classification of Functioning, Disability and Health: development of clinical assessment schedules for specified rehabilitation services. *Eur J Phys Rehabil Med.* 2017;53:319–332.

68. Selb M, Gimigliano F, Prodinger B, et al. Toward an International Classification of Functioning, Disability and Health clinical data collection tool: the Italian experience of developing simple, intuitive descriptions of the Rehabilitation Set categories. *Eur J Phys Rehabil Med.* 2017;53:290–298.

69. Gimigliano F, Selb M, Mukaino M, et al. Strengthening rehabilitation in health systems worldwide by implementing information on functioning in rehabilitation practice, quality management and policy. *J Int Soc Phys Rehabil Med.* 2018 [Epub ahead of print]

70. Swiss National Science Foundation. NRP 74 "Smarter Health Care". *Enhancing Continuous Quality Improvement and Supported Clinical Decision Making by Standardized Reporting of Functioning.* Available from: http://www.nfp74.ch/en

71. Gutenbrunner C, Bickenbach J, Kiekens C, et al. ISPRM discussion paper: proposing dimensions for an international classification system for service organization in health-related rehabilitation. *J Rehabil Med.* 2015;47:809–815.

72. Kiekens C, Meyer T, Gimigliano F, et al. European initiative for the application of the International Classification of Service Organization in Health-related Rehabilitation (ICSO-R). *Eur J Phys Rehabil Med.* 2017;53:308–318.

73. Ewert T, Grill E, Bartholomeyczik S, et al. ICF Core Set for patients with neurological conditions in the acute hospital. *Disabil Rehabil.* 2005;27:367–373.

74. Boldt C, Grill E, Wildner M, et al. ICF Core Set for patients with cardiopulmonary conditions in the acute hospital. *Disabil Rehabil.* 2005;27:375–380.

75. Stoll T, Brach M, Huber EO, et al. ICF Core Set for patients with musculoskeletal conditions in the acute hospital. *Disabil Rehabil.* 2005;27:381–387.

76. Grill E, Strobl R, Muller M, et al. ICF Core Sets for early post-acute rehabilitation facilities. *J Rehabil Med.* 2011;43:131–138.

77. Stier-Jarmer M, Grill E, Ewert T, et al. ICF Core Set for patients with neurological conditions in early post-acute rehabilitation facilities. *Disabil Rehabil.* 2005;27: 389–395.

78. Wildner M, Quittan M, Portenier L, et al. ICF Core Set for patients with cardiopulmonary conditions in early post-acute rehabilitation facilities. *Disabil Rehabil.* 2005;27:397–404.

79. Scheuringer M, Stucki G, Huber EO, et al. ICF Core Set for patients with musculoskeletal conditions in early post-acute rehabilitation facilities. *Disabil Rehabil.* 2005;27:405–410.

80. Grill E, Hermes R, Swoboda W, et al. ICF Core Set for geriatric patients in early post-acute rehabilitation facilities. *Disabil Rehabil.* 2005;27:411–417.

81. Kirchberger I, Cieza A, Biering-Sorensen F, et al. ICF Core Sets for individuals with spinal cord injury in the early post-acute context. *Spinal Cord.* 2010;48: 297–304.

82. Cieza A, Kirchberger I, Biering-Sorensen F, et al. ICF Core Sets for individuals with spinal cord injury in the long-term context. *Spinal Cord.* 2010;48:305–312.

83. Ballert C, Oberhauser C, Biering-Sorensen F, et al. Explanatory power does not equal clinical importance: study of the use of the Brief ICF Core Sets for spinal cord injury with a purely statistical approach. *Spinal Cord.* 2012;50:734–339.

84. Laxe S, Zasler N, Selb M, et al. Development of the International Classification of Functioning, Disability and Health core sets for traumatic brain injury: an international consensus process. *Brain Inj.* 2013;27:379–387.

85. United Nations. *Convention on the Rights of Persons with Disabilities, G.A. Res. 2006. [Internet];* 2006. Available from: http://www.un.org/esa/socdev/enable/rights/convtexte.htm [cited March 24, 2017].

86. World Health Organization. *Model Disability Survey. [Internet];* 2017. Available from: http://www.who.int/disabilities/data/mds/en/ [cited March 24, 2017].

87. Bostan C, Oberhauser C, Stucki G, et al. Which environmental factors are associated with lived health when controlling for biological health? A multilevel analysis. *BMC Public Health.* 2015;15:508.

88. Rauch A, Cieza A, Stucki G. How to apply the International Classification of Functioning, Disability and Health (ICF) for rehabilitation management in clinical practice. *Eur J Phys Rehabil Med.* 2008;44:329–342.

89. Rauch A, Bickenbach J, Reinhardt J, et al. The utility of the ICF to identify and evaluate problems and needs in participation in spinal cord injury. *Top Spinal Cord Inj Rehabil.* 2010;15:72–86.

90. Stucki G, Rauch A. The International Classification of Functioning, Disability and Health (ICF), a unifying model for physical and rehabilitation medicine (PRM). In: Didier J-P, Bigand E, eds. *Rethinking Physical and Rehabilitation Medicine. New Technologies Induce New Learning Strategies.* Paris, France: Springer Publishing; 2010:19–52.

91. Rauch A, Scheel-Sailer A. Applying the International Classification of Functioning, Disability and Health (ICF) to rehabilitation goal-setting. In: Siegert R, Levack W, eds. *Rehabilitation Goal Setting: Theory, Practice and Evidence.* Boca Raton, FL: CRC Press; 2014:161–180.

92. Selb M, Glässel A, Escorpizo R. ICF-based tools in rehabilitation toward return to work: facilitating interprofessional communication and comprehensive documentation. In: Escorpizo R, Brage S, Homa D, et al., eds. *Handbook of Vocational Rehabilitation and Disability Evaluation: Application and Implementation of the ICF.* New York, NY: Springer International Publishing; 2015:471–493.

93. Stucki G, Ewert T, Cieza A. Value and application of the ICF in rehabilitation medicine. *Disabil Rehabil.* 2002;24:932–938.

94. Swiss Paraplegic Research. *Translating Interventions into Real-Life Gains—A Rehab-Cycle Approach. [Internet];* 2017. Available from: http://www.icf-casestudies.org [cited March 24, 2017].

95. Rauch A, Escorpizo R, Riddle DL, et al. Using a case report of a patient with spinal cord injury to illustrate the application of the International Classification of Functioning, Disability and Health during multidisciplinary patient management. *Phys Ther.* 2010;90:1039–1052.

96. Glässel A, Rauch A, Selb M, et al. A case study on the application of the International Classification of Functioning, Disability and Health (ICF)-based tools for vocational rehabilitation in spinal cord injury. *Work.* 2012;41:465–474.

97. Peter C, Rauch A, Cieza A, et al. Stress, internal resources and functioning in a person with spinal cord disease. *NeuroRehabilitation.* 2012;30:119–130.

98. Finger ME, Selb M, De Bie R, et al. Using the International Classification of Functioning, Disability and Health in physiotherapy in multidisciplinary vocational rehabilitation: a case study of low back pain. *Physiother Res Int.* 2015;20:231–241.

99. Swiss Paraplegic Research. Sports in rehabilitation. *Translating Interventions into Real-Life Gains—A Rehab-Cycle Approach. [Internet];* 2016. Available from: http://www.icf-casestudies.org [cited March 24, 2017].

100. Steiner W, Ryser L, Huber E, et al. Use of the ICF model as a clinical problem-solving tool in physical therapy and rehabilitation medicine. *Phys Ther.* 2002;82:1098–1107.

101. World Health Organization. *International Classification of Health Interventions (ICHI). [Internet];* 2016. Available from: www.who.int/classifications/ichi/en/ [cited March 24, 2017].

102. Dorjbal D, Cieza A, Gmünder HP, et al. Strengthening quality of care through standardized reporting based on the World Health Organization's reference classifications. *Int J Qual Health Care.* 2016;28:626–633.

103. Madden R. International classification of health interventions. Lecture slides. Australia: National Centre for Classification of Health; 2006. Available from: https://www.icf.org.tw/upload/files/5-Richard%20Madden-ICHI%20August%20 2013-Taiwan-20130821.pdf [cited March 24, 2017].

104. Hurn J, Kneebone I, Cropley M. Goal setting as an outcome measure: a systematic review. *Clin Rehabil.* 2006;20:756–772.

105. Grimby G, Tennant A, Tesio L. The use of raw scores from ordinal scales: time to end malpractice? *J Rehabil Med.* 2012;44:97–98.

106. World Health Organization. *Monitoring and Evaluation of Health Systems Strengthening: An Operational Framework.* Geneva, Switzerland: WHO Press; 2009. Available from: http://www.who.int/healthinfo/HSS_MandE_framework_Nov_2009.pdf

107. Olsen L, Aisner D, McGinnis JM, eds. *The Learning Healthcare System: Workshop Summary.* Washington, DC: National Academies Press; 2007.

108. Krumholz HM, Bourne PE, Kuntz RE, et al. *Data Acquisition, Curation, and Use for a Continuously Learning Health System. A Vital Direction for Health and Health Care [Discussion Paper].* Washington, DC: National Academy of Medicine. Available from: https://nam.edu/wp-content/uploads/2016/09/Data-Acquisition-Curation-and-Use-for-a-Continuously-Learning-Health-System.pdf [cited March 24, 2017].

109. Stucki G, Post MWM, eds. The Swiss Spinal Cord Injury (SwiSCI) Cohort Study. *Am J Phys Med Rehabil.* 2011;90:S1–S79.

110. Bickenbach J, Tennant A, Stucki G, eds. Describing the lived experience of Swiss persons with spinal cord injury. *J Rehabil Med.* 2016;48:113–244.

111. Bickenbach J, ed. The International SCI Survey and the Learning Health System for SCI. *Am J Phys Med Rehabil* 2017;96:S1–S126.

112. World Health Organization. *Health Facility and Community Data Toolkit.* Geneva, Switzerland: WHO; 2014. Available from: http://www.who.int/healthinfo/facility_information_systems/Facility_Community_Data_Toolkit_final.pdf

113. Galloway RV, Granger CV, Karmarkar AM, et al. The uniform data system for medical rehabilitation report of patients with debility discharged from inpatient rehabilitation programs in 2000–2010. *Am J Phys Med Rehabil.* 2013;92:14–27.

114. U.S. Department of Health and Human Services, Centers for Medicare & Medicaid Services (CMS). *Inpatient Rehabilitation Facility—Patient Assessment Instrument (IRF-PAI).* Available from: https://www.cms.gov/medicare/medicare-fee-for-servicepayment/inpatientrehabfacpps/irfpai.html [cited March 24, 2017].

115. Gage B, Constantine R, Aggarwal J, et al. *The Development and Testing of the Continuity Assessment Record and Evaluation (CARE) Item Set: Final Report on the Development of the CARE Item Set. Vol. 1;* 2012. Available from: https://www.cms.gov/Medicare/Quality24Initiatives-Patient-Assessment-Instruments/Post-Acute-Care-Quality-Initiatives/Downloads/The-Development-and-Testing-of-the-Continuity-Assessment-Record-and-Evaluation-CARE-Item-Set-Final-Report-on-the-Development-of-the-CARE-Item-Set-Volume-1-of-3.pdf

116. U.S. Department of Health and Human Services, Centers for Medicare & Medicaid Services. 42 CFR Part 412. Medicare program; inpatient rehabilitation facility prospective payment system for Federal Fiscal Year 2016; Final Rule. *Fed Regist.* 2015;80(151).

117. World Health Organization. Concept note. In: *Rehabilitation 2030: A Call for Action. [Internet];* 2017. Available from: http://www.who.int/disabilities/care/rehab-2030/en/ [cited March 24, 2017].

118. Imamura M, Gutenbrunner C, Stucki G, et al. The international society of physical and rehabilitation medicine: the way forward—II. *J Rehabil Med.* 2014;46:97–107.

119. Khan F, Amatya B, de Groote W, et al. Capacity-building in clinical skills of rehabilitation workforce in low- and middle-income countries. *J Rehabil Med.* 2018;50:472–479.

120. Rentsch HP, Bucher P, Dommen Nyffeler I, et al. The implementation of the 'International Classification of Functioning, Disability and Health' (ICF) in daily practice of neurorehabilitation: an interdisciplinary project at the Kantonsspital of Lucerne, Switzerland. *Disabil Rehabil.* 2003;25:411–421.

121. de Brouwer CPM, van Amelsvoort LGPM, Heerkens YF, et al. Implementing the ICF in Occupational Health; building a curriculum as an exemplary case. *Work.* 2017;57:173–186.

122. European Physical and Rehabilitation. White book on physical and rehabilitation medicine in Europe. *Eur J Phys Rehabil Med.* 2018;54:125–321.

123. Stallinga HA, Roodbol PF, Annema C, et al. Functioning assessment vs. conventional medical assessment: a comparative study on health professionals' clinical decision-making and the fit with patient's own perspective of health. *J Clin Nurs.* 2014;23:1044–1054.

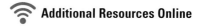 **Additional Resources Online**

James E. Graham
Steve R. Fisher
Kenneth J. Ottenbacher

CHAPTER **10**

Systematically Assessing and Improving the Quality of Physical Medicine and Rehabilitation

INTRODUCTION

Much has transpired since the prior edition of this textbook was published. None was more prominent than the changes related to measuring, reporting, and improving quality in health care. Although quality has always been a priority in medical rehabilitation, it is not an exaggeration to state that the collective interest in quality is at an all-time high. Recent health care reform has not only motivated health care administrators and providers to evaluate the perceived quality of the services they provide, but it has also made the term quality a frequent headline in the media as well as a common topic of conversation in the general public. Subsequently, rehabilitation providers, as well as the field as a whole, are now feeling the pressure to demonstrate their value under this prevalent quality lens.

Several recent health care reform initiatives directly target the costs and/or quality of postacute rehabilitation services. The Centers for Medicare and Medicaid Services (CMS) Innovation Center Web site (1) is a good resource for information on prior, ongoing, and pending demonstration projects. We highlight three of the more influential policies in this paragraph.

- Title III of the 2010 Affordable Care Act—Improving the Quality & Efficiency of Health Care—required the CMS to establish quality measures, develop quality reporting and value-based purchasing programs, and explore new patient care models (e.g., shared savings programs, bundled payments, etc.) (2).
- The Improving Medicare Post-Acute Care Transformation (IMPACT) Act of 2014 mandated the reporting of standardized quality measures across the four major postacute settings: inpatient rehabilitation facilities, skilled nursing facilities, long-term acute care hospitals, and home health agencies (3).
- The 2015 Medicare Access and Children's Health Insurance Program (CHIP) Reauthorization Act introduced two quality payment programs for Medicare Part B providers along with new incentives for cardiac rehabilitation utilization and additional procedures covered under the comprehensive care for joint replacement model (4).

It is difficult to assess the impact of these different, often over-lapping, reform initiatives. It is clear, however, that reimbursement is switching from a volume-based approach to a more quality-based one. The CMS aimed to have 50% of all Medicare fee-for-service payments made via alternative payment models by 2018 (5).

Patient-centered care is woven into the fabric of many of these regulatory initiatives and now occupies center stage in any discussions regarding quality and value (6). The intentions of this movement are worthy: strengthen the patient-clinician relationship, promote communication about things that matter, and facilitate patients' involvement in their own care. As such, "patient centeredness" has quite rapidly transformed our clinical encounters with patients, the outcomes they and their caregivers expect, and patients' access to their own medical record information (7,8). These same trends have also led to paradigm shifts in federally funded health research. The active engagement of stakeholders in the selection, design, funding, and conduct of research is now commonplace. A patient-centered focus can be employed by health care providers in any specialty, but it is particularly relevant to rehabilitation-related disciplines (9).

Physical rehabilitation is arguably more grounded in patient-clinician interactions and mutual participation than many other medical disciplines. Prescription medication and surgery are both passive interventions from the patient's perspective. Patients may take medications for extended periods with little clinician interaction. Surgical procedures are performed on the patient by the surgeon. Conversely, ongoing feedback, goal setting, and treatment modifications are inherent to the rehabilitation process. Much of the growth in patient-centered care and research could simply be viewed as other disciplines adopting some of the long-standing, fundamental principles of rehabilitation medicine.

As the culture of quality and patient-centered care continues to grow, rehabilitation needs to be knowledgeable, proactive, and flexible in its approach to assessing and improving the quality of care provided. Unquestionably, quality assessment and implementation efforts should be developed by professionals who understand the rehabilitation evidence base and informed by professionals engaged in clinical practice. The interests of other major stakeholders, including patients, caregivers, payers, and government agencies, must also be represented, even though their values may differ (10–12). The influence, prosperity, and even the survival of rehabilitation as a specialty may hinge on its ability to develop and implement evidence-based monitoring and management systems relevant to consumers, payers, administrators, and policy makers.

This chapter begins with an overview of the fundamental elements in assessing quality. These include the different types of quality measures, the objectives underlying different forms of quality assessment, and basics of the quality reporting process. We then review traditional approaches to improving rehabilitation program quality and also introduce some relatively new terminology and processes to achieve that goal. Next, we provide brief descriptions of the dominant general health care organization and rehabilitation-specific accreditation agencies. Lastly, we discuss expectations and offer suggestions for the field moving forward.

DEFINING QUALITY

Quality is a ubiquitous term, but one that is defined in many different ways. Regarding quality of health care, definitions and concepts can vary based on the principal perspectives for a given health care encounter. For example, one viewpoint may emphasize the provider's perspective in terms of practice procedures, standards of care, and/or guideline adherence when delivering care, whereas another may emphasize the patient's perspective in terms of clinical experiences and achieving desired outcomes when receiving care.

More than 25 years ago, the Institute of Medicine offered two definitions for quality health care:

1. The degree to which health services for individuals and populations increase the likelihood of desired health outcomes and are consistent with current professional knowledge (13).
2. Care that is safe, effective, patient-centered, timely, efficient, and equitable (14).

The Agency for Health care Research and Quality (AHRQ), the federal government's lead agency for improving the quality, safety, efficiency, and effectiveness of health care, more recently defined quality health care as "doing the right thing for the right patient, at the right time, in the right way to achieve the best possible results" (15). All three definitions provide broad perspectives and capture the positive connotations of quality. However, they also illustrate the lack of specificity inherent in conceptual definitions.

Inclusive definitions and theory-based conceptualizations are well suited for academic discussions and provide the foundation for developing practical quality measures. However, it is unrealistic to assume a singular measure or even a handful of measures can adequately cover the quality spectrum across health care disciplines or systems (16). Fundamental differences in clinical encounters, patient and provider expectations, treatment types, patient and provider responsibilities, and relevant outcomes, among other distinctions, preclude a one-measure-fits-all approach in health care. Thus, specificity and clinical utility are paramount when applying the construct of quality to health care. The next section defines basic concepts and terms related to operationalizing health care quality measures.

TYPES OF QUALITY MEASURES

More than 50 years ago, Avedis Donabedian developed a framework for assessing quality in health care that is still widely applied today (17). The Donabedian model classifies measures for assessing and comparing quality as structures, processes, or outcomes (**Fig. 10-1**).

Structural measures represent the physical and organizational characteristics of care settings. These measures convey a health care provider's or system's capacity for delivering high-quality care; for example, the facilities, equipment, personnel, and financial resources supporting the care provided.

Process measures capture what providers do to maintain or improve the health of their patients. These measures are not limited to direct elements of clinical care. They can also encompass organizational, administrative, and financing aspects of health care delivery. However, publicly reported process measures commonly reflect standard of care and/or established guidelines for clinical practice (16). Examples include the percentage of patients who received preventive services such as immunizations or percentage of Inpatient Rehabilitation Facility (IRF) patients who receive an overall care plan within 4 days of admission. Process measures are typically the first and most frequent type of measure in different health care quality reporting programs.

Outcome measures reveal the impact that care has on the health status of individuals and populations. More practically, outcome measures describe patient experiences and the end results of care. It is important to understand that a given outcome is the result of a myriad of factors, some of which are directly tied to provider quality and others that are beyond provider control. Nevertheless, outcomes are more patient-centered and seemingly more valued by patients and caregivers than the underlying structural or process measures, which are more directly under provider control. Familiar examples of quality outcome measures in acute care include mortality and hospital readmission rates. Outcomes may also include patient satisfaction with the types, timeliness, and/or targets of care. Rehabilitation is explicitly focused on improving and maintaining individuals' functioning, independence, and health-related quality of life. To date, each postacute setting has used a different standardized assessment tools: Inpatient Rehabilitation Facility-Patient Assessment Instrument (IRF-PAI) instrument for inpatient rehabilitation, Minimum Data Set (MDS) for skilled nursing, and Outcome and Assessment Information Set (OASIS) for home health. However, the IMPACT Act (3) mandated that CMS develop a unified functional measurement system for use across all postacute settings. As of the writing of this chapter, CMS was evaluating the utility of common self-care and mobility measures

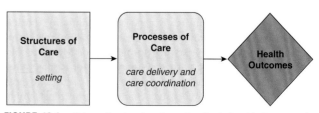

FIGURE 10-1. Schematic showing the ordered relationship between the three concepts in the Donabedian model.

developed from items in the Continuity and Assessment Record and Evaluation (CARE) tool. Updates on functional status measures and a link to the original report from RTI International can be found on the Medicare functional measures Web site (18).

Beyond the three core concepts in the Donabedian model, there are several other types of measures that are commonly used in quality assessment. Some of these measures are simply combinations of the prior concepts, whereas others incorporate additional elements of health care delivery and resources into the measure. The paragraphs below provide brief descriptions of two other types of frequently used measures.

Effectiveness measures are created by tying together processes and outcomes. Effectiveness implies that there is a criterion with which to compare the observed outcomes from a given care process. The simplest example being comparing the improvements from treatment "a" with the natural recovery improvements achieved without formal care. In recent years, natural history and even placebo comparators have fallen out of favor and been replaced by **comparative effectiveness research** designs. Comparative effectiveness research compares the benefits (and harms) of at least two plausible care processes in real-world settings (19). In the context of this chapter on assessing and improving quality, we emphasize the effectiveness in meeting a desired goal or benchmark. For example, a facility may want to determine if adding a simple home evaluation could increase its home discharge rate to 75% from the current 71% attained with existing care processes.

Efficiency measures convey outcomes in the context of cost constraints. Assessing and improving care quality would be easy if money were not an issue. However, resources are always limited. As health care funding continues to tighten, demonstrating high-quality cost-effective rehabilitative care is more important than ever. Accurate costs of care for a given condition are difficult to calculate. Costs for a specific treatment or a particular inpatient stay are relatively straightforward; however, a person's care needs typically extend well beyond a single intervention or discharge. Variability in defining the duration and related services for an episode of care can have dramatic or even contradicting influences on cost assessments. Subsequently, measures of service use (e.g., length of stay, treatments units) are often used as surrogates for detailed cost calculations. Simple examples include functional status efficiency (change in functional independence measure [FIM] Instrument ratings from admission to discharge divided by number of days in rehabilitation) and home time efficiency (costs of the initial postacute rehabilitation stay divided by the total number of days in the community over the first 6 months following hospital discharge). A more complex, and often debated, measure is quality adjusted life years (QALYs), which factors in a person's functional abilities, quality of life, and life expectancy based on the care received (20).

The "Triple Aim" of health care includes three broad goals: (a) improving care experiences, (b) improving population health, and (c) reducing per capita costs (21). Ideally, different health care disciplines, health systems, providers, and the patients they serve should be involved in the decisions regarding which specific measures are relevant and important for monitoring and improving their efforts to achieve the triple aim. **Table 10-1** shows the 2018 list of CMS quality measures specific to inpatient rehabilitation facilities (22). As of October 2018, there were 3 process and 9 outcome measures in the IRF quality reporting program. Additional measures are being considered with pending implementation dates.

As **Table 10-1** shows, many established quality outcome measures are focused on minimizing negative events (e.g., infections, falls, and readmissions). Thus, one must be vigilant to view quality as an indicator of total patient experiences and not simply the avoidance of adverse events. The *Quality Improvement* section, later in this chapter, further distinguishes between targeting adverse events and truly enhancing care quality.

TABLE 10-1	2018 Center for Medicare and Medicaid Services Quality Measures for Inpatient Rehabilitation Facilities	
Measure Title[a]		**Type**
Influenza vaccination coverage among health care personnel		Process
Percent of patients who were assessed and appropriately given the seasonal influenza vaccine		Process
Patients with admission and discharge functional assessments and care plan addressing function		Process
Catheter-associated urinary tract infection (CAUTI) outcome measure		Outcome
Percent of patients with pressure ulcers that are new or worsened		Outcome
Hospital-onset methicillin-resistant *Staphylococcus aureus* (MRSA) bacteremia outcome measure		Outcome
Hospital-onset *Clostridium difficile* infection (CDI) outcome measure		Outcome
Percent of patients experiencing one or more falls with major injury		Outcome
Discharge to community		Outcome
Potentially preventable 30-d postdischarge readmission measure		Outcome
Potentially preventable within stay readmission measure		Outcome
Medicare spending per beneficiary		Cost (outcome)

[a]The National Quality Form provides detailed information on the development and approval of measures in the IRF Quality Reporting Program (https://www.qualityforum.org).

ASSESSING QUALITY

This section discusses systems of measurement, monitoring, and interpretation focused on outcomes of care. We include both internal and external quality assessment systems. Rehabilitation is provided in many settings, including homes, outpatient clinics, transitional care facilities, nursing homes, and inpatient rehabilitation facilities. Most of our examples deal with inpatient rehabilitation facilities. However, the principles and concepts apply to other rehabilitation settings. Rehabilitation facilities—largely under the guidance of the Commission on Accreditation of Rehabilitation Facilities (CARF)—now have several decades of experience with program evaluation and quality assurance systems and the resulting knowledge provides a basis for developing or enhancing program monitoring and clinical management activities.

Program Evaluation

Program Evaluation is the systematic collection and analysis of information about some or all aspects of a health service program to inform decisions about that program (23). Most evaluations are aimed at providing an overview of program outcomes. While this information can be used for public reporting purposes, it is primarily given to the program staff with the expectation for improved program management and better patient outcomes—aka, "outcomes management."

Program evaluation refers to a variety of information-gathering activities designed to aid in program development or functioning (i.e., formative evaluation) or to decide whether a program as a whole is worthwhile (i.e., summative evaluation). Many approaches to program evaluation have been employed over the last three decades (24). These systems have multiple uses, including marketing, profitability, program planning and development, research, prognosis, utilization review, and improved clinical planning and treatment.

Standard program evaluation systems in rehabilitation have three components: design, goals, and reports (25). While this basic model is still widely used, updating has occurred as part of CARF's emphasis on outcomes management. CARF offers training, guidance, and materials on outcomes management. Anyone developing, implementing, or using a program evaluation or quality improvement system in rehabilitation should consult the CARF Web site (26) for the most recent standards manual and other resources.

CARF standards require the measurement of program performance in the domains of effectiveness (outcomes), efficiency (relationship between outcomes and resources used), service access (e.g., number of days from referral to admission, convenience of the hours and location of operation), and satisfaction (experience of the persons served and other stakeholders). Data to assess these domains are measured at admission, discharge, and follow-up, depending on the appropriate time for each domain. Outcomes are assessed after discharge. Follow-up data collection usually takes place 3 months after discharge but other periods can be justified.

Figure 10-2 shows the fundamental components of a general program evaluation system for inpatient rehabilitation programs. The sparseness of measures (italicized) in the process box and the larger set of admission (i.e., input) and outcomes (i.e., discharge and follow-up) measures show the emphasis of conventional program evaluations. Functional status measures, such as the IRF-PAI, constitute the primary input (admission, baseline) and output (discharge, follow-up) measures. Cost and length of stay are classified here as process or input measures because they indicate the effort or resources underlying the services provided. Program evaluation systems also need

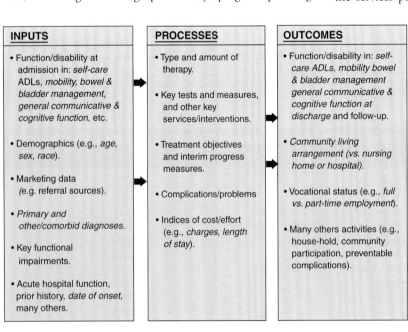

FIGURE 10-2. Basic program evaluation framework for rehabilitation programs. Items from the Inpatient Rehabilitation Facilities-Patient Assessment Instrument (IRF-PAI) are shown in italics.

INPUTS

- Function/disability at admission in: *self-care ADLs, mobility, bowel & bladder management, general communicative & cognitive function,* etc.
- Demographics (e.g., *age, sex, race*).
- Marketing data (e.g. referral sources).
- *Primary and other/comorbid diagnoses.*
- Key functional impairments.
- Acute hospital function, prior history, *date of onset,* many others.

PROCESSES

- Type and amount of therapy.
- Key tests and measures, and other key services/interventions.
- Treatment objectives and interim progress measures.
- Complications/problems
- Indices of cost/effort (e.g., *charges, length of stay*).

OUTCOMES

- Function/disability in: *self-care ADLs, mobility bowel & bladder management general communicative & cognitive function at discharge* and follow-up.
- *Community living arrangement (vs. nursing home or hospital).*
- Vocational status (e.g., *full vs. part-time employment*).
- Many others activities (e.g., house-hold, community participation, preventable complications).

SUPPLEMENTARY MEASURES

- *Payment source,* region of country, and many other descriptors.
- Date and cause of death.

supplementary measures used for general descriptive or comparative purposes. Demographic variables (e.g., age, gender, race) are used as input or independent variables. Although they are typically not good measures of case severity, demographic variables do help segment the population for other analyses (e.g., access to care, service type). Data on and reasons for rehospitalization and death are also essential supplementary measures in medical rehabilitation program evaluations.

The IRF-PAI data set contains essential measures for general inpatient rehabilitation program evaluations: demographic information, impairment group and comorbidities, functional status ratings at admission and discharge, and length of stay. The Uniform Data System for Medical Rehabilitation, eRehabData, ITHealthTrack, MedTell Outcomes, and other organizations produce national normative benchmarks using IRF-PAI data from subscribing facilities. These national norms are valuable for broad comparisons and for observing trends over time. However, the utility is limited by the degree to which the available benchmark data reflect the specific rehabilitation facility's objectives and population. Without stratifying by or accurate adjustments for case mix and functional severity, outcome comparisons can be misleading.

Lastly, the value of any program evaluation is only as good as the willingness to respond to the findings. A common response to unmet expectations is to simply change those expectations. Program evaluations provide insight on extracting information from clinical data systems, realistic outcome expectations, and monitoring and improving performance metrics, but they do not guarantee appropriate action to that insight. The next section discusses quality assurance, which helps to "assure" a commitment to improving health care quality.

Quality Assurance

Quality assurance can be defined as all activities related to defining, assessing, monitoring, and improving the quality of health care. These activities can be performed as part of the accreditation of facilities, supervision of health providers, or other efforts to improve the performance of health providers and the quality of health services (27). The term has a negative connotation for some who view it as external policing and micro management of providers and health systems. However, quality assurance activities of some type are needed to assure the public that standards of care are being met.

Program evaluation and quality assurance are complimentary efforts with differing targets. Program evaluation focuses on stated objectives and is concerned with identifying and evaluating the structure, processes, effectiveness, efficiency, and impact of the program. Quality assurance generally focuses on patient-specific practices of providers and evaluates these practices with regard to standards expected by the peer group or benchmarks of exemplary practice agreed upon by the profession.

Predefined standards are central to ensuring quality in medical care (28). Although efforts to systematically ensure quality in medical care go back to the first quarter of the 20th century, pressure for accountability has increased in recent decades, driven by explosive growth of costs, and by higher expectations of medical care (28). The federal government and the Joint Commission have been major forces behind quality assurance for hospital care. CARF has played an important role in defining quality specifically for rehabilitation.

Monitoring the quality of specific services provided does not guarantee that a different type of service might provide superior benefits to patients or whether the person served has major unmet service needs. Studies of quality in acute care hospitals have reported that errors of omission (e.g., a physician not detecting a major diagnostic problem) were more common than errors of commission (not providing the correct treatment for the diagnosis) (29). Errors of omission of needed rehabilitative treatments may be frequent as well, especially given today's cost and length of stay constraints. The results of inpatient rehabilitation, for example, will be compromised if quality follow-up care is not provided. A wider consideration of patient needs might lead to quality improvement efforts that address patient referral, adding or changing service mix, and education of payers regarding service needs. Patients, their families, and disability advocates can be influential allies in such education.

Obviously, the overarching intent of quality assurance is not to establish an active system for penalizing low-performing health care providers. Rather, the intent is to encourage self-assessment, increase transparency, spur innovation, and improve the health care experiences and outcomes for all patients (30). The next section describes the principles of a few quality improvement models that pick up where program evaluation and quality assurance leave off by helping programs implement change to improve care quality.

Quality Improvement

Traditional quality improvement models share the belief that established routines facilitate effectiveness and efficiency. The root causes of problems are more commonly at the level of the system or the sequences of care processes than at the individual or even department level. The goal is to identify and remove the errors, or at least unnecessary variation, in the sequence of care activities (31). The aim is to improve systems, not blame individuals. Improved protocols for activities and processes need to be developed and implemented as a key element of quality improvement (32). Global organizational commitment is essential. This philosophy has moved health care toward improving routine processes.

Two established models of quality improvement include **Total Quality Management** and **Continuous Quality Improvement** (33). These models emphasize the importance of knowledge of effective processes and participation by the staff directly involved in the process. Participation includes fact finding, focusing on preventing problems, and selecting measures that relate directly to the problem. The emphasis is on understanding the total system and involvement of everyone to diagnose, plan, and fix problems to improve systems. Both the specific problem and systems in which it is embedded need attention (34). Continuous quality improvement emphasizes review of systems and sequences rather than discrete inspections. One must acquire extensive knowledge about the system, not just identify errors or outliers as in traditional quality assurance. When variations exceed normally observed limits, knowledge of the system is needed to infer the cause and correct problematic processes.

The effectiveness of improving routine processes, compared to simply eliminating a focal problem or the worst performers, is graphically displayed in **Figure 10.3**. This conventional view assumes that measured quality or results

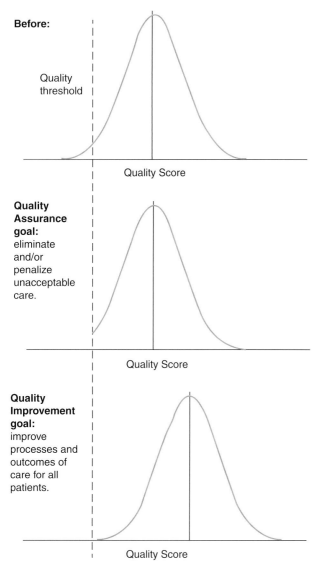

Before:

Quality threshold

Quality Score

Quality Assurance goal: eliminate and/or penalize unacceptable care.

Quality Score

Quality Improvement goal: improve processes and outcomes of care for all patients.

Quality Score

FIGURE 10-3.   Differences between traditional quality assurance and quality improvement approaches.

are distributed normally. An approach aimed at eliminating unacceptable care would eliminate poor care for only a small fraction of patients (the small left tail of the distribution). An approach aimed at improving the processes of care would improve results for most patients and, conceivably, could shift the entire quality performance distribution beyond the unacceptable threshold.

In the late 1990s, a quality improvement system specifically for clinical practice was developed and termed **Clinical Practice Improvement (CPI)** (35,36). It is a data-driven, bottom-up approach involving data collection on processes of care, relevant outcomes, and patient characteristics, including indicators of severity. Clinicians who choose different practices from those in the protocol are given the opportunity to present their reasoning to the team so that the protocol can be modified or consensus can be reached. The goal of the process is to enable clinicians to improve severity-adjusted outcomes within cost limits or to maintain relevant outcomes while decreasing costs. Sophisticated multivariate statistics are

used to statistically control for factors that confound process-outcome relationships for selected subsets of patients. Process variations are lessened through ongoing feedback from statistical analyses, discussion, and consensus.

Proponents of CPI argue that clinical practice guidelines are often based on a consensus of experts, and available scientific evidence is often limited or based on selected patient groups and programs that vary from those seen in practice. CPI studies have identified actionable factors that are associated with severity-adjusted outcomes (e.g., earlier admission of stroke patients to rehabilitation) (37). Thus, the validity of CPI depends on the accuracy of the statistical adjusters employed. Compared to typical randomized clinical trials, CPI has less internal validity, but greater external validity; that is, greater generalization to practice.

Quality improvement integrates knowledge, processes, outcomes, and action to improve care. The paragraphs below provide brief descriptions of common terms used in quality assessment and improvement efforts.

Norms are average population-based values from actual clinical practice that can be used as benchmarks for relevant providers or programs. Population does not necessarily mean everyone. Rather, norms are most clinically useful when they are specific to a patient diagnosis or other discrete patient characteristics. Rehabilitation-related examples include average length of stay, average functional status gain, and average hours of physical therapy. Norms apply to processes as well as outcomes. Rehabilitation professionals need benchmarks with which to compare their staffing, education, costs, initial evaluation, intervention types and intensities, patient satisfaction, and both short- and long-term outcomes. Furthermore, facility- or program-specific norms can be used to evaluate progress over time and/or to convey what is achievable in top-performing programs.

Criteria are statements that define appropriate or correct clinical care (28). Some distinguish between a criterion and a standard, using the former as the more general dimension and the latter as the specific numeric cut-point (38). Criteria are typically developed on the basis of professional experience and scientific literature. Criteria and standards may describe structure, process, or outcome. An example of a process-related criterion or standard is the assertion that inpatients in medical rehabilitation should receive 3 hours of combined therapy (physical, occupational, and speech and language) per day.

Sentinel events refer to single, remarkable occurrences that are highly problematic or socially unacceptable. In practice, motivation to improve quality of care frequently depends on sentinel events (39). Sentinel events require a response (40). The point of systematic quality improvement is to go beyond concern for negative outliers alone.

A **threshold** indicates a preestablished point in an indicator that should trigger more in-depth investigation to determine whether a problem or opportunity to improve care exists (28). As an example, a threshold of 5% might be set for rehabilitation patients discharged back to acute care and 15% to a nursing home. For sentinel events, such as death or suicide within rehabilitation, a threshold of 0% could be justifiable; however, every case needs to be individually reviewed. In general, thresholds of 100% success or 0% problems are unrealistic. Setting thresholds at less-than-perfect levels avoids disproportionate use of time to evaluate random events (28). Quality improvement efforts in rehabilitation are usually better spent on assessing and preventing frequently occurring or significant problems.

Quality Improvement involves applying appropriate methods of evaluation and outcomes assessment to close the gap between current and expected levels of quality as defined not only by professional standards but by consumers and other stakeholders. Advances in health information technology have reduced the burden of quality assessment and improvement (41).

QUALITY REPORTING

Public reporting of provider quality metrics has increased substantially over the past decade. Historically, provider and performance information was private for internal use only. The *Affordable Care Act* required the Secretary of Health and Human Services to establish quality reporting programs for virtually all sectors of health care that receive federal reimbursement. Section 3004 outlines the quality reporting mandate specific to inpatient rehabilitation facilities (2). Subsequent legislation, including the *IMPACT Act* (3), has further refined and expanded postacute provider quality reporting programs. Despite the dramatic increase in seemingly consumer-focused reporting efforts, some argue that the rush to public reporting has not provided what health care consumers value in making informed care decisions and is largely being ignored by the public (42). That is not to suggest that public reporting will soon run its course. Rather, public reporting programs will continue to evolve, becoming more consumer-driven and influential in care decisions. Providers, health systems, researchers, and professional organizations need to understand and help shape rehabilitation-related quality reporting programs moving forward. This section provides brief overviews of current efforts, fundamental elements, and challenges in creating fair quality performance ratings for public reporting.

Current Public Reporting Systems

The CMS maintains several consumer-friendly, setting-specific "compare" Web sites. These Web sites allow consumers to search for providers, learn about the services they offer, and make side-by-side comparisons on the quality of care they provide. The CMS also provides helpful tips on choosing providers and health coverage plans. The overall goal is to educate and empower patients to make more informed health care decisions. The seven compare Web sites in operation as of July 2017 are listed below:

- Hospital Compare (https://www.medicare.gov/hospitalcompare/)
- Inpatient Rehabilitation Facility Compare (https://www.medicare.gov/inpatientrehabilitationfacilitycompare/)
- Nursing Home Compare (https://www.medicare.gov/nursinghomecompare/)
- Long-Term Care Hospital Compare (https://www.medicare.gov/longtermcarehospitalcompare/)
- Home Health Compare (https://www.medicare.gov/homehealthcompare/)
- Dialysis Facility Compare (https://www.medicare.gov/dialysisfacilitycompare/)
- Physician (and other clinicians) Compare (https://www.medicare.gov/physiciancompare/)

Consumer Assessment of Health Providers and Systems (CAHPS) (43) was developed with funding from the Agency for Health Care Research and Quality to evaluate health care experiences from the viewpoint of consumers or patients. The CAHPS has evolved to a family of standardized surveys on multiple types of care and reports from the CAHPS are widely disseminated (44). CAHPS surveys on disability and rehabilitation have not yet been developed.

The National Committee on Quality Assurance (NCQA) (45) was formed to address quality issues among managed health care plans. Without objective measures and credible data, competition between such plans is possible only on the basis of cost. The NCQA accredits health plans and its Health care Effectiveness Data and Information Set (HEDIS) (46) is used by more than 90% of health care plans in the United States. The number of HEDIS quality indicators has increased over time. The current (2017) version includes 81 variables, including indicators of effectiveness, access, satisfaction, plan stability, intensity of care utilization, and structural descriptors. A few outcome indicators or surveys are specified (e.g., Medicare Health Outcome Survey), but most are process indicators. Quality indicators are specified for a number of chronic conditions and for disease management programs, but not for the neurological, traumatic, or orthopedic conditions commonly seen in inpatient rehabilitation hospitals. HEDIS data are compiled into a national database, and report cards are issued on health plans. It is important to note that health plan accreditation and much of the reporting is voluntary. Health management organizations with lower quality-of-care scores have tended to stop disclosing their quality data (47). In sum, adequate health plan report cards have not yet been developed for disability and rehabilitation, but CAHPS and HEDIS provide a foundation for future progress.

Risk Standardization

Complex illnesses, multiple morbidity, functional limitations, health behaviors, and other risk factors make some patients more costly and resource intensive and more likely to experience poor outcomes, regardless of care quality or efficiency (48). The need for severity or risk adjustment is central to quality reporting (49). Quality reporting systems that are unadjusted or poorly adjusted are likely to produce misleading information. While all factors cannot be controlled statistically, known confounding factors can be measured, and their effects can be projected. Knowledge of at least basic statistical principles is needed to interpret performance data.

Risk adjustment methodology has primarily focused on acute care hospital outcomes. Although, cost- or resource-related risk adjustment is well established in rehabilitation, due in large part to Medicare's move to prospective payment systems for postacute care. Function-related groups (FRGs) from the FIM instrument were developed to adjust inpatient medical rehabilitation caseload for factors affecting length of stay (50–53). Relabeled case mix groups (CMGs), these groups are the basis for Medicare reimbursement for inpatient rehabilitation programs in the United States. CMGs group patients primarily by admission functional status and impairment group. These functional categories correlate better with rehabilitation-related resource utilization than diagnosis-based classifications.

However, risk adjustment for more patient-centered rehabilitation outcomes is less established. Lisa Iezzoni, who literally wrote the book on *Risk Adjustment for Measuring Health Care Outcomes* (54), states that "Risk adjusting rehabilitation outcomes is more difficult than risk adjusting other clinical results, such as outcomes of many acute care services" (48).

The QualityNet Web site (55) includes detailed methodology reports for all measures included in the hospital inpatient and outpatient quality reporting programs, the physician quality reporting system, and other non–rehab-related settings and services. The principles and methodology for many of the measures in the inpatient rehabilitation quality reporting program (see **Table 10-1**) are based on the established risk-adjustment procedures for acute care quality reporting. The National Quality Forum Web site (56) provides detailed methodology and background reports for "endorsed" measures and some measures under consideration. A simple search by setting (e.g., inpatient rehabilitation) yields setting-specific quality measures and reports.

In terms of traditional regression model diagnostics such as variance explained or c-statistic, risk adjustment models for clinical outcomes typically do not perform too well. By design, these models are limited to conditions and characteristics present on admission; do not include provider-level factors, process-related variables (e.g., length of stay or treatment type), or health behavior information (e.g., body mass index, smoking status); and traditionally omit patient- and community-level socioeconomic indicators. Proponents of current risk-standardization procedures argue that baseline patient characteristics alone should not fully explain differences in outcomes. Rather, the remaining variation in outcomes is due to variability in the quality of care across providers. Nevertheless, risk-standardized outcome rankings for acute hospitals (57) and inpatient rehabilitation facilities (58) are sensitive to the adjustment methodology.

Sample size is also a necessary consideration when comparing provider performances. A single bad outcome may well be a fluke, whereas a pattern of outcomes below severity-adjusted norms indicates a possible process problem needing further investigation. Furthermore, nonspecialist physicians may encounter only a small number of patients with a specific disease so provider profiles may not be valid, and individual providers could game the system by avoiding just a few severe, high-cost, or poorly adherent patients. Most, if not all, publicly reported quality measures require a minimum case number for a given provider's ranking to be included.

LEARNING HEALTH SYSTEMS

There have been tremendous advances in our capacity to manage serious and often fatal medical conditions in the past two decades (59). Over this same time period, there have been equally dramatic advances in information technology both at the patient level and across our health care system as a whole. Paradoxically, this same health care system continues to rank low on such fundamentals as quality, outcomes, cost, and equity (60). Opportunities to improve quality, for example, developing knowledge, translating new information into medical evidence, applying the new evidence to patient care, are often marred by inefficiencies that result in waste—and sometimes

harm to patients (59). Recognition of these shortcomings has resulted in greater attention directed toward improving human health through more system-level innovations by addressing what are increasingly recognized as system-level problems (59).

A number of recent trends make, for the first time, intervening at the system level possible. These include the consolidation of ambulatory, in-patient, and postacute care settings of care into integrated delivery systems (61,62); the evolution of health information systems (63,64); and greater attention to population health management. Vast computational power is also increasingly affordable, and connectivity allows information to be accessed in real time. Human and organizational capabilities also offer new and expanded ways to improve the reliability and efficiency of the care provided (65). And, importantly, health care organizations recognize that effective care must be delivered by collaborative teams of clinicians, each member playing a vital role (65).

In response to these challenges and opportunities, The National Academies of Science, Engineering and Medicine (NASEM) convened a blue-ribbon committee to recommend ways health care delivery organizations, both small and large, can begin *systematically* gathering and creating evidence to improve their care delivery in real time and create a continuously learning health care system (59). The report recognized that while health care must accommodate many competing priorities and human factors unlike those in other industries, the health care *system* as a whole could learn from industry how to better meet specific needs, expand choices, and reduce costs. In short, the report contended that Americans would be better served by a nimbler health care system that is consistently reliable and improves by avoiding past mistakes and adopting newfound successes (59). Developing, measuring, and monitoring quality metrics relevant to patient-centered outcomes is an essential component of this process.

Definition

The NASEM has described a learning health care system as an organization that "is designed to generate and apply the best evidence for the collaborative health care choices of each patient and provider; to drive the process of discovery as a natural outgrowth of patient care; and to ensure innovation, quality, safety, and value in health care" (59).

Characteristics of the Learning Health System

In practice, the learning health system concept involves a structural commitment to a bidirectional feedback loop whereby data collection is embedded into care delivery processes, and care is changed in response to evidence generated (66). The NASEM's vision of a Learning Health System includes integrating science and informatics, patient-clinician partnerships, incentives, and culture to facilitate continuous learning, best care, and lower cost. To help guide organizations in making the transition, the NASEM has identified the following key characteristics integral to a true Learning Health Care System as shown in **Box 10-1**

Most fundamentally, these defining characteristics are based on the concept of rigorous self-improvement, which historically has been separated from the generation of knowledge and learning in real-world practice (67).

NASEM Key Characteristics to Learning Health Care System(s)

Science and Informatics
- Real-time access to knowledge—A learning health care system continuously and reliably captures, curates, and delivers the best available evidence to guide, support, tailor, and improve clinical decision-making and care safety and quality.
- Digital capture of the care experience—A learning health care system captures the care experience on digital platforms for real-time generation and application of knowledge for care improvement.

Patient-Clinician Partnerships
- Engaged, empowered patients—A learning health care system is anchored on patient needs and perspectives and promotes the inclusion of patients, families, and other caregivers as vital members of the continuously learning care team.

Incentives
- Incentives aligned for value—In a learning health care system, incentives are actively aligned to encourage continuous improvement, identify and reduce waste, and reward high-value care.
- Full transparency—A learning health care system systematically monitors the safety, quality, processes, prices, costs, and outcomes of care, and makes information available for care improvement and informed choices and decision-making by clinicians, patients, and their families.

Culture
- Leadership-instilled culture of learning—A learning health care system is stewarded by leadership committed to a culture of teamwork, collaboration, and adaptability in support of continuous learning as a core aim.
- Supportive system competencies—In a learning health care system, complex care operations and processes are constantly refined through ongoing team training and skill building, systems analysis and information development, and creation of the feedback loops for continuous learning and system improvement.

Rehabilitation and the Learning Health System

Information on the structure of care, the process of care and health outcomes (Donabedian model) described at the beginning of this chapter is fundamental for the learning health system. This information is also essential to improve the health system's response to people's functional needs during the course of rehabilitation (68). The delivery of successful rehabilitation services requires an integrated information system and the infrastructure to deliver the right treatment to the right patient, at the right time, in the right way to produce the right outcome (69). Our health care payment system has prevented the sharing of information in the past by creating segregated clinical silos where the fee-for-service payment model prevented partnerships across acute care, postacute care, and community care settings. The introduction of value-based payment models, in conjunction with patient-centered outcomes and legislations such as the IMPACT Act, are providing important opportunities for physical medicine and rehabilitation professionals to become leaders in developing learning health systems. The routine, informed, and systematic collection of standardized information regarding a person's

functional performance and status is now recognized as valuable by the larger medical and health care community. Data on functional status is essential in care transitions and collaboration across acute and postacute settings. A better understanding of functional potential is essential to a successful learning health system where recovery and independence are the goals for patients, providers, and payers (68).

Traditionally, health information has been understood in terms of biomedical data focusing on the health indicators of mortality and morbidity (70). Increasingly, however, information about functioning—as conceptualized by the WHO's International Classification of Functioning, Disability and Health (ICF) (71)—has been acknowledged as necessary to truly understand a person's health. Functioning incorporates biological health described in terms of impairments in body functions and capacity limitations as well as a person's actual performance across domains of activities and participation in interaction with the physical, built, attitudinal and social environment. Physical functioning information is an important part of the data stream across most health care settings, but it is essential when implementing and scaling up strategies for rehabilitative care (70).

A central goal of rehabilitation is to optimize functional health in the presence of disease, injury, and other debilitating conditions, within the larger context of a person's social life, available resources, and how that person interacts with his or her environment (72,73). Stucki and Bickenbach (68) illustrate in **Table 10-2** how functioning information can be used for the continuous improvement of functional outcomes in a learning health system across three distinct levels. At the clinical level, improvements are in the functioning of individual patients; at the meso-level, improvements are focused on sustainable rehabilitation services and continuity of care across settings; and at the macro level, suitable rehabilitation policies guide comprehensive rehabilitation programming to meet population needs. Stucki contends that continuous and sustainable improvement across all three of these health system levels are needed to have a system that truly "learns" from itself and requires the routine collection, monitoring, and analysis of information about functioning and its determinants.

To improve quality of care across all health care settings, valid physical functioning data will be critical for successful learning health systems and will help ensure that the innovations that arise from the natural conduct of patient care are meaningful to patients and their lives.

Implementation Science

Learning health care systems are designed to improve care over time using continuous quality improvement strategies and integrating the latest research into real world patient care. Implementation science is intended to support exactly this mission. Implementation research is the scientific study of methods to promote the systematic uptake of research findings and other evidence-based practices into routine medical care, and, hence, to improve the quality and effectiveness of health service delivery (74). The increased availability of personal devices (e.g., smartphones, body worn sensor technology) and electronic data capture tools over this past decade has positioned this relatively new field to have a significant impact

TABLE 10-2   **Continuous Improvement of the Health System's Response to Population and Individual Functioning Needs: Macro-, Meso-, and Micro Levels**

Health System Level and Explicit Goals	Process of Continuous Improvement of the Health System's Response to Population and Individual Functioning Needs
Macro level: **Rehabilitation policies guiding rehabilitation programming**	
Developing rehabilitation policies addressing a country's population functioning needs	• Monitoring country functioning needs with general population and subpopulation surveys • Evaluating rehabilitation policies against the backdrop of how a population's functioning needs are met • Analysis and potential modification of rehabilitation policies in light of evaluation results
Establishing comprehensive rehabilitation service programs addressing the needs of specific subpopulations along the continuum of care in a defined geographical area	• Monitoring functioning outcomes achieved across rehabilitation service programs • Improvement of rehabilitation programming in light of monitoring results, results reported by other countries, and scientific evidence from quasi-experimental studies comparing rehabilitation programming across geographical areas and over time
Meso level: **Optimizing rehabilitation programs through delivery of optimal individual services**	
Optimizing the operational management of a rehabilitation service program through provision of a set of individual rehabilitation services	• Benchmarking functioning outcomes across individual rehabilitation services (adjusted for case mix) • Identification of modifiable inputs associated with favorable functioning outcomes (e.g., physical infrastructure and organization of the rehabilitation service; work force; use of information, products, and procedure inputs) • Anonymous feedback to individual rehabilitation services
Optimizing rehabilitation service provision	• Monitoring functioning outcomes over time • Revision of rehabilitation services based on benchmark comparisons and new scientific evidence on best rehabilitation service provision (sequential quasi-experiments)
Micro level: **Improved management for individual patients receiving consecutive rehabilitation services**	
Documenting a person's functioning across consecutive rehabilitation services	• Functioning-informed clinical decision-making during consecutive rehabilitation services (i.e., assignment of the patient to consecutive rehabilitation services; assignment of clinical interventions provided by rehabilitation professionals; monitoring of functioning outcomes)
Devising and adjusting an individual rehabilitation plan in partnership with the patient or his/her proxy	• Clinical decision-making in sequential rehabilitation cycles • Assessment of functioning and specification of goals for the long-term (expected functioning level of a person returning to or living in the community); mid-term (expected functioning level at the end of consecutive rehabilitation services); and short-term (expected functioning upon completion of the next rehabilitation cycle) • Assigning rehabilitation professionals to clinical interventions aimed at functioning targets related to the short-term functioning goals • Evaluation of short-, mid-, and long-term functioning goal achievement against a predicted functioning trajectory (calculated with cumulative data of patients with similar health conditions, functioning, and personal characteristics) • Review and plan for the next rehabilitation cycle in light of mid-term and long-term goals as specified in the rehabilitation plan

on the study of health care professional and organizational behavior.

As such, implementation science has the potential to narrow the average 17-year latency between the initial publication of a research finding and its potential application in real-world clinical practice (75). Like rehabilitation itself, implementation science is inherently interdisciplinary. And it is an increasingly important area of emphasis for the rehabilitation sciences. The National Institutes of Health, AHRQ, Department of Veterans Affairs (VA), and Patient-Centered Outcomes Research Institute all sponsor ongoing funding opportunities in this area, focusing on identifying strategies that support the adoption, implementation, and ongoing improvement of evidence-based interventions and the optimal application of new scientific knowledge to benefit biomedical and health care outcomes.

There is a limited but growing body of research into the implementation of evidence-based programs relevant to physical medicine and rehabilitation. Available research for stroke rehabilitation, for example, has grown significantly in recent years. High-quality clinical trials supported by motor learning

and neuroplasticity basic science literature provide strong evidence for intensive repetitive task-oriented training after stroke (76,77). However, there is also evidence that stroke rehabilitation, in its present form, is not achieving the required intensity to maximize recovery (78). The field of implementation science has developed out of the recognition that a more systematic approach is needed to improve real world knowledge translation.

In an effort to bridge the evidence-practice gap that exists in stroke rehabilitation, Connell et al. (79) conducted a formative evaluation of the implementation of a hand and arm exercise program shown to be effective in a previously conducted randomized controlled trial and experienced unusually rapid uptake into clinical practice. The purpose of the evaluation was to inform the development and implementation of other similar interventions. It was found that although the program studied had translated into clinical practice, it was not consistently used in the way in which it was shown to be effective. The formative evaluation subsequently informed the development of novel interventions for upper limb rehabilitation after stroke. In another study, Connell et al. described an intervention to change the behaviors of health care professionals responsible for implementing evidence-based strategies to increase provision of upper limb repetitive task-oriented training in stroke rehabilitation (80). The intervention was collaborative and iterative with four stages of development emerging: (a) establishing an intervention development group; (b) structured discussions to understand the problem, prioritize and analyze target behaviors; (c) collaborative design of theoretically underpinned intervention components; and (d) piloting and refining of intervention components. This study was a clear example of interventions designed to implement behavior change in health professionals toward greater utilization of known science. It provided a general framework and taxonomy for replication, refinement, and clinical use.

Strategies to improve the routine uptake of research findings are strategically important for the advancement of quality care in physical medicine and rehabilitation—and health care in general. Poor translation of research trials into day-to-day patient care represents an invisible ceiling on the potential for research to enhance function, independence, and quality of life. Implementation science is important to the advancement of best care in rehabilitation because it identifies the behavior of health care professionals and health care organizations as key sources of variance requiring empirical and theoretical understanding before effective uptake can be achieved (81).

Stakeholder Engagement

With the growth of learning health systems and implementation science, the generation and dissemination of knowledge is gradually being transformed to include stakeholders (i.e., potential knowledge users such as patients). This transition is occurring in the field of rehabilitation research (82,83). The inclusion of stakeholders in the research process is now often mandated by federal funding agencies (84). But there are also pragmatic reasons for collaborating with the end users of new information or procedures. These include justifying the use of a given framework, recruitment, and the identification of more relevant research questions (82,85,86). The intended result being the creation of knowledge that is more readily transferable, relevant and usable to solving real-world problems, and thereby promoting its use in practice and helping to close the knowledge-to-practice-gap (83,86,87).

Involving stakeholders in the rehabilitation process could accelerate the uptake and implementation of knowledge to improve interventions, evidence-based practice, and policies influencing the research and care for individuals with disabilities (86). A scoping review on this topic found that engagement does facilitate uptake of research findings by increasing stakeholders' awareness of the evidence, the resources available, and their own ability to act upon a situation (86). However, the authors of the review also found that factors influencing opportunities for stakeholder engagement need to be better understood. For example, both barriers and facilitators for engaging stakeholders are primarily associated with financial and time constraints as well as cultural and language issues. More research is needed to identify which engagement strategies work best in specific circumstances. More systematic integration of stakeholder engagement is likely particularly fruitful in the field physical medicine and rehabilitation where there is already a strong history of care collaboration between stakeholder (i.e., patient) and rehabilitation professional. Greater

insight into these already existing bidirectional processes could lead to rapid actual practice changes and improved care.

ACCREDITATION

The Joint Commission (formerly the Joint Commission on Accreditation of Health Care Organizations [JCAHO]) is an independent, not-for-profit organization that accredits and certifies nearly 21,000 health care organizations and programs in the United States (88). The Joint Commission accreditation and certification is recognized nationwide as a symbol of quality that reflects an organization's commitment to meeting certain performance standards. Their stated mission is "to continuously improve health care for the public, in collaboration with other stakeholders, by evaluating health care organizations and inspiring them to excel in providing safe and effective care of the highest quality and value."

CARF assists rehabilitation providers in improving the quality of their services, demonstrating value, and meeting internationally recognized organizational and program standards (26). The accreditation process applies sets of standards to service areas and business practices and includes an on-site survey. Accreditation is an ongoing process, signaling to the public that a provider is committed to continuously improving service delivery, encouraging feedback, and serving the community. Accreditation also demonstrates a provider's commitment to enhance performance, manage risk, and share clinical outcomes. A rigorous accreditation process helps ensure that facilities (and individual providers) are remaining up-to-date with clinical practice guidelines and the findings of implementation research relevant to their areas of practice.

SUMMARY

Quality and value should be viewed in terms of results, not inputs. In turn, they should be measured and evaluated based on outcomes, not volume of services provided (16). Recent health care reform initiatives are changing the way payers, providers, and patients view health care quality and value. It is widely recognized that in the U.S. health care system, payment drives practice. Payment and practice are currently in a state of transition. Since passage of the Patient Protection and Affordable Care Act in 2010 (2), we have been moving away from a fee-for-service reimbursement system. In the traditional fee-for-service payment model, practitioners, hospitals, and other health facilities are reimbursed based on the number of procedures or services they provide (1,5). The major financial incentive for health care professionals and facilities in a fee-for-service payment system is volume. An objective of health care reform is to change the payment approach from fee-for-service to a model where reimbursement is directly related to patient improvement and quality outcomes (1,5). In this new model, reimbursement is based on the value of care as measured by quality outcomes (e.g., discharge to community), not the volume of services received. The new approach is referred to as value-based health care and is being developed and implemented by the CMS (5).

A challenge in moving to a reimbursement system based on value is how to identify, define, and measure value and quality in health outcomes. This is a challenge that physical medicine and rehabilitation has been dealing with for decades. While the current debate in defining value-based health care is complex, and sometimes contradictory, it represents an important opportunity for the field of physical medicine and rehabilitation to demonstrate the importance of functional outcomes and independence as a patient-centered quality measure (89). Persons with disabilities and chronic conditions are frequent consumers of health resources and rehabilitation services. They are knowledgeable consumers and can serve as influential stakeholders in promoting the importance of functional outcomes and how they should be measured, monitored, and integrated into payment models based on value (quality) and away from volume (48).

Work is needed to develop practical performance information systems that monitor routine care processes and outcomes, and integrate findings from quality improvement initiatives and more formal research projects. Such information systems will enable clinical professionals and patients to make better care decisions and to provide clear reports to administrators, payers, and policy makers. Developing and using the results of such systems to assure and improve the quality and efficiency of rehabilitation programs is a primary challenge to the field and its stakeholders, but it is now more feasible than ever before.

Multiple approaches are needed to assure and improve the quality and efficiency of rehabilitative care. Fortunately, the focus of quality improvement monitoring is shifting from simply documenting poor care toward identifying value and quality outcomes and integrating these outcomes into the payment models that will guide future practice. The evolution of patient-centered program evaluation and the advent of learning health systems represent opportunities for physical medicine and rehabilitation to advance value-based health care and quality outcomes using our tradition and expertise in function to promote recovery and independence.

REFERENCES

1. Centers for Medicare & Medicaid Services. *The CMS Innovation Center*; 2017. Updated: 2017. Available from: https://innovation.cms.gov/. Accessed on July 27, 2017.
2. Patient Protection and Affordable Care Act (Public Law 111-148), 111th Congress, 2010.
3. Improving Medicare Post-Acute Care Transformation Act of 2014 (Public Law 113-185), 113th Congress, 2014.
4. Medicare Access and CHIP Reauthorization Act of 2015 (Public Law 114-10), 114th Congress, 2015.
5. Centers for Medicare & Medicaid Services. *Health Care Payment Learning and Action Network*; 2017. Updated: September 5, 2017. Available from: https://innovation.cms.gov/initiatives/Health-Care-Payment-Learning-and-Action-Network/. Accessed on December 7, 2018.
6. Xu Y, Wells PS. Getting (along) with the guidelines: reconciling patient autonomy and quality improvement through shared decision making. *Acad Med*. 2016;91(7):925–929.
7. Chawla NV, Davis DA. Bringing big data to personalized healthcare: a patient-centered framework. *J Gen Intern Med*. 2013;28(suppl 3):S660–S665.
8. Clancy CM. Patient engagement in health care. *Health Serv Res*. 2011;46(2):389–393.
9. Mroz TM, Pitonyak JS, Fogelberg D, et al. Client centeredness and health reform: key issues for occupational therapy. *Am J Occup Ther*. 2015;69(5):1–8.
10. Blumenthal D. Part 1: Quality of care—what is it? *N Engl J Med*. 1996;335(12):891–894.
11. Blumenthal D. Quality of health care. Part 4: The origins of the quality-of-care debate. *N Engl J Med*. 1996;335(15):1146–1149.
12. Blumenthal D, Epstein AM. Quality of health care. Part 6: The role of physicians in the future of quality management. *N Engl J Med*. 1996;335(17):1328–1331.
13. Institute of Medicine. *Medicare: A Strategy for Quality Assurance, Volume 1*. Washington, DC: Institute of Medicine; 1990.
14. Institute of Medicine. *Medicare: A Strategy for Quality Assurance, Volume II: Sources and Methods*. Washington, DC: Institute of Medicine; 1990.
15. Agency for Healthcare Research and Quality. *Guide to Health Care Quality: How to Know it When You See It*. Rockville, MD: Agency for Healthcare Research and Quality; 2005.
16. Porter ME. What is value in health care? *N Engl J Med*. 2010;363(26):2477–2481.
17. Donabedian A. Evaluating the quality of medical care. *Milbank Mem Fund Q*. 1966;44(3 suppl):166–206.
18. Centers for Medicare & Medicaid Services. *Functional Measures*; 2014. Updated: January 13, 2015. Available from: https://www.cms.gov/Medicare/Quality-Initiatives-Patient-Assessment-Instruments/Post-Acute-Care-Quality-Initiatives/Functional-Measures-.html. Accessed on July 26, 2017.
19. Kowalski CJ, Mrdjenovich AJ. Comparative effectiveness research: decision-based evidence. *Perspect Biol Med*. 2014;57(2):224–248.
20. Rasanen P, Roine E, Sintonen H, et al. Use of quality-adjusted life years for the estimation of effectiveness of health care: a systematic literature review. *Int J Technol Assess Health Care*. 2006;22(2):235–241.
21. Berwick DM, Nolan TW, Whittington J. The triple aim: care, health, and cost. *Health Aff*. 2008;27(3):759–769.
22. Centers for Medicare & Medicaid Services. IRF Compare: About the data. Available from: https://www.medicare.gov/inpatientrehabilitationfacilitycompare/#about/theData. Accessed on December 7, 2018.
23. Schnelker DL, Rumrill PD. Program evaluation in rehabilitation. *Work*. 2001;16(2):171–175.
24. Hall J, Freeman M, Roulston K. Right timing in formative program evaluation. *Eval Program Plann*. 2014;45:151–156.
25. Glueckauf RL. Program evaluation guidelines for the rehabilitation professional. *Adv Clin Rehabil*. 1990;3:250–266.
26. CARF International. *CARF International: Resources*; 2017. Updated: 2017. Available from: http://www.carf.org/Resources/. Accessed on July 27, 2017.
27. Lohr KN, Donaldson MS, Harris-Wehling J. Medicare: a strategy for quality assurance, V: Quality of care in a changing health care environment. *QRB Qual Rev Bull*. 1992;18(4):120–126.
28. Fauman MA. Quality assurance monitoring in psychiatry. *Am J Psychiatry*. 1989;146(9):1121–1130.
29. Brennan TA, Leape LL, Laird NM, et al. Incidence of adverse events and negligence in hospitalized patients. Results of the Harvard Medical Practice Study I. *N Engl J Med*. 1991;324(6):370–376.
30. Gray CS. Quality assurance in a rehabilitation facility: a decentralized approach. *QRB Qual Rev Bull*. 1988;14(1):9–14.
31. Grossman RG. Quality improvement: an overview. *J Perinat Neonatal Nurs*. 1998;12(1):42–50.
32. Varkey P, Antonio K. Change management for effective quality improvement: a primer. *Am J Med Qual*. 2010;25(4):268–273.
33. Kirk R. The big picture. Total quality management and continuous quality improvement. *J Nurs Admin*. 1992;22(4):24–31.
34. Berlowitz DR, Frantz RA. Implementing best practices in pressure ulcer care: the role of continuous quality improvement. *J Am Med Dir Assoc*. 2007;8(3 suppl):S37–S41.
35. Horn SD. Overcoming obstacles to effective treatment: use of clinical practice improvement methodology. *J Clin Psychiatry*. 1997;58(suppl 1):15–19.
36. Horn SD. Quality, clinical practice improvement, and the episode of care. *Manag Care J*. 2001;9(3):10–24.
37. Horn SD, DeJong G, Smout RJ, et al. Stroke rehabilitation patients, practice, and outcomes: is earlier and more aggressive therapy better? *Arch Phys Med Rehabil*. 2005;86(12 suppl 2):S101–S114.
38. Donabedian A. Criteria and standards for quality assessment and monitoring. *QRB Qual Rev Bull*. 1986;12(3):99–108.
39. Gupta P, Varkey P. Developing a tool for assessing competency in root cause analysis. *Jt Comm J Qual Patient Saf*. 2009;35(1):36–42.
40. Berman S. The AMA clinical quality improvement forum on addressing patient safety. *Jt Comm J Qual Improv*. 2000;26(7):428–433.
41. Clancy CM, Cronin K. Evidence-based decision making: global evidence, local decisions. *Health Aff*. 2005;24(1):151–162.
42. Huckman RS, Kelley MA. Public reporting, consumerism, and patient empowerment. *N Engl J Med*. 2013;369(20):1875–1877.
43. Agency for Healthcare Research and Quality. *About CAHPS*; 2016. Updated: October 2016. Available from: http://www.ahrq.gov/cahps/about-cahps/index.html. Accessed on July 25, 2017.
44. Agency for Healthcare Research and Quality. *Profiles of Comparative Reports on Health Care Quality and Costs*; 2016. Updated: December 2016. Available from: http://www.ahrq.gov/cahps/consumer-reporting/rcc/index.html. Accessed on July 25, 2017.
45. National Committee for Quality Assurance. *NCQA: Measuring Quality. Improving Health Care*; 2017. Updated: July 17, 2017. Available from: http://www.ncqa.org/. Accessed on July 26, 2017.
46. National Committee for Quality Assurance. *HEDIS & Performance Measurement*; 2017. Updated. Available from: http://www.ncqa.org/hedis-quality-measurement. Accessed on July 26, 2017.
47. McCormick D, Himmelstein DU, Woolhandler S, et al. Relationship between low quality-of-care scores and HMOs' subsequent public disclosure of quality-of-care scores. *JAMA*. 2002;288(12):1484–1490.
48. Iezzoni LI. Risk adjusting rehabilitation outcomes: an overview of methodologic issues. *Am J Phys Med Rehabil*. 2004;83(4):316–326.
49. Deutsch A, Pardasaney P, Iriondo-Perez J, et al. Development of a risk-adjustment model for the inpatient rehabilitation facility discharge self-care functional status quality measure. *Med Care*. 2017;55(7):706–715.

50. Stineman MG, Hamilton BB, Granger CV, et al. Four methods for characterizing disability in the formation of function related groups. *Arch Phys Med Rehabil.* 1994;75(12):1277–1283.

51. Stineman MG, Escarce JJ, Goin JE, et al. A case-mix classification system for medical rehabilitation. *Med Care.* 1994;32(4):366–379.

52. Stineman MG. Case-mix measurement in medical rehabilitation. *Arch Phys Med Rehabil.* 1995;76(12):1163–1170.

53. Stineman MG, Tassoni CJ, Escarce JJ, et al. Development of function-related groups version 2.0: a classification system for medical rehabilitation. *Health Serv Res.* 1997;32(4):529–548.

54. Iezzoni LI. *Risk Adjustment for Measuring Health Care Outcomes.* 4th ed. Chicago, IL: Health Administration Press; 2012.

55. QualityNet. *QualityNet*; 2017. Updated: 2017. Available from: https://www.qualitynet.org/. Accessed on July 26, 2017.

56. National Quality Forum. *Measures, Reports & Tools*; 2017. Updated: 2017. Available from: https://www.qualityforum.org/Measures_Reports_Tools.aspx. Accessed on July 26, 2017.

57. Iezzoni LI, Shwartz M, Ash AS, et al. Using severity-adjusted stroke mortality rates to judge hospitals. *Int J Qual Health Care.* 1995;7(2):81–94.

58. Graham JE, Prvu Bettger J, Fisher SR, et al. Duration to admission and hospital transfers affect facility rankings from the postacute 30-day rehospitalization quality measure. *Health Serv Res.* 2017;52(3):1024–1039.

59. Institute of Medicine Committee on the Learning Health Care System in America. *Best Care at Lower Cost: The Path to Continuously Learning Health Care in America.* Washington, DC: Institute of Medicine of the National Academies; 2012.

60. GHAaQCEa, Collaborators GHAaQ. Healthcare Access and Quality Index based on mortality from causes amenable to personal health care in 195 countries and territories, 1990–2015: a novel analysis from the Global Burden of Disease Study 2015. *Lancet.* 2017;390(10091):231–266.

61. Enthoven AC. Integrated delivery systems: the cure for fragmentation. *Am J Manag Care.* 2009;15(10 suppl):S284–S290.

62. Feldstein DA, Hess R, McGinn T, et al. Design and implementation of electronic health record integrated clinical prediction rules (iCPR): a randomized trial in diverse primary care settings. *Implement Sci.* 2017;12(1):37.

63. Winter A, Haux R, Ammenwerth E, et al. *Health Information Systems, Architectures and Strategies.* Health Informatics; 2011.

64. Jha A, Pronovost P. Toward a safer health care system: the critical need to improve measurement. *JAMA.* 2016;315(17):1831–1832.

65. Agency for Healthcare Quality & Research. *Learning Health Systems.* Updated: November 2017. Available from: https://www.ahrq.gov/professionals/systems/learning-health-systems/index.html. Accessed on December 8, 2018.

66. Morain SR, Kass NE. Ethics issues arising in the transition to learning health care systems: results from interviews with leaders from 25 health systems. *EGEMS.* 2016;4(2):1212.

67. Pronovost PJ, Mathews SC, Chute CG, et al. Creating a purpose-driven learning and improving health system: The John Hopkins Medicine quality and safety experience. *Learn Health Syst.* 2017;1:e10018.

68. Stucki G, Bickenbach J. Functioning information in the learning health system. *Eur J Phys Rehabil Med.* 2017;53(1):139–143.

69. World Health Organization. *Monitoring and Evaluation of Health Systems Strengthening: An Operational Framework.* Geneva, Switzerland: World Health Organization; 2009.

70. Stucki G, Bickenbach J, Melvin J. Strengthening rehabilitation in health systems worldwide by integrating information on functioning in national health information systems. *Am J Phys Med Rehabil.* 2017;96(9):677–681.

71. WHO. *ICF: International Classification of Functioning, Disability and Health.* Geneva, Switzerland: WHO; 2001.

72. Gutenbrunner C, Fialka-Moser V, Li LS, et al. World Congresses of the International Society of Physical and Rehabilitation Medicine 2013–2015: the way forward—from Beijing to Berlin. *J Rehabil Med.* 2014;46(8):721–729.

73. Prodinger B, Reinhardt JD, Selb M, et al. Towards system-wide implementation of the International Classification of Functioning, Disability and Health (ICF) in routine practice: developing simple, intuitive descriptions of ICF categories in the ICF Generic and Rehabilitation Set. *J Rehabil Med.* 2016;48(6):508–514.

74. Eccles MP, Mittman BS. Welcome to Implementation Science. *Implement Sci.* 2006;1(1):1–3.

75. Morris ZS, Wooding S, Grant J. The answer is 17 years, what is the question: understanding time lags in translational research. *J R Soc Med.* 2011;104(12):510–520.

76. Nudo RJ. Recovery after brain injury: mechanisms and principles. *Front Hum Neurosci.* 2013;7:887.

77. Veerbeek JM, van Wegen E, van Peppen R, et al. What is the evidence for physical therapy poststroke? A systematic review and meta-analysis. *PLoS One.* 2014;9(2):e87987.

78. Lohse KR, Lang CE, Boyd LA. Is more better? Using metadata to explore dose–response relationships in stroke rehabilitation. *Stroke.* 2014;45(7):2053–2058.

79. Connell L, McMahon NE, Harris JE, et al. A formative evaluation of the implementation of an upper limb stroke rehabilitation intervention in clinical practice: a qualitative interview study. *Implement Sci.* 2014;12(9).

80. Connell LA, McMahon NE, Redfern J, et al. Development of a behaviour change intervention to increase upper limb exercise in stroke rehabilitation. *Implement Sci.* 2015;10:34.

81. Board E. *Implementation Science.* Updated. Available from: https://implementation-science.biomedcentral.com/about. Accessed on June 20.

82. Bowen SJ, Graham ID. From knowledge translation to engaged scholarship: promoting research relevance and utilization. *Arch Phys Med Rehabil.* 2013;94 (1 suppl):S3–S8.

83. Menon A, Korner-Bitensky N, Kastner M, et al. Strategies for rehabilitation professionals to move evidence-based knowledge into practice: a systematic review. *J Rehabil Med.* 2009;41(13):1024–1032.

84. (PCORI) P-CORI. Updated. Available from: https://www.pcori.org/. Accessed on June 20.

85. Morris C, Shilling V, McHugh C, et al. Why it is crucial to involve families in all stages of childhood disability research. *Dev Med Child Neurol.* 2011;53(8):769–771.

86. Camden C, Shikako-Thomas K, Nguyen T, et al. Engaging stakeholders in rehabilitation research: a scoping review of strategies used in partnerships and evaluation of impacts. *Disabil Rehabil.* 2015;37(15):1390–1400.

87. Straus SE, Tetroe J, Graham I. Defining knowledge translation. *CMAJ.* 2009;181(3–4):165–168.

88. The Joint Commission. *The Joint Commission*; 2017. Updated: 2017. Available from: https://www.jointcommission.org/. Accessed on July 30, 2017.

89. Institute of Medicine. *Crossing the Quality Chasm: A New Health System for the 21st Century.* Washington, DC: Institute of Medicine; 2001.

CHAPTER 11

Stephen P. Gulley   Abrahm J. Behnam
Elizabeth K. Rasch   Leighton Chan

Epidemiology of Disability in the United States and Internationally: Implications for Policy and Practice

Epidemiology, not unlike rehabilitation, sits at a point of intersection between the individual and the community. As derived from the Greek words epi, meaning on or upon; demos, meaning people; and logos, meaning the study of, epidemiology is the scientific study of the frequency, patterns, and determinants of health-related states and events at the population level (1). As a cornerstone of public health, epidemiologic methods and studies first arose to combat communicable diseases and epidemics such as the spread of cholera through contaminated drinking water in the 1800s (2). Many of the basic statistical and mapping techniques developed during these early efforts at public health remain a part of epidemiology today, but both the methods and the scope of inquiry in this field have expanded considerably. Modern epidemiology is a multidisciplinary field that draws upon the knowledge and techniques not only of biology and medicine but of biostatistics and informatics, and the social and behavioral sciences as well (1,2). Today, epidemiologists are certainly still studying the spread, determinants, and containment of life-threatening infectious diseases such as Ebola, H1N1, or the Zika virus (3). However, they are also studying such diverse topics as hip fracture among the elderly (4), seatbelt use (5), mental illness and gun violence (6), the recent rise in autism rates (7), and, more broadly, the social determinants of health (8). Each of these and many other topics taken up by epidemiologists touches on disability in a wide variety of ways.

In this chapter, we consider the overlap of epidemiology and disability research with a specific focus on rehabilitation and with examples drawn from both the United States and international sources. We begin with a recent history of disability theory and measurement before briefly reviewing a current gold standard in this field, the International Classification of Functioning, Disability and Health (ICF). We continue by considering the purposes of measurement and how these drive both the definitions and methods used to identify and assess disability. Next, we provide a macrolevel view of the current prevalence and distribution of disability in the population as organized within four domains drawn from the ICF: body function and structure, activities and participation, personal factors, and the environment. With the goal of demonstrating the relevance and application of epidemiologic knowledge,

we conclude the chapter with an examination of people with disabilities in the health care system. This includes discussions of the clinical and health policy implications of this chapter for the allied fields of rehabilitation whether in the United States or internationally.

CONCEPTUALIZING AND MEASURING DISABILITY AT THE POPULATION LEVEL

Prior to the 1960s, to the extent that disability was studied at the population level, it was generally understood as synonymous with, or a direct result of, medical pathology. The prevention or containment of specific conditions associated with morbidity (a term that conflated a diseased state, disability, and/or poor health) or mortality represented the focal points of most public health research studies (9). By that time, prevalence estimates of a wide and ever-expanding list of health conditions were being compiled in the international scientific literature. Moving beyond infectious diseases such as polio, the growing public health apparatus began to systematically surveil genetic conditions such as Down's syndrome and spina bifida, as well as chronic medical conditions that might be disabling, such as diabetes or heart disease (1,10). From a more modern perspective, many of the individuals identified in these early studies could have benefitted from improved social treatment, community-based services, and civil rights protections. But at the time, the primary focus was on prevention and containment of disease (9).

The 1960s marked the beginnings of a paradigm shift in the social and scientific understanding of disability. As the nascent movements to secure community-based services, educational reforms, and civil rights protections for people with physical disabilities, intellectual disabilities, and mental illnesses gained momentum in the United States and internationally (11,12), increasingly expansive theoretical models of disability were also developed. Beginning with the work of Saad Nagi (13–15), the biologic, functional, and societal determinants bound up in the expression of disability were named, debated, and explicated. Crucially, Nagi noted that sociocultural and physical environments themselves could be disabling because of stigma or other socially imposed barriers (13–15).

Subsequently, the World Health Organization developed the International Classification of Impairments, Disabilities, and Handicaps (ICIDH), which was released to the public in 1980 (16). Despite several differences in terms, the ICIDH nevertheless categorized the biologic, functional, and societal elements involved in disability measurement in a manner that paralleled the earlier work of Nagi and his contemporaries. As a classification system intended not only to guide scientific measurement, but clinical and policy development, the ICIDH included a coding system for particular impairments, disabilities, and "handicapping situations" (16).

The 1990s would see continued theoretical expansion of the domains involved in disability measurement. Verbrugge and Jette would synthesize elements of both the ICIDH and Nagi's work to develop a sociomedical model of disability (17). This model framed the main disability "pathway" as four steps, leading from pathology, to impairment, to functional limitations, to disability while specifying the risk factors, intraindividual factors, and extraindividual factors that mediate or moderate the extent and impact of each step in the pathway upon the person. In this way, two individuals with identical pathologies might nevertheless have very different experiences with impairment, functional limitations, and disability based upon such things as their ages, health status and conditions, lifestyles, psychosocial adaptation and coping, access to and use of rehabilitation services and other medical care, the availability of assistive devices, external supports, and the accessibility of the built, physical, and social environments in which they live—to name but a few. Works by the Institute of Medicine (IOM) in 1991 and 1997 (18) and the National Center for Medical Rehabilitation Research (NCMRR) in 1993 (19), along with a new release of the ICIDH (2) from the WHO in 1996 (20), gave additional consideration to the possible range and order of these factors. The IOM concluded that disability is best described as "a function of the interaction of the person with the environment" (18, p. 64).

This scholarship constituted a paradigm shift in the epidemiology of disability. Perhaps the most crucial contributions to the field from the 1960s through the 1990s were a conceptual realignment of the medical, social, and environmental aspects of disability; a biopsychosocial approach to the definition and measurement of these concepts; and a life-course perspective that validated disability as an expected, if perhaps sometimes difficult, part of the human experience.

Modern Disability Theory and the ICF

In the 2000s, as a matter of theory, the paradigm shift from the medical to the social model continued to push disability beyond matters of prevention, diagnosis, or containment of diseases and toward the identification, support, and protection of marginalized groups who, as *people with disabilities*, encounter barriers to participation in society. Following 9 years of revision efforts, the World Health Organization Collaborating Center for the Family of International Classifications presented a successor to the ICIDH-2, the ICF (21). Approved by the World Health Assembly in 2001, the ICF is a multipurpose classification system designed to serve various disciplines

and sectors across different countries and cultures. The aims of the ICF are to:

- Provide a scientific basis for understanding and studying health and health-related states, outcomes, determinants, and changes in health status and functioning
- Establish a common language for describing health and health-related states in order to improve communication between different users, such as health care workers, researchers, policy-makers, and the public, including people with disabilities
- Permit comparison of data across countries, health care disciplines, services, and time
- Provide a systematic coding scheme for health information systems (21)

The ICF complements the WHO International Classification of Diseases (ICD). Where the latter provides a diagnostic taxonomy and coding system for the identification of specific health conditions, the ICF is neutral in regard to etiology and focuses instead upon *functioning and disability*, which are umbrella terms that describe the interaction of the person and the environment from a biopsychosocial standpoint (21–23). Importantly, the ICF is not intended to define people as either disabled or not disabled. Instead, the ICF is applicable to all people and recognizes that disability exists over a series of continua bound or facilitated by contextual factors. The ICF includes chapters and codes that specify:

- *Body structures* (e.g., the structures involved in body functions, such as the brain and nervous system, the eye and ear, etc.) and *functions* (e.g., mental, sensory, vocal, movement, neuromuscular, metabolic, cardiovascular, etc.)
- *Activities and participation* (e.g., learning and applying knowledge, general tasks, communication, mobility, self-care, relationships, domestic life, major life areas such as employment, community life, etc.) (21)

In turn, contextual factors are listed in two domains, including *personal factors* (such as gender, age, or other demographics) and *environmental factors* (including the natural environment and human-made changes to it, products and technologies, support and relationships, social attitudes, services, systems, and policies). These domains influence each other in the production of function or disability, as further described in Chapter 9.

PURPOSE DRIVES MEASUREMENT

If, as the ICF posits, disability and function are multidimensional and dynamic concepts, it follows that there can be no *one* correct measure of disability at either the person or the population level. As medical sociologist and disability scholar Irving Zola explained:

> Having a disability is not a fixed status, but rather, a continually changing, evolving and interactive process. It is not something that one is or is not, but instead is a set of characteristics everyone shares to varying degrees and in varying forms and combinations. This does not mean that disability is unmeasurable. Instead, its conception, measurement and counting differ validly with the purposes for which such numbers are needed. The clearer the outcomes we seek, the clearer it will be what conceptions and measurements are necessary (24).

The purposes of disability measurement are many, but, at the least, include population prevalence, distributions and demographics, clinical assessment, needs assessment, resource allocation, and equalization of opportunities (25). In each of these different areas, disability researchers will necessarily begin with questions posed in different ways or at different levels and will make numerous choices about how best to analyze their data and report their findings (26). It should be unsurprising, then, that there is a wide variance not only in gross disability prevalence rates in the United States and internationally, but in the subject matter under consideration in this field (27). Next, we briefly consider the aforementioned purposes of disability measurement.

Population Prevalence, Distributions, and Demographics

The surveillance of particular health conditions, at least those with clear diagnostic criteria such as stroke, brain injury, spinal cord injury, amputation, or burns, is, relatively speaking, a straightforward matter. *Prevalence* (the number of cases in a given population at a point in time) and *incidence* (the number of new cases diagnosed over a time period, such as per year) can be expressed in proportions, percentages, or rates and can be drawn from many possible sources, including disease registries, medical records, administrative data, and surveys (1,28). The international epidemiologic literature is replete with incidence and prevalence estimates of all manner of health and mental health conditions, along with risk factors for their development (often expressed as *odds ratios*, *relative risks*, or *hazard ratios*) and demographic correlates (28).

However, at the population level, measuring the prevalence and correlates of disability is not straightforward and cannot be reduced to the presence of singular health conditions. Important here are the definitional choices researchers make in regard to the inclusion of diagnostic or other sample selection criteria in their study; the specific functional, activity and/or participation measures they employ; how they attend to *comorbidity* or *secondary conditions*; and the scale cut points and subgroups they create to represent their study populations (26,28).

Each of these choices flows from the purpose of the study and particularly whether disability is situated as an *independent* or *dependent* variable. Traditionally, disability has been a dependent variable, akin to morbidity or mortality, something to be reduced or contained. But increasingly, disability is understood as a series of independent variables, a set of markers that describe a population group (or groups) in its own right. Researchers must therefore decide which combinations of measures will best operationalize disability for the study at hand. Commonly used measures of disability at the population level (25,26,28) are those that assess

- Diagnostic information (particular conditions, ICD-9 or 10-CM codes, chronic conditions, comorbidity)
- Mental health status (including short screeners for psychological difficulties or distress)
- Functional limitations (limitations in seeing, hearing, walking, bending, etc.)
- Cognitive limitations (difficulties with memory or decision-making, need of supervision for safety, etc.)

- Limitations in major activities (work, school, community activities, etc.)
- Assistive device use (wheelchairs, canes, communication devices, etc.)
- Activities of daily living (ADLs, need for help or supervision with bathing, dressing, toileting, transferring, continence, and eating)
- Instrumental activities of daily living (IADLs, need for help or supervision with shopping, cooking, housekeeping, laundry, transportation, taking medications, using a telephone)
- Bed days (number of days in which at least half the day was spent in bed)
- Program participation (such as receipt of income supports or public insurance)
- Self-identification (as a person with a disability or as having a particular form of disability)

Much of what we now know about the education, work, community participation, health care, and health disparities of people with disabilities comes from large-scale national surveys that include some combination of these indicators. Both in the United States and internationally, the measures relevant to people with disabilities have varied considerably in these surveys, as has the way analysts have used these measures and as have the resulting estimates (25,26,28).

Clinical Assessment

Diagnosis, treatment, and monitoring of an individual are typically the provinces of clinicians, but epidemiology certainly has had a role to play in these matters, particularly in the development of clinical instruments, where individual level information is compared, and sometimes scored, against specific population-level norms. Among many such instruments, a prime example would be the Functional Independence Measure (FIM) that rates individuals across a series of measures such as self-care, transfers, locomotion, communication, and social cognition (13 motor tasks and 5 cognitive tasks for a total of 18 items). For an overview of the FIM and other clinical/functional measures, see Reference (29). The purpose of the FIM is to evaluate the amount of assistance required by a person with a disability to perform basic life activities. In each area, the amount of assistance required is assessed on a seven-point scale, ranging from complete independence to the need for total assistance with the activity. The FIM thus contains a practical mix of ICF functions and activities, and its measures do include at least some reference to environmental elements, such as social interaction. While the FIM is primarily used to assist clinicians to track individual progress in rehabilitation, it has also been used to describe the characteristics of patient panels and to assess case mix for reimbursement (30,31).

Needs Assessment, Resource Allocation, and Equalization of Opportunities

The field of epidemiology has been increasingly called upon, by government bodies, NGOs, and international authorities, to assist with the development of measures and strategies to better document and improve the lived experience of disability. A transformative moment came in this regard when the United Nations Convention on the Rights of Persons with Disabilities went into force in 2008. With 160 signatories, the purpose of the Convention is "to promote, protect and ensure the full and equal enjoyment of all human rights and fundamental freedoms by all persons with disabilities, and to promote respect for their inherent dignity" (32). Under the convention, people with disabilities are defined as those who have long-term physical, mental, intellectual, or sensory impairments, which, in interaction with various barriers, may hinder their full and effective participation in society on an equal basis with others (32). Among the guiding principles in the Convention are full and effective participation and inclusion in society, acceptance of persons with disabilities as part of human diversity, equalization of opportunity, and access to the physical environment, transportation, technology, and public facilities or services.

Serving as a kind of capstone to the paradigm shift described earlier, the Convention pushes nations to monitor the well-being and participation of citizens with disabilities, to study their needs, and to allocate resources accordingly (32). An example of the kind of measurement development the Convention necessitates can be found in the work of the Washington Group on Disability Statistics under the auspices of the United Nations Statistics Division (33). Their first product was a short set of disability questions (six items) that are being increasingly adopted in national surveys across the world in order to produce more consistent prevalence estimates.

It is important to note that the stated purpose of the Washington Group work is to provide data that will assist societies in their efforts to equalize opportunities for people living with disabilities (25,33). This stands in some contrast to other measurement approaches, particularly those concerned with the efficient allocation of medical resources on the basis of disease burden. For example, disability-adjusted life years, or DALYs, were developed as a way to quantify the impact of health conditions in the population by calculating not only years of life lost due to early death but to the number of years lived with disability (34–36). The measure reflects the burden of various health-related states as informed by medical experts and as quantified against the general public's beliefs and preferences regarding health and functioning (34–36). DALYs have been widely adopted as a tool in health services research at both national and international levels, such as through the Global Burden of Disease Studies supported by the World Bank and the World Health Organization (34). However, the notion that societies would place less value on the experience of living with a disability versus that of "ideal health" has also raised ethical, moral, and measurement concerns (35,36). While the advent of DALYs has produced an impressive volume of internationally comparative data on the burden of disease, it is critical that this approach not be conflated or confused with disability research, which, like the Washington Group's work, is designed to identify persons at risk of participation restrictions. It is the *purpose* of measurement that matters most of all.

ESTIMATES OF DISABILITY IN THE UNITED STATES AND INTERNATIONALLY

In this section, we provide a wide-angle lens on contemporary estimates of the prevalence, incidence, correlates, and outcomes potentially associated with disability. We begin with more traditional, disease-focused epidemiologic studies on the prevalence and incidence of conditions frequently seen in US rehabilitation settings. We then contrast these findings with those obtained from studies that operationally define disability on the basis of body functions, structures, and/or simple activities in which people engage. Next, we consider hybrid estimates that often include more involved activities and participation, such as school, work, or community life. Finally, we examine the personal and environmental factors that mediate or moderate function/disability, with an eye to participation restrictions that may hinder the health or community integration of people with disabilities.

Prevalence and Incidence of Common Conditions in US Rehabilitation Settings

In many ways, the knowledge and practice of rehabilitation is organized by diagnostic category. As such, knowing more about the population distributions of the key conditions treated in rehabilitation settings is important. We provide an overview of epidemiologic studies on eight such conditions in **Table 11-1**. The findings in this table are taken from a scoping literature review of the US medical and epidemiologic literature (64). Generally, studies such as these can be helpful in assessing the sheer numbers of people affected by particular conditions and, in some ways, the reach and scope of particular rehabilitation interventions or programs (65). It is useful, for example, to note that osteoarthritis and back pain each affect over 1 in 5 adults in the population and that substantial numbers of such individuals will also report health problems or activity limitations (40,66). Rehabilitation hospitals and particularly outpatient settings thus need to be well-prepared to treat the many individuals with these conditions. On the other hand, sheer numbers and the demand they create are not the only relevant metric for the rehabilitation fields.

Consider multiple sclerosis, a condition where prevalence is measured as a fraction of a percentage point in the adult population and where the impact on function and activities can change drastically, if sometimes very slowly, over time (67). Individuals with MS can often manage their conditions for many years before the need for rehabilitation may arise—and then possibly come and go—over many more years. Some will ultimately require the full armamentarium of our allied fields, including physiatry, PT, OT, speech, respiratory, as well as a host of community-based services. Others will require only a subset of these supports now and then (68). As a small, geographically diverse, dynamic numeric minority, there are many reasons to be concerned with the availability, quantity, quality, and timing of rehabilitation services available in the communities where individuals who have MS live, whether in the United States or internationally (69). In this way, *both high and low* prevalence conditions can be of concern.

Students of the ICF, while acknowledging the importance of disease prevalence and incidence, may be hesitant to draw causal connections between diagnosis at the individual level and functional, activity, or participation outcomes at the population level. This is for a variety of reasons, including the wide range of potential functional impacts associated with a given diagnosis (70), comorbidities that may alter an individual's functional profile or activities (24,71), the differing trajectories over time that may arise as the affected individual interacts with the environment (28), as well as the wide variety of measures used to assess disability (26).

TABLE 11-1	Eight Frequently Seen Conditions in US Rehabilitation: Prevalence, Incidence, and Associated Limitations		
Condition	**Prevalence**	**Incidence**	**Activity, Participation, or Other Limitations**
Back pain	59.1 million adults (age >18 years) have had back pain within the last 3 months (37). Of all those in the United States aged >18 years living in the community, 28.9% have had low back pain and 15.5% have had neck pain within the last 3 months (38)	139/100,000 person-years (39)	24.7% of people with back pain self-report functional limitations (40). 7.1 million adults aged >18 years have activity limitation due to chronic back conditions (37)
Osteoarthritis	49.9 million adults aged >17 years in 2009 (41) 26.9 million adults aged >25 years in 2005 (37) 21.6% of adults (42)	Hip, 88/100,000 person-years; knee, 240/100,000 person-years; hand, 100/100,000 person-years (43)	42% of people with osteoarthritis report arthritis-attributable activity limitations (41)
Rheumatoid arthritis	1.3 million adults aged >18 years in 2005 (44). 2% of adults in North America (45). 0.5%–1.0% of the general population (46)	41/100,000 person-years (47)	30% more likely to need help with personal care, people with RA are twice as likely to have a health-related activity limitation (48)
Stroke	6.8 million adults aged >20 years; 2.8% of adult population (49)	795,000/year, 610,000/year for first stroke (49)	Among stroke survivors aged >65 years, 26% were dependent on activities of daily living, 50% had hemiparesis, 30% were unable to walk without assistance, 19% had aphasia, 26% were in a nursing home 6 months poststroke (50)
Traumatic brain injury	3.32 million with long-term disability, 1.1% of total population in 2005 (51)	538.2 cases per 100,000 persons, 1,565,000 in 2003 (52)	43% of persons discharged after acute TBI hospitalizations develop long-term disability (52)
Amputation	1.6 million in 2005 (53)	30,000–50,000 lower limb amputations per year (53) 330/100,000 in people with diabetes (54)	31% of patients unable to live independently at 24 months; 49% loss of ambulation (55). 43%–74% 5-year mortality after lower extremity amputation (56)
Multiple sclerosis	400,000 (57); 350,000 (58); 58–95 per 100,000 individuals (59)	10,400 cases per year, 3.6/100,000 person-years in women, 2.0/100,000 person-years in men (57)	Average time from disease onset to difficulty walking is 8 years; 15 years for cane use; 30 years for wheelchair use (60)
Spinal cord injury	236,000–327,000 in 2012 (61)	43–77 per million, 12,000–20,000 per year (62)	Functional recovery after SCI depends on severity and spinal level of injury (63)

Reprinted from Ma VY, Chan L, Carruthers K. Incidence, prevalence, costs, and impact on disability of common conditions requiring rehabilitation in the United States. *Arch Phys Med Rehabil.* 2014;95(5):986–995, with permission from Elsevier. Ref. (64)

Function and Activities

As opposed to research that essentially relies upon medical conditions as the unit of analysis, much of disability epidemiology is increasingly focused upon how bodies function and give rise to the activities in which people engage (28). This shift in focus can still allow for estimation of prevalence, incidence, or risk factors. For example, in 2013, the U.S. Centers for Disease Control and Prevention adopted a standardized definition of paralysis developed by an expert panel and funded the Paralysis Prevalence and Health Disparities Survey (PPHDS) (72). Its primary goal was *not* to estimate the prevalence of spinal cord injury, multiple sclerosis, TBI, stroke, or other conditions that may be associated with paralysis; instead, this research shifted to a functional, cross-diagnosis description of *paralysis* itself in order to track prevalence, causes, and health effects among the US population. The results from this survey revealed that paralysis itself is far more common than previously recognized, affecting an estimated 5.4 million people in the United States, two thirds of whom are between the ages of 18 and 64 years (73). The findings go well beyond the leading medical causes to include health disparities, secondary conditions, access to care, and

measures of well-being among people living with this shared functional limitation.

Population-level research on individuals living with mental illness has also recently profited from more functionally oriented measurement. Epidemiologists have begun to screen for a common set of emotional-functional signs and symptoms that are indicative of serious psychological distress (SPD), regardless of specific diagnosis or etiology (74,75). In the United States, a recent study found that 3.2% of all working-age adults are in SPD at a point in time (76). As is also the case with paralysis, with this shift to a more functional view, we now know quite a bit more about the health, health care, and health disparities among people with SPD both in the United States and internationally.

Turning to more general, cross-diagnosis estimates of disability, most national surveys that identify people with disabilities include some combination of measures from both the functioning and activity domains of the ICF or from somewhere in between (25,26). In the United States, a key measure of disability now found in multiple surveys is that first fielded in the American Community Survey in 2008, referred to as the ACS-6 (77). Under the Affordable Care Act, the ACS-6 became a new national standard, with the intent of providing comparable disability data in federal surveys. Purposefully brief, it includes six questions:

- **Hearing** (asked of all ages): Is this person deaf or does he/she have serious difficulty hearing? Y/N
- **Vision** (asked of all ages): Is this person blind or does he/she have serious difficulty seeing even when wearing glasses? Y/N
- **Cognitive** (asked of persons ages 5 or older): Because of a physical, mental, or emotional condition, does this person have serious difficulty concentrating, remembering, or making decisions? Y/N
- **Ambulation** (asked of persons ages 5 or older): Does this person have serious difficulty walking or climbing stairs? Y/N
- **Self-care** (asked of persons ages 5 or older): Does this person have difficulty dressing or bathing? Y/N
- **Independent living** (asked of persons ages 15 or older): Because of a physical, mental, or emotional condition, does this person have difficulty doing errands alone such as visiting a doctor's office or shopping? Y/N

Some of these measures are more reflective of functions, such as seeing, while others capture relatively simple activities that people often do for themselves, such as bathing, dressing (both ADLs), or running errands (an IADL). In this way, while the ACS-6 identifies individuals nondiagnostically, it remains tightly focused on the individual, not the broader environment.

In the 2015 American Community Survey, of a total population of 316 million civilian, noninstitutionalized persons, 39.9 million individuals, or 12.6%, were estimated to have at least one of these difficulties, though individuals often reported more than one. More specifically, these national estimates indicate that 3.5% have a hearing difficulty, 2.3% have a vision difficulty, 6.2% have a cognitive difficulty, 6.6% have an ambulatory difficulty, 2.5% have a self-care difficulty, and 4.6% have an independent living difficulty (78). All in all, it is probably safe to say that the ACS estimates are conservative. For instance, using much broader criteria that straddle multiple domains of the ICF, the overall prevalence of disability was estimated to be 54.4 million, or 18.7% of the noninstitutionalized population in an official U.S. Census report using data from the 2010 Survey of Income and Program Participation (79).

International Estimates Based on Functioning and Activities

If there are substantial variations in the definition and measurement of disability in research conducted in the United States, these are only compounded when we widen our scope to the international stage. As a part of its ongoing efforts to promulgate the UN Washington Group's short set of internationally comparable disability questions, that group queried national statistic offices across the world about their current censuses and national data collection efforts on disability (25). Sixty-five countries responded and included all manner of instruments covering impairments, functioning, activities, participation, and various personal and environmental factors. Response categories in the instruments also varied widely, from dichotomous to many kinds of scales, as did skip patterns in

the questions and as did the cut points and algorithms used to determine disability. It is also crucial to remember that these data come from countries that differ not only in language and environment, but in culture and belief systems about disability. So while we can observe that the national disability prevalence estimates reported in this query ranged from under 1% to over 12%, the question remains: prevalence of what?

Until such time as the Washington Group's disability questions are better adopted internationally, there are few current sources of internationally comparable disability prevalence data. While the Global Burden of Disease Study (34) certainly provides a rich source of data using similar questions across countries, that line of research is concerned with disease burden, not functional disability *per se*. Probably the best such data that are currently available come from the World Health Survey (WHS), conducted by the WHO in 2002–2004. Though now dated, in a retrospective analysis of these data, Mitra and Sambamoorthi aligned the existing measures in the WHS with the Washington Group short set (80). The result is likely the closest emulation we currently have of what future censuses will reveal when using the WG set. In the study by Mitra and Sambamoorthi, disability was defined as at least one severe or extreme difficulty in seeing, concentrating or remembering, moving around, or self-care. Across 54 participating countries, they calculated an overall disability prevalence of 14%, ranging from a low of 2.3% (Ireland) to a high of 30% (South Africa). These data are presented in 📶 **eTable 11-1**, alongside the distributions of the number and severity of the reported limitations.

Hybrid Estimates of Disability

A strong argument can be made for the promulgation of consistent measures and estimates of disability from one study, and one country, to the next. Particularly when the estimates are based upon simple functions and activities (e.g., seeing, moving about, dressing, bathing, etc.) that are of near-universal importance and that are closely related to individual capacity, the resulting population groups become increasingly interpretable and comparable across countries, cultures, and languages. However, a strong argument can *also* be made that broader, context-sensitive definitions and measures are a necessary part of the epidemiology of disability. As such, other domains, including program participation, assistive device use, or even complex measures of social participation, are sometimes used as *definitional* elements of disability. In this section, we examine some of the advantages and disadvantages of these hybrid estimates, with a focus on children and youth with disabilities.

We certainly do not expect toddlers or preschoolers to function in the same ways or care for themselves as adults do. Yet we also know that babies born with Down's syndrome, spina bifida, and a host of other medical conditions will have *some* degree of functional limitation, and likely *some* degree of activity limitation, as they continue to grow and develop. In this way, disability measurement for the very young heavily depends upon diagnostic categorization (when possible), age-specific developmental milestones, and parental observation and report (81). However, we also expect that as children mature and reach the teenage years, their functional abilities and the activities in which they engage will expand considerably. This means that the criteria used to gauge childhood disability vary dramatically by age, as do prevalence rates (81).

For example, data from the U.S. Survey of Income and Program Participation (SIPP), mentioned earlier, show that 2.3% of children under age 3 have a disability, while 3.6% of children aged 3 to 5 years have a disability, but that children aged 6 to 14 years have a disability prevalence of 12.2% (79). This sudden quadrupling in prevalence for those aged 6 to 14 is the result not of some rapid increase in illness or injury but of the expanded criteria used to operationalize disability from the available measures in SIPP for that age group. For children aged 5 or younger, the criteria used were necessarily circumscribed, including moving arms or legs (under 3 only); walking, running, or playing (age 3+); and having a developmental delay (under 6 years). By contrast, for children aged 6 to 14, the criteria included a very wide array of items, from speech, hearing, and communication to schoolwork difficulties, behavior problems, and many more such complex functions or activities. Disability prevalence expanded accordingly.

Beyond broad census data, the choice of disability measures is also heavily influenced by the programmatic, policy or other contexts in which household surveys are designed and fielded. A good example is the 2012 National Longitudinal Transition Study (NLTS) (82). Including both parental and youth surveys, this study is nationally representative of public school students aged 13 to 21 and allows for the direct comparison of students who receive, or do not receive, special education services through an Individualized Education Plan (IEP) as required under the Individuals with Disabilities Education Act (IDEA). In this way, the entire study (including the sampling frame) is built around a legal definition of childhood disability enshrined in IDEA, which includes 13 categories of childhood impairment under which children with disabilities are eligible to receive services. We review the prevalence of these impairments, as well as findings on function and activities, among these youth in **Figure 11-1**.

As shown, there is no bright line that distinguishes children with and without IEPs on the basis of their functional or activity limitations—many children without IEPs have such limitations, too. Further, the ways that children function and the activities they do for themselves are not only a function of their possible impairments, but of their developmental trajectories and the expectations and resources of their parents or communities.

International Measures on Childhood Disability

Internationally comparable prevalence data on young persons are sparse, in large part because of methodologic differences between studies. While there are many data sources that do include information on children with specific medical conditions and functional or activity limitations, most of the published figures are culled from larger data sets where the primary focus was adults (81). Cappa et al. identified 716 large-scale population-based quantitative surveys and studies that collected nationally representative prevalence data on disability across 198 countries (185 UN Member States in addition to 13 countries that were not official UN Member States) (81). These data sources included censuses (the most common data source) and household surveys such as the Multiple Indicator Cluster Surveys (MCIS) supported by UNICEF, Demographic and Health Surveys funded by USAID, WHS conducted by WHO, targeted disability surveys, and questionnaires developed by the Washington Group. These sources were screened for the inclusion of childhood disability data and the instruments used to collect it were examined.

Across countries, the authors found that the questions ranged from a simple generic question on whether anyone in the household was "disabled" to complex hybrid questions including both diagnostic and biopsychosocial elements across functioning, activities, and participation. As a result, Cappa et al. reported disability prevalence rates for children, which ranged from as low as 1% to as high as 50%. Nor did the obtained prevalence rates necessarily track with the living conditions, health, or developmental resources available to children in these countries; some of the lowest prevalence rates were actually found in some of the poorest (or even war-torn) nations, raising questions over the validity and reliability of the instruments.

Personal and Environmental Factors and Their Impact on People with Disabilities

It is crucial for rehabilitation professionals to know that health, function, and disability are not equally distributed in the population. In this section, we briefly highlight epidemiologic and other studies that demonstrate the role of personal and environmental factors as they produce or reduce disability, beginning with sociodemographics. Turning to U.S. Census findings from the 2010 SIPP (79), it is important to remember that these estimates are based on a relatively broad definition that cuts across many domains of the ICF. However, of greater concern than the specific point estimates are the general relationships between disability and age, gender, education, employment, and income/poverty status. While the magnitude of these relationships will obviously differ from one study to the next, the relationships themselves are well documented and can be seen across surveys (28).

Age

Disability increases rather dramatically with age, from 10.2% among youth aged 15 to 24 to 19.7% among persons aged 45 to 54, to 70.5% of persons aged 80 and over. Particularly with the "graying of America," this can lead to a misconception that disability is primarily a concern for elders. To the contrary, persons over aged 65 constitute just 15% of the US population, whereas the working age (18 to 64) make up over 60%. In sheer numbers, there are more working-aged people with disabilities than persons over aged 65 who have disabilities. Severe disability, which includes the need for assistance with ADLs and/or IADLs in the SIPP study, is also higher in sheer numbers among the working age, but more highly concentrated among persons over 65.

Sex

Overall, the prevalence of disability among females (19.8%) is slightly higher than among males (17.4%). Some of this may owe to differences in age distributions; with women outliving men, they make up a higher proportion of the elderly, where disability is more concentrated. However, disability among children is generally higher in males than females.

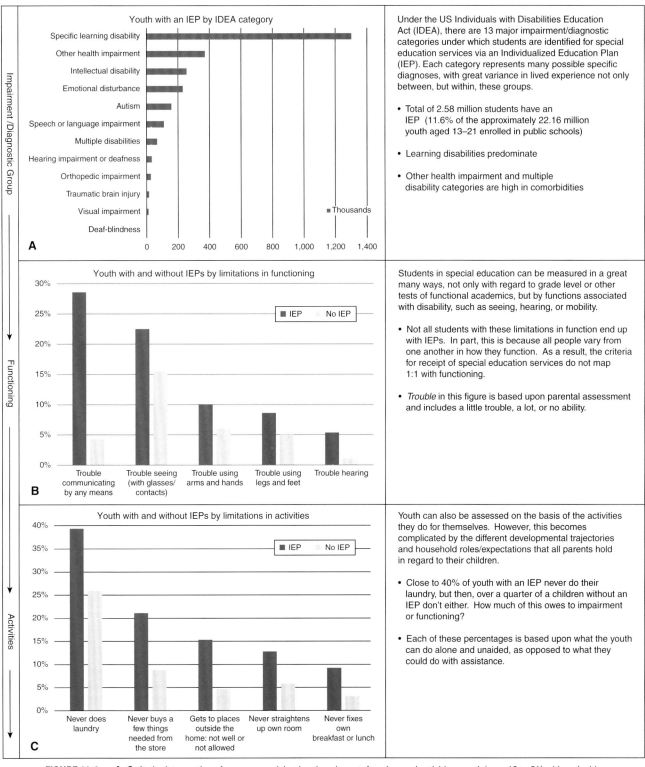

FIGURE 11-1. **A–C:** At the intersection of program participation, impairment, function, and activities: youth (ages 13 to 21) with and without individualized education plans in US Public Schools, 2012. (From Lipscomb S, Haimson J, Liu AY, et al. *Preparing for Life After High School: The Characteristics and Experiences of Youth in Special Education. Findings from the National Longitudinal Transition Study 2012 Volume 1: Comparisons with Other Youth.* Washington, DC: U.S. Department of Education, Institute of Education Sciences, National Center for Education Evaluation and Regional Assistance; 2017.)

Educational Attainment

Among those aged 25 to 64, while just 8.8% of persons without disabilities did not complete high school, 16.2% of people with disabilities did not do so. Conversely, where 34.1% of individuals without disabilities held a bachelor degree or higher, just 16.8% of people with disabilities held such a degree. Perhaps a testament to the requirement of a public education for all children with disabilities mandated in 1975, these figures are an improvement over those for individuals over the age of 65, most of whom born before any such guarantee; in that age group, 23.6% of people with disabilities did not complete high school. Education is particularly important among people with disabilities in as much as it often gives rise to enhanced health literacy and self-advocacy, the development of employment and other skills that compensate for functional limitations, as well as social capital (82).

Employment

The proper measurement of employment among people with disabilities is controversial, since it is sometimes situated as an independent measure (difficulty finding or keeping a job or limited in the kind or amount of work that can be performed) and sometimes used as a dependent measure (actual employment status at a point in time or over time). In some studies, it is used as both an independent and dependent measure simultaneously, as is the case with the SIPP estimates presented here, which include difficulty finding a job or remaining employed among the other criteria that establish disability status. That note made, where 79.1% of working-age (21 to 64) people without disabilities were employed at a point in time, just 41.1% of people with disabilities were so employed in 2010. Individuals with disabilities were also more likely to stay unemployed long term (2 years or more) than their counterparts without them.

Income and Poverty

Among the most consistent findings across surveys are that poverty and disability are bidirectionally related—with higher poverty comes higher exposure to risk of disability and with disability comes higher exposure to risk of poverty. Furthermore, as with education, the relationship between disability and income/poverty is complex in that the latter tends to narrow access to the medical, social, or environmental resources needed to prevent participation restrictions. When working, people with disabilities generally earn less (median monthly income of $1,961) than do people without disabilities ($2,724). Due in part to lower marriage rates, family incomes of adults with disabilities sit at about 60% of those in families of nondisabled individuals. The poverty rate follows suit, with 25.1% of working-age people with disabilities living at or below the federal poverty line, compared with 14.3% among their nondisabled counterparts. For elders (65+), perhaps owing to accrued savings and social security retirement benefits, these percentages improve (to 10.4% and 5.0%, respectively).

Race and Ethnicity

We strike a cautionary note about the distribution of disability across race and ethnicity. Historically, there has been a good deal of inconsistency in these prevalence rates, owing not only to differing measures of disability, but different categorizations of racial and ethnic groups as well as differing cultural values and beliefs about disability, health, and racial identification among survey respondents (83). Furthermore, race and ethnicity also sit at the intersection of a variety of social determinants of health and demographic or economic differences between people—age, gender, education, employment, and poverty among them (9). The risk, then, is assuming a direct relationship between race/ethnicity and disability and we caution the reader against such an assumption. That critical note made, after adjusting for age, the disability prevalence rates from the 2010 SIPP data were non-Hispanic, White, 17.6%; non-Hispanic, Black, 22.2%; non-Hispanic, Asian, 14.5%; and Hispanic/Latino (any race), 17.8.

International Demographics of Disability

Internationally, it is also the case that disability prevalence rises with age and is significantly and substantially associated with education, employment, and poverty, but with potentially stronger differences based on sex. In **Figure 11-2**, we depict findings from the World Health Survey that aggregates data from 59 participating countries (84). Here, disability is also defined broadly including affect, cognition, interpersonal relationships, mobility, pain, sleep and energy, self-care, and vision.

It is particularly important to note the difference in disability prevalence between high-income countries (like the United States), 11.8%, and low-income countries, 18.0% (so defined on the basis of gross national income per capita). This difference carries through the remaining demographic categories, such that while women have higher rates of disability than men overall, women in low-income countries have *substantially* higher disability rates (22%) than do men in high-income countries (9%). Similarly, persons aged 60 and over in low-income countries (43.4% with disabilities) are certainly more likely than their same-age counterparts in high-income countries (29.5%) to report a disability, but the difference is even more remarkable when the point of comparison is younger adults (age 18 to 49) in high-income countries, at just 6.4%. Household wealth, measured in quintiles, follows this pattern as well. The richest quintile individuals in low-income countries have a reported 13.3% disability prevalence, which is equivalent to that found in the second poorest quintile in high-income countries.

In the second and third panels of **Figure 11-2**, we compare respondents of all participating countries on measures of education and employment, doing so on the basis of disability status, age group, and sex. Women with disabilities have substantially lower rates of primary education completion (41.7%) than nondisabled men (61.3%). Similarly, individuals with disabilities aged 60 and over have much lower primary education rates (32.3%) than younger adults (18 to 49) without disabilities (67.4%). But perhaps the most striking of these findings is the difference in employment rates on the basis of sex and disability across the globe. Just 20% of women with disabilities reported that they were employed or looking for work, compared to almost 65% of nondisabled men. It is also telling that the employment rate for men with disabilities sits at 52.8%. While certainly lower than the rate for nondisabled men, taken together,

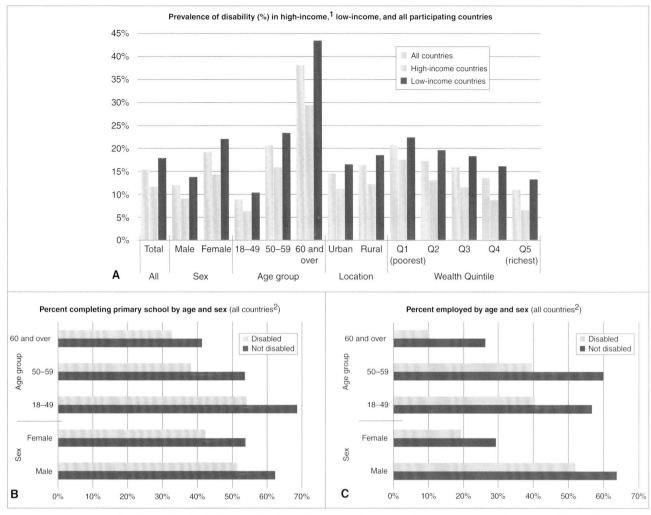

FIGURE 11-2. **A–C:** International sociodemographics of disability: sex, age, location, wealth, education, and employment over 59 countries. Notes: (1) Countries are divided between low-income and high-income according to their 2004 gross national income (GNI) per capita. The dividing point between low and high is a GNI of US$ 3255. (2) 51 (of 59) countries contributed to the education and employment figures. (From *World Report on Disability*. Geneva, Switzerland: World Health Organization; 2011:28, 207, 238. Data tables 2.1, 7.1 and 8.2. Available from: http://www.who.int/disabilities/world_report/2011/en/. Accessed on March 4, 2017, with permission of the World Health Organization. Data was originally collected in the *2002–2004 World Health Survey*.)

these numbers tend to indicate that impairment alone does not account for the low employment participation of people with disabilities.

The Environment Around the Person

From an epidemiologic standpoint, no matter what the country of residence, lack of access to needed resources, from basics like food, water, and sanitation to housing and economic support, education, public programs and accommodations, health care, and employment opportunities, can be simultaneously causes, consequences, and/or contributors of/to disability (8,9,11,17,18,24–26,28,84). Over time, individuals who are poorly resourced in these determinants face greater risk of acquiring physical and/or mental health conditions that may produce functional or activity limitations. Once living with disability, these determinants can also influence not only the development of secondary conditions, but mediate or moderate the relationship between functioning and participation in personal, family, social, work, or civic life. In turn,

environmental barriers, from the lack of assistive devices and technologies, inaccessible buildings, insufficient rehabilitation services, prejudicial or paternalistic public attitudes, and discriminatory practices in school or the workplace, also produce disability in their own right.

The Committee on Living Well with Chronic Disease of the Institute of Medicine published a Call for Public Health in 2012 that merits direct mention in this regard (85). Consistent with the ICF, it provides a carefully researched, macrolevel framework for the advancement of health and well-being among persons already living with chronic disease and/or disability. The framework from this Call for Public Health is shown in **Figure 11-3**.

Three primary domains can be seen in **Figure 11-3**. The first domain covers determinants of health, ranging from biology and genes to behavior and coping responses, to the sociocultural context and the environments in which people live. The second domain includes policies and interventions at the individual and population levels (as affected through health

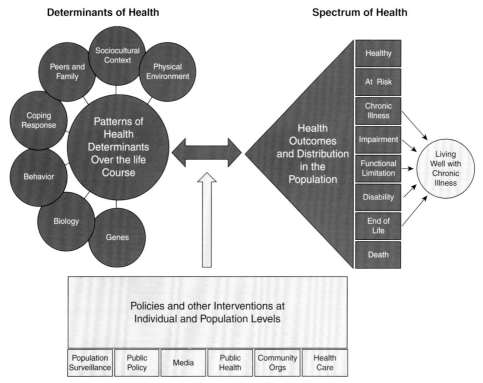

Determinants of Health

Spectrum of Health

FIGURE 11-3.   An integrated framework for living well with chronic illness. (Republished with permission of National Academies Press from Institute of Medicine Board on Population Health and Public Health Practice. *Living Well with Chronic Illness: A Call for Public Health Action.* Washington, DC: National Academies Press, 2012; permission conveyed through Copyright Clearance Center, Inc.)

care, public health initiatives, community organizations, etc.). The final domain is referred to as the spectrum of health, for which the IOM describes population subgroups ranging from healthy, to "at risk," to chronic illness without impairment, to functional limitations, and to disability.

In order to provide an example of the interaction of both personal and environmental factors in the production of disability, we return to a study briefly mentioned earlier in this chapter, on serious psychological distress (SPD) (76). Higher SPD prevalence was found among women versus men, middle-aged adults versus younger adults, Hispanics and non-Hispanic Blacks versus non-Hispanic Whites, participants with the lowest income, participants with less than a high school education compared with a college degree or higher, and persons with two or more other chronic conditions, such as COPD, diabetes, heart disease, stroke, or cancer. These differences potentially reflect not only possible social and health determinants of SPD, but, crucially, the resources and contexts within which individuals cope with SPD once it develops. Factors external to the individual, which influence the availability and uptake of treatment and support, are particularly salient in this regard. Weissman et al. found that a greater proportion of adults with SPD than adults without SPD had no health insurance coverage, delays in health care, insufficient money for health care, insufficient money to buy medications, insufficient money for mental health care, and changes in place of health care. They also found that compared to persons without SPD, people with SPD were far more likely to report limitations in ADLs as well as limitations in ability to work. A key question to consider, then, is how many of these limitations resulted not just from SPD but from the environment, available resources, or the policies and interventions (or lack thereof) suggested in **Figure 11-3**.

PEOPLE WITH DISABILITIES, CHRONIC CONDITIONS, HEALTH AND HEALTH CARE POLICY

It is true that across many measures of health and health care, people with disabilities—and with chronic conditions—often report compromised health. However, in an era when wheelchair users complete marathons an hour faster than able-bodied runners, when people with significant intellectual disabilities have begun to go to college, and when people with type 1 diabetes are now living into their 70s and 80s, it should be clear not only that many such people are healthy, but that health, function, and participation are each relative and multidimensional states, affecting *all* people.

It is important to know that chronic conditions and disability are overlapping phenomena. In health services research, increasing attention has been paid to defining and measuring this overlap and to identifying meaningful subgroups along the spectrum of health (see **Fig. 11-3**) (86–89). Studies on Adults with Chronic Healthcare Needs (ACHCN) in the United States, defined as "Adults (age 18 to 65) with [1] ongoing physical, cognitive, or mental health conditions or difficulties functioning who [2] need health or related support services of a type or amount beyond that needed by adults of the same sex and similar age," provide a relevant example (87,88,90). To identify the chronic health care need population in a secondary data analysis, the authors began with an exhaustive, validated list of chronic medical and mental health conditions and applied it to the International Classification of Disease (ICD-9-CM) codes provided in the Medical Expenditure Panel Survey (MEPS) (87). This list includes each reported medical or mental health condition expected to last at least 12 months and to result in a need for ongoing intervention (including regularly prescribed medications, therapies from health professionals, specialized medical equipment or protocols affecting diet or physical activity) and/or limitations (including age-appropriate task performance, ADLs, IADLS, or social inter-

actions). Persons reporting one or more of the listed conditions were flagged as potentially having chronic health care needs, whereas individuals without these conditions comprised a contrast group. ACHCN were then divided into three subgroups on the basis of the presence and extent of functional difficulties and activity limitations. In **Figure 11-4**, we highlight findings

Measures	With vs. Without CHCN		ACHCN Subgroups		
Prevalence, sociodemographics, health and health care use among persons with and without CHCNs and among ACHCN subgroups by limitation status					
	Adults Without CHCN	ACHCN (All)	No Limitation	Limitation Not Affecting ADL/IADL	ADL/IADL Limitations
Prevalence (weighted percent)	48.2%	51.8%	37.9%	10.6%	3.3%
Sociodemographics and resources:					
Mean age	36.7	44.6	43.2	48.5	48.2
Percent female	44.6%	57.0%	56.2%	58.8%	60.5%
Percent no high school degree or GED	16.7%	12.5%	9.7%	17.8%	27.3%
Percent poor or near poor (<125% FPL)	14.0%	14.2%	9.3%	24.1%	37.8%
Health-related measure:					
Poor or fair overall health at one or more rounds	8.8%	28.6%	16.3%	56.9%	79.4%
Poor or fair mental health at one or more rounds	4.9%	18.0%	9.7%	35.1%	58.3%
Body mass index ≥30	19.6%	31.8%	28.0%	41.9%	42.6%
Moderate-vigorous physical activity <3 times/week	39.2%	45.1%	40.4%	54.1%	68.9%
Currently smoke	23.6%	24.1%	20.9%	31.9%	35.8%
Health care use					
Percent with any ambulatory visit during year	56.9%	85.9%	83.8%	91.4%	93.8%
Among persons with 1+ visit(s), mean visits	4.8	9.5	7.2	14.1	20.8
Percent with any hospitalization during year	4.5%	8.5%	5.8%	12.8%	25.5%
Among persons with 1+ hospitalizations, mean hospitalizations during year	1.1	1.3	1.2	1.3	1.6
Percent with any ER visit during year	8.7%	17.0%	13.7%	24.4%	32.9%
Among persons with 1+ ER visits, mean ER visits during year	1.2	1.5	1.3	1.5	2.0
Percent with any home health during year	—	2.0%	0.4%	2.3%	20.1%
Among persons with any home health, mean provider during year	—	74.5	11.2	20.3	107.6
Percent with any prescribed medicine year	41.9%	86.5%	84.9%	90.2%	94.1%
Among persons with any prescribed medicine, mean number of fills/refills during year	5.3	17.5	13.3	24.3	36.9

A

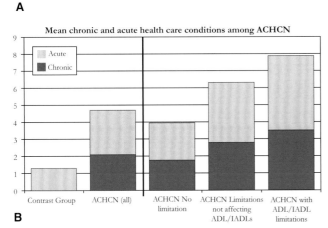

B

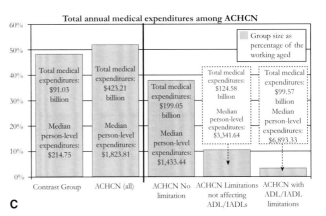

C

FIGURE 11-4. **A–C:** Working-age adults with chronic health care needs in the United States. (From Gulley SP, Rasch EK, Chan L. If we build it, who will come? Working-age adults with chronic health care needs and the medical home. *Med Care*. 2011;49:149–155. Available from: http://journals.lww.com/lww-medicalcare/Abstract/2011/02000/If_We_Build_It,_Who_Will_Come___Working_Age_Adults.7.aspx. Reprinted from Wolters Kluwer Health, Inc., with permission.)

from this study, with an emphasis on what they reveal about the relationships between and among health, chronic conditions, disability, and health service use.

Prevalence

The first and most important note to make regards the prevalence of ACHCN among the US working age. It was found that 91 million had chronic health care needs, approximately 52% of that age group overall. Although 67 million individuals (73% of ACHCN) had no limitations in functioning or activities, the remaining 25 million (27% of ACHCN) had at least some degree of limitation. Six million persons reported that they did need the help or supervision of another person in ADLs/IADLs.

Health and Health Conditions

As shown in **Figure 11-4**, *multiple* chronic and acute conditions are the norm among ACHCN. Both rise in the presence of functional or activity limitations, particularly for persons with ADL or IADL limitations. Relatedly, though not necessarily as a direct result, ACHCN also have lower markers of health than their counterparts without CHCNs, including self-reported overall health and mental health, while reporting higher BMI and lower rates of exercise. Again, the limitations associated with disability co-occur with progressively compromised health; almost 80% of persons with ADL/IADL limitations report fair to poor overall health and over half of such individuals report fair to poor mental health.

Health Service Use

Across virtually every type of care analyzed, ACHCN had significantly higher percentages of service use and mean visit/use rates than did adults without chronic health care needs. Furthermore, within the ACHCN group, utilization rates were significantly higher among ACHCN with limitations than without.

Expenditures and Access to Care

On average, four times as much was spent on the ACHCN population ($423 billion) than on the population without chronic health care needs ($91 billion) despite the fact that these two groups are close to the same size. However, the bulk of the costs among ACHCN were spent on the two smaller groups with limitations, who, together, accounted for some 224 billion in annual expenditures. The smallest of the groups, ACHCN with ADL/IADL limitations, represents only 3% of the working age, but, with 100 billion in expenditures, accounted for more total dollars than did the *entire* non-ACHCN contrast group.

Intersections

There are, undoubtedly, relationships between and among health, disability, and health care, but they are complex and multidimensional. First, while it is possible to make some delineations between chronic health conditions and the limitations associated with disability, these are overlapping phenomena that are influenced by a great many factors both inside and outside the human body. Indeed, even when limitations are not experienced, people with such conditions as diabetes or depression may require significant and ongoing medical treatment or related supports to avoid such limitations or health crises over time.

Second, it must be reiterated that people with disabilities typically have *multiple* chronic conditions. One, or several, of these conditions may contribute directly to a given limitation in function, activity, or participation—but then some limitations may be only peripherally related to a health "condition," such as in the case of deafness from birth or a status post lower leg amputation. These and other such examples may be more related to functional or structural differences among all people and how people accommodate or manage such differences than they are to health conditions in need of a medical response. That said, it is undeniably the case that people with disabilities report high rates of multiple chronic and acute conditions.

Third, it should be stressed that people with disabilities have, in the aggregate, a great deal of interaction with the health care system. In the United States, and abroad, that system is not always physically, programmatically, or financially accessible to people with disabilities (or chronic conditions) when they need it (76,84,88). Furthermore, the US health care system is in many ways "siloed" by diagnosis and medical specialty, leading to concerns over the coordination, settings, and timing of care available to individuals with chronic conditions and disabilities, even when well-insured (87). We take up these issues next, with a special focus upon rehabilitation.

IMPLICATIONS FOR REHABILITATION PRACTICE AND HEALTH POLICY IN THE UNITED STATES AND INTERNATIONALLY

Given the sheer breadth, scope, and prevalence of chronic conditions and disabilities just described, it is critical to note that individuals seen in US inpatient rehabilitation settings are *not* representative of the communities from which they come. Rather, the subpopulations commonly served in rehabilitation settings are selected and treated diagnostically. They are admitted on the basis of the medical need for and potential benefit from rehabilitation. They are typically required to demonstrate that they can tolerate therapy and show medical improvement in order to remain inpatients. They are also usually required to provide proof of ability to pay for services, whether through insurance or out of pocket. As such, they do not reflect the full distribution of children or adults with chronic conditions and/or disabilities living in the United States.

This same observation holds on the outpatient side of rehabilitation as well. While many factors influence access to and use of postacute care rehabilitation services, broad classes include financial, personal, structural, and attitudinal indicators, with structure of the payment system and availability reflecting major drivers (91–94). Hence, people with disabilities and chronic conditions are far more diverse than those served in rehabilitation settings at any given point in time. The services upon which they rely go far beyond rehabilitation as well, to include care coordination, ready access to medical specialists, home- and community-based long-term care services, mental health, and a range of other kinds of traditional and nontraditional physical, social, or occupational supports (28,87,89). Given that the fundamental goal of rehabilitation is to maximize the chances that clients will transition to and live well in the community—and will avoid readmissions—it is incumbent upon rehabilitation practitioners to be well-acquainted with this full range of community-based services, with the characteristics of people with disabilities living in the community, and with the implications of epidemiology for public health. This may be especially the case for practitioners who, day in and day out, see patients with disabilities when they are in a particularly difficult phase of illness or injury. This can lead to a distorted sense of the "burden" of disability and a narrowed view of the potential quality of a life lived well as a person, not as a patient, with a disability in the community.

Rehabilitation in the Patient-Centered Medical Neighborhood

Primary care reform in the United States and other industrialized nations has faced many challenges and barriers to providing effective health care. Individuals with complex medical issues that are multiple, chronic, and pervasive, whether disabled or not, can require a toolset beyond what a primary care practice can provide. It is well established that the proper balance and coordination of care between various providers is necessary to achieve optimal health care that addresses the needs of the whole person (95–97). With this in mind, it has been shown that health outcomes improve not only with increased provider continuity but also with interactive communication among primary care physicians, specialists, and rehabilitation providers (98,99).

The Patient-Centered Medical Home (PCMH) is central to health care reform in the United States. This model was developed by the American Academy of Family Physicians, the American Academy of Pediatrics, the American College of Physicians, and the American Osteopathic Association to drive transformative health system innovation. In short, the PCMH is a physician-directed practice providing care that is accessible, continuous, comprehensive, coordinated, and delivered in the context of family and community. The PCMH is idealized as the central hub connecting patients to a broad range of resources defined as the medical neighborhood (100). This neighborhood includes hospitals, nursing homes, specialists, and many other health care professionals and community-based providers.

Focusing on individuals with disabilities, McColl et al. investigated PCMH service delivery programs that offered both primary care and rehabilitation (101). They identified six different models that were designed to improve coordination and outcomes across these disciplines (see 🛜 **eTable 11-2**). McColl et al. found that each of these approaches has advantages and disadvantages depending in part upon the needs and characteristics of the communities in which they are embedded and the resources and infrastructure available to support the program. They also found eight common themes that either supported or impeded the integration of rehabilitation services in primary care settings, including the extent and nature of the team approach, interprofessional trust, leadership structure, communication mechanisms, compensation, accountability, referrals, and an individual- versus population-based approach.

A potential barrier in the medical neighborhood for people with disabilities and chronic conditions arises when primary care or rehabilitation providers cannot schedule or manage emergent or emergency medical needs in a timely manner. The relationship between emergency department use and people with disabilities has been studied among the working-age population in the United States (102). Rasch et al. reported that almost 40% of total annual ED visits in the United States

were made by people with disabilities. This study raised questions over how many such ED visits were appropriate and how many could have been prevented with better upstream access to proper primary or rehabilitative care. It also raised questions about what happens downstream from an ED visit and what measures might be taken to prevent more such visits in the weeks or months to come. Given the secondary conditions that accompany many types of disabilities (pressure sores, urinary tract infections, contractures, pneumonia, etc.), better prevention and management of these issues among PWDs in the medical neighborhood are increasingly the shared province of primary care providers and rehabilitation professionals.

U.S. Health Care Reform and People with Chronic Conditions or Disabilities

As demonstrated earlier, people with chronic conditions and disabilities experience high rates not only of emergency department visits, but hospitalizations, community-based services, and other forms of ongoing treatment that are frequently expensive for individuals and for the health care system as a whole (87,88,102). The hope remains that proactive, patient-centered care will prevail and produce not only better population health and functioning, but cost savings. However, no matter how effective delivery-side reforms may prove to be, when the distributions of disability and chronic conditions in our population are carefully studied, and when the range of services and supports affected individuals depend upon are made plain, it is clear that these population groups will continue to be high need and high cost. Looking to the future, the regulatory framework in which private and public insurance operate will play a key role in the financing, and perhaps even the availability, of services needed by people with chronic conditions and disabilities. These regulations will, in one way or another, determine the extent to which private payers will be able to deny coverage on the basis of pre-existing conditions, refuse guaranteed renewal of coverage, curtail essential health benefits, cap lifetime monetary benefits, or reduce coverage for mental health and substance abuse services—to name but a few (103). Similarly, on the public side, future regulations will determine the size, scope, and comprehensiveness of safety net programs as well as the variability in eligibility for those programs and the benefits available from one state to the next. Whether public or private, these reforms (or lack thereof) will affect all Americans. In an era marked by the advancing age of the baby boomers, it is people with ongoing and elevated needs for care, such as those with chronic conditions and disabilities, who may experience the impact of health care reform most directly (88).

Rehabilitation in an International Context

Many of the issues described in these last two sections—including the high prevalence and overlap of chronic conditions and disabilities in the population; the associated needs for health, health care, and social services; the exacerbating effects of inaccessible or discriminatory environments; and the importance of timely, patient-centered, and well-coordinated care—apply not only to the United States, but across the globe (84). However, and as troubled as the US healthcare system may seem at present, it is critical to remember that this country remains one of the wealthiest nations in the world with significant investments in education, civil rights, health care, and safety net programs. The United States also has formalized standards for the accreditation of rehabilitation hospitals, dedicated rehabilitation professional and scientific organizations, model systems of care for specific diagnoses such as TBI or SCI, and state and national networks of Aging and Disability Resource Centers, Independent Living Centers, and Councils on Developmental Disability. These many points of infrastructure shape the environment in which US citizens with disabilities live—and the quantity and quality of rehabilitation services and technologies available to them—respectively. However, such infrastructure is not always, or in some instances, even usually available to the citizens of other countries, particularly in developing parts of the world.

A global survey of the implementation of the United Nations Standard Rules on the Equalization of Opportunities for Persons with Disabilities (84), in 114 countries, found the following:

- In 57 of 114 (50%) countries, no legislation on rehabilitation for people with disabilities was passed.
- In 48 (42%) countries that responded to the survey, formal rehabilitation policies were not adopted.
- In 46 (40%) countries, formal rehabilitation programs were not established.
- In 41 (36%) countries, there was no government funding for assistive devices.
- In 37 (33%) countries, there was no specific budgetary process for rehabilitation services.

In review of these findings and other international sources, the World Health Organization concluded that while many countries have substantial legislation and related policies and programs for rehabilitation, about as many do not (84). This is particularly the case in poorer nations—and in some instances, the poorer regions and localities of wealthier nations as well. Even among the 35 member countries of the Organisation for Economic Co-operation and Development (OECD), which include many of the most advanced economies in the world, public spending on rehabilitation as a part of labor market programs averaged just 0.02% of GDP. Overall, the WHO attributed this dearth of rehabilitation services and investment around the world to six key factors:

- Lack of strategic planning, resulting in uneven distribution of service capacity and infrastructure
- Lack of health infrastructure, including hospitals, clinics, or facilities
- Lack of agencies to administer, coordinate, and monitor services
- Inadequate health information systems and communication strategies
- In systems that do have necessary infrastructure, complex referral systems that limit access to rehabilitation
- Absence of engagement with people with disabilities and the organizations that represent them

SUMMARY

In many ways, the fields of epidemiology, rehabilitation, and disability research have followed parallel, if unique, developmental arcs over the past several decades. Each discipline has its own unique focus, methods, and praxis. Where epidemiology primarily concerns itself with the frequency, patterns, and determinants of health-related states in order to produce knowledge that benefits public health, the field of rehabilitation has a more applied focus upon interventions at the individual-condition level, which preserve or improve functional abilities and health for the person. For their part, disability researchers have focused more squarely on mezzo and macro level societal factors and public policies that alternatively increase or decrease participation in major life activities and overall well-being for people living with disabilities in the community. However, each of these fields has also had to contend, in one way or another, with the increasingly well-understood nature of disability. This is, at once:

- Ubiquitous, dynamic, multidimensional, and an expected part of the human experience over the life course
- Biopsychosocial with far-reaching effects, both negative *and* positive, on the activities in which people participate
- Concerned with structural and functional differences between people, some of which medical and some of which not
- Coproduced by impairment at the individual level, the extent of resources and opportunities at the mezzo and macro levels, and participation restrictions at all levels
- Intersectionally related with social determinants of health such as poverty and education as well as demographics such as age, gender, or race/ethnicity
- Related to health in complex ways, particularly given the distribution of chronic health and mental health conditions among people with—and without—disabilities
- Frequently accompanied by elevated needs for health care, related services, and community-based supports for which there is a dearth of investment, infrastructure, and/or coordination in many countries, regions, or localities
- *Always involved with the interaction of the person and the environment*

Given this multidimensional nature of disability, it is not surprising that the fields mentioned above define and measure disability in different ways or for different purposes. Nor is it surprising that these disciplines focus upon differing subgroups of people with disabilities or produce differing estimates of prevalence or incidence of conditions, functional limitations, activity limitations, or participation restrictions. Perhaps it *should* be the case that the responses these fields suggest differ as well, whether they include disability prevention strategies grounded in epidemiologic knowledge, rehabilitation interventions to reduce the extent or impact of functional limitations for people with specific diagnoses, or the deconstruction of physical or attitudinal barriers that restrict the participation of people living with disability.

In review of what was covered in this chapter, if there is one dimension of disability that has served to triangulate these three fields, it is the increasingly shared appreciation for the role of the environment in producing and shaping the experience of disability. From an epidemiologic point of view, the prevalence of disability was shown to increase in the United States and internationally, when not just individuals, but communities and even nations have fewer economic resources or less health care infrastructure. From a rehabilitation standpoint, it was shown that functional limitations can be exacerbated when individuals do not have insurance coverage or well-coordinated access to community-based services and supports in the medical neighborhood. From the perspective of disability researchers, it was noted that environmental barriers, be they physical, policy based, and/or the result of stigma, delimit the activities in which people with disabilities can engage while also threatening health and well-being.

This shared focus on the environment as a key unit of analysis also has implications for the future production of knowledge in these three fields. As demonstrated in this chapter, much of what we currently know about disability comes from clinical, programmatic, administrative, or survey data sources. These sources typically rely upon the individual or the condition as the unit of analysis and are variously aggregated to describe disability populations of interest. Yet, even as each of these fields acknowledges the importance of the environment around the person, the development of direct environmental measures of participation restrictions (or facilitators) is still in its infancy. Where measures do exist, they are typically employed in smaller-scale, topical studies conducted by disability researchers. The development of regional and national systems and methods of surveillance, and internationally comparatives measures that permit the direct evaluation and estimation of the physical, attitudinal, technologic, and legal accessibility of *communities*, is a paramount goal for the future.

ACKNOWLEDGMENTS

This work was funded by the National Institutes of Health (NIH) intramural research program. The views expressed in this chapter are those of the authors and do not necessarily reflect the official policy or position of the NIH or the US government. The authors have no financial or other conflicts of interest to report pertaining to this chapter.

REFERENCES

1. CDC. *Principles of Epidemiology in Public Health Practice.* Atlanta, GA: U.S. Department of Health and Human Services, Centers for Disease Control; 2012.
2. Fine P, Victora CG, Rothman KJ, et al. John Snow's legacy: epidemiology without borders. *Lancet.* 2013;381:1302–1311.
3. Bennett JE, Dolin R, Blaser MJ. *Mandell, Douglas, and Bennett's Principles and Practice of Infectious Diseases.* 8th ed. Philadelphia, PA: Elsevier/Saunders; 2015.
4. Friedman SM, Mendelson DA. Epidemiology of fragility fractures. *Clin Geriatr Med.* 2014;30:175–181.
5. CDC. Vital signs: nonfatal, motor vehicle occupant injuries (2009) and seat belt use (2008) among adults in the United States. *Morb Mortal Wkly Rep.* 2011;59:1681–1686.
6. Swanson JW, McGinty EE, Fazel S, et al. Mental illness and reduction of gun violence and suicide: bringing epidemiologic research to policy. *Ann Epidemiol.* 2015;25:366–376.
7. Blumberg SJ, Bramlett MD, Kogan MD, et al. Changes in prevalence of parent-reported autism spectrum disorder in school-aged U.S. children: 2007 to 2011–2012. *Natl Health Stat Report.* 2013;(65):1–11.
8. Braveman P, Gottlieb L. The social determinants of health: it's time to consider the causes of the causes. *Public Health Rep.* 2014;129(suppl 2):19–31.
9. Berkman LF, Kawachi I, Glymour MM. *Social Epidemiology.* 2nd ed. Oxford, UK: Oxford University Press; 2014.
10. Declich S, Carter AO. Public health surveillance: historical origins, methods and evaluation. *Bull World Health Organ.* 1994;72:285–304.
11. Charlton JI. *Nothing About Us Without Us: Disability Oppression and Empowerment.* Berkeley, CA: University of California Press; 1998.
12. Shapiro JP. *No Pity: People with Disabilities Forging a New Civil Rights Movement.* New York: Times Books; 1994.
13. Nagi SZ. A study in the evaluation of disability and rehabilitation potential: concepts, methods, and procedures. *Am J Public Health Nations Health.* 1964;54:1568–1579.
14. Nagi SZ. Some conceptual issues in disability and rehabilitation. In: Sussman M, ed. *Sociology and Rehabilitation.* Washington, DC: American Sociological Association; 1965.
15. Nagi SZ. An epidemiology of disability among adults in the United States. *Milbank Mem Fund Q Health Soc.* 1976;54:439–467.
16. World Health Organization. *International Classification of Impairments, Disabilities, and Handicaps: A Manual of Classification Relating to the Consequences of Disease.* Albany, NY: World Health Organization; 1980.
17. Verbrugge LM, Jette AM. The disablement process. *Soc Sci Med.* 1994;38:1–14.
18. Brandt EN, Pope AM. *Enabling America: Assessing the Role of Rehabilitation Science and Engineering.* Washington, DC: National Academy Press; 1997.
19. National Institute of Child Health and Human Development. *Research Plan for the National Center for Medical Rehabilitation Research.* Bethesda, MD: U.S. Department of Health and Human Services, National Institutes of Health; 1993.
20. Gray DB, Hendershot GE. The ICIDH-2: developments for a new era of outcomes research. *Arch Phys Med Rehabil.* 2000;81:S10–S14.
21. World Health Organization. *International Classification of Functioning, Disability and Health: ICF.* Geneva, Switzerland: World Health Organization; 2001.
22. Alford VM, Ewen S, Webb GR, et al. The use of the International Classification of Functioning, Disability and Health to understand the health and functioning experiences of people with chronic conditions from the person perspective: a systematic review. *Disabil Rehabil.* 2015;37:655–666.
23. Cerniauskaite M, Quintas R, Boldt C, et al. Systematic literature review on ICF from 2001 to 2009: its use, implementation and operationalisation. *Disabil Rehabil.* 2011;33:281–309.
24. Zola IK. Disability statistics, what we count and what it tells us. *J Disabil Pol Stud.* 1993;4:9–39.
25. Altman BM. *International Measurement of Disability: Purpose, Method and Application.* New York: Springer Berlin Heidelberg; 2016.
26. Altman BM. Disability definitions, models, classification schemes and applications. In: Albrecht GL, Seelman KD, Bury M, eds. *Handbook of Disability Studies.* Thousand Oaks, CA: Sage Publications; 2001:97–116.
27. Iezzoni LI, Freedman VA. Turning the disability tide: the importance of definitions. *JAMA.* 2008;299:332–334.
28. Adams E, Krahn G, Horner-Johnson W, et al. Fundamentals of disability epidemiology. In: Drum C, Krahn G, Bersani H, eds. *Disability and Public Health.* Washington, DC: American Public Health Association; 2009:105–124.
29. White DK, Wilson JC, Keysor JJ. Measures of adult general functional status: SF-36 Physical Functioning Subscale (PF-10), Health Assessment Questionnaire (HAQ), Modified Health Assessment Questionnaire (MHAQ), Katz Index of Independence in activities of daily living, Functional Independence Measure (FIM), and Osteoarthritis-Function-Computer Adaptive Test (OA-Function-CAT). *Arthritis Care Res (Hoboken).* 2011;63(suppl 11):S297–S307.
30. Stineman MG, Escarce JJ, Goin JE, et al. A case-mix classification system for medical rehabilitation. *Med Care.* 1994;32:366–379.
31. Stineman MG, Granger CV. A modular case-mix classification system for medical rehabilitation illustrated. *Health Care Financ Rev.* 1997;19:87–103.
32. United Nations Division for Social Policy and Development. *Convention on the Rights of Persons with Disabilities (CRPD).* United Nations; 2006. Available from: https://www.un.org/development/desa/disabilities/convention-on-the-rights-of-persons-with-disabilities.html. Accessed March 27, 2017.
33. Madans JH, Loeb ME, Altman BM. Measuring disability and monitoring the UN Convention on the Rights of Persons with Disabilities: the work of the Washington Group on Disability Statistics. *BMC Public Health.* 2011;11(suppl 4):S4.
34. Murray CJ, Barber RM, Foreman KJ, et al. Global, regional, and national disability-adjusted life years (DALYs) for 306 diseases and injuries and healthy life expectancy (HALE) for 188 countries, 1990–2013: quantifying the epidemiological transition. *Lancet.* 2015;386:2145–2191.
35. Grosse SD, Lollar DJ, Campbell VA, et al. Disability and disability-adjusted life years: not the same. *Public Health Rep.* 2009;124:197–202.
36. Anand S, Hanson K. Disability-adjusted life years: a critical review. *J Health Econ.* 1997;16:685–702.
37. Lawrence RC, Felson DT, Helmick CG, et al. Estimates of the prevalence of arthritis and other rheumatic conditions in the United States: Part II. *Arthritis Rheum.* 2007;58:26–35.
38. National Center for Health Statistics. *Health, United States, 2011: With Special Feature on Socioeconomic Status and Health.* Hyattsville, MD: National Center for Health Statistics; 2012.
39. Waterman BR, Belmont PJ, Schoenfeld AJ. Low back pain in the United States: incidence and risk factors for presentation in the emergency setting. *Spine J.* 2012;12:63–70.
40. Martin BI. Expenditures and health status among adults with back and neck problems. *JAMA.* 2008;299:656.
41. CDC. Prevalence of doctor-diagnosed arthritis and arthritis-attributable activity limitation—United States, 2007–2009. *Morb Mortal Wkly Rep.* 2010;59:1261–1265.
42. Hootman JM, Helmick CG, Brady TJ. A public health approach to addressing arthritis in older adults: the most common cause of disability. *Am J Public Health.* 2012;102:426–433.
43. Oliveria SA, Felson DT, Reed JI, et al. Incidence of symptomatic hand, hip, and knee osteoarthritis among patients in a health maintenance organization. *Arthritis Rheum.* 1995;38:1134–1141.
44. Helmick CG, Felson DT, Lawrence RC, et al. Estimates of the prevalence of arthritis and other rheumatic conditions in the United States: Part I. *Arthritis Rheum.* 2007;58:15–25.
45. Jacobs P, Bissonnette R, Guenther LC. Socioeconomic burden of immune-mediated inflammatory diseases: focusing on work productivity and disability. *J Rheumatol Suppl.* 2011;88:55–61.
46. Silman A, Hochberg, MC. *Epidemiology of Rheumatic Disorders.* New York: Oxford University Press; 2001.

47. Myasoedova E, Crowson CS, Kremers HM, et al. Is the incidence of rheumatoid arthritis rising? Results from Olmsted County, Minnesota, 1955–2007. *Arthritis Rheum*. 2010;62:1576–1582.

48. Dominick KL, Ahern FM, Gold CH, et al. Health-related quality of life among older adults with arthritis. *Health Qual Life Outcomes*. 2004;2:5.

49. Go AS, Mozaffarian D, Roger VL, et al. Heart disease and stroke statistics—2013 update: a report from the American Heart Association. *Circulation*. 2013;127:e6–e245.

50. Kelly-Hayes M, Beiser A, Kase CS, et al. The influence of gender and age on disability following ischemic stroke: the Framingham study. *J Stroke Cerebrovasc Dis*. 2003;12:119–126.

51. Zaloshnja E, Miller T, Langlois JA, et al. Prevalence of long-term disability from traumatic brain injury in the civilian population of the United States, 2005. *J Head Trauma Rehabil*. 2008;23:394–400.

52. Rutland-Brown W, Langlois JA, Thomas KE, et al. Incidence of traumatic brain injury in the United States, 2003. *J Head Trauma Rehabil*. 2006;21:544–548.

53. Ziegler-Graham K, MacKenzie EJ, Ephraim PL, et al. Estimating the prevalence of limb loss in the United States: 2005 to 2050. *Arch Phys Med Rehabil*. 2008;89:422–429.

54. CDC. Hospital discharge rates for nontraumatic lower extremity amputation per 1,000 diabetic population, United States, 1988–2009. *Ctr Dis Control Prev*. 2012. Available from: http://www.cdc.gov/diabetes/statistics/lea/fig3.htm. Accessed June 12, 2013.

55. Taylor SM, Kalbaugh CA, Blackhurst DW, et al. Preoperative clinical factors predict postoperative functional outcomes after major lower limb amputation: an analysis of 553 consecutive patients. *J Vasc Surg*. 2005;42:227–234.

56. Robbins JM, Strauss G, Aron D, et al. Mortality rates and diabetic foot ulcers. *J Am Podiatr Med Assoc*. 2008;98:489–493.

57. National Multiple Sclerosis Society. *Multiple Sclerosis Prevalence*. National Multiple Sclerosis Society; 2009. Available from: http://www.nationalmssociety.org/about-the-society/ms-prevalence/index.aspx. Accessed June 10, 2013.

58. Frohman EM. Multiple sclerosis. *Med Clin North Am*. 2003;87:867–897.

59. Noonan CW, Williamson DM, Henry JP, et al. The prevalence of multiple sclerosis in 3 US communities. *Prev Chronic Dis*. 2010;7:A12.

60. Fox R. *Multiple Sclerosis*. Cleveland, OH: Cleveland Clinic Foundation Disease Management Project; 2010.

61. National Spinal Cord Injury Statistical Center. *Spinal Cord Injury Facts and Figures at a Glance*. Birmingham, AL: National Spinal Cord Injury Statistical Center; 2013.

62. Bernhard M, Gries A, Kremer P, et al. Spinal cord injury (SCI)—prehospital management. *Resuscitation*. 2005;66:127–139.

63. Braddom R. *Physical Medicine and Rehabilitation*. 2nd ed. Philadelphia, PA: WB Saunders; 2000.

64. Ma VY, Chan L, Carruthers KJ. Incidence, prevalence, costs, and impact on disability of common conditions requiring rehabilitation in the United States: stroke, spinal cord injury, traumatic brain injury, multiple sclerosis, osteoarthritis, rheumatoid arthritis, limb loss, and back pain. *Arch Phys Med Rehabil*. 2014;95:986–995 e1.

65. Verbrugge LM, Patrick DL. Seven chronic conditions: their impact on US adults' activity levels and use of medical services. *Am J Public Health*. 1995;85:173–182.

66. CDC. Prevalence of doctor-diagnosed arthritis and arthritis-attributable activity limitation—United States, 2010–2012. *Morb Mortal Wkly Rep*. 2013;62:869–873.

67. Kasser SL, Goldstein A, Wood PK, et al. Symptom variability, affect and physical activity in ambulatory persons with multiple sclerosis: understanding patterns and time-bound relationships. *Disabil Health J*. 2017;10:207–213.

68. Ytterberg C, Johansson S, Gottberg K, et al. Perceived needs and satisfaction with care in people with multiple sclerosis: a two-year prospective study. *BMC Neurol*. 2008;8:36.

69. Beer S, Khan F, Kesselring J. Rehabilitation interventions in multiple sclerosis: an overview. *J Neurol*. 2012;259:1994–2008.

70. Braddom RL, Chan L, Harrast MA. *Physical Medicine and Rehabilitation*. 4th ed. Philadelphia, PA: Saunders/Elsevier; 2011.

71. Levy SE, Giarelli E, Lee LC, et al. Autism spectrum disorder and co-occurring developmental, psychiatric, and medical conditions among children in multiple populations of the United States. *J Dev Behav Pediatr*. 2010;31:267–275.

72. Fox MH, Krahn GL, Sinclair LB, et al. Using the international classification of functioning, disability and health to expand understanding of paralysis in the United States through improved surveillance. *Disabil Health J*. 2015;8:457–463.

73. Armour BS, Courtney-Long EA, Fox MH, et al. Prevalence and causes of paralysis—United States, 2013. *Am J Public Health*. 2016;106:1855–1857.

74. Kessler RC, Barker PR, Colpe LJ, et al. Screening for serious mental illness in the general population. *Arch Gen Psychiatry*. 2003;60:184–189.

75. Kessler RC, Green JG, Gruber MJ, et al. Screening for serious mental illness in the general population with the K6 screening scale: results from the WHO World Mental Health (WMH) survey initiative. *Int J Methods Psychiatr Res*. 2010;19(suppl 1):4–22.

76. Weissman J, Russell D, Jay M, et al. Disparities in health care utilization and functional limitations among adults with serious psychological distress, 2006–2014. *Psychiatr Serv*. 2017;68(7):653–659.

77. McMenamin TM, Hipple SF. *The Development of Questions on Disability for the Current Population Survey*. U.S. Bureau of Labor Statistics; 2014. Available from: https://doi.org/10.21916/mlr.2014.15. Accessed March 4, 2017.

78. Disability Statistics & Demographics Rehabilitation Research & Training Center. *Annual Disability Statistics Compendium*. Institute on Disability at the University of New Hampshire; 2016. Available from: https://disabilitycompendium.org/sites/default/files/user-uploads/2016%20Annual%20Disability%20Statistics%20Compendium1.pdf. Accessed March 8, 2017.

79. Brault MW. *Americans with Disabilities, 2010: Household Economic Studies*. Washington, DC: U.S. Dept. of Commerce, Economics and Statistics Administration, U.S. Census Bureau; 2012.

80. Mitra S, Sambamoorthi U. Disability prevalence among adults: estimates for 54 countries and progress toward a global estimate. *Disabil Rehabil*. 2014;36:940–947.

81. Cappa C, Petrowski, N, Njelesani J. Navigating the landscape of child disability measurement: a review of available data collection instruments. *Eur J Disabil Res*. 2015;9:317–330.

82. Lipscomb S, Haimson J, Liu AY, et al. *Preparing for Life After High School: The Characteristics and Experiences of Youth in Special Education. Findings from the National Longitudinal Transition Study 2012 Volume 1: Comparisons with Other Youth*. Washington, DC: U.S. Department of Education, Institute of Education Sciences, National Center for Education Evaluation and Regional Assistance; 2017.

83. Gulley SP, Rasch EK, Chan L. Difference, disparity, and disability: a comparison of health, insurance coverage, and health service use on the basis of race/ethnicity among US adults with disabilities, 2006–2008. *Med Care*. 2014;52:S9–S16.

84. World Health Organisation. *World Report on Disability*. Geneva, Switzerland: World Health Organization; 2011.

85. Institute of Medicine Board on Population Health and Public Health Practice. *Living Well with Chronic Illness: A Call for Public Health Action*. Washington, DC: The National Academies Press; 2012.

86. Gulley SP, Rasch EK, Chan L. The complex web of health: relationships among chronic conditions, disability, and health services. *Public Health Rep*. 2011;126:495–507.

87. Gulley SP, Rasch EK, Chan L. If we build it, who will come? Working-age adults with chronic health care needs and the medical home. *Med Care*. 2011;49:149–155.

88. Gulley SP, Rasch EK, Chan L. Ongoing coverage for ongoing care: access, utilization, and out-of-pocket spending among uninsured working-aged adults with chronic health care needs. *Am J Public Health*. 2011;101:368–375.

89. Reichard A, Gulley SP, Rasch EK, et al. Diagnosis isn't enough: understanding the connections between high health care utilization, chronic conditions and disabilities among U.S. working age adults. *Disabil Health J*. 2015;8:535–546.

90. Gulley SP, Rasch EK, Altman BM, et al. Introducing the Adults with Chronic Healthcare Needs (ACHCN) definition and screening instrument: rationale, supporting evidence and testing. *Disabil Health J*. 2018;11(2):204–213.

91. Buntin MB. Access to postacute rehabilitation. *Arch Phys Med Rehabil*. 2007;88:1488–1493.

92. Buntin MB, Garten AD, Paddock S, et al. How much is postacute care use affected by its availability? *Health Serv Res*. 2005;40:413–434.

93. Chan L. The state-of-the-science: challenges in designing postacute care payment policy. *Arch Phys Med Rehabil*. 2007;88:1522–1525.

94. Ottenbacher KJ, Graham JE. The state-of-the-science: access to postacute care rehabilitation services. A review. *Arch Phys Med Rehabil*. 2007;88:1513–1521.

95. Rosenblatt RA, Hart LG, Baldwin L-M, et al. The generalist role of specialty physicians. *JAMA*. 1998;279:1364.

96. Stange KC. The problem of fragmentation and the need for integrative solutions. *Ann Fam Med*. 2009;7:100–103.

97. Stange KC, Ferrer RL. The paradox of primary care. *Ann Fam Med*. 2009;7:293–299.

98. Foy R. Meta-analysis: effect of interactive communication between collaborating primary care physicians and specialists. *Ann Intern Med*. 2010;152:247.

99. Van Walraven C, Oake N, Jennings A, et al. The association between continuity of care and outcomes: a systematic and critical review. *J Eval Clin Pract*. 2010;16:947–956.

100. American Academy of Family Physicians; American Academy of Pediatrics; American College of Physicians; American Osteopathic Association. *Joint Principles of the Patient-Centered Medical Home*. 2007.

101. McColl MA, Shortt S, Godwin M, et al. Models for integrating rehabilitation and primary care: a scoping study. *Arch Phys Med Rehabil*. 2009;90:1523–1531.

102. Rasch EK, Gulley SP, Chan L. Use of emergency departments among working age adults with disabilities: a problem of access and service needs. *Health Serv Res*. 2013;48:1334–1358.

103. National Disability Navigator Resource Collaborative. *Preserve the Protections Provided by the Affordable Care Act*. 2017. Available from: https://nationaldisabilitynavigator.org/wp-content/uploads/Materials/NDNRC-Statement_Preserve-ACA-Protections_Nov-2016.pdf. Accessed May 7, 2017.

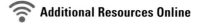 **Additional Resources Online**

CHAPTER **12**

Daniel E. Rohe
Thida Han

Psychological Aspects of Rehabilitation

This chapter reviews the history and current status of rehabilitation psychology. This is followed by a description of the direct and indirect services provided by rehabilitation psychologists. Frequently used psychological measures are described, and their importance for rehabilitation planning is explained. The final section examines theories of adjustment to disability.

REHABILITATION PSYCHOLOGY: HISTORY AND CURRENT STATUS

History

Rehabilitation psychology focuses on the study and application of psychological knowledge and skills on behalf of individuals with disabilities and chronic health conditions to maximize health and welfare, independence and choice, functional abilities, and social role participation (1). The field of rehabilitation psychology received initial impetus from veterans returning from the world wars in the first half of the last century. After World War II, the Veterans Administration focused on the psychological needs of the physically disabled, which led to the acceptance of psychologists as mental health providers. During this time, occupational therapy, physical therapy, and physical medicine and rehabilitation also became established disciplines. Thus, the birth and maturation of the disciplines constituting the rehabilitation team have overlapping histories (2).

As the number of psychologists working in rehabilitation settings grew, the need for a professional forum arose, and the Division of Rehabilitation Psychology was created within the American Psychological Association (APA) in 1958.

Rehabilitation psychology is unique by having value-based assumptions and beliefs that define the specialty. The "value-laden beliefs and principles" of rehabilitation psychology capture "the distinctive character of rehabilitation as a movement and philosophy" (3). These beliefs and principles are described in (4). Recently, the 20 value-laden beliefs were consolidated into 6 core Foundational Principles that are described

in **Table 12-1** (5). These Foundational Principles have made rehabilitation psychology the dynamic, person-centered, social justice–affirming, science-based psychological specialty that it is (4,6). The value-laden beliefs and principles were visionary and presaged the disability rights movement, the independent living movement, and participant action research.

Current Status

Rehabilitation psychologists have struggled with their identity since the field's inception, and a comprehensive review of the field's development is described by Sherwin (2).

Rehabilitation psychologists typically have doctoral degrees in clinical or counseling psychology. The training and credentialing of rehabilitation psychologists has changed dramatically over the past 20 years due to three factors.

First, the APA adopted a model of education in which the graduate-level curriculum is generic, with specialization occurring at the postdoctoral level. The Division of Rehabilitation Psychology published guidelines for postdoctoral training in rehabilitation psychology in 1995 (7). In 2007, Stiers and Stucky (8) described the need for a standardized curriculum and program evaluation tools. This led to the "Baltimore Conference" in 2012, which developed consensus guidelines for the structure and process of rehabilitation psychology postdoctoral training programs. Currently, there are 15 officially recognized programs (9,10).

The second major factor was establishment of the American Board of Rehabilitation Psychology (ABRP; www.abrp.org) in 1995. The ABRP is a member board of the American Board of Professional Psychology (ABPP), an organization of psychologists that accredits subspecialties. The ABRP provides a comprehensive rationale for specialty definition and competency-based practice standards (11,12). These standards include foundational competencies (generic to all doctoral level psychologists) and functional competencies unique to the field of rehabilitation psychology. The foundational competencies include the domains of interpersonal interactions, individual and cultural diversity, ethical and legal foundations,

TABLE 12-1	Foundational Principles of Rehabilitation Psychology
The Person-Environment Relation	Attributions about people with disabilities tend to focus on presumed dispositional rather than available situational characteristics. Environmental constraints usually matter more than personality factors to living with a disability.
The Insider-Outsider Distinction	People with disabilities (insiders) know what life with a chronic condition is like (e.g., sometimes challenging but usually manageable) whereas casual observers (outsiders) who lack relevant experience presume that disability is defining, all encompassing, and decidedly negative.
Adjustment to Disability	Coping with a disability or chronic illness is an ongoing dynamic process, one dependent on making constructive changes to the social and the physical environment.
Psychosocial Assets	People with disabilities possess or can acquire personal or psychological qualities that can ameliorate challenges posed by disability and also enrich daily living.
Self-Perception of Bodily States	Experience of bodily states (e.g., pain, fatigue, distress) is based on people's perception of the phenomenon, not exclusively the actual sensations. Changing attitudes, expectations, or environmental conditions can constructively alter perceptions.
Human Dignity	Regardless of the source or severity of a disability or chronic health condition, all people deserve respect, encouragement, and to be treated with dignity.

Reprinted with permission from Dunn DS, Ehde DM, Wegener ST. The foundational principles as psychological lodestars: theoretical inspiration and empirical direction in rehabilitation psychology. *Rehabil Psychol.* 2016;61:1–6.

and professional identification. The functional competencies include the domains of assessment, intervention, consultation, consumer protection, and professional development (13). Board certification requires postdoctoral training in rehabilitation psychology and 3 years of relevant experience.

The third major factor was certification of rehabilitation psychology as a specialty by the APA Commission for the Recognition of Specialties and Proficiencies in Professional Psychology (CRSPPP) in 2015 (http://www.apa.org/ed/graduate/specialize/rehabilitation.aspx). Specialty recognition by the APA was a major milestone that enabled rehabilitation psychologists to solidify their unique professional identity. In summary, the three recent developments of clearly defined training standards, board certification, and specialty recognition provide a platform for continued growth and evolution of the field of rehabilitation psychology.

Paralleling the growth of the field of rehabilitation psychology has been a paradigm shift by the World Health Organization and the National Institute on Disability, Independent Living, and Rehabilitation Research from a biomedical to a social model of disability. This paradigm shift aligns with and reinforces the "foundational principles" of rehabilitation psychology (14).

The direct and indirect services described in the following section reflect services typically found within an inpatient medical rehabilitation setting. Similar services are provided in outpatient settings. As service delivery shifts to outpatient, community, telehealth, and critical care settings, adaptations in these services continue to evolve (15,16). The 2011 World Report on Disability highlights the relevance of rehabilitation psychology in addressing the needs of the disabled (17). The value of rehabilitation psychology services is acknowledged by the Commission on the Accreditation of Rehabilitation Facilities through their mandated availability of the rehabilitation psychologist as part of the rehabilitation team in both acute and subacute rehabilitation facilities. Rehabilitation psychology's focus on enhancing the quality of life for those with chronic health conditions and disability remains the central goal despite changes in health care delivery. Eventually, the health care system will include universal coverage with a focus on prevention, multidisciplinary health care team communication, and measuring outcomes (18).

DIRECT SERVICES

The Clinical Interview

The psychologist's first contact with a patient is pivotal in the development of a therapeutic relationship. This may occur before transfer to a rehabilitation unit, as rehabilitation psychologists are beginning to intervene in critical care units prior to transfer (15,19,20). The patient's expectations of meeting with the psychologist are determined by previous exposure to mental health professionals and communication from other team members, especially the physician. During the introduction, the psychologist will explain that comprehensive rehabilitation includes help with problematic thoughts and feelings associated with chronic illness or the onset of disability. Frequently, patients are relieved to discover that contact with the psychologist is a routine part of comprehensive rehabilitation.

The initial interview may last an hour or more. Patients with cognitive impairment may be seen only long enough for a general determination of their information-processing capacity and emotional state. Further assessment will await improvement in their cognitive status or contact with an informed family member. The length of the initial interview with non–cognitively impaired patients depends on the complexity of the medical or social issues. There are two major goals for the initial interview. First, a comprehensive history of the patient's social background is obtained. **Box 12-1** lists frequently asked biographical questions. These data provide insight into previous learning experiences that may affect rehabilitation-related attitudes and behaviors. Second, the psychologist attempts to understand the disability as the patient sees it, with the most critical question being "what is the meaning of the disability for the patient and his or her life?" As the U.S. population becomes older and more diverse, understanding the meaning of disability through the unique cultural background of the patient is imperative (21,22). The foundation for a meaningful therapeutic relationship is laid by taking sufficient time to elicit the patient's perspective.

Patients often face a medical situation that they do not fully comprehend. Rehabilitation psychologists spend a significant

---

BOX 12-1

Psychosocial Information Sought During Initial Interview

- Data on family of origin
- Names, ages, occupations, marital status, and residence of parents and siblings
- Religious training
- Stability of family during early development
- History of major mental disorder in immediate and extended family, including any history of sexual abuse, chemical dependency, suicide, or psychiatric hospitalization
- Relevant patient information
- Educational background and school achievement
- Occupation and vocational history
- Avocational activities and hobbies
- History of adjustment to structured environments, such as school, work, and military service
- Social adjustment, including any previous arrests, chemical dependency treatment, or psychiatric diagnosis
- Prior association with hospitals and health care
- Preinjury stresses at the time of injury
- Most difficult loss the patient has had to adjust to previously; success in that task
- Prior associations with people who have a disability
- Family Structure
- Names, ages, and quality of relationship with spouse and children
- Background of dating and sexual relationship with current spouse
- Marital adjustment
- Understanding the patient's perspective
- The patient's understanding of the cause and probable course of the disability
- The patient's initial thoughts at the onset of the disability (if traumatic)
- The patient's most pressing immediate concern
- How well the patient thinks he or she is coping with the situation
- The patient's perception of how the disability will change lifestyle, including relationships, vocational future, and self-concept
- The patient's understanding of the behavioral expectations in the rehabilitation unit compared with those in the acute care unit of the hospital
- The degree to which the patient's sense of self-esteem or employment is related to physique or physical skills
- The patient's comfort in meeting with a psychologist
- Techniques used to cope with stressful events in the past
- Techniques used to get and maintain a sense of control over the environment

---

amount of time providing psychoeducation to the patients to help them understand their medical condition and its implications for their future (23–25). Anxiety and fear often block communication between the patient and the rehabilitation team. The opportunity to have one's perspective, including cognitive and emotional aspects, aired in a supportive and clarifying manner is uniquely therapeutic.

The rehabilitation psychologist occupies a difficult role. Although a team member, the psychologist has a professional responsibility to maintain the confidentiality of the therapeutic relationship. The patient may confide information that is personally sensitive and inappropriate to share with other team members. If directly asked by other team members about such information, the psychologist may need to explain that the information is confidential. General information of a less sensitive nature is provided in the form of an initial interview note. Subsequent therapeutic contacts are reported in the medical chart. The frequency of these contacts depends on therapeutic goals, psychological distress, the potential for behavioral decompensation, team members' concerns, and staffing levels.

Standardized Assessment

Given the time-consuming and subjective nature of clinical interviews, standardized tests are used by rehabilitation psychologists to speed assessment and enhance interventions (26). Frequently used instruments for the measurement of personality, mood, intellectual ability, and academic achievement are discussed. The domains of neuropsychological and substance use assessments are covered in more detail.

Personality

A personality test refers to a measure of personal characteristics and may include emotional status, interpersonal relations, motivation, interests, and attitudes. Personality measurement has generated controversy over two issues. The first concerns the stability of personality traits across situations as opposed to the situational specificity of behavior (27). The second issue involves the degree to which a given personality characteristic reflects a transitory state rather than a stable underlying trait. Johnson-Greene and Touradji (28) review the role of personality in rehabilitation outcomes and adjustment to disability. The most frequently used personality inventory designed to measure psychopathology is the Minnesota Multiphasic Personality Inventory-2 (MMPI-2), also available as the Restructured Form (MMPI-2-RF). A second measure is the Personality Assessment Inventory (PAI). Two measures of nonpathologic or "normal" personality that are relevant to rehabilitation are the NEO Personality Inventory 3 (NEO-PI-3) and the Strong Interest Inventory (SII).

Minnesota Multiphasic Personality Inventory-2

The MMPI-2 is the revised version of the MMPI; the most widely used and thoroughly researched objective measure of personality (29–31). The MMPI-2 is composed of statements describing thoughts, feelings, ideas, attitudes, physical and emotional symptoms, and previous life experiences. The MMPI-2 was originally designed to yield information about personality factors related to the major psychiatric syndromes. The 567 true-false questions are grouped into 10 clinical scales (📶 eTable 12-1) that reflect important aspects of personality despite their obsolete psychiatric titles. The items composing each scale were determined statistically. An item was included only if a carefully diagnosed group of patients (e.g., those with depression) answered that question in a manner statistically different from that of other carefully diagnosed groups of patients (e.g., those with schizophrenia) and from the normal standardization sample.

The 10 clinical scales are interpreted with the aid of four validity scales (see 📶 eTable 12-1) that provide information on the client's response style such as literacy, cooperation, malingering, comprehension, and defensiveness. There are special scales to help predict rehabilitation motivation, headache proneness, and tendencies toward the development of alcoholism. Additionally, there are norms on persons with diagnoses such as multiple sclerosis and spinal cord injury (SCI) (32). Norms are reported as standard scores with a mean of 50 and a standard deviation of 10. A score of 65 or greater is the point at which the normal and the pathologic groups are most reliably discriminated.

The MMPI-2 requires an eighth-grade reading level and is intended for adults 18 years of age and older. A version of the MMPI entitled the MMPI-A is intended for use with adolescents (33). The MMPI-2 requires about 90 minutes to complete. Although many computerized scoring services are available, this does not obviate the need for interpretation by an experienced psychologist. A variety of factors—including race, socioeconomic status, unique family circumstances, ethnic background, and physical disability—may distort the MMPI-2 profile (34). Appropriate interpretation of the MMPI-2 with medical and rehabilitation patients requires knowledge of these normative biases (35).

Minnesota Multiphasic Personality Inventory-2 Restructured Form

The MMPI-2-RF represents the continuing evolution of the MMPI (36). The original 10 MMPI clinical scales were problematic because of their intercorrelations, item overlap, and heterogeneous item content. To address these problems, a set of nine Restructured Clinical Scales (RCS) was derived (🛜 eTable 12-2) by identifying the major distinctive "core" components of each clinical scale. Tellegen et al. (37) provided data documenting the improved psychometric properties of the RCS that included improved reliability, reduced scale intercorrelations, and improved convergent and discriminant validity. Once the RCS were devised, 23 additional specific problem scales were constructed with titles such as malaise, suicidal/death ideation, anger proneness, substance abuse, shyness, and ideas of persecution. The MMPI-2-RF has a total of 8 validity scales and 3 higher order scales, entitled emotional/internalizing dysfunction, thought dysfunction, and behavioral/externalizing dysfunction. The MMPI-2-RF contains 338 items, requires 35 to 50 minutes to complete, and is written at a sixth-grade reading level.

Personality Assessment Inventory

The PAI (38) is a 344-item self-report inventory that assesses multiple domains of personality and psychopathology in adults. Items are answered on a 4-point Likert scale: *very true*; *mainly true*; *slightly true*; and *false, not at all true*. The PAI is suitable for individuals aged 18 and older who have at least a fourth-grade reading level. The test requires 50 to 60 minutes to complete.

The strengths of the PAI are numerous. First, the theory-driven, construct validation approach used in scale development and item selection is outstanding. Scales were designed to reflect both the breadth and depth of the mood or personality characteristic being measured. Second, the PAI meets and surpasses accepted reliability and validity test construction standards. Third, the clinical and nonclinical normative sampling was carefully conducted and is representative of the U.S. population. Finally, a significant number of scales are directly relevant to rehabilitation populations, including

those reflective of mood states (Anxiety, Depression, Mania), bodily states (Somatic Complaints), behavioral characteristics (Borderline Features, Antisocial Features) and substance abuse (Alcohol Problems, Drug Problems). The PAI is widely used because of its theoretical construction, low reading level, brevity, excellent psychometric properties, robust norming, clinical utility, and developing research base.

NEO Personality Inventory 3

The NEO-PI-3 reflects the culmination of decades of personality research that concludes that personality traits can be summarized by five factors termed the "five-factor model" (39,40). The NEO-PI-3 was designed to measure the five factors: Neuroticism, Extraversion, Openness, Agreeableness, and Conscientiousness. Each factor scale has six facet scales. Neuroticism refers to a propensity to experience negative affect such as anxiety, anger, and depression. This domain reflects self-consciousness, poor coping, irrational ideas, feelings of vulnerability, and difficulties controlling urges. Extraversion relates to interpersonal warmth, gregariousness, assertiveness, activity, excitement seeking, and the tendency to experience positive emotions. Openness pertains to depth of imagination, aesthetic sensitivity, intensity of feelings, preference for variety, intellectual curiosity, and independence in judgment. Agreeableness includes the characteristics of trust, straightforwardness, altruism, methods of handling interpersonal conflict, humbleness, and sympathy for others. Finally, conscientiousness encompasses competence, organization, reliability, achievement striving, self-discipline, and deliberation before acting.

The scale's 240 items are rated on a 5-point continuum from "strongly disagree" to "strongly agree." The inventory can now be used with persons 12 years of age and older. Separate norms are available for adolescents (age 12 to 20) and adults (age 21 and older). The inventory requires a fifth-grade reading level and 30 to 40 minutes for completion. The NEO-PI-3 has a self-report (Form S) and an observer rating form (Form R). This dual-form feature is unique among personality measures and is especially relevant to rehabilitation research. Also noteworthy, the NEO-PI-3 items do not contain references to physical abilities or sensations that could distort a physically disabled subject's responses.

There are two limitations to the NEO-PI-3. It assumes an honest respondent; no subtle items or validity scales are provided. In addition, while the inventory is intended to measure stable personality characteristics (traits), when completed in a state of unusual distress the results may partially reflect a transitory mood (state).

The NEO-PI-3 and its previous versions have been used extensively in research. The Web site www.parinc.com features a bibliography of over 2,500 studies using the instrument. This research has included participants from a wide variety of disabilities and chronic health conditions including burns, chronic pain, myocardial infarction, systemic lupus erythematosus, multiple sclerosis, diabetes, chronic fatigue, cancer, traumatic brain injury (TBI), and SCI. For example, Rohe and Krause administered the NEO-PI-R to males with traumatic SCI 16 years after injury (41). The subjects scored lower on the scales of conscientiousness, assertiveness, and activity, and higher on the scales of excitement seeking and fantasy. These results had negative implications for adherence to rehabilitation regimens but positive implications for long-term coping. A subsequent study discovered that elevated scores on the depression scale were associated with poorer adjustment, whereas elevated scores on the scales of warmth and positive emotions were associated with superior outcomes (42).

The Strong Interest Inventory

The SII is traditionally considered a measure of vocational interests; however, research has supported its use as a measure of personality (43). The SII is one of the most thoroughly researched, highly respected, and frequently used psychological tests. The SII asks the respondent to indicate his or her level of interest on a 5-point Likert scale ranging from "strongly like" to "strongly dislike" for occupations, subject areas, activities, leisure activities, and people. The last section asks the respondent to rate his or her possession of nine personal characteristics. The test requires 35 to 40 minutes to complete and is written at an eighth- to ninth-grade reading level (44).

The General Occupational Themes, one of the four types of scales on the SII, are based on trait theory as derived by Holland (45). Holland drew on factor-analytic studies of personality and interests to produce a typology of six basic personality types. These types are titled realistic, investigative, artistic, social, enterprising, and conventional. Rohe and Athelstan administered the SII to a national sample of persons with SCI (46). Contrary to previous research, they found unique personality characteristics associated with persons having SCI of traumatic onset. These characteristics included an interest in activities requiring physical interaction with things, such as machinery, and a disinterest in activities that require intense or complex interaction with either data or people. Malec used the Eysenck Personality Inventory with people having SCI of traumatic onset and discovered a pattern of personality characteristics congruent with that found in Rohe and Athelstan's study (47).

Rohe's review of the literature suggested that when a disability is of traumatic onset and secondary to the individual's behavior, statements in the literature about the lack of a relationship between disability and personality characteristics appear to be inaccurate (48). He noted that the previous literature either used pathology-oriented measures (e.g., MMPI) or studied individuals whose disability was not the result of trauma associated with their behavior. An additional study sought to determine whether those personality characteristics associated with people having SCI would change after years of living with the disability. The data indicated that personality characteristics remained constant over an average of 10 years (49). Rohe and Krause conducted a follow-up study to the aforementioned personality stability study. They found that males with traumatic SCI displayed marked consistency in personality characteristics over an 11-year follow-up period (50).

The MMPI-2, MMPI-2-RF, PAI, NEO-PI-3, and SII represent five measures of personality relevant to clinical rehabilitation settings that can help answer diagnostic and management questions. For example, a patient's willingness to comply with medical interventions or the hospital environment may be discerned through the use of personality measures. Knowledge of personality characteristics can help prevent ill-advised interventions and maximize patient compliance in the treatment environment.

Mood

Problematic mood in patients is one of the most common concerns among rehabilitation team members and a frequent reason for psychological assessment. While some change in mood is expected with adjustment to injury, the presence of severe mood symptoms can interfere with a patient's ability to participate in his or her rehabilitation program. Depression is an imprecise term used to describe an affective state that ranges from "being down" to major depressive disorder (MDD). The incidence and prevalence of MDD in rehabilitation populations has been the focus of significant research and debate. Assessing depression immediately after disability onset is complicated by such medical and environmental factors as sleep disruption, pain, and decreased appetite. A rehabilitation psychologist can assist the treatment team using assessment and clinical interview to differentiate between mood changes related to adjustment and those that indicate the presence of clinically significant depression or anxiety. Three brief and psychometrically robust screening instruments that are helpful in rehabilitation settings include the Patient Health Questionnaire-9 (PHQ-9) (51), the Beck Depression Inventory–Fast Screen (BDI-FS) to assess symptoms of depression, and the Generalized Anxiety Disorder-7 (GAD-7) to assess symptoms of anxiety. The PHQ-9 and the GAD-7 were developed and validated in health care settings. Anxiety and depressive disorders have high comorbidity but are distinct entities; thus, both types of measures are needed to effectively identify patients who would benefit from treatment (52). Early identification and treatment of these mood symptoms can help patients in rehabilitation to maximize their recovery. The PHQ-9 and the GAD-7 are free, are translated into multiple languages, and can be downloaded on the PHQ Web site (www.phqscreeners.com).

Patient Health Questionnaire-9

The PHQ-9 is a brief measure that asks patients to indicate how often they have been bothered by nine symptoms of depression over the past 2 weeks (**Box 12-2**). Each of the nine items is marked on a scale of 0, 1, 2, or 3 based on frequency of these symptoms. The total score ranges from 0 to 27. A cut-point of 10 is recommended to draw attention to a condition that may be clinically significant and would warrant further evaluation. Severity of depressive symptoms can further be classified as mild (5–9), moderate (10–14), moderately severe (15–19), or severe (20–27). This measure is sensitive to change over time (53). The PHQ-9 was developed for medical patients with high rates of nonspecific physical symptoms. Since the PHQ-9 contains somatic items that might confound accurate diagnosis, it is necessary that the clinician review the responses to ensure that any positive somatic responses are not due to medically based symptoms or normal bereavement. The PHQ-9 is a helpful instrument for detecting depressive symptoms in rehabilitation populations (54,55).

Beck Depression Inventory–Fast Screen for Medical Patients

The BDI-FS for medical patients (56) is a self-report inventory that screens for depression in adults and adolescents. The items were extracted from the original 21-item Beck Depression Inventory-II (57) and focus on the cognitive and affective components of depression, systematically excluding the somatically

---

BOX 12-2

PHQ-9 Items

Over the *last 2 weeks*, how often have you been bothered by any of the following problems?

Response options: (0) not at all, (1) several days, (2) more than half the days, (3) nearly every day

1. Little interest or pleasure in doing things
2. Feeling down, depressed, or hopeless
3. Trouble falling or staying asleep, or sleeping too much
4. Feeling tired or having little energy
5. Poor appetite or overeating
6. Feeling bad about yourself—or that you are a failure or have let yourself or your family down
7. Trouble concentrating on things, such as reading the newspaper or watching television
8. Moving or speaking so slowly that other people could have noticed? Or the opposite—being so fidgety or restless that you have been moving around a lot more than usual
9. Thoughts that you would be better off dead or of hurting yourself in some way

---

Developed by Drs. Robert L. Spitzer, Janet B.W. Williams, Kurt Kroenke and colleagues, with an educational grant from Pfizer Inc. No permission required to reproduce, translate, display, or distribute.

focused items. The BDI-FS consists of seven groups of four statements that focus on sadness, pessimism, past failure, loss of pleasure, self-dislike, self-criticalness, and suicidal thoughts. A score of 4 falls in the mildly depressed range while a score of 8 is average for persons with MDD. The inventory requires 5 minutes to complete and has acceptable reliability and validity data. The correlation between the 7-item and the 21-item inventories is 0.91. Research has supported its use in persons with multiple sclerosis (58) and stroke (59).

Generalized Anxiety Disorder-7

The GAD-7 is a 7-item screening measure for common anxiety symptoms. Items on the GAD-7 were based on the DSM-IV criteria for generalized anxiety (**Box 12-3**) (52). The GAD-7 has good sensitivity and specificity as a screening measure for panic disorder, social anxiety, and posttraumatic stress disorder (60). Items are marked 0, 1, 2, or 3 based on how frequently the patient has been bothered by each symptom. The resulting total score ranges from 0 to 21. Patients who score

---

BOX 12-3

GAD-7 Items

Over the *last 2 weeks*, how often have you been bothered by the following problems?

Response options: (0) not at all, (1) several days, (2) more than half the days, (3) nearly every day

1. Feeling nervous, anxious, or on edge
2. Not being able to stop or control worrying
3. Worrying too much about different things
4. Trouble relaxing
5. Being so restless that it is hard to stay still
6. Becoming easily annoyed or irritable
7. Feeling afraid as if something awful might happen

Developed by Drs. Robert L. Spitzer, Janet B.W. Williams, Kurt Kroenke and colleagues, with an educational grant from Pfizer Inc. No permission required to reproduce, translate, display, or distribute.

over 10 are experiencing clinically significant levels of anxiety, and further evaluation is warranted. Cut points of 5, 10, and 15 can also be used to identify mild, moderate, and severe levels of anxiety, respectively. The GAD-7 has been utilized in rehabilitation populations, including individuals with multiple sclerosis (61).

Intellectual Ability

Intellectual ability tests provide a summary score that serves as a global index of a person's general problem-solving ability, frequently referred to as an IQ or intellectual quotient score. This summary score is validated against a broad criterion such as scholastic achievement or occupational success. Although such tests are constructed of a number of subtests that sample facets of intellectual functioning, they are usually weighted toward tasks requiring verbal ability. The most frequently encountered measure of intellectual ability is the Wechsler Adult Intelligence Scale, IV (WAIS-IV) (62).

Wechsler Adult Intelligence Scale, IV

The WAIS-IV is the fourth edition of the WAIS, a test of intelligence and cognitive abilities that requires 60 to 90 minutes to complete and must be administered by a trained examiner. The large normative sample ranges from ages 16 to 90, and is stratified by gender, race/ethnicity, educational level, and region of the country (63). The WAIS-IV consists of 15 subtests, 10 of which are core subtests used in the calculation of a composite score. The 5 supplemental subtests can be used to broaden the range of cognitive skills sampled and substituted for core subtests when clinically indicated. 📶 eTable 12-3 lists these subtests and what they measure in order of administration. All WAIS-IV subtest scores are corrected for age and standardized with a mean of 10 and a standard deviation of 3. The test exceeds all standards of reliability and validity and correlates highly with other measures of cognitive ability.

The WAIS-IV subtests are organized into four index scales: Verbal Comprehension Index (VCI), Perceptual Reasoning Index (PRI), Working Memory Index (WMI), and Processing Speed Index (PSI). The index scores are derived using core subtest scores within that scale. As with the traditional IQ scores, index scores have a mean of 100 and a standard deviation of 15. Each index score also contributes to the Full Scale IQ (FSIQ), a measure of general intellectual ability.

In addition to the five composite scores, the General Ability Index (GAI), which is derived using only sum of scaled scores from the Verbal Comprehension and Perceptual Reasoning subtests, is available as an optional composite score on the WAIS-IV. The GAI can provide a summary score that is less sensitive to the influence of working memory and processing speed. This can be useful in the presence of neuropsychological deficits, where performances in these domains are more likely to be impaired. In general, the FSIQ is considered the most valid measure of overall cognitive ability, as working memory and processing speed are vital components in a comprehensive evaluation of cognitive ability.

Compared to earlier versions of the test, the WAIS-IV uses larger visual stimuli, reduced vocabulary level of verbal instructions, decreased administration time, more teaching items to ensure understanding of tasks, and less emphasis on motor demands or time bonus points awarded for shorter completion. These changes are ideal for assessing older patients and those with sensory and motor impairments.

TABLE 12-2	IQ Score, Percentile Ranges, and Classifications for the Wechsler Adult Intelligence Scale	
IQ Score	**Percentile Range**	**Classification**
130 and above	98 or greater	Very superior
120–129	91–97	Superior
110–119	74–89	High average
90–109	25–73	Average
80–89	9–23	Low average
70–79	2–8	Borderline
69 and below	<2	Extremely low

Given the emotional significance of IQ scores, psychologists usually convert both IQ scores and discussions about them into either percentiles or classifications (**Table 12-2**). When the physician is confronted with questions about test results from patients, the use of either percentiles or classifications is recommended. Measures of intellectual ability help the physiatrist set appropriate expectations about the rate and complexity of learning legitimately expected from the patient. They also serve as the cornerstone for determining the presence of organic brain dysfunction and provide guidance for postdismissal vocational planning.

Academic Achievement

A frequently overlooked but nonetheless important factor within rehabilitation settings is academic achievement. Reading and mathematics achievement are of particular concern not only during inpatient rehabilitation but also for longer-range educational and vocational planning. The patient's reading level is a potential limiting factor in tasks ranging from filling out hospital menus to incorporating ideas presented in patient education materials. The average reading level in the United States is at the sixth grade, the level required to read a newspaper. Patient education materials, however, often reflect the reading levels of the professionals who devise them. As the patients' reading level falls below the national average, progressively greater reliance on oral instruction and audiovisual materials becomes necessary. Patients are often expected to use mathematics when recording fluid intake and taking correct dosages of medications. Two frequently used measures of reading and mathematical achievement are the Wide Range Achievement Test-4 (WRAT-4) and the Woodcock-Johnson Psycho-Educational Battery-IV.

Wide Range Achievement Test-4

The WRAT-4 is the current edition of the WRAT (64). The test provides assessment of reading, spelling, and mathematics achievement by assessing correct word pronunciation, appropriately completing sentences with missing words, correct spelling, and basic math skills. The WRAT-4 can be administered to individuals ages 5 through 94. The entire test can be administered in 30 to 45 minutes, and results are presented in the form of standard scores, percentiles, stanines, grade equivalents, and Rasch ability scale scores. The WRAT-4 is reliable, and the stratified national sample of 3,000 individuals is representative of the U.S. population in terms of age, gender, ethnicity, geographic region, and educational attainment.

Woodcock-Johnson IV

The fourth edition of the Woodcock-Johnson (WJ-IV) was published in 2014 and consists of three distinct, co-normed batteries: Tests of Achievement, Tests of Cognitive Abilities, and Tests of Oral Language (65). The WJ-IV is designed to measure general intellectual ability, broad and narrow cognitive abilities based on the Cattell-Horn-Carroll theory of cognitive abilities (66), academic aptitudes, and academic knowledge. The three batteries may be used alone or in combination with tests and clusters from the other batteries (67). The current normative data were based on a nationally representative sample of 7,416 individuals ranging from 2 to over 90 years of age from geographically diverse communities. Alternate forms and options for evaluating Spanish speakers are also available. Simplified test administration and interpretation procedures help with assessment of individuals with disabilities.

In a rehabilitation setting, the WJ-IV Test of Achievement (68) can be particularly helpful for evaluations related to return to school or work. The battery is composed of 11 standard subtests and 9 extended subtests grouped into four broad curricular areas: reading, mathematics, writing, and academic knowledge. Five standard subtests are used to determine reading achievement: letter-word identification, passage comprehension, word attack, oral reading, and sentence reading fluency. The resulting score reflects basic or broad reading skills, reading comprehension, fluency, and rate. Mathematics achievement is based on three standard subtests: applied problems, calculation, and math fluency. Writing achievement is based on three standard subtests: spelling, writing samples, and sentence writing fluency. Achievement scores are reported in age- and grade-normed percentiles. The WJ-IV Test of Cognitive Abilities (69) can serve as an alternative to the WAIS-IV when a broad-based, well-constructed measure of intellectual ability is desired. A fluid-crystallized cognitive composite is available for comparison to other measures of academic achievement, linguistic competency, and cognitive processing to determine relative strengths and weaknesses across all domains. Finally, the WJ-IV Test of Oral Language (70) was developed to examine the influence of language on a student's academic and cognitive performance using tests from the previous cognitive and achievement batteries plus new tests that specifically measure narrow aspects of language. Several studies have demonstrated the WJ-IV scores to be correlated with other measures of cognitive abilities, oral language abilities, and academic achievement (71).

Neuropsychological Assessment

Individuals with cognitive dysfunction represent one of the largest groups receiving rehabilitation services. For many, the deficits are transient. For some, cognitive deficits are permanent and not only will complicate learning independent living skills but also determine future living arrangements, social interactions, and vocational prospects. In both situations, the rehabilitation psychologist or neuropsychologist is often asked to clarify the nature and type of cognitive deficits. This section describes five screening measures to evaluate cognitive status: Galveston Orientation and Amnesia Test (GOAT), Orientation Log (O-LOG), Montreal Cognitive Assessment (MoCA), Cognistat, and the Repeatable Battery for the Assessment of Neuropsychological Status (RBANS). Next, the structure and process of comprehensive neuropsychological assessment is described.

Screening Measures of Cognitive Status

The physician frequently encounters patients who may not benefit from an intensive rehabilitation program due to organic brain dysfunction. Screening measures of variable length enable the rehabilitation psychologist to rapidly evaluate the patient's cognitive status and communicate this information to the rehabilitation team.

The Galveston Orientation and Amnesia Test

The GOAT was developed by Levin et al. (72) and measures amnesia and disorientation after head injury. The scale consists of 10 questions that focus on temporal orientation, recall of biographical information, and memory of recent events. The final score is computed by subtracting the total number of error points from 100. The GOAT can be given at bedside to patients who are verbally responsive and comprehensible. This measure was standardized on a group of 50 young adults (median age 23) who had recovered from mild TBI, usually consisting of a momentary loss of consciousness. Scores below those received by members of the control group (≤65) are designated impaired, scores between 66 and 75 are designated borderline-abnormal, and those above 75 are considered normal. The greatest scoring difficulty occurs where points are assigned for the patient's accuracy in recalling events before trauma. The GOAT also provides an objective measurement of emergence from posttraumatic amnesia (PTA), as needed (73). Validity data for the GOAT were generated by comparing the length of PTA with the variables of initial neurologic impairment and scores on the Glasgow Outcome Scale. In both cases, the GOAT score discriminated according to the severity of head injury. Scaling recovery of cognitive function in the noncomatose patient permits meaningful discussion with the family and rehabilitation team members. Emergence from PTA is an important indicator that more comprehensive neuropsychological testing can be administered to assist with rehabilitation and postdischarge planning. The GOAT is less appropriate for individuals with nontraumatic brain injuries, as some questions pertain directly to the trauma. A modified multiple-choice version (the AGOAT) has been developed for aphasic individuals, so that impaired verbal expression does not confound the evaluation of disorientation or amnesia (74). On the AGOAT, a score of 90 corresponds to the standard GOAT cutoff of 75.

The Orientation Log

The Orientation Log is a quantitative measure of orientation that can be completed bedside in 3 to 15 minutes, depending on the amount of cueing required. The O-Log was developed to address some of the limitations of the GOAT and is appropriate for use with a variety of populations (e.g., TBI, CVA, tumor, infectious disease, and degenerative diseases). The test was normed on 90 individuals completing inpatient rehabilitation for mild-to-moderate or severe TBI, and has excellent interrater reliability and internal consistency in ABI populations (75). The O-Log can be used for serial assessment of orientation to document changes over time, with a graph available on the scoresheet. The measure consists of 10 questions that evaluate a patient's awareness of place, time, and situation. During administration of the O-Log, the evaluator is expected to cue at the next highest level when an incorrect response is provided. For questions that evaluate orientation to situation, the patient must demonstrate awareness that an event has taken place (e.g., motor vehicle accident, stroke, etc.) and the impact of that event (e.g., a brain injury was sustained). Total points range from 0 to 30. A score of 25 or greater represents normal orientation. The O-Log has been correlated with the GOAT and estimation of PTA duration in a TBI population (76,77). The measure is available free, and no equipment or specific training is required.

The Montreal Cognitive Assessment

The MoCA was the first brief screening measure specifically designed to detect mild cognitive impairment (MCI), an intermediary state between normal cognitive aging and dementia (78). Nasreddine et al. devised the MoCA to generate helpful information about cognitive domains frequently impacted in those with MCI in a minimum amount of time (79). The MoCA is a one-page, 30-point instrument that requires 10 minutes to administer. Tasks include five-item verbal learning and delay recall, clock drawing, cube copy, alphanumeric sequencing, phonemic fluency, verbal abstraction, sustained attention on a tapping task, serial subtraction, digits forwards and backwards, three-item confrontation naming, sentence repetition, and orientation to time and place. The MoCA was found to have high sensitivity and specificity for detecting MCI (80,81). It is available for free (www.mocatest.org) and has been translated into 17 languages. Persons scoring 26 or higher are in the nonimpaired range, 26 to 21 are in the MCI range, and below 21 are in the Alzheimer's disease range. The MoCA has much to offer the rehabilitation inpatient setting where rapid and reliable screening for subtle cognitive dysfunction is frequently requested.

The Cognistat

The Cognistat (82), formerly known as the Neurobehavioral Cognitive Status Exam, was developed to rapidly assess orientation, attention, language, construction (visuospatial), memory, calculation, and reasoning (executive function) abilities. The test is standardized for use with adolescents (12 to 17 years of age) and adults (18 to 84 years of age), and typically takes 15 to 30 minutes to administer depending on the level of impairment. The Cognistat employs a screen and metric approach in most domains. Test results are presented on a graphic profile that identifies whether performance in each domain falls in the average or impaired (mild, moderate, or severe) range. It can be used to screen for impairment in individual domains of cognitive function, as opposed to the overall summation score output by most cognitive screening measures (83). Several studies have supported the utility of the Cognistat with medical and neurologic populations (83–85), and performance during TBI inpatient rehabilitation has been significantly related to clinical outcomes 1 year after injury (86).

Several limitations of the Cognistat have been identified including limited normative data (87), ceiling effects, and low reliability in healthy, community-dwelling individuals (88), and tentative interpretation of performance is recommended for individuals with lower education (89). The scale profile is not useful for distinguishing between different types of dementias (90) or different locations of stroke (85). The measure may be relatively insensitive for detecting specific or subtle cognitive impairments after brain injury (88). Concerns have also been raised about the accuracy of the screen and metric approach, and administration of all metric items can decrease the likelihood of false negatives and provide a better estimate of cognitive functioning in individuals with CVA (87,91).

New computerized and online versions of the Cognistat were recently released, with improved features including guidance during testing, automatic scoring, creation of an electronic data record for longitudinal assessment, and data sharing among clinical groups. Two additional memory word lists are available to facilitate repeated testing. In addition, the examiner is asked to identify the presence of factors that could potentially influence test performance (e.g., sensory impairment, pain, mood symptoms, preexisting learning disorder, sleep, or CNS-active medications), to decrease the likelihood that examiners will arrive at a false-positive result. Other improvements include a 5-minute version of the test (Cognistat Five), a MCI index to reflect the risk of MCI and dementia, and availability of the test in 11 languages.

The Repeatable Battery for the Assessment of Neuropsychological Status

The RBANS is a brief battery that fills an important niche between brief screening measures of cognitive status and comprehensive neuropsychological assessment. The RBANS is an individually administered instrument that requires about 30 minutes to complete. The RBANS can be used for ages 12 to 89 and was normed on a stratified, nationally representative sample of healthy individuals (92). The 12 subtests are subdivided into five cognitive domains: immediate memory, visuospatial reasoning, language, attention, and delayed recall. A total scale score is also generated. Alternate forms and iPad-based administration are also available. The RBANS is useful for a broad-based but intermediate level of screening for cognitive deficits in acute care settings and for tracking improvements or declines in cognitive function over time.

Goals of Neuropsychological Assessment

The primary goal of the neuropsychological assessment is to describe brain-behavior relationships (93,94). In addition, there is increased focus on developing new methods for assessing rehabilitation potential, functional competence, and valid cognitive remediation procedures for patients with brain damage (95–99). For example, Sherer et al. (100) demonstrated how early brief cognitive assessment combined with severity of head injury indicators can more reliably predict long-term employment outcome. Miller and Donders (101) demonstrated that neuropsychological assessment during acute rehabilitation significantly improved the prediction of educational outcomes in children with TBI 2 years later. Unfortunately, most neuropsychological tests were designed with diagnosis, not prediction or remediation, as their major goal (102,103), and optimal prediction will require new approaches to the measurement of environments and careful attention to the ecologic validity of neuropsychological tests (102,104).

During inpatient rehabilitation, diagnosing the presence of brain damage is often of reduced importance as brain damage is frequently the reason for admission to the rehabilitation unit. Rehabilitation team members are more concerned with the degree to which the patient will be able to understand and profit from rehabilitation services or function in their home environments. Administration of a lengthy test battery may not be possible due to the recent onset of impairment, fatigue, or shortened lengths of stay in acute rehabilitation. In these cases, the rehabilitation psychologist may administer screening measures as described in the previous section to

inform the patient, family, and rehabilitation team about the patient's current cognitive functioning. These findings may be communicated during team rounds and/or in the medical record. Cognitive, behavioral, or emotional barriers to patient discharge may also be identified. A comprehensive battery of neuropsychological tests may be administered on an outpatient basis to more fully assess cognitive function for treatment planning and provide guidance on such issues as supervision, return to driving, and return to work. No single test can answer all questions about the patient's ability to function in complex environments; therefore, an experienced psychologist will select appropriate tests and interpret the findings in the context of the individual's history, behavioral presentation, and medical and psychological information.

The Structure and Process of Comprehensive Neuropsychological Assessment

In outpatient rehabilitation, there is no established standard for follow-up neuropsychological assessment, and it is determined based on individual need. Persons with acquired brain injury commonly undergo neuropsychological assessment 3 to 6 months after onset because issues of independence are often raised during that time (105). For persons who have sustained a TBI, repeat neuropsychological assessments may be suggested at 3 to 6 months, 1 year, and 2 years postinjury (106). Steps should be taken to minimize the likelihood of "practice effects," which can hinder the identification of improvement, by using alternate forms of a test, substituting equivalent tests, or lengthening the interval between evaluations (105). Comprehensive neuropsychological assessment includes a series of tests to assess a broad range of cognitive domains, to identify areas of strengths and weaknesses. Particular attention is paid to areas that are known to be impaired following the brain injury. The most common domains of cognition assessed after a brain injury are general intellectual functioning, attention, processing speed, language, memory, executive function, and psychomotor abilities (107). A brief overview follows.

General Intellectual Functioning. To understand the presence of cognitive impairment after a brain injury, the clinician must estimate the injured person's premorbid functioning for comparison (108). Tests of intellectual functioning are used to sample performance across a diverse range of mental functions, some of which are known to be resistant to the effects of injury. Tests of general intellectual functioning include the previously described WAIS-IV (62), the Wechsler Intelligence Scale for Children, Fifth Edition (WISC-V) (109), and the Wechsler Abbreviated Scale of Intelligence, Second Edition (WASI-II) (110).

Attention and Concentration. Attention is the process through which we receive and process information in our environment (111). Individuals whose attention is impaired may have difficulty focusing for long periods of time, ignoring distractions, completing tasks with multiple steps, or learning new information (107). There are several aspects of attention examined during neuropsychological testing, including orientation, concentration, sustained attention/vigilance, working memory, and divided attention. Commonly used measures include the Digit Span subtest of the WAIS-IV, Symbol Digit Modalities Test (SDMT) (112), Conner's Continuous Performance Test (113), and Trail Making Test—Part A (114).

Processing Speed. After a brain injury, individuals often have difficulties processing information as quickly as they could before (115). Individuals with reduced processing speed may have delayed reaction time or require additional time to complete tasks. Commonly used test of processing speed include Coding and Symbol Search subtests of the WAIS-IV (62), and the Paced Auditory Serial Attention Test (116).

Visuospatial Functioning. Visuospatial functioning describes a person's ability to process and interpret visual information about where objects are in space (117). Impaired visuospatial functioning can manifest in challenges interacting with a person's environment, resulting in clumsiness or issues with navigation. Commonly used tests of visuospatial functioning include Judgment of Line Orientation (118), Visual Form Discrimination (119), Hooper Visual Organization Test (HVOT) (120), and tasks of visual scanning.

Language. After a brain injury, individuals may have difficulties with verbal communication due to deficits in expressive or receptive language. This may include difficulty understanding conversations or instructions, maintaining conversation, finding words easily, and expressing their needs (107). Commonly used tests include the Boston Naming Test (121), Peabody Picture Vocabulary Test (122), Controlled Oral Word Association Test (COWAT) (123), Verbal Fluency (124), and Token Test (125).

Memory. Memory is a vital cognitive function, as impairments in this domain can result in dependency, isolation, and compromised safety. Individuals with memory deficits may have difficulties learning and retaining new information, which can affect attendance and compliance with medical treatment. Memory tests examine encoding, storage, and retrieval of visual and verbal (written or spoken) information. Commonly used tests of verbal memory include the Logical Memory subtest of the Wechsler Memory Scale, Fourth Edition (WMS-IV) (126), California Verbal Learning Test (CVLT-II) (127), Rey Auditory Verbal Learning Test (RAVLT) (128), and the Hopkins Verbal Learning Test—Revised (HVLT-R) (129). Commonly used tests of visual memory include the Visual Reproduction subtest of the WMS-IV (126), Brief Visuospatial Memory Test—Revised (BVMT-R) (130), and Rey-Osterrieth Complex Figure Test (131).

Executive Function. Executive function is the ability to "engage successfully in independent, purposive, self-serving behavior" (132) (p. 31). It is an umbrella term used to describe high-level cognitive processes, including planning and organization, inhibition, self-monitoring, reasoning, problem-solving, and cognitive flexibility (111). Impaired executive functions can affect all aspects of a person's ability to function effectively in his or her personal or vocational life. Commonly used measures of executive function include the Behavioral Dyscontrol Scale (BDS) (133), Behavioral Assessment of the Dysexecutive Syndrome (BADS) (134), Delis-Kaplan Executive Function System (DKEFS) (135), Trail Making Test—Part B, Category Test (114), Stroop Test (136) and Wisconsin Card Sorting Test (137).

Psychomotor Abilities. Individuals with impaired psychomotor abilities may struggle with tests that involve fine or gross motor skills, including dexterity, control, or coordination. Examining manual dexterity can also provide a quick assessment of the diffuseness of the brain injury based on differential performance of the dominant versus nondominant hand (107). Commonly used tests include the Grooved Pegboard Test (111), Purdue Pegboard Test (138), Grip Strength Test (111), and Finger-Tapping Test (111).

The above list of domains and tests is by no means exhaustive. Tests of symptom validity may be included, particularly when issues of secondary gain are present (139). Self-report tests of mood, personality, or neurobehavioral symptoms may also be administered. Many of the tests described above utilize more than one cognitive domain (for example, vision and motor abilities are typically used for any paper-and-pencil tasks), and different parts of the test or different scores may represent distinct abilities (117). Valid test interpretation requires a thoroughly trained psychologist. In addition to the quantitative information obtained from neuropsychological assessment, testing also yields valuable qualitative information. In the rehabilitation setting, this might include practical and functional improvements, or insights about the most effective methods to use for remediation of cognitive deficits. Given the current trend toward reduced lengths of inpatient rehabilitation, a common approach is to perform a brief assessment of cognitive function before discharge from inpatient rehabilitation and a comprehensive assessment in the weeks to months after discharge. This brief initial assessment provides a "benchmark" of current levels of cognition and can provide guidance about the amount of supervision needed for the patient. Although neuropsychological assessment has proved effective in detecting cognitive dysfunction (140), translating test results into ecologically valid rehabilitation recommendations has proved more elusive (102,141).

Assessment of Substance Use

Background

In 1985, Rohe and DePompolo identified the failure of rehabilitation professionals to address the issue of substance use among those with disabilities (142). Follow-up research found improved screening but continued poor staff training (143,144). Throughout this section, alcohol and drug abuse are considered jointly. The focus, however, is on alcohol, the more frequently abused substance. Bombardier and Turner reviewed alcohol and drug use in persons with disabilities (145). The recent epidemic of opioid abuse has further highlighted the necessity of including substance use assessment as a routine part of rehabilitation program.

The importance of alcohol screening is related to both the drug's impact on bodily functions and behavioral aberrations caused by its excessive use (146,147). In rehabilitation patients, alcohol ingestion may potentiate the action of prescribed medications intended to control blood clot formation and reduce spasticity, or act in an additive manner with muscle relaxants such as diazepam (Valium) and baclofen (Lioresal). Altered consciousness may result in reduced vigilance in health maintenance behaviors. If alcohol is ingested in the form of beer, the increased fluid volume could compromise a bladder retraining program.

The cognitive and behavioral aberrations associated with drug intoxication can also be related to the onset of a disability. Rohe and DePompolo noted that vehicular crashes and falls while intoxicated account for a large proportion of rehabilitation unit admissions (142). In a series of studies, Heinemann and colleagues found that 39% of their spinal cord–injured patients were intoxicated at injury onset (148) and drinking patterns persisted immediately post injury and long term (149). Corrigan's literature review found that roughly two thirds of head-injured patients have a history of substance abuse that precedes their injury, and alcohol intoxication is present in one third to one half of hospitalizations (150). Rivara et al. found that 47% of general trauma patients had a positive blood alcohol level and that 36% were intoxicated (151). The preceding research suggests that individuals admitted to rehabilitation units with traumatic CNS injuries are not a random sample of the drinking public. Assessment and intervention with this population represents an opportunity to reduce future medical, social, and personal costs. It has been argued that rehabilitation professionals, under scrutiny from third-party payers, cannot afford to have a significant proportion of their patients display poor long-term outcomes secondary to failure to address substance abuse (150).

The screening for substance abuse in all rehabilitation patients, especially those with trauma, must become a standard of care. Although one survey of rehabilitation unit administrators indicated that substance abuse screening has become common, Schmidt and Gavin found that only 4% of persons receiving initial TBI rehabilitation were screened for substance abuse (143,152). Thus, there is inconsistency between administrators' perception of the adequacy of chemical health screening occurring in their facilities versus actual practice. Unfortunately, staff training on this issue remains sorely lacking, with only 23% of rehabilitation unit administrators reporting that staff were provided education (143). Obtaining accessible substance abuse treatment for those with physical disabilities remains difficult (153). Perhaps the most overlooked substance abuse issue is screening and intervention for nicotine dependence in those with disabilities. Basford, Rohe, and DePompolo point out that rates of smoking may be higher in those with disabilities compared to the general population, and the health consequences in terms of lung function and wound healing may be particularly devastating to this population (143).

Screening for Chemical Dependency

The Center for Substance Abuse Prevention has indicated that individual attitudes about alcohol use are diverse, are strongly held, and determine the perception of another person's use (154). The two most frequent problems encountered during screening are viewing alcohol as a moral problem and using the interviewer's personal pattern of use as the standard for comparison. Important aspects of interviewing about alcohol use are (a) getting a detailed history; (b) demonstrating nonjudgmental acceptance; (c) asking direct, specific, and factual questions; (d) maintaining persistence; (e) never discussing alibis; and (f) titrating hostility (155). A promising approach to helping people change their alcohol use is through "motivational interviewing," a technique based on Prochaska's stages of change model and described later in the chapter (156,157). Two measures useful in assessing alcohol use are the CAGE Questionnaire and the Alcohol Use Disorders Identification Test (AUDIT).

The CAGE Questionnaire. The CAGE Questionnaire was developed on a sample of medical and surgical inpatients to find the least number of questions that would reliably identify those suffering from alcohol use disorder. The four CAGE questions are as follows:

1. Have you ever felt you ought to cut down on your drinking?
2. Have people annoyed you by criticizing your drinking?
3. Have you ever felt bad or guilty about your drinking?
4. Have you ever had a drink first thing in the morning to steady your nerves or to get rid of a hangover (i.e., an eye-opener)?

Ewing summarized the scale's development and data on four normative samples (158). A positive response to any of the questions raises the suspicion that alcohol use disorder is present. Two positive responses identified 97% of his alcoholic sample correctly, and only 4% of his nonalcoholic sample incorrectly. Three or more responses are clearly symptomatic of alcohol dependence. The sensitivity of the CAGE ranges from 60% to 95%, and its specificity ranges from 40% to 95% (159).

The Alcohol Use Disorders Identification Test. The AUDIT was developed by the World Health Organization to detect alcohol problems in primary medical care settings. The AUDIT consists of 10 multiple-choice questions examining alcohol consumption, drinking behaviors, and alcohol-related problems. The AUDIT requires 2 minutes to administer and 1 minute to score, with a recommended cutoff score of 8. Self-report and interview versions are both available. The measure can be freely downloaded from www.auditscreen.org in a variety of languages. Sensitivities are typically above 90%, with specificities in the 80% to 90% range (160).

In summary, the field of rehabilitation has yet to fulfill its responsibility in the screening and treatment of substance use disorders, particularly with alcohol and nicotine. Research data suggest that patients with traumatic CNS injuries have a high probability of alcohol abuse. Rehabilitation psychologists are a valuable resource in screening for substance use disorders. This intervention, early in the rehabilitation process, is a crucial aspect of the prevention of future medical complications. For example, Bombardier et al. studied individuals with recent SCI and TBI in the inpatient setting, and found that the majority of at-risk drinkers were considering changes in their alcohol use. Intervening shortly after the onset of disability can provide a window of opportunity to reduce postinjury alcohol abuse and related impairments (161,162).

Assessment of Patient-Reported Outcomes

The Patient-Reported Outcomes Measurement Information System

The Patient-Reported Outcomes Measurement Information System (PROMIS) was created by the National Institutes of Health (NIH) to improve the assessment of clinical outcomes (163). Valid, reliable, and generalizable patient outcome measures that also captured subjective aspects of the patient experience were desired. Using a multicenter research design, the NIH pursued an efficient, psychometrically robust, and publicly available system suitable for use with a wide range of chronic diseases and demographic characteristics (164). Investigators from the University of Washington ensured that accessibility issues were considered and tested throughout the stages of development (165). Phase II studies were funded from 2009 to 2014, incorporating longitudinal analyses, greater sociodemographic diversity, increased emphasis on pediatric populations, and evaluation of item banks for clinical research and population science (166).

Currently, the PROMIS system can be used to evaluate approximately 70 domains of physical, mental, and social health, including pain, sleep disturbance, sexual function, emotional distress, substance use, companionship, meaning and purpose, and ability to participate in social roles and activities (167). The PROMIS has been translated in over 40 languages and is suitable for adults and children, the general population, and those living with chronic conditions. The PROMIS provides several options for ease of administration, including paper measures available for download, electronic versions administered by computer or application item banks, short forms, and computer adaptive tests. Standardized scoring is available so that scores from different measures can be compared and interpreted. While PROMIS self-report measures were intended for independent completion, if respondents are unable to answer independently (i.e., young children, individuals with cognitive or physical impairment), a trusted individual can act as a "proxy."

Therapeutic Interventions

Cognitive Rehabilitation

"Cognitive rehabilitation" encompasses a broad range of interventions aimed at helping individuals whose cognition has been affected by an illness or injury to maximize their functioning through nonpharmacologic and nonsurgical interventions (168,169). Surveys of rehabilitation facilities in North America reveal that cognitive rehabilitation is a component of treatment for acquired brain injury treatment in most, if not all, facilities (170,171). While a comprehensive history of the field is beyond the scope of this chapter, pioneers in the field have published several resources on the history (170,172,173) and specific approaches (174–176) to cognitive rehabilitation. In inpatient and outpatient rehabilitation settings, cognitive rehabilitation may be implemented with the patient by an occupational therapist, speech-language pathologist, or rehabilitation psychologist (177). Broadly, cognitive rehabilitation practices fall into two categories. Remediation approaches aim to restore lost or impaired abilities. Compensation approaches focus on adaptation, teaching ways to "work around" a residual weakness by changing an individual's environment, approach to a task, or behavior. Often, use of both remediation and compensation strategies are utilized to maximize the functionality that can be achieved (178–180).

Since the field of cognitive rehabilitation was largely developed based on "expert opinion," there have been growing demands for scientifically based evidence supporting the effectiveness of cognitive rehabilitation (95,181). In response, several large-scale meta-analytic reviews have been conducted, with particular focus on prospective randomized controlled trials. The first comprehensive review was published in 1998 and based on the NIH Consensus Conference on Rehabilitation of Persons with TBI. This review found few rigorous studies on the effectiveness of cognitive rehabilitation, and that most studies were heterogeneous in terms of their subjects, study designs, and outcomes. Some evidence did support the use of compensatory strategies, such as memory books. Effective interventions typically (a) were structured, systematic, goal directed, and individualized and (b) involved learning, practice, social contact, and a relevant context (182). The National Institutes on Disability and Rehabilitation Research (NIDRR) commissioned a review of the literature from 1998 to 2004 to describe the "state of the science." The panel found evidence supporting the effectiveness of comprehensive holistic cognitive rehabilitation and specific neuropsychological interventions for deficits in memory, attention, and executive functioning (183).

The Brain Injury Interdisciplinary Special Interest Group (BI-ISIG) of the American Congress of Rehabilitation Medicine (ACRM) also formed the Cognitive Rehabilitation Task Force to advance the field through evidence-based reviews and develop recommendations for clinical practice. This multidisciplinary group has written a total of three evidence-based reviews that have collectively reviewed the literature through 2008 (95,181,184). Three levels of recommendations were described: Practice Standards, Practice Guidelines, and Practice Options. Practice Standards are based on the strongest body of evidence and are outlined in **Table 12-3**. Practice Guidelines and Practice Options were written for interventions that may be helpful but are based on less evidence. The ACRM BI-ISIG group has published the Cognitive Rehabilitation Manual (185) and offers training workshops to help interdisciplinary rehabilitation professionals implement evidence-based interventions for impairments of attention, memory, executive functions, hemispatial neglect, and social communication.

Concomitantly, the Institute of Medicine (IOM) was commissioned by the Department of Defense (DoD) to evaluate cognitive rehabilitation therapy for implementation with veterans with TBI. The IOM report, Cognitive Rehabilitation Therapy for Traumatic Brain Injury: Evaluating the Evidence (186), concluded that there is little continuity in the research on the effectiveness of cognitive rehabilitation therapy. The authors concluded that only a small amount of evidence supports the effectiveness of cognitive rehabilitation, although the evidence that does exist generally indicates some effectiveness. Importantly, more stringent criteria were used to evaluate the literature in this report than those used by the ACRM BI-ISIG group, and the divergence in conclusions may be attributed to the difference in metric. Ultimately, the committee supported the ongoing use of cognitive rehabilitation for TBI, and emphasized that there is crucial need for additional research to be conducted.

In summary, cognitive rehabilitation refers to a broad set of interventions used to remediate or compensate for impaired cognitive abilities. Although the field has historically relied on "expert opinion," there is a growing body of research supporting the efficacy of interventions to assist persons with acquired brain injury. There remains a clear need for more research on the effectiveness and efficacy of cognitive rehabilitation as a means of improving functioning after acquired brain injury.

Individual Psychotherapy

Psychotherapy is a generic term denoting psychological interventions that ameliorate emotional and behavioral difficulties. Although there are more than 130 varieties of psychotherapy, psychotherapy research has become increasingly sophisticated in understanding key variables (187). Regardless of the type of therapy practiced, effective therapists have been shown to

TABLE 12-3	Practice Standards of the American Congress of Rehabilitation Medicine Brain Injury Interdisciplinary Special Interest Group Cognitive Rehabilitation Task Force	
Practice Standards		
Modality	**Intervention**	**Recommendation**
Attention	Direct attention training and metacognitive training for development of compensatory strategies and foster generalization to real-world tasks.	Recommended during postacute rehabilitation after TBI. Insufficient evidence exists to distinguish the effects of specific attention training during acute recovery and rehabilitation from spontaneous recovery or from more general cognitive interventions.
Visuospatial and praxis	Visuospatial rehabilitation that includes visual scanning training	Recommended for left visual neglect after right hemisphere stroke.
Visuospatial and praxis	Specific gestural or strategy training	Recommended for apraxia during acute rehabilitation for left hemisphere stroke.
Language and communication	Cognitive-linguistic therapies	Recommended during acute and postacute rehabilitation for language deficits secondary to left hemisphere stroke.
Language and communication	Specific interventions for functional communication deficits, including pragmatic conversational skills	Recommended for social communication skills after TBI.
Memory	Memory strategy training	Recommended for mild memory impairments from TBI, including the use of internalized strategies (e.g., visual imagery) and external memory compensations (e.g., notebooks).
Executive function	Meta-cognitive strategy training (self-monitoring and self-regulation)	Recommended for deficits in executive functioning after TBI, including impairments of emotional self-regulation, and as a component of interventions for deficits in attention, neglect, and memory.
Multimodal	Comprehensive-holistic neuropsychological rehabilitation	Recommended during postacute rehabilitation to reduce cognitive and functional disability for persons with moderate to severe TBI.

Adapted from Cicerone KD, Langenbahn DM, Braden C, et al. Evidence-based cognitive rehabilitation: updated review of the literature from 2003 through 2008. *Arch Phys Med Rehabil.* 2011;92:519–530. doi:10.1016/j.apmr.2010.11.015.

communicate genuineness, unconditional positive regard, and empathy. As opposed to friendship, the therapist provides an atmosphere of acceptance, respect, understanding, warmth, and help in conjunction with deliberate efforts to avoid criticizing, judging, or reacting emotionally with the patient. The creation of this atmosphere results in a framework unmatched by any other human relationship, one conducive to therapeutic change.

The three basic assumptions underlying psychotherapy are as follows:

1. The person seeking services desires change.
2. The dysfunctional affect, behavior, or cognition is understood and amenable to change.
3. The process is a collaborative endeavor that assumes active client participation.

Psychotherapeutic intervention is often contraindicated in patients on whom it must be forced or in those with significant communication or learning impediments. Additionally, if the difficulties are due to factors solely in the patient's environment (e.g., long hospitalization, unpleasant medical interventions, prejudice, nonunderstanding staff), the focus of the psychotherapist's intervention may shift from the patient to the environment (188).

Psychologists frequently apply techniques termed *cognitive-behavioral*. There are several common elements of cognitive-behavioral therapy (189). Interventions are active, time limited, and fairly structured. The patient is assisted in recognizing the connections among cognition, affect, and behavior, together with their joint consequences, and is encouraged to become aware of and monitor the role that negative thoughts and images play in the maintenance of maladaptive behavior.

Because of the pressing practical problems faced by rehabilitation inpatients and the increasingly short periods of hospitalization, rehabilitation psychologists tend to use brief forms of therapy to achieve limited, focused, and readily attainable goals. These goals often include amelioration of the most disabling symptoms, reestablishment of previous levels of functioning, and development of enhanced coping skills.

Common Psychotherapeutic Interventions in Rehabilitation

The role of the Rehabilitation psychologist includes helping individuals with adjustment to disability, changes to identity, health-related stress, family stress and burden, existential issues, bereavement, depression, anxiety, and anger (190). Depressive disorders are more prevalent in people with MS (191), amputation (192), SCI (193), stroke (194), and TBI (195). In addition to facing the challenges of a catastrophic injury, patients may need to develop new coping skills, when ways they previously used to cope (e.g., engaging in exercise, distraction through pleasurable activities, substance use) may not be available due to physical, cognitive, or medical limitations. Interventions may include group, individual, or family therapy. Rehabilitation psychologists frequently have difficulties engaging the clients who may be uninterested or unwilling to participate (190). Those who do engage in psychotherapeutic interventions show several positive outcomes, including improved functional and emotional outcomes (196).

Motivational Interviewing

Motivational interviewing (MI) (156) is a patient-centered, directive style of counseling that enhances intrinsic motivation by helping the patient explore and resolve ambivalence. Problems in motivation have been consistently identified as a primary barrier to successful rehabilitation outcomes (197), as patients in rehabilitation often need to change their current behavior in order to manage new medical issues, or to adjust to a physical disability or a cognitive impairment. After a catastrophic injury, several factors may contribute to low motivation and feelings of dependence and inadequacy. MI is based on the premise that individuals are at different levels of readiness for change and that how the therapist interacts with the patient can increase or decrease the patient's motivation. Four basic therapeutic skills are used in MI: (a) expressing empathy, (b) rolling with resistance, (c) supporting self-efficacy, and (d) developing discrepancy between a current problematic behavior and the patient's values or hopes for the future. Since a patient who is ambivalent about making a change is likely to become resistant or defensive if he or she feels that another person is taking sides or imposing change, MI uses a collaborative approach in which the counselor remains congruent with the patient's level of readiness to help the patient change. Key therapeutic strategies include open-ended questions, affirmations, reflective listening, summary statements, and eliciting change talk from the patient. Ultimately, it is still the patient's willingness to change that drives the process; MI counselors do not argue, debate, or impose their views on the patient if the individual does not perceive difficulties or problems with his or her behavior. Several reviews and meta-analyses support the efficacy and applicability of MI (198). Originally developed for treatment of addictive behaviors, MI has been shown to be useful in helping to change of health behaviors (199,200) because it facilitates brief, focused, motivational conversations about health issues. In rehabilitation, MI interventions may help with such topics as perceived burden, side effects of prescribed pain medication, lack of income, or change in identity (201). MI is a promising intervention for rehabilitation patients (144,202,203).

Acceptance and Commitment Therapy

Acceptance and Commitment Therapy (ACT) (204) is an empirically supported psychological intervention designed to increase psychological flexibility through acceptance, mindfulness, and commitment to behavioral change. The basic premise of ACT is that psychological pain is a natural part of human life, and it is our efforts to avoid unpleasant internal processes (e.g., thoughts, feelings, or sensations), known as experiential avoidance, that lead to unnecessary suffering, even debilitating depression or anxiety (205). Influenced by Eastern philosophies, ACT teaches patients that they can live a fulfilling and meaningful life by being open to even the most difficult internal experiences, such as anxiety, anger, fear, or pain, instead of struggling to control these emotions. In ACT, psychological flexibility is enhanced through six core principles: (a) acceptance of thoughts and feelings without attempt to change them, (b) using cognitive defusion to reduce the power that our

thoughts have over us, (c) being present and nonjudgmental with experiences as they occur, (d) practicing mindfulness using one's self as context, (e) identifying and understanding our core values, and (f) using committed action to initiate behavioral change consistent with these values. In contrast to most types of psychotherapy, the goal of ACT is not to reduce or eliminate symptoms, but individuals do show a reduction of symptoms as a by-product of this approach (206). Acceptance-based approaches are particularly helpful for treatment of persons with chronic pain (207,208), in contrast to control-based strategies, which can exacerbate the problem (204,209). Rather than trying to avoid pain, acceptance-based strategies promote "an active willingness to engage in meaningful activities in life regardless of pain-related sensations, thoughts, and other related feelings that might otherwise hinder that engagement" (210) (p. 6). Similarly, ACT is useful in rehabilitation because many challenges faced by patients cannot be changed, such as coping with chronic pain, or social anxiety associated with their appearance. Often, patients report a need to control symptoms before they can attain a valued life, leading to narrow and inflexible behaviors. ACT can help individuals with chronic illness and disability (CID) live full and meaningful lives despite their symptoms by increasing their behavioral repertoire (211).

Positive Psychology

Positive psychology is the study of those factors that make life worth living, enable people to successfully confront challenges, and facilitate extracting meaning from daily life (212–214). The term "positive psychology" was introduced by Martin Seligman; this approach focuses on identifying and nurturing a person's strengths rather than his or her deficiencies (215,216). Positive psychology emphasizes prevention and is based on the premise that positive traits act as buffers against psychopathology (217). Most studies examining the efficacy of positive psychology interventions that focused on recognizing positive experiences, character strengths, gratitude, or acts of kindness were found to be beneficial (218–220). To date, there is a paucity of positive psychology research in rehabilitation settings.

Dunn and Dougherty (221) argue for connecting rehabilitation psychology's foundational principles and strengths to the emerging field of positive psychology, thus enriching both fields. Both rehabilitation psychology and positive psychology share an emphasis on personal strengths, and it would be valuable to understand what helps people thrive with chronic illness or disability (222). Ehde (214) suggests that three positive psychology constructs may be particularly relevant to rehabilitation: resilience, posttraumatic growth, and positive emotions. Rehabilitation psychology has long recognized the potential for positive growth as a result of a disability (4,223). Dunn, Uswatte, and Elliott (222) suggest that possible ways to promote resilience and positive growth after disability include reminding individuals of their continuing "assets" (e.g., skills, interpersonal strengths, hobbies and interests, and social networks) rather than highlighting assets that were lost (224). Nierenberg et al. (225) proposed well-being therapy (WBT) (226) as a psychotherapeutic intervention for persons with disability that is consistent with the foundational principles of rehabilitation psychology and has proven efficacy as a buffer against the development of some negative states. WBT focuses on improving an individual's suboptimal levels of psychological well-being in six dimensions: autonomy, personal growth, environmental mastery, purpose in life, positive relations, and self-acceptance (227). The application of positive psychology in rehabilitation is in its infancy. Additional research is needed to evaluate the efficacy of these approaches in rehabilitation populations. Furthermore, it is important for rehabilitation professionals to recognize that potential positive aspects of CID should never be imposed upon clients, as there is no right way for individuals to respond to a disability and each individual's personal process of adjustment must be honored (222).

Behavioral Management and Operant Conditioning Techniques

In contrast to many specialty areas of medicine, in rehabilitation medicine there is systematic interaction between the medical and the behavioral sciences. Because of their relevance to rehabilitation, the principles underlying behavior modification are described in detail. Included are the topics of behavioral contracting and misconceptions about behavior modification. The following material is drawn from the writings of Martin and Pear (228), Kazdin (229), and Brockway and Fordyce (230).

Types of Reinforcers

There are three types of reinforcers. *Primary* or *unconditioned reinforcers* are present at birth. They include food, water, sexual stimulation, rest after activity and activity after rest, a band of temperatures, air, and cessation of aversive stimuli. *Conditioned reinforcers* are stimuli that have been repeatedly paired with primary reinforcers. They are idiosyncratic and based on the learning history of the person. *Generalized reinforcers* are stimuli that have been paired with two or more conditioned reinforcers. The prime example of a generalized reinforcer is money; however, verbal responses such as "thank you," "correct," and "great" also are in this category. In addition to the three types of reinforcers, the Premack principle states that any high-frequency behavior can be used to reinforce a low-frequency behavior. For example, a high-frequency behavior such as watching television can be made contingent on performing a low-frequency behavior such as stretching exercises.

Behavioral Contracts

Behavioral contracts, also known as contingency contracts, are written agreements between people who desire a change in behavior. The contract precisely indicates the relationship between behaviors and their consequences. The contract serves four important functions. First, it ensures that the rehabilitation team and the patient agree on goals and procedures. Second, because the goals are specified behaviorally, evidence is readily available regarding fulfillment of the contract. Third, the patient has a clear picture of what behaviors are expected if he or she is to remain in the rehabilitation program. Fourth, the signing of a document functions as a powerful indicator of commitment and helps ensure compliance with the agreement.

Common Misconceptions About Behavior Modifications

Behavior modification arouses concerns usually because of a misunderstanding of its underlying principles. Kazdin presented a succinct overview of common objections, two of which are iterated here (231). A frequent objection is that use of tangible reinforcers is the same as bribery. Bribery can be differentiated from reinforcement, because bribery is used to increase behavior that is considered illegal or immoral and usually involves delivery of the payoff before performance of the behavior, not after, as in behavior modification. Bribery and reinforcement share the similarity of being ways of influencing behavior, but that is where the similarity ends.

A second objection is that behavior modification is "coercive." Although behavior modification is inherently controlling and designed to alter behavior, multiple safeguards prevent its misapplication. These safeguards include involving the patient when contingencies are negotiated, constructing programs that rely on positive reinforcement rather than negative reinforcement or punishment, and making response requirements for reinforcement lenient at the beginning of the program. The use of behavioral modification in rehabilitation units requires careful training of staff. A limiting factor in many inpatient rehabilitation units is the lack of stability in team membership, especially where nursing personnel change frequently.

INDIRECT SERVICES

The rehabilitation psychologist's core goal is to enhance the quality of rehabilitation outcomes for patients. Indirect services such as maximizing team interaction skills, staff development, administration, and research provide avenues for enhancing patient outcomes that are as important as direct patient services.

The rehabilitation team is a unique structure in the delivery of health care (232). Nowhere else are so many professionals with diverse training backgrounds expected to communicate in a clear, timely, and comprehensive manner. This communication may become tenuous because of different professional terminologies, overlap in roles, and the pressures of productivity in a competitive health care environment. The psychologist can enhance patient outcomes by facilitating cohesion of the rehabilitation team (233). This task can be accomplished through a variety of methods, including chairing committees to improve interdisciplinary cooperation and leading staff meetings to clarify overlap in professional roles. The rehabilitation psychologist's knowledge of distinguishing normal from abnormal behavior in adjustment to trauma and disability is frequently utilized for staff education. Although some in-service topics focus on patient variables, such as practical management suggestions and brain-behavior relationships, other topics include staff concerns such as stress and communication skills.

Rehabilitation psychologists trained at the doctoral level have extensive expertise in research design and statistical methods. As such, they frequently consult with other team members interested in conducting research. They may coordinate research or direct research committees. The research expertise of psychologists is reflected in their presence on editorial boards of numerous rehabilitation-related publications. They are also found in local, state, and national organizations whose function is to promote quality rehabilitation and social justice for the physically disabled.

Models of Psychological Adaptation to Chronic Illness and Disability

Models of psychological adaptation (PA) to CID grew out of the diverse training backgrounds of rehabilitation psychologists. The models described below represent distinct approaches to understanding PA to CID. After introducing the Moral/Medical/Minority Model, a critical review of the Stage Model is provided. This is followed by discussion of the Social, the Behavioral, and the Coping Skills Models. For detailed information on PA models, see Rath and Elliott (234) and Livneh and Martz (235).

The Moral, Medical, Minority Model

As described by Rhoda Olkin (188), perhaps the first model of PA to CID was the moral model. In this model, CID is believed to be caused by a moral lapse or failure of faith, resulting in divine retribution. Thus, CID enhances social conformity by reminding believers to not stray from their religious beliefs. Beginning in the mid-1800s, application of the scientific method increased understanding of the causes of CID. This led to the medical model assuming a dominant role in explaining CID. In the medical model, CID is due to a deficit or dysfunction of a bodily system. It fits the commonsense notion that the primary source of suffering associated with disability is the disability itself. Hence, the focus of the medical model is removal or amelioration of the disability through medical interventions. A more recent model, the minority model, shifts the focus from characteristics of the individual (moral or bodily function failure) to a focus on the environment. In the minority model, a failure in the environment, including the social environment (i.e., negative attitudes toward those with CID) and the built environment (i.e., inaccessible transportation and buildings) is the primary sources of difficulties with PA to CID. The minority model overlaps with the social model of disability described below.

Before leaving the medical model, additional points are worth stating. Although the medical model is easy to grasp, and is currently the most commonly held model in modern societies, it neglects the psychology of the individual with the CID. For example, some people remain incapacitated despite successful medical interventions for CID. When this was recognized in the early 1900s, theorizing shifted to the principles of dynamic psychology, which focused on internal events such as motivation. In these instances, continued incapacitation, despite seemingly successful medical interventions, was conceptualized in mental health terms. As time progressed, dynamic psychology models, especially the classic psychoanalytic model with its emphasis on psychopathology, proved insufficient to account for the diversity of outcomes. Professionals came to recognize that physical and social barriers, barriers external to the patient, produce a major source of adjustment problems. Emphasis on sociologic concepts such as the "sick role" (236) and "illness behavior" (237) ensued. These sociologic theories added to the understanding of adjustment to disability on a societal level (238). The ascendance of learning theory in the science of psychology, with its emphasis on the sensitivity of behavior to its consequences, led to an emphasis on the overt behavior of the individual rather than intrapsychic events. Models that attempt to simultaneously take into account the internal events of the person and the external demands of the environment are termed integrative or ecologic models.

The Stage Model

The stage model evolved from the work of Kubler-Ross (239) in the field of death and dying. This model was subsequently applied to theorizing about PA to CID. The model purports that people undergoing a life crisis follow a predictable, orderly path of emotional response. Although contemporary research on the stage model applied to bereavement has limited support (240), the stage model continues to be viewed as established truth by both the lay public and professionals.

The stage model was subsequently applied to those with trauma and disability with multiple rehabilitation psychologists making either implicit or explicit reference to a stage model of adjustment to disability (241,242).

There are several variations of the stage model. Most of these variations posit that individuals go through a series of three to five steps that begin with shock and end with adaptation. In the current bereavement literature, these stages are labeled as follows: disbelief, anger, yearning, depression, and acceptance (243). While important differences exist between the death and dying research and disability research, there are enough commonalities to consider them as overlapping.

Three common assumptions underlie the stage model. First, people respond to the onset of disability in specific and predictable ways. Second, they go through a series of stages over time. Third, they eventually accept or resolve their emotional crises.

Regarding the first assumption, Silver and Wortman's literature reviews concluded that there is little evidence supporting the belief that people react in specific and predictable ways to undesirable life events (244,245). A variety of reactions occur: some individuals experience shock; others react with paralyzing anxiety, while others appear calm and collected (246). In short, initial reactions are complex and likely a reflection of personality, learning history, coping styles, and the meaning of the event to the individual.

The second assumption of stage models, that people follow a predictable pattern of emotional response after the onset of a disability, is present in the professional literature of nurses, social workers, clergy, health care professionals, and psychologists. Wortman and Silver were unable to discover any studies specifically testing whether people go through a series of stages over time (245). In the case of death, Holland and Niemeyers' (240) review found at best limited support for progression through stages over time. Holland and Niemeyer suggested that "sense-making," described below, was a much stronger predictor of grief than time since loss. Earlier studies that involved serial assessment of mood in persons with SCI failed to find support for progression through stages over time (247,248).

Silver and Wortman summarized the data by stating, "Perhaps the most striking feature of available research, considered as a whole, is the variability in the nature and sequence of people's emotional reactions and coping mechanisms as they attempt to resolve their crises" (244). However, the authors note that there are deep-seated assumptions about how people "should" react to loss. These assumptions include (a) that individuals suffering a loss are supposed to go through a period of intense distress; (b) failure to experience intense distress is suggestive of a problem; (c) successful adjustment requires that the individual "work through" his or her feelings; (d) continued attachment to the deceased (in the case of CID, attachment to previous levels of body function) is viewed as pathologic; and (e) within a year or two, people will recover from their loss and return to earlier levels of functioning (245). They note that individuals who do not comply with these assumptions may incur negative reactions from their peers.

The third assumption, that persons who have suffered a major undesirable life event eventually accept or resolve their emotional crises, is not supported by research. Based on existing research, the expectation of resolution or acceptance appears unwarranted for traumatic life events such as severe burns, SCI, cancer, death of a spouse, and rape (244,249). For example, Shadish et al. studied a cross-sectional sample of patients with SCI and found that those who had been disabled for as long as 38 years continued to think about and miss physically impossible activities (250).

Wortman et al. provide a theoretical framework that suggests that the impact of a major undesirable life event is determined by whether the event can be incorporated into an individual's view of the world (251). The term worldview denotes the system of beliefs, assumptions, or expectations related to oneself, others, and the world that provides a sense of coherence and meaning (252). Losses that are sudden, uncontrollable, and random may shatter people's assumptions about the world. Thus, the extent to which an individual's worldview is violated will determine the intensity of the disequilibrium and distress that the individual experiences. The degree to which they can reconcile the event with their preexisting worldview or create a new worldview that adequately accounts for the event will determine their long-term adjustment. This reconciliation process is referred to as "sense making" or meaning making (240,253).

The Social Model

The Social Model of PA to CID is based on the work of Kurt Lewin (254,255) whose research was instrumental in the concomitant development of the fields of social psychology and rehabilitation psychology. His graduate students included seminal researchers in rehabilitation psychology who applied "Lewinian Field Theory" to the problems in living encountered by those with CID (4,241,256). According to the Lewinian equation B = f (P,E), any observed behavior (B) is a joint function of the interaction of the person (P) and his or her environment (E). In the social model, it is argued that PA to CID is a reciprocal, iterative process determined by the interaction of two types of variables. The first are intraindividual variables, which include the severity of the CID and psychological aspects of the person (e.g., cognitive ability, personality) coupled with their beliefs about the CID. The second are external variables that include physical, social and vocational aspects of the environment. In the social model, the experience of disability and the resulting behavior of the person with a CID is based on the person in the environment (257,258). Therefore, understanding PA to CID can only occur when the context of the individual's external environment is taken into account. As summarized by Livneh and Martz (235) (p. 49) "The strengths of the somatopsychological interactive model stem from its clinically intuitive approach to human behavior, its attention to contextual factors, and the body of research findings it has generated over the past few decades." A comprehensive description of the social model of PA to CID is available in Dunn's influential text, The Social Psychology of Disability (258,259). Dunn covers the topics of psychosocial concepts for understanding disability, stigma and stereotyping, coping, disability identity, positive psychology, and the ecology of disability. He also applies the Foundational Principles to disability issues in contemporary society.

Behavioral Model

The behavioral model of disability adjustment emphasizes the importance of external factors, with reduced interest in the patient's cognitions and a primary focus on observable behaviors (228,229,260). Wilbert Fordyce is known as the father of the behavioral management of chronic pain and the application of learning theory to rehabilitation problems (230,261–263). Fordyce's classic article, "Pain and Suffering," carefully delineates the importance of distinguishing between these two terms and the pivotal role of using applied behavioral analysis when prescribing pain medications (264). This article is a "must read" for any clinician who prescribes pain medication. Contemporary applications of the behavioral model include the use of biofeedback as an empirically based intervention for increasing function (265), and the use of constraint-induced movement therapy to help individuals recover physical function (266). The behavioral model has also been systematically applied to cognitive rehabilitation (267).

According to the behavioral model of adjustment to disability, individuals who are newly disabled face four tasks: remaining in the rehabilitation environment, eliminating disability-incongruent behaviors, acquiring disability-congruent behaviors, and maintaining the output of disability-congruent behaviors.

Remaining in the Rehabilitation Environment

The onset of physical disability and entry into the rehabilitation environment are equivalent to punishment, defined as the loss of access to positive reinforcers or the response-contingent onset of aversive stimuli. Thus, the newly disabled are initially operating in a punishment paradigm. Two types of behavior follow the onset of aversive stimuli: escape/avoidance or aggression. In the rehabilitation setting, escape or avoidance behaviors may include daydreaming, verbal disclaimers of disability, unauthorized forays off the medical unit, and refusal to participate in scheduled treatments. Aggressive behaviors may consist of rebellious behavior or verbal and at times physical attack. If avoidant or aggressive behaviors are not understood and dealt with therapeutically, rehabilitation may end prematurely.

The intervention strategy for these problems requires discovering and reducing aversive aspects of the rehabilitation environment, and reinforcing active participation in the rehabilitation program. Selecting and graphing a mutually agreed-upon indicator of rehabilitation progress can help the patient focus on tangible improvements. The treatment team must understand that patient reactions of hostility are common and should be tolerated, within limits. Team members should never respond to these patient behaviors with counter-hostility, as this increases the risk that the rehabilitation environment and treatment staff may become conditioned aversive stimuli. Instead, systematically ignoring undesirable behavior and establishing therapeutic rapport increases the probability that the patient will remain engaged in his or her rehabilitation program.

Eliminating Disability-Incongruent Behavior

The reduction of disability-incongruent behaviors and the acquisition of disability-congruent behaviors is equivalent to "psychosocial adaptation." Disability-incongruent behaviors are decreased by withdrawing reinforcers after their occurrence, a process known as extinction. Paradoxically, a temporary increase in the rate of disability-incongruent behavior is typical after the initial withdrawal of reinforcers. This is true for both verbal and performance behaviors.

The patient's verbal behavior is likely to change more slowly than performance behavior. For example, statements indicating a belief in the eventual return of physical function may take years to extinguish. The staff should neither reinforce nor punish unrealistic verbalizations. Rather, a verbal response suggesting the need to maintain hope tempered with a focus on the present is least likely to offend the patient. Unrealistic patient verbalizations are more frequent at the start of rehabilitation and may reflect the beginning of extinction. Providing detailed explanations about the anticipated recovery of functional abilities will help decrease unrealistic patient or family verbalizations and keep everyone focused on achievable functional goals. This is especially important for family members, who may erroneously believe that the proper way to help the disabled family member cope is by agreeing with unrealistic statements about eventual recovery of function.

Acquiring Disability-Congruent Behaviors

Difficulties in the acquisition of disability-congruent behaviors are typically conceptualized to be problems in "motivation." Typically, this term is applied when patients have failed to reach levels of performance set by the rehabilitation staff. Learning theory rejects this formulation because it relies on inference about the internal state of the person. The behavioral approach is to adjust contingencies to increase the rate of desired behavior or reduce the rate of behaviors competing with the desired behavior. Most disability-congruent behaviors are initially of low frequency, strength, and value. Steps to change this situation include establishing reinforcing relationships with the treatment staff, enhancing long-term reinforcers for disability-congruent behaviors, and introducing contingency management interventions that promote the acquisition of disability-congruent behaviors.

Maintaining the Output of Disability-Congruent Behaviors

The final and most important step in adjustment to disability is to maintain the output of disability-appropriate behaviors. Rehabilitation will ultimately be unsuccessful if the behaviors learned in the rehabilitation unit are not transferred to the home environment (268). Although the patient may have the ability to perform a task, the probability of its continued occurrence depends on contingencies operating in the home environment. Disability-congruent behaviors, such as propelling a wheelchair, maintaining a fluid schedule, and using gait aids are unlikely to be reinforcing in themselves.

Two strategies for improving generalization are to bring disability-congruent behaviors under the control of reinforcers that occur naturally in the environment, and reprogram the patient's home environment to deliver appropriate reinforcement contingently. The first strategy is promoted through interventions designed to reengage the patient in meaningful avocational and vocational activities after dismissal. Vocational counseling and therapeutic recreation are therefore important parts of inpatient rehabilitation. Gradual and systematic rehearsal of newly learned skills in the home environment also encourages generalization. The second strategy is promoted through such interventions as home modifications, assigning a family member to monitor and reinforce home therapy programs, and contracting with the patient for continued compliance. The developing fields of telehealth and digital technologies are dramatically increasing opportunities for generalization of rehabilitation interventions (269–271). Unfortunately, in some cases other contingencies are also present that prevent generalization. For example, the patient may receive reinforcers in the form of increased attention or financial rewards from litigation, known as secondary gain. Inability to control sources of secondary gain may prevent generalization of disability-congruent behaviors to the home environment. Family interventions are critical to prevent these problems.

Coping Skills Model

The coping skills model (272), which emphasizes both cognitive and behavioral factors, is based on the crisis theory originally formulated by Lindemann (273). Crisis theory asserts that people require a sense of social and psychological equilibrium. After a traumatic event, a state of crisis and disorganization occurs. At the time of the crisis, a person's characteristic patterns of behavior are ineffectual in establishing equilibrium. This state of disequilibrium is always temporary, and a new balance is achieved within days to weeks. Snyder's edited text on coping research is a must read for understanding both the theoretical constructs and the practical steps that underlie successful adaptation to loss and change (212). Snyder's seminal contributions to "hope theory" are closely linked with the coping skills model (274). Moos has developed an inclusive model of PA to CID; the reader is referred to his Crisis and Coping Model (275).

Moos' coping skills model comprises seven major adaptive tasks and seven major coping skills. The coping skills are elaborated in the following discussion.

Denying or Minimizing the Seriousness of a Crisis

This coping skill may be directed at the illness or at its significance and helps to reduce negative emotions to manageable levels. This reduction enhances the mental clarity needed for effective action in emergency situations. The likelihood of implementing a greater range of coping responses is also increased. The downside of denial is lack of engagement in the rehabilitation process (276).

Seeking Relevant Information

Often, misunderstanding of medical diagnoses and procedures causes emotional distress. Understanding often reduces anxiety and provides a sense of control. Gathering information gives the patient and family a concrete task and the accompanying feeling of purposefulness. One longitudinal study of people with chronic illness showed that information-seeking has salubrious effects on adjustment (277).

Requesting Reassurance and Emotional Support

The literature shows that perceived social support, adjustment during a crisis, and improved health outcomes are interrelated (278–280). Components of social support include perceiving that one is cared for, being encouraged to openly express beliefs and feelings, and being provided material aid. Social support may enhance coping by reducing counterproductive emotional states, building self-esteem, and increasing receptivity to new information. Cobb suggested that social support enhances health outcome either directly through neuroendocrine pathways or indirectly through increased patient compliance (281).

He cited evidence showing that patients who receive social support are more likely to stay in treatment and follow their physicians' recommendations. Turner found a reliable association between social support and psychological well-being, especially during stressful circumstances (282).

Learning Specific Illness-Related Procedures

Learning specific illness-related procedures is a skill that reaffirms personal competence and enhances self-esteem, which is often undermined by physical disability. Bulman and Wortman asked social workers and nurses on a rehabilitation unit to define good and poor coping in patients with SCI (283). Both groups agreed that good coping included the willingness to learn physical skills that would minimize disability. Conversely, the definition of poor coping included an unwillingness to improve the condition or attend physical therapy.

Setting Concrete Limited Goals

Limited goal setting breaks a large task into small and more readily mastered components. As each component is mastered, self-reinforcement accrues and sets the stage for further learning. Limited goal-setting decreases feelings of being overwhelmed and enhances the opportunity to achieve something considered meaningful.

Rehearsing Alternative Outcomes

Activities such as mental rehearsal, anticipation, discussions with significant others, and incorporation of medical information are involved in this skill. Here the patient considers possible outcomes and determines the most fruitful manner of handling each. Recalling previous periods of stress and how these were successfully managed is an example of this coping skill. The patient engages in behaviors that alleviate feelings of anxiety, tension, fear, and uncertainty. A cognitive road map is delineated to provide guidance on how any of a variety of possible future stressors will be minimized.

Finding a General Purpose or Pattern of Meaning in the Course of Events

Physical disability is a crisis that can destroy a person's belief that the world is a predictable, meaningful, and understandable place. There is a compelling psychological need to believe that the world is just (284) and to make sense out of a crisis experience. The previously discussed concept of worldview and meaning making, with their focus on coherence and meaning, is relevant in this context. Some theorists claim that the search for meaning is a basic human motivation (285). Bulman and Wortman studied 29 subjects with SCI and concluded that the "ability to perceive an orderly relationship between one's behaviors and one's outcomes is important for effective coping" (283). Krause, in a 15-year prospective study of persons with SCI, found that survival was directly related to higher activity levels and being employed (286).

SUMMARY

This chapter reviewed the history and current status of rehabilitation psychology, followed by an overview of services offered by the rehabilitation psychologist and theories of adjustment to disability. Although the rehabilitation psychologist provides a wide variety of direct and indirect services, specific skills are particularly relevant to rehabilitation, including psychological assessment, behavior modification, and research. Rehabilitation environments represent settings in which people under physical and emotional distress are asked to learn. Standardized measurement of personality, mood, intellectual ability, academic achievement, neuropsychological integrity, and substance use provide a reliable base on which to set rehabilitation goals.

Rehabilitation is concerned with ensuring that a patient can perform specific activities. Whether this person will actually do so is determined by contingencies in the rehabilitation unit and home environment. The rehabilitation psychologist's behavioral modification skills permit the careful assessment and harnessing of these contingencies in the service of the patient.

Progress in any scientific field depends on quality research. Such research is of particular concern for rehabilitation because outcomes are determined by a complex set of physical and social variables. Doctoral-level psychologists have extensive training in research and program evaluation. This training stresses asking practical research questions relevant to clinical problems. This training often leads them to leadership roles in clinical and research settings.

Theories of adjustment to disability are diverse, reflecting a history of the diverse training backgrounds of rehabilitation psychologists. The earliest model, termed the Moral Model, evolved into the Medical Model and now the Minority Model. Thus a shift from a moral, to a physical, to a social focus has occurred over time. Stage theory remains a widely believed, but unsubstantiated model that suggests that adjustment to a crisis follows a predictable and sequential pattern. Alternative models include the social model, the behavioral model, and the coping skills model. Contemporary research on the concepts of coping, hope, positive psychology, resilience, and well-being provide compelling theoretical perspectives for understanding the process of adjustment to disability and chronic illness. The field of rehabilitation psychology remains one of the most dynamic and socially relevant fields of psychology. Its relevance only increases as the rates of CID increase in the United States and across the world.

REFERENCES

1. Scherer MJ, Blair KL, Banks ME, et al. Rehabilitation psychology. In: Craighead WE, Nemeroff CB, eds. *The Concise Corsini Encyclopedia of Psychology and Behavioral Science*. 3rd ed. Hoboken, NJ: John Wiley & Sons, Inc.; 2004:801–802.
2. Sherwin E. A field in flux: the history of rehabilitation psychology. In: Kennedy P, ed. *The Oxford Handbook of Rehabilitation Psychology*. New York: Oxford University Press; 2012:10–31.
3. Wright BA. *Psychology and Rehabilitation*. Washington, DC: American Psychological Association; 1959.
4. Wright BA. *Physical Disability, A Psychosocial Approach*. 2nd ed. New York: Demos Publications; 1983.
5. Dunn DS, Ehde DM, Wegener ST. The foundational principles as psychological lodestars: theoretical inspiration and empirical direction in rehabilitation psychology. *Rehabil Psychol*. 2016;61:1–6. doi:10.1037/rep0000082.
6. Bentley JA, Bruyere SM, LeBlanc J, et al. Globalizing rehabilitation psychology: application of foundational principles to global health and rehabilitation challenges. *Rehabil Psychol*. 2016;61:65–73. doi:10.1037/rep0000068.
7. Patterson DR, Hanson SL. Joint Division 22 and ACRM guidelines for postdoctoral training in rehabilitation psychology. *Rehabil Psychol*. 1995;40:299–310.
8. Stiers W, Stucky K. A survey of rehabilitation psychology clinical training in the United States. *Rehabil Psychol*. 2007;53:536–543.
9. Stiers W, Barisa M, Stucky K, et al. Guidelines for competency development and measurement in rehabilitation psychology postdoctoral training. *Rehabil Psychol*. 2015;60:111–122. doi:10.1037/a0038353.
10. Stiers W, Hanson S, Turner AP, et al.; Council of Rehabilitation Psychology Postdoctoral Training Programs. Guidelines for postdoctoral training in rehabilitation psychology. *Rehabil Psychol*. 2012;57:267–279. doi:10.1037/a0030774.

11. Cox RH. Fellows address: excellence in rehabilitation psychology—the ABPP diplomate in rehabilitation psychology. *Rehabil Psychol.* 1998;43:348–352.

12. Hibbard MR, Cox D. Competencies of a rehabilitation psychologist. In: Frank RG, Rosenthal M, Caplan B, eds: *Handbook of Rehabilitation Psychology.* 2nd ed. Washington, DC: American Psychological Association; 2010:467–475.

13. Kerkhoff TR, Hanson SL. *Ethics Field Guide: Applications to Rehabilitation Psychology.* New York: Oxford University Press; 2013.

14. World Health Organization. *ICIDH-2: International Classification of Functioning and Disability.* Geneva, Switzerland: World Health Organization; 2000.

15. Jackson JC, Jutte JE. Rehabilitating a missed opportunity: integration of rehabilitation psychology into the care of critically ill patients, survivors, and caregivers. *Rehabil Psychol.* 2016;61:115–119. doi:10.1037/rep0000091.

16. Wade SL, Wolfe CR. Telehealth interventions in rehabilitation psychology: postcards from the edge. *Rehabil Psychol.* 2005;50:323–324. http://dx.doi.org/10.1037/0090-5550.50.4.323

17. MacLachlan M, Mannan H. The World Report on Disability and its implications for rehabilitation psychology. *Rehabil Psychol.* 2014;59:117–124. doi:10.1037/a0036715.

18. Heinemann AW. Putting outcome measurement in context: a rehabilitation psychology perspective. *Rehabil Psychol.* 2005;50:6–14.

19. Merbitz NH, Westie K, Dammeyer JA, et al. After critical care: challenges in the transition to inpatient rehabilitation. *Rehabil Psychol.* 2016;61:186–200. doi:10.1037/rep0000072.

20. Stucky K, Jutte JE, Warren AM, et al. A survey of psychology practice in critical-care settings. *Rehabil Psychol.* 2016;61:201–209. doi:10.1037/rep0000071.

21. Sue DW, Sue D. *Counseling for the Culturally Diverse: Theory and Practice.* 4th ed. New York: Wiley; 2003.

22. Lomay VT, Hinkebein JH. Cultural considerations when providing rehabilitation services to American Indians. *Rehabil Psychol.* 2006;51:36–42.

23. Huston T, Gassaway J, Wilson C, et al. The SCIRehab project: treatment time spent in SCI rehabilitation. Psychology treatment time during inpatient spinal cord injury rehabilitation. *J Spinal Cord Med.* 2011;34:196–204. doi:10.1179/1079026 11X12971826988219.

24. Lahey S, Beaulieu C, Sandbach K, et al. The role of the psychologist with disorders of consciousness in inpatient pediatric neurorehabilitation: a case series. *Rehabil Psychol.* 2017;62:238–248. doi:10.1037/rep0000156.

25. Wegener ST, Adams LL, Rohe D. Promoting optimal functioning in spinal cord injury: the role of rehabilitation psychology. *Handb Clin Neurol.* 2012;109:297–314. doi:10.1016/B978-0-444-52137-8.00019-X.

26. Plake BS, Impara JC, eds. *The Fourteenth Mental Measurements Yearbook.* Lincoln, OR: The Buros Institute of Mental Measurements; 2001.

27. Epstein S, O'Brien EJ. The person-situation debate in historical and current perspective. *Psychol Bull.* 1985;98:513–537.

28. Johnson-Greene D, Touradji P. Assessment of personality and psychopathology. In: Frank RG, Rosenthal M, Caplan B, eds: *Handbook of Rehabilitation Psychology.* 2nd ed. Washington, DC: American Psychological Association; 2010:195–211.

29. Nichols DS. *Essentials of MMPI-2 Assessment.* New York: J. Wiley; 2001.

30. Butcher JN. *MMPI-2: Minnesota Multiphasic Personality Inventory-2: Manual for Administration, Scoring, and Interpretation.* Rev ed. Minneapolis, MN: University of Minnesota Press; 2001.

31. Graham JR. *MMPI-2: Assessing Personality and Psychopathology.* 5th ed. New York: Oxford Press; 2012.

32. Levitt EE, Gotts EE. *The Clinical Application of MMPI Special Scales.* 2nd ed. Hillsdale, NJ: Lawrence Erlbaum Associates, Inc.; 1995.

33. Butcher JN. *MMPI-A: Minnesota Multiphasic Personality Inventory-Adolescent: Manual for Administration, Scoring, and Interpretation.* Minneapolis, MN: University of Minnesota Press: distributed by National Computer Systems Inc.; 1992.

34. Rodevich MA, Wanlass RL. The moderating effect of spinal cord injury on MMPI-2 profiles: a clinically derived T score correction procedure. *Rehabil Psychol.* 1995;40:181–190.

35. Porcelli P, McGrath RE. Introduction to the special issue on personality assessment in medical settings [comment]. *J Pers Assess.* 2007;89:211–215.

36. Ben-Porath YS, Tellegen A. *Minnesota Multiphasic Personality Inventory-2 Restructured Form;* 2008. Available from: http://www.pearsonassessments.com/tests/mmpi-2-rf.htm

37. Tellegen A, Ben-Porath YS, McNulty JL, et al. *MMPI-2 Restructured Clinical (RC) Scales: Development, Validation, and Interpretation.* Minneapolis, MN: University of Minnesota Press; 2003.

38. Morey LC. *The Personality Assessment Inventory Professional Manual.* Lutz, FL: Psychological Assessment Resources; 2007.

39. Digman JM. Personality structure: emergence of the five-factor model. *Annu Rev Psychol.* 1990;41:417–440.

40. Goldberg LR. The structure of phenotypic personality traits. *Am Psychol.* 1993;48:26–34.

41. Rohe DE, Krause JS. The five-factor model of personality: findings in males with spinal cord injury. *Assessment.* 1999;6:203–213.

42. Krause JS, Rohe DE. Personality and life adjustment after spinal cord injury: an exploratory study. *Rehabil Psychol.* 1998;43:118–130.

43. Costa PT, McCrae RR, Holland JL. Personality and vocational interests in an adult sample. *J Appl Psychol.* 1984;69:390–400.

44. Donnay DA, Morris ML, Schaubhut NA, et al. *Strong Interest Inventory Manual.* Mountain View, CA: Consulting Psychology Press; 2005.

45. Holland JL. *Making Vocational Choices: A Theory of Vocational Personalities and Work Environments.* 3rd ed. Odessa, FL: Psychological Assessment Resources; 1997.

46. Rohe DE, Athelstan GT. Vocational interests of persons with spinal cord injury. *J Couns Psychol.* 1982;29:283–291.

47. Malec J. Personality factors associated with severe traumatic disability. *Rehabil Psychol.* 1985;30:165–172.

48. Rohe DE. Personality and spinal cord injury. *Top Spinal Cord Injury.* 1996;2:1–10.

49. Rohe DE, Athelstan GT. Change in vocational interests after spinal cord injury. *Rehabil Psychol.* 1985;30:131–143.

50. Rohe DE, Krause J. Stability of interests after severe physical disability: an 11-year longitudinal study. *J Vocat Behav.* 1998;52:45–58.

51. Spitzer RL, Kroenke K, Williams JB. Validation and utility of a self-report version of PRIME-MD: the PHQ primary care study. Primary Care Evaluation of Mental Disorders. Patient Health Questionnaire. *JAMA.* 1999;282:1737–1744.

52. Spitzer RL, Kroenke K, Williams JB, et al. A brief measure for assessing generalized anxiety disorder: the GAD-7. *Arch Intern Med.* 2006;166:1092–1097. doi:10.1001/archinte.166.10.1092.

53. Lowe B, Kroenke K, Herzog W, et al. Measuring depression outcome with a brief self-report instrument: sensitivity to change of the Patient Health Questionnaire (PHQ-9). *J Affect Disord.* 2004;81:61–66. doi:10.1016/S0165-0327(03)00198-8.

54. Bombardier CH, Richards JS, Krause JS, et al. Symptoms of major depression in people with spinal cord injury: implications for screening. *Arch Phys Med Rehabil.* 2004;85:1749–1756.

55. Williams LS, Brizendine EJ, Plue L, et al. Performance of the PHQ-9 as a screening tool for depression after stroke. *Stroke.* 2005;36:635–638. doi:10.1161/01.STR.0000155688.18207.33.

56. Beck AT, Steer RA, Brown GK. *Manual for the Beck Depression Inventory—Fast Screen for Medical Patients.* San Antonio, TX: Psychological Corporation; 2000.

57. Beck AT. *BDI-II, Beck Depression Inventory: Manual.* 2nd ed. San Antonio, TX: Harcourt Brace; 1996.

58. Benedict RH, Fishman I, McClellan MM, et al. Validity of the Beck Depression Inventory-Fast Screen in multiple sclerosis. *Mult Scler.* 2003;9:393–396.

59. Healey AK, Kneebone II, Carroll M, et al. A preliminary investigation of the reliability and validity of the Brief Assessment Schedule Depression Cards and the Beck Depression Inventory-Fast Screen to screen for depression in older stroke survivors. *Int J Geriatr Psychiatry.* 2008;23:531–536. doi:10.1002/gps.1933.

60. Kroenke K, Spitzer RL, Williams JB, et al. Anxiety disorders in primary care: prevalence, impairment, comorbidity, and detection. *Ann Intern Med.* 2007;146:317–325.

61. Terrill AL, Hartoonian N, Beier M, et al. The 7-item generalized anxiety disorder scale as a tool for measuring generalized anxiety in multiple sclerosis. *Int J MS Care.* 2015;17:49–56. doi:10.7224/1537-2073.2014-008.

62. Wechsler D. *Wechsler Adult Intelligence Scale.* 4th ed. San Antonio, TX: Pearson; 2008.

63. Wechsler D. *Wechsler Adult Intelligence Scale—Fourth Edition: Technical and Interpretive Manual.* San Antonio, TX: Pearson; 2008.

64. Wilkinson GS, Robertson GJ. *Wide Range Achievement Test 4 (WRAT4).* 4th ed. Bloomington, MN: Pearson; 2006.

65. Schrank FA, McGrew KS, Mather N. *Woodcock-Johnson IV.* Rolling Meadows, IL: Riverside; 2014.

66. Schneider WJ, McGrew KS. The Cattell-Horn-Carroll model of intelligence. In: Flanagan DP, Harrison PL, eds. *Contemporary Intellectual Assessment: Theories, Tests, and Issues.* 3rd ed. New York: Guilford Press; 2012.

67. LaForte EM, McGrew KS, Schrank FA. *WJ IV Technical Abstract (Woodcock-Johnson IV Assessment Service Bulletin No. 2).* Rolling Meadows, IL: Riverside; 2014.

68. Schrank FA, Mather N, McGrew KS. *Woodcock-Johnson IV Tests of Achievement.* Rolling Meadows, IL: Riverside; 2014.

69. Schrank FA, McGrew KS, Mather N. *Woodcock-Johnson IV Tests of Cognitive Abilities.* Rolling Meadows, IL: Riverside; 2014.

70. Schrank FA, Mather N, McGrew KS. *Woodcock-Johnson IV Tests of Oral Language.* Rolling Meadows, IL: Riverside; 2014.

71. McGrew KS, LaForte EM, Schrank FA. *Techincal Manual: Woodcock-Johnson IV.* Rolling Meadows, IL: Riverside; 2014.

72. Levin HS, O'Donnell VM, Grossman RG. The Galveston Orientation and Amnesia Test. A practical scale to assess cognition after head injury. *J Nerv Ment Dis.* 1979;167:675–684.

73. Bode RK, Heinemann AW, Semik P. Measurement properties of the Galveston Orientation and Amnesia Test (GOAT) and improvement patterns during inpatient rehabilitation. *J Head Trauma Rehabil.* 2000;15:637–655.

74. Jain NS, Layton BS, Murray PK. Are aphasic patients who fail the GOAT in PTA? A modified Galveston Orientation and Amnesia Test for persons with aphasia. *Clin Neuropsychol.* 2000;14:13–17. doi:10.1076/1385-4046(200002)14:1;1-8;FT013.

75. Jackson WT, Novack TA, Dowler RN. Effective serial measurement of cognitive orientation in rehabilitation: the Orientation Log. *Arch Phys Med Rehabil.* 1998;79:718–720.

76. Kean J, Abell M, Malec JF, et al. Rasch analysis of the orientation log and reconsideration of the latent construct during inpatient rehabilitation. *J Head Trauma Rehabil.* 2011;26:364–374. doi:10.1097/HTR.0b013e3181ea4e2c.

77. Novack TA, Dowler RN, Bush BA, et al. Validity of the Orientation Log, relative to the Galveston Orientation and Amnesia Test. *J Head Trauma Rehabil.* 2000;15:957–961.

78. Petersen RC, Doody R, Kurz A, et al. Current concepts in mild cognitive impairment. *Arch Neurol.* 2001;58:1985–1992.

79. Nasreddine ZS, Phillips NA, Bedirian V, et al. The Montreal Cognitive Assessment, MoCA: a brief screening tool for mild cognitive impairment. *J Am Geriatr Soc.* 2005;53:695–699. doi:10.1111/j.1532-5415.2005.53221.x.

80. Smith T, Gildeh N, Holmes C. The Montreal Cognitive Assessment: validity and utility in a memory clinic setting. *Can J Psychiatry*. 2007;52:329–332.

81. Zadikoff C, Fox S, Tang Wai DF, et al. A comparison of MMSE to MoCA in identifying cognitive deficits in Parkinson's disease. *Mov Disord*. 2007;23:297–299.

82. Kiernan RJ, Mueller J, Langston JW, et al. The Neurobehavioral Cognitive Status Examination: a brief but quantitative approach to cognitive assessment. *Ann Intern Med*. 1987;107:481–485.

83. Schwamm LH, Van Dyke C, Kiernan RJ, et al. The Neurobehavioral Cognitive Status Examination: comparison with the Cognitive Capacity Screening Examination and the Mini-Mental State Examination in a neurosurgical population. *Ann Intern Med*. 1987;107:486–491.

84. Fladby T, Schuster M, Gronli O, et al. Organic brain disease in psychogeriatric patients: impact of symptoms and screening methods on the diagnostic process. *J Geriatr Psychiatry Neurol*. 1999;12:16–20. doi:10.1177/089198879901200105.

85. Osmon DC, Smet IC, Winegarden B, et al. Neurobehavioral Cognitive Status Examination: its use with unilateral stroke patients in a rehabilitation setting. *Arch Phys Med Rehabil*. 1992;73:414–418.

86. Poon WS, Zhu XL, Ng SC, et al. Predicting one year clinical outcome in traumatic brain injury (TBI) at the beginning of rehabilitation. *Acta Neurochir Suppl*. 2005;93:207–208.

87. Drane DL, Yuspeh RL, Huthwaite JS, et al. Healthy older adult performance on a modified version of the Cognistat (NCSE): demographic issues and preliminary normative data. *J Clin Exp Neuropsychol*. 2003;25:133–144. doi:10.1076/jcen.25.1.133.13628.

88. Doninger NA, Ehde DM, Bode RK, et al. Measurement properties of the neurobehavioral cognitive status examination (Cognistat) in traumatic brain injury. *Rehabil Psychol*. 2006;51:281–288.

89. Macaulay C, Battista M, Lebby PC, et al. Geriatric performance on the Neurobehavioral Cognitive Status Examination (Cognistat). What is normal? *Arch Clin Neuropsychol*. 2003;18:463–471.

90. van Gorp WG, Marcotte TD, Sultzer D, et al. Screening for dementia: comparison of three commonly used instruments. *J Clin Exp Neuropsychol*. 1999;21:29–38. doi:10.1076/jcen.21.1.29.939.

91. Oehlert ME, Hass SD, Freeman MR, et al. The Neurobehavioral Cognitive Status Examination: accuracy of the "screen-metric" approach in a clinical sample. *J Clin Psychol*. 1997;53:733–737.

92. Randolph C. *Repeatable Battery for the Assessment of Neuropsychological Status Manual*. San Antonio, TX: The Psychological Corporation; 1998.

93. Boll TJ. The Halstead-Reitan neuropsychological battery. In: Filskov SB, Boll TJ, eds. *Handbook of Clinical Neuropsychology*. New York: John Wiley & Sons; 1981:577–607.

94. Filskov SB, Goldstein SG. Diagnostic validity of the Halstead-Reitan neuropsychological battery. *J Consult Clin Psychol*. 1974;42:382–388.

95. Cicerone KD, Dahlberg C, Kalmar K, et al. Evidence-based cognitive rehabilitation: recommendations for clinical practice. *Arch Phys Med Rehabil*. 2000;81:1596–1615.

96. Conway T, Crosson B. Neuropsychological assessment. In: Frank RG, Elliott TR, eds. *Handbook of Rehabilitation Psychology*. Washington, DC: American Psychological Association; 2009:327–343.

97. Dunn EJ, Searight HR, Grisso T, et al. The relation of the Halstead-Reitan neuropsychological battery to functional daily living skills in geriatric patients. *Arch Clin Neuropsychol*. 1990;5:103–117.

98. Heinrichs R. Current and emergent applications of neuropsychological assessment: problems of validity and utility. *Prof Psychol Res Pract*. 1990;21:171–176.

99. Wilson BA, McLellan DL. *Rehabilitation Studies Handbook*. Cambridge, UK/New York: Cambridge University Press; 1997.

100. Sherer M, Sander AM, Nick TG, et al. Early cognitive status and productivity outcome after traumatic brain injury: findings from the TBI model systems. *Arch Phys Med Rehabil*. 2002;83:183–192.

101. Miller LJ, Donders J. Prediction of educational outcome after traumatic brain injury. *Rehabil Psychol*. 2003;48:237–241.

102. Marcotte TD, Grant I, eds. *Neuropsychology of Everyday Functioning*. New York: The Guildford Press; 2009.

103. Heaton RK, Pendleton MG. Use of neuropsychological tests to predict adult patients' everyday functioning. *J Consult Clin Psychol*. 1981;49:807–821.

104. Sbordone RJ. The ecological validity of neuropsychological testing. In: Horton AM, Wedding D, Webster J, eds. *The Neuropsychology Handbook: Vol. 1. Foundations and Assessment*. New York: Springer; 1997:365–392.

105. Novack TA, Sherer M, Penna S. Neuropsychological practice in rehabilitation. In: Frank RG, Rosenthal M, Caplan B, eds. *Handbook of Rehabilitation Psychology*. 2nd ed. Washington, DC: American Psychological Association; 2010.

106. Sherer M, Novack TA. Neuropsychological assessment after traumatic brain injury in adults. In: Prigatano GP, Pliskin NH, eds. *Neuropsychology and Cost Outcome Research: A Beginning*. New York: Psychology Press; 2003:39–60.

107. Tsaousides T, Gordon WA. Cognitive rehabilitation following traumatic brain injury: assessment to treatment. *Mt Sinai J Med*. 2009;76:173–181. doi:10.1002/msj.20099.

108. Kolb B, Whishaw IQ. *Fundamentals of Human Neuropsychology*. London: Macmillan; 2009.

109. PsychCorp. *Wechsler Intelligence Scale for Children*. 5th ed. San Antonio, TX: Pearson; 2014.

110. Wechsler D, Hsiao-Pin C. *WASI-II: Wechsler Abbreviated Scale of Intelligence*. San Antonio, TX: Pearson; 2011.

111. Strauss E, Sherman E, Spreen O. *A Compendium of Neuropsychological Tests: Administration, Norms, and Commentary*. 3rd ed. New York: Oxford University Press; 2006.

112. Smith A. *Symbol Digit Modalities Test*. Los Angeles, CA: Western Psychological Services; 1991.

113. Conners CK. *Conner's Continuous Performance Test (CPT II) Computer Programs for Windows: Technical Manual and Software Guide (Ver. 5)*. North Tonawanda, NY: Multi-Health Systems, Inc.; 2000.

114. Reitan RM. Validity of the trail making test as an indicator of organic brain damage. *Percept Mot Skills*. 1958;8:271–276.

115. Mathias JL, Wheaton P. Changes in attention and information-processing speed following severe traumatic brain injury: a meta-analytic review. *Neuropsychology*. 2007;21:212.

116. Gronwall DMA. Paced auditory serial-addition task: a measure of recovery from concussion. *Percept Mot Skills*. 1977;44:367–373.

117. Lezak MD, Howieson DB, Bigler ED, et al. *Neuropsychological Assessment*. 5th ed. New York: Oxford University Press; 2012.

118. Benton A, Hannay HJ, Varney NR. Visual perception of line direction in patients with unilateral brain disease. *Neurology*. 1975;25:907–910.

119. Benton AL, Sivan AB, Hamsher KD, et al. *Contributions to Neuropsychological Assessment: A Clinical Manual*. 2nd ed. New York: Oxford University Press; 1994.

120. Hooper HE. *Hooper Visual Organization Test Manual*. Los Angeles, CA: Western Psychological Services; 1983.

121. Kaplan EF, Goodglass H, Weintraub S. *The Boston Naming Test*. 2nd ed. Philadelphia, PA: Lea & Febiger; 1983.

122. Dunn LM, Dunn DM. *Peabody Picture Vocabulary Test, Fourth Edition (PPVT-4)*. San Antonio, TX: Pearson; 2007.

123. Benton LA, Hamsher KD, Sivan AB. Controlled oral word association test. Multilingual aphasia examination, 3rd ed. Lutz, FL: Psychological Assessment Resources; 1994.

124. Rosen WG. Verbal fluency in aging and dementia. *J Clin Neuropsychol*. 1980;2:135–146.

125. Benton LA, Hamsher KD, Sivan AB. *Multilingual Aphasia Examination*. 3rd ed. Iowa City, IA: AJA Associates; 1994.

126. PsychCorp. *Wechsler Memory Scale*. 4th ed. San Antonio, TX: Pearson; 2009.

127. Delis DC, Kramer JH, Kaplan E, et al. *California Verbal Learning Test—Second Edition (CVLT-II)*. San Antonio, TX: Psychological Corporation; 2000.

128. Schmidt M. *Rey Auditory Verbal Learning Test: A Handbook*. Los Angeles, CA: Western Psychological Services; 1996.

129. Benedict RHB, Schretlen D, Groniger L, et al. Hopkins verbal learning test—revised: normative data and analysis of inter-form and test-retest reliability. *Clin Neuropsychol*. 1998;12:43–55.

130. Benedict RHB. *The Brief Visual Memory Test—Revised*. Lutz, FL: Psychological Assessment Resources; 1997.

131. Osterrieth PA. Le test de copie d'une figure complexe [trans. J. Corwin & F. W. Bylsma, *Clin Neuropsychol*. 1993;7:9–15]. *Arch Psychol*. 1944;30:206–356.

132. Lezak MD, Howieson DB, Loring DW. *Neuropsychological Assessment*. 4th ed. New York: Oxford University Press; 2004.

133. Grigsby J, Kaye K. *Behavioral Dyscontrol Scale: Manual*. 2nd ed. Denver, CO: University of Colorado; 1996.

134. Wilson BA, Alderman N, Burgess PW, et al. *Behavioural Assessment of the Dysexecutive Syndrome*. Bury St. Edmunds, UK: Thames Valley Test; 1996.

135. Delis DC, Kaplan F, Kramer JH. *Delis-Kaplan Executive Function System*. San Antonio, TX: The Psychological Corporation; 2001.

136. Jensen AR, Rohwer WD. The Stroop color-word test: a review. *Acta Psychol (Amst)*. 1966;25:36–93.

137. Heaton RK, Chelune GJ, Talley JL, et al. *Wisconsin Card Sorting Test: Revised and Expanded*. Odessa, FL: Psychological Assessment Resources; 1993.

138. Tiffin J. *Purdue Pegboard Examiner's Manual*. Rosemont, IL: London House; 1968.

139. Bush SS, Ruff RM, Tröster AI, et al. Symptom validity assessment: practice issues and medical necessity: NAN Policy & Planning Committee. *Arch Clin Neuropsychol*. 2005;20:419–426.

140. Anonymous. Assessment: neuropsychological testing of adults. Considerations for neurologists. Report of the Therapeutics and Technology Assessment Subcommittee of the American Academy of Neurology. *Neurology*. 1996;47:592–599.

141. Hoskin KM, Jackson M, Crrowe SF. Money management after acquired brain dysfunction: the validty of neuropsychological assessment. *Rehabil Psychol*. 2005;50:355–365.

142. Rohe DE, DePompolo RW. Substance abuse policies in rehabilitation medicine departments. *Arch Phys Med Rehabil*. 1985;66:701–703.

143. Basford JR, Rohe DE, Barnes CP, et al. Substance abuse attitudes and policies in US rehabilitation training programs: a comparison of 1985 and 2000. *Arch Phys Med Rehabil*. 2002;83:517–522.

144. Cardoso ED, Pruett SR, Chan F, et al. Substance abuse training among rehabilitation psychologists: practice of APA Division 22 members. *Rehabil Psychol*. 2006;51:175–178.

145. Bombardier CH, Turner AP. Alcohol and other drug use in traumatic disability. In: Frank RG, Rosenthal M, Caplan B, eds. *Handbook of Rehabilitation Psychology*. 2nd ed. Washington, DC: American Psychological Association; 2010:241–258.

146. Eckardt MJ, File SE, Gessa GL, et al. Effects of moderate alcohol consumption on the central nervous system. *Alcohol Clin Exp Res*. 1998;22:998–1040.

147. Eckardt MJ, Harford TC, Kaelber CT, et al. Health hazards associated with alcohol consumption. *JAMA*. 1981;246:648–666.

148. Heinemann AW, Mamott BD, Schnoll S. Substance use by persons with recent spinal cord injuries. *Rehabil Psychol*. 1990;35:217–228.

149. Heinemann AW, Schmidt MF, Semik P. Drinking patterns, drinking expectancies, and coping after spinal cord injury. *Rehabil Couns Bull*. 1994;38:134–153.

150. Corrigan JD. Substance abuse as a mediating factor in outcome from traumatic brain injury. *Arch Phys Med Rehabil*. 1995;76:302–309.

151. Rivara FP, Jurkovich GJ, Gurney JG, et al. The magnitude of acute and chronic alcohol abuse in trauma patients. *Arch Surg*. 1993;128:907–912; discussion 912–913.

152. Schmidt MF, Heinemann AW, Semik P. The efficacy of inservice training on substance abuse and spinal cord injury issues. *Top Spinal Cord Inj*. 1996;2:11–20.

153. Cherry L. *Summary Report. Alcohol, Drugs and Disability II: Second National Policy and Leadership Development Symposium*. San Mateo, CA: Institute on Alcohol, Drugs and Disability; 1994.

154. Center for Substance Abuse Prevention. *Rehabilitation Specialists Prevention Training System*. Rockville, MD: Center for Substance Abuse Prevention, United States Department of Health and Human Services; 1994.

155. Weinberg JR. Interview techniques for diagnosing alcoholism. *Am Fam Physician*. 1974;9:107–115.

156. Miller WR, Rollnick S. *Motivational Interviewing: Helping People Change*. 3rd ed. New York: Guilford Press; 2013.

157. Prochaska JO, DiClemente CC, Norcross JC. In search of how people change: applications to addictive behaviors. *Am Psychol*. 1992;47:1102–1114.

158. Ewing JA. Detecting alcoholism. The CAGE questionnaire. *JAMA*. 1984;252:1905–1907.

159. Cooney NL, Zweben A, Fleming MF. Screening for alcohol problems and at-risk drinking in health-care settings. In: Hester R, Miller WR, eds. *Handbook of Alcoholism Treatment Approaches: Effective Alternatives*. 2nd ed. Needham Heights, MA: Allyn & Bacon, Inc.; 1995:45–60.

160. Allen JP, Litten RZ, Fertig JB, et al. A review of research on the Alcohol Use Disorders Identification Test (AUDIT). *Alcohol Clin Exp Res*. 1997;21:613–619.

161. Bombardier CH, Ehde D, Kilmer J. Readiness to change alcohol drinking habits after traumatic brain injury. *Arch Phys Med Rehabil*. 1997;78:592–596.

162. Bombardier CH, Rimmele CT. Alcohol use and readiness to change after spinal cord injury. *Arch Phys Med Rehabil*. 1998;79:1110–1115.

163. Ader DN. Developing the patient-reported outcomes measurement information system (PROMIS). *Med Care*. 2007;45:S1–S2.

164. Reeve BB, Hays RD, Bjorner JB, et al. Psychometric evaluation and calibration of health-related quality of life item banks: plans for the Patient-Reported Outcomes Measurement Information System (PROMIS). *Med Care*. 2007;45:S22–S31. doi:10.1097/01.mlr.0000250483.85507.04.

165. Harniss M, Amtmann D, Cook D, et al. Considerations for developing interfaces for collecting patient-reported outcomes that allow the inclusion of individuals with disabilities. *Med Care*. 2007;45:S48–S54. doi:10.1097/01.mlr.0000250822.41093.ca.

166. Health Measures. *PROMIS™ (Patient-Reported Outcomes Measurement Information System)*. Chicago, IL: Northwestern University; 2017. Available from: http://www.healthmeasures.net/explore-measurement-systems/promis

167. National Institutes of Health. *Patient-Reported Outcomes Measurement Information System (PROMIS)*. Bethesda, MD: National Institutes of Health; 2017. Available from: https://commonfund.nih.gov/promis/index

168. Prigatano GP. A history of cognitive rehabilitation. In: Halligan PW, Wade DT, eds. *The Effectiveness of Rehabilitation for Cognitive Deficits*. New York: Oxford University Press; 2005:3–10.

169. Wilson BA. Toward a comprehensive model of cognitive rehabilitation. *Neuropsychol Rehabil*. 2002;12:97–110.

170. Mazmanian PE, Kreutzer JS, Devany CW, et al. A survey of accredited and other rehabilitation facilities: education, training and cognitive rehabilitation in brain-injury programmes. *Brain Inj*. 1993;7:319–331.

171. Stringer A. Cognitive rehabilitation practice patterns: a survey of American Hospital Association Rehabilitation Programs. *Clin Neuropsychol*. 2003;17:34–44. doi:10.1076/clin.17.1.34.15625.

172. Parente R, Stapleton M. History and systems of cognitive rehabilitation. *NeuroRehabilitation*. 1997;8:3–11. doi:10.3233/NRE-1997-8102.

173. Gordon WA. Cognitive rehabilitation. In: Silver JM, McAllister TW, Yudofsky SC, eds. *Textbook of Traumatic Brain Injury*. 2nd ed. Arlington, VA: American Psychiatric Publishing, Inc.; 2011:579–586.

174. Ben-Yishay Y, Diller L. *Handbook of Holistic Neuropsychological Rehabilitation: Outpatient Rehabilitation of Traumatic Brain Injury*. Oxford, UK: Oxford University Press; 2011.

175. Sohlberg MM, Turkstra LS. *Optimizing Cognitive Rehabilitation: Effective Instructional Methods*. New York: Guilford Press; 2011.

176. Wilson BA. *Memory Rehabilitation: Integrating Theory and Practice*. New York: Guilford Press; 2009.

177. Bergquist TF, Malec JF. Psychology: current practice and training issues in treatment of cognitive dysfunction. *NeuroRehabilitation*. 1997;8:49–56. doi:10.3233/NRE-1997-8107.

178. Dirette DK, Hinojosa J, Carnevale GJ. Comparison of remedial and compensatory interventions for adults with acquired brain injuries. *J Head Trauma Rehabil*. 1999;14:595–601.

179. Law M, Sidebottom L, Bewick K, et al. *Recommendations for Best Practice in Cognitive Rehabilitation Therapy: Acquired Brain Injury*. The Society for Cognitive Rehabilitation, Inc.; 2004. Available from: https://www.societyforcognitiverehab.org/membership-and-certification/documents/EditedRecsBestPrac.pdf

180. Sohlberg MM, Mateer CA, eds. *Cognitive Rehabilitation: An Integrative Neuropsychological Approach*. New York: Guilford Press; 2001.

181. Cicerone KD, Dahlberg C, Malec JF, et al. Evidence-based cognitive rehabilitation: updated review of the literature from 1998 through 2002. *Arch Phys Med Rehabil*. 2005;86:1681–1692. doi:10.1016/j.apmr.2005.03.024.

182. Ragnarsson KT. Results of the NIH consensus conference on "rehabilitation of persons with traumatic brain injury". *Restor Neurol Neurosci*. 2002;20:103–108.

183. Gordon WA, Zafonte R, Cicerone K, et al. Traumatic brain injury rehabilitation: state of the science. *Am J Phys Med Rehabil*. 2006;85:343–382. doi:10.1097/01.phm.0000202106.01654.61.

184. Cicerone KD, Langenbahn DM, Braden C, et al. Evidence-based cognitive rehabilitation: updated review of the literature from 2003 through 2008. *Arch Phys Med Rehabil*. 2011;92:519–530. doi:10.1016/j.apmr.2010.11.015.

185. Haskins EC, Cicerone KD, Dams-O'Connor K, et al. *Cognitive Rehabilitation Manual: Translating Evidence-Based Recommendations into Practice*. Reston, VA: ACRM Publishing; 2012.

186. Koehler R, Wilhelm E, Shoulson I, eds. *Cognitive Rehabilitation Therapy for Traumatic Brain Injury: Evaluating the Evidence*. Washington, DC: National Academies Press; 2012.

187. Roth A, Fonagy P. *What Works for Whom: A Critical Review of Psychotherapy Research*. 2nd ed. New York: Guilford Publications, Inc.; 2005.

188. Olkin R. *What Psychotherapists Should know about Disability*. New York: Guilford Press; 1999.

189. Turk DC, Meichenbaum D, Genest M. *Pain and Behavioral Medicine: A Cognitive-Behavioral Perspective*. New York: Guilford Press; 1983.

190. Rusin MJ, Uomoto JM. Psychotherapeutic interventions. In: Frank RG, Rosenthal M, Caplan B, eds. *Handbook of Rehabilitation Psychology*. Washington, DC: American Psychological Association; 2010:259–271.

191. Ehde DM, Bombardier CH. Depression in persons with multiple sclerosis. *Phys Med Rehabil Clin N Am*. 2005;16:437–448.

192. Darnall BD, Ephraim P, Wegener ST, et al. Depressive symptoms and mental health service utilization among persons with limb loss: results of a national survey. *Arch Phys Med Rehabil*. 2005;86:650–658.

193. Elliott TR, Frank RG. Depression following spinal cord injury. *Arch Phys Med Rehabil*. 1996;77:816–823.

194. Dafer RM, Rao M, Shareef A, et al. Poststroke depression. *Top Stroke Rehabil*. 2008;15:13–21.

195. Rosenthal M, Christensen BK, Ross TP. Depression following traumatic brain injury. *Arch Phys Med Rehabil*. 1998;79:90–103.

196. Prigatano GP, Klonoff PS, O'Brien KP, et al. Productivity after neuropsychologically oriented milieu rehabilitation. *J Head Trauma Rehabil*. 1994;9:91–102.

197. Thoreson RW, Smits SJ, Butler AJ, et al. Counseling problems associated with client characteristics. *Wis Stud Vocat Rehabil Monogr*. 1968;3:46.

198. Burke BL, Arkowitz H, Menchola M. The efficacy of motivational interviewing: a meta-analysis of controlled clinical trials. *J Consult Clin Psychol*. 2003;71:843–861. doi:10.1037/0022-006X.71.5.843.

199. Lal S, Korner-Bitensky N. Motivational interviewing: a novel intervention for translating rehabilitation research into practice. *Disabil Rehabil*. 2013;35:919–923.

200. Rollnick S, Mason P, Butler C. *Health Behavior Change: A Guide for Practitioners*. Edinburgh, UK: Churchill Livingstone; 1999.

201. Wagner CC, McMahon BT. Motivational interviewing and rehabilitation counseling practice. *Rehabil Couns Bull*. 2004;47:152–161.

202. Bombardier CH, Rimmele CT. Motivational interviewing to prevent alcohol abuse after traumatic brain injury: a case series. *Rehabil Psychol*. 1999;44:52–67.

203. Cheng D, Qu Z, Huang J, et al. Motivational interviewing for improving recovery after stroke. *Cochrane Database Syst Rev*. 2015;(6):CD011398. doi:10.1002/14651858.CD011398.pub2.

204. Hayes SC, Strosahl KD, Wilson KG. *Acceptance and Commitment Therapy: An Experiential Approach to Behavior Change*. New York: Guilford Press; 1999.

205. Harris R. *ACT Made Simple: An Easy-to-Read Primer on Acceptance and Commitment Therapy*. Oakland, CA: New Harbinger Publications; 2009.

206. Bach PA, Moran DJ. *ACT in Practice: Case Conceptualization in Acceptance and Commitment Therapy*. Oakland, CA: New Harbinger Publications; 2008.

207. Dahl J, Luciano C, Wilson K. *Acceptance and Commitment Therapy for Chronic Pain*. Reno, NV: Context Press; 2005.

208. Robinson P, Wicksell RK, Olsson GL. ACT with chronic pain patients. In: Hayes SC, Strosahl KD, eds. *A Practical Guide to Acceptance and Commitment Therapy*. New York: Springer US; 2004:315–345.

209. Gutiérrez O, Luciano C, Rodríguez M, et al. Comparison between an acceptance-based and a cognitive-control-based protocol for coping with pain. *Behav Ther*. 2004;35:767–783.

210. McCracken LM, Carson JW, Eccleston C, et al. Acceptance and change in the context of chronic pain. *Pain*. 2004;109:4–7.

211. Kangas M, McDonald S. Is it time to act? The potential of acceptance and commitment therapy for psychological problems following acquired brain injury. *Neuropsychol Rehabil*. 2011;21:250–276.

212. Snyder CR. *Coping: The Psychology of What Works*. New York: Oxford; 1999.

213. Csikszentmihalyi M, Csikszentmihalyi IS. *A Life Worth Living: Contributions to Positive Psychology*. Oxford: Oxford University Press; 2006.

214. Ehde DM. Application of positive psychology to rehabilitation psychology. In: Frank RG, Rosenthal M, Caplan B, eds. *Handbook of Rehabilitation Psychology*. 2nd ed. Washington, DC: American Psychological Association; 2010.

215. Seligman ME. Positive psychology, positive prevention, and positive therapy. In: Snyder CR, Lopez SJ, eds. *Handbook of Positive Psychology*. New York: Oxford University Press; 2002:3–12.

216. Seligman MEP, Csikszentmihalyi M. Positive psychology: an introduction. *Am Psychol*. 2000;55:5–14.

217. Duckworth AL, Steen TA, Seligman ME. Positive psychology in clinical practice. *Annu Rev Clin Psychol*. 2005;1:629–651.

218. Burton CM, King LA. The health benefits of writing about intensely positive experiences. *J Res Pers.* 2004;38:150–163.

219. Emmons RA, McCullough ME. Counting blessings versus burdens: an experimental investigation of gratitude and subjective well-being in daily life. *J Pers Soc Psychol.* 2003;84:377.

220. Lyubomirsky S, Sheldon KM, Schkade D. Pursuing happiness: the architecture of sustainable change. *Rev Gen Psychol.* 2005;9:111.

221. Dunn DS, Dougherty SB. Prospects for a positive psychology of rehabilitation. *Rehabil Psychol.* 2005;50:305–311.

222. Dunn DS, Uswatte G, Elliott TR. Happiness, resilience, and positive growth following physical disability: issues for understanding, research, and therapeutic intervention. In: Lopez SJ, Snyder CR, eds. *Oxford Handbook of Positive Psychology.* 2nd ed. New York: Oxford University Press; 2009:651–664.

223. Elliott TR, Kurylo M, Rivera P. Positive growth following acquired physical disability. In: Lopez SJ, Snyder CR, eds. *Handbook of Positive Psychology.* New York: Oxford University Press; 2002:687–699.

224. Keany KMH, Glueckauf RL. Disability and value change: an overview and reanalysis of acceptance of loss theory. *Rehabil Psychol.* 1993;38:199–210.

225. Nierenberg B, Mayersohn G, Serpa S, et al. Application of well-being therapy to people with disability and chronic illness. *Rehabil Psychol.* 2016;61:32.

226. Fava GA, Ruini C. Development and characteristics of a well-being enhancing psychotherapeutic strategy: well-being therapy. *J Behav Ther Exp Psychiatry.* 2003;34:45–63.

227. Ryff CD, Keyes CLM. The structure of psychological well-being revisited. *J Pers Soc Psychol.* 1995;69:719.

228. Martin G, Pear JJ. *Behavior Modification: What it is and How to do it.* Milton Park, Oxfordshire, UK: Psychology Press; 2015.

229. Kazdin AE. *Behavior Modification in Applied Settings.* Long Grove, IL: Waveland Press, Inc.; 2012.

230. Brockway JA, Fordyce WE. Psychological assessment and management. In: Kottke FJ, Lehmann JF, eds. *Krusen's Handbook of Physical Medicine and Rehabilitation.* 4th ed. Philadelphia, PA: WB Saunders; 1990:153–170.

231. Kazdin AE. *Behavior Modification in Applied Settings.* 6th ed. Belmont, CA: Wadsworth/Thomson Learning; 2001.

232. Butt L, Caplan BC. The rehabilitation team. In: Frank RG, Rosenthal M, Caplan B, eds. *Handbook of Rehabilitation Psychology.* 2nd ed. Washington, DC: American Psychological Association; 2010:451–457.

233. Diller L. Fostering the interdisciplinary team, fostering research in a society in transition. *Arch Phys Med Rehabil.* 1990;71:275–278.

234. Rath JF, Elliott TR. Psychological models in rehabilitation psychology. In: Kennedy P, ed. *The Oxford Handbook of Rehabilitation Psychology.* Oxford, UK/New York: Oxford University Press; 2012:32–46.

235. Livneh H, Martz E. Adjustment to chronic illness and disabilities: theoretical perspectives, empirical findings, and unresolved issues. In: Kennedy P, ed. *The Oxford Handbook of Rehabilitation Psychology.* New York: Oxford University Press, Inc.; 2012:47–87.

236. Parsons T. Illness and the role of the physician: a sociological perspective. In: Stoeckle JD, ed. *Encounters between Patients and Doctors: An Anthology. MIT Press Series on the Humanistic and Social Dimensions of Medicine. Vol. 5.* Cambridge, MA: The MIT Press; 1987:147–156.

237. Mechanic D. The concept of illness behavior. *J Chron Dis.* 1962;15:189–194.

238. Kutner B. The social psychology of disability. In: Neff WS, ed. *Rehabilitation Psychology.* Washington, DC: American Psychological Association; 1971:143–167.

239. Kubler-Ross E. *On Death and Dying.* New York: The Macmillan Company; 1969.

240. Holland JM, Neimeyer RA. An examination of stage theory of grief among individuals bereaved by natural and violent causes: a meaning-oriented contribution. *Omega (Westport).* 2010;61:103–120. doi:10.2190/OM.61.2.b.

241. Dembo T, Leviton GL, Wright BA. Adjustment to misfortune: a problem of social-psychological rehabilitation. *Rehabil Psychol.* 1975;22:1–100.

242. Shontz FC. Psychological adjustment to physical disability: trends in theories. *Arch Phys Med Rehabil.* 1978;59:251–254.

243. Maciejewski PK, Zhang B, Block SD, et al. An empirical examination of the stage theory of grief. *JAMA.* 2007;297:716–723. doi:10.1001/jama.297.7.716.

244. Silver RC, Wortman CB. Coping with undesirable life events. In: Garber J, Seligman MEP, eds. *Human Helplessness: Theory and Applications.* New York: Academic Press; 1980:279–340.

245. Wortman CB, Silver RC. The myths of coping with loss revisited. In: Stroebe MS, Hansson RO, eds. *Handbook of Bereavement Research: Consequences, Coping, and Care.* Washington, DC: American Psychological Association; 2001:405–429.

246. Tyhurst JS. Individual reactions to community disaster; the natural history of psychiatric phenomena. *Am J Psychiatry.* 1951;107:764–769.

247. Dinardo QE. Psychological adjustment to spinal cord injury. *Diss Abstr Int.* 1972;32:4206–4207.

248. Lawson NC. Depression after spinal cord injury: a multimeasure longitudinal study. *Diss Abstr Int.* 1976;37:1439.

249. Davis CG, Wortman CB, Lehman DR, et al. Searching for meaning in loss: are clinical assumptions correct? *Death Stud.* 2000;24:497–540.

250. Shadish WR, Hickman D, Arrick M. Psychological problems of spinal cord injury patients: emotional distress as a function of time and locus of control. *J Consult Clin Psychol.* 1981;49:297.

251. Wortman CB, Silver RC, Kessler RC. The meaning of loss and adjustment to bereavement. In: Stroebe MS, Stroebe W, Hansson RO, eds. *Handbook of Bereavement: Theory, Research, and Intervention.* New York: Cambridge University Press; 1993:349–366.

252. Janoff-Bulman R. *Shattered Assumptions: Towards a New Psychology of Trauma.* New York: Free Press; 1992.

253. Park CL. Making sense of the meaning literature: an integrative review of meaning making and its effects on adjustment to stressful life events. *Psychol Bull.* 2010;136:257–301. doi:10.1037/a0018301.

254. Lewin K, Heider F, Heider GM. *Principles of Topological Psychology.* 1st ed. New York/London, UK: McGraw-Hill Book Company, Inc.; 1936.

255. Lewin KA. *Resolving Social Conflicts and Field Theory in Social Science.* Washington, DC: American Psychological Association; 1997.

256. Meyerson L. The social psychology of the physical disability: 1948 and 1988. *J Soc Issues.* 1988;44:173–188.

257. Dunn DS, Andrews EE. Person-first and identity-first language: developing psychologists' cultural competence using disability language. *Am Psychol.* 2015;70:255–264. doi:10.1037/a0038636.

258. Dunn DS, Burcaw S. Disability identity: exploring narrative accounts of disability. *Rehabil Psychol.* 2013;58:148–157.

259. Dunn DM. *The Social Psychology of Disability.* New York: Oxford University Press; 2015.

260. Hersen M, Eisler RM, Miller PM, eds. *Progress in Behavior Modification (Vol. 7).* Cambridge, MA: Academic Press; 2016.

261. Fordyce WE. *Behavioral Methods for Chronic Pain and Illness.* St. Louis, MO: Mosby; 1976.

262. Berni R, Fordyce WE. *Behavior Modification and the Nursing Process.* 2nd ed. St. Louis, MO: Mosby; 1977.

263. Patterson DR. Behavioral methods for chronic pain and illness: a reconsideration and appreciation. *Rehabil Psychol.* 2005;50:312.

264. Fordyce WE. Pain and suffering. *Am Psychol.* 1988;43:276–283.

265. Wolf SL, Huang H. Evolution of biofeedback in physical medicine and rehabilitation. In: Fronterra WR, ed. *Physical Medicine and Rehabilitation, Principles and Practice.* 5th ed. New York: Lippincott Williams & Wilkins; 2010:1937–1952.

266. Uswatte G, Taub E. Implications of the learned nonuse formulation for measuring rehabilitation outcomes: lessons from constraint-induced movement therapy. *Rehabil Psychol.* 2005;50:34–42.

267. McGlynn SM. Behavioral approaches to neuropsychological rehabilitation. *Psychol Bull.* 1990;108:420–441.

268. Davidoff G, Schultz JS, Lieb T, et al. Rehospitalization after initial rehabilitation for acute spinal cord injury: incidence and risk factors. *Arch Phys Med Rehabil.* 1990;71:121–124.

269. Dallery J, Kurti A, Erb P. A new frontier: integrating behavioral and digital technology to promote health behavior. *Behav Anal.* 2015;38:19–49. doi:10.1007/s40614-014-0017-y.

270. Morris JH, Macgillivray S, McFarlane S. Interventions to promote long-term participation in physical activity after stroke: a systematic review of the literature. *Arch Phys Med Rehabil.* 2014;95:956–967. doi:10.1016/j.apmr.2013.12.016.

271. Varnfield M, Karunanithi M, Lee CK, et al. Smartphone-based home care model improved use of cardiac rehabilitation in postmyocardial infarction patients: results from a randomised controlled trial. *Heart.* 2014;100:1770–1779. doi:10.1136/heartjnl-2014-305783.

272. Moos RH, Tsu VD, Schaefer JA. *Coping with Physical Illness.* New York: Plenum Medical Book Co.; 1977.

273. Lindemann E. Symptomatology and management of acute grief. *Am J Psychiatry.* 1944;101:141–148.

274. Snyder CR, Lehman KA. Hope for rehabilitation and vice versa. *Rehabil Psychol.* 2006;51:89–112.

275. Moos R, Holahan C. Adaptive tasks and methods of coping with illness and disability. In: Martz E, Livneh H, eds. *Coping with Chronic Illness and Disability: Theoretical, Empirical and Clinical Aspects.* New York: Springer; 2007:107–126.

276. Ramanathan-Elion DM, McWhorter JW, Wegener ST, et al. The role of psychological facilitators and barriers to therapeutic engagement in acute, inpatient rehabilitation. *Rehabil Psychol.* 2016;61:277–287. doi:10.1037/rep0000095.

277. Felton BJ, Revenson TA. Coping with chronic illness: a study of illness controllability and the influence of coping strategies on psychological adjustment. *J Consult Clin Psychol.* 1984;52:343–353.

278. Cutrona C, Russell D, Rose J. Social support and adaptation to stress by the elderly. *Psychol Aging.* 1986;1:47–54.

279. Gottlieb BH. Social support as a focus for integrative research in psychology. *Am Psychol.* 1983;38:278–287.

280. Schaefer C, Coyne JC, Lazarus RS. The health-related functions of social support. *J Behav Med.* 1981;4:381–406.

281. Cobb S. Social support as a moderator of life stress. *Psychosom Med.* 1976;38:300–314.

282. Turner RJ. Social support as a contingency in psychological well-being. *J Health Soc Behav.* 1981;22:357–367.

283. Bulman RJ, Wortman CB. Attributions of blame and coping in the "real world": severe accident victims react to their lot. *J Pers Soc Psychol.* 1977;35:351–363.

284. Lerner MJ. *The Belief in a Just World: A Fundamental Delusion.* New York: Plenum Press; 1980.

285. Frankl VE. *Man's Search for Meaning; An Introduction to Logotherapy.* Boston, MA: Beacon Press; 1963.

286. Krause JS. Survival following spinal cord injury: a fifteen-year prospective study. *Rehabil Psychol.* 1991;36:89–98.

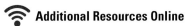 **Additional Resources Online**

CHAPTER 13

Marlís González
Fernández
Rachel W. Mulheren

Joseph P. Pillion
Rajani Sebastian
Donna C. Tippett

Speech, Language, Swallowing, and Auditory Rehabilitation

The ability to communicate is crucial for human interactions. Exchanging information and ideas is facilitated by intact speech, language, cognition, and hearing systems. Many of these interactions occur in social environments where meals are also shared. Consequently, we will discuss these processes and mechanisms to ultimately develop an understanding of the functions that allow us to enjoy an afternoon conversation over a cup of coffee or catching up with family during a holiday meal.

Human communication is dynamic, multidimensional, and continuously influenced by physiologic, psychological, and environmental factors. Although complex, the components of communication can be simplified into four steps:
- Encoding: the speaker creates the message in his or her mind
- Transmittal: the speaker sends the message
- Reception: the listener receives the message
- Decoding: the listener breaks down the message in his or her mind

This chapter serves to improve the understanding of human communication by describing the processes of speech, language, cognition, and hearing. Additionally, swallowing is reviewed due to the shared anatomical and physiologic substrates with speech production and as eating commonly occurs concurrent to communication efforts. We will discuss these topics with a focus on rehabilitation and treatment interventions when any of these functions is affected.

SPEECH PRODUCTION

The term *speech* refers to motor acts that result in the production of sounds through the coordination of respiration, phonation, resonance, articulation, and prosody. Anatomically, it involves the respiratory mechanism, laryngeal mechanism, soft palate (velum), tongue, lips, face, teeth, and jaw (1). Although these processes work concurrently with each other to achieve the end result of speech, it is often easier to understand the complexity of speech production by reviewing each process separately.

Respiration

Breathing involves *ventilation* and *respiration*. *Ventilation* is the movement of air through the upper and lower respiratory tracts. *Respiration* is the exchange of gases (oxygen and carbon dioxide) between the air breathed in and the cells of the body.

The respiratory mechanism provides the energy source for speech production. Speech production occurs during exhalation. During speech production, the amount of time for inhalation is often reduced while the amount of exhalation time is increased during one respiratory cycle.

Phonation

Phonation (voicing) is the product of the vibration of the vocal folds within the larynx. The vocal folds vibrate as air passes through the glottis (the space between the vocal folds). Phonation is achieved through the Bernoulli effect and tissue elasticity. The Bernoulli effect dictates that at a constant volume flow of air (or fluid), at a point of constriction (the glottis), there will be a decrease in air pressure perpendicular to the flow and an increase in velocity of flow. When this drop in pressure becomes sufficiently large, the vocal folds begin oscillating. This oscillation causes vibration, which is often referred to as the engine of the voicing mechanism. Vocal fold motion occurs in a wavelike fashion with lateral undulations as well as superior and inferior movements. The oscillation of the vocal folds serves to modulate the pressure and flow of the air through the larynx. This airflow is modulated and is the main source of voiced sounds. The vocal folds adduct (close) to produce voiced sounds and abduct (open) to produce voiceless sounds. When the vocal folds adduct, subglottic air pressure of 4 to 8 cmH2O is generated, and the vocal folds vibrate to produce phonation (2). During speech production, phonation is initiated and terminated repeatedly. Phonation is characterized by pitch and loudness. Pitch physiologically correlates with frequency or the number of cycles of vocal fold vibration per second (measured in Hertz, Hz). Pitch increases as frequency increases and decreases as frequency deceases. Loudness is the physiologic correlate of intensity (measured in decibels, dB). Medial compression of the vocal folds, achieved through the muscles of adduction and subglottic pressure, contribute to changes in loudness. Vocal registers describe different modes of vocal fold vibration. Modal register or modal phonation is the register used in daily conversation. Typical female voices are 225 Hz (range 155 to 334 Hz), and typical male voices are 128 Hz (range 85 to 196 Hz). Conversational loudness is 70 to 80 dB (SPL) (3).

Resonation

Resonance is the modification of phonation that is determined by the size and shape of the nasal, oral, and pharyngeal cavities. The velopharyngeal mechanism consists of a muscular valve that extends from the posterior surface of the hard palate to the posterior pharyngeal wall and includes the velum (soft palate), lateral pharyngeal walls (sides of the throat), and the posterior pharyngeal wall (back wall of the throat). During speech, velopharyngeal closure separates the oral and nasal cavities as is needed to produce oral speech phonemes. Only three sounds in the English language, /m/, /n/, and /ng/, are produced with an open velopharyngeal port. Velopharyngeal closure is achieved primarily through retraction and elevation of the velum by the velar elevators (levator veli palatini, tensor veli palatine, muscularis uvula) to appose the posterior and lateral pharyngeal walls. In addition, the lateral pharyngeal wall moves toward midline and the posterior pharyngeal wall moves anteriorly to create closure (4).

Articulation

Articulation is the process of shaping phonation (produced by the vocal folds) into speech sounds. The shape of oral cavity is changed by mobile or immobile articulatory structures. The mobile articulators include the velum, tongue, lips, cheeks, and mandible (lower jaw). The immobile articulators are the teeth, hard palate, and alveolar ridge of the maxillae (upper jaw) (5). The coordinated movements of the articulators produce specific phonemes. The addition or elimination of a voicing component from the larynx, during sound production, dictates whether a consonant is voiced or voiceless.

Neural Control

Motor control for respiration, phonation, resonation, and articulation requires complex neural networking, regulation, and monitoring of muscle activity of both the central nervous system and the peripheral nervous system. Neural motor control of speech involves both the pyramidal (direct) and extrapyramidal (indirect) motor pathways. In the pyramidal system, corticospinal and corticobulbar tracts descend from the primary motor and premotor cortices, pass through the internal capsule, decussate in the brainstem, and innervate muscles to control voluntary movement. Upper motor neurons in the cortex control lower motor neurons in the peripheral nervous system. Afferent and efferent loops of the basal ganglia circuit regulate motor movements through a "damping effect." The cerebellar circuit facilitates coordinated sequential movement. In addition, sensory pathways regulate speech motor control (6). Cranial nerves for speech production include cranial nerve V (trigeminal), cranial nerve VII (facial), cranial nerve IX (glossopharyngeal), cranial nerve X (vagus), cranial nerve XI (accessory), and cranial nerve XII (hypoglossal). Spinal nerves innervate muscles of respiration; at cervical levels 3 through 5, the phrenic nerve innervates the diaphragm, and at thoracic levels 2 through 11, spinal nerves innervate the internal and external intercostals.

SPEECH DISORDERS (SEE ALSO CHAPTER 18)

Speech disorders can be a result of *neurologic* etiologies, such as stroke or progressive neurologic disease, or to *structural* etiologies, such as head and neck cancer, velopharyngeal insufficiency (VPI), or vocal fold pathology (e.g., vocal fold motion impairment, nodules, polyps).

Differential Diagnosis

Dysarthria and *apraxia of speech* (AOS) are distinct from other neurogenic communication disorders, such as aphasia. Dysarthria is reserved for *neurogenic* speech disorders rather than speech disorders due to *structural* etiologies. In addition, voice disorders, including abnormalities of vocal quality due to vocal fold lesions or vocal fold motion impairments (e.g., hoarseness, roughness), are also separate entities. However, perceptual voice deviations (e.g., vocal hoarseness, strain, low volume) may be considered within the realm of dysarthria and may be typical of certain etiologies.

Unlike *aphasia* (a language disorder affecting the domains of verbal expression, written expression, auditory comprehension, and reading comprehension), language content is preserved in dysarthria and AOS. *AOS* is a disorder characterized by impaired motor planning and programming. It is defined as an articulatory disorder resulting from impairment of programming the positioning of speech musculature and the sequencing of muscle movements for the volitional production of speech without weakness, slowness, or incoordination (7,8). In most dysarthrias, all speech systems, including respiration, phonation, resonation, and articulation, are involved, whereas in AOS, respiratory or phonatory involvement is rare. It should be recognized that patients often can have elements of both dysarthria and AOS, particularly those with bilateral brain damage.

Dysarthria

Dysarthria is caused by damage to the central or peripheral nervous system (7,9,10). Causes include central nervous system etiologies, such as stroke, Parkinson's disease, or brain tumors (see also Chapters 18-25); peripheral nervous system diseases, such as amyotrophic lateral sclerosis; disorders of the neuromuscular junction, such as myasthenia gravis; and muscular disorders, such as muscular dystrophy. Dysarthria can result from isolated cranial nerve lesions (such as the vagus [X] or hypoglossal [XII]).

The prevalence and incidence of dysarthria are not precisely known. Dysarthria can be a symptom of a neurologic disease process with a constellation of other symptoms, or it can stand alone in the setting of a disease. Prevalence of dysarthria associated with traumatic brain injury (TBI) varies, depending upon severity of TBI and time post onset. Prevalence of dysarthria in the acute phase of recovery is 65%, whereas in the postacute phase (outpatient rehabilitation), prevalence is 22% (11,12). Dysarthria is seen in 50% to 90% of individuals with parkinsonism with increased prevalence as the disease progresses (13). Additionally, dysarthria can be a herald sign of amyotrophic lateral sclerosis or can become present as the disease progresses.

The perceptual classification system developed at the Mayo Clinic in 1969 (7,9,10) is used extensively in clinical practice by speech-language pathologists. Each dysarthria type is represented by a perceived and distinguishable grouping of speech characteristics with a presumed underlying pathophysiology or locus of lesion. The major types of dysarthria are flaccid, spastic, hyperkinetic, hypokinetic, ataxic, unilateral upper motor neuron, and mixed.

Flaccid Dysarthria

Flaccid dysarthria is due to lower motor neuron damage. Its specific characteristics depend on which nerve is involved. Cranial nerves affecting articulation include trigeminal, facial, or hypoglossal. The vagus nerve contributes to voice and resonance quality. Spinal nerves can also be affected with resultant deficits in breath patterning for speech, often causing production of short phrases. Common perceptual deviations include monoloudness, breathy phonation, hypernasality, nasal emission, imprecise articulation, and monotone. Flaccid dysarthria can result from brainstem stroke, muscular dystrophy, and myasthenia gravis.

Spastic Dysarthria

Spastic dysarthria is due to upper motor neuron damage, usually bilateral lesions of upper motor neuron pathways that innervate the relevant cranial nerve and spinal nerve. It is characterized by reduced volume, strained-strangled phonation, low pitch, hypernasality, imprecise articulation, slow rate, and reduced or equal and excess stress. Etiologies include stroke, TBI, and progressive supranuclear palsy.

Ataxic Dysarthria

Ataxic dysarthria is associated with cerebellar damage, such as stroke or spinocerebellar syndromes. It is characterized by excess loudness, pitch variations, excess and equal stress, variable rate, and irregular articulatory breakdown.

Hypokinetic Dysarthria

Hypokinetic dysarthria is associated with damage to the extrapyramidal tract. The speech deviations in Parkinson's disease are typical of this dysarthria subtype. Classic features are low volume, breathy phonation, monotone, imprecise articulation, and excess rate of speech.

Hyperkinetic Dysarthria

Hyperkinetic dysarthria is also associated with damage to the extrapyramidal tract; however, unlike hypokinetic dysarthria, hyperkinetic dysarthria is distinguished by abnormal involuntary movements that affect the intended speech movements. Hyperkinetic dysarthria can be seen in association with Huntington's disease and cerebral palsy. Excess loudness, strained phonation, phonation breaks, hypernasality, imprecise articulation, and variable rate characterize this dysarthria subtype.

Unilateral Upper Motor Neuron Dysarthria

This dysarthria has an anatomical rather than a pathophysiologic label. It typically results from unilateral stroke affecting upper neuron pathways. Characteristics overlap with other dysarthria subtypes (14).

Mixed Dysarthria

Mixed dysarthria is due to damage to upper and lower motor neurons. Common diagnoses are multiple system atrophy and multiple sclerosis. Combinations of perceptual speech characteristics are present, for example, spastic/flaccid, spastic/ataxic, hypokinetic/spastic/ataxic.

Apraxia of Speech

AOS occurs in the absence of significant weakness and incoordination of muscles, with automatic and reflexive movements undisturbed. AOS is seen after left hemisphere stroke (15,16). Lesions in the premotor cortex are a frequent finding. AOS is also seen after damage to left subcortical structures. Less commonly, it is a sign of progressive neurologic disease (17–19). Developmental AOS occurs in children and is present from

birth. The etiology of childhood AOS is not clear, although abundant research focuses on genetic origins (20,21). There is debate as to whether AOS is a pure motor or linguistic (i.e., phonemic) disturbance (22–24); it is seen by some as a distinct condition that often coexists and complicates aphasia, whereas others regard the characteristics as part of the nonfluent Broca's aphasia. AOS carries a negative prognosis for recovery when there is a moderate to severe aphasia in tandem. When it occurs without the concomitant language disturbance, therapy can focus on retraining the ability to program sound patterns, to shift from one sound to another, and to use preserved melodic and rhythmic patterns to facilitate speech.

Head and Neck Cancer

Speech and voice impairments can be seen in the setting of head and neck cancer. Head and neck cancers develop in the mucosa of the lining of the upper aerodigestive tract. Although excessive tobacco and alcohol use remains a primary cause of head and neck cancer, the incidence of human papillomavirus–related head and neck cancer is increasing (25). Speech and voice impairments depend upon tumor size and site (e.g., oral tongue, floor of mouth, base of tongue, tonsil, hard palate, velum, jaw) as well as treatment modality (i.e., surgery, reconstruction, radiation therapy and/or chemotherapy). Increasingly, individuals with head and neck cancer are treated with organ preservation therapy rather than surgery. Although organ preservation therapy is desirable because structures are preserved, function may be compromised (26–28). Prostheses may be needed to correct intraoral surgical defects, such as a palatal obturator in the setting of maxillectomy (29). Individuals whose treatment required total laryngectomy may be candidates for tracheoesophageal voice prostheses to restore voice (30).

Velopharyngeal Insufficiency

VPI refers to a structural defect compromising velopharyngeal closures. This can be due to abnormalities of the velum and/or lymphoid tissue (tonsils and adenoids), cervical or cranial base abnormalities, cleft palate, and surgical interventions, such as maxillary advancement, tonsillectomy, and adenoidectomy. VPI is distinguished from velopharyngeal incompetence, a neurophysiologic disorder in which poor movement of the velopharyngeal structures results in incomplete velopharyngeal closure, and velopharyngeal mislearning resulting in misarticulation (31). In VPI, resonance is hypernasal and there may be nasal emission of air. Treatment may include surgery, intraoral prostheses, and postsurgical speech articulation therapy.

SPEECH DISORDERS IN CHILDREN (SEE ALSO CHAPTER 45)

As part of normal development, speech sounds emerge at different ages, with some sounds being learned earlier, such as /b, d, m, n/ and others learned later, such as /ch, j, l, s/. Speech sound disorders include problems with articulation (sound production) and phonologic processes (sound patterns). The cause of articulation and phonologic speech sound disorders in most children is unknown, although risk factors include male sex and familial history of speech and language disorders, whereas protective factors include maternal well-being and a persistent and sociable temperament (32,33).

VOICE DISORDER

A voice disorder is defined as voice quality, pitch, and loudness that differ or are inappropriate for an individual's age, gender, cultural background, or geographic location (34,35). Voice disorders can be due to structural abnormalities, such as vocal nodules; a neurogenic etiology, such as vocal fold motion impairment due to a lesion of cranial nerve X (vagus); or a functional etiology, such as muscle tension dysphonia. Intervention depends on the etiology and may include both medical/surgical and/or behavioral therapy. Behavioral therapy can be physiologic, designed to balance the systems of respiration, phonation, and resonation, or symptomatic and designed to treat perceptual deviations.

TRACHEOSTOMY AND MECHANICAL VENTILATION

Speech is precluded by inflation of the cuff of the tracheostomy cannula. When the cuff is inflated, inspiration and expiration occur at the level of the cannula. There is minimal to no airflow past the inflated cuff and through the larynx. Cuff deflation allows airflow to occur through the cannula and through the upper airways. After cuff deflation, various options can be employed to restore speech, including modifications of ventilator settings and tracheostomy speaking valves (36).

FLUENCY

Fluency disorders are characterized by a disruption in the ease and flow of connected speech. The most common and well-known type of fluency disorder is stuttering. Stuttering typically has its origins in childhood. Most children who stutter begin to do so around 2½ years of age (37). Stuttering is a very complex, dynamic, and somewhat controversial disorder in that theories and opinions abound regarding etiology, diagnosis, and treatment. The evaluating clinician must be very cautious with diagnosis for several reasons. One, stuttering resolves in 75% to 90% of small children who begin to stutter. Additionally, there is a spectrum of normal dysfluency that is reactive to environmental pressures but is not consistent with a stuttering diagnosis (38). Less commonly, dysfluency can be neurogenic or psychogenic (39–42).

SPEECH ASSESSMENT

Assessment of speech begins with the collection of information about the nature and onset of the speech disorder. This can be accomplished through review of the individual's medical and/or educational records and through interview of the patient/client, family members, and caregivers to investigate the specific nature of the speech disorder, onset, duration, course, and impact on daily function and quality of life.

Speech-language pathologists perform speech/oral motor examinations to assess respiration (respiratory mechanism), phonation (laryngeal mechanism), resonation (velum, pharynx), and articulation (lips, cheeks, jaw, teeth). The structural integrity and function of each component is assessed via non–speech- and speech-related tasks.

Formal tests, such as the Frenchay Dysarthria Test and the Apraxia Battery for Adults-2 (ABA-2), may be administered to characterize the speech impairment (43,44). Measures of speech intelligibility, such as the Assessment of Intelligibility of Dysarthric Speech, may also be used to assess performance at the connected speech level (45). Specialized questionnaires, such as the Quality of Communication Life Scale, probe the impact of communication disorders on various aspects of quality of life (46).

Instrumental approaches may be employed as well. For example, measurement of respiratory function may include acoustic measures of vocal intensity and utterance durations. Respiratory performance may also be assessed by estimating the subglottic air pressure generated by the speaker (47,48). Laryngeal structure and function can be visualized during endoscopy and stroboscopy. Instrumentation, such as the Nasometer II, Model 6450 (Kay Elemetrics Corp., Lincoln Park, NJ, USA), can be used to measure the presence of nasality in speech production by assessing acoustic output from the oral and nasal cavities and calculating an output ratio (49). Movement of the velopharyngeal mechanism can be observed through endoscopic visualization. Lingual strength against resistance can be measured using the Iowa Oral Performance Instrument (IOPI—Blaise Medical Inc.), a handheld, portable pneumatic pressure sensor that provides visual feedback of pressure generation via an array of light-emitting diodes.

TREATMENT OF SPEECH DISORDERS

Although additional research is needed, the evidence base is growing to support speech-language pathology intervention to treat speech disorders in children and adults. Several systematic reviews and treatment guidelines exist (50–52). Caution continues to be warranted in the treatment of AOS (53). Therapy can be delivered in individual or group settings. Goals are individualized and based on the performance on specific assessments as well as patient input so that the therapy approach is person centered (54). Treatment is multifaceted, including direct (e.g., performing nonspeech oral motor exercises, practicing communication strategies such as rate control and overarticulation) and indirect therapy approaches (e.g., patient/client education and counseling, environmental modifications, prostheses, and devices).

Treatment goals can vary based on the severity of the speech impairment and the underlying etiology.

Treatment approaches for individuals with progressive etiologies are different from treatment for those who have more favorable prognoses (55). Early in the disease process, patients are encouraged to maximize functional communication by paying specific attention to the clarity and precision of their speech. At some point, the patients need to modify their speaking patterns by controlling rate and consonant emphasis and by reducing the number of words per breath. In severe cases, AAC systems may be considered (56). These augmentation systems usually are chosen or designed to accommodate the lifestyle of the patient while serving his or her anticipated communication needs over the longest period of time. The role of oral motor exercise in the management of bulbar dysfunction in amyotrophic lateral sclerosis remains unclear (57). In contrast, in another neuro-degenerative disease, there are multiple citations documenting the successful treatment of dysarthria with Lee Silverman Voice Treatment (58,59).

Partnerships with other medical professionals can be vital to the success of behavioral therapy. For example, a maxillofacial prosthodontist may assist with managing resonant disorders such as velopharyngeal incompetence. Fabrication of a prosthetic device such as a palatal lift can assist with management of impaired velopharyngeal closure. Assessment of candidacy for the device is a coordinated effort between the speech-language pathologist and the prosthodontist. An appropriately fitted palatal lift will allow certain dysarthric speakers to better produce speech sounds that require air pressure buildup and can maximize intelligibility by improving prosody and contextual breath support. Collaboration with otolaryngologists is indicated in determining candidacy for placement of tracheo-esophageal prostheses (30). Collaboration with respiratory therapists and nurses, among other members of the medical team, is needed when applying tracheostomy speaking valves to restore speech in appropriate candidates (36). In addition, medical and surgical interventions facilitate and complement behavioral speech therapy, such as vocal fold injection medialization, laryngoplasty, pharyngoplasty, and botulinum toxin injections.

Thorough education and counseling of patients, family members, and caregivers are integral to the success of speech-language intervention. Understanding the rationale for treatment facilitates adherence to treatment, carryover of exercises, and generalization of therapy techniques. Counseling also prepares individuals for significant changes in communication. For example, thorough preoperative counseling is an important part of rehabilitation in advance of total laryngectomy, glossectomy, and other head and neck surgeries and in advance of decline in communication ability in degenerative diseases (60,61).

LANGUAGE

Language is an arbitrary system of signs or symbols used according to prescribed rules to convey meaning within a linguistic community (62). An understanding of the mechanisms responsible for the processing and formulation of language is critical to good rehabilitation practice. Traditional study of language has focused on specified sites being responsible for specific functions. Paul Broca's work showed that damage to anterior parts of the brain, particularly the left posterior inferior frontal cortex (Broca's area), is associated with language production problems, while Carl Wernicke's work showed that damage to more posterior regions in the temporal lobe (Wernicke's area) is associated with language comprehension problems (63,64). Based on the work of Carl Wernicke, Lichtheim formulated a three-component model of language in which Broca's and Wernicke's areas are interconnected via a hypothetical (not anatomically localized) "concept center" involved in semantic processing (65). This model became the standard reference for clinicians to predict aphasic syndromes from lesions of either a center or a connection. This laid the groundwork for Geschwind's seminal work on aphasia classification and associated lesion sites (66).

Development of functional imaging has broadened our view of language processing, and current theories on brain organization suggest that cognitive functions such as language are organized in widespread, segregated, and overlapping networks (67). Neuroimaging studies reveal that, although the left hemisphere shows more activation in the majority of neurologically normal adults, both cerebral hemispheres are activated during language tasks (68). More distant areas of the cortex, such as the inferior and anterior temporal cortices, the basal ganglia, and thalamus, are also activated during language tasks (69,70). An influential language processing model, the dual stream model, was proposed by Hickok and Poeppel for auditory language processing (71). Their model describes two processing routes, a dorsal stream and a ventral stream, that roughly support speech production and speech comprehension, respectively, in normal subjects.

Aphasia

Aphasia is an acquired disorder of all language modalities, including verbal expression, auditory comprehension, written expression, and reading comprehension. It interferes with the ability to manipulate the meaning (i.e., semantics) or order (i.e., syntax) of words, spoken or written. Three important points to emphasize in this definition include the following:

1. The term *aphasia* implies impairment in both receptive and expressive language modalities. Expression may be more severely involved than comprehension, and comprehension can appear grossly intact. If the testing instrument is sensitive to subtle change in language behavior, pathology can be identified in the more intact modality.
2. Aphasia is consistent only with focal disease, usually of the left hemisphere. Aphasic symptoms may be part of a diffuse pathologic condition. However, these patients evidence more than disruptions in their ability to manipulate linguistic symbols, such as disorientation. Prognosis and recovery for this group are markedly different from those who evidence aphasia alone.
3. Although it is well known that aphasia is usually a consequence of cortical disease, the identification and classification of more atypical aphasic syndromes are also associated with subcortical infarction and hemorrhage (72).

Aphasia Categorization

Classic aphasiology, based primarily on cerebrovascular lesions, has shown that aphasias can differ in their clinical manifestations depending on lesion location within the language network. The Boston classification system standardizes terminology by classifying disorders into those in which expressive skills are predominantly fluent and those in which they are predominantly nonfluent (73). The eight major types of aphasia in the Boston system include the more common forms of Broca's aphasia, Wernicke's aphasia, anomia, conduction aphasia, and global aphasia, as well as the less frequent transcortical types, transcortical motor and transcortical sensory (**Table 13-1**). Each of these aphasic syndromes has discrete symptoms and is correlated with a specific localized cortical lesion, some with subcortical extension.

TABLE 13-1	**Summary of the Boston Classification System of Aphasia**
Type	**Language Characteristics**
Nonfluent	
Broca's	Telegraphic, agrammatic expression with relatively spared comprehension. Often associated with apraxia of speech.
Transcortical motor	Limited language output similar to those of Broca's aphasia, but repetition is intact and agrammatism may be less pronounced.
Global	Severe impairment in comprehension and expression of language.
Mixed transcortical	Severe impairment in expression and comprehension but repetition intact.
Fluent	
Anomia	Language output is generally fluent except for hesitations and pauses associated with word retrieval deficits.
Conduction	Language output is fluent but paraphasic, comprehension of spoken language is intact, and repetition is severely impaired.
Wernicke's	Language output is fluent but is highly paraphasic. Comprehension is impaired.
Transcortical sensory	Language output is fluent but is highly paraphasic. Comprehension is impaired, but repetition is intact.

Nonfluent Aphasias

Broca's Aphasia

Broca's aphasia is caused by damage or dysfunction to the left posterior, inferior frontal gyrus, which includes Broca's area (Brodmann area 44 and 45). Often called "expressive aphasia," this aphasia is characterized by nonfluent spontaneous speech and sentence repetition with relatively spared comprehension. The term "Nonfluent speech" often includes reduced phrase length, impaired melody and articulatory agility, diminished words per minute, or agrammatic sentence production. Patients with Broca's aphasia tend to have good comprehension of single words and grammatically simple sentences but have trouble with grammatically complex sentences. Reading and writing also show a range of impairments. AOS frequently accompanies Broca's aphasia.

Transcortical Motor Aphasia

Transcortical motor aphasia is caused by lesions just anterior or superior to (surrounding) Broca's area, often caused by occlusion of the anterior cerebral artery or "watershed" areas between the anterior and middle cerebral artery (73,74). Language function is similar to those of Broca's aphasia with the exception that repetition is relatively preserved.

Global Aphasia

Global aphasia is typically associated with a large left hemisphere lesion. It is considered the most severe aphasia with significant deficits in all language modalities. Often, automatic expressions such as counting or profanity are preserved. Also, frequently these patients can use other modalities, such as facial expression and/or gesture, to communicate basic wants, needs, or feelings (75). Typically, the person has severely impaired comprehension of single words, sentences, and conversation, and very limited, if any, spoken output. Spontaneous speech, naming, and repetition may be limited to a single perseverative word (e.g., no, no, no) or nonword utterance. Reading and writing are also profoundly impaired. In most cases, both Broca's area and Wernicke's area are damaged or functionally compromised (76).

Mixed Transcortical Aphasia

Mixed transcortical aphasia is comparable to global aphasia, except that sentence repetition is spared. These individuals appear to be echolalic and have lesions surrounding Broca's and Wernicke's area, but sparing language cortex itself (77). Because of this localization, the syndrome is sometimes known as "isolation of the speech area," as it appears to disconnect speech and language from broadly distributed meanings of words.

Fluent Aphasias

Wernicke's Aphasia

Wernicke's aphasia is caused by damage or dysfunction to the left Wernicke's area (Brodmann area 22, in the posterior, superior temporal gyrus). Often called "receptive aphasia," this aphasia is characterized by fluent but relatively meaningless spontaneous speech and repetition and relatively poor comprehension of words, sentences, and conversation. Patients with this type of aphasia often produce sentences with intact grammar and rhythm of speech, but spoken language may be limited to jargon comprised of either real words or neologisms (nonwords such as "klimorata") or a combination of the two frequent paraphasias of both types and/or frequent neologisms or jargon. Due to poor auditory comprehension, error awareness is also poor, usually making for a less effective communicator than one with Broca's aphasia. Written output is typically similar to spoken output—written words with little or no content, often including nonword letter strings. Reading comprehension is typically no better than spoken comprehension.

Transcortical Sensory Aphasia

Transcortical sensory aphasia is caused by lesions involving areas surrounding Wernicke's area, in the watershed territories between the MCA and posterior cerebral artery (PCA), or the PCA territory (78). It is similar to Wernicke's aphasia, but repetition is relatively preserved.

Conduction Aphasia

Conduction aphasia is caused by a lesion in the arcuate fasciculus, a white matter tract that runs between Broca's and Wernicke's areas. In conduction aphasia, repetition is disproportionately impaired relative to auditory comprehension and verbal expression (75). Verbal output is generally grammatical and fluent but has episodes of halting speech during moments of word retrieval difficulty. Spelling and reading abilities may be spared.

Anomic Aphasia

Anomic aphasia is a form of aphasia characterized primarily by significant word retrieval problems (79). It is differentiated from the symptoms of anomia, which is typical in the most forms of aphasia. It typically is the mildest form of aphasia.

Speech is generally fluent except for hesitations and pauses associated with word retrieval deficits. Syntax is generally intact. The lesion sites can be anywhere within the left hemisphere language network, including the middle and inferior temporal gyri.

Other Aphasias

Alexia and Agraphia

Stroke can selectively impair reading and/or writing. Pure alexia refers to impaired reading in the presence of spared writing and relatively spared recognition of words spelled aloud. This syndrome often results from a combination of two lesions, both caused by occlusion or stenosis of the left PCA. A lesion in the left occipital cortex results in right homonymous hemianopsia, such that all visual information is initially processed in the right occipital cortex. A second lesion in the splenium of the corpus callosum prevents visual information in the right hemisphere from being transferred to the left hemisphere language cortex (80). Agraphia refers to impaired writing in the presence of spared reading. Damage or dysfunction in the left inferior parietal lobe, left mid-fusiform gyrus (or nearby area in the left Brodmann area 37 in the left occipitotemporal cortex) results in impairment in spelling (81).

Agnosia

Agnosia is the inability to interpret or recognize information when the end organ is intact. For example, a patient with auditory agnosia would have normal audiometric hearing thresholds but cannot interpret speech signals at the cortical level. Hence, auditory comprehension will be severely compromised. Patients with agnosia can be differentiated from those with aphasia because they will be impaired in only one modality. For example, the patient with auditory agnosia who has severe comprehension deficits can read the same words through the intact visual modality.

Aphasia Assessments

Tests for aphasia measure the patient's receptive and expressive language capacities by sampling different types of language skills through systematically controlled channels. For example, an examination of auditory comprehension skills might begin with single word comprehension task assessed via picture word matching and then proceed to more difficult tasks such as sequential commands. Tests of expression might range from simple repetition to naming to providing definitions or picture descriptions. Most test batteries currently in use provide a representative sample from which inferences can be made about performance in similar linguistic situations.

Some of the more commonly utilized aphasia assessments include the Boston Diagnostic Aphasia Examination, 3rd edition (BDAE (82)) and Western Aphasia Battery—Revised (WAB (83)). The 3rd edition of BDAE provides a comprehensive exploration of a range of communicative abilities. The BDAE contains 34 subtests that assess conversational and narrative speech, auditory comprehension, oral expression, repetition, reading, and writing. The BDAE consists of an extended standard form for an in-depth study of aphasia symptoms, including grammar and syntax, and a short form that takes only 30 to 45 minutes to complete. The Boston Naming Test is included in BDAE-3 (84). Like the BDAE-3, the WAB is designed to diagnose aphasic syndromes.

The WAB-Revised contains 32 tasks with eight subtests and measures spontaneous speech, auditory comprehension, repetition, and naming, as well as reading and writing. Additionally, most isolated aphasia test batteries do not depict an individual's functional communication performance. To determine one's overall communicative functional status, additional testing is often required. The functional assessment of communication skills for adults (ASHA-FACS) is a commonly used test to assess functional communication skills (85). ASHA-FACS has 43 items and assesses functional communication in four areas: social communication; communication of basic needs; reading, writing, and number concepts; and daily planning.

Approaches to Treatment

Aphasia treatment is both restitutive and compensatory. Therapy may vary in treatment regimen, theoretical approach, or delivery model. Principles of neuroplasticity support early and intense therapy; however, questions remain regarding specific intervention strategies given the variable nature of aphasia. Participants with aphasia, even those with similar types of lesions, represent a heterogeneous group. Because of this heterogeneity, outcomes of treatment may be unpredictable. In addition to building on the patient's communicative strengths, remediation should be directed toward helping the patient, family, and friends accept and adapt to the person's impairment. Education and training of the family members or close loved ones in how to facilitate communication is also very important.

Traditionally, clinicians base therapy largely on assessment data. This follows a medical model, which emphasizes impairment of function, and is therapist centered. Therapy tasks are developed to target specific domains, such as word retrieval at a single word level for aphasia treatment. Clinicians use stimulation techniques such as semantic and phonemic cues to treat word retrieval deficits. There has been a growing shift from a medical model to a social model of therapy, which encompasses equalizing the social relations of service delivery, the authentic involvement of users (patients), creation of engaging experiences, user control, and accountability (86). This approach encourages patient-centered care, focusing on development of goals that address individual needs and circumstances. A specific example of a patient-centered approach is the Life Participation Approach to Aphasia (87). This approach places the life concerns of those affected by aphasia at the center of all decision-making. It empowers the consumer to select and participate in the recovery process and to collaborate on the design of interventions that aim for a more rapid return to active life. Therefore, this intervention has the potential to reduce the consequences of disease and injury that contribute to long-term health costs (87).

Applications of the principles governing brain organization and reorganization may contribute to the development of more meaningful therapy approaches in aphasia rehabilitation. One promising training approach is the development of constrained induced language therapy that has demonstrated positive clinical outcomes for individuals with aphasia (88). Noninvasive brain stimulation techniques such as transcranial direct current stimulation (tDCS) offer a potentially important adjunctive approach to behavioral therapy (89). Protocols employing tDCS have shown to improve naming in individuals with chronic aphasia (90–92). Although the precise mechanism of tDCS is still emerging, the prospect of augmenting the effectiveness of behavioral therapy is attractive to clinicians, patients, their families, and caregivers (93).

Language Deficits in Primary Progressive Aphasia

Primary progressive aphasia (PPA) is a clinical syndrome characterized by insidious onset and gradual deterioration of language skills. Language is disproportionately impaired, without impairment in other cognitive domains other than praxis (94,95). A 2011 consensus described recommendations for recognizing three common forms of PPA: nonfluent/agrammatic variant PPA, semantic variant PPA, and logopenic variant PPA (96). The clinical characteristics of each of the three variants are given in 🛜 eTable 13-1 (97). Structural and functional imaging data confirm distinct regions of cortical atrophy associated with each PPA subtype (96,98,99). The semantic variant is associated with left greater than right anterior temporal lobe atrophy, whereas the nonfluent/agrammatic variant is associated with predominant abnormalities in the left posterior frontal and insular. In contrast, the logopenic variant is associated with left posterior perisylvian temporoparietal atrophy. Clinicopathologic studies have most often linked nonfluent progressive aphasia to tau-positive pathology, semantic dementia to ubiquitin-positive, TDP43-positive pathology and the logopenic form to Alzheimer's disease pathology (100–102).

Assessment of Primary Progressive Aphasia

Language skills can be assessed using the commonly utilized aphasia assessments like BDAE and WAB. Assessment of linguistic skills should be accomplished at regular intervals to chart progression. In addition to language testing, neuropsychological screening needs to be done to determine if patients meet criteria for PPA diagnosis. The Clinical Dementia Rating Scale and the Mini-Mental State Examination can be used to assess global aspects of functionality and cognition, respectively (103,104). The California Verbal Learning Test–Mental Status Version and a modified version of the Rey–Osterrieth complex figure with a 10-minute free recall delay trial can be used to assess verbal and nonverbal episodic memory (105). Modified Trail B test and backward digit span can be used to assess executive functioning (106).

Treatment of Primary Progressive Aphasia

Within the language rehabilitation literature, there is an abundance of studies on therapy after stroke, but intervention approaches to treating language deficits in patients with PPA are few (107). It is very important to educate patients and their caregiver/family regarding the nature of PPA and language disorders. Treatment in PPA can be divided into impairment-focused remediation techniques and participation-focused activities (108). The impairment-focused remediation techniques included semantic therapy, naming therapy, word finding strategies, fluency treatment, and nonverbal language-based treatments. The participation-focused activities included the teaching of total communication techniques and/or development of augmentative and alternative communication (AAC) including life books, personal portfolios, and/or communication books. Depression is frequently observed in patients with PPA and should be treated with appropriate

interventions (109). There is growing interest in using tDCS as a possible means to augment behavioral intervention effects and reduce the rate of decline in language (110–112). To date, there are only a few studies with small sample sizes, so results require caution in interpretation but offer hope for improved outcomes of combined language therapy and tDCS.

Communication Impairment After Right Hemisphere Damage

The communication problems that appear in individuals with right hemisphere damage (RHD) are not exclusively language based. RHD has been found to result in a myriad of impairments. These may include visual spatial neglect and other attention deficits as well as difficulties with memory and components of executive function such as problem solving, reasoning, organization, planning, and self-awareness (113,114). In addition, individuals with RHD may exhibit a wide range of communication impairments that can negatively impact functional performance in social and vocational settings (115,116). Communication impairments can include impairment in the pragmatic aspects of language such as difficulty interpreting abstract language such as metaphors, making inferences, and understanding jokes. Impairment is also observed in the nonverbal aspects of language such as problems understanding nonverbal cues and following the rules of communication (e.g., saying inappropriate things, not using facial expressions, talking at the wrong time). Disorders of prosody are commonly observed individuals with RHD. Speech production may sound flat or monotone, and the individual may have difficulty interpreting emotion and/or intent conveyed through prosody (117,118). Some patients experience anosognosia, an unawareness of the problems experienced, which makes remediation more challenging (119).

Assessment of Right Hemisphere Damage

Clinicians complete a variety of formal and informal evaluation procedures. Specifically, the patient's language (comprehension and expression) and cognitive processes (attention, memory, reasoning, problem solving) will be examined. The nature and severity of the cognitive-communication problem will depend on the extent of damage to the brain. Understanding patient's personality and functional status prior to neurologic injury is important; therefore, interview of close friends or family members is a critical element in assessment. Several batteries are appropriate for use in individuals with RHD. The Mini Inventory of Right Brain Injury—2nd edition allows quick screening for neurocognitive deficits associated with right hemisphere lesions and takes 25 to 30 minutes to complete (120). The test consists of 27 items distributed across 10 subsections from four general functional domains: (a) visuospatial/visuoperceptual and attentional processing, (b) lexical knowledge processing, (c) affective processing, and (d) behavioral processing. The Right Hemisphere Language Battery (RHLB) is another widely used comprehensive battery to help provide a quantitative and qualitative assessment of the language and communication impairments that can arise as a result of RHD (121). The RHLB consists of tests of lexical semantic comprehension; spoken metaphor appreciation; written metaphor appreciation; verbal humor appreciation; comprehension of inference; production of emphatic stress; and a comprehensive discourse analysis.

Treatment of Right Hemisphere Damage

The area of RHD cognitive-communication disorders is quite new, with the earliest systematic research only about 30 years old. There continues to be a variety of challenges to research and rehabilitation. Heterogeneity of symptom presentation is one major problem (122). Similar to aphasia treatment, most clinicians follow a medical model, which emphasizes impairment of function, and is therapist centered. However, there is an increasing interest in focusing on development of goals that address individual needs and circumstances. For example, multidimensional applied cognitive rehabilitation conceptualizes treatment as a process of addressing obstacles to patients' attainment of their own goals. In this view, deficits are appropriate for direct treatment only when they create meaningful obstacles to goal attainment. Other obstacles may be factors outside of the patients themselves (123). Treatment of cognitive-communication impairment in RHD should concentrate on three broad areas as follows:

1. The communication specialist should develop tasks that help the patient attend to contextual cues in an effort to reduce verbosity and improve topic maintenance, retell stories in a fashion that highlights the main points, and produce language that follows a logical sequence. Although these tasks appear related to the impairment, no data support success or failure using such strategies.

2. Education of the patient's family members on how the loss of pragmatic and affective languages can affect their perception of the patient's personality is important. It is important to train family members and caregivers how to provide contextual constraint; supply and guide use of cue cards and other prompts or organizers; learn to elicit appropriate responses, reduce and simplify input, and identify triggers and reinforcers of desired and undesirable behaviors. Rehabilitation successes will be diminished or lost if the patient's family members/caregivers do not understand the reasons for the adjustment to a new personality.

3. Many speech-language pathologists also address the cognitive processes that affect communication, such as attention, memory, executive functioning, and safety awareness/judgment. They do this through tasks that are individualized to address the specific deficit areas and can translate to optimizing function in real-world situations. For example, answering questions regarding a map can address visual attention, visual perceptual skills, left attention, and, depending on the complexity of the map and the questions, executive functions such as planning, problem solving, and reasoning. Even more functional is the actual use of a map to route find within an unfamiliar setting. This will address the aforementioned skills but will more greatly challenge attention, executive functioning, and safety awareness.

Communication Impairment After Traumatic Brain Injury (see also Chapter 19)

Patients with TBI will suffer some degree of cognitive-communication impairment. Brain tissue damage in TBI may be discrete and focal; typically, however, injury is diffuse and includes cortical and subcortical involvement. Patients who sustain discrete lesions may display language impairments that are similar to those that appear in individuals with aphasia following a stroke. Patients with diffuse damage may display cognitive-communication disorders, perceptual deficits, and executive deficits. Individuals with TBI may experience a variety of cognitive, communication, physical, emotional, social, and psychological difficulties. These difficulties can create profound disruption and challenges for both the individuals and their families. Cognitive deficits in TBI may include one or more of the following areas: attention, perception, recognition, learning, memory, and executive function (124,125). Working memory, the ability to hold and manipulate information in the mind over short periods of time, and declarative memory (e.g., stored facts, memory for past events, and memory for words), one type of long-term memory, are most affected. Implicit, or procedural, memory, which is the other form of long-term memory and includes habits, skills, and emotional associations, typically remains preserved. Communication deficits include impoverished, vague, tangential, or disorganized discourse; word finding problems particularly in conversation or generative contexts, pragmatic or social communication difficulties; and impaired comprehension in the presence of length, complexity, detail, or indirect content (implied, abstract, figurative, humorous) (126–129). Neuropsychiatric deficits such as mood and anxiety disorders, postconcussive syndrome, personality change, aggression, and psychosis are also common reported after TBI (130).

Language Assessment After TBI

Individuals with cognitive-communication impairment following TBI vary considerably in behavior, and this must be taken into consideration when planning assessment. Speech-language pathologists use standardized and nonstandardized tools for assessing cognitive-communication impairment following TBI. The Academy of Neurologic Communication Disorders and Sciences (ANCDS) has published practice guidelines for the assessment of cognitive-communication skills of people with TBI. After review of standardized tests frequently given by speech-language pathologists and/or recommended by test publishers and distributors for assessment of communication ability in people with TBI, a report was generated delineating best assessment tools with regard to test reliability and validity. These include the American Speech-Language and Hearing Association Functional Assessment of Communication Skills (ASHA-FACS), the Behavior Rating Inventory of Executive Function (BRIEF), the Communication Activities of Daily Living-2, the Repeatable Battery for the Assessment of Neuropsychological Status (RBANS), the Test of Language Competence—Expanded (TLC), and the WAB.

The ANCDS, however, also strongly states that standardized tests are only one component of the evaluation process, which must include multiple sources of information, including the person's preinjury characteristics, stage of development and recovery, and communication-related demands of personally meaningful everyday activities. Most clinicians will utilize a combination of formal and informal measures designed to capture the new onset of cognitive-communication deficits. Based on how these deficits impact the individual's function in daily life, an individualized treatment plan will be developed.

It should be noted that assessment remains particularly challenging in the very early stages of recovery. Speech-language pathologists often become involved once the patient has begun to demonstrate some degree of localized response, becoming minimally aware of his or her immediate surroundings.

Language Treatment After TBI

Growing evidence suggests that TBI rehabilitation should be guided by a philosophy that focuses on restoration, compensation, function, and participation in all aspects of daily life, including consideration of contextual factors, the unique life circumstances of the individual, and the quality of support provided by others (131). Treatment of TBI should focus on cognitive, communication, and social deficits. For example, treatment of cognitive deficits can focus on tasks that improve orientation and memory, help in developing selective attention and discrimination, and emphasize reasoning, executive functioning, and social functioning. Treatment of social communication can focus on tasks that improve discourse, pragmatics skills, nonverbal communication such as eye contact, facial expression, proxemics, or personal space. Treatment of language can focus on improving word retrieval deficits, comprehension of humor, and figurative language. Treatment should focus on maximizing functional communication, including improving the understanding and competence of communication partners, in contexts that are most relevant to the individual with TBI (132).

An important role of the speech-language pathologist throughout the continuum of care is family training. How to speak to the patient, utilize external aids, and modify the environment by managing stimulation are part of training. Also, how best to intervene to manage disruptive social behavior can be helpful information. Family members are sometimes required to live with someone with a new personality and ability to adapt can be very difficult. Referrals to psychology or social work are often necessary.

SWALLOWING IMPAIRMENTS

Swallowing serves several life-sustaining functions. In order to consume adequate nutrition and hydration by mouth, swallowing must be safely and efficiently executed. During swallowing, the airway must be protected to prevent material from entering the trachea and lungs. Swallowing clears residual food and liquid as well as pooled secretions from the oropharynx. Sensory pathways to the brainstem provide feedback that is used to execute a specific motor plan for swallowing. Abnormal swallowing, or dysphagia, is associated with significant morbidity and mortality and may lead to dehydration, malnutrition, aspiration pneumonia, or airway obstruction (133,134). Dysphagia may result from a wide range of etiologies, including stroke, progressive neurologic disease, TBI, or head and neck cancer. Swallowing rehabilitation is guided by the evaluation of impacted anatomy and physiology as well as functional outcomes.

PHYSIOLOGY OF SWALLOWING

Swallowing is a patterned and modifiable behavior controlled by a combination of over 30 muscles and nerves (135). It is coordinated with other patterned responses, such as respiration for airway protection and mastication for bolus processing (97,136). Several events occur simultaneously during swallowing; however, swallowing can be divided into phases based on bolus flow and physiology (137).

Anticipation Before the Swallow

Before a substance is placed in the oral cavity, visual and olfactory perception, recognition of the substance as nutritive, appetite, and other factors may shape its delivery to the oral cavity. The delivery of food or drink to the oral cavity requires suitable utensils and motor control for their manipulation. Environmental factors such as distractors also affect the preparation for eating and drinking (138).

Oral Preparatory Phase

The oral preparatory phase of swallowing differs between solids and liquids as solids must be broken down into smaller pieces before being transported to the pharynx and swallowed. During stage 1 transport, solid food is transferred to the lower teeth for mastication and is further broken down by saliva. Liquids are typically held on the surface of the tongue or in the lingual sulcus in the anterior oral cavity while the soft palate and tongue seal prevent the liquid from premature movement. The nasopharyngeal opening allows odor molecules to travel from the oral cavity to olfactory receptors.

Food in the mouth stimulates mechanoreceptors that activate the central pattern generator for mastication, producing sequential contraction and relaxation of the elevator and depressor muscles of the mandible and resulting in cyclic opening and closing of the mouth (139). Saliva is excreted from the salivary glands, helping to break down the food and stimulate the taste receptors. The physical consistency of the food is monitored continuously by oral mechanoreceptors. Typically, the particles of a solid bolus will be broken down to a comparable degree across individuals, though the duration and number of masticatory cycles tends to vary (140).

Oral Propulsive Phase

The oral propulsive phase begins as the bolus is transported posteriorly into the pharynx. At the onset of stage 2 oral transport of solids, the tongue tip contacts the anterior hard palate and a wave of contraction propagates posteriorly propelling the bolus into the oropharynx (141). Stage 2 transport may occur more than one time per bolus, with a portion of food remaining in the valleculae while chewing continues and before the swallow. Liquids are not masticated but are similarly transported to the oropharynx via lingual propulsion.

Pharyngeal Phase

When appropriate sensory input reaches the medullary central pattern generator for swallowing, a complex motor sequence is elicited to propel a bolus through the pharynx, around the larynx, through the upper esophageal sphincter (UES), and into the esophagus, all occurring within approximately 1 second in healthy adults (142). Changes to bolus properties such as volume or consistency can shift the timing and duration of events during this phase (143).

At the onset of the pharyngeal phase, several events occur simultaneously to guide the bolus to the stomach without entry into the airway. The soft palate elevates and moves posteriorly while the posterior pharyngeal wall contracts to seal the nasopharynx and to create sufficient pressures for bolus propulsion. A brief period of apnea occurs as the larynx is sealed via adduction of the true and false vocal folds, anterior tilting of the arytenoid cartilages, and epiglottic inversion. Additionally, anterosuperior elevation of the hyoid and larynx protect the airway by placing structures under the chin and away from the food path. The posterior tongue contacts the posterior pharyngeal wall, and a wavelike contraction of the pharyngeal walls pushes the bolus through the hypopharynx. The pharyngeal phase ends as the UES relaxes to accommodate the bolus. The hyoid and larynx return to their baseline positions, the larynx and velopharynx open, and the epiglottis returns to an upright position.

Esophageal Phase

As the UES relaxes, the bolus enters the esophagus, is propelled by peristalsis through the lower esophageal sphincter (LES), and into the stomach. Esophageal clearance is assisted by gravity but also requires adequate oropharyngeal pressures and relaxation of the LES. Reflux of stomach contents is prevented by tonic contraction of the LES and reflex esophageal swallowing that is triggered by esophageal distension (secondary peristalsis).

Evaluation of Swallowing

The evaluation of swallowing is conducted when a patient reports or displays signs or symptoms of dysphagia. The goal of the evaluation is to define functional and neurophysiologic impairment and to determine a safe and efficient method of nutrition and hydration based on the patient's current swallowing status. The evaluation should include a description of the complaint, medical history, and a clinical evaluation of swallowing, including examination of the peripheral motor and sensory system and trials of oral intake. Instrumental diagnostic studies such as videofluoroscopy and fiberoptic endoscopy provide imaging of swallowing anatomy, bolus flow, and allow for identification of the specific physiologic impairments that result in swallowing dysfunction.

Description of the Complaint

In many instances, the subjective complaint can direct the evaluation as well as inform the extent to which the issue affects the individual's quality of life. Notable complaints include a sensation of food sticking in the throat or chest, difficulty initiating swallowing, coughing or choking spells associated with eating, drooling or difficulty clearing oral secretions, weight loss, change in diet or eating habits, and sensation of reflux or regurgitation. Patients are requested to specify the types of foods and liquids with which they experience these symptoms to delineate the anatomy and physiology that may be affected. It is important to recognize that swallowing function changes with age. These changes are largely unrecognized by the individual, and in most cases, swallowing remains functional in spite of physiologic change (144).

Patients may complain of coughing or choking during drinking or eating. These symptoms suggest laryngeal penetration (entrance of the bolus into the larynx above the level of the vocal folds) and/or aspiration (passage of the bolus through the vocal folds and into the lower airway). Small amounts of penetration and aspiration may occur infrequently in healthy individuals (145). However, substantial and regular aspiration may significantly increase the risk of pneumonia. The risk of aspiration pneumonia is compounded in older adults by factors such as dependence in others for feeding and oral care, poor dentition, nonoral alimentation, complicated medical history and medication amount, and smoking (146).

A complaint of food sticking in the throat or chest may indicate residue or reflux. Potential causes including bulbar palsy, pharyngoesophageal diverticula, tumor, stricture, or esophageal dysmotility. The sensation of food sticking in the chest (thoracic dysphagia) is usually associated with disease of the esophagus or LES. A complaint of cervical dysphagia (food sticking in the neck) may be caused by dysfunction of the pharynx, esophagus, or either one of the esophageal sphincters.

Nasal regurgitation may result from weakness or incompetence of the soft palate (velum). Oral malodor may be associated with tumor, infection, mastication problems, poor oral hygiene, or pharyngeal retention of food and can suggest the presence of a diverticulum of the pharynx or esophagus. Odynophagia may be present in cases of cancer of the esophagus. Heartburn, acid or sour regurgitation, and regurgitation of digested food suggest gastroesophageal reflux disease. Reflux or vomiting of stomach contents can lead to respiratory complications such as aspiration pneumonitis. Weight loss or changes in eating habits may reflect an underlying problem with swallowing.

Changes in swallowing function may disrupt the social experience of eating during meals. The impact of dysphagia on quality of life can be probed with standardized questionnaires, such as the SWAL-QOL or the Dysphagia Handicap Index (147,148).

History

The case history is compiled from the patient's general health and social histories. Neurologic history may suggest contributing factors to dysphagia, such as stroke, head trauma, neuromuscular disorders, or degenerative diseases. Respiratory disorders and use of artificial airways can also contribute to dysphagia. All prior operations should be noted, especially those involving the head and neck. Current medications should be listed to rule out side effects such as sedation, muscle weakness, drying of mucous membranes, disorientation, or dyskinesia that contribute to dysphagia. Imaging studies of the aerodigestive tract and brain can inform etiology of dysphagia. Relevant laboratory studies may provide evidence for infection, nutritional deficiency (especially iron deficiency, which may cause esophageal webs), connective tissue disease, or muscle inflammation. Current diet, route of alimentation and hydration, oral health, and disorders affecting behavior or level of consciousness are important to dysphagia rehabilitation. Additionally, psychosocial factors, such as the setting in which an individual typically consumes meals, may have a significant impact on swallowing.

Clinical Evaluation of Swallowing

The clinical evaluation of swallowing includes examination of the upper aerodigestive tract and the cranial nerves as well as trials of different types of foods and liquids. The oral cavity is examined for dentition and occlusion, which inform mastication ability. Residue in the oral cavity prior to the introduction of food trials suggests a disorder of swallowing. The oral cavity is also examined for structural and mucosal integrity and oral hygiene.

The strength, symmetry, and range of motion of structures of the face, neck, and oral cavity are probed in isolated and purposeful movements. Asymmetry of the brow, shoulders, lips, tongue, or soft palate may indicate neurologic impairment that may impact swallowing function. Reduced lip strength may complicate containment of a bolus in the oral cavity. Reduced tongue strength or range of motion may limit oral management of a bolus. Mastication may be impacted by limited mandibular range of motion and strength. Reduced sensation of the face and oral cavity may result in reduced awareness of residue and altered motor plan for swallowing. Volitional cough is assessed as a measure of airway protection. Palpation of the surface of the neck above the thyroid notch can be used as an indirect measure of hyolaryngeal elevation during swallowing.

Once the physical examination is complete, different consistencies and sizes of foods and liquids are trialed to assess functional swallowing. The order of trials is determined by clinician preference and by patient history particularly current diet. Typically, a small amount of water is trialed first. Several aspects of the swallow are documented, including oral containment, timing of swallow initiation, nasal regurgitation, hyolaryngeal elevation, and oral residue. Signs and symptoms of penetration/aspiration include coughing, throat clearing, wet vocal quality, and respiratory changes. If signs and symptoms of dysphagia are noted, the clinician may trial further consistencies and volumes to determine a diet level that is most safe and efficient. Compensatory strategies such as presentation method (i.e., use of spoon, cup, straws, etc.), positioning, and postures may also be trialed. If penetration and aspiration are strongly suspected, the trials may be stopped until an instrumental evaluation can be completed. Instrumental evaluation may also be conducted if the clinical evaluation suggests impairment that cannot be sufficiently quantified. It is important to mention that in some cases silent aspiration (aspiration occurring without signs or symptoms) is present. Patients at high risk and those who have recurrent pneumonia or weight loss should be carefully evaluated using instrumental diagnostic studies to rule out silent aspiration.

Diagnostic Studies

The purpose of instrumental examination is to determine the mechanism of swallowing dysfunction while maintaining a safe method for alimentation and hydration. Additional goals include detection of structural defects, determining which physiologic components (e.g., bolus preparation, tongue control, initiation of the pharyngeal swallow, tongue base retraction, laryngeal closure, UES opening, esophageal clearance) are impaired, detecting the presence of and mechanism for aspiration, and testing of therapeutic and compensatory techniques based on the physiologic impairments that are recognized. Indications for instrumental examination include frequent choking episodes, difficulty managing secretions, wet vocal quality after a swallow, respiratory complications or recurrent pneumonia, and unexplained weight loss. Relative contraindications include inability to cooperate with the examination and severe respiratory dysfunction. Two methods are discussed in some detail below—the videofluoroscopic swallowing study (VFSS) and the fiberoptic endoscopic evaluation of swallowing (FEES).

Videofluoroscopy

The VFSS, sometimes referred to as a modified barium swallow study, is considered the gold standard for evaluation of oral or pharyngeal dysphagia. During this procedure, patients consume radiopaque liquids and foods for direct visualization of bolus flow, swallowing anatomy, and physiology. Measures of bolus control and propulsion, timing and coordination of swallowing events, laryngeal penetration or aspiration, and oropharyngeal residue can be obtained.

Collimation for VFSS in the lateral plane reduces radiation exposure and should be set to view from the lips to the vertebral column on the x-axis and the hard palate to the cervical esophagus on the y-axis. Frame rate should be no less than 30 frames per second to adequately visualize swallowing events with a duration of 1 second or less (149,150). Lower frame rates may compromise the information required for a clinically informative evaluation as most swallowing events occur in the span of a second.

Standardized protocols assist in minimizing the time of testing thus reducing radiation exposure and provide systematic documentation of findings and impairments. The Modified Barium Swallow Impairment Profile provides guidelines for stimulus delivery as well as a taxonomy of clinical ratings (151). Typically, the VFSS begins with a small amount of thin liquid barium or iohexol in the lateral plane. The evaluation progresses with different sizes and textures, including thin and thickened liquids, pudding or puree, and a cookie or cracker. An empirical approach is used to identify factors associated with functional and disordered swallowing, such as the consistency and volume of liquids/food, patient positioning, and the modality of bolus administration. The order and inclusion of trials during VFSS may vary between patients according to observed airway protection and bolus management. When possible, self-administration is preferred as it better approximates what the person does when drinking or eating in nonclinical environments.

To assess pharyngeal contraction and symmetry of bolus clearance, the patient is repositioned in the anteroposterior plane for additional evaluation. This view should include the width of the skull on the x-axis and the hard palate to the cervical esophagus on the y-axis. Esophageal function is also assessed in this position by following the course of the bolus through the LES. This projection allows for visualization of the vocal cords, and phonation can be used to screen for impaired vocal cord adduction.

With VFSS, one can view the trajectory of the bolus and swallowing anatomy and physiology during every swallowing phase. The presence of penetration or aspiration can be delineated before, during, or after the swallow. Trials of compensatory and rehabilitative techniques can be conducted during VFSS in order to assess their physiologic effects. Limitations of the VFSS include radiation exposure and modification of oral stimuli with barium contrast. Additionally, VFSS records the three-dimensional process of swallowing as a two-dimensional image, and certain anatomical structures such as the vocal folds and laryngeal cartilages may be difficult to distinguish.

Fiberoptic Endoscopic Evaluation of Swallowing

FEES is an alternative to VFSS that can be used to assess swallowing function. FEES can be performed at bedside, which is particularly useful when access to the fluoroscopy suite is limited. Unlike VFSS, FEES provides clear visualization of mucosal integrity and movement of structures in the larynx and pharynx, such as the vocal folds and arytenoid cartilages. Transnasal positioning of the endoscope precludes imaging of the oral cavity. During FEES, patients can consume any liquid or foods without the addition of barium. Green food coloring may be added for clear imaging of the bolus and residue. Similar to VFSS, a range of consistencies, textures, and strategies may be trialed to fully assess swallowing function. Although FEES can provide a clear view of penetration or aspiration before and after swallow execution, epiglottic inversion and pharyngeal wall contraction reflect light back to the endoscope ("white out") obscuring the view and prevent the detection of penetration or aspiration during the moment of swallowing. Esophageal function cannot be assessed with FEES beyond upper border of the UES. FEES can be repeated frequently due to no radiation exposure, though discomfort, gagging, and, in rare instances, laryngospasm may limit its application in some patients. As neither measure provides a full three-dimensional view of the entire aerodigestive tract, the results of VFSS and FEES may complement one another; however, FEES may lead to diagnosis of more severe dysphagia than VFSS in the same patient (152).

Other Diagnostic Studies

Several additional tests may be used to evaluate esophageal function. An esophagram, or barium swallow, assesses esophageal motility. Endoscopy can detect a variety of esophageal and LES disorders and provides the opportunity for diagnostic biopsy. Manometry of the pharynx and esophagus can measure pressures for bolus propulsion and motility.

MANAGEMENT OF SWALLOWING IMPAIRMENT

Recommendations for dysphagia management are based on identification of impairments and trials of compensatory strategies during evaluation. Diet modifications may be recommended with trials of more difficult consistencies during treatment sessions. Formal hierarchies of food textures and liquid consistencies are provided by the International Dysphagia Diet Standardization Initiative (**Fig. 13-1**) (153). The optimal diet level for a patient must balance swallowing efficiency, safety, and patient acceptance. Additional manipulations of bolus flavor and temperature may also promote functional feeding and swallowing.

If a patient is recommended for nonoral alimentation or supplementation, a multidisciplinary team should determine the type of feeding tube that is most appropriate. A nasogastric tube is used for no longer than 1 month and should be considered when fast recovery of swallowing function is expected. An endoscopic or surgically placed percutaneous gastrostomy or jejunostomy tube may be necessary for long-term tube feeding. Tube feeding may not eliminate aspiration in all patients and carries additional risks of placement difficulty and insult to surrounding mucosa and structures (154,155). Esophageal dysphagia may be managed by surgical interventions, such as botulinum toxin injection for hypertonic UES, dilation of the UES, or cricopharyngeal myotomy.

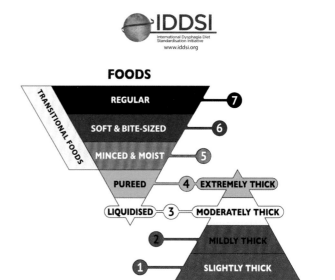

FIGURE 13-1. Formal hierarchies of food textures and liquid consistencies. (Copyright © The International Dysphagia Diet Standardisation Initiative 2016. Available from: http://iddsi.org/resources/framework/)

Based on the underlying physiologic deficit, certain postures may facilitate improved function:

- In some patients with laryngeal penetration/aspiration, **tucking the chin** to the chest enhances airway protection (156).
- In the case of unilateral pharyngeal weakness with significant pharyngeal residue, **turning the head to the weak side** directs the bolus toward the stronger side and reduces UES pressure (157). **Tilting the head to the strong side** can also be helpful to redirect the bolus to the stronger side.

Several exercises and maneuvers have been developed to improve swallowing function:

- The **supraglottic swallow** exercise combines breath-holding and swallowing followed by a cough to promote airway protection and UES opening (158,159).
- The **effortful swallow** is executed by squeezing the throat muscles for hyolaryngeal elevation, UES opening, airway protection, and pressure generation (160,161).
- During the **Mendelsohn maneuver**, patients are trained to prolong hyolaryngeal elevation, which also increases the duration of UES opening (162,163).
- The **Shaker exercise** is executed from the supine position as the patient nods the head forward and holds it up for 1 minute at a time to improve UES opening and suprahyoid strength (164).
- The **Masako maneuver** or tongue-hold exercise is completed by protruding and holding the anterior tongue between the teeth during swallowing. This exercises targets movement of the posterior pharyngeal wall (165).

Before implementation, the effect of postural maneuvers, diet modifications, or exercises should be evaluated during instrumental evaluation.

Recent advances in treatment techniques include surface electrical stimulation, respiratory training, and transcranial electrical stimulation. In patients with intact peripheral nervous system, surface electrical stimulation may facilitate contraction of the muscles involved in swallowing to improve hyolaryngeal elevation in dysphagia patients (166). Additionally, a low level of surface electrical stimulation program may reduce aspiration and residue in chronic dysphagia (167). The effect of stimulation may vary across patients, though it can be assessed individually during instrumental evaluation. The population of patients that benefit from electrical stimulation and the appropriate treatment programs remain under investigation. Respiratory training targeting expiratory muscle strength may improve airway protection during swallowing in patients with neurologic or degenerative etiologies of dysphagia; this treatment approach targets the submental muscles involved in hyolaryngeal elevation (168–170). In cases of neurologic dysphagia, transcranial electrical stimulation to the damaged or intact hemisphere may promote swallowing function by up-regulating neuronal activity in the swallowing network (171).

Throughout treatment, feedback can inform patients as to the accuracy of their exercises (172). Training strategies and exercises during instrumental evaluation provides visual feedback. Surface electromyography can allow the patient to compare the number and effort of swallows in a session. Verbal feedback from the clinician and training in self-monitoring also assist in therapy.

HEARING

Hearing loss is a very common public health problem; bilateral hearing loss is present in 12.7% of individuals in the United States 12 years and older (173). When unilateral hearing loss is included, 23.3% of individuals have hearing loss 25 dB HL (hearing level) or greater (173). With increasing life expectancy and the aging of the population as well as increasing noise exposure, the overall prevalence of hearing loss is anticipated to increase in the upcoming decades. The prevalence of hearing loss increases substantially with age. For individuals in the 60 to 69 decade, 44.9% are affected by hearing loss (173). The percentage increases to 68.1% for the 70 to 79 age group and 89.1% for individuals 80 and over (173). Hearing loss is a potentially disabling disorder that can affect communication with a resultant decline in psychosocial functioning, health-related quality of life, work productivity, and overall quality of life (174). The presence of hearing loss may have significant implications for cognitive function over the life span. Hearing loss has recently been shown to be independently related to changes in brain structure and function at cortical and brainstem levels (175,176). In aging individuals, changes in sensory function may be an early indicator of later occurring neurodegenerative disease (177). It has recently been shown that hearing loss is associated with an increased risk of dementia in aging adults (178). Hearing loss is frequently unrecognized, misunderstood, and all too often neglected, both by those who are affected and by health care providers.

Psychosocial Implications of Hearing Loss

The psychosocial impact of hearing loss is poorly understood and underappreciated. Even those who live with a person with hearing impairment rarely grasp the full extent to which this all-pervasive, invisible disability affects daily living. Until hearing loss is experienced directly or unless a very close acquaintance has impaired hearing, the ways in which a person depends on hearing remain largely underappreciated. Most aspects of daily life are affected by hearing loss in some way. Hearing loss impairs communication, often subtly at first, and increasingly so as the magnitude of the hearing loss increases. In addition, hearing loss restricts environmental awareness and can be a safety concern when it affects the ability to hear warning signals such as sirens and alarms. Hearing loss impacts relationships, employment opportunities, academics, and learning.

The two most commonly reported consequences of hearing loss are depression and social isolation. In addition, adverse effects on general well-being and on physical, cognitive, emotional, behavioral, and social functions have been reported. Social and emotional effects may be present even in those with only mild to moderate hearing loss. Inability to hear all or part of a conversation may create frustration, anger, and even paranoia. Over time, social connectivity and relationships may deteriorate, leaving the individual with hearing impairment in isolation and with a diminished quality of life. Hearing loss is associated with reduced abilities to perform activities of daily living as well as instrumental activities of daily living (174).

Misunderstanding and lack of sympathy for the hearing-impaired person seems to be integrated into our social bias. These attitudes are certainly quite different from our perceptions and treatment of blindness. Often the symptoms of hearing loss (e.g., not answering when spoken to, answering inappropriately, or requiring repetition) encourage other people to talk to and treat the person with hearing impairment as if his or her cognitive abilities were also diminished. This often leads to frustrating or truncated communication attempts.

A major goal of the health care practitioner is to help patients maintain or regain function. The capacity for independent living requires maintenance of functional health. Functional health refers not only to physical health but also to emotional, cognitive, and social health. Physicians are in an excellent position to identify treatable conditions that may compromise their patients' functional performance. Unfortunately, many health care professionals tend to view hearing loss as a benign problem that does not threaten functional health. Regular hearing assessments and management for persons aged 60 years and older should be considered a standard of care.

Anatomy and Physiology of the Ear

Anatomically, the ear is a complex organ, capable of transforming airborne sound waves into mechanical energy. This mechanical energy is then converted into electrochemical signals and then into neural impulses that are processed as auditory information. The peripheral portion of the auditory system is divided into three sections: the outer, middle, and inner ear. The outer ear is comprised of the auricle (pinna) and the external auditory canal. The auricle is a skin-covered cartilaginous structure and is the most visible portion of the outer ear. The 2.5- to 3-cm long external auditory canal provides an S-shaped tubal channel from the auricle leading to the tympanic membrane. The conical-shaped tympanic membrane is approximately 9 mm in length and separates the outer and middle ears. The middle ear is an air-filled space containing the ossicular chain (malleus, incus, and stapes) that links the tympanic membrane to the inner ear. The last bone in this chain, the stapes, is the smallest bone in the human body. It rests in the membranous oval window of the inner ear. The inner ear is divided into two primary components: the cochlea and vestibular labyrinth. The inner ear is responsible for sensorineural hearing (cochlea) and responding to linear and angular acceleration (vestibule/semicircular canals). The cochlea is a 32-mm long coil-shaped bony structure that contains three fluid-filled membranous cavities, the scala vestibuli, scala tympani, and scala media. Located within the scala media is the organ of Corti, the end organ for hearing, which has approximately 16,000 outer and inner hair cells that are located along the basilar membrane and are the primary auditory receptors. Located at the top of the outer and inner hair cells are hairlike projections called stereocilia. The basilar membrane is responsible for the initial stages of frequency analysis by the auditory system. The place of activation is instrumental in coding frequency information that is in turn preserved at all higher levels of the auditory pathway to cortical levels. The inner hair cells are activated by the motion of the basilar membrane and control the activation of the auditory nerve fibers. The outer hair cells have a different response to sound than the inner hair cells and through their elongation and shortening activity function primarily as an amplifier and add approximately 50 dB of sensitivity to the ear. At the base of the hair cells are approximately 30,000 sensory nerve fibers that project medially through the internal auditory canal, forming the cochlear branch of the eighth cranial nerve. These nerve fibers synapse at the ipsilateral cochlear nucleus located in the cerebellopontine angle at the junction of the pons, cerebellum, and medulla. This begins the central portion of the auditory system. Most auditory pathway fibers from the cochlear nucleus project via the trapezoid bodies to the superior olivary complex and then by way of the lateral lemniscus to the inferior colliculi. The next major synapse of the auditory tracts is at the medial geniculate bodies in the thalamus. From this point, fibers radiate to the primary auditory cortex located at Heschl's gyrus on the sylvian fissure in the temporal lobe.

Assessment of Auditory Function

Audiologic Evaluation

When a patient presents with a suspicion of hearing loss or a specific hearing complaint, diagnosis of the type and degree of hearing loss and the underlying etiology is typically the first goal in the assessment and management process. This begins with a detailed case history that includes questions about the duration of the hearing loss, whether the onset was sudden or gradual, and whether it is stable, progressive, or fluctuant. The patient should be queried about associated symptoms such as tinnitus, dizziness, ear pain or drainage, and aural fullness. In addition, questioning should review family history of hearing loss, as well as loud noise exposure, head trauma, ear surgery, and ototoxic drug use. Hearing questionnaires are also of considerable value in that information is obtained relating to the specific difficulties experienced by the individual and the individual's own perception of their difficulty with hearing. It is also helpful to query a significant other as to their perception of the patient's hearing status. The physical examination should include an otoscopic examination to ensure that the

external ear canal is healthy and unobstructed and that the tympanic membrane is translucent and intact. The status of the patient's hearing is determined through a series of audiologic tests. Based on the results of the audiologic examination, the patient's history, and physical examination findings, additional audiologic assessments as well as associated neurologic, laboratory, and imaging studies may be indicated. Only after the assessment has been completed and a diagnosis has been established should rehabilitation of the hearing loss be initiated.

Behavioral Hearing Assessment

Pure-Tone Audiometry

Determination of pure-tone thresholds across a wide frequency range for air conduction and bone conduction stimuli is the most basic component of the hearing test. Threshold is defined as the lowest level at which a person can detect an auditory stimulus 50% of the time. This information is used to establish the type, degree, and configuration of the hearing loss. Air conduction thresholds are determined in octave, and sometimes interoctave intervals (i.e., 750, 1,500, 3,000, or 6,000 Hz) over the frequency range of 250 through 8,000 Hz. For certain applications, such as ototoxic drug monitoring, assessment of frequencies above 8,000 Hz may also be included. Air conduction signals are presented via supra-aural or insert earphones, and the signal is transferred along the entire auditory pathway, including the outer, middle, and inner ear. Use of insert earphones has advantages in avoiding spurious findings due to poor placement or ear canal collapse when supra-aural earphones are utilized. Bone conduction thresholds are established for octave intervals between 250 and 4,000 Hz. For bone conduction measures, a bone oscillator is typically placed on the mastoid prominence of the test ear, while masking sounds are delivered to the nontest ear. The bone conduction oscillator causes the skull to vibrate resulting in direct stimulation of the cochlea, with minimal contribution of the outer and middle ears. Bone conduction thresholds reflect an individual's sensory hearing ability and are unencumbered by disorders affecting the outer and/or middle ear.

Pure-tone thresholds are represented graphically on an audiogram (**Fig. 13-2**) or in a tabular form. The frequency scale along the abscissa is measured in Hertz (Hz) for the octave and interoctave frequencies of 250 through 8,000 Hz. The intensity scale on the ordinate of the audiogram displays the HL of the signal in decibels (dB) ranging from a very faint level of –10 dB HL up to a very loud level of 110 to 120 dB HL.

Speech Audiometry

In addition to pure-tone thresholds, the basic audiologic evaluation includes measurement of the speech recognition threshold (SRT) and the assessment of word recognition performance. The SRT serves primarily as a reliability check of the pure-tone threshold levels. Familiar two-syllable spondee words (e.g., hotdog, cowboy, baseball) are presented, and the patient is asked to repeat back these words until they can no longer understand or hear them. The intensity level at which 50% of the words are correctly repeated is defined as the SRT. The SRT should be within 10 dB of the pure-tone average (PTA) of 500, 1,000, and 2,000 Hz or the average of the best two of these frequencies. The SRT provides a means to

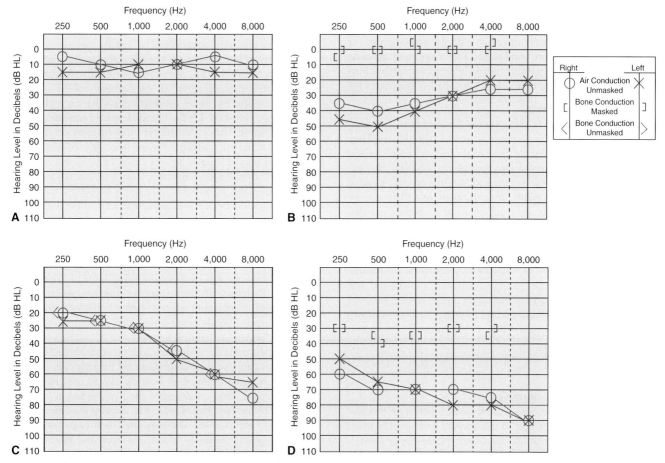

FIGURE 13-2. Examples of audiograms. **A:** Normal hearing in both ears. **B:** Mild conductive hearing loss—air conduction thresholds reveal a hearing impairment, but the bone conduction responses are within the normal range. Therefore, an air-bone gap is present. **C:** Sensorineural hearing loss—both the air conduction and the bone conduction thresholds are similarly depressed. **D:** Mixed hearing loss—although both the air conduction and the bone conduction thresholds are reduced, a greater impairment is evident for air conduction.

cross-check the validity of the pure-tone thresholds. When there is a difference between the SRT and the PTA of 10 dB or greater, the source of this discrepancy should be determined. Causes include functional hearing loss, unusual audiometric configurations, language or cognitive disorders, or patient misunderstanding of test instructions.

A hearing impairment may be reflected not only in a sensitivity loss but also in the reduced ability to understand speech, even when speech is sufficiently loud. Word recognition testing (speech discrimination) analyzes the patient's ability to understand speech using standardized lists of 25 to 50 single-syllable words. These lists are balanced to represent the phonetic content of everyday English speech. Word lists are presented to each ear separately, and the patient is asked to repeat back the test words. The test is initially presented at a comfortably loud level. Higher levels may be presented to determine the patient's best word recognition performance. Testing word recognition performance over a range of intensities may also provide useful diagnostic information as listening performance for more intense speech may be poorer in some individuals with certain forms of neural hearing loss. Individuals whose performance does not improve with increasingly more audible speech may not benefit with the introduction of hearing aid amplification. A basic hearing assessment should also include

some measure of speech processing in the background of noise or competing speech as it has been demonstrated that an individual's difficulty processing speech in the background of noise cannot be accurately predicted on the basis of a pure tone audiogram (179).

Physiologic Hearing Assessment

Immittance Measurements

Physiologic assessment of middle ear function is a routine part of the basic audiologic evaluation. Collectively referred to as immittance measurements, middle ear assessment includes tympanometry and acoustic reflex testing. Tympanometry provides information about the admittance, or compliance, of the middle ear transmission system and an estimate of middle ear pressure. This information is particularly useful in identifying and differentiating among middle ear disorders. The acoustic reflex occurs when a sufficiently intense sound is presented to the ear causing contraction of the stapedius muscle and stiffening of the ossicular chain. The reflex is bilateral and can be measured with stimuli presented ipsilateral or contralateral to the test ear. Evaluating the integrity of the acoustic reflex provides information regarding not only the middle ear function but also other components of the reflex arc including the cochlea, seventh and eighth cranial nerves, and the lower brainstem. Analysis of reflex patterns for signals presented ipsilateral or contralateral to the test ear can assist with determining the site of pathology for certain conditions. The absence of acoustic reflexes in young children can signal the need for further tests to rule out the presence of auditory neuropathy/dyssynchrony.

Otoacoustic Emissions

Otoacoustic emissions (OAEs) are low level sounds that emanate from the cochlea in response to sound stimulation. They are generated by healthy cochlear outer hair cells and impart insight into the functional integrity of the cochlea. In general, OAEs are observed in ears with normal to near-normal hearing sensitivity. However, measurement of OAEs can be greatly impacted by the presence of outer or middle ear disorders. OAEs are used in universal newborn hearing screening programs and in other cases in which patients are unable or unwilling to provide behavioral responses to sounds. They also provide an objective cross-check for behavioral test results, serve as an objective method of monitoring ototoxicity, and assist in the identification of both functional hearing loss and neurologic disorders of the auditory system such as auditory neuropathy/dyssynchrony. While OAEs provide adjunctive information in hearing evaluation, they do not replace the audiogram and cannot at this time predict adequately pure-tone sensitivity.

Auditory-Evoked Potentials

When the ear is stimulated with sounds, a series of bioelectric events occur, that begin in the cochlea and quickly reach cortical structures. Much like electroencephalography (EEG), auditory-evoked potentials can be recorded from surface electrodes placed on the scalp and in or near the ear canal. The auditory responses are extracted from ongoing EEG activity by time-locked computerized averaging during repeated stimulation with transient or tonal stimuli. The evoked potentials most commonly used for audiologic assessment include electrocochleography (ECochG), the auditory brainstem response (ABR), auditory steady-state response (ASSR), and auditory middle latency response (AMLR). The primary clinical application of ECochG, which measures electrical potentials generated in the cochlea, is identification and monitoring of Meniere's disease. The ABR is used in newborn hearing screening programs to estimate peripheral hearing sensitivity in pediatric and uncooperative patients, in otoneurologic diagnosis, and for intraoperative monitoring during cerebellopontine angle surgery in which the auditory system is at risk for iatrogenic insult. When the ABR is utilized to estimate peripheral auditory sensitivity, it is necessary to include frequency-specific stimuli and sometimes bone-conducted stimuli in order to estimate not only the degree of hearing loss but also the configuration and etiology of the hearing loss. The ASSR is used to estimate the degree, type, and configuration of peripheral hearing loss and appears to have a good predictive validity in relation to the behavioral audiogram, especially in cases of severe and profound hearing loss. Less frequently used, the AMLR is thought to be generated in the auditory thalamocortical pathway. It can be used to predict auditory thresholds but more typically is utilized to provide insight into neurologic diseases involving primary auditory pathways and auditory processing disorders.

Audiometric Test Interpretation and Types of Hearing Loss

The general anatomic location of a hearing impairment can be determined by comparing the air conduction and bone conduction thresholds for each ear individually. A *conductive* hearing loss is present when air conduction results demonstrate hearing loss but bone conduction results are within the normal range (see **Fig. 13-2**). The difference between air and bone conduction thresholds reflects the amount of conductive involvement and is called the *air-bone gap*. A conductive hearing loss may be caused by any disorder or dysfunction of the sound-conducting mechanisms from the external auditory canal through the middle ear. Although otoscopic examination may provide evidence of cerumen impaction, tympanic membrane perforation, or serous otitis media as the cause of a conductive hearing loss, there are also conductive pathologies that present with normal otoscopic examinations, such as otosclerosis or ossicular discontinuity. Tympanometry can provide useful information by describing the status of the middle ear system. Patients with conductive hearing loss typically have normal word recognition scores, because the sensorineural system is intact. Speech needs only to be presented at louder levels than normal to compensate for the conductive deficit. Consequently, patients with medically untreatable conductive hearing losses are excellent candidates for hearing aids.

When an equal amount of hearing loss is present by air conduction and bone conduction, the hearing loss is called a *sensorineural* loss (see **Fig. 13-2**). The hearing disorder could be located in the cochlea, the associated neural pathways, or both. The specific etiology of the sensorineural hearing loss cannot be determined by the audiometric results alone. Word recognition test results often provide important diagnostic insight into the site of lesion of sensorineural hearing loss. In general, cochlear involvement demonstrates speech discrimination scores that are reduced to a degree compatible with the degree of hearing loss. The greater the degree of sensory (cochlear) hearing loss, the poorer the word recognition. In addition, many individuals with cochlear hearing losses experience significant difficulty in processing speech in the background of noise or competing speech. On the other hand, neural auditory disorders often yield speech discrimination scores disproportionately poorer than would be expected from the pure-tone thresholds. That is, a 40-dB HL sensorineural hearing loss with a 72% word recognition score would be consistent with cochlear involvement, whereas a similar amount of hearing loss with only a 10% word recognition score would suggest the possibility of eighth cranial nerve, brainstem, or cortical involvement. From a rehabilitative standpoint, the better the speech discrimination score, the better the prognosis for hearing aid success, as there is less distortion in the auditory system. Tympanometry is most often normal in cases with sensorineural hearing loss, while acoustic reflex patterns may help to differentiate sensory from neural causes.

A loss of hearing sensitivity for bone conduction with a greater loss for air conduction represents a *mixed* hearing loss (see **Fig. 13-2**). A sensorineural hearing loss is present, as reflected by reduced bone conduction thresholds, and conductive loss also is present, as reflected by the air-bone gaps. Tympanograms may provide insight into middle ear problems contributing to the conductive component of a mixed hearing loss.

In addition to hearing loss resulting from damage or dysfunction of the peripheral hearing mechanisms, damage or dysfunction of the central auditory pathways can impact hearing abilities. Central auditory processing disorders most often are manifested as difficulty understanding speech in noise or situations in which the signal is degraded, such as a reverberant room. Auditory test results will frequently show normal hearing sensitivity and normal speech recognition ability in quiet. Performance declines are observed on degraded or difficult speech recognition tests including speech in noise and filtered speech, measures of frequency and temporal processing, dichotic listening, and/or on electrophysiologic measures of the central auditory pathways such as the ABR and AMLR. Common causes include head trauma, stroke, neurodevelopmental disorders, genetic factors, tumors, neurologic disease, and aging (180–186). While less amenable to traditional hearing aid amplification, people with auditory processing disorders may benefit from other types of assistive listening systems, as well as auditory training regimens or music training.

Degree and Configuration of Hearing Loss

The results obtained from the air conduction evaluation provide quantitative information as to the magnitude of hearing loss. The PTA is a three-frequency average of 500, 1,000, and 2,000 Hz, which is used to classify hearing. **Table 13-2** gives an example of one classification system based upon the PTA. In addition to type and degree of hearing loss, the configuration or shape of the pure-tone audiogram is helpful in describing and understanding the impact of a hearing loss. Classification schemes include flat, sloping, and rising configurations. A sloping audiogram has a greater amount of hearing loss in the high frequencies, whereas a rising configuration refers to a greater amount of hearing loss in the low frequencies.

As noted above, any type of audiometric classification system must be interpreted with caution because most are based on pure-tone air conduction thresholds alone and do not incorporate the effects of speech discrimination difficulties. Etiologic factors, the type of hearing loss, or hearing loss configuration are also significant factors in determining the degree to which a hearing loss impacts upon an individual's functioning. In addition, those with similar amounts of pure-tone hearing loss may be affected in very different ways, depending on lifestyles, hearing demands, cognition, and other psychosocial factors.

Causes of Hearing Loss

Hearing loss can be caused by or occur in conjunction with a variety of diseases and disorders, genetics, aging, trauma, or ototoxicity. The following provides an overview of the major causes of hearing loss including conditions affecting the outer, middle, and inner ear as well as the central auditory pathways.

Hereditary Hearing Loss

Hereditary hearing loss accounts for approximately 50% to 60% of hearing loss identified in newborns. Approximately 70% of genetic hearing loss is nonsyndromic, and approximately 30% is syndromic. Nonsyndromic hearing loss is most often sensorineural. As many as 40% of nonsyndromic hearing loss is caused by a mutation in the GJB2 gene. The GJB2 gene contains the instructions for the protein connexin 26, which is instrumental in cochlear function (187). Genetic transmission of hearing loss is recessive in approximately 70%, dominant in approximately 30%, x-linked in approximately 1%, and mitochondrial in approximately 1%. Nonsyndromic recessive hearing loss is most often congenital and profound, whereas nonsyndromic dominant hearing loss is more variable in presentation with congenital or delayed onset. There are at least 400 syndromes with hearing loss as a phenotypic feature. Syndromic hearing loss is quite variable in its presentation. It can be conductive, mixed, or sensorineural in origin, range from slight to profound, be stable or progressive, and involve one or both ears. The Hereditary Hearing Loss homepage provides a comprehensive review of the genetics of hereditary hearing loss (188).

Outer Ear

When hearing loss originates in the external auditory canal, it usually is related to obstruction in the form of cerumen (ear wax) or a foreign body. Accumulation and impaction of excess cerumen in the external ear canal is one of the most common reasons that patients seek care for hearing- and ear-related symptoms. Elderly, pediatric, and cognitively impaired individuals are at higher risk for cerumen impaction. The resultant conductive hearing loss from impacted cerumen ranges from slight to mild. Infections of the ear canal (otitis externa) can occur in acute, chronic, and malignant forms. They are most commonly caused by bacterial infection but more rarely may have a viral or fungal origin. Signs and symptoms include ear pain, drainage, edema, inflammation, itching, and aural fullness. If the infectious process causes the ear canal to become swollen shut, there is a resultant conductive hearing loss. Medical management includes treatment of pain and control of infection.

Middle Ear

Otitis media is an infection, or inflammation, of the middle ear usually with fluid (effusion) behind an intact tympanic membrane. Acute otitis media (AOM) occurs frequently in children and is the most common infection for which antibacterial agents are prescribed in the United States. When treated successfully with medications or middle ear surgery, AOM is alleviated or controlled, but when left untreated, complications of the disease may spread to involve intracranial or intratemporal structures. Otitis media with effusion (OME) indicates a situation where the middle ear is filled with fluid but typically without signs or symptoms of acute ear infection other than hearing loss. The audiometric presentation of a person with otitis media ranges from a slight to moderate conductive hearing loss, typically with a rising configuration. The tympanogram is flat indicating absence of middle ear system

TABLE 13-2	Classification System for Degree of Hearing Loss	
Pure-Tone Average	**Classification**
0–15 dB HL	Normal
16–25 dB HL	Slight
26–40 dB HL	Mild
41–55 dB HL	Moderate
56–70 dB HL	Moderately severe
71–90 dB HL	Severe
91 dB HL and above	Profound

mobility, and the stapedial reflexes are absent. OAEs may also be absent.

In addition to hearing loss, complications of otitis media include cholesteatoma, an inclusion of keratinizing squamous epithelium that proliferates within the temporal bone. A cholesteatoma can block sound transmission or cause erosion of the middle ear ossicles, resulting in a significant degree of conductive hearing loss. When a cholesteatoma erodes the temporal bone, it puts the patient at risk for mixed or sensorineural hearing loss, vertigo, and/or meningitis. Mastoid surgery is necessary to address a cholesteatoma. The primary surgical goal is to rid the ear of the cholesteatoma itself. Secondarily, reconstruction of the tympanic membrane and/or ossicles may be necessary to preserve or improve hearing. Following surgery, hearing aids may be required if a significant hearing loss remains.

Glomus tumors are the most common neoplasm of the middle ear (189). The most frequent initial symptoms are pulsatile tinnitus and hearing loss. On otoscopic examination, a glomus tympanicum appears as a red-blue mass behind or involving the tympanic membrane. Conductive hearing loss is the most common audiometric finding occurring in up to 75.9% of people with these tumors as the result of reduced ossicular mobility or destruction. As the tumor grows medially, there is cochlear involvement resulting in a mixed or sensorineural hearing loss. Surgical excision is the treatment of choice unless contraindicated by the patient's medical condition or tumor location and biology (189).

Otosclerosis is a progressive, focal disease of the ear in which there is excessive resorption of bone, which is replaced by soft new bone that gradually changes into a dense sclerotic mass. In its early stages, otosclerosis hinders transmission of sound by the ossicular chain due to fixation of the stapes footplate in the oval window. At this stage, the hearing loss is typically conductive and mild, and the patient is a good candidate for a stapedectomy, a corrective surgery in which the stapes is partially removed and replaced by a prosthesis. In its later stages, otosclerosis can invade the inner ear causing a mixed but primarily sensorineural hearing loss that can be of severe to profound degree. Hearing aid amplification is often beneficial for those who elect not to have surgery or who are not candidates for surgery.

Inner Ear

Presbycusis

Presbycusis is the term used to describe age-related hearing loss. The most common audiologic presentation of age-related hearing loss is a sloping, high-frequency sensorineural hearing loss. Hearing thresholds decline gradually with age, beginning as early as the third decade in men and the fifth decade in women. Age-related hearing loss may occur earlier in people with developmental disabilities or people with Down's syndrome (190). Concomitant to the loss of sensitivity is a reduction in the ability to understand speech, especially in background noise and reverberant rooms or when the speaker talks at a rapid rate or with accented speech. Reduced cognitive abilities can further compound these problems. Age-related changes in the ear include deterioration of structures within the inner ear, including the stria vascularis, cochlear hair cells, and dendritic fibers of the eighth nerve. In most cases,

age-related changes occur within the milieu of other potential causes of hearing loss, including genetic susceptibility, noise exposure, ototoxic drugs, and ear disease. Most people with presbycusis benefit from hearing aids used alone or in conjunction with other amplification devices.

Noise-Induced Hearing Loss

Exposure to high levels of sound can cause damage to the hair cells in the cochlea resulting in noise-induced hearing loss (NIHL). Approximately 24% Americans aged 20 to 69 have hearing loss attributable to noise exposure (191). NIHL in the pediatric populations has become a greater concern with evidence of NIHL in 16.8% of children aged 12 to 19 years of age in the most recent U.S. National survey (192). The prevalence of NIHL among youth is attributable to widespread use of personal music systems and failure to utilize noise protection devices. NIHL can occur suddenly after a single noise exposure but more commonly occurs gradually as the result of the accumulative effect of years of noise exposure. Harmful sounds include both impulse and continuous noises. The hearing loss begins in the high frequencies with a characteristic notch around 4,000 Hz. Over time with repeated exposure, NIHL spreads to the mid and low frequencies with deleterious effects on the ability to hear and understand speech, resulting in the need for amplification.

Ototoxic Drugs

There are a number of drugs that may be toxic to the inner ear and may cause hearing loss, tinnitus, balance dysfunction, or a combination of those symptoms. The most common ototoxic drugs include aminoglycoside antibiotics, cisplatin, high-dose salicylates, and loop diuretics. The typical ototoxic hearing loss is bilateral and sensorineural. It begins in the high frequencies and, with continued administration of the ototoxic agent, spreads to include lower frequencies while high-frequency hearing continues to decline. Eventually, the patient may experience significant communication difficulties necessitating use of amplification. In general, aminoglycosides cause a gradual onset of hearing loss, while cisplatin can cause a significant hearing loss after a single treatment. Aminoglycosides and cisplatin cause permanent hearing loss, while the hearing loss resulting from high-dose salicylates and loop diuretics is often reversible. Audiologic monitoring of hearing sensitivity should be undertaken in conjunction with administration of potentially ototoxic medications.

Infection and Immunologic Disorders

Labyrinthitis, an infection of the inner ear, is most commonly caused by direct extension from the middle ear; that is, as a complication of AOM or chronic suppurative otitis media with cholesteatoma. Congenitally acquired illnesses and complications of meningitis may also cause labyrinthitis. Inner ear infections are quite worrisome, as they often cause significant and even permanent sensorineural hearing loss or vertigo and can lead to meningitis, brain abscess, or death. Treatment includes antibiotics, steroids, and, in some cases, myringotomy and placement of middle ear ventilation tubes. Depending on the degree of resultant hearing loss, the patient may benefit from hearing aids, or in some cases, a cochlear implant may be necessary. Systemic infections such as acquired syphilis and Lyme's disease can also cause sensorineural hearing loss. Treatment consists of antibiotics with corticosteroids to manage the sensorineural hearing loss. Depending on the degree of hearing loss, hearing aids may be indicated.

Generalized inflammatory conditions and autoimmune illnesses occurring in the absence of infection may also affect the auditory system. They may affect the ear singularly as in autoimmune inner ear disease (AIED) or have typical systemic symptoms as exemplified by sarcoidosis, Wegener's granulomatosis, polychondritis, or systemic lupus erythematosus.

Trauma

Injury to the ear can occur as the result of head trauma in which damage may be limited to a single part of the ear, or it can be more pervasive involving the outer, middle, and inner ear as well as central structures. Longitudinal fractures of the temporal bone most often cause conductive or mixed hearing loss, while transverse fractures of the temporal bone most often result in a profound sensorineural hearing loss and vertigo. Self-cleaning or probing the ear canal with a foreign body, such as a cotton swab, is a frequent cause of ear canal lacerations, tympanic membrane ruptures, dislocation of the middle ear ossicles, and inner ear injuries. The external ear is also susceptible to injuries such as frostbite, lacerations, and burns.

Neoplasms

The most common tumor of the temporal bone is the acoustic neuroma (vestibular schwannoma) that accounts for 80% of intracranial tumors in the cerebellopontine angle. Vestibular schwannomas make up almost 10% of all intracranial tumors and most commonly arise from the vestibular portion of the eighth cranial nerve. Patients typically develop unilateral sensorineural hearing loss with poor speech discrimination, tinnitus, and sometimes vertigo. Treatment options include surgical resection to remove the tumor or highly focused radiation therapy. Although hearing preservation is possible in some patients, the primary goal is the removal of the neoplasm. Posttreatment benefit from a hearing aid may be possible in some cases.

Medical-Surgical Rehabilitation

Medical or surgical treatment of hearing loss is most often available for people with impairments involving the conductive mechanisms of the auditory system. Hearing impairment originating in the middle ear system may be treated with otologic surgery. Surgical procedures such as myringoplasty (i.e., repair of tympanic membrane perforation), tympanoplasty (i.e., tympanic membrane defect repair with ossicular reconstruction), stapedectomy for otosclerosis, and myringotomy with placement of ventilating tubes for middle ear effusion often can correct the conductive hearing loss.

Otologic surgery sometimes is required for treatment of life-threatening disease and not for hearing improvement. Pathologic conditions such as cholesteatoma, glomus tumor, or chronic middle ear disease often necessitate surgery. In addition, otoneurosurgery is necessary for sensorineural impairment caused by acoustic neuromas. Otologic treatment of congenital or hereditary sensorineural hearing loss, NIHL, presbycusis, and most other types of sensorineural impairments is not currently possible. Perhaps the greatest advancement in the surgical rehabilitation of sensorineural impairments is cochlear implant surgery for severe to profound hearing loss.

Hearing Aid Amplification

Hearing aids are the principal resource for improving communication and ameliorating hearing difficulties in people with sensorineural hearing loss, whereas hearing loss due to conductive disorders may often be improved with medical or surgical intervention. Significant improvements in hearing aid technology have resulted in greater flexibility in selecting and fitting hearing aids for most causes of hearing loss. The past decade has witnessed innovations resulting in a wide assortment of hearing aids, varying both in physical size and in technologic sophistication. Yet, despite the substantial benefits provided by hearing aids, only 15% of people with hearing loss own hearing instruments (193).

Hearing Aid Candidacy

It is a disservice to the patient to discourage a hearing aid trial because of the misconception that a hearing aid does not help "nerve deafness." While some physicians may tell their patients that they can probably "get by" without a hearing aid and should wait until the hearing loss progresses, consultation with an audiologist will provide the patient with an individualized opportunity to make amplification decisions that best suit their lifestyle and listening needs. Discouraging a hearing aid trial for an individual with communicative difficulties and a potentially remediable hearing loss serves only to invite isolation and frustration. Unless assurance and support are provided, hearing-impaired patients may unfortunately postpone and avoid the use of amplification. Referral to an audiologist for hearing assessment and hearing aid evaluation provides patients an opportunity to understand their hearing loss and its impact on daily function, as well as candidacy for the many types of amplification systems suitable for their individual needs.

Hearing Aid Selection and Fitting

Current hearing aid styles include devices that fit behind-the-ear, in-the-ear, in-the-canal, and completely-in-the-canal. There are also bone-anchored hearing aids for individuals with conductive hearing loss or one-sided hearing loss. Behind-the-ear hearing aids that feature a slim tube and an open-fitting have in recent years become increasingly popular. This type of fitting helps to eliminate the sensation of an occluded ear and has proven to be advantageous for those with mild to moderate hearing loss as well as hearing loss confined to the high frequencies. Selection of appropriate hearing aids must take into account factors such as the degree and type of hearing loss, loudness tolerance, communication needs, and manual dexterity.

Hearing aids include many features that enhance the amplified signal and tailor the sound to the specific needs of the individual hearing aid user. Compression circuitry amplifies softer speech and other sounds while providing little or no gain for louder sounds. In addition, automatic loudness-adjusting circuits automatically decrease amplification of continuous background sounds in an effort to improve speech understanding in noise. Binaural hearing aids communicate with each other and offer additional advantages in processing speech in the presence of background of noise. Frequency compression or frequency shifting modifies the bandwidth of the amplified signal so that it is within the patient's range of audibility. Most hearing aids allow for programs for use at the listener's discretion. One may choose broad frequency amplification for quiet environments, another program that eliminates low frequencies for noisier situations, or a program specifically suited for telephone use or listening to music. Individual programming of the hearing aid using computer software enables the audiologist to make significant modifications to meet the patient's needs. Hearing aids may include a user-operated remote control to facilitate program changes or volume changes. Fixed or adaptive directional microphones help to improve speech understanding by improving the signal-to-noise ratio. The multiplicity of adjustments afforded by digital hearing aids provides audiologists with many possible options for selecting the most optimal settings for each individual with hearing loss. However, this very flexibility may require multiple office visits and persistence on the part of the hearing impaired individual until their needs are addressed. Bluetooth technology enabling wireless communication between the hearing aid and other electronic devices such as cell phones, handheld external microphones, and MP3 players helps to keep the technology-savvy hearing aid user connected.

Assistive Listening Devices

Although substantial improvements have been achieved in hearing aid technology, factors such as distance from a speaker, background noise, reverberation, and declines in central auditory processing have deleterious effects on speech intelligibility that cannot be overcome through the use of hearing aids alone. Assistive listening devices (ALDs) comprise a number of situation-specific amplification systems designed for use in difficult listening environments. ALDs commonly use a microphone placed close to the desired sound source (e.g., a television, theater stage, or speaker's lectern from which sound is directly transmitted to the listener). Transmission methods include infrared light, FM radio waves, and induction loops. Such transmission of sound directly to the listener improves the signal-to-noise ratio. That is, the desired sounds are enhanced while competing extraneous noises are decreased, thus improving understanding. Public Law 101-336, the Americans with Disabilities Act (1990), requires assistive listening technology in places of public accommodation. ALDs in many churches, theaters, and classrooms enable hard-of-hearing persons to avoid the isolation imposed by the inability to hear a sermon, play, or public address.

Amplified telephones, low-frequency doorbells, amplified ringers, and closed-captioned TV decoders are just a few examples of the number of devices currently available for everyday use. Alarms are available with low-frequency signals for those persons with high-frequency hearing losses who cannot hear the higher pitch alarms. Flashing alarm clocks, alarm bed vibrators, and flashing smoke detectors are other alerting options available for severely hearing-impaired individuals.

Cochlear Implants

The cochlear implant is a surgically inserted auditory prosthesis designed to provide acoustic stimulation for people with bilateral severe to profound sensorineural hearing loss who derive little or no benefit from hearing aids. The implant bypasses the cochlear hair cells and provides direct electrical stimulation to the residual eighth nerve fibers. The FDA approved cochlear implants for adults in 1984 and for children as young as 2 years in 1990. In 2000, the age of eligibility was lowered to 12 months for children who have not obtained benefit from hearing aids. Over 219,000 patients over the world have received cochlear implants (194). Candidacy for a cochlear implant is evaluated by a team, including an otolaryngologist and audiologist. Prospective implant candidates require an extensive audiologic evaluation to document that hearing aids are not beneficial and an otologic evaluation to determine implant and surgical candidacy. The implant operation involves placing an electrode array into the cochlea and connecting it to an internal coil, which is placed under the skin behind the pinna and is aligned with an external coil placed behind the ear. After the healing period, the patient is fitted with an external microphone, speech processor, and transmitter. The microphone, usually worn at ear level, feeds electrical impulses to the speech processor that resembles a behind-the-ear hearing aid. The processor digitally encodes the sound and sends these electrical signals to the external coil, which transmits the signal to the internal coil and then to the electrodes in the cochlea. Current flows between the active electrodes, stimulating remaining eighth nerve fibers and producing a sensation of sound. The audiologist programs the speech processor to identify and establish a sound map that works best for the individual patient. Rehabilitation includes repeated visits to program and fine-tune the sound map and intensive auditory training. Patient commitment to the full rehabilitative process is vital to success with the implant.

While a cochlear implant does not provide normal hearing, users may derive many benefits including recognition of environmental sounds and ability to understand spoken language with, and in some cases without, speech reading cues. Benefits for children implanted early in life may include enhanced development of speech and language skills as well as improvement in overall literacy. Current evidence suggests that binaural implantation and bimodal fittings (combining a cochlear implant and hearing aid in opposite ears) has become the standard of care for pediatric cases. With universal screening for hearing loss, children identified early with severe to profound hearing loss who receive cochlear implants in conjunction with intensive early intervention services can achieve language outcomes comparable with normally hearing children at 4 to 7 years of age (195).

Speech Reading and Auditory Training

Hearing aids and other amplification systems provide the hearing-impaired individual with access to auditory information, but this alone does not guarantee comprehension. Supplementary information obtained through speech reading (lip reading) and auditory training to improve listening skills are important components of successful hearing rehabilitation.

Speech reading is the use of visual cues in the recognition of speech and incorporates the interpretation of facial expressions, body movements, and gestures. Everyone uses speech reading to some extent, although usually we are not conscious of the importance of visual input in helping us to recognize what is being said. Many people with hearing impairment, particularly those with gradually progressive hearing loss, develop this skill through necessity. Although a considerable amount of the speech signal can be perceived visually, only about one third of English speech sounds are clearly visible. Certain sounds (e.g., *f* and *th*) are relatively easy to see on the lips, whereas others, such as *k* and *g*, are not visible, and some (e.g., *p* and *b*) are indistinguishable from one another.

Auditory training teaches the hearing-impaired individual to make the most effective use of the limited auditory cues imposed by the hearing loss as well as the additional auditory information delivered by the hearing aid. While the benefits of auditory training programs have been documented, such programs have not been time- or cost-effective. Recently, computer-based, adaptive, auditory training programs have become available (e.g., Listening and Communication Enhancement) that provide a home-based, individualized approach to aural rehabilitation (196). Such programs have demonstrated some degree of success especially with new hearing aid users in improving listening performance in noisy listening conditions (196). However, the efficacy of many home-based auditory training programs for individuals with hearing loss has yet to be demonstrated conclusively (197).

Aural rehabilitation strategies also teach the hearing-impaired person to become a more assertive listener. Those who quietly accept hearing loss or not understanding speech merely invite continued social isolation. The hearing-impaired listener needs to inform others of his or her impairment and advise them as to the most effective means of communication. Self-help groups are available, most notably the Hearing Loss Association of America, which offers local groups, as well as an active national organization and journals.

Although management of hearing loss with hearing aid amplification, ALDs, cochlear implants, and aural rehabilitation therapy does not cure the impairment or restore hearing and communicative efficiency to normal, such approaches represent the best treatments available at this time. They will improve the ability of most people to communicate effectively and reduce the consequences of hearing loss.

ACKNOWLEDGMENTS

The authors wish to acknowledge the contributions of Beth Solomon, Carmen Brewer, Martin B. Brodsky, Jeffrey B. Palmer, and Jennifer Ryder (authors of *Speech Language, Swallowing, and Auditory Rehabilitation* of the previous edition). Much of their original published work has remained in this updated chapter. We would also like to acknowledge the contributions of Stephanie Kwiatkowski to format and prepare this chapter.

REFERENCES

1. Fogle P. Essentials of communication and its disorders. In: *Essentials of Communication Sciences and Disorders*. New York: Delmar Cengage Learning; 2013:117–132.
2. Baken R, Orlikoff R. *Clinical Measurement of Voice and Speech*. 2nd ed. San Diego, CA: Singular Publishing Group; 2000:297–336.
3. Williamson G. *Human Communication: A Linguistic Introduction*. 2nd ed. Billingham, UK: Speech-Language Services; 2006.
4. Perry JL. Anatomy and physiology of the velopharyngeal mechanism. *Semin Speech Lang*. 2011;32(2):83–92.
5. Seikel JA, Drumright DG, King DW. *Anatomy & Physiology for Speech, Language, and Hearing*. Boston, MA: Nelson Education; 2015.
6. Kent RD, Kent JF, Weismer G, et al. What dysarthrias can tell us about the neural control of speech. *J Phon*. 2000;28(3):273–302.
7. Darley FL, Aronson AE, Brown JR. *Motor Speech Disorders*. 1st ed. Philadelphia, PA: W.B. Saunders; 1975.
8. Kent RD, Rosenbek JC. Acoustic patterns of apraxia of speech. *J Speech Lang Hear Res*. 1983;26(2):231–249.
9. Darley FL, Aronson AE, Brown JR. Clusters of deviant speech dimensions in the dysarthrias. *J Speech Hear Res*. 1969;12(3):462–496.
10. Darley FL, Aronson AE, Brown JR. Differential diagnostic patterns of dysarthria. *J Speech Hear Res*. 1969;12(2):246–269.
11. Sarno MT, Buonaguro A, Levita E. Characteristics of verbal impairment in closed head injured patients. *Arch Phys Med Rehabil*. 1986;67(6):400–445.
12. Yorkston KM, Honsinger MJ, Mitsuda PM, et al. The relationship between speech and swallowing disorders in head injured patients. *J Head Trauma Rehabil*. 1989;4:1–16.
13. Logemann JA, Fisher HB, Boshes B, et al. Frequency and cooccurrence of vocal tract dysfunctions in the speech of a large sample of Parkinson patients. *J Speech Hear Disord*. 1978;43(1):47–57.
14. Duffy JR, Folger WN. Dysarthria associated with unilateral central nervous system lesions. *J Med Speech Lang Pathol*. 1996;4(2):57–70.
15. Hillis AE, Work M, Barker PB, et al. Re-examining the brain regions crucial for orchestrating speech articulation. *Brain*. 2004;127(Pt 7):1479–1487.
16. Dronkers NF. A new brain region for coordinating speech articulation. *Nature*. 1996;384(6605):159–161.
17. Ogar J, Slama H, Dronkers N, et al. Apraxia of speech: an overview. *Neurocase*. 2005;11(6):427–432.
18. Duffy JR. Apraxia of speech in degenerative neurologic disease. *Aphasiology*. 2006;20(6):511–527.
19. Josephs KA, Duffy JR, Strand EA, et al. Characterizing a neurodegenerative syndrome: primary progressive apraxia of speech. *Brain*. 2012;135:1522–1536.
20. Lewis BA, Freebairn LA, Hansen A, et al. Family pedigrees of children with suspected childhood apraxia of speech. *J Commun Disord*. 2004;37(2):157–175.
21. Shriberg LD, Lohmeier HL, Strand EA, et al. Encoding, memory, and transcoding deficits in childhood apraxia of speech. *Clin Linguist Phon*. 2012;26(5):445–482.
22. Duffy J, Buckingham H. Explanation in apraxia with consequences for the concept of apraxia of speech. *Brain Lang*. 1979;8(2):202–226.
23. Duffy RJ, Duffy JR, Pearson KL. Pantomime recognition in aphasics. *J Speech Lang Hear Res*. 1975;18(1):115–132.
24. Martin AD. Some objections to the term apraxia of speech. *J Speech Hear Disord*. 1974;39(1):53–64.
25. Chaturvedi AK, Engels EA, Pfeiffer RM, et al. Human papillomavirus and rising oropharyngeal cancer incidence in the United States. *J Clin Oncol*. 2011;29(32):4294–4301.
26. Dwivedi RC, Kazi RA, Agrawal N, et al. Evaluation of speech outcomes following treatment of oral and oropharyngeal cancers. *Cancer Treat Rev*. 2009;35(5):417–424.
27. Jacobi I, van der Molen L, Huiskens H, et al. Voice and speech outcomes of chemoradiation for advanced head and neck cancer: a systematic review. *Eur Arch Otorhinolaryngol*. 2010;267(10):1495–1505.
28. van der Molen L, van Rossum MA, Jacobi I, et al. Pre-and posttreatment voice and speech outcomes in patients with advanced head and neck cancer treated with chemoradiotherapy: expert listeners' and patient's perception. *J Voice*. 2012;26(5):664.e25–664.e33.
29. Salinas TJ. Prosthetic rehabilitation of defects of the head and neck. *Semin Plast Surg*. 2010;24(3):299–308.
30. Starmer HM, Tippett DC, Webster KT. Effects of laryngeal cancer on voice and swallowing. *Otolaryngol Clin North Am*. 2008;41(4):793–818.
31. Kummer AW. Types and causes of velopharyngeal dysfunction. *Semin Speech Lang*. 2011;32(2):150–158.
32. Campbell TF, Dollaghan CA, Rockette HE, et al. Risk factors for speech delay of unknown origin in 3-year-old children. *Child Dev*. 2003;74(2):346–357.
33. Fox A, Dodd B, Howard D. Risk factors for speech disorders in children. *Int J Lang Commun Disord*. 2002;37(2):117–131.
34. Aronson A, Bless D. *Clinical Voice Disorders*. New York, NY: Thieme Medical Publishers; 2009.
35. Boone D, McFarlane S, Von Berg S, et al. *The Voice and Voice Therapy*. Boston, MA: Allyn & Bacon; 2010.
36. Tippett DC. *Tracheostomy and Ventilator Dependency: Management of Breathing, Speaking, and Swallowing*. New York, NY: Thieme Medical Publishers; 2000.
37. Yairi E, Ambrose NG. *Early Childhood Stuttering for Clinicians by Clinicians*. Austin, TX: Pro-Ed; 2005.
38. Culatta R, Leeper L. The differential diagnosis of disfluency. *Nat Stud Speech Lang Hear Assoc J*. 1990;17:59–64.
39. Canter GJ. Observations on neurogenic stuttering: a contribution to differential diagnosis. *Int J Lang Commun Disord*. 1971;6(2):139–143.
40. Lundgren K, Helm-Estabrooks N, Klein R. Stuttering following acquired brain damage: a review of the literature. *J Neurolinguistics*. 2010;23(5):447–454.
41. Baumgartner J, Duffy JR. Psychogenic stuttering in adults with and without neurologic disease. *J Med Speech Lang Pathol*. 1997;5:75–96.
42. Tippett DC, Siebens AA. Distinguishing psychogenic from neurogenic dysfluency when neurologic and psychologic factors coexist. *J Fluency Disord*. 1991;16(1):3–12.
43. Enderby P, Palmer R. *FDA-2: Frenchay Dysarthria Assessment*. 2nd ed. Austin, TX: Pro-Ed; 2007.
44. Dabul BL, ed. *The Apraxia Battery for Adults*. Austin, TX: Pro-Ed; 2000.
45. Yorkston KM, Beukelman DR. *Assessment of Intelligibility of Dysarthric Speech*. Austin, TX: Pro-Ed; 1984.

46. Paul DR, Frattali CM, Holland AL, et al. *Quality of Communication Life Scale.* Rockville, MD: American Speech-Language-Hearing Association; 2005.

47. Netsell R, Hixon TJ. A noninvasive method for clinically estimating subglottal air pressure. *J Speech Hear Disord.* 1978;43(3):326–330.

48. Hixon TJ, Hoit JD. Physical examination of the rib cage wall by the speech-language pathologist. *Am J Speech Lang Pathol.* 2000;9(3):179–196.

49. Fletcher S, Adams L, McCutcheon M. Nasalance shaping routines. In: *Instruction Manual for the Nasometer Model 6200*; 1988.

50. Mitchell C, Bowen A, Tyson S, et al. Interventions for dysarthria due to stroke and other adult-acquired, non-progressive brain injury. *Cochrane Database Syst Rev.* 2017;1:CD002088.

51. Pennington L, Miller N, Robson S. Speech therapy for children with dysarthria acquired before three years of age. *Cochrane Database Syst Rev.* 2016(7).

52. Winstein CJ, Stein J, Arena R; American Heart Association Stroke Council, Council on Cardiovascular and Stroke Nursing, Council on Clinical Cardiology, and Council on Quality of Care and Outcomes Research. Guidelines for adult stroke rehabilitation and recovery: a guideline for healthcare professionals from the American Heart Association/American Stroke Association. *Stroke.* 2016;47(6):e98–e169.

53. Wambaugh JL, Nessler C, Cameron R, et al. Treatment for acquired apraxia of speech: examination of treatment intensity and practice schedule. *Am J Speech Lang Pathol.* 2013;22(1):84–102.

54. Atkins S, Ersser SJ. Clinical reasoning and patient-centred care. In: Higgs J, Jones M, Loftus S, Christensen N, eds. *Clinical Reasoning in the Health Professions.* Philadelphia, PA: Butterworth-Heinemann Elsevier; 2008:68–77.

55. Yorkston KM, Miller RM, Strand EA. *Management of Speech and Swallowing Disorders in Degenerative Diseases.* Austin, TX: Pro-Ed; 2004.

56. Fried-Oken M, Mooney A, Peters B. Supporting communication for patients with neurodegenerative disease. *NeuroRehabilitation.* 2015;37(1):69–87.

57. Plowman EK. Is there a role for exercise in the management of bulbar dysfunction in amyotrophic lateral sclerosis? *J Speech Lang Hear Res.* 2015;58(4):1151–1166.

58. Ramig LO, Sapir S, Fox C, et al. Changes in vocal loudness following intensive voice treatment (LSVT®) in individuals with Parkinson's disease: a comparison with untreated patients and normal age-matched controls. *Mov Disord.* 2001;16(1):79–83.

59. Sapir S, Spielman JL, Ramig LO, et al. Effects of intensive voice treatment (the Lee Silverman voice treatment [LSVT]) on vowel articulation in dysarthric individuals with idiopathic Parkinson disease: acoustic and perceptual findings. *J Speech Lang Hear Res.* 2007;50(4):899–912.

60. Shenson JA, Craig JN, Rohde SL. Effect of preoperative counseling on hospital length of stay and readmissions after total laryngectomy. *Otolaryngol Head Neck Surg.* 2017;156(2):289–298.

61. Andersen PM, Abrahams S, Borasio GD, et al. EFNS guidelines on the clinical management of amyotrophic lateral sclerosis (MALS)—revised report of an EFNS task force. *Eur J Neurol.* 2012;19(3):360–375.

62. Kent R. Normal aspects of articulation. In: Bernthal J, Bankson N, eds. *Articulation and Phonological Disorders.* Englewood Cliffs, NJ: Prentice-Hall; 1988:5–59.

63. Broca P. Sur la faculté du langage articulé. In: Sur la faculté du langage articulé. *Bull Soc Anthropol.* 1865:6:337–393.

64. Wernicke C. *Lehrbuch der gehirnkrankheiten.* Vol 2 Berlin, Germany: Theodore Fischer; 1881.

65. Lichtheim L. On aphasia. *Brain.* 1885;7:433–484.

66. Geschwind N. Disconnexion syndromes in animals and man. II. *Brain.* 1965;88(3):585–644.

67. Mesulam MM. Large-scale neurocognitive networks and distributed processing for attention, language, and memory. *Ann Neurol.* 1990;28(5):597–613.

68. Binder JR, Desai RH, Graves WW, et al. Where is the semantic system? A critical review and meta-analysis of 120 functional neuroimaging studies. *Cereb Cortex.* 2009;19(12):2767–2796.

69. Wise RJ. Language systems in normal and aphasic human subjects: functional imaging studies and inferences from animal studies. *Br Med Bull.* 2003;65:95–119.

70. Kraut MA, Kremen S, Moo LR, et al. Object activation in semantic memory from visual multimodal feature input. *J Cogn Neurosci.* 2002;14(1):37–47.

71. Hickok G, Poeppel D. The cortical organization of speech processing. *Nat Rev Neurosci.* 2007;8(5):393–402.

72. Robin DA, Schienberg S. Subcortical lesions and aphasia. *J Speech Hear Disord.* 1990;55(1):90–100.

73. Goodglass H, Kaplan E, Barresi B. *The Assessment of Aphasia and Related Disorders.* Philadelphia, PA: Lippincott Williams & Wilkins; 2001.

74. Freedman M, Alexander MP, Naeser MA. Anatomic basis of transcortical motor aphasia. *Neurology.* 1984;34(4):409–417.

75. Davis G. Causes of aphasia. In: Dragin S, ed. *Aphasiology: Disorders and Clinical Practice.* Needham Heights, MA: Allyn and Bacon; 2000:35–39.

76. Mazzocchi F, Vignolo LA. Localisation of lesions in aphasia: clinical-CT scan correlations in stroke patients. *Cortex.* 1979;15(4):627–653.

77. Rapcsak SZ, Krupp LB, Rubens AB, et al. Mixed transcortical aphasia without anatomic isolation of the speech area. *Stroke.* 1990;21(6):953–956.

78. Alexander MP, Hiltbrunner B, Fischer RS. Distributed anatomy of transcortical sensory aphasia. *Arch Neurol.* 1989;46(8):885–892.

79. Goodglass H, Wingfield A, eds. *Anomia: Neuroanatomical and Cognitive Correlates.* San Diego, CA: Academic Press; 1997.

80. Hillis AE. Aphasia: progress in the last quarter of a century. *Neurology.* 2007;69(2):200–213.

81. Hillis A. Alexia and agraphia in acute and chronic stroke. In: Godefroy O, ed. *The Behavioral and Cognitive Neurology of Stroke.* 2nd ed. New York: Cambridge University Press; 2013:86–100.

82. Goodglass H, Kaplan E. *Boston Diagnostic Aphasia Examination.* 3rd ed. Austin, TX: Pro-Ed; 2001.

83. Kertesz A. *Western Aphasia Battery—Revised (WAB-R).* Austin, TX: Pro-Ed; 2006.

84. Kaplan E, Goodglass H, Weintraub S. *Boston Naming Test.* Austin, TX: Pro-Ed; 2001.

85. Frattali CM, Thompson C, Holland AL, et al. *American Speech-Language-Hearing Association Functional Assessment of Communication Skills for Adults.* Rockville, MD: American Speech-Language-Hearing Association; 1995.

86. Byng S, Duchan JF. Social model philosophies and principles: their applications to therapies for aphasia. *Aphasiology.* 2005;19(10–11):906–922.

87. Chapey R, Duchan R, Linda J, et al. Language intervention strategies in aphasia and related neurogenic communication disorders. In: Chapey R, ed. *Life Participation Approach to Aphasia: A Statement of Values for the Future.* Philadelphia, PA: Lippincott Williams & Wilkins; 2001:279–289.

88. Pulvermuller F, Neininger B, Elbert T, et al. Constraint-induced therapy of chronic aphasia after stroke. *Stroke.* 2001;32(7):1621–1626.

89. Holland R, Crinion J. Can tDCS enhance treatment of aphasia after stroke? *Aphasiology.* 2012;26(9):1169–1191.

90. Baker JM, Rorden C, Fridriksson J. Using transcranial direct-current stimulation to treat stroke patients with aphasia. *Stroke.* 2010;41(6):1229–1236.

91. Fiori V, Coccia M, Marinelli CV, et al. Transcranial direct current stimulation improves word retrieval in healthy and nonfluent aphasic subjects. *J Cogn Neurosci.* 2011;23(9):2309–2323.

92. Shah-Basak PP, Norise C, Garcia G, et al. Individualized treatment with transcranial direct current stimulation in patients with chronic non-fluent aphasia due to stroke. *Front Hum Neurosci.* 2015;9:201.

93. Weiss SA, Bikson M. Open questions on the mechanisms of neuromodulation with applied and endogenous electric fields. *Front Hum Neurosci.* 2014;8:227.

94. Mesulam M. Primary progressive aphasia. *Ann Neurol.* 2001;49(4):425–432.

95. Mesulam M, Rogalski EJ, Wieneke C, et al. Primary progressive aphasia and the evolving neurology of the language network. *Nat Rev Neurol.* 2014;10(10):554–569.

96. Gorno-Tempini ML, Hillis AE, Weintraub S, et al. Classification of primary progressive aphasia and its variants. *Neurology.* 2011;76(11):1006–1014.

97. McFarland DH, Lund JP. An investigation of the coupling between respiration, mastication, and swallowing in the awake rabbit. *J Neurophysiol.* 1993;69(1):95–108.

98. Amici S, Gorno-Tempini ML, Ogar JM, et al. An overview on primary progressive aphasia and its variants. *Behav Neurol.* 2006;17(2):77–87.

99. Gorno-Tempini ML, Dronkers NF, Rankin KP, et al. Cognition and anatomy in three variants of primary progressive aphasia. *Ann Neurol.* 2004;55(3):335–346.

100. Josephs KA, Duffy JR, Strand EA, et al. Clinicopathological and imaging correlates of progressive aphasia and apraxia of speech. *Brain.* 2006;129(Pt 6):1385–1398.

101. Mesulam M, Wicklund A, Johnson N, et al. Alzheimer and frontotemporal pathology in subsets of primary progressive aphasia. *Ann Neurol.* 2008;63(6):709–719.

102. Knibb JA, Xuereb JH, Patterson K, et al. Clinical and pathological characterization of progressive aphasia. *Ann Neurol.* 2006;59(1):156–165.

103. Morris JC. The clinical dementia rating (CDR): current version and scoring rules. *Neurology.* 1993;43(11):2412–2414.

104. Folstein MF, Robins LN, Helzer JE. The mini-mental state examination. *Arch Gen Psychiatry.* 1983;40(7):812.

105. Delis DC, Kramer J, Kaplan E, et al. *CVLT-II: California Verbal Learning Test: Adult Version.* Bloomington, MN: Pearson; 2000.

106. Reitan RM. Validity of the trail making test as an indicator of organic brain damage. *Percept Mot Skills.* 1958;8(3):271–276.

107. Tippett DC, Hillis AE, Tsapkini K. Treatment of primary progressive aphasia. *Curr Treat Options Neurol.* 2015;17(8):1–11.

108. Taylor C, Kingma RM, Croot K, et al. Speech pathology services for primary progressive aphasia: exploring an emerging area of practice. *Aphasiology.* 2009;23(2):161–174.

109. Medina J, Weintraub S. Depression in primary progressive aphasia. *J Geriatr Psychiatry Neurol.* 2007;20(3):153–160.

110. Tsapkini K, Frangakis C, Gomez Y, et al. Augmentation of spelling therapy with transcranial direct current stimulation in primary progressive aphasia: preliminary results and challenges. *Aphasiology.* 2014;28(8–9):1112–1130.

111. Cotelli M, Manenti R, Petesi M, et al. Treatment of primary progressive aphasias by transcranial direct current stimulation combined with language training. *J Alzheimers Dis.* 2014;39(4):799–808.

112. Wang J, Wu D, Chen Y, et al. Effects of transcranial direct current stimulation on language improvement and cortical activation in nonfluent variant primary progressive aphasia. *Neurosci Lett.* 2013;549:29–33.

113. Myers P. *Right Hemisphere Damage: Disorders of Communication and Cognition.* San Diego, CA: Singular; 1999.

114. Tompkins C, Klepousniotou E, Scott G. Treatment of right hemisphere disorders. In: Papathanasiou I, Coppens P, Potagas C, eds. *Aphasia and Related Neurogenic Communication Disorders.* Sudbury, MA: Jones and Bartlett; 2013:345–364.

115. Blake ML. Clinical relevance of discourse characteristics after right hemisphere brain damage. *Am J Speech Lang Pathol.* 2006;15(3):255–267.

116. Lehman MT, Tompkins CA. Inferencing in adults with right hemisphere brain damage: an analysis of conflicting results. *Aphasiology.* 2000;14(5–6):485–499.

117. Baum SR, Dwivedi VD. Sensitivity to prosodic structure in left- and right-hemisphere-damaged individuals. *Brain Lang.* 2003;87(2):278–289.

118. Pell MD. Cerebral mechanisms for understanding emotional prosody in speech. *Brain Lang.* 2006;96(2):221–234.

119. Right hemisphere brain damage [homepage on the Internet]. Available from: http://www.asha.org/public/speech/disorders/RightBrainDamage.htm

120. Pimental PA, Kingsbury NA. *Mini Inventory of Right Brain Injury: Examiner's Manual.* Austin, TX: Pro-Ed; 2000.

121. Bryan K. *The Right Hemisphere Language Battery.* Hoboken, NJ: Wiley; 1995.

122. Tompkins CA. Rehabilitation for cognitive-communication disorders in right hemisphere brain damage. *Arch Phys Med Rehabil.* 2012;93(1):S61–S69.

123. McCue M, Chase S, Dowdy C, et al. *Functional Assessment of Individuals with Cognitive Disabilities: A Desk Reference for Rehabilitation.* Pittsburgh, PA: Center for Applied Neuropsychology; 1994.

124. Robert EH, Stuart CY, Jonathan MS. *Neuropsychiatry of traumatic brain injury.* In: Jonathan MS, Stuart CY, Robert EH, eds. Washington, DC: American Psychiatric Press; 1994.

125. Max W, MacKenzie EJ, Rice DP. Head injuries: costs and consequences. *J Head Trauma Rehabil.* 1991;6(2):76–91.

126. Coelho C, Grela B, Corso M, et al. Microlinguistic deficits in the narrative discourse of adults with traumatic brain injury. *Brain Inj.* 2005;19(13): 1139–1145.

127. Docking K, Murdoch BE, Jordan F. Interpretation and comprehension of linguistic humour by adolescents with head injury: a group analysis. *Brain Inj.* 1999;13(1):953–972.

128. King KA, Hough MS, Walker MM, et al. Mild traumatic brain injury: effects on naming in word retrieval and discourse. *Brain Inj.* 2006;20(7):725–732.

129. Dahlberg C, Hawley L, Morey C, et al. Social communication skills in persons with post-acute traumatic brain injury: three perspectives. *Brain Inj.* 2006;20(4): 425–435.

130. McAllister TW. Neuropsychiatric sequelae of head injuries. *Psychiatr Clin North Am.* 1992;15(2):395–413.

131. Wiseman-Hakes C, MacDonald S, Keightley M. Perspectives on evidence based practice in ABI rehabilitation. "Relevant research": who decides? *NeuroRehabilitation.* 2010;26(4):355–368.

132. MacDonald S, Wiseman-Hakes C. Knowledge translation in ABI rehabilitation: a model for consolidating and applying the evidence for cognitive-communication interventions. *Brain Inj.* 2010;24(3):486–508.

133. Martino R, Foley N, Bhogal S, et al. Dysphagia after stroke: incidence, diagnosis, and pulmonary complications. *Stroke.* 2005;36(12):2756–2763.

134. Altman KW, Yu GP, Schaefer SD. Consequence of dysphagia in the hospitalized patient: impact on prognosis and hospital resources. *Arch Otolaryngol Head Neck Surg.* 2010;136(8):784–789.

135. Jones B, ed. *Normal and Abnormal Swallowing: Imaging in Diagnosis and Therapy.* New York, NY: Springer Science and Business Media; 2003.

136. McFarland DH, Lund JP. Modification of mastication and respiration during swallowing in the adult human. *J Neurophysiol.* 1995;74(4):1509–1517.

137. Matsuo K, Palmer JB. Anatomy and physiology of feeding and swallowing: normal and abnormal. *Phys Med Rehabil Clin N Am.* 2008;19(4):691–707, vii.

138. Brodsky MB, McNeil MR, Martin-Harris B, et al. Effects of divided attention on swallowing in healthy participants. *Dysphagia.* 2012;27(3):307–317.

139. Dellow PG, Lund JP. Evidence for central timing of rhythmical mastication. *J Physiol.* 1971;215(1):1–13.

140. Mishellany A, Woda A, Labas R, et al. The challenge of mastication: preparing a bolus suitable for deglutition. *Dysphagia.* 2006;21(2):87–94.

141. Saitoh E, Shibata S, Matsuo K, et al. Chewing and food consistency: effects on bolus transport and swallow initiation. *Dysphagia.* 2007;22(2):100–107.

142. Cook IJ, Dodds WJ, Dantas RO, et al. Timing of videofluoroscopic, manometric events, and bolus transit during the oral and pharyngeal phases of swallowing. *Dysphagia.* 1989;4(1):8–15.

143. Dantas RO, Kern MK, Massey BT, et al. Effect of swallowed bolus variables on oral and pharyngeal phases of swallowing. *Am J Physiol.* 1990;258(5): G675–G681.

144. Gonzalez-Fernandez M, Humbert I, Winegrad H, et al. Dysphagia in old-old women: prevalence as determined according to self-report and the 3-ounce water swallowing test. *J Am Geriatr Soc.* 2014;62(4):716–720.

145. Butler SG, Stuart A, Kemp S. Flexible endoscopic evaluation of swallowing in healthy young and older adults. *Ann Otol Rhinol Laryngol.* 2009;118(2):99–106.

146. Langmore SE, Terpenning MS, Schork A, et al. Predictors of aspiration pneumonia: how important is dysphagia? *Dysphagia.* 1998;13(2):69–81.

147. McHorney CA, Bricker DE, Kramer AE, et al. The SWAL-QOL outcomes tool for oropharyngeal dysphagia in adults: I. Conceptual foundation and item development. *Dysphagia.* 2000;15(3):115–121.

148. Silbergleit AK, Schultz L, Jacobson BH, et al. The dysphagia handicap index: development and validation. *Dysphagia.* 2012;27(1):46–52.

149. Bonilha HS, Blair J, Carnes B, et al. Preliminary investigation of the effect of pulse rate on judgments of swallowing impairment and treatment recommendations. *Dysphagia.* 2013;28(4):528–538.

150. Cohen MD. Can we use pulsed fluoroscopy to decrease the radiation dose during video fluoroscopic feeding studies in children? *Clin Radiol.* 2009;64(1):70–73.

151. Martin-Harris B, Brodsky MB, Michel Y, et al. MBS measurement tool for swallow impairment—MBSImp: establishing a standard. *Dysphagia.* 2008;23(4):392–405.

152. Kelly AM, Drinnan MJ, Leslie P. Assessing penetration and aspiration: how do videofluoroscopy and fiberoptic endoscopic evaluation of swallowing compare? *Laryngoscope.* 2007;117(10):1723–1727.

153. The International Dysphagia Diet Standardisation Initiative; 2016. Available from: http://Iddsi.org/framework/

154. Metheny NA, Clouse RE, Chang YH, et al. Tracheobronchial aspiration of gastric contents in critically ill tube-fed patients: frequency, outcomes, and risk factors. *Crit Care Med.* 2006;34(4):1007–1015.

155. Ciocon JO, Silverstone FA, Graver LM, et al. Tube feedings in elderly patients. indications, benefits, and complications. *Arch Intern Med.* 1988;148(2):429–433.

156. Welch MV, Logemann JA, Rademaker AW, et al. Changes in pharyngeal dimensions effected by chin tuck. *Arch Phys Med Rehabil.* 1993;74(2):178–181.

157. Logemann JA, Kahrilas PJ, Kobara M, et al. The benefit of head rotation on pharyngoesophageal dysphagia. *Arch Phys Med Rehabil.* 1989;70(10):767–771.

158. Donzelli J, Brady S. The effects of breath-holding on vocal fold adduction: implications for safe swallowing. *Arch Otolaryngol Head Neck Surg.* 2004;130(2):208–210.

159. Martin BJ, Logemann JA, Shaker R, et al. Normal laryngeal valving patterns during three breath-hold maneuvers: a pilot investigation. *Dysphagia.* 1993;8:11–20.

160. Aviv JE, Martin JH, Sacco RL, et al. Supraglottic and pharyngeal sensory abnormalities in stroke patients with dysphagia. *Ann Otol Rhinol Laryngol.* 1996;105(2): 92–97.

161. Huckabee M, Butler SG, Barclay M, et al. Submental surface electromyographic measurement and pharyngeal pressures during normal and effortful swallowing. *Arch Phys Med Rehabil.* 2005;86(11):2144–2149.

162. McCullough GH, Kamarunas E, Mann GC, et al. Effects of mendelsohn maneuver on measures of swallowing duration post stroke. *Top Stroke Rehabil.* 2012;19(3):234–243.

163. McCullough GH, Kim Y. Effects of the mendelsohn maneuver on extent of hyoid movement and UES opening post-stroke. *Dysphagia.* 2013;28(4):511–519.

164. Shaker R, Kern M, Bardan E, et al. Augmentation of deglutitive upper esophageal sphincter opening in the elderly by exercise. *Am J Physiol.* 1997;272(6 Pt 1): G1518–G1522.

165. Fujiu M, Logemann JA, Pauloski BR. Increased postoperative posterior pharyngeal wall movement in patients with anterior oral cancer: preliminary findings and possible implications for treatment. *Am J Speech Lang Pathol.* 1995;4(2):24–30.

166. Leelamanit V, Limsakul C, Geater A. Synchronized electrical stimulation in treating pharyngeal dysphagia. *Laryngoscope.* 2002;112(12):2204–2210.

167. Ludlow CL, Humbert I, Saxon K, et al. Effects of surface electrical stimulation both at rest and during swallowing in chronic pharyngeal dysphagia. *Dysphagia.* 2007;22(1):1–10.

168. Troche MS, Okun MS, Rosenbek JC, et al. Aspiration and swallowing in Parkinson disease and rehabilitation with EMST: a randomized trial. *Neurology.* 2010;75(21):1912–1919.

169. Hegland KW, Davenport PW, Brandimore AE, et al. Rehabilitation of swallowing and cough functions following stroke: an expiratory muscle strength training trial. *Arch Phys Med Rehabil.* 2016;97(8):1345–1351.

170. Plowman EK, Watts SA, Tabor L, et al. Impact of expiratory strength training in amyotrophic lateral sclerosis. *Muscle Nerve.* 2016;54(1):48–53.

171. Pisegna JM, Kaneoka A, Pearson WG, et al. Effects of non-invasive brain stimulation on post-stroke dysphagia: a systematic review and meta-analysis of randomized controlled trials. *Clin Neurophysiol.* 2016;127(1):956–968.

172. Azola AM, Sunday KL, Humbert IA. Kinematic visual biofeedback improves accuracy of learning a swallowing maneuver and accuracy of clinician cues during training. *Dysphagia.* 2017;32(1):115–122.

173. Lin FR, Niparko JK, Ferrucci L. Hearing loss prevalence in the United States. *Arch Intern Med.* 2011;171(20):1851–1853.

174. Dalton DS, Cruickshanks KJ, Klein BE, et al. The impact of hearing loss on quality of life in older adults. *Gerontologist.* 2003;43(5):661–668.

175. Lin F, Ferrucci L, An Y, et al. Association of hearing impairment with brain volume changes in older adults. *Neuroimage.* 2014;90:84–92.

176. Chang Y, Lee S, Lee Y, et al. Auditory neural pathway evaluation on sensorineural hearing loss using diffusion tensor imaging. *Neuroreport.* 2004;15(11):1699–1703.

177. Albers MW, Gilmore GC, Kaye J, et al. At the interface of sensory and motor dysfunctions and Alzheimer's disease. *Alzheimers Dement.* 2015;11(1):70–98.

178. Deal JA, Betz J, Yaffe K, et al.; Health ABC Study Group. Hearing impairment and incident dementia and cognitive decline in older adults: the health ABC study. *J Gerontol A Biol Sci Med Sci.* 2017;72(5):703–709.

179. Killion MC, Niquette PA, Gudmundsen GI, et al. Development of a quick speech-in-noise test for measuring signal-to-noise ratio loss in normal-hearing and hearing-impaired listeners. *J Acoust Soc Am.* 2004;116(4):2395–2405.

180. Kraus N, Thompson EC, Krizman J, et al. Auditory biological marker of concussion in children. *Sci Rep.* 2016;6:39009.

181. Bamiou DE. Hearing disorders in stroke. *Handb Clin Neurol.* 2015;129:633–647.

182. Moore DR. Sources of pathology underlying listening disorders in children. *Int J Psychophysiol.* 2015;95(2):125–134.

183. Brewer CC, Zalewski CK, King KA, et al. Heritability of non-speech auditory processing skills. *Eur J Hum Genet.* 2016;24(8):1137–1144.

184. Batista PB, Lemos SMA, Rodrigues LOC, et al. Auditory temporal processing deficits and language disorders in patients with neurofibromatosis type 1. *J Commun Disord.* 2014;48:18–26.

185. Pillion JP, Shiffler DE, Hoon AH, et al. Severe auditory processing disorder secondary to viral meningoencephalitis. *Int J Audiol.* 2014;53(6):427–431.

186. Alain C, Zendel BR, Hutka S, et al. Turning down the noise: the benefit of musical training on the aging auditory brain. *Hear Res.* 2014;308:162–173.

187. Genetics of hearing loss [homepage on the Internet]. Available from: https://www.cdc.gov/ncbddd/hearingloss/genetics.html

188. Hereditary hearing loss [homepage on the Internet]. Available from: http://hereditaryhearingloss.org

189. Fayad JN, Keles B, Brackmann DE. Jugular foramen tumors: clinical characteristics and treatment outcomes. *Otol Neurotol.* 2010;31(2):299–305.

190. Buchanan LH. Early onset of presbycusis in Down syndrome. *Scand Audiol.* 1990;19(2):103–110.

191. Carroll YI. Vital signs: noise-induced hearing loss among adults—United States 2011–2012. *MMWR Morb Mortal Wkly Rep.* 2017;66(5):139–144.

192. Henderson E, Testa MA, Hartnick C. Prevalence of noise-induced hearing-threshold shifts and hearing loss among US youths. *Pediatrics.* 2011;127(1):e39–e46.

193. Lustig T, Olson S. *Hearing Loss and Healthy Aging.* Washington, DC: National Academic Press; 2014.

194. Cochlear implant quick facts [homepage on the Internet]. Available from: http://www.asha.org/public/hearing/Cochlear-Implant-Quick-Facts/

195. Yoshinaga-Itano C, Baca RL, Sedey AL. Describing the trajectory of language development in the presence of severe-to-profound hearing loss: a closer look at children with cochlear implants versus hearing aids. *Otol Neurotol.* 2010;31(8):1268–1274.

196. Olson AD, Preminger JE, Shinn JB. The effect of LACE DVD training in new and experienced hearing aid users. *J Am Acad Audiol.* 2013;24(3):214–230.

197. Henshaw H, Ferguson MA. Efficacy of individual computer-based auditory training for people with hearing loss: a systematic review of the evidence. *PLoS One.* 2013;8(5):e62836.

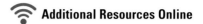 **Additional Resources Online**

CHAPTER 14

Debra B. Homa
David A. DeLambo

Vocational Rehabilitation, Independent Living, and Consumerism

According to a 2016 survey, approximately 20% of the US population report having a disability (1). Yet, individuals with disabilities have been underrepresented in the labor market, with recent surveys estimating that, at the end of 2016, more than two thirds of working-age people with disabilities were unemployed (1). Work plays a central role in life and is a common source of self-identify and financial independence (2). Since its beginning, a major goal of vocational rehabilitation in the United States has been to help people with disabilities become productive members of society through the activity of holding a job.

Vocational rehabilitation (VR) programs have been specifically designed to promote work opportunities for people with disabilities. Historically, the focus of VR services has been to assist persons with disabilities believed to have vocational potential. It was not until 1978 that legislation defining VR services also included provision of services for individuals without clear vocational goals (3). Title VII, Comprehensive Services for Independent Living (IL), an amendment to the Rehabilitation Act of 1973 (PL 93-112), authorizes services for people with severe disabilities, those who require multiple services over an extended period of time and persons whose disability prevents them from working or participating in other major life activities (4). This chapter provides an overview of both the VR and IL programs in the United States. Emphasis will be placed on the legislative history and purpose of VR and IL services as well as the differences between these two service paradigms. The authors describe VR program settings and staff, as well as the services that help individuals with disabilities achieve their goals. This chapter also provides a brief review of key research findings that document the effectiveness of VR services and implications for practice.

Although VR and IL are comprised in the same legislation, they have not always worked in tandem, as VR professionals have tended to view consumers of IL services as being unable to achieve gainful employment and therefore not likely to benefit from their efforts (3). In recent years, however, the goals and principles of VR and IL have begun to converge and are likely to continue to do so, especially as newer understandings of rehabilitation and disability become more widely accepted with the growing international impact of the International Classification of Functioning, Disability and Health (ICF). The ICF, which is described more fully in Chapter 9 of this volume, was endorsed by the World Health Organization

(WHO) in 2001 and provides a new framework for understanding health and health-related conditions (5).

The ICF conceptual model provides a holistic perspective of health that is consistent with contemporary rehabilitation philosophy, in which disability is seen as a consequence of the interaction of the person with the environment (6). In a further development of the ICF, the Physical and Rehabilitation Medicine section of the European Union of Medical Specialists adopted the ICF conceptual model, in which rehabilitation is understood as a health strategy to help people attain optimal functioning in their interaction with the environment (7,8). Within this model, individuals do not "have" disabilities; rather, they are "people with health conditions experiencing or likely to experience disability" (7). The United Nations Convention on the Rights of Persons with Disabilities has also endorsed an understanding of disability consistent with the ICF model, stating, "disability results from the interaction between persons with impairments and attitudinal and environmental barriers that hinders their full and effective participation in society on an equal basis with others," including maximum independence and the right to work (9).

PURPOSE AND CHARACTERISTICS OF VR AND IL SERVICES

Vocational Rehabilitation

The primary purpose of VR has been to help people with disabilities prepare for and obtain gainful employment, usually through competitive employment (e.g., paid work). VR programs provide rehabilitation services designed to maximize independence and employment and to promote full integration and participation in society (10). Rehabilitation counselors work with individuals who have a wide range of disabilities. These include physical disabilities, such as spinal cord injury (SCI), stroke, arthritis, multiple sclerosis, congenital or orthopedic difficulties, chronic pain, or amputations; cognitive disabilities, such as traumatic brain injury (TBI), organic brain syndromes, and developmental and learning disabilities; and psychiatric disorders, including major depression, bipolar disorder, and schizophrenia (4).

VR services are multidisciplinary, involving a wide range of professionals, such as physiatrists, physical therapists, occupational therapists, speech-language pathologists, psychologists, rehabilitation counselors, case managers, employment specialists, and special education teachers, among others (3,11). They may also be provided in a variety of settings, including the state-federal VR program (a public agency under the U.S. Department of Education), private, nonprofit community-based programs (e.g., Goodwill Industries, Easter Seals), rehabilitation hospitals, Veterans Administration system, for-profit rehabilitation firms, psychiatric rehabilitation programs, insurance companies, and employer disability management programs (12). Within the state-federal system, the VR process involves a collaborative relationship in which the rehabilitation counselor and individual with a disability work together to identify a feasible vocational goal and the services needed to achieve employment. This process generally involves: (a) individual assessment and planning, which may include interviewing, paper-and-pencil tests, and performance evaluation in real or simulated work situations; (b) comprehensive services, which may include counseling, education, vocational training, physical therapy, speech therapy, and assistive technology (AT); and (c) job placement, which may include on-the-job training or job trials, job development, job search training, supported employment, placement in permanent employment, and postemployment services. Private rehabilitation companies that work with individuals who have work-related disabilities provide or plan services such as vocational assessment, work capacity evaluation, job analysis, work hardening and reconditioning, vocational training, job accommodations, job-seeking skills, job placement, and employer development.

In the state-federal VR program, the service provision plan is formalized with an Individualized Plan for Employment (IPE), which is jointly developed by the individual and counselor. Once job placement has been achieved, follow-up services are continued for a minimum of 90 days to provide support and consultation to the new employee and to his or her employer. This helps to ensure that the employment situation is working out satisfactorily for all parties (4).

Independent Living

Living independently with a severe disability in a physical and social world that is often less than accommodating presents a lifetime of challenges. Attention to individual needs also is critical, as the impact of a severe disability may change at different life stages or in varying situations. For example, an individual who is relatively unhampered by disability in one area of life, or during one stage of development, may at another time or under different circumstances be completely overwhelmed by any one of the myriad challenges presented by a severe disability (4). The overriding goal of IL is the full inclusion and participation of individuals with disability in society. Moreover, IL services promote self-actualization of individuals with severe disabilities by helping them realize their ability "to gain greater control over their lives given certain support services and the removal of environmental barriers" (3).

IL services are most often provided by a national network of approximately 500 Centers for Independent Living (CILs) (also known as Independent Living Centers) across the country. CILs, as defined in the Rehabilitation Act, are "consumer-controlled, community-based, cross-disability, nonresidential private nonprofit agencies that are designed and operated within a local community by individuals with

disabilities and provide an array of independent living services" (13). CILs are required to provide the following core services:

1. Peer counseling and support.
2. Consumer and systems advocacy.
3. Information and referral.
4. Activities of living skills training.
5. Assist with the transition process from nursing homes and similar facilities to both home- and community-based living.
6. Help consumer with significant disabilities to remain/return in community and avoid institutional living.
7. Transition of adolescents with severe disabilities following secondary education to community living (i.e., postsecondary living).

In contrast to the public state-federal VR program, CILs are private, nonprofit, community-based organizations that are controlled by consumers to provide services and advocacy by and for persons with all types of disabilities. CILs are not residential programs per se; rather, they help individuals identify and achieve IL goals. In recent years, IL services have been increasingly recognized as being complementary to traditional VR (3). Due to medical advances, many persons with severe disabilities in the 1960s who only had hope for IL now are often employable. Thus, IL and VR are continuous elements of the larger rehabilitation process. While VR programs focus specifically on achieving employment-related goals, IL programs provide services that enable persons with severe disabilities to gain more autonomy in their lives. Their goal is to help individuals with disabilities to achieve their maximum potential within their communities and family units.

CILs serve as advocates for people with disabilities and address an array of national, state, and local issues. They strive to increase both physical and programmatic access to housing, employment, transportation, communities, recreational facilities, and social and health services. Services are often provided by individuals with disabilities. For example, a consumer with a recent SCI may be counseled by a seasoned one. Specific services typically include housing information, attendant care, reading or interpreting, and information about other goods and services necessary for IL. They may also include transportation, peer counseling, advocacy or political action, training in IL skills, equipment maintenance and repair such as wheelchair, and social and recreational services. VR programs may provide these services, but on a limited basis as a secondary or supplementary means of achieving the primary vocational objective. Rather, VR programs refer consumers for these services to the CILs, as stipulated in the Rehabilitation Act, as amended by the Workforce Innovation and Opportunity Act (WIOA) of 2014. Although the key features of IL legislation continue as they have for many years, WIOA implemented several significant changes. For example, CILs and their services are now housed in the Administration for Community Living (ACL) in the U.S. Department of Health and Human Services, while the state-federal VR program remains in the Department of Education. In addition, WIOA added the following changes (14):

1. Three additional core services have been added to the Center for Independent Living Core services. The core services 5 to 7 listed above show these additions (1 to 4 were the original CIL legislation).

2. Consumer control now refers to the consumer with a disability, not caregivers or parents of the consumer. This highlights the importance of autonomy and self-determination.
3. Personal assistance services encompass a full range of services that help consumers gain control over their lives and perform daily activities at the workplace, home, and community, including social relationships.

The VR and the IL paradigms share a consumer-centered approach, but they have different goals. In the VR process, the nature and extent of functional limitations, socioeconomic factors, and other factors are carefully assessed and reviewed to develop a vocational goal and plan for employment. VR has been criticized by many in the disability rights movement as being disempowering to people with disabilities due to its focus on providing services designed to "fix" the individual, rather than eliminate societal and environmental barriers that magnify or even create disability (15). The IL movement, in contrast, plays a significant role in recognizing disability as being the consequence of external barriers, rather than a "problem" within the individual (16). In the IL process, the concept of independence is subject to various definitions, depending on the unique need and desires of the individual. Success is defined through maximizing self-sufficiency to the greatest extent possible for as long as possible, with an emphasis on self-direction (17). The individual may be independent in some life situations but relatively "dependent" in others in terms of the level of services needed. Within IL, self-determination is the guiding principle; autonomy and level of independence may vary, depending on one's needs, but the individual maintains as much control as possible in decision-making (18). For example, a person with quadriplegia may be able to independently perform tasks at work (e.g., by using a voice recognition program on a computer to compensate for upper mobility limitations) but need more extensive assistance from a personal attendant in performing activities of daily living (ADL) at home. Though dependent in ADL, the person maintains self-determination.

In order to be considered eligible for VR services, the consumer must have a disability that presents a significant barrier to employment and have a feasible vocational goal (3,10).

Assessment is an important part of the VR process and is a required initial step to determine if the individual is eligible for services. Once eligibility is determined, assessment is essential to understanding the functional impact of disability on the consumer. Based on results of the assessment, the rehabilitation counselor and consumer identify a vocational objective and begin planning services needed to attain that objective.

IL services, on the other hand, acknowledge the effect of disability on the client, but do not require a thorough analysis of the client, nor the disability, as a prerequisite to the provision of services. In addition, IL services are totally separate from a consumer's eligibility for VR services. For example, a consumer may not desire to seek employment or VR services but be able to access IL services. The success of IL programs depends on the people and resources in the community for direction and support. Consumer involvement is assured through the governance structure of CILs, which must be managed by persons with disabilities; in addition, the CILs must ensure that a majority of the staff, including those responsible for decision-making, as well as the governing board, are persons with disabilities (13). IL services are aimed at addressing personal and environmental difficulties. In general, research has outlined the following areas of importance: self-image, well-being, functional limitations, health behaviors, interpersonal skills, and environmental barriers at both the system (e.g., regulations, physical access) and community (e.g., medical providers, social and family support) levels. In addition, research suggests that programs designed to teach IL skills (e.g., advocacy, housing and transportation, health care, social networking, and technology access) may be especially effective in helping individuals leave nursing homes and reintegrate to the community (19).

The appropriateness of IL services is based on the rights of people with disabilities for dignity, freedom, and control of their destiny. A major emphasis is that services assist with modifying the environment, not the person (3). **Table 14-1** highlights some of the differences between VR services in the state-federal system and IL services provided by CILs.

Consumer input provides the foundation of the IL movement (3). Yoshida et al. (20), utilizing feedback from consumers with SCI, developed a model highlighting the importance of *consumer input* in the rehabilitation process. This model is

TABLE 14-1 VR and IL Services

State-Federal Vocational Rehabilitation	Independent Living Centers
Public agency	Private, nonprofit community-based program managed by consumers
Assessment of functional impact of disability is required to determine eligibility for services	Assessment is not required to be eligible for services
Formal service plan (IPE)	No stringently defined service plan
Counselor and consumer work in partnership; must mutually agree on goals and services	Services are directed by consumers
Primary goal is gainful employment	Primary goals are related to IL, as defined by each consumer
Services provided by rehabilitation counselor	Services provided by individuals with disabilities
Consumer-centered	Consumer-centered
Employment is criterion of success	Maximized self-sufficiency is a criterion of success
Refer consumers to CILs for IL skills training	Provide IL skills training
Major services are directed to the goal of achieving an employment outcome	Advocacy is a major service
Focus on employment-related goals	Focus on improved autonomy

in alignment with IL and encompasses the following: (a) foster consumer autonomy by helping individuals take control of their lives in multiple areas (e.g., housing, IL plans, vocational goals, etc.) and promote informed decision-making, (b) enhance hopefulness by promoting activities that defeat hopelessness, (c) show caring and respect for the consumer and his/her individualism (individuals are unique and not numbers), and (d) apply the lived experience of disability. That is, consumers indicated the need for professionals to value the knowledge they can provide about the impact of the disability on their lives. Hence, according to these consumers with SCI, the aforementioned values (i.e., consumer care and respect, promoting consumer autonomy as well as hopefulness and application of the lived disability experience) are aligned with the IL movement and its philosophy.

Consumer sovereignty and empowerment are central to the IL movement. Persons with disabilities encounter an array of both physical and social discrimination. Empowerment is needed to battle discrimination in housing, employment, education, poverty, and social isolation (15). Empowerment is a form of self-determination where people with disabilities, via advocacy (self or institutional), have a right to determine their destiny. The Rehabilitation Act Amendments of 1998 also formalized consumer choice in the VR process and planning. *Consumer sovereignty*, sometimes referred as consumer involvement, asserts that people with disabilities can best judge their own interests and should ultimately determine what services are provided to them (16). This current rise of consumerism directly challenges the traditional service delivery system. There has been a gradual de-emphasis on professional decision-making with respect to case planning; accordingly, service provision plans are now drawn up jointly by the individual with the disability along with his or her counselor.

Because of the increased awareness created by advocacy skills training at CILs, many people with disabilities are better informed about their benefits and the regulations of the agencies with which they must interact (21).

LEGISLATIVE HISTORY

World Wars I and II as well as an array of legislation since the early 20th century have had a significant impact on VR programs and the IL movement (3). The United States VR program began in 1918 with the passage of the Soldiers' Rehabilitation Act. The Federal Board for Vocational Education, established in 1917 by the Smith-Hughes Act (PL 65-178), was authorized to create VR programs for veterans with disabilities, and the U.S. Department of Labor's task was to locate employment for these individuals (10). The Smith-Fess Act of 1920, VR legislation, was then passed to serve civilians with physical disabilities who were either totally or partially incapable of remunerative employment. State-federal fund matching was used for services, which included vocational guidance, vocational education, occupational adjustment, and placement. Although physical restoration was not emphasized, a prosthetic device would be provided if it was necessary for the person with a disability to complete vocational training (3). The 1920 bill had to be reauthorized every few years and consequently was frequently in jeopardy of being discontinued. Fortunately, the groundbreaking Social Security Act of 1935 included unemployment compensation, old age insurance, aid to dependent children, maternal and child health services, as well as other important programs. In addition, the VR program was made permanent so that an act of Congress would be required to dismantle the VR system. The Randolph-Sheppard Act of 1936 and Wagner-O'day Act of 1938 provided opportunities for individuals with visual impairment to operate vending stands on federal property and required the federal government to purchase certain products from workshops for the blind, respectively (3).

Between 1920 and 1943, VR provided services to only those with physical disabilities. The Barden-Lafollette Act of 1943 expanded services to individuals with intellectual disabilities, mental illness, and blindness. World War II was monumental in changing both the civilian and veteran rehabilitation systems. During the wartime industrial labor shortage, persons with disabilities demonstrated their ability to work. Furthermore, medical advances, such as the development of antibiotics, meant that many more military persons were able to survive. The Servicemen's Readjustment Act (PL 73-346) of 1944, known as the "GI Bill of Rights," guaranteed up to 4 years of tuition and a stipend for living expenses for returning veterans, whether disabled or not.

The Vocational Rehabilitation Act Amendment of 1954 (PL 83-565) laid the groundwork for a tremendous expansion of the rehabilitation programs. Important facets of this legislation included authorization for the use of federal funds to build and expand rehabilitation facilities, authorization of training grants to institutions for the education of new rehabilitation professionals, and extensive funding for research and demonstration projects to improve and disseminate knowledge of rehabilitation treatment. This legislation promoted the professionalization of VR by establishing graduate-level training programs throughout the United States. Research demonstration grants allowed state rehabilitation agencies or nonprofit agencies to conduct projects directed specifically at VR (3). Now, disability arenas such as the psychological, social, and behavioral components of disabilities were studied in a systematic manner. Results were then applied in training programs, policy, and rehabilitation service mandates (15).

The Rehabilitation Act of 1973 was a powerful piece of legislation and has had a major impact on VR programs that continues to the present day. Additional important features of the Act were the creation of the Individualized Written Rehabilitation Plans (now called the Individualized Plan for Employment or IPE) and consumer grievance procedures. These two innovative measures emphasized for the first time the notion of consumer empowerment, with simultaneous changes in language from "client" to "consumer." Now, clients were seen as consumers, and this change acknowledged that the traditional "paternalistic" attitude of the service provider was a barrier to rehabilitation. Consumers became more assertive than in the past and were empowered to make autonomous decisions with the assistance of trained VR professionals. In this paradigm, people with disabilities work as a team with the rehabilitation counselor, occupational therapist, physical therapist, physiatrist, and other medical professionals, signaling a change from the past, when they were expected to be compliant recipients of care (3,15,22,23).

Consumer advocacy was a powerful driving force on the tenets of the Rehabilitation Act of 1973. The Act included a number of provisions to address discrimination and environmental barriers, as follows: (a) Section 501, mandating that the federal government itself practices nondiscrimination in its hiring practice; (b) Section 502, establishing the Architectural and Transportation Compliance Board to enforce accessibility standards for persons with disabilities; (c) Section 503, prohibiting discrimination in the hiring process based on disability status (which applied only to federal contract recipients or subcontractors); and (d) Section 504, in which exclusion from participation from any federally sponsored program was prohibited for any qualified person with a disability. These programs included schools (elementary, secondary, postsecondary), hospitals, clinics, and welfare agencies. Accessibility of programs was emphasized. This legislation mandated that employers or institutions receiving federal funds were required to make "reasonable accommodations" for otherwise qualified people with disabilities. For employers, this meant job restructuring, workplace modifications, provision of specialized training, or ongoing support (3).

In 1974, the Rehabilitation Act of 1973 was amended to include a broader definition of the term "handicapped individual." The new definition emphasized limitations in major life activities rather than only vocational objectives. In 1978 (3,24), a number of amendments were made to the Rehabilitation Act of 1973, most importantly, Title VII entitled "Comprehensive Services for Independent Living." Its purpose was to authorize grants to states to provide independently living services for individuals with disabilities without emphasizing the employment component. A vocational outcome was not necessary for these services. In addition, a bill of rights section was included for those with disabilities, and the National Council on Independent Living was established. This amendment made centers for IL partners with the traditional rehabilitation program. The Rehabilitation Act Amendments of 1986 authorized state VR agencies to provide supported employment services to individuals with severe disabilities who were not capable of competitive employment. Consequently, long-term placement in workshops was viewed as a less than favorable option. This Amendment also increased the use of rehabilitation engineering to assist with independence (3).

The Americans with Disabilities Act (ADA; PL 101-336), a hallmark civil rights legislation for persons with disabilities, was passed in 1990 (15). Its purposes were to end discrimination against people with disabilities and to promote both their social and economic integration (24). To be covered under the ADA, either a mental or physical impairment exists that must "substantially limit" one or more major life activities (e.g., walk, eat, self-care, work, etc.) or the individual has a record of the impairment (e.g., cancer in remission, substance abuse in remission, records of mental illness, educational record depicting learning disability), or is regarded as disabled (e.g., the employer does not hire an individual for a sales position due to a facial birthmark). Contagious diseases (HIV/AIDS) were included in the law, though not in work situations where they may pose a "direct threat" to others. Other conditions such as pedophilia, kleptomania, compulsive gambling, and transvestism were not protected by the ADA. Subsequent court decisions determined that impairments that can be mitigated by corrective measures (mitigating measures) were not covered under the ADA. For example, high blood pressure and diabetes did not substantially limit major life activities when

medication regimes were followed. These court decisions had the effect of creating ambiguity in how the ADA was interpreted, raising concerns that its original antidiscrimination protections were being gradually eroded (3). As a consequence, the ADA Amendments Act was signed into law in September 2008. Taking effect in January 2009, the ADA Amendments Act is designed to protect the original ADA of 1990. The Amendments Act retains the ADA's definition of disability and maintains that the definition of disability should be viewed and interpreted in a "broad" manner. It offers clarification regarding what the law considers to be major life activities as well as mitigating measures. For example, it expands major life activities to include those that had not been specifically identified in the previous legislation, such as reading, bending, and communicating, and adds major bodily functions, such as the immune system and neurologic functions. Under the Amendments Act, mitigating measures, not including contacts or eyeglasses, will not be taken into account when determining disability status. An impairment that is either in remission or episodic is considered a disability if a major life activity would be substantially limited when the impairment is in an active state. In addition, one "regarded as" having a disability is not entitled to a reasonable accommodation (25).

The ADA prohibits discrimination against people with disabilities in employment (Title I), public services (Title II), public transportation (Title III), places of public accommodation (Title IV), and telecommunications (Title V). The primary purpose of Title I is to provide equal employment opportunities to qualified individuals with disabilities. Under Title I, the ADA prohibits discrimination because of disability in the hiring, promotion, job training, and firing process (15). A qualified individual with disabilities is one who can perform the essential functions (e.g., word processing skills for a newspaper writer) of a job with or without a reasonable accommodation (e.g., voice recognition computer software). Businesses with more than 15 employees are required to make reasonable accommodations for qualified candidates with disabilities unless such accommodations would impose "undue hardship." Such accommodations might include improving worksite accessibility, equipment modification, work schedule modification, or provision of interpreters. Undue hardship is determined by the organization's financial profile. Title II of the ADA prohibits discrimination against people with disabilities in state and local government programs such as the library, courtrooms, county museum, and public transportation that must be accessible. Individuals with disabilities should have equal access to these services, and reasonable accommodations must be provided for these services (3).

Title III of the ADA, the public services provision, prohibits discrimination against persons with disabilities when using public establishments such as theaters, hotels, auditoriums, museums, and private schools. Both barrier removal and reasonable accommodations that are readily achievable (in terms of financial impact) are required. Title III underscores the fundamental right of Americans to enjoy all public accommodations in society (3). The presence of a disability should not preclude one from this freedom. For example, an individual who uses a wheelchair would not be able to use a hotel during a family vacation if there is no ramp to the front door. Title IV is the component of the ADA addressing telecommunication and requires that individuals with hearing and/or speech impediments have equal access to telephone services at a cost comparable to those without disabilities (15). Services include the telecommunication device for the deaf (a keyboard is used to communicate via telephone lines) or a telephone relay service (in which a third-party operator relays messages from a nonspeaking patron to one who communicates through speech). Lastly, Title V prohibits retaliation or coercion toward individuals who use the ADA to protect their rights.

The Rehabilitation Act Amendments of 1992 emphasized consumer involvement in the policies and procedures of state VR agencies. These amendments emphasized employment outcomes for people with disabilities, commitment to IL services, informed choice, and consumer participation in VR process (3). In addition, Rehabilitation Advisory as well as Independent Living Councils were created and were required to be composed primarily of people with disabilities in order to provide guidance regarding agency policy and procedures. The order of selection process was also established for determining who would get services, with priority of services going to individuals whose disabilities were most severe. Eligibility requirements were changed in that it was now assumed that the person could benefit from VR services and achieve an employment outcome, unless it could be shown otherwise (10). Terminology was changed; instead of "handicapped," the term disabled was now used (15). Other amendment topics included support for transition from school to work, supported employment, on-the-job training, serving minorities, and personal care attendants.

In 1998, the Rehabilitation Act Amendments were incorporated within new legislation, the Workforce Investment Act (WIA; PL 105-220), which was designed to unify the workforce programs in the United States (3,10,15). The WIA was based on a "one-stop" concept of locating job training and education and employment services available at a single location. Programs were streamlined and consolidated to avoid problems that occurred in the past with disjointed services (10). Programs included unemployment assistance resources, vocational training, placement counseling, vocational assessment, and daycare services for individuals while they utilized the one-stop services. This law emphasized increased consumer control of the vocational planning process.

The Individualized Written Rehabilitation Plan was now called the IPE, and clients were expected to be active participants in plan development. The law put more emphasis on the need for qualified VR counselors to provide services. A master's degree in rehabilitation counseling and passing the certified rehabilitation counselor (CRC) examination were methods for establishing this qualified status (3).

In 1999, the Ticket to Work and Work Incentive Improvement Act (TWWIIA; PL 106-170) was passed, providing Supplemental Security Income (SSI) and Social Security Disability Insurance (SSDI) beneficiaries with a "ticket" they may use to obtain VR services from an employment network of their choice. This program is voluntary and consumers may choose their own rehabilitation service vendor, designated as an Employer Network, or EN. Vendors can be either private or public entities. For example, CILs, state VR agencies, educational institutions, and employment agencies are examples of potential employment networks. The TWWIIA also provided for the removal of work disincentives such as loss of medical coverage. Starting in October 2000, Medicare and Medicaid

coverage was expanded to more people with disabilities who were employed. With SSDI, a 9-month work trial (with a 3-month grace period) is allowed, so the person's benefits are not affected for 12 months. Extended medical coverage through Medicare is provided for up to 93 months following the trial work period for those who are working.

Consequently, employment rates can increase if individuals with disabilities do not believe they will lose benefits due to employment. These supplemental medical as well as Social Security benefits help remove important disincentives to employment for individuals with disabilities (3).

The Workforce Innovation and Opportunity Act (WIOA) updated and replaced the Workforce Investment Act (WIA). Although retaining many of key features of WIA designed to streamline and unify a range of federal workforce programs, WIOA also implemented significant changes that affect provision of services through the state-federal VR program. As in WIA, the Rehabilitation Act is included within WIOA as a partner among other workforce programs and amends the Rehabilitation Act of 1973. Most significantly, WIOA emphasizes transition services for youth with disabilities, requiring the state-federal VR program to reserve at least 15% of its budget to provide pre-employment transition services to students with disabilities. Pre-employment transition services include the following required activities: job exploration counseling, work-based learning experiences, counseling on options for postsecondary programs in colleges and universities, workplace readiness training, and self-advocacy training. Remaining funds may also be applied to activities to help students with disabilities make the transition from school to work or postsecondary education such as fostering IL skills, conducting research on evidence-based practices, providing training to VR counselors and school staff, and forming multiple partnerships with agencies and businesses (26). WIOA also places stronger emphasis on integrated employment as an outcome of VR services, along with a significantly reduced use of sheltered workshops. All workforce programs under WIOA, including the state-federal VR program, must share common performance measures, with an increased focus on high-quality employment outcomes, that is, helping more VR consumers achieve employment in jobs that offer better wages and benefits. In addition, the legislation strengthens efforts to work collaboratively with employers and to improve the effectiveness of job placement and related services (3).

THE CONSUMER MOVEMENT IN REHABILITATION

As the consumer (instead of patient/client) movement grew in the late 1960s to early 1970s, with its emphasis on advocacy and self-determination, the time was ready for the IL and disability rights movements. The driving force of IL was that individuals with severe disabilities were able to both direct and manage their lives. Furthermore, the services and supports that people with disabilities need are best delivered by individuals who themselves have disabilities and whose knowledge about both disability and services is derived from firsthand experience.

Empathy is a cornerstone of this model, with consumers serving and providing mentoring to other consumers. In this model, an individual with a disability may address the many concerns that a person with a newly acquired disability may encounter. Consumers may discuss adjustment to disability issues, adaptive equipment, and techniques for navigating the many service systems (4). The model follows that of organizations such as Alcoholics Anonymous, in which substance use disorders are best addressed by those who have gone through a similar path.

Little (27) noted that CILs promote consumer empowerment and independence through active involvement, self-determination, and education on disability in areas such as how reactions to persons with disability are based historically on group oppression rather than on their functional limitations. Personal control can be gained by making choices (autonomy) as much as possible in decisions and daily activities. Assistance from others is to be as minimal as possible. The construction of a collective identity is important, as is understanding the major underpinnings of the IL movement and centers. A number of consumers are unfamiliar with disability rights and the IL philosophy. Many consumers enter a CIL and ask about their living quarters. They do not know the mission and the core services of CIL. CILs can promote empowerment by providing collective identity training and activities that foster self-determination. An assertive consumer is more likely to make independent decisions that reflect both needs and wants. Activities that produce positive outcomes based on the consumers' input can enhance a sense of self-efficacy.

Empowerment of Consumers

Disability legislation continues to emphasize the fundamental right of individuals with disabilities to make decisions about their own lives (3). Since 1973, rehabilitation practice and legislation have been driven by consumer-counselor partnerships and consumer empowerment, which have been the underpinning of all rehabilitation legislation, as exemplified by the following:

- The 1978 Rehabilitation Act Amendments provided that individuals with disabilities be guaranteed more involvement in their rehabilitation plan.
- The 1986 Rehabilitation Act Amendments included support for individual consumer rights and revised the IPE format to include consumers' statements of their own rehabilitation goals.
- The 1990 ADA further strengthened consumer self-determination by ensuring rights in the areas of employment, transportation, public services, and public accommodations.
- The 1992 Amendments to the Rehabilitation Act also supported the movement toward self-determination.
- The Workforce Innovation and Opportunity Act of 2014 (3) gives individuals with disabilities increased access to high-quality workforce services as well as assists with competitive employment.

Consumer empowerment is the driving force behind our current rehabilitation policy and practice paradigm. Moreover, Niesz et al. (28) note that "consumer empowerment is now viewed by consumers, service providers, policymakers, and researchers, alike, as both a guiding philosophy *and* a desired outcome of vocational rehabilitation programing" (p. 124). Since its inception, the IL movement has viewed consumer

control as a necessary component of rehabilitation and direction, not only of the services needed by its individual constituents but also of the institutions and organizations that house its activities and administer its resources (3,15). Thus, the 1992 Amendments to the Rehabilitation Act required that a majority of CIL staff, management, and directors must be individuals with disabilities. This empowerment perspective sees the consumer as a competent change agent capable of identifying problems, finding solutions, and making independent decisions. Within this paradigm, the rehabilitation counselor serves as a guide or facilitator to problem solving and decision-making. Knowledge is viewed as power, and the counselor encourages the consumer to gather information to enhance knowledge. The rehabilitation counselor practices informed consent and continually drives the point that the consumer is a competent agent in charge of his or her change (15). Kosciulek (29) stressed that VR can be used to promote consumer empowerment by building a strong working alliance with the consumer, that is, an alliance that promotes autonomy and self-determination. When persons with disabilities have had fewer opportunities in the past to make decisions, this makes them less able to do so. Likewise, negative attitudes and low expectations of society at large "may result in a negative self-appraisal and negative worker self-concept" (p. 41) that impede career development.

Consumerism, Accessibility, and Assistive Technology

Social, environmental, and cultural barriers have long kept people with disabilities from having full access to work, education, and participation in their communities. Technologic advances have been recognized as a means of expanding opportunities for people with disabilities, helping them to surmount environmental barriers, enhance functional capacities, and maximize independence (30,31). Use of appropriate technology can improve the mobility, communication, and IL skills of people with disabilities, thus dramatically enhancing their ability to become full participants in American society. To this end, the Technology-Related Assistance for Individuals with Disabilities Act was passed in 1988 to promote the use of technology services for people with disabilities (30). The Tech Act officially defined AT as "any item, piece of equipment or product system, whether acquired commercially off the shelf, modified or customized, that is used to increase, maintain, or improve functional capabilities of individuals with disabilities" (30). AT can range from "low-tech" devices such as walkers or canes to "high-tech" devices such as speech synthesizers or stair-climbing wheelchairs. This law was replaced by the Assistive Technology Act of 1998 (often called the "Tech Act"), which advocated statewide coordination and utilization of AT services and development of consumer-responsive technology programs (3). The 2004 amendments to the Tech Act promoted improved AT services through a standardized, statewide implementation process, which included plans for providing AT training to rehabilitation counselors (32).

Other laws affecting the lives of individuals with disabilities have also included technology as an essential component. For example, the Telecommunications Act of 1996 (PL 104-104) addressed the civil rights of people with disabilities by mandating that telecommunications services and equipment be "designed, developed, and fabricated to be accessible to and usable by individuals with disabilities, if readily achievable" (33,34). AT helps fulfill the legislative mandate of the Rehabilitation Act of 1973 and its subsequent 1986 and 1992 Amendments, which reinforce the need for active consumer participation in the VR process and emphasize consumer choice, self-determination, and consumer empowerment (35). Consistent with the emphasis on consumer involvement, the 2014 Amendments to the Rehabilitation Act under WIOA mandate consideration of AT in provision of VR services (3). The importance of AT has also been increasingly recognized in provision of special education services to children with disabilities, as evidenced by the 1986 and 1990 amendments to the Individuals with Disabilities Education Act (IDEA), which mandated the inclusion of AT devices and services in education, and the 1997 Amendments to IDEA strengthened the role of AT in special education by requiring that AT services be considered for students who have an Individualized Education Program (IEP) (36).

The ADA expanded public awareness of physical barriers and established requirements for uniform, national accessibility standards. Consistent with the mandate of the ADA, the Architectural and Transportation Barriers Compliance Board issued guidelines for accessible design in 1991, which were modified and adopted by the U.S. Department of Justice and became enforceable ADA Standards for Accessible Design (37).

While AT has significantly expanded job opportunities and improved the quality of life (QOL) for many individuals with disabilities, the focus of AT services remains primarily on the individual, who must select and learn to use the assistive device. In contrast, the concept of "universal design" refers to the design of products to be useable by all people, as much as possible, without the need for individual adaptation or specialized design. Examples of universal design are pens and pencils with large rubber grips to minimize hand and wrist discomfort, products which are readily available in stores. Universal design and AT can be thought of as existing along a continuum, with universal design allowing access into the mainstream and AT meeting specific needs of the individual, with some overlap in products that can be either universal in design or AT (38).

AT's impact on the lives of people with disabilities is not limited to technology itself; it has also empowered consumers by enabling them to become full participants in selecting and making decisions about AT services and devices. AT has also made a significant contribution to current VR philosophy, helping to expand its view from normalization (where the person with a disability must adapt to becoming as "nondisabled" as possible) to an empowerment model, where individuals make their own decisions and enjoy full integration within the communities where they live and work (31).

In order to avoid AT abandonment and increase levels of consumer satisfaction, the consumer needs to be involved in the AT purchasing process (39). For example, consumers who were informed, that is, involved in the process of obtaining the device, tended to have AT satisfaction. If personal needs were not assessed properly, then there was less AT satisfaction. Thus, a needs assessment involving the consumer is encouraged. The Internet, using/auditioning a device (e.g., borrow from a local CIL), and talking with other users are all ways to feel informed. Therefore, the following practices are recommended: (a) provide information about an array of AT choices, (b) include the consumer in the entire purchasing process, (c) conduct a needs assessment of the person-environment and device, (d) ensure that the consumer meets current AT users and is able to try out devices before obtaining a device, and (e) provide follow-up to see if product is working effectively. The above strategies can help ensure that the consumer is both content with the product and will limit the chance of abandonment.

VR SERVICE SYSTEMS

Both VR and IL services foster consumer-driven services and are provided by systems of agencies and organizations that are often connected by common goals and principles, as well as funding mechanisms. The section below describes these systems in greater detail.

VR Systems

The state-federal VR program has been a major provider of VR services since the enactment of federal legislation almost 100 years ago. Private, for-profit rehabilitation firms also provide VR services, as do private, nonprofit community-based rehabilitation programs. Another important VR provider is the Veterans Administration, which offers VR services to veterans with service-connected disabilities (40). Increasingly, CILs are providing VR services, many in coordination with state VR agencies (4).

Rehabilitation Counselors

Although many CILs require that those providing services have firsthand experience with disability, rehabilitation counselors hired by state agencies or private rehabilitation firms are formally trained to provide counseling to people with disabilities. The rehabilitation counselor usually has a master's degree in rehabilitation counseling, although graduate degrees in guidance and counseling, or social work, are also common. However, rehabilitation counseling is unique among other counseling professions and is a specialization within the rehabilitation field (41). A rehabilitation counselor may be certified through the Commission on Rehabilitation Counselor Certification (CRCC) or licensed through his or her state. Although licensure or certification is not a standard requirement, state agencies may require it. The CRCC has defined the scope of practice for rehabilitation counseling as being a process that helps individuals with diverse disabilities "to achieve their personal, career, and IL goals in the most integrated setting possible through the application of the counseling process" (41). The rehabilitation counselor may employ a broad range of strategies in this process, including assessment; diagnosis and treatment planning; career counseling; individual and/or group counseling, with an emphasis on helping individuals adjust to the impact of disability; coordination of services; methods to eliminate environmental and/or attitudinal barriers; job analysis, job development, and placement services; and assistance with job accommodations.

State Vocational Rehabilitation Agencies

State VR agencies operate under federal legislation, the Rehabilitation Act Amendments, and are available in every state to individuals with disabilities. State agencies work with multiple community partners to provide outreach to individuals, as well as to implement services. These partners can include school systems, CILs, community mental health agencies, hospitals and health care clinics, substance abuse centers, local support groups, other state and county employment programs, and a host of social service agencies (4). State VR agencies may also contract with private rehabilitation firms or with community-based rehabilitation programs for an array of services, including vocational evaluation, job placement services, supported employment, and/or job coaching.

In the state VR agency, rehabilitation counselors and consumers work together in partnership to develop a rehabilitation plan, the IPE. Mandated by the Rehabilitation Act of 1973, the rehabilitation plan includes (a) a specific vocational goal and timelines for its achievement, (b) services necessary to achieve the goal, (c) secondary goals needed for goal achievement, (d) services and providers required for the secondary goals, (e) criteria and procedures for evaluating progress, (f) counselor and consumer responsibilities, and (g) an annual review for as long as the case is open (3,4). Objectives in the plan might include provision of a service such as treatment, training (e.g., college, on-the-job training), job placement, and specialized adaptive equipment or transportation.

Private Rehabilitation

Private rehabilitation generally refers to services provided by rehabilitation practitioners employed by private firms that bill a third-party payer for their services (42). In the late 1970s and 1980s, there was a tremendous growth in the number of private, for-profit rehabilitation firms, largely due to state workers' compensation legislation designed to foster rehabilitation of injured workers (43). As a consequence of this legislation, private rehabilitation firms emerged to meet the needs of insurance carriers and employers, who needed timely and efficient services (44,45). In addition, insurance companies were becoming increasingly concerned with controlling growing health care costs; they discovered that referring insured or ill workers early in the rehabilitation process could reduce their disability payments. Private rehabilitation firms tend to be more efficient in their approach to helping individuals return to work than their state VR counterparts. Rehabilitation counselors in the private sector have smaller caseloads than counselors in state VR agencies, and they focus primarily on vocational guidance and placement. Counselors working in the private sector require basic business skills, knowledge of the insurance industry, an understanding of the worker's compensation system, expertise in legal and medical case management, and the ability to provide vocational expert testimony (46). Many rehabilitation counselors in the private sector are self-employed or co-owners of small firms (47), although there has been a trend in recent years for smaller firms to merge with larger managed care organizations, insurance companies, and other health care entities. Private rehabilitation counselors often contract with insurance carriers to provide VR services to individuals who qualify for these services through worker's compensation, auto no-fault or long-term disability policies, and their services are provided within the insurers' parameters. Consequently, private rehabilitation firms are usually very responsive to the payer's goals and objectives. Because worker's compensation laws are governed by each state, rather than federal law, provision of VR services will vary among different states (3).

VR Services

Although services vary according to individual needs, the VR process consists primarily of four stages, which generally occur in sequence: (a) evaluation, (b) planning, (c) treatment (provision of services), and (d) termination, or achievement of the vocational goal, usually placement in a job. The rehabilitation counselor generally begins the evaluation phase by means of an initial interview with the consumer to obtain information, as well as to provide information to assist the consumer in making an informed choice. During the evaluation phase, additional information may be needed prior to rehabilitation planning and obtained through medical evaluation, psychological evaluation, vocational assessment, or related diagnostic services (3). Cultivating relationships with local employers to promote employment of people with disabilities also is an important component of the VR process. The following are services commonly offered by VR agencies during the VR process.

Vocational Assessment

VR begins with assessment of the consumer's vocational interests, abilities, and vocational potential. By providing information about an individual's strengths and weaknesses and identifying needed services, the vocational assessment helps the consumer and VR counselor set goals and establish a rehabilitation plan. Assessment may also be used to determine the consumer's potential to benefit from VR. Vocational assessment can help the counselor and consumer answer the following questions: (a) can you return to your former occupation? (b) would you be able to return to your previous occupation with job accommodations and AT? (c) which of your skills may be transferable to another occupation? and (d) what training or other services would help you become successfully employed?

Assessment is a multidisciplinary process that initially involves gathering data from a variety of sources, such as work and educational history, as well as medical records. For individuals who have received physical rehabilitation services, these records may include a medical examination and reports from the rehabilitation team, such as occupational and physical therapy. The VR counselor may also refer the consumer for additional assessment services, such as a psychological evaluation or a vocational evaluation. The psychological evaluation can provide helpful information regarding the individual's learning abilities, coping skills, and personality characteristics, while the vocational evaluation describes important work-related behaviors, capabilities, and interests.

Although the terms vocational evaluation and vocational assessment are often used interchangeably, vocational assessment is a general term that includes many different forms of evaluation. Vocational evaluation is defined specifically as a comprehensive assessment that utilizes a variety of tools, including paper-and-pencil tests, structured and unstructured interviews, and real or simulated work (48). With its focus on work-related abilities, a vocational evaluation may use work samples, situational assessments, and on-the-job evaluations. The work sample approach to measurement has been used most often in vocational evaluation, often through commercial work sample systems (e.g., VALPAR) designed to simulate specific jobs or a cluster of jobs; a vocational evaluation may also incorporate actual work samples from industry.

Using a variety of evaluation procedures can help verify other assessment data and thereby contribute to more accurate findings and recommendations (48). Cross-validating assessment data may be especially important for persons with disabilities, as concerns have been raised about the validity of paper-and-pencil tests for this population, particularly for individuals with severe disabilities (49). In addition, vocational evaluation may incorporate AT during the assessment process, for example, by modifying work samples or other test instruments and by making recommendations that include consideration of specific AT devices that would maximize the consumer's vocational potential (50). For example, the vocational evaluator may recommend speech recognition software to enable a consumer with limited hand function to perform a job requiring computer access.

Evaluation of an individual's functional skills is an important part of the assessment process and can be applied to various domains, such as IL skills, interpersonal communication, sensory awareness, emotional stability, learning ability, and stamina. Many functional skills can be observed as part of a situational assessment or on-the-job evaluation, as well as through more formal methods, such as work samples and inventories. Sophisticated systems designed to measure a wide range of physical capacities such as lifting strength are also available, such as the ERGOS II Work Simulator (51). These systems are more likely to be used as part of a functional capacity evaluation (FCE) conducted in a work conditioning program, hospital, or clinic, rather than during a vocational evaluation.

Job Placement

Job placement includes an array of services, such as job-seeking skills training, direct placement, job accommodation, supported employment, and job development. These services may be offered by rehabilitation counselors or by placement professionals (often called placement specialists or employment specialists). Job analysis is sometimes provided as a service in conjunction with job placement, though it may also occur as part of a vocational assessment. Employment readiness is an important consideration and may be affected by psychosocial factors, availability of accessible transportation, and medical status, including stability of the medical condition and capacities for stamina and endurance. Psychological readiness to work, including motivation, self-esteem, and coping resources, also must be addressed.

Once the individual is ready to seek employment, he or she must develop or refine the employment skills that will be required for success in the job search, which will largely be determined by past experience. For example, the individual who acquired a disability later in life and who has a long work history will likely need to refine job-seeking skills that include addressing disability issues with potential employers. The individual with virtually no work history will require far more extensive job-seeking skills training, which typically includes identifying and following up on job leads, resume writing, application completion, and interviewing skills (4).

Job placement activities can be viewed along a continuum, ranging from self-placement (usually called client-centered placement) to the counselor assuming all placement responsibility, often referred to as selective placement (52). The skills and personality traits of the job seeker, the nature of the

disability, local labor market conditions and opportunities, and even luck influence the extent of counselor involvement that may be needed. The rehabilitation plan will target the consumer's job goal, specify acceptable geographic and environmental criteria, consider the types of job accommodations needed, and specify follow-up and support services required. A primary role of the VR counselor or placement professional is to assist the consumer in developing job-seeking skills, using such tools as coaching and role playing or videotaping a mock job interview. In addition to job-seeking skills, he or she must also know how to respond to questions about disability, either on an application or in an interview. Knowledge of legal protections, such as those stipulated by the ADA, is critical for the individual with a disability who is seeking employment (4).

Consumers may also need help with identifying and learning how to request job accommodations. Although the individual must learn what types of accommodations are required, the VR counselor or placement specialist can often act as a consultant to the employer and help negotiate the accommodation process. As stipulated by the ADA, the employer is required to make reasonable accommodations, but this term is subject to various definitions.

Some employers view job accommodations as prohibitively expensive, although the majority of accommodations cost less than $500 (53). In fact, job accommodations can reduce worker's compensation and other costs. Some accommodations may be as simple as a rearrangement of equipment. For example, for individuals using wheelchairs, a height-adjustable desk, a voice-activated speakerphone and moving office supplies to accessible drawers are low cost and simple accommodations. Other examples of accommodations include job restructuring (e.g., trading off job tasks with other workers), flexible schedules, large print, allowing use of personal care attendants or service animals, and large-button phones.

Supported employment is another model of job placement that is particularly effective for individuals with severe disabilities, such as TBI, developmental disabilities, or significant cognitive limitations. In contrast to the traditional model of job placement, which assumes that the individual is job-ready and has been sufficiently trained before obtaining a job, supported employment uses a "place-train" approach. That is, the individual is placed in a regular, competitive job setting and given needed support, such as assistance from a job coach and/or work mentor, to provide training on the job and ensure success (54).

Once the consumer obtains employment, follow-up services with both consumer and employer help to ensure a successful outcome and are an important step in the job placement process. The rehabilitation counselor or placement professional may need to intervene either with the consumer, employer, or both, to solve problems as they occur. Further job accommodations may be needed to help resolve difficulties with performance. However, if the consumer is ultimately unable to perform the job, the consumer and counselor may agree that it would be best to discontinue the job, as VR involves a successful outcome for both the consumer and the employer. Placement professionals must establish positive relationships with employers, and ultimate employment success may require provision of long-term follow-up services (55).

Job development is also an important component of job placement services. People with disabilities continue to encounter discrimination from employers, who may object to hiring individuals with disabilities due to common employer "myths" about individuals with disabilities, such as a belief that they will increase their insurance rates, will be subject to accidents, or have problems with job performance or stability. Thus, rehabilitation counselors and placement professionals need to dispel these misconceptions and to actively promote the benefits to employers of hiring individuals with disabilities. Rehabilitation professionals must be visible and active in business organizations and build credibility within the community. Services that can be marketed include recruitment and referral of qualified applicants, consultant services (e.g., ADA compliance, job accommodation, and disability awareness training programs), employee assistance programming, and support and follow-up services (55). Many placement programs also develop business advisory boards constituted of employers and other important business contacts in their community to share ideas and develop strategies for improving employment opportunities for people with disabilities (56).

Job analysis can be critical to the ultimate success of job placement efforts. A thorough analysis of a particular job in a certain environment can assist the VR professional in identifying appropriate job accommodations or determining if a job is feasible for the consumer. For example, when providing services to an injured worker, the rehabilitation counselor may conduct an analysis of the worker's previous job or of alternate jobs being considered and provide this information to the worker's treating physician, who can then determine if the job is consistent with the individual's physical capacities. The job must be analyzed for the skills, knowledge, and abilities needed, characteristics of the work environment, and specific job tasks (57). An analysis of environmental factors may consider parking at the worksite, restrooms, cafeteria, and building accessibility. The physical demands of the job must be assessed, such as lifting, grasping, standing, walking, sitting, talking, hearing, writing, and reading. For people with cognitive or affective limitations, other critical factors might include the work atmosphere (e.g., busy or relaxed) and cognitive demands (e.g., memory, reasoning, problem solving). Job analysis requires that the rehabilitation counselor possesses considerable expertise in a variety of areas, including knowledge of disabilities, job accommodations, employer needs, accessibility standards, business practices, and the roles of labor and management (46).

EMPLOYMENT OUTCOMES: A REVIEW OF FINDINGS

An overview of rehabilitation studies on employment-outcomes among people with physical disabilities suggests a number of variables that may assist rehabilitation professionals in identifying those individuals who can best benefit from their services. This research can help rehabilitation professionals better understand both environmental and personal characteristics that promote or hinder employment outcomes for individuals with disabilities. Equipped with these research findings, professionals can design programs and/or implement specialized techniques and knowledge to help persons with disabilities be successful in the rehabilitation arena (3).

The past three decades have been marked by low employment of persons with disabilities, typically one third or less (3). The most recent data from the U.S. Bureau of Labor Statistics reflected significant gains in employment for persons with disabilities since the Great Recession. Despite these gains, the employment-to-population ratio (i.e., percentage of those who are working relative to the total population) for working-age individuals with disabilities was only 27% as of January 2017 and lagged far behind that of people without disabilities with an employment-to-population ratio of 72.4% (58).

The Kessler Foundation (59) surveyed individuals with disabilities to see if gaps in employment exist for persons with disabilities as compared to the general population since the passage of the Americans with Disabilities Act. Seventy-three percent of those unemployed individuals reported their disability was one of the reasons they were currently not working. Fifty-six percent could not find a job in their field of work. Likewise, 37% of those unemployed reported the inability to secure appropriate job accommodations had a negative impact on employment. Rubin et al. (3) noted perceived cost as a significant barrier and offered an array of technology resources, including Job Accommodation Network (JAN) (www.aksjan. org); Ability Hub (AH) (www.abilityhub.org), and Trace Research and Development Center (http://trace.umd.edu/). In addition, a range of potential funding resources are available for AT (e.g., Medicaid, Medicare, vocational rehabilitation, Plan to Achieve Self-Support, special education, Veterans Administration, etc.). Thus, VR professionals can help individuals utilize a variety of available resources to help mitigate the impact of the disability on their ability to obtain and maintain employment.

Chan et al. (60) found that clients participating in the state-federal VR program who had postsecondary education tended to have higher-quality employment. To ensure academic success, VR counselors can take steps to ensure that students with disabilities are provided with services that help them adjust to university life and foster success. Likewise, psychosocial issues related to college life can be addressed by VR counselors (e.g., study skills, adjustment issues, living arrangement preferences, support systems, etc.) to increase the likelihood of a successful college experience (3). Joining a club for social support, obtaining university counseling for adjustment issues, getting assistance with studying techniques, and securing tutoring services are all examples of assistance the VR professional could encourage and support. Oswald et al. (61) noted that rehabilitation professionals can increase the likelihood of employment for college students with disabilities. In this study, a university office of disability services (DS) provided a comprehensive vocational program for their students with disabilities to increase their success in gaining employment. The components of this program included the following strategies: (a) increase communication skills through face-to-face activities to improve communication (verbal, nonverbal) skills (e.g., mock interview with DS before official interview, participate in class discussions, join club, etc.); (b) self-awareness of disability in relation to employment (e.g., home or worksite accommodations, such as AT) and benefits analysis case appraisal (to determine what impact employment will have on disability benefits); (c) involvement in campus activities to hone professional skills; (d) experiential course enrollment (e.g., internship, field study, etc.); (e) build successful resumes via training and peer evaluation activities; (f) holistically review the student's profile before applying for job (consideration of a range of needs, such as accessible transportation, personal care attendant, home accessibility); and (g) job lead activities such as networking with peers, faculty, and family. The above activities are deemed important to increase employment outcomes for students with disabilities within college settings.

Not surprisingly, employed individuals with disabilities reported higher QOL as compared to their counterparts (62). The VR professional can therefore enhance individuals' QOL by utilizing evidenced-based practices that increase the likelihood of employment (62). Evidence-based practices such as postsecondary education, supported employment, and transition services have been found to enhance VR employment outcomes for consumers with disabilities (60).

Leahy et al. (63) described strategies that promote consumer motivation and consumer self-determination/autonomous decision-making as valuable tools within the VR treatment paradigm. These strategies include activities that promote clients' employment motivation and self-direction (e.g., motivational interviewing and mutual goal development with the counselor/client). Likewise, a large meta-analysis reviewing employment-related variables for individuals with SCIs determined that life satisfaction for those employed was robust. Thus, strategies to strengthen life satisfaction are encouraged in order to increase employment outcomes (64).

Individuals with severe TBIs who had fewer deficits in social communication skills tended to have higher employment rates than those who tend to violate conversational principles such as poor topic management, slow speech, and turn-taking difficulty. In addition, those who were employed tended to have increased self-awareness of their communication difficulties. These findings suggest that therapy directed to self-awareness and communication skills training could help improve employment rates for individuals with TBI (65). Likewise, a meta-analysis by Liaset and Loras (66) determined that the following four variables were linked to return to work (RTW) for consumers with acquired brain injury (ABI): (a) self-awareness (accept and be aware of strengths and weaknesses related to ABI), (b) empowerment (promote autonomous decision-making/self-efficacy), (c) motivation (desire to resume working), and (d) facilitation (e.g., modify work environment and work tasks).

Individuals with multiple sclerosis who had higher cognitive function tended to be employed more than their counterparts. That said, rehabilitation professionals can provide cognitive training (e.g., active listening, empathy, memory training, etc.) to these consumers. In addition, those who were younger, better educated, and who had less severe symptoms were more likely to be employed either full or part time as compared to those with more severe symptoms. These results suggest that approaches directed to help minimize symptoms and to provide education will increase the likelihood of successful employment (67). Individuals with bipolar disorders tended to have more favorable employment outcomes when cognitive performance (i.e., executive functioning and verbal memory) scores are higher, with less symptomology (i.e., depression symptoms). Manic symptoms did not negatively impact employment. Fewer hospitalizations were also linked to better employment outcomes. Hence, a cognitive skills training paradigm as well as a strengths-based approach can be utilized to decrease hospitalizations and focus on aspects that will increase the likelihood of a positive employment outcome (68). *Self-advocacy skills* among consumers as well as *employer*

support are considered key facilitators of employment for individuals with disabilities (69). An array of strategies are available to both increase client self-advocacy skills and job development to provide employer support (3).

Several studies have reported certain demographic factors such as race, gender, and disability severity and disability characteristics as factors related to vocational outcomes (70–72). In general, those with successful vocational outcomes tend to be Caucasian, young adults, well-educated, and had a successful career prior to the acquired disability (73–75). However, because consumer variables are easier to identify and measure than environmental variables, these research findings may at least partly reflect a lack of clear-cut strategies for assessing the impact of environmental factors on VR outcomes (76). As more research is conducted based on the conceptual model of the International Classification of Functioning, Disability and Health (ICF) discussed earlier, environmental facilitators and barriers can be specifically assessed for their impact on VR outcomes. For example, Young (77) examined variables associated with successful RTW for injured workers and identified a number of factors that facilitated successful employment, such as supportive relationships with coworkers, flexible working conditions, and positive relationships with family and health care providers.

Beveridge and Fabian (70) determined that when consumers' IPE is congruent with the employment outcome, they are more likely to earn higher wages. Although this finding was applicable to all consumers, it was particularly evident for those with cognitive disabilities. In addition, individuals with physical disabilities earned substantially more than persons with sensory and mental disabilities.

Age at the time of disability, premorbid employment status, work status, and psychological distress were also found to be significant predictors of successful employment for a group of people with TBI. In fact, learning as well as psychological disabilities coupled with TBI tended to have a negative impact on employment outcomes for this population (65,78). Individuals who are injured either at a very young age or over age 40 are less likely to be employed (72,79).

Psychosocial factors also appear to play an important role in employment outcomes for individuals with disabilities. For example, consumers' self-awareness is a key factor in returning to employment (80). Poor self-awareness, as well as unrealistic goals, is the primary reason why consumers fail to secure employment following provision of VR services. Motivation appears to predict employment status among an array of disability groups (73–75). Internal locus of control is frequently discussed as an important predictor of job search and employment success. This proactive stance tends to produce more successful outcomes compared to consumers who perceive themselves as being more externally controlled (81,82).

In a landmark study of the outcomes and effectiveness of the state-federal VR system, the Longitudinal Study of the Vocational Rehabilitation Services Program (LSVRSP) tracked consumers' progress over a period of 3 years (83). Of those participants who received services, 69% obtained an employment outcome, which is defined as either competitive or noncompetitive employment over a continuous 90-day period. Of those consumers with an employment outcome, 75% obtained competitive employment, while 25% received noncompetitive placements, which included supported employment, extended employment, homemaker, and unpaid family worker. The study identified a number of consumer characteristics, including type of disability, which had a significant impact on achievement of an employment outcome. For example, consumers with a hearing or orthopedic impairment were more likely to attain an employment outcome. Other characteristics associated with an employment outcome were working at the time of application, higher number of dependents, and higher self-esteem. In contrast, individuals receiving disability benefits (e.g., SSI, SSDI) were less likely to obtain employment. The LSVRSP also examined the relationship of VR services to employment outcome and found that job placement, on-the-job training, and business/vocational training were significant predictors of employment. That is, consumers who had received these services were more likely to be employed at follow-up 3 years later.

SUMMARY

Historically, VR and IL services often seemed to have different and sometimes opposing goals, with the early developers of IL seeing VR professionals as creating more barriers for individuals with disabilities through their paternalistic attitudes and origins in the medical model of disability. The consumer movement has been successful in effecting changes in policies, driving legislative mandates that have promoted consumer empowerment and facilitated the gradual merging of the goals of both VR and IL. Both VR and IL can be seen as serving essential and complementary roles in the rehabilitation process. VR and IL increasingly share a more holistic, ecologic understanding of disability that stresses the role of the environment in either magnifying or minimizing the impact of impairment. In VR, focus has been shifting from efforts to change the person with the disability to removing or modifying barriers in the environment that hinder the person from being an active participant in work and society. These programs also complement each other in many ways. With their goal-oriented approach to services, VR programs assist consumers in obtaining employment or furthering their education to expand future career opportunities. IL programs foster greater sense of accomplishment and control over one's own destiny. While promoting self-direction and self-sufficiency, they expand life opportunities and social identity for individuals with disabilities. By promoting independence, IL facilitates vocational options and thus can be seen to work in tandem with VR services.

In the past, the roles of VR and IL professionals also differed significantly but now are becoming more similar. Both rehabilitation and IL specialists are change agents who act as facilitators to help people with disabilities maximize their independence, participate as fully as possible in their communities, and advocate for their own needs and interests. However, VR and IL differ in the types of outcomes that each program emphasizes. VR programs define a successful outcome as employment, and preferably paid, competitive employment. Such an outcome is measurable, and outcome data from VR services can be gathered and statistically analyzed to assess its overall performance. At the same time, using employment as the sole criteria for success provides a narrow view of rehabilitation (84). In contrast, a successful outcome in IL is more individualized and broadly defined, as it is based on each consumer's needs and desires, and usually pertains to progress in areas that are more difficult to pinpoint and measure, such as QOL, coping skills, autonomy, and self-dignity. The ICF model offers a multidimensional perspective of health, in which persons with health conditions may or may not experience disability, depending on their interaction with the environment; this holds promise as a conceptual framework that could help unify VR and IL even further. For example, in the VR system, criteria based on the ICF could be used to measure indicators that reflect progress in other important aspects of life and more precisely assess program effectiveness, rather than relying solely on employment outcome (76). Such indicators could align closely with consumer goals of IL, such as improved QOL. In addition, ICF-based criteria could include environmental factors that have long been recognized by the IL movement as being critical in the lives of individuals who experience or are likely to experience disability.

REFERENCES

1. Whitehouse E, Ingram K, Silverstein B. *Work Matters: A Framework for States on Workforce Development for People with Disabilities.* Office of Disability Employment Policy; 2016. Available from: http://www.ncsl.org/research/labor-and-employment/work-matters-a-framework-for-states-on-workforce-development-for-people-with-disabilities.aspx. Accessed February 25, 2017.
2. Szymanski EM, Parker RM. Work and disability: basic constructs. In: Szymanski EM, Parker RM, eds. *Work and Disability.* 3rd ed. Austin, TX: Pro-Ed; 2010:1–15.
3. Rubin SE, Roessler RT, Rumrill JR, et al. *Foundations of the Vocational Rehabilitation Process.* 7th ed. Austin, TX: Pro-Ed; 2016.
4. Tate D, Kalpakjian C, Paasuke L, et al. Vocational rehabilitation, independent living and consumerism. In: DeLisa JA, Gans BM, Walsh NE, eds. *Physical Medicine and Rehabilitation: Principles and Practice.* 4th ed. Philadelphia, PA: Lippincott Williams & Wilkins; 2005:1073–1083.
5. World Health Organization. *The International Classification of Function, Disability and Health: ICF.* Geneva, Switzerland: World Health Organization; 2001.
6. Peterson DB, Rosenthal DA. The International Classification of Functioning, Disability and Health (ICF): a primer for rehabilitation educators. *Rehabil Educ.* 2005;19:81–94.
7. Stucki G, Cieza A, Melvin J. The International Classification of Functioning, Disability and Health: a unifying model for the conceptual description of the rehabilitation strategy. *J Rehabil Med.* 2007;39:279–285.
8. Stucki G, Melvin J. The International Classification of Functioning, Disability and Health: a unifying model for the conceptual description of physical and rehabilitation medicine. *J Rehabil Med.* 2007;39:286–292.
9. United Nations. *Convention on the Rights of Persons with Disabilities.* Available from: http://www.un.org/disabilities/documents/convention/convoptprot-e.pdf. Accessed February 15, 2017.
10. Patterson JB, Bruyere S, Szymanski EM, et al. Philosophical, historical, and legislative aspects of the rehabilitation counseling profession. In: Parker RM, Patterson JB, eds. *Rehabilitation Counseling: Basics and Beyond.* 5th ed. Austin, TX: Pro-Ed; 2012:27–53.
11. Marnetoft SU. Vocational rehabilitation. In: Escorpizo R, Brage S, Homa D, et al., eds. *Handbook of Vocational Rehabilitation and Disability Evaluation: Application and Implementation of the ICF.* Switzerland: Springer; 2015:73–103.
12. Fabian ES, MacDonald-Wilson KL. Professional practice in rehabilitation service delivery systems and related system resources. In: Parker RM, Patterson JB, eds. *Rehabilitation Counseling: Basics and Beyond.* 5th ed. Austin, TX: Pro-Ed; 2012:55–84.
13. U.S. Department of Education. *Centers for Independent Living.* Available from: www.ilru.org/projects/cil-net/cil-center-and-association-directory. Accessed February 15, 2017.
14. Federal Register. *Independent Living Services and Centers for Independent Final Rule.* Department of Health and Human Services; 2016. Available from: https://www.gpo.gov/fdsys/pkg/FR-2016-10-27/pdf/2016-25918.pdf. Accessed February 20, 2017.
15. Sales A. *Rehabilitation Counseling: An Empowerment Perspective.* Austin, TX: Pro-Ed; 2007.
16. DeJong G. *The Movement for Independent Living: Origins, Ideology, and Implications for Disability Research.* East Lansing, MI: Michigan State University; 1979.
17. DeLoach CP, Wilkins RD, Walker GW. *Independent Living: Philosophy, Process, and Services.* Baltimore, MD: University Park Press; 1983.
18. Proot, IM, Abu-Saad HH, Van Oorsouw GG, et al. Autonomy in stroke rehabilitation: the perceptions of care providers in nursing homes. *Nurs Ethics.* 2002;9:36–50.
19. Lee D, Hammel J, Wilson T. A community living management program for people with disabilities who have moved out of nursing homes: a pilot study. *Disabil Rehabil.* 2016;38:754–760.
20. Yoshida KK, Self HM, Renwick RM, et al. A value-based practice model of rehabilitation: consumers' recommendations in action. *Disabil Rehabil.* 2014;37:1825–1833.
21. Wright GN. *Total Rehabilitation.* New York: Little, Brown; 1980.

22. Nosek MA. Response to Kenneth R. Thomas commentary: some observations on the use of the word consumer. *J Rehabil.* 1993;59:9–10.

23. Thomas K. Commentary: some observations on the use of the word consumer. *J Rehabil.* 1993;59:6–8.

24. Peterson DB, Aguiar LJ. History and systems: United States. In: Riggar TF, Maki DR, eds. *Handbook of Rehabilitation Counseling.* New York: Springer; 2004:50–75.

25. U.S. Equal Employment Opportunity Commission. *Notice Concerning the Americans with Disabilities Act (ADA) Amendments Act of 2008.* Available from: https://www.eeoc.gov/laws/statutes/adaaa_notice.cfm. Accessed February 7, 2017.

26. U.S. Dept. of Education, Office of Special Education and Rehabilitative Services. *Vocational Rehabilitation Services and Supported Employment Services Programs: Federal FY 2017 Monitoring and Technical Assistance Guide.* Available from: https://www2.ed.gov/rschstat/eval/rehab/107-reports/2017/monitoring-and-technical-assistance-guide.pdf. Accessed February 21, 2017.

27. Little DL. Identity, efficacy and disabilities rights movement recruitment. *Disabil Stud Q.* 2010;30:2. Available from: http://eds.b.ebscohot.com/ehost/detail/detail?vid=12&sid=0622a8d5-1739-43dd-8d23-5848ed98d69b%40sessionmgr102&hid=120&bdata=JnNpdGU9ZWhvc3QtbGl2ZQ%3d%3d#AN=48487275&db=ehh. Accessed February 22, 2017.

28. Niesz T, Koch L, Rumrill PD. The empowerment of people with disabilities through qualitative research. *Work.* 2008;31:113–125.

29. Kosciulek JF. Empowering people with disabilities through vocational rehabilitation counseling. *Am Rehabil.* 2004;28:40–47.

30. Brodwin MG, Boland EA, Lane FJ, et al. Technology in rehabilitation counseling. In: Parker RM, Patterson JB, eds. *Rehabilitation Counseling: Basics and Beyond.* 5th ed. Austin, TX: Pro-Ed; 2012:333–355.

31. Scherer M. Introduction. In: Scherer M, ed. *Assistive Technology: Matching Device and Consumer for Successful Rehabilitation.* Washington, DC: American Psychological Association; 2002:3–13.

32. ATAP. *Amendment to the Assistive Technology Act of 1998: As amended 2004 Public Law 108-364.* Available from: http://www.resna.org/act-programs. Accessed February 15, 2017.

33. Gradel K. Funding and public policy. In: Olson D, DeRuyter F, eds. *Clinician's Guide to Assistive Technology.* St. Louis, MO: Mosby; 2002:75–88.

34. Federal Communications Commission. *Telecommunications Act of 1996.* Available from: https://www.fcc.gov/general/telecommunications-act-1996. Accessed February 15, 2017.

35. Breeding RR. The utility of proactive vocational assessments in advancing consumer empowerment. *Vocal Eval Career Assess Prof J.* 2006;2(2):39–56.

36. Bausch ME, Hasselbring TS. Assistive technology: are the necessary skills and knowledge being developed at the preservice and inservice levels? *Teach Educ Spec Educ.* 2004;27:97–104.

37. The Center for Universal Design, North Carolina State University. *Universal Design History.* Available from: https://www.ncsu.edu/ncsu/design/cud/about_ud/udhistory.htm. Accessed February 2, 2017.

38. The Center for Universal Design, North Carolina State University. *Universal Design Principles.* Available from: https://www.ncsu.edu/ncsu/design/cud/about_ud/udprinciples.htm. Accessed February 7, 2017.

39. Martin JK, Martin LG, Stumbo NJ, et al. The impact of consumer involvement on satisfaction with and use of assistive technology. *Disabil Rehabil Assist Technol.* 2011;6:225–242.

40. United States Department of Veterans Affairs. *Vocational Rehabilitation and Employment.* Available from: http://www.benefits.va.gov/vocrehab/. Accessed January 27, 2017.

41. Commission on Certification of Rehabilitation Counselors (CRCC). Available from: https://www.crccertification.com/. Accessed January 15, 2017.

42. Lynch RK, Lynch RT. Rehabilitation counseling in the private sector. In: Parker RM, Szymanski EM, eds. *Rehabilitation Counseling: Basics and Beyond.* 3rd ed. Austin, TX: Pro-Ed; 1998:71–105.

43. Havranek, JE. Foundations of forensic rehabilitation. In: Havranke JE, ed. *Advanced Issues in Forensic Rehabilitation.* Athens, GA: Elliot & Fitzpatrick; 2007:8–12.

44. Lewis J. Rehabilitation benefit system as a predicator of ethical standards. In: Deneen LJ, Hessellund TA, eds. *Counseling the Able Disabled.* San Francisco, CA: Rehab Publications; 1986:199–216.

45. Weed RO, Field TF. *Rehabilitation Consultant's Handbook.* 4th ed. Athens, GA: Elliot & Fitzpatrick; 2012.

46. Lynch R, Martin T. Rehabilitation counseling in the private sector: a training needs story. *J Rehabil.* 1982;48:51–73.

47. Matkin R. Rehabilitation services offered in the private sector: a pilot investigation. *J Rehabil.* 1982;48:31–33.

48. Smith F, Lombard R, Neubert D, et al. *Position Paper on the Interdisciplinary Council on Vocational Evaluation and Assessment.* Available from: https://vecap20.files.wordpress.com/2014/01/interdisciplinary_council.pdf. Accessed February 15, 2017.

49. Power P. *Guide to Vocational Assessment.* 5th ed. Austin, TX: Pro-Ed; 2013.

50. Vocational Evaluation and Career Assessment Professionals. *The Role of Assistive Technology in Assessment and Vocational Evaluation.* Available from: https://vecap.org/position-papers-and-seminal-works/vecap-the-role-of-assistive-technology-in-assessment. Accessed February 13, 2017.

51. Simwork Systems. Available from: http://www.simwork.com/Products.aspx. Accessed February 12, 2017.

52. Hagner D, Breault D. Job development and job-search support. In: Szymanski EM, Parker RM, eds. *Work and Disability.* 3rd ed. Austin, TX: Pro-Ed; 2010:363–388.

53. Job Accommodations Network. Available from: http://askjan.org/. Accessed January 20, 2017.

54. Hanley-Maxwell C, Maxwell K, Fabian E, et al. Supported employment. In: Szymanski EM, Parker RM, eds. *Work and Disability.* 3rd ed. Austin, TX: Pro-Ed; 2010: 415–453.

55. Gilbride D, Stensrud R. Job placement and employer consulting: services and strategies. In: Szymanski EM, Parker RM, eds. *Work and Disability.* 3rd ed. Austin, TX: Pro-Ed; 2010:325–362.

56. Luecking RG, Fabian ES, Tilson GP. *Working Relationships: Creating Career Opportunities for Job Seekers with Disabilities through Employer Partnerships.* Baltimore, MD: Brookes Publishing; 2004.

57. Patterson JB. Using occupational and labor market information in vocational counseling. In: Szymanski EM, Parker RM, eds. *Work and Disability.* 3rd ed. Austin, TX: Pro-Ed; 2010:245–280.

58. Brennan-Curry A. *nTIDE January 2017 Jobs Report: Solid Start to New Year for Americans with Disabilities.* Kessler Foundation and University of New Hampshire. Available from: http://researchondisability.org/national-disability-employment-survey/kessler-natempsurv-news/2017/02/03/ntide-january-2017-jobs-report-solid-start-to-new-year-for-americans-with-disabilities. Accessed February 27, 2017.

59. Kessler Foundation/NOD. *The ADA, 20 Years Later Executive Summary: Survey of Americans with Disabilities.* New York: Harris Interactive; 2010.

60. Chan F, Wang C-C, Fizgerald S, et al. Personal, environmental, and service-delivery determinants of employment quality for state vocational rehabilitation consumers: a multilevel analysis. *J Vocat Rehabil.* 2016;45:5–18.

61. Oswald GR, Huber MJ, Bonza A. Effective job seeking preparation and employment services for college students with disabilities. *J Postsecondary Educ Disabil.* 2015;28:375–382.

62. Young-An R, Kim WHK. Impact of employment and age on quality of life of individuals with disabilities: a multilevel analysis. *Rehabil Couns Bull.* 2016;59:112–120.

63. Leahy MJ, et al. An analysis of evidence-based practices in the public vocational rehabilitation program: gaps, future directions, and recommended steps to move forward. *J Vocat Rehabil.* 2014;41:147–163.

64. Kent ML, Dorstyn DS. Psychological variables associated with employment following spinal cord injury: a meta-analysis. *Spinal Cord.* 2014;52:722–728.

65. Douglas JM, Bracy CA, Snow PC. Return to work and social communication ability following severe traumatic brain injury. *J Speech Lang Hearing Res.* 2016;59:511–520.

66. Liaset IF, Loras H. Perceived factors in return to work after acquired brain injury: a qualitative meta-synthesis. *Scand J Occup Ther.* 2016;23:446–457.

67. Roessler RT, Rumrill PD, Li J, et al. Predictors of differential employment statuses of adults with multiple sclerosis. *J Vocat Rehabil.* 2015;42:141–152.

68. Tse S, Chan S, Ng KL, et al. Meta-analysis of predictors of favorable employment outcomes among individuals with bipolar disorder. *Bipolar Disord.* 2014;1;16:217–229.

69. Nevala N, Pehkonen I, Koskela I, et al. Workplace accommodation among persons with disabilities: a systematic review of its effectiveness and barriers or facilitators. *J Occup Rehabil.* 2015;25:432–448.

70. Beveridge S, Fabian E. Vocational outcomes: relationship between individualized plan for employment and employment outcomes. *Rehab Couns Bull.* 2007;50:238–246.

71. Hess D, Ripley D, McKinley W, et al. Predictors for return to work after spinal cord injury: a 3-year multicenter analysis. *Arch Phys Med Rehabil.* 2000;81:359–363.

72. Sevak P, Houtenville AJ, Brucker DL, et al. Individual characteristics and the disability employment gap. *J Disabil Policy Stud.* 2015;26:80–88.

73. DeVivo M, Rutt R, Stover S, et al. Employment after spinal cord injury. *Arch Phys Med Rehabil.* 1987;68:494–498.

74. Goldberg R, Freed M. Vocational development, interests, values, adjustment and rehabilitation outlook of spinal cord patients: four year follow-up. *Arch Phys Med Rehabil.* 1976;457:532.

75. Goldberg R, Bigwood A. Vocational adjustment after laryngectomy. *Arch Phys Med Rehabil.* 1975;56:521–524.

76. Homa DB. Using the International Classification of Functioning, Disability and Health (ICF) in job placement. *Work J Prev Assess Rehabil.* 2007;29:277–286.

77. Young AE. Return to work following disabling occupational injury—facilitators of employment continuation. *Scand J Work Environ Health.* 2010;36(6):473–483.

78. Johnstone B, Martin TA, Bounds TA, et al. The impact of concomitant disabilities on employment outcomes for state vocational rehabilitation clients with traumatic brain injury. *J Vocat Rehabil.* 2006;25:97–105.

79. Ponsford JL, Olver J, Curran C, et al. Predictors of employment status 2 years after traumatic brain injury. *Brain Inj.* 1995;9:11–20.

80. Fleming JM, Strong J, Lightbody S. Prospective memory rehabilitation for adults with traumatic brain injury: a compensatory training programme. *Brain Inj.* 2005; 19:1–13.

81. Roessler RT, Rubin SE. *Case Management and Rehabilitation Counseling.* 4th ed. Austin, TX: Pro-Ed; 2006.

82. Crisp R. Locus of control as a predictor of adjustment to spinal cord injury. *Aust Disabil Rev.* 1984;1(2):53–57.

83. Hayward BJ, Schmidt-Davis H. *Longitudinal Study of the Vocational Rehabilitation Services Program Second Final Report: VR Services and Outcomes [Revised Draft Report].* Research Triangle Park, NC: Research Triangle Institute; 2002.

84. Kilbury RF, Stotlar BJ, Eckert JM. Centers for independent living. In: Crimando W, Riggar TF, eds. *Community Resources.* 2nd ed. Long Grove, IL: Waveland Press; 2005:304–314.

CHAPTER 15

Danbi Lee
Allen W. Heinemann

Important to Measure Aspects of Participation and Environmental Factors in Medical Rehabilitation

Long after the passage of the Americans with Disabilities Act (ADA), people with disabilities continue to face inequality and disparities in community living, community participation, and work and economic participation. The most recent Kessler Foundation/National Organization on Disability survey of Americans with disabilities found that there are still large gaps between people with and without disabilities with regard to employment, household income, access to transportation, health care, access to Internet, socializing, going to restaurants, and satisfaction with life (1). These gaps in life participation are often the result of environmental barriers such as inaccessible features of the built and natural environment, lack of transportation, income inequality, discrimination, and stigma in conjunction with physical, cognitive, or functional limitations.

Until the International Classification of Functioning, Disability, and Health (ICF), participation had been described in terms such as community living, community integration, independent living, engagement, and life roles (2). The ICF (Fig. 15-1) presents participation as a major component of disability and health and the endpoint of rehabilitation services, which drew much attention on how to conceptualize this key outcome in rehabilitation practice and research (3). In addition, the ICF explicitly presents the influence of environmental factors in people's lives and participation, intensifying interest in developing more adequate and accurate measures of environmental factors and their effects on participation (see Chapter 9 for a detailed discussion of the ICF).

The use of participation measures as outcomes moves the focus of rehabilitation interventions to real-world outcomes that are relevant and meaningful in the daily lives of people with disabilities. While the use of participation instruments in clinical settings is yet limited, more clinical trials are using participation instruments as primary or secondary outcomes to evaluate the effects of interventions on people's lives (4). Participation and environmental assessments are also used to describe individual- and population-based participation levels or participation profiles that allow a better understanding of needs for interventions and supports (4,5).

This chapter reviews considerations for selecting instruments measuring participation and environmental factors in disability populations. We first review theoretical frameworks that conceptualize participation and environmental factors. We particularly focus on the ICF model, which has spurred

discussions in conceptualizing participation and environmental factors. Then, we introduce selected instruments that measure the two concepts and review how they can be best used.

CONCEPTUALIZING PARTICIPATION AND ENVIRONMENTAL FACTORS

Scholars from different fields have acknowledged the relationship between the environment and participation by examining how environmental factors influence human behaviors and engagement in activities. Theoretical frameworks such as ecologic models from behavioral and social sciences (6–9), the competence-press model from gerontology (10–12), person-occupation-environment models from occupational therapy (13–16), and the social model of disability from disability studies (17) have been developed and evolved to describe the dynamic and mutual interactions between people's performance and participation and their environments. These models also have informed and influenced the development of the ICF (3), which provides a components-of-health classification system that describes disability as the intersection of a health condition, activity limitations, participation restrictions, and personal and environmental contextual factors.

Participation

In the ICF model, participation is defined as an individual's involvement in life situations (3). There are nine domains that pertain to participation and activities: (a) learning and applying knowledge, (b) general tasks and demands, (c) communication, (d) mobility, (e) self-care, (f) domestic life, (g) interpersonal interactions and relationships, (h) major life areas, and (i) community, social, and civic life. While ICF offers a taxonomy for conceptualizing participation, the definition of participation as "involvement in life situations" has been critiqued for not providing sufficient details, leaving its users vulnerable to potentially idiosyncratic decisions (2,5,18). In addition, participation in the ICF focuses on the "doing" of an individual and does not take into account individual's subjective appraisals, roles, values, and unique meaning ascribed to participation. An emphasis on participation as performance overlooks one's ability to exert choice and control over life. People with disabilities

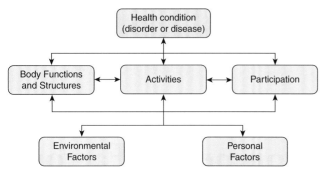

FIGURE 15-1. The International Classification of Functioning, Disability, and Health (ICF) model.

report that active and meaningful participation does not mean independent performance, but rather having a sense of control and power, choices, and opportunities to be part of an activity, context, or social group (19). For example, people may not feel or be restricted in their participation if they have their own way of engaging in an activity or if they have access to supports such as adaptive devices, personal assistance, and supportive social policies. People may not feel limited in their mode of participation if they choose not to participate in certain roles because those roles are unimportant. Therefore, participation is a nuanced, personal concept, reflecting the person's needs, resources, preferences, and social world.

Environmental Factors

The ICF describes environmental factors in terms of the physical, social, and attitudinal aspects of the environment in which people live and conduct their lives (3). The model distinguishes five domains of environmental factors: (a) products and technology, (b) natural environment and human-made changes to environment, (c) support and relationships, (d) attitudes, and (e) services, system, and policies learning. Aspects of the environment are categorized as barriers or facilitators to activities and participation. Often, the environmental factors act beyond barriers and facilitators. The interaction between participation and environmental factors is transactional, meaning that it is reciprocal and bidirectional in nature. People respond to their environments but also influence and modify environments to create opportunities for greater participation (5,20). In other words, the environment shapes people's lives and people change the environment to live well. Environmental factors can act as independent, confounding, moderating, and mediating factors to participation (21).

MEASURING PARTICIPATION

Multiple participation instruments have been developed to reflect research and clinical needs of various populations and settings. Although the term participation has not been used frequently in measurement until it was introduced in the ICF, instruments tapping similar concepts predate the ICF, including concepts such as community integration and handicap (22,23). Some instruments may be regarded as measuring participation because they include activities that occur in community settings or in a societal context or involve social components such as social interactions and leisure activities.

When selecting an instrument, users must consider carefully their conceptual framework, aspects of participation to measure (i.e., subjective, objective, or both), population of interest,

and the psychometric property of the instrument. We selected the participation instruments listed in **Box 15-1** because they operationalize participation clearly, demonstrate strong psychometric properties, were tested with more than one impairment group, and have been used by researchers other than the developer. The list includes seven instruments for adults (CIQ, CHART, CPI, IPA, KAP, PM-PAC, and PROMIS) and four instruments for children (CASP, CHORES, CAPE/PAC, and PEM-CY) that are tailored to the age-relevant aspects of life situations in which individuals may be involved, such as employment for adults and play and school participation for children. We categorized the participation instruments based on the content, type, and characteristics of each assessment

---

BOX 15-1

Participation Instruments for Adults and Children

Adults
- Activity Card Sort (ACS) (24)
- Assessment of Life Habits (LIFE-H) (25)
- Community Integration Questionnaire (CIQ) (22)
- Community Participation Indicators (CPI) (26)
- Craig Handicap Assessment and Reporting Technique (CHART) (27)
- Frenchay Activities Index (FAI) (28)
- Guernsey Community Participation and Leisure Assessment (GCPLA) (29)
- ICF Measure of Activity and Participation—Screener (IMPACT-S) (30)
- Impact on Participation and Autonomy (IPA) (31)
- Keele Assessment of Participation (KAP) (32)
- Nottingham Extended Activities of Daily Living (NEADL) (33)
- Participation Assessment with Recombined Tools-Objective (PART-O) (34)
- Participation Survey/Mobility (PARTS/M) (35)
- Participation Profile (PAR-PRO) (36)
- Participation Objective Participation Subjective (POPS) (37)
- Participation Measure for Post-Acute Care (PM-PAC) (38)
- Participation Scale (P-Scale) (39)
- Patient-Reported Outcomes Measurement Information System (PROMIS) Social health (40)

Children
- Activities Scale for Kids Performance (ASKp) (41)
- Assessment of Life Habits (LIFE-H) (42)
- Assistance to Participate Scale (APS) (43)
- Child and Adolescent Scale of Participation (CASP) (44)
- Children Helping Out: Responsibilities, Expectations, and Supports (CHORES) (45)
- Children Participation Questionnaire (CPQ) (46)
- Children's Assessment of Participation and Enjoyment/ Preferences for Activities of Children (CAPE/PAC) (47)
- Children's Leisure Assessment Scale (CLASS) (48)
- Participation and Environment Measure for Children and Youth (PEM-CY) (49)
- Participation in Childhood Occupations Questionnaire (PICO-Q) (50)
- Pediatric Activity Card Sort (PACS) (51)
- Pediatric Community Participation Questionnaire (PCPQ) (52)
- Pediatric Interest Profile (PIP) (53)
- Preschool Activity Card Sort (Preschool ACS) (54)

TABLE 15-1	Participation Instruments by Measurement Characteristics	
Objective	**Adults**	**Children**
Engagement	Community Integration Questionnaire (CIQ), Craig Handicap Assessment and Reporting Technique (CHART)	Children Helping Out: Responsibilities, Expectations, and Supports (CHORES), Children's Assessment of Participation and Enjoyment/Preferences for Activities of Children (CAPE/PAC)
Frequency	CHART, Community Participation Indicators (CPI), Keele Assessment of Participation (KAP)	CAPE/PAC, Participation and Environment Measure for Children and Youth (PEM-CY)
Level of assistance	CIQ, CHART	CHORES
Limitations	Participation Measure for Post-Acute Care (PM-PAC), Patient-Reported Outcomes Measurement Information System (PROMIS)	Child and Adolescent Scale of Participation (CASP)
Subjective	**Adults**	**Children**
Perceived difficulty	CHART, Impact on Participation and Autonomy (IPA), PROMIS	
Satisfaction	CPI	CAPE/PAC
Choice (importance)	CPI	CAPE/PAC
Control	CPI, IPA	

to assist clinicians and researchers select participation instruments for practice and research applications.

Because participation involves performance of activities as well as individuals' preferences and roles, participation instruments assess both objective and subjective aspects. Objective instruments assess the performance of an individual by the frequency, engagement, level of assistance needed, and restrictions; the subjective instruments assess perceived difficulties, satisfaction, importance, and sense of control over participation. Some instruments address both objective and subjective aspects of participation, while others focus only on one aspect. **Table 15-1** highlights the aspects of participation assessed by the participation instruments.

Table 15-2 shows the ICF domains covered by the participation instruments. The table also shows whether each instrument was developed for generic application with multiple populations or was developed for specific impairment groups. Many of the condition-specific instruments have been tested with other impairment groups and may be useful with people who have different types of impairments.

Tables 15-3 and **15-4** summarize the purpose, format, validity, reliability, and strengths and/or limitations of each selected instrument. We relied on the Rehabilitation Measures Database (https://www.sralab.org/rehabilitation-measures) for much of this information. This website regularly updates information to provide contemporary information about instruments suitable for populations receiving rehabilitation services.

MEASURING ENVIRONMENTAL FACTORS

Several instruments have been developed to measure the consequences of environmental factors on activities and participation; **Box 15-2** lists instruments measuring aspects of the environment. The typical measurement strategy is to ask respondents whether they experience environmental factors as barriers or facilitators to participation. **Table 15-5** lists aspects of environmental factors measured by the instruments listed in **Box 15-2**. Some instruments only assess environmental factors as barriers, supposing that absence of barriers counts as supports (78). While these types of instruments are useful in

TABLE 15-2		Each Instrument's Coverage of ICF Participation Domains						
Target	**Adults**	**Learning and Applying Knowledge**	**General Tasks and Demands**	**Communication**	**Mobility**	**Self-care**	**Domestic Life**	**Interpersonal Relationships**
Specific	CIQ		x		x		x	x
	CHART	x		x	x	x	x	x
Generic	CPI	x	x	x	x	x	x	x
	IPA				x	x	x	x
	KAP				x	x	x	x
	PM-PAC	x		x	x	x	x	x
	PROMIS		x				x	x
Target	**Children**	**Learning and Applying Knowledge**	**General Tasks and Demands**	**Communication**	**Mobility**	**Self-care**	**Domestic Life**	**Interpersonal Relationships**
Specific	CASP	x	x	x	x	x	x	x
Generic	CHORES		x	x	x		x	
	CAPE/PAC	x		x		x		x
	PEM-CY	x	x	x	x	x	x	x

All instruments measure "major life areas" and "community, social, and civic life" domains.

TABLE 15-3 Selected Participation Instruments for Adults

Measures	Purpose	Test Format	Reliability Test-Retest Reliability/ Internal Consistency Interrater Reliability	Tested Diagnosis/ Population	Validity Content Validity Criterion Validity Construct Validity	Comments
Community Integration Questionnaire (CIQ)	To assess the integration of people with disabilities into the community	15 items Three domains: • Home integration • Social integration • Productive activity Scoring: • Home integration • Social interaction • Productive activity • Total score (0–29) • Higher scores greater integration	**Stroke with aphasia** • Exc test-retest reliability (ICC = 0.96) (55) **TBI** • Adeq to exc test-retest reliability (ICC = 0.63–0.93) (56) • Exc interrater reliability $r = 0.74$–0.96 (between patients and family) (22) • Poor to exc internal consistency ($\alpha = 0.26$–0.95) (22,56,57) **Physical disability** • Poor to exc internal consistency ($\alpha = 0.45$–0.84) (58) **Older adults** • Exc test-retest reliability (ICC = 0.98) (59) • Adeq internal consistency ($\alpha = 0.79$) (59)	• Stroke with aphasia • Traumatic brain injury (TBI) • Acquired brain injury (ABI) • Brain tumor • Spinal cord injury (SCI) • Physical disability • Older adults	**TBI** • Content validity: created by rehabilitation experts, pilot tested, factor analysis resulted in three factors (22) • Criterion validity: 3 subscales measuring different domains (22); adeq corr with CHART ($r = 0.67$) and DRS ($r = 0.43$) (60) • Construct validity: 3 factors identified (61); adeq corr with corresponding subscales of Sydney Psychosocial Reintegration Scale ($r = 0.41$–0.60) (62); adeq corr with corresponding subscales of CHART ($r = 0.33$–0.67) (60) **SCI** • Criterion validity: poor to exc corr with CHART-SF ($r = 0.24$–0.79) (63)	• CIQ score reflects gender, age, education, and ethnicity in people with brain tumors (64).
Craig Handicap Assessment and Reporting Technique (CHART)	To assess the extent to which people with disabilities are able to function in the community	32 items Six domains: • Physical independence • Cognitive independence • Mobility • Occupation • Social integration • Economic self-efficacy Total score (0–600): higher scores greater participation	**SCI** • Exc test-retest reliability (ICC = 0.80–0.95) (27) • Poor to exc interrater reliability (between patient and proxy) ($r = 0.28$–0.84) (27) **Multiple diagnosis** • Exc test-retest reliability (ICC = 0.88–0.95) (65)	• Stroke • SCI • TBI • Multiple sclerosis (MS) • Burn • Amputation	**Amputation/SCI** • Criterion validity: poor to adeq corr with self-report FIM ($r = -0.04$ to 0.54) (27) **SCI** • Construct validity: employed persons reported higher subscores than unemployed persons (66) **TBI** • Adeq corr of CHART social integration subscale with Community Reintegration of Service member subscale ($r = 0.26$) (67)	• Short form (CHART-SF) is available in addition to 32-item-long form.
Community Participation Indicators (CPI)	To assess the extent to which individuals view their communities as valuing, respecting, and encouraging their participation	20 participation items (frequency, importance, and satisfaction question for each item) 48 enfranchisement items Domains: • Domestic, productive participation, social, leisure, and civic activities • Importance of participation • Control over participation Scores: • Frequency • Importance • Satisfaction • Total enfranchisement score transformed to a measure (0–100)	**Enfranchisement section** • Exc internal consistency ($\alpha = 0.96$), item-total corr ($r = 0.18$–0.73) (26)	• Multiple disability	**Enfranchisement section** • Construct validity: unidimensional; wheelchair users report lower enfranchisement, scores differed by disability severity (26)	• Online and telephone use following rehabilitation discharge is feasible for some rehabilitation patients. • Providing multiple modes of answering CPI questions enhances response rate (68).

Measure	Purpose	Description/Scores	Populations	Reliability	Validity	Strengths/Weaknesses
Impact on Participation and Autonomy (IPA)	To assess person-perceived disability and autonomy	39 items Five domains: • Autonomy indoors • Autonomy outdoors • Family roles • Social relationships • Paid work and education Scores: • Control (0–4) • Perceived difficulty (0–2)	Multiple impairments (neuromuscular, stroke, SCI, RA, fibromyalgia, MS) • Neuromuscular disease • Stroke • SCI • Rheumatoid arthritis • Fibromyalgia • Parkinson's disease • Older adults with disabilities	Multiple impairments (neuromuscular, stroke, SCI, RA, fibromyalgia, MS) • Exc test-retest reliability (ICC = 0.83–0.97) (31,69) • Exc internal consistency (α = 0.84–0.94) (23,31,69) SCI • Exc test-retest reliability (ICC = 0.83–0.88) (70) • Exc internal consistency (α = 0.90–0.96) (70)	Multiple impairments • Content validity: based on ICIDH-2, clinical experience of multidisciplinary research group, qualitative study with patients (23) • Construct validity: good fit to the model (normal fit index, 0.98; comparative fit index, 0.99) (69)	• IPA's psychometric properties are well documented for general disability and specific clinical groups. • Weaknesses include floor and ceiling effects and limited evidence of responsiveness (71).
Keele Assessment of participation (KAP)	To assess the level of participation in work, education, social activities, activities of daily living	15 items Score: • Total score (0–11)	• Joint pain • Psoriatic arthritis • Spinal conditions • Ankylosing spondylitis • Older adults	Joint pain (72) • Adeq test-retest reliability (ICC = 0.57–0.63) • Poor to adeq internal consistency (α = 0.57–0.74) • Interrater reliability not established	Older adults • Criterion validity: Increasing mobility restriction outside the home with increasing levels of knee pain and stiffness among older adults (32)	• KAP may be useful for epidemiologic studies that require a brief description of participation restrictions. • Ceiling effects and poor to adeq test-retest reliability may limit the KAP's utility.
Participation Measure for Post-Acute Care (PM-PAC)	To assess participation outcomes in outpatient or home care settings	51 items Seven domains • Mobility • Community, social and civic life • Role functioning • Self-care/domestic life • Home management and finances • Social relationships • Communication Scores: • Social and home participation • Community participation	• SCI • TBI • Musculoskeletal, neurologic, and medically complex disorders	Musculoskeletal, neurologic disorders (38) • Poor to adeq test-retest reliability (ICC = 0.61–0.86) • Adeq to exc internal consistency (α = 0.72–0.89)	• Content validity: development guided by ICIDH-2 and ICF, item review with focus groups with patients, pilot tested Musculoskeletal, neurologic disorders • Construct validity: CFA suggested seven-factor model, PCA results in two-factor solution (71); different scores among participants with different diagnosis (38)	• Good psychometric properties and minimal respondent burden make the PM-PAC a good choice for many applications. • PM-PAC may have limited utility for people with cognitive impairments.
Patient-Reported Outcomes Measurement Information System (PROMIS) Social Health items	To assess involvement in and satisfaction with one's usual social roles in life's situations and activities	Ability to participate in social roles and activities • 35 items (4, 6, 8 items) Satisfaction with social roles and activities • 44 items (4, 6, 8 items) Satisfaction with participation in social roles • 14 items (4, 6, 7, 8 items) Satisfaction with participation in discretionary social activities • 12 items	• General population • Chronic conditions (COPD, CHF, back pain, depressive disorder)	Ability items • High reliability coefficients (>0.98); acceptable item-total corr (0.65–0.85) (40) Satisfaction items • High reliability coefficients (>0.98); acceptable item-total corr (0.47–0.82) (40)	Ability and satisfaction items • Content validity: Delphi expert consensus, literature review, focus groups with people with chronic conditions (73) Satisfaction items • Construct validity: Good confirmatory factor analysis (CFI = 0.96, 0.97); unidimensional, good item fit (40)	• Sensitive to clinical change and changes in health status (74). • CAT and short form availability through http://www.healthmeasures.net and REDCap make PROMIS an attractive alternative.

Adeq, adequate; CAT, computerized adaptive testing; CFA, confirmatory factor analysis; Corr, correlation; DRS, disability rating scale; Exc, excellent; FIM, functional independence measure; ICC, intraclass correlation coefficient; PCA, principal component analysis.

TABLE 15-4 — Selected Participation Instruments for Children

Measures	Purpose	Test Format	Tested Diagnosis/Population	Reliability: Test-Retest Reliability, Internal Consistency, Interrater Reliability	Validity: Content Validity, Criterion Validity, Construct Validity	Comments
Child and Adolescent Scale of Participation (CASP)	To assess children's extent of participation and restrictions in home, school, and community life situations	20 items Four domains: • Home participation • School participation • Community participation • Home and community living activities Score: • Summary score (0–80)	• Children with ABI • Children with disabilities (ABI, CP, spina bifida, autism, learning disability, amputation, developmental delay, etc.)	Children with ABI • Exc test-retest reliability (ICC = 0.94) (44) Children with disabilities • Exc internal consistency (α = 0.96) • Person separation index (2.84), item separation index (6.71) (75)	Children with disabilities • Construct validity: scores differed by disability; hierarchy matching expected pattern of life situations (75); mod to high associations with PedsQoL and ABAS over 3 years (76)	• Multiple translations are available, including Spanish, French, German, Hebrew, and Mandarin. • An English and Spanish youth-report version is available for population-based studies of children and youth with TBI; psychometric evaluation is pending.
Children Helping Out: Responsibilities, Expectations, and Supports (CHORES)	To assess participation in household tasks and help needed to do household tasks	34 items Two domains: • Self-care household tasks • Family care household tasks Score: • Total performance sore (0–33) • Assistance score (0–100)	• Caregiver of children (6–14 years) without and with disabilities (cognitive and behavioral disorders, physical disabilities)	• Exc test-retest reliability (ICC = 0.92) (45) • Exc internal consistency (α = 0.96) (45) • High interrater reliability (parents-occupational therapists agreement = 80%) (77)	• Content validity: developed based on focus groups and expert input (45) • Construct validity: low association with CRI household responsibilities factor (77)	• CHORES focus on household tasks is narrower than other instruments.
Children's Assessment of Participation and Enjoyment and Preferences for Activities of Children (CAPE/PAC)	To assess a child's direct activity engagement and activity preferences	55 items Five domains: • Recreational • Active physical • Social • Skill-based • Self-improvement activities Scores • Overall participation score • Domain scores (formal/informal activities) • Participation scores for five types of activities	• Children (6–21 years) without and with disabilities	• Adeq test-retest reliability (0.72–0.81) (47) • Adeq internal consistency (0.67–0.84) (47)	• Content validity: developed by literature review, expert review, pilot testing (47) • Construct validity: intensity, enjoyment, and preference correlated with environmental, family, and child variables as expected (47)	• CAPE/PAC provides comprehensive assessment of activity preferences. • It is available for purchase from Pearson Education, Inc.
Participation and Environment Measure for Children and Youth (PEM-CY)	To assess participation frequency, extent of involvement, and desire for change in sets of activities typical for the home, school, or community	Participation section 25 items across three settings (home, school, community) Scores: • Frequency (0–100); percent maximum possible, percent participates ever • Level of involvement (1–5) • Percent desire for change (0–100)	• Children and youth (5–17 years) with and without disabilities	• Mod to good test-retest reliability (ICC = 0.58–0.79) (49) • Mod to good internal consistency (α = 0.59–0.83) (49)	• Construct validity: significant negative corr between desire for change with environmental supportiveness; group scores differed by disability (49)	• Multiple translations are available, including Dutch, German, Hebrew, Icelandic, Italian, Korean, Portuguese, Serbian, Turkish, French, Arabic, and Traditional Chinese.

ABAS, adaptive behavior assessment scale II; Adeq, adequate; Corr, correlation; CRI, child routine inventory; Exc, excellent; ICC, intraclass correlation coefficient; Mod, moderate; PedsQoL, pediatric quality of life inventory.

BOX 15-2	Environmental Instruments for Adults and Children

Adults
- Community Health Environment Checklist (CHEC) (81)
- Craig Hospital Inventory of Environmental Factors (CHIEF) (78)
- Facilitator And Barriers Survey of environmental influences on participation among people with lower limb Mobility impairments and limitations (FABS/M) (79)
- Home and Community Environment Instrument (HACE) (82)
- Measure of the Quality of the Environment (MQE) (83)
- Environmental Factors Item Banks (EFIB)
  - Built and Natural Environmental Features (84)
  - Access to Information and Technology (85)
  - Social Attitudes (86)
  - Systems, Services, and Policies (87)
  - Assistive Technology (88)

Children
- Craig Hospital Inventory of Environmental Factors-Children Parent version (CHIEF-CP) (89)
- Participation and Environment Measure for Children and Youth (PEM-CY) (90)
- Young Children's Participation and Environment Measure (YC-PEM) (91)

TABLE 15-5   Environmental Factor Instruments for Adults and Children

Objective	Adults	Children
Presence of environmental features	Community Health Environment Checklist (CHEC), Home and Community Environment Instrument (HACE)	
Subjective (Perceived)	**Adults**	**Children**
Frequency of encounter	Craig Hospital Inventory of Environmental Factors (CHIEF), Facilitator And Barriers Survey of environmental influences on participation among people with lower limb Mobility impairments and limitations (FABS/M), Environmental Factors Item Banks (EFIB)	Craig Hospital Inventory of Environmental Factors-Children Parent (CHIEF-CP) version
Magnitude/intensity	CHIEF, FABS/M, Measure of the Quality of the Environment (MQE)	CHIEF-CP
Impact of the environmental factor	CHIEF	Participation and Environment Measure for Children and Youth (PEM-CY), Young Children's Participation and Environment Measure (YC-PEM)
Accessibility	FABS/M	

identifying major barriers, some instruments identify environmental factors as both barriers and facilitators in different contexts (79,80). These instruments allow a fuller understanding of how environmental factors influence participation. These instruments use a variety of rating scales to describe environmental factors and their consequences. Objective instruments access the presence of environmental features regarding usability and accessibility and often use observational methods. Subjective instruments ask respondents to describe the frequency of encounters, magnitude, or intensity of environmental factors, and the overall consequences of environmental factors as perceived by individuals.

Table 15-6 lists the ICF domains covered by the environment instruments and the associated domains of measurement. All instruments can be used with general population samples, while the CHEC and FABS/M were developed for people with mobility impairments, and the EAMQ was developed for older adults.

We selected four environment instruments for adults (CHIEF, FABS/M, MQE, EFIB), listed in **Table 15-7**, and three instruments for children (CHIEF-CP, PEM-CY, YC-PEM), listed in **Table 15-8**, for a detailed review.

TABLE 15-6   Each Instrument's Coverage of ICF Environmental Factors

Target	Adults	Natural Environment and Human-Made Changes	Support and Relationships	Attitudes	Services, System, and Policies
Specific	CHEC	x			
	EAMQ	x			x
	FABS/M	x	x	x	x
Generic	CHIEF	x	x	x	x
	HACE			x	x
	MQE	x	x	x	x
	EFIB	x	x	x	x
Target	**Children**	**Natural Environment and Human-Made Changes**	**Support and Relationships**	**Attitudes**	**Services, System, and Policies**
Generic	CHIEF-CP	x	x	x	x
	PEM-CY	x	x	x	x
	YC-PEM	x	x	x	x

Note: All instruments measure the "products and technology" domain.

TABLE 15-7 Selected Environmental Factor Instruments for Adults

Measure	Purpose	Test Format	Tested Diagnosis/ Population	Reliability Test-Retest Reliability Internal Consistency Interrater Reliability	Validity Content Validity Criterion Validity Construct Validity	Comments
Craig Hospital Inventory of Environmental Factors (CHIEF)	To assess the extent the physical, social, and political environments act as barriers to participation	25 items Five domains: • Accessibility • Accommodations • Resource availability • Social support • Equality Scores: • Frequency (0–4) • Magnitude (0–2) • Impact score (0–8)	• Stroke • Cerebral palsy • Spinal cord injury (SCI) • Traumatic brain injury (TBI) • Multiple sclerosis • Amputation	SCI (78) • Exc test-retest reliability (ICC = 0.77–0.93) • Adeq interrater reliability (ICC = 0.62) (participant-proxy agreement) Multiple diagnosis (SCI, TBI, amputation) (78) • Adeq to exc internal consistency (α = 0.77–0.93)	Multiple diagnosis (78) • Content validity: created based on consensus of 4 subject matter experts • Construct validity: different scores across different impairment group TBI (92) • Criterion validity: adeq corr with Satisfaction with Life Scale and CHART total score	• Short form (CHIEF-SF) is available.
Facilitator And Barriers Survey of environmental influences on participation among people with lower limb Mobility impairments and limitations (FABS/M)	To assess the perceived impact of the environment on people with lower limb mobility impairment	65–133 items Six domains: • Primary mobility device • Home-built feature • Community-built and natural features • Community destination access • Community facilities access domain • Community support network	• Mobility impairment	Mobility impairment (79) • Exc test-retest reliability (r = 0.52–0.82) • Poor to exc internal consistency (α = 0.35–0.94)	Mobility impairment (79) • Content validity: created based on ICF • Construct validity: exc canonical corr with RNLI and PARTS/M	• FABS/M was designed for people with mobility impairments only.
Measure of the Quality of the Environment (MQE)	To assess the impact of environmental factors on social participation	109 items Nine domains: • Social network • Attitudes of family • Labor market • Income • Commercial services • Judicial services • Sociosanitary services • Educational services • Public infrastructure services Score: • Mean of obstacles (−3 to −1) and facilitator scores (1–3)	• Stroke • Can be used with any diagnosis	• Not established	• Content validity: created through input and guidance of rehabilitation professionals (83) • Criterion validity: adeq corr with LIFE-H total score (r = 0.42) (83)	• MQE provides broad coverage of ICF environmental codes. • MQE barrier and facilitator scores are correlated weakly, suggesting they measure distinct concepts (93).

| Environmental Factors Item Banks (EFIB) | To assess the environmental factor attributing to difficulties in performing activities | Natural and built environment items • 18 items Access to information and technology • 23 items Assistive technology • 14 items Social attitudes • 32 items Services, systems, and policy • 41 items | Neurologic disorders (stroke, SCI, TBI) | Natural and built environment items (84) • Adeq person separation reliability (0.70; $\alpha = 0.80$) • Good item separation reliability (0.97) Access to information and technology (85) • Good person separation reliability (0.83) and item separation reliability (0.99) Social attitudes (86) • Good person reliability (0.83) and item reliability (0.98) • High internal consistency ($\alpha = 0.97$) Services, systems, and policy (87) • 93.6% of participants showed Rasch reliability >0.7 | • Content validity: developed based on input from 10 content and outcome measurement experts and focus groups of people with stroke, TBI, SCI Natural and built environment items (84) • Construct validity: unidimensional; hierarchy; mod corr with CPI and PROMIS' participation in social roles and activities and satisfaction with social roles and activities Access to information and technology (85) • Construct validity: hierarchy; low to mod corr with PROMIS' social health scales, information support, and instrumental support ($r = 0.37$–0.46) and services, systems, and policies item bank ($r = 0.62$) Assistive technology (88) • Construct validity: device quality and type influence device benefit; device benefit influence participation Social attitudes (86) • Construct validity: unidimensionality Services, systems, and policy (87) • Construct validity: unidimensionality, good fit to the Rasch model, corr to CPI, PROMIS social participation items | • EFIB provides a brief but focused assessment of ICF environmental factors. • It is relatively new and been used by few investigators to date. |

Adeq, adequate; Corr, correlation; Exc, excellent; ICC, intraclass correlation coefficient; Mod, moderate; RNLI, reintegration to normal living index.

TABLE 15-8 | **Selected Environmental Factor Instruments for Children**

Measure	Purpose	Test Format	Tested Diagnosis/Population	Reliability Test-Retest Reliability Internal Consistency Interrater Reliability	Validity Content Validity Criterion Validity Construct Validity	Comments
Craig Hospital Inventory of Environmental Factors-Children Parent version (CHIEF-CP)	To assess the extent the physical, social, and political environments act as barriers to participation	10 items Domains: • Physical and structural • Services and assistance • School and work • Attitudes and support • Policies Scores: • Frequency (0–4) • Magnitude (0–2) • Impact score (0–8)	• Parents of children (2–12 years) with disability	• Adeq internal consistency (α = 0.76–0.78) (89) • Adeq test-retest reliability (ICC = 0.73) (89)	• Construct validity: mod to strong association with PEM-CY environmental supportiveness score and number of supports and barriers (89)	• CHIEF-CP provides continuity of measurement approach with adult CHIEF.
Participation and Environment Measure for Children and Youth (PEM-CY)	To assess perceived supports and barriers to participation within each setting	45 items across three settings (home, school, community) Domain • Environmental factors and activity demands • Resources Scores: • Environmental supportiveness (0–100) • Environmental supports (0–100) • Environmental resources (0–100)	• Children and youth (5–17 years) with and without disability	• Mod to good internal consistency (α = 0.67–0.91) (49) • Good test-retest reliability (ICC = 0.76–0.96) (49)	• Construct validity: mod to strong association with CHIEF-CP (90); group scores differed by income level (90)	• PEM-CY is available for purchase from CanChild. • Developers plan to develop an online survey version.
Young Children's Participation and Environment Measure (YC-PEM)	To assess the perceived supportiveness of the child's environment on participation	46 items across three settings (home, daycare/preschool, community) Scores: • Environmental supportiveness (0–100)	• Parents of young children (0–5 years) with and without developmental disability/delay	• High internal consistency (α = 0.92–0.96) (91) • Good to exc test-retest reliability (ICC = 0.91–0.94) (91)	• Construct validity: group scores differed by disability status (91)	• YC-PEM is the caregiver version of the PEM-CY for children 0–5 years.

Adeq, adequate; Exc, excellent; ICC, intraclass correlation coefficient; Mod, moderate.

We selected these instruments because they use self-report, assess environmental factors in the context of participation, cover all environmental domains of the ICF, and have been used by researchers other than the developer (93). The tables summarize the purpose, format, validity, reliability, and strengths and/or limitations of each instrument.

A challenge in measuring environmental factors is a phenomenon in which people with greater environmental supports tend to report greater participation, but because they experience more environmental exposure, they are likely to report more environmental barriers. In contrast, people who spend limited time outside their residence are less likely to be aware of meso- or macrolevel barriers, which might be misinterpreted as experiencing fewer barriers (5). Users may choose to utilize environmental measures in conjunction with participation measures to avoid such misinterpretation.

SUMMARY

Since the introduction of the ICF, we have achieved considerable progress in measurement of participation and environmental factors. This chapter highlights selected instruments that provide a comprehensive assessment and have at least the beginnings of a psychometric pedigree. The tables summarize information about participation and environmental instruments' characteristics, ICF domains covered, and psychometric properties that allow clinicians and researchers to evaluate and select suitable instruments. Clinicians and researchers should consider their own needs and the instruments' purpose, format, target population, strengths, and limitations when they select and apply instruments for practice and research applications.

REFERENCES

1. Kessler Foundation and National Organization on Disability. *The ADA, 20 Years Later: Executive Summary [Internet]*. New York, NY: Harris Interactive; 2010. Available from: http://www.2010disabilitysurveys.org/pdfs/surveysummary.pdf [cited January 26, 2017].
2. Dijkers M. Issues in the conceptualization and measurement of participation: an overview. *Arch Phys Med Rehabil*. 2010;91(9 suppl):S5–S16.
3. World Health Organization. *The International Classification of Functioning, Disability and Health*. 1st ed. Geneva, Switzerland: World Health Organization; 2001:299.
4. Whiteneck GG. Issues affecting the selection of participation measurement in outcomes research and clinical trials. *Arch Phys Med Rehabil*. 2010;91(9 suppl): S54–S59.
5. Whiteneck G, Dijkers MP. Difficult to measure constructs: conceptual and methodological issues concerning participation and environmental factors. *Arch Phys Med Rehabil*. 2009;90(11):S22–S35.
6. Lewin K, Heider F, Heider GM. *Principles of Topological Psychology*. New York, NY/London, UK: McGraw-Hill Book Company, Inc.; 1936.
7. Barker RG. *Ecological Psychology: Concepts and Methods for Studying the Environment of Human Behavior*. Stanford, CA: Stanford University Press; 1968:266.
8. Bronfenbrenner U. *The Ecology of Human Development*. Cambridge, MA: Harvard University Press; 1979:349.
9. Moos RH. Conceptualizations of human environments. *Am Psychol*. 1973;28(8):652–665.
10. Lawton P. Environment and aging theory revisited. In: Scheidt RJ, Windley PG, ed. *Environment and Aging Theory*. Westport, CT: Greenwood Press; 1998:1–31.
11. Lawton MP, Windley PG, Byerts TO. *Aging and the Environment: Theoretical Approaches*. New York: Springer; 1982:200.
12. Nahemow L, Lawton P. Toward an ecological theory of adaptation and aging. *Environ Des Res*. 1973;1:24–32.
13. Baum CM, Christiansen CH. Person-environment-occupation-performance: an occupation-based framework for practice. In: Baum CM, Christiansen CH, ed. *Occupational Therapy: Performance, Participation, and Well-Being*. 3rd ed. Thorofare, NJ: Slack Incorporated; 2005:243–266.
14. Townsend E, Polatajko HJ. *Enabling Occupation II: Advancing an Occupational Therapy Vision for Health, Well Being and Justice through Occupation*. Ottawa, ON: Canadian Association of Occupational Therapists; 2007.
15. Kielhofner G. *Model of Human Occupation: Theory and Application*. Baltimore, MD: Lippincott Williams & Wilkins; 2008.
16. Occupational therapy practice framework: domain and process (3rd Edition). *Am J Occup Ther*. 2014;68(suppl 1):S1–S48.
17. Oliver M. *The Individual and Social Model of Disability*. London, UK: Thames Polytechnic; 1990.
18. Hemmingsson H, Jonsson H. An occupational perspective on the concept of participation in the International Classification of Functioning, Disability and Health—some critical remarks. *Am J Occup Ther*. 2005;59(5):569–576.
19. Hammel J, Magasi S, Heinemann A, et al. What does participation mean? An insider perspective from people with disabilities. *Disabil Rehabil*. 2008;30(19):1445–1460.
20. Magasi S, Wong A, Gray DB, et al. Theoretical foundations for the measurement of environmental factors and their impact on participation among people with disabilities. *Arch Phys Med Rehabil*. 2015;96(4):569–577.
21. Wang PP, Badley EM, Gignac M. Exploring the role of contextual factors in disability models. *Disabil Rehabil*. 2006;28(2):135–140.
22. Willer B, Rosenthal M, Kreutzer JS, et al. Assessment of community integration following rehabilitation for traumatic brain injury. *J Head Trauma Rehabil*. 1993;8(2):75–87.
23. Cardol M, de Haan RJ, van den Bos GA, et al. The development of a handicap assessment questionnaire: the Impact on Participation and Autonomy (IPA). *Clin Rehabil*. 1999;13(5):411–419.
24. Katz N, Karpin H, Lak A, et al. Participation in occupational performance: reliability and validity of the Activity Card Sort. *OTJR (Thorofare NJ)*. 2003;23(1):10–17.
25. Noreau L, Fougeyrollas P, Vincent C. The LIFE-H: assessment of the quality of social participation. *Technol Disabil*. 2002;14(3):113–118.
26. Heinemann AW, Magasi S, Bode RK, et al. Measuring enfranchisement: importance of and control over participation by people with disabilities. *Arch Phys Med Rehabil*. 2013;94(11):2157–2165.
27. Whiteneck G, Charlifue S, Gerhart K, et al. Quantifying handicap: a new measure of long-term rehabilitation outcomes. *Arch Phys Med Rehabil*. 1992;73(6):519–526.
28. Schuling J, de Haan R, Limburg M, et al. The Frenchay Activities Index. Assessment of functional status in stroke patients. *Stroke*. 1993;24(8):1173–1177.
29. Baker PA. Measurement of community participation and use of leisure by service users with intellectual disabilities: the Guernsey Community Participation and Leisure Assessment (GCPLA). *J Appl Res Intellect Disabil*. 2000;13(3):169–185.
30. Post MWM, de Witte LP, Reichrath E, et al. Development and validation of IMPACT-S, an ICF-based questionnaire to measure activities and participation. *J Rehabil Med*. 2008;40(8):620–627.
31. Cardol M, de Haan RJ, de Jong BA, et al. Psychometric properties of the Impact on Participation and Autonomy Questionnaire. *Arch Phys Med Rehabil*. 2001;82(2):210–216.
32. Wilkie R, Peat G, Thomas E, et al. The Keele Assessment of Participation: a new instrument to measure participation restriction in population studies. Combined qualitative and quantitative examination of its psychometric properties. *Qual Life Res*. 2005;14(8):1889–1899.
33. Nicholl C, Lincoln N, Playford E. The reliability and validity of the Nottingham Extended Activities of Daily Living Scale in patients with multiple sclerosis. *Mult Scler*. 2002;8(5):372–376.
34. Bogner J, Bellon K, Kolakowsky-Hayner SA, et al. Participation assessment with recombined tools-objective (PART-O). *J Head Trauma Rehabil*. 2013;28(4): 337–339.
35. Gray DB, Hollingsworth HH, Stark SL, et al. Participation survey/mobility: psychometric properties of a measure of participation for people with mobility impairments and limitations. *Arch Phys Med Rehabil*. 2006;87(2):189–197.
36. Ostir GV, Granger CV, Black T, et al. Preliminary results for the PAR-PRO: a measure of home and community participation. *Arch Phys Med Rehabil*. 2006;87(8): 1043–1051.
37. Brown M, Dijkers MPJM, Gordon WA, et al. Participation objective, participation subjective. *J Head Trauma Rehabil*. 2004;19(6):459–481.
38. Gandek B, Sinclair SJ, Jette AM, et al. Development and initial psychometric evaluation of the participation measure for post-acute care (PM-PAC). *Am J Phys Med Rehabil*. 2007;86(1):57–71.
39. Brakel DWHV, Anderson AM, Mutatkar RK, et al. The Participation Scale: measuring a key concept in public health. *Disabil Rehabil*. 2006;28(4):193–203.
40. Hahn EA, DeVellis RF, Bode RK, et al. Measuring social health in the patient-reported outcomes measurement information system (PROMIS): item bank development and testing. *Qual Life Res*. 2010;19(7):1035–1044.
41. Young NL, Williams JI, Yoshida KK, et al. Measurement properties of the Activities Scale for Kids. *J Clin Epidemiol*. 2000;53(2):125–137.
42. Noreau L, Lepage C, Boissiere L, et al. Measuring participation in children with disabilities using the Assessment of Life Habits. *Dev Med Child Neurol*. 2007;49(9):666–671.
43. Bourke-Taylor H, Law M, Howie L, et al. Development of the Assistance to Participate Scale (APS) for children's play and leisure activities. *Child Care Health Dev*. 2009;35(5):738–745.
44. Bedell GM. Developing a follow-up survey focused on participation of children and youth with acquired brain injuries after discharge from inpatient rehabilitation. *NeuroRehabilitation*. 2004;19(3):191–205.
45. Dunn L. Validation of the CHORES: a measure of school-aged children's participation in household tasks. *Scand J Occup Ther*. 2004;11(4):179–190.
46. Rosenberg L, Jarus T, Bart O. Development and initial validation of the Children Participation Questionnaire (CPQ). *Disabil Rehabil*. 2010;32(20):1633–1644.

47. King GA, Law M, King S, et al. Measuring children's participation in recreation and leisure activities: construct validation of the CAPE and PAC. *Child Care Health Dev*. 2007;33(1):28–39.

48. Rosenblum S, Sachs D, Schreuer N. Reliability and validity of the Children's Leisure Assessment Scale. *Am J Occup Ther*. 2010;64(4):633–641.

49. Coster W, Bedell G, Law M, et al. Psychometric evaluation of the participation and environment measure for children and youth. *Dev Med Child Neurol*. 2011;53(11):1030–1037.

50. Bar-Shalita T, Yochman A, Shapiro-Rihtman T, et al. The Participation in Childhood Occupations Questionnaire (PICO-Q): a pilot study. *Phys Occup Ther Pediatr*. 2009;29(3):295–310.

51. Mandich AD, Polatajko HJ, Miller L, et al. *Pediatric Activity Card Sort (PACS)*. Ottawa, ON: Canadian Occupational Therapy Association; 2004.

52. Washington LA, Wilson S, Engel JM, et al. Development and preliminary evaluation of a pediatric measure of community integration: the Pediatric Community Participation Questionnaire (PCPQ). *Rehabil Psychol*. 2007;52(2):241–245.

53. Henry AD. *Pediatric Interest Profiles: Surveys of Play for Children and Adolescents, Kid Play Profile, Preteen Play Profile, Adolescent Leisure Interest Profile*. San Antonio, TX: Therapy Skill Builders; 2000.

54. Berg C, LaVesser P. The preschool activity card sort. *OTJR (Thorofare NJ)*. 2006;26(4):143–151.

55. Dalemans RJ, de Witte LP, Beurskens AJ, et al. Psychometric properties of the Community Integration Questionnaire adjusted for people with aphasia. *Arch Phys Med Rehabil*. 2010;91(3):395–399.

56. Andelic N, Arango-Lasprilla JC, Perrin PB, et al. Modeling of community integration trajectories in the first five years after traumatic brain injury. *J Neurotrauma*. 2016;33(1):95–100.

57. Corrigan JD, Deming R. Psychometric characteristics of the Community Integration Questionnaire: replication and extension. *J Head Trauma Rehabil*. 1995;10(4):41–53.

58. Hirsh AT, Braden AL, Craggs JG, et al. Psychometric properties of the community integration questionnaire in a heterogeneous sample of adults with physical disability. *Arch Phys Med Rehabil*. 2011;92(10):1602–1610.

59. Singh U, Sharma V. Validity and reliability of community integration questionnaire in elderly. *Int J Health Rehabil Sci*. 2015;4(1):1–9.

60. Zhang L, Abreu BC, Gonzales V, et al. Comparison of the Community Integration Questionnaire, the Craig Handicap Assessment and Reporting Technique, and the Disability Rating Scale in traumatic brain injury. *J Head Trauma Rehabil*. 2002;17(6):497–509.

61. Sander AM, Fuchs KL, High WM Jr, et al. The community integration questionnaire revisited: an assessment of factor structure and validity. *Arch Phys Med Rehabil*. 1999;80(10):1303–1308.

62. Kuipers P, Kendall M, Fleming J, et al. Comparison of the Sydney Psychosocial Reintegration Scale (SPRS) with the Community Integration Questionnaire (CIQ): psychometric properties. *Brain Inj*. 2004;18(2):161–177.

63. Gontkovsky ST, Russum P, Stokic DS. Comparison of the CIQ and chart short form in assessing community integration in individuals with chronic spinal cord injury: a pilot study. *NeuroRehabilitation*. 2009;24(2):185–192.

64. Kaplan CP. The Community Integration Questionnaire with new scoring guidelines: concurrent validity and need for appropriate norms. *Brain Inj*. 2001;15(8):725–731.

65. Walker N, Mellick D, Brooks CA, et al. Measuring participation across impairment groups using the Craig Handicap Assessment Reporting Technique. *Am J Phys Med Rehabil*. 2003;82(12):936–941.

66. Tozato F, Tobimatsu Y, Wang C-W, et al. Reliability and validity of the Craig Handicap Assessment and Reporting Technique for Japanese individuals with spinal cord injury. *Tohoku J Exp Med*. 2005;205(4):357–366.

67. Resnik L, Gray M, Borgia M. Measurement of community reintegration in sample of severely wounded service members. *J Rehabil Res Dev*. 2011;48(2):89–101.

68. Wong AWK, Heinemann AW, Miskovic A, et al. Feasibility of computerized adaptive testing for collection of patient-reported outcomes after inpatient rehabilitation. *Arch Phys Med Rehabil*. 2014;95(5):882–891.

69. Sibley A, Kersten P, Ward CD, et al. Measuring autonomy in disabled people: validation of a new scale in a UK population. *Clin Rehabil*. 2006;20(9):793–803.

70. Noonan VK, Kopec JA, Noreau L, et al. Comparing the reliability of five participation instruments in persons with spinal conditions. *J Rehabil Med*. 2010;42(8):735–743.

71. Magasi S, Post MW. A comparative review of contemporary participation measures' psychometric properties and content coverage. *Arch Phys Med Rehabil*. 2010;91(9):S17–S28.

72. Hermsen LAH, Terwee CB, Leone SS, et al. Social participation in older adults with joint pain and comorbidity; testing the measurement properties of the Dutch Keele Assessment of Participation. *BMJ Open*. 2013;3(8):e003181.

73. Bode RK, Hahn EA, DeVellis R, et al. Measuring participation: the Patient-Reported Outcomes Measurement Information System experience. *Arch Phys Med Rehabil*. 2010;91(9 suppl):S60–S65.

74. Hahn EA, Beaumont JL, Pilkonis PA, et al. The PROMIS satisfaction with social participation measures demonstrated responsiveness in diverse clinical populations. *J Clin Epidemiol*. 2016;73:135–141.

75. Bedell G. Further validation of the Child and Adolescent Scale of Participation (CASP). *Dev Neurorehabil*. 2009;12(5):342–351.

76. Golos A, Bedell G. Psychometric properties of the Child and Adolescent Scale of Participation (CASP) across a 3-year period for children and youth with traumatic brain injury. *NeuroRehabilitation*. 2016;38(4):311–319.

77. Dunn L, Magalhaes LC, Mancini MC. Internal structure of the Children Helping Out: Responsibilities, Expectations, and Supports (CHORES) measure. *Am J Occup Ther*. 2014;68(3):286–295.

78. Whiteneck GG, Harrison-Felix CL, Mellick D, et al. Quantifying environmental factors: a measure of physical, attitudinal, service, productivity, and policy barriers. *Arch Phys Med Rehabil*. 2004;85(8):1324–1335.

79. Gray DB, Hollingsworth HH, Stark S, et al. A subjective measure of environmental facilitators and barriers to participation for people with mobility limitations. *Disabil Rehabil*. 2008;30(6):434–457.

80. Fougeyrollas P, Noreau L, St-Mitchel G, et al. *Measure of the Quality of the Environment*. Lac St-Charles, Québec: International Network of the Disability Creation Process; Canadian Society for the International Classification of Impairments, Disabilities and Handicaps; 1999.

81. Stark S, Hollingsworth HH, Morgan KA, et al. Development of a measure of receptivity of the physical environment. *Disabil Rehabil*. 2007;29:123–137.

82. Keysor J, Jette A, Haley S. Development of the home and community environment (HACE) instrument. *J Rehabil Med*. 2005;37:37–44.

83. Rochette A, Desrosiers J, Noreau L. Association between personal and environmental factors and the occurrence of handicap situations following a stroke. *Disabil Rehabil*. 2001;23(13):559–569.

84. Heinemann AW, Lai J-S, Wong A, et al. Using the ICF's environmental factors framework to develop an item bank measuring built and natural environmental features affecting persons with disabilities. *Qual Life Res*. 2016;25(11):2775–2786.

85. Hahn EA, Garcia SF, Lai J-S, et al. Measuring access to information and technology: environmental factors affecting persons with neurologic disorders. *Arch Phys Med Rehabil*. 2016;97(8):1284–1294.

86. Garcia SF, Hahn EA, Magasi S, et al. Development of self-report measures of social attitudes that act as environmental barriers and facilitators for people with disabilities. *Arch Phys Med Rehabil*. 2015;96(4):596–603.

87. Lai J-S, Hammel J, Jerousek S, et al. An item bank to measure systems, services, and policies: environmental factors affecting people with disabilities. *Arch Phys Med Rehabil*. 2016;97(12):2102–2112.

88. Magasi S, Wong A, Miskovic A, et al. Mobility device quality impacts participation outcomes among people with disabilities: a structural equation modeling analysis. *Arch Phys Med Rehabil*. 2018;99(1):1–8.

89. McCauley D, Gorter JW, Russell DJ, et al. Assessment of environmental factors in disabled children 2–12 years: development and reliability of the Craig Hospital Inventory of Environmental Factors (CHIEF) for Children-Parent Version. *Child Care Health Dev*. 2013;39(3):337–344.

90. Khetani M, Marley J, Baker M, et al. Validity of the Participation and Environment Measure for Children and Youth (PEM-CY) for Health Impact Assessment (HIA) in sustainable development projects. *Disabil Health J*. 2014;7(2):226–235.

91. Khetani MA, Graham JE, Davies PL, et al. Psychometric properties of the young children's participation and environment measure. *Arch Phys Med Rehabil*. 2015;96(2):307–316.

92. Whiteneck GG, Gerhart KA, Cusick CP. Identifying environmental factors that influence the outcomes of people with traumatic brain injury. *J Head Trauma Rehabil*. 2004;19(3):191–204.

93. Heinemann AW, Miskovic A, Semik P, et al. Measuring environmental factors: unique and overlapping International Classification of Functioning, Disability and Health coverage of 5 instruments. *Arch Phys Med Rehabil*. 2016;97(12):2113–2122.

Ethical Issues in Rehabilitation Medicine

A 59-year-old man suffered a left hemispheric cerebrovascular accident. Two weeks later, he was admitted to a rehabilitation unit for treatment of deficits resulting from expressive language impairment and right-sided weakness. He did not agree with the self-care, mobility, and speech goals proposed by the rehabilitation team. Rather, he was anxious to return to his home and work. His wife of 30 years was apprehensive about caring for him in light of his level of disability and urged the team to continue therapy.

Patients, family members, and practitioners often disagree about the goals, processes, or utility of rehabilitation treatments. Health care practitioners face difficult dilemmas as they attempt to set a course that all parties will endorse. In this patient's case, practitioners were torn between honoring the patient's desire for discharge and respecting the concerns and wishes of his wife. They did not want to treat a patient who failed to provide informed consent, yet they realized that the patient's wife was not prepared to care for him at home. They knew that training would improve his functional abilities and enhance his eventual return home.

Rehabilitation practitioners confront moral quandaries often during the course of practice. A single moral principle— such as that of autonomy or beneficence—may fail to outweigh other principles, yet choices must be made. Practitioners must attempt to reconcile and assign priority to conflicting moral obligations (1). Decisions of a moral nature are distinguishable from those governed by law, technology, religion, or politics. They focus on what is proper rather than on what is possible or legally permissible. Considerations of etiquette, cost, and convenience play an insignificant role in moral decision-making.

The terms *moral* and *ethical* are closely related; both stress manners, customs, and character. Cicero apparently used the Latin word *moralis* to translate the Greek *ethikos* (2). Contemporary usage reflects a divergence of meaning, however. *Ethics* refers to theoretical and contemplative descriptions of values. *Morality* describes conduct—that is, whether behaviors are right or wrong. This chapter traces the development of ethical systems in medicine and discusses their application to rehabilitation practice. It describes moral conflicts inherent to issues frequently encountered in clinical rehabilitation practice and recommends approaches to resolve these dilemmas. Policy issues including resource allocation, health system reforms and costs, and responsibilities of rehabilitation professionals are discussed.

HISTORICAL DEVELOPMENT

Religious Influences

In the fifth century B.C., Hippocrates described scientific, technologic, and ethical aspects of medical care (3). The Hippocratic Oath is derived from the traditions of a religious sect known as the Pythagoreans. In swearing allegiance to the Oath, a small group of physicians on the Isle of Cos vowed secrecy and loyalty to their teachers and promised to seek the virtues of purity and holiness. Compelled to help patients and forbidden from harming them, physicians alone were qualified to determine how to treat sick patients.

Religious traditions influenced the development of medical ethics through the Middle Ages, when monks dominated medical practice, and beyond (4). Thereafter, Catholics incorporated principles of medical decision-making into their moral theology (3). Protestants, too, have examined specific ethical topics in detail and integrated concepts of medical ethics into a larger, systematic theology (3). Orthodox Jews have linked Talmudic and rabbinical teachings to the practice of medicine, with emphasis on the preservation and sanctity of life (3).

Secular Influences

During the Age of Enlightenment (late 17th century to early 19th century), the influence of religion on medical morality diminished as secular theories of philosophical reasoning arose. Controversy flourished as scholars studied, debated, and published a range of theories of medical care (3).

Codes of medical practice developed over time in response to medical challenges. In 1789, an epidemic of typhoid created chaos in a British hospital as staff members assumed onerous and unfamiliar responsibilities. As tension heightened and some staff resigned, a retired physician, Thomas Percival, sought to restore calm by designing a code of professional conduct. He instructed physicians to address the needs of individual patients in preference to those of the larger society and to show "tenderness with steadiness and condescension with authority" since they were to "inspire the minds of their patients with gratitude, respect, and confidence" (5). Percival's words were repeated in the first professional code of ethics of the American Medical Association published in 1847.

Recent Developments

Medical ethics evolved relatively little over the ensuing years. But more recently, particularly during the past 40 years, the practice of medicine has evolved dramatically. So, too, has medical ethics. Technologic advances have established a basis for medical treatment. Developments in health care and the biologic sciences have produced complex and difficult moral dilemmas that transcend discrete professional boundaries.

Daniel Callahan describes five factors that give rise to ethical tensions in health care (6). First, technologies such as renal dialysis, organ transplantation, genetic engineering, and embryonal transplantation have expanded our ability to intervene in nature. A strong social commitment to health care coupled with a compelling tendency to apply available technology has made it difficult to restrict use of technology.

Second, medical resources are costly. When medicine could do little to help people, care tended to be cheap. But now that improved neonatal, emergency, and acute care interventions save many lives, the chronicity and cost of disease have skyrocketed. For more than 40 years, health care costs have risen substantially faster than personal income or the overall economy (7). At $2 trillion annually, health care expenditures now exceed one sixth of the American economy (8).

Callahan cites an expanded role of the public as a third factor prompting recognition of ethical issues (6). The solitary and secretive aura of Hippocratic medicine has been supplanted by health care that is conducted in an increasingly public arena. More than 80% of Americans die in hospitals. Taxpayers fund health care entitlement programs and support medical research. Research on human subjects is regulated by federally mandated Institutional Review Boards. Legislation is in place to protect patients and assure their privacy.

The language of rights has evolved as well. Support for individual rights in American society and enhanced respect for the rights of racial minorities, women, and disabled persons have directed attention to patients' rights. In the medical context, respect for self-determination and personal dignity requires recognition that patients have a right to make their own decisions (3).

Finally, Callahan cites increasing concern about quality of life since many lives are now preserved and extended by medical interventions. We may wonder, however, what kind of life some survivors will lead (9). At times, the burdens of cure appear to outweigh its benefits (10).

Dramatic change has spread throughout the health care insurance industry in recent years. Mechanisms of reimbursement for health care have shifted due to the emergence of managed care and other for-profit systems. Expectations concerning the relationships and roles of payers, practitioners, and consumers have been profoundly altered.

Until the recent past, little formal attention was directed to ethical aspects of rehabilitative care. A number of explanations exist (11). Still a relatively young field, rehabilitation medicine has sought to acquire recognition and acceptance by the medical community (12). Its chronic care dilemmas may seem to lack the drama of life-and-death decisions. Often, patients are treated over an extended period of time by a broad range of practitioners, none of whom possesses clear or sole responsibility for addressing ethical issues.

Recognition of moral dilemmas inherent to chronic care has increased interest in ethical aspects of rehabilitation. Questions have been raised about duties of professionals, dynamics of professional-patient relationships, roles and expectations of family members, and goals of care (11,13–29). A discussion of fundamental ethical principles furnishes a conceptual framework to study issues relevant to rehabilitation medicine.

ETHICAL PRINCIPLES

Beneficence

The term *beneficence* connotes kindness, charity, and the doing of good; it refers to a moral obligation to help other people, refrain from harming them, and attempt to balance benefits with harms. In the health care setting, beneficence entails an obligation to promote the health and well-being of patients and to prevent disease, injury, pain, and suffering (2).

Whether beneficence can be assured is uncertain when patients' values conflict with traditional medical values of healing and care. Differences of opinion among patients, family members, and professionals about the best interests of patients or criteria for a good quality of life are not easily resolved. Discrepant interests may be difficult to balance within a moral framework. Beauchamp and McCullough suggest that "beneficence includes the obligation to balance benefits against harms, benefits against alternative benefits, and harms against alternative harms" (4).

Autonomy

The principle of *autonomy* is grounded in the notion of respect for the values and beliefs of other people. Individuals are entitled to privacy and to make decisions about their lives. They are perceived as possessing a right to self-determination that ensures freedom to make personal choices and resist the intervention of others. Within the context of health care, autonomy underlies the medical doctrine of informed consent. There is an obligation to inform patients accurately about their diagnoses and treatment alternatives, as well as to seek their permission before instituting treatment. Decisions are respected, even if they appear to be unwise (2,4).

Many authors describe tension between the principle of beneficence, which requires acting in a patient's best interests, and that of autonomy, which entails respecting patient choices (4,30). Balancing the two principles is a perpetual struggle for health care givers who consider certain decisions of patients to be harmful. It is not clear how to view patient behavior when patient choices seem at odds with information presented to them. To Englehardt, "the moral obligation to respect persons will often constrain physicians to acquiesce in patients' choices—choices that most likely will lead to the loss of important goods" (30). In everyday practice, health care givers may be tempted to act paternalistically by restricting patient freedom to make autonomous choices if those choices appear to compromise the patient's best interests.

Justice

The principle of *justice* concerns questions of what is due to whom and how to distribute the burdens and benefits of living in a society. An egalitarian model of distribution obliges society to provide all its members with a fair share of health care resources and to treat people equitably. However, scarcity of resources or competition for them can create conflict (2). Is it fairer for people to share social goods equally or for those who have less to be given more?

People in the United States have yet to define the basic medical services that will be provided for all citizens. For example, despite the fact that sexually transmitted diseases are relatively common and may present public health hazards, some people receive neither prevention nor treatment efforts. But other treatments, such as organ transplants or elective cosmetic surgery, appear to be readily available to some patients. Entitlement programs in certain states pay for procedures not funded in others. Emergency treatments may be generally available, but aftercare and rehabilitation to improve the lives saved may not be funded adequately. Millions of Americans, many of whom work, do not qualify for publicly funded insurance programs yet cannot afford to buy private health care insurance. Even for those who have insurance, reimbursement plans may provide vastly differing levels of coverage.

Concern for individual dignity and choice has overshadowed a holistic view of society's needs. Daniel Callahan ponders what kind of medicine is needed by a society that must address other needs, including education, housing, welfare, and culture (9). Determining how much health care to support spurs us to reflect on how we want to live within our larger society. Fundamental questions of meaning are not easy to answer. In contrast to other developed nations, which may possess a strong orientation to community, Americans have lagged in developing and implementing a sound health care delivery system based on a just social policy.

ETHICAL ISSUES OF CLINICAL PRACTICE

Overview of Rehabilitation

Acute care physicians attempt to save lives, relieve symptoms, reverse the course of pathologic processes, and discharge medically stable patients. Unlike acute care medicine, rehabilitation does not center on a sick patient whom treatment is expected to cure. Rather, rehabilitation practitioners treat dysfunctions that are chronic, often irreversible, and rarely curable. Residual disability may well persist throughout a person's life.

Medical rehabilitative care addresses impairment caused by pathologic processes that include disease, accident, and congenital abnormality. People with disabilities experience restricted ability to perform certain functions. When unable to execute activities important to role fulfillment, a person is said to be disabled (31). Rehabilitation therapy attempts to ameliorate impairments and disabilities by restoring skills and capabilities through functional retraining and environmental adaptation. Many professionals—including, but not limited to, physicians, nurses, psychologists, social workers, and educators, as well as physical, speech, occupational, recreational, and vocational therapists—contribute to this effort. They must reach beyond pathology and physiologic dysfunction to understand the unique familial, social, vocational, psychological, and financial dimensions of patients. Successful rehabilitation requires attention not only to medical but to nonmedical factors ranging from skin tolerance to household layout and availability of caregivers.

The need for a team of rehabilitation professionals and family members to engage in each patient's treatment leads to complex relationships that may be portrayed by three points of a triangle representing patient; family, generally including several people; and health care team, including practitioners of multiple disciplines. Those at each point share concerns with others but harbor unique considerations as well. Competing rights and obligations of patients, family members, and practitioners and blurred responsibilities and loyalties can cause confusion or conflict.

Following the seminal description of ethical issues in rehabilitation medicine in the Hastings Center Report in 1987, Kirschner studied ethical issues of greatest concern to rehabilitation clinicians (17,32). Practicing clinicians were asked to describe ethical conflicts encountered in daily practice. A broad range of clinicians listed four primary issues: reimbursement and allocation of scarce resources, determination

TABLE 16-1	Clinical Practice of Rehabilitation Care	
Clinical Practice Issues	**Policy Issues**
1. Selection of patients	1. Allocation of resources
2. Goal setting for patients	2. Medical insurance and implications for rehabilitation
3. Patient-practitioner relationships	3. Professional responsibilities
4. Professional and team issues	
5. Duties and rights of family members	
6. Quality of life and termination of treatment	

of rehabilitation goals, compromised decision-making capacity in patients, and concerns about confidentiality (32). They considered conflicts among the treatment team especially troubling. Practitioners expressed unease about balancing their obligations to payers with their roles as patient advocates. How to ensure justice in treatment decisions worried them.

In another study, registered nurses, many of whom held management positions, reported concern about misallocation of medical resources—including both overtreatment and suboptimal treatment of patients (33). They questioned how to assure an optimal balance of providing good and avoiding harm while respecting patient autonomy. Ethical issues identified in similar surveys (see **Table 16-1**) are discussed in this chapter within the context of clinical and policy dilemmas inherent to rehabilitation care.

Selection of Patients

Provision of medical care in the United States does not necessarily reflect need for it; in 2010, more than 48.6 million Americans lacked health insurance. In 2016, the number of uninsured Americans had dropped to 28.6 million as a result of coverage provided through the Affordable Care Act (ACA) that was approved by Congress in 2010 (34). Even for patients who are insured by Medicare, studies have shown that race, income level, and geography affect the care received (35). Many individuals may not be entitled to reimbursement for rehabilitation, nor is rehabilitative care guaranteed for those whose lives have been saved by acute care interventions.

Rehabilitation practitioners screen potential patients before selecting those who will receive treatment. Providers recognize that not all patients will benefit from rehabilitation therapy since some are too ill to participate in therapy or have impairments that are difficult to rehabilitate, while others have relatively insignificant functional impairment (36). Assessment of prospective patients requires practitioners to review information derived from hospital records and consult with referring and other treating professionals. They may also examine patients or interview family members.

Because treatment requires patients to solve problems by applying new approaches to their functional needs, patient ability to learn and retain information is considered crucial to successful rehabilitation. A person's age and predicted course of recovery also influence a decision to initiate care. Those patients who are anticipated to make significant progress are usually viewed as good candidates for rehabilitation despite severe dysfunction.

Practitioners explore nonmedical parameters in admission decisions. Particular attention is directed to whether family members are physically and emotionally available to help patients, because strong social support systems correlate with positive patient outcomes (37). Financial capacity is a powerful determinant of access to services since gains made during treatment are more likely to be retained if financial resources are available for further services or equipment as needed.

Features of the rehabilitation unit itself influence selection of patients. Some units specialize in treatment of specific disorders or impairments. Others emphasize training patients for work or independent living. Fluctuating bed availability or staffing patterns may affect selection such that surplus program capacity at a given time may prompt admission of patients who might otherwise be rejected (16).

Although practitioners are guided in the selection process by a patient's potential to benefit, some professionals may neglect evidence-based information regarding rehabilitation prognosis. Ability to pay and the burden of care that staff are likely to experience also influence decisions, yet the fact that admission criteria are not publicly disclosed not only confers significant flexibility on decision-makers but creates a potential for injustice as a result of bias or subjectivity. A lack of training with respect to moral dilemmas may cause practitioners to make judgments that reflect their personal belief systems and values (16). Decisions may also be influenced by perceptions that society desires to save money in its care for disabled persons or by practitioner bias about the likelihood of good rehabilitation outcomes in older patients (17). Decisions may be made without sufficient understanding of the body of evidence-based information regarding rehabilitation prognosis.

Dilemmas in selection abound. Who should be selected: a patient with considerable need but a relatively poor prognosis, or one with lesser need and disability but the likelihood of a better outcome? A young person who will apply his or her training throughout a lengthy life span, or an older person with few remaining years despite his contributions to society over a lifetime? How much treatment should be available to patients who bear responsibility for their disability or for those who have been noncompliant with past treatment?

Our current approach to patient selection seems to favor those already well-off. Engelhardt describes the impact of lotteries: a "natural lottery" of one's talents and abilities and diseases and illnesses and a "social lottery" that includes educational and work status, financial and insurance profiles, and social attractiveness (38). "Winners" can navigate complicated medical systems to gain assistance coping with disease, but "losers" may be uninformed about even the availability of services and resources. Patients disadvantaged by socioeconomic factors may experience restricted access to rehabilitation, but with absence of an explanation for this rejection, they are unlikely to challenge selection decisions effectively.

Potential for injustice inheres to a system that fails to provide clear criteria or standards for those who make difficult selection determinations. Although screening is necessary to assure that patients are medically stable and to demonstrate that they have remediable functional disabilities, the screening process has significant shortcomings. Practitioners should standardize selection guidelines and formulate them in writing. Reasons for rejecting patients, and a commitment to re-evaluating those patients in the future, should be assured.

Otherwise, a single decision made relatively early in the course of disease may preclude rehabilitative care entirely. A mechanism for patient appeals could provide valuable checks and balances to the selection process.

Goal Setting for Individual Patients

In order to develop patient treatment plans, staff members discuss the requirements of the postdischarge environment with patients and their family members. Initial treatment goals are outlined, reviewed, and adjusted during the course of therapy to ensure the relevance and feasibility of patient goals over time.

Authors who have addressed goal setting during patient care include Trieschman, who emphasizes the importance of consulting with patients and family members to cast and refine goals (22,24,25,39–42). She cautions caregivers to refrain from imposing goals on patients who may reject them in the long run anyway and stresses the importance of assuring transfer of skills from the rehabilitation setting to the home environment (42). Becker and associates emphasize the need to promote close interaction among family and staff members and to assure that the full team resolves discrepancies among treatment goals (39).

Although rehabilitation practitioners encourage patients to participate in designing their treatment program, this may be difficult for some patients. On admission to rehabilitation, many patients are exhausted by pain, weakness, fatigue, depression, or anxiety. Few come to terms with new or exacerbated disability and the demands of their condition absent real-life and home experiences that could illuminate their postdischarge needs (25,43). They may know little about what can be achieved from rehabilitation. The rehabilitation unit itself may be unsettling. Expected to socialize with strangers who may have visible scars and dysfunction at the very time that visits from friends and family are restricted by a demanding therapeutic schedule may cause patients to feel cutoff from all that is familiar.

People have different interpretations of data about probabilities and outcomes. One's approach to information regarding risks and benefits, pain, cost, health, and disability is influenced by his or her personal values. It is not uncommon for patients, family members, health care teams, and insurers to advocate for discrepant or even mutually exclusive goals. Patients are likely to want to make their own decisions; they know best what is personally meaningful and how exhausted or disheartened they feel. At the same time, they may feel indebted to family members who want to pursue different goals. Relatives may believe that their opinions should take priority since they will be serving as caregivers. Practitioners' experiences with disability may incline them to usurp decision-making power rather than to accept patient or family choices that appear likely to expend time, money, or effort unnecessarily. Tensions abound (25–27).

The principle of autonomy holds self-determination paramount regardless of whether patients make ill-advised choices. We know that patient autonomy can be compromised by limited knowledge of medicine. But the technical expertise possessed by practitioners does not imply moral authority. Professionals should refrain from imposing their personal values on patients who generally know best what makes sense for themselves. Experience demonstrates that in an unrestricted environment, former patients may refuse tasks that require extensive time, patience, or concentration. They may discard unattractive or cumbersome equipment and ignore recommendations for self-care and home exercise programs. Transportation, social networks, or finances may be insufficient to support interventions made in the rehabilitation setting (25).

Practitioners may not appreciate the potency of their recommendations for patients who have experienced profound, often abrupt, loss of physical ability. Patients require education about the costs, risks, and effectiveness of treatment options and benefit from an opportunity to explore fully the medical and functional ramifications of alternative treatment approaches (44). Clinicians should communicate the values, ethical norms, and institutional priorities that underlie their recommendations. Tauber believes that only sustained, deliberate efforts to elucidate values held by all interested parties and to delineate major conflicts among those values help to resolve the moral tensions that impact care of disabled persons (45).

Decision-Making Capacity of Patients

Relationships between rehabilitation patients and care providers are likely to be of long duration, in contrast to some acute care relationships (15). The nature of the moral rules and principles that determine exchange of information and provision of services in extended health care relationships bears exploration.

American laws and customs have evolved over time with respect to patient rights. An increasingly egalitarian relationship between patients and practitioners has displaced paternalism (17). A "contractual" model of care requires practitioners to tell patients the truth about their circumstances and to present options in an accurate and balanced manner. A professional duty to act beneficently toward patients is constrained by respect for patient autonomy. Physicians supply the medical care desired by autonomous people who make informed decisions about that care. Respect for confidentiality and patient privacy is deemed essential to the development of trusting and egalitarian relationships between patients and physicians.

Caplan describes factors that compromise the relevance of a contractual model to rehabilitation (15). Relationships in rehabilitation are multifaceted rather than restricted to a single practitioner and patient. Patients have multiple health care providers, and family members, too, that often assume an integral role in treatment. People who have experienced profound impairment need time to adjust to the reality of disability. Many are anguished by their functional losses. Facing an uncertain future and possessing little knowledge of ways that disability will impact their life choices, patients may feel unprepared to make important decisions. Similarly, family members are likely to be unfamiliar with issues that arise in the context of their loved ones' impairments.

Caplan describes the complex and evolving nature of relationships among patients and their rehabilitation providers. He argues that an effective and proper role of physicians in medical decision-making may entail more guidance on the part of professionals than a model that specifies the physician as a provider of information to an autonomous patient (15). He notes that the competence of patients during the earliest phases of rehabilitation treatment may be questionable and contends that rehabilitation professionals are justified in

overriding the autonomous wishes of patients at the outset of treatment (17,22,26,27). If patients have not yet adapted to impairment or come to understand their future possibilities, Caplan suggests that practitioners are justified in using persuasion to encourage even reluctant patients to participate in early rehabilitation. He recognizes that this approach tolerates more beneficence on the part of providers than customary in contemporary medicine but suggests that over the long run, it restores patient identity, capacity to cope, and autonomy (15). Caplan characterizes this as an "educational model" of care. He underscores the importance of earning the understanding and cooperation of patients at the same time that practitioners seek to understand patients' values and preferences as fully as possible.

Periodic assessment of patient capacities to make autonomous choices is essential. Practitioners must focus on restoring autonomy quickly so that patients will resume decision-making as they adjust to the consequences of impairment. An independent committee could be charged with assuring that patient autonomy is enhanced as soon as possible during treatment. Paternalism would be considered appropriate only as a bridge to restoring autonomy to patients, with practitioners recognizing that beneficence, however well intended, may compromise a patient's best interests over time (17).

Assessment of competency in patients with neuropsychological dysfunction requires presenting information in modalities and formats that patients are able to process. Simple tests such as the mini-mental status exam may be inadequate to discern patient capacity. More comprehensive evaluation, including determining specific competencies in appropriate contexts over time, may be needed to understand patient decision-making capacity. In the event that patients and caregivers disagree on a course of treatment, the values underlying those disagreements should be discerned and discussed thoughtfully, rather than providers assuming that a patient is incompetent. Competent patients understand potential benefits, risks, and consequences of treatment options and can communicate their decisions (44,46,47).

Moral Conflicts Among Professionals

Rehabilitation treatment is delivered by a multidisciplinary group of professionals who work together as a team. Amelioration of patients' functional deficits, psychosocial challenges, and vocational needs requires rehabilitation teams to provide coordinated and comprehensive treatment generally not offered by individual caregivers who work independently. Experienced teams have demonstrated the ability to provide efficient, organized services (19,22).

Patients and family members may be relatively unaccustomed to working intimately with so many practitioners in the health care setting. Distinguishing the responsibilities and lines of authority among team members may be challenging. Clarifying what each professional expects and needs to know is not easy for many patients. Acting consistently while working with a wide variety of professionals can be daunting for them as well.

Members of a rehabilitation team should recognize the vulnerability of patients to team pressure, no matter how subtle. Patients who are exhausted, frightened, or confused may be intimidated by professionals. Purtilo suggests that patients may feel compelled to follow recommendations with which they do not agree when outnumbered by the team (19). Sometimes, team members need to decide how to treat patient "secrets" or how to reconcile conflicting information gathered from patients and relatives.

Practitioners serve as teachers and guides to enhance patient function and assist adjustment to disability. Addressing the needs of many patients simultaneously requires the team to balance the conflicting interests of multiple patients. Institutional policies about patient schedules, smoking, or electronic devices, for example, may clash with the wishes of particular patients. The team must balance the interests of individuals with those of the collective and the guidelines of the institution (17).

Controversy about authority and responsibility can arise among team members as they recommend diverse and perhaps conflicting goals for patients or disagree about setting priorities among consensus goals. Certain team members may wish to work with patients in ways that conflict with those of their colleagues (48). A team in which authority is distributed may not have agreed on a method to resolve dissension. In addition, the fact that team members share lengthy and strenuous work hours may impose a sense of loyalty that makes some members uncomfortable questioning others.

Purtilo suggests that teams explore and clarify personal and shared values in order to develop a "common moral language" to frame ethical decisions (19). Team members should be trained about and practice effective team dynamics and should work within a framework of administrative guidelines that promote airing and resolution of conflicts (17,32). Accountable to the entire team for their actions, each member should be encouraged to raise questions about professional behaviors that seem to compromise patient interests. Team members must assure their accessibility to patients and families and strive to avoid intimidating them inadvertently. Even patients or families who are difficult to manage must be treated respectfully.

Professionals should explain to patients and their relatives how teams share responsibility and designate authority (17). Lines of communication should be clarified to alleviate patient uncertainty. Families should know what to expect in terms of decision-making. Practitioners should protect patient privacy and confidentiality to the extent possible while emphasizing to patients and relatives the need to share relevant information among those involved in a patient's care. Teams should strive to resolve the conflicts that inevitably arise among patients, family members, and professionals. They should seek advice and support from other professionals when such insight can advance rational decision-making (47). Ethics committees can be asked to provide a neutral forum for discussion and mediation.

Duties and Rights of Family Members

Family members frequently assume a vitally important role in the care of disabled relatives. The interest and commitment of relatives may determine whether a patient is admitted for rehabilitation. During treatment, family members are expected to meet with the team to learn caregiving skills, revise treatment goals, and establish postdischarge arrangements.

There is an expectation on the part of society that relatives will assist one another when needs arise. Family or family-like relationships are considered uniquely extensive and interconnected (17). Family members often undertake caretaking duties with the understanding that they are able to provide special emotional support and affection as well as the physical care that patients require (14).

The need for family caretaking has increased as the extent and cost of professional care have risen (49). Some rehabilitative care has shifted to home settings. Early discharge to home is thought to enhance patient autonomy while enabling patients to test their skills and the feasibility of their goals in a real-life setting. Outpatient or home settings are preferred by many patients and are less expensive than inpatient facilities.

A randomized, controlled trial of stroke patients with moderately severe disability contrasted routine hospital rehabilitation and early discharge with rehabilitation care provided at home. Patients in the latter group showed better recovery of activities of daily living, ambulation, motor capacity, manual dexterity, socialization, and satisfaction. They required half the resources of the hospitalized group and experienced no difficulties in the use of home help. No negative impact on family caregivers was noted (50).

Callahan has observed that many families discover that providing care to their disabled members is mutually satisfying and rewarding (14). Caretakers develop and hone skills and resources to adapt effectively to shifting demands. They may take pride in their ability to identify patient needs and to provide care sensitively and with compassion. Some family members are exceptionally responsive to a relative's situation and thus offer optimal care.

Other families experience difficulties, however. Unresolved tensions among patients and caregivers may interfere with satisfactory relationships. The demands of caring for a disabled person may exceed the capacities of some family members. Strain may result from limited financial resources or inadequate physical supports. Relatives may feel angry, sad, or depressed about the condition of their loved one. They may question whether they are prepared to cope over long years with the circumstances of a severely disabled person or one who has an uncertain prognosis. Facing an unanticipated situation that they have not chosen, their personal happiness or autonomy may feel threatened.

There is no simple formula to determine what family members ought to be expected to provide for patients or to identify the limits of duty. Some relatives may gladly dedicate the remainder of their days to caregiving, whereas others may view this as unjustified self-sacrifice (14). Family commitments are complicated by the fact that families today are smaller and more dispersed than in the past, making it difficult to share caregiving tasks among several relatives. Women may feel a special responsibility to become caretakers, but employment often restricts their availability to do so. Some families are not physically able to provide adequate care despite wishing to do so, whereas the financial or emotional resources of others are too meager. Some relatives are unwilling to relinquish personal plans, hopes, or dreams even if they are best qualified to address patient needs and vulnerabilities (14). Health care providers rarely have sufficient understanding about the lives and intimate relationships of specific patients and family members to know what to advise in difficult situations.

Practitioners may be uncertain about the amount of persuasion that is justified in an attempt to encourage potential caregivers to commit themselves to patients. When patient needs are minimal and family members poised to sacrifice relatively little, the patient's best interests may well entail encouraging relatives to fulfill family obligations. In circumstances of severe disability in which significant sacrifice will be required, however, strong persuasion does not appear justified. Callahan points out that our society neither rewards nor honors people who transcend their own needs to care for others. Such people are, in fact, more likely to meet with social isolation than with commendation and should not be expected to act as heroes (14).

Society has yet to develop mechanisms to reimburse the financial and psychological services that could minimize the burden on caregivers. It is critical that family members are furnished with tools to sustain them, including daycare centers, respite care, counseling, self-help groups, and adequate physical facilities (49). Only then can society expect any but the most extraordinary people to embrace an opportunity to care for a seriously disabled relative.

Termination of Rehabilitation Treatment

Many factors contribute to decisions to terminate treatment in the rehabilitation setting (17). Patients undergoing rehabilitation care are expected to make steady and measurable progress toward attaining their goals. When progress slows significantly or patients appear to have reached a plateau in degree of improvement, members of the treatment team may doubt whether continued therapy is justified. Such questions about efficacy of treatment are typically raised first by professionals rather than the family. At times, patients and their relatives seek goals that professionals no longer consider realistic or important. At other times, clinicians may be concerned that patients who are scheduled for discharge have received insufficient treatment (33).

Moral values of team members influence decisions to terminate treatment. Practitioners assess somewhat nebulous concepts, such as "benefit," "productivity," "functional improvement," and "integration into society," to delineate endpoints of treatment (39–41,51). Their subjective judgments about the capacity of patients to cope with impairment outside the rehabilitation setting and the validity of family members' requests for services and equipment affect their appraisals. Practitioner perceptions about acceptable levels of function do likewise, even though their personal values may differ substantially from those of patients (17). Not uncommonly, insurance providers determine the length and timing of treatment, which may not reflect a time frame that patients or practitioners consider reasonable. It is time-consuming for practitioners to advocate for public policies to assure adequate reimbursement by insurance plans for evidence-based rehabilitation therapy.

Our society lacks a common context that relates ambiguous concepts of health, function, and quality of life to cherished personal values such as autonomy and independence. Medical practitioners do not have the final word on quality of life, nor are their theoretical views—particularly if unexamined—necessarily more insightful than those of others.

Research about the quality of life of persons with disability indicates that adversity does not necessarily cause a person to appraise his quality of life negatively (52). In fact, persons who adapt to disability may be wholly satisfied with the meaningfulness of life (53). However, gaps between one's activities, aspirations, and accomplishments may impair quality of life

to the extent that significance is attached to those unattained wishes (54). To assure thoughtful decisions about terminating treatment, practitioners must understand the critical importance of patients' values in impacting patient assessments of elements that make their lives satisfying.

The progress of some patients during rehabilitation may be examined sooner than that of others. Patients who are considered noncompliant, uncooperative, or poorly motivated may be so difficult to manage that the team discusses discharge relatively early in the course of treatment. Other patients have limited insurance coverage. Professionals may feel pressured to use scarce institutional resources for new patients and thus decide to wean care from longer-term patients. A patient's home setting and his anticipated need for assistance at discharge also affect the timing of a decision to curtail care.

In recent years, it has become increasingly common for patients to begin rehabilitation care before they are able to participate fully in training. Because some patients may not be eligible for readmission following a temporary discharge, practitioners may be reluctant to interrupt treatment early. At other times, onset of medical complications results in transfer to acute care, regardless of progress made in rehabilitation. Whether to readmit patients for additional treatment can be a source of disagreement among both patients and professionals.

Even wise and morally sensitive caregivers feel challenged to allocate care wisely among patients. Sometimes, rehabilitation teams fail to explain the criteria that influence their decision to end treatment. At other times, patients and relatives may not appreciate the significance of the factors assessed. Surely, patients and their families have a right to know the parameters used to evaluate patient progress and the guidelines that determine whether treatment will be continued. Practitioners have a duty to document patient milestones in order to assure that objective data underlie decisions to stop care. Engaging patients and relatives in team discussions about termination of care is essential if their desires are to be honored (17).

ETHICAL IMPLICATIONS OF HEALTH CARE POLICY

Allocation of Health Care Resources

Over 125 million Americans live with chronic illness, disability, or functional limitations (55). Babies who would have died from complications of prematurity or congenital abnormality only a few years ago survive, often with significant disability. Many severely injured people overcome life-threatening conditions. Rapid medical triage and substantial technological advance enable victims of severe war wounds to survive. Americans today live considerably longer than their ancestors; by 2040, 23% of the population will be older than 65 years (56). Population growth, extended life span, and successful acute care interventions have rendered chronic disease increasingly prevalent. Persons with chronic disease frequently benefit from rehabilitation services to enhance their functional skills at work, at school, or in the home (49).

Costs of health care have increased annually since the 1980s. In 1950, approximately 5% of gross national product (GNP) was spent on health care; by 1998, health expenditures were 15% of the GNP, by far the highest level in the world and nearly double that of the nearest competitor nation (57,58).

Health spending now represents 16% of GNP (56). Even middle-income Americans worry that they may be excluded from necessary health care services because of inability to pay (59).

Our national appetite for medical care increases. Costs are driven by hospital-based services, complex technology, fee-for-service reimbursement plans, litigation concerns, and treatment of patients near the end of life (56). Treatment of severe injury is costly as well; some who survive trauma to the brain or spinal cord require care costing hundreds of thousands of dollars.

Studies show that although less healthy people are more likely than those who are healthy to qualify for public coverage, they are less likely to be insured. Minorities are uninsured in higher numbers than the white population. People who live in inner city or rural areas often have restricted access to care. Those who lack care have worse health than those who receive services, even controlling for factors such as increased stress and poor hygiene (59).

Churchill comments that, despite a sense of moral repugnance, Americans do ration health care according to ability to pay (56). Many uninsured people forego preventive care and basic services such as eyeglasses, hearing aids, and routine dental care. Even desperately needed care is typically sporadic for those without financial resources. The Commonwealth Fund's survey of 12,000 adults in seven developed countries (Australia, Canada, Germany, the Netherlands, New Zealand, the United Kingdom, and the United States) showed that Americans were most likely to complain of restricted access to care; 37% of those surveyed reported skipping doctor visits, tests, and prescriptions in the preceding year due to cost (60).

The most recent Commonwealth Fund survey sampled patients in 11 developed, high socioeconomic countries in 2013. American patients ranked last or near the bottom of the countries in ease of getting an appointment after regular working hours or when they were sick. Americans were the most likely to use the emergency room for care, with 39% of US adults having done so in the preceding 2 years. The United States had fewer general practitioners for its population than the comparison countries—half as many per 1,000 population as the next closest country, Sweden, and one fifth the proportion of France or Germany. Access of Americans was also limited by cost of care. More than one third said that costs prevented them from filling prescriptions, visiting the doctor, or having tests that had been ordered (61).

Interventions designed to extend life often overshadow those that enhance its quality. The heroism and drama of rescue medicine prevail over seemingly mundane preventive and primary care interventions. Our fragmented, uncoordinated system of private health insurance and publicly funded entitlement programs fails to address the medical needs of many, especially those who have chronic disease. Allocation decisions are made absent a larger context that would help to identify and weigh priorities (9).

A just society does not allocate health care to favor those who are insured, wealthy, and white. A morally acceptable heath care system must honor principles of equity and justice. We respect a community that offers mutual and reciprocal assistance to its members and honors its social obligations to care for those who are sick without discriminating among individuals. After all, no one is immune to unexpected disease or calamity—misfortune can, in fact, strengthen human bonds of mutual affection (56).

But what services should be offered in a society that cannot afford everything? Principles of utility would direct us to select services that provide the greatest good for the greatest number of people (2). Principles of justice imply that services should be based on need. Yet, assessment of need may be subjective, biased by highly individualistic desires, hopes, and preferences (9).

In an environment of finite resources, limits on health care should derive from generic guidelines that apply to common conditions. Personalized appeals for specialized services should be discouraged (56). Access to basic and primary care improves health outcome; use of more specialized care should depend on evidence regarding its effectiveness and an understanding of the efficiency with which it can be provided. Costly care of marginal benefit should be replaced by treatments that improve quality of life.

Some health care planners have concluded that poorly distributed medical services may compromise not only the health of those persons who have inadequate access to care but also those who receive excessive services. A 2004 federal study showed no differences in health outcomes across America regardless of substantial disparities in heath care spending among regions. For example, per capita spending in Utah was just 59% of that in Massachusetts, yet population health ratings were similar (62).

In a comparative study of patients conducted in Minneapolis, Miami, Portland, and Orange County, neither life expectancy nor quality of life in the last 6 months of life was improved by spending more on health care (63). Expenditures in Miami far exceeded those in Minneapolis, yet medical outcomes were similar. During the 6 months prior to death, Medicare costs in Miami were double that of Minneapolis. Miami patients visited medical specialists six times more frequently than those in Minneapolis, spent twice as much time in the hospital, and were admitted to intensive care units more than twice as often. Lifetime spending for a typical 65-year-old in Miami was $50,000 more than in Minneapolis. But no difference in outcomes was noted. The Congressional Budget Office estimates that less than half of all medical care in the United States is supported by sound evidence of its effectiveness (7). In fact, hospitalized patients may actually do worse than those who receive less treatment and experience fewer infections and other complications of treatment.

Evolution of Health Care Insurance

Despite benefiting from the most advanced medical technology in the world, Americans worry that such care may 1 day exceed their economic reach. Until recently, the last major change in federal health care policy had been the 1965 Medicare Act. In 1971, President Richard Nixon tried to forestall national interest in single-payer health insurance by proposing federal mandates for employer coverage and a Medicaid-like program available to those who were otherwise not insured with income-based sliding scale premiums. Although federal legislation with these provisions was never passed, increases in health costs over the next two decades drove states including Massachusetts, Vermont, Oregon, Minnesota, and Tennessee to implement mandates for coverage. These programs, however, proved costly and troublesome to implement as legislators repeatedly failed to enforce the mandates or to finance new coverage for the poor. Even those persons who faced fines were unable to purchase health insurance if they did not receive subsidies. The number of uninsured Americans continued to rise (64).

By the early 1990s, concern about inadequate health care coverage prompted President Bill Clinton to appoint a task force to draft reform measures ensuring universal and affordable health care. Although those reform efforts failed, the focus on health care costs propelled changes in systems of reimbursement, including managed care, that were intended to control medical costs.

Rates and duration of hospitalization decreased thereafter, but overall medical costs continue to grow. No reform effort included real cost controls (56,59).

One notable reform took place in Massachusetts in 2006, when the Republican governor and Democratic-controlled legislature enacted far-reaching health insurance reform. All residents were required to subscribe to health insurance or suffer a tax penalty. Employers were required to offer coverage or pay a small assessment if they did not do so. An expanded state/federal Medicaid program was made available to low-income individuals, who otherwise received subsidies to help purchase private insurance offered at substantially lower rates than in the past. By mid-2008, two thirds of persons who lacked health insurance at the outset of the program were covered; 40% now had private policies without government subsides. The cost of the program per person, shared between the state and redirected federal funds, was less than anticipated, although unexpectedly rapid enrollment increased the total budget for subsidized care (65).

Concerns about access, cost, and quality of health care continue to receive national political attention throughout the 2008 presidential campaign, reflecting voter concern. Physicians were not satisfied either. A panel of experts on medicine, academia, business, insurance, and politics was convened by the Massachusetts Medical Society and the *New England Journal of Medicine* in May 2008 to address physician concerns about primary care. The experts noted that the reimbursement system rewarded physicians and institutions for sophisticated technological procedures rather than for cognitive work and time spent with patients. They discussed the rewards that other countries realized from investments in electronic systems and health-related information technology and underscored the need for the academic health community to focus on the complex economic, research, and policy questions concerning improved access and quality of health care (66,67).

Public demand for health care reform continued after the election. President Barack Obama proposed the ACA, often dubbed "Obamacare," the most significant health care law since the creation of Medicare and Medicaid in the 1960s. The plan, modeled on the 2006 Massachusetts health reform, expanded Medicaid, made available income-based tax credits to help consumers purchase insurance on new health insurance exchanges, and implemented individual requirements to purchase health insurance or pay a penalty. Those with high incomes and "Cadillac" insurance were to be taxed, and larger employers were required to offer coverage to full-time employees. Political opponents filed the first of many lawsuits on the day that the law was passed in 2010. They argued that the requirement to purchase health insurance was unconstitutional and complained that states should not create health exchanges, despite the fact that this approach had been adopted pursuant to recommendations by Senate conservatives (34,68).

Although the two lawsuits that reached the Supreme Court were overturned, a Superior Court decision in 2012 exempted states from the requirement to expand Medicaid, and 19 governors refused to do so leaving approximately 3 million adults in those states without coverage (69). In subsequent years, Congress voted dozens of times to try to repeal the law. Although not successful, Congress did block transitional funding and cost-sharing subsidies needed to provide the insurance industry with financial relief as it stabilized the new market. The new marketplace failed to attract a large share of healthy young consumers to offset the sicker population now insured, although the uninsured rate of adults under 35 dropped 5% in 2016 alone (70). Over time, significant numbers of health insurers refused to participate in the health exchanges, reducing competition and increasing prices (34).

Nonetheless, over 20 million Americans have received health insurance, about 60% through Medicaid and 40% as a result of the law's premium subsidies for coverage purchased on the health exchanges. Enrollment continued to increase each year from 2013 to 2016 with the uninsured rate dropping in every state, particularly in states that had expanded Medicaid and created state health exchanges and strong outreach and enrollment programs (71). Overall, the uninsured rate dropped from 16% to 9% and from 48.6 million uninsured Americans in 2010 to 28.6 million in 2016 (34).

Controversy about health care coverage continued after the 2016 election. On March 7, 2017, Republicans proposed a health bill to replace the ACA far more oriented to the free market, rolling back Medicaid expansion and fundamentally altering the way the federal government funds Medicaid, which provides insurance to one in five Americans. It also eliminates the requirement for larger employers to offer coverage to full-time employees or pay an excise tax (72). The mandate for Americans to have health insurance is eliminated, as are, over time, the income-based tax credits that enable individuals to buy health insurance (73). Three of the ACA's most popular provisions would be continued: the prohibitions on barring insurance for pre-existing conditions and imposing lifetime coverage caps and the rule allowing young adults to remain on their parents' health plans until the age of 26. It also allows insurance companies to charge higher prices to older people (74). Due to insufficient tax credits, millions of people who are insured through the ACA will be at risk of losing their insurance, particularly people in their 50s and early 60s who will have higher insurance costs (75). Taxes on businesses and individuals making more than $200,000/year, a source of funding for ACA, would be eliminated.

There is no precedent for Congress to reverse a major social benefit program after it has reached millions of Americans (68). Influential groups representing hospitals, doctors, nurses, and retirees oppose the bill, stating their commitment to "ensuring health care coverage is available and affordable for all" (76). America's Health Insurance Plans, the health insurance lobby, has warned leaders that changes to Medicaid funding could harm care and coverage, including behavioral health services and treatment for opioid use disorders (74). Meanwhile, many conservatives have voiced the opinion that the new bill does not go far enough in dismantling the ACA (77). Regardless, persons in need of rehabilitation are very likely to continue to face restrictions of care based on insurance considerations.

Duties of Rehabilitation Professionals

Professionals who act as "gatekeepers" to managed-care services are torn between containing medical costs and advocating for resources likely to benefit individual patients. Seventy-five percent of physicians surveyed were concerned about the ethics of financial incentives intended to restrain testing, treatment, and medical referrals. Most of those surveyed—87%—believed that physicians should be empowered to discuss limitations of treatment coverage with patients (78).

Physicians worry that balancing the care of individual patients with stewardship of collective health care resources impairs their duty of loyalty to their patients. Many feel that their patients have lost trust in them over time. Caplan agrees that gatekeeping at the bedside undermines patient ability to trust caregivers. He advocates instituting public policies to assure ethical solutions to limitations on resources for patient care (78). Standardized treatment guidelines should be coupled with provisions that enable patients who find their treatment alternatives unreasonably limited to appeal those decisions (79).

Severely disabled patients may be particularly vulnerable to economic constraints. Patients with multisystem deficits who lack information about the potential benefits of rehabilitation care may be unable to overcome a bias to limit their treatment (79). Restricted access to care may fail to remedy characteristics of disease and disability that lead to social disadvantage. In a society that fosters individualism above mutual obligations to others, persons may be at particular risk if they are deemed incapable of contributing fully to society. A just health care system would not compromise quality and length of treatment for those who have chronic impairment (80).

Rehabilitation professionals have a duty to maintain personal and professional standards of competence in their field. Appropriate behaviors for professionals in many clinical fields are defined by discipline-specific codes of ethics. The commercial interests of health care providers who have complex business relationships with pharmaceutical, assistive device, and medical equipment companies invite increasing concern. Weber et al. describe the risks posed by pharmaceutical and biomedical businesses that provide gifts, free samples, equipment, medical devices, and educational and informational programs, dinners, and retreats for medical professionals (81). Research shows that such relationships impact physicians' prescribing behavior (82). Commercial sponsorship of research, equity ownership in biomedical companies, and paid consulting relationships can create a culture of entitlement among providers. Restrictions on industry relationships and requirements for disclosure are becoming common in medical schools and teaching hospitals (83). Professional codes of ethics and business conduct must be enforced to protect the interests of patients and the integrity of professionals in a landscape of commercial interests (84,85).

Reports indicate that treatment provided in certain "joint ventures" is more costly than that delivered at similar facilities not owned by doctors. A study of doctor-owned physical therapy facilities in Florida noted a lower quality of care, fewer licensed therapists, and shorter patient treatment sessions than occurred in nonphysician-owned facilities (86).

Other interprofessional issues may raise concerns (17). Dynamics within the treatment team can hamper the effectiveness of practitioners. Appropriate safeguards enable providers to question the recommendations or conduct of their coworkers or that of colleagues in other institutions. Individual team members may need support in disputing team norms or expectations. Practitioners should be permitted to decline roles with which they are personally uncomfortable, whether for reasons of professional expertise or personal values. They also have a duty to inform patients of treatments that have been recommended for potential benefit without scientific affirmation of efficacy.

Rehabilitation institutions should strive to serve persons with disabilities within the broader community. Institutions should widen and deepen their community engagement to reinforce integration of persons with disability and society. A virtuous institution conveys morally sound values by its responsiveness to families and broader social networks at the same time that it assures skillful care of patients in a fiscally responsible environment.

At times, disability results from preventable accidents or unwise lifestyle choices. For example, alcohol or cell phone use and excessive speed may precede traffic accidents, and road injuries are more serious when seat belts or car seats are not used. Absence of helmets worsens head injuries in motorcyclists and bicyclists. Firearms produce severely disabling injuries.

The knowledge that so many of their patients have sustained disability that was preventable should mobilize rehabilitation practitioners to advocate public policies to enhance injury prevention, including gun control, helmet laws, and severe penalties against drunk driving and excessive speed. Although balancing individual rights and responsibilities with needs of the larger society is always challenging, it would seem that practitioners have an obligation to advance public policies that prevent needless disability. Certainly, rehabilitation practitioners are able to vividly describe the devastating long-term ramifications of spinal cord injury and brain injury.

Medical institutions and professional societies now include ethics topics in their educational programs. If ethics education is to be considered as important for rehabilitation students as it is for students of other disciplines, faculty members need resources and time to familiarize themselves with the study of ethics. Certain professions and specialties (such as nursing, family practice, and internal medicine) have introduced an ethics requirement into their certification requirements. Rehabilitation accrediting agencies could do likewise (17). As the number of knowledgeable and committed instructors increases, rehabilitation practitioners might add formal certification requirements in ethics for students in specialty training programs.

Continuing education in rehabilitation should emphasize the study of ethics. Some rehabilitation institutions have initiated ethics grand rounds, and others have developed ethics committees similar to those in acute care hospitals to explore issues and advance understanding through discussion and educational workshops. Such programs increase the ethical literacy of professionals.

Journal editors can encourage examination of clinical case studies and scholarly writing about policy aspects of rehabilitation. Organizers of medical ethics conferences could sponsor symposia and panel discussions on intriguing rehabilitation topics. Rehabilitation professionals could collaborate with community organizations to enhance discussion about ethical care. Education about the ethical challenges that confront patients, families, and practitioners has been noted to be invaluable for advocacy groups, institutional trustees, staff, patients, and family members (17).

SUMMARY

Rehabilitation practitioners will continue to confront significant moral challenges in the future. They must strive to ensure excellence of patient care predicated on sound scientific research and must assure that patients are treated with compassion and respect in an era dominated by financial strain and rapid technological innovation. The extent to which providers accept differences among people and the manner in which they attend to and understand patients and families are critical in today's complex and intimidating health care environment. Providing reassurance and comfort in conjunction with competent care has never been more important.

Health care practitioners have a duty to recognize and address inequities of our current medical system. As rehabilitation practitioners examine the quality and availability of medical resources, they must respond to society's failure to provide access to basic medical resources to all Americans. Rehabilitation clinicians should identify conflicts of interest in their practices and set exacting standards for professional conduct in the face of business opportunities and other temptations. Practitioners have a responsibility to ponder the role of medical rehabilitation in an era of limited resources. Conscious of the fact that some medical needs will remain unmet in a society that has other important needs, they must recognize and limit care of marginal benefit or excessive cost. They must assist in the development of sound public policy as American society attempts to balance the needs of vulnerable individuals with those of the larger society.

REFERENCES

1. Ross WD. *The Right and the Good*. Oxford: Oxford University Press; 1930.
2. Beauchamp TL, Childress JF. *Principles of Biomedical Ethics*. New York: Oxford University Press; 1989.
3. Veatch RM. *A Theory of Medical Ethics*. New York: Basic Books; 1981.
4. Beauchamp TL, McCullough LB. *Medical Ethics: The Moral Responsibilities of Physicians*. Englewood Cliffs, NJ: Prentice Hall; 1984.
5. Percival T. *Percival's Medical Ethics*. [Originally published 1803.] Reprint, Leake CD, ed. Baltimore, MD: Lippincott Williams & Wilkins; 1927.
6. Callahan D. Personal communication (Telephone Conversation, January 21, 1998).
7. The high cost of health care. *New York Times*. 2007 November 25:9.
8. Oberlander J. Learning from failure in health care reform. *N Engl J Med*. 2007;357:1677–1679.
9. Callahan D. *What Kind of Life: The Limits of Medical Progress*. New York: Simon & Schuster; 1990.
10. Dutton DB. *Worse than the Disease: Pitfalls of Medical Progress*. Cambridge: Cambridge University Press; 1988.
11. Haas JF. Ethics in rehabilitation medicine. *Arch Phys Med Rehabil*. 1986;67:270–271.
12. deLateur BJ. Fostering research in the physiatrist's future. *Arch Phys Med Rehabil*. 1990;71:1–2.
13. Brody BA. Justice in allocation of public resources to disabled citizens. *Arch Phys Med Rehabil*. 1988;69:333–336.
14. Callahan D. Families as care givers: the limits of morality. *Arch Phys Med Rehabil*. 1988;69:323–328.
15. Caplan AL. Informed consent and provider-patient relationships in rehabilitation medicine. *Arch Phys Med Rehabil*. 1988;69:312–317.
16. Haas JF. Admission to rehabilitation centers: selection of patients. *Arch Phys Med Rehabil*. 1988;69:329–332.
17. Caplan AL, Callahan D, Haas J. Ethical and policy issues in rehabilitation medicine. *Hastings Cent Rep*. 1987;17(suppl 4):1–20.
18. Jennings B, Callahan D, Caplan AL. Ethical challenges of chronic illness. *Hastings Cent Rep*. 1988;18(special suppl):1–16.
19. Purtilo RB. Ethical issues in teamwork: the context of rehabilitation. *Arch Phys Med Rehabil*. 1988;69:318–322.
20. Haas JF, MacKenzie CA. The role of ethics in rehabilitation medicine. *Am J Phys Med Rehabil*. 1993;72:48–51.
21. Callahan D. Allocating health care resources: the vexing case of rehabilitation. *Am J Phys Med Rehabil*. 1993;72:101–105.
22. Meier RH III, Purtilo RB. Ethical issues and the patient-provider relationship. *Am J Phys Med Rehabil*. 1994;72:365–366.
23. Strax TE. Ethical issues of treating patients with AIDS in a rehabilitation setting. *Am J Phys Med Rehabil*. 1994;73:293–295.
24. Purtilo RB, Meier RH III. Team challenges: regulatory constraints and patient empowerment. *Am J Phys Med Rehabil*. 1993;72:327–330.
25. Haas J. Ethical considerations of goal setting for patient care in rehabilitation medicine. *Am J Phys Med Rehabil*. 1993;72:228–232.
26. Venesy BA. A clinician's guide to decision making capacity and ethically sound medical decisions. *Am J Phys Med Rehabil*. 1994;73:219–226.
27. Jennings B. Healing the self: the moral meaning of relationships in rehabilitation. *Am J Phys Med Rehabil*. 1993;72:401–404.
28. Haas JF. Ethical issues in physical medicine and rehabilitation: conclusion to a series. *Am J Phys Med Rehabil*. 1995;74(1 suppl):54–58.
29. Haas JF, Mattson Prince J. Ethics and managed care in rehabilitation medicine. *J Head Trauma Rehabil*. 1997;12:vii–xiii.
30. Englehardt HT Jr. *The Foundations of Medical Ethics*. New York: Oxford University Press; 1986.
31. Acton N. The world's response to disability: evolution of a philosophy. *Arch Phys Med Rehabil*. 1982;63:145–149.
32. Kirschner KL, Stocking C, Wagner LB, et al. Ethical issues identified by rehabilitation clinicians. *Arch Phys Med Rehabil*. 2001;82(suppl 2):S2–S8.
33. Redman BK, Fry ST. Ethical conflicts reported by certified registered rehabilitation nurses. *Rehabil Nurs*. 1998;23:179–184.
34. Gluck A, Blackman J. The future of Obamacare. *Philadelphia Inquirer*. 2016 March 5:C1.
35. Gornick M, Eggers P, Reilly TW, et al. Effects of race on mortality and use of services among Medicare beneficiaries. *N Engl J Med*. 1996;335:791–799.
36. Kottke FJ, Lehman JF, Stillwell GK. Preface. In: Kottke FJ, Stillwell GK, Lehman JF, eds. *Krusen's Handbook of Physical Medicine and Rehabilitation*. 3rd ed. Philadelphia, PA: WB Saunders; 1982:xi–xix.
37. De Vellis RF, Sauter SVH. Recognizing the challenges of prevention in rehabilitation. *Arch Phys Med Rehabil*. 1985;66:52–54.
38. Englehardt HT Jr, Rie MA. Intensive care units, scarce resources, and conflicting principles of justice. *JAMA*. 1986;255:1159–1164.
39. Becker MC, Abrams KS, Onder J. Goal setting: joint patient-staff method. *Arch Phys Med Rehabil*. 1974;55:87–89.
40. Kottke FJ. Future focus of rehabilitation medicine. *Arch Phys Med Rehabil*. 1980;61:1–6.
41. Wallace SG, Anderson AD. Imprisonment of patients in the course of rehabilitation. *Arch Phys Med Rehabil*. 1978;59:424–429.
42. Trieschmann RB. Coping with a disability: a sliding scale of goals. *Arch Phys Med Rehabil*. 1974;55:556–560.
43. Anderson TP. Educational frame of reference: an additional model for rehabilitation medicine. *Arch Phys Med Rehabil*. 1978;59:203–206.
44. Macciocchi SN, Stringer A. Assessing risk and harm: the convergence of ethical and empirical considerations. *Arch Phys Med Rehabil*. 2001;82(suppl 2):S15–S19.
45. Tauber AI. Putting ethics into the medical record. *Ann Intern Med*. 2002;36:559–563.
46. Callahan CD, Hagglund KJ. Comparing neuropsychological and psychiatric evaluation of competency in rehabilitation: a case example. *Arch Phys Med Rehabil*. 1995;76:909–912.
47. Malec JF. Ethical conflict resolution based on ethics of relationships for brain injury rehabilitation. *Brain Inj*. 1996;10:781–795.
48. Booth J, Davidson I, Winstanley J, et al. Observing washing and dressing of stroke patients: nursing intervention compared with occupational therapists. What is the difference? *J Adv Nurs*. 2001;33:98–105.
49. Lubin IM. *Chronic Illness: Impact and Interventions*. Boston, MA: Jones & Bartlett; 1990:200–217.
50. Holmqvist LW, von Koch L, de Pedro-Cuesta J. Use of healthcare, impact on family caregivers and patient satisfaction of rehabilitation at home after stroke in southwest Stockholm. *Scand J Rehabil Med*. 2000;32:173–179.
51. Rusk HA. Rehabilitation medicine: knowledge in search of understanding. *Arch Phys Med Rehabil*. 1978;59:156–160.
52. Diener E. Subjective well-being. *Psychol Bull*. 1984;95:542–575.
53. van Dijk AJ. Quality of life assessment: its integration in rehabilitation care through a model of daily living. *Scand J Rehabil Med*. 2000;32:104–110.
54. Montgomery H, Persson L-O. Importance and attainment of life values among disabled and non-disabled people. *Scand J Rehabil Med*. 1998;30:61–63.
55. Anderson G, Knickman JR. Changing the chronic care system to meet people's needs. *Health Aff (Millwood)*. 2001;20(6):46–60.
56. Churchill LR. *Rationing Health Care in America: Perceptions and Principles of Justice*. Notre Dame, IN: University of Notre Dame Press; 1987.
57. Mankiw NG. Beyond those health care numbers. *New York Times*. 2007 November 4:4.
58. Dalen JE. Health care in America. *Arch Intern Med*. 2000;160:2573–2576.
59. Bayer R, Caplan A, Daniels N, eds. *In Search of Equity: Health Needs and the Health Care System*. New York: Plenum; 1983.
60. America's lagging health care system. *New York Times*. 2007 November 8:A26.
61. Carroll A. Why U.S. still trails many Nations in access to care. *New York Times*. 2016 October 24:A16.

62. Pear R. States differ widely in spending on health care, study finds. *New York Times*. 2007 September 18:A28.

63. Kolata G. Research suggests more health care may not be better. *New York Times*. 2002 July 21:1.

64. Himmelstein DU, Woolhandler S. I am not a health reform. *New York Times*. 2007 December 15:A25.

65. The Massachusetts way. *New York Times*. 2008 August 30:A18.

66. Baker CD, Caplan A, Davis K, et al. Health of the nation—coverage for all Americans. *N Engl J Med*. 2008;359(8):777–780.

67. Morrissey S, Curfman GD, Drazen JM. Health of the nation—coverage for all Americans. *N Engl J Med*. 2008;359(8):855–856.

68. Goldstein A, DeBonis M, Snell K. House GOP releases its plan. *Philadelphia Inquirer*. 2016 March 7:A1.

69. Rosenbaum S. Medicaid and insuring the poor—where are we heading? *N Engl J Med*. 2016;375:1405–1407.

70. Sanger-Katz M, Bui Q. Visualizing Obamacare. Where people lack health insurance. *New York Times*. 2016 November 1:A18.

71. Frean M, Gruber J, Sommers BD. Disentangling the ACA's coverage effects—lessons for policymakers. *N Engl J Med*. 2016;375:1605–1608.

72. Park H. Republicans' changes to medicaid could have larger impact than their changes to Obamacare. *New York Times*. 2017 March 9:A16.

73. Pear R, Kaplan T. GOP health bill trades mandate for tax credits. *New York Times*. 2017 March 7:A1.

74. Sanger-Katz M. Meager support for blend of policy in replacement bill. *New York Times*. 2017 March 9:A16.

75. Goodnough A, Pear R, Kaplan T. Health groups unite to oppose Republican Bill. *New York Times*. 2017 March 9:A1.

76. Goodnough A, Abelson R. Analysts say millions risk losing coverage in GOP health plan. *New York Times*. 2017 March 8:A15.

77. Haberman M, Pear R. Trump jumps in trying to propel health care bill. *New York Times*. 2017 March 10:A1.

78. Caplan AL. The ethics of gatekeeping in rehabilitation medicine. *J Head Trauma Rehabil*. 1997;12:29–36.

79. Banja J. Values, function and managed care: an ethical analysis. *J Head Trauma Rehabil*. 1997;12:60–70.

80. Weber LJ, Wayland MT, Holton B. Health care professionals and industry: reducing conflicts of interest and established best practices. *Arch Phys Med Rehabil*. 2001;82(12 suppl 2):S20–S24.

81. Campbell EG. Doctors and drug companies—scrutinizing influential relationships. *N Engl J Med*. 2007;357:1796–1797.

82. Brennan TA, Rothman DJ, Blank L, et al. Health industry practices that create conflicts of interest: a policy proposal from academic medical centers. *JAMA*. 2006;295:429–433.

83. Angell M. Is academic medicine for sale? *N Engl J Med*. 2000;342:1516–1518.

84. Drazen JM, Curfman GD. Financial associations of authors. *N Engl J Med*. 2002;346:1901–1902.

85. Pear R. Study says fees are often higher when doctor has stake in clinic. *New York Times*. 1991 August 9:1.

86. Thobaben J. The moral character of rehabilitation institutions. *J Head Trauma Rehabil*. 1997;12:60–70.

International Aspects of the Practice of Physical Medicine and Rehabilitation[1]

Not chaos-like, together crushed and bruised, But, as the world harmoniously confused:
Where order in variety we see, And where, though all things differ, all agree.

Alexander Pope (1688–1744), Windsor Forest, 13

Physical medicine and rehabilitation (PMR), physical and rehabilitation medicine (PRM), rehabilitation medicine (RM), and physiatry are alternative terms used to describe "the primary medical specialty responsible for the prevention, medical diagnosis, treatment and rehabilitation management of persons of all ages with disabling health conditions and their co-morbidities, specifically addressing their impairments and activity limitations in order to facilitate their physical and cognitive functioning (including behavior), participation (including quality of life) and modifying personal and environmental factors" (1). A medical doctor specialized in PRM is named as physiatrist (1).

In his lecture at the first World Congress of the International Federation of Physical Medicine, Frank Krusen, in 1952, in London (United Kingdom), cited a consensus of the participants by saying, "Rehabilitation has become established as a new medical discipline which aims at restoration of the physically handicapped person...to normal life; that physicians should avoid an attitude of hopelessness or passive acceptance in the face of chronic illness or disability; that a dynamic approach to chronic illness frequently results in restoration of the chronically ill patient to a fair measure of self-sufficiency, self-respect and happiness; that physicians should be interested not only in adding years to life but also in adding life to years;...the physician should always consider the psychological as well physical problems" (2).

This chapter deals with several aspects of the development of the practice of PRM, including the role of the International Society of Physical and Rehabilitation Medicine (ISPRM) in the harmonization of the specialty worldwide.

HISTORY

PMR in its more modern modalities is nearly a century old. Its development as a medical specialty was linked to historical events that promoted a large number of disabilities, such as the World Wars in the first half of the last century, as well as the poliomyelitis epidemic. However, the use of physical agents, based on heat, cold and water, massage, and physical exercise, can be traced back to centuries before Christ. Archeologists discovered that, 100,000 years B.C., in Slovakia, Neanderthal women used to sink their bodies into thermal mineral springs (3). Spa treatments have been practiced by the Aztecs in Mexico and were very popular among the Greeks and the Romans.

The Americas

North America: United States and Canada

Within the United States and Canada, PMR is a medical specialty approved by the Accreditation Council for Graduate Medical Education that emphasizes prevention, diagnosis, and treatment of persons with disabilities who experience restrictions in functioning resulting from disease, injury, or symptom exacerbation. Practitioners of PMR are known as "physiatrists" and utilize a holistic and team-oriented treatment approach, which often combines medication, injections, exercise, physical modalities, and education customized to the patient's unique requirements (4). PMR specialists offer care for persons with neuromuscular disorders who have acute and chronic disabilities. The overriding goal of PMR is to optimize patient functioning in all domains of life, including the medical, emotional, social, and vocational spheres.

As in the most of Western Countries, the field of PMR, in the United States, traces its origins to the mid-20th century when a seismic shift in thinking among health care providers occurred. Due to the burgeoning numbers of wounded and injured soldiers emanating from the war, a new emphasis was placed on the value of comprehensive, team-oriented care for people with disabilities of all types. The critical importance of ministering to and caring for people with disabilities all across America soon came to be recognized as an essential societal and ethical obligation.

During the early days of PMR, the specialization was actually divided into two separate and distinct areas: "physical

---

[1]The medical specialty of Physical Medicine and Rehabilitation (PMR) is referred to as such in the USA and Canada. In other parts of the world (i.e., Europe, Asia, and many other international locations), the field is frequently referred to as Physical and Rehabilitation Medicine (PRM). For the purpose of uniformity and convention throughout this chapter, the specialty will be listed as PMR for when referring to the USA and Canada and PRM in other locations.

medicine" and "rehabilitation" (4). Frank Krusen (1898–1973), the author of the first rehabilitation textbook and the founder of the first residency training program in physical medicine (at the Mayo Clinic), is largely credited for his pioneering role in physical medicine, which focused on the use of electricity, heat, light, mechanotherapy, exercise, and other modalities in the alleviation of disease and disability. Frank Krusen was the first to originate the name "physiatrist," to differentiate physical medicine physicians from physical therapists.

Almost simultaneously, another physician, Howard Rusk (1901–1989), responding to the need for help with the medical and functional restoration of wounded, disabled soldiers returning from active duty, started the field of rehabilitation within the United States. His pioneering efforts resulted in the establishment of one of the first comprehensive inpatient rehabilitation hospitals—the Rusk Institute of Rehabilitation Medicine at the New York University.

Within the United States, physical medicine was recognized as a medical specialty in 1947, with the establishment of the American Board of Physical Medicine and, in 1949, the word "rehabilitation" was added to the name. Over the years, PMR as practiced in the United States has evolved steadily. During the 1980s and 1990s, inpatient rehabilitation remained the mainstay of physiatric practice. More recently, there has been an increased shift in emphasis toward outpatient services.

PMR has prospered as a medical specialization, not only in mainland United States but also in its territories. In Puerto Rico, for example, physiatry has grown by leaps and bounds. Herman Flax, one of the early pioneers of PMR in Puerto Rico, chronicled the history and development of the field over a 25-year period (5).

The pathway to becoming a board-certified physiatrist in the United States begins in medical school. After completing 4 years of medical school, the medical school graduate enters an internship, which is a 1-year sequence of coordinated rotations emphasizing basic medical skills within a transitional environment or an accredited training program in internal medicine, surgery, pediatrics, family medicine, obstetrics and gynecology, or some combination thereof. The 1-year internship period is followed by a 3-year residency training program in PMR. At the conclusion of the 3-year residency, the qualifying graduate takes a board exam administered by the American Board of Physical Medicine and Rehabilitation (ABPM&R). Once this exam is successfully completed, the graduate takes another exam, the oral board, at the conclusion of the first year of practice. Recertification is required of each graduate every 10 years.

An increasing number of PMR residency graduates are choosing to pursue accredited fellowship training in PMR subspecializations by the ABPM&R including Spinal Cord Injury (SCI), Pediatrics, Pain Medicine, Neuromuscular Medicine, Hospice and Palliative Care, Brain Injury, and Sports Medicine. Other nonaccredited fellowships exist in many areas. The typical duration of these fellowships is between 1 and 3 years.

With the aim of promoting the growth of education, training and research opportunities in PMR, in 1967, the Association of Academic Physiatrists (AAP) was founded by a group of academic physiatrists led by Ernest W. Johnson (6).

While the field as a whole continues to carry on its noble mission of providing quality, compassionate care for people with disabilities of all types, the specialization faces a major challenge from some insurers and third-party payers who have steadily decreased reimbursement. In addition, shrinkage of the allotted lengths of stay for a growing number of diagnostic categories has taken place. An illustrative example of this is that of an acute stroke patient who is allotted on average approximately 14 to 21 days of acute hospital rehabilitation prior to community discharge. Unlike many parts of the world, where such patients would be treated for 2 to 3 months, the US system of care offers much shorter lengths of stay.

Another major change and challenge has been the advent of prospective payment systems (7) for acute care hospitalization, which has led to a shifting of patient care from the acute rehabilitation setting where rehabilitation is delivered in a focused concentrated fashion for approximately 3 hours a day to a subacute environment where the rehabilitation is less intense and often is of a "nursing home style" vintage. Throughout the United States, in order to promote vertical integration of health delivery systems, hospitals have transformed acute care beds into subacute care beds. In addition, many hospitals have purchased subacute care facilities including nursing homes and convalescence centers, which serve a "surrogate rehabilitation" role.

Apart from the academic or hospital-based physiatric programs, an increasing number of private practice physiatrists (both solo practice and group practice) have now elected to focus a significant portion of their practice on pain management. This has occurred because of economic factors and arguably may pose a major threat to the roots and traditions of the field, since there may now be an evolving and diminishing number of available physiatrists to care for people with traditional disabilities such as stroke, SCI, and traumatic brain injury (TBI).

Within the educational and residency training realm, a growing and unprecedented number of graduating residents are pursuing fellowship training in PMR. Although some are restricting their practice, many still recognize the importance of remaining diversified and being prepared to care for persons with all types of disabilities. Since people with traditional disabilities (e.g., stroke, SCI, and TBI) occupy an essential and ever-growing portion of the health care bandwidth in the United States, rehabilitation "generalists" are very much in demand. A physiatrist's higher calling of transcendent care and impassioned advocacy for persons with disabilities was recently noted: "As practitioners of the healing art, we are often swept away by the mundane minutiae of providing expert technical care to our patients. Often overlooked (however) is the human side of caring—that transcendent sense of seeing life through the eyes of our patients" (8).

The field of PMR continues to thrive and prosper within the United States because of the synergy that it has engendered with other medical specialties and related rehabilitation disciplines. Since rehabilitation is recognized as a team effort, major bridges have been built with rehabilitation professionals across the spectrum including physical therapy, occupational therapy, speech and language pathology, recreational therapy, psychology, as well as rehabilitation nursing. More institutional and academic departments have integrated programs creating a fertile milieu for cross-disciplinary and trans-disciplinary integration.

Much like its Southern neighbor, Canada prides itself in providing quality, focused, functional-based care for citizens with disabilities. In Canada, after the completion of medical school (typically 4 years), physicians enter residency training through the Canadian Resident Matching Service.

The Royal College of Physicians and Surgeons of Canada (RCPSC) accredits the postgraduate education programs for physiatrists. The program consists of 5 years of specialty education. During the first year, residents complete their basic clinical training. This consists of several off-service rotations, including internal medicine, surgery, as well as additional 1-month electives. This is then followed by 4 years of training in both physiatry and additional rotations, which are pertinent to physiatry (neurology, orthopedics, rheumatology, etc.). During their final year, residents complete the Royal College certification examination. This consists of both a written component and an Objective Structured Clinical Examination. In contrast to the United States, both components of the examination are completed in the residents' final year. Following successful completion of this examination, the physician is awarded the designation: Fellow of the RCPSC.

Most physiatry residents also choose to complete 6 months of neuromuscular disease/electromyography training during their residency. This allows them to sit for the Canadian Society of Clinical Neurophysiologists Electromyography examination, which is administered to both physiatry and neurology residents. As Royal College certified specialists, all physiatrists must participate in the RCPSC Maintenance of Certification program and must accumulate 400 hours of continuous medical education (CME) credits over a 5-year cycle.

The Canadian Association of Physical Medicine and Rehabilitation (CAPM&R) (19) is the national organization for physiatrists in Canada. Its main goals are to promote education, scientific collaboration, and practice development among physiatrists. A 2006 survey by the CAPM&R indicated that 53% of physiatrists are in private practice. Of those, one third do not carry inpatients. Seventy-eight percent of physiatrists have clinical or academic university appointments. Similar to the United States, there has been a shift in the practice patterns of physiatrists to an outpatient focus. The inpatient system is moving toward a model where hospitalists/family physicians are the attending physicians of record and physiatrists act as the consultant.

In contrast to the United States, where health care is more managed care driven, Canada has a universal health care system. In this model, every citizen has equal access to health care and is fully insured by the government for all medically necessary care. This has both advantages and drawbacks with respect to the inpatient system. It ensures that anyone who benefits from rehabilitation services will be given the opportunity to participate in a program. Another advantage is that inpatient length of stay varies depending on the needs of the patient, and this is decided by the physiatrist and the rehabilitation team. For example, in the stroke population, the average length of stay in Canada is longer than that in the United States (40 days) (10). By contrast, a drawback of Canada's social system is that wait times can be prolonged compared to the United States; the time from onset of stroke to inpatient rehabilitation admission is an average of 29 days (median: 15 days).

Latin America

In Latin America, the main impetus for the development of PRM was the outburst of epidemics of transmissible illnesses such as poliomyelitis, which is now eradicated in many of this region's countries. This brought about an improvement in sanitary conditions and a rapid development of rehabilitation as a medical specialty. These phenomena emerged simultaneously in many Latin American countries.

European countries and the United States served as models for many of the Latin American rehabilitation systems. Therefore, the development of PRM followed the same pattern, being the area of expertise, initially, predominantly focused on aspects of physical medicine, and later on, RM started to develop as well. A continuous demand for the improvement in sanitary conditions and the possibilities for the development of the rehabilitation field at the national level hastened the development of these therapeutic modalities in this part of the world.

Scientific societies of PMR were being established in the individual countries of Latin America and the Caribbean in the 1940s and 1950s; consequently, the need of a Latin American Association that would bring these societies under one umbrella organization was recognized, and in 1961, the Asociación Médica Latinoamericana de Rehabilitación (AMLAR) was established (11).

Latin America spans a large area with respect to political, geographic, demographic, and epidemiologic aspects. This is the reason for the varied degrees in the implementation of the PRM and access to technology in the Latin American health systems. The demographic projections for Latin America and the Caribbean show that there will be progressive and dynamic changes during the course of the next 40 years. These trends show a shift in the demographic profile, with significant aging of the population, due to a decrease in the birth rate and an increase in life expectancy for those over 60 years of age.

This demographic change has a consequence from the epidemiologic point of view. A growth in the elderly population will increase the prevalence of chronic nontransmissible illnesses. There is also a multiplication in the occurrence of nontransmissible illnesses linked to trauma and habits of life (accidents, social violence, accidents at work, and addiction) that coexist in the region with the transmissible illnesses. The increased number of high-risk newborns, along with malnutrition, and the societal exclusion of indigenous ethnic groups (12), all contribute to the increase in the demand for qualified PRM practitioners. The growing need for rehabilitation professionals being trained to the highest standards and continuing their training after certification with a CME program, are the main focus of the Scientific Societies of Rehabilitation and Physical Medicine of each country and AMLAR (13).

PRM has developed in Latin American countries but not uniformly. The availability of rehabilitation facilities is found in 78% of the countries. There is specific legislation regarding rehabilitative medicine in 62% of them and implementation of specific programs in 51%. The field is further hindered by very limited documentation of relevant data and limited research work. The practitioners are either specialists in rehabilitation or technicians consisting mainly of physical therapists, in addition to speech-pathologists, psychologists, nurses, social workers, and occupational therapists. The medical schools and colleges offer little training and teaching in the field of rehabilitation. In addition to the abovementioned factors, there are additional roadblocks to the progress of PRM in Latin America. Some of those problems are that there are too few practitioners of PRM in most countries; people with disabilities have a hard time integrating themselves into society; the private sector plays a preeminent role in the health care systems and is reluctant to pay for rehabilitative medicine (12); and large sections of the population do not have accessibility to medical aid, let alone to rehabilitation facilities. There is a distinct association among disability, poverty, and social exclusion.

Rehabilitation in Uruguay prospered thanks to the efforts of a group of prominent Uruguayan professionals who completed their medical training abroad and the timely, determined, and intelligent action of others who understood the necessity to manage disability (14). Among the others, Álvaro Ferrari Forcade made great contributions to rehabilitation realizing that there was a need for a functional measurement tool to assess the patient's status. He developed a scale that registers the patient's functional clinical state in three basic categories: somatic, psychological, and social (15). It represented the first functional measure of disability developed in Latin America.

RM as a medical specialty was strengthened by unifying approaches to rehabilitative medicine, which took place at the study group on The Training of Specialists, summoned by the Pan American Health Organization (PAHO) in Santiago, Chile, in October 1969 (15).

There are three basic models of rehabilitative care in Latin America: (a) hospitals of acute care, (b) rehabilitation centers, and (c) community-based rehabilitation (CBR). Most countries have an emphasis on one of these models and subsequently affect the specialist's profile in each country. Uruguay is an example of a country that uses the rehabilitative model based on hospitals of acute care while promoting the interdisciplinary approach of the rehabilitation. They have recently started to work on rehabilitation centers related to pediatric care. Argentina and Chile have developed the models based on hospitals of acute care and rehabilitation centers. Nicaragua, El Salvador, Colombia, Argentina, and Guyana have developed the model based on CBR. Together with the help of nongovernmental organizations (NGOs), the respective governments are developing this model in Mexico, Ecuador, Peru, and Bolivia. Brazil is a remarkable example where all three models are used. The multidisciplinary diagnostic and therapeutic approach of disability treatment in Brazil has been an important factor in the development of rehabilitation in this country. The Rehabilitation Institute of the Hospital das Clinicas of Sao Paulo, the Associação Brasileira Beneficente de Reabilitação (ABBR) in Rio de Janeiro, and the Rehabilitation Institute of San Salvador were pivotal academic training sites in the specialty of rehabilitative medicine for Brazil and also for the region. In the early 1970s, Brazil was one of the first countries that developed a residency program in rehabilitation training (16). This residency program was used as a model for other such programs in others countries of the region.

The technology used in rehabilitation has improved from the 1990s in several countries, such as Argentina, Chile, Brazil, Colombia, and Mexico, especially in the field of orthopedic and neurologic rehabilitation. Improvements in these countries had a positive effect throughout the region, in the practice of the specialty, in the academic training programs, and in the makeup of the specialist's profile.

Recently, AMLAR has begun to work toward unifying the specialist doctor's profile in the different countries of Latin America. They are trying to achieve this through the Societies of PRM of the individual countries, as well as in the specialist doctor's CME, the professional certification, and certificate reexamination.

RM has developed differently in the various Latin American countries in accordance with various policies, legislative aspects, and technologic developments. In the last decade, Latin America has improved its epidemiologic data acquisition to make sure that the data are both more detailed and more uniformed for comparison purposes. A better understanding of the concept of disability in all its aspects starting from the problems in functioning, of integration and participation in society in general, and by using better epidemiologic sources seems to be the way toward standardizing and harmonizing the approaches used. This in turn will hopefully lead to the development of better policies and programs of rehabilitation and improve the integration of the medical rehabilitation specialty in each of the country's health care systems.

Europe, Eastern Mediterranean, and Africa

Europe and Eastern Mediterranean

In 1907, it was held in Rome the Second International Congress of Physio-Therapy, at the time mainly organized by radiologists (17). After the conference, several textbooks on physical therapy were published in Italy and in many other countries. In 1931, in Italy and in Germany, there was a push to deal with accidents in the workplace, which led to the development of functional restoration and prosthesis. The terms used at the time were physiotherapy and physical medicine. In the 1950s, the terms recovery and rehabilitation became popular as well. The areas of clinical application of rehabilitation expanded to include the management of disabled children, traumatic lesions and injuries, peripheral and central neurologic traumas, and degenerative diseases.

Education in rehabilitation was opened to both physicians and other rehabilitation-related professionals, such as masseurs and physiotherapists. In 1962, the European Union of Medical Specialists (UEMS) (18) recognized physical medicine as an autonomous discipline under the name of PRM. During that period, there was the development and the diffusion of many rehabilitative methodologies, such as Brunnstrom, Vojta, Bobath, Kabat, Salvini-Perfetti, Maigne, and others methods.

The development of the field was favored by the creation of the first national societies of PRM in Italy, France, Portugal, Belgium, and the Netherlands. Their development was parallel to the organization of the European political bodies. In 1963, the "Fédération Européenne de Médecine Physique et Réadaptation," that is, the European Federation of Physical Medicine and Rehabilitation (EFPMR) was founded in Brussels, with an officializing act by the Royal Belgian Bulletin. It initially grouped together the five national societies that were already present in the continent, and in 2003, it was transformed into a society, the European Society of Physical and Rehabilitation Medicine (ESPRM) (19), with 21 National European Societies included at the time, and 35 National Societies members now. In 1969, it was created the "Académie Médicale Européenne de Médecine de Réadaptation," that is, the European Academy of Rehabilitation Medicine (EARM) (20); in 1971 the PRM Section of the European Union of Medical Specialists (UEMS PRM) (21); and in 1991 the European College of PRM to act as the European Board (21).

The ESPRM has the following aims: (a) to be the leading scientific European Society for physicians in the field of PRM, (b) to improve the knowledge of fundamentals and the management of activities, participation, and contextual factors of people with a disability, and (c) to improve and maintain a strong connection between research and clinical practice in PRM (22). The society offers individual membership to all eligible PRM specialists and federated membership to the national PRM societies in Europe. The ESPRM organizes biennial scientific congresses.

The EARM is a European body including up to 50 senior PRM academicians across Europe. Members are invited on the basis of their distinguished contribution to the specialty, particularly to its humanitarian aspects. The aim of the Académie is to improve all areas of rehabilitation for the benefit of those who need it; its motto is "Societatis vir origo ac finis" (Man is both the source and the goal of society) (23).

The Section of UEMS PRM has as main purposes the promotion of PRM as a specialty in a professional capacity and the harmonization of the specialty at European level through specialist training and continuing professional development (CPD) through a validation and revalidation process. The European representatives work to develop clinical standards in practice and to help facilitate the required research. They are accountable (as with other specialties) to the UEMS and have started to work closely with the European Commission and the Council of Europe. They have three main committees under an Executive Committee: (a) the PRM Training and Education Committee (the European Board of PRM), (b) the Clinical Affairs Committee (responsible for the accreditation of the quality of clinical care in PRM), and (c) the Professional Practice Committee (responsible for defining and protecting the Field of Competence of the PRM physicians) (24).

One of the first areas of research in rehabilitation, developed in Europe, involved the treatment of scoliosis, the care and treatment of subjects with war amputations and work injuries, and the thousands of cases of poliomyelitis that were prevalent in the 1950s.

An important sprout to the growth of PRM in Europe, but not only, has been given by the publication of the International Classification of Impairment, Disability, and Handicap (ICIDH) in 1980 (25) but above all by the International Classification of Functioning, Disability, and Health (ICF), which was approved by the World Health Organization (WHO) in 2001 (26).

Rehabilitation, both on an individual and a population level, must represent the meeting point between scientific and epidemiologic evidence. Using indicators of health in different countries (e.g., the European community as a whole), it is possible to list the priorities of possible interventions in relation to their efficacy. The WHO's ICF is nowadays the best instrument, on both clinical and community levels, for integrating individual and population data. It offers a uniform methodology of interpretation and representation for all the determinants of the health status of a person and of a population. The European Union provides the means for representing and collating all the data on the health of its member countries, in scientific, administrative, social policy, cultural, educational, and occupational terms (27).

In 1989, the European Bodies of PRM published the first White Book of PRM (28), a second edition was prepared in 2006 (29,30), and a more recent edition has just come out (31). The White Book of PRM represents a reference text for PRM physicians in Europe.

In Italy and in other European countries, it has become central for PRM the Individual Rehabilitation Plan, which represents the pathway for reaching an optimal state of well-being, participation, and health, combining the skills and duties of the various members of the rehabilitation team and the different instruments and settings along the continuum of care. In Italy, in 2011, the Ministry of Health published, with the support of the Italian Society of PRM among others, the Italian Rehabilitation Plan that defines the guidelines for the development of the local rehabilitation policies including (a) the collection of disability and rehabilitation data, (b) the necessity to use the bio-psycho-social model of ICF as a framework for rehabilitation, (c) the team work, (d) the continuum of care, (e) the research in rehabilitation, and (f) the health and rehabilitation finances (32).

From an educational point of view, PRM is an independent medical specialty in almost all European countries, except Denmark and Malta, but its name and focus vary according to different national traditions and laws. Training usually lasts for between 4 and 6 years depending on the country. The number of specialists per inhabitants is not uniform throughout Europe. It ranges from a low of less than 0.5 per 100,000 inhabitants in the United Kingdom and Ireland to more than 4.5 per 100,000 inhabitants in Portugal and the Czech Republic. Specialists in PRM have the freedom of mobility across UEMS member states but require certification from the national training authorities, as any other medical specialty. Those with national certification are eligible to be certified by the European Board of PRM. The European Board of PRM has developed a comprehensive system of postgraduate education for PRM specialists that consists of the following: (a) a curriculum for postgraduate education containing basic knowledge and the application of PRM in specific health conditions; (b) a standardized training course of at least 4 years in a PRM department and detailed documentation in a uniform official logbook; (c) a single written annual examination throughout Europe; (d) a system of national managers for training and accreditation to foster good contacts with trainees in their country; (e) standard rules for the accreditation of trainers and a standard process of certification; (f) quality control of training sites performed by site visits of accredited specialists; and (g) CPD and CME within the UEMS. Recertification has to occur every 10 years. In April 2018, at its general meeting in Marrakesh, the UEMS Council approved the European Training Requirements in Physical and Rehabilitation Medicine (33).

A PRM specialist can either perform or prescribe the given interventions: (a) medical interventions (medications and practical procedures); (b) physical treatments (manual therapy, kinesiotherapy and exercise therapy, electrotherapy, and other types of physical treatments including ultrasound, heat and cold applications, phototherapy, hydrotherapy and balneotherapy, diathermy, massage therapy, and lymph therapy); (c) occupational therapy; (d) speech and language therapy, dysphagia management, and nutritional therapy; (e) neuropsychological interventions and psychological assessment and interventions, including counseling; (f) disability equipment, assistive technology, prosthetics, orthotics, and technical supports and aids; (g) patient education; and (h) rehabilitation nursing.

PRM specialists work in both public and private health services. This varies between different European countries, with Austria, Czech Republic, Greece, and Switzerland being the countries with the highest percentage of private practice.

An important event for the development of rehabilitation in the eastern Mediterranean area was the foundation of the Mediterranean Forum of Physical and Rehabilitation Medicine (MFPRM) (34). In the early 1990s, rehabilitation experts from around the Mediterranean Basin expressed their wish to promote PRM and rehabilitation services in the Mediterranean countries. They wanted to create an organization to unite them as a family, a mechanism for mutual help and for strengthening their relationships. The first step was taken in Israel by Haim Ring who proposed to the Israeli Association of PRM to organize the first Mediterranean Congress in Herzliya, Israel. This 1st Mediterranean Congress of PRM took place in May 1996. The symbol chosen for the Congress was a map of the Mediterranean Basin with a dove of peace flying above and the motto of "rehabilitation without frontiers" underneath. About 500 people from 42 countries from all world continents participated. The Mediterranean Basin was especially well represented with participants from 11 countries. During that congress, it was decided to hold a meeting every 2 years to reinforce the alliance among Mediterranean countries. The number of participants grew from one conference to another, and more importantly, the number of representatives from Mediterranean countries continued to grow steadily. During the 3rd Mediterranean Congress of PRM, in 2000, in Athens (Greece), the MFPRM was created, and during a general assembly of the 4th Mediterranean Congress, the MFPRM statute was accepted. MFPRM mission and goals are (a) to be the scientific Mediterranean body for physicians who work in the field of PRM in the countries surrounding the Mediterranean Sea as well as adjacent countries, (b) to facilitate the exchange of information regarding different aspects of rehabilitation research, multicenter trials, national and regional projects, and meetings and congresses throughout the Mediterranean Basin, (c) to organize the Mediterranean Congress of PRM in one of the countries that has active members in the Forum every 2 years, and (d) to cooperate with the national society of PRM to influence governments to support initiatives and collaborations in the field of PRM. The MFPRM membership is open to all qualified physicians specialized in PRM working in one of the countries bordering the Mediterranean Sea or in one of the adjacent countries. Membership is free to all (35,36). At an educational level, an important initiative born inside the MFPRM was the foundation of the Euro-Mediterranean Rehabilitation PRM School (37). Since its first edition in November 2005, the School is held each year in Siracusa (Italy), thanks to the efforts of its Director, Franco Cirillo, and to the financial contribution of Sicilian entities, the Italian Society of PRM and more recently of the PRM European Bodies. The Scientific Committee is made up of Italian and Euro-Mediterranean Members. The School lasts 4 days (usually from Monday to Thursday), and it is free of charge (including accommodation and food) for

a certain number of students, depending on the yearly budget. Every year, a different topic is selected, and experts on the topic are invited to hold both lectures and practical activities.

Several Middle-Eastern countries, such as Kuwait, Saudi Arabia, and Iraq, have been strongly engaged in the development of RM.

In Kuwait, there is a very active PMR Society that has organized several scientific events. There is a big hospital specialized in PRM with more than 80 beds dedicated to rehabilitation. It caters to persons with various physical disabilities from Kuwait and other Middle Eastern countries. It has several specialized services, and it is also a center for various academic activities. The PMR Hospital was granted accreditation in 2004 after having fulfilled the guidelines set by the Kuwaiti Ministry of Health. The First Conference of the PMR Society of Kuwait along with the First Regional Meeting of ISPRM was conducted in April 2000. There is an expansion of the diagnostic facilities in the hospital, which already has a fully equipped EMG and Urodynamics clinic, and a comprehensive cardiopulmonary rehabilitation program (38).

The Saudi Arabia specialists in PRM were responsible for the organization of an important symposium, endorsed by ISPRM, in February 2001, during which 25 speakers from Saudi Arabia and other countries gave lectures on numerous relevant topics, such as the development of stroke, TBI, and SCI rehabilitation (39). And in September 2014, there was the First International Conference for Pediatric Rehabilitation in Eastern Province, organized by the PRM Department of the King Fahad Specialist Hospital, Dammam, endorsed by ISPRM, with the presence of several international lecturers, including an ISPRM representative.

In 1982, in Baghdad (Iraq), a National Spinal Cord Injuries Centre with 130 beds was established, under the management of Kaydar M. Al-Chalabi, an ISPRM member (40). Initially, a Danish medical rehabilitation team worked together with the Iraqi team for 4 years to establish the working system. The success rate of this center was similar to other spinal centers even though many difficulties, such as shortage of medicines, assistive devices, and other supplies, were encountered. The hospital is academically linked to the College of Medicine of Baghdad University. Because of the war, the center had stopped operating for a while due to severe damages to the buildings. Rebuilding of the center was completed in 2004, and its operations resumed.

Africa

There is quite a difference in the development of rehabilitation services between North Africa and sub-Saharan Africa. If the development and the standards of PRM in North African countries can be assimilated to those of other Mediterranean countries (in 2015, the 11th Congress of the MFPRM was held in Egypt, and in 2019, the 13th Congress will be held in Morocco), the situation in the sub-Saharan ones is still faraway to meet the standards of rehabilitation set by the rest of the world.

In Morocco, the Mohamed V Military Hospital, in Rabat, has a well-organized rehabilitation department (41). In June 2016, the Morocco Health Minister sent a letter to the Health Regional Directors (Directeurs Regionaux du Ministère de la Santé) under the title "Renforcement de l'offre de soins de Rehabilitation en milieu hospitalier de 2ème et 3ème niveaux"

(Reinforcement of the offer of Rehabilitation care in 2nd and 3rd level hospitals). In this important document, the Health Minister stated that these hospitals, including the University hospitals, should implement a Rehabilitation Department. As a consequence, in Casablanca, a rehabilitation center was opened, as part of a health care program aimed to improve the lives of those with disabilities or suffering from certain health problems. The center is meant to offer rehabilitation and physiotherapy services to poor people with disabilities in order to encourage their independence (42).

Although in some places, such as South Africa, Zimbabwe, and Ethiopia, the rehabilitation services are better organized, in most of the other countries, the organizations most similar to a rehabilitation center are the centers for protection and rehabilitation of tortured victims, which often extend their services to nontortured individuals (43).

In South Africa, there are several centers offering medical rehabilitation services as well as private rehabilitation clinics dealing with all kinds of rehabilitation problems.

In Zimbabwe, public and private rehabilitation hospitals, schools, vocational training centers, and associations for and of people with disabilities provide key rehabilitation services. The Zimbabwean Ministry of Work and Social Welfare provides grants for the vocational training of people with disabilities who are registered with training centers in the country. The Ministry of Health and Child Welfare has rehabilitation units at each of the 15 referral hospitals in the country. Organizations for and of people with disabilities are more involved with vocational and psychosocial rehabilitation than with occupational and physical therapy (44).

In Ethiopia, in collaboration with an Austrian organization called the "Light for the World," a CBR program was established. The program is focused on giving proper care and follow-up to children who have clubfoot or hydrocephalus, to women who suffer from fistulas after obstructed labor, to children who become disabled due to obstructed labor or unsafe and unsuccessful abortions, and to others. The priorities of this program are to educate patients and medical providers and to convince the Ethiopian community of the value added by rehabilitation to patients' quality to life. The CBR program is not only a service program as they also train physiotherapy students. The University aims to produce graduates who are equally willing to work in urban and rural areas. In 2006, the first 80 physiotherapists graduated (45).

Asia and Oceania

The majority of the world's population, of which about 15% have some form of disability, reside in Asia. The wide variation in culture and economic development within the region has a significant impact upon the breadth and scope of rehabilitation services. In the developed countries of the region, the increasing demand for rehabilitation care is related to the aging population, particularly musculoskeletal disorders and stroke rehabilitation. Nevertheless, many Asian countries are developing countries and have limited health care and welfare service resources. Malnutrition, infectious disease, traffic and work accidents, natural disasters, and even wars continue to play important causative roles for disasters in the area (46). As a result of limited resources and limited expertise in rehabilitation, a CBR approach has been advocated and practiced in some developing countries in Asia (47–52).

Given the diversity of culture that it is also reflected in the practice of medical rehabilitation among the region, a formal collaboration has not been developed until recently. The ASEAN (West Asian region) Rehabilitation Medicine Association was established in 1998 and held its first Congress in Thailand in the same year. A subsequent meeting was held in 2002 in the Philippines. Between these two meetings, a Millennium Asian Symposium, sponsored by the Japanese Association of Rehabilitation, was held in Japan in 2001 (53). At this meeting, representatives from various Asian countries discussed the establishment of an Asian Society of Rehabilitation Medicine (ARMA). Thereafter, the Korea-Japan Joint Conference on Rehabilitation Medicine was held in Korea in 2002 and in Japan in 2004. These meetings, coupled with a rapid economic development in some Asian countries, prompted a growing interest to establish a regional society to facilitate the development and promotion of the PRM specialty. As a result, a regional society, the Asian Oceania Society of Physical and Rehabilitation Medicine (AOSPRM) (54), was officially established in Seoul (South Korea) during the 4th World Congress of ISPRM, in 2007, after initial task force meetings that were held in Sao Paulo (Brazil), and Zhuhai (China) in 2005 and 2006, respectively. Hereafter, AOSPRM has held biannual congresses, of which the first took place in 2008 in Nanjing (China). This first regional conference of the AOSPRM attracted more than 700 participants from its 19-member countries and included attendees from Europe and North and South America. During the conference, further closer collaboration among the countries in the region in terms of training, research, and exchange was put forward. A decision on a minor amendment of the official name of AOSPRM as "Asia-Oceanian Society of Physical and Rehabilitation Medicine" was also made during the Nanjing conference.

As in the rest of the world, in this area as well, different countries use different designations for PMR. The three most commonly used designations are RM, PMR, and PRM, with RM being the more commonly used term.

Japan and the Philippines established academic societies in the 1960s while two thirds of the other countries established their academic societies in 1980 or later. The specialty of RM is relatively new in this region. The percentage of physiatrists is 1% or less of the total number of practicing doctors in most countries (55,56). In some countries, the specialty was only established in the last few years, and some are still lacking sufficient physiatrists for the specialty and academic societies to develop.

The degree of maturity of training programs in the specialty of PRM also varies among the countries. Within the countries or administrative regions that have well-established training programs, there are also variations in the entry modalities and in the number of years required for the PMR training. In some countries, 2 to 3 years of general training in medicine along with passing an entry examination is required before commencing formal PMR training, after which a board certification examination is required for the final accreditation as a physiatrist. In general, the years spent in core training for RM varies from 3 to 5 years in most countries (55,56). Features of convergence and divergence of training programs between and within countries occur. For example, Australia and New Zealand share the same academic society and training system while China has a different training program in the mainland from her special administrative region, Hong Kong. Activities for CME or CPD have been established in most countries that have the board certification examination.

In some Asian countries, the practice of RM has been to some extent influenced by Eastern Medicine. Given the long history of Traditional Chinese Medicine (TCM) or Oriental Medicine in countries such as China, some components of these systems have been incorporated into the daily practice of RM. An international survey on stroke rehabilitation showed that in some of the Asian countries, Oriental Medicine techniques such as acupuncture and massage were more commonly used for stroke patients in comparison with countries in other parts of the world (57). This has triggered interest in the "East-meets-West" program where medical expertise is exchanged. The other important aspect of providing rehabilitation services to the disabled in some Asian countries has occurred through CBR. However, there have not been any formal training components in terms of CBR within the RM training programs in any of these countries. This will be one of the important areas of RM training to develop in the region.

With the advocacy of evidence-based medicine and practice, TCM and Oriental Medicine have opened up areas for research, which are leading to evidence for the role of TCM and Oriental Medicine in RM. Instead of separate practices of Western and Oriental Medicine, a combined approach for a "Universal Medicine" is an area of interest to be developed among the physiatrists in the region. This foreseeable development will likely be brought about by the strengthening of collaboration within the AOSPRM to facilitate RM specialty training and research in the region. Interregional collaborations such as between AOSPRM and ESPMR are also developing. Even though the RM specialty is relatively immature in the region, it will have a foreseeable bright future through a joint effort within the region and collaboration with other regions.

THE INTERNATIONAL SOCIETY OF PHYSICAL AND REHABILITATION MEDICINE

The ISPRM was established in November 1999 as the result of the merger of the International Rehabilitation Medicine Association (IRMA) and the International Federation of Physical and Rehabilitation Medicine (IFPRM) (58).

ISPRM serves as the global organization for PRM including (as per July 2018) 66 National Society members and over 35,000 individuals in the field of PRM (**Fig. 17-1**). It is an NGO, acting as a catalyst for international PRM research and has a humanitarian, professional, and scientific mandate (58).

The vision of the ISPRM is to be the leading Physical and Rehabilitation Medicine Society and medical voice for persons with disabilities in the world (59). The mission of ISPRM is to optimize functioning and health-related quality of life and minimize disability in persons with disability and/or medical problems throughout the world (60).

The official bodies of ISPRM are the Assembly of Delegates, the Assembly of Individual Members, the Executive Committee, the President's Cabinet, the Council of Past Presidents, and the International Education and Development Trust Fund (IEDF) (59). This structure is meant to ensure representation from both National PRM Societies and individual members and an equal representation of PRM specialists from all the three large world geographical areas: (a) the Americas; (b) Europe, Eastern Mediterranean, and Africa; and (c) Asia and Oceania (61) (see **Table 17-1**). These areas are used as a basis for rotation in the nomination of ISPRM leadership, election of representatives to the Assembly of Delegates, and the destination selection of the annual ISPRM World Congress.

The work of ISPRM is ensured by standing and ad hoc committees and task forces (59). There are three standing committees including (a) the Statutes Committee; (b) the Audit and Finance Committee; and (c) the Awards and Nominating Committee. The ad hoc committees are (a) the Clinical

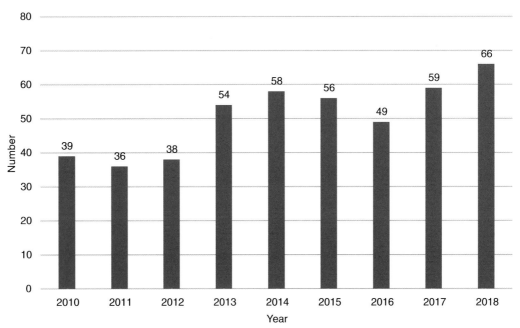

FIGURE 17-1. Number of national societies members of ISPRM.

TABLE 17-1	Number of National Societies in ISPRM by Geographical Area	
Geographical Area	**Number of National Societies**
The Americas	17
Europe, Eastern Mediterranean, and Africa	32
Asia and Oceania	17

Science and Research Committee; (b) the Congress Scientific Committee; (c) the Disaster Rehabilitation Committee; (d) the Education Committee; (e) the International Exchange Committee; (f) the Publications and Communications Committee; (g) the ISPRM-WHO Liaison Committee; and (h) the United Nations (UN) Liaison Committee. Moreover, there have been established two task forces: (a) the Ultrasound in PRM (USPRM) Task Force and (b) the Women and Health Task Force.

The Statutes Committee is aimed to assist the ISPRM in achieving its mission through maintaining up-to-date enabling governance documents. Its Chair and members are recommended by the President and approved by the Executive Committee (62).

The Audit and Finance Committee has the scope to supervise and make recommendations about the financial affairs of the Society. The Chair of this Committee is by Statutes the Treasurer of the ISPRM, and its members have to be recommended by the President and approved by the Executive Committee (63).

The Awards and Nominating Committee is responsible for the nomination of candidates for the offices of the Vice-President, Secretary, Treasurer, at-large Trustees of the IEDF Board of Trustees and the same members of the Awards and Nominating Committee; to make recommendations for Individual Honor Role Membership; and to prepare the criteria for the establishment of awards and prizes, recommend the type of awards (plaques, cash, other) and nominate candidates to receive them. The Committee is composed by six members nominated by the same committee and approved by the Assembly of Delegates. The Chair of the Committee is ex-officio the Immediate Past-President (64).

As for the ad hoc committees, Committee Chairs are generally recommended by ISPRM President and approved by the ISPRM Executive Committee with the only exception of the Congress Scientific Committee who is proposed by the Congress Local Organizing Committee (LOC) and approval by ISPRM President's Cabinet.

The Clinical Science and Research Committee is aimed to improve the quality of research in PRM, enhance the understanding of disability issues, and inform disability policy. It has been recently given the mission to produce ISPRM recommendations on several PRM topics.

The Congress Scientific Committee is responsible of ensuring a smooth and continuous organization and planning of ISPRM World Congresses and, in particular to identify the main themes of the congress, to define all aspects of the congress scientific/educational program, and to select the Review Committee, which is responsible for abstract reviews. It is composed of 23 members, 9 PRM experts chosen by the

Congress LOC, 9 experts chosen by the ISPRM President's Cabinet, the person who will be ISPRM President at the time of the congress, the current ISPRM President, and the Congress Scientific Committee Chairs from the last three congresses (65).

The Disaster Rehabilitation Committee is aimed to advocate PRM perspective in minimizing disability and optimizing functioning and health-related quality of life in persons who sustain traumatic injury and those with preexisting disability in a natural or man-made disaster (66).

The Education Committee has the scope to assist the Society in achieving its mission through providing its members educational and training opportunities (67).

The International Exchange Committee is aimed to serve as a central clearing house for unique educational and learning opportunities in PRM, across all continents (68).

The Publications and Communications Committee is aimed to coordinate the activities of ISPRM related to scientific publishing and information dissemination. To achieve its mission, the Committee is divided into four subcommittees: (a) Journals, aimed to liaise with the Chief Editor(s) and Editorial Board(s) of the official journal(s) and other journals linked to the Society; (b) News and Views, responsible to provide material for the publication of the electronic newsletter; (c) Web site, whose members in collaboration with the central office oversee and coordinate the operations of the ISPRM Web site; and (d) Social media network, a subcommittee recently introduced with the aim of using the main social media outlets to disseminate information about ISPRM, ISPRM World Congress, and other ISPRM-related news (69).

The ISPRM-WHO Liaison Committee is responsible of the relationship with WHO and, in particular, to provide input to the WHO on the issues it addresses that are of interest to the ISPRM and to present to the WHO any additional issues the ISPRM believes should be considered by the WHO. Given the importance of the collaboration with WHO, it has been recently decided that the official representative of ISPRM to WHO (main focal point) is the President of ISPRM and the Committee Chair is the ISPRM Designated Technical Officer to WHO (59).

The UN Liaison Committee has been established to assist ISPRM to optimize function and health-related quality of life for persons with disabilities through collaboration with the UN (70). In fact, ISPRM has recently been accredited as an NGO by the UN Conference of States Parties to the Convention on the Rights of Persons with Disabilities (COSP UNCRPD), thus becoming qualified to participate in the annual COSP UNCRPD meeting (59).

Other important external relationships of ISPRM have been established via Memoranda of Understanding—MoUs with various Scientific Societies and Regional PRM Societies, including AMLAR, ESPRM, EARM, PRM UEMS, MFPRM, ARMA, and AOSPRM (see **Box 17-1**). The aim of these agreements is to foster cooperation and coordination of activities at the international, regional, and national levels.

An important collaboration of ISPRM, aimed to favor research quality in rehabilitation as well as the dissemination of evidence, is with the recently established Cochrane Rehabilitation Field (71). This is a group inside Cochrane, formed by a global network of individuals, involved in

---

BOX 17-1

Regional Societies

Asia-Oceanian Society of Physical and Rehabilitation Medicine
Association of Southeast Asian Nations (ASEAN) Rehabilitation Medicine Association
Baltic and North Sea Forum on Physical and Rehabilitation Medicine
European Society of Physical and Rehabilitation Medicine
Latin American Association of Rehabilitation Medicine
Mediterranean Forum of Physical and Rehabilitation Medicine
Pan Arabic Association of Physical and Rehabilitation Medicine

---

the production, dissemination, and implementation of evidence-informed clinical practice in rehabilitation. The Cochrane Rehabilitation Field was established based on an initiative of ESPRM and the support of a number of organizations, including ISPRM. During the Assembly of Delegates at the 2017 ISPRM World Congress, ISPRM leadership signed a MoU with the Cochrane Rehabilitation Field Director. ISPRM has agreed to host Cochrane Rehabilitation Executive Committee and Advisory Board meetings during its annual World Congress and to give space for a dedicated scientific session in the Congress Program.

ISPRM World Congress is the main face-to-face meeting of the Society. The 1st ISPRM World Congress was held in 2001 in Amsterdam (The Netherlands) with 1,192 participants representing 61 different countries. Since 2013, the World Congress has become an annual event. In 2018, its 12th edition was held in Paris (France) with 4,005 participants coming from 104 different countries.

Starting in 2014, the ISPRM Developing Countries Summit is held yearly in China, under the auspice of ISPRM, with the aim of facilitating education in developing Asian countries.

Under the direction of the Publications and Communications Committee, ISPRM has created a "web of journals" defining specific criteria that journals must have to be in official relation with ISPRM (72). Three categories of journals have been identified: (a) official journal(s) of ISPRM including "The Journal of the International Society of Physical and Rehabilitation Medicine" (JISPRM) (73) and the "Journal of Rehabilitation Medicine" (JRM) (74); (b) journal(s) published in association with ISPRM as the "Annals of Rehabilitation Medicine" (ARM) (75), "The Annals of Physical and Rehabilitation Medicine" (76), and "The European Journal of Physical and Rehabilitation Medicine" (EJPRM) (77); and (c) journal(s) endorsed by ISPRM as "Acta Fisiatrica" (78), "Rehab in Review" (79), "The Chinese Journal of Rehabilitation Medicine" (80), and "The Portuguese Journal of Physical and Rehabilitation Medicine" (PJPRM) (81) (🛜 eFig. 17-1).

SUMMARY

There are some words whose meanings are so universally accepted that definition is unwarranted and might be considered pedantic by some. Physical medicine is such a term to some but not to others, for most specialists in physical medicine have their own idea of its meaning. But there are as many

definitions as there are countries, and within some countries there are many definitions, for this is a specialty that stems from many older specialties, each of which has its own national and international history.

Sidney Licht, 1960.

From the historical perspective (82,83), there is no doubt that PMR has come a long way since its inception and that the strengthening of a global organization such as ISPRM has been greatly contributing to its growth. Although differences still persist among regions and systems, there have been significant and rapid changes occurring in parallel across all the world regions, both in developed and developing countries. The increasing number of regional and world congresses and of international PRM journals have made great contributions to an international harmonization in residency and teaching programs, the understanding and building of common concepts and terms, the establishment of new rehabilitation systems, and the development of strategic plans to strengthen the stability of those systems in jeopardy.

Research in rehabilitation is thriving, and the quality of the research programs as well as their scope is dramatically improving, including animal experimental studies (84,85). One of the most salient features of the last years is the impressive recruitment, in number and mainly in quality of a cadre of active members who, whether they fill some formal position or not, are increasingly devoting themselves to the regional and international organizations. This has brought about a dramatic upgrade of standards of work and activities. By now, a kind of "international carrier" has been created in the rehabilitation realm. Above all, if to judge by the different regional reports, there is a bright future for PMR. The profession is closing the gaps among regions and is actively becoming global (86). It is the dawn of a new day.

ACKNOWLEDGMENT

The coauthors of this chapter wish to acknowledge posthumously the significant contributions of the late Professor Haim Ring in the initial iteration of this chapter. Professor Ring's leadership skills and academic contributions to International Physiatry will always be remembered and treasured.

REFERENCES

1. European Physical and Rehabilitation Medicine Bodies Alliance. White book on physical and rehabilitation medicine in Europe: introductions, executive summary, and methodology. *Eur J Phys Rehabil Med.* 2018;54(2):125–155.
2. Krusen FH. The second John Stanley Coulter memorial lecture. Report on the International Congress of Physical Medicine. *Arch Phys Med Rehabil.* 1952;33(11):651–660.
3. Vlček E. The fossil man of Gánovce, Czechoslovakia. *J R Anthropol Inst G B Irel.* 1955; 85(1/2):163–172.
4. Braddom RL. Epilogue: physical medicine and rehabilitation—or is it physical medicine versus rehabilitation. In: O'Young BJ, Mark Young MA, Stiens SA, eds. *Physical Medicine and Rehabilitation Secrets.* 3rd ed. Philadelphia, PA: Elsevier Publishers; 2007:704–710.
5. Flax HA. Twenty-five years of physical medicine and rehabilitation in Puerto Rico. *Arch Phys Med Rehabil.* 1972;53(4):149–153.
6. The history of PM&R. Available from: https://www.physiatry.org/page/History_PMR [cited September 18, 2018].
7. Lin W-C, Kane RL, Mehr DR, et al. Changes in the Use of Postacute Care during the Initial Medicare Payment Reforms. Does It Matter? *Health Serv Res.* 2006;41(4 Pt 1):1338–1356.

8. Young M. Review of still lives: narratives of spinal cord injury by Jonathan Cole. *JAMA*. 2005;293(4):497.
9. Canadian Association of Physical Medicine and Rehabilitation (CAPM&R). Available from: https://www.capmr.ca [cited September 18, 2018]
10. Canadian Institute for Health Information Dataset, October 2006 to September 2007.
11. Asociación Médica Latinoamericana de Rehabilitación (AMLAR). Available from: https://www.portalamlar.org [cited September 18, 2018].
12. Vasquez A. La discapacidad en America Latina. In: Amate E, Vasquez A, eds. *Discapacidad: lo que todos debemos saber*. Vol 9. Washington, DC: OPS; 2006:23.
13. Bolanos J. Mensajem da AMLAR. *Med Rehabil*. 2006;25(3):57.
14. Nunez BH. Origen y desarrollo de la Rehabiliacion en el Uruguay. *Med Rehabil*. 2006;25(1):22–23.
15. Ferrari Forcade A. Invalidez y Rehabilitacion. In: Ferrari Forcade A, De Castellet F, eds. *Fisiatria*. Montevideo: Editorial Delta; 1973:339–354.
16. Lianza S. Apresentacao: A Medicina de Reabilitacao—passado, presente e futuro. In: Lianza S, ed. *Medicina de Reabilitacao*. 3rd ed. Rio de Janeiro: Guanabara Koogan S.A; 2001.
17. Second International Congress of Physio-Therapy, Rome, 1907. *Arch Roentgen Ray*. 1907;12(1):2–3.
18. European Union of Medical Specialists (UEMS). Available from: https://www.uems.eu [cited September 18, 2018].
19. European Society of Physical and Rehabilitation Medicine (ESPRM). Available from: http://www.esprm.net [cited September 18, 2018].
20. European Academy of Rehabilitation Medicine (EARM). Available from: http://www.aemr.eu [cited September 18, 2018].
21. PRM Section of the European Union of Medical Specialists (UEMS PRM). Available from: https://www.euro-prm.org/index.php?lang=en [cited September 18, 2018].
22. European Society of Physical and Rehabilitation Medicine (ESPRM). *Aims & Goals*. Available from: http://www.esprm.net/about/G8KL/aims-amp-goals [cited September 18, 2018].
23. European Academy of Rehabilitation Medicine. *History of the Academy*. Available from: http://www.aemr.eu/index.php?option=com_content&task=view&id=12&Itemid=26 [cited September 18, 2018].
24. PRM Section of the European Union of Medical Specialists (UEMS PRM). Available from: https://www.euro-prm.org/index.php?option=com_content&view=category&layout=blog&id=39&Itemid=611&lang=en [cited September 18, 2018].
25. World Health Organization. *International Classification of Impairments, Disabilities, and Handicaps: A Manual of Classification Relating to the Consequences of Disease, Published in Accordance with Resolution WHA29.35 of the Twenty-ninth World Health Assembly, May 1976*. Geneva: World Health Organization; 1980. Available from: http://www.who.int/iris/handle/10665/41003
26. World Health Organization. *International Classification of Functioning, Disability and Health (ICF)*. Geneva: World Health Organization; 2001.
27. NHS. *National Health Service and Community Care Act*. Chapter 19. 1990. London: HMSO; 1990.
28. European Academy of Rehabilitation Medicine, E.F.O.P.A.R.M., European Union of Medical Specialists (Physical and Rehabilitation Medicine Section). *White Book on Physical and Rehabilitation Medicine*. U.C.D. Madrid; 1989.
29. White book on physical and rehabilitation medicine in Europe. *Eura Medicophys*. 2006;42(4):292–332.
30. White book on physical and rehabilitation medicine in Europe. *J Rehabil Med*. 2007;45(suppl):6–47.
31. White book on physical and rehabilitation medicine in Europe. *Eur J Phys Rehabil Med*. 2018;54(2):125–321.
32. Italian Health Ministry. Rehabilitation national plan: an Italian act. *Eur J Phys Rehabil Med*. 2011;47(4):621–638.
33. Union Européenne des Médecins Spécialistes. European Union of Medical Specialists. *Training Requirements for the Specialty of Physical and Rehabilitation Medicine. European Standards of Postgraduate Medical Specialist Training*. Available from: https://www.uems.eu/__data/assets/pdf_file/0010/64396/UEMS-2018.15-Council-Marrakesh-European-Training-Requirement-PRM-specialty.pdf [cited September 18, 2018].
34. Mediterranean Forum of Physical and Rehabilitation Medicine (MFPRM). Available from: http://www.mfprm.net/en/home/home [cited September 18, 2018].
35. Mediterranean Forum of Physical and Rehabilitation Medicine (MFPRM). *About the MFPRM*. Available from: http://www.mfprm.net/en/about-the-mfprm/about-the-mfprm [cited September 18, 2018].
36. European Physical and Rehabilitation Medicine Bodies Alliance. White Book on Physical and Rehabilitation Medicine (PRM) in Europe. Chapter 5. The PRM organizations in Europe: structure and activities. *Eur J Phys Rehabil Med*. 2018;54: 198–213. doi:10.23736/S1973-9087.18.05149-3.
37. Euro-Mediterranean Rehabilitation PRM School (EMRSS). Available from: http://www.emrss.it/ENG/index.html [cited September 18, 2018].
38. Abdulla E. *ISPRM News Views J*. 5:2002, 3:2005 and 7:2006.
39. Al Jadid M. *ISPRM News Views J*. 5:2002.
40. Al-Chalabi KM. *ISPRM News Views J*. 5:2004.
41. Mohamed V. *Military Hospital*. Available from: https://archnet.org/sites/4545 [cited September 18, 2018].
42. New Rehabilitation Center in Casablanca. Available from: https://www.morocco-worldnews.com/2017/06/218413/king-mohammed-vi-opens-new-rehabilitation-center-in-casablanca/ [cited September 18, 2018].
43. International Rehabilitation Council for Torture Victims (IRCT). *About the IRCT*. Available from: https://irct.org/index.php/who-we-are/about-the-irct [cited September 18, 2018].
44. Mpofu E, Harley D. Disability & rehabilitation in Zimbabwe: lessons & implications for rehabilitation practice in the U.S—Disability & Rehabilitation in Zimbabwe. *J Rehabil*. 2002;68(4):26–33.
45. Marieke B. *ISPRM News Views J*. 2005;7–8.
46. Helander E. *Prejudice and Dignity. An Introduction to Community-Based Rehabilitation*. New York: UNDP; 1999.
47. Lagerkvist B. Community-based rehabilitation—outcome for the disabled in the Philippines and Zimbabwe. *Disabil Rehabil*. 1992;14:44–50.
48. Thomas M. Community based rehabilitation in India—an emerging trend. *Indian J Pediatr*. 1992;59:401–406.
49. Kim YH, Jo NK. Community-based rehabilitation in South Korea. *Disabil Rehabil*. 1999;21:484–489.
50. Inthirat TR, Thonglith S. Community-based rehabilitation in the Lao People's Democratic Republic. *Disabil Rehabil*. 1999;21:469–473.
51. Hai TT, Chuong TV. Vietnam and activities of community-based rehabilitation. *Disabil Rehabil*. 1999;21:474–478.
52. Zhuo D, Kun ND. Community-based rehabilitation in the People's Republic of China. *Disabil Rehabil*. 1999;21:490–494.
53. Chino N, Ishigami S, Akai M, et al. Current status of rehabilitation medicine in Asia: a report from New Millennium Asia Symposium on Rehabilitation Medicine. *J Rehabil Med*. 2002;34:1–4.
54. Asian Oceania Society of Physical and Rehabilitation Medicine (AOSPRM). Available from: http://www.aosprm.org [cited September 18, 2018].
55. Han TR, Bang MS. Rehabilitation medicine: the Asian perspective. *Am J Phys Med Rehabil*. 2007;86:335–338.
56. Han TR, Evangelista TJP, Olver J, et al. Survey on Asian Oceania education and training in physical medicine & rehabilitation medicine. *J Rehabil Med*. 2008:46(suppl):28–29.
57. Li LS. Stroke rehabilitation: an international survey. *Neurorehabil Neural Repair*. 2006;20(1):86.
58. The International Society of Physical and Rehabilitation Medicine (ISPRM). *Discover the Society*. Available from: http://www.isprm.org/discover/the-society/ [cited September 18, 2018] [accepted for publication].
59. Jorge L, Francesca G, Jianan L, et al. The International Society of Physical and Rehabilitation Medicine: the past, present, and way forward-III. *J Int Soc Phys Rehabil Med*. 2018 [accepted for publication].
60. The International Society of Physical and Rehabilitation Medicine (ISPRM). *ISPRM Statutes*. Available from: http://www.isprm.org/wp-content/uploads/2012/09/Statutes-Version-approved-July-2018.pdf [cited September 18, 2018].
61. Stucki G, Reinhardt JD, von Groote PM, et al. Chapter 2: ISPRM's way forward. *J Rehabil Med*. 2009;41(10):798–809.
62. The International Society of Physical and Rehabilitation Medicine (ISPRM). *Statutes Committee Operational Guidelines*. Available from: http://www.isprm.org/wp-content/uploads/2018/09/ISPRM-Committee-operational-guidelines-Statutes-Committee-Mar-2018.pdf [cited September 18, 2018].
63. The International Society of Physical and Rehabilitation Medicine (ISPRM). *Audit and Finance Committee Operational Guidelines*. Available from: http://www.isprm.org/wp-content/uploads/2018/09/ISPRM-Committee-operational-guidelines-AF-Committee-Mar-2018.pdf [cited September 18, 2018].
64. The International Society of Physical and Rehabilitation Medicine (ISPRM). *Awards and Nominating Committee Operational Guidelines*. Available from: http://www.isprm.org/wp-content/uploads/2018/09/ISPRM-Committee-operational-guidelines-ANC-Sep-2018.pdf [cited September 18, 2018].
65. The International Society of Physical and Rehabilitation Medicine (ISPRM). *Congress Scientific Committee Operational Guidelines*. Available from: http://www.isprm.org/wp-content/uploads/2016/10/ISPRM-Committee-operational-guidelines-Congress-Scientific-Committee-Oct-2016.pdf [cited September 18, 2018].
66. The International Society of Physical and Rehabilitation Medicine (ISPRM). *Disaster Rehabilitation Committee Operational Guidelines*. Available from: http://www.isprm.org/wp-content/uploads/2016/08/ISPRM-Committee-operational-guidelines-Disaster-Rehabilitation-Committee-Aug-2016.pdf [cited September 18, 2018].
67. The International Society of Physical and Rehabilitation Medicine (ISPRM). *Education Committee Operational Guidelines*. Available from: http://www.isprm.org/wp-content/uploads/2015/09/ISPRM-Education-committee-Operational-guidelines.pdf [cited September 18, 2018].
68. Young MA, O'Young BJ. Promoting global physical & rehabilitation medicine educational exchange through ISPRM faculty-student exchange. *J Rehabil Med*. 2007;39(7):583–584.
69. The International Society of Physical and Rehabilitation Medicine (ISPRM). *Publications and Communications Committee Operational Guidelines*. Available from: http://www.isprm.org/wp-content/uploads/2018/08/ISPRM-Committee-operational-guidelines-PC-Committee-Aug-2018.pdf [cited September 18, 2018].
70. The International Society of Physical and Rehabilitation Medicine (ISPRM). *UN Liaison Committee Operational Guidelines*. Available from: http://www.isprm.org/wp-content/uploads/2018/09/ISPRM-Committee-operational-guidelines-UN-Liaison-Committee-Sep-2018.pdf [cited September 18, 2018].
71. Negrini S, Arienti C, Gimigliano F, et al. Cochrane rehabilitation: organization and functioning. *Am J Phys Med Rehabil*. 2018;97(1):68–71.

72. The International Society of Physical and Rehabilitation Medicine (ISPRM). *ISPRM Journals Policies and Guidelines*; 2016. Available from: http://www.isprm.org/wp-content/uploads/2015/01/Journals-Policies-and-guidelines.pdf [cited September 18, 2018].

73. The Journal of the International Society of Physical and Rehabilitation Medicine (JISPRM). JISPRM Website. Available from: http://www.jisprm.org [cited September 18, 2018].

74. Journal of Rehabilitation Medicine (JRM). JRM Website. Available from: https://www.medicaljournals.se/jrm/content/ [cited September 18, 2018].

75. Annals of Rehabilitation Medicine (ARM). ARM Website. Available from: http://www.e-arm.org/about/journal.html [cited September 18, 2018].

76. The Annals of Physical and Rehabilitation Medicine. The Annals of Physical and Rehabilitation Medicine Website. Available from: http://www.em-consulte.com/en/revue/rehab [cited September 18, 2018].

77. The European Journal of Physical and Rehabilitation Medicine (EJPRM). EJPRM Website. Available from: https://www.minervamedica.it/en/journals/europa-medico-physica/index.php [cited September 18, 2018].

78. Acta Fisiatrica. Acta Fisiatrica Website. Available from: http://www.actafisiatrica.org.br [cited September 18, 2018].

79. Rehab in Review. Rehab in Review Website. Available from: https://rehabinreview.com [cited September 18, 2018].

80. The Chinese Journal of Rehabilitation Medicine. The Chinese Journal of Rehabilitation Medicine Website. Available from: http://www.rehabi.com.cn [cited September 18, 2018].

81. The Portuguese Journal of Physical and Rehabilitation Medicine (PJPRM). PJPRM Website. Available from: https://spmfrjournal.org/index.php/spmfr [cited September 18, 2018].

82. Licht S. *World Directory of Physical Medicine Specialists. Physical MedicineLibrary.* Vol 6. Baltimore, MD: Waverly Press; 1960.

83. Chino N, Grimby G, Smith D, et al. International issues in rehabilitation medicine. In: DeLisa J, Gans BM, eds. *Rehabilitation Medicine—Principles and Practice.* 3rd ed. Philadelphia, PA/New York: Lippincott-Raven; 1998:47–54.

84. Ring H. Domains of research, development and strategic planning in rehabilitation medicine. *Editorial Eura Medicophys.* 2005;41(3):207–214.

85. Negrini S. DeLisa lecture. Evidence in rehabilitation medicine: between facts and prejudices. *Am J Phys Med Rehabil.* 2018 Aug 28. [Epub ahead of print].

86. Ring H. International rehabilitation medicine: closing the gaps and globalization of the profession (Invited Editorial). *Am J Phys Med Rehabil.* 2004;83(9):667–669.

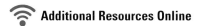 **Additional Resources Online**

PART III Major Conditions: Neuromuscular

CHAPTER 18

Joel Stein

Stroke Rehabilitation

Stroke has been recognized since antiquity, and it remains a major cause of disability. In this chapter, we review the causes, mechanisms, and symptoms of stroke, including a discussion of common stroke syndromes. We then address the evaluation of stroke cause and strategies to prevent recurrent stroke. A discussion of the process of recovery and rehabilitation after a stroke follows. Lastly, we discuss some of the long-term sequelae of stroke and their management.

DEFINITION

A stroke is the sudden occurrence of permanent damage to an area of the brain caused by a blocked blood vessel or bleeding within the brain. Other causes of focal brain damage, such as traumatic injury to the brain, demyelinating lesions, brain tumors, brain abscesses, and others, can produce strokelike symptoms and have similar rehabilitation needs but are not formally included in this definition.

Stroke is divided into two major categories: ischemic, generally caused by a vascular occlusion, and hemorrhagic, caused by bleeding within the parenchyma of the brain. Some classify nonparenchymal hemorrhage, such as subarachnoid hemorrhage (SAH) due to a ruptured intracranial aneurysm, as a form of hemorrhagic stroke as well.

A significant number of people who sustain a stroke do not reach medical attention due to a lack of symptoms or the failure to recognize the symptoms as requiring medical attention. (It is estimated that 28% of individuals aged 70 to 74 have had a silent cerebral infarction.) (1) The most common symptom of stroke is focal weakness, though stroke can produce a wide range of symptoms such as sensory loss, speech and language disturbance, visual loss, etc. The resultant neurologic deficits are generally referred to as *impairments*, which may or may not result in functional limitations.

The objectives of stroke rehabilitation are to achieve a maximum level of functional independence; facilitate neurologic recovery, minimize disability; successfully reintegrate back into home, family, and community; and reestablish a meaningful and gratifying life. Education of the stroke survivor and his or her family regarding secondary stroke prevention, including risk factor modification, and compliance with medical therapy for stroke prevention are responsibilities shared by the rehabilitation team. These goals are accomplished through exercise and other treatments to facilitate recovery and reduce impairments; functional training to compensate for residual impairments; and use of assistive devices, such as braces or wheelchair, to substitute for lost function.

Successful rehabilitation also requires management of the many psychosocial issues that surround integration of the patient back to home and community.

EPIDEMIOLOGY

Each year, approximately 795,000 Americans suffer a stroke, of which 610,000 are an initial event and the remainder are recurrent strokes (1). There are estimated to be about 6.6 million stroke survivors over the age of 20 in the United States (1). While the total number of strokes in the United States has been stable in recent years, there is a downward trend in the age-specific incidence of stroke that has been counterbalanced by the increased size of the older cohort most at risk for stroke. The death rate from stroke has fallen by 33.7% from 2003 to 2013 (with a reduction in the total number of stroke deaths of 18.2% [due to population growth and aging of the population]). Stroke has fallen to the fifth leading cause of death in the United States. Incidence is age related, with about 10% of stroke occurring among individuals 18 to 50 years of age. Ischemic stroke has increased among adolescents and young adults (aged 5 to 44 years) between 1995 and 2008 for unclear reasons. Stroke is more common among men than among women in younger cohorts, but more common among women for individuals over age 85 (1).

RISK FACTORS AND PREVENTION

Risk factors for ischemic stroke can be separated into two categories: those that are potentially modifiable and those that are nonmodifiable. The latter includes age, race/ethnicity, sex, and family history, whereas the potentially modifiable risk factors include hypertension, smoking, atrial fibrillation, diabetes, diet, obesity, sedentary lifestyle, and hyperlipidemia.

Risk factors for hemorrhagic stroke have also been identified, and while primary stroke prevention efforts generally focus on the risk factors for ischemic stroke, secondary prevention efforts for individuals who have already sustained a hemorrhagic stroke should include education with a particular focus on treating hypertension, refraining from excessive alcohol consumption, and avoiding the use of anticoagulant medications.

Risk Factors for Recurrent Stroke

The probability of stroke recurrence is highest early after a stroke. For survivors of an initial stroke, the annual risk of a second stroke is approximately 5%, with a 5-year cumulative risk of recurrence around 25% (2,3), although it may be as high as 42% (2). Risk factors (**Box 18-1**) for initial stroke also increase the risk of recurrence, especially hypertension, heart disease (e.g., atrial fibrillation), smoking, and diabetes mellitus (4,5). Heavy alcohol consumption is also a risk factor for recurrent stroke.

Mortality after stroke is high, with between 32% and 58% of initial survivors dead within 5 years after a first stroke, with survival varying based on age, sex, and race (1).

Leonberg and Elliott (4) were able to achieve 16% reduction in stroke recurrence rate by an energetic and sustained program of control of multiple risk factors. Therefore, efforts should be made to reduce risk of recurrent stroke and mortality by controlling risk factors.

TYPES OF STROKES

Cerebral Thrombosis

Thrombosis of the large extracranial and intracranial vessels as the result of atherosclerotic cerebrovascular disease accounts for approximately 30% of all cases of stroke (**Table 18-1**) (5). Atherosclerotic plaques are particularly prominent in the large vessels of the neck and at the base of the brain. Sudden occlusion of one of these large vessels, in the absence of good collateral circulation, usually results in a large brain infarction.

TABLE 18-1	Causes of Stroke	
Cause		**%**
Large vessel occlusion/infarction		32
Embolism		32
Small vessel occlusion, lacunar		18
Intracerebral hemorrhage		11
Subarachnoid hemorrhage		7

Reprinted with permission from Mohr JP, Caplan LR, Melski JW, et al. The Harvard cooperative stroke registry: a prospective study. *Neurology.* 1978;28(8):754–762.

Risk factors for atherosclerosis include hypertension, smoking, diabetes, and hyperlipidemia. In some cases, the gradual progressive stenosis of a major blood vessel provides sufficient time for collateral circulation to develop, and complete occlusion may be asymptomatic or produce fewer effects than might otherwise be expected.

Unlike embolic strokes, which tend to have an abrupt onset, atherothrombotic strokes often begin more subtly, and affected individuals may only become aware that they have weakness or other impairment when they attempt to walk or get out of bed. The extent of the clinical deficit usually worsens over some hours or sometimes days, followed by stabilization and then gradual improvement.

Cerebral Embolism

Embolism is responsible for about 30% of all cases of stroke. Emboli may arise from thrombi within the heart or on the heart valves, from paradoxical embolism, or from an ulcerated atherosclerotic plaque within an extracranial artery (**Box 18-2**). Cardiogenic embolism may occur from thrombus formation at the site of a recent myocardial infarction (MI), an area of myocardial hypokinesis, within the left atrium in patients with atrial fibrillation, or on diseased or prosthetic valves. Paradoxical embolism results from a deep vein thrombosis in the pelvis or leg that embolizes into the right side of the heart and then passes through a patent foramen ovale into the left atrium, and ultimately to the cerebral circulation.

Cerebral embolism presents with an abrupt onset that is due to sudden loss of arterial perfusion to a focal area of the brain. The blood flow and anatomy of the cerebral circulation favor passage of an embolism into the middle cerebral artery (MCA)

BOX 18-1

Modifiable Risk Factors for Stroke

Hypertension
Heart disease
   Ischemic/hypertensive
   Valvular
   Arrhythmias
Smoking
Diabetes mellitus
Elevated fibrinogen
Erythrocytosis
Hyperlipidemia

BOX 18-2

Sources of Cerebral Embolism

Cardiac
- Atrial fibrillation, other arrhythmias
- Mural thrombus—recent MI, hypokinesis, cardiomyopathy
- Bacterial endocarditis
- Valve prosthesis
- Nonbacterial valve vegetations
- Atrial myxoma

Large artery
- Atherosclerosis of the aorta and carotid arteries

Paradoxical
- Peripheral venous embolism with R-to-L cardiac shunt

territory, though any vascular territory may be affected. Many emboli are friable and may break into smaller pieces as they travel through the cerebral circulation, resulting in multiple smaller infarcts affecting several distal branches of the main vessel.

The initial clinical deficit may change rapidly. If the embolus undergoes lysis and fragmentation, the neurologic signs may fade rapidly. While treatment with anticoagulants is appropriate for long-term secondary prevention of recurrent stroke, immediate anticoagulation with heparin has been found to increase the risk of symptomatic hemorrhagic conversion (6). For this reason, anticoagulation therapy is frequently delayed from the acute onset for up to 2 weeks in individuals with large cardioembolic infarctions.

Lacunar Stroke

Lacunar lesions constitute approximately 20% of all strokes and are small, circumscribed lesions, at most 1.5 cm in diameter, resulting from occlusions in the deep penetrating branches of the large vessels that perfuse the subcortical structures, including internal capsule, basal ganglia, thalamus, and brainstem. Small lacunar infarcts may produce major neurologic deficits if they occur in key regions but generally cause more minor symptoms than do large vessel infarcts and may in fact be asymptomatic. Lacunar strokes are highly associated with hypertension and may result from either microatheroma or lipohyalinosis.

Cerebral Hemorrhage

Intracerebral hemorrhage (ICH) accounts for approximately 11% of all cases of stroke. The most common cause of cerebral hemorrhage is hypertension, and intracerebral hypertensive hemorrhage most commonly occurs at the site of small, deep, penetrating arteries. It is thought that hemorrhage occurs through rupture of microaneurysms (Charcot-Bouchard aneurysms) that develop in these vessels in hypertensive patients. The majority of lesions occur in the putamen or thalamus, and in about 10% of patients, the spontaneous hemorrhage occurs in the cerebellum.

Cerebral amyloid angiopathy is another important cause of cerebral hemorrhage, representing 5% to 20% of cases. It is most common after age 65, although it may occasionally affect individuals as early as age 45. Hemorrhages tend to be lobar rather than deep, and there is usually evidence of hemosiderin deposition on MRI imaging indicative of prior microhemorrhages at the time of initial clinical presentation. No specific treatments are yet available, aside from avoidance of medications that may predispose to bleeding and appropriate control of hypertension if present.

The clinical onset of the hemorrhage is often dramatic, with severe headache and rapidly progressive neurologic deficits. In patients with larger hemorrhages, consciousness becomes progressively impaired leading to coma. Brain displacement from the hematoma and cerebral edema may give rise to transtentorial herniation and death, generally within the first few days poststroke. While cerebral hemorrhage is associated with a higher mortality rate than infarction, there is some evidence that the neurologic deficit from a hemorrhage may recover to a greater degree than a comparable initial deficit from an infarction (7).

ICHs have been demonstrated to continue to expand after initial presentation in a substantial portion of patients.

A recent trial of recombinant activated factor VII reduced the growth of the hematomas but failed to show any improvement in functional status or reduction in mortality (8).

ICH is a well-recognized complication of anticoagulant therapy and may occur spontaneously or after minor trauma. For patients on warfarin, the risk is related to the degree of elevation of the INR. In one study, the adjusted odds ratio for sustaining an intracranial hemorrhage was 4.6 for INRs in the range of 3.5 to 3.9 (compared with individuals with INRs between 2.0 and 3.0) and increased to 8.8 for INRs above 4.0 (9).

Other causes of ICH include trauma, vasculitis, and bleeding into a tumor. Patients with a bleeding diathesis—for example, thrombocytopenia or coagulation disorders—may develop an intracranial hemorrhage.

Patients with acute cerebellar hemorrhages typically develop a sudden headache and inability to stand, along with nausea, vomiting, and vertigo. With large posterior fossa lesions, the hematoma and edema may occlude the fourth ventricle, causing acute hydrocephalus. Urgent decompression with evacuation of the hematoma can be lifesaving. Patients who survive surgical evacuation of a cerebellar hemorrhage, or who have a less severe lesion, usually make a good functional recovery, as do patients with cerebellar infarcts (10).

Subarachnoid Hemorrhage

In about 7% of all stroke patients, the lesion is an SAH, usually resulting from rupture of an arterial aneurysm at the base of the brain with bleeding into the subarachnoid space. Aneurysms develop from small defects in the wall of the arteries and slowly increase in size. The risk of rupture rises as the size of the aneurysm increases, and for this reason, intervention is generally advised for asymptomatic aneurysms greater than 10 mm in diameter (11). Major rupture of an aneurysm may be preceded by headache from a small bleed or by localized cranial nerve lesions caused by direct pressure by the expanding aneurysm. When rupture occurs, the clinical onset is usually dramatically abrupt. There is severe headache followed by vomiting and signs of meningeal irritation. Focal signs are usually not observed initially but may develop as a result of associated intracerebral bleeding or cerebral infarction occurring as a complication of arterial vasospasm. Coma frequently occurs, and as many as one third of patients may die acutely. Rebleeding is very common, and therefore, early surgical/invasive radiologic intervention has become routine, with the objective of obliterating the aneurysm to prevent recurrent hemorrhage. Blood in the subarachnoid space may cause arterial vasospasm, leading to localized areas of cerebral infarction with associated focal neurologic deficits. Nimodipine is routinely administered after SAH to reduce the likelihood and/or severity of vasospasm.

Hydrocephalus may develop immediately after SAH due to obstruction of the ventricular system from intraventricular hemorrhage, or as a later complication several weeks after the acute event as a result of arachnoiditis from blood in the CSF.

Obliteration of aneurysms may be performed surgically, by clipping the neck of the aneurysm or by the use of detachable coils placed through an angiographic approach to thrombose the aneurysm.

SAH or ICH may also result from bleeding from an arteriovenous malformation (AVM), which is a tangle of dilated vessels found on the surface of the brain or within the brain parenchyma. These lesions are congenital abnormalities and tend to bleed in childhood or young adulthood. In about half the cases, the hemorrhage is the first clinical indication of the lesion. In approximately one third of patients, the AVM presents as a seizure disorder or with chronic headaches. In most patients, the lesions eventually bleed. Most patients survive a single hemorrhagic event. The rate of rebleeding is about 6% in the first year and 2% to 3% per year thereafter. Treatment options include surgical excision of the AVM, proton beam therapy, or neurovascular ablation through embolization.

STROKE SYNDROMES

The relatively predictable anatomy of the brain's vascular supply, localization of particular functions to certain areas of the brain, and the predilection of stroke for certain vascular territories result in a number of commonly occurring ischemic stroke syndromes. These stroke syndromes can be recognized when they occur and assist in localization of the stroke lesion as well as in predicting functional outcome. While a myriad of stroke syndromes have been described, we discuss only a few of the most common ones in this chapter.

Internal Carotid Artery Syndrome

The clinical consequences of complete occlusion of an internal carotid artery vary from no observable deficit to catastrophic. In cases where there is good collateral circulation, no neurologic consequences may occur with carotid occlusion. By contrast, massive cerebral infarction in the distribution of the anterior and middle cerebral arteries may present with rapid obtundation, with dense contralateral motor and sensory deficits. In some cases (particularly in younger people), severe cerebral edema may lead to transtentorial herniation and death. In such cases, decompression of the swollen brain with craniectomy may be lifesaving.

Less extensive infarctions result in partial or total lesions in the distribution of the MCA. The anterior cerebral circulation may be preserved through flow from the opposite side via the anterior communicating artery.

Middle Cerebral Artery Syndromes

The internal carotid artery divides into the middle and anterior cerebral arteries. The MCA supplies the lateral aspect of the frontal, parietal, and temporal lobes and the underlying corona radiata, extending as deep as the putamen and the posterior limb of the internal capsule. As the main stem of the MCA passes out through the sylvian fissure, it gives rise to a series of small branches called lenticulostriate arteries, which penetrate deeply into the subcortical portion of the brain and perfuse the basal ganglia and internal capsule. At the lateral surface of the hemisphere, the MCA divides into upper and lower divisions, which perfuse the lateral surface of the hemisphere. When the MCA is occluded at its origin, a large cerebral infarction develops involving all the structures mentioned above. Because of the cerebral edema that usually accompanies such a large lesion with brain displacement, the patient frequently shows depressed consciousness, with head and eyes deviated to the side of the lesion, with contralateral hemiplegia, decreased sensation, and homonymous hemianopia. If the dominant hemisphere is involved, aphasia is usually present, which may be severe if the entire territory of the MCA is infarcted. As the

patient's mental status improves, other features become evident, namely, dysphagia, contralateral hemianopia, and, in patients with nondominant hemisphere lesions, perceptual deficits and neglect. Patients who survive the acute lesion regain control of head and eye movements, and normal level of consciousness is restored. However, severe deficits involving motor, visuospatial, and language function usually persist.

Occlusion of the MCA branches, except for the lenticulostriate, is almost always embolic in origin, and the associated infarctions are smaller and more peripherally located than those seen after occlusion of the MCA trunk. The superior division of the MCA supplies the rolandic and prerolandic areas, and an infarction in this territory will result in a dense sensory-motor deficit on the contralateral face, arm, and leg, with less involvement of the leg. As recovery occurs, the patient is usually able to walk with a spastic, hemiparetic gait. Little recovery occurs in motor function of the arm. If the left hemisphere is involved, there is usually severe aphasia initially with eventual improvement in comprehension, although an expressive aphasia is likely to persist. Small focal infarctions from occlusions of branches of the superior division will produce more limited deficits such as pure motor weakness of the contralateral arm and face, apraxia, or expressive aphasia.

The inferior division of the MCA supplies the parietal and temporal lobes, and lesions on the left side result in severe involvement of language comprehension. The optic radiation is usually involved, resulting in partial or complete contralateral homonymous hemianopia. Lesions affecting the right hemisphere often result in neglect of the left side of the body. Initially, the patient may completely ignore the affected side and even assert that his left upper extremity belongs to someone else. Such severe neglect often gradually improves but may be followed by a variety of persisting impairments such as deficits in attention, constructional apraxia, dressing apraxia, perceptual deficits, and aprosodia.

Several characteristic and rather common syndromes have been described when lacunar strokes occur in the distribution of the lenticulostriate branches of the MCA. Among the most common is a lesion in the internal capsule causing a pure motor hemiplegia. An anterior lesion in the internal capsule may cause dysarthria with hand clumsiness, and a lesion of the thalamus or adjacent internal capsule causes a contralateral sensory loss with or without weakness. The neurologic deficits in these lesions often show early and progressive recovery with good ultimate outcome.

Anterior Cerebral Artery Syndromes

Branches of the anterior cerebral arteries supply the median and paramedian regions of the frontal cortex and the strip of the lateral surface of the hemisphere along its superior border. There are deep penetrating branches that supply the head of the caudate nucleus and the anterior limb of the internal capsule. Occlusions of the anterior cerebral artery (ACA) are not common, but when they occur, there is contralateral hemiparesis with relative sparing of the hand and face and greater weakness of the leg. There is associated sensory loss of the leg and foot. Lesions affecting the left side may produce a transcortical motor aphasia characterized by diminution of spontaneous speech but preserved ability to repeat words. A grasp reflex is often present along with a sucking reflex and paratonic rigidity (also known as gegenhalten—muscle hypertonia presenting as an involuntary variable resistance during passive movement of a limb). Urinary incontinence is common. Large lesions of the frontal cortex often produce behavioral changes, such as lack of spontaneity, distractibility, and tendency to perseverate. Affected individuals may have diminished reasoning ability. Bilateral anterior cerebral artery infarctions may cause severe abulia (lack of initiation).

Vertebrobasilar Syndromes

The two vertebral arteries join at the junction of the medulla and pons to form the basilar artery. Together, the vertebral and basilar arteries supply the brainstem by paramedian and short circumferential branches and supply the cerebellum by long circumferential branches. The basilar artery terminates by bifurcating at the upper midbrain level to form the two posterior cerebral arteries. The posterior communicating arteries connect the middle to the posterior cerebral arteries, completing the circle of Willis.

Some general clinical features of lesions in the vertebrobasilar system should be noted. In contrast to lesions in the hemispheres, which are unilateral, lesions involving the pons and medulla often cross the midline and produce bilateral symptoms. When motor impairments are present, they are often bilateral, with asymmetric corticospinal signs, and they are frequently accompanied by cerebellar signs. Cranial nerve lesions are very frequent and occur ipsilateral to the main lesion. There may be dissociated sensory loss (involvement of the spinothalamic pathway with preservation of the dorsal column pathway or vice versa), dysarthria, dysphagia, disequilibrium and vertigo, and Horner's syndrome. Of particular note is absence of cortical deficits, such as aphasia and cognitive impairments. Visual field loss and visuospatial deficits may occur if the posterior cerebral artery is involved, but not with brainstem lesions. Identification of a specific cranial nerve deficit allows precise anatomic localization of the lesion.

Lacunar infarcts are common in the vertebrobasilar distribution, arising from occlusion of small penetrating branches of the basilar artery or posterior cerebral artery. In contrast to cerebral lacunae, most brainstem lacunae are symptomatic. There is a variety of characteristic brainstem syndromes associated with lesions at various levels in the brainstem. Pontine lacunar infarcts frequently result in a pure motor hemiparesis. The reader is referred to neurologic texts for a comprehensive discussion of these lesions.

Several brainstem syndromes are relatively common among patients referred for rehabilitation, and these are described in some detail.

The *lateral medullary syndrome* (Wallenberg's syndrome) is produced by an infarction in the lateral wedge of the medulla. It may occur as an occlusion of the vertebral artery or the posterior-inferior cerebellar artery. The clinical features of this syndrome, along with the corresponding anatomic structures involved, are impairment of contralateral pain and temperature (spinothalamic tract); ipsilateral Horner's syndrome consisting of miosis, ptosis, and decreased facial sweating (descending sympathetic tract); dysphagia, dysarthria, and dysphonia (ipsilateral paralysis of the palate and vocal cords); nystagmus, vertigo, nausea, and vomiting (vestibular nucleus); ipsilateral limb ataxia (spinocerebellar fibers); and ipsilateral impaired sensation of the face (sensory nucleus of the fifth nerve). Patients with this syndrome are frequently quite disabled initially because of

vertigo, disequilibrium, and ataxia, but they often make a good functional recovery.

Occlusion of the basilar artery may result in severe deficits with complete motor and sensory loss and cranial nerve signs from which patients do not recover. Patients are often comatose. *Locked-in syndrome* is an uncommon but devastating stroke syndrome involving the brainstem. The infarction in such cases affects the upper ventral pons, involving the bilateral corticospinal and corticobulbar pathways but sparing the reticular activating system and ascending sensory pathways. Patients have normal sensation and can see and hear but are unable to move or speak. Blinking and upward gaze are preserved, which provides a very limited but usable means for communication. The patient is alert and fully oriented. Some patients do not survive, and those who do are severely disabled and dependent. Slow improvement and partial recovery may occur in this group of patients, justifying appropriate levels of rehabilitation intervention.

Focal infarctions may occur in the midbrain and affect the descending corticospinal pathway, sometimes also involving the third cranial nerve nucleus (Weber's syndrome), resulting in ipsilateral third nerve palsy and paralysis of the contralateral arm and leg. Eye movement abnormalities are seen in a variety of brainstem stroke syndromes due to the location of the nuclei for these cranial nerves in the midbrain (third and fourth cranial nerves) and pons (sixth nerve) and their interconnections.

The posterior cerebral artery perfuses the thalamus through perforating arteries, as well as the temporal and occipital lobes with their subcortical structures, including the optic radiation. An occipital lobe infarction will cause a partial or complete contralateral hemianopia, and when these visual deficits involve the dominant hemisphere, there may be associated difficulty in reading or in naming objects. When the thalamus is involved, there is contralateral hemisensory loss. A lesion involving the thalamus may cause a syndrome characterized by contralateral hemianesthesia and central pain, although only about 25% of cases of central pain in stroke are caused by lesions of the thalamus. Other lesion sites reported to be associated with central pain are the brainstem and parietal lobe projections from the thalamus. In the thalamic syndrome, patients report unremitting, unpleasant, burning pain affecting the opposite side of the body. Examination of the patient reveals contralateral impairment of all sensory modalities, often with dysesthesia. There may be involvement of adjacent structures, such as the internal capsule (hemiparesis, ataxia) or basal ganglia (choreoathetosis).

EVALUATION OF THE STROKE ETIOLOGY

For many patients, a stroke represents only one facet of systemic atherosclerotic vascular disease. Such patients will often have multiple risk factors for an event, such as increased age, hypertension, diabetes, and smoking. Stroke, however, can occur in the absence of common risk factors or atherosclerosis.

The investigation undertaken to identify the cause of a stroke depends on the patient's age and presence or absence of risk factors. For example, a 79-year-old man with hypertension and a long history of smoking who sustains a lacunar infarct will not likely require assessment for a hypercoagulable state, whereas this may be an important component of the investigation of the cause of stroke in a 32-year-old woman without identifiable risk factors.

A basic evaluation of stroke cause includes a thorough physical and neurologic examination, cerebral imaging (CT or preferably MRI), an electrocardiogram, noninvasive carotid studies, and an echocardiogram (see Chapter 5, Imaging Techniques). In cases where there is concern regarding a possible cardiogenic embolism, a minimum of 24-hour electrocardiographic monitoring is appropriate, and longer periods of monitoring (e.g., the use of an implantable event recorder) increase the diagnostic yield. Transesophageal echocardiography provides superior imaging of the left atrium, the mitral valve, and the aortic arch. In cases where the possibility of a paradoxical embolism has been raised, the echocardiogram should include a "bubble" study to evaluate for right-to-left shunting, and studies for deep vein thrombosis are frequently performed. CT or MR angiography may be indicated when concerns regarding large vessel occlusion, stenosis, or dissection are present. Occasionally, conventional angiography may be indicated, although this is increasingly reserved for use during intravascular interventions.

In younger patients, evaluation frequently includes tests for a hypercoagulable state and screening for vasculitis or rheumatologic disorder (e.g., lupus).

STROKE IN CHILDREN AND YOUNG ADULTS

Stroke can occur at any age and is an important cause of disability in children and young adults. In a significant number of cases, 40% to 50%, no obvious risk factors—such as sources of cardiogenic emboli and atherosclerosis—are found. These patients should be thoroughly investigated for primary etiology of the stroke. A list of possible diagnoses is given in **Box 18-3**. Coagulation disorders may be inherited or acquired, but they may account for up to 20% of cases with thrombotic infarction in young adults. Deficiencies of antithrombin III, protein C, and protein S are among the most important coagulopathies, as each of these substances is part of the naturally occurring anticoagulant system. Each of these coagulopathies requires long-term treatment with warfarin.

BOX 18-3

Causes of Stroke in Children and Young Adults

Cerebral embolism
Trauma to extracranial arteries
   Thromboembolic occlusion
   Dissection
Subarachnoid hemorrhage
   Aneurysm
   Arteriovenous malformation
Sickle cell anemia
Vasculopathy
   Moyamoya disease
   Systemic lupus erythematosus
   Drug induced
   Vasculitis
Coagulopathy
   Deficiency of antithrombin III
   Deficiency of protein C
   Deficiency of protein S
Homocystinuria
Oral contraceptives
Postpartum
Drug induced

Carotid dissection may occur with minimal or no antecedent trauma and result in stroke in the MCA territory. Vertebral artery dissection may occur after high-velocity chiropractic manipulation of the cervical spine.

A variety of vasculitides may occur, some of which are part of multisystem autoimmune disease such as systemic lupus erythematosus. Another uncommon cause of stroke early in life is the inherited disorder homocystinuria, which predisposes individuals to early atherosclerosis. Lastly, stroke has been reported as an occasional complication occurring during pregnancy or in the postpartum period.

ACUTE STROKE MANAGEMENT

The goals of acute stroke management are (a) to limit or reverse neurologic damage through thrombolysis or neuroprotection and (b) to monitor and prevent secondary stroke complications such as elevated intracranial pressure.

Intravenous thrombolysis with recombinant tissue plasminogen activator is a well-established therapy and is most effective when given as early after stroke onset as possible (12,13). Efficacy has been found for administration as late as 4.5 hours poststroke (14). Mechanical thrombectomy has been found effective within the first 6 hours post stroke onset for individuals with proximal large artery occlusions in the anterior circulation (15–17). Efforts to increase the rapidity of thrombolytic therapy are ongoing, and recent innovations include the use of mobile CT scanners that can be housed in ambulances and brought to the patient to expedite care (18).

The development of an effective neuroprotective agent remains one of the major goals in acute stroke care but has thus far not been successful. Control of blood pressure, fever, and hyperglycemia has, however, been shown to improve outcome in acute stroke.

Excitotoxicity is believed to play a role in the death of ischemic neurons in the penumbra around an infarction. Dying cells release excitatory amino acids, particularly glutamate, which activate cell membrane channels, allowing toxic levels of calcium to accumulate inside cells that are injured but not yet dead. The elevated intracellular calcium initiates an array of neurochemical changes within the neurons that generate free radicals and result in cell death. Clinical trials of glutamate receptor antagonists and free radical scavengers for acute stroke have been disappointing in humans, despite evidence of efficacy in animal models.

SECONDARY STROKE PREVENTION

Secondary prevention involves a multipronged effort at risk factor reduction, which may involve behavioral change, such as smoking cessation, aerobic exercise, and dietary modifications in addition to optimizing treatment of associated medical risk factors, such as hypertension and diabetes (19).

Medical and occasionally surgical/procedural treatments are key components of stroke prevention.

Antiplatelet medications are appropriate for the majority of patients for secondary prevention of ischemic stroke. Aspirin in doses of 50 to 325 mg provides a reduction in stroke of approximately 25% (20). Gastrointestinal toxicity (bleeding, dyspepsia) is the most common side effect of aspirin, followed by allergies.

Clopidogrel is another antiplatelet agent with a different mechanism of action from aspirin. In clinical trials, its efficacy in preventing stroke is comparable to aspirin, though it is more costly. It is generally well tolerated, though its use has been associated with rare cases of thrombotic thrombocytopenic purpura. Combining clopidogrel and aspirin may provide benefit early after stroke (21), but over the long term, this combination appears to raise the risk of hemorrhagic complications without further reduction in stroke risk (22). Ticlopidine is a related drug, with similar efficacy. It has largely fallen out of use due to concerns regarding neutropenia (23).

Another agent, dipyridamole, has some efficacy when taken alone but is generally prescribed as part of a fixed-dose combination with aspirin (Aggrenox). In a large European trial, there was a 37% reduction in risk of stroke in patients prescribed both aspirin and dipyridamole (24), which compared favorably with treatment with aspirin alone. A recent study comparing dipyridamole with aspirin versus clopidogrel failed to show any difference in efficacy between these two therapies (25), and uncertainty regarding the ideal selection of antiplatelet agent persists (26).

Stroke can occur despite the use of antiplatelet agents. There is no consensus regarding the management of individuals who sustain a stroke despite preventive antiplatelet therapy, although substitution of combined aspirin plus dipyridamole therapy for aspirin monotherapy or substitution of clopidogrel for aspirin monotherapy is commonly instituted.

Warfarin use for stroke prevention is generally restricted to patients with atrial fibrillation or other known cardiac or other embolic source. For most indications, a target INR of 2 to 3 is used, although a higher range is needed for patients with certain types of mechanical heart valves. Newer oral anticoagulants, such as dabigatran, apixaban, rivaroxaban, and edoxaban, are effective alternatives to warfarin for stroke prevention in patients with atrial fibrillation or cardioembolic stroke and do not require the frequent laboratory testing needed for warfarin (27,28). These newer agents are more expensive than warfarin, impacting their affordability for some patients.

Statin medications have been demonstrated to reduce the risk of recurrent stroke, and are now generally included as part of secondary prevention, irrespective of the presence or absence of hyperlipidemia (29,30).

Carotid endarterectomy reduces the risk of stroke in those patients with single or multiple transient ischemic attacks (TIAs) and with 70% or greater stenosis of the ipsilateral internal carotid artery (31).

Patients with stenosis of 50% to 70% may be considered for surgery if symptomatic, that is, if they are having TIAs or a stroke ipsilateral to the carotid lesion. The evidence for carotid endarterectomy is less compelling for patients with asymptomatic carotid stenosis, with a recommendation that it be considered for asymptomatic patients with stenoses of 60% to 99% (32).

Carotid stenting is increasingly used as an alternative to carotid endarterectomy. Meta-analysis of the randomized controlled trials comparing carotid stenting with carotid endarterectomy indicates a somewhat higher risk of periprocedural stroke or death association with stenting in patients over age 70, but not for those below age 70 (33).

REHABILITATION DURING THE ACUTE PHASE

The care of stroke survivors is organized in a variety of different systems around the world. In many European countries, stroke units provide a combination of acute stroke management and subsequent intensive rehabilitation in a single unit. Studies of stroke units have consistently found improved outcomes when compared with care on general medical units (34). Interestingly, much of the benefits in mortality appear to relate to prevention and/or earlier recognition of medical complications of stroke and earlier mobilization (35).

In the United States, acute stroke care is often transitioned rapidly to rehabilitative care, often within a matter of days. Despite this, it is important that rehabilitation not be considered a separate phase of care, that only begins after acute medical intervention. Rather, it is an integral part of medical management and continues longitudinally through acute care, postacute care, and community reintegration. Although diagnosis and medical treatment are the principal focus of early treatment, rehabilitation measures should be offered concurrently. Many of these can be considered preventive in nature. For example, patients who are hemiplegic, lethargic, and incontinent are at high risk for developing pressure ulcers. Deliberate strategies should be followed to prevent skin breakdowns, including protection of skin from excessive moisture, the use of heel-protecting splints, maintenance of proper position with frequent turning, and daily inspection and routine skin cleansing (36).

Many patients with acute stroke have dysphagia and are at risk for aspiration and pneumonia (see Chapter 13, Speech, Language, Swallowing and Auditory Rehabilitation). In the able-bodied, aspiration usually results in vigorous coughing, but as many as 40% of patients with acute stroke experience silent aspiration. Protection against aspiration (and resulting pneumonia) includes avoiding oral feeding in patients who are not alert. Even in alert patients, the ability to swallow should be assessed carefully before oral intake of fluids or food is begun. This is done with a bedside screening assessment that can be efficiently completed by physician or nursing staff and generally includes taking a small drink of water and observing for coughing or change in vocal quality (37). If any doubt exists about aspiration, a swallowing videofluoroscopy examination or flexible endoscopic evaluation of swallowing (FEES) should be performed. During the acute phase, nasogastric tube feeding or gastrostomy tube placement may prove necessary. Patients who are lying flat in bed are at significant risk for regurgitation and aspiration, and the head of the bed should be kept elevated (38).

Impairment of bladder control is frequent following a stroke, which may initially cause a hypotonic bladder with overflow incontinence. If an indwelling catheter is used, it should be removed as soon as possible, with careful monitoring to insure that appropriate voiding resumes. For the occasional patient with persistent urinary retention after stroke, regular intermittent catheterization is preferable to an indwelling catheter (39).

Patients with hemiplegia are at high risk for development of contractures due to immobility. Spasticity, if present at this early stage, may contribute to the development of contractures through sustained posturing of the limbs. The harmful effects of immobility can be ameliorated by regular passive stretching and moving the joints through a full range of motion, preferably at least twice daily. While the use of resting hand splints remains widespread, studies have failed to demonstrate their utility (40,41). These may be considered as a component of care, but should be reevaluated periodically to determine if they are truly needed.

The risk of deep vein thrombosis is high, especially in patients with hemiplegia. Every patient should, therefore, have some form of deep vein thrombosis (DVT) prophylaxis, low molecular weight heparin, subcutaneous heparin, or external pneumatic compression boots.

Early mobilization is beneficial by reducing the risks of DVT, deconditioning, gastroesophageal regurgitation and aspiration pneumonia, contracture formation, skin breakdown, and orthostatic intolerance. Positive psychological benefits are also likely. Specific tasks include turning from side to side in bed and changing position, sitting up in bed, transferring to a wheelchair, standing, and walking. Mobilization also includes self-care activities such as self-feeding, grooming, and dressing. The timing and progression in these activities depend on the patient's condition. Despite the intuitive appeal of beginning these activities as soon as possible, the AVERT trial found that very early aggressive mobilization (within 24 hours poststroke) was associated with worse outcomes, and therefore mobilization efforts should be judicious within this time frame (39).

Evaluation for Rehabilitation Program

Evaluation of longer-term rehabilitation needs should occur within the first few days after stroke. Many stroke survivors will benefit from admission to an acute rehabilitation hospital or unit (also known as an inpatient rehabilitation facility, or IRF), and criteria for admission into such a program are listed in **Box 18-4**. Some individuals may be more appropriate for a subacute rehabilitation program (based on a skilled nursing facility, or SNF), which provides a less intense rehabilitation program with a lesser degree of medical supervision over a longer period of time. These programs are most appropriate for individuals who are unlikely to return home due to premorbid conditions (such as dementia), who are too frail to undergo an intensive rehabilitation program, or whose neurologic impairments are so profound as to prevent participation in a hospital-level program. The American Heart Association Stroke Rehabilitation Guideline recommends IRF care in preference to SNF care for stroke survivors who qualify for and have access to IRF care (42). Stroke survivors with isolated disabilities such as a partial aphasia, visual loss, or monoparesis may more appropriately receive rehabilitation on an outpatient basis or through a home care agency.

RECOVERY FROM STROKE

Compensation, Recovery, and Rehabilitation

Historically, rehabilitation focused primarily on instruction in compensatory techniques, such as ambulating with a cane and ankle-foot orthosis (AFO), or the use of one-handed dressing techniques. With the increasing recognition of the plasticity of the adult human brain and the ability of rehabilitation

---

BOX 18-4

Criteria for Admission to a Comprehensive Rehabilitation Program

Stable neurologic status
Significant persisting neurologic deficit
Identified disability affecting at least two of the following:
    mobility, self-care activities, communication, bowel or bladder control, or swallowing
Sufficient cognitive function to learn
Sufficient communicative ability to engage with the therapists
Physical ability to tolerate the active program (at least 3 h/d)
Achievable therapeutic goals

---

interventions to facilitate this recovery, there has been a growing component of therapy intended to maximize recovery of neurologic function (see Chapter 61, Neural Repair and Plasticity). These approaches are at some level complementary, inasmuch as the goal of rehabilitation should be to maximize neurologic recovery and then teach compensatory approaches to address whatever residual deficits exist. Unfortunately, treatments for improvement of recovery during the early phases of stroke often require intensive efforts, and their benefits, while appearing hopeful, are still difficult to assess. As a result, limitations in the duration and intensity of rehabilitation supported by third-party payers have resulted in a continued clinical emphasis toward compensatory approaches, even as the evidence demonstrating the opportunities to achieve partial neurologic recovery continues to grow. Resolution of this tension remains problematic in the current health care environment.

Recovery from Impairments

Hemiparesis and motor recovery have been the most studied of all stroke impairments. As many as 88% of patients diagnosed with an acute stroke have hemiparesis (43). In the majority of hemiparetic patients, the arm is more involved than the leg, and the degree of functional motor recovery in the arm is less than in the leg. There are several reasons for this preponderance. Perhaps the most important reason is that ischemic strokes, as noted above, occur in certain vascular territories more frequently than others. More specifically, strokes affecting the MCA territory are much more common than those affecting only the anterior cerebral artery territory. The higher flow through the MCA and the more direct path for embolism may underlie this predilection for the MCA. In patients who do experience ACA territory infarcts, the usual pattern of arm impairment exceeding leg impairment is reversed, with motor function best preserved in the distal upper limb.

Another factor contributing to the discrepant outcomes between the upper limb and the lower limb is the very distinct functional demands placed on the upper versus the lower limb. The lower limb can be reasonably functional if it is able to maintain an extended posture and have some gross volitional movements. By contrast, the upper limb relies on the exquisite fine motor control of the hand for functional tasks, and gross movements (as are often recovered in the proximal portion of the upper limb) do not result in a substantial level of function.

The severity of arm weakness at onset and the timing of the return of movement in the hand are both important predictors of eventual motor recovery in the arm (44–47). The prognosis for return of useful hand function is poor when there is complete arm paralysis at onset or no measurable grasp strength by 4 weeks. However, even among those patients with severe arm weakness at onset, as many as 11% may gain good recovery of hand function. Some other generalizations can be made. For patients showing some motor recovery in the hand by 4 weeks, as many as 70% will make a full or good recovery. Complete functional recovery, when it occurs, is usually complete within 3 months of onset. Imaging studies have demonstrated that the lesion load to the corticospinal tracts predicts recovery (48,49). The ability to evoke a motor response using transcranial magnetic stimulation is another predictor of recovery (50,51). These imaging and neurophysiologic parameters have not entered widespread clinical use, however.

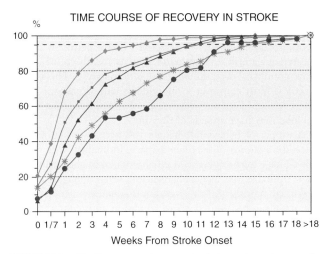

FIGURE 18-1. The time course of recovery in stroke survivors shown as the cumulated rate of patients having reached their best neurologic outcome. The course of recovery is given for patients whose initial stroke severity was mild, ♦; moderate, ▲; severe, *; very severe, ●. All patients are represented by ■.

The patterns of motor recovery have been described in detail in the Copenhagen Stroke Study (52). Summary data are shown in **Figure 18-1**. Ninety-five percent of stroke survivors reached their best neurologic level within 11 weeks of onset. Individuals with milder stroke recovered more quickly, and those with severe strokes reached their best neurologic level in 15 weeks on average. The course of motor recovery reaches a plateau after an early phase of progressive improvement, and only minor additional measurable improvement occurs after 6 months post onset (53). However, in some stroke survivors who have significant partial return of voluntary movement, recovery may continue over a longer period of time. However, recovery varies from person to person, and it is important that these data are not misinterpreted as dictating a fixed course. The observation that stroke survivors with apparently chronic stable motor deficits can experience improved motor function as the result of an intensive exercise program even years after a stroke also creates a conundrum for clinicians seeking to determine a reasonable therapeutic endpoint for motor rehabilitation efforts.

Aphasia occurs in about one third of patients with acute stroke, although a substantial portion of affected individuals will improve (see Chapter 13, Speech, Language, Swallowing and Auditory Rehabilitation). By 6 months or more after stroke, only 12% to 18% of stroke survivors have identifiable aphasia (54,55). The time course of recovery of language function is slower and more prolonged than motor abilities, with improvements continuing for more than a year in some cases (55). The course of recovery varies depending on the nature of the language impairments. Patients with Broca's (nonfluent) aphasia with large hemisphere lesions tend to have little recovery, whereas patients with smaller lesions (e.g., confined to the posterior frontal lobe) often show evolution into a milder form of aphasia with anomia and word-finding difficulty. Individuals with global aphasia (affecting both comprehension and verbal expression) tend to progress slowly, with comprehension often improving more than expressive ability. Communicative ability of stroke survivors who initially have global aphasia improves over a longer period of time, up to 1 year or more poststroke. Patients with global aphasia associated with large lesions may show only minor recovery, but those with smaller lesions may improve substantially. Language recovery in Wernicke's (fluent) aphasia is variable.

Hemispatial neglect commonly affects individuals with large infarcts in the right parietal lobe, resulting in inattention to objects and actions within the stroke survivor's left side of space. In some cases, this is associated with lack of awareness of impairments (e.g., hemiplegia) known as anosognosia and, in severe cases, lack of awareness of the left side of the body altogether. Substantial but not necessarily complete recovery is the norm, and the recovery from hemispatial neglect seems to generally follow a similar pattern of proportional recovery as hemiparesis after stroke (56).

About 20% of patients have a visual field defect. In general, the degree of visual improvement following stroke is modest, and if the field defect persists beyond a few weeks, late recovery is less likely.

Mechanisms of Neurologic Recovery

Neurologic improvement begins immediately after the stroke and is believed to result from a number of mechanisms (see Chapter 61, Neural Repair and Plasticity). Improvements seen in the first days to weeks after stroke appear to include recovery of function in portions of the ischemic penumbra and resolution of edema and associated mass effect. Overlapping with this early resolution and continuing for at least several months are the process of cerebral plasticity and functional reorganization of the cerebral cortex. Both animal and human studies with fMRI and other techniques have demonstrated alterations in cortical maps associated with this plasticity. Similarities exist between the processes of motor learning and motor recovery, and some overlap between these processes is likely. Some or all of the improvements in motor function observed with intensive training in chronic stroke survivors with apparently stable deficits may be a result of motor learning, rather than "motor recovery" *per se* (57).

Plasticity is strongly influenced by use, as shown in both animal and human studies (58). Research is ongoing to determine the optimal training program to achieve maximal motor recovery. While motor function has been the focus of much of the research on stroke recovery, it is likely that many of the principles established can be applied to other neurologic impairments resulting from stroke. (see Chapter 61 for more details about neuroplasticity.)

Specific Stroke Impairments and Their Rehabilitation

Cognition and Communication

The impact of stroke on cognition and communication depends on several factors, including the size and location of the lesion and the presence or absence of premorbid factors such as prior stroke(s), dementia, or other neurologic conditions. Particularly among older stroke survivors, there is a high prevalence of premorbid cognitive decline, often undiagnosed prior to the stroke.

Delirium is also common during the early phases of acute hospitalization and may result from infection, sleep disruption, fluid or electrolyte disturbances, or medication side effects. Elderly patients are at increased risk of delirium, although stroke patients can be affected at any age. This delirium is generally reversible and should be recognized so that the underlying cause can be treated, so that efforts to prognosticate are not based on faulty impressions of the magnitude of the deficits directly related to the stroke.

Stroke can also affect a person's ability to maintain an alert and attentive state. Large hemispheric strokes may cause drowsiness, as can some lesions affecting the brainstem. Stimulants are frequently employed as treatment (such as dextroamphetamine, methylphenidate, modafinil, or armodafinil), often with partial benefit. Most patients with reduced arousal after a stroke tend to improve substantially over a period of days to weeks.

A bedside mental status assessment is an essential part of the assessment of every stroke patient. The Mini-Mental State Examination (MMSE) developed by Folstein et al. (59) is a useful bedside tool that screens a variety of mental demands quickly and gives a well-validated measure of overall mental function, but is insensitive to visuospatial and executive function impairments compared with the alternative Montreal Cognitive Assessment (MoCA) (60). The NIH Stroke Scale (NIHSS) is another widely used measure that includes some elements of cognitive and language abilities. Formal neuropsychological testing may be useful to develop a comprehensive assessment of cognitive and linguistic functions but is usually best deferred until stroke survivors have completed a portion of their rehabilitation and are approaching a stable plateau in ability. Perceptual impairments, in which the primary sensory system is intact but the processing of the sensory information is impaired, are common among stroke survivors, particularly (but not exclusively) those with nondominant hemisphere lesions. Left hemispatial neglect may be accompanied by a right gaze preference in severe cases, but more subtle impairments may require formal testing to identify. Commonly used bedside tests for visual neglect include letter cancellation tasks, clock or figure drawing, or line bisection.

Hemispatial neglect may affect some forms of stimuli more than others, such as visual, tactile, or auditory. Therapies commonly include the use of visual and/or verbal cuing, including having the patient learn to cue himself or herself verbally to look to the left side. Fresnel prisms applied to eyeglasses are sometimes used to shift images further to the right in order to induce adaptation that persists after removal of the prisms. Small studies support the utility of this approach (61), but this technique is not in widespread use currently. Noninvasive brain stimulation using repetitive transcranial magnetic stimulation (rTMS) (62) or theta-burst stimulation (63) has been found useful in preliminary studies.

Strokes affecting the right parietal lobe also commonly cause deficits in constructional ability, and patients may be unable to copy or draw simple figures (or omit elements on the left side). Other bedside tests of perceptual function are failure to recognize palm writing (graphesthesia), inability to identify objects in the hand (astereognosis), and extinction of simultaneous bilateral cutaneous or visual stimulation.

Anosognosia, a lack of ability to recognize the deficits resulting from the stroke, is common among individuals with right parietal lesions and may include a lack of awareness of hemiplegia, a lack of insight regarding their need for continued hospitalization, and, in severe cases, an inability to recognize their hemiplegic limb(s) as their own.

The term *apraxia* describes the inability of an individual to execute an intended movement when basic motor and sensory functions are apparently preserved. Apraxia is a disorder of motor planning, rather than of coordination (such as ataxia) or of motor strength and control (such as hemiparesis). Ideomotor apraxia may be detected when a person is unable to carry out a task on command such as "comb your hair" or "wave goodbye," even though there is no paralysis. This type of apraxia is most common in individuals with dominant hemisphere strokes. Patients with lesions of the nondominant parietal lobe may have apraxia of dressing.

A variety of behavioral changes can occur after stroke and reflect the anatomy of the brain damage. Individuals with frontal lobe damage may display reduced attention and abulia. In more severe frontal lesions (generally bilateral), severe abulia may result in akinetic mutism. Apathy is common, manifesting as a lack of concern regarding one's personal condition and reduced insight and concern regarding the impact on friends or family.

Deficits in attention and executive function are very common following a stroke and can occur in association with frontal, parietal, or temporal lesions. Stroke survivors may show reduced ability to maintain attention to a task, inability to switch from one task to the next, or inability to filter out unimportant stimuli in the environment with resulting distractibility. Deficits in attention are commonly misinterpreted as memory impairments, as individuals who are not attending to stimuli and information provided will be unable to recall it at a later time.

Dementia, particularly in its milder forms, may have been present before a stroke and is often unrecognized and undiagnosed by clinicians during the early recovery period.

Stroke itself may cause multi-infarct dementia, and patients with multiple lesions, especially when bilateral, are more likely to show features of dementia. Numerous studies have shown that in patients with a history of stroke, those with more extensive white matter changes are at higher risk for dementia.

Poststroke depression is very common and is discussed in greater detail below. Emotional lability occurs in as many as 20% of patients poststroke and is more common in patients with right hemisphere lesions. Individuals with emotional lability often are unable to control or suppress their emotional response to common environmental stimuli and may cry or laugh very easily even though the stroke survivor recognizes that this response is inappropriate. Emotional lability (sometimes termed "emotional incontinence") is often mistaken for depression. Education of the stroke survivor and his or her family is particularly important, and many individuals find they can tolerate these symptoms reasonably well as long as they understand their cause. Emotional lability tends to improve with time and may respond partially to treatment with a combination of dextromethorphan/quinidine or selective serotonin reuptake inhibitor (SSRI) antidepressants (64–66).

Communication Disorders

Communication is a complex function involving reception, central processing, and expression of information (see Chapter 13). Communication occurs through the use of language and consists of a system of symbols that are combined to convey ideas, that is, letters, words, or gestures. Impairment of language is called *aphasia*, and its presence reflects an abnormality in the dominant hemisphere. *Speech*, on the other hand, is a term that refers to the motor mechanism involved in the production of spoken words, namely, breathing, phonation, and articulation. Dysphonia and dysarthria are disorders of speech.

The inflection and intonation of speech (prosody) are also important in communicating and may be impaired after right hemisphere stroke (aprosodia).

There are a number of aphasia classifications. In the simplest classification, aphasia is divided into two main categories: motor aphasia (sometimes called nonfluent, expressive, or anterior aphasia), characterized by nonfluent speech, and sensory aphasia (sometimes called fluent, receptive, posterior, or Wernicke's aphasia), characterized by fluent speech (see **Table 18-2**) (67). Anomic aphasia is a milder form of aphasia, where difficulty recalling the correct words or names is most prominent. Simple bedside tests can allow the clinician to categorize the communication disorder. Questions typically addressed during the bedside assessment of aphasia are provided in **Table 18-3**. Comprehensive evaluations of patients can be performed using formal aphasia tests. **Box 18-5** summarizes the more commonly used formal aphasia test instruments.

Language therapy is based on the detailed evaluation of the patient's cognitive and linguistic capabilities and deficits. In the early stages of rehabilitation, it is important for the therapist to help the patient establish a reliable means for basic yes/no communication. The therapist then progresses to specific techniques based on the patient's deficits.

Specific techniques have been described for improving comprehension, word or phoneme retrieval, and gestures to supplement verbal communication. Recovery of functional communication may have a more protracted course than motor recovery, and meaningful improvements may be seen in some stroke survivors 6 and 12 months after stroke and beyond. A meta-analysis found speech therapy effective for aphasia (68), although a Cochrane review (69) has found insufficient evidence to draw this conclusion. More recently, a dose-response effect has been identified, with more intensive therapy correlated with greater improvement (70). Newer methods of therapy, including constraint-induced aphasia therapy (involving intensive practice of speech tasks with which the stroke survivor has difficulty and avoiding the use of nonverbal communication) have shown some benefit (71,72).

Visual Deficits

Visual field deficits are common among patients with strokes in the MCA or posterior cerebral artery distributions. Bedside testing of visual fields, including examination for extinction with simultaneous stimulation, is an important element of the clinical evaluation of stroke patients undergoing rehabilitation.

TABLE 18-3	Bedside Aphasia Assessment
Questions	**Clinical Test**
Does the patient understand?	Give verbal commands; ask the patient to point to objects.
Is the patient able to talk?	Ask the patient to name objects, describe them, and count. Listen for spontaneous speech.
Can the patient repeat?	Ask the patient to repeat words.
Can the patient read?	Give commands in writing.
Can the patient write?	Ask the patient to copy or to write dictated words.

More formal visual field testing may prove useful in selected patients. Patients with isolated visual field deficits, but without concomitant hemispatial neglect, generally learn to compensate effectively. Initial reports of benefit from computer-based visual restoration therapy (73) have not been replicated in studies using more rigorous methods (74).

Strokes in the brainstem can cause extraocular palsies and associated diplopia. Patching is often useful to manage diplopia; patches may be alternated between eyes when appropriate to allow practice of extraocular movements and facilitate recovery of the paretic muscles.

Dysphagia

Dysphagia may affect 40% of patients with a unilateral hemispheric stroke (75) and is an important risk factor for pneumonitis and aspiration pneumonia (see Chapter 13, Speech, Language, Swallowing and Auditory Rehabilitation). It generally has a favorable prognosis (76,77) but may be more severe and persistent in patients with brainstem lesions or with bilateral hemispheric strokes (78).

Dysphagia may affect either or both the oral preparatory and pharyngeal phases of swallowing. Bedside evaluation of the patient includes observation of the function of the lips, tongue, cheeks, and jaw and elevation of the larynx during swallowing, as well as vocal quality. Having the patient swallow a small amount of water (30 to 90 mL) at the bedside provides considerable information about oral control, the timeliness of swallowing, presence or absence of a wet vocal quality, and the presence or absence of coughing. Patients who are drowsy should be considered unsafe for oral intake by virtue of their altered level of consciousness, and further assessment deferred until they are more awake.

TABLE 18-2	Classification of Aphasia			
Classification	**Fluency**	**Comprehension**	**Repetition**	**Naming**
Global	Poor	Poor	Poor	Poor
Broca	Poor	Good	Variable	Poor
Isolation	Poor	Poor	Good	Poor
Transcortical motor	Poor	Good	Good	Poor
Wernicke's	Good	Poor	Poor	Poor
Transcortical sensory	Good	Poor	Good	Poor
Conduction	Good	Good	Poor	Poor
Anomic	Good	Good	Good	Poor

Adapted by permission from Springer: Brandstater ME. Basic aspects of impairment evaluation in stroke patients. In: Chino N, Melvin JL, eds. *Functional Evaluation of Stroke Patients*. 1st ed. New York: Springer-Verlag; 1996:9–18.

BOX 18-5

Commonly Used Formal Aphasia Tests

- The Boston Diagnostic Aphasia Examination (14) produces a classification of the aphasic features observed in a particular patient. Besides classifying the aphasia, it also provides a score of the severity of the aphasia, which can be compared to aphasic patients in general (24).
- The Western Aphasia Battery (25) is somewhat similar to the Boston. It measures various parameters of spontaneous speech and examines comprehension, fluency, object naming, and repetition. It provides a total score called an aphasia quotient, which is a measure of the severity of the aphasia.
- The Porch Index of Communication Ability (PICA) is different from the other tests in that it evaluates verbal, gestural, and graphic responses. It is very structured in its format and must be given by a trained professional. It provides a useful statistical summary of the details of the language impairments and offers outcome prediction.
- The Functional Communication Profile (26) provides an overall rating of functional communication. It is not a diagnostic test. The score indicates severity and can be a useful indicator of recovery.

If an initial screening examination suggests dysphagia, a more extensive bedside evaluation by a speech and language pathologist (or, in some facilities, an occupational therapist) is generally advisable. Some patients aspirate "silently" (without coughing), and the overall results of the bedside assessment should guide decisions regarding more extensive assessment (79). A videofluoroscopic swallowing study (VFSS) (also called a modified barium swallow) provides detailed information about the swallowing mechanism and allows for direct visualization of aspiration. Moreover, modified food consistencies, such as thickened liquids, and compensatory swallowing maneuvers, such as a chin tuck, may be tested during the course of the fluoroscopic swallowing study to determine if they result in safer swallowing.

FEES is another technique that allows more direct visualization of the swallowing process and is used in some settings as an alternative to VFSS, particularly when VFSS is unavailable (e.g., at a nursing home) or logistically impractical (a patient who cannot be moved to the radiology suite for a VFSS for medical reasons). While it does not allow direct visualization of aspiration, FEES does provide considerable information that complements the bedside examination and avoids the radiation exposure present with VFSS.

Both compensatory and recovery strategies are useful for dysphagia. Modified food consistencies, such as pureed foods or thickened liquids, are widely used, as are physical maneuvers, such as a controlling food bolus size and pacing, or using a "chin tuck" or double swallow. It appears likely that practicing swallowing over time improves performance and may enhance the process of spontaneous recovery.

For patients who cannot swallow safely, a nasogastric, gastrostomy, or jejunostomy tube is indicated for enteral feedings. None of these tubes are entirely effective in preventing aspiration pneumonia, in part because oral secretions may be the source of aspiration pneumonia, rather than feedings. Nasogastric and gastrostomy tubes both permit aspiration through the mechanism of gastroesophageal reflux as well, especially when patients are placed flat in bed. The selection of a feeding tube depends on several factors, including patient preference, anticipated duration of the use of a feeding tube, and procedure-related risks. Nasogastric tubes often prove problematic for longer-term feeding due to frequent dislodgement, tube blockages, and patient discomfort, and therefore, gastrostomy tubes are often favored if the duration of the feeding tube use is expected to be lengthy. While most individuals

with hemispheric stroke recover good swallowing function, those with brainstem lesions or bilateral hemisphere lesions may progress more slowly, and some require indefinite use of a feeding tube. Some individuals recover the ability to ingest sufficient food before they are able to drink enough liquids to maintain adequate hydration—in these cases, a feeding tube may continue to be required for fluid supplementation on a shorter or long-term basis.

A surprising number of patients admitted for stroke rehabilitation are malnourished—as high as 22% in one report (80). Elderly patients may have marginal nutritional status prior to their stroke, and if not closely monitored during postacute rehabilitation, their fluid and nutritional status may be further compromised because of dysphagia, reliance on others for oral or tube feedings, lack of interest in food, depression, and problems with communication. The risk of malnutrition and dehydration is very real in even the most alert-appearing patient (particularly in older individuals on restricted diets or those with abulia or attentional deficits), and intake of fluid, protein, and total calories and body weight should be monitored closely in all patients. Oral nutritional supplements may have to be prescribed, and if a patient continues to have inadequate intake, enteral tube feeding may be necessary.

Motor Impairment

Strength, power (the speed with which force can be generated), motor control and coordination, muscle tone, and balance may all be affected by stroke. The most widely used clinical scale to assess strength is the Medical Research Council's (MRC) 6-point scale, 0 to 5, in which 0 represents complete paralysis, 3 is the ability to fully move the limb against gravity, and 5 indicates normal strength (81). This scale is useful in grading muscle strength in patients with lower motor neuron lesions or myopathies but is problematic for assessing stroke survivors. Stroke survivors will often be able to activate a muscle group to varying degrees depending on the position of the limb and coactivation of synergistic muscles. Thus, a stroke survivor may be able to generate considerable force when grasping in association with wrist and elbow flexion but have much less ability to selectively flex the fingers in isolation. Also, the failure of this scale to indicate the degree of motor control may lead to misinterpretation, as in the example of a patient who can generate considerable force, but who has limited motor control, and whose MRC score is recorded as normal or near normal. Despite these shortcomings, the MRC scale is widely used by clinicians, often supplemented by qualifying descriptions (e.g., "elbow flexion is 4/5 on MRC scale in a flexion synergy pattern with moderately reduced motor control"). Use of a dynamometer (82) to measure force generation requires more time and similarly fails to assess motor control and thus has a limited role in the clinical measurement of paresis in stroke survivors.

Brunnstrom (83) adopted a different approach for assessment of motor function in hemiplegic patients in which movement patterns are evaluated and motor function is rated according to stages of motor recovery (**Table 18**-4) (67). While this rating can be performed very quickly, the scale defines recovery only in broad categories. Moreover, not all hemiparetic stroke survivors progress through these "stages" sequentially, with some survivors skipping stages during their recovery. For these reasons, this scale has not achieved widespread clinical or research usage.

Despite the limitations of assessing and interpreting muscle strength in patients with upper motor neuron lesions, strength does correlate with performance on functional tasks (84). Fugl-Meyer et al. designed a more detailed and comprehensive motor scale in which 50 different movements and abilities were rated (85). The test evaluates strength, reflexes, and coordination, and a composite score is derived. The Fugl-Meyer scale is reliable, and repeat scores reflect motor recovery over time. The upper limb component of this scale is widely used in the research setting but has not been widely adopted by clinicians because it is time-consuming to complete. A variety of other motor scales have been developed to provide a more comprehensive picture of motor function (rather than merely impairment), which are primarily utilized in a research setting, such as the Wolf Motor Function Test (86), the Motor Activity Log (87), the Arm Research Action Test (88), and others.

Spasticity or muscle tone refers to the resistance felt when the examiner passively stretches a muscle by moving a limb and generally increases if the stretching is performed more quickly (velocity dependent). Abnormal increases in muscle tone are quite commonly seen in hemiparetic limbs, and patients with more severe spasticity tend to have less well-preserved motor control. Factors such as posture and limb position can affect spasticity and must be considered when measuring muscle tone. Scales for measuring spasticity remain of limited reliability, with the most widely used being the modified Ashworth scale (see Chapter 40, Spasticity) (89). Most spasticity can be managed conservatively with stretching and positioning. In cases where medical therapy is needed, treatment with oral antispasticity medications, such as baclofen or tizanidine, is

often ineffective and may cause sedation or cognitive impairments. The use of injection therapy (principally botulinum toxin, but also phenol or ethanol injection) is generally effective in reducing spasticity, although it does not ameliorate the underlying impairments in motor control. Occasionally, a more severely affected individual may benefit from an intrathecal baclofen pump.

Therapy for Motor Weakness
Early Phase and Supportive Care
In the early poststroke phase, the hemiparetic limb(s) may be completely paralyzed and are at high risk for the development of contractures or nerve pressure palsies. Therapy during this early phase should consist of proper positioning of the patient in bed and support of the arm in a wheelchair trough when sitting. Traction on the arm should be avoided when the patient is moved or transferred to a wheelchair. All joints of the affected limbs should be passively moved through a full range of motion at least once daily to prevent contractures.

If the limb(s) becomes quite spastic, frequent slow stretching can help to reduce tone. Spasticity usually dominates in the flexors of the upper limb and may hold the wrist and fingers in a constant position of excessive flexion and the lower limb in excessive extension. A static wrist-hand orthosis may be helpful in maintaining these upper limb joints in a functional position, but doesn't reduce the underlying spasticity (90). An AFO may be helpful for control of lower limb ankle positioning.

Motor Recovery
Motor recovery may become evident within hours to days after a stroke. A variety of approaches have been advocated to facilitate and enhance motor recovery, including traditional approaches, such as the neurodevelopmental technique advocated by Bobath (91), functionally oriented exercise training (such as practicing transfers and early ambulation), and a recent focus on repetitive task-oriented practice. The use of SSRIs in an effort to enhance motor recovery is used in some centers based on the results of the FLAME study (92), although larger definitive clinical trials of this treatment remain in progress at this time.

The optimal timing and dosing of motor rehabilitation remain uncertain. The VECTORS study found that early higher-dose upper limb motor therapy that incorporated constraint-induced movement therapy (CIMT) actually resulted in a poorer outcome when compared with a conventionally

TABLE 18-4	Brunnstrom Stages of Motor Recovery
Stage	**Characteristics**
Stage 1	No activation of the limb
Stage 2	Spasticity appears, and weak basic flexor and extensor synergies are present
Stage 3	Spasticity is prominent; the patient voluntarily moves the limb, but muscle activation is all within the synergy patterns
Stage 4	The patient begins to activate muscles selectively outside the flexor and extensor synergies
Stage 5	Spasticity decreases; most muscle activation is selective and independent from the limb synergies
Stage 6	Isolated movements are performed in a smooth, phasic, well-coordinated manner

Adapted by permission from Springer: Brandstater ME. Basic aspects of impairment evaluation in stroke patients. In: Chino N, Melvin JL, ed. *Functional Evaluation of Stroke Patients.* 1st ed. New York: Springer-Verlag; 1996:9–18.

dosed rehabilitation program (93). A recent study of increased upper limb therapy using task-oriented practice (ICARE) failed to demonstrate any benefit compared with conventional upper limb therapy poststroke (94).

While task practice forms the foundation of efforts to enhance motor recovery, a variety of other techniques have been studied, including CIMT, locomotor training, robot-aided rehabilitation, noninvasive brain stimulation (transcranial magnetic stimulation, transcranial direct-current stimulation), and stem cell therapies.

As originally described, CIMT utilizes an intensive short course (generally 2 weeks) of upper limb training with repetitive task-oriented practice and behavioral shaping techniques to enhance not only motor control of the upper limb but also incorporation into behavioral repertoires. The mechanism underlying this improved function remains uncertain. Taub (who developed this technique) initially hypothesized that this therapy was able to overcome a "learned nonuse" of the weak limb, in which the potential for improved motor function is present but not incorporated into actual usage (95–97). The identification of changes in cortical mapping using transcranial magnetic stimulation (58) and in activation of the primary and supplementary motor cortex using fMRI (98) suggests that cortical reorganization of the motor systems is an important underlying mechanism for the effects of this treatment. Other task-oriented practice techniques have also shown efficacy (99), and research on identifying the optimal exercise regiment is ongoing. Logistic and cost considerations have limited the availability of CIMT, as has the suitability of this therapy for only a narrow range of deficits. Modifications of CIMT have been developed in efforts to provide a more logistically feasible treatment program (100).

Robot-aided therapeutic exercise has several potential advantages over conventional therapies as it provides consistently delivered therapy and is particularly suitable for highly repetitive exercises. Most robotic systems provide assistance to users attempting movements and thus can be used by individuals with more severe paresis after stroke. Upper limb devices have been shown to provide benefit in both the acute (101,102) and chronic phases of stroke (103,104). Lower limb robotic systems have been developed for gait training, as discussed below ("Therapy for Mobility"). While these devices hold the promise of providing more efficient therapy, the current generation requires skilled assistance (from a therapist or aide) in setting the patient up and in supervision of treatment. With minor exceptions (104), robotic therapy has not been proven superior to comparably dosed conventional therapy. Robotic therapy is discussed in greater detail in Chapter 64.

Virtual reality and gaming systems have been proposed as another form of therapy to encourage movement and provide feedback to users. A meta-analysis found evidence of improved motor function (105). A subsequent multicenter randomized controlled trial failed to demonstrate benefit of a particular gaming intervention compared with more conventional upper limb motor activities (106). Given the low cost and minimal risk of incorporating commercially available gaming systems in rehabilitation, however, the use of these systems as an adjunct to conventional therapy is reasonable for motivated stroke survivors.

Electrical stimulation of the limb (sometimes termed therapeutic electrical stimulation or functional neuromuscular stimulation) has long been used in some form since the 1960s as a treatment for hemiparesis, with some recent evidence accumulating that it may be beneficial in restoring motor use to some extent (107). For the lower limb, these devices provide an alternative to ankle-foot orthoses and are preferred by some patients.

Implantable electrical stimulation systems have been developed for inadequate dorsiflexion in the lower limb, but not are currently available in the United States outside of clinical trials (108). Please see Chapter 54 for a more extensive discussion of this therapy.

Biofeedback using electromyographic (EMG) signals has been used in an attempt to improve motor control poststroke. Results of trials have been mixed, some showing benefit but others no better results than control therapy. While one review of clinical trials of biofeedback did find that biofeedback was somewhat effective (109), the magnitude of the benefits is small, and clinical use in the United States is relatively rare. Conventional EMG biofeedback involves recording surface EMG from the test muscle and using auditory or visual display of the EMG signal as feedback to the patient on the activity status of the muscle. The EMG signal supplements conventional re-education given by the therapist. A combination therapy in which therapeutic electrical stimulation is triggered by the EMG signal of the target muscle is available (110). In another approach, robotic devices that relay on surface EMG signals to control or trigger the device have been developed (111).

Mirror therapy, where the illusion of movement in the hemiplegic upper limb is produced through the use of a mirror, has been found beneficial in small studies (112), with a meta-analysis suggestive of benefit (113). Another, more invasive, approach, vagal nerve stimulation in combination with upper limb exercise, is being studied as another potential method of enhancing motor recovery (114).

Therapy for Mobility

In the early phase after stroke, some individuals will not have sufficient trunk control and hemiparetic leg strength to maintain upright posture for walking. These patients should receive initial therapy to develop gross trunk control and training in pregait activities such as posture, balance, and weight transfer to the hemiparetic leg. As recovery progresses, stroke survivors usually develop better gross motor skills and trunk balance and greater strength in the leg. Despite the presence of spasticity and the inability to selectively activate individual muscles, most stroke survivors will walk, although many will require an AFO and cane and will walk more slowly than previously. Individuals with less severe paresis may have an asymmetric gait but not require a brace for their affected leg. Many stroke survivors will require a cane for walking, which may be a standard cane or four pronged, depending on their balance impairments. While hemiparesis often makes it impossible to use a walker effectively, individuals with milder paresis or other stroke-related balance impairments such as ataxia may find a walker helpful.

There have been reports that hemiplegic patients benefit from intensive gait training when therapy consists of walking on a treadmill with body weight partially supported (PBWSTT) with a harness (115,116). The harness substitutes for poor trunk control, and the motor-driven treadmill forces locomotion. During early training, the patient is assisted by two or three therapists in controlling the trunk, pelvis, and weak leg. While preliminary studies of this approach were encouraging (117), a larger randomized controlled trial (the LEAPS trial) found no benefit to this technique compared to more conventional gait and balance training (118). Other devices to unweight patients during walking include devices using overhead tracks (e.g., ZeroG, Aretech, Ashburn, VA) or pneumatic support (e.g., AlterG, Fremont, CA).

Robotic therapy has been proposed as an alternative to PWBSTT training, in part because of the need for two or even three staff members to assist the patient during a treatment session. While the feasibility of this approach has been demonstrated (119), there is evidence that therapist-assisted locomotor training with a treadmill is more effective than robotic therapy (120), and, moreover, the results of the LEAPS trial (118) are not supportive of PBWSTT in this population in any case. At present, there is little evidence supporting this treatment outside of clinical trials.

Sensory Impairment and Central Pain

Sensory impairment may occur with or without accompanying motor weakness following a stroke, although loss of proprioception generally results in reduced motor performance even in the absence of weakness *per se*. Lesions of the thalamus may cause severe contralesional sensory loss and result in a central pain syndrome in some individuals. Central pain can occur, particularly with strokes involving the spinothalamic-cortical pathway. The pain usually begins a few weeks after stroke onset and is frequently poorly responsive to conventional analgesic medications, including opiate analgesics. The pain is classically described as burning in character, although other types of pain can predominate.

With lesions of the cortex, primary sensory modalities may be preserved, but the perception of these sensations may be both qualitatively altered and quantitatively reduced. Perceptual impairment, as often seen in parietal lobe lesions, frequently is manifested as inability to perceive stimulation of the affected side during simultaneous bilateral stimulation (extinction), reduced two-point discrimination, reduced object recognition (stereognosis), and impaired recognition of digits drawn in the palm (graphesthesia).

Regrettably, few interventions have been proposed to specifically treat sensory loss after stroke, although a variety of pharmacologic treatments have been studied for treatment of central pain poststroke. Tricyclic antidepressants have been best studied for this condition, although some patients do not have an adequate response, and anticholinergic side effects can be problematic (especially in the elderly). Anticonvulsants, such as gabapentin or lamotrigine, show some efficacy as well (121,122).

OUTCOME AND PROGNOSTICATION IN STROKE REHABILITATION

Patients, their families, and members of the health care team all benefit from an accurate prognosis to help inform decision-making. The prospects for survival, the degree of recovery that may be expected, and the extent of possible residual disability following rehabilitation are all important elements of prognosis.

The challenge in developing accurate prognostic models is not surprising, given the myriad of complex functions performed by the brain, the variability of stroke lesion location and size, the limitations of our assessment techniques, and the impact of many baseline factors on stroke recovery, such as age, comorbid conditions, personality and coping abilities, and social factors.

Predicting Disability and Functional Status

The key outcomes from a rehabilitation perspective are restoration of function and community reintegration. The central purpose of the rehabilitation program is to lessen ultimate disability; therefore, considerable attention has been directed at the identification of factors that will predict the functional outcome of the patient, especially with respect to walking and activities of daily living (ADLs).

The prognosis for recovery from lacunar lesions is usually excellent, although significant persisting deficits may occur when the lesion is strategically located. With large vessel infarctions, due either to thrombosis or embolism, prognosis is related to the volume of the lesion. Outcome is poorest when the lesion involves more than 10% of intracranial volume (123).

While many stroke survivors are initially unable to walk independently, 54% to 80% achieve this milestone within the first 3 months poststroke (although frequently requiring the assistance of a cane or AFO) (55,124). Data from the Framingham cohort reported by Gresham et al. (125) indicate that long-term survivors of stroke show good recovery of functional mobility, with 80% being independent in mobility.

Most patients with significant neurologic impairment who survive a stroke are initially dependent in basic ADLs, that is, bathing, dressing, feeding, toileting, grooming, transfers, and ambulation. The capacity of individuals to perform these activities is usually scored on ADL scales, such as the Functional Independence Measure (FIM^R) (126). Almost all patients show improved function in ADLs as recovery occurs. In most reports, between 47% and 76% of survivors achieve partial or total independence in ADLs (127–129). Basic ADL scales, such as the FIM, while sensitive to changes during the early phase of rehabilitation, have limited sensitivity at the upper end of the functional range and ceiling effects. Instrumental ADLs, such as the ability to prepare meals or perform housework, are not measured by the FIM yet represent an important component of reintegration into the community for stroke survivors.

Most authors who have attempted to determine which factors predict ultimate ADL functional outcome have used multivariate analysis. The single most useful predictor of functional outcome is the initial ADL assessment (most commonly the FIM score). Other important variables include age and sitting balance. A list of important variables predicting outcome is given in **Box 18-6**. Not all of these factors were shown in every study to statistically predict outcome status.

BOX 18-6

Factors Predicting Poor ADL Outcome

Advanced age
Comorbidities
   Myocardial infarction
   Diabetes mellitus
Severity of stroke
Severe weakness
   Poor sitting balance
   Visuospatial deficits
   Mental changes
   Incontinence
   Low initial ADL scores
   Time interval: onset to rehabilitation

ADL, activities of daily living.

The effect of age on outcome may partly be related to more frequent comorbid diseases and functional impairments, rather than merely a result of age *per se*.

Intuitively, it would seem reasonable to assume that patients with more severe neurologic deficits would have worse functional outcomes, but this is not necessarily the case when isolated neurologic impairments are considered. For example, analyses of predictive variables have failed to show that patients with sensory deficits have a poorer ultimate outcome than those with preserved sensation (130). When considering functional independence as the outcome measure of interest, the severity of the initial ADL score is generally one of the more reliable predictors of ultimate ADL function. On average, patients admitted for rehabilitation with lower ADL scores do not have as good a functional outcome as patients who initially had higher admission ADL scores. Most patients with FIM scores of greater than 80 are discharged home, although many other factors influence discharge disposition (131).

It is important that rehabilitation begins as early as possible. The Post-Stroke Rehabilitation Outcomes Project demonstrated that patients have better outcomes if they are admitted into a rehabilitation program early rather than later, regardless of severity of the stroke (132). In addition to enhancing recovery, early rehabilitation and mobilization appear to reduce the likelihood of secondary complications, such as contractures and deconditioning, and help patient motivation.

Social Variables

Stroke survivors with severe disabilities who need maximum physical assistance in ADLs and who have bowel or bladder incontinence are the most likely to require long-term institutional care (127). While functional status is the most important issue in determining discharge destination, psychosocial factors, especially prestroke family interaction (133) and the presence of an able spouse, also influence whether the patient returns home. A supportive family whose members are willing and able to provide significant physical care may be able to manage a severely disabled patient at home. By contrast, a patient with much less disability but no family support may require institutional care if not fully independent.

When a clinician is confronted with the challenge of evaluating an individual patient, guidelines for predicting functional outcome are useful but are not precise because multiple variables interact. A patient who might be judged as having a good prognosis for functional outcome may do poorly because of a negative psychosocial factor. The best estimate of prognosis can be made only after a thorough and comprehensive evaluation of the patient's medical, neurologic, functional, and psychosocial statuses.

MEDICAL MANAGEMENT DURING REHABILITATION

There is a high incidence of comorbid medical disorders among patients recovering from stroke, reflecting the age of the patient population and the fact that cerebrovascular disease is often part of a generalized disease process. If severe, or if poorly managed, these disorders may interfere with the patient's participation in the rehabilitation program and may adversely affect outcome. Similarly, medical complications frequently occur during the postacute phase of rehabilitation, affecting as many as 60% of patients and as many as 94% of patients with severe lesions (134). Common medical and neurologic complications are listed in **Table 18-5** (125,127–129). Some of the important and more frequent disorders are discussed briefly.

Cardiac Disease

In a large majority of patients, a stroke is an acute event in the course of a systemic disease, for example, atherosclerosis, hypertensive vascular disease, or cardiac disease causing embolic stroke. As many as 75% of stroke patients may show evidence of coexisting cardiovascular disease, including hypertension (estimates range from 50% to 84%) (135) and coronary artery disease (as many as 65%) (135). Another group of heart diseases causes a stroke through cardiogenic cerebral embolism. These diseases include atrial fibrillation and other arrhythmias from multiple causes, valvular disease, cardiomyopathy, endocarditis, or recent MI.

Concomitant heart disease has a negative impact on short-term and long-term survival and probably on functional outcome of stroke patients (136,137). Acute exacerbations of heart disease occur frequently during postacute stroke rehabilitation (136). Common problems include angina, uncontrolled hypertension, hypotension, MI, congestive heart failure, atrial fibrillation, and ventricular arrhythmias. Development of one of these complications may have minimal or no impact on the patient's progress or outcome if the problem is promptly diagnosed and appropriately treated. However, these complications often do impact the patient's capacity to participate fully in the therapeutic program. Congestive heart failure and angina

TABLE 18-5	Medical Complications During Postacute Stroke Rehabilitation
Complication	**Frequency (%)**
Medical	
Pulmonary aspiration, pneumonia	40
Urinary tract infection	40
Depression	30
Musculoskeletal pain, RSD	30
Falls	25
Malnutrition	16
Venous thromboembolism	6
Pressure ulcer	3
Neurologic	
Toxic or metabolic encephalopathy	10
Stroke progression	5
Seizure	4

RSD, reflex sympathetic dystrophy.
Data are from the following sources: Wade DT, Wood VA, Hewer RL. Recovery after stroke—the first 3 months. *J Neurol Neurosurg Psychiatry*. 1985;48:7–13; Feigenson JS, McDowell FH, Meese P, et al. Factors influencing outcome and length of stay in a stroke rehabilitation unit. Part 1. *Stroke*. 1977;8:651–656; Gresham GE, Fitzpatrick TE, Wolf PA, et al. The Framingham Study. Residual disability in survivors of stroke. *N Engl J Med*. 1975;293:954–956; Wade DT, Hewer RL. Functional abilities after stroke: measurement, natural history and prognosis. *J Neurol Neurosurg Psychiatry*. 1987;50:177–182; Dombovy ML, Basford JR, Whisnut JP, et al. Disability and use of rehabilitation services following stroke in Rochester Minnesota, 1975–1979. *Stroke*. 1987;18:830–836.

decrease exercise tolerance and reduce capacity to roll over in bed, transfer, and walk.

Urinary Tract

Urinary function can be affected in several ways by stroke, including urinary infection, urinary retention, and urge incontinence. At the time of the acute stroke, some patients develop urinary retention due to altered mental status or direct effects of the stroke on the neurologic control of micturition. Premorbid voiding dysfunction, often in the form of benign prostatic hypertrophy in men and stress incontinence in women, is a common comorbid condition in stroke patients and often becomes a more significant problem after a stroke due to the patient's decreased mobility or communication abilities.

Catheterization, often with an indwelling catheter, is common during the acute management of the stroke survivor. While this alleviates acute urinary retention, it may lead to urinary infection and interferes with reestablishment of a normal voiding pattern. Indwelling catheters should be removed as quickly as possible and intermittent catheterization substituted for individuals unable to void spontaneously. Noninvasive measurement of bladder volume using ultrasound is often helpful when managing individuals with impaired bladder function after stroke.

While urinary retention generally resolves quickly in affected stroke survivors, many stroke survivors develop urinary urgency and/or incontinence. Disinhibition of the bladder detrusor is common and results in urinary frequency and urgency that may result in incontinence in some individuals. Anticholinergic medications such as oxybutynin chloride (Ditropan) or tolterodine (Detrol) are useful to inhibit bladder contraction, although these may cause anticholinergic side effects, such as dry mouth, or confusion.

Musculoskeletal Pain and Complex Regional Pain Syndrome

Shoulder and arm pain is common following a stroke in survivors. It tends to develop early, several weeks to 6 months postonset, and some studies have found as many as 72% of individuals affected, especially those with more severe hemiplegia (138). More recent studies suggest a lower incidence, with one study finding 37% of patients on a stroke rehabilitation unit reporting pain (139). This apparent reduction in incidence may reflect more intensive and earlier rehabilitation programs incorporating range-of-motion exercises.

Although some patients may have preexisting shoulder problems, such as rotator cuff tendinitis, the pain in most patients with hemiplegia results from varying combinations of glenohumeral subluxation, spasticity, and contracture. Of these, subluxation is the commonly implicated cause. The role of subluxation in generating shoulder pain has been debated, and subluxation may occur without pain symptoms in many individuals.

Subluxation is evident on physical examination, and imaging studies are not generally useful unless other diagnoses are being considered. Treatment of a subluxed shoulder in poststroke patients can limit the subsequent development of shoulder pain (140). Some cases of shoulder pain appear related to

spasticity of shoulder girdle muscles (e.g., the subscapularis), although it is unclear how often this is the actual cause of pain versus an unrelated finding.

Preventative measures to reduce the likelihood of developing shoulder pain should be instituted early poststroke in patients with flaccid paralysis of the upper limb and clinically evident subluxation or with any symptoms of shoulder pain. Proper positioning includes supporting the arm in an arm trough or lapboard when seated and avoiding traction on the arm when transferring. Selective use of supportive slings during ambulation or standing is advisable, although their use negatively impacts balance.

Excessive use may contribute to undesirable reduction in opportunities to use the upper limb and potentially slow functional recovery and cause loss of range of motion. In cases where spasticity appears responsible for pain, the use of botulinum toxin or phenol injections may be appropriate (141).

The incidence of upper limb complex regional pain syndrome (CRPS, also known as reflex sympathetic dystrophy or shoulder-hand syndrome) remains controversial. Some studies have reported a high prevalence of 1 in 8 based on clinical criteria and up to 1 in 4 using bone scan criteria (142,143), but these figures appear inflated by inclusion of other causes of upper limb pain in hemiplegic stroke survivors, including patients with pain related to shoulder subluxation and some with central pain syndromes. Preventative measures, including frequent passive range of motion, desensitization with massage, and active incorporation of the paretic upper limb in the therapy program, are important and may have contributed to the apparent reduction in the frequency of this syndrome. Please see Chapter 40 for a discussion of treatments in established cases of CRPS.

Venous Thromboembolism

Most patients with significant immobility related to stroke should receive DVT prophylaxis, which should consist of either low-dose subcutaneous heparin or low molecular weight heparin, with the latter somewhat more effective in high-risk individuals. Treatment with low-dose low molecular weight heparin reduced the risk of DVT (odds ratio 0.34) without an increase in the risk of major intracranial or extracranial hemorrhage (144). In patients who cannot safely receive these medications, external pneumatic compression devices are an effective alternative, particularly in the acute hospital phase. Although many rehabilitation units attempt to use pneumatic compression in addition to or instead of pharmacologic treatment, their use in this setting is problematic due to the patients' involvement in out-of-bed activities. The optimal duration of prophylaxis remains uncertain, although most practitioners discontinue its use once patients are walking significant distances on a frequent basis or at the time of discharge to the community.

All patients with suspected DVT should undergo prompt investigation by venous duplex ultrasound imaging. Routine screening examinations are not generally used in this population at present. Symptoms may be subtle or absent, and therefore, physical examination is not reliable enough to confirm or exclude this diagnosis (145).

Patients with newly diagnosed DVT should immediately receive full-dose anticoagulation with low molecular weight heparin (or occasionally intravenous conventional heparin) until a therapeutic INR (between 2 and 3) can be achieved with the use of warfarin for at least 2 days or treatment is initiated with one of the newer oral anticoagulants (dabigatran, apixaban, etc.). Older recommendations for a period of bed rest for patients with acute DVT have been superseded, and most patients can continue activity as tolerated (146,147). In patients who cannot safely receive anticoagulation (most commonly those with a recent intracranial hemorrhage), an inferior vena cava filter should be inserted to prevent pulmonary embolism.

Depression

Depression is common following stroke and, depending on diagnostic criteria, has been reported in as many as 50% of patients (148,149). Some have reported a relationship between left frontal or bifrontal lesions and major depression (150), though this may be an artifact of the language function needed to complete the commonly used depression assessment scales that interferes with accurate measurement of depression in aphasic patients. Multiple theories exist for the high incidence of depression poststroke, which appears more common than would be expected merely as a result of the psychosocial stresses accompanying acquired disability. One hypothesis is that stroke may result in brain catecholamine depletion through lesion-induced damage to the frontal noradrenergic, dopaminergic, and serotonergic projections (151).

The diagnosis of poststroke depression may be complicated by the presence of normal sadness associated with the loss of independence, emotional lability that may result from stroke, and the high prevalence of symptoms often associated with depression (e.g., sleep disturbance, fatigue, altered appetite) that are known to result from stroke itself. Persistently depressed mood, loss of interest in socialization, and limited participation in the rehabilitation program are often more reliable indicators in this population (152).

Persisting depression correlates with delayed recovery and poorer ultimate outcome. Active treatment should be considered for all patients with significant clinical depression. Patients with poststroke depression generally respond well to standard antidepressant medications, with SSRIs commonly prescribed. SSRIs may also have the "side effect" of enhancing motor recovery, providing a dual rationale for their use (92). Some practitioners will also treat with a stimulant medication (typically methylphenidate) in an attempt to "boost" the response and achieve more rapid results.

Sexuality

Stroke survivors commonly experience sexual dysfunction (153), with reductions both in libido and sexual performance predominating, although occasionally stroke can cause hypersexuality. The precise mechanisms for sexual dysfunction after stroke have not been determined, but a combination of psychosocial and medical issues appears to be involved. Stroke is most common in people who are older, have hypertension, and/or have diabetes—all risk factors for sexual dysfunction even without a stroke. Iatrogenic causes of sexual dysfunction are also common in this population, as many commonly prescribed medications can interfere with sexual function, including antihypertensive medications and antidepressants (especially SSRIs). Anticonvulsant medications are well-established causes of reduced libido and sexual dysfunction (154).

Moreover, sexual dysfunction is common in the adult population at large, with as many as 40% to 45% of adult women and 20% to 30% of adult men having at least one manifestation (155). Thus, some of the sexual dysfunction observed in this population may not directly result from the stroke.

Regardless of the specific cause(s), the prevalence of sexual problems after stroke is estimated to be between 57% and 75% (156,157). Sexual dysfunction is also very common among the sexual partners of stroke survivors and is likely due to a combination of psychosocial stressors and the reduced sexual availability of their usual partner due to the sequelae of stroke.

Some stroke survivors and their sexual partners harbor fears (sometimes not expressed) that resumption of sexual activity might precipitate another stroke. While limited data are available to directly address this concern, most practitioners agree that resuming sexual activity is safe and appropriate after discharge from the hospital in the vast majority of cases. This is largely based on extrapolation from studies that have found a low risk of MI from resumption of sexual activity (158).

The natural history of sexual dysfunction after stroke appears favorable in most cases. In one study of men with stroke, 82% of those who experienced erectile dysfunction after stroke improved spontaneously within a few months. The degree of dependence in ADLs is a strong predictor of decreased sexual frequency among stroke survivors (159,160).

Phosphodiesterase-5 inhibitors, such as sildenafil (Viagra) and tadalafil (Cialis), are useful for selected men with poststroke erectile dysfunction. Caution should be exercised with regard to potential medication interactions, including α-blockers and nitrates.

Flibanserin is approved for treatment of reduced libido in women, but has not yet been studied for treatment of female stroke survivors with this symptom.

Generally speaking, physicians and other health care professionals caring for stroke survivors should inform stroke survivors of their willingness and availability to discuss sexuality after stroke and provide further information to patients and their sexual partners when desired. Embarrassment on the part of both the patient and the physician is often a barrier to discussing this subject, as are implicit assumptions about sexuality (e.g., a physician assuming that older stroke survivors are not sexually active). Reassurances regarding the safety of resuming sexual activity are a particularly critical aspect of this counseling. A structured 30-minute structured sexual rehabilitation program did not demonstrate any advantages over provision of written materials in one study, and more research is needed to understand patient preferences (161).

ONGOING CARE

The observations that continued improvement in motor function is possible in stroke survivors even years after the stroke have created both opportunity and challenge for rehabilitation providers. We do not yet know what the ideal rehabilitation program consists of, particularly with regard to intensity and duration of therapy. Uncertainty regarding the maximal achievable outcomes for stroke survivors both preserves hope for our patients and creates complexity for practitioners.

Furthermore, stroke survivors' other rehabilitation needs may extend for many years after the initial event. Late issues may include depression, spasticity, contracture, osteoporosis, weight gain, and deconditioning due to reduced activity. The gradual progression of some of these issues, such as gradual loss of range of motion resulting from spasticity and inadequate stretching, may result in functional loss without the patient seeking medical care. Patients with substantial residual disability from a stroke likely benefit from periodic physiatric assessment on an ongoing basis indefinitely.

REFERENCES

1. Mozaffarian D, Benjamin EJ, Go AS, et al. Executive summary: heart disease and stroke statistics-2016 update: a report from the American Heart Association. *Circulation.* 2016;133(4):447.
2. Sacco RL. Risk factors and outcomes for ischemic stroke. *Neurology.* 1995;45: S10–S14.
3. Viitanen M, Eriksson S, Asplund K. Risk of recurrent stroke, myocardial infarction and epilepsy during long-term follow-up after stroke. *Eur Neurol.* 1988;28:227–231.
4. Leonberg SC Jr, Elliott FA. Prevention of recurrent stroke. *Stroke.* 1981;12:731–735.
5. Mohr JP, Caplan LR, Melski JW, et al. The Harvard Cooperative Stroke Registry: a prospective registry. *Neurology.* 1978;28:754–762.
6. Paciaroni M, Agnelli G, Micheli S, et al. Efficacy and safety of anticoagulant treatment in acute cardioembolic stroke: a meta-analysis of randomized controlled trials [see comment]. *Stroke.* 2007;38:423–430.
7. Kelly PJ, Furie KL, Shafqat S, et al. Functional recovery following rehabilitation after hemorrhagic and ischemic stroke. *Arch Phys Med Rehabil.* 2003;84:968–972.
8. Mayer SA, Brun NC, Begtrup K, et al. Efficacy and safety of recombinant activated factor VII for acute intracerebral hemorrhage [see comment]. *N Engl J Med.* 2008;358:2127–2137.
9. Fang MC, Chang Y, Hylek EM, et al. Advanced age, anticoagulation intensity, and risk for intracranial hemorrhage among patients taking warfarin for atrial fibrillation [see comment] [summary for patients in *Ann Intern Med.* 2004;141(10):I38; PMID: 15545670]. *Ann Intern Med.* 2004;141:745–752.
10. Kelly PJ, Stein J, Shafqat S, et al. Functional recovery after rehabilitation for cerebellar stroke. *Stroke.* 2001;32:530–534.
11. Bederson JB, Awad IA, Wiebers DO, et al. Recommendations for the management of patients with unruptured intracranial aneurysms: a statement for healthcare professionals from the Stroke Council of the American Heart Association. *Circulation.* 2000;102:2300–2308.
12. Anonymous. Tissue plasminogen activator for acute ischemic stroke. The National Institute of Neurological Disorders and Stroke rt-PA Stroke Study Group [see comment]. *N Engl J Med.* 1995;333:1581–1587.
13. Jauch EC, et al. Guidelines for the early management of patients with acute ischemic stroke. *Stroke.* 2013;44(3):870–947.
14. Hacke W, Kaste M, Bluhmki E, et al. Thrombolysis with alteplase 3 to 4.5 hours after acute ischemic stroke [see comment]. *N Engl J Med.* 2008;359:1317–1329.
15. Berkhemer OA, Fransen PS, Beumer D, et al. A randomized trial of intraarterial treatment for acute ischemic stroke. *N Engl J Med.* 2015;372(1):11–20.
16. Goyal M, Demchuk AM, Menon BK, et al. Randomized assessment of rapid endovascular treatment of ischemic stroke. *N Engl J Med.* 2015;372(11):1019–1030.
17. Saver JL, Goyal M, Bonafe A, et al. Stent-retriever thrombectomy after intravenous t-PA vs. t-PA alone in stroke. *N Engl J Med.* 2015;372(24):2285–2295.
18. Walter S, Kostopoulos P, Haass A, et al. Diagnosis and treatment of patients with stroke in a mobile stroke unit versus in hospital: a randomised controlled trial. *Lancet Neurol.* 2012;11(5):397–404.
19. Kernan WN, et al. Guidelines for the prevention of stroke in patients with stroke and transient ischemic attack. *Stroke.* 2014;45(7):2160–2236.
20. Adams RJ, Albers G, Alberts MJ, et al. Update to the AHA/ASA recommendations for the prevention of stroke in patients with stroke and transient ischemic attack. *Stroke.* 2008;39:1647–1652.
21. Wang Y, Wang Y, Zhao X, et al. Clopidogrel with aspirin in acute minor stroke or transient ischemic attack. *N Engl J Med.* 2013;369(1):11–19.
22. Diener HC, Bogousslavsky J, Brass LM, et al. Aspirin and clopidogrel compared with clopidogrel alone after recent ischaemic stroke or transient ischaemic attack in high-risk patients (MATCH): randomised, double-blind, placebo-controlled trial [see comment]. *Lancet.* 2004;364:331–337.
23. Feinberg WM, Albers GW, Barnett HIM. Guidelines for the management of transient ischemic attacks. *Stroke.* 1994;25:1320–1335.
24. Diener HC, Cunha L, Forbes C, et al. European Stroke Prevention Study. 2. Dipyridamole and acetylsalicylic acid in the secondary prevention of stroke [see comment]. *J Neurol Sci.* 1996;143:1–13.
25. Sacco RL, Diener HC, Yusuf S, et al. Aspirin and extended-release dipyridamole versus clopidogrel for recurrent stroke [see comment]. *N Engl J Med.* 2008;359: 1238–1251.
26. Kent DM, Thaler DE, Kent DM, et al. Stroke prevention—insights from incoherence [comment]. *N Engl J Med.* 2008;359:1287–1289.
27. Patel MR, Mahaffey KW, Garg J, et al. Rivaroxaban versus warfarin in nonvalvular atrial fibrillation. *N Engl J Med.* 2011;365(10):883–891.
28. Connolly SJ, Ezekowitz MD, Yusuf S, et al. Dabigatran versus warfarin in patients with atrial fibrillation. *N Engl J Med.* 2009;361(12):1139–1151.
29. Stroke Prevention by Aggressive Reduction in Cholesterol Levels (SPARCL) Investigators. High-dose atorvastatin after stroke or transient ischemic attack. *N Engl J Med.* 2006;355:549–559.
30. Naci H, Brugts JJ, Fleurence R, et al. Comparative effects of statins on major cerebrovascular events: a multiple-treatments meta-analysis of placebo-controlled and active-comparator trials. *QJM.* 2013;106(4):299–306.
31. Barnett HJ, Taylor DW, Eliasziw M, et al. Benefit of carotid endarterectomy in patients with symptomatic moderate or severe stenosis. North American Symptomatic Carotid Endarterectomy Trial Collaborators. *N Engl J Med.* 1998;339:1415–1425.
32. Chaturvedi S, Bruno A, Feasby T, et al. Carotid endarterectomy—an evidence-based review: report of the Therapeutics and Technology Assessment Subcommittee of the American Academy of Neurology. *Neurology.* 2005;65:794–801.
33. Bonati LH, Lyrer P, Ederle J, et al. Percutaneous transluminal balloon angioplasty and stenting for carotid artery stenosis. *Cochrane Database Syst Rev.* 2012;(9):CD000515.
34. Collaboration SUT. Collaboration SUT: collaborative systematic review of the randomised trials of organized inpatient (stroke unit) care after stroke. *Br Med J.* 1997;314:1151–1159.
35. Langhorne P, Pollock A; Stroke Unit Trialists' Collaboration. What are the components of effective stroke unit care? *Age Ageing.* 2002;31:365–371.
36. Roth EJ. Medical complications encountered in stroke rehabilitation. *Phys Med Rehabil Clin N Am.* 1991;2:563–578.
37. DePippo KL, Holas MA, Reding MJ. The Burke dysphagia screening test: validation of its use in patients with stroke [see comment]. *Arch Phys Med Rehabil.* 1994;75:1284–1286.
38. Gresham GE, Duncan PW, Stason WB, et al. *Post-Stroke Rehabilitation: Clinical Practice Guideline No. 16.* Rockville, MD: U.S. Department of Health and Human Services. Public Health Service, Agency for Health Care Policy and Research. AHCPR Publication No. 95-0662; 1995.
39. AVERT Trial Collaboration Group; Bernhardt J, Langhorne P, Lindley RI, et al. Efficacy and safety of very early mobilisation within 24 h of stroke onset (AVERT): a randomised controlled trial. *Lancet.* 2015;386:46–55.
40. Harvey L, de Jong I, Goehl G, et al. Twelve weeks of nightly stretch does not reduce thumb web-space contractures in people with a neurological condition: a randomised controlled trial. *Aust J Physiother.* 2006;52:251–258.
41. Lannin NA, Cusick A, McCluskey A. Effects of splinting on wrist contracture after stroke: a randomized controlled trial. *Stroke.* 2007;38:111–116. doi: 10.1161/01.STR.0000251722.77088.12.
42. Winstein CJ, Stein J, Arena R, et al.; American Heart Association Stroke Council, Council on Cardiovascular and Stroke Nursing, Council on Clinical Cardiology, and Council on Quality of Care and Outcomes Research. Guidelines for adult stroke rehabilitation and recovery: a guideline for healthcare professionals from the American Heart Association/American Stroke Association. *Stroke.* 2016;47:e98–e169.
43. Foulkes MA, Wolf PA, Price TR, et al. The Stroke Data Bank: design, methods, and baseline characteristics. *Stroke.* 1988;19:547–554.
44. Nakayama H, Jorgensen HS, Raaschou HO, et al. Recovery of upper extremity function in stroke patients: the Copenhagen stroke study. *Arch Phys Med Rehabil.* 1994;75:394–398.
45. Bard G, Hirschberg GG. Recovery of voluntary motion in upper extremity following hemiplegia. *Arch Phys Med Rehabil.* 1965;46:567–572.
46. Gowland C. Management of hemiplegia upper limb. In: Brandstater ME, Basmajian JV, eds. *Stroke Rehabilitation.* Baltimore, MD: Williams & Wilkins; 1987:217–245.
47. Wade DT, Hewer RL, Wood VA, et al. The hemiplegic arm after stroke: measurement and recovery. *J Neurol Neurosurg Psychiatry.* 1983;46:521–524.
48. Feng W, Wang J, Chhatbar PY, et al. Corticospinal tract lesion load: an imaging biomarker for stroke motor outcomes. *Ann Neurol.* 2015;78(6):860–870.
49. Zhu LL, Lindenberg R, Alexander MP, et al. Lesion load of the corticospinal tract predicts motor impairment in chronic stroke. *Stroke.* 2010;41(5):910–915.
50. Byblow WD, Stinear CM, Barber PA, et al. Proportional recovery after stroke depends on corticomotor integrity. *Ann Neurol.* 2015;78(6):848–859.
51. Escudero JV, Sancho J, Bautista D, et al. Prognostic value of motor evoked potential obtained by transcranial magnetic brain stimulation in motor function recovery in patients with acute ischemic stroke. *Stroke.* 1998;29(9):1854–1859.
52. Jorgensen H, Nakayam H, Raaschou H. Stroke rehabilitation: outcome and speed of recovery. Part II: speed of recovery: the Copenhagen stroke study. *Arch Phys Med Rehabil.* 1995;3:65–70.
53. Kelly-Hayes M, Wolf PA, Kase CS. Time course of functional recovery after stroke: the Framingham study. *J Neurol Rehabil.* 1989;3:65–70.
54. Wade DT, Hewer RL, David RM, et al. Aphasia after stroke: natural history and associated deficits. *J Neurol Neurosurg Psychiatry.* 1986;49:11–16.
55. Skilbeck CE, Wade DT, Hewer RL, et al. Recovery after stroke. *J Neurol Neurosurg Psychiatry.* 1983;46:5–8.
56. Winters C, van Wegen EE, Daffertshofer A, et al. Generalizability of the maximum proportional recovery rule to visuospatial neglect early poststroke. *Neurorehabil Neural Repair.* 2017;31(4):334–342.
57. Krakauer JW. Motor learning: its relevance to stroke recovery and neurorehabilitation. *Curr Opin Neurol.* 2006;19:84–90.
58. Liepert J, Bauder H, Wolfgang HR, et al. Treatment-induced cortical reorganization after stroke in humans. *Stroke.* 2000;31:1210–1216.
59. Folstein MF, Folstein SE, McHugh PR. "Mini-mental state". A practical method for grading the cognitive state of patients for the clinician. *J Psychiatr Res.* 1975;12: 189–198.
60. Nasreddine ZS, Phillips NA, Bédirian V, et al. The Montreal Cognitive Assessment, MoCA: a brief screening tool for mild cognitive impairment. *Journal of the American Geriatrics Society.* 2005 April;53(4):695–699.

61. Fortis P, Maravita A, Gallucci M, et al. Rehabilitating patients with left spatial neglect by prism exposure during a visuomotor activity. *Neuropsychology.* 2010;24(6):681.
62. Kim BR, Chun MH, Kim DY, et al. Effect of high- and low-frequency repetitive transcranial magnetic stimulation on visuospatial neglect in patients with acute stroke: a double-blind, sham-controlled trial. *Arch Phys Med Rehabil.* 2013;94: 803–807. doi: 10.1016/j. apmr.2012.12.016.
63. Cazzoli D, Müri RM, Schumacher R, et al. Theta burst stimulation reduces disability during the activities of daily living in spatial neglect. *Brain.* 2012;135 (pt 11):3426–3439.
64. Seliger G, Hornstein A, Flax J. Fluoxetine improves emotional incontinence. *Brain Inj.* 1991;5:1–4.
65. Robinson RG, Parikh RM, Lipsey JR, et al. Pathological laughing and crying following stroke: validation of a measurement scale and a double-blind treatment study [see comment]. *Am J Psychiatry.* 1993;150:286–293.
66. Horrocks JA, Hackett ML, Anderson CS, et al. Pharmaceutical interventions for emotionalism after stroke. *Stroke.* 2004;35:2610–2611.
67. Brandstater ME. Basic aspects of impairment evaluation in stroke patients. In: Chino N, Melvin JL, eds. *Functional Evaluation of Stroke Patients.* New York, NY: Springer-Verlag; 1996:9–18.
68. Robey RR. A meta-analysis of clinical outcomes in the treatment of aphasia. *J Speech Lang Hear Res.* 1998;41:172–187.
69. Greener J, Enderby P, Whurr R. Speech and language therapy for aphasia following stroke. *Cochrane Database Syst Rev.* 2000;(6):CD000425.
70. Bhogal SK, Teasell R, Speechley M, et al. Intensity of aphasia therapy, impact on recovery [see comment]. *Stroke.* 2003;34:987–993.
71. Pulvermuller F, Neininger B, Elbert T, et al. Constraint-induced therapy of chronic aphasia after stroke. *Stroke.* 2001;32:1621–1626.
72. Woldag H, et al. Constraint-induced aphasia therapy in the acute stage: what is the key factor for efficacy? A randomized controlled study. *Neurorehabil Neural Repair.* 2017;31(1):72–80.
73. Kasten E, Wust S, Behrens-Baumann W, et al. Computer-based training for the treatment of partial blindness. *Nat Med.* 1998;4:1083–1087.
74. Reinhard J, Schreiber A, Schiefer U, et al. Does visual restitution training change absolute homonymous visual field defects? A fundus controlled study. *Br J Ophthalmol.* 2005;89(1):30–35.
75. Martino R, Foley N, Bhogal S, et al. Dysphagia after stroke: incidence, diagnosis, and pulmonary complications. *Stroke.* 2005;36:2756–2763.
76. Horner J, Massey EW, Riski JE, et al. Aspiration following stroke: clinical correlates and outcome. *Neurology.* 1988;38:1359–1362.
77. Teasell RW, Bach D, McRae M. Prevalence and recovery of aspiration poststroke: a retrospective analysis. *Dysphagia.* 1994;9:35–39.
78. Horner J, Massey EW, Brazer SR. Aspiration in bilateral stroke patients. *Neurology.* 1990;40:1686–1688.
79. Horner J, Massey EW. Silent aspiration following stroke. *Neurology.* 1988;38: 317–319.
80. Axelsson K, Asplund K, Norberg A, et al. Nutritional status in patients with acute stroke. *Acta Med Scand.* 1988;224:217–224.
81. Brain MRCGo. *Aids to the Examination of the Peripheral Nervous System.* London, UK: Bailliere Tindall; 1986.
82. Bohannon RW. Is the measurement of muscle strength appropriate in patients with brain lesions? A special communication [see comment]. *Phys Ther.* 1989;69: 225–236.
83. Brunnstrom S. *Movement Therapy in Hemiplegia: A Neurophysiological Approach.* New York, NY: Harper & Row; 1970.
84. Bohannon R. Correlation of lower limb strengths and other variables with standing performance in stroke patients. *Physiother Can.* 1989;41:198–202.
85. Fugl-Meyer AR, Jaasko L, Leyman I, et al. The post-stroke hemiplegic patient. 1. A method for evaluation of physical performance. *Scand J Rehabil Med.* 1975;7:13–31.
86. Wolf SL, Catlin PA, Ellis M, et al. Assessing Wolf motor function test as outcome measure for research in patients after stroke. *Stroke.* 2001;32:1635–1639.
87. Uswatte G, Taub E, Morris D, et al. The Motor Activity Log-28: assessing daily use of the hemiparetic arm after stroke. *Neurology.* 2006;67:1189–1194.
88. Hsieh CL, Hsueh IP, Chiang FM, et al. Inter-rater reliability and validity of the action research arm test in stroke patients. *Age Ageing.* 1998;27:107–113.
89. Bohannon RW, Smith MB. Interrater reliability of a modified Ashworth scale of muscle spasticity. *Phys Ther.* 1987;67:206–207.
90. Basaran A, Emre U, Karadavut KI, et al. Hand splinting for poststroke spasticity: a randomized controlled trial. *Top Stroke Rehabil.* 2012;19:329–337. doi: 10.1310/ tsr1904-329.
91. Bobath B. *Adult Hemiplegia: Evaluation and Treatment.* London, UK: Heinemann; 1976.
92. Chollet F, Tardy J, Albucher JF, et al. Fluoxetine for motor recovery after acute ischaemic stroke (FLAME): a randomised placebo-controlled trial. *Lancet Neurol.* 2011;10(2):123–130.
93. Dromerick AW, Lang CE, Birkenmeier RL, et al. Very early constraint-induced movement during stroke rehabilitation (VECTORS): a single-center RCT. *Neurology.* 2009;73(3):195–201.
94. Winstein CJ, Wolf SL, Dromerick AW, et al. Effect of a task-oriented rehabilitation program on upper extremity recovery following motor stroke: the ICARE randomized clinical trial. *JAMA.* 2016;315(6):571–581.
95. Wolf SL, Lecraw DE, Barton LA, et al. Forced use of hemiplegic upper extremities to reverse the effect of learned nonuse among chronic stroke and head-injured patients. *Exp Neurol.* 1989;104:125–132.
96. Taub E, Miller NE, Novack TA. A technique for improving chronic motor deficit after stroke. *Arch Phys Med Rehabil.* 1993;74:347–354.
97. Taub E, Wolf SL. Constraint induced movement techniques to facilitate upper extremity use in stroke patients. *Top Stroke Rehabil.* 1997;3:38–61.
98. Schaechter JD, Kraft E, Hilliard TS, et al. Motor recovery and cortical reorganization after constraint-induced movement therapy in stroke patients: a preliminary study. *Neurorehabil Neural Repair.* 2002;16:326–338.
99. Luft AR, McCombe-Waller S, Whitall J, et al. Repetitive bilateral arm training and motor recovery in chronic stroke: a randomized controlled trial [erratum appears in *JAMA.* 2004;292(20):2470]. *JAMA.* 2004;292:1853–1861.
100. Page SJ, Levine P, Leonard A, et al. Modified constraint-induced therapy in chronic stroke: results of a single-blinded randomized controlled trial [see comment]. *Phys Ther.* 2008;88:333–340.
101. Aisen ML, Krebs HI, Hogan N, et al. The effect of robot-assisted therapy and rehabilitative training on motor recovery following stroke. *Arch Neurol.* 1997;54:443–446.
102. Volpe BT, Krebs HI, Hogan N, et al. A novel approach to stroke rehabilitation: robot-aided sensorimotor stimulation. *Neurology.* 2000;54:1938–1944.
103. Fasoli SE, Krebs HI, Stein J, et al. Robotic therapy for chronic motor impairments after stroke: follow-up results. *Arch Phys Med Rehabil.* 2004;85:1106–1111.
104. Klamroth-Marganska V, Blanco J, Campen K, et al. Three-dimensional, task-specific robot therapy of the arm after stroke: a multicentre, parallel-group randomised trial. *Lancet Neurol.* 2014;13(2):159–166.
105. Saposnik G, Levin M; Stroke Outcome Research Canada (SORCan) Working Group. Virtual reality in stroke rehabilitation. *Stroke.* 2011;42(5):1380–1386.
106. Saposnik G, Cohen LG, Mamdani M, et al. Efficacy and safety of non-immersive virtual reality exercising in stroke rehabilitation (EVREST): a randomised, multicentre, single-blind, controlled trial. *Lancet Neurol.* 2016;15(10):1019–1027.
107. Daly JJ, Roenigk K, Holcomb J, et al. A randomized controlled trial of functional neuromuscular stimulation in chronic stroke subjects. *Stroke.* 2006;37:172–178.
108. Burridge J, Haugland M, Larsen B, et al. Phase II trial to evaluate the ActiGait implanted drop-foot stimulator in established hemiplegia. *J Rehabil Med.* 2007;39(3):212–218.
109. Schleenbaker RE, Mainous AG III. Electromyographic biofeedback for neuromuscular reeducation in the hemiplegic stroke patient: a meta-analysis [see comment]. *Arch Phys Med Rehabil.* 1993;74:1301–1304.
110. Kraft GH, Fitts SS, Hammond MC. Techniques to improve function of the arm and hand in chronic hemiplegia. *Arch Phys Med Rehabil.* 1992;73:220–227.
111. Stein J, Narendran K, McBean J, et al. Electromyography-controlled exoskeletal upper-limb-powered orthosis for exercise training after stroke [erratum appears in *Am J Phys Med Rehabil.* 2008;87(8):689]. *Am J Phys Med Rehabil.* 2007;86: 255–261.
112. Michielsen ME, Selles RW, van der Geest JN, et al. Motor recovery and cortical reorganization after mirror therapy in chronic stroke patients: a phase II randomized controlled trial. *Neurorehabil Neural Repair.* 2011;25(3):223–233.
113. Thieme H, Mehrholz J, Pohl M, et al. Mirror therapy for improving motor function after stroke. *Stroke.* 2013;44(1):e1–e2.
114. Dawson J, Pierce D, Dixit A, et al. Safety, feasibility, and efficacy of vagus nerve stimulation paired with upper-limb rehabilitation after ischemic stroke. *Stroke.* 2016;47(1):143–150.
115. Hesse S, Bertelt C, Jahnke MT, et al. Treadmill training with partial body weight support compared with physiotherapy in nonambulatory hemiparetic patients [see comment]. *Stroke.* 1995;26:976–981.
116. Hesse S, Bertelt C, Schaffrin A, et al. Restoration of gait in nonambulatory hemiparetic patients by treadmill training with partial body-weight support. *Arch Phys Med Rehabil.* 1994;75:1087–1093.
117. Pohl M, Mehrholz J, Ritschel C, et al. Speed-dependent treadmill training in ambulatory hemiparetic stroke patients: a randomized controlled trial [see comment]. *Stroke.* 2002;33:553–558.
118. Duncan PW, Sullivan KJ, Behrman AL, et al. Body-weight-supported treadmill rehabilitation after stroke. *N Engl J Med.* 2011;364(21):2026–2036.
119. Husemann B, Muller F, Krewer C, et al. Effects of locomotion training with assistance of a robot-driven gait orthosis in hemiparetic patients after stroke: a randomized controlled pilot study. *Stroke.* 2007;38:349–354.
120. Hornby TG, Campbell DD, Kahn JH, et al. Enhanced gait-related improvements after therapist- versus robotic-assisted locomotor training in subjects with chronic stroke: a randomized controlled study. *Stroke.* 2008;39:1786–1792.
121. Frese A, Husstedt IW, Ringelstein EB, et al. Pharmacologic treatment of central post-stroke pain. *Clin J Pain.* 2006;22:252–260.
122. Vestergaard K, Andersen G, Gottrup H, et al. Lamotrigine for central poststroke pain: a randomized controlled trial. *Neurology.* 2001;56:184–190.
123. Ganesan V, Ng V, Chong WK, et al. Lesion volume, lesion location, and outcome after middle cerebral artery territory stroke. *Arch Dis Child.* 1999;81:295–300.
124. Wade DT, Wood VA, Hewer RL. Recovery after stroke—the first 3 months. *J Neurol Neurosurg Psychiatry.* 1985;48:7–13.
125. Gresham GE, Fitzpatrick TE, Wolf PA, et al. Residual disability in survivors of stroke—the Framingham study. *N Engl J Med.* 1975;293:954–956.
126. Granger CV, Hamilton BB, Linacre JM, et al. Performance profiles of the functional independence measure. *Arch Phys Med Rehabil.* 1993;72:84–89.
127. Feigenson JS, McDowell FH, Meese P, et al. Factors influencing outcome and length of stay in a stroke rehabilitation unit. Part 1. Analysis of 248 unscreened patients—medical and functional prognostic indicators. *Stroke.* 1977;8:651–656.
128. Wade DT, Hewer RL. Functional abilities after stroke: measurement, natural history and prognosis. *J Neurol Neurosurg Psychiatry.* 1987;50:177–182.

129. Dombovy ML, Basford JR, Whisnant JP, et al. Disability and use of rehabilitation services following stroke in Rochester, Minnesota, 1975–1979. *Stroke*. 1987;18:830–836.
130. Wade DT, Skilbeck CE, Hewer RL. Predicting Barthel ADL score at 6 months after an acute stroke. *Arch Phys Med Rehabil*. 1983;64:24–28.
131. Ostwald SK, Swank PR, Khan MM, et al. Predictors of functional independence and stress level of stroke survivors at discharge from inpatient rehabilitation. *J Cardiovasc Nurs*. 2008;23:371–377.
132. Horn SD, DeJong G, Smout RJ, et al. Stroke rehabilitation patients, practice, and outcomes: is earlier and more aggressive therapy better? [see comment]. *Arch Phys Med Rehabil*. 2005;86:S101–S114.
133. Evans RL, Bishop DS, Matlock AL, et al. Family interaction and treatment adherence after stroke. *Arch Phys Med Rehabil*. 1987;68:513–517.
134. Kalra L, Yu G, Wilson K, et al. Medical complications during stroke rehabilitation. *Stroke*. 1995;26:990–994.
135. Hertzer NR, Young JR, Beven EG, et al. Coronary angiography in 506 patients with extracranial cerebrovascular disease. *Arch Intern Med*. 1985;145:849–852.
136. Roth EJ, Mueller K, Green D. Stroke rehabilitation outcome: impact of coronary artery disease. *Stroke*. 1988;19:42–47.
137. Roth EJ. Heart disease in patients with stroke. Part II: impact and implications for rehabilitation. *Arch Phys Med Rehabil*. 1994;75:94–101.
138. Van Ouwenaller C, Laplace PM, Chantraine A. Painful shoulder in hemiplegia. *Arch Phys Med Rehabil*. 1986;67:23–26.
139. Dromerick AW, Edwards DF, Kumar A, et al. Hemiplegic shoulder pain syndrome: frequency and characteristics during inpatient stroke rehabilitation. *Arch Phys Med Rehabil*. 2008;89:1589–1593.
140. Chae J, Yu DT, Walker ME, et al. Intramuscular electrical stimulation for hemiplegic shoulder pain: a 12-month follow-up of a multiple-center, randomized clinical trial. *Arch Phys Med Rehabil*. 2005;84:832–842.
141. Hecht JS. Subscapular nerve block in the painful hemiplegic shoulder. *Arch Phys Med Rehabil*. 1992;73:1036–1039.
142. Davis SW, Petrillo CR, Eichberg RD, et al. Shoulder-hand syndrome in a hemiplegic population: a 5-year retrospective study. *Arch Phys Med Rehabil*. 1977;58:353–356.
143. Tepperman PS, Greyson ND, Hilbert L, et al. Reflex sympathetic dystrophy in hemiplegia. *Arch Phys Med Rehabil*. 1984;65:442–447.
144. Kamphuisen PW, Agnelli G, Kamphuisen PW, et al. What is the optimal pharmacological prophylaxis for the prevention of deep-vein thrombosis and pulmonary embolism in patients with acute ischemic stroke? *Thromb Res*. 2007;119:265–274.
145. Brandstater ME, Roth EJ, Siebens HC. Venous thromboembolism in stroke: literature review and implications for clinical practice. *Arch Phys Med Rehabil*. 1992;73:S379–S391.
146. Kearon C, Kahn SR, Agnelli G, et al. Antithrombotic therapy for venous thromboembolic disease: American College of Chest Physicians Evidence-Based Clinical Practice Guidelines (8th Edition). *Chest*. 2008;133:454S–545S.
147. Aissaoui N, Martins E, Mouly S, et al. A meta-analysis of bed rest versus early ambulation in the management of pulmonary embolism, deep vein thrombosis, or both. *Int J Cardiol*. 2009;137(1):37–41.
148. Robinson RG, Starr LB, Kubos KL, et al. A two-year longitudinal study of post-stroke mood disorders: findings during the initial evaluation. *Stroke*. 1983;14:736–741.
149. Coll P, Erickson RJ. Mood disorders associated with stroke. *Phys Med Rehabil*. 1989;3:619–628.
150. Robinson RG, Szetela B. Mood change following left hemispheric brain injury. *Ann Neurol*. 1981;9:447–453.
151. Spalletta G, Caltagirone C. Depression and other neuropsychiatric complications after stroke. In: Stein J, Harvey RL, Macko R, et al., eds. *Stroke Recovery and Rehabilitation*. New York, NY: Demos Medical; 2009:2391–2400.
152. Lazarus LW, Moberg PJ, Langsley PR, et al. Methylphenidate and nortriptyline in the treatment of poststroke depression: a retrospective comparison. *Arch Phys Med Rehabil*. 1994;75:403–406.
153. Monga TN. Sexuality post stroke. *Phys Med Rehab State Art Rev*. 1993;7:225–236.
154. Devinsky O, Devinsky O. Neurologist-induced sexual dysfunction: enzyme-inducing antiepileptic drugs [comment]. *Neurology*. 2005;65:980–981.
155. Lewis RW, Fugl-Meyer KS, Bosch R, et al. Epidemiology/risk factors of sexual dysfunction. *J Sex Med*. 2004;1:35–39.
156. Korpelainen JT, Nieminen P, Myllyla VV. Sexual functioning among stroke patients and their spouses [see comment]. *Stroke*. 1999;30:715–719.
157. Monga TN, Lawson JS, Inglis J. Sexual dysfunction in stroke patients. *Arch Phys Med Rehabil*. 1986;67:19–22.
158. Muller JE, Mittleman MA, Maclure M, et al. Triggering myocardial infarction by sexual activity. Low absolute risk and prevention by regular physical exertion. Determinants of Myocardial Infarction Onset Study Investigators [see comment]. *JAMA*. 1996;275:1405–1409.
159. Sinyor D, Amato P, Kaloupek DG, et al. Post-stroke depression: relationships to functional impairment, coping strategies, and rehabilitation outcome. *Stroke*. 1986;17:1102–1107.
160. Kotila M, Numminen H, Waltimo O, et al. Depression after stroke: results of the Finnstroke study. *Stroke*. 1998;29:368–372.
161. Ng L, Sansom J, Zhang M, et al. Effectiveness of a structured sexual rehabilitation programme following stroke: a randomized controlled trial. *J Rehabil Med*. 2017;49:333–340.

CHAPTER 19

Steven R. Flanagan
Brian S. Im
Heidi N. Fusco

Prin Amorapanth
Erika L. Trovato

Traumatic Brain Injury

Traumatic brain injury (TBI) is a common condition throughout the world. It occurs from either a direct impact to the head or through forces that are indirectly transmitted to the brain that disrupt normal cerebral function. It impacts all age, racial, and gender groups and accounts for considerable morbidity and mortality. Although the reported incidence of TBI in the United States is very high, it is largely felt to be underreported, obscuring the immense impact it has on the lives of those injured, their families, the health care system, and society. The same is true throughout the world, particularly in developing countries that have even less capability of tracking TBI incidence. Problems related to TBI affect overall health, function, social roles, and family dynamics. Not surprisingly, it exerts a tremendous financial toll from direct medical cost, custodial care, and lost productivity.

The impact of TBI on any one person varies widely due to differences in injury severity, pathophysiology, acute and long-term medical management, age at the time of injury, gender, and very likely genetics. The presentation of TBI is extremely variable, given the wide array of physical, behavioral, and cognitive problems that present in innumerable combinations. This presents considerable challenges to clinicians who assess, diagnose, and treat people with TBI. These consequences of TBI may be short-lived as commonly occurs after an isolated concussion or can be long term with an increased risk of developing seemingly unrelated medical problems as one ages. While physical impairments are common and a source of considerable disability, particularly after moderate to severe injury, behavioral and cognitive problems are the common hallmarks of TBI and often present as the major barriers to successful community reintegration. These problems also impact the delivery of rehabilitation services, necessitating a comprehensive and holistic approach to treatment that requires the combined talents of health care practitioners from many disciplines, ideally led by a physiatrist with specialized training in brain injury medicine.

Several medical problems are either specific to TBI or occur with sufficient regularity after injury that physicians, primarily physiatrists, seek fellowship training to gain additional knowledge and skills to adequately recognize, diagnose, and treat patients appropriately. The adage, "you see what you look for and look for what you know," is pertinent when considering TBI. Recognizing the unique skills and knowledge required to optimally treat people with TBI, the American Board of Medical Specialties approved the subspecialty of brain injury medicine, which is awarded through the American Board of Physical Medicine and Rehabilitation for qualified candidates who successfully pass a written examination.

EPIDEMIOLOGY

TBI is common in the United States and throughout the world, accounting for considerable morbidity and mortality. Of the 30 million injury-related emergency department (ED) visits, hospitalizations, and deaths each year in the United States, 16% are attributable at least in part to TBI (1). Approximately 30% of trauma-related deaths are either directly or partly attributable to TBI (2). The overall reported incidence of TBI dramatically increased from 2007 to 2010, largely accounted by an increase in ED visits, while hospitalizations and death rates either remained stable or slightly decreased (3). The increase in reported incidence and ED visits most likely reflects greater public awareness of TBI resulting from media attention to sports- and military-related concussion in addition to national campaigns such as the CDC's HEADS UP program rather than an actual increase in the occurrence of TBI (3).

The majority of ED visits are for mild TBI, also referred to as concussion. Supporting greater awareness for the increased reported incidence of concussion is a study demonstrating a 62% increase in sports-related concussion ED visits from 2001 to 2009 (4). Nearly 90% of persons with TBI presenting to an ED are treated and released, and 11% are hospitalized and discharged, with the remaining 2% dying (1). Although substantial, these figures underestimate the true incidence of TBI as they rely only on ED/hospital visits and reported deaths and do not account for those with mild TBI who often do not receive hospital-based care, seek office-based treatment, or remain untreated. The data also fail to capture those seeking treatment at federal facilities (1). In addition to civilian injuries, Department of Defense data indicate that 235,000 servicemen and woman serving in the Army, Navy, Air Force, and Marine Corps sustained a TBI from 2000 to 2011 (5). Further compounding the problem is the challenge of making a conclusive diagnosis of mild TBI. Neither a definitive diagnostic test nor widely accepted definition exists for mild TBI, making it a clinical diagnosis subject to inaccuracies. Last, the Centers for Disease Control and Prevention has funded only 20 states to produce state-level TBI incidence estimates, thus limiting data coming from unfunded states (3).

While TBI impacts the young and old alike, its overall incidence is unevenly distributed across the age spectrum. The highest rate of injuries occurs in the young (children, adolescents, young adults) and the elderly. Children aged ≤4 have the highest rate of TBI-related ED visits, followed by adolescents, young adults, and the elderly. Adults ≥75 years old are much more likely to be hospitalized, have the highest mortality rate, and have the worse functional outcomes than any other age group (1,6,7). Men are more likely to be injured than women at all age groups, with an overall ratio of approximately 3:2 (1).

Reported TBIs due to falls have steadily increased since 1996 (1,8,9) and are the leading cause of TBI overall, occurring most commonly in the very young and the elderly. TBIs due to motor vehicle-traffic–related events have been decreasing but remain the second most commonly reported etiology and account for the highest incidence among adolescents and young adults. They are also the leading cause of TBI-related deaths. Colliding with a moving or stationary object is the next most common cause with assault being the least common of the four major etiologic categories (1). A significant percentage of TBI etiology is classified as either other or unknown, the latter because of failure to complete external cause codes in hospital and other settings (1,3). There has been increasing interest in sports and recreational TBI, although their incidence is not well established as they are currently reported under other categories such as falls or being struck by an object (3). Some limited data exist from ED and organized sporting activities but at present are insufficient to provide accurate information.

The prevalence of long-term disability related to TBI has been reported to range from 3.17 (10) to 5.3 million (11) in the United States. Prevalence varies by age with pediatric and elderly disability estimated at approximately 145,000 and 775,000, respectively (10). Both may be underestimations given the possibility that mild TBI and abusive head trauma in pediatric populations are underreported (12). In elderly groups, TBI-related disabilities may be mistakenly attributed to normal aging as well as age-related conditions such as dementia. TBI causes a tremendous economic burden, due to the costs of medical care and lost wages arising from absences and long-term disability. The combined cost in 2000 was estimated to be $60.43 billion (U.S. dollars) with productivity losses greater than that occurring for injury to any other body region (13). Existing disability rates, however, are only rough estimates as they were extrapolated from onetime estimates from only two states (3). Thus, there currently exists an inability to establish reliable national estimates, state-to-state comparisons, trends, recent accurate estimates, or differences between demographic groups (3).

TBI-related mortality has steadily decreased since 1988 (1,14), likely due in part to an overall decrease in motor vehicle collisions along with the mandatory use of seatbelts and placement of airbags. There has also been an increase in compliance with published guidelines for managing severe TBI, which, when applied, has been estimated to decrease mortality by 50% (15). In addition to older age, the degree of intoxication with alcohol at the time of injury, occurring in one fourth to one half of all injuries (16), is associated with higher mortality (17).

PATHOPHYSIOLOGY

Pathophysiology of TBI can be divided into broad categories based on whether the injury occurs at the time of impact or at a later time and whether injury is localized to a specific cerebral region or is widespread. Primary injury occurs or is initiated at the onset of trauma, while secondary injury occurs at a

later time point. Focal injury refers to fairly discreet regions of injury, whereas diffuse injuries are present over wide regions of the brain. Prevention of injury, such as by the mandatory use of safety belts and placement of airbags in motor vehicles, is the only means of decreasing the incidence or ameliorating the impact of primary injury. Cerebral damage occurring at times after the initial impact provides opportunities to ameliorate the impact of the injury and the potential to improve outcomes. This is further discussed in the "Acute Management" section of this chapter.

Primary injury includes focal contusions and traumatic axonal injury. The brain has a soft, gelatinous consistency *in vivo*. As a result of impact to the head or body, the brain will move within the cranial vault where its surface can impact the skull, resulting in contusions. Although the entire surface of the brain is susceptible to contusions, the rough inner surface of the skull where it approximates the inferior portion of the frontal lobes and the anterior tips of the temporal lobes makes these regions particularly vulnerable to injury. Coup-contrecoup describes contusions at opposite sides of the brain, occurring from the back-and-forth motion of the brain within the cranial vault at the time of injury. The size, location, and depth as well as whether contusion has occurred bilaterally provide an indication of injury severity. Contusions can result in focal motor and sensory impairment depending on their location but more frequently contribute to behavioral and cognitive difficulties. Contusions may undergo hemorrhagic conversion, contributing to edema and local ischemic changes that lead to further tissue destruction, neuronal necrosis, cavitation, and reactive gliosis (18) (**Fig. 19-1**). They can also lead to increases in intracranial pressure (ICP) that may require neurosurgical intervention or other aggressive treatments.

Diffuse axonal injury (DAI), also commonly referred to as traumatic axonal injury, is a major contributor to TBI morbidity and mortality. It occurs in acceleration-deceleration injuries, which involve forces that rapidly move the head in an angular and rotational manner. This results in rapid shearing of axons causing membrane instability, ionic disequilibrium, and cytoskeletal disruption (19–24) that initiate a cascade of events that ultimately leads to calcium-mediated neuronal injury and impaired axonal transport. Axonal transport is impaired further by disruption of the cytoskeletal structure of the neuron that normally supports movement of cellular components (19,25,26), leading to swelling and ultimately axonal disconnection and Wallerian degeneration. Although DAI occurs throughout the brain, there is a predilection to the midbrain, pons, corpus callosum, white matter tracts of the cerebral hemispheres including the internal capsule, the cerebellum (27,28), and at sites with differences in tissue density or where white matter tracts change direction (29). Collectively, these pathologic processes result in deafferentation due to synaptic loss, accounting for considerable morbidity, including immediate loss of consciousness (30) as well as alterations in behavior and cognition. Axonal injury is microscopic and thus is typically not visualized on standard neuroimaging studies, although indirect evidence may appear as petechial hemorrhages on CT and T1/T2-weighted MR images from microvascular disruption (**Fig. 19-2**). More advanced MRI technologies that are clinically available such as gradient echo

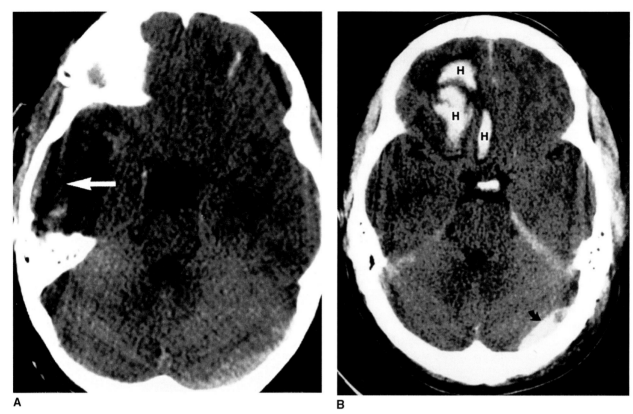

A

B

FIGURE 19-1. **A:** Cerebral contusion. This head computed tomography scan was performed on a 6-year-old boy who was found unresponsive and apneic after being a passenger in a high-speed motor vehicle collision. The *arrow* indicates a large area of hypodense nonhemorrhagic contusion in the right temporal lobe. (Reprinted with permission from Fleisher GR, Ludwig S, et al. *Textbook of Pediatric Emergency Medicine*. 5th ed. Philadelphia, PA: Lippincott Williams & Wilkins; 2005.) **B:** Cerebral contusions. The patient has hemorrhagic contusions (H = hemorrhage) on the base of the right frontal region with surrounding edema as well as a small left occipital epidural hematoma (*black arrow*). (Reprinted with permission from Pope TL, Harris J. *Harris & Harris' Radiology of Emergency Medicine*. 5th ed. Philadelphia, PA: Wolters Kluwer Health/Lippincott Williams & Wilkins; 2013.)

and susceptibility-weighted images can visualize microscopic hemorrhages associated with DAI (**Fig. 19-3**), while diffusion tensor imaging (DTI) has been shown to detect axonal disruption. Diffusion-weighted and fluid-attenuated inversion recovery (FLAIR) images have also been shown to be more sensitive in visualizing evidence of DAI than standard CT and T1/T2-weighted MR images.

DAI is seen histologically as axon retraction balls, representing the proximal portion of an axon that has disconnected from its distal segment (**Fig. 19-4**). Although once thought to occur at the time of injury, ultimate axonal disconnection typically occurs at some point after injury onset, providing an opportunity for researchers to discover means to alter the process prior to neuronal demise (31). DAI occurs across the

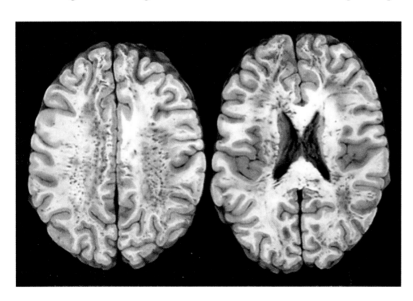

FIGURE 19-2. Diffuse white matter petechial hemorrhage seen in diffuse axonal injury (DAI) on gross section. (Reprinted with permission from Weiner WJ, Goetz CG, Shin RK. *Neurology for the Non-Neurologist*. 6th ed. Philadelphia, PA: Wolters Kluwer Health/Lippincott Williams & Wilkins 2010.)

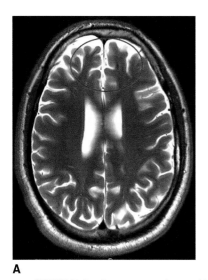
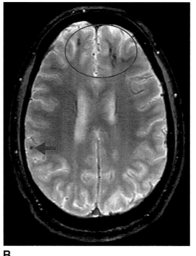
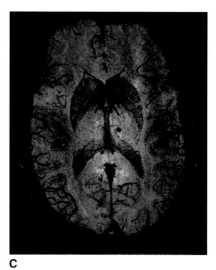

A B C

FIGURE 19-3. Remote traumatic axonal injury not evident on admission CT and only visualized with T2* gradient MRI. Axial T2-weighted **(A)** and T2* gradient **(B)** MR images obtained 1 year after the injury demonstrate numerous bilateral microhemorrhages within the subcortical white matter of the frontal lobes (*circle*) and a single focus within the right parietal subcortical white matter (*arrow*). Diffuse cerebral volume loss is also evident as judged by abnormal prominence of ventricles and sulci for a patient this age. As expected, the TAI lesions are more conspicuous on the T2* gradient sequence than on the T2 spin-echo sequence. (Reprinted with permission from Gean AD. *Brain Injury: Applications from War and Terrorism.* 1st ed. Philadelphia, PA: Wolters Kluwer Health/Lippincott Williams & Wilkins; 2014.) **C:** Susceptibility-weighted image (SWI) from a subject with traumatic brain injury. The venous vasculature appears dark on the images due to deoxygenated hemoglobin. A dark microbleed lesion appears in the left thalamus resulting from the traumatic brain injury. (Reprinted with permission of Smith WL, Farrell TA. *Radiology 101: The Basics and Fundamentals of Imaging.* 4th ed. Philadelphia, PA: Wolters Kluwer Health/Lippincott Williams & Wilkins; 2014.)

spectrum of TBI severity, as noted by histologic autopsy results revealing evidence in persons with mild TBI but who succumbed to other injuries (28,32).

Within minutes of TBI, there is an excessive release of excitatory amino acids, predominantly glutamate, the magnitude of which correlates with injury severity (33–38). Depolarized neurons release large quantities of glutamate, which is compounded by leakage from damaged astrocytes, and this impaired neuronal reuptake mechanisms. The excess glutamate in term initiates unregulated stimulation of predominantly N-methyl-D-aspartate glutamate receptors that leads to alterations in potassium transport and unregulated

influx of sodium and calcium. Toxic increases in intracellular calcium lead to activation of Ca^{++}-dependent proteases, generation of destructive oxygen and nitrogen compounds, and mitochondrial injury, which initiates apoptosis from increased mitochondrial permeability (39–41). Cellular energy failure ensues from the combination of widespread depolarization, mitochondrial damage, marked increases in glycolysis, and the massive energy requirements used in the cell's attempt to reestablish ionic homeostasis (42–44).

Secondary injury occurs at some point after the initial insult and provides an opportunity to prevent or ameliorate further damage through medical interventions. Increased

FIGURE 19-4. Diffuse axonal injury. Microscopic section of the cerebral cortex from a 25-year-old man who sustained a severe closed head injury. **Left:** Axon retraction ball (*arrow*) seen as an eosinophilic swelling on hematoxylin and eosin staining. **Right:** Retraction ball on Bielschowsky-stained specimen. (Source: Dr. S.R. Vandenberg.)

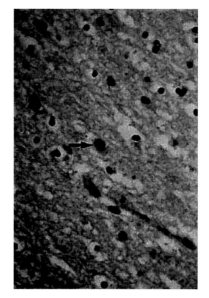
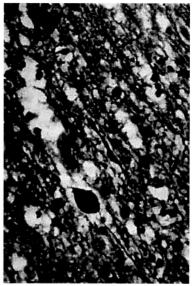

ICP is the main factor contributing to secondary injury by causing diffuse ischemia and potentially herniation. The brain is contained within the rigid confines of the skull. Cerebral swelling and intracranial hemorrhages (ICHs) contribute to elevated ICP, which if severe enough will displace the brain into adjacent compartments causing neurologic compromise as well as limit cerebral perfusion resulting in ischemia. The latter is often exacerbated following severe TBI due to alterations in cerebral blood flow (CBF) autoregulation. In the uninjured state, cerebrovascular resistance is regulated in response to changes in blood pressure that maintains adequate cerebral circulation. Impaired autoregulation subjects the degree of cerebral perfusion to that dictated by systemic blood pressure, potentially worsening ischemia during periods of hypotension. Therefore, a primary objective acutely after trauma is to maintain adequate cerebral perfusion. That is achieved by aggressively managing intracranial hypertension and ensuring adequate systemic blood pressure.

Both extraaxial and intraparenchymal hemorrhages can increase ICP and displace cerebral tissue. Extraaxial hemorrhages occur externally to cerebral parenchyma but within or directly adjacent to the meninges. Epidural hemorrhages (EDHs) typically occur in association with skull fractures that disrupt the middle meningeal artery or less frequently dural sinuses (**Fig. 19-5**). Subarachnoid hemorrhages predispose cerebral arteries to vasospasm and potentially poorer outcomes

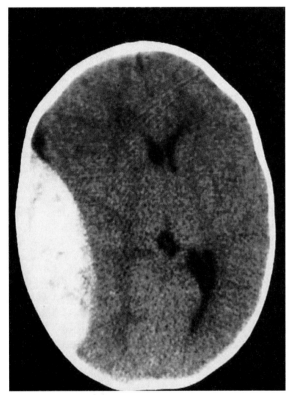

FIGURE 19-5. A large mass of white (blood) density convex toward the brain is characteristic of an epidural hemorrhage. Most of these occur because of traumatic tear of an artery and are surgical emergencies. The brain is shifted by the hematoma as evidenced by the shift of midline. (Reprinted with permission of Smith WL, Farrell TA. *Radiology 101: The Basics and Fundamentals of Imaging.* 4th ed. Philadelphia, PA: Wolters Kluwer Health/Lippincott Williams & Wilkins; 2014.)

after TBI (45) (**Fig. 19-6**). Subdural hemorrhages (SDHs) arise from disruption of bridging veins that are susceptible to shear forces. An acute large SDH manifests as a rapid deterioration of arousal or development of focal neurologic deficits (**Fig. 19-7**). However, the elderly have larger subdural spaces due to naturally occurring cerebral atrophy, thus permitting the presence of a limited subdural collection without obvious clinical deterioration. An SDH may also slowly expand in the elderly as a result of increased capillary permeability caused by degeneration, cytoplasmic protrusions and fenestration of endothelial cells (46), increased fibrinolysis (47), and abnormal coagulation (48). This in part accounts for the late neurologic deterioration often observed in elderly people who have a slowly expanding SDH.

ACUTE MANAGEMENT

Under normal physiologic conditions, cerebrovascular autoregulation permits adequate CBF over a wide range of blood pressures by altering vascular resistance. Thus, when systemic blood pressure is low, cerebrovascular resistance decreases permitting sufficient brain perfusion. Alternatively, high systemic blood pressure can result in increased vascular resistance, thus preventing cerebral hyperemia. Following TBI, normal cerebrovascular regulation is altered, subjecting brain perfusion to the status of systemic blood pressure. The brain is confined within the rigid confines of the skull. In response to injury, cerebral edema often occurs, frequently accompanied by ICHs. This results in increased ICP against which systemic blood pressure must overcome to adequately perfuse the brain. When accompanied by altered cerebrovascular autoregulation, the brain becomes susceptible to cerebral ischemia, particularly in the presence of systemic hypotension. Thus, the main goal of acute management of severe TBI is to limit secondary brain injury, which is largely focused on maintaining adequate CBF.

The adequacy of brain perfusion can be measured by cerebral perfusion pressure (CPP). CPP is defined as the difference between mean arterial pressure (MAP) and ICP. In the absence of normal cerebral vascular autoregulation, prevention of cerebral ischemia is achieved by measuring and then either medically or surgically managing both MAP and ICP. Management typically involves a balanced approach of decreasing elevated ICP as well as maintaining MAP at levels that promote sufficient CPP but avoids the deleterious effects of prolonged systemic hypertension. Low MAP subjects the injured brain to ischemia, while maintaining blood pressure too high can result in cerebral hyperemia and other deleterious effects. The Brain Trauma Foundation and the American Association of Neurological Surgeons (AANS) developed guidelines for managing severe TBI, which includes steps to prevent secondary injury and improve outcomes (49). In addition to surgical evacuation of mass occupying ICHs, several means to decrease ICP are described.

Treatment is guided by either close monitoring of clinical signs indicating the presence of elevated ICP or more directly by measuring ICP via an ICP bolt. When using direct measurements, current guidelines recommend initiating treatment when ICP exceeds 22 mm Hg and maintaining CPP between 60 and 70 mm Hg. ICP higher than 22 mm Hg has been associated with increased mortality (50), while keeping CPP greater than 70 has been associated with the development of

FIGURE 19-6. Traumatic subarachnoid hemorrhage. Images from four different TBI patients. **A:** Traumatic subarachnoid hemorrhage (tSAH) is common in the peripheral sulci adjacent to a site of impact (*arrows*). A frequently overlooked site of tSAH is in the interpeduncular cistern (**B**, *arrow*), which may be the only clue to TBI. tSAH will be hyperintense on FLAIR (**C**, *arrows*) and can also be visible on SWI (**D**, *dotted arrows*). (Reprinted from Sanelli PC, Schaefer P, Loevner LA. *Neuroimaging the Essentials.* 1st ed. Philadelphia, PA: Wolters Kluwer; 2016.)

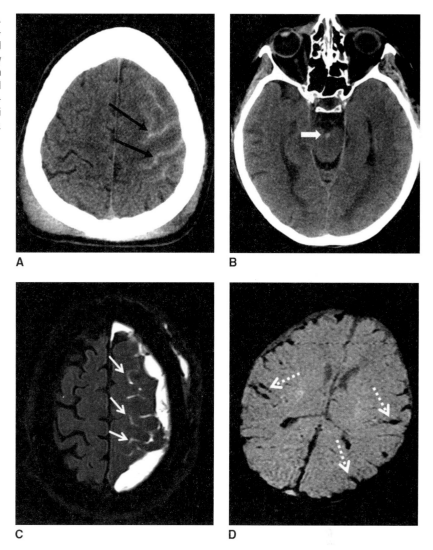

adult respiratory distress syndrome (51). Systolic blood pressure should be maintained ≥100 mm Hg for patients aged 50 to 69 and ≥110 mm Hg for those aged 15 to 49 and greater than 70 (52). Intravenous hyperosmolar therapy with either hypertonic saline or mannitol will reduce cerebral edema by drawing fluid from the brain. Placing an ICP monitor in the ventricular system will permit draining of cerebrospinal fluid (CSF), which has been shown to reduce ICP. However, it is currently recommended in only those patients with Glasgow Coma Scale (GCS) scores of less than 6, as one study indicated increased mortality when CSF drainage is used in less severe injuries (53). Decompressive hemicraniectomy, a surgical procedure that removes a large portion of the skull and opens the underlying dura mater, eliminates restricted cerebral expansion the skull imposes on a swelling brain, thus decreasing ICP. Studies examining its effects on mortality and outcomes have been mixed, although methodologic issues have limited the interpretability of the findings (49,54–57).

In the past, barbiturates and hyperventilation were widely used to reduce ICP but are now resorted to only in very limited situations because of side effects that restrict their benefits. Barbiturates increase the risk of systemic hypotension, decreasing cardiac output and increasing intrapulmonary shunting that can lead to hypoxemia. Current recommendations suggest

their use in cases of increased ICP refractory to standard medical and surgical management with the caveat that hemodynamic stability be achieved and monitored prior to and during treatment (49). Hyperventilation decreases $PaCO_2$, resulting in decreased CBF. Thus, its use is only recommended as a temporizing measure to prevent herniation and is avoided during the first 24 hours postinjury when CBF is often critically reduced (49). Normal ventilation is the goal following TBI to prevent ischemia and cerebral hyperemia, the latter that could result from hypoventilation causing increased $PaCO_2$ and increased ICP. Steroids are contraindicated in managing ICP following TBI. Although frequently used to reduce cerebral edema in many neurologic conditions and following neurosurgical procedures, they are not used following TBI as they were found to increase mortality and worsen outcomes (58).

ASSESSMENTS

Injury Severity

Reliably assessing injury severity ideally provides a means to offer information pertaining to immediate and long-term prognosis, to follow progression of the condition, and to accurately share information between healthcare providers. In order to gain widespread use, an assessment needs to be

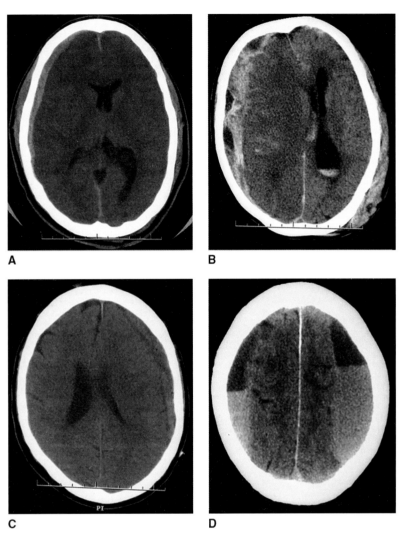

A

B

C

D

FIGURE 19-7.   CT scans of subdural hematomas. **A:** Right-sided acute subdural hematoma with the typical crescent shape. **B:** Right-sided acute subdural hematoma with low-density areas within representing unclotted serum and blood. Note the significant mass effect with midline shift to the left. There is also intraventricular hemorrhage within the left lateral ventricle. **C:** Left-sided subacute subdural hematoma isodense to brain parenchyma. **D:** Bilateral acute on chronic subdural hematomas with fluid-fluid levels. (Reprinted with permission from Griggs RC, Joynt RJ. *Baker and Joynt's Clinical Neurology on CD-ROM.* Philadelphia, PA; Lippincott Williams & Wilkins; 2004.)

easy to use, valid, and reliable. Several tools are available to assess the severity of TBI as well as to provide some degree of prognostic information regarding mortality and long-term functional outcomes. The GCS was developed by Jennett and Teasdale in the early 1970s as a standardized means to assess and document injury severity and level of consciousness (59). It describes three components of the physical examination that are meant to quantitatively describe the level of consciousness and thus injury severity. The three subscale scores are based on the patient's best motor, verbal, and eye response (**Fig. 19-8**).

The total score is the sum of all the subscale scores and ranges from 3 to 15. Injury severity is considered mild for scores 13 to 15, moderate for 9 to 12, and severe for 3 to 8. Although initially describing coma as scores ≤8, more specific guidelines for defining altered levels of consciousness were subsequently developed and are described later in this chapter. The GCS is easily used by multiple healthcare practitioners and provides reliable information regarding the depth of unconsciousness in persons with TBI. It remains the most widely used tool to assess injury severity in the acute setting and is useful for monitoring changes in the neurologic condition of persons with TBI. However, there are limitations of the GCS that restrict its utility. Chemical paralysis and early intubation prevent accurate scoring, as does intoxication with alcohol or recreational drug use that can artificially lower scores. When

patients are intubated, GCS is scored using only the eye and motor subscales followed by a "T," indicating intubation and inability to assess the verbal component of the score.

Glasgow Coma Scale	Best possible total score 15	Worst possible total score 3
Monitored Performance	**Reaction**	**Score**
Eye opening	Spontaneous	4
	Open when spoken to	3
	Open at pain stimulus	2
	No reaction	1
Verbal performance	Coherent	5
	Confused, disoriented	4
	Disconnected words	3
	Unintelligible sounds	2
	No verbal reaction	1
Motor responsiveness	Follows instructions	6
	Intentional pain-avoidance	5
	Large motor movement	4
	Flexor synergism	3
	Extensor synergism	2
	No reaction	1

FIGURE 19-8.   The Glasgow Coma Scale (GCS). The GCS is scored between 3 and 15, with 3 being the worst score and 15 being the best score. (Reprinted from Teasdale G, Jennett B. Assessment of coma and impaired consciousness. A practical scale. *Lancet.* 1974; 2(7872):81–84. Copyright © 1984 Elsevier. With permission.)

TABLE 19-1 Full Outline of Unresponsiveness

Domain	0	1	2	3	4
Eye response	Eyes stay closed to pain	Eyes closed but open to pain	Eyes closed but open to loud voice	Eyes open but no tracking	Eyes open, tracking or blink to command
Motor response	No response to pain or myoclonus	Extensor response	Flexion response	Localized to pain	Follows motor commands
Brainstem response	Absent pupil, corneal, and cough reflex	Pupil and corneal reflex absent	Pupil or corneal reflex absent	One pupil fixed and dilated	Pupil and corneal reflex present
Respiration	Intubated, breathes at ventilator rate or apnea	Intubated, breathes above ventilator rate	Not intubated, irregular breathing	Not intubated, Cheyne-Stokes respirations	Not intubated, regular breathing

The Full Outline of UnResponsiveness (FOUR) is a relatively new tool to assess depth of unconsciousness. It assesses four components of the physical examination, including eye responses, motor responses, brainstem reflexes, and respiration. Each is scored from 0 to 4 with a total score ranging from 0 to 16 (**Table 19-1**). It does not rely on verbal responses, thus eliminating the intubation limitation imposed on the GCS. It's been shown to have good interrater reliability and may provide greater neurologic detail than the GCS, including being able to better recognize different stages of herniation (60). Studies have shown that the FOUR score has at least comparable ability to predict early mortality as the GCS (60,61) as well as predicting unfavorable outcome 3 months post injury (62). Although the FOUR does not have the intubation limitation of the GCS, it shares the same limitation imposed by chemical paralysis and intoxication.

Neuroimaging

Initial management of moderate to severe TBI, as well as selected cases of mild TBI, invariably involves neuroimaging studies to identify and quantify macroscopic lesions that either require an immediate surgical intervention or a baseline against which future studies can be compared to assess for change. Computed tomography (CT) remains the imaging modality of choice to acutely assess lesions requiring immediate surgical

management. Nonhemorrhagic contusions are identified by regions of hypodensity typically seen in areas known to have high susceptibility to injury, such as the inferior poles of the frontal lobes and anterior tips of the temporal lobes. Associated edema or hemorrhagic conversion of bland contusions may necessitate neurosurgical intervention to manage intracranial hypertension (see **Fig. 19-1**).

Extraaxial hemorrhages are identified by their unique shape, associated injuries, and their location in relation to the three layers of the meninges (**Fig. 19-9**). EDHs lie within the epidural space defined by the skull and the dura mater. In the uninjured condition, the epidural space is a potential space as the dura strongly adheres to the skull. Following trauma and typically in association with a skull fracture, the middle meningeal artery or, less frequently, a dural sinus can be disrupted. The resulting hemorrhage tears the dura off the skull except at the areas of bony sutures, thus producing the typical elliptical or biconvex shape of EDHs (see **Fig. 19-5**). The subdural space is defined by the boundaries of the dura and arachnoid mater. Hemorrhages here result from disruption of bridging veins, filling the subdural space, and have a typical crescent shape (see **Fig. 19-7**). The subarachnoid space is defined by the arachnoid and pia mater. The pia mater is adherent to the brain; thus, hemorrhages here are typically seen within the cerebral sulci (see **Fig. 19-6**).

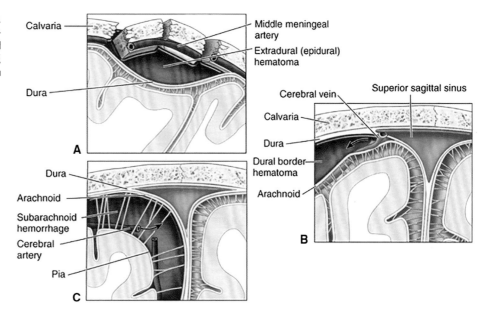

FIGURE 19-9. Intracranial hemorrhages. **A:** Epidural hemorrhage. **B:** Subdural hemorrhage. **C:** Subarachnoid hemorrhage. (Reprinted with permission from Moore KL, Dalley AF, Agur AMR. *Clinically Oriented Anatomy.* 8th ed. Baltimore, MD: Wolters Kluwer; 2017.)

Traditional imaging techniques, such as CT and conventional magnetic resonance imaging (MRI), have proven to be highly effective in identifying macroscopic lesions, which is a necessary component in managing acute trauma. However, they have marked limitations in assessing microscopic lesions and cerebral physiology, such as those associated with DAI and metabolic alteration. Furthermore, they offer little insight into the normal physiology associated with behavior and cognition. Newer MR technologies, such as gradient echo, susceptibility-weighted, functional, and MR spectroscopy, can detect both microscopic injuries and physiologic alteration that may account for TBI-related morbidities not visible on traditionally standard images. This is particularly true in mild TBI where standard imaging studies typically fail to detect pathology despite clinical evidence of impaired physical, cognitive, and emotional function.

Structural/Chemical Imaging

DAI is felt to be a major contributor to morbidity following TBI, yet because it occurs at a micro- rather than macroscopic level, it is poorly imaged on standard CT and MRI scans. Diffusion-weighted MRI detects the speed of water molecule diffusion within biologic tissues. It can identify and differentiate cytotoxic from vasogenic edema, the former manifested by restricted diffusion and associated with TBI lesions and outcomes (63). DTI generates images by taking advantage of the variability of both the speed and direction of water diffusion *in vivo*. Water diffuses faster along an axon, as opposed to across it, a phenomenon known as anisotropy. Values are reported as fractional anisotropy (FA), ranging from 0 to 1 with higher values indicating a greater degree of diffusion that is restricted to the parallel axis of a white matter tract. Mean diffusivity (MD) refers to the degree of water diffusion perpendicular to the axis of the axon. Uninjured white matter tracts manifest large FA values and low MD, which can be assessed by diffusion tensor technology. This permits an *in vivo* investigation of fiber tract integrity that has been correlated with histopathologic evidence of DAI (64). DTI has been shown to provide evidence of axonal injury in the presence of normal standard MR imaging (65), the extent and quantity of white matter injury (66), and the location of maximum white matter tract abnormalities associated with motor impairment post-TBI (67). FA values have been correlated with both injury severity and outcomes (68–70).

DTI in association with other diffusion-weighted images permits a greater understanding of the pathophysiologic process of axonal injury. It does so by examining the individual components and time course responsible for decreased anisotropy, such as edema and axonal truncation, potentially identifying a therapeutic window for future treatments designed to ameliorate DAI (71). Using DTI technology, images of fiber tracts can be generated providing additional information about neuronal injury, brain anatomy, and cerebral function. Both DTI and fiber tract imaging are used for research and are not readily accepted as clinical tools.

Gradient echo and susceptibility-weighted MRI can detect microscopic deposition of hemosiderin and other degradation products of hemoglobin in the brain that are indicators of DAI not imaged by CT (see **Fig. 19-3**). Magnetic resonance spectroscopy (MRS), which uses different software but whose hardware is similar to standard MRI, analyzes the concentrations of various metabolites in specific cerebral regions, which in pathologic states differ from healthy tissue. Data are presented from either a single volume of the brain, known as single-voxel spectroscopy, or a 2D or 3D analysis obtained simultaneously over a wider region, known as magnetic resonance spectroscopy imaging (MRSI). *N*-acetylaspartic acid (NAA) is present only in neuronal tissue and is one of several key cerebral metabolites measured by MRS. Lower than normal levels of NAA are indicative of either neuronal loss or abnormal changes in cellular function (72), which is associated with poorer outcomes post-TBI even in the presence of normal-appearing standard neuroimages (73). Other metabolites of interest measured by MRS include creatine (energy utilization marker), choline (marker of cell membrane disruption, inflammation, and changes in myelination), myoinositol (astrocyte marker), glutamate, and lactate, which along with NAA have been correlated with various outcomes when obtained at various times post-TBI (74–77).

MRS is one potential tool to assess for injury after mild TBI, revealing whole-brain reductions in NAA associated with cerebral atrophy despite the absence of focal lesions detected on conventional MRI. This provides evidence that mild TBI can result in widespread damage (78) and has been correlated with outcomes (77). MRS data can provide information on TBI-induced physiologic changes, cerebral regions susceptible to injury, individual susceptibility to injury based on characteristics such as age (78), and the predictive role of metabolic alterations on outcomes post-TBI not feasible with conventional imaging. Longitudinal MRS studies can examine the extent and location of concentration changes over time in association with specific cognitive abilities. This provides information regarding the physiologic and chemical modifications that impact either favorably or unfavorably on recovery occurring over time post injury (79). With greater understanding provided by MRS regarding the molecular changes associated with the acute and reparative processes of TBI and at what time postinjury these changes occur, comes the possibility of developing treatments to ameliorate pathologic alterations and improve outcomes.

SPECIAL POPULATIONS

Disorders of Consciousness

Jennett and Plum described the persistent vegetative state (VS) as a condition manifested by wakefulness but without awareness in the early 1970s (80). Since then, several definitions have been developed to more fully describe and classify disorders of consciousness (DOC) that include diagnostic criteria and assessment tools. Coma is described as a state of unwakefulness in which the eyes remain closed without evidence of sleep-wake cycles or purposeful voluntary activity. Responses to noxious stimulation are manifested as reflexive, while there is absence of verbalization and ability to follow commands and to communicate. Following trauma, the true comatose state is generally short-lived, with patients either dying or emerging into another level of either unconsciousness or consciousness.

The VS, as initially described by Jennett and Plum, is succinctly describes as a condition where a person appears to be awake yet manifests no discernible evidence of awareness. Sleep-wake cycles are preserved as noted by EEG recordings and eyes will spontaneously open. However, there is no evidence of purposeful or voluntary motor activity, verbalization, communication, or emotional reaction in response to appropriate stimulation.

There are two important prognosticators regarding recovery from VS: etiology and time elapsed from injury. TBI has a notably better prognosis for emergence into a higher state of consciousness than nontraumatic causes such as anoxia, ischemia, or other metabolic derangements (81,82). Fifty-two percent of persons in VS due to TBI 1 month postinjury have been shown to emerge into a higher state of consciousness, such as minimally conscious by 1 year, whereas only 11% of those caused by nontraumatic etiologies emerge (81). Similarly, 16% of persons in VS 6 months after TBI have been shown to emerge at 1 year, whereas none did after nontraumatic causes in a meta-analysis of 423 patients (81). The qualitative term, persistent, was added to the VS to connote unconsciousness that was sustained over time, whereas permanent inferred it was irreversible. Thus, the term permanent VS was initially developed because of the poor prognosis for recovery as time passed and was applied to those in VS at various times post injury based on etiology (80). However, recovery of consciousness is feasible even more than 1 year after onset in some cases with a traumatic etiology. Therefore, the Aspen Neurobehavioral Group (ANG) recommended replacing the qualitative "persistent" term with descriptors indicating traumatic versus nontraumatic etiology and the time since onset (83).

Recognizing the progression of recovery of consciousness, the ANG further expanded the definition of conditions falling within the realm of DOC. They acknowledged the existence of an altered state of consciousness in which there was minimal or intermittent but definitive behavioral evidence of conscious awareness. Initially described as the minimally responsive state, the group later renamed it the minimally conscious state (MCS) to better reflect responses that were consciously mediated rather than reflexive. Behavioral evidence suggesting the presence of MCS includes at least one of the following: simple command following, intelligible verbalizations, recognizable verbal or gestural "yes/no" responses without regard to accuracy, or movement or emotional responses triggered by relevant environmental stimuli not attributable to reflex activity (83). Emergence from MCS is heralded by reliable and consistent demonstration of interactive communication and functional object use. Similar to VS, prognosis for recovery from MCS is more likely following a traumatic rather than nontraumatic etiology (84) (**Table 19-2**).

Studies have demonstrated that accurately diagnosing DOC in people incapable of speaking or following commands is challenging and ranges from 30% to 40% (85–87). Serial examinations are necessary in order to account for alterations in arousal that may intermittently interfere with a person's ability to comprehend and follow commands. Assessments should ideally occur at different times of day over several days in order to increase the likelihood of examining a patient during a time they are awake or adequately aroused. Determining the ability to follow commands also depends on the complexity of the command itself and the consistency at which it is followed. Asking a person to close their eyes may provide a false-positive response given people in VS will periodically blink. However, asking a person a more complex command that would not be considered a spontaneous act, such as "lift

TABLE 19-2 Behavioral Features of Disorders of Consciousness

Behavior	Coma	Vegetative State	Minimally Conscious State
Eye opening	None	Spontaneous	Spontaneous
Spontaneous movement	None	Reflexive/ patterned	Automatic/object manipulation
Response to pain	Posturing/ none	Posturing/ withdrawal	Localization
Visual response	None	Startle/pursuit (rare)	Object recognition/ pursuit
Affective response	None	Random	Contingent
Commands	None	None	Inconsistent
Verbalization	None	Random vocalization	Intelligible words
Communication	None	None	Unreliable

Reprinted from Hirschberg R, Giacino JT. The vegetative and minimally conscious states: diagnosis, prognosis and treatment. *Neurol Clin.* 2011;29(4):773–786. Copyright © 2011 Elsevier. With permission.

two fingers," even if performed very rarely to command, would be a strong indication of a purposeful act that accurately differentiates MCS from VS. Further complicating the difficulty in differentiating VS from MCS are motor impairments that may prevent patients from following motor commands despite having intact ability to accurately perceive and understand them. Studies using fMRI have demonstrated intact abilities of some people clinically classified as VS to comprehend and mentally follow commands (88–90). Several tools are available to assess people in DOC, although the Coma Recovery Scale-Revised was determined to be the most acceptable instrument by the Disorder of Consciousness Task Force of the American Congress of Rehabilitation Medicine (91). The scale consists of six subscales assessing auditory, visual, motor, oromotor/verbal, communication, and arousal functions that are arranged in a hierarchal format progressing from brainstem-mediated to cortical functions.

TBI Sustained at Younger Ages

Children experience many of the same problems as adults with TBI, although there are differences regarding pathophysiology, assessments, interventions, and outcomes that warrant special attention. The brains of children differ from those of adults with regard to water content, extent of myelination, CBF, skull properties, and number of synapses, which likely impact how their brain responds to trauma (92–95). The short- and long-term effects of trauma on a developing brain can manifest differently than similar injury sustained in adults. Specialized assessment tools, such as the Pediatric GCS or the Children's Orientation and Amnesia Test (COAT), are more appropriate for the developmental age of younger children than their adult versions and can therefore better assess a child's true status (**Fig. 19-10**). Depending on their development age at the time of injury, children may experience TBI-related problems many years after a seemingly good early recovery. This requires that injured children be closely monitored as they grow into adolescence and adulthood when problems with behavior and/or acquisition of new cognitive skills may become evident (96–99).

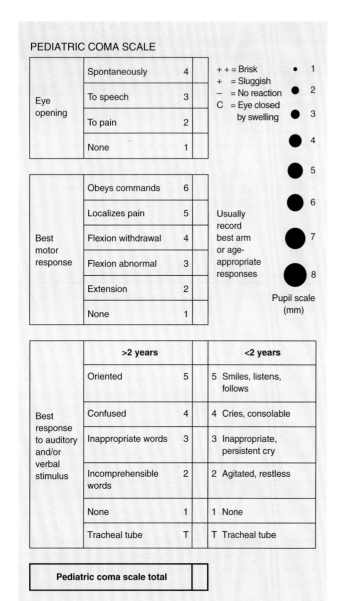

FIGURE 19-10. Pediatric Glasgow Coma Scale (GCS). The Pediatric GCS provides for developmentally appropriate cues to assess level of consciousness (LOC) in infants and children. Numeric values are assigned to the levels of response and the sum provides an overall picture, as well as an objective measure, of the child's LOC. The lower the score, the less responsive the child. (Reprinted with permission from Ricci SS, Kyle T, Carman S. *Maternity and Pediatric Nursing.* 3rd ed. Philadelphia, PA: Wolters Kluwer; 2016.)

Children and adolescents have the highest rates of TBI, which are likely underestimated. Similar to older individuals, many children and adolescents with mild TBI are unknown to the health care system (1), and it has been suggested that abusive head trauma is particularly underreported (12). The rates of presentation to EDs are highest among those aged 0 to 4 and 15 to 19 years of age (1). Falls account for the majority of ED visits for children 0 to 14 years old, with motor vehicle– or traffic-related events accounting for most of the visits in children 15 to 19 (1). Nonaccidental TBI occurring from shaking impact has an alarming reported incidence of 17 per 100,000 in children less than 2 years of ages and is also

likely underreported (12). TBI-related death rates are highest among 15- to 19-year-olds, largely due to motor vehicle– and traffic-related injuries (1). Existing estimate of children and adolescents living with a chronic problem related to TBI in the United States is 145,000, but is likely to be higher given the previously described underreporting of TBI (12).

TBI accounts for considerable problems in children, particularly in the domains of physical functioning, cognitive and academic skills, behavior, and socialization (100–102).

Cognitive impairments are most commonly seen in the realms of language, memory, perceptual motor skills, attention, memory, and learning (97,100,102). Executive dysfunction also frequently occurs, particularly in association with injury to the frontal lobes (103). Most children with mild TBI recover well without long-term cognitive or behavioral problems (104), although those with more severe TBI are most likely to have long-term problems (105). Mild pediatric TBI has also been associated with persistent problems (106,107) and accounts for a large burden of TBI-related disability in children (106). The home and family environment has repeatedly been shown to play a significant role in outcomes following TBI, with poorer family coping skills, lower socioeconomic status, fewer resources, and unfavorable home environments contributing to worse outcomes (100,101,107).

The immediate consequences of TBI in children and adolescent impact are similar to those in other age groups, but, depending on the developmental age at the time of injury, may have differing presentations and sequelae over the course of time. In general, younger children have been shown to have poorer cognitive and motor recovery than their similarly injured older counterparts, which is seemingly contrary to the theory that younger children have greater neural plasticity potential than their older peers. This may be due to the relative immaturity of the developing brain that prevents the acquisition of skills needed later to develop more complex cognitive abilities (108,109). While many children appear to have good recoveries, problems often develop years later, typically manifested by academic difficulties, behavioral problems, social isolation, and criminal activity (96–98,110). When they occur, these problems are often misattributed to other causes (111), likely in part due to the time elapsed from the injury and the onset of the maladaptive behavior. Psychiatric disorders occur commonly after pediatric TBI of all injury severities, including mild TBI (112,113). Similar to other outcomes, family functioning was a significant predictor of developing a psychiatric disorder (113). The rate of psychiatric diagnoses reported to increase after pediatric TBI includes personality change, attention-deficit/hyperactivity disorder, oppositional defiant disorder, posttraumatic stress disorder, and anxiety. Post-TBI depression appears to be associated with either a pre-TBI history of depression, other risk factors such as a first-degree relative with depression, or being socially disadvantaged (114,115). A relationship between pediatric TBI and later development of bipolar disorder and psychosis remains problematical (114).

Children and adolescents with TBI will often require educational accommodations upon return to school, regardless of injury severity. Although those with concussion will likely require short-term modifications, those with more severe TBI often require sustained programming.

TBI-related disabilities in the realms of cognition, motor skills, and behavioral issues will impact school performance and ability to learn and socialize. Approximately 20,000 children and adolescents return to school each year with TBI-related disabilities requiring specialized services (116), although this may be an underrepresentation as many are classified under alternative diagnoses, often related to a pre-TBI learning disorder, failure to recognize TBI as the etiology of their disability, or variation in state classification categories (116,117). Proper identification of children with TBI is critically important as cognitive development may lag as injured children age, resulting in academic failure, thus requiring that they be followed closely as their education progresses.

TBI Sustained at Older Ages

Although the pathophysiologic changes associated with TBI can occur in any age group, advanced age at the time of injury predisposes to particular findings. The risk of subdural hematomas increases with advancing age because the bridging veins become more susceptible to shearing forces as the brain naturally atrophies over time (48,118). SDHs may enlarge quickly, resulting in a rapid neurologic deterioration shortly after trauma, or they may expand slowly, resulting in a more insidious decline in physical and cognitive functioning. This slow deterioration is more commonly observed in older persons because of their relatively large subdural space. This permits a greater volume of fluid to accumulate before causing significant mass effect on the brain, often resulting in either delayed, minimal, or no deterioration of neurologic function. Many elderly will develop SDHs after a seemingly trivial injury or a fall without direct trauma to the head, with many unable to recall the inciting event (119,120).

In addition to differences in susceptibility to subdural bleeding, other factors distinguish older people with TBI from their younger counterparts. Incidence rates, gender, race, etiology of injury, length of hospitalization, hospital discharge disposition, medical complications, functional outcomes, and mortality all vary with age at the time of injury. TBI has a multimodal age distribution, with those ≥75 years of age having among the highest incidence (1). They also have the highest rates of TBI-related hospitalizations (1,121,122), with recent trends indicating a substantial increase in trauma center admission for elderly with TBI (123). An alarming analysis indicates the rate of TBI-related hospitalization and ED visits for the elderly exceeds their growth in the population (123), suggesting there will be a considerable growth in the overall rate of TBI given the rapid expansion of this segment of the population.

Outcome studies reveal a significant and consistent adverse impact of advancing age on functional skills, cognitive abilities, length of hospitalization, medical charges, and hospital disposition after TBI compared to their equally injured younger counterparts (7,124–126). Undesirable outcomes are potentially related to numerous factors including poorer overall health status of the elderly. Elderly with TBI have higher rates of comorbidities affecting the cerebrovascular, cardiorespiratory, and musculoskeletal systems and are more likely to have impairments in cognitive function and the special senses (127), all contributing to added challenges presented by TBI. Higher use of anticoagulant and antiplatelet medications in the elderly increases the risk of expanding ICHs (128). Furthermore, the effects of injury on an aging brain that exacerbates cerebral

atrophy, neuronal shrinkage, reduced synaptic density, and decreased cerebral plasticity (129,130) likely contribute to poorer outcomes. However, it is also known that significant functional and cognitive improvements are achievable in the elderly as the majority of older patients admitted to inpatient rehabilitation are capable of being discharged to a community setting, noting that they require longer recovery times (6). However, the initiation of the Prospective Payment System (PPS) for Medicare beneficiaries beginning in 2002 by the Centers for Medicare and Medicaid Services (CMS) financially restricted the length of acute inpatient rehabilitation hospitalization, thus curtailing the maximal benefits that may be achieved by elderly patients and limiting the outcomes attained. Under PPS, reimbursement to rehabilitation facilities has been shown to be significantly less than their costs for treating individuals with TBI (131). This likely has an adverse impact on how and where the elderly with TBI receive needed rehabilitation services with aggressive rehabilitation potentially viewed as too costly to provide in many centers.

Age is an independent risk factor for mortality after TBI (132), which is strengthened when combined with GCS (133). The death rate is higher for older adults than younger adults across all levels of TBI severity (3,7,134–136). Although overall acute TBI-related mortality has been declining, deaths associated with fall-related TBIs have been steadily increasing over the past several decades and are the leading cause of TBI-related deaths for individuals ≥75 years of age (1,14). Likely contributing to the reported rise in TBI-related death rates in the elderly are better identification of people with TBI and more detailed coding on death certificates. Other factors include medication side effects, such as antihypertensive, antiplatelet, and anticoagulant drugs (137,138); greater incidence of complications and preexisting comorbidities (139); and a greater likelihood of dying from secondary organ failure (140,141). The most common causes of death in the elderly early after TBI are related to nervous system diseases, mental disorders, and respiratory diseases including aspiration pneumonia.

Given this sharp increase in age-related mortality, further investigation of factors associated with the onset of TBI in the elderly is warranted, particularly as the population ages. In addition, prevention programs are needed to help reduce TBI-related risk factors. For example, proactive strategies, such as fall prevention and refresher driving programs as well as monitoring medication compliance, may be beneficial. However, elderly individuals with severe TBI who are discharged from the hospital typically live at least several more years, although minimal neurologic or functional improvement is noted over time (142).

Special considerations are required when prescribing treatment to the elderly, particularly after any central nervous system (CNS) injury. Pharmacologic effects are often unpredictable or more pronounced compared with younger individuals and may predispose the elderly persons to altered mental states, greater fall risk, and additional injury. The axiom "start low and go slow" with drug treatment is important in elderly individuals with TBI, who, as result of their injury, have problems associated with cognition and ambulation in addition to other age-related comorbidities. As a result, they are more susceptible to the adverse effects of many pharmacologic agents. Extra consideration is required when planning discharge from the hospital because spouses of elderly individuals with TBI are more likely to be physically or cognitively impaired themselves than those of younger individuals and may not be capable of caring for a disabled loved one. Greater use of home care services is often needed, and if the caretaker is unavailable or unable to provide a safe environment, care in appropriate skilled nursing facilities may be necessary.

Aging with Traumatic Brain Injury

While the acute problems of TBI are generally well-known, the long-term sequelae of living with TBI have only recently been a focus of systematic scientific inquiry. It has been estimated that up to 5.3 million Americans live with long-term problems associated with TBI (11). The National Academy of Medicine (NAM), formerly known as the Institute of Medicine, convened a panel to examine the long-term health problems related to people living with TBI (143). The results of this extensive 2009 review strongly indicated that TBI is for many people the beginning of a chronic, often lifelong, medical condition. Evidence indicates that people with TBI who survive beyond hospital discharge are at increased risk for psychiatric disease, neuroendocrine dysfunction, sleep disorders, neurodegenerative disease, seizures, and cognitive decline. Risk of mortality has been found to be more than twice that of the general population, with life expectancy reported to decrease from 6 to 9 years following moderate to severe TBI (144–146). These chronic sequelae lead to decreased quality of life for survivors and increased stress on their families and add significant burden on the health care system. It has been suggested that the long-term sequelae of TBI be collectively considered a chronic disease (147).

The risk of developing dementia after TBI remains controversial. Several studies have found an association between sustaining a TBI and the development of dementia many years later (148–151), while others have not (152–154). However, after examining all the available evidence at the time of their extensive review, the NAM concluded that there is an association between TBI severe enough to cause loss of consciousness and the development of dementia later in life (143). Recent evidence suggests the existence of chronic traumatic encephalopathy (CTE), a condition reported to occur after repetitive trauma to the brain. CTE reportedly results in a combination of physical, cognitive, and affective problems that have been associated with specific neuropathologic findings in the brains of a convenience sample of people who are predominantly former professional athletes (155,156). The clinical picture and suggested histopathologic findings of CTE are similar to but distinct enough from other dementing conditions to consider it a potentially unique condition. Similarly, the clinical presentation, course, and subtle differences in cognitive findings in people with dementia who have previously sustained TBI compared to those who have no history of TBI indicate a neurodegenerative phenotype that is distinct from other known dementia subtypes (157,158). This suggests that the etiology and manifestations of dementia resulting from TBI are distinct from previously described conditions that are worthy of continued study and potentially unique treatments.

Many adults experience significant psychiatric disorders after TBI, with rates considerably higher than the general population. The most prevalent psychiatric diagnosis is major depression, with prevalence rates varying between 13%

at 1 year post injury (159) and greater than 60% (160) during the first decade after TBI. Anxiety disorders are the next most common psychiatric diagnosis, with frequencies varying between 18% and 60% (160–162). These long-term psychiatric sequelae not only pose additional challenges to community re-entry and quality of life but have also been viewed as more seriously handicapping than the cognitive or physical consequences of TBI (160). Proactive monitoring of mood in these individuals is needed along with psychological support to minimize the severity of psychiatric sequelae.

CONCUSSION

Definition

Concussion is currently defined by the International Conference on Concussion in Sport (ICCS) as a complex pathophysiologic process affecting the brain, induced by biomechanical forces (163). While acknowledging the basis for symptoms in a neural disturbance within the brain, the current definition is relatively agnostic as to the precise presentation of the injury. Concussion is a type of mild TBI that is typically not associated with the extended loss of consciousness typical of moderate or severe TBI, as graded by the GCS, with functional impairments typically displaying a time-limited course. Recent data have demonstrated that loss of consciousness occurs in less than 10% of sports-related injuries and posttraumatic amnesia only between 25% and 30% of cases (164–166). Thus, another notable aspect of the current definition of concussion is the absence of further gradations or subclassifications such as loss of consciousness or posttraumatic amnesia, which have historically been prominent features of the diagnosis of concussion (167–170). Due to lack of clinical utility with regard to prognosis and a lack of professional consensus with regard to which grading or classification schemes were most useful, concussion currently represents a single diagnosis.

Epidemiology of Concussion

Reported incidence of concussion in the United States varies from 1.6 to 3.8 million (171–173). As previously mentioned, a significant percentage of concussions likely go unreported due to a multitude of factors, including limited understanding of its symptoms, a lack of awareness for the seriousness of the diagnosis, and incentives for underreporting (173–176). Many people with concussion may also seek medical care in places other than hospital settings where concussions may not be screened for, not reported or simply seek no treatment at all. In the elderly, likely furthering the underreporting is misattribution of signs and symptoms of concussion to normal aging processes, rather than to concussion. A lack of fast, objective testing methods for concussion also plays a role in its underdiagnosis. Nearly all team and some individual sports display significant rates of concussion, with the greatest numbers of concussion found in football, wrestling, soccer, and girls' basketball (177–179). Football should be noted as having one of the highest rates of both participation and concussion, with the National Football League (NFL) reporting a concussion nearly every other game and with 60% of retired NFL players reporting at least one concussion in their career (180,181). The data also suggest that females have a greater incidence of concussion when controlled for type of sport, with proposed hypotheses explaining this difference including differences in cervical neck muscle strength, greater tendency for women to report symptoms, and the nature of gameplay in female versions of the sports (179,182,183).

Acute Concussion

The signs and symptoms of concussion span a wide range, with no one sign or symptom pathognomonic or diagnostic.

Symptoms are often split into several domains, commonly including somatic, cognitive, emotional, and sleep-related (164,165,184–189). The most commonly reported include headache, dizziness, fatigue, and feeling "slowed down" (164,188–190). Symptoms may take some time to declare themselves, thus underscoring the importance of having trained personnel available for clinical evaluation following suspected concussion when possible. Recent evidence suggests that persisting in physical activity following initial concussive injury may worsen symptoms and prolong recovery (191). Notwithstanding complicating factors, most patients with concussion report resolution of symptoms within 7 to 10 days, though neuropsychological performance and neurophysiologic changes may persist well after this period (166,192–198). Symptoms may be exacerbated by either cognitive or physical exertion, and so current recommendations include a brief initial period of relative cognitive and physical rest (163).

Postconcussion Symptoms/Syndrome

In approximately 10% to 30% of concussions, symptoms will persist up to a month or longer (193,199). There is some disagreement with regard to whether the presence of persistent symptoms following concussion represents a unitary syndrome or rather reflects the underlying heterogeneity of the individual injury. Much of the literature recognizes postconcussion syndrome to include the presence of at least three symptoms appearing within 3 weeks of the initial injury, and persisting for at least 3 months, with persistent postconcussive syndrome (PPCS) generally defined as symptoms lasting past this 3- to 6-month period (200). ICD-10 criteria define postconcussion syndrome by the presence of three or more of the following eight symptoms: (a) headache, (b) dizziness, (c) fatigue, (d) irritability, (e) insomnia, (f) impaired concentration, (g) memory difficulties, and (h) intolerance of stress, emotion, or alcohol, in the setting of concussive injury.

According to the *Diagnostic and Statistical Manual of Mental Disorders*, Fifth Edition (DSM-5), postconcussion syndrome refers to either mild or major neurocognitive disorder (NCD) presenting immediately following TBI and persisting past the acute postinjury period (201). Some factors associated with persistent concussion symptoms have been identified and include initial self-reported symptom severity, prolonged headache, and concentration deficits (202). There are some data to suggest that ongoing litigation or secondary gain involvement may increase the severity and duration of persistent symptoms (203,204).

Mechanism of Injury of Concussion

Current data suggest that both linear and rotational accelerations of the head are primary risk factors for concussive injury. A number of theoretical models of how accelerative forces may result in brain injury have been investigated at a number of levels ranging from animals and cadavers to computer models (205–207). Furthermore, while direct impacts to the head may obviously produce an acute increase in both linear and rotational accelerations, indirect impacts involving inertial movements (as sustained in "whiplash" injuries) may also load the head in such a way that results in concussion. Head acceleration is thought to result in strain patterns on brain tissue, which may cause injury to white matter tracts via DAI, previously described in this chapter. An exact threshold in terms of peak accelerative forces that result in a concussive injury has not yet been identified. Part of the difficulty in making this determination pertains to the challenge of accurate and direct measurement of force dynamics within the brain during an injury. As a proxy, investigators are currently refining sensor technologies and force analysis algorithms in order to better quantify acceleration of the head.

These sensors have provided more specific data allowing the calculation of risk of concussion associated with impacts to specific areas of the head to the effect of protective equipment on mitigating changes in white matter integrity (208,209). There are some data to suggest that, contrary to moderate and severe TBI, the location and magnitude of force of head impact currently do not appear to have any clear relationship with measures of recovery in concussion (210,211). However, investigators have identified several biomechanical factors that may influence the impact forces associated with concussion. These include the stability of the head in relationship to the neck and shoulders, as well as individual differences in brain tissue vulnerability. Recent work suggests that increased cervical neck strength may play a role in mitigating impact forces (212,213).

Anticipating head impacts may decrease the risk of concussion by allowing time to activate the cervical musculature, thus stabilizing the head (214,215).

Concussion Pathophysiology

From a pathophysiologic standpoint, DAI is thought to be the main structural mechanism underlying concussion and its resultant functional impairments. Animal work supports a multilevel cascade of metabolic changes following the acute axonal injury underlying concussive brain injury (216–219), similar to what occurs in more severe TBI and is described earlier in this chapter. This includes disturbance of the ionic environment of neurons due to indiscriminate depolarization, which results in glutamate-mediated excitotoxic injury.

Further studies using proton MRS have also demonstrated metabolite profiles indicative of neuronal damage (220,221). Insofar as restoration of membrane potential is thought to normally account for the majority of basal energy expenditure in the cerebral cortex, unchecked excitatory activity following concussive injury may impose a large mismatch between cerebral perfusion and glucose utilization (216–218,222,223). The concept of postconcussion metabolic mismatch, exacerbated by impairments of cerebral autoregulation, forms the theoretic basis for graduated exercise protocols for concussion diagnosis and management developed by Leddy and others (224,225). While neuroimaging studies such as CT and MRI are often noted in the clinical history of concussion, these are typically normal in the majority of concussed persons, as concussion is thought to result in structural and functional changes that are detected only with more advanced imaging methods (226). These methods may include MRI protocols previously described in this chapter, as well as changes in functional activity and functional connectivity (227–231). Resting-state fMRI, which demonstrates patterns of brain connectivity while the subject is not engaged in any particular cognitive task, has shown changes in what has been called the default mode network (DMN) (232–235). Task-based fMRI studies have demonstrated changes in both episodic and working memory networks, depending on the task that subjects are asked to perform. It is unclear whether these changes in functional activity reflect increased pathologic activity by areas damaged in concussion or increased compensatory activity by nearby uninjured areas (232,236,237).

Clinical Evaluation of Concussion

Concussion is currently a clinical diagnosis that results from synthesizing a history of the injury, symptomatology, physical examination findings, and data provided by clinical assessment tools. As a matter of course, immediate medical evaluation following a suspected concussion should specifically assess for concerning emergent neurologic pathologies such as intracranial bleeding, skull and facial fracture, or cervical spinal cord injury, with "red flags" including alterations in consciousness, neck pain, loss of sensation or motor control, and abnormal posturing. Having attended to emergent concerns, further evaluation specific to concussion should include a specific history that notes the presence of prior concussions, neurologic or psychiatric diagnoses, and family history of migraines, as these factors predict prolonged or more severe symptomatology (235). Symptoms may be quantified through the use of standardized symptom checklists, such as found in the fifth edition of the Sports Concussion Assessment Tool (SCAT-5), which asks patients to rate the intensity of 22 symptoms (238). Given the multitude of symptoms that can be associated with concussion, the use of a standardized checklist ensures that symptoms are not missed.

Assessment can also serve as an opportunity to grossly observe the speed of cognitive processing, language function, and attention.

An exam specific to concussion should include focused assessments of cognition, balance, and visual functioning in addition to standard physical exam items such as cranial nerve function, motor strength, and coordination. Further expansion of the exam is typically done using standardized clinical tools. The Standardized Assessment of Concussion (SAC) is a widely used battery of brief cognitive tasks that is reportedly sensitive for detecting concussion (194,195,239,240). The tasks of the SAC specifically assess memory formation, delayed recall, and attention. In order to assess balance, the Balance Error Scoring System (BESS), performed in its original formation on a foam mat or "modified" by the omission of the mat, is a useful instrument to assess balance function (241,242). The BESS assesses patients' stability in three different static stances (double leg, single leg, and tandem stance ("sharpened Romberg"). These two scales are embedded into the SCAT-5. In addition, the King-Devick (KD) and the Mobile Universal Lexicon Evaluation System (MULES) tests are well-studied and validated screening tools for concussion that leverage the wide representation of visual function in the brain by asking patients to rapidly name numbers (KD) (243,244) or photographs of objects (MULES) presented as an array on cards or on electronic displays (245,246).

These tests as a whole are easily deployed in acute game-play environments, as well as outpatient clinical settings, and provide useful objective information regarding the functioning of persons suspected of having a concussion. In combination with graded symptom checklists, this multipronged approach to the evaluation of concussion has been demonstrated to be highly reliable for both diagnosis and management of concussion (166,192,193).

Management and Treatment

Current recommendations following acute concussion include immediate removal from the circumstances of injury following a suspected concussion, to avoid further brain injury or a worsened symptom burden and longer recovery (163,191). The person should then be evaluated by a clinical professional experienced in the diagnosis of concussion, followed by no same-day return-to-play (163). In addition to mitigating symptom burden, the emphasis on no same-day return-to-play is also motivated by concerns for second-impact syndrome (SIS), which is a potentially lethal consequence of sustaining a second concussion shortly after the initial injury. SIS is thought to be the result of an acute loss of cerebral hemodynamic autoregulation, resulting in malignant cerebral edema, with nearly 50% mortality and 100% morbidity (247,248). However, data on SIS are relatively scarce, with only 35 possible cases identified over 23 years (249,250). Once medically stable, an initial brief period of relative cognitive and physical rest following an acute concussive injury (2 to 3 days) followed by gradual reintroduction of activity (163,251,252) is typically recommended. An increasing amount of research suggests that, contrary to prior recommendations, prolonged periods of rest in the manner of "cocooning" may actually result in worsened symptom burden for a longer period of time (253–255). Athletes may return to play following the "graduated return-to-play" protocol, which incorporates a stepwise progressive increase in the level of physical exertion over the 7 to 10 days, culminating in activity under return-to-play conditions (163).

In addition to management recommendations focused on metabolic recovery of the damaged brain, concussion treatment may also include specific symptomatic treatment through the judicious use of medications or focused therapies. Dizziness and balance impairment are common after concussion, with etiologies such as benign paroxysmal positional vertigo (BPPV) representing a very treatable condition that can result in significant symptomatic relief (256). Mood symptoms, such as depression and anxiety, may be treated with antidepressants such as sertraline (257,258). Disturbances of visual function may be precisely characterized by a neuro-optometrist or neuro-ophthalmologist and then accommodated by way of vision therapy (259). Improving sleep through optimization of sleep hygiene practices along with reinforcement of circadian rhythms with melatonin or other sleep-promoting agents is crucial for recovery as well (260).

As people recover and return to activity, it is important to consider secondary prevention of further concussions, as patients with a history of concussion are at a three- to fivefold increased risk of sustaining another injury (199,261–264). This may include consideration of factors ranging from successful treatment of symptoms that may limit optimal performance to quality and intensity of activity. If a person presents with multiple concussions as a result of a particular activity, clear discussion of that activity's risk/benefit ratio is warranted.

OUTCOME MEASURES

As a TBI often leads to cognitive and physical functional deficits as well as behavioral difficulties, outcome assessments need to be multifaceted. This requires the use of various scales and assessment tools focusing on different aspects of recovery to provide a comprehensive assessment. Although it is not possible to use every outcome scale and measure, there are some more commonly utilized tools that can provide information across several domains.

A good guide to some of the more widely recognized outcome measures can be found by looking at those used by the Traumatic Brain Injury Model Systems (TBIMS) of Care. The TBIMS, sponsored by the National Institute on Disability, Independent Living, and Rehabilitation Research (NIDILRR), is a multicenter program focusing on collecting longitudinal data and producing both individual center and collaborative research on TBI. Overall, TBIMS data from the 2016 national data and statistical center's factsheet show that persons with TBI as a whole make the most significant functional improvement through the course of their inpatient rehabilitation course, with recovery tending to plateau, typically over 1 to 2 years after injury. Approximately one third of persons with TBI require some level of supervision 2 years following their injury. Long-term employment rates following TBI for subjects enrolled in the TBIMS are approximately half of their rate prior to injury. Studies suggest that persons with TBI have a shorter life expectancy as a whole than the general population, but there are variations in the rate of decline in health and function (265). Outcome measures used by the program, as well as some of their limitations, are highlighted below.

The Functional Independence Measure (FIM) and FIM ratio (FIM change divided by length of inpatient rehabilitation, also referred to as FIM efficiency) have been widely used to measure progress and quality of improvement in the rehabilitation setting. The FIM measures the assistance level needed for 18 functional skills (266). Although it does include a small number of cognitive and communication skills, it is more heavily weighted toward physical function. As a result, it has been criticized for its limited scope of cognitive and behavioral assessments, which are particularly important for brain-injured patients. As an example, those who make significant cognitive gains following a brain injury may demonstrate very little change in their FIM score, thus not reflecting their overall improvement.

The Functional Assessment Measure (FAM) was created to address this shortcoming by including assessments of cognitive, behavioral, communication, and community reintegration skills not evaluated in the FIM. Despite these added assessments, critics claim the FAM remains an inadequate tool to sufficiently address these domains (267).

The Disability Rating Scale (DRS) measures general functional abilities and can be used to track recovery from coma through community living (268). It lacks comprehensive detailed assessments for specific functional tasks but can be used to follow the overall level of disability as a person recovers from a brain injury. Critics state the DRS has a ceiling effect in patients with subtle mild impairments (269).

TABLE 19-3 Glasgow Outcome Scale and Glasgow Outcome Scale: Extended

Glasgow Outcome Scale
1. Death
2. Persistent vegetative state
3. Severe disability: conscious but disabled
4. Moderate disability: disabled but independent
5. Good recovery: able to return to work or school

Glasgow Outcome Scale: Extended
1. Death
2. Persistent vegetative state
3. Low severe disability: cannot be left unattended for >8 h
4. Upper severe disability: can be left unattended for >8 h
5. Lower moderate disability: cannot return to work
6. Upper moderate disability: can return to work with special arrangements
7. Lower good recovery: remaining deficits are disabling
8. Upper good recovery: remaining deficits are not disabling

The Glasgow Outcome Scale (GOS) is a simple five-point scale that measures disability and describes general categories of functional outcome from death and VS at the lower end to severe disability, moderate disability, and good recovery on the other end (270). In an attempt to more specifically categorize the functional level of patients with recovery beyond the VS, the Glasgow Outcome Scale was extended (GOS-E) to include upper and lower levels for severe disability, moderate disability, and good recovery to create an eight-point scale (271) (**Table 19-3**). It does not provide a detailed assessment of recovery and lacks sensitivity to assess small but clinically important changes in outcomes.

The Rancho Los Amigos Levels of Cognitive Functioning is a well-known tool used to classify persons with TBI in general stages of typical recovery from TBI. Although it does not provide an individualized objective assessment of a patient, it can be used to monitor progress and formulate treatment programs. Originally, it was developed with 8 stages, but a later revision increased it to 10 that incorporate more detailed descriptions at the higher functioning levels. There is no scoring system for the Rancho Levels tool, as persons with TBI are assigned a level based on their observed predominant cognitive abilities and behaviors (**Table 19-4**).

TABLE 19-4 Rancho Los Amigos Levels of Cognitive Functioning-Revised

Level	Description
I	**No response**
II	**Generalized response**
III	**Localized response**
IV	**Confused and agitated**
V	**Confused and inappropriate**
VI	**Confused and appropriate**
VII	**Automatic and appropriate**
VIII	**Purposeful and appropriate, standby assistance**
IX	**Purposeful and appropriate, standby assistance on request**
X	**Purposeful and appropriate, modified independence**

The Community Integration Questionnaire (CIQ) measures how independently and frequently a person with TBI participates in social, household, and community activities. It provides an assessment of how well a person has integrated into the community. It is a 15-item scale each with multiple-choice options for scoring (272). A ceiling effect for its usage in assessing people in the community has been reported as well (269). The Participation Assessment with Recombined Tools-Objective (PART-O) is a measure of participation and societal functioning that is derived from the CIQ and two other measures, the Participation Objective and Participation Subjective. It was originally a 24-item measure but was revised to 17 items (273). It has been used to investigate long-term outcomes and effectiveness of interventions regarding reintegration into society.

The Supervision Rating Scale (SRS) is a 13-item scale used to describe and categorize the level of supervision a person is receiving (274). It provides descriptions of the intensity and duration of supervision they receive and indicates their burden of care. Of note, when done correctly, the rating given is for the care the person actually receives and not what is felt to be needed.

The Satisfaction with Life Scale (SWLS) is a five-item tool rated by seven points ranging from strongly agree to strongly disagree. It assesses satisfaction with life as a whole by measuring global cognitive judgments as opposed to emotions. Scores of 5, 10, 15, 20, 25, and 30 are used as cutoff measures for outcomes ranging from extremely dissatisfied to extremely satisfied (275).

Posttraumatic amnesia (PTA) is the duration of time following a TBI that a person is in a state of confusion, disoriented, and unable to carryover information and events occurring after the injury. The Orientation Log (O-Log) and Galveston Orientation and Amnesia Test (GOAT) were developed to assess orientation and track recovery through the posttraumatic amnestic state via improvement in orientation (276,277). A pediatric version, the COAT, was developed to better determine PTA in an age-appropriate manner. A modified multiple-choice version (AGOAT) was also developed to better assess PTA in the setting of aphasia. Tracking improvement in orientation can be helpful as the recovery time-out of PTA is one of the strongest predictors of functional recovery after TBI, with longer periods associated with poorer outcomes.

The posttraumatic confusional state (PCS) is preferred by some practitioners over PTA, as it better describes a state of confusion posttrauma, rather than one that focuses predominantly on amnesia (278). Similar to PTA, PCS provides an index of injury severity and is predictive of outcomes (279–281).

TBI can negatively impact both behavioral control and mental health. Poor behavioral control and agitated behavior can significantly affect a person's safety and independence with daily activities. Psychological sequelae of TBI are commonly seen and can exacerbate TBI-related cognitive and physical impairments as well as hinder reintegration into society.

The Agitated Behavior Scale (ABS) was developed to monitor and track the severity of the agitation a person may exhibit following a brain injury (282). It is most often used for those in confusional states. During a period of observation, an evaluator ranks 14 specific behaviors as being present or absent and the degree to which it is present. Each behavior is scored from 1 being absent up to 4 indicating it is present to an extreme degree. Total scores range from 14 to 56, with higher scores indicative of more severe levels of agitation. Subscores from specific items are combined to provide a numerical assessment of disinhibition, aggression, and lability (**Fig. 19-11**). As agitation monitoring is dependent on capturing all episodes, the challenge with using this scale as well as most other agitation monitoring tools is maintaining diligence in documentation to avoid missing an event, as may happen when those charged with completing the form are not present during an episode. It is a useful tool to monitor the effectiveness of an intervention aimed at ameliorating a specific maladaptive behavior.

Mood disorders are common after TBI, with several commonly used tools to assess their presence and severity. The Generalized Anxiety Disorder Seven-Item Scale (GAD-7) assesses the frequency with which patients experience seven different types of generalized anxiety.

Scores of 5, 10, and 15 are used as cutoff measures for grading mild, moderate, and severe anxiety. A score of 10 or greater indicates further evaluation is warranted (283). The Patient Health Questionnaire Nine-Item Scale (PHQ-9) assesses the frequency with which patients experience nine different symptoms of depression. Scores of 5, 10, 15, and 20 are used as cutoff measures for grading mild, moderate, moderately severe, and severe depression. It is used to monitor the severity of depression and was derived from a larger patient health questionnaire (283,284).

COGNITIVE IMPAIRMENTS

Cognitive problems related to TBI are extremely common across all levels of injury severity and account for a considerable degree of an individual's disability. They are also potent predictors of patients' ability to return to gainful employment and independent living (285). Cognitive problems are manifested in multiple domains, most commonly impacting attention, memory, reaction time, working memory, and executive skills. Both the focal and diffuse nature of TBI pathophysiology help to explain why cognitive processes are so commonly impaired. For example, focal injuries involving the frontal lobe, commonly impacted by contusion, likely contribute to impaired executive skills that normally rely on intact functioning of the prefrontal cortex. Nearly all cognitive skills rely on interrelated neural networks that are disrupted by DAI, resulting in disconnection and inefficient functioning. The broad spectrum of TBI-related cognitive impairments is also due in part to the interrelated nature of cognition.

Normal memory and executive skills in part rely on intact attention, while attention and working memory are sometimes considered overlapping processes. Addressing cognitive impairments requires thoughtful analysis through neuropsychological assessment, observation of its impact on daily function, cognitive remediation, and possibly pharmacologic intervention.

Formalized neuropsychological assessment is important to identify areas of cognitive problems as well as areas of preserved cognitive strengths. Numerous standardized tests that assess multiple domains of cognitive abilities are needed to identify and define the nature and scope of the impairments, including relative strengths and weaknesses. This requires interpretation of test results in view of estimated pre-TBI cognitive abilities assessed by using standardized word reading tests, such as the Wechsler Test of Adult Reading, as well as by knowledge of a

FIGURE 19-11. Agitated Behavior Scale.

AGITATED BEHAVIOR SCALE

Patient _____   Period of Observation:

                                                        a.m.
Observ. Environ. _____   From: _____ p.m. ___/___/___

                                                        a.m.
Rater/Disc. _____   To: _____ p.m. ___/___/___

At the end of the observation period indicate whether the behavior described in each item was present and, if so, to what degree: slight, moderate or extreme. Use the following numerical values and criteria for your ratings.

1 = absent: the behavior is not present.

2 = present to a slight degree: the behavior is present but does not prevent the conduct of other, contextually appropriate behavior. (The individual may redirect spontaneously, or the continuation of the agitated behavior does not disrupt appropriate behavior.)

3 = present to a moderate degree: the individual needs to be redirected from an agitated to an appropriate behavior, but benefits from such cueing.

4 = present to an extreme degree: the individual is not able to engage in appropriate behavior due to the interference of the agitated behavior, even when external cueing or redirection is provided.

DO NOT LEAVE BLANKS.

_____   1. Short attention span, easy distractibility, inability to concentrate.
_____   2. Impulsive, impatient, low tolerance for pain or frustration.
_____   3. Uncooperative, resistant to care, demanding.
_____   4. Violent and/or threatening violence toward people or property.
_____   5. Explosive and/or unpredictable anger.
_____   6. Rocking, rubbing, moaning or other self-stimulating behavior.
_____   7. Pulling at tubes, restraints, etc.
_____   8. Wandering from treatment areas.
_____   9. Restlessness, pacing, excessive movement.
_____ 10. Repetitive behaviors, motor and/or verbal.
_____ 11. Rapid, loud, or excessive talking.
_____ 12. Sudden changes of mood.
_____ 13. Easily initiated or excessive crying and/or laughter.
_____ 14. Self-abusiveness, physical and/or verbal.

_____ **Total Score**

patient's employment and educational background. Once the standardized testing and thoughtful interpretation of results are completed, a cognitive rehabilitation program is developed that aims to ameliorate the impact of cognitive dysfunction on daily life. This is typically achieved by developing strategies that compensate for areas of identified impairments, although some interventions have demonstrated efficacy in improving performance on specific neuropsychological tests (286).

Cognitive remediation is provided in multiple ways. Process-specific remediation directs retraining of specific cognitive skills through repeated trials of stimulation of the specific skill, with the goal of reorganizing higher-level neurologic and cognitive processes (287).

Functional skills training focuses on enhancing a person's abilities in context-specific areas that result in retraining in skills needed for everyday life as opposed to ameliorating the underlying cognitive impairment. Metacognitive approaches address issues pertaining to awareness of cognitive problems, self-monitoring of errors, and self-regulation with the goal of using compensatory strategies in the appropriate situation, such as using a daily schedule in response to a self-recognized memory or planning impairment. Multiple techniques have been described and found to be effective in compensating for specific cognitive impairments. Three comprehensive reviews

examining multiple cognitive therapy modalities support specific interventions for attention, memory, social communication skills, executive function, and comprehensive-holistic neuropsychological rehabilitation after TBI (288–290).

Pharmacologic intervention is an additional means to potentially augment cognitive performance after TBI. They are generally recommended as an adjuvant rather than primary treatment and are best used in conjunction with rather than as an alternative to remediation strategies. Impacting neurotransmitter function is the principle means of pharmacologically altering cognitive skills and thus requires an understanding of related neuroanatomy and neurophysiology. An important principle is to first limit the use of medications that potentially adversely impact cognitive skills whenever feasible and medically tolerable. These include anticonvulsants (291), dopaminergic antagonists (292,293), benzodiazepines (292,294), anticholinergic medications (295), and opiates (292). The catecholaminergic and cholinergic neurotransmitter systems underlie attention function and can be modulated by medications. The strongest evidence to enhance attention is for methylphenidate (296–298).

Acetylcholinesterase inhibitors have been shown to improve memory function in those with moderate to severe memory disorders, but not those with mild impairments. Evidence supporting medications for many other cognitive skills is limited, although guidelines have been published based on existing evidence (298).

POSTTRAUMATIC AGITATION

Agitation has been described as aggression, restlessness, impulsivity, and combative behavior, but can include any behavior that prevents a person with TBI from participating in rehabilitation therapies and assimilating into the community. Agitation has an incidence of roughly 33% after TBI (299–301) and places a patient at risk of harming themselves or others, including caretakers, nursing staff, and people in the community.

Treating agitation starts with describing and documenting behaviors as objectively as possible. The ABS, previously described in this chapter, provides an objective assessment of aggressive behavior. It can be both used to assess the degree of agitation present during a prescribed period of time and a means to gauge the effectiveness of treatments to ameliorate it. Agitation can also be described using the Rancho Los Amigos Levels of Cognitive Functioning, which describes the wakefulness and confusional level of the patient. The Modified Overt Aggression Scale (MOAS) rates four aspects of aggressive behavior, including verbal aggression, aggression against property, autoaggression, and physical aggression. It can be used by multiple caregivers, including nurses and family members, which are useful to track agitation and evaluate the efficacy of a therapy and interventions.

Initial management of agitation includes identifying and correcting or omitting neurologic, metabolic, infectious, endocrine, and painful stimuli that the person with TBI may be experiencing. For example, untreated seizure disorders, constipation, or a urinary tract infection may manifest as agitation in patients with impaired neurologic function. Unexpected medication effects can also contribute to agitation, including those with paradoxical side effects such as diphenhydramine, levetiracetam, or benzodiazepines.

Environment modification is a multifaceted approach to limit agitation and predominantly involves creating a level of sensory stimulation tolerable to patients as they recover. In the acute setting, this typically includes enforcing a calm and quiet environment, limiting the number of clinicians and visitors at any given time, and tolerating a level of patient restlessness that does not impact safe mobility. Patients also benefit by being frequently reoriented during each clinician interaction. Patient safety measures include increasing the frequency of nursing checks, providing direct 1:1 observation, and bed/room modifications that enhance safety and control for excessive stimulation. Seatbelts and mittens are considered physical restraints and thus require daily documented assessment of need and effectiveness. Wrist restraints, side rails on beds, chest Poseys, and netbeds are no longer recommended as they can contribute to agitation and injury. During hospitalization, a specific portion of a nursing unit can be locked to better control the environment and prevent elopement of patients with impaired cognitive skills (299).

Antipsychotics and benzodiazepines should be reserved for use of acute psychiatric dysfunction and unsafe behavior escalation. In more chronic use, haloperidol and risperidone have been demonstrated to hinder spatial learning and motor recovery (302). Likewise, chronic administration of benzodiazepine has been demonstrated to impair cognitive function (303–305). Anticholinergic agents can cause paradoxical agitation in patients with cognitive impairment due to their anticholinergic effects (306,307). Although there is no perfect agent in controlling agitation, a Cochrane review provided the most support for nonselective beta-blockers (propranolol and pindolol) in the treatment of agitation (308). Dosing is multiple times per day with holding parameters for decreased heart rate and hypotension. Side effects can include sleepiness and depression and are contraindicated in asthma and heart block. In single-site randomized control trial of 38 patients, amantadine administration (100 mg 2 times per day) demonstrated reduction in irritability but not aggression (309). In a larger design of this study (multisite), there was no significant effect on irritability reduction. Anecdotally, valproic acid has been beneficial in reducing agitation, but studies are limited (310). When using valproic acid, the clinician must follow valproic acid levels, white blood cell count, liver enzymes, and ammonia levels periodically.

GENETIC AND MOLECULAR BIOLOGIC MARKERS

Research into potential genetic markers, or genes that help to identify or classify individuals into groups, that predispose persons with TBI toward more or less severe injury and better or worse recovery is of significant interest to many different elements of society including the military, sports organizations, and the health community at large. These markers may provide insight toward prognosis for recovery. Biologic markers, or biomarkers, are objective indicators that can be assessed from persons with TBI that provide insight into their current medical state. A biomarker can be anything from blood pressure as a marker of heart function to imaging or molecular assessments for various pathologic processes. Identifying biomarkers such as serum or CSF molecules or specific findings on neuroimaging studies that indicate if a TBI has occurred and the extent of injury also has widespread research appeal. This would potentially help predict outcomes and possibly direct more specific interventions based on individual responses to injury.

A detailed assessment of the research ongoing regarding genetic and molecular biologic markers associated with TBI and TBI recovery is beyond the scope of this chapter, but there are some general themes and trends worth mentioning. The presence of certain isoforms of the apolipoprotein E allele has gained a substantial amount of attention as a potential indicator for a person's susceptibility to brain injury and neuroplasticity response. The E4 allele has been associated with poorer outcomes post-TBI (311,312). Assessing the up-regulation or down-regulation of various other genes has potential applications as biomarkers as well.

Studying the various changes in inflammatory and immune response factors after a TBI is also of great interest. Numerous proteins including those in the classes of interleukins, enzymes, interferons, receptors, S100 proteins, and amino acids are being studied for their potential role as an indicator for various aspects of TBI. Currently, there is no identified marker that has gained wide acceptance for use in standard clinical assessment or practice.

MEDICAL COMPLICATIONS OF TRAUMATIC BRAIN INJURY

Medical complications are frequent after brain injury and are known to increase hospital length of stay as well as worsen functional outcome (313). Such complications may include and are not limited to seizures, autonomic nervous system dysfunction, hydrocephalus, endocrine dysfunction, heterotopic ossification (HO), cranial nerve dysfunction, venous thrombosis and embolism, spasticity, bowel and bladder dysfunction, and pressure injuries. The primary aim of care is to treat and prevent these systemic complications, thus modifying morbidity and mortality after TBI (314).

Posttraumatic Seizures and Epilepsy

Posttraumatic seizures and posttraumatic epilepsy are common complications of TBI. Posttraumatic seizures (PTS) are single or recurrent seizures that occur after an individual sustains a TBI. Posttraumatic epilepsy (PTE) is a disorder characterized by recurrent late seizure episodes not attributable to another obvious cause in patients with a history of TBI (315). PTS can be classified by when they occur in relation to the initial injury. Immediate PTS occur within 24 hours of the traumatic event, early seizures occur between 24 hours and 7 days postinjury, and late seizures occur any time after 7 days postinjury. PTS can be further classified according to their clinical and electroencephalographic (EEG) characteristics. Focal seizures are thought to occur in a localized region of one cerebral hemisphere, whereas generalized seizures occur from bilateral symmetrical locations without focal onset. Focal seizures can be further categorized based on maintenance or loss of consciousness at the time of the injury. Partial seizures refer to those seizures where consciousness is maintained, while complex seizures refer to those seizures where consciousness is lost. Focal onset seizures are observed in slightly more than half of all people with PTS and appear more frequently in adults and patients with early seizures (316), focal lesions on CT (317), penetrating TBI (318), and nonpenetrating TBI of greater severity (317).

The incidence of PTS varies according to the severity of injury, the time since injury, and the presence of risk factors. Approximately one half to two thirds of persons with TBI who suffer from PTS will experience seizure onset within the first 12 months and 75% to 80% by the end of 2 years (319). TBI accounts for about 20% of structural epilepsy observed in the general population and 5% of all epilepsy (320). Structural epilepsy encompasses a distinct structural brain abnormality that has been acquired or may be of genetic origin. While treatment focuses on amelioration of seizures, there is always the risk of recurrences. Recent evidence suggests that although patients with early PTS will experience a late seizure in 20% to 30% of cases, seizure onset after the first week is associated with a much higher likelihood of recurrence (321). Immediate PTS are generally believed to carry little to no increased risk of recurrence (316). Between one fifth and one third of persons with late PTS will experience frequent recurrences, often refractory to conventional antiepileptic drug (AED) therapy (321).

Seizure activity is an important cause of hospitalization and death in persons with severe TBI (144), and recurrent PTS may adversely affect children and adults who sustain a TBI (322). Therefore, treatment of PTS and PTE is important

in order to decrease the occurrence of complications and consequences, including cognitive and behavioral dysfunction. Evidence indicates that disinhibited and/or aggressive behavior as well as irritability is significantly more frequent and severe during rehabilitation in persons with PTE compared to those who are seizure free. Likewise, PTS is correlated with significantly poorer outcome, as measured by the GOS, DRS, FIM, and the subscales of the neurobehavioral rating scale at 1 year after severe TBI (323).

Risk factors that increase an individual's susceptibility to PTE include age younger than 5 years or older than 65 years, alcoholism, and family history of seizures (324). Inheriting the apolipoprotein E (ApoE) epsilon 4 genotype has also been proposed as a risk factor (325). Injury-related factors that increase the risk of PTE include severe trauma, penetrating head injuries, intracranial hematoma, linear or depressed skull fracture, hemorrhagic contusion, coma lasting more than 24 hours, early PTS, and history of prior TBI. There tends to be cumulative focal neuroimaging or EEG abnormalities in the acute postinjury period in these individuals (326).

Seizure prophylaxis with antiepileptic medications (AED) has been shown to reduce the incidence of early PTS but not late PTS (327). A systematic review examining the effectiveness of prophylaxis indicated there is no clinical evidence that AED prophylaxis of early seizures reduces the occurrence of late PTS or has any effect on death or neurologic disability (328).

As part of their clinical guidelines, the American Academy of Neurology (AAN) concluded that prophylaxis with phenytoin is effective in reducing the risk of early seizures in persons with severe TBI. However, AED prophylaxis with phenytoin, carbamazepine, or valproate is not effective in the prevention of late seizures in persons with severe TBI (316). Administration of an AED for the first week after neurosurgery is a routine practice and is recommended by the Brain Trauma Foundation and the AANS (49). Evidence shows phenytoin is effective in decreasing the risk of early PTS in patients with severe TBI (329). However, a recent study suggested that levetiracetam is safe and efficacious and results in better long-term outcomes than phenytoin, based on the DRS score and the Glasgow Outcome Scale score (329), and appears to be gaining popularity (330).

Most clinical seizures can be diagnosed based on clinical observations made by trained professionals. EEG provides valuable information in focus localization, seizure persistence, and severity prognostication once PTS have been observed. Additionally, EEG may identify the presence of subclinical seizures among patients with altered levels of consciousness (331).

Long-term EEG monitoring techniques include ambulatory EEG, which allows patients to continue activities of daily living without interruption in their normal environment, while inpatient video-EEG (VEEG) monitoring provides a direct opportunity to obtain artifact-free EEG while observing clinical behavior (332). Prolonged VEEG may help to distinguish psychogenic attacks from epilepsy, which has been reported to occur in 20% to 30% of refractory PTE in persons with moderate to severe TBI (333). Furthermore, EEG can provide useful information when deciding whether to taper antiepileptic medications in patients who have a history of early PTS.

Should a patient be deemed appropriate for treatment with an AED, the type of PTS, route, frequency and choice of drug administration, anticipated side effects, and comorbidities should all be considered. Adverse effects of AEDs may limit their use and warrant dosing adjustment, the need to switch to an alternative drug, or the need for polytherapy to achieve adequate seizure control. Cognitive side effects are of great concern in persons with TBI, which should be considered when choosing an AED. Carbamazepine has been described as a useful agent for the treatment of partial seizures while valproic acid as a reasonable choice for generalized seizures (334,335). Phenobarbital was commonly used in the past, but is now seldom used due to its adverse effects on cognition and behavior (336). Likewise, phenytoin has fallen from favor mainly due to its adverse effect on cognition compared to carbamazepine or valproate (337). Second-generation agents such as levetiracetam, lamotrigine, and topiramate are increasingly used in the clinical setting despite lack of evidence demonstrating their superiority over the older AEDs, particularly with regard to PTS. There is evidence suggesting no difference in the effectiveness and safety of the older compared to newer AEDs in persons with epilepsy, noting that the older medications (phenytoin, carbamazepine, and valproic acid) are more likely to result in a greater number of adverse events (338).

There are no specific guidelines regarding the timing of when or if to withdraw antiepileptic medications used in patients for PTE. However, many clinicians consider withdrawal of AEDs in patients who have been seizure-free for 2 years (339). Likewise, there are no recommendations over what time period to withdraw AED medications if the decision is made to do so, although conservative views recommend tapering over a period of 1 year (340).

For those patients who continue to experience medically refractory seizures, surgical intervention should be considered. The AAN, in association with the American Epilepsy Society, and the AANS support the benefits of anteromesial temporal lobe resection for disabling complex partial seizures and recommend referral of these patients to an epilepsy surgery center (341). Likewise, surgical excision of the seizure focus also provides an important treatment option for carefully selected patients with refractory PTE (342). In cases where patients are refractory to medications and prefer to not have surgical resection, vagus nerve stimulation (VNS) is an alternative therapy option. The AAN Therapeutics and Technology Subcommittee classified VNS as safe and effective for intractable partial seizures (343).

Autonomic Dysfunction

The autonomic nervous system is made up of the sympathetic and parasympathetic systems, which promote homeostasis in response to daily bodily challenges. TBI can cause autonomic dysfunction resulting in hypertension, fever, tachycardia, tachypnea, pupillary dilation, and extensor posturing.

Incidence of this condition varies widely in the published literature, likely due to the fact that there are many different names describing it, including paroxysmal sympathetic storms, autonomic dysfunction syndrome, dysautonomia, sympathetic or autonomic storming, and paroxysmal autonomic instability with dystonia (PAID). There are also no widely accepted diagnostic criteria defining it. Recently, efforts have focused on more precisely characterizing this syndrome, including clarifying its definition, nomenclature, and diagnostic criteria.

This resulted in recommending that the term "paroxysmal sympathetic hyperactivity" (PSH) replace previous terms to describe the "syndrome, recognized in a subgroup of survivors of severe acquired brain injury, of simultaneous, paroxysmal transient increases in sympathetic (elevated heart rate, blood pressure, respiratory rate, temperature, sweating) and motor (posturing) activity" (344).

TBI is the most commonly reported condition causing PSH, with a reported incidence ranging from 8% to 30% in moderate and severe cases admitted to an intensive care unit (345). It rarely occurs in other acute neurologic conditions. They are more frequent in younger people and are associated with prolonged duration of fever (346). The wide range of reported incidence is likely due to the lack of clarity in defining PSH. In a prospective cohort study, dysautonomic subjects had a significantly worse outcome, a greater period of hospitalization, and higher estimated costs compared to nondysautonomic survivors of TBI (345).

While there are several theories regarding the etiology of PSH, there appears to be greater evidence for a disconnection pathogenesis. This means that the usual balance of CNS excitatory and inhibitory drives becomes disrupted, which causes autonomic dysfunction (347). The general conclusion supported by a small number of autopsy and pathophysiologic studies suggests a relative disconnection of pathways at or around the level of the midbrain although no single lesion or pattern of lesions has been identified (348).

A diagnosis of PSH is one of exclusion, because there are no pathognomonic tests or findings. PSH is defined by the transient presence of four of the following six criteria in the absence of other potential causes such as uncontrolled sepsis or airway obstruction: fever, tachycardia (heart rate >120 beats/min or >100 beats/min if treated with beta-blocker), hypertension (systolic blood pressure >160 mm Hg or pulse pressure >80 mm Hg), tachypnea (respiratory rate >30 breaths/min), excessive diaphoresis, and extensor posturing or severe dystonia (345,346).

Pupillary dilatation and intense flushing may also be present (**Table 19-5**). The paroxysms usually begin 5 to 7 days after the injury but may start earlier. The episodes follow a relatively regular pattern, occurring on average one to three times per day. The duration of each episode can range from less than 1 hour up to 10 hours. Total duration of the disorder varies widely, ranging from 1 to 2 weeks to several months. Over time, episodes tend to become less frequent but more prolonged (346).

TABLE 19-5	Signs of Paroxysmal Sympathetic Hyperactivity
Tachycardia	>120 beats/min (or >100 beats/min on beta-blockers)
Tachypnea	>30 breaths/min
Blood pressure	Systolic BP > 160 mm Hg or pulse pressure >80 mm Hg
Fever	
Excessive Diaphoresis	
Pupillary dilation	
Extensor posturing	
Intense flushing	

General principles in the management of PSH include adequate hydration, exclusion of mimicking conditions (e.g., infection, pulmonary embolism [PE], hydrocephalus, epilepsy), effective analgesia, and avoidance of any identified triggers (349). If symptoms persist, medications may be needed. Because a wide array of neurotransmitters is involved in the pathways of autonomic control, several medications may be considered to ameliorate the manifestation of PSH. Limited studies exist supporting medication efficacy, most of which were conducted in intensive care settings, making the interventions used difficult to adapt in a rehabilitation setting where this syndrome typically occurs. Thus, the establishment of guidelines and best-practice protocols has proven difficult. However, more evidence exists on the potential effectiveness of morphine sulfate and nonselective beta-blockers (e.g., propranolol) (350). Intrathecal baclofen (ITB) may be effective in refractory cases. Bromocriptine and clonidine are helpful in some patients, but their efficacy is less consistent (351). Early recognition and adequate treatment of PSH are important to decrease hospitalization and promote recovery.

Posttraumatic Hydrocephalus

Hydrocephalus is defined as an active distension of the ventricular system of the brain resulting from inadequate passage of CSF from its point of production within the cerebral ventricles to its point of absorption into the systemic circulation (352). This definition is specific to hydrocephalus in that it excludes other abnormalities of CSF dynamics such as benign intracranial hypertension in which the ventricles are not enlarged. It also excludes brain atrophy or hydrocephalus *ex vacuo* in which the ventricular dilatation is not an active process of distension (**Fig. 19-12**).

The incidence of posttraumatic hydrocephalus (PTH) varies among published studies, most likely due to variance in its definition, but has been reported in up to 45% of persons with severe TBI (353). PTH is often diagnosed during inpatient rehabilitation, with some evidence indicating that up to 40% of cases are diagnosed in that setting (354). One study supports that most cases of PTH occurred in the early stages of inpatient rehabilitation, with 25% diagnosed within 2 weeks, 50% within 3 weeks, and 75% within 8 weeks of rehabilitation. Two patients developed PTH between discharge and 1 year following injury (355).

Risk factors for developing PTH include ICH, meningitis, and craniectomy (352,356,357). Advanced age, severe disability, and DOC on admission are independent predictors of developing PTH during rehabilitation. VS upon referral to rehabilitation raised the relative risk for PTH more than twofold (355). It is a common disorder following TBI, with one study finding 8% of patients admitted to an acute TBI inpatient rehabilitation program were diagnosed with PTH. Acute neuroanatomic characteristics of injury observed on CT imaging in that study included subarachnoid hemorrhage or subdural fluid collection in 93% of the patients with PTH, intraventricular hemorrhage in 30%, midline shift in 52%, and compression of the basal cisterns in 83%. Subcortical contusions were observed in 32% and cortical contusions in 97% of patients (358). Hydrocephalus can be classified as being

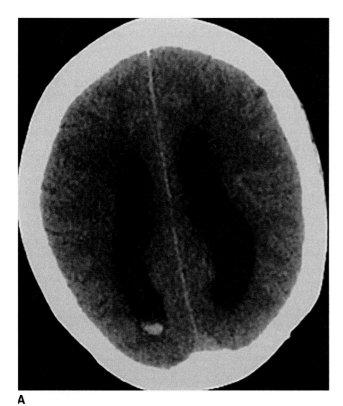
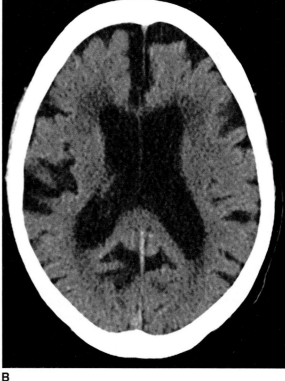

A   **B**

FIGURE 19-12.   A: CT image demonstrating widening of the ventricle with effacement of the sulci. The ventricles are enlarged due to communicating hydrocephalus. (Reprinted with permission from Weiner WJ, Goetz CG, Shin RK. *Neurology for the Non-Neurologist.* 6th ed. Philadelphia, PA: Wolters Kluwer Health/Lippincott Williams & Wilkins; 2010.) **B:** CT image of the head demonstrates cerebral atrophy as noted by the prominence of the ventricles and sulci and absence of transependymal edema.

communicating, also known as nonobstructive, or noncommunicating, also known as obstructive. In communicating hydrocephalus, the ventricles are connected and CSF is able to freely flow through the system. The condition arises from obstructed resorption of blood products, protein, or fibrosis at the level of the arachnoid granulations, which interferes with the absorption of CSF (352,356). Communicating hydrocephalus is the most common type of PTH, observed by enlargement of all components of the ventricular system (352,357). Noncommunicating hydrocephalus occurs when CSF flow is obstructed either within the ventricular system or upon its entrance/exit revealed on imaging by enlargement of only specific components of the ventricular system corresponding to the location of the obstruction.

The onset of PTH varies from weeks to 1 year after TBI, but most commonly within the first 3 months after injury, when persons with severe brain injury are treated in an inpatient setting.

Hydrocephalus can present with signs and symptoms associated with elevated ICP, including headache, nausea, vomiting, lethargy, and altered mental status. It may also present with findings consistent with normal pressure hydrocephalus, including ataxia, urinary incontinence, and dementia. Bulging at a craniectomy site is often observed, or one may note the combination of hypertension, bradycardia, and hypoventilation, known as the Cushing triad. Suspicion for PTH begins with clinical observation of the signs and symptoms previously mentioned. It may also be suspected when patients cease to progress in their recovery or if their function and/or arousal worsens. When PTH is present, CT and MRI imaging typically reveal ventriculomegaly, although this finding alone is insufficient to make a definitive diagnosis, as it may represent cerebral atrophy, also known as hydrocephalus *ex vacuo*. Ventricular configurations favoring dynamic hydrocephalus include enlargement of the temporal horns, convex shape of the frontal horns, widening of the frontal horn radius, and frontal horn location closer to midline narrowing the "ventricular angle" (359). Sulcal effacement, periventricular lucency, and transependymal fluid support the diagnosis of hydrocephalus. More invasive tests exist, including radioisotope cisternography, lumbar infusion studies, CSF tap test. A tap test involves a lumbar puncture with drainage of CSF, followed by clinical evaluations to determine the presence or absence of transient improvements in functional abilities. Improvements post tap test indicate placement of a ventricular shunt will be clinically beneficial. A lumbar catheter drainage trial for a period of 3 to 5 days has been shown to have a greater sensitivity and predictive value of shunt success than a simple tap test (360).

Treatment of PTH depends on a number of factors, including clinical presentation, medical comorbidities, severity of symptoms, and patient tolerance. Symptoms may be temporarily improved with administrations of carbonic anhydrase inhibitors such as acetazolamide or furosemide. Patients may also benefit from the temporizing effects of serial lumbar punctures or external ventricular drains. Definitive treatment is with surgical placement of a shunt to enable proper and adequate removal of fluid from the ventricular system. There are four main types of shunts available including ventriculoperitoneal (VP), ventriculoatrial, ventriculopleural, and lumboperitoneal. VP shunts are most commonly used for treatment of PTH. Shunt complications are not rare and include failure to adequately drain CSF, infection, seizures, and subdural hematomas, the latter occurring from overdrainage.

Neuroendocrine Disorders

Awareness of posttraumatic hypopituitarism is becoming better known as a complication of TBI that might contribute to morbidity and poor recovery. In a systematic review of neuroendocrine dysfunction following brain injury, the pooled prevalence of hypopituitarism in the chronic phase after TBI and aneurysmal SAH was 27.5% and 47%, respectively. Evidence also suggested that hypopituitarism is greater in persons with severe compared with those with mild or moderate TBI. Additionally, patients with posttraumatic hypopituitarism showed an impaired quality of life and an adverse metabolic profile (361). This is consistent with research findings demonstrating prompt diagnosis and treatment of endocrine complications following TBI facilitate the rehabilitation process (362).

The central neuroendocrine system is made up of the hypothalamus and the anterior and posterior lobes of the pituitary gland. The hypothalamus is a section of the forebrain below the thalamus that coordinates the interactions of the neuroendocrine system. The pituitary gland (hypophysis) sits in the sella turcica, which is a bony cavity within the sphenoid bone and is connected to the hypothalamus by the pituitary stalk. The larger anterior lobe of the pituitary (adenohypophysis) stores and releases a number of hormones under the influence of the hypothalamus, including follicle-stimulating hormone (FSH), luteinizing hormone (LH), adrenocorticotropic hormone (ACTH), thyroid-stimulating hormone (TSH), prolactin, and growth hormone (GH). The smaller posterior lobe of the pituitary (neurohypophysis) is responsible for the storage and release of oxytocin and antidiuretic hormone (ADH), also known as vasopressin. These hormones are produced by the hypothalamus and then travel to the posterior pituitary via the pituitary stalk, where they are eventually released. This makes these two hormones especially susceptible to neuronal damage at the level of the hypothalamus and stalk, as well as the pituitary gland itself (**Fig. 19-13**).

Determining who and when to screen for hypopituitarism is not well established as little scientific evidence exists guiding clinicians. In acute TBI, screening and treatment should commence whenever clinically indicated. In chronic TBI of moderate to severe severity, clinicians may choose to follow the consensus guidelines, which recommended that all people undergo endocrine function evaluation at 3 months and at 1 year postinjury. The recommended screening includes morning cortisol level, free T4, TSH, insulin-like growth factor (IGF)-1, FSH, LH, testosterone (for men), estradiol (for women), prolactin, and urinary free cortisol. If indicated, more specialized testing, including GH and cortisol stimulation tests, can be performed to more accurately diagnose an endocrine abnormality (363).

One of the most common neuroendocrine disorders encountered in TBI patients is the syndrome of inappropriate antidiuretic hormone secretion (SIADH). This syndrome is suspected in the setting of hyponatremia, which requires investigation to differentiate from other causes of low serum sodium. The classic criteria for diagnosing SIADH were first introduced by Bartter and Schwartz in 1967 and include

FIGURE 19-13. The pituitary gland, the relationship of the hypothalamus to pituitary action, and the hormones secreted by the anterior, middle, and posterior pituitary lobes. (Reprinted with permission from Rosdahl CB, Kowalski MT. *Textbook of Basic Nursing.* 10th ed. Philadelphia, PA: Wolters Kluwer Health/Lippincott Williams & Wilkins; 2012.)

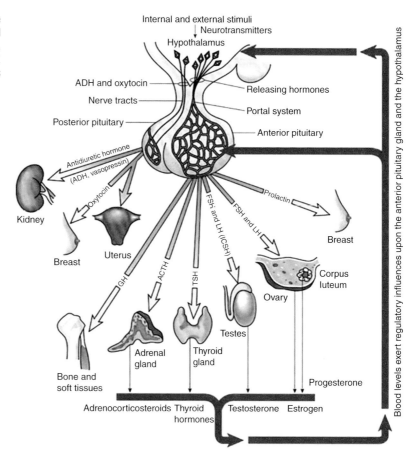

hyponatremia with corresponding serum hypo-osmolality, continued renal excretion of Na⁺, urine less than maximally dilute, absence of clinical evidence of volume depletion (normal skin turgor, blood pressure within the reference range), absence of other causes of hyponatremia (adrenal insufficiency, hypothyroidism, cardiac failure, pituitary insufficiency, renal disease with salt wastage, hepatic disease, drugs that impair renal water excretion), and correction of hyponatremia by fluid restriction (364). Head trauma can disrupt posterior pituitary function and is among the reasons why ADH is secreted at inappropriate levels despite plasma hypo-osmolality and normal or increased plasma volume.

Symptoms will vary depending on the severity and rate of development of hyponatremia, which are typically variably present in cases of mild (Na 130 to 134 mmol/L) or gradually developing SIADH. If symptoms do exist, they are likely to be nonspecific, such as nausea, anorexia, and malaise. In severe (Na < 130 mmol/L) or acute-onset SIADH, the patient may demonstrate symptoms of cerebral edema such as headache, muscle weakness, seizures, or altered mental status. There may also be an overall increase in body weight, but peripheral and pulmonary edema, dry mucous membranes, reduced skin turgor, and orthostatic hypotension are usually absent (364).

Once SIADH is clinically suspected, additional laboratory testing including serum and urine osmolality as well as urine sodium should be ordered to support its diagnosis. Hallmark laboratory findings include hyponatremia (serum Na⁺ < 135 mEq/L) with concomitant serum hypo-osmolality and high urine osmolality.

The treatment of SIADH and how rapidly the hyponatremia should be corrected depend on several factors, including the degree of hyponatremia and patient symptoms, and on whether it is acute or chronic. A mainstay of treatment in most cases is fluid restriction to about 1.0 to 1.2 L per 24 hours with daily serum sodium monitoring. Strictly monitoring fluid inputs and outputs helps to ensure fluid intake is less than the combined loss through urine output and insensible loss. This can also be further monitored by recording daily weights. Should the patient demonstrate more severe symptoms or develop symptoms acutely such as convulsion or altered mental status, 3% hypertonic saline can be infused over several hours with careful clinical and laboratory monitoring. However, it is important to not raise the sodium level more than 10 mEq/L over 24 hours in order to avoid development of pontine myelinolysis. For cases of chronic SIADH, medications may be needed. Vasopressin receptor antagonists work by reducing the number of aquaporin-2 water channels in the renal collecting duct, thus decreasing the water permeability of the collecting duct. Conivaptan and tolvaptan are currently the only vasopressin receptor antagonists that are commercially available in the United States and FDA approved for the treatment of euvolemic hyponatremia in hospitalized patients (365). Loop diuretics such as furosemide are usually used in conjunction with normal saline to replenish the Na⁺ excreted with the diuresis. Osmotic diuretics such as urea and mannitol are also treatment options. Urea is typically used in the treatment of refractory SIADH, in patients noncompliant with other therapies, or when other therapies are not available. Additionally, demeclocycline can be used as it induces diabetes insipidus by impairing the generation and action of cAMP, thus interfering with the action of arginine vasopressin on the collecting duct.

Another cause of hyponatremia in persons with TBI is cerebral salt wasting (CSW). This is characterized by extracellular volume depletion caused by a renal sodium transport abnormality in patients with intracranial disease and normal adrenal and thyroid function (366). CSW typically occurs in the setting of acute CNS disease or trauma. Conditions leading to cerebral salt-wasting syndrome include head injury, brain tumor, intracranial surgery, stroke, intracerebral hemorrhage, tuberculous meningitis, and craniosynostosis repair. However, CSW can also occur in the absence of cerebral disease (367). The exact mechanism underlying CSW remains unclear but is thought that a defect in renal sodium transport is the precipitating event (368). The precise incidence of CSW is not well established, with published reports varying widely from 0.8% to 34.6% following TBI, likely due to methodologic differences used in these reports (369).

Hyponatremia in CSW will present with some similar signs and symptoms described in SIADH, including lethargy, agitation, headache, altered consciousness, seizures, and coma. Similarly, the severity of symptoms typically reflects the magnitude and rapidity of the decrease in serum sodium concentration. The differentiation of SIADH from CSW depends on an accurate estimation of extracellular volume. Unfortunately, no single physical finding can accurately and reproducibly measure this volume. Therefore, indirect signs of hypovolemia should be investigated, including orthostatic hypotension, increased capillary refill time, decreased skin turgor, dry mucous membranes, and a sunken anterior fontanel. These signs usually appear only when the degree of dehydration is moderate to severe. Similar to SIADH, the laboratory finding in CSW includes elevated urinary sodium concentrations and low serum osmolality. The main differentiating factor between the two conditions is the extracellular fluid volume, which is low in CSW.

Management of CSW syndrome centers on correction of intravascular volume depletion and hyponatremia, as well as on replacement of ongoing urinary sodium loss, usually with intravenous (IV) hypertonic saline solutions (370). It is of utmost importance to distinguish CSW syndrome from SIADH because improper treatment (i.e., fluid restriction) may lead to worsening intravascular volume depletion, which would potentially jeopardize cerebral perfusion by lowering system blood pressure.

Hypernatremia following acute TBI warrants a workup to rule out diabetes insipidus (DI). There are two types, pituitary/central and nephrogenic. Pituitary or central DI is associated with TBI and it is believed to occur from injury to the neurohypophysis. Oftentimes, it is associated with skull fractures near the sella turcica, which may tear the stalk of the pituitary gland, disrupting ADH secretion from the posterior pituitary gland. With low levels of ADH, there is excessive volume depletion from renal water loss, leading to hypernatremia and plasma hyperosmolarity.

Patients will typically present with signs of dehydration due to passing high volumes of dilute urine, including excessive thirst and polydipsia. Laboratory workup includes a 24-hour urine collection for determination of urine volume and urinary specific gravity, which is typically less than 1.005 in patients

with DI. Serum and urine studies reveal a high serum sodium (>145 mEq/L) and high serum osmolality (>280 mOsm/kg) combined with a low urine osmolality (<300 mOsm/kg).

The drug of choice for treatment of DI is desmopressin acetate (DDAVP), which is an analog of ADH that has a prolonged antidiuretic effect (371). DDAVP is available in subcutaneous, intravenous, intranasal, and oral preparations. In cases of partial ADH deficiency, chlorpropamide can be administered, which improves renal response to ADH.

Heterotopic Ossification

HO is the formation of mature lamellar bone in extraskeletal soft tissue, typically forming near large proximal joints, which is painful and severely restricts joint range of motion. It can occur at any time after sustaining a TBI, but most commonly within the first 6 months, with a peak incidence in the 2nd month. The precise incidence of HO after TBI is unclear, with reports ranging from 11% to 73.3%, largely due to differences in patient populations and diagnostic criteria used in various studies. Incidence of clinically significant HO is somewhat better defined as between 10% and 20% (319,372). TBI-associated HO is associated with significantly longer inpatient rehabilitation hospitalizations and poorer FIM scores. More specifically, both admission and discharge FIM scores are lower, mostly accounted by ADL and mobility subscores, when compared with matched persons with TBI without clinical stigmata of HO (373).

Several factors have been associated with a higher risk for developing HO in persons with TBI, but are inconsistently reported. Reported factors include overall injury severity (not specific to brain trauma), coma duration, mechanical ventilation, spasticity, coexisting fractures, demographic characteristics, pressure skin injuries, and edema. A recent study indicated that prolonged coma and duration of mechanical ventilation, coexistent surgically treated bone fractures, and clinical signs of autonomic dysregulation were associated with a higher risk for developing HO (374). These characteristics likely in part explain the poorer functional gains achieved in afflicted patients and adversely impact mobility. Therefore, ambulation and both regular and cautious mobilization of the joints are of paramount importance in the early period of the rehabilitation process to preserve joint range of motion (375).

At time of presentation, pain and decreased range of motion are the two most common symptoms and signs. Other clinical signs include local swelling, erythema, warmth in the joint, muscle guarding, and low-grade fever (376). The hip is the most common site of HO after TBI, followed by the elbows, shoulders, and knees (377–380). Diagnosing HO first begins with a clinical suspicion based on its clinical presentation and ruling out other causes such as infection, venous thromboembolism (VTE), or undiagnosed orthopedic injury. An elevated serum alkaline phosphatase (SAP) may be found during early formation of HO. SAP is a sensitive indicator, increasing in the advance of symptoms and radiographic findings. Levels become abnormal approximately 2 weeks after onset and reach a peak, typically 3.5 times normal around 8 weeks later (378). Unfortunately, SAP has poor specificity, as it can be elevated for multiple other reasons (e.g., surgical intervention for fractures, hepatotoxicity). Although not specific for HO, patients with HO may have elevated creatinine kinase levels, which may be helpful in treatment planning and evaluation of

FIGURE 19-14. A: Anteroposterior radiograph of the pelvis of a 40-year-old rancher who was involved in a light plane crash in which he sustained a fracture-dislocation of the right hip and fracture of the left femoral neck. He also had a concomitant head injury and was comatose for 2 weeks. Note the significant heterotopic ossification, which virtually eliminated hip joint motion. **B:** Photograph of the same patient at 1 year after excision of heterotopic bone. The patient had recovered 90 degrees of flexion of the hip and had minimal restriction of rotation and abduction. He was very satisfied with his result. (Reprinted with permission from Callaghan JJ, Clohisy J, Beaule P, et al. *The Adult Hip: Hip Arthroplasty Surgery.* 3rd ed. Philadelphia, PA: Wolters Kluwer; 2016.)

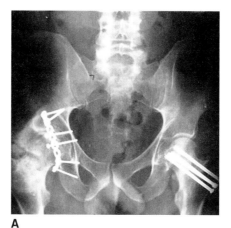

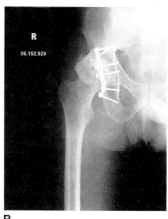

A   B

response to treatment (379). Ultrasonography has been used in the early diagnosis of HO about the hip joints. However, it is an operator-dependent examination, and no data are available on the value of ultrasonography in the diagnosis of HO in other joints (377). Plain radiographs are often unremarkable early in the process of bone formation, revealing evidence of HO weeks to months later (**Fig. 19-14**). The most sensitive imaging modality for early detection and assessing the maturity of HO is the three-phase technetium-99m (99mTc) methylene diphosphonate bone scan (376). CT and MRI may be useful in delineating local anatomy prior to resection, but the role of these imaging modalities in the evaluation of other aspects of HO has not been well established (379).

It is of upmost importance to take measures to prevent HO from adversely impacting joint range of motion once it occurs. This is done with ROM exercises, controlling spasticity, and use of NSAIDs if no contraindications exist. Once HO begins to develop, there are no treatment options to prevent or reverse its process. Management is aimed at limiting its progression and maximizing function of the affected joint with aggressive range of motion and therapeutic interventions once acute inflammatory signs have subsided.

Treatment of HO in TBI is largely extrapolated from studies examining its presence in spinal cord injury and following total hip arthroplasty (THA). Indomethacin remains the gold standard for HO prophylaxis following THA, although other NSAIDs, including naproxen and diclofenac, are equally as effective and can be considered as alternative first-line treatments (377). Indomethacin prescribed for 3 weeks in a dose of 75 mg/d after spinal cord injury reduced the incidence of HO by a factor of 2 to 3. For most patients undergoing THA, a 7-day course of indomethacin has been recommended as a prophylaxis against HO (377).

Surgical excision of HO should be considered in cases where the intervention is anticipated to improve function, such as standing posture and ability to sit or ambulate or independently perform activities of daily living. Excision should also be considered for patients in whom an underlying bone mass contributes to repeated pressure injuries (379). Planned excision typically occurs 12 to 18 months postinjury to allow for maturation of HO. Garland has recommended different schedules for surgical intervention, depending on the etiology of the condition underlying the HO: 6 months after direct traumatic musculoskeletal injury, 1 year after spinal cord injury, and 1.5

years after TBI. The ideal candidate for surgical resection of HO before 18 months will have no joint pain or swelling, a normal alkaline phosphatase level, and a three-phase bone scan indicating mature HO (372,380). Complications of surgical removal of HO include hemorrhage, wound healing problems, cellulitis, infection including osteomyelitis, and possible recurrence of HO (377).

Cranial Nerve Dysfunction

Cranial nerve injuries can be overlooked or even missed during the acute management and stabilization of a trauma patient. As the rehabilitation provider, it is imperative to be able to diagnose these pathologies as cranial nerve dysfunction can affect participation in rehab, vision, swallowing, and communication. The presence of multiple cranial nerve injuries, fractures, and facial deformities can make it difficult to identify the cranial nerve involved. The following sections will review each of the nerve injuries and potential treatment options.

Persons with injury to the olfactory nerve (CN I) will complain of impaired or total loss of smell and will also often notice loss of taste sensation. CN I injury occurs due to tearing of the thin nerve filaments that cross the cribriform plate. The incidence of CN I injury is 7% in all persons with TBI (381–383). Bedside testing for CN I integrity typically involves having a patient identify a common aromatic substance, such as ground coffee. Noxious substances, such as ammonia, are not used as they can also stimulate CN V, resulting in a false-negative test result.

CN I injury may improve spontaneously; however, treatment focuses on compensatory measures such as using smoke alarms and checking food expiration dates, thus avoiding environmental dangers.

Optic nerve (CN II) injuries present with visual impairments, manifested as blurred or spotty vision, visual field cuts, or blindness. The incidence is 5% of all persons with TBI (382). CN II injury can easily be confused with parietal lesion that causes hemi-inattention or occipital cortex injuries, which will cause a hemianopia or quadrantanopia. Terson's syndrome is a vitreous or intraocular hemorrhage associated with trauma and contributes to vision impairments. Assessments of CN II injury include a comprehensive eye and fundus exam and as needed visual-evoked potentials. In a person with severe injuries and inability to participate in an exam, the clinician may only be able to ascertain a gross visual assessment, such as identification of colorful pictures or objects. As recovery ensues, permitting improved participation in the examination process, a more thorough ophthalmologic assessment can be obtained, ideally by a neuro-optometrist or neuro-ophthalmologist. Patients with specific visual problems may benefit from special lenses and training to compensate for identified deficits (384).

Extraocular movements are affected by injury to any of the three nerves controlling eye movement, CN III, IV, and VI, or to their brainstem nuclei. CN III innervates the majority of muscles that move the eye and raise the eyelid, as well as the muscles that constrict the pupil. Injury to CN III causes diplopia and a divergent strabismus, ptosis, and a fixed, dilated pupil of the ipsilateral nerve injured. The reported incidence ranges widely following TBI, from 17% to 71%, reflective of the manner of how the data were collected (385,386). The trochlear nerve (CN IV) innervates the superior oblique muscle, which, although moves the eye in a complex manner, is most concisely described as moving it downward and inward. Of all the cranial nerves, CN IV is the only one that emerges from the dorsal aspect of the brain, giving it the longest intracranial course, and is therefore more susceptible to injury from increased ICP. Injury presents as a vertical or torsional diplopia, which occurs when the patient attempts to gaze downward and is often noticed when negotiating stairs or reading. Patients with CN IV injury often unconsciously compensate by tilting the top of the head down and toward the unaffected side, thus avoiding diplopia. The incidence is rare, reported at 1.4% of all persons with TBI (387).

The abducens nerve (CN VI) innervates the lateral rectus muscle. Injury to this nerve causes the eye to be adducted at rest, resulting in horizontal diplopia. Incidence is reported as high as 4.1% (387). Treatment of these nerve injuries includes treating the underlying disorder (i.e., tumor, hydrocephalus, cerebral edema), vision therapy, eyelid taping, and patching. Injuries to CN III, IV, and VI, either in isolation or in combination, may be treated with the thoughtful use of botulinum toxin (BT) injections or corrective surgery, but should only be considered after spontaneous recovery has plateaued (6 to 12 months) (388).

The trigeminal nerve (CN V) is the largest of the cranial nerves. It has three main branches, including the ophthalmic nerve (V1), maxillary nerve (V2), and mandibular nerve (V3). All three branches have sensory components with only the mandibular branch having additional motor function. Loss of corneal and facial sensation or facial neuropathic pain is indicative of trigeminal nerve injury and has an incidence of 0.4% to 2% after TBI (389). Treatment involves using eye lubrication and protective glasses, as well as neuropathic medications to reduce pain. Facial nerve (CN VII) injuries co-occurring with TBI are typically due to temporal bone fractures and result in facial weakness, loss of taste to the anterior two thirds of the tongue, hyperacusis, and impaired tear production. Upper or central motor neuron damage can be distinguished from lower or peripheral nerve injury as the latter results in paralysis of both the upper and lower muscles of the face, resulting in an inability to lower the eyelid. This places patients at immediate risk of corneal ulceration. Treatment includes eye lubrication, gold weight implantation to the eyelid, or tarsorrhaphy.

Acoustic nerve (CN VIII) injuries can present as hearing loss, vertigo, and tinnitus and result from the initial trauma or temporal bone fracture. Hearing loss can be described as conductive, which occurs from injury to the outer or middle ear structures (malleus, incus, and stapes), and sensorineural, which occurs from injury to the nerve or mixed. There is a greater incidence of hearing loss in the presence of a temporal bone fracture (390). Sensorineural hearing loss and tinnitus are becoming more prevalent in veterans with blast-related TBI (391). In case of hearing loss after TBI, spontaneous recovery may occur, although surgical correction of the fractures or nerve injury may be indicated. Vestibular therapy may be beneficial in the setting of CN VIII injury resulting in balance dysfunction (392).

Isolated injuries to CN IX to XII are rare following TBI. The glossopharyngeal nerve (CN IX) contains both sensory and motor fibers. It provides sensory function to the tonsils, posterior tongue, carotid bodies, carotid sinus, parasympathetic function to the parotid gland and otic ganglion, and motor function to the stylopharyngeal muscle. Injury presents as loss of taste to the posterior third of the tongue with the uvula deviating toward the contralateral side, decreased salivation, dysphagia, and loss of the gag reflex. Incidence is 0.5% to 1.6% of all TBI (389), with treatment directed by a speech-language pathologist. The vagus nerve (CN X) is also composed of both sensory and motor fibers and has the most extensive course and distribution of all the cranial nerves. Injuries present with loss of the gag reflex, dysphagia, hypophonia, and vocal cord paralysis with incidence of roughly 0.1% (389). CN X most commonly occurs with blunt trauma and fracture to the occipital condyles. Treatment involves speech therapy and vocal cord augmentation.

The spinal accessory nerve (CN XI) has only motor fibers, innervating the trapezius and sternocleidomastoid muscles. Injury presents as the inability to turn the head to the opposite side and ipsilateral shoulder droop. Treatment includes aggressive physical therapy and positioning, reserving surgical options in select cases. The hypoglossal nerve (CN XII) is a purely motor nerve that innervates the extrinsic and intrinsic muscles of the tongue with the exception of the palatoglossus. Patients with injury to this nerve present with dysarthria and dysphagia, with the tongue deviated to the side of the lesion. Injury to CN XII occurs most commonly from penetrating neck wounds and is treated with specific exercises.

Spasticity

Spasticity is defined as velocity-dependent increased resistance to passive stretch and occurs after injury to the CNS (see Chapter 40). In a retrospective study of 122 persons with severe TBI, incidence of spasticity was found to be as high as 70% (313). Spasticity is just one of the upper motor neuron signs that occur when there is a lesion to the CNS with other signs including clonus, dystonia, muscle stiffness, and joint contracture (393,394).

Spasticity is thought to be due to signal mishandling at the spinal cord level combined with lack of inhibition of the stretch reflex from the supraspinal cord level (394). In certain clinical situations, spasticity can be beneficial in facilitating mobility, promoting venous return, maintaining muscle bulk and bone mass, and preventing deep venous thrombosis (299).

However, spasticity is often problematic as it can be painful, cause deformities of the limb and joint, hinder function and mobility, and adversely affect proper positioning and hygiene (395).

TABLE 19-6	Modified Ashworth Scale and Tardieu Scale

Modified Ashworth Scale

Grade	Description
0	No increase in muscle tone
1	Slight increase in muscle tone, manifested by a catch or minimal resistance at the end of the range of motion when the affected part is moved in flexion or extension
1+	Slight increase in muscle tone, manifested by a catch followed by minimal resistance through the remainder (<1/2) of the range of motion
2	Marked increase in muscle tone through most of the range of motion, but the affected part is easily moved
3	Considerable increase in muscle tone, passive movement is difficult
4	Affected part is rigid in flexion or extension

Tardieu Scale

Score	Description
0	No resistance to passive range of motion
1	Slight resistance to passive range of motion
2	Clear catch at precise angle, interrupting passive range of motion, followed by release
3	Fatigable clonus (<10 s while pressure is maintained) occurring at a precise angle followed by release
4	Unfatigable clonus (>10 s while pressure is maintained) occurring at a precise angle followed by release
5	Affected part is not movable

Modified Ashworth Scale: Assessed while passively moving a joint through its available range of motion; Tardieu Scale: Scores obtained at three speeds: V1 as slow as possible, V2 as limb falling under force of gravity, and V3 as fast possible. Angle of muscle reaction (catch or clonus) recorded as R1. Range of motion of joint recorded as R2 under conditions of V1.

Evaluation of spasticity starts with physical examination of joint position and range of motion, muscle tone, muscle stretch reflexes, strength, and motor coordination. The Tardieu Scale and Modified Ashworth Scale (MAS) are commonly used to objectively measure and document spasticity (**Table 19-6**) (395,396). The clinician must then set the goals of treatment with patients and their caregivers (395). Treatment is multidisciplinary and involves nonpharmacologic and pharmacologic interventions as well as correction of underlying noxious stimuli (e.g., metabolic or infectious etiologies). Muscle stretching is the first-line therapy for spasticity and, while often directed by a skilled rehabilitation therapist, should be the responsibility of all caregivers including family members and the patient themselves if possible. Stretching is achieved though several means and includes prolonged positioning typically using static or dynamic orthoses, as well as passive, active, isokinetic, and isotonic stretching. These all promote maintaining or increasing the length of the muscle tendon unit and decreasing motor unit excitability (395,397). Other nonpharmacologic modalities include neuromuscular electrical stimulation (NEMS) and use of robotics such as the Lokomat (395,396).

Pharmacologic treatment includes central and peripheral acting agents. Baclofen is a GABA-B receptor agonist that acts at the pre- and postsynaptic nerve terminals resulting in inhibition of spinal reflexes. Baclofen is a first-line pharmacologic treatment in spinal cord injury and multiple sclerosis and has been extended for use in TBI (299). Side effects often limit maximal dosing (up to 80 mg total per day), which include confusion, fatigue, dry mouth, urinary retention, and constipation (299). TBI-related problems including impaired cognition and arousal are often exacerbated with oral baclofen, limiting its usefulness in this population. Abrupt cessation can cause withdrawal and seizure.

Diazepam and clonazepam are benzodiazepines that act near the GABA-A receptor. Side effects of benzodiazepines include sedation and cognitive impairments, with negative effects on new learning, which often prevent their use in brain injury (299). Tizanidine is a centrally acting alpha-2 adrenergic agonist and decreases intraspinal glutamate, thus depressing the spasticity pathway. Tizanidine side effects include sedation, dry mouth, weakness, orthostasis, and transaminitis, and dosing is limited in the presence of renal insufficiency (395,397). Dantrolene sodium inhibits muscle contractility by inhibiting release of calcium from the sarcoplasmic reticulum, but can cause generalized muscle weakness. The main caution with dantrolene is its potential to cause irreversible liver toxicity at doses greater than 200 to 300 mg/d (299,398). Finally, gabapentin has been studied for its use in non-TBI spasticity cases and has the added benefit of treating neuropathic pain. The mechanism of action of gabapentin in decreasing spasticity is not well delineated, noting that dosing is limited by side effects that include fainting, somnolence, nystagmus, headache, and tremor.

BT injections are effective in treating spasticity and work locally at the site where the muscles are injected. Unlike enteral antispasticity mediations, it does not cause sedation or confusion and when dosed appropriately will not cause systemic weakness. BT inhibits the release of acetylcholine at the neuromuscular junction, thus preventing activation of the corresponding motor units. Different forms of guidance can be used to assist with localization of the spastic muscle including electrical stimulation, electromyography, and ultrasound. Effects of BT injection generally last 3 months and thus must be regularly repeated in order to maintain control of spasticity. Side effects include muscle weakness, injection site irritation, bleeding, and bruising, and if injected near the neck, dysphagia may develop. Several formulations of BT are currently available, with their effectiveness in treating spasticity and contribution to achieving patients' personal goals well documented in multiple randomized controlled trials (395). Also injected peripherally, phenol has been used for chemodenervation by causing neurolysis. This effect is not limited to motor fibers and thus can cause dysesthesia when injected in close proximity to sensory nerves. It can also cause soft tissue fibrosis but is considerably less costly than BT (395).

For treatment of more severe widespread spasticity, ITB is useful. Dosed in micrograms, the drug is delivered directly to the intrathecal space continuously through a catheter attached to a small pump implanted into the subcutaneous layer of the abdomen. It has been demonstrated to reduce MAS scores even when a patient has been treated with maximal doses of oral baclofen (399). Lower doses of baclofen are used when administered intrathecally, which causes decreased side effects compared with oral baclofen (400). The pump requires maintenance with setting adjustments, percutaneous refills at least every 6 months, and battery changes every 5 to 7 years (400). This level of maintenance may be difficult for patients with a decreased support system and impaired mobility. Thus, it is important to first establish the ability and willingness of patients to follow up prior to implantation of the pump as neglecting to refill can result in withdrawal with increase spasticity, risk of seizure, organ failure, and death.

Joint contractures can occur after brain injury and are thought to be due to shortening of the muscle tendon ligaments and joint capsules and commonly result from inadequately treated spasticity (401). Common patterns of contracture are shoulder adduction and internal rotation, hip and knee flexion, and ankle plantar flexion. Prevention of contractures is most important, achieved by stretching joints through their functional range of motion several times a day (401). Contractures are treated with prolonged static stretch, with serial casting with a skilled therapy team, and with adequate spasticity management (401). If contractures are severe, are minimally responsive to conservative measures, and are limiting functional gains, surgical release may be considered (402).

Venous Thrombosis and Embolism

Deep vein thrombosis (DVT) and PE are common after TBI, with the latter a potentially life-threatening consequence of VTE. PE is the third leading cause of death in trauma patients after day 3 (403), yet fear of expanding ICH in the TBI population is a major hindrance in initiating DVT prophylaxis. The incidence of DVT in TBI when DVT prophylaxis is not used is 54% (404).

While DVT prophylaxis includes both mechanical and chemical prophylaxes, standard care is with chemoprophylaxis. Mechanical prophylaxis includes using intermittent pneumatic compression (IPC) or compression stockings to prevent blood pooling in the lower extremities. In persons with TBI receiving mechanical prophylaxis alone, incidence of DVT was reported as 31% and PE as 3% (405). Those with advanced age, dehydration, and severe brain injury and who are immobile or hemiparetic are at highest risk for DVT (406).

Pharmacologic VTE prophylaxis with subcutaneous anticoagulation has also been proven effective in preventing DVT. Both unfractionated heparin (UFH) and low molecular weight heparin (LMWH) in varying doses have been prospectively studied. In trauma patients, LMWH has been found to be superior over UFH in preventing DVT (404). In addition,

UFH has been found to have an increase rate of ICH and PE compared to LMWH (407).

In practice, there is concern that chemoprophylaxis will cause or exacerbate ICH following TBI. However, a recent meta-analysis concludes that starting chemoprophylaxis within the first 72 hours postinjury reduces the risk of VTE without exacerbating ICH (408).

Inferior vena cava (IVC) filters theoretically have the benefit of reducing PE without increasing the risk of ICH. However, complications of IVC include its migration away from the site of implantation, erosion, and thrombosis, contributing to postthrombotic syndrome. In practice, IVC filter placement is reserved for patients with contraindication to mechanical and chemoprophylaxis (409).

Bowel and Bladder Dysfunction

After brain injury, bowel dysfunction includes but is not limited to constipation and incontinence (410), adversely influencing quality of life, functional outcomes, and disposition destination (411). Bowel dysfunction can be due to decreased mobility, dysphagia (resulting in decreased fiber and fluid intake), dysfunctional intestinal contractility, and deficits in cognition, consciousness, and communication (412).

Evaluation and treatment of bowel dysfunction after brain injury require the clinician to evaluate the pattern of a patient's bowel movements and perform an adequate clinical exam. Measures to improve regular bowel function focus on establishing an evacuation schedule (usually after breakfast or dinner) combined with dietary adjustments to increase fiber and fluid. Psyllium husk is a bulk-producing laxative and fiber supplement that increases stool bulk, resulting in firming or solidifying very loose stools or softening very hard small stools. Docusate sodium and polyethylene glycol are stool softeners that increase the amount of water in the stool making passage easier. Senna and bisacodyl are stimulant laxatives that irritate bowel tissues and promote evacuation. Enemas are useful when there is an impaction. Finally, simethicone is useful in treating gastrointestinal discomfort by decreasing stomach and intestinal gas bubble surface tension and aiding gas elimination.

Urinary dysfunction has been associated with impaired cognition, aphasia, and motor deficits (413) and contributes to decreased quality of life, skin breakdown, discomfort, social isolation, not living in the community, and higher mortality rates (414). In assessing dysfunction, the pattern of voiding needs to be determined, as well as laboratory and clinical examinations that assess if the patent is adequately hydrated or has a urinary infection. Bedside determination of bladder evacuation effectiveness can be achieved through ultrasound measurement of bladder urine volume or by direct catheterization. Formal urodynamic studies (UDS), performed by a skilled clinician, provide useful information pertaining to bladder filling pressure and sphincter activity that can be used to identify causes of bladder dysfunction and guide treatment. A UDS is helpful if micturition history, physical exam, and determination of postvoid residual volumes do not declare the cause of incontinence or retention.

In detrusor overactivity, a patient demonstrates frequent low-volume incontinence episodes, where the detrusor muscle contracts at lower than normal bladder volumes. The patient may feel frequent and urgent needs to void, with loss of bladder control. Timed voiding is deemed the gold standard in treating detrusor overactivity, with decreased incontinence episodes markedly decreasing (414,415). In timed voiding, the patient is assisted in voiding at short intervals (every 2 to 3 hours), thus preventing uncontrolled detrusor contraction as the bladder fills with urine. The length of time between voids is only increased once continence is maintained between these intervals. Timed voiding may also be used in conjunction with an anticholinergic medication such as oxybutynin. However, timed voiding alone, or timed voiding with oxybutynin, has been demonstrated to be more effective than oxybutynin alone (413,415). In addition, anticholinergic medications should be prescribed with caution in the brain injury population as these medications can exacerbate constipation, dry mouth, drowsiness, and cognitive impairment.

Urinary retention poses immediate danger to the patient as it can quickly lead to bladder infection, bladder overdistension, ureter reflux, hydronephrosis, and renal failure. Causes of urinary retention include outflow obstruction due to an enlarged prostate or urethral stricture and detrusor-sphincter dyssynergia (DSD). DSD, which more commonly occurs after spinal cord injury than isolated TBI, occurs when there is loss of coordinated contraction of the detrusor muscle and relaxation of the internal and external urethral sphincters. A patient may still have incontinence when they have retention due to overflow from an overdistended bladder and detrusor overactivity. Clean intermittent catheterization is preferred over indwelling catheters for the treatment of urinary retention. The patient will need to be catheterized on a schedule to avoid overfilling. Finally, if there is bladder outlet obstruction, such as an enlarged prostate, alpha-blockers such as doxazosin and tamsulosin have been demonstrated to improve urinary flow and reduce PVR (414), but care should be taken as these medications can cause orthostasis.

Pressure Injuries

Pressure injuries are areas of damaged skin and underlying tissue that form over bony prominences or weight-bearing surfaces. Patients with TBI are at risk for pressure injuries due to impaired mobility, decreased nutrition, altered level of consciousness and sensation, and bowel and bladder incontinence (416). The most common areas of pressure injuries in patients occur over bony prominences where pressure on the skin is greatest, including the occiput, scapula, sacrum, buttocks, and heels. Pressure injuries development after brain injury has demonstrated increased mortality (417).

Treatment of pressure injuries requires multidisciplinary management with modification of support surfaces, optimization of nutrition, wound dressing and applications, positioning, and surgical repair (416). Wound care clinicians are specialized in prescribing the proper dressing and seating/bedding type for the patient, which in part is determined by the type of injuries (necrotic, dry, moist, etc.) Despite the advances in dressings, it is imperative to first focus on correcting the underlying issues identified earlier.

ETHICAL CONSIDERATIONS

For all patients, the principles of beneficence, nonmaleficence, and autonomy are important medical ethical considerations in any situation (see Chapter 16). This is certainly true in the care of TBI patients. However, cognitive deficits and behavioral changes often associated with TBI frequently complicate ethical decision-making for this population. A fourth principle, justice, is even more challenging to address rigorously, especially in the health care system that exists within the United States.

In the United States, respecting a patient's autonomy, the right of a patient to make their own decisions, is a core requirement in medical care. Even if the decision may appear detrimental to their well-being, patients have the right to decide what medical treatments they will undergo if they do so without coercion and demonstrate clear consistent decision-making with full understanding of the situation and treatment options. However, these conditions should not be taken lightly in regard to persons with TBI. Cognitive deficits as a result of TBI often lead to impaired awareness of the environment and situation, impaired ability to understand consequences of decisions being made, impaired communication skills, and impulsive responses to situations. Due to these complications, it is important to determine if a patient is capable to make any given decision before doing or not doing anything in the name of autonomy.

Appelbaum and Grisso (418) outlined four conditions that must be met to determine if a patient has capacity to make a decision. The patient must be able to express a choice, understand the situation and information provided, demonstrate reasoning to reach a decision, and appreciate the consequences of this decision. Obtaining informed consent that meets each of these conditions is an important practice in delivering ethical medical care.

As persons with TBI have varying levels of cognitive impairment and ability to process and understand information, the clinician's assessment of decision-making capacity should be performed for each specific situation or question being asked. For patients with severe cognitive or communication deficits, this process may be very quick and straightforward. For those with less severe impairments, they may have capacity to make certain, more basic decisions but fail to meet the conditions for decisional capacity regarding more complicated matters. Furthermore, improvement in cognitive skills associated with recovery from a TBI necessitates ongoing reevaluation of decisional capacity as patients progress through their recovery course. Determinations regarding the capacity of patients to make specific medical decisions for themselves on a case-by-case basis fall within the clinician's scope of practice. However, more formal and binding competency determinations require legal proceedings and may result in the appointment of a guardian to assume decision-making responsibilities.

The behavioral changes that may occur as a result of TBI reveal further potential challenges to ethical medical care. A person with TBI may make a decision that does not align with conventional thought or the majority of society's values. Yet, prior written evidence or family and friends may provide support that this was consistent with the patient's beliefs prior to the brain injury. In this situation, it must be considered whether the patient lacks decisional capacity or if a bias based on conventional thought is clouding the picture. This determination becomes even more complicated if the patient had a preinjury psychiatric condition or personality disorder. Even under these conditions, respect for autonomy should be considered and weighed heavily against confounding factors. It is also important to consider that even if a health care proxy or next of kin makes a decision for a patient who is demonstrating lack of decisional capacity for that decision, every effort should be made to ensure that decision aligns with the patient's prior belief system.

Conversely, a patient may demonstrate decisional capacity, but the decision they make appears inconsistent with prior beliefs as per written evidence or family and friends. This situation is less easily navigated as it touches on issues of identity and sense of self after a TBI for which there are no easy answers. For nonurgent matters, waiting until the patient recovers may provide clarity or confidence regarding a decision. Situations where a patient and the patient's support system including next of kin or health care proxy are in agreement regarding a decision also helps provide confidence in that decision. However, when the two parties are at odds or a situation requires more urgent attention, they only serve to complicate matters. Seeking the advice of ethicists or an ethics board and reviewing the principles of medical ethics help to provide guidance in these situations.

The principles of nonmaleficence and beneficence are also important considerations in providing ethical medical care. Nonmaleficence is the responsibility to avoid actions that will be detrimental to a patient's well-being. Beneficence refers to taking actions for the benefit of a patient's well-being. Although not the same concept, these two principles often work together in guiding ethical medical care. They may appear straightforward, but in reality, there are very few decisions made that have no potential risk for negative consequences. It is important to weigh the risks and benefits of each decision made and ensure that all decisions are guided by the goals of providing net benefit while making every effort to avoid harm to a patient. In certain circumstances, this may require foregoing treatment that may potentially help a patient if the benefit is not sufficiently significant and the potential complications from that treatment are highly likely or potentially of great severity. In TBI management, these principles are frequently tested as the evidence base for many treatments is limited or mixed. For instance, commonly used medications in TBI management such as valproic acid for agitation management and trazodone for insomnia management lack large population studies supporting their use for these issues (298). Additionally, many treatments utilized in brain injury medicine are undertaken in attempts to improve function or quality of life but are not needed to maintain medical stability.

In these situations, the focus of the treatment should be clearly understood by the patient, or patient's decision-makers, if they lack decisional capacity. Their goals of care must also be clearly understood as this context is an important factor in weighing beneficence versus nonmaleficence. If a patient's goals do not align with the potential benefit of a treatment, the principle of beneficence may not be met for undergoing that treatment for this patient.

The principle of justice adds another layer of complexity in regard to medical ethics, especially in the United States health care system. Justice refers to fairness and, in the context of medicine, the fair treatment of patients. The definition of what is fair is where there may be controversy.

For instance, most people believe that two patients characteristically equal in every way should be treated equally. However, patients are often not equal, such as in regard to

prognosis, resource requirements, ability to benefit from a given treatment, and benefit versus burden to society. In this context, the question becomes what is fair treatment for each of these patients if their varying conditions are taken into account.

There are also different kinds of justice, specifically distributive, corrective, and compensatory justice. Although they are all possibly relevant to medical ethics and TBI care in some ways, the most relevant kind of justice to this discussion is distributive justice. Distributive justice refers to the distribution of resources and responsibilities fairly across society. Again, what is considered fair is important to define. In TBI care, where there are innumerous treatments being endorsed by various entities as potentially beneficial and very few rigorously studied treatments with strong evidence of their benefit, it is difficult to determine what would be considered unjust to deny as a treatment option, especially when financial considerations are included. In our society, access to resources in TBI rehabilitation care is also often unequal for those with and without insurance or even with different levels of insurance coverage or financial means. Is it fair to provide unequal care in this situation or should resources be distributed equally regardless of the burden on society in the form of tax dollar usage. Other considerations are whether greater resource usage in the rehabilitation setting would have an impact on decreasing the burden of care on society over the long term and whether this alters what would be considered fair relative to distributive justice. These are important philosophical questions without easy answers.

The principles of autonomy, nonmaleficence, beneficence, and justice are often discussed in regard to medical ethics. Each of these principles is also relevant to ethical considerations in TBI management. In our society, a high value is placed on respecting autonomy and providing care in a way that adheres to the principles of nonmaleficence and beneficence. TBI complicates the delivery of care in relation to these principles as cognitive deficits and behavioral changes associated with brain injury often put into question if a patient has decisional capacity. Beyond this determination, it is often difficult to navigate what qualifies as the most appropriate decision in regard to doing what is best for any given patient. In these situations, careful evaluation is necessary to adhere to the principles of medical ethics. Distributive justice and how it should relate to our society are also a topic of much debate in our health care system. Controversy over what is considered fair is at the heart of this debate. In TBI care, where the population is heterogeneous, resource utilization is high, and a solid evidence base for treatment is limited, determining what is fair is even more difficult.

SUMMARY

TBI is a common disorder, afflicting millions of people throughout the world. It has an enormous impact on those who are injured, their families, the health care system, and society. Although reported incidence rates are very high, they almost certainly underestimate the true burden of the problem, which is further exacerbated by the aging population whose reported incidence is rising. While overall death rates are falling with the exception of elderly injured through falls, the overall prevalence of people living with long-term

TBI-related disability will almost certainly increase in the future. In addition to the well-known consequences of acute injury, long-term problems including psychiatric disorders, neurodegenerative conditions, other medical problems, and early mortality underscore a growing recognition that TBI is a chronic, often lifelong condition.

Treatment presents numerous challenges for clinicians in rehabilitation, given the unique and very varied presentation of patients with TBI, who, in addition to motor problems, typically have concurrent challenges in the realms of cognition and behavior that adds complexity to their overall management. Despite a growing body of knowledge related to outcomes, genetics, and biologic markers, accurately diagnosing mild TBI and predicting outcomes regardless of severity remain an inexact science. What is certain is that clinicians treating people with TBI need to have a comprehensive understanding of their conditions, including identifying and diagnosing their associated morbidities, the impact their injuries have on their overall physical and psychological health, and the knowledge and skill to effectively intervene to ameliorate their adverse consequences.

REFERENCES

1. Faul M, Xu L, Wald MM, et al. *Traumatic Brain Injury in the United States: Emergency Department Visits, Hospitalizations, and Deaths 2002–2006.* Atlanta, GA: Centers for Disease Control and Prevention, National Center for Injury Prevention and Control; 2010.
2. Centers for Disease Control and Prevention QuickStats. Injury and traumatic brain injury (TBI)—related deaths by age group—United States, 2006. *MMWR Morb Mortal Wkly Rep.* 2010;59:303.
3. Centers for Disease Control and Prevention. *Report to Congress on Traumatic Brain Injury in the United Sates. Epidemiology and Rehabilitation.* Atlanta, GA: National Center for Injury Prevention and Control; Division of Unintentional Injury Prevention; 2014.
4. Centers for Disease Control and Prevention. Nonfatal traumatic brain injuries related to sports and recreation activities among persons aged ≤19 years—United States, 2001-2009. *MMWR Morb Mortal Wkly Rep.* 2011;60:1337–1342.
5. CDC, NIH, DOD, and VA Leadership Panel. *Report to Congress on Traumatic Brain Injury in the United States. Understanding the Public Health Problem among Current and Former Military Personnel.* Atlanta, GA: Centers for Disease Control and Prevention (CDC), the National Institutes of Health (NIH), the Department of Defense (DOD), and the Department of Veterans Affairs (VA); 2013.
6. Cifu DX, Kreutzer JS, Marwitz JH, et al. Functional outcomes of older adults with traumatic brain injury: a prospective, multicenter analysis. *Arch Phys Med Rehabil.* 1996;77(9):883–888.
7. Susman M, DiRusso SM, Sullivan T, et al. Traumatic brain injury in the elderly: increased mortality and worse functional outcome at discharge despite lower injury severity. *J Trauma.* 2002;53(2):219–223.
8. Coronado VG, Xu L, Basavaraju SV, et al. Surveillance for traumatic brain injury-related deaths—United States, 1997–2007. Centers for Disease Control and Prevention (CDC). *MMWR Surveill Summ.* 2011;60(5):1–32.
9. Stevens JA, Adekoya N. Brain injury resulting from falls among elderly persons. *JAMA.* 2001;286(21):2665–2666.
10. Zaloshnja E, Miller T, Langlois JA, et al. Prevalence of long-term disability from traumatic brain injury in the civilian population of the United States, 2005. *J Head Trauma Rehabil.* 2008;23(6):394–400.
11. Thurman DJ, Alverson C, Dunn KA, et al. Traumatic brain injury in the United States: a public health perspective. *J Head Trauma Rehabil.* 1999;14(6):602–615.
12. Theodore AD, Chang JJ, Runyan DK, et al. Epidemiologic features of the physical and sexual maltreatment of children in the Carolinas. *Pediatrics.* 2005;115(3):e331–e337.
13. Finkelstein E, Corso PS, Miller TR. *The Incidence and Economic Burden of Injuries in the United State.* New York: Oxford University Press; 2006
14. Adekoya N, Thurman DJ, White OD, et al. Surveillance for traumatic brain injury deaths—United States 1988-1998. *MMWR Surveill Summ.* 2002;51(10):1–14.
15. Hersorffer DC, Ghajar J. Marked improvement in adherence to traumatic brain injury guidelines in United States trauma centers. *J Trauma.* 2007;63(4):841–848.
16. Shandaro JR, Rivara FP, Wang J, et al. Alcohol and risk of mortality in patients with traumatic brain injury. *J Trauma.* 2009;66(6):1584–1590.
17. Tien HC, Tremblay LN, Rizoli SB, et al. Association between alcohol and mortality in patients with severe traumatic head injury. *Arch Surg.* 2006;141(12):1185–1191.
18. McGinn MJ, Povlishock JT. Pathophysiology of traumatic brain injury. *Neurosurg Clin N Am.* 2016;27(4):397–407.
19. Marmarou CR, Walker SA, Davis CL, et al. Quantitative analysis of the relationship between intra-axonal neurofilament compaction and impaired axonal transport following diffuse traumatic brain injury. *J Neurotrauma.* 2005;22(10):1066–1080.
20. Buki A, Siman R, Trojanowski JQ, et al. The role of calpain-mediated spectrin proteolysis in traumatically induced axonal injury. *J Neuropathol Exp Neurol.* 1999;58(4):365–375.
21. Smith DH, Hicks R, Povlishock JT. Therapy development for diffuse axonal injury. *J Neurotrauma.* 2013;30(5):307–323.
22. Buki A, Povlishock JT. All roads lead to disconnection? Traumatic axonal injury revisited. *Acta Neurochir (Wien).* 2006;148(2):181–193.
23. Povlishock JT, Kontos HA. The role of oxygen radicals in the pathobiology of traumatic brain injury. *Hum Cell.* 1992;5(4):345–353.
24. Povlishock JT, Becker DP, Cheng CL, et al. Axonal change in minor head injury. *J Neuropathol Exp Neurol.* 1983;42(3):225–242.
25. Bain AC, Meaney DF. Tissue-level thresholds for axonal damage in an experimental model of central nervous system white matter in jury. *J Biomech Eng.* 2000;122(6):615–622.
26. Tang-Schomer MD, Patel AR, Baas PW, et al. Mechanical braking of microtubules in axons during dynamic stretch injury underlies delayed elasticity, microtubule disassembly, and axon degeneration. *FASEB J.* 2010;24(5):1401–1410.
27. Sahuquillo J, Vilalta J, Lamarca J, et al. Diffuse axonal injury after severe head trauma. *Acta Neurochir Suppl.* 1989;101(3–4):149–158.
28. Adams JH, Doyle D, Ford I, et al. Diffuse axonal injury in head injury: definition, diagnosis and grading. *Histopathology.* 1989;15(1):49–59.
29. Povlishock JT. Pathobiology of traumatically induced axonal injury in animals and man. *Ann Emerg Med.* 1993;22(6):980–986.
30. Denny-Brown D, Russel WR. Experimental cerebral contusion. *Brain.* 1941;64:93–164.
31. Povlishock JT. Pathophysiology of neural injury: therapeutic opportunities and challenges. *Clin Neurosurg.* 2000;10:46:113–126.
32. Oppenheimer DR. Microscopic lesions in the brain following head injury. *J Neurol Neurosurg Psychiatry.* 1968;31(4):299–306.
33. Katayama Y, Becker DP, Tamura T, et al. Massive increases in extracellular potassium and the indiscriminate release of glutamate following concussive brain injury. *J Neurosurg.* 1990;73(6):889–900.
34. Koura SS, Doppenberg EM, Marmarou A, et al. Relationship between excitatory amino acid release and outcome after severe human head injury. *Acta Neurochir Suppl.* 1998;71:244–246.
35. Bullock R, Zauner A, Myseros JS, et al. Evidence for prolonged release of excitatory amino acids in severe human head trauma. Relationship to clinical events. *Ann N Y Acad Sci.* 1995;765:290–297.
36. Chamoun R, Suki D, Gopinath SP, et al. Role of extracellular glutamate measured by cerebral microdialysis in severe traumatic brain injury. *J Neurosurg.* 2010;113(3):564–570.
37. Faden AI, Demediuk P, Panter SS, et al. The role of excitatory amino acids and NMDA receptors in traumatic brain injury. *Science.* 1989;244(4906):798–800.
38. Palmer AM, Marion DW, Botscheller ML, et al. Traumatic brain injury-induced excitotoxicity assessed in a controlled cortical impact model. *J Neurochem.* 1993;61(6):2015–2024.
39. Saatman KE, Creed J, Raghupathi R. Calpain as a therapeutic target in traumatic brain injury. *Neurotherapeutics.* 2010;7(1):31–42.
40. Cheng G, Kong RH, Zhang LM, et al. Mitochondria in traumatic brain injury and mitochondrial-targeted multipotential therapeutic strategies. *Br J Pharmacol.* 2012;167(4):699–719.
41. Weber JT. Altered calcium signaling following traumatic brain injury. *Front Pharmacol.* 2012;3:60.
42. Feuerstein D, Manning A, Hashemi P, et al. Dynamic metabolic response to multiple spreading depolarizations in patients with acute brain injury: an online microdialysis study. *J Cereb Blood Flow Metab.* 2010;30(7):1343–1355.
43. Hartings JA, Watanabe T, Bullock MR, et al. Spreading depolarizations have prolonged direct current shifts and are associated with poor outcome in brain trauma. *Brain.* 2011;134(Pt 5):1529–1540.
44. Hinzman JM, DiNapoli VA, Mahoney EJ, et al. Spreading depolarizations mediate excitotoxicity in the development of acute cortical lesions. *Exp Neurol.* 2015;267:243–253.
45. Servadei F, Murray GD, Teasdale GM, et al. Traumatic subarachnoid hemorrhage: demographic and clinical study of 750 patients from the European Brain Injury Consortium survey of head injuries. *Neurosurgery.* 2002;50(2):261–267.
46. Sato S, Suzuki J. Ultrastructural observations of the capsule of chronic subdural hematoma in carious clinical stages. *J Neurosurg.* 1975;43(5):569–578.
47. Ito H, Yamamoto S, Saito K, et al. Quantitative estimation of hemorrhage in chronic subdural hematoma using the 51Cr erythrocyte labeling method. *J Neurosurg.* 1987;66(6):862–864.
48. Traynelis VC. Chronic subdural hematomas in the elderly. *Clin Geriatr Med.* 1991;7(3):583–598.
49. Carney N, Totten AM, O'Reilly C, et al. Guidelines for the management of severe traumatic brain injury. Available from: https://braintrauma.org/uploads/03/12/Guidelines_for_Management_of_Severe_TBI_4th_Edition.pdf. Accessed March 16, 2017
50. Sorrentino E, Diedler J, Kasprowicz M, et al. Critical thresholds for cerebrovascular reactivity after traumatic brain injury. *Neurocrit Care.* 2012;16(2):258–266.
51. Robertson CS, Valadaka AB, Hannay HJ, et al. Prevention of secondary ischemic insults after severe head injury. *Crit Care Med.* 1999;27(10):2086–2095.
52. Berry C, Ley EJ, Burkur M, et al. Redefining hypotension in traumatic brain injury. *Injury.* 2012;43(11):1833–1837.

53. Nwachuku EL, Puccio AM, Fetzick A, et al. Intermittent versus continuous cerebro-spinal fluid drainage management in adult severe traumatic brain injury: assessment of intracranial pressure burden. *Neurocrit Care.* 2014;20(1):49–53.

54. Cooper DJ, Rosenfeld JV, Murray L, et al. Decompressive craniectomy in diffuse traumatic brain injury. *N Engl J Med.* 2011;264(16):1493–1502.

55. Jiang JY, Xu W, Li WP, et al. Efficacy of standard trauma craniectomy for refractory intracranial hypertension with severe traumatic brain injury: multicenter, prospective, randomized controlled study. *J Neurotrauma.* 2005;22(6):623–628.

56. Qiu W, Guo C, Shen H, et al. Effects if unilateral decompressive craniectomy on patients with unilateral acute post-traumatic brain swelling after traumatic brain injury. *Crit Care Med.* 2009;13(6):R185.

57. Kolias AG, Kirkpatrick PJ, Hutchinson PJ. Decompressive craniectomy: past, present and future. *Nat Rev Neurol.* 2013;9(7):405–415.

58. Roberts I, Yates D, Sandercock P, et al. Effects of intravenous corticosteroids on death within 14 days in 10,008 adults with clinically significant head injury. (MRC CRASH trial): randomised placebo-controlled trial. *Lancet.* 2004;364(9442):1321–1328.

59. Jennett B, Teasdale G. Aspects of coma after severe head injury. *Lancet.* 1977;1(8017):878–881.

60. Widjicks EF, Bamlet WR, Maramatton BV, et al. Validation of a new coma scale: the FOUR score. *Ann Neurol.* 2005;58(4):585–593.

61. Nyam TE, Ao KH, Hung SY, et al. FOUR score predicts early outcome in patients after traumatic brain injury. *Neurocrit Care.* 2017;26(2):225–231.

62. Kasprowicz M, Burzynska M, Melcer T, et al. A comparison of the Full Outline of UnResponsiveness (FOUR) score and Glasgow Coma Score (GCS) in predictive modelling in traumatic brain injury. *Br J Neurosurg.* 2016;30(2):211–220.

63. Schaefer PW, Huisman TA, Sorenson AG, et al. Diffusion-weighted MR imaging in closed head injury: high correlation with initial Glasgow coma scale score and score on modified Rankin scale at discharge. *Radiology.* 2004;233(1):58–66.

64. Mac Donald CL, Dikranian K, Bayly P, et al. Diffusion tensor imaging reliably detects experimental traumatic axonal injury and indicates approximate time of injury. *J Neurosci.* 2007;27(44):11869–11876.

65. Nakayama N, Okumura A, Shinoda J, et al. Evidence for white matter disruption in traumatic brain injury without macroscopic lesions. *J Neurol Neurosurg Psychiatry.* 2006;77(7):850–855.

66. Xu J, Rasmussen IA, Lagopoulos J, et al. Diffuse axonal injury in severe traumatic brain injury visualized using high-resolution diffusion tensor imaging. *J Neurotrauma.* 2007;24(5):753–765.

67. Yasokawa YT, Shinoda J, Okumura A, et al. Correlation between diffusion-tensor magnetic resonance imaging and motor-evoked potential in chronic severe diffuse axonal injury. *J Neurotrauma.* 2007;24(1):163–173.

68. Benson RR, Meda SA, Vasudevan S, et al. Global white matter analysis of diffusion tensor images is predictive of injury severity in traumatic brain injury. *J Neurotrauma.* 2007;24(3):446–459.

69. Huisman TA, Schwamm LH, Schaefer PW, et al. Diffusion tensor imaging as potential biomarker of white matter injury in diffuse axonal injury. *AJNR Am J Neuroradiol.* 2004;25(3):370–376.

70. Wozniak JR, Krach L, Ward E, et al. Neurocognitive and neuroimaging correlates of pediatric traumatic brain injury: a diffusion tensor imaging (DTI) study. *Arch Clin Neuropsychol.* 2007;22(5):555–568.

71. Newcombe VF, Williams GB, Nortje J, et al. Analysis of acute traumatic axonal injury using diffusion tensor imaging. *Br J Neurosurg.* 2007;21(4):340–348.

72. Demougeot C, Garnier P, Mossiat C, et al. *N*-Acetylaspartate, a marker of both cellular dysfunction and neuronal loss: its relevance to studies of acute brain injury. *J Neurochem.* 2001;77(2):408–415.

73. Garnett MR, Blamire AM, Corkill RG, et al. Early proton magnetic resonance spectroscopy in normal-appearing brain correlates with outcome in patients following traumatic brain injury. *Brain.* 2000;123(Pt 10):2046–2054.

74. Marino S, Zei E, Battaglini M, et al. Acute metabolic brain changes following traumatic brain injury and their relevance to clinical severity and outcome. *J Neurol Neurosurg Psychiatry.* 2007;78(5):501–507.

75. Shutter L, Tong KA, Holshouser BA. Proton MRS in acute traumatic brain injury: role for glutamate/glutamine and choline for outcome prediction. *J Neurotrauma.* 2004;21(12):1693–1705.

76. Signoretti S, Marmarou A, Fatouros P, et al. Application of chemical shift imaging for measurement of NAA in head injured patients. *Acta Neurochir Suppl.* 2002;81:373–375.

77. Kirov II, Tal A, Babb JS, et al. Proton MR spectroscopy correlates diffuse axonal abnormalities with post-concussive symptoms in mild traumatic brain injury. *J Neurotrauma.* 2013;30(13):1200–1204.

78. Cohen BA, Inglese M, Rusinek H, et al. Proton MR spectroscopy and MRI-volumetry in mild traumatic brain injury. *AJNR Am J Neuroradiol.* 2007;28(5):907–913.

79. Yeo RA, Phillips JP, Jung RE, et al. Magnetic resonance spectroscopy detects brain injury and predicts cognitive functioning in children with brain injuries. *J Neurotrauma.* 2006;23(10):1427–1435.

80. Jennett B, Plum F. Persistent vegetative state after brain damage: a syndrome in search of a name. *Lancet.* 1972;1(7753):734–737.

81. Medical aspects of the persistent vegetative state. The Multi-Society Task Force on PVS. *N Engl J Med.* 1994;330(21):1499–1508.

82. Katz DI, Polyak M, Coughlan D, et al. Natural history of recovery from brain injury after prolonged disorder of consciousness: outcome of patients admitted to inpatient rehabilitation with 1–4 year follow-up. *Prog Brain Res.* 2009;177:73–88.

83. Giacino JT, Ashwal S, Childs W, et al. The minimally conscious state: definition and diagnostic criteria. *Neurology.* 2002;58(3):349–353.

84. Giacino JT, Kalmar K. The vegetative and minimally conscious state: a comparison of clinical features and functional outcome. *J Head Trauma Rehabil.* 1997;12(4):36–51.

85. Schnakers C, Vanhaudenhuyse A, Giacino J, et al. Diagnostic accuracy of the vegetative and minimally conscious states: clinical consensus versus standardized neurobehavioral assessment. *BMC Neurol.* 2009;9:35.

86. Childs NL, Mercer WN, Childs HW. Accuracy of diagnosis of persistent vegetative state. *Neurology.* 1993;43(8):1465–1467.

87. Andrews K, Murphy L, Munday R, et al. Misdiagnosis of the vegetative state in a rehabilitation unit. *BMJ.* 1996;313(7048):13–16.

88. Owen AM, Coleman MR, Boly M, et al. Detecting awareness in the vegetative state. *Science.* 2006;313(5792):1402.

89. Coleman MR, Davis MH, Rodd JM, et al. Towards the routine use of brain imaging to aid the clinical diagnosis of disorders of consciousness. *Brain.* 2009;132(Pt 9):2541–2552.

90. Monti MM, Vanhaudenhuyse A, Coleman MR, et al. Willful modulation of brain activity in disorders of consciousness. *N Engl J Med.* 2010;362(7):579–589.

91. Seel RT, Sherer J, Whyte J, et al. Assessment scales for disorders of consciousness: evidence-based recommendations for clinical practice and research. *Arch Phys Med Rehabil.* 2010;91(12):1795–1813.

92. Chugani HT. Positron emission tomography: principles and applications in pediatrics. *Mead Johnson Symp Perinat Dev Med.* 1987;(25):15–18.

93. Prins ML, Hovda SA. Developing experimental models to address traumatic brain injury in children. *J Neurotrauma.* 2003;20(2):123–137.

94. Thibault KL, Margulies SS. Age-dependent material properties of the porcine cerebrum. Effect on pediatric inertial head injury criteria. *J Biomech.* 1998;31(12):1119–1126.

95. Guskiewicz KM, Valovich McLeod TC. Pediatric sports-related concussion, *PM R.* 2001;3(4):353–364.

96. Ewing-Cobbs L, Barnes M, Fletcher JM, et al. Modeling of longitudinal academic achievement score after pediatric traumatic brain injury. *Dev Neuropsychol.* 2004;25(1–2):107–133.

97. Gerrard-Morris A, Taylor HG, Yeates KO, et al. Cognitive development after traumatic brain injury in young children. *J Int Neuropsychol Soc.* 2010;16(1):157–168.

98. Hendryx PM, Verduyn WH. Diagnosis and treatment strategies for the latent sequelae of head trauma in children. *J Cognitive Rehabil.* 1995;13(3):8–12.

99. Williams WH, Cordan G, Mewse AJ, et al. Self-reported traumatic brain injury in male young offenders: a risk factor for re-offending, poor mental health and violence? *Neuropsychol Rehabil.* 2010;20(6):801–812.

100. Anderson VA, Catroppa C, Dudgeon P, et al. Understanding predictors of functional recovery and outcomes 30 months following early childhood injury. *Neuropsychology.* 2006;20(1):42–57.

101. Yeates KO, Swift E, Taylor HG, et al. Short- and long-term social outcomes following pediatric traumatic brain injury. *J Int Neuropsychol Soc.* 2004;10(3):412–426.

102. Yeates KO, Taylor HG. Behavior problems in school and their educational correlates among children with traumatic brain injury. *Exceptionality.* 2006;14(3):141–154.

103. Taylor HG, Swartwout MD, Yeates KO, et al. Traumatic brain injury in young children: post-acute effects on cognitive and school readiness skills. *J Int Neuropsychol Soc.* 2008;14(5):734–745.

104. Carroll JL, Cassidy JD, Pelosos PM, et al.; for WHO Collaborating Centre Task Force on Mild Traumatic Brain Injury. Prognosis for mild traumatic brain injury: results of the WHO Collaborating Centre Task Force on Mild Traumatic Brain Injury. *J Rehabil Med.* 2004;(suppl 43):84–105.

105. Nadebaum C, Anderson V, Catroppa C. Executive function outcomes following traumatic brain injury in young children: a five year follow up. *Dev Neuropsychol.* 2007;32(2):703–728.

106. Rivara FP, Koepsell TD, Wang J, et al. Incidence of disability among children 12 months after traumatic brain injury. *Am J Public Health.* 2010;102(11):2074–2079.

107. Wade SL, Zhang N, Yeates KO, et al. Social environmental moderators of long-term functional outcomes of early childhood brain injury. *JAMA Pediatr.* 2016;170(4):343–349.

108. Anderson V, Catroppa C, Morse S, et al. Functional plasticity or vulnerability after early traumatic brain injury? *Pediatrics.* 2005;116(6):1374–1382.

109. Kriel RL, Krach LE, Panser LA. Closed head injury: comparison of children younger and older than 6 years of age. *Pediatr Neurol.* 1989;5(5):296–300.

110. William WH, Cordan, G, Mewse AJ, et al. Self-reported traumatic brain injury in male young offenders: a risk factor for re-offending, poor mental health and violence? *Neuropsychol Rehabil.* 2010;20(6):801–812.

111. Wade SL, Walz, NC, Carey J, et al. A randomized trial of teen online problem solving for improving executive function deficits following pediatric traumatic brain injury. *J Head Trauma Rehabil.* 2010;25(6):409–415.

112. Brown G, Chadwick O, Schaffer D, et al. A prospective study of children with head injuries, III: psychiatric sequelae. *Psychol Med.* 1981;11(1):63–78.

113. Max JE, Robin DA, Lindgren SD, et al. Traumatic brain injury in children and adolescents: psychiatric disorders at 2 years. *J Am Acad Child Adolesc Psychiatry.* 1997;36(9):1278–1285.

114. Max JE. Children and adolescents. In: Silver JS, McAllister TW, Yudofsky SC, eds. *Textbook of Traumatic Brain Injury.* 2nd ed. Washington, DC/London, England: American Psychiatric Publishing, Inc.; 2011:439–450.

115. Kirkwood M, Janusz J, Yeates KO, et al. Prevalence and correlates of depressive symptoms following traumatic brain injury in children. *Child Neuropsychol.* 2000;6(3):195–208.

116. Ylvisaker M, Todis B, Glang A, et al. Educating students with TBI: themes and recommendations. *J Head Trauma Rehabil.* 2001;16(1):76–93.

117. Cronin AF. Traumatic brain injury in children: issues in community function. *Am J Occup Ther.* 2001;55(4):377–384.

118. Ellis GL. Subdural hematoma in the elderly. *Emerg Med Clin North Am.* 1990;8(2):281–294.

119. Feldman RG, Pincus JH, McEntee WJ. Cerebrovascular accident or subdural fluid collection? *Arch Intern Med.* 1963;112:966–976.

120. Rozzelle CJ, Wofford JL, Branch CL. Predictors of hospital mortality in older patients with subdural hematoma. *J Am Geriatr Soc.* 1995;43(3):240–244.

121. Rutland-Brown W, Langlois JA, Thomas KE, et al. Incidence of traumatic brain injury in the United States, 2003. *J Head Trauma Rehabil.* 2006;21(6):544–548.

122. Colantonio A, Saverino C, Zagorski B, et al. Hospitalizations and emergency department visits for TBI in Ontario. *Can J Neurol Sci.* 2010;37(6):783–790.

123. Dams-O'Connor K, Cuthbert JP, Whyte J, et al. Traumatic brain injury among older adults at level I and II trauma centers. *J Neurotrauma.* 2013;30(24):2001–2013.

124. Ponsford J, Cameron P, Fitzgerald M, et al. Long-term outcomes after uncomplicated mild traumatic brain injury: a comparison with trauma control. *J Neurotrauma.* 2011;28(6):937–946.

125. Marquez de la Plata CD, Hart T, Hammond FM, et al. Impact of age on long-term recovery from traumatic brain injury. *Arch Phys Med Rehabil.* 2008;89(5):896–903.

126. Mosenthal AC, Livingston DH, Lavery RF, et al. The effect of age on functional outcome in mild traumatic brain injury: 6-month report of a prospective multicenter trial. *J Trauma.* 2004;56(5):1042–1048.

127. Thompson HJ, McCormick WC, Kagan SH. Traumatic brain injury in older adults: epidemiology, outcomes, and future implications. *J Am Geriatr Soc.* 2006;54(10):1590–1595.

128. Brewer ES, Reznikov B, Liberman RF, et al. Incidence and predictors of intracranial hemorrhage after minor head trauma in patients taking anticoagulant and antiplatelet medication. *J Trauma Acute Care Surg.* 2011;70(1):e1–e5.

129. Dijkers M, Cantor J, Hibbard M, et al. The consequences of TBI in the elderly: a systematic review. *Brain Inj Prof.* 2008;5:14–18.

130. Fjell AM, Walhovd KB. Structural brain changes in aging: courses, causes and cognitive consequences. *Rev Neurosci.* 2010;21(3):187–221.

131. Hoffman JM, Doctor JN, Chan L, et al. Potential impact of the new Medicare prospective payment system on reimbursement for traumatic brain injury inpatient rehabilitation. *Arch Phys Med Rehabil.* 2003;84(8):1165–1172.

132. Mosenthal AC, Lavery RF, Addis M, et al. Isolated traumatic brain injury: age is an independent predictor of mortality and early outcome. *J Trauma.* 2002;52(5):907–911.

133. Quigley MR, Vidovich D, Cantella D, et al. Defining the limits of survivorship after very severe head injury. *J Trauma.* 1997;42(1):7–10.

134. Harrison-Felix C, Whiteneck G, Devivo M, et al. Mortality following rehabilitation in the Traumatic Brain Injury Model Systems of Care. *NeuroRehabilitation.* 2004;19(1):45–54.

135. Ventura T, Harrison-Felix C, Carlson N, et al. Mortality after discharge from acute care hospitalization with traumatic brain injury: a population-based study. *Arch Phys Med Rehabil.* 2010;91(1):20–29.

136. Ritchie PD, Cameron PA, Ugoni A, et al. A study of the functional outcome and mortality in elderly patients with head injuries. *J Clin Neurosci.* 2000;7(4):301–304.

137. Tinetti ME, Doucette J, Claus E, et al. Risk factors for serious injury during falls by older person in the community. *J Am Geriatr Soc.* 1995;43(11):1214–1221.

138. Speechley M, Tinetti M. Falls and injuries in frail and vigorous community elderly persons. *J Am Geriatr Soc.* 1991;39(1):46–52.

139. Perdue PW, Watts DD, Kaufman CR, et al. Differences in mortality between elderly and younger adult trauma patients: geriatric status increases risk of delayed death. *J Trauma.* 1998;45(4):805–810.

140. Pennings JL, Bachulis BL, Simons CT, et al. Survival after severe brain injury in the aged. *Arch Surg.* 1993;128(7):787–793.

141. Harrison-Felix C, Kolakowsky-Hayner SA, Hammond FM, et al. Mortality after surviving traumatic brain injury: risks based on age groups. *J Head Trauma Rehabil.* 2012;27(6):e45–e56.

142. Kilaru S, Garb J, Emhoff T, et al. Long-term functional status and mortality of elderly patients with severe closed head injuries. *J Trauma.* 1996;41(6):957–963.

143. Committee on Gulf War and Health: Brain Injury in Veterans and Long-Term Health. Gulf war and health: volume 7: long-term consequences of traumatic brain injury. Available from: http://nap.edu/catalog/12436.html. Accessed March 19, 2017

144. Harrison-Felix C, Oretz C, Hammond FM, et al. Life expectancy after inpatient rehabilitation for traumatic brain injury in the United States. *J Neurotrauma.* 2015;32(23):1893–1901.

145. Brooks JC, Shavelle RM, Strauss DJ, et al. Long-term survival after traumatic brain injury Part II: life expectancy. *Arch Phys Med Rehabil.* 2015;96(6):1000–1005.

146. Harrison-Felix C, Kreider SE, Arango-Lasprilla JC, et al. Life expectancy following rehabilitation: a NIDRR Traumatic Brain Injury Model Systems study. *J Head Trauma Rehabil.* 2012;27(6):E69–E80.

147. Masel BE, DeWitt DS. Traumatic brain injury: a disease process, not an event. *J Neurotrauma.* 2010;27(8):1529–1540.

148. Schofield PW, Tang M, Marder K, et al. Alzheimer's disease after remote head injury: an incidence study. *J Neurol Neurosurg Psychiatry.* 1997;2(2):119–124.

149. O'Meara ES, Kukull WA, Sheppard L, et al. Head injury and risk of Alzheimer's disease by apolipoprotein E genotype. *Am J Epidemiol.* 1997;146(5):373–384.

150. Fleminger S, Oliver DL, Lovestone S, et al. Head injury as a risk factor for Alzheimer's disease: the evidence 10 years on: a partial replication. *J Neurol Neurosurg Psychiatry.* 2003;74(7):857–862.

151. Mortimer JA, van Duijn CM, Chandra V, et al. Head trauma as a risk factor for Alzheimer's disease: a collaborative re-analysis of case-control studies. EURODEM Risk Factors Research Group. *Int J Epidemiol.* 1991;20(suppl 2):S28–S35.

152. Mehta KM, Ott A, Kalmijn S, et al. Head trauma and risk of dementia and Alzheimer's disease: the Rotterdam study. *Neurology.* 1999;53(9):1959–1962.

153. Katzman R, Aronson M, Fuld P, et al. Development of dementing illnesses in an 80-year-old volunteer cohort. *Ann Neurol.* 1989;25(4):317–324.

154. Williams DB, Annegers JF, Kokmen E, et al. Brain injury and neurologic sequelae: a cohort study of dementia, parkinsonism, and amyotrophic lateral sclerosis. *Neurology.* 1991;41(10):1554–1557.

155. McKee A, Cantu RC, Nowinski CJ, et al. Chronic traumatic encephalopathy in athletes: progressive tauopathy after repetitive head injury. *J Neuropathol Exp Neurol.* 2009;68(7):709–735.

156. McKee AC, Stern RA, Nowinski CJ, et al. The spectrum of disease in chronic traumatic encephalopathy. *Brain.* 2013;136(Pt 1):43–64.

157. Dams-O'Connor K, Spielman L, Hammond FM, et al. An exploration of clinical dementia phenotypes among individuals with and without traumatic brain injury. *NeuroRehabilitation.* 2013:32(2):199–209.

158. Sayed N, Culver C, Dams-O'Connor K, et al. Clinical phenotype of dementia after traumatic brain injury. *J Neurotrauma.* 2013;30(13):1117–1122.

159. Deb S, Lyons I, Koutzoukis C, et al. Rate of psychiatric illness 1 year after traumatic brain injury. *Am J Psychiatry.* 1999;156(3):374–378.

160. Hibbard MR, Uysal S, Kepler K, et al. Axis I psychopathology in individuals with traumatic brain injury. *J Head Trauma Rehabil.* 1998;13(4):24–39.

161. Brooks N, Campsie L, Symington C, et al. The five year outcome of severe blunt head injury: a relative's view. *J Neurol Neurosurg Psychiatry.* 1986;49(7):764–770.

162. Schoenhuber R, Gentilini M. Anxiety and depression after mild head injury: a case control study. *J Neurol Neurosurg Psychiatry.* 1988;51(5):722–724.

163. McCrory P, Meeuwisse W, Dvořák J, et al. Consensus statement on concussion in sport-the 5(th) international conference on concussion in sport held in Berlin, October 2016. *Br J Sports Med.* 2017;51(11):838–847.

164. Dikmen S, Machamer J, Fann JR, et al. Rates of symptom reporting following traumatic brain injury. *J Int Neuropsychol Soc.* 2010;16(3):401–411.

165. Meehan W, d'Hemecourt P, Comstock RD. High school concussions in the 2008–2009 academic year: mechanism, symptoms, and management. *Am J Sports Med.* 2010;38(12):2405–2409.

166. McCrea M, Guskiewicz KM, Marshall SW, et al. Acute effects and recovery time following concussion in collegiate football players: The NCAA Concussion Study. *JAMA.* 2003;290(19):2556–2563.

167. The American Congress of Rehabilitation Medicine. Definition of mild traumatic brain injury. *J Head Trauma Rehabil.* 1993;8(3):86.

168. Vos PE, Battistin L, Birbamer G, et al. EFNS guideline on mild traumatic brain injury: report of an EFNS task force. *Eur J Neurol.* 2002;9(3):207–219.

169. Cantu RC. Posttraumatic retrograde and anterograde amnesia: pathophysiology and implications in grading and safe return to play. *J Athl Train.* 2001;36(3):244–248.

170. Colorado Medical Society. *Report of the Sports Medicine Committee: Guidelines for the Management of Concussions in Sport (Revised).* Denver, CO: Colorado Medical Society; 1991.

171. Langlois JA, Rutland-Brown W, Wald MM. The epidemiology and impact of traumatic brain injury: a brief overview. *J Head Trauma Rehabil.* 2006;21(5):375–378.

172. Hyder AA, Wunderlich CA, Puvanachandra P, et al. The impact of traumatic brain injuries: a global perspective. *NeuroRehabilitation.* 2007;22(5):341–353.

173. McCrea M, et al. Unreported concussion in high school football players: Implications for prevention. *Clin J Sport Med.* 2004;14(1):13–17.

174. Register-Mihalik JK, et al. Knowledge, attitude, and concussion-reporting behaviors among high school athletes: a preliminary study. *J Athl Train.* 2013;48(5):645–653.

175. Marin JR, et al. Trends in visits for traumatic brain injury to emergency departments in the United States. *JAMA.* 2014;311(18):1917–1919.

176. Bakhos LL. Emergency department visits for concussion in young child athletes. *Pediatrics.* 2010;126(3):e550–e556.

177. Marar M, McIlvain NM, Fields SK, et al. Epidemiology of concussions among United States high school athletes in 20 sports. *Am J Sports Med.* 2012;40(4):747–755.

178. Powell JW, Barber-Foss KD. Traumatic brain injury in high school athletes. *JAMA.* 1999;282(10):958–963.

179. Lincoln AE, Caswell SV, Almquist JL, et al. Trends in concussion incidence in high school sports: a prospective 11-year study. *Am J Sports Med.* 2011;39(5):958–963.

180. Pellman EJ, Powell JW, Viano DC, et al. Concussion in professional football: epidemiological features of game injuries and review of the literature—Part 3. *Neurosurgery.* 2004;54(1):81–94.

181. Guskiewicz KM, Marshall SW, Bailes J, et al. Recurrent concussion and risk of depression in retired professional football players. *Med Sci Sports Exerc.* 2007;39(6):903–909.

182. Dick RW. Is there a gender difference in concussion incidence and outcomes? *Br J Sports Med.* 2009;43(suppl 1):i46–i50.

183. Gessel LM, Fields SK, Collins CL, et al. Concussions among United States high school and collegiate athletes. *J Athl Train.* 2007;42(4):495–503.

184. Eisenberg MA, Meehan W III, Mannix R. Duration and course of post-concussive symptoms. *Pediatrics.* 2014;133(6):999–1006.

185. Makdissi M, Darby D, Maruff P, et al. Natural history of concussion in sport: markers of severity and implications for management. *Am J Sports Med.* 2010;38(3):464–471.

186. Stovner LJ, Schrader H, Mickeviciene D, et al. Headache after concussion. *Eur J Neurol.* 2009;16(1):112–120.

187. Englander J, Hall K, Stimpson T, et al. Mild traumatic brain injury in an insured population: Subjective complaints and return to employment. *Brain Inj.* 1992;6(2):161–166.

188. Lucas S, Hoffman JM, Bell KR, et al. A prospective study of prevalence and characterization of headache following mild traumatic brain injury. *Cephalalgia*. 2013;34(2):93–102.

189. Lovell MR. Measurement of symptoms following sports-related concussion: reliability and normative data for the post-concussion scale. *Appl Neuropsychol*. 2006;13(3):166–174.

190. Kraus J, Schaffer K, Ayers K, et al. Physical complaints, medical service use, and social and employment changes following mild traumatic brain injury: a 6-month longitudinal study. *J Head Trauma Rehabil*. 2005;20(3):239–256.

191. Elbin RJ, Sufrinko A, Schatz P, et al. Removal from play after concussion and recovery time. *Pediatrics*. 2016;138(3).

192. McCrea M, Barr WB, Guskiewicz K, et al. Standard regression-based methods for measuring recovery after sport- related concussion. *J Int Neuropsychol Soc*. 2005;11(1):58–69.

193. McCrea M, Guskiewicz K, Randolph C, et al. Incidence, clinical course, and predictors of prolonged recovery time following sport-related concussion in high school and college athletes. *J Int Neuropsychol Soc*. 2013;19(1):22–33.

194. Echemendia RJ, Putukian M, Mackin RS, et al. Neuropsychological test performance prior to and following sports-related mild traumatic brain injury. *Clin J Sport Med*. 2001;11(1):23–31.

195. Barr WB, McCrea M. Sensitivity and specificity of standardized neurocognitive testing immediately following sports concussion. *J Int Neuropsychol Soc*. 2001;7(6):693–702.

196. Belanger HG, Vanderploeg RD. The neuropsychological impact of sports-related concussion: a meta-analysis. *J Int Neuropsychol Soc*. 2005;11(4):345–357.

197. Collins MW, Lovell MR, Mckeag DB. Relationship between concussion and neuropsychological performance in college football players. *JAMA*. 1999;282(10):964–970.

198. Mathias JL, Beall JA, Bigler ED. Neuropsychological and information processing deficits following mild traumatic brain injury. *J Int Neuropsychol Soc*. 2004;10(2):286–297.

199. Guskiewicz KM, McCrea M, Marshall SW, et al. Cumulative effects associated with recurrent concussion in collegiate football players: The NCAA concussion study. *JAMA*. 2003;290(19):2549–2555.

200. Alexander MP. Mild traumatic brain injury: pathophysiology, natural history, and clinical management. *Neurology*. 1995;45(7):1253–1260.

201. *Diagnostic and Statistical Manual of Mental Disorders: DSM-5*. Washington, DC: American Psychiatric Association; 2013.

202. Yang CC, Tu YK, Hua MS, et al. The association between the postconcussion symptoms and clinical outcomes for patients with mild traumatic brain injury. *J Trauma*. 2007;62(3):657–663.

203. Paniak C, Reynolds S, Toller-Lobe G, et al. A longitudinal study of the relationship between financial compensation and symptoms after treated mild traumatic brain injury. *J Clin Exp Neuropsychol*. 2002;24(2):187–193.

204. McKinlay WW, Brooks DN, Bond MR. Post-concussional symptoms, financial compensation and outcome of severe blunt head injury. *J Neurol Neurosurg Psychiatry*. 1983;46(12):1084–1091.

205. Ono K, Kanno M. Influences of the physical parameters on the risk to neck injuries in low impact speed rear-end collisions. *Accid Anal Prev*. 1996;28(4):493–499.

206. Viano DC, King AI, Melvin JW, et al. Injury biomechanics research: an essential element in the prevention of trauma. *J Biomech*. 1989;22(5):403–417.

207. Viano DC, Lovsund ER. Biomechanics of brain and spinal-cord injury: analysis of neuropathologic and neurophysiology experiments. *J Crash Prev Inj Control*. 1999;1(1):35–43.

208. Myer GD, Yuan W, Barber Foss KD, et al. Analysis of head impact exposure and brain microstructure response in a season-long application of a jugular vein compression collar: a prospective, neuroimaging investigation in American football. *Br J Sports Med*. 2016;50(20):1276–1285.

209. Guskiewicz KM, Mihalik JP, Shankar V, et al. Measurement of head impacts in collegiate football players: relationship between head impact biomechanics and acute clinical outcome after concussion. *Neurosurgery*. 2007;61(6):1244–1252.

210. Holbourn AHS. The mechanics of brain injuries. *Br Med Bull*. 1943;3(6):147–149.

211. Ommaya AK, Gennarelli TA. Cerebral concussion and traumatic unconsciousness. Correlation of experimental and clinical observations of blunt head injuries. *Brain*. 1974;97(4):633–654.

212. Schmidt JD, Guskiewicz KM, Blackburn JT, et al. The influence of cervical muscle characteristics on head impact biomechanics in football. *Am J Sports Med*. 2014;42(9):2056–2066.

213. Eckner JT, Oh YK, Joshi MS, et al. Effect of neck muscle strength and anticipatory cervical muscle activation on the kinematic response of the head to impulsive loads. *Am J Sports Med*. 2014;42(3):566–576.

214. Mihalik J, Guskiewicz KM, Marshall SW, et al. Does cervical muscle strength in youth ice hockey players affect head impact biomechanics? *Clin J Sport Med*. 2011;21(5):416–421.

215. Mansell J, Tierney RT, Sitler MR, et al. Resistance training and head-neck segment dynamic stabilization in male and female collegiate soccer players. *J Athl Train*. 2005;40(4):310–319.

216. Giza CC, Hovda DA. The neurometabolic cascade of concussion. *J Athl Train*. 2001;36(3):228–235.

217. Prins ML, Hales A, Reger M, et al. Repeat traumatic brain injury in the juvenile rat is associated with increased axonal injury and cognitive impairments. *Dev Neurosci*. 2010;32(5–6):510–518.

218. Barkhoudarian G, Hovda DA, Giza CC. The molecular pathophysiology of concussive brain injury. *Clin Sports Med*. 2011;30(1):33–48.

219. Johnson VE, Stewart W, Smith DH. Axonal pathology in traumatic brain injury. *Exp Neurol*. 2013;246:35–43.

220. Vagnozzi R, Signoretti S, Cristofori L, et al. Assessment of metabolic brain damage and recovery following mild traumatic brain injury: a multicentre, proton magnetic resonance spectroscopic study in concussed patients. *Brain*. 2010;133(11):3232–3242.

221. Gasparovic C, Yeo R, Mannell M, et al. Neurometabolite concentrations in gray and white matter in mild traumatic brain injury: an 1H-magnetic resonance spectroscopy study. *J Neurotrauma*. 2009;26(10):1635–1643.

222. Attwell D, Laughlin SB. An energy budget for signaling in the grey matter of the brain. *J Cereb Blood Flow Metab*. 2001;21(10):1133–1145.

223. Attwell D, Iadecola C. The neural basis of functional brain imaging signals. *Trends Neurosci*. 2002;25(12):621–625.

224. Leddy JJ, Baker JG, Kozlowski K, et al. Reliability of a graded exercise test for assessing recovery from concussion. *Clin J Sport Med*. 2011;21(2):89–94.

225. Cordingley D, Girardin R, Reimer K, et al. Graded aerobic treadmill testing in pediatric sports-related concussion: safety, clinical use, and patient outcomes. *J Neurosurg Pediatr*. 2016;25(6):693–702.

226. Jagoda AS, Bazarian JJ, Bruns JJ Jr, et al. Clinical policy: neuroimaging and decisionmaking in adult mild traumatic brain injury in the acute setting. *Ann Emerg Med*. 2008;52(6):714–748.

227. Cubon VA, Putukian M, Boyer C, et al. A diffusion tensor imaging study on the white matter skeleton in individuals with sports-related concussion. *J Neurotrauma*. 2011;28(2):189–201.

228. Grossman EJ, Jensen JH, Babb JS, et al. Thalamus and cognitive impairment in mild traumatic brain injury: a diffusional kurtosis imaging study. *J Neurotrauma*. 2012;29(13):2318–2327.

229. Grossman EJ, Jensen JH, Babb JS, et al. Cognitive impairment in mild traumatic brain injury: a longitudinal diffusional kurtosis and perfusion imaging study. *Am J Neuroradiol*. 2013;34(5):951–957.

230. Kumar R, Husain M, Gupta RK, et al. Serial changes in the white matter diffusion tensor imaging metrics in moderate traumatic brain injury and correlation with neuro-cognitive function. *J Neurotrauma*. 2009;26(4):481–495.

231. Messe A, Caplain S, Paradot G, et al. Diffusion tensor imaging and white matter lesions at the subacute stage in mild traumatic brain injury with persistent neurobehavioral impairment. *Hum Brain Mapp*. 2011;32(6):999–1011.

232. Palacios EM, Sala-Llonch R, Junque C, et al. Resting-state functional magnetic resonance imaging activity and connectivity and cognitive outcome in traumatic brain injury. *JAMA Neurol*. 2013;70(7):845–851.

233. Sharp DJ, Beckmann CF, Greenwood R, et al. Default mode network functional and structural connectivity after traumatic brain injury. *Brain*. 2011;134(Pt 8):2233–2247.

234. Zhang K, Johnson B, Gay M, et al. Default mode network in concussed individuals in response to the YMCA physical stress test. *J Neurotrauma*. 2012;29(5):756–765.

235. Morgan CD, Zuckerman SL, Lee, YM, et al. 114 Risk factors for post-concussion syndrome in an exclusively sport- related concussion group: case control study. *Neurosurgery*. 2014;1(196):88.

236. Palacios EM, Sala-Llonch R, Junque C, et al. White matter integrity related to functional working memory networks in traumatic brain injury. *Neurology*. 2012;78(12):852–860.

237. Ford JH, Giovanello KS, Guskiewicz KM. Episodic memory in former professional football players with a history of concussion: an event-related functional neuroimaging study. *J Neurotrauma*. 2013;30(20):1683–1701.

238. Echemendia RJ, Meeuwisse W, McCrory P, et al. The Sport Concussion Assessment Tool 5th Edition (SCAT5): background and rationale. *Br J Sports Med*. 2017;51(11):848–850.

239. McCrea M, Kelly JP, Kluge J, et al. Standardized assessment of concussion in football players. *Neurology*. 1997;48(3):586–588.

240. McCrea M. Standardized mental status testing on the sideline after sport-related concussion. *J Athl Train*. 2001;36(3):274–279.

241. Riemann BL, Guskiewicz KM. Effects of mild head injury on postural stability as measured through clinical balance testing. *J Athl Train*. 2000;35(1):19–25.

242. Guskiewicz KM, Ross SE, Marshall SW. Postural stability and neuropsychological deficits after concussion in collegiate athletes. *J Athl Train*. 2001;36(3):263–273.

243. Galetta KM, Brandes LE, Maki K, et al. The King-Device test and sports-related concussion: study of a rapid visual screening tool in a collegiate cohort. *J Neurol Sci*. 2011;309(1–2):34–39.

244. Galetta KM, Barrett J, Allen M, et al. The King-Device test as a determinant of head trauma and concussion in boxers and MMA fighters. *Neurology*. 2011;76(17):1456–1462.

245. Cobbs L, Hasanaj L, Amorapanth P, et al. Mobile Universal Lexicon Evaluation System (MULES) test: a new measure of rapid picture naming for concussion. *J Neurol Sci*. 2017;372:393–398.

246. Akhand O, Galetta MS, Cobbs L, et al. The new Mobile Lexicon Evaluation System (MULES): a test of rapid picture naming for concussion sized for the sidelines. *J Neurol Sci*. 2018;387:199–204.

247. Wetjen NM, Pichelmann MA, Atkinson JL. Second impact syndrome: concussion and second injury brain complications. *J Am Coll Surg*. 2010;211(4):553–557.

248. Cantu RC, Gean AD. Second-impact syndrome and a small subdural hematoma: an uncommon catastrophic result of repetitive head injury with a characteristic imaging appearance. *J Neurotrauma*. 2010;27(9):1557–1564.

249. Bey T, Ostick B. Second impact syndrome. *West J Emerg Med*. 2009;10(1):6–10.

250. Cantu RC. Second-impact syndrome. *Clin Sports Med*. 2008;17(1):37–44.

251. Harmon KG, Drezner JA, Gammons M, et al. American Medical Society for Sports Medicine position statement: Concussion in sport. *Br J Sports Med.* 2013;47(1): 15–26.

252. Broglio SP, Cantu RC, Gioia GA, et al. National Athletic Trainers' Association position statement: management of sport concussion. *J Athl Train.* 2014;49(2):245–265.

253. Majerske CW, Mihalik JP, Ren D, et al. Concussion in sports: postconcussive activity levels, symptoms, and neurocognitive performance. *J Athl Train.* 2008;43(3):265–274.

254. Brown NJ, Mannix RC, O'Brien MJ, et al. Effect of cognitive activity level on duration of post-concussion symptoms. *Pediatrics.* 2014;133(2):e299–e304.

255. Moser RS, Glatts C, Schatz P. Efficacy of immediate and delayed cognitive and physical rest for treatment of sports-related concussion. *J Pediatr.* 2012;161(5):922–926.

256. Lau BC, Kontos AP, Collins MW, et al. Which on-field signs/symptoms predict protracted recovery from sport-related concussion among high school football players? *Am J Sports Med.* 2011;39:2311–2318.

257. Jorge RE, Acion L, Burin DI, et al. Sertraline for preventing mood disorders following traumatic brain injury: a randomized clinical trial. *JAMA Psychiat.* 2016;73(10):1041–1047.

258. Ashman TA, Cantor JB, Gordon WA, et al. A randomized controlled trial of sertraline for the treatment of depression in persons with traumatic brain injury. *Arch Phys Med Rehabil.* 2009;90(5):733–740.

259. Thiagarajan P, Ciuffreda KJ, Capo-Aponte JE, et al. Oculomotor neurorehabilitation for reading in mild traumatic brain injury (mTBI): an integrative approach. *NeuroRehabilitation.* 2014;34(1):129–146.

260. Kemp S, Biswas R, Neumann V, et al. The value of melatonin for sleep disorders occurring post-head injury: a pilot RCT. *Brain Inj.* 2004;18(9):911–919.

261. Guskiewicz KM, Weaver NL, Padua DA, et al. Epidemiology of concussion in collegiate and high school football players. *Am J Sports Med.* 2000;28(5):643–650.

262. Schulz MR, Marshall SW, Mueller FO, et al. Incidence and risk factors for concussion in high school athletes, North Carolina, 1996–1999. *Am J Epidemiol.* 2004;160(10):937–944.

263. Noble JM, Hesdorffer DC. Sport-related concussions: a review of epidemiology, challenges in diagnosis, and potential risk factors. *Neuropsychol Rev.* 2013;23(4): 273–284.

264. Benson BW, Meeuwisse WH, Rizos J, et al. A prospective study of concussions among National Hockey League players during regular season games: The NHL-NHLPA Concussion Program. *CMAJ.* 2011;183(8):905–911.

265. Dams-O'Connor K, Pretz C, Billah T, et al. Global outcome trajectories after TBI among survivors and nonsurvivors: a National Institute on Disability and Rehabilitation Research Traumatic Brain Injury Model Systems Study. *J Head Trauma Rehabil.* 2015;30(4):E1–E10.

266. Keith RA, Granger CV, Hamilton BB, et al. The functional independence measure: a new tool for rehabilitation. *Adv Clin Rehabil.* 1987;1:6–18.

267. Linn RT, Blair RS, Granger CV, et al. Does the functional assessment measure (FAM) extend the functional independence measure (FIM) instrument? A rasch analysis of stroke inpatients. *J Outcome Meas.* 1999;3(4):339–359.

268. Rappaport M, Hall KM, Hopkins K, et al. Disability rating scale for severe head trauma: coma to community. *Arch Phys Med Rehabil.* 1982;63(3):118–123.

269. Hall KM, Mann N, High W, et al. Functional measures after traumatic brain injury: ceiling effects of FIM, FIM+FAM, DRS and CIQ. *J Head Trauma Rehabil.* 1996;11(5):27–39.

270. Jennett B, Bond M. Assessment of outcome after severe brain damage. *Lancet.* 1975;1(7905):480–484.

271. Teasdale GM, Pettigrew LEL, Wilson JTL, et al. Analyzing outcome of treatment of severe head injury: a review and update on advancing the use of the Glasgow Outcome Scale. *J Neurotrauma.* 1998;15(8):587–597.

272. Willer B, Rosenthal M, Kreutzer JS, et al. Assessment of community integration following rehabilitation for traumatic brain injury. *J Head Trauma Rehabil.* 1993;8(2):75–87.

273. Whiteneck G, Dijkers M, Heinemann AW, et al. Development of the participation assessment with recombined tools–objective for use with individuals with traumatic brain injury. *Arch Phys Med Rehabil.* 2011;92(4):542–551.

274. Boake C. Supervision rating scale: a measure of functional outcome from brain injury. *Arch Phys Med Rehabil.* 1996;77(8):765–772.

275. Diener E, Emmons R, Larsen J, et al. The satisfaction with life scale. *J Pers Assess.* 1985;49(1), 71–75.

276. Jackson WT, Novack TA, Dowler RN. Effective serial measurement of cognitive orientation in rehabilitation: The Orientation Log. *Arch Phys Med Rehabil.* 1998;79(6):718–720.

277. Levin HS, O'Donnell VM, Grossman RG. The Galveston Orientation and Amnesia Test. A practical scale to assess cognition after head injury. *J Nerv Ment Dis.* 1979;167(11):675–684.

278. Stuss DT, Binns MA, Carruth FG, et al. The acute period of recovery from traumatic brain injury: posttraumatic amnesia or posttraumatic confusional state? *J Neurosurg.* 1999;90(4):635–643.

279. Ellenberg JH, Levin HS, Saydjari C. Posttraumatic amnesia as a predictor of outcome after severe closed head injury. *Arch Neurol.* 1996;53(8):782–791.

280. Sherer M, Sander A, Nick TG, et al. Early cognitive status and productivity outcome after traumatic brain injury: findings from the TBI model systems. *Arch Phys Med Rehabil.* 2002;83(2):183–192.

281. Nakase-Richardson R, Yablon SA, Sherer M. Prospective comparison of acute confusion severity with duration of post-traumatic amnesia in predicting employment outcome after traumatic brain injury. *J Neurol Neurosurg Psychiatry.* 2007;78(8): 872–876.

282. Corrigan JD. Development of a scale for assessment of agitation following traumatic brain injury. *J Clin Exp Neuropsychol.* 1989;11(2):261–277.

283. Spitzer RL, Kroenke K, Williams JB. Validation and utility of a self-report version of PRIME-MD: the PHQ primary care study. Primary Care Evaluation of Mental Disorders. Patient Health Questionnaire. *JAMA.* 1999;282(18):1737–1744.

284. Kroenke, K, Spitzer RL, Williams JBW. The PHQ-9 validity of a brief depression severity measure. *J Gen Intern Med.* 2001;16(9):606–613.

285. Drake AI, Gray N, Yoder S, et al. Factors' predicting return to work following mild traumatic brain injury: a discriminant analysis. *J Head Trauma Rehabil.* 2000;15(5):1103–1112.

286. Sohlberg MM, McLaughlin KA, Pavese A, et al. Evaluation of attention process training and brain injury education in persons with acquired brain injury. *J Clin Exp Neuropsychol.* 2000;22(5):656–676.

287. Cicerone KD. Cognitive rehabilitation. In: Zasler ND, Katz DI, Zafonte RD, eds. *Brain Injury Medicine: Principles and Practice.* 2nd ed. New York: Demos Medical Publishing; 2012:1021–1032.

288. Cicerone KD, Langenbahn DM, Braden C, et al. Evidence-based cognitive rehabilitation: updated review of the literature from 2003 through 2008. *Arch Phys Med Rehabil.* 2011;92(4):519–530.

289. Cicerone KD, Dahlberg C, Malec JF, et al. Evidence-based cognitive rehabilitation: updated review of the literature from 1998 through 2002. *Arch Phys Med Rehabil.* 2005;86(8):1681–1692.

290. Cicerone KD, Dahlberg C, Kalmar K, et al. Evidence-based cognitive rehabilitation: recommendations for clinical practice. *Arch Phys Med Rehabil.* 2000;81(12): 1596–1615.

291. Schierhout G, Roberts I. Anti-epileptic drugs for preventing seizures following acute traumatic brain injury. *Cochrane Database Syst Rev.* 2001;(4):CD000173.

292. Mysiew WJ, Bogner JA, Corrigan JD, et al. The impact of acute care medications on rehabilitation outcome after traumatic brain injury. *Brain Inj.* 2006;20(9):905–911.

293. Roa N, Jellinek HM, Woolston DC. Agitation in closed head injury: haloperidol effects on rehabilitation outcome. *Arch Phys Med Rehabil.* 1985;66(1):30–34.

294. Bleiberg J, Garmoe W, Cederquist J, et al. Effects of Dexedrine on performance consistency following brain injury: a double-blind placebo crossover case-study. *Neuropsychiatry Neuropsychol Behav Neurol.* 1993;6(4):245–248.

295. Fortin MO, Rouch I, Dauphinot V, et al. Effects of anticholinergic drugs on verbal episodic memory function in the elderly: a retrospective, cross-sectional study. *Drugs Aging.* 2011;28(3):195–204.

296. Arciniegas DB, Sliver JM. Pharmacotherapy of posttraumatic cognitive impairments. *Behav Neurol.* 2006;17(1):25–42.

297. Chew E. Zafonte RD. Pharmacological management of neurobehavioral disorders following traumatic brain injury—a state-of-the-art review. *J Rehabil Res Dev.* 2009;46(6):851–879.

298. Neurobehavioral Guidelines Working Group; Warden DL, Gordon B, et al. Guidelines for the pharmacologic treatment of neurobehavioral sequelae of traumatic brain injury. *J Neurotrauma.* 2006;23(10):1468–1501.

299. Bhatnagar S, Laccarino MA, Zafonte R. Pharmacotherapy in rehabilitation of post-acute traumatic brain injury. *Brain Res.* 2016;1640(Pt A):164–1179.

300. Tateno A, Jorge RE, Robinson RG. Clinical correlates of aggressive behavior after traumatic brain injury. *J Neuropsychiatry Clin Neurosci.* 2003;15(2):155–160.

301. Baguley IJ, Cooper J, Felmingham K. Aggressive behavior following traumatic brain injury: how common is common? *J Head Trauma Rehabil.* 2006;21(1):45–56.

302. Hoffman AN, Cheng JP, Zafonte RD, et al. Administration of haloperidol and risperidone after neurobehavioral testing hinders the recovery of traumatic brain injury-induced deficits. *Life Sci.* 2008;83(17–18):602–607.

303. Larson EB, Zollman FS. The effect of sleep medications on cognitive recovery from traumatic brain injury. *J Head Trauma Rehabil.* 2010;25(1):61–67.

304. Bryczkowski SB, Lopreiato MC, Yonclas PP, et al. Risk factors for delirium in older trauma patients admitted to the surgical intensive care unit. *J Trauma Acute Care Surg.* 2014;77(6):944–951.

305. Potential benefits of reducing medication-related anticholinergic burden for demented older adults: a prospective cohort study. *Geriatr Gerontol Int.* 2013;13(3):694–700.

306. Rothberg MB, Herzig SJ, Pekow PS, et al. Association between sedating medications and delirium in older inpatients. *J Am Geriatr Soc.* 2013;61(6):923–930.

307. Ochs KL, Zell-Kanter M, Mycyk MB. Toxikon Consortium. Hot, blind, and mad: avoidable geriatric anticholinergic delirium. *Am J Emerg Med.* 2012;30(3):514. e1–514.e3.

308. Fleminger S, Greenwood RJ, Oliver DL. Pharmacological management for agitation and aggression in people with acquired brain injury. *Cochrane Database Syst Rev.* 2006;(4):CD003299.

309. Hammond FM, Bickett AK, Norton JH, et al. Effectiveness of amantadine hydrochloride in the reduction of chronic traumatic brain injury irritability and aggression. *J Head Trauma Rehabil.* 2014;29(5):391–399.

310. Chatham Showalter PE, Kimmel DN. Agitated symptom response to divalproex following acute brain injury. *J Neuropsychiatry Clin Neurosci.* 2000;12(3):395–397.

311. Teasdale G, Jennett B. Assessment of coma and impaired consciousness. A practical scale. *Lancet.* 1974;2(7872):81–84.

312. Maiti TK, Konar S, Bir S, et al. Role of apolipoprotein E polymorphism as a prognostic marker in traumatic brain injury and neurodegenerative disease: a critical review. *Neurosurg Focus.* 2015;39(5):E3.

313. Nakase-Richardson R, McNamee S, Howe LL, et al. Descriptive characteristics and rehabilitation outcomes in active duty military personnel and veterans with disorders of consciousness with combat- and noncombat-related brain injury. *Arch Phys Med Rehabil.* 2013;94(10):1861–1869.

314. Lim HB, Smith M. Systemic complications after head injury: a clinical review. *Anaesthesia*. 2007;62(5):474–482.

315. Practice parameter: antiepileptic drug treatment of posttraumatic seizures. Brain Injury Special Interest Group of the American Academy of Physical Medicine and Rehabilitation. *Arch Phys Med Rehabil*. 1998;79(5):594–597.

316. Chang BS, Lowenstein DH. Practice parameter: antiepileptic drug prophylaxis in severe traumatic brain injury: report of the Quality Standards Subcommittee of the American Academy of Neurology. *Neurology*. 2003;60(1):10–16.

317. Da Silva AM, Nunes B, Vaz AR, et al. Posttraumatic epilepsy in civilians: clinical and electroencephalographic studies. *Acta Neurochir Suppl (Wien)*. 1992;55:56–63.

318. Salazar AM, Jabbari B, Vance SC, et al. Epilepsy after penetrating head injury. I. Clinical correlates: a report of the Vietnam Head Injury Study. *Neurology*. 1985;35(10):1406–1414.

319. Cuccurullo S. *Physical Medicine and Rehabilitation Board Review*. 3rd ed. New York: Demos Medical Publishing; 2014.

320. Hauser WA, Annegers JF, Kurland LT. Prevalence of epilepsy in Rochester, Minnesota: 1940–1980. *Epilepsia*. 1991;32(4):429–445.

321. Haltiner AM, Temkin NR, Dikmen SS. Risk of seizure recurrence after the first late posttraumatic seizure. *Arch Phys Med Rehabil*. 1997;78(8):835–840.

322. Zasler, ND, Katz, DI, Zafonte RD, et al. *"Brain Injury Medicine, 2nd Edition", Principles and Practice*. New York: Demos Medical Publishing; 2012.

323. Mazzini L, Cossa FM, Angelino E, et al. Posttraumatic epilepsy: neuroradiologic and neuropsychological assessment of long-term outcome. *Epilepsia*. 2003;44(4):569–574.

324. Frey LC. Epidemiology of posttraumatic epilepsy: a critical review. *Epilepsia*. 2003;44(suppl 10):11–17.

325. Diaz-Arrastia R, Gong Y, Fair S, et al. Increased risk of late posttraumatic seizures associated with inheritance of APOE epsilon4 allele. *Arch Neurol*. 2003;60(6):818–822.

326. Annegers JF, Hauser WA, Coan SP, et al. A population-based study of seizures after traumatic brain injuries. *N Engl J Med*. 1998;338(1):20–24.

327. Temkin NR, Dikmen SS, Wilensky AJ, et al. A randomized, double-blind study of phenytoin for the prevention of post-traumatic seizures. *N Engl J Med*. 1990;323(8):497–502.

328. Schierhout G, Roberts I. Prophylactic antiepileptic agents after head injury: a systematic review. *J Neurol Neurosurg Psychiatry*. 1998;64(1):108–112.

329. Szaflarski JP, Sangha KS, Lindsell CJ, et al. Prospective, randomized, single-blinded comparative trial of intravenous levetiracetam versus phenytoin for seizure prophylaxis. *Neurocrit Care*. 2010;12(2):165–172.

330. Inaba K, Menaker J, Branco BC, et al. A prospective multicenter comparison of levetiracetam versus phenytoin for early posttraumatic seizure prophylaxis. *J Trauma Acute Care Surg*. 2013;74(3):766–771.

331. Vespa PM, Nuwer MR, Nenov V, et al. Increased incidence and impact of nonconvulsive and convulsive seizures after traumatic brain injury as detected by continuous electroencephalographic monitoring. *J Neurosurg*. 1999;91(5):750–760.

332. American Academy of Neurology, Therapeutics and Technology Assessment Subcommittee. Assessment: intensive EEG/video monitoring for epilepsy. *Neurology*. 1989;39(11):1101–1102.

333. Hudak AM, Trivedi K, Harper CR, et al. Evaluation of seizure-like episodes in survivors of moderate and severe traumatic brain injury. *J Head Trauma Rehabil*. 2004;19(4):290–295.

334. Karceski S, Morrell M, Carpenter D. The expert consensus guidelines series: treatment of epilepsy. *Epilepsy Behav*. 2001;2:A1–A50.

335. Pellock JM. Who should receive prophylactic antiepileptic drug following head injury? *Brain Inj*. 1989;3:107–108.

336. Feely M. Fortnightly review: drug treatment of epilepsy. *BMJ*. 1999;318(7176):106–109.

337. Brodie MJ, Dichter MA. Established antiepileptic drugs. *Seizure*. 1997;6(3):159–174.

338. Talati R, Scholle JM, Phung OJ, et al. *Effectiveness and Safety of Antiepileptic Medications in Patients with Epilepsy. Comparative Effectiveness Review No. 40. (Prepared by the University of Connecticut/Hartford Hospital Evidence-based Practice Center under Contract No. 20-2007-10067-I.) AHRQ Publication No. 11(12)-EHC082-EF*. Rockville, MD: Agency for Healthcare Research and Quality; 2011.

339. Randomised study of antiepileptic drug withdrawal in patients in remission. Medical Research Council Antiepileptic Drug Withdrawal Study Group. *Lancet*. 1991;337(8751):1175–1180.

340. Westover MB, Cormier J, Bianchi MT, et al. Revising the "Rule of Three" for inferring seizure freedom. *Epilepsia*. 2012;53(2):368–376.

341. Engel J, Wiebe S, French J, et al. Practice parameter: temporal lobe and localized neocortical resections for epilepsy: report of the Quality Standards Subcommittee of the American Academy of Neurology, in association with the American Epilepsy Society and the American Association of Neurological Surgeons. *Neurology*. 2003;60(4):538–547.

342. Diaz-Arrastia R, Agostini MA, Frol AB, et al. Neurophysiologic and neuroradiologic features of intractable epilepsy after traumatic brain injury in adults. *Arch Neurol*. 2000;57(11):1611–1666.

343. Fisher RS, Handforth A. Reassessment: vagus nerve stimulation for epilepsy: a report of the Therapeutics and Technology Assessment Subcommittee of the American Academy of Neurology. *Neurology*. 1999;53(4):666–669.

344. Baguley IJ, Perkes IE, Fernandez-Ortega JF, et al. Paroxysmal sympathetic hyperactivity after acquired brain injury: consensus on conceptual definition, nomenclature, and diagnostic criteria. *J Neurotrauma*. 2014;31(17):1515–1520.

345. Baguley IJ, Slewa-Younan S, Heriseanu RE, et al. The incidence of dysautonomia and its relationship with autonomic arousal following traumatic brain injury. *Brain Inj*. 2007;21(11):1175–1181.

346. Rabinstein AA. Paroxysmal sympathetic hyperactivity in the neurological intensive care unit. *Neurol Res*. 2007;29(7):680–682.

347. Baguely IJ. The excitatory:inhibitory ratio model (EIR model): an integrative explanation of acute autonomic overactivity syndromes. *Med Hypotheses*. 2008;70(1):26–35.

348. Bengtsson BA, Abs R, Bennmarker H, et al. The effects of treatment and the individual responsiveness to growth hormone (GH) replacement therapy in 665 GH-deficient adults. KIMS Study Group and the KIMS International Board. *J Clin Endocrinol Metab*. 1999;84(11):3929–3935.

349. Rabinstein AA, Benarroch EE. Treatment of paroxysmal sympathetic hyperactivity. *Curr Treat Options Neurol*. 2008;10(2):151–157.

350. Chioléro RL, Breitenstein E, Thorin D, et al. Effects of propranolol on resting metabolic rate after severe head injury. *Crit Care Med*. 1989;17(4):328–334.

351. Payen D, Quintin L, Plaisance P, et al. Head injury: clonidine decreases plasma catecholamines. *Crit Care Med*. 1990;18(4):392–395.

352. Rekate HL. A contemporary definition and classification of hydrocephalus. *Semin Pediatr Neurol*. 2009;16(1):9–15.

353. Mazzini L, Campini R, Angelino E, et al. Posttraumatic hydrocephalus: a clinical, neuroradiologic, and neuropsychologic assessment of long-term outcome. *Arch Phys Med Rehabil*. 2003;84(11):1637–1641.

354. Denes Z, Barsi P, Szel I, et al. Complication during postacute rehabilitation: patients with posttraumatic hydrocephalus. *Int J Rehabil Res*. 2011;34(3):222–226.

355. Kammersgaard LP, Linnemann M, Tibæk M. Hydrocephalus following severe traumatic brain injury in adults. Incidence, timing, and clinical predictors during rehabilitation. *NeuroRehabilitation*. 2013;33(3):473–480.

356. Long DF. Hydrocephalus. In: Zollman FS, ed. *Manual of Traumatic Brain Injury Management*. New York: Demos Medical Publishing; 2011:303–308.

357. Waziri A, Fusco D, Meyer SA, et al. Postoperative hydrocephalus in patients undergoing decompressive hemicraniectomy for ischemic or hemorrhagic stroke. *Neurosurgery*. 2007;61(3):489–493.

358. Weintraub AH, Gerber DJ, Kowalski RG. Posttraumatic hydrocephalus as a confounding influence on brain injury rehabilitation: incidence, clinical characteristics, and outcomes. *Arch Phys Med Rehabil*. 2017;98(2):312–319.

359. Barkovich AJ, Edwards MS. Applications of neuroimaging in hydrocephalus. *Pediatr Neurosurg*. 1992;18(2):65–83.

360. Marmarou A, Bergsneider M, Klinge P, et al. The value of supplemental prognostic tests for the preoperative assessment of idiopathic normal-pressure hydrocephalus. *Neurosurgery*. 2005;57(3 suppl):S17–S28.

361. Schneider HJ, Kreitschmann-Andermahr I, Ghigo E, et al. Hypothalamopituitary dysfunction following traumatic brain injury and aneurysmal subarachnoid hemorrhage: a systematic review. *JAMA*. 2007;298(12):1429–1438.

362. Mesquita J, Varela A, Medina JL. Trauma and the endocrine system. *Endocrinol Nutr*. 2010;57(10):492–499.

363. Ghigo E, Masel B, Aimaretti G, et al. Consensus guidelines on screening for hypopituitarism following traumatic brain injury. *Brain Inj*. 2005;19(9):711–724.

364. Bartter FC, Schwartz WB. The syndrome of inappropriate secretion of antidiuretic hormone. *Am J Med*. 1967;42(5):790–806.

365. Gross P. Treatment of hyponatremia. *Intern Med*. 2008;47(10):885–891.

366. Peters JP, Welt LG, Sims EA, et al. A salt-wasting syndrome associated with cerebral disease. *Trans Assoc Am Physicians*. 1950;63:57–64.

367. Maesaka JK, Imbriano LJ, Ali NM, et al. Is it cerebral or renal salt wasting? *Kidney Int*. 2009;76(9):934–938.

368. Yee AH, Burns JD, Wijdicks EFM. Cerebral salt wasting: pathophysiology, diagnosis, and treatment. *Neurosurg Clin N Am*. 2010;21:339–352.

369. Leonard J, Garrett RE, Salottolo K, et al. Cerebral salt wasting after traumatic brain injury: a review of the literature. *Scand J Trauma Resusc Emerg Med*. 2015;23:98.

370. Rahman M, Friedman WA. Hyponatremia in neurosurgical patients: clinical guidelines development. *Neurosurgery*. 2009;65(5):925–935.

371. Richardson DW, Robinson AG. Desmopressin. *Ann Intern Med*. 1985;103(2):228–239.

372. Garland DE. A clinical perspective on common forms of acquired heterotopic ossification. *Clin Orthop Relat Res*. 1991;(263):13–29.

373. Johns JS, Cifu DX, Keyser-Marcus L, et al. Impact of clinically significant heterotopic ossification on functional outcome after traumatic brain injury. *J Head Trauma Rehabil*. 1999;14(3):269–276.

374. van Kampen PJ, Martina JD, Vos PE, et al. Potential risk factors for developing heterotopic ossification in patients with severe traumatic brain injury. *J Head Trauma Rehabil*. 2011;26(5):384–391.

375. Dizdar D, Tiftik T, Kara M, et al. Risk factors for developing heterotopic ossification in patients with traumatic brain injury. *Brain Inj*. 2013;27(7–8):807–811.

376. Freed JH, Hahn H, Menter R, et al. The use of the three-phase bone scan in the early diagnosis of heterotopic ossification (HO) and in the evaluation of Didronel therapy. *Paraplegia*. 1982;20(4):208–216.

377. Mavrogenis AF, Soucacos PN, Papagelopoulos PJ. Heterotopic ossification revisited. *Orthopedics*. 2011;34(3):177.

378. Orzel JA, Rudd TG. Heterotopic bone formation: clinical, laboratory, and imaging correlation. *J Nucl Med*. 1985;26(2):125–132.

379. Subbarao JV, Garrison SJ. Heterotopic ossification: diagnosis and management, current concepts and controversies. *J Spinal Cord Med*. 1999;22(4):273–283.

380. Shehab D, Elgazzar AH, Collier BD. Heterotopic ossification. *J Nucl Med.* 2002;43(3):346–353.

381. Sumner D. Post-traumatic ageusia. *Brain.* 1967;90(1):187–202.

382. Rovit RL, Murali R. Injuries to the cranial nerves. In: Cooper PR, ed. *Head Injury.* 3rd ed. Baltimore, MD: Lippincott Williams & Wilkins; 1993:10.

383. Reiter ER, DiNardo LJ, Costanzo RM. Effects of head injury on olfaction and taste. *Otolaryngol Clin North Am.* 2004;37(6):1167–1184.

384. Kerkhoff G. Rehabilitation of visuospatial cognition and visual exploration in neglect: a cross-over study. *Restor Neurol Neurosci.* 1998;12(1):27–40.

385. Sabates NR, Gonce MA, Farris BK. Neuro-ophthalmological findings in closed head trauma. *J Clin Neuroophthalmol.* 1991;11(4):273–277.

386. Tokuno T, Nakazawa K, Yoshida S, et al. [Primary oculomotor nerve palsy due to head injury: analysis of 10 cases]. [Article in Japanese]. *No Shinkei Geka.* 1995;23(6):497–501.

387. Keane JR. Neuro-ophthalmic signs and symptoms of hysteria. *Neurology.* 1982;32(7):757–762.

388. Lagrèze WA. Neuro-ophthalmology of trauma. *Curr Opin Ophthalmol.* 1998;9(6):33–39.

389. Keane JR, Baloh RW. Posttraumatic cranial neuropathies. *Neurol Clin.* 1992;10(4):849–867.

390. Podoshin L, Fradis M. Hearing loss after head injury. *Arch Otolaryngol.* 1975;101(1):15–18.

391. Lew HL, Jerger JF, Guillory SB, et al. Auditory dysfunction in traumatic brain injury. *J Rehabil Res Dev.* 2007;44(7):921–928.

392. Gottshall K. Vestibular rehabilitation after mild traumatic brain injury with vestibular pathology. *NeuroRehabilitation.* 2011;29(2):167–171.

393. Harrison RA, Field TS. Post stroke pain: identification, assessment, and therapy. *Cerebrovasc Dis.* 2015;39(3–4):190–201.

394. Lance J. Spasticity: disorders motor control. In: Feldman RG, Young RP, Koella WP eds. *Symposium Synopsis.* Miami, FL: Year Book Medical Publishers; 1980.

395. Sunnerhagen KS, Olver J, Francisco GE. Assessing and treating functional impairment in post stroke spasticity. *Neurology.* 2013;80(3 suppl 2):S35–S44.

396. Bethoux F. Spasticity management after stroke. *Phys Med Rehabil Clin N Am.* 2015;26(4):625–639.

397. Nakao S, Takata S, Uemura H, et al. Relationship between Barthel Index scores during the acute phase of rehabilitation and subsequent ADL in stroke patients. *J Med Invest.* 2010;57:81–88.

398. Nesbitt J, Moxham S, Ramadurai G, et al. Improving pain assessment and management in stroke patients. *BMJ Qual Improv Rep.* 2015;4(1). pii: u203375.w3105.

399. Posteraro F, Calandriello B, Galli R, et al. Timing of intrathecal baclofen therapy in persons with acquired brain injury: influence on outcome. *Brain Inj.* 2013;27(13–14):1671–1675.

400. McCormick ZL, Chu SK, Binler D, et al. Intrathecal versus oral baclofen: a matched cohort study of spasticity, pain, sleep, fatigue, and quality of life. *PM R.* 2016;8(6):553–562.

401. Ada L, Goddard E, McCully J, et al. Thirty minutes of positioning reduces the development of shoulder external rotation contracture after stroke: a randomized controlled trial. *Arch Phys Med Rehabil.* 2005;86(2):230–234.

402. Tafti MA, Cramer SC, Gupta R. Orthopaedic management of the upper extremity of stroke patients. *J Am Acad Orthop Surg.* 2008;16(8):462–470.

403. Acosta JA, Yang JC, Winchell RJ, et al. Lethal injuries and time to death in a level I trauma center. *J Am Coll Surg.* 1998;186(5):528–533.

404. Geerts WH, Code KI, Jay RM, et al. A prospective study of venous thromboembolism after major trauma. *N Engl J Med.* 1994;331(24):1601–1606.

405. Ekeh AP, Dominguez KM, Markert RJ, et al. Incidence and risk factors for deep venous thrombosis after moderate and severe brain injury. *J Trauma.* 2010;68(4):912–915.

406. Kelly J, Rudd A, Lewis RR, et al. Screening for proximal deep vein thrombosis after acute ischemic stroke: a prospective study using clinical factors and plasma D-dimers. *J Thromb Haemost.* 2004;2(8):1321–1326.

407. Minshall CT, Eriksson EA, Leon SM, et al. Safety and efficacy heparin or enoxaparin prophylaxis in blunt trauma patients with a head abbreviate injury severity score >2. *J Trauma.* 2011;71(2):396–399.

408. Jamjoom AA, Jamjoom AB. Safety and efficacy of early pharmacological thromboprophylaxis in traumatic brain injury: systematic review and meta-analysis. *J Neurotrauma.* 2013;30(7):503–511.

409. Foreman PM, Schmalz PG, Griessenauer CJ. Chemoprophylaxis for venous thromboembolism in traumatic brain injury: a review and evidence-based protocol. *Clin Neurol Neurosurg.* 2014;123:109–116.

410. Engler, TM, Dourado, CC, Amâncio TG, et al. Stroke: bowel dysfunction in patients admitted for rehabilitation. *Open Nurs J.* 2014;8:43–47.

411. Camara-Lemarroy CR, Ibarra-Yruega, BE, Gongora-Rivera F. Gastrointestinal complications after ischemic stroke. *J Neurol Sci.* 2014;346(1–2):20–25.

412. Lim SF, Ong SY, Tan YL, et al. Incidence and predictors of new-onset constipation during acute hospitalisation after stroke. *Int J Clin Pract.* 2015;69(4),422–428.

413. Gelber DA, Good DC, Laven LJ, et al. Causes of urinary incontinence after acute hemispheric stroke. *Stroke.* 1993;24(3):378–382.

414. McKenzi P, Badlani GH. The incidence and etiology of overactive bladder in patients after cerebrovascular accident. *Curr Urol Rep.* 2012;13(5):402–406.

415. Ostaszkiewicz J, Johnston L, Roe B. Habit retraining for the management of urinary incontinence in adults. *Cochrane Database Syst Rev.* 2004;(1):CD002801.

416. Tânia MN, de Engler C, Thais GD. *Dressing Materials for the Treatment of Pressure Ulcers in Patients in Long-Term Care Facilities: A Review of the Comparative Clinical Effectiveness and Guidelines [Internet].* Ottawa, ON: Canadian Agency for Drugs and Technologies in Health; 2013.

417. Lee SY, Chou CL, Hsu SP, et al. Outcomes after stroke in patients with previous pressure ulcer: a nationwide matched retrospective cohort study. *J Stroke Cerebrovasc Dis.* 2016;25(1), 220–227.

418. Appelbaum PS, Grisso T. Assessing patients' capacities to consent to treatment. *N Engl J Med.* 1988;319(25):1635–1638.

CHAPTER 20

Francois A. Bethoux
Mary Alissa Willis

Multiple Sclerosis

Multiple sclerosis (MS) is a complex, multifactorial central nervous system (CNS) disease. While its diagnosis as well as the prescription and monitoring of disease-modifying therapies (DMTs) are usually handled by neurologists, the comprehensive management of the disease and its consequences requires a multidisciplinary team, including rehabilitation professionals. As MS is a chronic and often progressive disorder, the focus is not only on improving function where necessary but also on maintaining function where possible. A firm understanding of the underlying pathophysiology of the disease as well as the role and rationale of its treatment is key to the rehabilitative treatment of MS.

MS is the most common cause of nontraumatic disability affecting young adults in the Northern Hemisphere (1). Onset is usually in the 20s to 40s (2) though the onset and course vary considerably from patient to patient. Care needs change over time as a result of relapses and/or progressive impairment. A team approach to maintain and improve function is critical. The number of medications approved by the United States Food and Drug Administration (FDA) for treatment of relapsing MS has been increasing steadily, up from 6 in 2007 to 15 in 2017, and there are more in development. Despite a significant increase in the number of medications available for treatment of MS, none provides a cure or an alternative to rehabilitative approaches to MS care.

DEMOGRAPHICS AND EPIDEMIOLOGY

MS is a common disorder in North America. Prevalence varies in the United States and Canada with a range from approximately 40 to 220 per 100,000 population (3). With few exceptions, the prevalence of MS increases with increasing distance from the equator—north or south (4).

Theories to explain this distribution include vitamin D deficiency due to reduced sunlight, dairy products, genetic factors, and exposures to a variety of environmental factors (5). The prevalence of MS is higher among persons of Northern European ancestry (6) though it can occur in persons of any race or ethnicity. Infections have been linked to MS, but no one infection has emerged as a specific cause or precipitant of disease activity (7). Recent reports suggest that the incidence of MS has increased over time, although improved education and access to health care, the advent of DMTs and the refinement of diagnostic criteria have also led to better identification of the disease (8). Even though MS is not as prevalent as many other neurologic disorders, the costs associated with this lifelong disease are considerable, with the direct cost of medications being the main driver for individuals with low disability, and indirect costs due to loss of productivity and informal care being the main drivers for individuals with higher level of disability (9).

ETIOLOGY

MS is considered to be an "autoimmune" disease (10). It occurs two to three times as often in women as in men (11). While MS is not considered to be a genetic disorder, some families do share genetic factors—such as HLA-DR2—that may increase susceptibility to MS (12). The risk of concordant MS is 30% with monozygotic twins, 5% with dizygotic twins, and between 2% and 4% for first-degree family members of people with MS (13). Multiple genetic linkage studies have confirmed a linkage with the major histocompatibility region, as well as less well-defined linkages to other zones that code for interleukins (14). The role of environmental factors, in addition to genetic factors, is suggested by the fact that individuals who move to an area with a different incidence of MS tend to "acquire" the incidence of the new area, particularly when the move occurs during childhood. The specific cause of MS remains unknown.

PATHOLOGY, PATHOGENESIS, AND PATHOPHYSIOLOGY

Pathology and Pathogenesis

The hallmark of MS pathology is the presence of multifocal plaques (lesions) of demyelination in the cerebral hemispheres, optic nerves, brainstem, and spinal cord (15). The early plaque has a demarcated area of demyelination with incomplete axonal injury, inflammatory infiltrates composed of lymphocytes and macrophages, and evidence of astrocytic proliferation and gliosis (16). Ultrastructural analysis of axons has shown an early reduction in axonal fibers and axonal transections in new demyelinating regions (17).

In acute active lesions, gadolinium leaks into tissue parenchyma due to an interruption of the blood-brain barrier (BBB) that accompanies the inflammatory response (18). Perivenular lymphocytic infiltrates are evident in areas of demyelination (19). Macrophages are the most prominent inflammatory cells in the lesion, and many are filled with myelin debris (20).

With progression of the pathologic process, chronic inactive lesions are less inflammatory and become hypocellular, with relatively quiescent oligodendrocyte precursor cells (21).

Degeneration occurs, as oligodendrocytes are destroyed and astrocytes proliferate. As demyelination occurs, there can also be some degree of remyelination in the lesion (22). However, as the disease progresses, demyelination at the plaque margin takes place in the newly remyelinated areas and leads to expansion of the lesion. This eventually results in permanent scarring.

Pathophysiology of MS

The clinical symptoms of MS are often due to loss of axonal conduction. Demyelination of segments of conducting axons causes conduction block, which varies depending on the extent of demyelination and whether compensatory mechanisms have intervened. Conduction block in experimental demyelination occurs at sites of demyelination and does not occur in otherwise unaffected segments (23). The block appears to be most severe in the first few days after experimental demyelination (24). Acutely demyelinated axolemma has a relatively low sodium channel density that may be insufficient for the action potential to be propagated effectively (25).

The safety factor is a measure of the excess current allowing conduction divided by the minimum current necessary to depolarize an axon (26). In normal myelinated axons, this is usually a factor of three to five times. In demyelinated axons, this is reduced, often measured at just above one.

Small changes in environmental factors can thus cause axonal block in such fibers (reduced safety factor). This may be the basis for worsening MS symptoms with fever and with exercise, both of which may reduce the safety factor to the point where conduction block occurs.

Restoration of conduction occurs in demyelinated axons after a few days or weeks. This is likely related to the appearance of sodium channels along the demyelinated portion of the axon to allow microsaltatory conduction along these demyelinated segments, mimicking the saltatory conduction along myelinated axons but over considerably shorter distances (27). Remyelination occurs with improved conduction in previously demyelinated segments (28).

Recovery of function may be due to resolution of inflammation or the pressure of edema, removal of humoral factors, reattachment of paranodal myelin, or rerouting of nerve transmission through alternative pathways (brain plasticity) (29). Remyelination may also be a key component in the restoration phase, which usually requires days to weeks (30). Patients frequently note that with repeated activity, they develop weakness, especially with walking. In experimental demyelination, a train of stimuli over time will elicit intermittent conduction block (23). This correlates with hyperpolarization of the membrane (31).

TYPES OF MS

An international panel was convened in the late 1990s to develop a common classification of subtypes of MS (32). This classification is useful as a way to group patients and remains widely used, but more recently proposed phenotypic descriptions may define more precisely an individual patient's course (33).

Relapsing-Remitting MS

Relapsing-remitting MS (RRMS) is characterized by discrete relapses of new or worsened neurologic symptoms that emerge over a few days and may resolve over a 4- to 8-week period with or without corticosteroid treatment. "True" relapses (symptoms lasting more than 24 hours and without alternate cause) must be differentiated from "pseudorelapses," during which symptom worsening is triggered by an infection or other physiologic stress and typically resolves after the cause is treated. Patients often approach their prerelapse baseline, but most have some residual impairment, and relapses have been linked to the accumulation of disability in individuals with RRMS (34). RRMS is the most common form of MS at the time of diagnosis (35). RRMS frequently begins with optic neuritis (ON)—transient unilateral visual impairment lasting days to weeks, which may be associated with retrobulbar pain (36). Others with RRMS may initially experience tingling or weakness of a limb; paresthesias are the most common initial symptom of MS (37). In general, patients with sensory symptoms, and those whose symptoms fully remit after early exacerbations, demonstrate better long-term prognosis (37). FDA-approved medications for RRMS reduce rate of relapses, reduce measures of MRI activity, and may slow progression of disability (📶 **eTable 20-1**) (38–46).

Secondary Progressive MS

A significant proportion of RRMS patients convert to secondary progressive multiple sclerosis (SPMS) at a variable time in the course of their disease. SPMS is characterized by gradual worsening in between discrete relapses. They may generally have fewer relapses and fewer new MRI lesions than during the relapsing-remitting phase and may eventually exhibit progression without relapses. The medications for RRMS may still be useful for those patients with recent relapses or MRI change. However, in older patients who do not have continued relapse activity, the beneficial effect of these medications is less pronounced (47). Most patients with SPMS have accrued deficits such as gait disturbance and spasticity, which may benefit from rehabilitative approaches.

Primary Progressive MS

Primary progressive multiple sclerosis (PPMS) patients are often older at onset and have a progressive course without attacks. They tend to have fewer MRI lesions than do RRMS or SPMS patients. PPMS occurs in about 10% to 15% of patients with MS. PPMS tends to affect both sexes equally, unlike RRMS (48). It usually becomes clinically apparent when patients are in their 50s (49). PPMS more often starts with motor symptoms, often an asymmetric paraparesis, and tends to progress more rapidly, validating observations that patients starting with motor symptoms fare less well (vs. sensory symptoms), regardless of disease type (49).

Ocrelizumab is the only FDA-approved immunomodulating agent for PPMS (50). Like all medications used for RRMS, ocrelizumab prevents inflammation. This agent slows disability progression in some patients with PPMS but does not restore lost function.

OTHER ASSOCIATED DEMYELINATING DISORDERS

Optic Neuritis

Many patients with MS will present with ON, a sudden unilateral loss of vision, which can vary from a slight central scotoma to complete loss of light perception (36). In one long-term study of ON, 57% eventually developed MS (51). Both ON and ON/MS patients respond favorably to intravenous (IV) methylprednisolone (36). A Cochrane analysis of corticosteroid use for ON concluded that there is no evidence of a long-term benefit of high- or low-dose steroids; the improvement seen with high-dose corticosteroids in the ON trials appears to be limited to short-term outcomes (52). Data on patients with clinical isolated syndromes (CIS) such as isolated ON have shown that patients with multiple brain lesions on MRI are at higher risk of progressing to clinical MS within 1 to 2 years after presentation (53). Obtaining a brain MRI in patients with ON or other CIS is therefore an effective risk stratification methodology and potentially guides later therapy.

Transverse Myelitis

Transverse myelitis (TM) is an inflammatory disorder of the spinal cord. Some patients have rapid progression to a relatively complete spinal cord syndrome with paralysis, sensory level, and bowel and bladder involvement. Other patients have asymmetric or incomplete motor or sensory symptoms. TM may be an initial manifestation of MS, part of another immune-mediated neurologic disorder (neuromyelitis optica, neurosarcoidosis, lupus), a result of infection, or idiopathic. Up to one third of cases remain idiopathic despite extensive serologic and cerebrospinal fluid (CSF) testing. Key rehabilitation issues in TM include mobility, spasticity, bowel and bladder management, and avoiding decubitus ulceration and deep venous thrombosis during the acute illness.

Neuromyelitis Optica (Devic's Disease)

Neuromyelitis optica (NMO), or NMO spectrum disorder (NMOSD), is now recognized as a clinical entity distinct from MS. The traditional concept of NMO consists of the subacute combination of relatively severe ON and TM with sparing of the brain. The classification of NMO has undergone several revisions (54) since the identification of the NMO-IgG antibody, which targets the aquaporin-4 water channel and is positive in 70% of clinically defined NMO but is rarely positive in MS. Episodes of neurologic impairment in NMO—classically ON and TM—are typically more severe, and recovery is less complete than MS relapses. Plasma exchange is used to treat NMO relapses that do not respond to high-dose corticosteroids. The spinal cord lesions tend to be longer (three or more cord segments) than typical MS lesions in the cord (usually one segment only). CSF may show a striking pleocytosis or a neutrophilic predominance, which would be unusual for MS. Prevention of relapses requires lifelong immune suppression. It

is important to be alert for clinical and imaging features suggestive of NMO, as its prognosis and treatment do not fully overlap with those of MS, as explained above.

DIAGNOSIS OF MS

The most common presenting course for MS is relapsing symptoms affecting different neurologic structures occurring over time ("lesions distributed in time and space"). Common symptoms include fatigue, ataxia, weakness, numbness and tingling, bladder dysfunction, spasticity, cognitive problems, depression, ON, and pain. Notwithstanding multiple revisions over time, the diagnosis of MS still requires the presence of signs and symptoms separated in space and time, or the presence of progressive symptoms with appropriate paraclinical evidence of demyelination (55–57).

Diagnostic Criteria

Over the years, several sets of diagnostic criteria have been developed. In the 1960s, Schumacher et al. based the diagnosis of MS entirely on clinical findings (55). In the early 1980s, these were modified by Poser et al. to allow paraclinical data to substitute for some clinical criteria (56).

The diagnosis of MS remains primarily clinical with MRI characteristics facilitating early diagnosis (57). Characteristic MRI findings in MS include periventricular, juxtacortical, subcortical, infratentorial, and spinal cord lesions. The MRI can be used to demonstrate dissemination in space, replacing examination findings in two areas. The revised McDonald criteria allow for consistent diagnostic criteria to be applied and are helpful in epidemiologic studies as well as patient recruitment into clinical trials.

Magnetic Resonance Imaging

MRI has become the most important paraclinical tool in the diagnosis and monitoring of MS and related diseases (57–59). A variety of MRI measures have been used to analyze MS in terms of diagnosis, progression, the acute lesion, subtypes of MS, and monitoring treatment trials (59).

MRI has also been crucial in modifying our concepts of disease pathogenesis and course in MS (**Fig. 20-1**). In the 1980s,

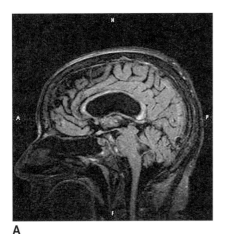
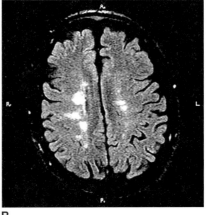
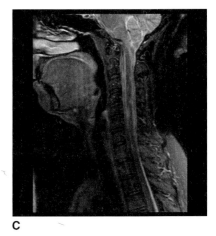

A   **B**   **C**

FIGURE 20-1. **A:** Sagittal T1-weighted image 0.93 T brain. A 57-year-old female with secondary progressive MS. Note thinning of corpus callosum. **B:** Axial T2 Flair image 1.5 T brain. A 37-year-old male with 2-year history of relapsing MS. Multiple paraventricular oval-shaped lesions. **C:** Sagittal T2 Flair 1.0 T cervical cord. A 24-year-old female with Lhermitte's sign and neurogenic bladder. Multiple single-segment or smaller lesions consistent with demyelination.

sequential MRI trials showed that new lesion formation occurs 5 to 10 times as often as there were new clinical events, altering the understanding of disease activity during clinically quiescent times (60). In addition, MRI has supported the notion of early axonal injury with MS lesions, which was first introduced based on pathologic studies. Longitudinal MRI measures of atrophy have shown slow but definite atrophy with time in patients with otherwise relapsing MS (61). Finally, MRI imaging particularly with FLAIR (fluid-attenuated inversion recovery) has shown that cortical lesions are common in MS, a fact that went unrecognized prior to these imaging techniques (62).

Conventional MRI imaging identifies MS lesions as T2 hyperintense periventricular, oval-shaped lesions, sometimes oriented perpendicularly to the ventricles. Lesions of the corpus callosum are common and extend in a fingerlike pattern, known as "Dawson's fingers" (59). With disease progression, lesions may coalesce. With more chronic and severe disease, brain atrophy becomes apparent. T1 hypointense lesions (black holes) are correlated with axonal loss in the affected areas (63).

For several weeks after the occurrence of the breakdown in the BBB, affected brain will be permeable to gadolinium. Consequently, MRIs taken shortly after the IV injection of gadolinium will show "enhancement" or opaque regions on T1-weighted images. A characteristic enhancement pattern for MS is the "open ring sign," where gadolinium enhances in an incomplete peripheral pattern, often pointing away from the lateral ventricles (64).

Other techniques that at present have a primarily research application include brain parenchymal fraction, magnetization transfer ratio, diffusion tensor imaging (DTI), and MR spectroscopy. These techniques may be most helpful in documenting axonal tract fibers loss and in predicting disability.

Evoked Potentials

Evoked potentials—visual, somatosensory, and brainstem auditory—are a method for evaluating central components of sensory pathways using summation and averaging of repeated peripheral stimulation (65). American Academy of Neurology guidelines suggested that visual evoked potentials are probably useful to identify patients at increased risk for developing clinically definite MS; somatosensory evoked potentials are possibly useful to identify patients at increased risk for developing clinically definite MS; and there is insufficient evidence to recommend brainstem evoked potentials as a useful test to identify patient at increased risk for developing clinical definite MS (66). There are no data to support repeated evoked potential testing for monitoring of ongoing disease.

Ocular Coherence Tomography

Ocular coherence tomography (OCT) is a technique that allows imaging of the retinal nerve fiber layer (RNFL) thickness (67). OCT is a sensitive, safe, and reproducible measure that allows analysis of features such as nerve fiber loss, ganglion cell loss, and macular edema. Its role in clinical trials and clinical decision-making is still being evaluated (68).

Lumbar Puncture

Lumbar puncture and CSF analysis are less often performed today, as improvements in imaging have generally replaced this invasive procedure. However, when done, identification of oligoclonal bands and increased IgG synthesis are associated with a diagnosis of MS (69). These findings indicate activity of the immune system in and around the CNS compartment and as such are not specific for MS. Other diseases such as lupus, Lyme disease, and neurosarcoidosis also may show oligoclonal banding. Studies of the diagnostic accuracy of MRI, evoked potentials, and CSF have shown that if two of three of these tests are positive, the third does not add significantly to the diagnosis (70). Neurologists are reducing the frequency of CSF tests in patients with otherwise typical MS and in whom MRI findings are characteristic. CSF studies are most useful in atypical presentations, where the MRI is nonspecific, and where other diagnoses are being considered.

Electrodiagnostic Testing

In general, there is no role for electromyography and nerve conduction testing in MS, as the peripheral nervous system is usually spared in MS. There are rare patients with central and peripheral demyelination in which these tests would be useful (71).

MEDICAL MANAGEMENT

Corticosteroids

Corticosteroids and adrenocorticotropic hormone (ACTH) have been used in MS therapy for years, well before randomized controlled trials were undertaken in MS therapy. An early randomized trial of ACTH versus placebo for exacerbations of MS showed improvements in disability scores at 4 weeks in patients treated with ACTH compared with patients treated with placebo (72). Over the past 20 years, various studies have shown a similar short-term effect of steroid therapy during exacerbations. A systematic review found a sufficient body of evidence to support the use of IV methylprednisolone in acute exacerbations of MS (73). The usual place for IV steroids is for acute exacerbations that cause functional deficits. The use of steroids has to be balanced against the considerable long-term risks, which include occasional anaphylaxis against IV methylprednisolone, osteoporosis, cataracts, aseptic necrosis of the hips or shoulders, and diabetes mellitus.

Disease-Modifying Therapies

Fifteen medications are FDA approved for treating relapsing forms of MS, and more medications are in development (**Table 20-1**). The early medications—interferon beta (IFN-β) and glatiramer acetate—are injectable agents with modest efficacy in preventing relapses and MRI changes (74–78).

Although oral medications are now available, these latter two medications remain widely used due to their safety profiles. Common side effects of the interferons include flulike symptoms following the injections (74–76). Patients with spasticity may experience a worsening in spasticity after the injections. Skin injection site reactions are the most common side effect with glatiramer acetate (77,78). An idiosyncratic reaction with chest tightness and shortness of breath lasting a few minutes occurs in 1/3,000 injections.

Three oral medications are available. Fingolimod is a sphingosine-1-phosphate receptor modulator approved in 2010. The first dose of this once-daily medication is associated with a transient decrease in heart rate (79). Dimethyl fumarate is a

TABLE 20-1	Disease-Modifying Therapies for Relapsing MS		
Agent	**Year Approved in the US**	**Route**	**Dosing Frequency**
Interferon beta-1b (Betaseron/Extavia)	1993/2009	SC	Every other day
Interferon beta-1a (Avonex)	1996	IM	Weekly
Glatiramer acetate (Copaxone)	1996	SC	Daily
(Copaxone 40)	2014	SC	3 times per week
(Glatopa)	2015	SC	Daily
Interferon beta-1a (Rebif)	2000	SC	3 times per week
Pegylated interferon beta-1a (Plegridy)	2014	SC	Every 2 wk
Fingolimod (Gilenya)	2010	PO	Daily
Dimethyl fumarate (Tecfidera)	2013	PO	Twice daily
Teriflunomide (Aubagio)	2012	PO	Daily
Mitoxantrone (Novantrone)	2000	IV	Every 3 mo
Natalizumab (Tysabri)	2004	IV	Every 4 wk
Daclizumab[a] (Zinbryta)	2016	SC	Monthly
Alemtuzumab (Lemtrada)	2014	IV	Annually
Ocrelizumab (Ocrevus)	2017	IV	Days 1 and 15 then every 6 mo

[a]Voluntarily withdrawn from the market in 2018.

SC, subcutaneous; IM, intramuscular; PO, oral; IV, intravenous.

twice-daily oral agent approved in 2013. Common side effects include gastrointestinal symptoms and flushing (80). The efficacy of fingolimod and dimethyl fumarate is similar with both showing reduced rate of relapses and MRI change compared to interferon (79,80). Teriflunomide is a once-daily pill that inhibits an enzyme required for pyrimidine synthesis. Like the interferons and glatiramer, this medication has modest efficacy (81). Side effects of teriflunomide include diarrhea and hair thinning.

Mitoxantrone is an intravenous agent with limited use due to risk for decreased cardiac function and treatment-related leukemia (82). Natalizumab, which is given as a monthly IV injection, has potent efficacy with a reduction in relapse frequency by approximately 70% and reduction in MRI new gadolinium-enhancing lesions at year 2 by 92% when compared to placebo (83). Use of this medication is also limited by potential for a serious complication: progressive multifocal leukoencephalopathy (PML). While often not fatal, PML related to natalizumab use results in neurologic deficits in addition to those present from MS (84).

More recently approved therapies include a monthly injection and two IV therapies.

Daclizumab, an interleukin-2 receptor blocker given as monthly subcutaneous injections, appears to have similar efficacy to the oral agents (85). This agent was voluntarily withdrawn in March 2018 due to safety concerns. Alemtuzumab is a highly effective agent given as an initial course of two annual infusions—5 days in year 1 and 3 days in year 2 (86). Use of this medication is limited by risk for development of secondary autoimmune conditions, and monthly labs must be strictly monitored. Ocrelizumab has been approved for both relapsing and PPMS. This humanized anti-CD20 monoclonal antibody is administered every 6 months after an initial series of two biweekly infusions (87). Mild infusion reactions are common. Long-term safety—including risk for breast cancer—remains to be determined.

The approach to using a DMT varies among neurologists and must be individualized for each patient. DMT should be started early in the disease course (88). Relapses or new MRI lesions after 6 months of therapy may indicate breakthrough disease provided the patient is compliant with medication. Breakthrough disease or failure of DMT may increase the risk for disability. Thus, a change in therapy is often considered.

REHABILITATION

Rehabilitation is an important component of the management of patients with MS. An expert opinion paper published by the National MS Society summarized general recommendations for the use of rehabilitation in MS (89). In practice, rehabilitation professionals are faced with serious challenges when attempting to apply rehabilitative interventions to MS patients.

MS is overall a progressive neurologic disease, which does not follow the traditional model of rehabilitation, with the notable exception of severe disease exacerbations. The best timing for rehabilitation interventions is not well defined. Too often, patients are referred late, when impairments are fixed and opportunities for functional improvement are limited. Payors usually allow a small number of therapy sessions every year when many MS patients have ongoing needs, and demonstration of progress is required to continue therapy, when preventing functional loss is essential in reducing the individual and societal costs of the disease.

Variability and unpredictability make it difficult to apply standard rehabilitation protocols in MS. Clinical presentations are highly heterogeneous, and intricate impairments are an obstacle to functional compensation. Symptoms and functional performance vary over time, even within the course of a day, but not always with a consistent pattern, giving a feeling of "trying to hit a moving target." Furthermore, transient worsening of MS symptoms is frequently encountered with exertion and may compromise patient adherence to therapy sessions and home exercise programs. Finally, it is not uncommon to note a discrepancy between patient complaints and clinical findings (e.g., high level of concern with mild observed deficits, or apparent lack of insight or awareness of significant physical or cognitive limitations), which may impact goal setting and outcomes.

Evidence Supporting the Use of Rehabilitation in MS

In the expert opinion paper cited above, the National MS Society acknowledged a need for stronger evidence to support treatment recommendations. Recently, the Guideline Development, Dissemination, and Implementation Subcommittee of the American Academy of Neurology published a review of the evidence on rehabilitation in MS (90). The authors found evidence suggesting the effectiveness of multidisciplinary outpatient rehabilitation, outpatient or home physical therapy, inpatient exercise followed by home exercise, balance training, and respiratory rehabilitation. The need for well-designed trials of rehabilitation interventions was emphasized. In a review of systematic reviews on rehabilitation in MS, Khan and Amatya reported strong evidence for improvement of activity and participation with physical therapy and for improvement of patient-reported fatigue with exercise-based educational programs (91). In one meta-analysis, there was a small but significant improvement of walking outcomes with physiotherapy compared with usual care (92). In summary, the body of evidence regarding the effects of rehabilitation in MS is rapidly growing, although well-designed clinical trials with long-term follow-up are needed to refine clinical care.

Neuroplasticity

There is emerging evidence suggesting that some of the effects of rehabilitation are mediated by CNS plasticity. Cerebral functional reorganization as a result of CNS damage from MS has been demonstrated. Compared to healthy controls, individuals with MS generally demonstrate increased activation in relation to a specific task (including the recruitment of areas not usually activated in healthy controls) while activation is decreased in other areas, suggesting adaptive reorganization (93). Alterations of white matter microstructure have also been demonstrated on DTI, with decreased fractional anisotropy and increased transverse diffusivity. Despite the widespread damage caused by MS, functional reorganization and improvement in white matter microstructure were demonstrated after motor rehabilitation (94,95) and cognitive training (96).

Exercise Training

Deconditioning has been identified as a significant contributing factor to fatigue in MS (97). The benefits of aerobic and resistance exercise training on fitness, activity level, subjective fatigue, and perceived health status have been demonstrated in randomized controlled studies (98). A recent meta-analysis showed a small but statistically significant improvement of walking performance (speed and endurance) with various modalities of exercise training (99). Current recommendations for exercise in individuals with MS and moderate disability include 30 minutes of aerobic exercise, and strength training for major muscle groups, at least twice per week (ideally not on the same day to avoid overexertion) (100). In practice, it is often difficult for patients to initiate a sustainable exercise routine without the guidance of a rehabilitation professional, to find the appropriate type, intensity, and duration of exercises, and to encourage the patient through a usually difficult initial period for the first few weeks. Short intensive activity and exercise programs, such as the CAN DO Multiple Sclerosis program, are also an option.

Recovery After Exacerbations

Even when treated with high-dose corticosteroids, MS exacerbations often leave patients with residual impairments. In fact, exacerbations have been identified as the main cause of accrual of disability in relapsing forms of the disease (34). Inpatient or outpatient multidisciplinary rehabilitation may also enhance functional recovery (101), physical activity, and self-efficacy (102).

Rehabilitation of Chronic Disability

Several controlled trials showed objective and/or subjective benefits from multidisciplinary inpatient or outpatient rehabilitation, mostly in patients with a progressive disease course (103). However, the carryover of these benefits after the end of the rehabilitation program varies. There is no definitive evidence to support an effect of exercise or rehabilitation on disease progression (104).

Disease-Specific Outcome Measures for MS Rehabilitation

Generic outcome measures used in rehabilitation, such as the Barthel Index and the Functional Independence Measure (FIM), can be applied to MS patients. However, these measures do not cover important aspects of the disease (e.g., fatigue, visual disturbance), lack sensitivity to small but significant changes over time, or exhibit a ceiling effect (particularly with regard to cognitive disability). Many disease-specific instruments, although often not developed and validated in a rehabilitation setting, can be useful in clinical practice and in research studies (🛜 **eTable 20-1**).

SYMPTOM MANAGEMENT

MS is a condition that leads to multiple symptoms affecting function and well-being. The management of these chronic symptoms often includes nonpharmacologic treatments, including lifestyle modifications and rehabilitation interventions.

Heat Intolerance

Worsening or recurrence of preexisting neurologic symptoms with heat (from a hot environment or from elevated body temperature) is a very common phenomenon and was even used to support the diagnosis of MS in the past (105). Reduced safety factor for neurologic transmission due to demyelinated or partially demyelinated axons is a likely mechanism (see Pathophysiology). Heat intolerance can limit a patient's potential to participate in rehabilitation and exercise. Adjusting air or water temperature, using fans, cooling vests, or heat extraction units, and the medical recommendation of air-conditioning units in the home, are all practical and valid management tools, although high-level evidence for the effectiveness of cooling equipment was found to be lacking (89).

Transient Neurologic Events

Transient neurologic events (TNEs) constitute a common but underrecognized problem in MS. TNEs were reported in one series in as many as 20% of patients (106) and consist of stereotyped, brief (seconds), frequent (up to hundreds of times a day) events involving neurologic symptomatology. Dystonic posturing of a limb, weakness, visual disturbances, dysarthria, abnormal sensations, and muscle spasm can all be seen, often in combination. These events are often not reported by patients without direct questioning, as they do not conform to the general pattern for a relapse of MS. They are likely due to ephaptic transmission between adjacent demyelinated fibers and are not a cortically based seizure phenomenon. They sometimes occur over a period of weeks and resolve and may represent a new demyelinating event. If needed, treatment with low-dose antiepileptic medication can be effective (e.g., carbamazepine, topiramate).

Spasticity

Spasticity (defined as a velocity-dependent increase in stretch reflexes (107)) and decreased motor performance (paresis, loss of dexterity), both of which are components of the upper motor neuron syndrome, frequently coexist in MS patients, and represent a major source of disability (see Chapter 40). Spasticity in MS is usually considered of spinal origin, although features of cerebral origin spasticity are also encountered.

In a recently published survey of over 10,000 participants in the North American Consortium of MS (NARCOMS) Patient Registry, over 80% of the participants reported experiencing spasticity-related symptoms, and over one third were moderately or greatly bothered by these symptoms. More severe spasticity was associated with worse disability and mobility (108). Even though outcome measures and interventions used in other CNS conditions can all be applied to MS patients, evaluating and treating spasticity in MS can be challenging. Furthermore, side effects from symptomatic therapies (particularly sedation and weakness) can make it difficult to reach effective doses. Clinical practice guidelines for the management of spasticity in MS have been developed based on a review of the literature and expert consensus (109).

Overall, there is limited published evidence to support the efficacy of most antispasticity agents in MS, and there are methodologic concerns with most studies (110). Some of the treatments are used off-label for this indication. Controlled clinical trials have demonstrated the efficacy of oral baclofen (111), tizanidine (112), gabapentin (113), benzodiazepines (114), and dantrolene sodium (115) in patients with MS. The benefits usually consisted of symptom relief (e.g., stiffness, spasms, spasticity-related pain), decreased resistance to passive movement, and improved range of motion. Objective functional benefits (e.g., on ambulation), however, were either not assessed or not found. Increased weakness, and sometimes functional deterioration, were reported with baclofen and benzodiazepines (114), but these occurred less frequently with tizanidine (112). Reports of liver toxicity with some of these agents (particularly dantrolene and tizanidine) must be kept in mind, particularly when patients are on potentially hepatotoxic DMTs, such as IFN-β, azathioprine, cyclophosphamide, and mitoxantrone. Levetiracetam was reported to be helpful with phasic phenomena associated with spasticity (116).

Cannabinoids have been recently introduced in the management of MS-related spasticity. An endocannabinoid modulator administered as an oromucosal spray (delta-9-tetrahydrocannabinol [THC]/cannabidiol [CBD], nabiximols) is approved in some European countries and in Canada for moderate to severe MS-related spasticity resistant to other treatments, based on the results of several large clinical trials (117). The most consistent benefits from this medication were demonstrated on patient-reported spasticity using the spasticity numeric rating scale (118).

Dizziness and fatigue were the most commonly reported side effects in clinical trials and observational studies. Long-term safety remains unclear (119).

Chemodenervation with botulinum toxin (BT) can be used to treat focal spasticity, or diffuse spasticity with focal problems (120). Unfortunately, large clinical trials of BT were mainly focused on poststroke spasticity, but the authors of a recent literature review concluded that the efficacy and safety of BT appears comparable in MS-related spasticity (121). However, criteria for patient selection and dosing algorithms need to be more carefully studied in the context of MS. The same applies to chemical neurolysis with phenol or alcohol, another local treatment.

Intrathecal baclofen (ITB) therapy is the most frequently used surgical treatment for spasticity in MS. There is a fairly large body of evidence regarding its efficacy, side effects, and complications, although most of the evidence is derived from uncontrolled observational studies (122). However, the risk of inducing weakness is significant, and for this reason, ITB therapy has been used mostly in nonambulatory MS patients with severe lower extremity spasms and contractures. The benefits of ITB in this patient group include relief of discomfort and pain related to spasticity, enhanced ease of care, improved posture, and improved ability to transfer (122). ITB can also be utilized in ambulatory MS patients without causing loss of function (123). Benefits in this patient group include not only relief of spasticity-related symptoms and objective reduction of hypertonia but also subjective improvement of function and quality of life (124) and objective improvement of gait parameters (125). Opiates and clonidine have also been used intrathecally to treat intractable pain and spasticity in MS, alone or more frequently in combination with baclofen (126).

Weakness

Decreased voluntary motor output in the extremities and axial muscles can be observed with or without spasticity. Multiple factors may account for the observed weakness, including decreased motor control from the CNS, immobility and deconditioning, spasticity, chronic elongation of muscles due to positioning, heat, and fatigue. Increased weakness with effort is thought to be related to nerve conduction blocks in the CNS but could also be related to muscle fatigue with impaired muscle excitability and metabolism (127). In addition, other symptoms such as pain or cognitive impairment may inhibit motor performance.

Fluctuations in motor performance are the hallmark of MS, which complicate testing and treatment planning. In addition to muscle testing, or handheld dynamometry (128), functional testing is essential, and in a busy clinical practice may consist of simple tests such as the Timed 25-Foot Walk or the Nine-Hole Peg Test. Motor fatigue can be evaluated with tests of walking endurance, such as the 6-minute (129) or 2-minute (130) walk tests.

There are few interventions aimed directly at muscle weakness. Improvement of muscle strength has been reported after aerobic and progressive resistance training (131). These exercise programs must be highly customized to the specific limitations of MS patients, particularly in terms of intensity and duration of exercises. Since the increase in body temperature due to physical activity is thought to be at least in part responsible for motor fatigue, pre-exercise cooling may improve performance and increase the benefits of exercise (132). Treatments for spasticity may improve muscle strength output by reducing the cocontraction of antagonist muscle groups, particularly when administered as local injections. In the context of an exacerbation of MS, high-dose steroids may enhance muscle strength as they hasten neurologic recovery.

4-Aminopyridine (4-AP) is a potassium channel blocker, which facilitates conduction in demyelinated axons. An extended release form of 4-AP is approved by the FDA (Ampyra, dalfampridine-extended release [dalfampridine-ER]) to improve walking in patients with MS, based on significant improvement in walking speed in two phase III clinical trials. Beneficial effects on lower extremity muscle strength were also noted (133). The rate of patients responding to the drug in the trials (based on sustained improvement of walking speed) was 35% and 43%.

Dalfampridine-ER is administered at the dose of one 10-mg tablet twice daily (approximately 12 hours apart), with or without food. A history of seizure and moderate or severe renal impairment are contraindications to this medication. Side effects occurring at a rate greater than 2% and more frequent with the drug compared to placebo were urinary tract infection, insomnia, dizziness, headache, nausea, asthenia, back pain, balance disorder, MS relapse, paresthesia, nasopharyngitis, constipation, dyspepsia, and pharyngolaryngeal pain. The risk of seizure (in the absence of history of seizure) is low at the recommended dose. Long-term open-label safety studies showed the same safety profile (134).

Assistive devices and orthoses, in addition to their benefits in terms of safety, help compensate for weakness by reducing the energetic demands of activities and by replacing the action of weak muscles. The hip flexion assist device (HFAD) was developed as an active device to aid hip flexion during walking. The HFAD consists of a proximal waist attachment, a medial and a lateral dynamic tension band, and a distal connector that attaches to the shoelaces. All the components are adjustable. An uncontrolled pilot study of the HFAD in 21 ambulatory MS patients showed significant improvement in pain, walking speed, walking endurance, as well as muscle strength in the "affected" leg (135).

Functional electrical stimulation (FES) is another way to compensate for a lack of strength output in an active manner, by causing the contraction of select muscles to enhance function. Several FES devices for foot drop (e.g., Odstock Dropped Foot Stimulator [ODFS], NDI Medical, Cleveland, OH [USA]; NESS L300, Bioness Inc., Valencia, CA [USA]; WalkAide, Innovative Neurotronics, Austin, TX [USA]) are currently used in MS patients. Published evidence shows improved walking speed with FES for foot drop in individuals with MS (136). Recently, an implanted FES device for foot drop has been introduced (137).

Fatigue

Fatigue is one of the most common symptoms of MS and was associated with limited activity in 78% of patients in one survey (138). Fatigue is a subjective symptom defined as "lack of physical and/or mental energy, which is perceived by the individual or caregiver as interfering with usual and desired activities" (97). In general, the magnitude of perceived fatigue does not correlate well with decline in observed motor or cognitive performance, which is usually called fatigability (139). Primary MS fatigue may be a direct effect of immunologic activity in the brain, similar to the fatigue associated with viral illness (140). In addition, functional MRI studies have shown that MS patients activate more brain areas than able-bodied healthy controls to perform the same task, and some studies suggest that this phenomenon correlates with fatigue (93). Fatigue in MS does not seem to correlate with common brain MRI measures of disease burden or atrophy (141). Perceived fatigue does correlate with depression, which also contributes to fatigue (142). Fatigue measurement scales (e.g., Fatigue Severity Scale and Modified Fatigue Impact scale) are useful to track outcomes (143).

Clinical practice guidelines for the evaluation and management of fatigue in MS are available (97). A thorough baseline assessment is essential, both to characterize the symptom and to detect treatable secondary causes or contributing factors such as medications, poor sleep, depression, infection, and thyroid dysfunction. Behavior modifications are an essential component of fatigue management and include strategies to optimize energy utilization throughout the day (timing of activities, rest periods and naps, and use of assistive devices to decrease the energetic cost of activities) and exercise (144). Self-management programs focused on behavior modification have been proposed (145). The symptomatic medications for MS fatigue are generally used off-label and mainly include amantadine and modafinil. While some studies suggest that these medications improve MS fatigue, results are inconsistent and meta-analyses suggest that rehabilitation-oriented strategies are more effective than pharmacologic treatments (146). Alternative treatments such as yoga (147) or mindfulness training (148) may also be helpful.

Bladder Dysfunction

Bladder dysfunction affects up to 90% of MS patients and correlates with disease severity and disability, but not always with disease duration (149) (see Chapter 22). Urinary symptoms affect daily activities, employment, social life, and quality of life in general (150). Furthermore, urinary tract infections, usually secondary to urinary retention, can cause worsening of MS symptoms and increased disease activity.

Although there are wide variations in the reported prevalence and incidence of urinary symptoms in MS, urgency and frequency are consistently noted as the most frequent, followed by incontinence, hesitancy, and retention (151). While the presence of urinary symptoms is highly correlated with abnormal test results, bladder dysfunction can be found in the absence of complaints. Workup for neurogenic bladder dysfunction usually includes urinalysis and urine culture, postvoiding residual (PVR) volume measurement, and urodynamic testing. A renal ultrasound and other upper urinary tract imaging studies may be ordered, particularly in patients with detrusor-sphincter dyssynergia (DSD) or indwelling catheter, but upper urinary tract complications are relatively rare in MS compared to other neurologic conditions (149).

Education and behavior modifications, with teaching of "bladder hygiene" (e.g., adequate fluid intake; avoiding bladder stimulants such as caffeine, aspartame, and alcohol), are often helpful in reducing urinary symptoms, particularly those related to detrusor overactivity. Other management options include pelvic exercises (152), medications, catheters (preferably intermittent catheterization [IC], sometimes indwelling catheter), and less frequently surgical interventions.

Detrusor overactivity, the most common bladder function disorder in MS, is often treated with anticholinergic medications, such as hyoscyamine, oxybutynin, tolterodine, solifenacin, trospium, darifenacin, mirabegron, or fesoterodine, although they have not all been well studied in MS (153). Common side effects of antimuscarinics constitute the main limitation to the use of these medications and may be less severe with extended-release formulations (154). Desmopressin acetate (DDAVP) nasal spray or tablet may be useful in reducing nocturia and enuresis in MS patients (155). BT-A injections in the detrusor muscle were shown to be effective on urinary incontinence due to detrusor overactivity with a median time of 42 weeks before repeat injections, although they may cause temporary urinary retention requiring IC (156). Positive results have been reported with sacral neuromodulation in carefully selected MS patients (157). Surgical treatment options are considered when conservative management failed and include augmentation cystoplasty (in most cases with an abdominal catheterizable stoma) and sacral denervation.

DSD consists of sphincter contraction coinciding with detrusor contraction, leading to incomplete bladder emptying. DSD often occurs in combination with detrusor hyperreflexia; therefore, it is recommended to measure the PVR before initiating treatment with anticholinergics in patients who experience urgency and incontinence but do not already perform IC. Impaired bladder emptying (due to DSD or to detrusor underactivity) can be treated with alpha blockers such as terazosin or tamsulosin, although there have been contradictory reports on their efficacy (153). Bethanechol is usually not considered effective in MS. There are anecdotal reports of the efficacy of BT injections into the sphincter in MS patients with urinary retention. A randomized placebo-controlled trial failed to show a significant change in PVR after a single injection of BT-A in the sphincter, although voiding volume and detrusor pressures were significantly improved (158). Sphincterotomy or the placement of a urethral stent can be performed, for example when IC is not feasible, but requires adequate detrusor contractility to be fully effective. IC is the most common treatment for detrusor hypocontractility. Surgical interventions for urinary retention include the placement of a suprapubic catheter, which may be easier to manage than an indwelling Foley catheter, and incontinent urinary diversion.

Bowel Dysfunction

Bowel dysfunction, although common in MS, has been less studied than bladder dysfunction. Clinical management recommendations have been recently published (159). Constipation is the most commonly reported symptom of bowel dysfunction in MS, followed by fecal urgency and incontinence (160). The pathophysiology of neurogenic

bowel dysfunction in MS is not fully elucidated, although it is thought to be mainly related to spinal cord involvement (161). There are many factors contributing to bowel dysfunction, including immobility, inadequate diet and fluid intake, and side effects of medications. Patient and caregiver education is key to a successful bowel management program. In addition to remediating the factors listed above, fiber supplements, bulk-forming agents, and stool softeners are often helpful and may be supplemented with suppositories and enemas. Anticholinergic medications may help with fecal urgency and incontinence.

Sexual Dysfunction

Sexual dysfunction is frequent in MS patients, who often wish to remain sexually active (162). Sexual dysfunction was found to be correlated with lesion burden in the brain (163). While the primary effects of MS on the CNS are thought to be the main cause of sexual dysfunction, secondary and tertiary consequences of MS, including concomitant neurologic symptoms (fatigue, decreased sensation, spasticity), depression, and marital relationship problems, often contribute to sexual dysfunction. Men report primarily erectile dysfunction (ED), as well as decreased libido, ejaculation or orgasmic dysfunction, and impaired genital sensation. Common complaints in women include decreased desire, decreased lubrication, orgasmic dysfunction, dyspareunia, and decreased vaginal sensation (164). A thorough interview (including validated questionnaires) and examination, including the evaluation of perineal sensation, and in women pelvic examination, guide treatment planning. Paraclinical testing is not often performed.

Education and counseling are useful in both sexes, as a good relationship is key to intimacy. Phosphodiesterase-5 inhibitors (sildenafil, vardenafil, tadalafil) are often prescribed for the treatment of male ED. Other, less often used approaches include vibratory stimulation, vacuum pumps, papaverine or prostaglandin E1 injections, and implanted penile prostheses.

Pharmacologic treatment options for female sexual dysfunction are more limited due to a lack of evidence. A small double-blind trial of sildenafil in women with MS showed a significant improvement of vaginal lubrication (165). The management of other contributing symptoms, vibratory stimulation, and adequate sexual positioning can be helpful.

Tremor

Tremor, the most common movement disorder in MS (after spasticity), is often associated with ataxia and may include rest, postural, and action components ("rubral tremor") (166). Tremor is most commonly reported in the upper extremities. The pathophysiology of this very debilitating symptom is not completely elucidated, although the role of the thalamus has been more extensively studied. Tremor severity and the outcome of interventions have often been measured with Fahn's Tremor Rating Scale. Rehabilitation interventions include the use of assistive devices and technologies and wrist weights (which can be difficult to use if weakness and fatigability are present). Pharmacologic treatments are often disappointing, although some positive results were reported with isoniazid, glutethimide, primidone, levetiracetam, carbamazepine, oral tetrahydrocannabinol, clonazepam, and propranolol. Thalamotomy and deep brain stimulation have been used in

MS patients with severe tremor (167). Overall, the use of these surgical techniques remains limited in MS. Evidence regarding their efficacy is limited and mostly consists of case reports and case series using various assessment tools. Long-term outcomes have been less often studied and appear modest.

Pain

The old saying "MS doesn't cause pain" is contradicted by clinical experience and numerous publications (see Chapter 39). Up to 81% of MS patients experience pain at some time in the course of their disease (168). Pain is often multifactorial and multifaceted in MS. It is sometimes thought to be a direct consequence of the disease process, such as neuropathic pain and pain related to inflammation and upper motor neuron damage. Musculoskeletal pain and headaches are also common.

Neuropathic Pain

Central neuropathic pain is frequently encountered in MS (169). It may present as dysesthesia, allodynia, and/or neuralgia and is often associated with other sensory disturbances. Partial TM can be associated with a painful band sensation around the trunk, sometimes called the "MS hug." Chronic dysesthetic pain is often described as burning, but patients are sometimes at a loss when trying to characterize their pain. The pain is thought to originate from lesions in the CNS. Anticonvulsants and antidepressants (tricyclic and selective serotonin reuptake inhibitors [SSRIs]) are commonly used to treat neuropathic pain in MS, despite limited evidence to demonstrate their efficacy in this population. Duloxetine was found to be effective on central neuropathic pain in two recent small clinical trials (170). The potential side effects of these medications, particularly sedation, should not be overlooked (171). The use of opioids is increasingly controversial due to lack of definitive evidence and to the potential for misuse (172). Cannabis and cannabinoids may be effective in reducing central pain in MS (119).

Trigeminal neuralgia is experienced by up to 15% of MS patients in the course of their disease, usually involving the second and third divisions of the trigeminal nerve, and may precede the diagnosis in some patients (173). This syndrome is believed to arise from ephaptic transmission of nerve conduction, which occurs with demyelination in the area around the trigeminal nerve entry zone. Carbamazepine and other anticonvulsants are usually effective. When the pain is refractory to oral medications, treatment options include glycerol injections, balloon ablation of the trigeminal nerve, and radiofrequency thermal or surgical rhizotomy.

Pain Related to Upper Motor Neuron Damage

Spasticity can be associated with pain. Nocturnal painful spasms have been described in MS. These are defined as transient painful extensor or flexor spasms of the legs, lasting seconds to minutes, often occurring at night, and referred to by many patients as "Charley horses." These may significantly interfere with sleep and increase daytime fatigue. An open-label trial of gabapentin at night showed that 20 of 22 patients experienced reduction in their nocturnal painful spasms with an acceptable side effect profile (174). Cannabinoids may also be helpful with painful spasms (119).

Pain Related to Inflammation

Retro- and periorbital pain, aggravated or triggered by eye movement, often occurs in the context of ON and usually improves with corticosteroid treatment. Retro-orbital pain without visual disturbance is of unclear significance and may respond to steroidal or nonsteroidal anti-inflammatory agents.

Musculoskeletal Pain

Back, neck, and upper and lower extremity pain of musculoskeletal origin are commonly encountered in the general population and as a consequence may occur concomitant to MS, particularly as a result of aging. This issue should not be neglected because it represents a source of added disability, discomfort, and medical complications. Indeed, MS and its treatments increase the risk of musculoskeletal problems. For example, abnormal posture and body mechanics as a result of weakness, spasticity, and/or loss of coordination may cause excessive joint stress. Falls related to neurologic impairments can cause fractures and other injuries.

Corticosteroid treatments increase the risk of aseptic necrosis of the femoral head and in combination with immobility are a risk factor for osteoporosis and subsequent complications. Even if the diagnosis of musculoskeletal problems is straightforward, confusion may arise when it is combined with other types of pain, or when several etiologies are possible. For example, radicular pain can arise from demyelination as well as nerve root compression. When in doubt, additional testing and referral to a musculoskeletal specialist are helpful.

Headache

Headache is a common complaint among MS patients and was more commonly reported by MS patients than by healthy controls in several studies (175). Migraine and tension-type headaches are the most commonly reported types of headache by MS patients, although a pathophysiologic link has not been fully demonstrated. Focal facial pain syndromes (e.g., trigeminal neuralgia) and retro-orbital pain, particularly with eye movements, are more specifically encountered in MS. Since MS patients often take multiple medications, headache might be related to drug side effects. The management of migraine and tension-type headaches in MS is generally not different from the general population.

Visual Impairment

Visual disturbance occurs in a little over one fourth of all MS patients and often fluctuates, similar to other MS symptoms, making it more difficult for the patient to adapt. Unfortunately, there is no treatment for the residual visual loss after ON. Even when visual acuity is satisfactory, contrast sensitivity and color perception may be impaired. Night driving may be compromised. Patients should undergo yearly eye examination surveillance for conditions amenable to treatment or correction. The use of steroids may increase the risk of developing cataracts, and uveitis is encountered in 1% of patients with definite MS. Large-print reading materials and computer-based magnification systems may be helpful in patients with severe visual compromise. Patients with photophobia will benefit from the use of sunglasses. Corrective surgery is rarely recommended in MS patients with diplopia. Alternative interventions include the use of an eye patch and prisms. Oscillopsia sometimes responds to anticonvulsants or baclofen (176).

Depression

Depression, common in patients with MS, is considered both a symptom of MS and a comorbidity. A large population survey of 739 MS patients in King County, Washington, found the point prevalence of significant depressive symptoms to be 41.8% (177). An increased risk of suicide was reported in the MS population (178), although more recent publications find no increase in suicide risk (179). The causality of depression in MS is multifactorial and includes CNS damage, immunologic and hormonal dysfunction, MS symptom burden, medication side effects, and psychosocial factors (180). The risk of depression may be increased with IFN therapy, although supporting evidence was found to be of questionable methodologic quality (181). Depression often contributes to fatigue and perceived cognitive difficulties. A symptomatic triad of fatigue, pain, and depression has been identified in MS and other neurologic disorders, due to the frequent co-occurrence of these symptoms. The overlap between some of the somatic manifestations of depression and MS symptoms may affect scores on some depression severity scales. Monitoring for the presence of depression as well as a proactive approach to its treatment is crucial. In an evidence-based guideline published by the American Academy of Neurology in 2014, no recommendations were made regarding pharmacologic or nonpharmacologic interventions for depression, due to insufficient evidence (182). A placebo-controlled randomized clinical trial of paroxetine for major depression in MS patients showed no significant effect (183). Nevertheless, antidepressant medications are widely used. Some antidepressants are considered "energizing" (e.g., paroxetine, bupropion) and may be of interest in the presence of severe fatigue. Nonpharmacologic interventions include psychotherapy and counseling and cognitive behavioral therapy. Exercise may have short-term beneficial effects on mood. Depression is thought to be underdiagnosed and undertreated in MS, although recent reports suggest that a larger percentage of depressed MS patients receive treatment (184).

Cognitive Impairment

Cognitive impairment represents a significant problem in persons with MS. Comprehensive neuropsychological (NP) testing suggests that over 40% of MS patients show cognitive impairment to at least some degree (185). Common complaints include forgetfulness, decreased attention/concentration, difficulty with multitasking, and "cognitive fatigue." While some patients will exhibit obvious cognitive deficits and may meet the diagnostic criteria for dementia, in many cases, the standard interview and testing during a routine visit will not detect significant abnormalities. Comprehensive NP testing typically demonstrates selective deficits in attention, information-processing speed, working memory, verbal and visuospatial memory, and executive functions (186).

Recently, the Brief International Cognitive Assessment for Multiple Sclerosis (BICAMS) was validated in several countries (187). The BICAMS takes up to 15 minutes and does not require neuropsychological training to administer. Single tests such as the Paced Auditory Serial Addition Test and the Symbol Digit Modalities Test have been suggested as screening tools and outcome measures in clinical trials. Self-report measures of perceived cognitive difficulties were found to correlate better with depression and fatigue scores than with performance on neuropsychological testing (188).

The pathophysiology of cognitive deficits in MS is not fully elucidated, although advanced imaging techniques (e.g., fMRI, DTI) have led to the identification of structural and functional correlates to cognitive impairment (96).

The management of cognitive impairment often starts with educating (and often reassuring) the patient about their specific deficits and addressing contributing factors, such as depression, fatigue, heat intolerance, and medications. Sleep disorders, particularly obstructive sleep apnea, should not be overlooked. Rehabilitation interventions traditionally rely on the use of compensatory strategies (e.g., pacing, memory aides) and environmental adaptations. There is an emerging literature on cognitive training in MS (189). Acetylcholinesterase inhibitors used to treat Alzheimer's disease (e.g., donepezil, memantine), although not FDA approved in MS, may be helpful (190).

Speech and Swallowing Problems

More than one in five MS patients reports problems with speech or communication (191) (see Chapter 13). Dysarthria, decreased voice intensity, cognitive impairments, fatigue, and depression may all contribute to decreased communication. Language disorders have been described in MS, although at least some of them appear to be related to deficits in executive functions (192).

Dysphagia is also relatively frequent and may range from intermittent mild problems to chronic aspiration requiring percutaneous endoscopic gastrostomy (PEG) tube placement.

SOCIAL, VOCATIONAL, AND FINANCIAL MANAGEMENT

Similar to many chronic conditions, MS affects the interaction between the patient and the outside world (193). Caregiver burden has been reported in MS, with female caregivers (or care partners) reporting a higher level of burden and increased psychological concerns, while male caregivers report more physical concerns (194). Caregiver burden is increased by the presence of psychiatric and cognitive impairments (195). Some characteristics of MS complicate management: the disease is typically diagnosed in early adulthood, when the patients are still in the process of building their personal and professional life; the evolution of the disease is unpredictable and symptoms fluctuate, making it difficult for the patient to adjust and plan ahead; DMTs are expensive, and even with health insurance, an increasing portion of the cost is left to the patient; and functional limitations often result from a combination of impairments and subjective symptoms, which may not be fully ascertained by a standard neurologic examination. Even if maintaining employment is desirable for social, psychological, and financial reasons, the worsening of MS symptoms with stress at work, the difficulty of getting reasonable accommodations in the workplace, and the negative impact of fatigue from work on family and leisure activities may force the patient to stop working and apply for disability benefits (196).

WELLNESS

Patients with MS develop the same pathologies that afflict the general population, and the impact of comorbidities on disability has been recently highlighted in several publications (197). In addition, MS (and sometimes treatments for MS) may increase the risk for secondary medical issues, which in turn may have an impact on MS symptoms. For example, urinary tract infections due to neurogenic bladder often cause a worsening of MS symptoms; decreased mobility causes osteoporosis and increases the risk of obesity. However, individuals with MS may have a tendency to neglect systematic screening for common health problems because they are focused on managing MS and its consequences. At a more advanced stage of the disease, physical disability may represent an obstacle to accessing primary care services (198). It is essential that MS patients see a primary care physician on a regular basis and be referred to the appropriate specialty when needed. Also, basic wellness recommendations (e.g., diet, exercise) can help improve general health and decrease the severity of MS symptoms (199).

CONCLUSION

MS is a complex, long-term, unpredictable, functionally and emotionally taxing disease. It is arguably one of the most difficult neurologic diseases to manage. The number of choices for DMTs have greatly increased, and some of the newer therapies may cause severe complications. While decisions regarding DMTs are made between the patient and a neurologist, rehabilitation professionals often have more frequent contact with patients and may become aware of changes in neurologic status suggesting disease worsening, or of potential side effects or complications, and communication of these concerns to the neurology treating team is essential.

Rehabilitation is still underutilized in MS, and MS rehabilitation is not as well-defined as spinal cord injury or stroke rehabilitation. However, a growing body of evidence shows that rehabilitation interventions can improve function and reduce symptom severity. While rehabilitation is still not considered to have a direct impact on the disease process, it can address indirect consequences of MS (such as loss of strength and endurance due to deconditioning) and help with the management of comorbidities that have been linked to higher levels of disability (e.g., musculoskeletal and cardiovascular comorbidity). The principles commonly used for disease management can and should be applied to symptom management and rehabilitation: diagnose (or identify the problem), start appropriate treatment early, and monitor and adjust the treatment strategy over time.

REFERENCES

1. Goodkin D. Treatment of progressive forms of multiple sclerosis. In: Burks J, Johnson KP, eds. *Multiple Sclerosis: Diagnosis, Medical Management, and Rehabilitation*. New York: Demos Medical Publishing; 2000:177–192.
2. Amato MP, Ponziani G. A prospective study on the prognosis of multiple sclerosis. *Neurol Sci*. 2000;21(suppl):831–838.
3. Kurtzke JF, Wallin M. Epidemiology. In: Burks J, Johnson KP, eds. *Multiple Sclerosis: Diagnosis, Medical Management, and Rehabilitation*. New York: Demos Medical Publishing; 2000:49–71.
4. Riise T, Wolfson C. The epidemiologic study of exogenous factors in the etiology of multiple sclerosis. *Neurology*. 1997;49(suppl 2):S1–S82.
5. Marrie RA. Environmental risk factors in multiple sclerosis aetiology. *Lancet Neurol*. 2004;3:709–718.
6. Baranzini SE, Oksenberg JR, Hauser SL. New insights into the genetics of multiple sclerosis. *J Rehabil Res Dev*. 2002;39(2):201–209.
7. Bach JF. The effect of infections on susceptibility to autoimmune and allergic diseases. *N Engl J Med*. 2002;347(12):911–920.
8. Grytten N, Torkildsen Ø, Myhr KM. Time trends in the incidence and prevalence of multiple sclerosis in Norway during eight decades. *Acta Neurol Scand*. 2015;132(199):29–36.
9. Ernstsson O, Gyllensten H, Alexanderson K, et al. Cost of illness of multiple sclerosis—a systematic review. *PLoS One*. 2016;11(7):e0159129.
10. Sørensen TL, Ransohoff RM. Etiology and pathogenesis of multiple sclerosis. *Semin Neurol*. 1998;18(3):287–294.
11. Weinshenker BG, Bass B, Rice GP, et al. The natural history of multiple sclerosis: a geographically based study. 1. Clinical course and disability. *Brain*. 1989;112: 133–146.
12. Barcellos LF, Oksenberg JR, Green AJ, et al. Genetic basis for clinical expression in multiple sclerosis. *Brain*. 2002;125(pt 1):150–158.
13. Sadovnick AS, Ebers GC, Dyment DA, et al. The Canadian Collaborative Study Group. Evidence for genetic basis of multiple sclerosis. *Lancet*. 1996;347: 1728–1730.
14. Marrosu MG. Susceptibility to multiple sclerosis: the role of interleukin genes. *Lancet Neurol*. 2007;6:846–847.
15. Lassman H, Wekerle H. The pathology of multiple sclerosis. In: Compston A, et al., eds. *McAlpines Multiple Sclerosis*. 4th ed. Philadelphia, PA: Churchill Livingston; 2005.
16. Barnett MH, Prineas JW. Relapsing and remitting multiple sclerosis: pathology of the newly formed lesion. *Ann Neurol*. 2004;55:458–468.
17. Trapp BD, Ransohoff R, Rudick R. Axonal pathology in multiple sclerosis: relationship to neurologic disability. *Curr Opin Neurol*. 1999;12:295–302.
18. McLean BN, Zeman AZ, Barned D, et al. Patterns of blood brain barrier impairment and clinical features in multiple sclerosis. *J Neurol Neurosurg Psychiatry*. 1993;56:356–360.
19. Adams CW, Poston RN, Buk SJ, et al. Inflammatory vasculitis in multiple sclerosis. *J Neurol Sci*. 1985;69:269–283.
20. Brück W, Sommermeier N, Bergmann M, et al. Macrophages in multiple sclerosis. *Immunobiology*. 1996;195(4–5):588–600.
21. Wolswijk G. Chronic stage multiple sclerosis lesions contain a relatively quiescent population of oligodendrocyte precursor cells. *J Neurosci*. 1998;18:601–609.
22. Hommes OR. Remyelination in human CNS lesions. *Prog Brain Res*. 1980;53: 39–63.
23. McDonald WI, Sears TA. Effect of demyelination on conduction in the central nervous system. *Nature*. 1969;221:182–183.
24. Waxman SG, Ritchie JM. Molecular dissection of the myelinated axon. *Ann Neurol*. 1993;33:121–136.
25. Utzschneider DA, Thio C, Sontheimer H, et al. Action potential conduction and sodium channel content in the optic nerve of the myelin-deficient rat. *Proc R Soc Lond*. 1993;B254:2–50.
26. Rushton WAH. Initiation of the propagated disturbance. *Proc R Soc Lond*. 1937;B124:210–243.
27. Novakovic SD, Deerinck TJ, Levinson SR, et al. Clusters of axonal Na+ channels adjacent to remyelinating Schwann cells. *J Neurocytol*. 1996;25:403–412.
28. Prineas JW, Barnard RO, Kwon EE. Multiple sclerosis: remyelination of nascent lesions. *Ann Neurol*. 1993;33:137–151.
29. Reddy H, Narayanan S, Matthews PM, et al. Relating axonal injury to functional recovery in multiple sclerosis. *Neurology*. 2000;54:236.
30. Ludwin SK. An autoradiographic study of cellular proliferation in remyelination of the central nervous system. *Am J Pathol*. 1979;95:683–696.
31. Bostock H, Grafe P. Activity-dependent excitability changes in normal and demyelinated rat spinal root axons. *J Physiol (Lond)*. 1985;365:239–257.
32. Lublin FD, Reingold SC. Defining the clinical course of multiple sclerosis: results of an international survey. *Neurology*. 1996;46:907–911.
33. Lublin FD, Reingold SC, Cohen JA, et al. Defining the clinical course of multiple sclerosis: the 2013 revisions. *Neurology*. 2014;83:278–286.
34. Lublin FD, Baier M, Cutter G. Effect of relapses on development of residual deficit in multiple sclerosis. *Neurology*. 2003;61(11):1528–1532.
35. Weinshenker BG. Natural history of multiple sclerosis. *Ann Neurol*. 1994;36(S1):S6–S11.
36. Beck R, Cleary P, Anderson MJ, et al. A randomized, controlled trial of corticosteroids in the treatment of acute optic neuritis. *N Engl J Med*. 1992;326(9):581–598.
37. Myhr KM, Riise T, Vedeler C, et al. Disability and prognosis in multiple sclerosis demographic and clinical variables important for the ability to walk and the awarding of disability pension. *Mult Scler*. 2001;7:59–65.
38. Solari A, Amato M, Bergamaschi R, et al. Accuracy of self-assessment of the minimal record of disability in patients with multiple sclerosis. *Acta Neurol Scand*. 1993;87:43–46.
39. Fischer J, Rudick R, Cutter G, et al. The multiple sclerosis functional composite measure (MSFC): an integrated approach to MS clinical outcome assessment. *Mult Scler*. 1999;5:244–250.
40. Syndulko K, Tourtelotte WW, Baumhefner RW, et al. Neuroperformance evaluation of multiple sclerosis disease progression in a clinical trial: implications for neurological outcomes. *J Neurol Rehabil*. 1993;7:153–176.
41. Sipe JC, Knobler RL, Braheny SL, et al. A neurologic rating scale (NRS) for use in multiple sclerosis. *Neurology*. 1984;34(10):1368–1372.
42. Hauser SL, Dawson DM, Lehrich JR, et al. Intensive immunosuppression in progressive multiple sclerosis: a randomized, three-arm study of high-dose intravenous cyclophosphamide, plasma exchange, and ACTH. *N Engl J Med*. 1983;308:173–180.
43. Hobart J, Lamping D, Fitzpatrick R, et al. The Multiple Sclerosis Impact Scale (MSIS-29): a new patient-based outcome measure. *Brain*. 2001;124:962–973.
44. Hobart JC, Riazi A, Lamping DL, et al. Measuring the impact of MS on walking ability: the 12-Item MS Walking Scale (MSWS-12). *Neurology*. 2003;60:31–36.
45. Vickrey BG, Hays RD, Harooni R, et al. A health-related quality of life measure for multiple sclerosis. *Qual Life Res*. 1995;4:187–206.

46. Ritvo PG, Fisher JS, Miller DM, et al. *Multiple Sclerosis Quality of Life Inventory: A Users Manual.* New York: National Multiple Sclerosis Society; 1997.
47. Willis MA, Fox RJ. Progressive multiple sclerosis. *Continuum.* 2016;22:785–798.
48. McDonnell GV, Hawkins SA. Clinical study of primary progressive multiple sclerosis in Northern Ireland, UK. *J Neurol Neurosurg Psychiatry.* 1998;64(4):451–454.
49. Thompson AJ, Polman CH, Milleret DH, et al. Primary progressive multiple sclerosis. *Brain.* 1997;120:1085–1096.
50. Montalban X, Hauser SL, Kappos L, et al. Ocrelizumab versus placebo in primary progressive multiple sclerosis. *N Engl J Med.* 2017;376:209–220.
51. Francis DA, Compston DA, Batchelor JR, et al. A reassessment of the risk of multiple sclerosis developing in patients with optic neuritis after extended follow-up. *J Neurol Neurosurg Psychiatry.* 1987;50(6):758–765.
52. Vedula SS, Bordney-Foise S, Gal RL, et al. Corticosteroids for treating optic neuritis. *Cochrane Database Syst Rev.* 2007;(1):CD001430.
53. O'Riordan JI, Thompson AJ, Kingsley DP, et al. The prognostic value of brain MRI in clinically isolated syndromes of the CNS. A 10-year follow-up. *Brain.* 1998;121:495–503.
54. Wingerchuk DM, Banwell B, Bennett JL, et al. International consensus diagnostic criteria for neuromyelitis optica spectrum disorders. *Neurology.* 2015;85:177–189.
55. Schumacher G, Beebe G, Kibler R. Problems of experimental trials of therapy in multiple sclerosis: report by the panel on the evaluation of experimental trials of therapy in multiple sclerosis. *Ann N Y Acad Sci.* 1965;122:552–568.
56. Poser CM, Paty DW, Scheinberg L, et al. New diagnostic criteria for multiple sclerosis: guidelines for research protocols. *Ann Neurol.* 1983;13(3):227–231.
57. Thompson AJ, Banwell BL, Barkhof F, et al. Diagnosis of multiple sclerosis: 2017 revisions of the McDonald criteria. *Lancet Neurol.* 2018;17(2):162–173.
58. Filippi M, Tortorella C, Rovaris M. Magnetic resonance imaging of multiple sclerosis. *J Neuroimaging.* 2002;12:289–301.
59. Fazekas F, Barkhof F, Filippi M, et al. The contribution of magnetic resonance imaging to the diagnosis of multiple sclerosis. *Neurology.* 1999;53(3):448–456.
60. Harris JO, Frank JA, Patronas N, et al. Serial gadolinium-enhanced magnetic resonance imaging scans in patients with early, relapsing-remitting multiple sclerosis: implications for clinical trials and natural history. *Ann Neurol.* 1991;29:548–555.
61. Chard DT, Griffin CM, Parker GJ, et al. Brain atrophy in clinically early relapsing-remitting multiple sclerosis. *Brain.* 2002;125(pt 2):327–337.
62. Calabrese M, De Stefano N, Atzori M, et al. Detection of cortical inflammatory lesions by double inversion recovery magnetic resonance imaging in patients with multiple sclerosis. *Arch Neurol.* 2007;10:1416–2422.
63. Bagnato F, Jeffries N, Richert ND, et al. Evolution of T1 black holes in patients with multiple sclerosis imaged monthly for 4 years. *Brain.* 2003;126:1782–1789.
64. Masdeu JC, Quinto C, Olivera C, et al. Open-ring imaging sign: highly specific for atypical brain demyelination. *Neurology.* 2000;54:1427–1433.
65. Matthews WB, Small DG. Serial recordings of visual and somatosensory evoked potentials in multiple sclerosis. *J Neurol Sci.* 1979;40:11–21.
66. Gronseth GS, Ashman EJ. Practice parameter: the usefulness of evoked potentials in identifying clinically silent lesions in patients with suspected multiple sclerosis (an evidence- based review). Report of the Quality Standards Subcommittee of the American Academy of Neurology. *Neurology.* 2000;54:1720–1725.
67. Chen J, Lee L. Clinical applications and new developments of optical coherence tomography: an evidence-based review. *Clin Exp Optom.* 2007;90:317–335.
68. Frohman E, Costello F, Zivadinov R, et al. Optical coherence tomography in multiple sclerosis. *Lancet Neurol.* 2006;5:853–863.
69. Massaro AR, Tonali P. Cerebrospinal fluid markers in multiple sclerosis: an overview. *Mult Scler.* 1998;4(1):1–4.
70. O'Connor P; Canadian Multiple Sclerosis Working Group. Key issues in the diagnosis and treatment of multiple sclerosis: an overview. *Neurology.* 2002;59(6 suppl 3):S1–S33.
71. Pollock M, Calder C, Allpress S. Acute combined central and peripheral inflammatory demyelination. *J Neurol Neurosurg Psychiatry.* 2004;75:1784–1786.
72. Rose A, Kuzma J, Kurtzke JF, et al. Cooperative study in the evaluation of therapy in multiple sclerosis: ACTH vs. placebo. Final report. *Neurology.* 1970;20(5):1–59.
73. Filippini G, Brusaferri F, Sibley WA, et al. Corticosteroids or ACTH for acute exacerbations in multiple sclerosis. *Cochrane Database Syst Rev.* 2000;(4):CD001331.
74. Paty DW, Li DK. Interferon beta-1b is effective in relapsing-remitting multiple sclerosis. II. MRI analysis results of a multicenter, randomized, double-blind, placebo-controlled trial. UBC MS/MRI Study Group and the IFNB Multiple Sclerosis Study Group. *Neurology.* 1993;43(4):662–667.
75. Jacobs LD, Cookfair DL, Rudick RA, et al. Intramuscular interferon beta-1a for disease progression in relapsing multiple sclerosis. The Multiple Sclerosis Collaborative Research Group (MSCRG). *Ann Neurol.* 1996;39(3):285–294.
76. PRISMS (Prevention of Relapses and Disability by Interferon beta-1a Subcutaneously in Multiple Sclerosis) Study Group. Randomised double-blind placebo-controlled study of interferon beta-1a in relapsing/remitting multiple sclerosis. *Lancet.* 1998;352(9139):1498–1504.
77. Johnson KP, Brooks BR, Cohen JA, et al. The Copolymer 1 Multiple Sclerosis Study Group. Copolymer 1 reduces relapse rate and improves disability in relapsing-remitting multiple sclerosis: results of a phase III multicenter, double-blind placebo-controlled trial. *Neurology.* 1995;45(7):1268–1276.
78. Conmi G, Filippi M, Wolinsky JS. European/Canadian multicenter, double-blind, randomized, placebo-controlled study of the effects of glatiramer acetate on magnetic resonance imaging-measured disease activity and burden in patients with relapsing multiple sclerosis. European/Canadian Glatiramer Acetate Study Group. *Ann Neurol.* 2001;49(3):290–297.
79. Cohen JA, Barkhof F, Comi G, et al. Oral fingolimod or intramuscular interferon for relapsing multiple sclerosis. *N Engl J Med.* 2010;362:402–415.
80. Fox RJ, Miller DH, Phillips JT, et al. Placebo-controlled phase 3 study of oral BG-12 or glatiramer in multiple sclerosis. *N Engl J Med.* 2012;367:1087–1097.
81. O'Connor P, Wolinsky JS, Confavreux C, et al. Randomized trial of oral teriflunomide for relapsing multiple sclerosis. *N Engl J Med.* 2011;365:1293–1303.
82. Martinelli Boneschi F, Vacchi L, Rovaris M, et al. Mitoxantrone for multiple sclerosis. *Cochrane Database Syst Rev.* 2013;(5):CD002127.
83. Miller DH, Khan OA, Sheremata WA, et al. A controlled trial of natalizumab for relapsing multiple sclerosis. *N Engl J Med.* 2003;348(1):15–23.
84. Bloomgren G, Richman S, Hotermans C, et al. Risk of natalizumab-associated progressive multifocal leukoencephalopathy. *N Engl J Med.* 2012;366:1870–1880.
85. Kappos L, Wiendl H, Selmaj K, et al. Daclizumab HYP versus interferon beta-1a in relapsing multiple sclerosis. *N Engl J Med.* 2015;373:1418–1428.
86. Coles AJ, Twyman CL, Arnold DL, et al. Alemtuzumab for patients with relapsing multiple sclerosis after disease-modifying therapy: a randomised controlled phase 3 trial. *Lancet.* 2012;380:1829–1839.
87. Hauser SL, Bar-Or A, Comi G, et al. Ocrelizumab versus interferon beta-1a in relapsing multiple sclerosis. *N Engl J Med.* 2017;376:221–234.
88. National Clinical Advisory Board of the National Multiple Sclerosis Society. Disease management consensus statement. 2008. Available from: http://www.nationalmssociety.org/PRC
89. Medical Advisory Board of the National Multiple Sclerosis Society. *Rehabilitation: Recommendations for Persons with Multiple Sclerosis.* New York: National Multiple Sclerosis Society; 2005:10.
90. Haselkorn JK, Hughes C, Rae-Grant A, et al. Summary of comprehensive systematic review: rehabilitation in multiple sclerosis: report of the Guideline Development, Dissemination, and Implementation Subcommittee of the American Academy of Neurology. *Neurology.* 2015;85(21):1896–1903.
91. Khan F, Amatya B. Rehabilitation in multiple sclerosis: a systematic review of systematic reviews. *Arch Phys Med Rehabil.* 2017;98(2):353–367.
92. Learmonth YC, Ensari I, Motl RW. Physiotherapy and walking outcomes in adults with multiple sclerosis: systematic review and meta-analysis. *Phys Ther Rev.* 2016;21(3-6):160–172.
93. Rocca MA, Filippi M. Functional MRI in multiple sclerosis. *J Neuroimaging.* 2007;17(suppl 1):36S–41S.
94. Bonzano L, Tacchino A, Brichetto G. Upper limb motor rehabilitation impacts white matter microstructure in multiple sclerosis. *Neuroimage.* 2014;90:107–116.
95. Rasova K, Prochazkova M, Tintera J, et al. Motor programme activating therapy influences adaptive brain functions in multiple sclerosis: clinical and MRI study. *Int J Rehabil Res.* 2015;38(1):49–54.
96. Chiaravalloti ND, Genova HM, DeLuca J. Cognitive rehabilitation in multiple sclerosis: the role of plasticity. *Front Neurol.* 2015;6:67.
97. MS Council for Clinical Practice Guidelines. *Fatigue and Multiple Sclerosis: Evidence Based Management Strategies for Fatigue in Multiple Sclerosis.* Washington, DC: Paralyzed Veterans of America; 1998:33.
98. Mostert S, Kesselring J. Effects of a short-term exercise training program on aerobic fitness, fatigue, health perception and activity level of subjects with multiple sclerosis. *Mult Scler.* 2002;8(2):161–168.
99. Pearson M, Dieberg G, Smart N. Exercise as a therapy for improvement of walking ability in adults with multiple sclerosis: a meta-analysis. *Arch Phys Med Rehabil.* 2015;96(7):1339.e7–1348.e7.
100. Latimer-Cheung AE, Pilutti LA, Hicks AL, et al. Effects of exercise training on fitness, mobility, fatigue, and health-related quality of life among adults with multiple sclerosis: a systematic review to inform guideline development. *Arch Phys Med Rehabil.* 2013;94(9):1800.e3–1828.e3.
101. Asano M, Raszewski R, Finlayson M. Rehabilitation interventions for the management of multiple sclerosis relapse: a short scoping review. *Int J MS Care.* 2014;16(2):99–104.
102. Nedeljkovic U, Dackovic J, Tepavcevic DK, et al. Multidisciplinary rehabilitation and steroids in the management of multiple sclerosis relapses: a randomized controlled trial. *Arch Med Sci.* 2016;12(2):380–389.
103. Campbell E, Coulter EH, Mattison PG, et al. Physiotherapy rehabilitation for people with progressive multiple sclerosis: a systematic review. *Arch Phys Med Rehabil.* 2016;97(1):141.e3–151.e3.
104. Dalgas U, Stenager E. Exercise and disease progression in multiple sclerosis: can exercise slow down the progression of multiple sclerosis? *Ther Adv Neurol Disord.* 2012;5(2):81–95.
105. Berger JR, Sheremata WA. Persistent neurological deficit precipitated by hot bath test in multiple sclerosis. *JAMA.* 1983;249(13):1751–1753.
106. Rae-Grant AD, Eckert NJ, Bartz S, et al. Sensory symptoms of multiple sclerosis: a hidden reservoir of morbidity. *Mult Scler.* 1999;5:179–183.
107. Lance J. Symposium synopsis. In: Feldman RG, Young RR, Koella WP, eds. *Spasticity: Disordered Motor Control.* Chicago, IL: Year Book Medical Publishers; 1980:485–494.
108. Bethoux F, Marrie RA. A cross-sectional study of the impact of spasticity on daily activities in multiple sclerosis. *Patient.* 2016;9(6):537–546.
109. Multiple Sclerosis Council for Clinical Practice Guidelines. *Spasticity Management in Multiple Sclerosis.* Consortium of Multiple Sclerosis Centers; 2003.
110. Shakespeare DT, Boggild M, Young C. Anti-spasticity agents for multiple sclerosis. *Cochrane Database Syst Rev* 2003;(4):CD001332.
111. Orsnes G, Sorensen P, Larsen T, et al. Effect of baclofen on gait in spastic MS patients. *Acta Neurol Scand.* 2000;101:244–248.

112. The United Kingdom Tizanidine Study Group. A double-blind placebo-controlled trial of tizanidine in the treatment of spasticity caused by multiple sclerosis. *Neurology.* 1994;44:70–79.

113. Cutter N, Scott D, Johnson J, et al. Gabapentin effect of spasticity in multiple sclerosis: a placebo-controlled, randomized trial. *Arch Phys Med Rehabil.* 2000;81:164–169.

114. From A, Heltberg A. A double-blind trial with baclofen and diazepam in spasticity due to multiple sclerosis. *Acta Neurol Scand.* 1975;51:158–166.

115. Gelenberg A, Poskanzer D. The effect of dantrolene sodium on spasticity in multiple sclerosis. *Neurology.* 1973;23:1313–1315.

116. Hawker K, Frohman E, Racke M. Levetiracetam for phasic spasticity in multiple sclerosis. *Arch Neurol.* 2003;60:1172–1174.

117. Zettl UK, Rommer P, Hipp P, et al. Evidence for the efficacy and effectiveness of THC- CBD oromucosal spray in symptom management of patients with spasticity due to multiple sclerosis. *Ther Adv Neurol Disord.* 2016;9:9–30.

118. Patti F, Messina S, Solaro C. Efficacy and safety of cannabinoid oromucosal spray for multiple sclerosis spasticity. *J Neurol Neurosurg Psychiatry.* 2016;87:944–951.

119. Koppel BS, Brust JC, Fife T, et al. Systematic review: efficacy and safety of medical marijuana in selected neurologic disorders: report of the Guideline Development Subcommittee of the American Academy of Neurology. *Neurology.* 2014;82(17):1556–1563.

120. Simpson DM, Hallet M, Ashman EJ, et al. Practice guideline update summary: botulinum neurotoxin for the treatment of blepharospasm, cervical dystonia, adult spasticity, and headache: report of the Guideline Development Subcommittee of the American Academy of Neurology. *Neurology.* 2016;86:1818–1826.

121. Dressler D, Bhidayasiri R, Bohlega S, et al. Botulinum toxin therapy for treatment of spasticity in multiple sclerosis: review and recommendations of the IAB-Interdisciplinary Working Group for Movement Disorders task force. *J Neurol.* 2017;264(1):112–120.

122. Stempien L, Tsai T. Intrathecal baclofen pump use for spasticity. *Am J Phys Med Rehabil.* 2000;79:536–541.

123. Lee BS, Jones J, Lang M, et al. Early outcomes after intrathecal baclofen therapy in ambulatory multiple sclerosis patients. *J Neurosurg.* 2018;129:1056–1062.

124. Stough D, Bethoux F. Satisfaction and outcomes one and six months after intrathecal baclofen pump placement in ambulatory multiple sclerosis patients. *Arch Phys Med Rehabil.* 2005;86(10):E13.

125. Bethoux F, Sutliff M, Stough D. Effect of intrathecal baclofen therapy on gait performance in ambulatory multiple sclerosis patients. *Arch Phys Med Rehabil.* 2005;86(10):E20.

126. Delehanty L, Sadiq S. Use of combination intrathecal baclofen and morphine in MS patients with intractable pain and spasticity. *Neurology.* 2001;56:A99.

127. Sharma KR, Kent-Braun J, Mynhier MA, et al. Evidence of an abnormal intramuscular component of fatigue in MS. *Muscle Nerve.* 1995;18:1403–1411.

128. Newsome SD, Wang JI, Kang JY, et al. Quantitative measures detect sensory and motor impairments in multiple sclerosis. *J Neurol Sci.* 2011;305(1-2):103–111.

129. Goldman MD, Marrie RA, Cohen JA. Evaluation of the six-minute walk in multiple sclerosis subjects and healthy controls. *Mult Scler.* 2008;14(3):383–390.

130. Gijbels D, Eijnde BO, Feys P. Comparison of the 2- and 6-minute walk test in multiple sclerosis. *Mult Scler.* 2011;17(10):1269–1272.

131. Platta ME, Ensari I, Motl RW, et al. Effect of exercise training on fitness in multiple sclerosis: a meta-analysis. *Arch Phys Med Rehabil.* 2016;97(9):1564–1572.

132. Alquist AD, Kraft G. Optimization of the exercise stimulus by pre-cooling in multiple sclerosis. *Int J MS Care.* 2002;4(2):82–83.

133. Goodman AD, Brown TR, Schapiro RT, et al. A pooled analysis of two phase 3 clinical trials of dalfampridine in patients with multiple sclerosis. *Int J MS Care.* 2014;16(3):153–160.

134. Goodman AD, Bethoux F, Brown TR, et al. Long-term safety and efficacy of dalfampridine for walking impairment in patients with multiple sclerosis: results of open-label extensions of two Phase 3 clinical trials. *Mult Scler.* 2015;21(10):1322–1331.

135. Sutliff M, Naft J, Stough D, et al. Efficacy and safety of a hip flexion assist orthosis in ambulatory multiple sclerosis patients. *Arch Phys Med Rehabil.* 2008;89(8):1611–1617.

136. Miller L, McFadyen A, Lord AC, et al. Functional electrical stimulation for foot drop in multiple sclerosis: a systematic review and meta-analysis of the effect on gait speed. *Arch Phys Med Rehabil.* 2017;98(7):1435–1452.

137. Taylor PN, Wilkinson Hart IA, Khan MS, et al. Correction of footdrop due to multiple sclerosis using the stimustep implanted dropped foot stimulator. *Int J MS Care.* 2016;18(5):239–247.

138. Freal JE, Kraft GH, Coryell JK. Symptomatic fatigue in multiple sclerosis. *Arch Phys Med Rehabil.* 1984;65(3):135–138.

139. Loy BD, Taylor RL, Fling BW, et al. Relationship between perceived fatigue and performance fatigability in people with multiple sclerosis: a systematic review and meta-analysis. *J Psychosom Res.* 2017;100:1–7.

140. Heesen C, Nawrath L, Reich C, et al. Fatigue in multiple sclerosis: an example of cytokine mediated sickness behavior? *J Neurol Neurosurg Psychiatry.* 2006;77:34–39.

141. Biberacher V, Schmidt P, Selter RC, et al. Fatigue in multiple sclerosis: associations with clinical, MRI and CSF parameters. *Mult Scler.* 2018;24:1115–1125.

142. Gunzler DD, Perzynski A, Morris N, et al. Disentangling Multiple Sclerosis and depression: an adjusted depression screening score for patient-centered care. *J Behav Med.* 2015;38(2):237–250.

143. Fisk JD, Ritvo PG, Ross L, et al. Measuring the functional impact of fatigue: initial validation of the fatigue impact scale. *Clin Infect Dis.* 1994;18(suppl 1):S79–S83.

144. Pilutti LA, Greenlee TA, Motl RW, et al. Effects of exercise training on fatigue in multiple sclerosis: a meta-analysis. *Psychosom Med.* 2013;75(6):575–580.

145. Hugos CL, Copperman LF, Fuller BE, et al. Clinical trial of a formal group fatigue program in multiple sclerosis. *Mult Scler.* 2010;16(6):724–732.

146. Asano M, Finlayson ML. Meta-analysis of three different types of fatigue management interventions for people with multiple sclerosis: exercise, education, and medication. *Mult Scler Int.* 2014;2014:798285.

147. Oken BS, Kishiyama S, Zajdel D, et al. Randomized controlled trial of yoga and exercise in multiple sclerosis. *Neurology.* 2004;62:2058–2064.

148. Ulrichsen KM, Kaufmann T, Dorum ES, et al. Clinical utility of mindfulness training in the treatment of fatigue after stroke, traumatic brain injury and multiple sclerosis: a systematic literature review and meta-analysis. *Front Psychol.* 2016;7:912.

149. Koldewijn EL, Homme OR, Lemmens WA, et al. Relationship between lower urinary tract abnormalities and disease-related parameters in multiple sclerosis. *J Urol.* 1995;154:169–173.

150. Khalaf KM, Coyne KS, Globe DR, et al. The impact of lower urinary tract symptoms on health-related quality of life among patients with multiple sclerosis. *Neurourol Urodyn.* 2016;35(1):48–54.

151. Aharony SM, Lam O, Corcos J. Evaluation of lower urinary tract symptoms in multiple sclerosis patients: review of the literature and current guidelines. *Can Urol Assoc J.* 2017;11(1-2):61–64.

152. Lúcio AC, Campos RM, Perissinotto MC, et al. Pelvic floor muscle training in the treatment of lower urinary tract dysfunction in women with multiple sclerosis. *Neurourol Urodyn.* 2010;29:1410–1413.

153. Aharony SM, Lam O, Corcos J. Treatment of lower urinary tract symptoms in multiple sclerosis patients: review of the literature and current guidelines. *Can Urol Assoc J.* 2017;11(3-4):E110–E115.

154. Diokno AC, Appell RA, Sand PK, et al. Prospective, randomized, double-blind study of the efficacy and tolerability of the extended-release formulations of oxybutinin and tolterodine for overactive bladder: results of the OPERA trial. *Mayo Clin Proc.* 2003;78:687–695.

155. Bosma R, Wynia K, Havlikova E, et al. Efficacy of desmopressin in patients with multiple sclerosis suffering from bladder dysfunction: a meta–analysis. *Acta Neurol Scand.* 2005;112:1–5.

156. Cruz F, Herschorn S, Aliotta P, et al. Efficacy and safety of onabotulinumtoxinA in patients with urinary incontinence due to neurogenic detrusor overactivity: a randomized, double-blind, placebo-controlled trial. *Eur Urol.* 2011;60:742–750.

157. Peters KM, Kandagatla P, Killinger KA, et al. Clinical outcomes of sacral neuromodulation in patients with neurologic conditions. *Urology.* 2013;81:738–744.

158. Gallien P, Reymann JM, Amarenco G, et al. Placebo controlled, randomised, double blind study of the effects of botulinum A toxin on detrusor sphincter dyssynergia in multiple sclerosis patients. *J Neurol Neurosurg Psychiatry.* 2005;76(12):1670–1676.

159. Cotterill N, Madersbacher H, Wyndaele JJ, et al. Neurogenic bowel dysfunction: clinical management recommendations of the Neurologic Incontinence Committee of the Fifth International Consultation on Incontinence 2013. *Neurourol Urodyn.* 2018;37:46–53.

160. Chia YW, Fowler CJ, Kamm MA, et al. Prevalence of bowel dysfunction in patients with multiple sclerosis and bladder dysfunction. *J Neurol.* 1995;242(2):105–108.

161. Preziosi G, Raptis DA, Raeburn A, et al. Autonomic rectal dysfunction in patients with multiple sclerosis and bowel symptoms is secondary to spinal cord disease. *Dis Colon Rectum.* 2014;57(4):514–521.

162. DasGupta R, Fowler CJ. Bladder, bowel and sexual dysfunction in multiple sclerosis: management strategies. *Drugs.* 2003;63(2):153–166.

163. Zorzon M, Zivadinov R, Locatelli L, et al. Correlation of sexual dysfunction and brain magnetic resonance imaging in multiple sclerosis. *Mult Scler.* 2003;9(1):108–110.

164. Cordeau D, Courtois F. Sexual disorders in women with MS: assessment and management. *Ann Phys Rehabil Med.* 2014;57(5):337–347.

165. DasGupta R, Wiseman OJ, Kanabar G, et al. Efficacy of Sildenafil in the treatment of female sexual dysfunction due to multiple sclerosis. *J Urol.* 2004;171:1189–1193.

166. Mehanna R, Jankovic J. Movement disorders in multiple sclerosis and other demyelinating diseases. *J Neurol Sci.* 2013;328(1-2):1–8.

167. Yap L, Kouyialis A, Varma TR. Stereotactic neurosurgery for disabling tremor in multiple sclerosis: thalamotomy or deep brain stimulation? *Br J Neurosurg.* 2007;21(4):349–354.

168. Svendsen KB, Jensen TS, Overvad K, et al. Pain in patients with multiple sclerosis: a population-based survey. *Arch Neurol.* 2003;60:1089–1094.

169. Osterberg A, Boivie J, Thuomas A. Central pain in multiple sclerosis—prevalence and clinical characteristics. *Eur J Pain.* 2005;9:531–542.

170. Brown TR, Slee A. A randomized placebo-controlled trial of duloxetine for central pain in multiple sclerosis. *Int J MS Care.* 2015;17(2):83–89.

171. Solaro C, Brichetto G, Battaglia MA, et al. Antiepileptic medications in multiple sclerosis: adverse effects in a three-year follow-up study. *Neurol Sci.* 2005;25(6):307–310.

172. Kalman S, Osterberg A, Sorensen J, et al. Morphine responsiveness in a group of well-defined multiple sclerosis patients: a study with i.v. morphine. *Eur J Pain.* 2002;6(1):69–80.

173. Fallata A, Salter A, Tyry T, et al. Trigeminal neuralgia commonly precedes the diagnosis of multiple sclerosis. *Int J MS Care.* 2017;19:240–246.

174. Solaro C, Messmer Uccelli MM, Guglieri P, et al. Gabapentin is effective in treating nocturnal painful spasms in multiple sclerosis. *Mult Scler.* 2000;6:192–193.

175. La Mantia L, Prone V. Headache in multiple sclerosis and autoimmune disorders. *Neurol Sci.* 2015;36(suppl 1):75–78.

176. Chen L, Gordon LK. Ocular manifestations of multiple sclerosis. *Curr Opin Ophthalmol.* 2005;16(5):315–320.

177. Chwastiak L, Ehde D, Gibbons L, et al. Depression and severity of illness in multiple sclerosis: epidemiologic study of a large community sample. *Am J Psychiatry.* 2002;159(11):1862–1868.

178. Fredrikson S, Cheng Q, Jiang G-X, et al. Elevated suicide risk among patients with multiple sclerosis in Sweden. *Neuroepidemiology.* 2003;22:146–152.

179. Kalson-Ray S, Edan G, Leray E; SURVIMUS Study Group. An excessive risk of suicide may no longer be a reality for multiple sclerosis patients. *Mult Scler.* 2017;23(6):864–871.

180. Feinstein A, Magalhaes S, Richard JF, et al. The link between multiple sclerosis and depression. *Nat Rev Neurol.* 2014;10(9):507–517.

181. Feinstein A. Multiple sclerosis, disease modifying treatments and depression: a critical methodological review. *Mult Scler.* 2000;6:343–348.

182. Minden SL, Feinstein A, Kalb RC, et al. Evidence-based guideline: assessment and management of psychiatric disorders in individuals with MS: report of the Guideline Development Subcommittee of the American Academy of Neurology. *Neurology.* 2014;82(2):174–181.

183. Ehde DM, Kraft GH, Chwastiak L, et al. Efficacy of paroxetine in treating major depressive disorder in persons with multiple sclerosis. *Gen Hosp Psychiatry.* 2008;30(1):40–48.

184. Raissi A, Bulloch AGM, Fiest KM, et al. Exploration of undertreatment and patterns of treatment of depression in multiple sclerosis. *Int J MS Care.* 2015;17(6):292–300.

185. Rao S, Leo G, Bernardin L, et al. Cognitive dysfunction in multiple sclerosis: I. Frequency, patterns and prediction. *Neurology.* 1991;41:685–691.

186. Hoffmann S, Tittgemeyer M, von Cramon DY. Cognitive impairment in multiple sclerosis. *Curr Opin Neurol.* 2007;20(3):275–280.

187. Langdon DW, Amato MP, Boringa J. Recommendations for a Brief International Cognitive Assessment for Multiple Sclerosis (BICAMS). *Mult Scler.* 2012;18(6):891–898.

188. Strober LB, Binder A, Nikelshpur OM, et al. The perceived deficits questionnaire: perception, deficit, or distress? *Int J MS Care.* 2016;18(4):183–190.

189. das Nair R, Martin KJ, Lincoln NB. Memory rehabilitation for people with multiple sclerosis. *Cochrane Database Syst Rev.* 2016;(3):CD008754.

190. Krupp LB, Christodoulou C, Melville P, et al. Donepezil improved memory in multiple sclerosis in a randomized clinical trial. *Neurology.* 2004;63:1579–1585.

191. Beukelman DR, Kraft GH, Freal J. Expressive communication disorders in persons with multiple sclerosis: a survey. *Arch Phys Med Rehabil.* 1985;66(10):675–677.

192. Renauld S, Mohamed-Saïd L, Macoir J. Language disorders in multiple sclerosis: a systematic review. *Mult Scler Relat Disord.* 2016;10:103–111.

193. Schwartz L, Kraft GH. The role of spouse responses to disability and family environment in multiple sclerosis. *Am J Phys Med Rehabil.* 1999;78(6):525–532.

194. McKenzie T, Quig ME, Tyry T, et al. Care partners and multiple sclerosis. *Int J MS Care.* 2015;17(6):253–260.

195. Figved N, Myhr KM, Larsen JP, et al. Caregiver burden in multiple sclerosis: the impact of neuropsychiatric symptoms. *J Neurol Neurosurg Psychiatry.* 2007;78(10):1097–1102.

196. Johnson KL, Fraser RT. Mitigating the impact of multiple sclerosis on employment. *Phys Med Rehabil Clin N Am.* 2005;16(2):571–582.

197. Marrie RA. Comorbidity in multiple sclerosis: implications for patient care. *Nat Rev Neurol.* 2017;13(6):375–382.

198. Dobos K, Healy B, Houtchens M. Access to preventive health care in severely disabled women with multiple sclerosis. *Int J MS Care.* 2015;17(4):200–205.

199. Moss BP, Rensel MR, Hersh CM. Wellness and the role of comorbidities in multiple sclerosis. *Neurotherapeutics.* 2017;14:999–1017.

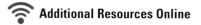 **Additional Resources Online**

CHAPTER 21

Vu Q. C. Nguyen
Mark A. Hirsch
Nicole F. Rup

Comprehensive Rehabilitation of Parkinson Disease and Movement Disorders

Rehabilitation medicine, with its focus on optimizing functional status regardless of the condition, is a specialty uniquely qualified to address progressively degenerative neurologic movement disorders. These conditions are among the most amenable to a comprehensive, interdisciplinary rehabilitation approach. This chapter will focus on the disorders of movement with a review of current understandings of idiopathic Parkinson disease. Specific functional manifestations and complications of these movement disorders will be surveyed with a discussion of the integrated rehabilitation and exercise approach to their management. The chapter will finish with an appraisal of the value of technology and interventions such as chemodenervation.

Parkinson disease is a complex, chronic, progressive, and highly disabling neurodegenerative condition that increases in incidence with age and is characterized by a diverse set of motor and nonmotor features. It is the second most common neurodegenerative disorder following Alzheimer's disease (1). It affects approximately 1 million people with 60,000 new diagnoses each year in the United States and estimated 6.2 million people worldwide. There is a sharp increase in incidence starting at age 50 and peaking by age 80 with the mean age at diagnosis being 61. The prevalence is 1% in persons aged 60 years or older and approaches 4% in those aged 80 years or older. One in 20 patients are diagnosed before 60 years of age and are considered to be "young-onset Parkinson disease" (YOPD) (2,3). Affected men outnumber women 2:1 with males having the higher rates every decade, while females develop Parkinson disease at lower rates and later in life. This is attributed to the neuroprotective effects of estrogen on the nigrostriatal dopaminergic system. When considering ethnic background, the highest rate is observed in Hispanic individuals, followed by non-Hispanic Whites, Asians, and African American persons (4,5).

Major drivers of Parkinson disease-related cost are disease severity and progression. In the United States, medical care for Parkinson disease is currently $15.5 billion annually in direct (e.g., health care costs) and indirect costs (e.g., income loss) and is expected to rapidly rise due to significant increase in population aging and Parkinson disease-related early retirement (6). Current economic models predict that reducing Parkinson disease progression rates could result in substantial savings in U.S. health care expenditures. Slowing progression by 20% could save the U.S. health care system $75,891 per patient, including lost income. Halting progression could save the U.S. health care system $442,429 per Parkinson disease patient (7). Physical medicine and rehabilitation interventions, including promotion of a more active lifestyle, are likely to contribute to these efforts. Life expectancy is decreased compared to the general population with the average time from symptom onset to death being 16 years and the average age at death being 81. The United States has the fourth highest annual death rate from Parkinson disease in the world. Factors associated with earlier deaths include having a later diagnosis in life, worse motor severity, dementia, and psychotic symptoms (5,8). Age, gender, and Tinetti Gait Score are independent predictors of Parkinson disease mortality, as well as the degree of gait, balance, and postural function impairment; ability to climb and descend stairs; and ability to change postural set.

Parkinson disease was first described in 1817 by English physician James Parkinson who wrote an essay at age 62 on the "shaking palsy" or "paralysis agitans" (9). It is a diagnosis made on a clinical basis for management and by autopsy findings of striatal dopamine neuron loss with Lewy bodies (LB) for confirmation. The hallmark features of Parkinson disease are grouped into a Parkinson syndrome that include bradykinesia, resting tremors, and rigidity, with or without postural instability. Postural instability was a classically described feature; however, due to its late disease onset, it is usually not present at the time of diagnosis. Another feature of Parkinson disease is the existence of "on" and "off" states. "On" states refer to the effective management of motor symptoms by medication. "Off" states describe refractory motor symptoms and functional impairment. Additionally, parkinsonism expressions can be seen with various neurodegenerative disorders that will be discussed later in the chapter. Overall, all patients with Parkinson disease have parkinsonism but not all parkinsonism is Parkinson disease (4).

BASIC ANATOMY AND PATHOPHYSIOLOGY

The progressive deterioration in motor function of Parkinson disease is caused by the loss of nigrostriatal dopaminergic neurons in the substantia nigra pars compacta and ventral tegmentum with the most prominent loss identified in the ventral lateral substantia nigra. By the time of motor dysfunction and diagnosis, the patient has already suffered a 60% to 80% neuronal loss (10). Anatomically, the caudate nucleus and the putamen are grouped together as the striatum. The striatum and the subthalamic nucleus serve as the receptive entity for all motor projections into the basal ganglia. They received excitatory input from the cerebral cortex, midline thalamic nuclei, hippocampus, amygdala, and primary olfactory cortex. The striatum also receives dopaminergic input from the substantia nigra pars compacta and serotonergic input from the midbrain raphe nuclei (11). The basal ganglia-thalamocortical structures in turn modulate the efferent output to optimize normal physical movement (1). There are two dopaminergic pathways involved in the modulation. The excitatory pathway is direct, involves dopaminergic D1 receptors, and projects to the globus pallidus and substantia nigra reticulata. The inhibitory pathway is indirect, involves dopaminergic D2 receptors, and projects to connections between the external globus pallidus with the striatum and the subthalamic nucleus. The net effect of the basal ganglia on voluntary movement is the inhibition of competing motor patterns and the focused facilitation of the cortically selected voluntary movement **(Fig. 21-1)** (12).

The loss of dopamine production from neuronal cellular loss leads to a deactivation of the excitatory pathway and a hyperactivation of the inhibitory pathway, which inhibits voluntary motor activity (13). Research suggests that environmental and genetic neuroinflammatory factors in the enteric, peripheral, and central nervous systems provoke dysfunction in neuronal mitochondria, which results in accumulation of miscoded proteins particularly alpha-synuclein misfolding. The aggregation of alpha-synuclein leads to accumulation of critical neurotransmitter enzymes, loss of cytoplasmic tyrosine hydroxylase (TH), and decrease in

choline acetyltransferase. These events increase oxidative stress and degeneration of cellular integrity. Additionally, the misfolding of alpha-synuclein activates astrocytes and microglia, glial cells that respond to tissue injury. This supports the concept that an immuno-inflammatory response contributes to neurodegeneration in Parkinson disease (14–17).

Thinly or sparsely myelinated axons, derived from projection neurons, are morphologically long and thin. This makes them particularly susceptible to injuries caused by alpha-synuclein misfolding associated with unfavorable environments. Projection neurons are typically from the glutamatergic, gamma-aminobutyric acidergic, dopaminergic, noradrenergic, serotonergic, histaminergic, and cholinergic pathways (18). Alpha-synuclein misfolding leads to aggregate formations in these projection neurons in the enteric, peripheral, and central nervous systems. The aggregates are disseminated trans-synaptically from neuron to neuron, leading to a progressively widening web of neuronal degeneration and death (1,13,17). Evidence suggests that the enteric nervous system plays a major role in the initiation of the degeneration cascade, with the vagus nerve serving as the major conduit from the gastrointestinal tract to the brainstem. Other representative pathways include the autonomic nervous system and spinal cord centers with projections to the brainstem nuclei (17).

RISK FACTORS

Factors linked to an increased incidence of Parkinson disease are grouped into medical conditions, social habits, environmental exposure, and genetics. Medical conditions include diets high in caloric content, elevated serum cholesterol, head trauma, and postinfectious states. Traumatic brain injury (TBI) is strongly associated with Parkinson disease in patients who have the long Rep1 alleles of the alpha-synuclein gene (SNCA Rep1). Patients with TBI and SNCA Rep1 were diagnosed with Parkinson disease on average 5 years earlier than those with neither risk factors (19). The social habits identified are consumption of methcathinone, methamphetamines, and amphetamines. These drugs create a threefold rise in risk level. Environmental exposures consist of pesticides (insecticides, fungicides, rodenticides, and herbicides), milk consumption, methanol, organic solvents, carbon disulfide, cyanide, and lack of physical activity. Among pesticides, paraquat and rotenone increase the risk. Paraquat creates formation of reactive oxygen species, which accelerates alpha-synuclein misfolding, disrupts cellular membrane conductance, and speeds up protein aggregation (20). Rotenone inhibits mitochondrial I complex, increases alpha-synuclein fibril formation, and escalates alpha-synuclein misfolding, aggregation, modification, and toxicity (21). Finally, gene mutations cited with Parkinson disease are SNCA; eukaryotic translation initiation factor 4 gamma 1 (EIF4G1) gene; glucocerebrosidase, an enzyme that is deficient in Gaucher's disease, (GBA) gene; leucine-rich repeat kinase 2 (LRRK2) gene loci; PTEN-induced putative kinase 1 (PINK1) gene loci; superoxide dismutase 2 (SOD2) gene; and vacuolar protein sorting 35 (VPS35) homolog gene (4). A mutation of LRRK2 encoding dardarin (PARK8) has been shown to be the most common genetic form of Parkinson disease accounting for 2% of cases. The penetrance is incomplete, and manifestations are based on environmental exposure and activation (22).

Several factors are deemed protective against Parkinson disease. Studies confirmed that cigarette smoking lowers the

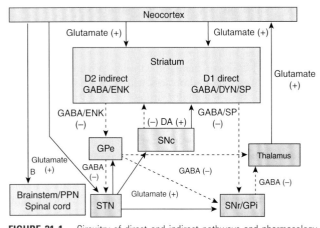

FIGURE 21-1. Circuitry of direct and indirect pathways and pharmacology of the basal ganglia. The direct pathway projects gamma-aminobutyric acid (GABA)-mediated inhibitory input directly to the output nuclei of substantia nigra reticulata (SNr) and globus pallidus interna (GPi). The indirect pathway sends an inhibitory GABA projection to the globus pallidus externa (GPe), which subsequently projects GABA-mediated inhibitory input on the subthalamic nucleus (STN). The STN output to the SNr/GPi is an excitatory glutamate projection. *Solid arrows* reflect excitatory pathways and *dashed arrows* inhibitory pathways. DA, dopamine; D1, D1 dopamine receptor; D2, D2 dopamine receptor; DYN, dynorphin; ENK, enkephalin; PPN, pedunculopontine nucleus; SNc, substantia nigra zona compacta; SP, substance P. (Modified from Alexander GE, Crutcher MD. Functional architecture of basal ganglia circuits: neural substrates of parallel processing. *Trends Neurosci.* 1990;13(7):266–271.)

risk. The protective feature seems to be the duration of smoking. Those who smoked longer had less chances of developing Parkinson disease. Smokers for 40 or more years were noted to lower their odds ratio (OR) down to as low as 0.30. On the other hand, a higher level of smoking did not confer any added protective benefit. Evidence suggests that the neuroprotective aspect of nicotine is seen through nicotinic acetylcholine receptors (nAchRs) increased expression when exposed to nicotine. Through the nAchR increased expression, nicotine also seems to be protective against dopaminergic deficits caused by methamphetamine abuse (23). Another factor associated with lowered risk is caffeine consumption. Coffee drinkers with moderate intake of 3.1 to 5 cups per day have an OR of 0.45. Alcohol consumption is also protective. Moderate alcohol use between 3.1 and 7 units per week has an OR of 0.60. A higher consumption level did not confer any additional protective benefit (24,25). Epidemiologic studies have found an inverse association between exercise and Parkinson disease risk. Sports activities and high levels of moderate to vigorous physical activity (≥180 MET-hours per week) in young adulthood appear to lower Parkinson disease risk; however, it is still unclear whether low physical activity levels cause Parkinson disease signs to appear or whether patients become less physically active after their diagnosis. It is intriguing that low amounts of physical activity in young adulthood are statistically associated with neurodegenerative disease and considered another important reason for physiatrists to promote physical activity to all patients who do not display contraindications to exercise.

PATHOLOGIC STAGES OF PARKINSON DISEASE

In 2003, Braak and colleagues advanced the concept of a 20-year preclinical phase affecting the brainstem. They described a peripheral to central nervous system pathologic progression. Misfolding leads to aggregates of alpha-synuclein protein fibrils, which are the core components of LB. LB are spherical protein masses that accumulate in neuronal cytoplasm displacing normal functional cellular components. LB are transsynaptically transferred from one neuron to the next (13,17). Evidence suggests that LB accumulations start in the enteric and autonomic nervous systems with involvement of the gastrointestinal tracts and the oral cavity (salivary glands). According to Braak, they spread via the nuclei of the glossopharyngeal nerve, vagus nerve, and the olfactory nerve. Thereafter, these protein aggregates are distributed in an ascending pattern affecting the reticular formation, the lower raphe nuclei, and the locus coeruleus. The next regions to be affected are the midbrain tegmentum, the basal forebrain, and the substantia nigra pars compacta. The disease penetrates the amygdala, the intralaminar thalamic nuclei, and the hippocampal CA2 section. At this stage, motor functional deficits are expressed phenotypically. Emotional deficits are experienced when the pathology extends to the cingulate and temporal cortex. In the same manner, cognitive deficits are seen with involvement of the frontal and parietal cortex (⏚ **eTable 21-1**).

NONMOTOR PRESENTATION

Parkinson disease has a premotor stage, called prodromal phase, with clinical expressions caused by enteric and autonomic nervous system involvement prior to spreading to the substantia nigra. The prodromal phase may occur up to 30 years before motor syndromes are evident.

Historically, nonmotor features include depression or mood fluctuations, fatigue or excessive daytime somnolence, rapid eye movement (REM) sleep disturbance, anosmia, and constipation. Recent data recognize visuospatial and cognitive features such as executive dysfunction manifesting as disrupted memory retrieval, attention, planning, multitasking, and concentration performance (26). Long-term epidemiologic data suggest that 80% of patients develop dementia. Additionally, cerebrospinal fluid levels of alpha-synuclein and brain-derived neurotrophic factor (BDNF) polymorphisms have been shown to be predictive of cognitive impairment and decline (27). REM sleep behavior disorder is characterized by dream enactment behavior during sleep. The sleeping patient experiences laughing, crying, or yelling; complex voluntary movements; falling out of bed; and violent behaviors leading to injury (28). REM sleep behavior disorder is a strong predictor with 80% eventually developing synuclein-mediated neurodegenerative diseases and 62% being diagnosed with Parkinson disease. There is a 5 to 29 years range with a mean of 14.2 years from REM sleep behavior disorder to parkinsonism or dementia onset (29). Anosmia or olfactory nuclei degeneration is another early nonmotor feature of Parkinson disease. Up to 100% of patients experience olfactory dysfunction (30). Constipation predates Parkinson disease by as much as 15 years. Men with less than one bowel movement per day were four times more likely to develop Parkinson disease (30). Finally, as the majority of patients do not volunteer symptoms of apathy, pain, sexual dysfunction, bowel incontinence, constipation, or sleep disorders, these must be surveyed.

MOTOR PRESENTATION

Parkinson disease is considered a heterogeneous condition. Patients do not express every nonmotor and motor feature. However, all patients eventually experience motor decline and frequently succumb to aspiration pneumonia as a cause of death. Mhyre derived the acronym TRAP to describe parkinsonism core motor features: tremor at rest, rigidity, akinesia (bradykinesia and hypokinesia), and postural instability (13). Resting tremor is a presenting symptom in 70% to 90% of Parkinson disease. It is evident at rest and suppressed with movement. It is an involuntary, often unnoticed, rhythmic movement of 4- to 6-Hz oscillations. A common term associated with the tremor is "pill rolling," describing the rubbing of the thumb and index finger. Rigidity is manifested as increased tone in both agonist and antagonistic muscle groups at rest with the relaxed limb resistant to passive range of motion in flexion or extension. It presents unilaterally at first and occurs in up to 90% of patients. Bradykinesia is usually misnamed by combining bradykinesia, which is slowness of movement, with hypokinesia, which is decreased movement amplitude. It leads to progressive reduction in the speed of initiating and amplitude of movement. The loss of fine motor control and dexterity manifests in the difficulty with activities like buttoning shirts and tying shoelaces. The progressive small amplitude and delayed movements lead to decreased facial expressions, hypomimia, hypophonia, and micrographia. Eventually, a freezing gait occurs in up to 90% of patients. Finally, axial motor signs are displayed as postural instability with difficulty adjusting to postural changes, turning en bloc, and gait impairment. Progression leads to loss of postural reflexes;

dyssynchrony among reciprocally innervated leg musculature during movement initiation; reduced peak torque production in knee extension, knee flexion, and ankle dorsiflexion; a stooped posture; fear of falling; freezing; and an increased fall risk (31). The gait impairment is marked by slow, short-shuffling steps, with a narrow base of support associated with decreased arm swing. The patient experiences festination or retropulsion. Dual tasking, such as walking and concurrent talking, becomes more difficult.

DIAGNOSTIC EVALUATION AND CLINICAL MONITORING

In 1992, Hughes and colleagues introduced a set of diagnostic criteria that were subsequently adopted to be the United Kingdom Parkinson Disease Society (UKPDS) Brain Bank Clinical Diagnostic Criteria (🛜 **eTable 21-2**). This has been the most widely used diagnostic criteria for Parkinson disease and was utilized in Europe and North America.

With modern imaging technology, more promising diagnostic tools are introduced. Dopamine transporters (DAT) are presynaptic proteins that regulate dopamine production in the striatum. They are found in high concentration in the putamen and caudate nucleus. A reduction in DAT is consistent with Parkinson disease (32). In January 2011, the Food and Drug Administration (FDA) approved the use of DaTscan to assist the confirmation of Parkinson disease (33). DaTscan utilizes radioisotope ioflupane I-123 markers to highlight striatal dopamine activity via single-photon emission computed tomography (SPECT) brain imaging. A normal brain image shows symmetric "comma" or "crescent-shaped" images of bilateral putamen and caudate nuclei (golf ball on a pin). As disease state progresses, one or both hemispheric images show a truncated comma or "period" shape and is reflective of diminished striatal dopamine production in the putamen with activity only in the caudate nuclei. Absence of SPECT activity denotes advanced condition where activity is now lost to both the putamen and the caudate nuclei. Of note, partial restoration in bilateral posterior putamen binding and symmetrical

binding in the caudate nucleus has been documented with DaTscan in a Parkinson disease patient following participation in an ultramarathon race (34).

In recent years, due to its age and the fact that it only addresses motor impairments, the UKPDS Brain Bank Clinical Diagnostic Criteria is felt to be outdated. To address the global effects of Parkinson disease, the International Parkinson and Movement Disorder Society (MDS) Task Force established a new set of diagnostic criteria in 2015 (**Fig. 21-2**). The task force focused on establishing a more comprehensive set of criteria that reflects current understanding of Parkinson disease as a multisystem, slowly progressive neurodegenerative condition, often with a genetic component, that affects all parts of the nervous system. The first criterion is the presence of parkinsonism, defined as bradykinesia, resting tremors, and rigidity, with or without postural instability. After confirmation of parkinsonism, the MDS Diagnostic Criteria for Parkinson disease is utilized to establish "clinically probable Parkinson disease" versus "clinically established Parkinson disease." A *probable* condition exists with (a) absence of absolute exclusion criteria, (b) presence of no more than two red flags, and (c) each red flag must have at least one counterbalanced supportive criteria. An *established* condition exists with (a) absence of absolute exclusion criteria, (b) presence of at least two supportive criteria, and (c) no red flags. **Figure 21-2** outlines the criteria.

Once diagnosis is made, monitoring the patient's status and minimizing progression are important. Several scales exist to monitor clinical changes and rate the level of disability. In 1967, Margaret Hoehn and Melvin Yahr (H&Y) developed criteria to rate the level of disability with parkinsonism (36). They utilized the term "parkinsonism" to allow a broader evaluation of Parkinson disease and related movement disorders. A modified H&Y scale was later introduced to increase sensitivity between axial and limb involvement as well as describe functional status. This was widely used until the 1980s. In 1987, Stanley Fahn and colleagues developed the Unified Parkinson Disease Rating Scale (UPDRS), and it became the most commonly utilized clinical tracking scale for Parkinson disease (37). In 2001, the MDS sponsored a critical review of the

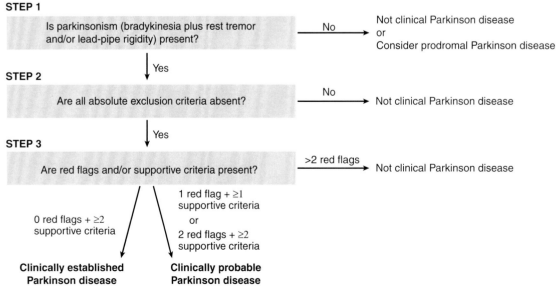

FIGURE 21-2. MDS clinical diagnostic criteria for Parkinson disease. (Reprinted by permission from Nature: Kalia L, Lang A. Evolving basic pathologic and clinical concepts in PD. *Nat Rev Neurol.* 2016;12(2):65–66. Copyright © 2016 Springer Nature. Ref. (35).)

UPDRS to improve its utilization. This resulted in a revision of the UPDRS and subsequently the creation of the MDS-UPDRS (38). The new scale added nonmotor elements of cognitive impairment, hallucination and psychosis, depressed mood, anxious mood, apathy, and features of dopamine dysregulation syndrome such as excessive, risky, or addictive behaviors (gambling, abnormal sex drive, repetitive activities, drug use, or hyperphagia). Clinical anchors were added to provide consistency across the measures. Additionally, a new focus on measuring mild impairments with demarcations of "slight" and "mild" was added. The entire MDS-UPDRS scale can be found on the International Parkinson and Movement Disorder Society's web site (39).

Differential diagnoses of Parkinson disease include conditions that express parkinsonism. Previously identified insults that manifest parkinsonism include exposure to the potent neurotoxin 1-methyl-4-phenyl-1,2,3,6-tetrahydropyridine (MPTP). In the early 1980s, a cohort of people using an illicitly produced meperidine (Demerol) analog tainted with MPTP developed severe, irreversible parkinsonism. The MPTP crosses the blood-brain barrier and is oxidized into 1-methyl-4-phenylpyridinium (MPP+), a neurotoxin. The MPP+ inhibits mitochondrial complex I activity, which destroys striatal dopamine neurons (40). The dopamine D2 receptor antagonists can induce or exacerbate parkinsonism. These include typical antipsychotics (haloperidol, thioridazine, chlorpromazine), atypical antipsychotics (risperidone, olanzapine), and gastrointestinal agents (prochlorperazine, promethazine, and metoclopramide). Less frequent causes include tetrabenazine, reserpine, methyldopa, flunarizine, cinnarizine, verapamil, valproic acid, and lithium.

MEDICAL MANAGEMENT

Pharmacology

Levodopa

Since exogenous dopamine cannot cross the blood-brain barrier, levodopa is the gold standard for the treatment of Parkinson disease. It is a dopamine precursor that crosses the blood-brain barrier and is converted to dopamine in the substantia nigra pars compacta. The dopamine is then stored presynaptically in dopaminergic neurons. Aromatic amino acid decarboxylase (AAAD) is the enzyme responsible for converting levodopa to dopamine throughout the body. After ingestion, levodopa is highly metabolized in the gastrointestinal system by AAAD leaving only 30% residual capable of reaching systemic circulation. To minimize the effects of AAAD, levodopa is combined with carbidopa, which is a peripherally acting AAAD inhibitor. In combination with carbidopa, levodopa bioavailability is tripled. Additionally, by decreasing the peripheral conversion of levodopa, carbidopa decreases the peripheral dopamine side effects of nausea, vomiting, and hypotension. Levodopa's half-life is about 1 hour, and it is metabolized in the gastrointestinal tract, kidneys, and liver with 70% excreted through urine.

In 2015, the FDA approved an intestinal gel formulation of carbidopa-levodopa. Due to the erratic nature of the gastrointestinal tract and gastric emptying in advanced disease, medication malabsorption is common. The intestinal gel formulation enhances absorption with the direct delivery of the medication into the proximal jejunum via percutaneous endoscopic gastrojejunostomy tube (41). Food and protein intake affect levodopa absorption. Daily protein intake should be reduced to 0.8 g/kg body weight. When combined with any other dopaminergic medications, carbidopa-levodopa dosing should be decreased by 10% to 30%. Levodopa does increase the risk of developing dyskinesia and motor complications. Therefore, there is argument for a delay in initiation of levodopa until onset of more advanced disease, when motor symptom progression affects the patient's daily function.

Dopamine Agonists

Dopamine agonists are the second most effective medications for Parkinson disease. Dopamine D2 and D3 receptor agonists bind with dopamine receptors postsynaptically to increase dopamine transmission. Compared to levodopa, dopamine agonists have less risks for dyskinesia and motor fluctuations but increased side effects of hallucination, psychosis, hypotension, peripheral edema, excessive daytime somnolence, and impulse control disorders. Use in patients older than 70 years of age should be cautious or avoided. All patients should have blood pressure, heart rate, alertness, and weight monitoring while taking dopamine agonists (42,43).

Most commonly used and recommended first-line agents include ropinirole (oral), pramipexole (oral), and rotigotine (transdermal patch). Ropinirole has a 6-hour half-life and is hepatically metabolized. Side effects are gastrointestinal (nausea, vomiting, dyspepsia, abdominal pain, and constipation) and nervous system effects (dizziness, somnolence, headache, syncope, confusion, hallucination, impulse control, and sleep attacks). Pramipexole has an 8-hour half-life in young adults and 12 hours in elderly and is excreted unchanged in the urine. Renal dosing is recommended with renal compromise. Side effects include nausea, abdominal discomfort, constipation, dizziness, somnolence, headache, hallucination, impulse control, dyskinesia, orthostatic hypotension, xerostomia, peripheral edema, and muscle spasms. Rotigotine has an initial 3-hour half-life and terminal 7-hour half-life after patch removal. It is metabolized by conjugation and N-dealkylation. Side effects include nausea, vomiting, anorexia, somnolence, dizziness, dyskinesia, hyperhidrosis, local site skin reaction, visual disturbance, and peripheral edema. Precautions include avoidance with sulfa allergy and removal prior to MRI as the patch contains aluminum (44). With advanced disease, subcutaneous apomorphine via continuous pump can be utilized with rescue treatment for hypomobility and "off" episodes. It is injected into the abdomen, upper arm, or upper leg. Its half-life is 40 minutes with significant first-pass metabolism. Side effects include nausea, vomiting, drowsiness, somnolence, dizziness, orthostatic hypotension, hallucination, confusion, dyskinesia, rhinorrhea, and peripheral edema. Precaution is avoidance of coingestion with serotonin inhibitors to avoid hypotension (44).

Second-line drugs include the ergot derivative dopamine agonists cabergoline and bromocriptine. These options are for patients who have lost benefits or tolerability to first-line agents. Bromocriptine mesylate is an oral agent with 5- to 15-hour half-life and is metabolized in the liver. Side effects include nausea, vomiting, abdominal discomfort, involuntary movements, ataxia, hallucination, confusion, "on/off" phenomenon, dizziness, syncope, hypotension, drowsiness, insomnia, depression, visual disturbance, shortness of breath, constipation, vertigo, and asthenia. Long-term use increases pleural fibrosis (44). Monoamine oxidase B (MAO-B) inhibitors such as selegiline and rasagiline block the breakdown of dopamine.

They are effective as monotherapy for early disease or adjuvant therapy with levodopa in the latter course of Parkinson disease. Selegiline is an oral agent with a 10-hour half-life and is broken down by CYP450 to amphetamines. Rasagiline has a 3-hour half-life and is metabolized by CYP1A2. Side effects for both drugs include hypertensive crisis if high dose, nausea, weight loss, dyspepsia, hypotension, bradycardia, dizziness, headache, hallucination, vivid dreams, insomnia, flu-like symptoms, dyskinesia, dystonia, rash, and photosensitivity (45).

Catechol-*O*-Methyltransferase Inhibitors

Catechol-*O*-methyltransferase (COMT) acts peripherally to break down levodopa to an ineffective metabolite 3-*O*-methyldopa (3-OMD). COMT inhibitors, in combination with levodopa, increase its bioavailability. Entacapone has a 2-hour half-life and is metabolized via glucuronidation. Side effects include exacerbation of levodopa's adverse effects, brown/orange urine, and diarrhea. Changes in blood pressure and mental status are possible complications. Tolcapone has a 3-hour half-life and is metabolized via glucuronidation, CYP2A6, and CYP3A4. Side effects are similar to entacapone with possible transaminitis and hepatic failure. Opicapone is a once-daily, third-generation COMT inhibitor with improved "off" state. Side effects include dyskinesia, insomnia, and constipation (44).

Other Pharmacotherapy and Investigational Agents

Anticholinergic agents, benztropine and trihexyphenidyl, are helpful for severe tremor or dystonia in younger patients early in the course. Nonselective cholinergic receptor blockade is significant, and side effects include cognitive impairment, exacerbation of dementia, delirium, sedation, hallucination, constipation, xerostomia, blurred vision, and urinary retention. Higher dosing is associated with hypotension and palpitations. Effects are magnified in the elderly and should be avoided (43). Parkinson disease has been linked to overactivation of glutamate in the basal ganglia leading to oxidative stress and cell death. Amantadine is an *N*-methyl-D-aspartate (NMDA) antagonist, which augments presynaptic dopamine release and NMDA glutamatergic antagonism. It is the only agent shown to suppress levodopa-induced dyskinesia. Side effects include pedal edema and livedo reticularis. It is excreted through the kidneys. In frail elderly or those with renal insufficiency, amantadine may cause confusion, hallucination, and worsened motor symptoms (13). Riluzole exerts its effects via NMDA receptor antagonism and has been approved for amyotrophic lateral sclerosis but has yet to show efficacy with Parkinson disease (45). Acetylcholinesterase inhibitors include rivastigmine, donepezil, galantamine, and memantine. Rivastigmine is the only medication approved by the FDA for the treatment of mild to moderate Parkinson disease dementia (46). Adenosine A2A receptors are colocalized on dopamine D2 receptors and is believed to be hyperactive in Parkinson disease. Istradefylline is an adenosine A2A receptor antagonist shown to improve "off" time as a levodopa adjunct. Safinamide, an alpha-aminoamide, is an adjunct to levodopa or dopamine agonists through its effects on MAO inhibition, sodium channel antagonism, and inhibition of glutamate release (47). Finally, cannabidiol is the primary nonpsychoactive component of cannabis. It significantly decreases psychosis, improves REM sleep behavior disorder, and eliminates nightmares (48,49).

CLINICAL MANAGEMENT

Deep Brain Stimulation Surgery

Early surgical interventions were ablative in nature. Thalamotomy was utilized to treat tremors and pallidotomy was used to manage levodopa-induced dyskinesia. These procedures are still beneficial; however, due to the permanency of the intervention, they are limited to only a select population. Deep brain stimulation surgery (DBS) has become the surgical treatment of choice for advanced Parkinson disease when medical management fails to control motor symptoms. The primary loci of stimulation are the subthalamic nucleus and the globus pallidus. DBS is advantageous over ablative surgery as it allows modification of the stimulation (or removal of the stimulator) adapting to changing symptoms as Parkinson disease progresses. Bilateral implantation is a possible cost-effective option to treat bilateral motor symptoms (43); however, there are risks to bilateral stimulation of the subthalamic nuclei, regarding cognitive impairment and general risks of equipment failure leading to increased hospitalizations and emergency room utilization (50). DBS does not slow disease progression. It is most effective for the management of motor symptoms such as bradykinesia, freezing, dyskinesia from levodopa, rigidity, gait instability, and tremor. This improves activities of daily living (ADLs) and mobility. Stimulation of the subthalamic nucleus is cost-effective and most beneficial for severe "on" and "off" symptoms. Stimulation of the globus pallidus pars interna is effective for dyskinesia and offers long-term stability of effects. DBS has not been effective for nonmotor symptoms such as cognitive impairment, mood disorders, speech impairment, or autonomic dysfunctions (51,52). Adverse effects are generally manageable and reversible. They include infections (6.1%), migration or misplacement of the stimulator leads (5.1%), lead breakage (5%), intracranial hemorrhage (3%), and skin erosion (1.3%). Other complications possibly associated with deep brain stimulation include eyelid opening apraxia (1.8% to 30%), dysarthria or hypophonia (4% to 17%), gait disturbances (14%), postural instability (12.5%), weight gain (8.4%), and decline in verbal fluency (14%). As of 2016, more than 100,000 patients have undergone DBS surgery for Parkinson disease and other movement disorders. Ten-year outcome studies support the durable benefits of DBS on motor fluctuations, dyskinesia, tremor, rigidity, and bradykinesia (53).

REHABILITATION

The interdisciplinary treatment team improves access to providers and ensures Parkinson disease patients receive individually tailored, evidence-based, cost-effective care throughout their disease course. It fosters collaborative care among patient and providers while reducing overall costs. The team includes a movement disorder neurologist, physiatrist, physical therapist, occupational therapist, speech language pathologist, neuropsychologist, pharmacist, neurosurgeon, sexologist, fitness professional, Parkinson disease nurse specialist, and nutritionist, who work as a team to "codesign" care that is individually tailoring to the needs of individuals at all stages of Parkinson disease (54–57). Social work and involvement of the patient's care partner help with care plan design and management of social issues. Physiatrists and the rehabilitation team assist in the care of persons with Parkinson disease by targeting and managing various deficits or impairments of the condition. This section highlights active and exercise principles that rehabilitation professionals can utilize to minimize the impact of impairments and functional limitations that affect the well-being and disability of those with Parkinson disease. At all stages of Parkinson disease, beginning at diagnosis for those who do not have contraindications, initiation of therapy and exercise programs is recommended.

Physical Inactivity in Parkinson Disease

Increasingly, physical activity is recognized to be beneficial in Parkinson disease. Unfortunately, most home-dwelling Parkinson disease patients (>80%) remain less physically active than adults with stroke or multiple sclerosis (58). They have about a 30% reduction in weekly physical activity when compared to healthy age-matched controls (59). For Parkinson disease, physical activity decreases with axial motor dysfunction, age, disease progression, and severity. This diminishes strength and endurance, promoting further inactivity and comorbidity. Without daily physical activity, the degenerative disease process progresses more rapidly, increasing morbidity as well as burden and cost of care. Motivating patients with neurodegenerative conditions to become more physically active is challenging, as many patients may experience motor, mental, and emotional symptoms including gait impairment, depression, apathy, anxiety, low outcome expectation, lack of insight, and low self-efficacy (60,61). The largest study to date on physical activity promotion in Parkinson disease, the Dutch ParkFit study, assigned sedentary patients with Parkinson disease to coaching sessions to increase outdoor sports activities (ParkFit) using benchmarks established by the American College of Sports Medicine (five times per week moderate exercise for 30 minutes or three times per week intensive exercise for 20 minutes) or a matched general physiotherapy intervention (62). The results showed that the ParkFit program increased the amount of weekly physical activity on ambulatory activity, timed up and go score, and distance on the 6-minute walk test (63). Additionally, participants in ParkFit increased their weekly participation in outdoor sports activities by 24%. Evidence suggests that exercise should be used as a physiologic tool in the treatment of patients at all stages of Parkinson disease. Prior to beginning an exercise program, a screening for contraindications to exercise is recommended due to the high incidence of cerebrovascular and heart disease in Parkinson disease (64,65).

Anti-Parkinson medication and exercise likely utilize similar pathways to promote symptomatic relief in Parkinson disease. Accumulating evidence suggests exercise promotes endogenous brain repair mechanisms with far greater effect on the cardinal features of the disease than previously believed. Animal models indicate inactivity or stress is prodegenerative, while exercise induces brain repair or reorganization (neuroplasticity) and accompanying behavioral recovery. Mechanisms of exercise-induced plasticity include striatal neurogenesis, synaptogenesis, angiogenesis, and improved overall synaptic efficiency with increased localized dopamine release in motor circuits (dorsal striatum), greater dopaminergic diffusion, and time in synapse (via down-regulation of dopamine transporter [DAT] and TH and changes in the glutamate storage system) (61,66). Many of these mechanisms are triggered by exercise and by the up-regulation of endogenous neurotrophic factors, including BDNF and glial cell–derived neurotrophic factor (GDNF). In animal models of Parkinson disease (focused on enrichment, forced limb use, and treadmill training), exercise has been shown

to improve mitochondrial function and ATP levels, increase BDNF levels, restore TH-labeled neurons, increase net dopamine neuron count or slow dopaminergic neuron loss in substantia nigra pars compacta, and modulate genes important to striatal function (67–69).

Low corticomotor excitability is a marker for the severity of Parkinson disease. In human Parkinson disease studies, exercise-induced changes in the brain include increased corticomotor excitability during intense treadmill training with or without use of a partial body weight support harness when a goal of 3.0 metabolic equivalents (METS) and/or 75% of the age-adjusted maximum heart rate was reached for each training session lasting up to 45 minutes in duration. Another positive change includes increased dopamine D2 receptor density within the dorsal striatum (putamen) following 24 training sessions of progressive treadmill running starting at 75% of age-adjusted maximal heart rate for up to 45-minute duration over 2 months. This is important as D2 receptors are a significant source of corticostriatal glutaminergic input modulation, and D2 receptor activation is associated with striatal medium spiny neuron activity. Still other beneficial neuronal changes include up-regulation of serum BDNF during interval training with a stationary cycle, rapid (within ≥90 minutes) balance training–induced changes in brain gray matter volume in connected lateralized parietal-basal ganglia and cerebellar circuitry, and improvement in bilateral putamen and caudate dopaminergic uptake after running a 100-km ultramarathon (34,70,71).

From 2004 to 2011, the largest physical therapy (PT) trial for Parkinson disease in the world was the ParkinsonNet Trial. It reported five key findings: ParkinsonNet participation (a) reduced home care utilization and improved care delivered within the community closer to patients' homes with cost containment and beneficial clinical outcome (hip fracture rate cut in half); (b) improved knowledge and adherence to guidelines for evidence-based physiotherapy by practicing PT; (c) increased referrals into PT by doctors; (d) boosted the patient volumes per therapist, thereby increasing their Parkinson disease expertise; and (e) provided greater patient-provider collaboration, reducing anxiety and stress, which is a prodegenerative feature in Parkinson disease (72,73). In recent years, implementation of ParkinsonNet has improved the quality of Parkinson disease care around the world (74–76).

Key messages for implementing ParkinsonNet include the following: (a) Parkinson disease patients and care partners want more involvement in multidisciplinary care networks as "health coaches" and (b) patients who are more involved in their care have better health literacy, are more compliant, perceive higher satisfaction with care, and achieve better health outcomes (77). Patients' perceptions of their most troubling symptoms show wide interindividual variability and often differ from clinicians' views. Therefore, it is important for the physiatrist to involve patients directly in "codesigning" their care during clinical encounters. An example is encouraging patients to identify and rank the importance of their quality of life and goals of PT. Providers, who are encouraged to coidentify problematic areas, display enhanced patient/provider communication. Additionally, incorporating patient-identified goals into the treatment plan has proven to improve adherence to the physiatrist's therapy recommendations and progress toward PT goals (78). In addition, the personalized treatment approach meets the patients' diverse expectations about what constitutes high-quality treatment (62,63,70–72,84,99,111,113,120–124) (🛜 **eTable 21-3**).

Gait Dysfunction and Balance

Gait dysfunction is the primary presenting sign in 18% of patients with Parkinson disease (117,118). Shortened step length is the focal disturbance of gait, and the classic gait pattern is characterized by shuffling steps (79,119). Reduced hip, knee, and ankle flexion range of motion, decreased arm swing, limited trunk rotation, and increased forward flexed trunk are typical kinematic changes affecting Parkinson disease gait (80,81). Many patients demonstrate episodic hesitation to initiate gait or instances of "freezing" where they stop and cannot initiate movement (82). The second parkinsonian gait pattern is festination, characterized by small steps, increasing in speed and frequency with a forward trunk posture (83). Festination will place the patient's feet involuntarily behind their center of gravity requiring rapid and involuntary corrective steps that are small and forward resulting in a cycle of propulsion and retropulsion (84). Decreased arm swing and slow en bloc turns are also commonly seen in Parkinson disease (84). Average gait speed is estimated at 0.88 m/s in H&Y stage 3 to 4 as compared to normative standards for gait speed required to use a pedestrian crosswalk at 0.94 to 1.2 m/s (85,86). Reduced walking speed is an independent risk factor for mortality with OR of 16.28 (87). These gait abnormalities place persons living with Parkinson disease at varying risks for loss of balance or falls (81,88).

Although people with Parkinson disease may certainly be able to perform straight-line walking, their overall gait is hampered by hypokinesia, rigidity, postural imbalance, and the fear of falling, especially in advanced stages of the disease (81,89–91). Fear of falling has long been noted to increase the risk of future falls (92). In a 2009 prospective analysis by Mak, the Activities-specific Balance Confidence (ABC) scale was a significant predictor of recurrent falls. An ABC scale with results greater than 69 demonstrated 93% sensitivity in predicting future falls in the coming 12 months (92). Gait rehabilitation in Parkinson disease should aim to increase stride length and step length, widen the base of support, improve heel-toe progression, and increase arm swing. Historically, this has been effective in overground training. New strategies have also emerged including the use of partial body weight–supported treadmill training (PBWSTT). Other promising training include cross-training with dance, virtual reality, and martial arts. Gait training frequently incorporates the use of both auditory and visual cueing to improve initiation and limit freezing. It often extends to include balance training (see also Chapter 4).

A 2013 randomized controlled trial (RCT) comparing a 5-week course of three times per week sessions of either individually adjusted treadmill training versus overground walking demonstrated improvement in preferred walking speeds in both groups, but only the treadmill training program showed improvement in stride length. Treadmill training also showed improvement in the timed "up and go" (TUG) test and static posturography. Improvement in gait parameters persisted at 1-month follow-up assessments (93). PBWSTT has also demonstrated improvement in on-phase UPDRS scores and gait performance measures (2-minute treadmill walking and 10-m walk test). In 2014, Ganesan showed significant improvements in UPDRS motor score and balance indices when compared to nonexercising controls on stable medications and to conventional gait training (walking a straight path, increasing arm swing, and turning with auditory cueing for longer steps) (94). Cochrane's 2014 review of different therapeutic approaches in

Parkinson disease included six studies examining gait speed. In all the reviewed studies, except one, the largest improvement in gait speed was seen in the intervention arm with cueing or treadmill training or both. The one study that did not show this did not include these therapies (95). In 2014, Hass determined the minimal clinically important difference (MCID) in gait speed to be 0.06 m/s (85). More work is needed to solidify the MCID for gait speed in people with Parkinson disease.

The National Parkinson Foundation statistics showed 38% of patients will fall within a 1-year period and many will fall repeatedly throughout the day (96). Studies have noted prior falls, freezing episodes, poor balance, disease severity, and reduced leg strength as predictors for falls in Parkinson disease (97). Self-selected gait speed less than 1.1 m/s increases risk of falls with Parkinson disease. PT aimed at gait training may then help patients with gait normalization and decrease risk of falls (98). In a study of patients varying in disease severity from H&Y stages 1 to 4 with mean score of 2.6, 59% of patients experienced at least one fall in a given 6-month period. The study showed falls were most closely associated with three predictors: at least one fall in the previous 12 months (OR 5.8), freezing of gait in the past month (OR 2.4), and self-selected gait speed less than 1.1 m/s (OR 1.9) (98). In 2012, Li showed that Tai Chi training reduces balance impairments in mild to moderate Parkinson disease as compared to resistance training versus stretching. Tai Chi was shown to reduce the number of falls in participants but no better than those in resistance training, with improvements maintained at 3 months (99). McGinley demonstrated the number of falls were significantly lower in the 8-week intervention phase of progressive strength training (95,100).

Movement Initiation and Freezing

The person with Parkinson disease typically possesses slow movement initiation that may result from delayed activation of the motor cortex, impeding the ability to initiate and execute normal movement (101). Although the corticospinal system is intact, the abnormal motor commands result in bradykinesia affecting implementation and execution of motor tasks. These impairments are exacerbated with high-complexity tasks. Highly refined motor activities such as handwriting require switching between motor components, and the limited ability of people with Parkinson disease to adapt to changing task conditions makes this difficult. Indeed, it appears that slow initiation of movement, or paucity of movement, may be an adaptive strategy by those with Parkinson disease to conserve energy and/or maintain function (102,103). A freezing episode is often observed with turning, walking through a doorway threshold, or stepping around or over objects (80,83,104). The freezing is often described as a shuffling with small steps or trembling as opposed to a complete akinesia (105). Freezing is commonly seen when performing dual tasks, reaching an open space, or ambulating in complete darkness (106–109). Such episodes most often last less than 10 seconds but can be longer with disease progression (108). Freezing can be improved with a combination of walking exercise and somatosensory, visual, or auditory cues. Examples include a beating metronome; "the laser shoe," which provides a continuous ambulatory visual cue to the patient by projecting a laser line orthogonally in front of the patients' contralateral foot just prior to the swing phase; or stepping over laser lights on a U-step (110). Conscious movement strategies designed to increase step amplitude, retain step rhythm, shift weight laterally, direct attention to gait, encourage wide turning arcs, and maintain sufficient exercise levels have all been recommended as treatment strategies for freezing (111). Studies also suggest that patients with freezing retain the ability to exercise on a stationary bicycle, regular bicycle, or walk-cycle. Freezing in the home is troublesome. In the home, treatment strategies including weight shifting exercises, using instructional cues to encourage taking larger steps, encouraging higher effort to lift the foot to clear obstacles, and using commercially available three-dimensional staircase carpets or tiles have shown great promise (112,120–124).

Bradykinesia

Slowed and reduced movements or bradykinesia is perhaps the most characteristic impairment in Parkinson disease. The prevalence of bradykinesia approaches 77% to 98% of all patients with Parkinson disease. Medications do help bradykinesia (84). A few studies have examined the effect of exercise on bradykinesia. These studies have used action observation, cycling, music and PT, and resistance training. A trial of 20 participants has shown that a 12-week program of high-intensity eccentric exercise improves bradykinesia: 10-m walk, TUG, PDQ-39, and muscle force (98). One study investigated the benefits of resistance exercise for the upper limb on bradykinesia in 48 patients with mild to moderate Parkinson disease. The results showed a faster movement velocity and increased duration and magnitude of upper limb agonist burst activity when objectively assessed by EMG (114). Another study investigated the effect of high-intensity power training on bradykinesia in 26 patients with mild to moderate Parkinson disease and concluded that power training reduces upper and lower limb bradykinesia and improves quality of life (115).

Dyskinesia and Dystonia

While medications can control and improve motor symptoms, they can lead to adverse effects. A common complication after 7 or 8 years of levodopa therapy is involuntary large amplitude, fidgety movement called dyskinesia. Most commonly, dyskinesias are seen when the plasma concentration of levodopa is at its highest. This is referred to as "peak-dose" dyskinesia. It is believed to result from abnormal neuronal firing patterns in response to pulsatile stimulation of dopamine receptors (116). In the early stages, it can be managed by reducing the dose or frequency of levodopa. This typically results in a worsening of the symptoms of Parkinson disease, such as rest tremor, bradykinesia, and rigidity. If dyskinesias are relatively mild and not bothersome or dangerous to the patient, then most people prefer to move too much rather than too little. If dyskinesias become large in amplitude, to the extent that they risk injury to the patient, then they must be treated. Treatment options include manipulating levodopa or adding amantadine to the regimen. If dyskinesia is persistent and accompanied by pervasive parkinsonian symptoms or severe motor fluctuations, consideration can be made for neurosurgery referral for DBS.

Dystonia (involuntary muscular contraction causing abnormal posture) commonly coexist with Parkinson disease. The most common site is the foot, with toe flexion and foot inversion. This is usually seen at the end of a levodopa dose, when plasma concentrations are at their lowest. With the ingestion of another dose of levodopa, the dystonia is relieved. Dystonia may also occur as a peak-dose effect. Unfortunately, peak-dose dystonia is not as easily treated. If dystonia presents as a focal problem, then local therapy with botulinum toxin injection is an option.

Dysphagia

Up to 75% of people with Parkinson disease experience dysphagia and esophageal dysmotility (125–130). Only 20% to 40% of Parkinson disease patients are aware of their dysphagia and less than 10% of patients report symptoms (131). Abnormalities in striated muscles under dopaminergic control and smooth muscles under autonomic influence contribute to this complicated impairment. Videofluoroscopic swallowing evaluations help to determine which specific phases of swallowing are impaired and can allow trialing of compensatory strategies. Modified barium swallows under fluoroscopy have shown that the most common abnormalities are motility problems, hypopharyngeal stasis, aspiration, and deficient positioning of the esophagus (132,133). Common patterns in Parkinson disease-related dysphagia of the oral phase often include repetitive pump movements of the tongue, oral residue, and/or premature spillage. In the pharyngeal phase, patients can show residue in the valleculae, somatosensory deficits, and/or reduced rates of spontaneous swallows as well as hypomotility, spasms, and/or multiple contractions in the esophageal phase. Given patient's infrequent reporting of swallowing impairments, use of Parkinson disease-standardized questionnaires such as the Swallowing Disturbance Questionnaire (sensitivity 80.5% and specificity 82%) and the Munich Dysphagia Test-Parkinson disease (sensitivity 81.3% and specificity 71%) is recommended (131). Speech-language pathology training includes oral-motor exercises and compensatory strategies to prevent penetration and aspiration. Oral-motor exercises, airway protecting maneuvers, and postural compensation are important. Compensatory maneuvers incorporate thickened liquids/solids, chin tuck, and multiple swallows. Other options include expiratory muscle strength training. The effects of DBS and levodopa on dysphagia remain debatable (134) (see also Chapter 13).

Sialorrhea

Sialorrhea is commonly seen in Parkinson disease with incidence of 70% to 78% (135). Drooling can be related to either excessive saliva production or insufficient salivary clearance. There seem to be data suggesting this may be more of a swallowing issue than salivary overproduction in Parkinson disease (136). Drooling can contribute to aspiration and subsequent aspiration pneumonia. Treatment can be trialed starting with the use of chewing gum or hard candy, oral or topical anticholinergics, as well as medications such as glycopyrrolate. Intraparotid injections of botulinum toxin injections can also be helpful and radiotherapy may be required in rare cases (134,136).

Nutrition

Weight loss is common in Parkinson disease and correlates with worsened quality of life. This may be at least in part due to impaired olfaction and gustatory sensory. Malnourishment is associated with loss of appetite, dysphagia, early satiety, and constipation. Vitamin D is important for normal basal ganglia function. Vitamin D deficiency is common and may also contribute to the higher rate of osteoporosis seen in Parkinson disease. Levodopa effectiveness has been tied to B_6, B_{12}, folate, and homocysteine deficiencies. Compulsive eating is related to dopamine agonist use and is associated with weight gain. Finally, weight gain has been reported following DBS at the subthalamic nuclei in 13% of patients (134,136). Protein intake should be monitored and limited because amino acids compete with levodopa absorption. Patients should take levodopa 1 hour before or after a meal to facilitate absorption. This is of concern in the later stages of the disease with severe dyskinesia. Vitamin supplements with D, B$_{12}$, and folate, as well as calcium, should be considered to maintain well-balanced and adequate nutrition (137). When an individual cannot meet his or her caloric and fluid requirements, a gastrostomy feeding tube is considered.

Delayed Gastric Emptying

Parkinson disease patients frequently experience early satiety, nausea, vomiting, bloating, or abdominal distension secondary to delayed gastric emptying. Reduced peristalsis and gastroesophageal reflux present as complaints of "heartburn" or indigestion. This increases risk for poor nutritional intake. As levodopa is absorbed from the small intestine, gastroparesis can result in delayed or complete loss of the benefit of levodopa (136). Anti-Parkinson drugs themselves may also contribute to delayed gastric emptying. Unfortunately, promotility agents, such as metoclopramide, may worsen dyskinesia (132). Treatment of gastroparesis can include small frequent meals, avoiding high fat and fiber foods, and exercise (134). Alternative forms of levodopa administration include effervescent, liquid, gel, and pump forms (136).

Constipation

Constipation is thought to be one of the earliest signs/symptoms of the disease occurring as early as 15.3 years before motor features. Population-based study has reported the risk of development of Parkinson disease increases with constipation severity (hazard ratio from 3.3 to 4.2) (136). The cause is multifactorial, including altered sympathetic innervation of the gastrointestinal tract, delayed colonic transit, medications such as opioids and even Sinemet, overall limited mobility, and impaired hydration (136). Nonpharmacologic treatments include adequate hydration, increased physical activity, and high-fiber diets. Daily osmotic agent such as polyethylene glycol or lactulose can be helpful. Dyssynergic defecation can also be seen in Parkinson disease and can be improved with biofeedback/pelvic floor rehabilitation (136).

Bladder Dysfunction

Some of the most common bladder abnormalities in Parkinson disease are overactive bladder symptoms such as nocturia, frequency, and urgency with little or no postvoid residuals. The prevalence of these lower urinary tract symptoms ranges from 38% to 71% (138). The most prevalent symptom reported is nocturia, which is seen in more than 60% of patients with urinary complaints. Urinary symptoms in Parkinson disease are thought to be secondary to disruption of the dopaminergic circuit that normally suppresses the micturition reflex (138). In some patients, detrusor hyporeflexia and urinary sphincter problems occur and urinary retention may be an issue. Urodynamic studies may be needed to diagnose the nature of the problem. The effect of levodopa on urinary symptoms is unclear and may be unpredictable (138). Behavioral management is first line and includes adaptive equipment such as urinal or bedside commode, avoidance of triggers, adjustment of timing of dietary intake, and timed voiding. Given mobility impairment, patient education on early response to urges allows sufficient time to reach the restroom. Biofeedback can improve urinary sphincter control. Pharmacologic agents, such as peripherally acting anticholinergics, can address urinary symptoms; however, use

is limited secondary to side effect profiles, which include confusion, constipation, and dry mouth. A voiding diary should be performed to help providers identify potential treatment strategies. Voiding diary should have bladder capacity through maximum voided volume, presence/absence of polyuria, relationship of voided volume with incontinence, grading of urinary urgency, and voided volume. Intermittent catheterization may be required in cases where urinary retention occurs (139). A key differentiation occurs between patients with multisystem atrophy (MSA) versus Parkinson disease with bladder dysfunction. MSA patients typically experience urinary dysfunction (among other autonomic dysfunctions) much earlier in the disease course and more commonly have large postvoid residuals with urinary sphincter dysfunction. Patients with Parkinson disease typically develop lower urinary tract symptoms after emergence of motor symptoms. Levodopa has not been effective with MSA, whereas there is some benefit with Parkinson disease although this is not predictable (138,139).

Cognition

Cognitive impairment is present in most patients at diagnosis; however, the progression of cognitive impairment is usually slow. The cognitive domains that are most often affected include attention, memory, and learning; executive; and visual-spatial functions (140). Verbal function and the ability to reason seem to be spared, although information processing may be slower. In comparison with Alzheimer's disease, Parkinson disease dementia more often affects visuospatial and executive functions rather than memory impairment (141). Researchers found that 36% of people who were newly diagnosed with Parkinson disease have some form of cognitive impairment (142). Additional features of cognitive impairment in Parkinson disease often include visual hallucinations and paranoia (141). The development of Parkinson disease dementia does not follow a predictable time course. There is a distinction for patients who develop dementia within 1 year of parkinsonism to be diagnosed as dementia with LB (141). There are likely pathologic differences between dementia with LB and Parkinson disease dementia related to the patterns of Lewy body distribution (140). The Sydney Multicenter Study showed 83% of patients who survive 20 years with Parkinson disease would develop dementia. This finding was supported by multiple other large cohort studies with the mean duration from onset of Parkinson disease to development of dementia reported as 10 years (140,141). Recent studies have associated sleep disturbance including REM behavior disorder in patients with Parkinson disease with worse cognitive performance and risk of dementia (141).

In 2007, a Movement Disorder Society task force examined clinical diagnostic criteria for dementia in Parkinson disease and found the risk of dementia to be increased up to six times in those with Parkinson disease, with a point prevalence near 30%. The task force cites older age, more severe parkinsonism, and akinetic form of Parkinson disease to be associated with higher risk of dementia in those with Parkinson disease. The main pathologic correlate was Lewy body–type degeneration in cerebral cortex and limbic structures. The presence of Parkinson disease dementia has been associated with a higher mortality rate (140). A 2015 meta-analysis from neurology looked at the effect of cognitive training on cognition and behavior of patients with mild to moderate Parkinson disease. Cognitive training involved structured and theoretical-driven teaching strategies or guided practice on tasks targeting cognitive domains; this can be electronic or paper based. Overall, there was a small but significant improvement for overall cognition, working memory, processing speed, and executive function. Cognitive therapy is important especially given the lack of efficacy seen in pharmacologic treatment. Except for rivastigmine, there are no specific drugs to treat impaired cognition in Parkinson disease (143). Studies have investigated the benefits of aerobic and anaerobic exercise training on cognitive function in patients with Parkinson disease (144–147). A study of aerobic treadmill training showed a beneficial effect on executive function (144). The largest study, to date, evaluated the benefits of a multimodal physical exercise program on working memory and attention among nondemented patients with mild to moderate Parkinson disease while *off* medication. The researchers concluded that exercise improved memory and frontal lobe–based executive function (146).

Sleep Disturbances/Fatigue

Sleep disorders are among nonmotor symptoms of Parkinson disease. Common sleep disorders include excessive daytime sleepiness, insomnia, restless leg syndrome, and REM sleep behavior (148). The etiology of hypersomnia or excessive daytime sleepiness is thought to be multifactorial including the disease process itself, medications, age-related sleep architecture changes, and coexistence of primary sleep disorders such as obstructive sleep apnea. Consideration can be made for behavioral management such as exercise, consistent sleep-wake schedule, consistent bedtime routine, and avoidance of electronic devices at least 1 hour before bedtime. In addition, pharmacologic interventions should be considered, including reduction of dopaminergic medications, medication changes, and consideration of stimulants such as modafinil (148). Caffeine has recently been studied but not yet recommended as possible treatment for excessive daytime sleepiness in Parkinson disease patients (149,150). Patients with Parkinson disease often complain of difficulty falling asleep, remaining asleep, and early awakening. Treatment of any coexisting mood disorders such as depression or anxiety or nighttime motor symptoms may help with insomnia and sleep quality. Consideration can be made for melatonin as a pharmacologic treatment along with cognitive behavioral therapy for insomnia, although more data are needed to support the use of both in patients with Parkinson disease (148,149). Several studies have found an increased prevalence of restless legs syndrome (RLS) in patients with Parkinson disease; however, the characterization of RLS versus akathisia, motor restlessness, and wearing off seen in Parkinson disease can be difficult to differentiate. Iron deficiency, pregnancy, and end-stage renal disease with dialysis may potentiate or predispose to RLS (148). Many of the dopaminergic agents used to treat Parkinson have also been independently demonstrated to be effective in treating RLS; however, most research focuses on treatment strategies in healthy subjects and not in those specifically with Parkinson disease. Recommendations from evidence-based treatment in the non-Parkinson literature are likely applicable here as well and include assessment for iron deficiency and contributing agents such as antidepressants, when appropriate (151).

Among patients with established Parkinson disease seen at tertiary care centers, the prevalence of polysomnography-defined REM sleep behavior disorder is approximately 39% to 46%. REM sleep behavior disorder is characterized by loss of normal atonia that occurs during REM sleep and is associated with dream enactment (151). Protecting the patient and any bed partners should be the first step in REM sleep behavior disorder management. Sleep environment modifications include placing a mattress on the floor, moving fragile items out of reach, and placing bed away from windows or glass. Clonazepam is the first-line treatment for REM behavior disorder, with melatonin and pramipexole suggested as potentially useful (148). REM sleep behavior disorder can both precede the motor manifestations of Parkinson disease and develop after its onset and has been one of the strongest clinical predictors of future synucleinopathy including Parkinson disease, dementia with LB, or MSA (151). Only three studies have investigated the benefits of exercise on sleep in patients with Parkinson disease (56,152,153). One of these studies investigated the effects of resistance training on sleep quality and muscle strength in patients with moderate Parkinson disease. The results showed a beneficial effect of training on sleep quality (152). The other study evaluated the effectiveness of Qigong on sleep in patients with mild to moderate Parkinson disease (153). The results showed sleep quality improvement in a variety of standardized sleep scales, improved gait performance, and functional mobility at 6-month follow-up.

Osteoporosis/Bone Mass Density

Studies confirm serum 25-hydroxy vitamin D levels are low in Parkinson disease. Patients with Parkinson disease are less active and remain indoors more often than controls, which possibly leads to vitamin D deficiency. Vitamin D supplementation with 1,200 IU daily may prevent worsening of disease progression as measured by H&Y staging and UPDRS. Higher vitamin D levels may be associated with better motor function and, in animal models, has been shown to be neuroprotective, slowing neurotoxin-induced loss of dopaminergic neurons. Vitamin D is of key importance for basal ganglia function (154). Several meta-analyses have shown Parkinson disease patients to be at higher risk of osteoporosis than healthy controls (155,156). The Global Longitudinal Study of Osteoporosis in Women (GLOW) found Parkinson disease to be the strongest single predictor of fracture risk with age-adjusted hazard ratio of 2.2 (95% CI 1.6 to 3.1). This was compared to other studied factors including multiple sclerosis, COPD, osteoarthritis, cancer, and heart disease (157). Ozturk has shown patients with Parkinson disease to have lower bone density as measured by DEXA scans compared to age-matched controls (158). The study also confirmed a lower vitamin D level than expected in patients with Parkinson disease based on age-matched controls. The osteoporosis risk may be related to alterations in homocysteine levels, a known side effect of levodopa, which has been implicated as a potential risk factor for fractures (155,159). Whether increased risk of osteoporosis occurs secondary to medication side effects, reduced mobility and activity, weight loss, vitamin deficiency (D, B_{12}, K, folate), or alternative factors remains unclear (159) (see also Chapter 31).

A 2014 meta-analysis of six studies suggests that patients with Parkinson disease have 2.66-fold (95% CI 2.10 to 3.36) higher risk of fracture as compared to their counterparts (160). Another study showed patients with Parkinson disease have a higher risk of fragility fractures than age-matched controls. Similar findings have been seen in the United Kingdom database and a large German health insurance company database (159). Tan postulates the mechanism of association between Parkinson disease and fracture may be in part due to lower than expected bone mineral density and increased fall risk in these patients (160). Idjadi has shown hip fracture patients with Parkinson disease experienced longer hospital stays and were more frequently discharged to skilled nursing facility from acute care. Patients with Parkinson disease and hip fracture also declined more in ADLs but not as much in instrumental ADLs at 1-year follow-up as compared to other community-dwelling patients with hip fractures (161).

Psychiatric and Emotional Manifestations

A 2008 systematic review of 104 studies demonstrated a weighted prevalence of major depressive disorder of 17% in Parkinson disease, minor depression 22%, and dysthymia 13%. Clinically significant depressive symptoms were present in 35% of patients irrespective of the presence of a DSM-defined depressive disorder (162). Dopamine replacement, the cornerstone of treatment for Parkinson disease, can also result in psychiatric complications (163). As levodopa replacement is increased, some people may experience hallucinations, delusions, agitation, mania, or confusion. Newly diagnosed, untreated patients with Parkinson disease were followed over a 24-month period and noted to have higher rates of depression, anxiety, fatigue, and apathy. Initiation of dopamine replacement therapy for at least 1 year's time was associated with increase in psychiatric symptoms including impulse control disorders and excessive daytime sleepiness (164). Apathy, or the loss of motivation, interest, or effortful behavior, is a symptom seen more commonly in patients with Parkinson disease, and its presence is not necessarily associated with depression (165).

Depression in Parkinson disease has been shown to be independent of disease severity and duration (166–169). Parkinson disease-associated depression is unique in that it is not commonly associated with feelings of guilt, self-blame, or worthlessness (170). Depressed patients with Parkinson disease experience higher rates of anxiety and have lower rates of suicide despite higher rates of suicidal thoughts. It is unclear as to the extent to which "reactive depression," or one's depressive symptoms as related to the chronic disease, exists as compared to neurochemically based or intrinsic depression. Both likely play a role. Those with Parkinson disease indeed exhibit more depressive symptoms than do other chronic disease counterparts, showing that intrinsic processes likely predominate in Parkinson disease (171,172). Depression in Parkinson disease has been associated with lower scores on scales of self-care, more significant motor impairments, more cognitive symptoms, and lower quality of life (162,170). The overlap of apathy, cognitive impairment, psychomotor retardation or agitation, fatigue, and sleep dysfunction seen in both Parkinson disease and major depression can cloud the depression assessment and lead to underdiagnosis (170). An MDS commissioned task force to identify the use of depression scales in Parkinson disease published its findings in 2007. The task force recommended the Hamilton Rating Scale for Depression (HAM-D), Beck Depression Inventory (BDI), Geriatric Depression Scale (GDS), Hospital Anxiety and Depression Scale (HADS), as well as Montgomery-Asberg Depression Rating Scale (MADRS). For assessment of severity of depressive symptoms, the HAM-D, MADRS, BDI, and Zung self-rating depression scale (SDS) were recommended (170).

There are limited data pointing to specific medications for treatment of depression in Parkinson disease. A 2012 study by Richard suggested venlafaxine or paroxetine might be an efficacious treatment for depression in Parkinson disease. However, there is also a 2009 study by Menza comparing nortriptyline, paroxetine CR, and placebo demonstrating nortriptyline but not paroxetine as superior to placebo for change in HAM-D-17 score, although low sample size and short duration are limits to this study (173,174). A 2011 study also showed benefit for a 10-week course of cognitive-behavioral therapy versus clinical monitoring on HAM-D-17 score reduction in Parkinson disease (175).

Psychosocial and Behavioral Concerns

A 2016 study showed requiring assistance for ADLs, gait difficulties, number of nonmotor symptoms, fatigue, depression, low self-efficacy, motor symptoms, pain, disease severity, freezing episodes, female gender, and motor fluctuations as negative impactors of life satisfaction. In late-stage disease (H&Y stages 4 and 5), the number of nonmotor symptoms, self-efficacy, walking difficulties, and fatigue was associated with life satisfaction (176). In 2009, Hackney has shown a positive significant difference in health-related quality of life in those who participated in tango dance versus no benefit seen in waltz/foxtrot, tai chi, and control groups (177). Ebersbach's 2010 study did not demonstrate a difference in quality of life between a prescription of Lee Silverman Voice Treatment (LVST) BIG, Nordic walking, and control exercises; however, the study may have been underpowered for this (178). An interesting Swedish cohort is currently underway looking at 223 individuals first in 2013 and again planned for 2016 including assessments of their disease severity, mobility, falls and fear of falling, need for assistive devices, life satisfaction, as well as characterizations of their home environment and self-care skills. Further published information on the home and health in people aging with Parkinson disease study is anticipated (179).

Pain

Pain occurs in 60% of Parkinson disease patients and occurs two to three times more commonly than in age-matched control. This often predates motor symptoms and is not felt to be clearly associated with disease duration, gender, or age. Pain in patients with Parkinson disease can be classified into five domains: musculoskeletal, dystonic, central, associated with akathisia, or neuropathic/radicular (180). Limb rigidity is the most common cause of pain in patients with Parkinson disease (181). Headaches are also frequent and characterized by deep, throbbing, occipital, or neck pain (182). Fractures should be ruled out whenever a person with Parkinson disease experiences a fall. Pain most often occurs on the side most affected by motor symptoms or the side where motor symptoms first appeared. Risk factors for the development of pain are noted as the presence of motor fluctuations and severity of motor symptoms. Pain can be associated with the off periods of levodopa treatment (180). Treatment of the parkinsonian symptoms with the goal of improving mobility and flexibility of the affected limbs can help alleviate primary pain. Secondary pain may present as abdominal discomfort resulting from constipation or shoulder and limb pain due to complex regional pain syndrome. Painful limb dystonia may be helped by botulinum toxin injections.

Cardiovascular Disease/Cerebrovascular Disease

Some nonmotor symptoms of Parkinson disease often include orthostasis. There is evidence that cardiac sympathetic denervation occurs early in the Parkinson disease course, later progressing to autonomic dysfunction and orthostasis. Data suggest these patients should use caution in their exercise regimens due to risk of inadequate heart rate elevation needed for submaximal exercise (183). Treatment of orthostasis includes nonpharmacologic measures such as sleeping in head-up position, eating small frequent meals, liberalized fluid and salt intake, as well as support stockings. Medications have also been suggested including midodrine and fludrocortisone; however, there are insufficient data to recommend their use (135,184). Ergot-derived dopamine agonists, such as pergolide and cabergoline, have been associated with significant increased risk of valvular heart disease. It is thought that these medications induce fibrosis in valve leaflets and in the mitral subvalvular apparatus leading to thickening, retraction, and stiffening of valves with resulting incomplete leaf closure and regurgitation. Looking at echocardiographic prevalence of valve regurgitation in patients taking dopamine agonists (both ergot derived and non–ergot derived) compared to controls, Zanetti demonstrated the risk of clinically important valve regurgitation to be significantly higher in patients taking pergolide or cabergoline and suggested an association between cumulative dose and severity of valve regurgitation. There was no increased risk in non–ergot-derived dopamine agonists as compared to controls. There was a significantly increased mean mitral tenting area, which was used as a measurement of leaflet stiffening and apical displacement of leaflets, seen in both ergot- and non–ergot-derived dopamine agonists. This study suggests that dopamine agonists may require cardiac monitoring (185).

Therapeutic Approaches and Modalities

PT and exercise have been shown to be helpful to patients with Parkinson disease. The 2014 European Physiotherapy guidelines for Parkinson disease suggest exercise may be neuroprotective and, citing improvement in corticomotor excitability in patients with Parkinson disease, suggestive of neuroplasticity (84,186). A 2001 RCT of group PT showed benefit for the ADL section of the UPDRS as well as improvement in patient's self-selected comfortable walking speed. These improvements were noted both short term and were seen at 6 month follow-up (187). There are several methodologies unique to Parkinson therapy that will be reviewed here. LSVT BIG focuses on intensive exercise of high-amplitude movements to specifically tackle amplitude of movements (188). The speech component, LSVT LOUD, focuses on speech volume and intelligibility over 16 sessions over 1 month (189). LSVT LOUD has been demonstrated to show a 2-year retention of improved loudness (190). According to the 2014 European PT guidelines, conventional physiotherapy is defined as PT-supervised active exercise interventions targeting gait, balance, transfers, and physical capacity. There is a focus on large-amplitude functional task exercises, positive feedback, and a progressive increase in intensity and complexity (84). BWSTT has been used with benefit in patients with Parkinson disease. Nordic walking has been trialed with benefit as has yoga, martial arts, and dance including Argentine tango, ballet, and Irish set dancing.

A 2012 Cochrane review showed benefit and efficacy for short-term rehabilitation (<3 months) for Parkinson disease and suggested there was no treatment difference between the types of physiotherapy interventions (191). The 2014 European Physiotherapy guidelines suggest gait speed is improved with both conventional PT, cueing, and treadmill training. They note strong evidence for UPDRS section III

score improvements for both conventional therapy and tai chi (84). A 2014 Cochrane review compared therapy techniques in the Parkinson disease population summated a total of 43 RCTs. This was an update to a 2001 review that was unable to find enough evidence to support or refute one intervention over another (84). UPDRS motor subscale was shown to improve significantly in the LSVT BIG group by a decrease of 5.05 points versus the Nordic walking and home exercise in the Ebersbach 2010 study, which both increased by 0.53 and 1.68, respectively (178). UPDRS motor scores also showed significant improvement in Rigdel's 2009 study with forced-use exercise group with a decrease by 16.6 points versus the group who exercised at a voluntary pace (192). The MCID is thought to be between 2.3 and 5 for the motor score according to Cochrane review by Tomlinson and colleagues (95).

Orthoses and Adaptive Equipment

Kegelmeyer in 2013 examined the effects of five different assistive devices versus none on gait and maneuvering around obstacles (193). Patients were noted to have approximately 50% fall rate in the prior 6 months and were not dependent on assistive devices prior to the study. They were required to ambulate 10 m independently. The devices trialed included a cane, standard walker, 2-wheeled walker, 4-wheeled walker, and U-step walker with a laser. Freezing occurred with all devices but was seen most frequently with the 2-wheeled walker. The 4-wheeled walker was felt to provide the best safety and nearest normal gait patterns.

Auditory and Visual Cueing

Visual and auditory cueing have been demonstrated to improve gait parameters. A 2013 meta-analysis on the effect of cueing on gait parameters demonstrated auditory cueing such as the beat of a metronome, music, or counting to produce improvements in cadence, stride length, and velocity, whereas visual cueing, such as laser pointers, adaptive glasses, or lines on the floor, was significant for improvements in stride length alone. There were only 3 studies of the 26 included that examined both visual and auditory feedback; these studies showed significant improvement in cadence but again not for stride length or velocity. These data suggest auditory cueing may be more beneficial on normalizing gait parameters than visual alone (194).

OTHER MOVEMENT DISORDERS

The most common difficulty rehabilitation professionals encounter when faced with movement disorders is correctly classifying them **(Box 21-1)** (195) (e.g., Is this dystonia or simply spasticity? Does this patient have a tic or focal myoclonus?). In contrast to the importance of correct classification, identifying the underlying etiology of a given movement disorder (e.g., ischemic, anoxic, traumatic) is often less important in its management. Regardless of the specific cause, the individual movement disorders are often managed similarly (except for medication-induced movement disorders).

The Parkinson Plus Syndromes

The Parkinson plus syndromes include multiple system atrophy (MSA), progressive supranuclear palsy (PSP), and diffuse Lewy body disease (DLBD). In the first 1 to 2 years of illness, these disorders mimic Parkinson disease. It is only with careful

---

BOX 21-1

Movement Disorders

Chorea
Brief, rapid, forceful, dysrhythmic, discrete, purposeless, flinging of limb

Athetosis
Slow, writhing movements and inability to maintain position of limb or body part

Ballismus
Large amplitude, flinging movement of limb (usually proximal)

Dystonia
Sustained muscle contraction that leads to repetitive twisting movements of variable speed and abnormal posture

Tremor
Rhythmic, oscillatory movements of a body part

Tic
Intermittent, repetitive, stereotypical, abrupt, jerky, typically affecting the face and head

Stereotypy
Purposeless, uniformly repetitive, voluntary, movement of whole body areas

Akathisia
Subjective restlessness, compulsion to move about

Myoclonus
Sudden, brief, irregular, contraction of a group of muscles

---

clinical follow-up and monitoring of an individual's response, or lack of a response, to dopamine replacement that a reasonable clinical diagnosis can be made. MSA is characterized by urinary incontinence, reduced sweating, and orthostatic hypotension (196). In MSA, these symptoms occur within the first 3 to 5 years of disease onset. In Parkinson disease, these symptoms may occur but only 10 to 15 years after disease onset. Clinically, those with MSA do not improve with dopamine replacement. PSP is characterized by the inability to exercise voluntary movement of the eyes (197). Another feature is a marked change in personality; affected individuals become apathetic and may appear to be depressed. PSP causes marked gait difficulty with frequent falls within 1 or 2 years after symptom onset. Thus, gait abnormalities appear more rapidly in those with PSP than in those with Parkinson disease.

DLBD is characterized by a marked decline in intellectual function, visual hallucinations, and signs of bradykinesia, rigidity, and possibly rest tremor (198). In DLBD, the dementia and visual hallucinations progress rapidly within the first 3 years of symptom onset. The bradykinesia and rigidity progress more slowly. Treatment is limited as dopamine replacement, which would alleviate the motor symptoms of bradykinesia and rigidity, worsens the visual hallucinations, and can produce an acute worsening of the underlying dementia. A common feature to all the Parkinson plus syndromes is that the symptoms do not improve with dopamine. This is in stark contrast to Parkinson disease, in which the symptoms do improve significantly with dopamine replacement. It is this lack of response to dopamine, as well as the monitoring of the progression of symptoms, that helps to distinguish these syndromes from Parkinson disease and from one another.

Tremors

Tremors are regular, oscillatory movements produced by alternating but synchronous contractions of antagonistic muscles (199–201). The rhythmic quality distinguishes them from other involuntary movement disorders (202,203). Tremors are classified as resting, essential, or action. Resting tremors occur when the affected limb is at rest with relaxed muscles. These tremors are typically seen in those with Parkinson disease or one of the Parkinson plus syndromes. Essential are visible and persistent tremors occurring when the arms or head are in a specific position or are moving. Most cases of essential tremor are hereditary and are ameliorated with alcohol, benzodiazepines, propranolol, or primidone. Action tremors exist with any voluntary muscle contraction. Specifically, an "intention tremor" is a subtype of action tremor, in that the type of muscle contraction is kinetic as opposed to isometric or postural (204).

Dystonia

Dystonia refers to a sustained muscle contraction that causes repetitive, twisting movements of variable speed, leading to abnormal posture. Dystonia may be focal, segmental, multifocal, or generalized (205–208). Focal dystonia involves single body parts (e.g., blepharospasm, "writer's cramp"), whereas the segmental variety affects two or more contiguous regions (e.g., craniocervical). Multifocal dystonia consists of abnormalities in noncontiguous body parts. Generalized dystonia involves segmental crural dystonia and at least one other body part. Unilateral dystonia is also called hemidystonia. Regardless of anatomic distribution, dystonic contractions typically begin intermittently and become severe and persistent, leading to sustained abnormal postures. Secondary dystonia is associated with neurologic disorders, such as brain injury, cerebral tumor, and infections (209–211). Secondary dystonias may also be caused by medications, such as phenothiazines and sertraline (212).

Impairment of basal ganglia output is thought to play a role in the genesis of dystonia (213). In a series of subjects with hemidystonia, 73% had prior hemiparesis or basal ganglia lesions on imaging studies (214). Lesions in the putamen have been linked to hemidystonia, whereas bilateral putaminal involvement may be responsible for generalized dystonia (205). Torticollis and hand dystonia are thought to result from involvement of the head of the caudate nucleus and thalamus, respectively (214). Disease of the thalamus and subthalamus and derangement of hypothalamic function have also been suspected (215,216). The current lack of understanding of the exact pathophysiology of dystonia has made it difficult to define specific pharmacologic therapy. Treatment has become a "trial and error" process, often leading to frustration for the patient and clinician (206,207,217). Oral medications used to treat the various dystonias include dopamine agonists, antagonists, and depletors; anticholinergics; and GABA agonists (benzodiazepines [$GABA_A$] and baclofen [$GABA_B$]). These systemic medications have numerous adverse effects. Local injection of botulinum toxin is a safe and efficacious alternative, particularly for focal dystonias. The efficacy of PT techniques, such as soft tissue mobilization, cervical muscle strengthening and stretching, and orthotic intervention, has not been well studied to date. Similarly, limited success has been achieved through behavioral modifications, including hypnosis, biofeedback, and relaxation techniques.

Cervical Dystonia

Cervical dystonia, the most common focal dystonia, involves the sternocleidomastoid, trapezius, and posterior cervical muscles. It gives rise to patterned, repetitive, and spasmodic movement that causes the head to twist (rotational torticollis), extend (retrocollis), flex (anterocollis), or tilt toward the shoulder (laterocollis). One or more of these head movements may occur simultaneously. Walking or standing worsens the condition, but the patient may be able to return the head to midline by placing the hand on the jaw or chin. The neck movement may be associated with blepharospasm, lip or chewing movements, and tremor. Because they play a role in maintaining normal head posture, the basal ganglia and the vestibuloocular reflex pathway have been implicated in the development of cervical dystonia (218). Disturbances of neurotransmitter systems have also been described in dystonias (219). Abnormalities in blink reflex recovery have suggested involvement of the brainstem (220). Earlier cervical and upper limb trauma has also been implicated in the development of cervical dystonia (221–223). With respect to treatment, baclofen, benzodiazepines, anticholinergics, carbamazepine, and dopamine agonists or antagonists have been trialed; but side effects may limit their use. Local injection of botulinum toxin into the affected muscles (i.e., sternocleidomastoid, trapezius, splenius capitis) has been successful and not associated with significant complications. In few cases, dysphagia may develop due to local spread of the toxin to neighboring pharyngeal and laryngeal muscles.

Chorea, Athetosis, and Ballismus

Chorea, derived from the Greek word for dance, is an involuntary movement that is brief, rapid, forceful, and dysrhythmic (224). Choreic movements are discrete and purposeless and involve distal body regions such as the hands and feet. Athetosis refers to writhing, snakelike involuntary movements of large and proximal muscle groups, such as the entire arm or leg. The contralateral subthalamic nucleus, caudate nucleus, and putamen may be responsible for chorea (225–228). Bilateral thalamic involvement has been described as well. Choreic movements have been evident in Sydenham's chorea, hyperthyroidism, cerebral arteritis, polycythemia vera, systemic lupus erythematosus, Huntington disease, and phenothiazine intake (211,229). The movements in athetosis are typically slower than choreiform movements. They are characterized by writhing movements and the inability to maintain the position of virtually any body part (e.g., fingers, wrists, toes). Although the limbs are most commonly affected, the axial musculature may be involved as well. Athetoid movements may be seen in Wilson's disease, cerebral palsy, and basal ganglia disease, or drug induced. When it appears with chorea, it is referred to as choreoathetosis. In contrast to chorea, movements related to ballismus are of large amplitude and involve the proximal limbs. The movements are often sudden, with no clear pattern. Ballismus is frequently unilateral and is commonly referred to as hemiballismus. Involvement of the contralateral subthalamic nucleus has been suggested, but other subcortical structures may also be involved (226–228,230,231). It is thought that a lesion in the contralateral subthalamic nucleus disrupts the inhibitory pathways to the globus pallidus, leading to dopamine hyperactivity in the striatum (232). Bilateral involvement (biballism) is seen in bilateral basal ganglia disease (233). Ballismus has also been associated with metabolic abnormalities, such as hyperglycemia, neoplasms, systemic lupus erythematosus, and encephalitis (227,234).

Antiepileptic drugs, such as phenobarbital and valproic acid, may be of benefit in chorea, athetosis, and hemiballismus. In hemiballismus, dopamine antagonists, such as haloperidol and phenothiazines, and dopamine-depleting agents, such as reserpine and tetrabenazine, may be helpful (231). GABA agonists, such as clonazepam, may also ameliorate chorea in that GABA appears to mediate the inhibitory action of the subthalamic nucleus (231). Stereotactic thalamotomy may be considered in severe conditions refractory to medications (235).

Tics, Stereotypy, and Akathisia

Tics are intermittent, stereotypical, repetitive, jerky movements. Although the individual is aware of such movements, he or she finds it difficult to resist performing the action (236). Tics can be either motor or vocal. Many tics are associated with purposeful tasks such as eye blinking and throat clearing. They generally can be volitionally suppressed to some extent. Tics may be classified as simple, such as grimacing, or complex, as in the many tics of Gilles de la Tourette's syndrome (237). In general, tics disappear during sleep and worsen during stressful situations. Stereotypy is purposeless, uniformly repetitive, voluntary movement of whole body areas. Examples include head nodding, head banging, body rocking, and arm jerking, seen in individuals with intellectual disabilities and amphetamine addiction (238).

Akathisia is defined as inner restlessness and compulsion to move about. Although subjective by definition, it may manifest as the inability to stand or sit still or as an urge to pace constantly. In some, the only finding is toe tapping or leg shaking. Akathisia is often seen early after TBI, when it is difficult to distinguish from other behavioral sequelae, such as agitation. Akathisia is thought to result from dopamine blockade in the frontal area (239). Thus, antidopaminergic medications, such as neuroleptics, may induce this disorder. Dopamine agonists, such as ropinirole, are sometimes used. Clomipramine, clonidine, propranolol, clozapine, and piracetam (240,241) may be helpful. Neuroleptic-induced akathisia may be treated with amantadine but best treated by reducing or discontinuing the offending drug (242).

Psychogenic Movement Disorders

Psychogenic movement disorders (PMD) result from various psychiatric conditions. Up to 9% of conditions presenting with neurologic symptoms are believed to have no "organic" basis, with motor disorders being the more common symptoms (243,244). An evaluation of self-reporting of disability in patients with PMD versus those with Parkinson disease revealed that the severity of perceived disability was equivalent in both populations (245). In a series of patients with movement disorders, 3.3% were diagnosed as having clinically documented PMD (244). Common PMD expressions are tremor, dystonia, myoclonus, tics, chorea, hemiballismus, and parkinsonism (246). One feature suggestive of PMD is inconsistent or fluctuating clinical presentation of symptoms. PMD usually have an acute onset and static course characterized by spontaneous remissions. They are worsened by attention and dampened by distraction. They are no more responsive to medications than placebo. When PMD are entertained, attempts should be made to make a psychiatric diagnosis even if the diagnoses of PMD are based on neurologic examination. Common psychiatric diagnoses include conversion, malingering, somatoform disorder, factitious disorder, depression, and anxiety. Associated psychiatric diagnosis (usually depression), precipitating events, and secondary gain are obvious in up to 60% of cases of PMD. Behavioral management, support, and encouragement, in addition to rehabilitation, are efficacious in managing psychogenic gait disorders; however, when symptoms persist ≥12 months, long-term disability is likely (247).

Drug-Induced Movement Disorders

Medications are common causes of movement disorders and should be considered in the evaluation of movement disorders (238). Neuroleptics are among the most common that can directly trigger movement disorders. Extrapyramidal syndromes, including akathisia, parkinsonism, dystonia, and tardive dyskinesia, represent untoward motor side effects of antipsychotic drug therapy. The mechanism is thought to involve postsynaptic blockade of dopamine receptors (241,248,249). Acute extrapyramidal syndromes present within a few days following administration of neuroleptics and may persist days after withdrawal of the offending agent. Although considered different manifestations of the same underlying etiology, drug-induced akathisia, dystonia, and parkinsonism have unique motor and mental symptoms that help distinguish one from another (249). A less common extrapyramidal reaction to neuroleptics is acute laryngeal dystonia (238).

Tardive dyskinesia, characterized by orofacial dyskinesia, dystonia, and choreoathetosis, is thought to result from hypersensitivity of dopamine receptors in the basal ganglia (due to prolonged postsynaptic receptor blockade by neuroleptics). Advanced age, female gender, history of alcohol or substance abuse, diabetes, and smoking are considered risk factors for tardive dyskinesia in older individuals (248). In contrast to tardive dyskinesia, the parkinsonian side effect is thought to arise from blockade of dopamine receptors in the striatum. Other drugs have been implicated in the development of movement disorders. For instance, lithium, methyldopa, and metoclopramide may bring about parkinsonism (250). Choreoathetosis may result from tricyclic antidepressants, oral contraceptives, amphetamines, pemoline, and lithium (251). Diphenhydramine and flecainide have been reported to cause dystonia; asterixis has been associated with carbamazepine; and phenytoin has been implicated in the development of choreoathetosis (252–255). **Box 21-2** lists drugs commonly encountered in physiatric and neurologic practice that may induce movement disorders.

OTHER TREATMENT CONSIDERATIONS

Botulinum Toxin Injection

Local intramuscular injection of botulinum toxin is arguably the most important advance in the nonsurgical management of dystonia and other movement disorders. Derived from *Clostridium botulinum* serotypes A and B, the neurotoxin affects neuromuscular transmission by blocking the release of acetylcholine. Injected intramuscularly, the toxin results in partial chemodenervation. Clinical effects are seen 24 to 72 hours after injection, and peak effects occur 4 to 6 weeks later. The average duration of effect is 3 to 4 months. Injections are guided by surface anatomy, electromyography, electrical stimulation, or ultrasound. Early indications for treatment were blepharospasm and strabismus. Over the years, it has been utilized to treat various dystonias: cervical dystonia

---

BOX 21-2

Some Medications That May Induce Movement Disorders

Dopamine antagonists
Haloperidol
Metoclopramide
Dopamine agonists
Levodopa
Antihypertensives
Methyldopa
Monoamine oxidase inhibitors
Antiepileptics
Phenytoin
Carbamazepine
Valproic acid
Gabapentin
Felbamate
Adrenergic agents
Amphetamines
Methylphenidate
Caffeine
β-Adrenergic agonists
Others
Antihistaminics
Tricyclic antidepressants
Buspirone
Lithium
Cimetidine
Oral contraceptives
Cocaine
Selective serotonin reuptake inhibitors

Adapted from Jain SS, Francisco GE. Parkinson disease and other movement disorders. In: DeLisa JA, ed. *Rehabilitation Medicine: Principles and Practice*. 3rd ed. Philadelphia, PA: Lippincott Williams & Wilkins; 1988:1035–1041, Ref. (256).

(spasmodic torticollis), hemifacial spasm, orolingual dystonia, cranial dystonia, limb dystonia, and "occupational cramps" (257–260). Because it affects neuromuscular transmission, the toxin is contraindicated in disorders of neuromuscular junction, such as myasthenia gravis and myasthenic syndrome. However, successful use in the treatment of spasmodic torticollis in a patient with myasthenia gravis has been reported (261). Possible adverse effects include excessive weakness in the injected and adjacent muscles. Rare flu-like symptoms and allergic reactions have been described. Readministration of the toxin within 3 months of the previous injection is discouraged to avoid potential development of antibodies.

Intrathecal Baclofen Pump

Intrathecal baclofen may be helpful in alleviating focal limb and axial dystonia (262,263). Early reports suggest beneficial effects; however, its efficacy has not been supported by trials. Furthermore, outcomes from intrathecal baclofen therapy have not been compared directly with those from oral medications, botulinum toxin, and neurosurgical techniques. The pump is an alternative when oral medications are ineffective and their side effects are intolerable or when the severity of the condition requires more than the recommended dose of botulinum toxin. Intervention requires the neurosurgical placement of the pump. Physiatrists may participate in screening patients with movement disorders who might benefit from intrathecal baclofen. Trained physiatrists also play a critical role in postimplantation rehabilitation care by monitoring response and complications and prescribing appropriate therapy interventions. Patients who respond to a trial dose of intrathecal baclofen are considered for surgical implantation of the infusion system. The pump, with the drug reservoir, is placed in the abdominal wall and connected to a catheter that has been introduced to the intrathecal space, usually at the lower thoracic level. An external programmer adjusts the dose, rate, and mode of drug delivery by radiotelemetry. The drug reservoir can be refilled through transcutaneous insertion of a Huber-type needle into the reservoir port. Simple dose titration and safe concurrent use with other therapies, such as oral drugs and botulinum toxin, are among the advantages of intrathecal baclofen. Common adverse effects include drowsiness, weakness, and dizziness, which subside with dose reduction. Pump-related problems include catheter kink, fracture, dislodgment, and disconnection, which are corrected surgically.

REFERENCES

1. National Institute of Neurological Disorders and Stroke. *Parkinson's Disease: Challenges, Progress, and Promise.* Available from: http://www.ninds.nih.gov/disorders/parkinsons_disease/parkinsons_research.htm. Accessed August 1, 2017.
2. Hirsch L, Jette N, Frolkis A, et al. The incidence of Parkinson's disease: a systematic review and meta-analysis. *Neuroepidemiology.* 2016;46(4):292–300.
3. Pringsheim T, Jette N, Frolkis A, et al. The prevalence of Parkinson's disease: a systematic review and meta-analysis. *Mov Disord.* 2014;29(13):1583–1590.
4. DeMaagd G, Philip A. Parkinson's disease and its management. Part 1: Disease entity, risk factors, pathophysiology, clinical presentation, and diagnosis. *P T.* 2015;40(8):504–532.
5. Van Den Eeden SK, Tanner CM, Bernstein AL, et al. Incidence of Parkinson's disease: variation by age, gender, and race/ethnicity. *Am J Epidemiol.* 2003;157(11):1015–1022.
6. Johnson S, Davis M, Kaltenboeck A, et al. Early retirement and income loss in patients with early and advanced Parkinson's disease. *Appl Health Econ Health Policy.* 2011;9(6):367–376.
7. Johnson SJ, Diener MD, Kaltenboeck A, et al. An economic model of Parkinson's disease: implications for slowing progression in the United States. *Mov Disord.* 2013;28(3):319–326.
8. Forsaa EB, Larsen JP, Wentzel-Larsen T, et al. What predicts mortality in Parkinson disease? A prospective population-based long-term study. *Neurology.* 2010;75(14):1270–1276.
9. Parkinson J. *An Essay on the Shaking Palsy.* London: Whittingham and Rowland; 1817.
10. Braak H, Del Tredici K. Invited article: nervous system pathology in sporadic Parkinson's disease. *Neurology.* 2008;70(2):1916–1925.
11. Alexander GE, Crutcher MD. Functional architecture of basal ganglia circuits: neural substrates of parallel processing. *Trends Neurosci.* 1990;13(7):266–271.
12. Mink JW. The basal ganglia: focused selection and inhibition of competing motor programs. *Prog Neurobiol.* 1996;50(4):381–425.
13. Mhyre TH, Boyd JT, Hamill RW, et al. Parkinson's disease. *Subcell Biochem.* 2012;65:389–455.
14. Camilleri A, Vassallo N. The centrality of mitochondria in the pathogenesis and treatment of Parkinson's disease. *CNS Neurosci Ther.* 2014;20(7):591–602.
15. Celardo I, Martins LM, Gandhi S. Unravelling mitochondrial pathways to Parkinson's disease. *Br J Pharmacol.* 2014;171(8):1943–1957.
16. Dexter DT, Jenner P. Parkinson disease: from pathology to molecular disease mechanisms. *Free Radic Biol Med.* 2013;62:132–144.
17. Del Tredici K, Braak H. Sporadic Parkinson's disease: development and distribution of alpha-synuclein pathology. *Neuropathol Appl Neurobiol.* 2015;42(1):33–50.
18. Dickson DW, Braak H, Duda JE, et al. Neuropathological assessment of Parkinson's disease: refining the diagnostic criteria. *Lancet Neurol.* 2009;8(12):1150–1157.
19. Goldman SM, Kamel F, Ross GW, et al. Head injury, alpha-synuclein Rep1 and Parkinson's disease. *Ann Neurol.* 2012;71(1):40–48.
20. Feng LR, Maguire-Zeiss KA. Dopamine and paraquat enhance alpha-synuclein-induced alterations in membrane conductance. *Neurotox Res.* 2011;20(4):387–401.
21. Lu L, Gu L, Liang Y, et al. Dual effects of alpha-synuclein on neurotoxicity induced by low dosage of rotenone are dependent on exposure time in dopaminergic neuroblastoma cells. *Sci China Life Sci.* 2010;53(5):590–597.
22. Khan NL, Jain S, Lynch JM, et al. Mutations in the gene LRRK2 encoding dardarin (PARK8) cause familial Parkinson's disease: clinical, pathological, olfactory and functional imaging and genetic data. *Brain.* 2005;128(Pt 12):2786–2796.
23. Vieira-Brock PL, McFadden LM, Nielsen SM, et al. Chronic nicotine exposure attenuates methamphetamine-induced dopaminergic deficits. *J Pharmacol Exp Ther.* 2015;355(3):463–472.
24. Kenborg L, Lassen CF, Ritz B, et al. Lifestyle, family history, and risk of idiopathic Parkinson disease: a large Danish case-control study. *Am J Epidemiol.* 2015;181(10):808–816.
25. Liu R, Guo X, Park Y, et al. Caffeine intake, smoking, and risk of Parkinson disease in men and women. *Am J Epidemiol.* 2012;175(11):1200–1207.
26. Williams DR, Litvan I. Parkinsonian syndromes. *Continuum.* 2013;19(5):1189–1212.
27. Stewart T, Liu C, Ginghina C, et al. Cerebrospinal fluid alpha-synuclein predicts cognitive decline in Parkinson disease progression in the DATATOP cohort. *Am J Pathol.* 2014;184(4):966–975.
28. Postuma RB, Gagnon JF, Bertrand JA, et al. Parkinson risk in idiopathic REM sleep behavior disorder: preparing for neuroprotective trials. *Neurology.* 2015;84(11):1104–1113.
29. Schenck CH, Boeve BF, Mahowald MW. Delayed emergence of a parkinsonian disorder or dementia in 81% of older men initially diagnosed with idiopathic rapid eye movement sleep behavior disorder: a 16-year update on a previously reported series. *Sleep Med.* 2013;14(8):744–748.
30. Langston JW. The Parkinson's complex: parkinsonism is just the tip of the iceberg. *Ann Neurol.* 2006;59(4):591–596.
31. Toole T, Park SB, Hirsch MA, et al. The multicomponent nature of equilibrium in persons with Parkinson's disease: a regression approach. *J Neural Transm.* 1996;103:561–580.
32. Vaughan RA, Foster JD. Mechanisms of dopamine transporter regulation in normal and disease states. *Trends Pharmacol Sci.* 2013;34(9):489–496.
33. Okun M. *What's hot in PD? An update on DAT scanning for Parkinson's disease diagnosis.* Available from: https://parkinson.org/blog/whats-hot/update-DAT-scanning. Accessed March 12, 2019.
34. Daviet JC, Roy X, Quelven-Bertin I, et al. Parkinson's patient runs an ultra-marathon: a case report. *Eur J Phys Rehabil Med.* 2014;50:447–451.
35. Kalia L, Lang A. Evolving basic pathologic and clinical concepts in PD. *Nat Rev Neurol.* 2016;12:65–66.
36. Hoehn M, Yahr M. Parkinsonism: onset, progression and mortality. *Neurology.* 1967;17(5):427–442.
37. Fahn S, Elton RL; UPDRS Program Members. Unified Parkinson's disease rating scale. In: Fahn S, Marsden CD, Goldstein M, et al., eds. *Recent Developments in Parkinson's Disease.* Vol. 2. Florham Park, NJ: Macmillan Healthcare Information; 1987:153–163, 293–304.
38. Goetz CG, Tilley BC, et al. Movement Disorder Society-Sponsored Revision of the Unified Parkinson's Disease Rating Scale (MDS-UPDRS): scale presentation and clinimetric testing results. *Mov Disord.* 2008;23(15):2129–2170.
39. International Parkinson and Movement Disorder Society. *MDS Rating Scales.* 2017. Available from: http://www.movementdisorders.org/MDS/Education/Rating-Scales.htm. Accessed January 20, 2017.
40. Ballard PA, Tetrud JW, Langston JW. Permanent human parkinsonism due to 1-methyl-4-phenyl-1,2,3, 6-tetrahydropyridine (MPTP): seven cases. *Neurology.* 1985;35(7):949–956.
41. Fernandez HH, Standaert DG, Hauser RA, et al. Levodopa-carbidopa intestinal gel in advanced Parkinson's disease: final 12-month, open-label results. *Mov Disord.* 2015;30(4):500–509.
42. Ferreira JJ, Katzenschlager R, Bloem BR, et al. Summary of the recommendations of the EFNS/MDS-ES review on therapeutic management of Parkinson's disease. *Eur J Neurol.* 2013;20(1):5–15.
43. Grimes D, Gordon J, Snelgrove B, et al. Canadian guidelines on Parkinson's disease. *Can J Neurol Sci.* 2012;39(suppl 4):S1–S30.
44. DeMaagd G, Phillip A. Parkinson's disease and its management. Part 2: Introduction to the pharmacotherapy of Parkinson's disease, with a focus on the use of dopaminergic agents. *P T.* 2015;40(9):590–600.
45. DeMaagd G, Phillip A. Parkinson's disease and its management. Part 3: Nondopaminergic and nonpharmacological therapy options. *P T.* 2015;40(10):668–679.
46. Giugni JC, Okun MS. Treatment of advanced Parkinson's disease. *Curr Opin Neurol.* 2014;27(4):450–460.
47. Drugs.com [Internet]. *Xadago Information from Drugs.com.* c2000-2019. [Cited: 22 January 2017]. Available from: https://www.drugs.com/history/xadago.html.
48. Zuardi AW, Crippa J, Hallak J, et al. Cannabidiol for the treatment of psychosis in Parkinson's disease. *J Psychopharmacol.* 2009;23(8):979–983.
49. Chagas MH, Eckeli AL, Zuardi AW, et al. Cannabidiol can improve complex sleep-related behaviors associated with rapid eye movement sleep behavior disorder in Parkinson's disease patients: a case series. *J Clin Pharm Ther.* 2014;39(5):564–566.
50. Hassan A, Wu SS, Dai Y, et al. High rates and risk factors for emergency room visits and hospitalization in Parkinson's disease. *Parkinsonism Relat Disord.* 2013;19(11):949–954.
51. Perlmutter JS, Mink JW. Deep brain stimulation. *Annu Rev Neurosci.* 2006;29:1–598.
52. Moro E, Lozano AM, Pollak P, et al. Long-term results of a multicenter study on subthalamic and pallidal stimulation in Parkinson's disease. *Mov Disord.* 2010;25(5):578–586.
53. Fasano A, Lozano AM. Deep brain stimulation for movement disorders: 2015 and beyond. *Curr Opin Neurol.* 2015;28(4):423–436.
54. Bloem BR, van Laar T, Keus SHJ. *Multidisciplinary Guideline "Parkinson's Disease".* Alphen aan den Rijn, The Netherlands: Van Zuiden Communications; 2010.

55. Post B, van der Eijk M, Munneke M, et al. Multidisciplinary care for Parkinson's disease: not if, but how! *Pract Neurol.* 2011;11:58–61.

56. Frazzitta G, Maestri R, Ferrazzoli D, et al. Multidisciplinary intensive rehabilitation treatment improves sleep quality in Parkinson's disease. *J Clin Mov Disord.* 2015;2:11.

57. van der Marck MA, Bloem BR, Borm GF, et al. Effectiveness of multidisciplinary care for Parkinson's disease: a randomized, controlled trial. *Mov Disord.* 2013;28(5):605–611.

58. Hassan A, Wu SS, Schmidt P, et al. What are the issues facing Parkinson's disease patients at ten years of disease and beyond?: data from the NPF-QII study. *Parkinsonism Relat Disord.* 2012;18(suppl 3):S10–S14.

59. van Nimwegen M, Speelman AD, Hofman-van Rossum EJ, et al. Physical inactivity in Parkinson's disease. *J Neurol.* 2011;258(12):2214–2221.

60. Ellis T, Boudreau JK, DeAngelis TR, et al. Barriers to exercise in people with Parkinson disease. *Phys Ther.* 2013;93:628–636.

61. Hirsch MA, Farley BG. Exercise, neuroplasticity and Parkinson's disease. *Eur J Phys Rehabil Med.* 2009;45(2):215–229.

62. van Nimwegen M, Speelman AD, Smulders K, et al. Design and baseline characteristics of the ParkFit study, a randomized controlled trial evaluating the effectiveness of a multifaceted behavioral program to increase physical activity in Parkinson patients. *BMC Neurol.* 2010;10:70.

63. van Nimwegen M, Speelman AD, Overeem S, et al. Promotion of physical activity and fitness in sedentary patients with Parkinson's disease: randomised controlled trial. *BMJ.* 2013;346:f576.

64. Nanhoe-Mahabier W, De Laat KF, Visser JE, et al. Parkinson disease and comorbid cerebrovascular disease. *Nat Rev Neurol.* 2009;5:533–541.

65. Visser M, Marinus J, van Hilten JJ, et al. Assessing comorbidity in patients with Parkinson's disease. *Mov Disord.* 2004;19(7):824–828.

66. Petzinger GM, Fisher BE, McEwen S, et al. Exercise-enhanced neuroplasticity targeting motor and cognitive circuitry in Parkinson's disease. *Lancet Neurol.* 2013;12(7):716–726.

67. Tuon T, Valvassori SS, Lopes-Borges J, et al. Physical training exerts neuroprotective effects in the regulation of neurochemical factors in an animal model of Parkinson's disease. *Neuroscience.* 2012;227:305–312.

68. Dutra MF, Jaeger M, Ilha J, et al. Exercise improves motor deficits and alters striatal GFAP expression in a 6-OHDA-induced rat model of Parkinson's disease. *Neurol Sci.* 2012;33(5):1137–1144.

69. VanLeeuwen JE, Petzinger GM, Walsh JP, et al. Altered AMPA receptor expression with treadmill exercise in the 1-methyl-4-phenyl-1,2,3,6-tetrahydropyridine-lesioned mouse model of basal ganglia injury. *J Neurosci Res.* 2010;88(3):650–668.

70. Fisher BE, Wu AD, Salem GJ, et al. The effect of exercise training in improving motor performance and corticomotor excitability in persons with early Parkinson's disease. *Arch Phys Med Rehabil.* 2008;89(7):1221–1229.

71. Fisher BE, Li Q, Nacca A, et al. Treadmill exercise elevates striatal dopamine D2 receptor binding potential in patients with early Parkinson's disease. *Neuroreport.* 2013;24:509–514.

72. Munneke M, Nijkrake MJ, Keus SH, et al. Efficacy of community-based physiotherapy networks for patients with Parkinson's disease: a cluster-randomised trial. *Lancet Neurol.* 2010;9(1):46–54.

73. Beersen N, Berg M, van Galen M, et al. *Onderzoek naar de meerwaarde van ParkinsonNet [Research into the Added Value of ParkinsonNet].* The Netherlands: KPMG-Plexus, Vektis; 2011:1–42.

74. Keus SHJ, Oude Nijhuis LB, Nijkrake MJ, et al. Improving community healthcare for patients with Parkinson's disease: the Dutch model. *Parkinsons Dis.* 2012;2012:543426, 7 pages.

75. Keus SHJ, Munneke M, Nijkrake MJ, et al. Evidence-based, patient-centered physiotherapy for people with Parkinson's: a pilot implementation of the Dutch ParkinsonNet concept in Germany. *Mov Disord.* 2015;30(suppl 1):S373.

76. Hirsch MA, Iyer SS, Sanjak M. Developing a regional community-based exercise network for Parkinson's disease. World Congress on Parkinson's Disease and Related Disorders; 2013; Geneva, Switzerland.

77. Grosset KA, Grosset DG. Patient-perceived involvement and satisfaction in Parkinson's disease: effect on therapy decisions and quality of life. *Mov Disord.* 2005;20:616–619.

78. Nijkrake MJ, Keus SHJ, Quist-Anholts GWL, et al. Evaluation of a patient-specific index as an outcome measure for physiotherapy in Parkinson's disease. *Eur J Phys Rehabil Med.* 2009;45:507–512.

79. Brown P, Steiger M. Basal ganglia gait disorders. In: Bronstein AM, Brandt T, Woollacott MH, eds. *Clinical Disorders of Balance, Posture and Gait.* London: Arnold; 1996:156–167.

80. Huxham F, Baker R, Morris ME, et al. Head and trunk rotation during walking turns in Parkinson's disease. *Mov Disord.* 2008;23(10):1391–1397.

81. Boonstra TA, van der Kooij H, Munneke M, et al. Gait disorders and balance disturbances in Parkinson's disease: clinical update and pathophysiology. *Curr Opin Neurol.* 2008;24(4):461–471.

82. Plotnik M, Giladi N, Hausdorff JM. Bilateral coordination of walking and freezing of gait in Parkinson's disease. *Eur J Neurosci.* 2008;27(8):1999–2006.

83. Knutsson E. An analysis of Parkinsonian gait. *Brain.* 1972;95(3):475–486.

84. Keus SHJ, Munneke M, Graziano M, et al. *European Physiotherapy Guideline for Parkinson's Disease.* The Netherlands: KNGF/ParkinsonNet; 2014.

85. Hass CJ, Bishop M, Moscovich M, et al. Defining the clinically meaningful difference in gait speed in persons with Parkinson disease. *J Neurol Phys Ther.* 2014;38(4):233–238.

86. A History of Pedestrian Signal Walking Speed Assumptions. Seattle, Washington: 3rd Urban Street Symposium; 2007.

87. Matinolli M, Korpelainen JT, Sotaniemi KA, et al. Recurrent falls and mortality in Parkinson's disease: a prospective two-year follow-up study. *Acta Neurol Scand.* 2011;123(3):193–200.

88. Ashburn A, Stack E, Ballinger C, et al. The circumstances of falls among people with Parkinson's disease and the use of Falls Diaries to facilitate reporting. *Disabil Rehabil.* 2008;30(16):1–8.

89. Dietz V, Zijlstra W, Assaiante C, et al. Balance control in Parkinson's disease. *Gait Posture.* 1993;1:77–84.

90. McIntosh GC, Brown SH, Rice RR, et al. Rhythmic auditory-motor facilitation of gait patterns in patients with Parkinson's disease. *J Neurol Neurosurg Psychiatry.* 1997;62(1):22–26.

91. Morris M, Iansek R, Matyas T, et al. Abnormalities in the stride length-cadence relation in parkinsonian gait. *Mov Disord.* 1998;13(1):61–69.

92. Mak MKY, Pang MYC. Fear of falling is independently associated with recurrent falls in patients with Parkinson's disease: a 1-year prospective study. *J Neurol.* 2009;256:1689.

93. Bello O, Sanchez JA, Lopez-Alonso V, et al. The effects of treadmill or overground walking training program on gait in Parkinson's disease. *Gait Posture.* 2013;38(4):590–595.

94. Ganesan M, Sathyaprabha TN, Gupta A, et al. Effect of partial weighted supported treadmill gait training on balance in patients with Parkinson disease. *PM R.* 2014;6(1):22–33.

95. Tomlinson CL, Herd CP, Clarke CE, et al. Physiotherapy for Parkinson's disease: a comparison of techniques (Review). *Cochrane Database Syst Rev.* 2014;(6):CD002815.

96. Csuy J, Grondin N. *Falls Prevention Workbook.* National Parkinson's Foundation; Lee Memorial Health System Rehabilitation Services Older Adult Services; and Southwest Community Foundation. Available from: https://www.parkinson.org/sites/default/files/NPF_Manual_FallsPrevention.pdf. Accessed January 22, 2017.

97. Hirsch MA, Toole T, Maitland CG, et al. The Effects of balance training and high-intensity resistance training on persons with idiopathic Parkinson's disease. *Arch Phys Med Rehabil.* 2003;84(8):1109–1117.

98. Paul SS, Canning CG, Sherrington C, et al. Three simple clinical tests to accurately predict falls in people with Parkinson's disease. *Mov Disord.* 2013;28(5):655–662.

99. Li F, Fitzgerald K. Tai Chi and postural stability in patients with Parkinson's disease. *N Engl J Med.* 2012;366(6):511–519.

100. McGinley JL, Martin C, Huxham FE, et al. Feasibility, safety, and compliance in a randomized controlled trial of physical therapy for Parkinson's disease. *Parkinsons Dis.* 2012;2012:795294.

101. Muenter MD, Sharpless NS, Tyce GM, et al. Patterns of dystonia ("I-D-I" and "D-I-D-") in response to l-dopa therapy for Parkinson's disease. *Mayo Clin Proc.* 1977;52(3):163–174.

102. Carter J. Exercise. In: Johnson A, ed. *Young Parkinson's Handbook.* New York: American Parkinson Disease Association; 1995:29–33.

103. Comella CL, Stebbins GT, Brown-Toms N, et al. Physical therapy and Parkinson's disease: a controlled clinical trial. *Neurology.* 1994;44(3 pt 1):376–378.

104. Huxham F, Baker R, Morris ME, et al. Footstep adjustments used to turn during walking in Parkinson's disease. *Mov Disord.* 2008;23(6):817–823.

105. Giladi N. Freezing of gait. Clinical overview. *Adv Neurol.* 2001;87:191–197.

106. Ehgoetz Martens KA, Pieruccini-Faria F, Almeida QJ. Could sensory mechanisms be a core factor that underlies freezing of gait in underlies freezing of gait in Parkinson's disease? *PLoS One.* 2013;8(5):e62602.

107. Morris ME. Locomotor training in people with Parkinson disease. *Phys Ther.* 2006;86(10):1426–1435.

108. Schaafsma JD, Balash Y, Gurevich T, et al. Characterization of freezing of gait subtypes and the response of each to levodopa in Parkinson's disease. *Eur J Neurol.* 2003;10(4):391–398.

109. Snijders AH, van de Warrenburg BP, Giladi N, et al. Neurological gait disorders in elderly people: clinical approach and classification. *Lancet Neurol.* 2007;6(1):63–74.

110. Ferraye MU, et al. The laser-shoe: a new form of continuous ambulatory cueing for patients with Parkinson's disease. *Parkinsonism Relat Disord.* 2016;29:127–128. doi: 10.1016/j.parkreldis.2016.05.004

111. Nonnekes J, Snijders AH, Nutt JG, et al. Freezing of gait: a practical approach to management. *Lancet Neurol.* 2015;14(7):768–778.

112. Janssen S, Soneji M, Nonnekes J, et al. A painted staircase illusion to alleviate freezing of gait in Parkinson's disease. *J Neurol.* 2016;263(8):1661–1662.

113. Dibble LE, Hale TF, Marcus RL, et al. High intensity eccentric resistance training decreases bradykinesia and improves Quality Of Life in persons with Parkinson's disease: a preliminary study. *Parkinsonism Relat Disord.* 2009;15(10):752–757.

114. David FJ, Robichaud JA, Vaillancourt DE, et al. Progressive resistance exercise restores some properties of the triphasic EMG pattern and improves bradykinesia: the PRET-PD randomized controlled trial. *J Neurophysiol.* 2016;116(5):2298–2311.

115. Ni M, Signorile JF, Balachandran A, et al. Power training induced change in bradykinesia and muscle power in Parkinson's disease. *Parkinsonism Relat Disord.* 2016;23:37–44.

116. Olanow CW, Watts RL, Koller WC. An algorithm (decision tree) for the management of Parkinson's disease (2001): treatment guidelines. *Neurology.* 2001;56(11 suppl 5):S1–S88.

117. Morris ME, Huxham F, McGinley J, et al. The biomechanics and motor control of gait in Parkinson disease. *Clin Biomech (Bristol, Avon).* 2001;16(6):459–470.

118. Bronstein A, Hood J, Gresty M, et al. Visual control of balance in cerebellar and Parkinsonian syndromes. *Brain.* 1990;113:767–779.

119. Parkinson Study Group. DATATOP: a multicenter controlled clinical trial in early Parkinson's disease. *Arch Neurol.* 1989;46(10):1052–1060.

120. Stummer C, Dibilio V, Overeem S, et al. The walk-bicycle: a new assistive device for Parkinson's patients with freezing of gait? *Parkinsonism Relat Disord.* 2015;21(7):755–757.

121. Snijders AH, Bloem BR. Images in clinical medicine. Cycling for freezing of gait. *N Engl J Med.* 2010;362(13):e46.

122. Snijders AH, Toni I, Ruzicka E, et al. Bicycling breaks the ice for freezers of gait. *Mov Disord.* 2011;26(3):367–371.

123. Snijders AH, van Kesteren M, Bloem BR. Cycling is less affected than walking in freezers of gait. *J Neurol Neurosurg Psychiatry.* 2012;83(5):575–576.

124. Luhnes CA, Earhart GM. The impact of attentional, auditory, and combined cues on walking during single and cognitive dual tasks in Parkinson disease. *Gait Posture.* 2011;33(3):478–483.

125. Logemann JA, Blonsky ER, Boshes B. Dysphagia in parkinsonism [editorial]. *JAMA.* 1975;231(1):69–70.

126. Robbins J. Normal swallowing and aging. *Semin Neurol.* 1996;16(4):309–317.

127. Leopold NA, Kagel MC. Pharyngo-esophageal dysphagia in Parkinson's disease. *Dysphagia.* 1997;12(1):11–18.

128. Beyer PL, Palarino MY, Michalek D, et al. Weight change and body composition in patients with Parkinson's disease. *J Am Diet Assoc.* 1995;95(9):979–983.

129. Nutt JG, Carter JH. Sensory symptoms in parkinsonism related to central dopaminergic function. *Lancet.* 1984;2(8400):456–457.

130. Eadie M, Tyler J. Alimentary disorders in parkinsonism. *Australas Ann Med.* 1965;14:13–22.

131. Suttrup I, Warnecke T. Dysphagia in Parkinson's disease. *Dysphagia.* 2016;31: 24–32.

132. Jost WH. Gastrointestinal motility problems in patients with Parkinson's disease. Effects of antiparkinsonian treatment and guidelines for management. *Drugs Aging.* 1997;10(4):249–258.

133. Edwards L, Quigley EM, Hofman R, et al. Gastrointestinal symptoms in Parkinson disease: 18-month follow-up study. *Mov Disord.* 1993;8(1):83–86.

134. Mukherjee A, Biswas A, Das SK. Gut dysfunction in Parkinson's disease. *World J Gastroenterol.* 2016;22(25):5742–5752.

135. Kim JS, Sung HY. Gastrointestinal autonomic dysfunction in patients with Parkinson's disease. *J Mov Disord.* 2015;8(2):76–82.

136. Fasano A, Visanji N, Liu L, et al. Gastrointestinal dysfunction in Parkinson's disease. *Lancet Neurol.* 2015;14(6):625–639.

137. Nutt J, Carter J. Dietary issues in the treatment of Parkinson's disease. In: Koller WC, Paulson G, eds. *Handbook of Parkinson's Disease.* New York: M. Dekker; 1987:531–553.

138. Sakakibara R, Tateno F, Nagao T, et al. Bladder function of patients with Parkinson's disease. *Int J Urol.* 2014;21(7):638–646.

139. Badri AV, Purohit RS, Skenazy J, et al. A review of lower urinary tract symptoms in patients with Parkinson's disease. *Curr Urol Rep.* 2014;15(9):435.

140. Emre M, Aarsland D, Brown R, et al. Clinical diagnostic criteria for dementia associated with Parkinson's disease. *Mov Disord.* 2007;22(12):1689–1707.

141. Davis AA, Racette B. Parkinson disease and cognitive impairment: five new things. *Neurol Clin Pract.* 2016;6:452–458.

142. Foltynie T, Brayne CEG, Robbins TW, et al. The CamPaIGN study. The cognitive ability of an incident cohort of Parkinson's patients in the UK. *Brain.* 2004;127:50–60.

143. Leung I, Walton C, Hallock H, et al. Cognitive training in Parkinson disease. *Neurology.* 2015;85(21):1843–1851.

144. Picelli A, Varalta V, Melotti C, et al. Effects of treadmill training on cognitive and motor features of patients with mild to moderate Parkinson's disease: a pilot, single blind, randomized controlled trial. *Funct Neurol.* 2016;31(1):25–31.

145. Altmann LJP, Stegemoller E, Hazamy AA, et al. Aerobic exercise improves mood, cognition, and language function in Parkinson's disease: results of a controlled study. *J Int Neuropsychol Soc.* 2016;22(9):978–989.

146. David FJ, Robichaud JA, Leurgans SE, et al. Exercise improves cognition in Parkinson's disease: the PRET-PD randomized, clinical trial. *Mov Disord.* 2015;30(12):1657–1663.

147. Tanaka K, de Quadros AC, Santo RF, et al. Benefits of physical exercise on executive functions in older people with Parkinson's disease. *Brain Cogn.* 2009;69(2): 435–441.

148. Gulyani S, Salas R, Mari Z, et al. Evaluating and managing sleep disorders in the Parkinson's disease clinic. *Basal Ganglia.* 2016;6(3):165–172.

149. Seppi K, Weintraub D, Coelho M, et al. Update: treatments for Non-motor Symptoms of Parkinson's disease–December 2012. *Evidenced Based Medicine Publications.* Movement Disorder Society; 2013. Available from: http://www.movementdisorders.org/MDS-Files1/PDFs/EBM-Papers/EBM-NMS-Updated15Jan2014.pdf. Accessed March 14, 2019.

150. Postuma RB, Lang AE, Munhoz RP, et al. Caffeine for treatment of Parkinson disease: a randomized controlled trial. *Neurology.* 2012;79(7):651–658.

151. Chahine LM, Amara AW, Videnovic A. A systematic review of the literature on disorders of sleep and wakefulness in Parkinson's disease from 2005 to 2015. *Sleep Med Rev.* 2017;35:33–50.

152. Silva-Batista C, Campos de Brito L, Corcos DM, et al. Resistance training improves sleep quality in subjects with moderate Parkinson's disease. *J Strength Cond Res.* 2017;31(8):2270–2277.

153. Xiao CM, Zhuang YC. Effect of health Baduanjin Qigong for mild to moderate Parkinson's disease. *Geriatr Gerontol Int.* 2016;16(8):911–919.

154. Rimmelzwaan L, van Schoor N, Lips P. Systematic review of the relationship between vitamin D and Parkinson's disease. *J Park Dis.* 2016;6(1):29–37.

155. Torsney KM, Noyce AJ, Doherty KM, et al. Bone health in Parkinson's disease: a systematic review and meta-analysis. *J Neurol Neurosurg Psychiatry.* 2014;85(10):1159–1166.

156. Zhao Y, Shen L, Ji HF. Osteoporosis risk and bone mineral density levels in patients with Parkinson's disease: a meta-analysis. *Bone.* 2013;52(1):498–505.

157. Dennison EM, Compston JE, Flahive J, et al. Effect of co-morbidities on fracture risk: findings from the Global Longitudinal Study of Osteoporosis in Women (GLOW). *Bone.* 2012;50(6):1288–1293.

158. Ozturk EA, Gundogdu I, Tonuk B, et al. Bone mass and vitamin D levels in Parkinson's disease: is there any difference between genders? *J Phys Ther Sci.* 2016;28:2204–2209.

159. Malochet-Guinamand S, Durif F, Thomas T. Parkinson's disease: a risk factor for osteoporosis. *Joint Bone Spine.* 2015;82(6):406–410.

160. Tan L, Wang Y, Zhou L, et al. Parkinson's disease and risk of fracture: a meta-analysis of prospective cohort studies. *PLoS One.* 2014;9(4):e94379.

161. Idjadi JA, Aharonoff GB, Su H, et al. Hip fracture outcomes in patients with Parkinson's disease. *Am J Orthop (Belle Mead NJ).* 2005;34(7):341–346.

162. Reijnders JS, Ehrt U, Weber WE, et al. A systematic review of prevalence studies of depression in Parkinson's disease. *Mov Disord.* 2008;23(2):183–189.

163. Cognitive and Emotional Aspects of Parkinson's Disease. National Institute of Neurological Disorders and Stroke, National Institute on Aging, and National Institute of Mental Health Working Group Meeting. January 24 to 25, 2001 (Unpublished Summary).

164. de la Riva P, Smith K, Xie SX, et al. Course of psychiatric symptoms and global cognition in early Parkinson disease. *Neurology.* 2014;83(12):1096–1103.

165. Kirsch-Darrow L, Fernandez HF, Marsiske M. Dissociating apathy and depression in Parkinson disease. *Neurology.* 2006;67(1):33–38.

166. Poewe W, Luginger E. Depression in Parkinson's disease: impediments to recognition and treatment options. *Neurology.* 1999;52(7 suppl 3):S2–S6.

167. Serratrice G, Michel B. Pain in Parkinson's disease patients. *Rev Rhum Engl Ed.* 1999;66(6):331–338.

168. Snider S, Sandyk R. Sensory dysfunction. In: Koller WC, ed. *Handbook of Parkinson's Disease.* New York: Dekker; 1987:171–180.

169. Waseem S, Gwinn-Hardy K. Pain in Parkinson's disease. Common yet seldom recognized symptom is treatable. *Postgrad Med.* 2001;110(6):33–40, 46.

170. Schrag A, Barone P, Brown RG, et al. Depression rating scales in Parkinson's disease: critique and recommendations. *Mov Disord.* 2007;22(8):1077–1092.

171. Ehmann TS, Beninger RJ, Gawel MJ, et al. Depressive symptoms in Parkinson's disease: a comparison with disabled control subjects. *J Geriatr Psychiatry Neurol.* 1990;3:3–9.

172. Menza MA, Mark MH. Parkinson's disease and depression: the relationship to disability and personality. *J Neuropsychiatry Clin Neurosci.* 1994;6:165–169.

173. Richard IH, McDermott MP, Kurlan R, et al. A randomized, double-blind, placebo-controlled trial of antidepressants in Parkinson disease. *Neurology.* 2012;78(16):1229–1236.

174. Menza M, Dobkin RD, Marin H, et al. A controlled trial of antidepressants in patients with Parkinson disease and depression. *Neurology.* 2009;72(10):886–892.

175. Dobkin RD, Menza M, Allen LA, et al. Cognitive-behavioral therapy for depression in Parkinson's disease: a randomized, controlled trial. *Am J Psychiatry.* 2011;168(10):1066–1074.

176. Rosqvist K, Hagell P, Odin P, et al. Factors associated with life satisfaction in Parkinson's disease. *Acta Neurol Scand.* 2017;136(1):64–71.

177. Hackney M, Earhart G. Health-related quality of life and alternative forms of exercise in Parkinson disease. *Parkinsonism Relat Disord.* 2009;15(9):644–648.

178. Ebersbach G, Ebersbach A, Edler D, et al. Comparing exercise in Parkinson's disease—the Berlin LSVT®BIG study. *Mov Disord.* 2010;25:1902–1908.

179. Nilsson MH, Iwarsson S. Home and health in people ageing with Parkinson's disease: study protocol for a prospective longitudinal cohort survey study. *BMC Neurol.* 2013;13:142.

180. Young Blood MR, Ferro MM, Munhoz RP, et al. Classification and characteristics of pain associated with Parkinson's disease. *Parkinsons Dis.* 2016;2016:6067132.

181. Vaserman-Lehuede N, Verin M. Shoulder pain in patients with Parkinson's disease. *Rev Rhum Engl Ed.* 1999;66(4):220–223.

182. Snider SR, Fahn S, Isgreen WP, et al. Primary sensory symptoms in parkinsonism. *Neurology.* 1976;26(5):423–429.

183. Speelman AD, Groothuis JT, van Nimwegen M, et al. Cardiovascular responses during a submaximal exercise test in patients with Parkinson's disease. *J Parkinsons Dis.* 2012;2(3):241–247.

184. Seppi K, Weintraub D, Coelho M, et al. The movement disorder society evidence-based medicine review update: treatments for the non-motor symptoms of Parkinson's disease. *Mov Disord.* 2011;(26):S42–S80.

185. Zanetti R, Antonini A, Gatto G, et al. Valvular heart disease and the use of dopamine agonists for Parkinson's disease. *N Engl J Med.* 2007;356:39–46.

186. Speelman AD, van de Warrenburg BP, van Nimwegen M, et al. How might physical activity benefit patients with Parkinson disease? *Nat Rev Neurol.* 2011;7(9):528–534.

187. Ellis T, de Goede CJ, Feldman RG, et al. Efficacy of a physical therapy program in patients with Parkinson's disease: a randomized controlled trial. *Arch Phys Med Rehabil.* 2005;86(4):626–632.

188. Available from: https://www.lsvtglobal.com/patient-resources/what-is-lsvt-big

189. Available from: https://www.lsvtglobal.com/patient-resources/what-is-lsvt-loud

190. Ramig LO, Sapir S, Countryman S, et al. Intensive voice treatment (LSVT) for patients with Parkinson's disease: a 2 year follow up. *J Neurol Neurosurg Psychiatry.* 2001;71:493–498.

191. Tomlinson CL, Patel S, Meek C, et al. Physiotherapy versus no intervention in Parkinson's disease. *Cochrane Database Syst Rev.* 2012;11(7):CD002817.

192. Rigdel AL, Vitek JL, Alberts JL. Forced, not voluntary, exercise improves motor function in Parkinson's disease patients. *Neurorehabil Neural Repair.* 2009;23(6):600–608.

193. Kegelmeyer DA, Parthasarathy S, Kostyk SK, et al. Assistive devices alter gait patterns in Parkinson disease: advantages of the four-wheeled walker. *Gait Posture.* 2013;38(1):20–24.

194. Spaulding S, Barber B, Colby M, et al. Cuing and gait improvement among people with Parkinson's disease: a meta-analysis. *Arch Phys Med Rehabil.* 2013;94(3):562–570.

195. Sanger TD, Delgado MR, Gaebler-Spira D, et al. Task force on childhood motor disorders classification and definition of disorders causing hypertonia in childhood. *Pediatrics.* 2003;111:e89–e97.

196. Bhidayasiri R, Ling H. Multiple system atrophy. *Neurologist.* 2008;14(4):224–237.

197. Williams DR, Lees AJ. Progressive supranuclear palsy: clinicopathological concepts and diagnostic challenges. *Lancet Neurol.* 2009;8(3):270–279.

198. Josif S, Graham K. Diagnosis and treatment of dementia with Lewy bodies. *JAAPA.* 2008;21(5):22–26.

199. Evidente VG. Understanding essential tremor. Differential diagnosis and options for treatment. *Postgrad Med.* 2000;108(5):138–140, 143–146, 149.

200. Benabid AL, Pollak P, Gao D, et al. Chronic electrical stimulation of the ventralis intermedius nucleus of the thalamus as a treatment of movement disorders. *J Neurosurg.* 1996;84(2):203–214.

201. Camicioli R. Movement disorders in geriatric rehabilitation. *Clin Geriatr Med.* 1993;9(4):765–781.

202. Findley LJ. Tremor: differential diagnosis and pharmacology. In: Jankovic J, Tolosa E, eds. *Parkinson's Disease and Movement Disorders.* Baltimore, MD: Williams & Wilkins; 1993:293–314.

203. Jacob PC, Pratap CR. Posttraumatic rubral tremor responsive to clonazepam. *Mov Disord.* 1998;13(6):977–978.

204. Bhidayasiri R. Differential diagnosis of common tremor syndromes. *Postgrad Med J.* 2005;81:756–762.

205. Jankovic J. Can peripheral trauma induce dystonia and other movement disorders? Yes! *Mov Disord.* 2001;16(1):7–12.

206. Weiner WJ. Can peripheral trauma induce dystonia? No! *Mov Disord.* 2001;16(1):13–22.

207. Janavs JL, Aminoff MJ. Dystonia and chorea in acquired systemic disorders. *J Neurol Neurosurg Psychiatry.* 1998;65(4):436–445.

208. Stanislav SW, Childs NL. Dystonia associated with sertraline. *J Clin Psychopharmacol.* 1999;19(1):98–100.

209. Marsden CD, Rothwell JC. The physiology of idiopathic dystonia. *Can J Neurol Sci.* 1987;14(3 suppl):521–527.

210. Obeso JA, Gimenez-Roldan S. Clinicopathological correlation in symptomatic dystonia. *Adv Neurol.* 1988;50:113–122.

211. Lee MS, Marsden CD. Movement disorders following lesions of the thalamus or subthalamic region. *Mov Disord.* 1994;9(5):493–507.

212. Sandyk R, Bamford CR. The hypothalamic luteinizing hormone releasing hormone "pulse generator" and the opioid system in Tourette's syndrome. *Int J Neurosci.* 1988;41(1–2):81–82.

213. Adler CH. Strategies for controlling dystonia. Overview of therapies that may alleviate symptoms. *Postgrad Med.* 2000;108(5):151–156, 159.

214. Sandyk R. Treatment of writer's cramp with sodium valproate and baclofen. A case report. *S Afr Med J.* 1983;63(18):702–703.

215. Seibel MO, Date ES, Zeiner H, et al. Rehabilitation of patients with Hallervorden-Spatz syndrome. *Arch Phys Med Rehabil.* 1993;74(3):328–329.

216. Truong DD, Sandroni P, van den NS, et al. Diphenhydramine is effective in the treatment of idiopathic dystonia. *Arch Neurol.* 1995;52(4):405–407.

217. Jankovic J. Botulinum toxin in movement disorders. *Curr Opin Neurol.* 1994;7(4):358–366.

218. Hornykiewicz O, Kish SJ, Becker LE, et al. Biochemical evidence for brain neurotransmitter changes in idiopathic torsion dystonia (dystonia musculorum deformans). *Adv Neurol.* 1988;50:157–165.

219. Jankovic J, Leder S, Warner D, et al. Cervical dystonia: clinical findings and associated movement disorders. *Neurology.* 1991;41(7):1088–1091.

220. Jankovic J, Shale H. Dystonia in musicians. *Semin Neurol.* 1989;9(2):131–135.

221. Hunter D. *The Diseases of Occupations.* London: Hodder & Stoughton; 1978 (Abstract).

222. Higgins DS Jr. Chorea and its disorders. *Neurol Clin.* 2001;19(3):707–722, vii.

223. Vonsattel JP, Myers RH, Stevens TJ, et al. Neuropathological classification of Huntington's disease. *J Neuropathol Exp Neurol.* 1985;44(6):559–577.

224. Burnett L, Jankovic J. Chorea and ballism. *Curr Opin Neurol Neurosurg.* 1992;5(3):308–313.

225. Quinn N, Schrag A. Huntington's disease and other choreas. *J Neurol.* 1998;245(11):709–716.

226. Provenzale JM, Glass JP. Hemiballismus: CT and MR findings. *J Comput Assist Tomogr.* 1995;19(4):537–540.

227. Kant R, Zeiler D. Hemiballismus following closed head injury. *Brain Inj.* 1996;10(2):155–158.

228. Berardelli A. Transcranial magnetic stimulation in movement disorders. *Electroencephalogr Clin Neurophysiol Suppl.* 1999;51:276–280.

229. Lietz TE, Huff JS. Hemiballismus as a presenting sign of hyperglycemia. *Am J Emerg Med.* 1995;13(6):647–648.

230. Gupta R, Emili A, Pan G, et al. Characterization of the interaction between the acidic activation domain of VP16 and the RNA polymerase II initiation factor TFIIB. *Nucleic Acids Res.* 1996;24(12):2324–2330.

231. Levesque MF, Markham C, Nakasato N. MR-guided ventral intermediate thalamotomy for posttraumatic hemiballismus. *Stereotact Funct Neurosurg.* 1992;58(1–4):88.

232. Trelles L, Trelles JO, Castro C, et al. Successful treatment of two cases of intention tremor with clonazepam. *Ann Neurol.* 1984;16(5):621.

233. Cardoso F, Jankovic J. Peripherally induced tremor and parkinsonism. *Arch Neurol.* 1995;52(3):263–270.

234. Tsubokawa T, Katayama Y, Yamamoto T. Control of persistent hemiballismus by chronic thalamic stimulation. Report of two cases. *J Neurosurg.* 1995;82(3):501–505.

235. Stewart JT. Akathisia following traumatic brain injury: treatment with bromocriptine. *J Neurol Neurosurg Psychiatry.* 1989;52(10):1200–1201.

236. Borison RL, Davis JM. Amantadine in Tourette syndrome. *Curr Psychiatr Ther.* 1983;22:127–130.

237. Lipinski JF, Zubenko GS, Barreira P, et al. Propranolol in the treatment of neuroleptic-induced akathisia. *Lancet.* 1983;2(8351):685–686.

238. Kock RJ, Pi EH. Acute laryngeal dystonic reactions to neuroleptics. *Psychosomatics.* 1989;30(4):359–364.

239. Kabes J, Sikora J, Pisvejc J, et al. Effect of piracetam on extrapyramidal side effects induced by neuroleptic drugs. *Int Pharmacopsychiatry.* 1982;17(3):185–192.

240. Wirshing WC, Phelan CK, van Putten T, et al. Effects of clozapine on treatment-resistant akathisia and concomitant tardive dyskinesia. *J Clin Psychopharmacol.* 1990;10(5):371–373.

241. Marsden CD, Obeso JA, Rothwell JC. Clinical neurophysiology of muscle jerks: myoclonus, chorea, and tics. *Adv Neurol.* 1983;39:865–881.

242. Caviness JN. Primary care guide to myoclonus and chorea. Characteristics, causes, and clinical options. *Postgrad Med.* 2000;108(5):163–172.

243. Eldridge R, Riklan M, Cooper IS. The limited role of psychotherapy in torsion dystonia. Experience with 44 cases. *JAMA.* 1969;210(4):705–708.

244. Ranawaya R, Riley D, Lang A. Psychogenic dyskinesias in patients with organic movement disorders. *Mov Disord.* 1990;5(2):127–133.

245. Anderson KE, Gruber-Baldini AL, Vaughan CG. Impact of psychogenic movement disorders versus Parkinson's on disability, quality of life, and psychopathology. *Mov Disord.* 2007;22:2204–2209.

246. Jiminez-Jiminez FJ, Garcia-Ruiz PJ, Molina JA. Drug induced movement disorders. *Drug Saf.* 1997;16(3):180–204.

247. Sudarsky, L. Psychogenic gait disorders *Semin Neurol.* 2006;26:351–356.

248. Jeste DV, Caligiuri MP, Paulsen JS, et al. Risk of tardive dyskinesia in older patients. A prospective longitudinal study of 266 outpatients. *Arch Gen Psychiatry.* 1995;52(9):756–765.

249. Miller LG, Jankovic J. Neurologic approach to drug-induced movement disorders: a study of 125 patients. *South Med J.* 1990;83(5):525–532.

250. Caviness JN, Forsyth PA, Layton DD, et al. The movement disorder of adult opsoclonus. *Mov Disord.* 1995;10(1):22–27.

251. Podskalny GD, Factor SA. Chorea caused by lithium intoxication: a case report and literature review. *Mov Disord.* 1996;11(6):733–737.

252. Santora J, Rozek S, Samie MR. Diphenhydramine-induced dystonia. *Clin Pharm.* 1989;8(7):471.

253. Miller LG, Jankovic J. Persistent dystonia possibly induced by flecainide. *Mov Disord.* 1992;7(1):62–63.

254. Harrison MB, Lyons GR, Landow ER. Phenytoin and dyskinesias: a report of two cases and review of the literature. *Mov Disord.* 1993;8(1):19–27.

255. Childers MK, Holland D. Psychomotor agitation following gabapentin use in brain injury. *Brain Inj.* 1997;11(7):537–540.

256. Jain SS, Francisco GE. Parkinson's disease and other movement disorders. In: DeLisa JA, ed. *Rehabilitation Medicine: Principles and Practice.* 3rd ed. Philadelphia, PA: Lippincott Williams & Wilkins; 1988:1035–1041.

257. Thaut MH, McIntosh GC, Rice RR. Rhythmic auditory stimulation in gait training for Parkinson's disease patients. *Mov Disord.* 1996;11(2):193–200.

258. Marchese R, Diverio M, Zucchi F. The role of sensory cues in the rehabilitation of parkinsonian patients: a comparison of two physical therapy protocols. *Mov Disord.* 2000;15(5):879–883.

259. Van den BP, Francart J, Mourin S, et al. Five-year experience in the treatment of focal movement disorders with low-dose Dysport botulinum toxin. *Muscle Nerve.* 1995;18(7):720–729.

260. Mountain RE, Murray JA, Quaba A. Management of facial synkinesis with *Clostridium botulinum* toxin injection. *Clin Otolaryngol.* 1992;17(3):223–224.

261. Emmerson J. Botulinum toxin for spasmodic torticollis in a patient with myasthenia gravis. *Mov Disord.* 1994;9(3):367.

262. Penn RD, Gianino JM, York MM. Intrathecal baclofen for motor disorders. *Mov Disord.* 1995;10(5):675–677.

263. Narayan RK, Loubser PG, Jankovic J, et al. Intrathecal baclofen for intractable axial dystonia. *Neurology.* 1991;41(7):1141–1142.

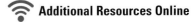 **Additional Resources Online**

CHAPTER 22

Ronald K. Reeves
Morgan Brubaker
Steven Craig Kirshblum

Rehabilitation of Spinal Cord Injury

The earliest reference to spinal cord injury (SCI) is found in the *Edwin Smith Surgical Papyrus*, written between 2,500 and 3,000 B.C., as "an ailment not to be treated" (1). Much has changed in the last 50 years in spinal cord care as it relates to increasing survival, life expectancy, community reintegration, and quality of life (QOL). Major advances include the specialized spinal cord centers of care; model SCI centers funded by the National Institute on Disability, Independent Living, and Rehabilitation Research (NIDILRR), establishment and growth of organizations and journals dedicated to SCI; and the development of the subspecialty of SCI Medicine in 1998. Advances continue in understanding the pathophysiology of the injury, as well in trialing interventions for persons with acute, subacute, and chronic SCI to improve neurologic and functional outcome. The goal remains to improve independence while searching for a potential cure.

EPIDEMIOLOGY OF TRAUMATIC SCI

Incidence and Prevalence

The National SCI Statistical Center (NSCISC) database has been in existence since 1973 and captures approximately 13% of all new traumatic SCIs that occur in the United States each year and has been used to develop an epidemiologic profile (2). When compared to population-based studies, persons in this database are representative of all SCIs except that more severe injuries, nonwhites, and injuries due to acts of violence are slightly overrepresented. The incidence of traumatic SCI in the United States is approximately 54 new cases per million population or approximately 17,000 cases per year (2). Worldwide, there are an estimated 179,000 new cases of traumatic SCI (3), with the incidence of SCI in the rest of the world consistently lower than in the United States (3). The prevalence in the United States is estimated at 282,000 persons (2).

Age, Gender, and Race

While SCI has primarily affected young men, the average age at injury has steadily increased from 29 years during the 1970s to 42 years currently (2,4). Since 2000, greater than 11.5% of persons injured are older than 60 (2). Reasons for the observed trend toward older age at injury may include changes in the referral patterns to model SCI systems and the location of the systems that contribute data to the NSCISC, survival rates of older persons at the scene of the accident, or age-specific incidence rates including falls. Approximately 5% of traumatic SCI occur below the age of 15. In adults, men suffer traumatic SCI more commonly than do women, at a 4:1 ratio, while in the pediatric population, the difference is less dramatic. State registries and NSCISC data reveal higher incidence rates of SCI for African Americans than Whites.

Etiology and Time of Injury

The NSCISC reports that motor vehicle crashes (MVCs) including automobile, motorcycle, and bicycle rank first (since 2010, MVCs account for 38% of cases), followed by falls (30%), acts of violence (13.5%) (primarily, gunshot wounds [GSWs]), and recreational sporting activities (9%). Other data report that falls have become the leading cause of SCI (5,6). Consistently, falls are the leading cause of traumatic SCI for person over the age 45. Falls are most often from low heights, resulting in a cervical lesion (7). With aging, there is an increased frequency of cervical spinal stenosis, placing the elderly population at a greater risk of SCI with relatively minor trauma. MVCs account for a lower percentage of cases among men than women, while men have a higher percentage of SCIs that are due to GSW, diving mishaps, and motorcycle crashes. The likelihood of SCI from an MVC is higher in nonsedan cars (e.g., sport utility vehicles) involved in rollover crashes (8).

Acts of violence caused 13.3% of SCIs prior to 1980, and peaked between 1990 and 1999 at 24.8%, before declining to 13.5% since 2010. Violence causing SCI is more common in minority groups. Diving injuries account for the majority of SCI due to recreational sports, followed by snow skiing, surfing, wrestling, and football. The sport as a cause of SCI varies by country (9). Recreational sports and acts of violence decrease with advancing age as a cause of injury.

In children, the incidence of SCI in the United States is 1.99 cases per 100,000. MVCs are the leading cause, and in children involved in an MVC, two thirds are reported as not wearing a seat belt. Alcohol and drugs are reportedly involved in 30% of all pediatric cases. Boys are twice as likely to have an SCI as girls, with an overall mean age of 14.6 years. Incidence of pediatric SCI varies by region, with the South and Midwest regions having almost twice as many as in the Northeast (10).

Traumatic SCI occurs with greater frequency on weekends, with the greatest incidence on Saturday. Seasonal variation exists, with peak incidence occurring in July followed closely by August and June. The seasonal pattern is more pronounced in the northern part of the United States.

Associated Injuries

Spinal cord injuries are often accompanied by other significant injuries. The most common include broken bones (i.e., ribs, long bones), loss of consciousness, and traumatic pneumothorax. The nature and frequency of these injuries are, typically, associated with the etiology of the SCI. For example, pneumo-thorax occurs more frequently with GSW as compared with other causes of SCI. Noncontiguous spinal injuries (a lesion separated by at least one normal intervening vertebra from a spine fracture or subluxation/dislocation) occur in 12% to 28% of cases as documented by magnetic resonance imaging (MRI) (11,12).

Neurologic Level and Extent of Lesion

Traumatic SCI, most commonly, causes cervical lesions (approximately 58%) followed by thoracic and then lumbo-sacral lesions. The C5 segment is the most common lesion level with T12 the most common level for paraplegia. Since 2010, the most frequent neurologic category at discharge from rehabilitation of persons reported to the NSCISC data-base is incomplete tetraplegia (45%), followed by incomplete paraplegia (21.3%), complete paraplegia (20%), and complete tetraplegia (13.3%) (2). Pediatric SCI more often results in paraplegia and neurologically complete injuries than does adult SCI. Less than 1% of persons experience complete neurologic recovery at discharge. The percentage of persons with incom-plete tetraplegia has recently increased while that of complete paraplegia and tetraplegia has decreased.

The etiology of injury is strongly associated with the level and severity of the injury. Most recreational sports–related injuries, falls, and approximately 50% of MVC result in tet-raplegia, whereas acts of violence usually result in paraplegia. Neurologically complete injuries are more likely to occur as a result of acts of violence and among younger age groups. Thoracic injuries are most likely to be neurologically complete, while lower-level lesions are incomplete injuries. Cervical inju-ries are most commonly classified as either ASIA Impairment Scale (AIS) A or D.

Marital and Occupational Status After SCI

Given that there is still a relatively youthful age of many per-sons who sustain an SCI, it is not surprising that slightly more than half (51.4%) are single when injured. Divorce is increased as compared to the general population among those who were married at the time of injury, especially in the first 3 years after injury, as well as those who marry after injury. The likelihood of getting married after injury is also reduced (2,13,14).

More than half (58.1%) the persons with SCI, admitted to a model SCI system, reported being employed at the time of their injury (2). Approximately 12.4% and 27.7% of per-sons with SCI are employed postinjury by years 1 and 10, respectively, but the percentage varies substantially by neu-rologic level and extent of injury. A higher level of injury and increased injury severity are associated with a reduced chance of returning to gainful employment. By postinjury year 10, most persons who have returned to work have full-time rather than part-time jobs. Predictors of returning to work include greater formal education, being of younger age (with employment rates declining particularly after age 50), male sex, Caucasian, being married, being employed at the time of injury, AIS D injury, having greater motivation to return to work, nonviolent SCI etiology, ability to drive, lower level of social security disability benefits, and a greater elapsed time postinjury. Persons who return to work within the first year of injury usually return to the same job and employer, while those who return to work after 1 year usually acquire a different job with a different employer, often after retraining.

Hospitalization

Average days hospitalized in the acute care unit for those who enter a model SCI system immediately following injury have declined from 24 days in the 1970s to 11 days currently (2). Similar downward trends are noted for days in the rehabilita-tion unit (from 98 to 35 days) (2). Overall, mean days hos-pitalized (during acute care and rehabilitation) are greater for persons with neurologically complete injuries.

Life Expectancy

Mortality rates are significantly higher during the first year after injury than during subsequent years, particularly for severely injured persons. Over the last three decades, there has been a 40% decline in mortality during the first 2 years after injury. However, the average life expectancy for persons with SCI has not improved much since the 1980s and remains significantly below life expectancies of persons without SCI (2,15). Predictors of mortality after injury include male gen-der, advanced age, ventilator dependence, injured by an act of violence, high injury level (particularly C4 or above), a neurologically complete injury, poor self-rated adjustment to disability, poor community integration, poor economic status indicators, and having either Medicare or Medicaid third-party sponsorship of care (15–17).

Life expectancy estimates (**Table 22-1**) are typically based on neurologic level of injury (NLI), degree of injury com-pleteness, age at injury, and ventilator dependency (2). For persons with complete injuries, mortality rates are higher for those with high tetraplegia (C1-3) than for those with mid or low tetraplegia, and the latter have higher mortality than those with paraplegia. The distinction between injury grades is more important for those with the highest levels of injury, but not for those with lower injuries. For persons with paraplegia, there is no significant difference between AIS grades of A, B, or

TABLE 22-1	Life Expectancy (Years) for Postinjury by Severity of Injury and Age at Injury (for Persons Surviving at Least 1 Year Postinjury)					
Age at Injury	No SCI	Motor Functional at Any Level	Para	Low Tetra (C5-8)	High Tetra (C1-4)	Ventilator-Dependent at Any Level
20	59.6	53.4	46.4	41.3	35.3	18.1
40	40.7	35.6	30.3	25.8	22.2	13.0
60	23.2	19.8	16.5	14.1	12.5	7.9

Source: National Spinal Cord Injury Statistical Center. Facts and figures. *J Spinal Cord Med.* 2016;39:370–371.

C injuries. Those with higher paraplegia (T1-6) have a higher mortality than do those with lower injuries.

Causes of Death

Diseases of the respiratory system are the leading cause of death following SCI, with pneumonia being the most common (2). Heart disease ranks second, followed by septicemia (usually associated with pressure injuries [PIs] or urinary tract or respiratory infections) and cancer. The most common location of cancer is the lung, followed by the bladder, prostate, and colon/rectum.

Pneumonia is by far the leading cause of death for persons with tetraplegia, while heart disease, septicemia, and suicide are more common among persons with paraplegia. The suicide rate is highest in younger patients and in persons with paraplegia. Heart disease is the primary cause of death in persons injured for greater than 30 years and in patients over 60 and in persons with neurologically motor incomplete (AIS D) injuries at any neurologic level. While genitourinary (GU) disease (i.e., renal failure) was the leading cause of death 30 years ago, this has declined dramatically, most likely due to advances in urologic management.

Lifetime Costs

The average yearly expenses (health care costs and living expenses) and the estimated lifetime costs that are directly attributable to SCI vary greatly based on education, neurologic impairment, and preinjury employment history (2). First-year cost estimates include $1,079,412, $779,969, $526,066, and $352,279 for persons with (ASIA Impairment Scale A, B, and C) high tetraplegia (C1-4), low tetraplegia (C5-8), paraplegia, and motor functional at any level AIS D, respectively, with each subsequent year's estimated expenses at $187,443, $114,988, $69,688, and $42,789, respectively. Estimated lifetime costs by age at injury are: $4,789,384 at age 25 and $2,632,164 at age 50 for persons with C-1-4 high tetraplegia. For C-5-8 ABC low tetraplegia the lifetime cost of injury at age 25 are $3,499,423 and $2,152,458 if injured at age 50. For persons with AIS ABC paraplegia the lifetime cost of injury at age 25 are $2,341,458 and $1,536,976 if injured at age 50. For persons with AIS D motor functional SCI at any level the estimates are $1,600,058 and $1,129,365 for age 25 and 50, respectively. (2,18).

ACUTE MEDICAL AND SURGICAL MANAGEMENT

The treatment of a traumatic SCI begins at the scene (19). An injury to the spinal column should be suspected whenever trauma occurs. As such, all trauma victims should have their spine immobilized, preferably with a rigid cervical collar with supportive blocks on a backboard, with straps to secure the entire spine in patients with a potential spinal injury, and should be transferred onto a firm padded surface while maintaining spinal alignment to prevent skin breakdown. Movement should be via logrolling until spinal injury has been ruled out. Traditional cardiopulmonary resuscitation (CPR) methods should be utilized, minimizing trauma to a potentially unstable cervical spine including utilizing the jaw-thrust maneuver to access the airway. After injury, prompt resuscitation, stabilization of the spine, and avoidance of additional neurologic injury and medical complications are of greatest importance. During the first seconds after SCI, there is release of catecholamines with an initial hypertensive phase. This is rapidly followed by a state of spinal shock, defined as flaccid paralysis and extinction of muscle stretch reflexes below the injury level, although this may not occur in all patients. Ditunno et al. proposed four phases of spinal shock from initial loss of reflex activity to hyperreflexia (20). Neurogenic shock, as part of the spinal shock syndrome, is a direct result of a reduction in sympathetic activity below the level of injury; consists of hypotension, bradycardia, and hypothermia; and is common in the acute postinjury period. Parasympathetic (PS) activity predominates, especially in persons with injuries at or above the T6 level. Treatment of hypotension involves fluid resuscitation (usually 1 to 2 L) to produce adequate urine output of greater than 30 cc/h. In neurogenic shock, further fluid administration must proceed cautiously, as the patient is at risk for neurogenic pulmonary edema, and vasopressors are utilized. Maintenance of mean arterial pressure at approximately 85 mm Hg during the first week postinjury has been associated with improved neurologic outcomes (21).

Bradycardia is common in the acute period in cervical spinal level injury and may be treated, if below 40 to 44 per minute or if symptomatic, with intravenous (IV) atropine (0.1 to 1 mg) or prevented with atropine given prior to any maneuver that may cause further vagal stimulation (i.e., nasotracheal suctioning). While significant bradycardia typically resolves within 6 weeks, episodes of persistent bradycardia beyond this time may occur in some severe injuries. Some patients may require implantation of a cardiac pacemaker to facilitate safe mobilization (22).

Respiratory assessment is critical for acute SCI patients and should include arterial blood gases and measurement of forced vital capacity (VC) as an assessment of respiratory muscle strength (23). A VC of less than 1 L indicates ventilatory compromise, and the patient usually requires assisted ventilation. Serial assessments should be obtained for those with borderline values. A nasogastric tube should be inserted during the initial assessment period to prevent emesis and potential aspiration. A Foley catheter should be inserted for urinary drainage and facilitates accurate assessment of urine output. It should be left in place until the patient is hemodynamically stable and strict attention to fluid status is no longer required (19).

Upon presentation to the emergency department, a baseline neurologic examination should be performed, maintaining spinal precautions. Imaging studies including x-rays, computed tomography (CT) scan, or MRI should be employed to assess spinal fracture, instability, and/or spinal cord pathology. A standard trauma series includes cross-table laterals and AP views of the cervical and thoracolumbar spine. Because of the incidence of noncontiguous fractures, once one fracture is identified, careful inspection of the rest of the spine is imperative. CT scans often provide improved visualization of the C1 and C7 vertebrae, while MRI provides optimal visualization of the neuronal structures. The spine should remain immobilized until an injury has been definitively excluded or the spine is stabilized either surgically or by application of an appropriate orthotic device. In patients with a stiff spine and midline tenderness, the clinician should suspect a fracture (even if plain x-ray is negative), especially in the presence of spondylosis, ankylosing spondylitis, or diffuse interstitial skeletal hyperostosis (DISH) (19). Forty-seven percent of patients with spine trauma and 64% of patients with SCI have concomitant injuries, including head, chest, rib, and long bone fractures (24). Therefore, a thorough assessment of the total patient is imperative.

Stab wounds and GSWs generally do not produce spinal instability and therefore usually do not require surgical stabilization or orthotic immobilization. Objects that are embedded around the spinal canal (i.e., knife) should be left in place with removal performed in the operating room under direct visualization of the spinal canal. Bullets that pass through the abdominal viscera are treated with broad-spectrum antibiotics and tetanus prophylaxis. Bullets do not have to be removed; however, they can be if accessible while performing another surgical procedure.

The issue of IV methylprednisolone (MP) administration in traumatic SCI has been debated (25). Mechanisms of action for MP include improving blood flow to the spinal cord, preventing lipid peroxidation, free radical scavenger, and having anti-inflammatory function. The National Acute SCI Study (NASCIS) 2 reported that IV MP given within 8 hours of injury (30 mg/kg bolus and 5.4 mg/kg/h for 23 hours) improves neurologic recovery at 6 weeks, 6 months, and 1 year, although functional recovery was not clearly studied (26). NASCIS 3 reported that if initiated within 3 hours of SCI, MP should be continued for 24 hours, whereas if initiated at 3 to 8 hours after SCI, it should be continued for 48 hours (27). The benefits and safety of utilizing the NASCIS protocol have been questioned, due to the fact that the findings have not been consistently replicated, concerns regarding methodology and analysis, as well as possibly increased morbidity and mortality in persons administered steroids (28–31). The neurosurgical guidelines in 2013 state that high-dose MP is not recommended and "are associated with harmful side effects including death" (32). Other articles have shown alternative opinions and this issue continues to be discussed in the literature, and the protocol seemingly is hospital dependent (33,34).

Additional recommendations after the acute injury include transferring the SCI patient to a specialized center as soon as possible to decrease complications and hospital length of stay (LOS) (19,35). Patients with acute SCI, especially high-level tetraplegia, should be assessed for evidence of concomitant traumatic brain injury (TBI; see also Chapter 19) (i.e., assessing for loss of consciousness or posttraumatic amnesia [PTA]). Early stabilizations should be considered for extraspinal fractures. In cases of high-energy injuries, aortic injury should be evaluated. For anesthesia, avoid the use of succinylcholine after the first 48 hours postinjury (potentially fatal hyperkalemic response). While priapism is frequently seen, it is usually self-limited and does not require treatment. Lastly, it is important to maintain normoglycemia in critically ill, mechanically ventilated patients (19).

Not all SCIs are associated with a spinal fracture or dislocation and may result from forced extreme range of spinal movement without mechanical abnormality. A high index of suspicion for SCIWORA (SCI without radiologic abnormality) is important when evaluating adolescents with sports-related neck trauma or victims of child abuse (especially in children who may be suffering from physical abuse) (19).

SPINAL STABILITY AND PRINCIPLES OF SPINAL STABILIZATION

White and Panjabi proposed the most widely accepted theory on spinal instability defining it as "the loss of the ability of the spine, under physiologic loads, to maintain its pattern of displacement so that there is no initial or additional neurological deficit, no major deformity, and no incapacitating pain" (36). This definition is applicable at all levels of the axial spine. Currently, there are various classifications to characterize damage to the spinal axis. Radiographic criteria have been established for the diagnosis of clinical instability of the spine. Denis described the widely accepted "three-column theory" for thoracolumbar fractures, where the spine is divided into three columns (🛜 eFig. 22-1). The anterior column comprises the anterior vertebral body, the anterior longitudinal ligament, and the anterior half of the annulus fibrosus. The middle column consists of the posterior vertebral body, the posterior longitudinal ligament, and the posterior half of the annulus fibrosus. The posterior column includes all the posterior elements (including the pedicles). In this three-column theory of Denis, spinal instability is present if any two of the three columns are violated (37). Additional classifications systems have been established for the cervical spine (38) and thoracolumbar spine (39) that mainly focuses on morphology and mechanism of injury and is useful for communication among health care providers and better definitions from a research perspective.

Injuries that are primarily ligamentous, such as facet dislocations, are unstable and require internal stabilization procedures. The primary objective of surgical intervention is to decompress the spinal cord and regain stability of the spinal axis to optimize neurologic recovery. If surgery is performed, either an anterior or a posterior approach may accomplish this. The approach chosen depends on the expertise of the operating surgeon and the specific pathophysiology of the injury. Since the most common etiology of SCI occurs from retropulsion of bone and/or disk material from a ventral location into the spinal canal, an anterior approach may be preferable. Anterior surgery, however, is associated with increased complications including recurrent laryngeal nerve lesions leading to speech and swallowing disorders. After adequate neural decompression is accomplished, the spine is stabilized and fused. Fusion is typically performed by using autologous bone, which is most frequently harvested from the iliac crest. The fibula can also be used as a donor site for autograft bone; however, this is usually reserved for cases that require more than a single level of fusion. Surgical hardware is utilized to help fixate bones to allow a fusion to occur. The hardware, however, is only a temporary fixation device that facilitates the eventual long-term bony fusion.

The role and timing of spinal surgery including decompression have been trending toward intervening early. Early spinal decompression within 24 hours, and perhaps within 8 hours, may improve neurologic recovery, particularly in patients with incomplete injuries (40–44). Earlier surgery overall seems to reduce LOS in the acute hospital, facilitates rehabilitation, decreases hospital costs, and often reduces postoperative complications. The indication for emergent surgical treatment is progressive neurologic deterioration. For persons with central cord syndrome (CCS), although several studies have reported favorable neurologic recovery after conservative management

(45,46), recent studies show a clear trend toward a preference for surgical decompression (47,48).

Postoperatively, or if surgery is not required, an orthosis is often prescribed and maintained for approximately 1 to 3 months. The type of spinal orthotic chosen depends on the level of spinal injury. Generally, for the occipito-C2 levels, the Halo-vest may be used, although some surgeons will utilize a head-cervical orthosis (HCO) (e.g., Miami J Collar or Aspen Collar). An HCO is utilized for the C3-7 levels; for the T1-3 levels, a cervicothoracic orthosis is used (i.e., extended HCO or Yale brace). From T4 through L2, a thoracolumbar spinal orthotic (TLSO) is utilized; however, at L3 and below, a lumbosacral orthotic (LSO) with the incorporation of one hip/thigh (spica attachment to a LSO or TLSO) that will ensure satisfactory immobilization of the low lumbar and sacral spine is required.

ANATOMY, NEUROANATOMY, AND VASCULAR SUPPLY

A thorough understanding of the vertebral and spinal cord anatomy is critical to the understanding of spinal cord medicine, and the reader should consult anatomy texts for additional information. By adulthood, the spinal cord occupies only the upper two thirds of the vertebral column with its caudal end located at the lower border of the first lumbar (L1) vertebra (level of L1-2 intervertebral disk) (**Fig. 22-1**). Because there are eight cervical nerve roots and only seven cervical vertebrae, the C8 nerve root exits through the intervertebral foramen just rostral to the first thoracic vertebra. The spinal cord segments, especially in the thoracic and lumbar regions, do not line up with their corresponding vertebral level, which explains why a fracture of T12, for instance, results in a L1-2 NLI. At the

caudal end, the spinal cord is conical in shape and is known as the conus medullaris. The lumbar and sacral nerve roots descend some distance within the vertebral canal to exit from their respective intervertebral foramina. These nerve roots resemble a horse's tail and are termed the cauda equina (CE).

The spinal cord receives its blood supply from one anterior and two posterior spinal arteries (PSAs) as well as anterior and posterior radicular arteries. The anterior spinal artery (ASA) arises in the upper cervical region and is formed by the union of two branches of the vertebral arteries. The ASA supplies the anterior two thirds of the spinal cord including the gray matter and anterior and anterolateral white matter. Disruption of cord perfusion from the ASA gives rise to the anterior cord syndrome (ACS) described later in the chapter. The PSAs supply the posterior one third of the spinal cord consisting of posterolateral and posterior white matter of the spinal cord.

The internal structure of the spinal cord is such that a transverse section of the spinal cord reveals a butterfly-shaped central gray matter surrounded by white matter. The gray matter of the spinal cord contains cell bodies and primarily neurons, dendrites, and myelinated and unmyelinated axons. Autonomic neurons are located laterally and exit by the ventral root and innervate smooth muscle. Lower motor neurons (LMNs) are located ventrally, exit by the ventral roots, and innervate striated muscle. The white matter consists of ascending and descending bundles of myelinated and unmyelinated axons (tracts or fasciculi). The ascending pathways relay sensory information to the brain, while the descending pathways relay motor information from the brain.

Sensory tracts are composed of axons from peripheral sensory nerves whose cell bodies are located in the dorsal root ganglion (DRG) and ascend toward the brainstem. Receptors for pain and temperature enter the spinal cord and synapse in the dorsal horn of the gray matter. The fibers cross over within one to two vertebral segments, then travel in the lateral spinothalamic tract, and ascend to the ventral posterolateral (VPL) nucleus of the thalamus. Pressure and light touch (LT) fibers enter the cord in the same fashion and pass into the ipsilateral dorsal white column and bifurcate. One branch immediately enters the dorsal horn gray matter, synapses, and crosses over within one to two segments, while the other branch remains ipsilateral and ascends in the dorsal column for as many as 10 spinal segments. The ipsilateral branch ultimately enters the dorsal horn, synapses, and crosses over to join the other branch in the ventral white column, forming the ventral spinothalamic tract. These axons travel in the same pathway as the lateral tract to reach the postcentral gyrus, which interprets these sensations.

The posterior columns transmit three different sensations: proprioception, fine touch, and vibration sense. Their nerve fibers reach the DRG and immediately pass into the ipsilateral dorsal white columns and ascend to the medulla. Axons that enter the cord at the sacral, lumbar, and lower thoracic levels are situated in the medial part of the dorsal column (i.e., the lower part of the body) called the fasciculus gracilis. Those axons that enter at the thoracic (above T6) and cervical levels are situated in the lateral part of the column (from the upper part of the body) and are termed the fasciculus cuneatus. Axons of each fasciculus synapse in the medulla and form a bundle termed the medial lemniscus, which ascends to the postcentral gyrus. The spinocerebellar tract is a set of axonal fibers originating in the spinal cord and terminating in the

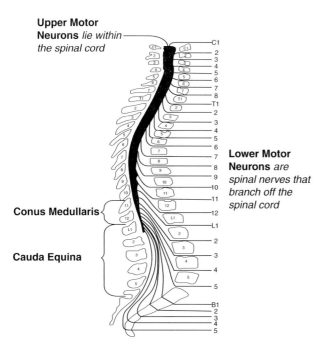

Upper Motor Neurons *lie within the spinal cord*

Lower Motor Neurons *are spinal nerves that branch off the spinal cord*

Conus Medullaris

Cauda Equina

The **spinal cord** ends between L-1 and L-2. The **nerves** continue to descend in the spinal column, existing between the vertebrae and through the sacrum.

FIGURE 22-1. Spinal vertebrae and nerve roots.

ipsilateral cerebellum that conveys information to the cerebellum about limb and joint positions (proprioception).

The lateral corticospinal tract is the main tract for voluntary muscle activity. Its origin is the precentral gyrus of the frontal lobe of the brain. Their axons descend through the internal capsule to the medulla oblongata. Approximately 80% to 90% of the axons cross at the pyramidal decussation to the contralateral side of the medulla and descend in the lateral white columns of the spinal cord, in the lateral corticospinal tract. At each level of the spinal cord, the axons from the lateral tract peel off and enter the gray matter of the ventral horn and synapse with secondary neurons. The 10% to 20% of uncrossed axons that continue down on the same side of the cord travel in the ventral corticospinal tract. The axons of the ventral tract then cross over at the corresponding level of muscles that it innervates. Both tracts travel from the precentral gyrus to the ventral horn as a single uninterrupted neuron and are termed upper motor neurons (UMNs), while the secondary neurons that they synapse on are termed LMNs.

NEUROLOGIC ASSESSMENT

The most accurate way to document impairment in a person with an SCI is by performing a standardized neurologic examination, as endorsed by the International Standards for Neurological Classification of SCI (ISNCSCI) (41). These standards provide basic definitions of the most common terms used by clinicians in the assessment of SCI and describe the neurologic examination. Key terms are defined in 🛜 **eTable 22-1**. The examination is composed of sensory and motor components and is performed with the patient in the supine position to be able to compare initial and follow-up examinations. The information from this examination is recorded on a standardized flow sheet (**Fig. 22-2**) and helps determine the sensory, motor, and NLI and sensory and motor index scores and to classify the impairment. An online course for examination and classification utilizing the Standards is available through the ASIA Web site (www.asia-spinalinjury.org).

Sensory Examination

The sensory examination is performed separately for LT and sharp/dull discrimination modalities. Each of 28 dermatomes (see **Fig. 22-2**) is tested and graded 0 for absent, 1 for impaired, 2 for normal (or intact), or NT for not testable. The face is used as the reference point for testing sensation in each dermatome. A grade of 2 indicates the sensation is equal to that of the face. For the LT examination, a cotton-tip applicator is used. A score of 1 is recorded if the sensation is less than on the face and a 0 if there is no sensation. For the sharp/dull discrimination, a clean safety pin is used, and a grade

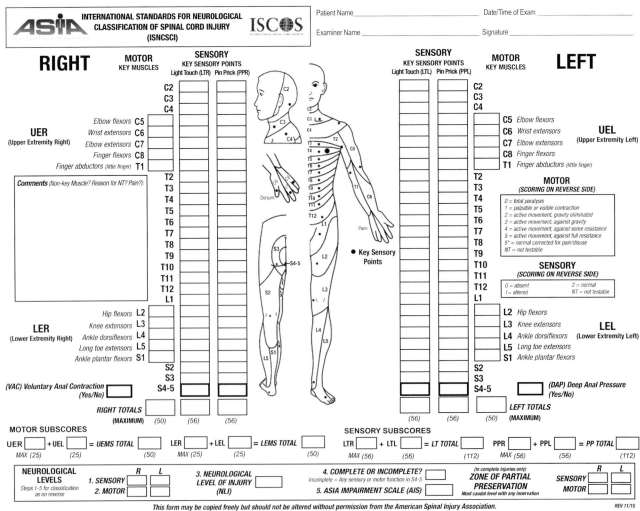

FIGURE 22-2. ASIA flow sheet. (© 2011 American Spinal Injury Association. Reprinted with permission.)

of 1 indicates the ability to discriminate sharp from dull; however, the sensation is qualitatively different as compared to the face (i.e., either hypo- or hyperesthetic). If the patient cannot feel the pin, or discriminate the sharp from the dull aspect of the safety pin, the score is 0. If accurate sensory testing is unable to be performed due to extenuating circumstances (i.e., dermatomal covering burns, casts, amputations, etc.), the level is designated as not testable, or "NT," or an alternate location within the dermatome can be tested and noted. If there is a question whether the patient can definitively discriminate between the pin and dull edges, 8 out of 10 correct answers is considered accurate, as this reduces the probability of correct guessing to less than 5.0%.

The lowest sacral segment, S4-5 (anal musculocutaneous junction), should be tested with the pin and cotton swab as well. To test for deep anal pressure (DAP), a rectal digital examination is performed. The patient is asked to report any sensory awareness, touch, or pressure, with firm pressure of the examiner's digit on the rectal wall. DAP is recorded as either present (yes) or absent (no). If a patient has intact sensation to LT or sharp/dull differentiation at S4/S5, DAP is not required for classification in the current ISNCSCI examination. However, the motor portion of the anorectal examination should be performed to assess for motor sparing (described below) (49).

The *sensory level* is defined as the most caudal level where sensations for LT and PP are both graded as 2 (normal) for both sides of the body. If the LT level is C6 and PP is C5, the overall sensory level is C5. In a case where sensory loss begins at or just above the nipple line (T4 dermatome), often a patient is credited with the T3 dermatome being spared. If the sensation is absent in the T1 and T2 dermatomes despite the presence of some sensation at the T3 dermatome, it is recommended that the T3 dermatome be scored as absent. It is felt that this sparing above the nipple line is from C4 innervation and represents what is termed the C4 "cape" or "shelf."

Motor Examination

The motor examination is conducted using conventional manual muscle testing (MMT) technique (on a scale from 0 to 5) in ten key muscle groups, five in the upper limb (C5-T1 myotomes) and five in the lower limb (L2-S1), on each side of the body (eTable 22-1). Key muscles were chosen based upon their myotomal innervations and ability to be tested in the supine position. Most muscles are innervated by two root levels (e.g., the elbow flexors are innervated from C5 to C6). When a key muscle tests initially as a grade 5, it is presumed to be fully innervated by the contributions from the two roots. If a muscle initially grades a 3/5, it is presumed to have full innervation of its more proximal segment (in the case of the elbow flexors, innervation from the C5 myotome). Voluntary anal contraction is tested by sensing contraction of the external anal sphincter (EAS) around the examiner's finger and graded as either present or absent.

When examining a patient with an acute injury below T8, the hip should not be flexed passively or actively beyond 90 degrees as this may place too great a kyphotic stress on the lumbar spine. Therefore, it may only be possible to test hip flexor muscle strength isometrically. If pain limits full patient effort and the examiner feels that the initial contraction given represents normal strength, the muscle should be graded as 5* while indicating the reason for this scoring (e.g., pain).

The *motor level* is defined as the most caudal motor level with a score of ≥3, with the more rostral key muscles grading a 5. For injuries with no corresponding motor level (i.e., above C5, T2-L1, below S1), the last normal sensory level is used. For example, a person with normal strength in all key muscles of the UEs, 0/5 strength in the key muscles of the LEs, with a T4 sensory level, would be assigned a motor level of T4. Similarly, in a case where the elbow flexors (C5 level) grade 3/5 on both sides, with a sensory level on the left at C4 and on the right C3, the motor level on the left would be C5 and on the right C3. This is due to the C4 dermatome on the right being scored as impaired—it is presumed that the C4 myotome is also impaired. Therefore, the motor level is designated as C3, since the patient does not meet the criteria of having a key muscle ≥3/5, with the levels above (in this case C4) scoring as normal. On the left side, the C4 dermatome is normal, so the C4 myotome is considered normal and as a result, the left motor level is C5.

The NLI is the most caudal level, at which both motor and sensory modalities are intact on both sides of the body. The motor and sensory levels are the same in less than 50% of complete injuries, and the motor level may be multiple levels below the sensory level at 1-year postinjury (50). In cases where there is no key muscle level available (i.e., cervical levels at and above C5; T2-L1; and sacral levels below S2), the NLI is that which corresponds to the sensory level.

If there are non–SCI-related causes of weakness, this should be documented and taken into account when classifying the injury. For example, in a patient with a T8 fracture and complete paraplegia who also has a left brachial plexus injury, notation should be made that the sensory and motor deficits in the left arm are due to brachial plexus injury, not SCI, and the patient may still be classified with a NLI of T8.

ASIA Impairment Scale (AIS) Classification

The International Standards have evolved over the past 30 years and have become accepted as the most appropriate method to describe the neurologic impairment of SCI for clinical and research use and have been incorporated into the International Core SCI Data Set. In 1982, the ASIA first published the *Standards for Neurological Classification of SCI*, adopting the Frankel Scale (51). The Standards were replaced in 1992 by the AIS (52) and revised a number of times since (1996, 2000, and 2011) (53–56) with an update in 2015 (49).

The AIS is used to classify the SCI, separating the injury into a neurologically complete versus incomplete injury. A neurologically *complete* injury is defined as an injury with the individual having no "sacral sparing." *Sacral sparing* refers to having one or more of the following residual findings: LT or PP in the S4-5 dermatome (can be on either side, impaired or intact), DAP, or voluntary anal contraction preserved. If any of these components are present, the individual has sacral sparing and therefore has a neurologically *incomplete* injury. Patients who have an incomplete injury initially (i.e., sacral sparing) have a significantly better prognosis for motor recovery than do those without preservation of the lower sacral segments.

 eTable 22-2 describes the steps to classify the SCI and **Table 22-2** outlines the AIS. An online training course is available that provides a detailed explanation of the examination elements (www.asia-spinalinjury.org). As periodic updates to the ISNCSCI classification occur, the reader is encouraged to visit the ASIA Learning Center for the most up to date

TABLE 22-2	**ASIA Impairment Scale**

A = Complete: No motor or sensory function is preserved in the sacral segments S4-5.

B = Sensory Incomplete: Sensory but not motor function is preserved at the most caudal sacral segments S4-S5, AND no motor function is preserved more than three levels below the motor level on either side of the body.

C = Motor Incomplete: Motor function is preserved at the most caudal sacral segments (S4-S5) on voluntary anal contraction (VAC) **OR** the patient meets the criteria for sensory incomplete status (sensory function preserved at the most caudal sacral segments (S4-S5) by LT, *sharp/dull discrimination* or DAP), with sparing of motor function more than three levels below the motor level on either side of the body. This includes key or non-key muscle functions more than 3 levels below the motor level to determine motor incomplete status. For AIS C – less than half of key muscle functions below the single NLI have a muscle grade ≥ 3.

D = Motor Incomplete: Motor incomplete status as defined above, with at least half (half or more) of key muscle functions below the single NLI having a muscle grade ≥ 3.

E = Normal: If sensation and motor function as tested with the ISNCSCI are graded as normal in all segments, and the patient had prior deficits, then the AIS grade is E. Someone without a SCI does not receive an AIS grade.

Note: For an individual to receive a grade of C or D, he/she must be incomplete, that is, have sensory or motor function in the sacral segments S4-5. In addition, the individual must have either (a) voluntary anal sphincter contraction or (b) sparing of motor function more than three levels below the motor level.

Source: Kirshblum S, Waring W III. Updates for the International Standards for Neurological Classification of Spinal Cord Injury *Phys Med Rehabil Clin N Am.* 2014;25(3):505–517.

classification rules. The *zone of partial preservation* (ZPP) refers to the dermatomes and myotomes caudal to the NLI that remain partially innervated in persons with a neurologically complete injury (AIS A). The ZPP should be recorded as the most caudal segment with some sensory and/or motor sparing but only in persons with a neurologically complete injury.

Incomplete SCI Syndromes

Incomplete SCI syndromes include CCS and Brown-Sequard, anterior cord, conus medullaris, and CE syndromes (CES) and can result from traumatic as well as NT injuries (57). CCS is the most common, accounting for approximately 50% of incomplete injuries and 9% of all traumatic SCIs. CCS is characterized by motor weakness in the UE greater than the LE, in association with sacral sparing. CCS most frequently occurs in older persons with cervical spondylosis who suffer a hyperextension injury from a fall, but it may also occur in persons of any age and is associated with other etiologies, predisposing factors, and injury mechanisms (58). The postulated mechanism of the injury involves compression of the cord both anteriorly and posteriorly by degenerative changes of the bony structures, with inward bulging of the ligamentum flavum during hyperextension in an already narrowed spinal canal.

CCS generally has a favorable prognosis for functional recovery. Recovery occurs earliest and to the greatest extent in the LEs, followed by bowel and bladder function, proximal UE, and then distal hand function. Prognosis for functional recovery of ambulation, ADL, and bowel and bladder function is dependent upon the patient's age (< or >50 years of age), with a less optimistic prognosis in older patients (>50 years old) relative to younger patients (57,59–61). Specifically,

younger patients are more successful in becoming independent in ambulation (87% to 97% vs. 31% to 41%), bladder function (83% vs. 29%), and dressing (77% vs. 12%) than older patients. Older newly injured individuals, however, with an initial classification of AIS D tetraplegia, have a good prognosis for recovery of independent ambulation.

Brown-Sequard syndrome (BSS) is defined as a lesion similar to a hemisection of the spinal cord and accounts for 2% to 4% of all traumatic SCIs (57,62–64). In the classic presentation, there is (a) ipsilateral loss of all sensory modalities at the level of the lesion; (b) ipsilateral flaccid paralysis at the level of the lesion; (c) ipsilateral loss of position, sense, and vibration below the lesion; (d) contralateral loss of pain and temperature below the lesion; and (e) ipsilateral motor loss below the level of the lesion. This is due to the crossing of the spinothalamic tracts in the spinal cord, as opposed to the corticospinal and dorsal columns that cross the brainstem. The pure form of BSS is rare and the Brown-Sequard plus syndrome is more common (BSPS) (65), which refers to a relative ipsilateral hemiplegia with a relative contralateral hemianalgesia. Although BSS has traditionally been associated with knife injuries, a variety of etiologies, including closed spinal injuries with or without vertebral fractures, may be the cause (66).

Recovery usually takes place in the ipsilateral proximal extensors and then in the distal flexors (67,68). Motor recovery of any extremity having a pain/temp sensory deficit occurs before the opposite extremity. Seventy-five to ninety percent of patients ambulate independently at discharge from rehabilitation, and nearly 70% perform functional skills and activities of daily living independently. The most important predictor of function is whether the upper or lower limb is the predominant site of weakness: when the upper limb is weaker than the lower limb, patients are more likely to ambulate at discharge. Recovery of bowel and bladder function is also favorable.

The *anterior cord syndrome* involves a lesion affecting the anterior two thirds of the spinal cord while preserving the posterior columns. This may occur with flexion injuries, from retropulsed disk or bone fragments compressing the cord, with direct injury to the anterior spinal cord, or with lesions of the ASA that provides blood supply to the anterior spinal cord. It is frequently seen after aortic aneurysm procedures. There is a variable loss of motor as well as PP sensation with a relative preservation of LT, proprioception, and deep-pressure sensation.

Posterior cord syndrome (PCS) has been omitted from recent versions of the International Standards and is the least common of the SCI clinical syndromes with an incidence of less than 1%. There is a loss of proprioception and vibration sense, but with preservation of muscle strength, temperature, and pain sensation due to a selective lesion of the posterior columns. PCS has been linked to neck hyperextension injuries, PSA occlusion, tumors, disk compression, and vitamin B_{12} deficiency. Prognosis for ambulation is guarded, secondary to the proprioceptive deficits.

Conus medullaris and cauda equina (CE) injuries include the segment above the conus medullaris that is termed the epiconus, consisting of spinal cord segments L4-S1. Lesions of the epiconus will affect the lower lumbar roots supplying muscles of the lower part of the leg and foot, with sparing of reflex function of sacral segments. The bulbocavernosus (BC) reflex and micturition reflexes are preserved, representing an UMN or suprasacral lesion. Spasticity will most likely develop in sacral innervated segments (e.g., toe flexors, ankle plantar flexors, and hamstring muscles). Recovery is similar to other UMN spinal cord injuries. Conus medullaris lesions present with UMN and LMN aspects. Lesions affecting neural segments S2 and below will present with LMN deficits of the anal sphincter and bladder due to damage of the anterior horn cells of S2-4. Bladder and rectal reflexes are diminished or absent, depending on the exact level and extent of the lesion. Motor strength in the legs and feet may remain intact if the nerve roots (L3-S2) are not affected, that is, "root escape." Trauma and tumors are among the most common etiologies responsible for this condition.

Injuries below the L1 vertebral level usually affect the CE or nerve rootlets supplying the lumbar and sacral segments producing motor weakness and atrophy of the LEs (L2-S2) with bowel and bladder involvement (S2-4), impotence, and areflexia of the ankle and plantar reflexes. CES is a LMN injury. In CES, there is a loss of anal and BC reflexes. CE injuries have a better prognosis relative to UMN injuries for neurologic recovery, most likely due to the fact that the nerve roots are more resilient to injury as they are histologically peripheral nerves and therefore regeneration can occur. CE injuries may represent a neurapraxia or axonotmesis and demonstrate progressive recovery over a course of weeks and months. CES can occur as a result of trauma, tumors, spinal stenosis, disk compression, infection, or postsurgical epidural hematoma (57).

Separation of CE and conus lesions in clinical practice is difficult, because some of the clinical features of these lesions overlap. Pain is uncommon in conus lesions but is frequently a complaint in CES. Sensory abnormalities occur in a saddle distribution in conus lesions, and, if there is sparing, there is usually dissociated loss with a greater loss of pain and temperature while sparing touch sensation. In CE lesions, sensory loss occurs more in a root distribution and is not dissociated.

NONTRAUMATIC SPINAL CORD INJURY

Nontraumatic spinal cord injury (NT SCI) is an important population of patients in spinal cord medicine and includes etiologies such as spinal stenosis, neoplasm, multiple sclerosis (MS) (see Chapter 20), transverse myelitis (TM), infection (viral, bacterial, fungal, parasitic), vascular ischemia, radiation myelopathy, motor neuron diseases, syringomyelia, vitamin B_{12} deficiency, and others. Our understanding of spinal cord diseases is rapidly evolving and treatments are constantly improving. The International Spinal Cord Society has proposed a classification system for NT SCI to facilitate data comparison across centers in this rapidly evolving area (69). Spinal stenosis and tumors are the most common causes of NT SCI presenting for inpatient rehabilitation in North America, Europe, and Australia; however, in some nations, infections are the most import cause of nontraumatic myelopathy (70,71). As compared to persons with traumatic-related SCI, individuals with NT SCI are more likely to be older, female, and married and usually have a less severe neurologic impairment with motor incomplete paraplegia (70–73). There is a lower incidence of secondary medical complications including spasticity, orthostasis, deep vein thrombosis (DVT), PIs, autonomic dysreflexia (AD), and wound infections during rehabilitation in patients with NT SCI (74,75). However, because NT SCI affects older individuals, they may have other premorbid medical issues that impact their rehabilitation. In general, patients with NT SCI benefit from inpatient rehabilitation, but the length of stay for NT SCI is shorter than TSCI with similar

home discharge rates (70). Functional status, gender, age and NT SCI etiology all predict survival (76).

It appears the most common cause of nontraumatic myelopathy is age-related changes in the spine resulting in spinal stenosis, neural compression, and gradual symptoms. Fortunately, neurologic and functional improvement occurs and patients benefit from inpatient rehabilitation (77). Neurogenic bladder and bowel symptoms, neuropathic pain, and spasticity are common and often require management during inpatient rehabilitation (73).

The second most common cause of NT SCI in the United States is tumors. Spinal cord tumors can be primary or metastatic, intradural, or extradural. Depending on the referral bias impacting individual centers, the type of tumor can vary. However, metastatic disease is the most common cause of tumor-related myelopathy, and survival after inpatient rehabilitation for metastatic disease is relatively short (76,78). Because of this, the focus of inpatient rehabilitation is to help the patient and family manage at home with the highest QOL feasible without spending too much time in the hospital. The majority of spine tumors are metastatic in origin and 95% are extradural. Approximately 70% of spinal metastasis occurs in the thoracic spine, with clinical presentation of pain, which is typically worse at night and in the supine position. The strongest predictors of functional outcome are the tumor type and the preoperative neurologic status (79).

In contrast, patients with primary tumors of the spine, meninges, or neural tissues such as meningiomas and ependymomas appear to have excellent survival durations after inpatient rehabilitation (76). In this case, the inpatient rehabilitation treatment program is similar to the program for someone with an incomplete traumatic SCI. Tumors such as sarcomas, or chordomas, may require extensive surgical resections followed by radiation and chemotherapy. However, with optimal surgical resection, survival increases and rehabilitation after surgery plays an important role in patient care (80,81). Aggressive intramedullary astrocytomas may similarly require radiation and chemotherapy. At times, inpatient rehabilitation will need to be modified to accommodate these treatments. In some cases, discharge from inpatient rehabilitation may be necessary before chemotherapy or radiation can be started.

The understanding of inflammatory disorders of the spinal cord is an evolving area. Historically, the term transverse myelitis encompassed a broad group of disorders of acute and subacute infectious and inflammatory disorders, which has made it difficult to establish a rehabilitation prognosis (82). Gradually, distinct clinical entities within this broad category are being understood, much in the way our understanding of tumor type informs prognosis and treatment options. Multiple sclerosis (MS), acute disseminated encephalomyelitis (ADEM), and neuromyelitis optica (NMO) are distinct inflammatory conditions affecting the spinal cord. MS generally presents with brain lesions and short asymmetric spinal cord lesions, and there is no specific biomarker associated with MS. In contrast, NMO usually presents with longitudinally extensive spinal cord MRI imaging abnormalities spanning three or more vertebral levels. As our understanding evolves, diagnostic criteria are periodically revised (83). It was previously referred to as Devic's disease (84) and was the first CNS inflammatory syndrome to have a specific serologic biomarker, the aquaporin-4 autoantibody (85) (AQP4). Titers of anti-AQP4, an antibody to an astrocyte water channel protein in spinal cord gray matter, have shown to correlate with the length of longitudinally extensive spinal cord lesions and clinical disease activity (86). While NMO was initially thought to be a condition specific to the optic nerves and spinal cord, it is now recognized as a diffuse disorder of the CNS. Because it is now recognized to be part of a spectrum of AQP4 channelopathies, the term neuromyelitis optica spectrum disorder (NMOSD) is now being used for cases of CNS inflammation with AQP4 autoantibody seropositivity (87). Presently, acute attacks of NMO, MS, and ADEM are treated with 1,000 mg IV MP daily for 5 days. Depending upon the response to IV steroids, secondary treatment of NMO and ADEM may include therapeutic plasma exchange and IV immunoglobulin. These treatments may need to be continued during inpatient rehabilitation. Fortunately, they are well tolerated and generally do not impact therapy participation except for the scheduling ramifications. Occasionally, steroids will be maintained for extended periods of time and *Pneumocystis* prophylaxis is necessary. In distinction from MS, NMO is treated with immunosuppression to prevent recurrent attacks whereas MS is treated with neuromodulatory agents. ADEM is generally a monophasic illness that acutely affects multiple regions of the central nervous system (CNS). But its prognosis is better than that of MS and NMO. Seropositivity for an antibody to myelin oligodendrocyte glycoprotein (MOG) has been shown to predict a monophasic illness and better recovery (88). MS exacerbations often resolve, and the disability due to MS appears to be primarily due to the chronic progression over time. As MS exacerbation prevention improves, inpatient rehabilitation for MS attacks is becoming uncommon. Instead, outpatient rehabilitative care and longitudinal follow-up are critical.

Infection-related myelopathy is the most common cause of NT SCI in some centers (70). SCI from epidural abscess is the most common infection-related cause of myelopathy, and *Staphylococcus aureus* is the most common pathogen (89–91). Similar to most SCI causes, men are more commonly affected than women, and like most NT SCI etiologies, the average age is approximately 60 years. Because epidural abscesses result from bacteremia, the 17 thoracolumbar vertebras are more commonly affected than the 7 cervical vertebras. Therefore, incomplete paraplegia is the most common neurologic deficit. Mosquito-based transmission of viral infections such as Zika and West Nile virus can present with acute fulminant paralysis just as polio did in the early 20th century. While relatively uncommon in North America, Europe, and Australia, tuberculosis is a major cause of myelopathy in some countries (92). Similar to most SCI, the severity of the neurologic deficit at the time of presentation predicts recovery (92). While rare, infection-related myelopathy can present as a chronic condition such as in the case of neurosyphilis, and a CSF examination is necessary to make the diagnosis.

The last major category of NT SCI is vascular causes. This group includes extrinsic cord compression due to epidural hematoma, ischemia, vasculitis, and vascular malformations. The percentage of patients with vascular NT SCI varies dramatically between centers (70). Epidural hematomas and ischemic lesions present with abrupt-onset deficits, whereas vascular malformations and dural arteriovenous fistulas present with insidious neurologic deterioration. Anticoagulation is a common cause of epidural hematomas and medical/surgical procedures are a common cause of ischemic SCI. Because dural arteriovenous fistulas and vascular malformations may cause venous hypertension, patients with these conditions may present with an unusual symptom of recurrent transient leg weakness due to exercise as the increased blood flow from exercise exacerbates the venous hypertension. Similar to other NT SCI groups, those with vascular myelopathy are older than those with TSCI (93). Possibly due to the relatively low incidence of vascular NT SCI, reported outcomes vary (70,93). An unusual but increasingly recognized possible cause for ischemic SCI is fibrocartilaginous embolism (FCE). This was originally described from autopsy findings in veterinary medicine; it is the most common cause of ischemic myelopathy in dogs (94). The initial case reports in humans were also due to autopsy findings of embolized fragments of nucleus pulposus in the arterial supply to the spinal cord (95,96). In contrast to most causes of NT SCI, the average age is similar to TSCI and women are more commonly affected than men. Distinguishing FCE from other acute-onset NT SCI can be challenging and diagnostic criteria have recently been proposed (97).

A potpourri of additional atypical causes of NT SCI such as metabolic, nutritional, and toxic myelopathies are important elements of the differential diagnosis for subacute and chronic progressive myelopathy, especially in at-risk populations. Individuals with a history of: obesity surgery, alcohol abuse, radiation treatment, methotrexate exposure, or excessive zinc exposure are at risk (98,99). Subacute combined degeneration of the spinal cord from B12 deficiency classically presents with gait ataxia and spasticity. Proprioceptive deficits on examination and signal abnormality in the posterior columns on MRI imaging are noted. Copper deficiency is rare, but can present similarly (100). Replacement of the identified nutritional deficiency may result in some degree of clinical improvement. Late radiation myelopathy is a delayed complication of radiation that develops months or years after treatment. The incidence of this complication is correlated with the total radiation dose, the dose fraction, and the length of the spinal cord irradiated. The injury predominantly affects the white matter in the lateral spinal cord and is often insidiously progressive. The diagnosis of late radiation myelopathy remains one of exclusion, and prognosis for significant recovery is poor.

THE SPINAL CORD FUNCTIONAL EVALUATION AND MANAGEMENT

The International Standards are the most widely accepted instrument of impairment, and interrater reliability is very good overall (101). The International Classification for Surgery of the Hand in Tetraplegia (102) is most commonly used when dealing with upper limb reconstruction procedures. The Autonomic Standards have also been developed to document autonomic functions, including blood pressure (BP), heart rate, and temperature regulation; bladder function; bowel function; and sexual function and are recommended in association with the ISNCSCI (103,104).

Individuals with the same SCI level and severity may have different levels of activity performance due to differences in adaptive equipment, personal assistance, and accessibility of their environment. Chapter 7 provides a detailed examination of functional evaluation. After SCI, function can be measured by a number of tests including the Grasp and Release Test (105), Capabilities of UE (CUE) instrument (106,107), Functional Independence Measure (FIM), Canadian Occupational

Performance Measure, Quadriplegia Index of Function (QIF), Spinal Cord Independence Measure (SCIM), and the Graded Redefined Assessment of Strength, Sensibility, and Prehension (GRASSP) (108–113). The FIM as a generic instrument has shortcomings when applied to SCI. The GRASSP and SCIM III are currently most often used especially for measuring functional ability in tetraplegia.

To measure walking in a standardized environment, the Timed Get Up and Go test, 6-minute walk test, and 10-m walk have been utilized (114,115). Forrest has reviewed benefits of these measures (116). The Walking Scale for SCI (WISCI) is a valid scale that ranks walking based on various combinations of braces, assistive devices, and level of personal assistance (117,118).

REHABILITATION OF SCI

Rehabilitation begins in the intensive care setting and includes addressing the SCI-specific needs to help the individual meet their potential in terms of medical, physical, social, emotional, recreational, vocational, and functional recovery (119). If early medical complications can be prevented, the inpatient rehabilitation course is facilitated, and the total cost of care is lessened.

The medical aspects of the SCI specialist's acute recommendations can be formulated into a problem list (eTable 22-3). The most important aspects include bowel, bladder, and pulmonary management; deep venous thrombosis; GI prophylaxis; and proper positioning in bed to prevent contractures and skin breakdown. Chapter 50 discusses exercise to prevent contractures, and Chapter 58 discusses orthotics. Each of these plays a key role in early SCI care. Once medically stable, the patient should be transferred to a specialized spinal cord rehabilitation unit.

A specialized SCI center offers access to experienced SCI physicians and therapists, including psychology, vocational and SCI educational services, an active peer support program, and an opportunity to undergo rehabilitation with other patients who have similar impairments (120,121). A comprehensive SCI education program is essential for educating the patients and their families about SCI-related issues. Additional opportunities available at larger SCI centers include availability of trial equipment for mobility and accessibility to high-level assistive technology. The interdisciplinary approach of the rehabilitation team, including the patient and family, is important for the optimal care of the individual with SCI. A sample rehabilitation prescription is listed in eTable 22-4. As the LOS shortens in acute rehabilitation, coordination and communication with the entire team is needed to allow for a timely and safe discharge. Frequent team conferences with an early home evaluation are recommended.

Functional Goals

Once the patient's motor level of injury, AIS, and prognosis for neurologic recovery are determined at the onset of rehabilitation, short- and long-term functional goals are formulated and a therapy prescription is established. General functional outcomes and equipment needs based on the level of injury are listed in **Table 22-3** and **eTable 22-5** (122).

The projected long-term goals are a starting point for the rehabilitation prescription. The rehabilitation program should be individualized to meet each person's strengths, weaknesses, and individual circumstances. Discharge planning should

be discussed as early as the first team conference, assuring a timely, but most importantly, a safe discharge. The ideal outcome may not always be achieved for each patient, as there is a significant amount of variability in individual outcomes despite similar levels of injury based upon the age, gender, and medical comorbidities.

C1-4 Level

Persons with motor levels above C3 will usually require long-term ventilator assistance, whereas most individuals with lesions at C4 will be able to wean off the ventilator. Respiratory equipment including a ventilator, a method for secretion management (i.e., suction machine or mechanical device), backup ventilator and batteries, and a generator in case of power failure should be obtained. Contact should be made with the local power company and emergency services to alert them of the patient's needs prior to discharge.

Rehabilitation goals for persons with high cervical SCI primarily include prevention of secondary medical complications, education and training of the patient and family members, prescription of appropriate durable medical equipment (DME), and environmental modification. The patient should be independent in instructing others in providing care including weight shifts, range of motion (ROM), positioning, donning orthoses, and transfers and in setting up their environmental control unit (ECU). Additional goals include independence in power wheelchair mobility, using breath control, mouth stick, head array, tongue, or chin control mechanisms. The wheelchair should be equipped with a pressure relief cushion and recline and/or tilt features for independent pressure relief. If the patient can control a power chair, then both a power chair and a manual positional wheelchair with a high back and tilt or recline should be prescribed for use as a backup wheelchair for assisted mobility in the home and in the community as needed (122). Once properly set up, persons at these levels of injury should be independent in using assistive technology. This includes lower-level technology devices (i.e., adapted phones and page turners) and higher-level devices (known as electronic aids of daily living [e-ADL]) that control one or more electronic appliances (i.e., television, radio, lights) via voice activation or switch access. These will allow for independence in communication and controlling their local environment. A type of lift to assist in transfers and a padded commode/shower chair should be prescribed. An attendant-operated van with a lift and tie-down or accessible public transportation is important for community mobility.

Restoring respiratory function for persons with high level of injuries (C2 and above) has been achieved by the use of various electrical stimulation options (see Chapter 55). These procedures may assist in weaning off of the ventilator and enhance speech production and improve QOL.

Persons with a NLI at C4 who have some elbow flexion and deltoid strength may be able to use a mobile arm support (MAS) or balanced forearm orthosis (BFO) to assist with feeding, grooming, and hygiene. Once the elbow flexors have antigravity strength with adequate endurance, these devices are no longer needed. A long straw or a bottle that the person can easily access to drink fluids should be obtained as early as possible.

The benefit of specialized acute inpatient rehabilitation for persons with such high levels of injury is justifiable despite their possible inability to initially tolerate 3 hours a day of

TABLE 22-3	Projected Functional Outcomes at 1 Year Postinjury by Level				
	C1-4	C5	C6	C7	C8-T1
Feeding	Dependent	Independent with adaptive equipment after set up	Independent with or w/o adaptive equipment	Independent	Independent
Grooming	Dependent	Min assist with equip. after set up	Some assist to independent with adaptive equipment	Independent with adaptive equipment	Independent
UE dressing	Dependent	Requires assistance	Independent	Independent	Independent
LE dressing	Dependent	Dependent	Requires assistance	Some assist to independent with adaptive equipment	Usually independent
Bathing	Dependent	Dependent	Some assist to independent with equipment	Some assist to independent with equipment	Independent with equipment
Bed mobility	Dependent	Assists	Assists	Independent to some assist	Independent
Weight shifts	Independent in power Dependent in manual wheelchair	Assists unless in power wheelchair	Independent	Independent	Independent
Transfers	Dependent	Maximum assist	Some assist to independent on level surfaces	Independent with or without board for level surfaces	Independent
Wheelchair propulsion	Independent with power Dependent in manual	Independent in power; independent to some assist in manual with adaptations on level surfaces	Independent—manual with coated rims on level surfaces	Independent—except curbs and uneven terrain	Independent
Driving	Unable	Independent with adaptations	Independent adaptations	Car with hand controls or adapted van	Car with hand control or adapted van

Potential Outcomes for Complete Paraplegics

	T2-9	T10-L2	L3-S5
ADL (grooming, feeding, dressing, bathing)	Independent	Independent	Independent
B/B	Independent	Independent	Independent
Transfers	Independent	Independent	Independent
Ambulation	Standing in frame, tilt table, or standing wheelchair Exercise only	Household ambulation with orthoses Can trial ambulation outdoors	Community ambulation is possible
Braces	Bilateral KAFO forearm crutches or walker	KAFOs, with forearm crutches	Possibly KAFO or AFOs, with canes/crutches

therapy and having what may seem as limited goals. The SCI medical and nursing care during the early period after injury are crucial for monitoring, treating, and preventing medical complications that can lead to future morbidity and mortality. Patient and family education, emotional and social support, and exposure to advanced technology that may allow independence in the proper environment (i.e., power mobility, assistive technology) may be the difference between returning to their family/community and living in a long-term facility.

C5 Level

The C5 motor level adds the key muscle group of the elbow flexors (biceps), as well as the deltoids, rhomboids, and partial innervation of the brachialis, brachioradialis (BR), supraspinatus, infraspinatus, and serratus anterior. It is important during the acute period after SCI to prevent elbow flexion and forearm supination contractures caused by unopposed flexion activity by stretching, splinting, and if needed antispasticity

injections. A long opponens splint, with a pocket for inserting different utensils (i.e., Universal cuff), is important to assist with many tasks including feeding, hygiene, grooming, and writing. Most functional activities will require the use of assistive devices; however, tendon transfers may be considered after neurologic recovery is complete.

The addition of the elbow flexors should allow for use of a joystick for a power wheelchair and can allow manual wheelchair propulsion on level surfaces with either rim projections (lugs) or plastic-coated hand rims with a protective glove. A power wheelchair, with power tilt, is usually still required in addition to the manual wheelchair. Push rim–activated power-assist wheelchairs may also be advantageous. These are manual wheelchairs that have a motor linked to each rear hub. With each manual propulsion stroke by the user, there is supplementary power provided by the motor. Therefore, the force required by the user for propulsion over the same distance is decreased when compared to a regular manual wheelchair. This feature is particularly useful for those with tetraplegia or those with paraplegia and overuse injury causing shoulder pain. The use of power-assist wheelchairs can improve the ability to perform ADL in persons with tetraplegia, when compared to the use of regular manual wheelchairs (123,124).

Persons with this level of injury will require almost total assistance for their bowel program. A padded commode/shower chair is recommended as the gravity from the upright position assists with the program and the padding helps to prevent skin breakdown. Bladder management is a decision based upon discussion with the SCI specialist and urologist, urodynamic results, amount of assistance available, and lifestyle circumstances. Intermittent catheterization (IC) usually cannot be performed independently and will need to be performed by another person. If using a leg drainage bag, electronic devices to help empty the bag are available. Driving a specially modified van is possible at this level, with a lift for access allowing the patient to be fully independent in this activity.

C6 Level

The C6 level adds the key muscle group that performs wrist extension (extensor carpi radialis), as well as partially innervating the supinator, pronator teres, and latissimus dorsi. Active wrist extension can allow for tenodesis, the opposition of the thumb and index finger with flexion as the tendons are stretched with wrist extension. One should avoid overly stretching the finger flexors initially after injury ("selective tightening") in C5 and C6 motor level patients to avoid potentially losing the tenodesis action. Tenodesis may allow some individuals with this level of injury to perform activities without splints, that is, feeding. Tenodesis splints can be fabricated but are frequently discarded by patients.

Feeding, grooming, and UE hygiene are usually independent after assistance with setting up the utensils; however, clothing modifications such as Velcro closures on shoes, loops on zippers, and pullover garments are recommended. Assistance for meal preparation and for other homemaking tasks is still required. Transfers may be possible using a transfer board and with loops for LE management, but most often require assistance. Although persons with a C6 motor level can propel a manual wheelchair with plastic-coated rims, a power wheelchair is often required for long distances, especially if the individual will be returning to the workplace. Power-assist wheels may be of benefit as well. IC may be possible for males after assistance for setup with assistive devices (125), but this technique is more difficult for females.

C7 and C8 Levels

The C7 motor level adds the elbow extensors (triceps) as the key muscle group and C8 the long finger flexors. The C7 level is considered the key level for becoming independent in most activities at the wheelchair level, including weight shifts, transfers between level surfaces, feeding, grooming, upper body dressing, and light meal preparation (126). Uneven surface transfers, lower body dressing, and house cleaning may require some assistance. The independent use of a car is possible if the individual can transfer and load/unload their wheelchair.

IC in males can be performed although it is more difficult for females, especially if LE spasticity is present. Surgical options for females including a continent urinary diversion with an umbilical stoma can allow for a cosmetic means to

catheterize easily (127). Bowel care on a padded commode seat, especially suppository insertion, may still require assistance or the use of adaptive devices (i.e., suppository inserter).

T1-12 Thoracic Levels

Individuals with all levels of paraplegia should be independent with basic ADL including LE dressing and mobility skills at the wheelchair level on even and uneven surfaces. This includes advanced wheelchair techniques such as curbs, ramps, wheelies (balancing the wheelchair on the two rear wheels), and floor to wheelchair transfers. Bowel and bladder management should be independent.

For most individuals with higher levels of complete thoracic injury, community ambulation is not a functional long-term goal. The lower the level of injury, the greater the trunk control due to abdominal and paraspinal muscle innervation. For lower levels of thoracic injuries, there is improved trunk control to allow for ambulation training with bilateral LE orthoses, as an exercise and for short distance household ambulation, once they have mastered basic wheelchair mobility skills.

L1-2 Levels

Muscles gained at these levels include the hip flexors and part of the quadriceps. While the person may be able to ambulate for short distances, a wheelchair will still be required for functional mobility needs. Bladder care is usually by IC. Individuals with these levels of injury can drive a car with hand controls.

L3-4 Levels

The knee extensors are fully innervated with some strength of ankle dorsiflexion (L4 myotome). Ambulation usually requires ankle-foot orthoses (AFOs) with canes and crutches. Bowel and bladder management should be independent. These injuries are, typically, LMN in nature, and bowel management is usually by contraction of abdominal muscles and manual disimpaction. Suppositories will not be effective because of the loss of sacral reflexes. Bladder management is usually performed via IC or Valsalva maneuver if postvoid residuals (PVRs) are within normal limits, and urologic workup reveals no contraindication to this method. Absorbent pads can be used.

L5 and Below

These individuals should be independent in all activities unless there are associated problems, that is, severe pain, cardiac conditions, etc.

Specific Activities in Therapy
Range of Motion

Shoulder ROM is important to prevent pain in persons with all levels of injury. In persons with C5 and C6 motor levels, ROM should be especially addressed to diminish the development of elbow flexion and supination contractures. As previously mentioned, for those individuals with active wrist extension and weak or no finger function, the finger flexors should not be fully stretched, but, instead, allowed to tighten somewhat and naturally curl to improve grip strength and function utilizing a "tenodesis" action. Lying prone when medically able is helpful in preventing and stretching the hip flexors. Prevention of heel cord tightness and contracture is important for proper positioning of the feet on the wheelchair footplate. Stretching of the lumbar spine is initiated when tightness or spasticity interferes with function, but is often avoided to provide the patient with increased postural stability and balance in the short and long sitting positions.

Pressure Reliefs

Pressure reliefs are essential to prevent the occurrence of pressure injuries (PIs). When supine, turning is initially performed every 2 hours and is progressively extended with close monitoring for signs of erythema that does not quickly dissipate (i.e., early-stage one pressure sore). The use of a mirror will greatly enhance the ability to monitor the sacral area and ischial tuberosities (ITs). Persons with high-level injuries (at C5 and above) will usually require a wheelchair with a tilt and/or recline mechanism. Some individuals with a C5 motor level can perform an anterior weight shift (with loops attached to the back of the wheelchair to assist in returning to the upright position) or a lateral weight shift. These weight shifts are more effective in pressure relief than having someone tip the wheelchair backward to 35 or 65 degrees (128). The small frontward lean however was shown to be ineffective in reducing pressure or increasing blood flow (129). Individuals with an injury at C7 and below are usually able to perform independent push-up pressure relief, although other types of weight shifts are still recommended. A pressure relief should be performed for at least 2 minutes every 20 to 30 minutes while in the wheelchair (130,131). Computerized pressure mapping can be used to locate areas of high pressure in the patient's wheelchair cushion and serve as a teaching tool to demonstrate the pressure relief technique that provides the best results. The use of a tilt system for pressure relief is best when sustained for greater than 3 minutes and at an angle of greater than 25 degrees to relieve pressure and improve tissue perfusion at the ITs (132).

Transfers

Initially, transfer training can be started on the mat, with subsequent progression to functional surfaces. Transfer training involves both the patient and the care providers. A lift transfer (one or two persons) is for individuals who are dependent for transfers. These can be performed with a lift that may be manual or electric: free standing, rolling, or attached to a structure (i.e., ceiling). Stand-pivot transfers are for patients who can weight-bear through the LEs with sufficient extension ROM in the hips and knees. Transfer (often referred to as "sliding") board transfers allow transfer between seated surfaces, with the use of a board that bridges the gap between them. One should, however, be careful not to slide across the board, preventing shearing forces leading to skin breakdown. The board is a sturdy, smooth, flat surface that is made of wood or plastic and comes in different sizes, styles, and handgrips for different transfer situations. The use of the board may decrease the pressure on the shoulders relative to a sit-pivot transfer. Sit-pivot transfers are performed by patients with a strong upper body, good short sitting balance, and good control of the head and shoulder movements. An overhead swivel trapeze bar can be attached to the bed, with the person lifting their body up swinging across to another surface. This can be a source of shoulder pain and is not recommended to be used on a consistent basis. Floor-to-chair/chair-to-floor transfers are particularly useful in accidental situations such as a fall, when the individual can then return to the wheelchair independently.

This is a physically demanding technique, requiring strong upper body strength in both the arms and the shoulders.

When transferring into the wheelchair, positioning is critical. The wheelchair should be positioned next to the surface being transferred to, at about a 30 to 45 degrees angle to it. The brakes should be locked and the footrest and armrests should be out of the way. The transfer technique and method used should take into account the presence of PIs at surfaces such as the sacrum and the IT.

Generally speaking, individuals with paraplegia should be independent of transfers, whereas those with tetraplegia may have varying levels of transfer independence. In most instances, those with a NLI at or below C7 can perform independent transfers, with or without the use of a transfer board, though some individuals with a C6 injury may be independent with the board. Individuals with a C5 injury are expected to seek the assistance of one person with or without a transfer board, whereas individuals with an injury at or above C4 will be dependent. The exact transfer technique used by individuals with SCI varies tremendously. Devices such as cushions to raise the seat height, frames, and mechanical devices that can also assist individuals with SCI to stand up may be very helpful in transfers.

Standing

Standing with the use of a tilt table or standing frame, after an acute SCI, decreases hypercalciuria and may retard or lessen bone loss (133); however, it has not been shown to reverse osteoporosis in chronic SCI. Standing should proceed with caution in patients with chronic SCI since bone mineral density is often at or below fracture threshold (134). Additional physiologic benefits of standing include a decrease in spasticity, enhancing bowel and bladder programs secondary to the effect of gravity and preventing PIs by facilitating pressure relief on normally weight-bearing areas (135,136). Tilt tables can be used early in the rehabilitation process in the treatment of orthostatic hypotension (OH).

Ambulation

There are four general levels of ambulation: community, household, ambulation for exercise, and nonambulatory (137). Community ambulation requires independence in performing transfers, capable of going from the sit to stand position, and ambulating unassisted in and outside the home for reasonable distances (>150 ft) with or without braces and assistive devices. Household ambulation is the ability to ambulate only within the home with relative independence, but may require assistance for transfers. Ambulation for exercise is for a person who requires significant assistance for ambulation.

Physiologic benefits of walking includes potentially decreasing the progression of osteoporosis, reducing urinary calcinosis and spasticity, aiding in digestion and improving the bowel program because of the effect of gravity, and preventing PIs as with standing (138,139). In addition, standing and walking enable reaching objects not obtainable from the wheelchair level and afford access to areas that are not wheelchair accessible, such as through narrow doorways or into a bathroom that is not appropriately modified. While ambulation following SCI has physiologic and psychological benefits, it also has significant drawbacks including increased energy consumption, with decreased speed of ambulation when compared to the relatively normal energy expenditure and velocity of wheelchair use; weight bearing through the UEs that may predispose an individual to shoulder, elbow, and wrist problems; and poor long-term follow-through (140–142).

Community ambulation requires bilateral hip flexor strength greater than 3/5 and one knee extensor to be at least 3/5, with a maximum amount of bracing of one long leg and one short leg brace (137). Prognostication for ambulation can begin early after injury and is determined by age and the neurological examination (143–147). While multiple studies have looked at this, but one of the simplest models was described by Van Middendorp et al., (148). That model uses age, and L3 and S1 sensory and motor function motor function assessed within the first 14 days to estimate the prognosis for ambulation one year post injury. Forty-six percent of persons with incomplete tetraplegia advance to community ambulation at 1 year, with an additional 14% performing household ambulation. Patients with initially motor incomplete injuries have a greater chance of ambulation than those with initial sensory incomplete injuries. For those with AIS B, PP sparing offers a better prognosis for regaining the ability to ambulate. Approximately 5% of complete paraplegics (the lower the level of injury, the greater the chance of ambulating) and 76% of incomplete paraplegics regain community ambulation. The percentage of persons with incomplete tetraplegia able to achieve community ambulation is lower than for incomplete paraplegia with equivalent lower extremity motor strength (LEMS), because the UE strength may be compromised and insufficient to enable assistive device ambulation if required. AIS grades at inpatient rehabilitation admission are helpful in predicting walking at discharge. Approximately 28% of persons with AIS C and 67% with AIS D at rehabilitation admission will regain the ability to ambulate by discharge. While level of injury does not significantly affect walking, older age does have a negative effect on the recovery of walking (146–148).

A number of orthotic options exist to assist in ambulation, including mechanical orthoses, functional ES (FES), and hybrid orthoses (a combination of a mechanical orthosis and FES) (149). The knee-ankle-foot orthoses (KAFOs) are most frequently prescribed for ambulation. Other devices used occasionally include the Parawalker, the reciprocal gait orthosis (RGO), advanced RGO (ARGO), hip-knee-ankle-foot orthoses (HKAFOs), and the hip guidance orthosis (HGO) that may enable persons with thoracic level paraplegia to ambulate. The Parastep system was the first example of a FES system for walking (149,150). Since then, robotic exoskeletons and advanced gait training strategies have become available, which are covered in Chapters 4, 55, 58, and 63. Over the last decade, several trials have investigated gait training approaches, and neither partial body weight–supported gait training nor robotic ambulation has been consistently shown to be superior to conventional over ground walking therapy for the rehabilitation of the patients with acute and chronic SCI (151–153).

Assisted Technology Devices

Assisted technology devices (ATDs) are covered in detail in Chapter 56. Following SCI, one can use any body part to activate a switch as long as they can perform the activity consistently. Reliable activating sites include the head, chin, mouth, shoulder, arm, or hand. Voice activation is also an option. Prior to prescription, it is important to identify the patient's capabilities (i.e., cognitive status and functional movements)

and needed tasks, the patient's goals, as well as any environmental barriers that may be present (154).

The use of brain-based command signals for controlling assistive technology, robotics, or neuroprostheses is showing increasing potential in rehabilitation research and may prove to be useful for persons with high-level tetraplegia. Brain signals are collected and processed through electrodes that may be placed or implanted at different levels. Once a signal is processed, it can potentially be used to control a number of devices, including computers linked to neuroprosthetic or robotic devices for assistance with ADL (155,156). There is no clinical product available for brain-based command signals at present and more research is necessary for its application.

HOME MODIFICATIONS FOR PEOPLE WITH SCI

A number of general guidelines and recommendations for making the home accessible are listed in 📶 **eTable 22-6**. A home evaluation or a floor plan of the residence should be completed early as an important aspect of the rehabilitation process to allow the injured individual to return home. The key pieces of information to know when performing the home evaluation are the patient's level of injury and mobility status, their prognosis for functional recovery, social situation for return to home, and financial considerations. The main areas to be evaluated include the entrances, bedroom, bathroom, and kitchen and general safety issues ensuring that there is safe wheelchair access and egress and space to maneuver a wheelchair in the home. The home should be free from fire, health, and safety hazards and have an adequate heating, cooling, and electrical supply to meet the needs of additional medical equipment that must be present.

DRIVING AFTER SCI

Most individuals with a motor level at or below C5 have the potential to return to independent driving with the appropriate adaptive equipment. The driver rehabilitation specialist evaluates the patient, assists in choosing the proper vehicle, and recommends modifications required including proper controls, lifts, lockdown, and tie-down devices.

A person with complete paraplegia and no additional complications will probably require mechanical hand controls and a few additional minor pieces of equipment to operate a car with an automatic transmission. The evaluation and training for such individuals can usually occur within 3 months of injury. Individuals with tetraplegia are usually evaluated at a later time postinjury (up to 1 year) to allow for neurologic recovery to plateau, since any gain in motor function can mean a difference in equipment required. Higher-level injuries (C5 and some C6) require more extensive adaptations allowing for acceleration, breaking, and steering. For lower-level tetraplegia, steering may be facilitated by a spinner knob or other devices. In all cases, the person should be medically stable and be psychologically ready to return to the road.

A driving assessment should be performed and includes a current and past driving history, current medications, a vision screen, physical skills testing (i.e., ROM, strength, sensory and proprioception testing, balance, spasticity, transfer, and wheelchair loading skills), wheelchair or mobility equipment required, and reaction time (157,158). If the individual has a history of brain trauma, cognitive and perceptual screens should also be included. The behind-the-wheel assessment involves vehicle entry and exit and operation of primary and secondary controls. Training time can range from a few hours for mechanical hand controls and standard steering to over 40 hours for joystick drivers.

For most persons with paraplegia, an automatic transmission car is an option if there are no problems with transfers. Transfer aides are available that can raise the person up to the level of a full-size truck seat, but these are costly. If transfers or chair loading is more difficult, then vans should be considered. Loading devices can assist the client in loading the wheelchair. Options include car top devices that fold the manual wheelchair and stow it in a rooftop carrier or a lift that can stow the folding chair behind the driver's seat. Most persons with tetraplegia choose a modified van with power door openers and a ramp or lift. Persons with a NLI above C5 will require a van to accommodate their transportation needs, but will not be able to drive independently. It is usually easier to transport the person seated in their wheelchair that is already set up to provide the proper support. A structurally modified full-size van or lowered-floor minivan will usually be required. For the dependent passenger, the lowered floor drops their eye height to a point where they may be able to see out the side windows.

MEDICAL ISSUES AFTER SCI

Cardiovascular System Conditions

Thromboembolic Disorders

Thromboembolic disorders, including DVT and pulmonary embolism (PE), are common medical complications after SCI. The incidence of DVT during the acute postinjury period has varied depending on the method of detection used for screening and whether prophylaxis is utilized and has been reported in approximately 64% of patients (range of 47% to 100%) (159–163). Model system data reported an incidence of 9.8% for DVT and 2.6% for PE during acute rehabilitation (161). More recent data from Taiwan confirm the marked increase in VTE risk after SCI and noted the DVT risk was 16.9 times higher after SCI than the general population risk (164). The development of DVT occurs most frequently during the first 2 weeks (approximately 80% of cases) following injury. PE previously was reported to occur approximately 5% to 8% of patients in the first year and was the third leading cause of death in all SCI patients in the first year postinjury (162). However, more recent data from the National Spinal Cord Injury Statistical Center report that the mortality rate due to PE has diminished to 3.3%, now accounting for the sixth leading cause of death in the first year after SCI (165). As time post injury increases, the risk of VTE decreases. A recent large database reported that the risks of VTE in the first 3 months, at 6 months, and at 1 year after injury risk were 34%, 1.1%, and 0.4%, respectively (166).

Among major trauma patients, those with an SCI have been shown to have the highest risk of DVT, with an odds ratio of 8.6 compared to trauma patients without SCI (163). Certain risk factors include paraplegia greater than tetraplegia, complete greater than incomplete injury, concomitant fractures of the lower extremities and pelvis, and previous history of VTE. Others factors that have not been consistently found to be related include gender, obesity, nonorthopedic injuries, and surgical management.

The high incidence of DVT/PE in persons with SCI is related to Virchow's triad that includes stasis, intimal injury, and hypercoagulability, which are all sequelae of acute neurologic injury. Suspicion should be high and diagnostic testing ordered to make the proper diagnosis if suspected. Clinical signs of a DVT may include unilateral edema, low-grade fever, and pain/tenderness in a patient with an incomplete injury. However, the physical examination is limited in SCI because edema may be present secondary to immobilization and the patient may have loss of sensation.

The most recent Consortium Guidelines in SCI (163) have the following recommendations. Mechanical thromboprophylaxis with intermittent pneumatic compression devices (PCDs) with or without graduated compression stockings (GCSs) should be applied as soon as feasible after acute SCI when not contraindicated by lower extremity injury. Low molecular weight heparin (LMWH) should be used as thromboprophylaxis in the acute care phase following SCI once there is no evidence of active bleeding. Low-dose or adjusted-dose unfractionated heparin is not recommended for the prevention of venous thromboembolism in SCI (unless LMWH is not available or contraindicated). Oral vitamin K antagonists (such as warfarin) are also not recommended to be used as thromboprophylaxis in the early, acute care phase following SCI. Although there are no trials as of yet reported in SCI, direct oral anticoagulants (DOACs) may be considered as thromboprophylaxis during the rehabilitation phase following SCI.

For duration of prophylaxis, it is recommended that anticoagulant thromboprophylaxis continue at least 8 weeks in SCI patients with limited mobility. Although the optimal duration of thromboprophylaxis following SCI remains unclear and should be individualized, consideration for longer-duration prophylaxis include motor complete injuries, lower extremity fractures, older age, previous VTE, cancer, and obesity.

Inferior vena cava (IVC) filters are not recommended to be used as primary thromboprophylaxis in SCI; however, a temporary IVD filter can be used for patients with an acute proximal DVT and an absolute contraindication to therapeutic anticoagulation. Placement of a temporary IVC filter is appropriate until anticoagulation can be initiated. Prophylactic IVC filters are not recommended in SCI because evidence supporting filter benefit (reduction in PE or mortality) is absent; complication rates associated with filter use exceed the rates of the disease that filters are designed to prevent; current filters are not safe when left in place for the long term; and there are significant unjustified costs associated with these devices (167,168).

Routine Doppler ultrasonography (DUS) is not recommended for clinically unapparent DVT during their acute care hospitalization nor on admission to rehabilitation.

In children with acute SCI, mechanical prophylaxis with GCSs and/or PCDs is recommended, and adolescents (greater than age 12 years) receive anticoagulant thromboprophylaxis, especially if they have additional risk factors such as lower extremity or pelvic fractures. Lastly, for persons with chronic SCI, prophylaxis is recommended if hospitalized for medical illnesses or surgical procedures during the period of increased risk (164).

Anemia

Anemia is common following acute SCI and is usually normochromic and normocytic (169). Serum iron, TIBC, and transferrin are usually low. Although the exact cause is not known, bleeding may be a factor in some cases. By 1 year postinjury, anemia improves in the majority of patients, and if it persists, it is usually associated with chronic inflammatory complications (170). A study of persons with chronic SCI found that average prevalence rates of anemia and hypoalbuminemia were 34% and 6%, respectively, with a higher rate in those preceding mortality usually secondary to sepsis, cancer, and pulmonary and cardiovascular diseases (CVDs) (171).

Orthostatic Hypotension

OH occurs when there is a decrease in systolic BP (SBP) by 20 mm Hg or a decrease in diastolic blood pressure (DBP) of greater than 10 mm Hg or more (172). Many patients with acute SCI have a baseline SBP of ≤90 mm Hg, making symptoms a more reliable parameter to follow in diagnosis and treatment. SCI patients often experience symptomatic hypotension with position changes, especially moving from supine to more upright positions. Associated symptoms include lightheadedness, dizziness, ringing of the ears, fatigue, tachycardia, and sometimes syncope. In one study, OH occurred during 74% of therapy treatments in patients with acute SCI, with accompanying signs and symptoms noted on 59% of occasions and were perceived as limiting treatment on 43% of occasions (173). OH can last for several weeks after the injury, often delaying the rehabilitative process. OH occurs more frequently in persons with cervical level and neurologically complete injuries. When bed rest is prolonged, the degree of orthostasis tends to be more severe (174). OH intensifies after eating, exposure to warm environments, defecation, and rapid bladder emptying (175). Symptoms are related to a reduction in cerebral perfusion rather than a specific peripheral BP level.

Habituation to the symptoms of OH occurs slowly although the resting BP rarely returns to preinjury values, especially in person with tetraplegia and those with injuries above T6. The exact mechanism is unknown, but theories include increased sensitivity of baroreceptors and catecholamine receptors in the vessel walls, development of spasticity, improved autoregulation of cerebral vascular perfusion, and adaptations of the renin-angiotensin system (176). Patients should be cautioned to avoid rapid changes in position. Simple adjustments, such as raising the head for several minutes prior to transferring out of bed, can be effective in decreasing episodes of OH.

Physical methods, including compression wraps to the legs and an abdominal binder donned prior to sitting up, repeated postural changes on a tilt table or a high-back reclining wheelchair, as well as FES, may be helpful in treatment (177) although studies are limited. Maintaining adequate fluid intake is important, and one should not be started on fluid restriction for an IC bladder program until the symptoms have improved. Avoiding diuretics such as alcohol and caffeine and partaking in small meals to minimize postprandial hypotension are recommended. Sleeping with the bed head raised by 10 to 20 degrees should be encouraged to increase plasma volume and orthostatic tolerance.

Pharmacologic agents are added to the treatment regimen if the above interventions do not resolve the symptoms.

The most common pharmacologic intervention is midodrine hydrochloride (2.5 to 10 mg three times per day), and if this is ineffective, then initiate a salt-retaining mineralocorticoid such as fludrocortisone (0.05 to 0.1 mg daily) (178,179). The medication should be given approximately 1 hour prior to activity known to cause hypotensive episodes. Patients should be monitored closely for hypertension when taking these medications. Other medications including salt tablets (sodium chloride 1 g four times per day), ephedrine, L-threo-3,4-dihydroxyphenylserine (L-DOPS), and L-NAME have been infrequently used (178,180).

Chronic low resting BP may interfere with participation in activities that may have a deleterious effect on the patient's long-term health, as low resting systolic BP (<110 mm Hg) is associated with fatigue and can lead to deficits in cognitive performance and perhaps other medical complications (179,181). In February 2014, the Food and Drug Administration (FDA) approved droxidopa, a synthetic amino acid acting as a precursor of norepinephrine, for the treatment of OH of neurologic nature and has been studied in SCI (182,183).

Autonomic Dysreflexia

AD, also known as autonomic hyperreflexia, is a composite of symptoms, most notably a sudden rise in BP, is seen in SCI patients with injuries at or above T6, and is due to autonomic dysfunction. Individuals who are neurologically complete and at higher levels of injury are apt to have more severe symptoms (184–188). The incidence in susceptible patients varies between 48% and 90%, but rarely presents within the first few weeks after injury, and nearly all patients who develop AD will do so within the first year.

Typically, a noxious stimulus below travels via the peripheral nerves to the spinal cord and ascends in the spinothalamic tracts and dorsal columns where sympathetic neurons in the intermediolateral cell columns are stimulated. This triggers an unregulated sympathetic nervous system cascade, leading to focal vasoconstriction. Classically, if the NLI is at or above T6, this vasoconstriction can involve the splanchnic vessels (innervated by nerves originating from T5-L2) and leads to the progressive hypertension, which typifies AD. The hypertension from AD is defined as a rise of >20 mm Hg above baseline.

The most common source is from the bladder, either from overdistension or infection, with the second most common source being the bowel (i.e., fecal impaction). These account for over 80% of all cases. Other causes include PIs, ingrown toenails, abdominal emergencies, fractures, and body positioning. In females, AD can occur during labor and delivery (189) and in males during stimulation techniques for ejaculation.

Symptoms include most commonly a headache that is pounding in nature and found in the frontal and occipital areas, followed by sweating and flushing above the level of lesion. Baroreceptors from the carotid sinus and aortic arch detect the elevated BP and relay impulses to the vasomotor center in the brainstem that attempts to compensate by slowing the heart rate via impulses through the vagus nerve. Signals meant to inhibit the sympathetic system are blocked at the spinal cord lesion (**Fig. 22-3**).

Signs and symptoms reflect sympathetic overflow, and the consequent compensatory reaction mediated by the PS nervous system. The sympathetic discharge causes hypertension

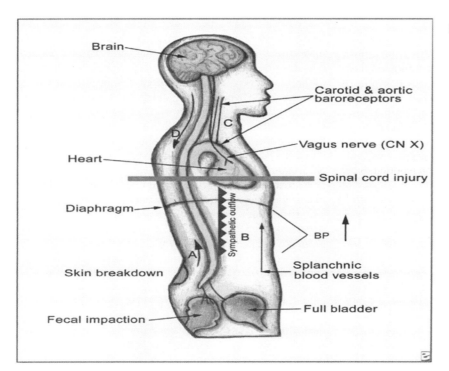

FIGURE 22-3. Autonomic dysreflexia.

and piloerection. The PS response causes headache, pupillary constriction, sinus congestion, and bradycardia. While classically bradycardia can occur, tachycardia is more commonly seen. More serious and even life-threatening symptoms may occur including cardiac arrhythmias, seizures, intracranial hemorrhage, pulmonary edema, and myocardial infarction.

AD requires immediate attention, with the goal to remove the inciting stimulus and reduce the BP. The BP and pulse should be monitored every 2 to 5 minutes until stabilized. A rapid survey of the patient for the causes should be initiated. The first intervention upon diagnosis is to sit the patient upright with loosening of all tight-fitting clothes. The bladder should next be checked for overdistension by flushing an indwelling catheter if one is present or catheterizing the patient if without one. If the catheter is blocked, gentle irrigation with a small amount of fluid, at body temperature, is used. If available, Xylocaine gel (2%) should be used prior to catheterization. If the bladder is the source, the BP should quickly return to baseline. If the pressure remains elevated (i.e., systolic BP >150 mm Hg), pharmacologic management should be initiated prior to checking for fecal impaction. If so, one should use an antihypertensive agent with rapid onset and short duration while the causes of AD are being investigated. Prior to rectal examination, Xylocaine gel is recommended to be placed within the anorectal area. If impaction is not present, other possible sources should then be sought, including PIs, ingrown toenails, infections, fractures, DVT, and HO.

Medications used for AD most commonly include nitrate gels (e.g., nitroglycerine paste) and less frequently clonidine, nifedipine, terazosin, β-blockers, phenoxybenzamine, and hydralazine. The use of nitrates is beneficial as they can be easily applied, titrated, and removed immediately if a source is later found. If using nifedipine, chew and swallow is the recommended route, rather than sublingual. The BP should be monitored frequently because hypotension may occur,

especially if the source is found rapidly. The individual should be monitored for recurrent symptoms for at least 2 hours after resolution of the AD episode to ensure that it does not recur. If there is poor response to treatment and/or if the cause of the AD has not been identified, the patient should be hospitalized for monitoring, maintenance of pharmacologic control of BP, and investigation of other possible causes of the AD. For most women with AD during labor and delivery, epidural anesthesia is preferred and effective.

Cardiovascular Disease, Obesity, and Diabetes after SCI

Metabolic syndrome, a constellation of central obesity, dyslipidemia, hypertension, and insulin resistance, is associated with a proinflammatory and prothrombotic state that directly promotes CVD (190).

Cardiovascular disease is a leading cause of mortality and morbidity in chronic SCI. In contrast to the able-bodied population, CVD occurs more frequently and at earlier ages in the SCI population (191,192). Several factors contribute to this increased incidence, including relatively sedentary lifestyle, poor dietary habits, dyslipidemia, and increased prevalence of obesity and diabetes mellitus. Those with tetraplegia and neurologically complete injuries are at highest risk (193). The prevalence of CVD has been reported between 25% and 50% (191,192,194).

The pathophysiology of CVD in persons with SCI is multifactorial. Changes in body composition occur and include decreased fat-free body mass and a relative increase in adipose tissue. The relative decrease of fat-free body mass contributes to lowered high-density lipoprotein (HDL) levels, impaired glucose metabolism, and progressive insulin resistance (190,195). Given the prevalence of CVD in the SCI population, early recognition of risk factors is crucial to initiate early interventions, which can modify these risks.

Changes in lipid metabolism develop early after SCI and progress overtime. The major disruption seen in men after SCI is a profound reduction in HDL-c. Bauman et al. reported that in men with paraplegia, 63% had HDL-c values less than 40 mg/dL, 44% had values less than 35 mg/dL, and 19% had values less than 30 mg/dL (196). Reduced HDL-c levels are associated with higher NLI, motor complete injuries, and increased abdominal circumference (197,198). In contrast to men, premenopausal women have HDL-c levels similar to the general population (199). Serum LDL, total cholesterol, and TG in men and women with SCI have also been reported to be similar to that of the general population (196).

Using criteria for the general population, Nash et al. found that 34% of individuals with SCI had metabolic syndrome (200). Nevertheless, it is likely that general metabolic syndrome criteria or other common screening tools for CVD risk do not fully capture the changes in body composition, lipid profiles, glucose homeostasis, and BP after SCI. Therefore, modifications have been suggested for this specific population (201,202).

Interventions to decrease the risk of cardiovascular events should initially focus on modifiable risk factor reduction including smoking cessation, weight loss, dietary modification, and increased physical activity levels (see also Chapter 49). Although individuals with SCI consume fewer kilocalories than the general population, they have been shown to consume levels of fat that exceed recommendations and likely still have a daily calorie surplus due to the significant reduction in energy expenditure (203,204).

Those with hypertension, dyslipidemia, or hyperglycemia that persists after attempted behavior modification should receive appropriate pharmacotherapy. A structured exercise regimen is recommended (205). Arm ergometry (high intensity with a target HR of 70% to 80% of max predicted) and FES have shown efficacy in improving glucose tolerance and lipid profiles in persons with SCI (206–208).

Acute exercise responses and capacity for exercise conditioning are related to the level and completeness of the spinal lesion. Patients with complete SCI at or above T4 have diminished cardiac acceleration with maximal heart rates less than 130 beats/min (209). The exercise capacity of these persons is limited by reductions in cardiac output and circulation to the exercising musculature. Persons with paraplegia also have reduced exercise capacity and increased heart rate responses (compared with the nondisabled), which have been associated with circulatory limitations within the paralyzed tissues. Statins should be considered for treatment of lipid alterations in patients with SCI (210).

The true incidence of obesity within SCI is likely underreported given the measures used to typically measure adiposity. Estimates (using % body fat) conclude that two thirds of persons with SCI are obese (202). Unfortunately, the presence of paralysis makes effective weight loss more difficult for wheelchair users. Recommendations for CV exercise include exercise at least three times per week (more to facilitate weight loss) for up to 90 min/d incorporating cardiovascular conditioning and strength training. Caution should be taken to avoid overuse injuries to the UEs commonly seen in this population. Obesity has been associated with breast and colon cancer, CTS, stroke, coronary artery disease, diabetes mellitus, hypertension, dyslipidemia, obstructive sleep apnea, and PIs (202,211).

Diabetes mellitus has been reported to occur in approximately 20% of individuals with chronic SCI. Studies have shown that oral glucose tolerance testing may detect insulin resistance earlier than fasting blood glucose measures (212,213). Early detection is helpful in initiating early treatment, a key component to minimize the long-term complications associated with diabetes mellitus including chronic skin ulcers, peripheral vascular disease, heart attacks, and strokes. Symptoms of hyperglycemia include polydipsia and polyuria. In the SCI patient population, polyuria may include increased IC volumes, new-onset urinary incontinence, or AD. The measurement of the hemoglobin A1C is also helpful in making the diagnosis of diabetes mellitus and monitoring the efficacy of treatment.

THE GASTROINTESTINAL SYSTEM

Anatomic and Physiologic Considerations: Regulation of Gastrointestinal Function

Fortunately, many of the organs, tissues, and cells of the gastrointestinal system operate autonomously. Regulatory influences include the parasympathetic and sympathetic nervous systems, the enteric system within the gut, and endocrine, myogenic, and intraluminal cues. Upper motor neuron bowel dysfunction occurs with lesions between the pons and the sacral spinal cord. This is the type of dysfunction most common in patients with C1 through T10 SCI. Associated deficits in function include sensory deficit for perception of fullness, a spastic pelvic floor that retains stool, and less effective peristaltic patterns (214). The gastrocolic response is an increase in peristalsis in the large and small intestine that occurs after a meal. It is preserved after SCI, although it may be less robust compared to able-bodied controls (215). Colonic propulsion of the fecal contents requires motility. After SCI, in the absence of regular spontaneous or willful defecation, transit and motility are dependent on regular scheduled bowel care. Rectal distension in itself can reflexively inhibit peristalsis and affect alimentary function as proximal as the stomach, preventing gastric emptying. A bowel program is a unique plan designed to effectively eliminate stool and prevent incontinence. The components are fluid intake, diet, exercise, medications, and scheduled bowel care (216). Bowel care is the procedure for assisted defecation. Through empirical manipulation of diet, hydration, medications, and stimulation techniques, a balance is maintained between continence and evacuation.

Fecal Continence

Fecal continence is achieved with a combination of structures that work together to prevent inadvertent passage of stool. These barriers are removable to allow bowel evacuation to occur. The current state, continence or evacuation, depends on the balance between those forces that favor expulsion of stool and those that resist it (**Fig. 22-4**). Expulsive forces include intra-abdominal pressure, colorectal contraction, elastic forces, and gravity. Resistive forces include the anorectal angle, anal canal tone contributed by the internal anal sphincter (IAS) and external anal sphincter (EAS), and friction. Stool consistency is a pivotal factor that can shift the balance in either direction. Small, hard stool is evacuated less completely and with more difficulty than soft, bulky stool (217,218). Whereas even subjects with normal continence mechanisms may be incontinent

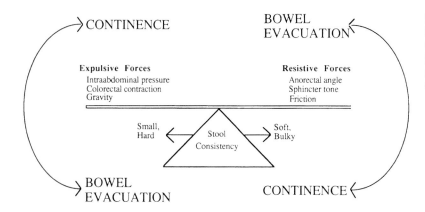

FIGURE 22-4. Balance of forces favoring continence or bowel evacuation. Physical character of stool is the pivotal variable that can shift the balance in either direction. Small, hard stool shifts the fulcrum to the left, and more force is required to evacuate. Soft, bulky stool causes the fulcrum to shift the opposite way.

when faced with large volumes of liquid stool as in during an acute diarrheal illness.

Intraluminal Content

The intraluminal contents can affect gastrointestinal function through alteration of the physical characteristics of stool, bacterial action, and the effects of various substances on mucosal receptors. The physical characteristics of the fecal mass have an important effect on colonic motility and defecation efficiency. The typical Western diet, deficient in fiber, results in small, hard, often scybalous stool that is difficult for the colon to propel and the rectum to evacuate. The effect of stool consistency on rectal evacuation has been well studied in able-bodied subjects (217,218). Dry, hard stool is not compressible, breaks apart, and contributes to high friction against the colonic wall. These stools produce difficulty with evacuation.

Addition of vegetable fiber to the diet increases stool volume and moisture content, which increases plasticity and decreases transit time (219). With increased dietary fiber, fecal microbial mass also increases (220). Bacterial fermentation of indigestible fiber within the colon generates short-chain fatty acids. These short-chain fatty acids are passively absorbed by colonic mucosa and may be oxidized as an important energy source (221). Bacteria also are important in the metabolism of bile salts. Bile salts stimulate colonic motility; as a result, agents that bind bile salts such as cholestyramine can be helpful if the stool is too loose.

Furthermore, the luminal content also can affect gastrointestinal function by the stimulation of specific mucosal receptors. Five types of gastrointestinal sensory receptors are known to exist. These respond to mechanical, chemical, osmotic, thermal, or painful stimuli.

Intrinsic Neural Regulation

The enteric nervous system is embedded in the wall of the gut and runs its entire length, from the pharynx to the anus. Meissner's plexus is distributed throughout the submucosa and transmits local sensory and motor signals to Auerbach's plexus, autonomic ganglia, and the spinal cord. Auerbach's plexus (intramuscular myenteric) is distributed between the longitudinal and circular muscle layers. The enteric nervous system integrates sensory information from the contents and coordinates local and distant secretion and peristalsis. Ablation of all enteric nervous activity by the neurotoxin tetrodotoxin causes the colon to contract, the rectum to undergo tonic and phasic contractions, and the IAS to contract tonically (222). Thus,

it appears that the major effect of the enteric nervous system on the lower gastrointestinal tract is to provide an inhibitory influence.

Extrinsic Neural Regulation

Extrinsic neural influences provide overall coordination of intestinal reflexes as well as integration of the gastrointestinal tract with the whole person (**Fig. 22-5**).

The gastrointestinal tract receives both parasympathetic and sympathetic nervous system innervations. The function of the parasympathetic efferents is complex. Separate groups of vagal preganglionic fibers may innervate inhibitory or excitatory neurons in the same organ. Injury to the inferior splanchnic nerve (parasympathetic S2-4) results in impaired defecation and constipation (223). The function of the

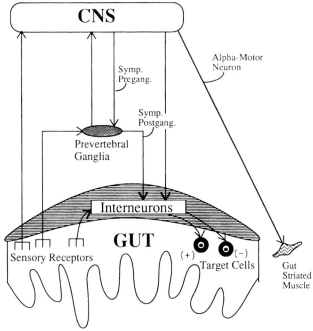

FIGURE 22-5. General organization of the enteric nervous system. Sensory fibers in the gut send afferents to the central nervous system (CNS) through the vagus nerve (cell bodies in nodose ganglia) or the sympathetic nerves (cell bodies in the dorsal root ganglia), prevertebral ganglia, and interneurons within the gut wall. Input may be processed and efferent fibers sent to effector cells at all three levels. The only efferent neurons that do not involve the enteric nervous system are the α-motor neurons that innervate the striated muscle at both ends of the gut (i.e., cricopharyngeus and external anal sphincter).

sympathetic nerves is generally to cause inhibition of motor and secretory activity and contraction of gastrointestinal sphincters. Sympathetic stimulation leads to adynamic ileus and decreased bowel activity. Although surgical sympathectomy has little clinical effect on bowel function in humans, diarrhea has been reported in animal models (224).

The striated muscle of the EAS is innervated by α-motor neurons directly from the CNS. The cell bodies of the α-motor neurons to the EAS are located in the anterior horn cells of spinal segments S2 through S4. Their axons are carried in the pudendal nerve. Injuries to the pudendal nerves or the sacral cord produce flaccid paralysis of the pelvic floor along with the external sphincter.

Anorectum

The anal canal provides the primary mechanism for fecal continence and is the barrier that must be traversed for evacuation to occur. The *internal anal sphincter* (IAS) is the specialized thickening of the circular smooth muscle layer of the rectum that maintains a continuous state of maximal contraction. It is responsible for the majority of resting tone in the anal canal (225).

Normal internal anal canal resting pressures range from 50 to 100 cm H_2O. This resting tone is not altered after SCI (226). The *external anal sphincter* is a striated muscle that is continuous with the pelvic floor and is innervated by the pudendal nerves bilaterally. The EAS, along with muscles of the pelvic floor, displays the unusual property of continuous electrical activity in both waking and sleeping states (227). Presumably, this special property allows the EAS and pelvic floor to maintain continence without conscious will and during sleep. Although the EAS plays a small role in the resting state, contraction of the EAS can double anal canal pressure for short periods of time. External sphincter function is felt to be important during events that are an acute threat to continence, such as coughing, acute rectal contraction, or assuming an upright position.

The puborectalis muscle originates from behind the pubic symphysis and extends posteriorly to loop around the rectum just proximal to the anal canal. The puborectalis tugs the rectum anteriorly and creates an angle between the rectum and the anal canal, the *anorectal angle*. This kink in the fecal pathway aids in continence (228,229). Conversely, failure of the puborectalis to relax appropriately, with persistence of an acute anorectal angle, has been associated with inability to defecate (230). The IAS, the EAS, and the puborectalis work together synergistically to maintain continence and are collectively named the *anal sphincter mechanism*.

The mucosa at the proximal end of the rectum and anal canal (anorectal junction) is rich in sensory receptors. This allows for socially critical judgments about the phases of the matter therein: liquid, solid, and gaseous material. The rectoanal inhibitory or sampling reflex allows a sample of the rectal contents to come into contact with this sensory zone. The *rectoanal inhibitory reflex* consists of a transient relaxation of the IAS stimulated by a rise in rectal pressure. A simultaneous increase in EAS tone, *the guarding reflex*, occurs to preserve continence while sensory receptors of the anorectal junction appraise the contents. The rectoanal inhibitory reflex occurs during sleep and throughout the day, usually at a subconscious level.

Early GI Complications after SCI

Immediately after an SCI, an adynamic ileus is usually present and typically resolves within a week. Gastric decompression via nasogastric tube with intermittent suction may be necessary for persistent abdominal distension. Parenteral nutrition should be considered when the ileus lasts longer than 3 days. In cases where the ileus lasts longer, erythromycin and/or metoclopramide can be used to stimulate peristalsis (231). Neostigmine has also been effective in refractory cases of pseudo-obstruction (232).

Individuals with SCI have a higher risk of developing peptic ulcers compared with the general trauma population (233). The incidence is approximately 5% to 7%, although an incidence as high as 24% has been reported (234,235). Most ulcers occur acutely, within a few days from injury. Higher-level and more severe injuries (neurologically complete) have the greatest risk. The use of stress ulcer prophylaxis is recommended (histamine 2 blockers or proton pump inhibitors [PPIs]) usually for 4 weeks unless other risk factors are present (19). PPIs are more effective in preventing upper GI bleeding in high-risk patients; however, it may increase the rate of *Clostridium difficile* infections.

Individuals with SCI also have a higher risk (25% to 30%) of developing biliary stasis and gallstone disease compared to able-bodied persons (236,237). Impaired gallbladder motility has been implicated as the cause. Patients with lesions above T10 have impaired filling of the gallbladder and lower fasting volumes, which may make the bile more lithogenic. Due to altered sensation after SCI, the diagnosis may be more challenging. However, the majority of patients still presents with traditional symptoms, often with radiation of the pain to the right shoulder, and may still have findings such as right upper quadrant abdominal pain and tenderness (236,238). A high index of suspicion, as well as laboratory and radiographic tests, are essential in making a timely diagnosis.

Superior mesenteric artery (SMA) syndrome is a condition where the third segment of the duodenum is compressed between the SMA and the aorta. It occurs rarely, though more commonly in persons with tetraplegia, with an incidence of less than 0.33%. The patient experiences nausea, vomiting, abdominal tightness, and bloating, which is made worse after a meal or by lying supine. The diagnosis is made definitively with an upper GI series. Risk factors that may predispose patients to this condition include weight loss, use of a spinal orthotic, and immobilization in the supine position. Patients may gain some relief by lying on the left side and by taking metoclopramide (239).

Acute abdominal emergencies are often a challenge to diagnose, especially in patients with higher-level SCI because of the absence of the usual signs and symptoms of abdominal pathology. It is, therefore, important to have a high suspicion in evaluating patients with SCI presenting with fever, abdominal pain, and/or pain radiating to the shoulders and an elevated white blood cell count. Performing specialized lab tests, such as abdominal ultrasonography or CT scan early, is often helpful to confirm the diagnosis. Pancreatitis should be considered, especially in acute patients with persistent ileus or recurrence of an adynamic ileus (240). The clinical recognition of acute pancreatitis is hampered by diminished or lost visceral sensitivity and therefore is based on laboratory investigations. Acute pancreatitis in the setting of high-level SCI may result from a combination of locally mediated sphincter of Oddi dysfunction and vagal dominant innervation of the pancreatic gland in autonomic failure (241).

Clinical Evaluation

As with any patient, the evaluation begins with a complete history and physical examination. A request for symptoms guides the evaluation. Symptoms typically are vague; clues to their origin may be derived from a careful search for a relationship to exacerbating or remitting factors. The effect of body position, time of day, eating, bowel care, medications, and urinary function should be elicited (216). The presence of associated symptoms, such as AD, abdominal wall spasticity, fever, and weight change, should be noted. A gastrointestinal review of symptoms further clarifies function. A careful query of premorbid bowel function should be made, because neurologic lesions may alter the way that preexisting problems are manifest. Recognition of the impact of the symptom on the patient's ability to carry out important life activities is essential; neurogenic bowel dysfunction is notorious for detrimental impact on QOL (242). Finally, the components of the bowel program should be systematically evaluated. A history of the type of diet—with special emphasis on fluid and fiber intake and use of laxatives, stool softeners, fiber supplements, and medications with anticholinergic properties—should be obtained. The frequency, duration, and technique of bowel care are elicited, as well as problems with stool consistency, lack of stool in the rectum at the time of stimulation, incontinence, and bleeding.

The physical examination is not only an assessment of the colon and pelvic floor but also includes a survey for associated pathology, sensory/motor impairments, and activity limitations that could affect bowel care (243). Abdominal examination allows for motor assessment of the abdominal wall, percussion for tympany, palpation of the colon for impaction, and elicitation of symptoms (216). Pelvic floor innervation and function should be appraised with neurologic and rectal examination. The anocutaneous reflex is recognized with EAS contraction on anal skin contact. The bulbocavernosus reflex is elicited with penile head squeeze or clitoral pressure and the recognition of an increase in anal sphincter tone. Both these reflexes suggest an intact sensory (S3-4) to motor (S2) reflex arch (214). The rectal examination should assess for sensation, voluntary contraction, puborectalis tone, masses in the rectal vault, and stool consistency. The examination is an opportunity for education and explanation of options for various techniques of bowel care. The Consortium for Spinal Cord Injury Medicine has published recommendations on "Neurogenic Bowel Management in Adults with SCI." These give recommendations for assessment, management monitoring, and education concerning neurogenic bowel. The full text can be downloaded at PVA.org or reviewed in *The Journal of Spinal Cord Medicine* (216).

Bowel Evacuation Mechanics

In neurologically intact people, the sequence of defecation begins with the perception of rectal fullness. This often occurs in response to a giant migratory contraction that pushes stool into the rectum. Rectal distension may be perceived at volumes as low as 10 mL by stretch receptors in the rectal wall,

the puborectalis muscle (244), and the pelvic floor. Continued rectal distension triggers rectal contraction and the rectoanal inhibitory reflex. (245) If the choice is made to defecate, the sitting position is assumed. Sitting makes the angle between the rectum and anal canal less acute (246). In the able bodied, a rise in intra-abdominal and perhaps intrarectal pressure is generated by closing the glottis to retain a full breath in the chest. The abdominal muscles are contracted and the diaphragm is pulled down. Neurologically intact people often are able to increase intrarectal pressure by 100 cm H_2O or more with a Valsalva maneuver. Persons with upper motor neuron SCI often initiate bowel evacuation with digital stimulation. Digital rectal stimulation is done by introducing the entire length of the gloved and lubricated finger into the rectum and dilating the distal rectum by moving in a circular funnel pattern. This key unlocks the sphincter mechanism, stretches the puborectalis, and provides a stimulus for peristalsis (216,243,247). Digital rectal stimulation results in the transient loss of approximately 75% of resting anal tone and presumably further straightens the anorectal angle. Expulsive force is added by performance of a Valsalva maneuver as well as the addition of external abdominal compression. The ability to elevate intra-abdominal pressure with the use of these techniques is closely related to the level and completeness of SCI. Patients with C5-6 level injuries rarely can generate intra-abdominal pressures greater than 10 cm H_2O.

Once evacuation is initiated, the entire left colon may empty by mass peristaltic action, or the fecal bolus may be passed bit by bit. The presence of an anocolic reflex (i.e., stool passing through the anus causes colonic contraction) has been postulated but not proven. Stool consistency is probably the major determinant of the pattern of defecation. Stool consistency is of even greater importance in SCI patients, in whom the balance between expulsive and resistive forces is so tenuous.

Gastrointestinal Problems After Spinal Cord Injury

Gastrointestinal symptoms are very common in the chronic phase after SCI. Colonic and pelvic floor functions are entwined in etiquette and governed by social norms. The need for scheduled bowel care and fears of unanticipated evacuation are life limiting (242). Difficult bowel evacuation was said to be present in patients who required more than 60 min/d for their bowel care or needed manual disimpaction more than once a week. The impact of problems with bowel evacuation on QOL is formidable. In patients with difficult bowel evacuation, bowel care routinely occupies a significant part of the day, greatly restricted diets are adopted to minimize symptoms, and emergency trips to a physician for disimpaction are common. Episodes of dysreflexia, rectal bleeding, and incontinence from overtreatment with laxatives also occur frequently.

There are a few surgical options to improve success in neurogenic bowel management should conventional bowel care be ineffective (248). The decision for surgical adaptation requires interdisciplinary evaluation (216) to explore implications of surgical risk (249), body image, and functional outcome. Transanal irrigation has been demonstrated to reduce constipation and improve continence and QOL (250). An anterograde continence enema (ACE) procedure may be an option for adult patients with neurogenic bowel recalcitrant to a bowel program. Originally designed for children with myelomeningocele, it also significantly decreases toileting time and improves QOL (251,252). The appendicocecostomy stoma is constructed by bringing the appendix through the abdominal wall. This stoma is irrigated with a 100 to 500 mL of saline to trigger defecation. Colostomy is also an elective procedure that can improve independence in bowel care and enhance QOL (249,253,254). It has been performed with good success in the subgroup of these patients with the most severe disability (249). In patients with severe difficulty with evacuation, unresponsive to alterations in the bowel program, colostomy can shorten the time needed for bowel care and enhance self-efficacy and QOL (253,255). Many patients have reported that they retrospectively wished that these alternatives were offered earlier (255,256).

Medical and Rehabilitation Management of the Neurogenic Bowel

The approach of evaluation and intervention to improve gastrointestinal function after SCI should be interdisciplinary and address all domains of disablement (214). A bowel management plan considers the following components: diet, fluid intake, medications, physical activity, and a schedule for bowel care. Bowel care is the procedure for assisted defecation with one or more of the following components: positioning, assistive devices, rectal simulation or trigger for defecation, and assistive maneuvers (abdominal massage) (214,216).

All components of the bowel program should be designed for maximal performance. People with SCI, particularly those with tetraplegia, have very little capability to overcome resistive forces and expel stool with bowel care. Stool consistence should be titrated with diet and medications (see **Fig. 22-4**). Adjustments in the bowel program that may be trivial in the nondisabled population can shift the balance significantly. Stool consistency is a pivotal variable. A diet containing 15 to 30 g of dietary fiber per day should be encouraged (214,216). Wheat bran and psyllium make the stool more pliable by increasing the fecal water content (257). Other helpful interventions include upright bowel care to utilize gravity, abdominal binders, daily osmotic laxatives, increased frequency of bowel care, more frequent digital stimulation, and stronger triggering medications.

Avoidance of colorectal overdistension is desirable because rectal distension is known to decrease intestinal transit by the colocolic reflex. Frequent bowel care (i.e., every 1 to 2 days) will avoid colonic distension with stool and may also enhance colonic transit. Timing bowel care after a large meal to take advantage of the gastrocolic response or giving an oral laxative the day before may improve bowel care results. Fluid intake should be adequate to maintain soft stools and is recommended at 2 to 3 L/d, depending upon bladder management and restrictions. An effective bowel management program is important to both the physical and psychological well-being of the SCI patient. More than one third of persons with paraplegia ranked the loss of bowel and bladder control as the most significant functional loss associated with injury (258). Stool incontinence can be devastating to patients, leading to social isolation, loss of income secondary to work absenteeism, depression, and decreased QOL (214,242,259). The bowel program individualization often requires trial and error. The level of injury, previous bowel habits, lifestyle of the patient, and availability of caregivers should be taken into account when planning a bowel program.

The bowel program will vary depending on the type of neurogenic bowel dysfunction, that is, UMN versus LMN bowel. Patients with UMN injuries may have decreased GI motility, especially in the descending colon, but they will have normal to increased resting rectal tone and GI-related reflexes remain intact. These include the gastrocolic and rectocolic reflexes. To utilize the gastrocolic reflex (contraction of the colon occurring with gastric distension), patients should be instructed to perform their bowel program 20 to 30 minutes after eating. Caffeine may act as a stimulant and may be used prior to a bowel program to help facilitate fecal evacuation. Dietary or supplemental fiber acts as a bulking agent and can enhance colonic transit time. It is suggested that the daily intake of fiber be at 30 g/d.

The basic bowel care procedure for UMN neurogenic bowel has been broken down into steps (📶 **eTable 22-7**). An integral part of the bowel program is digital stimulation, which is performed by inserting a gloved lubricated finger into the rectum and slowly rotating the finger in a circular motion in a clockwise direction until relaxation of the bowel wall is felt or stool or flatus passes (approximately 1 minute). This initiates the rectocolic reflex: contraction of the colon occurring with stimulation of the rectal mucosa. This will trigger evacuation of stool in the lower rectal vault. Once the vault is empty, a suppository is inserted to stimulate contraction of the lower colon and evacuation of stool located higher in the descending colon. Repeat digital stimulation (three to five times) should be performed every 10 to 15 minutes to check for stool, which may remain in the rectal vault until there is closure around the finger by the internal sphincter or there are no results after two stimulations. Ideally, the bowel program should be performed at the same time of day to facilitate "retraining" of the bowel. Patients injured for more than 1 year are more likely to perform the bowel program every other day and in the morning. Persons with tetraplegia report requiring more assistance and more time overall for the program (260). If a person is having difficulty with AD during digital stimulation, pretreatment with topical application of viscous 2% lidocaine may be beneficial.

For patients who remain constipated, laxatives such as lactulose, polyethylene glycol, bisacodyl tablets, milk of magnesium, or cascara may replace or be used in combination with components of the 3-2-1 program. The use of oral agents should be individualized, with the ultimate goal of minimizing medications as the time from injury increases. Only one change to the bowel program regimen should be at a time, and at least three bowel cycles should be completed to realize the effects of the change. While large-volume enemas are occasionally indicated for episodes of constipation, they are not recommended for chronic use. Bisacodyl is an active ingredient in most suppository preparations (261,262). They stimulate the sensory nerve endings, resulting in local- and conal-mediated reflex increases in peristalsis, frequently signaled by flatus. It generally takes 15 to 60 minutes for passage of the first flatus, which is followed shortly thereafter by stool flow (214). Suppositories with a water-soluble base (Magic Bullet) have been shown to dissolve more quickly and significantly shorten the time to complete a bowel program compared with standard vegetable oil-based preparations (263). Docusate sodium minienemas may allow for the most rapid bowel evacuation (262). Recently approved medications lubiprostone, linaclotide, and plecanatide may prove to be very helpful for severe neurogenic bowel-related evacuation difficulty, but these have not been studied in SCI yet.

Patients with LMN bowel typically have SCI lesions affecting the conus or cauda equina. Anal canal tone is reduced, anocutaneous bulbocavernosus reflexes are absent, and the pelvic floor may passively descend. In LMN lesions, continence is often lost due to weakness of the pelvic floor muscles with a flaccid EAS. Because spinal-mediated reflexes are absent, digital stimulation and contact irritant suppositories are largely ineffective, necessitating manual disimpaction. The stool is kept firm by use of bulking agents to aid manual disimpaction. LMN bowel care typically consists of digital rectal stimulation and manual evacuation after the morning and evening meals. A study of bowel care patterns of persons with SCI revealed that the average frequency of bowel care in persons with LMN bowel was twice per day, and the frequency of those with UMN bowels averaged three times per week (264). Assistive techniques such as Valsalva maneuver, abdominal massage in a clockwise direction starting in the right lower quadrant and progressing along the course of the colon, increase in physical activity, and completing the bowel program in a commode chair may facilitate the process.

UROLOGIC SYSTEM ISSUES

Prior to the 1970s, renal disease was the leading cause of mortality in chronic SCI. Since the advent of IC programs and improved urologic care, the prevalence of renal disease has decreased dramatically. Despite this, neurogenic bladder continues to be a risk for development of renal disease if not properly managed. Understanding the anatomy and physiology of urinary tract function and how this is affected by SCI is essential for providers and patients with SCI to help prevent these complications.

Anatomy and Physiology of the Urinary System

Upper Urinary Tract

The kidney is composed of two parts: the renal parenchyma and collecting system. The ureters travel down from the ureteropelvic junction to the bladder and traverse obliquely between the muscular and submucosal layers of the bladder wall before opening into the bladder. This allows urine to flow into the bladder, but prevent reflux into the ureter (265) (eFig. 22-2).

Lower Urinary Tract

The bladder is composed of the bladder body, or detrusor, and bladder base, including the trigone and bladder neck. The detrusor is composed of smooth muscle bundles that freely crisscross and interlace with each other. The trigone is located at the inferior base of the bladder and extends from the ureteral orifices to the bladder neck (265) (eFig. 22-2).

The urethra has been thought to have two distinct sphincters, internal and external. The internal sphincter is the junction of the bladder neck and proximal urethra, composed of connective tissue and smooth muscle, and is under involuntary control (266). The external urethral sphincter is composed of striated muscle and is under voluntary control. Continence is maintained by adequate tone of the urinary sphincters and pelvic floor musculature (267).

Neuroanatomy of the Lower Urinary Tract

Urine storage and emptying is a complex function of interactions among the CNS and peripheral nervous system (PNS). The CNS coordinates and controls micturition via signals traveling between the spinal cord and brain. The PNS mediates bladder storage and contraction via the parasympathetic, sympathetic, and somatic innervation of the lower urinary tract (eFig. 22-3). The classic neurotransmitters in the bladder are acetylcholine and norepinephrine, but there are other transmitters that may work independently or help modulate these.

PS nerves originate in the intermediolateral gray matter from the S2-4 spinal cord segments. Preganglionic nerves travel through the pelvic nerves to ganglia immediately adjacent to or within the detrusor muscle and then through short postganglionics to the smooth muscle cholinergic receptors in the bladder, activated by acetylcholine. These signals cause bladder contraction (268,269).

Sympathetic nerves originate in the intermediolateral gray column from the T11-L2 spinal cord segments. Sympathetic impulses travel a short distance to the lumbar sympathetic paravertebral ganglia and then along the long postganglionic hypogastric nerve to synapse at α-receptors in the bladder base and urethra and β-receptors in the bladder (**Fig. 22-6**). α-Receptor stimulation causes smooth muscle contraction, increasing bladder and sphincter outlet resistance. β-Receptor stimulation causes smooth muscle relaxation, relaxing the bladder (268–270) (see **Fig. 22-6**).

The sensory innervation of the bladder occurs via the pelvic nerve to the sacral spinal cord and transmits mechanoreceptive input essential for voiding. The internal urethral sphincter is under control of the autonomic system and has a large number of sympathetic α-receptors, which cause closure when stimulated. The external urethral sphincter is under somatic innervation, allowing it to be closed at will (266,271).

Normal Voiding Physiology

Micturition has two phases: the filling (storage) phase and emptying (voiding) phase. During filling, there is a progressive increase in sympathetic stimulation of β-receptors in the bladder body causing relaxation and stimulation of α-receptors at the bladder base and urethra causing contraction. When a bladder is full and has normal compliance, intravesical pressures are between 0 and 6 cm H_2O and should not rise above 15 cm H_2O (272). When voiding occurs, there is cessation of urethral sphincter muscle activity, followed by detrusor contraction.

Types of Neurogenic Bladder Dysfunction

Individuals with SCI may have concomitant brain injury, which may also affect bladder function. The type of bladder dysfunction will depend upon the degree of brain and SCI. The expected bladder dysfunction of an isolated suprapontine lesion is detrusor hyperreflexia with preserved coordination of the bladder and urinary sphincter.

Traumatic suprasacral SCI results in an initial period of spinal shock, in which there is hyporeflexia below the level of injury and detrusor areflexia. During this phase, the bladder is acontractile. Recovery of bladder function usually follows recovery of skeletal muscle reflexes. Uninhibited bladder contractions gradually return after 6 to 8 weeks (273).

FIGURE 22-6. Location of bladder receptors. Bladder storage is maintained by simultaneous sympathetic α-adrenergic receptor (contraction) **(A)** and β-adrenergic receptor (relaxation) stimulation **(B)**. Bladder emptying occurs with parasympathetic cholinergic receptor stimulation **(C)**.

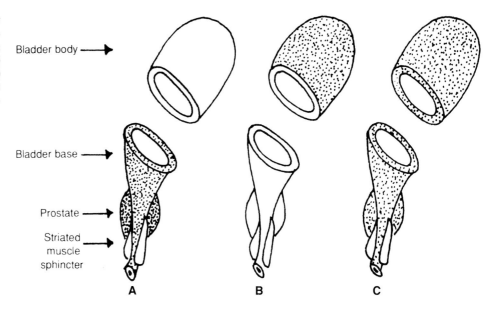

Bladder body →

Bladder base →

Prostate →

Striated muscle sphincter →

A **B** **C**

After spinal shock resolves, patients with complete suprasacral spinal cord lesions often develop detrusor hyperreflexia with detrusor-sphincter dyssynergia (DSD). DSD occurs when the urinary sphincter contracts simultaneously when the detrusor muscle contracts. If not treated, this places the bladder at risk for vesicoureteral reflux and upper urinary tract damage. In cases of partial or incomplete lesions of the suprasacral cord, detrusor hyperreflexia and DSD can occur in varying degrees (274).

Damage to the sacral cord or roots generally results in an acontractile bladder and varied degrees of sphincter dysfunction. Decreased bladder compliance may also occur, so these individuals also require urologic evaluation to ensure there is no risk of damage to their upper urinary tract (275).

Neurourologic Evaluation

History and Physical Examination

The patient's evaluation should capture issues that contribute to their urologic function prior to injury (e.g., diabetes, prostate surgery, etc.) and the ability to manage the physical and cognitive demands of bladder management after SCI. Social support can also play an important role in bladder management options and should be discussed.

Diagnostic Testing

Although there is no agreement regarding the tests and testing frequency, there is agreement that regular upper and lower tract evaluation is necessary for patients with SCI. The American Paraplegia Society and American Urological Association have developed urologic evaluation recommendations (276,277).

Once a patient is medically stabilized after acute injury, baseline urologic assessment should be performed. Blood urea nitrogen, creatinine, cystatin C, and creatinine clearance are easy, inexpensive tests to evaluate renal function. Of note however, individuals with chronic SCI frequently have less muscle mass than able-bodied individuals, so their serum creatinine is less than that of able-bodied individuals. Diagnostic tests to evaluate the upper urinary tract include renal ultrasound, computerized tomography (CT), intravenous pyelogram (IVP), 24-hour urine creatinine clearance, and quantitative

mercaptoacetyltriglycine (MAG) 3 renal scan. Renal ultrasound is helpful for detecting hydronephrosis and kidney stones. If further anatomic definition is needed to evaluate for stones or tumors, CT should be considered. IVP evaluates both anatomy and function, but has a number of disadvantages including allergic reactions, radiation exposure, and patient inconvenience. A quantitative MAG 3 radioisotope renal scan evaluates renal function and has been found to be a safe and effective modality (278,279).

Lower urinary tract tests include cystogram, cystoscopy, and urodynamics (UDS). A cystogram can assess bladder anatomy and voiding function and identify reflux. Cystoscopy can assess for causes of hematuria, recurrent symptomatic UTIs, recurrent asymptomatic bacteriuria with a stone-forming organism (e.g., *Proteus mirabilis*), difficulty with catheter passage such as stricture, and bladder calculi. Those with indwelling catheters should have more frequent cystoscopic examinations to evaluate and remove bladder stones and to assess for possible cancerous lesions, which can be biopsied at the same time (280).

UDS assesses bladder and urinary sphincter function during bladder filling and emptying. UDS for neurogenic bladder should be performed once the individual is out of the spinal shock or during initial urologic evaluation. This type of testing is essential to determine bladder function as individuals' voiding symptoms often do not correlate with the type of voiding dysfunction. Following initial testing, it can be performed as needed. UDS includes a number of tests and should include complex cystometrogram (CMG), pressure flow analysis, external urinary sphincter electromyography (EMG), fluoroscopy at the time of UDS (videourodynamics), and PVR testing. UDS testing is performed with pressure sensors in the bladder and rectum and monitors pressures during bladder filling and voiding (if the person is able) (📶 **eFig. 22-4**). Normal UDS findings are demonstrated in 📶 **eFigure 22-5**, and abnormal findings consistent with different patterns of neurogenic bladder dysfunction are demonstrated in 📶 **eFigure 22-6**.

BP monitoring should be performed during UDS as testing may cause AD. Urine culture should be performed and bacteriuria should be treated with antibiotics prior to performing UDS to prevent bacteremia (277).

Management of the Neurogenic Bladder

The main goals of neurogenic bladder management include (a) preventing upper tract complications (e.g., deterioration of renal function, hydronephrosis, and pyelonephritis), (b) preventing lower tract complications (e.g., cystitis, bladder stones, vesicoureteral reflux), and (c) developing a bladder management program that will allow the individual to reintegrate most easily back into the community. Maintaining a balanced bladder with relatively low voiding pressures (50 to 60 cm H_2O) and low PVR volumes (100 cc or less) after bladder emptying will help achieve these goals.

Bladder Drainage Methods

Intermittent Catheterization

IC is the preferred method for urinary drainage in individuals with urinary retention secondary to SCI and adequate upper limb function to perform it themselves. IC should be performed every 4 to 6 hours with the goal to catheterize frequently enough to keep the bladder from becoming overdistended (<500 mL). Individuals should restrict fluid intake to 2 L/d to keep bladder volumes controlled. IC is not recommended for individuals who are unable to perform IC; have abnormal urethral anatomy, small bladder capacity (<200 mL), poor cognition, and little motivation; are unable to adhere to the catheterization time schedule or fluid restriction; or develop AD with bladder filling despite treatment (280).

Indwelling Catheterization

Indwelling catheterization should be considered for individuals with SCI who have limited upper limb function, high fluid intake, cognitive impairment or substance abuse, elevated detrusor pressures, and lack of success with other less invasive bladder management methods (280). A major advantage of using an indwelling catheter is increased independence and less reliance on a caregiver for bladder management. The catheter tubing should be secured with an anchor on an individual's leg or abdomen to prevent tension at the urethral meatus. The catheter size should be limited to 14 to 16 Fr and be changed every 2 to 4 weeks.

Medical complications are higher with an indwelling urinary catheter compared with IC. These include bladder or renal calculi, hematuria, urethral erosions and strictures, penile-scrotal fistulas, epididymitis, pyelonephritis, bacteremia, bladder fibrosis, and may be a cause of bladder cancer (281). The risk of bladder cancer has been reported to occur after 10 years of indwelling catheter use (280).

If an indwelling catheter is going to be used long term, individuals may switch to a suprapubic catheter (SPC). SPCs pass directly into the bladder, not through the urethra, and use a larger diameter catheter (22 to 26 Fr). Advantages of a SPC include the following: it can be changed without undressing, the tubing is less likely to become kinked, it can be more comfortable, it is less likely to interfere with sexual activity, it is much easier to clean, and it is reversible. Although SPCs have similar bladder risks as they are also indwelling catheters, they have less risk of prostatitis, urethritis, epididymo-orchitism, and urethral irritation, stricture, and erosion because they do not pass through the urethra (280,281).

Condom Catheterization and Other Methods of Voiding

The following voiding methods should only be considered after comprehensive urologic evaluation to ensure an individual does not have high intravesical pressures. Timed, Valsalva, and Credé voiding do not require catheterization, but sometimes do require the use of an external condom catheter, as described below.

Timed voiding can be helpful in individuals with mild-to-moderate incontinence and normal bladder function, but an underactive urethral sphincter mechanism. The patient voids at regular time intervals to avoid leaking. This can be combined with increasing intravesical pressure manually (i.e., Credé maneuver) or intra-abdominal pressure (i.e., Valsalva voiding). These methods may allow bladder emptying in individuals with an underactive or areflexic detrusor and with lower motor lesions or sphincterotomy (280). These maneuvers may cause exacerbation of hemorrhoids, rectal prolapse, hernia, and worsening DSD if present (282). Vesicoureteral reflux and high detrusor pressures are contraindications to these types of voiding.

Reflex (spontaneous) voiding can be considered in men with an intact sacral micturition reflex. This occurs when spontaneous uninhibited contractions cause voiding. Men who reflexly void usually have DSD and treatments for the sphincter are often necessary. These include α-blockers, urethral stents, botulinum toxin injections into the sphincter, and sphincterotomy (280). These options are discussed in more detail below. These men need to have their upper tracts and lower tracts monitored as elevated voiding pressures cause problems including vesicoureteral reflux, kidney or bladder stones or infection, deterioration of bladder or renal function, as well as AD (283–286).

External condom catheters can be used for men who perform the above voiding maneuvers. These should only be used if the bladder is able to contract and empty with minimal PVR (<100 mL). The skin needs to be monitored carefully as individuals that use condom catheters are at risk for skin breakdown due to decreased penile sensation.

Pharmacologic Management

Treatment of Neurogenic Detrusor Overactivity

Antimuscarinic medications are first-line medications for management of neurogenic detrusor overactivity. These medications stabilize and relax the detrusor muscle, which reduce overactivity and improve bladder compliance, which helps prevent bladder and kidney damage. There are a number of oral antimuscarinic medications used in clinical practice. These include oxybutynin, tolterodine, trospium, darifenacin, solifenacin, and fesoterodine (287,288). Oxybutynin, tolterodine, trospium, and darifenacin have been studied extensively and have been shown to be well-tolerated and effective treatments (287,289).

Commonly noted adverse effects of antimuscarinic medications include dry mouth and constipation, which can interfere with patient medication compliance. These occur more frequently with the nonselective antimuscarinics such as oxybutynin (287–289). More recently reported is the potential for cognitive impairment with the nonselective muscarinic agents, and this needs to be considered when selecting a treatment, especially for patients with a history of brain injury or cognitive impairment. Antimuscarinics should not be used in patients with narrow-angle glaucoma unless approved by an ophthalmologist, and caution is advised with use in patients with impaired gastric emptying (288). The use of transdermal oxybutynin has been shown to have less side effects than the oral formulation of oxybutynin.

Mirabegron is a newer medication being used in SCI individuals that mediates relaxation of the detrusor muscle via beta-3 adrenoreceptor stimulation (288). Initial studies in patients with SCI have shown decreased maximum detrusor pressure, improved capacity and compliance of the bladder, and decreased incontinence episodes (290,291). More evaluation is still needed to determine if this medication should be a primary treatment or an add-on therapy (288).

Tricyclic antidepressants sometimes are used alone or in combination with anticholinergic agents. These medications are thought to have peripheral and central anticholinergic effects. They have been found to suppress uninhibited bladder contractions, increase bladder capacity, and increase urethral resistance (292).

Intravesical instillation of medications is sometimes used because of side effects from oral anticholinergic medications. The major advantage of these is minimal to no systemic side effects due to less systemic absorption. Although these medications can be effective, individuals may abandon using them because most medications have a short duration of action and they are labor intensive to administer. Medications that have been used for intravesical installation include lidocaine, oxybutynin, capsaicin, and resiniferatoxin.

Another modality more commonly being used is botulinum-A toxin injected into the bladder wall. Botulinum toxin inhibits acetylcholine release at the neuromuscular junction, which blocks neuromuscular contraction and relaxes spastic or overactive muscles. Doses ranging between 100 and 300 units have been found to suppress an overactive detrusor (293–295). It may take 1 to 4 weeks to reach maximal effect, which can last for 3 to 9 months, so the injections usually need to be repeated. Systematic reviews have shown botulinum toxin injections into the detrusor provide clinically significant improvement in neurogenic detrusor overactivity and are well-tolerated (287,293–295). These should be avoided in individuals with neuromuscular disease, allergy to botulinum toxin, or taking an aminoglycoside (280). If a patient is also having botulinum toxin injections for upper or lower limb spasticity, injections in these regions and the bladder need to be coordinated to avoid inadvertent botulinum toxin overdose.

Treatment for Sphincter Outlet Obstruction and Overactive Sphincter

Alpha-adrenergic blocking agents have been shown to be effective at improving bladder emptying in individuals with prostate outlet obstruction and detrusor sphincter dyssynergia (296,297). OH is a potential side effect of these agents, especially in individuals with cervical level SCI. Careful consideration should be given prior to starting these medications, especially if the individual is also taking phosphodiesterase inhibitors for erectile dysfunction.

Botulinum toxin injections into the sphincter mechanism are used as a treatment for DSD. These injections have been shown to be an effective treatment for an overactive sphincter with few adverse effects (287). Botulinum toxin injections are especially useful in individuals who have symptomatic hypotension, adverse effects to α-blockers, or difficulty with medication compliance.

Treatment for an Incompetent Urinary Sphincter

Individuals with lower motor neuron SCI may have a weak or incompetent sphincter. Before treatment options to increase sphincter pressure are used, it is essential that detrusor overactivity or poor bladder compliance be ruled out. Otherwise, increasing the urethral sphincter tone to prevent urinary incontinence may increase intravesical pressure, which may result in back pressure, poor drainage from the upper tracts, and upper tract damage.

Periurethral collagen injection therapy is FDA approved for those with intrinsic urethral sphincter deficiency. Clinical trials have focused primarily on non-SCI individuals, but it can be helpful in SCI individuals who have decreased sphincter tone.

Treatment of Neurogenic Detrusor Underactivity or Areflexia

Bethanechol chloride, which provides relatively selective stimulation of the bladder and bowel and is resistant to rapid hydrolysis by acetylcholinesterase, can be used to augment bladder contractions in non-SCI individuals. Although it has been used in SCI individuals, studies have not shown it to be effective to induce bladder contractions in detrusor areflexia, but it has been shown to increase sphincter pressures. Therefore, this should only be considered in individuals with bladder hypocontractility and coordinated sphincter function (298). It should not be used in individuals with DSD or bladder outlet obstruction (299–301).

Surgical Neurogenic Bladder Management

Surgical management of the neurogenic bladder should only be considered if other conservative methods are ineffective or have intolerable side effects. Complete urologic evaluation, including evaluation of the upper and lower urinary tract anatomy and function, should be performed to determine what type of surgical management could be considered safe and effective.

Continent and Noncontinent Urinary Diversion

Urinary diversion is an option for surgical management of the neurogenic bladder. Although there are many types of diversions, those used in neurogenic bladder can be grouped into two types: continent and noncontinent diversion.

Continent diversions are generally the first choice for diversions and may be used in those who need to have their urinary stream diverted and have adequate hand function to perform IC. Continent diversions are divided into two types: (a) orthotopic diversions, in which the bowel reservoir is anastomosed to the urethra, and (b) a continent catheterizable pouch.

Orthotopic diversions are used to increase bladder capacity and people will catheterize through their urethra. For continent catheterizable pouches, the stoma can be placed in a location that makes catheterization easier, such as within the umbilicus so that a person does not have to undress to catheterize. The most commonly used bowel segment for these diversions is the ileocecal valve. The right colon is used for the pouch, and the terminal ileum or appendix is used to create the catheterizable limb (302,303). Potential complications of diversions using the colon are stricture, mucus production, urinary leakage, and malabsorption of bile salts (304).

The most common reason for noncontinent urinary diversions in those with SCI is to divert the urinary stream away from the perineum because of impaired healing of a decubitus PI due to urinary incontinence, urethral stricture, or fistula. It is also considered for individuals who are unable to perform IC. There should be caution with considering urinary diversions with in SCI individuals who are too debilitated to undergo a major surgical procedure or have one of the following conditions: inflammatory bowel disease, pelvic irradiation, severe abdominal adhesions from previous surgery, or compromised renal function (280).

The most common noncontinent diversion is an ileal conduit. Ten to fifteen centimeters of the ileum, along with its mesentery, is isolated from the ileum. The isolated segment of ileum is closed off at one end, and the other end is brought out through the abdominal wall and everted as a nipple stoma. The ureters are implanted into the ileum for drainage.

Bladder Augmentation

Bladder augmentation is a surgical technique frequently used to create a large bladder capacity with low intravesical pressures and for those who would like to perform IC. Bladder augmentation should be avoided in individuals with inflammatory bowel disease, pelvic irradiation, severe abdominal adhesions from previous surgery, and compromised renal function (280).

Prior to considering bladder augmentation, an extensive preoperative evaluation is important, including history of gastrointestinal problems, screening laboratory work including liver and renal function (serum creatinine has to be <2.0 mg/dL), and comprehensive urologic evaluation, as there can be metabolic complications secondary to the procedure (302–309). Performing bladder autoaugmentation is another option that does not produce metabolic abnormalities, but is a technically difficulty procedure (309).

Long-term follow-up of bladder augmentations and urinary diversions includes regular monitoring of the upper tracts and careful monitoring of blood chemistries and renal function. Cystoscopy is used to monitor for stones or tumors (302,303).

Transurethral Sphincterotomy and Endourethral Stents

Although not as commonly used anymore, transurethral sphincterotomy (TURS) and endourethral stents are options to decrease sphincter outlet resistance.

TURS is a well-established treatment for men with SCI and DSD that requires use of a condom catheter. This can be considered if a male wants to reflex void, has vesicoureteral reflux or upper or lower tract complications, or cannot tolerate medications to decrease detrusor pressures (280). TURS should be avoided in males who cannot wear a condom catheter. Although TURS can improve dysreflexic symptoms and decrease residual urine and infections (310), this procedure has numerous potential negative consequences and is an irreversible procedure. These include significant intraoperative and perioperative bleeding, clot retention, prolonged drainage with a large diameter catheter, urethral stricture, erectile and ejaculatory dysfunction, and the need for reoperation in 30% to 60% of cases.

Another option to decrease sphincter outlet resistance is placement of a urethral stent, which holds the sphincter open. The procedure is potentially reversible with removal of the stent. This treatment is effective in decreasing voiding pressures and PVR urine volumes without loss of erectile function. Complications include hematuria, penile edema, urethral trauma or pain, stone encrustation, tissue growth into the stent, stent migration, persistent AD, subsequent operation, and urethral stricture (280,311,312).

Artificial Urinary Sphincters and Urethral Slings

The goal of these procedures is to increase bladder outlet resistance in individuals with an incompetent urinary sphincter. These should only be performed after urologic evaluation to ensure there is no evidence of high intravesical pressures or vesicoureteral reflux.

An artificial urinary sphincter consists of (a) a urethral cuff surrounding the proximal urethra that is able to be inflated and deflated, (b) a balloon that acts as a reservoir for the fluid in the cuff when deflated, and (c) a pump that deflates or inflates via shunting fluid from the cuff to the balloon. A urethral sling uses synthetic, autologous, or donated tissue to form a sling around the urethra. Both of these procedures have high success rates, but are not without complications and the potential need for reoperation (313).

Neurostimulation

Investigators continue to try to improve voiding through the use of neurostimulation, which is an option for neurogenic bladder management if the sacral reflex arc is intact. There are multiple targets for electrical stimulation to enhance neurogenic bladder function, and this has been used both to facilitate storage by decreasing uninhibited bladder contractions and improve voiding by helping to trigger uninhibited contractions. Techniques include placing electrodes on the bladder itself, pelvic nerves, conus medullaris, sacral nerves, sacral anterior roots, or posterior tibial nerve. Of these, sacral anterior root stimulation has been the most successful (314). Chapter 54 covers this topic in detail.

Pediatric Bladder Management Considerations

The same pharmacologic principles discussed above also apply for children, but the age of the child needs to be considered.

Clean IC has been shown to be an effective treatment for children with failure to empty. Often, an anticholinergic medication is also required (oxybutynin, 1.0 mg/y of age twice daily). Both parents and children adjust to IC if started when the child is a newborn. Children usually can begin performing their own IC at 5 years old.

In those who are unable to have a successful IC program due to problems such as significant urinary incontinence due to poor sphincter tone, small bladder capacity, or difficulty catheterizing the urethra, an alternative is to create a continent urinary diversion with either the Mitrofanoff principle (appendicovesicostomy) or Monti tube (ileovesicostomy). Concomitant bladder augmentation and urethral sling placement are frequently needed. While complications can occur, there are successful long-term outcomes and durability of continent urinary diversions in children with neurogenic bladders. Potential complications include bladder calculi, stomal stenosis, stomal bleeding, small bowel obstruction, and superficial wound dehiscence (315).

Complications of the Neurogenic Bladder

Urinary Tract Infections

There is a lack of consensus in the literature and among health care professionals regarding the definition of a true urinary tract infection (UTI) versus bacterial colonization in a person with a neurogenic bladder secondary to SCI. It is important that a person being treated has a true UTI. Those being treated who do not have a true UTI will likely have unnecessary urine cultures, have risk side effects of antibiotics, and potentially develop resistant organisms, which will be difficult to treat if they develop a true UTI. No matter what type of neurogenic bladder management, bacteriuria is common and usually represents colonization, not a bladder infection. The literature sometimes calls this an asymptomatic UTI. To help clarify this misunderstanding, the NIDRR has defined three criteria necessary to diagnose a UTI in an individual with an SCI with neurogenic bladder: (a) presence of bacteria in the urine (bacteriuria), (b) increase in white blood cells in the urine (pyuria), and (c) onset of new symptoms (316). Because many SCI patients have decreased or no bladder sensation, they may present with less specific signs and symptoms, such as weakness or malaise, increased spasticity, new onset of urinary incontinence, urinary retention, or AD. UTIs also should be considered in the differential diagnosis of new cognitive changes in a patient with a concomitant brain injury. It is very unlikely that a significant fever is due to a bladder infection. If a person complains of a high fever, pyelonephritis, or nonurinary cause, such as an infected pressure ulcer should be considered.

Antibiotic Treatment

Currently, there is a general consensus not to treat asymptomatic bacteriuria or use prophylactic antibiotics to prevent UTI (317). Multiple studies have shown a decrease in bacteriuria with the use of prophylactic antibiotics, but no significant difference in the rate of clinical infection (318–320). There are some circumstances where prophylactic antibiotics are acceptable for use, including urine sterilization for procedures such as cystoscopy or UDS to prevent bacteremia and if the bladder contains urease-producing pathogens (e.g., *Proteus*, *Pseudomonas*, *Klebsiella*, *Providencia*). It is unknown whether prophylactic antibiotics should be used in patients with recurrent clinical infections, anatomic abnormalities such as vesicoureteral reflux, or hydronephrosis, but they are sometimes used in these situations. In addition to the cost and potential side effects of antibiotics, a major concern of prophylactic antibiotics is the development of resistant organisms.

Once a urine culture has been obtained and UTI has been diagnosed, empiric oral antibiotic treatment can be started for patients with symptoms while waiting for the culture results. Patients usually do well with a 7-day course of antibiotics. Patients with significant fever are likely to have upper tract involvement (i.e., pyelonephritis) and, therefore, should be continued on antibiotics longer than patients with bladder infections. In addition, these patients should undergo a urologic evaluation for cause of urosepsis. It is important to have an indwelling urinary catheter in place during IV or oral fluid hydration to keep the bladder decompressed.

Potential complications from bladder infections include epididymitis, prostatic or scrotal abscess, sepsis, or an ascending infection to the upper tracts. Potential complications from

pyelonephritis include chronic pyelonephritis, renal scarring, progressive renal deterioration, renal calculi if there is a urea-splitting organism such as *Proteus*, papillary necrosis, renal or retroperitoneal abscess, or bacteremia and sepsis.

The best method for prevention of UTI is maintaining a balanced bladder by ensuring low-pressure storage and regular complete emptying of the bladder at low pressures. Various approaches have been trialed to prevent UTIs, including cranberry supplements, methenamine hippurate, L-methionine, and bladder irrigation, but none have been shown to be effective and there is little scientific evidence to support their use (287).

Vesicoureteral Reflux

Vesicoureteral reflux is associated with renal deterioration after SCI and there is an association between the degree of reflux and renal damage (321,322). In individuals with neurogenic voiding dysfunctions, high intravesical pressures are thought to be a major cause of reflux. Other causes include recurrent cystitis, pyelonephritis, and anatomic changes in the oblique course of the intravesical ureter caused by bladder thickening and trabeculation. The mainstay of treatment in those with reflux and voiding dysfunction is to lower intravesical pressures and eradicate infections.

Bladder and Renal Calculi

Bladder calculi are the second most common cause of morbidity, following UTIs, in those with SCI (323). The risk of stone formation is higher in those who use an indwelling urinary catheter versus IC (324–326). In a large retrospective study of 500 patients, the absolute annual risk of stone formation in patients with an indwelling catheter was 4% compared with 0.2% for those on intermittent self-catheterization. After having formed a stone, the risk of forming a subsequent stone quadrupled to 16% per year (326). The standard treatment of bladder calculi involves cystoscopy and the breaking up and removal of the stones under direct visualization.

Approximately 8% of patients with SCI develop renal calculi (327), which place individuals at high risk for renal deterioration (328). Stones are typically associated with UTIs, especially when bacteria are urease-producing since urease alkalinizes the urine and promotes crystallization of struvite and calcium phosphate stones. The most common stones previously reported are infection-related stones with struvite (magnesium ammonium phosphate), followed by calcium oxalate and phosphate stones, although this trend may be changing (329). Staghorn calculi are more common with struvite stones and, without treatment, carry a 50% chance of losing the involved kidney (330). Other risk factors for renal calculi include higher injury level and neurologically complete quadriplegia, prior history of bladder or renal calculi, vesicoureteral reflux, indwelling catheterization, and high serum calcium values (327,331,332).

Clinical presentation of renal calculi includes flank pain, nausea, emesis, hematuria, hyperhidrosis, AD, or recurrent UTIs. Evaluation includes stone analysis, serum studies (BUN, creatinine, calcium, and phosphorus), urinalysis (including urine pH), and 24-hour urine collection for total volume and measuring calcium, oxalate, citrate, magnesium, uric acid, sodium, potassium, and phosphorus. Imaging options includes a KUB x-ray, which can visualize calcium stones (struvite stones are not as dense), ultrasound, CT, and intravenous pyelogram (IVP).

Treatment for renal calculi includes medical stabilization with fluids, treatment of infection, and pain management. Surgical treatment for stones includes extracorporeal shock wave lithotripsy, percutaneous nephrolithotomy, ureteroscopy, and open nephrolithotomy. Once stones are present, there is a recurrence rate of 15% to 72% over a 5-year period.

Prevention of stones is best accomplished by catheter changes every 2 to 4 weeks and treatment of stone-forming organisms such as *Proteus*.

Hydronephrosis and Renal Deterioration

Ureteral dilation occurs as a result of ureteral peristalsis being unable to overcome increased pressures along its path (333). Ureteral dilation can occur for several reasons including brisk diuresis, mechanical obstruction from a stone or stricture, poor bladder wall compliance, DSD, bladder outlet obstruction, or certain types of UTIs. One should be concerned about ureteral dilation as this can lead to hydronephrosis and renal failure.

Renal failure was previously the leading cause of death following SCI. Careful monitoring of the upper and lower urinary tracts combined with effective bladder management programs has markedly reduced the incidence of renal failure. Risk factors for renal deterioration include the risks described above for ureteral dilation as well as recurrent decubitus ulcers and tetraplegia (322,328,333).

Bladder Cancer

Individuals who have indwelling catheters or bladder augmentations have been reported to have higher risk for bladder cancer than their able-bodied counterparts (334,335). Among those with indwelling catheters, this increased risk may only be for squamous cell cancer, which is an extremely rare form of bladder cancer (336). Possible causes of cancer development may include chronic irritation from UTIs, urine stasis, bladder calculi, or exposure of the bowel mucosal to urine following bladder augmentation or urinary diversion (334,335). Yearly cystoscopy should be performed in individuals with indwelling catheters for more than 10 years. Persistent hematuria or constitutional symptoms consistent with underlying malignancy should be screened immediately (335).

A recent meta-analysis was performed looking at bladder cancer in individuals with SCI. They found a 6% incidence of bladder cancer, with 36.8% of these individuals with squamous cell carcinoma and 46.3% with transitional cell carcinoma. The interval between SCI and diagnosis of bladder cancer was 24 years, and the length of indwelling urinary catheter use in the patient population ranged from 6 to 29 years. In terms of diagnosis, cystoscopy had a sensitivity of 64% and cytology had a sensitivity of 36.3% for detecting bladder cancer (337).

MUSCULOSKELETAL SYSTEM DISORDERS

Immobilization Hypercalcemia

After acute immobilization, calciuria increases within 2 weeks, reaching a maximum between 1 and 6 months after injury. The immobilization from the acute SCI stimulates osteoclastic bone resorption causing calcium loss from the bones and hypercalciuria, with hypercalcemia resulting when calcium resorption exceeds the capacity of urinary excretion. The incidence of hypercalcemia (level >10.5) in SCI is approximately 10% to 23%. Signs and symptoms usually present between 1

and 2 months postinjury, but may occur as early as 2 weeks and up to 6 months after injury (338). Symptoms may be vague and include acute onset of nausea, vomiting, fatigue, abdominal discomfort, constipation, anorexia, diffuse musculoskeletal pain, polydipsia, polyuria (which could result in dehydration), and behavioral changes including lethargy, confusion, or even psychosis. Ingesting a high-calcium diet does not increase either urinary or serum calcium concentration. For diagnosis, a serum calcium level should be evaluated, with correction for a low serum albumin if present. Ionized calcium can also be measured.

Treatment includes early mobilization and hydration. IV fluid (normal saline at 100 to 150 cc/h), as tolerated, to increase the calcium excretion. A Foley catheter is recommended due to the volume of fluid being administered. Many of the symptoms will quickly resolve as the serum calcium level drops.

Once the patient is hydrated, furosemide may be given to enhance calcium excretion, but often continued aggressive hydration alone is used. Calcium-sparing diuretics such as hydrochlorothiazide are contraindicated because of their hypercalcemic effects.

Bisphosphonates such as pamidronate (30 to 90 mg IV administered over 4 to 24 hours) are effective, with the advantage of only requiring one dose, and have a rapid onset (339,340). This treatment rapidly lowers serum calcium within 3 days with the symptoms improving quickly as the serum calcium level drops, and at that point, IV fluids can be discontinued. The serum calcium falls to a nadir within 7 days and may remain normal for several weeks or longer. Some may require repeat treatment, so continued monitoring of calcium levels following treatment is recommended. Standing has been reported to decrease hypercalciuria (133,341). Other medications that have been used include calcitonin, etidronate, and glucocorticoids (133,342). Treatment for asymptomatic hypercalcemia is recommended as prolonged hypercalcemia may cause nephrocalcinosis.

Osteoporosis

Following injury, there is a marked increase in osteoclastic activity leading to net bone resorption. Bone loss is most active in the first 14 months postinjury, with a slower loss over the next few years, placing patients at an increased risk early after injury of developing pathologic fractures (134,343,344). Bone loss occurs in the LEs at a rate of 2% to 4% per month (345,346), with a more rapid loss in the distal femur and proximal tibia as compared with the proximal and midshaft femur. There is a greater loss of trabecular bone as opposed to cortical bone and as such greater loss at the metaphysis compared to the diaphysis and long bones. By 2 to 3 years post injury, 25% to 50% of BMD may be lost in the LEs with continued loss up to 3% per year. There is no difference in bone loss in the LEs between persons with paraplegia or tetraplegia (343). The greatest risk factors for osteoporosis, especially at the knee, include a neurologically complete injury, lower body mass index (BMI), and greater age (347).

Treatments for bone loss after SCI have included weight-bearing, FES, and pharmacologic intervention (348,349). Therapeutic interventions including the use of standing tables, ambulation, and FES have produced mixed results (349–353). While there may be a dose-response effect in utilizing FES, the precise requirements needed to obtain clinically useful outcomes are yet to be determined. In chronic SCI, FES intervention greater than 3 d/wk of more than a 3-month duration has shown to significantly increase in knee-region BMD, but effects are only maintained if FES is continued (349). The use of FES in a person with chronic SCI and low BMD may lead to fracture, and caution should be taken (354).

Treatment of bone loss after SCI includes addressing secondary causes of osteoporosis, lifestyle modifications, supplementation, rehabilitation interventions, and consideration of pharmacologic intervention. This includes counseling patients on the effects of smoking, excessive caffeine, and alcohol on bone health (355). In patients with chronic SCI, after the rapid phase of bone resorption is complete, supplementation with calcium 1,000 mg/d is recommended for patients with reduced BMD and no-premorbid or post-SCI history of renal or bladder calculi (355). As vitamin D deficiency is very common after SCI and can negatively impact bone health, levels should be assessed and corrected with supplementation (356). The effects of lifestyle modifications and supplementation on reducing bone loss and fracture risk have not been fully studied in this population.

Studies to determine the efficacy of bisphosphonates in treating bone loss in acute and chronic SCI have conflicting results leading to differences in clinical approach (355,357–360). Similarly, several recent systematic reviews on the use of bisphosphonates for the treatment of bone loss after SCI have come to different conclusions (361–364). The effect of bisphosphonates in preventing fractures after SCI has not been studied. Promising new treatments on the horizon are discussed further in Chapter 31.

Fracture

Fractures below the level of injury are a well-known complication of bone loss after SCI. The prevalence of fractures in the chronic SCI population is approximately 25% to 46% (365,366) although this is likely an underestimate as patient may not recognize the presence of fracture and may not seek medical attention. Fractures increase over time with the mean time to first fracture approximately 9 years (367).

Fractures are more common in women and persons with neurologic complete injuries and in paraplegia relative to tetraplegia (162,365,366,368). Most fractures are due to falls during transfers, but fractures can result from minor stresses (e.g., long-sitting or ROM) or without any known etiology and referred to as fragility fractures (caused by injury that would be insufficient to fracture normal bone) (369). Supracondylar femur fractures are the most common fractures, followed by the distal tibia, proximal tibia, femoral shaft, femoral neck, and humerus, respectively. Symptoms of acute fracture include fever, acute pain, swelling, or increased spasticity. A plain x-ray will usually give a definitive diagnosis.

For individuals who are ambulatory, management is similar to the non-SCI population. For fractures in chronic patients with SCI who do not use their lower limbs for functional mobility, the main goals of treatment are to minimize complications, allow for healing with satisfactory alignment, and preserve prefracture function. Most fractures are treated nonoperatively with soft padded splints (366). A well-padded knee immobilizer is useful for femoral supracondylar, femoral shaft, and proximal tibial fractures; a well-padded ankle immobilizer

can be used for distal tibial fractures. In nonambulatory patients, some degree of shortening and angulation is acceptable. The patient should be allowed to sit within a few days. Callus formation is usually evident in 3 to 4 weeks; however, ROM is initiated at 6 to 8 weeks, with weight bearing delayed for a longer period. While nonunion of fractures occurs (2% to 10%), this is not clinically significant in those who do not weight-bear through their lower limbs.

Surgery, circumferential casting, and external fixation are usually not indicated in the SCI population because of potential complications due to low bone mass, risk of osteomyelitis, recurrent bacteremia, and skin breakdown. Surgery may be indicated when conservative methods will not control rotational deformity, for proximal femur fractures, in patients with severe muscle spasm, if vascular supply is in danger, and in whom shortening and angulation will result in unacceptable function or cosmesis. Femoral neck and subtrochanteric fractures are the most difficult to manage, and internal fixation may be considered if a minimal device such as an intramedullary rod can be used.

Heterotopic Ossification

HO is the formation of lamellar bone within the soft tissue surrounding a joint. The incidence ranges between 13% and 57% and is usually found in the first 6 months (peak at 2 months) after injury. HO may occur beyond 1 year and is usually associated with a newly developed PI, DVT, or fracture. Risk factors for HO include older age (children and adolescents have a lower incidence), neurologic complete lesions, male gender, spasticity, DVT, and pressure sores (370). These risk factors may be cumulative.

Most of the cases of HO will have only radiologic findings and are not clinically significant. Up to 20% will present with a limitation of the ROM, with up to 8% progressing to joint ankylosis. Only joints below the NLI will develop heterotopic bone, with the most common location being the hips (anteromedial aspect), followed by the knees and then shoulders. The joint may appear warm and swollen and must therefore be differentiated from a septic joint, cellulitis, DVT, fractures, and inflammatory arthritis. The patient may experience pain, malaise, low-grade fever, and an increase in spasticity. In severe cases, adjacent neurovascular structures may be compromised leading to distal extremity swelling and nerve entrapment (371).

The pathogenesis underlying the development HO after SCI is not completely understood, but it is most commonly believed that a combination of proprioceptive dysfunction related to CNS disruption, local inflammatory changes 2 degrees to trauma, spasticity, immobilization hypercalcemia, and humoral factors may lead to the migration of mesenchymal osteoprogenitor cells into the joint space (372,373). Damage to the sympathetic tracts may also promote HO by increasing the local vascularity and blood perfusion around the joint. At least two processes have an important role in the development of HO after SCI: the activation of pluripotential mesenchymal cells in the soft tissue and the local production of bone morphogenetic protein (BMP). Mesenchymal cells in muscle may switch their differentiation from fibroprogenitor to osteoprogenitor pathway under the influence of BMP and then proliferate into bone-forming cells. The specific factors involved in the activation of mesenchymal cells in muscle and local induction of BMP expression are still unknown. The histology of HO is similar to normotopic mature bone with well-developed cortical and trabecular structures. The bone has a high metabolic rate, adding new bone at more than three times the rate of normal bone (374).

The extent of tissue involvement by HO varies. In some patients, only a small amount of bone develops around the joint not causing joint dysfunction, while in others massive ossification can be found resulting in severe functional limitations or ankylosis of the joint.

Long-term complications of HO include loss of ability to sit secondary to reduced ROM, chronic pain, development of pressure ulcers, DVT, and an increase in spasticity, and, in severe cases, adjacent neurovascular structures may be compromised leading to distal extremity swelling and nerve entrapment. HO may also present several years after the initial SCI associated with a newly acquired PI, DVT, or fracture.

Laboratory tests are sensitive but are not specific markers for HO. Serum alkaline phosphatase levels start to increase prior to clinical and radiographic presentation, but may not exceed normal levels for several weeks. Because levels do not correlate with the amount or degree of bone activity, they should not be used to judge the maturity of the new bone or predict its recurrence. An elevation of serum creatinine phosphokinase (CPK) may be a more reliable predictor of HO (375,376). While nonspecific markers of inflammation such as C-reactive protein (CRP) and the erythrocyte sedimentation rate (ESR) can be useful in following disease activity (377), any cause of systemic inflammation (e.g., infection, PIs) may result in these elevations. CRP is a more reliable predictor of disease activity, with normalization of the CRP correlating with resolution of the inflammatory phase of HO. Urinary excretion of hydroxyproline and collagen metabolites correlates with alkaline phosphatase levels and can also serve as indirect markers for the presence of HO.

A triple-phase bone scan is the most sensitive imaging study in diagnosing early HO and can detect disease activity before calcification becomes apparent on plain x-ray. The first two phases of the bone scan measure the increase in blood flow to a joint during the early inflammatory period. The third phase, or static bone phase, is more specific since it measures the incorporation of the radionuclide into the bony matrix but may take another 3 weeks before it is positive (378). Bone scans are also the most useful technique to assess maturity of the heterotopic bone. Plain x-rays become positive approximately 2 to 6 weeks after a triple-phase bone scan first reveals HO or 1 to 10 weeks after clinical presentation (379). Ultrasonography may be positive early and has the advantage of being a relatively inexpensive examination without requiring radiation (380). MRI, with an increased T2 signal (edema) in muscles, fascia, and subcutaneous tissue, can be helpful in diagnosing HO acutely (381). CT scan may be used to determine the volume of bone needed for planning surgical resection. Multiple grading systems for classifying HO have been proposed (382).

The Brooker classification describes the progression of the ossification on an anteroposterior radiograph and is only applied for HO around the hip (383). Finerman and Stover describe five different grades for HO around the hip based on radiographic evaluation (384). Garland and coworkers proposed a radiographic classification composed of five groups for preoperative grading based on the extent of bone formation

in soft tissue. These included 1, minimal; 2, mild; 3, moderate; 4, severe; and 5, ankyloses (385). This classification can be used for any location of HO. Mavrogenis et al. recommended a description based on the location of HO to better estimate prognosis (386).

On the basis of radiographic findings and clinical course, Garland proposed two classes of HO (385). Class I patients have radiographic progression of HO and elevated serum ALP for 5 to 6 months with HO thereafter becoming inert. Class II is characterized by a radiographic progression of HO with a persistent activity on the bone scan for an extended period of time. Patients in class II are more likely to ultimately require surgery.

Treatment options include ROM with gentle stretching, bisphosphonates, NSAIDs if not contraindicated, as well as possible radiation therapy and surgical excision later in the course. Once HO is diagnosed, it is not recommended to perform an aggressive ROM program that can induce additional tissue microtrauma, possibly leading to an increased formation of HO (387). Careful and gentle mobilization of the affected joints is however recommended to prevent further loss of ROM and does not appear to accelerate HO formation (388). After the acute inflammatory period, ROM with gentle and sustained pressure to slowly increase or maintain range may be performed. Low-load prolonged stretching at end range may increase ROM without causing tissue damage with the goal to maintain ROM within a functional range. More frequent but shorter duration of range may be helpful. The application of ice may help reduce inflammation. If pain is encountered, tissue trauma may be occurring. The acute phase of HO is a relative contraindication for the use of FES (389).

Prophylaxis of HO in SCI patients has been studied using several agents including etidronate and indomethacin (75 mg daily for 3 weeks within 5 weeks of injury), with less HO formation as compared with placebo (390,391). Warfarin may also be an effective agent by inhibiting the formation of osteocalcin (392). Despite the available therapeutic options, prophylaxis is not routinely used because of the relatively low incidence of morbidity and potential interference with bone healing post spinal fusion surgery.

Treatment with bisphosphonates has been shown to decrease the rate of new bone formation in patients with HO; however, it has no effect on bone, which has already been deposited. This drug blocks the late phase of bone formation, the stage of mineralization, preventing the conversion of amorphous calcium phosphate to hydroxyapatite. There is no definitive protocol; however, a current recommendation is for oral administration of etidronate 20 mg/kg/d for 6 months if the CPK level is elevated at the time of diagnosis or 20 mg/kg/d for 3 months, followed by 10 mg/kg/d for an additional 3 months if the initial CPK level is normal (393). With this regimen, there is faster resolution of edema with less rebound formation after the medication is discontinued. If the initial CPK is elevated, or CRP greater than 8, some recommend addition of a NSAID until the CRP less than 2 or CPK normalizes (377).

The most common side effect of etidronate is gastrointestinal, including nausea and vomiting in 10% to 20% of patients. Administering the medication in divided doses 1 to 2 hours before meals is recommended. Clinical trials with newer-generation bisphosphonates are ongoing. Although IV administration of etidronate reportedly led to quicker resolution of edema with less rebound formation after the medication was discontinued (394), this formulation is no longer available. NSAIDs have been studied in the treatment of HO (391,395), although often limited in use because of the GI complications especially in the initial periods post-SCI.

Pulse low-intensity electromagnetic field therapy (PLIMF) utilizes magnetic fields to increase oxygen levels and decrease toxic by-products of inflammation by increasing local blood flow and has been shown to be effective in preventing HO post-SCI, (396) although not frequently used at this time. Radiation therapy in a variety of doses has been described for patients with early HO formation (397). The long-term risks however have not been studied. Given the possibility of long-term complications, radiation treatment is usually not utilized as a primary treatment.

Surgical excision is reserved for patients with severely limited ROM that causes significant functional limitations in mobility or ADL or directly resulting medical complications, such as PIs. Surgical indications for removal of HO around the elbow and shoulder are for improvements in feeding, hygiene, and dressing and for clinical evidence of progressive ulnar nerve compression (398,399). Most clinicians recommend waiting until after the ectopic bone is mature by bone scan, which may take up to 12 to 18 months to occur, although early surgery has been described (399). MRI or CT scan best determines preoperative localization of HO.

Various surgical approaches have been utilized for the resection of HO. Wedge resection is the most common procedure; however, it is frequently associated with a significant blood loss. Other complications include wound infection, neurologic or vascular injury, and recurrence of the HO. After resection, it is beneficial to start gentle ROM at 72 hours postoperatively and wait 1 to 2 weeks until soft tissue swelling subsides until active physical therapy is commenced. Post-op treatment includes NSAIDs for 6 weeks and/or etidronate (20 mg/kg/d) for 3 to 12 months and/or radiation (379,400–403). While radiation decreases the degree of recurrence of HO, complications include delayed wound healing, osteonecrosis, and the risk of developing sarcoma. In a small study ($n = 5$), individuals who received pamidronate pre- and postsurgery for HO had no recurrence, offering some evidence that pamidronate can halt progression of HO after surgical resection (402). While recurrence of HO after resection is common (379,401,402), the measure of success of the surgery is by the functional improvement, that is, wheelchair sitting, grooming, hygiene, feeding, and mobility capabilities.

UE Neuromusculoskeletal Pain

The upper limbs in persons with SCI are used for weight-bearing activities including weight shifts, transfers, and wheelchair propulsion as well as for ADL, thereby increasing the chances of overuse syndromes. Chapter 29 provides a comprehensive review of upper limb musculoskeletal disorders. Shoulder pain is the most commonly reported painful joint after SCI (404). Approximately 30% to 50% of patients complain of shoulder pain severe enough to interfere with function, with the prevalence increasing with time from injury (405,406). Pain during the first year after injury is more common in tetraplegics, but in later years, it is more common in paraplegics. Since the person with SCI relies extensively on

their upper limbs, any further loss of upper limb function because of pain may have adverse effects on functional independence (407,408).

Two thirds of shoulder pain is due to chronic impingement syndrome and approximately half involves rotator cuff pathology. Other causes that are specific to SCI include muscle imbalance, spasticity, contractures, HO, and the presence of a syrinx. Acute atraumatic pain should trigger consideration of referred pain from peptic ulcer disease, angina, and an acute abdominal problem. In addition to the typical evaluation for upper limb pain outlined in Chapter 29, the evaluation of a person with SCI should include an evaluation of the patient's posture, function (i.e., pressure reliefs, wheelchair mobility, ADL, transfers), and home/work environment. The Wheelchair User's Shoulder Pain Index (WUSPI) is a 15-item self-report instrument, with a range of 0 to 15 that measures shoulder pain intensity during various ADL utilizing a visual analog scale (VAS) (408,409). This is often used to monitor the effectiveness of treatment.

Shoulder pain treatment generally adheres to routine musculoskeletal care. Relative rest utilizing compensatory techniques such as a transfer board rather than performing lateral transfers or performing lateral or anterior weight shifts rather than push-up weight shifts may be an important part of musculoskeletal injury management for a person with SCI. After the pain has subsided, emphasis should be focused on preventing further injury by obtaining a balance in strength and flexibility of the musculature surrounding the shoulder (410,411). The most often described muscle imbalance is the tightening of anterior muscles without development of proper strength in posterior stabilizing muscles (405). A proper wheelchair and back support will also play a role in preventing shoulder pain. Surgery is not typically performed for patients with rotator cuff tears, as patients require prolonged immobilization postoperatively, creating a period of extreme disability and loss of independent function (405,412). However, there may be some benefit for pain, and a small study reported improved strength and ROM with surgery and therefore can be considered for those who fail conservative management, who are compliant, and in whom postoperative immobilization is not a limiting factor (413).

Overuse injuries may also affect the elbow (32%), wrist, and hand (45%), including the development of carpal tunnel syndrome (CTS), ulnar nerve entrapment, de Quervain syndrome, and stress fractures (407). The most common source of elbow pain is overuse of the extensor and flexor tendons as they attach to the medial epicondyle. Ulnar neuropathy can lead to intrinsic hand weakness and medial hand numbness and can impact ADL (405). The incidence of CTS is between 40% and 80%, affecting persons with paraplegia more often (414), and with a higher incidence at longer times postinjury (415). This may be due to recurrent stress from transfers, wheelchair propulsion, and pressure reliefs. In addition to typical CTS treatment, the use of padded gloves may decrease the trauma of wheelchair propulsion. Surgical release may be required, with the postoperative recovery time being weighed against the long-term benefits of the procedure (416).

Spine pain is also common. Considerations should include spasticity, adjacent segment degeneration, vertebral osteomyelitis, and Charcot spondyloarthropathy (417). Chapters 27 and 28 address disorders of the spine.

SURGICAL INTERVENTIONS OF THE UPPER EXTREMITY IN TETRAPLEGIA

Surgical interventions can improve the functional ability in appropriately selected persons with tetraplegia. Tendon transfers, nerve transfers, arthrodeses, and implantation of an upper extremity (UE) neuroprosthesis system are procedures that can be utilized alone, or more commonly, in combination, to restore upper limb function after cervical SCI (418). As a general rule, delaying for 6 to 12 months after SCI allows adequate time for neurologic stabilization. Components of the preoperative evaluation include measurements of UE strength, sensation, ROM, and spasticity. Vocational and recreational activities should also be noted (419). Discussing the anticipated outcomes and the postoperative recovery plan prior to the procedure allows patients and clinicians to establish realistic expectations.

The International Classification of Surgery of the Hand in Tetraplegia has been utilized to standardize communication regarding upper limb restoration surgery after SCI (420,421) (**Table 22-4**). In contrast to the International Standards For Neurological Classification of Spinal Cord Injury, functional muscle strength is considered grade 4 or 5 rather than 3 or greater (422). This is because muscles used for transfer generally lose one motor grade, and therefore, those with a grade of 3 or less prior to surgery may not have sufficient strength for functional tasks following the transfer. Spasticity should be minimal or absent in the muscle being considered for transfer. In order to restore elbow extension with posterior deltoid or biceps-to-triceps transfer, there should be functional ROM at the shoulder and minimal elbow flexion contracture (423).

Behavioral evaluation of potential surgical candidates is extremely important as the recovery phase will place limitations on their current regimen by introducing a period of immobilization, activity restriction, and rehabilitation. Patients must be prepared and able to adhere to all phases of the recovery plan. During recovery, patients will require more assistance from caregivers, modification of work/leisure activities, and adaptive strategies for ADL/mobility. There is a long history of upper limb surgery after tetraplegia and a number of options have been described (424,425). Unfortunately, these techniques may not be offered to many patients that can benefit (426,427). The most common procedures for persons with a C5 level include the transfer of the BR to the extensor carpi radialis brevis (ECRB) to restore active wrist extension, thus providing passive pinch and grip (improvements in lifting objects, feeding, grooming, and hygiene are gained), and deltoid to triceps to restore elbow extension (428,429). This latter transfer enables patients to stabilize themselves while sitting, and to reach out with the shoulder abducted from the body, improving grooming, personal hygiene, writing, and self-feeding (430). The goal, however, should not be to improve the ability to perform transfers, since the latissimus dorsi, the prime shoulder depressor muscle, is lacking. A biceps-to-triceps transfer can also be performed (431,432) and some surgeons prefer this transfer.

The Moberg "key grip" procedure may be performed to restore the lateral or "key" grip in patients without a natural tenodesis (433,434). Improvements in functional activities include grooming, eating, writing, and desktop skills and these are maintained over time (435). Transfer of an active muscle, like the BR or others, to the flexor pollicis longus (FPL) to provide lateral pinch and to the finger flexors to provide grasp provides better function and is preferable to Moberg's simple FPL tenodesis (436–438). Posterior deltoid-to-triceps transfer may also be performed in C6 patients. This procedure is recommended prior to hand reconstruction or simultaneously without diminishing outcomes (439). A supination contracture of the forearm that may occur in individuals with C5 and C6 motor injuries can be corrected by rerouting of the biceps brachii around the radial neck (440).

At the C7 level, the goal is to restore active grasp and improve hand control. Transfer of the BR to FPL can achieve restoration of thumb flexion. Restoration of finger flexion is achieved through transfer of ECRL or flexor carpi ulnaris to the flexor digitorum profundus (FDP). At the C8 level, an intrinsic minus or "claw hand" posture results. A lumbrical bar that prevents hyperextension of the metacarpal phalangeal may improve a patient's function, and surgery is rarely indicated.

Traditionally, postoperative immobilization of the extremity in a cast is usually between 1 and 3 months, but now some surgeons begin immediate muscle activation training to prevent atrophy and adhesions (426). In either situation, the patient should be instructed in proper elevation techniques to control edema. Once the patient is cleared for ROM, a removable thermoplastic splint is fabricated to protect the tendon transfers from overstretching. Scar management may include breaking down adhesions and desensitization techniques. Biofeedback and therapeutic ES can help reeducate muscles following tendon transfer (441) Activities are graded progressively by performance time and resistance applied, eliminating any that create heavy resistance to the tendons until after 3 months. Data suggest that benefits from transfer procedures are maintained and patient satisfaction remains high (442,443).

Neuroprostheses implanted in patients with C5 or C6 tetraplegia have been shown to improve upper extremity function

TABLE 22-4	Modified International Classification for Surgery of the Hand in Tetraplegia
Motor Group	**Functional Muscles**[a]
0	Weak or absent BR (grade 3 or less)
1	BR
2	BR, ECRL
3	BR, ECRL, ECRB
4	BR, ECRL, ECRB, PT
5	BR, ECRL, ECRB, PT, FCR
6	BR, ECRL, ECRB, PT, FCR, finger extensors
7	BR, ECRL, ECRB, PT, FCR, finger extensors, thumb extensors
8	BR, ECRL, ECRB, PT, FCR, finger extensors, thumb extensors, finger flexors
9	Lacks intrinsics only
Sensory	
0	Two-point discrimination in the thumb >10 mm
Cu	Two-point discrimination in the thumb <10 mm

[a]Functional muscle: Grade 4 or 5.
BR, brachioradialis; ECRL, extensor carpi radialis longus; ECRB, extensor carpi radialis brevis; PT, pronator teres; FCR, flexor carpi radialis.
Reprinted from Mc Dowell CL, Moberg EA, House JH. The Second International Conference on Surgical Rehabilitation of the upper limb in traumatic quadriplegia. *Hand Surg.* 1986;11(4):604–608. Copyright © 1986 Elsevier. With permission.

(444–446). Chapter 54 describes FES device advances in detail (447–449). Despite the tremendous promise of many evolving technologies, significant obstacles exist in bringing new technologies to the clinic (450).

PRESSURE INJURIES

Pressure injuries are one of the most common and serious complications of SCI, acutely after injury and through the patients' lifetime. Up to 80% of persons with SCI will at some time develop a PI (451–453). During the acute stage after injury, approximately one third of patients develop a PI, although the incidence may be lower for patients cared for at specialized SCI centers (454–457). Pressure injuries can have a profound consequence on the patients' daily activities and QOL, as well as significant direct and indirect economic costs. Diseases of the skin are the second most common cause of rehospitalization of persons with chronic SCI, with persons with ASIA Impairment Scale (AIS) A, B, or C paraplegia more likely to be hospitalized than those with any level of tetraplegia or AIS D paraplegia (458). The National Pressure Ulcer Advisory Panel (NPUAP) revised the terminology of "pressure ulcer" to "pressure injury" in April 2016 (459), which is therefore being used in this section.

A PI can present as intact skin or an open ulcer and may be painful. The injury occurs as a result of intense and/or prolonged pressure or pressure in combination with shear (459,460). There is an inverse relationship between the amount of pressure and the duration of the pressure necessary to cause ulceration; intense pressure applied for a short duration can be as damaging as lower intensity pressure for extended periods. When pressure is placed on a body surface, the greatest pressure is to the tissues overlying the bone, with muscle being more sensitive to the effects of pressure than the skin. Shear, the application of force tangential to the skin surface, occurs when the skin remains stationary and the underlying tissue shifts and can result from varied activities, for example, sliding rather than lifting during transfers.

There have been many risk factors studied for the development of PIs that include demographic and psychosocial variables with some inconsistencies in their findings (461). During the acute rehabilitation phase, the presence of a PI on admission and possibly a lower FIM score are the greatest risk factors for developing a new PI during the hospitalization (455,457). Overall, longer duration of SCI and having a previous PI are significant risk factors for developing future ulcers. Other variables associated include male gender, use of tobacco and alcohol, and poor nutrition. Medical comorbidities, including cardiac disease, diabetes mellitus, vascular disease, immune deficiencies, collagen vascular diseases, malignancies, psychosis, and pulmonary disease, are also factors associated with PI development and may contribute to poor wound healing.

Long-standing ulcers (20 years or more) can, although rarely (<0.5%), develop Marjolin's ulcers, a type of squamous cell carcinoma. Biopsy can identify the carcinoma that is suspected clinically with pain, increasing discharge, verrucous hyperplasia, and bleeding (462).

The NPUAP is the most common staging classification used and is detailed in **Table 22-5**. Specific changes included the term *pressure injury* replacing *pressure ulcer* as this was felt to more accurately describe PIs to both intact and ulcerated skin.

In the previous staging system, stage 1 and deep tissue injury described injured intact skin, while the other stages described open ulcers. This reportedly led to confusion because the definitions for each of the stages referred to the injuries as *pressure ulcers*. Arabic numbers replaced Roman numerals. The term *suspected* was removed from the Deep Tissue Injury diagnostic label, and additional PI definitions added included Medical Device Related Pressure Injury and Mucosal Membrane Pressure Injury.

A comprehensive educational program for SCI patients and their family/caregivers is essential, including information on etiology, risk factors, proper positioning, equipment (e.g., cushions), complications, and principles of wound prevention, skin care, treatment, and when to seek medical attention. Prevention recommendations include examining the skin over bony prominences at least daily with the use of a mirror as needed, shifting body weight in bed and wheelchair on a regular basis, keeping the skin clean and dry if there is incontinence, having an individually prescribed wheelchair and pressure redistribution cushion or power tilt/recline mechanism, ensuring all equipment is maintained and functioning properly, maintaining a nutritionally complete diet and appropriate body weight, stopping smoking, and limiting alcohol intake (451,463).

Since PIs occur over bony prominences, the site of injury development depends upon the position. When sitting, the ITs are at greatest risk, while in side lying, the greater trochanters become at risk, and in the supine position, the sacrum, heels, and occiput (especially in infants) are at risk for PI development. Accordingly, the most common sites of PIs after SCI change based on the amount of time spent in a given position. Acutely after injury, the most common sites are the sacrum, followed by the heels and ischium. At 1 year, the most common sites are the sacrum, ischium, heels, and trochanters and at 2 years postinjury, the ischium, sacrum, and trochanters. When in bed, an appropriate mattress should be sought. Pillows can be used to provide additional padding or provide pressure reduction over bony prominences. Most commonly prescribed early after injury is a turn frequency in bed every 2 hours. Once discharged, it is common to extend the 2-hour turn schedule although there is no documented protocol for this. The prone position has a large surface area of low-pressure and is recommended in the chronic patients as tolerated.

Weight shifting, redistributing the pressure off of the IT to other areas to allow for reperfusion of the ischial areas, is extremely important when the patient is seated in the wheelchair and can be performed by the patient via a number of techniques including an anterior, lateral, or push up weight shift. If the patient is unable to perform their own weight shift, a caregiver can assist or tilt the chair posteriorly so that the patient's weight is no longer on their IT.

It is recommended that weight shifts be performed every approximately 15 minutes for greater than 2 minutes to allow for adequate tissue reperfusion (130,464,465). When performing a tilt weight shift without any recline mechanism, a minimum of 45 degrees is required for adequate pressure distribution (466).

Cushion selection is extremely important. No one cushion is suitable for all individuals with SCI, and prescription should be based on a combination of pressure mapping results, clinical knowledge of the prescriber, and patient preferences.

TABLE 22-5	Classification of Pressure Injuries of the National Pressure Ulcer Advisory Panel (NPUAP)
Stage	**Description**
Stage 1	**Nonblanchable erythema of intact skin** Intact skin with a localized area of nonblanchable erythema, which may appear differently in darkly pigmented skin. Presence of blanchable erythema or changes in sensation, temperature, or firmness may precede visual changes. Color changes do not include purple or maroon discoloration; these may indicate deep tissue pressure injury.
Stage 2	**Partial-thickness skin loss with exposed dermis** Partial-thickness loss of skin with exposed dermis. The wound bed is viable, pink or red, and moist and may also present as an intact or ruptured serum-filled blister. Adipose (fat) is not visible and deeper tissues are not visible. Granulation tissue, slough, and eschar are not present. These injuries commonly result from adverse microclimate and shear in the skin over the pelvis and shear in the heel. This stage should not be used to describe moisture-associated skin damage (MASD) including incontinence-associated dermatitis (IAD), intertriginous dermatitis (ITD), medical adhesive–related skin injury (MARSI), or traumatic wounds (skin tears, burns, abrasions).
Stage 3	**Full-thickness skin loss** Full-thickness loss of skin, in which adipose (fat) is visible in the ulcer and granulation tissue and epibole (rolled wound edges) are often present. Slough and/or eschar may be visible. The depth of tissue damage varies by anatomical location; areas of significant adiposity can develop deep wounds. Undermining and tunneling may occur. Fascia, muscle, tendon, ligament, cartilage, and bone are not exposed. If slough or eschar obscures the extent of tissue loss, this is an unstageable pressure injury.
Stage 4	**Full-thickness skin and tissue loss** Full-thickness skin and tissue loss with exposed or directly palpable fascia, muscle, tendon, ligament, cartilage, or bone in the ulcer. Slough and/or eschar may be visible. Epibole (rolled edges), undermining, and/or tunneling often occurs. Depth varies by anatomical location. If slough or eschar obscures the extent of tissue loss, this is an unstageable pressure injury.
Unstageable	**Obscured full-thickness skin and tissue loss** Full-thickness skin and tissue loss in which the extent of tissue damage within the ulcer cannot be confirmed because it is obscured by slough or eschar. If slough or eschar is removed, a stage 3 or stage 4 pressure injury will be revealed. Stable eschar (i.e., dry, adherent, intact without erythema or fluctuance) on an ischemic limb or the heel(s) should not be removed.
Deep tissue injury	**Persistent nonblanchable deep red, maroon, or purple discoloration** Intact or nonintact skin with localized area of persistent nonblanchable deep red, maroon, purple discoloration or epidermal separation revealing a dark wound bed or blood-filled blister. Pain and temperature change often precede skin color changes. Discoloration may appear differently in darkly pigmented skin. This injury results from intense and/or prolonged pressure and shear forces at the bone-muscle interface. The wound may evolve rapidly to reveal the actual extent of tissue injury or may resolve without tissue loss. If necrotic tissue, subcutaneous tissue, granulation tissue, fascia, muscle, or other underlying structures are visible, this indicates a full-thickness pressure injury (unstageable, stage 3, or stage 4). Do not use DTPI to describe vascular, traumatic, neuropathic, or dermatologic conditions.
Medical device–related pressure injury	**This describes an etiology.** Medical device–related pressure injuries result from the use of devices designed and applied for diagnostic or therapeutic purposes. The resultant pressure injury generally conforms to the pattern or shape of the device. The injury should be staged using the staging system.
Mucosal membrane pressure injury	Mucosal membrane pressure injury is found on mucous membranes with a history of a medical device in use at the location of the injury. Due to the anatomy of the tissue, these injuries cannot be staged.

The general principles of PI treatment are similar to non-SCI population and include the importance to relieve pressure; eliminate reversible underlying predisposing conditions; avoid friction, shear, and tissue maceration; keep the wound bed moist; manage excessive drainage; and debride devitalized tissue (451,467). In general, stage 1 and 2 PIs are usually treated with local care nonsurgically. Stage 3 and 4 PIs, because of their high rate of recurrence as well as the long duration necessary for wound closure, often require surgical intervention. Involvement of a wound care team early after a PI (especially grades 3 and 4) has developed is important. A key issue is to eliminate direct pressure over the PI through positioning techniques and appropriate support surfaces. Limiting sitting time in individuals with IT injuries is important.

If the PI does not heal, surgery may be required. Musculocutaneous and fasciocutaneous flaps are the procedure of choice for SCI patients who require surgical closure of the PI. Because of their blood supply, these flaps are better able to withstand pressure and shear and can be particularly useful in osteomyelitis, by bringing highly vascularized muscle tissue into the area of infection. The decision to use a particular flap or type depends on the surgeons' expertise and the size and location of the injury. It is important to approach issues that impair postoperative healing that include smoking, spasticity, nutritional concerns, and bacterial colonization (contamination from urine and feces). If there is a great deal of stool incontinence interfering with the wound, or suspected to interfere with postoperative healing of PIs over the sacrum and ITs, a temporary diverting colostomy may be considered, although most PIs heal postoperatively without such procedures (468).

At the sacral area, the gluteus maximus muscle may be used entirely or in portions. At the ischium, a posterior thigh fasciocutaneous flap, inferior gluteus maximus myocutaneous flap, hamstring V-Y advancement flap, and tensor fascia lata fasciocutaneous flap can all be used to cover defects in this region. Prophylactic unilateral or bilateral ischiectomy is not recommended. At the greater trochanter, the tensor fascia lata fasciocutaneous flap is considered the flap of choice, although alternatives include the use of the vastus lateralis, inferior gluteus maximus, and rectus femoris muscles.

Postoperatively, strict bed rest is prescribed on a low-air-loss mattress or an air-fluidized bed, maintaining pressure off the surgical site as much as possible. For repairs of the sacrum or IT, the head of the bed should not be elevated greater than 15 degrees since this position increases the risk of shear on the repaired ulcer site. There is no consensus in the literature on the necessary length of immobilization postflap and varies based on the size of the flap as well as the individual protocols and ranges from 2 to 6 weeks. Once healing occurs, passive ROM of the hips in preparation for sitting can be initiated. Once the hip ROM is at 90 degrees without stress on the surgical site, sitting is initiated in short intervals, that is, 15 minutes, and then with return to bed for evaluation of the surgical site. A progressive sitting program ensues, with an increase in sitting by 15 minutes once to twice per day. While institutional protocols vary, usually over a course of 2 to 3 weeks, the patient can progress to sitting up to 5 h/d with completing the full protocol up to 8½ weeks (469). Postoperative complications are common. In a recent study of postflap complications, they found that the overall rate was 21%, with suture dehiscence the most common (31%) followed by infection (25%) (470).

Pressure injury recurrence is common and most frequently recurs at the ITs. Smoking, diabetes mellitus, and cardiovascular disease are associated with the highest rates of recurrence.

RESPIRATORY SYSTEM CONSIDERATIONS

Respiratory failure is the leading cause of death in acute and chronic SCI (471,472). Approximately two thirds of all acute SCI patients will experience a complication of the pulmonary system including atelectasis, pneumonia, and/or respiratory failure requiring mechanical ventilation (473). The primary muscle for inspiration is the diaphragm, which receives its innervation from the phrenic nerve (C3-5), and contributes to 65% of the VC in able-bodied individuals. Additional muscles involved in inspiration include the external intercostals and accessory muscles including the scalenes, sternocleidomastoid, trapezius, and pectoralis. However, these alone are insufficient to maintain adequate oxygenation. Expiration is largely a passive activity caused by recoil of the chest wall. A forceful expiration, such as that required for effective cough, requires contraction of the abdominal and thoracic musculature, innervated by the thoracic level nerve roots (T1-11). The pattern of pulmonary dysfunction most commonly seen in SCI is one of restriction rather than obstruction.

The VC in the newly injured individual with tetraplegia is reduced but improves over time due to increased strength and the development of intercostal and abdominal tone that stabilizes the rib cage and enhances the mechanical effect of the diaphragm (474–476). The typical loss of VC in persons with a complete C5 motor lesion and above is roughly 50%, for C6-8 one third, and for T1-7 only slightly below the lower limits of normal (477–479).

Epidemiologic studies indicate that 20% to 25% of acutely injured SCI patients will require mechanical ventilation. Ventilation is usually initiated at lower tidal volumes (TVs) 6 to 8 cc/kg of ideal body weight based on general ICU management, but many specialists in SCI suggest the volumes to be adjusted upward (10 to 20 cc/kg) while closely monitoring the patient pressures. Higher TV in the SCI population has been found to be safe and may result in faster clearing of atelectasis with better results in assisting with weaning off the ventilator (475,480–482). Oxygen should only be used as a temporary measure, as most patients have healthy lungs. If the oxygen saturation is low, the patient usually has secretions that need to be cleared or an insufficient TV.

Once patients are intubated, forced VC is a key parameter to follow. A VC of approximately 15 to 20 mg/kg is a good predictor of successful weaning from the ventilator (477). Patients with a neurologically complete NLI of C2 and above will have no function of the diaphragm and will need some type of ventilatory assistance immediately. While patients with injuries at the C4 or C5 level may initially require MV, most will be successfully weaned from the ventilator (483).

Weaning is usually attempted when the patient has a VC approximating 10 mL/kg body weight (481,484). The progressive free-breathing technique is the recommended weaning protocol, which consists of removing the patient from ventilator support with a gradual increase in time off the ventilator (472,485,486). This allows the patient to rest in between trials, to gradually build up their strength, and to maintain expansion of the lungs in between the weaning trials. Other methods, including the use of noninvasive means of ventilation, have been utilized. A peak cough flow of 160 L/min correlates with successful decannulation in persons with neuromuscular disease (487).

For patients who remain ventilator-dependent, electrical stimulation of diaphragm contraction may allow weaning from positive pressure ventilation for at least a portion of the day. Chapter 55 includes a detailed discussion of electrical stimulation for respiratory function. Noninvasive means of ventilation including intermittent positive pressure ventilation (IPPV) via mouthpiece, intermittent abdominal pressure ventilator, continuous positive airway pressure (CPAP), and biphasic PAP (BiPAP) can also be employed for persons with SCI.

In the cervical and high thoracic level–injured patients, the effective management of pulmonary secretions is critical. Manually assisted cough (i.e., "quad coughing") is performed by providing an upward thrust on the abdomen while the patient attempts to exhale. Due to possible displacement of an IVC filter, it is best to not use "quad coughing" in patients who have a new IVC filter placed (488). Prior to performing a cough, secretions should be mobilized by percussion or use of devices similar to the "pneumovest" or "rocking bed," which loosen secretions by gentle vibration to the chest wall. Routine tracheal suctioning can also be used to extract secretions, but one should observe for reflex bradycardia secondary to vagal stimulation. The use of a mechanical insufflation/exsufflation

(MI-E) device is beneficial in managing secretions and can be used via tracheostomy, face mask, or mouthpiece. The MI-E delivers a deep insufflation (positive pressure) to the airway that is immediately followed by an exsufflation (negative pressure). The rapid shift in pressure produces a high expiratory flow rate from the lungs, simulating a cough. Advantages of MI-E over suctioning include the following: it has better ability to clear secretions from the left lung, larger mucous plugs can be removed, and it is more comfortable and better tolerated by patients (489).

VC in tetraplegia is affected by the position of the patient, with a 15% decrease in the upright position relative to supine. The diaphragm, like other muscles, is at a mechanical disadvantage near its end range. In SCI patients with midthoracic level injuries and higher, the diaphragm tends to remain partially collapsed, placing it at a mechanical disadvantage and increasing the residual volume. An abdominal binder improves the respiratory function in the sitting position by placing the diaphragm in a more efficient position (490,491). The use of inspiratory resistance muscle training, abdominal weights, and incentive spirometry can improve pulmonary function (492). Glossopharyngeal breathing (GPB) is a technique that involves rapidly taking small gulps, 6 to 9 gulps of 60 to 200 mL each, and using the tongue and pharyngeal muscles to project the air past the glottis into the lungs. Many patients can use this technique to augment VC to assist with coughing or prolong ventilator free time (493).

Diseases of the respiratory system are the leading cause of death in chronic SCI, with the majority specifically due to pneumonia. Individuals with a history of ventilator usage at disease onset, a history of repeated atelectasis or pneumonia, a VC less than 2 L, nocturnal hypercapnia, or a mean SaO_2 less than 95% are at risk to develop late-onset respiratory insufficiency. Immunization for pneumonia (every 5 years) and influenza (yearly) is important for persons with SCI as they are considered to be a high-risk population (494).

Sleep Apnea

The rate of sleep apnea has been reported to occur in more than half of SCI patients that initiates even in their first year post injury (495–500). Common features include loud snoring, disrupted sleep, witnessed apnea, nocturnal gasping and choking, daytime sleepiness, and fatigue. Certain risk factors have been described although not consistent among all reports and are more commonly seen in older men with a short, thick neck and neurologically complete tetraplegia. Certain medications (i.e., antispasticity and antiarrhythmics) and length of time from injury may also play a role. In SCI patients, the sleep apnea is primarily obstructive, although a smaller percentage of patients demonstrate central sleep apnea. Complications include daytime sleepiness and cognitive changes including poor attention, concentration, complex problem solving, short-term recall, and judgment. In addition, there is an increased risk for the development of hypertension, pulmonary hypertension, congestive heart failure, depression, and mortality.

It is advisable to review questions with the patient regarding sleep disturbance, snoring, and daytime somnolence. However, the questionnaire alone is not enough and persons with sleep disorders should undergo a more formal polysomnography sleep study. A home monitoring program is being evaluated (500) for effectiveness as it is difficult for persons with SCI to access a sleep laboratory (499). Treatment includes assisted ventilation at night and possible use of medications directed toward relief of upper airway symptoms.

NEUROLOGIC ISSUES

Dual Diagnosis: TBI Concurrent with Acute SCI

The incidence of concomitant TBI in those with a primary SCI is reported between 24% and 60% (501,502). Historical factors such as mechanism of injury (i.e., high velocity impact), loss of consciousness, prolonged extrication and/or intubation at the scene, higher NLI, presence of PTA, and impaired initial Glasgow Coma Scale (GCS) score should alert medical personnel of the possibility of a concomitant TBI (see Chapter 19).

Fortunately, most TBI associated with SCI is mild and does not appear to impact outcomes at 1 year after injury (501). However, when the TBI is severe, the individual with a dual diagnosis presents a challenge to the rehabilitation team (503). Deficits may be seen in attention, concentration, and memory. These may interfere with new learning and problem solving. The patient may exhibit agitation, aggression, disinhibition, and depression. This is problematic as SCI rehabilitation requires intensive new learning, with the ability to master new skills in terms of mobility and self-care and adapt to a new lifestyle to be able to integrate into the community.

Medical management of problems common to the SCI population such as pain, DVT prophylaxis, spasticity, and neurogenic bladder requires special consideration in the dual-diagnosis patient. SCI care providers need to take into account the fact that some medications routinely used in SCI may have an adverse impact on the recovering brain (i.e., baclofen and benzodiazepines). Special care should be taken to utilize medications with minimal cognitive impact. The evaluation of acute issues can be more complicated in a patient with SCI and TBI dual diagnosis. Fever may represent infection, poikilothermia, or "central fever," which occurs in TBI. Elevated BP may signal the presence of AD in those with SCI at or above the T6 level. However, those with concomitant TBI may experience transient elevation of BP secondary to a centrally driven "sympathetic storm." If initial interventions to calm AD do not improve the patient's BP, pharmacotherapy should be initiated. Agitation is common in those with TBI and should be managed similarly in those with dual diagnosis. Behavioral interventions such as redirection and decreasing environmental stimulation are first-line treatments. Pharmacotherapy is appropriate when behavioral modifications are ineffective.

In those with TBI, acquisition of new information is often challenging and may benefit from simple task repetition in therapy until individual skills can be completed with minimal prompting from the therapist. The therapeutic environment itself may also differ, as persons with TBI may perform better in less stimulating environments (i.e., with fewer visual and auditory distractions, with close supervision by the treating therapist). Cognitive therapy strategies should be reinforced by all members of the treating team such as reminding patients to utilize memory books and orientation cues with each clinical encounter. Neuropsychological evaluation is extremely important.

Concurrent moderate to severe TBI clearly impacts rehabilitation outcomes among individuals with paraplegia (504). Additionally, greater adjustment difficulties, smaller functional gains (as measured by the motor FIM), and variable impact on rehabilitation LOS have been noted (501,504–508). Medical morbidities may be increased. For example, there could be an increased risk of PI due to the inability of the patient to remember to perform a pressure relief and bladder and bowel difficulties due to the inability to perform these programs adequately.

Pain After SCI

Pain after SCI is common enough to be considered an expected condition (509). In the acute phase, pain is usually related to damage to the soft tissue and skeletal system from the initial trauma. After the injuries are appropriately treated, this type of pain usually subsides. However, between 47% and 96% of patients will develop pain thereafter (405,510–513). Model system data indicate that pain prevalence is up to 81% at 1 year after injury and 82.7% at 25 years. Pain is rated as severe in 20% to 33% of persons with pain after SCI. The presence of chronic pain is a significant contributor to decreased QOL, lower levels of psychological functioning and social integration, and an increased interference with ADL (514). The impact of pain on QOL may be greater than that of the injury itself (515).

Several different SCI pain classifications (516–518) have recently been unified (519,520). There are two basic categories of pain after SCI: nociceptive and neuropathic. Additional important SCI pain characteristics can be found in the International SCI Pain Datasets (521–523). As a major category, musculoskeletal or nociceptive pain is more common, occurring in more than half of people with SCI, and neuropathic pain is prevalent in 40% to 50% of persons after SCI (524). Musculoskeletal pain refers to the pain originating from damage to tissue and bone structures and may include overuse syndromes, fractures, and compression syndromes. Neuropathic pain (also called neurologic or central pain) is directly attributable to spinal cord damage and can be divided into multiple subtypes by the level of injury (at the zone of injury or below) and etiology. It is often described as burning, tingling, cramping, shock-like, or a sensation of intolerable coldness. Neuropathic pain is more refractory to treatment than musculoskeletal pain and can occur at any time following injury, even years following the initial injury, with a low frequency of spontaneous recovery.

Chapter 39 provides a detailed discussion of pain management. A Cochrane review found relatively little evidence to substantiate the benefit of nonpharmacologic interventions for chronic pain after SCI (525). Anticonvulsants, most notably gabapentin and pregabalin, are first-line agents and have shown effectiveness in patients with SCI-related neuropathic pain (526,527) as well as anxiety, sleep dysfunction, and depression (528). Because of the strength of the evidence supporting gabapentin and pregabalin, they are strongly preferred first-line options (529,530). Additionally, duloxetine, a relative new selective serotonin and norepinephrine reuptake inhibitor, has demonstrated efficacy in SCI-related neuropathic pain (531).

Surgical treatments including spine fusions or nerve decompression are useful for treating pain originating from spine instability or syringomyelia. Several studies have not found any advantage to spinal cord stimulation (532,533). Dorsal root entry zone lesions are thought to be indicated for some cases of neuropathic pain at the level of injury, while those with below-level neuropathic pain had poor results (534).

Posttraumatic Syringomyelia

The most common cause of progressive myelopathy after an SCI is posttraumatic syringomyelia (PTS). PTS may develop at any time, from 2 months to decades postinjury (535–538). PTS presents as neurologic decline in up to 8% of patients, but is more frequently first seen on MRI as an elongated cavity in a much higher percentage of cases (up to 50%). The pathogenesis is unknown, but the cavity begins at the level of the cord injury in the gray matter between the dorsal horns and posterior columns. PTS usually presents at 5 to 15 years postinjury and is more common and may occur earlier in persons with neurologically complete SCI (AIS A), in cervical followed by thoracic compared with lumbar SCI, and in those injured after age greater than 30 (538–540). Initiating factors include cord hematoma, residual spinal canal stenosis or compression, and spinal kyphotic deformity. The cyst may extend rostrally and/or caudally, compressing the cord, by dissecting through the intermediate gray matter, and may result from increases in subarachnoid fluid pressure due to intra-abdominal or intrathoracic pressure increases (i.e., cough, sneeze, straining or Valsalva, weight lifting, forward-lean pressure release, and quad coughing).

Early signs and symptoms of PTS are often nonspecific and variable; some patients with a markedly elongated syrinx may even have minimal symptoms. The most common presenting symptom is aching, burning pain that increases with cough, sneeze, and straining, usually located at the site of the original injury or may radiate to the neck or upper limbs. The earliest sign is an ascending loss of deep tendon reflexes. An ascending sensory level is common, typically with a dissociated loss of pain and temperature sensation, but intact touch, position, and vibration sense. Loss of pain sensation can lead to a Charcot joint. Weakness occurs, but rarely in isolation. Additional findings may include spasticity changes, hyperhidrosis, AD, fatigue, bladder changes, worsening OH, scoliosis, respiratory changes, and a myriad of other symptoms.

MRI with gadolinium is the gold standard for diagnosing PTS. A syrinx may spontaneously resolve, progress, and then plateau or progress continuously. Neurologic monitoring is essential, and serial MRI imaging may be helpful. Conservative treatment includes pain control, activity restrictions, maintaining head of bed elevation greater than 20 degrees, and providing rehabilitation interventions as needed (i.e., functional training and adaptive equipment). Activity restrictions include avoiding maneuvers that increase intrathoracic/abdominal pressure, that is, high-force exercise, Valsalva, Credé, and quad coughing with direct compression over the IVC, and avoiding anterior weight reliefs and weight lifting, especially if these activities exacerbate symptoms. Surgical treatment is usually indicated if there is an ongoing neurologic (motor) decline or severe intractable pain. Surgical treatments include shunting (syringo-subarachnoid, syringo-pleural, or syringo-peritoneal), reconstructing the subarachnoid space with dissection of arachnoiditis/meningeal scarring and duraplasty, and cordectomy (541–543). Surgery yields improved strength and improved pain control in some but not all, whereas sensory recovery is not usually as favorable. Reduction of syrinx size on postoperative MRI usually predicts a good surgical result; however, complete resolution of the syrinx is not necessary for a good clinical outcome. Recurrence of neurologic *symptoms is common* (*up to 50%*).

Spasticity

The incidence of spasticity in UMN-related SCI is approximately 70%, with roughly half the patients requiring pharmacologic intervention (544,545). While spasticity may occasionally contribute to improved function (i.e., transfers, standing, ambulation, and assisting in ADL), it more often leads to various complications including contractures, pain, impaired function, and decreased QOL. Spasticity occurs more frequently in persons with cervical and upper thoracic SCI than in those with lower thoracic and lumbosacral SCI.

Chapter 40 provides a comprehensive review of spasticity management. The most common clinical scales used to assess spasticity in SCI include the Ashworth scale (AS) (546), modified Ashworth scale (MAS) (547), the Penn Spasm Frequency Scale (PSFS) (548), Spinal Cord Assessment Tool for Spasticity (SCATS) (549), VAS, self-rated scale of spasticity (550), and the Wartenberg Pendulum Test (551). Different scales measure different aspects of spasticity and individual tools correlate weakly with each other (552).

Before initiating treatment, potential nociceptive sources should be evaluated and if present, they should be treated. Common causes include UTI, bladder calculi, PIs, abdominal pathology, ingrown toenails, hemorrhoids, and bowel impaction. Changes in spasticity in an otherwise stable patient may also be an important presenting sign in syringomyelia (535). Spasticity-related interventions should be aimed at what matters most to the patient, improving comfort and function, and allowing the individual to participate in life activities.

Stretching is a mainstay of treatment for SCI-related spasticity (553) and should be done twice a day or more. Standing activities, including use of tilt table or standing frame, provide prolonged stretch to joints and may reduce spasticity as well. Modalities have been used including cold and ES, usually with short-term benefits. Posture and positioning are extremely important for tone reduction. Adequate low-back support in the wheelchair to maintain lumbar lordosis and a positive seat plane angle or "dump," with a reduction in seat-to-back angle, encourages proper upright posture and may reduce extensor tone. Splinting and orthotic management of joints at risk for contracture may also be helpful in reducing tone (553,554).

There are numerous medications for persons with SCI-related spasticity (555,556). Baclofen is the most commonly utilized. The person's age, comorbidities, cognitive status, and goals should be carefully considered when choosing a medication for spasticity. Unfortunately, some evidence suggests spasticity medications may slow functional recovery after SCI, and this too should be factored into treatment decisions (557). Chapter 41 offers additional information in a comprehensive review of spasticity management.

Thermoregulation

The hypothalamus is the brain's central temperature processor for controlling core and body temperature through regulation of blood flow via the autonomic (sympathetic and parasympathetic) nervous system. The hypothalamus will cause shivering and vasoconstriction with arteriovenous shunting of blood flow from the skin when core temperature falls below 37°C and sweating and vasodilation when it senses temperature above 37°C.

SCI above the T6 level affects temperature regulation of the body by interrupting both temperature sensing and spinal autonomic nervous system control of the periphery. This results in the patients being partially poikilothermic, in that they may have difficulty maintaining a normal core temperature in response to environmental change in temperature (558,559). SCI may also reduce or provide abnormal temperature sensations to the brain. Therefore, a person with SCI particularly at cervical levels may feel cold even though core temperature may be normal because of increased or abnormal activity of thermal information.

Many drugs can play a role in hypothermia in people with SCI. Medications that may aggravate hypothermia include antispasticity agents (baclofen, tizanidine), benzodiazepines, tricyclic antidepressants, serotonin uptake blocker, alcohol, and narcotics. Medications that may reduce hypothermia include oxybutynin, gabapentin, and antidepressants that are norepinephrine and serotonin uptake inhibitors.

Hypothermia can cause significant complications including compromising respiration and cardiac arrhythmias and therefore should be prevented. Long-term treatments of hypothermia are preventive with the most important approach to keep warm. Secondly, alcohol should be avoided as it causes vasodilation and heat loss and should be avoided when cold conditions are anticipated. Patients with chronic tetraplegia may also have subnormal body temperatures (<97.7°F) in a normal ambient environment (560).

Similarly, persons with SCI may present with a high temperature while in a warm environment, and they should be cautioned to wear appropriate clothing depending on the setting/environment they are in, as well as frequently drink cold fluids, have a fan, and water spray their face and exposed skin.

PSYCHOLOGICAL ISSUES

SCI is a life-altering event for patients and their families. It is, therefore, not surprising that patients have a myriad of adjustment issues post injury (see also Chapter 12).

Depressive disorders are the most common form of psychological distress after SCI, estimated to affect 20% to 45% of those injured, and usually occur within the first month (561–564). Risk factors for depression include a prior history or family history of depression, pain, female gender, lack of social support, multiplicity of life stresses, concurrent medical illness, and alcohol or substance abuse. Additional factors include having a complete neurologic injury, medical comorbidity with TBI, a low level of autonomy, poor education, unemployment, poor social network and family support, few financial resources, architectural barriers, vocational difficulties, and the need for personal and transportation assistance. Chapter 12 discusses psychological aspects of rehabilitation in more detail.

The suicide rate for individuals with SCI is approximately five times the age-/sex-specific suicide rate in the United States. It is the leading cause of death in individuals with SCI in the youngest age groups and is highest 1 to 5 years post injury (565–567). The suicide rate is higher for those "marginally" injured (incomplete injuries) who have a near-complete recovery (568). In addition to depression, lack of social support, history of suicide attempt, and a feasible plan for inflicting harm to self are risk factors for suicide. Substance abuse, which is increased in the SCI population, is also a major risk factor for suicide. It is imperative that physicians and other health care personnel continue to monitor patients for depression well after the acute phase of injury.

Anxiety and posttraumatic stress disorder (PTSD) have been reported in up to 20% of persons with SCI (569). Symptoms of PTSD may be higher in those with features of depression and/or anxiety (570).

The treatment for psychological disturbances after SCI includes counseling, exercise, and pharmacologic intervention. Cognitive-behavioral therapy has been shown to be helpful in multiple studies (571–574). Similarly, regular exercise also has a favorable impact on mood after SCI (575–578). Chapter 12 offers additional information regarding the psychological aspects of rehabilitation medicine.

Substance Abuse

Substance abuse is frequently encountered in SCI. The CAGE, a four-question screening device for alcoholism, is a reliable instrument with the SCI population (579). At-risk drinkers and substance users tend to be younger, single, male, and less educated. Those with higher CAGE scores have a higher incidence of medical complications, including more pain, PIs, and lower satisfaction with life (580,581).

Alcohol and drug misuse contributes to SCI by increasing risk taking while intoxicated; hampers learning and rehabilitation gains; interferes with self-care; places persons at risk for complications; contributes to depression, mortality, and morbidity; and limits long-term outcomes and capacity for independent living (580–583). Heavy drinkers prior to injury spend less time in educational and vocational activities while in a rehabilitation hospital, and alcohol users are less motivated to participate in their rehabilitation than nondrinkers (584). Substance abuse prevention and treatment programs should be included as part of the SCI rehabilitation.

SEXUALITY AND FERTILITY

While men and women remain interested in sexual activity after SCI, their level of desire and frequency of activity decreases (seed also Chapter 46) (585). Regaining sexual function is extremely important and is an area of unmet need for persons with SCI (585–587). It is reported to be the highest priority among individuals with paraplegia and the second highest priority, after regaining arm and hand function, among individuals with tetraplegia (586). As such, discussion with patients at the appropriate time is extremely important.

The degree of erectile dysfunction in men depends upon the level and severity of the SCI. A man with an UMN lesion will typically have preserved reflexogenic erections, with a lower capacity for psychogenic erections. Greater than 90% of men with complete and incomplete UMN lesions can achieve reflexogenic erections, while less than 10% of men with complete UMN injuries and approximately 50% of those with an incomplete UMN lesion may be able to achieve psychogenic erections (588). Often, the reflexogenic erections are unreliable, poorly sustained, and often are insufficiently rigid to achieve successful intercourse. For persons with a complete LMN lesion, approximately 12% can achieve reflexogenic erections, with approximately 25% being able to achieve psychogenic erections (588). Approximately 90% of patients with an incomplete LMN injury can achieve an erection. Intrathecal baclofen, as well as other medications, may cause difficulties with erection and sexual function.

There are several treatment options available for erectile dysfunction and include oral phosphodiesterase PDE-5 inhibitors, penile implants, vacuum erection devices, vasoactive intracavernosal injections, and intraurethral alprostadil. Most commonly, men with SCI will have their erectile dysfunction treated or managed with a PDE-5 inhibitor (585) including sildenafil (Viagra) and vardenafil (Levitra) and tadalafil (Cialis) (589–591). These medications appear to have similar safety and efficacy profiles, although side effect profile may vary. As PDE-5 inhibitors operate on the nitric oxide–induced cyclic GMP system, they are less effective in men with LMN lesions where reflexogenic erections are rare. PDE-5 inhibitors do not initiate the erection (as do intracavernosal injections), but help maintain erections via maintenance of intracavernosal levels of cyclic GMP. PDE-5 inhibitors are contraindicated in patients taking nitrates (because of hypotension) for angina or coronary artery disease, and as such patients at risk for AD should be so cautioned. Men with tetraplegia or high-level paraplegia should be cautioned about the possibility of experiencing postural hypotension for several hours after use.

Vacuum erection devices (pump with constriction band) can be an effective noninvasive method of managing erectile dysfunction in men with SCI (592). Although fairly safe and effective, the device is not used frequently because of the process required for use.

Intracorporeal injections with prostaglandin E1 (alprostadil) can induce an erection in those with UMN and LMN injuries, with a response rate of over 90% (593). Intracavernosal alprostadil injections work rapidly and are not dependent on the nitric oxide-PDE-5 system of maintaining high intracavernous levels of cyclic GMP (594). Adverse effects include hypotension, bleeding, bruising, pain and fibrosis at the injection site, and priapism, especially if the dose is not carefully titrated. As with the vacuum pump, men with poor hand function may have difficulty administering the injections without help or may be dependent on a partner who is trained and willing to perform the injection. This should not be used in persons with sickle cell disease. Alprostadil has also been formulated as a small suppository (MUSE) that can be administered intraurethrally (595). While less invasive, intraurethral preparations are not effective for treatment of erectile dysfunction in men with SCI (585).

Most men with SCI have difficulty fathering children without some assistance, with less than 10% of couples achieving successful spontaneous pregnancies (596). Erectile dysfunction, ejaculatory dysfunction, and semen abnormalities are the chief contributors to this condition. Despite this, men with SCI should maintain realistic expectations of becoming a biologic father.

Successful ejaculations only occur in approximately 5% of men with complete UMN lesions and 18% of those with LMN lesions (597). The percentage is higher in those with incomplete injuries. To obtain sperm in men who do not ejaculate, penile vibratory stimulation (PVS) and, if unsuccessful, electroejaculation (EEJ) can be attempted. These methods are more effective in men with a level of injury T10 or above (with an intact bulbocavernosus response) as compared to men with a level of injury T11 and below (598,599). They may induce AD and patients should be monitored and pretreated as needed for this.

If these methods are unsuccessful, there are a number of surgical techniques available to obtain sperm. These include testicular sperm extraction, testicular sperm aspiration, microsurgical epididymal sperm aspiration, percutaneous epididymal sperm aspiration, and aspiration of sperm from the vas deferens (588). With the advancement of reproductive medicine techniques, reasonable pregnancy rates have been obtained in couples with SCI male partners.

For women with SCI, there are a number of physical and psychological barriers to engaging in sexual activity (585,600,601). Longer duration and lower level of injury are positive predictors of participation in sexual intercourse (602).

Genital arousal in women can be achieved via psychogenic or reflexogenic pathways and is diminished in approximately 25% to 50% women with SCI (603). Spared pinprick and sensory function in the T11-L2 dermatomes in women with SCI has been associated with the ability to have psychogenic genital vasocongestion (psychogenic arousal) and a greater degree of genital responsiveness than subjects with minimal or no sensory preservation in those dermatomes (604,605). Reflex genital arousal (manual genital stimulation) has been associated with intact reflex function in the S2-4 dermatomes (606). In women with complete SCI above T6, psychogenic arousal can occur in the absence of genital vasocongestion. Approximately 50% of women report developing new areas of arousal above their level of injury, including the head, neck, and torso (607). It is believed that the vagus nerve may serve as a genital sensory pathway that bypasses the spinal cord and conveys afferent activity that can lead to orgasm (608,609).

More than 50% of women with SCI report frequent sexual activity, and almost half of all women with SCI are able to achieve orgasm, although time to orgasm is prolonged compared to women without SCI (610–612). Women with intact bulbocavernosus and/or anal wink reflexes are usually able to experience orgasm, whereas women without S2-5 sensation or absent bulbocavernosus and anal wink reflexes (LMN injuries) have significantly reduced ability. Of note, sildenafil does not appear to result in clinically meaningful benefits in women who have sexual arousal disorder as a result of SCI (585,613).

SCI does not affect female fertility once menses returns. Immediately following SCI, amenorrhea occurs in 85% of women with cervical and high thoracic injuries and 50% to 60% of women overall. Within 6 months and 1 year postinjury, 50% and 90% of women have return of menstruation. The completeness of injury does not appear to influence the menstrual cycle. Women with SCI experience menopause at similar ages to women without SCI. Once normal menstruation resumes, women with SCI can become pregnant with similar success rates as the general population. Methods of birth control should be discussed with the patient's gynecologist taking into account risks (e.g., risk of thromboembolism) versus benefits of each option.

Pregnancy presents a unique set of potential problems including the development of pressure ulcers, recurrent UTIs, increased spasticity, or decreased pulmonary function. There is a slightly increased incidence of preterm labor in SCI women (614,615). AD may develop in susceptible women during labor. Preeclampsia can be difficult to distinguish from AD; however, once the diagnosis of AD has been made, epidural anesthesia is the treatment of choice and should continue at least 12 hours after delivery or until the AD resolves.

The rate of spontaneous vaginal delivery has been reported at approximately 37%, with an additional 31% of deliveries by assisted vaginal delivery, the remaining 32% delivered by cesarean delivery (616). The rate of spontaneous vaginal delivery is probably higher in patients with a level of injury below T6, whereas patients with higher-level injuries are more likely to develop AD and require assisted deliveries.

LONG-TERM FOLLOW-UP

Long-term follow-up with an SCI specialist is extremely important. Initially, visits should occur more often; as the patient and support system gain comfort and expertise, the visit frequency can be decreased. Follow-up allows for monitoring of medical issues, reevaluation of the therapy program, and updating goals and equipment prescriptions. As patients go home from inpatient hospitalization earlier, medical issues that previously were experienced in the hospital now may develop while at home (617). This includes bowel, bladder, and spasticity changes and the possible development of HO, hypercalcemia, and AD. After medical issues have stabilized and outpatient therapy has concluded, visits can transition to as needed with annual comprehensive follow-up visits. Persons with SCI require regular and comprehensive health care throughout their lifetime. This includes routine health monitoring and care for non-SCI medical issues as well as for SCI-specific problems. The altered physiology and the absence of many typical symptoms for common problems following SCI pose a unique challenge for health care providers.

Recommendations for the general medical screening should be followed in persons with SCI, including screening for colon cancer and diabetes, mammography, and lipid panel. Unfortunately, people with SCI are less likely to receive preventive health screening (618). The preparation for colon cancer screening can be especially challenging due to altered continence after SCI. While relatively new, stool sample testing for colon cancer may prove especially useful for people with neurogenic bowel. Due to the expected changes in bone density after SCI, screening for osteoporosis will need to be started earlier than usual. In some instances, SCI physicians may manage all the routine health care screening, but usually partnership with a primary care provider allows for both the SCI-specific and general care needs to be addressed.

At times, readmission to the rehabilitation hospital for medical (e.g., PI, AD) or rehabilitation issues may be needed. Following acute hospitalization, the person with SCI may require a "refresher course" in rehabilitation techniques that can best be taught in an intensive inpatient setting. Secondary medical complications are extremely common in patients with chronic SCI. The most common reasons for rehospitalization include GU complications, PIs, and respiratory complications (162,458).

THE FUTURE

Improved understanding of spinal cord neurobiology, technologic developments, and innovative treatment approaches will continue yield increased opportunities to restore function after SCI. Certainly, the quest for cure is as strong as ever. Over the last decade, stem cell technologies, gene therapy, understanding the microbiome, and advanced robotics have all been shown to have enormous potential in SCI care. Spinal cord stimulation appears particularly promising. Basic science research continues to make progress with the ultimate goal of a cure for SCI. The key factors related to spinal cord healing include minimizing secondary effects of injury, neutralizing the effects of substrates that inhibit CNS regeneration, delivery of regeneration-promoting substances to the injured spinal cord, allowing a bridge to which the spinal cord axons can attach and grow along after injury, and enhancing axonal growth after injury. In addition to medications and procedures, rehabilitation is also a crucial part of any cure treatment strategy. Rehabilitation professionals should be involved in the research but remain committed to the patients and their needs. Caring for the acute and long-term medical issues, as well as assisting the patient to be active in all domains including social, recreational, and vocational activities, is what rehabilitation is all about!

ACKNOWLEDGEMENTS

We want to express our deepest appreciation to the outstanding contributions of the following authors whose foundational efforts on previous versions made this chapter possible: Kath Bogie, Monifa Brooks, Chester H. Ho, Todd A. Linsenmeyer, Steven A. Steins, and James M. Stone.

REFERENCES

1. Elsberg LA. The Edwin Smith Surgical Papyrus and the diagnosis and treatment of injuries of the skull and spine 5000 years ago. *Ann Med Hist.* 1931;3:271.
2. National Spinal Cord Injury Statistical Center. Facts and figures. *J Spinal Cord Med.* 2017;40:126–127.
3. Lee BB, Cripps RA, Fitzharris M, et al. The global map for traumatic spinal cord injury epidemiology: update 2011, global incidence rate. *Spinal Cord.* 2014;52(2):110–116.
4. Chen Y, He Y, DeVivo MJ. Changing demographics and injury profile of new traumatic spinal cord injuries in the United States, 1972-2014. *Arch Phys Med Rehabil.* 2016;97(10):1610–1619.
5. Jain NB, Ayers GD, Peterson EN, et al. Traumatic spinal cord injury in the United States, 1993–2012. *JAMA.* 2015;313(22):2236–2243.
6. Selvarajah S, Hammond ER, Haider AH, et al. The burden of acute traumatic spinal cord injury among adults in the united states: an update. *J Neurotrauma.* 2014;31(3):228–238.
7. Hagen EM, Aarli JA, Gronning M. The clinical significance of spinal cord injuries in patients older than 60 years of age. *Acta Neurol Scand.* 2005;112:42–47.
8. O'Connor PJ. Injury to the spinal cord in motor vehicle traffic crashes. *Accid Anal Prev.* 2002;34:477–485.
9. Chan CWL, Eng JJ, Tator CH, et al. Spinal Cord Injury Research Evidence Team. Epidemiology of sport-related spinal injuries: a systematic review. *J Spinal Cord Med.* 2016;39(3):255–264.
10. Vitale MG, Goss JM, Matsumoto H, et al. Epidemiology of pediatric spinal cord injury in the United States: years 1997–2000. *J Pediatr Orthop.* 2006;26:745–749.
11. Choi SJ, Shin MJ, Kim SM, et al. Non-contiguous spinal injury in cervical spinal trauma: evaluation with cervical spine MRI. *Korean J Radiol.* 2004;5:219–224.
12. Vaccaro AR, An HS, Betz RR, et al. The management of acute spinal trauma: prehospital and in-hospital emergency care. *Instr Course Lect.* 1997;46:113–125.
13. DeVivo MJ, Richards JS. Marriage rates among persons with spinal cord injury. *Rehabil Psych.* 1996;41:321–339.
14. DeVivo MJ, Hawkins LN, Richards JS, et al. Outcomes of post-spinal cord injury marriages. *Arch Phys Med Rehabil.* 1995;76:130–138.
15. Strauss DJ, DeVivo MJ, Paculda DR, et al. Trends in life expectancy after spinal cord injury. *Arch Phys Med Rehabil.* 2006;87:1079–1085.
16. DeVivo MJ, Krause JS, Lammertse DP. Recent trends in mortality and causes of death among persons with spinal cord injury. *Arch Phys Med Rehabil.* 1999;80:1411–1419.
17. DeVivo MJ, Stover SL. Long-term survival and causes of death. In: Stover SL, DeLisa JA, Whiteneck GG, eds. *Spinal Cord Injury: Clinical Outcomes from the Model Systems.* Gaithersburg, MD: Aspen; 1995:289–316.
18. Cao Y, Chen Y, DeVivo M. Lifetime direct costs after spinal cord injury. *Top Spinal Cord Inj Rehabil.* 2011;16(4):10–16.
19. Consortium for Spinal Cord Medicine. *Early Acute Management in Adults with Spinal Cord Injury: Clinical Practice Guidelines for Health-care Professionals.* Washington, DC: Paralyzed Veterans of America; 2008.
20. Ditunno JF, Little JW, Tessler A, et al. Spinal shock revisited: a four phase model. *Spinal Cord.* 2004;42:383–395.
21. Hawryluk G, Whetstone W, Saigal R, et al. Mean arterial blood pressure correlates with neurological recovery after human spinal cord injury: analysis of high frequency physiologic data. *J Neurotrauma.* 2015;32(24):1958–1967.
22. Gilgoff IS, Ward SLD, Holn AR. Cardiac pacemaker in high spinal cord injury. *Arch Phys Med Rehabil.* 1991;72:601–603.
23. Berly M, Shem K. Respiratory management during the first five days after spinal cord injury. *J Spinal Cord Med.* 2007;30:309–318.
24. Savitsky E, Votey S. Emergency department approach to acute thoracolumbar spine trauma. *J Emerg Med.* 1997;15:49–60.
25. Bowers CA, Kundu B, Hawryluk GW. Methylprednisolone for acute spinal cord injury: an increasingly philosophical debate. *Neural Regen Res.* 2016;11(6):882–885.
26. Bracken M, Holford T. Effects of timing of methylprednisolone or naloxone administration on recovery of segmental and long-tract neurological function in NASCIS 2. *J Neurosurg.* 1993;80:954–955.
27. Bracken MB, Shepard MJ, Holford TR, et al. Administration of methylprednisolone for 24 or 48 hours or tirilazad mesylate for 48 hours in the treatment of acute spinal cord injury: results of the Third National Acute Spinal Cord Injury Randomized Controlled Trial. National Acute Spinal Cord Injury Study. *JAMA.* 1997;277:1597–1604.
28. Heary RF, Vaccaro AR, Mesa JJ, et al. Steroids and gunshot wounds to the spine. *Neurosurgery.* 1997;41:576–583.
29. Nesathurai S. Steroids and spinal cord injury: revisiting the NASCIS2 and NASCIS3 trials. *J Trauma.* 1998;45:1088–1093.
30. Hurlbert RJ. Methylprednisolone for acute spinal cord injury: an inappropriate standard of care. *J Neurosurg.* 2000;93(1 suppl):1–7.
31. Evaniew N, Belley-Côté EP, Fallah N, et al. Methylprednisolone for the treatment of patients with acute spinal cord injuries: a systematic review and meta-analysis. *J Neurotrauma.* 2016;33(5):468–481.
32. Hurlbert RJ, Hadley MN, Walters BC, et al. Pharmacological therapy for acute spinal cord injury. *Neurosurgery.* 2013;72(suppl 2):93–105.
33. Bracken MB. Steroids for acute spinal cord injury. *Cochrane Database Syst Rev.* 2012;(1):CD001046.
34. Bowers CA, Kundu B, Rosenbluth J, et al. Patients with spinal cord injuries favor administration of methylprednisolone. *PLoS One.* 2016;11(1):e0145991.
35. Herzer KR, Chen Y, Heinemann AW, et al. Association between time to rehabilitation and outcomes after traumatic spinal cord injury. *Arch Phys Med Rehabil.* 2016;97(10):1620–1627.
36. White AA, Panjabi MM. *Clinical Biomechanics of the Spine.* 2nd ed. Philadelphia, PA: Lippincott Williams & Wilkins; 1990.
37. Denis F. The three column spine and its significance in the classification of acute thoracolumbar spinal injuries. *Spine.* 1938;8:817–831.
38. Vaccaro AR, Koerner JD, Radcliff KE, et al. AOSpine subaxial cervical spine injury classification system. *Eur Spine J.* 2016;25:2173–2184.
39. Vaccaro AR, Oner C, Kepler CK, et al. AOSpine thoracolumbar spine injury classification system: fracture description, neurological status, and key modifiers. *Spine.* 2013;38:2028–2037.
40. Campagnolo D, Heary R. Acute medical and surgical management of spinal cord injury. In: Kirshblum SC, Campagnolo D, DeLisa JE, eds. *Spinal Cord Medicine.* Philadelphia, PA: Lippincott Williams & Wilkins; 2002:96–107.
41. Fehlings MG, Vaccaro A, Wilson JR, et al. Early versus delayed decompression for traumatic cervical spinal cord injury: results of the Surgical Timing in Acute Spinal Cord Injury Study (STASCIS). *PLoS One.* 2012;7(2):e32037.
42. van Middendorp JJ, Hosman AJ, Doi SA. The effects of the timing of spinal surgery after traumatic spinal cord injury: a systematic review and meta-analysis. *J Neurotrauma.* 2013;30(21):1781–1794.
43. Gupta DK, Vaghani G, Siddiqui S, et al. Early versus delayed decompression in acute subaxial cervical spinal cord injury: a prospective outcome study at a Level I trauma center from India. *Asian J Neurosurg.* 2015;10(3):158–165.
44. Bourassa-Moreau É, Mac-Thiong JM, Li A, et al. Do patients with complete spinal cord injury benefit from early surgical decompression? Analysis of neurological improvement in a prospective cohort study. *J Neurotrauma.* 2016;33(3):301–306.
45. Newey ML, Sen PK, Fraser RD. The long-term outcome after central cord syndrome: a study of the natural history. *J Bone Joint Surg Br.* 2000;82:851–855.
46. Ishida Y, Tominaga T. Predictors of neurologic recovery in acute central cervical cord injury with only upper extremity impairment. *Spine.* 2002;27:1652–1658.
47. Yoshihara H, Yoneoka D. Trends in the treatment for traumatic central cord syndrome without bone injury in the United States from 2000 to 2009. *J Trauma Acute Care Surg.* 2013;75:453–458.
48. Brodell DW, Jain A, Elfar JC, et al. National trends in the management of central cord syndrome: an analysis of 16,134 patients. *Spine J.* 2015;15:435–442.
49. American Spinal Injury Association. *International Standards for Neurological Classification of Spinal Cord Injury.* Atlanta, GA: ASIA. Revised 2011; updated 2015.
50. Marino RJ, Rider-Foster D, Maissel G, et al. Superiority of motor level over single neurological level in categorizing tetraplegia. *Paraplegia.* 1995;33:510–513.

51. Frankel HL, Hancock DO, Hyslop G, et al. The value of postural reduction in initial management of closed injuries of the spine with paraplegia and tetraplegia. *Paraplegia.* 1969;7:179–192.

52. American Spinal Injury Association. *International Standards for Neurological Classification of Spinal Cord Injury.* Chicago, IL: ASIA; 1992.

53. American Spinal Injury Association. *International Standards for Neurological Classification of Spinal Cord Injury.* Chicago, IL: ASIA; 1996.

54. American Spinal Injury Association. *International Standards for Neurological Classification of Spinal Cord Injury.* Chicago, IL: ASIA; 2000.

55. Kirshblum SC, Burns S, Biering-Sorensen F, et al. International standards for neurological classification of spinal cord injury. *J Spinal Cord Med.* 2011;34(6):535–546.

56. Kirshblum SC, Waring W, Biering-Sorensen F, et al. Reference for the 2011 revision of the International Standards for Neurological Classification of Spinal Cord Injury. *J Spinal Cord Med.* 2011;34(6):547–554.

57. McKinley W, Santos K, Meade M, et al. Incidence and outcomes of spinal cord injury clinical syndromes. *J Spinal Cord Med.* 2007;30:215–224.

58. Schneider RC, Cherry GR, Patek H. Syndrome of acute central cervical spinal cord injury with special reference to mechanisms involved in hyper-extension injuries of cervical spine. *J Neurosurg.* 1954;11:546–577.

59. Penrod LE, Hegde SK, Ditunno JF. Age effect on prognosis for functional recovery in acute, traumatic central cord syndrome. *Arch Phys Med Rehabil.* 1990;71:963–968.

60. Roth EJ, Lawler MH, Yarkony GM. Traumatic central cord syndrome: clinical features and functional outcomes. *Arch Phys Med Rehabil.* 1990;71:18–23.

61. Burns SP, Golding DG, Rolle WA, et al. Recovery of ambulation in motor incomplete tetraplegia. *Arch Phys Med Rehabil.* 1997;78:1169–1172.

62. Bohlman HH. Acute fractures and dislocations of the cervical spine: an analysis of three hundred hospitalized patients and review of the literature. *J Bone Joint Surg.* 1979;61A:1119–1142.

63. Bosch A, Stauffer ES, Nickel VL. Incomplete traumatic quadriplegia—a ten year review. *JAMA.* 1971;216:473–478.

64. Brown-Sequard CE. Lectures on the physiology and pathology of the central nervous system and the treatment of organic nervous affections. *Lancet.* 1868;2:593–595, 659–662, 755–757, 821–823.

65. Roth EJ, Park T, Pang T, et al. Traumatic cervical Brown-Sequard and Brown-Sequard plus syndromes: the spectrum of presentations and outcomes. *Paraplegia.* 1991;29:582–589.

66. Tersall R, Turner B. Brown-Sequard and his syndrome. *Lancet* 2000;356:61–63.

67. Graziani V, Tessler A, Ditunno JF. Incomplete tetraplegia: sequence of lower extremity motor recovery. *J Neurotrauma.* 1995;12:121.

68. Little JW, Halar E. Temporal course of motor recovery after Brown-Sequard spinal cord injuries. *Paraplegia.* 1985;23:39–46.

69. New PW, Marshall R. International Spinal Cord Injury Data Sets for non-traumatic spinal cord injury. *Spinal Cord.* 2014;52(2):123–132.

70. New PW, Reeves RK, Smith E, et al. International retrospective comparison of inpatient rehabilitation for patients with spinal cord dysfunction epidemiology and clinical outcomes. *Arch Phys Med Rehabil.* 2015;96(6):1080–1087.

71. New PW, Reeves RK, Smith E, et al. International retrospective comparison of inpatient rehabilitation for patients with spinal cord dysfunction: differences according to etiology. *Arch Phys Med Rehabil.* 2016;97(3):380–385.

72. McKinley WO, Seel RT, Gardi RK, et al. Nontraumatic vs. traumatic spinal cord injury: a rehabilitation outcome comparison. *Am J Phys Med Rehabil.* 2001;80(9):639–639; quiz 700, 716.

73. McKinley WO, Tellis AA, Cifu DX, et al. Rehabilitation outcome of individuals with nontraumatic myelopathy resulting from spinal stenosis. *J Spinal Cord Med.* 1998;21(2):131–136.

74. McKinley WO, Teskbury M, Godbout CJ. Comparison of medical complications following non-traumatic spinal cord injury. *J Spinal Cord Med.* 2002;25(2):88–93.

75. New PW, Rawicki HB, Bailey MJ. Nontraumatic spinal cord injury: demographic characteristics and complications. *Arch Phys Med Rehabil.* 2002;83(7):993–1001.

76. Hatch B, Wood-Wentz T, Therneau T, et al. Factors predictive of survival and estimated years of life lost in the decade following nontraumatic and traumatic spinal cord injury. *Spinal Cord.* 2017;55(6):540–544.

77. Ronen J, Goldin D, Itzkovich M, et al. Outcomes in patients admitted for rehabilitation with spinal cord or cauda equina lesions following degenerative spinal stenosis. *Disabil Rehabil.* 2005;27(15):884–889.

78. McKinley WO, Conti-Wyneken AR, Vokac CN, et al. Rehabilitative functional outcome of patients with neoplastic spinal cord compression. *Arch Phys Med Rehabil.* 1996;77(9):892–895.

79. Sandalcioglu IE, Gasser T, Asgari S, et al. Functional outcome after surgical treatment of intramedullary spinal cord tumors: experience with 78 patients. *Spinal Cord.* 2005;43(1):34–41.

80. Schwab JH, Healey JH, Rose P, et al. The surgical management of sacral chordomas. *Spine (Phila Pa 1976).* 2009;34(24):2700–2704.

81. Dekutoski MB, Clark MJ, Rose P, et al. Osteosarcoma of the spine: prognostic variables for local recurrence and overall survival, a multicenter ambispective study. *J Neurosurg Spine.* 2016;25(1):59–68.

82. Gupta A, Kumar SN, Taly AB. Neurological and functional recovery in acute transverse myelitis patients with inpatient rehabilitation and magnetic resonance imaging correlates. *Spinal Cord.* 2016;54(10):804–808.

83. Wingerchuk DM, Banwell B, Bennett JL, et al. International panel for NMO diagnosis. International consensus diagnostic criteria for neuromyelitis spectrum disorders. *Neurology.* 2015;85(2):177–189.

84. Devic C. Myélite subaiguë compliquée de nevrite optique. *Bull Med.* 1894;35: 18–30.

85. Lennon VA, Wingerchuk DM, Kryzer TJ, et al. A serum autoantibody marker of neuromyelitis optica: distinction from multiple sclerosis. *Lancet.* 2004;364(9451): 2106–2112.

86. Takahashi T, Fujihara K, Nakashima I, et al. Anti-aquaporin-4 antibody is involved in the pathogenesis of NMO: a study on antibody titre. *Brain.* 2007;130 (Pt 5):1235–1243.

87. Pittock S, Lucchinetti CF. Neuromyelitis optica and the evolving spectrum of autoimmune aquaporin-4 channelopathies: a decade later. *Ann N Y Acad Sci.* 2016;1366(1):20–39.

88. Sato DK, Callegaro D, Lana-Peixoto MA, et al. Distinction between MOG antibody positive and AQP4 antibody positive NMO spectrum disorders. *Neurology.* 2014;82(6):474–481.

89. McKinley W, Merrel C, Meade M, et al. Rehabilitation outcomes after infection related spinal cord disease: a retrospective analysis. *Am J Phys Med Rehabil.* 2008;87(4):275–280.

90. New PW, Astrakhantseva I. Rehabilitation outcomes following infections causing spinal cord myelopathy. *Spinal Cord.* 2014;52(6):444–448.

91. Brubaker ML, Luetmer MT, Reeves RK. Clinical features and inpatient rehabilitation outcomes of infection related myelopathy. *Spinal Cord* 2017;55:264–268.

92. Sharma A, Chhabra HS, Chabra T, et al. Demographics of tuberculosis of spine and factors affecting neurological improvement in patients suffering from tuberculosis of spine: a retrospective analysis of 312 cases. *Spinal Cord.* 2017;55:59–63.

93. McKinley W, Sinha A, Ketchum J, et al. Comparison of rehabilitation outcomes following vascular related and traumatic spinal cord injury. *J Spinal Cord Med.* 2011;34:410–415.

94. De Risio L. A review of fibrocartilaginous embolic myelopathy and different types of peracute non compressive intervertebral disk extrusions in dogs and cats. *Front Vet Sci.* 2015;2:24.

95. Naiman JL, Donohue WL, Prichard JS. Fatal nucleus pulposus embolism of the spinal cord after trauma. *Neurology.* 1961;11:83–87.

96. Han JJ, Massagli TL, Jaffe KM. Fibrocartilagenous embolism—an uncommon cause of spinal cord infarction: a case report and review of the literature. *Arch Phys Med Rehabil.* 2004;85(1):153–157.

97. Mateen FJ, Monrad PA, Leep Hunderfund AN, et al. Clinically suspected fibrocartilaginous embolism: clinical characteristics, treatments, and outcomes. *Eur J Neurol.* 2011;18(2):218–225.

98. Juhasz-Pocsine K, Rudnicki SA, Archer RL, et al. Neurological complications of gastric bypass surgery for morbid obesity. *Neurology.* 2007;68(21):1843–1850.

99. Kumar N. Copper deficiency myelopathy (human swayback). *Mayo Clin Proc.* 2006;81(10):1371–1384.

100. Kumar N, Gross J, Ahlskog JE. Copper deficiency myelopathy produces a clinical picture like subacute combined degeneration. *Neurology.* 2004;63(1):33–39.

101. Marino R. Domains of outcomes in spinal cord injury for clinical trials to improve neurological function. *J Rehabil Res Dev.* 2007;44:113–122.

102. Mc Dowell CL, Moberg EA, House JH. The second international conference on surgical rehabilitation of the upper limb in traumatic quadriplegia. *Hand Surg.* 1986;11A:604–608.

103. Krassioukov AV, Karlsson AK, Wecht JM, et al. Assessment of autonomic dysfunction following spinal cord injury: rationale for additions to international standards for neurological assessment. *J Rehabil Res Dev.* 2007;44:103–112.

104. Krassioukov A, Biering-Sørensen F, Donovan W, et al. International standards to document remaining autonomic function after spinal cord injury. *J Spinal Cord Med.* 2012;35:202–211.

105. Woulle KS, Van Doren CL, Thorpe GB, et al. Development of a quantitative hand grasp and release test for patients with tetraplegia using a hand neuroprosthesis. *J Hand Surg Am.* 1994;19:209–218.

106. Marino RJ, Shea JA, Steinman MG. The capabilities of upper extremity instrument: reliability and validity of a measure of functional limitation in tetraplegia. *Arch Phys Med Rehabil.* 1998;79:1512–1521.

107. Marino RJ, Kern SB, Leiby B, et al. Reliability and validity of the capabilities of upper extremity test (CUE-T) in subjects with chronic spinal cord injury. *J Spinal Cord Med.* 2015;38(4):498–504.

108. Kahn JH, Tappan R, Newman CP, et al. Outcome measure recommendations from the Spinal Cord Injury EDGE Task Force. *Phys Ther.* 2016;96(11):1832–1842.

109. Kalsi-Ryan S, Beaton D, Ahn H, et al. Responsiveness, sensitivity, and minimally detectable difference of the graded and redefined assessment of strength, sensibility, and prehension, Version 1.0. *J Neurotrauma.* 2016;33(3):307–314.

110. Law M, Baptiste S, McColl M, et al. The Canadian occupational performance measure: an outcome measure for occupational therapy. *Can J Occup Ther.* 1990;57:82–87.

111. Hall KM, Werner P. Characteristics of the functional independence measure in traumatic spinal cord injury. *Arch Phys Med Rehabil.* 1999;80:1471–1476.

112. Gresham GE, Labi MLC, Dittmar SS, et al. The quadriplegia index of function (QIF): sensitivity and reliability demonstrated in a study of thirty quadriplegic patients. *Paraplegia.* 1986;24:38–44.

113. Catz A, Itzkovitz M, Agranov E, et al. SCIM-spinal cord independence measure: a new disability scale for patients with spinal cord lesions. *Spinal Cord.* 1997;35: 850–856.

114. Van Hedel HJ, Wirz M, Dietz V. Assessing walking ability in subjects with spinal cord injury: validity and reliability of 3 walking tests. *Arch Phys Med Rehabil.* 2005;86:190–196.

115. Aigner A, Curt A, Tanadini LG, et al. Concurrent validity of single and groups of walking assessments following acute spinal cord injury. *Spinal Cord.* 2017;55: 435–440.

116. Forrest GF, Hutchinson K, Lorenz DJ, et al. Are the 10 meter and 6 minute walk tests redundant in patients with spinal cord injury? *PLoS One.* 2014;9(5):e94108.

117. Ditunno PL, Ditunno JF. Walking index for spinal cord injury (WISCI II): scale revision. *Spinal Cord.* 2001;39:654–656.

118. Ditunno JF, Barbeau H, Dobkin BH, et al. Validity of the walking scale for spinal cord injury and other domains of function in a multicenter clinical trial. *Neurorehabil Neural Repair.* 2007;21:539–550.

119. Ho CH, Wuermser LA, Priebe MM, et al. Spinal cord injury medicine: epidemiology and classification. *Arch Phys Med Rehabil.* 2007;88(suppl 1):S49–S54.

120. Maharaj MM, Stanford RE, Lee BB, et al. The effects of early or direct admission to a specialised spinal injury unit on outcomes after acute traumatic spinal cord injury. *Spinal Cord.* 2017;55:518–524.

121. Maharaj MM, Hogan JA, Phan K, et al. The role of specialist units to provide focused care and complication avoidance following traumatic spinal cord injury: a systematic review. *Eur Spine J.* 2016;25(6):1813–1820.

122. Consortium for Spinal Cord Medicine. *Outcomes Following Traumatic Spinal Cord Injury: Clinical Practice Guidelines for Health-care Professionals.* Washington, DC: Paralyzed Veterans of America; 1999.

123. Algood SD, Cooper RA, Fitzgeraold SG, et al. Effect of a Pushrim-activated power-assist wheelchair on the functional capabilities of persons with tetraplegia. *Arch Phys Med Rehabil.* 2005;86:380–386.

124. Nash MS, Koppens D, van Haaren M, et al. Power-assisted wheels ease energy costs and perceptual responses to wheelchair propulsion in persons with shoulder pain and spinal cord injury. *Arch Phys Med Rehabil.* 2008;89(11):2080–2085.

125. Adler US, Kirshblum SC. Assistive device for intermittent self-catheterization in men with tetraplegia. *J Spinal Cord Med.* 2003;26:155–158.

126. Long C, Lawton EB. Functional significance of spinal cord lesion level. *Arch Phys Med Rehabil.* 1955;36:249–255.

127. Moreno JG, Chancellor MB, Karasick S, et al. Improved quality of life and sexually with continent urinary diversion in quadriplegic women with umbilical stoma. *Arch Phys Med Rehabil.* 1995;76:758–762.

128. Henderson JL, Price SH, Brandstater ME, et al. Efficacy of three measures to relieve pressure in seated persons with spinal cord injury. *Arch Phys Med Rehabil.* 1994;75:535–539.

129. Sonenblum SE, Vonk TE, Janssen TW, et al. Effects of wheelchair cushions and pressure relief maneuvers on ischial interface pressure and blood flow in people with spinal cord injury. *Arch Phys Med Rehabil.* 2014;95(7):1350–1357.

130. Coggrave MJ, Rose LS. A specialist seating assessment clinic: changing pressure relief practice. *Spinal Cord.* 2003;41:692–695.

131. RESNA Position on the Application of Tilt, Recline, and Elevating Legrests for Wheelchairs: 2015 Current State of the Literature. Available from: http://www.resna.org/knowledge-center/position-papers-and-provision-guides

132. Jan Y, Crane BA, Liao F, et al. Comparison of muscle and skin perfusion over the ischial tuberosities in response to wheelchair tilt-in-space and recline angles in people with spinal cord injury. *Arch Phys Med Rehabil.* 2013;94(10):1990–1996.

133. Kaplan PE, Roden W, Gilbert E, et al. Reduction of hypercalciuria in tetraplegia after weight-bearing and strengthening exercises. *Paraplegia.* 1981;19:289–293.

134. Szollar S, Martin EM, Sartoris DJ, et al. Bone mineral density and indexes of bone metabolism in spinal cord injury. *Am J Phys Med Rehabil.* 1998;77:28–35.

135. Bohannon RW. Tilt table standing for reducing spasticity after spinal cord injury. *Arch Phys Med Rehabil.* 1993;74:1121–1122.

136. Kunkel CF, Scremin AME, Eisenberg B, et al. Effect of "standing" on spasticity, contracture and osteoporosis in paralyzed males. *Arch Phys Med Rehabil.* 1993;74:73–78.

137. Hussey RW, Stauffer ES. Spinal cord injury: requirements for ambulation. *Arch Phys Med Rehabil.* 1973;54:544–547.

138. Rosenstein BD, Greene WB, Herrington RT, et al. Bone density in myelomeningocele: the effects of ambulatory status and other factors. *Dev Med Child Neurol.* 1987;29:486–494.

139. Ogilvie C, Bowker P, Rowley DI. The physiological benefits of paraplegic orthotically aided walking. *Paraplegia.* 1993;31:111–115.

140. Waters RL, Lunsford BR. Energy cost of paraplegic locomotion. *J Bone Joint Surg.* 1985;67A:1245–1250.

141. Waters RL, Mulroy S. The energy expenditure of normal and pathologic gait. *Gait Posture.* 1999;9:207–231.

142. Huang CT, Kuhlemeier KV, Moore NB, et al. Energy cost of ambulation in paraplegic patients using Craig-Scott braces. *Arch Phys Med Rehabil.* 1979;60:595–600.

143. Waters RL, Adkins R, Yakura JS, et al. Motor and sensory recovery following complete tetraplegia. *Arch Phys Med Rehabil.* 1993;74:242–247.

144. Waters RL, Adkins RH, Yakura JS, et al. Motor and sensory recovery following incomplete tetraplegia. *Arch Phys Med Rehabil.* 1994;75:306–311.

145. Waters RL, Adkins RH, Yakura JS, et al. Motor and sensory recovery following incomplete paraplegia. *Arch Phys Med Rehabil.* 1994;75:67–72.

146. Kay ED, Deutch A, Wuermser LA. Predicting walking at discharge from inpatient rehabilitation after a traumatic. *Arch Phys Med Rehabil.* 2007;88(6):745–750.

147. Oleson CV, Marino RJ, Leibly BE, et al. Influence of age alone, and age combined with pinprick on recovery of walking function in motor complete, sensory incomplete spinal cord injury. *Arch Phys Med Rehabil.* 2016;97(10):1635–1641.

148. Van Middendorp JJ, Hosman AJF, Donders ART, et al. A clinical prediction rule for ambulation outcomes after traumatic spinal cord injury: a longitudinal cohort study. *Lancet.* 2011;377:1004–1010.

149. Nene AV, Hermens HJ, Zilvold G. Paraplegic locomotion: a review. *Spinal Cord.* 1996;34:507–524.

150. Chaplin E. Functional neuromuscular stimulation for mobility in people with spinal cord injuries: the parastep I system. *J Spinal Cord Med.* 1996;19:99–105.

151. Field-Fote EC, Lindley SD, Sherman AL. Locomotor training approaches for individuals with spinal cord injury: a preliminary report of walking-related outcomes. *J Neurol Phys Ther.* 2005;29:127–137.

152. Nui X, Varoqui M, Kindig M, et al. Prediction of gait recovery in spinal cord injured individuals trained with robotic gait orthosis. *J Neuroeng Rehabil.* 2014;11:42. doi:10.1186/1743-0003-11-42

153. Mehrholz J, Harvey LA, Thomas S, et al. Is body-weight supported treadmill training or robotic-assisted gait training superior to overground gait training and other forms of physiotherapy in people with spinal cord injury? A systematic review. *Spinal Cord.* 2017;55:722–729.

154. Graf M, Holle A. Environmental control unit considerations for the person with high level tetraplegia. *Top Spinal Cord Inj.* 1997;2:30–40.

155. Hochberg LR, Serruya MD, Friehs GM, et al. Neuronal ensemble control of prosthetic devices by a human with tetraplegia. *Nature.* 2006;442:164–171.

156. Wang W, Collinger JL, Degenhart AD, et al. An electrocorticographic brain interface in an individual with tetraplegia. *PLoS One.* 2013;8:e55344.

157. Monga TN, Ostermann H, Kerrigan A. Driving: a clinical perspective on rehabilitation technology. *Phys Med Rehabil State Art Rev.* 1997;11:69–92.

158. Kirshblum SC, Bloomgarden J, Nead C, et al. Rehabilitation after spinal cord injury. In: Kirshblum SC, Campagnolo D, eds. *Spinal Cord Medicine.* 2nd ed. Philadelphia, PA: Lippincott Williams & Wilkins; 2011:309–340.

159. Green D. Diagnosis, prevalence, and management of thromboembolism in patients with spinal cord injury. *J Spinal Cord Med.* 2003;26:329–334.

160. Chen D. Treatment and prevention of thromboembolism after spinal cord injury. *Top Spinal Cord Inj Rehabil.* 2003;9:14–25.

161. Chen D, Apple DF Jr, Hudson LM, et al. Medical complications during acute rehabilitation following spinal cord injury—current experience of the model systems. *Arch Phys Med Rehabil.* 1999;80:1397–1401.

162. McKinley WO, Jackson AB, Cardenas DD, et al. Long-term medical complications after traumatic spinal cord injury: a regional model systems analysis. *Arch Phys Med Rehabil.* 1999;80:1402–1410.

163. Consortium of Spinal Cord Medicine. *Clinical Practice Guidelines: Prevention of Thromboembolism in Spinal Cord Injury.* 3rd ed. Washington, DC: Paralyzed Veterans of America; 2016.

164. Chung WS, Lin CL, Chang SN, et al. Increased risk of deep vein thrombosis and pulmonary thromboembolism in patients with spinal cord injury: a nationwide cohort prospective study. *Thromb Res.* 2014;133:579–584.

165. National Spinal Cord Injury Statistical Center. *2014 Annual Statistical Report for the Spinal Cord Injury Model Systems Public Version.* Birmingham, AL: University of Alabama at Birmingham. Available from: https://www.nscisc.uab.edu/reports.aspx

166. Godat LN, Kobayashi L, Chang DC, et al. Can we ever stop worrying about venous thromboembolism after trauma? *J Trauma Acute Care Surg.* 2015;78(3):475–481.

167. Gorman P, Qadri SFA, Roa-Patel A. Prophylactic inferior vena cava filter placement may increase the relative risk of deep venous thrombosis after acute spinal cord injury. *J Trauma.* 2009;66:707–712.

168. Nicholson W, Nicholson WJ, Tolerico P, et al. Prevalence of fracture and fragment embolization of Bard retrievable vena cava filters and clinical implications including cardiac perforation and tamponade. *Arch Intern Med.* 2010;170:1827–1831.

169. Hirsch GH, Menard MR, Anton HA. Anemia after traumatic spinal cord injury. *Arch Phys Med Rehabil.* 1991;72:195–201.

170. Lipetz JS, Kirshblum SC, O'Connor KC, et al. Anemia and serum protein deficiencies in patients with traumatic spinal cord injury. *J Spinal Cord Med.* 1997;20:335–340.

171. Frisbie JH. Anemia and hypoalbuminemia of chronic spinal cord injury: prevalence and prognostic significance. *Spinal Cord.* 2010;48(7):566–569.

172. The Consensus Committee of the American Autonomic Society and American Academy of Neurology. Consensus statement on the definition of orthostatic hypotension, pure autonomic failure and multiple system atrophy. *Neurology.* 1996;46:1470.

173. Illman A, Stiller K, Williams M. The prevalence of orthostatic hypotension during physiotherapy treatment in patients with an acute spinal cord injury. *Spinal Cord.* 2000;38:741–747.

174. Mathias CJ, Christensen NJ, Corbett JL, et al. Plasma catecholamines, plasma rennin activity and plasma aldosterone in tetraplegics man, horizontal and tilted. *Clin Sci Mol Med.* 1975;49:291–299.

175. Maury M. About orthostatic hypotension in tetraplegic individuals reflections and experience. *Spinal Cord.* 1998;36:87–90.

176. Teasell RW, Arnold MO, Krassioukov A, et al. Cardiovascular consequences of loss of supraspinal control of the sympathetic nervous system after spinal cord injury. *Arch Phys Med Rehabil.* 2000;81:506–516.

177. Mills PB, Fung CK, Travlos A, et al. Nonpharmacologic management of orthostatic hypotension: a systematic review. *Arch Phys Med Rehabil.* 2015;96(2):366–375.

178. Krassioukov A, Eng JJ, Warburton DE, et al. A systematic review of the management of orthostatic hypotension after spinal cord injury. *Arch Phys Med Rehabil.* 2009;90(5):876–885.

179. Wecht JM, Rosado-Rivera D, Handrakis JP, et al. Effects of midodrine hydrochloride on blood pressure and cerebral blood flow during orthostasis in persons with chronic tetraplegia. *Arch Phys Med Rehabil.* 2010;91(9):1429–1435.

180. Wecht JM, Weir JP, Radulovic M, et al. Effects of midodrine and L-NAME on systemic and cerebral hemodynamics during cognitive activation in spinal cord injury and intact controls. *Physiol Rep.* 2016;4(3):e12683.

181. Claydon VE, Steeves JD, Krassioukov A. Orthostatic hypotension following spinal cord injury: understanding clinical pathophysiology. *Spinal Cord.* 2006;44:341–351.

182. Wecht JM, Rosado-Rivera D, Weir JP, et al. Hemodynamic effects os l- Threo-3,4-Dihydroxyphenylserine (Droxidopa) in hypotensive individuals with spinal cord injury. *Arch Phys Med Rehabil.* 2013;94(10):2006–2012.

183. Canosa-Hermida E, Mondelo-García C, Ferreiro-Velasco ME, et al. Refractory orthostatic hypotension in a patient with a spinal cord injury: treatment with droxidopa. *J Spinal Cord Med.* 2017;24:1–4.

184. Erickson RP. Autonomic hyperreflexia: pathophysiology and medical management. *Arch Phys Med Rehabil.* 1980;70:234–241.

185. Campagnolo DI, Merli GJ. Autonomic and cardiovascular complications of spinal cord injury. In: Kirshblum S, ed. *Spinal Cord Medicine.* Philadelphia, PA: Lippincott Williams & Wilkins; 2002:126.

186. Garstang SV, Miller-Smith SA. Autonomic nervous system dysfunction after spinal cord injury. *Phys Med Rehabil Clin N Am.* 2007;18(2):275–296.

187. Krassioukov A, Blackmer J, Teasell RW, et al. Autonomic dysreflexia following spinal cord injury. In: Eng JJ, Teasell RW, Miller WC, et al., eds. *Spinal Cord Injury Rehabilitation Evidence.* Version 5.0. Vancouver; 2014:1–35.

188. Consortium of Spinal Cord Medicine. Clinical practice guidelines: acute management of autonomic dysreflexia. *J Spinal Cord Med.* 2002;25(suppl 1):S67–S88.

189. McGregor JA, Meeuwsen J. Autonomic hyperreflexia: a mortal danger for spinal cord-damaged women in labor. *Am J Obstet Gynecol.* 1985;151:330–333.

190. Bauman WA, Spungen AM. Carbohydrate and lipid metabolism in chronic spinal cord injury. *J Spinal Cord Med.* 2001;24:266–277.

191. Yekuteil M, Brooks ME, Ohry A, et al. The prevalence of hypertension, ischemic heart disease and diabetes in traumatic spinal cord-injured patients and amputees. *Paraplegia.* 1989;27:58–62.

192. Bauman WA, Adkins RH, Waters RL. Cardiovascular risk factors: prevalence in 300 subjects with SCI. *J Spinal Cord Med.* 1996;19:56A.

193. Bauman WA, Adkins RH, Spungen AM, et al. The effect of residual neurological deficit on oral glucose tolerance in persons with chronic spinal cord injury. *Spinal Cord.* 1999;37:765–771.

194. Myers J, Lee M, Kiratli J. Cardiovascular disease in spinal cord injury: an overview of prevalence, risk, evaluation, and management. *Am J Phys Med Rehabil.* 2007;86:142–152.

195. Bauman WA, Spungen AM, Zhong YG, et al. Depressed serum high density lipoprotein cholesterol levels in veterans with spinal cord injury. *Paraplegia.* 1992;30:697–703.

196. Bauman WA, Adkins RH, Spungen AM, et al. The effect of residual neurological deficit on serum lipoproteins in individuals with chronic spinal cord injury. *Spinal Cord.* 1998;36:13–17.

197. Illner K, Brinkmann G, Heller M, et al. Metabolically active components of fat free mass and resting energy expenditure in nonobese adults. *Am J Physiol Endocrinol Metab.* 2000;278(2):E308–E315.

198. Bauman WA, Adkins RH, Spungen AM, et al. Is immobilization associated with an abnormal lipoprotein profile? Observations from a diverse cohort. *Spinal Cord.* 1999;37(7):485–493.

199. Bauman WA, Spungen AM. Disorders of carbohydrate and lipid metabolism in veterans with paraplegia or quadriplegia: a model of premature aging. *Metabolism.* 1994;43(6):749–756.

200. Nash MS, Mendez AJ. A guideline-driven assessment of need for cardiovascular disease risk intervention in persons with chronic paraplegia. *Arch Phys Med Rehabil.* 2007;88:751–757.

201. Maruyama Y, Mizuguchi M, Yaginuma T, et al. Serum leptin, abdominal obesity and the metabolic syndrome in individuals with chronic spinal cord injury. *Spinal Cord.* 2008;46(7):494–499.

202. Gater DR. Obesity after spinal cord injury. *Phys Med Rehabil Clin N Am.* 2007;18(2):333–351.

203. Perret C, Stoffel-Kurt N. Comparison of nutritional intake between individuals with acute and chronic spinal cord injury. *J Spinal Cord Med.* 2011;34(6):569–575.

204. Khalil RE, Gorgey AS, Janisko M, et al. The role of nutrition in health status after spinal cord injury. *Aging Dis.* 2013;4(1):14–22.

205. Nash MS, van de Ven I, van Elk N, et al. Effects of circuit resistance training on fitness attributes and upper-extremity pain in middle-aged men with paraplegia. *Arch Phys Med Rehabil.* 2007;88:70–75.

206. Jeon JY, Weiss CB, Steadward RD, et al. Improved glucose tolerance and insulin sensitivity after electrical stimulation-assisted cycling in people with spinal cord injury. *Spinal Cord.* 2002;40:110–117.

207. El-Sayed MS, Younesian A. Lipid profiles are influenced by arm cranking exercise and training in individuals with spinal cord injury. *Spinal Cord.* 2005;43:299–305.

208. Hooker SP, Wells CC. Effects of low and moderate activity training on spinal cord persons. *Med Sci Sports Exerc.* 1989;21:18–22.

209. Jacobs PL, Nash MS. Exercise recommendations for individuals with spinal cord injury. *Sports Med.* 2004;34:727–751.

210. Stillman MD, Aston CE, Rabadi MH. Mortality benefit of statin use in traumatic spinal cord injury: a retrospective analysis. *Spinal Cord.* 2016;54(4):298–302.

211. Weaver FM, Collins EG, Kurichi J, et al. Prevalence of obesity and high blood pressure in veterans with spinal cord injuries and disorders: a retrospective review. *Am J Phys Med Rehabil.* 2007;86:22–29.

212. Duckworth WC, Solomon SS, Jallepalli P, et al. Glucose intolerance due to insulin resistance in patients with spinal cord injuries. *Diabetes.* 1980;29:906–910.

213. Duckworth WC, Jallepalli P, Solomon SS. Glucose intolerance in spinal cord injury. *Arch Phys Med Rehabil.* 1983;64:107–110.

214. Stiens SA, Bergman SB, Goetz LL. Neurogenic bowel dysfunction after spinal cord injury: clinical evaluation and rehabilitative management. *Arch Phys Med Rehabil.* 1997;78:S86–S102.

215. Walter A, Morren GL, Ryn AK, et al. Rectal pressure response to a meal in patients with high spinal cord injury. *Arch Phys Med Rehabil.* 2003;84:108–110.

216. Consortium for Spinal Cord Medicine. Clinical Practice Guideline: neurogenic bowel management in adults with spinal cord injury. *J Spinal Cord Med.* 1998;21:248–293.

217. Bannister J, Gibbons C, Read N. Preservation of fecal continence during rises in intraabdominal pressure: is there a role for the flap valve? *Gut.* 1987;28:1242–1245.

218. Ambroze W, Bell A, Pemberton J, et al. The effect of stool consistency on rectal and neorectal emptying. *Gastroenterology.* 1989;96(suppl 5):A11.

219. Findlay J, Smith A, Mitchell W, et al. Effects of unprocessed bran on colon function in normal subjects and in diverticular disease. *Lancet.* 1974;1:146.

220. Cummings J. Constipation, dietary fibre and the control of large bowel function. *Postgrad Med J.* 1984;60:811–819.

221. Bond J, Currier B, Buchwald H, et al. Colonic conservation of malabsorbed carbohydrate. *J Gastroenterol.* 1980;78:444–449.

222. Goyal R, Crist J. Neurology of the gut. In: Sleisenger MH, Fordtran JS, eds. *Gastrointestinal Disease: Pathophysiology, Diagnosis, Management.* 4th ed. Philadelphia, PA: WB Saunders; 1989:21–47.

223. Devroede G, Arhan P, Duguay C, et al. Traumatic constipation. *Gastroenterology.* 1979;77:1258–1267.

224. Graffner H, Ekelund M, Hakanson R, et al. Effects of upper abdominal sympathectomy on gastric acid, serum gastrin, and catecholamines in the rat gut. *Scand J Gastroenterol.* 1984;19:711–716.

225. Duthie HL, Watts JM. Contribution of the external anal sphincter to the pressure zone in the anal canal. *Gut.* 1965;6:64–68.

226. Frenckner B. Function of the anal sphincters in spinal man. *Gut.* 1975;16:638–644.

227. Parks A, Porter N, Melzack J. Experimental study of the reflex mechanism controlling the muscles of the pelvic floor. *Dis Colon Rectum.* 1962;5:407–414.

228. Madoff R, Williams J, Caushaj P. Fecal incontinence. *N Engl J Med.* 1992;326:1002–1007.

229. Schweiger M. Method for determining individual contributions of voluntary and involuntary anal sphincters to resting tone. *Dis Colon Rectum.* 1979;22:415–416.

230. Wallace W, Madden W. Partial puborectalis resection: a new surgical technique for anorectal dysfunction. *South Med J.* 1969;62:1121–1126.

231. Clanton LJ Jr, Bender J. Refractory spinal cord injury induced gastroparesis: resolution with erythromycin lactobionate: a case report. *J Spinal Cord Med.* 1999;22:236–238.

232. Althausen PL, Gupta MC, Benson DR, et al. The use of neostigmine to treat postoperative ileus in orthopedic spinal patients. *J Spinal Disord.* 2001;14:541–545.

233. Soderstrom CA, Ducker TB. Increased susceptibility of patients with cervical cord lesions to peptic gastrointestinal complications. *J Trauma.* 1985;25:1030–1038.

234. Kiwerski J. Bleeding from the alimentary canal during the management of spinal cord injury patients. *Paraplegia.* 1986;24:92–96.

235. Gore RM, Minzter RA, Calenoff L. Gastrointestinal complications of spinal cord injury. *Spine.* 1981;6:538–544.

236. Moonka R, Stiens SA, Resnick WJ, et al. Prevalence and natural history of gallstones in spinal cord injured persons. *J Am Coll Surg.* 1999;189:274–281.

237. Rotter KP, Larrain CG. Gallstones in spinal cord injury (SCI): a late medical complication? *Spinal Cord.* 2003;41:105–108.

238. Tola VB, Chamberlain S, Kostyk SK, et al. Symptomatic gallstones in patients with spinal cord injury. *J Gastrointest Surg.* 2000;4:642–647.

239. Roth EJ, Fenton LI, Gaebler-Spira DJ, et al. Superior mesenteric artery syndrome in acute traumatic quadriplegia: care reports and literature review. *Arch Phys Med Rehabil.* 1991;72:417–420.

240. Berlly MH, Wilmot CB. Acute abdominal emergencies during the first four weeks after spinal cord injury. *Arch Phys Med Rehabil.* 1984;65:687–690.

241. Nobel D, Baumberger M, Eser P, et al. Nontraumatic pancreatitis in spinal cord injury. *Spine.* 2002;27:E228–E232.

242. Roach MJ, Frost FS, Creasey G. Social and personal consequences of acquired bowel. *J Spinal Cord Med.* 2000;23:263–269.

243. Stiens S, Fajardo N, Korsten M. The gastrointestinal system after spinal cord injury. In: Lin VW, ed. *Spinal Cord Medicine.* 1st ed. New York: Demos; 2002;2:549–570.

244. Rasmussen O. Anorectal function. *Dis Colon Rectum.* 1994;37:386–403.

245. Read N, Timms J. Defecation and the pathophysiology of constipation. *Clin Gastroenterol.* 1986;15:937–965.

246. Barkel D, Pemberton J, Pezim M, et al. Scintigraphic assessment of the anorectal angle in health and after ileal pouch–anal anastomosis. *Ann Surg.* 1988;208:42–49.

247. Sun WM, MacDonagh R, Forster D, et al. Anorectal function in patients with complete spinal transection before and after sacral posterior rhizotomy. *Gastroenterology.* 1995;108:990–998.

248. Pfeifer J, Agachan F, Wexner S. Surgery for constipation: a review. *Dis Colon Rectum.* 1996;39:444–460.

249. Stone JM, Wolfe VA, Nino-Murcia M, et al. Colostomy as treatment for complications of spinal cord injury. *Arch Phys Med Rehabil.* 1990;71:514–518.

250. Christensen P, Bazzocchi G, Coggrave M, et al. A randomized, controlled trial of transanal irrigation versus conservative bowel management in spinal cord-injured patients. *Gastroenterology.* 2006;131:738–747.

251. Shandling B, Gilmore R. The enema continence catheter in spina bifida: successful bowel management. *J Pediatr Surg.* 1987;22:271–273.

252. Yang C, Stiens S. Antegrade continence enema for the treatment of neurogenic constipation and fecal incontinence after spinal cord injury. *Arch Phys Med Rehabil.* 2000;81:683–685.

253. Saltzstein R, Romano J. The efficacy of colostomy as a bowel management alternative in selected spinal cord injured patients. *J Am Paraplegia Soc.* 1990;13:9–13.

254. Kirk PM, King RB, Temple R. Long term follow-up of bowel management after spinal cord injury. *SCI Nurs.* 1997;14:556–553.

255. Rosito O, Nino-Murcia M, Wolfe VA, et al. The effects of colostomy on the quality of life in patients with spinal cord injury: a retrospective analysis. *J Spinal Cord Med.* 2002;25(3):174–183.

256. Kelly SR, Shashidharan M, Borwell B, et al. The role of intestinal stoma in patients with spinal cord injury. *Spinal Cord.* 1999;37:211–214.

257. Cameron KJ, Nyulasi IB, Collier GR, et al. Assessment of the effect of increased dietary fibre intake on bowel function in patients with spinal cord injury. *Spinal Cord.* 1996;34:277–283.

258. Hanson RW, Franklin MR. Sexual loss in relation to other functional losses for spinal cord injured males. *Arch Phys Med Rehabil.* 1976;57:291–293.

259. Paralyzed Veterans of America. *Neurogenic Bowel Management in Adults with Spinal Cord Injury: A Clinical Practice Guideline.* Washington, DC: Paralyzed Veterans of America; 1998.

260. Kirshblum S, Gulati M, O'Connor K, et al. Bowel function in spinal cord injured patients. *Arch Phys Med Rehabil.* 1998;79:20–23.

261. Stiens S. Reduction in bowel program duration with polyethylene glycol based bisacodyl suppositories. *Arch Phys Med Rehabil.* 1995;76:674–677.

262. House J, Stiens S. Pharmacologically initiated defecation for persons with spinal cord injury: effectiveness of three agents. *Arch Phys Med Rehabil.* 1997;78:1062–1065.

263. Stiens SA, Lutrel W, Binard JE. Polyethylene glycol versus vegetable oil based bisacodyl suppositories to initiate side-lying bowel care: a clinical trial in persons with spinal cord injury. *Spinal Cord.* 1998;36:777–781.

264. Yim SY, Yoon SH, Lee IY, et al. A comparison of bowel care patterns in patients with spinal cord injury: upper motor neuron bowel vs lower motor neuron bowel. *Spinal Cord.* 2001;39(4):204–207.

265. Brooks JD. Anatomy of the lower urinary tract. In: Walsh PC, Retik AB, Vaughan ED, et al., eds. *Campbell's Urology.* 8th ed. Philadelphia, PA: WB Saunders; 2002:56–70.

266. Myers RP, Goellner JR, Cahill DR. Prostate shape, external striated urethral sphincter and radical prostatectomy: the apical dissection. *J Urol.* 1987;138:543–547.

267. Delancey JO. Structure and function of the continence mechanism relative to stress incontinence. In: Leach GE, Paulson DF, eds. *Problems in Urology*, vol. 1. Female Urology. Philadelphia, PA: JB Lippincott; 1991:1–9.

268. Fletcher TF, Bradley WE. Neuroanatomy of the bladder-urethra. *J Urol.* 1978;119:153–160.

269. Benson GS, McConnell JA, Wood JG. Adrenergic innervation of the human bladder body. *J Urol.* 1979;122:189–191.

270. Elbadawi A. Autonomic muscular innervation of the vesical outlet and its role in micturition. In: Hinman F Jr, ed. *Benign Prostatic Hypertrophy.* New York: Springer Verlag; 1983:330–348.

271. de Groat WC. Mechanism underlying the recovery of lower urinary tract function following spinal cord injury. *Paraplegia.* 1995;33:493–505.

272. Barrett DM, Wein AJ. Voiding dysfunction: diagnosis, classification and management. In: Gillenwater JY, Grayhack JT, Howards SS, et al., eds. *Adult and Pediatric Urology.* 2nd ed. St Louis, MO: Mosby Year Book; 1991:1001–1099.

273. Yalla SV, Fam BA. Spinal cord injury. In: Krane RJ, Siroky MB, eds. *Clinical Neurourology.* 2nd ed. Boston, MA: Little, Brown & Co; 1991:319–331.

274. Kaplan SA, Chancellor MB, Blaivas JG. Bladder and sphincter behavior in patients with spinal cord lesions. *J Urol.* 1991;146:113–117.

275. Shan MM, Carfield JC, Jenkins JD. Lumbar spondylosis and neuropathic bladder investigations of 73 patients with chronic urinary symptoms. *BMJ.* 1976;1:645.

276. Linsenmeyer TA, Culkin D. APS Recommendations for the urological evaluation of patients with spinal cord injury. *J Spinal Cord Med.* 1999;22(2):139–142.

277. Winters JC, Dmochowski RR, Goldman HB, et al. *Adult Urodynamics: AUA/ SUFU Guideline.* Published 2012. Available from: http://www.auanet.org/guidelines/urodynamics. Accessed April 20, 2017.

278. Bih LI, Changlai SP, Ho CC, et al. Application of radioisotope renography with technetium-99m mercaptoacetyltriglycine on patients with spinal cord injuries. *Arch Phys Med Rehabil.* 1994;75(9):982–986.

279. Phillips JR, Jadvar H, Sullivan G, et al. Effect of radionuclide renograms on treatment of patients with spinal cord injuries. *AJR Am J Roentgenol.* 1997;169(4):1045–1047.

280. Consortium for Spinal Cord Medicine. Bladder management for adults with spinal cord injury: a clinical practice guideline for health-care providers. *J Spinal Cord Med.* 2006;29(5):527–573.

281. Weld KJ, Dmochowski RR. Effect of bladder management on urological complications in spinal cord injured patients. *J Urol.* 2000;163:768–772.

282. Barbalias GA, Klauber GT, Blaivas JG. Critical evaluation of the Crede maneuver: a urodynamic study of 207 patients. *J Urol.* 1983;130:720–723.

283. Kim YH, Katten MW, Boone TB. Bladder leak point pressure: the measure for sphincterotomy success in spinal cord injured patients with external detrusor-sphincter dyssynergia. *J Urol.* 1998;159:493–497.

284. Killorin W, Gray M, Bennet JK, et al. The value of urodynamics and bladder management in predicting upper urinary tract complications in male spinal cord injury patients. *Paraplegia.* 1992;30:437–441.

285. Gerridzen RG, Thijssen AM, Dehoux E. Risk factors for upper tract deterioration in chronic spinal cord injury patients. *J Urol.* 1992;147:416–418.

286. Linsenmeyer TA, Horton J, Benevento J. Impact of alpha-1 blockers in men with spinal cord injury and upper tract stasis. *J Spinal Cord Med.* 2002;25(2):124–128.

287. Pannek J, Blok B, Castro-Diaz D, et al. *Guidelines on Neurogenic Lower Urinary Tract Dysfunction.* European Association of Urology. Published 2013. Available from: https://uroweb.org/wp-content/uploads/20_Neurogenic-LUTD_LR.pdf. Accessed May 7, 2017.

288. Ginsberg DA, Schneider LK, Watanabe TK. Improving outcomes in patients with refractory idiopathic and neurogenic detrusor overactivity: management strategies. *Arch Phys Med Rehabil.* 2015;96(9 suppl 4):S341–S357.

289. Madersbacher H, Murtz G, Stohrer M. Neurogenic detrusor overactivity in adults: A review on efficacy, tolerability and safety of oral antimuscarinics. *Spinal Cord.* 2013;51:432–441.

290. Wollner J, Pannek J. Initial experience with the treatment of neurogenic detrusor overactivity with a new beta-3 agonist (mirabegron) in patients with spinal cord injury. *Spinal Cord.* 2016;54:78–82.

291. Wada N, Okazaki S, Kobayashi S, et al. Efficacy of combination therapy with mirabegron for anticholinergic-resistant neurogenic bladder: videourodynamic evaluation. *Hinyokika Kiyo.* 2015;61(1):7–11.

292. Baldessarini RJ. Drugs and the treatment of psychiatric disorders. In: Gillman AG, Rall TW, Nies AS, et al., eds. *Goodman and Gilman's the Pharmacologic Basis of Therapeutics.* 8th ed. New York: Pergamon Press; 1990:383–435.

293. Nitti VW. Botulinum toxin for the treatment of idiopathic and neurogenic overactive bladder: state of the art. *Rev Urol.* 2006;8(4):198–208.

294. Schurch B. Botulinum toxin for the management of bladder dysfunction. *Drugs.* 2006;66(10):1301–1318.

295. Karsenty G, Denys P, Amarenco G, et al. Chartier-Kastler Botulinum toxin A (Botox) intradetrusor injections in adults with neurogenic detrusor overactivity/neurogenic overactive bladder: a systematic literature review. *Eur Urol.* 2008;53(2):275–287.

296. Lepor H. Alpha blockers for the treatment of benign prostatic hypertrophy. *Probl Urol.* 1991;5:419–429.

297. Scott MB, Morrow JW. Phenoxybenzamine in neurogenic bladder dysfunction after spinal cord injury: I. Voiding dysfunction. *J Urol.* 1978;119:480–482.

298. Finkbeiner AE. Is bethanechol chloride clinically effective in promoting bladder emptying? A literature review. *J Urol.* 1985;134:443–449.

299. Light KJ, Scott FB. Bethanechol chloride and the traumatic cord bladder. *J Urol.* 1982;128:85–87.

300. Sporer A, Leyson JFJ, Martin BF. Effects of bethanechol chloride on the external urethral sphincter in spinal cord injury patients. *J Urol.* 1978;120:62–66.

301. Taylor P. Cholinergic agonists. In: Gilman AC, Rall TW, Nies AS, et al., eds. *Goodman and Gilman's the Pharmacological Basis of Therapeutics.* 8th ed. New York: Pergamon Press; 1990:122–130.

302. Gray GJ, Yang C. Surgical procedures of the bladder after spinal cord injuries. *Top Spinal Cord Med.* 2000;11(1):61–69.

303. McDougal WS. Use of intestinal segments and urinary diversion. In: Walsh PC, Retik AB, Vaughan ED, et al., eds. *Cambell's Urology.* 7th ed. Philadelphia, PA: WB Saunders Co; 1998:3121–3157.

304. Anderson B, Mitchell M. Management of electrolyte disturbances following urinary diversion and bladder augmentation. *AUA News.* 2000;5(8):1–7.

305. Sakano S, Yoshihiro S, Joko K, et al. Adenocarcinoma developing in an ileal conduit. *J Urol.* 1995;153:146–148.

306. Golomb J, Klutke CG, Lewin KJ, et al. Bladder neoplasms associated with augmentation cystoplasty: report of 2 cases and literature review. *J Urol.* 1989;142:377–380.

307. Mast P, Hoebeke P, Wyndaele JJ, et al. Experience with augmentation cystoplasty: a review. *Paraplegia.* 1995;33:560–564.

308. Kuo HC. Clinical outcomes and quality of life after enterocystoplasty for contracted bladders. *Urol Int.* 1997;58(3):160–165.

309. Stohrer M, Kramer G, Gopel M, et al. Bladder autoaugmentation in adult patients with neurogenic voiding dysfunction. *Spinal Cord.* 1997;35(7):456–462.

310. Perkash I. Modified approach to sphincterotomy in spinal cord injury patients. *Paraplegia.* 1976;13:247–260.

311. Chancellor MB, Rivas DA, Linsenmeyer T, et al. Multicenter trial in North America of Urolume urinary sphincter prosthesis. *J Urol.* 1994;152:924–930.

312. Hamid R, Arya M, Patel HR, et al. The mesh wallstent in the treatment of detrusor external sphincter dyssynergia in men with spinal cord injury: a 12-year follow-up. *BJU Int.* 2003;91(1):51–53.

313. Farag F, Koens M, Sievert KD, et al. Surgical treatment of neurogenic stress urinary incontinence: a systematic review of quality assessment and surgical outcomes. *Neurourol Urodyn.* 2016;35:21–25.

314. Brindley GS, Polkey CE, Rushton DN. Sacral anterior root stimulator for bladder control in paraplegia. *Paraplegia.* 1982;20:365–381.

315. Chulamorkodt NN, Estrada CR, Chaviano AH. Continent urinary diversion: 10-year experience of Shriners Hospitals for Children in Chicago. *J Spinal Cord Med.* 2004;27(suppl 1):S84–S87.

316. The prevention and management of urinary tract infections among people with spinal cord injuries. National Institute on Disabilities and Rehabilitation Research, Consensus Conference Statement, January 27–29, 1992. *J Am Paraplegia Soc.* 1992;15:194–204.

317. Morton SC, Shekelle PG, Adams JL, et al. Antimicrobial prophylaxis for urinary tract infection in persons with spinal cord dysfunction. *Arch Phys Med Rehabil.* 2002;83:129–138.

318. Maynard FM, Diokno AC. Urinary infection and complications during clean intermittent catheterization following spinal cord injury. *J Urol.* 1984;132:943–946.

319. Anderson RU. Non sterile intermittent catheterization with antibiotic prophylaxis in the acute spinal cord injured male patient. *J Urol.* 1980;124:392–394.

320. Merritt JLM, Erickson RP, Opitz JL. Bacteriuria during follow up in patients with spinal cord injury: Part II. Efficacy of antimicrobial suppressants. *Arch Phys Med Rehabil.* 1982;63:413–415.

321. Price M, Kottke FJ. Renal function in patients with spinal cord injury: the eighth year of a ten year continuing study. *Arch Phys Med Rehabil.* 1975;56:76–79.

322. Fellows GJ, Silver JR. Long term follow up of paraplegic patients with vesico-ureteric reflux. *Paraplegia*. 1976;14:130–134.

323. Cardenas D, Farrell-Roberts L, Sipski M, et al. Management of gastrointestinal, genitourinary and sexual function. In: Stover SL, DeLisa JA, Whiteneck GG, eds. *Spinal Cord Injury Clinical Outcomes From the Model Systems*. Gaithersburg, MD: Aspen Publications; 1995: 129–130.

324. DeVivo MJ, Fine PR, Cutter GR, et al. The risk of bladder calculi in patients with spinal cord injuries. *Arch Intern Med*. 1985;145:428–430.

325. Linsenmeyer MA, Linsenmeyer TA. Accuracy of predicting bladder stones based on catheter encrustation in individuals with spinal cord injury. *J Spinal Cord Med*. 2006;29(4):402–405.

326. Ord J, Lunn D, Reynard J. Bladder management and risk of bladder stone formation in spinal cord injured patients. *J Urol*. 2003;170(5):1734–1737.

327. DeVivo MJ, Fine PR. Predicting renal calculus occurrence in spinal cord injury patients. *Arch Phys Med Rehabil*. 1986;67:722–775.

328. Kuhlemeier KV, Lloyd LK, Stover SL. Long term followup of renal function after spinal cord injury. *J Urol*. 1985;134:510–513.

329. Matlaga BR, Kim SC, Watkins SL, et al. Changing composition of renal calculi in patients with neurogenic bladder. *J Urol*. 2006;175:1716–1719.

330. Singh M, Chapman R, Tresidder GC, et al. Fate of unoperated staghorn calculus. *Br J Urol*. 1973;45:581–585.

331. Ku JH, Jung TY, Lee JK, et al. Risk factors for urinary stone formation in men with spinal cord injury: a 17-year follow-up study. *BJU Int*. 2006;97:790–793.

332. Hansen RB, Biering-Sørensen F, Kristensen JK. Urinary calculi following traumatic spinal cord injury. *Scand J Urol Nephrol*. 2007;41:115–119.

333. Staskin DR. Hydroureteronephrosis after spinal cord injury. *Urol Clin North Am*. 1991;18:309–316.

334. West DA, Cummings JM, Longo WE, et al. Role of chronic catheterization in the development of bladder cancer in patients with spinal cord injury. *Urology*. 1999;53(2):292–297.

335. Kaufman JM, Fam B, Jacobs SC, et al. Bladder cancer and squamous metaplasia in spinal cord injury patients. *J Urol*. 1977;118:967–971.

336. Subramonian K, Cartwright RA, Harnden J, et al. Bladder cancer in patients with spinal cord injuries. *BJU Int*. 2004;93:739–742.

337. Gui-Zhong L, Li-Bo M. Bladder cancer in individuals with spinal cord injuries: a meta-analysis. *Spinal Cord*. 2017;55(4):341–345.

338. Maynard FM. Immobilization hypercalcemia following spinal cord injury. *Arch Phys Med Rehabil*. 1986;67:41–44.

339. Massagli TL, Cardenas DD. Immobilization hypercalcemia treatment with pamidronate disodium after spinal cord injury. *Arch Phys Med Rehabil*. 1999;80:998–1000.

340. Kedlaya D, Brandstater ME, Lee JK. Immobilization hypercalcemia in incomplete paraplegia: successful treatment with pamidronate. *Arch Phys Med Rehabil*. 1998;79:222–225.

341. de Bruin ED, Frey-Rindova P, Herzog RE, et al. Changes of tibia bone properties after spinal cord injury: effects of early intervention. *Arch Phys Med Rehabil*. 1999;80(2):214–220.

342. Meythaler JM, Tuel SM, Cross LL. Successful treatment of immobilization hypercalcemia using calcitonin and etidronate. *Arch Phys Med Rehabil*. 1993;74: 316–319.

343. Garland DE, Stewart CA, Adkins RH, et al. Osteoporosis after spinal cord injury. *J Orthop Res*. 1992;10:371–378.

344. Biering-Sorensen F, Bohr H. Bone mineral content of the lumbar spine and lower extremities years after spinal cord lesion. *Paraplegia*. 1988;26:293–301.

345. Wilmet E, Ismail A, Heilporn A, et al. Longitudinal study of bone mineral content and soft tissue composition after spinal cord section. *Paraplegia*. 1995;33(11): 674–677.

346. Edwards WB, Schnitzer TJ, Troy KL. Bone mineral and stiffness loss at the distal femur and proximal tibia in acute spinal cord injury. *Osteoporosis Int*. 2014;25:1005–1015.

347. Garland DE, Adkins RH, Scott M, et al. Risk factors for osteoporosis at the knee in the spinal cord injury population. *J Spinal Cord Med*. 2004:202–269.

348. Giangregorio L, McCartney N. Bone loss and muscle atrophy in spinal cord injury: epidemiology, fracture prediction, and rehabilitation strategies. *J Spinal Cord Med*. 2006;29:489–500.

349. Dolbow DR, Gorgery AS, Daniels JA, et al. The effects of spinal cord injury and exercise on bone mass: a literature review. *NeuroRehabilitation*. 2011;29(3):261–269.

350. Belanger M, Stein R, Wheeler G, et al. Electrical stimulation: can it increase muscle strength and reverse osteoporosis in spinal cord injured individuals. *Arch Phys Med Rehabil*. 2000;81:1090–1098.

351. Ben M, Harvey L, Denis S, et al. Does 12 weeks of regular standing prevent loss of ankle mobility and bone mineral density in people with recent spinal cord injuries? *Aust J Physiother*. 2005;51:251–256.

352. Chen SC, Lai CH, Chan WP, et al. Increases in bone mineral density after functional electrical stimulation cycling exercises in spinal cord injured patients. *Disabil Rehabil*. 2005;27:1337–1341.

353. Clark JM, Jelbart M, Rischbieth H, et al. Physiological effects of lower extremity functional electrical stimulation in early spinal cord injury: lack of efficacy to prevent bone loss. *Spinal Cord*. 2007;45:78–85.

354. Harktopp A, Murphy R, Mohr T, et al. Bone fracture during electrical stimulation of the quadriceps in a spinal cord injured subject. *Arch Phys Med Rehabil*. 1998;79(9):1133–1136.

355. Craven BC, Robertson LA, McGillivray CF, et al. Detection and treatment of sublesional osteoporosis among patients with chronic spinal cord injury: proposed paradigms. *Top Spinal Cord Inj Rehabil*. 2009;14(4):1–22.

356. Bauman WA, Morrison NG, Spungen AM. Vitamin D replacement in persons with spinal cord injury. *J Spinal Cord Med*. 2005;28(3):203–207.

357. Bauman WA, Cardozo CP. Osteoporosis in individuals with spinal cord injury. *PM R*. 2015;7(2):188–201; quiz 201.

358. Bauman WA, Wecht JM, Kirshblum S, et al. Effect of pamidronate administration on bone in patients with acute spinal cord injury. *J Rehabil Res Dev*. 2005;42:305–313.

359. Shapiro J, Smith B, Beck T, et al. Treatment with zoledronic acid ameliorates negative geometric changes in the proximal femur following acute spinal cord injury. *Calcif Tissue Int*. 2007;80:316–322.

360. Bauman WA, Cirnigliaro CM, La Fountaine MF, et al. Zoledronic acid administration failed to prevent bone loss at the knee in persons with acute spinal cord injury: an observational cohort study. *J Bone Miner Metab*. 2015;33(4):410–421.

361. Craven C, Lynch CL, Eng JJ. Bone health following spinal cord injury. In: Eng JJ, Teasell RW, Miller WC, et al., eds. *Spinal Cord Injury Rehabilitation Evidence*. Version 5.0. Vancouver; 2014:1–37.

362. Biering-Sorensen F, Hansen B, Lee BS. Non-pharmacological treatment and prevention of bone loss after spinal cord injury: a systematic review. *Spinal Cord*. 2009;47(7):508–518.

363. Ashe MC, Craven BC, Eng JJ, et al. Prevention and treatment of bone loss after a spinal cord injury: a systematic review. *Top Spinal Cord Inj Rehabil*. 2007;13(1):123–145.

364. Bryson JE, Gourlay ML. Bisphosphonate use in acute and chronic spinal cord injury: a systematic review. *J Spinal Cord Med*. 2009;32(3):215–225.

365. Comarr AE, Hutchinson RH, Bors E. Extremity fractures of patients with spinal cord injuries. *Am J Surg*. 1962;103:732–739.

366. Freehafer AA. Limb fractures in patients with spinal cord injury. *Arch Phys Med Rehabil*. 1995;76:823–827.

367. Zehnder Y, Luthi M, Michel D, et al. Long term changes in bone metabolism, bone mineral density, quantitative ultrasound parameters, and fracture incidence after spinal cord injury: a cross sectional observational study in 100 paraplegic men. *Osteoporosis Int*. 2004;15(3):180–189.

368. Vertergard P, Krogh K, Rejnmark L, et al. Fracture rates and risk factors for fractures in patients with spinal cord injury. *Spinal Cord*. 1998;36:790–796.

369. Nelson A, Ahmed S, Harrow J, et al. Fall-related fractures in persons with spinal cord impairment: a descriptive analysis. *SCI Nurs*. 2003;20:30–37.

370. Subbarao JV, Garrison SJ. Heterotopic ossification: diagnosis and management, current concepts and controversies. *J Spinal Cord Med*. 1999;22:273–283.

371. Colachis SC III, Clinchot DM, Venesy D. Neurovascular complications of heterotopic ossification following spinal cord injury. *Paraplegia*. 1993;31:51–57.

372. Citak M, Suero EM, Backhaus M, et al. Risk factors for heterotopic ossification in patients with spinal cord injury: a case-control study of 264 patients. *Spine*. 2012;37(23):1953–1957.

373. Pape HC, Marsh S, Morley JR, et al. Current concepts in the development of heterotopic ossification. *J Bone Joint Surg Br*. 2004;86B(6):783–787.

374. McIntyre A, Thompson S, Mehta S, et al. Heterotopic ossification following spinal cord injury. In: Eng JJ, Teasell RW, Miller WC, et al., eds. *Spinal Cord Injury Rehabilitation Evidence (SCIRE)*. Version 5.0; 2014:1–19.

375. Singh RS, Craig MC, Katholi CR, et al. Predictive value of creatine phosphokinase and alkaline phosphatase in identification of heterotopic ossification in patients after spinal cord injury. *Arch Phys Med Rehabil*. 2003;84:1584–1588.

376. Sherman AL, Williams J, Patrick L, et al. The value of serum creatine kinase in early diagnosis of heterotopic ossification. *J Spinal Cord Med*. 2003;26: 227–231.

377. Estores I, Harrington A, Banovac K. C-reactive protein and ESR rate in patients with HO. *J Spinal Cord Med*. 2004;27:434–437.

378. Freed JH, Hahn H, Menter R, et al. Use of the three phase bone scan in the early diagnosis of heterotopic ossification and in the evaluation of didronel therapy. *Paraplegia*. 1982;20:208–216.

379. van Kuijk AA, Geurts ACH, van Kuppevelt HJM. Neurogenic heterotopic ossification in spinal cord injury. *Spinal Cord*. 2002;40(7):313–326.

380. Cassar-Pulicino VN, McCleland M, Badwan DAH, et al. Sonographic diagnosis of heterotopic bone formation in spinal cord patients. *Paraplegia*. 1993;31: 40–50.

381. Wick L, Berger M, Knecht H. Magnetic resonance signal alterations in the acute onset of heterotopic ossification in patients with spinal cord injury. *Eur Radiol*. 2005;15(9):1867–1875.

382. Alibrahim F, McIntyre A, Serrato J, et al. Heterotopic ossification following spinal cord injury. In: Eng JJ, Teasell RW, Miller WC, et al., eds. *Spinal Cord Injury Rehabilitation Evidence*. Version 6.0; 2016:1–20.

383. Brooker AF, Bowerman JW, Robinson RA, et al. Ectopic ossification following total hip-replacement—incidence and a method of classification. *J Bone Joint Surg Am*. 1973;55(8):1629–1632.

384. Finerman GAM, Stover SL. Heterotopic ossification following hip-replacement or spinal-cord injury—2 clinical-studies with EHDP. *Metab Bone Dis Relat Res*. 1981;3(4–5):337–342.

385. Garland DE, Orwin JF. Resection of heterotopic ossification in patients with spinal-cord injuries. *Clin Orthop Relat Res*. 1989;242:169–176.

386. Mavrogenis AF, Guerra G, Staals EL, et al. A classification method for neurogenic heterotopic ossification of the hip. *J Orthop Traumatol*. 2012;13(2):69–78.

387. Crawford C, Varghese G, Mani MM, et al. Heterotopic ossification: Are range of motion exercises contraindicated? *J Burn Care Rehabil*. 1986;7:323–327.

388. Subbarao JV, Nemchausky B, Gratzer M. Resection of heterotopic ossification and Didronel therapy—regaining wheelchair independence in the spinal cord injured patient. *J Am Paraplegia Soc*. 1987;10:3–7.

389. Snoecx M, Demuynck M, Vanlaere M. Association between muscle trauma and heterotopic ossification in spinal-cord injured patients—reflections on their causal relationship and the diagnostic-value of ultrasonography. *Paraplegia.* 1995;33(8):464–468.

390. Stover SL, Hahn HR, Miller JM III. Disodium etidronate in the prevention of heterotopic ossification following spinal cord injury (preliminary report). *Paraplegia.* 1976;14(2):146–156.

391. Banovac K, Williams JM, Patrick LD, et al. Prevention of heterotopic ossification after spinal cord injury with indomethacin. *Spinal Cord.* 2001;39(7):370–374.

392. Buschbacher R, McKinley W, Buschbacher L, et al. Warfarin in prevention of heterotopic ossification. *Am J Phys Med Rehabil.* 1992;71:86–91.

393. Banovac K, Sherman AL, Estrores IM, et al. Prevention and treatment of heterotopic ossification after spinal cord injury. *J Spinal Cord Med.* 2004;27(4):376–382.

394. Banovac K, Gonzalez F, Wade N, et al. Intravenous disodium etidronate therapy in spinal-cord injury patients with heterotopic ossification. *Paraplegia.* 1993;31(10):660–666.

395. Banovac K, Williams JM, Patrick LD, et al. Prevention of heterotopic ossification after spinal cord injury with COX-2 selective inhibitor (rofecoxib). *Spinal Cord.* 2004;42(12):707–710.

396. Durović A, Miljković D, Brdareski Z, et al. Pulse low-intensity electromagnetic field as prophylaxis of heterotopic ossification in patients with traumatic spinal cord injury. *Vojnosanit Pregl.* 2009;66(1):22–28.

397. Sautter-Bihl ML, Liebermeister E, Nanassy A. Radiotherapy as a local treatment option for heterotopic ossifications in patients with spinal cord injury. *Spinal Cord.* 2000;38(1):33–36.

398. Banaovac K, Renfree K, Hornicek F. Heterotopic ossification after brain and spinal cord injury. *Crit Rev Phys Rehabil Med.* 1998;10:223–256.

399. McAuliffe JA, Wolfson AH. Early excision of heterotopic ossification about the elbow followed by radiation therapy. *J Bone Joint Surg Am.* 1997;79A(5):749–755.

400. van Kuijk AA, van Kuppevelt HJM, van der Schaaf DB. Osteonecrosis after treatment for heterotopic ossification in spinal cord injury with the combination of surgery, irradiation, and an NSAID. *Spinal Cord.* 2000;38(5):319–324.

401. Freebourn TM, Barber DB, Able AC. The treatment of immature heterotopic ossification in spinal cord injury with combination surgery, radiation therapy and NSAID. *Spinal Cord.* 1999;37(1):50–53.

402. Schuetz P, Mueller B, Christ-Crain M, et al. Amino-bisphosphonates in heterotopic ossification: first experience in five consecutive cases. *Spinal Cord.* 2005;43(10):604–610.

403. Meiners T, Abel R, Bohm V, et al. Resection of heterotopic ossification of the hip in spinal cord injured patients. *Spinal Cord.* 1997;35(7):443–445.

404. Dyson-Hudson TA, Kirshblum SC. Shoulder pain in chronic spinal cord injury. Part I: epidemiology, etiology, and pathomechanics. *J Spinal Cord Med.* 2004;27: 4–17.

405. Irwin RW, Restrepo A, Sherman A. Musculoskeletal pain in persons with spinal cord injury. *Top Spinal Cord Inj Rehabil.* 2007;13:43–57.

406. Curtis KA, Drysdale GA, Lanza RD, et al. Shoulder pain in wheelchair users with tetraplegia and paraplegia. *Arch Phys Med Rehabil.* 1999;80:453–457.

407. Goldstein B. Musculoskeletal complications after spinal cord injury. *Phys Med Rehabil Clin N Am.* 2000;11:91–108.

408. Curtis KA, Roach KE, Applegate EB, et al. Development of the Wheelchair User's Shoulder Pain Index (WUSPI). *Paraplegia.* 1995;33:290–293.

409. Curtis KA, Roach KE, Applegate EB, et al. Reliability and validity of the wheelchair user's shoulder pain index (WUSPI). *Paraplegia.* 1995;33:595–601.

410. Curtis KA, Tyner TM, Zachary L, et al. Effect of a standard exercise protocol on shoulder pain in long-term wheelchair users. *Spinal Cord.* 1999;37:421–429.

411. Hastings J, Goldstein B. Paraplegia and the shoulder. *Phys Med Rehabil Clin N Am.* 2004;15:699–718.

412. Robinson MD, Hussey RW, Ha CY. Surgical decompression of impingement in the weight bearing shoulder. *Arch Phys Med Rehabil.* 1993;74:324–327.

413. Popowitz RL, Zvijac JE, Uribe JW, et al. Rotator cuff repair in spinal cord injury patients. *J Shoulder Elbow Surg.* 2003;12:327–332.

414. Yang J, Boninger ML, Leath JD, et al. Carpal tunnel syndrome in manual wheelchair users with spinal cord injury. *Am J Phys Med Rehabil.* 2009;88:1007–1016.

415. Nemchausky BA, Ubilluz RM. Upper extremity neuropathies in patients with spinal cord injuries. *J Spinal Cord Med.* 1995;18:95–97.

416. Kirshblum S, Druin E, Planten K. Musculoskeletal conditions in chronic spinal cord injury. *Top Spinal Cord Inj Rehabil.* 1997;2:23–35.

417. Standaert C, Cardenas DD, Anderson P. Charcot spine as a late complication of traumatic spinal cord injury. *Arch Phys Med Rehabil.* 1997;78:221–225.

418. Waters RL, Muccitelli LM. Tendon transfers to improve function of patients with tetraplegia. In: Kirshblum SC, Campagnolo D, DeLisa JE, eds. *Spinal Cord Medicine.* Philadelphia, PA: Lippincott Williams & Wilkins; 2002:424–438.

419. Pedretti LW. Occupational performance: a model for practice in physical dysfunction. In: Pedretti LW, ed. *Occupational Therapy Practice Skills for Physical Dysfunction.* 4th ed. St. Louis, MO: Mosby; 1996:3–12.

420. McDowell CL, Moberg EA, House JH. Third International Conference on surgical rehabilitation of the upper limb in tetraplegia. *J Hand Surg Am.* 1989;4(6): 1064–1066.

421. McDowell CL, Moberg EA, Smith AG. International conference on surgical rehabilitation of the upper limb in tetraplegia. *J Hand Surg Am.* 1979;4(4): 387–390.

422. Moberg E, Freehafer AA, Lamb DK, et al. International federation of societies for surgery of the hand. A report from the committee on spinal injuries 1980. *Scand J Rehabil Med.* 1982;14:3–5.

423. Moberg E. Surgical rehabilitation of the upper limb in tetraplegia. *Paraplegia.* 1990;28:330–334.

424. Lipscomb PR, Elkins EC, Henderson ED. Tendon transfers to restore function of hands in tetraplegia, especially after fracture dislocation of the sixth cervical vertebra on the seventh. *J Bone Joint Surg Am.* 1958;40-A(5):1071–1080.

425. Friden J, Gohritz A. Tetraplegia management update. *J Hand Surg Am.* 2015;40:2489–2500.

426. Friden J, Reinholdt C. Current concepts in reconstruction of hand function in tetraplegia. *Scand J Surg.* 2008;97:341–346.

427. Zlotolow DA. The role of the upper extremity surgeon in the management of tetraplegia. *J Hand Surg Am.* 2011;36A:929–935.

428. Freehafer AA. Tendon transfers in patients with cervical spinal cord injury. *J Hand Surg Am.* 1991;16A:804–809.

429. Johnson DL, Gellman H, Waters RL, et al. Brachioradialis transfer for wrist extension in tetraplegic patients who have fifth-cervical-level neurological function. *J Bone Joint Surg.* 1996;78A:1063–1067.

430. Raczka R, Braun R, Waters RL. Posterior deltoid-to-triceps transfer in quadriplegia. *Clin Orthop.* 1984;187:163–167.

431. Revol M, Briand E, Servant JM. Biceps-to-triceps transfer in tetraplegia. The medial route. *J Hand Surg Br.* 1999;24:235–237.

432. Kuz JE, Van Heest AE, House JH. Biceps-to-triceps transfer in tetraplegic patients: report of the medial routing technique and follow-up of three cases. *J Hand Surg Am.* 1999;24(1):161–172.

433. Moberg E. *The Upper Limb in Tetraplegia: A "New Approach" to Surgical Rehabilitation.* Stuttgart, NY: George Thieme; 1978.

434. Moberg EA. The present state of surgical rehabilitation for the upper limb in tetraplegia. *Paraplegia.* 1987;25:351–356.

435. Reiser TV, Waters RL. Long term follow up of the Moberg key grip procedure. *J Hand Surg Am.* 1986;11A:724–728.

436. Water R, Moore K, Graboff S, et al. Brachioradialis to flexor pollicis longus tendon transfer for active lateral pinch in the tetraplegic. *J Hand Surg Am.* 1985;10A(3):385–391.

437. House JH, Shannon M. Restoration of strong grasp and lateral pinch in tetraplegia: a comparison of two methods of thumb control in each patient. *Hand Surg.* 1985;10A:22–29.

438. Gansel J, Waters RL, Geilman H. Pronator teres to flexor digitorum profundus transfer in quadriplegia. *J Bone Joint Surg.* 1990;72A:427–432.

439. Paul SD, Gellman H, Waters R, et al. Single-stage reconstruction of key pinch and extension of the elbow in tetraplegic patients. *J Bone Joint Surg.* 1994;76(A): 1451–1456.

440. Gellman H, Kan D, Waters RL, et al. Rerouting of the biceps brachii for paralytic supination contracture of the forearm in tetraplegia due to trauma. *J Bone Joint Surg.* 1994;76A:398–402.

441. Gellman H. The hand and upper limb in tetraplegia. *Curr Orthop.* 1991;5: 233–238.

442. Vastamaki M. Short-term versus long-term comparative results after reconstructive upper-limb surgery in tetraplegic patients. *J Hand Surg Am.* 2006;31:1490–1494.

443. Wuolle KS, Bryden AM, Peckham PH, et al. Satisfaction with upper-extremity surgery in individuals with tetraplegia. *Arch Phys Med Rehabil.* 2003;84:1145–1149.

444. Peckham PH, Keith MW, Kilgore KL, et al. Implantable Neuroprosthesis Research Group. Efficacy of an implanted neuroprosthesis for restoring hand grasp in tetraplegia: a multicenter study. *Arch Phys Med Rehabil.* 2001;82:1380–1388.

445. Mulcahay MJ, Beta RR, Smith BT, et al. Implanted functional electrical stimulation hand system in adolescents with spinal injuries: an evaluation. *Arch Phys Med Rehabil.* 1997;78:597–607.

446. Hobby J, Taylor PN, Esnouf J. Restoration of tetraplegic hand function by use of the Neurocontrol Freehand System. *J Hand Surg Am.* 2001;26:459–464.

447. Kilgore KL, Peckham PH, Keith MW, et al. Advanced control alternatives for upper extremity neuroprosthetic systems (abstract). *J Spinal Cord Med.* 2002;25: 228–229.

448. Memberg WD, Polasek KH, Hart RL, et al. Implanted neuroprosthesis for restoring arm and hand function in people with high level tetraplegia. *Arch Phys Med Rehabil.* 2014;95(6):1201–1211.

449. Fox IK. Nerve Transfers in Tetraplegia. *Hand Clin.* 2016;32(2):227–242.

450. Peckham PH, Kilgore KL. Challenges and opportunities in restoring function after paralysis. *IEEE Trans Biomed Eng.* 2013;60(3):602–609.

451. Consortium for Spinal Cord Medicine. Pressure ulcer prevention and treatment following spinal cord injury: a clinical practice guideline for health care professionals. 2000:1–77.

452. Kirshblum S, O'Connor K, Radar C. Pressure ulcers and spinal cord injury. In: Kirshblum SC, Campagnolo D, eds. *Spinal Cord Medicine.* 2nd ed. Philadelphia, PA: Lippincott Williams & Wilkins; 2011:242–264.

453. Chen Y, DeVivo MJ, Jackson AB. Pressure ulcer prevalence in people with spinal cord injury: age-period-duration effects. *Arch Phys Med Rehabil.* 2005;86: 1208–1213.

454. Ploumis A, Kolli S, Patrick M, et al. Length of stay and medical stability for spinal cord-injured patients on admission to an inpatient rehabilitation hospital: a comparison between a model SCI trauma center and non-SCI trauma center. *Spinal Cord.* 2011;49(3):411–415.

455. Verschueren JH, Post MW, de Groot S, et al. Occurrence and predictors of pressure ulcers during primary in-patient spinal cord injury rehabilitation. *Spinal Cord.* 2011;49:106–112.

456. DeJong G, Hsieh CJ, Brown P, et al. Factors associated with pressure ulcers in spinal cord injury rehabilitation. *Am J Phys Med Rehabil.* 2014;93:971–986.

457. Scheel-Sailer A, Wyss A, Boldt C, et al. Prevalence, location, grade of pressure ulcers and association with specific patient characteristics in adult spinal cord injury patients during the hospital stay: a prospective cohort study. *Spinal Cord.* 2013;51:828–833.

458. Cardenas DD, Hoffman JM, Kirshblum S, et al. Etiology and incidence of rehospitalization after traumatic spinal cord injury: a multicenter analysis. *Arch Phys Med Rehabil.* 2004;85(11):1757–1763.

459. National Pressure Ulcer Advisory Panel (NPUAP). Pressure ulcers prevalence, cost and risk assessment: consensus development conference statement. *Decubitus.* 1989;2:24–28.

460. National Pressure Ulcer Advisory Panel. Pressure Ulcer Stages Revised by NPUAP. 2016. Available from: http://www.npuap.org/resources/educational-and-clinical-resources/pressure-injury-staging-illustrations/. Accessed June 1, 2016.

461. Hsieh J, McIntyre A, Wolfe D, et al. Pressure ulcers following spinal cord injury. In: Eng JJ, Teasell RW, Miller WC, et al., eds. *Spinal Cord Injury Rehabilitation Evidence.* Version 5.0; 2014:1–90.

462. Dumurgier C, Pujol G, Chevalley J, et al. Pressure sore carcinoma: a late but fulminant complication of pressure sores in spinal cord injury patients: case reports. *Paraplegia.* 1991;29:390–395.

463. Regan MA, Teasell RW, Wolfe DL, et al. A systemic review of therapeutic interventions for pressure ulcers after spinal cord injury. *Arch Phys Med Rehabil.* 2009;19:213–231.

464. Makhsous M, Priebe M, Bankard J, et al. Measuring tissue perfusion during pressure relief maneuvers: insights into preventing pressure ulcers. *J Spinal Cord Med.* 2007;30(5):497–507.

465. Jan YK, Jones MA, Rabadi MH, et al. Effect of wheelchair tilt-in-space and recline angles on skin perfusion over the ischial tuberosity in people with spinal cord injury. *Arch Phys Med Rehabil.* 2010;91(11):1758–1764.

466. Hobson DA. Comparative effects of posture on pressure and shear at the body-seat interface. *J Rehabil Res Dev.* 1992;15:21–31.

467. Jones KR, Fennie K, Lenihan A. Evidence-based management of chronic wounds. *Adv Skin Wound Care.* 2007;20(11):591–600.

468. de la Fuente SG, Levin LS, Reynolds JD, et al. Elective stoma construction improves outcomes in medically intractable pressure ulcers. *Dis Colon Rectum.* 2003;46(11):1525–1530.

469. Kruger EA, Pires M, Ngann Y, et al. Comprehensive management of pressure ulcers in spinal cord injury: current concepts and future trends. *J Spinal Cord Med.* 2013;36:572–585.

470. Biglari B, Buchler A, Reitzel T, et al. A retrospective study on flap complication after pressure ulcer surgery in spinal cord injured patients. *Spinal Cord.* 2014;52:80–83.

471. Soden RJ, Walsh J, Middleton JW, et al. Causes of death after spinal cord injury. *Spinal Cord.* 2000;38:604–610.

472. Consortium for Spinal Cord Medicine. Respiratory management following spinal cord injury: a clinical practice guideline for health-care professionals. *J Spinal Cord Med.* 2005;28:259–293.

473. Jackson AB, Groomes TE. Incidence of respiratory complications following spinal cord injury. *Arch Phys Med Rehabil.* 1994;75:270–275.

474. Mansel JK, Norman JR. Respiratory complications and management of spinal cord injuries. *Chest.* 1990;97:1446–1452.

475. Ledsome JR, Sharp JM. Pulmonary function in acute cervical cord injury. *Am Rev Respir Dis.* 1981;124:41–44.

476. Morgan MD, Gourly AR, Silver JR, et al. The contribution of the rib cage to breathing in tetraplegia. *Thorax.* 1985;40:613–617.

477. Roth EJ, Nussbaum SB, Berkowitz M, et al. Pulmonary function testing in spinal cord injury: correlation with vital capacity. *Paraplegia.* 1995;33:454–457.

478. Almenoff PL, Spungen AM, Lesser M, et al. Pulmonary function survey in spinal cord injury: influence of smoking and level and completeness of injury. *Lung.* 1995;173:297–306.

479. Linn WS, Adkins RH, Gong H Jr, et al. Pulmonary function in chronic spinal cord injury: a cross-sectional survey of 222 southern California adult outpatients. *Arch Phys Med Rehabil.* 2000;81:757–763.

480. Peterson WP, Barbalata L, Brooks CA. The effect of tidal volumes on the time to wean persons with high tetraplegia from ventilators. *Spinal Cord.* 1999;37:284–288.

481. Petersen WP, Kirshblum SC. Respiratory management in spinal cord injury. In: Kirshblum SC, Campagnolo D, DeLisa JE, eds. *Spinal Cord Medicine.* Philadelphia, PA: Lippincott Williams & Wilkins; 2002:135–154.

482. Fenton JJ, Warner ML, Lammertse D, et al. A comparison of high vs standard tidal volumes in ventilator weaning for individuals with subacute spinal cord injuries: a site specific randomized clinical trial. *Spinal Cord.* 2016;54(3):234–238.

483. Wicks AB, Menter RR. Long-term outlook in quadriplegic patients with initial ventilator dependency. *Chest.* 1986;90:406–410.

484. Gardner BP, Watt JW, Krishnan KR. The artificial ventilation of acute spinal cord damaged patients: a retrospective study of forty-four patients. *Paraplegia.* 1986;24:208–220.

485. Peterson P, Brooks CA, Mellick D, et al. Protocol for ventilator management in high tetraplegia. *Top Spinal Cord Inj Rehabil.* 1997;2:101–106.

486. Peterson W, Charlifue W, Gerhart A, et al. Two methods of weaning persons with quadriplegia from mechanical ventilators. *Paraplegia.* 1994;32:98–103.

487. Bach JR. Indications for tracheostomy and decannulation of tracheostomized ventilator users. *Monaldi Arch Chest Dis.* 1995;50:223–227.

488. Kinney TB, Rose SC, Valji K, et al. Does Cervical spinal cord injury induce a higher incidence of complications after prophylactic Greenfield filter usage? *J Vasc Interv Radiol.* 1996;7:907–915.

489. Garstang SV, Kirshblum SC, Wood KE. Patient preference for in-exsufflation for secretion management in spinal cord injury. *J Spinal Cord Med.* 2000;23:80–85.

490. Estenne M, DeTroyer A. Mechanism of the postural dependence of vital capacity in tetraplegic subjects. *Am Rev Respir Dis.* 1987;135:367–371.

491. Maloney FP. Pulmonary function in quadriplegia: effects of a corset. *Arch Phys Med Rehabil.* 1979;60:261–265.

492. Lin KW, Chuang CC, Wu HD, et al. Abdominal weight and inspiratory resistance: their immediate effects on inspiratory muscle functions during maximal voluntary breathing in chronic tetraplegic patients. *Arch Phys Med Rehabil.* 1999;80:741–745.

493. Bach JR, Alba AS. Non-invasive options for ventilatory support of the traumatic high level quadriplegic. *Chest.* 1990;98:613–619.

494. Weaver FM, Goldstein B, Evans CT, et al. Influenza vaccination among veterans with spinal cord injury: Part 2. Increasing vaccination rates. *J Spinal Cord Med.* 2003;26:210–218.

495. Ludec BE, Dagher JH, Mayer P, et al. Estimated prevalence of obstructive sleep apnea-hypopnea syndrome after cervical cord injury. *Arch Phys Med Rehabil.* 2007;88:333–337.

496. Burns SP, Rad MY, Bryant S, et al. Long-term treatment of sleep apnea in persons with spinal cord injury. *Am J Phys Med Rehabil.* 2005;84:620–626.

497. Berlowitz D, Brown D, Campbell D, et al. A longitudinal evaluation of sleep and breathing in the first year after cervical spinal cord injury. *Arch Phys Med Rehabil.* 2005;86:1193–1199.

498. Sankari A, Martin JL, Bascom AT, et al. Identification and treatment of sleep-disordered breathing in chronic spinal cord injury. *Spinal Cord.* 2015;53(2):145–149.

499. Chiodo AE, Sitrin RG, Bauman KA. Sleep disordered breathing in spinal cord injury: a systematic review. *J Spinal Cord Med.* 2016;39(4):374–382.

500. Bauman KA, Kurili A, Schotland HM, et al. Simplified approach to diagnosing sleep-disordered breathing and nocturnal hypercapnia in individuals with spinal cord injury. *Arch Phys Med Rehabil.* 2016;97(3):363–371.

501. Bombardier CH, Lee DC, Tan DL, et al. Comorbid traumatic brain injury and spinal cord injury: screening validity and effect on outcomes. *Arch Phys Med Rehabil.* 2016;97:1628–1634.

502. Macciocchi S, Seel RT, Thompson N, et al. Spinal cord injury and co-occurring traumatic brain injury: assessment and incidence. *Arch Phys Med Rehabil.* 2008;89:1350–1357.

503. Sommer JL, Witkiiwicz PM. The therapeutic challenges of dual diagnosis: TBI/SCI. *Brain Inj.* 2004;18:1297–1308.

504. Macciocchi S, Seel RT, Warshowsky A, et al. Co-Occurring traumatic brain injury and acute spinal cord injury rehabilitation outcomes. *Arch Phys Med Rehabil.* 2012;93:1788–1794.

505. Brown L, Hagglund K, Bua G, et al. Spinal cord injury and concomitant traumatic brain injury. *Am J Phys Med Rehabil.* 1988;67:211–216.

506. Brown M, Vandergoot D. Quality of life for individuals with traumatic brain injury: comparison with others living in the community. *J Head Trauma Rehabil.* 1998;13:1–23.

507. Kreuter M, Sullivan M, Dahlof A, et al. Partner relationships, functioning, mood and global quality of life in person with spinal cord injury and traumatic brain injury. *Spinal Cord.* 1998;36:252–261.

508. Macciocchi SN, Bowman B, Coker J, et al. Effect of co-morbid traumatic brain injury on functional outcome of persons with spinal cord injuries. *Am J Phys Med Rehabil.* 2004;83:22–26.

509. Ullrich PM. Pain following spinal cord injury. *Phys Med Rehabil Clin N Am.* 2007;18:217–233.

510. Yerzierski RP. Pain following spinal cord injury: the clinical problem and experimental studies. *Pain.* 1996;68:185–194.

511. Cardenas DD, Jensen MP. Treatments for chronic pain in persons with spinal cord injury: a survey study. *J Spinal Cord Med.* 2006;29:109–117.

512. Finnerup NB, Johannesen IL, Sindrup SH, et al. Pain and dysesthesia in patients with spinal cord injury: a postal survey. *Spinal Cord.* 2001;39:256–262.

513. Jensen TS, Hoffman AJ, Cardenas DD. Chronic pain in individuals with spinal cord injury: a survey and longitudinal study. *Spinal Cord.* 2005;43:704–712.

514. Budh CN, Osteraker AL. Life satisfaction in individuals with a spinal cord injury and pain. *Clin Rehabil.* 2007;21:89–96.

515. Westgren N, Levi R. Quality of life and traumatic spinal cord injury. *Arch Phys Med Rehabil.* 1998;79:1433–1439.

516. Siddall PJ, Yezierski RP, Loeser JD. Pain following spinal cord injury: clinical features, prevalence, and taxonomy. *IASP News.* 2000;3:3–7. Available from: http://www.iasp-pain.org/AM/Template.cfm?Section=Technical_Corner&Template=/CM/ContentDisplay.cfm&ContentID=2179

517. Bryce TN, Rgnarsson KT. Pain management in persons with spinal cord injury. In: Lin VW, Cardenas DD, Cutter NC, et al., eds. *Spinal Cord Medicine: Principles and Practice.* New York: Demos Medical Publishing; 2003:441–460.

518. Cardenas DD, Turner JA, Warms CA, et al. Classification of chronic pain associated with spinal cord injury. *Arch Phys Med Rehabil.* 2002;83:1708–1714.

519. Bryce TN, Biering-Sorensen F, Finnerup NB, et al. International Spinal Cord Injury Pain Classification: part 1. Background and description. *Spinal Cord.* 2012;50:413–417.

520. Bryce TN, Biering-Sorensen F, Finnerup NB, et al. International Spinal Cord Injury Pain Classification: part 2. Initial validation using vignettes. *Spinal Cord.* 2012;50:404–412.

521. Widerström-Noga E, Biering-Sørensen F, Bryce TN, et al. The international spinal cord injury pain basic data set (version 2.0). *Spinal Cord.* 2014;52(4):282–286.

522. Widerström-Noga E, Biering-Sørensen F, Bryce TN, et al. The international spinal cord injury pain basic data set. *Spinal Cord.* 2008;46(12):818–823.

523. Widerström-Noga E, Biering-Sørensen F, Bryce TN, et al. The International Spinal Cord Injury Pain Extended Data Set (Version 1.0). *Spinal Cord.* 2016;54(11):1036–1046.

524. Finnerup NB. Pain in patients with spinal cord injury. *Pain.* 2013;54:S71–S76.

525. Boldt I, Eriks-Hoogland I, Brinkhof MW, et al. Non-pharmacological interventions for chronic pain in people with spinal cord injury. *Cochrane Database Syst Rev.* 2014;(11):CD009177.

526. Levendoglu F, Ogun CO, Ozerbil O, et al. Gabapentin is a first line drug for the treatment of neuropathic pain in spinal cord injury. *Spine.* 2004;29:743–751.

527. Siddall PJ, Cousins MJ, Otte A, et al. Pregabalin in central neuropathic pain associated with spinal cord injury: a placebo-controlled trial. *Neurology.* 2006;67:1792–1800.

528. Mehta S, McIntyre A, Dijkers M, et al. Gabapentinoids are effective in decreasing neuropathic pain and other secondary outcomes after spinal cord injury: a meta-analysis. *Arch Phys Med Rehabil.* 2014;95:2180–2186.

529. Guy SD, Mehta S, Casalino A, et al. The CanPain SCI clinical practice guidelines for rehabilitation management of neuropathic pain after spinal cord injury: recommendations for treatment. *Spinal Cord.* 2016;54:S14–S23.

530. Mehta S, McIntyre A, Janzen S, et al. Systematic review of pharmacologic treatments of pain after spinal cord injury: an update. *Arch Phys Med Rehabil.* 2016;97:1381–1391.

531. Vranken JH, Hollmann MW, van der Vegt MN, et al. Duloxetine in patients with central neuropathic pain caused by spinal cord injury or stroke: a randomized, double blind, placebo controlled trial. *Pain.* 2011;152:267–273.

532. Cioni B, Meglio M, Pentimalli L, et al. Spinal cord stimulation in the treatment of paraplegic pain. *J Neurosurg.* 1995;82:35–39.

533. Vaarwerk I, Staal M. Spinal cord stimulation in chronic pain syndromes. *Spinal Cord.* 1998;36:671–682.

534. Friedman AH, Nashold BS Jr. DREZ lesions for relief of pain related to spinal cord injury. *J Neurosurg.* 1986;65:465–469.

535. Schurch B, Wichmann W, Rossier AB. Post traumatic syringomyelia (cystic myelopathy): a prospective study of 449 patients with spinal cord injury. *J Neurol Neurosurg Psychiatry.* 1996;60:61–67.

536. Rossier AB, Foo D, Shillito J, et al. Post-traumatic syringomyelia: incidence, clinical presentation, electrophysiological studies, syrinx protein and results of conservative and operative treatment. *Brain.* 1985;108:439–461.

537. Vannemreddy SS, Rowed DW, Bharatwal N. Posttraumatic syringomyelia: predisposing factors. *Br J Neurosurg.* 2002;16:276–283.

538. Krebs J, Koch HG, Hartmann K, et al. The characteristics of posttraumatic syringomyelia. *Spinal Cord.* 2016;54:463–466.

539. Karam Y, Hitchon PW, Mhanna NE, et al. Post-traumatic syringomyelia: outcome predictors. *Clin Neurol Neurosurg.* 2014;124:44–50.

540. Ko HY, Kim W, Kim SY, et al. Factors associated with early onset post-traumatic syringomyelia. *Spinal Cord.* 2012;50:695–698.

541. Sgouros S, Williams B. Management and outcome of posttraumatic syringomyelia. *J Neurosurg.* 1996;85:197–205.

542. Batzdorf U, Klekamp J, Johnson JP. A critical appraisal of syrinx cavity shunting procedures. *J Neurosurg.* 1998;89:382–388.

543. Laxton AW, Perrin RG. Cordectomy for the treatment of posttraumatic syringomyelia. Report of four cases and review of the literature. *J Neurosurg Spine.* 2006;4:174–178.

544. Maynard FM, Karunas R, Waring WW. Epidemiology of spasticity following traumatic spinal cord injury. *Arch Phys Med Rehabil.* 1990;71:566–569.

545. Levi R, Hultling C, Seiger A. The Stockholm Spinal Cord Injury Study: 2. Associations between clinical patient characteristics and post-acute medical problems. *Paraplegia.* 1995;33:585–594.

546. Ashworth B. Preliminary trial of carisoprodol in multiple sclerosis. *Practitioner.* 1964;192:540–542.

547. Bohannon RW, Smith MB. Interrater reliability of a modified Ashworth scale of muscle spasticity. *Phys Ther.* 1987;67:206–207.

548. Penn RD. Intrathecal baclofen for severe spasticity. *Ann N Y Acad Sci.* 1988;531:157–166.

549. Adams MM, Martin Ginis KA, Hicks AL. The spinal cord injury spasticity evaluation tool: development and evaluation. *Arch Phys Med Rehabil.* 2007;88:1185–1192.

550. Skold C. Spasticity in spinal cord injury: self and clinically rated fluctuations and intervention induced changes. *Arch Phys Med Rehabil.* 2000;81:144–149.

551. Wartenburg R. Pendulousness of the legs as a diagnostic test. *Neurology.* 1951;1:18–24.

552. Hseih JT, Wolfe DL, Miller WC, et al. Spasticity outcome measures in spinal cord injury: psychometric properties and clinical utility. *Spinal Cord.* 2008;42(2):86–95.

553. Kirshblum S. Treatment alternatives for spinal cord injury related spasticity. *J Spinal Cord Med.* 1999;22:199–217.

554. Carlson SJ. A neurophysiologic analysis of inhibitive casting. *Phys Occup Ther Pediatr.* 1985;4:31–42.

555. Hsieh JTC, Connolly SJ, McIntyre A, et al. Spasticity following spinal cord injury. In: Eng JJ, Teasell RW, Miller WC, et al., eds. *Spinal Cord Injury Rehabilitation Evidence.* Version 6.0. 2016.

556. Taricco M, Pagliacci MC, Telaro E, et al. Pharmacological interventions for spasticity following spinal cord injury: results of a Cochrane systematic review. *Eura Medicophys.* 2006;42(1):5–15.

557. Theriault ER, Huang V, Whiteneck G, et al. Antispasmodic medications may be associated with reduced recovery during inpatient rehabilitation after traumatic spinal cord injury. *J Spinal Cord Med.* 2016;39:1–9.

558. Schmidt KD, Chan CW. Thermoregulation and fever in normal persons and in those with spinal cord injuries. *Mayo Clin Proc.* 1992;67:469–475.

559. Menard MR, Hahn G. Acute and chronic hypothermia in a man with spinal cord injury: environmental and pharmacologic causes. *Arch Phys Med Rehabil.* 1991;72:421–424.

560. Khan S, Plummer M, Martinez-Arizala A, et al. Hypothermia in patients with chronic spinal cord injury. *J Spinal Cord Med.* 2007;30:27–30.

561. Krause JS, Kemo B, Coker J. Depression after spinal cord injury: relation to gender, ethnicity, aging and socioeconomic indicators. *Arch Phys Med Rehabil.* 2000;81:1099–1109.

562. Consortium of Spinal Cord Medicine. *Depression Following Spinal Cord Injury: A Clinical Practice Guideline For Primary Care Physicians.* Washington, DC: Paralyzed Veterans of America; 1998.

563. Fichtenbaum J, Kirshblum SC. Psychological adaptations after spinal cord injury. In: Kirshblum SC, Campagnolo D, DeLisa JE, eds. *Spinal Cord Medicine.* Philadelphia, PA: Lippincott Williams & Wilkins; 2002:299–311.

564. Dryden DM, Saunders LD, Rowe BH, et al. Depression following traumatic spinal cord injury. *Neuroepidemiology.* 2005;25:55–61.

565. DeVivo MJ, Black KJ, Richards JS, et al. Suicide following spinal cord injury. *Paraplegia.* 1991;29:620–627.

566. Heinemann AW. Spinal cord injury. In: Goreczny AJ, ed. *Handbook of Health and Rehabilitation Psychology.* New York: Plenum Press; 1995:341–360.

567. Charlifue SW, Gerhart K. Behavioral and demographic predictors of suicide following traumatic spinal cord injury. *Arch Phys Med Rehabil.* 1991;72:448–492.

568. Hartkopp A, Bronnum-Hansen H, Seidenschnur A, et al. Suicide in a spinal cord injured population: its relation to functional status. *Arch Phys Med Rehabil.* 1998;79:1356–1361.

569. Nielsen MS. Post-traumatic stress disorder and emotional distress in persons with spinal cord lesion. *Spinal Cord.* 2003;41:296–302.

570. Kennedy P, Evans MJ. Evaluation of post traumatic distress in the first 6 months following SCI. *Spinal Cord.* 2001;39:381–386.

571. Dorstyn D, Mathias J, Denison L. Efficacy of cognitive behavior therapy for the management of psychological outcomes following spinal cord injury: a meta-analysis. *J Health Psychol.* 2010;16:374–391.

572. Dorstyn D, Mathias J, Denison L, et al. Effectiveness of telephone counselling in managing psychological outcomes after spinal cord injury: a preliminary study. *Arch Phys Med Rehabil.* 2012;93:2100–2108.

573. Heutink M, Post MW, Bongers-Janssen HM, et al. The CONECSI trial: results of a randomized controlled trial of a multidisciplinary cognitive behavioral program for coping with chronic neuropathic pain after spinal cord injury. *Pain.* 2012;153:120–128.

574. Schultz R, Czaja SJ, Lustig A, et al. Improving quality of life of caregivers of persons with spinal cord injury: a randomized controlled trial. *Rehabil Psychol.* 2009;54:1–15.

575. Ginis KAM, Latimer AE, McKechnie K, et al. Using exercise to enhance subjective well-being among people with spinal cord injury: the mediating influences of stress and pain. *Rehabil Psychol.* 2003;48:157–164.

576. Hicks AL, Martin KA, Ditor DS, et al. Long-term exercise training in persons with spinal cord injury: effects on strength, arm ergometry performance and psychological well-being. *Spinal Cord.* 2003;41:34–43.

577. Latimer AE, Ginis KA, Hicks AL, et al. An examination of the mechanisms of exercise induced change in psychological well-being among people with spinal cord injury. *J Rehabil Res Dev.* 2004;41:643–652.

578. Kennedy P, Taylor N, Hindson L. A pilot investigation of a psychosocial activity course for people with spinal cord injuries. *Psychol Health Med.* 2006;11:91–99.

579. Tate DG. Alcohol use among spinal cord-injured patients. *Arch Phys Med Rehabil.* 1993;72:192–195.

580. Heinemann AW, Hawkins D. Substance abuse and medical complications following spinal cord injury. *Rehabil Psychol.* 1995;40:125–140.

581. Tate DG, Forschheimer MB, Krasue JS, et al. Patterns of alcohol and substance use and abuse in persons with spinal cord injury: risk factors and correlates. *Arch Phys Med Rehabil.* 2004;85:1837–1847.

582. Young ME, Rintala DH, Rossi D, et al. Alcohol and marijuana use in a community-based sample of persons with spinal cord injury. *Arch Phys Med Rehabil.* 1995;76:525–532.

583. Bombardier CH, Stroud MW, Esselman PC, et al. Do preinjury alcohol problems predict poorer rehabilitation progress in persons with spinal cord injury? *Arch Phys Med Rehabil.* 2004;85:1488–1492.

584. Heinemann AW, Goranson N, Ginsburg K, et al. Alcohol use and activity patterns following spinal cord injury. *Rehabil Psychol.* 1989;34:191–205.

585. Elliott S, McBride K. Sexual and reproductive health following spinal cord injury. In: Eng JJ, Teasell RW, Miller WC, et al., eds. *Spinal Cord Injury Rehabilitation Evidence.* Version 5.0. Vancouver; 2014:1–84.

586. Anderson KD. Targeting recovery: priorities of the spinal cord-injured population. *J Neurotrauma.* 2004;21:1371–1383.

587. Kennedy P, Lude P, Taylor N. Quality of life, social participation, appraisals and coping post spinal cord injury: a review of four community samples. *Spinal Cord.* 2006;44:95–105.

588. Brakett NL, Lynne CM, Sonksen J, et al. Sexual function and fertility after spinal cord injury. In: Kirshblum SC, Campagnolo D, eds. *Spinal Cord Medicine.* 2nd ed. Philadelphia, PA: Lippincott Williams & Wilkins; 2011:410–426.

589. Soler JM, Previnaire JG, Denys P, et al. Phosphodiesterase inhibitors in the treatment of erectile dysfunction in spinal cord-injured men. *Spinal Cord.* 2007;45:169–173.

590. Del Popolo G, Li Marzi V, Mondaini N, et al. Time/duration effectiveness of sildenafil versus tadalafil in the treatment of erectile dysfunction in male spinal cord-injured patients. *Spinal Cord.* 2004;42:643–648.

591. Maytom MC, Ferry FA, Dinsmore WW, et al. A two-part pilot study of sildenafil (VIAGRA) in men with erectile dysfunction caused by spinal cord injury. *Spinal Cord.* 1999;37:110–116.

592. Lloyd EE, Toth LL, Perkash I. Vacuum tumescence: an option for spinal cord injured males with erectile dysfunction. *SCI Nurs.* 1989;6:25–28.

593. Lloyd LK, Richards JS. Intracavernous pharmacotherapy for management of erectile dysfunction in spinal cord injury. *Paraplegia.* 1989;27:457–464.

594. Monga M, Bernie J, Rajasekaran M. Male infertility and erectile dysfunction in spinal cord injury: a review. *Arch Phys Med Rehabil.* 1999;80:1331–1339.

595. Padma-Nathan H, Hellstrom WJ, Kaiser FE, et al. Treatment of men with erectile dysfunction with transurethral alprostadil. Medicated Urethral System for Erection (MUSE) Study Group. *N Engl J Med.* 1997;336:1–7.

596. Bennett CJ, Seager SW, Vasher EA, et al. Sexual dysfunction and electroejaculation in men with spinal cord injury: review. *J Urol.* 1998;139:453–456.

597. Brown DJ, Hill ST, Baker HW. Male fertility and sexual function after spinal cord injury. *Prog Brain Res.* 2006;152:427–439.

598. Kafetsoulis A, Brackett NL, Ibrahim E, et al. Current trends in the treatment of infertility in men with spinal cord injury. *Fertil Steril.* 2006;86:781–789.

599. Bird VG, Brackett NL, Lynne CM, et al. Reflexes and somatic responses as predictors of ejaculation by penile vibratory stimulation in men with spinal cord injury. *Spinal Cord.* 2001;39:514–519.

600. Julia PE, Othman AS. Barriers to sexual activity: counseling spinal cord injured women in Malaysia. *Spinal Cord.* 2011;49:791–794.

601. Kreuter M, Taft C, Siösteen A, et al. Women's sexual functioning and sex life after spinal cord injury. *Spinal Cord.* 2011;49:154–160.

602. Jackson AB, Wadley V. A multicenter study of women's self-reported reproductive health after spinal cord injury. *Arch Phys Med Rehabil.* 1999;80:1420–1428.

603. Sipski ML. Spinal cord injury: what is the effect on sexual response? *J Am Paraplegia Soc.* 1991;14:40–43.

604. Sipski ML, Alexander CJ, Rosen R. Sexual arousal and orgasm in women: effects of spinal cord injury. *Ann Neurol.* 2001;49:35–44.

605. Sipski ML, Alexander CJ, Rosen RC. Physiologic parameters associated with sexual arousal in women with incomplete spinal cord injuries. *Arch Phys Med Rehabil.* 1997;78:305–313.

606. Sipski ML, Alexander CJ, Rosen RC. Physiological parameters associated with psychogenic sexual arousal in women with complete spinal cord injuries. *Arch Phys Med Rehabil.* 1995;76:811–818.

607. Anderson KD, Borisoff JF, Johnson RD, et al. Spinal cord injury influences psychogenic as well as physical components of female sexual ability. *Spinal Cord.* 2007;45:349–359.

608. Komisaruk BR, Whipple B, Crawford A, et al. Brain activation during vaginocervical self-stimulation and orgasm in women with complete spinal cord injury: fMRI evidence of mediation by the vagus nerves. *Brain Res.* 2004;1024:77–88.

609. Whipple B, Komisaruk BR. Sexuality and women with complete spinal cord injury. *Spinal Cord.* 1997;35:136–138.

610. Charlifue SW, Gerhart KA, Menter RR, et al. Sexual issues of women with spinal cord injuries. *Paraplegia.* 1992;30:192–199.

611. Sipski M, Alexander C, Rosen R. Orgasm in women with spinal cord injuries: a laboratory assessment. *Arch Phys Med Rehabil.* 1995;76(12):1097–1102.

612. Sipski ML, Rosen RC, Alexander CJ, et al. Sildenafil effects on sexual and cardiovascular responses in women with spinal cord injury. *Urology.* 2000;55:812–815.

613. Alexander MS, Rosen RC, Steinberg S, et al. Sildenafil in women with sexual arousal disorder following spinal cord injury. *Spinal Cord.* 2011;49:273–279.

614. Baker ER, Cardenas DD. Pregnancy in spinal cord injured women. *Arch Phys Med Rehabil.* 1996;77:501–507.

615. Camune BD. Challenges in the management of the pregnant woman with spinal cord injury. *J Perinat Neonatal Nurs.* 2013;27(3):225–231.

616. Pereira L. Obstetric management of the patient with spinal cord injury. *Obstet Gynecol Surv.* 2003;58:678–687.

617. Stillman MD, Barber J, Burns S, et al. Complications of spinal cord injury over the first year after discharge from inpatient rehabilitation. *Arch Phys Med Rehabil.* 2017;98(9):1800–1805.

618. Stillman MD, Frost KL, Smalley C, et al. Health care utilization and barriers experienced by individuals with spinal cord injury. *Arch Phys Med Rehabil.* 2014;95(6):1114–1126.

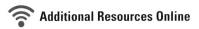 **Additional Resources Online**

CHAPTER 23

Nanette C. Joyce   Ileana Michelle Howard
Dorothy Weiss Tolchin   Sabrina Paganoni

Motor Neuron Disease

The emergence of physical medicine and rehabilitation as a specialty in the mid-20th century is inextricably linked to motor neuron disease (MND) because of the effects of the polio epidemic. While poliomyelitis in the United States has nearly been reduced to a historical footnote, thanks to effective vaccination and public health efforts, the value of rehabilitation for other MNDs has now been firmly established.

The term "motor neuron disease" (MND) is often used as a synonym for amyotrophic lateral sclerosis (ALS), and in the United States, ALS is often used as an umbrella term for adult MND that encompasses less common variants such as primary lateral sclerosis (PLS), progressive muscular atrophy (PMA), and progressive bulbar palsy (PBP) (**Fig. 23-1**). PLS is defined as a condition involving purely upper motor neuron (UMN) features. Conversely, PMA presents with pure lower motor neuron (LMN) symptoms and signs. PBP is restricted to the bulbar region (see **Fig. 23-1**). Despite initial presentation with one of these isolated upper or lower motor neuron or bulbar disorders, affected individuals may later evolve to manifest a classic mixed UMN/LMN syndrome typical of ALS on clinical or pathological examination. In its classic form, ALS results from a combination of both UMN and LMN dysfunction involving multiple body regions. Other diseases that fall under the category of MND but have distinct clinical presentations and prognosis include spinal muscular atrophy (SMA), which has both pediatric and adult variants, and spinobulbar muscular atrophy (SBMA), an X-linked disease. Finally, MND can be caused by infectious agents such as the polio virus or the West Nile virus (not covered in this chapter).

In the adult population, ALS is far more common than the other disorders. Thus, ALS will constitute most of the focus of this chapter, which will start with a description of the diseases, including anatomy, physiology, epidemiology, and genetics. This is followed by diagnostic workup, pharmacologic management, and rehabilitation strategies most of which may be applied to any of the adult MNDs.

BASIC ANATOMY AND PHYSIOLOGY

As the name of this disease category implies, the motor nervous system is the primary site of pathology in the MNDs. The motor system is composed of the UMNs that give rise to the corticospinal and corticobulbar tracts and the LMNs that originate in the anterior horn cells. Motor impulses are generated in the UMNs in the motor cortex. Their axons pass deep into the corona radiata and the internal capsule and then continue through the brainstem where the majority decussate in the pyramids of the medulla. Corticobulbar neurons proceed to synapse at the nuclei of the brainstem, while corticospinal axons descend in the lateral corticospinal tracts of the spinal cord. These axons terminate in the anterior horns of the spinal cord where they synapse with the LMNs. The axons of the LMNs carry impulses from the spinal cord to the skeletal muscles.

EPIDEMIOLOGY

Amyotrophic Lateral Sclerosis

ALS is the most common of the adult MNDs. Analysis of European population–based registries has provided incidence rates of 2.6/100,000 person-years and prevalence rates of 7 to 9/100,000 persons. As ALS is a nonreportable disease in the United States, no national database exists with complete information regarding disease prevalence and risk factors. Instead, much of the epidemiologic data regarding ALS in the United States comes from Medicare, Medicaid, Veterans Health Administration, and Veterans Benefit Administration claims data. A voluntary national online ALS Registry is operated under the auspices of the Agency for Toxic Substances and Disease Registry (ATSDR), providing an opportunity to gather more complete information regarding the incidence and prevalence of ALS, and for individuals with ALS to provide information about environmental, lifestyle, occupational, and other potential risk factors (1). There are an estimated 5,000 to 6,000 new diagnoses of ALS every year in the United States. PLS and PMA are often included in these numbers; it is estimated that PLS and PMA make up 1% to 3% and 10% of the cases, respectively (2,3). ALS most commonly strikes between 40 and 60 years of age

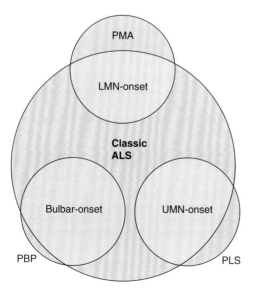

FIGURE 23-1. Schematic representation of adult MNDs.

PMA

LMN-onset

Classic
ALS

Bulbar-onset

UMN-onset

PBP

PLS

(4). Fifty percent of people with ALS (pALS) die within 3 years of onset of symptoms and 90% die within 5 years (4). About 20,000 Americans may currently be affected by ALS with highest prevalence among white non-Hispanic males.

Cigarette smoking has been associated with ALS in large prospective cohorts (5,6); this association appears to persist in recent findings of the National ALS Registry (7). Military service also appears to be associated with higher rates of ALS. In 2006, the Institute of Medicine (now known as the National Academy of Medicine) released the report: "Amyotrophic Lateral Sclerosis in Veterans: Review of the Scientific Literature" reviewing epidemiologic studies relating military service and diagnosis of ALS. Based on the available evidence, the report concluded that there was "limited and suggestive evidence of an association between military service and later development of ALS" (8).

Additional potential risk factors under consideration for ALS include traumatic brain injury and athletics. There is a correlation between history of traumatic brain injury and diagnosis of ALS, although it remains unclear as to whether emerging ALS symptoms are the cause rather than the result of the injury. A meta-analysis on the subject revealed an overall odds ratio of 1.45 (95% CI 1.21–1.74) for developing ALS with any prior history of head injury, although the strongest correlation was for head injuries nearest the time of diagnosis (9). While several epidemiologic studies have cited increased risk of ALS in professional athletes and athletic populations, other population studies have demonstrated a protective effect of exercise on mortality (10). Therefore, the association between ALS and strenuous exercise remains nebulous. Several other potential risk factors have been explored in the literature with conflicting results, including environmental toxins, history of trauma, history of electrical shock, and others (11–14).

Spinal Muscular Atrophy

SMA is an autosomal recessive disease and is the leading genetic cause of infant death. Carrier frequencies are estimated at 1 in 40 to 1 in 60 and SMA affects an estimated 10 per 100,000 live births. The prevalence of SMA in the general population is estimated at 1.2 per 100,000. Most SMA cases have onset in childhood (15).

Spinobulbar Muscular Atrophy (SBMA or Kennedy Disease)

The incidence of SBMA, an X-linked disease, is estimated at approximately one tenth of that of ALS or 0.19 per 100,000 males, with onset in adulthood.

PATHOPHYSIOLOGY AND GENETICS

Amyotrophic Lateral Sclerosis

Although great progress has been made in identifying key steps in pathophysiology, the exact disease mechanisms underlying ALS remain elusive. The discovery in 1993 that mutations in the superoxide dismutase type 1 (SOD1) gene are associated with some cases of ALS (16) suggested that oxidative injury may play a role in the process of motor neuron death (17). A number of additional putative mechanisms have been proposed including mitochondrial dysfunction, cytoskeletal derangements, microglial activation, and excitotoxicity (18). In support of the latter is the finding that riluzole, an Food and Drug Administration (FDA)-approved drug for ALS, affects

neurotransmission of glutamate, the major excitatory neurotransmitter in the central nervous system (19). The survival benefit of riluzole therapy, however, is modest (on the order of 3 months of increased survival compared to placebo). Several key developments, including the identification of ubiquilin protein in familial ALS (fALS) and sporadic ALS (sALS) (20), and the presence of ubiquitinated TAR DNA-binding protein 43 (TDP-43) (21) accumulations in both frontotemporal dementia (FTD) and ALS have shed light on common pathways in the disease process. Despite much research, however, no unifying hypothesis for ALS pathogenesis has so far emerged.

ALS appears to begin as a focal disease that starts in either the brain or the spinal cord and spreads to adjacent regions. Death of motor neurons in the cortex and spinal cord leads to degeneration of axons, atrophy of the spinal cord and ventral roots, and atrophy of distal muscles. Both UMNs and LMNs are affected. The cascade of events resulting in neuronal death is unclear, but pathologic studies demonstrate increased intracellular inclusions, including TDP-43 and ubiquitinated inclusions (22). Recently, it has been recognized that extramotor systems, such as temporal circuits and behavioral and executive frontal circuits, can also be affected in ALS, challenging the traditional vision of ALS as a pure motor disease (23).

ALS has been traditionally classified as either sporadic ALS (sALS) (about 90% of cases) or familial ALS (fALS) (the remaining 10%). Mutations in SOD1 account for about 2% of all ALS cases and about 20% of fALS. Increasing efforts over the last 20 years have been made to understand the genetic component of ALS: the number of ALS genes continues to grow with the most common genetic cause of ALS being a hexanucleotide repeat (GGGGCC) expansion in an intron of the chromosome 9 open reading frame 72 (C9orf72) gene, which is responsible for about 40% of fALS and a sizable portion of sALS (up to 10% depending on the ethnic background) (24). ALS-related genes are implicated in several intracellular processes, which has added to our understanding of disease pathophysiology (25,26).

Spinal Muscular Atrophy

SMA is an autosomal recessive disease that results from mutations in the survival motor neuron (SMN) gene. Although we know that the SMN protein is expressed widely in many tissues throughout the body, its function is still not completely understood at this time (27).

Genetic studies have now established that SMA is caused by mutations in the SMN1 gene, with all patients having at least one copy of the SMN2 gene. At least one copy of the SMN2 must be present in the setting of homozygous SMN1 mutations; otherwise, embryonic lethality occurs. The copy number of SMN2 varies in the population, and this variation appears to have important modifying effects on SMA disease severity (28). A higher number of SMN2 copies results in less severe clinical SMA phenotype. However, variability in SMA phenotype and disease severity can exist with a given SMN2 copy number.

Most cases of SMA have onset in childhood. Adult-onset SMA is also caused by homozygous mutations in the SMN1 gene, though there are rare cases of adult-onset SMA that are due to autosomal dominant mutations in other genes.

Spinobulbar Muscular Atrophy

The genetic mechanism underlying SBMA was elucidated in 1991: the disease results from an X-linked recessive mutation producing a CAG expansion in the androgen receptor gene.

Unaffected individuals have a CAG repeat size that ranges between 5 and 35, while symptomatic individuals always have a repeat size of at least 37 glutamines (29).

CLINICAL PRESENTATION

Amyotrophic Lateral Sclerosis

Typical ALS is characterized by mixed UMN and LMN symptoms and signs—including weakness, atrophy, fasciculations, hyperreflexia, and spasticity. Several studies have documented the extensive spectrum of phenotypic heterogeneity in this disorder (30–34). Exclusively UMN and LMN variants of ALS are described along the spectrum of MNDs (see **Fig. 23-1**).

In classic ALS, initial symptoms of weakness may present, in the limbs, bulbar muscles, or, more rarely, in the respiratory muscles. Most often, ALS presents with asymmetric, painless, progressive limb weakness (60% of cases). Symptoms of muscle weakness may be quite insidious and develop slowly. Bulbar-onset disease presenting with dysarthria or dysphagia occurs in approximately 30% of cases; this usually presents in older individuals. Respiratory-onset weakness in isolation is a rare presentation, accounting for less than 3% of cases in one study (35). Most often, symptoms will progress to adjacent myotomes and body regions; however, some variants of ALS demonstrate prolonged periods of disease isolated to a single body region—including flail arm (brachial monomelic amyotrophy), flail leg, brachial amyotrophic diplegia (BAD), and leg amyotrophic diplegia.

The evaluation of a patient suspected of having ALS begins with a detailed history, general physical examination, and neurologic examination. The nonmotor cranial nerve function, sensory examination, and cerebellar examinations should be normal. Eye movements and bowel and bladder function are typically spared.

On history or exam (either bedside exam or in the context of formal neuropsychological testing), one may detect cognitive and/or behavioral changes that are now recognized as part of the ALS/FTD disease spectrum (36). While traditional cognitive screens may not be sensitive for changes associated with FTD, the ALS Cognitive Behavioral Scale and ALS Caregiver Behavioral Questionnaire are convenient tools that can be used by clinicians to screen for impairments (36). Cognitive or behavioral impairment can precede muscle weakness or manifest with disease progression as ALS is increasingly recognized as a multisystem disorder, which includes both clinical and neuropathologic features of FTD (37). Pseudobulbar affect is often seen in ALS as an UMN syndrome. Patients experience inappropriate laughter or crying, which is not concordant with their mood and can be socially embarrassing.

Bulbar weakness due to motor neuron loss in the brainstem affects speech, swallowing, and ability to manage secretions. Although only a third of patients present with bulbar weakness initially at disease onset (bulbar-onset ALS), most will develop bulbar weakness in later stages of the disease. Speech disturbances may include spastic, flaccid, or mixed dysarthria. Signs of spastic dysarthria include a strained and strangled quality of speech, reduced rate, low pitch, imprecise consonant pronunciation, vowel distortion, and breaks in pitch. LMN dysfunction creates a flaccid dysarthria in which speech has a nasal and/or wet quality; pitch and intensity are monotone, phrases abnormally are short, and inspiration is audible.

Normal swallow involves an intricate coordination of approximately 50 pairs of muscles to transport food and liquid from the mouth to the stomach. Complaints of difficulty chewing and swallowing, nasal regurgitation, or coughing when drinking liquids, may all indicate dysphagia. Individuals may also describe fatigue with eating. On physical examination, the following tests may be used to assess facial and bulbar muscle function: ability to pocket air in the cheeks, whistle, jaw opening and lip closure strength, and phonation of a variety of syllables. The tongue should be examined for fasciculations and atrophy and tongue strength and range of motion assessed. The gag reflex and jaw jerk should be assessed to look for UMN dysfunction. Saliva production is generally unaffected by ALS, but drooling and aspiration are common consequences of bulbar weakness due to dysphagia. Respiratory tract secretions may be thickened due to impaired fluid intake, which further compounds the difficulty clearing the airway.

On limb examination, one is looking for evidence of mixed UMN and LMN dysfunction. LMN pathology is evidenced by muscle atrophy, fasciculations, and muscle cramping. Cramping may occur anywhere in the body, including the thighs, arms, and abdomen (38). Atrophy of the hand intrinsic muscles is common; however, finger flexor strength is often preserved, a helpful distinguishing factor from inclusion body myositis (39). Head drop is a manifestation of muscle weakness often seen in ALS although it can be seen in other neuromuscular disorders (ALS and myasthenia gravis are the two most common neuromuscular causes of head drop). UMN pathology may result in loss of dexterity or a feeling of stiffness in the limbs. UMN signs on exam include spasticity and hyperreflexia, indicated by abnormal spread of reflexes and clonus or by the presence of brisk reflexes despite muscle atrophy due to LMN loss. Pathologic reflexes such as the Babinski sign, Hoffmann sign, or hyperactive jaw jerk, are highly suggestive of UMN dysfunction.

Although motor weakness of the limbs is often the most recognizable effect of ALS, respiratory weakness arguably has the most profound impact on function and survival. Early symptoms of respiratory weakness may be subtle and involve orthopnea or sleep-disordered breathing. Sleep-disordered breathing and nocturnal hypoventilation are common in individuals with ALS, even in the setting of preserved daytime function. Symptoms may include air hunger, snoring, choking episodes, orthopnea, restlessness, insomnia or daytime hypersomnolence, morning headaches, drowsiness, and fatigue. These symptoms should prompt further evaluation (40). The basic function of the lung tissue for gas exchange is unaffected by ALS in the absence of microaspiration (which may induce some impairment in gas exchange). In contrast, motor neuron degeneration in ALS impairs inspiratory, expiratory, and upper airway musculature. Inspiratory muscle weakness involving the diaphragm, intercostals, and accessory muscles of respiration, results in reduced vital capacity. In the absence of premorbid pulmonary pathology, spirometry generally reveals evidence of a restrictive respiratory impairment. On average, vital capacity decreases at a rate of 2% to 4% per month in individuals with ALS (41). The restrictive respiratory impairment ultimately results in hypercarbic respiratory failure, as well as decreased cough effectiveness and ability to clear secretions. Decreased ability to clear secretions places the individual with ALS at risk of respiratory complications.

Recent surveys of pALS have revealed a high prevalence of secondary symptoms; in particular, fatigue, muscle stiffness and cramps, and pain are commonly reported (42). Weight loss is another common feature of this disease. Weight loss is common and associated with poorer prognosis (43–45). While it is easy to ascribe weight loss solely to dysphagia, there are several other factors that can influence weight. ALS is thought to induce a hypermetabolic state owing to several factors: increased energy expenditure of weak muscles for functional tasks, increased muscle activity from spasticity and fasciculations, and muscle catabolism. These have the effect of increasing the basal metabolic rate and caloric demand (46). In addition, upper extremity and bulbar weakness may limit the individual's self-feeding due to fatigue. Many patients with ALS feel an overwhelming sense of muscle fatigue (47). Pain is reported in about half of all patients as a consequence of muscle imbalance and progressive loss of muscle mass and mobility (48). Common musculoskeletal complaints include shoulder pain, adhesive capsulitis, neck and back pain, ankle plantar flexion contractures, and claw hand.

Average life expectancy with ALS is 2 to 5 years following diagnosis. The most common immediate cause of death in ALS as determined by postmortem examinations is respiratory failure, followed by heart failure and pulmonary embolism (49). Poor prognostic factors include older age at the time of onset, bulbar and/or pulmonary dysfunction early in the clinical course of the disease, and short time period from symptom onset to diagnosis (50,51).

Adult-Onset Spinal Muscular Atrophy

There are many forms of SMA, all of which involve selective destruction of anterior horn cells (LMNs). The most common forms are often referred to as types I, II, and III. These are disorders of childhood and are inherited as autosomal recessive traits (14). *Adult-onset* SMA patients (SMA type IV) typically present in the third to fourth decade. Inheritance can be either recessive (SMN-related) (52) or dominant (53). The disease is characterized by progressive, proximal symmetric weakness. Patients complain of proximal leg and hip girdle weakness due to LMN dysfunction and degeneration. Proximal arm weakness, tongue fasciculations, and hand tremor can be present. *Adult-onset* SMA is a much milder form than childhood-onset SMAs and has a normal life span.

Spinobulbar Muscular Atrophy

SBMA, also known as Kennedy disease, is an X-linked, recessive, adult-onset disease of the anterior horn cells. LMNs are involved with slowly progressive weakness of the proximal and bulbar muscles and diffuse fasciculations, often prominently involving the lower face and tongue. Unlike other MNDs, there is often an associated, but generally asymptomatic, sensory neuropathy that is often detected incidentally when nerve conduction studies are performed as part of the diagnostic process. The disease is multisystemic as it results from mutations of the androgen receptor gene on the X chromosome; signs and symptoms may therefore include gynecomastia, testicular atrophy, and reduced fertility. Although gross muscle weakness generally does not present until the third decade, earliest manifestations of SBMA may present in adolescence or young adulthood, including gynecomastia, muscle exhaustion, cramps, or creatine kinase (CK) elevation (54).

Individuals with SBMA have slower disease progression than ALS, but life expectancy has been estimated to be approximately 12 to 15 years shorter than the general population, with most common cause of death being pneumonia and respiratory failure (55). Given the overlap in clinical presentation, SBMA can be commonly mistaken for atypical ALS (56). In contrast to ALS, however, individuals with SBMA generally experience much slower progression of symptoms and absence of UMN signs and symptoms.

DIAGNOSIS

In the absence of reliable biomarkers, ALS remains a clinical diagnosis supported by electrodiagnostic (EDX) findings. The diagnosis of ALS and other forms of adult MND therefore is primarily a process of exclusion. With the exception of genetic testing revealing a mutation in a known ALS-causing gene, there is no individual test that can confirm the diagnosis. Patients with early or limited disease may prove challenging to diagnose; the average time to establish a firm diagnosis of ALS is about 12 months (57). When ALS is suspected, one must generate a differential diagnosis that varies greatly based on individual clinical presentation (**Table 23-1**) and then work to exclude processes mimicking ALS. Results from most laboratory tests are generally within normal limits, except for a mild elevation of CK levels and abnormal EDX results. Differential diagnosis and laboratory studies that can be used to rule out potential disease mimics are listed in **Table 23-1**. Of note, the proposed diagnostic studies should be used only as clinically indicated, and it is certainly not necessary to perform all of these studies in every patient. Oftentimes, it is possible to diagnose ALS based on clinical grounds with supportive EDX data and a handful of adjunct laboratory tests, which are selected based on clinical presentation. Recent data suggest that cortical hyperexcitability is among the earliest pathologic changes seen in ALS patients, which may translate into useful clinical biomarkers in the future (58). The El Escorial criteria are used in a research setting to classify the certainty of the ALS diagnosis and are useful for enrollment into clinical trials (59).

A portion of MND cases can be confirmed by genetic testing. These include about 70% of fALS and 10% of sALS patients carrying ALS genes that are testable with currently available gene panels, patients with Kennedy disease, and adult-onset SMA cases related to SMN1 mutations.

Electrodiagnostic Testing

EDX testing can be helpful to confirm a clinically suspected diagnosis of MND, to exclude competing and possibly treatable diagnoses (such as multifocal motor neuropathy with conduction blocks), and to define the extent of the disease process. Motor nerve conduction studies may reveal decreased amplitudes with relatively preserved latencies and conduction velocities. With significant loss of amplitude, a 25% drop in conduction velocity is allowable, given the possible loss of the fastest conducting nerve fibers. Sensory nerve conduction studies are generally normal in ALS. In contrast, in SBMA pathologic involvement of the dorsal root ganglia commonly results in sensory nerve conduction abnormalities (60).

Needle electrode exam provides the most information for detailing the extent of the disease and providing EDX data in support of the diagnosis. Needle electromyography (EMG) assesses LMN involvement, including emerging subclinical disease. Abnormal spontaneous activity, including fibrillation potentials, positive sharp waves, and fasciculations, may be observed. Motor unit action potentials may exhibit polyphasia, increased amplitude and duration, and reduced recruitment.

TABLE 23-1	Differential Diagnosis and Laboratory Testing for Motor Neuron Disease	
Clinical Presentation	**Differential Considerations**	**Laboratory Testing**
Bulbar-onset	Myasthenia gravis	Acetylcholine receptor and muscle-specific kinase (MuSK) antibodies
	Brainstem tumor	Brain magnetic resonance imaging (MRI)
Lower motor neuron predominant	Multifocal motor neuropathy	Ganglioside-monosialic acid (GM1) antibodies
	Spinobulbar muscular atrophy (Kennedy's disease)	Genetic testing
	Spinal muscular atrophy	Genetic testing
	Hypothyroidism	Thyroid-stimulating hormone
	Paraproteinemias	Serum protein electrophoresis/immunofixation
	Paraneoplastic	Antibody panel (serum, cerebrospinal fluid [CSF])
	Inclusion body myositis	Muscle biopsy
	Lyme disease/West Nile virus/polio/syphilis	Serology
	Tay-Sachs disease	Hexosaminidase A level
	Heavy metal intoxication	24-h urine collection for heavy metals
Upper motor neuron predominant	Copper deficiency	Serum copper and zinc
	B_{12} deficiency	Vitamin B_{12}, methylmalonic acid, homocysteine
	Human immunodeficiency virus (HIV)	HIV
	Tropical spastic paraparesis	Human T-cell lymphotropic virus 1 serology
	Adrenomyeloneuropathy	Very long-chain fatty acids
	Hereditary spastic paraplegia (HSP)	Genetic testing
	Multiple sclerosis	Brain and spine MRI
Mixed	Spine disease	Spine MRI

EDX criteria to support the clinical suspicion of ALS have evolved over time. The most commonly used criteria are known as the El Escorial criteria-Revised. They were established, and then revised, by the World Federation of Neurology in an effort to define consensus criteria for enrollment into clinical trials and research studies related to ALS (59). The criteria outlined threshold requirements to establish a diagnosis of definite, probable, probable laboratory-supported, or possible ALS (the category of suspected ALS that was included in the original El Escorial criteria was deleted from the revised version) (**Table 23-2**). According to the El Escorial criteria, the diagnosis of ALS requires the *presence* of LMN degeneration (by clinical, electrophysiologic, or neuropathologic examination), and evidence of UMN degeneration by clinical examination, AND progressive spread of symptoms or signs within a region or to other regions (59). At the same time, the criteria require the *absence* of electrophysiologic, radiologic, or pathologic evidence of disease processes that might mimic the observed signs of LMN and/or UMN degeneration (59). EDX studies can be used to provide laboratory evidence of LMN dysfunction: in order to meet EDX criteria, one must obtain evidence of both active denervation (defined as fibrillations and positive sharp waves) and chronic reinnervation (defined as long-duration, large-amplitude motor units with reduced recruitment) in two out of four separate body regions (bulbar, cervical, thoracic, and lumbosacral) (59). Of note, these changes must be seen in at least two muscles innervated by different roots and peripheral nerves when the cervical and lumbosacral regions are examined. In the bulbar region, changes in one muscle would suffice. In the thoracic region, changes either in the paraspinal muscles at or below the T6 level or in the abdominal muscles are acceptable.

The El Escorial criteria were established mostly for research purposes and trial enrollment and are strict: it was estimated that about 20% of pALS would die without ever meeting threshold criteria for diagnosis. In an attempt to increase the sensitivity of diagnostic criteria, the Awaji criteria were

developed in 2008. These criteria allow fasciculation potentials to be considered equivalent to fibrillations as signs of acute denervation (61). While the Awaji criteria may have increased sensitivity for the diagnosis of ALS while maintaining acceptable specificity (62), they have not been widely adopted by the research community.

TABLE 23-2	El Escorial Criteria-Revised
Diagnostic Category	**Requirements**
Clinically definite ALS	UMN + LMN signs on clinical exam in three body regions
Clinically probable ALS	UMN + LMN signs on clinical exam in two body regions, with some UMN signs rostral to the LMN signs
Clinically probable ALS—laboratory-supported	UMN + LMN signs on clinical exam in one body region
	OR
	UMN signs alone in one region
	AND
	LMN signs defined by EMG criteria are present in at least two regions
Possible ALS	UMN + LMN signs in one body region
	OR
	UMN signs in two or more body regions
	OR
	LMN signs rostral to UMN signs
	AND
	the diagnosis of clinically probable ALS—laboratory-supported cannot be proven

Body regions: bulbar, cervical, thoracic, lumbosacral.

MANAGEMENT

Pharmacologic Treatment and Research

There is a lack of effective disease-modifying treatments for ALS. The first FDA-approved medication for ALS, riluzole, offers a modest therapeutic effect, does not materially improve strength or function, and prolongs survival by only a few months (63–65). Yet, ALS research has brought about several breakthrough discoveries (65,66). The pace of discovery in ALS has greatly accelerated over the last 20 years, and a second drug, edaravone, was recently approved by the FDA to slow down disease progression (**Fig. 23-2**) (66). While recent preclinical discoveries have yet to translate into effective treatments, several factors contribute to a renewed sense of hope. First and foremost, the ALS research community is extremely collaborative and has developed infrastructure resources to optimize translational research (67–72). This is supported by an active patient community (73,74) that has galvanized the field. It is estimated that there are about 20 active drug trials for ALS at the moment, with an ever-growing pipeline of candidate compounds and a myriad of clinical research projects including large-scale genomics and deep phenotyping studies. It is hoped that these efforts, combined with new knowledge about genetic underpinnings and disease molecular mechanisms, will result in novel ways to target the disease in the near future. Ultimately, given the multiple pathophysiologic mechanisms that are at play in ALS, it is likely that a combination of drugs targeting different pathways will be needed to effectively slow down or stop motor neuron loss (75).

While effective disease-modifying treatments are still in development, several ALS-related symptoms including mood changes, pain, spasticity, cramps, fatigue, excess oral secretions, and pseudobulbar affect can be effectively treated by pharmacologic and nonpharmacologic means (**Table 23-3**). Patients frequently inquire about complementary and alternative treatments to manage the disease process as well as symptoms (77). ALSUntangled (ALSUntangled.com) provides excellent reviews of these and off-label treatments. There is survey-based

TABLE 23-3	Treatment Options for ALS-Related Symptoms
Symptom	**Possible Treatments**
Depression	SSRIs, SNRIs, bupropion, tricyclics Cognitive-behavioral therapy
Pseudobulbar affect	Nuedexta (dextromethorphan/quinine)
Pain	Medications: Topical analgesics, acetaminophen, NSAIDs, gabapentin, pregabalin, opioids, steroid injections (frozen shoulder) Other: Stretching and range-of-motion exercises, massage, TENS, ice/heat, acupuncture, trigger point injections
Cramps	Baclofen, gabapentin, cannabinoids. A recent trial suggested that mexiletine may be effective at relieving cramps in ALS (76)
Sialorrhea	Medications: Glycopyrrolate, amitriptyline, atropine drops (SL), scopolamine transdermal patch, hyoscyamine Other: Botulinum toxin or radiation to salivary glands
Difficulty removing secretions	Mechanical inexsufflation (MIE) device or cough assist device, guaifenesin

NSAIDs, nonsteroidal anti-inflammatory drugs; SL, sublingual; SSRIs, selective serotonin reuptake inhibitors; SNRIs, serotonin-norepinephrine reuptake inhibitors; TENS, transcutaneous electrical nerve stimulation.

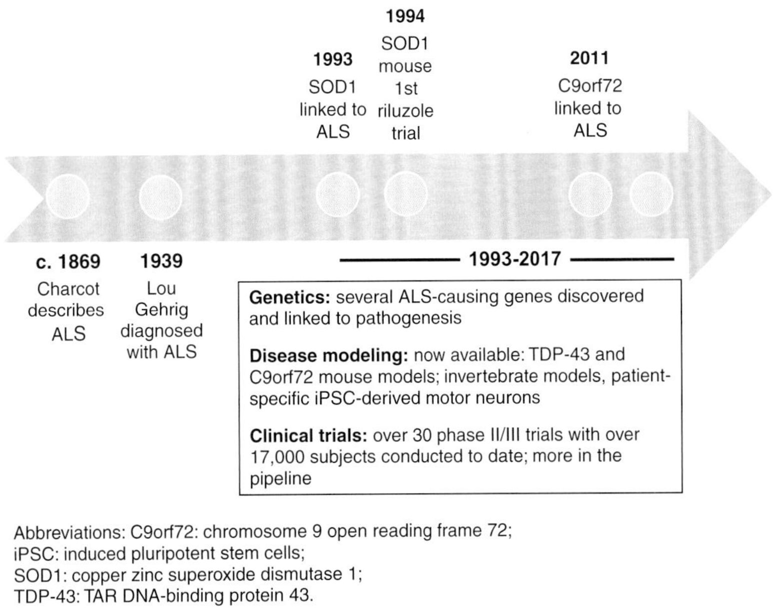

evidence suggesting that medicinal cannabis may alleviate some of the symptoms associated with ALS (78) due to its properties including analgesia, antispasticity, muscle relaxation, bronchodilation, saliva reduction, appetite stimulation, and sleep induction (79). These anecdotal reports have been substantiated by data from animal models (80,81). The potential of cannabinoid therapeutics as disease-modifying or symptom control agents in ALS warrants further investigation (80,81). Coordinated care of these symptoms and management of disease progression are best addressed in the context of the ALS multidisciplinary clinic.

FIGURE 23-2. Timelines of ALS research. (Adapted from *NeuroRehabilitation*, 37, Paganoni S, Karam C, Joyce N, et al. Comprehensive rehabilitative care across the spectrum of amyotrophic lateral sclerosis, 53–68. Copyright 2015, with permission from IOS Press. The publication is available at IOS Press through http://dx.doi.org/10.3233/NRE-151240)

Abbreviations: C9orf72: chromosome 9 open reading frame 72;
iPSC: induced pluripotent stem cells;
SOD1: copper zinc superoxide dismutase 1;
TDP-43: TAR DNA-binding protein 43.

MULTIDISCIPLINARY CARE

To meet the complex and rapidly changing needs of the ALS patient, a multidisciplinary care model, based on the 2009 ALS practice parameters of the American Association of Neurology, has emerged as the optimal treatment paradigm (82).

The shift toward multidisciplinary care has been supported by literature reporting prolonged survival, improved quality of life, and reduced hospitalizations when comparisons are made between traditional single practitioner and multidisciplinary clinic models (83–85). The Amyotrophic Lateral Sclerosis Association (ALSA), a patient advocacy group, bestows the designation of an ALSA Clinical Center of Excellence to sites who pass an onsite review confirming they have an experienced, comprehensive multidisciplinary team available for patients during single visits and whom also provide access to ALS research (see http://www.alsa.org/community/centers-clinics/centers-and-clinics-descriptions.html accessed on 2/1/17). Currently, there are 51 centers across the United States that have achieved this designation. In California, the ALSA partnered with clinical centers and lobbyists to pass Bill SB1503, giving all Californians diagnosed with ALS the right to have access to multidisciplinary care. Other ALS clinics are sponsored by the Muscular Dystrophy Association (MDA) or other nonprofits. Most ALS clinics tend to be located in academic centers and patients may have to travel a few hours to reach the closest multidisciplinary clinic.

The multidisciplinary team includes a neuromuscular specialist (generally a neurologist or a physiatrist) and a team of health care professionals such as physical therapists (PT), occupational therapists (OT), respiratory therapists, nurses, dieticians, speech-language pathologists, social workers, and psychologists (86). Clinics may also have orthotists and durable medical equipment providers available for patients during their appointments. An expanded interdisciplinary specialty physician team is also necessary to provide comprehensive care for the ALS patient and often includes a pulmonologist for management of ALS-associated restrictive lung disease and a gastroenterologist or interventional radiologist to perform gastrostomy for improved nutritional support.

To meet the American Academy of Neurology (AAN) practice parameters and quality metrics (87), the following medical concerns should be addressed during the multidisciplinary appointment: pulmonary function testing, management of noninvasive or invasive ventilation, discussion or management of gastrostomy use for maintaining nutrition, management and use of riluzole for disease modification, scoring of the ALS functional rating scale (ALSFRS), safe mobility and fall screening, sialorrhea assessment, screening for cognitive impairment, and discussion regarding and completion of advanced directives and planning for end-stage care. The typical multidisciplinary clinic appointment is longer than the traditional appointment with reports showing that each practitioner spends on average about 30 minutes with each patient (88). However, if one considers the time that would otherwise be spent by the patient and caregiver preparing to attend and traveling to and from individual appointments to see each practitioner, the multidisciplinary clinic model significantly reduces the patient's health care burden. Rigorous assessments regarding the cost of delivering care by the multidisciplinary clinic model and whether the benefits outweigh these costs are beginning to appear in the literature (88).

Respiratory Function: Assessment and Management

Monitoring and support of respiratory function is of primary importance in the ALS multidisciplinary clinic and is achieved by a close collaboration among the neuromuscular medicine physician, the pulmonologist, and the respiratory therapist. The role of the respiratory therapist in the multidisciplinary ALS clinic includes clinical evaluation for evidence of ALS-associated restrictive lung disease, performance of pulmonary function tests, and provision of recommendations for secretion clearance and ventilatory support. Ventilatory support includes noninvasive and invasive options as will be described below, and the respiratory therapist can assist with both management and equipment recommendations (e.g., trialing different nasal masks for best fit and comfort to increase tolerability).

Respiratory failure is the most common cause of death in ALS. It occurs due to muscle weakness that causes failure of the respiratory pump—a mechanical problem. Serial monitoring of pulmonary function is necessary, and pulmonary function testing should be performed at each appointment until the patient is no longer able to tolerate performing the tests. Multiple modality testing is considered the most effective strategy (89,90). In ALS, the use of five tests is considered the most sensitive way to detect early respiratory failure and in turn initiate noninvasive ventilation (NIV) as early as possible. NIV has been associated with improved survival (89). The panel of tests (90) include the following:

- Upright and supine forced vital capacity (FVC); AAN guidelines recommend initiation of NIV at FVC of 50% predicted.
- Upright and supine maximum inspiratory pressure (MIP); AAN guidelines recommend initiation of NIV at MIP of greater than –60 cmH$_2$O (centimeter of water).
- Overnight oximetry; Centers for Medicare and Medicaid Services (CMS) recommend initiation of NIV when SpO$_2$ drops below 88% for more than 5 minutes during nocturnal pulse oximetry testing. [Centers for Medicare & Medicaid Services, "LCD for Respiratory Assist Devices (L11504, L5023, L11493)," U.S. Department of Health and Human Services, (revision effective date 2/4/2011).]

In addition, a sniff nasal inspiratory pressure (SNIP) greater than (i.e., closer to zero) –40 cmH$_2$O or a PaCO$_2$ greater than 45 mm Hg meets AAN and CMS guidelines, respectively, for initiation of NIV. Lastly, the AAN guidelines suggest that lung function testing can be used to predict survival in pALS. Survival of less than 3 months has been associated with a SNIP of greater than –30 cmH$_2$O (i.e., closer to zero), daytime oxygen saturation less than 95%, or nocturnal saturation less than 93%.

Assessment for adequate secretion clearance is done with peak cough flow (PCF) testing using a peak flow meter. Secretion clearance techniques should be initiated when the PCF is less than 270 L/min. Augmented cough support can be achieved using manual-assisted cough or mechanical inexsufflation (MIE) device. The MIE device improves both the inhale and exhale components of a cough with delivery of positive pressure airflow followed by negative pressure flow through a mask, mobilizing secretions. MIE devices provide the following major benefits:

- Secretion management with reduction in mucous plugging–related macroatelectasis
- Reduction of chronic microatelectasis
- Reduction in chest wall stiffness, reducing the work of breathing

When initiating cough assistance with an MIE, it is helpful to titrate both the negative and positive pressure settings. Starting pressures of +25 to –25 cmH$_2$O can be gradually increased to +40 and –40 cmH$_2$O, as tolerated. Caution should be used when prescribing the MIE to a patient with hypotonic bulbar dysfunction, as the negative pressure may cause airway collapse. For these patients, high-frequency chest wall oscillation (HFCWO) and bag mask breath stacking with manual-assisted cough maneuvers and suction can be used.

NIV is strongly recommended to improve disease outcomes as well as the patient's quality of life. Assisted ventilation therapy, whether invasive or noninvasive, is the most effective life-prolonging therapy we have for treatment in ALS (64). Bilevel positive airway pressure devices, which provide fluctuating pressures of airflow, are chosen over continuous pressure devices. The newer bilevel devices offer multiple setting options and can automatically adjust, within the prescribed setting ranges. Generally, for pALS, the goal is to reach a high pressure span between the expiratory positive airway pressure (EPAP) and the minimum inspiratory positive airway pressure (IPAP) over time. Patients with restrictive lung disease have difficulty exhaling over high EPAP settings and may retain carbon dioxide (CO$_2$) if the EPAP setting is too high. Unless the patient has an obstructive component, the starting EPAP pressure should be low, around 3 to 4 cmH$_2$O. If titrating the device without a formal sleep study, a starting minimum IPAP setting of 8 cmH$_2$O ranging to 12 cmH$_2$O will provide some support. It is generally safe to start with an initial tidal volume of 6 mL/kg and a backup respiratory rate of 8 to 10 breaths per minute. The respiratory therapist will help monitor the adequacy of settings, which can be accomplished with sleep studies or in home nocturnal pulse oximetry studies. Patients transitioning to 24-hour NIV benefit from a volume-cycled ventilator. These devices offer greater mobility as they are equipped with rechargeable batteries and can be mounted to a power wheelchair.

Tracheostomy with mechanical ventilation (also called tracheostomy-invasive ventilation, or TIV) is also a recommended intervention according to the AAN (64). Those patients with bulbar or thoracic-onset disease, or severe restrictive lung disease with low lung volumes, are more likely to choose TIV. Prior to starting TIV, the patient, caregivers, and clinical team should define the conditions that would trigger cessation of TIV (e.g., some patients state they want to discontinue the intervention if they are unable to communicate/locked-in). It is important to describe that ALS will progress even while a patient is kept alive with TIV and that duration of life on TIV cannot be well predicted (can be months to years based on disease progression and the development of life-threatening complications such as pulmonary embolism, infections, open skin lesions). Brain-computer interface technology is emerging for this population (83).

Supplemental oxygen is generally avoided, as it may suppress respiratory drive, exacerbate alveolar hypoventilation, and ultimately lead to carbon dioxide retention and premature respiratory arrest (91,92). Supplemental oxygen is recommended only for pALS with concomitant pulmonary disease, which can be bled into the bilevel device after first improving saturations as much as possible with NIV, or as a comfort measure in the terminal stage of disease.

Dysphagia

Dysphagia is a major cause of malnutrition in pALS. The ALS speech and language pathologist (SLP) and dietitian are responsible for evaluating the effectiveness of a swallow and making recommendations to improve safe eating and nutritional intake. Dysphagia is present in 45% of patients with bulbar-onset disease at diagnosis, and nearly 81% of all pALS will experience dysphagia (93). Due to the involvement of cranial nerves IX, X, and XII, patients with bulbar weakness develop disruption in tongue, pharyngeal, and esophageal function. As a result, these patients have difficulty talking, chewing, and swallowing. The weakened oral activities ultimately result in reduced calorie and fluid intake as patients become fearful of choking or are unable to spend the increased time it takes to complete a meal safely. These findings illustrate the importance of having both a registered dietitian and speech therapist as members of the multidisciplinary ALS team.

Swallowing is a complicated task requiring coordination and precise timing of bulbar muscle activity (see Chapter 13). There are four phases in a normal swallow: the oral preparatory and propulsive phases, the pharyngeal, and esophageal phases. The oral phases, which prepare a food bolus and then propel the bolus into the oropharynx for swallow, require good tongue control, which is often impaired in bulbar ALS. The pharyngeal phase follows the oral phases and requires the rapid coordination of movements involving the soft palate, larynx, vocal folds, and epiglottis. The oropharyngeal phases of swallow are the first to be affected in ALS and often cause aspiration when abnormal. The earliest evidence of dysphagia in pALS is difficulty swallowing thin liquids such as water, coffee, and tea without a postswallow cough.

There are multiple techniques used to evaluate the oropharyngeal phases of swallow and aspiration risk:

- 3-Ounce Water Swallow Test—Observe the patient consume water noting postswallow cough, salivary pooling, increased dysarthria, and wet speech.
- Video Fluoroscopy Swallowing Study (VFSS)—Also known as a modified barium swallow study, it assesses the effects of food consistency and postural change on swallow while capturing evidence of aspiration and motor abnormalities.
- Flexible Fiber-Optic Endoscopic Swallow Study (FEES)—Transnasal laryngoscope is used to assess pharyngeal swallowing and aspiration and can identify pharyngeal food retention.

To accommodate swallow dysfunction, swallowing techniques and food consistency changes are often recommended with the goal to reduce the risk of aspiration and optimize nutritional status. Recommendations may include postural maneuvers such as head-tilt–chin-tuck or behavioral modification such as breath holding, to help avoid the collection and pocketing of residual food and aspiration. Dietary modification is a commonly used treatment strategy that addresses both the viscosity of liquids and the texture of solids to improve swallow safety and reduce the need for thorough chewing in the weakened patient.

Several surgical procedures have been employed as a definitive treatment to prevent aspiration though their use in ALS has been limited: laryngotracheal separation, tracheoesophageal diversion, and total laryngectomy (94). These surgeries may be appropriate for the individual who has lost function of the larynx—both for phonation and protection of the lower airway. In each surgery, the trachea is diverted to a stoma in the neck, while the oropharynx remains connected to the esophagus, permitting the passage of food into the stomach and preventing aspiration of food, liquid, or saliva into the lower airway. While drastic, this procedure allows the possibility of safe oral intake to continue despite weakness of bulbar muscles (95).

Nutritional Status

Weight loss is nearly ubiquitous in ALS and presents significant challenges for patients. Nutritional status is monitored in the clinic by the physician and the ALS dietitian. The ALS dietitian monitors weight and provides recommendations to meet the unique caloric needs of the ALS patient.

The reasons underlying weight loss in ALS are multifactorial and include but are not limited to muscle wasting, hypermetabolism, respiratory failure, dysphagia, and reduced intake due to upper limb weakness. Low body mass index (BMI) and rapid weight loss are associated with more rapid disease progression (44,45,96,97). While the prevalence varies somewhat among studies, it seems that over half of all pALS meet criteria for malnutrition with a BMI of less than 18.5 kg/m². Individuals meeting criteria for malnutrition have a 7.7-fold increased risk of mortality (98). In a recent report by Korner et al., weight loss had a negative impact on quality of life with perception of reduced physical functioning and vitality (99). Of the 121 pALS studied, those who had lost weight and were subsequently placed on high calorie supplementation with or without gastrostomy (*n* = 23) reported weight stabilization or gain. Eighty-five percent of those who chose gastrostomy reported an improvement in quality of life (99).

There are varying recommendations for the optimal timing of gastrostomy placement. Patient understanding and readiness are of course necessary, and placement before the gastrostomy is fully necessary allows time to adjust to its presence while still enjoying oral nutritional intake. The AAN recommends gastrostomy placement when the FVC is equal to or greater than 50% predicted, in order to reduce associated respiratory-related surgical risks (64). Radiographically inserted gastrostomy (RIG) is considered the safest approach for tube placement in those with FVC less than 50% predicted.

Recently, Dorst et al. published findings from a multicenter, prospective study assessing the safety of percutaneous endoscopic gastrostomy (PEG) placement in 89 pALS and found the procedure to be generally safe with 1.1% mortality in the periprocedure period with FVCs below 50% predicted (91). Of note, the authors also recommend a single periprocedure prophylactic injection of antibiotics, slow initiation of nutritional supplementation (<200 kcal/d), and aiming for target of high calorie nutritional supplementation (100). In addition,

the authors concluded that the use of NIV in the periprocedural period further decreased the respiratory risks associated with PEG, allowing safe placement later in the disease course.

Another strategy used for determining the timing of gastrostomy placement is one based on percent baseline body weight lost, with recommendations for placement when a patient loses 10% of their baseline weight (64). A recent series comparing outcomes among patients with weight loss above and below 20% of their baseline weight demonstrated an associated decrease in survival post gastrostomy or RIG by 149 days in the group with weight loss of greater than 20% of their baseline.

Predicting the caloric needs of the ALS patient is complicated due to the related hypermetabolism of ALS, which is not completely understood. There is growing evidence that points to impaired glucose metabolism and mitochondrial dysfunction (101). While the Harris-Benedict equation has traditionally been used to predict the caloric needs of patients in the clinic setting, the equation is well known to be inadequate for the ALS patient. To address this concern, Shimizu et al. recently completed a study using doubly labeled water to determine total energy expenditure of pALS and developed an equation they believe is more accurate at predicting their caloric need, using both the Harris-Benedict Equation and the ALS Functional Rating Scale-Revised (ALSFRS-R) score: total energy expenditure = (1.67 × resting metabolic rate as predicted by the Harris-Benedict equation) + (11.8 × ALSFRS-R) – 680 (102).

REHABILITATION AND PALLIATIVE CARE

Role for The Physiatrist

While there is currently no cure for any form of degenerative MND, there is much that physiatrists can do to meaningfully address the physical and psychosocial impact of these progressive diseases (103). We will focus in this section on ALS, although some of the principles described may apply to other MNDs as well.

The most comprehensive management of ALS is achieved through collaborative neurology, rehabilitation, and palliative clinical care from the time of diagnosis (103). Typically, neurology care is most intensive early in the disease course, focused on diagnosis and medication management, and palliative care most intensive when there is a focus on spiritual support, advanced pain and dyspnea management, and planning for and managing death and family bereavement (86,104–106). Rehabilitation interventions span the course of the disease and are designed to prevent complications (e.g., stretching to prevent contractures in weak limbs), optimize quality of life (e.g., conserve energy to allow for participation in social activities), compensate for lost function (e.g., alternative communication devices for patients with anarthria), and anticipate future needs (e.g., educating families about available interventions and the factors involved in decision-making) (86). Rehabilitation and palliative care specialists overlap most in providing symptom management, organizing psychosocial support for patients and families, supporting decision-making, and engaging patients and families with community support services (103,106).

There is no uniform, evidence-based guideline for rehabilitation interventions and their timing; rehabilitation interventions require careful individual assessment and individualized solutions. Interdisciplinary clinics, as described earlier in this chapter, are recommended as the medical home for patients with ALS and their families, ideally managed by a neuromuscular specialist (neurologist or physiatrist) (107). A function-based assessment should be repeated at each office visit (every 3 months, or more often as necessary) and by phone or telehealth when patients can no longer travel to clinic. A rehabilitation plan of care for a patient with ALS should include recommendations in the following domains: exercise, patient and family education/safety, equipment/modifications, symptom management, patient- and family-centered decision-making, review of advance directives, and consideration of any needs that would benefit from collaboration with palliative care (103,106).

Formally Assessing Rehabilitation Needs

The physiatrist in ALS care can provide a problem-based, functionally oriented approach to a constantly changing set of impairments and challenges, along with anticipatory guidance for managing impending functional decline (86,103). Identifying and addressing constantly changing needs can be clinically challenging, and witnessing a patient's progressive decline can be emotionally challenging. Using an assessment tool at each visit can direct providers to current needs and, in turn, point to necessary interventions and provide professional satisfaction with care (108). A useful tool for monitoring changes in function is the ALS Functional Rating Scale-Revised (ALSFRS-R). This is a 12-question self-report questionnaire, frequently used as an outcome measure in research studies, that can also be used in the clinic to provide an overview of a patient's functional status. In each domain (speech, salivation, writing, cutting food/handling utensils, dressing/hygiene, turning in bed/adjusting bedclothes, walking, climbing stairs, dyspnea, orthopnea, respiratory insufficiency), respondents choose a response from 0 to 4, with 0 being normal function and 4 representing complete loss of function/dependence on others (109). Two additional staging tools have recently been designed to help clinicians assess progression of disease and could be used in the clinic to monitor progression and evaluate rehabilitation needs: the King's College and Milano-Torino staging systems. The King's College system is based on progressive involvement of body regions (110), and the Milano-Torino system is based on progressive loss of independence in walking/self-care, swallowing, communication, and breathing (111).

In 1978, Sinaki and Mulder described six stages of ALS to be used for guiding rehabilitation management (112), and in 1998, Dal Bello-Haas et al. described an augmented set of therapy considerations for each stage (113):

- Stage I is characterized by independence in mobility and activities of daily living (ADLs). Therapy focuses on patient and family education, energy conservation, and home safety. Active range-of-motion, aerobic, and resistance exercise is recommended as tolerated.
- Stage II is characterized by moderate weakness and minimally decreased independence. Therapy often includes bracing and range of motion with active/active-assisted/passive as applicable.
- Stage III is equated with severe weakness in some muscle groups. Patients are often ambulatory but have increasing leg weakness. Therapy includes planning for wheelchair. A cervical collar may be necessary to compensate for neck extensor weakness. The therapeutic focus is on function.

- Stage IV is wheelchair use. Therapy at this stage includes monitoring the skin for pressure areas and modifying seating and mattresses for pressure relief.
- Stage V is marked by difficulty with transfers and repositioning. Therapy includes transfer training and positioning to reduce pain occurring as a consequence of immobility.
- Stage VI is dependence for all ADLs and use of respiratory support. Therapy is focused on quality of life and training caregivers for extensive patient needs.

Psychological support, education, and connection with community resources are recommended throughout the course of the disease (112,113).

The physiatrist works in close collaboration with physical, occupational, and speech therapists to implement and direct the rehabilitation plan. Physical and occupational therapists help address motor abnormalities including muscle weakness, spasticity, and contractures that cause impairments of gait, transfers, and ADLs. SLPs evaluate dysphagia and communication needs. The progression of disease in ALS can rapidly take the ALS patient from independence to dependence, and the phenotypic variability between patients means that each individual's pattern of functional loss will be unique, requiring serial assessments to meet the patient's needs.

Rehabilitation Interventions

Exercise

Patients often ask about the role of exercise in slowing muscle loss and the safety of performing premorbid exercise activities. Evaluation of the most rigorous existing data on exercise in ALS suggests that a moderate aerobic and gentle strengthening program may improve function, as compared with a stretching program alone, although more research is needed to confirm this effect (114,115). Importantly, no adverse effects of moderate exercise programs were seen (116,117).

Based on clinical experience, for patients cleared medically to exercise, we recommend an exercise program supervised by a PT with experience in caring for patients with ALS, to include a daily exercise regimen and fitting for assistive and mobility devices as needed (103). Physical activity can maintain cardiovascular fitness and can prevent disuse atrophy from compounding disease-related atrophy. Practical exercise recommendations for flexibility, strengthening, aerobic, and balance exercises are described in **Table 23-4** (103). The intensity of the exercise program should be decreased if a patient experiences symptoms of overuse, namely, muscle soreness 24 to 48 hours after exercise, major muscle cramping or heaviness, or prolonged shortness of breath (118).

Over time, the focus of physical therapy will change from maximizing use of remaining muscles to compensating for weak muscles using mobility and other equipment to optimize comfort and quality of life (113). As most insurance providers only cover a fixed number of sessions per year, a patient should use physical therapy visits intermittently to address new needs and revise a home program, rather than in one continuous burst at the beginning of the disease course. When modified activity is necessary, community-based adaptive sports provide a nice combination of social engagement, support, and exercise, and patients can also consider low-impact aquatic therapy and body weight–supported treadmill therapy (119). Beyond

TABLE 23-4	Practical Exercise Recommendations		
Exercise	**Description**	**Benefits**	**Practical Considerations**
Flexibility	Stretching, range of motion	Part of the standard of care for prevention and management of contractures; might also help reduce pain and spasticity	Encourage regular stretching and range-of-motion exercises early in the course of disease. Caregiver participation is needed when muscle weakness prevents the patient from performing program independently.
Strengthening	Repeated muscle actions against resistance	Potential role in maintaining muscle strength and delaying onset of functional impairment	Avoid high-resistance exercise. A practical approach is to find a weight that the patient can lift comfortably 20 times. Then, ask the patient to perform 2–3 sets of 10 repetitions each with that weight. Progression to heavier loads depends on the stage of disease. Do not exercise muscles that do not have antigravity strength. Avoid eccentric exercise.
Aerobic	Dynamic activity using large muscle groups	Potential role in reducing deconditioning and improving functional independence, mood, sleep, spasticity, and quality of life	Select a mode of exercise with minimal risk of injury from falling (e.g., recumbent stationary bike as opposed to treadmill). Aerobic exercise should be performed at a moderate, submaximum level. A practical approach is to begin with bouts of 10 minutes of exercise 2–3 times a week and progress as tolerated. If the patient cannot talk comfortably during exercise, the program is too vigorous.
Balance	Balance training using different modalities	Potential role in fall risk reduction	Perform under supervision of a physical therapist.

From Majmudar S, Wu J, Paganoni S. Rehabilitation in amyotrophic lateral sclerosis: why it matters. *Muscle Nerve*. 2014,50(1):4–13. Copyright © 2014 Wiley Periodicals, Inc. Reprinted by permission of John Wiley & Sons, Inc.

physical decline, engagement in safe exercise activity may be limited by mood or cognitive changes, and these factors must be considered if a patient experiences decreased interest or engagement.

Respiratory exercise to strengthen muscles of respiration is an important, often overlooked, component of a comprehensive exercise program as well. Respiratory therapists can offer inspiratory and expiratory muscle training, lung volume recruitment training, and manually assisted cough, which may improve muscle strength (120,121).

Energy Conservation

As extremity and diaphragmatic muscles weaken, strategies for ambulating and performing activities as efficiently as possible will help maximize autonomy, social engagement, safety, and enjoyment of daily life. Energy conservation techniques include planning ahead, prioritizing activities, balancing short bursts of activity with rest, avoiding unnecessary movements, obtaining a disability placard and/or paratransit access, arranging workspaces efficiently, wearing lightweight clothing, and utilizing appropriate equipment. Many energy conservation techniques can be practiced during PT and OT sessions.

Transfers and Functional Mobility

Daily functional mobility includes bed mobility and transfers. Repositioning in bed and moving from one surface to another safely are important because injury to a patient can result in substantial physical decline. Injury to a caregiver can reduce the caregiver's ability to provide care. As extremity or respiratory weakness progresses or mobility equipment is changed, patients and caregivers should be trained on safe bed mobility and transfer techniques. Collaboration with physical and occupational therapists can optimize patient-specific recommendations for techniques and equipment. Generally, bed mobility aids include overhead trapezes and adjustable hospital beds. For pALS, fully electric hospital beds are the best option especially for patients with advanced disease when the use of trapeze devices may become difficult and may even lead

to musculoskeletal injury. Transfer aids include slideboards, transfer belts, and adjustable height seating. A major principle in assisted functional mobility is teaching the patient to talk a caregiver through repositioning and transfers, enabling the patient to remain in control of their care, comfort, and bodies, as much as possible.

Equipment

Orthoses

Orthoses are commonly prescribed for positioning, preventing deformity, improving function, decreasing pain, and conserving energy in weak muscle groups. Common orthoses used for patients with ALS are cervical orthoses to compensate for next extensor weakness, hand orthoses (splints) to compensate for intrinsic hand muscle weakness, and ankle-foot orthoses (AFOs) to compensate for ankle dorsiflexion weakness. Key principles in prescribing orthoses are (a) evaluation and fitting by an experienced therapist/orthotist, (b) customization where necessary to ensure comfort and use, (c) focused function-based physical or occupational therapy training with a new orthosis, and (d) frequent skin checks under the orthosis to check for proper fit and skin integrity. **Tables 23-5** and **23-6** describe hand orthoses and ankle-foot orthoses commonly used in ALS care (103).

Ambulatory Aids

As ALS progresses, lower extremity orthoses alone may be insufficient to provide safe ambulation. Respiratory dysfunction may limit ambulatory endurance as well. Assisted ambulation with canes, crutches, or walkers may be possible initially, with the anticipation that in most cases, wheeled mobility with a power wheelchair and caregiver assistance will ultimately be required.

Canes, crutches, and walkers require trunk and upper extremity strength, and specific device selection is based upon the amount of body weight support needed, rate of progression, upper extremity strength, and patient preferences. When

TABLE 23-5	Hand Orthoses (Splints) Used Most Commonly in ALS Care	
Type of Splint	**Description**	**Use**
Resting hand splint	Lightweight; may be used during the day and/or at night to maintain proper muscle length in patients with wrist and intrinsic hand muscle weakness	Prevention of wrist and finger flexion contractures
Anticlaw	Limits metacarpophalangeal (MCP) extension and improve grasp by keeping the joints flexed	Reduction of "claw hand" deformity; improvement of grasp
Volar cock-up	Supports the wrist in 20–30 degrees of extension	Improvement of grasp in people with wrist extensor weakness
Short opponens	Keeps the thumb in an abducted and opposed position	Improvement of grasp in people with thumb abduction and extension weakness

From Majmudar S, Wu J, Paganoni S. Rehabilitation in amyotrophic lateral sclerosis: why it matters. *Muscle Nerve.* 2014,50(1):4–13. Copyright © 2014 Wiley Periodicals, Inc. Reprinted by permission of John Wiley & Sons, Inc.

hand strength is adequate for pressing grip brakes, a four-wheeled walker with hand brakes and a seat is commonly used for stability, ease of pushing, and ease of resting. Scooters are generally not used for patients with ALS for several reasons: they require substantial trunk stability, they cannot be modified for disease progression, and insurance coverage may preclude coverage for an eventual power wheelchair.

When a wheelchair is necessary and a patient is able to transfer between sitting surfaces, a manual chair may allow the most flexibility at first for self-propelling, pushing by a caregiver, and transporting in a car. We recommend that a lightweight (<36 lb) or ultralightweight (<30 lb) manual chair be rented or borrowed from an organization such as the ALS Association or Muscular Dystrophy Association or purchased out of pocket. Most insurance providers cover only one wheelchair over the course of several years, and the covered chair should be the power chair, which can cost upwards of $25,000.

A power wheelchair should be anticipated when manual wheelchair use begins. Ideally, a patient will be seen in a specialty wheelchair and seating clinic, and a detailed wheelchair prescription will be written by the patient's doctor in consultation with the clinic (122). Specific documentation of patient need, assessed in-person by the prescribing physician, is also required for insurance coverage. The physician must include why a manual wheelchair is insufficient and that the patient can use a power wheelchair safely. Generally, a person with ALS requires a CMS Class C wheelchair (the most modifiable, allows for pressure relief and ventilator accommodations). Features to be specified on the wheelchair prescription

include seat size; back height; head, neck, trunk, and extremity supports; seat cushion type; modes of pressure relief; seat belts; type of drive (front, mid-, or rear wheel); user interface (e.g., joystick, mini joystick, head array, sip-and-puff, eye gaze control); accommodations for spasticity or contractures; and additional equipment to be attached (e.g., communication devices).

A physiatrist can play a key role in expediting a patient's receipt of a wheelchair by completing paperwork thoroughly and rapidly and advocating for the patient's needs with the insurance company and wheelchair vendors. The process can take several months for the power wheelchair to be approved by insurance, built, and delivered to the patient.

Public transportation systems are required to provide accessible transport for individuals who have mobility or other impairments. Options typically include ramped buses with wheelchair ties to secure the chair to the bus, ramped subway cars, and paratransit vehicles that transport clients directly between client-requested destinations. A patient may need a physician's letter of necessity to register for paratransit services.

The main principles of mobility equipment prescription are the following: (a) prescribe and begin fitting before the patient fully requires a device, in order to allow the patient to train on equipment and allow time for paperwork processing; (b) write a detailed prescription in collaboration with a trained specialist in an orthosis/wheelchair clinic—equipment should be individualized to the patient and accommodate weakness, spasticity, contractures, and other concerns; (c) for wheelchairs, anticipate future needs, for example, allow room for a

TABLE 23-6	Ankle-Foot Orthoses (AFOs) Used Most Commonly in ALS Care	
Type of AFO	**Description**	**Use**
Posterior leaf spring	Medial and lateral trim lines are placed posterior to the malleoli; somewhat flexible	Mild-to-moderate foot drop
Carbon-fiber lateral or posterior strut dorsiflexion assist brace	Lightweight, unobtrusive	Moderate foot drop (also helps with knee control)
Floor reaction orthoses (FROs), such as the ToeOFF braces	Built to leverage ground reaction forces to offer a "push" at toe off to assist with propulsion and compensate for ankle plantar flexion weakness; they also create a knee extension moment to help counteract quadriceps weakness and tendency to knee buckling	Mild-to-moderate foot drop with quadriceps weakness; they also help compensate for ankle plantar flexion weakness
Hinged (articulated)	Include an ankle joint; allow sit-to-stand transfers more easily than solid AFOs; antispasticity features (such as a plantar flexion stop) can be incorporated as needed	Moderate foot drop ± spasticity. Sufficient knee extensor strength needed for optimal use

From Majmudar S, Wu J, Paganoni S. Rehabilitation in amyotrophic lateral sclerosis: why it matters. *Muscle Nerve.* 2014,50(1):4–13. Copyright © 2014 Wiley Periodicals, Inc. Reprinted by permission of John Wiley & Sons, Inc.

lap tray or ventilator tubing even if neither is not yet needed; (d) be mindful of insurance and timing of hospice referrals as most insurance allows only one wheelchair every 5 years and hospice does not pay for wheelchairs or most other durable medical equipment; (e) after new equipment arrives, a patient and family should be trained with it under the guidance of an experienced therapist; (f) monitor frequently for comfort and skin integrity, and modify the wheelchair as necessary; (g) power wheelchair use may require additional modifications to the home and vehicle, including ramps; (h) power wheelchairs frequently need repair—a backup manual wheelchair is recommended; and (i) transition to assisted mobility can be emotionally difficult, challenging to a patient's self-perception, and physically restrictive (e.g., patient can no longer access parts of his or her home). It is important to incorporate open communication and supportive counseling into this phase of care.

Assistive Devices for Activities of Daily Living

In ALS, weakness, fatigue, contractures, and pain can limit independence with ADLs (self-care) and more complex instrumental ADLs (home management tasks such as housework, childcare, meal preparation, driving, financial management, turning appliances on and off). Activity modifications to promote participation in these tasks include altering the task itself, utilizing assistive technology to perform the task, and modifying the environment in which to perform the task. Using eating/cooking as an example, altering a task for a person with limited fine motor coordination could be mashing a banana instead of slicing it; assistive technology for fruit preparation could include a rocker knife to compensate for hand weakness and a plate guard to reduce spilling; environmental modification could include removing cabinets from under kitchen counters to facilitate access to food preparation space.

Assistive devices come in prefabricated versions and can also be modified or created from scratch, typically by occupational therapists. To get the best use from a device, the device needs to be positioned appropriately and utilized when a patient is awake and attentive. Patients and caregivers are often creative problem-solvers when faced with challenges in the home, and we can learn many lessons from them that we can share with other patients and caregivers. **Table 23-7** lists sample assistive devices for basic ADLs and their uses.

Home Renovations, Home Safety, and Emergency Preparedness

For patients with hand weakness, modifications to existing devices that can prolong independence in accessing the home include key extenders to make a key larger for easier grip, doorknob extenders to convert doorknobs into levers for easier use, and voice-activated control over window shades, thermostats, lights, and other home features. Typical home modifications to accommodate wheelchairs include remodeling bathrooms to allow full wheelchair turning radius and wheeled entry into a shower, installing ramps outside the home, offsetting door hinges to allow for wider door openings, and retrofitting a first floor room (e.g., living room) into a bedroom. Medicare and private insurance typically do not cover home renovations, but in some cases, Medicaid will cover renovations/modifications.

The Americans with Disabilities Act specifies architectural standards for creating accessible public facilities. These standards should also be used to the greatest extent possible when making home accessibility modifications, as they provide adequate wheelchair turning radius (60 in.), appropriate switch heights (30 to 36 in. from the floor to be reachable from a seated position), and safe ramp inclines (1 ft height for 12 ft of length). Regulations for accessible design can be found at ADA.gov.

Modifications for home safety are important because falls and injuries can result in substantial functional decline. General home safety tips include removing loose rugs and clearing pathways for walking, installing good lighting, keeping walkways free of small pets that run and jump, and adding grab bars in bathrooms and other areas. Installing ramps or stair lifts early where possible can prevent falls on stairs as weakness progresses. A PT or OT home visit for safety evaluation can result in useful situation-specific recommendations.

Planning for emergencies such as loss of power, home fire, or weather-related evacuation can reduce anxiety and provide immense practical and possibly lifesaving benefit. General recommendations include registering with local utility companies to be placed on a priority list for backup power during outages, obtaining a backup generator for lifts and ventilators if possible, and keeping a list of medications and advance directives with a patient and posted in the home at all times.

TABLE 23-7	**Sample Assistive Devices for ADLs**	
Activity	**Devices**	**Use**
Feeding	Universal cuff	Holding utensils, compensating for weak intrinsic hand muscle
	Scoop dishes, plate bumpers	Allow manipulation of food and minimize spilling
Grooming	Shoulder-mounted shampoo rinse trays	Facilitate hair washing over a sink while sitting in wheelchair
	Thick and/or long-handled toothbrushes, combs, toenail clippers; nail brushes with suction cup bases	Compensate for hand weakness and decreased balance or spine range of motion
Bathing	Bath mitts	Compensate for hand weakness
	Shower benches, grab bars	Compensate for weakness, conserve energy, promote safety (note, towel racks should not be used as grab bars as they typically cannot support body weight)
Dressing and undressing	Button looper, modified zipper pulls, elastic shoelaces	Compensate for hand weakness and impaired coordination
	Dressing stick	Compensate for arm weakness; used pulling the side of a shirt across the body
Toileting	Commode chairs, raised toilet seats	Facilitating safe transfers; prolonging independence

The Red Cross publishes a booklet and detailed checklist for emergency preparedness for people with disabilities—Preparing for Disaster for People with Disabilities and other Special Needs.

Communication

It is expected that nearly all individuals with ALS will develop dysarthria, progressing to anarthria. Both speech intelligibility and prosody are affected, and communication effectiveness is impaired long before a patient is anarthric. The inability to communicate, with its associated loss of autonomy and social interaction, is a major fear in newly diagnosed patients. It is important to educate patients about the range of options available for supporting communication over the course of the disease. It is equally important to ensure that patients have excellent speech-language therapy monitoring and care so that communication is always maximized (see Chapter 13).

A speech-language pathologist, alternative and augmentative communication specialist, and an orthotist are key rehabilitation team members in helping individuals interact with others and control their surroundings. Rehabilitation focuses initially on optimizing intelligibility through avoiding overuse, minimizing background noise, slowing speech rate, overarticulating words, and helping patient and caregiver develop a system for confirming understanding (123). Dysarthria in ALS does not respond well to articulation training, is not corrected by traditional speech therapy exercises, and may even worsen speech intelligibility due to fatigue.

As dysarthria progresses, a variety of low and high technology alternative and augmentative communication aids can be prescribed, as listed in **Table 23-8**. Low technology solutions are often easier to use than higher technology devices and should be used as long as possible. A relatively inexpensive option, and an upgrade from the dusty whiteboard, is the boogie board—an electronic tablet with a stylus for writing. As long as the patient has adequate hand function, the boogie board is simple and easy to use. Another simple and popular option is the texting feature on a cell phone. Asynchronous communication such as e-mail, Text Telephone (TTY) systems (if dysarthria and enough preserved hand function), and social media programs should be encouraged, as communication is not limited by slow or difficult-to-understand speech. A growing number of communications programs for mobile devices in both PC and Apple formats, such as the MyTalkTools mobile app (support@mytalk.zendesk.com), are becoming available as well. Both low and high technology communication options are listed in **Table 23-8**.

Pain Management

Pain is not a common presenting feature of ALS though it frequently occurs as a complication of disease progression (126,127) and is not adequately managed especially as patients with ALS near end of life (128,129). Pain can result from improper positioning in an orthosis or wheelchair, musculoskeletal complications of immobility, cramps, neuropathic syndromes, spasticity, pressure ulcers, and unrelated conditions, such as arthritis. **Figure 23-3** shows multiple potential sources of pain. Pain can be exacerbated by depression, poor sleep quality, and fatigue. Pain management includes etiology-specific pharmacologic management, joint injections

TABLE 23-8	Communication Technology
Low technology	• Word/letter/picture boards (patient-selected options or partner-assisted scanning acknowledged by patient eyeblink or other response) • Palatal lifts • Binary choice eye gaze communication system developed between patient and speech therapist or caregiver • Cell phone texting, social media • Mobile and tablet apps
High technology	• LiteWriter with word prediction • Portable voice amplifiers • Voice banking with playback (speech samples banked while speech still intelligible) • Text-to-speech synthesizers (can be controlled by hand, eye gaze, infrared signal; can be mounted to wheelchair)
Emerging technology	• Brain-computer interfaces (124,125)

as appropriate, proper equipment fitting and use, proper bed positioning and transfers, and palliative care consultation for intractable pain requiring opioid medications in large doses (**Table 23-3**).

Quality of Life

In general, quality of life among pALS tends to be underestimated by both caregivers and clinicians (130,131). Patients with ALS report fairly stable quality of life over time, not related to changes in strength or physical function. It can be diminished by certain experiences, such as initial speech impairment (132) and pain (48), but generally quality of life in ALS seems to be related most to social and existential factors such as social support, financial situation, and spirituality (133–136). This is important because a patient's expression of dissatisfaction or sadness should not be assumed to be simply related to progression of disease, and other manageable etiologies should be sought.

Caregivers, on the other hand, do seem to experience worsening quality of life as a patient's physical function declines (137,138). Primary caregivers for pALS are typically spouses. The spousal role changes dramatically across the trajectory of ALS. The unaffected spouse loses a partner in intimacy, financial support, and shared family responsibilities. He or she acquires responsibilities for patient care and comfort, home modifications, and decision-making in multiple domains. Social interactions outside the home become less frequent, attention is diverted from other family members, and responsibilities and routines continually change. The financial cost of caring for a patient with ALS in the home can be tens of thousands of dollars a year or more, factoring in supplies, assistance, home modifications, medications, and medical bills. These factors can result in feelings of stress, guilt, anxiety, and depression.

Comprehensive rehabilitation care for a patient with ALS includes addressing caregiver burden. Recommendations include validating caregiver concerns, encouraging self-care, and partnering with caregivers as experts in a patient's care. Strategies from a mindfulness approach (139) might be helpful for some families as well.

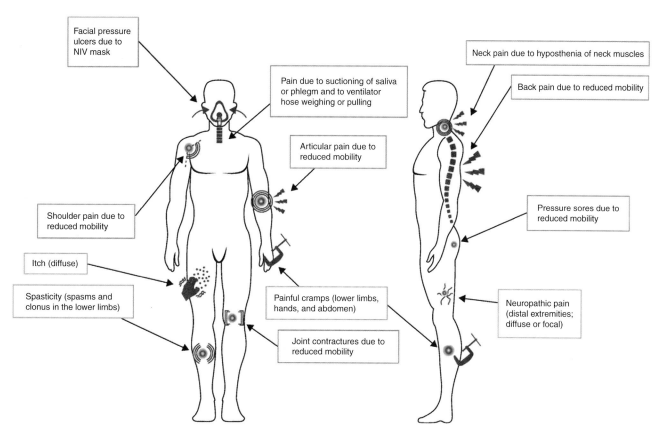

FIGURE 23-3. Types of pain in ALS. (Reprinted from Chio A, Mora G, Lauria G. Pain in amyotrophic lateral sclerosis. *Lancet Neurol.* 2017;16(2):144–157. Copyright © 2016 Elsevier. With permission.)

Importantly, facilitating the introduction of home care services has great potential for alleviating caregiver stress. In a study of home care for patients with ALS, even caregivers with additional assistance spent a median of 11 hours/day performing patient care. Forty-two percent of primary caregivers surveyed felt physically unwell and 48% felt psychologically unwell (140). Given the expense of hiring assistance in the home, a social worker or other resource expert can be very helpful in connecting a caregiver with appropriate resources.

A recent study of neurologists showed that experience in palliative care enabled neurologists to better estimate quality of life for those patients with ALS using feeding tubes and invasive ventilation (131). This suggests that physiatrists too can benefit from, and should seek, palliative care training and experience to improve their care for patients with ALS and other neuromuscular diseases. Palliative care training can sharpen expertise in eliciting patient preferences and guiding management consistent with patient values, experiences, and preferences.

Palliative Care

Palliative care is both a philosophy of care and a subspecialty of medicine (see also Chapter 36). Like rehabilitation care, the focus is on comfort and quality of life, although palliative care focuses primarily on treating patients with life-limiting illnesses. Palliative care can be offered concurrently with disease-modifying treatment and participation in clinical trials.

Principles of palliative care relevant to caring for pALS and their families include understanding a patient's values and goals; supporting decision-making; educating patients and families; managing advanced symptoms of pain, dyspnea, oral secretions, and anxiety; helping patients avoid emergent unplanned hospitalizations; navigating ethical concerns; helping patients create closure and legacy; helping to plan for the dying process; managing symptoms of active dying; transitioning to hospice; and supporting patients and families experiencing grief.

Substantial functional decline requiring new equipment such as power wheelchair, major decline in pulmonary function, weight loss of 10% or more, recurrent infections, poorly healing skin lesions, onset of communication or cognitive challenges, medical need for decisions regarding intervention use (e.g., PEG, NIV, TIV), and a specific request by patient or family are each appropriate times to convene a patient/family meeting and have an open discussion about recent changes and anticipated future changes. For example, increasing leg weakness in an ambulatory patient might trigger planning for wheelchair fitting; the new stage might also trigger patient/family questions about topics ranging from wheelchair use to life expectancy. The neuromuscular specialist may choose to facilitate such meetings in collaboration with palliative care or other supportive care providers and should use a "breaking bad news" framework. This includes being seated with the patient/family, making eye contact, asking families what they know and what they'd like to know, deferring calls/pages in order to focus on the conversation, bearing witness to sadness, and helping to make a plan going forward that includes follow-up by phone or in person within days/weeks. The pace of discussions, if medical status allows, should be guided by the patient (105,141,142). If a patient specifically declines feeding tube or long-term mechanical ventilation at a time when either is deemed medically necessary, a focused palliative care approach and/or consultation should be initiated, with consideration of a role for hospice services (143).

Decision-Making

Many difficult decisions are required of patients through the course of their disease. Starting with diagnosis, a patient must decide how much information they want at a time and how they want to receive it. Before communication and cognition impair decision-making, and before the medical needs for interventions become emergent, advance decisions about nutrition and ventilation must be discussed. Decisions for these interventions are generally based on a patient's values, religious beliefs, goals (e.g., to be alive for a child's wedding), and availability of home support, although the perspective of the patient's physician affects decision-making too. It is important for physicians to be cognizant of this during decision-making conversations.

Directives about resuscitation must be determined and posted in the home in the event of emergency. Many states have specific Physician Orders for Life-Sustaining Treatment/ Medical Orders for Life-Sustaining Treatment (POLST/ MOLST) forms, which provide out-of-hospital emergency treatment/do not resuscitate (DNR) orders for emergency medical personnel and in addition can be used as a tool for discussion between health care providers and families. Wishes for aggressiveness of general care must be documented as well. For example, while the patient is still relatively healthy, queries such as "If you were to get a serious infection, where would you like to be treated?" and "Do you want all available medical interventions, including those that may be life prolonging?" will help open discussions about locations and types of care desired and define preferences (144).

A patient may inquire about physician-assisted suicide. In Washington state, where individuals can receive lethal medication under the Death with Dignity Act, 5% of patients who died of ALS sought medications, and among those obtaining a prescription for lethal medication, 77% of the patients used them (145). Major reasons included loss of autonomy, loss of ability to engage in enjoyable activities, loss of dignity, loss of control of body function, burden on others, inadequate pain control, and financial implications of treatment (145). An extensive discussion of requests for physician-assisted death is beyond the scope of this chapter, but principles of doctor-patient conversation about this topic include (a) understanding a patient's reasons and assuring that symptoms such as pain and depression are managed and fears about end of life are adequately addressed (e.g., many patients fear air hunger or asphyxiation; in reality, most patients die peacefully, and should bothersome symptoms arise, medical management is available); (b) physicians should become familiar with local rules and laws about physician-assisted death; and (c) physicians should respectfully refer to other providers if they do not feel comfortable with the conversations.

Early in the course of disease, a health care directive should be defined and durable power of attorney assigned. These decisions should be revisited every few months, as wishes can change over time. Conversations should include the opportunity for patients and families to describe their concerns—commonly, a patient has concerns about becoming a physical and financial burden to family and friends; a long-term planning discussion that allows these issues to be resolved can reduce anxiety and facilitate planning (146). Offering end-of-life planning assistance at least annually (including advance directives, invasive ventilation, and hospice) is recommended by the American Academy of Neurology (87).

Hospice and End-of-Life Care

Hospice care is an insurance benefit a patient can elect when prognosis is 6 months or less, which focuses on comfort and end of life. Hospice provides multidisciplinary symptom management, psychosocial and spiritual support, medical supplies (but typically not mobility or other expensive durable medical equipment), identification of the process of active dying, provision of pharmacologic management to provide comfort during the dying process, planning for avoidance of unwanted emergent hospitalizations, and family bereavement support. A patient can have tube feeding and noninvasive positive pressure ventilation while receiving hospice services, as these are considered comfort measures. Hospice care often occurs in the patient's home per patient wishes, but can be provided in inpatient hospice or ALS-specific facilities as well. While hospice does provide psychosocial support for the family, it does not provide many hours of home care assistance.

In many cases, it can be difficult to estimate life expectancy due to a relatively prolonged dying process in ALS, making it difficult to document a 6-month prognosis to meet eligibility for hospice criteria. As hospice services can ease distress and promote a peaceful death, one should consider a patient with ALS to be in the terminal phase and eligible for hospice if there is rapid decline over a 12-month period along with major respiratory impairment, nutritional impairment, or life-threatening complication (recurrent aspiration pneumonia, decubitus ulcers, upper urinary tract infections [UTIs], sepsis, fever after antibiotics). It can be clearer that the patient is approaching death when major interventions are declined or withdrawn. In those cases, we recommend initiating hospice quickly, as long as patient and caregiver are in agreement. Sometimes, it can take several conversations on separate occasions in order to give patients and families time and support in thinking about end of life. It is important to focus on the value of hospice in optimizing home care and providing a comfortable death in the location of the patient's choice.

The primary cause of death in ALS is respiratory failure, whether or not a patient is using invasive ventilation. Most patients with ALS die peacefully. Distressing symptoms can occur—especially cough, congestion, pain, dyspnea, insomnia, anxiety, and fear (147). These can be managed pharmacologically by hospice providers. If a patient decides not to have a feeding tube placed, aggressive comfort measures also include allowing small amounts of oral intake for pleasure if possible, providing good oral hygiene, and managing of dry mouth (148). If a patient declines or withdraws noninvasive or invasive ventilation when it would be required for sustaining life, breathlessness, cough, secretions, and anxiety can be managed aggressively pharmacologically with benzodiazepines and opioids, and sedation can be available if symptoms cannot be comfortably managed (148,149).

It is absolutely appropriate (and welcomed by patients and families) for a rehabilitation doctor to continue to be involved in care when a patient is receiving hospice care. This provides continuity for patient, caregivers, and clinician and allows ongoing personalized clinical input to the hospice team. Some physicians attend funeral services when possible, to provide closure and continuity for both clinician and family.

SUMMARY

ALS is a progressive disease, with no known cure. Patients with ALS present with multiple symptoms and increasing evolving needs over the trajectory of the disease (typically 3 to 5 years). An experienced multidisciplinary team can make a significant impact on the lives of patients and caregivers at each stage of the disease by treating disease-related symptoms, offering a variety of rehabilitation strategies that can enhance function and quality of life, and fostering collaboration among neurology, physiatry, palliative care, and the host of critically necessary allied health providers who provide direct education and care to patients and caregivers. As new scientific breakthroughs bring us ever closer to finding disease-modifying treatments, it is anticipated that the life span of pALS will increase and the need for ALS rehabilitation interventions will continue to grow.

All of the MNDs are relentlessly progressive diseases that rob patients of independence and families of time and experiences together. While discussion of ALS, as the most common of the MNDs, occupies the majority of this chapter, the principles of its treatment outlined apply to the other MNDs as well.

ACKNOWLEDGMENTS

This chapter is dedicated in remembrance of Dr. Lisa Stroud Krivickas, a pioneer for physiatrists caring for persons with ALS. We are fortunate to have been mentored and inspired by Dr. Krivickas and strive to continue her work as physiatrists dedicated to finding a cure and enhancing rehabilitation options for ALS.

REFERENCES

1. Mehta P, Antao V, Kaye W, et al. Prevalence of amyotrophic lateral sclerosis—United States, 2010-2011. *MMWR Suppl.* 2014;63:1–14.
2. Chancellor AM, Warlow CP. Adult onset motor neuron disease: worldwide mortality, incidence and distribution since 1950. *J Neurol Neurosurg Psychiatry.* 1992;55:1106–1115.
3. Blasco H, Patin F, Andres CR, et al. Amyotrophic Lateral Sclerosis, 2016: existing therapies and the ongoing search for neuroprotection. *Expert Opin Pharmacother.* 2016;17:1669–1682.
4. Chio A, Logroscino G, Hardiman O, et al. Prognostic factors in ALS: a critical review. *Amyotroph Lateral Scler.* 2009;10:310–323.
5. Wang H, O'Reilly EJ, Weisskopf MG, et al. Smoking and risk of amyotrophic lateral sclerosis: a pooled analysis of 5 prospective cohorts. *Arch Neurol.* 2011;68:207–213.
6. Gallo V, Bueno-De-Mesquita HB, Vermeulen R, et al. Smoking and risk for amyotrophic lateral sclerosis: analysis of the EPIC cohort. *Ann Neurol.* 2009;65: 378–385.
7. Bryan L, Kaye W, Antao V, et al. Preliminary results of national amyotrophic lateral sclerosis (ALS) registry risk factor survey data. *PLoS One.* 2016;11:e0153683.
8. Institute of Medicine (U.S.); Committee on the Review of the Scientific Literature on Amyotrophic Lateral Sclerosis in Veterans. *Amyotrophic Lateral Sclerosis in Veterans: Review of the Scientific Literature.* Washington, DC: National Academies Press; 2006.
9. Watanabe Y, Watanabe T. Meta-analytic evaluation of the association between head injury and risk of amyotrophic lateral sclerosis. *Eur J Epidemiol.* 2017 Oct;32(10):867–879.
10. Gallo V, Vanacore N, Bueno-de-Mesquita HB, et al. Physical activity and risk of Amyotrophic Lateral Sclerosis in a prospective cohort study. *Eur J Epidemiol.* 2016;31:255–266.
11. Armon C. Occurrence of amyotrophic lateral sclerosis among Gulf War veterans. *Neurology.* 2004;62:1027; author reply 1027–1029.
12. Chio A, Benzi G, Dossena M, et al. Severely increased risk of amyotrophic lateral sclerosis among Italian professional football players. *Brain.* 2005;128: 472–476.
13. Valenti M, Pontieri FE, Conti F, et al. Amyotrophic lateral sclerosis and sports: a case-control study. *Eur J Neurol.* 2005;12:223–225.
14. Wang MD, Little J, Gomes J, et al. Identification of risk factors associated with onset and progression of amyotrophic lateral sclerosis using systematic review and meta-analysis. *Neurotoxicology.* 2016;61:101–130.
15. Carter GT, Abresch RT, Fowler WM Jr, et al. Profiles of neuromuscular diseases. Spinal muscular atrophy. *Am J Phys Med Rehabil.* 1995;74:S150–S159.
16. Rosen DR, Siddique T, Patterson D, et al. Mutations in Cu/Zn superoxide dismutase gene are associated with familial amyotrophic lateral sclerosis. *Nature.* 1993;362: 59–62.
17. D'Amico E, Factor-Litvak P, Santella RM, et al. Clinical perspective on oxidative stress in sporadic amyotrophic lateral sclerosis. *Free Radic Biol Med.* 2013;65:509–527.
18. Taylor JP, Brown RH Jr, Cleveland DW. Decoding ALS: from genes to mechanism. *Nature.* 2016;539:197–206.
19. Blasco H, Mavel S, Corcia P, et al. The glutamate hypothesis in ALS: pathophysiology and drug development. *Curr Med Chem.* 2014;21:3551–3575.
20. Deng HX, Chen W, Hong ST, et al. Mutations in UBQLN2 cause dominant X-linked juvenile and adult-onset ALS and ALS/dementia. *Nature.* 2011;477: 211–215.
21. Strong MJ, Volkening K, Hammond R, et al. TDP43 is a human low molecular weight neurofilament (hNFL) mRNA-binding protein. *Mol Cell Neurosci.* 2007;35:320–327.
22. Vucic S, Rothstein JD, Kiernan MC. Advances in treating amyotrophic lateral sclerosis: insights from pathophysiological studies. *Trends Neurosci.* 2014;37:433–442.
23. Ng AS, Rademakers R, Miller BL. Frontotemporal dementia: a bridge between dementia and neuromuscular disease. *Ann N Y Acad Sci.* 2015;1338:71–93.
24. Renton AE, Chio A, Traynor BJ. State of play in amyotrophic lateral sclerosis genetics. *Nat Neurosci.* 2014;17:17–23.
25. Turner MR, Hardiman O, Benatar M, et al. Controversies and priorities in amyotrophic lateral sclerosis. *Lancet Neurol.* 2013;12:310–322.
26. Al-Chalabi A, van den Berg LH, Veldink J. Gene discovery in amyotrophic lateral sclerosis: implications for clinical management. *Nat Rev Neurol.* 2017;13:96–104.
27. Hausmanowa-Petrusewicz I, Vrbova G. Spinal muscular atrophy: a delayed development hypothesis. *Neuroreport.* 2005;16:657–661.
28. Swoboda KJ, Prior TW, Scott CB, et al. Natural history of denervation in SMA: relation to age, SMN2 copy number, and function. *Ann Neurol.* 2005;57:704–712.
29. Boda B, Mas C, Giudicelli C, et al. Survival motor neuron SMN1 and SMN2 gene promoters: identical sequences and differential expression in neurons and non-neuronal cells. *Eur J Hum Genet.* 2004;12:729–737.
30. Burrell JR, Vucic S, Kiernan MC. Isolated bulbar phenotype of amyotrophic lateral sclerosis. *Amyotroph Lateral Scler.* 2011;12:283–289.
31. Chio A, Calvo A, Moglia C, et al.; PARALS study group. Phenotypic heterogeneity of amyotrophic lateral sclerosis: a population based study. *J Neurol Neurosurg Psychiatry.* 2011;82:740–746.
32. Ravits J, Appel S, Baloh RH, et al. Deciphering amyotrophic lateral sclerosis: what phenotype, neuropathology and genetics are telling us about pathogenesis. *Amyotroph Lateral Scler Frontotemporal Degener.* 2013;14(suppl 1):5–18.
33. Swinnen B, Robberecht W. The phenotypic variability of amyotrophic lateral sclerosis. *Nat Rev Neurol.* 2014;10:661–670.
34. Wolf J, Safer A, Wohrle JC, et al. Variability and prognostic relevance of different phenotypes in amyotrophic lateral sclerosis—data from a population-based registry. *J Neurol Sci.* 2014;345:164–167.
35. Shoesmith CL, Findlater K, Rowe A, et al. Prognosis of amyotrophic lateral sclerosis with respiratory onset. *J Neurol Neurosurg Psychiatry.* 2007;78:629–631.
36. Woolley SC, Jonathan SK. Cognitive and behavioral impairment in amyotrophic lateral sclerosis. *Phys Med Rehabil Clin N Am.* 2008;19:607–617, xi.
37. Strong MJ, Grace GM, Freedman M, et al. Consensus criteria for the diagnosis of frontotemporal cognitive and behavioural syndromes in amyotrophic lateral sclerosis. *Amyotroph Lateral Scler.* 2009;10:131–146.
38. Stephens HE, Joyce NC, Oskarsson B. National study of muscle cramps in ALS in the USA. *Amyotroph Lateral Scler Frontotemporal Degener.* 2017;18:32–36.
39. Amato AA, Barohn RJ. Inclusion body myositis: old and new concepts. *J Neurol Neurosurg Psychiatry.* 2009;80:1186–1193.
40. Benditt JO, Boitano L. Respiratory treatment of amyotrophic lateral sclerosis. *Phys Med Rehabil Clin N Am.* 2008;19:559–572, x.
41. Schiffman PL, Belsh JM. Pulmonary function at diagnosis of amyotrophic lateral sclerosis. Rate of deterioration. *Chest.* 1993;103:508–513.
42. Nicholson K, Murphy A, McDonnell E, et al. Improving symptom management for people with amyotrophic lateral sclerosis. *Muscle & nerve.* 2018 Jan;57(1):20–24.
43. Marin B, Arcuti S, Jesus P, et al. Population-based evidence that survival in amyotrophic lateral sclerosis is related to weight loss at diagnosis. *Neurodegener Dis.* 2016;16:225–234.
44. Paganoni S, Deng J, Jaffa M, et al. What does body mass index measure in amyotrophic lateral sclerosis and why should we care? *Muscle Nerve.* 2012;45:612.
45. Paganoni S, Deng J, Jaffa M, et al. Body mass index, not dyslipidemia, is an independent predictor of survival in amyotrophic lateral sclerosis. *Muscle Nerve.* 2011;44:20–24.
46. Kasarskis EJ, Mendiondo MS, Matthews DE, et al. Estimating daily energy expenditure in individuals with amyotrophic lateral sclerosis. *Am J Clin Nutr.* 2014;99: 792–803.

47. Sharma KR, Miller RG. Electrical and mechanical properties of skeletal muscle underlying increased fatigue in patients with amyotrophic lateral sclerosis. *Muscle Nerve*. 1996;19:1391–1400.

48. Chio A, Mora G, Lauria G. Pain in amyotrophic lateral sclerosis. *Lancet Neurol*. 2017;16:144–157.

49. Corcia P, Pradat PF, Salachas F, et al. Causes of death in a post-mortem series of ALS patients. *Amyotroph Lateral Scler*. 2008;9:59–62.

50. Norris F, Shepherd R, Denys E, et al. Onset, natural history and outcome in idiopathic adult motor neuron disease. *J Neurol Sci*. 1993;118:48–55.

51. Ringel SP, Murphy JR, Alderson MK, et al. The natural history of amyotrophic lateral sclerosis. *Neurology*. 1993;43:1316–1322.

52. Fischbeck KH, Ionasescu V, Ritter AW, et al. Localization of the gene for X-linked spinal muscular atrophy. *Neurology*. 1986;36:1595–1598.

53. MacKenzie AE, Jacob P, Surh L, et al. Genetic heterogeneity in spinal muscular atrophy: a linkage analysis-based assessment. *Neurology*. 1994;44:919–924.

54. Sperfeld AD, Karitzky J, Brummer D, et al. X-linked bulbospinal neuronopathy: Kennedy disease. *Arch Neurol*. 2002;59:1921–1926.

55. Atsuta N, Watanabe H, Ito M, et al. Natural history of spinal and bulbar muscular atrophy (SBMA): a study of 223 Japanese patients. *Brain*. 2006;129: 1446–1455.

56. Parboosingh JS, Figlewicz DA, Krizus A, et al. Spinobulbar muscular atrophy can mimic ALS: the importance of genetic testing in male patients with atypical ALS. *Neurology*. 1997;49:568–572.

57. Paganoni S, Macklin EA, Lee A, et al. Diagnostic timelines and delays in diagnosing amyotrophic lateral sclerosis (ALS). *Amyotroph Lateral Scler Frontotemporal Degener*. 2014;15:453–456.

58. Vucic S, Kiernan MC. Transcranial magnetic stimulation for the assessment of neurodegenerative disease. *Neurotherapeutics*. 2017;14:91–106.

59. Brooks BR, Miller RG, Swash M, et al.; World Federation of Neurology Research Group on Motor Neuron D. El Escorial revisited: revised criteria for the diagnosis of amyotrophic lateral sclerosis. *Amyotroph Lateral Scler Other Motor Neuron Disord*. 2000;1:293–299.

60. Ferrante MA, Wilbourn AJ. The characteristic electrodiagnostic features of Kennedy's disease. *Muscle Nerve*. 1997;20:323–329.

61. de Carvalho M, Dengler R, Eisen A, et al. Electrodiagnostic criteria for diagnosis of ALS. *Clin Neurophysiol*. 2008;119:497–503.

62. Geevasinga N, Menon P, Scherman DB, et al. Diagnostic criteria in amyotrophic lateral sclerosis: a multicenter prospective study. *Neurology*. 2016;87:684–690.

63. Miller RG, Mitchell JD, Moore DH. Riluzole for amyotrophic lateral sclerosis (ALS)/ motor neuron disease (MND). *Cochrane Database Syst Rev*. 2012;(2):CD001447.

64. Miller RG, Jackson CE, Kasarskis EJ, et al. Practice parameter update: the care of the patient with amyotrophic lateral sclerosis: drug, nutritional, and respiratory therapies (an evidence-based review): report of the Quality Standards Subcommittee of the American Academy of Neurology. *Neurology*. 2009;73:1218–1226.

65. Rooney J, Byrne S, Heverin M, et al. Survival analysis of irish amyotrophic lateral sclerosis patients diagnosed from 1995-2010. *PLoS One*. 2013;8:e74733.

66. Writing G, Edaravone ALSSG. Safety and efficacy of edaravone in well defined patients with amyotrophic lateral sclerosis: a randomised, double-blind, placebo-controlled trial. *Lancet Neurol*. 2017;16:505–512.

67. Sherman AV, Gubitz AK, Al-Chalabi A, et al. Infrastructure resources for clinical research in amyotrophic lateral sclerosis. *Amyotroph Lateral Scler Frontotemporal Degener*. 2013;14(suppl 1):53–61.

68. Otto M, Bowser R, Turner M, et al. Roadmap and standard operating procedures for biobanking and discovery of neurochemical markers in ALS. *Amyotroph Lateral Scler*. 2012;13:1–10.

69. Beghi E, Chio A, Couratier P, et al. The epidemiology and treatment of ALS: focus on the heterogeneity of the disease and critical appraisal of therapeutic trials. *Amyotroph Lateral Scler*. 2011;12:1–10.

70. Atassi N, Yerramilli-Rao P, Szymonifka J, et al. Analysis of start-up, retention, and adherence in ALS clinical trials. *Neurology*. 2013;81:1350–1355.

71. Cudkowicz ME, Katz J, Moore DH, et al. Toward more efficient clinical trials for amyotrophic lateral sclerosis. *Amyotroph Lateral Scler*. 2010;11:259–265.

72. Paganoni S, Cudkowicz M, Berry JD. Outcome measures in amyotrophic lateral sclerosis clinical trials. *Clin Investig (Lond)*. 2014;4:605–618.

73. Chad DA, Bidichandani S, Bruijn L, et al. Funding agencies and disease organizations: resources and recommendations to facilitate ALS clinical research. *Amyotroph Lateral Scler Frontotemporal Degener*. 2013;14(suppl 1):62–66.

74. Vaidya M. Ice bucket challenge cash may help derisk ALS drug research. *Nat Med*. 2014;20:1080.

75. Weiss MD, Weydt P, Carter GT. Current pharmacological management of amyotrophic [corrected] lateral sclerosis and a role for rational polypharmacy. *Expert Opin Pharmacother*. 2004;5:735–746.

76. Weiss MD, Macklin EA, Simmons Z, et al. A randomized trial of mexiletine in ALS: safety and effects on muscle cramps and progression. *Neurology*. 2016;86: 1474–1481.

77. Bedlack RS, Joyce N, Carter GT, et al. Complementary and alternative therapies in amyotrophic lateral sclerosis. *Neurol Clin*. 2015;33:909–936.

78. Amtmann D, Weydt P, Johnson KL, et al. Survey of cannabis use in patients with amyotrophic lateral sclerosis. *Am J Hosp Palliat Care*. 2004;21:95–104.

79. Carter GT, Rosen BS. Marijuana in the management of amyotrophic lateral sclerosis. *Am J Hosp Palliat Care*. 2001;18:264–270.

80. Giacoppo S, Mazzon E. Can cannabinoids be a potential therapeutic tool in amyotrophic lateral sclerosis? *Neural Regen Res*. 2016;11:1896–1899.

81. Carter GT, Abood ME, Aggarwal SK, et al. Cannabis and amyotrophic lateral sclerosis: hypothetical and practical applications, and a call for clinical trials. *Am J Hosp Palliat Care*. 2010;27:347–356.

82. Miller RG, Jackson CE, Kasarskis EJ, et al. Practice parameter update: the care of the patient with amyotrophic lateral sclerosis: multidisciplinary care, symptom management, and cognitive/behavioral impairment (an evidence-based review): report of the Quality Standards Subcommittee of the American Academy of Neurology. *Neurology*. 2009;73:1227–1233.

83. Traynor BJ, Alexander M, Corr B, et al. Effect of a multidisciplinary amyotrophic lateral sclerosis (ALS) clinic on ALS survival: a population based study, 1996-2000. *J Neurol Neurosurg Psychiatry*. 2003;74:1258–1261.

84. Chio A, Bottacchi E, Buffa C, et al.; PARALS. Positive effects of tertiary centres for amyotrophic lateral sclerosis on outcome and use of hospital facilities. *J Neurol Neurosurg Psychiatry*. 2006;77:948–950.

85. Van den Berg JP, Kalmijn S, Lindeman E, et al. Multidisciplinary ALS care improves quality of life in patients with ALS. *Neurology*. 2005;65:1264–1267.

86. Paganoni S, Karam C, Joyce N, et al. Comprehensive rehabilitative care across the spectrum of amyotrophic lateral sclerosis. *NeuroRehabilitation*. 2015;37:53–68.

87. Miller RG, Brooks BR, Swain-Eng RJ, et al. Quality improvement in neurology: amyotrophic lateral sclerosis quality measures: report of the quality measurement and reporting subcommittee of the American Academy of Neurology. *Neurology*. 2013;81:2136–2140.

88. Boylan K, Levine T, Lomen-Hoerth C, et al. Prospective study of cost of care at multidisciplinary ALS centers adhering to American Academy of Neurology (AAN) ALS practice parameters. *Amyotroph Lateral Scler Frontotemporal Degener*. 2015;17:119–127.

89. Lechtzin N, Scott Y, Busse AM, et al. Early use of non-invasive ventilation prolongs survival in subjects with ALS. *Amyotroph Lateral Scler*. 2007;8:185–188.

90. Gruis KL, Lechtzin N. Respiratory therapies for amyotrophic lateral sclerosis: a primer. *Muscle Nerve*. 2012;46:313–331.

91. Gay PC, Edmonds LC. Severe hypercapnia after low-flow oxygen therapy in patients with neuromuscular disease and diaphragmatic dysfunction. *Mayo Clin Proc*. 1995;70:327–330.

92. Jackson CE, Rosenfeld J, Moore DH, et al. A preliminary evaluation of a prospective study of pulmonary function studies and symptoms of hypoventilation in ALS/MND patients. *J Neurol Sci*. 2001;191:75–78.

93. Traynor BJ, Codd MB, Corr B, et al. Incidence and prevalence of ALS in Ireland, 1995-1997: a population-based study. *Neurology*. 1999;52:504–509.

94. Tomita T, Tanaka K, Shinden S, et al. Tracheoesophageal diversion versus total laryngectomy for intractable aspiration. *J Laryngol Otol*. 2004;118:15–18.

95. Garvey CM, Boylan KB, Salassa JR, et al. Total laryngectomy in patients with advanced bulbar symptoms of amyotrophic lateral sclerosis. *Amyotroph Lateral Scler*. 2009;10:470–475.

96. Calvo A, Moglia C, Lunetta C, et al. Factors predicting survival in ALS: a multi-center Italian study. *J Neurol*. 2017;264:54–63.

97. Reich-Slotky R, Andrews J, Cheng B, et al. Body mass index (BMI) as predictor of ALSFRS-R score decline in ALS patients. *Amyotroph Lateral Scler Frontotemporal Degener*. 2013;14:212–216.

98. Heffernan C, Jenkinson C, Holmes T, et al. Nutritional management in MND/ALS patients: an evidence based review. *Amyotroph Lateral Scler Other Motor Neuron Disord*. 2004;5:72–83.

99. Korner S, Hendricks M, Kollewe K, et al. Weight loss, dysphagia and supplement intake in patients with amyotrophic lateral sclerosis (ALS): impact on quality of life and therapeutic options. *BMC Neurol*. 2013;13:84.

100. Dorst J, Dupuis L, Petri S, et al. Percutaneous endoscopic gastrostomy in amyotrophic lateral sclerosis: a prospective observational study. *J Neurol*. 2015;262: 849–858.

101. Tefera TW, Borges K. Metabolic dysfunctions in amyotrophic lateral sclerosis pathogenesis and potential metabolic treatments. *Front Neurosci*. 2016;10:611.

102. Shimizu T, Ishikawa-Takata K, Sakata A, et al. The measurement and estimation of total energy expenditure in Japanese patients with ALS: a doubly labelled water method study. *Amyotroph Lateral Scler Frontotemporal Degener*. 2017;18:37–45.

103. Majmudar S, Wu J, Paganoni S. Rehabilitation in amyotrophic lateral sclerosis: why it matters. *Muscle Nerve*. 2014;50:4–13.

104. Turner-Stokes L, Sykes N, Silber E, et al. From diagnosis to death: exploring the interface between neurology, rehabilitation and palliative care in managing people with long-term neurological conditions. *Clin Med (Lond)*. 2007;7:129–136.

105. Connolly S, Galvin M, Hardiman O. End-of-life management in patients with amyotrophic lateral sclerosis. *Lancet Neurol*. 2015;14:435–442.

106. Karam CY, Paganoni S, Joyce N, et al. Palliative care issues in amyotrophic lateral sclerosis: an evidenced-based review. *Am J Hosp Palliat Care*. 2016;33:84–92.

107. McDonald CM, Fowler WM Jr. The role of the neuromuscular medicine and physiatry specialists in the multidisciplinary management of neuromuscular disease. *Phys Med Rehabil Clin N Am*. 2012;23:475–493.

108. Hogden A, Greenfield D, Caga J, et al. Development of patient decision support tools for motor neuron disease using stakeholder consultation: a study protocol. *BMJ Open*. 2016;6:e010532.

109. Cedarbaum JM, Stambler N, Malta E, et al. The ALSFRS-R: a revised ALS functional rating scale that incorporates assessments of respiratory function. BDNF ALS Study Group (Phase III). *J Neurol Sci*. 1999;169:13–21.

110. Tramacere I, Dalla Bella E, Chio A, et al. The MITOS system predicts long-term survival in amyotrophic lateral sclerosis. *J Neurol Neurosurg Psychiatry*. 2015;86: 1180–1185.

111. Ferraro D, Consonni D, Fini N; Emilia Romagna Registry for ALSG, et al. Amyotrophic lateral sclerosis: a comparison of two staging systems in a population-based study. *Eur J Neurol*. 2016;23:1426–1432.
112. Sinaki M, Mulder DW. Rehabilitation techniques for patients with amyotrophic lateral sclerosis. *Mayo Clin Proc*. 1978;53:173–178.
113. Dal Bello-Haas V, Kloos AD, Mitsumoto H. Physical therapy for a patient through six stages of amyotrophic lateral sclerosis. *Phys Ther*. 1998;78:1312–1324.
114. Lunetta C, Lizio A, Sansone VA, et al. Strictly monitored exercise programs reduce motor deterioration in ALS: preliminary results of a randomized controlled trial. *J Neurol*. 2016;263:52–60.
115. Bello-Haas VD, Florence JM, Kloos AD, et al. A randomized controlled trial of resistance exercise in individuals with ALS. *Neurology*. 2007;68:2003–2007.
116. Ng L, Khan F, Young CA, et al. Symptomatic treatments for amyotrophic lateral sclerosis/motor neuron disease. *Cochrane Database Syst Rev*. 2017;(1):CD011776.
117. Dal Bello-Haas V, Florence JM. Therapeutic exercise for people with amyotrophic lateral sclerosis or motor neuron disease. *Cochrane Database Syst Rev*. 2013;(2):CD005229.
118. Kilmer DD, McCrory MA, Wright NC, et al. The effect of a high resistance exercise program in slowly progressive neuromuscular disease. *Arch Phys Med Rehabil*. 1994;75:560–563.
119. Anziska Y, Sternberg A. Exercise in neuromuscular disease. *Muscle Nerve*. 2013;48:3–20.
120. Macpherson CE, Bassile CC. Pulmonary physical therapy techniques to enhance survival in amyotrophic lateral sclerosis: a systematic review. *J Neurol Phys Ther*. 2016;40:165–175.
121. Plowman EK, Watts SA, Tabor L, et al. Impact of expiratory strength training in amyotrophic lateral sclerosis. *Muscle Nerve*. 2016;54:48–53.
122. Ward AL, Sanjak M, Duffy K, et al. Power wheelchair prescription, utilization, satisfaction, and cost for patients with amyotrophic lateral sclerosis: preliminary data for evidence-based guidelines. *Arch Phys Med Rehabil*. 2010;91:268–272.
123. Brownlee A, Palovcak M. The role of augmentative communication devices in the medical management of ALS. *NeuroRehabilitation*. 2007;22:445–450.
124. Nijboer F, Sellers EW, Mellinger J, et al. A P300-based brain-computer interface for people with amyotrophic lateral sclerosis. *Clin Neurophysiol*. 2008;119:1909–1916.
125. Vansteensel MJ, Pels EG, Bleichner MG, et al. Fully implanted brain-computer interface in a locked-in patient with ALS. *N Engl J Med*. 2016;375:2060–2066.
126. Ganzini L, Johnston WS, Silveira MJ. The final month of life in patients with ALS. *Neurology*. 2002;59:428–431.
127. Hanisch F, Skudlarek A, Berndt J, et al. Characteristics of pain in amyotrophic lateral sclerosis. *Brain Behav*. 2015;5:e00296.
128. Goy ER, Carter J, Ganzini L. Neurologic disease at the end of life: caregiver descriptions of Parkinson disease and amyotrophic lateral sclerosis. *J Palliat Med*. 2008;11:548–554.
129. Oliver D. The quality of care and symptom control--the effects on the terminal phase of ALS/MND. *J Neurol Sci*. 1996;139(suppl):134–136.
130. Trail M, Nelson ND, Van JN, et al. A study comparing patients with amyotrophic lateral sclerosis and their caregivers on measures of quality of life, depression, and their attitudes toward treatment options. *J Neurol Sci*. 2003;209:79–85.
131. Aho-Ozhan HE, Bohm S, Keller J, et al. Experience matters: neurologists' perspectives on ALS patients' well-being. *J Neurol*. 2017;264(4):639–646.
132. Felgoise SH, Zaccheo V, Duff J, et al. Verbal communication impacts quality of life in patients with amyotrophic lateral sclerosis. *Amyotroph Lateral Scler Frontotemporal Degener*. 2016;17:179–183.
133. Bromberg MB. Quality of life in amyotrophic lateral sclerosis. *Phys Med Rehabil Clin N Am*. 2008;19:591–605, x–xi.
134. Nelson ND, Trail M, Van JN, et al. Quality of life in patients with amyotrophic lateral sclerosis: perceptions, coping resources, and illness characteristics. *J Palliat Med*. 2003;6:417–424.
135. Robbins RA, Simmons Z, Bremer BA, et al. Quality of life in ALS is maintained as physical function declines. *Neurology*. 2001;56:442–444.
136. Simmons Z, Bremer BA, Robbins RA, et al. Quality of life in ALS depends on factors other than strength and physical function. *Neurology*. 2000;55:388–392.
137. Pagnini F, Rossi G, Lunetta C, et al. Burden, depression, and anxiety in caregivers of people with amyotrophic lateral sclerosis. *Psychol Health Med*. 2010;15:685–693.
138. Chio A, Gauthier A, Calvo A, et al. Caregiver burden and patients' perception of being a burden in ALS. *Neurology*. 2005;64:1780–1782.
139. Pagnini F, Phillips D, Bosma CM, et al. Mindfulness as a protective factor for the burden of caregivers of amyotrophic lateral sclerosis patients. *J Clin Psychol*. 2016;72:101–111.
140. Krivickas LS, Shockley L, Mitsumoto H. Home care of patients with amyotrophic lateral sclerosis (ALS). *J Neurol Sci*. 1997;152(suppl 1):S82–S89.
141. Elman LB, Houghton DJ, Wu GF, et al. Palliative care in amyotrophic lateral sclerosis, Parkinson's disease, and multiple sclerosis. *J Palliat Med*. 2007;10:433–457.
142. Seeber AA, Pols AJ, Hijdra A, et al. Experiences and reflections of patients with motor neuron disease on breaking the news in a two-tiered appointment: a qualitative study. *BMJ Support Palliat Care*. 2016, February 2.
143. McCluskey L. Amyotrophic Lateral Sclerosis: ethical issues from diagnosis to end of life. *NeuroRehabilitation*. 2007;22:463–472.
144. Carter GT, Joyce NC, Abresch AL, et al. Using palliative care in progressive neuromuscular disease to maximize quality of life. *Phys Med Rehabil Clin N Am*. 2012;23:903–909.
145. Wang LH, Elliott MA, Jung Henson L, et al. Death with dignity in Washington patients with amyotrophic lateral sclerosis. *Neurology*. 2016;87:2117–2122.
146. Benditt JO, Smith TS, Tonelli MR. Empowering the individual with ALS at the end-of-life: disease-specific advance care planning. *Muscle Nerve*. 2001;24:1706–1709.
147. Mandler RN, Anderson FA Jr, Miller RG, et al. The ALS patient care database: insights into end-of-life care in ALS. *Amyotroph Lateral Scler Other Motor Neuron Disord*. 2001;2:203–208.
148. Hobson EV, McDermott CJ. Supportive and symptomatic management of amyotrophic lateral sclerosis. *Nat Rev Neurol*. 2016;12:526–538.
149. Kettemann D, Funke A, Maier A, et al. Clinical characteristics and course of dying in patients with amyotrophic lateral sclerosis withdrawing from long-term ventilation. *Amyotroph Lateral Scler Frontotemporal Degener*. 2017;18:53–59.

CHAPTER 24

Mark A. Thomas
Stephanie Rand

Peripheral Neuropathy

The intent of this chapter is to provide a comprehensive look at the breadth of diseases affecting the peripheral nerves and their consequences with a focus on the how and the why of pathology and treatment. Although there is a tremendous variety in peripheral nerve pathology, it is reflected in a limited number of clinical responses. These responses, pain, weakness, autonomic dysfunction, sensory changes, and deformity impact daily function and quality of life and are addressed in a physiatric context throughout the chapter.

PERIPHERAL NEUROANATOMY AND NEUROPHYSIOLOGY

The peripheral nerve is vulnerable to a variety of insults but has a great capacity for repair and regeneration. The peripheral nerve includes the cell body, axons and dendrites, the cell membrane (neurolemma), the endoneurium, the perineurium, the mesoneurium, the epineurium, and the Schwann cell. These structures are central to the classification, pathophysiology, and treatment of peripheral neuropathy (📶 **eFigure 24-1**). Nerve fibers are categorized by their caliber and myelination, with the fastest signal conduction achieved by the largest myelinated fibers (📶 **eTable 24-1**).

Type A fibers (alpha through delta) are the thickest myelinated fibers and have the fastest conduction (4 to 120 m/s). They mediate motor, muscle spindle, and skin activity. The smaller type B fibers are myelinated, conduct at 3 to 15 m/s, and are preganglionic autonomic efferents. Small fibers, type C, have a diameter of 0.1 to 2 μm and conduction velocity of 0.5 to 4 m/s. These are the postganglionic autonomic efferents and afferents that also regulate visceral activity (vasomotor, cardiac, digestive, respiratory). They can be selectively affected in small fiber neuropathy.

The cell body of motor nerve fibers is the anterior horn cell. The cell body of sensory nerves is located in the dorsal root ganglion. In contrast to the somatic fibers, autonomic nerve fibers have both preganglionic and postganglionic neurons, with the cell body of the postganglionic neuron lying in the periphery and extending through unmyelinated C fibers.

The axolemma, or cell membrane, contains the axoplasm, which has tracts for both antegrade and retrograde flow. The tracts are maintained by electrical polarity, and flow occurs at 1 to 3 mm/d, one rate-limiting aspect of nerve regeneration. Flow can occur more rapidly in response to injury.

The axolemma of myelinated nerve fibers is enclosed by the Schwann cell, which elaborates the lipoprotein myelin. Normal Schwann cell function is the key factor in maintaining or regenerating myelinated fibers.

The Schwann cell internode space (node of Ranvier) is the site of membrane depolarization, saltatory conduction, and axonal branching. In unmyelinated nerve fibers, the relationship of nerve fibers is less complex, and several fibers may be contained in one trough. Such fibers propagate signals through continuous depolarization along the axolemma (eddy depolarization).

The endoneurium contains the axon and Schwann cell in a grouped arrangement of fascicles. These fascicles are in turn contained by the perineurium, which maintains a positive intrafascicular pressure. This structure presents a barrier to diffusion, the blood-nerve barrier. When the perineurium is compromised, diffusion produces axonal swelling, which impairs signal conduction.

External to the perineurium, the epineurium is a loose collection of collagen and elastin fibers that contains and supports the fascicles of a peripheral nerve and its vascular supply. Its organization is elaborate in the proximal nerve and becomes progressively less complicated in more distal nerve segments. The external epineurium surrounds the peripheral nerve and is largely responsible for its resistance to mechanical disruption. Its elastic properties allow a degree of deformation beyond which rupture occurs. This is why a stretched nerve is more readily injured than when at its resting length.

Axon fascicles divide and fuse with other fascicles in the epineurium. Communication between fascicles occurs every 0.5 to 15 mm, more frequently in the proximal peripheral nerve. They branch between 20 and 100 times before reaching the motor endplate.

The mesoneurium supports the capillary network that supplies the nerve fibers through the epineurium. The mesoneurium is easily compromised, and this accounts for the peripheral nerve's susceptibility to ischemia.

In addition to stem cell differentiation and organization, genetics dictate the metabolic processes of the peripheral nerve. The synthesis of glycoproteins and glycan is involved in the myelination and regulations of axons (defective in Charcot-Marie-Tooth disease) (1). Normal sphingolipid metabolism protects the cell surface from the environment and is involved in cell recognition and signaling in the processes of proliferation, differentiation, stress response, necrosis, inflammation, senescence, apoptosis, and autophagy. Palmitoylation plays a role in axon growth and integrity, degeneration, regeneration, and anterograde and retrograde signaling (2).

The peripheral nerves are supplied by vessels distributed through the mesoneurium and epineurium called vasa nervorum. These vessels form longitudinal anastomoses on the surface of the nerves. Endoneurial blood flow is directly proportional to the number of endoneurial capillaries. Capillary density varies according to site and corresponds to the nerve's susceptibility to ischemic damage (3).

A number of age-related physiologic changes occur in the peripheral nervous system (4). The number of anterior horn cells decreases. The capacity for neuronal sprouting, biosynthesis, transport, and proliferation declines. Schwann cell synthesis of trophic factors decreases. The net result is slowing of protective reflexes and decrement in proprioception, vibratory sense, and stretch reflexes. Pain and temperature recognition thresholds increase.

EPIDEMIOLOGY

The precise incidence, prevalence, disability rate, and cost of peripheral neuropathy in the United States are unknown. The prevalence has been reported as 8% for persons 55 years or older and up to 2.4% in the general population (5). The prevalence of small fiber neuropathy may be as high as 53 per 100,000 (6).

The prevalence of peripheral neuropathy in patients with type 2 diabetes may exceed 26% (5). The prevalence of diabetes in the US population is currently about 10%, increasing each year. Diabetic neuropathy is the most common complication with a lifetime prevalence of almost 50% (7). In 2003, with an estimated number of patients exceeding 20 million, the annual cost of diabetic peripheral neuropathy (DPN) exceeded 10.9 billion dollars (8).

The annual cost of patient care and disability payments for acute idiopathic demyelinating polyneuropathy (Guillain-Barré syndrome) is approximately $1.7 billion. An estimated 11% of these patients have permanent disability (9).

Approximately 60% to 70% of patients with vasculitic disease have a peripheral neuropathy. Of these, 65% have mild to moderate disability, 13% moderately severe disability, and 4% severe disability (10).

Traumatic peripheral nerve injury costs about $150 billion annually in the United States with 8.5 million restricted activity days and 5 million disability days in 2004. Over 200,000 peripheral nerve repairs were performed in that same year (11).

PATHOPHYSIOLOGY

Risk factors for, and the pathogenesis of, peripheral neuropathy encompass a broad array of mechanical, metabolic, comorbid, genetic, and epigenetic factors that disrupt homeostasis within the peripheral nerve. Enhanced activity of negative regulators is one such factor. Impaired axonal regeneration from abnormal chromosome 10 directed phosphatase and tensin production or from impaired signalers, promotors, or regulators (12,13). The failure to maintain myelin and axon homeostasis or promote recovery may be pronounced. Positive regulators may be down-regulated, such as growth factors Insulin Like Growth Factor 1 (IGF-1), Fibroblast Growth Factor (FGF), Epidermal Growth Factor (EGF), Erythropoietin (EPO), which prevent neuronal injury during oxidative stress, modulate Wnt signaling, block proapoptotic pathways, and maintain neuronal integrity (14). Abnormal levels and activity of transcriptional regulators (such as YAP/TAZ) will affect both peripheral nerve development and myelin maintenance (15).

Estradiol production or G-protein–coupled estrogen receptor density (16) may be insufficient and fail to attenuate abnormal vasodilatation, provide an antinociceptive effect (17), or promote Schwann cell proliferation and myelination (18). Mutations in small heat shock proteins can result in an axonal distal hereditary motor neuropathy.

Neural inflammation is characteristic of many peripheral neuropathies, such as those that are immune or toxin induced. There is an increase in proinflammatory cytokine expression and changes in immune signaling pathways (19). Peripheral neuropathy can be an early symptom of systemic vasculitis (20).

Abnormal Schwann cell function may play a role in the pathogenesis of certain peripheral neuropathies. Schwannopathy is implicated in the pathogenesis of diabetic neuropathy with effects on axons and microvessels (21). Lipid-lowering medications can impact Schwann cell elaboration of myelin and are a risk factor for peripheral neuropathy (22).

Impaired physiology affects peripheral nerve signal conduction. Neurapraxia is a local conduction block due to transient demyelination and rarely affects sensory or autonomic fibers. Thick myelinated nerves are most affected. Neurapraxia commonly results from compression of the peripheral nerve. These lesions heal by Schwann cell repair, and normal conduction is generally resumed in 1 to 2 months (12). Axonotmesis is a more significant injury and results in wallerian degeneration. An axonotmetic lesion leaves the endoneurial tube intact. Axonotmesis frequently follows a traction injury or a severe nerve compression. The prognosis for regeneration is good, particularly for shorter or distal nerve segments. The prognosis following proximal injury is less certain as the length of necessary regeneration is a primary limiting factor to recovery. Neurotmesis is complete severance of the peripheral nerve, and recovery is unlikely unless neurorrhaphy is performed. Healing of a neurotmetic lesion often results in the misconnection of nerve fibers and incomplete reinnervation.

Peripheral nerve injury can result from compression, crush injury, laceration, stretch/traction, ischemia, thermal injury, or high-velocity trauma. Damage can also be caused by infection, scar tissue formation, fracture callus, or vasculopathy.

Compression injury of a peripheral nerve generally results in focal demyelination. This causes a conduction block. Recovery depends upon remyelination. With all peripheral nerve lesions that leave the axon intact, there is axonal transport of tumor necrosis factor alpha (TNF alpha) to the lesion and a concomitant reorganization of peripheral nerve TNF receptors (23).

A crush injury provokes segmental demyelination, but the Schwann cell tube is commonly preserved and recovery can occur. A laceration injury due to blunt or penetrating trauma produces a well-localized lesion, usually millimeters in size. A stretch of the peripheral nerve beyond 10% to 20% of its resting length increases the risk of axonotmesis (24). This is the common mechanism of injury during joint dislocations. Stretch alone may provoke a mild conduction block, which recovers in hours. A more severe stretch will interrupt axons and connective tissue, cause hemorrhage, and might require surgical repair.

Thermal vascular injury can cause necrosis of all tissues. Large myelinated fibers are most susceptible to cold injury. Damage to the blood-nerve barrier results in endoneurial edema and increased intraneurial pressure with a resulting focal conduction block. If the pathology is progressive, axonal transport ceases and the axon degenerates within a few days.

Degeneration and Regeneration

Primary, or retrograde, degeneration proceeds from the site of injury to the next proximal node of Ranvier and is a consequence of trauma. It occurs less frequently than secondary (wallerian) degeneration.

Wallerian degeneration is antegrade, progressing distally from the point of injury. Degeneration begins on the 2nd or 3rd day after injury with retraction of myelin. Nerve fragmentation on day 2 to 3 precedes neurofibrillar degeneration. The nerve body swells. Neuron edema continues for 10 to 20 days. These changes are more pronounced and longer lasting with proximal nerve lesions. The Schwann cells at the site of injury activate and participate in the removal of myelin debris by the end of the 1st week after injury.

Schwann cells are essential for nerve repair. They not only support the migrating axon but also secrete neurotrophic factors to promote nerve growth (25). Neural crest or mesenchymal stem cells can differentiate into Schwann cells to promote peripheral nerve regeneration.

Axonal regeneration and remyelination progress in a sequence that begins with the activation of Schwann cells in the empty endoneurial tube. Axonal sprouts appear and progress down the endoneurial tube. These regenerating axons are guided along the perineurium by neutropins. They are directed toward the largest surviving distal fascicles (24).

The peripheral nerve can form a neuroma during the repair process. This may be a nerve stump neuroma (neuroma in continuity), which is usually located lateral to the nerve trunk. It forms as axonal/fascicular continuity is reestablished. A laterally located neuroma indicates partial neurotmesis with preserved ability to conduct signals. When the neuroma is imbedded in scar tissue, the prognosis for recovery is worse. A fusiform-shaped neuroma is likely to be in continuity while a bulbous or dumbbell-shaped neuroma is indicative of widespread neurotmesis. The latter should be treated by excision and neurorrhaphy. If more than 50% of the nerve diameter is within a neuroma, function will be impaired and the neuroma should be resected (26).

Unmyelinated axonal sprouts initially unite with the distal peripheral nerve remnant and then remyelination begins. Both the nerve sheath and axon increase in diameter. If there is a gap in continuity greater than 2 mm, reconnection is much less likely. In such instances, the immature neurite (sprout) dies back or forms a neuroma.

After reconnection, there is a shrinking area of sensory loss with an enlarging area of partial sensation as anastomotic branches with other nerves form (27). Involvement of autonomic fibers causes anhidrosis and impaired pilomotor and vasomotor activity. If the skin wrinkles on immersion in water, or if sweating is present, the peripheral nerve reconnection is inaccurate or incomplete. The production of neuropeptides (galanin and pituitary adenylate cyclase–activating peptide) promotes neurite outgrowth but can result in excessive branching during repair (28).

With further recovery, there is a return of pain and temperature sensation, a return of sudomotor function, and later a return of light touch, vibratory sensation, and stereognosis. Two-point discrimination is a good predictor of a return of global sensory function (26).

Classification

Peripheral neuropathy can be classified based upon location, etiology, pathology (of the nerve or the genetic error), time since onset, or clinical presentation (**Table 24-1**). It may be generalized, patchy, proximal, or distal in location. Etiologies include trauma, metabolic disease, malnutrition, infection, autoimmune disease, collagen-vascular disease, genetic error, toxic exposure (including medication), thermal injury, or ischemia.

The neuropathy can affect the axon and/or the myelin sheath. The disease may be confined to a single nerve (mononeuropathy), involve multiple nerves (polyneuropathy), and be symmetric or asymmetric. The neuropathy can be acute or chronic although this may be unclear when there is an insidious onset and delayed diagnosis. Depending upon the nerve involved, the clinical presentation will include weakness, paresthesia, hyperesthesia, anesthesia, or changes in autonomic function such as circulation or hidrosis.

The Seddon classification of peripheral nerve pathology is clinically relevant. It can be used to predict functional outcome and suggest appropriate care. There are three degrees of nerve pathology: neurapraxia, axonotmesis, and neurotmesis (**Table 24-1**).

DIAGNOSIS

The diagnosis of peripheral nerve injury is based on the history, clinical examination, and the electrodiagnostic evaluation. Imaging may also play a role in identifying a specific nerve lesion.

Clinical Findings

Symptoms relate to the nerve dysfunction. Weakness, cramps, numbness, paresthesias, and pain are common complaints. Patients may also complain of problems with walking or

TABLE 24-1	Correlations of the Seddon Classification of Peripheral Nerve Pathology				
Class	**Cause**	**Consequence**	**Usual Site Affected**	**Sunderland Classification of Nerve Injury**	**Prognosis**
Neurapraxia	Compression	Conduction block	Thick myelinated motor nerves	I Nerve fiber intact	Healing in 1–2 mo
Axonotmesis	Traction, severe compression	Wallerian degeneration	Myelinated motor and sensory nerves	II Nerve fiber intact III Endoneurium disrupted IV Endoneurium, perineurium disrupted	Good for healing of short/distal segments Repair likely needed for Sunderland III and IV lesions
Neurotmesis	Trauma transection	Complete disruption of nerve continuity	Any	V Endoneurium, perineurium, epineurium disrupted	Poor, even with surgery

activities of daily living (ADL) due to clumsiness, imbalance, or gait abnormalities. Other possible symptoms include dizziness, light-headedness, digestive problems, abnormal sweating, or urinary, bowel, or cardiac irregularities. A variety of specific and sensitive questionnaires have been validated for peripheral neuropathies, such as the Small-Fiber Symptom Survey (29) or questionnaires for polyneuropathy due to diabetes or chemotherapy. Manual muscle testing can reveal weakness in a peripheral nerve distribution. Muscle atrophy can reach 50% to 70% of the muscle bulk after about 2 months. Measuring limb girth helps detect a subtle loss of muscle mass or track changes. Weakness can produce abnormalities in gait and impair the ability to reach, grab, lift, or carry.

The sensory examination can delineate impaired sharp or light touch or two-point discrimination. Other sensory modalities are more qualitatively assessed, such as temperature and vibration.

Involvement of autonomic fibers is evidenced by a loss of sweating and impaired pilomotor and vasomotor action. If the skin wrinkles on immersion in water, or if sweating is present, the peripheral nerve damage is incomplete.

A nerve percussion sign is indicative of demyelination and remyelination. When the sign progresses from the proximal to the distal nerve, recovery is taking place. This distally advancing Tinel's sign occurs as the nerve recovers from a Sunderland II or III lesion (30).

The best diagnostic tool to characterize or confirm the presence of peripheral neuropathy remains the electrodiagnostic examination (see Chapter 3 on Electrodiagnosis). Nerve conduction studies quantify sensory, motor, and mixed nerve function in the distribution of symptoms or the lesion. Evidence of focal demyelination includes prolongation of distal latencies and slow or absent conduction. In axonopathy, amplitudes of the evoked response are low or absent.

The electrodiagnostic examination is valuable for both diagnosis and prognosis. Nerve conduction studies may be normal until wallerian degeneration takes place. Neurapraxia is less likely than a more severe injury if sensory conduction is absent beyond 7 to 10 days. 🛜 **eTable 24-2** summarizes electrodiagnostic findings following nerve injury.

Testing
Diagnostic testing for small fiber neuropathy may include quantitative sensory testing, measuring temperature and vibratory sensation, and quantitative sudomotor axon reflex testing. A distal leg skin punch biopsy (3 mm) measures epidermal nerve fiber density (31). Intraepidermal nerve fiber density below the 0.5 quantile for age (5% or less of mean normal fiber density) indicates small fiber peripheral neuropathy. Imaging modalities include ultrasound, magnetic resonance imaging (MRI), functional imaging, and imaging specific for associated injuries (see Chapter 5 on Imaging Techniques). MRI studies can supplement the diagnostic workup by characterizing spatial patterns of the neuropathy, assessing proximal nerve structures such as plexi, assessing nerve fascicles, and viewing posttrauma or perioperative changes in the peripheral nerve structure (32). Structural changes can be detected by MRI at about the fourth postinjury day. MRI has good sensitivity and specificity for axonotmetic or neurotmetic lesions. Increased signal in nerve fascicles is highly sensitive for subtle nerve lesions. MRI can also measure nerve caliber (33). Neurapraxia yields normal MRI findings.

Magnetic resonance neurography and even plain films for associated injuries, such as fracture or dislocation, may be useful. Laser Doppler flowmetry can demonstrate sympathetic involvement when examination reveals an abnormal vascular response (34).

Laboratory screening can help identify the etiology of a peripheral neuropathy. Routine studies include serum glucose, hemoglobin, leukocytes, platelets, erythrocyte sedimentation rate, thyroid studies, creatinine, and serum protein electrophoresis. Testing is directed to a specific disease as suggested by the history and examination.

There are also certain biomarkers that can be helpful in prognostication and tracking. Serum IL-27 (pathogenic) and IL-35 (protective) may correspond to severity and outcome in Guillain-Barré syndrome (acute inflammatory demyelinating polyneuropathy [AIDP] and acute motor axonal neuropathy [AMAN]) (35). Estrogen levels in postmenopausal women correlate with the risk for peripheral neuropathy (36), and about 10% of patients with a chronic sensorimotor neuropathy of unknown origin have an associated monoclonal gammopathy, typically of undetermined significance (MGUS) (37).

NONTRAUMATIC PERIPHERAL NEUROPATHIES

The peripheral nerve axon is vulnerable to toxic, metabolic, endocrine, and genetic insults. The myelin sheath is most commonly affected by autoimmune, nutritional, or genetic disorders and toxic or metabolic disease. In the United States, diabetes and alcohol abuse are the most frequent agents of peripheral nerve injury. Fifteen to twenty percent of nontraumatic peripheral nerve injuries are idiopathic (38).

Toxic, Nutritional, Metabolic, and Endocrine Peripheral Neuropathies
Toxic peripheral neuropathy results from exposure to a variety of organic and inorganic toxins, medications, and heavy metals (🛜 **eTable 24-3**). Some toxic peripheral neuropathies resolve with appropriate treatment. Many commonly prescribed therapeutic drugs, environmental pollutants, industrial solvents, and other workplace chemicals can be neurotoxic. Most toxins produce distal axonal degeneration in the longer peripheral nerves although there are toxins that damage the cell body directly or induce primary demyelination (39). Cisplatin and suramin, for example, result in apoptosis of neurons in the dorsal root ganglion.

Therapeutic drugs that can cause neuropathy include alfa interferon, amiodarone, amitriptyline, chloramphenicol, chloroquine, cimetidine, colchicine, corticosteroids, cisplatin, dapsone, didanosine, diphenylhydantoin, disulfiram, ethambutol, hydralazine, isoniazid, lithium, metronidazole, nitrofurantoin, nitrous oxide, paclitaxel, phenytoin, pyridoxine, sodium cyanate, suramin, tetanus toxoid, thalidomide, and vincristine (38). Neurotoxic organic compounds include acrylamide, carbon disulfide, dichlorophenoxyacetic acid, ethyl alcohol, ethylene oxide, methylbutyl ketone, and triorthocresyl phosphate. Heavy metals that may be neurotoxic include antimony, arsenic, gold, lead, mercury, and thallium.

Metabolic peripheral neuropathies typically present with sensory loss in a stocking and glove distribution. This is followed by weakness in the same distribution. The presentation may be protracted and insidious, particularly with nutritional or endocrine etiologies. Recovery can take months or years following appropriate treatment (40).

Vitamin deficiencies in B_1, thiamine (beriberi or pellagra), riboflavin (B_2), pyridoxine (B_6), B_{12} (pernicious anemia), and protein or calorie deficiency can produce an axonopathy. Diabetes, thyroid, and parathyroid disease are the most common endocrinopathies that damage the peripheral nerve axon.

DPN affects between 5% and 50% of diabetics in the United States. The incidence of peripheral neuropathy increases with age, duration of diabetes, mean serum glucose, smoking, HTN, height, and hyperlipidemia. The average annual incidence is 2%, and 0.56% have severe symptoms and deficits. The prevalence among people with diabetes for longer than 25 years rises to 50%. HLA genotypes might be genetic markers for the prediction or management of peripheral neuropathy in diabetic patients (41).

DPN is associated with decreased peripheral nerve vascularity and a paucity of angiogenic and neurotrophic factors (42). Impaired endogenous fibrinolysis and impaired glucose metabolism contribute to microvascular ischemia of the peripheral nerve. The vascular changes are mediated by the polyol pathway. Sorbitol and aldose reductase deposit glucose in tissues that are insulin independent (retina, kidney, nerve). Accumulation of sorbitol produces osmotic stress on the cell membrane while at the same time decreasing nitric oxide and vasodilation. The net result is microvascular disease due to vasoconstriction, thickening of the capillary basement membrane, endothelial hyperplasia, a decrease in oxygen tension, and hypoxia.

Hyperglycemia damages neurons, Schwann cells, and endothelial cells of the vasa nervorum. It produces oxidative stress, generates reactive oxygen species and glycation end product production leading to impaired sensory, motor, and autonomic nerve function (42). There is endoneurial and epineurial lymphocyte infiltration that disrupts signal conduction (43). Abnormal insulin signaling can also impair myelin protein regulation (44).

In addition to the symmetrical, length-dependent sensorimotor polyneuropathy, diabetes can cause an autonomic neuropathy, cranial neuropathy, mononeuritis multiplex, mononeuropathy, or radiculoplexus neuropathy. There is also treatment-induced neuropathy in diabetes. Further, multiple forms of neuropathy can coexist in diabetic patients. Neuropathic pain affects up to 20% to 30% of patients with DPN (7).

The most common complaint is of tingling or burning paresthesia in the feet, ankles, and calves. Due to distal weakness, postural control shifts from the ankle to hip thereby increasing the work of remaining upright. Autonomic neuropathy causes arteriovenous shunting and tissue hypoxia in the feet as well as in other organ systems. Strict control of serum glucose will retard the development or progression of diabetic neuropathy (45,46). Antioxidant therapy, aldose reductase inhibitors, alpha-lipoic acid, and gamma-linolenic acid may have some application in the treatment of diabetic neuropathy. Brain-derived nerve growth factor (NGF), recombinant NGF, neurotrophin 3, granulocyte-stimulating factor, and other peptides have been used to treat diabetic neuropathy with limited success

(47,48). Infusion of small neurotrophic nonneural peptides ("dual-action peptides") might increase nerve conduction velocity (49).

Both poor glucose control and rapid treatment of hyperglycemia can be associated with an increased risk of neuropathy, possibly due to arteriovenous shunting with endoneurial hypoxia of small fibers. Treatment-induced small fiber neuropathy presents with neuropathic pain and/or autonomic dysfunction within 8 weeks of a large improvement in glycemic control. It is most common in type 1 diabetes mellitus (DM) treated with insulin (7).

Small Fiber Neuropathy

Small fiber neuropathy is a feature of diseases such as Fabry's or Ehler-Danlos Syndrome but is more frequently a complication of another disease such as DM, hypothyroidism, Sjögren's syndrome, Lupus or other vasculitis, sarcoidosis, nutritional deficiency, celiac disease, Lyme disease, HIV infection, amyloidosis, or fibromyalgia (50). No cause of small fiber neuropathy is identifiable in 40% of cases (51).

Small fiber neuropathy produces dysfunction in nociception, temperature sensation, and autonomic regulation. Typical complaints include dysesthesias, pain, abnormal hot and cold sensation, and a variety of gastrointestinal, urinary, and cardiovascular complaints. Symptoms are most typically nerve length dependent, starting in the feet and progressing proximally, although a patchy, nonlength dependent or widespread distribution is not unusual. Examination can be unrevealing or relate to the specific fibers affected (6). Allodynia may be present.

Hereditary Peripheral Neuropathies

The classification of hereditary peripheral neuropathies can be confusing as it is variably based upon genetics, distribution of clinical findings, prominence of motor, sensory, or autonomic involvement, neuropathology, or associated disease. The hereditary peripheral neuropathies 🛜 **eTable 24-4** include the hereditary motor and sensory neuropathies (HMSNs) types I and II (Charcot-Marie-Tooth [CMT] disease), type III (Dejerine-Sottas disease), type IV (Refsum's disease), and HMSN types V to VII. Inheritance of an HMSN is usually autosomal dominant with variable penetration. Autosomal recessive and X-linked diseases occur less frequently and generally have a poorer prognosis (🛜 **eTable 24-5**). The mutations in HMSN affect genes that encode myelin proteins. Several abnormalities have been identified. These include duplication of chromosome 17p11.2, resulting in abnormalities of peripheral myelin protein 22 (52). Mutations can produce abnormal endoplasmic proteins that lead to Schwann cell apoptosis (53). The type of myelin gene mutation determines the disease severity. Deletion of myelin protein zero results in the most severe disease. Deletion of the 17p11.2 chromosome results in a hereditary neuropathy with susceptibility to pressure palsies. Point mutation of the PO gene and defects of the connexin 32 gene occur in X-linked forms of HMSN (54). Type Ia CMT disease results from a defect in chromosome 17. In type Ib CMT disease, the defect is located in chromosome 1. Mutations in the MFN2 gene are the most common cause of the axonal type, CMT2 (55). In 30% of CMT type II disease, there is a defect in mitofusin 2 genes with a decoupling of mitochondria in the axon, leading to decreased oxidative phosphorylation (56).

The prevalence of the most common HMSN, type I and II CMT disease, ranges from 1 per 50,000 to 1 per 250,000. The clinical manifestations are variable. The slowly progressive weakness is symmetric and more pronounced in distal musculature. In type I disease, the myelin is affected and onset is within the first decade of life. In type II disease, the axon is most affected and onset is usually within the second decade. In both types, the onset can be insidious and the patient asymptomatic until much later. The distribution of sensory deficit parallels that of the motor deficit. Loss of balance and tripping due to foot drop can be the presenting complaints and deformities such as equinovarus, calcaneovalgus, and pes cavus can be evident. Pain is uncommon.

CMT type II inheritance is more heterogeneous than in type I, with wider phenotypic variation. The resulting disability ranges from very mild to severe. There is less hypertrophic change in myelin and more neuronal or axonal involvement in type II disease (52–56). HMSN type III (Dejerine-Sottas disease) is an inherited hypertrophic peripheral neuropathy with prominent demyelination and remyelination. Neurapraxia is typical of this disease (57). Patients present with delay in motor development, difficulty running and jumping, and weakness affecting the arms as well as legs.

HMSN type IV (Refsum's disease) is characterized by altered mitochondria within the Schwann cell. A similar abnormality is described in other HMSN types (58). HMSN type V is associated with prominent spinocerebellar degeneration, type VI with optic atrophy, and type VII occurs with retinitis pigmentosa.

Other inherited peripheral neuropathies include Friedreich's ataxia, pressure-sensitive hereditary neuropathy, and various diseases that alter the structure or function of peripheral nerves such as acute intermittent porphyria, Roussy-Lévy syndrome, Riley-Day syndrome, Fabry disease, and Pelizaeus-Merzbacher disease. These neuropathies produce segmental demyelination and remyelination of the peripheral nerve with slowed signal conduction (59–63). Large myelinated motor fibers are the most severely affected. Weakness and atrophy in the distal leg muscles can reach 60% to 80% (60). Sensory loss and areflexia are notable. Atrophy and weakness in the upper extremities are less prominent.

Infectious Peripheral Neuropathy

Peripheral neuropathy can occur in association with infection due to immune overactivation or be related to the toxic effect of a therapeutic agent. In certain instances, peripheral nerve damage results directly from microbial infection and neuroinflammation or vasculitis. These are potentially treatable. The most common viral diseases that affect the peripheral nerve are human immunodeficiency virus (HIV), cytomegalovirus, Zika virus, Epstein-Barr virus, herpes zoster, hepatitis C, poliomyelitis, parvovirus, and rabies. West Nile viral infection can produce lesions in the anterior horn cell and motor axon similar to acute poliomyelitis (61).

Up to 16% of people with recently diagnosed HIV infection and 50% of patients with chronic HIV have some form of peripheral neuropathy, and neurologic disease can be the first manifestation of disease (62). The most common symptom is stocking-glove paresthesia or hypesthesia due to a distal symmetric polyneuropathy.

Other HIV-related peripheral neuropathies include AIDP, chronic inflammatory demyelinating polyneuropathy (CIDP), mononeuritis multiplex, lumbar polyradiculopathy, and lymphomatous neuropathy (63,64). The degree of neurologic impairment parallels the plasma HIV1 RNA level (64). Antiretroviral agents can also produce a peripheral neuropathy.

Bacterial diseases that affect the peripheral nerve include Lyme disease, leprosy, and diphtheria. The typical presentation is sensory and motor impairment due to distal symmetric polyneuropathy, although mononeuropathy and radiculopathy are also seen. Infection with *Borrelia* (Lyme disease) can produce several patterns of peripheral neuropathy. The most common pattern occurs late in the disease course. It is a large fiber axonopathy affecting multiple sensory nerves (65). Compromise of the endoneurial vascular supply can produce a mononeuritis multiplex (66). Worldwide, Leprosy remains a common infection that directly damages the peripheral nerve. Less frequently, peripheral neuropathy may be a complication of infection by *Campylobacter*, *Brucella*, or *Clostridium* (67).

Treatment primarily rests upon effective antibiotic or antiviral therapy. Hyperbaric O_2 can salvage peripheral nerve fibers from infection as well as ischemic, toxic, or antibody-mediated degeneration (68). Hyperbaric O_2 can improve symptoms of neuropathy in HIV patients (69). Trophic or growth factors, such as recombinant NGF used to treat HIV-related neuropathy, might enhance nerve recovery (70) following resolution of the infection.

Critical Illness Polyneuropathy

Critical illness polyneuropathy (CIP) can present as a failure to wean from mechanical ventilation (71). In septic multisystem organ failure, the systemic inflammatory response syndrome or high fever leads to a polyneuropathy of mixed or motor nerves. Chronic liver or pulmonary disease, cryoglobulinemia, giant cell arteritis, gout, and necrotizing angiopathy (72,73) and high-dose intravenous steroids have also been implicated in the pathogenesis of CIP. Electrodiagnostic studies are key in the diagnosis and monitoring of CIP since the clinical findings of CIP can be obscured by the primary medical condition, steroids, neuromuscular blocking agents, or concomitant compression neuropathies. The differential diagnosis includes critical illness–associated transient neuromuscular blockage, thick-filament myopathy, and necrotizing myopathy.

CIP results from cytokine and free radical release during sepsis, which impairs peripheral nerve microcirculation (74). Noninflammatory axonal degeneration and related atrophy in distal motor fibers are typical although there is often weakness of the proximal muscles and diaphragm as well. Sensory fibers are minimally affected. CIP produces moderate to severe weakness in all limb, facial, and paraspinal muscles. Atrophy is prominent. Loss of deep tendon reflexes is inconsistent. Serial serum creatine kinase levels and serial electrodiagnostic testing are helpful in monitoring the disease course.

Recovery time from CIP ranges from 3 weeks to 6 months (75). Peroneal nerve distribution weakness is the most common long-term deficit. The prognosis is good if the patient survives the precipitating critical illness, although weakness and reduced quality of life may persist.

Immune-Mediated Peripheral Neuropathies

Immune-mediated peripheral neuropathies are typically postinfectious or associated with hematopoietic and rheumatic diseases (76). Multiorgan failure and malignancy can provoke a similar response involving both inflammation and direct nerve damage. The neuropathies can be acute or chronic and involve sensory, motor, and mixed nerves.

Immune-mediated demyelinating protein attacks myelin and produces vasculitis and ischemia (77). The inflammatory mechanism is both cellular and humeral (78). TNF-alpha modulates the immune response, particularly in T-cell–mediated tissue injury. The acute demyelination characteristic of AIDP results from postinfection antibodies that recognize glycolipids and gangliosides GM1, GD12, and GD16. Lymphocytic infiltration of the spinal roots and peripheral nerves aids macrophages in myelin stripping.

AIDP (Guillain-Barré syndrome) is a postinfection demyelination of the peripheral nerve with perineurial and axonal damage. There is a breakdown of the blood-nerve barrier and segmental macrophage–mediated damage of the myelin sheath. Inflammation and demyelination result in varying degrees of axonal degeneration, and neurapraxia is prominent. Sixty-seven percent of patients with AIDP have a history of preceding viral infection, immunization, surgery, or a disease affecting the immune system. AIDP presents with acute-onset weakness, hypotonia, and areflexia. The weakness is progressive and involves the extremities. Bulbar and facial muscles can be affected. Autonomic dysfunction and sensory symptoms are usually mild (78). Respiratory failure occurs in up to 30% of cases within 1 to 2 weeks after disease onset (79). Recovery generally takes 3 to 18 months. Residual weakness is common and usually mild.

The Miller Fisher syndrome is a relatively benign AIDP variant occurring in about 5% of cases. It is characterized by ophthalmoplegia, areflexia, and ataxia. Antibodies to GQ1b are common. Acute motor axonal neuropathy (AMAN) is an axonal variant that usually follows infection with *Campylobacter jejuni*. Wallerian degeneration occurs, but myelin is not affected. The antibody mediators include GM1, GD1a, and GD16 (79). Acute motor sensory axonal neuropathy (AMSAN) is another clinical syndrome characterized by axonopathy. There is also a sensory variant of AIDP and, most rare, an acute pandysautonomia.

The medical management of AIDP includes the administration of high-dose immunoglobulins, plasmapheresis, or plasma exchange (80,81). Treatment reduces the duration of paralysis and intubation, particularly in the most severe cases. Cerebrospinal fluid (CSF) filtration of antibody complexes potentially reduces peripheral nerve damage. Corticosteroid therapy has no proven efficacy.

CIDP is a T-cell–mediated autoimmune peripheral neuropathy. It involves motor and sensory fibers. Disability results from weakness of both proximal and distal muscles. Cramps and fasciculations are common in the upper extremities (82).

The differential diagnosis of CIDP includes HMSN and amyotrophic lateral sclerosis. Histologic changes characteristic of CIDP include mononuclear cell infiltrates, prominent endoneurial edema, and wide interfascicle variability. CIDP can be associated with malignancy, particularly melanoma, due to immunoreactivity with surface antigens present in both myelin and the tumor (83).

The medical management of CIDP includes high-dose intravenous immunoglobulins, immunosuppressive drugs, or immune adsorption (84). Treatment with steroids is probably not effective. There is evidence that CIDP responds well to stem cell therapy (85).

Paraproteinemic peripheral neuropathy (📶 eTable 24-6) most commonly occurs as a monoclonal gammopathy of undetermined significance (MGUS) although it can be associated with hematologic disorders that produce paraproteins (immunoglobulins). These include multiple myeloma, cryoglobulinemia, lymphoma, amyloidosis, Waldenstrom macroglobulinemia (associated with IgM monoclonal gammopathy), and POEMS syndrome (38). Various malignancies such as bronchogenic carcinoma, ovarian, testicular, penile, gastric, oral cavity and meningeal cancers, oat cell carcinoma, and osteosclerotic myeloma are also associated with paraproteinemic neuropathy. Despite the variability in the clinical presentation and progression, there is often significant resulting morbidity (86). Neuropathy can precede or follow the antibody-producing condition.

The neuropathy typically is a length-dependent axonal loss sensorimotor polyneuropathy. It most affects sensation and causes numbness, allodynia, and hyperpathia. Cramps and mild distal weakness occur. Other variants include distal demyelinating symmetric neuropathy and chronic inflammatory demyelinating neuropathy.

Other immune neuropathies include multifocal acquired demyelinating sensory and motor neuropathy (Lewis-Sumner syndrome, MADSAM), distal acquired demyelinating symmetric neuropathy, multifocal motor neuropathy (87,88), and subacute inflammatory demyelinating polyneuropathy (SIDP).

Tumors of the Peripheral Nerve Sheath

The nerve sheath tumors that can undergo malignant transformation include schwannomas and neurofibromas. In neurofibromatosis (NF) type 1 (NF1 gene mutation), there is decreased neurofibromin production and loss of the tumor suppressor gene on chromosome 22. Pain is present 30% of the time. Malignant transformation is most common with NF type 1 (10%) and should be suspected when there is rapid enlargement of the nerve tumor (89,90).

Nerve Entrapment/Compression Syndromes

Nerve entrapment/compression syndromes are common and can involve almost any peripheral nerve (📶 eTable 24-7). Long peripheral nerves such as the median, ulnar, radial, fibular, and tibial nerves are most vulnerable, especially in their distal segments. Compression can be acute or chronic and result from external compression, swelling of the nerve or compression of the vascular supply with ischemia. Excessive pressure and rigidity in fascial compartments results in segmental demyelination with neurapraxia. Changes in the intraneurial circulation, impairment of axonal transport, and changes in vascular permeability contribute to edema formation and impede signal conduction (91). A rise in pressure within a contained site (e.g., fluid retention before menses or tendon thickening/edema from overuse), rigid containment (carpal tunnel borders), a pathologic increase in nerve caliber (edema or hypertrophic remyelination), stretching or tethering the nerve, or the presence of anomalous muscle or bone in a confined space predispose the nerve to injury. The best diagnostic tests to confirm and evaluate an entrapment neuropathy are the electrodiagnostic examination and ultrasound (92).

Thoracic outlet syndrome produces symptoms in ulnar and/or median nerve distributions. There can be intrinsic hand weakness and sensory impairment in a C8-T1 distribution.

Compression of the neurovascular bundle typically occurs between the scalene muscle heads or by an accessory rib or Pancoast tumor. Treatment may include ultrasound-guided injection of an anesthetic, botulinum toxin injection of the scalenes, physical therapy, and even endoscopic or open surgery when conservative care fails (93,94). Therapy emphasizes shoulder and neck range of motion, posture, and strengthening of the shoulder girdle.

The median nerve is susceptible to entrapment at several sites, including the carpal tunnel, supracondylar process/ligament of Struthers, and the bicipital aponeurosis/lacertus fibrosus.

Pronator syndrome involves the median nerve in the forearm and results in predominantly sensory loss in the median nerve distribution of the hand and the thenar eminence. The anterior interosseus nerve (AIN) syndrome is characterized by loss of motor function of the muscles innervated by the AIN in the forearm.

The most common entrapment syndrome is carpal tunnel syndrome (CTS) (95). The patient may awaken with hand or finger pain and paresthesias and complain of hand clumsiness and dropping objects. In approximately 50% of patients, there is no clear etiology. More than 50% of patients eventually have bilateral complaints (96). CTS can follow repetitive trauma, pregnancy, rheumatoid arthritis, anomalies of muscle or tendon, gout, myxedema, amyloid deposition, trauma with fracture, or scleroderma.

Findings include diminished touch and two-point discrimination and weakness in a distal median nerve distribution. There is sensory sparing of the thenar eminence (median palmar cutaneous nerve) and of the skin in the ulnar and superficial radial nerve distributions. The thenar muscles can atrophy. Abductor pollicis brevis muscle weakness can be present, but there is no weakness of the median-innervated forearm muscles. Provocative tests produce or worsen paresthesias in the median digital nerve distribution. The Tinel's, or nerve percussion, sign is elicited by tapping over the median nerve at the flexor retinaculum. Distal paresthesias indicate demyelination/remyelination. When Phalen's maneuver (the wrist in complete flexion) or reverse Phalen's maneuver (maximum dorsiflexion) reproduce the symptoms, median entrapment in the carpal tunnel is likely, as it is when direct compression over the distal edge of the carpal tunnel provokes paresthesias.

CTS is treated with use of a volar wrist splint to limit motion and place the wrist in a neutral position. Local corticosteroid injection into the carpal tunnel and medications for neuropathic pain can be helpful. Massage, stretch of the transverse carpal ligament, and tendon-gliding exercises are useful. Ergonomic modifications place the wrist in a neutral position during work to reduce carpal tunnel symptoms. When conservative treatment fails or when acute CTS is due to a wrist fracture or dislocation with injury to the median nerve, surgery is considered. A good outcome requires complete section of the transverse carpal ligament. The approach may be either open or endoscopic. The open has a lower risk of complications. The endoscopic release results in earlier return to work and ADL but has a higher incidence of recurrence (97).

Ulnar nerve entrapment or compression can occur at several points along its length. The most frequent sites include the elbow (within the ulnar sulcus or more distally between the heads of the flexor carpi ulnaris), in the cubital tunnel, and at the wrist (Guyon's tunnel, between the hook of the hamate and pisiform). Compression can occur within the hypothenar eminence following repetitive strain injury. The ulnar nerve can also be compressed between the elbow and wrist when it exits anomalously through the flexor carpi ulnaris. Weakness may be limited to the ulnar intrinsic hand muscles or involve the ulnar forearm muscles, flexor digitorum profundus (ulnar), and the flexor carpi ulnaris depending upon the site of compression. Sensory deficits in the ulnar hand dorsum help to differentiate proximal entrapment from compression within Guyon's tunnel.

Radial nerve compression can occur at several places. Examination findings correlate well with the site of compression. Weakness can occur in the elbow, wrist, or finger extensors. Sensory loss can involve the posterior arm, forearm, or hand. Weakness of the triceps is compatible with entrapment proximal to the circumflex portion of the nerve at the midhumeral level. Brachioradialis weakness with normal triceps strength suggests a lesion distal to the circumflex portion of the nerve. Sparing of the extensor carpi radialis indicates entrapment proximal to the supinator margin, at the arcade of Frohse. A posterior interosseus nerve compression involves the flexor carpi ulnaris and long finger extensors without sensory involvement. A superficial radial nerve lesion produces sensory findings without weakness.

Splinting may be helpful if recovery is anticipated. Dynamic orthoses can provide wrist and finger extension, but power grasp remains compromised due to loss of tenodesis. Surgical release is most commonly needed when the nerve is compressed at the arcade of Frohse.

Lateral femoral cutaneous nerve (LFCN) compression (meralgia paresthetica, Bernhardt-Roth Syndrome) is most common in middle age, and there is a gender predisposition for males. It presents as pain or irritation over the anterior or anterolateral thigh and results from injury, compression, or disease of the LFCN. Entrapment can occur near the spinal column, within the abdominal cavity as the nerve courses along the pelvis or as it exits the pelvis (the most common site). It can also be caused by superficial compression near the iliac crest and anterior superior iliac spine. Tight clothing, belts with a heavy load (typically related to occupation), trauma (such as compression by a seatbelt during rapid deceleration), gynecologic compression (related to menstrual cycle, endometriosis, or fetal compression), and obesity are typical causes (98). Less likely etiologies include pelvic fracture, pelvic osteotomy, hysterectomy, tumor, hemorrhage, and abscess.

Hip extension may increase, and flexion decrease, angulation and tension of the LFCN and symptoms. Meralgia paresthetica is bilateral in about 20% of cases. Treatment includes correction of any leg length discrepancy (to minimize hip hyperextension on the affected side), manual release of superficial entrapment, electroacupuncture, and pulsed radiofrequency application. Corticosteroid injection or alcohol neurolysis, typically ultrasound guided, may be indicated. If surgery is necessary, nerve transection and nerve decompression have similar success rates (99).

The most common site of peroneal nerve compression is behind the fibular head. Ankle dorsiflexor, foot evertor and toe extensor weakness, and hypesthesia in the leg and foot are typical findings. Sensory loss occurs in both deep and superficial peroneal nerve distributions. The common peroneal nerve sensory territory at the proximal half of the lateral leg is spared, as are muscles innervated proximal to the knee. Treatment may include prescription of an appropriate ankle-foot orthosis, range-of-motion exercises, and strengthening exercises.

The most common entrapment of the tibial nerve occurs at the tarsal tunnel. There is pain and/or paresthesia of the medial heel and plantar foot. The medial arch is variably involved depending upon the saphenous nerve sensory territory. There may be a history of foot injury or deformity such as pes planus. A nerve percussion sign may be present at the tarsal tunnel. Foot orthoses can compensate for weakness and may help to relieve associated pain. Surgical release of the laciniate ligament is an option when conservative treatment is insufficient.

TRAUMATIC PERIPHERAL NERVE INJURY

Traumatic peripheral nerve injury can result from compression, crush injury, laceration, stretch/traction, ischemia, thermal injury, or high-velocity trauma. Infection, scar tissue formation, fracture callus, or vasculopathy can further injure the peripheral nerve. Peripheral nerves vary in their vulnerability to trauma. Fiber-type composition, size of the nerve, number of nerve fascicles, amount of soft tissue protective cushioning, course of the nerve (on bone, through fascia or muscle), and tethering all affect the nerves' ability to sustain and recover from injury. Scar formation, heterotopic ossification, and fracture callus can tether the peripheral nerve.

The most traumatic injury is transection due to blunt or penetrating trauma. There may be a delay in diagnosis due to adjacent tissue injury.

Fracture and fracture/dislocation carry a high risk of associated nerve damage. Nerve injury after shoulder dislocation occurs in 48% of cases. The incidence of radial nerve damage following humeral fracture is 11% (100). Ulnar neurapraxia is the most commonly identified nerve lesion associated with fracture dislocation at the elbow. Dislocation of the hip is associated with a nerve injury rate of 3%, and the rate associated with knee dislocation is 18% (101).

Compression injury of a peripheral nerve generally results in focal demyelination with a conduction block. Recovery depends upon remyelination. A crush injury provokes segmental demyelination, but the Schwann cell tube is commonly preserved and recovery can occur. A laceration injury due to blunt or penetrating trauma produces a well-localized lesion, usually millimeters in size.

A stretch of the peripheral nerve beyond 10% to 20% of its resting length increases the risk of axonotmesis (24). This is the common mechanism of injury during joint dislocations. Mild stretch–related conduction block recovers in hours. Severe stretch will interrupt axons and connective tissue, cause hemorrhage, and might require surgical repair.

Cold injury can cause necrosis of all tissues. Large myelinated fibers are the most susceptible to cold injury. Damage to the blood-nerve barrier results in endoneurial edema and increased intraneurial pressure with a focal conduction block. If the pathology is progressive, axonal transport ceases and the axon degenerates within a few days.

Iatrogenic injury can result from compression and tension of the affected nerve following surgical manipulation, retractor placement, or hematoma (101). Plating of forearm fractures results in a nerve injury in 1% to 10% of cases. Damage has

also been reported during elbow and shoulder arthroscopy. The incidence of nerve palsy following primary hip arthroplasties in a tertiary care setting is 0.3%. Identified risk factors include lumbar disease, young age, and smoking (101).

TREATMENT

Conservative Management of Disease

The acute management of a peripheral neuropathy focuses on treating the associated disease, providing adequate analgesia, and preventing complications (**Box 24-1**). Examples of such treatment include CSF filtration, antiretroviral therapy, chemotherapy agents and biologics, intravenous immune globulin, plasmapheresis, and stem cells (38). The treatment of underlying disease should also address comorbid conditions that lead to fluid retention or thickening of tissues surrounding a nerve. There may be a need to correct nutritional deficiencies, eliminate toxic exposure, or suppress an immune response.

Ascorbic acid, curcumin, and cannabinoids have been studied for their impact on the injured peripheral nerve through a genetic or direct effect. The goal of treatment is to enhance nerve survival and regeneration, promote neural anabolism, reduce oxidative stress, or delay apoptosis. The value of each treatment option varies, and new strategies are regularly being proposed (102–106).

Stem cell therapy may be an increasingly valuable tool to promote peripheral nerve regeneration. There is evidence that functional Schwann cells can be obtained by seeding with stem cell precursors. Mesenchymal stem cells also secrete neurotrophic factors, angiogenic factors, cytokines, and immunomodulatory substances that may be especially beneficial in treating diabetic neuropathy (44). They improve the potential for a peripheral nerve to bridge a short gap in continuity (107,108). Neural crest stem cells have a propensity for differentiating into Schwann cells that effectively promote axon regeneration (109).

Antimuscarinic receptor drugs such as pirenzepine and muscarinic toxin 7 (MT7) have been used and improve indices of peripheral neuropathy such as depletion of sensory nerve terminals, thermal hypoalgesia, and nerve conduction slowing. Improvement has been seen in animal models of DPN and HIV chemotherapy–induced peripheral neuropathy (109).

BOX 24-1

Initial Management of Peripheral Neuropathy

- Avoid or modify aggravating activities—ergonomic modifications
- Treatment of underlying medical conditions
- Splinting—resting splints: to minimize nerve compression secondary to joint position, muscle/tendon overuse, or stretch of the nerve
- Minimize external compression
- Orthotic devices to restore joint motion or position—generally, ankle and foot
- Reduce swelling and/or edema
- Anti-inflammatory and/or pain medications
- Corticosteroid injection
- Physical therapy: modalities, massage, exercise
- Surgical decompression or transposition of nerve

Pharmacologic treatment most commonly addresses symptoms of pain or autonomic dysfunction (see Chapter 52 on Pharmacotherapy). When symptoms of dysautonomia are pronounced and disruptive, there are several classes of medication that can be helpful. These medications for orthostatic hypotension or tachycardia, difficulty with bladder function, and hyperhidrosis are typically employed off-label. They include alpha-1 agonists, beta-adrenergic blockers, acetylcholinesterase inhibitors, mineralocorticoids, anticholinergic agents, botulinum toxin, and anticholinergic agents. They are used cautiously and can have serious potential side effects.

The selection of analgesics for long-term use takes into account potential cumulative drug-related adverse effects. The long-term use of opioids is discouraged. Other analgesics, local anesthetics, or corticosteroid injections and nerve stimulation (transcutaneous, spinal cord) are used to address peripheral neuropathic pain.

Analgesics include tricyclic antidepressants, selective serotonin/serotonin-norepinephrine reuptake inhibitors, nonsteroidal anti-inflammatory drugs (including transdermal preparations), opioids, topical counterirritants, topical capsaicin, alpha-lipoic acid, botulinum toxin A, marijuana, anticonvulsants, and antispasticity agents (110,111). In the setting of chronic moderate to severe neuropathic pain, the Canadian Pain Society (2007) has recommended that first-line treatment includes gabapentin and pregabalin, tricyclic antidepressants, and serotonin noradrenaline reuptake inhibitors (112). If these fail, tramadol and controlled-release opioid analgesics are recommended as second-line agents. Cannabinoids are recommended as alternative treatment (113). If other agents fail, drugs such as methadone, anticonvulsants with lesser evidence of efficacy (lamotrigine, lacosamide), tapentadol, and botulinum toxin can be considered.

Anticonvulsants modulate sodium channels and suppress ectopic or ephaptic discharge in neuropathic pain. Gabapentin and pregabalin have demonstrated efficacy in decreasing pain, improving sleep, and enhancing mood and quality of life for patients with postherpetic or diabetic neuropathy. Specific sodium channel subtype inhibitors acting on peripheral nociceptive neurons or modified T-type voltage-gated calcium channel blockers are promising targets for future pharmaceutical options to manage neuropathic pain. Monoclonal antibodies against NGF, sodium channels, specific receptors, and cytokines are also under study as therapeutic options.

Antidepressants are helpful for pain and pain-related depression. The tricyclics and the SNRI medications treat pain. Stimulatory peptides (short-chain amino acids derived from cytokine proteins or growth factors) encourage healing, alleviate pain, and may prevent neuron death (114).

Another component of conservative treatment is physical therapy. Transcutaneous electrical stimulation, pulsed radiofrequency stimulation, pulsed galvanic stimulation, and heat and cold modalities (115–117) are treatments reported to provide relief from neuropathic pain. Mobilization of a painful limb segment and normal use of a limb is important, particularly as chronic regional pain syndromes may complicate a peripheral neuropathy (118). Conservative treatment options for entrapment/compression syndromes relieve pressure/nerve compression and reduce inflammation and edema. Treatment should also address comorbid conditions that lead to fluid retention or tissue thickening such as in myxedema, gout, or acromegaly. Strategies include splinting, medications, massage, and tendon

mobilization. Splints can restrict motion of a joint and reduce the intermittent increase in pressure on a nerve, improve hand position, and function or prevent motion that could produce a stretch injury of the nerve. Avoid use of bupivacaine/local anesthetics following injury of a peripheral motor nerve as this can exacerbate cell death (119).

Surgery

Surgical release is indicated when nonoperative management fails, and decompression is necessary to preserve viability of the nerve or in the presence of an anomaly or foreign object causing acute nerve compression.

The ability of the peripheral nerve to recover from trauma is facilitated or inhibited by intrinsic factors such as age, condition of surrounding tissue, nutrition, time since injury and type of injury, the specific peripheral nerve involved, and the level of lesion. In general, well-nourished younger patients with recent injury of the distal nerve do best. Similarly, extrinsic factors such as the quality of medical, surgical, and postoperative management enhance or inhibit healing (24).

Negative prognosticators for successful nerve repair include advanced age, nerve injury due to dislocation, delay of repair beyond 5 months, prior radiation therapy, nerve discontinuity (gap) exceeding 2.5 cm, proximal nerve injury, and a poor condition of the nerve endings (26).

Exploratory surgery can expose the extent and severity of the lesion when the clinical and electrodiagnostic examinations are inconclusive. Repair is done for Sunderland grade 3 to 5 lesions. Early repair is desirable whenever possible as maximal nerve regeneration occurs at about 3 weeks after injury (12). Surgery is also considered when there is no return of function at about 2 months after injury (4 months for the brachial plexus) or when partial loss of function shows no improvement after several weeks. The purpose of surgical repair is to improve peripheral nerve recovery and function.

There are two basic approaches to reestablishing nerve continuity: macrorepair (reconnecting the nerve ends by epineurial suture or graft) and microscopic repair (suturing individual nerve bundles) (120). The four key components of peripheral nerve repair include support cells, a scaffold for axonal migration, growth factors, and optimization of the extracellular matrix (25). Schwann cells or stem cells can be implanted along the matrix and neurotrophic factors added to enhance the speed and quality of axon growth (121).

Immediate or primary repair is performed within 8 to 12 hours on clean lacerations. Delayed or secondary repair is more usual after major trauma, blunt transection, wound contamination, or complete neurotmesis without clear nerve margins. This is performed at least 1 month after injury. The delay in repair allows better definition of the lesion and reduces the risk of infection.

Macroneurorrhaphy reestablishes the continuity of the epineurium. Epiperineurial repair, fascicular or perineurial nerve repair, and interfascicular nerve repair are also done, but there is no consistent evidence that these approaches improve clinical outcomes. Epineurium neurorrhaphy with direct epineurial suturing can lead to neuroma formation. Fascicular groups must be large enough to anchor sutures, and proper tensioning of the repaired nerve is essential (122).

A peripheral nerve graft is needed when the gap between nerve endings is greater than 2 cm (123). Nerve conduits are derived from various sources. Grafts and conduits are biologic or synthetic tubes that are nondegradable or biodegradable. They can be filled with scaffolds containing neurotrophic factors and seeded with Schwann cells or stem cells. Microenvironmental factors regulate the neuroinflammatory response and affect the accuracy and direction of axonal regeneration. Nerve conduits are enriched with neurotrophic factors, building a microenvironment, which enhances axonal regeneration. Autologous grafts are largely unavailable, and their harvest results in morbidity, scarring, sensory loss, and harvest neuroma. Constructs should be flexible and of biologic origin (artery, vein, muscle, or collagen) for short gaps. Degradable material (collagen, chitin, polymers, hydrogel) is preferred to nondegradable conduits, which can cause inflammation of surrounding tissue with nerve compression (124).

Trophic factors that enhance nerve regeneration through a graft or tube include neurocytokines (NGF), brain-derived neurotrophic factor (BDNF), ciliary neurotrophic factor, and neurotrophin-3, -4, -5, and -6 (125). Trophic factors work by preventing fibroblast activity and inhibiting protease activity.

Neurolysis may be needed to remove scar tissue. In order to bridge a gap in nerve continuity, surgical alternatives to grafting include nerve mobilization, nerve transposition, tissue expansion (126), joint flexion, and bone shortening (127). When peripheral nerve repair and regeneration are not options, nerve transfers might provide an alternate means to restore function in the upper extremity (128–131).

FUNCTIONAL EVALUATION AND REHABILITATION

The functional evaluation of a patient with peripheral neuropathy begins with the history and physical examination. The examination should identify the distribution of motor and sensory deficits. The history should include the patient's report on bowel, bladder, and sexual function as well as a self-assessment of basic and instrumental ADL performance and vocational and avocation activities. There are validated tools that can supplement the physical examination. There are instruments to measure function that are disease specific, such as those for diabetic or chemotherapy-induced peripheral neuropathy or neuropathic pain. Generic questionnaires to assess function

are also useful (132–134). Serial assessment of function can document progress during treatment and help to determine if a patient's care is effective or needs to be modified.

Specific patterns of weakness should prompt further investigation into specific activities. Proximal weakness can impair overhead reach or transfers. Distal weakness can affect fine motor tasks or gait. Mobility and ADL performance should be assessed by direct observation whenever possible. Peripheral neuropathy can have a profound impact on vocation. Numbness, tingling, and weakness can lead to a deterioration in the quality and productivity of work. Neuropathic pain can be severe, persistent and limit the ability to work. If autonomic fiber involvement is severe, symptoms can limit work tolerance.

Patients with impaired sensation may have difficulty with fine motor or precision tasks. In combination with diabetes or other vascular risk factors, the neuropathy may limit a worker's performance in jobs requiring prolonged standing and walking due to the risk of skin breakdown. Impaired balance or weakness increases the risk of falling and requires work accommodations or restriction. Weakness may compromise a worker's ability to consistently grasp, lift, carry, or hold onto tools and other objects. Working at heights or with hazardous equipment may be unsafe.

Entrapment neuropathies and compression neuropathies can develop from work-related activity and produce disability. CTS is the most frequent example. Negative predictors for return to work include strenuous work, an occupational history of repetitive hand movements, involvement in a worker's compensation case, and use of vibrating tools. Treatment includes control of inflammation, ergonomic assessment, and modification of the tools used or the workstation.

Work capacity and disability are dictated by the combined effects of a peripheral neuropathy and any comorbidities. A functional capacity evaluation can be very helpful in the determination of a patient's status. It can identify deficits that might improve with an appropriate rehabilitation plan.

Rehabilitation efforts address symptoms and disability (**Table 24-2**). Treatment includes a broad range of therapeutic modalities that address inflammation, pain, weakness, loss of endurance, and mobility and ADL-related disabilities.

Exercise is a frequent component of the rehabilitation program. The type, intensity, and progression of exercise are

TABLE 24-2	Rehabilitation Strategies for Peripheral Neuropathy		
Problem		**Functional Consequence**	**Rehabilitation Intervention**
Weakness	**Proximal**	Rising from chair, jumping, stairs, difficulty lifting/carrying, and reaching	Progressive resistance exercises
	Distal	Foot drop/slap, poor toe clearance, weak grasp, or pinch	Ankle-foot or supramalleolar orthosis, splint, functional orthosis, tool or equipment modification
Generalized weakness and deconditioning		Loss of endurance, fatigue	General conditioning exercises, education in energy conservation techniques and sleep hygiene
Distal sensory loss		Loss of proprioception, imbalance, impaired fine motor control	Fine motor exercises, assistive devices (e.g., cane)
Impaired motor control		As above	
Autonomic dysfunction		Abnormal sweating, cold intolerance, bowel, bladder and cardiorespiratory symptoms	Educate regarding selection of gloves, clothing, antiperspirant, diet, relaxation exercises
Pain		Decreased activity	Analgesics, nerve stimulation, nerve blocks, surgery
Deformity			Splints, foot orthotics, bracing, surgery

dictated by the goals of treatment and patient health status and tolerance. Endurance training can compensate for neurotrophin deficiency and potentially improve peripheral nerve function in diabetic neuropathy. Strength and endurance training improves ADL performance (135). Strength training alone, focusing on weak areas, will improve leg strength and ADL performance, particularly for proximal muscles. Key exercise targets to improve mobility include the hip flexors and quadriceps. There is also evidence that exercise benefits sensory as well as motor nerve deficits (136).

Splinting and bracing is useful for restricting joint or tendon motion, reducing intermittent pressure on the nerve, and avoiding exacerbating postures or activities. Bracing, adaptive equipment, ambulation aids, or wheelchairs may be necessary to improve mobility or the use of an affected extremity. Safety measures include hand railings, transfer aids, and environmental optimization with removal of obstacles, adequate lighting, and protective shoes. Orthotics can compensate for more distal weakness. Strategies that mobilize tissues and reduce adhesions (massage, ultrasound, exercise) are useful in entrapment neuropathies before considering surgical release.

Weakness from an HMSN frequently impairs ambulation and falls are common. Rehabilitation interventions focus on maintaining a safe and effective gait. Bracing, particularly ankle-foot orthoses, usually provide adequate support. If contractures require surgical release, postoperative bracing or splinting is essential. Attention to footwear is important because equinus/cavus deformities typically occur. A comfortable protective shoe with adequate depth and a reinforced medial counter helps to avoid pain, skin breakdown, and progressive deformity. Exercise is most effective for strengthening the proximal muscles of the lower extremities (137).

The rehabilitation management of AIDP focuses on the prevention of contractures, skin breakdown, pneumonia, and depression. Communication devices, a trapeze, pressure relief mattresses and bed rails are helpful during the acute phase of the disease. AIDP presents with evolving weakness so exercise, bracing, adaptive equipment and vocational retraining are not appropriate until the patient is clinically stable. Retraining ADLs, wheelchair and ambulation training, and bracing are necessary to address residual impairment and disability.

Rehabilitation efforts for CIP patients focus on preventing decubitus ulceration, contractures, and compression neuropathies. Strengthening exercise, mobility and ADL retraining, orthotics, and adaptive equipment should be provided at appropriate stages of recovery. Early mobilization of critically ill patients improves overall outcome and reduces residual disability (138). Following peripheral nerve surgery, active range of motion of related joints is begun and splinting is provided as necessary. Early passive mobilization following surgery is controversial. Usually the operated limb is immobilized for 4 to 6 weeks, apart from providing limited range of motion to prevent or limit joint contracture (139). Early tactile stimulation may enhance recovery of sensory function (127). Hyperbaric oxygen can decrease endoneurial edema, pressure, and improve vascular compromise (74).

MANAGEMENT OF COMPLICATIONS

Complications such as skin breakdown, amputation, Charcot joint, and urinary tract infection are commonly associated with diabetic, amyloid, and hereditary sensory neuropathies.

Other neuropathies result in foot deformities, kyphoscoliosis, and loss of hair or ulceration in the affected area. Imaging might reveal loss of bone density, pathologic fracture, or neuropathic arthropathy.

Pain, burns, skin trauma, infection, falls with injury, skin breakdown, and amputation are potential complications of a sensory neuropathy. Patients should be educated regarding footwear, skin and foot care, and the need to maintain adequate glycemic control in cases of diabetic neuropathy. Shoes should be wide, deep, and have an open throat design (a Blucher last is preferred to the Balmoral last). There should be adequate medial counter and arch support. Shoe orthotics can improve pain and ambulation when foot deformity or dynamic instability results from intrinsic muscle weakness.

Conditions that can complicate the postoperative course after nerve repair include chronic pain, complex regional pain syndromes type 1 and 2, neuroma formation, peripheral nerve entrapment syndromes, weakness, sensory loss, and atrophic skin changes. If neurosurgery fails, tendon transfers can sometimes offer the patient a partial restitution of function.

The peripheral nervous system is an essential component of motor control and sensory experience. When normal operations of the system are disrupted, the consequences include pain, disability, and impaired quality of life. Physiatric care is directed toward optimal function and patient satisfaction. The ability to address the impairments and disabilities related to peripheral neuropathy is based upon knowledge of the clinical aspects of the disease enhanced by understanding the underlying pathology. This allows focused treatment and anticipatory care and ideally results in a patient achieving their best possible physical performance and quality of life.

REFERENCES

1. Yoshimura T, Hayashi A, Handa-Narumi M, et al. GlcNAc6ST-1 regulates sulfation of N-glycans and myelination in the peripheral nervous system. *Sci Rep*. 2017;7:42257.
2. Holland SM, Thomas GM. Roles of palmitoylation in axon growth, degeneration and regeneration. *J Neurosci Res*. 2017;95(8):1528–1539.
3. Kozu H, Tamura E, Parry GJ. Endoneurial blood supply to peripheral nerves is not uniform. *J Neurol Sci*. 1992;111(2):204–208.
4. Vrancken AF, Franssen H, Wokke JH, et al. Chronic idiopathic axonal polyneuropathy and successful aging of the peripheral nervous system. *Arch Neurol*. 2002;59(4):533–540.
5. Azhary I, Farooq M, Bhanushali M, et al. Peripheral neuropathy: differential diagnosis and management. *Am Fam Physician*. 2010;81(7):887–892.
6. Chan AC, Wilder-Smith EP. Small fiber neuropathy: getting bigger! *Muscle Nerve*. 2016;53(5):671–682.
7. Juster-Switlyk K, Smith AG. Updates in diabetic peripheral neuropathy. *F1000Res*. 2016;5:F1000 Faculty Rev-738. doi: 10.12688/f1000research.7898.1.
8. Gordois A, Scuffham P, Shearer A, et al. The health care cost of diabetic peripheral neuropathy in the US. *Diabetes Care*. 2003;26(6):1790–1795.
9. Frenzen PD. Economic cost of Guillain Barre syndrome in the US. *Neurology*. 2008;71:21–29.
10. Medhi D. Vasculitis neuropathy. 2006. Available from: https://emedicine.medscape.com/
11. Tian L, Prabhakarn M, Ramakrishna S. Strategies for regeneration of components of nervous system: scaffolds, cells and biomolecules. *Regen Biomater*. 2015;2(1):31–45.
12. Terres DJ. Wound healing, nerve. *eMedicine*. 2002:3(6, sec.2):1–10.
13. Sango K, Mizukami H, Horie H, et al. Impaired axonal regeneration in diabetes. Perspective on the underlying mechanism from in vivo and in vitro experimental studies. *Front Endocrinol*. 2017;8:12.
14. Maiese K. Novel applications of trophic factors, Wnt and WISP for neuronal repair and regeneration in metabolic disease. *Neural Regen Res*. 2015;10(4):518–528.
15. Grove M, Kim H, Santerre M, et al. YAP/TAZ initiate and maintain Schwann cell myelination. *Elife*. 2017;6:e20982.
16. Atua I, Kurutas EB. G protein-coupled estrogen receptor levels after peripheral nerve injury in an experimental rat model. *World Neurosurg*. 2015;84(6):1903–1906.
17. Pan Y, Chen F, Huang S, et al. TRPA1 and TRPM8 receptors may promote local vasodilation that aggravates oxaliplatin-induced peripheral neuropathy amenable to 17B estradiol treatment. *Curr Neurovasc Res*. 2016;13(4):309–317.
18. Chen Y, Guo W, Xu L, et al. 17Bestradiol promotes Schwann cell proliferation and differentiation, accelerating early remyelination in a mouse peripheral nerve injury model. *Biomed Res Int*. 2016;2016:7891202.

19. Lees JG, Makker PG, Tonkin RS, et al. Immune-mediated processes implicated in chemotherapy-induced peripheral neuropathy. *Eur J Cancer*. 2017;73:22–29.

20. Roh YH, Koh YD, Noh JH. Low median nerve palsy as initial manifestation of Churg-Strauss syndrome. *J Hand Surg [Am]*. 2017;42(6):478.e1–478.e4.

21. Goncalves NP, Vaegter CB, Andersen H, et al. Schwann cell interactions with axons and microvessels in diabetic neuropathy. *Nat Rev Neurol*. 2017;13(3):135–147.

22. Gaist D, Garcia Rodriguez LA, et al. Are users of lipid-lowering drugs at increased risk of peripheral neuropathy? *Eur J Clin Pharmacol*. 2001;56(12):931–933.

23. Shubayev VI, Myers RR. Axonal transport of TNF-alpha in painful neuropathy: distribution of ligand tracer and TNF receptors. *J Neuroimmunol*. 2001;114 (1–2):48–56.

24. Pollock M. Nerve regeneration. *Curr Opin Neurol*. 1995;(5):354–358.

25. Zhu Q, Lu Q, Rong G, et al. Prospect of human pluripotent stem cell-derived neural crest stem cells in clinical application. *Stem Cells Int*. 2016;2016. Article 7695836.

26. Orthoteers, Nerve Injuries: General Principles. Available from: www.orthoteers.co.uk/nrujpn-j33/m/orthnerveinj.htm

27. Sharon I, Fishfeld C. Acute nerve injury. *eMedicine*. 2002;3(6):1–21.

28. Suarez V, Guntinas-Lichius O, Streppel M, et al. The axotomy-induced neuropeptides galanin and pituitary adenylate cyclase-activating peptide promote axonal sprouting of primary afferent and cranial motor neurones. *Eur J Neurosci*. 2006;24:1555–1564.

29. Treisser R, Lodahl M, Lang M et al. Initial development and validation of a patient-reported symptom survey for small-fiber polyneuropathy. *J Pain*. 2017;18(5): 556–563.

30. Terris DJ, Wound healing, nerve. *eMedicine*. 2002;3(6).

31. Hovaguimian A, Gibbons CH. Diagnosis and treatment of pain in small-fiber neuropathy. *Curr Pain Headache Rep*. 2011;14(3):193–200.

32. Godel T, Weiler M. Clinical indications for high-resolution MRI diagnostics of the peripheral nervous system. *Radiologe*. 2017;57(3):148–156.

33. Baumer P. Diagnostic criteria in MR neurography. *Radiologe*. 2017;57(3):176–183.

34. Hilz MJ, Hecht MJ, Berghoff M, et al. Abnormal vasoreaction to arousal stimuli—an early sign of diabetic sympathetic neuropathy demonstrated by laser Doppler flowmetry. *J Clin Neurophysiol*. 2000;17(4):419–425.

35. Zhang LJ, Guo HY, Zhang DQ. Analysis of serum interleukin-27 and interleukin-35 concentrations in patients with Guillain-Barre syndrome. *Clin Chim Acta*. 2017;468:5–9.

36. Singh A, Asif N, Singh PH. et al. Motor nerve conduction velocity in post-menopausal women with peripheral neuropathy. *J Clin Diagn Res*. 2016;10(12): CC13–CC16.

37. Rison R, Beydoun S. Paraproteinemic neuropathy: a practical review. *BMC Neurol*. 2016;16:13.

38. Poncelet AN. An algorithm for the evaluation of peripheral neuropathy. *Am Fam Physician*. 1998;57(4):755–764. Available from: www.aafp.org

39. Ludolph AC, Spencer PS. Toxic neuropathies and their treatment. *Baillieres Clin Neurol*. 1995;4(3):505–527.

40. Wein TH, Albers JW. Diabetic neuropathies. *Phys Med Rehabil Clin N Am*. 2001;12(2):307–320.

41. Marzban A. Kiani J, Hajilooi M, et al. HLA class II alleles and risk for peripheral neuropathy in type 2 diabetes patients. *Neural Regen Res*. 2016;11(11):1839–1844.

42. Zhu JY, Zhang Z, Qian GS. Mesenchymal stem cells to treat diabetic neuropathy: a long and strenuous way from bench to the clinic. *Cell Death Discov*. 2016;2:16055.

43. Dyck PJ, Windebank AJ. Diabetic and nondiabetic lumbosacral radiculoplexus neuropathies: new insights into pathophysiology and treatment. *Muscle Nerve*. 2002;25(4):477–491.

44. Manu MS, Rachana KS, Advirao GM. Altered expression of IRS2 and GRB2 in demyelination of peripheral neurons: implications in diabetic neuropathy. *Neuropeptides*. 2017;62:71–79.

45. King RH. The role of glycation in the pathogenesis of diabetic polyneuropathy. *Mol Pathol*. 2001;54(6):400–408.

46. Perkins BA, Greene DA, Bril V. Gylcemic control is related to the morphological severity of diabetic sensorimotor polyneuropathy. *Diabetes Care*. 2001;24(4): 748–752.

47. Wellmer A, Misra VP, Sharief MK, et al. A double-blind placebo controlled clinical trial of recombinant human brain-derived neurotrophic factor (rhBDNF) in diabetic polyneuropathy. *J Peripher Nerv Syst*. 2001;6(4):204–210.

48. Schmidt RE, Dorsey DA, Beaudet LN, et al. Effect of NGF and neurotrophin-3 treatment on experimental diabetic autonomic neuropathy. *J Neuropathol Exp Neurol*. 2001;60(3):263–273.

49. Tam J, Diamond J, Maysinger D. Dual-action peptides: a new strategy in the treatment of diabetes-associated neuropathy. *Drug Discov Today*. 2006;11(5–6):254–260.

50. Caro XJ, Winter EF. The role and importance of small fiber neuropathy in fibromyalgia pain. *Curr Pain Headache Rep*. 2015;19(12):55.

51. Devigili G, Tugnoli V, Penza P, et al. The diagnostic criteria for small fibre neuropathy; from symptoms to neuropathology. *Brain*. 2008;131(7):1912–1925.

52. Gabreels Festen A, Gabreels F. Hereditary demyelinating motor and sensory neuropathy. *Brain Pathol*. 1993;3(2):135–146.

53. Uncini A, Di Guglielmo G, Di Muzio A, et al. Differential electrophysiological features of neuropathies associated with 17p11.2 deletion and duplication. *Muscle Nerve*. 1995;18(6):628–635.

54. Harding AF. From the syndrome of Charcot, Marie and Tooth to disorders of peripheral myelin proteins. *Brain*. 1995;118(pt 3):809–818.

55. Schon K, Spasic-Boskovic O, Brugger K, et al. Mosaicism for a pathogenic MFN2 mutation causes minimal clinical features of CMT2A in the parent of a severely affected child. *Neurogenetics*. 2017;18(1):49–55.

56. Loiseaa D, Chevrollier A, Verny C, et al. Mitochondrial coupling defect in Charcot-Marie-Tooth type 2A disease. *Ann Neurol*. 2007;61(4):315–323.

57. Gabreels-Festen AA, Gabreels FJ, Jennekens FG, et al. The status of HMSN type III. *Neuromuscul Disord*. 1994;4(1):63–69.

58. Schroder JM. Neuropathy associated with mitochondrial disorders. *Brain Pathol*. 1993;3(2):177–190.

59. Hanemann CO. Hereditary demyelinating neuropathies: from gene to disease. *Neurogenetics*. 2001;3(2):53–57.

60. Carter GT, Abresch RT, Fowler WM Jr., et al. Profiles of neuromuscular diseases: hereditary motor and sensory neuropathy, types I and II. *Am J Phys Med Rehabil*. 1995;74(5 suppl):S140–S149.

61. Acute flaccid paralysis syndrome associated with West Nile Virus infection—Mississippi and Louisiana, Jul–Aug 2002. *MMWR Morb Mortal Wkly Rep*. 2002;51(37):825.

62. Sharma SR, Hussain M, Habung H. Neurological manifestations of HIV-AIDS at a tertiary care institute in North Eastern India. *Neurol India*. 2017;65(1):64–68.

63. Verma A. Epidemiology and clinical features of HIV-1 associated neuropathies. *J Peripher Nerv Syst*. 2001;6(1):8–13.

64. Simpson DM, Haidich AB, Schifitto G, et al. Severity of HIV-associated neuropathy is associated with plasma HIV-1 RNA levels. *AIDS*. 2002;16(3):407–412.

65. Kindstrand E, Nilsson BY, Hovmark A, et al. Polyneuropathy in late lyme borreliosis—a clinical, neurophysiologic and morphological description. *Acta Neurol Scand*. 2000;101(1):47–52.

66. Jalladeau E, Pradat PF, Maisonobe T, et al. Multiple mononeuropathy and inflammatory syndrome manifested in lyme disease. *Rev Neurol (Paris)*. 2001;157(10):1290–1292.

67. Brizzi K, Lyons J. Peripheral nervous system manifestations of infectious diseases. *Neurohospitalist*. 2014;4(4):230–240.

68. Kihara M, McManis PG, Schmelzer JD, et al. Experimental ischemic neuropathy: salvage with hyperbaric oxygenation. *Ann Neurol*. 1995;37(1):89–94.

69. Jordan WC. The effectiveness of intermittent hyperbaric O_2 in relieving drug-induced HIV-associated neuropathy. *J Natl Med Assoc*. 1998;90(6):355–358.

70. Schifitto G, Yiannoutsos C, Simpson DM, et al. Long term treatment with recombinant nerve growth factor for HIV-associated sensory neuropathy. *Neurology*. 2001;57(7):1313–1316.

71. Hund EF, Fogel W, Krieger D, et al. Critical illness polyneuropathy: clinical findings and outcomes of a frequent cause of neuromuscular weaning failure. *Crit Care Med*. 1996;24(8):1328–1333.

72. Gemignani F, Melli G, Inglese C, et al. Cryoglobulinemia is a frequent cause of peripheral neuropathy in undiagnosed referral patients. *J Peripher Nerv Syst*. 2002;7(1):59–64.

73. Young GB. Neurologic complications of systemic critical illness. *Neurol Clin*. 1995;13(3):645–658.

74. Wijdicks EF, Litchy WJ, Harrison BA, et al. The clinical spectrum of critical illness polyneuropathy. *Mayo Clin Proc*. 1994;69(10):955–959.

75. Bolton CF, Young GB, Zochodne DW. The neurological complications of sepsis. *Ann Neurol*. 1993;33(1):94–100.

76. Martinez AR, Faber I, Nucci A, et al. Autoimmune neuropathies associated to rheumatic diseases. *Autoimmun Rev*. 2017;16(4):335–342.

77. Stubgen JP. Tumor necrosis factor-alpha antagonists and neuropathy. *Muscle Nerve*. 2007.

78. Davids H. Guillain Barre syndrome. 2006. Available from: https://emedicine.medscape.com/

79. Lisak RP. The immunology of neuromuscular disease. In: Walton JN, ed. *Disorders of Voluntary Muscle*. 5th ed. London: Churchill Livingstone; 1988:628–665.

80. Wollinsky KH, Hulser PJ, Brinkmeier H, et al. Filtration of cerebrospinal fluid in acute inflammatory demyelinating polyneuropathy (Guillain-Barre syndrome). *Ann Med Interne (Paris)*. 1994;145(7):451–458.

81. van der Meche FG, van Doorn PA, Jacobs BC. Inflammatory neuropathies—pathogenesis and the role of intravenous immune globulin. *J Clin Immunol*. 1995;15 (6 suppl):63S–69S.

82. Leger JM. Multifocal motor neuropathy and chronic inflammatory demyelinating polyradiculoneuropathy. *Curr Opin Neurol*. 1995;8(5):359–363.

83. Bird SJ, Brown MJ, Shy ME, et al. Chronic inflammatory demyelinating polyradiculoneuropathy associated with malignant melanoma. *Neurology*. 1996;46(3):822–824.

84. Toepfer M, Schroeder M, Muller-Felber W, et al. Successful management of polyneuropathy associated with IgM gammopathy of undetermined significance with antibody-based immunoadsorption. *Clin Nephrol*. 2000;53(5):404–407.

85. Remeny P, Masszi T, Borbényi Z, et al. CIDP cured by allogeneic hematopoietic stem cell transplantation. *Eur J Neurol*. 2007;14(8):e1–e2.

86. D'Sa S, Kersten MJ, Castillo JJ. Investigation and management of IgM and Waldenstrom-associated peripheral neuropathies: recommendations from the IWWWM-8 consensus panel. *Br J Haematol*. 2017;176(5):728–742.

87. Saperstein DS, Katz JS, Amato AA, et al. Clinical spectrum of chronic acquired demyelinating polyneuropathies. *Muscle Nerve*. 2001;24(3):311–324.

88. Notermans NC, Franssen H, Eurerlings M, et al. Diagnostic criteria for demyelinating polyneuropathy associated with monoclonal gammopathy. *Muscle Nerve*. 2000;23:73–79.

89. Shimada S, Tzuzuki T, Kuroda M, et al. Nestin expression as a new marker in malignant peripheral nerve sheath tumors. *Pathol Int*. 2007;57(2):60–67.

90. Roth TM, Ramamurthy P, Ebisu F, et al. A mouse embryonic stem cell model of Schwann cell differentiation for studies of the role of neurofibromatosis type 1 in Schwann cell development and tumor formation. *Glia*. 2007;55(11):1123–1133.

91. Lundborg G, Dahlin LB. The Pathophysiology of nerve compression. *Hand Clin*. 1992;8(2):215–227.

92. Chang KV, Lin CP, Lin CS, et al. Sonographic tracking of trunk nerves: essential for ultrasound-guided pain management and research. *J Pain Res.* 2017;10: 79–88.

93. Vaidya Y, Vaithianathan R. An unusual case of neurogenic thoracic outlet syndrome. *Int J Surg Case Rep.* 2017;31:139–141.

94. Godoy IR, Donahue DM, Torriani M. Botulinum toxin injections in musculoskeletal disorders. *Semin Musculoskelet Radiol.* 2016;20(5):441–452.

95. Dawson DM, Hallett M, Wilbourn AJ. *Entrapment Neuropathies.* Philadelphia, PA: Lippincott-Raven; 1999.

96. Bagatur AE, Zorer G. The carpal tunnel syndrome is a bilateral disorder. *J Bone Joint Surg Br.* 2001;83:655–658.

97. Gerritsen AA, Uitdehaag BM, van Geldere D, et al. Systematic review of randomized clinical trials of surgical treatment for carpal tunnel syndrome. *Br J Surg.* 2001;88:1285–1295.

98. Knapik JJ, Reynolds K, Orr R, et al. Load carriage-related paresthesias (Part 2): meralgia paresthetica. *J Spec Oper Med.* 2017;17(1):94–100.

99. Payne R, Seaman S, Sieg E, et al. Evaluated the evidence: is neurolysis of neurectomy a better treatment for meralgia paresthetica. *Acta Neurochir.* 2017;159(5):931–936.

100. Kim DH, Kam AC, Chandika P, et al. Surgical management and outcome in patients with radial nerve lesions. *J Neurosurg.* 2001;95(4):573–583.

101. Su EP. Post-operative neuropathy after total hip arthroplasty. *Bone Joint J.* 2017; 99-B:46–49.

102. Carter GT, Weiss MD, Han JJ, et al. Charcot-Marie-Tooth disease. *Curr Treat Options Neurol.* 2008;10(2):94–102.

103. Kaya F, Belin S, Burgeois P, et al. Ascorbic acid inhibits PMP 22 expression by reducing cAMP levels. *Neuromuscul Disord.* 2007;17:248–253.

104. Khajavi M, Shiga K, Wiszniewski W, et al. Oral curcumin mitigates the clinical and neuropathologic phenotype of the Trembler-J mouse: a potential therapy for inherited neuropathy. *Am J Hum Genet.* 2007;81(3):438–453.

105. Guzman M, Sanchez C, Galve-Roperh I. Control of the cell survival/death decision by cannabinoids. *J Mol Med.* 2001;78:613–625.

106. Hampson AJ, Grimaldi M, Axelrod J, et al. Cannabidiol and (–) delta9-tetrahydrocannabinol are neuroprotective antioxidants. *Proc Natl Acad Sci U S A.* 1998;95:8268–8273.

107. Hu J, Zhu QT, Liu XL, et al. Repair of extended peripheral nerve lesions in rhesus monkeys using acellular allogenic nerve grafts implanted with autologous mesenchymal stem cells. *Exp Neurol.* 2007;204(2):658–666.

108. McKenzie IA, Biernaskie J, Toma JG, et al. Skin-derived precursors generate myelinating Schwann cells for the injured and dysmyelinated nervous system. *J Neurosci.* 2006;26(24):6651–6660.

109. Calcutt NA, Smith DR, Frizzi K, et al. Selective antagonism of muscarinic receptors in neuroprotective in peripheral neuropathy. *J Clin Invest.* 2017;127(2): 608–622.

110. Tajti J, Szok D, Majlath Z, et al. Alleviation of pain in painful diabetic neuropathy. *Expert Opin Drug Metab Toxicol.* 2016;12(7):753–764.

111. Cakici N, Fakkel TM, van Neck JW, et al. Systematic review of treatments for diabetic peripheral neuropathy. *Diabet Med.* 2016;22(11):1466–1478.

112. Moulin D, Boulanger A, Clark AJ, et al. Pharmacological management of chronic neuropathic pain: revised consensus statement from the Canadian Pain Society. *Pain Res Manag.* 2014;19(6):328–335.

113. Meng H, Johnston B, Englesakis M, et al. Selective cannabinoids for chronic neuropathic pain: a systematic review and meta-analysis. *Anesth Analg.* 2017;125(5):1638–1652.

114. Nolan RC, Raynor AJ, Berry NM, et al. Self-reported physical activity using the international physical activity questionnaire (IPAQ) in Australian adults with type 2 diabetes, with and without peripheral neuropathy. *Can J Diabetes.* 2016;40(6): 576–579.

115. Apfel SC, Kessler JA. Neurotrophic factors in the treatment of peripheral neuropathy. *Ciba Found Symp.* 1996;196:98–112. Elsevier Science at www.elsevier.com

116. Hamza MA, White PF, Craig WF, et al. Percutaneous electrical nerve stimulation: a novel analgesic therapy for diabetic neuropathic pain. *Diabetes Care.* 2000;23(3):365–370.

117. Munglani R. The longer term effect of pulsed radiofrequency for neuropathic pain. *Pain.* 1999;80(1–2):437–439.

118. Girgis FL, Parry CB. Management of causalgia after peripheral nerve injury. *Int Disabil Stud.* 1989;11(1):15–20.

119. Byram Sc, Byram SW, Miller NM, et al. Bupivacaine increases the rate of motoneuron death following peripheral nerve injury. *Restor Neurol Neurosci.* 2017;35(1):129–135.

120. Borgens RB. Cellular engineering: molecular repair of membranes to rescue cells of the damaged nervous system. *Neurosurgery.* 2001;49(2):370–379.

121. Fowler JR, Lavasani M, Nuard J, et al. Biologic strategies to improve nerve regeneration after peripheral nerve repair. *J Reconstr Microsurg.* 2015;31(4):243–248.

122. Zhang F, Inserra M, Richards L, et al. Quantification of nerve tension after nerve repair: correlations with nerve deficits and nerve regeneration. *J Reconstr Microsurg.* 2001;17(5):445–451.

123. McCallister WV, Cober SR, Norman A, et al. Using intact nerve to bridge peripheral nerve defects: an alternative to the use of nerve grafts. *J Hand Surg [Am].* 2001;26(2):315–325.

124. Muheremu A, Ao Q. Past, present and future of nerve conduits in the treatment of peripheral nerve injury. *Biomed Res Int.* 2015;2015:237507.

125. Yin Q, Kemp GJ, Yu LG, et al. Neurotrophin-4 delivered by fibrin glue promotes peripheral nerve regeneration. *Muscle Nerve.* 2001;24(3):345–351.

126. Ohkaya S, Hirata H, Uehida A. Repair of nerve gap with the elongation of Wallerian degenerated nerve by tissue expansion. *Microsurgery.* 2000;20(3):126–130.

127. Meek MF, Coert JH. Clinical use of nerve conduits in peripheral-nerve repair: review of the literature. *J Reconstr Microsurg.* 2002;18(2):97–109.

128. Patterson JM. High ulnar nerve injuries: nerve transfers to restore function. *Hand Clin.* 2016;32(2):219–226.

129. Soldado F, Bertelli JA, Ghizoni MF. High median nerve injury: motor and sensory nerve transfers to restore function. *Hand Clin.* 2016;32(2):209–217.

130. Bulstra LE, Shin AY. Nerve transfers to restore elbow function. *Hand Clin.* 2016;32(2):165–174.

131. Leechavengvongs S, Malungpaishorpe K, Uerpairojkit C, et al. Nerve transfers to restore shoulder function. *Hand Clin.* 2016;32(2):153–164.

132. Peripheral Neuropathy Medical Disability Guidelines. Available from: http://www.mdguidelines.com/peripheral-neuropathy

133. Van Nooten FE, Trundell D, Staniewska D, et al. Scoring and responsiveness of the self-assessment of treatment version Ii questionnaire in patients with painful diabetic peripheral neuropathy. *Value Health.* 2015;18(7):A706–A707.

134. Hamdan A, Luna JD, Del Pozo E, et al. Diagnostic accuracy of two questionnaires for the detection of neuropathic pain in the Spanish population. *Eur J Pain.* 2014;18(1):101–109.

135. Corrado B, Ciardi G, Bargigli C. Rehabilitation management of the Charcot-Marie-Tooth Syndrome, a systematic review of the literature. *Medicine (Baltimore).* 2016;95(17):e3278.

136. Cooper MA, Kluding PM, Wright DE. Emerging relationships between exercise, sensory nerves and neuropathic pain. *Front Neurosci.* 2016;10:372.

137. Benstead TJ, Grant IA. Progress in clinical neurosciences: Charcot-Marie-Tooth disease and related inherited peripheral neuropathies. *Can J Neurol Sci.* 2001;28(3):199–214.

138. Hashem MD, Parker AM, Needham DM. Early mobilization and rehabilitation of patients who are critically ill. *Chest.* 2016;150(3):722–731.

139. Chao RP, Braun SA, Ta KT, et al. Early passive mobilization after digital nerve repair and grafting in a fresh cadaver. *Plast Reconstr Surg.* 2001;108(2):386–391.

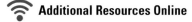 **Additional Resources Online**

Myopathy

Representing a diverse group of disorders primarily affecting skeletal muscle, myopathies are an important cause of disability affecting patient mobility, self-care, and independence. In addition to weakness, many myopathies have associated dysfunction in other organ systems, such as the cardiac and pulmonary systems. The disability associated with muscle disease depends on the specific type, extent of clinical involvement, and rate of progression.

The number and type of different muscle disorders under the umbrella term myopathy are vast and expanding. With our increasing knowledge about genetic and molecular basis for these disorders, classification and nomenclature regarding myopathies are constantly being reevaluated and modified. A detailed discussion of all the different myopathies is beyond the scope of this chapter; however, this chapter is intended to provide the physical medicine and rehabilitation specialist with an overview of diagnostic approach, clinical characteristics, and care and management of patients with myopathies, with emphasis on few of the most common diagnoses that a physiatrist may encounter.

Although most myopathies remain largely incurable, as is the case for most neuromuscular diseases at this time, they are not untreatable. Rehabilitation specialists have an important role in the care of patients with myopathies to maximize their functional capacities, prolong or maintain independent locomotion and function, prevent physical deformity and medical complications, and provide access for integration into the community with quality of life in mind. The comprehensive management of all the varied clinical problems associated with myopathies and other neuromuscular diseases often requires specialists from neurology, cardiology, pulmonology, and orthopedic surgery as well as clinical specialists in physical therapy, occupational therapy, speech therapy, and orthotics. Coordination of this difficult and demanding task may be best handled by a neuromuscular and rehabilitation medicine specialist knowledgeable in various myopathies. It is important for the rehabilitation physician to understand these diseases in order to appropriately treat the functional problems caused by muscle weakness as well as provide comprehensive interdisciplinary rehabilitation through awareness of other manifestations of the disease.

DEFINITION AND CATEGORIES OF MYOPATHY

In the peripheral nervous system, a primary defect may occur at the level of the anterior horn cell, peripheral nerve, neuromuscular junction, or muscle. A disease process in which the primary abnormality is at the level of the muscle itself is termed *myopathy*. A brief overview of the various myopathies is presented in this section to help the reader classify numerous myopathies in an orderly fashion. A more detailed discussion of the individual myopathies pertinent to rehabilitation specialists is found in the subsequent sections.

There are three basic categories of myopathy: hereditary, acquired, and myopathies associated with systemic disease (Table 25-1). In the *hereditary myopathies*, all of the myopathies have their inheritance pattern characterized or gene mutations identified. This category of myopathy is further subdivided into muscular dystrophies, congenital, distal, metabolic, and mitochondrial myopathies. In general, the muscular dystrophies present with significant structural defect of the muscle cell due to mutations in genes crucial for its normal function. Typically, the muscular dystrophies are accompanied by progressive muscle fiber degeneration, atrophy, and inflammation as noted by histopathologic evaluation. The specific muscular dystrophies that are more commonly encountered, with their characteristic inheritance pattern, affected genes, and mutations are listed (eTable 25-1). Congenital myopathies are a group of relatively nonprogressive muscle diseases that present during infancy or early childhood and are classified largely based on clinical features and muscle biopsy morphologic findings. Distal myopathies, as the name implies, have more pronounced weakness involving distal limb muscles rather than the typical proximal weakness seen with majority of other myopathies. Metabolic myopathies are caused by gene mutations that result in either abnormal glycogen or lipid metabolism. Usually, deficiency of an enzyme results from a gene mutation and causes an abnormal accumulation of substrate or a deficiency of the product of the enzymatic pathway. Mitochondrial myopathies are a group of muscle disorders with maternal inheritance pattern associated with abnormal structure and function of mitochondria. Since mitochondria are important in energy production throughout the body, other organ system involvements are also common including the nervous, cardiac, gastrointestinal, pulmonary, and endocrine systems. Diagnosis is often based on a combination of clinical findings and associated biochemical defects, along with histologic abnormality noted as "ragged red fibers" on the modified Gomori trichrome stain. Another group of myopathies called channelopathies include primary muscle disorders caused by inherited abnormalities of various ion channels found on cell membranes. These include myotonia congenita, paramyotonia congenita, and primary hyperkalemic and hypokalemic periodic paralysis.

TABLE 25-1

Hereditary Myopathies	Acquired Myopathies
Muscular dystrophies	**Inflammatory myopathies**
Duchenne muscular dystrophy (DMD)	Polymyositis (PM)
Becker muscular dystrophy (BMD)	Dermatomyositis (DM)
Myotonic muscular dystrophy (DM1 and DM2)	Inclusion body myositis (IBM)
Facioscapulohumeral muscular dystrophy (FSHD)	**Toxic myopathies**
Limb-girdle muscular dystrophy (LGMD)	Corticosteroid myopathies
Congenital muscular dystrophy (CMD)	Lipid-lowering agent myopathies
Oculopharyngeal muscular dystrophy (OPMD)	Alcohol-related myopathies
Emery-Dreifuss muscular dystrophy (EDMD)	Myopathies related to other medications
Congenital myopathies	**Endocrine myopathies**
Central core, nemaline, centronuclear, multicore	Myopathies with glucocorticoid abnormalities
Fiber-type disproportion, reducing body	Myopathies with thyroid disease
Fingerprint, cytoplasmic body, myofibrillar	Myopathies with parathyroid disease
Metabolic myopathies	Myopathies associated with pituitary dysfunction
Disorders of glycogenoses	Myopathies related to electrolyte disturbance
Disorders of lipid metabolism	**Infectious and granulomatous myopathies**
Respiratory chain defects	Viral, bacterial, fungal, tuberculous, parasitic
Distal myopathies	Sarcoid myopathy
Welander, Markesbery-Griggs-Udd, Nonaka, Miyoshi, Laing	
Mitochondrial myopathies	**Myopathies associated with systemic disease**
Kearns-Sayre's syndrome, progressive external ophthalmoplegia (PEO), mitochondrial encephalo-myopathy lactic acidosis stroke (MELAS), myoclonic epilepsy ragged red fibers (MERRF)	Critical illness myopathy
Neuropathy ataxia retinitis pigmentosa (NARP), myopathy and external ophthalmoplegia neuropathy gastrointestinal encephalopathy (MNGIE), Leber's hereditary optic neuropathy (LHON), Leigh's syndrome	Electrolyte disturbances
Channelopathies	
Myotonia congenita	Paraneoplastic
Paramyotonia congenita	
Primary hyperkalemic and hypokalemic periodic paralysis	

The second category, *acquired myopathies*, consists of inflammatory, endocrine, toxic, granulomatous, and infectious myopathies. Under inflammatory myopathies are polymyositis (PM), dermatomyositis (DM), and inclusion body myositis (IBM). Muscle disorders associated with various endocrinopathies are now well recognized. These include myopathies associated with thyroid dysfunction (hyperthyroidism or hypothyroidism), adrenal disease, pituitary dysfunction, and parathyroid dysfunction (hyperparathyroidism or hypoparathyroidism). Myopathies can also result from electrolyte disturbances, including abnormalities of serum potassium, sodium, calcium, magnesium, and phosphorus. Under the toxic myopathy category, the most common agents associated with myopathy include HMG-CoA reductase inhibitors (cholesterol-lowering agents), corticosteroids, fibric acid derivatives (lipid- and cholesterol-lowering agents), chloroquine and amiodarone (amphiphilic drugs), colchicine and vincristine (antimicrotubular agents), zidovudine (HIV medication), and alcohol. Of the toxic myopathies, alcohol-related myopathy is thought to be the most common with both acute and chronic manifestations, often associated with heavy and prolonged alcohol use. Although typically asymptomatic in terms of muscle manifestation, sarcoidosis can present in the form of a granulomatous myopathy. Lastly, infectious myopathies are associated with essentially all types of infectious agents including viral (coxsackievirus, HIV, HTLV-1), bacterial, fungal, tuberculous, as well as parasites.

The last category is *myopathies associated with systemic disease*. Under this category are myopathies that have significant systemic processes that result in derangement of muscle function and health. The most common etiologies are severe multiorgan failure with sepsis, electrolyte disturbances associated with systemic disease, and underlying neoplasms.

Clinical features and progression vary within and between these categories as pathophysiology of each muscle disorder is different. Some of the myopathies, partly due to their time course of progression, involvement of other organ systems, prevalence in the population, and the availability of rehabilitative treatment options, may be more or less pertinent to rehabilitation specialists. However, in order to devise an appropriate rehabilitation plan, the rehabilitation physician should understand the expected disabilities and prognosis associated with the specific cause of myopathy.

EVALUATION OF THE PATIENT WITH SUSPECTED MYOPATHY

History

The primary symptom of a patient with suspected myopathy is weakness, defined as a reduction in maximal force generated by a muscle or muscle group (**Box 25-1**). This weakness may be fairly acute or insidious. Because the weakness is typically in the proximal musculature, certain functional problems should

---

BOX 25-1

Clinical Features and Laboratory Findings Suggestive of Myopathies

Proximal symmetric weakness
Normal sensation
Normal or mildly diminished tendon reflexes
Elevation of serum CK
EMG demonstrating brief, low-amplitude, polyphasic potentials
Normal nerve conduction studies
Muscle biopsy with muscle fiber necrosis and regeneration, with central nuclei

---

BOX 25-2

Key Physical Examination Points for Suspected Myopathy

Proximal > distal weakness, including neck and facial muscles
Observation of facial features
Sensation—should be normal
Muscle tendon reflexes preserved or mildly decreased
Presence of clinical myotonia
Waddling gait with Gower's sign on standing
Positioning of the shoulder girdle

---

alert the clinician to the possibility of myopathy: difficulty getting up from a chair or toilet seat, trouble descending and climbing stairs, or difficulty with overhead activities, such as dressing, grooming, or reaching cabinets (📶 **eBox 25-1**). Symptoms suggesting distal weakness, such as problems opening jars, may be prominent with certain myopathies. The symptom of muscle fatigue, defined as the inability to sustain a given level of force for a certain period, is often difficult to assess. Although it may be associated with myopathy, when fatigue is the predominant symptom, other pathologic processes, such as neuromuscular junction disease and upper motor neuron disease, are more likely.

Muscle pain, or myalgia, is a common presenting symptom, particularly in the inflammatory myopathies. However, the absence of pain should not distract the clinician from strongly considering the diagnosis of myopathy. When myalgias are the predominant symptom without demonstrated weakness, other disorders are more likely. History of myoglobinuria associated with weakness or fatigue symptoms should be sought and can help in the workup of muscle disorders, especially the metabolic myopathies. The presence of paresthesias or dysesthesias on history is certainly helpful because they make the presence of myopathy very unlikely. A rare patient might interpret myalgias with descriptors sounding like sensory symptoms, distracting the clinician.

One of the most critical pieces of information is the family history. Whenever a myopathy is suspected that may have a genetic cause, a detailed family history and pedigree chart are essential. In an X-linked recessive disorder such as Duchenne muscular dystrophy (DMD), men on the maternal side of the family are affected about 50% of the time and women are carriers in an equal percentage. Autosomal recessive disorders, such as many limb-girdle syndromes, frequently have no family members involved, making the diagnosis of a familial disorder more difficult. In an autosomal dominant disorder such as myotonic muscular dystrophy or facioscapulohumeral dystrophy (FSHD), typically 50% of offspring within a pedigree are affected. Sporadic cases resulting from new genetic defects occur with most autosomal dominant and sex-linked dystrophies, making a dystrophy possible even in the absence of a suspicious family history.

In a child presenting with weakness, a developmental history should include milestones of age for head control, independent sitting, standing, and walking. Additional factors related to ambulation include toe walking, excessive lordosis, falls, and running ability.

Physical Examination

Examination of the patient with suspected myopathy begins with observation (**Box 25-2**). In myopathies, muscle atrophy may not be obvious until late in the disease because of a wide normal range of variation in the population and the typical symmetry of muscular involvement. Calf enlargement may be noted in dystrophic myopathies, particularly in DMD and Becker muscular dystrophy (BMD). This "pseudohypertrophy" is caused by increased fat and connective tissue volume, rather than muscle fiber hypertrophy (1) (**Fig. 25-1**). Observation of facial features, such as a long thin face with temporal and masseter wasting with frontal balding, is typical for myotonic muscular dystrophy.

Other physical examination findings that may be particularly helpful in the evaluation of myopathies are the presence and distribution of rash, contractures, and ligamentous laxity.

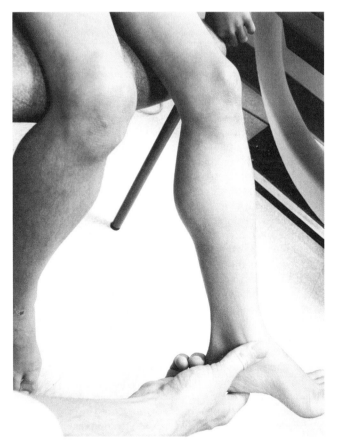

FIGURE 25-1.   Calf pseudohypertrophy in an 8-year-old boy with DMD.

These may be useful when considering diagnoses such as DM, Emery-Dreifuss muscular dystrophy (EDMD), and muscle diseases with associated collagen dysfunctions. Cardiac examination is also important as some myopathies have an associated conduction abnormality or a cardiomyopathy. Examination of the pulmonary system can provide clues to an accompanying restrictive lung disease process or an aspiration pneumonia secondary to swallowing difficulties.

Because weakness is the predominant symptom, determination of muscle strength is critical. Unfortunately, the manual muscle test typically used by clinicians is only a very rough measure of strength. It is well known that up to 50% strength loss may occur before a muscle is graded as 4/5 using the Medical Research Council (MRC) scale (2). The more powerful pelvic proximal muscles are particularly difficult to measure because the patient should be able to overcome the examiner's resistance. The handheld dynamometer is a quantitative device to measure strength, but it shares the same limitation when strong muscles are being tested. It has been shown to provide reliable data in persons with neuropathic weakness (3). Because of a wide range of normality, the handheld dynamometer is probably better suited to measure serial strength than to quantify a specific muscle group as "normal" or "abnormal."

Probably the most reasonable method to test strength in the clinic is to observe repetitive maneuvers, such as rising from a squat, repeatedly standing on the toes, or raising the arms overhead with resistance. The clinician should observe for Gower's sign: The patient rises from a low surface by pushing against the knees and moving the hands up the thighs to substitute for knee and hip extensor weakness.

Facial and neck muscle weakness predominates in several myopathies such as FSHD. The ability to "bury" the eyelashes or the ability of the examiner to easily overcome forced eye closure (because of orbicularis oculi weakness) and difficulty whistling (because of orbicularis oris weakness) are reasonable screening tests. The presence of ptosis or ophthalmoplegia should also be noted. The neck flexor muscles are usually much more affected than the neck extensors and are the earliest muscle group to show abnormality in DMD (4).

Myotonia, a state of delayed relaxation or sustained contraction of muscle, is common to the myotonic muscular disorders. Action myotonia may be demonstrated by asking the patient to grip the examiner's fingers tightly and then quickly attempt to relax. Extension of the fingers will be difficult. Alternatively, percussion myotonia may be elicited by tapping the thenar eminence with a reflex hammer, causing a local involuntary contraction of the thenar muscles. Muscle tendon reflexes are generally preserved in myopathies until there is profound loss of strength, an important differentiating factor from neuropathic disorders.

Careful observation of gait is very helpful in evaluation of the patient with myopathy, and a classic pattern of gait progression may be noted in progressive dystrophic myopathies. One of the earliest features in patients with myopathy is hyperlordosis of the lower back, a compensation for hip extensor weakness by maintaining the weight line behind the hip joints. Waddling is typical during gait because of weakness of the hip abductor musculature, resulting in the necessity to bring the trunk over the weight-bearing limb during stance phase, the so-called gluteus medius lurch. When knee extensor weakness becomes significant enough to cause knee buckling, the ankle is postured into progressive plantar flexion, producing a knee extension moment at heel strike and positioning the weight line anterior to the knee during later stance, which stabilizes the knee. This pattern predominates in DMD and BMD. In other myopathies, "back knee" or genu recurvatum during stance phase provides stability by bringing the weight line in front of the knee joint. In the unusual myopathy in which distal weakness predominates, such as myotonic muscular dystrophy and an occasional FSHD, weakness of the ankle dorsiflexors and evertors occurs early. These patients may ambulate with steppage gait and foot slap at floor contact, very similar to the neuropathic disorders.

Positioning of the shoulder musculature and scapulae may be helpful in discerning myopathy. In FSHD and limb-girdle muscular dystrophy (LGMD), involvement of the latissimus dorsi, lower trapezius, rhomboids, and serratus anterior results in superior and lateral displacement of the scapula, giving the shoulders a forward-sloped appearance. There is associated scapular winging of the medial border, and the upward positioning of the scapula into the trapezius can mimic hypertrophy of this muscle.

Laboratory Evaluation

The most important blood study for suspected myopathy is measurement of serum creatine kinase (CK). With muscle fiber injury, this enzyme leaks into the serum. Particularly high elevations of CK (50 to 100 times normal) may be found in acute inflammatory myopathies and the early stages of DMD and BMD. The more slowly progressive dystrophies may have mild to moderate elevations in CK. However, CK is not the ideal screening test for all myopathies because the congenital myopathies, slowly progressive dystrophies, chronic inflammatory myopathies, and myopathies of systemic disease may have normal values. The clinician should be cautious not to overinterpret one mildly elevated CK level, because it may be elevated in healthy persons for several days after vigorous exercise. Conversely, once there is significant muscular atrophy, CK values may be low or normal based on the paucity of remaining muscle tissue to release the enzyme. Other serum transaminases, aldolase, and lactate dehydrogenase are often elevated in myopathy but are much less specific because they are found in liver in equally high amounts. In the metabolic myopathies, measurement of blood lactate and pyruvate may be helpful, particularly arterial lactate levels during ischemic or exercise stress. With abnormalities of glycogen metabolism, there will be no rise in lactate because patients cannot catabolize glycogen.

Electrodiagnosis

Electrodiagnostic studies (electromyography [EMG]) can be extremely important in the evaluation of the patient with myopathy to localize the pathology to the muscle rather than nerve or anterior horn cell. The pattern of EMG findings may indicate the best muscle for biopsy, and certain abnormalities on the EMG occasionally suggest a specific myopathic disease. However, electrodiagnostic studies in myopathy may be normal as well, so a myopathic disorder is not ruled out by normal EMG studies.

Nerve conduction studies should be normal in myopathic disorders, with the exception of a low compound motor action potential obtained when recording over muscles with severe atrophy. With needle EMG, the presence of abnormal spontaneous activity (positive sharp wave/fibrillation potentials) is dependent on whether the myopathy is causing active muscle fiber degeneration. For example, the inflammatory myopathies and rapidly progressive dystrophies frequently demonstrate abnormal spontaneous activity, whereas it is not often encountered in the slowly progressive dystrophies or myopathies associated with systemic disease.

The hallmark needle EMG finding suggesting myopathy is the presence of low-amplitude, often polyphasic, brief-duration potentials with voluntary contraction. Because recruitment of each additional motor unit only slightly augments strength, the electromyographer often notes an excessive number of motor units for a given strength of contraction (early recruitment pattern). These findings may be subtle or absent, particularly in slowly progressive disorders. Particularly important muscles to evaluate with possible myopathy include the paraspinal, supraspinatus and infraspinatus, glutei, and iliopsoas muscles.

Muscle Biopsy

The ideal muscle for biopsy is weak but not profoundly atrophic (see Chapter 2). Electrodiagnostic abnormalities increase the likelihood that the muscle will demonstrate useful findings, although one should not biopsy a muscle that has recently been evaluated with a needle electrode because of possible needle-induced fiber damage (see Chapter 2). The most accessible muscles include the vastus lateralis in the lower limb and the deltoid or biceps brachii in the upper limb. Histologic findings suggestive of myopathy include fiber necrosis, central nuclei indicative of regeneration, atrophied fibers, inflammatory infiltrates, and proliferation of connective tissue and fibrosis. Certain congenital myopathies, including centronuclear or myotubular, central core, and nemaline rod, have distinctive histologic and electron microscopy findings. In addition to histologic studies, immunohistochemical techniques can provide information about the amounts of dystrophin and other structural membrane proteins.

Molecular Genetic Studies

Recent advances in molecular genetic techniques have resulted in remarkable increases in the knowledge of various myopathies. The chromosomal location, causal gene, and mutations have been identified in many neuromuscular disorders and are frequently helpful in diagnostic evaluation. An example of the impact of molecular genetic studies is the evaluation for possible DMD or BMD. Both disorders are caused by mutations in an extremely large gene located on the X chromosome. The protein product of the gene, known as *dystrophin*, was determined to be an important component of the muscle membrane cytoskeleton, contributing to the stability of the muscle fiber (5). For diagnosis, a clinically available gene deletion study from a blood sample is diagnostic of a dystrophinopathy, but it is able to detect mutations present in only about 65% of DMD patients and 80% of BMD patients. Additional DNA analysis to detect smaller mutations in the dystrophin gene increases the detection rate to approximately 90% of patients with DMD (6). However, a positive test does not clearly distinguish between DMD and BMD. A muscle biopsy for immunohistochemical analysis of the dystrophin protein is necessary

in patients testing negative for the mutation or to differentiate between a patient with a particularly severe form of BMD and a patient with a milder form of DMD. Absent dystrophin or levels less than 3% is consistent with DMD, whereas in BMD, the dystrophin may have an abnormal molecular weight or decrease in quantity.

The number of commercially available genetic tests has grown tremendously over the past several years and continues to expand. In addition, there are numerous research laboratories that specialize in specific myopathies and can even offer genetic testing for research purposes, when commercial tests are not available. An updated review of various genetic disorders as well as a list of clinical and research laboratories offering genetic tests for various myopathies or neuromuscular disorders can be found at https://www.ncbi.nlm.nih.gov/gtr/. Although genetic tests occupy an important place among diagnostic tools now available to a clinician, it should not replace a careful history, thorough physical examination, and clinical common sense in the evaluation of a patient with myopathy.

CLINICAL FEATURES OF SPECIFIC MYOPATHIC DISORDERS

Dystrophic Hereditary Myopathies

Duchenne Muscular Dystrophy

DMD is an X-linked disorder with the chromosomal abnormality at the Xp21 gene locus (7). As noted above, the gene codes for the protein dystrophin, an important cytoskeletal component of the muscle cell membrane. It appears that absence of dystrophin makes the muscle cell highly susceptible to mechanical stress, with eventual muscle fiber loss and replacement with fibrotic tissue (5,8).

DMD is the most common form of childhood muscular dystrophy, with an incidence of approximately 1:3,500 to 5,000 male births (9). Although a male inheritance pattern is typical, as many as one third of cases may be due to new mutations, without any previous family history. Typical initial symptoms include abnormal gait, frequent falls, and difficulty climbing steps. Hypotonia and delayed motor milestones occur in earlier onset cases, but in 75% to 80% of cases, onset is noted before age 4 (4). The abnormal gait is often noted by toe walking, which is a compensatory adaptation to knee extensor weakness, or increased lumbar lordosis as a compensation for hip extensor weakness. Another indication of pelvic girdle weakness is Gower's sign, demonstrated as the child rises from the floor. The patient generally begins by assuming a four-point stance, then brings the knees into extension while leaning the upper limbs forward, and sequentially moves the hands up the thighs until upright stance is achieved **(Fig. 25-2A–D)**.

On examination, the earliest weakness is seen in the neck flexors, typically during the preschool years. Weakness of the proximal musculature of the shoulder and pelvic girdle is next, with steady progression, although the patient and family may feel that functional loss does not occur gradually but rather quite suddenly. This may relate to a critical point in weakness or range of motion when compensatory actions can no longer suffice to perform a task. Quantitative strength testing shows greater than 40% to 50% loss of strength by age 6 years (4),

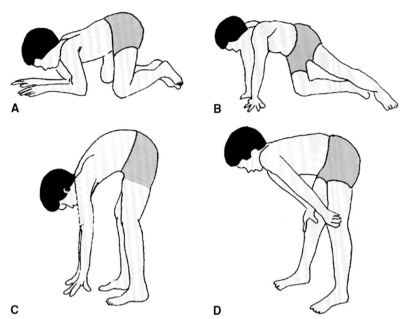

FIGURE 25-2. A–D: Gower's sign in a boy with DMD that is due to pelvic girdle weakness. (Reprinted with permission from Rosdahl CB, Kowalski MT. *Textbook of Basic Nursing.* 10th ed. Philadelphia, PA: Wolters Kluwer Health/Lippincott Williams & Wilkins; 2012.)

with fairly linear progression from ages 5 to 13 measured by manual muscle testing. Weakness appears to plateau after age 14 to 15, but this is probably a function of a floor effect and lack of sensitivity of the manual muscle testing scale (10,11).

Rehabilitation concerns are summarized in **Box 25-3**. In patients not aggressively treated, the average age to wheelchair use is 10, with a range of 7 to 13 years of age. Prediction of transition to wheelchair use may be helped by using timed motor performance tests. In one natural history study, all DMD subjects who took more than 12 seconds to ambulate 30 ft lost the ability to ambulate within 1 year (4). Immobilization, even for an acute illness, may lead to permanent loss of ambulatory ability during this phase of the disease.

Unlike many myopathic disorders, joint contractures are a major concern in DMD. Nearly all affected boys older than 13 years have contractures (4,12,13), and these contractures most commonly occur first in the ankle plantar flexors, iliotibial bands, and hip flexors, with subsequent involvement of the knee flexors and elbow and wrist flexors. There does not appear to be a strong correlation between less than antigravity strength for a muscle group and the severity of joint contracture, nor for strength imbalance between antagonists across a joint (4). Clearly, lower extremity contractures become a problem after transition to a wheelchair for a significant part

of the day. Natural history data suggest that progressive weakness, rather than heel-cord contractures, is associated with loss of ambulation as plantar-flexion contractures greater than 15 degrees are uncommon until after wheelchair reliance (4) (**Fig. 25-3**).

Scoliosis (see Chapter 28) is a major clinical concern in DMD, and its prevalence is strongly related to age. Although significant curves often coincide with transition into wheelchair mobility, there does not appear to be a cause-and-effect relationship between scoliosis and wheelchair use (4,14). Rather, factors such as the adolescent growth spurt and progressive involvement of the trunk musculature may be responsible for progression of scoliosis during the adolescent years. There is some evidence that severity of scoliosis may be predicted by the type of curve and early pulmonary function measurements (15). When the curves do not involve significant kyphosis or hyperlordosis and peak forced vital capacity (FVC) is greater than 2 L, severe progressive scoliosis appears less likely.

It is now clear that bracing does not slow the progression of spinal deformity (12,16,17). Decision-making for surgical management of scoliosis is closely related to pulmonary function. Although FVC volumes increase during the first decade of life close to 100% predicted with DMD, maximal static airway pressure (both maximal inspiratory and expiratory pressures) is impaired by 5 to 10 years of age. After a plateau in the early part of the second decade, there is progressive, fairly linear decline of FVC during adolescence (4). A higher peak FVC obtained at age 10 to 12 may predict less severe restrictive lung disease and spinal deformity developing over the next few years (4). An FVC below 40% predicted may contraindicate spinal instrumentation for scoliosis because of increased perioperative mortality; however, with current improved pulmonary care, this is not an absolute contraindication (18). Symptomatic respiratory failure in DMD typically manifests in later adolescence. Management of this complication is covered more in detail at a later section.

BOX 25-3

Rehabilitation Concerns in DMD

Maintaining mobility, range of motion, and strength during childhood
Progressive scoliosis
Progressive restrictive lung disease
Cardiac dysrhythmias and cardiomyopathy
Obesity (early adolescence) and cachexia (late adolescence)
Psychosocial adjustment and social interaction

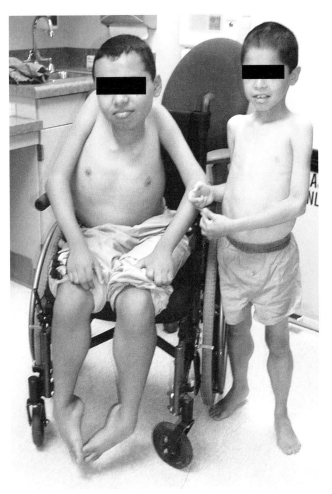

FIGURE 25-3. Brothers, ages 8 and 15, with DMD. In the older brother (*left*), note the presence of profound muscular wasting, scoliosis, and multiple joint contractures. The younger brother (*right*) demonstrates scapular retraction, increased lumbar lordosis, and stance phase plantar flexion (toe walking) to maintain a weight line posterior to the hip and anterior to the extended knee.

It is not surprising that cardiac function is affected in DMD, because the dystrophin protein has been shown to be present in both the myocardium and Purkinje fibers (19). Most DMD patients older than age 13 demonstrate electrocardiogram (ECG) abnormalities (4). The first abnormalities noted are Q waves in the lateral leads, followed by elevated ST segments, poor R-wave progression, increased R/S ratio, and resting tachycardia and conduction defects (4). ECG findings have been used to predict death from cardiomyopathy and include R wave in lead V, less than 0.6 mV; R wave in lead V_5, less than 1.1 mV; R wave in lead V_6, less than 1.0 mV; abnormal T waves in leads II, III, aVF, V_5, and V_6; cardiac conduction defects; premature ventricular contractions; and sinus tachycardia (20). Sudden death from ventricular ectopy, a complication of the cardiomyopathy and left ventricular dysfunction, is well described in DMD (21,22). However, progressive congestive heart failure is a more frequent sequela, and some investigators estimate that 40% to 50% of DMD patients die from this complication (23,24). Cardiomyopathy is usually noted after 10 years of age and occurs in nearly all patients by age 18 (25). Cardiomyopathy is typically followed clinically with echocardiography, and the onset of systolic dysfunction

is associated with a poor short-term prognosis (26). Once patients with DMD reach adolescence, regular screening with ECG, echocardiography, and Holter monitoring is prudent.

Considering the presence of a dystrophin isoform in brain tissue (27), it is not surprising that DMD patients show mildly decreased IQ scores compared with their peers and normative data (4). There may be a specific deficit with tasks requiring attention to complex verbal information, regardless of IQ (28). Mild impairments are noted on neuropsychological testing as well (4), without a specific area of strength or weakness.

Obesity from reduced physical activity is a major concern in DMD, particularly at the onset of wheelchair dependence (29,30). Since many patients are now placed on corticosteroid treatment, weight gain is the most frequently reported side effect. At later stages of the disease (ages 17 to 21), significant weight loss becomes the predominant nutritional concern (4,30). This probably results from nutritional compromise along with increased protein and calorie requirements during the later stages of DMD (31,32), partially as a result of the increased work of breathing from restrictive lung disease.

At this time, there is no curative treatment available for DMD. Oral corticosteroids have been shown to increase muscle mass, increase strength, and slow muscle deterioration. However, the mechanism of its action is still unclear. Recent studies demonstrate additional potential benefits of corticosteroids including amelioration of cardiac, pulmonary, and scoliosis complications in DMD (33–35). Research involving other pharmacoagents that can increase muscle bulk and strength as well as research into the stem cell and gene therapy are ongoing (36,37).

Becker Muscular Dystrophy

BMD is similar to DMD as an X-linked recessive disorder. It has a similar pattern of muscle weakness but generally presents with a later onset and a slower rate of progression (🛜 **eTable 25-2**). Like DMD, the disorder has an abnormality in the gene location (Xp21) coding for the protein dystrophin. However, in this case, dystrophin levels are usually 20% to 80% of normal or have the presence of the protein with an abnormal molecular weight. Mutation analysis of BMD has shown that majority are "in-frame" deletions, while DMD results are from "frame-shift" mutations. BMD is less common than DMD, with an overall prevalence recently estimated as 24 per million (38).

Without dystrophin analysis, it may be difficult to clinically discriminate between DMD and BMD. Although age of onset typically occurs later in BMD, there is significant overlap with DMD (39). The degree of CK elevation does not discriminate between the two diseases. The most useful clinical diagnostic discriminator is the ability to ambulate into adolescence. It is unusual for a patient with BMD to be wheelchair dependent before late adolescence, whereas even DMD outliers are dependent on the wheelchair for mobility by age 16. In fact, some BMD patients may be ambulatory well into middle age and beyond. There may be two distinct patterns of progression in BMD. In the first type, age of onset averages 7.7, and most patients have difficulty climbing stairs by age 20. In the more common milder form, age of onset averages 12, and there is no problem climbing stairs at age 20. The former group also seems to have a much higher rate of ECG abnormalities (40). The percentage of normal dystrophin cannot be used to predict clinical course with any certainty in BMD (41).

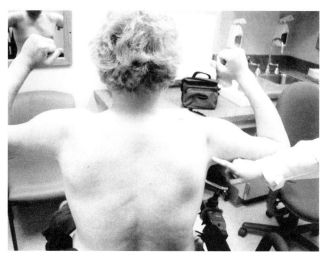

FIGURE 25-4. A 36-year-old man with BMD with pseudohypertrophy of the posterior deltoid and infraspinatus resulting in a posterior axillary depression sign.

Findings on examination of the BMD patient mirror DMD, although milder. The neck flexors and proximal lower limb muscles are affected early, particularly the hip and knee extensors (39). Subsequently, there is gradual involvement of the proximal upper limb muscles (**Fig. 25-4**). Extensors are generally weaker than flexors (39). Calf enlargement occurs, and presence of Gower's sign is indicative of the proximal muscle weakness. On standing, there is increased lumbar lordosis, and hip abductor weakness results in a waddling gait with trunk lean over the weight-bearing limb.

Contractures are not a significant early functional problem in BMD (39,40), becoming problematic only after wheelchair dependence. The joint locations for contractures are typical for one assuming the sitting posture, occurring in the hip flexors, knee flexors, and ankle plantar flexors. Significant scoliosis is much less common than DMD, and BMD patients rarely require spinal instrumentation (39,40).

One particular clinical concern in BMD is the potential for significant cardiac disease out of proportion to other manifestations of the myopathy (40,42–46). ECG abnormalities can be detected in about 75% of BMD patients (39,47). Most common abnormalities include abnormal Q waves, right or left ventricular hypertrophy, right bundle branch block, and nonspecific T-wave changes. Echocardiography demonstrates left ventricular dilatation in 37% of BMD patients, and 63% have subnormal systolic function that is due to global cardiac hypokinesis (47). Cardiac transplantation may even be necessary in some patients (48,49). The degree of cardiac compromise may not be reflected by clinical symptoms, and these patients should be screened at regular intervals with ECG and echocardiographic studies.

Unlike DMD, significant pulmonary dysfunction is not a hallmark of BMD. FVC does not fall below the predicted level until the third to fifth decade of life. Because of relatively greater involvement of the intercostals and abdominal musculature compared with the diaphragm, maximum expiratory pressure is compromised at an earlier age than maximal inspiratory pressure (MIP), similar to DMD (39).

There are no consistent abnormalities on cognitive and neuropsychological testing in BMD other than a mild reduction in some patients (39).

Myotonic Muscular Dystrophy (DM1 and DM2)

There are two subtypes of myotonic muscular dystrophy, DM1 and DM2 (dystrophia myotonica type 1 and type 2). Both are muscular dystrophies that share similar clinical features of myotonia and distinctive effects on other organ systems. However, DM1 and DM2 are genetically separate entities with different genes involved. DM1 is caused by abnormal expansion of the CTG trinucleotide repeats in the dystrophia myotonica protein kinase (DMPK) gene on chromosome 19q13.3, while DM2 is caused by an abnormal expansion of the CCTG repeats in the zinc finger protein 9 (ZNF9) gene on chromosome 3q21 (50–52).

Myotonic muscular dystrophy type 1 (DM1) is the most common slowly progressive dystrophy in adults, with an incidence of 1/8,000 (9), while DM2 is much less common and thought to account for only about 2% of myotonic muscular dystrophy patients. Both are multisystem disorders affecting skeletal muscle, smooth muscle, myocardium, brain, and ocular structures (**Box 25-4**). This may manifest clinically with cataracts, cardiac conduction defects, endocrine abnormalities, swallowing dysfunction, and skeletal muscle weakness and myotonia.

Inheritance pattern for both DM1 and DM2 is autosomal dominant. As noted above, phenotype of DM1 results from abnormal expansion of CTG trinucleotide repeats within the DMPK gene (50,51). Normal individuals have fewer than 37 CTG repeats, whereas myotonic muscular dystrophy patients may have from 50 to several thousand repeats. The age of onset is inversely correlated with the number of repeats (50–52). With mild, late-onset myotonic muscular dystrophy, there may only be 50 to 150 repeats, whereas congenital myotonic muscular dystrophy may have greater than 1,000 repeats. The congenital form of myotonic muscular dystrophy is typically found only with DM1. The expanded region seems to further expand in subsequent generations, with increased severity of phenotype, in genetic anticipation. Currently, molecular genetic tests are commercially available for both DM1 and DM2 to determine the respective CTG or CCTG repeat expansions.

Patients with myotonic muscular dystrophy often have a characteristic facies. Long-standing myotonic muscular dystrophy is generally associated with a long, thin face, with temporal and masseter wasting. This is sometimes described as "lugubrious facies." Ptosis can be prominent in these patients and contribute to the characteristic facies. Frontal balding at a young age is common in men.

The pattern of weakness in DM1 may be an unusual exception to the typical proximal greater than distal pattern in myopathies. The distal muscles may be affected to a greater extent,

---

BOX 25-4

Rehabilitation Concerns in Myotonic Muscular Dystrophies

Progressive weakness, often in a distal > proximal distribution
Clinical myotonia, with difficulty in releasing grip
Cardiac conduction defects
Swallowing dysfunction
Cataracts
Nocturnal hypoventilation/sleep apnea

particularly early in the disease. This manifests as footdrop that is due to involvement of the ankle dorsiflexors, ankle invertors, and evertors and grip weakness from affected hand muscles (53). DM2 is different from DM1 in that proximal greater than distal distribution of weakness is noted. However, eventually, the neck, shoulder, and hip girdle muscles all become progressively weak in both DM1 and DM2. Significant contractures are unusual in myotonic muscular dystrophies, and scoliosis is usually a clinical problem only in congenital myotonic muscular dystrophy of DM1 (53).

A distinctive feature of myotonic muscular dystrophy among the dystrophies is the presence of myotonia, a state of delayed relaxation or prolonged contraction of muscle. This may be demonstrated by percussion of the thenar eminence with a reflex hammer, causing sustained flexion and adduction of the thumb. Grip myotonia is provoked by having the patient sustain a tight grip and then suddenly attempt to relax. Delayed opening of the fingers will occur. Myotonic "crescendo-decrescendo" discharges are also easily elicited with diagnostic needle EMG, although not specific for myotonic muscular dystrophy. Weakness and myotonia may exist in different proportions in an individual patient, with functional problems often from only one or the other manifestation of myotonic muscular dystrophy.

Cardiac abnormalities are common in both DM1 and DM2. Approximately 70% to 75% of patients demonstrate ECG and echocardiographic abnormalities (54). Cardiac conduction defects are the primary concern, with prolongations of the PR interval, abnormal axis, and infranodal conduction abnormalities leading to potential cardiac morbidity and the possibility of sudden death in a small percentage (55). A cardiac pacemaker may be indicated. Regular cardiac evaluation is recommended, particularly for those patients with dyspnea, palpitations, chest pain, or other cardiac symptoms.

When myotonic muscular dystrophy manifests in infancy as congenital myotonic muscular dystrophy, involvement of the respiratory musculature may cause significant respiratory distress. In noncongenital myotonic muscular dystrophy, restrictive lung disease causes significant morbidity later in life for many patients with DM1 (53). Nocturnal hypoventilation and sleep apnea may occur, and clinicians should take a careful history to elicit symptoms common to these disorders: morning headache, frequent nightmares, excessive snoring, difficulty sleeping, and daytime somnolence.

Smooth muscle involvement most frequently manifests as difficulty swallowing and constipation, particularly in congenital myotonic muscular dystrophy. However, videofluoroscopy during swallowing reveals prolonged bolus transit times in adults with myotonic muscular dystrophy, placing them at risk for aspiration (56). Although a higher incidence of frank diabetes mellitus is controversial in myotonic muscular dystrophy, insulin insensitivity is a relatively common finding. Other endocrine abnormalities including primary gonadal dysfunction with infertility and thyroid dysfunction are also seen in patients with myotonic muscular dystrophy and should be evaluated when suspected. Posterior subcapsular cataract is present in almost all DM1 and DM2 patients and requires ophthalmologic follow-up with eventual cataract removal if visual acuity worsens.

Cognitive deficits are most profound in the congenital myotonic muscular dystrophy population, with a reduced IQ often in the mentally retarded range (53,57). In noncongenital DM1, there is a wide range of scores with intelligence testing (53), and there appears to be some correlation between cognitive function and the number of CTG repeats at the myotonic muscular dystrophy gene locus.

Facioscapulohumeral Muscular Dystrophy

FSHD was identified as a distinctive muscular dystrophy because of the predilection for slowly progressive muscular weakness in the facial and shoulder girdle musculature. It is the second most common inherited muscular dystrophy in adult population with a prevalence estimate of 10 to 20 per million (9). It is nearly always inherited as an autosomal dominant disorder, with the chromosomal abnormality identified at the 4q35 gene locus (58), with reduced DNA fragment size at the telomere region (59). The reduction in DNA fragment size is due to deletions of a repeat sequence called D4Z4, and the specific mechanism of disease is currently being elucidated (60). Currently, a highly specific and sensitive genetic test is commercially available for the diagnosis of FSHD.

The distinctive clinical feature of FSHD is the presence of facial weakness, primarily involving the orbicularis oris, zygomaticus, and orbicularis oculi. These manifest as difficulty with eye closure (but not ptosis) and expressionless face (**Fig. 25-5**). The patient will typically have difficulty burying the lashes and pursing the lips, drinking through a straw, or whistling. Onset of symptoms is typically in adolescence or early adulthood. There are no distinctive findings on muscle biopsy, with histology frequently demonstrating mild findings of atrophied fibers along with hypertrophied fibers. Serum CK may be normal or only slightly elevated. Molecular genetic testing is available when the diagnosis requires confirmation.

In the shoulder girdle, the scapulae are typically displaced laterally and superiorly, resulting from combined weakness of the serratus anterior, rhomboids, latissimus dorsi, and lower

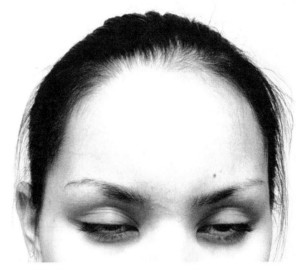

FIGURE 25-5. Attempted eye closure in a 21-year-old woman with facioscapulohumeral muscular dystrophy. Eye closure is weak and facial expression reduced.

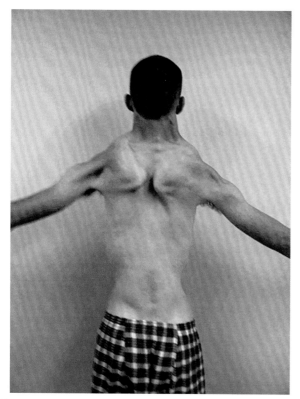

FIGURE 25-6. Shoulder girdle appearance in a young man with facioscapulohumeral muscular dystrophy. Shoulder abductor weakness and high-riding scapulae may give the appearance of trapezius hypertrophy. (Reprinted with permission from Campbell WW. *DeJong's The Neurologic Examination.* 7th ed. Philadelphia, PA: Wolters Kluwer Health/Lippincott Williams & Wilkins; 2013.)

trapezius (**Fig. 25-6**). Profound winging of the medial border of the scapula is common. Unlike most other muscular dystrophies, asymmetry of muscular involvement is common (61). Some authors feel this may be a manifestation of overwork weakness on the more affected side (62), but this is controversial. Although shoulder abductors and external rotators are typically involved, in some cases, deltoid strength may be quite good if the scapula is stabilized. Elbow flexors and extensor involvement is common. In the lower extremities, the proximal musculature of the hip girdle is typically affected, often later in the disease course. However, there also appears to be a predilection for early involvement of the ankle dorsiflexors. About 20% of FSHD patients will eventually require either a power wheelchair or a scooter for mobility (63).

Coats' syndrome is an early-onset variant of FSHD associated with sensorineural hearing loss. Muscle weakness typically begins in infancy, with progressive weakness and wheelchair dependence by late second or third decade. There is also an associated progressive exudative telangiectasia of the retina, requiring early recognition to prevent permanent visual loss. Interestingly, audiometric studies may demonstrate high-frequency hearing loss in more common forms of FSHD patients as well (64–66).

Significant contractures are uncommon in FSHD (61), and spinal deformity typically presents as hyperlordosis, scoliosis, or a combination. Although hyperlordosis to compensate for hip extensor weakness may be severe in some patients, the

scoliosis rarely progresses to the point of requiring surgical instrumentation.

Cardiac complications in FSHD are rare, although some studies report cardiac abnormalities including cardiac fibrosis (67) and cardiac conduction defects (68). Mild restrictive lung disease is present in nearly half of patients with the expiratory muscles affected to a greater extent than inspiratory muscles, similar to other dystrophic disorders (61). In the absence of significant bulbar or respiratory involvement, the life expectancy of FSHD patients is normal.

Limb-Girdle Muscular Dystrophies

Before the advent of genetic testing, a group of patients commonly sharing a slowly progressive pattern of proximal greater than distal muscular weakness with either autosomal dominant (type 1) or autosomal recessive (type 2) inheritance were considered to have *limb-girdle muscular dystrophies*. Recent advances in molecular and genetic analyses have now identified a number of distinct genetic abnormalities with mutations in these patients. Currently, 34 subtypes of LGMD are recognized (69). Eight have autosomal dominant inheritance pattern (LGMD type 1, A to H) and 26 with autosomal recessive inheritance (LGMD type 2, A to Z). A detailed discussion of all subtypes of LGMD is beyond the scope of this chapter; however, the interested reader is directed to a recent review for more information (70). The term LGMD is still used as a general category of myopathy because of similarities in clinical presentation and progression.

It is important to keep in mind that "limb girdle weakness" is not unique to LGMDs. Other disorders such as BMD, myotonic muscular dystrophy type 2, EDMD, or late-onset spinal muscular atrophy should also be considered in the differential diagnosis. Determining the precise subtype of LGMDs is often difficult and may not be possible in majority of cases; however, a detailed symptom history, family history, mode of inheritance, and presence of associated clinical features may help narrow the differential diagnoses.

It is now known that some of the autosomal recessive LGMDs are associated with abnormalities in genes coding for components of the sarcoglycan complex, intimately involved with the dystrophin protein in supporting the cytoskeletal structure of the muscle cell membrane (71). Although muscular weakness may eventually be profound, significant contractures and restrictive lung disease are unusual (72). In the United States, the LGMD 2C to F (sarcoglycanopathies) along with LGMD 2B (dysferlinopathy) and LGMD 2A (calpainopathy) are the most common limb-girdle dystrophies encountered; however, the distribution and prevalence of different subtypes of LGMD may differ around the world (73).

The cardiac involvement is rare and typically less than the dystrophinopathies such as DMD and BMD. However, depending on the LGMD subtypes (LGMD 1A to D, LGMD 2C to F, and LGMD 2I), it can be significant and warrants a close follow-up with cardiology consultation and regular ECG, echocardiography, and Holter monitoring. Respiratory involvement may also be a feature of the above subtypes of LGMD later in the disease course.

One subgroup of sarcoglycanopathy with a more rapid course is known as severe childhood autosomal recessive muscular dystrophy (SCARMD). These patients may mimic

DMD early in the disease, with childhood onset and a similar pattern of weakness. However, it occurs equally in males and females and has a slower progression. Loss of ambulation generally occurs between 10 and 20 years.

Nondystrophic Hereditary Myopathies

Congenital Myopathies

The term *congenital myopathy* is used for a group of heterogeneous autosomal recessive disorders that typically present as hypotonia in infancy, can clearly be localized to muscle, and have weakness that is nonprogressive or slowly progressive. Frequently, there are delayed motor milestones in early childhood. Mental retardation may be profound in some syndromes. The weakness is usually in a proximal hip and shoulder girdle pattern. Because there is no progressive loss of muscle fibers, these disorders are not generally classified as dystrophic. The diagnosis for each specific disorder is based on histologic and electron microscopic muscle biopsy findings. Examples include central core myopathy, nemaline myopathy, and myotubular (centronuclear) myopathy.

Metabolic Myopathies

In patients with defects in glycogen, lipid, or purine metabolism, a common primary symptom is exercise intolerance or exertional muscle pain. There may be no fixed weakness on examination. Symptoms with activity include fatigue, myalgia, and muscle stiffness. When exercise is intense, patients may note a brownish-red color of the urine from myoglobinuria that is due to frank rhabdomyolysis. In some metabolic myopathies, progressive muscle weakness may predominate over dynamic symptoms and mimic a muscular dystrophy. Examples of metabolic myopathies include acid maltase deficiency (Pompe disease), myophosphorylase deficiency (McArdle's disease), and carnitine deficiency.

Pompe disease (acid maltase deficiency, glycogen storage disease type 2) is a disorder of glycogen metabolism, with defects in the lysosomal acid maltase pathway. There are three autosomal recessive forms of acid maltase deficiency, the first presenting shortly after birth as hypotonia, with death by 2 years. The childhood-onset form is associated with delayed motor milestones and proximal weakness, with death by about age 20. In the adult variety of acid maltase deficiency, there is slow progression of proximal weakness beginning in the third or fourth decade. The clinical presentation may mimic limb-girdle dystrophy or PM. A potential treatment in the form of enzyme replacement therapy (ERT) is currently being evaluated in clinical trials. A guideline for diagnostic evaluation and management is available (74). With a potential treatment now on the horizon, it is important to consider the Pompe disease in the differential diagnosis of a patient with limb-girdle weakness, respiratory insufficiency without significant cardiac involvement, and findings suggestive of metabolic myopathy. Pompe disease represents one of only a handful of potentially treatable neuromuscular disorders at this time, and there is a commercially available diagnostic test.

McArdle's disease is usually inherited in an autosomal recessive pattern, more commonly in males. Because of the inability to metabolize glycogen, there is exercise intolerance, easy fatigability, and stiffness of the exercised muscles. Physical findings may be normal between episodes, although some patients develop progressive proximal weakness. There are now protocols using nonischemic forearm exercise test in the evaluation of patients for McArdle's disease (75).

Carnitine deficiency is the most common disorder of lipid metabolism. There are primary and secondary forms: the primary form has severely decreased plasma and tissue carnitine levels, and the secondary form has mild deficiency. Lack of carnitine impairs long-chain fatty acid metabolism in the mitochondria, thereby reducing energy production by the muscle cell. Oral L-carnitine supplementation may be helpful in some cases.

ACQUIRED MYOPATHIES

Inflammatory Myopathies

The hallmark of an inflammatory myopathy is the predominance of inflammatory cells on muscle biopsy. There are three primary types: DM, PM, and IBM. Although each is distinct, this group of myopathies is thought to involve immune-mediated processes possibly triggered by environmental factors in genetically susceptible individuals. DM and PM may be associated with disorders of the heart and lung as well as neoplasms. In addition, an inflammatory myopathy may be present as part of a multisystem disorder in other connective tissue diseases, most commonly scleroderma, systemic lupus erythematosus, mixed connective tissue disease, and Sjogren's syndrome. Overall, the age of onset for idiopathic inflammatory myopathies is bimodal, with peaks between 10 and 15 years of age in children and between 45 and 60 years of age in adults. Women are affected twice as often, with the exception of IBM, which is twice as common in men. It is important to diagnose accurately and in timely fashion for both DM and PM, since treatment is available and prognosis depends on early initiation of immunotherapy.

Dermatomyositis

Characteristic features of DM include muscle weakness that may present acutely, subacutely, or insidiously, along with a characteristic rash. This violaceous, scaling rash typically involves the eyelids and occurs with periorbital edema, termed a *heliotrope rash*. Other common locations for the rash are the dorsum of the hands, extensor surfaces of the knees and elbows, and ankles. Myalgias may or may not be present. The weakness initially involves the proximal musculature and may progress to the distal muscles. Pharyngeal muscle involvement is evident from the frequent finding of dysphagia or dysphonia. Other manifestations include cardiac dysrhythmias and cardiomyopathy, joint arthralgias, and interstitial lung disease. In adults, there appears to be an association between DM and occult carcinoma, and a judicious workup for carcinoma is advisable in newly diagnosed patients.

Childhood DM differs somewhat from the adult version because of the higher incidence of vasculitis, ectopic calcification in the subcutaneous tissues or muscle, and lipodystrophy. Corticosteroids alone are often highly effective in both inducing a remission and preventing a recurrence and can usually be gradually withdrawn. Adults with DM do not respond to corticosteroids quite so predictably, and other immunosuppressive agents are often required. It may be difficult to fully discontinue pharmacologic treatment.

Polymyositis

The diagnosis of PM is often more difficult than that of DM, because no distinctive rash is present. It rarely occurs before age 20. Proximal limb and neck flexor muscle weakness presenting subacutely or insidiously should raise suspicion for PM. Myalgias are present in as many as one third of patients but are not generally the predominant symptom. CK elevation usually occurs at some point in the disease but may be normal in advanced cases with significant muscle atrophy. In general, serum CK level is a reasonable indicator of disease severity. Potential cardiac and pulmonary manifestations are similar to DM. Underlying carcinoma may less commonly occur than with DM. Treatment with corticosteroids supplemented by other immunosuppressive medications is the primary means of pharmacologic management.

Inclusion Body Myositis

A third type of inflammatory myopathy with a different pattern of involvement and course was identified in the 1970s. It was termed *inclusion body myositis* because of the presence of both inflammatory cells and vacuolated muscle fibers with nuclear and cytoplasmic fibrillary inclusions. IBM is now recognized as the most common myopathy in patients aged more than 50 years (76). Males are affected more than females. IBM has distinctive involvement of both proximal and distal musculature. In particular, the wrist and finger flexors are often more affected than the extensors, and the quadriceps may be affected out of proportion to other muscle groups. About one third have dysphagia, and the disease may be mistaken for amyotrophic lateral sclerosis because the age of onset is frequently after 50. IBM is relentlessly progressive in most cases, sometimes to the point of requiring a wheelchair for mobility. Unfortunately, it is not responsive to immunosuppressive medications, and treatment primarily involves appropriate assistive devices (77).

Toxic Myopathies

Medications and toxins can have various effects on muscle and its function. They can either directly injure muscle cells or indirectly via electrolyte disturbances, muscle ischemia, excessive muscle activity, and immune mechanisms. The muscle effects of medications and toxins may be focal or generalized, and it can occur acutely or after prolonged exposure.

Corticosteroid Atrophy and "Steroid Myopathy"

Although muscle weakness is an infrequent symptom of patients with endogenous hypercortisolism (Cushing's syndrome), long-standing administration of exogenous corticosteroids is a common cause of proximal greater than distal muscular weakness and atrophy. Prednisone dosages higher than 30 mg/day increase vulnerability compared with lower dosages or an alternate-day regimen (78). The extent of weakness does not necessarily correlate with the duration of drug treatment. CK levels are generally normal or reduced, and muscle biopsy demonstrates type 2 greater than type 1 fiber atrophy. This is probably due to reduced muscle protein synthesis rather than increased catabolism. There is some evidence that resistance exercise training may help reduce or prevent steroid-induced myopathy (79).

Statin-Associated and Medication-Related Myopathies

The HMG-CoA reductase inhibitors (often called collectively as the "-statin" medications) have been developed as treatment for hypercholesterolemia. Statins are now among the most commonly prescribed medications in the world. For majority of patients receiving statin medications, there are no significant muscle complaints or myotoxic consequences. However, it is estimated that incidence of statin-induced myotoxicity (SIM) is approximately 7% to 29% in clinical practice depending upon the report (80). Although statins are generally well tolerated, a range of muscle-related symptoms from mild to very severe may be present. Some patients may present with vague muscle complaints of mild weakness (especially in legs) and/or transient muscle ache (myalgias) that may or may not be accompanied by elevated serum CK levels. Other muscle complaints can include sense of stiffness, cramps, muscle tenderness, and joint pain. Moreover, in some patients, an isolated elevation in serum CK may be the only presenting abnormality without any other signs or symptoms of SIM. The exact mechanism of statin-associated muscle myotoxicity is unclear, but it is thought to be multifactorial, including direct effects of the drug itself on muscle cells as well as a more severe manifestation through an immune-mediated mechanism possibly interacting with environmental factors and perhaps more prone in genetically susceptible individuals. Typically, with mild symptoms of myalgia and mildly elevated CK (<4 times the upper limit of normal level, ULN), statin medication may be continued with close monitoring (depending on risk/benefit of the medication on the overall health of the patient) or a change to a different agent may be considered. For patients with severe myalgia or objective muscle weakness noted in physical examination, as well as a significant CK elevation (>4× ULN), statin should be discontinued. In these cases, the symptoms rarely progress to a necrotizing myopathy and for the most part undergo a self-limited course. Stopping the offending medication typically leads to resolution of symptoms and return of serum CK to normal levels within several weeks. Rechallenge with another statin and starting at a lower dose with gradual increase may reduce the likelihood of SIM. Medical workup as well as review of systems should also be undertaken to evaluate for concomitant potentially correctable factors exacerbating the SIM, such as alcohol intake, hypothyroidism, and low vitamin D level. When necrotizing myopathy does occur, acute to subacute proximal weakness, prominent muscle tenderness, and significantly elevated serum CK (>10× ULN) can be seen. In severe cases, rhabdomyolysis and myoglobinuria can also occur. Recently, it has been also recognized that there is a very severe form of SIM called statin-associated autoimmune myopathy that is very rare (affecting approximately 2 or 3 out of 100,000 patients treated with statins) (81). This statin-associated immune myopathy is characterized by the presence of autoimmune antibodies against 3-hydroxy-3-methylglutaryl coenzyme A reductase (HMGCR), the pharmacologic target of statins. This rare and very severe form of statin-associated myopathy presents with progressive muscle weakness, significant CK elevation (typically >10× ULN), and muscle necrosis on biopsy. Unlike most patients who experience self-limited muscle side effects from statin and recover after discontinuation of the medication, those with statin-associated autoimmune myopathy with anti-HMGCR antibodies have a more protracted disease course. Therefore, testing for these antibodies may help differentiate those with self-limited statin myopathy from those with a progressive statin-associated autoimmune myopathy who typically require immunosuppressive therapy. Additionally, other cholesterol- and lipid-lowering agents that are fibric acid derivatives may cause myopathy. Amphiphilic agents (used as antimalarial and antirheumatic medications) and antimicrotubular agents (such as colchicines and vincristine) have also been shown to cause myopathies.

Alcohol-Related Myopathies

Alcohol-related myopathies are thought to be the most common among toxic myopathies. Muscle effects of alcohol are diverse and span from acute necrotizing myopathy with myoglobinuria to chronic atrophic myopathy. The common symptoms of acute alcoholic myopathy are diffuse muscle cramps, myalgia, muscle swelling, and weakness. The exact mechanisms of alcohol-related myopathies are unknown at this time. However, severity of alcoholic myopathies appears to be related to a history of heavy, either acute or prolonged alcohol intake. Treatment is withdrawal of alcohol and correction of any electrolyte disturbances.

Endocrine Myopathy

Thyroid Disorders

Symptoms of muscle pain, cramps, or spasms are frequent in untreated hypothyroidism. However, only about one third of patients have demonstrable muscle weakness (82). In these patients, subtle proximal weakness with hyporeflexia and delayed relaxation of reflexes is evident. A PM-like syndrome with more profound proximal weakness and elevation of muscle enzymes may also occur (83). CK may be elevated 10- to 100-fold. Muscle histology is nonspecific, and the weakness resolves with appropriate thyroid hormone replacement. Thyrotoxicosis may present with symptoms of muscle weakness and proximal weakness, atrophy, and preserved or even brisk reflexes on examination. CK level is usually normal or low, and muscle biopsy may be normal or show predominant atrophy of type 2 fibers. The etiology is probably from increased catabolism of muscle tissue. Treatment of thyrotoxicosis improves the myopathy.

Infectious Myopathy

HIV Infection

HIV infection may be associated with an inflammatory myopathy or myositis, generally in patients with acquired immunodeficiency syndrome (AIDS). The clinical presentation is similar to idiopathic PM, with symmetric proximal weakness and elevation of serum CK. This disorder needs to be distinguished from the myotoxicity of zidovudine as well as the generalized weakness that may occur with advancing HIV infection.

Myopathies Associated with Systemic Disease

Many major illnesses are associated with muscle compromise, not generally demonstrable by manual muscle testing but resulting in poor muscle endurance and reduced motor performance with functional tasks. This is not generally classified as a "myopathic" disorder. However, certain systemic diseases or conditions do have a particular predilection to involve muscle and may be considered myopathies.

With severe illness, often in the ICU setting, patients can develop critical illness myopathy, critical illness polyneuropathy, or a combination of these syndromes (84,85). Critical illness myopathy may develop in patients who received high doses of corticosteroids with or without neuromuscular blocking agents or who have sepsis with multiorgan system failure. Necrotizing myopathy may be associated with underlying neoplasm, especially adenocarcinoma or the gastrointestinal system or lung cancer.

Electrolyte disturbances associated with systemic illness of various causes can produce myopathy. Hypokalemia is the most common electrolyte disturbance producing muscle weakness. This may be related to the use of diuretics or chronic diarrhea. Weakness is usually proximal, and CK elevation corresponds to the level of weakness. Frank rhabdomyolysis may be present, with muscle fiber necrosis noted on muscle biopsy. Clinical resolution occurs with correction of the hypokalemia. Other electrolyte abnormalities, which may be associated with muscle weakness, include hypocalcemia and hypercalcemia, hypophosphatemia, hyponatremia, and hypermagnesemia.

REHABILITATION CONCERNS AND STRATEGIES IN MYOPATHIC DISORDERS

Weakness and Resistance Training

The primary clinical manifestation of myopathies is muscle weakness. With the exception of certain inflammatory and metabolic myopathies, there is currently no effective pharmacologic management. Thus, the primary physiatric goal is to maintain strength, function, and independence. By using appropriate bracing, gait aids, and other assistive devices, functional mobility may be prolonged. Because of the proximal predilection of weakness, coming from sit to stand, managing stairs, and completing overhead activities such as dressing are primary functional problems.

An essential tool to maintain strength in most chronic diseases is resistance exercise. This is a controversial issue in myopathies (86,87). There is not clear evidence that persons with myopathy respond to strengthening exercise in a similar fashion as the able-bodied, and significant concern about excessively exercising weak muscles prevents widespread acceptance by clinicians. Unfortunately, probably because of caution and concern by caring providers, this population often adopts a sedentary lifestyle, resulting in a component of disuse weakness (88).

Traditional concern about excessive exercise in myopathy primarily stems from case reports and circumstantial evidence noted in individual patients (62,89,90). However, newer knowledge about the function of dystrophin and related glycoproteins does provide additional concern. These proteins appear to be essential in maintaining the cytoskeletal framework of the muscle fiber during muscle contraction (71,91). In animal models of dystrophin-deficient dystrophy, there is increased damage to muscle using eccentric contractions, which particularly stress these cytoskeletal elements (92,93).

Thus, it is conceivable that intensive muscle contractions, particularly when including an eccentric component, may damage myopathic muscle to a greater extent than in the able-bodied. This is a particular concern in those diseases known to involve structural proteins of the muscle cell, such as DMD, BMD, and many of the limb-girdle syndromes. A recent study demonstrated a similar response to an acute bout of eccentric contractions in myopathic subjects and controls (94), but the effect over a longer time period is unknown.

The role of exercise differs between rapidly progressive disorders such as DMD and the more slowly progressive or static myopathies. In DMD, there is a rapid progression of strength loss when measured using qualitative (manual muscle testing) and quantitative (isokinetic dynamometry) methods (4,95). Considering this natural history, maintenance of strength would be the primary rehabilitation goal. Although hampered by methodologic limitations, several investigations have demonstrated the ability to maintain or even slightly improve strength in DMD using resistance exercise (95–97). No protocol has demonstrated signs of weakness. In DMD, resistance exercise activities are probably best encouraged by incorporating them into normal play and games of the child rather than a weight-lifting program (98).

In slowly progressive or static myopathies, the goal of resistance exercise is to increase strength, thereby giving the patient increased capacity to perform daily functions. A number of investigations combining patients with slowly progressive myopathies along with other peripheral neuromuscular disorders demonstrate modest benefits of strengthening exercise in slowly progressive disorders (99–103). Whether strength gains occur through direct hypertrophy of diseased muscle fibers or through reducing the effects of disuse weakness is not known. A systematic review of the literature found only two randomized, controlled trials of resistance exercise (in myotonic muscular dystrophy and FSHD) fulfilling inclusion criteria. The only conclusion drawn was that moderate-resistance strength training appeared to do no harm in these disorders, but there was insufficient evidence for benefit (104).

Therefore, unanswered questions include the appropriate regimen and whether increased strength translates into an improved ability to perform daily work tasks. There is some evidence that compared with a moderate-resistance strengthening program, a high-resistance training program offers no additional strength benefits (101,102). The moderate-resistance program included three sets of four to eight repetitions at 30% to 40% maximal strength of the knee extensors, with a similar regimen of 10% to 20% maximal strength training of the elbow flexors. No controlled investigations have demonstrated evidence of weakness associated with excessive exercise in muscular dystrophy.

Traditionally, patients with inflammatory myopathies were discouraged from physical activity due to fear of exacerbating muscle inflammation. Although sample sizes are small, more recent studies suggest that moderate-intensity resistance exercise may improve strength and function without signs of increased muscle inflammation (105). Response to exercise may vary depending on disease activity, medications, and degree of disability. Patients with stable, chronic inflammatory myopathy may be able to tolerate more intensive strengthening regimens (10 maximal muscle contractions 3 d/wk) without untoward effects (106).

Aerobic Training

Aerobic exercise training in myopathies has received scant research attention. Involvement of the cardiac and pulmonary musculature in both dystrophic and inflammatory myopathies may reduce cardiopulmonary fitness, compounding the effects of deconditioning. Decreased aerobic capacity compared with controls has been demonstrated in both adult patients with inflammatory myosis (107) and juvenile DM (108). Combining multiple neuromuscular diseases, several investigators have demonstrated improved oxygen uptake (109) or reduced heart rate at a submaximal workload after stationary bicycle training (110). Focusing specifically on patients with LGMD type 2I, moderate-intensity cycle endurance training was found to be safe and result in improved work capacity (111). Similarly, aerobic exercise in patients with FSHD and myotonic muscular dystrophy improved maximal oxygen uptake without signs of muscle damage (112,113). Improved oxygen uptake in subjects with inflammatory myosis was reported in two investigations combining strength and aerobic training (stationary cycling and step aerobics) not specifically designed to improve aerobic performance (114,115). There have been no randomized, controlled studies of aerobic exercise meeting Cochrane review criteria for recommendations in muscle disease (104).

Because maximal aerobic capacity is rarely the limiting factor in performing daily work tasks (116), improving muscular strength and endurance through resistance training will more likely enhance the ability to perform physical work tasks. However, an aerobic training program may help modify cardiovascular risk, because epidemiologic studies show that the physically inactive lifestyle so common in myopathic patients is associated with twice the risk of coronary artery disease in an able-bodied population (117). Swimming in warm water is a particularly useful activity to maintain aerobic capacity in myopathic patients.

Management of Cardiac Complications

Symptomatic cardiac complications associated with myopathies are primarily seen in DMD, BMD, myotonic muscular dystrophy (DM1 and DM2), EDMD, certain LGMDs, and mitochondrial myopathies (118,119). Asymptomatic electrocardiographic abnormalities are common in the inflammatory myopathies, although significant supraventricular arrhythmias, cardiomyopathy, and congestive heart failure may occur.

In managing patients with chronic myopathies, yearly ECG screening is warranted as it is generally the first cardiac test to become abnormal (120). The dystrophin protein is normally found in the Purkinje fibers of the heart, but its absence likely contributes to the rhythm abnormalities seen in the DMD and BMD patients. When the ECG is abnormal, echocardiography is indicated, also on a yearly basis, as well as involvement of the cardiology specialist. At times, cardiac conduction abnormalities and arrhythmias associated with myopathies can be severe enough to require a pacemaker, such as in DMD and BMD, myotonic muscular dystrophy, and EDMD. Cardiomyopathy is treated in the standard fashion, using angiotensin-converting enzymes when ejection fraction is less than 35% (121), as well as digitalis and diuretics with symptomatic heart failure (122). However, special caution with kaliuretic diuretics is warranted, because hypokalemia may exacerbate weakness (123,124).

The clinician should not confuse the presence of cor pulmonale that is due to chronic respiratory failure with intrinsic cardiomyopathy. Correction of hypoxemia and respiratory failure should be performed before treating cardiomyopathy. As detailed below, this usually requires mechanical ventilatory assistance rather than provision of supplemental oxygen, which may be inappropriate and perhaps even detrimental in patients with CO_2 retention.

Management of Pulmonary Complications (see also Chapter 34)

Breathing disorders are the leading cause of mortality in neuromuscular diseases (125). The causes of respiratory failure include direct respiratory muscle involvement from the skeletal myopathy, alteration in respiratory mechanics, poor secretion management, infections, and occasionally a problem with central control of respiration. However, with improved pulmonary care, patients with progressive neuromuscular diseases and pulmonary system involvement are living longer. In DMD, the average life expectancy has increased from 19 to 25 years, with increasing numbers of patients in their 30s (126).

Measurements of respiratory muscle strength and function have allowed clinicians to better determine the need for ventilation and cough assistance. Serial FVC measurements have demonstrated to be highly predictive of respiratory impairment and survival. An FVC of less than 1 L has shown to be the best negative predictor of survival in DMD, with mean survival of 3.1 years and 5-year survival of approximately 8% if ventilatory support is not provided (127). Other spirometric measurements including MIP, maximal expiratory pressure (MEP), and peak cough flow are also useful in the assessment of respiratory muscle weakness. When these values decline (peak cough flow < 160 L/min or MEP < 45 cmH$_2$O), they can indicate poor airway clearance function and hastened respiratory failure (128,129). Manual techniques or mechanical insufflator-exsufflators (cough-assist machines) can help in improving the airway clearance and secretion management. Intrapulmonary percussive devices and ventilators are also available to help mobilize secretions and improve pulmonary hygiene.

Progressive respiratory muscular weakness leads to restrictive lung disease manifesting as hypoventilation, hypercarbia, and ultimately respiratory failure when FVC dwindles to less than 30% predicted (130). The work of breathing is affected by the presence of pulmonary secretions, increased elastic and resistive loads, and kyphoscoliosis. In DMD, the presence of chronic hypercarbia and hypoxemia reduces central respiratory drive to these conditions, which may result in apnea during sleep and further worsening of the hypercapnia (131).

There may be a role for inspiratory muscle training through breathing against resistance in DMD. However, the current research data on the efficacy of respiratory muscle training are conflicting, and no recommendation is available at this time. A study demonstrated improvement in MIP and 12-second maximal voluntary ventilation after 24 months of inspiratory muscle training (132). Others have also reported increased ventilatory strength and endurance (133–135). However, several investigations found no significant improvements in respiratory function (136,137). In addition, it was recently found that nitric oxide release in exercising muscle as a protective mechanism is impaired in DMD (138). It has been postulated that already dystrophic muscle may be further damaged during respiratory muscle training protocols. If instituted, one should not wait until the later stages of the disease, when respiratory muscles are already working to near their fatigue threshold (139).

Other general measures for patients with restrictive lung disease include yearly influenza vaccination and a pneumococcal vaccination unless there are contraindications. Maintenance of an optimal body weight through proper nutrition (avoiding obesity or cachexia) is crucial. A consensus statement regarding respiratory care of patients with DMD is available (140).

Indications for Ventilatory Support

Signs and symptoms suggesting respiratory impairment include those related to sleep-disordered breathing (nightmares, morning headache, and daytime drowsiness) as well as respiratory dysfunction (exertional dyspnea, orthopnea, generalized fatigue, and paradoxical breathing patterns) (140–142) (⚲ eBox 25-2). A polysomnography with continuous CO_2 monitoring is helpful in determining sleep-related hypoventilation associated with myopathies. However, a nocturnal pulse oximetry in the home environment can serve as a screening tool for sleep-related oxyhemoglobin desaturation and alveolar hypoventilation when polysomnography is unavailable (143).

Several studies have examined the indices useful to predict the need for ventilatory support. Vital capacity and MIP are generally the most useful pulmonary tests. Hypercapnia generally may occur when vital capacity falls to 500 to 700 mL (141), or with a vital capacity less than 55% predicted when the MIP is less than 30% predicted (130). When monitoring a patient with progressive myopathy, general warning signs for the impending need for mechanical ventilation include severe restrictive lung disease (vital capacity < 45% predicted), respiratory muscle weakness (MIP < 30% predicted), dyspnea at rest, and hypercapnia (144).

Methods of Ventilatory Support in Myopathies

Respiratory failure often presents insidiously in chronic myopathic disorders. Noninvasive methods of managing early respiratory failure are quite effective in maintaining adequate respiratory function and usually first instituted during the nocturnal period, with demonstrated improvements in PAO$_2$ and reduction in PaCO$_2$ (145–149). These benefits may be carrying over into periods off the ventilator and may result in improved daytime alertness and functional ability. Investigators report that ventilator-assisted individuals with DMD have similar life satisfaction scores to the general population (150) and similar levels of health perception and social function to ventilator users with nonprogressive conditions (151).

Noninvasive positive pressure ventilation (NIPPV) may be delivered via mouthpiece with or without a lip seal, via nasal mask, or via full-face mask. In any method, the most important factor is to obtain a good seal. Nasal intermittent positive pressure methods (nasal mask, nasal pillow) are particularly convenient for nighttime use while mouthpiece interface may be preferred during daytime. Nocturnal NIPPV with bilevel positive airway pressure (BiPAP) has demonstrated its efficacy in use with sleep-disordered breathing and nighttime hypoventilation in DMD (152–154). In general, BiPAP mode of ventilation rather than the continuous positive airway pressure (CPAP) is appropriate for majority of restrictive lung volume processes as seen with myopathies. Frequent monitoring for adequate mask fit and appropriate ventilator pressure level settings is necessary.

Negative pressure ventilators apply a negative pressure to the surface of the chest and abdomen, expanding the chest wall and lungs. The cuirass, or chest shell, is the prototypical negative pressure device and is occasionally used but limited by the need for a snug fit to avoid air leaks. Some patients requiring intermittent ventilatory support may be amenable to the pneumobelt, an inflatable rubber bladder strapped around the abdomen. During inflation of the device, abdominal contents are displaced upward, resulting in upward displacement of the diaphragm and passive exhalation. When the device is deflated, descent of the diaphragm then results in spontaneous inhalation. One drawback is that the patient must be seated at a greater than 30-degree angle from horizontal, making nocturnal use impractical. However, it may increase speech volume and allow time off other methods of ventilation.

Continuous invasive ventilatory support via tracheostomy can be considered when contraindications and patient aversion to noninvasive ventilation are present or when noninvasive ventilation is not feasible due to severe bulbar weakness or dysfunction. For those patients with myopathy and tracheostomy requiring full-time ventilatory support, portable ventilators can be attached to power wheelchairs, markedly improving quality of life in the community. However, recent technologic advances in noninvasive ventilation have continued to encourage more patients and clinicians to opt for noninvasive ventilation methods rather than invasive ventilation via tracheostomy, even for those patients requiring 24-hour ventilatory support (155–157). With improved portability due to smaller size, longer battery life, ease of operation, better performance, and customization of ventilator settings that can be tailored to an individual's needs, noninvasive ventilation method has become increasingly more popular for individuals with various neuromuscular conditions (158).

Limb Contractures and Bracing

Many chronic myopathic disorders are associated with limb contractures in later stages of the disease, usually occurring with wheelchair dependence. Contractures may be myogenic, arthrogenic, or from soft tissue shortening. Potentially important factors in the development of contractures in myopathies include (159) replacement of normal muscle tissue with collagen and fatty tissue, resulting in shortened muscle length; inability to obtain full range of motion of a joint; imbalance of agonist and antagonist muscle strength across a joint; static positioning in sitting; compensatory postural changes to stabilize joints for standing, most frequently seen in the equinus positioning of the ankles in DMD to keep the ground reaction force in front of the knee; and inability to obtain good muscle stretch in multijoint muscle groups, such as the hamstrings, tensor fasciae latae, and gastrocnemius.

Prevention and Management of Contractures

In some myopathies such as DMD, contractures are inevitable with wheelchair reliance, despite aggressive stretching programs. Range-of-motion programs are most useful in ambulatory patients with mild contractures. In DMD, an early stretching program has been shown to slow the progression

of contractures (160–162). A minimum of 2 to 3 hours/day standing and walking may be necessary, along with a passive stretching program to avoid contracture development (163). Proper stretching technique is essential. The stretched position should be held for a slow count of 15, and each exercise should be repeated 10 to 15 times during a session. The gastrocnemius-soleus group, hamstrings, and iliotibial bands are particularly important to stretch in younger DMD patients (164). Written instruction materials for the family effectively supplement verbal instruction. Physical modalities, such as heat to augment stretching, have not been adequately studied to recommend their use. Probably the most important component of contracture development in the weaker myopathic patient is the static position of the joint throughout each day and night.

The use of nighttime resting splints or ankle-foot orthoses to prevent plantar-flexor contractures is controversial. Some authors support their use (160), whereas others feel they are ineffective (164,165). A randomized trial in ambulatory DMD patients of stretching versus stretching and night resting splints demonstrated a 23% annual delay of heel-cord contracture in the combined group, although dropout rate was high (166). However, there is no evidence that delaying contracture development prolongs ambulation. Once contractures are present, early release of the hip flexors, iliotibial bands, and Achilles tendon lengthening do not appear to have beneficial effects on strength and function in DMD (167).

Bracing for Ambulation

Because of the proximal predilection of weakness in most myopathies, bracing for ambulation becomes much more complex and controversial than distal disorders. The greatest controversy is with DMD (🛜 eTable 25-3). At the time when upright ambulation becomes difficult in DMD, hip and knee flexion contractures are usually mild (4,160), but the heel cords and iliotibial bands often require surgical release if braced ambulation is to be successful (168,169). Bracing then consists of bilateral knee-ankle-foot orthoses with solid ankles set at 90 degrees, drop-lock knee joints, and ischial weight-bearing upper thigh components to help maintain the upright posture with reduced lumbar lordosis.

Clearly, continued standing and limited ambulating with the braces provide good stretch to the hip, knee, and ankle musculature. Heel-cord and knee flexion contractures are less pronounced at age 16 in patients who continue daily standing (164). Although reported in the literature (170), it is not clearly known if scoliosis becomes less pronounced with the use of lower extremity bracing. However, a slowing in the progression of contractures by itself does not prolong standing and ambulation, because weakness, not contractures, is primarily responsible for the transition to wheelchair reliance (159). In addition, using braces requires significant energy expenditure on the part of the patient, requires ongoing physical therapy, and increases the risk of falls. Clearly, quality of life issues require detailed discussions with the patient and family before proceeding with aggressive surgical and orthotic management in rapidly progressing muscular dystrophy. A systematic review of the effectiveness of knee-ankle-foot orthoses in DMD reports probable prolongation of standing but not necessarily functional ambulation (171).

Management of Spinal Deformity

Spinal deformity in neuromuscular diseases and myopathies can be very severe and progress to result in multiple problems. Severe scoliosis and pelvic obliquity can lead to pain, poor sitting balance and upright seating position, difficulty in attendant care, skin ulcers, and potential exacerbation of restrictive lung disease. Although various different myopathies can be associated with progressive spinal deformity, the most common are those that are in the hereditary myopathy category and those that are relatively more severe in disease phenotype. These include DMD, congenital muscular dystrophy (CMD), congenital myotonic muscular dystrophy, and SCARMD. Scoliosis may also be an occasional concern in facioscapulohumeral muscular dystrophy and congenital myopathies.

In DMD, scoliosis affects 75% to 90% of nonambulatory patients (4,172). The prevalence of scoliosis has shown to be closely related to age and usually becomes noticeable between the ages of 10 and 14. Although the severity of the spinal curve increases with the length of time in wheelchair, no causal relationship has been established between scoliosis progression and wheelchair use. It is likely that both loss of ambulation and increasing spinal deformity represent disease severity and progression and are related to factors such as age, adolescent growth spurt, and weak truncal muscle. Routine screening for scoliosis with radiography before the transition to wheelchair is usually not productive. Once transitioned to wheelchair, scoliosis progression can be monitored with serial radiographs every 4 to 6 months. The reported degree of curve progression is variable (11 to 42 degrees/year) but can progress rapidly, so close follow-up is needed.

Spinal bracing in DMD does not change the natural history of the scoliosis, with continued progression despite brace usage (12,16,17). Modification of wheelchair seating system to slow the scoliosis progression has been ineffective (173). Other approaches, such as spinal exercises, manipulation, and electrical stimulation of paraspinal musculature, are also unproven. Recent studies in DMD suggest that the progression of scoliosis may be slowed with treatment with corticosteroids; however, greater side effects related to long-term corticosteroids use were also noted (33,172). At this time, the only effective treatment for progressive spinal deformity in severe myopathy remains surgical spinal instrumentation.

Indication for surgical intervention and optimal timing depends on the degree of scoliosis and cardiopulmonary status of the patient. It is generally agreed that surgical intervention should be sought when the Cobb angle is between 30 and 50 degrees (15,174,175). Preoperative pulmonary function testing is essential, and surgery should probably not be performed with FVC less than 30% predicted. Although a recent study demonstrated no clinically significant increase in operative and postoperative complications for those patients with FVC less than 30%, a careful preoperative risk assessment and planning as well as routine postoperative aggressive ventilatory support are stressed to minimize morbidity (176). Nocturnal pulse oximetry can provide valuable information about potential postoperative ventilation need. In those patients at risk, preoperative mask fitting and initiation of nocturnal NIPPV can improve postoperative respiratory recovery. Cardiology consultation, including preoperative ECG and echocardiography, is also important to evaluate for conduction abnormalities

and cardiomyopathy. Impaired left ventricular function and cardiomyopathy are risk factors for dysrhythmias and sudden death. A potential complication of malignant hyperthermia during anesthesia is not specific to DMD. It can also occur in other myopathies and should be kept in mind for those patients undergoing anesthesia. Postoperative management after scoliosis surgery includes early involvement of therapies, mobilization out of bed when clinically stable, pain control, ventilatory support as needed, and appropriate pulmonary toilet.

Although some improvement in spinal deformity may be expected with surgical instrumentation, it is still unclear whether the procedure leads to improved or sustained pulmonary function. Progressive loss of vital capacity in DMD results from disease of the respiratory musculature, although there is probably a component from the scoliosis as well. Some studies support preserved pulmonary function and survival (17), whereas others note no change in pulmonary decline and age at death in their DMD patients (4,177). It is important to keep in mind that the primary goals for prevention of scoliosis and corrective surgery are to provide the patients with improved sitting balance, which can help to maintain use of wheelchair, facilitate nursing care, and enhance their quality of life.

Body Composition and Metabolic Issues

Loss of skeletal muscle mass, gain of excess body fat, and changes in physical activity and energy metabolism are common to both rapidly progressive and slowly progressive myopathies. Excess body weight places greater burden on already weakened skeletal muscle, reduces mobility, and may increase the work of breathing. In one study on DMD, 40% of patients were overweight (weight-for-age > 90th percentile) between ages 9 and 17, 40% were underweight (weight-for-age < 10th percentile) between ages 13 and 17, whereas 65% were underweight older than age 17 (4). This supports a divergence in weight in early adolescence but a tendency toward underweight in later stages of the disease. Because of the replacement of muscle tissue by fat, at a given weight-for-age, the DMD individual will have a lower percentage of lean tissue. Although it is unclear why only certain individuals with DMD develop obesity, the weight loss in later stages of DMD may be from higher energy and protein requirements (31) with inadequate caloric intake to meet nutritional needs. Placement of a percutaneous feeding tube may be beneficial to provide rapid provision of calories and fluids, even if the patient can still swallow. Oral intake for enjoyment is still possible. Adequate nutritional intake may be a concern in slowly progressive myopathies as well. In a study of adults with non–dystrophin-related muscular dystrophies, there was inadequate intake of various micronutrients and macronutrients, with significant correlations between copper, water-soluble vitamins, and strength measures (178).

The relationships between metabolism, energy expenditure, and chronic disease risk are now being considered in persons with neuromuscular diseases. Several studies have shown a lower basal metabolic rate for patients with slowly progressive myopathies (88,179,180). In a study combining patients with a number of slowly progressive neuromuscular diseases, the neuromuscular disease subjects were shown to have reduced 24-hour energy expenditure as a result of reduced physical activity and a higher percentage of fat mass than controls (88). A similar population was found to have a high risk for developing chronic diseases resulting from obesity and a sedentary lifestyle (181). Using pedometer-derived activity goals combined with dietary intervention, persons with slowly progressive neuromuscular diseases can increase physical activity and reduce caloric intake, although improved health outcomes have not yet been shown (182).

Quality of Life/Psychosocial Issues

A survey on patients with neuromuscular diseases, including chronic myopathies, supports the notion that as a group, the quality of life of individuals with neuromuscular disease in various disease stages is not much different from that of the able-bodied (183). However, analysis of certain components of quality of life is of interest. Although level of impairment and disability did not predict life satisfaction, certain factors such as lack of information about the disease, poor coordination of services, negative attitudes, and decreased expectations of their potential were identified as important issues. The ability to attain independence, either through themselves or through personal care assistants, was an important key to quality of life. Support groups often serve as an excellent resource for psychological support and identifying other resources in the community. A recent study demonstrates that those patients who are single, childless, and with an earlier-onset neuromuscular disease may have their quality of life impacted more by their impairments and disabilities than previously thought (184). Psychosocial issues are summarized in 🛜 **eBox 25-3**. It is important for the rehabilitation specialist to be attuned to these factors in their care of patients with myopathies, so that therapeutic interventions can be timely and effective.

Clinicians may underestimate the presence of pain in their patients with myopathies. The causes of pain are multifactorial and may be treatable, often related to joint degenerative conditions and myofascial origin rather than directly from the myopathy. A survey in slowly progressive neuromuscular diseases found that the frequency and severity of pain reported in these disorders were comparable to persons with osteoarthritis and chronic low back pain (185). Appropriate assessment and treatment of pain may significantly improve quality of life and should be part of overall physiatric management.

In a recent survey of employment among those with neuromuscular diseases including muscular dystrophies, the major barrier to employment was lack of education (186). Level of disability and physical impairment were not critical factors. Unemployment is a particular problem in myotonic muscular dystrophy, possibly related to nonphysical factors. Although much more work needs to be done to determine ways to improve quality of life with chronic diseases such as myopathy, it is incumbent on the rehabilitation specialist to see the person beyond the disease, one in which others may view as "untreatable." There are always interventions to be made to improve quality of life, even diseases that have no cure.

CONCLUSION

Although great strides in genetics and molecular biology have helped us improve our understanding of many muscle diseases, the treatment for these and most other neuromuscular diseases remains supportive rather than curative. An important component of this treatment involves appropriate and judicious use of physical activity, assistive devices, and other common physiatric interventions. Knowledge of these diseases also provides the basis of expectant management to prevent secondary complications. With this knowledge, the physician can orchestrate a rehabilitation plan matching the goals of the patient and family. With proper care, many persons with myopathy have the potential to have a reasonable quality of life.

ACKNOWLEDGMENT

This chapter is dedicated to Dr. David D. Kilmer, who contributed significantly to this chapter but passed away prior to its completion and publication. Supported in part by Grant H133B090001 from the National Institute of Disability and Rehabilitation Research (NIDRR).

REFERENCES

1. Cros D, Harnden P, Pellisier JF, et al. Muscle hypertrophy in Duchenne muscular dystrophy: a pathological and morphometric study. *J Neurol*. 1989;236:43–47.
2. Beasley WC. Quantitative muscle testing: principles and applications to research and clinical services. *Arch Phys Med Rehabil*. 1961;42:398–425.
3. Kilmer DD, McCrory MA, Wright NC, et al. Hand-held dynamometry reliability in persons with neuropathic weakness. *Arch Phys Med Rehabil*. 1997;78:1364–1368.
4. McDonald CM, Abresch RT, Carter GT, et al. Profiles of neuromuscular diseases: Duchenne muscular dystrophy. *Am J Phys Med Rehabil*. 1995;74:S70–S92.
5. Pasternak C, Wong S, Elson EL. Mechanical function of dystrophin in muscle cells. *J Cell Biol*. 1995;128:355–361.
6. Mendell JR, Buzin CH, Feng J, et al. Diagnosis of Duchenne dystrophy by enhanced detection of small mutations. *Neurology*. 2001;57:645–650.
7. Koenig M, Hoffman EP, Bertelson CJ, et al. Complete cloning of the Duchenne muscular dystrophy gene (Duchenne muscular dystrophy) cDNA and preliminary genomic organization of the MD gene in normal and affected individuals. *Cell*. 1987;50:509–517.
8. Petrof BJ, Shrager JB, Stedman HH, et al. Dystrophin protects the sarcolemma from stresses developed during muscle contraction. *Proc Natl Acad Sci U S A*. 1993;90:3710–3714.
9. Emery AE. Population frequencies of inherited neuromuscular diseases: a world survey. *Neuromuscul Disord*. 1991;1:19–29.
10. Kilmer DD, Abresch RT, Fowler WM Jr. Serial manual muscle testing in Duchenne muscular dystrophy. *Arch Phys Med Rehabil*. 1993;74:1168–1171.
11. Mendell JR, Provence MA, Moxley RT, et al. Clinical investigation of Duchenne muscular dystrophy: a methodology for therapeutic trials based on natural history controls. *Arch Neurol*. 1987;44:808–811.
12. Brooke MH, Fenichel GM, Griggs RC, et al. Duchenne muscular dystrophy: patterns of clinical progression and effects of supportive therapy. *Neurology*. 1989;39:475–481.
13. Johnson ER, Fowler WM Jr, Lieberman JS. Contractures in neuromuscular disease. *Arch Phys Med Rehabil*. 1992;73:807–810.
14. Lord J, Behrman B, Varzos N, et al. Scoliosis associated with Duchenne muscular dystrophy. *Arch Phys Med Rehabil*. 1990;71:13–17.
15. Oda T, Shimizu N, Yonenobu K, et al. Longitudinal study of spinal deformity in Duchenne muscular dystrophy. *J Pediatr Orthop*. 1993;13:478–488.
16. Cambridge W, Dennan J. Scoliosis associated with Duchenne muscular dystrophy. *J Pediatr Orthop*. 1987;7:436–440.
17. Galasko CSB, Delaney C, Morris P. Spinal stabilization in Duchenne muscular dystrophy. *J Bone Joint Surg*. 1992;74B:210–214.
18. Rideau Y, Gloriaon B, Delaubier A, et al. The treatment of scoliosis in Duchenne muscular dystrophy. *Muscle Nerve*. 1984;7:281–286.
19. Bies RD, Friedman D, Roberts R, et al. Expression and localization of dystrophin in human cardiac Purkinje fibers. *Circulation*. 1992;86:147–153.
20. Akita H, Matsuoka S, Kuroda Y. Predictive electrocardiographic score for evaluating prognosis in patients with Duchenne's muscular dystrophy. *Tokushima J Exp Med*. 1993;40(1–2):55–60.
21. Chenard AA, Becane HM, Tertrain F, et al. Systolic time intervals in Duchenne muscular dystrophy: evaluation of left ventricular performance. *Clin Cardiol*. 1988;11:407–411.
22. Yanagisawa A, Miyagawa M, Yotsukura M, et al. The prevalence and prognostic significance of arrhythmias in Duchenne type muscular dystrophy. *Am Heart J*. 1992;124:1244–1250.
23. Gilroy J, Cahalan J, Berman R, et al. Cardiac and pulmonary complications in Duchenne's progressive muscular dystrophy. *Circulation*. 1963;27:484–493.
24. Leth A, Wulff K. Myocardiopathy in Duchenne progressive muscular dystrophy. *Acta Paediatr Scand*. 1976;65:28–32.
25. Nigro G, Comi LI, Politano L, et al. The incidence and evolution of cardiomyopathy in Duchenne muscular dystrophy. *Int J Cardiol*. 1990;26:271–277.

26. Nagai T. Prognostic evaluation of congestive heart failure in patients with Duchenne muscular dystrophy: retrospective study using non-invasive cardiac function tests. *Jpn Circ J.* 1989;53:406–415.

27. Nudel U, Zuk D, Einat P, et al. Duchenne muscular dystrophy gene product is not identical in muscle and brain. *Nature.* 1989;337:76–78.

28. Hinton VJ, De Vivo DC, Nereo NE, et al. Poor verbal working memory across intellectual level in boys with Duchenne dystrophy. *Neurology.* 2000;54:2127–2132.

29. Scott OM, Hyde SA, Goddard C, et al. Quantitation of muscle function in children: a prospective study. *Muscle Nerve.* 1982;5:291–301.

30. Willig TN, Carlier L, Legrand M, et al. Nutritional assessment in Duchenne muscular dystrophy. *Dev Med Child Neurol.* 1993;35:1074–1082.

31. Okada K, Manabe S, Sakamoto S, et al. Protein and energy metabolism in patients with progressive muscular dystrophy. *J Nutr Sci Vitaminol (Tokyo).* 1992;38:141–154.

32. Okada K, Manabe S, Sakamoto S, et al. Predictions of energy intake and energy allowance of patients with Duchenne muscular dystrophy and their validity. *J Nutr Sci Vitaminol (Tokyo).* 1992;38:155–161.

33. Alman BA, Raza SN, Biggar WD. Steroid treatment and the development of scoliosis in males with Duchenne muscular dystrophy. *J Bone Joint Surg Am.* 2004;86A(3):519–524.

34. Markham LW, Spicer RL, Khoury PR, et al. Steroid therapy and cardiac function in Duchenne muscular dystrophy. *Pediatr Cardiol.* 2005;26(6):768–771.

35. Balaban B, Matthews DJ, Clayton GH, et al. Corticosteroid treatment and functional improvement in Duchenne muscular dystrophy: long-term effect. *Am J Phys Med Rehabil.* 2005;84(11):843–850.

36. Echevarría L, Aupy P, Goyenvalle A. Exon-skipping advances for Duchenne muscular dystrophy. *Hum Mol Genet.* 2018;27(R2):R163–R172. doi: 10.1093/hmg/ddy171.

37. Mah JK. An overview of recent therapeutics advances for Duchenne muscular dystrophy. *Methods Mol Biol.* 2018;1687:3–17.

38. Bushby KMD, Thambyayah M, Gardner-Medwin D. Prevalence and incidence of Becker muscular dystrophy. *Lancet.* 1991;337:1022–1024.

39. McDonald CM, Abresch RT, Carter GT, et al. Profiles of neuromuscular diseases: Becker's muscular dystrophy. *Am J Phys Med Rehabil.* 1995;74:S93–S103.

40. Bushby KMD, Gardner-Medwin D. The clinical, genetic and dystrophin characteristics of Becker muscular dystrophy: I. Natural history. *J Neurol.* 1993;240:98–104.

41. Bushby KMD, Gardner-Medwin D, Nicholson LVB, et al. The clinical, genetic and dystrophin characteristics of Becker muscular dystrophy: II. Correlation of phenotype with genetic and protein abnormalities. *J Neurol.* 1993;240:105–112.

42. Bradley WG, Jones MZ, Mussini JM, et al. Becker-type muscular dystrophy. *Muscle Nerve.* 1978;1:111–132.

43. Ringel SP, Carroll JE, Schold C. The spectrum of mild X-linked recessive muscular dystrophy. *Arch Neurol.* 1977;34:408–416.

44. Lazzeroni E, Favaro L, Botti G. Dilated cardiomyopathy with regional myocardial hypoperfusion in Becker's muscular dystrophy. *Int J Cardiol.* 1989;22:126–129.

45. Yoshida K, Ikeda S, Nakamura A, et al. Molecular analysis of the Duchenne muscular dystrophy gene in patients with Becker muscular dystrophy presenting with dilated cardiomyopathy. *Muscle Nerve.* 1993;16:1161–1166.

46. Sakata C, Sunohara N, Sunohara N, et al. Cardiomyopathy in Becker muscular dystrophy. *Rinsho Shinkeigaku.* 1990;30:952–955.

47. Steare SE, Benatar A, Dubowitz V. Subclinical cardiomyopathy in Becker muscular dystrophy. *Br Heart J.* 1992;68:304–308.

48. Quinlivan RM, Dubowitz V. Cardiac transplantation in Becker muscular dystrophy. *Neuromuscul Disord.* 1992;2:165–167.

49. Casazza F, Brambilla G, Salvato A, et al. Cardiac transplantation in Becker muscular dystrophy. *J Neurol.* 1988;235:496–498.

50. Harley H, Rundle SA, MacMillan JC, et al. Size of the unstable CTG repeat sequence in relation to phenotype and parental transmission in myotonic dystrophy. *Am J Hum Genet.* 1993;52:1164–1174.

51. Hunter A, Tsilfidis C, Mettler G, et al. The correlation of age of onset with CTG trinucleotide repeat amplification in myotonic dystrophy. *J Med Genet.* 1992;29:774–779.

52. Bachinski LL, Udd B, Meola G, et al. Confirmation of the type 2 myotonic dystrophy (CCTG)n expansion mutation in patients with proximal myotonic myopathy/proximal myotonic dystrophy of different European origins: a single shared haplotype indicates an ancestral founder effect. *Am J Hum Genet.* 2003;73(4):835–848.

53. Johnson ER, Abresch RT, Carter GT, et al. Profiles of neuromuscular diseases: myotonic dystrophy. *Am J Phys Med Rehabil.* 1995;74:S104–S116.

54. Redman JB, Fenwick RG, Fu Y, et al. Relationship between parental trinucleotide CTG repeat length and severity of myotonic dystrophy in offspring. *JAMA.* 1993;269:1960–1965.

55. Moorman JR, Coleman RE, Packer D, et al. Cardiac involvement in myotonic muscular dystrophy. *Medicine.* 1985;64:371–387.

56. Leonard RJ, Kendall KA, Johnson R, et al. Swallowing in myotonic muscular dystrophy: a videofluoroscopic study. *Arch Phys Med Rehabil.* 2001;82:979–985.

57. Tuikka RA, Laaksonen RK, Somer HVK. Cognitive function in myotonic muscular dystrophy: a follow-up study. *Eur Neurol.* 1993;33:436–441.

58. Wijmenga C, Frants RR, Hewitt JE, et al. Molecular genetics of facioscapulohumeral muscular dystrophy. *Neuromuscul Disord.* 1993;3:487–491.

59. Wijmenga C, Hewitt JE, Sankuijl LA, et al. Chromosome 4q DNA rearrangements associated with facioscapulohumeral muscular dystrophy. *Nat Genet.* 1992;2(1):26–30.

60. Tawil R, van der Maarel SM, Tapscott SJ. Facioscapulohumeral dystrophy: the path to consensus on pathophysiology. *Skeletes Muscle.* 2014;4:12. doi: 10.1186/2044-5040-4-12. eCollection 2014. Review.

61. Kilmer DD, Abresch RT, McCrory MA, et al. Profiles of neuromuscular diseases: facioscapulohumeral muscular dystrophy. *Am J Phys Med Rehabil.* 1995;74:S131–S139.

62. Johnson EW, Braddom R. Over-work weakness in facioscapulohumeral muscular dystrophy. *Arch Phys Med Rehabil.* 1971;52:333–336.

63. Tawil R, Van Der Maaer SM. Facioscapulohumeral muscular dystrophy. *Muscle Nerve.* 2006;34(1):1–15.

64. Meyerson MD, Lewis E, Ill K. Facioscapulohumeral muscular dystrophy and accompanying hearing loss. *Arch Otolaryngol.* 1984;110:261–266.

65. Padberg GW, Brouwer OF, deKeizer RJ, et al. On the significance of retinal vascular disease and hearing loss in facioscapulohumeral muscular dystrophy. *Muscle Nerve.* 1995;2:S73–S80.

66. Verhagen WI, Huygen PL, Padberg GW. The auditory, vestibular and oculomotor system in facioscapulohumeral dystrophy. *Acta Otolaryngol.* 1995;520(pt 1):140–142.

67. Yamamoto S, Matsushima H, Suzuki A, et al. A comparative study of thallium-201 single photon emission computed tomography and electrocardiography in Duchenne and other types of muscular dystrophy. *Am J Cardiol.* 1988;61:836–843.

68. Matsuo S, Oku Y, Oshibuchi R, et al. Systolic time intervals in progressive muscular dystrophy. *Jpn Heart J.* 1979;20:23–32.

69. Liewluck T, Milone M. Untangling the complexity of limb-girdle muscular dystrophies. *Muscle Nerve.* 2018;58(2):167–177. doi: 10.1002/mus.26077. Review.

70. Pegoraro E, Hoffman EP. Limb-girdle muscular dystrophy overview. In: Adam MP, Ardinger HH, Pagon RA, et al., eds. *GeneReviews® [Internet].* Seattle, WA: University of Washington, Seattle; 1993–2018. Available from: http://www.ncbi.nlm.nih.gov/books/NBK1408 [initial posting June 8, 2000; updated August 30, 2012].

71. Lim LE, Campbell KP. The sarcoglycan complex in limb-girdle muscular dystrophy. *Curr Opin Neurol.* 1998;11:443–452.

72. McDonald CM, Johnson ER, Abresch RT, et al. Profiles of neuromuscular diseases: limb-girdle syndromes. *Am J Phys Med Rehabil.* 1995;74:S117–S130.

73. Moore SA, Shilling CJ, Westra S, et al. Limb girdle muscular dystrophy in the United States. *J Neuropathol Exp Neurol.* 2006;65(10):995–1003.

74. Kishnani PS, Steiner RD, Bali D, et al. Pompe disease diagnosis and management guideline. *Genet Med.* 2006;8(5):267–288.

75. Kazemi-Esfarjani P, Skomorowska E, Jensen TD, et al. A nonischemic forearm exercise test for McArdle disease. *Ann Neurol.* 2002;52(2):153–159.

76. Askanas V, Engel WK. Inclusion body myositis, a multifactorial muscle disease associated with aging: current concepts of pathogenesis. *Curr Opin Rheumatol.* 2007;19(6):550–559.

77. Schmidt K, Schmidt J. Inclusion body myositis: advancements in diagnosis, pathomechanisms, and treatment. *Curr Opin Rheumatol.* 2017;29(6):632–638. doi: 10.1097/BOR.0000000000000436. Review.

78. Bowyer SL, LaMothe MP, Hollister JR. Steroid myopathy: incidence and detection in a population with asthma. *J Allergy Clin Immunol.* 1985;76:234–242.

79. Braith RW, Welsch MA, Mills RM Jr, et al. Resistance exercise prevents glucocorticoid-induced myopathy in heart transplant recipients. *Med Sci Sports Exerc.* 1998;30:483–489.

80. du Souich P, Roederer G, Dufour R. Myotoxicity of statins: mechanism of action. *Pharmacol Ther.* 2017;175:1–16. doi: 10.1016/j.pharmthera.2017.02.029. Review.

81. Christopher-Stine L, Casciola-Rosen LA, Hong G, et al. A novel autoantibody recognizing 200-kd and 100-kd proteins is associated with an immune-mediated necrotizing myopathy. *Arthritis Rheum.* 2010;62(9):2757–2766. doi: 10.1002/art.27572.

82. Kissel JT, Mendell JR. The endocrine myopathies. In: Rowland LP, DiMauro S, eds. *Handbook of Clinical Neurology: Myopathies.* Vol 18. Amsterdam, UK: Elsevier Science Publishers; 1992:527–551.

83. Madariaga MG, Gamarra N, Dempsey S, et al. Polymyositis-like syndrome in hypothyroidism: review of cases reported over the past twenty-five years. *Thyroid.* 2002;12:331–336.

84. Stevens RD, Dowdy DW, Michaels RK, et al. Neuromuscular dysfunction acquired in critical illness: a systematic review. *Intensive Care Med.* 2007;33(11):1876–1891.

85. Williams S, Horrocks IA, Ouvrier RA, et al. Critical illness polyneuropathy and myopathy in pediatric intensive care: a review. *Pediatr Crit Care Med.* 2007;8(1):18–22.

86. Fowler WM Jr, Taylor M. Rehabilitation management of muscular dystrophy and related disorders: I. The role of exercise. *Arch Phys Med Rehabil.* 1982;63:319–321.

87. Vignos PJ Jr. Physical models of rehabilitation in neuromuscular disease. *Muscle Nerve.* 1983;6:323–338.

88. McCrory MA, Kim HR, Wright NC, et al. Energy expenditure, physical activity and body composition of ambulatory adults with hereditary neuromuscular disease. *Am J Clin Nutr.* 1998;67:1162–1169.

89. Bonsett CA. Pseudohypertrophic muscular dystrophy: distribution of degenerative features as revealed by anatomical study. *Neurology.* 1963;13:728–738.

90. Wagner M, Vignos PJ Jr, Fonow D. Serial isokinetic evaluations used for a patient with scapuloperoneal muscular dystrophy: a case report. *Phys Ther.* 1986;66:1110–1113.

91. Ervasti JM. A role for the dystrophin-glycoprotein complex as a transmembrane linker between laminin and actin. *J Cell Biol.* 1993;122:809–823.

92. Franco A Jr, Lansman JB. Calcium entry through stretch-inactivated ion channels in mdx myotubes. *Nature.* 1990;344:670–673.

93. Turner PR, Fong PY, Denetclaw WF, et al. Increased calcium influx in dystrophic muscle. *J Cell Biol.* 1991;115:1701–1712.

94. Kilmer DD, Aitkens S, Wright NC, et al. Response to high-intensity eccentric muscle contractions in persons with myopathic disease. *Muscle Nerve.* 2001;24:1181–1187.

95. Scott OM, Hyde SA, Goddard C, et al. Effect of exercise in Duchenne muscular dystrophy: controlled six-month feasibility study of effects of two different regimes of exercises in children with Duchenne dystrophy. *Physiotherapy.* 1981;67:174–176.

96. Vignos PJ Jr, Watkins MP. Effect of exercise in muscular dystrophy. *JAMA*. 1966;197:843–848.

97. DeLateur BJ, Giaconi RM. Effect on maximal strength of submaximal exercise in Duchenne muscular dystrophy. *Am J Phys Med*. 1979;58:26–36.

98. Kilmer DD, McDonald CM. Childhood progressive neuromuscular disease. In: Goldberg B, ed. *Sports and Exercise for Children with Chronic Health Conditions*. Champaign, IL: Human Kinetics; 1995:109–121.

99. Milner-Brown HS, Miller RG. Muscle strengthening through high-resistance weight training in patients with neuromuscular disorders. *Arch Phys Med Rehabil*. 1988;69:14–19.

100. McCartney N, Moroz D, Garner SH, et al. The effects of strength training in patients with selected neuromuscular disorders. *Med Sci Sports Exerc*. 1988;20:362–368.

101. Aitkens SG, McCrory MA, Kilmer DD, et al. Moderate resistance exercise program: its effect in slowly progressive neuromuscular disease. *Arch Phys Med Rehabil*. 1993;74:711–715.

102. Kilmer DD, McCrory MA, Wright NC. The effect of a high resistance exercise program in slowly progressive neuromuscular disease. *Arch Phys Med Rehabil*. 1994;75:560–563.

103. Tollback A, Eriksson S, Wredenberg A, et al. Effects of high-resistance training in patients with myotonic dystrophy. *Scand J Rehabil Med*. 1999;31:9–16.

104. Van der Kooi EL, Lindeman E, Riphagen I. Strength training and aerobic exercise training for muscle disease. *Cochrane Database Syst Rev*. 2005;(1):CD003907.

105. Alexanderson H, Lundberg IE. The role of exercise in the rehabilitation of idiopathic inflammatory myopathies. *Curr Opin Rheumatol*. 2005;17:164–171.

106. Alexanderson H, Dastmalchi M, Esbjornsson-Liljedahl M, et al. Benefits of intensive resistance training in patients with chronic polymyositis or dermatomyositis. *Arthritis Rheum*. 2007;57:768–777.

107. Wiesinger GF, Quittan M, Nuhr M, et al. Aerobic capacity in adult dermatomyositis/polymyositis patients and healthy controls. *Arch Phys Med Rehabil*. 2000;81:1–5.

108. Hicks JE, Drinkard B, Summers RM, et al. Decreased aerobic capacity in children with juvenile dermatomyositis. *Arthritis Rheum*. 2002;15:118–123.

109. Florence JM, Brooke MH, Hagberg JM, et al. Endurance exercise in neuromuscular disease. In: Serratrice G, ed. *Neuromuscular Diseases*. New York: Raven Press; 1984:577–581.

110. Wright NC, Kilmer DD, McCrory MA. Aerobic walking in slowly progressive neuromuscular disease: effect of a 12-week program. *Arch Phys Med Rehabil*. 1996;77:64–69.

111. Sveen ML, Jeppesen TD, Hauerslev S, et al. Endurance training: an effective and safe treatment for patients with LGMD21. *Neurology*. 2007;68:59–61.

112. Olsen DB, Omgreen MC, Vissing J. Aerobic training improves exercise performance in fascioscapulohumeral muscular dystrophy. *Neurology*. 2005;64:1064–1066.

113. Orngreen MC, Olsen DB, Vissing J. Aerobic training in patients with myotonic dystrophy type I. *Ann Neurol*. 2005;57:754–757.

114. Wiesinger GF, Quittan M, Aringer M, et al. Improvement of physical fitness and muscle strength in polymyositis/dermatomyositis patients by a training programme. *Br J Rheumatol*. 1998;37:196–200.

115. Wiesinger GF, Quittan M, Graninger M, et al. Benefit of 6 months long-term physical training in polymyositis/dermatomyositis patients. *Br J Rheumatol*. 1998;37:1338–1342.

116. Bar-Or O. Role of exercise in the assessment and management of neuromuscular disease in children. *Med Sci Sports Exerc*. 1996;28:421–427.

117. Miller TD, Balady GJ, Fletcher GF. Exercise and its role in the prevention and rehabilitation of cardiovascular disease. *Ann Behav Med*. 1997;19:220–229.

118. Finsterer J, Stollberger C, Blazek G, et al. Cardiac involvement over 10 years in myotonic and Becker muscular dystrophy and mitochondrial disorder. *Int J Cardiol*. 2007;119(2):176–184.

119. English KM, Gibbs JL. Cardiac monitoring and treatment for children and adolescents with neuromuscular disorders. *Dev Med Child Neurol*. 2006;48(10):863–864.

120. Barona Zamora P, Narbona Gacia J, Alvarez Gomez M, et al. Chronologic study of signs of myocardiopathy in progressive muscular dystrophy. *An Esp Pediatr*. 1993;38:173–177.

121. The SOLVD Investigators. Effect of enalapril on survival in patients with reduced left ventricular ejection fractions and congestive heart failure: the SOLVD investigators. *N Engl J Med*. 1991;325:293–302.

122. The Digitalis Investigation Group. The effect of digoxin on mortality and morbidity in patients with heart failure: the digitalis investigation group. *N Engl J Med*. 1997;336:525–533.

123. Knochel JP. Diuretic-induced hypokalemia. *Am J Med*. 1984;77:18–27.

124. Bland WH, Lederer M, Cassen B. The significance of decreased body potassium concentrations in patients with muscular dystrophy and nondystrophic relatives. *N Engl J Med*. 1967;276:1349–1352.

125. Bergofsky EH. Respiratory failure in disorders of the thoracic cage. *Am Rev Respir Dis*. 1979;119:643–669.

126. Eagle M, Baudouin S, Chandler C, et al. Survival in Duchenne muscular dystrophy: improvements in life expectancy since 1967 and the impact of home nocturnal ventilation. *Neuromuscul Disord*. 2002;12:926–929.

127. Phillips MF, Quinlivan RC, Edwards RH, et al. Changes in spirometry over time as a prognostic marker in patients with Duchenne muscular dystrophy. *Am J Respir Crit Care Med*. 2001;164:2191–2194.

128. Bach JR, Ishikawa Y, Kim H. Prevention of pulmonary morbidity for patients with Duchenne muscular dystrophy. *Chest*. 1997;112:1024–1028.

129. Szeinberg A, Tabachnik E, Rashed N, et al. Cough capacity in patients with muscular dystrophy. *Chest*. 1988;94:1232–1235.

130. Braun NMT, Aurora NS, Rochester DF. Respiratory muscle and pulmonary function in polymyositis and other proximal myopathies. *Thorax*. 1983;38:316–323.

131. Bach JR. Pathophysiology of paralytic/restrictive pulmonary syndromes. In: Bach JR, ed. *Pulmonary Rehabilitation: The Obstructive and Paralytic Conditions*. Philadelphia, PA: Hanley & Belfus; 1996:275–283.

132. Koessler W, Wanke T, Winkler G, et al. 2 years' experience with inspiratory muscle training in patients with neuromuscular disorders. *Chest*. 2001;120:765–769.

133. Vilozni D, Bar-Yishay E, Gur I, et al. Computerized respiratory muscle training in children with Duchenne muscular dystrophy. *Neuromuscul Disord*. 1994;4:249–255.

134. Wanke T, Toifl K, Merkle M, et al. Inspiratory muscle training in patients with Duchenne muscular dystrophy. *Chest*. 1994;105:475–482.

135. Gozal D, Thiriet P. Respiratory muscle training in neuromuscular disease: long-term effects on strength and load perception. *Med Sci Sports Exerc*. 1999;31:1522–1527.

136. Rodillo E, Noble-Jamieson CM, Aber V, et al. Respiratory muscle training in Duchenne muscular dystrophy. *Arch Dis Child*. 1989;64:736–738.

137. Stern LM, Martin AJ, Jones N, et al. Training inspiratory resistance in Duchenne dystrophy using adapted computer games. *Dev Med Child Neurol*. 1989;31:494–500.

138. Sander M, Chavoshan B, Harris S, et al. Functional muscle ischemia in neuronal nitric oxide synthase-deficient skeletal muscle of children with Duchenne muscular dystrophy. *Proc Natl Acad Sci U S A*. 2000;97:13818–13823.

139. Smith PEM, Calverley PMA, Edwards RHT, et al. Practical considerations of respiratory care of patients with muscular dystrophy. *N Engl J Med*. 1987;316:1197–1205.

140. Finder JD, Birnkrant D, Carl J, et al.; American Thoracic Society. Respiratory care of the patient with Duchenne muscular dystrophy: ATS consensus statement. *Am J Respir Crit Care Med*. 2004;170(4):456–465.

141. Baydur A, Gilgoff I, Prentice W, et al. Decline in respiratory function and experience with long-term assisted ventilation in advanced Duchenne's muscular dystrophy. *Chest*. 1990;97:884–889.

142. Simonds AK. Recent advances in respiratory care for neuromuscular disease. *Chest*. 2006;130(6):1879–1886.

143. Kirk VG, Flemons WW, Adams C, et al. Sleep-disordered breathing in Duchenne muscular dystrophy: a preliminary study of the role of portable monitoring. *Pediatr Pulmonol*. 2000;29:135–140.

144. Benditt JO. Management of pulmonary complications in neuromuscular diseases. *Phys Med Rehabil Clin N Am*. 1998;9:167–185.

145. Splaingard ML, Frates RC Jr, Harrison GM, et al. Home positive-pressure ventilation: twenty years' experience. *Chest*. 1983;84:376–382.

146. Ellis ER, Bye PT, Bruderer JW, et al. Treatment of respiratory failure during sleep in patients with neuromuscular disease. *Am Rev Respir Dis*. 1987;135:148–152.

147. Heckmatt JZ, Loh L, Dubowitz V. Night-time nasal ventilation in neuromuscular disease. *Lancet*. 1990;335:579–582.

148. Kerby GR, Mayer LS, Pingleton SK. Nocturnal positive pressure ventilation via nasal mask. *Am Rev Respir Dis*. 1987;135:738–740.

149. Waldhorn RE. Nocturnal nasal intermittent positive pressure ventilation with bilevel positive airway pressure (BiPAP) in respiratory failure. *Chest*. 1992;101:516–521.

150. Bach JR, Campagnolo DI, Hoeman S. Life satisfaction of individuals with Duchenne muscular dystrophy using long-term mechanical ventilatory support. *Am J Phys Med Rehabil*. 1991;70:129–135.

151. Simonds AK, Muntoni F, Heather S, et al. Impact of nasal ventilation on survival in hypercapnic Duchenne muscular dystrophy. *Thorax*. 1998;53:949–952.

152. Hill NS, Redline S, Carskadon MA, et al. Sleep-disordered breathing in patients with Duchenne muscular dystrophy using negative pressure ventilators. *Chest*. 1992;102:1656–1662.

153. Guilleminault C, Philip P, Robinson A. Sleep and neuromuscular disease: bilevel positive airway pressure by nasal mask as a treatment for sleep disordered breathing in patients with neuromuscular disease. *J Neurol Neurosurg Psychiatry*. 1998;65:225–232.

154. Padman R, Lawles S, Von Nessen S. Use of BiPAP by nasal mask in the treatment of respiratory insufficiency in pediatric patients: preliminary investigation. *Pediatr Pulmonol*. 1994;17:119–123.

155. Bach JR. Noninvasive positive pressure ventilatory support begins during sleep. *Sleep Med Clin*. 2017;12(4):607–615.

156. Pinto T, Chatwin M, Banfi P, et al. Mouthpiece ventilation and complementary techniques in patients with neuromuscular disease: a brief clinical review and update. *Chron Respir Dis*. 2017;14(2):187–193.

157. Simonds AK. Home mechanical ventilation: an overview. *Ann Am Thorac Soc*. 2016;13(11):2035–2044.

158. Hess DR. Noninvasive ventilation for neuromuscular disease. *Clin Chest Med*. 2018;39(2):437–447. doi: 10.1016/j.ccm.2018.01.014. Review.

159. McDonald CM. Limb contractures in progressive neuromuscular disease and the role of stretching, orthotics, and surgery. *Phys Med Rehabil Clin N Am*. 1998;9:187–211.

160. Scott OM, Hyde SA, Goddard C, et al. Prevention of deformity in Duchenne muscular dystrophy: a prospective study of passive stretching and splintage. *Physiotherapy*. 1981;67:177–180.

161. Seeger BR, Caudrey DJ, Little JD. Progression of equinus deformity in Duchenne muscular dystrophy. *Arch Phys Med Rehabil*. 1985;66:286–288.

162. Williams EA, Read L, Ellis A, et al. The management of equinus deformity in Duchenne muscular dystrophy. *J Bone Joint Surg*. 1984;66B:546–550.

163. Vignos PJ Jr. Rehabilitation in the myopathies. In: Vinken PJ, Bruyn GW, eds. *Handbook of Clinical Neurology*. Amsterdam, UK: North Holland Publishing; 1980:457–500.

164. Vignos PJ Jr. Management of musculoskeletal complications in neuromuscular disease: limb contractures and the role of stretching, braces and surgery. *Phys Med Rehabil State Art Rev.* 1988;2:509–536.

165. Fowler WM Jr. Rehabilitation management of muscular dystrophy and related disorders: II. Comprehensive care. *Arch Phys Med Rehabil.* 1982;63:322–328.

166. Hyde SA, Flytrup I, Glent S, et al. A randomized comparative study of two methods for controlling tendo Achilles contracture in Duchenne muscular dystrophy. *Neuromuscul Disord.* 2000;10:257–263.

167. Manzur AY, Hyde SA, Rodillo E, et al. A randomized controlled trial of early surgery in Duchenne muscular dystrophy. *Neuromuscul Disord.* 1992;2:379–387.

168. Siegel IM, Miller JE, Ray RD. Subcutaneous lower limb tenotomy in the treatment of pseudohypertrophic muscular dystrophy: description of technique and presentation of twenty-one cases. *J Bone Joint Surg.* 1986;50A:1437–1443.

169. Spencer GE, Vignos PJ Jr. Bracing for ambulation in childhood progressive muscular dystrophy. *J Bone Joint Surg.* 1962;44A:234.

170. Rodillo EB, Fernandez-Bermejo E, Heckmatt JZ, et al. Prevention of rapidly progressive scoliosis in Duchenne muscular dystrophy by prolongation of walking with orthoses. *J Child Neurol.* 1988;3:269–274.

171. Bakker JP, de Groot IJ, Beckerman H, et al. The effects of knee-ankle-foot orthoses in the treatment of Duchenne muscular dystrophy: review of the literature. *Clin Rehabil.* 2000;14:343–359.

172. Kinali M, Messina S, Mercuri E, et al. Management of scoliosis in Duchenne muscular dystrophy: a large 10-year retrospective study. *Dev Med Child Neurol.* 2006;48(6):513–518.

173. Seeger BR, Sutherland AD, Clark MS. Orthotic management of scoliosis in Duchenne muscular dystrophy. *Arch Phys Med Rehabil.* 1984;65(2):83–86.

174. Granata C, Merlini L, Cervellati S, et al. Long-term results of spine surgery in Duchenne muscular dystrophy. *Neuromuscul Disord.* 1996;6:61–68.

175. Miller F, Moseley CF, Koreska J. Spinal fusion in Duchenne muscular dystrophy. *Dev Med Child Neurol.* 1992;34:775–786.

176. Harper CM, Ambler G, Edge G. The prognostic value of pre-operative predicted forced vital capacity in corrective spinal surgery for Duchenne's muscular dystrophy. *Anaesthesia.* 2004;59(12):1160–1162.

177. Miller R, Chalmers A, Dao H, et al. The effect of spine fusion on respiratory function in Duchenne muscular dystrophy. *Neurology.* 1991;41:38–40.

178. Motlagh B, MacDonald JR, Tamopolsky MA. Nutritional inadequacy in adults with muscular dystrophy. *Muscle Nerve.* 2005;31:713–718.

179. Jozefowicz RF, Welle SL, Nair KS, et al. Basal metabolic rate in myotonic dystrophy: evidence against hypometabolism. *Neurology.* 1987;37:1021–1025.

180. Welle S, Jozefowicz R, Forbes G, et al. Effect of testosterone on metabolic rate and body composition in normal men and men with muscular dystrophy. *J Clin Endocrinol Metab.* 1992;74:332–335.

181. Aitkens S, Kilmer DD, Wright NC, et al. Metabolic syndrome in neuromuscular disease. *Arch Phys Med Rehabil.* 2005;86:1030–1036.

182. Kilmer DD, Wright NC, Aitkens S. Impact of a home-based activity and dietary intervention in people with slowly progressive neuromuscular diseases. *Arch Phys Med Rehabil.* 2005;86:2150–2156.

183. Abresch RT, Seyden NK, Wineinger MA. Quality of life: issues for persons with neuromuscular diseases. *Phys Med Rehabil Clin N Am.* 1998;9:233–248.

184. Bostrom K, Ahlstrom G. Quality of life in patients with muscular dystrophy and their next of kin. *Int J Rehabil Res.* 2005;28(2):103–109.

185. Abresch RT, Jensen MP, Carter GT, et al. Assessment of pain and health-related quality of life in slowly progressive neuromuscular disease. *Am J Hosp Palliat Care.* 2002;19:39–48.

186. Fowler WM Jr, Abresch RT, Koch TR, et al. Employment profiles in neuromuscular diseases. *Arch Phys Med Rehabil.* 1997;76:26–37.

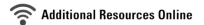 **Additional Resources Online**

CHAPTER **26**

Matthew T. Santa Barbara
Gwendolyn Sowa

Disorders of the Cervical Spine

The intricately designed and highly mobile cervical spine is a critical structure biomechanically that when damaged is a significant source of disability, pain, and health care expenditures. Approximately 95% of individuals will experience cervical pain by the age of 65 (1). Severe episodes of neck discomfort will affect 10% of the population at some point in their lives. The annual incidence of significant cervical pain has been estimated at 12.3% (2).

The incidence and degree of impaired functioning associated with cervical spine disorders have resulted in increased research into the pathophysiology of cervical spine disorders and different treatment modalities, including a wide variety of invasive interventions. This chapter will review common cervical spine disorders, as well as an overview of anatomy, biomechanics, rehabilitative approaches, and treatments.

ANATOMY AND BIOMECHANICS

The cervical spine is composed of seven vertebrae and five intervertebral discs. The C2 through C7 bodies articulate anteriorly through the intervertebral discs and uncovertebral joints, also known as the joints of Luschka, and posteriorly through the zygapophyseal joints (**Fig. 26-1**). The C1 and C2 segments are anatomically unique. The occipito-atlanto-axial or Oc-C1-C2 complex is a specialized upper cervical segment that allows for a significant range of motion between the head and upper torso (3). The articulations of this segment are composed of synovial joints with no intervertebral discs. The basic structure of this segment is a biconcave ring of C1 interposed between the convex condyles of the occiput (Oc) above and the C2 lateral masses below. The odontoid, or dens, projects upward from the C2 vertebrae, providing a post to which the C1 ring and Oc are directly anchored (4). The Oc is attached to the odontoid predominantly by the alar ligaments and also by the less significant apical and upper arms of the cruciform ligament (5). The C1 ring is bound to the odontoid by the sturdy transverse arm of the cruciform ligament as well as the accessory C1-2 ligaments and the C1-2 joint capsules (6) (**Fig. 26-2**).

In the lower cervical spine, the intervertebral discs contribute to approximately one fourth of the height of the cervical column (7,8). The cervical disc is thicker anteriorly than posteriorly, which contributes to the cervical spine's lordotic curvature (9). The cervical disc allows for a greater degree of motion than do the discs in the lumbar region, as the disc-to-vertebral body height ratio in the cervical region is 2:5, compared with a 1:3 ratio in the lumbar spine. The anterior longitudinal ligament runs along the anterior vertebral body and discs, providing structural support in limiting cervical extension. The posterior longitudinal ligament supports the disc and body posteriorly, stretching in flexion and relaxing with extension. The superficial ligamentum nuchae is a dense midline band that extends from the Oc to the spinous process of C7. Proceeding ventrally in the midsagittal plane, the supraspinous ligament, interspinous ligament, and ligamentum flavum are encountered in order, each contributing to the stability of the cervical spine (4). The ligamentum flavum contributes significantly to multidimensional force resistance, particularly in response to flexion and lateral bending. The cervical facets are also important contributors, specifically in resistance to axial rotation and lateral bending (10). Injuries to these structures may contribute to abnormal load distribution and hypermobility within the cervical spine.

The external component of the intervertebral disc is composed of the annulus fibrosus, which consists of multiple lamellae dominated by type I and II collagen. The annulus encapsulates the internal nucleus pulposus. The fiber direction of the annular lamellae alternates, with each consecutive layer oriented opposite to the adjacent fibers (9). This structural arrangement uniquely allows the annulus to accommodate angular motion while providing stability against torsion and shear. Abnormal forces experienced by the annulus are an important precipitant of disc pathology. Excessive mechanical stress and prolonged duration of loading contribute to the release of inflammatory cytokines that are associated with pain and furthering of the disc degenerative cascade (11).

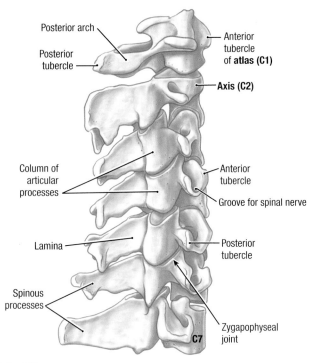

Lateral View

FIGURE 26-1. Articulated cervical vertebrae: lateral view. (Reprinted with permission from Agur AM, Dalley AF. *Grant's Atlas of Anatomy.* 14th ed. Baltimore, MD: Wolters Kluwer; 2016.)

The nucleus pulposus is a semifluid gel, composed predominantly of water, which represents 40% to 60% of the intervertebral disc and allows for deformation and accommodation of movement as well as compressive loading (7). It also contains large amounts of type II collagen and is rich in proteoglycans, which imbibe water contributing to its ability to resist compressive forces (11). With aging, the nucleus is slowly replaced by fibrocartilage, with associated decreases in water and proteoglycan content and disc height. As degeneration progresses, the distinction between the nucleus and surrounding annulus begins to lessen.

Innervation of the normal intervertebral disc is limited to the outer one third to half of the annulus fibrosus (12,13). The anterior disc is innervated by branches of the vertebral nerves and sympathetic trunks. The posterior disc, posterior longitudinal ligament, anterior dura, and dural root sleeves are innervated by a posterior plexus derived from the sinuvertebral nerves (14) (📶 **eFig. 26-1**).

The intervertebral discs are separated from the vertebral bodies by the end plates (8,15). The end plates are composed of hyaline and fibrocartilage and form a permeable surface through which nutrients may pass between the cancellous bone of the vertebral body and the intervertebral discs. The end plates are vascularized during fetal life, but their vessels involute during the first 10 to 15 years of development (16). Thereafter, the essentially avascular intervertebral disc receives its nourishment through the end plates and vessels circumscribing the outer annular fibers (7,9). These changes to the endplates may contribute to the age-related degenerative changes to the disc through alterations in solute transport and disc mechanics (17).

The uncovertebral joints or joints of Luschka are anterior articulations found between the third through seventh vertebrae that share in load bearing and are often affected by degenerative change (7). The zygapophyseal ("z") joints are planar synovial joints, which are created by the inferior and superior articular processes of adjacent vertebrae. Each z joint is composed of circular or ovoid facets that are covered by articular cartilage and enclosed by a fibrous joint capsule (18). The zygapophyseal joint may include fibroadipose menisci located at the ventral and dorsal joint poles. These menisci are thought to be drawn from the joint cavity during joint gliding to cover those articular surfaces that become exposed during such motions (19) (📶 **eFig. 26-2**).

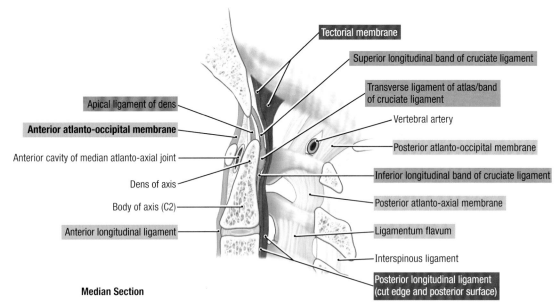

Median Section

FIGURE 26-2. Median section of Oc C1-2 complex. (Reprinted with permission from Agur AM, Dalley AF. *Grant's Atlas of Anatomy.* 14th ed. Baltimore, MD: Wolters Kluwer; 2016.)

From C2-3 through C5-6, the zygapophyseal joints are angled at approximately 45 degrees, with the longitudinal axis of the cervical spine, with a typically steeper angle at C6-7 (20). The superior articular processes are progressively taller at the more caudal segments, with the upper ends of the joints extending further above the level of the segmental intervertebral disc. The orientation of the zygapophyseal joints allows them to resist both forward and downward displacement of the vertebral body. As the zygapophyseal joint of the upper cervical segments are relatively more horizontally oriented, they contribute more to bearing axial loads than do the more caudal segments. The orientation of the zygapophyseal joints dictates the nature and magnitudes of movement in the cervical spine (18).

The primary motion of the Oc-C1-C2 complex is flexion and extension at both Oc-C1 and C1-2, axial rotation only at C1-2, and minimal lateral bending at Oc-C1 (4). The Oc-C1 articulation allows for approximately 10 degrees of flexion and 25 degrees of extension. Rotation of 45 degrees in either rotation can be observed at the C1-2 joint (21,22). A useful approximation of the range of motion allowed by each segment between C2-3 and C7-T1 is 10 degrees of total range from flexion to extension, as well as 10 degrees of lateral bending and axial rotation to each side. Flexion and extension and axial rotation tend to be the greatest in the midcervical region, decreasing both above and below. Lateral bending is typically greatest at C2-3 and diminishes caudally (23). Normal range of motion of the neck has been estimated at 60 degrees of flexion, 75 degrees of extension, and 45 and 80 degrees of bilateral side bending and rotation (24). Instability of the cervical region has been defined as a horizontal displacement of the vertebral body during flexion and extension of greater than 3.5 mm or angular change of greater than 11 degrees (25).

The neural elements of the cervical spine include the spinal cord, dorsal and ventral roots, spinal nerves, and dorsal and ventral rami. The dural and arachnoid mater sleeves contain the ventral and dorsal roots and ultimately blend with the spinal nerve epineurium. The spinal nerves are formed by the joining of the ventral and dorsal roots. Each spinal nerve exits the spinal canal through the intervertebral foramen, which is bordered by the uncovertebral joint anteromedially, the zygapophyseal joint posteriorly, and superiorly and inferiorly by the pedicles of the respective vertebral bodies. The most cephalad and first true neural foramen is located at the C2-3 level. This foramen has the largest area, with a progressive reduction in foraminal size observed more caudally (8). The spinal nerve is a mixed nerve that resides within the neural foramen and is accompanied by the radicular arteries and veins (26). The C3 through C7 nerves exit above their respective pedicles, whereas the C8 spinal nerve exits beneath the pedicle of C7. The C1 nerve rests on the posterior arch of C1, where it divides into dorsal and ventral rami, and the C2 nerve exits the thecal sac and descends obliquely across the dorsal aspect of the atlantoaxial joint (27). Upon exiting the intervertebral foramen, the spinal nerves divide into dorsal and ventral rami. The C5-T1 ventral rami contribute to the brachial plexus. The C1-4 ventral rami constitute the cervical plexus, which innervates the cervical musculature and cutaneous structures of the ear, face, and neck. The C1 and C2 ventral rami innervate the atlantooccipital and atlantoaxial joints, respectively (14).

The cervical zygapophyseal joints are innervated by articular branches originating from the medial branches of the cervical dorsal rami. Each cervical zygapophyseal joint receives a dual innervation from the medial branches arising from the dorsal rami above and below. The medial branches of the C3 dorsal ramus are unique. A deep C3 medial branch contributes to the C3-4 joint innervations, whereas the larger superficial medial branch of C3, also known as the third occipital nerve, innervates the C2-3 joint (18). Beyond the C2-3 joint, the third occipital nerve innervates the semispinalis capitis and supplies cutaneous sensation to the suboccipital region. This is the only dorsal ramus below C2 that has a cutaneous distribution (28).

AXIAL PAIN AND SYMPTOM REFERRAL

Axial or mechanical neck pain is a nonspecific term referring to a variety of neck pain disorders, including degenerative disc disease, spondylosis, and whiplash-associated disorders. This is distinct from cervical radiculopathy, in which the cervical nerve root is the primary pain generator, which will be discussed below.

Pathophysiology

Cervical spondylosis describes the degenerative change that affects the five articulations of the cervical segment, including the intervertebral discs, the bilateral zygapophyseal joints, and the uncovertebral joints of Luschka (29). The degenerative cascade is thought to begin with loss of disc height and an approximation of the uncovertebral joints as well as a disruption of the normal zygapophyseal joint biomechanics. These anatomic changes are often preceded by progressive loss of proteoglycans within the nucleus proposes, which triggers disc dehydration leading to altered biomechanics. Uncovertebral and zygapophyseal joint hypertrophy, osteophyte formation, annular disruption, and ligamentum flavum hypertrophy contribute to the ensuing phases of degenerative change (30–32).

Degenerative disc disease is most commonly observed at C5-6, followed by C6-7. These intervertebral discs might be more commonly affected because of increased segmental motion at these spinal segments (33,34). An injured disc, resulting from degenerative change or more acute trauma, can produce local and referred symptoms (12). The outer third of the annulus fibrosus houses nerve endings that can be stimulated during injury. It has been suggested that degenerative or traumatic alteration of the internal architecture of the annulus can result in pain production through stimulation of local mechanoreceptors and nociceptors (12,33). Furthermore, these degenerative changes may create an environment rich in inflammatory mediators. Increased levels of inflammatory mediators have been identified in degenerative and herniated discs (35). This cytokine-rich milieu is favorable to neoinnervation and neovascularization, which may also contribute to pain in the degenerating disc (36). The ability of the annulus to mediate pain has also been demonstrated during surgery through mechanical and electrical stimulation of cervical intervertebral discs (34). Annular defects allow for the migration of nuclear material, which further stimulates an inflammatory response that can then affect the outer annulus, dura mater, posterior longitudinal ligament, dorsal root ganglion, and spinal nerve (37).

Using cervical discography, characteristic discogenic pain patterns have been described (34,38,39). In a study of 807

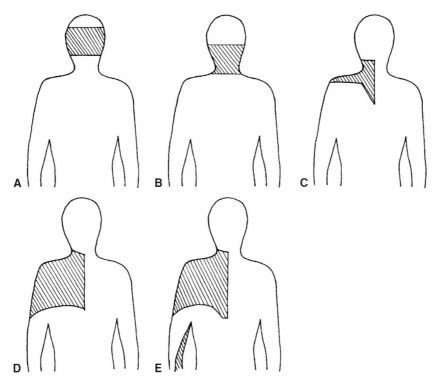

FIGURE 26-3. Pattern of pain described during cervical discography at each cervical level: C2-3 **(A)**, C3-4 **(B)**, C4-5 **(C)**, C5-6 **(D)**, and C6-7 **(E)**. For illustration purposes only, pain is depicted in a unilateral fashion to the left for C4-5 through C6-7. (Reprinted with permission from Grubb SA, Kelly CK. Cervical discography: clinical implications from 12 years of experience. *Spine*. 2000;25(11):1382–1389.)

disc injections, 404 concordant pain responses were used to describe pain referral patterns. Pain referral to the scapular region was observed to arise from disc stimulation at the C3-4 through C7-T1 levels. The C5-6 and more caudal segments were noted to refer symptoms to the upper limb, and C6-7 stimulation was unique in that pain was referred to the anterior chest wall (38) (**Fig. 26-3**). Of note, cervical discography has been shown to produce pain patterns in up to 70% of asymptomatic control patients. The evidence for cervical discography as a diagnostic tool is mixed, and there is no evidence correlating its use with functional outcomes (40). Additionally, the correlation between cervical disc magnetic resonance imaging (MRI) abnormalities and pain-generating potential observed through discography has been shown to be poor (39).

The z joints can also become active pain generators in the setting of degenerative change or following trauma. These posterior elements are particularly vulnerable to injury during a whiplash event, in which an abrupt flexion and extension movement occurs to the cervical spine. Whiplash-associated disorders have increased in incidence over the last decade and are a significant source of disability (41–44).

As defined by diagnostic blocks, chronic cervical zygapophyseal joint pain lasting longer than 3 months has an estimated frequency of 54% to 60% in cases of whiplash injuries (43,44). In this chronic neck pain population, the C2-3 joint has been observed to be most frequently symptomatic, followed by C5-6 (43,44). Studies in a limited number of asymptomatic and symptomatic volunteers have suggested particular resultant pain patterns from intra-articular zygapophyseal joint stimulation and anesthetization (45–47). Pain arising from C2-3 stimulation was described as referred to the upper neck and occipital region, whereas C3-4 and C4-5 joint pain was

observed to affect the mid- and lower cervical region, extending toward the superior scapular border. Pain from C5-6 stimulation was observed to extend toward the shoulder, whereas C6-7 pain radiated over the more caudal scapular region (**Fig. 26-4**). Based on observed overlap, pain referral

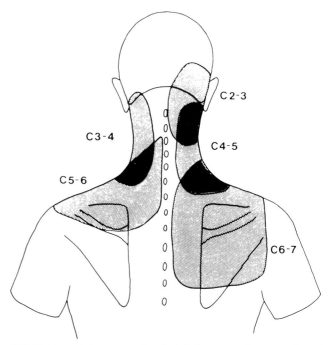

FIGURE 26-4. Pain patterns described during provocative zygapophyseal joint injection. (Reprinted with permission from Dwyer A, Aprill C, Bogduk N. Cervical zygapophyseal joint pain patterns 1: a study in normal volunteers. *Spine*. 1990;15(6):453–457.)

patterns arising from primary axial zygapophyseal joint or discogenic pain generators can be difficult to distinguish clinically from one another and from radicular pain. Diagnostic medial branch blocks can be utilized to clarify the zygapophyseal joint as the pain generator in cases of whiplash-associated disorder or axial neck pain (48).

Of those patients with chronic neck pain, 58% to 88% describe significant cervicogenic headaches, defined as pain referred to the head from a bony or soft tissue source (42–44). Cervicogenic headaches are frequently encountered in whiplash disorders due to innervation of the zygapophyseal joints from the first three cervical nerves, which can produce referred pain to the head and face region. The C2-3 zygapophyseal joint is the most frequent pain generator in cervicogenic headaches, with an estimated frequency of 50–53% in those individuals with a chief symptom of headache following whiplash (42,44,49). The Oc-C1 joints (42,50–52) and C1-2 joints (50,51) have similarly been described as active nociceptors in cervicogenic headaches. Although often not observed radiographically, zygapophyseal joint fractures, intra-articular hemorrhage, and capsular tears have been observed in pathologic studies (42–44,53–59).

History

Axial pain encompasses a wide variety of disorders, including discogenic pain and cervical facet syndrome, and thus the subjective report provided by the patient is variable. The key in distinguishing discogenic and facet-mediated pain from neurogenic pain is the predominance of pain localized to the axial region. Patients should be screened for red flags, or indicators of severe underlying systemic disease or spinal cord compromise. Potential red flags include recent trauma, history of or symptoms indicating malignancy, bowel and bladder dysfunction, saddle anesthesia, gait and balance dysfunction, progressive weakness, intravenous drug use, and known history or symptoms indicating ankylosing spondylitis or inflammatory arthritis (40).

Patients with primarily discogenic pain may report pain limited to the neck with associated muscle tightness and spasms that are worse with holding the neck in one position for a prolonged period of time. Cervical facet-mediated pain may manifest as midline or slightly offset cervical spine pain with referral to the shoulders and scapula (41). Patients with cervical facet pain may recount a history of recent whiplash event. These patients may also report pain with activities involving extension and protraction of the head.

Referred pain is pain perceived in a region other than the actual pain generator. Pain referral patterns arise as the brain is unable to decipher the true pain origin secondary to convergence at the level of the spinal cord and thalamus. Referred pain is typically experienced as deep, diffuse, and poorly localized pain (14). Any of the innervated structures of the cervical spine can contribute to local pain as well as symptom referral. Injury to the cervical musculature and ligamentous structures can also result in local and regional pain, but neither have been extensively investigated as pain generators (60,61).

The examination of the neck in patients with suspected axial neck pain should be comprehensive in order to clarify the diagnosis and evaluate for other potential neck pain generators. Range of motion of the cervical spine and palpation of the surrounding musculature as well as a neurologic examination, including manual muscle testing, reflexes, and sensation should be included. Spurling's maneuver is useful to evaluate for radiculopathy. Hoffmann's sign should also be included to assess potential upper motor neuron pathology. Examination of the shoulder is needed in cases of referred neck pain as disorders of the shoulder joints and/or rotator cuff can mimic symptoms arising from the cervical spine. The examination of a patient with pure axial neck pain may reveal decreased or painful range of motion along with a normal neurologic exam (62).

Radiology

Radiographic evidence of degenerative change (see also Chapter 5) is appreciated in 10% of individuals by the age of 25, 35% by the age of 40, and in up to 95% by the age of 65 (1,2). Plain film imaging in asymptomatic subjects reveals degenerative change affecting the cervical spine in 70% of women and 95% of men between the ages of 60 and 65 (63). It is essential to remember that although there is commonly radiographic evidence of degenerative disease, including loss of disc space height and osteophytes, in individuals presenting with cervical pain, not all individuals with degenerative findings are symptomatic and the presence of these changes does not accurately identify the pain generator (63,64). CT scans of the cervical spine are warranted in cases of trauma when fracture is suspected but are not required for patients presenting with axial neck pain alone. MRIs of the cervical spine are also not required as first-line workup, unless there are important symptoms on history or exam. Similar to plain films, there is a high false-positive rate with cervical MRIs with up to 30% of asymptomatic individuals demonstrating disc protrusions or extrusions (62,65).

Cervical provocation discography is another diagnostic tool occasionally utilized in the workup of axial neck pain. This test involves the use of image guidance to inject contrast material into the nucleus pulposus followed by assessment of disc morphology on CT scan or plain films. Concordant pain provocation is monitored during injection and then considered in combination with pathologic features noted on images (66). Indications include further evaluation of a radiologically abnormal disc, investigation of severe symptoms without MRI or CT correlate, and clarification of symptomatic level when imaging reveals multilevel disc disease (66).

The Spine Intervention Society (SIS) criteria for a positive provocation discography test include concordant pain with absence of pain at two other normal/control cervical levels (67). However, there is an overall lack of consensus on what constitutes a positive response in the literature (68). A 2012 systematic review of the utility of cervical discography in chronic neck pain demonstrated limited evidence for the diagnostic accuracy of this test (68). Furthermore, similar to plain films and MRI, there is a suspected high false-positive rate for cervical provocative discography, although this rate may be overestimated given inconsistent definitions of positive results. An estimation of the false-positive rate ranges from 5% to 27%, although the true value may be lower when SIS guidelines for a positive result are utilized (68). *The limited reliability of discography along with the invasive nature of the procedure limits its utility, and it is most commonly used currently in select surgical planning cases.*

Noninvasive Treatment

The treatment of axial neck pain typically begins with a trial of noninvasive techniques, including physical therapy. The physical therapy prescription should mark the initiation of an ongoing dialogue between the physician and the therapist. Its purpose is to introduce the patient to the treating therapist and provide the therapist with pertinent physical and radiologic findings. The prescribing physician should, whenever possible, avoid the assignment of more generic diagnoses such as "sprain/strain," or treatment recommendations such as "evaluate and treat." *Though a spine physical therapist will perform an independent assessment to arrive at a diagnosis, information provided by the physician regarding his/her assessment and objective diagnostic testing results are vital communication to relay precautions and improve outcomes.* Sufficient detail about findings and recommendations will provide the starting point for open communication and therapeutic partnership between the treating physician and therapist, and regular communication is vital throughout the episode of care.

Physical therapy and modalities are frequently prescribed for the patient with cervical pain and whiplash injuries, with both patient populations demonstrating similar responses to these approaches (69). A wide range of therapeutic exercise programs have been employed in the treatment of axial neck pain. Clinical outcomes can be optimized by proceeding with a comprehensive diagnosis and symptom-specific approach and with the judicious use of modalities only when necessary to facilitate active treatment. The patient's general state of aerobic fitness as well as strengthening of the neck and chest musculature should also be included in a physical therapy program for axial neck pain. According to the Task Force on Neck Pain's 2000–2010 best evidence synthesis, physical therapy including the McKenzie protocol resulted in better recovery from whiplash-associated disorders than passive modalities or collar use. Physical therapy and exercise interventions also showed positive results for axial neck pain (70).

Exercise interventions, in particular programs targeting strengthening of the deep cervical flexors consisting of the longus colli and longus capitis muscles, have shown efficacy in relieving mechanical neck pain in the acute and chronic stages (71). An example of a deep cervical flexor strengthening program consists of a 10-minute warm-up period of sets of static (static [isometric]) holds in cervical flexion, followed by a dynamic strengthening program consisting of sets of dynamic (isotonic) full flexion and extension movements of the neck with incremental increases in resistance when a predetermined number of repetitions are achieved (72). A 2017 systematic review identified eight studies ranging from moderate to good quality that demonstrated the effectiveness of low-load craniocervical flexion exercise programs for the deep cervical flexors. Subjects in the low-load craniocervical flexion exercise groups demonstrated decreased neck pain and reduced levels of functional disability along with significant improvements in strength and endurance of the deep cervical flexors (73). These findings should be considered by physicians and therapists when designing a rehabilitation program for a patient with acute or chronic axial neck pain.

The clinician should limit the application of modalities to the acute injury phase with a primary objective of pain modification to facilitate therapy. Both superficial heat and ice have the potential to serve as an analgesic and to reduce muscle spasm. Neural firing rates have been demonstrated to change in response to changes in temperature (74). Both an elevation and a reduction of muscle temperature resulting from the application of superficial heat and cold have been correlated with decreased gamma motor neuron activity (75,76). These changes in nerve firing rates are thought to contribute to a reduction in muscle spasm (77). Although superficial heat is often applied for comfort measures, application of ice is preferred in the acute phase of injury because of its greater depth of penetration and its analgesic and anti-inflammatory effects (78). Local regular icing can result in vasoconstriction and a reduction in the release of nociceptive and inflammatory mediators such as prostaglandins (79). The use of heat or icing modalities can be repeated several times daily. The decision to use heat or ice can be predominantly determined by which is perceived by the patient as most analgesic.

Ultrasound is perhaps one of the most commonly overused physical therapy modalities (see also Chapter 51). A review of 35 randomized controlled trials published between 1975 and 1999 studying the effectiveness of therapeutic ultrasound revealed that there was little evidence that active therapeutic ultrasound was more effective than placebo in treating people with pain arising from a wide range of musculoskeletal injuries or for promoting soft-tissue healing (80).

Electric stimulation consisting of both low- and high-rate transcutaneous electrical nerve stimulation and interferential current is often similarly used in an effort to reduce pain and inflammation (see also Chapter 54). Dermatomally applied percutaneous neuromodulation therapy and transcutaneous electrical nerve stimulation, in addition to ice and heat, have demonstrated immediate pain relief and acute decreases in disability index scores (70). However, the use of modalities in the treatment of cervical disorders should be time limited and should not serve as a substitute for a more active rehabilitation approach.

Manipulation is a passive movement that is applied to a joint or structure beyond normal physiologic limits with the intent of improving range of motion or reducing a derangement (81). Some believe that manipulative procedures to the zygapophyseal joints enhance afferent signals from mechanoreceptors to the peripheral and central nervous system (82). This normalization of afferent impulses is hypothesized to reduce muscle guarding, improve muscle tone and local tissue metabolism, and lead to increased range of motion and pain reduction (78). Before performing spinal manipulation, the clinician must rule out cervical instability and vertebral artery insufficiency, as high-velocity movements could place the patient at risk for neurologic compromise or vascular insult (83). Manipulation should also likely be avoided in patients with radicular pathology or significant neural foraminal or central canal compromise. It is also recommended that spinal manipulation only be performed by skilled clinicians with comprehensive understanding of spinal disorders. The common adverse effects of spinal manipulative therapy include local and radiating discomfort, headache, and fatigue, the majority of which resolve within 1 day (84). However, severe adverse effects of these manipulations include vertebrobasilar artery stroke. The precise incidence of this catastrophic adverse effect is unknown, with a wide variability of estimations from 1 in 200,000 cervical manipulations to 1 in 5.85 million (85,86).

A 2015 Cochrane review of manipulation indicated that the literature for these interventions was low to very low quality (87). Manipulation was shown to be beneficial for immediate pain relief, but this was not sustained at follow-up (87). There is also a lack of consensus on indications and exclusion criteria for manipulative therapy. Furthermore, the risk of vertebral artery dissection must be weighed in consideration of the relatively poor evidence of long-term efficacy of cervical manipulation.

Acupuncture for the treatment of neck pain is likely more effective than sham treatments (70). This intervention may be particularly useful and cost effective for those with greater than 6 months of axial neck pain (88,89). Acupuncture also produced superior posttreatment pain scores when compared to trigger point injections for neck pain (90).

Cervical Injections for Axial Neck Pain

Cervical injections with corticosteroids may be considered after a patient has failed to respond to an initial noninvasive approach to axial neck pain (see also Chapter 53). A 2015 systematic review of cervical epidural injections identified only one high-quality, randomized, double-blinded controlled trial evaluating the efficacy of cervical epidural injections in discogenic neck pain despite multiple uncontrolled studies that demonstrated effectiveness (91). This RCT demonstrated improved pain and functional outcomes in patients with cervical discogenic pain treated with cervical epidural injections, with or without steroids, at 2-year follow-up (92). In a recent observational, retrospective study, interlaminar and transforminal approaches for cervical injections demonstrated similar levels of effectiveness. However, the interlaminar approach is preferred due to concern for anterior spinal artery syndrome given the proximity of the arterial system with the transforaminal approach (93). Additional randomized controlled trials are needed to reach consensus on the efficacy of cervical epidural injections for discogenic pain.

A systematic review demonstrated fair evidence for radiofrequency neurotomy and cervical medial branch blocks for axial neck pain, signifying that limited studies have shown positive effects, but more well-designed trials are needed for consensus on effectiveness. Pain is expected to return following neurotomy, as distal axons innervating the zygapophyseal joint are likely to regenerate (94).

Radiofrequency ablation of the C2-3 facet has shown greater duration of pain relief than steroid in cases of cervicogenic headache (49). The third occipital nerve is the superficial medial branch of the C3 dorsal primary ramus and innervates the C2-3 zygapophyseal joint. When this nerve is confirmed as the pain generator in cervicogenic headaches with anesthetic blocks, radiofrequency neurotomy is reported to be effective in 88% of cases (95). Initial visualization and blockade of the third occipital nerve can be accurately achieved with a combination of ultrasound and fluoroscopic guidance (96).

The 2000–2010 Neck Pain Task Force best evidence synthesis did not find any well-designed clinical trials or cohort studies for the use of open surgical techniques for treatment of neck pain with degenerative pathology alone. There are several case series on cervical fusion for axial neck pain, but none of these were met inclusion criteria for the Task Force's evidence appraisal (97).

RADICULOPATHY

Epidemiology

Cervical radiculopathy can arise from pathologic compressive processes affecting the nerve root, including acute disc herniation, degenerative foraminal stenosis, trauma, or tumor (98–101). The annual incidence of cervical radicular pain is 5.5/100,000 (102). The nerve roots most commonly involved by cervical radiculopathy are C6 and C7, with most studies suggesting C7 syndromes as the most common (98,103–106). Patients younger than 55 years are more likely to present with radiculopathy arising from acute disc herniations, whereas those older than 55 years are more likely to demonstrate symptoms arising from degenerative foraminal or central canal stenosis (29).

Pathophysiology

The cervical nerve root can be compressed in the neural foramen by the intervertebral disc, degenerative change affecting the zygapophyseal or uncovertebral joint, or in a combined fashion (107–110) (**Fig. 26-5**). With disc degeneration, tears in the annulus can allow for disc herniations, or displacement of nucleus pulposus of fragmented annulus beyond the intervertebral disc space. Disc herniations have been characterized based on type and location (111,112). The types of disc herniations are classified based on the shape of the displaced disc material (**Fig. 26-6**) (113). A disc protrusion occurs when the distance between the edges of the herniated material in any plane is less than the distance between the edges of the herniated material at the border of the disc space. A disc extrusion occurs when the distance between the edges of the herniated material is greater than the distance between the edges of the base of the material at the disc space. Disc sequestration occurs when disc material fragments from the disc (113).

The three locations of disc herniations described are intraforaminal, posterolateral, and central. Intraforaminal herniations are the most common and may result in an acute radiculopathy affecting the nerve root exiting through the respective foramen. For example, an intraforaminal herniation of disc material at the C4-5 level could result in a C5 radiculopathy. The posterolateral disc herniation occurs because the rhomboidal shape of the posterior longitudinal ligament tends to direct disc material laterally. These herniations are located

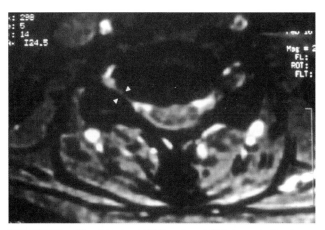

FIGURE 26-5. T2-weighted axial MRI section at C5-6 demonstrating degenerative spondylosis and resultant advanced right-sided neural foraminal stenosis, delineated by *arrowheads*, in a patient with a C6 radiculopathy.

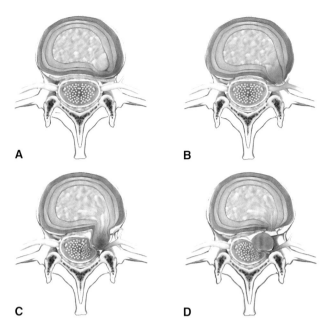

FIGURE 26-6. Types of disc herniations are characterized based on the shape of the herniated material in relation to the outer annulus. A disc bulge (**A**) is not considered a true herniation as disc material remains remains within the outer border of the annulus. Note that the distance between the edges of the herniated material in a protrusion (**B**) is less than the distance between the edges of the outer annulus where the herniation begins, while the opposite is true with an extrusion (**C**). A sequestration (**D**) represents a complete fragmentation of disc material. (Reprinted with permission from Rhee J, Boden SD, Wiesel SW. *Operative Techniques in Spine Surgery.* 2nd ed. Philadelphia, PA: Wolters Kluwer; 2016.)

between the lateral edge of the posterior longitudinal ligament and the posterior aspect of the uncinate process. The central disc herniation passes through the substance of the posterior longitudinal ligament. These lesions are more likely to result in central canal compromise and spinal cord compression. Central herniations are believed to be more likely to occur in the later stages of cervical degeneration when uncovertebral joint hypertrophy serves as a barrier to the more lateral migration of disc material (114).

After disc herniation, the resultant injury to the nerve roots likely arises from combined mechanical and biochemical pathophysiologic processes. A study in which cervical disc specimens removed surgically from patients with radiculopathy were compared with discs from a traumatic control group found significantly increased levels of matrix metalloproteinase, nitric oxide, prostaglandins, and interleukins in the radiculopathy group (35), and these biochemical markers have been implicated in the pathologic process of cervical radiculopathy (115–119).

History

Patients with radiculopathy typically present with complaints of pain, weakness, paresthesias, or a combination of sensorimotor deficits (98). The majority of patients describe cervical and upper-extremity pain that began without trauma or a particular inciting event (104,105). Most studies suggest that pain affects the upper limb more commonly than the neck, although most often both are involved (105,120). Coughing, sneezing, or a Valsalva maneuver may lead to symptomatic worsening. The reports of pain might also incorporate the anterior chest wall, resulting in a syndrome of pseudoangina pectoris (100,121–123). It is often difficult to determine the

symptomatic level based on the patient's pain description alone. The distribution of symptoms might not follow the classic dermatomal patterns as defined by Keegan and Garrett (124) or Foerster (125). The limitations of these mapping studies include the assignment of dermatomal distribution based predominantly on the loss of sensation or hyposensitivity arising from compressive injuries. Each of these classic studies describes considerable dermatomal overlap. Dermatomal pain patterns, arising from selective cervical spinal nerve stimulation, have been described and may be more representative of the pain and paresthesia patterns clinically observed in radiculopathy (126). Using fluoroscopically guided cervical nerve root stimulation, pain patterns were described after the stimulation of 134 roots in 87 subjects. Pain distribution distal to the elbow was found in only 14% of C5 stimulations. C6 stimulation affected the ulnar hand in 67%, C7 uniquely resulted in anterior head symptoms and most commonly referred pain to the chest, and C8 affected the thumb in 14%. No nerve root pain distribution was observed to be confined to the classically defined dermatomes in greater than 50% of stimulations (126) (**Fig. 26-7**). Some of the discrepancy between clinical

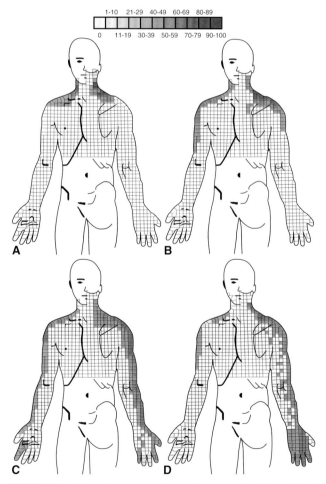

FIGURE 26-7. Percent occurrence of symptom provocation for each body map section during C4-7 spinal nerve stimulation. Ventral and dorsal thorax and limb demonstrated. **A:** C4 dynatome; **B:** C5 dynatome; **C:** C6 dynatome; and **D:** C7 dynatome. (Reprinted with permission from Slipman CW, Plastaras CT, Palmitier RA, et al. Symptom provocation of fluoroscopically guided cervical nerve root stimulation: are dynatomal maps identical to dermatomal maps? *Spine.* 1998;23(20):2235–2242.)

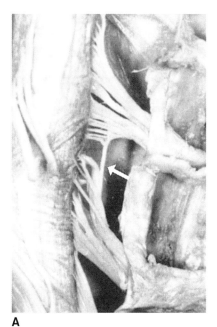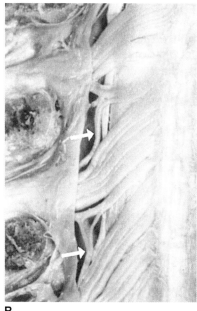

A   **B**

FIGURE 26-8. *Arrows* demonstrating ventral **(A)** and more commonly observed dorsal **(B)** intradural intersegmental anastomoses between nerve roots of the cervical spine. (Reprinted with permission from Tanaka N, Fujimoto Y, An HS, et al. The anatomic relation among the nerve roots, intervertebral foramina, and intervertebral discs of the cervical spine. *Spine.* 2000;25(3):286–291.)

presentation and the more classic dermatomal maps might also be explained by intrathecal cervical dorsal root intersegmental anastomosis, which can be present in as many as 61% of individuals (127–129) (**Fig. 26-8**). Additionally, pain in radiculopathy might arise in part from a myotomal or myalgic pain component arising from ventral nerve root irritation (130).

When examining the patient with suspected cervical radiculopathy, it is essential that the clinician remains mindful of extraspinal disorders that can mimic nerve root pathology. A brachial plexopathy or neuralgic amyotrophy with upper-trunk involvement can appear similar to a radiculopathy of C5 or C6 origin (131–133). More localized disorders affecting the upper limb can similarly result in regional pain, including subacromial bursitis, lateral epicondylosis, and bicipital tendinosis (98). More distal neural entrapments affecting the median, radial, or ulnar nerve should also be considered. A median neuropathy at the wrist can result in pain extending as proximal as the cervical region (98). When cervical radiculopathy and myelopathy coexist, such as in amyotrophic lateral sclerosis and syringomyelia, the examiner should seek signs of possible combined cord and root compression (98,134).

Muscle girth should be carefully inspected for any evidence of atrophy that might be consistent with a more chronic radiculopathy. C5 and C6 involvements can lead to wasting of the biceps and periscapular musculature. Loss of triceps girth can be observed in the setting of a C7 radiculopathy. Atrophy of the hand intrinsics might be observed in patients with C8 or T1 pathology. Manual muscle testing has been suggested to be a more sensitive means of isolating a level of segmental pathology than either reflex or sensory testing. It is important to note that variations in the contributions of the spinal nerves to the cords and branches of the brachial plexus can lead to an altered pattern of muscular innervation in the upper limb (98,106).

Reflex testing of the upper extremity should include the bicep, tricep, brachioradialis, and Hoffmann's response. Lower-extremity reflex testing and gait analysis should be included to evaluate for hyperreflexia or ataxia, which are consistent with cervical cord compromise.

Active cervical range of motion can be recorded and observed for symptom provocation in a particular plane. In particular, extension and ipsilateral side bending are more likely to result in a reproduction of radicular symptoms. Spurling's maneuver incorporates rotation and side-bending of the head toward the affected side, and this can be combined with axial compression. The goal of this maneuver is to diminish the foraminal area and reproduce radicular symptoms (29). This neck compression test was initially defined by Spurling and Scoville in the 1940s at a time when cervical radicular syndromes were first recognized (135). This maneuver has been demonstrated to have a high specificity but a low sensitivity (136). Such maneuvers should be performed with caution in patients with a suspected radicular syndrome, as this could lead to further neural irritation. In those patients demonstrating a reproduction of radicular symptoms with active cervical extension or ipsilateral side-bending, this provocative test should be avoided (98). The shoulder abduction relief sign has the patient place the affected hand on the top of the head. This position of upper-extremity abduction reduces stress on the nerve root affected by a disc herniation and relieves pain (137,138). Upper limb neural tension testing applies mechanical stress to nerves through upper-extremity movements (139). For example, shoulder depression, 110-degree shoulder abduction, shoulder external rotations, wrist and finger extension, and elbow extension have been shown in cadaver studies to produce inferolateral displacement and strain in cervical nerve roots (140). A neural tension test is considered positive when concordant pain is produced and has demonstrated high sensitivity but low specificity (139,141).

A complete exam should also include passive ranging of the shoulder and impingement maneuvers. Tinel's testing at the supraclavicular fossa, elbow, and wrist and carpal tunnel stress maneuvers, such as Phalen's testing and carpal compression, might reveal a proximal entrapment neuropathy or carpal tunnel syndrome. Observing for a pain response during palpation of the medial and lateral epicondyle can be helpful in ruling out a contributing focal tendinosis. Thoracic outlet maneuvers should also be considered to rule out a contributing lower-trunk plexopathy or dynamic vascular insufficiency, also referred to as "neurogenic" or "vascular" thoracic outlet syndromes. These regional exam techniques are included in the complete examination of a patient with suspected radiculopathy and might enlighten the examiner to a contributing musculoskeletal disorder or more distal neuropathic process.

Radiologic Findings

Plain films can provide information regarding anatomic pathology but are not necessary in every individual presenting with cervical or radicular pain. In addition to anteroposterior and lateral images, flexion and extension views can prove of value in patients with recent trauma, suspected instability, or in cases of ankylosing spondylitis or RA (98).

MRI can provide additional information regarding soft tissues or neuroforaminal compromise, but a high incidence of abnormalities has been observed on cervical MRI of asymptomatic individuals (142–147). Boden et al. observed significant abnormalities in 19% of 63 asymptomatic patients (148). In those younger than age 40 years, 14% had a herniated disc or neural foraminal stenosis, and similar abnormalities were observed in 25% of individuals older than age 40 years (112). An investigation of cervical myelography has identified nerve root filling defects in 21% of asymptomatic subjects (149).

As there is a significant prevalence of such abnormalities in asymptomatic subjects, advanced cervical spine imaging in symptomatic individuals must be interpreted carefully to determine if a correlation exists between radiographic pathology and clinical findings (150,151). Advanced imaging should be limited to situations in which it will alter the therapeutic plan or when red flag signs are present. Also of interest is the natural radiographic history of symptomatic disc pathology in the cervical spine. A study following disc herniations in 21 patients with radiculopathy found that the largest lesions decreased in size the most, with 16 of 21 lesions reducing in size by 35% to 100% at 15-month follow-up CT (152). In similar studies observing patients with serial MRI, 40% to 92% of patients demonstrated radiographic regression (153,154). More lateral and extruded discs were less likely to resolve (**Fig. 26-9**).

Electrodiagnostics

Electromyography (EMG) and nerve conduction studies (NCS) can help to localize the level of a cervical radiculopathy and differentiate such a presentation from a brachial plexopathy, more distal entrapment, or peripheral neuropathic process (see also Chapter 3). EMG is also useful in cases when interventional management is being considered and the physical exam findings are inconclusive of the level of pathology. However, such testing is not necessary in all patients presenting with cervical radicular syndromes. The earliest abnormality that might be observed in the setting of motor root compromise is reduced voluntary recruitment observed during needle exam. Abnormal activity at rest in the form of positive sharp waves or fibrillation potentials, indicative of axonal loss, might not be observed until at least 18 to 21 days after the onset of a radicular syndrome (155). EMG abnormalities have been

shown to correlate well with myelographic abnormalities and operative pathology (156). Needle examination of seven limb muscles is likely adequate for the identification of segmental pathology (157). It is important to note, though, that the segmental sensitivity and specificity of EMG abnormalities might only approach 67% and 50% (158).

Cervical radiculopathy can be diagnosed clinically in patients with a suggestive pain distribution and/or a myotomal strength deficit, reflex abnormality, or sensory loss. Imaging can help clarify a diagnosis when the history is less clear. If the cervical radiographs and clinical findings are less conclusive, electrodiagnostic studies might prove helpful in confirming a level of radicular pathology when a myotomal denervation pattern is observed. If radicular pain remains within the differential and these diagnostic criteria are not satisfied, a diagnostic selective nerve root block might be employed, particularly in cases when multilevel pathology is identified on MRI and the precise pain generator root level is unclear on exam (159). A 2007 systematic review concluded that the positive predictive value of these injections is low, but they do have a significant negative predictive value (160).

Noninvasive Treatment

There is no consensus on a nonoperative treatment algorithm for cervical radiculopathy (70,97,161,162). Several first-line approaches are similarly employed in cases of axial pain and cervical radiculopathy, such as an emphasis on physical therapy and exercise interventions. Well-designed studies comparing nonoperative treatment to surgical interventions are sparse, with a 2010 Cochrane Database Systematic Review identifying only one randomized controlled trial meeting review standards comparing the two interventions (163). This study demonstrated short-term benefits for those treated with surgery at 3-month follow-up, but outcomes at 1-year follow-up were not significantly different between the operative and nonoperative groups (164). The nonoperative group included both physical therapy and cervical collar subdivisions, with the physical therapy group showing improved functional outcomes at follow-up compared to the collar group (164).

A review of multiple retrospective and uncontrolled studies of nonsurgically treated cervical radiculopathy revealed satisfactory outcomes in 80% to 90% of patients, although time to complete recovery may not occur for up to 24 to 36 months (105,164–167). A 2016 systematic review indicated that oral NSAIDs are likely more effective than placebo for the management of neck pain and whiplash disorders, although those with cervical radiculopathy were not studied as a separate subgroup (168). A recent double-blind, placebo-controlled, randomized trial comparing the short-term effectiveness of oral prednisone to placebo demonstrated the effectiveness of a short course of prednisone in patients with cervical radiculopathy, although both the prednisone group and placebo group in this study received acetaminophen as well. Both groups had significantly reduced pain scores and improved functional scores from baseline. However, the prednisone group improved by a significantly greater amount (169). Medications that target the neuropathic component of cervical radiculopathy include tricyclic antidepressants (TCAs) such as amitriptyline and antiepileptic medications such as gabapentin and pregabalin (170). Studies evaluating the effectiveness of these medications in patients suffering from cervical radiculopathy specifically are lacking.

FIGURE 26-9. Sagittal **(A)** and successively sliced axial **(B)** MRI performed 1 month (1M), 3 months (3M), and 5 months (5M) after the onset of a C5 radiculopathy in a 56-year-old man. Radiographic regression of a lateral extrusion with superior and inferior extension is demonstrated. (Reprinted with permission from Mochida K, Komori H, Okawa A, et al. Regression of cervical disc Regression of cervical disc herniation observed on magnetic resonance images. *Spine.* 1998;23(9):990–997.)

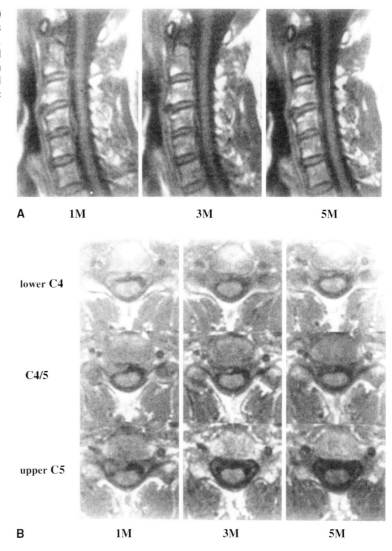

In a retrospective study of 26 consecutive patients treated nonsurgically, 20 achieved good to excellent results with an average of 2.3 years of follow-up with varied treatment regimens of oral analgesics, collars, traction, oral steroids, epidural injections, and physical therapy (171). In a prospective study of 155 patients with cervical radiculopathy, one third were treated surgically, whereas two thirds were prescribed medical treatment that included oral analgesics and steroids, traction, and epidural injection. At 1-year follow-up, significant improvements in pain and functional status were observed in both groups, with a greater degree of improvement in the surgical group. Twenty-six percent of the surgical group continued to experience severe pain (172). Lees and Turner studied 57 patients with a diagnosis of cervical radiculopathy for a period of up to 19 years (1). Patients in this study pursued a variety of treatments, including rest, manipulation, therapeutic exercise, and soft-collar use. Of these 57 patients, 45% described one primary pain episode without a future symptomatic recurrence. Of the remaining patients, 30% described a continuation of mild symptoms, and 25% reported a persistence of significant symptoms or worsening. Of the 57 patients, 32 remained significantly improved, whereas 18 described their condition as static or symptomatic. In their series of patients with radiculopathy, none became myelopathic.

Similar to axial neck pain, the physical therapy prescription and open communication between the prescribing physician and treating therapist are vital in the noninvasive, initial treatment of radicular neck pain. The patient's overall physical conditioning as well as strengthening of the cervical musculature should be addressed in a similar manner to axial neck pain. The McKenzie method is a commonly utilized physical therapy approach for cervical radiculopathy that enables the evaluating clinician to assign a directional preference of motion and instruct the patient in repetitive movements that can decrease spinal pain associated with soft-tissue dysfunctions, structural derangements, or postural syndromes (173). Treatment is based on the individual's signs and symptoms during the movement assessment. Specific spinal motion can affect the patient's baseline symptoms by increasing, decreasing, producing, abolishing, centralizing, or peripheralizing pain. It is also of particular importance to observe whether pain production is evident during a given movement or at end range. Information gathered from the initial mechanical assessment will enable the clinician to tailor the rehabilitation program to the patient's needs (173).

The goal of mobilization is to relieve pain and restore the normal range of motion of the involved soft tissues and joints (174). Mobilizations are often required to facilitate reduction of spinal derangements and can also expedite restoration of motion in spinal dysfunctions. There is evidence to suggest that manual diagnosis techniques may be more reliable if the treating clinician relies on provoking the patient's typical symptoms rather than relying on positional or palpatory findings alone (175–180). The therapist should continuously communicate with the patient in order to correlate pain provocation with the direction of mobilizing force and resistance.

Geoffery Maitland has described four grades of passive movement to restore spinal motion (181,182). Grade I mobilizations are performed using small oscillations at the beginning of range of motion. Grade II mobilizations are large oscillations that are performed during resistance-free range of motion. Grade III mobilizations are large oscillations performed at 50% of joint resistance during range of motion. Grade IV mobilizations are described as small oscillations similarly performed at 50% of joint resistance. A plus and minus system is also incorporated into this system to provide a specific grade of mobilization. Every plus or minus equals 25%; that is, a mobilization graded at 3+ is equivalent to a force of 75% of joint resistance while using large oscillations, and a grade of 3− is equivalent to a force of 25% of joint resistance while using large oscillations. However, similar to spinal manipulation, systematic reviews suggest that the literature supporting mobilization techniques are low to very low quality and thus should not be the focal point of a noninvasive, rehabilitation program for cervical radiculopathy (87).

Although soft cervical collars can improve patient comfort, long-term clinical outcomes are likely not affected by collar use (183,184). In the absence of significant instability, it has been recommended that collars not be used continually for greater than 72 hours because their use can lead to soft tissue tightening and a delay in range-of-motion restoration (184–186). Improperly fitted collars can also predispose patients to aberrant cervical motion and increase risk of secondary injury (187). The Neck Pain Task Force's best evidence synthesis found little to no benefit of cervical collars when these were compared to active therapies and rest (70).

Traction is often used in patients presenting with cervical radiculopathy. The literature is lacking a prospective, randomized, controlled study comparing traction with other rehabilitation approaches in the treatment of radiculopathy, and the efficacy of traction in improving treatment outcomes has not been demonstrated (188–192). A reduction in the signs and symptoms associated with spinal nerve root impingement has been reported with traction use, particularly if applied shortly after the onset of radicular pain (193). It has been suggested that if a sufficient traction force is applied, the size of the neural foramen may temporarily be increased, reducing pressure on a spinal nerve root and potentially contributing to the healing process (194–196). The clinician is encouraged to apply manual traction to assess the likely therapeutic response to force before introducing mechanical devices. The application of traction might only be considered in those patients unable to reduce radicular symptoms through more independent mechanical exercises.

Maximum posterior elongation of the cervical spine is achieved during traction when the neck and angle of pull are in a position of 24 degrees of flexion (197). Over-the-door traction units are properly used with the patient facing the door with 20 to 30 degrees of neck flexion (197,198). Home traction devices have also been designed to apply cervical distractive forces in the recumbent position, and these might allow for more secure and reproducible patient positioning. Mechanical traction may be administered statically, with a uniform force throughout the treatment session, or intermittently, with the force varying throughout the session. It is generally recommended that static traction be performed if the area being treated is more acutely inflamed, if the patient's symptoms are easily aggravated by motion, or if the patient's symptoms are related to disc protrusion (199). The force of traction should always be kept low during the initial traction session in order to decrease the risk of reactive muscle guarding and to further confirm if mechanical traction is appropriate. The recommended initial mechanical force for cervical traction is between 8 and 10 lb (74). Fifteen pounds of force will introduce muscle stretching, whereas 25 lb of force is the minimum force required to achieve vertebral separation. Cervical traction may be of additional benefit when combined with exercise (200). Traction use is contraindicated in patients with myelopathy, instability, and RA and should be introduced with caution in elderly patients who may be at greater risk for vascular injury (191,201).

Instruction in proper positioning at the work station represents an important component in the rehabilitation of patients with cervical disorders. Regardless of the therapeutic exercise program employed or the patient's diligence with home exercise efforts, sustained spinal posturing out of the neutral zone can lead to further aggravation of the affected tissues and a perpetuation of symptoms. The sedentary worker spending most of the day seated at a desk is more likely to encounter proper positioning challenges. In general, the patient should be instructed to avoid, whenever possible, those positions that typically aggravate his or her cervical or limb pain.

The recommended positioning at the desk or computer station is usually prescribed with approximately 90 degrees of hip, knee, and elbow flexion (202) (**Fig. 26-10**). Proper distance from the computer monitor is an arm's length measurement, which is unique to each individual. The upper third of the computer screen should be situated at eye level. Individuals that require bifocal eyeglasses should be instructed to position reading materials in such a fashion as to avoid sustained cervical extension postures (203). In addition, the wrist or elbow, and preferably both, should be maintained in a supported position. This support contributes to total neutral positioning of the body and ultimately can lead to decreased stresses on peripheral nerves passing through the elbow and carpal tunnel.

Cervical Injections for Radiculopathy

Cervical epidural steroid injections can be considered in cases of cervical radiculopathy with severe pain or symptoms that have failed to respond to an initial trial of spine-specific physical therapy, oral anti-inflammatory agents, and analgesics. There are two approaches for cervical injections, interlaminar and transforaminal (**Fig. 26-11**). Transforaminal injections offer the advantage of injecting the desired medication around the pain generating dorsal root ganglion (204). However, comparison studies between these two techniques in the cervical spine have demonstrated similar levels of efficacy (205). The interlaminar approach is thus preferred, although not exclusively used, given the risk of anterior spinal artery syndrome with the transforaminal approach (206).

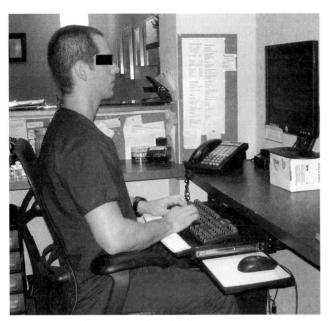

FIGURE 26-10. Correct ergonomic positioning.

The choice of steroid must also be considered prior to cervical injection. Dexamethasone, which is a nonparticulate steroid, is the only steroid formulation that has not been implicated in brain or spinal cord infarctions following cervical transforaminal epidural steroid injections (207,208). The FDA issued a black box warning for triamcinolone, which is a particulate steroid, in 2011 citing case reports of paralysis, stroke, and death when this steroid formulation was injected via a transforaminal approach into the cervical spine. Particulate steroid particles adhere together and may exceed the diameter

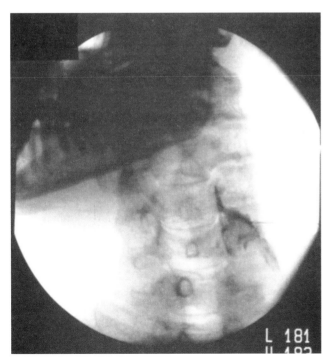

FIGURE 26-11. Contrast-enhanced left C6 transforaminal selective spinal injection.

of the spinal arteriole system, thus leading to vascular compromise. Nonparticulate steroids are more easily passed through the arterial system given their increased water solubility and are considered a safer and equally effective injectable medication for cervical indications.

Several of the studies on cervical epidural steroid injections have limitations. The 2000–2010 Neck Pain Task Force's best evidence synthesis on interventions for neck pain identified only one randomized controlled trial meeting their inclusion criteria (97). This study demonstrated potential short-term symptomatic improvement of cervical radicular symptoms with corticosteroids (209). A 2014 multi-center, randomized study comparing epidural steroid injections, conservative treatment, or combination treatment consisting of gabapentin and/or nortriptyline plus physical therapy for cervical radicular pain demonstrated short-term improvement of symptoms in the combination group, but these results were not sustained at 6 months (210). Overall, there is a lack of well-designed randomized controlled trials of cervical epidural injections under fluoroscopic guidance in treatment of radicular neck pain despite the frequency with which these procedures are performed.

Minor complications associated with cervical epidural injections include vasovagal reactions, transient neurologic deficits, hypersensitivity reactions and skin rashes. Major complications include the before mentioned anterior spinal artery syndrome, stroke, spinal cord injury, cortical blindness, seizures and bleeding. As a result of these potentially severe complications along with mixed evidence on efficacy, cervical injections are currently not approved by the Food and Drug Administration and are performed off label. Furthermore, the FDA issued a letter in 2014 warning about the potential serious adverse events of injections of corticosteroids into the epidural space throughout the spine and required the addition of a warning to the drug labels of injectable corticosteroids. (https://www.fda.gov/Drugs/DrugSafety/ucm394280.htm)

Surgical Treatment

For those patients whose debilitating pain persists despite a full trial of nonsurgical treatments, surgical intervention may be considered. Surgery should be considered without delay in those patients with a pronounced and rapidly progressive neurologic deficit. Significant weakness, atrophy, and numbness that present without pain are also relative indicators for surgical intervention (211,212). Anterior and posterior approaches have both been utilized for the operative treatment of radiculopathy with choice of procedure determined by patient anatomy, physician preference and type of nerve root compression.

Anterior cervical discectomy fusion (ACDF) and cervical disc arthroplasty (CDA) are both anterior approaches used in the treatment of cervical radiculopathy. Of these, ACDF is the more frequently utilized (213). The advantages of this approach include the ability to remove anteriorly offending structures without disturbing the cord, resultant neural foraminal distraction, distraction of the segment with an associated reduction in ligamentum flavum buckling, and segmental stabilization (29). Disadvantages of ACDF include graft donor site pain, the need for postprocedural immobilization, the possibility of graft dislodgement, and subsequent adjacent segment degeneration. When used for radiculopathy, ACDF has been described to result in excellent outcomes in 53% to 91% of patients. When compared to nonsurgical treatment, ACDF may offer more rapid symptom improvement, although long-term outcomes do not differ significantly (213–216). Multilevel surgery is associated with poorer outcomes (213–216). ACDF is contraindicated in patients with congenital stenosis, stenosis arising predominantly from posterior structures, and disease at greater than three levels (217). Furthermore, the risk of pseudoarthrosis increases with the number of levels included in the procedure (218).

Cervical disc replacement/arthroplasty (CDA) is a surgical technique that has increased recently given its advantage of maintaining cervical flexion and extension and thus potentially preventing the development of pseudoarthrosis, although studies comparing this technique to cervical fusion have yielded mixed results (218–220). Studies are exploring expanding CDA to multilevel radiculopathy (221). CDA and ACDF share common adverse effects, but CDA also carries a risk of heterotropic ossification, the clinical consequences of which have not been documented (222). Further studies on CDA with a wider variety of patients are needed to clarify the effectiveness and indications for this procedure as well as the incidence of severe adverse effects, such as displacement.

Laminoforaminotomy is an alternative posterior surgical approach to the patient with radiculopathy. This approach is particularly indicated in patients with lateral disc herniation or zygapophyseal joint arthrosis who present without significant neck or periscapular pain (29). The advantages with this approach include an avoidance of spinal destabilization and fusion-related complications. There is also no need for postoperative immobilization and vital anterior structures, such as the carotid and vertebral arteries, recurrent laryngeal nerve and esophagus are avoided (110). Disadvantages include a greater level of postoperative neck pain compared with ACDF during the recovery period and an inability to decompress the cord. This approach is contraindicated in patients with cord compression or cervical kyphosis. Success rates as high as 90% have been reported for this procedure in terms of improved pain, weakness, and function (223).

MYELOPATHY

Pathophysiology

Myelopathic symptoms occur when the spinal cord is affected by central canal stenosis. Disease entities that can present in a similar fashion to cervical myelopathy include motor neuron disease, multiple sclerosis, and other demyelinating conditions, peripheral and entrapment neuropathies, intracranial pathology, spinal cord tumors, or syrinxes (29). Neurologic symptoms of cervical myelopathy can arise during the cervical degenerative cascade from stenotic compromise of the central canal and spinal cord. Similar to findings in the lumbar spine, narrowing of the cervical central canal can arise from developmental abnormalities or acquired change. Cervical spondylosis remains the most common form of central canal compromise and resultant myelopathy. Disc space narrowing leads to a loss of the normal cervical lordosis and buckling of the posteriorly located ligamentum flavum. Calcification of the ligamentum

flavum resulting in myelopathy has also been documented (224). Combined with flaval buckling, osteophytes from the uncovertebral joints, zygapophyseal joints, and vertebral bodies contribute to the central canal compromise (225). Spinal cord compression arising from spondylosis is typically slowly progressive. Patients are often noted to have significant radiographic compression while remaining asymptomatic. The cord is apparently able to withstand significant chronic deformation without resultant dysfunction (226). In addition to direct compressive effects, dynamic stressors, vascular insufficiency, and ischemia likely contribute to the pathophysiology of myelopathy.

In cervical extension, the central canal diameter decreases, and the cord may be pinched between the anterior osteophytic vertebral bodies, discs, hypertrophied posterior elements and ligamentum flavum. During flexion, although the central canal may widen, the cord can become tethered over spondylotic anterior elements (225,226). Instability may also contribute to spinal cord impingement. As spinal segments are stiffened by spondylotic change, adjacent motion segments might also develop relative hypermobility and even subluxation. Myelopathy can also evolve in the setting of ossification of the posterior longitudinal ligament, which can occur at one or multiple levels. The ossified posterior longitudinal ligament can develop into a bulbous mass that contributes to anterior cord compression. Asian populations, such as the Japanese, have a particularly high incidence of ossification of the posterior longitudinal ligament as compared with other populations. The etiology of this condition remains less clear, but there is likely an associated genetic influence (226).

The corticospinal tracts are typically involved early in the evolution of myelopathy, resulting in lower-limb weakness. Subsequent posterior column dysfunction results in ataxia manifesting as a wide-based gait (29). A classification system has been proposed that includes five cervical myelopathic syndromes (227). According to this categorization, the most common presentation is the transverse lesion syndrome. In this scenario, the upper limbs are relatively spared with symptoms arising in the lower extremities from corticospinal tract, spinothalamic tract, and posterior column involvement. In the motor system syndrome, symptoms can resemble those of amyotrophic lateral sclerosis. In this scenario, the corticospinal tracts and anterior horn cells are affected by the compressive injury. The patient characteristically presents without sensory symptoms, and upper- and lower-limb weakness can present in combination with spasticity and gait disturbances. The third variant is a central cord syndrome, which is similar to the posttraumatic incomplete spinal cord injury. In these patients, upper-limb involvement predominates, and the prevailing hand weakness has a poor potential for recovery. The upper-limb syndrome of myelopathy has also been described as cervical spondylotic amyotrophy and myelopathy hand (228,229) (**Fig. 26-12**). In the fourth presentation, Brown-Sequard syndrome, unilateral cord compression and corticospinal tract involvement results in an ipsilateral hemiparesis, and spinothalamic tract compromise results in contralateral sensory disturbances. In the brachialgia cord syndrome, long tract signs present in combination with radicular pain arising from spinal nerve root compression (29,227).

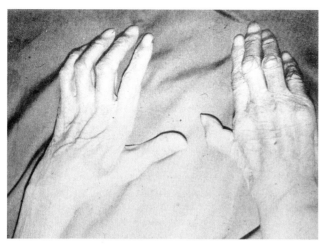

FIGURE 26-12. Amyotrophic hand of cervical spondylotic myelopathy. (Reprinted with permission from Ebara S, Yonenobu K, Fujiwara K, et al. Myelopathy hand characterized by muscle wasting: a different type of myelopathy hand in patients with cervical spondylosis. *Spine.* 1988;13(7):785–791.)

History

The clinical presentation of myelopathy can be quite variable (230). Patients commonly describe paresthesias that can occur in a fairly diffuse and nondermatomal distribution in the upper extremities. Many patients are not aware of their weakness but do describe subtle difficulties with balance and gait alteration. Gait and balance difficulties become more pronounced as cord compression and myelopathy become moderate to severe. Fine motor coordination of the hands is adversely affected and is manifested as difficulty manipulating buttons or handwriting abnormalities. Patients might report an inability to rapidly open and close the hand (231). Arm weakness may be unilateral or bilateral. Proximal lower-limb weakness usually prevails over a loss of more distal strength. For example, patients might describe difficulty arising from a chair, but a foot drop would be a rarer presentation. In this regard, cervical myelopathy presents distinctly to the weakness associated with lumbar spinal stenosis. Bowel and bladder abnormalities may occur in more severe compressive syndromes, but these are less common. Although patients may present with neck pain, as many as 50% will not. Furthermore, as many as 15% of individuals with more advanced myelopathy do not report cervical discomfort, often leading to a delayed diagnosis (226,227,232). Individuals with associated radicular involvement may be more likely to report upper-extremity pain (29).

Physical Examination

In examining the patient with suspected myelopathy, cervical extension may be restricted and painful for patients with cord or nerve root compression (226). L'Hermitte's sign, initially described in 1932, is performed by passively flexing the neck with the patient in the seated position and causing an electric-type sensation that progresses along the trunk and to the upper and lower limbs (233). This may be appreciated in 10% of patients with spondylotic myelopathy. A positive response can also be observed in individuals with multiple sclerosis and spinal tumors (227,234). Wasting of the shoulder girdle musculature might be appreciated in patients with stenosis at the C4-6 levels secondary to loss of local anterior

horn cell function. Similarly, fasciculations might be noted in the upper-limb musculature, and wasting of the intrinsic hand musculature may be observed (226).

The patient can be asked to hold the fingers extended and adducted. If the two ulnar digits are observed to flex and abduct within 30 to 60 seconds, this is referred to as a finger escape sign, which may be indicative of a myelopathic process. Additionally, the patient should be able to rapidly open and close the hand repetitively up to 20 times in a 10-second interval. A clumsier performance of this grip-and-release test may also be consistent with cervical cord compression (226). Sensory exam for sharp sensation in the upper and lower extremities can help to demonstrate both diffuse and dermatomal patterns of sensory loss. Vibratory testing, which assesses function of the posterior columns, might demonstrate abnormalities in the setting of more long-standing and severe myelopathy. Reflex testing may reveal hyperreflexia in both the upper and lower limbs. If there is associated cervical root compromise, hyporeflexia might be identified at the respective level in the upper extremities. Long tract signs can be found and include ankle clonus, a Babinski response, and Hoffmann's sign. The inverted radial reflex is another pathologic reflex that can be observed in the setting of myelopathy. Specifically, tapping the brachioradialis tendon results in a hypoactive brachioradialis reflex and hyperactive finger flexion. This is felt to represent cord compromise and a concomitant C5 root lesion resulting in spasticity distal to the level of compression and a hypoactive response at the level of nerve root involvement. In patients with more cephalad cord compromise, at the C3 level or above, a caudally directed tap on the acromion might result in a scapulohumeral reflex, marked by elevation of the scapula and abduction of the humerus (29,235).

Gait should also be assessed for the ability to heel and toe walk, as well as heel-to-toe ambulation. Romberg testing, during which the patient stands with the eyes closed and the arms held forward, is a test of position sense. Loss of balance during this exam maneuver may be consistent with posterior column dysfunction (226). If indicated, electrodiagnostic studies might prove helpful in distinguishing a myelopathic presentation from other potential diagnoses contributing to the constellation of symptoms.

Radiologic Findings

Although plain radiographs can demonstrate degenerative changes associated with aging and spondylosis, this imaging modality does not offer visualization of the neural elements. In lateral plain films of patients with cervical spondylosis, anterior osteophytes are often larger than those appreciated posteriorly but typically do not cause symptoms. Posterior osteophytes are more clinically relevant because of the possibility of associated neural compression. The presence of such plain film findings should be regarded with caution, as degenerative change is commonly observed in asymptomatic subjects and increases in frequency with increasing age. In certain cases, ossification of the posterior longitudinal ligament can be visualized on lateral images as a bar of bone extending along the posterior aspect of the vertebral bodies. Flexion-extension views are necessary to diagnose instability that may not be evident on a neutral lateral view (226).

The typical cervical lordosis measures 21 degrees, ±13 degrees. Cervical lordosis decreases with age and degenerative change. Additionally, 9% of asymptomatic individuals can demonstrate a cervical kyphosis. The normal adult cervical canal demonstrates a midsagittal diameter of 17 to 18 mm (range from 13 to 20 mm). This measurement is taken from a point at the posterior vertebral body margin to a corresponding point on the laminar line. Cord compromise is believed to occur when the central canal is narrowed to between 10 and 13 mm. At this stage, stenosis is defined as relative. Absolute stenosis is defined by a central canal with an anteroposterior dimension of less than 10 mm. Such canal compromise is highly correlated with spinal cord compression. Cervical extension maneuvers further reduce the canal diameter, and the cord can be dynamically compressed with such maneuvers.

The most accurate means of determining spinal canal dimensions is by CT scan. Ratios have also been described that compare the central canal size to the width of the vertebral body. A ratio of less than 0.85 has been defined as consistent with stenosis, with a ratio of less than 0.8 predisposing the patient to myelopathy. It is believed that such comparisons of vertebral body and canal dimensions are not as reliable in larger individuals (29,63,236,237). MRI is the standard imaging modality in the assessment of patients with cervical myelopathy. The advantages of MRI imaging include superior visualization of the disc and neural elements, as well as the ability to visualize intrinsic changes within the cord (29). Cord atrophy might be observed in cases of more long-standing cord compression; MRI also allows for identification of parenchymal changes, such as syrinx formation and abnormal signal within the cord, which may be representative of myelomalacia (**Fig. 26-13**). The disadvantages of MRI include a more limited visualization of the neural foramen and a relative inability to distinguish between soft and hard disc materials

and an ossified posterior longitudinal ligament. Therefore, some practitioners prefer CT myelography, which can offer greater differentiation of soft-tissue and osseous structures in the assessment of patients with cervical disorders (29).

Abnormal signal within the cord does not necessarily correlate with clinical outcome, but it does serve to identify pathologic cord change (226). Increased T2 cord signal likely represents a wide spectrum of compressive pathology and is not considered a useful predictor of clinical outcome (238–240). In patients with significant upper-limb weakness and atrophy, also known as cervical spondylotic amyotrophy, high T2 signal intensity has been observed within the cord in the region of the anterior horn cells (**Fig. 26-14**). Such findings suggest that the lower motor neuron component, including upper-limb weakness and atrophy, in these individuals might arise from anterior horn cell damage induced by dynamic cord compression and circulatory compromise (228).

Pathologic cord findings from myelopathic patients include white and gray matter destruction with demyelinating changes ascending and descending from the site of injury (225,226). An examination of pathologic specimens and correlation with the degree of cord compression has revealed degeneration of the lateral white mater tracts in mild to moderate compression and necrosis of the central gray matter in more severe compressive injuries. Interestingly, the anterior white columns remain relatively spared, even in more severe cord compression. Histologic changes observed include axonal demyelination followed by cell body necrosis and scarring or gliosis. Cystic cavitation can also be observed within the gray matter. This central destruction is believed to arise from ischemic changes arising from cord deformation (241). Bulging disc material and anteriorly located spurs might also compress the anterior

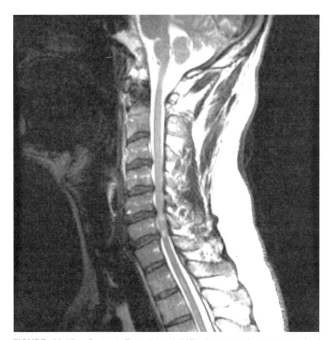

FIGURE 26-13. Sagittal T2-weighted MRI demonstrating a neutralized lordosis and cord compression from C5-6 to C6-7, with associated increased signal intensity within the cord inferior to the C5-6 disc and posterior to the intervertebral disc space at C6-7. (Reprinted from Kim DH, Vaccaro AR. Surgical treatment of cervical myelopathy. In: Slipman CS, Derby R, Simeone FA, et al., eds. *Interventional Spine—An Algorithmic Approach.* Philadelphia, PA; 2008:753–766. Copyright © 2008 Elsevier. With permission.)

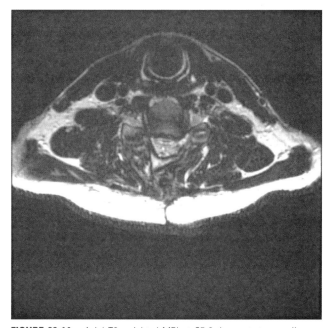

FIGURE 26-14. Axial T2-weighted MRI at C5-6 demonstrates small areas of high-signal intensity within the spinal cord, inclusive of the regions of the bilateral anterior horn cells. (Reprinted from Kim DH, Vaccaro AR. Surgical treatment of cervical myelopathy. In: Slipman CS, Derby R, Simeone FA, et al., eds. *Interventional Spine—An Algorithmic Approach.* Philadelphia, PA; 2008:753–766. Copyright © 2008 Elsevier. With permission.)

spinal artery, contributing to a vascular myelopathy (225,226). The vascular supply to the gray matter has been shown to arise from arterioles branching from the anterior spinal artery. With compression of the cord in the anterior to posterior plane, these branches are subject to mechanical distortion, which can lead to relative ischemia of the gray and medial white matter (242). Atherosclerosis and intimal fibrosis have also been observed in the regional spinal arteries (226).

Natural History

The natural history of cervical myelopathy is variable. Certain patients experience a progressive deterioration, while others experience static symptoms for months to years. Age greater than 60 years as well as bilateral and more severe myelopathic symptoms at initial presentation are associated with worse prognosis and more rapid progression (243–245).

Patients with radiologic evidence of cord compression, but no signs of myelopathy, can be observed and monitored both clinically and radiologically. There is no evidence that minor trauma is a risk factor for cord compromise in patients with radiographic evidence of cervical spondylotic myelopathy (162). For those individuals with milder myelopathic symptoms, such as hyperreflexia and subtle gait abnormalities, the anticipated clinical course suggested by the literature should be reviewed with the patient. If the patient has not demonstrated a progressive deterioration, there may be a role for nonoperative management with neurologic reevaluation every 6 to 12 months (153). However, nonoperative interventions, such as medications, immobilization, physical therapy, and spinal injections have not been shown to be beneficial for cervical myelopathy (162).

Surgical Treatment

Most authors recommend surgical intervention for patients with moderate to severe myelopathy, although a 2013 prospective multicenter study of surgical decompression for cervical spondylotic myelopathy demonstrated improved neurologic and functional outcomes as well as quality of life for surgical patients regardless of disease severity (246). For patients with similar levels of myelopathic symptoms, operative intervention might be recommended earlier in those individuals with more pronounced radiologic abnormalities, including cord atrophy, abnormal cord signal, or cervical kyphosis. The degree of ultimate recovery typically correlates with the severity of preoperative myelopathy, in addition to larger transverse cord area, younger age, single rather than multiple levels of involvement, and shorter symptom duration (226,232,243).

Both anterior and posterior surgical approaches have been employed in the treatment of cervical myelopathy. Similar to cervical radiculopathy, ACDF is the most utilized anterior approach for cervical myelopathy. Expected outcomes after ACDF in cases of cervical myelopathy include improved ambulation, increased upper-extremity strength, and overall motor recovery (226,232). Posterior approach options include multilevel laminectomy, laminectomy with fusion, and laminoplasty. These approaches are indicated in multilevel cord compression without kyphosis. Posterior approaches produce larger increases in spinal canal diameter and decrease the risk of dysphagia but were associated with greater postoperative neck pain when compared to anterior approaches (247). The surgical approach to the myelopathic patient is determined by the nature of the central canal compromise and the experience of the treating surgeon. Factors considered in choosing the most appropriate procedure include the number of pathologic levels, the sagittal alignment of the cervical spine, the location of the compressive lesion, and the presence of instability (222).

SUMMARY

Disorders of the cervical spine are a significant source of functional decline and disability. While numerous interventional and surgical techniques are available for axial neck pain and cervical radiculopathy, an initial noninvasive approach with an emphasis on physical therapy, strengthening exercises, and correction of improper biomechanics with modalities and oral analgesics as needed remains first line. More well-designed studies are needed to fully evaluate the efficacy and safety profile of epidural steroid injections for cervical axial pain and cervical radiculopathy. Cervical myelopathy represents a more severe manifestation of cervical pathology, with no current evidence advocating for noninvasive approaches when treatment is needed. The cervical spine is a complex structure with a variety of associated pathologies, and optimal treatment will require additional research to maximize function and limit associated disability.

REFERENCES

1. Lees F, Turner JWA. Natural history and prognosis of cervical spondylosis. *Br Med J.* 1963;2:1607–1610.
2. Gore DR, Sepic SB, Gardner GM, et al. Neck pain: a long term follow up of 205 patients. *Spine.* 1987;12:1–5.
3. Bernhardt M, Hynes RA, Blum HW, et al. Cervical spondylotic myelopathy. *J Bone Joint Surg.* 1993;75A:119–128.
4. Krag MH. Biomechanics of the cervical spine: I. General trauma. In: Frymoyer JW, ed. *The Adult Spine—Principles and Practice.* 2nd ed. Philadelphia, PA: Lippincott-Raven; 1997:1075–1119.
5. Smith MD, Phillips WA, Hensinger RN. Complications of fusion to the upper cervical spine. *Spine.* 1991;16(7):702–706.
6. Schneiderman GA, Hambly M. Spinal orthoses. In: Hochschuler SH, Cutler HB, Guyer RD, eds. *Rehabilitation of the Spine—Science and Practice.* St. Louis, MO: Mosby; 1993:213–222.
7. Rogers C, Joshi A, Dreyfuss P. Cervical intrinsic disc pain and radiculopathy. *Spine State Art Rev.* 1998;12(2):323–356.
8. Oliver J, Middleditch A. *Functional Anatomy of the Spine.* Oxford: Butterworth-Heinemann Ltd, Reed International Books; 1991.
9. An HS. Anatomy of the cervical spine. In: An HS, ed. *Surgery of the Cervical Spine.* Baltimore, MD: Lippincott Williams & Wilkins; 1994:1–39.
10. Hartman RA, Tisherman RE, Wang C, et al. Mechanical role of the posterior column components in the cervical spine. *Eur Spine J.* 2016;25(7):2129–2138.
11. Leckie S, Sowa G. Emerging technologies for degenerative disk disease: potential synergy between biochemical signaling and spinal biomechanics. *PM R.* 2009;1(5):466–470.
12. Bogduk N. The innervation of the cervical intervertebral discs. *Spine.* 1988;13:2–8.
13. Ferlic DC. The nerve supply of the cervical intervertebral discs in man. *Bull Johns Hopkins Hosp.* 1963;113:347–351.
14. Bogduk N. Innervation and pain patterns of the cervical spine. In: Grant R, ed. *Clinics of Physical Therapy: Physical Therapy of the Cervical and Thoracic Spine.* 2nd ed. New York: Churchill Livingstone; 1994:65–76.
15. Urban JP, Holm S, Maroudas A, et al. Nutrition of the intervertebral disc: effect of fluid flow on solute transport. *Clin Orthop.* 1982;170:296–302.
16. Taylor JR, Twomey LT. Vertebral column development and its relation to adult pathology. *Aust J Physiother.* 1985;31:83.
17. DeLucca JF, Cortes DH, Jacobs NT, et al. Human cartilage endplate permeability varies with degeneration and intervertebral disc site. *J Biomech.* 2016;49(4):550–557.
18. Lord SM, Barnsley L, Bogduk N. Cervical zygapophyseal joint pain in whiplash injuries. *Spine State Art Rev.* 1998;12(2):301–322.
19. Mercer S, Bogduk N. Intra-articular inclusions of the cervical synovial joints. *Br J Rheumatol.* 1993;32:705–710.
20. Nowitzke A, Westaway M, Bogduk N. Cervical zygapophyseal joints: geometrical parameters and relationship to cervical kinematics. *Clin Biomech.* 1994;9:342–348.
21. Dvorak J, Panjabi M, Gerber D, et al. Functional diagnostics of the rotary instability of the upper cervical spine: an experimental study in cadavers. *Spine.* 1987;12:187.
22. Dvorak J, Panjabi M, Novotny J, et al. In vivo flexion/extension of the normal cervical spine. *J Orthop Res.* 1991;9:828–834.
23. Mestdagh H. Morphological aspects and biomechanical properties of the vertebroaxial joint (C2-3). *Acta Morphol Neerl Scand.* 1976;14:19–30.

24. Lind B, Schlbom H, Nordwall A, et al. Normal range of motion in cervical spine. *Arch Phys Med Rehabil*. 1989;70:692–695.

25. White AA, Panjabi MM. Update on the evaluation of instability of the lower cervical spine. *Instr Course Lect*. 1987;36:513–530.

26. Bland JH. *Disorders of the Cervical Spine*. Philadelphia, PA: WB Saunders; 1987.

27. Bogduk N. Local anesthetic blocks of the second cervical ganglion: a technique with application in occipital headache. *Cephalalgia*. 1981;1:41–50.

28. Bogduk N. The clinical anatomy of the cervical dorsal rami. *Spine*. 1982;7:319–330.

29. Truumees E, Herkowitz HN. Cervical spondylotic myelopathy and radiculopathy. *Instr Course Lect*. 2000;49:339–360.

30. Adams CB, Logue V. Studies in cervical spondylotic myelopathy. *Brain*. 1971;94:557–594.

31. Friberg S, Hirsch C. Anatomical and clinical studies on lumbar disc degeneration. *Acta Orthop Scand*. 1949;19:222–242.

32. Harris RI, MacNab I. Structural changes in the lumbar intervertebral discs: their relationship to low back pain and sciatica. *J Bone Joint Surg*. 1954;36B:304–322.

33. Crock HV. A reappraisal of intervertebral disc lesions. *Med J Aust*. 1970;1:983.

34. Cloward RB. Cervical discography: a contribution to the aetiology and mechanism of neck, shoulder, and arm pain. *Ann Surg*. 1959;150:1052.

35. Kang JD, Georgescu HI, McIntyre-Larkin L, et al. Herniated cervical intervertebral discs spontaneously produce matrix metalloproteinases, nitric oxide, interleukin 6, and prostaglandin E2. *Spine*. 1995;20:2373–2378.

36. Ito K, Creemers L. Mechanisms of intervertebral disk degeneration/injury and pain: a review. *Global Spine J*. 2013;3(3):145–152.

37. Bogduk N. Neck pain: an update. *Aust Fam Physician*. 1988;17:75.

38. Grubb SA, Kelley CK. Cervical discography: clinical implications from 12 years of experience. *Spine*. 2000;25(11):1382–1389.

39. Schellhas KP, Smith MD, Gundry CR, et al. Cervical discogenic pain: prospective correlation of magnetic resonance imaging and discography in asymptomatic subjects and pain sufferers. *Spine*. 1996;21(3):300–312.

40. Nordin M, Carragee EJ, Hogg-Johnson S. Assessment of neck pain and its associated disorders: results of the Bone and Joint Decade 2000-2010 Task Force on Neck Pain and Its Associated Disorders. *Spine*. 2008;33(4):S101–S122.

41. Sarrami P, Armstrong E, Naylor JM, et al. Factors predicting outcome in whiplash injury: a systematic meta-review of prognostic factors. *J Orthop Traumatol*. 2017;18(1):9–16.

42. Lord SM, Barnsley L, Wallis BJ, et al. Third occipital nerve headache: a prevalence study. *J Neurol Neurosurg Psychiatry*. 1994;57:1187–1190.

43. Barnsely L, Lord SM, Wallis BJ, et al. The prevalence of chronic cervical zygapophyseal joint pain after whiplash. *Spine*. 1995;20:20–26.

44. Lord SM, Barnsley L, Wallis BJ, et al. Chronic cervical zygapophyseal joint pain after whiplash: a placebo-controlled prevalence study. *Spine*. 1996;21:1737–1745.

45. Aprill C, Dwyer A, Bogduk N. Cervical zygapophyseal joint pain patterns. II. A clinical evaluation. *Spine*. 1990;15:458–461.

46. Dwyer A, Aprill C, Bogduk N. Cervical zygapophyseal joint pain patterns. I. A study in normal volunteers. *Spine*. 1990;15:453–457.

47. Fukui S, Ohesto K, Shiotani M, et al. Referred pain distribution of the cervical zygapophyseal joints and cervical dorsal rami. *Pain*. 1996;68:79–83.

48. Bogduk B. On the rational use of diagnostic blocks for spinal pain. *Neurosurg Quart*. 2009;19(2):88–100.

49. Mehnert MJ, Freedman MK. Update on the role of z-joint injection and radiofrequency neurotomy for cervicogenic headache. *PM R*. 2013;5:221–227.

50. Ehni GE, Benner B. Occipital neuralgia and the C1-2 arthrosis syndrome. *J Neurosurg*. 1984;61:961–965.

51. McCormick CA. Arthrography of the atlanto-axial (C1-2) joints: techniques and results. *J Intervent Radiol*. 1987;2:9–13.

52. Dreyfuss P, Michaelson M, Fletcher D. Atlanto-occipital and lateral atlantoaxial joint pain patterns. *Spine*. 1994;19:1125–1131.

53. Binet EF, Moro JJ, Marangola JP, et al. Cervical spine tomography in trauma. *Spine*. 1977;2:163–172.

54. Abel MS. Moderately severe whiplash injuries of the cervical spine and their roentgenologic diagnosis. *Clin Orthop*. 1958;12:189–208.

55. Woodring JH, Goldstein SJ. Fractures of the articular process of the cervical spine. *Am J Roentgenol*. 1982;139:341–344.

56. Jonsson H Jr, Bring G, Rausching W, et al. Hidden cervical spine injuries in traffic accident victims. *J Spinal Disord*. 1991;4:251–263.

57. Taulor JR, Twomey LT. Acute injuries to cervical joints: an autopsy study of neck sprain. *Spine*. 1993;18:1115–1122.

58. Wickstrom J, Martinez JL, Rodriguez R Jr. The cervical sprain syndrome: experimental acceleration injuries to the head and neck. In: Selzer ML, Gikas PW, Huelke DF, eds. *The Prevention of Highway Injury*. Ann Arbor, MI: Highway Safety Research Institute; 1967:182–187.

59. Buonocore E, Hartman JT, Nelson CL. Cineradiograms of cervical spine in diagnosis of soft tissue injuries. *JAMA*. 1966;198:143–147.

60. Feinstein B. Referred pain from paravertebral structures. In: Buerger AA, Tobis JS, eds. *Approaches to the Validation of Manipulative Therapy*. Springfield, IL: Charles C. Thomas; 1977:139–174.

61. Deng YC. Anthropomorphic dummy neck modeling and injury considerations. *Accid Anal Prev*. 1989;21:85–100.

62. Boden SD, McCowin PR, Davis DO, et al. Abnormal magnetic-resonance scans of the cervical spine in asymptomatic subjects. A prospective investigation. *J Bone Joint Surg Am*. 1990;72(8):1178–1184.

63. Gore DR, Sepic SB, Gardner GM. Roentgenographic findings of the cervical spine in asymptomatic people. *Spine*. 1986;11(6):521–524.

64. Garfin SR. Cervical degenerative disorders: etiology, presentation, and imaging studies. *Instr Course Lect*. 2000;49:335–338.

65. Teresi LM, Lufkin RB, Reicher MA, et al. Asymptomatic degenerative disk disease and spondylosis of the cervical spine: MR imaging. *Radiology*. 1987;164(1):83–88.

66. Peh WCG. Provocative discography: current status. *Biomed Imaging Interv J*. 2005;1(1):e2.

67. Malik KM, Cohen SP, Walega DR. Diagnostic criteria and treatment of discogenic pain: a systematic review of recent clinical literature. *Spine*. 2013;13(11):1675–1689.

68. Onyewu O, Manchikanti L, Falco FJ. An update of the appraisal of the accuracy and utility of cervical discography in chronic neck pain. *Pain Physician*. 2012;15(6):E777–E806.

69. Castaldo M, Catena A, Chiarotto A. Do subjects with whiplash-associated disorders respond differently in the short-term to manual therapy and exercise than those with mechanical neck pain? *Pain Med*. 2017;18:791–803. doi:10.1093/pm/pnw266.

70. Hurwitz EL, Carragee EJ, van der Velde G. Treatment of neck pain: noninvasive interventions: results of the Bone and Joint Decade 2000-2010 Task Force on Neck Pain and Its Associated Disorders. *Spine*. 2008;33(4):S123–S152.

71. Kay TM, Gross A, Goldsmith C, et al. Exercises for mechanical neck disorders. *Cochrane Database Syst Rev*. 2005;(3):CD004250.

72. Chiu TT, Lam TH, Hedley AJ. A randomized controlled trial of the efficacy of exercise for patients with chronic neck pain. *Spine*. 2004;30(1):E1–E7.

73. Arimi A, Bandpei MA, Javanshir K. The effect of different exercise programs on sive and function of deep cervical flexor muscles in patients with chronic nonspecific neck pain: a systematic review of randomized controlled trials. *Am J Phys Med Rehabil*. 2017;96(8):582–588. doi:10.1097/PHM.0000000000000721.

74. Cameron MH. *Physical Agents in Rehabilitation*. Philadelphia, PA: W.B. Saunders Company; 1999.

75. Lehmann JF, Delateur BJ. Therapeutic heat. In: Lehmann JF, ed. *Therapeutic Heat and Cold*. 4th ed. Baltimore, MD: Lippincott Williams & Wilkins; 1990.

76. Rennie GA, Michlovitz SL. Biophysical principles of heating and superficial heating agents. In: Michlovitz SL, ed. *Thermal Agents in Rehabilitation*. Philadelphia, PA: FA Davis; 1996.

77. Fountain FP, Gersten JW, Senger O. Decrease in muscle spasm produced by ultrasound, hot packs and IR. *Arch Phys Med Rehabil*. 1960;41:293–299.

78. Falco F, Malanga G. Rehabilitation of whiplash injuries. *Spine State Art Rev*. 1998;12(2):453–467.

79. Lehmann J, DeLauter BJ. Diathermy and superficial heat and cold therapy. In: Kottke EJ, Stillwell GK, Lehmann JF, eds. *Krusen's Handbook of Physical Medicine and Rehabilitation*. Philadelphia, PA: WB Saunders; 1982:275–350.

80. Robertson VJ, Baker KG. A review of therapeutic ultrasound: effectiveness studies. *Phys Ther*. 2001;81(7):1339–1350.

81. Laslett M. Use of manipulative therapy for mechanical pain of spinal origin. *Orthop Rev*. 1987;16:8.

82. Roeske R. The new vertebral subluxation. *J Chiropractic*. 1993;30:19–24.

83. Miller R, Burton R. Stroke following chiropractic manipulation of the spine. *JAMA*. 1974;229:189.

84. Senstad O, Leboeuf-Yde C, Borchgrevink C. Predictors of side effects to spinal manipulative therapy. *J Manipulative Physiol Ther*. 1996;19(7):441–445.

85. Michaeli A. Reported occurrence and nature of complications following manipulative therapy in South Africa. *Aust J Physiother*. 1993;39(4):309–315.

86. Haldeman S, Kohlbeck FJ, McGregor M. Stroke, cerebral artery dissection, and cervical spine manipulation therapy. *J Neurol*. 2002;249(8):1098–1104.

87. Gross A, Langevin P, Burnie SJ. Manipulation and mobilization for neck pain contrasted against an inactive control or another active treatment. *Cochrane Database Syst Rev*. 2015;(9):CD004249.

88. Witt CM, Jena S, Brinkhaus B. Acupuncture for patients with chronic neck pain. *Pain*. 2006;125(1–2):98–106.

89. Willich SN, Reinhold T, Selim D. Cost-effectiveness of acupuncture treatment in patients with chronic neck pain. *Pain*. 2006;125(1–2):107–112.

90. Irnich D, Behrens N, Gleditsch JM. Immediate effects of dry needling and acupuncture at distant points in chronic neck pain: results of a randomized, double-blind, sham-controlled crossover trial. *Pain*. 2002;99(1–2):83–89.

91. Manchikanti L, Nampiaparampil DE, Candido KD, et al. Do cervical epidural injections provide long-term relief in neck and upper extremity pain? A systematic review. *Pain Physician*. 2015;18(1):39–60.

92. Manchikanti L, Cash KA, Pampati V. Two-year follow-up results of fluoroscopic cervical epidural injections in chronic axial or discogenic neck pain: a randomized, double-blind, controlled trial. *Int J Med Sci*. 2014;11(4):309–320.

93. Lee JH, Lee SH. Comparison of clinical efficacy between interlaminar and transforaminal epidural injection in patients with axial neck pain due to cervical disc herniation. *Medicine*. 2016;95(4):E2568.

94. Lord SM, Barnsley L, Bogduk N. Percutaneous radiofrequency neurotomy in the treatment of cervical zygapophyseal joint pain: a caution. *Neurosurgery*. 1995;36:732–739.

95. Bogduk N, Govind J. Cervicogenic headache: an assessment of the evidence on clinical diagnosis, invasive tests, and treatment. *Lancet Neurol*. 2009;8(10):959–968.

96. Eichenberger U, Greher M, Kapral S. Sonographic visualization and ultrasound-guided block of the third occipital nerve: prospective for a new method to diagnose C2-C3 zygapophysial joint pain. *Anesthesiology*. 2006;104(2):303–308.

97. Carragee EJ, Hurwitz EL, Cheng I. Treatment of neck pain: injections and surgical interventions: results of the Bone and Joint Decade 2000-2010 Task Force on Neck Pain and Its Associated Disorders. *Spine*. 2008;33(4 suppl):S153–S169.

98. Ellenberg MR, Honet JC, Treanor WJ. Cervical radiculopathy. *Arch Phys Med Rehabil*. 1994;75:342–352.

99. Ockene IS, Shay MJ, Alpert JS, et al. Unexplained chest wall pain in patients with normal coronary arteriograms. *N Engl J Med.* 1980;3030:1249–1252.
100. Mixter WJ, Ayer JB. Herniation or rupture of the intervertebral disc into the spinal canal. *N Engl J Med.* 1935;9:386–393.
101. Semmes RE, Murphy MF. The syndrome of unilateral rupture of the sixth cervical intervertebral disk with compression of the seventh cervical nerve root: a report of four cases with symptoms simulating coronary disease. *JAMA.* 1943;121:1209–1214.
102. Kondo K, Molgaard CA, Kurland LT, et al. Protruded intervertebral cervical disk: incidence and affected cervical level: Rochester, Minnesota, 1950 through 1974. *Minn Med.* 1981;64(12):751–753.
103. Heiskari M. Comparative retrospective study of patients operated for cervical disc herniation and spondylosis. *Ann Clin Res.* 1986;18(47):57–63.
104. Odom GL, Finney W, Woodhall B. Cervical disk lesions. *JAMA.* 1958;166:23–38.
105. Honet JC, Puri K. Cervical radiculitis: treatment an results in 82 patients. *Arch Phys Med Rehabil.* 1976;57:12–16.
106. Yoss RE, Corbin KB, McCarthy CS, et al. Significance of symptoms and signs in localization of involved root in cervical disc protrusion. *Neurology.* 1957;7:673–683.
107. Hunt WE, Miller CA. Management of cervical radiculopathy. *Clin Neurosurg.* 1986;33(29):485–502.
108. Yu YL, Woo E, Huang CY. Cervical spondylitic myelopathy and radiculopathy. *Acta Neurol Scand.* 1987;75:367–373.
109. Adams C. Cervical spondylotic radiculopathy and myelopathy. In: Vinken PJ, Bruyn GW, eds. *Handbook of Clinical Neurology.* Amsterdam: North-Holland; 1977:97–112.
110. Dillan W, Booth R, Cuckler J, et al. Cervical radiculopathy: a review. *Spine.* 1986;11:988–991.
111. Stookey B. Compression of spinal cord and nerve roots by herniation of the nucleus pulposus in the cervical region. *Arch Surg.* 1940;40:417–432.
112. Rothman RH, Marvel JP Jr. The acute cervical disc. *Clin Orthop.* 1975;109:59–68.
113. Appel B. Nomenclature and classification of lumbar disc pathology. *Neuroradiology.* 2001;43(12):1124–1125.
114. Simpson JM, An HS. Degenerative disc disease of the cervical spine. In: An HS, Simpson JS, eds. *Surgery of the Cervical Spine.* London: Martin Dunitz; 1994: 181–194.
115. Marshall LL. Chemical irritation of nerve root in disc prolapse. *Lancet.* 1973;2:230.
116. Rydevik B, Brown MD, Lundborg G. Pathoanatomy and pathophysiology of nerve root compression. *Spine.* 1984;9:7–15.
117. Howe JF, Loeser JD, Calvin WH. Mechanosensitivity of dorsal root ganglia and chronically injured axons: a physiologic basis for the radicular pain of nerve root compression. *Pain.* 1977;3:25–41.
118. Olmarker K, Rydevik B, Nordburg C. Autologous nucleus pulposus induces neurophysiologic and histologic changes in porcine cauda equina nerve roots. *Spine.* 1993;18:1425–1432.
119. Lee HM, Weinstein JN, Meller ST, et al. The role of steroids and their effects on phospholipase A2: an animal model of radiculopathy. *Spine.* 1998;23:1191–1196.
120. Lundsford LD, Bissonette DJ, Jannetta PJ, et al. Anterior surgery for cervical disc disease. Part 1: treatment of lateral cervical disc herniation in 253 cases. *J Neurosurg.* 1980;53:1–11.
121. Nachlas IW. Pseudo-angina pectoris originating in the cervical spine. *JAMA.* 1934;103:323.
122. Booth RE Jr, Rothman RH. Cervical angina. *Spine.* 1976;1:28–32.
123. LeBan MM, Meerschaert JR, Taylor RS. Breast pain: a symptom of cervical radiculopathy. *Arch Phys Med Rehabil.* 1979;60:315–317.
124. Keegan JJ, Garrett FD. The segmental distribution of the cutaneous nerves in the limbs of man. *Anat Rec.* 1948;102:409–437.
125. Foerster O. The dermatomes in man. *Brain.* 1933;102:1–39.
126. Slipman CW, Plastaras CT, Palmitier RA, et al. Symptom provocation of fluoroscopically guided cervical nerve root stimulation: are dynatomal maps identical to dermatomal maps? *Spine.* 1998;23(20):2235–2242.
127. Moriishi J, Otani K, Tanaka K, et al. The intersegmental anastomoses between spinal nerve roots. *Anat Rec.* 1989;224:110–116.
128. Schwartz HG. Anastomoses between cervical nerve roots. *Neurosurgery.* 1956;13:190–194.
129. Tanaka N. The anatomic relation among nerve roots, intervertebral foramina, and intervertebral discs of the cervical spine. *Spine.* 2000;25:286–291.
130. Frykholm HJ, Norlen G, Skoglund CR. On pain sensations produced by stimulation of ventral roots in man. *Acta Physiol Scand.* 1953;29(S106):455.
131. Favero KJ, Hawkins RH, Jones MW. Neuralgic amyotrophy. *J Bone Joint Surg.* 1987;69B:195–198.
132. England JD, Sumner AJ. Neuralgic amyotrophy: an increasingly diverse entity. *Muscle Nerve.* 1987;10:60–68.
133. Dyck PJ, Thomas PK, Lambert EH, et al., eds. *Peripheral Neuropathy.* 2nd ed. Philadelphia, PA: Saunders; 1984.
134. Modic MT, Masaryk TJ, Ross JS, eds. *Magnetic Resonance Imaging of the Spine.* New York: Yearbook; 1989.
135. Spurling RG, Scoville WB. Lateral rupture of the cervical intervertebral discs: a common cause of shoulder and arm pain. *Surg Gynecol Obstet.* 1944;78:350–358.
136. Viikari-Juntura E, Porras M, Laasonen EM. Validity of clinical tests in the diagnosis of root compression in cervical disc disease. *Spine.* 1989;14:253–257.
137. Davidson RI, Dunn EJ, Metzmaker JN. The shoulder abduction test in the diagnosis of radicular pain in cervical extradural compressive monoradiculopathies. *Spine.* 1981;6:441–446.
138. Beatty RM, Fowler FD, Hanson EJ Jr. The abducted arm as a sign of ruptured cervical disc. *Neurosurgery.* 1987;21:731–732.
139. Butler DS. Adverse mechanical torsion in the nervous system: a model for assessment and treatment. *Aust J Physiother.* 1989;35(4):227–238.
140. Lohman CM, Gilbert KK, Sobczak S, et al. 2015 young investigator award winner: cervical nerve root displacement and strain during upper limb neural tension testing. *Spine.* 2015;40(11):793–800.
141. Rubinstein SM, Pool JJM, Maurits W, et al. A systematic review of the diagnostic accuracy of provocative tests of the neck for diagnosing cervical radiculopathy. *Eur Spine J.* 2007;16:307–309.
142. Manelfe C. Imaging of the spine and spinal cord. *Radiology.* 1991;3:5–15.
143. Daniels DL, Grogan JP, Johansen JG, et al. Cervical radiculopathy: computed tomography and myelography compared. *Radiology.* 1984;151:109–113.
144. Modic MT, Masaryk TJ, Mulopulos GP, et al. Cervical radiculopathy: prospective evaluation with surface coil MR imaging, CT with metrizamide, and metrizamide myelography. *Radiology.* 1986;161:753–759.
145. Larsson E-M, Holtas S, Cronqvist S, et al. Comparison of myelography, CT myelography and magnetic resonance imaging in cervical spondylosis and disk herniation: pre- and postoperative findings. *Acta Radiol.* 1989;30:233–239.
146. Nakstad PH, Hald JK, Bakke SJ, et al. MRI in cervical disk herniation. *Neuroradiology.* 1989;31:382–385.
147. Wilson DW, Pezzuti RT, Place JN. Magnetic resonance imaging in the preoperative evaluation of cervical radiculopathy. *Neurosurgery.* 1991;28:175–179.
148. Boden SD, McCowin PR, Davis DO, et al. Abnormal magnetic resonance scans of the cervical spine in asymptomatic subjects: a prospective investigation. *J Bone Joint Surg.* 1990;72A:1178–1184.
149. Hitselberger WE, Witten RM. Abnormal myelograms in asymptomatic patients. *J Neurosurg.* 1968;28:204–206.
150. Simon JE, Lukin RR. Diskogenic disease of the cervical spine. *Semin Roentgenol.* 1988;23(2):118–124.
151. Bates D, Ruggieri P. Imaging modalities for evaluation of the spine. *Radiol Clin North Am.* 1991;29(4):675–690.
152. Maigne JY, Deligne L. Computed tomographic follow-up study of 21 cases of nonoperatively treated cervical intervertebral soft disc herniation. *Spine.* 1994;19:189–191.
153. Bush K, Chaudhuri R, Hillier S, et al. The pathomorphologic changes that accompany the resolution of cervical radiculopathy: a prospective study with repeat magnetic resonance imaging. *Spine.* 1997;22(2):183–187.
154. Mochida K, Komori H, Okawa A, et al. Regression of cervical disc herniation observed on magnetic resonance imaging. *Spine.* 1998;23:990–997.
155. Eisen H. Electrodiagnosis of radiculopathies. *Neurol Clin.* 1985;3(3):495–510.
156. Marinacci AA. A correlation between operative findings in cervical herniated disc with electromyelograms and opaque myelograms. *Electromyography.* 1966;6:5–20.
157. Lauder TD, Dillingham TR. The cervical radiculopathy screen: optimizing the number of muscles studied. *Muscle Nerve.* 1996;19:662–665.
158. Leblhuber FF, Reisecker H. Diagnostic value of different electrophysiologic tests in cervical disc prolapse. *Neurology.* 1988;38:1879–1881.
159. Anderberg L, Annertz M, Rydholm U. Selective diagnostic nerve root block for the evaluation of radicular pain in the multilevel degenerated cervical spine. *Eur Spine J.* 2006;15(6):794–801.
160. Datta S, Everett CR, Tescot AM, et al. An updated systematic review of the diagnostic utility of selective nerve root blocks. *Pain Physician.* 2007;10(1):113–128.
161. Woods BI, Hilibrand AS. Cervical radiculopathy: epidemiology, etiology, diagnosis, and treatment. *J Spinal Disord Tech.* 2015;28(5):E251–E259.
162. Iyer S, Kim HJ. Cervical radiculopathy. *Curr Rev Musculoskelet Med.* 2016;9(3):272–280.
163. Nikolaidis I, Fouyas IP, Sandercock PA. Surgery for cervical radiculopathy or myelopathy. *Cochrane Database Syst Rev.* 2010;(1):CD001466.
164. Persson LC, Carlsson CA, Carlsson JY. Long-lasting cervical radicular pain managed with surgery, physiotherapy, or a cervical collar: a prospective, randomized study. *Spine.* 1997;22(7):751–758.
165. Colachis SC, Strohm BR, Ganter EL. Cervical spine motion in normal women: radiographic study of effect of cervical collars. *Arch Phys Med Rehabil.* 1973;54:161–169.
166. Rubin D. Cervical radiculitis: diagnosis and treatment. *Arch Phys Med Rehabil.* 1960;41:580–586.
167. Wong JJ, Cote P, Quesnele JJ. The course and prognostic factors of symptomatic cervical disc herniation with radiculopathy: a systematic review of the literature. *Spine J.* 2014;14(8):1781–1789.
168. Wong JJ, Cote P, Ameis A. Are non-steroidal anti-inflammatory drugs effective for the management of neck pain and associated disorders, whiplash-associated disorders, or non-specific low back pain? A systematic review of systematic reviews by the Ontario Protocol for Traffic Injury Management (OPTIMa) Collaboration. *Eur Spine J.* 2016;25(1):34–61.
169. Ghasemi M, Masaeli A, Rezvani M. Oral prednisolone in the treatment of cervical radiculopathy: a randomized placebo controlled trial. *J Res Med Sci.* 2013;18(1): S43–S46.
170. Colloca L, Ludman T, Bouhassira D. Neuropathic pain. *Nat Rev Dis Primers.* 2017;3:17002.
171. Saal JS, Saal JA, Yurth ER. Nonoperative management of herniated cervical intervertebral disc with radiculopathy. *Spine.* 1996;21:1877–1883.
172. Sampath P, Bendebba M, Davis JD, et al. Outcome in patients with cervical radiculopathy: prospective multicenter study with independent clinical review. *Spine.* 1999;24:591–597.
173. McKenzie R. *The Cervical and Thoracic Spine: Mechanical Diagnosis and Therapy.* Waikanae, New Zealand: Spinal Publications; 1990.
174. Saal JS. Flexibility training. *Phys Med Rehabil State Art Rev.* 1987;1:537–554.
175. Mataya T, Bach T. The reliability of selected techniques in clinical arthrometrics. *Aust J Physiother.* 1985;31(5):175–179.
176. Maher C, Adams R. Reliability of pain and stiffness assessment in clinical manual lumbar spine examination. *Phys Ther.* 1994;74(9):801.

177. McCombe PF, Fairbank JCT, Cockersole BC, et al. Reproducibility of physical signs in low-back pain. *Spine.* 1989;14(9):908–918.

178. Spratt KF, Lehman TR, Weinstein JN, et al. A new approach to the low-back physical examination; behavioral assessment of mechanical signs. *Spine.* 1990;15(2):96–102.

179. Kilby J, Stignant M, Roberts A. The reliability of back pain assessment by physiotherapists using a "Mckenzie algorithm." *Physiotherapy.* 1990;76(9):579–583.

180. Potter NA, Rothstein JM. Intertester reliability for selected clinical tests of the sacroiliac joint. *Phys Ther.* 1985;65(11):1671–1675.

181. Maitland GD. *Peripheral Manipulation.* 3rd ed. London: Butterworth-Heinemann; 1991.

182. Maitland GD. *Vertebral Manipulation.* 5th ed. London: Butterworth-Heinemann; 1986.

183. Naylor JR, Mulley GP. Surgical collars: a survey of their prescription and use. *Br J Rheumatol.* 1991;30:282–284.

184. Pennie BH, Agambar LJ. Whiplash injuries: trial of early management. *J Bone Joint Surg.* 1990;72B:277–279.

185. McKinney LA. Early mobilization of acute sprain of the neck. *BMJ.* 1989;299:1006–1008.

186. Mealy K, Brennan H, Fenelon GC. Early mobilization of acute whiplash injury. *BMJ.* 1986;292:1656–1657.

187. Bell KM, Frazier EC, Shively CM. Assessing range of motion to evaluate the adverse effects of ill-fitting cervical orthoses. *Spine J.* 2009;9(3):225–231.

188. Tan JC, Nordin M. Role of physical therapy in the treatment of cervical disk disease. *Orthop Clin North Am.* 1992;23(3):435–449.

189. Caldwell JW, Krusen EM. Effectiveness of cervical traction in treatment of neck problems: evaluation of various methods. *Arch Phys Med Rehabil.* 1962;43:214–221.

190. Goldie I, Landquist A. Evaluation of the effects of different forms of physiotherapy in cervical pain. *Scand J Rehabil Med.* 1970;2(2):117–121.

191. Hinterbuchner C. Traction. In: Basmajian JV, ed. *Manipulation, Traction, and Massage.* 3rd ed. Baltimore, MD: Lippincott Williams & Wilkins; 1985:175–195.

192. Rath W. Cervical traction: a clinical perspective. *Orthop Rev.* 1984;13:430–449.

193. Mathews JA, Mills SB, Jenkins VM, et al. Back pain and sciatica: controlled trials of manipulation, traction, sclerosant, and epidural injections. *Br J Rheumatol.* 1987;26:416–423.

194. Judovich B. Lumbar traction therapy. *JAMA.* 1955;159:549.

195. Twomey LT. Sustained lumbar traction: an experimental study of long spine segments. *Spine.* 1985;10:146–149.

196. Saunders HD, Saunders R, eds. *Treatment and Prevention of Musculoskeletal Disorders.* Bloomington, MN: Educational Opportunities; 1993.

197. Colachis SC, Strohm BR. A study of tractive forces and angle of pull on vertebral interspaces in the cervical spine. *Arch Phys Med Rehabil.* 1965;46:820–824.

198. Colachis SC, Strohm BR. Cervical traction: relationship of traction time to varied tractive force with constant angle. *Arch Phys Med Rehabil.* 1965;46:815–819.

199. Maitland GD, ed. *Vertebral Manipulation.* 5th ed. London: Butterworth; 1986.

200. Fritz JM, Thackeray A, Brennan GP. Exercise only, exercise with mechanical traction, or exercise with over-door traction for patients with cervical radiculopathy, with or without consideration of status on a previously described subgrouping rule: a randomized clinical trial. *J Orthop Sports Phys Ther.* 2014;44(2):45–57.

201. Colachis SC, Strohm BR. Effect of duration of intermittent cervical traction on vertebral separation. *Arch Phys Med Rehabil.* 1966;47:353–359.

202. Sweeny T, Prentice C, Saal JA, et al. Cervicothoracic muscular stabilizing technique. *Phys Rehabil Art Rev.* 1990;4:335–360.

203. Johnson EW, Wolfe CV. Bifocal spectacles in the etiology of cervical radiculopathy. *Arch Phys Med Rehabil.* 1972;53:201–205.

204. Anderberg L, Annertz M, Persson L. Transforaminal steroid injections for the treatment of cervical radiculopathy: a prospective and randomized study. *Eur Spine J.* 2007;16(3):321–328.

205. Huston CW. Cervical epidural steroid injections in the management of cervical radiculitis: interlaminar versus transforaminal. A review. *Curr Rev Musculoskelet Med.* 2009;2(1):30–42.

206. Epstein NE. The risks of epidural and transforaminal steroid injections in the Spine: commentary and a comprehensive review of the literature. *Surg Neurol Int.* 2013;4(2):S74–S93.

207. Lee JW, Park KW, Chung SK. Cervical transforaminal epidural steroid injections for the management of cervical radiculopathy: a comparative study of particulate versus non-particulate steroids. *Skeletal Radiol.* 2009;38(11):1077–1082.

208. Scanlon GC, Moeller-Bertram T, Romanowsky SM. Cervical transforaminal epidural steroid injections: more dangerous than we think? *Spine.* 2007;32(11):1249–1256.

209. Stav A, Ovadia L, Sternberg A. Cervical epidural steroid injection for cervicobrachialgia. *Acta Anaesthesiol Scand.* 1993;37(6):562-566.

210. Cohen SP, Hayek S, Semenov Y. Epidural steroid injections, conservative treatment, or combination treatment for cervical radicular pain: a multicenter, randomized, comparative-effectivness study. *Anesthesiology.* 2014;121(5):1045–1055.

211. Ellenberg MR, Honet JC. Clinical pearls in cervical radiculopathy. *Phys Med Rehabil Clin N Am.* 1996;7:487–568.

212. Andersson GB, Brown MD, Dvorack J, et al. Consensus summary of the diagnosis and treatment of lumbar disc herniation. *Spine.* 1996;21S:75–78.

213. Lunsford LD, Bissonette DJ, Jannetta PJ, et al. Anterior surgery for cervical disc disease: Part 1. Treatment of lateral cervical disc herniation in 253 cases. *J Neurosurg.* 1980;53:1–11.

214. Robinson RA, Walker AE, Ferlic DC, et al. The results of anterior interbody fusion of the cervical spine. *J Bone Joint Surg.* 1962;44A:1569–1587.

215. Boni M, Cherubino P, Denaro V, et al. Multiple subtotal somatectomy: technique and evaluation of a series of 39 cases. *Spine.* 1984;9:358–362.

216. Brigham CD, Tsahakis PJ. Anterior cervical foraminotomy and fusion: surgical technique and results. *Spine.* 1995;20:766–770.

217. Connolly ES, Seymour RJ, Adams JE. Clinical evaluation of anterior cervical fusion for degenerative cervical disc disease. *J Neurosurg.* 1965;23:431–437.

218. Verma K, Gandhi S, Maltenfort M. Rate of adjacent segment disease in cervical disc arthroplasty versus single-level fusion: meta-analysis of prospective studies. *Spine.* 2013;38(26):2253–2257.

219. Zigler JE, Delamarter R, Murrey D. ProDisc-C and anterior cervical discectomy and fusion as surgical treatment for single-level cervical symptomatic degenerative disc disease: five year results of a food and drug administration study. *Spine.* 2013;38(3):203–209.

220. Qureshi SA, McAnany S, Goz V. Cost-effectiveness analysis: comparing single-level cervical disc replacement and single-level anterior cervical discectomy and fusion: clinical article. *J Neurosurg Spine.* 2013;19(5):546–554.

221. Davis RJ, Nunley PD, Kim KD. Two-level total disc replacement with Mobi-C cervical artificial disc versus anterior discectomy and fusion: a prospective, randomized, controlled multicenter clinical trial with 4-year follow-up results. *J Neurosurg Spine.* 2015;22:15–25.

222. Kong L, Ma Q, Meng F, Cao J, Yu K, Shen Y. The prevalence of heterotopic ossification among patients after cervical artificial disc replacement: a systematic review and meta-analysis. *Medicine (Baltimore).* 2017;96:e7163.

223. Church EW, Halpern CH, Faught RW. Cervical laminoforaminotomy for radiculopathy: symptomatic and functional outcomes in a large cohort with long-term follow up. *Surg Neurol Int.* 2014;5(15):S536–S543.

224. Roet M, Spoor JK, de Waal M. Extensive calcification of the ligamentum flavum causing cervical myelopathy in a Caucasian woman. *Springerplus.* 2016;5(1):1927.

225. Ono K, Ota H, Tada K, et al. Cervical myelopathy secondary to multiple spondylotic protrusions: a clinicopathologic study. *Spine.* 1977;2:109–125.

226. Emery SE. Cervical spondylotic myelopathy: diagnosis and treatment. *J Am Acad Orthop Surg.* 2001;9(6):376–388.

227. Crandall PH, Batzdorf U. Cervical spondylotic myelopathy. *J Neurosurg.* 1966;25:57–66.

228. Kameyama T, Ando T, Yanagi Y, et al. Cervical spondylotic amyotrophy: magnetic resonance imaging demonstration of intrinsic cord pathology. *Spine.* 1998;23:448–452.

229. Ebara S, Yonenobu K, Fujiwara K, et al. Myelopathy hand characterized by muscle wasting: a different type of myelopathy hand in patients with cervical spondylosis. *Spine.* 1988;13:785–791.

230. Gorter K. Influence of laminectomy on the course of cervical myelopathy. *Acta Neurochir (Wien).* 1976;33:265–281.

231. Ono K, Ebara S, Fuji T, et al. Myelopathy hand: new clinical signs of cervical cord damage. *J Bone Joint Surg.* 1987;69B:215–219.

232. Emery SE, Bohlman HH, Bolesta MJ, et al. Anterior cervical decompression and arthrodesis for the treatment of cervical spondylotic myelopathy: two to seventeen year follow up. *J Bone Joint Surg Am.* 1998;80:941–951.

233. L'Hermitte J. Etude de la commation de la moele. *Rev Neural.* 1932;1:210–239.

234. Parminder SP. Management of cervical pain. In: Delisa JA, ed. *Rehabilitation Medicine: Principles and Practice.* Philadelphia, PA: Lippincott Williams & Wilkins; 1988:753.

235. Shimizu T, Shimada H, Shirakura K. Scapulohumeral reflex (Shimizu): its clinical significance and testing maneuver. *Spine.* 1993;18:2182–2190.

236. Pavlov H, Torg JS, Robie B, et al. Cervical spinal stenosis: determination with vertebral body ratio method. *Radiology.* 1987;164:771–775.

237. Wolf BS, Khilnani M, Malis L. The sagittal diameter of the bony cervical spinal canal and its significance in cervical spondylosis. *J Mt Sinai Hosp N Y.* 1956;23:283–292.

238. Morio Y, Teshima R, Nagashima H, et al. Correlation between operative outcomes of cervical compression myelopathy and MRI of the spinal cord. *Spine.* 2001;26(11):1238–1245.

239. Chen CJ, Iyu RK, Lee ST, et al. Intramedullary high signal intensity on T2-weighted MR images in cervical spondylotic myelopathy: prediction of prognosis with type of intensity. *Radiology.* 2001;221:789–794.

240. Matsumoto M, Toyama Y, Ishikawa M, et al. Increased signal intensity of the spinal cord on magnetic resonance images in cervical compressive myelopathy. Does it predict the outcome of conservative treatment. *Spine.* 2000;25:677–682.

241. Ogino H, Tada K, Okada K, et al. Canal diameter, anteroposterior compression ration, and spondylotic myelopathy of the cervical spine. *Spine.* 1983;8:1–15.

242. Breig A, Turnbull I, Hassler O. Effects of mechanical stresses on the spinal cord in cervical spondylosis: a study on fresh cadaver material. *J Neurosurg.* 1966;25:45–56.

243. Fujiwara K, Yonenobu K, Ebara S, et al. The prognosis of surgery for cervical compression myelopathy: an analysis of factors involved. *J Bone Joint Surg.* 1989;71B:393–398.

244. Nurick S. The natural history and the results of surgical treatment of the spinal cord disorder associated with cervical spondylosis. *Brain.* 1972;95:101–108.

245. Epstein JA, Epstein NE. The surgical management of cervical spinal stenosis, spondylosis, and myeloradiculopathy by means of the posterior approach. In: Sherk HH, Dunn EJ, Eismont FJ, et al., eds. *The Cervical Spine.* 2nd ed. Philadelphia, PA: JB Lippincott; 1989:625–643.

246. Fehlings MG, Wilson JR, Kopjar B. Efficacy and safety of surgical decompression in patients with cervical spondylotic myelopathy: results of the AOSpine North America prospective multi-center study. *J Bone Joint Surg Am.* 2013;95(18):1651–1658.

247. Lawrence BD, Jacobs WB, Norvell DC. Anterior versus posterior approach for treatment of cervical spondylotic myelopathy: a systematic review. *Spine.* 2013;38(22S):173–182.

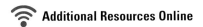 **Additional Resources Online**

CHAPTER 27

Stefano Negrini   Michele Romano
Fabio Zaina   Carlo Trevisan

Rehabilitation of Lumbar Spine Disorders: An Evidence-Based Clinical Practice Approach

The approach to low back pain (LBP) has changed dramatically in the past decades, while medicine has changed also (1–4). Formerly, according to a classical disease model, all LBP classifications considered a pathoanatomic basis and consequently proposed treatments; but the increasing burden on society in terms of costs and disability (5), presumably due to inappropriate treatment and medical approach, leads to a revolution in the understanding of the problem (4,6). Accordingly, LBP is now classified as secondary (<10% of cases) and primary, or idiopathic, or simply LBP; the latter is then divided according to the localization of symptoms (LBP and sciatica) and the duration of pain (acute, subacute, and chronic) (3,7–11). Generally speaking, in this model, LBP is recognized as a biopsychosocial syndrome (4,12). Consequently, the importance of the discipline of physical medicine and rehabilitation (PM&R), as one with particular focus on biopsychosocial approaches according to the International Classification of Functioning (ICF) (13–20), has greatly increased in this field (21,22). As is always the case in medicine, these advancements require time to reach the clinical everyday world (10,23–27). Today, the clinical reality is a mix of different approaches, usually driven by what each single specialty, doctor, and/or allied professional knows and offers in terms of treatments, more than by a coherent and systematic evidence-based approach (28,29). Considering the world of PM&R and its inevitably multiprofessional reality (14,30), combined with the almost complete outpatient reality of LBP treatment, the confusion seems even higher than in other specialties (31–35). Moreover, considering the widespread recognition of LBP as a biopsychosocial syndrome, and consequently the crucial role PM&R should have in its treatment, this confusion must be cleared away. That is the main aim of this chapter.

This chapter is fully evidence-based, but it is also totally focused on what to do in the clinical everyday world once the evidence is known: in reality, it is an evidence-based clinical practice tool. Therefore, we will start from some clinical-scientific premises, including assessment and outcome criteria, the actual scientific evidence on treatments of PM&R interest, and also the diagnostic-therapeutic pathways (flowcharts) (9) to be followed. In fact, another unavoidable premise is that in LBP rehabilitation, as well as in all other PM&R approaches to patients who are diagnosed with a specific disease, a correct disease diagnosis is the first step and must be achieved. We cannot rehabilitate the patient if we do not start with diagnosis, and only after that can we look for a mandatory biopsychosocial picture of the patient, possibly inside the mainframe of ICF (17,18,36–38). Finally, we will have an evidence-based description of the single clinical LBP pictures of PM&R interest, concluding with the rehabilitation approach to each of them.

The last important premise is one of terminology: rehabilitation is neither a pain-orientated (PO) nor a conservative treatment. From our perspective, the term "conservative treatment" should be abandoned because it is based on the past, when the only need was to define whether an LBP was surgical or not (21,22). The term "conservative" is not the positive affirmation of what we have to be in regard to our patients. Instead, it is only the negation of surgery, as if this were the gold standard. In the so-called field of conservative treatment, there are abundant treatments that focus on pain ("medications, manual therapy, and physical therapy"); these have been traditionally used for years, and continue to be used, sometimes according to some evidence. However, with the increased scientific understanding of the limits of this pain-oriented approach (4,5,39), more complex rehabilitation approaches focusing on increasing function, on recovering activities and participation, and on rising quality of life have emerged and developed: we will call them functioning-orientated (FO) approaches and they represent a rehabilitation approach (40–42). These FO approaches are based on WHO's understanding of functioning (13), representing the comprehensive view taken by PM&R (14–20,30). In most patients, this is far more appropriate, and it should be the main concern of PM&R specialists, who have the best conceptual tools with which to appropriately rehabilitate LBP patients (13,14,22,30,37,38). This does not lead us to ignore medications, manual therapy, or physical therapy treatments, which in some or many cases must be applied, but the differentiation is crucial to achieving a better understanding of our everyday behaviors, including their advantages and limitations. Moreover, there is growing evidence that some of them can be very effective in the acute LBP, allowing to make patient subgrouping for a personalized approach.

ASSESSMENT, DECISION-MAKING PROCESS, AND REHABILITATION TREATMENT TOOLS

Assessment and Outcome Criteria

An appropriate diagnostic workup is the cornerstone of an effective treatment. It is founded on taking the most accurate medical history and conducting a thorough physical examination (8–10), both of which are useful in forging a good doctor-patient relationship. The first objective of assessing the patient who is experiencing back pain is to identify the patient who presents with serious spinal pathology (tumor, infection, fracture, etc.). It is possible to establish a well-defined pathology in only about 15% of patients who present with LBP (43). Among patients suffering from LBP and sciatica for a period of approximately 4 weeks, Deyo et al., as well as Udén, were able to identify the following: herniated disk (4% to 5%), lumbar spinal stenosis (LSS) (4% to 5%), spinal fractures (4%), metastatic tumor or osteomyelitis (1%), and visceral pathologies such as aortic aneurysms, kidney disorders, or gynecologic disorders (<1%).

According to Waddell (44), when dealing with a patient suffering from LBP, the first step is to identify any possible serious spinal pathologies (primitive or metastatic neoplasia, infections or inflammatory diseases such as ankylosing spondylitis, osteoporotic fractures, cauda equina syndrome, or any of various neurologic diseases). An assessment of the pain is then conducted in order to determine whether it originates in the nerve root (sciatica from a prolapsed disk, spinal stenosis, or surgical scarring):

- On one side of one of the lower limbs, generally radiating below the knee, down to the ankle and the foot
- Very often more intense than LBP
- Hypoesthesia or paresthesia with the same distribution
- Positive signs of radicular irritation
- Motor, sensory, or reflex changes related to a single nerve root

Assessing LBP means evaluating pain symptoms, with all the ensuing uncertainties that this entails. It is especially difficult to objectively assess the severity of the pain due to the complex neurophysiologic sensory mechanisms and the psychoemotional assimilation that occurs in the experience of pain, and which cannot be differentiated by the person experiencing it (45). Regarding duration of the pain, the updated universally accepted classification is as follows (3,5,8,11,46):

- Acute LBP (ALBP): up to 4 weeks
- Chronic LBP (CLBP): over 6 months
- Subacute LBP (SALBP): from 1 to 6 months

A recent study has shown the presumable transition between ALBP and SALBP in 14 days (47), while others propose 90 days as the starting point of CLBP (9). As the symptoms of pain persist, there is a shift from a pathology of a physiologic nature with biologic ramifications to one characterized by psychosocial implications. The assessment at this stage no longer simply concerns a disorder but also disability and diminished quality of life.

Scientific Evidence on Assessment

Generally in the medical field, the basic requirements for any diagnostic test are its accuracy, safety, and reproducibility (48–50). Accuracy comprises the twin parameters of specificity and sensitivity: specificity refers to the ability of the test to

be positive only when a pathology is present, while sensitivity is the characteristic of being positive whenever the pathology is present. Moreover, to ascertain the accuracy of a diagnostic test, it is necessary to have a gold standard against which to measure the sensitivity and specificity. For spinal pathologies, in some cases, the gold standard is the presence or absence of defined tissue pathology confirmed through a surgical procedure, while in other instances it is the confirmation or relief of pain. In all these cases, given the difficulty in obtaining an objective assessment of pain, the true accuracy of any test that provokes or alleviates pain carries an intrinsic uncertainty (51).

Various clinical guidelines (CGs) (8,9,52) stress the importance of taking a detailed medical history and a comprehensive physical examination of the patient, and they emphasize that during the first visit in particular, the physicians should dedicate their full attention to the patient and spend the appropriate amount of time needed to earn the individual's trust. Indeed, evidence shows that an appropriate clinical approach can only have a beneficial impact on the pain and on allaying the patient's fears (53).

Due to its biopsychosocial characteristics, an important future advancement in LBP assessment could be represented in the near future by the application of the ICF (15–20) and mainly its core set (36–38,54–56).

Red and Yellow Flags

To improve the accuracy of excluding serious spinal pathologies, as well as to reassure the patient, almost all existing CGs (57) have recommended that a series of risk factors called "red flags" (**Table 27-1**) be assessed as the patient's medical history is taken down. The presence of one or more of these flags would determine whether there is a need for a targeted diagnostic confirmation and subsequent consultation with a specialist, but the reliability of many of them seems questionable (57). Recently, two systematic reviews have reported that there is a lack of evidence to support or refute individual red flag, suggesting to use a combination of them as a pragmatic indication for further examination both for spinal fractures and for malignancy (58,59), and further.

Other CGs (58) have identified other risk factors, being indicators of the possible evolution in chronicity of pain, that have been called "yellow flags" (60), whose presence, if found in ALBP or SALBP, indicates the need to take into account psychosocial factors and apply early therapeutic strategies in a cognitive-behavioral approach (see **Table 27-1**).

Medical History and Physical Examination

The first level of diagnostic triage during the history taking is to identify "red flags" and assess potential "yellow flags" (61).

Several studies have focused on how a physical examination is performed in regard to the range of motion of the lumbar spine, muscle strength, and provoking or relieving pain symptoms with specific movements. The McKenzie technique for determining which movements can cause the centralization of pain and what courses to take has not found unanimity in the literature for indicating prognosis (62–64).

A study by Simmonds et al. (65) has established the reliability, validity, and good clinical use of nine physical evaluations comparing asymptomatic subjects and LBP patients. Also, a modest correlation with the degree of disability was detected through a questionnaire. No evidence of clinical benefit has been obtained in the analysis of muscle strength carried out by

TABLE 27-1	**In the Diagnostic Process of LBP Patients, It Is Important Since the Beginning to Search for Red Flags (Risk Factors for Secondary LBP Due to Important Pathologies): In Subacute Cases, It Is Crucial to Search for Yellow Flags (Risk Factors for Chronicization of LBP)**

Red Flags (Risk Factors for Secondary LBP Due to Important Pathologies)

Back pain in children <18 y with considerable pain or onset >55 y
History of violent trauma
Mild trauma in an aged patient
Constant progressive pain at night
History of cancer
Systemic steroids
Drug abuse, human immunodeficiency virus infection
Weight loss
Systemic illness
Persisting severe restriction of motion
Intense pain or minimal motion
Structural deformity
Difficulty with micturition
Loss of anal sphincter tone or fecal incontinence; saddle anesthesia
Widespread progressive motor weakness or gait disturbance
Inflammatory disorders (ankylosing spondylitis) suspected
    Gradual onset <40 y
    Marked morning stiffness
    Persisting limitation of motion
    Peripheral joint involvement
    Iritis, skin rushes, colitis, urethral discharge
    Family history

Yellow Flags (Risk Factors for Chronicization of Acute and SALBP)

Personal	Age (U form correlation)
	Female gender
	Minor ethnicity
	Low income
	Low education
Medical	High BMI
	Previous surgery
	Impairment
	Neurologic deficit
	Radicular impingement (SLR, Wassermann tests)
Pain related	Duration
	Intensity
	Leg pain
	Pain in lateral flexion and/or in flexion-extension
	Difficulties in sitting
Impairment disability related	High referred impairment
	High functional limitation at 4 wk
	High disability (Roland-Morris, Oswestry, Sickness Impact Profile)
	Perceived risk of not recovering
Psychosocial	Not appropriate signs and symptoms
	Avoidance behavior
	Psychological burden
	Vital energy reduction
	Reduced emotional confronting capacity
	Social isolation
	Depression (SCL-90, Zung, Beck Depression Inventory)
	Somatization (SCL-90)
	Reduced coping strategies (CPCT)
Work related	High requests
	Reduced control on own work
	Monotony
	Low satisfaction
Treatments	Treatment before retiring from work
	Disability compensation
	Heat and cold therapies
	Physiotherapy
	Back school

Adapted from Negrini S, Giovannoni S, Minozzi S, et al. Diagnostic therapeutic flow-charts for low back pain patients: the Italian clinical guidelines. *Eura Medicophys.* 2006;42(2):151–170.

various machines (66). In fact, a good correlation of testing and retesting has shown that the Biering-Sörensen test is simpler to conduct and is of greater benefit in clinical practice. Regarding muscle fatigue, Taimela et al. (67) have shown that LBP sufferers first get tired, whereupon the fatigue reduces the quality of movement, and consequently the muscle fatigue lessens the kinesthesia. Muscle fatigue, therefore, is a risk factor.

Clinical trials, as well as various national CGs, have taught us that a fundamental point of the evaluation is physical contact with the patient: palpation of the vertebral structure provoking pain and the direct assessment of regional and segment motion are an integral part of a complete physical examination. The most reliable tests are those that provoke pain, while less reliable diagnostic testing is that which is done by palpating the soft tissues (68). Regional motion testing is also more reliable than segmental motion testing, and intraexaminer reliability is greater than interexaminer reliability (68).

If, on the one hand, there is a lack of definition of the specific structural causes in a great number of LBP sufferers, on the other hand the practice tends to identify specific subgroups of subjects affected by LBP. While we have no evidence for a clinical diagnosis of LBP due to facet joint pathology (69), we have some tools to clinical suspect lumbar instability. Among the various tests, the passive lumbar extension scored the highest values for sensitivity and specificity (70).

LBP and Leg Pain

Regarding the pain that radiates to a lower limb below the knee, there is not enough evidence for history and clinical symptoms to guide the diagnosis (71). Diagnostic performance of most physical tests (paresis or muscle weakness, muscle wasting, impaired reflexes, sensory deficits) is poor, and the results of different studies are partially justified by the different setting and available populations, a lack of a standardized classification criterion for disk herniation, and the variable psychometric properties of the testing procedures (**Table 27-2**) (72,73). In surgical populations characterized by a high prevalence of disk herniation (58% to 98%), the straight leg raising (SLR) test showed high sensitivity (pooled estimate 0.92, 95% CI: 0.87 to 0.95) with widely varying specificity (0.10 to 1.00, pooled estimate 0.28, 95% CI: 0.18 to 0.40) (72). Results of studies using imaging showed more heterogeneity and poorer sensitivity (72). The crossed SLR showed high specificity (pooled estimate 0.90, 95% CI: 0.85 to 0.94) with consistently low sensitivity (pooled estimate 0.28, 95% CI: 0.22 to 0.35) (72). Combining positive test results increased the specificity of physical tests (72).

Diagnostic Imaging

The choice of an imaging examination for diagnostic purposes should only be based on an evaluation of the symptoms, medical history taking, and physical examination (74) (see Chapter 5). The purpose of diagnostic imaging is to verify the suspicion of a serious pathology due to red flags or a herniated disk due to symptoms ascribed to nerve-root pain. In the case of LBP or simple sciatica, and in the absence of red flags, diagnostic imaging is not required within 30 days of the onset of symptoms (3,8,9).

Regarding radiographic examinations, all the current CGs agree on refuting their diagnostic or therapeutic value in the absence of red flags and discourage any routine use, since among radiographic findings, only a disk space narrowing, spondylolisthesis (SL), and spondylolysis showed a significant association with LBP (**Table 27-3**) (75). The noninvasiveness

TABLE 27-2	Findings in Patients with History of a Well-Described Lumbar Nerve Root Pain of Sufficient Predictive Value for Finding a Disk Hernia at Neuroradiographic Examination
Finding	**Prediction Strength**
Crossed SLR reproducing pain in the symptomatic leg	+++
SLR <60 degrees (SLR reproduces leg pain)	++
Ankle dorsiflexion weakness	+
Great toe weakness	+
Impaired ankle reflex	+
Sensory loss, pins and needles, paresthesia	+
Patellar reflex weakness	+
Ankle reflex weakness	+
Severe radicular pain	++
Pain causing awakening at night	++
Severe lumbar motion restriction	++
Loss of lordosis and/or sciatic scoliosis	++
Unilateral leg pain worse than back pain	++
Radiation into the foot	+
Pain drawing (exact dermatome depicted)	(+)

Adapted from Negrini S, Giovannoni S, Minozzi S, et al. Diagnostic therapeutic flowcharts for low back pain patients: the Italian clinical guidelines. *Eura Medicophys.* 2006;42(2):151–170.

and characteristics unique to MRI in satisfactorily evaluating both soft and bone tissues allow it to be a more comprehensive tool for the diagnostic imaging of an LBP patient. That being said, there is no evidence that its use provides any real advantage in the treatment of LBP without irradiation (76). Many studies have shown that the presence of disk anomalies (bulges, swelling, hernia) in the vertebral canal, the foramen, and the vertebral structures is found in asymptomatic subjects; nevertheless, new imaging techniques seem promising and could be more helpful in the future (77). Consequently, Roland and van Tulder (78) recommended, somewhat provocatively, that radiologists add the following to the reports along with their referrals: "This finding may be unrelated to patient symptoms because it is often seen in asymptomatic subjects."

TABLE 27-3	Studies on the Association Between Radiographic Findings and Nonspecific LBP Judged to be Valid		
Radiographic Finding	**No. of Studies**	**Odds Ratio**	**Results**
Disk degeneration	12	1.2–3.3	Moderately positive
Spondylosis	3	1.2–2.0	Negative
Spondylolysis and spondylolisthesis	6	0.82–1	Negative
Spina bifida	2	0.5–0.6	Negative
Transitional vertebrae	3	0.5–0.8	Negative
Scheuermann's disease	2	0.8–3.6	Unclear

Adapted from Negrini S, Giovannoni S, Minozzi S, et al. Diagnostic therapeutic flowcharts for low back pain patients: the Italian clinical guidelines. *Eura Medicophys.* 2006;42(2):151–170.

The MRI is a highly sensitive exam, and hence there is a risk of obtaining many false positives. We must bear this in mind in clinical practice so that costs can be kept down and unnecessary surgical procedures avoided.

Psychosocial Factors, Disability, and Quality of Life

The assessment of a patient with LBP must not be limited to a physical examination but should also include an analysis of psychosocial factors that play a crucial role in the chronicity of pain, delays in returning to work, and the success of the treatment (see Chapter 12). Evidence shows that some conditions—such as low level of job satisfaction, poor work motivation, disability compensation, and dissatisfaction with previous treatment—are risk factors for chronicity and/or the relapse of LBP. Psychological discomfort, depression, somatization, and cognitive factors such as catastrophism are predictors of chronicity/disability (79) and are very frequent in acute LBP (80). Although the symptoms of mental stress in asymptomatic subjects can be predictors (81), the main indicator for LBP is a positive medical history (82).

Persistent pain always entails a certain degree of disability. The measurement for disability in LBP can be gauged through means of dedicated and scientifically validated questionnaires such as the Oswestry LBP Disability Questionnaire, the Roland-Morris Questionnaire, and the Core Outcome Measurement Instrument (COMI) (83–88). Some data have shown a weak but significant correlation among pain, disability, and quality of life (89). Thus, it appears that the persistence of pain and disability worsens the quality of life to an appreciable extent. Clearly, the impact of pain and disability on decreasing the quality of life depends more on their duration than their intensity. Moreover, even a clinically significant variation in the degree of pain can bring about nearly imperceptible changes in disability and quality of life. We must, therefore, adopt the concept of the minimal clinically important difference (90,91), that is, the slightest change in an evaluation scale that will be perceived by the patient as an improvement in his or her condition. It is important to stress the benefit of such a concept as a better outcome criterion because it is aimed at the patient from a functional and psychosocial perspective. However, it is a well-known fact that today there is also the need to evaluate a treatment's efficiency in terms of managing the costs of health care.

This section concludes with a word about younger patient, since there is an increased incidence of LBP among children and adolescents, even if the QoL is usually not significantly impaired (92,93). Among the defined risk factors in a school population of 10,000 subjects are the excessive weight of backpacks, the sitting level of students compared to that of the teacher, and the heights of chairs and desks (94). Starting with the premise that a better predictor of LBP is precisely a positive medical history and the awareness that children and adolescents exhibit significant differences regarding medical history, physical examination, and diagnosis compared to the adult population (95), it would appear altogether appropriate that new studies be conducted so as to bring this subgroup to the fore and thereby formulate better treatment and avoid the relapse of LBP in adulthood.

Diagnostic-Therapeutic Flowcharts

The Quebec Task Force started in 1987 (96) published the first systematic CG that is a summary of the existing evidence on LBP treatment. More recently, with the objective of painting in a simple way the everyday clinical behaviors, those published in 2006 in *Europa Medicophysica* (9) (now the *European Journal of Physical and Rehabilitation Medicine*) (97) appear very interesting. The "Diagnostic-Therapeutic Flowcharts for LBP Patients" (DTP) have been developed as real flowcharts (**Figs. 27-1** to **27-7**), in order to provide a complete idea of what should be done and to cover, through expert multidisciplinary consensus, the multiple gray areas in which the actual evidence does not offer answers. Moreover, these DTP have other unique characteristics in terms of PM&R (21) that are reported below. In **Figures 27-2** to **27-7**, the most interesting flowcharts of the DTP are given to the reader, while in the open-access version of the *European Journal of Physical and Rehabilitation Medicine* (EJPM&R) (www.ejPM&R.org), they can be viewed for further details.

The DTP have been developed through a systematic search of the literature and a multidisciplinary consensus of all Italian scientific societies engaged in this field. The classical distinction between ALBP, SALBP, and CLBP is at the base of the

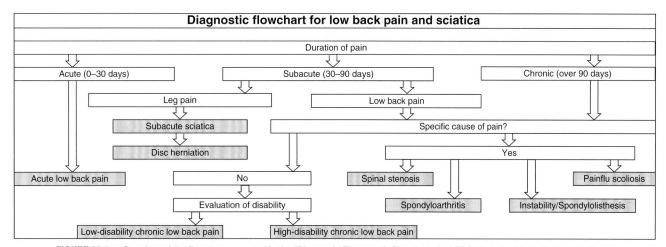

FIGURE 27-1. Overview of the flowcharts reported in the "Diagnostic-Therapeutic Flowcharts for LBP Patients" published in 2006 in *Europa Medicophysica*, now the *European Journal of Physical and Rehabilitation Medicine*. The classification of LBP used can be easily gathered (Reprinted by permission of Edizioni Minerva Medica from Negrini S, Giovannoni S, Minozzi S, et al. Diagnostic therapeutic flow-charts for low back pain patients: the Italian clinical guidelines. *Eura Medicophys.* 2006;42(2):151–170.)

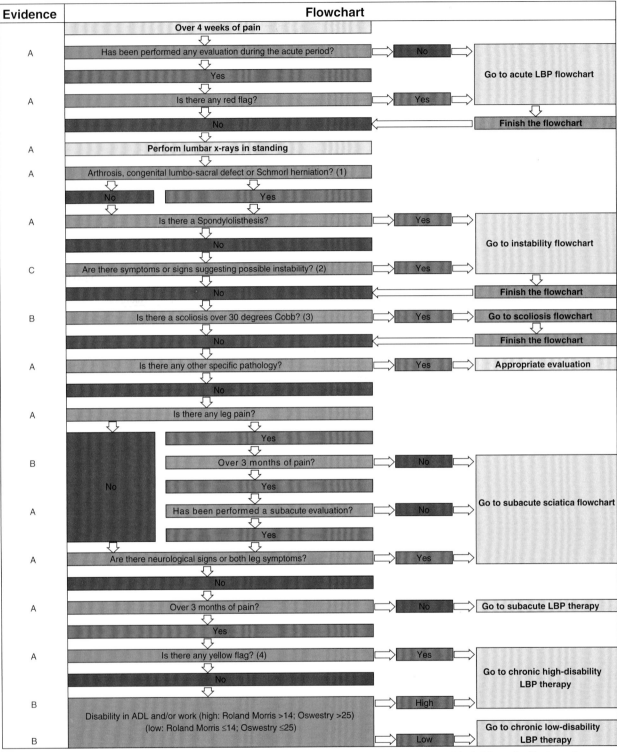

1. Arthrosis: discopathy, osteophitosis, reduction of discal space, and/or vertebral endplates thickening. Usually these are radiological diagnosis without any relevance.
2. Neuro-muscular spinal instability (different from the osteo-ligamentous one) has not been defined in the literature. It's possible to consider the following criteria:
   • sharp and brief acute pain following sudden position changes and/or efforts
   • pain during stabilization tests: e.g. sudden release after isometric contraction of hip muscles (flexion, adduction, abduction), trunk destabilization
3. Scoliosis over 30 degrees can progress in adulthood and needs specialistic control.
4. See Table 27-1.

FIGURE 27-2.   Subacute and CLBP diagnostic flowchart. (Reprinted by permission of Edizioni Minerva Medica from Negrini S, Giovannoni S, Minozzi S, et al. Diagnostic therapeutic flow-charts for low back pain patients: the Italian clinical guidelines. *Eura Medicophys.* 2006; 42(2):151–170.)

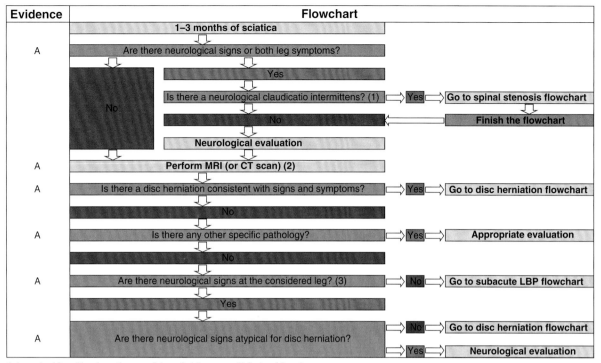

1. Leg pain while walking always the same distance that disappears with flexion of the spine.

2. CT scan is second choice screening exam.

3. Reduced strength, sensibility or reflexes with a metameric distribution and/or crossed SLR.

FIGURE 27-3. Subacute sciatica diagnostic flowchart. (Reprinted by permission of Edizioni Minerva Medica from Negrini S, Giovannoni S, Minozzi S, et al. Diagnostic therapeutic flow-charts for low back pain patients: the Italian clinical guidelines. *Eura Medicophys.* 2006;42(2):151–170.)

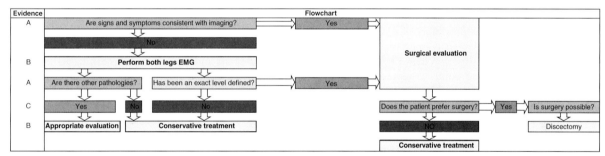

FIGURE 27-4. DH diagnostic flowchart. (Reprinted by permission of Edizioni Minerva Medica from Negrini S, Giovannoni S, Minozzi S, et al. Diagnostic therapeutic flow-charts for low back pain patients: the Italian clinical guidelines. *Eura Medicophys.* 2006;42(2):151–170.)

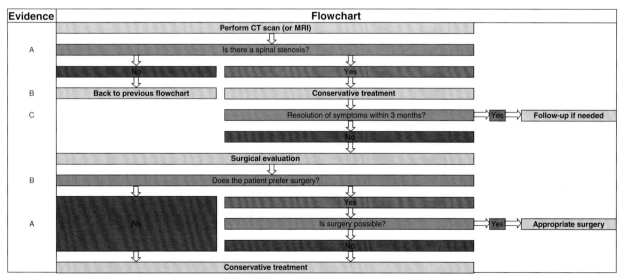

FIGURE 27-5. Spinal stenosis diagnostic flowchart. (Reprinted by permission of Edizioni Minerva Medica from Negrini S, Giovannoni S, Minozzi S, et al. Diagnostic therapeutic flow-charts for low back pain patients: the Italian clinical guidelines. *Eura Medicophys.* 2006;42(2):151–170.)

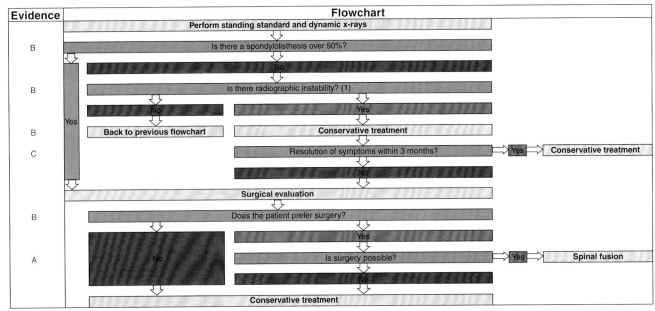

1. Over 3 mm of mobility or over 10 degrees of intervertebral angle.

FIGURE 27-6.   Spinal instability and spondylolisthesis diagnostic flowchart. (Reprinted by permission of Edizioni Minerva Medica from Negrini S, Giovannoni S, Minozzi S, et al. Diagnostic therapeutic flow-charts for low back pain patients: the Italian clinical guidelines. *Eura Medicophys.* 2006;42(2):151-170.)

DTP. Even though a recurrent form of LBP was hypothesized at the start of the DTP project, the absence of literature and the lack of any evidence on the possibility of differentiating a recurrent episode from a single first episode of LBP made it necessary to eliminate this classification item (9).

One of the most interesting points is represented in the flowchart in **Figure 27-2**. In fact, while preparing the DTP, it was discussed how to grade the importance of the different rehabilitation approaches possible for SALBP and CLBP patients. It was agreed that, from the viewpoint of rehabilitation and also prevention, the most important patients were the SALBP ones, where it was still possible to try avoiding

chronicity, which is the worst end of the story, because it is extremely rare that a patient will exit from CLBP. In the meantime, which CLBP patient would deserve the highest attention so to reduce the burden of the biopsychosocial situation for them and for society? According to the literature, such a choice has been defined using the level of disability as a way to discriminate among patients (9,21). This is a totally new conceptual development, but it is consistent with the actual knowledge of CLBP (22). Moreover, the actual disease-specific disability questionnaires have already defined cutoff levels in order to distinguish high-disability and low-disability patients (48,86). This conceptual step forward provides

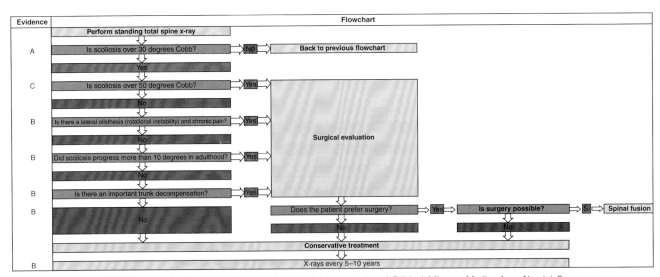

FIGURE 27-7.   AS diagnostic flowchart. (Reprinted by permission of Edizioni Minerva Medica from Negrini S, Giovannoni S, Minozzi S, et al. Diagnostic therapeutic flow-charts for low back pain patients: the Italian clinical guidelines. *Eura Medicophys.* 2006;42(2):151–170.)

a means by which to classify the various possible treatments (see **Fig.** 27-2).

Another important point of the DTP has been to recognize the importance of not only the therapy proposed but also the other elements constituting a complete approach to LBP patients. This starts with the biopsychosocial theory, which is the basis of a modern approach to LBP patients (3,4). It clearly contradicts the usual disease-oriented approach, where only therapy could be considered enough. This is correct and

typical of CGs for specific diseases, but it is incorrectly maintained for analogy in the field of LBP. Consequently, in the DTP all therapeutic schemes (**Tables 27-4** through **27-8**), including those on secondary LBP, consider counseling, work

TABLE 27-4	**SALBP Treatment**
Evidence	**Contents**
	Aim of Treatment
A	Patient at high risk of chronicity. The main aim of treatment is early, specific intervention on biopsychosocial risk factors of chronicity
A	Symptomatic therapy could be useful, but multidisciplinary psychosocial intervention is necessary to avoid chronicization
A	**Counseling**
	Recovery can be slow
	There is no significant pathology
	Avoid bed rest
	Not useful for further diagnostic examinations
	Learn pain control
	Learn pain management
B	**Work and ADL Interventions**
	Continue/resume gradually
	Eventually change/reduce work activities
	Control posture
	Reduce for a while physical efforts, if necessary
	Reduce stress
A	**Physical Activity Counseling**
	Immediately, low-impact aerobic physical activity
	Start gradually, preferred physical activity
	Practice regularly, at least twice a week
B	**Painkiller Therapy (1–5)**
A	Paracetamol with or without opioids
A	NSAIDs
A	Muscle relaxants
C	Manual therapy
C	Physical therapy
C	Pain-kill exercises
B	**Expert Multidisciplinary Team Intervention (4, 5)**
A	Complete diagnostic reevaluation
B	Painkiller therapies
C	Individual cognitive-behavioral therapy
C	Back school in-group (education + exercises)
C	Individual specific exercises
C	Multidisciplinary treatment with workplace inspection

1. Painkiller therapy should be proposed only when necessary.
2. Perform a complete treatment.
3. Follow the specific indications of each treatment.
4. Cost-effectiveness priority listing.
5. Choice recommended according to cost-effectiveness, patient preferences, disponibility, and previous results.

Reprinted by permission of Edizioni Minerva Medica from Negrini S, Giovannoni S, Minozzi S, et al. Diagnostic therapeutic flow-charts for low back pain patients: the Italian clinical guidelines. *Eura Medicophys.* 2006;42(2):151–170.

TABLE 27-5	**CLBP Treatment**
Evidence	**Contents**
	Aim of Treatment
A	Chronic pain resolution occurs in <5% of patients. In case of low disability, the aim of treatment is reducing actual disability and avoiding its progression through instruments to manage the problem (active approach by the patient) and control pain
A	**Counseling**
	There is no significant pathology
	It is difficult to eliminate pain completely
	Pain can be reduced
	It is possible to improve quality of life and reduce disability
	Learn pain management
	Reduce stress
	Be fit
	Work is not enemy
	Physical exercises are important and useful
A	**Work and ADL Interventions**
	Continue/resume gradually
	Eventually change/reduce work activities
	Control posture
	Reduce stress
A	**Physical Activity Counseling**
	Start gradually, preferred physical activity
	Practice regularly, at least twice a week
A	**Expert Physician Evaluation**
	Complete diagnostic reevaluation
	Physical fitness evaluation (biologic)
	Behavioral evaluation (psychological)
	Disability evaluation (biopsychosocial)
	Expert Multidisciplinary Team Intervention
	See Table 27-6
B	Chronic LBP therapy changes according to patient disability level (low or high)
C	In case of low disability, a nonexpert approach is possible
C	There is no evidence of efficacy in the literature of a nonexpert approach, but it could be preferred in terms of cost/benefit ratio
C	A multidisciplinary approach is complex; nevertheless, it is preferable in case of: High disability Low disability but early chronicization (it is still possible to solve the problem) Low disability, no previous trial of this approach and highly motivated patient
C	Multidisciplinary approach is not recommended in case of low disability and Complex treatment difficult because of cognitive, psychological, or motivational factors The patient does not believe in a possible solution

Reprinted by permission of Edizioni Minerva Medica from Negrini S, Giovannoni S, Minozzi S, et al. Diagnostic therapeutic flow-charts for low back pain patients: the Italian clinical guidelines. *Eura Medicophys.* 2006;42(2):151–170.

TABLE 27-6	High-Disability and Chronic Low-Disability LBP Treatment			
High Disability			**Low Disability**	
Evidence	Contents	Evidence	Contents	
A	**Multidisciplinary Rehabilitation (1, 2)**	A	**Multidisciplinary Rehabilitation (1, 2)**	
A	Functional recovery therapy with cognitive-behavioral approach		Back school in-group (education + exercises)	
A	Individual cognitive-behavioral therapy		Individual specific exercises	
B	Specific individual exercises		Individual cognitive-behavioral therapy	
A	Back school in-group (education + exercises)		Functional recovery therapy with cognitive-behavioral approach	
C	**Painkiller Therapy (3–6)**	C	**Painkiller Therapy (3–6)**	
A	Paracetamol with or without opioid	A	Paracetamol with or without opioid	
A	NSAIDs	A	NSAIDs	
A	Antidepressants	A	Antidepressants	
B	Muscle relaxants	A	Muscle relaxants	
A	Pain-kill exercises	A	Manipulation/mobilization	
	Manipulation/mobilization	A	Massage	
	Massage	B	Pain-kill exercises	
	Surgery (7)			
C	Spinal fusion			

1. Cost-effectiveness priority listing.
2. Choice recommended according to cost-effectiveness, patient preferences, disponibility, and previous results.
3. Painkiller therapy should be proposed only when necessary.
4. Perform a complete treatment.
5. Follow the specific indications of each treatment.
6. Painkiller therapy kills only pain, but is not therapeutic.
7. Only after 2 years of unsuccessful appropriate rehabilitation and according to patient's choice.
For definition of high and low disability, look at the text and Figure 27-1.
Adapted from Negrini S, Giovannoni S, Minozzi S, et al. Diagnostic therapeutic flow-charts for low back pain patients: the Italian clinical guidelines. *Eura Medicophys.* 2006;42(2):151–170.

and activities of daily living (ADL) interventions, physical activity counseling, medical therapy, and specific rehabilitation. It emphasizes again the importance of all these elements in approaching what is not a "simple" disease but is instead a biopsychosocial syndrome.

Secondary LBP is usually not included in CGs (10), eventually with the exception of disk herniation (DH): in the DTP, there are also specific flowcharts for spinal stenosis, spondylolisthesis and spinal instability, adult scoliosis (AS), and spondyloarthritis. Excluding the last one, where a specific rheumatologic approach is proposed, in the others the main ideas were as follows:

- Identify specific cutoffs for the eventual proposal of surgery.
- Apart from rare medical urgencies, postpone in any case surgery after an appropriate complete rehabilitation process.
- Verify the absence of contraindications to surgery.
- Fully inform the patient regarding the advantages and disadvantages so as to allow an individual, informed choice.

For each secondary LBP clinical picture, specific rehabilitation is listed according to the actual literature. For example,

the best types of exercises are proposed even if there is no definitive proof in the literature today, but this is obviously discussed according to the strength of evidence.

Rehabilitation Approach: Treatment Tools

Actual Evidence in the Literature

Many therapies are proposed in LBP management in everyday clinical practice. For some therapies, there are no data at all or limited evidence at best. Occasionally, the only rationale of prescription is traditional, while for others we can rely on more consistent findings. We distinguish the treatment options as pain-oriented treatments (oral drugs and injections, physical therapies, manipulations), rehabilitation approaches, and educational interventions (9). This distinction could now appear to some readers less than totally justified: in fact, most of the PO approaches propose themselves as "normalizers" of physiology and/or "etiologic" (34,62,98–102), but to date there are no scientific proofs of these hypotheses. Moreover, according to the actual literature, we will consider together ALBP and SALBP because there are not enough papers to make a real distinction between the two.

TABLE 27-7	DH Treatment
Evidence	**Contents**
A	**Counseling**
	Herniation recovers naturally, but very slowly
	The problems are pain and a possible mild neurologic residual damage
	Neurologic damage recovery is slow, progressive, and independent from treatment
	Learn pain control
	Learn pain management
A	**Work and ADL Interventions**
	Continue/resume gradually
	Control posture
	Eventually change/reduce work activities
	Stress reduction
	Mandatory denunciation, if exposed to professional risks (1)
B	**Physical Activity Counseling**
B	Immediately, low-impact aerobic physical activity
C	**Anti-Inflammatory Therapy**
C	Steroids (2)
C	NSAIDs
A	**Painkiller Therapy (3–6)**
A	Paracetamol with or without opioid
A	NSAIDs
C	Manual therapy (mild mobilization, mild massage)
C	Pain-kill exercises
C	Physical therapy
B	**Rehabilitation**
B	Specific individual exercises
B	Individual cognitive-behavioral therapy

1. Professional risk: load mobilization, trunk movements, and vibrations.
2. Only one short-time treatment, not repeated.
3. Perform a complete treatment.
4. Follow the specific indications of each treatment.
5. Cost-effectiveness priority listing.
6. Choice recommended according to cost-effectiveness, patient preferences, disponibility, and previous results.
Reprinted by permission of Edizioni Minerva Medica from Negrini S, Giovannoni S, Minozzi S, et al. Diagnostic therapeutic flow-charts for low back pain patients: the Italian clinical guidelines. *Eura Medicophys.* 2006;42(2):151–170.

Acute and Subacute LBP

Pain Management

Nonsteroidal anti-inflammatory drugs (NSAIDs) have been shown to be more effective than placebo concerning a general effect on ALBP (see also Chapter 52). However, no single NSAID molecule overcame the others in terms of effectiveness. There is moderate evidence that NSAIDs are not more effective than paracetamol for ALBP, and paracetamol had fewer side effects. Traditional NSAIDs seem to have more gastric side effects compared to COX-2, but there are no differences in terms of efficacy. In any case, the effect ranges are small. There is high-quality evidence that paracetamol

(4 g/d) is no better than placebo for relieving acute LBP in either the short or longer term, with 20% of patients reporting side effects (103). Benzodiazepines, as well as central muscle relaxants other than benzodiazepines, were shown to be more effective than placebo on ALBP (104).

There is low- to very low-quality evidence suggesting that manipulation is no more effective in the treatment of patients with acute LBP than inert interventions, sham (or fake) manipulation, or when added to another treatment such as standard medical care. Manipulation also appears to be no more effective than other recommended therapies. Manipulation appears to be safe when compared to other treatment options, but other considerations include costs of care (105). There is moderate evidence that lumbar supports are not more effective than no intervention or training in preventing LBP, and there is conflicting evidence about whether they are effective as supplements to other preventive interventions. It remains unclear whether lumbar supports are more effective than no or other interventions for the treatment of LBP (106).

Concerning steroid injections, oral colchicine, acupuncture, electromyographic biofeedback, lumbar supports, transcutaneous electrical nerve stimulation (TENS), traction, thermic effect–based therapies (ultrasound, ice, heat), and insoles (there is strong evidence that insoles are not effective for the prevention of LBP), no relevant data are available to support their use as LBP treatments (107–111). Massage improves acute and subacute LBP in the short-term follow-up, and some herbal medicines seem to reduce pain more than placebo, but the quality of evidence supporting these approaches is very (112).

Educational Interventions

Advice to stay active is effective and sufficient for the long-term improvement of function in ALBP (113,114). The indication to rest in bed is less effective than the indication to stay active (115). There is strong evidence that an individual 2.5-hour session of oral education is more effective on short- and long-term return to work than no intervention. Educational interventions that were less intensive were not more effective than no intervention (116). It is uncertain if back schools are effective for acute and subacute nonspecific LBP as there is only very low-quality evidence available (117).

Function-Oriented Rehabilitation Approaches

Exercises showed no effect in the first 2 weeks of LBP, but they were shown to be effective in SALBP in the occupational setting (118). There is some evidence that the McKenzie method is more effective than passive therapy for ALBP. However, the magnitude of the difference suggests the absence of clinically significant effects (64).

Chronic LBP

Function-Oriented Rehabilitation Approaches

There is moderate-quality evidence that multidisciplinary biopsychosocial rehabilitation (MBR) results in larger improvements in pain and daily function than usual care or treatments

TABLE 27-8	Secondary LBP (Spinal Stenosis, Spinal Instability, and AS) Treatment				
Spinal Stenosis		**Spinal Instability**		**Adult Scoliosis**	
Evidence	Content	Evidence	Content	Evidence	Content
C	**Counseling**	C	**Counseling**	C	**Counseling**
	Difficult resolution of spinal stenosis symptoms		Distinction between structural and neuromotor vertebral instability		A scoliosis over 30 degrees can progress even during adulthood
	Spinal stenosis natural history is not well known		Improvement of stabilization capacity can reduce pain		If the scoliosis already progressed, it likely will keep on progressing
	A progressive flexion of the spine is possible with time		During long time, reactive arthrosic rigidity gives positive prognosis		In the long term, a forward flexion of scoliosis with difficulties in maintaining a normal posture in elder age is possible
	Control progressive flexion of the spine		Learn how to control and prevent pain		Aesthetics worsen with progression of scoliosis
	Learn pain control and prevention		It is necessary to face not to undergo pain		Respiratory capacity must be regularly checked and cardiopulmonary apparatus should be constantly trained
	Learn pain management				Exercises can help for pain and provide short-term improvements, but there is no evidence that they can stop progression in the long term
					Exercises must be continuous in time
					Learn pain control and prevention
					Learn pain management
	Work and ADL Interventions		**Work and ADL Interventions**		**Work and ADL Interventions**
A	Avoid long walks; use a bicycle	A	Avoid excessive loads and repeated end of ROM reaching	B	Avoid excessive loads
	Physical Activity Counseling		**Physical Activity Counseling**		**Physical Activity Counseling**
B	Mild aerobic activity without impact	B	Mild aerobic activity without high-ROM and impact	B	Aerobic activity
	Painkiller Therapy		**Painkiller Therapy**	B	**Painkiller Therapy**
A	See chronic LBP	A	See chronic LBP (Table 27-5), but avoid spinal mobilization and manipulation (1)		See chronic LBP (Table 27-5), but avoid spinal mobilization and manipulation (1)
	Rehabilitation		**Rehabilitation**		**Rehabilitation**
C	ROM increasing exercises and progressively increased gait	C	Regular and continuous stabilizing exercises (22)	C	Regular and continuous stabilizing exercises (2)
C	Lumbar supports	C	Lumbar supports	B	Lumbar supports
B	Rigid orthosis	B	Rigid orthosis, eventually	B	Rigid orthosis

1. Mobilization means performing repeated maneuvers till the end of ROM that imply an increase of ROM during time.
2. Stabilizing exercises increase spinal neuromotor control ability and are based on the improvement of proprioception, kinesthesia, spinal coordination, precise neuromotor control of movement, and strengthening of stabilizing muscles (particularly multifidus and transversus).
Adapted from Negrini S, Giovannoni S, Minozzi S, et al. Diagnostic therapeutic flow-charts for low back pain patients: the Italian clinical guidelines. *Eura Medicophys.* 2006;42(2):151–170.

aimed only at physical factors. There is also moderate evidence that multidisciplinary treatment doubled the likelihood that people were able to work in the following 6 to 12 months compared to treatments aimed at physical factors. Multidisciplinary treatment programs are often quite intensive and expensive, so they are probably most appropriate for people with quite severe or complex problems (119).

For patients with CLBP, there is moderate-quality evidence that in the short term, operant therapy (that involves the removal of positive reinforcement of pain behaviors and the promotion of healthy behaviors) is more effective than waiting-list, and behavioral therapy is more effective than usual care for pain relief, but no specific type of behavioral therapy is more effective than another. In the intermediate to long term, there is little or no difference between behavioral therapy and group exercises for pain or depressive symptoms. Further research is likely to have an important impact on our confidence in the estimates of effect and may change the estimates (120).

Educational Interventions

The effectiveness of individual education is still unclear (116). However, there is moderate evidence suggesting that back schools, in an occupational setting, reduce pain and improve function and return-to-work status in the short term and intermediate term as compared to exercises, manipulation, myofascial therapy, advice, placebo, or waiting-list controls for patients with chronic and recurrent LBP (121).

Regarding CLBP, there is strong evidence to support the use of advice to remain active, in addition to specific advice relating to the most appropriate exercise and/or functional activities by which to promote active self-management (114).

Pain Management

No clear evidence exists to the effect that antidepressants are more effective than placebo in the management of patients with CLBP. These findings do not imply that severely depressed patients with LBP should not be treated with antidepressants (122). There is some evidence (very low to moderate quality) for short-term efficacy (for both pain and function) of opioids to treat CLBP compared to placebo (123).

Both TENS and traction, as a single treatment for LBP, are probably not effective (109,124). Low-level laser therapy (LLLT), in contrast to a sham treatment, may be beneficial for pain relief and improved disability in patients with SALBP or CLBP, although the treatment effects are small. However, when LLLT is added to exercise and compared to exercise therapy, either with or without sham treatments, there appears to be little or no difference between the groups in terms of pain and disability (125).

The evidence is conflictive about the efficacy of prolotherapy injections for patients with CLBP. When used alone, prolotherapy is not an effective treatment for CLBP, but combined with spinal manipulation, exercise, and other cointerventions, it may improve CLBP and decrease disability (126).

Rehabilitation Tools

The rehabilitation treatment tools used in the field of LBP have three different backgrounds: mainly physical (exercises), mainly psychological (cognitive-behavioral approaches), and finally social (education approaches). These are only tools that can be combined in a thorough rehabilitation of the individual patient so as to achieve the best results. They should not be considered separately but only as ingredients in the correct mix designed to achieve the best individual rehabilitation. In fact, there is moderate evidence that intensive MBR with a functional restoration approach is useful for CLBP (119): in this case, the complete rehab package includes exercises (functional restoration) (127,128) together with psychological (cognitive-behavioral) (120) and social approaches to the patient (40), which allows to achieve the best results.

Exercises

The use of exercises as a therapeutic tool for chronic LBP is quite common in most countries of the West (129), despite scientific evidence that shows its efficacy to be quite inconsistent. In a 2000 Cochrane review, the authors highlight the modest effectiveness of exercises in treatment for patients with CLBP while noting its effectiveness in reducing work absenteeism in patients with SALBP. In ALBP, the benefits of exercises are considered to be as effective as conservative treatment or nontreatment (118).

The low effectiveness of exercises, as reported in a great number of studies published in scientific journals, is in contrast to the benefits perceived by patients and experts in the treatment of LBP. This discrepancy may be due to the fact that in a great number of these studies with high scientific impact, the subjects are randomly chosen and placed in various treatment groups without being first classified into subgroups based on the criteria of pain characteristics (130–133). Such a method, being conceptually flawed from the outset, can skew the outcome of clinical trial results. Because classification based on a proposed relevant pathology is possible in at least 10% of cases (134), one of the objectives of a diagnostic procedure would be to allow the collection of data useful in placing subjects in homogeneous groups in order to prescribe the most appropriate treatment (130). If it is not possible to classify according to etiology, presumably it will be possible for functional characteristics or others that are now under scientific exploration. Recently, some attempts have been made to define prediction rules and subgrouping to assign to each patient the most appropriate treatment, being this a specific set of exercises or a manual approach. So far we don't know which one is the most reliable, but we feel it is appropriate to follow up with more research about this topic to reach a final clinical flowchart to approach patients (135). Until then, we have to wait before being able to state clearly what the evidence on exercises can be.

Moreover, this may explain why various types of exercise—albeit with very different physiologic origins—have all shown benefits in treating LBP, particularly CLBP (118,129,136). A few years ago, an open question in the treatment of patients with LBP was to explore whether trunk-flexion exercises would be more efficient than trunk-extension exercises. Studies did not completely resolve this question because the choice of prescribing a preferred course of exercises could not be entrusted to randomness but instead through a careful examination of subjects based on the characteristics of the symptom and its modification. An in-depth meta-analytical study examined precisely the types of exercises that were potentially the most effective in the treatment of CLBP (118,129,136). While promising results emerged from the study, in both the areas of muscle stretching and strengthening, its main conclusion was that much more research would be needed before a better definition of protocols could be reached and that the best course is most likely that of subclassifying patients. Core stability seems no more effective than other exercise (137), while some evidence has been published in favor of motor control exercise in CLBP (138), but not in ALBP (139).

The objectives of exercise (**Fig. 27-8**) could include
- Reducing symptoms
- Regaining function, reducing disability and fears related to movement, and encouraging regular physical activity in SALBP and/or CLBP
- Preventing relapse

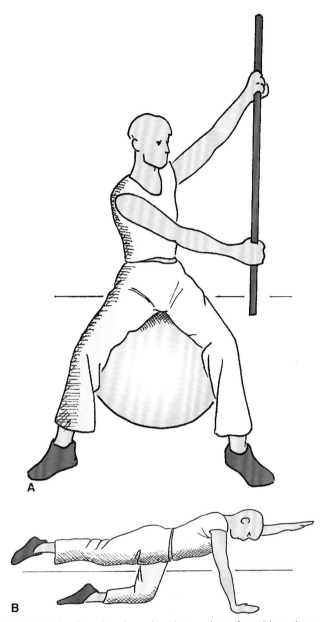

FIGURE 27-8. Examples of exercises that can be performed by patients with LBP with different aims. **A:** Development of kinesiophobia is one of the main elements to avoid in CLBP management: for this reason, the patient must experiment kind of movement as far as complex. **B:** Trunk and pelvis imbalancing exercise to improve coordination and motor control of the spine.

Reducing the sensation of pain could be linked to biologic changes in tissues, thanks to increased blood circulation, improved mechanics of the joints in question due to the stimulation of joint capsules and their ligaments, better function of stabilizer muscles, and a neurologic desensitization of tissues, thanks to the repetition of movement (140).

In SALBP and CLBP, along with pain, the patient must also face various other problems. Many studies have shown that "pain-related fear" has a negative impact on some basic spinal functions, such as elasticity and strength (141). This condition increases the risk of a progressive worsening of disability and the development of a deconditioning syndrome, which could

be an additional obstacle to improving conditions. Another typical behavior is that a CLBP patient may exhibit "avoidance behavior": the patient fears incurring back damage and adopts motor behavior marked by excessive caution (142), which further worsens motor neurologic quality. An intensive, targeted exercise program could reduce the risk of kinesiophobia and have a positive impact on the related disability (143,144). In this respect, there are proofs that a graded increased functional training has good results in SALBP (145–147), but this methodology can quite easily be extended to CLBP patients (118,129) allowing the achievement of cognitive-behavioral goals as well (120).

There are many studies that have shown how the characteristics of the muscles that maintain the stability of the spine change after an episode of LBP. The lumbar multifidus muscle exhibits a delayed activation (148) and a decrease in the transversal size on the side of the pain (149). It has been observed notably that in the absence of specific treatment, these deficits remain, even when the LBP disappears. The high incidence of recurrence in LBP the year after the first episode could be due to precisely this functional weakness in the stabilizer muscles. Some studies have supported this hypothesis by showing how a program of functional reactivation of these muscles could work as a safeguard against future episodes. A year after an episode, a group of subjects who had participated in a specific program for strengthening the lumbar multifidus muscle had a 30% rate of relapse compared to 84% in the group of patients who had not participated. Even a follow-up 3 years later revealed a significant difference in the results, with a 35% rate of relapse in the group tested compared to 75% in the control group (150).

The same results were observed for adolescent LBP (151,152). The choice of favoring a program of stabilizing exercises to prevent the relapse of LBP is not clearly supported by scientific literature. In the case of recurrent nonspecific LBP, a program of general exercise reduces disability more effectively than does a program centered on stabilizing the spine, which should only be an option for cases having obvious signs of instability.

Finally, the so-called functional rehabilitation approach is discussed (41,127,153). This gained popularity in the recent past and has been proposed as an inpatient intensive training of 3 to 5 weeks (154,155) or as a long-term training program, mainly machine-guided outpatient training (67,128,156). The main theory at the basis of this approach is derived from sports medicine (141) and considers function more than pain: in fact, results are best in the functional disability domains than on the pain itself that is in any case decreased (41). Even without considering that any kind of rehabilitation by definition must be "functional" (22), this approach has shown good results (41) and must be adopted as a concept, even if other settings (i.e., outpatient without specific machines) can be considered apart from the ones presented in the literature.

Cognitive-Behavioral Approach

Cognitive-behavioral intervention is commonly used in the treatment of disabling CLBP, and it originates from a new viewpoint in regard to chronic pain. The traditional medical approach considers pain as a cause of illness and consequent disability according to an established illness model (4,12). This provides a circle in which physical damage causes pain that will eventually cause impairment, and the impairment will ultimately induce a disability. Nevertheless, while acute pain has a biologic means of alarm to signal tissue damage, chronic pain lacks this characteristic; it is not only influenced by somatic pathology but also by psychological and social factors (44). Moving from this consideration, Waddell (**Fig. 27-9**) theorized a new model of illness for LBP, known as biopsychosocial model, in which various aspects can determine and explain chronic pain.

They are as follows:

- *Physical dysfunction*: It depends on an imbalance between the demands of physical ability and real body capacities that are not ready to provide the required performances.
- *Belief and coping*: Human thought and the way of perceiving pain play a crucial role in determining how the patient manages his or her health problem. Frequently, patients with CLBP are persuaded that they suffer from a serious pathology and are therefore hardly considered curable. They have incorrect assumptions about the possibility of recovery, often due to previous failed treatment. This leads them to adopt a discouraged approach to the problem and to new proposed treatments. The different strategy for coping with pain can explain why certain patients overcome the acute phase, while others come to suffer from CLBP. There are two means of response to pain: actively face it (copers) or undergo it (noncopers). Pain-related fear, catastrophizing beliefs, and lack of psychological and cognitive instruments with which to oppose painful symptoms lead the patient to assume an avoidance behavior from the same pain. This means the reduction of physical activity, work, and social relationships until one arrives at a physical and psychological deconditioning.

- *Distress*: Increased pain perception, emotional stimulus, and psychological factors are deeply linked, and they can give rise to a vicious circle. Feelings of fear, anxiety, anger, and depression are common in patients of this kind.
- *Illness behavior*: It is heavily conditioned from prejudices about the pathology, future treatments, and the ability of medical care to resolve the pain.
- *Social relationship*: Social networks such as family, friends, and colleagues can influence the emotional status, development of illness beliefs, and coping strategy. A favorable family activity can help to face and overcome pain, while an accommodating ground to illness will increase it. This model provides a multidisciplinary approach to the problem that requires, above all, a multidisciplinary treatment through the use of different techniques appropriate for the individual subject, such as his or her psychological state.

Two systematic Cochrane reviews (120), and additional trials (145,146,157), all of which are considered high-quality studies, showed there is moderate evidence that behavioral treatment is more effective for pain, functional status, and behavioral outcomes than placebo, no treatment, and waiting-list control, most of all when it is intensive, and that a graded activity program using a behavioral approach is more effective than traditional care for returning to work. One low-quality trial (158) found there is no difference between the effects of behavioral therapy and exercise therapy in terms of pain, functional status, or depression for as long as a year after treatment.

The goal of the cognitive-behavioral approach to non-specific CLBP is the ability to modify wrong beliefs about health status and changing the perception of health. Weisenberg (159) and Meichenbaum, who in 1977 first introduced this model, support the importance of change in the health pattern by a cognitive incentive, seeking to modify the patient's relationship with the chronic pain by offering him/her the possibility of reacting to pain through an awareness of the real problem. This approach must be presented to the patient like a process of correct learning, in the passage from an illness behavior to a wellness behavior. Generally, three behavioral treatment approaches can be distinguished (160,161):

- Operant treatment, which is based on the operant conditioning principles of Skinner (151) and, applied to pain by Fordyce (152), consists of the positive reinforcement of healthy behaviors
- Cognitive treatment, which aims to identify and modify the patient's cognitions regarding his/her pain and disability
- Respondent treatment, which aims to modify the physiologic response system directly

The first therapeutic aim is to forecast the positive effects of treatment results by acting on external events. This approach allows the patient to move from a control pain model, typical of the acute phase while improving behavioral and functional ability through communication, education, and motivation, which are methodologic instruments peculiar to the cognitive-behavioral model. Communication

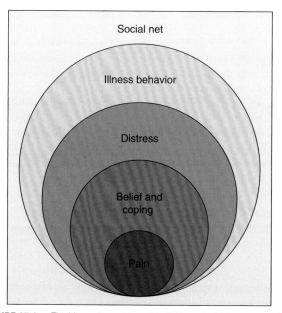

FIGURE 27-9. The biopsychosocial model of illness for LBP as proposed by Waddell (4): various aspects can determine and explain chronic pain.

must be efficacious and bidirectional in order to educate the patient in viewing his or her health condition from the correct perspective. Physicians and therapists should ensure that the patient understands his/her problem and that they are ready to help. Only in this way they can gain the patient's confidence, which is necessary to ensure good compliance with the treatment. The advantage of the educational program is to offer the patient explanations about the true extent of the problem through easy lessons about anatomy and physiology until the patient can be clearly informed in regard to CLBP. It is useful to encourage the patient to manage his/her pain instead of simply suffering and giving him/her simple means to be applied in his/her everyday life. This is done by explaining how this active approach to LBP influences, in a crucial way, the perception of pain and the disability correlated to it. This does not signify the minimization of the problem, but instead it helps the patient face it and rid self from incorrect beliefs and the behaviors of pain avoidance that only serve to strengthen the pain.

The methodology applied is not simply "learn to change" but also "test the change." To follow this model, it is necessary to establish, before treatment begins, certain realistic aims and to document the improvements through self-evaluation techniques for involving the patient so that he/she will be responsible for the change. The operating setup of this theoretical warning is to test during daily living what the patient learns and to make him/her aware of improvements. Central to diagnostic evaluation is an understanding of the deep interactions between the physical and psychosocial factors, and how they can support themselves according to a vicious circle, since disability in this kind of patient also means chronic pain, physical dysfunction, and illness behavior.

Educational Tools

A primary objective of LBP management is to provide the patient with accurate information. LBP treatment strategies have changed through the past few decades, thanks to the results of various clinical trials conducted during this period. An emblematic example of this is the general consensus regarding the recommendation of remaining active as much as possible during cases of ALBP (162). However, while it is an important element of LBP primary care, this consensus is not a widely held belief, and many people continue to believe their patients need rest.

Accordingly, an updated collection of data to adequately address the issue is an important tool in modifying popular beliefs. In the case of ALBP, it is crucial to reassure the patient and inform him or her of the appropriate methods for managing symptoms (114). In the case of SALBP, the information must be particularly targeted toward the prevention of chronicity by providing the patient with useful advice on how to identify any behavior that could delay healing (114). As for CLBP, the information should include advice on how to manage pain, control catastrophism, and decrease avoidance behavior (114,120).

Back schools have been proposed in the past as a possible important tool for LBP treatment (114), and for a period of time, they were quite popular. However, they have been widely criticized (163) because the original proposals

(164–167) were mainly based on ergonomic assumptions and a disease-oriented model of illness that was clearly overcome by the actual biopsychosocial one. Nevertheless, the back school can be considered a therapeutic tool that can be filled with the most actual contents and/or according to the individual needs and/or clinical realities, more than a schematically uniform treatment. In everyday clinics, this is the reality, because there are as many back schools as there are therapists applying them. Today, there are some proofs of efficacy, mainly in specific professional settings (121). As a therapeutic tool, if it is used as a cognitive-behavioral exercise-based group approach to nonspecific CLBP, the back school can be important as a low-cost approach to large numbers of patients (9), while there is not enough evidence in acute and subacute (117).

Media is another interesting information tool for educational purposes. With a multimedia information campaign, a significant change can be observed in popular beliefs, with a considerable number of people abandoning the notion that they need rest when experiencing pain and instead embracing the correct idea of remaining active (168). This change in behavior is cost-effective and continues for several years after the end of the information campaign (25).

Lastly, various studies have shown that a crucial element in reducing the cost of LBP primary care management is the awareness of getting family physicians to adopt the right behavior (164,169), in which a multimedia campaign could play a part.

Main Pain Management Tools of PM&R Interest

These approaches have different backgrounds, according to the pathoanatomic hypotheses proposed by the different authors and schools who have developed or use each of the tools. Some have a certain efficacy, but not in all patients: In an evidence-based clinical practice view, they should be regarded not for their theory but only for their efficacy. Moreover, to date there is no consensus on how to choose each single treatment for each single patient (9). Presumably, and as far as we know today, the best way is through trial and error, starting with what is preferred by the patient and the treating physician. What should be avoided is absolute approach, coming from the idea of superiority of the medication treatment proposed versus any other and based on specific diagnoses (diagnostic labels) (170,171) not scientifically sound: in fact, it has been shown that such a medical style highly increases the probability of chronicization (102,170,172), constituting an important, iatrogenic yellow flag.

Manual Approaches

Hands are probably the most ancient tool man has employed in bringing relief for LBP. Both written evidence and artistic representations show that manual methods were highly valued even when very simple techniques were used, because there was little knowledge of anatomy and the mechanisms of joint physiology. Over the centuries, the progress of knowledge and wider experience have led to the development of various manual techniques for the treatment of LBP.

The term "manual therapy" includes techniques aimed primarily at the treatment of soft tissues, such as massage, mobilization techniques carried out to increase the range of motion, and techniques based on the application of small-amplitude high-velocity thrusts, such as manipulation (173). Theories proposed on the way of action of manual therapies are almost as many as the different schools (34); terminologies such as "ostheopathic lesion" and "minor vertebral derangement," all supposing little injuries of the mobile segment mainly at the zygapophyseal joints, have been proposed; nonetheless, until any of these possible lesions will be proved, this treatment is definitely a PO one.

Massage is undoubtedly the most ancient and widely used form of manual therapy. It is practiced in every region of the world and through a variety of techniques. Massage has also spurred considerable scientific interest, and this is shown in the large number of systematic reviews conducted by Cochrane to explore the effectiveness of its use. Massage has proved to be beneficial in the short-term effect on pain in acute, subacute, and chronic LBP and function in subacute and chronic LBP (174). Osteopathy and manipulation are two other manual therapy techniques widely used to fight LBP. One recent review shows the benefits of osteopathy for acute and chronic LBP (175).

Manipulations are no more effective in the treatment of patients with acute LBP than inert interventions, sham manipulations, or when added to another treatment such as standard medical care. Manipulations also appear to be no more effective than other recommended therapies with the advantage of being safe when compared to other treatment options (105). In CLBP, it has a clinically nonsignificant benefit on pain with respect to other treatments (176). Considering the low benefits and high cost, the effectiveness of these treatments is also low. However, it should be noted that when therapeutic techniques are characterized by a close relationship between the patient and the therapist—as in the case of manual therapy—even in those cases of treatment failure, only 50% of the patients require alternative therapies, most likely because the ties forged with the therapist enable the patient to better face the symptoms and disability (177).

Modalities of Physical Therapy

Modalities of physical therapy include a wide variety of devices that apply physical principles in treating many problems in rehabilitative medicine. It is frequently proposed in LBP management in everyday clinical practice, sometimes alone but sometimes as part of a more complex approach. Despite the specific principle behind the action of each device, it can be considered a PO therapy because they act mainly on pain perception and transmission, even if they are supposed to possibly act on cell membrane or on inflammation.

Electricity is probably the main physical principle applied in this field, and within this group TENS is probably the form most commonly used (178). The development and application of TENS were based on the gate control theory conceptualized by Melzack and Wall (45). According to this theory, the stimulation of large-diameter (A-β) primary sensory afferents activates inhibitory interneurons in the substantia gelatinosa of the

spinal cord dorsal horn, thereby accentuating the transmission of nociceptive signals from small-diameter A-D and C fibers (45,172,173). Supraspinal mechanisms involving the endogenous opioid system have also been described (179–182). In summary, the postulated effect of TENS is to "close the gate" and dampen the perception of pain (45). Despite its rationale and well-documented biologic effects, TENS as a single treatment for LBP is probably ineffective (109,124). Other forms of electrical therapy have been proposed, and some papers have been published (183,184), even if we still lack a substantial basis for them.

Ultrasound has for many years been used in the treatment of musculoskeletal conditions. Laboratory research has demonstrated the application of ultrasound results in the promotion of cellular metabolic rate and increased viscoelastic properties of collagen (185). In animal studies, an exposure to 1 MHz ultrasound at 50 J/cm² is reported to be sufficient for the increase of tissue temperature (186). This rise in temperature is assumed to be the mediating mechanism for tissue repair, enhancement of soft tissue extensibility, promotion of muscle relaxation, augmentation of blood flow, and alleviation of inflammatory reactions of soft tissue (185,187). Despite the theoretical benefits and widespread use, conclusive evidence on the effectiveness of ultrasound therapy in CLBP is not yet available (188).

The low-level laser therapy (LLLT) is currently used by some as a therapeutic intervention for musculoskeletal disorders such as LBP (189,190). LLLT is a light-source treatment that generates light of a specific wavelength. It emits no heat, sound, or vibration. Instead of producing a thermal effect, LLLT may act through nonthermal or photochemical reactions in cells. It is also referred to as photobiology or biostimulation (191,192). LLLT is thought to affect fibroblast function and accelerate the repair of connective tissue (193). It has also been reported that LLLT has anti-inflammatory effects due to its action in reducing prostaglandin synthesis (194). Some studies suggest that LLLT has a beneficial anti-inflammatory and pain-attenuation effect in humans (195). A possible mechanism of the effect of LLLT on pain relief is its anti-inflammatory and connective-tissue repair process, which has been shown in some *in vitro* and *in vivo* studies (194,196). The effectiveness of laser therapy in LBP is still unclear (125).

Pulsed magnetic field therapy (PMFT) is a simple, noninvasive technique used extensively for the treatment of muscle pain (197). This technique is based on changes in the cell membrane induced by magnetic fields (MF) and, to a limited extent, the electric field. Exposure to pulsed MF has been shown to have a therapeutic benefit in both animals and humans. MF exposure does not affect basic human perception but can increase pain thresholds in a manner indicative of an analgesic response (197). Nevertheless, there is no evidence to recommend it in CLBP.

All the aforementioned physical therapies have some basic research studies and have been widely applied, but conclusive research on their efficacy is lacking. These approaches can be considered in the PO phase of an integrated rehabilitative process, but until there is further proof, they should be avoided as stand-alone LBP treatments.

Drugs

Pharmacologic treatment is the first way to control pain in patients with LBP (see also Chapter 52). There are various kinds of medications, and each one has a unique balance of risks and benefits. A systematic Cochrane review (104) of NSAIDs—which are widely used in LBP—demonstrated that there is a moderate evidence that NSAIDs are not more effective than other drugs for ALBP, and there is a strong evidence that various types of NSAIDs (including COX-2 NSAIDs) are equally effective. For CLBP, there is low-quality evidence that NSAIDs are slightly more effective than placebo (104). COX-2 NSAIDs had statistically significantly fewer side effects than traditional NSAIDs, but recent studies have shown that COX-2 inhibitors are associated with increased cardiovascular risk in specific patient populations.

The use of muscle relaxants (198) in the management of nonspecific LBP is controversial even if they seem to be effective. However, the adverse effects—particularly the effects on the central nervous system—require caution in the use of muscle relaxants. The potential for tolerance and withdrawal, combined with the risk of misuse and dependency, leads clinicians to restrict the prescription of opioids, even if they are commonly used for CLBP and may be efficacious for short-term pain relief. The long-term efficacy (>16 weeks) is unclear (199,200). A Cochrane review (122) reported that there is no clear evidence that antidepressants are more effective than placebo, even if such findings do not imply that severely depressed patients with LBP should not be treated with antidepressants.

A pharmacologic strategy for the treatment of LBP, particularly in regard to leg pain, is the epidural injection of corticosteroids (98). Further details can be retrieved in Chapter 53. A review of evidence for an American Pain Society/American College of Physicians (201) summarized this knowledge in terms of good short-term evidence with moderate effectiveness for NSAIDs, acetaminophen, and skeletal muscle relaxant (for ALBP), while the minimal one proposed on tricyclic antidepressant for CLBP has been overcome, according to the last Cochrane review (122). They also found a reasonable amount of evidence that opioids, tramadol, benzodiazepines, and gabapentin (for radiculopathy) are effective for pain relief as opposed to systemic corticosteroids, which the evidence strongly suggested was ineffective. The authors found that evidence is insufficient to identify one medication as offering a clear overall net advantage due to the complex trade-offs between benefits and objectives. This leads to the choice of one or more medications after a specific analysis for each patient, taking into account the comorbidity and other drugs just assumed.

Low Back Pain

We definitively recognize, according to the actual knowledge, the term "LBP" as a diagnosis instead of being merely a symptom. LBP diagnosis is made by exclusion through a triage (5): in such cases, other terms such as "sprain," "injury," "trouble," and "lumbago" have been used for years, in most cases supposing and supporting the idea of different specific pathoanatomic background. Today, the scientific community has abandoned this approach: the most up-to-date

classification of LBP is based on the localization and on the duration of pain (3,8–10). Even if this could appear as an epidemiologic framework unduly applied to the clinical field, actually it is the only real way to differentiate patients with different prognoses and pathologies. Hopefully, in the future, it will be possible to deepen this broad classification, but it is already a good way to arrive at clinical and rehabilitative everyday choices.

Research thus continues its gradual progress toward the subclassification of different syndromes, mainly with the objective of increasing the quality of approach (63,131,133). However, this process will take years to reach a satisfactory conclusion.

The incidence, prevalence, and costs of LBP are incredibly high (60,202–208). ALBP life prevalence is more than 80% of the population, year prevalence counts up to 30%, and costs in terms of absenteeism rank second in importance, following only cold and flu. However, over 90% of ALBP resolve in less than 30 days; on the other side, CLBP is an everyday experience for 4% to 7% of the population. It consumes 75% to 80% of the entire enormous costs of LBP and less than 5% of patients achieve a complete resolution of pain. SALBP has scarcely been studied and today we have no reliable epidemiologic data, even if this stage of pathology should deserve the highest attention.

Acute LBP

Definition and Pathogenesis

ALBP is defined as pain or discomfort in the lumbar region, on one or both sides, eventually irradiating to the buttocks and lasting no more than a month (3,8,9,52). All the factors that contribute to the development of ALBP are poorly understood (102,170). When an acute bony or nerve injury has been excluded, the differential diagnosis turns toward the evaluation of soft tissue. Muscles, ligaments, apophyseal joints, together with disks eventually and/or vessels, and/or the sympathetic nervous system can be the origin of pain. Nevertheless, the hypotheses are as numerous as the authors who have studied them.

Clinical Presentation

ALBP is clinically multiform: it can appear suddenly when one encounters a significant physical effort, or it can appear without an apparent cause. It can start insidiously, or it can arrive at the complete lumbar blockage. It can start on one side and move to the other or remain fixed in time. Independently from the quantity of pain, it can last from several minutes to several weeks. Apparently, the level of pain has no correlation with the anatomical lesion and its recovery.

Diagnosis, Classification, and Prognosis

Diagnosis is made by exclusion, and it must be done only through clinical examination (3,8,9,52). Red flags must be carefully excluded (see **Table 27-1**), and if there are no warning signs, the health risk and the costs of imaging and other exams will not be justified (3,8,9,52). Today, a validated subclassification based on spine structure has not been established, even if scientific efforts are under way in this respect (130,132). Prognosis is very good: ALBP is autoresolving in most of the cases, usually in less than a month (59,60,206,209). Most of the time, ALBP is recurrent (209–211). Even if there is a clinical widespread suspicion, there is no proof that it implies a progressive worsening of the clinical situation (9).

Treatment Approaches

The main objective of therapy in ALBP is, in fact, to reassure the patient and provide accurate preventive information (3,8,9,52). Medication treatment is useful but secondary, even in the eyes of patients (212).

Rehabilitation Approach

There are very few issues on which the international scientific community has reached a general consensus. One of these issues is the right behavior to adopt in cases of ALBP. The key recommendation is to remain as active as possible and to avoid bed rest (210,213). Caring for a patient suffering from ALBP should, however, take into account two important factors related to prevention simultaneously: avoiding chronicity and regaining any fitness lost during the period of acute pain, which may open the way to frequent relapses.

The real issue with LBP entails the progression from an isolated episode into chronic pain. This transformation depends on a complex series of not always identifiable psychosocial factors, "yellow flags" (60) that must be carefully taken into consideration and which could enable the health care provider to distinguish between a single episode of LBP and the transformation into a chronic disorder (214).

Many studies reveal how LBP brings about a rapid change in the function of the paravertebral and stabilizer muscles (149,215,216). It was noted, in particular, how rehabilitation of the musculature is not spontaneous with the disappearance of the symptoms, and it is believed that this deficit may be one of the reasons for the frequent relapses reported after an episode of LBP (150). Studies have shown that the rate of relapse drops drastically when the patient participates in a rehabilitation program focused specifically on the stabilizer muscles. A short-term follow-up (1 year) shows that the relapse rate drops from 87% in the group that did not participate in a specific program to 30% in the group that did follow the program. This same gap also holds for the medium term. The probability of experiencing LBP 3 years following the first episode is 35% in subjects who participated in a specific exercise program, compared to 75% in subjects who returned to their daily routine without exercise (150,217).

Subacute LBP

This is the less known type of LBP, and research in this field is really lacking, even if in recent years it has progressively flourished due to the understanding of the key role of this stage of LBP.

Definition and Pathogenesis

SALBP is defined as pain or discomfort in the lumbar region, on one or both sides, eventually irradiating to the buttocks and lasting more than 1 month but less than 6 months (3,8,9,52). Some authors distinguish a subacute phase (1 to 3 months) and a subchronic phase (4 to 6 months), but there is neither epidemiologic proof nor a real clinical decision based on that distinction. The pathogenesis of SALBP is complex. As far as we know, it is a real intermediate stage, being the passage between ALBP and CLBP. In this period, apparently there is something that impedes the spontaneous resolution of ALBP, maintains the previous situation, makes it more complex, and gradually drives the patient, through a series of vicious cycles, to CLBP (4,12,218). These factors have been studied in these years and therefore recognized as the chronicization risk factors (see **Table 27-1**) (79,219–223). According to the definition of biopsychosocial syndrome, they can be divided into biologic, psychological, and social factors. Moreover, certain other distinctions, as shown in the table, can be made. What can be supposed, according to the actual knowledge, is that an organic and definite cause of pain, which is manifested in the acute phase, cannot reach a resolution because of pre-existing factors and/or newly developed that appears in predisposed personal/social contextual factors. In this way, the resolution becomes more difficult. The patient usually starts a pilgrimage between different specialists and professionals, each one giving his/her own etiologic opinion, proposing a treatment, and using his/her own diagnostic labels (170,171). All this makes the situation progressively worse because it encourages the patient's feeling of having a bad pathology that is impossible to understand and cannot be treated in a definitive way.

Clinical Presentation

Apparently, the SALBP patient is not very different from the ALBP patient, even if a careful history taking and a good clinical examination can usually let the expert physician discover the stigmata of chronicization. A key factor is to look for the time passed since the inception of LBP, and another one is to let the patient speak freely about his or her problem. This way, if there are psychological and/or social disturbances, they usually come out quite easily, and the presence of relatives and their interrelations can offer other clues. What must be clearly pointed out is that these patients are usually quite the same on the surface, but with due time and careful evaluation, it is possible to slowly discover a multiform, individual manifestation of SALBP. Ultimately, this constitutes the real clinical presentation.

Diagnosis, Classification, and Prognosis

Diagnosis, as is the case in all LBP situations, is made by exclusion. Nevertheless, it is widely recognized that further evaluation is needed at this stage, because true spinal pathologies must be excluded (3,8,52). Standing (and eventually dynamic) x-rays in the case of LBP, or MRI (and/or TC) in the case of sciatica, and eventually other hematologic and/or neurophysiologic exams according to each individual evaluation can be proposed (3,8,9,51,52). Nevertheless, these examinations should not be repeated continuously once the supposed pathology has been ruled out (51,224). As soon as a definite disease can be excluded, the patient should be evaluated carefully in a biopsychosocial way so as structural disorder has been excluded; the patient should be evaluated for biopsychosocial risk factors that will need to be addressed during their treatment, so that the patient can be treated accordingly.

Treatment Approaches

SALBP is mainly of PM&R interest **(Table 27-4)** (9,21). In fact, it is the situation in which it is still possible to avoid CLBP. However, this necessitates a definite rehabilitative approach. In this situation, maintaining a medication treatment attitude that is usual in the disease-oriented specialties and in some "interventional" approaches, without being able to solve the problem definitively but instead using diagnostic labels, is a recognized risk factor of chronicization and should be avoided. Only a true biopsychosocial approach can lead to a possible resolution.

Rehabilitation Approach

The approach to the SALBP patient is not easy because of the already painted multiform characteristics of these patients. Moreover, there is clearly a lack of research and the evidence is quite weak for all types of treatments (225). Nevertheless, a clear-cut clinical behavior emerges from research and the knowledge we have regarding ALBP and CLBP.

The first choice is to decide whether there is a need for medication treatment. There is evidence regarding its efficacy (225), even if drugs do not significantly decrease the disability (226), but this solution should be considered carefully because most often it is what the patient has always received, which usually means short-term results with no final resolution. Some patients will not be satisfied by this answer, while others already run the risk of finishing in the "Saint Graal" vicious cycle (the infinite but sometimes impossible research for the "final solution" of their pain, possibly passive and without any individual effort) that physician behaviors can start and maintain. Consequently, a medication treatment can be proposed but should avoid any diagnostic label. Instead, one should carefully explain that this is not the final solution but a treatment with possible short-term benefits that can be added to the compulsory rehabilitation treatment.

Rehabilitation is the most important approach, combining educational, cognitive-behavioral, and physical exercise treatments according to the individual needs (40,227–230). Generally, patients in the first subacute stage are more in need of educational approaches than individual cognitive-behavioral ones, while the opposite appears more appropriate in later stages (subchronic ones), where the painful situation can be more established with many psychological and social vicious cycles already in effect (9). Nevertheless, these choices must be totally individual, as it happens for the physical exercise approach whereby the evaluation leads to the exercise.

The approach to SALBP must definitely comprise a team. This is because a multiprofessional contribution facilitates a better understanding of the different risk factors involved, while maintaining coherent messages from different professionals has a crucial reinforcement role that allows the best results to be obtained. The multiprofessional evaluation must focus on the different risk factors of chronicity (see **Table 27-1**), so as to individually

face these factors and prevent the establishment of the CLBP syndrome. Consequently, the physical, psychological, and social approach will change on an individual basis. This gives SALBP treatment the considerable adaptability required by the situation itself.

The efficacy of a psychological approach (231) to SALBP, even in the hands of specialists other than psychologists, has clearly been shown. However, it should be in the background instead of being the main goal, because most often the patient will not accept a direct psychological intervention and/or a treatment that is totally psychological. This is particularly so in SALBP, when the psychological implication of pain has not yet been fully understood by the patient and his or her relatives.

Chronic LBP

Definition and Pathogenesis

CLBP is a pain with or without functional limitation in the posterior region, including the area between the inferior limit of the costal arch and the inferior buttock fold that lasts more than 6 months (see also Chapter 39). Chronic sciatica is a pain in one or both legs that lasts more than 6 months. Given the absence of real differences between the two symptom presentations in terms of pathogenesis and clinical approach, they can be considered together (9). Even if the only difference between acute and chronic pain definitions seems to be the persistence of pain, their pathogeneses and clinical pictures are quite different. In the literature, three frequently used models regarding the development and maintenance of CLBP functional limitations are described (153):

- The physical deconditioning model, which assumes that loss of muscle strength, endurance, and aerobic capacity is responsible for reduced activity levels and hence functional limitations (100)
- The cognitive-behavioral model, which postulates that functional limitations result from the maladaptive beliefs and avoidance behaviors that are maintained by learning processes (161,232)
- The biopsychosocial model, which assumes that the loss of functional abilities results from the deconditioning and the cognitive-behavioral model (233)

CLBP, as far as we know today, can be defined as a biopsychosocial syndrome (4,12,39) in which all the aspects of the syndrome have developed over time: The patient is enveloped in a series of vicious cycles that emerge from SALBP through a full development of the chronicity risk factors for LBP (see **Table 27-1**). When pain is not resolved, altered behavioral answers inevitably develop (4,234,235), even if sometimes these are already present in the patient due to contextual factors (13). Pain also leads to a peripheral and central sensitization that increases pain *per se* (236–240). Moreover, pain can lead to a physical deconditioning, that is, the loss of fitness or dysfunction, meaning altered mobility, strength, endurance, and coordination (99,100,127,140,156,241,242). Finally, long-lasting pain has social consequences because it changes work and familiar and hobby behaviors (157,219,243). All these factors interrelate with each other, leading to a continuous reverberation and redundancy that together increase the problem in all respects, meaning the physical, psychological, and social. Looking at this entire picture, the CLBP patient's lower back simply does not work anymore, partly physically and partly due to the incorrect behavioral and psychological responses. Eventually, this situation leads to social consequences that exacerbate the problem.

Clinical Presentation

Usually, a CLBP patient whose pain has persisted for years will present a mix of hope, disappointment, disillusion, fear, and sometimes desperation. Most of the times, he or she has already undergone numerous medical examinations, had various diagnoses, and faithfully engaged in many therapies, but nothing has been able to solve the problem. When entering your facility, such a person used to say something like, "This is my last hope." In CLBP patients, the pain usually becomes the center of their life. They are so used to experiencing pain that it has become a sort of mate in their everyday life. They think about it every day, and they plan their lives according to the pain behavior and daily cadence. They are not able to imagine a life without pain, and this becomes a sort of preoccupation. Thus, the fear of pain also becomes a mate, since the patient has experienced it so much. Consequently, such a patient develops a fear-avoidance behavior (243,244). It also happens that limitations due to the fear of pain are much more disabling than the real intensity of the pain. CLBP patients are more sensitive to the risk of feeling pain, so they frequently limit their activities in order to prevent pain. This leads to a "nonuse syndrome," sometimes called deconditioning syndrome (154,245), which is a progressive loss of physical abilities that can maintain and contribute to CLBP (100) even if there is an absence of current data to support this concept (99).

Diagnosis, Classification, and Prognosis

Again, diagnosis is made by exclusion (see **Fig. 27-2**). Usually, CLBP patient has already undergone a number of Rx, CT, MRI procedures and many others, so that no further exams are really necessary in order to define a diagnosis. If the chronic situation is quite new and there has been no SALBP evaluation, then this must be done (9). Quite often one will notice that the patient has been to many different MDs, therapists, and health professionals in search of a definitive answer to the problem, and usually such a patient has received as many diagnoses, exams prescriptions, and therapies as there were consultations. Almost every time they are disappointed by the outcome, which has been provisional at best or nothing at worst. Actually, the main reasons for these scant outcomes are inadequate treatments that were merely PO instead of FO therapies.

A major topic in LBP treatment is the attempt to subgroup patients (63,130–133). It is generally agreed that LBP is a common final pathway of many different clinical pictures, of different problems of the back that, complicated by chronicity factors, have led to a more complex clinical situation with a disability sometimes quite important (22). The possibility of subgrouping patients in a reliable way could be the opportunity to provide for each one a more personalized and specific treatment. To date, no subgrouping shared by LBP experts has been made.

A subgroup of CLBP patients has been described using the deconditioning syndrome term, meaning patients in whom the physical aspects of dysfunction and deconditioning prevail (99,100,127,140,156,241,242). Nevertheless, this syndrome is not completely defined. Apparently the more useful approach is to subgroup the patients on the basis of disability (9,21). This is done using specific questionnaires, that is, the Roland Morris (246) (cutoff 14 points (86)) and the "Oswestry Disability Questionnaire" (88) (cutoff 25 points (86)) (see **Fig. 27-2**). They were designed for LBP patients and are now disseminated worldwide, and have been translated and validated in many languages. The usefulness of this classification relies on the ability and opportunity to choose patients requiring a multidisciplinary approach and those who can be initially treated with a less-expensive approach (9,21).

CLBP resolves completely in very few patients (210). Thus, the patient should be informed about the difficulties in reaching a complete restitution to wellness, and should be provided with tools to manage the problem. There is scientific consensus that the predictors of prolonged disability are more psychosocial than biomedical in nature (79,219,247–249). It has been shown that fear-avoidance beliefs about work and physical activity, catastrophizing the lack of belief in one's own ability to manage pain, cope and function, and self-efficacy beliefs are all significantly related to disability in patients with chronic pain.

Treatment Approaches

A CLBP patient is a typical rehabilitation patient because of the disability deriving from long-lasting pain (9,21,22). At this stage the attention should not be centered only on pain, because pain itself is only part of the picture. It also consists of loss of function, physical deconditioning, and fear-avoidance behaviors. For many years it has been clearly demonstrated that the attention should be focused on function more than on pain (102,250). A medication treatment alone is destined to fail, and usually many different approaches have been proposed and performed without lasting results in each CLBP patient. This point should be clearly explained to patients, since the call for the quickest possible solution to pain is common, and pills are the symbol of every quick solution. A PO therapy can be a useful adjunct to rehabilitation treatment, especially in high-disability LBP, but it cannot grant by itself a lasting improvement of pain and disability. Some patients use NSAIDs, muscle relaxants, or sometimes opioids or steroids every day, believing this is the only way to survive pain. Usually, when they try to reduce the amount of drugs they discover their pain is nearly the same. The literature data clearly show that drugs are effective in CLBP only in the short term, but a psychological addiction can lead to abuse (104,201).

The Rehabilitative Approach

The rehabilitation tools that are effective in CLBP include biopsychosocial inpatient approaches (42), cognitive-behavioral approaches (120), exercises of different kinds (136), and educational interventions (121). All these differ in their cost/benefit ratios, even if they have generally been shown to be effective in selected patients. They can be considered as different rehabilitation tools in the hands of the treating physician: the choice of the more adequate depends on individual features of the single patient. There is quite a range of clinical presentations among CLBP patients, since physical deconditioning and dysfunction, fear-avoidance beliefs, social and psychological factors, and functional limitations can combine in many ways. Therefore, we should choose the less "invasive" and less costly treatment as well as the most effective treatment possible on an individual basis, even if there is no scientific way to distinguish groups of patients according to disability (9).

Regarding high-disability CLBP (9), one should propose as the most effective rehabilitation treatment a cognitive-behavioral approach with specific exercises, aimed at recovering the physical limitations of the back, improving function, and giving the patient the right coping strategies. In low-disability CLBP, the suggested intervention is a back school in-group with exercises and education (9); if that does not work, other steps forward include an individual approach with specific exercises, individual cognitive-behavioral therapy, and a cognitive-behavioral approach with specific exercises. According to the DTP (9), a higher level of disability justifies the choice of higher cost and individual effort for therapy, while a lower one could benefit from an approach that is generally considered less effective.

General Guidelines

Despite the foregoing, there are some basic points coming from the literature to be maintained in all CLBP patients, whichever treatment is proposed. The main claim of an LBP patient is to somehow solve his or her problem, which is nearly constant pain, and hopefully to do it quickly. In the meantime, the patient is not so convinced that a solution is possible, because he/she has already tried many different approaches without achieving a final solution. Because a complete recovery is quite unlikely, even after a long time, the first step of any rehabilitation approach to CLBP should be informing the patient of this prognosis. It should be made clear that the goal of treatment is not to miraculously eliminate the pain but to improve quality of life and reduce the disability by giving the patient the right tools with which to manage CLBP. Obviously, hope must not be erased, but realistic goals must be set at the beginning in order to avoid another disillusion. Moreover, the patient will totally understand that these are realistic goals and the patient himself, due to previous experience, would not believe otherwise.

It has been demonstrated that coping patients have a different response to pain with respect to noncoping patients, who abnormally activate brain areas linked to the emotional processing of pain (236,251–254). Findlay, in a paper presented at the ISSLS Meeting in 2007, has shown that noncopers are "passive patients," while copers are able to actively manage pain more adequately. It follows that each patient should be the primary actor in his own rehabilitation instead of being part of the audience. Patients are not used to being active during treatments in general, in any disease but in LBP particularly, and sometimes they react by showing disappointment: they want to be taken care of using a pill or a drug, by a physician, or through passive maneuvers by a physiotherapist, a chiropractor, or an osteopath. They want to receive some passive

treatments and avoid doing anything independently. Indeed, changing their minds on becoming protagonists of the treatment leads to better results.

Good counseling of the patient can achieve many preliminary good results. The patient should be reassured that he or she has no significant malignant pathology and that even if we cannot completely eliminate pain, we can reduce its intensity and decrease the number of acute episodes. Moreover, they must know that managing the situation by becoming copers, reducing physical dysfunction, and deconditioning will lead to a reduced disability and ultimately improve their quality of life. This will allow patient to regain many activities he had once abandoned due to fear avoidance. The patient can gradually start working again and engage in general physical activity, eliminating some of the established vicious cycles (see **Fig. 27-10**) and instead achieving a virtuous cycle.

The team approach is another important point in this discussion. There is evidence that a multiprofessional treatment has the best efficacy in the above cases (120). The psychological attitude of the patient, meaning fear and disbelief, can be best challenged by different professionals who follow the same method and use the same language for progressive reinforcement. Moreover, such patients are by definition multifaceted. They have many different issues to face, and different professionals can give different contributions to solve the puzzle in the best way possible.

Cognitive-Behavioral Approach to Physical Exercise

According to the literature, we envision a cognitive-behavioral approach based on specific exercises, since it deals with the psychosocial and physical aspects of CLBP. Moreover, exercises are a very good and accepted way to reach a psychological recovery (118,120,145,147). The fear-avoidance behavior must be faced through a reassuring and courageous challenge to what is considered the main problem: movement. This approach can be used when the patient shows relevant psychosocial and physical limitations without a clear predominance of one aspect over another. The physiotherapist inside the rehabilitation team will choose where to concentrate the efforts according to the individual needs and reactions to treatment, both on the

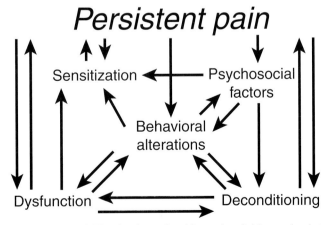

FIGURE 27-10. CLBP patient is enveloped in a series of vicious cycles that emerge from the subacute stage through a full development of the chronicity risk factors for LBP. A simplification (though inevitably complex) of all these processes is represented here.

physical (exercises) and psychosocial aspects (counseling). The most typical case in which this approach should be the gold standard is the high-disability CLBP patient (see **Table 27-6**) (9). Usually, in these patients, physical impairment is strictly connected to psychological and social limitations, so there is not a clear predominance of one single aspect. A clear causal relationship between these aspects is generally missing, because what we see is the final outcome of a vicious cycle in which pain limits physical activity, thus rendering movements more difficult and painful with each occurrence. Fear-avoidance beliefs are a crucial factor in generating and aggravating this cycle. Social and other elements are always part of the picture, but this sequence is so deeply bound that one cannot find the beginning.

Usually, a long period of outpatient rehabilitation (months) is needed in order to reach a satisfying result (127,128,255); alternative can be inpatient rehabilitation that neverthe-less must be adequately prepared in advance to reach the best results (154,155,242,256). Patients are not very trustful of therapists at the beginning, generally because they have already tried many therapies without significant results. It is very difficult for a patient to clearly understand the difference between this treatment and a general physiotherapy he or she has already experimented. It is necessary to emphasize that this approach is more complex, team-driven, since it also deals with fear-avoidance beliefs and wrong behaviors, which are second-ary to long-lasting pain. The patient should feel that the team trusts him and does not think he is crazy or a hypochondriac. Therefore, every professional must balance words and expla-nations in the proper way. It is highly relevant to this pur-pose that the cognitive-behavioral treatment is performed by a physiotherapist. This makes the patient feel more comfortable, since he or she is generally not prepared for a real psychologist to handle this part of the treatment.

This approach is quite expensive, both physically and psy-chologically, and cannot be used in all patients. It is not rec-ommended when cognitive, behavioral, or motivational factors are present or when the patient does not believe in the possibil-ity of a solution (9).

Cognitive-Behavioral Approach

When psychosocial aspects are predominant and the general physical condition and function are almost preserved, we can choose a simple cognitive-behavioral treatment. The differ-ence from the previous one is the lack of a specific physical approach with exercises. Usually, the patient who can benefit from this approach is quite young and has good overall physical function but relevant fear-avoidance beliefs and is quite upset about LBP and the prospect for the future. Poor information from the media or a physician, who is not fully prepared, along with a general health-related fear or even real hypochondria, can lead this patient to chronicity, despite a physical limitation that, by itself, is not so relevant. The patient needs to be reas-sured about his/her future and health and should be encour-aged to return to sports without thinking too much about the previous experience of LBP.

Physical Exercise Approach

On the other hand, a simple exercise approach that is spe-cifically developed for the patient and is gradually increased (118,129,145,147) can be proposed when the physical aspects are relevant and the psychosocial aspects are less important.

Even if a specific psychological treatment is not provided through this approach, the therapist should provide appro-priate general counseling about back-related problems. This approach should be proposed to the patient who lacks psycho-logical and social chronicity factors but is physically decondi-tioned and limited by dysfunction. A typical example is the older patient who does not have particular chronic stigmata but has undergone a relative loss of function consequent upon the progressive decrease in his or her level of physical activity. It is quite difficult for such a patient to start moving again, and often he or she will feel embarrassed about not being used to performing exercises, sports, or physical activity in a gym. Usually, these patients achieve good results and recover to a good functional level, but they still need a maintenance proto-col that will preserve the benefits.

Cognitive-Behavioral Back School

A back school in-group with exercises and education is the least burdensome rehabilitative approach for CLBP. As with all group treatments, it has the advantage of being less expen-sive, and it gives the patient a point of comparison by being in contact with other persons with the same problem. The main limitation is that it cannot be as specific as an individual treatment. Nevertheless, it can provide good information and a valid psychosocial support for such patients. Its main indica-tion is low-disability CLBP (see **Table 27-6**) (9), when the quality of life is not so impaired that a more aggressive treat-ment would be required. In the case of a high-disability CLBP, this approach can be used too, particularly when the possibility or opportunity for a stronger treatment is absent.

Conclusion

Generally, all these rehabilitation tools should last several months in an outpatient setting or must be intensive in an inpatient one for several weeks. This is the minimum needed to achieve a real change, to stop the progression of chronic-ity and revert it to some extent, and thereby return to a bet-ter quality of life. If specific causes of LBP are not known, a maintenance protocol would not be necessary; however, it is important to stop the treatment by reducing the medication of the patient, since he must have acquired effective tools with which to manage his problem. The best maintenance proto-col is a physical activity, whether general or through specific machines (156), performed regularly a couple of times each week. Loss of maintenance in CLBP can drive to relapses of the problem (156).

Rehabilitative treatments have demonstrated their effective-ness in reducing disability and pain intensity. A precise evalua-tion of the patient's features can allow the physician to choose the best rehabilitation tool in terms of cost/benefit ratio. Even if the most effective rehabilitation strategy is a multidisciplinary approach with cognitive-behavioral treatment including spe-cific exercises, there are cases in which other strategies can be more effective, or perhaps equally effective but less expensive.

Secondary LBP

This section considers the spinal diseases that are recognized as causes of LBP. It must be clearly stated that there is a big difference between imaging diagnosis and clinical diagnosis. According to the actual literature, the clinical diagnosis of sec-ondary LBP should be defined when there are symptoms and signs confirming that the imaging is meaningful and strictly related to the clinical picture (3,8,9,46,52). If this is not the case, the best interpretation of the imaging is the presence of specific risk factors for the problems. In contrast, the worst interpretation of the imaging finding is giving the patient a "diagnostic label" (169,171) that can propel him toward chronicization.

Sciatica and DH

As with LBP, the approach to sciatica has also changed with time: if at the clinical evaluation there are no neurologic signs (weakness, ipo-/anesthesia, loss of reflexes, radicular impingement), only subacute sciatica is managed differently from LBP (9) (see **Fig. 27-2**). Consequently, this paragraph will consider subacute sciatica and DH (see **Figs. 27-3** and **27-4**).

Definition and Pathogenesis

Sciatica is generally defined as a pain in the lower back and hip, radiating in the distribution of the sciatic nerve (257). It affects many people, and the annual prevalence of disk-related sciatica in the general population is estimated at 2.2% (258).

Sciatica, in the majority of cases, is caused by irritation of the sensory root or dorsal root ganglion of a spinal nerve. A conflict between the intervertebral disk and the nearby neural structures is the origin of irritation, but lumbar stenosis and tumors are other possible causes (46). When irritation arises, it causes ectopic nerve impulses, which are perceived as pain in the distribution of the axon.

There are two distinctive but not mutually exclusive pathomechanisms for neural irritation. First, the nerve roots, which are subject to sustained compression for long periods, may become sensitized to mechanical stimulation and show pathologic changes such as focal demyelination, intraneural edema, wallerian degeneration, and axonal damage. Second, the irritation of the nerve might occur for a chemically mediated noncellular inflammatory reaction due to the perineural spread of nucleus pulposus, which is inflammatogenic and leukotactic (101,259).

Clinical Presentation

The typical clinical picture of sciatica is radicular pain: a deep, severe pain that starts low on one side of the back and then shoots down the buttock and leg when certain movements are attempted. Radicular pain is perceived in the territory innervated by the affected nerve root in the lower extremity when L4-5/S1 nerve roots are involved or in the anterior thigh when L2-3 are involved. Pain does not always follow the corresponding dermatomes, so it is sensory loss that indicates the affected segment.

Usually, lumbar radicular pain travels through the lower limb along a narrow band. It is perceived as sharp, shooting, or lancinating. It can be experienced superficially and deeply, worsens with coughing and other maneuvers that increase the pressure around the nerve, and radiates to the foot.

The pain is usually worse with prolonged sitting and standing. Bending backward can also increase the pain.

The lumbar spine may present an altered range of motion with limited forward flexion and spasm of the paraspinal muscles. Occasionally, the somatic pain can exist as a dull, aching pain.

If axonal damage is severe, weakness in the leg or the foot may occur, leading to neurogenic claudication. When there is

bladder dysfunction with urinary retention or overflow incontinence, saddle anesthesia, and unilateral or bilateral leg pain and weakness, a cauda equina syndrome is present.

Diagnosis, Classification, and Prognosis

Sciatica is mainly diagnosed through history taking and physical examination (see **Figs. 27-2, 27-3**, and **Table 27-2**). By definition, the patient mentions radiating pain in the leg and may also report sensory symptoms. Occasionally, the patient will also have LBP, but this is usually less severe than the leg pain.

The first task of medical history and the physical examination is to rule out the suspicions of tumor, infection, significant trauma, or dangerous nonspinal pathology mimicking a back problem. The red flags are a list of relevant risk factors and signs by which an underlying severe disease (260) can be suspected (see **Table 27-1**).

A severe neurologic compromise, limping or coordination problems, severe guarding of lumbar motion on all planes, vertebral point tenderness to palpation, or spinal cord dysfunction are the most relevant findings in the physical examination, which may suggest relevant underlying diseases.

The neurologic examination can focus on a few tests that seek evidence of nerve-root impairment, peripheral neuropathy, or spinal cord dysfunction (see **Table 27-2**).

More than 90% of all clinically significant lower extremity radiculopathy is due to DH and involves the L5 or S1 nerve root at the L4-5 or L5-S1 disk level.

The neurologic examination includes sensory examination, testing for muscle strength and trophism, reflexes, and clinical tests for sciatic tension.

Sensory examination is performed by testing with a light touch or pressure in the medial (L4), dorsal (L5), and lateral (S1) aspects of the foot. Muscle strength is tested through the patient's ability to toe-walk (calf muscles, mostly the S1 nerve root), heel-walk (ankle and toe dorsiflexor muscles, L5, and some L4 nerve roots), or perform a single squat-and-rise (quadriceps muscles, mostly L4 nerve root). Muscle atrophy can be detected through circumferential measurements of the calf and thigh bilaterally, and the difference may be significant when there is a difference of more than 2 cm in the measurements of the two limbs at the same level.

Reflexes may test the S1 nerve root (ankle jerk reflex) or the L4 nerve root (knee-jerk reflex). Up-going toes, in response to stroking the plantar footpad (Babinski or plantar response), may indicate upper motor neuron abnormalities (such as myelopathy or demyelinating disease).

The SLR test that reproduces the patient's pain indicates the nerve root is irritable related to inflammation, tension, compression, or any combination of these settings. Pain below the knee at less than 70 degrees of SLR, aggravated by dorsiflexion of the ankle and relieved by ankle plantar flexion or external limb rotation, is suggestive of tension in the L5 or S1 nerve root related to DH.

Because the sensitivity of the SLR test is estimated as 91% with a corresponding specificity of 26%, if a patient reports the typical radiating pain in one leg combined with a positive result on one or more neurologic tests indicating nerve-root tension or neurologic deficit, the diagnosis of sciatica is justified (46).

Regarding acute sciatica, imaging may be indicated if the results influence further management or infer the suspicion of an underlying disease (infections, malignancies) rather than DH. Diagnostic imaging may also be indicated in patients with severe symptoms who fail to respond to conservative care after 6 to 8 weeks (46).

The clinical course of acute sciatica is favorable, and most pain and related disability resolve within few weeks. Therefore, in most cases, the prognosis is good, but at the same time, up to 30% of patients continue to have pain for at least a year (46).

Surgical Treatment: Indication and Limits

The broad consensus is that a cauda equina syndrome is an absolute indication for immediate surgery, but the surgical treatment of sciatica is still a matter of debate. Its goal is to remove DH and eventually part of the disk or foraminal stenosis, thereby eliminating the suspected cause of the sciatica. Surgery may relieve leg pain, but it has no effect on LBP.

In 2006, the extensive SPORT trial including 1,244 patients compared surgery to medical treatment: 501 patients participated in a RCT and 743 in a prospective cohort study in which patients chose either surgery or medical treatment (261,262).

Unfortunately, in the randomized controlled trial, adherence to the assigned treatment was limited. Within the first 3 months, 30% of patients in the medical group had undergone surgery, whereas 50% of patients in the surgical group had improved to such an extent that surgery was not performed.

At 8-year follow-up, statistically significant advantages were seen for surgery in intent-to-treat analyses for the randomized cohort only for secondary outcomes (sciatica bothersomeness, satisfaction with symptoms, and self-rated improvement) (263). In long-term follow-up, the observed effects were relatively small and not statistically significant for primary outcomes (bodily pain, physical function, Oswestry Disability Index). The conclusions were that carefully selected patients who underwent surgery for a lumbar disk herniation achieved greater improvement than nonoperatively treated patients with little to no degradation of outcomes in either group up to 8 years.

The last Cochrane review on conventional microdiscectomy for lumbar disk prolapse has stated that surgical discectomy for carefully selected patients with sciatica due to lumbar disk prolapse provides more rapid relief from the acute attack than conservative management, although any positive or negative effect on the lifetime natural history of the underlying disk disease remains unclear (264).

A recent clinical guideline of the North American Spine Society's gave a grade of recommendation B to the statements that discectomy provides a more effective symptom relief than medical/interventional care for patients with lumbar disk herniation with radiculopathy whose symptoms warrant surgical intervention, while in patients with less severe symptoms, surgery or medical/interventional care appears to be effective for both short- and long-term relief (265).

In the last years, different interventional spine procedures such as intradiscal electrothermal annuloplasty and chemical or mechanical percutaneous discectomy were introduced for the treatment of lumbar disk herniation with radiculopathy. The North American Spine Society's guidelines stated that there is an insufficient evidence to make recommendation for or against intradiscal ozone, automated percutaneous discectomy,

plasma disk decompression/nucleoplasty, intradiscal high-pressure saline injection, and percutaneous electrothermal disk decompression (265).

Surgery, in conclusion, appears more suitable for a carefully selected percentage of patients with uncontrolled pain or deteriorating neurologic symptoms.

Rehabilitative Approach

DH was, for years, thought of as a disease of surgical interest. Only recently has proof been accumulated to show that spontaneous recovery is common, many times with improvement of the DH itself (266–269). This has also been proved in the context of specific approaches to rehabilitation (270). In the meantime, proof has accumulated that DH is also quite common in asymptomatic people (266,269), leading to a different understanding of the sciatica symptom. Nowadays, an imaging technique is not considered useful in the 1st month of symptoms (acute sciatica) if the neurologic symptoms are mild or absent, because the spontaneous evolution can be rapid and in most cases autoresolving (8,9,46). This means it is necessary to understand which kind of rehabilitation program could be most useful in such patients, and now some studies are under way regarding specific conservative and rehabilitative treatments (63,270,271) (**Table 27-7**).

PO Approaches

Medication treatment (see also Chapter 52) is certainly a first choice in these cases, where usually we confront important neurologic pain. According to the actual evidence, we have some proof of efficacy for NSAIDs (272) and short periods of bed rest (115). On the other hand, even without the existence today of any real evidence, manual therapies and manipulation, physical therapies, bed rest for long periods of time, and steroids are commonly employed. The choice of the type of medication treatment in these cases should follow a progression to be chosen according to the individual risk/benefit ratio and the patient's preferences.

Pharmacologic Treatment

Because most guidelines recommend a course of conservative care before surgery is considered, pharmacologic treatment could have a crucial role in DH.

In the past, the main pathoanatomic hypothesis for sciatica in the context of a DH was compression, but in the last decade, the inflammatory hypothesis has gradually become more significant and today appears to prevail (273,274). Therefore, both analgesic and anti-inflammatory drugs have been tested as potential treatment, and the evidence on their role has recently reported on a review and meta-analysis on drugs for relief of pain in patients with sciatica (275).

NSAIDs. Four trials compared orally administered NSAIDs with placebo for acute sciatica. Data for pooling were available from all three studies. A small and nonsignificant pooled effect size was observed for pain (overall and leg pain) in the immediate-term follow-up, but the quality of evidence for this pooling was rated "low quality."

Five studies compared one type of NSAID with the other, but none of these studies showed one NSAID to be better than the other.

In three separate trials, diclofenac showed no difference in outcomes compared with antidepressant or electroacupuncture but did worse than caudal epidural injections of corticosteroids for pain and disability in the immediate follow-up. In one trial, ketoprofen was no better than a combination of corticosteroids for pain in the immediate follow-up.

Therefore, there is some low-quality support for the use of NSAIDs to relieve pain in the short term in patients with acute sciatica (275).

Corticosteroids. Three trials in patients with acute sciatica tested the effect of corticosteroids compared with placebo.

For the immediate term, pooling of data showed no effect of steroids on leg pain with a moderate quality of evidence. For the short term, pooling showed a significant effect of steroids on pain with a moderate quality of evidence. Therefore, there is some moderate-quality support for the use of corticosteroids to relieve pain in the short term in patients with acute sciatica (275).

Antidepressants, Anticonvulsants, and Opioid Analgesics. Three trials investigated the efficacy of antidepressants, anticonvulsants, and opioid analgesics. The quality of evidence for all these medications was considered "low quality" or "very low quality." Anticonvulsants in patients with chronic symptoms of sciatica showed no better immediate effects than placebo for disability and leg or back pain. In contrast, data from another trial showed significant overall pain relieving effect with the anticonvulsant gabapentin in the short term compared with placebo.

One crossover study with four periods investigated the relative efficacy of opioid analgesics (sustained-release morphine 15 mg/d), antidepressants (nortriptyline 25 mg/d), and a combination of both and placebo in patients with chronic sciatica. In this trial, antidepressants, opioid analgesics, and a combination of both had no significant effect compared with placebo in the immediate term for disability or leg or back pain (275).

Tumor Necrosis Factor-α Inhibitors. The interaction of activated macrophages with intervertebral disk cells in the herniated disks produced tumor necrosis factor-alpha (TNF-α) and other inflammatory cytokines. Therefore, TNF-α is considered an inflammatory factor involved in the pathophysiologic mechanism underlying disk herniation–induced sciatica (276,277). In the past decade, different studies tested TNF-α inhibitors to treat sciatica.

In terms of the natural course of the disease, compared with the control condition, TNF-α inhibitors neither significantly relieved lower back and leg pain nor enhanced the proportion of patients who felt overall satisfaction or were able to return to work at the short-term and long-term follow-ups. The only demonstrated effect was a reduction the risk ratio of discectomy or radicular block at medium-term follow-up. Therefore, TNF-α inhibitors showed limited clinical value in the treatment of sciatica caused by herniated disks (278).

In conclusion, there is at best only low-quality evidence to judge the efficacy and tolerability of drugs commonly prescribed for the management of sciatica. The available evidence does not clearly show favorable effects of NSAIDs, corticosteroids, antidepressants, opioid analgesics, or TNF-α inhibitors in the immediate term, even compared with placebo.

Rehabilitation and/or Medication/Anti-Inflammatory Exercises

Considering the various types of rehabilitation strategies, again we must think about what they really do. In fact, there are some exercise treatments that are proposed mainly in terms of a medication approach (64), while other strategies such as education and cognitive-behavioral support have broader objectives. In any case, confronting with a DH and an acute sciatica is a disease-oriented treatment more than a biopsychosocial rehabilitative approach. Accordingly, a conservative treatment spine expert could be the specialist to consider, and these many times are PM&R doctors. Therefore, it relates to our field, but we have to understand what we are really doing, meaning whether it is a rehabilitation or a medication treatment.

Research on rehabilitation is in the earliest stage. The last systematic review on effectiveness of conservative treatments for the lumbosacral radicular syndrome was concluded with the absence of any real evidence (279). A more recent review on structured exercise showed that supervised exercise programs provide small, superior effects compared with advice to stay active on leg pain in the short term only for patients experiencing sciatica. In the long term, exercise programs provide similar pain and disability outcomes to advice to stay active (280,282).

When compared to surgery, rehabilitation has almost always been proposed in terms of "standard care" (261,262,264), an expression that means nothing more than "whatever a more or less expert physiotherapist wanted/was able to offer." The same occurred in a RCT comparing physiotherapy to bed rest and the continuation of ADL, which showed that neither of the two interventions had any effect (281). We cannot rely on such methodologies as the means to understand something real. In a retrospective review of patients with good results, mobilization and general exercises have shown better efficacy than spasm-reduction interventions (282,285). In the literature, we cannot find much data, due to the fact that this field of research is very young.

The McKenzie approach (62–64,283) is a physiotherapy method that theoretically focused on DH or, better, on disk behavior as the possible source of all LBP problems. The main merits of this method include the discovery of the importance of the centralization phenomenon (62,134,284,285) and the discovery and systematization of a mechanical diagnosis to individualize exercises according to pain behavior (62,63). Centralization is the response of pain that occurs with repeated movements, such pain moving toward the midline and the back. It is a prognostic factor and a determinant clue to develop pain-killing exercises (62,134,284,285). The subclassification of McKenzie, stemming from repeated movements and answers of pain, has proved important in terms of exercise choice (63), and today it is used by others in their own development of subclassification methods (130,132). This technique has not yet provided definitive answers on its efficacy (64), but it must be looked carefully as a possible pain-killing tool with the advantage of being administered by a physiotherapist who could also offer other rehabilitative advice. Obviously, cost is the main limitation, as compared to other medication treatments.

According to the DH pathophysiology and natural history, the first objective of rehabilitation—when facing an acute sciatica and/or a DH trying to avoid surgery—should be to help spontaneous resorption and, if possible, to increase the speed of this process. On the other hand, one must avoid increasing pain and the problem itself. In this respect, movement is known as a means to increase blood flow: consequently, whichever movement that does not increase pain or tissue damage can be useful to accelerate the washout of the inflammatory and proteolytic enzymes while increasing oxygenation, nutrient caption, and the arrival of macrophages, thereby reducing inflammation and facilitating a rapid DH resorption. Accordingly, the McKenzie approach, more than being a way to mechanically drive the disk back into position, could be a way to mobilize the spine and symptomatic disk without causing an increase in pain. Therefore, it could facilitate an immediate washout of inflammatory agents and a progressive reduction of the pathologic situation. If this is true, it could explain why the physiotherapy approach that showed the best results in a retrospective analysis of sciatica treatment was joint mobilization (282).

Setting aside any other consideration, central to a rehabilitation approach to DH is education and a cognitive-behavioral counseling with the goal of encouraging DH resorption and reducing the risk of increased symptoms, but also of chronicization and ultimately increasing the patient's self-care. Knowing what to do and what to avoid should always be part of a complete treatment in these cases, but if we also add what can be expected in the near future and beyond—meaning what a DH is and what its prognosis is—the fact that DH is not a chronic condition but an acute one, etc., will be a sure help for the patient (9). Moreover, in the case of neurologic damage, the patient must clearly understand the timing of recovery and what it can mean to his or her everyday life.

A good approach to DH should, therefore, include a medication treatment combined with joint mobilization and/or active exercises performed in a pain-free way, looking for the centralization of symptoms so as to speed up the autonomous and spontaneous recovery of the situation. Counseling and information are crucial, as are work and ADL interventions. This will stand until we have more data regarding what should be done.

Lumbar Spinal Stenosis

Definition and Pathogenesis

LSS is defined as any type of narrowing of the lumbar spinal canal, causing compression of its content (**Fig. 27-11**). This narrowing causes direct mechanical compression on the neural elements or on their blood supply, which may lead to

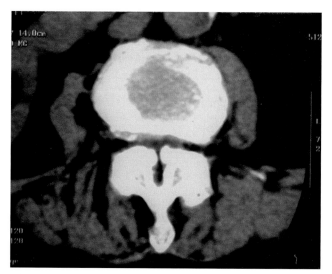

FIGURE 27-11. Severe stenosis of the spine. CT scan image showing central stenosis by congenital pedicle shortness and facet degenerative hypertrophy.

symptoms (286,287,289,290). The symptoms can decrease the patient's quality of life and cause him or her to seek treatment.

LSS may occur at different places in the spinal canal, sometimes in more than one location at the same time. In central canal stenosis, the nerve roots in the cauda equina may be compressed. Lateral recess stenosis and foraminal stenosis may cause compression of the nerve roots leaving the spine (288,289).

The presence of a narrow canal in radiographic imaging does not define the syndrome. Instead, a diagnosis of LSS is defined by symptoms and clinical findings that must be supported by radiographic evidence.

LSS results from degenerative, developmental, or congenital disorders. The degenerative type is often due to arthritic changes: disk degeneration, facet degeneration and hypertrophy, degenerative SL and ligamentum flavum hypertrophy, and calcification can cause LSS alone or in combination or can further compromise the space of canal that is already small (290,291). The degenerative type occurs most often, particularly, in patients over 50 years of age (288,289,291,292). The congenital type may occur earlier in life, and LSS is a result of congenitally anatomic changes or malformations, for example, an excessive scoliosis or excessive lordotic curvature (286,287,292). Developmental LSS is a condition in which the narrow spinal canal is caused by a growth disturbance of the posterior elements (293).

Clinical Presentation

LSS patients frequently present with few objective physical findings. Approximately 65% of patients have decreased walking ability, but up to 95% of patients treated surgically have only subjective symptoms, chiefly pain (294,295).

Patients with LSS report three types of complaints: LBP, leg symptoms, and neurogenic claudication. Leg symptoms are due to a radiculopathy with an aching or sharp pain and/or symptoms of pain, burning, numbness, and paresthesia following a specific dermatomal distribution in one lower extremity. The fifth lumbar nerve root associated with L5 stenosis is most often involved in this type of LSS.

Regarding neurogenic claudication, patients complain of cramping, weakness, pain, numbness, and tingling. These do not follow a specific dermatomal distribution but are most often experienced in both lower extremities. Occasionally, the patient will complain of bladder dysfunction and sexual difficulties. In LSS with less dermatomally specific neurogenic claudication, nerve roots below L5 are most commonly involved. In several patients, radiculopathy and neurogenic claudication coexist in a mixed type of LSS (296). Full-blown cauda equina syndrome only occurs in rare instances (153).

Because both the central canal and foraminal dimensions increase in flexion and diminish in extension, patients with LSS experience the exacerbation of symptoms with extension and improvement with flexion, meaning the symptoms are provoked by the act of standing but relieved when the patient is seated.

Diagnosis, Classification, and Prognosis

The tendency in diagnosing LSS is to focus on imaging studies (see **Fig. 27-5**). However, it has been reported that in approximately 30% of asymptomatic subjects, lumbar spinal abnormalities can be seen on imaging studies (297–299). In asymptomatic individuals, 60 years old or more, LSS was detected on MRI in 21% of cases by Boden et al. (298). In a study by Jensen et al., the percentages of spinal abnormalities over 30% were reported (269).

Due to the discrepancies between clinical symptoms and imaging findings (293,300), there is a difference between the clinical and radiologic diagnosis of LSS. Therefore, clinical and radiologic findings should be considered together when diagnosing this disease.

Regarding patient history, the key factors that seem most strongly associated with the diagnosis of LSS are a higher age, severe pain in the lower extremities, and the absence of pain when seated (301). The physical findings most strongly associated with the diagnosis were a wide-based gait, an abnormal Romberg test, thigh pain following 30 seconds of lumbar extension, and neuromuscular deficit (301). Treadmill walking is also useful for diagnosis: a combination of time to onset of symptoms and recovery time after treadmill walking or a longer walking time during inclined treadmill walking is suggestive of LSS (302). A combination of these key diagnostic factors has been proposed as a diagnostic algorithm for clinical practice to assess the likelihood of LSS, to guide and facilitate the clinical decision-making process (301,303–305).

Once the diagnosis of LSS is suspected due to history and clinical findings, the anatomical structures can be evaluated through CT or MRI, which, in a recent meta-analysis, seem to have comparable accuracy. Myelography should be avoided due to its invasiveness and lack of superior accuracy versus CT or MRI (302).

Both CT and MRI allow a precise measurement of canal diameter. An anteroposterior (AP) canal diameter of less than 10 mm constitutes absolute stenosis, whereas an upper limit of less than 13 mm denotes relative stenosis (306–308).

According to the study of Geisser et al., patients with smaller canals report greater perceived disability, but AP spinal canal diameter was not significantly associated with other clinical symptoms (309).

LSS, in radiologic terms, has been classified by the location of the stenosis into central, lateral recess, and foraminal stenosis. Theoretically, central stenosis gives rise to cauda equina compression and neurogenic claudication, whereas lateral recess (or foraminal) stenosis is associated with radiculopathy.

Electromyography and nerve conduction studies may be useful in the diagnosis of LSS because fibrillation potentials could discriminate clinical LSS from other disorders with excellent specificity and could detect alternative or comorbid disorders (310).

The few studies of the natural history of LSS generally seem to indicate a relatively benign course (311–315). Anatomy is seldom related to the severity of symptoms and probably other factors come into play. Segmental hypermobility, local neurovascular compromise, venous congestion, foraminal stenosis, or facet joint effusion may explain pain exacerbation and disability. Generally, LSS is a fluctuating syndrome with an overall improvement, and it is in a continuum with LBP and the absence of symptoms.

Surgical Treatment: Indication and Limits

LSS is the most common reason requiring lumbar spine surgery in adults older than 65 years (316). The patient's subjective experience of disablement must be an important part of the indication for surgery, since anatomic and neurologic deficits do not predict future function (see **Fig. 27-5**).

The aim of the operation is to improve the quality of life, and surgical candidates include patients who have persistent severe leg symptoms and functional limitations.

Different studies have suggested the benefit of surgery in selected candidates. Atlas et al. reported a greater improvement in surgically treated patients compared to nonsurgically treated patients in both the 1- and 4-year evaluations (317,318). Similar results were reported in a prospective 10-year study, in which considerably better treatment results were found in a group of patients randomized for surgical treatment compared to a group randomized for conservative treatment (319). The recently released guidelines of the North American Spine Society stated with a grade of recommendation B that decompressive surgery is suggested to improve outcomes in patients with moderate to severe symptoms of LSS and with a grade of recommendation C that medical/interventional treatment may be considered for patients with moderate symptoms of LSS (320).

Conversely, the last Cochrane review on surgical versus nonsurgical treatment for LSS concluded that, due to the low quality of current evidence, it's not possible to establish whether a surgical or a conservative approach is better for LSS; nevertheless, given the high rates of side effects associated with surgery, clinicians should be cautious when proposing surgery for LSS, and patients should be properly informed about the risks (321).

Finally, surgery is only valuable for leg pain, while it does not necessarily relieve LBP (322–324).

Depression, cardiovascular comorbidity, disorder influencing walking ability, and scoliosis are predictors of poorer subjective outcome after surgery, and they may be considered in the decision-making process for surgical indication (325).

Less aggressive surgical techniques that provide for adequate decompression have recently been reported. These procedures have been described as fenestration, laminotomy, selective decompression, and laminarthrectomy and are purported to improve postoperative morbidity, provide early mobility, and reduce the hospital stay. However, their long-term impact on disability has not been determined.

A systematic review and meta-analysis on interspinous spacer showed that, although patients may obtain some benefits from interspinous spacers implanted through a minimally invasive technique, their use is associated with a higher incidence of reoperation and higher cost (326).

Rehabilitative Approach

According to the earlier definition, when a patient has an imaging diagnosis of LSS without any clinical sign, he/she should be considered as carrying a specific risk factor for LBP, but nothing more. In the literature, there are studies comparing surgery to the conservative approach, but they are mainly observational, and crossover between groups due to patient's choice has been quite common. Usually, in the literature the tested rehabilitation programs are not well described (312,317–319,321). Generally, it is possible to find some "expert opinions" that, in any case, are not in full agreement with one another (317,327–329).

We can consider two main possible exercise approaches to LSS (**Table 27-8**): one is aimed at directly facing the pathology and trying to achieve improvements with treatment; the other focuses on allowing better management of an already stable situation, even if the possible future increase of problems can be the long-term result. The first protocol should be pursued whenever possible, while the second can be considered when the first one fails.

LSS is partly due to new bone formation and partly due to the thickening of soft tissues (289,306). Only in the latter is it possible to try to allow better blood flow while walking and avoid (or delay) the development of symptoms. In this respect, the elasticity of soft tissues is the main objective, along with guaranteeing the best physiology through appropriate movement. On one hand, this means manual therapy, mobilization techniques (327), and exercises to increase the range of motion, while on the other hand, it means neuromotor control, proprioception, strength, and endurance training. In the meantime, achieving a good capability of counteracting gravity force so as to slightly elongate the lumbar spine and provide more space for neural tissues can be another goal of exercises. This can be achieved through postural education and an increased endurance of deep stabilizing muscles, as well as with various activities in elongation. In this regard, specific muscular impairments have been shown in LSS patients (310,330), and these could definitively contribute to the symptoms. In this exercise approach, it is also important to educate the patient in maintaining a good erect posture while walking, because we are trying to renormalize the pathoanatomic situation as much as possible and avoid a progressively forward-bent posture, which is quite typical of long-standing LSS patients (311).

The other possible program is the one most discussed in the literature (317,327,329) and should be proposed in the worst cases and/or if the previous one fails. By contrast to the previous program, this one aims to increase the gait autonomy by teaching the patient to move in flexion, because flexion increases the space for blood flow and can allow one to move better than extension in LSS (293,331). This program has been evaluated in the literature and short-term results have been presented (332). Nevertheless, in this case we can ultimately facilitate the progressive flexion of the spine, or we can with time reduce autonomy and require that the patient use a cane to move from one place to the other.

Apart from these specific programs, aerobic training can increase the peripheral oxygen uptake, thereby reducing symptoms and increasing the patient's maximum walking distance (329,333). Another alternative procedure, or eventually a first step toward achieving the programs previously described, can include body weight support treadmill training (328). Additionally, water-based exercises and traction have been proposed, as well as neural mobilization techniques (327) despite the absence of evidence in the literature. Orthosis and lumbar supports have been proposed, but again no data exist in the literature (327).

As is always the case with LBP patients, counseling is a crucial point (9). Key messages should include knowledge of the pathology, its main symptoms, and its prognosis in terms of pain and the ADL. Particularly, the possible evolution in a flexed posture (FP) must be explained with the aim of avoiding it. Moreover, pain control and prevention are crucial, as are strategies for pain management. ADL can be adapted according to the need, and the use of a bicycle instead

of walking is suggested. Or, when needed, the use of a cane could be proposed.

Lumbar Spine Instability and Spondylolisthesis

Definition and Pathogenesis

Instability of the lumbar spine is a controversial topic. Despite several efforts, an accepted definition of lumbar spine instability (LSI) is not yet available.

A reasonable definition has been proposed by Pope and Panjabi (334) and Frymoyer and Selby (335). Instability can be defined as an abnormal response to applied loads, characterized kinematically by abnormal movement in the motion segment beyond normal constraints (335). This abnormal movement can be explained in terms of damage to the restraining structures (i.e., facet joints, disks, ligaments, and muscles) that, if damaged or lax, will encourage altered equilibrium and thus instability (334).

LSI is considered to represent one of the potential conditions causing nonspecific LBP (334).

Traditionally, the occurrence of SL in subjects with CLBP has been considered one of the most obvious manifestations of LSI (**Fig. 27-12**) (336,337). Furthermore, several studies (338,339) have reported increased and abnormal intersegmental motion in subjects with CLBP and in the absence of other radiologic findings.

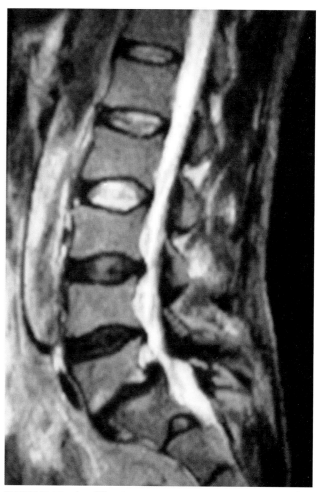

FIGURE 27-12. Instability of the spine. MRI image of first grade L5-S1 spondylolisthesis with disk degeneration of L3-4, L4-5, and L5-S1.

Clinical Presentation

Nonspecific LBP and sciatica are the most frequent clinical presentations of LSI and SL. Higher incidences of SL might be seen in people involved in repetitious alternate loading activities such as gymnastics, weight lifting, and football.

Numerous anamnestic and clinical findings are proposed to suggest instability: frequent recurrent episodes of LBP, short-term relief from manipulation, a history of trauma, improvement of symptoms with a rigid brace or external fixation, palpation for the presence of a "step-off" between adjacent spinous processes, aberrant motions such as an "instability catch," or increased mobility with passive intervertebral motion testing. Generally, the validity of these findings has not been reported.

A published questionnaire completed by patients diagnosed with LSI described back pain symptoms as "recurrent" (70%), "constant" (55%), "catching" (45%), "locking" (20%), "giving way" (20%), and/or "accompanied by a feeling of instability" (35%) (342).

Data by subjects diagnosed with LSI involved in clinical trials revealed that half of the subjects developed their LBP condition secondary to a single event injury, while the other half developed LBP gradually in relation to multiple minor traumatic incidents (343).

In another questionnaire completed by physical therapists, identification of muscle dysfunction, motor control abnormalities, and loss of strength were the greatest indicators of clinical lumbar instability. The descriptors of poor lumbopelvic control include segmental hinging or pivoting with movement, muscle guarding/spasm, poor coordination/neuromuscular control, decreased strength and endurance of local muscles at the level of segmental instability were the top three component scores (340).

In another study, the two most predictive factors of radiographic instability from the history and physical examination were lumbar flexion ROM and a lack of hypomobility during lumbar intervertebral motion testing. The presence of both findings increased the probability of instability from 50% to 93% (340).

In a study about the correlation between LSI and clinical symptoms, the translation of the lumbar segment had a greater influence than angulation on lumbar symptoms, and the combination of translation and angulation was associated with worse symptoms and the persistence of pain (341).

Diagnosis, Classification, and Prognosis

A systematic clinical history and physical examination should be performed to characterize the LBP, distinguish referred from radicular symptoms, document sagittal alignment and spinal mobility, and establish the presence of any neurologic deficit, paying particular attention to the function of the nerve roots exiting at the level of the olisthetic vertebrae (see **Fig. 27-6**).

Spine instability may be classified into two categories: radiologic appreciable instability and clinical instability. Radiologic instability reflects marked disruption of passive osseoligamentous anatomical constraints, as in the case of spondylolisthesis. Clinical instability is more challenging to diagnose and may involve discrepancies in radiographic findings.

The imaging analysis begins with conventional radiology, with anteroposterior, lateral, and flexion-extension radiographs. A number of radiographic indices can be made from the standing lateral radiograph, including the degree of slippage, slip angle, sacral inclination, sacrohorizontal angle, and lumbar index. CT and MRI are useful advanced imaging methods, particularly in the preoperative planning stage, for better defining both the bony and soft tissue anatomies, respectively.

Knutsson originally described a method for diagnosing segmental instability using lateral radiographs with the patient performing maximum lumbar flexion and extension (342). The amount of sagittal plane translation and rotation occurring at individual spinal motion segments is calculated (343–345).

White and Panjabi defined criteria for diagnosing instability from flexion-extension radiographs as sagittal plane translation greater than 4.5 mm or greater than 15% of the vertebral body width or sagittal plane rotation greater than 15 degrees at L1-2, L2-3, or L3-4, greater than 20 degrees at L4-5, or greater than 25 degrees at L5-S1 (346). Although concerns about the validity of flexion-extension radiographs have been raised (347,348), this method has become the standard by which lumbar instability is diagnosed.

At the lumbosacral junction, stability is dependent on the spatial orientation of L5 to the sacrum, lumbosacral angle, sacral slope, and pelvic incidence as well as an intact osteo-discal-ligamentous complex. Because spinal parameters are dependent on pelvic parameters, alterations in local spatial orientation, such as SL, can produce global spinal imbalance. Some spondylolistheses progress to severe deformity, while others progress very little. The pelvic incidence seems to be one of the most important factors linked with a higher degree of slippage.

Given the aging population, degenerative SL is getting more and more common. It occurs in individuals older than 50 years; it occurs four times more frequently in women and is most commonly seen at L4-5 (349–351). Rarely, however, does the slip exceed 25% to 30% of the width of the subjacent vertebra (352).

Surgical Treatment: Indication and Limits

Management decisions for adults with LSI need to take into account the severity and duration of symptoms and patient comorbidities. Those patients with intolerable back and/or leg pain recalcitrant to a prolonged conservative treatment program could be candidates for surgery (see **Fig. 27-6**).

In patients with SL, progression of the slippage occurred only in about 30% of cases. Over 70% of the patients who were initially neurologically intact did not deteriorate over time, and these patients may be treated conservatively. Conversely, most patients with a history of neurogenic claudication or vesicorectal symptoms deteriorated with poor final outcome, and these patients should preferably have surgical treatment (350).

In case of SL, indications for surgical treatment are persistent or recurrent back and/or leg pain or neurogenic claudication, with significant reduction of quality of life, despite at least 3 months of nonoperative treatment, progressive neurologic deficit, or bladder or bowel symptoms (353).

Because there is no consensus as to what constitutes the optimal surgical treatment or what constitutes the more appropriate nonoperative program, the decision to recommend surgical treatment to an adult patient with LSI must be carefully individualized.

Spine fusion is the selected procedure for LSI. It was initially performed to stabilize vertebral fractures, spinal tuberculosis, and deformities such as scoliosis. In recent years, however, a majority has been performed for degenerative spinal conditions. The rationale for fusion is that it should reduce abnormal motion and, therefore, reduce pain. The efficacy of fusion in this context remains uncertain (354–356).

Regarding SL, the mainstay of surgical treatment is decompression and there is no general agreement about the indications for fusion and instrumentation. The goals for decompression are to relieve radicular symptoms and neurogenic claudication, the goals for fusion are to relieve LBP by elimination of instability, and the goals for instrumentation are to promote fusion and to correct listhesis or kyphotic deformity.

Two considerations rise doubts on the efficiency of surgery. First, the long-term outcome of surgery is uncertain: most studies are predominantly retrospective and most certainly describe a wide variety of surgical indications and surgical techniques. Second is the reoperation rate: in a recent study among over 24,000 patients after lumbar surgery, the 11-year cumulative incidence of reoperation was 19.0% with a higher incidence among patients whose initial operation involved a fusion (357).

Rehabilitative Approach

An important contribution to understand clinical instability was provided by Panjabi (358), who proposed the existence of three separate but interrelated subsystems that act to control intersegmental spine stability: the passive subsystem (e.g., ligaments, vertebrae, disks), the active subsystem (musculature), and the neural subsystem (e.g., sensory receptors, cortical, and subcortical controls). Instability can result from a deficit in one of these components, and, according to Panjabi's (359) definition, it consists in a significant decrease in the capacity of the stabilizing system to maintain the intervertebral neutral zones within the physiologic limits. The intervertebral neutral zone (359) is the zone, within the "range of motion," of high flexibility, laxity within which the spinal motion is produced with minimal internal resistance. The components of the stabilizing system are functionally (360) interdependent so that compensation for system dysfunction may occur. Instability could be a result of tissue damage, making the segment more difficult to stabilize, insufficient muscular strength or endurance, or poor muscular control; instability is usually a combination of all three. This is the ratio for rehabilitation program in the patient with spinal instability due whether to a functional, neuromuscular instability or SL (see **Table 27-8**). The major source of spinal stability and the component that can be enhanced from a rehabilitation approach is the second one (361), meaning the musculature, which appears particularly effective in the neutral zone, when passive structures assume only a minor role. Trunk-stabilizing muscles are also defined as a core stabilizing system that is described (361) like a box with the diaphragm on top, pelvic floor on bottom, abdominals in front, and paraspinal and gluteal muscles in back. Core musculature is required for the spine (362) to move freely throughout its entire range of motion, and it also serves as a functional center of the kinetic chain by connecting the upper and lower extremities. This musculature is divided in the local deep unisegmental muscle (363) (transversus abdominis and multifidus), whose function consists mainly in stabilization, and global, superficial, mul-

tisegmental muscles (external oblique, erector spinae, rectus abdominis, psoas) intended mainly to produce control movement of the trunk. Moreover, in healthy individuals, fibers of the multifidus and transversus abdominis are the first fibers to become active when a limb is moved in response to visual stimulus (364), and the timing of superficial fiber activation depends also on the direction the limb is moved to assist with control of spinal orientation. Nevertheless, the neuromuscular subsystem coordinates muscle activity to respond to both expected and unexpected forces. This system must activate the correct muscle at the right time (365) by the right amount to protect the spine from injury and also allow the desired movement. Poor neuromuscular control may explain the onset of ALBP (360,366), even though there is no external load. Pain may be due to an adjustment mistake by one or more muscle in terms of magnitude and timing of responses caused by faulty afferent information.

In the acute phase, the first aim consists in providing a good control of pain (367) by pharmacologic treatment or physical modalities and some easy exercises to minimize pain, avoiding spinal manipulation or traction; according to cognitive-behavioral approach, physician will explain what is happening to the spine (distinguishing between a mechanical instability, due, e.g., to a SL or a neuromuscular one; informing patient that the degenerative SL natural history shows an improvement as the disk space collapses and progression of the slippage occurred only in 34% of the cases) and what patient can do to manage pain instead of undergo it. It is also useful teaching to avoid heavy and sudden loads and extreme flexion and extension movement of the spine; patients with SL must know the risk factors of worsening (like hyperextension movements, high-level physical activity) and main problems that may present like nerve-root pain and neurologic claudication. An aerobic conditioning will be encouraged, such as swimming, walking, or stationary bicycling, that promotes spinal flexion and avoids wear and tear associated with impact aerobic exercises such as running (367). Lumbar support may be used in the acute phase only a few hours per day in order to help the spine to support itself, but with the beginning of stabilizing exercises, it will gradually be removed. A rigid brace (368), in selected cases of SL, can provide a way to control worsening of listhesis and sometimes also a reduction.

In the chronic phase, treatment consists of an intensive continuous stabilizing program (**Fig. 27-13**) with a deep cognitive-behavioral intervention. Lumbar stabilization exercises aim (360) at a sensorimotor reprogrammation of the spine stabilizer muscle intended to improve their motor control skills and delay of response and consequently to compensate for weakness of the passive stabilization system. Stiffness is achieved with specific patterns of muscle activity, which differ depending on the position of the joint and the load on the spine. Core muscle endurance seems to be more important than total strength (67). This is due to the fact that in normal circumstances, only a small amount (approximately 10% of maximal contraction) is needed to provide segmental stability. The first phase of the exercise program previews specific isometric transversus abdominis-multifidus cocontractions (361) while maintaining the spine in a static neutral position. Exercises are based on the drawing-in action, called abdominal hollowing, presented by Richardson (361) who recommends performing exercises for 10 minutes 10 times a

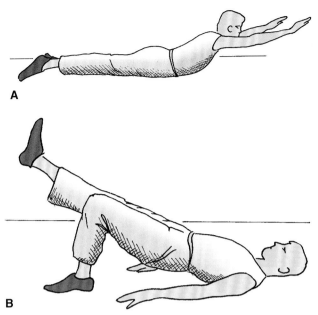

FIGURE 27-13. Stabilizing exercises. **A:** Strengthening of back muscles to improve spine stabilization function. **B:** In this exercise, loss of pelvis support allows to excite stabilization muscle complex.

day while maintaining a normal breath. It can be performed by abdominal hollowing in a prone position, eventually with diagonal elevation of the arm and leg, or in a four-point kneeling position, which facilitates maintenance of neutral lordosis and a sensation of transversus abdominis muscle contraction. The therapist will use techniques of facilitation such as muscular palpation or visual feedback. The second stage requires cocontraction in situation where patients feel "unstable" and experience or anticipate pain. The third stage of training includes functional demands of daily requiring a low degree of attention for adequate contraction. However, exercises can then progress from training isolated muscle to training the core as an integrated unit to facilitate functional activity. The neutral spine, considered like a pain-free position that is touted as the position of power and balance, has been advocated as a safe place to begin exercises. Neuromuscular control can be enhanced through a combination of joint stability (cocontraction) exercises, balance training, perturbation (proprioceptive) training, and polymeric (jump) and also via wobble boards, roller boards, and physio ball. O'Sullivan et al. (369) found that individuals with CLBP and a radiologic diagnosis of SL, who underwent a 10-week specific exercise program, showed a statistically significant reduction in pain intensity and functional disability levels, which was maintained at 30-month follow-up.

Vertebral Deformities in Adults

Definition and Pathogenesis

The aging spine might develop two characteristic deformities: scoliosis and Flexed Posture (FP). Scoliosis in the adult is a disorder that involves a convergence of deformity and degenerative disease in the spine. It is defined as a spinal deformity in a skeletally mature patient with a Cobb angle of more than 10 degrees in the coronal plane (370). Independently from this definition, scoliosis can worsen in adulthood when it exceeds

30-degree Cobb, and this evolution when it exceeds 50 degrees (371–375). The pathomechanism in these cases of AS is quite predictable: The primum movens is an asymmetric load or degeneration. Asymmetric degeneration leads to increased asymmetric load and therefore to a progression of the degeneration and deformity. The progression of a curve might be further supported by osteoporosis, particularly in postmenopausal women. The destruction of facet joints, joint capsules, disks, and ligaments may create monosegmental or multisegmental instability and finally LSS. There is also a *de novo* scoliosis (370) directly caused by asymmetric degeneration in a previously straight spine. Even if quite painful, this condition usually does not lead to a wide increase in Cobb angle over time (376).

FP is defined by thoracic kyphosis, protrusion of the head, and, in more severe cases, knee flexion. The pathophysiology of FP in the elderly is most likely multifactorial: low bone mineral density, vertebral fractures, intervertebral disk degeneration, and back extensor strength, which decreases with age, are the most frequently encountered factors (377).

Clinical Presentation

The patient with significant AS may be relatively asymptomatic or severely disabled by his or her deformity.

The most frequent clinical problem of AS is LBP (370,378,379). LBP at the site of the curve can be localized either at the apex, on the prominence/hump, or in its concavity. It can be combined with radicular leg pain. It can be the expression of a muscular fatigue or of a genuine mechanical instability.

When the lumbar curve is accompanied by the loss of lumbar lordosis, the overloaded and stressed paravertebral back muscles may become a source of diffuse, permanent muscular pain. The pain, however, is generally present when the patient is upright, especially when standing and sitting, presenting as a so-called axial LBP, and the patients often indicate that they can control their pain well when lying down flat or on their side and when the spine is relieved of its axial load.

The second important symptom of AS is radicular pain and claudication symptoms when standing or walking (380). The radicular pain may be due to a localized compression or root traction, whereas claudication may be due to single- or multiple-level LSS.

The third important clinical presentation is a real neurologic deficit, including individual roots, several roots, or the whole cauda equina with apparent bladder and rectal sphincter problems. However, an objective neurologic deficit is rare, and when present it is due to a significantly compromised space in the spinal canal with relatively acute aggravation and decompensation.

The fourth relevant symptom or sign is a progression of curvature. It usually becomes relevant when the curve has reached a certain degree and/or when osteoporotic asymmetric collapse could be relevant as a contributor to such curvature. Once the curvature has reached a certain degree, the progression will automatically follow due to the axial mechanical overload of individual facet joints and/or osteoporotic vertebral bodies. In case of evolution, usually AS progressively drives the spine laterally and ultimately in anterior flexion in the elderly, causing the need for a cane when walking.

Concerning FP, the kyphotic changes of the spine may cause local pain for vertebral overloading, inappropriate stretching of the ligaments and muscles, as well as overstress on the paravertebral back muscles (377,381). Compensatory hyperlordosis in the lumbar spine can cause LBP, and a forward-bending posture has been suggested to be associated with sacral and pelvic pain. FP also alters the load distribution on vertebral joint surfaces, leading to an increased spondylosis and vertebral body deformities when osteoporosis is present. Patients with severe FP show greater depression, reduced motivation, muscle impairment with a weaker spine extensor and ankle plantar flexor, lower scores in the balance and gait tests, a slower and wider base of support, and diminished ability in the ADL (377).

Diagnosis, Classification, and Prognosis

The diagnosis of AS is made on conventional x-rays (see **Fig. 27-7**). It is classified into four major groups (370):

- *Type 1*: Primary degenerative scoliosis, mostly on the basis of a disk and/or facet joint arthritis, affecting those structures asymmetrically with predominantly LBP symptoms, often accompanied with signs of LSS or without such signs. These curvatures are often classified as *de novo* scoliosis.
- *Type 2*: Idiopathic adolescent scoliosis of the thoracic and/or lumbar spine, which progresses in adult life and is usually combined with secondary degeneration and/or imbalance. Such patients may develop secondary degeneration and progression of the adjacent curve.
- *Type 3a*: Secondary adult curvature in the context of an oblique pelvis, for example, due to a leg length discrepancy or hip pathology, or as a secondary curve in idiopathic; as neuromuscular and congenital scoliosis or as asymmetrical anomalies at the lumbosacral junction.
- *Type 3b*: Secondary adult curvature in the context of a metabolic bone disease (mostly osteoporosis) combined with asymmetric arthritic disease and/or vertebral fractures.

In AS, sagittal balance seems to be the most important and reliable radiographic predictor of clinical health status, as patients with positive sagittal imbalance report worse self-assessment in pain, function, and self-image domains (381). Age also influences the natural history of AS. Thoracic kyphosis increases with age, whereas lumbar lordosis decreases, leading to a net effect trending toward positive global sagittal balance with advancing age (382,383,385,386).

Coronal imbalance seems to be associated with deterioration in pain and function scores for nonoperated patients, but only when it is greater than 4 cm (381).

Other radiographic parameters correlated with pain in AS were lateral vertebral olisthy, L3 and L4 endplate obliquity angles, lumbar lordosis, and thoracolumbar kyphosis (384).

Beyond the standard clinical examination, patients with symptomatic AS may sometimes require interventional radiologic procedures, such as sequential discograms, facet blocks, and epidural blocks to evaluate pain source. Finally, in elderly people with degenerative scoliosis and symptoms of claudication, leg pain, and multilevel LSS, motor evoked potentials (MEPs) may be helpful to identify the level responsible for the clinical presentation.

Regarding FP, kyphosis and vertebral deformities could be evaluated on lateral conventional x-rays. Kyphosis is measured by the traditional Cobb angle where the angle is derived from the slope of the superior vertebral endplate of T4 and the inferior vertebral endplate of T9.

Intervening vertebral deformity could be quantified by morphometry, which compares the height of the anterior, middle, and posterior parts of each individual vertebral body. When one of these heights is more than 20% lower than one of the other heights, the occurrence of a vertebral fracture is assumed (385). Because the number and the severity of vertebral fractures are both of prognostic value regarding pain, disability, and risk of further fractures, a cumulative semiquantitative index of the number and severity of vertebral deformities occurring between T4 and L5 has been developed (386,387).

Surgical Treatment: Indication and Limits

In AS and FP, surgery is an extreme option when the nonsurgical measures have no effect or do not promise any relevant long-term improvement.

Planning the surgical procedure requires a clear understanding of the prominent symptoms or clinical signs, and it is also influenced by the patient's general health, age, conditions of bone quality, and expectations.

The possible surgical technique can be divided into posterior, anterior, or combined procedures. In all these procedures, a simple decompression or stabilization can be done, or both can be combined. In some cases, additional correction may be performed by osteotomies or by sequential segmental correction through instrumentation (370).

Spinal surgery in these conditions is very demanding because it frequently deals with fragile elderly with poor bone quality. In these cases, reoperation rate and complications are significantly above the average for spinal surgery (370,388,389).

Rehabilitative Approach

Any treatment of LBP caused by vertebral deformity in adults must address two essential elements (see **Table 27-8**): degenerative instability and the reduction or loss of the physiologic curvature of the lumbar segment in the sagittal plane. In fact, findings from various studies (384,390) have confirmed that there is no direct correlation between the degree of pain, the Cobb's angle of curvature, and the cause of scoliosis (degenerative, *de novo*, etc.). Schwab et al. (391), however, noted a statistically significant correlation between the angle of L3 and L4 in the frontal plane, the extent of lumbar lordosis measured from L1 to S1, and pain and disability. The discomfort felt by the patient increased with the widening of the spinal angle and the decrease in lumbar lordosis.

Scoliotic curves over 30-degree Cobb at the end of skeletal maturity often evolve slowly and insidiously, involving both the anatomical structure of the curve and the functional status of the patient (373). This worsening seems to be a postural collapse that, at least initially, is not a real deformity because it is not structured. However, over time the permanent asymmetric load tends to modify the vertebral structure and can no longer be recovered. The development of curvature is accompanied in a linear way by an increase in CLBP and psychological suffering and, in the most serious cases, by a reduction of cardiopulmonary function (392).

Scoliosis Progression

Scoliosis is the most disabling deformity of the spine among adults (375). In addition to the concern for present disabilities, there is also the awareness that, as time passes, the condition will probably grow worse. Furthermore, when the major curve is at the lumbar and thoracolumbar levels, besides the worsening of rotation and lateral curvature, there is the risk of a collapse into a disabling total round back and flexed anterior or lateral posture.

We find in the literature a growing amount of data confirming the possibility that exercise alone can in some cases slow down the development of scoliotic curvature, not only in the child but also in the adult (**Fig. 27-14**) (393). The reduction of scoliotic curvature certainly does not indicate a reduction of deformity but a recovery from the postural collapse, which is present in the upright posture. From a study by Torell and Nachemson, there is evidence that in adolescents, regardless of the magnitude of curvature, the mean difference between a standing radiography and a supine one is 9-degree Cobb (394). There are no data in the literature to indicate precisely what this difference is (Duval-Beaupère called it "postural collapse") (395) in adult scoliotic patients. Probably, the recovery of this collapse is the key with which to avoid any worsening of adult curvature. On the other hand, the functional, cosmetic, and psychosocial damage caused by scoliosis is directly proportional to the magnitude of curvature (396), so an initial improvement, followed by stability over time, must be considered a remarkable success in the therapeutic treatment of AS.

The goals at the neuromotor and biomechanical levels are the recovery of postural collapse, postural control, and vertebral stability. The following are included as objectives of rehabilitative treatment:

- Becoming aware of pathology consequences and recovery possibilities for postural collapse
- Muscular strengthening and vertebral stabilization, always done in autocorrection, that is, in the position of maximum postural collapse recovery
- Global improvement of patient's function, even with a partial recovery of possible deficits in the joint range of motion and of muscular retractions, if present
- Development of balance
- Postural integration, which includes the neuromotor integration of correct postures and an ergonomic education program
- Functional improvement, with aerobic and respiratory exercises in the case of reduced cardiopulmonary function
- Cognitive-behavioral approach, even in the absence of pain

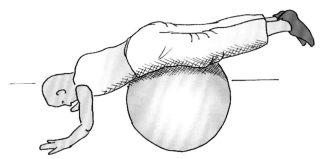

FIGURE 27-14. Improvement of balance and muscle stabilization function are two of the main points of adult scoliotic spine treatment.

Back Pain and Adult Scoliosis

The literature on spinal pain and scoliosis in adults is fairly uniform. In adult scoliotic subjects, researchers have found that the incidence of lumbar pain was similar to that of subjects without vertebral deviation (397), but the prevalence was higher (372,389,393,398). This pain seems to be more frequent in women after pregnancy or after a period of spinal mechanical overload (399), even if researchers have found no risk of debilitating LBP in adult patients whose lumbar scoliosis has not been treated. Moreover, there is a similar rate of surgery for lumbar pain in patients, either with or without scoliosis (400). Even if the symptom of pain is the main cause of surgical treatment requests for stabilization purposes, its extent cannot be correlated to the magnitude of curvature (401). Instead, there is a significant relationship between pain and the magnitude of lumbar lordosis. In fact, the increase of pain and reduction in quality of life are directly proportional to the flattening of the lumbar curve (391). For this reason, in the treatment of an adult patient with scoliosis and persistent lumbar pain, one of our goals is to recover/maintain sagittal curves with particular attention to the research of a good lumbar lordosis.

Strength-endurance training exercises that emphasize the extension of the spine can be particularly useful. In any case, the three-dimensional nature of scoliotic deviation requires that we pay attention to the starting position, which should be chosen after performing several tests to find the one most appropriate for the patient.

The scoliotic patient, like all subjects who report CLBP, also tends to develop a progressive fear-avoidance behavior, that is, a growing reduction of his/her activities for the sake of avoiding pain. In the acute phase, this fear-avoidance behavior, as exemplified by rest, claudication, or stick usage, has a protective effect against pain, given the reduced stress on the recovering structure.

Consequently, this behavior can persist in order to avoid pain, but it can also cause a progressive "disuse syndrome." Therefore, the treatment schedule for a patient who experiences CLBP must be organized from the cognitive-behavioral perspective.

Back Pain and Hyperkyphosis

Hyperkyphosis resulting from Scheuermann's disease, and from idiopathic or postural hyperkyphosis among adults, involves a pronounced rigidity of the thoracic section that leads to dysfunctional strain on the spinal segments retaining mobility, meaning the cervical spine and lumbar spine. While the mediodorsal spine benefits from a type of "natural" arthrodesis, which is just as efficient as surgery, the increased pressure on the transition areas of the lordotic curvatures above and below the thoracic kyphosis can cause localized stress and eventually lead the patient to experience cervical and LBP. Additionally, the apex of the kyphosis itself can at times become a locus of sharp pain that is difficult to manage. Rehabilitative measures should include exercises to control posture and recover function similar for those for nonspecific LBP.

SUMMARY

Today's approach to LBP requires deep knowledge of the actual evidence and the clinical specifics of the individual circumstance. A superficial, nonexpert approach to these problems is no longer acceptable. That is particularly the case in our specialty, because the evolution of knowledge in the literature, if not the expert consensus, indicates a PM&R leadership role in the LBP field. In fact, excluding ALBP, a rehabilitative team approach eventually combined with medication treatments (but clearly distinguishing the two) is mandatory in most of the cases (21,22).

ACKNOWLEDGMENT

We wish to thank for their help Salvatore Atanasio, Claudia Fusco, and Francesco Negrini.

REFERENCES

1. Deyo RA, Weinstein JN. Low back pain. *N Engl J Med*. 2001;344(5):363–370.
2. Deyo RA. Low-back pain. *Sci Am*. 1998;279(2):48–53.
3. Balagué F, Mannion AF, Pellisé F, et al. Clinical update: low back pain. *Lancet*. 2007;369(9563):726–728.
4. Waddell G. 1987 Volvo award in clinical sciences. A new clinical model for the treatment of low-back pain. *Spine*. 1987;12(7):632–644.
5. Back Pain. *Committee on Back Pain*. London: HMSO-CSAG; 1994.
6. Deyo RA. Acute low back pain: a new paradigm for management. *BMJ*. 1996;313(7069):1343–1344.
7. Arnau JM, Pellisé F, Vallano A, et al. Editorial Comment: European guidelines for low back pain—a necessary step forward and an opportunity not to be missed. *Eur Spine J*. 2006;15(suppl 2):S131–S133.
8. Airaksinen O, Brox JI, Cedraschi C, et al. Chapter 4. European guidelines for the management of low back pain. *Eur Spine J*. 2006;15:S192–S300.
9. Negrini S, Giovannoni S, Minozzi S, et al. Diagnostic therapeutic flow-charts for low back pain patients: the Italian clinical guidelines. *Eura Medicophys*. 2006;42(2):151–170.
10. Arnau JM, Vallano A, Lopez A, et al. A critical review of guidelines for low back pain treatment. *Eur Spine J*. 2006;15(5):543–553.
11. Clinical Practice Guideline 14. Acute Lower Back Problems In Adults. Available from: http://www.chiro.org/LINKS/GUIDELINES/Acute_Lower_Back_Problems_in_Adults.html [cited February 14, 2017].
12. Waddell G. Biopsychosocial analysis of low back pain. *Baillieres Clin Rheumatol*. 1992;6(3):523–557.
13. OMS Organizzazione Mondiale della Sanità. *ICF Classificazione Internazionale del Funzionamento, della Disabilità e della Salute*. Gardolo, TN: Erickson; 2001:234.
14. Section of Physical and Rehabilitation Medicine Union Européenne des Médecins Spécialistes (UEMS), European Board of Physical and Rehabilitation Medicine, Académie Européenne de Médecine de Réadaptation, European Society for Physical and Rehabilitation Medicine. White book on physical and rehabilitation medicine in Europe. *Eura Medicophys*. 2006;42(4):292–332.
15. Stucki G, Ewert T, Cieza A. Value and application of the ICF in rehabilitation medicine. *Disabil Rehabil*. 2003;25(11–12):628–634.
16. Stucki G, Reinhardt JD, Grimby G, et al. Developing research capacity in human functioning and rehabilitation research from the comprehensive perspective based on the ICF-model. *Eur J Phys Rehabil Med*. 2008;44(3):343–351.
17. Rauch A, Cieza A, Stucki G. How to apply the International Classification of Functioning, Disability and Health (ICF) for rehabilitation management in clinical practice. *Eur J Phys Rehabil Med*. 2008;44(3):329–342.
18. Stucki G, Kostanjsek N, Ustün B, et al. ICF-based classification and measurement of functioning. *Eur J Phys Rehabil Med*. 2008;44(3):315–328.
19. Cieza A, Stucki G. The International Classification of Functioning Disability and Health: its development process and content validity. *Eur J Phys Rehabil Med*. 2008;44(3):303–313.
20. Stucki G, Cieza A. The International Classification of Functioning, Disability and Health (ICF) in physical and rehabilitation medicine. *Eur J Phys Rehabil Med*. 2008;44(3):299–302.
21. Negrini S. Usefulness of disability to sub-classify chronic low back pain and the crucial role of rehabilitation. *Eura Medicophys*. 2006;42(3):173–175.
22. Negrini S. The low back pain puzzle today. *Eura Medicophys*. 2004;40(1):1–8.
23. Negrini S, Politano E, Carabalona R, et al. General practitioners' management of low back pain: impact of clinical guidelines in a non-English-speaking country. *Spine*. 2001;26(24):2727–2733; discussion 2734.
24. Buchbinder R, Gross DP, Werner EL, et al. Understanding the characteristics of effective mass media campaigns for back pain and methodological challenges in evaluating their effects. *Spine*. 2008;33(1):74–80.
25. Buchbinder R, Jolley D. Improvements in general practitioner beliefs and stated management of back pain persist 4.5 years after the cessation of a public health media campaign. *Spine*. 2007;32(5):E156–E162.
26. McKenzie JE, French SD, O'Connor DA, et al. IMPLEmenting a clinical practice guideline for acute low back pain evidence-based manageMENT in general practice (IMPLEMENT): cluster randomised controlled trial study protocol. *Implement Sci*. 2008;3:11.
27. Bero LA, Grilli R, Grimshaw JM, et al. Closing the gap between research and practice: an overview of systematic reviews of interventions to promote the implementation of research findings. The Cochrane Effective Practice and Organization of Care Review Group. *BMJ*. 1998;317(7156):465–468.
28. Armstrong MP, McDonough S, Baxter GD. Clinical guidelines versus clinical practice in the management of low back pain. *Int J Clin Pract*. 2003;57(1):9–13.
29. Volinn E, Mayer J, Diehr P, et al. Small area analysis of surgery for low-back pain. *Spine*. 1992;17(5):575–581.
30. White Book on Physical and Rehabilitation Medicine in Europe. *J Rehabil Med*. 2007;(45 suppl):6–47.
31. Ferguson FC, Brownlee M, Webster V. A Delphi study investigating consensus among expert physiotherapists in relation to the management of low back pain. *Musculoskeletal Care*. 2008;6(4):197–210.
32. Pincus T, Foster NE, Vogel S, et al. Attitudes to back pain amongst musculoskeletal practitioners: a comparison of professional groups and practice settings using the ABS-mp. *Man Ther*. 2007;12(2):167–175.
33. Pincus T, Vogel S, Breen A, et al. Persistent back pain—why do physical therapy clinicians continue treatment? A mixed methods study of chiropractors, osteopaths and physiotherapists. *Eur J Pain*. 2006;10(1):67–76.
34. van de Veen EA, de Vet HCW, Pool JJM, et al. Variance in manual treatment of nonspecific low back pain between orthomanual physicians, manual therapists, and chiropractors. *J Manipulative Physiol Ther*. 2005;28(2):108–116.
35. Daykin AR, Richardson B. Physiotherapists' pain beliefs and their influence on the management of patients with chronic low back pain. *Spine*. 2004;29(7):783–795.
36. Schwarzkopf SR, Ewert T, Dreinhöfer KE, et al. Towards an ICF Core Set for chronic musculoskeletal conditions: commonalities across ICF Core Sets for osteoarthritis, rheumatoid arthritis, osteoporosis, low back pain and chronic widespread pain. *Clin Rheumatol*. 2008;27(11):1355–1361.
37. Weigl M, Cieza A, Kostanjsek N, et al. The ICF comprehensively covers the spectrum of health problems encountered by health professionals in patients with musculoskeletal conditions. *Rheumatology (Oxford)*. 2006;45(10):1247–1254.
38. Cieza A, Stucki G, Weigl M, et al. ICF Core Sets for low back pain. *J Rehabil Med*. 2004;(44 suppl):69–74.
39. Waddell G. Low back pain: a twentieth century health care enigma. *Spine*. 1996; 21(24):2820–2825.
40. Karjalainen K, Malmivaara A, van Tulder M, et al. Multidisciplinary biopsychosocial rehabilitation for subacute low back pain among working age adults. *Cochrane Database Syst Rev*. 2003;(2):CD002193.
41. Schonstein E, Kenny DT, Keating J, et al. Work conditioning, work hardening and functional restoration for workers with back and neck pain. *Cochrane Database Syst Rev*. 2003;(1):CD001822.
42. Guzmán J, Esmail R, Karjalainen K, et al. Multidisciplinary bio-psycho-social rehabilitation for chronic low back pain. *Cochrane Database Syst Rev*. 2002;(1):CD000963.
43. Deyo RA. Early diagnostic evaluation of low back pain. *J Gen Intern Med*. 1986; 1(5):328–338.
44. Waddell G. *The Back Pain Revolution*. 2nd ed. Edinburgh; New York: Churchill Livingstone; 2004.
45. Melzack R, Wall PD. Pain mechanisms: a new theory. *Science*. 1965;150(3699): 971–979.
46. Koes BW, van Tulder MW, Peul WC. Diagnosis and treatment of sciatica. *BMJ*. 2007;334(7607):1313–1317.
47. Kovacs FM, Abraira V, Zamora J, et al. The transition from acute to subacute and chronic low back pain: a study based on determinants of quality of life and prediction of chronic disability. *Spine*. 2005;30(15):1786–1792.
48. Bombardier C. Outcome assessments in the evaluation of treatment of spinal disorders: summary and general recommendations. *Spine*. 2000;25(24):3100–3103.
49. Deyo RA, Battie M, Beurskens AJ, et al. Outcome measures for low back pain research. A proposal for standardized use. *Spine*. 1998;23(18):2003–2013.
50. Franchignoni F, Ring H. Measuring change in rehabilitation medicine. *Eura Medicophys*. 2006;42(1):1–3.
51. Saal JS. General principles of diagnostic testing as related to painful lumbar spine disorders: a critical appraisal of current diagnostic techniques. *Spine*. 2002;27(22):2538–2545; discussion 2546.
52. Koes BW, van Tulder MW, Ostelo R, et al. Clinical guidelines for the management of low back pain in primary care: an international comparison. *Spine*. 2001;26(22):2504–2513; discussion 2513–2514.
53. Cherkin DC, MacCornack FA. Patient evaluations of low back pain care from family physicians and chiropractors. *West J Med*. 1989;150(3):351–355.
54. Sigl T, Cieza A, Brockow T, et al. Content comparison of low back pain-specific measures based on the International Classification of Functioning, Disability and Health (ICF). *Clin J Pain*. 2006;22(2):147–153.
55. Cieza A, Ewert T, Ustün TB, et al. Development of ICF Core Sets for patients with chronic conditions. *J Rehabil Med*. 2004;(44 suppl):9–11.
56. Weigl M, Cieza A, Andersen C, et al. Identification of relevant ICF categories in patients with chronic health conditions: a Delphi exercise. *J Rehabil Med*. 2004;(44 suppl):12–21.
57. Verhagen AP, Downie A, Popal N, et al. Red flags presented in current low back pain guidelines: a review. *Eur Spine J*. 2016;25(9):2788–2802.
58. Henschke N, Maher CG, Refshauge KM. A systematic review identifies five "red flags" to screen for vertebral fracture in patients with low back pain. *J Clin Epidemiol*. 2008;61(2):110–118.
59. Henschke N, Maher CG, Ostelo RWJG, et al. Red flags to screen for malignancy in patients with low-back pain. *Cochrane Database Syst Rev*. 2013;(2):CD008686.

60. Krismer M, van Tulder M; Low Back Pain Group of the Bone and Joint Health Strategies for Europe Project. Strategies for prevention and management of musculoskeletal conditions. Low back pain (non-specific). *Best Pract Res Clin Rheumatol.* 2007;21(1):77–91.

61. Rubinstein SM, van Tulder M. A best-evidence review of diagnostic procedures for neck and low-back pain. *Best Pract Res Clin Rheumatol.* 2008;22(3):471–482.

62. Donelson R, Aprill C, Medcalf R, et al. A prospective study of centralization of lumbar and referred pain. A predictor of symptomatic discs and annular competence. *Spine.* 1997;22(10):1115–1122.

63. Long A, Donelson R, Fung T. Does it matter which exercise? A randomized control trial of exercise for low back pain. *Spine.* 2004;29(23):2593–2602.

64. Machado LA, de Souza MV, Ferreira PH, et al. The McKenzie method for low back pain: a systematic review of the literature with a meta-analysis approach. *Spine.* 2006;31(9):E254–E262.

65. Simmonds MJ, Olson SL, Jones S, et al. Psychometric characteristics and clinical usefulness of physical performance tests in patients with low back pain. *Spine.* 1998;23(22):2412–2421.

66. Newton M, Waddell G. Trunk strength testing with iso-machines. Part 1: Review of a decade of scientific evidence. *Spine.* 1993;18(7):801–811.

67. Taimela S, Kankaanpää M, Luoto S. The effect of lumbar fatigue on the ability to sense a change in lumbar position. A controlled study. *Spine.* 1999;24(13):1322–1327.

68. Seffinger MA, Najm WI, Mishra SI, et al. Reliability of spinal palpation for diagnosis of back and neck pain: a systematic review of the literature. *Spine.* 2004;29(19):E413–E425.

69. Maas ET, Juch JNS, Ostelo RWJG, et al. Systematic review of patient history and physical examination to diagnose chronic low back pain originating from the facet joints. *Eur J Pain.* 2017;21(3):403–414.

70. Alqarni AM, Schneiders AG, Hendrick PA. Clinical tests to diagnose lumbar segmental instability: a systematic review. *J Orthop Sports Phys Ther.* 2011;41(3):130–140.

71. Shultz S, Averell K, Eickelman A, et al. Diagnostic accuracy of self-report and subjective history in the diagnosis of low back pain with non-specific lower extremity symptoms: a systematic review. *Man Ther.* 2015;20(1):18–27.

72. van der Windt DA, Simons E, Riphagen II, et al. Physical examination for lumbar radiculopathy due to disc herniation in patients with low-back pain. *Cochrane Database Syst Rev.* 2010;(2):CD007431.

73. Al Nezari NH, Schneiders AG, Hendrick PA. Neurological examination of the peripheral nervous system to diagnose lumbar spinal disc herniation with suspected radiculopathy: a systematic review and meta-analysis. *Spine J.* 2013;13(6):657–674.

74. Chou R, Qaseem A, Owens DK, et al. Diagnostic imaging for low back pain: advice for high-value health care from the American College of Physicians. *Ann Intern Med.* 2011;154(3):181–189.

75. Raastad J, Reiman M, Coeytaux R, et al. The association between low back pain and radiographic features: a systematic review with meta-analysis. *Arthritis Rheumatol.* 2014;(Abstract number 186):S78–S79.

76. Chou R, Qaseem A, Snow V, et al. Diagnosis and treatment of low back pain: a joint clinical practice guideline from the American College of Physicians and the American Pain Society. *Ann Intern Med.* 2007;147(7):478–491.

77. Samartzis D, Borthakur A, Belfer I, et al. Novel diagnostic and prognostic methods for disc degeneration and low back pain. *Spine J.* 2015;15(9):1919–1932.

78. Roland M, van Tulder M. Should radiologists change the way they report plain radiography of the spine? *Lancet.* 1998;352(9123):229–230.

79. Pincus T, Burton AK, Vogel S, et al. A systematic review of psychological factors as predictors of chronicity/disability in prospective cohorts of low back pain. *Spine.* 2002;27(5):E109–E120.

80. Shaw WS, Hartvigsen J, Woiszwillo MJ, et al. Psychological distress in acute low back pain: a review of measurement scales and levels of distress reported in the first 2 months after pain onset. *Arch Phys Med Rehabil.* 2016;97(9):1573–1587.

81. Croft PR, Papageorgiou AC, Ferry S, et al. Psychologic distress and low back pain. Evidence from a prospective study in the general population. *Spine.* 1995;20(24):2731–2737.

82. Mannion AF, Dolan P, Adams MA. Psychological questionnaires: do "abnormal" scores precede or follow first-time low back pain? *Spine.* 1996;21(22):2603–2611.

83. Fairbank JCT. Use and abuse of Oswestry Disability Index. *Spine.* 2007;32(25):2787–2789.

84. Ferrer M, Pellisé F, Escudero O, et al. Validation of a minimum outcome core set in the evaluation of patients with back pain. *Spine.* 2006;31(12):1372–1379; discussion 1380.

85. Mannion AF, Boneschi M, Teli M, et al. Reliability and validity of the cross-culturally adapted Italian version of the Core Outcome Measures Index. *Eur Spine J.* 2012;21(suppl 6):S737–S749.

86. Roland M, Fairbank J. The roland-morris disability questionnaire and the oswestry disability questionnaire. *Spine.* 2000;25(24):3115–3124.

87. Fairbank JC, Pynsent PB. The oswestry disability index. *Spine.* 2000;25(22):2940–2952; discussion 2952.

88. Fairbank JC, Couper J, Davies JB, et al. The Oswestry low back pain disability questionnaire. *Physiotherapy.* 1980;66(8):271–273.

89. Kovacs FM, Abraira V, Zamora J, et al. Correlation between pain, disability, and quality of life in patients with common low back pain. *Spine.* 2004;29(2):206–210.

90. Hägg O, Fritzell P, Nordwall A, et al. The clinical importance of changes in outcome scores after treatment for chronic low back pain. *Eur Spine J.* 2003;12(1):12–20.

91. van der Roer N, Ostelo RWJG, Bekkering GE, et al. Minimal clinically important change for pain intensity, functional status, and general health status in patients with nonspecific low back pain. *Spine.* 2006;31(5):578–582.

92. Balagué F. 2010 ISSLS presidential address: juvenile low back pain: some reflections. *Spine.* 2011;36(11):837–841.

93. Balagué F, Ferrer M, Rajmil L, et al. Assessing the association between low back pain, quality of life, and life events as reported by schoolchildren in a population-based study. *Eur J Pediatr.* 2012;171(3):507–514.

94. Limon S, Valinsky LJ, Ben-Shalom Y. Children at risk: risk factors for low back pain in the elementary school environment. *Spine.* 2004;29(6):697–702.

95. Clifford SN, Fritz JM. Children and adolescents with low back pain: a descriptive study of physical examination and outcome measurement. *J Orthop Sports Phys Ther.* 2003;33(9):513–522.

96. Scientific approach to the assessment and management of activity-related spinal disorders. A monograph for clinicians. Report of the Quebec Task Force on Spinal Disorders. *Spine.* 1987;12(7 suppl):S1–S59.

97. Negrini S. European Journal of Physical and Rehabilitation Medicine: a new clinical rehabilitation journal, an update of our 44 year old Latin name (Europa Medicophysica). *Eur J Phys Rehabil Med.* 2008;44(1):1–2.

98. Novak S, Nemeth WC. The basis for recommending repeating epidural steroid injections for radicular low back pain: a literature review. *Arch Phys Med Rehabil.* 2008;89(3):543–552.

99. Bousema EJ, Verbunt JA, Seelen HAM, et al. Disuse and physical deconditioning in the first year after the onset of back pain. *Pain.* 2007;130(3):279–286.

100. Verbunt JA, Seelen HA, Vlaeyen JW, et al. Disuse and deconditioning in chronic low back pain: concepts and hypotheses on contributing mechanisms. *Eur J Pain.* 2003;7(1):9–21.

101. Olmarker K, Blomquist J, Strömberg J, et al. Inflammatogenic properties of nucleus pulposus. *Spine.* 1995;20(6):665–669.

102. Nachemson AL. Newest knowledge of low back pain. A critical look. *Clin Orthop.* 1992;(279):8–20.

103. Saragiotto BT, Machado GC, Ferreira ML, et al. Paracetamol for low back pain. *Cochrane Database Syst Rev.* 2016;(6):CD012230. John Wiley & Sons, Ltd. Available from: http://onlinelibrary.wiley.com/doi/10.1002/14651858.CD012230/abstract. Accessed February 18, 2017.

104. Enthoven WT, Roelofs PD, Deyo RA, et al. Non-steroidal anti-inflammatory drugs for chronic low back pain. *Cochrane Database Syst Rev.* 2016;(2):CD012087. John Wiley & Sons, Ltd. Available from: http://onlinelibrary.wiley.com/doi/10.1002/14651858.CD012087/abstract [cited April 5, 2017].

105. Rubinstein SM, Terwee CB, Assendelft WJ, et al. Spinal manipulative therapy for acute low-back pain. *Cochrane Database Syst Rev.* 2012;(9):CD008880. John Wiley & Sons, Ltd. Available from: http://onlinelibrary.wiley.com/doi/10.1002/14651858.CD008880.pub2/abstract [cited February 18, 2017].

106. van Duijvenbode ICD, Jellema P, van Poppel MNM, et al. Lumbar supports for prevention and treatment of low back pain. *Cochrane Database Syst Rev.* 2008;(2):CD001823.

107. van Tulder MW, Furlan AD, Gagnier JJ. Complementary and alternative therapies for low back pain. *Best Pract Res Clin Rheumatol.* 2005;19(4):639–654.

108. Furlan AD, van Tulder M, Cherkin D, et al. Acupuncture and dry-needling for low back pain: an updated systematic review within the framework of the cochrane collaboration. *Spine.* 2005;30(8):944–963.

109. Khadilkar A, Milne S, Brosseau L, et al. Transcutaneous electrical nerve stimulation (TENS) for chronic low-back pain. *Cochrane Database Syst Rev.* 2005;(3):CD003008.

110. Sahar T, Cohen MJ, Ne'eman V, et al. Insoles for prevention and treatment of back pain. *Cochrane Database Syst Rev.* 2007;(4):CD005275.

111. French SD, Cameron M, Walker BF, et al. Superficial heat or cold for low back pain. *Cochrane Database Syst Rev.* 2006;(1):CD004750.

112. Oltean H, Robbins C, van Tulder MW, et al. Herbal medicine for low-back pain. *Cochrane Database Syst Rev.* 2014;(12):CD004504. John Wiley & Sons, Ltd. Available from: http://onlinelibrary.wiley.com/doi/10.1002/14651858.CD004504.pub4/abstract [cited February 18, 2017].

113. van Tulder MW, Koes B, Malmivaara A. Outcome of non-invasive treatment modalities on back pain: an evidence-based review. *Eur Spine J.* 2006;15(suppl 1):S64–S81.

114. Liddle SD, Gracey JH, Baxter GD. Advice for the management of low back pain: a systematic review of randomised controlled trials. *Man Ther.* 2007;12(4):310–327.

115. Hagen KB, Hilde G, Jamtvedt G, et al. Bed rest for acute low-back pain and sciatica. *Cochrane Database Syst Rev.* 2004;(4):CD001254.

116. Engers A, Jellema P, Wensing M, et al. Individual patient education for low back pain. *Cochrane Database Syst Rev.* 2008;(1):CD004057.

117. Poquet N, Lin C-WC, Heymans MW, et al. Back schools for acute and subacute non-specific low-back pain. *Cochrane Database Syst Rev.* 2016;(4):CD008325. John Wiley & Sons, Ltd. Available from: http://onlinelibrary.wiley.com/doi/10.1002/14651858.CD008325.pub2/abstract [cited February 18, 2017].

118. Hayden JA, van Tulder MW, Malmivaara A, et al. Exercise therapy for treatment of non-specific low back pain. *Cochrane Database Syst Rev.* 2005;(3):CD000335.

119. Kamper SJ, Apeldoorn AT, Chiarotto A, et al. Multidisciplinary biopsychosocial rehabilitation for chronic low back pain. *Cochrane Database Syst Rev.* 2014;(9):CD000963. John Wiley & Sons, Ltd. Available from: http://onlinelibrary.wiley.com/doi/10.1002/14651858.CD000963.pub3/abstract [cited February 18, 2017].

120. Henschke N, Ostelo RW, van Tulder MW, et al. Behavioural treatment for chronic low-back pain. *Cochrane Database Syst Rev.* 2010;(7):CD002014.

121. Heymans MW, van Tulder MW, Esmail R, et al. Back schools for nonspecific low back pain: a systematic review within the framework of the Cochrane Collaboration Back Review Group. *Spine.* 2005;30(19):2153–2163.

122. Urquhart DM, Hoving JL, Assendelft WWJJ, et al. Antidepressants for non-specific low back pain. *Cochrane Database Syst Rev.* 2008;(1):CD001703.

123. Chaparro LE, Furlan AD, Deshpande A, et al. Opioids compared to placebo or other treatments for chronic low-back pain. *Cochrane Database Syst Rev.* 2013;(8):CD004959. John Wiley & Sons, Ltd. Available from: http://onlinelibrary.wiley.com/doi/10.1002/14651858.CD004959.pub4/abstract [cited February 18, 2017].

124. Wegner I, Widyahening IS, van Tulder MW, et al. Traction for low-back pain with or without sciatica. *Cochrane Database Syst Rev.* 2013;(8):CD003010.

125. Yousefi-Nooraie R, Schonstein E, Heidari K, et al. Low level laser therapy for non-specific low-back pain. *Cochrane Database Syst Rev.* 2008;(2):CD005107.

126. Dagenais S, Yelland MJ, Del Mar C, et al. Prolotherapy injections for chronic low-back pain. *Cochrane Database Syst Rev.* 2007;(2):CD004059.

127. Taimela S, Negrini S, Paroli C. Functional rehabilitation of low back disorders. *Eura Medicophys.* 2004;40(1):29–36.

128. Taimela S, Härkäpää K. Strength, mobility, their changes, and pain reduction in active functional restoration for chronic low back disorders. *J Spinal Disord.* 1996;9(4):306–312.

129. Hayden JA, van Tulder MW, Malmivaara AV, et al. Meta-analysis: exercise therapy for nonspecific low back pain. *Ann Intern Med.* 2005;142(9):765–775.

130. Fritz JM, Cleland JA, Childs JD. Subgrouping patients with low back pain: evolution of a classification approach to physical therapy. *J Orthop Sports Phys Ther.* 2007;37(6):290–302.

131. Brennan GP, Fritz JM, Hunter SJ, et al. Identifying subgroups of patients with acute/subacute "nonspecific" low back pain: results of a randomized clinical trial. *Spine.* 2006;31(6):623–631.

132. Fritz JM, Brennan GP, Clifford SN, et al. An examination of the reliability of a classification algorithm for subgrouping patients with low back pain. *Spine.* 2006;31(1):77–82.

133. Donelson R. Evidence-based low back pain classification. Improving care at its foundation. *Eura Medicophys.* 2004;40(1):37–44.

134. Aina A, May S, Clare H. The centralization phenomenon of spinal symptoms—a systematic review. *Man Ther.* 2004;9(3):134–143.

135. Saragiotto BT, Maher CG, Moseley AM, et al. A systematic review reveals that the credibility of subgroup claims in low back pain trials was low. *J Clin Epidemiol.* 2016;79:3–9.

136. Hayden JA, van Tulder MW, Tomlinson G. Systematic review: strategies for using exercise therapy to improve outcomes in chronic low back pain. *Ann Intern Med.* 2005;142(9):776–785.

137. Smith BE, Littlewood C, May S. An update of stabilisation exercises for low back pain: a systematic review with meta-analysis. *BMC Musculoskelet Disord.* 2014;15:416.

138. Saragiotto BT, Maher CG, Yamato TP, et al. Motor control exercise for chronic non-specific low-back pain. *Cochrane Database Syst Rev.* 2016;(1):CD012004. John Wiley & Sons, Ltd. Available from: http://onlinelibrary.wiley.com/doi/10.1002/14651858.CD012004/abstract [cited March 30, 2017].

139. Macedo LG, Saragiotto BT, Yamato TP, et al. Motor control exercise for acute non-specific low-back pain. *Cochrane Database Syst Rev.* 2016;(2):CD012085. John Wiley & Sons, Ltd. Available from: http://onlinelibrary.wiley.com/doi/10.1002/14651858.CD012085/abstract [cited March 24, 2016].

140. Rainville J, Hartigan C, Martinez E, et al. Exercise as a treatment for chronic low back pain. *Spine J.* 2004;4(1):106–115.

141. Thomas JS, France CR. The relationship between pain-related fear and lumbar flexion during natural recovery from low back pain. *Eur Spine J.* 2008;17(1):97–103.

142. Thomas JS, France CR, Lavender SA, et al. Effects of fear of movement on spine velocity and acceleration after recovery from low back pain. *Spine.* 2008;33(5):564–570.

143. Kernan T, Rainville J. Observed outcomes associated with a quota-based exercise approach on measures of kinesiophobia in patients with chronic low back pain. *J Orthop Sports Phys Ther.* 2007;37(11):679–687.

144. Cohen I, Rainville J. Aggressive exercise as treatment for chronic low back pain. *Sports Med.* 2002;32(1):75–82.

145. Staal JB, Hlobil H, Twisk JWR, et al. Graded activity for low back pain in occupational health care: a randomized, controlled trial. *Ann Intern Med.* 2004;140(2):77–84.

146. van den Hout JHC, Vlaeyen JWS, Heuts PHTG, et al. Secondary prevention of work-related disability in nonspecific low back pain: does problem-solving therapy help? A randomized clinical trial. *Clin J Pain.* 2003;19(2):87–96.

147. Lindström I, Ohlund C, Eek C, et al. The effect of graded activity on patients with subacute low back pain: a randomized prospective clinical study with an operant-conditioning behavioral approach. *Phys Ther.* 1992;72(4):279–290; discussion 291–293.

148. Hides JA, Stokes MJ, Saide M, et al. Evidence of lumbar multifidus muscle wasting ipsilateral to symptoms in patients with acute/subacute low back pain. *Spine.* 1994;19(2):165–172.

149. Hides JA, Richardson CA, Jull GA. Multifidus muscle recovery is not automatic after resolution of acute, first-episode low back pain. *Spine.* 1996;21(23):2763–2769.

150. Hides JA, Jull GA, Richardson CA. Long-term effects of specific stabilizing exercises for first-episode low back pain. *Spine.* 2001;26(11):E243–E248.

151. Jones M, Stratton G, Reilly T, et al. The efficacy of exercise as an intervention to treat recurrent nonspecific low back pain in adolescents. *Pediatr Exerc Sci.* 2007;19(3):349–359.

152. Jones MA, Stratton G, Reilly T, et al. Recurrent non-specific low-back pain in adolescents: the role of exercise. *Ergonomics.* 2007;50(10):1680–1688.

153. Smeets RJ, Vlaeyen JW, Hidding A, et al. Active rehabilitation for chronic low back pain: cognitive-behavioral, physical, or both? First direct post-treatment results from a randomized controlled trial [ISRCTN22714229]. *BMC Musculoskelet Disord.* 2006;7:5.

154. Kohles S, Barnes D, Gatchel RJ, et al. Improved physical performance outcomes after functional restoration treatment in patients with chronic low-back pain. Early versus recent training results. *Spine.* 1990;15(12):1321–1324.

155. Mayer TG, Gatchel RJ, Mayer H, et al. A prospective two-year study of functional restoration in industrial low back injury. An objective assessment procedure. *JAMA.* 1987;258(13):1763–1767.

156. Taimela S, Diederich C, Hubsch M, et al. The role of physical exercise and inactivity in pain recurrence and absenteeism from work after active outpatient rehabilitation for recurrent or chronic low back pain: a follow-up study. *Spine.* 2000;25(14):1809–1816.

157. Spinhoven P, Ter Kuile M, Kole-Snijders AMJ, et al. Catastrophizing and internal pain control as mediators of outcome in the multidisciplinary treatment of chronic low back pain. *Eur J Pain.* 2004;8(3):211–219.

158. Turner JA, Clancy S, McQuade KJ, et al. Effectiveness of behavioral therapy for chronic low back pain: a component analysis. *J Consult Clin Psychol.* 1990;58(5):573–579.

159. Weisenberg MI. Pain and pain control. *Psychol Bull.* 1977;84(5):1008–1044.

160. Turk DC, Flor H. Etiological theories and treatments for chronic back pain. II. Psychological models and interventions. *Pain.* 1984;19(3):209–233.

161. Vlaeyen JW, Kole-Snijders AM, Boeren RG, et al. Fear of movement/(re)injury in chronic low back pain and its relation to behavioral performance. *Pain.* 1995;62(3):363–372.

162. Dahm KT, Brurberg KG, Jamtvedt G, et al. Advice to rest in bed versus advice to stay active for acute low-back pain and sciatica. *Cochrane Database Syst Rev.* 2010;(6):CD007612.

163. Hall H, Hadler NM. Controversy. Low back school. Education or exercise? *Spine.* 1995;20(9):1097–1098.

164. Forssell MZ. The Swedish back school. *Physiotherapy.* 1980;66(4):112–114.

165. Lankhorst GJ, Van de Stadt RJ, Vogelaar TW, et al. The effect of the Swedish Back School in chronic idiopathic low back pain. A prospective controlled study. *Scand J Rehabil Med.* 1983;15(3):141–145.

166. Hall H, Iceton JA. Back school. An overview with specific reference to the Canadian Back Education Units. *Clin Orthop.* 1983;(179):10–17.

167. Linton SJ, Kamwendo K. Low back schools. A critical review. *Phys Ther.* 1987;67(9):1375–1383.

168. Waddell G, O'Connor M, Boorman S, et al. Working Backs Scotland: a public and professional health education campaign for back pain. *Spine.* 2007;32(19):2139–2143.

169. Cherkin D, Deyo RA, Berg AO, et al. Evaluation of a physician education intervention to improve primary care for low-back pain. I. Impact on physicians. *Spine.* 1991;16(10):1168–1172.

170. Nachemson A. Back pain: delimiting the problem in the next millennium. *Int J Law Psychiatry.* 1999;22(5–6):473–490.

171. Cedraschi C, Nordin M, Nachemson AL, et al. Health care providers should use a common language in relation to low back pain patients. *Baillieres Clin Rheumatol.* 1998;12(1):1–15.

172. Nachemson A. Chronic pain—the end of the welfare state? *Qual Life Res.* 1994;3(suppl 1):S11–S17.

173. Harvey E, Burton AK, Moffett JK, et al. Spinal manipulation for low-back pain: a treatment package agreed to by the UK chiropractic, osteopathy and physiotherapy professional associations. *Man Ther.* 2003;8(1):46–51.

174. Furlan AD, Giraldo M, Baskwill A, et al. Massage for low-back pain. *Cochrane Database Syst Rev.* 2015;(9):CD001929. John Wiley & Sons, Ltd. Available from: http://onlinelibrary.wiley.com/doi/10.1002/14651858.CD001929.pub3/abstract [cited February 18, 2017].

175. Franke H, Franke J-D, Fryer G. Osteopathic manipulative treatment for nonspecific low back pain: a systematic review and meta-analysis. *BMC Musculoskelet Disord.* 2014;15:286.

176. Rubinstein SM, van Middelkoop M, Assendelft WJ, et al. Spinal manipulative therapy for chronic low-back pain. *Cochrane Database Syst Rev.* 2011;(2):CD008112. John Wiley & Sons, Ltd. Available from: http://onlinelibrary.wiley.com/doi/10.1002/14651858.CD008112.pub2/abstract [cited April 5, 2017].

177. Burton AK, McClune TD, Clarke RD, et al. Long-term follow-up of patients with low back pain attending for manipulative care: outcomes and predictors. *Man Ther.* 2004;9(1):30–35.

178. Wu L-C, Weng P-W, Chen C-H, et al. Literature review and meta-analysis of transcutaneous electrical nerve stimulation in treating chronic back pain. *Reg Anesth Pain Med.* 2018;43:425–433.

179. Han JS, Chen XH, Sun SL, et al. Effect of low- and high-frequency TENS on Met-enkephalin-Arg-Phe and dynorphin A immunoreactivity in human lumbar CSF. *Pain.* 1991;47(3):295–298.

180. Hughes GS, Lichstein PR, Whitlock D, et al. Response of plasma beta-endorphins to transcutaneous electrical nerve stimulation in healthy subjects. *Phys Ther.* 1984;64(7):1062–1066.

181. Kalra A, Urban MO, Sluka KA. Blockade of opioid receptors in rostral ventral medulla prevents antihyperalgesia produced by transcutaneous electrical nerve stimulation (TENS). *J Pharmacol Exp Ther*. 2001;298(1):257–263.

182. Salar G, Job I, Mingrino S, et al. Effect of transcutaneous electrotherapy on CSF beta-endorphin content in patients without pain problems. *Pain*. 1981;10(2):169–172.

183. Zambito A, Bianchini D, Gatti D, et al. Interferential and horizontal therapies in chronic low back pain due to multiple vertebral fractures: a randomized, double blind, clinical study. *Osteoporos Int*. 2007;18(11):1541–1545.

184. Poitras S, Brosseau L. Evidence-informed management of chronic low back pain with transcutaneous electrical nerve stimulation, interferential current, electrical muscle stimulation, ultrasound, and thermotherapy. *Spine J*. 2008;8(1):226–233.

185. Maxwell L. Therapeutic ultrasound: its effects on the cellular and molecular mechanisms of inflammation and repair. *Physiotherapy*. 1992;78(6):421–426.

186. Hedrick WR, Hykes DL, Starchman DE. *Ultrasound Physics and Instrumentation*. Boston: Mosby; 1995:412.

187. Falconer J, Hayes KW, Chang RW. Effect of ultrasound on mobility in osteoarthritis of the knee. A randomized clinical trial. *Arthritis Care Res*. 1992;5(1):29–35.

188. Ebadi S, Henschke N, Nakhostin Ansari N, et al. Therapeutic ultrasound for chronic low-back pain. *Cochrane Database Syst Rev*. 2014;(3):CD009169.

189. Beckerman H, de Bie RA, Bouter LM, et al. The efficacy of laser therapy for musculoskeletal and skin disorders: a criteria-based meta-analysis of randomized clinical trials. *Phys Ther*. 1992;72(7):483–491.

190. Bjordal JM, Couppé C, Chow RT, et al. A systematic review of low level laser therapy with location-specific doses for pain from chronic joint disorders. *Aust J Physiother*. 2003;49(2):107–116.

191. Basford JR. Low-energy laser therapy: controversies and new research findings. *Lasers Surg Med*. 1989;9(1):1–5.

192. Baxter G, Bell A, Allen J, et al. Low level laser therapy: current clinical practice in Northern Ireland. *Physiotherapy*. 1991;77(3):171–178.

193. Kreisler M, Christoffers AB, Al-Haj H, et al. Low level 809-nm diode laser-induced in vitro stimulation of the proliferation of human gingival fibroblasts. *Lasers Surg Med*. 2002;30(5):365–369.

194. Sakurai Y, Yamaguchi M, Abiko Y. Inhibitory effect of low-level laser irradiation on LPS-stimulated prostaglandin E2 production and cyclooxygenase-2 in human gingival fibroblasts. *Eur J Oral Sci*. 2000;108(1):29–34.

195. Ceccherelli F, Altafini L, Lo Castro G, et al. Diode laser in cervical myofascial pain: a double-blind study versus placebo. *Clin J Pain*. 1989;5(4):301–304.

196. Skinner SM, Gage JP, Wilce PA, et al. A preliminary study of the effects of laser radiation on collagen metabolism in cell culture. *Aust Dent J*. 1996;41(3):188–192.

197. Shupak NM, Prato FS, Thomas AW. Human exposure to a specific pulsed magnetic field: effects on thermal sensory and pain thresholds. *Neurosci Lett*. 2004;363(2):157–162.

198. van Tulder MW, Touray T, Furlan AD, et al. Muscle relaxants for non-specific low back pain. *Cochrane Database Syst Rev*. 2003;(2):CD004252.

199. Martell BA, O'Connor PG, Kerns RD, et al. Systematic review: opioid treatment for chronic back pain: prevalence, efficacy, and association with addiction. *Ann Intern Med*. 2007;146(2):116–127.

200. Deshpande A, Furlan A, Mailis-Gagnon A, et al. Opioids for chronic low-back pain. *Cochrane Database Syst Rev*. 2007;(3):CD004959.

201. Chou R, Huffman LH; American Pain Society, American College of Physicians. Medications for acute and chronic low back pain: a review of the evidence for an American Pain Society/American College of Physicians clinical practice guideline. *Ann Intern Med*. 2007;147(7):505–514.

202. Kuijer W, Groothoff JW, Brouwer S, et al. Prediction of sickness absence in patients with chronic low back pain: a systematic review. *J Occup Rehabil*. 2006;16(3):439–467.

203. Volinn E, Nishikitani M, Volinn W, et al. Back pain claim rates in Japan and the United States: framing the puzzle. *Spine*. 2005;30(6):697–704.

204. Hansson T, Jensen I. Swedish Council on Technology Assessment in Health Care (SBU). Chapter 6. Sickness absence due to back and neck disorders. *Scand J Public Health Suppl*. 2004;63:109–151.

205. Walker BF. The prevalence of low back pain: a systematic review of the literature from 1966 to 1998. *J Spinal Disord*. 2000;13(3):205–217.

206. Bressler HB, Keyes WJ, Rochon PA, et al. The prevalence of low back pain in the elderly. A systematic review of the literature. *Spine*. 1999;24(17):1813–1819.

207. Volinn E. The epidemiology of low back pain in the rest of the world. A review of surveys in low- and middle-income countries. *Spine*. 1997;22(15):1747–1754.

208. Leboeuf-Yde C, Lauritsen JM. The prevalence of low back pain in the literature. A structured review of 26 Nordic studies from 1954 to 1993. *Spine*. 1995;20(19):2112–2118.

209. Pengel LHM, Herbert RD, Maher CG, et al. Acute low back pain: systematic review of its prognosis. *BMJ*. 2003;327(7410):323.

210. Dunn KM, Croft PR. Epidemiology and natural history of low back pain. *Eura Medicophys*. 2004;40(1):9–13.

211. van den Hoogen HJ, Koes BW, Devillé W, et al. The prognosis of low back pain in general practice. *Spine*. 1997;22(13):1515–1521.

212. Verbeek J, Sengers M-J, Riemens L, et al. Patient expectations of treatment for back pain: a systematic review of qualitative and quantitative studies. *Spine*. 2004;29(20):2309–2318.

213. Shen FH, Samartzis D, Andersson GBJ. Nonsurgical management of acute and chronic low back pain. *J Am Acad Orthop Surg*. 2006;14(8):477–487.

214. Kinkade S. Evaluation and treatment of acute low back pain. *Am Fam Physician*. 2007;75(8):1181–1188.

215. Lee S, Chan CK, Lam T, et al. Relationship between low back pain and lumbar multifidus size at different postures. *Spine*. 2006;31(19):2258–2262.

216. Hodges P, Holm AK, Hansson T, et al. Rapid atrophy of the lumbar multifidus follows experimental disc or nerve root injury. *Spine*. 2006;31(25):2926–2933.

217. Sung PS. Multifidi muscles median frequency before and after spinal stabilization exercises. *Arch Phys Med Rehabil*. 2003;84(9):1313–1318.

218. Waddell G. How patients react to low back pain. *Acta Orthop Scand Suppl*. 1993;251:21–24.

219. Hilfiker R, Bachmann LM, Heitz CA-M, et al. Value of predictive instruments to determine persisting restriction of function in patients with subacute non-specific low back pain. Systematic review. *Eur Spine J*. 2007;16(11):1755–1775.

220. Linton SJ. A review of psychological risk factors in back and neck pain. *Spine*. 2000;25(9):1148–1156.

221. Hoogendoorn WE, van Poppel MN, Bongers PM, et al. Systematic review of psychosocial factors at work and private life as risk factors for back pain. *Spine*. 2000;25(16):2114–2125.

222. Leboeuf-Yde C. Body weight and low back pain. A systematic literature review of 56 journal articles reporting on 65 epidemiologic studies. *Spine*. 2000;25(2):226–237.

223. Leboeuf-Yde C. Smoking and low back pain. A systematic literature review of 41 journal articles reporting 47 epidemiologic studies. *Spine*. 1999;24(14):1463–1470.

224. Jarvik JG, Deyo RA. Diagnostic evaluation of low back pain with emphasis on imaging. *Ann Intern Med*. 2002;137(7):586–597.

225. Pengel HM, Maher CG, Refshauge KM. Systematic review of conservative interventions for subacute low back pain. *Clin Rehabil*. 2002;16(8):811–820.

226. Rossignol M, Allaert FA, Rozenberg S, et al. Measuring the contribution of pharmacological treatment to advice to stay active in patients with subacute low-back pain: a randomised controlled trial. *Pharmacoepidemiol Drug Saf*. 2005;14(12):861–867.

227. Göhner W, Schlicht W. Preventing chronic back pain: evaluation of a theory-based cognitive-behavioural training programme for patients with subacute back pain. *Patient Educ Couns*. 2006;64(1–3):87–95.

228. Karjalainen K, Malmivaara A, van Tulder M, et al. Multidisciplinary biopsychosocial rehabilitation for subacute low back pain in working-age adults: a systematic review within the framework of the Cochrane Collaboration Back Review Group. *Spine*. 2001;26(3):262–269.

229. Wright A, Lloyd-Davies A, Williams S, et al. Individual active treatment combined with group exercise for acute and subacute low back pain. *Spine*. 2005;30(11):1235–1241.

230. Schiltenwolf M, Buchner M, Heindl B, et al. Comparison of a biopsychosocial therapy (BT) with a conventional biomedical therapy (MT) of subacute low back pain in the first episode of sick leave: a randomized controlled trial. *Eur Spine J*. 2006;15(7):1083–1092.

231. Pengel LHM, Refshauge KM, Maher CG, et al. Physiotherapist-directed exercise, advice, or both for subacute low back pain: a randomized trial. *Ann Intern Med*. 2007;146(11):787–796.

232. Turk DC, Okifuji A. Psychological factors in chronic pain: evolution and revolution. *J Consult Clin Psychol*. 2002;70(3):678–690.

233. Main CJ, Waddell G. Behavioral responses to examination. A reappraisal of the interpretation of "nonorganic signs." *Spine*. 1998;23(21):2367–2371.

234. Waddell G, Main CJ, Morris EW, et al. Chronic low-back pain, psychologic distress, and illness behavior. *Spine*. 1984;9(2):209–213.

235. Waddell G, McCulloch JA, Kummel E, et al. Nonorganic physical signs in low-back pain. *Spine*. 1980;5(2):117–125.

236. Diers M, Koeppe C, Diesch E, et al. Central processing of acute muscle pain in chronic low back pain patients: an EEG mapping study. *J Clin Neurophysiol*. 2007;24(1):76–83.

237. O'Neill S, Manniche C, Graven-Nielsen T, et al. Generalized deep-tissue hyperalgesia in patients with chronic low-back pain. *Eur J Pain*. 2007;11(4):415–420.

238. Winkelstein BA. Mechanisms of central sensitization, neuroimmunology & injury biomechanics in persistent pain: implications for musculoskeletal disorders. *J Electromyogr Kinesiol*. 2004;14(1):87–93.

239. Cavanaugh JM, Ozaktay AC, Yamashita T, et al. Mechanisms of low back pain: a neurophysiologic and neuroanatomic study. *Clin Orthop*. 1997;(335):166–180.

240. Cavanaugh JM. Neural mechanisms of lumbar pain. *Spine*. 1995;20(16):1804–1809.

241. Maigne JY. Towards a model of back pain. The 3 circles of pain. *Eura Medicophys*. 2004;40(1):21–27.

242. Mayer TG, Gatchel RJ, Kishino N, et al. A prospective short-term study of chronic low back pain patients utilizing novel objective functional measurement. *Pain*. 1986;25(1):53–68.

243. Vlaeyen JW, Linton SJ. Fear-avoidance and its consequences in chronic musculoskeletal pain: a state of the art. *Pain*. 2000;85(3):317–332.

244. Fritz JM, George SZ, Delitto A. The role of fear-avoidance beliefs in acute low back pain: relationships with current and future disability and work status. *Pain*. 2001;94(1):7–15.

245. Protas EJ, Mayer TG, Dersh J, et al. Relevance of aerobic capacity measurements in the treatment of chronic work-related spinal disorders. *Spine*. 2004;29(19):2158–2166; discussion 2167.

246. Roland M, Morris R. A study of the natural history of low-back pain. Part II: development of guidelines for trials of treatment in primary care. *Spine*. 1983;8(2):145–150.

247. Vendrig AA. Prognostic factors and treatment-related changes associated with return to work in the multimodal treatment of chronic back pain. *J Behav Med*. 1999;22(3):217–232.

248. Polatin PB, Gatchel RJ, Barnes D, et al. A psychosociomedical prediction model of response to treatment by chronically disabled workers with low-back pain. *Spine.* 1989;14(9):956–961.

249. Barnes D, Smith D, Gatchel RJ, et al. Psychosocioeconomic predictors of treatment success/failure in chronic low-back pain patients. *Spine.* 1989;14(4):427–430.

250. Nachemson AL. Advances in low-back pain. *Clin Orthop.* 1985;(200):266–278.

251. Buckalew N, Haut MW, Morrow L, et al. Chronic pain is associated with brain volume loss in older adults: preliminary evidence. *Pain Med.* 2008;9(2):240–248.

252. Langevin HM, Sherman KJ. Pathophysiological model for chronic low back pain integrating connective tissue and nervous system mechanisms. *Med Hypotheses.* 2007;68(1):74–80.

253. Thunberg J, Lyskov E, Korotkov A, et al. Brain processing of tonic muscle pain induced by infusion of hypertonic saline. *Eur J Pain.* 2005;9(2):185–194.

254. Hodges P, Cresswell A, Thorstensson A. Preparatory trunk motion accompanies rapid upper limb movement. *Exp Brain Res.* 1999;124(1):69–79.

255. Kankaanpää M, Taimela S, Laaksonen D, et al. Back and hip extensor fatigability in chronic low back pain patients and controls. *Arch Phys Med Rehabil.* 1998;79(4):412–417.

256. Gatchel RJ, Mayer TG. Evidence-informed management of chronic low back pain with functional restoration. *Spine J.* 2008;8(1):65–69.

257. Buijs E, Visser L, Groen G. Sciatica and the sacroiliac joint: a forgotten concept. *Br J Anaesth.* 2007;99(5):713–716.

258. Younes M, Béjia I, Aguir Z, et al. Prevalence and risk factors of disk-related sciatica in an urban population in Tunisia. *Joint Bone Spine.* 2006;73(5):538–542.

259. McCarron RF, Wimpee MW, Hudkins PG, et al. The inflammatory effect of nucleus pulposus. A possible element in the pathogenesis of low-back pain. *Spine.* 1987;12(8):760–764.

260. Bogduk N, Govind J. *Medical Management of Acute Lumbar Radicular Pain : An Evidence-Based Approach/Nikolai Bogduk, Jayantilal Govind.* Newcastle, NSW: Newcastle Bone and Joint Institute, Royal Newcastle Hospital; 1999.

261. Weinstein JN, Tosteson TD, Lurie JD, et al. Surgical vs nonoperative treatment for lumbar disk herniation: the Spine Patient Outcomes Research Trial (SPORT): a randomized trial. *JAMA.* 2006;296(20):2441–2450.

262. Weinstein JN, Lurie JD, Tosteson TD, et al. Surgical vs nonoperative treatment for lumbar disk herniation: the Spine Patient Outcomes Research Trial (SPORT) observational cohort. *JAMA.* 2006;296(20):2451–2459.

263. Lurie JD, Tosteson TD, Tosteson ANA, et al. Surgical versus nonoperative treatment for lumbar disc herniation: eight-year results for the spine patient outcomes research trial. *Spine.* 2014;39(1):3–16.

264. Gibson JNA, Waddell G. Surgical interventions for lumbar disc prolapse: updated Cochrane review. *Spine.* 2007;32(16):1735–1747.

265. Kreiner DS, Hwang SW, Easa JE, et al. An evidence-based clinical guideline for the diagnosis and treatment of lumbar disc herniation with radiculopathy. *Spine J.* 2014;14(1):180–191.

266. Boos N, Semmer N, Elfering A, et al. Natural history of individuals with asymptomatic disc abnormalities in magnetic resonance imaging: predictors of low back pain-related medical consultation and work incapacity. *Spine.* 2000;25(12):1484–1492.

267. Boos N, Rieder R, Schade V, et al. 1995 Volvo Award in clinical sciences. The diagnostic accuracy of magnetic resonance imaging, work perception, and psychosocial factors in identifying symptomatic disc herniations. *Spine.* 1995;20(24): 2613–2625.

268. Autio RA, Karppinen J, Niinimäki J, et al. Determinants of spontaneous resorption of intervertebral disc herniations. *Spine.* 2006;31(11):1247–1252.

269. Jensen MC, Brant-Zawadzki MN, Obuchowski N, et al. Magnetic resonance imaging of the lumbar spine in people without back pain. *N Engl J Med.* 1994;331(2):69–73.

270. Jensen TS, Albert HB, Soerensen JS, et al. Natural course of disc morphology in patients with sciatica: an MRI study using a standardized qualitative classification system. *Spine.* 2006;31(14):1605–1612; discussion 1613.

271. Jensen TS, Albert HB, Sorensen JS, et al. Magnetic resonance imaging findings as predictors of clinical outcome in patients with sciatica receiving active conservative treatment. *J Manipulative Physiol Ther.* 2007;30(2):98–108.

272. Roelofs PDDM, Deyo RA, Koes BW, et al. Non-steroidal anti-inflammatory drugs for low back pain. *Cochrane Database Syst Rev.* 2008;(1):CD000396.

273. Kato T, Haro H, Komori H, et al. Sequential dynamics of inflammatory cytokine, angiogenesis inducing factor and matrix degrading enzymes during spontaneous resorption of the herniated disc. *J Orthop Res.* 2004;22(4):895–900.

274. Mulleman D, Mammou S, Griffoul I, et al. Pathophysiology of disk-related sciatica. I.—Evidence supporting a chemical component. *Joint Bone Spine.* 2006;73(2):151–158.

275. Pinto RZ, Maher CG, Ferreira ML, et al. Drugs for relief of pain in patients with sciatica: systematic review and meta-analysis. *BMJ.* 2012;344:e497.

276. Kawakami M, Tamaki T, Matsumoto T, et al. Role of leukocytes in radicular pain secondary to herniated nucleus pulposus. *Clin Orthop.* 2000;(376):268–277.

277. Chia S, Qadan M, Newton R, et al. Intra-arterial tumor necrosis factor-alpha impairs endothelium-dependent vasodilatation and stimulates local tissue plasminogen activator release in humans. *Arterioscler Thromb Vasc Biol.* 2003;23(4):695–701.

278. Wang YF, Chen PY, Chang W, et al. Clinical significance of tumor necrosis factor-α inhibitors in the treatment of sciatica: a systematic review and meta-analysis. *PLoS One.* 2014;9(7):e103147.

279. Luijsterburg PAJ, Verhagen AP, Ostelo RWJG, et al. Effectiveness of conservative treatments for the lumbosacral radicular syndrome: a systematic review. *Eur Spine J.* 2007;16(7):881–899.

280. Fernandez M, Hartvigsen J, Ferreira ML, et al. Advice to stay active or structured exercise in the management of sciatica: a systematic review and meta-analysis. *Spine (Phila Pa 1976).* 2015;40:1457–1466.

281. Hofstee DJ, Gijtenbeek JMM, Hoogland PH, et al. Westeinde sciatica trial: randomized controlled study of bed rest and physiotherapy for acute sciatica. *J Neurosurg.* 2002;96(1 suppl):45–49.

282. Jewell DV, Riddle DL. Interventions that increase or decrease the likelihood of a meaningful improvement in physical health in patients with sciatica. *Phys Ther.* 2005;85(11):1139–1150.

283. Donelson R. Reliability of the McKenzie assessment. *J Orthop Sports Phys Ther.* 2000;30(12):770–775.

284. Long AL. The centralization phenomenon. Its usefulness as a predictor or outcome in conservative treatment of chronic law back pain (a pilot study). *Spine.* 1995;20(23):2513–2520; discussion 2521.

285. Donelson R, Silva G, Murphy K. Centralization phenomenon. Its usefulness in evaluating and treating referred pain. *Spine.* 1990;15(3):211–213.

286. Arnoldi CC, Brodsky AE, Cauchoix J, et al. Lumbar spinal stenosis and nerve root entrapment syndromes. Definition and classification. *Clin Orthop.* 1976;(115): 4–5.

287. Epstein NE, Maldonado VC, Cusick JF. Symptomatic lumbar spinal stenosis. *Surg Neurol.* 1998;50(1):3–10.

288. Alvarez JA, Hardy RH. Lumbar spine stenosis: a common cause of back and leg pain. *Am Fam Physician.* 1998;57(8):1825–1834, 1839–1840.

289. Szpalski M, Gunzburg R. Lumbar spinal stenosis in the elderly: an overview. *Eur Spine J.* 2003;12(suppl 2):S170–S175.

290. Kent DL, Haynor DR, Larson EB, et al. Diagnosis of lumbar spinal stenosis in adults: a metaanalysis of the accuracy of CT, MR, and myelography. *Am J Roentgenol.* 1992;158(5):1135–1144.

291. Postacchini F. The diagnosis of lumbar stenosis. Analysis of clinical and radiographic findings in 43 cases. *Ital J Orthop Traumatol.* 1985;11(1):5–21.

292. Tan SB. Spinal canal stenosis. *Singapore Med J.* 2003;44(4):168–169.

293. Amundsen T, Weber H, Lilleås F, et al. Lumbar spinal stenosis. Clinical and radiologic features. *Spine.* 1995;20(10):1178–1186.

294. Jönsson B, Strömqvist B. Symptoms and signs in degeneration of the lumbar spine. A prospective, consecutive study of 300 operated patients. *J Bone Joint Surg Br.* 1993;75(3):381–385.

295. Pheasant HC, Dyck P. Failed lumbar disc surgery: cause, assessment, treatment. *Clin Orthop.* 1982;(164):93–109.

296. Rauschning W. Pathoanatomy of lumbar disc degeneration and stenosis. *Acta Orthop Scand Suppl.* 1993;251:3–12.

297. Hitselberger WE, Witten RM. Abnormal myelograms in asymptomatic patients. *J Neurosurg.* 1968;28(3):204–206.

298. Boden SD, Davis DO, Dina TS, et al. Abnormal magnetic-resonance scans of the lumbar spine in asymptomatic subjects. A prospective investigation. *J Bone Joint Surg Am.* 1990;72(3):403–408.

299. Wiesel SW, Tsourmas N, Feffer HL, et al. A study of computer-assisted tomography. I. The incidence of positive CAT scans in an asymptomatic group of patients. *Spine.* 1984;9(6):549–551.

300. Beattie PF, Meyers SP, Stratford P, et al. Associations between patient report of symptoms and anatomic impairment visible on lumbar magnetic resonance imaging. *Spine.* 2000;25(7):819–828.

301. Katz JN, Dalgas M, Stucki G, et al. Degenerative lumbar spinal stenosis. Diagnostic value of the history and physical examination. *Arthritis Rheum.* 1995;38(9): 1236–1241.

302. de Graaf I, Prak A, Bierma-Zeinstra S, et al. Diagnosis of lumbar spinal stenosis: a systematic review of the accuracy of diagnostic tests. *Spine.* 2006;31(10): 1168–1176.

303. Katz JN, Dalgas M, Stucki G, et al. Diagnosis of lumbar spinal stenosis. *Rheum Dis Clin North Am.* 1994;20(2):471–483.

304. Stucki G, Liang MH, Fossel AH, et al. Relative responsiveness of condition-specific and generic health status measures in degenerative lumbar spinal stenosis. *J Clin Epidemiol.* 1995;48(11):1369–1378.

305. Stucki G, Daltroy L, Liang MH, et al. Measurement properties of a self-administered outcome measure in lumbar spinal stenosis. *Spine.* 1996;21(7):796–803.

306. Botwin KP, Gruber RD. Lumbar spinal stenosis: anatomy and pathogenesis. *Phys Med Rehabil Clin N Am.* 2003;14(1):1–15, v.

307. Verbiest H. A radicular syndrome from developmental narrowing of the lumbar vertebral canal. *J Bone Joint Surg Br.* 1954;36–B(2):230–237.

308. Ullrich CG, Binet EF, Sanecki MG, et al. Quantitative assessment of the lumbar spinal canal by computed tomography. *Radiology.* 1980;134(1):137–143.

309. Geisser ME, Haig AJ, Tong HC, et al. Spinal canal size and clinical symptoms among persons diagnosed with lumbar spinal stenosis. *Clin J Pain.* 2007;23(9):780–785.

310. Haig AJ, Geisser ME, Tong HC, et al. Electromyographic and magnetic resonance imaging to predict lumbar stenosis, low-back pain, and no back symptoms. *J Bone Joint Surg Am.* 2007;89(2):358–366.

311. Benoist M. The natural history of lumbar degenerative spinal stenosis. *Joint Bone Spine.* 2002;69(5):450–457.

312. Herno A, Airaksinen O, Saari T, et al. Lumbar spinal stenosis: a matched-pair study of operated and non-operated patients. *Br J Neurosurg.* 1996;10(5):461–465.

313. Johnsson KE, Rosén I, Udén A. The natural course of lumbar spinal stenosis. *Clin Orthop.* 1992;(279):82–86.

314. Porter RW, Hibbert C, Evans C. The natural history of root entrapment syndrome. *Spine.* 1984;9(4):418–421.

315. Johnsson KE, Udén A, Rosén I. The effect of decompression on the natural course of spinal stenosis. A comparison of surgically treated and untreated patients. *Spine.* 1991;16(6):615–619.

316. Mazanec DJ, Podichetty VK, Hsia A. Lumbar canal stenosis: start with nonsurgical therapy. *Cleve Clin J Med.* 2002;69(11):909–917.

317. Atlas SJ, Keller RB, Robson D, et al. Surgical and nonsurgical management of lumbar spinal stenosis: four-year outcomes from the maine lumbar spine study. *Spine.* 2000;25(5):556–562.

318. Atlas SJ, Deyo RA, Keller RB, et al. The Maine Lumbar Spine Study, Part III. 1-year outcomes of surgical and nonsurgical management of lumbar spinal stenosis. *Spine.* 1996;21(15):1787–1794; discussion 1794–1795.

319. Amundsen T, Weber H, Nordal HJ, et al. Lumbar spinal stenosis: conservative or surgical management?: a prospective 10-year study. *Spine.* 2000;25(11):1424–1435; discussion 1435–1436.

320. Kreiner DS, Shaffer WO, Baisden JL, et al. An evidence-based clinical guideline for the diagnosis and treatment of degenerative lumbar spinal stenosis (update). *Spine J.* 2013;13(7):734–743.

321. Zaina F, Tomkins-Lane C, Carragee E, et al. Surgical versus non-surgical treatment for lumbar spinal stenosis. *Cochrane Database Syst Rev.* 2016;(1):CD010264.

322. Katz JN, Stucki G, Lipson SJ, et al. Predictors of surgical outcome in degenerative lumbar spinal stenosis. *Spine.* 1999;24(21):2229–2233.

323. Deyo RA. Back surgery—who needs it? *N Engl J Med.* 2007;356(22):2239–2243.

324. van Tulder MW, Koes B, Seitsalo S, et al. Outcome of invasive treatment modalities on back pain and sciatica: an evidence-based review. *Eur Spine J.* 2006;15(suppl 1):S82–S92.

325. Aalto TJ, Malmivaara A, Kovacs F, et al. Preoperative predictors for postoperative clinical outcome in lumbar spinal stenosis: systematic review. *Spine.* 2006;31(18):E648–E663.

326. Wu AM, Zhou Y, Li QL, et al. Interspinous spacer versus traditional decompressive surgery for lumbar spinal stenosis: a systematic review and meta-analysis. *PLoS One.* 2014;9(5):e97142.

327. Vo AN, Kamen LB, Shih VC, et al. Rehabilitation of orthopedic and rheumatologic disorders. 5. Lumbar spinal stenosis. *Arch Phys Med Rehabil.* 2005;86(3 suppl 1):S69–S76.

328. Fritz JM, Erhard RE, Vignovic M. A nonsurgical treatment approach for patients with lumbar spinal stenosis. *Phys Ther.* 1997;77(9):962–973.

329. Fritz JM, Delitto A, Welch WC, et al. Lumbar spinal stenosis: a review of current concepts in evaluation, management, and outcome measurements. *Arch Phys Med Rehabil.* 1998;79(6):700–708.

330. Leinonen V, Määttä S, Taimela S, et al. Paraspinal muscle denervation, paradoxically good lumbar endurance, and an abnormal flexion-extension cycle in lumbar spinal stenosis. *Spine.* 2003;28(4):324–331.

331. Suda Y, Saitou M, Shibasaki K, et al. Gait analysis of patients with neurogenic intermittent claudication. *Spine.* 2002;27(22):2509–2513.

332. Simotas AC, Dorey FJ, Hansraj KK, et al. Nonoperative treatment for lumbar spinal stenosis. Clinical and outcome results and a 3-year survivorship analysis. *Spine.* 2000;25(2):197–203; discussions 203–204.

333. Atlas SJ, Delitto A. Spinal stenosis: surgical versus nonsurgical treatment. *Clin Orthop.* 2006;443:198–207.

334. Pope MH, Panjabi M. Biomechanical definitions of spinal instability. *Spine.* 1985;10(3):255–256.

335. Frymoyer JW, Selby DK. Segmental instability. Rationale for treatment. *Spine.* 1985;10(3):280–286.

336. Nachemson AL. Instability of the lumbar spine. Pathology, treatment, and clinical evaluation. *Neurosurg Clin N Am.* 1991;2(4):785–790.

337. Pope MH, Frymoyer JW, Krag MH. Diagnosing instability. *Clin Orthop.* 1992;(279):60–67.

338. Lindgren KA, Sihvonen T, Leino E, et al. Exercise therapy effects on functional radiographic findings and segmental electromyographic activity in lumbar spine instability. *Arch Phys Med Rehabil.* 1993;74(9):933–939.

339. Sihvonen T, Partanen J, Hänninen O, et al. Electric behavior of low back muscles during lumbar pelvic rhythm in low back pain patients and healthy controls. *Arch Phys Med Rehabil.* 1991;72(13):1080–1087.

340. Fritz JM, Piva SR, Childs JD. Accuracy of the clinical examination to predict radiographic instability of the lumbar spine. *Eur Spine J.* 2005;14(8):743–750.

341. Iguchi T, Kanemura A, Kasahara K, et al. Lumbar instability and clinical symptoms: which is the more critical factor for symptoms: sagittal translation or segment angulation? *J Spinal Disord Tech.* 2004;17(4):284–290.

342. Knutsson F. The instability associated with disk degeneration in the lumbar spine. *Acta Radiol.* 1944;(25):593–609.

343. Posner I, White AA, Edwards WT, et al. A biomechanical analysis of the clinical stability of the lumbar and lumbosacral spine. *Spine.* 1982;7(4):374–389.

344. Dupuis PR, Yong-Hing K, Cassidy JD, et al. Radiologic diagnosis of degenerative lumbar spinal instability. *Spine.* 1985;10(3):262–276.

345. Dvořák J, Panjabi MM, Novotny JE, et al. Clinical validation of functional flexion-extension roentgenograms of the lumbar spine. *Spine.* 1991;16(8):943–950.

346. White AA, Panjabi MM. *Clinical Biomechanics of the Spine.* 2nd ed. Philadelphia, PA: Lippincott Williams & Wilkins; 1990:752.

347. Hayes MA, Howard TC, Gruel CR, et al. Roentgenographic evaluation of lumbar spine flexion-extension in asymptomatic individuals. *Spine.* 1989;14(3):327–331.

348. Boden SD, Wiesel SW. Lumbosacral segmental motion in normal individuals. Have we been measuring instability properly? *Spine.* 1990;15(6):571–576.

349. Rosenberg NJ. Degenerative spondylolisthesis. Predisposing factors. *J Bone Joint Surg Am.* 1975;57(4):467–474.

350. Matsunaga S, Ijiri K, Hayashi K. Nonsurgically managed patients with degenerative spondylolisthesis: a 10- to 18-year follow-up study. *J Neurosurg.* 2000;93(2 Suppl):194–198.

351. Bird HA, Eastmond CJ, Hudson A, et al. Is generalized joint laxity a factor in spondylolisthesis? *Scand J Rheumatol.* 1980;9(4):203–205.

352. Matsunaga S, Sakou T, Morizono Y, et al. Natural history of degenerative spondylolisthesis. Pathogenesis and natural course of the slippage. *Spine.* 1990;15(11):1204–1210.

353. Sengupta DK, Herkowitz HN. Degenerative spondylolisthesis: review of current trends and controversies. *Spine.* 2005;30(6 suppl):S71–S81.

354. Fritzell P, Hägg O, Wessberg P, et al. 2001 Volvo Award Winner in Clinical Studies: lumbar fusion versus nonsurgical treatment for chronic low back pain: a multicenter randomized controlled trial from the Swedish Lumbar Spine Study Group. *Spine.* 2001;26(23):2521–2532; discussion 2532–2534.

355. Brox JI, Sørensen R, Friis A, et al. Randomized clinical trial of lumbar instrumented fusion and cognitive intervention and exercises in patients with chronic low back pain and disc degeneration. *Spine.* 2003;28(17):1913–1921.

356. Fairbank J, Frost H, Wilson-MacDonald J, et al. Randomised controlled trial to compare surgical stabilisation of the lumbar spine with an intensive rehabilitation programme for patients with chronic low back pain: the MRC spine stabilisation trial. *BMJ.* 2005;330(7502):1233.

357. Martin BI, Mirza SK, Comstock BA, et al. Reoperation rates following lumbar spine surgery and the influence of spinal fusion procedures. *Spine.* 2007;32(3):382–387.

358. Panjabi MM. Clinical spinal instability and low back pain. *J Electromyogr Kinesiol.* 2003;13(4):371–379.

359. Panjabi MM. The stabilizing system of the spine. Part II. Neutral zone and instability hypothesis. *J Spinal Disord.* 1992;5(4):390–396; discussion 397.

360. Demoulin C, Distrée V, Tomasella M, et al. Lumbar functional instability: a critical appraisal of the literature. *Ann Readapt Med Phys.* 2007;50(8):677–684, 669–76.

361. Richardson C, Jull G, Hodges PW, et al. *Therapeutic Exercises for Spinal Segmental Stabilization in Low Back Pain: Scientific Basis and Clinical Approach.* 1st ed. Edinburgh: Churchill Livingstone; 1998:192.

362. Krabak B, Kennedy DJ. Functional rehabilitation of lumbar spine injuries in the athlete. *Sports Med Arthrosc Rev.* 2008;16(1):47–54.

363. Danneels LA, Vanderstraeten GG, Cambier DC, et al. A functional subdivision of hip, abdominal, and back muscles during asymmetric lifting. *Spine.* 2001;26(6):E114–E121.

364. Moseley GL, Hodges PW, Gandevia SC. Deep and superficial fibers of the lumbar multifidus muscle are differentially active during voluntary arm movements. *Spine.* 2002;27(2):E29–E36.

365. Barr KP, Griggs M, Cadby T. Lumbar stabilization: core concepts and current literature, Part 1. *Am J Phys Med Rehabil.* 2005;84(6):473–480.

366. Hodges PW, Richardson CA. Inefficient muscular stabilization of the lumbar spine associated with low back pain. A motor control evaluation of transversus abdominis. *Spine.* 1996;21(22):2640–2650.

367. Vibert BT, Sliva CD, Herkowitz HN. Treatment of instability and spondylolisthesis: surgical versus nonsurgical treatment. *Clin Orthop.* 2006;443:222–227.

368. Bell DF, Ehrlich MG, Zaleske DJ. Brace treatment for symptomatic spondylolisthesis. *Clin Orthop.* 1988;(236):192–198.

369. O'Sullivan PB, Phyty GD, Twomey LT, et al. Evaluation of specific stabilizing exercise in the treatment of chronic low back pain with radiologic diagnosis of spondylolysis or spondylolisthesis. *Spine.* 1997;22(24):2959–2967.

370. Aebi M. The adult scoliosis. *Eur Spine J.* 2005;14(10):925–948.

371. Marty-Poumarat C, Scattin L, Marpeau M, et al. Natural history of progressive adult scoliosis. *Spine.* 2007;32(11):1227–1234; discussion 1235.

372. Hawes MC. Health and function of patients with untreated idiopathic scoliosis. *JAMA.* 2003;289(20):2644; author reply 2644–2645.

373. Negrini S, Grivas TB, Kotwicki T, et al. Why do we treat adolescent idiopathic scoliosis? What we want to obtain and to avoid for our patients. SOSORT 2005 Consensus paper. *Scoliosis.* 2006;1:4.

374. Sponseller PD. Sizing up scoliosis. *JAMA.* 2003;289(5):608–609.

375. Weinstein SL, Dolan LA, Spratt KF, et al. Health and function of patients with untreated idiopathic scoliosis: a 50-year natural history study. *JAMA.* 2003;289(5):559–567.

376. Kobayashi T, Atsuta Y, Takemitsu M, et al. A prospective study of de novo scoliosis in a community based cohort. *Spine.* 2006;31(2):178–182.

377. Balzini L, Vannucchi L, Benvenuti F, et al. Clinical characteristics of flexed posture in elderly women. *J Am Geriatr Soc.* 2003;51(10):1419–1426.

378. Epstein JA, Epstein BS, Jones MD. Symptomatic lumbar scoliosis with degenerative changes in the elderly. *Spine.* 1979;4(6):542–547.

379. Jackson RP, Simmons EH, Stripinis D. Incidence and severity of back pain in adult idiopathic scoliosis. *Spine.* 1983;8(7):749–756.

380. Simmons EH, Jackson RP. The management of nerve root entrapment syndromes associated with the collapsing scoliosis of idiopathic lumbar and thoracolumbar curves. *Spine.* 1979;4(6):533–541.

381. Glassman SD, Berven S, Bridwell K, et al. Correlation of radiographic parameters and clinical symptoms in adult scoliosis. *Spine.* 2005;30(6):682–688.

382. Gelb DE, Lenke LG, Bridwell KH, et al. An analysis of sagittal spinal alignment in 100 asymptomatic middle and older aged volunteers. *Spine.* 1995;20(12):1351–1358.

383. Hammerberg EM, Wood KB. Sagittal profile of the elderly. *J Spinal Disord Tech.* 2003;16(1):44–50.

384. Schwab FJ, Smith VA, Biserni M, et al. Adult scoliosis: a quantitative radiographic and clinical analysis. *Spine.* 2002;27(4):387–392.

385. Black DM, Palermo L, Nevitt MC, et al. Defining incident vertebral deformity: a prospective comparison of several approaches. The Study of Osteoporotic Fractures Research Group. *J Bone Miner Res.* 1999;14(1):90–101.

386. Minne HW, Leidig G, Wüster C, et al. A newly developed spine deformity index (SDI) to quantitate vertebral crush fractures in patients with osteoporosis. *Bone Miner.* 1988;3(4):335–349.

387. Genant HK, Wu CY, van Kuijk C, et al. Vertebral fracture assessment using a semi-quantitative technique. *J Bone Miner Res.* 1993;8(9):1137–1148.

388. Hawes MC, O'Brien JP. A century of spine surgery: what can patients expect? *Disabil Rehabil.* 2008;30(10):808–817.

389. Hawes M. Impact of spine surgery on signs and symptoms of spinal deformity. *Pediatr Rehabil.* 2006;9(4):318–339.

390. Simmons ED, Kowalski JM, Simmons EH. The results of surgical treatment for adult scoliosis. *Spine.* 1993;18(6):718–724.

391. Schwab F, el-Fegoun AB, Gamez L, et al. A lumbar classification of scoliosis in the adult patient: preliminary approach. *Spine.* 2005;30(14):1670–1673.

392. Kearon C, Viviani GR, Kirkley A, et al. Factors determining pulmonary function in adolescent idiopathic thoracic scoliosis. *Am Rev Respir Dis.* 1993;148(2):288–294.

393. Hawes MC. The use of exercises in the treatment of scoliosis: an evidence-based critical review of the literature. *Pediatr Rehabil.* 2003;6(3–4):171–182.

394. Torell G, Nachemson A, Haderspeck-Grib K, et al. Standing and supine Cobb measures in girls with idiopathic scoliosis. *Spine.* 1985;10(5):425–427.

395. Duval-Beaupère G, Lespargot A, Grossiord A. Flexibility of scoliosis. What does it mean? Is this terminology appropriate? *Spine.* 1985;10(5):428–432.

396. Freidel K, Petermann F, Reichel D, et al. Quality of life in women with idiopathic scoliosis. *Spine.* 2002;27(4):E87–E91.

397. Kostuik JP. Recent advances in the treatment of painful adult scoliosis. *Clin Orthop.* 1980;(147):238–252.

398. Hawes MC, O'brien JP. The transformation of spinal curvature into spinal deformity: pathological processes and implications for treatment. *Scoliosis.* 2006; 1(1):3.

399. Ascani E, Bartolozzi P, Logroscino CA, et al. Natural history of untreated idiopathic scoliosis after skeletal maturity. *Spine.* 1986;11(8):784–789.

400. Nachemson A. Adult scoliosis and back pain. *Spine.* 1979;4(6):513–517.

401. Simmons ED, Simmons EH. Spinal stenosis with scoliosis. *Spine.* 1992;17 (6 suppl):S117–S120.

CHAPTER 28

Stefano Negrini
Sabrina Donzelli
Alessandra Negrini

Michele Romano
Fabio Zaina

Idiopathic Scoliosis

DEFINITION

Scoliosis is a three-dimensional deformity of the spine and the trunk (1). While it is commonly seen as a spinal curve in the frontal plane, research has shown that a true scoliosis is associated with a rotation in the horizontal plane and a distortion of the normal curves on the sagittal plane; the latter usually drives the spine to a flat back (reduction of kyphosis and lordosis) (2–5). While scoliosis can result from a specific etiology, in up to 85% to 90% of cases, it is not possible to identify a cause: this is called idiopathic scoliosis (IS) (6,7). The most common form of scoliosis occurs during adolescence (adolescent idiopathic scoliosis—AIS), that is also the period of worse progression of an established IS; nevertheless, it is now known that IS appears in all ages, from infant to the elderly. In this chapter, we will review the general concepts and rehabilitation approach to IS with a greater focus on AIS, but including also all the other types.

IDIOPATHIC SCOLIOSIS

Etiology and Pathogenesis

The knowledge on etiology of IS is still poor: many hypotheses have been considered, and the controversy persists (8). The multifactorial nature of the etiology of IS has led to a variety of hypotheses in this field. The main available theories can be categorized in two main groups. The first group deals with the possibility of a primary disturbance in the development of the spine, spine biomechanics, and growth. The second group addresses possible causative factors outside the spine. If we consider only intrinsic factors, they can be divided into asymmetric bone growth, bone deformation, and abnormal active or passive spinal tissue system, which are strongly related to the biomechanics of the spine. According to the law of Heuter and Volkmann, increased compressive forces at the epiphyseal plates reduce growth, and increased distractive forces result in accelerated growth. Therefore, asymmetric loading of the epiphyseal plates results in asymmetric growth and wedging of the vertebrae (9,10). These mechanical theories have been tested in animal models and could explain the development and progression of the deformity in humans (11). Based on these results, the growth disturbances seem to be secondary to the deformity rather than primary. An earlier growth peak in IS subjects has been advocated to play a role in scoliosis progression and evolution (12,13). The roles of intervertebral disk and spinal ligaments contributing to the development of scoliosis remains unclear as only *in vitro* and animal models (14,15) have been studied.

Some studies in both animal models and humans have tried to correlate vestibular system dysfunction to IS (16). Despite an association between the two having been documented, no clear causal effect has been demonstrated (17). Several studies have described the role of a genetic predisposition in the origin of IS (18). Twin studies have documented a concordance rate of 73% in 37 pairs of monozygotic twins and 36% in 31 pairs of dizygotic twins (19). Many different chromosome resulted having a role in the scoliosis etiology but due to the large number of chromosome involved in its origin it is difficult to draw clinically relevant conclusion. According to the genetic researches the environmental effects play a role in the manifestation of the pathology (18). Also the X chromosomes seem involved, and this would explain the higher prevalence of IS in females (20).

Some hormones may have a role in the origin and development of IS: melatonin, calmodulin, and leptin. Melatonin has a role in bone metabolism (21–23). High levels of calmodulin in platelets have been correlated to scoliosis severity (24). Leptin has been reported to be a risk factor for IS onset (25–27). Stokes has described the concept of mechanical modulation of vertebral body growth in the pathogenesis of progressive scoliosis (10,28,29). The *vicious cycle hypothesis of pathogenesis* formulated by Stokes assumes that a small preexisting scoliosis curve initiates a mechanically modulated alteration of vertebral body growth, which in turn causes worsening of scoliosis (10,30).

Diagnosis

Scoliosis is diagnosed combining the clinical finding of a prominence in forward bending with the radiographic finding of a curve in the frontal plane (1). If only one of these two signs is present scoliosis cannot be diagnosed: a prominence without curve could be due to other trunk asymmetries; a curve without prominence is a scoliotic postural attitude.

Classification

The chronologic, angular, and topographic classifications receive the largest agreement among experts in scoliosis conservative treatment (1,31) **(Table 28-1)**. "Early-onset scoliosis" is alternatively used to classify together infantile idiopathic scoliosis (IIS) and juvenile idiopathic scoliosis (JIS). Other topographic classification systems are used mainly in surgical settings (32–35). Finally, a specific classification has been proposed for Adult Scoliosis Deformity (ASD) that is based on curve type and magnitude using a specific index based on sagittal pelvic and spine parameters: this can be applied also in rehabilitation, since it has been shown to be reliable and correlates with quality of life (36).

TABLE 28-1	**Classifications of Idiopathic Scoliosis during Growth**							
Chronologic		**Angular**				**Topographic**		
Age at diagnosis (y/mo)		**Cobb degrees**					**Apex**	
							From	**To**
Infantile	0–2/11	Low	Low	20 or less		Cervical	—	Disk C6-7
Juvenile	3–9/11	Moderate	Moderate	21–35		Cervicothoracic	C7	T1
Adolescent	10–17/11		Moderate to severe	36–40		Thoracic	Disk T1-2	Disk T11-12
Adult	18–	Severe	Severe	41–50		Thoracolumbar	T12	L1
			Severe to very severe	51–55		Lumbar	Disk L1-2	—
		Very severe		56 or more				

Data from Negrini S, Donzelli S, Aulisa AG, et al. 2016 SOSORT guidelines: orthopaedic and rehabilitation treatment of idiopathic scoliosis during growth. *Scoliosis Spinal Disord.* 2018;13:3, Ref. (1).

Natural History

Broadly speaking, understanding the natural history of a disease enables physicians to anticipate prognosis and to identify opportunities for prevention and control. Unfortunately, concerning the natural history of IS, there is marked variability. The rate of progression ranges from 10.3% to 100%, and the rapidity of progression ranges from 2.3 to 6.4 degrees per year (37–40).

High rate of progression (58% of the observation group) has been shown by the Bracing in Adolescent Idiopathic Scoliosis Trial (BrAIST) as a risk factor for the primary outcome, which was curve progression to 50 degrees at skeletal maturity (41). After the spinal growth is complete, the risk of progression in adulthood starts for curves larger than 30 degrees and becomes highest for curves exceeding 50 degrees (1,42).

Evaluation

Clinical Evaluation

The clinical assessment plays a very important role in diagnosis, prognosis, prescription, and follow-up of the disease. The main goals are early detection, evaluation of the progression potential for the definition of an early and appropriate conservative treatment.

Certain clinical parameters are evaluated quantitatively (e.g., Bunnell angle of trunk rotation [ATR] using an inclinometer, rib hump height or trunk list), while others are evaluated semiquantitatively by means of ordinal numbers (e.g., curve flexibility or height differences of the shoulders and pelvis). In the approach to scoliosis, the patient's clinical history plays a fundamental role and is the first step in any clinical evaluation. The first visit differs from subsequent visits because possible causes of secondary scoliosis must be excluded. In this respect, it is important to inquire about associated signs and symptoms. It is important to know whether another family member has developed scoliosis and/or there are genetic or familiar diseases that can cause a secondary scoliosis. Pregnancy, maternal exposure to risk factors, delivery, and psychophysical development should be carefully evaluated. For a girl, the age of menarche is another relevant element to determine the progression potential of scoliosis. It is also important to consider sports activity and its frequency. Minor neurologic signs, traumatic brain injury, and vertebral pain are some other relevant factors that should be investigated.

In subsequent visits, history focuses mainly on compliance to treatment. It is important to help the patient understand the importance of the treatment. Questions like, "When do you wear your brace and when do you remove it?" or "How many times each week do you perform your exercises, and how long does it take?" can be helpful. Temperature sensors, like Thermobrace (43,44), have been developed to allow one to track the actual brace wear.

Some questionnaires have been developed to more easily and objectively monitor various treatment aspects related to function, pain, body aesthetics, and psychological impact. The most used are SRS-22 (45), the Bad Sobernheim Stress Questionnaire (BSSQbrace) (46) and the Brace Questionnaire (BrQ) (47). More recent Rasch analysis compatible questionnaires have also been developed, including the SRS-7 (48) and ISYQOL (49).

Overall observation and evaluation of the patient is required to assess the most affected somatic areas and posture alterations. The patient should be evaluated in standing position, with straight legs and habitual posture. At the side of the patient, it is possible to evaluate the ante/retroversion of the pelvis, the abdominal prominence, the ante/retroposition of the trunk, and the anteposition of the head. Frontally, rib cage abnormalities such as pectus excavatum or carinatum can be noted, while from the back the symmetry of the shoulders, scapulae, thorax, waist, and head positioning can be evaluated.

Recently, a clinical scale for objective aesthetic evaluation has been developed, the "TRunk Aesthetic Clinical Evaluation" (TRACE). It is based on four subscales: shoulders (0-3), scapulae (0-2), hemithorax (0-2), and waist (0-4). Each point is fully described and gives an ordinal scale for increasing asymmetry (50). Aesthetics is important in scoliosis, since it is considered a major goal of conservative treatment by SOSORT experts (51) and one of the most relevant indications for surgery among surgeons (52). Since repeatability and sensitivity of the measurements are known, it is now possible to use this instrument for everyday clinical evaluation and to monitor the aesthetic changes achieved with treatment.

The evaluation of leg-length discrepancy is important when altered pelvic position leads to frontal imbalance. Usually in this field, it is typically measured in standing. A plumb line is used to assess the sagittal and frontal profiles of the spine. To check the frontal decompensation, the plumb line is set along the medial sacral crest, and the discrepancy from the plumb line is measured at C7. In patients with scoliosis, it is important to also evaluate sagittal balance in the coronal plane. In the sagittal profile, the distance from the plumb line is measured at the spinous processes of C7, and L3 with respect to the most prominent point of the dorsal kyphosis (**Fig. 28-1**). For the evaluation of kyphosis, the Sagittal Index given by C7 + L3 is used, and for lordosis, L3 distance is used. Plumb line measurement is reliable and sensible for intraobserver evaluation (53–55).

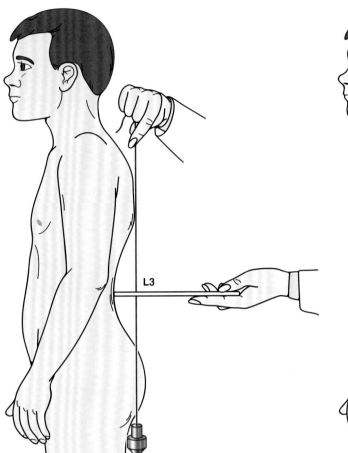
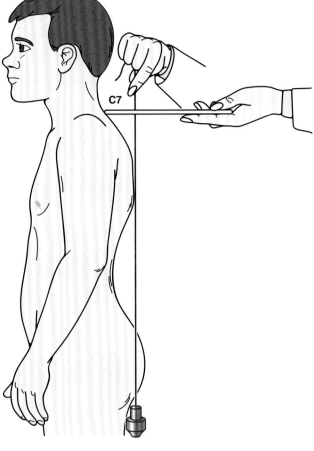

FIGURE 28-1. Measurement of plumb line distances.

The forward bending test, the classic screening test for scoliosis, allows the measurement of the ATR, one of the most relevant measurements in the clinical evaluation of scoliosis (56). This parameter is fundamental for monitoring the effects of the treatment, even without radiographic evaluation. The ATR measurement is performed using a dedicated instrument called a scoliometer: the patient is asked to forward-bend with arms dangling and palms pressed together. The scoliometer is placed on the back and used to measure the most leaning point of each hump (**Fig. 28-2**). In this position, it is also possible to measure the height of the hump (HH) (57,58): it is necessary to elevate the scoliometer on the side opposite to the hump,

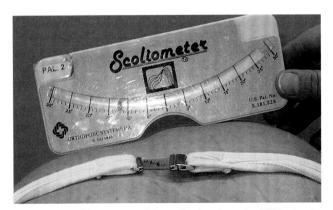

FIGURE 28-2. Measurement of the angle of trunk rotation (ATR) using the Bunnell scoliometer.

thus positioning it to 0 degree and measuring the height with a ruler. The ATR and HH correlate with the Cobb angle.

Curve rigidity is another important parameter that adds information relevant to prognosis and therapeutic choices. While bending forward, the patient is asked to side-bend on one side and then the other. If the curve is not rigid or structured, it is possible to invert the hump; if it does not change, the curve is very rigid.

Tests are available as means to exclude a possible secondary scoliosis, and these tests provide certain general information. The Romberg test and the Unterberger (Fukuda) test are useful for screening. The clinical assessment of gait and posture can also be used in ambiguous cases, but it should preferably be concluded with a neurologic examination, which should evaluate reflexes (including the abdominal ones), motor and sensory testing, balance, and Babinski's sign.

The evaluation of strength and extensibility of some muscular groups (like abdominals, hamstrings, and pectoralis) are useful general parameters; the evaluation of spinal rigidity in extension is performed in prone position. Finally, height and weight measurements (with body mass index calculation) are important to monitor skeletal growth and the correlated risk of scoliosis progression.

Imaging

To date, the gold standard to identify and modify and monitor scoliosis has been standing frontal and lateral full-spine x-rays, with systematic radiographic imaging performed throughout the individual's course of treatment (31). It is recommended not to perform x-rays if the Adam's test (which is the measurement of the hump using a scoliometer while the patient is bending forward with arm and head relaxed) is negative and the scoliometer value is below 5 degrees, unless otherwise justified in the opinion of a clinician specialized in conservative treatment of spinal deformities (31). X-ray is needed not only for diagnosis during first consultation but also for treatment decisions at follow-ups. In fact, it is possible to document the severity of the curvature, determine the skeletal maturity, monitor progression and treatment results, and search for nonidiopathic causes of scoliosis. It is recommended that frontal radiographic studies be made posteroanteriorly, using digital films, including visualization of the femoral heads and protection of the gonads. Standing position without the use of support aids or indication of correct posture should be adopted, unless otherwise justified (59). To reduce the invasiveness of follow-up, it is recommended that no more than one radiographic study per year is performed, unless it is truly necessary (31). It is also recommended to use the EOS system (60), a novel technology in which orthogonal anteroposterior and lateral low-dose x-rays are used for a 3D detailed semiautomatic reconstruction of the spine (61).

The x-ray examination evaluates localization of the curve, morphology alterations, and residual growth and allows one to measure the frontal and lateral curves, and rotation. By convention, all spinal films are viewed as if looking at the patient from the back—the patient's right side is on the viewer's right side. The observation of the x-rays in the frontal and sagittal plane shows the body vertebrae and rib conformation: this allows one to identify congenital scoliosis, which can be characterized by congenital morphologic deformities like partial or complete failure of formation, failure of segmentation, multiple alterations, or rib fusion. For the curve, one should identify the apex vertebra/ disk (that is the most horizontal) and the end vertebrae (that are the most tilted in the frontal plane). Through apex localization, it is possible to define the topographic classification (**Table 28-1**).

To measure scoliosis severity, the Cobb angle measurement is used; this is measured from the superior end plate of the most

cephalad end vertebra (the upper end vertebra) to the inferior end plate of the most caudal end vertebra (the lower end vertebra) in the curve. The angle, measured with a goniometer, is made by the two perpendicular lines to these vertebrae (**Fig. 28-3**). Due to inherent measurement error, to define significant changes, a curvature variation of 5 degrees or more is needed (31). In case of variation below this threshold, the curve is considered stable (31). It is also possible to evaluate in the frontal plane the vertebral slopes (62–64): the Cobb angle corresponds to the sum of the two vertebral slopes (see **Fig. 28-3**). The slopes can be evaluated with the scoliometer (until 25 degrees): it is recognized that an intraobserver variability of 3 to 5 degrees and an interobserver variability of 6 to 7 degrees exist (65).

The second step of the evaluation in the frontal plane is the measurement of rotation. To evaluate the rotation, there are various methods. The Nash and Moe method (66) is based on deviation of pedicle shadows of the vertebrae according to five grades. The Cobb method is based on the spinous process: the space between the center and the lateral edge of the body is divided into three sections representing the 3 degrees of rotation, while the fourth is reached when the spinous process is out of the vertebral body. Finally, rotation can be measured in degrees through a grid named the Perdriolle torsiometer (67–69). The grid is put on the radiograph, with the lateral margin of the convex side of the vertebra of interest, with the straight margin in the grid. The intercept line of the pedicle measures the magnitude of the rotation.

Skeletal maturity is assessed through the Risser scale, which is based on the level of ossification and fusion of the iliac crest apophyses. Risser described five stages: stage 0 (no ossification center at the level of iliac crest apophysism), stage 1 (apophysis under 25% of the iliac crest), stage 2 (apophysis over 25% to 50% of the iliac crest), stage 3 (apophysis over 50% to 75% of the iliac crest), stage 4 (apophysis over >75% of the iliac crest), and stage 5 (complete ossification and fusion of the iliac crest apophysis). In Europe, another Risser staging system prevails due to the description by Stagnara (70): stage 1 is the appearance of the apophysis, stage 2 is the partial coverage of

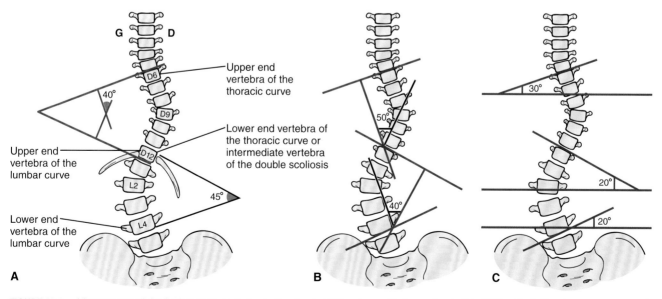

FIGURE 28-3. Measurement of the Cobb degrees according to the classical **(A)** and a modified according to Cotrel **(B)** method. Also slopes measurement is shown **(C)**: In this case, Cobb degrees of the curves are given by the sum of the two slopes of each curve.

the iliac crest, stage 3 is the complete cover without fusion, and stage 4 is when the fusion starts. To estimate peak of growth velocity is also useful to observe the triradiate cartilage between ilium, ischium, and pubis as a marker of growth velocity (71). The "Risser plus" scale is the result of the confluence between the original Risser staging and the European version, which includes also the triradiate cartilage fusion, that has been shown to be a useful and prognostic subdivision of Risser staging 0 (**Table 28-2**) (72).

The analysis of lateral projection is fundamental to complete the diagnostic process and for the correct clinical decision (3,73). Cervical lordosis, thoracic kyphosis, and lumbar lordosis angle are calculated with the Cobb method considering, respectively, the angle between Cl and Tl, between Tl and the thoracolumbar inflexion point (normally should be T12), and between this inflexion point and S1.

Other important sagittal parameters to be included are the pelvic angles that correlate each other and are used to define the sagittal balance of the spine.

The pelvic parameters include the following:
- Sacral slope: the angle between the horizontal reference line and the S1 end plate
- Pelvic tilt: the angle between the vertebral reference line and the line joining the center of femoral heads and the center of the S1 end plate
- Pelvic incidence: the angle between the line joining the hip axis and the center of S1 end plate and the line orthogonal to the S1 end plate

All these parameters are shown in **Figure 28-4**.

Treatments

Treatment Selection

IS during growth is treated to avoid problems in adulthood (51,74,75) that arise when scoliosis exceeds 30 degrees Cobb: over this threshold, the risks of back pain and progression in adulthood increase (42,76,77). Another important threshold is 50 degrees, which is proposed by consensus as the limit to propose surgery—in fact above this level, problems

in adulthood are always present (72). According to these two thresholds, it is possible to define the goals of IS treatment.

We need also to consider the natural history of IS. Duval-Beaupère (78) showed the role of Risser sign and age as predictors of scoliosis progression. Typically the highest risk of progression is in the prepubertal phase, when Risser sign is between 0 and 1. Scoliosis treatment has been defined as a step-by-step approach, where a higher step implies more efficacy but also more difficulties for the patient: this concept has been accepted by the current guidelines (1).

Braces

Brace therapy was developed to stop curve progression. According to the current guidelines, braces are prescribed for curves exceeding 20 degrees Cobb discovered during growth. The primary aim of brace treatment is to reach the end of growth below 30-degree threshold (the best possible result able to guarantee the best function and quality of life in adulthood) or at least avoid surgical treatment (31). The role of bracing in scoliosis conservative treatment was debated due to the very low quality of evidences in favor of bracing (74). The bracing in Adolescent Randomized Trial (BrAIST study) provided a high level of evidence of bracing in reducing curve progression and avoiding surgery (79). A linear relationship between success and brace dosage was found. Considering the prospective observational trials, Lusini showed that brace treatment is useful for patients with curves above 45 degrees Cobb and still growing, reducing the rate of surgery (80). Despite the difficulties in creating stronger evidence endorsing brace therapy, an effort to standardize treatment protocols and brace construction arose in the last decades (31,81), pointing out the importance of expertise of the treating physician and orthotist as well as defining a minimum threshold of expertise required to provide scoliosis conservative treatment (82). There are many different types of braces used all around the world; mainly in Europe and North America, a recently published paper gives an overview of the braces used and highlights the currently available evidence supporting their efficacy, together with a summary of

TABLE 28-2	**Risser Plus Staging, Resuming the Original and European Versions of Risser Test**		
"Risser+" Staging	**Triradiate Cartilage Ossification**	**US Risser Staging**	**European Risser Staging**
0-	No	0	0
0	Yes	0	0
1		1	1
0%–25% coverage		0%–25% coverage	Initial ossification
2		2	2
25%–50% coverage		25%–50% coverage	Partial coverage
3		3	
50%–75% coverage		50%–75% coverage	
3/4		4	3
75%–100% coverage		75%–100% coverage	Complete coverage
4			4
Start of fusion			Start of fusion
5		5	5
Complete fusion		Complete fusion	Complete fusion

From Negrini S, Hresko TM, O'Brien JP, et al. Recommendations for research studies on treatment of idiopathic scoliosis: consensus 2014 between SOSORT and SRS non-operative management committee. *Scoliosis*. 2015;10:8. http://creativecommons.org/licenses/by/4.0/ Ref. (72).

FIGURE 28-4. **A:** Main sagittal parameters: thoracic kyphosis (*TK*), lumbar lordosis (*LL*). **B:** Sacral slope (*SS*), pelvic tilt (*PT*), pelvic incidence (*PI*), and spinosacral angle (*SSA*).

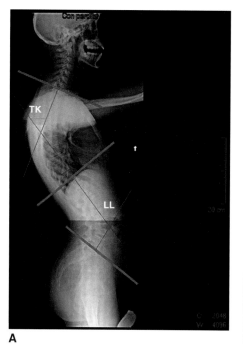
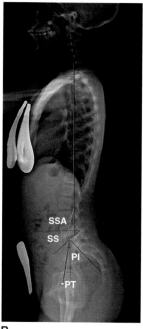

A   **B**

the biomechanical principles at the basis of their functioning and construction (83).

Brace Wearing and Weaning.

The more hours per day the brace is worn, the greater the effect in preventing progression (79,84). Rowe et al. (85), in a meta-analysis of the efficacy of nonoperative management of scoliosis, found that the most effective brace regimen was 23 hours per day. Adherence (86) is consequently a key factor for brace treatment success. The main problem in scoliosis treatment is that adherence is not always easy to obtain (87). This can depend both on the brace design and comfort as well as on the commitment of the treating team (88,89). When the team is really committed and the goal of the treatment is shared with patients, a high level of adherence can be achieved (90). In recent years, some devices have been developed to objectively monitor compliance (91,92) and are routinely used in clinical practice (90,93). These devices allow a precise measurement of brace wear and can help the patient to increase adherence (57,94). The brace should be worn until skeletal maturity. Most bracing regimens utilize a weaning period after maturity over 6 to 12 months, usually finishing with nighttime brace wear. Nevertheless, more gradual and long-term weaning has been shown to be effective in high-degree curves (61,80,95,96).

Physiotherapic Scoliosis-Specific Exercises

Recently, a number of scientific studies have supported the efficacy of exercise in prevention that is supported now by several randomized controlled trials (RCTs) (97–102).

The general term used to refer to the exercise approaches used for IS treatment is physiotherapic scoliosis-specific exercises (PSSE) (1). The objective of PSSE in the treatment of scoliosis is secondary prevention, that is, to stop or slow down progression of curves. The most important elements to consider in an exercise program specifically developed for scoliosis (103) include 3D autocorrection, stabilization, and theoretical information for the patient and family. The 3D

autocorrection approach uses a conscious series of active movements performed to reach the best possible realignment of the scoliosis curves carried out by the patient himself. The self-correction can be performed in an active or passive way. With "passive" self-correction, the patient performs the corrective movement with the help of external tools or thanks to specific positions of the body that drive the correction. **Figure 28-5** shows examples that explain this concept. In **Figure 28-5A**, the position of the left arm of the patient and the hand resting on the wall allow to help the realignment of a hypothetical right thoracic curve. In **Figure 28-5B**, the lying position on the left and the use of a support under the apex of a hypothetical left lumbar curve will help the realignment. In "active self-correction," the patient performs movements to obtain the best optimal realignment of the scoliotic curve without using external tools or specific position of the body.

Figure 28-6 shows a patient that performs an active self-correction of a right thoracic curve (**Fig. 28-6A**, relaxed position; **Fig. 28-6B**, self-correction).

An ambitious objective of a PSSE program for the treatment of scoliosis is to contribute to the breaking of the "vicious circle" suggested by Stokes (28–30,104). This process describes the relationship between the consequential progressive vertebrae deformation and the worsening of the curves. The PSSE should be used to start a process of a "virtuous circle" (proposed by Rigo for braces (105) and that we propose also for exercises) to counteract this unwanted mechanism.

PSSE for the treatment of scoliosis can be interpreted in two different ways. First exercise can represent the achievement of the best possible self-correction and then keeping it for several seconds to target stability. An example of this interpretation is given by the Schroth method (106).

A different concept of specific movement for the treatment of scoliosis provides that exercise and self-correction are two distinct elements. These two elements are combined with the aim to use the exercise as a tool to progressively train the patient to be more and more able to use the self-correction. This means

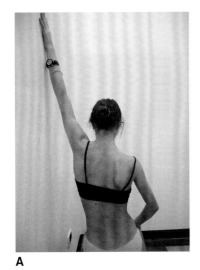
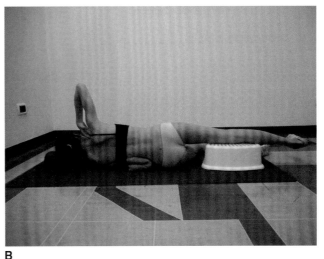

A **B**

FIGURE 28-5. Self-correction according to "passive" concept (see the text). **A:** Self-correction helped by the position of the arm and the patient's hand. **B:** Self-correction helped by the lying position of the patient and the passive support under the apex of the curve.

that the final objective of the treatment is to train the best ability of the patient to handle the self-correction also during some activities of daily life. For this reason, both self-correction and exercises are strictly carried out without external aid and in physiological postures. The method of treatment using this concept is the SEAS (Scientific Exercises Approach to Scoliosis) (64).

Surgical Treatment

In case the nonsurgical treatment of scoliosis fails, spinal surgery should be considered. This is recommended when the curve progresses to over 45 to 50 degrees, to avoid problems in adulthood due to progressive trunk imbalance. The goals of spinal surgery include preventing further progression of the curve, reducing the deformities, and maintaining trunk balance. Surgery description is beyond the scope of this chapter, and we will give only some general notes.

Surgical treatment for scoliosis can be divided into fusion and fusionless surgery. To obtain realignment and stabilization of the spine, modern surgical approaches use instrumentation, rods, screws, hooks, and/or wires placed in the spine. The standard surgical approach for treatment of scoliosis is posterior fusion with instrumentation. The instrumentation includes anchors, to connect the rod and the spine, segmental pedicle screw constructs or hybrid constructs using pedicle screws, hooks, and wires.

Today there are no standard protocols for rehabilitation after a spinal surgical treatment. The primary aim is to restore the patient to full function as early as possible, without compromising the spinal surgery. Early mobilization is recommended to prevent deconditioning and other postoperative morbidities, such as related respiratory diseases. The physical and rehabilitation medicine (PRM) physician should decide

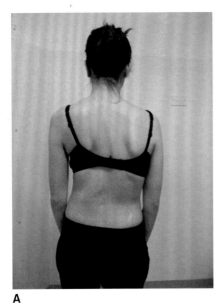
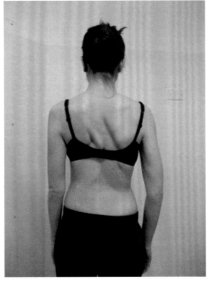
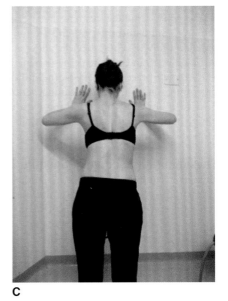

A **B** **C**

FIGURE 28-6. SEAS exercises are based on an "active" concept of self-correction (see the text). **A:** Patient with right thoracic scoliosis in relaxation. **B:** Same patient in active self-correction. **C:** Patient performing the exercise in active self-correction.

step-by-step timing of postoperative rehabilitation to help return the patient to daily life function and prevent secondary deformities.

Clinical management of spinal curvature requires a good understanding of spinal anatomy, physiology, and biomechanics. Clinical examination with measurable outcomes, including radiographs, should allow PRM physicians to better understand their patients' spinal curvature and the pathophysiology of that condition and how it is affecting the spine. With this knowledge, the PRM physician should be able to advise his or her patients regarding surgical treatment and to develop an appropriate rehabilitation program to control and reduce the patients' spinal curvature and optimize their quality of life.

Other Therapeutic Options

Manual Therapy

Manual therapy is one of the treatments applied especially in countries where chiropractic medicine is commonly practiced. In 2008, the first systematic review focused on the effectiveness of manual therapy as a treatment of IS patients (107). No conclusions were possible because only two trials were found. In 2016, another systematic review showed that most of the published studies were case reports or case series, and the very few available trials had a very poor methodology. Another important problem with IS literature is the outcomes reported. Until now, only two studies have described outcomes as recommended in the SRS-SOSORT guidelines. The currently available scientific data are not sufficient to draw conclusions about the efficacy of manual therapy as an effective technique for the treatment of IS.

Orthodontic Approaches

Some theories propose a correlation between scoliosis and dental occlusion.

A recent review showed that there are data to support a correlation between malocclusion and scoliosis (108). The quality of papers included in this review is very low: no RCTs are available, only longitudinal studies without a control group and with cross-sectional design. In the published studies, the samples are very small, usually 20 to 30 subjects; the diagnosis of scoliosis is sometimes questionable since incomplete date are reported; and frequently no radiographies are available (109). One RCT tested the effect of early orthodontic treatment in juvenile population with unilateral posterior cross-bite. The results showed no change in the postural parameters after 1 year of treatment (110). In conclusion, some data have shown a correlation between a posterior cross-bite and scoliosis, but no conclusions can be made because of the low quality of the papers.

Shoe Lift and Insoles

There is no evidence to correlate a leg-lift length discrepancy and the development or progress of IS; therefore, they are not recommended as a treatment for IS in isolation. There is no evidence that insoles can treat or prevent scoliosis; therefore they are not recommended as a treatment.

Sport and Scoliosis

Controversies on the relationship between sports activities and scoliosis have always existed. existed. In the past, sports activities have been used and prescribed as a treatment for IS

or were considered responsible for scoliosis progression or for scoliosis onset. Currently, we know that PSSE act to contrast the biomechanical alterations induced by scoliosis in the three spatial planes, while sports activities play a pivotal role in social interaction, education, and improving coordination, muscle, development, and general well-being (31–59,61–111). Sports considered dangerous for scoliosis include competitive dancers and gymnasts, in whom a higher prevalence of scoliosis was found (112–114). Swimming has been prescribed to treat scoliosis, but some recent data show that it might have a negative impact on the growing spine; in fact an increasing prevalence of trunk asymmetries was found in competitive swimmers (115). Finally, asymmetric sports were traditionally thought to be harmful for scoliosis progression, but recent data about tennis rejected this idea, showing similar prevalence of trunk asymmetry compared with general population (116).

Current evidence shows that different sports can influence body growth in different ways; competitive athletes with scoliosis should be treated carefully by considering the potential negative effects of the sports performed (112–116).

There is not a specific sport to be prescribed to patients undergoing treatment for spinal deformities, but there is a strong agreement among experts that sports activities play a pivotal role in growth and that patients treated for spinal deformities should be encouraged to perform the sport they like on a regular basis.

OTHER SCOLIOSIS DURING GROWTH

Infantile Idiopathic Scoliosis (IIS) and Juvenile Idiopathic Scoliosis (JIS)

The main differences among IIS, JIS and AIS are related to epidemiology, natural history and response to treatment (117–119). Since the curves occur at a younger age, there is a higher risk of severe deformity (117), whereas in adolescent type the risk of progression is much lower (7,117,120,121). The same has been shown for IIS (122), even if these are the only patients who can have self-resolving curves (123,124). Min Mehta described the Rib Vertebra Angle as a specific sign to differentiate self-resolving from evolutionary curves (125). Rate of secondary curves and left thoracic curves is higher in IIS.

Long-term follow-up and bracing effects for JIS and IIS cannot be found in the literature. The study by Min Mehta suggested the importance of casting (124) and is still considered a valuable treatment (126–128). Robinson followed 89 patients (braced full-time with a Milwaukee or Boston or part-time) to skeletal maturity. Sixty-seven percent progressed to spinal fusion (120). Jarvis investigated the effectiveness of part-time bracing for JIS to skeletal maturity and reported 51% of patients improved (129). Other studies showed better results with lower rates of progression even in 16 early-onset forms of scoliosis (130), and they can be justified by treatment effectiveness and patient management as suggested by Donzelli, who found the JIS can have a very similar presentation to AIS, with similar results (90).

Congenital Scoliosis

Congenital scoliosis is defined as skeletal anomalies of the spine that are present at birth.

These anomalies, which can include multiple levels, are the result of a failure of formation or segmentation (or both) during vertebral development. Congenital spinal anomalies are described according to the part of the vertebra that is malformed or connected. Depending on the structure of the anomaly, the child may exhibit scoliosis (a curve to the right or left), kyphosis (round back), or lordosis (sway back) (131). However, not all congenital anomalies fit neatly into these categories. There are often elements of more than one deformity, particularly scoliosis and kyphosis occurring together.

Because these spinal deformities are present *in utero*, they are often first identified on fetal ultrasound (132). In 60% of cases, there can be neurologic, cardiovascular, and genitourinary system anomalies associated to the spinal ones, as these are the organ systems that develop at the same gestational time (5th to 6th week) (133,134). Scoliosis can be associated with neurologic conditions, muscular abnormalities, and global syndromes.

An incidence of 0.5 to 1/1,000 births has been estimated for congenital scoliosis (135). The first congenital scoliosis classification was made by Winter and collaborators in 1988 studying a series of 234 patients (136). This classification relies on the radiographic findings. The types of malformations described by Winter are defined as a formation, segmentation or mixed defect. Moe classified congenital scoliosis according to morphologic characteristics on plain AP frontal and lateral images as an embryologic defect into formation failure, segmentation failure, and a mixed type. This classification also includes several other factors, such as the level of formation failure and the presence or absence of intervertebral disk space.

The natural history of congenital scoliosis is generally benign (71), in fact only 37% of the children had curves greater than 30 degrees at maturity. Winter and McMaster and Ohtsuka (136,137) reported that the rate of deterioration and the severity of final deformity were predictable according to the type of anomaly and curve location. Upper thoracic curves tend to be less severe than thoracolumbar curves. Curve progression occurs more rapidly during the first 5 years of life and, again, during the adolescent growth period of puberty; these two periods represent the most rapid stages of spine growth (71,138).

Neuromuscular scoliosis is a spine deformity secondary to other pathologies in the central nervous system. Scoliosis is considered neuromuscular when associated with muscular dystrophy, cerebral palsy, spinal amyotrophy, and other diseases related to the closure of the tube, like, for example, myelomeningocele. Neuromuscular curves are often associated with pelvic obliquity, a condition in which the child's pelvis is unevenly tilted with one side higher than the other. Frequently, kyphosis is also concurrently present. Compared with IS, neuromuscular scoliosis is much more likely to produce curves that progress and continue progressing into adulthood. Curve progression and trunk imbalances are more severe in patients who are not able to walk.

Children with neuromuscular scoliosis usually do not experience any pain from the condition. Most children with neuromuscular scoliosis have poor balance and poor coordination of their trunk, neck, and head. Neuromuscular scoliosis can lead to thoracic insufficiency syndrome, seating problems, and hygiene challenges. The incidence of neuromuscular scoliosis

can widely vary (17,18). The likelihood and severity of the curves tends to increase with the degree of neuromuscular involvement.

Syndromic Scoliosis

Scoliosis can occur as part of many syndromic diseases (both genetic and nongenetic syndromes). Examples include Marfan's syndrome (138,139), Ehlers-Danlos syndrome (138), muscular dystrophy (140), osteochondrodystrophy (dwarfism) (141), neurofibromatosis (NF) (142), Noonan's syndrome (143), VATER/VACTERL syndrome (144), Angelman's syndrome (145), Rett's (146), Prader-Willi (147), osteogenesis imperfecta (148), trisomy 21 (Down's syndrome) (149), and other connective tissue disorders (138).

The symptoms in these cases are highly variable based on the underlying syndrome and degree of scoliosis. Usually scoliosis is not painful but when severe can cause discomfort and/or pain. When a child is diagnosed with a syndrome known to cause scoliosis, screening for scoliosis would begin earlier. Examination of the back, including x-rays, will be performed on a regular basis. Regarding prognosis, the natures of the causal syndromes are so varied that the curves progression varies too. Some syndromes also affect growth, and this must be taken into account when considering the involved risk factors for progression.

Therefore, "connective tissue laxity" involved in Marfan's or Ehnler-Danlos syndromes, or the need to use growth hormone in syndromes like Prader-Willi plays a role in scoliosis progression and in scoliosis therapy results. A close assessment and follow-up together with a team approach with a syndrome specialist is strongly encouraged and will help to manage effects of scoliosis and ensure the best possible results.

Treatments

Observation is usually the first method of treatment for a young child with a spinal deformity. Treatment is based on the age of the patient, progression of the curve, and the location and type of anomaly. In secondary forms, nonoperative treatment should be prescribed and managed by a multidisciplinary team to ensure that all clinical areas receive the proper treatment.

If congenital anomalies create a compensation with an overall balance of the curves, the risk of progression is reduced. If there is a single congenital anomaly causing a big imbalance, treatment must be planned. Overall, PSSE alone has no real effects and can focus only on balancing the spine. If the curve is progressive, a full-time brace is needed to prevent scoliosis progression with the main goal to delay the need for surgery or in the best cases to avoid surgery. Bracing is sometimes used to prevent progression of secondary curves that develop above or below the congenital curve. The type of brace is mostly related to the localization of the congenital deformity. Brace results have been reported only anecdotally. In our experience, they can help balancing the spine and remodel the deformity. In case of patients not able to walk, bracing will be used less frequently and wheelchair modifications will be used.

Surgical goals are to prevent curve progression, improve sitting or standing balance and tolerance (in nonambulators), reduce repositioning, and reduce pain. The options for surgical treatment include *in situ* fusion and resection with correction of the deformity (150). The risk of neurologic injury with surgical treatment of patients with congenital spinal deformities is greater than that in patients with idiopathic spinal deformity (151). The type of spinal stabilization depends on the age of the patient, ambulatory status, and underlying condition.

ADULT SCOLIOSIS

Etiology, Classification, and Natural History

Adult Spinal Deformities (ASD) is a spinal deformity diagnosed after skeletal maturity, regardless of etiology or age at development. ASD can be classified into three groups: curves that develop prior to skeletal maturity, curves that develop after skeletal maturity, and curves that develop in adults after surgery or trauma. Currently, three classification systems have been developed for ASD: Aebi (152), Schwab (153), and SRS (154). The last two joined recently in a single classification (155). Risk factors that are responsible for continued curve progression in adult life have also been determined. Generally, it is reasonable to assume that most curves over 45 to 50 degrees at skeletal maturity may progress, from 0.5 to 1–3 degrees Cobb per year (156).

One of the most important reasons we must treat scoliosis during growth is the risk for back pain in adult life (42). It is in fact known that scoliosis in adult patients can become painful and functionally impairing (157,158). In the last decade, many papers have focused on the correlation between sagittal spinal parameters and health-related quality-of-life tests in the general population and in patients with different spinal pathologies including scoliosis (159–162).

Evaluations

Clinical assessment of the patient is an essential element of the evaluation of ASD. Clinical evaluation should include history, discussion of concerns, and a review of comorbidities. When pain is reported, it is important to document the quality, intensity, location, and timing of pain. Physical examination should include assessment of the deformity and a neurologic examination (163).

Standing is the most revealing posture for spinal deformity in which sagittal and coronal alignment can be assessed by dropping a plumb line through the middle of C7; supine/prone position can be useful in order to evaluate spinal stiffness and muscle contractures; in forward-bending position, hump size can be evaluated by measuring ATR and HH. Pelvic retroversion and hip and knee flexion are compensatory measures of positive sagittal malalignment that should be recorded in clinical assessment and should be linked to the radiographic evaluation (the position of the hips and knees in space may not be apparent on conventional radiographs) (163,164).

Imaging studies are crucial to the evaluation of ASD: posteroanterior and lateral spine radiographs in a free-standing posture are the gold standard, while advanced imaging studies, such as MRI and CT, are indicated to assess for surgical planning and for neurologic compromise (163) and quality of life (160,165–168).

Therapeutic Approach

The scientific literature concerning ASD treatment is sparse. The main tested therapeutic approaches recognize the same rationale and objectives: reduce pain and prevent or slow down progression for those adults with curve at risk of progression.

Therefore, ASD natural history guides the therapeutic choices (156,169). In cases of adults with curves below 30 degrees Cobb, there are no significant risks and a wait-and-see approach is recommended: these patients can conduct a normal healthy life style and should undergo a follow-up visit at least every 5 years, with an x-ray every 5 to 10 years. In case of back pain, scoliosis has a minor role but should be considered and evaluated by expert professionals. For curves exceeding the 30-degree threshold, the monitoring period can change from 5 to 3 years to 1 year according to curve severity, or to the other associated symptoms. For curves exceeding 50 degrees, a follow-up visit can be recommended every year, and an x-ray every 3 to 5 years can be useful to catch any sign of progression. (170,171). Adults with scoliosis should be encouraged to maintain regular physical activity and regular follow-up visits. In cases of pain or other symptoms like an increase in fatigue and a subjective worsening of the aesthetic of the trunk, the situation should be evaluated by an expert physician in the field of scoliosis treatment.

ASD progresses in some cases during adulthood. According to our current knowledge, scoliosis curve magnitude is the main trigger for progression; it is unknown which other factors are involved in the breakout of curves' progression, and long-term follow-up studies are needed to increase our knowledge. Pregnancy and labor can be considered a potential risk factor for scoliosis progression as well as menopause (156,172–174). In this view, it is correct to recommend a follow-up visit and/or exercises to prevent scoliosis progression in those patients with more severe curves who are approaching pregnancy or menopause. In case of pain occurring in these conditions, it is important to ask for an evaluation from an expert in the field. The available evidence for treatment modalities in adults with scoliosis includes exercises, braces, and surgery.

In a retrospective cohort of 34 adults with scoliosis after an average period of 2 years of exercise treatment, 68% of the patients experienced an improvement in their scoliosis (175). Monticone's randomized trial showed that the SEAS program was superior to general physiotherapy in reducing disability of ads. Changes were maintained for at least 1 year (176). Palazzo showed the efficacy of rigid braces in reducing curve progression (177). Two other types of braces have been tested in adults: the peak brace showed good short-term results in reducing pain and disability in a small sample of prospectively collected patients with severe ASD (178), and the Spinecor brace improved pain in 77% of patients in a group of 30 scoliosis subjects monitored for 18 to 28 months. In adults, scoliosis surgery is recommended in case of important spinal imbalance and pain not responding to conservative treatment (160,179).

SUMMARY

Idiopathic scoliosis is an expanding field of interest for PRM physicians that need our attention because nowadays surgical specialties focus almost only on surgery. It is a challenging field where development of specific competences is needed but requires specific education (1,31,82). Moreover, the evidence regarding PRM approach is steadily growing (1,31), and this requires dedication for further growth. A specific international society, SOSORT, exists today and is the best forum to grow the required competences.

ACKNOWLEDGMENTS

We wish to thank for their help: Oriana Amata, Francesca Di Felice, Claudia Fusco, Salvatore Minnella, and Andrea Zonta.

REFERENCES

1. Negrini S, Donzelli S, Aulisa AG, et al. 2016 SOSORT guidelines: orthopaedic and rehabilitation treatment of idiopathic scoliosis during growth. *Scoliosis Spinal Disord.* 2018;13:3.
2. Clément J-L, Geoffray A, Yagoubi F, et al. Relationship between thoracic hypokyphosis, lumbar lordosis and sagittal pelvic parameters in adolescent idiopathic scoliosis. *Eur Spine J.* 2013;22(11):2414–2420.
3. Gutman G, Labelle H, Barchi S, et al. Normal sagittal parameters of global spinal balance in children and adolescents: a prospective study of 646 asymptomatic subjects. *Eur Spine J.* 2016;25(11):3650–3657.
4. Mac-Thiong J-M, Labelle H, Roussouly P. Pediatric sagittal alignment. *Eur Spine J.* 2011;20(suppl 5):586–590.
5. Mac-Thiong J-M, Labelle H, Berthonnaud E, et al. Sagittal spinopelvic balance in normal children and adolescents. *Eur Spine J.* 2007;16(2):227–234.
6. Hresko MT. Clinical practice. Idiopathic scoliosis in adolescents. *N Engl J Med.* 2013;368(9):834–841.
7. Weinstein SL, Dolan LA, Cheng JCY, et al. Adolescent idiopathic scoliosis. *Lancet.* 2008;371(9623):1527–1537.
8. Kouwenhoven J-WM, Castelein RM. The pathogenesis of adolescent idiopathic scoliosis: review of the literature. *Spine.* 2008;33(26):2898–2908.
9. Pope MH, Stokes IA, Moreland M. The biomechanics of scoliosis. *Crit Rev Biomed Eng.* 1984;11(3):157–188.
10. Stokes IAF, Burwell RG, Dangerfield PH, et al. Biomechanical spinal growth modulation and progressive adolescent scoliosis—a test of the "vicious cycle" pathogenetic hypothesis: summary of an electronic focus group debate of the IBSE. *Scoliosis.* 2006;1:16.
11. Mente PL, Aronsson DD, Stokes IA, et al. Mechanical modulation of growth for the correction of vertebral wedge deformities. *J Orthop Res.* 1999;17(4):518–524.
12. Nissinen M, Heliövaara M, Seitsamo J, et al. Anthropometric measurements and the incidence of low back pain in a cohort of pubertal children. *Spine.* 1994;19(12):1367–1370.
13. Poussa MS, Heliövaara MM, Seitsamo JT, et al. Development of spinal posture in a cohort of children from the age of 11 to 22 years. *Eur Spine J.* 2005;14(8):738–742.
14. Venn G, Mehta MH, Mason RM. Characterisation of collagen from normal and scoliotic human spinal ligament. *Biochim Biophys Acta.* 1983;757(2):259–267.
15. Hee HT, Zhang J, Wong HK. An in vitro study of dynamic cyclic compressive stress on human inner annulus fibrosus and nucleus pulposus cells. *Spine J.* 2010;10(9):795–801.
16. Hawasli AH, Hullar TE, Dorward IG. Idiopathic scoliosis and the vestibular system. *Eur Spine J.* 2015;24(2):227–233.
17. Catanzariti J-F, Agnani O, Guyot M-A, et al. Does adolescent idiopathic scoliosis relate to vestibular disorders? A systematic review. *Ann Phys Rehabil Med.* 2014;57(6–7):465–479.
18. Wajchenberg M, Astur N, Kanas M, et al. Adolescent idiopathic scoliosis: current concepts on neurological and muscular etiologies. *Scoliosis Spinal Disord.* 2016;11:4.
19. Kesling KL, Reinker KA. Scoliosis in twins. A meta-analysis of the literature and report of six cases. *Spine.* 1997;22(17):2009–2014; discussion 2015.
20. Justice CM, Miller NH, Marosy B, et al. Familial idiopathic scoliosis: evidence of an X-linked susceptibility locus. *Spine.* 2003;28(6):589–594.
21. Machida M, Dubousset J, Yamada T, et al. Serum melatonin levels in adolescent idiopathic scoliosis prediction and prevention for curve progression—a prospective study. *J Pineal Res.* 2009;46(3):344–348.
22. Moreau A, Wang DS, Forget S, et al. Melatonin signaling dysfunction in adolescent idiopathic scoliosis. *Spine.* 2004;29(16):1772–1781.
23. Man GCW, Wai MGC, Wang WWJ, et al. A review of pinealectomy-induced melatonin-deficient animal models for the study of etiopathogenesis of adolescent idiopathic scoliosis. *Int J Mol Sci.* 2014;15(9):16484–16499.
24. Lowe TG, Burwell RG, Dangerfield PH. Platelet calmodulin levels in adolescent idiopathic scoliosis (AIS): can they predict curve progression and severity? Summary of an electronic focus group debate of the IBSE. *Eur Spine J.* 2004;13(3):257–265.
25. Clark EM, Taylor HJ, Harding I, et al. Association between components of body composition and scoliosis: a prospective cohort study reporting differences identifiable before the onset of scoliosis. *J Bone Miner Res.* 2014;29(8):1729–1736.
26. Tam EMS, Yu FWP, Hung VWY, et al. Are volumetric bone mineral density and bone micro-architecture associated with leptin and soluble leptin receptor levels in adolescent idiopathic scoliosis?—A case-control study. *PLoS ONE.* 2014;9(2):e87939. Available from: http://www.ncbi.nlm.nih.gov/pmc/articles/PMC3916359/
27. Liang G, Gao W, Liang A, et al. Normal leptin expression, lower adipogenic ability, decreased leptin receptor and hyposensitivity to leptin in adolescent idiopathic scoliosis. *PLoS One.* 2012;7(5):e36648.
28. Stokes IAF. Mechanical modulation of spinal growth and progression of adolescent scoliosis. *Stud Health Technol Inform.* 2008;135:75–83.
29. Stokes IAF. Analysis and simulation of progressive adolescent scoliosis by biomechanical growth modulation. *Eur Spine J.* 2007;16(10):1621–1628.
30. Stokes I, Gardner-Morse M. The role of muscles and effects of load on growth. *Stud Health Technol Inform.* 2002;91:314–317.
31. Negrini S, Aulisa AG, Aulisa L, et al. 2011 SOSORT guidelines: orthopaedic and rehabilitation treatment of idiopathic scoliosis during growth. *Scoliosis.* 2012; 7(1):3.
32. Lenke LG, Betz RR, Clements D, et al. Curve prevalence of a new classification of operative adolescent idiopathic scoliosis: does classification correlate with treatment? *Spine.* 2002;27(6):604–611.
33. Lenke LG, Edwards CC, Bridwell KH. The Lenke classification of adolescent idiopathic scoliosis: how it organizes curve patterns as a template to perform selective fusions of the spine. *Spine.* 2003;28(20):S199–S207.
34. Lenke LG, Betz RR, Harms J, et al. Adolescent idiopathic scoliosis: a new classification to determine extent of spinal arthrodesis. *J Bone Joint Surg Am.* 2001; 83-A(8):1169–1181.
35. King HA. Selection of fusion levels for posterior instrumentation and fusion in idiopathic scoliosis. *Orthop Clin North Am.* 1988;19(2):247–255.
36. Terran J, Schwab F, Shaffrey CI, et al. The SRS-Schwab adult spinal deformity classification: assessment and clinical correlations based on a prospective operative and nonoperative cohort. *Neurosurgery.* 2013;73(4):559–568.
37. Rogala EJ, Drummond DS, Gurr J. Scoliosis: incidence and natural history. A prospective epidemiological study. *J Bone Joint Surg Am.* 1978;60(2):173–176.
38. Wiemann JM, Shah SA, Price CT. Nighttime bracing versus observation for early adolescent idiopathic scoliosis. *J Pediatr Orthop.* 2014;34(6):603–606.
39. Duval-Beaupere G. Threshold values for supine and standing Cobb angles and rib hump measurements: prognostic factors for scoliosis. *Eur Spine J.* 1996;5(2):79–84.
40. Goldberg CJ, Dowling FE, Fogarty EE. Adolescent idiopathic scoliosis: is rising growth rate the triggering factor in progression? *Eur Spine J.* 1993;2(1):29–36.
41. Weinstein SL, Dolan LA, Wright JG, et al. Effects of bracing in adolescents with idiopathic scoliosis. *N Engl J Med.* 2013;369(16):1512–1521.
42. Weinstein SL, Dolan LA, Spratt KF, et al. Health and function of patients with untreated idiopathic scoliosis: a 50-year natural history study. *JAMA.* 2003;289(5):559–567.
43. Donzelli S, Zaina F, Negrini S. In defense of adolescents: They really do use braces for the hours prescribed, if good help is provided. Results from a prospective everyday clinic cohort using thermobrace. *Scoliosis.* 2012;7(1):12.
44. Donzelli S, Zaina F, Martinez G, et al. Adolescents with idiopathic scoliosis and their parents have a positive attitude towards the Thermobrace monitor: results from a survey. *Scoliosis Spinal Disord.* 2017;12:12.
45. Asher MA, Min Lai S, Burton DC. Further development and validation of the Scoliosis Research Society (SRS) outcomes instrument. *Spine.* 2000;25(18):2381–2386.
46. Botens-Helmus C, Klein R, Stephan C. The reliability of the Bad Sobernheim Stress Questionnaire (BSSQbrace) in adolescents with scoliosis during brace treatment. *Scoliosis.* 2006;1:22.
47. Vasiliadis E, Grivas TB, Gkoltsiou K. Development and preliminary validation of Brace Questionnaire (BrQ): a new instrument for measuring quality of life of brace treated scoliotics. *Scoliosis.* 2006;1:7.
48. Caronni A, Zaina F, Negrini S. Improving the measurement of health-related quality of life in adolescent with idiopathic scoliosis: the SRS-7, a Rasch-developed short form of the SRS-22 questionnaire. *Res Dev Disabil.* 2014;35(4):784–799.
49. Caronni A, Sciumè L, Donzelli S, Zaina F, Negrini S. ISYQOL: a rasch-consistent questionnaire for measuring health-related quality of life in adolescents with spinal deformities. *Spine J.* 2017 Sep;17(9):1364-1372. doi: 10.1016/j.spinee.2017.05.022. Epub 2017 May 18.
50. Zaina F, Negrini S, Atanasio S. TRACE (Trunk Aesthetic Clinical Evaluation), a routine clinical tool to evaluate aesthetics in scoliosis patients: development from the Aesthetic Index (AI) and repeatability. *Scoliosis.* 2009;4:3.
51. Negrini S, Grivas TB, Kotwicki T, et al. Why do we treat adolescent idiopathic scoliosis? What we want to obtain and to avoid for our patients. SOSORT 2005 Consensus paper. *Scoliosis.* 2006;1:4.
52. Donaldson S, Stephens D, Howard A, et al. Surgical decision making in adolescent idiopathic scoliosis. *Spine.* 2007;32(14):1526–1532.
53. Negrini S, Donzelli S, Zaina F, et al. Complete validation of plumbline distances as a screening tool for sagittal plane deformities. *Scoliosis.* 2012;7(suppl 1):O16.
54. Zaina F, Negrini S, Romano M, et al. Repeatability of different methods to collect in everyday clinics the sagittal profile of patients with adolescent idiopathic scoliosis. *Scoliosis.* 2007;2(suppl 1):S44.
55. Grosso C, Negrini S, Boniolo A, et al. The validity of clinical examination in adolescent spinal deformities. *Stud Health Technol Inform.* 2002;91:123–125.
56. Bunnell WP. An objective criterion for scoliosis screening. *J Bone Joint Surg Am.* 1984;66(9):1381–1387.
57. Ferraro C, Venturin A, Ferraro M, et al. Hump height in idiopathic scoliosis measured using a humpmeter in growing subjects: the relationship between the hump height and the Cobb angle and the effect of age on the hump height. *Eur J Phys Rehabil Med.* 2016;53(3):377–389.
58. Aulisa AG, Guzzanti V, Perisano C, et al. Correlation between hump dimensions and curve severity in idiopathic scoliosis before and after conservative treatment. *Spine (Phila Pa 1976).* 2018;43(2):114–119.
59. Knott P, Pappo E, Cameron M, et al. SOSORT 2012 consensus paper: reducing x-ray exposure in pediatric patients with scoliosis. *Scoliosis.* 2014;9:4.
60. Pedersen PH, Petersen AG, Østgaard SE, et al. EOS® micro-dose protocol: first full-spine radiation dose measurements in anthropomorphic phantoms and comparisons with EOS standard-dose and conventional digital radiology (CR). *Spine (Phila Pa 1976).* 2018 April 18.

61. Wade R, Yang H, McKenna C, et al. A systematic review of the clinical effectiveness of EOS 2D/3D X-ray imaging system. *Eur Spine J*. 2013;22(2):296–304.

62. Negrini S, Atanasio S, Donzelli S, et al. "Slopes": a new approach to scoliosis radiographic measurement and evaluation, related to the horizontal plane in a bodily view. *Scoliosis*. 2013;8(1):O29.

63. Negrini S, Marchini G, Tessadri F. Brace technology thematic series—the Sforzesco and Sibilla braces, and the SPoRT (Symmetric, Patient oriented, Rigid, Three-dimensional, active) concept. *Scoliosis*. 2011;6:8.

64. Romano M, Negrini A, Parzini S, et al. SEAS (Scientific Exercises Approach to Scoliosis): a modern and effective evidence based approach to physiotherapic specific scoliosis exercises. *Scoliosis*. 2015;10(1):3.

65. He J-W, Yan Z-H, Liu J, et al. Accuracy and repeatability of a new method for measuring scoliosis curvature. *Spine*. 2009;34(9):E323–E329.

66. Nash CL. Current concepts review: scoliosis bracing. *J Bone Joint Surg Am*. 1980; 62(5):848–852.

67. Perdriolle R, Boffelli N, Ousset M. *La Scoliose: Son Étude Tridimensionnelle*. Paris, France: Maloine; 1979.

68. Richards BS. Measurement error in assessment of vertebral rotation using the Perdriolle torsionmeter. *Spine*. 1992;17(5):513–517.

69. Omeroğlu H, Ozekin O, Biçimoğlu A. Measurement of vertebral rotation in idiopathic scoliosis using the Perdriolle torsionmeter: a clinical study on intraobserver and interobserver error. *Eur Spine J*. 1996;5(3):167–171.

70. Stagnara P. *Les Deformations Du Rachis*. Paris, France: Masson; 1985.

71. DiMeglio A, Dimeglio A, Canavese F, et al. Growth and adolescent idiopathic scoliosis: when and how much? *J Pediatr Orthop*. 2011;31(1 suppl):S28–S36.

72. Negrini S, Hresko TM, O'Brien JP, et al. Recommendations for research studies on treatment of idiopathic scoliosis: consensus 2014 between SOSORT and SRS non-operative management committee. *Scoliosis*. 2015;10:8.

73. Roussouly P, Pinheiro-Franco JL. Sagittal parameters of the spine: biomechanical approach. *Eur Spine J*. 2011;20(5):578–585.

74. Negrini S, Minozzi S, Bettany-Saltikov J, et al. Braces for idiopathic scoliosis in adolescents. *Cochrane Database Syst Rev*. 2010;(1):CD006850.

75. Negrini S, Minozzi S, Bettany-Saltikov J, et al. Braces for idiopathic scoliosis in adolescents. *Cochrane Database Syst Rev*. 2015;6:CD006850.

76. Mayo NE, Goldberg MS, Poitras B, et al. The Ste-Justine Adolescent Idiopathic Scoliosis Cohort Study. Part III: back pain. *Spine (Phila Pa 1976)*. 1994;19(14):1573–1581.

77. Weinstein SL, Zavala DC, Ponseti IV. Idiopathic scoliosis. Long-term follow-up and prognosis in untreated patients. *J Bone Joint Surg Am*. 1981;63(5):702–712.

78. Duval-Beaupère G. [The growth of scoliotics. Hypothesis and preliminary study]. *Acta Orthop Belg*. 1972;38(4):365–376.

79. Dolan LA, Wright JG, Weinstein SL. Effects of bracing in adolescents with idiopathic scoliosis. *N Engl J Med*. 2014;370(7):681.

80. Lusini M, Donzelli S, Minnella S, et al. Brace treatment is effective in idiopathic scoliosis over 45°: an observational prospective cohort controlled study. *Spine J*. 2013;14(9):1951–1956. Available from: http://linkinghub.elsevier.com/retrieve/pii/S1529943013019359

81. Rigo M, Negrini S, Weiss HR, et al. SOSORT consensus paper on brace action: TLSO biomechanics of correction (investigating the rationale for force vector selection). *Scoliosis*. 2006;1:11.

82. Negrini S, Grivas TB, Kotwicki T, et al. Guidelines on "Standards of management of idiopathic scoliosis with corrective braces in everyday clinics and in clinical research": SOSORT Consensus 2008. *Scoliosis*. 2009;4:2.

83. Coillard C, Vachon V, Circo AB, et al. Effectiveness of the SpineCor brace based on the new standardized criteria proposed by the scoliosis research society for adolescent idiopathic scoliosis. *J Pediatr Orthop*. 2007;27(4):375–379.

84. Brox JI, Lange JE, Gunderson RB, et al. Good brace compliance reduced curve progression and surgical rates in patients with idiopathic scoliosis. *Eur Spine J*. 2012;21(10):1957–1963.

85. Rowe DE, Bernstein SM, Riddick MF, et al. A meta-analysis of the efficacy of non-operative treatments for idiopathic scoliosis. *J Bone Joint Surg Am*. 1997;79(5):664–674.

86. Zaina F, Donzelli S, Negrini S. We cannot give up bracing for poor adherence to treatment: Letter to the Editor concerning the paper "The effectiveness of the SpineCor brace for the conservative treatment of adolescent idiopathic scoliosis. Comparison with the Boston brace". *Spine J*. 2016;16(8):1032–1033.

87. Nicholson GP, Ferguson-Pell MW, Smith K, et al. The objective measurement of spinal orthosis use for the treatment of adolescent idiopathic scoliosis. *Spine*. 2003;28(19):2243–2250; discussion 2250–2251.

88. Tavernaro M, Pellegrini A, Tessadri F, et al. Team care to cure adolescents with braces (avoiding low quality of life, pain and bad compliance): a case-control retrospective study. 2011 SOSORT Award winner. *Scoliosis*. 2012;7(1):17.

89. Rivett L, Rothberg A, Stewart A, et al. The relationship between quality of life and compliance to a brace protocol in adolescents with scoliosis: a comparative study. *BMC Musculoskelet Disord*. 2009;10:5.

90. Donzelli S, Zaina F, Lusini M, et al. In favour of the definition "adolescents with idiopathic scoliosis": juvenile and adolescent idiopathic scoliosis braced after ten years of age, do not show different end results. SOSORT award winner 2014. *Scoliosis*. 2014;9:7.

91. Takemitsu M, Bowen JR, Rahman T, et al. Compliance monitoring of brace treatment for patients with idiopathic scoliosis. *Spine*. 2004;29(18):2070–2074; discussion 2074.

92. Rahman T, Borkhuu B, Littleton AG, et al. Electronic monitoring of scoliosis brace wear compliance. *J Child Orthop*. 2010;4(4):343–347.

93. Rahman T, Sample W, Yorgova P, et al. Electronic monitoring of orthopedic brace compliance. *J Child Orthop*. 2015;9(5):365–369.

94. Miller DJ, Franzone JM, Matsumoto H, et al. Electronic monitoring improves brace-wearing compliance in patients with adolescent idiopathic scoliosis: a randomized clinical trial. *Spine*. 2012;37(9):717–721.

95. Negrini S, Donzelli S, Negrini A, Parzini S, Romano M, Zaina F. Specific exercises reduce the need for bracing in adolescents with idiopathic scoliosis: a practical clinical trial. *Ann Phys Rehabil Med*. 2018 Aug 24. pii: S1877-0657(18)31441-6. doi: 10.1016/j.rehab.2018.07.010.

96. Negrini S, Atanasio S, Zaina F, et al. End-growth results of bracing and exercises for adolescent idiopathic scoliosis. Prospective worst-case analysis. *Stud Health Technol Inform*. 2008;135:395–408.

97. Kuru T, Yeldan İ, Dereli EE, et al. The efficacy of three-dimensional Schroth exercises in adolescent idiopathic scoliosis: a randomised controlled clinical trial. *Clin Rehabil*. 2016;30(2):181–190.

98. Monticone M, Ambrosini E, Cazzaniga D, et al. Active self-correction and task-oriented exercises reduce spinal deformity and improve quality of life in subjects with mild adolescent idiopathic scoliosis. Results of a randomised controlled trial. *Eur Spine J*. 2014;23(6):1204–1214.

99. Schreiber S, Parent EC, Moez EK, et al. The effect of Schroth exercises added to the standard of care on the quality of life and muscle endurance in adolescents with idiopathic scoliosis-an assessor and statistician blinded randomized controlled trial: "SOSORT 2015 Award Winner." *Scoliosis*. 2015;10:24.

100. Romano M, Minozzi S, Bettany-Saltikov J, et al. Exercises for adolescent idiopathic scoliosis. *Cochrane Database Syst Rev*. 2012;8:CD007837.

101. Romano M, Minozzi S, Zaina F, et al. Exercises for adolescent idiopathic scoliosis: a Cochrane systematic review. *Spine*. 2013;38(14):E883–E893.

102. Negrini S, Bettany-Saltikov J, De Mauroy JC, et al. Letter to the Editor concerning: "Active self-correction and task-oriented exercises reduce spinal deformity and improve quality of life in subjects with mild adolescent idiopathic scoliosis. Results of a randomised controlled trial" by Monticone M, Ambrosini E, Cazzaniga D, Rocca B, Ferrante S (2014). Eur Spine J; DOI:10.1007/s00586-014-3241-y. *Eur Spine J*. 2014;23(10):2218–2220.

103. Weiss H-R, Negrini S, Hawes MC, et al. Physical exercises in the treatment of idiopathic scoliosis at risk of brace treatment—SOSORT consensus paper 2005. *Scoliosis*. 2006;1:6.

104. Stokes IA. Analysis of symmetry of vertebral body loading consequent to lateral spinal curvature. *Spine*. 1997;22(21):2495–2503.

105. Rigo MD, Grivas TB. "Rehabilitation schools for scoliosis" thematic series: describing the methods and results. *Scoliosis*. 2010;5:27.

106. Weiss H-R. The method of Katharina Schroth—history, principles and current development. *Scoliosis*. 2011;6:17.

107. Romano M, Negrini S. Manual therapy as a conservative treatment for adolescent idiopathic scoliosis: a systematic review. *Scoliosis*. 2008;3:2.

108. Saccucci M, Tettamanti L, Mummolo S, et al. Scoliosis and dental occlusion: a review of the literature. *Scoliosis*. 2011;6:15.

109. Korbmacher H, Koch L, Eggers-Stroeder G, et al. Associations between orthopaedic disturbances and unilateral crossbite in children with asymmetry of the upper cervical spine. *Eur J Orthod*. 2007;29(1):100–104.

110. Lippold C, Moiseenko T, Drerup B, et al. Spine deviations and orthodontic treatment of asymmetric malocclusions in children. *BMC Musculoskelet Disord*. 2012;13:151.

111. Negrini S, Donzelli S, Negrini F, et al. Bracing does not change the sport habits of patients. *Stud Health Technol Inform*. 2012;176:437–440.

112. Meyer C, Cammarata E, Haumont T, et al. Why do idiopathic scoliosis patients participate more in gymnastics? *Scand J Med Sci Sports*. 2006;16(4):231–236.

113. Tanchev PI, Dzherov AD, Parushev AD, et al. Scoliosis in rhythmic gymnasts. *Spine*. 2000;25(11):1367–1372.

114. Warren MP, Brooks-Gunn J, Hamilton LH, et al. Scoliosis and fractures in young ballet dancers. Relation to delayed menarche and secondary amenorrhea. *N Engl J Med*. 1986;314(21):1348–1353.

115. Zaina F, Donzelli S, Lusini M, et al. Swimming and spinal deformities: a cross-sectional study. *J Pediatr*. 2015;166(1):163–167.

116. Zaina F, Donzelli S, Lusini M, et al. Tennis is not dangerous for the spine during growth: results of a cross-sectional study. *Eur Spine J*. 2016;25(9):2938–2944.

117. Figueiredo UM, James JI. Juvenile idiopathic scoliosis. *J Bone Joint Surg Br*. 1981; 63-B(1):61–66.

118. Tolo VT, Gillespie R. The characteristics of juvenile idiopathic scoliosis and results of its treatment. *J Bone Joint Surg Br*. 1978;60-B(2):181–188.

119. Lenke LG, Dobbs MB. Management of juvenile idiopathic scoliosis. *J Bone Joint Surg Am*. 2007;89(suppl 1):55–63.

120. Robinson CM, McMaster MJ. Juvenile idiopathic scoliosis. Curve patterns and prognosis in one hundred and nine patients. *J Bone Joint Surg Am*. 1996;78(8):1140–1148.

121. Fernandes P, Weinstein SL. Natural history of early onset scoliosis. *J Bone Joint Surg Am*. 2007;89(suppl 1):21–33.

122. Scott JC, Morgan TH. The natural history and prognosis of infantile idiopathic scoliosis. *J Bone Joint Surg Br*. 1955;37-B(3):400–413.

123. Ferreira JH, de Janeiro R, James JI. Progressive and resolving infantile idiopathic scoliosis. The differential diagnosis. *J Bone Joint Surg Br*. 1972;54(4):648–655.

124. Mehta MH. Growth as a corrective force in the early treatment of progressive infantile scoliosis. *J Bone Joint Surg Br*. 2005;87(9):1237–1247.

125. Mehta MH. The rib-vertebra angle in the early diagnosis between resolving and progressive infantile scoliosis. *J Bone Joint Surg Br*. 1972;54(2):230–243.

126. Hassanzadeh H, Nandyala SV, Puvanesarajah V, et al. Serial Mehta cast utilization in infantile idiopathic scoliosis: evaluation of radiographic predictors. *J Pediatr Orthop*. 2015;37(6):387–391.

127. Sanders JO, D'Astous J, Fitzgerald M, et al. Derotational casting for progressive infantile scoliosis. *J Pediatr Orthop*. 2009;29(6):581–587.

128. Iorio J, Orlando G, Diefenbach C, et al. Serial casting for infantile idiopathic scoliosis: radiographic outcomes and factors associated with response to treatment. *J Pediatr Orthop*. 2017;37(5):311–316.

129. Jarvis J, Garbedian S, Swamy G. Juvenile idiopathic scoliosis: the effectiveness of part-time bracing. *Spine*. 2008;33(10):1074–1078.

130. Fusco C, Donzelli S, Lusini M, et al. Low rate of surgery in juvenile idiopathic scoliosis treated with a complete and tailored conservative approach: end-growth results from a retrospective cohort. *Scoliosis*. 2014;9:12.

131. Batra S, Ahuja S. Congenital scoliosis: management and future directions. *Acta Orthop Belg*. 2008;74(2):147–160.

132. Barnewolt CE, Estroff JA. Sonography of the fetal central nervous system. *Neuroimaging Clin N Am*. 2004;14(2):255–271, viii.

133. Beals RK, Robbins JR, Rolfe B. Anomalies associated with vertebral malformations. *Spine*. 1993;18(10):1329–1332.

134. Basu PS, Elsebaie H, Noordeen MHH. Congenital spinal deformity: a comprehensive assessment at presentation. *Spine*. 2002;27(20):2255–2259.

135. Shands AR, Eisberg HB. The incidence of scoliosis in the state of Delaware; a study of 50,000 minifilms of the chest made during a survey for tuberculosis. *J Bone Joint Surg Am*. 1955;37-A(6):1243–1249.

136. Winter RB. Congenital scoliosis. *Orthop Clin North Am*. 1988;19(2):395–408.

137. McMaster MJ, Ohtsuka K. The natural history of congenital scoliosis. A study of two hundred and fifty-one patients. *J Bone Joint Surg Am*. 1982;64(8):1128–1147.

138. Vyskocil V, Pavelka T. Differential diagnosis of connective tissue disorders, Marfan Ehlers-Danlos syndrome, osteogenesis imperfecta and benign joint hyperelasticity. *Osteoporos Int*. 2013;24(suppl 1):S06.

139. Zenner J, Hitzl W, Meier O, et al. Surgical outcomes of scoliosis surgery in Marfan syndrome. *J Spinal Disord Tech*. 2014;27(1):48–58.

140. Daher YH, Lonstein JE, Winter RB, et al. Spinal deformities in patients with muscular dystrophy other than Duchenne. A review of 11 patients having surgical treatment. *Spine*. 1985;10(7):614–617.

141. Bethem D, Winter RB, Lutter L, et al. Spinal disorders of dwarfism. Review of the literature and report of eighty cases. *J Bone Joint Surg Am*. 1981;63(9):1412–1425.

142. Calvert PT, Edgar MA, Webb PJ. Scoliosis in neurofibromatosis. The natural history with and without operation. *J Bone Joint Surg Br*. 1989;71-B(2):246–251.

143. Lee CK, Chang BS, Hong YM, et al. Spinal deformities in Noonan syndrome: a clinical review of sixty cases. *J Bone Joint Surg Am*. 2001;83-A(10):1495–1502.

144. Lawhon SM, MacEwen GD, Bunnell WP. Orthopaedic aspects of the VATER association. *J Bone Joint Surg Am*. 1986;68(3):424–429.

145. Sewell MD, Wallace C, Gibson A, et al. A retrospective review to assess whether spinal fusion and scoliosis correction improved activity and participation for children with Angelman syndrome. *Dev Neurorehabil*. 2016;19(5):315–320.

146. Downs J, Torode I, Wong K, et al. The natural history of scoliosis in females with Rett syndrome. *Spine*. 2016;41(10):856–863.

147. Cassidy SB, Schwartz S, Miller JL, et al. Prader-Willi syndrome. *Genet Med*. 2012;14(1):10–26.

148. Sato A, Ouellet J, Muneta T, et al. Scoliosis in osteogenesis imperfecta caused by COL1A1/COL1A2 mutations—genotype-phenotype correlations and effect of bisphosphonate treatment. *Bone*. 2016;86:53–57.

149. Milbrandt TA, Johnston CE. Down syndrome and scoliosis: a review of a 50-year experience at one institution. *Spine*. 2005;30(18):2051–2055.

150. Janicki JA, Alman B. Scoliosis: review of diagnosis and treatment. *Paediatr Child Health*. 2007;12(9):771–776.

151. Rinella A, Lenke L, Whitaker C, et al. Perioperative halo-gravity traction in the treatment of severe scoliosis and kyphosis. *Spine*. 2005;30(4):475–482.

152. Aebi M. The adult scoliosis. *Eur Spine J*. 2005;14(10):925–948.

153. Schwab F, Farcy J-P, Bridwell K, et al. A clinical impact classification of scoliosis in the adult. *Spine*. 2006;31(18):2109–2114.

154. Lowe T, Berven SH, Schwab FJ, et al. The SRS classification for adult spinal deformity: building on the King/Moe and Lenke classification systems. *Spine*. 2006;31(19 suppl):S119–S125.

155. Hallager DW, Hansen LV, Dragsted CR, et al. A comprehensive analysis of the SRS-Schwab adult spinal deformity classification and confounding variables: a prospective, non-US cross-sectional study in 292 patients. *Spine*. 2016;41(10):E589–E597.

156. Marty-Poumarat C, Scattin L, Marpeau M, et al. Natural history of progressive adult scoliosis. *Spine*. 2007;32(11):1227–1234; discussion 1235.

157. Schwab F, Dubey A, Pagala M, et al. Adult scoliosis: a health assessment analysis by SF-36. *Spine*. 2003;28(6):602–606.

158. Berven S, Deviren V, Demir-Deviren S, et al. Studies in the modified Scoliosis Research Society Outcomes Instrument in adults: validation, reliability, and discriminatory capacity. *Spine*. 2003;28(18):2164–2169; discussion 2169.

159. Glassman SD, Berven S, Bridwell K, et al. Correlation of radiographic parameters and clinical symptoms in adult scoliosis. *Spine*. 2005;30(6):682–688.

160. Glassman SD, Bridwell K, Dimar JR, et al. The impact of positive sagittal balance in adult spinal deformity. *Spine*. 2005;30(18):2024–2029.

161. Mac-Thiong J-M, Transfeldt EE, Mehbod AA, et al. Can c7 plumbline and gravity line predict health related quality of life in adult scoliosis? *Spine*. 2009;34(15):E519–E527.

162. Ploumis A, Liu H, Mehbod AA, et al. A correlation of radiographic and functional measurements in adult degenerative scoliosis. *Spine*. 2009;34(15):1581–1584.

163. Smith JS, Shaffrey CI, Fu K-MG, et al. Clinical and radiographic evaluation of the adult spinal deformity patient. *Neurosurg Clin N Am*. 2013;24(2):143–156.

164. Ames CP, Scheer JK, Lafage V, et al. Adult spinal deformity: epidemiology, health impact, evaluation, and management. *Spine Deform*. 2016;4(4):310–322.

165. Schwab F, Ungar B, Blondel B, et al. Scoliosis Research Society-Schwab adult spinal deformity classification: a validation study. *Spine*. 2012;37(12):1077–1082.

166. Bess S, Line B, Fu K-M, et al. The health impact of symptomatic adult spinal deformity: comparison of deformity types to United States population norms and chronic diseases. *Spine*. 2016;41(3):224–233.

167. Protopsaltis T, Schwab F, Bronsard N, et al. The t1 pelvic angle, a novel radiographic measure of global sagittal deformity, accounts for both spinal inclination and pelvic tilt and correlates with health-related quality of life. *J Bone Joint Surg Am*. 2014;96(19):1631–1640.

168. Schwab FJ, Blondel B, Bess S, et al. Radiographical spinopelvic parameters and disability in the setting of adult spinal deformity: a prospective multicenter analysis. *Spine*. 2013;38(13):E803–E812.

169. Bunnell WP. The natural history of idiopathic scoliosis. *Clin Orthop*. 1988;(229):20–25.

170. Danielsson AJ, Nachemson AL. Back pain and function 22 years after brace treatment for adolescent idiopathic scoliosis: a case-control study-part I. *Spine*. 2003;28(18):2078–2085; discussion 2086.

171. Nachemson A. Adult scoliosis and back pain. *Spine*. 1979;4(6):513–517.

172. Chopra S, Adhikari K, Agarwal N, et al. Kyphoscoliosis complicating pregnancy: maternal and neonatal outcome. *Arch Gynecol Obstet*. 2011;284(2):295–297.

173. Schroeder JE, Dettori JR, Ecker E, et al. Does pregnancy increase curve progression in women with scoliosis treated without surgery? *Evid Based Spine Care J*. 2011;2(3):43–50.

174. *Adolescent Idiopathic Scoliosis and Pregnancy: An Unsolved Paradigm*. Available from: http://www.ncbi.nlm.nih.gov/pubmed/?term=Adolescent+Idiopathic+Scoliosis+and+Pregnancy_An+Unsolved+Paradigm

175. Negrini A, Negrini MG, Donzelli S, et al. Scoliosis-Specific exercises can reduce the progression of severe curves in adult idiopathic scoliosis: a long-term cohort study. *Scoliosis*. 2015;10:20.

176. Monticone M, Ambrosini E, Cazzaniga D, et al. Adults with idiopathic scoliosis improve disability after motor and cognitive rehabilitation: results of a randomised controlled trial. *Eur Spine J*. 2016;25(10):3120–3129.

177. Palazzo C, Montigny JP, Barbot F, et al. Effects of bracing in adult with scoliosis: a retrospective study. *Arch Phys Med Rehabil*. 2017;98(1):187–190.

178. Zaina F, Poggio M, Donzelli S, et al. Can bracing help adults with chronic back pain and scoliosis? Short-term results from a pilot study. *Prosthet Orthot Int*. 2018;942(4):410–414.

179. Glassman SD, Carreon LY, Shaffrey CI, et al. The costs and benefits of nonoperative management for adult scoliosis. *Spine*. 2010;35(5):578–582.

CHAPTER 29

Nitin B. Jain
Chan Gao
Brian Richardson

Disorders of the Upper Limbs

Upper extremity pain is a leading cause of physician visits in the United States. This is particularly prevalent in sports and the workplace, contributing significantly to disability and lost productivity.

PATHOPHYSIOLOGY

Along the spectrum of potential conditions, injuries to the nerve and/or musculoskeletal system are most common. A detailed understanding of the relevant functional anatomy and potential mechanisms of injury allows for the most accurate diagnosis and successful treatment.

Tissue Injury/Repair

Injuries to upper limbs affect a diverse group of connective tissues, including ligament, tendon, muscle, cartilage, fascia, synovium, adipose, and bone. Connective tissues are susceptible to failure under conditions of stress and strain. The most common mechanisms of injury include acute trauma and repetitive overuse or overload. Musculotendinous structures are especially vulnerable to failure from sudden overloading, as with forceful muscular contractions, particularly when weakened as a result of concurrent illness (connective tissue disorders). The three phases of soft tissue healing include the cellular response to injury; repair and regeneration, as immature collagen is laid down; and scar remodeling, a process that may continue for years (1). Understanding this sequence of events has direct implications on the success of treatment and rehabilitation. The type of injury, age, vascularity, nutrition, genetic and hormonal factors, and activity level influence successful healing of soft tissues. Acute injuries typically have a sudden onset, are associated with a classic inflammatory reaction, and tend to follow a predictable course toward resolution. Chronic injuries (duration longer than 3 months) are often marked by an insidious onset of pain, progressive functional impairments, and a tendency toward reinjury. Advanced age is associated with decreased collagen synthesis and impaired tendon healing. Exercise improves both the mechanical and structural properties of tendon as opposed to inactivity, which favors collagen degradation and decreased tendon strength.

More commonly, repetitive overuse leads to cumulative trauma disorders (CTDs) characterized by an insidious onset of pain, and ultimately, structural failure. In addition, it can also be caused by poor sustained posture/biomechanics, vibrations, and/or repetitive forceful exertions. CTD is an umbrella term that includes multiple specific diagnoses and nonspecific conditions affecting primarily the upper limbs, shoulder, neck, and lower back. Furthermore, within each of these body regions,

there can be multiple types of CTD that involve pathology of the tendons, joints, muscles, or nerves. Among the most common CTDs are lumbar back pain, carpal tunnel syndrome (CTS), epicondylitis, neck/shoulder pain, and de Quervain tenosynovitis. CTDs constitute a large portion of occupational injuries. Although the workplace is the most common setting for development of CTD, these disorders can arise in any setting with prolonged exposure to the aforementioned mechanical stressors. The evidence for cumulative trauma in the pathogenesis of these conditions is discussed, and summary is provided in ⎙ **eTable 29-1**. In the context of persistent or uncontrolled stress, a cycle may occur in which structural maladaptations develop in the damaged tissue, setting the stage for further injury and chronic symptomatology which can in turn lead to pain or loss of motion. The most common site of overuse injury is the osteotendinous junction (2).

Although many hypotheses have been put forth, the pathophysiology of CTD is not completely understood. Cumulative biomechanical stresses can result in tissue alteration in tendons, muscles, joints, and nerves over time. In soft tissues, damage is marked by inflammation, collagen deposition, and tissue contraction, which can in turn lead to pain or loss of motion. Myalgia may be due to prolonged muscle contractions that lead to decreased local blood flow, deoxygenation, and metabolite buildup that manifest as muscle fatigue and soreness. The mechanism for tendon-related disorders may be related to inflammation and hypoxia. It has been demonstrated that repeated mechanical stresses release prostaglandin E2 (PGE2) from human fibroblasts *in vivo* (3). Exposure of rabbit patellar tendons to PGE2 resulted in degenerative changes. Therefore, tendon pathology may result from prolonged or recurring inflammation. Another possible precipitant is hypovascularity, which may predispose tendons to hypoxic degeneration and subsequent tendinopathy. Regardless of cause, tendinopathies have been shown to have disordered collagen arrangement and increased proteoglycan ground substance.

Several elements contribute to occupational CTD, including forceful exertions, repetition of a work task, awkward biomechanical postures, and vibration (4). The National Institute for Occupational Safety and Health (NIOSH), a division of the U.S. Department of Health, reviewed the epidemiologic evidence for each of these physical work factors for the major CTD subtypes. It is important to note that many CTDs will involve a combination of these factors.

- *Repetition or prolonged activities*: The NIOSH conducted a 1997 review that found moderate evidence for repetition as a cause of work-related musculoskeletal disorders in neck and shoulder pain, CTS, and hand/wrist tendonitis. It did not find sufficient evidence in lower back pain (LBP) or epicondylitis (4).

- *Forceful exertions*: There is epidemiologic evidence to support the role of forceful exertions in the workplace in contributing to neck, lumbar back, elbow, and hand/wrist pain (5).
- *Posture*: Sustained wrist and forearm flexion-extension or radial-ulnar deviation may induce friction between tendons and adjacent anatomic surfaces. A good example of this is frequent radial deviation of the wrist and subsequent development of de Quervain tenosynovitis (6).
- *Vibration*: Exposure to vibration occurs in a variety of contexts: using power tools, holding an object as it is processed in a machine (e.g., wood in a power saw), or using percussion tools (e.g., hammering a nail). Vibration has been implicated as the cause of hand-arm vibration syndrome (HAVS), a constellation of vascular and neurologic symptoms associated with high levels of exposure to vibration (7).

Several studies show that psychosocial factors contribute to disability in CTD, especially in cases involving cervical or lumbar spine pain. CTDs are costly to both employers and employees. They result not only in time lost from work but also in decreased productivity and poor employee morale, which in turn leads to further disability. One study used patients' self-report of upper extremity symptoms to show a positive correlation between depression and severity of carpal tunnel, de Quervain tenosynovitis, lateral elbow pain, and trigger finger (8). Another study found job strain to adversely affect successful return to employment in CTS patients (9). Given the association between psychosocial stressors and disability from CTD, psychosocial issues should be addressed appropriately for optimal recovery. In evaluating new CTD patients, clinicians should screen for psychosocial factors and psychiatric comorbidities and consult relevant mental health practitioners if indicated.

It is useful to approach the treatment and rehabilitation of upper extremity injuries through a conceptual framework that begins with establishing an accurate diagnosis and ultimately returns the patient to normal athletic or occupational performance (10) (📶 **eTable 29-2**). Ergonomic design plays a critical role as force requirements may increase based upon several factors including poor body mechanics, high torque or speed of power tools, and friction between objects and the worker (5).

Ligament

Ligament sprains have been classically defined as grades I, II, and III based on the degree of tissue damage and separation (📶 **eTable 29-3**). Grade I sprains demonstrate negligible loss of structural integrity, display minimal signs of inflammation, and generally recover quickly and completely. In grade II sprains, partial rupture of the ligament is associated with significant pain and inflammation. Functional recovery generally occurs within 4 to 6 weeks; however, pain is often experienced for months after the injury (11). Grade III injuries are often associated with prolonged healing time, chronic instability, susceptibility to recurrent sprains, and impaired proprioception of the involved joint.

Tendon

Tendons are susceptible to injury through the same mechanisms of tensile overload and repetitive overuse (12,13). Tendons are particularly vulnerable to failure when tension is

TABLE 29-1	Classification of Tendon Injuries
Injury	**Characteristics**
Paratenonitis or tenosynovitis	Inflammation of the paratenon with associated pain, swelling, and tenderness
Tendinitis	Inflammation of the tendon with associated vascular disruption and inflammation
Tendinosis	Intratendinous atrophy and degeneration with a relative absence of inflammation; a palpable nodule may be present over tendon
Paratenonitis with tendinosis	Acute inflammation superimposed on chronic tendinitis
Partial or complete rupture	Acute inflammation is often superimposed on chronic inflammation with tendinosis

applied quickly or obliquely, the tendon is tense before trauma, the attached muscle is maximally innervated, the muscle group is stretched by external stimuli, and the tendon is weak in comparison to its muscle (14). Tendon injuries, or tendinopathies, can be classified according to a sequence of overlapping pathologic conditions: inflammation, degeneration, and rupture (**Table 29-1**). When the structure is associated with a synovial lining, the condition is described as tenosynovitis. The term *tendinitis* refers to injuries and inflammation specifically involving tendon although there is debate on whether tendon pathology is accompanied by inflammation. *Tendinosis* describes a chronic process of intratendinous degeneration and atrophy, minimal or no inflammation, and loss of structural integrity, potentially leading to tendon failure (15,16). Inflammation of the paratendon may occur concomitantly with tendon atrophy, referred to as paratenonitis with tendinosis. A functional classification of traumatic tendinitis is particularly useful because the degree of disability correlates well with the extent of injury (📶 **eTable 29-4**). This grading system also provides objective parameters for following treatment and rehabilitation.

Muscle

Muscular injuries are particularly common in sports. These are typically classified as contusions, strains, avulsions, and delayed-onset muscle soreness. Contusions result as a direct blow and are graded as mild, moderate, or severe based on the degree of soft tissue swelling, motion restriction, and functional impairment (17–19). Muscular strains result from overstretching or peak contraction of the musculotendinous unit, particularly during eccentric muscular contractions. These injuries tend to occur more commonly at the musculotendinous junction. Delayed-onset muscle soreness typically occurs within the first 24 to 48 hours after an intense bout of exercise that often involves repeated eccentric muscular contractions. Both inflammatory and metabolic mechanisms have been proposed for muscle damage in this condition (20,21).

Cartilage (Articular Cartilage, Labrum)

Hyaline cartilage forms the articular surface and is the most relevant to skeleton system (22). It can be divided into four structurally different zones: superficial zone, transitional zone, the radial zone, and the calcified cartilage zone (23). The extracellular matrix (ECM) of cartilage tissue is abundant in collagen type II and proteoglycan. Chondrocytes possess limited healing capacity and surgical procedures attempting to expedite the cartilage repair, such as microfracturing of the subchondral bone, were found to cause the formation of fibrocartilaginous tissue instead of hyaline cartilage and inferior physiologic structure and properties (24,25). Fibrocartilage is typically incapable of heal unless the injury site is in the vascularized zone where angiogenesis and repair cascade can be initiated (26).

Peripheral Nerve

Peripheral nerves are encased by a layer of myelin formed by Schwann cells. Myelin accelerates conduction velocity by limiting the ionic transfer to the nodes of Ranvier and provides trophic support through release of neurotrophins, such as nerve growth factor (NGF) (27). Neurapraxia, often as a result of compressive and crush injury, is a result of myelin damage and characterized by focal conduction block. Although the myelin sheath is thinner and degraded, the nerve morphology is largely normal and neuromuscular junction is still present. Also, seen in this situation are Schwann cell proliferation, dedifferentiation, and increased metabolism suggesting attempt to remyelination (28,29). When axonal damage occurs, that is, loss of cell membrane integrity and breakdown of axonal cytoskeleton, Wallerian degeneration distal to the injury site ensues to form a microenvironment conducive for axonal regrowth and reinnervation (30).

Bone

Bone possesses excellent healing capacity that enables bone to heal with tissue indistinguishable from uninjured tissue (31). Both primary and secondary healing can be initiated in the fracture repair process (32): primary healing is the direct bridging of fracture ends with minimal callus formation (33), whereas secondary bone healing is the bridging of bone segments by abundant bone callus and followed by remodelling process (31). Secondary healing is the healing pattern seen under majority of circumstances and consists of intramembranous and endochondral ossifications (31). Osteogenic cells, osteoinductive signals, sufficient vascularization, and optimal mechanical environment are prerequisites for successful bone healing (34).

PERIPHERAL NEUROPATHY

Please refer to Chapter 24 for detailed discussion.

MUSCULOSKELETAL CONDITIONS

Shoulder

Shoulder injuries are one of the most common musculoskeletal causes to seek care (35). Injuries of the shoulder can be broadly classified as those that result from more acute processes, such as a direct trauma, those that occur from more repetitive tasks, and degenerative conditions. Certain occupations are significantly associated with the occurrence of shoulder pain, such as fish-processing worker (36,37), electricians (38), garment workers (39), hospital workers (40), and construction workers (41). Overall, rotator cuff injury has been reported as the third most common diagnosis encountered in workers, accounting for 8.3% of cases (42).

Anatomy and Kinesiology

The shoulder is composed of many joints, including the scapulothoracic joint, which is considered a functional joint. The glenohumeral joint is a synovial joint lined by the glenoid labrum, which provides a large contact surface to the glenoid fossa. The humeral head comes into contact with only about one third of the glenoid fossa at any one time. The capsule of the glenohumeral joint is divided into three functional bands that are considered ligaments, named the superior glenohumeral ligament (SGHL), middle glenohumeral ligament (MGHL), and inferior glenohumeral ligament (IGHL). Additional support is provided by the coracohumeral ligament (CHL) originating on the coracoid and inserting into the greater and lesser tuberosities. The acromioclavicular (AC) joint is another synovial joint made up of the distal aspect of the clavicle and the acromion and is supported by the coracoacromial ligament, the AC ligament, and the coracoclavicular (CC) ligament (composed of two smaller ligaments—the conoid and the trapezoid). Motion at the AC joint requires not only translation but also rotation for smooth movement of the shoulder. The last synovial joint involved in the shoulder is the sternoclavicular joint. The joint is bordered by the medial aspect of the clavicle and the manubrium of the sternum. There are four ligaments surrounding the joint: the anterior and posterior sternoclavicular ligaments, the costoclavicular ligament, and the interclavicular ligament.

The muscles of the shoulder and shoulder girdle can be divided into two major groups: those that stabilize the scapula and those that attach to the humerus. The stabilizers include the trapezius, levator scapula, rhomboids, serratus anterior, and pectoralis minor. These muscles allow for the stability of the shoulder girdle and provide a foundation for movement and force generation that is passed along the trunk into the arm for functional use. The muscles that attach to the humerus include the rotator cuff muscles (supraspinatus, infraspinatus, teres minor, and subscapularis), deltoid, teres major, pectoralis major, coracobrachialis, biceps brachii, and latissimus dorsi. These muscles provide the arm with most of its motion.

The muscles noted above can be divided into several functional groups. For example, internal rotation is accomplished by the subscapularis, latissimus dorsi, anterior fiber of the deltoid, pectoralis major, and teres major. External rotators include the infraspinatus, teres minor, and posterior fibers of the deltoid. Abductors include the deltoid, supraspinatus, trapezius, and serratus anterior. Adduction is accomplished by the subscapularis, infraspinatus, teres minor, pectoralis, latissimus dorsi, and teres major. Flexion of the arm involves the pectoralis major, biceps brachii, and anterior deltoid. Extension is accomplished by posterior deltoid, teres major, and latissimus dorsi. Some muscles may contribute to motion based on the initial position of the humerus. For example, if the humerus is in a flexed position, the pectoralis may assist in early extension to the neutral plane.

The rotator cuff resides in the subacromial space, which is defined by the acromion, subacromial bursa, and coracoacromial ligament above; the coracoid process at the medial border; and the humeral head below. The rotator cuff plays an especially important role in the case of overhead elevation of the arm, which requires tonic contraction to keep the humeral head anchored in the shallow glenoid fossa (43). This explains why rotator cuff tendinopathy is common in laborers who work with their arms overhead or athletes who throw repeatedly (2).

The shoulder is a complex structure that affords great mobility at the expense of stability. Its stability can be divided into static and dynamic components. Statically, the bony glenoid, cartilaginous labrum, glenohumeral ligaments, and joint capsule provide moderate stability. Dynamically, the rotator cuff muscles and biceps tendon function to assist with shoulder stability. Range of motion (ROM) of the shoulder is accomplished by glenohumeral and scapulothoracic motions. The first 30 degrees of abduction is initiated by the deltoid muscle followed by a 2:1 ratio of movement, with the glenohumeral joint responsible for 120 degrees and the scapulothoracic motion supplying the additional 60 degrees. The humerus, however, needs to be in an externally rotated position to be able to obtain full abduction; otherwise, the tuberosity on the humerus impinges on the undersurface of the acromion.

Several authors have evaluated the kinematics of the scapula and its interaction with the humerus. Borstad and Ludewig (44) looked at scapular motion in both symptomatic and asymptomatic individuals. Through electromagnetic tracking, they were able to evaluate scapular tipping and internal rotation. They noted that in symptomatic individuals there was less upward rotation at lower humeral elevations and increased tipping at higher elevations when compared to controls. These same scapular changes were also noted in patients with multidirectional instability (45).

Common conditions include glenohumeral instability (see Chapter 41 for detailed discussion), AC joint injury (see Chapter 41 for detailed discussion), and Rotator Cuff Disease.

Rotator Cuff Disease

Rotator cuff disease is a spectrum of disorders including subacromial/subdeltoid bursitis, rotator cuff tendinopathy, and partial- and full-thickness rotator cuff tears. Rotator cuff disorders are the underlying problems in 65% to 70% of patients with shoulder pain (46,47).

Pathogenesis. Repetitive motion from an abducted and externally rotated position to an internally rotated flexed position leads to the tuberosity of the humerus to come under the arch of the acromion or along the coracoacromial ligament. Progressive impingement of the rotator cuff tendons was described by Neer (48,49) and divided into three stages. The first is noted to have edema and hemorrhage along the supraspinatus insertion. The changes usually occur in younger individuals (12 to 25 years of age) and are typically reversible. Stage II is associated with fibrosis, thickening of the coracoacromial ligament, and bony changes of the acromion. The last stage is most commonly seen in people older than 40 years of age and is associated with partial or complete cuff tears. Overall, shoulder impingement, a mechanical compression process, often leads to rotator cuff tendinopathy.

Rotator cuff tears, categorized as partial- and full-thickness (50–52), can result from direct trauma or underlying tendon degeneration. Traumatic tears can happen at any age, but degenerative tears are commonly seen in patients older than 40 years. There is a 54% incidence of tears within the cuff in asymptomatic individuals older than 60 years (53). The rotator cuff tendons undergoing degenerative tear are characterized by increased fibroblast cellularity, neovascularity, thinning/loss of collagen matrix, and fatty infiltration (54).

Biomechanical studies have been done looking at scapular motion, specifically dyskinesis in the setting of impingement.

Scapular dyskinesis is defined by Kibler (55) as the loss of control in the motion of scapular with respect to external rotation and retraction. This results in an anterior tilt of the glenoid, loss of maximal rotator cuff muscle activation, and reduced rotation of the acromion. All of these factors contribute to clinical impingement.

Symptoms and Signs. Symptoms frequently associated with rotator cuff disorders are pain at the site along the tuberosity, night pain, exacerbation of the symptoms with lying on that shoulder at night, pain along the lateral aspect of the arm toward the insertion of the deltoid, and pain with overhead activities. There may also be loss of strength and motion secondary to the pain. The discomfort is worsened by activities at shoulder level or above.

It is a helpful to assess isometric strength of the individual rotator cuff muscles (i.e., resisted internal/external rotation of shoulder or abduction), and this test can be performed conveniently by using a portable hand-held dynamometer in the office (53). To isolate the supraspinatus, abduction is performed along the plane of the scapula (about 30% anterior to the frontal plane) with the arm internally rotated. Significant weakness will be noted if there is a full-thickness tear, and mild or no weakness is noted with partial tears, secondary to muscular compensation.

A painful arc is present (pain noted with abduction of the arm in the range of 60 to 120 degrees), and sometimes a drop arm test (pain on lowering the arm causing the individual to drop the arm rapidly) is noted. There are several special tests commonly used to evaluate individual rotator cuff muscle/tendon and impingement (**Table 29-2**) (48,56–66).

Diagnosis. In addition to history and physical examination, the cuff can be further evaluated with radiograph, MRI, MR arthrography, ultrasound, and diagnostic arthroscopy. Plain radiographic field may show calcified tendons and superior humeral head migration which could infer a chronic tear. MRI with T2-weighted images is highly sensitive and specific for a full-thickness tear, whereas its sensitivity is less for partial-thickness tears (67). Retraction of torn tendon can be staged by the position of medial edge of torn tendon visualized in coronal plane: stage I if over greater tuberosity, stage II if lateral to glenoid with humeral head exposed, stage III if at glenoid, and stage IV if medial to glenoid (68). In addition, the muscle atrophy and fatty infiltration of muscle bulk can also be appreciated by MRI (51). MR arthrography is excellent in terms of diagnostic sensitivity and specificity; however, it is invasive and indicated when other pathology is suspected, for example, labral tear (69). Ultrasound is gaining more popularity in the diagnosis of rotator cuff tear due to the comparable accuracy to MRI, dynamic examination, excellent portability in the office and less expense (67). Ultrasound shows rotator cuff tear as an area of hypoechogenicity and, similar to MRI, is less sensitive in identifying partial-thickness tears (67).

Treatment. Rotator cuff disease can be treated by either surgical or nonsurgical approach (70–72). Currently, surgical rotator cuff repair is almost exclusively done under arthroscopy. Nonoperative treatment encompasses a wide spectrum of options, namely activity and postural modification (73), topical/oral medication (71,74), physical therapy (75–80), modalities (acupuncture, manual therapy, ice, heat, iontophoresis, phonophoresis, transcutaneous electrical nerve stimulation, pulsed electromagnetic field, and ultrasound) (71,79,81–83), and

TABLE 29-2	Special Tests for Rotator Cuff		
Subject	**Test**	**Procedure**	**Interpretation**
Subscapularis	Lift-off test	The examiner assists the patient to get in a position where he/she touches their lower back with the arm fully extended and internally rotated	The test is positive if the patient is unable to lift the dorsum of his hand off his/her back.
	Passive lift-off test	The examiner brings the arm behind the body into maximal internal rotation (around the lower back region and pull it backwards away from the back).	The test is positive if the patient cannot maintain this position.
	Belly-press test	The examiner requests the patient to presses the abdomen with the hand flat and attempts to keep the arm in maximum internal rotation.	A positive test is when the elbow drops back behind the trunk.
	Belly-off sign	The examiner will passively bring the arm of the patient into flexion and maximum internal rotation with the elbow 90 degrees flexed. The elbow of the patient is supported by one hand of the examiner while the other hand brings the arm into maximum internal rotation placing the palm of the hand on the abdomen. The patient is then asked to keep the wrist straight and actively maintain the position of internal rotation as the examiner releases the wrist.	The test is positive if the patient cannot maintain the above position, lag occurs and the hand lifts off the abdomen.
	Bear Hug	The examiner requests the patient to place the palm of the involved side on the opposite shoulder, extend the fingers (so that the patient could not resist by grabbing the shoulder), and position the elbow anterior to the body. The examiner then asks the patient to hold that position (resisted internal rotation) as the examiner tries to pull the patient's hand from the shoulder with an external rotation force applied perpendicular to the forearm.	The test is positive if the patient could not hold the hand against the shoulder or if he or she shows weakness of resisted internal rotation of >20% compared with the opposite side.
Infraspinatus and Teres minor	External Rotation Lag Sign at 0 degrees	The patient is seated on an examination couch with his or her back to the physician. The elbow is passively flexed to 90 degrees, and the shoulder is held at 20 degrees elevation (in the scapular plane) and near maximum external rotation (i.e., maximum external rotation minus 5 degrees to avoid elastic recoil in the shoulder) by the examiner. The patient is then asked to actively maintain the position of external rotation as the examiner releases the wrist while maintaining support of the limb at the elbow.	The sign is positive when a lag, or angular drop, occurs.
	External Rotation Lag Sign at 90 degrees (drop sign)	The patient is seated on an examination couch with his or her back to the examiner, who holds the affected arm at 90 degrees of elevation (in the scapular plane) and at almost full external rotation, with the elbow flexed at 90 degrees. The patient is asked to actively maintain this position as the physician releases the wrist while supporting the elbow.	The sign is positive if a lag or "drop" occurs. (The maintenance of the position of external rotation of the shoulder is a function mainly of infraspinatus.)
	Hornblower's Sign	The examiner supports the patient's arm at 90 degrees of abduction in the scapular plane with elbow flexed at 90 degrees. The patient then attempts external rotation of the forearm against resistance of the examiner's hand.	The test is positive if the patient cannot externally rotate, then he or she assumes a characteristic position.
Supraspinatus	Jobe test (Empty can test)	It is performed by first assessing the deltoid with the arm at 90 degrees of abduction and neutral rotation. The shoulder is then internally rotated and angled forward 30 degrees; the thumbs should be pointing toward the floor. Manual muscle testing against resistance is performed with the examiner pushing down at the distal forearm.	The test is positive if there is weakness to resistance with the second maneuver as compared with the first maneuver.
	Full can test	With the arm in 90 degrees of elevation in the scapular plane and 45 degrees of external rotation, manual muscle testing against resistance is performed with the examiner pushing down at the distal forearm.	A positive test is when there is weakness to resistance.
	Drop arm test	The examiner abducts the patient's shoulder to 180 degrees passively and then observes as the patient slowly lowers the arm to the waist.	The test is positive if the arm drops to the side. A positive result indicates a tear of the rotator cuff.

Continued

TABLE 29-2	Special Tests for Rotator Cuff *(Continued)*		
Subject	**Test**	**Procedure**	**Interpretation**
Impingement	Neer sign	The patient is seated and the examiner stands behind him or her. Scapular rotation is prevented with one hand while the other hand raises the arm in forced forward elevation, causing the greater tuberosity to impinge against the acromion.	The test is positive if the maneuver produces pain.
	Hawkin sign	The examiner forward flexes the humerus to 90 degrees and forcibly internally rotates the shoulder. This maneuver drives the greater tuberosity farther under the coracoacromial ligament.	The test is positive if the maneuver produces pain.
	O'Brien sign	The examiner stands behind the patient. The patient is asked to forward flex the affected arm 90 degrees with the elbow in full extension. The patient then adducts the arm 10 to 15 degrees medial to the sagittal plane of the body. The arm is internally rotated so that the thumb is pointed downward. The examiner then applies a uniform downward force to the arm. With the arm in the same position, the palm is then fully supinated and the maneuver is repeated.	The test is positive if pain is elicited with the first maneuver and is reduced or eliminated with the second maneuver. Of note, pain or painful clicking described as within the glenohumeral joint itself is also indicative of labral abnormality. Pain localized to the acromioclavicular joint or on top of the shoulder is diagnostic of acromioclavicular joint abnormality.

procedures such as corticosteroid injection (84,85). Insufficient evidence is available to guide surgical versus conservative treatment. It is expert consensus that acute symptomatic traumatic tear should be treated by surgical repair (71).

Pharmacologic management aims at pain relief and facilitation of participation in therapy. The most commonly used oral medication with proven efficacy includes nonsteroidal anti-inflammatory drugs (NSAIDs), COX-2 inhibitors, and acetaminophen (86). Topical NSAIDs are increasingly favored due to its similar pain relief compared to systemic NSAIDs, and adverse effects compared to placebo (87). Injection of lidocaine and corticosteroid in rotator cuff disease was reported to show variable efficacy in pain control (88–90) with reported failure rate around 40% (91). No convincing data favors platelet rich plasma (PRP) injection in rotator cuff disease (92) despite its reported benefits in lateral epicondyle extensor tendinopathy and patellar tendinopathy (93). The rehabilitation therapy will be illustrated in the section below.

Tendinopathy of Long Head of Biceps

The biceps function as a flexor of the elbow and a supinator of the forearm, and there is also some activity with abduction of the arm when externally rotated. The long head of the biceps is integrally linked to shoulder function and may assist the rotator cuff muscles with counteracting anterior and superior forces at the humerus. Its origin is at the supraglenoid tubercle and the adjacent labrum. It courses within the capsule and along the bicipital groove between the tubercles and is held in place by the tendoligamentous biceps sling or pulley (94). Tendinopathy of the long head of biceps is a recognized shoulder pain generator and consists of a spectrum of conditions including inflammatory tendinitis and degenerative tendinosis (95).

Pathogenesis. Biceps tendinopathy can be caused by inflammation, degeneration, overuse, and direct/indirect trauma (94). The biceps tendon is frequently affected with other shoulder pathology, such as rotator cuff disease, superior labrum anterior and posterior (SLAP) lesion, and AC joint disorder. The synovial sheath of the biceps tendon is connected to the synovial lining of the glenohumeral joint and closely adjacent to rotator cuff tendons; therefore, it can become inflamed as a result

of inflammation occurring in nearby structures (96). Isolated bicipital tendinopathy may occur secondary to trauma, repetitive pressure and shear forces, and tendon instability (96,97). The tendon has been noted to be swollen, stenotic at the anatomically narrow sites, and frequently hemorrhagic. In addition, adhesions may develop in the area with ongoing inflammation. The role of the transverse humeral ligament as primary stabilizer for the long head of biceps has been questioned (98). It is a biceps sling or pulley, which is jointly formed by subscapularis tendon, supraspinatus tendon, CHL, and SGHL, that maintains the biceps within its groove (98,99). Distal to the tuberosities, the pectoralis major muscle insertion is the primary stabilizer for the long head of biceps (100).

Symptoms and Signs. Symptoms range from discomfort and weakness to a painful snap. Patients typically complain of anterior shoulder pain localized to the region of the bicipital groove. Point tenderness in the bicipital groove is a common finding. The tenderness is located approximately 6 to 7 cm distal to the anterolateral corner of the acromion with the humerus in 10 degrees of internal rotation and moves laterally as a result of external rotation of the arm. This tenderness in motion is highly specific for biceps pathology (95). When testing subpectoral long head of the biceps tendon, palpation is medial to the pectoralis major tendon insertion while patient internally rotates the arm against resistance (101). Palpation of the tendon and pain produced with resisted supination while the elbow is flexed and held against the trunk (Yergason's test) or with resistance of forward flexion with the elbow extended and supinated (Speed's test) are indicative of tendonitis. In the O'Brien active compression test, patient is asked to forward flex at 90 degrees and adduct the arm at 15 degrees. The arm is then internally rotated with thumb pointing downward and resists downward force applied by the examiner. This test is then repeated with palm facing upward. It is positive if pain is elicited in the first part but reduced in the second part. The O'Brien test is nonspecific to biceps tendinopathy and can be positive in SLAP and AC joint injury (66). Subluxation of the biceps tendon can be palpated when asked to perform full abduction and external rotation of the arm, and both the patient and examiner can feel a snapping sensation (97).

Rupture of the tendon most commonly affects the proximal portion of the long head and generates a Popeye sign (102).

Diagnosis. Radiograph is useful in identifying associated pathology, such as bony abnormalities and joint degeneration. MRI is very helpful in visualization of tenosynovitis, partial-thickness tear, and rupture (103). Ultrasound is accurate for identifying biceps dislocation/subluxation, rupture, and tear. Since other shoulder pathology frequently occurs in concert, the clinician should also investigate for rotator cuff tendinopathy, impingement, or shoulder instability.

Treatment. Mariani et al. (104) evaluated conservative versus surgical intervention and noted the following: there was no difference in residual pain, elbow motion, strength of elbow extension, forearm pronation, or grip strength; the nonsurgical group usually returned to activities, including work, more rapidly, albeit initially at a reduced capacity; and there was usually an associated loss of strength with elbow flexion (10%) and supination (20%), and many individuals were aware of this weakness.

The first-line treatment for biceps tendinopathy is conservative approaches that are generally successful in symptom relief and include rest, activity modification, NSAIDs, and physical therapy (94,95). Corticosteroid injection into the subacromial space, glenohumeral joint, and biceps tendon sheath can be attempted if the initial management does not lead improvement (105). Surgeries most commonly performed are biceps tenotomy and tenodesis (94).

Labral Tear

The glenoid labrum is a fibrocartilaginous structure that increases the depth of the glenoid to improve its stability. The superior labrum is clinically important as it is the site that the long head of the biceps attaches to the superior glenoid rim. SLAP tear is a common cause of shoulder pain and instability. The prevalence of labral injury was reported between 3.9% and 11.8% (106) and, in patients who had arthroscopy, as high as 26% (107).

Pathogenesis. SLAP tears are commonly caused by identifiable mechanisms such as forceful traction to the arm, direct compression load, and repetitive overhead throwing activities. Several cadaver studies suggested that the orientation of the biceps tendon during loading plays a very important role in the development of SLAP (108). Increased shoulder external rotation and posterior capsular contracture are recognized predisposing risk factors for throwing athletes to develop SLAP (109,110).

Symptoms and Signs. The pain is typically over the anterior shoulder, and clicking is sometimes noted with abduction and external rotation. A clunk test may be positive with translation of the humerus over the edge of the labrum and may indicate instability of the shoulder or a labral tear. O'Brien's test is relatively common test when SLAP tears are suspected. Sensitivity of the O'Brien's test appears to be limited in isolation (approximately 63%); however, in combination with other tests, the sensitivity is better (111). One study revealed 90% sensitivity of the O'Brien's test, when the compression test and apprehension tests were both positive. In isolation, the most sensitive and specific test for labral tears appears to be the biceps load test II described by Kim et al. (112). The test is performed in the supine position, and the arm is elevated to 120 degrees and externally rotated to its maximal point, with the elbow in 90-degree flexion and the forearm in the supinated position. The patient is asked to flex the elbow while resisting

the elbow flexion by the examiner. The test is considered positive if the patient complains of pain during the resisted elbow flexion. The test is negative if pain is not elicited or if the pre-existing pain during the elevation and external rotation of the arm is unchanged or diminished by the resisted elbow flexion. Dynamic labral shear test yields nearly 80% sensitivity in detecting isolated SLAP lesion (113). In this test, the examiner stands behind the patient and holds the patient's wrist with one hand while applying an anteriorly directed force on the proximal humerus near the joint line with the other hand. This test is positive if the patient reports pain or the examiner feels a click in the patient's posterior shoulder while the patient's shoulder is being elevated between 90 and 120 degrees.

Diagnosis. MR arthrogram is superior to MRI in identifying SLAP with sensitivity between 82% and 100% as well as specificity between 71% and 98% (114) and the test of choice if a labral tear is suspected. Ultrasound is not reliable in the assessment of the superior labrum, but the posterior labrum is well seen using a transverse approach; therefore, SLAP tears that extend into posterior portion of the labrum may be demonstrated on ultrasound (114).

SLAP tears were classified into four types (I to IV) by Snyder et al. based on the extent and morphology of the tear at the superior labrum and biceps anchor (**Table 29-3**) (115). This classification remains widely used in practice.

Treatment. Nonoperative treatment should be offered initially which entails rest from provocative activities, NSAIDs, stretching to improve posterior capsular flexibility, and strengthening exercise of rotator cuff and scapular stabilizers (108,116). More than 60% of overhead-throwing athletes treated with a nonoperative regimen for a SLAP tear were able to return to play at the same or better level than before the injury (117). Operative intervention is considered if nonsurgical treatment modalities fail and there is strong suspicion that SLAP is account for the symptoms (116).

Adhesive Capsulitis (Frozen Shoulder)

Adhesive capsulitis is a common shoulder condition that is associated with pain and loss of range of motion in the glenohumeral joint. Its incidence is approximately 2% to 5% in the general population and peaks between the ages of 40 and 60 (118). Middle-aged women and diabetic patients appear to be at a higher risk for spontaneous idiopathic adhesive capsulitis.

Pathogenesis. The pathophysiology of frozen shoulder can be either idiopathic or associated with internal derangement such as trauma, tendonitis, and tears. Histologically, a biologic cascade underlies adhesive capsulitis that includes fibroblastic proliferation, inflammatory contracture, capsular hyperplasia, and fibrosis (119).

TABLE 29-3	Classification of SLAP Lesion
Type I	Superior labral fraying with localized degeneration
Type II	Detachment of the superior labrum and biceps anchor from the glenoid
Type III	Bucket-handle tear of the superior labrum with an intact biceps anchor
Type IV	Bucket-handle tear of the superior labrum with an extension of labral tear into the biceps tendon

Symptoms and Signs. Idiopathic adhesive capsulitis is a self-limiting syndrome that can be divided into four different stages and has a natural recovery lasting up to 2 years (118,120). Stage 1. Painful stage (<3 months): pain and multiplanar loss of range of motion with external rotation and abduction being the most affected. Stage 2. Freezing stage (3 to 9 months): severe nocturnal pain and significant loss of active/passive ROM. Stage 3. Frozen stage (9 to 14 months): shoulder stiffness and pain at the end of motion or at night. Stage 4. Thawing stage (15 to 24 months): minimal pain and gradual recovery of ROM.

Diagnosis. Adhesive capsulitis is a clinical diagnosis. Patients have shoulder pain and active and passive limitation in range of motion. If an MRI is obtained, features of adhesive capsulitis include extracapsular edema, joint capsule thickening, abnormal size of axillary recess, and obliteration of subcoracoid fat triangle (121).

Treatment. Treatment is aimed at pain relief and gradual restoration in range of motion. The use of NSAIDs at the early inflammatory stage was reported effective in providing short-term pain relief (122). Oral steroids may play a role in the acute management of adhesive capsulitis. According to Buchbinder and the Cochrane reviews, oral steroids provide significant short-term benefits in pain, range of movement of the shoulder, and function in adhesive capsulitis, but the effect may not be maintained beyond 6 weeks (123). Corticosteroid injection offers rapid pain relief and improvement in ROM in the short term, particularly in the first 6 weeks. By using an image-guided technique, either fluoroscope or ultrasound, the accuracy of injection is increased and thus may lead to better outcome (124). Suprascapular nerve block was shown in RCT to be effective in pain relief but not beneficial in terms of ROM (125). Physiotherapy is a pivotal component of conservative care to prevent capsular contraction and regaining ROM. It is the first-line treatment for the freezing phase of adhesive capsulitis and should be initiated once symptoms allow, as intensive physical rehabilitation beyond the pain limits can be counter-productive (126). Distention arthrography, an injection of saline and/or steroid or air into shoulder joint to break up the adhesion, was reported by some authors to be safe and effective treatment (127). Distention of the capsule requires larger volumes to be injected (25 to 35 mL is the typical joint capacity). Initial infusion of lidocaine (3 to 5 mL) may make distention easier and less painful. Manipulation under anesthesia (MUA) may also be considered (122). In this procedure, forced elevation and abduction are used to release the inferior capsule, while forced external rotation is used to tear the CHL (128). The safety of MUA is a concern as several iatrogenic complications were reported; therefore, injection is recommended rather than MUA (129). Surgical release is usually reserved for refractory cases.

Glenohumeral Arthritis

Glenohumeral arthritis is a progressive condition that causes shoulder pain, joint stiffness, and considerable disability. It affects up to one third of the patients older than 60 years (130).

Pathogenesis. In patient over 60 years, most of the glenohumeral arthritis is primary osteoarthritis (OA), that is, degeneration (131). In the younger patient group, the most likely diagnosis includes instability, capsulorrhaphy arthropathy, posttraumatic arthritis, osteonecrosis, infection, and rheumatoid arthritis (RA).

Symptoms and Signs. Most common complaints are shoulder pain, limited movement, impaired function, and sometimes mechanical symptoms, such as popping, locking, and catching. Physical examination can reveal tenderness, loss of range of motion (both active and passive), bony crepitus, joint swelling, and sensible grinding or popping. When axial load is applied to compress the humeral head toward the glenoid cavity, pain can be induced by rotating the arm internally and externally. It is equally important to evaluate concomitant pathology of affected rotator cuff musculature.

Diagnosis. Plain radiograph is essential in the diagnostic workup. Pathologic changes of arthritis can be well visualized and include joint space narrowing, subchondral sclerosis, bone cyst, and osteophytes. Also, abnormal bony alignment and soft tissue calcification can be appreciated. A dislocated humeral head that migrates upward to the acromion suggests underlying rotator cuff tear. CT is the imaging modality to assess bony structure especially for surgical planning. MRI can be used to evaluate for a cartilage lesion (sensitivity 87%, specificity 81%) (132), subchondral bone edema, and pathologic changes of surrounding soft tissue.

Treatment. The goals of treatment of glenohumeral arthritis are reducing pain and improving function. Conservative management is the first-line option, particularly for patients with mild-to-moderate arthritis or modest impairment of function despite more severe radiographic appearance. Rest with an optional period of immobilization, and application of ice can help to relieve pain. Oral NSAIDs are the mainstay of pharmacologic treatment; however, its long-term use is discouraged due to the systemic adverse effects. The efficacy of glucosamine and chondroitin is debatable, and most studies do not show benefit. Activity modification and occupational changes could be considered to reduce the mechanical stress and repetitive motions suffered by the degenerating joint. Physical therapy can promote the ROM, strength, and general well-being of the patients. Intra-articular injections can provide symptomatic relief (130). Ultrasound guidance was shown to improve the accuracy of needle placement (133). Surgical treatment should be considered for patients who have persistent significant symptoms unresponsive to conservative treatment or progressive glenoid bone erosion.

General Principles of Shoulder Rehabilitation

The goal of a shoulder rehabilitation program is to restore normal range of motion and strength and decrease pain in the involved joint in order to return the patient to his or her daily activities, work-related tasks, or sport. Rehabilitation of the shoulder should include a thorough evaluation of the shoulder girdle complex as well as the cervical and thoracic spine. Cervical pathologies may mimic shoulder pathologies, and it is important to rule out any cervical involvement when completing the evaluation. Both cervical and thoracic immobility can also affect the range of motion of the shoulder girdle complex and should be assessed for any restrictions.

Manual or hands-on techniques may be included in the treatment of the shoulder to restore range of motion to the involved structures. Both passive range of motion (PROM) and active assisted range of motion (AAROM), along with soft tissue mobilizations or joint mobilization techniques may be performed to restore normal mobility to the affected joint. Stretches to the shoulder girdle, particularly stretches to the pectoralis minor muscle and posterior capsule, are performed in order to improve the scapular position and kinematics of the shoulder.

Once range of motion has been restored, strength may be addressed (Refer to Chapter 49 for detailed discussion). Strengthening of the scapular stabilizers should be included and should target the serratus anterior, lower, and middle trapezius muscles in order to restore normal scapulohumeral rhythm. Rotator cuff strengthening exercises should also be included. Resistance can be used and may include the use of dumbbells or resistance bands. The amount of resistance or the intensity of the exercise should be challenging to the patient but at the same time not causing aggravation or inflammation to the shoulder. Determining the appropriate amount of resistance should be determined by observation of the patient's response and where the patient is in the healing process.

Plyometric exercises may be included once normal range of motion and strength has been restored in order to prepare athletes to return to their sport. Most movements in sports require the use of speed and strength such as throwing a ball or serving a tennis ball. These movements are an essential part of the athlete's program and should be performed in order to prevent reinjury.

Elbow

Soft tissue injuries adjacent to the elbow are relatively common. Proper biomechanical functioning of the elbow is critical to ensure coordinated movement patterns and force transmission throughout the upper extremity. Assessment of the elbow likewise requires a functional understanding of the distal and proximal components in the upper extremity kinetic chain. In the context of elbow injuries, it is not unusual to observe motion restriction due to joint contracture and musculotendinous shortening or weakness involving the shoulder, cervical spine, wrist, and digits. The success of rehabilitation is often based on normalizing function throughout the involved extremity.

Anatomy and Kinesiology

The elbow joint is structurally complex. Although commonly referred to as a hinged joint, various articulations contribute to its dynamic movement. The ulnar-humeral joint is the primary articulation and contributes greatly to joint stability. It is a typical, single-axis, hinged joint allowing for 150 degrees of flexion. A few degrees of hyperextension are often seen, primarily in women, related to relative ligamentous laxity. The radio-humeral and proximal radioulnar articulations allow for axial rotation and can be considered pivot-type joints (134). Up to 75 degrees of forearm pronation and 85 degrees of supination are conveyed through these articulations. The radial and ulnar collateral ligaments, olecranon fossa, and anterior joint capsule act as the main static stabilizers of the elbow. Dynamic stability is conveyed through neuromuscular control about the elbow, with the biceps, triceps, pronator teres, and supinator providing the main stabilizing function. The radial, median, and ulnar nerves all become relatively accessible around the elbow and are susceptible to injury through direct trauma, repetitive overuse, compressive forces, or entrapment. These syndromes are often overlooked in the context of chronic elbow pain.

Common conditions are epicondylopathy (see Chapter 41 for detailed discussion) and olecranon bursitis.

In sports, olecranon bursitis is more commonly seen in wrestling, weight lifting, and gymnastics. It is also observed in skateboarders and rollerbladers who do not wear elbow protection.

Pathogenesis. The location of the olecranon bursa, being superficial to the triceps insertion and olecranon, makes it susceptible to injury from acute trauma and repetitive friction.

Symptoms and Signs. Patients with acute olecranon bursitis present with pain and swelling, normal elbow range of motion, and pain reproduction with passive elbow flexion beyond 90 degrees. Chronic conditions may not be painful, and the bursa often feels thickened and boggy.

Diagnosis. The differential diagnosis includes posterior elbow impingement syndrome, triceps tendinitis, and fracture of the olecranon. Patients with systemic arthropathies often develop bursal reactions, but rarely the elbow is involved alone. It is important to rule out an infected bursa and fracture of the olecranon or trochlea. A suspected infected bursa should be aspirated and analyzed before instituting appropriate antibiotic therapy.

Treatment. Treatment includes pressure relief over the elbow, cryotherapy, anti-inflammatory drugs, and compression, particularly in the acute phase. Aspiration may also be indicated in a severely swollen sterile bursa, and in chronic conditions, surgical excision may be necessary.

Triceps Tendinitis

Triceps tendinitis is commonly seen in boxers, pitchers, weight lifters, bowlers, and gymnasts.

Pathogenesis. Triceps tendinitis generally occurs as a result of repetitive overuse or extension overload at the elbow. The injury, associated with inflammation and microtrauma, typically occurs at the insertion of the triceps to the olecranon process.

Symptoms and Signs. Pain is reproduced with resisted elbow extension and passive elbow flexion with shoulder forward flexion. In the throwing athlete, loss of flexibility may be seen in elbow flexion and shoulder internal rotation. In atypical cases, patients will report a snapping sensation at the elbow caused by subluxation of the medial head of the triceps over the medial epicondyle.

Diagnosis. Triceps tendinitis is distinguished from subluxation of the ulnar nerve at the medial elbow owing to the absence of sensory symptoms in the hand.

Treatment. The treatment of triceps tendinitis requires activity modification; therapeutic modalities including cryotherapy, ultrasound, or phonophoresis; electrical stimulation, and soft tissue manipulation. Therapeutic exercise emphasizes flexibility training through the kinetic chain with a focus on elbow flexion and shoulder flexion and internal rotation. Progressive resistance training and a graded return to activity are addressed, monitoring for any increase in symptoms. An orthosis, limiting full extension of the elbow, may be useful during this period of reconditioning.

Elbow Arthritis

Elbow arthritis is a debilitating condition that causes pain, weakness, and loss of motion. It can be classified as primary and secondary according to the etiology.

Pathogenesis. Elbow arthritis is most commonly caused by trauma and RA. Other causes include primary OA, septic arthritis, crystalline arthropathy, and hemophilia (135). Unlike OA in other joints, primary OA of the elbow is rare and affects less than 2% in general population (136). Primary OA was found associated with heavy use of the upper limb, such as weight lifting. Posttraumatic arthritis caused by cartilage damage and/or residual joint surface incongruencies secondary instability, abnormal fracture healing, suboptimal position of hardware, and complication of infection (137).

Primary OA of the elbow is characterized by osteophyte formation and joint capsular contracture; however, the articular cartilage is preserved relatively well, and joint space is maintained. Articular pathologies of posttraumatic arthritis can be isolated to specific area of the elbow or may affect the entire joint (138).

Symptoms and Signs. Different etiology, that is, RA versus OA versus trauma, may lead to slightly different clinical presentations. Generally, patients complain about pain and limited ROM of elbow and forearm. It is helpful to clarify the relationship of pain with elbow movement. Impingement-type pain, pain at the terminal motion, is due to the osteophyte formation and capsular contracture. Pain throughout the entire motion suggests joint surface damage. Pain at rest is concerning for infection, tumor, cervical radiculopathy, and reflex sympathetic dystrophy (138,139). In the early stage of primary OA, there may be impingement symptoms: loss of terminal elbow extension and impingement pain (139). Symptomatic instability may be seen in prolonged RA and posttraumatic arthritis (135). Loose bodies in the joint lead to "catching" or "locking" of the elbow.

Besides routine elbow examination, attention should be paid to assessment of ulnar nerve regarding irritability, subluxation, sensory, and motor function. Range of motion and its relationship with pain should be carefully evaluated. Complete loss of ROM is rare in arthritis and warrants suspicion of heterotopic ossification. Muscle strength and ligamentous stability are documented.

Diagnosis. Pain radiograph plays an essential role in diagnosis and planning for treatment. Normally obtained views are anteroposterior, lateral with elbow flexed at 90 degrees, and radiocapitellar oblique views. Based on the radiograph, primary OA of elbow is divided into three classes which are implicated in the choice of surgical treatment. Class I is characterized by marginal arthritic spurring of the ulnotrochlear joint with normal radiocapitellar joint. Class II is marginal ulnotrochlear arthritis as well as arthritic change in radiocapitellar joint. Class III shows changes in the previous two classes with addition of radiocapitellar subluxation (140). The radiographic presentation of RA is noted for general space narrowing, periarticular erosion, and osteopenia.

CT and MRI are not routinely performed unless there is need to visualize the intra-articular loose bodies, substantial bony deformity, and suspected heterotopic ossification. When peripheral neuropathy is clinically present, EMG is sometimes indicated to evaluate the extent and severity of nerve injury. Joint aspiration should be done when infection is thought to be the cause of arthritis.

Treatment. The diagnosis of RA warrants early and aggressive treatment with disease-modifying antirheumatic drugs and biologic agents (141). Early stage of OA where patients report mild pain and minimal motion loss is amenable for nonoperative treatment that includes rest, NSAIDs, activity modification, physical therapy with dynamic hinged and static progressive splinting, and corticosteroid injection (135). More evidence is needed to show that viscosupplementation is effective in elbow arthritis. Surgery is reserved for intermediate or late stages of OA, patients with complaint of stiffness with terminal pain (i.e., impingement) or pain throughout the entire arc of motion, and those who do not respond to nonoperative treatment. There are several surgical options including synovectomy, debridement, hemiarthroplasty, distraction interposition arthroplasty, and total elbow arthroplasty (TEA). The choice of surgical intervention is determined jointly by age, functional demand, etiology, neurologic comorbidity, and severity of arthritis (138,139).

General Principles of Elbow Rehabilitation

Rehabilitation of the elbow may involve either an occupational therapist or a physical therapist. The initial goal of an elbow rehabilitation program is to decrease the pain and swelling in the joint. The use of physical modalities, such as cryotherapy, may be utilized in order to control the pain and inflammation. Bracing or splinting may also be beneficial early in the rehabilitation process in order to allow for tissue healing. If the patient's elbow is immobilized, it will be important to initiate early mobilization, when appropriate, in order to improve range of motion and prevent stiffness in the joint. Mobilization techniques may include PROM, soft tissue mobilization techniques, and joint mobilizations. Both active range of motion and AAROM exercises should be included and may be a part of the patient's home exercise program. If the patient has difficulty regaining range of motion, a static progressive splint may be utilized in order to regain the missing range of motion.

Initiating a strengthening program for the rotator cuff and scapula stabilizers is important in order to prevent atrophy at the shoulder girdle. Once range of motion has improved at the elbow, the patient may begin strengthening the biceps, triceps, wrist, and hand. Resistance may include either dumbbells or resistance bands and should be progressed upon the patient's tolerance of the particular exercise. Rhythmic exercises for the upper extremity may be initiated in order to restore neuromuscular control and proprioception to the entire upper extremity. If the patient is returning to sport, a sport-specific exercise program as well as a plyometric program should be initiated to prevent reinjury. Exercises should be selected based upon the specific sport or task the patient will be resuming.

Hand and Wrist

Our hands are our primary tools for interacting with our environment. One may argue that the most significant function of the shoulder, elbow, and wrist is to position the hand in space. Once the hand is positioned, it is able to proceed with its functional task. Therefore, any abnormalities of hand function are important to evaluate and when possible treat, because of the critical role that our hands play in our daily routines.

Anatomy and Kinesiology

The anatomy of the human hand is extremely complex, with many intricate mechanisms that allow us to grip a tennis racket, hold a pencil, or play the piano. Relevant anatomy will be discussed later.

Common conditions include triangular fibrocartilage complex (TFCC) injuries and distal radioulnar joint (DRUJ) instability.

TFCC Injuries and DRUJ Instability

TFCC is a complicated anatomical structure located in the ulnar side of the wrist and composed of triangular fibrocartilage articular disc, the superficial and deep dorsal/volar radioulnar ligament, meniscus homolog, ulnar collateral ligament, and the sheath of extensor carpi ulnaris (ECU) (142). The superficial section of radioulnar ligament is continuous with ECU subsheath while the deep section, also known as ligamentum subcruentum, inserts into the fovea and the base of ulnar styloid (143). The physiologic function of TFCC is to stabilize DRUJ and absorb load of wrist (144). Injuries to TFCC are commonly seen in athletes in sports such as tennis, golf, hockey, boxing, and pole vaulting (144).

Pathogenesis. The injuries to TFCC may result from either acute trauma or repetitive load bearing and rotational stresses (144). The central/radial articular part of TFCC is avascular, and the peripheral ligamentous portion is more vascular; therefore, central/radial portion is limited in healing in comparison to the peripheral region (145). TFCC, together with pronator quadratus and bony articulation between radius and ulna, stabilizes DRUJ. The dorsal superficial and volar deep radioulnar ligaments tighten and stabilize DRUJ in pronation; the volar superficial and dorsal deep ligaments stabilize DRUJ in supination (146).

Symptoms and Signs. Patient may recall a traumatic injury event that leads to the pathology of TFCC and DRUJ; however, there could be no inciting event in the chronic and degenerative injuries. The pain localized to the ulnar side of wrist and exacerbated by loading the wrist or pronation/supination. Tenderness in the ulnar fovea area, that is, ulnar fovea sign, indicates ulnotriquetral ligament injury (147). Other examination maneuvers to evaluate TFCC include piano key test, ulnocarpal stress test, DRUJ ballottement (143).

Diagnosis. Plain radiograph is the initial workup to help identifying bone and joint pathologies, particularly ulnar variance, presence of styloid fracture, and gapping between the distal radius and ulna. Positive ulnar variance, measured in clenched fist pronation PA view, predisposes to ulnar impaction and degeneration of TFCC (148). MR arthrography is the definitive imaging of choice and possesses superior diagnostic accuracy compared to MRI in the central TFCC tears (95.8% vs. 77.1%) and peripheral TFCC tear (95.8% vs. 87.5%) (149). Of note, abnormalities of TFCC were found significantly more prevalent in the age group greater than 50 years by conventional MRI (150).

Treatment. For chronic tear without DRUJ instability, nonoperative treatment is the first-line option which includes bracing, taping, activity modification, and corticosteroid injections (151). Surgery is indicated if symptoms persist despite conservative management or if the DRUJ is unstable (144). Acute TFCC tear, most commonly sustained from traumatic event, is amenable to surgical debridement (central lesion) or repair (peripheral lesion) (144).

ECU Injury

Please refer to Chapter 41 for detailed discussion.

Carpal Instability

Please refer to Chapter 41 for detailed discussion.

Kienböck Disease

Kienböck disease, avascular necrosis of the lunate, is a progressive disease that leads to wrist pain and dysfunction. It most commonly affects men between the ages of 20 and 40 years (152). It is caused by a combination of factors (vascular, anatomic, and traumatic) and follows a predictable pattern: lunate collapse, fragmentation, carpal change, and degeneration (153).

Pathogenesis. The exact etiology of Kienböck disease remains unknown, but it is considered multifactorial resulting from anatomic/mechanical factors, vascular interruption, and traumatic insults (154). Vascular supply may be compromised by fracture, ligament collapse, systemic disease, or primary circulatory collapse. Repetitive microtrauma, but not a single traumatic event, was found to be associated with the development of Kienböck disease (153).

Symptoms and Signs. The typical symptom is that of middorsal wrist pain; besides, other symptoms include decreased motion, swelling, and weakness in the affected hand. On physical exam, there is point tenderness to palpation over the dorsum of the lunate and radiolunate facet. An effusion or bogginess overlying the radiocarpal joint can also be present.

Diagnosis. In the early stage of the disease, x-rays may be normal. With disease worsening, radiograph can show cystic change, increased lunate density, lunate collapse, and fragmentation. At advanced stages, secondary changes can be visualized including the proximal migration of the capitate and lunate with dorsal intercalated segment instability (DISI), and degenerative changes. On radiograph, DISI is evaluated by measuring scapholunate angle on lateral view while lunate collapse and carpal OA can be evaluated by measuring carpal height ratio that is obtained by dividing carpal height (distance between the distal articular surface of the capitate to the lunate fossa of the distal radius) by the length of the third metacarpal and approximately 0.53 in normal individuals. Three-phase bone scan shows an area of decreased uptake at the lunate in all phases of the scan, indicating a lack of blood flow. MRI can detect early disease and shows a decreased T1 and T2 signal at the lunate or what appears to be a black lunate (155). It is of note that perilunate dislocation and ulnar impaction syndrome appear similar to Kienböck disease on MRI; however, they are focal and nonprogressive lesions.

Disease staging system proposed by Lichtman is the most frequently used and is helpful in guiding treatment options (**Table 29-4**) (152,153).

Treatment. Conservative treatment with cast immobilization for 3 months should be attempted in stage I disease (156). Most authors suggest surgery for Kienböck disease; however, the reported outcome of conservative treatment is controversial (153). A study comparing surgical versus nonsurgical treatment at 65 months found no difference in the outcome but change in social activities and loss of function in nearly 25% of the patients treated surgically (157). Although it was found most of the patients undergoing nonoperative treatment show radiographic progression of the disease in the long-term follow-up, only less than 25% of the patients were symptomatic (158). For those having conservative trial, routine monitoring should be performed. If there is progression of symptoms or radiographs, surgical intervention should be initiated. Many surgical procedures have been described, including joint leveling (either shortening the radius or lengthening the ulna) (159), various intercarpal fusions (160), silastic arthroplasty (161), or vascularized bone grafts (162). Most importantly, Kienböck should be treated immediately to limit further compression of the lunate and collapse of the carpus.

	TABLE 29-4	**Staging of Kienböck Disease**			
Stages	**Symptoms**	**Radiograph**	**MRI**	**Bone scan**
I	Nonspecific wrist pain	Normal ± compression fracture lines	Uniform decrease in signal on both T1 and T2	Decreased signal uptake
II	Swelling, stiffness, progressive pain	Lunate sclerosis, ± fracture lines	As above	As above
IIIA	Symptoms suggesting instability, such as clunking with radial and ulnar deviation; progressive pain; decreased strength	Lunate collapse (widened lunate in anteroposterior plane viewed on lateral view) with maintenance of carpal height and alignment (scapholunate angle preserved at –10 to 10 degrees)	As above	As above
IIIB	Similar to above	Lunate collapse plus one of the following: loss of carpal height, proximal capitate migration, flexed and rotated scaphoid	As above	As above
IV	Stiffness, constant pain, swelling	As above + degeneration changes	As above	As above

De Quervain Tenosynovitis

Please refer to Chapter 41 for detailed discussion.

Trigger Finger

Please refer to Chapter 41 for detailed discussion.

Hand Fractures, Dislocations, and Injuries to Ligaments and Tendons

Please refer to Chapter 41 for detailed discussion.

Degenerative Joint Disease

Basilar thumb OA is the most common symptomatic arthropathy of the hand. Thirty-three percent of postmenopausal women older than 50 years have radiographic evidence of OA of the thumb carpometacarpal (CMC) joint (163). The etiology of CMC arthritis is likely to be multifactorial, including genetic, environmental, and physiologic contributions (164).

Pathogenesis. The thumb CMC joint is a double-saddle configuration. This configuration allows for movement in multiple planes such as flexion-extension, adduction-abduction, and pronation-supination. Sixteen ligaments have been described stabilizing the trapezium and the CMC joint (165). The most important of these is thought to be the so-called beak ligament or deep anterior oblique ligament. Ligamentous laxity plus axial loading of the joint are thought to be major contributors to the development of OA at the base of the thumb. However, there may also be a link between hand OA and obesity (166).

Symptoms and Signs. The sequelae of OA, such as instability or pain of the first metacarpophalangeal (MCP) joint, may contribute to pain and prehensile abnormalities.

Diagnosis. Classification of the thumb OA is radiographic and is graded according to the change in the trapeziometacarpal space, degree of synovitis, and subluxation. Stage 1 is associated with a normal joint space, whereas stages 2 to 4 have a decreased joint space. Stage 3 has obligatory osteophyte changes and sclerosis of the joint. Stage 4 has all of the observations plus involvement of the scaphotrapezial joint (167). Symptoms vary with each stage.

Treatment. In the treatment of basilar thumb degenerative joint disease (DJD), one tries to manage the symptoms. The patient may acquire new prehensile patterns and adaptive equipment in order to minimize symptoms and maximize function. The CMC joint biomechanics is such that any pinch force generated at the thumb and index finger is greatly magnified at the CMC joint interface. In fact, 1 kg of pinch force translates to 12 kg of intra-articular pressure; thus, one strives to minimize fingertip-to-fingertip pinch activities (168). When pinching cannot be avoided, one tries to increase the size of the objects being pinched. In other words, the greater the distance between the thumb and the fingertip, the less pressure on the CMC joint; therefore, enlarging the grip of tools or objects that are being gripped decreases the pressure at the base of the thumb. Twisting activities also stress the CMC joint by causing a torque or twisting force on the joint. Therefore, various gadgets such as key holders and electric can openers may be helpful. In addition, one may use pens, kitchen utensils, or gardening implements with built-up grips.

Splints are used to help stabilize the thumb, reducing pain and enabling more symptom-free function. There are two commonly used splints for this problem: a short opponens splint which is hand based and crosses the first MCP joint; and a long opponens splint which is forearm based, supports the wrist, and crosses the interphalangeal joint. Patients typically best tolerate the long opponens, forearm-based splint at night and prefer the less obstructive hand-based splint for daytime activities. These splints usually put the thumb in palmar abduction with the MCP in 30 degrees of flexion. Several authors have documented benefits from splinting in stabilizing the joint and providing pain relief (164,169). Others have found studies of the efficacy of splints to be methodologically weak and unconvincing (169). Splints usually are not successful in symptom reduction when there is fixed deformity of the joint. A review of the evidence for splinting the CMC joint in arthritis is available (170).

Many patients use pain-relieving modalities such as contrast baths, hot-water soaks, or paraffin baths. Anti-inflammatory medications are often used for pain control. In addition, one may consider corticosteroid injections into the CMC joint (171). If the patient has involvement of the scapho-trapezio-trapezoid (STT) joint, this may be injected at the same time with a single needle stick.

As a last resort, some patients may consider surgical options for basilar thumb DJD. The most common procedure used to treat this problem is ligamentous reconstruction of the joint (172). The trapezium is wholly or partially excised. The base of the first metacarpal is then reattached to the carpus using a tendon slip from the flexor carpi radialis (FCR), the abductor pollicis longus (APL), or the extensor pollicis brevis (EPB). Various techniques are used to weave the tendon between the bases of the first and second metacarpals with the distal scaphoid. Some variations also employ the remaining tendon slip as a cushion to fill in the gap left by the trapezium. This is also called the ligamentous reconstruction tendon interposition (LRTI) or the "anchovy" procedure. Although the tendon reconstruction procedures help restore mobility of the thumb and reduce pain, they are not suited for heavy activities or manual labor. The patients requiring a large amount of grip strength and durability would be better served by arthrodesis of the joint (173,174). This allows for quicker recovery and preservation of grip strength. The tendon reconstruction method requires 6 months of recovery and often only results in 60% to 70% of normal grip and pinch strength (175). Various interposition arthroplasty procedures are less common and are not as well established as tendon or fusion procedures.

Dupuytren Contracture

Dupuytren contracture is a thickening of the palmar fascia. It affects men 7 to 15 times more than women and is thought to be an autosomal dominant inheritance, with variable penetration. Usually, Dupuytrens affects whites of northern European descent, and its prevalence increases with age (176,177). The fascial thickening progresses ulnarly to radially and can result in flexion deformities of the MCP, proximal interphalangeal (PIP), and, occasionally, the distal interphalangeal (DIP) joint.

Pathogenesis. Dupuytren contracture is a benign hypertrophy of the fascia. It usually begins insidiously as small imperceptible nodules in the area of the palmar crease. It can progress to thick cords that form along the fascia tension lines of the palm (178). The underlying tendons, synovial sheaths, and skin layers are not affected (179).

The pathophysiology of Dupuytrens is not fully understood; there is, however, a higher incidence in alcoholic, diabetic, and epileptic patients, and there is thought to be a correlation with tobacco use (180). A clear association between Dupuytrens and trauma or work activities has not been identified (181). The palmar fascia thickening is caused by an abnormal proliferation of fibroblasts. This proliferation is closely correlated with that observed in scar formation and healing. Three stages in the nodule and cord formation have been described. The first stage is proliferation. During this stage, the numbers of myofibroblasts within the palmar fascia spontaneously increase. The second stage is involution, when the myofibroblasts align along the tension lines of the palm and digits. The fascia enlarges owing to contraction of the myofibroblastic activity. In the third phase, the myofibroblasts resolve, leaving contracting collagen, which is perceived as nodules and matures into cords (182).

Symptoms and Signs. Many individuals with this condition are unaware of its presence. Usually, it is first noted when the palmar nodules and cords become tender with pressure (178). Activities that require frequent or strenuous gripping often result in tenderness near the nodules or cords. The palmar fascia of the small finger is the most commonly affected in 70% of individuals with this condition (183). This is typically followed in succession by the fascia of the ring, middle, thumb, and index fingers.

Diagnosis. Dupuytren contracture is a clinical diagnosis. The hallmark of clinical evaluation is the palpable nodules and cords in the palmar fascia, most notably in the small finger. Hypertrophic changes of the skin are also appreciated. Joint deformity, including flexion contractures of the MCP, PIP, and DIP, is usually present in advanced conditions. Transverse or web space contractures may also occur. These contractures can result in significant functional limitations necessitating treatment. Other pathologic processes with a similar presentation include intrinsic joint contractures, palmar ganglion inclusion cysts, stenosing tenosynovitis, occupational hyperkeratosis, callus formation, soft tissue giant cell tumors, epithelial sarcomas, and early changes of RA (178).

Treatment. Multiple treatment regimes for this condition have been described, including splinting, radiation, and use of disulfides, vitamin E, antigout medications, physical therapy, and ultrasonic therapy. These therapies have shown minimal effectiveness (184). Treatment of advanced Dupuytrens is surgical fasciectomy. This is recommended when the patient can no longer perform a "tabletop test" (185). In this test, the individual places the palm on a flat surface and attempts to extend the involved finger actively. A positive test is noted if the MCP joint cannot be placed flat against the surface. This usually correlates with a greater than 30-degree fixed flexion contracture of the MCP joint. The goal of surgery is to restore function, not to cure the disease (186).

Recently, there has been a great deal of interest in percutaneous or enzymatic fasciotomies as an alternative to surgical fasciectomy. Hurst and Badalamente (184) have demonstrated that by injecting collagenase into the fibrous cords, joint contractures can be improved. They report that 90% enjoyed excellent results at an average of 9-month follow-up. Although no long-term studies have been completed, this procedure does offer promise.

Postoperative surgical rehabilitation is extremely important following fasciectomy, with concentration on maintaining skin integrity, restoration of joint range of motion, and overall improvement of function (187). Despite surgical treatment, this condition can be quite recalcitrant, and reoccurrence rates range from 28% to 80% (183).

Focal Dystonia (Writer's Cramp)

Writer's cramp and musician's cramp are both focal dystonias that affect a discrete anatomical area. They are characterized by disabling cramps, contractions, or spasms during specific activities (188). When not so engaged, the hand appears and functions normally. It tends to affect young adult males.

Pathogenesis. Dystonia may occur sporadically in the population or may be genetically transmitted. The gene for early-onset dystonia (DYT1) has been sequenced. Approximately, 10% of people with dystonia have a family history of tremor or dystonia (189). Others report that a higher percentage of those affected have a family history of dystonia (190). The pathophysiology of dystonia is not entirely understood. However, there seems to be some evidence for abnormalities in the basal ganglia (188) or problems with cortical organization (191). There is a neurophysiologic defect in the ability to produce and process neurotransmitters, including (a) gamma-amino-butyric acid (*GABA*), an inhibitory substance that helps the brain maintain muscle control; (b) dopamine, an inhibitory chemical that influences the brain's control of movement; and (c) acetylcholine, norepinephrine, and serotonin.

Symptoms and Signs. It is usually idiopathic and not a result of overt trauma, although it may follow a traumatic episode. The flexors are more commonly involved than the extensors. Among the flexors, the flexor digitorum superficialis (FDS), flexor digitorum profundus (FDP), flexor pollicis longus (FPL), and the lumbricals may be involved. The extensor pollicis longus, extensor indicis, and digitorum communis may be involved among the extensors. Patients frequently have mirror dystonia, demonstrated by inducing the writer's cramp in the dominant hand even when attempting to write with the nondominant (146). Focal dystonias tend to remain focal and do not become generalized dystonias over time.

Diagnosis. Electrodiagnostic studies show a cocontraction of muscle and a loss of alternation of agonist/antagonist muscle contractions. There are prolonged bursts of muscle contractions and overflow contraction seen in those muscles not activated by the motor task (192).

Treatment. Treatments have been aimed at correcting these possible pathologic situations. GABA-regulating drugs such as the muscle relaxants diazepam, lorazepam, clonazepam, and baclofen have been used with modest success. Deep brain stimulation (193) and proprioceptive retraining (194,195) have anecdotally been reported as successful.

Currently, it appears that botulinum toxin offers the most reliable relief for focal dystonia, with minimal risk (196). Selection of patients for this treatment should include a careful neuromusculoskeletal examination. Once the diagnosis of focal dystonia is confirmed, the selection of the muscles that are to be injected is made. Often, these muscles can be identified by observing the patient performing the inciting tasks. However, it may be useful to use EMG to identify all those that are activated, including the deeper muscles that may not be obvious clinically. A starting dose of 2.5 units of botulinum toxin type A for small muscles and up to 50 units for larger muscles is usually injected. The botulinum toxin can be diluted into a larger volume for ease of administration. The use of EMG or ultrasound to guide injections increases the accuracy of correctly identifying the contracting muscles (197). The benefits are usually seen within 1 week and may last for a few months. Repeated injections are safe and are often needed to sustain the benefits (198). A secondary effect of botulinum type A injections is associated muscle weakness, which may respond to muscle strengthening. A small proportion of patients receiving continued treatment may develop antibodies to type A. These patients may respond to botulinum type B or F (199,200).

Hand-Arm Vibration Syndrome

HAVS is a constellation of vascular and neuromuscular symptoms associated with high levels of exposure to vibration. This is typically an occupational disorder that results from both increased duration and intensity of exposure to handling vibrating tools or objects, such as jackhammers, drills, or chain saws.

Pathogenesis. Although it is difficult to quantify the threshold intensity or the amount of operating time needed to cause HAVS, a positive correlation of symptoms with cumulative exposure has been shown (201). This disorder is most prevalent in forestry workers, construction workers, stone cutters, and shipyard workers (201,202).

Symptoms and Signs. Onset of HAVS can occur as rapidly as within 3 months of full-time, daily vibration exposure (203). The clinical presentation of HAVS includes vascular, sensorineural, and musculoskeletal symptoms. The vascular component consists of Raynaud phenomenon and may be triggered by a cold environment. There is initial digital blanching (associated with vasoconstriction), followed by cyanotic discoloration that eventually resolves into erythema when blood vessels dilate allowing reperfusion. During this bright red phase of reactive hyperemia, there may be significant pain in the wrist, hands, or fingers. Not all patients will experience all three phases, as some only have the initial blanching phase. The duration of these symptoms varies greatly from minutes to hours. Neurologically, symptoms include tingling paresthesias or numbness. Patients may also note intermittent aching pain in their hands. Grip strength may be reduced due to weakness of the finger flexors or intrinsic hand muscles. In chronic cases, skin ulceration may develop, usually at the fingertips.

Diagnosis. There are various tests for the diagnosis of HAVS. Physical exam should include two-point discrimination and vibration perception testing, which can uncover sensorineural dysfunction (204–206). Duplex ultrasonography checks the patency of arteries of the upper limbs. Cold provocation testing utilizes the fact that patients with Raynaud's secondary to HAVS often have prolonged coolness of digits after cold water immersion. Coughlin et al. demonstrated high sensitivity and specificity for cold provocation thermography, in which thermal measurements of the digits are made before and minutes after cold immersion of hands (85). Nerve conduction studies have found sensory nerve conduction velocity slowing in the digits in 36% and across the wrist in 20% of patients in advanced stages of HAVS (207). HAVS patients often have both median and ulnar neuropathies (208). Another objective measure involves recording finger systolic blood pressures (FSBPs) at baseline and again after exposure to cold. The cold temperatures result in greater vasoconstriction, which is measured by the FSBP decrease in symptomatic HAVS patients (209). Poole et al. found a specificity of 90% to 95% and sensitivity of 43.5% to 60% for this technique (210).

Treatment. Treatment of HAVS begins with limiting exposure to hand vibration, using antivibration gloves and coated tool handles, and ensuring proper technique in handling equipment (211). Avoidance of contact with cold objects or maintaining warm hands in cold environment can decrease bouts of Raynaud's. Smoking cessation is highly recommended because of its vasoconstrictive effects on peripheral arteries (203). Medications such as calcium channel blockers, nitrates, pentoxifylline, and NSAIDs may help reduce symptoms especially if used in combination (212,213).

General Principles of Hand and Wrist Rehabilitation

The goal for a wrist and hand rehabilitation program is to restore normal pain-free range of motion to the joints and normalize the strength in the upper extremity in order for the individual to return to his or her regular activities of daily living. Splinting or bracing may be indicated initially in order to decrease pain and allow the involved structures to heal. Range of motion exercises may be initiated and may consist of active or AAROM, PROM, soft tissue mobilization, and joint mobilization techniques. The patient should be educated on performing activities that do not exacerbate his or her symptoms.

The patient may also be educated on the use of cryotherapy to help control pain and swelling in the area.

Once the range of motion is normalized and the pain has decreased, the patient may begin to work on a strengthening program. Exercises for the wrist and hand may include wrist flexion and extension, digit flexion and extension, and thumb opposition. A strengthening program should be considered for the muscles that surround the elbow as well as the shoulder and scapula. Strengthening exercises should be kept in the pain-free range so that the surrounding tissues and joint structures are not overstressed. Once the patient has normalized strength and range of motion, the patient may begin a gradual return to his or her specific functional activity or sport.

ERGONOMICS

Per the International Ergonomics Association Council of 2000, ergonomics is "the scientific discipline concerned with the understanding of interactions among humans and other elements of a system, and the profession that applies theory, principles, data and methods to design in order to optimize human well-being and overall system performance." It requires an understanding of human abilities and the limitations imposed by the work environment, machines, tools, and specific job tasks.

Much of ergonomics relates to CTDs. Their role and mechanism of injury in musculoskeletal disorders has been discussed earlier in this chapter. In addition to the management principles for each of the respective disorders, ergonomic workplace modifications are increasingly utilized to prevent CTD. The Occupational Safety and Health Administration, a division of the U.S. Department of Labor, has published workplace guidelines for different industries including health care, retail groceries stores, shipyards, etc. The Center for Disease Control also has a concise summary of ergonomic considerations in a variety of workplace settings available at http://www.cdc.gov/od/ohs/ergonomics/ergohome. While an in-depth discussion of ergonomic evaluation and design is beyond the scope of this chapter, some general considerations are introduced in **Box 29-1**.

Many workplace environments have already implemented ergonomic design changes. Further research and studies are needed in this area to determine optimal positioning and ways to avoid repetitive strain.

BOX 29-1

Positions/Postures

- The worker should avoid extreme flexion of the elbow, extreme flexion or extension of the wrist, and sustained supination or pronation of the forearm.
- During repetitive work (e.g., typing), the upper extremity should be relaxed at the sides, with the elbows flexed no more than 70 to 90 degrees.
- Avoid prolonged maintenance of the elbow in the overhead position during repetitive or sustained activities.
- Avoid activities with sustained grip or pinch.
- Avoid repetitive radial or ulnar deviations of the wrist.
- Avoid sitting in the same position for extended periods of time. Take breaks to stretch and walk around.

REFERENCES

1. Leadbetter WB. Soft tissue athletic injury. In: Fu FH, Stone DA, eds. *Sports Injuries: Mechanism, Prevention, Treatment.* Baltimore, MD: Williams & Wilkins; 1994: 733–780.
2. Wilson JJ, Best TM. Common overuse tendon problems: a review and recommendations for treatment. *Am Fam Physician.* 2005;72(5):811–818.
3. Khan MH, Li Z, Wang JH. Repeated exposure of tendon to prostaglandin-E2 leads to localized tendon degeneration. *Clin J Sport Med.* 2005;15(1):27–33.
4. National Institute for Occupational Safety and Health. *Musculoskeletal Disorders and Workplace Factors: A Critical Review of Epidemiologic Evidence for Work-Related Musculoskeletal Disorders of the Neck, Upper Extremity, and Low Back.* Washington, DC: U.S. Department of Health & Human Services; 1997.
5. Johnson SL. Ergonomic hand tool design. *Hand Clin.* 1993;9(2):299–311.
6. Muckart RD. Stenosing tendovaginitis of abductor pollicis longus and extensor pollicis brevis at the radial styloid (de Quervain's disease). *Clin Orthop Relat Res.* 1964;33:201–208.
7. Armstrong TJ, Fine LJ, Radwin RG, et al. Ergonomics and the effects of vibration in hand-intensive work. *Scand J Work Environ Health.* 1987;13(4):286–289.
8. Ring D, Kadzielski J, Fabian L, et al. Self-reported upper extremity health status correlates with depression. *J Bone Joint Surg Am.* 2006;88(9):1983–1988. doi:10.2106/jbjs.e.00932.
9. Gimeno D, Amick BC III, Habeck RV, et al. The role of job strain on return to work after carpal tunnel surgery. *Occup Environ Med.* 2005;62(11):778–785. doi:10.1136/oem.2004.016931.
10. Herring SA, Kibler WB. A framework of rehabilitation. In: Kibler WB, Herring SA, Press JM, eds. *Functional Rehabilitation of Sports and Musculoskeletal Injuries.* Gaithersburg, MD: Aspen; 1998:1–8.
11. Frank C, Amiel D, Woo SL, et al. Normal ligament properties and ligament healing. *Clin Orthop Relat Res.* 1985;(196):15–25.
12. Kannus P. Etiology and pathophysiology of chronic tendon disorders in sports. *Scand J Med Sci Sports.* 1997;7(2):78–85.
13. Sharma P, Maffulli N. Biology of tendon injury: healing, modeling and remodeling. *J Musculoskelet Neuronal Interact.* 2006;6(2):181–190.
14. Barfred T. Experimental rupture of the Achilles tendon. Comparison of various types of experimental rupture in rats. *Acta Orthop Scand.* 1971;42(6):528–543.
15. Leadbetter WB. Cell-matrix response in tendon injury. *Clin Sports Med.* 1992;11(3):533–578.
16. Puddu G, Ippolito E, Postacchini F. A classification of Achilles tendon disease. *Am J Sports Med.* 1976;4(4):145–150. doi:10.1177/036354657600400404.
17. Garrett WE Jr. Muscle strain injuries: clinical and basic aspects. *Med Sci Sports Exerc.* 1990;22(4):436–443.
18. Cushner FD, Morwessel RM. Myositis ossificans traumatica. *Orthop Rev.* 1992;21(11):1319–1326.
19. Finnerman GAM, Shapiro MS. Sports induced soft tissue calcification. In: Leadbetter WB, Buckwalter JA, Gordon SL, eds. *Sports-Induced Inflammation: Clinical and Basic Science Concepts.* Park Ridge, IL: American Academy of Orthopedic Surgeons; 1990:257–275.
20. Armstrong RB. Mechanisms of exercise-induced delayed onset muscular soreness: a brief review. *Med Sci Sports Exerc.* 1984;16(6):529–538.
21. Tiidus PM, Ianuzzo CD. Effects of intensity and duration of muscular exercise on delayed soreness and serum enzyme activities. *Med Sci Sports Exerc.* 1983;15(6): 461–465.
22. Madry H, Grun UW, Knutsen G. Cartilage repair and joint preservation: medical and surgical treatment options. *Dtsch Arztebl Int.* 2011;108(40):669–677. doi:10.3238/arztebl.2011.0669.
23. Wong M, Carter DR. Articular cartilage functional histomorphology and mechanobiology: a research perspective. *Bone.* 2003;33(1):1–13.
24. Dowthwaite GP, Bishop JC, Redman SN, et al. The surface of articular cartilage contains a progenitor cell population. *J Cell Sci.* 2004;117(Pt 6):889–897. doi:10.1242/jcs.00912.
25. Mankin HJ. The reaction of articular cartilage to injury and osteoarthritis (second of two parts). *N Engl J Med.* 1974;291(25):1335–1340. doi:10.1056/nejm197412192912507.
26. Freemont AJ, Hoyland J. Lineage plasticity and cell biology of fibrocartilage and hyaline cartilage: its significance in cartilage repair and replacement. *Eur J Radiol.* 2006;57(1):32–36. doi:10.1016/j.ejrad.2005.08.008.
27. Menorca RM, Fussell TS, Elfar JC. Nerve physiology: mechanisms of injury and recovery. *Hand Clin.* 2013;29(3):317–330. doi:10.1016/j.hcl.2013.04.002.
28. Gupta R, Steward O. Chronic nerve compression induces concurrent apoptosis and proliferation of Schwann cells. *J Comp Neurol.* 2003;461(2):174–186. doi:10.1002/cne.10692.
29. Gupta R, Rummler LS, Palispis W, et al. Local down-regulation of myelin-associated glycoprotein permits axonal sprouting with chronic nerve compression injury. *Exp Neurol.* 2006;200(2):418–429. doi:10.1016/j.expneurol.2006.02.134.
30. Griffin JW, Hogan MV, Chhabra AB, et al. Peripheral nerve repair and reconstruction. *J Bone Joint Surg Am.* 2013;95(23):2144–2151. doi:10.2106/jbjs.l.00704.
31. Giannoudis PV, Jones E, Einhorn TA. Fracture healing and bone repair. *Injury.* 2011;42(6):549–550. doi:10.1016/j.injury.2011.03.037.
32. Einhorn TA. The cell and molecular biology of fracture healing. *Clin Orthop Relat Res.* 1998;(355 suppl):S7–S21.
33. McKibbin B. The biology of fracture healing in long bones. *J Bone Joint Surg Br.* 1978;60-B(2):150–162.

34. Alborzi A, Mac K, Glackin CA, et al. Endochondral and intramembranous fetal bone development: osteoblastic cell proliferation, and expression of alkaline phosphatase, m-twist, and histone H4. *J Craniofac Genet Dev Biol.* 1996;16(2):94–106.

35. Zakaria D, Robertson J, MacDermid JC, et al. Estimating the population at risk for Ontario Workplace Safety and Insurance Board-covered injuries or diseases. *Chronic Dis Can.* 2002;23(1):17–21.

36. Chiang HC, Ko YC, Chen SS, et al. Prevalence of shoulder and upper-limb disorders among workers in the fish-processing industry. *Scand J Work Environ Health.* 1993;19(2):126–131.

37. Ohlsson K, Attewell RG, Palsson B, et al. Repetitive industrial work and neck and upper limb disorders in females. *Am J Ind Med.* 1995;27(5):731–747.

38. Hunting KL, Welch LS, Cuccherini BA, et al. Musculoskeletal symptoms among electricians. *Am J Ind Med.* 1994;25(2):149–163.

39. Punnett L, Robins JM, Wegman DH, et al. Soft tissue disorders in the upper limbs of female garment workers. *Scand J Work Environ Health.* 1985;11(6):417–425.

40. Punnett L. Upper extremity musculoskeletal disorders in hospital workers. *J Hand Surg Am.* 1987;12(5 pt 2):858–862.

41. Holmstrom EB, Lindell J, Moritz U. Low back and neck/shoulder pain in construction workers: occupational workload and psychosocial risk factors. Part 2: Relationship to neck and shoulder pain. *Spine.* 1992;17(6):672–677.

42. English CJ, Maclaren WM, Court-Brown C, et al. Relations between upper limb soft tissue disorders and repetitive movements at work. *Am J Ind Med.* 1995;27(1):75–90.

43. Silliman JF, Hawkins RJ. Current concepts and recent advances in the athlete's shoulder. *Clin Sports Med.* 1991;10(4):693–705.

44. Borstad JD, Ludewig PM. Comparison of scapular kinematics between elevation and lowering of the arm in the scapular plane. *Clin Biomech (Bristol, Avon).* 2002;17(9–10):650–659.

45. Ogston JB, Ludewig PM. Differences in 3-dimensional shoulder kinematics between persons with multidirectional instability and asymptomatic controls. *Am J Sports Med.* 2007;35(8):1361–1370. doi:10.1177/0363546507300820.

46. Chard MD, Hazleman R, Hazleman BL, et al. Shoulder disorders in the elderly: a community survey. *Arthritis Rheum.* 1991;34(6):766–769.

47. Vecchio P, Kavanagh R, Hazleman BL, et al. Shoulder pain in a community-based rheumatology clinic. *Br J Rheumatol.* 1995;34(5):440–442.

48. Neer CS. Impingement lesions. *Clin Orthop Relat Res.* 1983;173:70–77.

49. Basic science and clinical application in the athlete's shoulder. *Clin Sports Med.* 1991;10(4):693–971.

50. Gomoll AH, Katz JN, Warner JJ, et al. Rotator cuff disorders: recognition and management among patients with shoulder pain. *Arthritis Rheum.* 2004;50(12):3751–3761. doi:10.1002/art.20668.

51. Opsha O, Malik A, Baltazar R, et al. MRI of the rotator cuff and internal derangement. *Eur J Radiol.* 2008;68(1):36–56. doi:10.1016/j.ejrad.2008.02.018.

52. Recht MP, Resnick D. Magnetic resonance-imaging studies of the shoulder. Diagnosis of lesions of the rotator cuff. *J Bone Joint Surg Am.* 1993;75(8):1244–1253.

53. Reid D, Polson K, Johnson L. Acromioclavicular joint separations grades I-III: a review of the literature and development of best practice guidelines. *Sports Med (Auckland, NZ).* 2012;42(8):681–696. doi:10.2165/11633460-000000000-00000.

54. Dean BJ, Franklin SL, Carr AJ. A systematic review of the histological and molecular changes in rotator cuff disease. *Bone Joint Res.* 2012;1(7):158–166. doi:10.1302/2046-3758.17.2000115.

55. Kibler WB. Scapular involvement in impingement: signs and symptoms. *Instr Course Lect.* 2006;55:35–43.

56. Jain NB, Wilcox RB III, Katz JN, et al. Clinical examination of the rotator cuff. *PM R.* 2013;5(1):45–56. doi:10.1016/j.pmrj.2012.08.019.

57. Gerber C, Krushell RJ. Isolated rupture of the tendon of the subscapularis muscle. Clinical features in 16 cases. *J Bone Joint Surg.* 1991;73(3):389–394.

58. Gerber C, Hersche O, Farron A. Isolated rupture of the subscapularis tendon. *J Bone Joint Surg Am.* 1996;78(7):1015–1023.

59. Scheibel M, Magosch P, Pritsch M, et al. The belly-off sign: a new clinical diagnostic sign for subscapularis lesions. *Arthroscopy.* 2005;21(10):1229–1235. doi:10.1016/j.arthro.2005.06.021.

60. Barth JR, Burkhart SS, De Beer JF. The bear-hug test: a new and sensitive test for diagnosing a subscapularis tear. *Arthroscopy.* 2006;22(10):1076–1084. doi:10.1016/j.arthro.2006.05.005.

61. Hertel R, Ballmer FT, Lombert SM, et al. Lag signs in the diagnosis of rotator cuff rupture. *J Shoulder Elbow Surg.* 1996;5(4):307–313.

62. Walch G, Boulahia A, Calderone S, et al. The 'dropping' and 'hornblower's' signs in evaluation of rotator-cuff tears. *J Bone Joint Surg.* 1998;80(4):624–628.

63. Jobe FW, Jobe CM. Painful athletic injuries of the shoulder. *Clin Orthop Relat Res.* 1983;(173):117–124.

64. Kelly BT, Kadrmas WR, Speer KP. The manual muscle examination for rotator cuff strength. An electromyographic investigation. *Am J Sports Med.* 1996;24(5):581–588. doi:10.1177/036354659602400504.

65. Hawkins RJ, Kennedy JC. Impingement syndrome in athletes. *Am J Sports Med.* 1980;8(3):151–158. doi:10.1177/036354658000800302.

66. O'Brien SJ, Pagnani MJ, Fealy S, et al. The active compression test: a new and effective test for diagnosing labral tears and acromioclavicular joint abnormality. *Am J Sports Med.* 1998;26(5):610–613. doi:10.1177/03635465980260050201.

67. de Jesus JO, Parker L, Frangos AJ, et al. Accuracy of MRI, MR arthrography, and ultrasound in the diagnosis of rotator cuff tears: a meta-analysis. *AJR Am J Roentgenol.* 2009;192(6):1701–1707. doi:10.2214/ajr.08.1241.

68. Boileau P, Brassart N, Watkinson DJ, et al. Arthroscopic repair of full-thickness tears of the supraspinatus: does the tendon really heal? *J Bone Joint Surg Am.* 2005;87(6):1229–1240. doi:10.2106/jbjs.d.02035.

69. Jain NB, Collins J, Newman JS, et al. Reliability of magnetic resonance imaging assessment of rotator cuff: the ROW study. *PM R.* 2015;7(3):245.e3–254.e3; quiz 54. doi:10.1016/j.pmrj.2014.08.949.

70. Matsen FA III. Clinical practice. Rotator-cuff failure. *N Engl J Med.* 2008;358(20):2138–2147. doi:10.1056/NEJMcp0800814.

71. Pedowitz RA, Yamaguchi K, Ahmad CS, et al. American Academy of Orthopaedic Surgeons Clinical Practice Guideline on optimizing the management of rotator cuff problems. *J Bone Joint Surg Am.* 2012;94(2):163–167.

72. Williams GR Jr, Rockwood CA Jr, Bigliani LU, et al. Rotator cuff tears: why do we repair them? *J Bone Joint Surg Am.* 2004;86-A(12):2764–2776.

73. Lewis JS, Wright C, Green A. Subacromial impingement syndrome: the effect of changing posture on shoulder range of movement. *J Orthop Sports Phys Ther.* 2005;35(2):72–87. doi:10.2519/jospt.2005.35.2.72.

74. Cumpston M, Johnston RV, Wengier L, et al. Topical glyceryl trinitrate for rotator cuff disease. *Cochrane Database Syst Rev.* 2009;(3):CD006355. doi:10.1002/14651858.CD006355.pub2.

75. Ainsworth R, Lewis JS. Exercise therapy for the conservative management of full thickness tears of the rotator cuff: a systematic review. *Br J Sports Med.* 2007;41(4):200–210. doi:10.1136/bjsm.2006.032524.

76. Bennell K, Coburn S, Wee E, et al. Efficacy and cost-effectiveness of a physiotherapy program for chronic rotator cuff pathology: a protocol for a randomised, double-blind, placebo-controlled trial. *BMC Musculoskelet Disord.* 2007;8:86. doi:10.1186/1471-2474-8-86.

77. Hertling D, Kessler RM. *The Shoulder and Shoulder Girdle. Management of Common Musculoskeletal Disorders: Physical Therapy Principles and Methods.* Philadelphia, PA: Lippincott; 1990.

78. Kuhn JE. Exercise in the treatment of rotator cuff impingement: a systematic review and a synthesized evidence-based rehabilitation protocol. *J Shoulder Elbow Surg.* 2009;18(1):138–160. doi:10.1016/j.jse.2008.06.004.

79. Green S, Buchbinder R, Hetrick S. Physiotherapy interventions for shoulder pain. *Cochrane Database Syst Rev.* 2003;(2):CD004258. doi:10.1002/14651858.CD004258.

80. Misamore GW, Ziegler DW, Rushton JL II. Repair of the rotator cuff. A comparison of results in two populations of patients. *J Bone Joint Surg Am.* 1995;77(9):1335–1339.

81. Engebretsen K, Grotle M, Bautz-Holter E, et al. Radial extracorporeal shockwave treatment compared with supervised exercises in patients with subacromial pain syndrome: single blind randomised study. *BMJ.* 2009;339:b3360. doi:10.1136/bmj.b3360.

82. Buchbinder R, Johnson MP, Roos JF. Shock wave therapy for rotator cuff disease with or without calcification. *Cochrane Database Syst Rev.* 2011;(1):CD008962. doi:10.1002/14651858.cd008962.

83. Green S, Buchbinder R, Hetrick S. Acupuncture for shoulder pain. *Cochrane Database Syst Rev.* 2005;(2):CD005319. doi:10.1002/14651858.CD005319.

84. Gialanella B, Prometti P. Effects of corticosteroids injection in rotator cuff tears. *Pain Med.* 2011;12(10):1559–1565. doi:10.1111/j.1526-4637.2011.01238.x.

85. Coughlin PA, Chetter IC, Kent PJ, et al. The analysis of sensitivity, specificity, positive predictive value and negative predictive value of cold provocation thermography in the objective diagnosis of the hand-arm vibration syndrome. *Occupational Medicine.* 2001;(51)2:75–85.

86. Itoi E, Tabata S. Conservative treatment of rotator cuff tears. *Clin Orthop Relat Res.* 1992;(275):165–173.

87. Derry S, Moore RA, Rabbie R. Topical NSAIDs for chronic musculoskeletal pain in adults. *Cochrane Database Syst Rev.* 2012;(9):CD007400. doi:10.1002/14651858.CD007400.pub2.

88. Mellor SJ, Patel VR. Steroid injections are helpful in rotator cuff tendinopathy. *BMJ.* 2002;324(7328):51.

89. Alvarez CM, Litchfield R, Jackowski D, et al. A prospective, double-blind, randomized clinical trial comparing subacromial injection of betamethasone and xylocaine to xylocaine alone in chronic rotator cuff tendinosis. *Am J Sports Med.* 2005;33(2):255–262. doi:10.1177/0363546504267345.

90. Coombes BK, Bisset L, Vicenzino B. Efficacy and safety of corticosteroid injections and other injections for management of tendinopathy: a systematic review of randomised controlled trials. *Lancet.* 2010;376(9754):1751–1767. doi:10.1016/s0140-6736(10)61160-9.

91. Contreras F, Brown HC, Marx RG. Predictors of success of corticosteroid injection for the management of rotator cuff disease. *HSS J.* 2013;9(1):2–5. doi:10.1007/s11420-012-9316-6.

92. Kesikburun S, Tan AK, Yilmaz B, et al. Platelet-rich plasma injections in the treatment of chronic rotator cuff tendinopathy: a randomized controlled trial with 1-year follow-up. *Am J Sports Med.* 2013;41(11):2609–2616. doi:10.1177/0363546513496542.

93. Mautner K, Kneer L. Treatment of tendinopathies with platelet-rich plasma. *Phys Med Rehabil Clin N Am.* 2014;25(4):865–880. doi:10.1016/j.pmr.2014.06.008.

94. Nho SJ, Strauss EJ, Lenart BA, et al. Long head of the biceps tendinopathy: diagnosis and management. *J Am Acad Orthop Surg.* 2010;18(11):645–656.

95. Mellano CR, Shin JJ, Yanke AB, et al. Disorders of the long head of the biceps tendon. *Instr Course Lect.* 2015;64:567–576.

96. Sethi N, Wright R, Yamaguchi K. Disorders of the long head of the biceps tendon. *J Shoulder Elbow Surg.* 1999;8(6):644–654.

97. Yamaguchi K. *Disorders of the Biceps Tendon.* Philadelphia, PA: Lippincott Williams & Wilkins; 1999.

98. Gleason PD, Beall DP, Sanders TG, et al. The transverse humeral ligament: a separate anatomical structure or a continuation of the osseous attachment of the rotator cuff? *Am J Sports Med.* 2006;34(1):72–77. doi:10.1177/0363546505278698.

99. Walch G, Nove-Josserand L, Levigne C, et al. Tears of the supraspinatus tendon associated with "hidden" lesions of the rotator interval. *J Shoulder Elbow Surg.* 1994;3(6):353–360. doi:10.1016/s1058-2746(09)80020-7.

100. Romeo AA, Mazzocca AD, Tauro JC. Arthroscopic biceps tenodesis. *Arthroscopy.* 2004;20(2):206–213. doi:10.1016/j.arthro.2003.11.033.

101. Mazzocca AD, Rios CG, Romeo AA, et al. Subpectoral biceps tenodesis with interference screw fixation. *Arthroscopy.* 2005;21(7):896. doi:10.1016/j.arthro.2005.04.002.

102. Kelly AM, Drakos MC, Fealy S, et al. Arthroscopic release of the long head of the biceps tendon: functional outcome and clinical results. *Am J Sports Med.* 2005;33(2):208–213. doi:10.1177/0363546504269555.

103. Mohtadi NG, Vellet AD, Clark ML, et al. A prospective, double-blind comparison of magnetic resonance imaging and arthroscopy in the evaluation of patients presenting with shoulder pain. *J Shoulder Elbow Surg.* 2004;13(3):258–265. doi:10.1016/s1058274604000205.

104. Mariani EM, Cofield RH, Askew LJ, et al. Rupture of the tendon of the long head of the biceps brachii. Surgical versus nonsurgical treatment. *Clin Orthop Relat Res.* 1988;(228):233–239.

105. Tallia AF, Cardone DA. Diagnostic and therapeutic injection of the shoulder region. *Am Fam Physician.* 2003;67(6):1271–1278.

106. Aydin N, Sirin E, Arya A. Superior labrum anterior to posterior lesions of the shoulder: diagnosis and arthroscopic management. *World J Orthop.* 2014;5(3):344–350. doi:10.5312/wjo.v5.i3.344.

107. Kim TK, Queale WS, Cosgarea AJ, et al. Clinical features of the different types of SLAP lesions: an analysis of one hundred and thirty-nine cases. *J Bone Joint Surg Am.* 2003;85-A(1):66–71.

108. Keener JD, Brophy RH. Superior labral tears of the shoulder: pathogenesis, evaluation, and treatment. *J Am Acad Orthop Surg.* 2009;17(10):627–637.

109. Burkhart SS, Morgan CD, Kibler WB. The disabled throwing shoulder: spectrum of pathology. Part II: evaluation and treatment of SLAP lesions in throwers. *Arthroscopy.* 2003;19(5):531–539. doi:10.1053/jars.2003.50139.

110. Burkhart SS, Morgan CD. The peel-back mechanism: its role in producing and extending posterior type II SLAP lesions and its effect on SLAP repair rehabilitation. *Arthroscopy.* 1998;14(6):637–640.

111. Hegedus EJ, Goode A, Campbell S, et al. Physical examination tests of the shoulder: a systematic review with meta-analysis of individual tests. *Br J Sports Med.* 2008;42(2):80–92; discussion 92. doi:10.1136/bjsm.2007.038406.

112. Oh JH, Kim JY, Kim WS, et al. The evaluation of various physical examinations for the diagnosis of type II superior labrum anterior and posterior lesion. *Am J Sports Med.* 2008;36(2):353–359. doi:10.1177/0363546507308363.

113. Sodha S, Srikumaran U, Choi K, et al. Clinical assessment of the dynamic labral shear test for superior labrum anterior and posterior lesions. *Am J Sports Med.* 2017;45(4):775–781. doi:10.1177/0363546517690349.

114. Rowbotham EL, Grainger AJ. Superior labrum anterior to posterior lesions and the superior labrum. *Semin Musculoskelet Radiol.* 2015;19(3):269–276. doi:10.1055/s-0035-1549320.

115. Snyder SJ, Karzel RP, Del Pizzo W, et al. SLAP lesions of the shoulder. *Arthroscopy.* 1990;6(4):274–279.

116. Knesek M, Skendzel JG, Dines JS, et al. Diagnosis and management of superior labral anterior posterior tears in throwing athletes. *Am J Sports Med.* 2012;41(2):444–460. doi:10.1177/0363546512466067.

117. Edwards SL, Lee JA, Bell JE, et al. Nonoperative treatment of superior labrum anterior posterior tears: improvements in pain, function, and quality of life. *Am J Sports Med.* 2010;38(7):1456–1461. doi:10.1177/0363546510370937.

118. Zuckerman JD, Rokito A. Frozen shoulder: a consensus definition. *J Shoulder Elbow Surg.* 2011;20(2):322–325. doi:10.1016/j.jse.2010.07.008.

119. Uppal HS, Evans JP, Smith C. Frozen shoulder: a systematic review of therapeutic options. *World J Orthop.* 2015;6(2):263–268. doi:10.5312/wjo.v6.i2.263.

120. Neviaser RJ, Neviaser TJ. The frozen shoulder. Diagnosis and management. *Clin Orthop Relat Res.* 1987;(223):59–64.

121. Park S, Lee D-H, Yoon S-H, et al. Evaluation of adhesive capsulitis of the shoulder with fat-suppressed T2-weighted MRI: association between clinical features and MRI findings. *Am J Roentgenol.* 2016;207(1):135–141. doi:10.2214/AJR.15.15200.

122. Hsu JE, Anakwenze OA, Warrender WJ, et al. Current review of adhesive capsulitis. *J Shoulder Elbow Surg.* 2011;20(3):502–514. doi:10.1016/j.jse.2010.08.023.

123. Buchbinder R, Green S, Youd JM, et al. Oral steroids for adhesive capsulitis. *Cochrane Database Syst Rev.* 2006;(4):CD006189. doi:10.1002/14651858.cd006189.

124. Song A, Higgins LD, Newman J, et al. Glenohumeral corticosteroid injections in adhesive capsulitis: a systematic search and review. *PM R.* 2014;6(12):1143–1156. doi:10.1016/j.pmrj.2014.06.015.

125. Dahan TH, Fortin L, Pelletier M, et al. Double blind randomized clinical trial examining the efficacy of bupivacaine suprascapular nerve blocks in frozen shoulder. *J Rheumatol.* 2000;27(6):1464–1469.

126. Diercks RL, Stevens M. Gentle thawing of the frozen shoulder: a prospective study of supervised neglect versus intensive physical therapy in seventy-seven patients with frozen shoulder syndrome followed up for two years. *J Shoulder Elbow Surg.* 2004;13(5):499–502. doi:10.1016/s1058274604000825.

127. Clement RG, Ray AG, Davidson C, et al. Frozen shoulder: long-term outcome following arthrographic distension. *Acta Orthop Belg.* 2013;79(4):368–374.

128. Georgiannos D, Markopoulos G, Devetzi E, et al. Adhesive capsulitis of the shoulder. Is there consensus regarding the treatment? A comprehensive review. *Open Orthop J.* 2017;11:65–76. doi:10.2174/1874325001711010065.

129. Loew M, Heichel TO, Lehner B. Intraarticular lesions in primary frozen shoulder after manipulation under general anesthesia. *J Shoulder Elbow Surg.* 2005;14(1):16–21. doi:10.1016/j.jse.2004.04.004.

130. Menge TJ, Boykin RE, Byram IR, et al. A comprehensive approach to glenohumeral arthritis. *South Med J.* 2014;107(9):567–573. doi:10.14423/smj.0000000000000166.

131. Denard PJ, Wirth MA, Orfaly RM. Management of glenohumeral arthritis in the young adult. *J Bone Joint Surg Am.* 2011;93(9):885–892. doi:10.2106/jbjs.j.00960.

132. Hayes ML, Collins MS, Morgan JA, et al. Efficacy of diagnostic magnetic resonance imaging for articular cartilage lesions of the glenohumeral joint in patients with instability. *Skeletal Radiol.* 2010;39(12):1199–1204. doi:10.1007/s00256-010-0922-4.

133. Daley EL, Bajaj S, Bisson LJ, et al. Improving injection accuracy of the elbow, knee, and shoulder: does injection site and imaging make a difference? A systematic review. *Am J Sports Med.* 2011;39(3):656–662. doi:10.1177/0363546510390610.

134. Pacelli LL, Guzman M, Botte MJ. Elbow instability: the orthopedic approach. *Semin Musculoskelet Radiol.* 2005;9(1):56–66. doi:10.1055/s-2005-867103.

135. Papatheodorou LK, Baratz ME, Sotereanos DG. Elbow arthritis: current concepts. *J Hand Surg.* 2013;38(3):605–613. doi:10.1016/j.jhsa.2012.12.037.

136. Kozak TK, Adams RA, Morrey BF. Total elbow arthroplasty in primary osteoarthritis of the elbow. *J Arthroplasty.* 1998;13(7):837–842.

137. Biswas D, Wysocki RW, Cohen MS. Primary and posttraumatic arthritis of the elbow. *Arthritis.* 2013;2013:473259. doi:10.1155/2013/473259.

138. Sears BW, Puskas GJ, Morrey ME, et al. Posttraumatic elbow arthritis in the young adult: evaluation and management. *J Am Acad Orthop Surg.* 2012;20(11):704–714. doi:10.5435/jaaos-20-11-704.

139. Cheung EV, Adams R, Morrey BF. Primary osteoarthritis of the elbow: current treatment options. *J Am Acad Orthop Surg.* 2008;16(2):77–87.

140. Rettig LA, Hastings H II, Feinberg JR. Primary osteoarthritis of the elbow: lack of radiographic evidence for morphologic predisposition, results of operative debridement at intermediate follow-up, and basis for a new radiographic classification system. *J Shoulder Elbow Surg.* 2008;17(1):97–105. doi:10.1016/j.jse.2007.03.014.

141. Ishii K, Inaba Y, Mochida Y, et al. Good long-term outcome of synovectomy in advanced stages of the rheumatoid elbow. *Acta Orthop.* 2012;83(4):374–378. doi:10.3109/17453674.2012.702391.

142. Palmer AK, Werner FW. The triangular fibrocartilage complex of the wrist—anatomy and function. *J Hand Surg.* 1981;6(2):153–162.

143. Pang EQ, Yao J. Ulnar-sided wrist pain in the athlete (TFCC/DRUJ/ECU). *Curr Rev Muscoskelet Med.* 2017;10(1):53–61. doi:10.1007/s12178-017-9384-9.

144. Henderson CJ, Kobayashi KM. Ulnar-sided wrist pain in the athlete. *Orthop Clin North Am.* 2016;47(4):789–798. doi:10.1016/j.ocl.2016.05.017.

145. Bednar MS, Arnoczky SP, Weiland AJ. The microvasculature of the triangular fibrocartilage complex: its clinical significance. *J Hand Surg.* 1991;16(6):1101–1105.

146. Hagert CG. Distal radius fracture and the distal radioulnar joint—anatomical considerations. *Handchir Mikrochir Plast Chir.* 1994;26(1):22–26.

147. Tay SC, Tomita K, Berger RA. The "ulnar fovea sign" for defining ulnar wrist pain: an analysis of sensitivity and specificity. *J Hand Surg.* 2007;32(4):438–444. doi:10.1016/j.jhsa.2007.01.022.

148. Tomaino MM. The importance of the pronated grip x-ray view in evaluating ulnar variance. *J Hand Surg.* 2000;25(2):352–357. doi:10.1053/jhsu.2000.jhsu25a0352.

149. Lee YH, Choi YR, Kim S, et al. Intrinsic ligament and triangular fibrocartilage complex (TFCC) tears of the wrist: comparison of isovolumetric 3D-THRIVE sequence MR arthrography and conventional MR image at 3 T. *Magn Reson Imaging.* 2013;31(2):221–226. doi:10.1016/j.mri.2012.06.024.

150. Iordache SD, Rowan R, Garvin GJ, et al. Prevalence of triangular fibrocartilage complex abnormalities on MRI scans of asymptomatic wrists. *J Hand Surg.* 2012;37(1):98–103. doi:10.1016/j.jhsa.2011.10.006.

151. Jarrett CD, Baratz ME. The management of ulnocarpal abutment and degenerative triangular fibrocartilage complex tears in the competitive athlete. *Hand Clin.* 2012;28(3):329–337, ix. doi:10.1016/j.hcl.2012.05.018.

152. Lichtman DM, Mack GR, MacDonald RI, et al. Kienbock's disease: the role of silicone replacement arthroplasty. *J Bone Joint Surg Am.* 1977;59(7):899–908.

153. Cross D, Matullo KS. Kienbock disease. *Orthop Clin North Am.* 2014;45(1):141–152. doi:10.1016/j.ocl.2013.09.004.

154. Stamos BD, Leddy JP. Closed flexor tendon disruption in athletes. *Hand Clin.* 2000;16(3):359–365.

155. Allan CH, Joshi A, Lichtman DM. Kienbock's disease: diagnosis and treatment. *J Am Acad Orthop Surg.* 2001;9(2):128–136.

156. Jackson MD, Barry DT, Geiringer SR. Magnetic resonance imaging of avascular necrosis of the lunate. *Arch Phys Med Rehabil.* 1990;71(7):510–513.

157. Delaere O, Dury M, Molderez A, et al. Conservative versus operative treatment for Kienbock's disease. A retrospective study. *J Hand Surg Br.* 1998;23(1):33–36.

158. Kristensen SS, Thomassen E, Christensen F. Ulnar variance in Kienbock's disease. *J Hand Surg Br.* 1986;11(2):258–260.

159. Salmon J, Stanley JK, Trail IA. Kienbock's disease: conservative management versus radial shortening. *J Bone Joint Surg.* 2000;82(6):820–823.

160. Trail IA, Linscheid RL, Quenzer DE, et al. Ulnar lengthening and radial recession procedures for Kienbock's disease. Long-term clinical and radiographic follow-up. *J Hand Surg Br.* 1996;21(2):169–176.

161. Watson HK, Ryu J, DiBella A. An approach to Kienbock's disease: triscaphe arthrodesis. *J Hand Surg.* 1985;10(2):179–187.

162. Alexander AH, Turner MA, Alexander CE, et al. Lunate silicone replacement arthroplasty in Kienbock's disease: a long-term follow-up. *J Hand Surg.* 1990;15(3):401–407.

163. Armstrong AL, Hunter JB, Davis TR. The prevalence of degenerative arthritis of the base of the thumb in post-menopausal women. *J Hand Surg Br.* 1994;19(3):340–341.

164. Glickel SZ. Clinical assessment of the thumb trapeziometacarpal joint. *Hand Clin.* 2001;17(2):185–195.

165. Bettinger PC, Linscheid RL, Berger RA, et al. An anatomic study of the stabilizing ligaments of the trapezium and trapeziometacarpal joint. *J Hand Surg.* 1999;24(4):786–798.

166. Felson DT, Chaisson CE. Understanding the relationship between body weight and osteoarthritis. *Baillieres Clin Rheumatol.* 1997;11(4):671–681.

167. Eaton RG, Glickel SZ. Trapeziometacarpal osteoarthritis. Staging as a rationale for treatment. *Hand Clin.* 1987;3(4):455–471.

168. Cooney WP III, Chao EY. Biomechanical analysis of static forces in the thumb during hand function. *J Bone Joint Surg Am.* 1977;59(1):27–36.

169. Poole JU, Pellegrini VD Jr. Arthritis of the thumb basal joint complex. *J Hand Ther.* 2000;13(2):91–107.

170. Egan MY, Brousseau L. Splinting for osteoarthritis of the carpometacarpal joint: a review of the evidence. *Am J Occup Ther.* 2007;61(1):70–78.

171. Shin EK, Osterman AL. Treatment of thumb metacarpophalangeal and interphalangeal joint arthritis. *Hand Clin.* 2008;24(3):239–250, v. doi:10.1016/j.hcl.2008.03.007.

172. Tomaino MM. Ligament reconstruction tendon interposition arthroplasty for basal joint arthritis. Rationale, current technique, and clinical outcome. *Hand Clin.* 2001;17(2):207–221.

173. Klimo GF, Verma RB, Baratz ME. The treatment of trapeziometacarpal arthritis with arthrodesis. *Hand Clin.* 2001;17(2):261–270.

174. Illarramendi AA, Boretto JG, Gallucci GL, et al. Trapeziectomy and intermetacarpal ligament reconstruction with the extensor carpi radialis longus for osteoarthritis of the trapeziometacarpal joint: surgical technique and long-term results. *J Hand Surg.* 2006;31(8):1315–1321. doi:10.1016/j.jhsa.2006.07.002.

175. Rayan GM, Young BT. Ligament reconstruction arthroplasty for trapeziometacarpal arthrosis. *J Hand Surg.* 1997;22(6):1067–1076. doi:10.1016/s0363-5023(97)80051-2.

176. Burge P. Genetics of Dupuytren's disease. *Hand Clin.* 1999;15(1):63–71.

177. Ross DC. Epidemiology of Dupuytren's disease. *Hand Clin.* 1999;15(1):53–62, vi.

178. Rayan GM. Palmar fascial complex anatomy and pathology in Dupuytren's disease. *Hand Clin.* 1999;15(1):73–86, vi–vii.

179. Strickland JW, Leibovic SJ. Anatomy and pathogenesis of the digital cords and nodules. *Hand Clin.* 1991;7(4):645–657; discussion 59–60.

180. Yi IS, Johnson G, Moneim MS. Etiology of Dupuytren's disease. *Hand Clin.* 1999;15(1):43–51, vi.

181. Saar JD, Grothaus PC. Dupuytren's disease: an overview. *Plast Reconstr Surg.* 2000;106(1):125–134; quiz 35–36.

182. Tomasek JJ, Vaughan MB, Haaksma CJ. Cellular structure and biology of Dupuytren's disease. *Hand Clin.* 1999;15(1):21–34.

183. McFarlane RM, Botz FS, Cheung H. Epidemiology of surgical patients. In: McFarlane RM, McGrouther DA, Flint M, eds. *Dupuytren's Disease Biology and Treatment.* Edinburgh: Churchill Livingstone; 1990.

184. Hurst LC, Badalamente MA. Nonoperative treatment of Dupuytren's disease. *Hand Clin.* 1999;15(1):97–107, vii.

185. Trojian TH, Chu SM. Dupuytren's disease: diagnosis and treatment. *Am Fam Physician.* 2007;76(1):86–89.

186. McGrouther DA. Dupuytren's contracture. In: Green DP, Hotchkiss RN, Pederson WC, eds. *Green's Operative Hand Surgery.* New York, NY: Churchill Livingstone; 1990.

187. Mullins PA. Postsurgical rehabilitation of Dupuytren's disease. *Hand Clin.* 1999;15(1):167–174, viii.

188. Zeuner KE, Molloy FM. Abnormal reorganization in focal hand dystonia—sensory and motor training programs to retrain cortical function. *NeuroRehabilitation.* 2008;23(1):43–53.

189. Das CP, Prabhakar S, Truong D. Clinical profile of various sub-types of writer's cramp. *Parkinsonism Relat Disord.* 2007;13(7):421–424. doi:10.1016/j.parkreldis.2007.01.009.

190. Waddy HM, Fletcher NA, Harding AE, et al. A genetic study of idiopathic focal dystonias. *Ann Neurol.* 1991;29(3):320–324. doi:10.1002/ana.410290315.

191. Hallett M. Pathophysiology of writer's cramp. *Hum Mov Sci.* 2006;25(4–5):454–463. doi:10.1016/j.humov.2006.05.004.

192. Cohen LG, Hallett M. Hand cramps: clinical features and electromyographic patterns in a focal dystonia. *Neurology.* 1988;38(7):1005–1012.

193. Fukaya C, Katayama Y, Kano T, et al. Thalamic deep brain stimulation for writer's cramp. *J Neurosurg.* 2007;107(5):977–982. doi:10.3171/jns-07/11/0977.

194. Rosenkranz K, Butler K, Williamon A, et al. Sensorimotor reorganization by proprioceptive training in musician's dystonia and writer's cramp. *Neurology.* 2008;70(4):304–315. doi:10.1212/01.wnl.0000296829.66406.14.

195. Zeuner KE, Hallett M. Sensory training as treatment for focal hand dystonia: a 1-year follow-up. *Mov Disord.* 2003;18(9):1044–1047. doi:10.1002/mds.10490.

196. Simpson DM, Blitzer A, Brashear A, et al. Assessment: botulinum neurotoxin for the treatment of movement disorders (an evidence-based review): report of the Therapeutics and Technology Assessment Subcommittee of the American Academy of Neurology. *Neurology.* 2008;70(19):1699–1706. doi:10.1212/01.wnl.0000311389.26145.95.

197. Molloy FM, Shill HA, Kaelin-Lang A, et al. Accuracy of muscle localization without EMG: implications for treatment of limb dystonia. *Neurology.* 2002;58(5):805–807.

198. Karp BI. Botulinum toxin treatment of occupational and focal hand dystonia. *Mov Disord.* 2004;19 suppl 8:S116–S119. doi:10.1002/mds.20025.

199. Chen R, Karp BI, Hallett M. Botulinum toxin type F for treatment of dystonia: long-term experience. *Neurology.* 1998;51(5):1494–1496.

200. Dressler D, Bigalke H, Benecke R. Botulinum toxin type B in antibody-induced botulinum toxin type A therapy failure. *J Neurol.* 2003;250(8):967–969. doi:10.1007/s00415-003-1129-6.

201. Griffin MJ, Bovenzi M, Nelson CM. Dose-response patterns for vibration-induced white finger. *Occup Environ Med.* 2003;60(1):16–26.

202. Bovenzi M. Hand-arm vibration syndrome and dose-response relation for vibration induced white finger among quarry drillers and stonecarvers. Italian Study Group on Physical Hazards in the Stone Industry. *Occup Environ Med.* 1994;51(9):603–611.

203. Pelmear PL, Taylor W. Hand-arm vibration syndrome: clinical evaluation and prevention. *J Occup Med.* 1991;33(11):1144–1149.

204. Coughlin PA, Bonser R, Turton EP, et al. A comparison between two methods of aesthesiometric assessment in patients with hand-arm vibration syndrome. *Occup Med (Lond).* 2001;51(4):272–277.

205. Kurozawa Y, Nasu Y. Current perception thresholds in vibration-induced neuropathy. *Arch Environ Health.* 2001;56(3):254–256. doi:10.1080/00039890109604450.

206. Zamyslowska-Szmytke E. Efficacy of vibration, electric current and thermal perception tests in diagnosis of hand-arm vibration syndrome. *Int J Occup Med Environ Health.* 1998;11(3):247–254.

207. Sakakibara H, Hirata M, Hashiguchi T, et al. Affected segments of the median nerve detected by fractionated nerve conduction measurement in vibration-induced neuropathy. *Ind Health.* 1998;36(2):155–159.

208. Pelmear PL. The clinical assessment of hand-arm vibration syndrome. *Occup Med (Lond).* 2003;53(5):337–341.

209. Bovenzi M, D'Agostin F, Rui F, et al. A longitudinal study of finger systolic blood pressure and exposure to hand-transmitted vibration. *Int Arch Occup Environ Health.* 2008;81(5):613–623. doi:10.1007/s00420-007-0255-3.

210. Poole K, Elms J, Mason HJ. The diagnostic value of finger systolic blood pressure and cold-provocation testing for the vascular component of hand-arm vibration syndrome in health surveillance. *Occup Med (Lond).* 2004;54(8):520–527. doi:10.1093/occmed/kqh108.

211. Koton J. [Prevention of hand-arm vibration syndrome by using antivibration gloves]. *Med Pr.* 2002;53(5):423–431.

212. Pelmear PL, Taylor W. Hand-arm vibration syndrome. *J Fam Pract.* 1994;38(2):180–185.

213. Buell C, Tobinick E, Lamp K. Resolution of chronic pain and fingertip ulceration due to hand-arm vibration syndrome following combination pharmacotherapy. *Arch Dermatol.* 2007;143(10):1343–1344. doi:10.1001/archderm.143.10.1343.

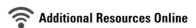 **Additional Resources Online**

CHAPTER 30

Stephen C. Johnson
Adrielle L. Fry

Eric T. Chen
Melinda S. Loveless

Disorders of the Lower Limbs

This chapter reviews the more common conditions that affect the lower extremities from the hip girdle to the feet as well as a brief review of the associated anatomy and physical examination. Each problem is reviewed within its region with the exception of osteoarthritis (OA), which will be discussed separately as the concepts are similar for all regions. While each region is reviewed separately, it is important to remember that through the kinetic chain (structures linked together by joints), a problem in one region can contribute to a problem in another. Thus, when examining a patient with a lower-extremity complaint, the entire kinetic chain should be taken into account. Conditions in the lower extremities can occur due to trauma, overuse, biomechanical deficits, or anatomical variants. Some of the conditions that are more specific to the active population will be reviewed in the Sports Medicine chapter (see Chapter 41).

HIP REGION

Pain around the hip girdle is a common musculoskeletal complaint. There are multiple sources that contribute to pain in the area including intra- and extra-articular pathology of the hip as well as referred pain from the lumbar spine, pelvis, peripheral nerves, or abdominal organs (1,2). It is important to first identify where the patient is experiencing pain, as patients will refer to pain in the buttock, lateral hip, and groin as "hip pain." A thorough history combined with a focused physical examination can often identify the source of pain, but diagnostic injections and imaging may be necessary clinical tools to identify or confirm a pain source in this region.

Anatomy

The hip girdle, including the bony pelvis and surrounding musculature, provides a link from the trunk to the lower body. It is important to be familiar with the bony anatomy as well as muscular attachment sites as these are common areas of pathology in the hip girdle. The synovial femoroacetabular (hip) joint is made of the cartilage-covered femoral head and bony acetabulum. The acetabulum is deepened by the fibrocartilage labrum, which serves to provide a fluid seal for the hip joint to maintain lubrication and hydrostatic pressure (3). The joint is surrounded by a capsule that attaches proximally at the acetabulum and distally in the region of the intertrochanteric line on the femur. The capsule is further reinforced by surrounding ligaments, which are the primary stabilizers in standing with the hip in extension (**Fig. 30-1**).

As in many regions of the body, there are more superficial and deeper layers of muscles that serve various functions.

Muscles in this region provide hip flexion, extension, abduction, adduction, internal rotation, and external rotation. Based on the position of the limb, the function of the muscle may vary. The pertinent muscles will be reviewed later in the chapter as they pertain to pathology.

Physical Examination

When evaluating pain located in the hip girdle, it is important to examine the lumbar spine and lower limb kinetic chain in addition to the hip (see Chapter 1). Inspection includes evaluation of posture and lower limb alignment in addition to evaluating gait to assess for a Trendelenburg, compensated Trendelenburg (ipsilateral trunk lean), or other abnormal gait pattern. Individuals with hip pain often demonstrate a compensated Trendelenburg pattern. Hip heights should also be compared by palpating the top of the iliac crests to evaluate for possible underlying scoliosis or leg-length discrepancy. Use of palpation is somewhat limited for hip examination as many structures of interest are deep; however, it can be valuable in individuals with pain over bony prominences where muscles/tendons attach especially the greater trochanter. It is also important to perform a neurologic examination including strength, sensation, and reflexes.

Hip range of motion (ROM) is tested with the hip flexed to 90 degrees (seated or supine) and with the hip in neutral with the knee flexed to 90 degrees (prone or supine). Flexion, extension, internal rotation, external rotation, abduction, and adduction are assessed. The tension of surrounding soft tissue structures (capsule, ligaments, muscles) changes with hip position, so there may be differences in rotational ROM with the hip flexed compared to neutral. Additionally, with active ROM, testing in the seated position is against gravity while it is gravity assisted in prone, which may lead to increased active ROM in prone. Lastly, total hip ROM and the distribution of motion into external versus internal rotation are variable between individuals (4,5). Therefore, it is important to examine and compare the ROM of both hips and to combine the ROM examination with special testing to further determine a possible source of pain. Additional evaluation of hip abduction ROM as well as hip abduction strength can be performed with the patient in a side-lying position.

There are multiple special physical examination maneuvers for the hips, which are reviewed in 🛜 **eTable 30-1**. All of the tests are considered positive if they reproduce the patient's groin and/or lateral hip pain. It is important to clarify during the examination where the patient experiences pain as other surrounding structures can also be stressed. For each test, the available sensitivity and specificity data are provided (6–8).

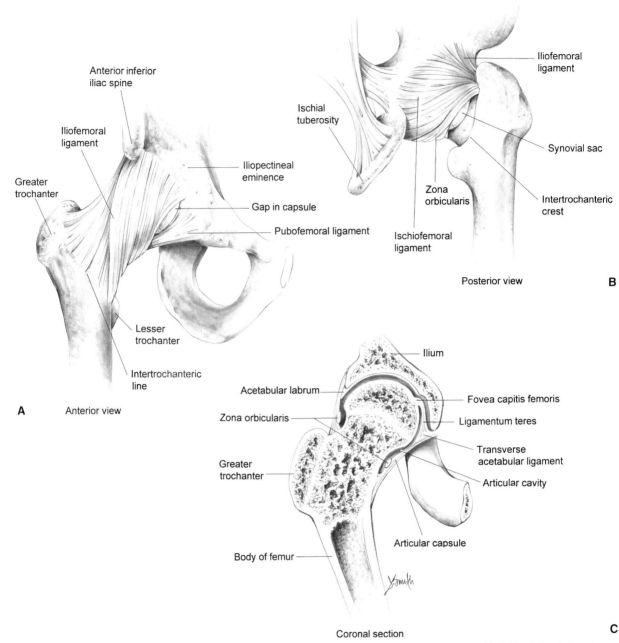

FIGURE 30-1. Anatomy of the hip joint and supporting structures. (Reprinted with permission from Callaghan JJ, Clohisy J, Beaule P, et al. *The Adult Hip.* 3rd ed. Philadelphia, PA: Wolters Kluwer Health, 2015.)

Intra-Articular Hip Pathology

Intra-articular problems involve the labrum, cartilage, and bone of the hip joint. Patients most commonly describe pain located in the groin, buttock, or lateral hip. However, pain from the hip refers to the anterior thigh, posterior thigh, knee, or even distal to the knee (9,10). The structural deformities reviewed below are all considered prearthritic hip conditions, but OA will be discussed separately at the end of the chapter.

Femoroacetabular Impingement and Developmental Dysplasia of the Hip

There are three forms of femoroacetabular impingement (FAI): cam, pincer, and mixed. Due to these abnormalities, repetitive collisions occur between the acetabulum and femur resulting

in impingement and potential damage to the surrounding structures. The cam deformity is an osseous prominence of the proximal femoral neck that results in decreased head-neck offset. Cam deformity produces shearing damage to the labrum and acetabular cartilage. The pincer deformity is overcoverage of the femoral head by the acetabulum. It results in degeneration and tearing of the labrum and contrecoup cartilage loss in the posteroinferior aspect of the hip joint. There can also be resulting ossification of the labrum. The mixed form of FAI involves both pincer and cam deformities. The etiology of FAI is unknown, but there are potential contributors including history of slipped capital femoral epiphysis (SCFE) or Legg-Calvé-Perthes disease (LCPD) as a child, hip dysplasia, and repetitive physeal stresses through trauma or sport participation during development. FAI is common in asymptomatic individuals, but exact rates are not known (11,12). Individuals with FAI present with groin pain that worsens with hip flexion, but pain can also be located at the lateral hip or buttock. There is often a sense of stiffness, mechanical symptoms of giving way or catching, and pain that can interfere with daily activities. On examination, there is positive flexion adduction internal rotation (FADDIR) or flexion abduction external rotation (FABER) test, pain with hip flexion, and often a loss of internal rotation range with the hip flexed.

On the other end of the spectrum, many young adults with complaints of hip pain have underlying developmental dysplasia of the hip (DDH). There is wide variety in the severity of dysplasia and symptoms. The dysplastic acetabulum is shallow, lateral, and anteverted with deficient coverage superiorly and anteriorly. The dysplastic femoral head is small with anteversion of the femoral neck and increased neck-shaft angle (coxa valga), and there is posterior displacement of the greater trochanter. The result is decreased contact area between the acetabulum and femoral head resulting in increased stresses. This may ultimately lead to degenerative changes and labral tears depending on the severity of dysplasia. Patients often present with groin pain that worsens with activity. If there is associated labral or chondral pathology, the patient may note mechanical symptoms. On examination, individuals with hip dysplasia often have increased hip ROM (13).

Initial evaluation for FAI or DDH is radiographs (x-rays) with anteroposterior (AP) view of the pelvis and lateral view of the hip (Dunn, lateral frog leg, or cross-table). These views evaluate for evidence of hip deformity (FAI, DDH, Legg Calvé-Perthes, SCFE), avascular necrosis (AVN), and hip OA (13–16).

FAI and DDH are considered prearthritic conditions with many studies demonstrating the progression to OA (17–19). Therefore, there has been a push to treat FAI and DDH surgically to reduce the progression to OA and prevent other secondary pathology. However, an initial trial of nonoperative treatment should be considered with treatment based on each individual's impairment. Treatments include education, activity modification, physical therapy, analgesic medications, and corticosteroid injections (20,21). If there is inadequate relief of symptoms with conservative management, surgical intervention may be pursued to correct the hip morphology and repair or resect damaged labrum and/or articular cartilage (13,20,21).

Acetabular Labral Tears

The acetabular labrum is a fibrocartilage structure that is triangular in cross section. It is attached to the acetabular rim at its base, and the hip capsule attaches to the exterior portion. The outer third of the labrum, at its attachment with the capsule, is well vascularized, but the inner portion is hypovascular. Additionally, due to the inferior mechanical properties of the anterosuperior labrum, most tears occur in that portion of the labrum. Tears of the labrum lead to reduced ability of the joint to maintain lubrication and hydrostatic pressure, which can lead to cartilage degeneration and OA. It is important to note that labral tears are commonly found in asymptomatic individuals (22).

Patients with labral tears often present with groin pain, but pain can be referred to the gluteal or trochanteric regions. Pain is worse with hip flexion and weight bearing. There is usually insidious onset, but in the case of trauma there may be more acute onset of pain. There can be mechanical symptoms such as giving way, clicking, catching, or popping in addition to pain.

Labral tears are classified as traumatic, degenerative, idiopathic, or congenital. It is important to ask about a history of pediatric hip pathology such as dysplasia, SCFE, or LCPD. Although classified as idiopathic, the majority (approximately 49% to 87%) of individuals with labral tears have findings of osseous dysmorphism consistent with FAI or dysplasia (3,23).

On examination, provocative hip tests that reproduce groin, lateral hip, and/or buttock pain suggest that pain is related to an intra-articular disorder. These tests include anterior impingement, FADDIR, and posterior impingement. The patient may have an antalgic gait or positive Trendelenburg sign. Radiographic evaluation begins with an AP view of the pelvis and a lateral view of the affected hip (Dunn, lateral frog leg, or cross-table). The next step in evaluation is often a diagnostic (anesthetic only) or diagnostic and therapeutic (anesthetic and corticosteroid) hip joint injection under ultrasound or fluoroscopic guidance. If this provides relief of the patient's usual hip pain, then magnetic resonance imaging (MRI) or magnetic resonance (MR) arthrogram can be obtained to evaluate for a suspected labral tear. MR arthrography is preferred over MRI to evaluate for labral tears, but 3.0-Tesla MRI has been found to be almost equivalent (24). The MRI can also provide a more detailed evaluation of the cartilage and may demonstrate evidence of early OA. Arthroscopy is the gold standard in evaluation of labral tears.

There have been few studies on nonoperative management of labral tears. However, it is recommended to trial a course of conservative management with activity modification, avoidance of provocative positions, physical therapy to strengthen weak hip muscles, and possibly an intra-articular corticosteroid injection first before pursuing surgery (23). Surgical treatment can be open or arthroscopic. Treatment of the labral tear can be a repair, refixation, or partial debridement. If there is FAI or other contributing bony pathology such as dysplasia, that must also be addressed to prevent future reinjury (3,23,25).

Osteonecrosis (AVN) of the Femoral Head

Osteonecrosis, also known as avascular necrosis (AVN), of the femoral head is caused by loss of blood supply and can result in destruction of the hip joint. The pathogenesis is likely multifactorial with contributions from genetics, chronic medical diseases, and other risk factors. Risk factors include trauma, excessive alcohol use, smoking, and corticosteroid use. Higher doses of steroid (≥2 g of prednisone or equivalent) increase the risk of developing osteonecrosis in the year after exposure (26). Small lesions may be asymptomatic, but most lesions progress to larger lesions and eventual collapse of the femoral head and destruction of the femoroacetabular joint. It is most common in individuals between the ages of 30 and 70 years (27,28).

When symptomatic, patients present with groin pain that may be referred to the buttock or knee. Examination may be normal, or there can be pain with internal rotation and reduced internal rotation range. Gait may be antalgic. Initial evaluation is with x-rays to evaluate for radiographic evidence of osteonecrosis and to rule out other pathology such as fracture or OA. X-rays may demonstrate crescent sign (subchondral lucency) or flattening of the femoral head. MRI is the gold standard for diagnosis and demonstrates edema in the femoral head. MRI can also rule out transient osteoporosis, which is a rare but self-limited condition that presents in the third trimester of pregnancy or in men in their fifth or sixth decades. On MRI in transient osteoporosis, there will be more diffuse bone marrow edema with spread into the femoral neck and intertrochanteric region.

Management of osteonecrosis is generally surgical, but for small or asymptomatic lesions, individuals may be managed nonsurgically with observation and protected weight bearing if needed. There is insufficient evidence to support the use of modalities or medications for treatment of osteonecrosis. Surgery consists of femoral head–preserving procedures or total hip arthroplasty. Femoral head–preserving procedures can be used in cases where there is no femoral head collapse. In older individuals, those with evidence of OA or involvement of the acetabulum, or in cases of femoral head collapse, total hip arthroplasty is recommended (28).

Extra-Articular Hip Pathology

Greater Trochanteric Pain Syndrome

Pain at the lateral hip, previously referred to solely as greater trochanteric bursitis, has been shown to have multiple etiologies. Therefore, the term greater trochanteric pain syndrome (GTPS) is used to encompass the many different underlying disorders. The disorder involves the tendons and bursae at the lateral hip, including the gluteus medius and minimus and three surrounding bursae (1,2,29). See **Figure 30-2** for posterior hip muscle anatomy and **Figure 30-3** for the anatomy of the lateral hip bursae and tendon insertions. The gluteus medius and minimus are thought of as the "rotator cuff of the hip" and exhibit similar pathology to the rotator cuff of the shoulder. The most common cause of GTPS is tendinopathy of the gluteus medius. Other pathology includes tendinopathy of the gluteus minimus, partial or full-thickness tears of the tendons, and calcific tendonitis. Tears are most commonly atraumatic, partial, and located at the undersurface of the tendon. Bursitis can be present but is rarely present in isolation. The involved bursae are the subgluteus maximus (trochanteric), subgluteus medius, and subgluteus minimus (2,29,30).

Patients present to clinic primarily with a complaint of lateral hip pain that can radiate into the lateral thigh but generally not distal to the knee. Most commonly, the pain increases when lying on the affected side. There can also be pain with weight bearing or prolonged sitting. On examination, there is tenderness to palpation over the greater trochanter. The patient may also have pain with the FABER test, a positive Trendelenburg sign, and weakness and/or pain with resisted hip external rotation with the hip flexed to 90 degrees and with resisted hip abduction with the hip extended (1,2).

X-rays are the first imaging study completed. These may show irregularity or enthesopathy of the greater trochanter or calcifications within the soft tissues that may represent calcifications within the tendons. X-rays are also useful in ruling out other pathology such as hip OA. To evaluate for pathology of the gluteal tendons and bursae, MRI or ultrasound can be obtained. MRI can also demonstrate pathology of the hip joint and may be preferred for that reason.

Conservative treatment is usually successful and consists of activity modification, analgesic medications, ice, heat, and physical therapy with a focus on hip girdle strengthening. If needed, steroid injections into the bursa can be utilized for short-term pain relief. Alternatively, percutaneous needle tenotomy with or without injection of autologous blood or platelet-rich plasma (PRP) can be considered. If conservative treatments fail, open or endoscopic surgical procedures are an option for treatment of tendinopathy, chronic bursitis, and tendon tears (1,2,29–31).

Snapping Hip (Coxa Saltans)

Snapping hip is an extra-articular hip disorder with external (coxa saltans externa) and internal (coxa saltans interna) variants. The more common external variety involves snapping of the posterior iliotibial band (ITB) or anterior aspect of gluteus maximus over the greater trochanter. As the hip is moved from flexion to extension, the snapping is noted laterally and can be visualized on examination. The internal variety is related to the iliopsoas tendon, and there are several mechanisms for snapping. Dynamic ultrasound imaging has found the most common etiology to be an interposition of a portion of the iliacus muscle under the psoas tendon during hip flexion, abduction, and external rotation. When the hip is then extended, the tendon snaps against the underlying bone as the iliacus muscle moves away. The other commonly proposed mechanism is snapping of the iliopsoas tendon over the iliopectineal eminence, but this has not been found frequently with ultrasound evaluation (32).

The primary symptom of snapping hip, aside from the snapping, is pain. In the absence of pain, no treatment is necessary. Usual conservative treatment involves addressing muscle tightness and improving neuromuscular control and muscle balance. If these treatments are unsuccessful, an injection of corticosteroid into the adjacent bursa can be performed. Surgery, lengthening or release of the affected tendon, is used in refractory cases (1,32,33).

Adductor Strain

Muscle strains are defined as tears in the muscle that can range from small mildly symptomatic tears to more significant partial tears and complete tears. The adductor longus muscle is the most frequently injured of the adductor muscles and is a common injury in soccer and ice hockey. Weak hip adductors, especially when compared to abductors, and prior adductor strain are risk factors for injury. On examination, there is tenderness to palpation along the adductor tendons or at their insertion on the pubis. Pain is reproduced with resisted hip adduction. X-rays can be used to rule out avulsion or fracture but are generally not necessary to make the diagnosis. If needed, MRI can be used to confirm the diagnosis and define the extent of injury and can assist in determining prognosis for return to play in injured athletes. Strains are graded from 1 to 3 with grade 1 involving minimal loss of strength and motion and grade 3 complete disruption of the muscle tendon unit. Rehabilitation begins with rest from both stretching and strengthening exercises until pain free with concentric adduction against gravity. The individual is then progressed through a strengthening program to regain normal function. To reduce the risk for initial injury or reinjury, an adductor strengthening program should be incorporated into preseason training for athletes (34,35).

Muscles of the Gluteal Region

A Superficial dissection

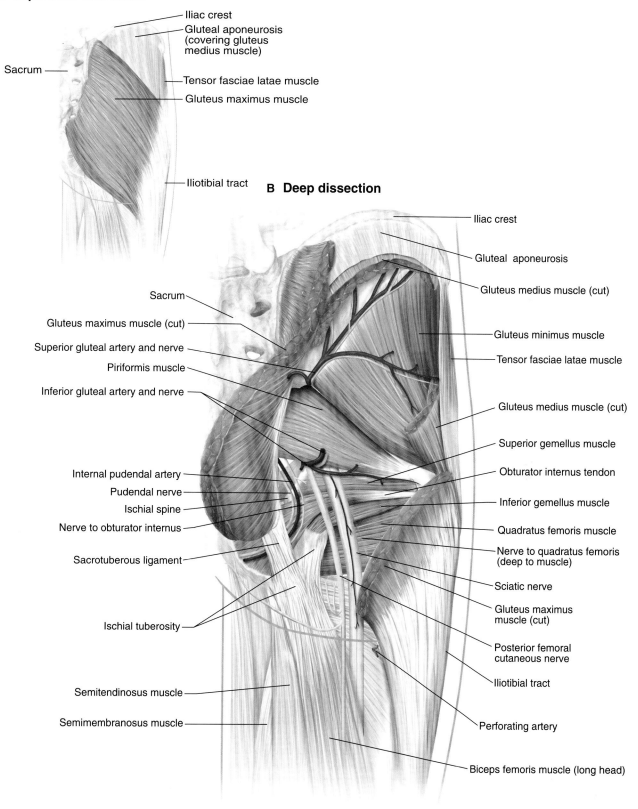

Iliac crest

Gluteal aponeurosis (covering gluteus medius muscle)

Sacrum

Tensor fasciae latae muscle

Gluteus maximus muscle

Iliotibial tract

B Deep dissection

Iliac crest

Gluteal aponeurosis

Gluteus medius muscle (cut)

Sacrum

Gluteus maximus muscle (cut)

Superior gluteal artery and nerve

Piriformis muscle

Inferior gluteal artery and nerve

Gluteus minimus muscle

Tensor fasciae latae muscle

Gluteus medius muscle (cut)

Superior gemellus muscle

Internal pudendal artery

Pudendal nerve

Ischial spine

Nerve to obturator internus

Sacrotuberous ligament

Obturator internus tendon

Inferior gemellus muscle

Quadratus femoris muscle

Nerve to quadratus femoris (deep to muscle)

Sciatic nerve

Gluteus maximus muscle (cut)

Ischial tuberosity

Posterior femoral cutaneous nerve

Iliotibial tract

Semitendinosus muscle

Semimembranosus muscle

Perforating artery

Biceps femoris muscle (long head)

FIGURE 30-2. Anatomy of the posterior hip muscles. (Reprinted with permission from Tank PW, Gest TR. *Lippincott Williams & Wilkins Atlas of Anatomy.* 1st ed. Baltimore, MD: Wolters Kluwer Health/Lippincott Williams & Wilkins; 2009.)

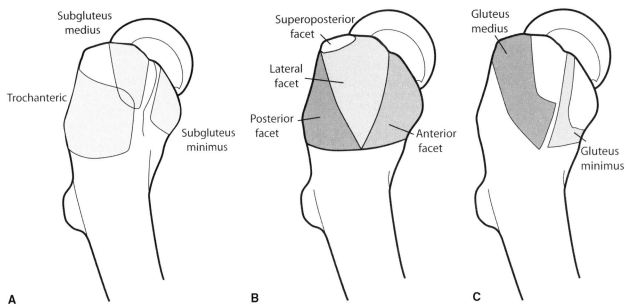

FIGURE 30-3. Anatomy of the greater trochanter bursae **(A)**, bony facets **(B)**, and tendon insertions **(C)**. (Reprinted from Domb BG. Partial-thickness tears of the gluteus medius: rationale and technique for trans-tendinous endoscopic repair. *Arthroscopy*. 2010;26(12):1697-1705. Copyright © 2010 Elsevier. With permission.)

Osteitis Pubis

Osteitis pubis is a condition of the pubic symphysis character-ized by joint disruption and pain. Pain is commonly located at the adductors, pubic symphysis, and lower abdomen and rarely radiates to the perineal region or scrotum. It has many etiologies, including sports, pregnancy, urologic or gynecologic procedures, and degeneration. It must be differentiated from osteomyelitis of the joint, which can occur spontaneously or after surgery. Mechanisms of injury to the pubic symphysis include repetitive stress from activity or increased stress related to pathology of the sacroiliac joints or limited hip rotation.

Pain is usually worsened by hip flexion or rotation. On examination, pain is reproduced with palpation of the pubic symphysis. X-rays demonstrate irregularity of the joint, includ-ing widening, irregular contour of the articular surfaces of the pubic bones, and sclerosis. Bone scan can show increased uptake at the pubic symphysis. MRI shows marrow edema, joint fluid, and periarticular edema early in the disease course and subchondral sclerosis and osteophytes in chronic disease. MRI can also be used to evaluate for soft tissue pathology related to athletic pubalgia. Treatment consists of activity mod-ification, nonsteroidal anti-inflammatory drugs (NSAIDs), and physical therapy. Corticosteroid injections can be utilized to provide short-term pain relief. If conservative treatments fail, surgery such as partial wedge resection or arthrodesis of the pubic symphysis can be considered (35–37).

Pediatric Conditions

Slipped Capital Femoral Epiphysis

SCFE is the most common hip condition in adolescents. It is characterized by movement of the femoral neck metaphy-sis anteriorly and superiorly in relation to the capital femoral epiphysis due to weakness of the growth plate. It is more com-mon in males than females, approximately 1.5:1. It presents most commonly in males between age 11 and 14 and females between age 10 and 12, with average age at presentation 12.2

years (12.7 in males, 11.2 in females). With earlier onset of ado-lescence in recent years, the age of presentation has decreased. Rates of SCFE are also higher in adolescents who are Black, Hispanic, and Polynesian. Risk factors for SCFE include obe-sity, endocrine disorders, and rapid growth spurts (38,39).

Patients can present with severe acute onset of pain or more gradual and mild symptoms. Pain can be located in the groin, thigh, or knee. SCFE is classified as stable if the patient can bear weight on the affected lower extremity with or without support and unstable if he or she is unable to bear weight. On examination, the patient is limping and has an externally rotated hip. There is limitation in internal rotation of the hip, and when the hip is passively flexed, it moves into external rotation. X-rays are diagnostic, and an AP view of the pelvis and bilateral frog-leg lateral views should be obtained as up to 60% of cases are bilateral. On the AP view, a line is drawn along the superior aspect of the femoral neck, and on the lateral view, a line is drawn along the anterior aspect of the femoral neck. These lines should intersect the femoral head; in SCFE, they do not. The physis may also appear blurred or widened. Treatment is non–weight bearing and referral to an orthopedic surgeon for early surgical intervention. Early intervention improves prognosis and reduces the risk of osteo-necrosis, which occurs primarily in unstable SCFE. Even with treatment, the patient may develop FAI with cam deformity and limited hip flexion and internal rotation (39).

Legg-Calvé-Perthes Disease

LCPD is pediatric ischemic necrosis of the femoral head that leads to deformity of the femoral head. The cause is unknown, but the underlying pathology is disruption of the blood supply to the femoral head. Maternal smoking during pregnancy and low birth weight are risk factors (40). It presents most com-monly between the ages of 5 and 8 and is 3 to 5 times more common in males. Ten to fifteen percent of cases are bilateral. Affected children present with insidious onset of mild pain at the hip or knee and a limp. On examination, they may have limited ROM with internal rotation and abduction. In more severe disease, there is more restriction in motion, and there may be a leg-length discrepancy.

X-rays are used for initial evaluation, but MRI may be necessary to make the diagnosis early in the disease course. Conservative treatments include observation, ROM, or bracing. In more advanced cases or in older children, osteotomy is performed. Long-term prognosis is better in those with a younger age at presentation or with a spherical femoral head on x-rays at maturity. Those with aspherical or flattened femoral heads are at increased risk for developing early OA of the hip (41).

Apophyseal Injuries

Avulsion Fractures
Bony avulsion injuries occur in adolescent athletes between the ages of 11 and 17. The unfused apophysis is weak relative to the muscle and tendon; therefore, a rapid muscle contraction produces separation of the apophysis rather than a tendon or muscle tear. See **Table 30-1** for bone attachment sites for involved muscles. Symptoms include acute onset of sharp pain when sprinting, jumping, or kicking. There is often a pop, and pain limits activity including ambulation. On examination, there is tenderness over the injured apophysis, pain with passive stretching, and pain with activation of the involved muscle. An x-ray of the pelvis is used to confirm the diagnosis and determine the amount of displacement. It is often helpful to compare to the contralateral side. MRI can be obtained if x-rays are nondiagnostic. In general, referral to an orthopedic surgeon is recommended if there is more than 2 cm of displacement. Initial nonsurgical treatment includes rest, ice, and protected weight bearing with crutches if needed. When there is pain-free ambulation, a stretching and strengthening program is initiated. This is followed by higher-impact activities as tolerated. Healing takes 4 to 12 weeks (27,35,42,43).

Apophysitis
Apophysitis, inflammation of the tendon-periosteal junction, is similar in presentation to avulsion injuries without the acute onset. It results from overuse and most commonly involves the sartorius or rectus femoris. Symptoms include gradual onset of dull hip pain that worsens with activity. On examination, there is pain with palpation of the affected apophysis or with resisted muscle activation. Tight hip and thigh muscles are risk factors. X-rays may demonstrate apophyseal widening and can help rule out other pathology. MRI, if necessary, will show edema at the site of tendon attachment. Apophysitis is treated with rest, ice, and gradual rehabilitation with stretching and strengthening (27,42).

TABLE 30-1	Muscles Involved in Apophyseal Injuries and Their Bony Attachments
Bony Attachment Site	**Muscle(s)**
Iliac crest	Abdominal muscles
Anterior superior iliac spine (ASIS)	Sartorius
Anterior inferior iliac spine (AIIS)	Rectus femoris
Ischial tuberosity	Hamstrings
Greater trochanter	Gluteus medius, gluteus minimus
Lesser trochanter	Iliopsoas

THIGH

The anterior and posterior thigh are common sites for musculoskeletal injuries, such as quadriceps muscle contusion, quadriceps muscle strain, hamstring tendinopathy, and hamstring strain (44–47). Referred pain from the lumbar spine, sacroiliac joint, and the hip are also common (9). Stress fractures of the femur are a rare cause of thigh pain. This section focuses on quadriceps and hamstring injuries.

Anatomy
The thigh can be divided into three main regions: anterior, medial, and posterior.

The anterior compartment includes the quadriceps femoris and sartorius muscles. The quadriceps femoris muscle occupies most of the compartment. It is composed of four muscle bellies: the rectus femoris, vastus medialis, vastus lateralis, and vastus intermedius. The sartorius is the longest muscle in the body, crossing the quadriceps muscle obliquely from cranial to caudal and from lateral to medial, running along the anteromedial aspect of the thigh to the pes anserine (eFig. 30.1).

There are five adductor muscles that make up the medial thigh. The anterior layer originates superolateral on the pubis and includes the pectineus, adductor brevis, and adductor longus. The adductor longus is most superficial, covering the adductor brevis. The posterior layer consists of the large adductor magnus, which inserts more caudally and is composed of two muscle bellies, which converge distally. The fifth, and most medial, adductor muscle is the gracilis (eFig. 30.2).

The posterior compartment is made up of three hamstring (ischiocrural) muscles: the biceps femoris, semimembranosus, and semitendinosus. All three originate from the ischial tuberosity and insert distally onto the medial tibia (semimembranosus, semitendinosus) or fibular head (biceps femoris). The distal tendon of the semitendinosus forms the pes anserine along with the sartorius and gracilis tendons. The biceps femoris is composed of a long head and a short head. The long head arises from the conjoint tendon proximally and travels lateral to the semitendinosus. The short head originates from the distal linea aspera and joins the long head to form a common distal tendon before inserting on the fibular head. The hamstring muscles' main actions include flexion at the knee and extension at the hip (eFig. 30.3).

Physical Examination
The goal of physical examination is to determine the location of injury and to assess ROM and muscle strength. As with physical examination of other regions, a systematic approach to assessment of the thigh should include inspection, palpation, ROM, neurovascular examination, and special tests. The examination begins with observation and inspection of the patient with standing, with walking, and while lying supine (anterior and medial thigh) or prone (posterior thigh). Palpation should be performed relevant to the area of injury. Active movements including lumbar flexion, lumbar extension, hip flexion, hip extension, knee flexion, and knee extension should be assessed followed by passive movements of the hip and knee. A neurologic examination should include testing of the lumbosacral myotomes and manual muscle testing of the hip and knee. Sensory examination should also be carried out for the L2-S1 dermatomes and testing the sensory distributions

of the obturator nerve, femoral nerve, lateral cutaneous nerve of thigh, and posterior cutaneous nerve of the thigh.

Special Tests

The popliteal angle may be used as a measure of hamstring flexibility. The popliteal angle or knee extension angle is measured with the patient supine and the hip flexed to 90 degrees. The examiner extends the knee until firm resistance is met while the hip is kept at 90 degrees. This can also be performed with the patient actively extending the knee. The popliteal angle is the angle between the lower leg and an imaginary line extending up from the flexed femur (48).

Quadriceps Contusion

Quadriceps contusion is a common injury in contact sports such as football and basketball. Sports that involve a ball traveling at high speed, such as lacrosse and field hockey, also have a high incidence (45). A quadriceps contusion is defined as an external blow to the anterior, medial, or lateral thigh in the area of the quadriceps femoris muscle belly (49).

Patients often report a direct blow to the anterior thigh followed by anterior thigh pain. There may be associated swelling. Physical examination confirms a localized area of tenderness. There is often increased pain with passive stretch and active contraction. The degree of passive knee flexion after 24 hours has been used to grade severity (50). Grade 1 (mild) injuries have localized tenderness on examination, greater than 90 degrees of knee flexion, no alteration in gait, and ability to do a deep knee bend. Grade 2 (moderate) injuries have swelling and tender muscle mass on examination, ≤90 degrees of knee flexion, antalgic gait, and inability to perform a knee bend, climb stairs, or rise from a chair without severe pain. Patients with a grade 3 (severe) injury have a markedly swollen and tender thigh and may have an associated knee effusion. Knee flexion is ≤45 degrees, and patients walk with a severe limp and prefer crutches (50). The severity of the contusion determines prognosis with mild injuries returning to sport in several days, while severe injuries may require a several weeks to return to play.

A quadriceps contusion is a clinical diagnosis based on the history and physical examination. Rarely is advanced imaging necessary unless quadriceps tendon rupture is suspected or if planned aspiration of a hematoma is being considered. X-rays are typically unremarkable in the acute setting. MRI will show edema throughout the involved muscle (51).

Treatment of quadriceps contusions initially consists of rest, ice, compression, and elevation (RICE) to limit or control hemorrhage. The knee is rested in a flexed position to maintain quadriceps muscle length, to provide compression to the underlying hematoma, and to limit knee stiffness (45). Immobilizing the knee in 120 degrees of flexion immediately after injury for the first 24 hours may be advantageous and shorten the time to full recovery and return to play (52). NSAIDs are often avoided for the first 48 to 72 hours to decrease further bleeding risk. For moderate to severe contusions, there is a risk of rebleed that is highest in the first 7 to 10 days. Precautions must be taken to avoid overstretching, heat, alcohol, and massage. When permitted by pain, the next stage of rehabilitation focuses on restoring pain-free ROM. Once full pain-free ROM at the hip and knee is restored, quadriceps strengthening and functional rehabilitation of the lower extremity begins. This is followed by a gradual return-to-play protocol. For mild to moderate injuries, a full recovery should be expected within 4 weeks of injury (49).

Complications are rare but should be considered in patients with prolonged recovery. A thigh hematoma may calcify resulting in myositis ossificans (MO). Incidence rates range from 9% to 20% of thigh contusions (53). The risk of developing MO is higher in moderate to severe contusions and in the setting of inappropriate initial treatment of the contusion with heat and massage. Rebleeding may also increase the risk of developing MO (45,53). MO typically presents as a painful, indurated mass that later becomes firm. Symptoms include increased morning pain, pain with activity, and night pain. MO can be seen on x-rays as early as 2 to 4 weeks following injury (45). Most patients regain full knee and hip motion and return to play without residual pain (45). Rarely, persistent symptoms may warrant surgical excision. This is performed once the mass is mature, typically not earlier than 6 months to 1 year (45,49,50).

Quadriceps Strain

The hamstrings, followed by the quadriceps, are the most frequently strained muscle groups among amateur and professional athletes. Muscle strains account for about 20% of all sport practice injuries with nearly half of all strains occurring within the anterior and posterior thigh (45). The strongest risk factor is a recent history of prior quadriceps strain. Fatigue may also increase susceptibility (54). Strains often occur following a sudden forceful eccentric contraction of the quadriceps during sprinting, jumping, or kicking. Strains are most common in the rectus femoris, which is more susceptible to strain as it crosses two joints (hip and knee) (45). Strains occur more commonly in the distal quadriceps muscle at the distal myotendinous junction of the rectus femoris but also occur frequently in the proximal rectus femoris. Distal rectus femoris strain injuries have a better prognosis as proximal rectus femoris injuries involving the central tendon have a significantly longer rehabilitation interval (55).

Patients may localize pain anywhere along the quadriceps muscle belly and walk with an antalgic gait. Swelling may be evident initially, and ecchymosis often develops within the first 24 hours. Palpation along the injured muscle should be performed, and knee flexion strength should be assessed in both the sitting and supine positions. Quadriceps muscle strains can be graded by degree of muscle fiber disruption, pain, quadriceps strength, and the presence or absence of a palpable defect (**Table 30-2**) (56).

Most strains do not require imaging, but MRI and ultrasound can be used to evaluate for partial or complete rupture. If the central tendon of the rectus femoris is involved on MRI, a significantly longer rehabilitation course is expected (55). A staged rehabilitation protocol, like the one described previously for quadriceps contusions, is recommended.

Hamstring Strain

Hamstring strains are the most common muscle strains (44,45,54,57). In professional athletes, acute hamstring strains account for up to 12% to 15% of all injuries (58). There is a high rate of recurrence with one in three athletes suffering recurrence often in the first 2 weeks after return to sport (44,45).

TABLE 30-2	Quadriceps Strain Grading System			
Grade	Fiber Disruption	Pain	Strength	Physical Exam
1	Minor	Mild	None or minimal loss	No palpable muscle defect
2	Severe	Moderate	Moderate loss	May feel palpable muscle defect
3	Complete	Severe	Complete loss	Palpable muscle defect

Modified by permission from Springer: Kary JM. Diagnosis and management of quadriceps strains and contusions. *Curr Rev Musculoskelet Med.* 2010;3(1–4):26–31. Copyright © 2010 Humana Press.

There are two distinct types of hamstring strains. Type I hamstring strains most commonly involve the long head of the biceps femoris at the proximal muscle-tendon junction. Type I injuries occur with high-speed running during terminal swing phase as a result of eccentric contraction of the hamstring muscle to slow the swinging limb in preparation for foot strike (44,59). Type II injuries commonly involve the proximal free tendon of the semimembranosus (60). Type II injuries occur during high kicking, dancing, or slide tackling due to excessive lengthening of the hamstring while the hip is flexed and knee extended. Recovery from type II injuries is often prolonged compared to type I (61).

Patients with hamstring strain often describe sudden onset of sharp, "twinge-like" posterior thigh pain. Type II injuries may result in an audible "pop." Athletes may be unable to continue activity and often avoid hip and knee flexion creating a stiff-legged gait (44,62).

During physical examination, inspection may reveal ecchymosis distal to the injury site. Direct palpation may localize the injury, and a palpable defect may be felt with complete ruptures. Passive straight leg raise and passive hip flexion with knee extension are used to assess flexibility. Pain with passive knee extension is expected with hamstring strain. Knee flexion and hip extension strength are assessed with the patient prone. Assessment should include the contralateral limb for comparison (44,62). Hamstring strains are classified into three grades based on the amount of musculotendinous unit disruption (**Table 30-3**) (45,63).

Hamstring strains are a clinical diagnosis, and generally advanced imaging is not needed for diagnosis. X-rays are not recommended unless there is concern for ischial avulsion injury. MRI may be obtained to differentiate between partial

TABLE 30-3	Hamstring Strain Grading System		
Grade	Fiber Disruption	Strength	Physical Exam
1 (mild)	<5%	None or minimal loss	No palpable defect
2 (moderate)	Partial tear	Moderate loss	May feel palpable muscle defect
3 (severe)	Complete rupture	Complete loss	Palpable muscle defect and/or hematoma

Modified from Zarins B, Ciullo JV. Acute muscle and tendon injuries in athletes. *Clin Sports Med.* 1983;2:167–182. Copyright © 1983 Elsevier. With permission.

and complete rupture and to rule out other injuries. As a result of edema, high signal intensity on T2-weighted MR images is seen within and around the affected hamstring muscle (64). On ultrasound, edema can also be visualized most commonly at the myotendinous junction (65).

Three phases of rehabilitation for hamstring strains has been described. Phase I involves RICE with the goal of decreasing pain, reducing edema, preventing scar formation, and regaining neuromuscular control. Isolated resistance training is avoided, and all exercises are performed within a protected ROM avoiding excessive stretching. Phase II includes increasing ROM, adding eccentric resistance exercises, and progressing neuromuscular training. Phase III begins when the athlete has full strength in the hamstring muscle and can jog forward and backward at 50% maximum speed without pain. Phase III adds sport-specific exercises (44). Return to play varies based on the type and grade of hamstring strain ranging from 8 days up to 50 weeks with type II injuries taking longer on average (44,62).

The use of corticosteroids in the treatment of hamstring strains has not been widely studied but is generally avoided as little is known regarding potential adverse effects. Overall, the limited data available for the use of PRP for the treatment of hamstring strain demonstrate no significant benefit compared to traditional rehabilitation for return to play or reinjury rates (66–70).

Hamstring Tendinopathy

The incidence of proximal hamstring tendinopathy (PHT) is unknown but thought to be more common in sprinters, long-distance runners, and endurance athletes (71). Tendinopathy is a chronic degenerative condition. Risk factors include overuse and weak hamstring musculature (44). The semimembranosus is the most commonly affected of the hamstring tendons (71).

Symptoms present insidiously with gradual increase in posterior thigh pain. The pain is usually described as a "tightness" in the posterior thigh or buttock near the ischial tuberosity. Symptoms are worse with sitting and during repetitive activities, such as running, that involve eccentric hamstring contraction. On physical examination, patients with PHT often have tenderness over the ischial tuberosity at the hamstring origin. Active hamstring stretch testing has been described with pain localizing to the hamstring origin. In subjects with PHT, loss of strength with knee flexion and hip extension is not expected (44,62).

MRI has higher sensitivity than does ultrasound for PHT. MRI findings include increased tendon cross-sectional area, increased signal heterogeneity at the hamstring origin, and sometimes reactive bony edema (72). On ultrasound, PHT shows tendon thickening, hypoechoic regions of tendon, and sometimes calcifications (72).

Eccentric exercise has been shown to be effective in the treatment of tendinopathy in general, and observational studies support its use for PHT (44,73,74). A small outcome study suggests that ultrasound-guided proximal hamstring tendon PRP injection is effective for the treatment of PHT (75). Larger, controlled studies have not been done to corroborate this treatment effect. Image-guided corticosteroid injections have shown improved pain levels and improved function at 1 month (76) and 21 months (72). However, corticosteroids are controversial as tendinopathy is a degenerative and not inflammatory process; thus, the use of an anti-inflammatory lacks face validity. Corticosteroids may also suppress tenocyte activity and collagen synthesis and increase the risk of tendon avulsion. There are limited data describing return-to-play guidelines for patients with PHT (44).

KNEE

Anatomy

The knee is the largest synovial joint in the body, formed collectively by the superior tibiofibular, patellofemoral, and tibiofemoral joints (77). The majority of flexion and extension occurs at the tibiofemoral joint. The menisci facilitate this articulation by deepening the surface area of the tibial plateau and improving tibiofemoral congruence. The cruciate ligaments provide AP stability to the knee and are named by the position of their distal insertions onto the intercondylar area. Anteriorly, the patellofemoral joint helps to facilitate flexion and extension; as the knee moves from extension into flexion, the contact between the patellar facets and femoral condyles increases to accommodate for increased stress experienced in full knee flexion (77) (**Fig. 30-4**).

Medial and lateral stability of the knee is achieved through static and dynamic stabilizers. The superficial medial collateral ligament (MCL) is the primary static stabilizer of the

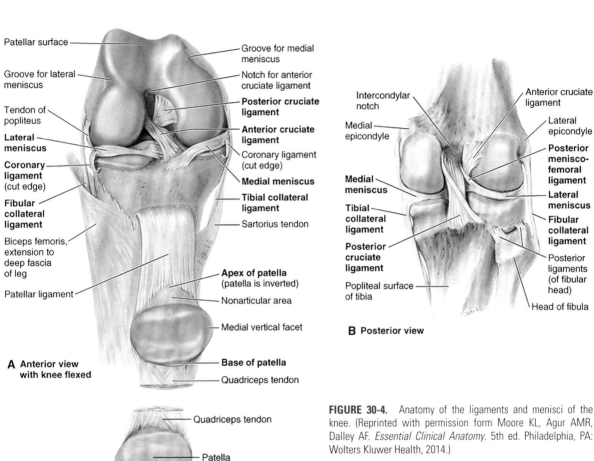

FIGURE 30-4. Anatomy of the ligaments and menisci of the knee. (Reprinted with permission form Moore KL, Agur AMR, Dalley AF. *Essential Clinical Anatomy*. 5th ed. Philadelphia, PA: Wolters Kluwer Health, 2014.)

medial knee, while the sartorius, gracilis, and semitendinosus, known collectively as the pes anserine tendon, serve as the primary dynamic stabilizers of the medial knee (78). The lateral ligamentous complex provides static stabilization to the lateral knee and consists of the lateral collateral ligament (LCL), popliteofibular, fabellofibular, and arcuate ligaments. Finally, the ITB provides dynamic lateral stabilization; it runs posterior to the lateral retinaculum and has distal insertions onto both the lateral femoral condyle and the tibia at Gerdy's tubercle (79).

Posteriorly, the popliteal fossa gives rise to several clinically important anatomic structures around the knee. The boundaries of the popliteal fossa are formed by the distal hamstring muscles and the proximal heads of the medial and lateral gastrocnemius. Important neurovascular structures that run through this fossa include the popliteal artery and vein, the tibial and common fibular nerves (CFNs), and medial and lateral sural nerves.

Physical Examination

Physical examination of the knee begins with inspection of the lower limb. The alignment of the knee as well as the position and tilt of the patella should be evaluated. Generalized or localized swelling may be present. Inspection of muscle girth should be compared side to side and will help to reveal subtle signs of muscle atrophy. Next, palpation of the knee is helpful to localize sites of pain and tenderness, as well as detecting swelling or effusion. Attention should be paid to palpate specific structures including the joint lines, patellar facets, superficial ligaments and tendons, and bony attachment sites. The clinician should take note of warmth or erythema around the knee, which may indicate local inflammation. Side-to-side comparison is particularly useful for detecting asymmetric swelling or effusion. The ballottement test uses one hand to milk fluid from the suprapatellar pouch while the other hand presses down on the patella. The patella's springing back indicates the presence of a larger effusion. Both active and passive ROM of the knee should be evaluated. Approximately 135 degrees of knee flexion and up to 5 to 10 degrees of hyperextension is normal (80). While ranging the knee through flexion and extension, the movement and tracking of the patella should be assessed. The clinician may observe the patella tilt laterally, anteroposteriorly, or rotate during ROM of the knee. Any loss of ROM may be due to a variety of causes including joint effusion, loose body, meniscal injury, or arthritic change. Increased ROM or increased laxity may indicate ligamentous injury.

A comprehensive knee examination also includes manual muscle testing at the hip, knee, and ankle. Manual muscle testing of the knee focuses primarily on knee flexors and extensors. Knee extension can be tested with the patient seated. Knee flexion can be tested with the patient prone or seated. Refer to 🛜 **eTable 30-2** for a summary of the special testing available for the knee with note of the pathology being tested, description of the test, and the sensitivity and specificity (80).

Ligamentous Injuries

Anterior Cruciate Ligament Injury

Most anterior cruciate ligament (ACL) injuries are noncontact, usually occurring during the act of landing or during a plant-and-cut maneuver (81). Several biomechanical and neuromuscular control factors have been identified as risk factors for ACL injuries, including increased knee abduction angle and knee abduction moments, reduced hip and knee flexion during cutting movements, increased knee valgus and internal rotation of the tibia, and increased quadriceps to hamstring activation ratio (82).

ACL injuries tend to be painful, and patients are unable to continue with activity following the injury. They will often report a "pop" or "crack," and feeling of the knee "going in and out of the socket." There is typically tenderness along the lateral joint line and restricted ROM. An effusion is often present and occurs almost immediately after injury. Special testing may reveal increased laxity and anterior translation of the tibia.

Initial imaging modalities should include AP and lateral x-rays of the knee to rule out acute fractures. Tibial eminence fractures and avulsion fractures of the tibia, also known as Segond fractures, are considered pathognomonic radiologic findings for ACL injuries. MRI is the imaging modality of choice in diagnosing ACL injuries and is 94% sensitivity and 100% specific for ACL tears (83).

Initial management focuses on controlling pain, swelling, and inflammation. This is followed by strengthening of the quadriceps, hamstrings, hip extensors, abductors, and calf muscles while also working on pain-free ROM. Debate remains regarding whether ACL injuries should be managed surgically or nonsurgically. One study demonstrated equivalent outcomes at 2 years when comparing surgical to nonsurgical management of acute ACL tears (84). Surgical repair may be favored when coexisting ligamentous or meniscal injuries are present or in an active patient who desires to return to cutting or jumping sports. In either case, the rehabilitation program should focus on minimizing swelling, restoring ROM, and normalizing gait mechanics.

Posterior Cruciate Ligament Injury

Injuries to the posterior cruciate ligament (PCL) generally occur due to hyperextension of the knee, a posteriorly directed force to the tibia on a flexed knee, forced hyperflexion of the knee, or knee dislocation. While only accounting for about 2% to 3% of sports-related knee injuries, PCL injuries have been reported in up to 40% of trauma patients with a knee effusion (85).

PCL injuries often present with vague and nonspecific knee discomfort. Acute injuries may present with effusion, stiffness, and pain in the posterior aspect of the knee. Pain may be exacerbated with squatting or kneeling. Patients may not complain of instability, unless there is concurrent ACL or MCL injury. The physical examination may reveal diminished ROM in knee flexion. Special testing may reveal increased laxity with posterior tibial translation.

Initial workup begins with x-ray examination of the knee. These views should include AP, lateral, notch, and sunrise views. Identification of a PCL avulsion injury is important because early operative repair of PCL avulsion injuries is associated with better outcomes (86). MRI remains the imaging modality of choice for diagnosing acute PCL injuries. MRI has been reported to have a sensitivity of 100% and specificity of 99% in detecting acute PCL injuries (87).

Partial PCL tears usually occur in isolation and do well with conservative nonsurgical management. Initial management focuses on reducing pain and inflammation followed by ROM and strengthening exercises. A rehabilitation program specifically targeting eccentric strengthening of the hamstring and quadriceps muscle groups may be beneficial (88).

Management of complete PCL tears begins with a period of immobilization in full extension and partial weight bearing for 2 to 4 weeks. After the initial period of immobilization, the patient can progress to full weight bearing and begin a progressive rehabilitation program focusing on quadriceps strengthening, closed kinetic chain, and open kinetic chain exercises. Most patients with complete PCL injuries who are managed conservatively return to their prior level of function at 3 months (86). However, patients who continue to have pain or are unable to return to prior level of function should be referred for surgical consultation.

Medial Collateral Ligament Injury

The MCL is one of the most commonly injured ligaments in the knee. The mechanism of MCL injury is typically a valgus stress to the knee; patients may report a direct blow to the outer aspect of the knee associated with a pop or tear and acute pain or tenderness along the medial aspect of the knee. An effusion may be present depending on time since onset of the injury. Valgus stress test should be performed on both the affected and unaffected knee to assess for laxity. This test should be repeated at both 0 and 30 degrees of knee flexion; increased laxity with 0 degrees of knee flexion may be suggestive of additional injuries of the knee including the cruciate ligaments or posterior capsule (89).

The need for initial imaging with plain films should be assessed based on the Ottawa Knee Rules: age 55 or older, tenderness at the fibular head, isolated patellar tenderness, inability to flex the knee greater than 90 degrees, and inability to bear weight for four steps immediately and at evaluation. Additionally, in the case of a contact injury, imaging is recommended. In most cases where isolated MCL tear is suspected, advanced imaging with MRI is not required. However, in cases where complete MCL tear is suspected, MRI may be useful for classification and treatment planning (89,90). Some authors have also recommended MRI in all patients with laxity greater than 10 mm to diagnose other intra-articular injuries (91).

Most MCL injuries can be managed conservatively. Conservative management focuses on early ROM and progressive strengthening exercises. Anti-inflammatory medication and ice may help to control initial pain and inflammation. A hinged knee brace can provide additional stability. Operative treatment may be indicated depending on the location and extent of MCL injury, most commonly in situations involving complete disruption of the ligament (90). Surgical consult may also be considered in the setting of large bony avulsion, tibial plateau fracture, complete tibial side avulsion in athletes, or presence of intra-articular ligamentous entrapment (89).

Lateral Collateral Ligament and Posterolateral Corner Injury

The posterolateral ligamentous complex provides lateral stability to the knee. LCL injuries rarely occur in isolation, and there must be concern for posterolateral corner (PLC) injuries, which involve other structures in the posterolateral ligamentous complex. Most PLC injuries occur due to acute trauma related to motor vehicle accident or sports injuries (92). When LCL and PLC injuries do occur, they are often associated with concomitant ACL or PCL injuries (93). The typical mechanism of injury occurs when a posterolateral or varus force is directed at the knee while the knee is in or near full extension (92).

Patients may complain of feeling the knee giving way into hyperextension or instability with twisting, pivoting, or cutting movement (92). There may be tenderness over the posterolateral knee or over the fibular head. Patients may demonstrate an abnormal gait pattern, favoring a flexed knee to avoid hyperextension during stance phase (94). Varus stress test should be performed at both 30 and 0 degrees. If instability is present at 0 degrees, additional ligamentous injuries may be present. Testing of the cruciate ligaments should also be performed.

Standard AP and lateral x-rays of the knee should be obtained to rule out fractures. Varus stress x-rays may be helpful to quantify the amount of lateral compartment varus gapping (95). MRI is the imaging modality of choice as it has been shown to be highly sensitive and specific for detecting injuries to the LCL and posterolateral structures of the knee (93).

Most LCL and PLC injuries with less than 10 mm of varus stress gapping can be managed nonoperatively. Published rehabilitation protocols call for an initial period of immobilization for 4 to 6 weeks, followed by progressive weight bearing, strengthening, and ROM (96,97). Patients with more than 10 mm of varus stress gapping should be referred for surgical repair, as these patients tend to have poor functional outcomes, persistent instability, and increased degenerative changes when managed nonoperatively (95,96,98).

Meniscus Injuries

The menisci are semilunar cartilage structures in the medial and lateral tibiofemoral compartments whose purpose is to deepen the surface area of the tibial plateau, allowing the tibia to receive the femur while improving tibiofemoral congruence (77). They also act to transfer loads across the knee joint and absorb shock during dynamic joint movements (99). Meniscal tears can be classified as acute or degenerative. Acute meniscus injuries are usually associated with trauma such as twisting or deep squatting. Degenerative meniscal tears are usually nontraumatic and considered part of the same disease process as OA of the knee (100).

Patients with either acute or degenerative meniscus tears will complain of knee pain associated with catching or locking. There may be medial or lateral joint line pain and tenderness on examination. Pain may be provoked with deep knee flexion. Special test maneuvers such as the McMurray test, Thessaly test, and the Apley grind test may be positive (80).

Initial imaging with weight-bearing x-rays of the knee is helpful for detecting OA and other possible bony sources of knee pain, such as fracture or tumor. MRI is sensitive and specific for detecting meniscal injuries and should be obtained for acute meniscus injuries to determine extent and type of tear (101). The use of MRI when degenerative meniscus injury is suspected should be reserved for cases where conservative management has failed and surgical intervention is considered (102).

Initial treatment is aimed at reducing symptoms of pain and inflammation. Rest, ice, and NSAIDs can be used for pain relief. Management of acute tears without mechanical symptoms and degenerative meniscus tears is generally non-operative. Patients should complete a rehabilitation program that includes strengthening, low-impact aerobic exercises, and neuromuscular re-education (103). Simple tears and tears in the peripheral vascular "red zone" are thought to have better healing potential than complex tears and tears in the central avascular "white zone." Acute tears with mechanical symptoms should be referred for surgical consultation. Surgical options include arthroscopic meniscal repair, meniscal debridement, and partial meniscectomy depending on the location and type of tear.

Baker's Cyst

Baker's cysts, also known as popliteal cysts, are found in the medial popliteal fossa and formed by distension of the gastrocnemius-semimembranosus bursa (104). Baker's cysts are known to communicate with the joint capsule and are thought to be an extension of the posterior joint capsule itself (105). Accumulation of fluid within the cyst is hypothesized to occur due to a one-way valve mechanism and allow for normalization of intracapsular pressure in the setting of joint effusion due to intra-articular pathology (104). Baker's cysts are commonly associated with meniscus injuries, ACL tears, chondral lesions, OA, rheumatoid arthritis, and gout (106,107).

Patients present with posterior knee swelling associated with vague posterior knee discomfort. These cysts may be an incidental finding in the setting of underlying knee pathology. Baker's cysts are usually round, smooth, and easily palpated on the medial aspect of the popliteal fossa. Other causes of popliteal masses include benign or malignant tumor, popliteal artery aneurysm, deep vein thrombosis, meniscal cyst, and ganglion cyst. Other disease processes such as osteochondromatosis, pigmented villonodular synovitis, and synovial sarcoma are also possible (104). On occasion, Baker's cysts can rupture and present acutely with calf pain and swelling. In this setting, clinicians should rule out deep vein thrombosis, pseudothrombophlebitis, and superficial thrombophlebitis, as these conditions can present in a similar manner and could potentially require more aggressive intervention.

MRI remains the gold standard in diagnostic imaging of masses around the knee. Baker's cysts appear as well defined and unilocular and extend posteriorly behind the knee. High-intensity signal indicating edema in adjacent soft tissues on T2 weighted images is suggestive of popliteal cyst rupture (108). Ultrasound offers a low cost and accurate alternative modality to MRI in identifying Baker's cysts. However, ultrasound is not reliable for intra-articular evaluation, and MRI should be used in cases where identification of underlying intra-articular pathology is desired (109).

Initial management of Baker's cysts is conservative and includes supportive measures targeted at controlling pain and inflammation. Ultrasound-guided aspiration of the cyst combined with either intra-articular or intra-cystic corticosteroid injection is commonly employed (110,111). Patients who fail to respond to conservative management or have recurrent symptoms may consider surgical intervention. There are a variety of surgical approaches employed in treating Baker's cysts, which include treating the underlying primary knee pathology, eliminating the valve mechanism arthroscopically, or suturing the communication altogether (104).

Patellofemoral Pain Syndrome

The term patellofemoral pain syndrome (PFPS) is used to describe anterior knee pain caused by overuse in the setting of altered biomechanics, malalignment of the lower extremity, and muscular imbalance at the hip and knee (112). PFPS is estimated to account for between 25% and 40% of all knee problems seen in sports medicine clinics. While PFPS occurs in patients of all ages, peak prevalence occurs in young, active patients between ages 12 and 17 (113).

Patients with PFPS present with gradual onset anterior or retropatellar knee pain that is worse with activities such as squatting, hopping, or jogging. This may be associated with report of knee crepitus or stiffness. Pain is usually absent when the patellofemoral joint is not loaded. There may be pain with patellar grind maneuver and functional testing with single-leg squat may reveal poor femoral shaft control.

PFPS is primarily a clinical diagnosis. Imaging of the knee may reveal other sources of pain or other knee pathology but is not specific for PFPS. The utility of MRI is limited due to poor diagnostic accuracy for low-grade cartilage lesions, poor correlation between lesions seen on MRI and patellofemoral symptoms, and high prevalence of cartilage lesions in asymptomatic athletic patients (114).

The mainstay of treatment for PFPS is a targeted physical therapy program focusing on strengthening the quadriceps and hip abductors (114). Patellar taping and patellar mobilization are adjunct modalities that have also been shown to be effective in reducing pain due to PFPS. Prefabricated foot orthotics with medial arch supports have also been shown to be beneficial (115). NSAIDs are often prescribed for short-term pain relief; however, evidence for their efficacy is limited (116).

Patellar Tendinopathy

Patellar tendinopathy refers to clinical overuse of the patellar tendon and is a common cause of anterior knee pain. This condition has also been referred to in the past as patellar tendinitis, which inaccurately characterizes the condition as patellar tendinopathy is a chronic noninflammatory, overuse injury (117). Patellar tendinopathy affects patients who expose the extensor mechanism of the knee to repeated and intense stress and has been well reported in athletes (118). The proposed pathogenesis of this condition is secondary to mismatch between ongoing microtrauma and the rate of tendon self-repair (97).

Patients with patellar tendinopathy usually present with anterior knee pain that is worse with activity and prolonged knee flexion. Pain can be localized over the anterior knee at the proximal origin of the patellar tendon on the inferior pole of the patella. Initial imaging with x-rays may show commonly associated findings, such as intratendinous calcifications or enthesophytes. Ultrasound and MRI are useful to demonstrate pathology of the tendon, including thickening, irregularity, and partial tears (119).

Treatment of patellar tendinopathy begins with activity modification and a period of relative rest to reduce pain. The mainstay of treatment is a rehabilitation program that emphasizes eccentric strengthening of the quadriceps (120). Evidence does not support the use of NSAIDs in the treatment of chronic overuse tendinopathies, as these conditions are noninflammatory in nature (121). There may be short-term benefit with corticosteroid injections, but these should be used with caution as the evidence supporting their use in patellar tendinopathy is mixed, and use may increase the risk for tendon rupture (122,123). The evidence for the use of PRP, extracorporeal shock wave therapy (ESWT), and injection with sclerosing medications remains mixed, and additional investigation is needed (120).

Iliotibial Band Friction Syndrome

ITB friction syndrome is an overuse condition that can cause lateral knee pain and is commonly seen in athletic populations (124). The ITB is the lateral thickening of the fascia of the thigh and is formed proximally by the fascia of the gluteus maximus and tensor fascia latae (TFL) (79). Distally, the ITB has insertions onto the lateral femoral condyle and the proximal anterolateral tibia at Gerdy's tubercle (79). Importantly, bursae underlie each of these distal tendinous insertions.

ITB friction syndrome is thought to be caused by repetitive anterior-posterior motion of the ITB over the lateral femoral condyle, leading to inflammation of the distal ITB and underlying bursae (124). Commonly occurring in runners and cyclists, training errors such as a rapid increase in training load, hill running, excessive striding, and increased mileage have been associated with injury (125). Biomechanical factors such as excessive genu varum, excessive internal tibial torsion, foot pronation, and hip abductor weakness have also been implicated (124).

Patients with ITB friction syndrome will present with lateral knee pain localizing to the lateral femoral condyle or to Gerdy's tubercle. Pain may occur during or just after repetitive flexion-extension activities. On examination, there is often tenderness over the corresponding bony insertions. The Noble compression test, in which pressure is applied over the lateral femoral condyle as the knee is passively flexed and extended, will reproduce pain at the lateral knee. The Ober test, performed with the patient side-lying and the knee flexed, may also demonstrate tightness of the ITB as the hip is passively brought into extension.

Imaging is not required for diagnosis of ITB friction syndrome. However, x-rays of the knee may be helpful for ruling out an alternative cause of knee pain such as OA. MRI may also be helpful to confirm the diagnosis if symptoms are refractory to conservative management.

Management is similar to that of most overuse injuries. Initial management begins with activity modification and rest. Ice can be used to reduce pain and inflammation. NSAIDs, when used in conjunction with other nonsurgical modalities, may be helpful in reducing pain (126). Local corticosteroid injection into the bursa has been shown to be effective (127). Rehabilitation should include a program that focuses on stretching of the ITB, TFL, and gluteus maximus along with strengthening of core and hip abductor muscles. Other interventions such as manual therapy, myofascial release, and use of a foam roller may be helpful. Obvious biomechanical derangements should be corrected and are patient specific.

Bursitis

There are many bursae that surround the knee joint (**Fig. 30-5**). Several of these can be affected as reviewed below.

Prepatellar Bursitis

Patients with prepatellar bursitis present with localized pain, swelling, and tenderness at the anterior knee. The two main bursae involved in prepatellar bursitis are the subcutaneous prepatellar bursa and the superficial infrapatellar bursa. Clinicians must differentiate between septic and nonseptic bursitis when presented with prepatellar bursitis. Both septic bursitis and nonseptic bursitis usually arise as a result of trauma. In the case of septic bursitis, trauma causes direct inoculation of bacteria into the bursal space. Miners, gardeners, carpet layers, and mechanics are at higher risk for developing both septic and nonseptic bursitis due to frequent, repeated blunt trauma to the anterior knee. Crystal-induced bursitis may also occur but usually presents in patients with a prior history of gout.

Differentiating between septic and nonseptic bursitis can be challenging based on clinical presentation alone. Bursal tenderness is more common in septic bursitis than nonseptic bursitis, about 90% and 45% of patients, respectively. Peribursal cellulitis and fever are also common findings in septic bursitis. Local warmth and erythema are usually present in both septic and crystal-induced bursitis but are rarely present in nonseptic traumatic or idiopathic bursitis (128). Ultimately, aspiration of the bursa should be performed and aspirate sent for Gram's stain, cell count, crystal analysis, and culture if there is clinical concern for septic bursitis.

Nonseptic bursitis should be treated with a compressive dressing and a 10- to 14-day course of NSAIDs (128). Corticosteroid injections are effective in reducing bursal effusion related to prepatellar bursitis but should be used with caution due to risk of skin atrophy, infection, and chronic pain over the injection site (129).

Pes Anserine Bursitis

Patients with pes anserine bursitis present with pain and tenderness over the medial aspect of the knee at the insertion of the pes anserine tendons on the tibia. Patients often report pain that is worse with ascending or descending stairs, localized tenderness at the pes anserine insertion and may occasionally report localized swelling. Diagnosis is based on clinical presentation, and additional imaging may not be necessary. Targeted physical therapy and corticosteroid injection to the pes anserine bursa have both been found to be effective therapies (130).

Osgood-Schlatter Syndrome and Sinding-Larsen-Johansson Syndrome

Osgood-Schlatter syndrome (OSS) and Sinding-Larsen-Johansson syndrome (SLJS) are two sources of anterior knee pain that occur most commonly in pediatric populations. OSS occurs due to repetitive strain of the patellar tendon on the secondary ossification center of the tibial tuberosity, while SLJS occurs due to repetitive strain of the patellar tendon on the inferior pole of the patella (131,132). OSS is considered an apophysitis; however, debate remains over whether SLJS is a true apophysitis, periostitis, chronic tendinitis, or osteochondrosis (133,134).

OSS usually presents during a period of rapid growth in pediatric patients: 12 to 15 years for boys and 8 to 12 years for girls (135). SLJS is a much more uncommon condition but also occurs during adolescence between the ages of 10 and

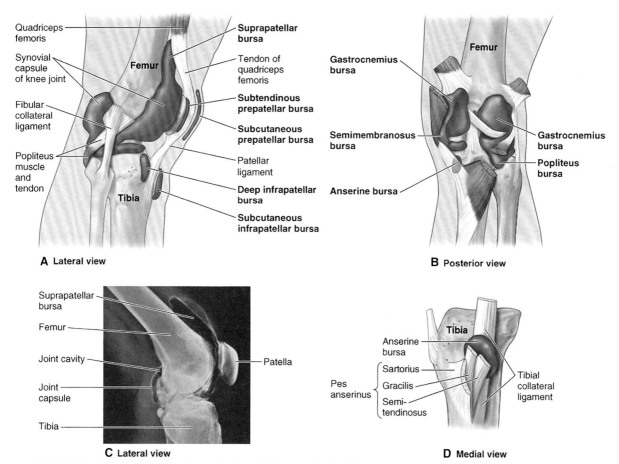

FIGURE 30-5. Anatomy of the knee bursae. (Reprinted with permission from Moore KL, Agur AMR, Dalley AF. *Essential Clinical Anatomy.* 5th ed. Philadelphia, PA: Wolters Kluwer; 2014.)

14 (133). Both conditions commonly occur in patients who are active or participating in sports (133). OSS and SLJS present with localized pain to either the tibial tuberosity or inferior pole of the patella, respectively. The onset of symptoms is gradual, starting with intermittent symptoms that progress to more constant pain. Pain is usually exacerbated by activity, particularly athletic activities involving jumping and deep flexion of the knee. Physical examination may reveal localized tenderness, swelling, and prominence over the tibial tuberosity or inferior patella. Pain may also be reproduced with resisted knee extension.

Both OSS and SLJS are clinical diagnoses; however, x-rays are helpful for ruling out other sources of pain such as acute tibial apophyseal fracture, infection, or tumor. On x-ray, irregularity of the apophysis with separation or fragmentation from the tibial tuberosity is consistent with OSS. In SLJS, lateral x-rays show speckled calcification in the patellar tendon adjacent to the lower pole of the patella (134). Ultrasound is a useful modality for imaging the infrapatellar tendon and may reveal patellar tendon swelling, intratendinous calcifications, as well as avulsion injuries (136).

Initial treatment of OSS and SLJS is similar. Reduction of pain and inflammation with relative rest from exacerbating activities, application of ice, and use of oral NSAIDs is recommended. Protective knee padding may be helpful in avoiding

local trauma and irritation. Casting is no longer recommended due to risk of quadriceps wasting (137). Physical therapy should focus on strengthening and flexibility of the quadriceps, hamstrings, ITB, and gastrocnemius (138). For 5% to 10% of patients, symptoms may persist despite conservative measures; surgical intervention may be considered after skeletal maturity occurs (137).

LOWER LEG

Lower leg injuries are a common presenting complaint in musculoskeletal practices. This section focuses on exertional leg pain (ELP), as it is particularly common in endurance and recreational athletes, as well as other common pathology in the lower leg. A retrospective study of over 2,000 running injuries reported an incidence of 12.8%. Another study of cross-country athletes reported that 82.4% had a prior history of ELP (139,140). ELP is defined as pain distal to the knee and proximal to the ankle joint that is associated with exertion (141). The etiology of the pain is often musculoskeletal, vascular, or neurologic in origin. The differential diagnosis of ELP includes medial tibial stress syndrome (MTSS), tibial bone stress injury (TBSI), chronic exertional compartment syndrome (CECS), popliteal artery entrapment syndrome (PAES), and peripheral entrapment neuropathies (140,142).

A thorough history, physical examination, and appropriate use of diagnostic testing are necessary for accurate diagnosis and treatment.

Anatomy

There are two compartments in the lower leg. These are the anterolateral and posteromedial compartments. They are separated by a strong interosseous membrane running from the medial tibia to the fibula and the posterior crural intermuscular septum, which is lateral to the fibula. The anterolateral compartment can be subdivided into the anterior compartment and lateral compartment separated by the anterior crural intermuscular septum, located between the extensor muscles and the fibular (peroneal) muscles. The posterolateral compartment can be subdivided into two compartments (or groups of muscles)—the superior and deep posterior compartments—separated by the transverse crural intermuscular septum (**Fig. 30-6**).

The anterolateral compartment of leg is located between the anterior edge of the tibia and the lateral aspect of the fibula. This compartment houses muscles involved in dorsiflexion, supination, and pronation of the ankle (📶 **eFigs. 30-4 and 30-5**). It is subdivided into the anterior compartment and lateral compartment. The anterior compartment muscles, from medial to lateral, are the tibialis anterior, extensor hallucis longus, and the extensor digitorum longus. The anterior neurovascular bundle, consisting of the anterior tibial artery/vein and deep fibular (peroneal) nerve, is located deep to the tibialis anterior. The lateral compartment muscles are the fibularis (peroneus) longus and the fibularis (peroneus) brevis. The lateral neurovascular bundle, consisting of the superficial fibular nerve (SFN), runs along the fibular shaft proximally and between the fibularis longus and extensor digitorum longus distally.

The posteromedial compartment of the lower leg is larger than the anterolateral compartment. It contains muscles acting as plantar flexors of the ankle and toes. The compartment is subdivided into the superficial and deep posterior compartments. The superficial posterior compartment muscles, from superficial to deep, are the gastrocnemius (medial and lateral heads) and soleus. Together these muscles are referred to as the triceps surae (📶 **eFig. 30-6**). The deep posterior compartment, muscles from medial to lateral, are the flexor digitorum longus, tibialis posterior, and flexor hallucis longus (📶 **eFig. 30-7**).

Physical Examination

Assessment of the lower leg begins with observation of a patient's limb alignment, normal gait pattern, and standing posture. Inspection of the ankle during static standing can reveal factors that increase the risk of developing lower leg problems such as pes cavus and pes planus. Functional pes planus is better evaluated during normal gait. Inspection also includes observation of any fascia defects with obvious muscle herniation. Palpation should be performed along the posteromedial tibia assessing for diffuse tenderness as found in MTSS or more localized tenderness in TBSI. Depending on the clinical presentation, palpation should also include the anterior tibia and fibula. ROM should be assessed at the lumbar spine, hip, knee, and ankle. Increases or limitations in joint ROM in the ankle and hip may increase the risk of developing lower leg injuries. A neurologic examination should include testing of the lumbosacral dermatomes and myotomes with specific testing of the ankle and foot. Sensory examination should also be carried out in the distribution of the superficial fibular, deep fibular, tibial, saphenous, and sural nerves. The vascular examination should include palpation of the popliteal, dorsalis pedis, and posterior tibial pulses.

Special Tests

The navicular drop test measures the difference in distance between the lower border of the loaded and unloaded navicular bone and the ground. The test is an indicator of midfoot pronation. There are no sensitivity or specificity data available. In two studies, the mean navicular drop distance was increased in runners with MTSS compared to asymptomatic athletes.

In one study, in patients suspected of having tibial stress fractures, a 128-Hz tuning fork was used to elicit pain by placing it on the anterior surface of the tibia (not at site of suspected fracture). Using bone scintigraphy within 30 days of the tuning fork test, it was found to be 75% sensitive and 67% specific (143).

Medial Tibial Stress Syndrome

MTSS, also known as shin splints, is most commonly defined as pain along the posteromedial border of the middle to distal thirds of the tibia that occurs during exercise, excluding pain from ischemic origin or stress fracture (144). In runners, the incidence of MTSS is between 13.6% and 20.0% (145). The exact cause of MTSS is unclear but may involve a periosteal traction reaction along the tibia from posterior compartment lower leg muscles (146–148). Studies show that patients with MTSS are less adapted than healthy controls to handle tibial loads (149). Low tibial bone density is found in MTSS patients compared with healthy controls (150). The decreased tibial bone density normalizes after recovery from MTSS (151). Thus, patients with low tibial bone density may not tolerate repetitive loading leading to MTSS or, alternatively, repetitive loading may lead to decreased bone density and ultimately MTSS.

MTSS is the most common cause of posteromedial tibial border pain in runners (142). The pain localizes to a diffuse region along the posteromedial border of the middle to distal third of the tibia. The patient usually reports pain that is absent at rest, begins with exercise, and may subside with continued exertion. As MTSS worsens, pain may not resolve during exercise and may be present after the activity ends (142). If pain is present at rest, TBSI or stress fracture must be ruled out (142,152). On physical examination, diffuse tenderness to palpation along the posteromedial border of the middle to distal tibia is the most sensitive finding (142). Intrinsic risk factors associated with MTSS include hyperpronation of the foot, female sex, and history of prior MTSS. Foot pronation can be evaluated using the navicular drop test (142,153).

In patients with uncomplicated MTSS, imaging is not indicated. If there is a concern for TBSI, imaging is necessary to rule out stress fracture. Plain radiography has limited value in the diagnosis of MTSS but may be helpful in ruling out stress fracture. Bone scintigraphy has historically been used in the diagnosis of MTSS but has been found to have a high false-positive rate, and its routine use in evaluating

Compartmental Organization of the Leg

A Orientation

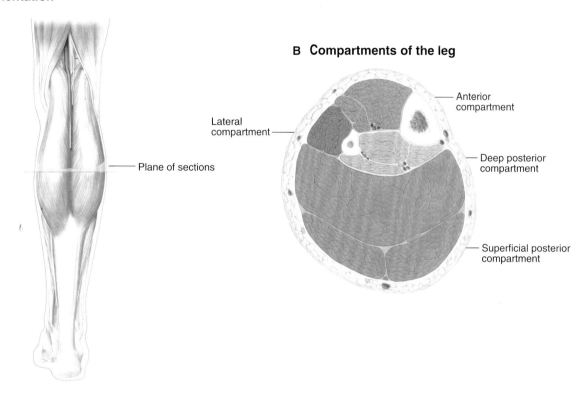

Plane of sections

B Compartments of the leg

Lateral compartment

Anterior compartment

Deep posterior compartment

Superficial posterior compartment

C Cross section

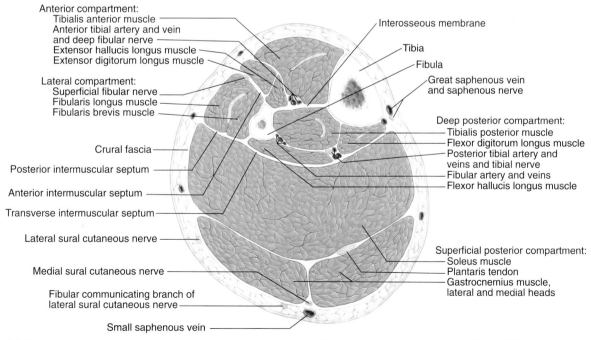

Anterior compartment:
Tibialis anterior muscle
Anterior tibial artery and vein and deep fibular nerve
Extensor hallucis longus muscle
Extensor digitorum longus muscle

Lateral compartment:
Superficial fibular nerve
Fibularis longus muscle
Fibularis brevis muscle

Crural fascia

Posterior intermuscular septum

Anterior intermuscular septum

Transverse intermuscular septum

Lateral sural cutaneous nerve

Medial sural cutaneous nerve

Fibular communicating branch of lateral sural cutaneous nerve

Small saphenous vein

Interosseous membrane

Tibia

Fibula

Great saphenous vein and saphenous nerve

Deep posterior compartment:
Tibialis posterior muscle
Flexor digitorum longus muscle
Posterior tibial artery and veins and tibial nerve
Fibular artery and veins
Flexor hallucis longus muscle

Superficial posterior compartment:
Soleus muscle
Plantaris tendon
Gastrocnemius muscle, lateral and medial heads

FIGURE 30-6. Cross-sectional anatomy of the left lower leg compartments. (Reprinted with permission from Tank PW, Gest TR. *Lippincott Williams & Wilkins Atlas of Anatomy.* 1st ed. Baltimore, MD: Wolters Kluwer Health/Lippincott Williams & Wilkins; 2009.)

MTSS is limited (154–156). MRI has been shown to accurately diagnose MTSS and distinguish between MTSS and TBSI (154). MTSS remains a clinical diagnosis, and diagnostic imaging should be used only when the diagnosis is in question (142,153).

Initial treatment of MTSS begins with activity modification. Aggravating activities must be avoided and biomechanical deficits addressed. If the navicular drop test is positive, overpronation should be treated (shoe wear, prefabricated or custom orthotics, taping, gait retraining). If an MRI has been completed, the grading scale developed by Fredericson (**Table 30-4**) can be used to guide length of rest and return to play (157). ESWT, combined with a graded running program, has been shown to shorten the duration of symptoms compared to control subjects (158). Rarely, when all conservative treatments have failed, surgery is indicated (142,153).

Tibial Bone Stress Injury

Bone stress injury may affect the cortical bone in the diaphysis or the cancellous bone in the metaphysis and epiphysis of long bones. The term TBSI is preferred over "stress fracture" as TBSI can occur in the absence of a true fracture on imaging (157). Diaphyseal TBSI has two types. The first affects the posterior tibial cortex and is thought to be due to compressive strain. The second affects the anterior tibial cortex and is due to tension strain (159). The pathophysiology is not well elucidated, but it has been proposed that repetitive strain to the tibia leads to microdamage of cortical or cancellous bone. This microdamage initiates a remodeling response by increasing osteoclastic activity before a deposition response (osteoblastic activity), which leads to weakening of the tibia and TBSI. TBSI occurs in patients with normal bone density, known as a fatigue-type stress injury, and in those with decreased bone mineral density, which is known as an insufficiency type stress injury. Fatigue-type injuries are more common in patients with decreased cross-sectional area of tibia and decreased lower leg muscle mass. Insufficiency-type injuries are more common among female athletes (140,160).

Athletes with TBSI present with well-localized tibial pain of insidious onset that worsens with activity. The defining feature of TBSI, which distinguishes it from MTSS, is pain after exertion that progresses to pain during exertion (157). In severe cases, pain can be present at night (160). Risk factors include recent increases in training intensity, frequency, and duration (140). In one study, running shoes over 6 months old were found to predispose to TBSI (161). In female athletes, risk factors for the female athlete triad (menstrual irregularities, disordered eating, and decrease in bone mineral density) should be assessed (140).

On physical examination, there is tenderness to palpation over a localized area of tibial bone. Swelling may or may not be present. The tuning fork test may elicit pain (143). Physical examination alone cannot rule out TBSI. Imaging is essential to the diagnosis. X-rays are recommended first as they may reveal a fracture, but sensitivity is low for TBSI. Use of bone scintigraphy and CT is limited due to low sensitivity (154). MRI is superior to other studies and may also help determine the management of TBSI (154,157).

The Fredericson MRI criteria (**Table 30-4**) are used to guide treatment. Grade III injuries require 6 to 9 weeks of nonimpact activity. Grade IV injuries are immobilized for 6 weeks in a cast, followed by 6 weeks of nonimpact activity (157). These recommendations hold true for most posterior diaphysis (compression side) TBSI's, but anterior (tension side) TBSI may take up to 6 months to heal with conservative treatments. In cases of delayed healing of anterior cortex TBSI, surgery may decrease recovery time. The most common procedure is intramedullary nailing with a return-to-play rate of 100% (159,162).

Preventative measures include screening for and treating the female athlete triad. Athlete and training staff education regarding symptoms of TBSI may decrease the time of symptom onset to diagnosis thereby improving prognosis (140). Vitamin D levels between 40 and 50 ng/mL have been shown to reduce the risk of TBSI (163). Prefabricated shock-absorbing insoles may also reduce the incidence of TBSI (164).

Chronic Exertional Compartment Syndrome

CECS in the lower leg(s) presents as pain brought on by activity and improved with rest. The cause is not well understood but involves an expanding compartment volume within a fixed fascial sheath resulting in increased compartment pressure that limits blood flow and compresses nerves (165). This may be due to impaired microcapillary capacity, abnormally increased blood flow, venous congestion, and edema (increased interstitial volume) (140,141,165). The pain caused by CECS is theorized to be related to muscle or nerve ischemia, direct stimulation of fascial and periosteal sensory nerves (direct pressure), and release of local kinins (140,141,165). The exact incidence is unknown as many patients simply modify their activities and do not present for evaluation. In athletes with undiagnosed lower leg pain, the incidence has been reported

TABLE 30-4	MRI Classification for MTSS and TBSI		
Grade	**Clinical Diagnosis**	**MRI**	**Rehabilitation**
1	Medial tibial stress syndrome	Periosteal edema on T2-weighted images only	2–3 wk nonimpact activity
2		Periosteal and bone marrow edema on T2-weighted images only	4–6 wk nonimpact activity
3	Tibial bone stress injury	Bone marrow edema on T1- and T2-weighted images +/- periosteal edema	6–9 wk nonimpact activity
4		Periosteal and bone marrow edema on T1- and T2-weighted images; Fracture line clearly visible on all sequences	6 wk of cast, followed by 6 wk of nonimpact activity

Modified from Fredericson M, et al. Tibial stress reaction in runners: correlation of clinical symptoms and scintigraphy with a new magnetic resonance imaging grading system. *Am J Sports Med.* 1995;23:472–481. Copyright © 1995 SAGE Publications.

to be between 14% and 27% (141). Males and females are equally affected, and the average age at diagnosis is between 26 and 28 years old (140). CECS affects lower leg compartments 95% of the time, but CECS in the thigh, forearm, and foot has also been described. CECS may occur in any of the four lower leg compartments (see **Fig. 30-6**). The anterior compartment (40% to 60%) and the deep posterior compartments (32% to 60%) are the most commonly affected, followed by the lateral compartment (12% to 35%), which frequently occurs with CECS of the anterior compartment. The superficial compartment is rarely involved (2% to 20%) (140).

Patients with CECS often describe symptom development after a specific volume of exertion. Symptoms may occur in any or all lower leg compartments and are bilateral in up to 82% of patients (141). The pain is described as a "fullness" or cramp-like sensation in the affected lower leg compartment. Neurologic symptoms (numbness, paresthesias, or weakness) may occur in the sensorimotor distribution of the nerve in the affected compartment. Symptoms stop immediately or soon after cessation of activity. As the condition worsens, recovery time after exertion may increase (140,141,166). In CECS, the physical examination is normal at rest. Following exertion, neurologic dysfunction in the sensorimotor distribution of the affected compartment nerve may be present. Stretching the muscles of the affected compartment may elicit pain. Edema has also been described (140,141,165). Fascial hernias may be present in CECS but are also seen in asymptomatic patients (140,167).

In patients with a convincing history of CECS, the diagnosis is confirmed with pre-exertional and postexertional intracompartmental pressure (ICP) testing. A side-port needle manometer is most commonly used. Static ICP measurements are taken at rest and then at 1 and 5 minutes postexertion. The modified Pedowitz criteria (**Table 30-5**) are often used for diagnosis although a recent meta-analysis suggests modifications to improve sensitivity and specificity (168,169).

Noninvasive testing methods are emerging (MRI, ultrasound, near-infrared spectroscopy), but further research is needed before they can be recommended for clinical use (140,165). Conservative treatment of CECS is typically activity modification and refraining from the aggravating activity. Limited evidence suggests that changing to a forefoot running technique may reduce symptoms (140). As described in two case reports, another nonsurgical treatment option is injection of botulinum toxin A into muscles of the affected compartments. There are not yet enough data to support widespread clinical use of botulinum toxin A for CECS (140). When conservative treatments fail, the mainstay of treatment for CECS is surgical fasciotomy with the best outcome obtained in isolated anterior compartment CECS (success range between 81% and 100%) (170).

Popliteal Artery Entrapment Syndrome

PAES involves anatomic or functional entrapment of the popliteal artery in the popliteal fossa. Anatomic PAES may occur due to an aberrant course of the popliteal artery with entrapment by several anatomic variants including the medial head of the gastrocnemius, accessory slip of the medial gastrocnemius, fibrous bands arising from the medial gastrocnemius, and the popliteus muscle. Other variants are also possible (171). Functional PAES is thought to occur due to entrapment from a hypertrophied gastrocnemius. PAES presents as pain in the proximal posterior calf with exertion. Associated signs include paresthesias in the tibial nerve distribution and less frequently calf swelling (172).

The physical examination is often normal at rest. A diminution of the tibial and dorsalis pedis pulse may be seen with passive ankle dorsiflexion and active plantar flexion with the knee extended, but these findings are also present in asymptomatic individuals (140,172).

Ankle brachial index (ABI) testing should be completed in the assessment of PAES. Provocation maneuvers (passive ankle dorsiflexion, active plantar flexion with knee extended) should also be done with ABI testing, looking for a decrease in the ABI. Conventional angiography and Doppler ultrasonography have been used in the past to evaluate for PAES. Both lack the ability to adequately define the surrounding anatomy. MRI with angiography (MRA) or CT with CT angiography (CTA) is preferred as they both allow assessment of the popliteal artery and soft tissue anatomy allowing for diagnosis of anatomic PAES (173). There is a high false-positive rate with advanced imaging for PAES with one small study of 13 asymptomatic patients showing a false-positive rate of 69% with MRA (174). The presentation of functional PAES has similarities to CECS, and compartment pressure testing should be considered if entertaining this diagnosis.

The mainstay of treatment for PAES is surgical. For anatomic PAES, numerous techniques have been described that involve mobilization of the medial gastrocnemius attachment or body. With functional PAES, the surgery is fasciotomy of the medial gastrocnemius with take-down of the soleus tibial attachments. If the popliteal artery is damaged, bypass surgery is preferred. Success rates have been reported close to 100% if the popliteal artery is intact (173). Return to play is gradual over about 6 weeks (140).

Lower Leg Peripheral Entrapment Neuropathies

Lower leg entrapment neuropathies most commonly involve the CFN, SFN, deep fibular nerve (DFN), or saphenous nerve (SN). Of these, CFN is the most common. CFN is often caused by compression of the CFN as it crosses the fibular neck (175). CFN has also been seen following tibiofibular joint dislocations and in runners due to repetitive inversion and eversion at the ankle. SFN, DFN, and SN are less common and not covered in this section. With entrapment neuropathies, symptoms are often present at rest but may increase with exertion.

On physical examination, neuropathy involving the CFN may present as weakness with ankle dorsiflexion, ankle eversion, and great toe extension (140,175). Sensory impairments are present over the anterolateral lower leg and the dorsum of the foot.

TABLE 30-5	Modified Pedowitz Criteria for CECS		
	Preexercise (Rest)	1 min Postexercise	5 min Postexercise
Static pressure (mm Hg)	≥15	≥30	≥20

Pre-exertional and postexertional physical examinations are helpful if symptoms are only present with activity.

Diagnostic evaluation may include electrodiagnostic testing. Electrodiagnostic testing should be employed when objective neurologic loss is seen on physical examination or when axonal damage is suspected. In the setting of a normal physical examination, electrodiagnostic testing may be of limited value (141). Diagnostic musculoskeletal ultrasound at the entrapment site may show dilation of the nerve proximal to the fibular neck (176). If clinical suspicion of common fibular neuropathy is high, and the ultrasound evaluation is normal, an MRI and/or MRI neurogram can be obtained to further define the surrounding anatomy and to assess the nerve for dilatation at the fibular neck (177).

In the absence of axonal damage and with a normal physical examination, conservative treatments can be tried. These can include an ultrasound-guided nerve block with hydrodissection at the entrapment site, neuropathic pain medications, and addressing modifiable causes such as running technique (141). In patients with axonal damage on electrodiagnostic testing, common fibular neuropathy decompression by surgical neurolysis with or without fascial release is recommended (175).

Medial Gastrocnemius Tear

Calf pain is a common complaint occurring frequently in recreational athletes. Males aged 40 to 60 years are at highest risk of injury to the triceps surae. In runners, master's athletes have a higher rate of injury (178). In calf muscle injuries, the medial head of the gastrocnemius is most commonly involved (179). Patients often present with pain and swelling in the calf. The location of injury is often at the fascial intersection of the medial gastrocnemius and soleus as they merge with the proximal Achilles tendon (180). For most gastrocnemius injuries, there is an acute, definable injury that occurs after sprinting or jumping. The knee is often extended while the ankle is flexed followed by a ballistic movement and eccentric contraction of the calf. This is contrasted by soleus injuries, which are often insidious onset in the setting of overuse (178).

On examination, there may be swelling, bruising, tenderness to palpation, pain with resisted plantar flexion, and a palpable or visible defect. Tenderness is often localized at the distal insertion of the medial head of the gastrocnemius into the proximal Achilles fascia. A Thompson's test should be performed to ensure the Achilles tendon is intact and not ruptured (181). Rarely, bleeding and hematoma from a medial gastrocnemius tear can lead to acute compartment syndrome. In these cases, evaluate for pain, paresthesias, pallor, pulselessness, and poikilothermia (178).

Imaging is not required for diagnosis. Diagnostic musculoskeletal ultrasound may be used to confirm the diagnosis and to determine the severity of damage (178). Depending on the severity of tear, return to play ranges from 3 to 4 weeks up to 3 to 4 months. Initial treatment includes RICE. The goal is to reduce hematoma formation and decrease swelling. In severe cases, a short period of crutch walking may be indicated. Compression sleeves may speed return to running by several days (182). Heel lifts often improve pain with walking following calf injuries. When pain has improved, progressing to standard eccentric calf raises or heavy slow resistance training (concentric/eccentric) have both been shown to be effective as a treatment (183). When the patient can walk without pain and perform single-leg calf raises with minimal pain, gradual return to running is indicated.

ANKLE

Ankle injuries are common presenting complaints to emergency rooms and physician offices with approximately 650,000 visits to the emergency room each year in the United States (184). The ankle joint is vulnerable to injury due to its weight-bearing function and construction of the articulation of the joint. Injuries to the ankle can affect athletes and sedentary persons alike, and a recent systematic review found the point prevalence of ankle pain in middle to older aged persons to be 24% of that population (185). Understanding the ankle joint from an anatomical perspective as well as some of the common conditions that can affect it is essential due to its high prevalence of pathology.

Anatomy

The ankle joint is made up of the distal tibiofibular articulation (tibiofibular syndesmosis) and the talocrural articulation (ankle mortise) (**Fig. 30-7**). The tibia and fibula are bound together by the syndesmosis, which is formed by the anterior inferior tibiofibular ligament, the posterior inferior tibiofibular ligament, and the interosseous membrane. The talus fits into the mortise formed by the tibia and fibula and is a wedge shaped bone that is narrower posteriorly than anteriorly. The dorsiflexed ankle is stable due to the wider anterior portion of the talus, and the plantar flexed ankle is less stable due to the narrow posterior talus allowing more movement. The ankle joint is supported by various ligaments with the strong deltoid ligament medially, and the anterior talofibular ligament, posterior talofibular ligament, and calcaneofibular ligament laterally (**Fig. 30-8**). The main motions of this joint are dorsiflexion and plantar flexion.

The other joint of the ankle region is the subtalar joint, which is the interface between the talus and calcaneus. There are three articular facets between the talus and calcaneus with the anterior and middle often congruous and the posterior being larger and separate. The sustentaculum tali forms the floor of the middle facet. The main ligament of this joint is the interosseous talocalcaneal ligament; it runs through the sinus tarsi, which is a canal between the articulations of the two bones. Four other ligaments are involved as well: the anterior, posterior, lateral, and medial talocalcaneal ligaments. The subtalar joint does not play a role in dorsiflexion or plantar flexion, but instead is crucial for inversion and eversion.

The most important tendon of the ankle is the Achilles tendon, which is formed by the gastrocnemius and soleus muscles. It attaches onto the calcaneus and is an important plantar flexor of the ankle. Other important muscles of the ankle—the tibialis anterior, tibialis posterior, and fibularis (peroneus) longus and brevis—insert further distally in the foot. These are discussed in the foot anatomy section.

Physical Examination

Assessment of the ankle joint should always begin with careful inspection and observation of the patient's static posture, gait, and shoe wear patterns. The patient should be examined with bare feet for better observation. The skin should be evaluated for any ecchymosis, erythema, pressure sores, calluses, and blisters.

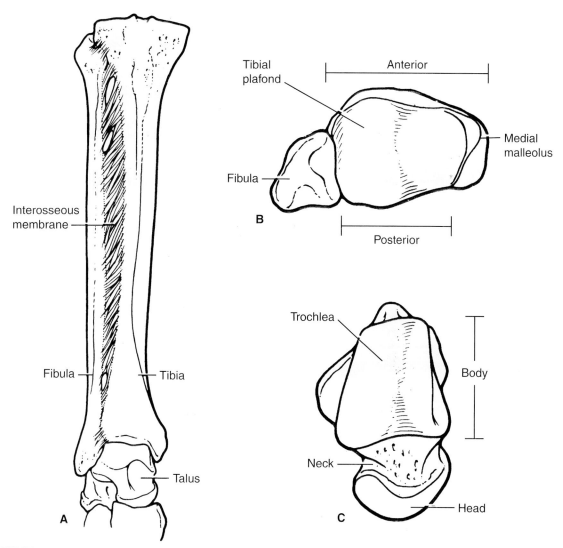

FIGURE 30-7. Bony anatomy of the ankle. Mortise view **(A)**, inferior–superior view of the tibiofibular side of the joint **(B)**, and superior–inferior view of the talus **(C)**. (Reprinted with permission from Court-Brown C, Heckman JD, McKee M, et al. *Rockwood and Green's Fractures in Adults*. 8th ed. Philadelphia, PA: Wolters Kluwer; 2014.)

The height of the medial arch should be noted, which can help place a patient into categories such as cavovarus or planovalgus alignment. This can be important when considering a differential diagnosis as each of these alignments have been associated with numerous complaints. Particular care should be placed on evaluating the alignment of the subtalar joint as well. There is a lot of overlap of foot and ankle conditions and they should often be examined together. Please see the foot section for further information on examination of the foot.

Next, palpation should be undertaken with a systematic approach. Bones, joints, and soft tissue structures of importance should all be palpated to determine if they are a source of pain. Observation of ROM of the ankle joint in dorsiflexion, plantar flexion, inversion, and eversion should be performed both with active and passive motion. Manual muscle testing should be performed for these motions as well. Neurologic and vascular evaluation should also be undertaken.

Lastly, special testing should be performed to help rule in and out pathology. Refer to 📶 **eTable 30-3** for a summary of the special testing available for the ankle with note of the pathology being tested, description of the test, and the sensitivity and specificity (186).

Achilles Tendinopathy

Tendinopathy is a general term to describe any condition in or around a tendon causing pain (187). Historically, the term "tendonitis" was used in this place and this term implies an underlying pathophysiology of inflammation. There has recently been research and evidence to suggest that degeneration of the tendon architecture, development of neovascularization, and some component of inflammation all contribute to the problem at hand, now often called tendinosis or tendinopathy as it will be called in this chapter (188). Injury to the Achilles tendon can result from overuse, poor foot and ankle biomechanics, or a combination. It can occur at one of three locations in the tendon: the mid-portion (2 to 6 cm proximal to insertion), at the insertion on the calcaneus, or at the myotendinous junction. The latter will not be a focus of this section; it often heals with rest and physical therapy by 4 to 6 weeks. There is a watershed area in the mid-portion of the

Ankle Joint and Joints of the Foot

A Medial view

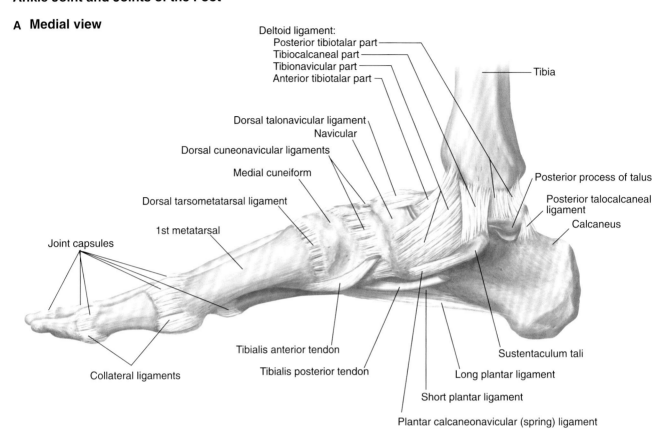

B Lateral view

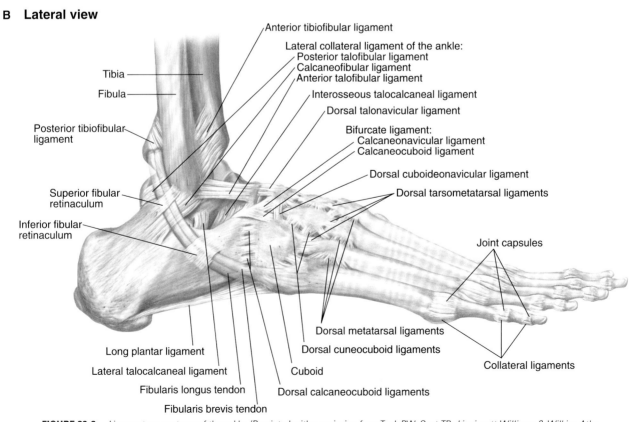

FIGURE 30-8.   Ligamentous anatomy of the ankle. (Reprinted with permission from Tank PW, Gest TR. *Lippincott Williams & Wilkins Atlas of Anatomy*. 1st ed. Baltimore, MD: Wolters Kluwer Health/Lippincott Williams & Wilkins; 2009.)

tendon that predisposes it to injury at this location (188). Insertional Achilles tendinopathy may be contributed to by an abnormal bony prominence on the posterior superior lateral aspect of the calcaneus known as Haglund's deformity.

On examination, swelling can be apparent at the area of pathology in the tendon. Pain is reproduced with palpation along the tendon, resisted heel raise, or by hopping or jumping. It is important to rule out a complete rupture of the tendon, which is treated differently and discussed later. Imaging can be used to supplement physical examination findings; MRI and ultrasound are often modalities of choice for investigation of the extent of tendon pathology. It is worth noting that neither of these imaging studies is 100% sensitive or specific and cannot reliably predict outcomes, so it is prudent to also use clinical suspicion (189).

The majority of patients can overcome a painful Achilles tendinopathy with conservative measures alone, although the evidence to support these measures is lacking. Treatment involves a period of rest, treatment of underlying biomechanical deficits, orthotic treatment with a heel lift or a controlled ankle motion (CAM) walking boot, and a stretching and strengthening program. There has not been substantial benefit shown in the use of NSAIDs for treatment of tendinopathies, but it could be considered as a short-term adjunct for analgesia (190). Steroid injections in and around the tendon have more recently fallen out of favor due to concern for weakening of the tendon and possible rupture as well as a lack of evidence for long-term benefit (191).

For the treatment of tendon disorders, it is often recommended to perform eccentric exercises. This concept began with Stanish et al. in 1986 for general tendon issues, and a specific program for Achilles tendinopathy was developed by Alfredson and published in 1998 (192,193). This program, which proved successful in rehabilitating painful Achilles tendinopathy, consisted of twice daily sets of eccentric exercises (slow heel lowering) done on the edge of a stair to allow full ankle ROM with gradual increase in loading weight over a 12-week course (190,193). This was later modified for individuals with insertional Achilles tendinopathy; unlike mid-portion tendinopathy, eccentric exercises for insertional tendinopathy should be done on a flat surface to avoid dorsiflexion (194). More recently, a strengthening program utilizing heavy slow resistance has been shown to be equally efficacious (183). Determining a program that works for patients and their lifestyle is a key component to their success and compliance.

If the interventions mentioned thus far are unsuccessful, ESWT, injection of sclerosing agents, tendon scraping, percutaneous tenotomy, injection of autologous blood or PRP, and surgery are other options. The body of literature evaluating these modalities is not robust (191). There is also no consensus on length of time to attempt conservative care prior to considering surgical referral (195).

Achilles Tendon Rupture

The rate of Achilles tendon rupture has been on the rise with peak incidence between 40 to 50 years of age. Around 80% of cases are related to sports or athletics (196). The location and function of the tendon combined with its mid-portion watershed zone make it susceptible to rupture. The American Academy of Orthopedic Surgeons (AAOS)

published guidelines for the diagnosis and management of acute Achilles tendon ruptures in 2010 (197). Diagnosis should be made on history and physical examination with reduced plantar flexion strength, Thompson's test, and palpable defect being their recommended examination maneuvers. They were unable to recommend for or against the use of MRI or ultrasound to confirm the diagnosis due to lack of sufficient evidence (197).

Management of acute ruptures is controversial. While studies show a greater rerupture rate for nonoperative management, they also demonstrated a higher complication rate with surgical repair, including deep infection, scar complaints, and sensory nerve disturbances (198). However, with early mobilization, there may be no difference in rerupture rate for both management options (199). There is no consensus on how to set up an early mobilization program as multiple studies have different time frames and recommendations for when to start exercising and weight bearing, but the evidence does appear to demonstrate that most approaches are beneficial (199–201). More traditional approaches utilize 8 weeks in a cast or walking boot for nonoperative management and postoperatively; this is followed by 4 weeks with a heel lift (202).

Chronic Achilles tendon ruptures can be managed by either operative repair or nonoperative management similar to acute ruptures, with more in favor of operative repair to improve function (181). In a low-demand patient or in those who cannot undergo surgery, an ankle foot orthosis (AFO) can be used to increase long-term function (181).

Tibialis Posterior Tendinopathy and Dysfunction

The tibialis posterior originates from the lateral posterior aspect of the tibia, medial aspect of the body of the fibula, and interosseous membrane of the leg (203). The tendon courses under the medial malleolus and into the foot, with the majority of the tendon inserting on the navicular tuberosity and a smaller portion onto the tarsal bones except the talus. It functions as a plantar flexor and invertor of the foot as well as a strong supinator of the subtalar and midtarsal joints. Additionally, it dynamically supports the medial longitudinal arch (204). Posterior tibial tendon dysfunction is the most common cause of acquired flat foot deformity in adults (205,206).

The tibialis posterior tendon has an area of hypovascularity at the mid-portion just distal to the medial malleolus that is an area of vulnerability (207). However, there is often pathology distal to this area as well (208). Tendon changes can be caused by chronic degeneration or an acute trauma such as puncture or laceration wounds and severe eversion ankle sprains (209,210). Other factors such as inflammatory arthritis, diabetes mellitus, obesity, prior local steroid exposure, and biomechanical factors such as equinus or pes planus have been known to contribute to tibialis posterior tendon dysfunction (207,208,211,212).

Tibialis posterior tendon dysfunction presentation has been divided into stages (213). Stage I is medial ankle pain, mild swelling, possibly painful heel raise, and importantly, no deformity. There will likely be pain and swelling along the tendon with painful resisted inversion. Stage II includes progressive flattening of the medial longitudinal arch and an abducted midfoot, but the hindfoot is still flexible. The tendon itself in this stage is functionally incompetent and possibly completely disrupted, thus patients can often have a difficult time

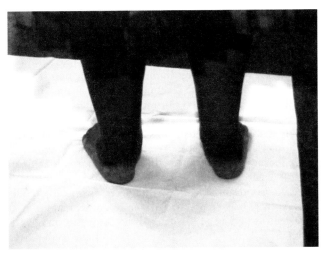

FIGURE 30-9. The "too many toes" sign.

performing a heel raise. Stage III includes a fixed hindfoot deformity. Collapse of the arch leads to a "too many toes" sign on examination, whereby the toes are visualized lateral to the leg when looking at the patient from behind (see **Fig. 30-9**). Additional examination findings include an apropulsive gait, limited heel lift and toe off, and excessive wear on the medial posterior aspect of the shoe (203).

Radiographic evaluation is not required in order to diagnose dysfunction of the tibialis posterior tendon as it can be based on clinical evaluation (208). However, imaging can be helpful to evaluate for any arthritic changes in the ankle or subtalar joint, degree of deformity, and to further evaluate the tendon itself. Standard weight-bearing dorsoplantar, oblique, and lateral x-rays can be ordered in patients displaying weakness or with long-standing deformities. MRI and ultrasound can help confirm the presence of tenosynovitis and intrasubstance tears (208).

Treatment varies based on the stage of clinical presentation and patient activity level. Despite the high prevalence of this issue, there are no current intervention guidelines (206,214). Early and appropriate conservative treatment is essential to prevent progression of this issue, which can result in long-term disabling consequences (214). Conservative modalities include custom foot orthotics to control poor biomechanics and support the medial longitudinal arch, ankle braces, AFOs, orthopedic shoes with medial heel wedges, or CAM walking boot. A strengthening program of foot adduction combined with foot orthoses has also been effective in reducing pain and increasing function in those with stage I or II posterior tibial tendon dysfunction. Surgery is sometimes the only option for full correction in late stage II or stage III cases (206). Surgical options include tendon transfers, soft tissue reconstructions, or limited arthrodesis (208).

Fibularis (Peroneal) Tendinopathies, Tears, and Dislocations

The fibularis brevis originates from the lateral distal two thirds of the fibula, and it is the strongest abductor of the foot as well as a plantar flexor and everter (215). The fibularis longus originates at the proximal two thirds of the lateral fibula and is a plantar flexor and everter of the foot. Both tendons pass through a tunnel created by the superior fibular retinaculum

and then pass inferior to the lateral malleolus. At the tip of the malleolus, the tendons split. Fibularis longus courses under the cuboid and foot to insert onto the lateral plantar base of the first metatarsal and first cuneiform. The fibularis brevis inserts onto the lateral base of the fifth metatarsal (216).

Fibularis tendon dysfunction can be divided into three categories that can be interrelated: tendinopathy, tendon tears, and subluxation or dislocation (216). These injuries can occur traumatically from laceration/puncture wound or forced inversion ankle sprains, or they can occur insidiously from a combination of overuse and irritation related to being in a tight space bordered by the calcaneus (217). Other contributing factors include having a supinated foot, gout, rheumatoid arthritis, or diabetes mellitus (217).

Fibularis brevis tears are common, but the incidence of clinically significant tears remains unknown. Although fibularis longus tears are not as common, they can dramatically affect foot function and can be seen in combination with fibularis brevis tears. History and physical examination can often be diagnostic. Pain to palpation along the course of the tendons or swelling can be noted. Resisted eversion is often painful but is not always weak on manual muscle testing even with full tendon tears. Having the patient plantar flex can help determine if fibularis longus is affected due to its insertion site on the first metatarsal. If tendon dislocation is suspected, there can also be pain with palpation and visible swelling at the lateral ankle. One or both tendons can dislocate, and in chronic cases, the dislocation usually produces symptoms of ankle instability with a painful snap (216,217).

X-rays are used to evaluate for fractures, os peroneum, or lateral malleolar avulsions. Arthritis and other degenerative changes can be seen on x-ray with chronic issues. MRI and ultrasound more specifically evaluate the integrity of the tendons and have similar sensitivity and specificity on cadaveric studies, with the caveat being that ultrasound can be examiner dependent (216).

For most patients with tendinopathy or tears, starting with conservative treatment is appropriate. This includes activity modification, bracing or orthotics, NSAIDs for pain relief, and working on a rehabilitation program with physical therapy. There are no studies of eccentric exercises for fibularis tendons, but this type of program can be considered as well. Corticosteroid injections are not recommended due to concern for weakening and possible rupture of the tendon (217).

For those that have failed nonoperative management, surgery can be considered. Different surgical options include tendon debridement, tenodesis, tendon transfer, and lateralizing calcaneal osteotomy (216). Additionally, for acute tendon dislocation, surgical repair of the retinaculum is often recommended depending on the activity level of the patient. In patients with chronic dislocation with pain or dysfunction, reconstructive surgery is an option as well (217).

Ankle Ligament Sprains and Associated Fractures

Acute ankle injuries are one of the most common injuries to affect both athletes and sedentary persons and can account for an estimated 2 million injuries per year and approximately 650,000 visits to the emergency room (184,218). The vast majority of these injuries involve damage to the lateral ligament complex from an acute inversion of the ankle. The anterior talofibular ligament is by far the most commonly injured of the ligaments, followed by the calcaneofibular ligament, and the posterior talofibular ligament, which is rarely involved with severe sprains and dislocations (184). An inversion injury usually occurs with the foot plantar flexed and then inverted, as often seen with coming down on someone else's foot or a misstep coming off a curb or stair. In this position, the ankle joint is most vulnerable due to the configuration of the talus in the ankle mortise. Additionally, the anterior talofibular ligament is at its greatest tension in this position, which also leads to vulnerability (219).

A less common type of ankle sprain is a high ankle sprain or a syndesmotic sprain. The syndesmosis can be injured in severe inversion sprains, in isolation, or along with deltoid ligament injuries. A common mechanism is ankle dorsiflexion and eversion with internal rotation of the tibia and can be seen more commonly than lateral ankle sprains in collision sports or those that involve rigid immobilization of the ankle such as skiing (220). It is worth noting that the deltoid ligament is a very strong ligament and is rarely injured in isolation.

Ankle sprains are graded based on the amount of injury to the ligaments (219). Grade I is a sprain, or stretch, of the ligament with no tear and only minimal loss of functional ability without much pain, swelling, or ecchymosis. Grade II is a partial tear of the ligament with some functional disability with moderate pain, swelling, and ecchymosis. Grade III is a complete tear with increased functional disability, severe swelling, pain, and ecchymosis.

A good history and physical examination are important in diagnosing an ankle sprain with particular attention paid to the mechanism of injury and position of the ankle. Physical examination can be limited due to excessive pain and swelling during the initial assessment, and one can consider re-examination 3 to 5 days after injury. Tests of ligament laxity include the anterior drawer test for the anterior talofibular ligament, talar tilt test for the calcaneofibular ligament, and the tibiofibular squeeze test and eversion test for syndesmotic injuries (218). Side-to-side laxity or lack of a firm endpoint should raise suspicion for partial or complete tear.

The Ottawa foot and ankle rules are used to determine if x-rays are indicated. Ankle radiographs should be obtained if there was noted inability to bear weight for four steps either initially or at the time of evaluation or if there is tenderness to palpation along the posterior edge or tip of the distal 6 cm of the lateral or medial malleolus. Additionally, foot radiographs should be obtained if there is tenderness of the navicular or base of the fifth metatarsal or inability to take four steps with pain in the foot (221). One should also palpate the proximal fibula to evaluate for the possibility of a Maisonneuve (proximal fibular) fracture, which can occur with medial ankle injuries.

In the absence of fracture, initial treatment of an ankle sprain is a combination of protection, rest, cryotherapy, compression, elevation, and anti-inflammatory or analgesic medications. If not contraindicated, early weight bearing and mobilization along with beginning therapeutic exercises in the 1st week after a sprain produce significant improvements in ankle function (222). Progressing through a program of strengthening, proprioceptive retraining, and return to sport-specific activi-

ties has proven effective, and physical therapy can be used to guide the individual through these steps (223). A Cochrane review demonstrated that lace-up or semi-rigid ankle supports are more effective than tape or an elastic bandage and helped return patients to sport and work faster (224).

For grade III ankle sprains, surgery can be considered in an athlete to help achieve an earlier return to sport (218). However, a Cochrane review failed to demonstrate a benefit of surgery and found inherent risks associated with surgery and thus recommended avoiding surgery for acute lateral ankle sprains regardless of severity (184).

Special Considerations

High Ankle (Syndesmotic) Sprains

When a syndesmotic injury is suspected, radiographs are important to evaluate for concomitant fracture and to evaluate for the presence of diastasis. Diastasis is identified by an increased tibiofibular clear space of 6 mm or greater on an AP radiograph (220). MRI has high sensitivity and specificity to diagnose anterior and posterior inferior tibiofibular ligament tears (225). Current indications for surgical treatment of acute syndesmotic injuries include frank diastasis of the syndesmosis on radiographs or arthroscopic evidence of syndesmotic instability. For those who do not meet surgical criteria, a phased rehabilitation program is used. Initially, patients may require a splint or walking boot with at least protected weight bearing with crutches until they can tolerate further progression. Further rehabilitation can proceed in a similar fashion to that of the acute lateral ankle sprain, including progressing ROM, strengthening, proprioceptive training, and return to sport-specific activity as indicated (220).

Associated Fractures

Inversion ankle injuries can be associated with fractures of the lateral malleolus, while eversion injuries can cause medial malleolar fractures. Maisonneuve fractures can occur with external rotation combined with eversion of the ankle. Emergent orthopedic referral is indicated for fracture-dislocation, any vascular or neurologic compromise, intra-articular fractures, or an unstable ankle. An unstable ankle can occur with fractures of both lateral and medial malleoli (bimalleolar fractures), a trimalleolar fracture (bimalleolar plus posterior malleolus), or a malleolar fracture on one side with an associated ligament disruption on the opposite side (226). If a distal fibular fracture has occurred above the tibiotalar joint line, this should cause concern for associated syndesmotic disruption and consideration for surgical referral (226). Maisonneuve fractures should also receive orthopedic referral as surgery may be indicated.

For all other fractures, the ankle should be splinted at 90 degrees with the patient made non–weight bearing until further follow-up with a specialist. Isolated nondisplaced lateral malleolar fractures generally heal with a low risk for complications, and small nondisplaced avulsions can be treated with early mobilization similar to treatment of an ankle sprain. Isolated malleolar fractures and distal fibular shaft fractures can be managed with splinting acutely for 3 to 5 days and then transitioning to a short leg walking cast or CAM boot for 4 to 6 weeks for malleolar fractures and 6 to 8 weeks for distal fibular shaft fractures (226). Repeat radiographs should be obtained at 1 week for distal fibular fractures to assess positioning and at 4 weeks for malleolar fractures to assess healing. After immobilization, the patient should begin a progressive ROM, stretching, and strengthening rehabilitation program.

Fractures in the pediatric population should be managed differently due to the concern for fractures along the physis. Fractures of the distal fibular physis are the most common type of pediatric ankle fracture and generally heal well. The Salter-Harris classification system is useful to help guide management. Type I is a separation of the physis, and type II involves fracture above or proximal to the physis. Nondisplaced type I and II fractures usually heal well with 4 weeks of immobilization in a walking cast or CAM boot. Type III is a fracture below or distal to the physis, type IV is a fracture through the physis involving proximal and distal fractures, and type V is a compression type fracture of the growth plate. Types III to V and all displaced type I and II injuries should have orthopedic referral for consideration of operative management, but strict immobilization should be achieved while awaiting the orthopedic surgical consultation (226).

Osteochondral Defects of the Ankle

Osteochondral defects (OCDs) of the ankle are an important cause of residual ankle pain after a sprain or injury (227). These generally affect the talar dome but can also occur on the tibial plafond. They are defined as separation of a fragment of articular cartilage with or without subchondral bone. There are several potential causes of ankle OCDs including acute trauma, local AVN, systemic vasculopathies, endocrine or metabolic factors, chronic microtrauma (sometimes associated with chronic ankle instability), degenerative joint disease, joint malalignment, osteochondritis dissecans in the pediatric population, and genetic predispositions. OCDs are classified in four stages. Stage I is an area of osteochondral compression. Stage II is a partially loose fragment, while stage III is a completely detached fragment without displacement. Stage IV represents a completely detached and displaced fragment (228,229).

On history, patients report intermittent deep ankle pain that increases with weight-bearing activities. They may not recall a specific injury. Examination can be normal as some patients may have no tenderness or limitations in ROM (227). A high index of suspicion and imaging studies are required to effectively diagnose this condition. In a patient with history of acute ankle injury that has symptoms persisting beyond 3 to 6 weeks, an OCD should be suspected (230). OCD findings can be absent on x-rays, particularly early in the process but are a good initial study (231). Both CT and MRI are useful in assessing OCDs, but MRI can be more helpful with early-stage lesions and as a screening tool (227,229).

OCD lesions that are asymptomatic and incidentally found can be treated nonoperatively. Low-grade OCD or OCD lesions in the pediatric population may resolve with rest, ice, and reduced weight bearing. Recovery can be determined by pain status and serial imaging. Complete resolution of lesions is much more common in the pediatric population than in adults, and in adults, there is a relatively high rate of failure for nonoperative management. In cases of failed conservative management, surgery to revascularize the bony defect can be considered. These surgeries employ a combination of cartilage stabilization and pinning, retrograde drilling, microfracture,

and tissue transplantation. There has been some investigation into other nonoperative treatment strategies such as injections with hyaluronic acid (HA), PRP, or mesenchymal stem cells, or electromagnetic or ultrasound stimulation, but at this time, research is limited, and these are not yet standards of care (229).

FOOT

Foot problems are common among people of all ages. The prevalence has been reported as 15% to 40% depending on demographic distribution of the patient population (232–234). The toes and forefoot are the most common anatomical sites of pain, and disability is common in cases of foot pain in middle-aged and older individuals (185).

Anatomy

Each foot is composed of 26 bones and 55 joints (**Fig. 30-10**) with muscle attachments that have their origin within the foot or leg. The foot is divided into the forefoot, midfoot, and rearfoot-ankle complex. The forefoot is composed of the metatarsals and phalanges. The first metatarsal head distally articulates on the plantar surface with the tibial and fibular sesamoid bones, which are within the flexor hallucis brevis tendon. The midfoot consists of three cuneiform bones, the cuboid, and the navicular. The three cuneiforms articulate with the base of the first three metatarsals, and the cuboid articulates with the fourth and fifth metatarsals. Proximally, the cuneiforms articulate with the navicular, and laterally, the cuboid articulates with the navicular and lateral cuneiform. The navicular and cuboid proximally articulate with the talus and calcaneus forming the midtarsal joint. The Lisfranc joint is formed by the metatarsals, cuneiforms, and cuboid. The keystone of this joint is the second metatarsal cuneiform articulation. The configuration of the articulation between the metatarsals, cuneiforms, and cuboid helps form the transverse metatarsal arch. The muscles of the foot are divided into extrinsic and intrinsic groups. The extrinsic muscles arise in the leg and insert into the foot and are held in place by retinacula as they enter the foot. These muscles produce movements at the ankle as well as toe flexion and extension.

Physical Examination

Initial examination of the foot is similar to examination of the ankle discussed previously. There is a lot of overlap of foot and ankle conditions, and they should often be examined together. The bones, joints, and tendons of interest in the foot should be palpated to determine if they are a source of pain. Observation of ROM of the foot should be performed both with active and passive motion. The first metatarsophalangeal (MTP) joint ROM should also be assessed passively and actively, with functional dorsiflexion/extension range ≥70 degrees.

Lastly, special testing should be undertaken to help rule in and out pathology. The majority of the special testing for the foot in particular is in regard to evaluating for possible Morton's neuroma. One test evaluates for a "Mulder's click" by placing plantar pressure at the interspace in question and then squeezing the distal metatarsals together. A click can be felt or heard if a neuroma is present (sensitivity 62%, specificity 100%). Simply squeezing the involved intermetatarsal space at the level of the metatarsal heads, called the thumb-index

Skeleton of the Foot

A Dorsal view

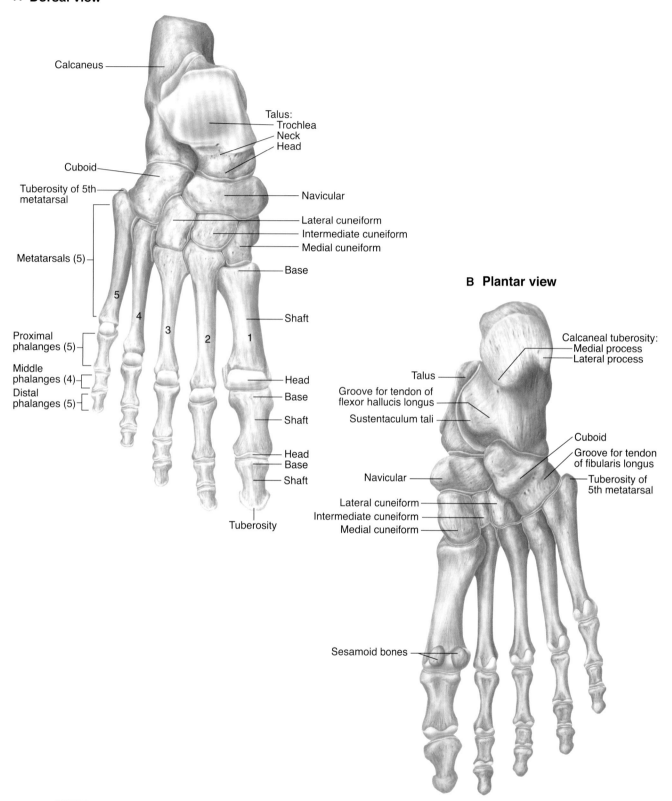

FIGURE 30-10. Bony anatomy of the foot. (Reprinted with permission from Tank PW, Gest TR. *Lippincott Williams & Wilkins Atlas of Anatomy.* 1st ed. Baltimore, MD: Wolters Kluwer Health/Lippincott Williams & Wilkins; 2009.)

finger squeeze test, can recreate pain in a positive test (sensitivity 96%, specificity 100%). The metatarsal squeeze test, which involves squeezing the forefoot at the level of the metatarsal heads, has a sensitivity of 41% and specificity of 0% for diagnosing a Morton's neuroma (186).

Plantar Fasciosis

The plantar fascia is a strong aponeurosis that originates on the medial process of the calcaneal tuberosity and fans out into the medial, central, and lateral slip. The fascia blends in with the flexor plate distally and has a connection with the plantar aspect of the toes. The central slip is the thickest. The plantar fascia acts as a windlass that is helpful for propulsion during gait and supports the arch of the foot. The main site of abnormality is near the origin of the plantar fascia at the medial tuberosity of the calcaneus and is a degenerative process similar to tendinopathy as described previously and less likely a purely inflammatory process as once thought.

The exact cause remains poorly understood. Limited data from case-control studies reveal possible contributing factors of obesity, occupations with prolonged standing, pes planus, reduced ankle dorsiflexion, and inferior calcaneal exostoses (heel spurs). There is a high incidence in runners, and there could be contributions from repetitive microtrauma, faulty running shoes, or the running surface, but evidence is limited (235).

Plantar fasciosis is a common cause of pain in the inferior heel, and diagnosis can be made based on clinical assessment alone (235). Patients often describe significant pain with the first step in the morning or after prolonged inactivity, and pain often worsens with prolonged standing or weight-bearing activity. On examination, there is tenderness over the medial plantar aspect of the heel. A tight Achilles tendon or pes planus deformity might be present. Standard radiographs may demonstrate a calcaneal spur, but this is not pathognomonic for this condition. MRI and ultrasound can demonstrate plantar fascia thickening and pathology but are not required for diagnosis.

Most patients respond favorably to conservative treatment, but there are very few high-quality, randomized, controlled trials that support the efficacy of various conservative treatment options (236). A combination of rest, activity modification, foot orthotics, night splints, deep transverse friction massage, stretching, ice, analgesics, and physical therapy is the initial conservative treatment. Physical therapy should focus on stretching the Achilles, strengthening the intrinsic muscles of the foot, and addressing other biomechanical factors that could be contributing.

If pain persists, other treatment options can be considered. Steroid injections have been shown to be associated with possible plantar fascia rupture or heel fat pad atrophy and often provide only short-term relief (235,237). Other options include autologous blood or PRP injections, ESWT, and percutaneous tenotomy. The body of literature evaluating these modalities is not robust, but they can be considered. The most invasive treatment option for recalcitrant cases is surgery.

Morton's Neuroma

Morton's neuroma is a compression entrapment neuropathy that commonly affects the third interdigital nerve of the foot between the third and fourth metatarsals (238). It less commonly affects the second interdigital nerve and rarely the first or fourth nerves. Classically, it is seen in 40- to 60-year-old

women, especially those who wear pointed or high-heeled shoes, but it occurs in a wide-ranging population (238). The pathophysiology most likely includes repetitive microtrauma and compression from the surrounding metatarsal heads. Anything that diminishes the space available to the nerve, such as a ganglion cyst, MTP synovitis, or trauma with swelling, can contribute.

Patients complain of pain in the forefoot with burning or numbness/tingling in the toes innervated by the affected nerve. Symptoms are aggravated by certain footwear and weight-bearing activity (238,239). Physical examination maneuvers that are most helpful are compression of the web space, metatarsal squeeze test, and evaluation for a Mulder's click (238,240). X-rays can be helpful to rule out any musculoskeletal pathology, but the neuroma itself is only visualized with ultrasound or MRI.

Treatment begins with conservative care such as wearing shoes with a wide toe box and avoiding high-heeled shoes. Additionally, a metatarsal pad or metatarsal bar can be used to offload the area. Corticosteroid injections can be used to relieve inflammation and pain. This has been cited as having a success rate ranging from 11% to 47%, but care should be taken to avoid overusing these injections as they are associated with atrophy of the plantar fat pad. Dilute alcohol injections or sclerosing agents have also been investigated with varying levels of efficacy, and lastly, surgical management is often recommended for those refractive to conservative care (239).

Hallux Valgus

Hallux valgus (bunion) is medial angulation of the first metatarsal and lateral deviation of the hallux. It is thought to be hereditary, but improper footwear can also play a role. It is a progressive deformity that can worsen with time, and footwear is a large contributor to the pain felt on the dorsomedial aspect of the first MTP joint. On examination, there is notable deformity and possibly erythema or a small bursa noted on the medial aspect of the joint. As this condition progresses, there is intrinsic instability in the first MTP joint, and the fibular sesamoid drifts laterally (241).

Weight-bearing radiographs reveal an increase in the intermetatarsal angle, lateral deviation of the sesamoids, and lateral deviation of the great toe. Initial conservative treatment with ice and NSAIDs for pain control and appropriate footwear with a wide toe box is appropriate. Off-the-shelf or custom foot orthoses can also be used. If these measures fail, surgical intervention can be considered, but surgery for an asymptomatic patient or for cosmesis is not recommended. The goal of surgery is reducing pain and improving function.

Sesamoiditis

Sesamoiditis is a generalized term for a painful condition of the sesamoid complex (242,243). It is more typically seen in younger women but can affect anyone. The differential diagnosis can include acute sesamoid fracture, AVN of a sesamoid, stress fracture, and OA of the first MTP joint. The sesamoids are located within the tendons of the flexor hallucis brevis and form a portion of the plantar plate. There are generally two sesamoids, the tibial (medial) and fibular (lateral), but a third can develop inferior to the hallux interphalangeal joint. Their function is to absorb and disperse weight-bearing shock from the metatarsal head and enhance the gliding function of the first MTP joint. They are less vascularized distally. Bipartite sesamoids can be present and more common in the tibial sesamoid.

With involvement of the sesamoids, clinical history often includes pain around the big toe during the toe off phase of gait, and patients avoid weight bearing on the involved sesamoid and load the lateral aspect of their foot. On examination, there is pain at end ROM of the first MTP joint with dorsiflexion and direct palpation or translation of the sesamoids. Weight-bearing radiographs that also include a sesamoid axial view allow for evaluation but can often appear normal. Further imaging with a bone scan, CT, or MRI can be helpful to evaluate for and rule out other pathology on the differential. Sesamoiditis can be devoid of findings as stated above, but there may be positive findings on MRI or bone scan (243,244).

Treatment should begin with activity modification, changes in footwear, avoidance of high-heeled shoes, foot orthotics, consideration of a metatarsal bar or pad, and NSAIDs. A corticosteroid or local anesthetic injection can be considered for both diagnostic and possibly therapeutic benefit but are contraindicated in cases of sesamoid fracture or AVN. If conservative measures fail, surgical excision can be considered. The tibial sesamoid is more commonly affected and resected (243).

Lisfranc Joint Injuries

Lisfranc joint injuries encompass dislocation and fracture-dislocation of the tarsometatarsal (Lisfranc) joint. Ligaments and capsular structures connect the second through fifth metatarsals, but there is an absence of connection between the first and second metatarsal bases. The Lisfranc ligament connects the medial cuneiform and the second metatarsal base. Injuries to this joint are often the result of a high-energy force. Direct injuries result from a crushing force, while indirect injuries

occur in the setting of a combination of twisting and axial forces when the metatarsals and foot are in a plantar-flexed position relative to the ground (245). Indirect injuries are more common (246,247). Examples of direct trauma are being stepped on by a horse or crushed under the wheel of a car, and indirect trauma can occur from a fall down stairs, car accidents, or athletic endeavors.

A high index of suspicion should be maintained for these injuries as they can be easily missed. Physical examination reveals swelling, ecchymosis, and pain of the forefoot. Ecchymosis at the plantar midfoot, termed plantar ecchymosis sign, may provide insight into the presence of this injury. An adduction or abduction deformity of the forefoot can be present. The patients generally cannot walk on their toes (248).

X-rays are necessary for diagnosis and should include multiple weight-bearing views. The medial border of the second metatarsal base should align with the medial border of the middle cuneiform, and the space between the first and second metatarsal bases should be less than 2 mm on an AP x-ray. On the oblique view, the lateral border of the third metatarsal and the lateral border of the lateral cuneiform should be aligned, and the medial border of the fourth metatarsal base should align with the medial border of the cuboid. Attention should also be directed at the cuboid, which may fracture and collapse. In the absence of displacement on x-ray but positive bone scan or MRI, nonsurgical management with 6 weeks of cast immobilization is pursued. In cases with any displacement, surgery is recommended (249).

Metatarsal Fractures

Fifth Metatarsal Base Fractures

Fractures of the base of the fifth metatarsal are the most common metatarsal fracture. There are two types of fractures that can occur at the base or proximal end of the fifth metatarsal: avulsion and Jones fractures (see **Fig. 30-11**). Avulsion

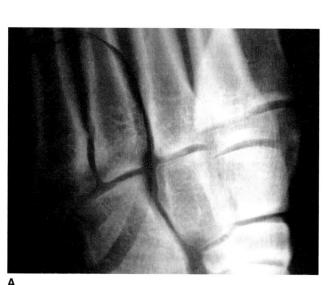
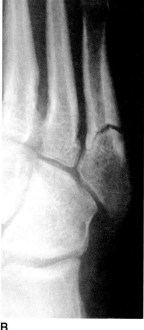

A   **B**

FIGURE 30-11. X-rays of 5th metatarsal fractures. Avulsion fracture **(A)** and Jones' fracture **(B)**.

fractures involve the most proximal portion and tuberosity of the fifth metatarsal, and they commonly occur in inversion ankle sprains due to the pull of the fibularis brevis tendon. Treatment for avulsion fractures is conservative with 6 to 8 weeks in a CAM boot with weight bearing as tolerated. If there is significant displacement, open reduction and internal fixation should be considered.

Jones fractures are transverse fractures at the junction of the diaphysis and metaphysis of the fifth metatarsal, about 1.5 to 3 cm distal to the fifth metatarsal tuberosity. Jones fractures are less stable than avulsion fractures because of the long lever arm of the metatarsal placing stress on the fracture site. Healing is also complicated by poor vascularity in this area of the metatarsal (250). Treatment depends on the activity level of the patient. In less active patients, attempts at conservative care with cast immobilization and non–weight bearing for a period of 6 to 8 weeks can be considered initially. For those patients with delayed union or nonunion, surgical treatment with or without bone grafting is recommended. In an athletic patient, early surgical fixation with intramedullary screw is usually recommended for shorter healing time and faster return to sports (251).

Lesser Metatarsal Fractures

The second, third, and fourth metatarsals are the most frequently fractured, and injuries are usually related to direct or indirect (repetitive) trauma (203). Clinical signs of a fracture include edema, ecchymosis, and pain in the area. It is important to evaluate for any vascular compromise. X-rays should be obtained with AP, medial oblique, and a lateral view for full evaluation.

Metatarsal neck fractures are most common and are often obliquely oriented. Emergent orthopedic referral should be undertaken for any signs of vascular compromise or an open fracture (226). If the fracture is displaced, then closed reduction should be attempted. Failure of closed reduction often necessitates intramedullary pinning to help prevent any metatarsal shortening or floating toe syndrome (203). For nondisplaced fractures, treatment is 6 to 8 weeks in a short-leg non–weight-bearing cast.

Metatarsal shaft fractures have similar requirements for orthopedic referral and reduction as neck fractures. Displacement of more than 3 to 4 mm is the cutoff for reduction. Nondisplaced metatarsal shaft fractures often heal well without cast immobilization, and a firm-soled shoe or CAM walking boot can be used for 4 to 6 weeks. Follow-up radiographs are obtained at 1 week to confirm alignment and again at 4 to 6 weeks to document healing (226).

Sever's Disease

Sever's disease is a traction apophysitis that causes pain at the insertion of the Achilles tendon on the secondary calcaneal ossification center. Sever's disease is thought to be an overuse injury caused by repetitive microtrauma from traction of the Achilles tendon and occurs from ages 6 to 12. It is seen most commonly in active children and can be associated with obesity, a period of growth, or an increase in activity.

The diagnosis is generally made clinically based on pain to palpation along the calcaneal apophysis or with compression of the calcaneus. The patient may have reproduction of typical pain with heel raise. Assessment for contributing biomechanical factors such as hallux valgus, pes planus, pes cavus, or tight heel cord is essential. It is challenging to differentiate Sever's disease from a normal calcaneal apophysis on radiographs, but they can be helpful to rule out fracture or coalition (252).

Sever's disease is self-limiting with resolution of pain after fusion of the calcaneus, but conservative treatment for pain reduction is appropriate. A combination of rest, activity modification, icing, heel lifts, heel cord stretching, and physical therapy can be helpful (252,253). Most children return to pain-free activity within 3 to 6 weeks (254).

LOWER-EXTREMITY OSTEOARTHRITIS

OA is a disorder of synovial joints involving degeneration of the cartilage and changes to subchondral bone (255). Common symptoms associated with OA include pain, limited ROM, and stiffness. Pain usually worsens with activity or bearing weight on the extremity and improves with rest. However, with more advanced OA, there can also be pain at rest. Many individuals also describe an increase in their symptoms with cold or wet weather. Associated periarticular changes include ligamentous laxity and weakness of supporting muscles, which can lead to instability (256–259). OA of the lower extremities is common and has increased in prevalence with aging of the population and increased prevalence of obesity (256,260,261).

Epidemiology

OA is a chronic disease and a common cause of disability especially in older individuals (262). In the lower extremities, the most commonly affected joints are the knees, hips, and feet in that order (256). The lifetime risk of symptomatic knee OA has been estimated between 7% and 17% with the highest rates in obese women. Peak incidence occurs between ages 55 and 64 (260,263). For the hip, estimates of symptomatic OA are between 5% to 10% (256,260,264). Prevalence of ankle and foot OA has not been studied as extensively, but it is estimated that ankle OA affects approximately 1% of the world's population (265). The prevalence of symptomatic foot OA in one population study was 16.7% for all joints in the foot with the first MTP joint most commonly affected (266).

Etiology, Pathology, and Pathophysiology

OA, or degenerative joint disease, is characterized by loss of articular cartilage with associated bony changes. OA is defined as primary, secondary, or posttraumatic. Primary OA is the failure of an otherwise normal joint. Posttraumatic and secondary OA are similar to primary in the pathology that affects the joint, but there is an underlying cause of joint degeneration. In the hips, knees, and first MTP of the foot, the majority of OA is primary (265,267). Conversely, OA of the ankle and midfoot is most commonly posttraumatic (257,267); therefore, it is important to ask patients about a prior history of trauma including minor sprains (259). In end-stage painful ankle OA, approximately 70% to 80% of cases are related to prior fracture, osteochondral injury, or ligament sprain (265,268). Despite the ankle being the most commonly injured joint in the body, the low rates of OA are thought to be secondary to characteristics of the articular cartilage in the ankle joint and the bony congruity of the joint (259,265).

The degenerative process begins with small tears (fibrillations) in the superficial zone of cartilage, which propagate by enzymatic breakdown of cartilage (269,270). This leads to larger areas of cartilage loss exposing the underlying subchondral bone. Eventually, the chondrocytes lose their ability to replicate, and the chemical makeup of the cartilage changes (271). Fibrous, cartilaginous, and osseous prominences called osteophytes eventually develop around the periphery of the joints but can also be located along the capsule insertions or on the joint surface. Cyst-like cavities containing myxoid, fibrous, or cartilaginous tissue eventually form within the bone. Usually both cartilage degeneration and subchondral bone remodeling are found by the time the patient is symptomatic (272). There are also changes in the synovial membrane and synovial fluid. This consists of increased water content, reduced hyaluronate concentration, and increased concentration of inflammatory mediators in the synovial fluid (273). The progression of OA is usually slow (256).

Risk Factors

There are many identified risk factors for the development of lower-extremity OA. Obesity, female sex, older age, genetics, and increased bone mineral density are associated with development of hip and knee OA. In the ankle, a prior injury is the greatest risk factor, but a prior traumatic knee injury is also a risk factor for developing knee OA (256–258). Repetitive and excessive joint loading also increase the risk of developing lower-extremity OA, but more moderate activity with cyclic joint loading is likely beneficial to joint health. There are also likely genetic and cultural contributions to the development of hip and knee OA as rates for knee OA in Chinese women are higher than in other populations, but rates for hip OA are lower (256). Risk factors specific to foot OA include having a long second toe, wide first metatarsal, wide proximal phalanx, long sesamoids, flat feet, high arches, and wearing high-heeled shoes (267).

Imaging

X-rays are often diagnostic for OA, but early changes affecting the cartilage may only be visible with MRI. For evaluation with x-rays, at least two views of the joint, AP and lateral, are obtained in a weight-bearing position. For the knee, it is beneficial to obtain a skyline/sunrise or Merchant view of the patella as well as a Rosenberg/notch view (postcroantcrior [PA] view with the knees at 45 degrees of flexion). In the ankle, the mortise view is also added.

The changes seen on x-ray include osteophytes, joint space narrowing, subchondral sclerosis, and subchondral cysts (see **Fig. 30-12**). With more advanced OA, bony deformity also occurs. There are several grading systems for OA for the hip, knee, ankle, and foot. The most commonly referenced is the Kellgren-Lawrence (K&L) grading scale, which ranges from 0 to 4. A grade of 0 indicates no radiographic evidence of OA. Osteophytes are present in grade 1 and joint space loss in grade 2. In grade 3, there is sclerosis, and in grade 4, there is more severe joint space narrowing and sclerosis with bony deformity. It is also important to note that there may be radiographic evidence of OA without symptoms, and the grade of OA on imaging does not always correlate to severity of symptoms (256,260).

Management

The management of OA is focused on improving pain, function, and quality of life. The initial focus should be on conservative measures, but surgery can be pursued when conservative

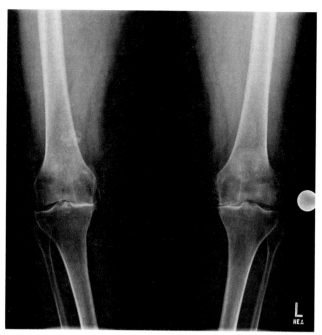

FIGURE 30-12. X-ray findings in severe osteoarthritis, including joint space narrowing, subchondral sclerosis, osteophytes, subchondral cysts, and loose bodies.

management has failed to provide an adequate level of pain relief and functional improvement for the patient. There are many organizational and committee guidelines regarding the nonoperative management of OA, which primarily focus on hip and knee OA. There is general agreement among these recommendations, which are reviewed below (103,255,261,262,274–277).

Nonpharmacologic

Education and Self-Management

When an individual is diagnosed with OA, the initial counseling should include a discussion of the etiology, natural history, and prognosis of OA. Patients should be educated on tools they can utilize to manage their symptoms. These include activity modification to reduce pain, appropriate exercise, use of supportive footwear, and heat or ice for pain relief. In the home, raised toilet seats, grab rails, walk-in showers, and higher seating surfaces can be helpful for those with hip and knee OA especially.

Weight Loss

Weight loss is recommended for all individuals who are overweight or obese, and those with a healthy body weight should be encouraged to maintain their weight. Weight loss has been shown to improve pain and disability related to OA. Some may require referral to a nutritionist or weight loss clinic for assistance.

Exercise and Physical Therapy

An individualized program is important for adherence to and maintenance of an exercise program. Patients should be encouraged to include both aerobic and strengthening exercises. Land-based and aquatic exercise programs are beneficial for improving pain and function. Low-impact exercises are often better tolerated as well as shorter bouts of exercise. Strengthening exercises should focus on the muscles around the affected joints as they are often weak in the setting of OA.

Physical therapy can be utilized to help patients develop an appropriate exercise and strengthening program that is well tolerated. Another exercise program with demonstrated benefit for knee OA is tai chi.

Orthotics

A variety of knee orthoses are available (see Chapter 57). Elastic or neoprene braces, which are often well tolerated, can be used to provide some compression and keep the joint warm. Patellar stabilizing braces or patellar taping can be helpful in the setting of patellofemoral OA. Braces with more supportive medial and lateral uprights or medial and lateral unloader knee braces are other options. These braces are bulkier and may be less tolerated.

In the past, shoe wedges were used more commonly—lateral wedge for medial compartment OA and vice versa—but these have had mixed reviews in recent recommendations. For those who do not tolerate a knee brace or whose leg shape does not allow the individual to wear a brace, a wedge insole can be a good alternative. A cushioned insole can also be used to provide decreased impact in the setting of knee and ankle OA.

For the ankle, a lace-up ankle support with a custom plastic AFO shell between layers of leather to support the foot and ankle is one option. Alternatively, a rocker bottom shoe with solid-ankle cushioned heel (SACH) or CAM boot can be used to reduce stress on the foot and ankle during ambulation (259,278).

For foot OA, a rigid foot orthosis can reduce joint stresses and loading during ambulation (258).

Assistive Devices

Utilizing a cane in the contralateral hand can reduce pain and improve function in the setting of hip and knee OA. For those concerned about the appearance of a cane, a good alternative is a walking stick or trekking poles. If there is not sufficient joint offloading with a cane or in the presence of bilateral OA, a walker can be used.

Pharmacologic

The medications most commonly used to reduce OA pain include acetaminophen and NSAIDs (see Chapter 52). It is important to remember that OA is a chronic condition, but these commonly recommended analgesic medications are not intended for long-term use and have the potential for negative health effects with prolonged use. Patients should be encouraged to take the medications on an as-needed basis rather than scheduled. An individual's medical comorbidities must also be taken into account when determining the most appropriate treatments. If a medication is ineffective, an alternative medication should be trialed; however, if it is partially effective, a second medication can be added (275,277).

Acetaminophen

Most guidelines recommend acetaminophen (paracetamol) as first-line therapy for managing pain related to OA. However, recent reviews have raised concerns about the efficacy and safety of acetaminophen with potential risk for gastrointestinal (GI), hepatic, and cardiovascular (CV) adverse effects (274,275,279,280). It remains a good option for analgesia when used within new dosing guidelines of up to 3 g/d on an as needed basis.

Nonsteroidal Anti-Inflammatory Drugs

NSAIDs are available in both oral and topical formulations. In the United States, there are many oral NSAIDs available both over the counter and prescription, but diclofenac is the only approved topical NSAID and is only available by prescription. While the various NSAIDs have been shown to provide equivalent benefit, some individuals may benefit more from one NSAID compared to others. Therefore, if one is ineffective, others can be considered.

NSAIDs carry risk of GI, CV, and renal adverse effects. Topical NSAIDs have little systemic absorption and therefore less GI and CV risk compared to oral formulations (281,282). However, they have limited penetration and therefore cannot be used for deeper joints such as the hip; but they can be used for the knee, ankle, and foot. The guidelines differ with regard to their recommendations for NSAIDs; several recommend topical NSAIDs over oral NSAIDs due to their improved safety profile, whereas others do not differentiate between the two. Oral NSAIDs should be avoided in individuals with known CV disease or GI ulcer or bleeding if possible (274,277,280,283,284).

Other Medications

When there is insufficient pain relief with acetaminophen or NSAIDs, or those medications cannot be used due to contraindications, tramadol or opioids can be considered. These medications can be used in combination with acetaminophen or NSAIDs for synergistic effect. Caution must be used when prescribing opioids given risk for possible serious adverse events.

Lastly, recent studies of duloxetine, a serotonin and norepinephrine reuptake inhibitor (SNRI), have shown benefit for chronic pain related to OA.

Nutraceuticals

Glucosamine and chondroitin, normal components of the extracellular matrix of articular cartilage, are available as supplements, but the evidence supporting their benefit for pain relief and slowing disease progression is mixed. In studies that have shown more benefit, the study medications were prescription-grade crystalline glucosamine sulfate and chondroitin sulfate (277). The published guidelines vary from recommending glucosamine and chondroitin as first-line treatment to stating that there is either uncertain or no benefit. Overall, these supplements are safe and well tolerated and can be considered for a 3- to 6-month trial and continued long term if beneficial.

Injectables

In addition to oral and topical medications, there are injectable medications utilized in the setting of OA. The primary medications are corticosteroids and HA, a component of synovial fluid and cartilage. In the United States, HA is approved as a biologic device for use in the knees only.

Corticosteroids are anti-inflammatories and have generally shown benefit for short-term pain relief in the hips, knees, ankles, and feet. Most guidelines recommend use of intra-articular steroids for flares of pain or when other treatments have not provided sufficient pain relief. Injections can be performed up to four times per year. HA has limited evidence for efficacy, and many of the guidelines now do not recommend the use of HA. If used and the patient has good relief of symptoms, injections can be repeated every 6 months.

Studies are being conducted on use of PRP and stem cells for OA, but there is not enough evidence at this time to recommend for or against the use of these treatments.

Surgery

When nonoperative treatments have failed and the patient has pain that is limiting function and producing a negative impact on quality of life, surgery can be considered. The primary surgery for OA is joint arthroplasty and is most commonly performed in the hip and knee. Arthroplasty is also an option for the ankle and joints within the foot. An alternative to arthroplasty in the foot and ankle is arthrodesis (fusion) (258,259).

In the setting of loose bodies or OCDs, joint arthroscopy can be performed. Additionally, in individuals with mechanical symptoms of joint locking or instability in the setting of a meniscus tear with OA, arthroscopy can be considered. However, in the absence of mechanical symptoms, arthroscopy is not generally recommended as it does not have a positive long-term benefit. Lastly, arthroscopy is not recommended solely for the treatment of OA (103).

REFERENCES

1. Strauss EJ, Nho SJ, Kelly BT. Greater trochanteric pain syndrome. *Sports Med Arthrosc Rev.* 2010;18:113–119.
2. Mallow M, Nazarian LN. Greater trochanteric pain syndrome diagnosis and treatment. *Phys Med Rehabil Clin N Am.* 2014;25:279–289.
3. Beaulé PE, O'Neill M, Rakhra K. Acetabular labral tears. *J Bone Joint Surg Am.* 2009;91–A:701–710.
4. Simoneau GG, Hoenig KJ, Lepley JE, et al. Influence of hip position and gender on active hip internal and external rotation. *J Orthop Sports Phys Ther.* 1998;28:158–164.
5. Kouyoumdjian P, Coulomb R, Sanchez T, et al. Clinical evaluation of hip joint rotation range of motion in adults. *Orthop Traumatol Surg Res.* 2012;98:17–23.
6. Krabak B, Sussman W, Byrd JWT. Physical examination of the pelvis and hip. In: Malanga GA, Mautner K, eds. *Musculoskeletal Physical Examination: An Evidence-Based Approach.* Philadelphia, PA: Elsevier; 2017.
7. Reiman MP, Goode AP, Hegedus EJ, et al. Diagnostic accuracy of clinical tests of the hip: a systematic review with meta-analysis. *Br J Sports Med.* 2013;47:893–902.
8. Prather H, Colorado B, Hunt D. Managing hip pain in the athlete. *Phys Med Rehabil Clin N Am.* 2014;25:789–812.
9. Lesher JM, Dreyfuss P, Hager N, et al. Hip joint pain referral patterns: a descriptive study. *Pain Med.* 2008;9:22–25.
10. Khan AM, Mcloughlin E, Giannakas K, et al. Hip osteoarthritis: where is the pain? *Ann R Coll Surg Engl.* 2004;86:119–121.
11. Frank JM, Harris JD, Erickson BJ, et al. Prevalence of femoroacetabular impingement imaging findings in asymptomatic volunteers: a systematic review. *Arthroscopy.* 2015;31:1199–1204.
12. Hack K, Di Primio G, Rakhra K, et al. Prevalence of cam-type femoroacetabular impingement morphology in asymptomatic volunteers. *J Bone Joint Surg Am.* 2010;92–A:2436–2444.
13. Sanchez-Sotelo J, Trousdale RT, Berry DJ, et al. Surgical treatment of developmental dysplasia of the hip in adults: I. Nonarthroplasty options. *J Am Acad Orthop Surg.* 2002;10:321–333.
14. Philippon MJ, Maxwell RB, Johnston TL, et al. Clinical presentation of femoroacetabular impingement. *Knee Surg Sports Traumatol Arthrosc.* 2007;15:1041–1047.
15. Leunig M, Beaulé PE, Ganz R. The concept of femoroacetabular impingement: current status and future perspectives. *Clin Orthop Relat Res.* 2009;467:616–622.
16. Bedi A, Kelly BT. Femoroacetabular impingement. *J Bone Joint Surg Am.* 2013;95:82–92.
17. Kowalczuk M, Yeung M, Simunovic N, et al. Does femoroacetabular impingement contribute to the development of hip osteoarthritis? A systematic review. *Sports Med Arthrosc Rev.* 2015;23:174–179.
18. Sankar WN, Nevitt M, Parvizi J, et al. Femoroacetabular impingement: defining the condition and its role in the pathophysiology of osteoarthritis. *J Am Acad Orthop Surg.* 2013;21:S7–S15.
19. Thomas GER, Palmer AJR, Batra RN, et al. Subclinical deformities of the hip are significant predictors of radiographic osteoarthritis and joint replacement in women. A 20 year longitudinal cohort study. *Osteoarthr Cartil.* 2014;22:1504–1510.
20. Wall PDH, Fernandez M, Griffin DR, et al. Nonoperative treatment for femoroacetabular impingement: a systematic review of the literature. *PM R.* 2013;5:418–426.
21. Griffin DR, Dickenson EJ, O'Donnell J, et al. The Warwick Agreement on femoroacetabular impingement syndrome (FAI syndrome): an international consensus statement. *Br J Sports Med.* 2016;50:1169–1176.
22. Lee AJJ, Armour P, Thind D, et al. The prevalence of acetabular labral tears and associated pathology in a young asymptomatic population. *Bone Joint J.* 2015;97–B:623–627.
23. Skendzel JG, Philippon MJ. Management of labral tears of the hip in young patients. *Orthop Clin North Am.* 2013;44:477–487.
24. Magee T. Comparison of 3.0-T MR vs 3.0-T MR arthrography of the hip for detection of acetabular labral tears and chondral defects in the same patient population. *Br J Radiol.* 2015;88:20140817.
25. Parvizi J, Bican O, Bender B, et al. Arthroscopy for labral tears in patients with developmental dysplasia of the hip: a cautionary note. *J Arthroplasty.* 2009;24:110–113.
26. Mont MA, Jones LC, Hungerford DS. Nontraumatic osteonecrosis of the femoral head: ten years later. *J Bone Joint Surg Am.* 2006;88:1117–1132.
27. Prather H. Pelvis and sacral dysfunction in sports and exercise. *Phys Med Rehabil Clin N Am.* 2000;11:805–836.
28. Zalavras CG, Lieberman JR. Osteonecrosis of the femoral head. *J Am Acad Orthop Surg.* 2014;22:455–464.
29. Domb BG, Nasser RM, Botser IB. Partial-thickness tears of the gluteus medius: rationale and technique for trans-tendinous endoscopic repair. *Arthroscopy.* 2010;26:1697–1705.
30. Klauser AS, Martinoli C, Tagliafico A, et al. Greater trochanteric pain syndrome. *Semin Musculoskelet Radiol.* 2013;17:43–48.
31. Redmond JM, Chen AW, Domb BG. Greater trochanteric pain syndrome. *J Am Acad Orthop Surg.* 2016;24:231–240.
32. Lee KS, Rosas HG, Phancao JP. Snapping hip: imaging and treatment. *Semin Musculoskelet Radiol.* 2013;17:286–294.
33. Yen Y-M, Lewis CL, Kim Y-J. Understanding and treating the snapping hip. *Sports Med Arthrosc Rev.* 2015;23:194–199.
34. Nicholas SJ, Tyler TF. Adductor muscle strains in sport. *Sports Med.* 2002;32:339–344.
35. Morelli V, Smith V. Groin injuries in athletes. *Am Fam Physician.* 2001;64:1405–1414.
36. Mandelbaum B, Mora SA. Osteitis pubis. *Oper Tech Sports Med.* 2005;13:62–67.
37. Kunduracioglu B, Yilmaz C, Yorubulut M, et al. Magnetic resonance findings of osteitis pubis. *J Magn Reson Imaging.* 2007;25:535–539.
38. Lehmann CL, Arons RR, Loder RT, et al. The epidemiology of slipped capital femoral epiphysis: an update. *J Pediatr Orthop.* 2006;26:286–290.
39. Gholve PA, Cameron DB, Millis MB. Slipped capital femoral epiphysis update. *Curr Opin Pediatr.* 2009;21:39–45.
40. Bahmanyar S, Montgomery SM, Weiss RJ, et al. Maternal smoking during pregnancy, other prenatal and perinatal factors, and the risk of Legg-Calvé-Perthes disease. *Pediatrics.* 2008;122:e459–e464.
41. Kim HKW. Legg-Calvé-Perthes disease. *J Am Acad Orthop Surg.* 2010;18:676–686.
42. Seto CK, Statuta SM, Solari IL. Pediatric running injuries. *Clin Sports Med.* 2010;29:499–511.
43. Sanders TG, Zlatkin MB. Avulsion injuries of the pelvis. *Semin Musculoskelet Radiol.* 2008;12:42–53.
44. Chu SK, Rho ME. Hamstring injuries in the athlete: diagnosis, treatment, and return to play. *Curr Sports Med Rep.* 2016;15:184–190.
45. Lamplot JD, Matava MJ. Thigh injuries in American football. *Am J Orthop.* 2016;45:E308–E318.
46. Jackson TJ, Starkey C, McElhiney D, et al. Epidemiology of hip injuries in the National Basketball Association: a 24-year overview. *Orthop J Sports Med.* 2013;1:1–7.
47. Heiderscheit B, McClinton S. Evaluation and management of hip and pelvis injuries. *Phys Med Rehabil Clin N Am.* 2016;27:1–29.
48. Reurink G, Goudswaard GJ, Oomen HG, et al. Reliability of the active and passive knee extension test in acute hamstring injuries. *Am J Sports Med.* 2013;41:1757–1761.
49. Ryan JB, Wheeler JH, Hopkinson WJ, et al. Quadriceps contusions. West Point update. *Am J Sports Med.* 1991;19:299–304.
50. Jackson DW, Feagin JA. Quadriceps contusions in young athletes. Relation of severity of injury to treatment and prognosis. *J Bone Joint Surg Am.* 1973;55:95–105.
51. Bencardino JT, Rosenberg ZS, Brown RR, et al. Traumatic musculotendinous injuries of the knee: diagnosis with MR imaging. *Radiographics.* 2000;20:S103–S120.
52. Aronen JG, Garrick JG, Chronister RD, et al. Quadriceps contusions: clinical results of immediate immobilization in 120 degrees of knee flexion. *Clin J Sport Med.* 2006;16:383–387.
53. King JB. Post-traumatic ectopic calcification in the muscles of athletes: a review. *Br J Sports Med.* 1998;32:287–290.
54. Orchard JW. Intrinsic and extrinsic risk factors for muscle strains in Australian football. *Am J Sports Med.* 2001;29:300–303.
55. Cross TM. Acute quadriceps muscle strains: magnetic resonance imaging features and prognosis. *Am J Sports Med.* 2004;32:710–719.
56. Kary JM. Diagnosis and management of quadriceps strains and contusions. *Curr Rev Musculoskelet Med.* 2010;3:26–31.
57. Orchard JW, Seward H, Orchard JJ. Results of 2 decades of injury surveillance and public release of data in the Australian football league. *Am J Sports Med.* 2013;41:734–741.
58. Orchard J, Seward H. Epidemiology of injuries in the Australian Football League, seasons 1997–2000. *Br J Sports Med.* 2002;36:39–45.
59. Chumanov ES, Heiderscheit BC, Thelen DG. Hamstring musculotendon dynamics during stance and swing phases of high speed running. *Med Sci Sports Exerc.* 2011;43:525–532.
60. Askling CM, Tengvar M, Saartok T, et al. Acute first-time hamstring strains during slow-speed stretching: clinical, magnetic resonance imaging, and recovery characteristics. *Am J Sports Med.* 2007;35:1716–1724.
61. Askling C, Saartok T, Thorstensson A. Type of acute hamstring strain affects flexibility, strength, and time to return to pre-injury level. *Br J Sports Med.* 2006;40:40–44.

62. Ali K, Leland JM. Hamstring strains and tears in the athlete. *Clin Sports Med.* 2012;31:263–272.

63. Zarins B, Ciullo JV. Acute muscle and tendon injuries in athletes. *Clin Sports Med.* 1983;2:167–182.

64. Connell DA, Schneider-Kolsky ME, Hoving JL, et al. Longitudinal study comparing sonographic and MRI assessments of acute and healing hamstring injuries. *Am J Roentgenol.* 2004;183:975–984.

65. Koulouris G, Connell D. Imaging of hamstring injuries: therapeutic implications. *Eur Radiol.* 2006;16:1478–1487.

66. Hamid MSA, Yusof A, Ali MRM. Platelet-rich plasma (PRP) for acute muscle injury: a systematic review. *PLoS One.* 2014;9:e90538.

67. Hamilton B, Tol JL, Almusa E, et al. Platelet-rich plasma does not enhance return to play in hamstring injuries: a randomised controlled trial. *Br J Sports Med.* 2015;49:943–950.

68. Reurink G, Goudswaard GJ, Moen MH, et al. Platelet-rich plasma injections in acute muscle injury. *N Engl J Med.* 2014;370:2546–2547.

69. Reurink G, Goudswaard GJ, Moen MH, et al. Rationale, secondary outcome scores and 1-year follow-up of a randomised trial of platelet-rich plasma injections in acute hamstring muscle injury: the Dutch Hamstring Injection Therapy study. *Br J Sports Med.* 2015;49:1206–1212.

70. Rettig AC, Meyer S, Bhadra AK. Platelet-rich plasma in addition to rehabilitation for acute hamstring injuries in NFL players: clinical effects and time to return to play. *Orthop J Sports Med.* 2006;1:1–5.

71. Lempainen L, Sarimo J, Mattila K, et al. Proximal hamstring tendinopathy: results of surgical management and histopathologic findings. *Am J Sports Med.* 2009;37:727–734.

72. Zissen MH, Wallace G, Stevens KJ, et al. High hamstring tendinopathy. *Am J Roentgenol.* 2010;195:993–998.

73. Cushman D, Rho ME. Conservative treatment of subacute proximal hamstring tendinopathy using eccentric exercises performed with a treadmill: a case report. *J Orthop Sports Phys Ther.* 2015;45:557–562.

74. Jayaseelan DJ, Moats N, Ricardo CR. Rehabilitation of proximal hamstring tendinopathy utilizing eccentric training, lumbopelvic stabilization, and trigger point dry needling: 2 case reports. *J Orthop Sports Phys Ther.* 2014;44:198–205.

75. Fader RR, Mitchell JJ, Traub S, et al. Platelet-rich plasma treatment improves outcomes for chronic proximal hamstring injuries in an athletic population. *Muscles Ligaments Tendons J.* 2014;4:461–466.

76. Nicholson LT, DiSegna S, Newman JS, et al. Fluoroscopically guided peritendinous corticosteroid injection for proximal hamstring tendinopathy: a retrospective review. *Orthop J Sports Med.* 2014;2:1–5.

77. Standring S, ed. *Gray's Anatomy.* 41st ed. Philadelphia, PA: Elsevier; 2016.

78. Warren LF, Marshall JL. The supporting structures and layers on the medial side of the knee: an anatomical analysis. *J Bone Joint Surg Am.* 1979;61:56–62.

79. Fairclough J, Hayashi K, Toumi H, et al. The functional anatomy of the iliotibial band during flexion and extension of the knee: implications for understanding iliotibial band syndrome. *J Anat.* 2006;208:309–316.

80. Beutler A, O'Connor FG. Physical examination of the knee. In: Malanga GA, Mautner K, eds. *Musculoskeletal Physical Examination: An Evidence-Based Approach.* Philadelphia, PA: Elsevier; 2017.

81. Boden BP, Dean GS, Feagin JA, et al. Mechanisms of anterior cruciate ligament injury. *Orthopedics.* 2000;23:573–578.

82. Kaeding CC, Léger-St-Jean B, Magnussen RA. Epidemiology and diagnosis of anterior cruciate ligament injuries. *Clin Sports Med.* 2017;36:1–8.

83. Lee JK, Yao L, Phelps CT, et al. Anterior cruciate ligament tears: MR imaging compared with arthroscopy and clinical tests. *Radiology.* 1988;166:861–864.

84. Ranstam J, Lohmander LS, Frobell R, et al. A randomized trial of treatment for acute anterior cruciate ligament tears. *N Engl J Med.* 2010;4:331–342.

85. Fanelli GC, Edson CJ. Posterior cruciate ligament injuries in trauma patients: part II. *Arthroscopy.* 1995;11:526–529.

86. Harner CD, Höher J. Evaluation and treatment of posterior cruciate ligament injuries. *Am J Sports Med.* 2006;26:471–482.

87. Vaz CES, De Camargo OP, De Santana PJ, et al. Accuracy of magnetic resonance in identifying traumatic intraarticular knee lesions. *Clinics.* 2005;60:445–450.

88. MacLean CL, Taunton JE, Clement DB, et al. Eccentric and concentric isokinetic moment characteristics in the quadriceps and hamstrings of the chronic isolated posterior cruciate ligament injured knee. *Br J Sports Med.* 1999;33:405–408.

89. Phisitkul P, James SL, Wolf BR, et al. MCL injuries of the knee: current concepts review. *Iowa Orthop J.* 2006;26:77–90.

90. Nakamura N, Horibe S, Toritsuka Y, et al. Acute grade III medial collateral ligament injury of the knee associated with anterior cruciate ligament tear. The usefulness of magnetic resonance imaging in determining a treatment regimen. *Am J Sports Med.* 2003;31:261–267.

91. Indelicato PA, Hermansdorfer J, Huegel M. Nonoperative management of complete tears of the medial collateral ligament of the knee in intercollegiate football players. *Clin Orthop Relat Res.* 1990;(256):174–177.

92. Covey DC. Injuries of the posterolateral corner of the knee. *J Bone Joint Surg Am.* 2001;83–A:106–118.

93. LaPrade RF, Wentorf FA, Fritts H, et al. A prospective magnetic resonance imaging study of the incidence of posterolateral and multiple ligament injuries in acute knee injuries presenting with a hemarthrosis. *Arthroscopy.* 2007;23:1341–1347.

94. Fleming RE, Blatz DJ, McCarroll JR. Posterior problems in the knee. Posterior cruciate insufficiency and posterolateral rotatory insufficiency. *Am J Sports Med.* 1981;9:107–113.

95. Crespo B, James EW, Metsavaht L, et al. Injuries to posterolateral corner of the knee: a comprehensive review from anatomy to surgical treatment. *Rev Bras Ortop.* 2015;50:613.

96. Krukhaug Y, Mølster A, Rodt A, et al. Lateral ligament injuries of the knee. *Knee Surg Sports Traumatol Arthrosc.* 1998;6:21–25.

97. Kannus P, Natri A. Etiology and pathophysiology of tendon ruptures in sports. *Scand J Med Sci Sports.* 1997;7:107–112.

98. Kannus P. Nonoperative treatment of grade II and III sprains of the lateral ligament compartment of the knee. *Am J Sports Med.* 1989;17:83–88.

99. Aagaard H, Verdonk R. Function of the normal meniscus and consequences of meniscal resection. *Scand J Med Sci Sports.* 1999;9:134–140.

100. Guermazi A, Niu J, Hayashi D, et al. Prevalence of abnormalities in knees detected by MRI in adults without knee osteoarthritis: population based observational study (Framingham Osteoarthritis Study). *BMJ.* 2012;345:e5339.

101. Subhas N, Sakamoto FA, Mariscalco MW, et al. Accuracy of MRI in the diagnosis of meniscal tears in older patients. *Am J Roentgenol.* 2012;198:575–580.

102. Beaufils P, Becker R, Kopf S, et al. Surgical management of degenerative meniscus lesions: the 2016 ESSKA meniscus consensus. *Knee Surg Sports Traumatol Arthrosc.* 2017;25:335–346.

103. Jevsevar DS. Treatment of osteoarthritis of the knee: evidence-based guideline, 2nd edition. *J Am Acad Orthop Surg.* 2013;21:571–576.

104. Herman AM, Marzo JM. Popliteal cysts: a current review. *Orthopedics.* 2014;14:e678–e684.

105. Lindgren PG, Willén R. Gastrocnemio-semimembranosus bursa and its relation to the knee joint. I. Anatomy and histology. *Acta Radiol Diagn (Stockh).* 1977;18:497–512.

106. Sansone V, de Ponti A, Paluello GM, et al. Popliteal cysts and associated disorders of the knee. Critical review with MR imaging. *Int Orthop.* 1995;19:275–279.

107. Liao S-T, Chiou C-S, Chang C-C. Pathology associated to the Baker's cysts: a musculoskeletal ultrasound study. *Clin Rheumatol.* 2010;29:1043–1047.

108. Marra MD, Crema MD, Chung M, et al. MRI features of cystic lesions around the knee. *Knee.* 2008;15:423–438.

109. Ward EE, Jacobson JA, Fessell DP, et al. Sonographic detection of Baker's cysts: comparison with MR imaging. *Am J Roentgenol.* 2001;176:373–380.

110. Acebes JC, Sánchez-Pernaute O, Díaz-Oca A, et al. Ultrasonographic assessment of Baker's cysts after intra-articular corticosteroid injection in knee osteoarthritis. *J Clin Ultrasound.* 2006;34:113–117.

111. Köroğlu M, Callıoğlu M, Eriş HN, et al. Ultrasound guided percutaneous treatment and follow-up of Baker's cyst in knee osteoarthritis. *Eur J Radiol.* 2012;81:3466–3471.

112. Teitge RA. Patellofemoral syndrome a paradigm for current surgical strategies. *Orthop Clin North Am.* 2008;39:287–311.

113. Witvrouw E, Callaghan MJ, Stefanik JJ, et al. Patellofemoral pain: consensus statement from the 3rd International Patellofemoral Pain Research Retreat held in Vancouver, September 2013. *Br J Sports Med.* 2014;48:411–414.

114. Crossley KM, Callaghan MJ, van Linschoten R. Patellofemoral pain. *Br Med J.* 2015;351:h3939.

115. Young B, Walker MJ, Strunce J, et al. Efficacy of nonsurgical interventions for anterior knee pain: systematic review and meta-analysis of randomized trials. *J Orthop Sports Phys Ther.* 2012;42:22–29.

116. Heintjes E, Berger MY, Bierma-Zeinstra SM, et al. Pharmacotherapy for patellofemoral pain syndrome. *Cochrane Database Syst Rev.* 2004;3:CD003470.

117. Peers KHE, Lysens RJJ. Patellar tendinopathy in athletes current diagnostic and therapeutic recommendations. *Sports Med.* 2005;35:71–87.

118. Ferretti A. Epidemiology of jumper's knee. *Sports Med.* 1986;3:289–295.

119. LLopis E, Padrón M. Anterior knee pain. *Eur J Radiol.* 2007;62:27–43.

120. Gaida JE, Cook J. Treatment options for patellar tendinopathy: critical review. *Curr Sports Med Rep.* 2011;10:255–270.

121. Åstrom M, Westlin N. No effect of piroxicam on Achilles tendinopathy. *Acta Orthop.* 1992;63:631–634.

122. Shrier I, Matheson GO, Kohl HW. Achilles tendonitis: are corticosteroid injections useful or harmful? *Clin J Sport Med.* 1996;6:245–250.

123. Nichols AW. Complications associated with the use of corticosteroids in the treatment of athletic injuries. *Clin J Sport Med.* 2005;15:370–375.

124. Strauss EJ, Kim S, Calcei JG, et al. Iliotibial band syndrome: evaluation and management. *J Am Acad Orthop Surg.* 2011;19:728–736.

125. Messier SP, Edwards DG, Martin DF, et al. Etiology of iliotibial band friction syndrome in distance runners. *Med Sci Sports Exerc.* 1995;27:951–960.

126. Ellis R, Hing W, Reid D. Iliotibial band friction syndrome—a systematic review. *Man Ther.* 2007;12:200–208.

127. Gunter P, Schwellnus MP. Local corticosteroid injection in iliotibial band friction syndrome in runners: a randomised controlled trial. *Br J Sports Med.* 2004;38:269–272.

128. McAfee JH, Smith DL. Olecranon and prepatellar bursitis. Diagnosis and treatment. *West J Med.* 1988;149:607–610.

129. Weinstein PS, Canoso JJ, Wohlgethan JR. Long-term follow-up of corticosteroid injection for traumatic olecranon bursitis. *Ann Rheum Dis.* 1984;43:44–46.

130. Sarifakioglu B, Afsar SI, Yalbuzdag SA, et al. Comparison of the efficacy of physical therapy and corticosteroid injection in the treatment of pes anserine tendinobursitis. *J Phys Ther Sci.* 2016;28:1993–1997.

131. Ogden JA, Southwick WO. Osgood-Schlatter's disease and tibial tuberosity development. *Clin Orthop Relat Res.* 1976;180–189.

132. Kajetanek C, Thaunat M, Guimaraes T, et al. Arthroscopic treatment of painful Sinding-Larsen-Johansson syndrome in a professional handball player. *Orthop Traumatol Surg Res.* 2016;102:677–680.

133. Iwamoto J, Takeda T, Sato Y, et al. Radiographic abnormalities of the inferior pole of the patella in juvenile athletes. *Keio J Med.* 2009;58:50–53.

134. Jackson AM. Anterior knee pain. *J Bone Joint Surg Br.* 2001;583:937–948.

135. Orava S, Malinen L, Karpakka J, et al. Results of surgical treatment of unresolved Osgood-Schlatter lesion. *Ann Chir Gynaecol.* 2000;89:298–302.

136. Peace KAL, Lee JC, Healy J. Imaging the infrapatellar tendon in the elite athlete. *Clin Radiol.* 2006;61:570–578.

137. Gholve PA, Scher DM, Khakharia S, et al. Osgood Schlatter syndrome. *Curr Opin Pediatr.* 2007;19:44–50.

138. Ross MD, Villard D. Disability levels of college-aged men with a history of Osgood-Schlatter disease. *J Strength Cond Res.* 2003;17:659–663.

139. Taunton JE, Ryan MB, Clement DB, et al. A retrospective case-control analysis of 2002 running injuries. *Br J Sports Med.* 2002;36:95–101.

140. Rajasekaran S, Finnoff JT. Exertional leg pain. *Phys Med Rehabil Clin N Am.* 2016;27:91–119.

141. Rajasekaran S, Kvinlaug K, Finnoff JT. Exertional leg pain in the athlete. *PM R.* 2012;4:985–1000.

142. Reshef N, Guelich DR. Medial tibial stress syndrome. *Clin Sports Med.* 2012;31:273–290.

143. Lesho EP. Can tuning forks replace bone scans for identification of tibial stress fractures? *Mil Med.* 1997;162:802–803.

144. Yates B, White S. The incidence and risk factors in the development of medial tibial stress syndrome among naval recruits. *Am J Sports Med.* 2004;32:772–780.

145. Lopes AD, Hespanhol LC, Yeung SS, et al. What are the main running related musculoskeletal injuries? *Sports Med.* 2012;42:892–905.

146. Devas MB. Stress fractures of the tibia in athletes or shin soreness. *J Bone Joint Surg Br.* 1958;40–B:227–239.

147. Saxena A, O'Brien T, Bunce D. Anatomic dissection of the tibialis posterior muscle and its correlation to medial tibial stress syndrome. *J Foot Surg.* 1990;29:105–108.

148. Bouché RT, Johnson CH. Medial tibial stress syndrome (tibial fasciitis): a proposed pathomechanical model involving fascial traction. *J Am Podiatr Med Assoc.* 2007;97:31–36.

149. Franklyn M, Oakes B, Field B, et al. Section modulus is the optimum geometric predictor for stress fractures and medial tibial stress syndrome in both male and female athletes. *Am J Sports Med.* 2008;36:1179–1189.

150. Magnusson HI, Westlin NE, Nyqvist F, et al. Abnormally decreased regional bone density in athletes with medial tibial stress syndrome. *Am J Sports Med.* 2001;29:712–715.

151. Magnusson HI, Ahlborg HG, Karlsson C, et al. Low regional tibial bone density in athletes with medial tibial stress syndrome normalizes after recovery from symptoms. *Am J Sports Med.* 2003;31:596–600.

152. Kortebein PM, Kaufman KR, Basford JR, et al. Medial tibial stress syndrome. *Med Sci Sports Exerc.* 2000;32:S27–S33.

153. Moen M, Tol J, Steunebrink M, et al. Medial tibial stress syndrome: a critical review. *Sports Med.* 2009;7:21–49.

154. Beck BR, Bergman AG, Miner M, et al. Tibial stress injury: relationship of radiographic, nuclear medicine bone scanning, MR imaging, and CT severity grades to clinical severity and time to healing. *Radiology.* 2012;263:811–818.

155. Chisin R, Milgrom C, Giladi M, et al. Clinical significance of nonfocal scintigraphic findings in suspected tibial stress fractures. *Clin Orthop Relat Res.* 1987;(220):200–205.

156. Batt ME, Ugalde V, Anderson MW, et al. A prospective controlled study of diagnostic imaging for acute shin splints. *Med Sci Sports Exerc.* 1998;30:1564–1571.

157. Fredericson M, Bergman AG, Hoffman KL, et al. Tibial stress reaction in runners: correlation of clinical symptoms and scintigraphy with a new magnetic resonance imaging grading system. *Am J Sports Med.* 1995;23:472–481.

158. Moen MH, Rayer S, Schipper M, et al. Shockwave treatment for medial tibial stress syndrome in athletes; a prospective controlled study. *Br J Sports Med.* 2012;46:253–257.

159. Robertson GAJ, Wood AM. Return to sports after stress fractures of the tibial diaphysis: a systematic review. *Br Med Bull.* 2015;114:95–111.

160. Harrast M, Colonno D. Stress fractures in runners. *Clin Sports Med.* 2012;31:291–306.

161. Gardner LI, Dziados JE, Jones BH, et al. Prevention of lower extremity stress fractures: a controlled trial of a shock absorbent insole. *Am J Public Health.* 1988;78:1563–1567.

162. Burrus MT, Werner BC, Starman JS, et al. Chronic leg pain in athletes. *Am J Sports Med.* 2014;43:1538–1547.

163. Shuler FD, Wingate MK, Moore GH, et al. Sports health benefits of vitamin D. *Sports Health.* 2012;4:496–501.

164. Rome K, Handoll HHG, Ashford R. Interventions for preventing and treating stress fractures and stress reactions of bone of the lower limbs in young adults. *Cochrane Database Syst Rev.* 2005;(2):CD000450.

165. Flick D, Flick R. Chronic exertional compartment syndrome. *Curr Sports Med Rep.* 2016;33:219–233.

166. Detmer DE, Sharpe K, Sufit RL, et al. Chronic compartment syndrome: diagnosis, management, and outcomes. *Am J Sports Med.* 1985;13:162–170.

167. Nguyen JT, Nguyen JL, Wheatley MJ, et al. Muscle hernias of the leg: a case report and comprehensive review of the literature. *Can J Plast Surg.* 2013;21:243–247.

168. Pedowitz RA, Hargens AR, Mubarak SJ, et al. Modified criteria for the objective diagnosis of chronic compartment syndrome of the leg. *Am J Sports Med.* 1990;18:35–40.

169. Roscoe D, Roberts AJ, Hulse D. Intramuscular compartment pressure measurement in chronic exertional compartment syndrome: new and improved diagnostic criteria. *Am J Sports Med.* 2015;43:392–398.

170. Packer JD, Day MS, Nguyen JT, et al. Functional outcomes and patient satisfaction after fasciotomy for chronic exertional compartment syndrome. *Am J Sports Med.* 2013;41:430–436.

171. Di Marzo L, Cavallaro A. Popliteal vascular entrapment. *World J Surg.* 2005;29:43–45.

172. Joy S, Raudales R. Popliteal artery entrapment syndrome. *Curr Rev Musculoskelet Med.* 2015;14:364–367.

173. Sinha S, Houghton J, Holt PJ, et al. Popliteal entrapment syndrome. *J Vasc Surg.* 2012;55:252.e30–262.e30.

174. Chernoff DM, Walker AT, Khorasani R, et al. Asymptomatic functional popliteal artery entrapment: demonstration at MR imaging. *Radiology.* 1995;195:176–180.

175. Anderson JC. Common fibular nerve compression anatomy, symptoms, clinical evaluation, and surgical decompression. *Clin Podiatr Med Surg.* 2016;33:283–291.

176. Visser LH, Hens V, Soethout M, et al. Diagnostic value of high-resolution sonography in common fibular neuropathy at the fibular head. *Muscle Nerve.* 2013;48:171–178.

177. Pineda D, Barroso F, Cháves H, et al. High resolution 3T magnetic resonance neurography of the peroneal nerve. *Radiologia.* 2014;56:107–117.

178. Fields KB, Rigby MD. Muscular calf injuries in runners. *Curr Sports Med Rep.* 2016;15:320–324.

179. Koulouris G, Ting AYI, Jhamb A, et al. Magnetic resonance imaging findings of injuries to the calf muscle complex. *Skeletal Radiol.* 2007;36:921–927.

180. Delgado GJ, Chung CB, Lektrakul N, et al. Tennis leg: clinical US study of 141 patients and anatomic investigation of four cadavers with MR imaging and US. *Radiology.* 2002;224:112–119.

181. Maffulli N, Ajis A. Management of chronic ruptures of the Achilles tendon. *J Bone Joint Surg Am.* 2008;90:1348–1360.

182. Kwak HS, Lee KB, Han YM. Ruptures of the medial head of the gastrocnemius ("tennis leg"): clinical outcome and compression effect. *Clin Imaging.* 2006;30:48–53.

183. Beyer R, Kongsgaard M, Hougs Kjær B, et al. Heavy slow resistance versus eccentric training as treatment for Achilles tendinopathy: a randomized controlled trial. *Am J Sports Med.* 2015;43:1704–1711.

184. Chaudhry H, Simunovic N, Petrisor B. Cochrane in CORR: surgical versus conservative treatment for acute injuries of the lateral ligament complex of the ankle in adults (review). *Clin Orthop Relat Res.* 2015;473:17–22.

185. Thomas MJ, Roddy E, Zhang W, et al. The population prevalence of foot and ankle pain in middle and old age: a systematic review. *Pain.* 2011;152:2870–2880.

186. Schumer RA, Hall MM, Amendola A. Physical examination of the foot and ankle. In: Malanga GA, Mautner KR, eds. *Musculoskeletal Physical Examination: An Evidence-Based Approach.* Philadelphia, PA: Elsevier; 2017.

187. Skjong CC, Meininger AK, Ho SSW. Tendinopathy treatment: where is the evidence? *Clin Sports Med.* 2012;31:329–350.

188. Abate M, Silbernagel KG, Siljeholm C, et al. Pathogenesis of tendinopathies: inflammation or degeneration? *Arthritis Res Ther.* 2009;11:235.

189. Khan KM, Forster BB, Robinson J, et al. Are ultrasound and magnetic resonance imaging of value in assessment of Achilles tendon disorders? A two year prospective study. *Br J Sports Med.* 2003;37:149–153.

190. Alfredson H, Cook J. A treatment algorithm for managing Achilles tendinopathy: new treatment options. *Br J Sports Med.* 2007;41:211–216.

191. Magnussen RA, Dunn WR, Thomson AB. Nonoperative treatment of midportion Achilles tendinopathy: a systematic review. *Clin J Sport Med.* 2009;19:54–64.

192. Stanish WD, Rubinovich RM, Curwin S. Eccentric exercise in chronic tendinitis. *Clin Orthop Relat Res.* 1986;65–68.

193. Alfredson H, Pietilä T, Jonsson P, et al. Heavy-load eccentric calf muscle training for the treatment of chronic Achilles tendinosis. *Am J Sports Med.* 1998;26:360–366.

194. Jonsson P, Alfredson H, Sunding K, et al. New regimen for eccentric calf-muscle training in patients with chronic insertional Achilles tendinopathy: results of a pilot study. *Br J Sports Med.* 2008;42:746–749.

195. Kearney R, Costa ML. Insertional Achilles tendinopathy management: a systematic review. *Foot Ankle Int.* 2010;31:689–694.

196. Leppilahti J, Puranen J, Orava S. Incidence of Achilles tendon rupture. *Acta Orthop Scand.* 1996;67:277–279.

197. Chiodo CP, Glazebrook M, Bluman EM, et al. Diagnosis and treatment of acute Achilles tendon rupture. *J Am Acad Orthop Surg.* 2010;18:503–510.

198. Wilkins R, Bisson LJ. Operative versus nonoperative management of acute Achilles tendon ruptures: a quantitative systematic review of randomized controlled trials. *Am J Sports Med.* 2012;40:2154–2160.

199. van der Eng DM, Schepers T, Goslings JC, et al. Rerupture rate after early weight-bearing in operative versus conservative treatment of Achilles tendon ruptures: a meta-analysis. *J Foot Ankle Surg.* 2013;52:622–628.

200. Suchak AA, Bostick GP, Beaupre LA, et al. The influence of early weight-bearing compared with non-weight-bearing after surgical repair of the Achilles tendon. *J Bone Joint Surg Am.* 2008;90:1876–1883.

201. Twaddle BC, Poon P. Early motion for Achilles tendon ruptures: is surgery important? A randomized, prospective study. *Am J Sports Med.* 2007;35:2033–2038.

202. Ingvar J, Encroth M. Nonoperative treatment of Achilles tendon rupture. *Sports Med.* 2005;76:597–601.

203. McGlamry E, Banks A. *McGlamry's Comprehensive Textbook of Foot and Ankle Surgery.* 3rd ed. Philadelphia, PA: Lippincott Williams & Wilkins; 2001.

204. Kaye RA, Jahss MH. Tibialis posterior: a review of anatomy and biomechanics in relation to support of the medial longitudinal arch. *Foot Ankle.* 1991;11:244–247.

205. Wapner KL, Chao W. Nonoperative treatment of posterior tibial tendon dysfunction. *Clin Orthop Relat Res.* 1999;(365):39–45.

206. Kulig K, Reischi SF, Pomrantz AB, et al. Nonsurgical management of posterior tibial tendon dysfunction with orthoses and resistive exercise: a randomized control trial. *Phys Ther.* 2009;89:26–37.

207. Holmes GBJ, Mann RA. Possible epidemiological factors associated with rupture of the posterior tibial tendon. *Foot Ankle.* 1992;13:70–79.

208. Pomeroy GC, Pike RH, Beals TC, et al. Acquired flatfoot in adults due to dysfunction of the posterior tibial tendon. *J Bone Joint Surg Am.* 1999;81:1173–1182.

209. Griffiths JC. Tendon injuries around the ankle. *J Bone Joint Surg Br.* 1965;47:686–689.

210. Marcus RE, Goodfellow DB, Pfister ME. The difficult diagnosis of posterior tibialis tendon rupture in sports injuries. *Orthopedics.* 1995;18:715–721.

211. Myerson M, Solomon G, Shereff M. Posterior tibial tendon dysfunction: its association with seronegative inflammatory disease. *Foot Ankle.* 1989;9:219–225.

212. Banks AS, McGlamry ED. Tibialis posterior tendon rupture. *J Am Podiatr Med Assoc.* 1987;77:170–176.

213. Johnson KA, Strom DE. Tibialis posterior tendon dysfunction. *Clin Orthop Relat Res.* 1989;196–206.

214. Bowring B, Chockalingam N. A clinical guideline for the conservative management of tibialis posterior tendon dysfunction. *Foot (Edinb).* 2009;19:211–217.

215. Sammarco GJ. Peroneal tendon injuries. *Orthop Clin North Am.* 1994;25:135–145.

216. Selmani E, Gjata V, Gjika E. Current concepts review: peroneal tendon disorders. *Foot Ankle Int.* 2006;27:221–228.

217. Sammarco GJ, Mangone PG. Diagnosis and treatment of peroneal tendon injuries. *Foot Ankle Surg.* 2000;6:197–205.

218. Ivins D. Acute ankle sprain: an update. *Am Fam Physician.* 2006;74(10):1714–1720.

219. Wexler RK. The injured ankle. *Am Fam Physician.* 1998;57:474–480.

220. Williams GN, Jones MH, Amendola A. Syndesmotic ankle sprains in athletes. *Am J Sports Med.* 2007;35:1197–1207.

221. Stiell I, Greenberg G, McKnight R, et al. A study to develop clinical decision rules for the use of radiography in acute ankle injuries. *Ann Emerg Med.* 1992;21:384–390.

222. Bleakley CM, O'Connor SR, Tully MA, et al. Effect of accelerated rehabilitation on function after ankle sprain: randomised controlled trial. *BMJ.* 2010;340:c1964.

223. Mattacola CG, Dwyer MK. Rehabilitation of the ankle after acute sprain or chronic instability. *J Athl Train.* 2002;37:413–429.

224. Kerkhoffs GM, Rowe BH, Assendelft WJ, et al. Immobilisation and functional treatment for acute lateral ankle ligament injuries in adults. *Cochrane Database Syst Rev.* 2002;3:CD003762.

225. Takao M, Ochi M, Oae K, et al. Diagnosis of a tear of the tibiofibular syndesmosis: the role of arthroscopy of the ankle. *J Bone Joint Surg Br.* 2003;85-B:324–329.

226. Eiff M, Hatch R, Higgins MK. *Fracture Management for Primary Care.* 3rd ed. Philadelphia, PA: Saunders/Elsevier; 2012.

227. Verhagen RAW, Maas M, Dijkgraaf MGW, et al. Prospective study on diagnostic strategies in osteochondral lesions of the talus—is MRI superior to helical CT? *J Bone Joint Surg Br.* 2005;87-B:41–46.

228. Berndt AL, Harty M. Transchondral fractures (osteochondritis dissecans) of the talus. *J Bone Joint Surg Am.* 1959;41-A:988–1020.

229. O'Loughlin PF, Heyworth BE, Kennedy JG. Current concepts in the diagnosis and treatment of osteochondral lesions of the ankle. *Am J Sports Med.* 2010;38:392–404.

230. Zengerink M, Szerb I, Hangody L, et al. Current concepts: treatment of osteochondral ankle defects. *Foot Ankle Clin.* 2006;11:331–359.

231. Kabbani YM, Mayer DP. Magnetic resonance imaging of osteochondral lesions of the talar dome. *J Am Podiatr Med Assoc.* 1994;84:192–195.

232. Black JR, Hale WE. Prevalence of foot complaints in the elderly. *J Am Podiatr Med Assoc.* 1987;77:308–311.

233. Karasick D, Wapner KL. Hallux valgus deformity: preoperative radiologic assessment. *AJR Am J Roentgenol.* 1990;155:119–123.

234. Pommering TL, Kluchurosky L, Hall SL. Ankle and foot injuries in pediatric and adult athletes. *Prim Care.* 2005;32:133–161.

235. Buchbinder R. Plantar fasciitis. *N Engl J Med.* 2004;350:2159–2166.

236. Crawford F, Thomson C. Interventions for treating plantar heel pain. *Cochrane Database Syst Rev.* 2003;(3):CD000416.

237. Tatli YZ, Kapasi S. The real risks of steroid injection for plantar fasciitis, with a review of conservative therapies. *Curr Rev Musculoskelet Med.* 2009;2:3–9.

238. Wu KK. Morton's interdigital neuroma: a clinical review of its etiology, treatment, and results. *J Foot Ankle Surg.* 1996;35:112–119.

239. Thomas JL, Blitch EL IV, Chaney DM, et al. Diagnosis and treatment of forefoot disorders. Section 3. Morton's intermetatarsal neuroma. *J Foot Ankle Surg.* 2009;48:251–256.

240. Mulder JD. The causative mechanism in Morton's metatarsalgia. *J Bone Joint Surg Br.* 1951;33-B:94–95.

241. Gerbert J. *Textbook of Bunion Surgery.* Philadelphia, PA: WB Saunders; 2001.

242. Boike A, Schnirring-Judge M, McMillin S. Sesamoid disorders of the first metatarsophalangeal joint. *Clin Podiatr Med Surg.* 2011;28:269–285.

243. Sims AL, Kurup HV. Painful sesamoid of the great toe. *World J Orthop.* 2014;5:146–150.

244. Yang R, Chu Y. Hallucal sesamoiditis manifested on bone scan. *Clin Nucl Med.* 2013;38:1019–1021.

245. Berg JH, Silveri CP, Harris M. Variant of the Lisfranc fracture-dislocation: a case report and review of the literature. *J Orthop Trauma.* 1998;12:366–369.

246. Arntz CT, Hansen ST Jr. Dislocations and fracture dislocations of the tarsometatarsal joints. *Orthop Clin North Am.* 1987;18:105–114.

247. Myerson MS, Fisher RT, Burgess AR, et al. Fracture dislocations of the tarsometatarsal joints: end results correlated with pathology and treatment. *Foot Ankle.* 1986;6:225–242.

248. Ross G, Cronin R, Hauzenblas J, et al. Plantar ecchymosis sign: a clinical aid to diagnosis of occult Lisfranc tarsometatarsal injuries. *J Orthop Trauma.* 1996;10:119–122.

249. Nunley JA, Vertullo CJ. Classification, investigation, and management of midfoot sprains: Lisfranc injuries in the athlete. *Am J Sports Med.* 2002;30:871–878.

250. Smith JW, Arnoczky SP, Hersh A. The intraosseous blood supply of the fifth metatarsal: implications for proximal fracture healing. *Foot Ankle.* 1992;13:143–152.

251. Cheung CN, Tun HL. Proximal fifth metatarsal fractures: anatomy, classification, treatment and complications. *Arch Trauma Res.* 2016;5:e33298.

252. Scharfbillig RW, Jones S, Scutter SD. Sever's disease: what does the literature really tell us? *J Am Podiatr Med Assoc.* 2008;98:212–223.

253. James AM, Williams CM, Haines TP. Effectiveness of interventions in reducing pain and maintaining physical activity in children and adolescents with calcaneal apophysitis (Sever's disease): a systematic review. *J Foot Ankle Res.* 2013;6:16.

254. Cassas KJ, Cassettari-Wayhs A. Childhood and adolescent sports-related overuse injuries. *Am Fam Physician.* 2006;73:1014–1022.

255. Sinusas K. Osteoarthritis: diagnosis and treatment. *Am Fam Physician.* 2012;1:49–56.

256. Litwic A, Edwards MH, Dennison EM, et al. Epidemiology and burden of osteoarthritis. *Br Med Bull.* 2013;105:185–199.

257. Barg A, Pagenstert GI, Hügle T, et al. Ankle osteoarthritis: etiology, diagnostics, and classification. *Foot Ankle Clin.* 2013;18:411–426.

258. Kalichman L, Hernández-Molina G. Midfoot and forefoot osteoarthritis. *Foot (Edinb).* 2014;24:128–134.

259. Grunfeld R, Aydogan U, Juliano P. Ankle arthritis: review of diagnosis and operative management. *Med Clin North Am.* 2014;98:267–289.

260. Neogi T, Zhang Y. Epidemiology of osteoarthritis. *Rheum Dis Clin North Am.* 2013;39:1–19.

261. Nelson AE, Allen KD, Golightly YM, et al. A systematic review of recommendations and guidelines for the management of osteoarthritis: the chronic osteoarthritis management initiative of the U.S. bone and joint initiative. *Semin Arthritis Rheum.* 2014;43:701–712.

262. Fernandes L, Hagen KB, Bijlsma JWJ, et al. EULAR recommendations for the non-pharmacological core management of hip and knee osteoarthritis. *Ann Rheum Dis.* 2013;72:1125–1135.

263. Losina E, Weinstein AM, Reichmann WM, et al. Lifetime risk and age at diagnosis of symptomatic knee osteoarthritis in the US. *Arthritis Care Res.* 2013;65:703–711.

264. Kim C, Linsenmeyer KD, Vlad SC, et al. Prevalence of radiographic and symptomatic hip osteoarthritis in an urban United States community: the Framingham osteoarthritis study. *Arthritis Rheumatol.* 2014;66:3013–3017.

265. Valderrabano V, Horisberger M, Russell I, et al. Etiology of ankle osteoarthritis. *Clin Orthop Relat Res.* 2009;467:1800–1806.

266. Roddy E, Thomas MJ, Marshall M, et al. The population prevalence of symptomatic radiographic foot osteoarthritis in community-dwelling older adults: cross-sectional findings from the Clinical Assessment Study of the Foot. *Ann Rheum Dis.* 2015;74:156–163.

267. Iagnocco A, Rizzo C, Gattamelata A, et al. Osteoarthritis of the foot: a review of the current state of knowledge. *Med Ultrason.* 2013;15:35–40.

268. Saltzman CL, Salamon ML, Blanchard GM, et al. Epidemiology of ankle arthritis: report of a consecutive series of 639 patients from a tertiary orthopaedic center. *Iowa Orthop J.* 1999;25:44–46.

269. Guilak F, Ratcliffe A, Lane N, et al. Mechanical and biochemical changes in the superficial zone of articular cartilage in canine experimental osteoarthritis. *J Orthop Res.* 1994;12:474–484.

270. Ehrlich MG, Armstrong AL, Treadwell BV, et al. The role of proteases in the pathogenesis of osteoarthritis. *J Rheumatol.* 1987;14:30–32.

271. Bollet AJ, Nance JL. Biochemical findings in normal and osteoarthritic articular cartilage. II. Chondroitin sulfate concentration and chain length, water, and ash content. *J Clin Invest.* 1966;45:1170–1177.

272. Radin EL, Rose RM. Role of subchondral bone in the initiation and progression of cartilage damage. *Clin Orthop Relat Res.* 1986;(213):34–40.

273. Balazs EA, Watson D, Duff IF, et al. Hyaluronic acid in synovial fluid. I. Molecular parameters of hyaluronic acid in normal and arthritic human fluids. *Arthritis Rheum.* 1967;10:357–376.

274. McAlindon TE, Bannuru RR, Sullivan MC, et al. OARSI guidelines for the non-surgical management of knee osteoarthritis. *Osteoarthr Cartil.* 2014;22:363–388.

275. National Institute for Health and Care Excellence. *Osteoarthritis: Care and Management in Adults.* NICE clinical guideline 177; 2014. Available from: https://www.nice.org.uk/guidance/cg177

276. Hochberg MC, Altman RD, April KT, et al. American College of Rheumatology 2012 recommendations for the use of nonpharmacologic and pharmacologic therapies in osteoarthritis of the hand, hip, and knee. *Arthritis Care Res.* 2012;64:465–474.

277. Bruyère O, Cooper C, Pelletier J-P, et al. A consensus statement on the European Society for Clinical and Economic Aspects of Osteoporosis and Osteoarthritis

(ESCEO) algorithm for the management of knee osteoarthritis-From evidence-based medicine to the real-life setting. *Semin Arthritis Rheum.* 2016;45:S3–S11.

278. Robinson AHN, Keith T. Osteoarthritis of the ankle. *Orthop Trauma.* 2016;30:59–67.

279. Zhang W, Nuki G, Moskowitz RW, et al. OARSI recommendations for the management of hip and knee osteoarthritis. Part III: Changes in evidence following systematic cumulative update of research published through January 2009. *Osteoarthr Cartil.* 2010;18:476–499.

280. Scarpignato C, Lanas A, Blandizzi C, et al. Safe prescribing of non-steroidal anti-inflammatory drugs in patients with osteoarthritis—an expert consensus addressing benefits as well as gastrointestinal and cardiovascular risks. *BMC Med.* 2015;13:55.

281. Derry S, Moore RA, Rabbie R. Topical NSAIDs for chronic musculoskeletal pain in adults. *Cochrane Database Syst Rev.* 2012;(9):CD007400.

282. Brewer AR, McCarberg B, Argoff CE. Update on the use of topical NSAIDs for the treatment of soft tissue and musculoskeletal pain: a review of recent data and current treatment options. *Phys Sportsmed.* 2010;38:62–70.

283. Nissen SE, Yeomans ND, Solomon DH, et al. Cardiovascular safety of celecoxib, naproxen, or ibuprofen for arthritis. *N Engl J Med.* 2016;375:2519–2529.

284. McGettigan P, Henry D. Cardiovascular risk with nonsteroidal anti-inflammatory drugs: systematic review of population-based controlled observational studies. *PLoS Med.* 2011;8:e1001098.

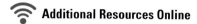 **Additional Resources Online**

Pamela Hansen
Rebecca Wilson Zingg

CHAPTER 31

The Prevention, Treatment, and Rehabilitation of Osteoporosis

Bone health is important to overall health and quality of life. Bones provide a frame that permits mobility, and protects internal organs from injury, while being a storehouse for minerals vital to the self-sustaining functions of daily life. Although osteoporosis is the most common bone disease, it continues to be underrecognized because there are no warning signs before fracture. It is often not treated, even after osteoporosis-related fractures have occurred. Disfigurement, chronic pain, depression, disability, and increased mortality can result (1).

In the United States, 53 million individuals currently have osteoporosis or osteopenia (2). The financial burden associated with bone mineral density (BMD) disease is significant and will only continue to rise. Based on Medicare population samples, annual costs associated with osteoporosis and osteoporosis-associated fractures were estimated at $22 billion in the US elderly in 2008. These costs reflect the 5% of Medicare recipients (1.6/30.2 million) treated for fracture and 24% with osteoporosis without fracture (3). These numbers continue to rise in light of the growing, American aging population. Forty-six million Americans were 65 or older in 2014 with anticipated growth to 98 million older persons in 2060 and a projected increase from 14.5% of the US population in 2014 to 21.7% by 2040 (4).

Early screening and implementation of exercise, diet, fall prevention, and pharmaceutical strategies will become increasingly crucial from a public health and economic standpoint with uptrending life expectancy. As osteoporotic fractures often result from a combination of reduced quantity and quality of the bone, relative neuromuscular instability, and environmental hazards, physiatrists have the expertise and opportunity to apply the multidisciplinary rehabilitation model to successfully address medical and functional factors integral to screening, prevention, and management of this serious public health issue.

DEFINITION

Bone is a live tissue capacitated in its skeletal versatility by both its flexibility and strength. It is composed primarily of collagen (the protein base for a soft framework) and calcium phosphate (the mineral source of bone strength and hardness) (2). Osteoporosis is a disease characterized by low bone mass and deterioration of the microarchitecture of bone tissue, particularly trabecular bone; this leads to increased bone fragility and fracture risk (**Fig. 31-1**). Fractures occur when applied loads are in excess of the capacity of the bone, which is dependent on the degree of bone mineralization

and architecture. Although bone mass is reduced in osteoporosis, the remaining bone demonstrates the normal composition of both organic (40%) and mineral components (60%).

The current procedure of greatest clinical utility for measuring bone density is the dual-energy x-ray absorptiometry or DXA. DXA testing can help in detection of low bone density (before fracture), confirmation of osteoporosis (once fracture occurs), prediction of chances of future fracture, and determination of rate of bone loss and effect of treatment through serial assessments (at intervals of a year or more) (2). In 1994, the World Health Organization (WHO) established the term *normal bone density* to designate bone density within one standard deviation (SD) of the mean for normal young adults and low bone density, or *osteopenia*, as the designation for those with bone density 1.0 to 2.5 SD below the mean for young adults. The number of SD from the normal young mean is designated as a T-score on the final DXA report. In the recent past, the diagnosis of osteoporosis was based solely on a bone mass measurement of 2.5 SD or more below this mean (i.e., T-score ≤ 2.5) (**Table 31-1**) (5). Another means of expressing bone density is as a comparison to persons of the same age, gender, and ethnicity; this is reported as one's Z-score and is clinically most useful in following bone mass in children and adults less than 50 years old. In 2008, the WHO expanded the designation of osteoporosis beyond only statistical determinants to include clinical criteria: those patients with osteopenia who have had a fragility fracture, particularly of the spine or hip, are also now defined as having osteoporosis (6).

When osteoporosis occurs without association with other conditions and in conjunction with postmenopausal and age-related changes, it is defined as *primary osteoporosis*; in women, it is referred to as *postmenopausal osteoporosis* and *senile osteoporosis* in men. Osteoporosis is also commonly seen in association with endocrine diseases, immobility, medications, and inflammation (7). These cases can be called *secondary osteoporosis*. These conditions have generalized bone mass reduction and increased risk for fracture in common (**Table 31-2**).

EPIDEMIOLOGY

General Population and Persons with Disability

The National Osteoporosis Foundation (NOF) estimated in 2008 that more than 12 million people in the United States would have osteoporosis by 2010 and 40 million would have low bone mass, or osteopenia (8). By the year 2020, these

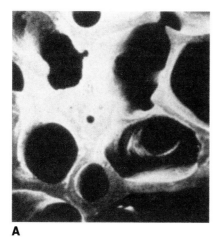 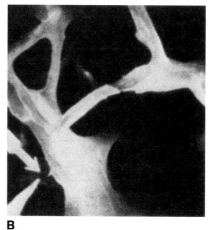

A   **B**

FIGURE 31-1. Micrographs of biopsy specimens of **(A)** normal bone and **(B)** osteoporotic bone. (Adapted from Demptster DW, Shane E, Horbert W. A simple method for correlative light and scanning electron microscopy of human iliac crest bone biopsies: qualitative observations in normal and osteoporotic subjects. *J Bone Miner Res.* 1986;1(1):15–21. Copyright © 1986 ASBMR. Reprinted by permission of John Wiley & Sons, Inc.)

numbers are expected to rise to 14 and 47 million, respectively. Unchecked, these changes could double or triple the number of hip fractures in the United States by 2040 (9). *It is important to remember that persons with osteopenia far outnumber those with osteoporosis; thus, more fractures occur in the osteopenic population* (10). Fractures are also more likely to occur in trauma patients who have preexisting low bone mass or osteoporosis (11).

Advancing age and female gender incur higher risk of bone density disease. From 2005 to 2010, 16.2% of US adults over 65 had osteoporosis at the lumbar spine or femoral neck and 48.3% of adults 65 and over had low bone mass (osteopenia) (12). Women account for approximately 80% of the total number of people in the United States with osteoporosis (13). When compared with other ethnic/racial groups, risk is increasing most rapidly among Hispanic women (14).

In 2005, there were greater than 2 million osteoporosis-related fractures in the United States, costing approximately $19 billion (with men accounting for 25% of fractures and 29% of costs). Overall fracture cost distribution is estimated to be 57% for inpatient care, 13% for outpatient care, and 30% for long-term care. Fracture percentages by skeletal site (in descending order) were the vertebral (27%), wrist (19%), hip (14%), and pelvic (7%), while other sites comprised 33% of fractures. Costs

related to fracture type were the *hip* (72%), vertebral (6%), pelvic (5%), wrist (3%), and other sites (14%). Women bore over 75% of the total costs of incident fracture ($12.8 billion), with women ≥65 contributing in overwhelming majority to the share of total costs (89%). This disproportion is due to a higher mix of more costly hip and pelvic fractures (34% in women ≥75 vs. 9% in women <65). Osteoporotic fractures and costs are estimated to rise greater than 48% by 2025 to greater than 3 million fractures costing $25.3 billion (15). In addition to fracture, osteoporosis is furthermore one of the highest ranking diseases to contribute to bedridden status and associated costly, medical complications (16).

One half of American women and up to 25% of men will have an osteoporotic fracture in their lifetime. Because of lower bone mass accrual in youth, and higher rate of bone loss in mid- and late life, women are more susceptible than men to osteoporosis (17). The prevalence of osteoporosis at the hip is 17% for white, 14% for Hispanic, and 6% for black postmenopausal women. While African Americans are less likely to have osteoporosis, once diagnosed, they have the same increased risk of fracture. After age 50, 20% of white and Asian women and 7% of men are diagnosed with osteoporosis compared to only 5% of non-Hispanic black females and 4% of males (18). After hip fracture, black women have a higher mortality than white women, thought to be due to in part to more advanced age and differences in medical care (19).

As mentioned, hip fractures constitute greater than 70% of the cost burden of fragility fractures in the United States. The importance of appropriate diagnosis and management of osteoporosis and fracture prevention is underscored by the fact that the lifetime risk of hip fracture in women is larger than the sum of lifetime risks of having breast, endometrial, and ovarian cancer combined (20).

In the past, osteoporosis has been largely neglected in men, but research shows it is an important clinical and public health problem. Based on current WHO diagnostic criteria for osteoporosis, its prevalence is 4%, 2%, and 3% among white, Mexican American, and black men aged 50 and older, respectively (21). It is now recognized that the prevalence of hip fracture in men is approximately one third to one half that of women of similar age. Mortality after fracture in men,

TABLE 31-1	Defining Bone Loss by BMD
Condition	**Definition**
Normal	BMD is within 1 SD of a "young normal" adult (T-score ≥ −1)
Osteopenia	BMD is between 1 and 2.5 SDs below that of a "young normal" adult (T-score between −1.0 and −2.5)
Osteoporosis	BMD is 2.5 SDs or more below that of a "young normal" adult (T-score ≤ 2.5)

SD, standard deviation.

Note: Definitions are based on WHO assessment of bone mass measurement at any skeletal site in white women. (From Tinetti ME, Liu WL, Claus EB. Predictors and prognosis of inability to get up after falls among elderly persons. *JAMA.* 1993;269:65–70.)

TABLE 31-2	**Classification of Osteoporosis**

A. Primary osteoporosis
1. Postmenopausal osteoporosis: women
2. Senile osteoporosis: elderly men
B. Secondary osteoporosis: secondary to inherited or acquired disease states, medications, or physiologic aberrations
1. Rheumatoid arthritis
2. End-stage renal disease
3. Hyperparathyroidism and acromegaly
4. Hyperthyroidism (endogenous and iatrogenic)
5. Diabetes mellitus
6. Malabsorption (i.e., partial gastrectomy; gastric bypass, celiac disease)
7. 25-OH and 1,25(OH)$_2$ vitamin D deficiency or toxicity
8. Alcoholism
9. Chronic liver disease
10. Genetic factors (i.e., osteogenesis imperfecta, Ehlers-Danlos syndrome, Marfan's disease)
11. Chronic obstructive pulmonary disease
12. Conditions associated with medication
    a. Glucocorticoids
    b. Heparin
    c. Anticonvulsants
    d. Selective serotonin reuptake inhibitors (SSRIs)
    e. Proton pump inhibitors
13. Conditions associated with hypoestrogen state
    a. Anorexia and bulimia
    b. Exercise-induced amenorrhea (i.e., FAT)
14. Conditions associated with disuse
    a. Tetraplegia/paraplegia/hemiplegia
    b. Immobilization
    c. Prolonged bed rest
15. Malnutrition
16. Chronic liver disease
17. Idiopathic hypercalciuria
18. Low testosterone or androgen insensitivity (Klinefelter and Turner syndromes)
19. Systemic mastocytosis
20. Adult hypophosphatasia
21. Malignancy (multiple myeloma, leukemia, lymphoma)

however, is consistently higher than that in women (22). *Although hip fracture rate in women is two to three times that of men, 1-year mortality after hip fracture for men is nearly twice that of women* (19). Although women lose bone mass rapidly during menopause, by age 70, calcium absorption has decreased in both sexes, resulting in an equal rate of bone loss by age 65 in men and women. After the age of 75 years, osteoporosis affects half the population, men and women equally.

Osteoporosis occurs commonly in the rehabilitation patient population in both its primary and secondary forms. Smeltzer et al. demonstrated that community-dwelling American women with disabilities (control group) had a higher incidence of osteoporosis (22.6% vs. 7%) and lower BMD (53.1% vs. 40%) than nondisabled postmenopausal women; only 50.9% of the controls were postmenopausal, with mean age of 50.6 (23). This corroborates findings by Nosek et al. that women with disabilities develop osteoporosis earlier (24). In Smeltzer's study, DXA screening of subjects showed that the highest incidence of osteoporosis was seen in women with spina bifida

(69.2%), spinal cord injury (SCI) (65%), postpoliomyelitis (44.2%), and cerebral palsy (40%). Risk factors included Caucasian race (87.6%), lack of exercise (64.6%), menopausal status (50.9%), and medication-associated risk (44.8%). Only one quarter of these women with disabilities had been previously screened for BMD, and only one third were taking calcium supplementation (23).

Secondary osteoporosis is not restricted to disabled adults; children with disabilities, including cerebral palsy and juvenile idiopathic arthritis, are also susceptible (25,26). Although screening and treatment protocols are not as well studied as in adults, these children are also at increased risk for low bone mass, osteoporosis, and fractures compared to their peers (27–29). Pediatric patients with cerebral palsy are particularly susceptible to spontaneous fractures (30).

Loss of bone mass with immobilization is most dramatically demonstrated in SCI patients, in whom sublesional bone mineral loss occurs in the lower limbs and pelvis in paraplegic patients and also in the upper limbs in tetraplegic patients. Dauty et al. showed in 2000 that sublesional BMD in SCI patients decreased 41% relative to controls at 1-year postinjury. It is most prominent at the tibia (−70%) and distal femur (−52%), the most common fracture sites (31). However, the spine bone mass does not significantly decrease (32).

The morbidity associated with osteoporotic fracture is high (33). In 1995, there were greater than one-half million hospitalizations and 800,000 emergency room encounters secondary to osteoporotic fractures. Of these, hip fractures were the most devastating (34). Hip fractures account for nearly 50% of all osteoporotic fracture–related hospitalizations in the United States, compared to 8% for vertebral fractures (35). In terms of resulting disability, WHO data show that, postfracture, one hip fracture is equivalent to four vertebral fractures, or twenty fractures at other sites (10).

Most of the social and economic burden of osteoporosis relates directly to hip fracture as well (18). Although some fracture patients suffer only temporary disability, many patients face deformity, loss of function, dependence, or institutionalization. Hip fracture almost invariably results in hospitalization and is a strong risk factor for acute complication (36). Fewer than 50% of hospitalized patients with hip fracture recover their prefracture competence in activities of daily living (ADLs); 80% are unable to perform at least one instrumental ADL, such as shopping or driving, and only 25% regain previous levels of social functioning (37,38). Of those who are ambulatory before hip fracture, studies have shown that 20% require long-term care afterward (13). *Hip fractures are now clearly associated with increased mortality as well; approximately 20% of these patients will die within 1 year of their fracture* (39).

Although less debilitating than hip fractures, fractures of the spine, wrist, and other sites are more common. Vertebral fractures are the most common (more than 700,000 per year in the United States) (13) and are largely responsible for the "dowager's hump" deformity. These fractures, when severe, may cause chronic back pain, loss of height, and disability (40), as well as balance dysfunction. They may additionally contribute to altered abdominal anatomy leading to abdominal distension, constipation, pain, and reduced appetite. Multiple thoracic fractures can lead to restrictive lung disease (41–43). These adverse changes may compromise the ability to perform ADLs resulting in functional impairment equal to that seen after hip fracture (44). Wrist fractures are more likely to result in short-term disability, due to resultant pain, loss of function, nerve entrapment (particularly carpal tunnel syndrome), bone deformity, and arthritis. Past studies have demonstrated a 30% risk of complex regional pain syndrome with wrist fractures (45,46).

ETIOLOGY AND RISK FACTORS

Fracture risk is dependent on the specifics of an individual's genetic profile, peak bone mass, and strength of the bone achieved in one's lifetime and the subsequent rate of bone loss. There are identified risk factors and causes of low bone mass and osteoporosis that contribute to this fracture risk model. In primary osteoporosis, multiple etiologic factors may act independently or in combination in an individual patient to produce diminished bone mass. In secondary osteoporosis, specific causes are identified. The presence of one or more of these factors in the elderly increases the risk of accelerated bone loss and subsequent fracture. The "weighting" of each of these risk factors in terms of relative importance as an etiologic factor is not always well defined, although estrogen depletion; calcium, vitamin D, and testosterone deficiency; smoking; advanced age; positive family history; diminished peak bone mass; diminished physical activity; and history of previous fractures are important. Corticosteroid use of 5 mg/d for a minimum of 3 months is also an important risk factor, as are such factors as excessive alcohol intake, cigarette smoking, use of antiepileptic medication, excessive thyroxine replacement, and falls (**Table 31-3**).

Secondary osteoporosis frequently results from a variety of endocrine conditions (such as glucocorticoid excess, hypogonadism, hyperparathyroidism, and type 1 diabetes), altered activity (CVA, SCI, immobilization), environmental factors (alcoholism, gastrectomy, celiac disease, medications), and inflammation (RA, IBD, ankylosing spondylitis).

Certain medications are commonly implicated in secondary osteoporosis, with glucocorticoids being the best known

through impact on both bone formation and resorption. Glucocorticoids most substantively impact bone mass through decrease in bone formation (via inhibition of osteoblasts and osteoblastic precursors, alteration of osteoblastic function, and increase in osteocyte apoptosis). Glucocorticoids additionally inhibit the secretion of androgen in the pituitary–gonadal and adrenal systems and increase osteoclastogenesis (leading to increased bone resorption) (7).

Other notable medications contributory to osteoporosis include aromatase inhibitors (AIs), gonadotropin-releasing hormone agonists, antiepileptic drugs (AEDs) (phenytoin, carbamazepine, and phenobarbital), antidepressants (similar for SSRIs and TCAs), antidiabetic medication (glitazones), and proton pump inhibitors (PPIs). The proposed mechanisms for impacting bone health are variable for different medications. AIs reduce total estrogen levels and contribute to increased bone resorption and fractures. Certain AEDs contribute to vitamin D catabolism, decreased calcium absorption, and resultant secondary hyperparathyroidism. PPIs contribute to increased risk of fracture, one proposed mechanism being through calcium malabsorption in the digestive tract (7).

Inflammation serves a significant role in secondary osteoporosis and bony remodeling through enhancement of osteoclastogenesis and decrease in bone formation. The risk of hip and vertebral fractures doubles with rheumatoid arthritis regardless of steroid use, and risk of vertebral fractures increases with ankylosing spondylitis, both driven by inflammation (47).

Immobilization (stroke, SCI) contributes to secondary osteoporosis through mechanisms that impact mechanical stimulation to the bones (bone resorption is increased without compensatory increase in bone formation). Bone loss is at sublesional levels with SCI and on the paretic side with stroke (7). Although the prevalence of osteoporosis in the traumatic brain injury population is not well studied, high risk for hypogonadism and immobility in this population is likely to predispose them to low bone mass (48).

PATHOGENESIS

Osteoporosis is a heterogeneous disease with multiple causes. Although the pathogenesis of bone mass loss in secondary osteoporosis may be readily apparent, the exact pathogenesis of primary osteoporosis may be more difficult to define. Low bone mass may be attributable to failure to achieve adequate bone mass at skeletal maturity (age 13 to 25 for women) and/or subsequent age-related and postmenopausal bone loss. Although low bone mass is principally associated with fracture, other determinants of fracture include the quality of the bone (e.g., trabecular architecture), the ability to heal trabecular microfractures, and the propensity to fall (49,50). The pathogenetic basis of inadequate bone mass, particularly in the elderly, also may be considered from the standpoint of tissue, cellular, and hormonal abnormalities.

Tissue Abnormalities

Although cellular and hormonal abnormalities undoubtedly contribute to osteopenia and osteoporosis, the basic abnormality in all types of osteoporosis is a disturbance of the normal bone remodeling sequence at the tissue level. Therefore, to fully understand the pathogenesis of osteoporosis, knowledge of bone remodeling is necessary.

TABLE 31-3	**Risk Factors for Osteoporotic Fractures**

Personal history of low-impact fracture
Current low BMD
Hip fracture of either parent
Caucasian race
Advanced age
Female sex
Dementia
Recurrent falls
Inadequate physical activity
Poor health/frailty
Current smoker
Low body weight
Estrogen deficiency
Corticosteroid use
Testosterone deficiency
Vitamin D deficiency
Low lifetime calcium intake
Alcoholism
Impaired eyesight despite correction

The bone is constantly turning over (remodeling). The skeleton is a reservoir for 99% of the body's calcium, and remodeling provides calcium to the organism without sacrificing the skeleton. In addition, remodeling allows bone mass to respond to increased and decreased muscle activity (e.g., bone mass is increased in a tennis player's dominant arm). The initial event in bone remodeling with normal bone turnover is an increase in bone resorption, as mediated by the osteoclast (the cell responsible for bone resorption). This event is typically followed within 40 to 60 days with an increase in bone formation, as mediated by the osteoblast (the cell responsible for bone formation). Bone resorption and formation are normally "coupled"; an increase or a decrease in resorption produces a corresponding increase or decrease in formation, so that the net change in bone mass is zero. In postmenopausal osteoporosis, and possibly in senile osteoporosis, bone resorption is increased without a corresponding increase in bone formation, thereby leading to a net loss in bone mass. In this case, bone remodeling is described as "negatively uncoupled." In other forms of osteoporosis, particularly those associated with corticosteroid-induced osteoporosis, a primary decrease in bone formation may occur. The end result is the same: a net loss of bone mass,

with concomitant increasing risk for fracture as bone density decreases. Abnormalities of bone remodeling at the tissue level will therefore contribute to the pathogenesis of osteoporosis.

Cellular Abnormalities

Conclusive evidence of cellular abnormalities contributing to the pathogenesis of primary osteoporosis is building. In its simplest terms, the rate of growth and activity of osteoblasts falls behind that of osteoclasts, resulting in a loss of bone density. It may be a failure of the osteoblast, as a result of either decreased cell number or decreased cell activity, which accompanies advancing age (but is not specific for osteoporosis) (see Chapter 47).

Cellular abnormalities that contribute to osteoporosis may also be attributable to factors outside of aging alone. RANKL (receptor activator of nuclear factor kB ligand) is a cytokine essential to osteoclast formation and activation (**Fig. 31-2A**). RANKL, expressed on bone-forming osteoblasts, activates its receptor RANK expressed on osteoclasts. Osteoprotegerin (OPG) counterbalances RANKL's physiologic effects, serving as a decoy receptor that inhibits osteoclast activity (**Fig. 31-2B**). The ratio of RANKL to OPG is enhanced by

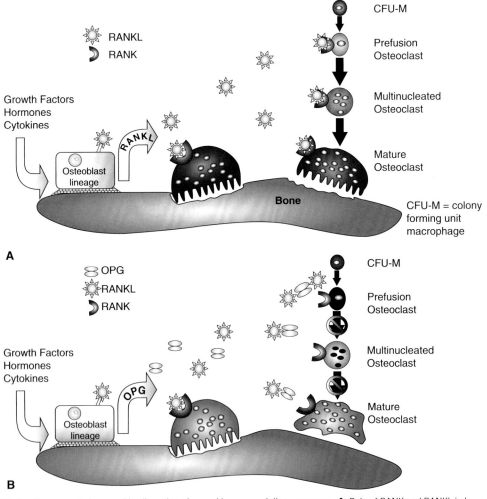

FIGURE 31-2. Osteoporosis is caused by disruption of normal bone remodeling sequences. **A:** Role of RANK and RANKL in bone remodeling. **B:** Regulation of RANK/RANKL binding by osteoprotegerin (OPG). (Adapted from Delmas PD. Clinical potential of RANKL inhibition for the management of postmenopausal osteoporosis and other metabolic bone diseases. *J Clin Densitom.* 2008;11:325–338; Boyle WJ, et al. Osteoclast differentiation and activation. *Nature.* 2003;423:337–342.)

glucocorticoid exposure, estrogen deficiency, T-cell activation (such as with rheumatoid arthritis), and skeletal malignancies leading to increased osteoclastogenesis. RANKL blockade therefore serves to prevent bone loss (51).

Understanding that RANKL is the final cytokine involved in the resorption process and that OPG is a natural antagonist of RANKL has led to evaluation of potential therapeutic treatments. Initially, there was an attempt to use OPG as a therapy to block RANKL. The problem was that antibodies against OPG developed, so this line of treatment was discontinued. Next, a monoclonal antibody against RANKL was developed and this proved to be very effective in blocking bone resorption. It led to the development of denosumab, which is now one of the therapeutic options for osteoporosis treatment. Bone biology research additionally shows that osteocytes produce sclerostin, which is an inhibitor of the anabolic signaling pathway. Recent development of a monoclonal antibody against sclerostin has shown remarkable anabolic activity. Bone density and fracture clinical trials are now underway. Newer treatments for osteoporosis are likely to be based on a clearer understanding of bone biology leading to the design of highly specific compounds hopefully with fewer side effects (52). Interestingly, RANKL is also being explored as a therapeutic target in treating bone cancers (53).

Hormonal Abnormalities

Many hormonal agents may affect bone cell function and bone mass. Although there are numerous age- and menopause-related alterations in the physiology of these hormones, a specific pathogenetic hormonal abnormality in osteoporosis (excluding the osteopenia associated with hypercorticism and hyperparathyroidism) has not been conclusively defined. Estrogen deficiency remains the most frequently incriminated factor in the pathogenesis of postmenopausal osteoporosis in women, while testosterone deficiency is considered a potential cause in younger men.

Estrogen deficiency of any etiology, including menopause, early oophorectomy (54), and functional hypogonadism associated with chronic strenuous exercise (female athlete triad [FAT]) (55), should be considered a prime risk factor for bone mass loss. Physiologically, estrogen has an intimate role in the regulation of bone health. Estrogen directly modulates resorption of trabecular bone through activation of estrogen receptors on bone cells, prolonging osteoblastic life span and shortening osteoclastic life span. Estrogen indirectly impacts bone health through suppression of cytokines such as interleukin-6 (IL-6) that stimulate bone resorption. Estrogen additionally increases OPG secretion, whereas estrogen deficiency increases RANKL expression in B lymphocytes, leading to binding of RANKL to RANK and osteoclastogenesis (56,57).

Estrogen deficiency alone is an incomplete pathogenetic explanation for osteoporosis because all postmenopausal women are relatively estrogen deficient, but not all develop osteoporosis. Parathyroid hormonal perturbations must additionally be considered; however, as with estrogen deficiency, these perturbations don't have universal, clear culpability in osteoporotic contribution. Parathyroid hormone (PTH), secreted by the parathyroid glands, helps to regulate blood calcium levels. With low calcium, PTH enhances release of calcium from bones (through indirect stimulation of bone resorption), absorption of calcium from the kidneys (and

decreased absorption of phosphate), and stimulation of conversion of 25-hydroxyvitamin D_3 to 1,25-dihydroxyvitamin D_3 (which in turn increases intestinal absorption of calcium). The serum level of immunoreactive PTH increases with aging and is increased in about 10% of postmenopausal osteoporotic women (58). In these women, the increase in PTH may be related causally to bone loss.

In most postmenopausal osteoporotic women, however, PTH levels are normal or low compared with those of normal elderly women. In these patients, the pathogenetic contribution of PTH abnormalities to osteoporosis is less clear. Estrogen deficiency results in increased skeletal responsiveness to PTH and increased bone resorption, a transient increase in the serum calcium level, and potentially a resultant decrease in PTH secretion. With such a decrease, reduced production of the active form of vitamin D (1,25-dihydroxyvitamin D_3) may occur, with a consequent decrease in intestinal calcium absorption.

A number of vitamin D abnormalities occur with aging, although an abnormality specific for osteoporosis (rather than simply aging) has not been defined. Decreased levels of 1,25-dihydroxyvitamin D_3 are noted with increasing age. A postulated defect in the osteoporotic elderly person of the renal 25(OH) vitamin D 1-α-hydroxylase enzyme in response to PTH has been suggested but not conclusively proven (59,60). Older people may simply not be able to make vitamin D in response to sunlight, compared to younger people. Nevertheless, calcium absorption does decrease with advancing age and is lower in postmenopausal osteoporotic women, and its decline is associated with increased risk for hip fracture.

Suffice it to say, in all postmenopausal women, bone resorption increases more than bone formation, and estrogen deficiency and perturbations in PTH and vitamin D are contributory. Other hormones that may play a role in skeletal loss with aging include testosterone, insulin-like growth factor I (IGF-I), and dehydroepiandrosterone sulfate (DHEAS). A deficiency of the hormone calcitonin also could contribute to ongoing bone loss, although it is unlikely that it exerts a major pathogenetic effect in osteoporosis. Calcitonin inhibits the production and activity of osteoclasts and thus decreases osteoclastic bone resorption. Serum levels of immunoreactive calcitonin decrease with age and are indeed lower in women than in men. In addition, decreased calcitonin secretion in response to calcium stimulation has been noted in some, but not all, osteoporotic populations (61,62). As we continue to learn more about the bone biology causing the pathogenesis of osteoporosis in an individual, newer targeted treatments that are individualized to the patient will likely become standard.

Genetic Abnormalities

The degree of peak bone mass achieved and the amount of bone loss as we age determine our risk of osteoporosis. Complex genetic and environmental factors determine these contributing factors. It is likely that a cohort of genes contribute to a predisposition to osteoporosis and that they differ with ethnic backgrounds (63). Definitive identification of all candidate genes is not established, but numerous gene susceptibilities are implicated, including abnormalities in receptors for the active form of vitamin D_3 (calcitriol), estradiol, and PTH as well as genes coding for transforming growth factor β (TGF-β) and IL-6. These genes are associated with achieving peak bone mass and bone remodeling processes and are active throughout the life span (64).

Stroke (See Chapter 18)

Paresis, reduced mobility and bone loading, endocrine changes, nutritional factors, and pharmacologic exposures all increase risk of poststroke osteoporosis. Immobilization-induced bony turnover and associated calcium mobilization cause alterations in the vitamin D-PTH axis through inhibition of PTH secretion. Decreased sunlight exposure due to impaired mobility further exacerbates vitamin D deficiency. Finally, malnutrition due to dysphagia, impaired mobility, cognitive deficits, depression, and social isolation contribute to nutritional deficiencies including vitamins D, K, and B_{12} and folate. Bone loss occurs typically on the paretic side; however, bone loss can additionally occur in the proximal, nonparetic femur. Bone loss commences days after cerebral vascular injury, with progression over the first 3 to 4 months and gradual slowing over the 1st year until steady state is reached. This can account for up to 14% bone mineral density loss at the proximal femur and 17% at the upper extremities over the 1st year poststroke (65). Kanis et al. demonstrated a greater than 7-fold fracture risk increase within the 1st year of hospitalization for stroke (66).

Spinal Cord Injury (See Chapter 22)

Although disuse is thought to play a role in the development of osteoporosis in this population, neural factors are also implicated, as is an impaired PTH-vitamin D axis and calcium/phosphate metabolism (67). There is no demineralization in supralesional areas following injury, and weight bearing in the spine is thought to limit loss of bone mass in vertebrae. Spasticity, degree of injury, female sex, age, and duration after injury negatively influence bone mass. Reduced intestinal absorption and increased renal elimination of calcium, inhibition of sex steroids, pituitary suppression of thyroid-stimulating hormone (TSH), insulin resistance, and IGFs may also contribute (68), but the majority of patients with SCI have decreased bone mass below the lesion. Animal models have demonstrated increased osteoclast activity, with severe bone loss (48% trabecular and 35% cortical), decreased mineral apposition, and growth plate abnormalities consistent with osteoblast dysfunction (69) and elevated RANKL mRNA induction (70).

In his study of the spinal cord–injured population, Szollar et al. found that serum levels of calcium and calcitonin could not be correlated with changes in bone mass. However, in this study, the PTH level decreased in the 1st year after injury and started to increase 1 to 9 years after injury. Osteoblast activity decreased immediately after injury in these patients, with consequent dramatic increases in bone degradation. In fact, loss of BMD in the proximal femur was measurable at 12 months following injury in all 176 persons with paraplegia or tetraplegia. Of significance, risk for fracture increased between years 1 and 9 after injury in the 20- to 39-year age group, but continued increasing to year 19 after injury in the 40- to 59-year age group before plateau. This study also showed that BMD in the spine actually increased from weight bearing 1 to 9 years after injury in all study participants, though becoming significant only in those with paraplegia in the 20- to 39-year age group 10 to 19 years after injury (32).

Fractures occurred in this population most frequently in the pelvis and lower extremities, particularly the tibia, and

correlated with sites of most bone density loss. Similar to the general population, women with SCI tend to develop osteoporosis more frequently than men with SCI.

CLINICAL EVALUATION FOR OSTEOPOROSIS

Although the first clinical indication of osteoporosis, either primary or secondary, is usually a fracture, it is optimal to screen and treat patients, both male and female, prior to first fracture.

Quantitating Bone Mass

A number of clinical parameters positively correlate with bone mass, such as paraspinal muscle strength in postmenopausal women and grip strength in premenopausal women and men. Although these are useful methods, they do not substitute for precise quantitation (71). Plain radiographs of the spine are relatively insensitive in quantitating bone mass because 30% to 35% of bone mass must be lost before demineralization is detected. They are, however, sensitive and reliable to assess for fractures of the spine when unexpected height loss is noted or when fractures are suspected in axial or peripheral bone.

Several noninvasive procedures have been developed over the past 50 years to quantitate bone mass (bone density). The current procedure of greatest clinical utility, DXA, is noninvasive, quantifies primarily trabecular (cancellous) bone at the spine and hip with an acceptable precision and accuracy, is simple to perform at a reasonable cost, and is associated with low radiation exposure. Most importantly, it predicts which patients are at risk for subsequent fracture and can be repeated to assess therapeutic response to treatment. The DXA technique also satisfies requirements for ionizing radiation safety to the greatest degree, as bone density measurements can be obtained within 30 seconds to 2 minutes with a radiation exposure of approximately 10 mrad—one sixth the exposure of a chest x-ray—with 99% precision and approximately 97% accuracy. CT measurements of the spine provide an exclusive assessment of trabecular bone, and actual volumetric density, but the technique is compromised by high radiation exposure and lower precision.

WHO recommendations for baseline and follow-up testing are based on DXA measurements at axial sites (spine and hip). For patients in whom the spine cannot be measured, the forearm is substituted. The spine and the distal forearm contain primarily trabecular bone, metabolically more active than cortical bone, preferentially altered in osteoporosis, and thus most affected by medications used in the treatment of osteoporosis. The hip and parts of the forearm also have cortical bone. The vertebrae and hips are also the fracture sites likely to cause the most disability. WHO guidelines are adapted to the epidemiology of individual countries and are well described in special position papers by the NOF Guide Committee (6,72). As WHO DXA standards were established from research of white, postmenopausal women, some controversy exists in interpretation of DXA for men, premenopausal females, non-white populations, and children. The International Society for Clinical Densitometry (ISCD) recommends the use of a uniform, Caucasian, female normative database for women of all ethnicities and the use of a uniform, Caucasian, female reference for men of all ethnic groups (73). Although peripheral measurements with other techniques such as pDXA, pQCT, and ultrasound may predict hip and spine fracture similar to

DXA, they have less clinical utility than axial measurements. Because of low cost, portability, and lack of radiation exposure, peripheral measurements with ultrasound have evolved primarily as a screening tool, which, when positive, instigates further clinical evaluation and DXA screening (74).

Revised 2008 WHO guidelines for DXA screening and treatment shifted from a T-score–only basis for treatment to evidence-based assessment of the 10-year risk for fracture at hip and other sites, based on age, gender, race, bone density values, and known osteoporosis and fracture risks. Guidelines were then adapted to demographic and health care profiles of individual countries (6,72). Interpretation of these guidelines, though, can vary among diverse governmental and medical specialty organizations.

In 2011, the U.S. Preventative Task Force recommended osteoporosis screening for all women 65 or older and for younger women with fracture risk equal to or greater than a 65-year-old white woman without additional risk factors. No recommendation was made for men without previous known fracture or secondary cause of osteoporosis (75). In addition to this, the ISCD (2015) recommends bone mineral density testing in men 70 and older, menopausal women, postmenopausal women younger than 65, men less than 70 with a known risk factor for low bone mass (low body weight, prior fracture, high-risk medication use, or disease associated with bone loss), adults with a fragility fracture or disease/condition associated with low bone mass, and anyone being considered for or treated with pharmacologic therapy (to monitor effect). The WHO reference standard for osteoporosis is a T-score of −2.5 at the femoral neck where the T-score is calculated from the female, white, 20- to 29-year-old reference group. According to the ISCD, T-scores are preferred for reporting bone mineral density in postmenopausal women and men 50 and older; however, Z-scores are preferred in reporting BMD in females prior to menopause and men less than 50 (particularly important in children); BMD alone cannot be used to diagnose osteoporosis in men under 50 (73).

Protocols for DXA and laboratory screening in children and young adults with chronic disability (i.e., cerebral palsy or SCI), and with medical conditions associated with osteoporosis such as eating disorders and FAT, are not well established, but the ISCD has published recommendations. The ISCD recommends DXA assessment in children/adolescents with primary bone disease or at risk for secondary bone disease if the patient may benefit from intervention. In such cases, the total body less head and the posterior-anterior spine are the preferred skeletal sites for BMD assessment (the hip is not preferred due to skeletal variability with development) (76). Fragility fractures in these populations warrant at least baseline DXA assessment. Screening, interpretation of results, and treatment for loss of bone density must be individualized until more research can be done in these populations.

The FRAX WHO Fracture Risk Assessment Tool (http://www.shef.ac.uk/FRAX/tool.jsp), developed at the University of Sheffield, in England by Kanis et al. assists the clinician in treatment guidelines for patients with low BMD (osteopenia, DXA T-score between −1.0 and −2.5) without previous pharmaceutical intervention (77). After inserting data reflecting patients' gender, age, race, body weight, and height, known osteoporosis risk factors, and femoral neck bone density (in g/cm²) with the manufacturer of DXA equipment, the FRAX

tool establishes a treatment threshold in accordance with WHO guidelines. In the United States, if the data indicate a 10-year fracture risk at the hip of ≥3%, or at other major sites of ≥20%, prescription medications should be considered (78). If the patient is not started on pharmacologic therapy, subsequent screening by FRAX or with DXA is recommended at 2 years, although some low-risk patients can be assessed at much longer intervals. For those patients who are at risk for fracture and begin therapy, a follow-up DXA is suggested at 2 years, to assess response to treatment. If femoral neck BMD is not available (e.g., in a patient with bilateral hip surgery), the FRAX tool must determine fracture risk by body mass index (BMI).

Bone Markers

Serum and urine markers of bone resorption and formation are diagnostic modalities used primarily to monitor efficacy of prescription therapy. In this sense, the markers may be complementary to bone density assessment. These markers show an individual patient's response to therapy earlier than BMD changes, sometimes within 24 hours. Current rate of bone resorption is most commonly assessed with a urinary marker n-telopeptide of type I collagen (NTX) and c-telopeptides of type I collagen (CTX) (79). Serum levels of NTX and CTX can also be tested. Both spot urine and serum markers are best checked in the morning after fasting to try to minimize variance, but all bone turnover markers have considerable day-to-day variability, which makes clinical interpretation in an individual difficult. One recommendation is to check a spot urine NTX and serum CTX at baseline and repeat in 6 months after starting treatment. If there is greater than a 50% decrease in urine NTX or greater than 30% decrease for serum CTX, the drug is considered to be having the desired effect. Likewise, they can be used to help determine the duration of "drug holiday."

Clinical Evaluation of the Patient at Risk for Osteoporosis

Patients at risk for osteoporosis require careful evaluation, consisting of the following elements. A thorough history is required to determine the presence of risk factors for osteoporosis such as menopausal status, family history of hip fracture, and certain medications (**Table 31-4**) and to exclude medical conditions leading to secondary osteoporosis (see **Table 31-2**). A separate intake questionnaire for osteoporosis to expand standard intake history intake can be helpful. History of previous fragility fractures and sites of persistent pain (i.e., atraumatic vertebral compression fracture) must be identified. Identify any history of falls or associated risk factors such as poor vision, bladder urgency, or peripheral neuropathy (**Table 31-5**). Document any loss of height from early adulthood (average loss of 2 to 3 in. from the occiput to the sacrum is expected between the ages of 40 and 80 (80), and include in DXA order if greater than 1.5 in. Assess current level of physical activity and exercise, and past history of eating disorders, in all patients. Social behaviors such as tobacco abuse or excessive alcohol are both positively correlated with bone loss and should be noted (81). The importance of the social history cannot be overemphasized, especially in the elderly, who may have history of frequent falls, require assistive devices or personnel in their living environment, or need consideration for transitional care unit placement. Inadequate daily calcium intake and exercise, vitamin D deficiency, corticosteroid use,

TABLE 31-4   Etiologic Factors Contributing to the Risk of Osteopenia/Osteoporosis

1. Estrogen depletion
   a. Postmenopausal state (natural or artificial)
   b. Exercise-induced amenorrhea and anorexia nervosa
2. Calcium deficiency
   a. Inadequate calcium intake
   b. Malabsorption
   c. Lactose intolerance
3. Diminished peak bone mass at skeletal maturity; varies with sex (women > men), race (whites > blacks), and heredity
4. Diminished physical activity
5. Testosterone depletion
6. Aging
7. Low body weight (adipose tissue is the major source of extragonadal estrogen production postmenopause)
8. Alcoholism and smoking
9. Excessive coffee intake (>4–6 cups daily); excessive dietary protein or salt intake (increased calcium loss in the urine)
10. Medications: corticosteroids, thyroid hormone, and phenytoin

Data from the National Osteoporosis Foundation, Prevention, NOF.org.

diabetes mellitus, and multiple myeloma are common in the elderly. Inquire into pending dental procedures, as dental extractions could delay start-up of bisphosphonates, the most commonly prescribed medication class for osteoporosis, due to risk of osteonecrosis of the jaw (82,83). History of certain malignancies may be a relative contraindication for teriparatide, a potent anabolic treatment option.

A thorough physical examination establishes cognitive status, assesses oral hygiene and hydration status, and excludes causes of secondary osteoporosis (e.g., hemiplegia, rheumatoid arthritis, anorexia, SCI). One must assess for preexisting fractures; for example, multiple vertebral fractures can induce severe kyphosis, with anteroposterior widening of the rib cage, increasing its proximity to the iliac crests and inducing abdominal protuberance (80). Document any risks for fall (i.e., visual disturbance, neurologic deficits, contractures, leg length discrepancy, poor balance with transfers, gait abnormalities, and improper use of assistive devices). Evaluate the potential for safe weight-bearing and resistive exercise (i.e., cognitive status, cardiopulmonary status, posture, degree of kyphosis, balance, and pain with active and resisted motion).

TABLE 31-5   Major Risk Factors for Falls

	Risk Reduction Strategies
	See corrective strategies below
Demographic	
Advanced age	
Female gender	
Previous falls	
Functional deficits	
Environmental	
Insufficient lighting	Light hallways, stairs, entrances, bathroom
Obstacles in walking path	Clear clutter/loose cords; move furniture
Loose throw rugs	Anchor or eliminate rugs
Lack of assistive devices in bathroom	Install grab bars; high commode seat
Slippery outdoor conditions	Sturdy shoes; assistive device
Wet bathroom and kitchen floors	Nonskid mats; grab bars; tub bench/chair
Improperly fitting shoes, slippers	Encourage use of sturdy, low-heeled shoes
Uneven terrain, cellar stairs	Stair rails; cane/walker
House pets	
Neuromuscular	
Poor balance	High-level balance challenge exercises
	Cane or walker; tai chi
Sarcopenia	Resistive exercise; optimize vitamin D levels
Kyphosis	Optimize myofascial release/postural training
Reduced proprioception	Sturdy shoewear; balance training; cane/walker
Impairments: transfer/mobility	Mobility training
Medical	
Poor vision	Annual visual examination
Urinary urge incontinence	Medication; timed voids; avoid PM fluids
Orthostatic hypotension	Hydrate; optimize medications
Medication (i.e., for pain, HTN, seizures)	Annual medication review
Depression, anxiety, agitation	Counseling support; medications
Alcohol (>3 drinks/d)	Counseling; abstinence
Malnutrition	Nutritionist; home health nursing consult
Fear of falling	Mobility training; counseling

Adapted from data from the National Osteoporosis Foundation, 2002–2009.

Document height and weight, contracture limitations, and leg length discrepancies after measurement. Assess the general mobility of the spine and joints of the extremities, as well as abdominal, spinal, and extremity muscle strength. Verify sites of pain (i.e., vertebrae T8-L2 are associated with osteoporosis, whereas fractures at T6 or above are more likely associated with malignancy) (80). Assess for tibial tenderness in thin, female runners, especially with irregular or absent menses, as seen in FAT. Identify any risks for intolerance of prescription medications; for instance, poor dentition, history of gastric disorder such as GERD, gastritis or peptic ulcer, or diffuse myalgias can delay or preclude bisphosphonate use.

Proximal muscle weakness and chronic corticosteroid use will require special exercise focus. Proprioception, balance, transfers, and gait must be evaluated. Proper use and design of assistive devices should also be addressed. Specific physical performance measures that correlate with higher bone mass density in the hip and spine, wrist, or whole body in postmenopausal women include longer step length, normal and brisk gait speeds and step length, longer single-leg stance, and grip strength (84). Evaluation of these parameters and improving where possible with resistive exercises may improve bone mass parameters.

A basic laboratory evaluation is listed in **Table 31-6**. In primary osteoporosis, results of laboratory tests typically are normal (except 25-hydroxyvitamin D); the primary role of blood and urine tests is therefore to exclude other diseases and, in a few cases with bone markers, to establish baseline bone turnover rate. For example, multiple myeloma should be suspected with anemia, abnormal serum protein electrophoresis (SPEP), and elevated B-cell population in complete blood cell count. Vitamin D deficiency is best evaluated by serum 25-hydroxyvitamin D. Serum IgA antitissue transglutaminase and IgA endomysial antibody, if positive, can be an indication of malabsorption (i.e., celiac disease). Low urinary calcium-to-creatinine ratio and a 24-hour urinary calcium are less specific measures of malabsorption in some cases.

Severe vitamin D deficiency causes osteomalacia, with bone pain and poor mineralization of the bone. More commonly, milder degrees of vitamin D deficiency lead to decreased gut absorption of calcium and in some cases secondary hyperparathyroidism, causing loss of bone mineral. Many osteoporosis patients have some degree of vitamin D inadequacy. Vitamin D deficiency also has an effect on muscle, leading to decreased

TABLE 31-6	Basic Osteoporosis Laboratory Tests

Complete blood cell count
Serum chemistry (renal electrolytes, liver enzymes, BUN, creatinine, calcium, total protein/albumin, alkaline phosphatase, and phosphorus)
Vitamin D-25 hydroxy
Intact PTH
Serum protein electrophoresis
Thyroid function test
24-h urine calcium
Urine markers for bone resorption-urine NTX[a]

[a]Serum NTX can be substituted.

lower body strength and increased propensity to fall. If 24-hour urine calcium value is low, inadequate calcium intake or absorption, or vitamin D deficiency, is likely. If urine calcium value is high, either dietary calcium excess or idiopathic hypercalciuria is a possibility. If the serum calcium is elevated, measurement of PTH is the most important test to do. Primary hyperparathyroidism leads to bone loss and must be differentiated from familial hypocalciuric hypercalcemia (FHH), a benign abnormality of the calcium receptor. Patients with FHH have mild elevations of serum calcium and PTH but very low urinary calcium excretion. It should be noted that patients with primary hyperparathyroidism may have vitamin D deficiency, leading to secondary hyperparathyroidism as well (see **Table 31-7**).

DXA screening is of value in the individual patient with history of spine or hip fragility fracture, or two or more risk factors for low bone mass. (See **Fig. 31-3** for defining DXA screening candidates.) If osteoporosis is found by DXA, treatment is indicated. For those patients with osteopenia, the WHO FRAX questionnaire[1] can be used to determine if prescription medications are needed for improving bone mass. If DXA/FRAX analysis indicates that fracture risk is 3% or more at the hip, or 20% or more at other sites, more aggressive prophylactic therapy (e.g., bisphosphonate) is recommended. If fracture risk does not meet these thresholds, increased exercise, a diet rich in calcium, and calcium and vitamin D supplements may be sufficient fracture prophylaxis, in conjunction with fall reduction training. Such patients should have a repeat DXA in 2 years, with

[1]Available at: http://www.shef.ac.uk/FRAX/tool.jsp

TABLE 31-7	Laboratory Tests in Disorders of Calcium Metabolism

Disorder	Serum Calcium	Serum Phosphate	Vitamin D Hydroxy	PTH	1,25(OH)$_2$ Vitamin D	Urine Calcium	Renal Function
Primary hyperparathyroidism	↑	↓	Variable	↑	↑	Normal ↑	Variable
Familial hypocalciuric hypercalcemia	↑	Variable	Variable	↑	Normal	↓↓	Variable
Hypercalcemia of malignancy	↑	Variable	Variable	↓	Normal	↑	Variable
Vitamin D deficiency	↓ or normal	↓ or normal	↓↓	↑ or normal	Usually normal	↓	Variable
Renal osteodystrophy	↓	↑	Variable	↑↑	↓	↓	↓↓
Primary hypoparathyroidism	↓	↑	Variable	↓	↓	↓	Variable

Note: While 25(OH) vitamin D levels are variable in many disorders, low levels are very common in general. Renal function is often normal in the various disorders, but it may be decreased. Patients may have more than one disorder. For example, some patients with primary hypoparathyroidism may also be vitamin D insufficient, leading to further elevation of serum PTH.

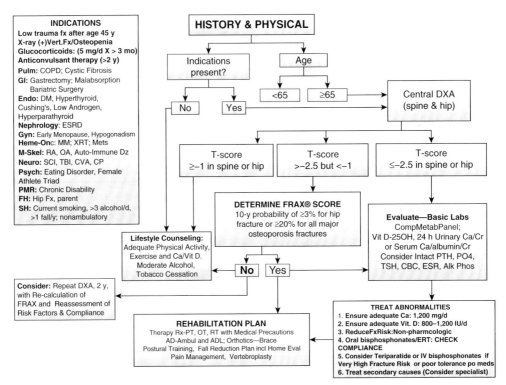

FIGURE 31-3. Osteoporosis management algorithm.

recalculation of the fracture risk via the FRAX tool at that time if osteopenia persists.

Iliac crest bone biopsy is used primarily to exclude osteomalacia or other metabolic bone diseases, such as is seen with late-stage renal failure. Although such biopsies can be used to define high and low bone turnover, this is not usual practice at this time for the typical patient with osteoporosis.

Educational materials can be provided to all patients to reinforce the importance of maintaining bone health, understanding the sequelae of untreated osteoporosis, identifying sources of dietary calcium, and improving fall risk in the home at the time of office visit (http://www.nof.org/).

PREVENTIVE STRATEGIES FOR PATIENTS AT RISK

Efforts to improve bone health have focused on prevention and treatment protocols. Prevention programs focus on adequate nutritional status, including optimization of calcium, vitamin D and protein intake, and monitoring for excessive fats or carbohydrate intake. Avoidance of lifestyles known to result in bone loss, including cigarette smoking, excessive alcohol, and possibly carbonated beverage intake, is also important. Weight-bearing and strengthening exercises, as well as fall prevention strategies in the home and community, are equally important.

Because bone mass is the principal, although not the only, determinant of fracture risk, preservation or improvement of bone mass via pharmacologic means is associated with a reduced risk of fracture. The rationale of the various therapeutic agents available for preserving or improving bone mass density or bone mass is based on knowledge of bone remodeling.

In normal bone, there is no net change in the amount of bone mass present, as ongoing bone remodeling is a balance between bone resorption and the process of bone formation. In most forms of osteoporosis, however, a perturbation of bone remodeling occurs. Bone resorption increases over normal levels, and bone formation does not compensate for this increase, with a net loss of bone mass overall.

Nutritional Adjuncts

Calcium

Dietary and supplemental calcium intake is a mainstay of osteoporosis prevention and treatment. The Surgeon General's Report on Bone Health and Osteoporosis (2015) recommends calcium intake of 1,200 mg/d for women over 50 and 1,000 mg/d for men over 50; children require 700 to 1,300 mg/d, dependent on age (**Table 31-8**). Food sources such as dairy products, dark green vegetables, salmon, and enriched cereals are rich in calcium (85). (See **Table 31-9** for a more detailed list of food and beverage sources of calcium.)

Calcium supplementation alone has been documented to produce sustained reduction in the rate of loss of total body BMD in healthy postmenopausal women (86). In healthy, older, nonosteoporotic men, a recent study documented less falls and increased BMD of 1% to 1.5% at all sites in men receiving 1,200 mg calcium supplement daily over those receiving placebo. However, vascular events tended to be more common in the experimental group during the 2-year study (87). Calcium supplementation is inexpensive, relatively simple to ingest, and generally safe for most patients (i.e., in the absence of end-stage renal disease, a history of previous kidney stones, or idiopathic hypercalciuria). Despite the relative ease of obtaining daily calcium requirements, average dietary intake

TABLE 31-8	Recommended Daily Calcium Intake
Age or Life Stage	**Adequate Calcium Intake (mg/d)**
0–6 mo (human milk content)	210
7–12 mo (human milk + solid food)	270
1–3 y	500
4–8 y	800
9–18 y	1,300
19–50 y	1,000
>50 y	1,200
Pregnancy or lactation	
≤18 y	1,300
19–50 y	1,000

Source: Institute of Medicine. *Dietary Reference Intakes: Calcium, Phosphorus, Magnesium, Vitamin D, and Fluoride.* Washington, DC: The National Academies Press; 1997.

is approximately 700 mg/d (87). In the past studies, no more than 1% of men and women more than 70 years of age are meeting their calcium requirements from food sources (88).

The immobilization that occurs with hemiplegia and paraplegia, if coupled with excessive calcium intake, may result in elevated urinary calcium levels. A predisposition for kidney stones and nephrolithiasis may then be seen. In general, a urinary calcium excretion of up to 250 mg/d is acceptable in individuals without a history of kidney stones (89–92). High sodium intake, as is commonly seen in the United States, can lead to increased urinary calcium loss. Early studies of calcium metabolism suggest that 1 additional gram of sodium per day above Recommended Daily Allowance (RDA) decreases bone density by 1% per year in women (93,94).

Vitamin D

Vitamin D facilitates absorption of calcium and mineralization of the bone. It is found in the liver, fatty fish, egg yolks, and as an additive in foods such as milk, orange juice, and cereals. It can be taken as a supplement and is also synthesized in the skin through sunlight exposure. With sunlight exposure, 7-dehydrocholesterol in the skin is converted to previtamin D_3 through absorption of UVB radiation and isomerizes to vitamin D_3. Vitamin D_3 is subsequently metabolized in the liver to 25-hydroxyvitamin D_3 and by the kidneys to 1,25-dihydroxyvitamin D_3 (biologically active form, which help regulate calcium and phosphate metabolism). 1,25-Dihydroxyvitamin D_3 helps increase absorption of intestinal calcium and phosphate, stimulates the healthy remodeling of bone, and increases calcium absorption in the renal distal tubule (95). Vitamin D_3 generated from the skin lasts two to three times longer in

TABLE 31-9	Selected Food Sources of Calcium	
Food, Standard Amount	**Calcium (mg)**	**Calories**
Fortified ready-to-eat cereals (various), 1 oz	236–1,043	88–106
Plain yogurt, nonfat (13-g protein/8 oz), 8-oz container (low-fat[a])	452 (415)	127 (143)
Soy beverage, calcium fortified, 1 cup	368	98
Fruit yogurt, low-fat (10-g protein/8 oz), 8 oz	345	232
Orange juice, fortified, 1 cup	308–344	85
Swiss cheese, 1.5 oz	336	162
Sardines, Atlantic, in oil, drained, 3 oz	325	177
Fat-free (skim) milk, 1 cup[a]	306	83
1% low-fat milk, 1 cup (whole milk[a])	290 (276)	102 (146)
Plain yogurt, whole milk (8-g protein/8 oz), 8-oz container[a]	275	138
Tofu, firm, prepared with nigari[b], ½ cup	253	88
Mozzarella cheese, whole milk, 1.5 oz	215	128
Pink salmon, canned, with bone, 3 oz	181	118
Collards, cooked from frozen, ½ cup	180	31
Molasses, blackstrap, 1 tbsp	172	47
Soybeans, cooked, ½ cup, green (mature)	130 (88)	127 (149)
Ocean perch, Atlantic, cooked, 3 oz	116	103
Oatmeal, plain or flavored, instant, fortified, 1 prepared packet	99–110	97–157
Pizza, cheese	100	255
White beans, canned, ½ cup	96	153
Broccoli (raw), 1 cup	90	25
Okra, cooked from frozen, ½ cup	88	26
Ice cream, vanilla, ½ cup	85	135

[a]Calcium content varies slightly by fat content; the more fat, the less calcium the food contains.
[b]Calcium content is for tofu processed with a calcium salt; other salts do not provide significant calcium. See http://www.nal.usda.gov/fnic/foodcomp/Data/SR20/nutrlist/sr20a301.pdf for a more comprehensive list of foods containing calcium.
Source: Nutrient values from Agricultural Research Service (ARS) Nutrient Database for Standard Reference, Release 17.
Adapted from 2002 revision of USDA Home and Garden Bulletin No. 72, Nutritive Value of Foods. Food sources of calcium ranked by mg of calcium and calories per standard amount. Bioavailability may vary. (All dairy are ≥20% of AI for adults 19 to 50, which is 1,000 mg/d.)

circulation compared to oral ingestion and is bound to vitamin D–binding protein 100% of the time, whereas ingested vitamin D_3 is bound to this protein only 60% of the time (40% is rapidly cleared). Many factors affect cutaneous vitamin D_3 synthesis. These include latitude and solar zenith angle (decreased vitamin D_3 production in the winter, especially at latitudes above and below 33 degrees), altitude (more production at higher altitude), air pollution (reduced effectiveness of sun exposure), skin pigment (decreased penetration of UVB radiation with darker skin), age (7-dehydrocholesterol concentrations inversely relate to age), and sunscreen. Sunscreen, designed to absorb UVB radiation, impacts vitamin D synthesis depending on strength. SPF 30 absorbs 95% to 98% of solar UVB radiation and therefore reduces skin production of vitamin D_3 by the same amount. Most cells in the body have vitamin D receptors, and deficiency can lead to many chronic diseases (autoimmune disease, some cancers, cardiovascular disease, infectious disease, and type 2 diabetes among them) (96).

The National Academy of Medicine (formerly Institute of Medicine) recommends a dietary allowance of 600 IU/d of vitamin D for individuals 70 and under and 800 IU/d for both males and females greater than 70 (with the upper level of daily intake being 4,000 IU/d) (97). Cholecalciferol (vitamin D_3) is probably the preferred form of vitamin D supplement, but ergocalciferol (vitamin D_2) can also be used as an oral dose of 50,000 IU weekly for 4 to 12 weeks as replacement therapy when very low–vitamin D levels are found. The active form of vitamin D (1,25-dihydroxyvitamin D_3 or calcitriol) is also beneficial in osteoporosis and is commonly prescribed as a supplement for patients who lack the 1-α-hydroxylase enzyme because of severe renal impairment.

Severe deficiency can lead to secondary hyperparathyroidism, osteomalacia, or rickets and is associated with increased risk of osteoporotic fracture (98,99). As these supplements increase calcium absorption at the gut level, their use can result in an increased risk for hypercalciuria, nephrolithiasis, or even nephrocalcinosis in patients at risk. Increased urinary calcium is the first sign of such toxicity and is easily evaluated with a 24-hour urine sample. Many institutionalized and housebound elderly patients are deficient in vitamin D and can benefit from its administration (91,92,100,101). In general, total daily administration of vitamin D should not exceed 2,000 IU (102). As calcium and vitamin D are critical to the action of bisphosphonates, normal levels must be verified prior to the start of bisphosphonate therapy.

Protein

Along with calcium and vitamin D supplementation, protein supplementation has been shown to improve healing and decrease mortality in persons who have sustained hip fractures. In a study by Schurch et al. (103), elderly patients received dietary protein supplements of 20 g/d for 6 months following hip fracture. Much of the rapid bone loss that usually occurs in the contralateral hip during the year after a fracture was avoided in these patients. The RDA for protein can usually be achieved with two to three servings of meat or beans and two to three servings of milk and cheese per day (104). Too much protein, however, may be harmful, as it can incur an acid load; calcium from the bone is a major source of serum alkaline buffering in this instance.

Exercise

A lifelong dedication to physical activity and exercise (60 minutes daily for all children aged 8 and older and 30 minutes for adults) (105) is recommended (see also Chapters 43 and 49). Therapeutic exercise is an essential element of the rehabilitation program for patients with osteoporosis and should be tailored to the patient's level of fitness and anticipated propensity to fracture. Exercise increases muscle and bone strength, joint flexibility, and balance; it also helps with fall prevention. Although genetic factors can determine a large proportion of bone mass and structure, up to 50% to 90%, controllable lifestyle factors contribute as well (106). A thorough history and physical examination and, if appropriate, bone density testing can address deficits and define exercise precautions to avoid injury. An exercise program should incorporate both short- and long-term goals, which must be reviewed with the patient. Patient education concerning proper posture, body mechanics, and increasing strength and aerobic capacity is an essential component of both short-term and long-term interventions. Osteoporosis is a disease that is progressive and, if unchecked, can cause severe disability. In patients with physical disabilities, inactivity can be especially harmful because of a propensity for further deterioration with aging and concomitant health problems. The PASIPD questionnaire (Physical Activity Scale for Individuals with Physical Disabilities) can be useful in assessing levels of activity in the persons with disability, such as home maintenance function, moderate and vigorous sport and recreation activities, occupation, and transportation (107).

Current cardiorespiratory exercise recommendations are for adults to get at least 150 minutes of moderate-intensity exercise weekly. This exercise should be coupled with resistance exercise addressing each major muscle group, flexibility exercise, and neuromotor exercise (balance, coordination, agility, proprioceptive activity, and gait), all to be done 2 to 3 days/week (108).

For optimal bone health, an exercise program should include weight-bearing activities for 45 minutes three or four times per week or weight lifting for 20 to 30 minutes two to three times per week (80). Weight-bearing, low-impact activities include walking or treadmill use; jogging, tennis, and soccer are high-impact activities. Swimming is beneficial from a cardiovascular standpoint, but is not a weight-bearing sport, and thus does not contribute to bone mass (109). Swimming does maintain muscle mass, however, which contributes to fall reduction. Balance training should be included to prevent falls for patients with fall risks (see **Table 31-7**). Regular exercise has been shown to improve bone mass (0.5% to 3.0%), with 20% to 45% reduction in hip fractures in older populations with moderate-to-vigorous physical activity (80,110–112).

Life Span Bone Phases

Bone health is determined by many factors (113). Increased physical activity, especially weight-bearing and resistive exercise, stimulates bone building via the piezoelectric effect of contracted muscle on the bone. In defining general life phases in which bone changes are likely to occur, the clinician can target screening and exercise recommendations more easily. During childhood and adolescence, the bone undergoes a *growth phase*, especially during puberty. This is followed by a *maintenance phase* during young and middle adulthood. A *midlife phase*, ages

50 to 70, can be characterized as a bone loss phase; after age 70, a *frailty phase* is more likely (see Chapter 47). An important time to consider is the menopausal transition period in women. The average decrease in BMD during this transition (114) is about 10%. This is just the average, but 25% of these women are classified as fast bone losers measured by rates of bone loss and bone resorption markers (115). This explains why 15% to 20% of women may suffer fractures in their early 60s.

CDC surveillance data report only about 1 in 5 Americans (21%) and less than 3 in 10 high school students meet physical activity recommendations (116). Globally, the WHO reports that 1 in 4 adults is not active enough and over 80% of the world's adolescent population is not sufficiently active. Insufficient physical activity is sited as a key risk factor for noncommunicable diseases (such as cardiovascular disease, cancer, and diabetes) and a worldwide leading risk factor for death (117).

Physical activity recommendations for children under 18 include 60 minutes/day of moderate- to vigorous-intensity activity in addition to muscle- and bone-strengthening activities 3 days/week. Recommendations for adults are 150 minutes/week of moderate-intensity or 75 minutes/week of vigorous-intensity activity in addition to muscle strengthening (118). As Americans age, their participation in physical activity declines, with women persistently lagging behind men: 61% of adults report never engaging in vigorous physical activity, with 66% of women compared to 56% of men included in this category of inactivity (119). Lower levels of physical activity (lack of vigorous exercise) are correlated with lower levels of education (80% of those without high school diploma vs. 43% of those with bachelor's degree or higher) and lower income (72% of poor families compared with 52% of families classified as not poor) (120).

The most critical period of bone growth is thought to be during puberty and adolescence, with the greatest gains, on average 25% to 30% of adult bone mass, developing between age 12 to 14 in girls and 13 to 15 in boys (121). Most of these gains reflect increased bone length and size, not bone density (122). Bone mass gained during this period was found to typically equal to the amount lost later in adult life (123). As bone mineralization lags behind growth in length, fracture rates increase during periods of rapid growth (124). In a school-based program that emphasized jumping activities over 7 months, only early pubertal girls improved in bone mass (1.5% to 3.1% at the femoral neck and lumbar spine when compared with controls), with no benefit noted in the late pre-pubertal experimental group of girls (125).

Exercise need not be strenuous to confer benefit (126–128). The gentle, slow movements involved in the practice of tai chi have been gaining in popularity with the elderly. Benefits have been reported in balance, strength, cardiovascular fitness, respiratory function and flexibility, and decreased injury. Wolf et al. reported a 47.5% decrease in multiple falls in assisted living residents aged 70 to 97 during a 1-year program for elderly patients (129). Li et al. demonstrated a 55% reduction in multiple falls and reduced injury from fall (7% vs. 18% in controls) with a three-time weekly tai chi program during a 6-month period (130). Later studies demonstrated delayed bone density loss in postmenopausal female tai chi practitioners (131–133). Early research in whole-body vibration also shows preliminary benefit in balance in residents of long-term facilities (134), muscle strength (135,136), and bone mass (136).

Exercise Principles

The following general principles should be considered when recommending therapeutic exercise (137).

Principle of Specificity

Exercise should stress the specific physiologic system being trained; modality, dose, frequency, and intensity must be optimized for osteogenic benefit in addressing osteoporosis. Recommendations therefore must consider the benefit of dynamic exercises (cyclic rather than continuous), exercise that induces relatively high bone strain or deformation, exercise that can be applied rapidly, and exercise that applies diverse loading (multidirectional movements as opposed to patterned loading as with running). Weight-bearing sports with diverse loading such as gymnastics, ballet, powerlifting, tennis, and figure skating have demonstrated superior bone mass in athletes compared to sports that require lower impact or non–weight bearing. In light of this, moderate- to high-impact weight-bearing activities (hopping, running, jumping, and high-impact aerobics), balance training, and high-intensity progressive resistance training (PRT) should be included to optimize osteogenesis, safety, and fall prevention. PRT should be recommended at least twice a week, should address large muscles across the spine and hips, and should optimize magnitude of loading (80% to 85% of the 1 repetition maximum). Technique, incremental increase in loading, and avoidance of activities that may contribute to falls should be emphasized with supervised progression of an exercise plan, especially in high-risk individuals (with osteoporosis or previous fracture). Postural exercises (including spinal extensor exercises) should be integrated to oppose the kyphotic forces associated with disk degeneration and vertebral fracture.

Exercise programs for patients with arthritis, very low bone mass, and multiple fractures should optimize skeletal protection while building strength, balance, conditioning, and flexibility. Modifications for arthritis may include low- to moderate-impact activities (with reduction or elimination of high ground reaction forces) and moderate- to high-intensity PRT (138). High-impact exercises additionally may not be appropriate for the frailty-phase patient population. Isometric, core-strengthening exercises with the spine in neutral position should be emphasized in all patients. Spinal flexion and twisting should be avoided in patients with compression fracture; these modifications may additionally be considered in the frail and those with abnormal bone density (139).

Principle of Reversibility

The positive effect of exercise will slowly be lost if the program is discontinued. Hence, a lifelong dedication to exercise and physical activity is necessary for optimal bone health, as changes associated with aging can have profound physical and clinical consequences. On average, adults lose 5% of muscle mass per decade after age 30, with potentially more rapid decline after age 65 (140). However, many patients with sarcopenia (age-related loss of skeletal muscle, strength, and/or function) and impaired balance remain highly functional. This muscle loss may be reversed by exercise, as shown by Frontera et al. (141). A comprehensive exercise program must increase bone mass and muscle strength (142) with continued variety to prevent abandonment of exercise goals. It is important to emphasize strengthening the bone while it still has adaptive ability; this is particularly important in persons with disability and the elderly. While passive standing is not recommended for active adults for exercise, in a person with severe disability such as SCI, the use of a standing frame or standing wheelchair is a rehabilitative strategy shown to prevent bone loss (143).

Principle of Progression
To increase bone mass, the stimulus must exceed previous bone-loading activity. Thus, there must be a progressive increase in the intensity of the exercise for continued improvement. Kerr's study of resistive exercises at the hip demonstrated that exercise benefits are site specific and result from progressive resistance exercise with maximum loading as opposed to an endurance regimen (144). To avoid injury, however, applied loads must be within the capacity of the bone to sustain mechanical stress. Progressive resistance is important for both bone health and improved functional capacity (145). Slowly increasing time or intensity of exercise by 10% weekly decreases risk of injury (146).

Principle of Initial Values
Those who initially have low capacity will have the greatest functional improvement from a given program (147). Nevertheless, it is important for inactive participants to begin with short exercise sessions of low intensity and progress systematically to limit risk of injury.

Principle of Diminishing Returns
There is a biologic ceiling to exercise-induced improvements in function. As this ceiling is approached, greater effort is needed to achieve minimal gain.

Optimal calcium intake is thought to be synergistic with physical activity throughout life in improving bone mass (148–150) and should be encouraged in all patient populations where medical contraindications do not coexist. In meta-analysis of randomized clinical trials, Shea et al. concluded that calcium supplements in postmenopausal women reduced bone loss by 2%, with an approximate 23% reduction in spine fractures (151). Vitamin D supplements may reduce spine fractures by as much as 7% (152). Exercise must also be supported with adequate caloric intake for energy expended for all patients, as indicated by adequate glycemic index. Weight loss, which sacrifices adipose tissue and depletes estrogen production stores sufficiently to cause amenorrhea in females, increases the risk of osteoporosis and stress fractures. More than 3 months without menstruation should prompt clinical evaluation in these patients (see "Female Athlete Triad [FAT]," below).

The prevention of falls and fractures through an ongoing exercise program that maintains proper nutrition, strength, and aerobic capacity should be coupled with adjunctive measures such as the provision of adequate support for the spine, pain management, and psychological support when developing objectives for long-term goals.

Fall Reduction Strategies
Over one fourth of community-dwelling persons 65 years of age and older will fall each year (153); this number doubles for residents in nursing homes (154). Although less than 1% of falls result in fracture, according to the Northeast Hip Fracture Study Group, 90% of hip fractures are due to a fall (155). The propensity to fall may be as important as bone mass, given the frequency and severity of falls in this age group. Falls have many etiologies, including decreased neuromuscular coordination of the elderly (resulting in an inability to prevent loss of balance or break a fall's impact), mental status issues such as confusion and dizziness with medication, and environmental factors such as poor lighting and loose rugs. New research has examined differences in frequency, mechanism, and risk factors for falling between men and women (156,157). The loss of muscle mass can be as much as 3% to 5% per decade after age 30 and is also commonly associated with falls and fracture in the elderly. Fiatarone Singh et al. found 71% of elderly hip fracture patients had reduced muscle mass (158).

Degree of demineralization of the bone and the trauma of falling are well established as risk factors for fracture. There are rare reports of spontaneous hip fracture, although one historical study in 1981 demonstrated that 11% of fractures were spontaneous, with 25% of them associated with standing or sitting transfers and 60% during simple ambulation (159). More research is needed in this area. These studies support the notion that fractures of the proximal femur can be the result of muscle forces acting on the hip exceeding the mechanical ability of the femur to withstand stress (160). Because hip fractures have multifactorial causes (161), interventions must aim not only at increasing BMD at the hips but also at increasing muscular strength, balance, and flexibility and reducing the forces of impact when a fall occurs.

A successful program aimed at preventing falls includes education on how to eliminate identifiable fall risks and implementation of an exercise regimen that focuses on balance, gait training, coordination and function, and muscle strengthening (162–164). Preservation of autonomy after a fracture can be aided by modifications made to the home environment before the patient is released from the hospital. Home visits from an occupational therapist have also been shown to be helpful in this regard (165).

Falls in long-term care facilities present very specific challenges. According to the CDC, approximately 5% of adults aged 65 and older live in nursing homes in the United States, and about three out of four of these residents fall each year, which is twice the rate of older community dwellers. About 2% to 6% of these falls result in death. The most common causes of these falls are similar to those of community dwellers listed above. The most effective strategies to prevent falls include postfall assessment and follow-through on findings; staff education; medication review; environmental changes such as raised toilet seats, lower bed height, and hallway handrails; hip pads; and bed alarms. Physical restraints do not lower fall risk and, in fact, may increase the risk of injury and death with falls (157).

Mechanisms of Falls
Although much attention has been given to methods for increasing bone density, the mechanisms behind falls are less studied (159,166–169). The severity of the fall is an independent risk factor for hip fracture (170) and is related to many factors, including the direction of the fall and the specific anatomic location of major impact (168). Whereas young adults tend to fall to the side or backward, the elderly tend to fall sideways or drop in place, especially those with unsteady gaits (166). It is falls to the side that result in major impact forces that greatly exceed the mechanical strength of the proximal femur and therefore result in fracture.

The risk of falling appears to increase linearly with the number of risk factors present. The most consistent predictors for falling include balance and gait abnormalities, impaired vision, decreased ADL function, polypharmacy, and cognitive impairment (171). Sedative use, particularly polypharmacy, is associated with falling independent of other risk factors. Benzodiazepines, phenothiazines, and antidepressants are used frequently in the elderly for dementia and depression, and use of these medications is associated with increased falling—particularly when taken in their longer-acting forms. Diuretics and antihypertensive agents are also associated with an increased risk of falling, as they can induce postural hypotension. An annual review of current medications, especially antihypertensives, psychotropics, sedatives, analgesics, antihistamines, and diuretics, should be included in fall risk assessment screening. **Table 31-5** lists other major risk factors, including environmental hazards.

For a fall to result in hip fracture, there must be impact near the hip that is not reduced by body mechanisms or absorbed by soft tissue structures. General conditioning exercises, appropriate provision of assistive devices, adequate footwear, modification of medications, and attention to other risk factors for falling are targeted at preventing the instability that results in a loss of balance (172). There is ample evidence of the benefit of exercise increasing bone mass and preventing falls. These programs must be maintained, however, for continued benefit to accrue to bone mass and muscle strength (173). Several important determinants govern the forces applied to the femur as a result of falling. These forces include the person's weight, thickness of subcutaneous tissue, height of the fall, configuration of the body during the fall, velocity at which the hip strikes the impact surface, and nature of the impact surface. Contraction of the quadriceps and other muscles of the lower limb is likely to reduce velocity at impact and reduce impact forces at the proximal femur in falls to the side. Exercise programs aimed at increasing lower extremity strength may therefore prevent hip fracture by reducing fall severity (144,171,173–176).

Meta-analysis by Moayyeri et al. demonstrated that moderate-to-vigorous physical activity is associated with hip fracture risk reduction of 38% in women and 45% in men (177). Low body weight and low BMI are associated with an increased risk of hip fracture in elderly men and women (161,170,174,175). Although the impact force most closely correlates with the individual's weight, velocity on impact is most associated with height. Thus, although an individual may be heavier and the resultant force of impact more, he or she may have more padding over the trochanter in addition to stronger bone, thereby preventing fracture.

While the benefits of physical activity and exercise are well described, it is less clear which exercises are most efficacious in preventing falls and decreasing risk of osteoporotic fractures (178,179). Carter et al. addressed the effects of improved resistance and agility training, but found no benefit in reducing fall risk in osteoporotic women aged 65 to 75. Although trunk stabilization exercises were included in this "Osteofit" exercise program, only knee extension strength was evaluated as a measure of improvement in fall risk (180). Liu-Ambose et al. found decreased fall risk (20% to 57%) with regular exercise in women with low bone mass aged 75 to 85, with the greatest benefit from resistive exercise group (57.3%) followed by the agility training group (47.5%) followed by the stretching exercise group (20.2%) (181).

There is a clear need for further research in clarifying the relationship between specific exercise protocols and their contribution to fall and fracture reduction.

Recognition that increases in soft tissue thickness around the hip substantially reduce peak force to the trochanter at fall impact has led to the development of hip protectors. Fractures have been prevented in women wearing hip protectors, and Lauritzen concludes that the use of hip protectors could reduce fracture by 53% (176). The Cochrane Database System Reviews of 2003 and 2007 indicated many trials have identified strategies to prevent falls (162,182), but standardization is lacking for outcome measures. The 2005 Cochrane review by Parker and Gillespie, however, showed no clear benefit from hip protectors in preventing fractures, citing poor compliance due to discomfort and practicality as important factors (183). Pads are designed in two primary configurations: a simple pad that covers the trochanter and reduces impact force by absorbing energy in the pad material and one based on shunting energy from the fall away from the trochanter (184). The latter pad is designed in an inverted U shape and is filled with a colloidal-like substance that hardens on impact, permitting 68% reduction in peak force at the hip with impact. Softer pads tend to promote more compliance with wear (185).

Psychosocial Considerations

Psychological issues have been noted to contribute significantly to disability in the osteoporotic patient after fracture. Depression is the most common psychological problem identified in these patients. A study of community-dwelling postmenopausal women found that those with osteoporosis had significantly higher depression scores than did those with normal bone density (186). Anxiety, fear, and other emotional reactions also affect postfracture outcome. In a study of 200 women recovering from hip fractures, those with high depression scores following surgery were more likely to experience poorer recovery of function (187). In a 1993 study of 100 women with osteoporosis-induced vertebral fracture, women noted emotions as having greater importance than physical functioning, leisure and social activities, and ADLs (188). In this group, most reported fear of falling, fear of new fractures, frustration, anger, and feeling overwhelmed. Vertebral fracture patients also suffered loss of self-esteem, isolation, vulnerability, and embarrassment related to physical appearance (145).

There is increasing evidence that women with depression are more susceptible to low bone mass, with both antidepressant medications and imbalance of immune system inflammatory proteins implicated (189). Inflammatory proteins are induced by adrenalin, which is frequently elevated in depressed patients. Of these proteins, IL-6 is known to promote bone loss (190). Dudgeon et al. investigated the relationship of physical disability and chronic pain to changes in lifestyle. They found patients learned to suppress pain complaints to some degree because of perceived negative social consequences in the form of isolation, rejection, and consequent depression. Patients' methods for coping with pain included distraction techniques (e.g., listening to music), which conferred some sense of control in a health care system in which the nature of their pain was not well understood, not addressed adequately, and peripheralized by health care providers (191).

PHARMACOLOGIC AGENTS

The ability of Food and Drug Administration (FDA)-approved pharmacologic agents to prevent or treat osteoporosis has been studied best in postmenopausal women; fracture data are more limited for men and for corticosteroid-induced osteoporosis. Thus, prescription treatments at present demonstrate fracture risk reduction best in those with osteoporosis by DXA and/ or fragility fracture history, compared with osteopenic patients without fractures. Benefits and risks of therapy must be individualized to each patient. The therapeutic agents available for the treatment and prevention of osteoporosis are classified as decreasing bone resorption (antiresorptive agents) or stimulating bone formation (anabolic agents). The end result of each is the same: to preserve or improve bone mass and thereby prevent fractures. As noted in **Tables 31-10** and **31-11**, most U.S. FDA-approved therapeutic agents decrease bone resorption. Reduction of hip fracture may lead to a reduction in mortality. Lyles et al. showed a 28% reduction in deaths from annual infusion of zoledronic acid within 90 days after repair of hip fragility fracture (192). A study by Gilchrist et al. with alendronate 70-mg weekly dosing in acute SCI patients demonstrated significant differences over placebo controls in total body BMD (+5.3%) and total hip BMD (+17.6%) at 1 year (193).

Antiresorptive Agents

Bisphosphonates

The FDA-approved bisphosphonates, alendronate, risedronate, ibandronate, and zoledronic acid, have the ability to preserve and increase bone mass at the spine, hip, and other sites to varying degrees and, in most cases, prevent fractures at these sites. The FDA has approved their use for the prevention and treatment of osteoporosis for postmenopausal women and men in most cases. The use of these medications in pediatric populations is promising, particularly in juvenile idiopathic arthritis, but more studies are needed (194,195). Their mechanism of action is well studied: they bind to the surface of the bone and are taken up by osteoclasts during the bone resorption process. They subsequently precipitate early cell death by blocking essential lipid compounds within the osteoclast,

slowing the resorption process. (See **Tables 31-10** and **31-11** for summary of dosing, safety, and efficacy of medications in this class and other treatments.)

Long half-life allows some bisphosphonates to accumulate and persist in the bone, which promotes maintenance of bone density gains even after treatment is stopped. This permits treatment "holidays," provided DXA and bone turnover markers remain stable. When ingested orally, these drugs must be taken at least one-half hour before any food, drink, or other medication in the morning for maximal absorption, and the patient must maintain an upright position during that time to avoid the risk of esophageal irritation and, rarely, ulceration. Other side effects include visual disturbances, musculoskeletal pain, and difficulty swallowing. While in one British study there was a higher risk of atrial fibrillation with zoledronic acid compared to placebo (1.3% vs. 0.4%), this risk is still under investigation with other bisphosphonates and has not led to any FDA-induced change in prescription recommendations (196). Bisphosphonates should be prescribed with caution in patients with severe renal dysfunction and are not considered safe for pregnant women (197). Hypocalcemia is a recognized consequence of bisphosphonate administration, most often with IV infusion. All patients who are initiating treatment with these medications should have adequate calcium and vitamin D intake. Compliance with medication dosing must be monitored. Siris et al. found only 43% of women over age 45 were compliant with refills of bisphosphonate prescriptions, and only 20% were without gaps in refills at 2 years; only compliant patients had significant reductions (20% to 45%) in fractures (198). The need for concomitant calcium and vitamin D supplementation must additionally be stressed to patients to maximize efficacy of the bisphosphonates, as noncompliance with supplements is also common and reported as low as 40% (199). There is a newer formulation of bisphosphonate, which has been approved (delayed-release risedronate), with pH-sensitive enteric coating that helps the drug to bypass the esophagus and stomach, allowing for absorption in the small intestine and therefore potentially increasing oral medication compliance. This drug can be taken after breakfast. It is once-weekly dosing and has shown to be as effective as risedronate 5 mg IR daily in increasing spine and hip BMD (200).

TABLE 31-10	**Bisphosphonate Comparison**			
Name	**Treatment Dose (per d/wk/mo)**	**Increased BMD Sites[a,b]**	**Decreased Fracture Sites[a,b]**	**FDA Indications**
Alendronate	10/70/na[c]	Spine, hip	Spine, hip	P[d], T, M, G
Ibandronate	2.5/na[c]/150 (3 mg IV/3 mo)		Spine	P, T
Risedronate	5/35/150	Spine, hip	Spine	P, T, M, G
			Nonspine	
			Hip	
Zoledronic acid	5 mg IV yearly	Hip	Spine, nonspine, hip	T, M, G, F

[a]Note: Definitions are based on WHO assessment of bone mass measurement at any skeletal site in white women (198); data cited for increased BMD and decreased fracture sites are not from comparable studies.

[b]In postmenopausal women.

[c]na, not available.

[d]Dose 5/35/na.

F, posthip fragility fracture; G, treatment for glucocorticoid-induced osteoporosis, male or female; M, treatment of men with osteoporosis; P, prevention of postmenopausal osteoporosis; T, treatment of postmenopausal osteoporosis.

Data adapted from NOF Clinician's Guide to Prevention and Treatment of Osteoporosis.

TABLE 31-11	Nutritional and Pharmacologic Treatments for Osteoporosis		
Medication	**Usual Dosage**	**Mode of Action**	**Side Effects > Placebo ($\geq$5%)**
Calcium	1,200 mg/d	Decreased bone resorption	Increased urinary calcium
Vitamin D$_2$	800–1,200 IU/d	Increased calcium absorption	(low risk) hypercalcemia
Or D$_3$	—	In the GI tract	
Bisphosphonates		Decreased bone resorption	Esophageal irritation (PO), osteonecrosis of the jaw (IV predominantly, in cancer patients), atypical femoral fractures
Alendronate (Fosamax)	10 mg daily or 70 mg weekly (space) PO (mg daily or 35 mg weekly for osteopenia)		
Risedronate (Actonel)	5 mg daily, 35 mg weekly or 150 mg monthly		
Ibandronate (Boniva)	150 mg PO monthly or 3 mg IV every 3 mo		
Zoledronic acid (Reclast)[a]	5 mg IV over 15 min yearly		
Postmenopausal women			
Teriparatide (Forteo)	20 µg daily SQ (max. 18–24 mo Rx)	Increased bone mineralization	Leg cramps; dizziness
Calcitonin (Miacalcin)	200 MR IU/d (nasal spray)	Decreased bone resorption	Nasal irritation (rare)
Estrogen with or without progesterone	0.625 mg/d for 21–30 d (cycled 21 of 30 d)	Decreased bone resorption	Possible increased risk of cancer, high blood pressure, deep vein thrombosis, stroke, heart disease, thromboembolic disease
Estrogen agonist/antagonist			
Raloxifene (Evista)	60 mg/daily	Decreased bone resorption	Hot flashes, leg cramps, deep vein thrombosis
RANKL inhibition Denosumab (Prolia)	60 mg SQ twice yearly	Decreased bone resorption via RANKL inhibition	Musculoskeletal pain, elevated cholesterol, cystitis pancreatitis

[a]FDA approved

There have been long-term safety concerns regarding osteonecrosis of the jaw and atypical femur fractures. These are both very rare adverse events (1 in 50,000 to 1 in 150,000) and are related to the duration of treatment. Ninety-four percent of the case reports of osteonecrosis of the jaw with this class of drug are associated with cancer patients receiving multiple doses of IV bisphosphonates (83). The atypical femur fractures usually occur as transverse or oblique fractures in the proximal or mid femoral diaphysis. They may occur spontaneously and have delayed healing. These fractures occur in patients who have received prolonged bisphosphonate therapy, which has raised the question of whether long-term treatment causes oversuppression of bone remodeling and impaired ability to repair microfractures with increased fragility. These concerns raise the questions about optimum duration of bisphosphonate therapy and when to consider a drug holiday.

The duration of treatment and the length of holiday should be individualized based on fracture risk. For those with mild fracture risk, it is recommended to treat with bisphosphonates for 5 years. With moderate fracture risk, the recommendation is to treat for 5 to 10 years and with severe fracture risk to treat for 10 years. If at these time points BMD is stable, it is reasonable to consider a drug holiday. After initiation of a drug holiday, risk reassessment should be done after 1 year for risedronate (lower skeletal affinity), 1 to 2 years for alendronate, and 2 to 3 years for zoledronic acid by measuring BMD (every 1 to 2 years) and/or bone turnover markers (annually). In those who are at high fracture risk, one should consider adding teriparatide or raloxifene during the drug holiday.

RANKL Inhibition

Research on the remodeling mechanisms involving osteoblasts and osteoclasts has resulted in the development of a newer category of antiresorptive medication, an inhibitor of RANKL. Denosumab decreases bone resorption by inhibiting the earliest stages of osteoclast maturation. The antibody prevents RANKL from interacting with the receptor RANK, truncating the earliest stages of the osteoclast maturation cascade (see **Fig. 31-2**). Denosumab is administered via subcutaneous injection (60 mg) twice yearly and is currently approved for the treatment of osteoporosis. There is slow absorption via the SC route with a median time to maximal absorption of 10 days. After maximal concentration, serum denosumab concentrations decline over 4 to 5 months (201). In the FREEDOM trial, 7,868 postmenopausal women with osteoporosis were randomly assigned to denosumab or placebo for 3 years. Denosumab increased BMD of the lumbar spine and total hip compared with placebo (9.2% vs. 0% and 4.0% vs. −2.0%, respectively) and reduced the risk of new vertebral fractures by 68% and hip fractures by 40%, both statistically significant (202). In the FREEDOM extension trial (203) of 4,550 women, the FREEDOM group was continued on 3 additional years of denosumab where the placebo group initiated denosumab for 3 years. Lumbar spine and hip BMD continued to increase significantly at the end of 6 years (15.2% and 7.2%, respectively). In the crossover group, lumbar spine and hip BMD increased by 9.4% and 4.8%, respectively.

In a phase II study, discontinuation of therapy led to return toward baseline values for both BMD (6.4% decrease in BMD 12 months after discontinuation) and bone turnover markers, which generally returned to baseline values (204). This is important to note because in contrast to bisphosphonates where the duration is long-lived, the effects after discontinuing denosumab and other therapies are short-lived, and an alternative form of treatment should be considered to maintain the desired effect on the bone.

The most common side effects include respiratory and urinary tract infections, cataracts, constipation, rashes, and joint pain. In the 6-year extension trial, there were six cases of osteonecrosis of the jaw and one case of atypical fracture. Hypocalcemia and anaphylaxis have been reported. It is recommended all patients using denosumab receive calcium 1,000 mg daily and at least 400 IU of vitamin D daily to avoid hypocalcemia complications. Of note, the DAPS (Denosumab Adherence Preference Satisfactions) study comparing denosumab or alendronate in alternating years showed a significantly greater adherence to therapy with denosumab, and 92.4% of subjects expressed preference for denosumab over alendronate (205).

Hormone Therapy

Estrogen

Estrogen is important to bone development throughout life for both men and women. Because it acts on both reproductive and nonreproductive tissues in the body, consideration for use of its exogenous forms, alone or in combination with progesterone, must balance its benefits with the individual patient's medical and family history. It was first approved by the FDA for postmenopausal osteoporosis in 1972, after approval in 1942 for relief of menopausal symptoms (197). A trial by the Women's Health Initiative (WHI) (206) reported the first definitive data supporting a benefit of postmenopausal hormones in the prevention of fractures at the hip and spine by at least one third compared to placebo. One arm of this placebo-controlled trial involved the administration of an estrogen/progestin (HT) combination tablet (0.625-mg estrogen, 2.5-mg progestin vs. placebo) to approximately 17,000 postmenopausal women with an intact uterus. A second arm of the study evaluated estrogen alone (ET) in women who had had hysterectomies (207). Both arms were halted early because evidence of harm was found. HT resulted in a small but measurable risk of heart attack, stroke, venous thromboembolism, and breast cancer. Positive findings included a reduced risk of colorectal cancer and fractures. In the ET arm, there was not an increase in the risk for heart attack or breast cancer. There was slight increase in stroke risk and there was a reduction in fractures. The use of HT and ET declined after the WHI trial with the concern that the risks may outweigh the benefits. Notably, however, the average age of women in the WHI study was 63; therefore, the results may not apply to early postmenopausal women.

A secondary reanalysis (208) by age group or years post menopause showed that the above-outlined cardiovascular events occurred primarily in women older than 70 years and not in younger women. In women within 10 years of menopause, there was a reduced risk of heart attack and reduced mortality suggesting that the timing of initiation of HT is important for the prevention of heart disease. In a review article (209), it was concluded that hormone replacement therapy (HRT) is very effective in relieving menopausal symptoms and prevention of osteoporosis while maintaining a good safety profile.

Estrogen supplementation continues to be an important part of the overall treatment of osteoporosis in women. Given the totality of the findings, ET/HT remains somewhat controversial but can still be considered a first-line choice for prevention of bone loss and fracture in the early postmenopausal period for a period of 5 years. In women with a low risk of adverse events associated with ET/HRT, it is felt treatment can be continued with an acceptable risk/benefit ratio. Hormone therapy may be especially important in the first 3 to 4 years after menopause as this is the time bone resorption is highest and response to treatment is most significant.

Studies have shown that withdrawal of estrogen produces rapid loss of BMD: within 1 year, any increase in BMD accumulated over the prior 3 to 4 years disappeared (210). It has been proposed that the most effective way to treat the acute bone loss in postmenopausal women is by using a high dose of HT/ET for 6 months to rapidly reduce bone resorption and then reduce the dose in subsequent years.

HRT in women is FDA approved for prevention of osteoporosis only and is to be taken in conjunction with calcium and vitamin D. Research with lower-dose hormone therapy and newer "designer estrogens" offers promise of beneficial effects without the detrimental side effects.

SERMs

Selective estrogen receptor modulators (SERMs) are now called *estrogen agonist/antagonists* and have been developed to provide beneficial effects similar to those obtained with estrogen, but without the adverse effects. They have an agonistic effect on bone and lipoprotein production, while being antagonistic toward breast tissue, without effect on uterine mucosa. Raloxifene is FDA approved in this class for the treatment of postmenopausal osteoporosis and prevention of bone loss in recently postmenopausal women (211). The use of raloxifene provides modest increases in bone mass, but reduction in the risk of vertebral fracture is 40% to 50%. To date, studies have not shown a reduction in nonvertebral fractures (44). It also appears to reduce the risk of estrogen-dependent breast cancer.

Bazedoxifene is a third-generation SERM. In late 2013, it was approved as part of the combination drug DUAVEE (20-mg bazedoxifene with 0.45-mg conjugated estrogens) for the prevention of postmenopausal osteoporosis and treatment of hot flashes. In clinical trials, it has been shown to increase BMD at both the hip and spine and demonstrated efficacy in reducing fractures at these two sites (212). It is also being studied for possible treatment of breast and pancreatic cancer.

Lasofoxifene is another third-generation SERM with excellent oral bioavailability. In a randomized controlled study looking at two doses of lasofoxifene (0.25 and 0.5 mg daily) over 3 years, results showed increased spine BMD by 3.0% and 3.1%, respectively, and increased femoral neck BMD by 2.9% and 3.0%, respectively. The low-dose group had a reduction in spine fractures by 31%. The higher-dose group had a reduction in spine fractures by 42% and nonvertebral fracture by 22%. The lower-dose group had a reduction of breast cancer of 49%, while the higher-dose group achieved a reduction of 81% (213).

The greatest concerns with using SERMs are an increased risk of thrombotic and thromboembolic events, which is comparable to what is observed with HRT. The incidence of thrombotic events is higher during the first 2 years of treatment and progressively decreases (214). Other side effects include vasomotor instability and leg cramps.

Combination Antiresorptive Therapies

The efficacy and safety of combined bisphosphonates with either hormone therapy or SERMs are being studied; as they have different mechanisms of action, there may be potential for an additive effect when used together. Bone et al. showed an 8% increase in spine BMD in combination, compared to 6% with either alone (215). However, as there is no proven additive effect on fracture reduction, these combination therapies are currently considered experimental (216).

The DATA (Denosumab and Teriparatide Administration) study was a 2-year RCT in 94 postmenopausal women with osteoporosis in which subjects were randomized in a 1:1:1 ratio to receive 20 µg teriparatide daily, 60 mg SC denosumab q6 months, or both. At 12 months, lumbar spine BMD increased more in the combination group than in the teriparatide or denosumab groups (9.1%, 6.2%, and 5.5%, respectively). Total hip BMD showed the same trend (combination 4.9%, teriparatide 0.7%, denosumab 2.5%). CTX showed maximal suppression in the denosumab and combination groups, and bone formation markers were measurable in the combination group in contrast to unmeasurable in the denosumab group (217). These findings are in contrast to studies combining bisphosphonates with teriparatide, which have shown poorer efficacy with combined therapy compared to monotherapy (218).

Calcitonin

Calcitonin is a natural hormone secreted by parafollicular cells within the thyroid gland and has an inhibitive effect on osteoclasts. Salmon calcitonin has been most widely used because its affinity is 40 times higher than human calcitonin for the human calcitonin receptor. The PROOF trial noted a decrease in spine fractures by 33% with 200 IU daily dose of nasal spray although no reduction was noted with doses of 100 or 400 IU (219). Subsequent studies showed no significant difference in nonspine fracture rates after 5 years. It may have limited potential to decrease pain after acute compression fracture in the spine.

Calcitonin was initially felt to have few side effects of significance: nasal congestion, nosebleeds, and nausea; however, two FDA advisory committees have concluded that use of a nasal spray formulation of the peptide hormone salmon calcitonin is associated with a slight but significant increased risk of cancer. Due to these findings, the FDA's advisory panel in 2013 recommended that marketing of calcitonin salmon for the treatment of osteoporosis in women greater than 5 years after menopause be stopped. In 2012, the European Medicines Agency recommended that calcitonin salmon not be used to treat osteoporosis after determining the risk of cancer was 2.4% higher in those using the nasal spray compared to placebo.

Anabolic Agents

Teriparatide

The FDA approved the use of teriparatide, a recombinant human PTH fragment (PTH 1 to 34) for the treatment of osteoporosis in 2002 after initial studies showed increased absorption of calcium and phosphorus, and a remarkable increase in bone turnover, with bone formation outweighing bone resorption (220). It is administered by subcutaneous injection daily (20 µg) in a preassembled multiple-dose pen device. It has an anabolic effect on the bone through thickening of the bone cortex and increasing connections within the bone matrix. It is approved for treatment of postmenopausal osteoporosis and for men with idiopathic or hypogonadal osteoporosis who are at high risk for fracture and for those who have failed or are intolerant of previous treatment (214). In postmenopausal women with osteoporosis, BMD increased by 9.7% in the spine and 2.6% at the hip, with fracture reduction of 65% at the spine and 53% at nonspine sites (221). Data for fracture risk improvement in men have not been established, but a 1998 study showed BMD increases of 5.9% in the spine and 1.2% at the hip in this population (222). Common side effects include dizziness and leg cramps. Although the approved dose regimen has not been found to increase risk of osteosarcoma in humans as has been observed in laboratory animal studies, this medicine is presently not prescribed for patients with a history of bone carcinoma or bone metastases. Nor is it thought safe in pediatric patients or adult patients with hypercalcemia, Paget's disease, or kidney disease (223). Neither efficacy nor safety of treatment beyond 2 years is established (224). In the European Study of Forsteo (EUROFORS), women who had received 1 year of teriparatide were randomly assigned to either receive a 2nd year of teriparatide or switching to either raloxifene or placebo (225). BMD in women who received teriparatide for a 2nd year continued to increase, whereas BMD was maintained in women who received raloxifene and decreased in women who received placebo. Knowing this, when PTH treatment is discontinued, an antiresorptive should be used to preserve or increase gains in BMD following PTH treatment.

Testosterone

Testosterone is of value in the treatment of secondary osteoporosis in hypogonadal men. Prostate-specific antigen and serum lipid status should be monitored during treatment.

Anabolic steroids may actually have a beneficial effect on bone mass; however, their side effects include liver toxicity, masculinization, and increased cholesterol levels, which prohibits their use in osteoporosis.

Cytokines

In theory, a number of cytokines may function as growth factors (TGF-β, IGF-I, etc.) with potential benefit in osteoporosis. Their benefits as established by clinical trials, however, are not presently common in clinical practice, although IGF-I and DHEAS may be used to assess bone health in pediatric populations in the future (i.e., anorexia nervosa and cerebral palsy) (226).

Non–FDA-Approved Drugs

Current data suggest that high-dose sodium fluoride, which is a positive bone former, may actually worsen osteoporosis by increasing the risk of nonspine fracture. Whether sodium fluoride in newer formulations, including a low-dose sustained-release preparation, will prove of benefit is unclear. Sodium fluoride must be viewed as an experimental therapy with some concerns regarding its overall benefit in osteoporosis (227–229).

Strontium ranelate (SR) is another bone former that is absorbed onto the bone surface and is incorporated into bone, changing the crystal structure without affecting mineralization (230). SR increases bone formation markers, reduces bone resorption markers, and increased BMD. In a 4-year trial of osteoporotic women, SR decreased the incidence of vertebral fractures by 33% (231). Side effects of SR are concerning and include a possible association with cardiovascular events, especially myocardial infarction. There is a possible association with venous thromboembolism (232). There have also been rare but severe skin reactions (233).

REHABILITATION MANAGEMENT POSTFRACTURE

Osteoporosis is a silent disease that can progress from minimal impairment of the skeleton's capacity to bear stress to a disease characterized by frailty, fracture, deformity, chronic pain, handicap, and loss of independence. Patients present with an individualized spectrum of complaints warranting different degrees of investigation and intervention (see **Fig. 31-3**). Rehabilitation management depends on accurate determination of the degree of bone loss, the risk factors for osteoporosis, the degree of frailty and propensity to fall, the capacity for participation in ADLs and safe exercise, and pain impairment level. All patients with chronic disability should be investigated for secondary causes of osteoporosis with comprehensive treatment initiated where warranted.

Imaging of symptomatic skeletal sites to evaluate for the presence of fractures and ascertain degree of associated deformity may be required. Plain radiographs often suffice to determine site of fracture, but if negative, MRI may be needed to detect first signs of inflammation associated with vertebral microfractures of individual trabeculae. This can determine acuity of compression fracture or occult hip fracture. MRI is also useful if neurologic involvement is suspected with new compression fracture. For example, severe vertebral collapse can precipitate foraminal narrowing and nerve impingement, or retropulsed bone fragments may compromise spinal cord function. MRI can also identify avascular necrosis, disk herniation, and facet pathology postfracture. When MRI is contraindicated or poorly tolerated, CT scan can be performed; it is particularly helpful in identifying metastatic disease and fracture lines that may be potential routes for cement extravasation with vertebroplasty. Skeletal scintigraphy can be also helpful in differentiating acute from chronic compression fracture sites, fracture pain from arthritic complaints, and bone malignancy.

Bone mass measurement with DXA is of value in determining the goals and intensity of the therapeutic exercise program postfracture. However, if not available, the diagnosis of fragility fracture at the spine or hip also establishes the diagnosis of osteoporosis to guide medical precautions during the postfracture rehabilitation phase. When the fracture is healed, DXA can be obtained in most patients and can provide a baseline to monitor response to treatment over time. (See **Fig. 31-3**, **Tables 31-6** and **31-7**, and Clinical Evaluation, above, for appropriate screening and treatment guidelines.) Rehabilitation goals include pain reduction; improvement or maintenance of bone mass, muscle strength, and flexibility; and establishment of medical precautions for safe exercise, fall reduction (see **Table 31-5**), and maximum recovery of independence. Strategies to achieve these goals should also address secondary causes for osteoporosis and any deformity, pain, or contractures while improving core and peripheral muscle strength, balance, and gait.

The plan of care should include appropriate diagnostic tests and pain management strategies, prescriptions where appropriate for osteoporosis medications or supplements (see **Tables 31-10** and **31-11**), rehabilitation therapy, assistive devices and home modification to prepare the patient for maximum independence in exercise, fall reduction, and safe ADLs. Clearly define all medical precautions for patient and therapists to prevent injury or medical complications during exercise and ADLs; recommend diet and lifestyle behaviors to optimize bone health (see **Fig. 31-3**).

Commonly, older patients present with many significant risk factors for low bone mass, and history of previous fractures, with acute or chronic disability. As has been discussed, fractures can occur in virtually any bone, but often occur in one of the three common sites, distal radius, proximal femur, and/or vertebra due to the biomechanical strategies of falling. The pain associated with these fractures is usually severe but self-limiting. The loss of function resulting from these fractures can be significant, affecting mobility and ADLs, and may lead to loss of independence and to subsequent institutionalization.

As stressed above, screening for calcium intake and vitamin D deficiency is very important in the elderly and in persons with disability. This is both due to the prevalence of vitamin D deficiency in these populations and the synergistic benefit of calcium and vitamin D in exercise and fall reduction programs. Weight-bearing and progressive resistance exercises targeted to areas most commonly fractured can increase bone formation at those sites, with consideration of the general fragility of the skeleton guiding an individualized program to optimize safety.

Vertebral Fracture

Rehabilitation Course

Up to 33% of vertebral fractures are silent (**Table 31-12**). Although fractures of the proximal femur and distal forearm are associated with significant pain, fractures of the vertebrae can be associated with minimal trauma, such as coughing or straining on the commode, and can be asymptomatic (145). Shen and Kim in 2007 estimated that only 20% to 25% of vertebral compression fracture patients seek medical attention (234). Diagnostic procedures, most frequently the radionuclide bone scan or MRI with STIR (short-tau inversion recovery), may be used in evaluating the acuity of vertebral fractures noted on plain radiographs, particularly with active pain complaints at the site.

Vertebral fractures in the osteoporotic patient typically involve the anterior portion of the vertebral body and occur most frequently at the thoracolumbar junction, T8 through L2 (235). This portion of the spine is made of predominantly

TABLE 31-12	Loss of Quality of Life Years in Osteoporosis	
Event	**QALYs Lost Due to Event**	**Rationale**
Hip fracture		
Acute event	0.0833	Complete loss of quality of life for 1 mo (=1/12)
Rehabilitation or short-stay hospital (9 d)	0.0237	Complete loss of quality for 9 d (=9/365)
Readmitted (8 d)	0.0219	Complete loss of quality for 8 d (=8/365)
Home care services (6 mo)	0.25	Quality of life reduced by 0.5 for 6 mo (=0.5 × 6/12)
Nonmedical home care (6 mo)	0.25	Quality of life reduced by 0.5 for 6 mo (=0.5 × 6/12)
Posthospital physician visits	0.011	Quality of life reduced by 0.5 for 8 d (=0.5 × 8/365)
ER, ambulance	0.0027	Complete loss of quality for 1 d (=1/365)
Wrist fracture, acute event	0.0404	Quality reduced by 0.3 for 7 wk (=0.3 × 7/52)
Vertebral fracture, acute event	0.0324	33%: clinically silent with no loss of quality
		57%: quality of life reduced by 0.5 for 1 mo
		10%: complete loss of quality for 1 wk and then loss of quality by 0.5 for an additional 7 wk {= (0.57 × 0.5) + 0.1 × (1 × 1/52) + (0.5 × 7/25)}

ER, emergency room.
Data from the National Osteoporosis Foundation (45).

cancellous bone (65% to 75% trabecular and 25% to 35% cortical). The midradius, by contrast, is about 95% cortical bone in content. In primary osteoporosis, one sees about 40% decrease in the density of trabecular bone by 75 years of age (236).

Most patients with compression fractures present with acute or chronic back pain and complain of sharp pain that increases with movement, particularly bed mobility and transfers, and is alleviated with rest. After acute fracture, patients can complain of pain with even basic ADLs like walking, combing hair, or donning clothing. Severe and frequently disabling pain may persist for 2 to 3 weeks, but usually subsides by 6 to 8 weeks from the time of fracture. It is unlikely that osteoporosis produces acute severe pain in the absence of a fracture. Spine pain can also be secondary to mechanical derangement of the spine such as kyphosis, especially when severe. Paraspinal muscle spasm, arthritis, nerve impingement, or costal-iliac impingement syndrome, a painful rubbing of the rib cage against the iliac crest, can also be sources of pain (237). Signs and symptoms of vertebral fracture may be mimicked by neoplasm, herpes zoster, polymyalgia rheumatica, pancreatic disorders, and abdominal aortic aneurysm. It is important to investigate and treat the pain complaint promptly. If the patient experiences pain over prolonged periods, he or she may suffer consequences such as depression, sleep disturbance, and functional decline. The persistence of pain beyond 6 months at the site of a previous vertebral fracture may suggest causes other than original osteoporotic fracture; alternative etiologies of back pain in this group should be reconsidered, including progressed loss of height at original fracture site.

Plain film x-rays have poor sensitivity in diagnosis of osteoporotic sacral fractures (called *sacral insufficiency fractures*, or *SIF*). There may be other associated fractures including rib fractures in addition to the sacral fracture in many cases. Therefore, a technetium-99 bone scan may be helpful in identifying such fractures, as well as their acuity. The classic "H" or "Honda" sign seen on bone scan, representing combined bilateral vertical and horizontal sacral fractures, is present inconsistently and may vary from 15% to 68% (238). MRI

demonstrating bone marrow edema as low-signal intensity on T1-weighted images and high-signal intensity on T2-weighted images and the T2-weighted STIR images is particularly sensitive (239). However, CT is regarded as the gold standard in diagnosing occult fractures.

The osteoporotic patient complaining of acute pain resulting from vertebral fracture should be managed initially with rest, immobilization of fracture site, and analgesic agents. Because vertebral fractures generally heal well, management is directed at pain control and providing adequate rest and immobilization of the fracture site (**Table 31-13**). The unwanted side effects associated with analgesic agents may complicate treatment. Common pharmacologic interventions for acute fractures include narcotics such as codeine, but in some cases, transdermal applications (diclofenac, lidocaine) or oral tramadol may suffice. Within 3 to 4 weeks, weaning trials with other analgesic agents such as acetaminophen or nonsteroidal anti-inflammatory drugs (NSAIDs) should be attempted, in conjunction with other pain therapies. NSAIDs, however, must be used sparingly and with caution in the elderly. Primary pain management should incorporate rest, orthoses, and physical agents, with pharmacologic agents serving as adjunctive therapy. A program of progressive activity is indicated after brief initial bed rest. Because of mechanical forces translated into the spine with bed mobility and transfers, these movements are typically more painful than ambulation at the onset of the rehabilitative phase postfracture. The use of a sheepskin, egg crate, or gel flotation pad on the mattress frequently enhances patient comfort. A stool softener and laxative will help prevent straining with bowel movements. Use of a bedside commode may prove easier than a bedpan and requires less energy expenditure. Progressive transfer and ambulation training should be provided by the therapist, followed by a gentle progressive resistance exercise program for the limbs. Resistance exercises are unlikely to cause fracture in osteoporotic bones of the limbs, but can cause a new fracture or progression of acute compression fracture if resistance forces are translated into the spine. Slow introduction of isometric

TABLE 31-13 **Rehabilitation Management of Back Pain in Patients with Vertebral Fracture**

Acute back pain

Limit bed rest during the day; encourage good sleep and nutrition habits

Recommend analgesics to facilitate optimal function; utilize opiates with caution

Consider transdermal medicines to limit sedation (i.e., lidocaine or NSAID patch)

Prescribe medications for constipation if needed, if natural remedies fail

Consider back brace (i.e., CASH brace) or rigid TLSO if risk for cord compression

Monitor for signs of radiculopathy and spinal cord compression at site of fracture

Teach proper bed positioning and mobility techniques, and emphasize spine-neutral principles during transfers, ADLs, and exercise

Train caregivers to assist patients safely with minimal spine loading

Prescribe appropriate ambulation assistive device where needed

Coordinate physical therapy and occupational therapy services as appropriate

Chronic back pain

Improve posture, transfers, and gait pattern to limit vertebral compression forces

Consider postural support orthotic to decrease ligament stretch

Adjust analgesics, as pain warrants; establish opiate management contract with patient

Prescribe a sound, ongoing therapeutic exercise program

Consider vertebroplasty if conservative measures fail to improve pain profile

Evaluate and treat psychological and social consequences: consider relaxation techniques, biofeedback, support groups, and self-management skills training

Adapted from Sinaki M. Musculoskeletal challenges of osteoporosis. *Aging.* 1998;10:249–262; Sinaki M. *Musculoskeletal Rehabilitation in Osteoporosis: Etiology, Diagnosis and Management.* 2nd ed. Philadelphia, PA: Lippincott-Raven; 1995.

exercises for the abdomen and back muscles is considered safe. Strict adherence to neutral spinal positioning during exercise is recommended.

A fracture of the spine can result in three to five times increased risk of further spine fracture and a 1.2 to 1.9 increased death rate (240). Clusters of vertebral fractures may occur in patients aged 50 and older, in rapid progression. The cause of this most aggressive form of osteoporosis is unclear, but may be associated with an accelerated trabecular bone loss soon after menopause, malnutrition, immobility, and possibly in some cases in vertebrae adjacent to previous sites of vertebroplasty (see below). After a number of fracture events in the spine, the collapsed and/or anteriorly wedged vertebrae may lead to deformity of the back. This may result in subsequent kyphosis, loss of height, and chronic pain in the area of the thoracolumbar junction, secondary to mechanical deformity and paraspinal muscle spasm. This chronic back pain is typically of lesser intensity than the pain associated with the acute fracture event; it radiates laterally, is associated with exertion, and is relieved to a certain extent

with rest. In addition, with progressive spinal deformity and height loss, an abdominal protuberance and resultant gastrointestinal discomfort (bloating and constipation) may occur, as well as some degree of pulmonary insufficiency secondary to thoracic cage deformity. In patients with multiple fractures, and severe spinal kyphosis, costal-iliac impingement syndrome may result.

Although chronic back pain is a common complaint of the elderly, the extent to which osteoporosis contributes to this pain is questionable. In a study involving 242 women 55 years of age, 30% had complaints of back pain, but there was no relationship between this pain and spinal curvature. In a group of older women (60 to 79 years of age), back pain affected a similar proportion (30%) but was twice as likely to occur in women with kyphosis or a loss in height exceeding 4 cm (241). There is not an absolute relationship, therefore, between osteoporosis and kyphosis. It is recognized that kyphosis may be secondary to chronic poor posture and age-related changes in muscles, ligaments, and intervertebral disks. Seventy percent of women over 60 years of age may demonstrate kyphosis without evidence of vertebral deformity. With aging, there is a progression of kyphosis (242), but back pain does not appear to be associated with the kyphosis unless vertebral deformity is such that there is a reduction in the height of the vertebral body greater than 4 SDs from normal (241).

Investigations into causes of back pain using bone scintigraphy showed a high incidence of facet joint disease in osteoporotic women with previous vertebral fracture, most prominently at the level of the vertebral collapse. Smaller lesions were commonly found in the facets above and below this level. Back pain with neurologic symptoms in the lower extremities may occur when vertebral fracture results in retropulsed fragments or neuroforaminal narrowing, causing nerve impingement and radicular symptoms (243).

The pain of costal-iliac impingement syndrome is particularly difficult to treat. It is typically localized to the site of actual mechanical irritation, but can refer to the lower back and into the leg. Lateral bending and rotation can elicit this pain. Diagnosis is made by provocation of pain when palpating the lower ribs and the iliac crest contact site and with lateral bending and rotation of spine. Injection of lidocaine into the margin of the iliac crest and lower ribs can be both diagnostic and therapeutic. Postural training, strengthening of abdominal and lumbar musculature, and the use of a wide, soft belt or CASH (cruciate anterior sternal hyperextension) brace have been reported as beneficial in relieving symptoms by lifting the ribs to avoid contact with the iliac crest. Concomitant trial with transdermal pain medications such as diclofenac or lidocaine should be considered, but narcotic medications may be needed. In severe cases, resection of the lower ribs has been beneficial (244).

In summary, the management of chronic back pain associated with osteoporotic vertebral fracture should include a program of strengthening paravertebral, abdominal, and gluteal muscles and optimization of balance, flexibility, and posture. Relief of stress on the spine through the use of proper body mechanics is encouraged. In severe cases, an orthosis can be of benefit. An assessment of ADLs may lead to the use of other techniques and devices that can help the patient avoid situations that aggravate pain. The strategic placement of a pillow or towel roll behind the back frequently increases sitting tolerance in patients with kyphosis. Physical agents such as heat, ice, transcutaneous electrical nerve stimulation, and acupuncture can be of benefit. Hypnosis, behavioral modification, biofeedback, and counseling have also been of benefit in the treatment of chronic pain.

Back Supports and Bracing

The degree and types of skeletal pain and disability among patients with osteoporosis present a complicated challenge to provide adequate mechanical support for the spine (245). When many solutions are available to answer a given problem, it usually indicates that there is no single, good solution. Such is the case with mechanical supports for the osteoporotic spine. These orthoses may be used for pain relief and stabilization of the spine in both acute fracture and long-term care and to promote healing and improve function. In the long-term treatment of the osteoporotic spine, orthoses may prevent further fracture.

When prescribing a brace or corset, one must understand the biomechanics of the spine, the types and causes of vertebral fractures, and the principles of bracing, including indications and hazards of individual orthoses (246) (see Chapter 57). It is important to understand the functions of the lower thoracic and upper lumbar spine, where most compression fractures occur. The articulation of the thoracic vertebrae with the ribs, as well as the overlapping of the spinous processes, significantly limits its mobility in flexion and extension; rotation is relatively free, however. The lumbar spine has limited lateral flexion and axial rotation secondary to the relatively vertical orientation of the facet joints, so flexion and extension account for the majority of its movement. One must also understand the kinematic function or "coupling" that occurs in the thoracolumbar spine (247). While considering these functions of the spine, it is important to remember that movements that cause loading of the vertebral bodies increase the risk of fracture if bone density cannot support the resulting increase in applied force. Hence, bracing to help prevent this additional loading of the vertebral bodies must restrict flexion, which loads the anterior column of vertebrae. Restriction of flexion is therefore one goal of bracing, in conjunction with decreased pain, increased function, and prevention of soft tissue shortening, which may contribute to deformity.

There are several commonly used orthoses to stabilize osteoporotic vertebral fractures. These include a postural training support (PTS; a weighted kypho-orthosis), a thoracolumbar support such as the CASH brace, a lumbosacral corset, and a thoracolumbosacral orthosis (TLSO). All orthoses work on the principle of a three-point force system. Generally, the more rigid orthoses are used for acute thoracolumbar fractures, whereas the nonrigid orthoses such as the PTS and lumbosacral corset are used more commonly in the management of stable fractures and painful conditions. All orthoses described may not adequately prevent gravity-related axial compression, which may ultimately result in new fracture. Continuous and chronic use of spinal orthotics is generally discouraged because of the increased likelihood of weakening or atrophy of the trunk muscles and reduced spinal mobility. Weakness of the

supporting musculature may in time predispose to increased risk of vertebral fracture.

The PTS has been described as an inexpensive, unobtrusive device that promotes improvement in posture and decreases back pain by producing a force posteriorly below the inferior angles of the scapulae or by acting as a proprioceptive reinforcement (248). A TLSO such as the rigid clamshell brace is a long spinal orthosis that provides virtual fixation from the pelvis through the shoulders and is commonly prescribed when vertebral fracture results in retropulsed fragments or severe spinal stenosis that could compromise the spinal cord. Also, the lumbosacral region of the spine is one of the most difficult areas of the body to immobilize, requiring more than a simple lumbosacral orthosis after retropulsion has occurred. Although the TLSO affords the greatest immobility, it is cumbersome and hot, and noncompliance with wearing it is very common. When neurologic compromise is not an imminent risk, a semirigid TLSO such as Spinomed or CASH brace is often used after vertebral fracture. Custom-fitted rigid TLSOs are also more expensive than the PTS and CASH brace.

The inexpensive abdominal corset has also been used to decrease pain and increase function after an acutely painful vertebral fracture. It restricts movement via both mechanical and sensory feedback. This orthosis may also generate heat, pressure, or a massage-like effect that may be soothing for muscles in spasm. The use of corsets may relieve pain by increasing hydrostatic support of the spine through increased intra-abdominal pressure, thereby placing an anteriorly directed force on the vertebral bodies. Again, this device can be hot, but it is not as bulky as a TLSO or CASH brace, it can be worn under clothing, and it has a higher compliance rate in patients with uncomplicated lumbar fracture.

Kaplan et al. conducted a pilot study to compare the effects of back supports on back strength in women aged 40 and older with diagnosis of osteopenia or osteoporosis who were randomly assigned to one of the three groups: postural exercises (PE) alone, PE and conventional thoracolumbar support (CTLS), or PE and PTS. Compliance was poor among those who wore the TLS. The PTS and PE groups increased back strength significantly, implying that the more rigid CTLS inhibited strengthening of this area—a known complication of rigid bracing across any joint (249). Lynn and Sinaki found that kyphotic, osteoporotic patients had more postural sway and greater reliance on their hips to provide balance than those with normal posture, who based balancing strategies in their ankles (250). Subsequently, they demonstrated that use of the PTS in these patients improved balance and decreased pain with only 1 month of PTS even in the absence of strong back muscles (251). The weighted PTS is thought to reduce pain by encouraging correct gravitational alignment and reduce strain to compensating muscles. In combination with back extensor muscle-strengthening exercises, the weighted PTS can contribute to the management of kyphotic pain.

In summary, rigid TLSO bracing is typically prescribed after vertebral compression fracture with retropulsed fragments and associated risk of neurologic impairment. Noncompliance with wear is common, and associated risks must be discussed with patients. Other supports such as a nonrigid TLSO brace or a lumbosacral corset are better tolerated and can be valuable after uncomplicated osteoporotic fracture. They reduce pain and facilitate early recovery of functional mobility and ADL function. The PTS can be useful in improving chronic pain and balance deficits in patients with kyphosis, but is not typically used after vertebral fracture. All spinal orthotics are thought to diminish excessive loading of the vertebral bodies, but chronic use is not encouraged, so as to promote strengthening of intrinsic back muscles to support the skeleton.

Vertebroplasty and Kyphoplasty

Vertebroplasty and its derivative kyphoplasty are spinal procedures first introduced in 1984 and 1998, respectively, in which a radio-opaque bone cement, polymethyl methacry-late, is injected into vertebral fractures with an 8- to 13-gauge bone needle under fluoroscopy or CT guidance. **Figure 31-4** shows the outcome of injection, in a L4 compression fracture after vertebroplasty. Kyphoplasty requires slightly more time, as space for cement is created first by inserting an inflatable balloon tamp prior to injection. The procedure can be inpatient or outpatient, in part dependent on medical status of the patient at the time of procedure. These procedures are thought to stabilize the anterior column and any endplate fractures of the compressed vertebrae in order to restore vertebral height, spinal alignment, and function to the greatest degree possible (252).

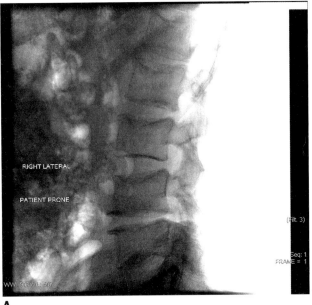

A

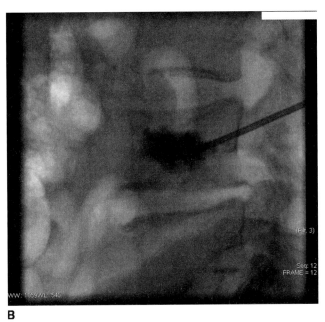

B

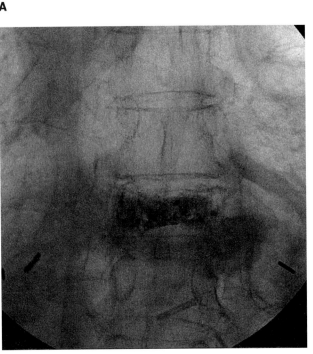

C

FIGURE 31-4. Plain radiographs, L4 compression fracture: **(A)** before vertebroplasty, **(B)** during vertebroplasty, and **(C)** after vertebroplasty. (Courtesy from Veteran's Administration Central California HealthCare System, UCSF-Fresno.)

Based on initial open trial studies, there appeared to be strong evidence for efficacy in relieving pain from compression fractures. However, a Cochrane review published in 2015 (253) showed moderate-quality evidence demonstrating that vertebroplasty does not provide more clinically important benefits (in pain, quality of life, or function) than a placebo procedure. The review did not support a role for vertebroplasty in routine treatment of osteoporotic vertebral fractures. There were no demonstrable, clinically important benefits compared with a sham procedure and subgroup analyses indicated that results did not differ according to duration of pain less than 6 weeks versus greater than 6 weeks. The quality was rated as moderate rather than high due to the small number of trials and participants. There is still uncertainty about the effect of vertebroplasty on the risk of new vertebral fractures or other serious adverse events compared with placebo. In regard to kyphoplasty, evidence does not support a benefit of kyphoplasty over vertebroplasty with respect to pain, but the procedures may differ in restoring lost vertebral height and in safety issues like cement extravasation. As with vertebroplasty, several unblinded studies have suggested a benefit from balloon kyphoplasty. To date, we are aware of no blinded studies that have been performed, and since the procedure is a derivative of vertebroplasty, the unsuccessful results of the blinded vertebroplasty studies have cast doubt upon the benefit of kyphoplasty.

Although 700,000 vertebral compression fractures occur in the United States annually, one must clearly establish by a thorough history, physical examination, and correlative radiologic study that the compression fracture site in question is indeed the locus of debilitating pain. This is especially important because the typical age group of patients that develop osteoporotic vertebral fractures is also prone to degenerative joint disease of the spine and consequent back pain. Although the thoracolumbar vertebrae are the most likely sites for intervention, vertebral augmentation can also be performed at the cervical spine. An evolving intervention, sacroplasty, attempts to replicate the success of vertebral augmentation procedures for SIF (254).

Given the above evidence, there is question as to when or whether to use these procedures. Currently, for many insurance companies, kyphoplasty and vertebroplasty may be considered medically necessary for the following indications: osteoporotic or osteolytic compression fractures of the thoracic or lumbar vertebrae resulting in persistent debilitating pain, which has not responded to standard medical treatment (initial bed rest with progressive activity, analgesics, physical therapy, bracing and exercises to correct postural deformity and increase muscle tone, and use of pharmacologic agents); osteolytic metastasis with severe back pain related to destruction of the vertebral body; multiple myeloma with severe back pain related to destruction of the vertebral body; painful and/or aggressive vertebral hemangiomas (or eosinophilic granulomas of the spine); painful vertebral fracture associated with osteonecrosis (Kummell disease); reinforcement, or stabilization, of vertebral body prior to surgery; and steroid-induced fractures. Percutaneous sacroplasty in the treatment of SIF is still considered investigational. There is a lack of peer-reviewed literature demonstrating the effects of sacroplasty on health outcomes. The evidence to date is limited to individual

case reports, and no randomized controlled trials regarding its safety and efficacy or improved patient outcomes have been published in the scientific peer-reviewed literature to our knowledge.

Absolute contraindications for these procedures include uncorrected coagulopathy, preexisting systemic or spine infection, and ongoing neurologic deficits secondary to the fracture site. Reported complications include extravasation of cement, bleeding, infection and neural injury, fracture, cement embolism, and predisposition to subsequent vertebral fractures at fragile adjacent vertebrae (12% to 52%) (255).

A multidisciplinary team approach is beneficial to ensuring maintenance of function in this population. Nonpharmacologic interventions should be preferentially used to manage chronic back pain. This program should be supplemented by encouraging adjustments in lifestyle, medication use, physical agents, orthoses, and other therapies considered useful for chronic pain. These interventions are used only after ruling out other causes of back pain in the elderly and after assessing the degree to which depression is contributing to the symptoms.

Hip Fracture

Hip fractures may be divided into three categories according to the anatomic area in which they occur. Intracapsular fractures (femoral neck fractures) are located distal to the femoral head but proximal to the greater and lesser trochanters. These fractures frequently disrupt the blood supply to the femoral head and are therefore associated with nonunion and osteonecrosis of the femoral head and typically require hemiarthroplasty for stabilization of the joint (256). Fractures occurring between the greater and the lesser trochanter are not associated with the complications seen in the intracapsular region. However, they are associated with malunion and shortening of the leg as a result of osteoporotic bone and the deforming forces exerted on this area of the proximal femur. Intertrochanteric and femoral neck fractures occur with equal frequency and together account for 90% of hip fractures. Subtrochanteric fractures occur just below the lesser trochanter and are responsible for only 5% to 10% of all hip fractures. Because 90% of peripheral osteoporotic fractures result from a fall, radiographs should also exclude fracture of the pubic ramus, acetabulum, and greater trochanter. Pain in this area after fall can also be associated with trochanteric bursitis and sacroiliac dysfunction. In all patients, the goal of treatment is to return the patient, pain-free, to maximum level of mobility as soon as possible, address fall risks, and implement appropriate screening and treatment for underlying bone disease.

Per orthopedic recommendation, surgery should commence within 24 to 48 hours after fracture. All displaced femoral neck fractures should be managed with hip replacement (257). Surgical management may include internal fixation or joint replacement depending on fracture location. Poor bone quality may render treatment unsuccessful or lead to complications (258).

Rehabilitation begins on the 1st day after surgery with a progressive ambulation program. Special precautions to prevent deep venous thrombosis with anticoagulant medication (such as enoxaparin or warfarin) and early mobilization are routine.

Most patients begin walking on the 1st or 2nd postoperative day, with weight-bearing status established by the orthopedic surgeon. When long-term stability of the surgical fixation is in question, weight-bearing status is decreased to minimize the possibility of hardware failure. Duke and Keating showed that mobility on day 2 following surgery was a significant predictor of independence at 2 weeks; independent mobility was defined as the ability to walk at least 15 m with a walker and transfer to and from bed independently (259).

In a study involving a large patient population aged 65 years or older, Cree et al. found that almost all patients with cognitive impairment who had sustained a hip fracture were functionally dependent 3 months after the fracture and had acquired a new disability in transfers between chair and bed (260). Most of those who functioned independently prior to fracture functioned independently afterward, with postfracture assistance most often needed in bathing and dressing. In those patients who were considered to be of high mental status, postfracture dependence correlated with advanced age, a greater number of comorbidities, hip pain, previous employment in a high prestige occupation, and poorer self-related health (261). Magaziner et al. found little change in the areas of greatest disability in the respective 12- and 24-month follow-ups to hip fracture in previously independent patients: climbing five stairs (90% and 91%), toilet transfers (66% and 63%), and tub and shower transfers (83% at both intervals) (262).

The proportion of patients that discharge home after hip fracture ranges from 40% to 90%, although many patients remain institutionalized (263,264). Factors associated with permanent institutionalization are assistance with ADLs, age greater than 80 years, lack of involvement of family members, incontinence, and insufficient physical therapy at a skilled nursing facility (263). In a hospital-based comprehensive rehabilitation unit, more than 90% of these patients are discharged home. Although this high percentage has clearly been influenced by the selection process, the scope and intensity of rehabilitation services and the ability to manage acute exacerbation of comorbidities in close geographic relationship with an acute medical-surgical hospital may promote higher function. Discharge home is positively associated with presence of another person in the home, ability to walk independently before the fracture, ability to perform ADLs (263,264), absence of preexisting dementia, younger age, and preexisting social network (265).

The risk of death after a hip fracture is increased by a factor of 2.8 within the first 3 months after fracture, and is more likely in those in poor health (266), with mortality rate after 1 year approximately 20% in the NHANES I study. In fact, analysis of NHANES I data showed that with each SD decrease in bone density (e.g., each T-score decrease of −1.0), mortality increased by 10% to 40% (267). Increased mortality with hip fracture is also associated with institutionalization, preexisting medical conditions, surgical intervention before stabilization of coexisting medical conditions, poorly controlled systemic disorders, complications of surgery (268), increasing age and male gender (22), and black race in females (19).

These patients often require the care of a physiatrist, physical therapist, occupational therapist, nurses, and social workers (269,270). The benefits of this multidisciplinary approach have been documented as resulting in fewer transfers for acute emergencies, fewer postoperative complications, improved ambulation at the time of discharge, and fewer discharges to nursing homes (263–265). Recent trends in health care delivery have challenged resources and have made rehabilitation strategies difficult to implement. The emphasis on shortened hospital stays has had a negative effect on patients with hip fractures. The number of patients remaining in a nursing home after 1 year is now much higher than before the initiation of the prospective payment system (239). There are increased costs to insurers and to patients as a result of the acceleration of patients through a system of care that does not account for patients' individuality, degree of impairment or disability, existing comorbidities, and social resources. The largest cost to the patient is loss of independence as a direct result of denial of access to the proper scope and intensity of rehabilitative services.

Wrist Fracture

Fractures of the wrist are the most common type of fractures in women less than 75 years of age. A prior wrist fracture doubles the risk of any future osteoporotic fracture in postmenopausal women and triples the risk for a second wrist fracture (271). These fractures increase in number after menopause, and although they usually occur in relatively healthy active women, they may be the first sign of an underlying problem such as low bone mass. The primary goal of treatment is return to pain-free, normal function of the hand and wrist. Initial casting does not usually extend above the elbow. During the period of immobilization, usually 6 to 8 weeks, strength and flexibility should be maintained in the upper extremities. Active and passive range-of-motion exercises should be provided for the fingers and shoulder on the affected side, with close monitoring for signs and symptoms of median nerve impingement (carpal tunnel syndrome) secondary to cast impingement with postfracture edema. These exercises should be continued after cast removal, with wrist, forearm, and elbow range-of-motion and strengthening exercises added. At that time, a local wrist splint may be used to support and protect the wrist. As a result of the wrist fracture, particularly on the dominant side, the patient may require assistance with ADLs such as getting dressed, combing hair, and brushing teeth.

MacDermid et al. reported the rate of improvement to normal pain-free function after distal radius fractures to be highest in the first 6 months after the fracture, with gains generally leveling off during the next 6 months (272). Of note, even with well-healed fractures, pain may persist because of ligament or triangular fibrocartilage complex (TFCC) injuries, which are common and can often be missed in the initial workup for a wrist fracture (273–275).

FEMALE ATHLETE TRIAD

With the advent of Title IX in the early 1970s, high school age girls' participation in organized sports has increased 1,000% (276). As energy expenditures increase with more intensive training, caloric intake must be increased accordingly. Carbohydrates should compose approximately 60% of daily caloric intake by American Dietetic Association guidelines, with fats comprising 25% to 30% and proteins 15%. Carbohydrates are therefore the primary source of muscle energy, and adequate total caloric intake prevents sacrifice of body fat and proteins. Although vitamins, minerals, and water also are essential for health, they do not provide energy.

Failure to increase caloric intake with training can precipitate weight loss and sacrifice adipose tissue for training needs. This can deplete estrogen stores sufficiently to cause amenorrhea in female athletes and increase the risk of osteoporosis and stress fractures, especially in conjunction with eating disorders. The FAT refers to this syndrome where an eating disorder, amenorrhea/oligomenorrhea, and decreased bone mineral density exist. Eating disorders have been reported as high as 62% in college female athletes and are becoming more common in adolescents. Although secondary amenorrhea in the general population is approximately 5%, it can increase to 10% to 20% in college athletes and 50% in elite athletes (277). Delayed menarche or absent menses for more than 3 months, particularly during times of increased training, should prompt clinical evaluation, including history of intentional weight loss strategies (i.e., diuretics, bulimia or anorexia, laxatives, avoidance of "fear foods"), distorted body image, and refractory pain sites. Evaluation with a nutritionist is recommended, as well as with a psychologist or a psychiatrist if eating disorder is suspected. Inpatient treatment should be considered in patient's refractory to treatment efforts. Monitoring for bulimia in light- and middle-weight category male wrestlers, especially prior to competition, is also needed. Although these athletes are not as likely to fracture, there is concern they will be at increased risk of fracture as they age, if bulimic behavior coexists with the bone formation phase of adolescence.

In addition to basic osteoporosis laboratory tests (see **Table 31-6**), hormonal evaluation (pregnancy test, TSH, follicle-stimulating hormone [FSH], and prolactin) is required in these patients, including estradiol level checked between days 2 and 4 of expected menstrual cycle. Any deficiencies must be addressed clinically. During childhood and adolescence, it is normal to see ongoing bone growth at bone metaphyses by plain radiographs and corresponding elevation of bone turnover markers such as urine or serum NTX. This precludes their use to monitor treatment efficacy in this population. Although IGF-I and DHEAS are useful markers in FAT research, at present they cannot be used clinically in young patients at high risk, such as is seen in anorexia nervosa or cerebral palsy (226). Similarly, applicability of DXA T-scores for bone mass assessment is not recommended in pediatric populations; Z-score monitoring is under investigation and will likely prove useful clinically in the future.

With FAT, stress fractures usually occur at the tibia or hip. If plain radiographs are negative, MRI is needed, as it can differentiate best between fracture and soft tissue injury, such as anterior tibialis muscle tear. Calcium and vitamin D supplementation, oral contraceptive therapy, and a minimum 6-week non–weight bearing in the fractured extremity are the standard of care in this population. Bed rest in hospitalized, anorexic patients should be used with caution, so as to limit further bone loss. Resistance exercise regimens for the other limbs are recommended during the bone healing phase, provided the patient follows strict nutritional guidelines for caloric intake for energy expenditures. Return to regular exercise and competitive sports requires close monitoring of caloric intake and weight, with nutritional and mental health counseling if needed. Although oral contraceptives can be used to regulate

menses and improve bone mass in these patients, irreversible osteoporosis is common.

ELECTRONIC MEDICAL RECORD SYSTEMS COORDINATION

More comprehensive osteoporosis screening and treatment will require expanded utilization of existing medical and electronic resources to improve communication between physicians and their patients. Multiple studies in Europe and America have shown that electronic medical record utilization, in strict compliance with patient privacy guidelines, has had good-to-excellent results in improving management of low bone mass (278–281). The best results to date in the United States have been in private health maintenance organizations. Newman et al. reported in 2003 that EMR targeting within a small, rural Pennsylvania Health Maintenance Organization of at-risk women 55 and older for DXA screening and osteoporosis treatment resulted in reduced hip fractures over a 5-year period in women 65 and older, with $1.5 million savings per annum over baseline in direct costs of care (282). Later, EMR targeting of those patients who required chronic glucocorticoid medication resulted in 96% compliance with calcium, vitamin D, and prescription medication where indicated, significant improvement in bone density at hip and spine, and improved exercise frequency and vitamin D levels (283). A comprehensive screening, education, and treatment program in California for patients aged 65 or older at risk for osteoporosis reduced hip fractures by 37%, saving a larger private health plan approximately $30 million over 5 years (284). Studies have also demonstrated the benefit of a nurse coordinator or manager to improve appropriate treatment and decrease hip fractures (285) and provide patient education (286).

SUMMARY

Osteoporosis is a disease that is characterized by low bone mass and deterioration of the bony microarchitecture potentially contributory to fracture and resultant disability, morbidity, and mortality. Physical medicine and rehabilitation expertise can be of great value in the management of patients with osteoporosis. Integrating traditional rehabilitation interventions (i.e., pain management, posture and exercise programs, and fall reduction strategies) with nutritional and pharmaceutical optimization (decreasing polypharmacy and targeting treatment of osteoporosis) can improve management of bone health, decrease risk of falling, and augment overall functional recovery should fracture occur. The benefits of assistive devices such as canes, walkers, and wheelchairs for those with disturbed balance or deficits in gait should also be emphasized as frailty develops with aging and disability. Targeting persons with chronic disability, who are at increased risk of bone loss compared to their more mobile peers, is particularly needed.

By utilizing both medical and traditional rehabilitation strategies, physiatrists can play a unique role in the interdisciplinary model to optimize screening and treatment efforts within the medical community. The implementation and coordination of these efforts in all inpatient rehabilitation settings, particularly during the seminal postfracture period, could prevent further fracture and reduce disability resulting from impairments in bone mass and structure, muscle strength, and coordination. To advocate for our patients in order to increase the likelihood of independent community dwelling, and to improve the quality of life for those in extended care facilities who have increased risk of falls, is at the core of our mission as physiatrists.

REFERENCES

1. U.S. Department of Health and Human Services. *Bone Health and Osteoporosis: A Report of the Surgeon General.* Rockville, MD: U.S. Department of Health and Human Services, Office of the Surgeon General; 2004:5.
2. *Osteoporosis Overview.* Niamsnihgov; 2017. Available from: https://www.niams.nih.gov/health_info/bone/osteoporosis/overview.asp. Accessed December 8, 2016.
3. Blume S, Curtis J. Medical costs of osteoporosis in the elderly medicare population. *Osteoporos Int.* 2011;22(6):1835–1844.
4. Administration on Aging. *Aging Statistics.* Aoaaclgov; 2017. Available from: https://aoa.acl.gov/Aging_Statistics/index.aspx. Accessed December 8, 2016.
5. World Health Organization. *Assessment of Fracture Risk and its Application to Screening for Postmenopausal Osteoporosis. WHO Technical Report Series 843.* Geneva, Switzerland: WHO; 1994.
6. Dawson-Hughes B, Tosteson ANA, Melton LJ III, et al.; National Osteoporosis Foundation Guide Committee. Implications of absolute fracture risk assessment for osteoporosis practice guidelines in the USA. *Osteoporos Int.* 2008;19(4):449–458.
7. Kok C, Sambrook PN. Secondary osteoporosis in patients with an osteoporotic fracture. *Best Pract Res Clin Rheumatol.* 2009;23(6):769–779. doi:10.1016/j.berh.2009.09.006.
8. National Osteoporosis Foundation. *America's Bone Health: The State of Osteoporosis and Low Bone Mass.* Washington, DC: National Osteoporosis Foundation; 2002. Available from: www.nof.org/advocacy/prevalence/index.htm. Accessed August 1, 2010.
9. Schneider EL, Guralnik J. The aging of America: impact on health care costs. *JAMA.* 1990;263:2335–2340.
10. Kanis J, Black D, Cooper C, et al. A new approach to the development of assessment guidelines for osteoporosis. *Osteoporos Int.* 2002;13(7):527–536.
11. Mackey DC, Lui LY, Cawthon PM, et al. High trauma fractures and low bone mineral density in older women and men. *JAMA.* 2007;298:2381–2388.
12. Looker A, Fenk S. *Percentage of Adults Aged 65 and over with Osteoporosis or Low Bone Mass at the Femur Neck or Lumbar Spine: United States, 2005–2010*; 2015.
13. National Osteoporosis Foundation. *Fast Facts on Osteoporosis.* Washington, DC: National Osteoporosis Foundation; 2008. Available from: www.nof.org/osteoporosis/disease.htm. Accessed August 1, 2010.
14. Zingmond DS, Melton LJ III, Silverman SL, et al. Increasing hip fracture incidence in California Hispanics, 1983 to 2000. *Osteoporos Int.* 2004;15(8):603–610.
15. Burge R, Dawson-Hughes B, Solomon D, et al. Incidence and economic burden of osteoporosis-related fractures in the United States, 2005–2025. *J Bone Miner Res.* 2007;22(3):465–475.
16. WHO Scientific Group on the Assessment of Osteoporosis at Primary Health Care Level. Summary Meeting Report. Brussels, Belgium, 5-7 May 2004. Copyright by WHO in 2007. Available from: http://www.who.int/chp/topics/Osteoporosis.pdf. Accessed December 8, 2016.
17. U.S. Department of Health and Human Services. *Bone Health and Osteoporosis: A Report of the Surgeon General.* Rockville, MD: U.S. Department of Health and Human Services, Office of the Surgeon General; 2004:78.
18. Looker AC, Johnston CC Jr, Wahner HW, et al. Prevalence of low femoral bone density in older U.S. women from NHANES III. *J Bone Miner Res.* 1997;12:1761–1768.
19. Jacobsen SJ, Goldberg J, Miles TP, et al. Race and sex differences in mortality following fracture of the hip. *Am J Public Health.* 1992;82(8):1147–1150.
20. King AB, Tosteson AN, Wong JB, et al. *J Bone Miner Res.* 2009;24(4):681–692.
21. U.S. Department of Health and Human Services. *Bone Health and Osteoporosis: A Report of the Surgeon General.* Rockville, MD: U.S. Department of Health and Human Services, Office of the Surgeon General; 2004:80.
22. Center JR, Nguyen TV, Schneider D, et al. Mortality after all major types of osteoporotic fracture in men and women: an observational study. *Lancet.* 1999;353:878–882.
23. Smeltzer SC, Zimerman V, Capriotti T. Osteoporosis risks and low bone mineral density in women with physical disabilities. *Arch Phys Med Rehabil.* 2005;86(3):582–586.
24. Nosek M, Howland CA, Rintala DH, et al. *National Study of Women with Physical Disabilities.* Houston, TX: Center for Research on Women with Disabilities; 1997.
25. Bacharach LK. Osteoporosis and measurement of bone mass in children and adolescents. *Endocrinol Metab Clin North Am.* 2005;34(30):521–535, vii.
26. Thornton J, Ashcroft D, O'Neill T, et al. A systematic review of the effectiveness of strategies for reducing fracture risk in children with juvenile idiopathic arthritis with additional data on long-term risk of fracture and cost of disease management. *Health Technol Assess.* 2008;12(3):xi–xiv, 1–208.
27. Iwasaki T, Takei K, Nakamura S, et al. Secondary osteoporosis in long-term bedridden patients with cerebral palsy. *Pediatr Int.* 2008;50(3):269–275.
28. Kilpinen-Loisa P, Nenonen H, Pihko H, et al. High-dose vitamin D supplementation in children with cerebral palsy or neuromuscular disorder. *Neuropediatrics.* 2007;38(4):167–172.

29. Caulton JM, Ward KA, Alsop CW, et al. A randomised controlled trial of standing programme on bone mineral density in non-ambulant children with cerebral palsy. *Arch Dis Child.* 2004;89(2):131–135.
30. Wick JY. Spontaneous fracture: multiple causes. *Consult Pharm.* 2009;24(2):100–102, 105–108, 110–112.
31. Dauty M, Perrouin Verbe B, Maugars Y. Supralesional and sublesional bone mineral density in spinal cord-injured patients. *Bone.* 2000;27(2):305–309.
32. Szollar SM, Martin EM, Parthemore JG, et al. Densitometric patterns of spinal cord injury associated bone loss. *Spinal Cord.* 1997;35(6):374–382.
33. Tosteson AN, Hammond CS. Quality-of-life assessment in osteoporosis: health-status and preference-based measures. *Pharmacoeconomics.* 2002;20(5):289–303.
34. U.S. Department of Health and Human Services. *Bone Health and Osteoporosis: A Report of the Surgeon General.* Rockville, MD: U.S. Department of Health and Human Services, Office of the Surgeon General; 2004:91.
35. U.S. Department of Health and Human Services. *Bone Health and Osteoporosis: A Report of the Surgeon General (Table 5-1).* Rockville MD: U.S. Department of Health and Human Services, Office of the Surgeon General; 2004:92.
36. Graves EJ, Kozak LJ. Detailed diagnoses and procedures: National Hospital Discharge Survey, 1996. *Vital Health Stat 13.* 1998;(138):i–iii, 1–151.
37. U.S. Congress Office of Technology Assessment. *Effectiveness and Costs of Osteoporosis Screening and Hormone Replacement Therapy. Vol. 1. Cost Effectiveness Analysis. OTA-BP-H-160.* Washington, DC: U.S. Government Printing Office; 1995.
38. Greendale GA, et al. Late physical and functional effects of osteoporotic fracture in women: the Rancho Bernardo study. *J Am Geriatr Soc.* 1995;43(9):955–961.
39. Leibson CL, Tosteson AN, Gabriel SE, et al. Mortality, disability and nursing home use for persons with and without hip fracture: a population-based study. *J Am Geriatr Soc.* 2002;50(10):1644–1650.
40. Ettinger B, Black DM, Nevitt MC, et al. Contribution of vertebral deformities to chronic back pain and disability. The Study of Osteoporotic Fractures Research Group. *J Bone Miner Res.* 1992;7:449–456.
41. Leech JA, Dulberg C, Kellie S, et al. Relationship of lung function to severity of osteoporosis in women. *Am Rev Respir Dis.* 1990;141:68–71.
42. Culham EG, Jomenez HAI, King CE. Thoracic kyphosis, rib mobility, and lung volumes in normal women and women with osteoporosis. *Spine.* 1994;11:1230–1255.
43. Schlaich C, Minne HW, Bruckner T, et al. Reduced pulmonary function in patients with spinal osteoporotic fractures. *Osteoporos Int.* 1998;8:261–267.
44. National Osteoporosis Foundation. *Health Professional's Rehabilitation Guide for Osteoporosis.* Washington, DC: National Osteoporosis Foundation; 2002.
45. Atkins RM, Duckworth T, Kanis JA. Features of algodystrophy after Colles' fracture. *J Bone Joint Surg Br.* 1990;72:105–110.
46. Bickerstaff DR, Kanis JA. Algodystrophy: an under-recognized complication of minor trauma. *Br J Rheumatol.* 1994;33:240–248.
47. Briot K, Roux C. Glucocorticoid-induced osteoporosis. *RMD Open.* 2015;8(1):769–779.
48. Agha A, Thompson CJ. High risk of hypogonadism after traumatic brain injury: clinical implications. *Pituitary.* 2005;8(3–4):245–249.
49. Parfitt AM, Matthews CHE, Villanueva AR, et al. Relationships between surface, volume, and thickness of iliac trabecular bone in aging and in osteoporosis. *J Clin Invest.* 1983;72:1396–1409.
50. Frost HM. The pathomechanics of osteoporoses. *Clin Orthop Relat Res.* 1985;200:198–226.
51. Hofbauer LC, Schoppet M. Clinical implications of the osteoprotegerin/RANKL/RANK system for bone and vascular diseases. *JAMA.* 2004;292(4):490–495. doi:10.1001/jama.292.4.490.
52. Tella SH, Gallagher JC. Prevention and treatment of postmenopausal osteoporosis. *J Steroid Biochem Mol Biol.* 2014;142:155–170.
53. Chen Y, Di Grappa MA, Molyneux SD, et al. RANKL blockade prevents and treats aggressive osteosarcomas. *Sci Transl Med.* 2015;9(7):317. doi:10.1126/scitranslmed.aad0295.
54. Richelson LS, Wahner HW, Melton LJ, et al. Relative contributions of aging and estrogen deficiency to postmenopausal bone loss. *N Engl J Med.* 1984;311:1273–1275.
55. Drinkwater BL, Nilson K, Chesnut CH, et al. Bone mineral content of amenorrheic athletes. *N Engl J Med.* 1984;311:277–281.
56. Shen Y, Gray DL, Martinez DS. Combined pharmacologic therapy in postmenopausal osteoporosis. *Endocrinol Metab Clin North Am.* 2017;46(1):193–206. doi:10.1016/j.ecl.2016.09.008.
57. Hofbauer L. The roles of osteoprotegerin and osteoprotegerin ligand in the paracrine regulation of bone resorption. *J Bone Miner Res.* 2000;15:2–12.
58. Marcus R, Madvig P, Young G. Age-related changes in parathyroid hormone and parathyroid hormone action in normal humans. *J Clin Endocrinol Metab.* 1984;58:223–230.
59. Riggs BL, Hamstra A, DeLuca HF. Assessment of 25-hydroxy vitamin D α-hydroxylase reserve in postmenopausal osteoporosis by administration of parathyroid extract. *J Clin Endocrinol Metab.* 1981;53:833–835.
60. Slovik DM, Adams JS, Neer RM, et al. Deficient production of 1,25 dihydroxyvitamin D in elderly osteoporotic patients. *N Engl J Med.* 1981;25:372–374.
61. Taggart HM, Chesnut CH, Ivey JL, et al. Deficient calcitonin response to calcium stimulation in postmenopausal osteoporosis? *Lancet.* 1982;2:475–477.
62. Tiegs RD, Body JJ, Wahner HW, et al. Calcitonin secretion in postmenopausal osteoporosis. *N Engl J Med.* 1985;12:1097–1100.
63. Tai ES, Gillies PJ, eds. *Forum of Nutrition. Vol. 60. Nutrigenomics—Opportunities in Asia.* Basel, Switzerland: Karger; 2007:158.

64. Rizzoli R, Bonjour JP, Ferrari SL. Osteoporosis, genetics and hormones. *J Mol Endocrinol*. 2001;26(2):79–94.

65. Carda S. Osteoporosis after stroke: a review of the causes and potential treatments. *Cerebrovasc Dis*. 2009;28:191–200.

66. Kanis J. Acute and long-term increase in fracture risk after hospitalization for stroke. *Stroke*. 2001;32(3):702–706.

67. Jiang, SD, Jiang LS, Dai LY. Mechanisms of osteoporosis in spinal cord injury. *Clin Endocrinol (Oxf)*. 2006;65(5):555–565.

68. Jiang SD, Dai LY, Jiang LS. Osteoporosis after spinal cord injury. *Osteoporos Int*. 2006;17(2):180–192.

69. Morse L, Tang YD, Pham L, et al. Spinal cord injury causes rapid osteoclastic resorption and growth plate abnormalities in growing rats (SCI-induced bone loss in growing rats). *Osteoporos Int*. 2008;19(5):645–652.

70. Jiang SD, Jiang LS, Dai LY. Effects of spinal cord injury on osteoblastogenesis, osteoclastogenesis and gene expression profiling in osteoblasts in young rats. *Osteoporos Int*. 2007;18(3):339–349.

71. Gosfield E III, Bonner FJ Jr. Evaluating bone mineral density in osteoporosis. *Am J Phys Med Rehabil*. 2000;79:283–291.

72. Tosteson ANA, Melton LJ III, Dawson-Hughes B, et al.; National Osteoporosis Foundation Guide Committee. Cost-effective osteoporosis treatment thresholds: the United States perspective. *Osteoporos Int*. 2008;19(4):437–447.

73. *2015 ISCD Official Positions—Adult*. ISCD; 2015. Available from: http://www.iscd.org/official-positions/2015-iscd-official-positions-adult/. Accessed February 19, 2017.

74. Njeh CF, Boivin CM, Langton CM. The role of ultrasound in assessment of osteoporosis: a review. *Osteoporos Int*. 1997;7:7–22.

75. *Clinical Summary Osteoporosis: Screening*. US Preventive Services; 2017. Available from: https://www.uspreventiveservicestaskforce.org/Page/Document/ClinicalSummaryFinal/osteoporosis-screening. Accessed February 9, 2017.

76. *2015 ISCD Official Positions—Adult*. ISCD; 2015. Available from: http://www.iscd.org/official-positions/2015-iscd-official-positions-pediatric/. Accessed February 19, 2017.

77. McCloskey EV, Johansson H, Oden A, et al. Ten-year fracture probability identifies women who will benefit from clodronate therapy-additional results from a double-blind, placebo-controlled randomised study. *Osteoporos Int*. 2009;20(5):811–817.

78. *Fracture Risk Assessment Tool*. Available from: www.shef.ac.uk/FRAX/. Accessed August 1, 2010.

79. Chesnut CH III, Bell NH, Clark GS, et al. Hormone replacement therapy in postmenopausal women: urinary N-telopeptide of type I collagen monitors therapeutic effect and predicts response of bone marrow density. *Am J Med*. 1997;102:29–37.

80. Kaplan RJ, Vo AN, Stitik TP. Rehabilitation of orthopedic and rheumatologic disorders. 1. Osteoporosis assessment, treatment and rehabilitation. *Arch Phys Med Rehabil*. 2005;86(S1):S40.

81. Ward KD, Klesges RC. A meta-analysis of the effects of cigarette smoking on bone mineral density. *Calcif Tissue Int*. 2001;68(5):259–270.

82. Khosla S, Burr D, Cauley J, et al. Bisphosphonate-associated osteonecrosis of the jaw: report of a task force of the American Society for Bone and Mineral Research. *J Bone Miner Res*. 2007;22(10):1479–1491.

83. Woo SB, Hellstein JW, Kalmar Jr. Narrative [corrected] review: bisphosphonates and osteonecrosis of the jaws. *Ann Intern Med*. 2006;144(10):753–761.

84. Lindsey C, Brownbill RA, Bohannon RA, et al. Association of physical performance measures with bone mineral density in postmenopausal women. *Arch Phys Med Rehabil*. 2005;86(6):1102–1107.

85. *The Surgeon General's Report on Bone Health and Osteoporosis: What It Means to You*. NIH; 2017. Available from: https://www.niams.nih.gov/health_info/bone/SGR/surgeon_generals_report.asp. Accessed February 9, 2017.

86. Reid IR, Ames RW, Evans MC, et al. Long-term effects of calcium supplementation on bone loss and fractures in postmenopausal women: a randomized controlled trial. *Am J Med*. 1995;98:331–335.

87. Reid IR, Ames R, Mason B, et al. Randomized controlled trial of calcium supplementation in healthy nonosteoporotic, older men. *Arch Intern Med*. 2008;168(20):2276–2282.

88. Nusser SM, Carriquiry AL, Dodd KW, et al. A semiparametric transformation approach to estimating usual daily intake distributions. *J Am Stat Assoc*. 1996;91:1440–1449.

89. Orimo H, Shiraki M, Hayashi T, et al. Reduced occurrence of vertebral crush fractures in senile osteoporosis treated with 1α-hydroxy vitamin D_3. *J Bone Miner Res*. 1987;3:47–52.

90. Chevalley T, Rizzoli R, Nydegger V, et al. Effects of calcium supplements on femoral bone mineral density and vertebral fracture rate in vitamin D replete elderly patients. *Osteoporos Int*. 1994;4:245–252.

91. Chapuy MC, Arlot ME, Duboeuf F, et al. Vitamin D_3 and calcium to prevent hip fractures in elderly women. *N Engl J Med*. 1992;327:1637–1642.

92. Chapuy MC, Arlot ME, Delmas PD, et al. Effect of calcium and cholecalciferol treatment for three years on hip fractures in elderly women. *Br Med J*. 1994;308:1081–1082.

93. Devine A, et al. A longitudinal study of the effect of sodium and calcium intakes on regional bone density of postmenopausal women. *Am J Clin Nutr*. 1995;62(4):740–745.

94. Shortt KC, et al. Influence of dietary sodium intake on urinary calcium excretion in selected Irish individuals. *Eur J Clin Nutr*. 1988;42(7):595–603.

95. DeLuca H. The metabolism and functions of vitamin D. *Adv Exp Med Biol*. 1986;196:361–375.

96. Wacker M, Holick M. Sunlight and vitamin D: a global perspective for health. *Dermatoendocrinology*. 2013;1(5):51–108. doi:10.4161/derm.24494.

97. *DRIs for Calcium and Vitamin D*. The National Academies of Science, Engineering, and Medicine; 2017. Available from: http://www.nationalacademies.org/hmd/Reports/2010/Dietary-Reference-Intakes-for-Calcium-and-Vitamin-D/DRI-Values.aspx. Accessed February 10, 2017.

98. Delaney MF, et al. Epidemiology, etiology and diagnosis of osteoporosis. *Am J Obstet Gynecol*. 2006;194(2 suppl):S3–S11.

99. U.S. Department of Health and Human Services. *Bone Health and Osteoporosis: A Report of the Surgeon General*. Rockville, MD: U.S. Department of Health and Human Services, Office of the Surgeon General; 2004:223.

100. Dawson-Hughes B, Harris SS, Krall EA, et al. Rates of bone loss in postmenopausal women randomly assigned to one of two dosages of vitamin D_{1-4}. *Am J Clin Nutr*. 1995;61:1140–1150.

101. Ooms ME, Roos JC, Bezemer PD, et al. Prevention of bone loss by vitamin D supplementation in elderly women: a randomized double-blind trial. *J Clin Endocrinol Metab*. 1995;80:1052–1058.

102. U.S. Department of Health and Human Services. *Bone Health and Osteoporosis: A Report of the Surgeon General*. Rockville, MD: U.S. Department of Health and Human Services, Office of the Surgeon General; 2004:222.

103. Schurch MA, Rizzoli R, Slosman D, et al. Protein supplements increase serum insulin-like growth factor-1 levels and attenuate proximal femur bone loss in patients with recent hip fracture: a randomized, double-blind, placebo-controlled trial. *Ann Intern Med*. 1998;128:801–809.

104. Institute of Medicine. *Dietary Reference Intakes for Energy, Carbohydrate, Fiber, Fat, Fatty Acids, Cholesterol, Protein, and Amino Acids*. Washington, DC: National Academies Press; 2005.

105. U.S. Department of Health and Human Services. *Bone Health and Osteoporosis: A Report of the Surgeon General*. Rockville, MD: U.S. Department of Health and Human Services, Office of the Surgeon General; 2004:124.

106. Recker RR, Deng H-W. Role of genetics in osteoporosis. *Endocrine*. 2002;17(1):55–66.

107. Washburn RA, Zhu W, McAuley E, et al. The physical activity scale for individuals with physical disabilities: development and evaluation. *Arch Phys Med Rehabil*. 2002;83(2):193–200.

108. *ACSM Issues New Recommendations on Quantity and Quality of Exercise*. ACSM. Available from: http://www.acsm.org/about-acsm/media-room/news-releases/2011/08/01/acsm-issues-new-recommendations-on-quantity-and-quality-of-exercise. Accessed February 10, 2017.

109. U.S. Department of Health and Human Services. *Bone Health and Osteoporosis: A Report of the Surgeon General*. Rockville, MD: U.S. Department of Health and Human Services, Office of the Surgeon General; 2004:173.

110. Lin JT, Lane JM. Nonmedical management of osteoporosis. *Curr Opin Rheumatol*. 2002;14(4):441–466.

111. Bonaiuti D, Shea B, Iovine R, et al. Exercise for preventing and treating osteoporosis in postmenopausal women. *Cochrane Database Syst Rev*. 2002;(3):CD000333.

112. Layne JE, Nelson ME. The effects of progressive resistance training on bone density: a review. *Med Sci Sports Exerc*. 1999;31:25–30.

113. U.S. Department of Health and Human Services. *Bone Health and Osteoporosis: A Report of the Surgeon General*. Rockville, MD: U.S. Department of Health and Human Services, Office of the Surgeon General; 2004:112, 118–119.

114. Shinchuk L, Morse L, Huancahuari N, et al. Vitamin D deficiency and osteoporosis in rehabilitation inpatients. *Arch Phys Med Rehabil*. 2006;87(7):904–908.

115. Garnero P, Sornay-Rendu E, Duboeuf F, et al. Markers of bone turnover predict postmenopausal forearm bone loss over 4 years: the OFELY study. *J Bone Miner Res*. 1999;14(9):1614–1621.

116. *Facts about Physical Activity*. CDC; 2014. Available from: https://www.cdc.gov/physicalactivity/data/facts.htm. Accessed February 8, 2018.

117. *Physical Activity*. World Health Organization; 2018. Available from: http://www.who.int/mediacentre/factsheets/fs385/en/. Accessed January 29, 2018.

118. *Physical Activity Basics*. CDC; 2015. Available from: https://www.cdc.gov/physicalactivity/basics/index.htm. Accessed February 10, 2017.

119. *Adults*. CDC; 1999. Available from: http://www.cdc.gov/nccdphp/sgr/adults.htm. Accessed August 1, 2010.

120. *National Health Interview Survey*. National Center for Health Statistics; 2008. Available from: http://www.cdc.gov/nchs/about/major/nhis. Accessed November 1, 2009.

121. Weaver CM. The role of nutrition on optimizing peak bone mass. *Asia Pac J Clin Nutr*. 2008;17(supp1):135–137.

122. Katzman DK, Bachrach LK, Carter DR, et al. Clinical and anthropometric correlates of bone mineral acquisition in healthy adolescent girls. *J Clin Endocrinol Metab*. 1991;73(6):1332–1339.

123. Bailey DA, Martin AD, McKay HA, et al. Calcium accretion in girls and boys during puberty: a longitudinal analysis. *J Bone Miner Res*. 2000;15(11):2245–2250.

124. Khosla S, Melton LJ III, Dekutoski MB, et al. Incidence of childhood distal forearm fractures over 30 years: a population-based study. *JAMA*. 2003;290(11):1479–1485.

125. Mackelvie KJ, McKay HA, Khan KM, et al. A school-based exercise intervention augments bone mineral accrual in early pubertal girls. *J Pediatr*. 2001;139(4):501–508.

126. Marcus R, Jamal S, Cosman F. Exercise and osteoporosis. In: Cummings S, Cosman F, Jamal S, eds. *Osteoporosis: An Evidence Based Approach to the Prevention of Fractures*. Philadelphia, PA: American College of Physicians; 2002.

127. Taaffe DR, Pruitt L, Pyka G, et al. Comparative effects of high- and low-intensity training on thigh muscle strength, fiber area, and tissue composition in elderly women. *Clin Physiol*. 1996;16:381–392.

128. Taaffe DR, Duret C, Wheeler S, et al. Once-weekly resistance exercise improves muscle strength and neuromuscular performance in older adults. *J Am Geriatr Soc*. 1999;47:1208–1214.

129. Wolf SL, Barnhart HX, Kutner NG, et al. Reducing frailty and falls in older persons: an investigation of Tai Chi and computerized balance training. *J Am Geriatr Soc*. 1996;44:489–497.

130. Li F, Harmer P, Fisher KJ, et al. Tai Chi and fall reductions in older adults: a randomized controlled trial. *J Gerontol A Biol Sci Med Sci*. 2005;60(2):187–194.

131. Qin L, Au S, Choy W, et al. Regular Tai Chi Chuan exercise may retard bone loss in postmenopausal women: a case–control study. *Arch Phys Med Rehabil*. 2002;83(10):1355–1359.

132. Chan K, Qin L, Lau M, et al. A randomized, prospective study of the effects of Tai Chi Chuan exercise on bone mineral density in postmenopausal women. *Arch Phys Med Rehabil*. 2004;85(5):717–722.

133. Wayne PM, Kiel DP, Krebs DE, et al. The effects of Tai Chi on bone mineral density in postmenopausal women: a systematic review. *Arch Phys Med Rehabil*. 2007;88(5):673–680.

134. Bautmans I, Van Hees E, Lemper JC, et al. The feasibility of whole body vibration in institutionalized elderly persons and its influence on muscle performance, balance and mobility: a randomised controlled trial. *BMC Geriatr*. 2005;5:17.

135. Roelants M, Delecluse C, Verschueren SM. Whole-body-vibration training increases knee-extension strength and speed of movement in older women. *J Am Geriatr Soc*. 2004;52(6):901–908.

136. Verschueren SM, Roelants M, Delecluse C, et al. Effect of 6-month whole body vibration training on hip density, muscle strength, and postural control in postmenopausal women: a randomized controlled pilot study. *J Bone Miner Res*. 2004;19(3):352–359.

137. Kraemer WJ, Adams K, Cafarelli E, et al. American College of Sports Medicine position stand. Progression models in resistance training for healthy adults. *Med Sci Sports Exerc*. 2002;34(2):364–380.

138. Breck B. Exercise and Sports Science Australia (ESSA) position statement on exercise prescription for the prevention and management of osteoporosis. *J Sci Med Sport*. 2017;20(5):438–445. doi:10.1016/j.jsams.2016.10.001.

139. Sinaki M, Mikkelsen BA. Postmenopausal spinal osteoporosis: flexion versus extension exercises. *Arch Phys Med Rehabil*. 1984;65(10):593–596.

140. U.S. Department of Health and Human Services. *Bone Health and Osteoporosis: A Report of the Surgeon General*. Rockville, MD: U.S. Department of Health and Human Services, Office of the Surgeon General; 2004:129.

141. Frontera W, Meredith CN, O'Reilly KP, et al. Strength conditioning in older men: skeletal muscle function and mass. *J Appl Physiol*. 1988;64:1038–1044.

142. Sinaki M, Wahner HW, Bergstralh EJ, et al. Three year controlled, randomized trial of the effect of dose-specified loading and strengthening exercises on bone mineral density of spine and femur in nonathletic, physically active women. *Bone*. 1996;19(3):233–244.

143. National Osteoporosis Foundation. *Scientific Advisory Board. Position Paper on Exercise and Osteoporosis*. Washington, DC: National Osteoporosis Foundation; 1991.

144. Kerr D, Morton A, Dick I, et al. Exercise effects on bone mass in postmenopausal women are site-specific and load dependent. *J Bone Miner Res*. 1996;11:218–225.

145. Paier GS. Specter of the crone: the experience of vertebral fracture. *ANS Adv Nurs Sci*. 1996;18:27–36.

146. U.S. Department of Health and Human Services. *Bone Health and Osteoporosis: A Report of the Surgeon General*. Rockville, MD: U.S. Department of Health and Human Services, Office of the Surgeon General; 2004:172.

147. Evans WW, Campbell WW. Sarcopenia and age-related changes in body composition and functional capacity. *J Nutr*. 1993;123(2 suppl):465–468.

148. Specker BL. Evidence for an interaction between calcium intake and physical activity on changes in bone mineral density. *J Bone Miner Res*. 1996;11(10): 1539–1544.

149. Specker BL, Mulligan L, Ho M. Longitudinal study of calcium intake, physical activity, and bone mineral content in infants 6–18 months of age. *J Bone Miner Res*. 1999;14(4):569–576.

150. Specker B, Binkley T. Randomized trial of physical activity and calcium supplementation on bone mineral content in 3- to 5-year-old children. *J Bone Miner Res*. 2003;18(5):885–892.

151. Shea B, Wells G, Cranney A, et al. Meta-analyses of therapies for postmenopausal osteoporosis. VII: Meta-analysis of calcium supplementation for the prevention of postmenopausal osteoporosis. *Endocr Rev*. 2002;23(4):552–559.

152. Papadimitropoulos E, Wells G, Shea B, et al. Meta-analyses of therapies for postmenopausal osteoporosis. VIII: Meta-analysis of the efficacy of vitamin D treatment in preventing osteoporosis in postmenopausal women. *Endocr Rev*. 2002;23(4):560–569.

153. Ganz DA, Bao Y, Shekelle PG, et al. Will my patient fall? *JAMA*. 2007;297(1): 77–86.

154. Rubenstein LZ. Falls in older people: epidemiology, risk factors and strategies for prevention. *Age Ageing*. 2006;35(S2):ii37–ii41.

155. Grisso JA, Kelsey JL, Strom BL, et al. Risk factors for falls as a cause of hip fracture in women. The Northeast Hip Fracture Study Group. *N Engl J Med*. 1991;324(19):1326–1331.

156. *Injury Prevention & Control*. CDC; 2016. Available from: http://www.cdc.gov/ncipc/factsheets/nursing.htm. Accessed February 28, 2017.

157. http://www.cdc.gov/ncipc/factsheets/nursing.htm. Accessed August 1, 2010.

158. Fiatarone Singh MA, Singh NA, Hansen RD, et al. Methodology and baseline characteristics for the sarcopenia and hip fracture study: a 5-year prospective study. *J Gerontol A Biol Sci Med Sci*. 2009;64(5):568–574.

159. Sloan J, Holloway O. Fractured neck of the femur: the cause of the fall? *Injury*. 1981;13:230–232.

160. Yang K, Shen K, Demetropoulos CK, et al. The relationship between loading conditions and fracture patterns of the proximal femur. *J Biomech Eng*. 1996;118(4):575–578.

161. Felson DT, Zhang Y, Hannan MT, et al. Effects of weight and body mass index on bone mineral density in men and women: the Framingham study. *J Bone Miner Res*. 1993;8:567–573.

162. Howe TE, Rochester L, Jackson A, et al. Exercise for improving balance in older people. *Cochrane Database Syst Rev*. 2007;(4):CD004963.

163. Orr R, Raymond J, Fiatarone-Singh M. Efficacy of progressive resistance training on balance performance in older adults: a systematic review of randomized controlled trials. *Sports Med*. 2008;38(4):317–343.

164. Faber MJ, Bosscher RJ, Chin A, et al. Effects of exercise programs on falls and mobility in frail and pre-frail older adults: a multicenter randomized controlled trial. *Arch Phys Med Rehabil*. 2006;87(7):885–896.

165. Pardessus V, Puisieux F, Di Pompeo C, et al. Benefits of home visits for falls and autonomy in the elderly: a randomized trial study. *Am J Phys Med Rehabil*. 2002;81:247–252.

166. Cumming S, Klineberg R. Fall frequency and characteristics and the risk of hip fractures. *J Am Geriatr Soc*. 1994;42:774–778.

167. Lotz JC, Cheal EJ, Hayes WC. Stress distributions within the proximal femur during gait and falls: implications for osteoporotic fracture. *Osteoporos Int*. 1995;5:252–261.

168. Ford CM, Keaveny TM, Hayes WC. The effect of impact direction on the structural capacity of the proximal femur during falls. *J Bone Miner Res*. 1996;11:322–383.

169. Kroonenberg AJ, Hayes WC, McMahon TA. Dynamic models for sideways falls from standing height. *J Biomed Eng*. 1995;117:309–318.

170. Greenspan SL, Myers ER, Maitland LA, et al. Fall severity and bone mineral density as risk factors for hip fracture in ambulatory elderly. *JAMA*. 1994;271:128–133.

171. Tinetti ME, Liu WL, Claus EB. Predictors and prognosis of inability to get up after falls among elderly persons. *JAMA*. 1993;269:65–70.

172. Tinetti ME, Baker D, Garrett P, et al. Yale FICSIT: risk factor abatement strategy for fall prevention. *J Am Geriatr Soc*. 1993;41:315–320.

173. Tinetti ME, Baker DI, McAvay G, et al. A multifactorial intervention to reduce the risk of falling among elderly people living in the community. *N Engl J Med*. 1994;331:821–827.

174. Farmer ME, Harris T, Madans JH, et al. Anthropometric indicators and hip fracture. The NHANES I epidemiologic follow-up study. *J Am Geriatr Soc*. 1989;37: 9–16.

175. Perez Cano R, Galan F, Disen G. Risk factors for hip fracture in Spanish and Turkish women. *Bone*. 1993;14(suppl):69–72.

176. Lauritzen JS. Protection against hip fractures by energy absorption. *Dan Med Bull*. 1992;39:91–93.

177. Moayyeri A, et al. The association between physical activity and osteoporotic fractures: a review of the evidence and implications for future research. *Ann Epidemiol*. 2008;18(11):827–835.

178. Lord SR, Ward JA, Williams P, et al. The effect of a 12-month exercise trial on balance, strength, and falls in older women: a randomized controlled trial. *J Am Geriatr Soc*. 1995;43(11):1198–1206.

179. Carter ND, Kannus P, Khan KM. Exercise in the prevention of falls in older people: a systematic literature review examining the rationale and the evidence. *Sports Med*. 2001;31(6):427–438.

180. Carter ND, Khan KM, Petit MA, et al. Results of a 10-week community based strength and balance training programme to reduce fall risk factors: a randomized controlled trial in 65–75 year old women with osteoporosis. *Br J Sports Med*. 2001;35(5):348–351.

181. Liu-Ambose TY, Khan KM, Eng JJ, et al. The beneficial effects of group-based exercise on fall risk profile and physical activity persist 1 year post-intervention in older women with low bone mass: follow-up after withdrawal of exercise. *J Am Geriatr Soc*. 2005;53(10):1767–1773.

182. Gillespie LD, Gillespie WJ, Robertson MC, et al. Interventions for preventing falls in elderly people. *Cochrane Database Syst Rev*. 2003;(4):CD000340.

183. Parker MJ, Gillespie WJ, Gillespie LD. Hip protectors for preventing hip fractures in older people. *Cochrane Database SystRev*. 2005;(3):CD0012555.

184. Bentzen H, Forsen L, Becker C, et al. Uptake and adherence with soft- and hard-shelled hip protectors in Norwegian nursing homes: a cluster randomised trial. *Osteoporos Int*. 2008;19:101–111.

185. Robinovitch SN, Hayes WC, McHahan TA. Energy-shunting hip padding system attenuates femoral impact force in a simulated fall. *J Biomech Eng*. 1995;17: 409–413.

186. Coehlo R, Silva C, Maia A, et al. Bone mineral density and depression: a community study in women. *J Psychosom Res*. 1999;46:329–350.

187. Mossey JM, Mutran E, Knoh K, et al. Determinants of recovery 12 months after hip fracture: the importance of psychological factors. *Am J Public Health*. 1989;79:279–286.

188. Cook DJ, Gugatt GH, Adachi JD, et al. Quality of life issues in women with vertebral fractures due to osteoporosis. *Arthritis Rheum*. 1993;36:750–756.

189. Mezuk B, Eaton WW, Golden SH. Depression and osteoporosis: epidemiology and potential mediating pathways. *Osteoporos Int*. 2008;19:1–12.

190. Eskandari F, Martinez PE, Torvik S, et al. Low bone mass in premenopausal women with depression. *Arch Intern Med.* 2007;167(21):2329–2336.

191. Dudgeon BJ, Gerrard BC, Jensen MP, et al. Physical disability and the experience of chronic pain. *Arch Phys Med Rehabil.* 2002;83:229–235.

192. Lyles KW, et al. Zoledronic acid in reducing clinical fracture and mortality after hip fracture. *N Engl J Med.* 2007;357:nihpa40967.

193. Gilchrist NL, Frampton CM, Acland RH, et al. Alendronate prevents bone loss in patients with acute spinal cord injury: a randomized double-blind, placebo-controlled study. *J Clin Endocrinol Metab.* 2007;92(4):1385–1390.

194. Thornton J, Ashcroft D, O'Neill T, et al. A systematic review of the effectiveness of strategies for reducing fracture risk in children with juvenile idiopathic arthritis with additional data on long-term risk of fracture and cost of disease management. *Health Technol Assess.* 2008;12(3):iii–iv, xi–xiv, 1–208.

195. Ward L, Tricco AC, Phuong P, et al. Bisphosphonate therapy for children and adolescents with secondary osteoporosis. *Cochrane Database Syst Rev.* 2007;(4): CD005304.

196. Sorensen HT, Christensen S, Mehnert F, et al. Use of bisphosphonates among women and risk of atrial fibrillation and flutter: population based case–control study. *Br Med J.* 2008;336(7648):813–816.

197. U.S. Department of Health and Human Services. *Bone Health and Osteoporosis: A Report of the Surgeon General.* Rockville, MD: U.S. Department of Health and Human Services, Office of the Surgeon General; 2004:229.

198. Siris ES, Harris ST, Rosen CJ, et al. Adherence to bisphosphonate therapy and fracture rates in osteoporotic women: relationship to vertebral and non-vertebral fractures from two US claims databases. *Mayo Clin Proc.* 2006;81: 1013–1022.

199. Giusti A, Barone A, Razzano M, et al. Persistence with calcium and vitamin D in elderly patients after hip fracture. *J Bone Miner Metab.* 2009;27(1):95–100.

200. McClung M, Balske A, Burgio D, et al. Treatment of postmenopausal osteoporosis with delayed release risedronate 35 mg weekly for 2 years. *Osteoporos Int.* 2013;24(1):301–310.

201. Amgen, Inc. *Prolia (Denosumab) Prescribing Information.* 2010. Updated 2014.

202. Cummings S, Ensrud K, Delmas P. Denosumab for prevention of fractures in postmenopausal women with osteoporosis. *N Engl J Med.* 2009;361(8):756–765.

203. Bone H, Chapurlat R, Brandi M. The effect of 3 or 6 years of denosumab exposure in women with postmenopausal osteoporosis: results from the FREEDOM extension. *J Clin Endocrinol Metab.* 2013;98(11):4483–4492.

204. Miller P, Bolognese M, Lewiecki E. Effect of denosumab on bone density and turnover in postmenopausal women with low bone mass after long-term continued, discontinued, and restarting of therapy: a randomized blinded phase 2 clinical trial. *Bone.* 2008;43(2):222–229.

205. Freemantle N, Satram-Hoang A, Tang E. Final results of the DAPS (denosumab adherence preference satisfaction) study: a 24-month, randomized, crossover comparison with alendronate in postmenopausal women. *Osteoporos Int.* 2012;23(1): 317–326. doi: 10.1007/s00198-011-1780-1. Epub 2011 Sep 17.

206. Rossouw JE, Anderson GL, Prentice RL et al.; Writing Group for the Women's Health Initiative Investigators. Risks and benefits of estrogen plus progestin in healthy postmenopausal women: principal results from the women's health initiative randomized controlled trial. *JAMA.* 2002;288:321–333.

207. Anderson GL, Limacher M, Assaf AR, et al. Effects of conjugated equine estrogen in postmenopausal women with hysterectomy: the WHI randomized controlled trial. *JAMA.* 2004;291(14):1701–1712.

208. Manson J, Hsia J, Johnson K. Estrogen plus progestin and the risk of coronary heart disease. *N Engl J Med.* 2003;349:523–534.

209. Stevenson J, Panay N, Pexman-Fieth C. Oral estradiol and dydrogesterone combination therapy in postmenopausal women: review of efficacy and safety. *Maturitas.* 2013;76(1):10–21.

210. Karim R, Dell R, Greene D, et al. Hip fracture in postmenopausal women after cessation of hormone therapy: results from a prospective study in a large health management organization. *Menopause.* 2011;18(11):1172–1177

211. Hodgson SF, Watts NB, Bilezikian JP, et al. American Association of Clinical Endocrinologists medical guidelines for clinical practice for the prevention and treatment of postmenopausal osteoporosis: 2001 edition, with selected updates for 2003. *Endocr Pract.* 2003;9(6):544–564.

212. Miller P, Chines A, Christiansen C. Effects of bazedoxifene on BMD and bone turnover in postmenopausal women: 2-yr results of a randomized, double-blind, placebo-, and active-controlled study. *J Bone Miner Res.* 2008;23(4):525–535.

213. Cummings S, Ensrud K, Delmas P. Lasofoxifene in postmenopausal women with osteoporosis. *N Engl J Med.* 2010;362(8):686–696.

214. Grady D, Wenger N, Herrington D. Postmenopausal hormone therapy increases risk for venous thromboembolic disease. The Heart and Estrogen/Progestin Replacement Study. *Ann Intern Med.* 2000;132:689–696.

215. Bone HG, Greenspan SL, McKeever C, et al. Alendronate and estrogen effects in postmenopausal women with low bone mineral density. Alendronate/Estrogen Study Group. *J Clin Endocrinol Metab.* 2000;85(2):720–726.

216. U.S. Department of Health and Human Services. *Bone Health and Osteoporosis: A Report of the Surgeon General.* Rockville, MD: U.S. Department of Health and Human Services, Office of the Surgeon General; 2004:234.

217. Tsai J, Uihlein A, Lee H. Teriparatide and denosumab, alone or combined, in women with postmenopausal osteoporosis: the DATA study randomised trial. *Lancet.* 2013;382(9886):50–56.

218. Finkelstein J, Wyland J, Lee H. Effects of teriparatide, alendronate, or both in women with postmenopausal osteoporosis. *J Clin Endocrinol Metab.* 2010;95(4): 1838–1845.

219. Chesnut CH III, Silverman S, Andriano K, et al. A randomized trial of nasal spray salmon calcitonin in postmenopausal women with established osteoporosis: the prevent recurrence of osteoporotic fractures study. PROOF Study Group. *Am J Med.* 2000;109(4):267–276.

220. Reeve J, Hesp R, Williams D, et al. Anabolic effect of low doses of human parathyroid hormone on the skeleton in postmenopausal osteoporosis. *Lancet.* 1976;1(7968):103.

221. Neer RM, et al. Effect of parathyroid hormone (1–34) on fractures and bone mineral density in postmenopausal women with osteoporosis. *N Engl J Med.* 2001;344(19):1434–1441.

222. Orwoll E, Ettinger M, Weiss S, et al. Alendronate for the treatment of osteoporosis in men. *N Engl J Med.* 2000;343(9):604–610.

223. Department of Health and Human Services. *Bone Health and Osteoporosis: A Report of the Surgeon General.* Rockville, MD: Department of Health and Human Services; 2004:235.

224. Fraser WD, Ahmad AM, Vora JP, et al. The physiology of the circadian rhythm of parathyroid hormone and its potential as a treatment for osteoporosis. *Curr Opin Nephrol Hypertens.* 2004;13(4):437–444.

225. Eastell R, Nickelsen T, Martin F. Sequential treatment of severe postmenopausal osteoporosis after teriparatide: final results of the randomized, controlled European Study of Forsteo (EUROFORS). *J Bone Miner Res.* 2009;24:726.

226. Gordon CM, Goodman E, Emans SJ, et al. Physiologic regulators of bone turnover in young women with anorexia nervosa. *J Pediatr.* 2002;141(1): 64–70.

227. Kleerekoper M, Peterson EL, Nelson DA, et al. A randomized trial of sodium fluoride as a treatment for postmenopausal osteoporosis. *Osteoporos Int.* 1991;1: 155–161.

228. Pak CYC, Sakhaee K, Adams-Huet B, et al. Treatment of postmenopausal osteoporosis with slow-release sodium fluoride: final report of a randomized controlled trial. *Ann Intern Med.* 1995;123:401–408.

229. Riggs BL, Hodgson SF, O'Fallon WM, et al. Effect of fluoride treatment on the fracture rate in postmenopausal women with osteoporosis. *N Engl J Med.* 1990;332:802–809.

230. Boivin G, Deloffre P, Perrat B, et al. Strontium distribution and interactions with bone mineral in monkey iliac bone after strontium salt (S12911) administration. *J Bone Miner Res.* 1996;11:1302–1311.

231. Meunier PJ, Roux C, Ortolani S, et al. Effects of long-term strontium ranelate treatment on vertebral fracture risk in postmenopausal women with osteoporosis. *Osteoporos Int.* 2009;20:1663–1673.

232. European Medicines Agency. PSUR Assessment Report for Strontium Ranelate; 2013.

233. Musette P, Brandi ML, Cacoub P, et al. Treatment of osteoporosis: recognizing and managing cutaneous adverse reactions and drug-induced hypersensitivity. *Osteoporos Int.* 2010;21:723–732.

234. Shen M, Kim Y. Osteoporotic vertebral compression fractures: a review of current surgical management techniques. *Am J Orthop.* 2007;36(5):241–248.

235. Goltzman D. *L'actualité Thérapeutique.* Vol 2. Basel, Switzerland: Sandoz; 1985.

236. Remagen W. *Osteoporosis.* Basel, Switzerland: Sandoz; 1991.

237. Wynne AT, Nelson MA, Nordin BEC. Costoiliac impingement syndrome. *J Bone Joint Surg Br.* 1985;67:124–125.

238. Gotis-Graham I, Mcguigan L, Diamond T, et al. Sacral insufficiency fractures in the elderly. *J Bone Joint Surg Br.* 1994;76:882–886.

239. Blake SP, Connors AM. Pictorial review sacral insufficiency fracture. *Br J Radiol.* 2004;77:891–896.

240. Melton LJ III. Excess mortality following vertebral fracture. *J Am Geriatr Soc.* 2000;48(3):338–339.

241. Ettinger B, Black DM, Palermo L, et al. Kyphosis in older women and its relation to back pain, disability and osteopenia: the study of osteoporosis fractures. *Osteoporos Int.* 1994;4:55–60.

242. Gandy S, Payne R. Back pain in the elderly: updated diagnosis and management. *Geriatrics.* 1986;41:59–72.

243. Ryan PJ, Evans P, Gibson T, et al. Osteoporosis and chronic back pain: a study with single-photon emission computed tomography bone scintigraphy. *J Bone Miner Res.* 1992;7:455–460.

244. Hirschberg GG, Williams KA, Byrd JG. Medical management of iliocostal pain. *Geriatrics.* 1992;47:62–66.

245. Frost HM. Managing the skeletal pain and disability of osteoporosis. *Orthop Clin North Am.* 1972;3:561–570.

246. Stevenson JC, Lindsay R, eds. *Osteoporosis.* London, UK: Chapman & Hall; 1998:339–346.

247. Stillo JV, Stein AB, Ragnarson KT. Low back orthoses. *Phys Med Rehabil Clin N Am.* 1992;3:57–94.

248. Kaplan RS, Sinaki M. Posture training support: preliminary report on a series of patients with diminished symptomatic complications of osteoporosis. *Mayo Clin Proc.* 1993;68:1171–1176.

249. Kaplan RS, Sinaki M, Hameister MD. Effect of back supports on back strength in patients with osteoporosis: a pilot study. *Mayo Clin Proc.* 1996;71:235–241.

250. Lynn SG, Sinaki M, Westerlind KC. Balance characteristics of persons with osteoporosis. *Arch Phys Med Rehabil.* 1997;78:273–277.

251. Sinaki M, Lynn SG. Reducing the risk of falls through proprioceptive dynamic posture training in osteoporotic women with kyphotic posturing: a randomized pilot study. *Am J Phys Med Rehabil.* 2002;81:241–246.

252. Ortiz AO. Vertebral body reconstruction: review and update on vertebroplasty and kyphoplasty. *Appl Radiol.* 2008;37(12):10–24.

253. Buchbinder R, Golmohammadi K, Johnston RV, et al. Percutaneous vertebroplasty for osteoporotic vertebral compression fracture. *Cochrane Database Syst Rev.* 2015;(4):CD006349. doi:10.1002/14651858.CD006349.pub2.

254. Frey ME, Depalma MJ, Cifu DX, et al. Percutaneous sacroplasty for osteoporotic sacral insufficiency fractures: a prospective, multicenter, observational pilot study. *Spine J.* 2008;8(2):367–373.

255. Ortiz AO. Vertebral body reconstruction: review and update on vertebroplasty and kyphoplasty. *Appl Radiol.* 2008;37(12):8.

256. Barnes R, Brown JT, Garden RS, et al. Subcapital fractures of the femur: a prospective review. *J Bone Joint Surg Br.* 1976;58:2–24.

257. Moroni A, et al. Surgical treatment and management of hip fracture patients. *Arch Orthop Trauma Surg.* 2014;134(2):277–281. doi:10.1007/s00402-011-1441-z.

258. Leung F, Liu F, Morrey C, et al. Osteoporotic hip fractures: current issues and evolving concepts of surgical management. *ScientificWorldJournal.* 2013;2013:793138. doi:10.1155/2013/793138.

259. Duke RG, Keating JL. An investigation of factors predictive of independence in transfers and ambulation after hip fracture. *Arch Phys Med Rehabil.* 2002;83:158–164.

260. Cree M, Carriere KC, Soskolne CL, et al. Functional dependence after hip fracture. *Am J Phys Med Rehabil.* 2001;80:736–743.

261. Ceder L, Thorngren KG, Walden B. Prognostic indicators and early home rehabilitation in elderly patients with hip fractures. *Clin Orthop Relat Res.* 1980;152:173–184.

262. Magaziner J, Hawkes W, Hebel JR, et al. Recovery from hip fracture in eight areas of function. *J Gerontol A Biol Sci Med Sci.* 2000;55(9):M498–M507.

263. White BL, Fisher WD, Lauriss CA. Rate of mortality for elderly patients after fracture of the hip in the 1980's. *J Bone Joint Surg Am.* 1987;69:1335–1340.

264. Zuckerman JD, Sakales SR, Fabrien DR, et al. Hip fractures in geriatric patients. Results of an interdisciplinary hospital care program. *Clin Orthop Relat Res.* 1992;274:213–225.

265. Fitzgerald JF, Moore PS, Dittus RS. The case of elderly patients with hip fracture: changes since implementation of the prospective payment system. *N Engl J Med.* 1988;319:1392–1397.

266. Richmond J, Aharonoff GB, Zuckerman JD, et al. Mortality risk after hip fracture. *J Orthop Trauma.* 2003;17(1):53–56.

267. Mussolino ME, Madans JH, Gillum RF. Bone mineral density and mortality in women and men: the NHANES I epidemiologic follow-up study. *Ann Epidemiol.* 2003;13(10):692–697.

268. Kenyor JE, McCarthy RE, Lowell JD, et al. Hip fracture mortality: relation to age, treatment, preoperative illness, time of surgery and complications. *Clin Orthop Relat Res.* 1984;186:45–56.

269. Boncor SK, Tinetti ME, Spechley M, et al. Factors associated with short- versus long-term skilled nursing facility placement among community living hip fracture patients. *J Am Geriatr Soc.* 1990;38:1139–1144.

270. Pryor GA, Nyles JW, Williams DR, et al. Team management of the elderly patient with hip fracture. *Lancet.* 1988;1:401–403.

271. Barrett-Connor E, Sajjan SG, Siris ES, et al. Wrist fracture as a predictor of future fractures in younger versus older postmenopausal women: result from the National Osteoporosis Risk Assessment. *Osteoporos Int.* 2008;19(5):607–613.

272. MacDermid JC, Richards RS, Roth JH. Distal radius fracture: a prospective outcome study of 275 patients. *J Hand Ther.* 2001;14: 154–169.

273. Fischer M, Denzler C, Sennwald G. Carpal ligament lesions associated with fresh distal radius fractures: arthroscopic study of 54 cases [German]. *Swiss Surg.* 1996;2:269–272.

274. Richards RS, Bennett JD, Roth JH, et al. Arthroscopic diagnosis of intra-articular soft tissue injuries associated with distal radius fractures. *J Hand Surg Am.* 1997;22:772–776.

275. Lindau T, Amer M, Hagberg L. Intraarticular lesions in distal radius fractures of the radius in young adults: a descriptive arthroscopic study in 50 patients. *J Hand Surg Br.* 1997;22:638–643.

276. Gill J, Miller SL. Female athletes. In: Schepsis AA, Busconi BD, eds. *Sports Medicine.* Philadelphia, PA: Lippincott Williams & Wilkins; 2006:P51–P60.

277. Kaziz K. The female athlete triad. *Adolesc Med.* 2003;14:87–95.

278. McLellan AR, et al. The osteoporosis-orthopedic liaison nurse: a model for effecting secondary prevention of osteoporotic fractures in an orthopedic and accident and emergency setting. *J Bone Miner Res.* 2000;15(suppl 1):S439.

279. Jaglal SB, et al. Development of an integrated-care delivery model for post-fracture care in Ontario, Canada. *Osteoporos Int.* 2006;17(9):1337–1345.

280. Bogoch ER, et al. Effective initiation of osteoporosis diagnosis and treatment for patients with a fragility fracture in an orthopaedic environment. *J Bone Joint Surg Am.* 2006;88:25–34.

281. Hawker G, et al. The impact of a simple fracture clinic intervention in improving the diagnosis and treatment of osteoporosis in fragility fracture patients. *Osteoporos Int.* 2003;14(2):171–178.

282. Newman ED, Ayoub WT, Starkey RH, et al. Osteoporosis disease management in a rural health care population: hip fracture reduction and reduced costs in postmenopausal women after 5 years. *Osteoporos Int.* 2003;14(2):146–151.

283. Newman ED, Matzko CK, Olenginski TP, et al. Glucocorticoid-induced osteoporosis program (GIOP): a novel, comprehensive, and highly successful care program with improved outcomes at 1 year. *Osteoporos Int.* 2006;17(9):1428–1434.

284. Inacio MCS, Funahashi TT, Downs D, Ninh C, Dell R, Chen G. Effect of an osteoporosis management program on hip fracture rates: an analysis of 527,266 patients. American Academy of Orthopaedic Surgeons Annual Meeting: Abstract 474. Medscape Medical News; 2009.

285. Majumdar SR, Lier DA, Beaupre LA, et al. Osteoporosis case manager for patients with hip fractures: results of a cost-effectiveness analysis conducted alongside a randomized trial. *Arch Intern Med.* 2009;169(1):25–31.

286. Tosi LL, Gliklich R, Kannan K, et al. The American Orthopaedic Association's "Own the Bone" initiative to prevent secondary fractures. *J Bone Joint Surg Am.* 2008;90:63–73.

CHAPTER 32

Ramona Raya
Galen O. Joe
Lynn H. Gerber

Rheumatic Diseases

Rheumatic diseases are having an increasing impact on mortality and morbidity (1). It is estimated that musculoskeletal disorders are the most frequent cause of disability in developed countries (2). Currently, 46 million people are affected by arthritis, and this number is predicted to rise to 67 million by 2030 (3). These individuals often sustain impairments, functional losses, and disability. The annual cost in medical care and lost wages is $128 billion (4).

Twenty-first-century physicians who care for these patients must be aware of current pharmacologic and rehabilitation strategies to control disease, limit impairment, preserve or enhance function, reduce disability, and support quality of life (5). Additionally, they must be aware that people with arthritis diagnoses are likely to have at least one additional comorbidity (6). Additional comorbidities are very likely to impact physical and emotional health and negatively impact social and behavioral functioning (7).

New trends have developed in the management of inflammatory arthritis: (a) early use of disease-modifying antirheumatic drugs (DMARDs) and biologics in combination has demonstrated better control of disease activity and reduction in disability (8), (b) a transition from physician-administered care to active patient engagement, with patient-centered outcomes as part of treatment goals results in better functional outcomes and better control of disease activity (9), (c) a change from prescribing rest to one of advocating appropriate rest and exercise and activity, (d) an increased use of rehabilitation early in the disease course, (e) a greater use of complementary and alternative therapies by patients and health care providers, and (f) an increased interest in which rehabilitation measures are available and effective in preventing disability and achieving restoration of function for arthritis patients.

The specialty of rheumatology is dedicated to the understanding and control of disease activity. The current understanding of rheumatic diseases has significantly advanced over the past decade. Much evidence has accumulated to identify important contributions of genetics, environment, and genetic-environmental interaction in the pathogenesis of rheumatic diseases (10). As of this writing, these findings only partially explain the disease expression and phenotype. Additionally, they often do not explain the functional impact of the disease. Nonetheless, this improved understanding of pathogenesis has had significant impact on therapeutics and has led to the development of biologically active substances that impact disease activity and immune regulation and improve disease outcomes.

Rehabilitation medicine has its roots in maintenance and restoration of function as well as prevention of dysfunction. This is achieved by having a keen knowledge of the impairments associated with the various rheumatic diseases and the formulation of individualized treatment plans conjointly with patients. The rehabilitation goals of the patients with rheumatic diseases were found to be wide-ranging, with healthy lifestyle as the most prominent focus (11).

The following are some of the methods employed to maximize patient function using education; physical modalities of heat, cold, and electricity for symptom management; manual therapies; exercise; assistive and adaptive devices; energy conservation; joint protection; and vocational planning. The success of rehabilitation interventions requires the ability to explain interventions and elicit patient (and often family) participation in the process.

The care of patients with arthritis takes a multidisciplinary team effort with the patient in the center helping to define goals and feasible processes that will lead to good outcomes (12). The best treatment plans incorporate medical, rehabilitation, and orthopedic interventions based on early intervention and coordinated care appropriately timed (13).

This chapter addresses a spectrum of inflammatory diseases, their impact on the entire person, as well as specific joints and organ systems. It discusses risk and benefits of pharmacologic and nonpharmacologic treatment strategies.

Rheumatic diseases may involve a single or multiple joints, periarticular structures, and other organ systems. The process may be acute and resolve (e.g., septic joint) or may become chronic (e.g., rheumatoid arthritis [RA]). Arthritis may be symmetrical (RA) or asymmetrical (e.g., seronegative arthritides, psoriatic arthritis [PSA], gout) and may affect women disproportionately (RA) or men (e.g., ankylosing spondylitis [AS], reactive arthritis). Inflammatory arthritis may involve all the joint structures: synovium, cartilage, tendons, capsule, bone, and surrounding muscle and skin. Rheumatic diseases are often systemic, associated with fever and weight loss. Examples are RA, juvenile rheumatoid arthritis (JRA), systemic lupus erythematosus (SLE), polymyositis dermatomyositis (DM-PM), progressive systemic sclerosis (PSS), mixed connective tissue disease (MCTD), or vasculitides. These diseases are usually chronic, remitting, and relapsing; they are variable in their course and affect the lungs, kidney, heart, and central nervous system. They require long-term treatments with pharmacologic agents, which may have a significant impact on appearance, sleep, and psychological, cognitive, physical, and sexual function and may need long-term monitoring by the rehabilitation team.

This chapter describes elements of the initial evaluation, early treatment intervention, and long-term management for patients with rheumatic diseases. This chapter will reference established clinical guidelines and seasoned clinical judgment.

ARTHRITIC DISEASES

Classification and Clinical Findings

Classification of arthritides is important for assessing prognosis and long-term care needs. The key is to identify whether the disorder is inflammatory or not, symmetric or not, and associated with systemic/extra-articular manifestations (**Fig. 32-1**). Classification according to etiology may also help distinguish among the various types of arthritic conditions.

Inflammatory arthritis falls into four different groups and may be monoarticular or polyarticular (14–16):

1. Inflammatory connective tissue disease (e.g., RA, JIA, SLE, PSS, DM-PM, MCTD, and vasculitides)
2. Inflammatory crystal-induced disease (e.g., gout, pseudogout, and basic calcium phosphate)
3. Inflammation induced by infectious agents (e.g., bacterial, viral, spirochete, tuberculous, and fungal arthritis)
4. Seronegative spondyloarthropathies (e.g., AS, PSA, reactive arthritis, and inflammatory bowel disease–associated arthritis [IBD])

Noninflammatory arthritis may be classified as:

1. Degenerative, posttraumatic, or overuse (e.g., osteoarthritis [OA], posttraumatic aseptic necrosis [AN])
2. Inherited or metabolic (e.g., lipid storage disease, hemochromatosis, ochronosis, hypogammaglobulinemia, hemoglobinopathies, and hypothyroidism)

Clinical features that suggest inflammatory rather than noninflammatory disease include acute painful onset, fever, erythema of the skin over the joint or joints involved, warmth of the joint or joints, and tenderness that usually parallels the degree of inflammation. These diseases are often accompanied by morning stiffness that improves with movement as the day progresses. Fatigue frequently accompanies rheumatic disease and is thought to be a correlate of disease activity. The rehabilitation team is often consulted with respect to a number of functional problems, and fatigue is one of the most common. It is included as one of the core sets for outcomes (17).

Laboratory and x-ray findings that suggest an inflammatory process include an increased peripheral white blood cell count with left shift, an elevated erythrocyte sedimentation rate (ESR), a group II joint fluid (**Table 32-1**), and x-ray demonstration of soft tissue swelling, periostitis, bony erosions, or uniform cartilage loss (**Table 32-2**). Joint fluid is an important contributor to the proper classification of arthritis and should be evaluated for crystals such as monosodium urate (MSU) and hydroxyapatite.

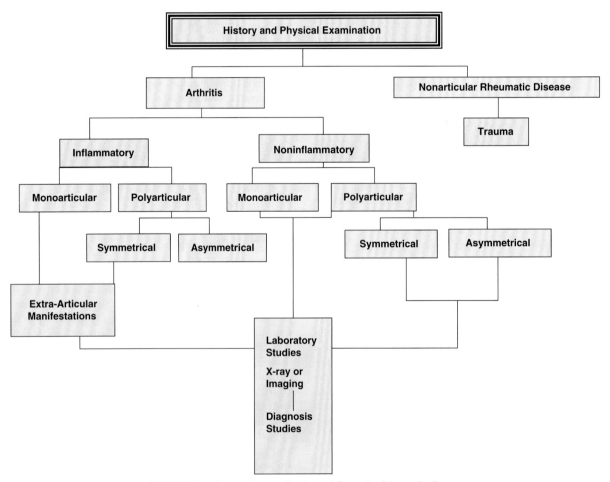

FIGURE 32-1.   Steps in the classification and diagnosis of rheumatic disease.

TABLE 32-1   Synovial Fluid Analysis

Fluid Group	Color	Clarity	Viscosity	Mucin Clot	Cells/mm³	Percentage of White Blood Cells that Are Polymorphonuclear Leukocytes
Normal	Pale yellow	Transparent	High	Good	<25%	<10%
Group 1 (noninflammatory)	Yellow or straw	Transparent	High	Good	<2,000	<25%
Group II (moderately inflammatory)	Yellow or straw	Transparent to opaque, slightly Cloudy	Variably decreased	Fair to poor	3,000–50,000	>70%
Group III (highly inflammatory, septic)	Variable; yellow-gray, purulent	Opaque, cloudy	Low	Poor	50,000–100,000 (usually 100,000 or more)	>75%, usually close to 100%
Group IV (hemorrhagic)	Red	Opaque	High	Good	Up to normal count in blood	May be the same as normal blood

TABLE 32-2   Radiographic Findings in Rheumatic Diseases

Disease	Anatomic Distribution	Types of Changes Seen
Rheumatoid arthritis	Symmetric:	Juxta-articular osteoporosis, fusiform soft tissue swelling marginal erosion, bony cysts
	Most frequent: MCP, MTP, wrist, PIP	Subluxation (swan-neck/Boutonniere/ulnar deviation)
	Often: Knee, hip, ankle, shoulder, C-spine	Late: bony eburnation, compressive erosions, surface resorption
Spondylarthropathies	Asymmetric:	Soft tissue swelling, sausage fingers (i.e., Reactive's, PSA)
AS	Most frequent:	New bone formation, fluffy periosteal bone, and syndesmophytes
Reactive	Sacroiliac joint, heel	Enthesopathic ossification or erosion or both
PSA	Vertebral column, hip, shoulder	Bony ankylosis
	Knee, ankle	Severe—arthritis mutilans
	MCP, PIP, DIP, MTP	
Septic	Asymmetric:	Soft tissue swelling—periarticular
	Knee, ankle, wrist, hip, small joints	Joint space enlargement
		Periosteal elevation
		Late: bony destruction
	Asymmetric:	Soft tissue swelling
Gout	First MTP, small joint, knee, elbow > feet and hands	Soft tissue speckled calcification, gouty tophi
		Erosion of bone with marginal overhangs
Pseudogout	Symmetric:	Chondrocalcinosis
	Knee, wrist, hip>>	Subchondral cysts
	Intervertebral disks, shoulder (glenoid labrum and acetabulum)	
SLE	Symmetric:	Calcific deposits
	Small joints of hands, feet, wrists	Subchondral lucency (i.e., crescent sign/osteonecrosis)
	Articular osteonecrosis:	Subchondral sclerosis
	Hip, knee, shoulder, ankle	Subchondral collapse and remodeling of bone/tuft resorption
PSS	Symmetric:	Late: joint space loss
	Small joints of hands and feet	Acro-osteolysis (i.e., bone resorption)
		Soft tissue calcification
		Sausage digits
Juvenile chronic arthritis (JIA seronegative chronic RA, Still's disease)	Femoral condyle, humeral head, radial head	Epiphyseal enlargement, flattening, and abnormal diaphyseal growth
	Phalanges, MCP, MTP	Osteopenia, osteoporosis, soft tissue swelling
	Femur, tibia, fibula, radius, C-spine	Periostitis and apophyseal narrowing
Vasculitis	Symmetric: Small/medium joints of hand/feet	Soft tissue swelling, nonerosive

AS, ankylosing spondylitis; PSA, psoriatic arthritis; PIP, proximal interphalangeal; Reactive Reiter's Disease; DIP, distal interphalangeal joint; SLE, systemic lupus erythematosus; PSS, progressive systemic sclerosis; MCP, metacarpal phalangeal; MTP, metatarsal phalangeal; >, greater than; >>, much greater than.

TABLE 32-3	Extra-Articular Manifestations of Rheumatic Diseases	
System	**Disease**	
Skin	Juvenile idiopathic arthritis	
	Psoriatic arthritis	
	Reactive arthritis	
	Colitic arthritis	
	Sarcoid arthritis	
	Septic arthritis (especially *Neisseria gonorrhoeae* and *meningitides*)	
	Hyperlipoproteinemia	
	Systemic lupus erythematosus	
	Amyloidosis	
	Dermatomyositis	
	Vasculitis	
Nasopharynx and ear	Reactive arthritis	
	Rheumatoid arthritis	
Eye	Juvenile idiopathic arthritis	
	Reiter's syndrome	
	Rheumatoid arthritis	
	Sarcoid arthritis	
	Vasculitis	
Gastrointestinal tract	Colitic arthritis	
	Scleroderma	
	Progressive systemic sclerosis	
Heart and circulation	Amyloidosis	
	Polymyositis	
	Juvenile idiopathic arthritis	
	Reiter's syndrome	
	Ankylosing spondylitis	
	Vasculitis	
Respiratory tract	Sarcoidosis	
	Polymyositis	
	Rheumatoid arthritis	
	Vasculitis	
	Progressive systemic sclerosis	
Nervous system	Systemic lupus erythematosus	
	Rheumatoid arthritis	
	Vasculitis	
Renal system	Amyloidosis	
	Gout	
	Systemic lupus erythematosus	
	Progressive systemic sclerosis	
	Vasculitis	
Hematologic system	Rheumatoid arthritis	
	Systemic lupus erythematosus	

A number of these diseases have systemic or extra-articular manifestations (**Table 32-3**), many of which should be addressed in addition to treatment of the arthritis itself and are often the deciding factor for pharmacologic choice. The physiatrist must be aware of the impact of a chronic, unpredictable illness on various life stages.

Many types of arthritis have a specific distribution in terms of age, gender, race, and geographic appearance. Severity of disease may vary with age and gender. Genetics and occupation also may be influencing factors. It is helpful to be familiar with those portions of the population that are more susceptible to certain diseases (**Table 32-4**) (18).

SPECIFIC CONDITIONS

Rheumatoid Arthritis

Rheumatoid arthritis is the most common inflammatory arthropathy and is often difficult to diagnose in its early stages. The etiology of RA remains unknown, although much has been learned in the past two decades about the inflammatory process, its relationship to the immune system, molecular genetic regulation (19), and environmental exposures (i.e., smoking and gluten products) (20). Of the two most common hypotheses about etiology, one is that RA is an autoimmune disorder; the other is that specific external agents initiate the response, which then is perpetuated or amplified by the immune host response. Data in support of the first hypothesis are derived from the fact that antibodies against autologous immunoglobulin G are present in many patients with RA, which may be the primary abnormality in the regulation of cells that control immunoglobulin synthesis. Rheumatoid factor (RF) and anticyclic citrullinated peptides (CCP) have been associated with more severe disease and almost exclusively with extra-articular disease (20,21).

This primary defect may alter the control mechanisms, so that stimulation and control of these events are unbalanced and the response to endogenous immune products goes awry.

A more likely etiology of RA is that specific external antigens initiate inflammation, and in the susceptible host, this leads to continual disease activity. All efforts to associate an infectious agent with RA have failed, despite sophisticated electron microscopy and molecular biology techniques. Exposure to cigarette smoke is an additional environmental factor believed to play a role in increasing the risk for development of RA (22,23).

Infectious synovitis follows a more direct path. Some invade joint space (e.g., *Mycobacterium*, *Staphylococcus*, *parvovirus*) and cause synovitis; others initiate a local immune response, which may be self-limited or persistent (e.g., rubella or Lyme disease, an example of a spirochete-initiated disease that may lead to chronic arthritis). Another mechanism may result from gastrointestinal (GI) infection (e.g., *Shigella*, *Salmonella*, *Yersinia*). No organism is recovered from the joint, although an inflammatory process is initiated by a remote infection.

Several components need to be acknowledged in the understanding of this process: an inciting agent, most likely exogenous and possibly a wide range of antigens; a genetic susceptibility; and an abnormality in the host immune response. Smoking has been associated with an increased risk of RA (23).

The mechanism of tissue injury in RA has been demonstrated to include the following components of the immune system and its associated mediators of inflammation. In the affected host, a stimulus initiates an inflammatory response directed against self or nonself, which sets into motion complement, leukocyte phagocytosis, lysosomal enzyme release, and several small mediators that may initiate clotting and fibrolysis. In the joint, the local reactions are helper T-cell (in particular CD4 T cells) mediators that are attracted to macrophages and dendritic cells. Antibody synthesis is initiated, thus perpetuating the immunologic activities already begun. Cytokines (including TNF-alpha, IL-1, and IL-6) play a key role in the perpetuation of synovial inflammation. Many have been found in the RA synovium (24). These cytokines are targets for clinical drug trial intervention. Some of the joint

TABLE 32-4	Demographic Characteristics of Inflammatory Arthritis				
Disease	Incidence (per 100,000)	Prevalence (per 1,000)	Peak Visit (Years)	Gender	Frequency by Race
RA	32.7	10 (1%)	25–50	2.5:1 Female	Higher in whites and Native Americans (Pima Indians)
JIA	3.5–13.9	1–2	1–3	2:1 Female	Lower in African Americans, Asian, and Japanese
SLE	2–8	0.5–1	15–40	9:1 Female	Three times higher in blacks, Chinese; increased in Haida, North American Indian
AS	7.3	1.5	25–44	3:1 Male	Higher in Central European
PM	1.0	0.1		2.5:1 Female	Three times higher in black females
PSS	0.9–1.9	0.29	30–50	4:1 Female	Increased in Southern United States. Higher among African Americans
Gout	>120	27.5	45–65	10:1 Male	African Americans. Asian-Pacific Islanders
Vasculitis		Various with subtypes			

RA, rheumatoid arthritis; AS, ankylosing spondylitis; JIA, juvenile idiopathic arthritis; PM, polymyositis; SLE, systemic lupus erythematosus; PSS, progressive systemic sclerosis.

mononuclear cells can produce proteinases, prostaglandins (PG), and other small mediators of inflammation.

Tissue inflammation causes the synovial membrane to become hyperplastic, and neoangiogenesis occurs, with production of chemokines that increase the influx of more inflammatory cells. Synovial fluid enzymes directly affect articular cartilage. Bone erosions develop when the synovial membrane has invaded the cartilage. Production of metalloproteinases, fibroblasts, and monocytic phagocytes produced by the synovium is controlled by cytokines (IL$_1$, TNF$_2$, and TGF-β). These cytokines influence chondrocytes to produce less collagen and proteoglycan and increase collagenase synthesis, which degrades type II collagen (25).

As the high-intensity inflammation subsides in the joint, repair takes place, often with the proliferation of fibroblasts and scar tissue. Although it is unclear what triggers all this, once the process is in place, it often continues for a longer period than would be expected to successfully clear antigen. Hence, the host immunoregulatory system, which is genetically controlled, must be abnormal.

Clinical presentation often begins with subtle findings and symptoms, including arthralgia, morning stiffness with involvement of small joints of the hands and feet. Fatigue is often a significant feature (16). As the disease progresses, other joints may be involved, often with rubor (redness), dolor (pain), and calor (warmth), and deformities may soon follow. People with RA may have systemic manifestations with other organ damage (pleural and cardiac involvements are not uncommon) and inappropriate reduction in thymic function (26). RA is a clinical diagnosis that relies upon distribution and nature of joint symptoms. The diagnosis can be confirmed if there is a positive RF (an autoantibody of IgM directed against the Fc portion of IgG). Not all with RA will have a positive RF. People with +RF and/or anticitrulline antibody are likely to have more aggressive disease (27).

Systemic Lupus Erythematosus

SLE is a systemic disease that is associated with abnormalities of immune regulation and immune complex–mediated tissue injury. It has been called a classic autoimmune disease as a result of an abundance of autoantibodies generated against

cytoplasmic and nuclear cellular components. The hallmark is IgG antibodies to double-stranded DNA. The etiology of SLE is obscure, but viral inclusion bodies have been implicated because of electron microscopic observations made in lymphocytes and vessel walls. Virus has never been isolated in patients with SLE; even those diseases with documented infectious etiologies are often multifactorial. Family members with SLE are more likely to have immunologic abnormalities than are controls. Hormonal influences are important in the expression of SLE, and women in the childbearing years appear to be at greater risk. Women taking progestational oral contraceptives are at higher risk than those taking estrogen-based oral contraceptives.

The pathogenesis of SLE depends on abnormalities in humoral and cellular immunity. Lymphopenia is common and is inversely related to disease activity. B lymphocytes are normal in number but are hyperactive. T lymphocytes are often decreased, most markedly in the T-suppressor lymphocyte subpopulation. Natural killer cell activity is diminished, but there are an increased number of lymphocytotoxic antibodies (28).

Clinically, SLE patients can present with very mild symptoms including fatigue, Raynaud's syndrome, arthralgias, and skin rashes to severe multiorgan involvement with glomerulonephritis, pericarditis, serositis, and cerebritis. Women of childbearing years are frequently affected, and SLE may manifest itself for the first time during pregnancy with these symptoms. The most common arthritis manifested by these patients is a nonerosive arthritis usually involving both small and large joints that rarely leads to reversible deformities, known as Jaccoud's arthropathy.

Progressive Systemic Sclerosis

Progressive systemic sclerosis is a progressive disorder in which microvascular obliterative lesions in multiple organs terminate in fibrosis and atrophy. The hallmark of this disease is induration of the skin. Patients with PSS have capillary abnormalities and small artery lesions, which appear late with organ involvement. However, major organ involvement of the lung and kidneys is not uncommon. The pathogenesis of organ involvement is most likely due to injury to the endothelial cell lining of vessels. Disturbing the lining activates the clotting system, with the release of vasoactive peptides. These factors stimulate smooth muscle cells to migrate, proliferate, and deposit in connective tissue, which results in the proliferative vascular lesion of PSS. The etiologic agent is obscure, and no strong hypotheses exist as to its nature (29).

Clinically, PSS patients often present with Raynaud's phenomenon that can therefore lead to digital ischemic ulcers. They can also develop sclerosis of their skin leading to claw hands and joint contractures. Inability to open the mouth adequately may occur in later stages along with esophageal dysmotility, pulmonary hypertension, interstitial lung disease (ILD), and renal failure.

Idiopathic Inflammatory Myopathies

Polymyositis (PM), dermatomyositis (DM), inclusion body myositis (IBM), and autoimmune necrotizing myositis are part of a heterogeneous group of diseases characterized by inflammation of muscle and skin, often associated with profound weakness of all striated muscle, including the heart and elevated levels of skeletal muscle enzymes (30).

Two leading hypotheses may explain the etiology of DM-PM: viral infection and abnormal recognition of self. Immunoglobulins have been demonstrated in vessel walls, especially in intramuscular blood vessels, suggesting that these deposits are immune complexes to muscle. These deposits are seen in a variety of muscle-wasting conditions and may be nonspecific. Cellular immunity is abnormal with DM-PM, as demonstrated by myotoxic activity of the lymphocytes in patients with DM-PM. Skeletal muscle antigens cause lymphocytes of patients with DM-PM to proliferate, suggesting that the lymphocytes are inappropriately responding to these antigens (31).

Clinically, inflammatory myopathy often causes a proximal muscle weakness, Raynaud's disease, and occasionally ILD as well. Some of the medications, steroids in particular, are also associated with muscle atrophy. These inflammatory disorders often have overlapping signs and symptoms. For example, PSS may associate with myositis, and RA and SLE findings may overlap. Screening antibodies for diagnostic and prognostic purposes may help treatment planning (32) (**Table 32-5**).

Crystal-Induced Synovitis

Crystal-induced synovitis can be caused by uric acid, calcium pyrophosphate, hydroxyapatite, and cholesterol crystals. Best understood is gout, a clinical syndrome caused by an overproduction of uric acid (hyperuricemia). As the concentration of urate in the blood increases, MSU crystals can precipitate in the tissues and synovium leading to acute gout flares. It has been shown that injecting urate crystals subcutaneously will cause tophus formation, and when urate is injected into joints, gouty attacks will ensue. Other factors involved in the pathogenesis of the gouty attack include elevated temperature—which increases joint urate concentration—lowered pH, trauma, dehydration, and aging (33).

Pseudogout, or calcium pyrophosphate dihydrate deposition (CPPD), can be hereditary or sporadic. The etiologic agent is the calcium pyrophosphate crystal, which is formed secondary to a disorder of local pyrophosphate metabolism. The crystals adhere to leukocytes, and often immunoglobulin is absorbed, which stimulates phagocytosis and the perpetuation of inflammatory arthritis. These calcium-containing crystals get deposited in the pericellular matrix of cartilage and can present as chondrocalcinosis, which is evident on radiographs (33).

Clinically, crystalline arthropathies often present with acute, intermittent attacks of most often monoarticular inflammation that will self-resolve within 7 to 10 days. They are likely to need pain management during the acute phase. These attacks are followed by intercritical periods of quiescent disease. Frequency and joint location of attacks vary from patient to patient. However, MSU crystals have a higher prevalence for the first metatarsal phalangeal (MTP) joint and knee, whereas CPPD crystals can cause flares of wrists and knees more commonly.

Spondyloarthropathies

Spondyloarthropathies are inflammatory polyarticular disorders that primarily involve the sacroiliac joints, vertebral column, and, to a lesser extent, larger, peripheral joints (shoulder and hip) (34,35). In addition to spinal abnormalities, the eyes, GI tract, cardiovascular system, lungs, kidney and skin may be affected. These arthritides share a number of additional features, including mucocutaneous lesions, sacroiliitis, heel pain, and the HLA-B27 antigen. Antecedent GI infection, caused by *Salmonella*, *Shigella*, and *Yersinia*, has stimulated interest that these diseases may be caused by a Gram-negative organism. The most convincing data in support of this came from the well-documented *Shigella* epidemics, in which reactive arthritis occurred in 344 of 150,000 infected persons in one study (36) and in 9 of 602 in another study (37). No case occurred in anyone who was not infected. Arthritis with some additional features of reactive arthritis has followed *Salmonella* and *Yersinia* infections. In PSA and AS, the data are less convincing, but evidence has linked the development of guttate psoriasis and streptococcal infection (38).

The presence of HLA B27 antigen appears to be the crucial link in expression of AS. Antecedent urethritis has also been associated with acute arthritis, and *Chlamydia* is the organism most frequently identified (34,39). The etiology of some spondyloarthropathies may be an infective agent, possibly Gram-negative bacteria, that interacts with a susceptible gene host: B27 in AS and reactive arthritis and perhaps B27, B38, and C6 in PSA (40). The pathology occurs at the entheses (insertion of tendon to bone). The axial spine may fuse due to anterior spinal ligament ossification. If peripheral joints are involved, there is erosion and periosteal new bone growth without periarticular osteoporosis, as seen in RA.

TABLE 32-5	Antibodies Associated with Rheumatic Diseases	
Disease	**Antigens**	**Antinuclear Antigen Pattern**
SLE, Sjogren's syndrome, scleroderma, polymyositis	ENA, RNP, Ro/SSA, La/SSB, SCL-70, Jo-1	Speckled
SLE	Ds-DNA	Homogeneous
Scleroderma	RNP, Sm	Peripheral
Polymyositis, scleroderma	RNP (To and U3)	None

Clinically, seronegative spondyloarthropathies often cause sacroiliitis in all four subgroups, which often leads to chronic low back pain in this patient population. As patients develop further pain and limitations of spinal movement, they can develop fusion of the spinal vertebrae leading to what is known as "bamboo" spine on imaging. PSA patients typically have inflammatory arthritis of the knees, DIPs, and feet along with psoriatic plaques over the scalp and extensor surfaces of the olecranons and knees. IBD-associated arthritis and reactive arthritis most often present with large mono- to oligoarthritis.

Infectious Arthritis

A wide variety of infectious agents can cause arthritis secondary to the infection itself or as a consequence of the host's immunologic response. The organisms can be viral (e.g., hepatitis, rubella, mumps, herpes), bacterial (e.g., Gram-positive *Staphylococcus*, *Streptococcus*, and *Pneumococcus*; Gram-negative *Neisseria* and *Haemophilus influenzae*; *Pseudomonas*, *Mycobacterium tuberculosis*), spirochete (Lyme disease), or fungal. Recently, interest has developed in the role of hepatitis C and the development of an RA-like arthritis (41).

Vasculitis

Vasculitis, or inflammation of the blood vessels, may occur as a primary process or secondary to an underlying disease. Primary vasculitis is classified by vessel size involvement: large vessel (LVV), medium vessel (MVV), and small vessel vasculitis (SVV) (42) (**Fig. 32-2**). Secondary vasculitis can occur in association with various infections, other CTDs (SLE, RA), malignancies, or medication induced (**Table 32-6**). The etiology of primary vasculitis is unknown. In several SVV, autoantibodies, particularly ANCAs or anti-GBM antibodies, have been found to play a role in direct tissue injury, especially of the vessel walls of various organs including renal, pulmonary, and neurovascular bundles (43,44). In LVV, such as in

giant cell arteritis (GCA)—a clinical condition defined by acute visual loss, headaches, and jaw pain—the pathophysiology is not known and no autoantibodies have been discovered. Increasing age, genetic factors (HLA-DR4), and infection are thought to have causative roles (45). Both the humoral and cellular immune systems have been implicated in the pathogenesis. On vessel biopsy in GCA, multinucleated giant cells, T lymphocytes, and macrophages are found in the media and internal elastic membrane causing fragmentation and intimal thickening of the vessel walls (46). It is hypothesized that a viral infection or other factors first trigger monocyte activation in a susceptible host, which then infiltrates the adventitia and recruits further macrophages and lymphocytes (47). This cellular response results in the production of inflammatory mediators, tissue injury, and the stimulation of repair mechanisms in the media that can lead to fibrosis, scarring, and narrowing of the artery (42).

APPROACH TO PATIENTS WITH RHEUMATIC DISEASES

A detailed history, physical examination, and laboratory and x-ray findings are essential to the proper diagnosis and management of rheumatic diseases. Many schemes have been developed in an attempt to construct an organized approach to the classification of rheumatic diseases, including algorithms that sort signs and symptoms around the presence or absence of inflammation, symmetry, and number of involved joints. However, these categories are not very helpful in sorting out the underlying pathophysiologic processes that need therapeutic intervention. A practical approach is suggested by James Fries, in which eight specific types of musculoskeletal pathology are distinguished (48). Evaluations for each type are summarized in **Table 32-7**. A more recent approach to patient evaluation incorporating the World Health Organization (WHO) biopsychosocial model and using functional measures may be useful (**Table 32-8**). This approach will seek out not only the

FIGURE 32-2. Diagram depicting the usual distribution of vessel involvement by large vessel vasculitis, medium vessel vasculitis, and small vessel vasculitis. All three major categories of vasculitis can affect any size artery, although large vessel vasculitis most often affects large arteries. Medium vessel vasculitis predominantly affects medium arteries, but small arteries may be affected. Small vessel vasculitis predominantly affects venules and capillaries. Immune complex small vessel vasculitis rarely affects arteries. Note that ANCA (antineutrophil cytoplasmic antibody)-associated vasculitis affects a broader spectrum of vessels than does immune complex vasculitis.

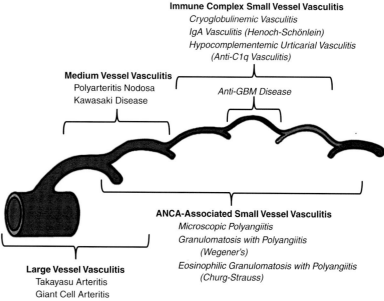

Immune Complex Small Vessel Vasculitis
Cryoglobulinemic Vasculitis
IgA Vasculitis (Henoch-Schönlein)
Hypocomplementemic Urticarial Vasculitis
(Anti-C1q Vasculitis)

Medium Vessel Vasculitis
Polyarteritis Nodosa
Kawasaki Disease

Anti-GBM Disease

ANCA-Associated Small Vessel Vasculitis
Microscopic Polyangiitis
Granulomatosis with Polyangiitis
(Wegener's)
Eosinophilic Granulomatosis with Polyangiitis
(Churg-Strauss)

Large Vessel Vasculitis
Takayasu Arteritis
Giant Cell Arteritis

TABLE 32-6	Definitions of Vasculitis

CHCC2012 Name	CHCC2012 Definition
Large vessel vasculitis (LVV)	Vasculitis affecting large arteries more often than other vasculitides. Large arteries are the aorta and its major branches. Any size artery may be affected.
Takayasu arteritis (TAK)	Arteritis, often granulomatous, predominantly affecting the aorta and/or its major branches. Onset usually in patients younger than 50 years.
Giant cell arteritis (GCA)	Arteritis, often granulomatous, usually affecting the aorta and/or its major branches, with a predilection for the branches of the carotid and vertebral arteries. Often involves the temporal artery. Onset usually in patients older than 50 years and often associated with polymyalgia rheumatica.
Medium vessel vasculitis (MVV)	Vasculitis predominantly affecting medium arteries defined as the main visceral arteries and their branches. Any size artery may be affected. Inflammatory aneurysms and stenoses are common.
Polyarteritis nodosa (PAN)	Necrotizing arteritis of medium or small arteries without glomerulonephritis or vasculitis in arterioles, capillaries, or venules and not associated with antineutrophil cytoplasmic antibodies (ANCAs).
Kawasaki disease (KD)	Arteritis associated with the mucocutaneous lymph node syndrome and predominantly affecting medium and small arteries. Coronary arteries are often involved. Aorta and large arteries may be involved. Usually occurs in infants and young children.
Small vessel vasculitis (SVV)	Vasculitis predominantly affecting small vessels, defined as small intraparenchymal arteries, arterioles, capillaries, and venules. Medium arteries and veins may be affected.
ANCA-associated vasculitis (AAV)	Necrotizing vasculitis, with few or no immune deposits, predominantly affecting small vessels (i.e., capillaries, venules, arterioles, and small arteries), associated with myeloperoxidase (MPO) ANCA or proteinase 3 (PR3) ANCA. Not all patients have ANCA. Add a prefix indicating ANCA reactivity, for example, MPO-ANCA, PR3-ANCA, ANCA-negative.
Microscopic polyangiitis (MPA)	Necrotizing vasculitis, with few or no immune deposits, predominantly affecting small vessels (i.e., capillaries, venules, or arterioles). Necrotizing arteritis involving small and medium arteries may be present. Necrotizing glomerulonephritis is very common. Pulmonary capillaritis often occurs. Granulomatous inflammation is absent.
Granulomatosis with polyangiitis (Wegener's) (GPA)	Necrotizing granulomatous inflammation usually involving the upper and lower respiratory tract, and necrotizing vasculitis affecting predominantly small to medium vessels (e.g., capillaries, venules, arterioles, arteries, and veins). Necrotizing glomerulonephritis is common.
Eosinophilic granulomatosis with polyangiitis (Churg-Strauss) (EGPA)	Eosinophil-rich and necrotizing granulomatous inflammation often involving the respiratory tract, and necrotizing vasculitis predominantly affecting small to medium vessels, and associated with asthma and eosinophilia. ANCA is more frequent when glomerulonephritis is present.
Immune complex vasculitis	Vasculitis with moderate to marked vessel wall deposits of immunoglobulin and/or complement components predominantly affecting small vessels (i.e., capillaries, venules, arterioles, and small arteries). Glomerulonephritis is frequent.
Anti–glomerular basement membrane (anti-GBM) disease	Vasculitis affecting glomerular capillaries, pulmonary capillaries, or both, with GBM deposition of anti-GBM autoantibodies. Lung involvement causes pulmonary hemorrhage, and renal involvement causes glomerulonephritis with necrosis and crescents.
Cryoglobulinemic vasculitis (CV)	Vasculitis with cryoglobulin immune deposits affecting small vessels (predominantly capillaries, venules, or arterioles) and associated with serum cryoglobulins. Skin, glomeruli, and peripheral nerves are often involved.
IgA vasculitis (Henoch-Schönlein) (IgAV)	Vasculitis, with IgA1-dominant immune deposits, affecting small vessels (predominantly capillaries, venules, or arterioles). Often involves the skin and gastrointestinal tract and frequently causes arthritis. Glomerulonephritis indistinguishable from IgA nephropathy may occur.
Hypocomplementemic urticarial vasculitis (HUV) (anti-C1q vasculitis)	Vasculitis accompanied by urticaria and hypocomplementemia affecting small vessels (i.e., capillaries, venules, or arterioles) and associated with anti-C1q antibodies. Glomerulonephritis, arthritis, obstructive pulmonary disease, and ocular inflammation are common.
Variable vessel vasculitis (VVV)	Vasculitis with no predominant type of vessel involved that can affect vessels of any size (small, medium, and large) and type (arteries, veins, and capillaries).
Behçet's disease (BD)	Vasculitis occurring in patients with Behçet's disease that can affect arteries or veins. Behçet's disease is characterized by recurrent oral and/or genital aphthous ulcers accompanied by cutaneous, ocular, articular, gastrointestinal, and/or central nervous system inflammatory lesions. Small vessel vasculitis, thromboangiitis, thrombosis, arteritis, and arterial aneurysms may occur.
Cogan's syndrome (CS)	Vasculitis occurring in patients with Cogan's syndrome. Cogan's syndrome characterized by ocular inflammatory lesions, including interstitial keratitis, uveitis, and episcleritis and inner ear disease, including sensorineural hearing loss and vestibular dysfunction. Vasculitic manifestations may include arteritis (affecting small, medium, or large arteries), aortitis, aortic aneurysms, and aortic and mitral valvulitis.
Single-organ vasculitis (SOV)	Vasculitis in arteries or veins of any size in a single organ that has no features that indicate that it is a limited expression of a systemic vasculitis. The involved organ and vessel type should be included in the name (e.g., cutaneous small vessel vasculitis, testicular arteritis, central nervous system vasculitis). Vasculitis distribution may be unifocal or multifocal (diffuse) within an organ. Some patients originally diagnosed as having SOV will develop additional disease manifestations that warrant redefining the case as one of the systemic vasculitides (e.g., cutaneous arteritis later becoming systemic polyarteritis nodosa, etc.).
Vasculitis associated with systemic disease	Vasculitis that is associated with and may be secondary to (caused by) a systemic disease. The name (diagnosis) should have a prefix term specifying the systemic disease (e.g., rheumatoid vasculitis, lupus vasculitis, etc.).
Vasculitis associated with probable etiology	Vasculitis that is associated with a probable specific etiology. The name (diagnosis) should have a prefix term specifying the association (e.g., hydralazine-associated microscopic polyangiitis, hepatitis B virus–associated vasculitis, hepatitis C virus–associated cryoglobulinemic vasculitis, etc.).

Definitions for vasculitides adopted by the 2012 International Chapel Hill Consensus Conference on the Nomenclature of Vasculitides (CHCC2012) (42).

TABLE 32-7	Evaluation of Rheumatic Diseases		
Pathology	**Examples**	**Laboratory Tests**	**Other Organs Involved**
Synovitis	Rheumatoid arthritis	RF, CCP, x-rays	Lung, heart, skin nodules
	Psoriatic arthritis/reactive arthritis	X-rays	Skin
	Primary vasculitis (rarely)	ANCAs, cryo, GBM	
		MRA/CT angio	
Enthesopathy	Ankylosing spondylitis	HLA-B27, sacroiliac	Heart
		Joint, x-rays, MRI	
	Psoriatic arthritis/reactive arthritis		Skin, mucous membrane
Crystal arthritis	Gout	Serum uric acid, joint fluid	Skin, kidney
	Pseudogout		
Joint infection	Bacterial	Joint culture, joint fluid	Vaginal infection
	Viral		Bacteremia
	Fungal		Hepatitis
Joint effusion	Trauma	Joint fluid	
	Reactive arthritis		
	Metabolic/endocrine disorders		Thyroid livers
Secondary vasculitis	Scleroderma	Muscle biopsy	Any organ
	DM–PM	EMG	
	SLE	Antinuclear antibody	Heart
	Polymyalgia	Erythrocyte sedimentation rate	
		CRP	
Tissue conditions			
Local	Tendinitis		
Generalized	Fibrositis		

primary etiology and how the disease process affects the organ or system but also the associated effects on the patient and his or her interactions with the environment (http://www.who.int/classifications/icf/en/).

History and Examination

A detailed description of the symptom onset, prodromal symptoms, setting, pattern, and sequence will greatly aid in establishing a differential diagnosis. Exacerbating or remitting factors, functional impairments, and therapeutic effects should also be documented (49).

The following are the most frequent presenting symptoms:

Pain. Although often difficult to define, anatomic location and symmetry, character (e.g., burning, aching), and severity or intensity (graded by a numeric 10-point scale) should be included. This is particularly common in arthritides, not in PSS or DM-PM.

Fatigue may be one of the earliest symptoms of an inflammatory disease and one of the most ubiquitous. Some patients may have these complaints even though pain and swelling have been objectively controlled. Fatigue is a critical contributor to decision-making about pharmacologic management. It is also a frequently associated finding in comorbid conditions such as diabetes, congestive failure, and lung disease. Several medical conditions are frequently associated with rheumatic diseases, including anemia, thyroid disease, pulmonary fibrosis, and renal failure. Assessment of these associated findings and treatment of comorbid conditions are critical.

TABLE 32-8	Functional Measures in Rheumatic Diseases							
	MMT	**Range of Motion**	**Pain**	**Fatigue**	**ADLs**	**Ambulation**	**Cognition**	**Role/Social Interaction**
OA		+++	++		+	++		
RA	+	++	++	+++	++	++		++++
Spondyloarthropathies		+++	++		+	+		++
DM-PM	++			+++	++	++		++++
PSS		++	++	+	++			++
SLE	+			+++	+	+	++	++++
Gout (crystals)			+++			++		
Fibromyalgia			+++	+++				++++

Key: +, possibly useful evaluation; ++, recommended evaluation; +++, strongly recommended; ++++, must evaluate.
MMT, manual muscle test; OA, osteoarthritis; PSS, progressive systemic sclerosis; RA, rheumatoid arthritis; DM-PM, dermatomyositis-polymyositis; SLE, systemic lupus erythematosus; OA, osteoarthritis; RA, rheumatoid arthritis; PSS, progressive systemic scoliosis; ADLs, activities of daily living.

Stiffness may be seen as well. This may be described as a "gel" phenomenon where after periods of recumbency or general inactivity, joint motion is difficult. In some cases, this may be as short as 20 to 30 minutes but typically is greater than 1 hour. Timing, duration, and location of stiffness should be noted. In the diagnostic criteria of RA, morning stiffness must last at least 1 hour.

Range-of-motion (ROM) limitations may accompany complaints of stiffness. These symptoms in the rheumatologic population are usually not transient and should not be confused with gelling or stiffness. Noting the duration of the problem may help to differentiate an acute from a chronic process, such as nonreducible joint subluxation. The most important is to determine if the loss of ROM is fixed or likely to be successfully ranged. Passive and active ROM testing should be performed to rule out weakness as an etiology for ROM limitation.

Joint swelling should be carefully assessed by rubor, dolor, calor, and size of effusion. The acute inflammatory effusion should be treated with cold. Arthrocentesis is recommended for diagnostic purposes.

Weakness is important to differentiate from fatigue. Careful documentation of patient reports on muscle groups involved and relationship to functional limitations is needed. Proximal muscle weakness may be indicative of inflammatory myopathy such as PM. Persistent versus intermittent complaints of weakness may indicate other processes, such as neuromuscular disease (e.g., Guillain-Barré syndrome).

Biomechanics

Evaluation of mobility can be performed with visual gait analysis or automated measures. The former has been standardized and the latter have been significantly advanced with video-based high-speed systems. There is an increased ability to reliably measure motion in three dimensions: in real time, ground reaction forces, and pressures on the bottoms of the feet to calculate moments of force at various joints. These procedures are now more available and being performed fairly frequently. In addition, newer instrumentation has been developed to describe foot pressure profiles and describe forces and their influences on the foot (50). Gait abnormalities for several of the rheumatic diseases have been noted. The RA gait has been termed *apropulsive* because of the absence of push-off from the ball of the foot. Similarly, studies of differences in gait before and after surgical procedures have been reported that describe which biomechanical changes occur as a result (51).

Laboratory Tests

The laboratory evaluation of blood, urine, and synovial fluid, coupled with radiographic evaluations, history, and physical examination information, can usually help to establish a proper diagnosis. The following initial determinations are made: complete blood count, ESR, SMA 12 (sequential multiple analyzer), RF, anti-CCP, and antinuclear antibody (ANA). Further specific autoantibodies can be tested if the initial ANA screen is positive, which helps categorize various CTDs including Sjögren's syndrome, SLE, PSS, MCTD, and DM-PM (52). The acute-phase reactants (C-reactive protein [CRP], serum amyloidal [SAA], and ESR) should be monitored, as they may be part of the early defense or adaptive mechanisms that precede the immune response. Although nonspecific, moderate elevation in CRP, ESR, and serum amylase can be seen in systemic diseases. For vasculitis, ANCA,

anti-GBM, cryoglobulins, and serum IgA levels may be helpful in diagnosing small/medium vessel vasculitis (**Table 32-6**).

There has been significant progress in understanding potential genetic contributions to disease susceptibility and inheritance patterns both from twin studies and the genome-wide association project (53). Genetic typing has been used for diagnostic purposes (e.g., HLA-B27 for AS and sacroiliitis, DHR 4+ for RA, and molecules that regulate immune pathways such as STAT4). Joint fluid is easy to obtain in the presence of effusion. Analysis of fluid is essential in the diagnosis of crystal-induced arthritis and infection, and it is helpful in differentiating traumatic from inflammatory arthritis. However, rarely will the diagnosis of RA, OA, PSA, or AS be made on the basis of joint fluid alone. Rather, the fluid helps confirm a diagnosis. Joint taps must be done when a question of infection is raised and should be made before injecting steroid or other material into the joint. Classification of joint fluid into categories will help differentiate inflammatory, noninflammatory, septic, and hemorrhagic arthritis (**Table 32-1**).

Radiographic Assessment

Radiography is often the most valuable technique for differentiating among arthritides. Carefully selected radiograph series with the proper projections, addition of stress, and weight-bearing views will add valuable information about the extent of soft tissue, articular surface, or bony changes. Marginal erosion of bone with juxta-articular osteoporosis and uniform joint space narrowing is the hallmark of RA. Nonuniform joint space loss in association with bony sclerosis and marginal osteophytes is the characteristic change in OA. Spondyloarthropathies classically have involvement of the sacroiliac joints, either symmetric, as in AS, or asymmetric, as in reactive arthritis and PSA. Bony changes include periosteal new bone formation and ankylosis. Gout and pseudogout often involve only a few joints. In gout, there are soft tissue tophaceous deposits and marginal erosion with large bony overhangs, and in pseudogout, there can be calcinosis in fibrocartilage (chondrocalcinosis). Early in joint infection, the x-ray films may be negative, or there may be some joint space widening. If the process continues and osteomyelitis develops, periosteal reaction can occur, which may indicate progressive infection or bony destruction. **Table 32-2** presents typical radiographic findings in patients with rheumatic diseases.

Additional imaging such as computed tomography (CT), which gives good structural definition of soft tissue and bone, is often combined with arthrography to study axial structures in disorders such as sacroiliitis. Magnetic resonance imaging (MRI) allows further differentiation of soft tissue and fluid as well as use of variable imaging planes and combination. Gadolinium for contrast is of great benefit in the evaluation of joint effusions, tendinopathies, and myositis (54). Ultrasound has become more useful in evaluating early disease and to help assess for ongoing synovitis in this patient population as well (55). Angiography via CT, MRI, or conventional angiogram can be very useful and often diagnostic in cases of vasculitis (**Table 32-2**).

Surgical Biopsy

Various tissue biopsies are often used to confirm a diagnosis, especially in cases of inflammatory myositis, vasculitis, sarcoidosis, and occasionally infectious or malignancy-associated conditions (56). For the various inflammatory myopathies, muscle biopsies are the gold standard in diagnosis, whereas often a skin/renal or lung biopsy can confirm various vasculitides (57). In sarcoidosis, often a lymph node or bone marrow biopsy is used (58).

Functional Assessment

Rehabilitation assessment for patients with rheumatic diseases includes both impairment and functional measures. Goniometry, the measurement of joint ROM, is standardized and widely used, as is manual muscle testing (MMT). A new 10-point MMT with specific grade definitions has been devised and offers more sensitivity in the strength range that is most important to know for assessment of capability for independence (59). Quantifiable measures of spine motion are particularly useful for patients with rheumatic diseases (60). They can help chart progressive loss of spinal mobility, which prompts interventions designed to preserve posture as well as chest expansion programs, as in the management of patients with spondyloarthropathies.

Patients with arthritis often have stiffness rather than pain that limits function. Both symptoms are difficult to measure. However, duration of morning stiffness may be quantified. Pain can be measured in terms of severity in a descriptive way (e.g., mild, moderate, severe) or by use of a visual analog scale (61), which is quite reliable. Measures of degree of joint tenderness, swelling, deformity, relative instability, or crepitus with active and passive movement are also useful in defining rheumatic disease processes.

Fatigue is a frequent problem for patients with rheumatic disease. Its cause is multifactorial: medication, chronic inflammation, abnormal posture and gait that are energy inefficient, abnormalities of the sleep cycle, and atrophy of muscle secondary to disease or chronic pain. Fatigue is difficult to quantify. A visual analog of fatigue has been used with some success, but it has an imprecise reference. A multidimensional assessment of fatigue (62) has been devised and validated in this population. The Fatigue Severity Scale has also been used to assess this parameter (63). The Human Activity Profile is an instrument designed to measure amount of activity and those activities that an individual is no longer able to perform. It also has a dyspnea scale. Specific activities have been correlated with metabolic equivalents required for performance (64).

Despite reliable, sensitive indices of strength, ROM, and grip strength, other measures are needed for evaluation of patients with rheumatic disease. The American Rheumatism Association in 1949 devised a functional scale for patients with RA. This scale, a simple, global assessment that rated patients'

functional status as independent (i.e., class I), able to perform with pain (i.e., class II), able to do some activities (i.e., class III), and unable to perform (i.e., class IV), was revised in 1992 (65).

Two generations of functional assessments have been used in evaluating patients with rheumatic disease. The first set looked primarily at performance of patients in ambulation, self-care, and other activities of daily living (ADLs). Most had some testing of reliability and validity and were relatively easy to use. The problem with them was that they defined function very narrowly and excluded psychological, social, and vocational functions. The newer functional indices are more comprehensive and offer a broader view of patients' functioning. These global, multidimensional tools had been designed for the arthritis population, children, and adults and have demonstrated validity and reliability (66,67).

When rheumatologists were asked which functional measures were important to use in evaluation of patients with rheumatic diseases, the consensus was mobility, pain, self-care, and role activity (68). The evaluations needed may vary, because some rheumatic diseases involve only joints (e.g., OA); others, primarily the kidneys, skin, and central nervous system (e.g., SLE); and still others, different organ systems, such as cardiovascular and pulmonary systems. **Table 32-8** identifies standard functional measures likely to be needed for each of the rheumatic diseases. Other useful scales include the Wisconsin Brief Pain Questionnaire, the Sickness Impact Profile (69), Stanford Health Assessment Questionnaire (HAQ) (70), Short Form Survey 36 Version 2 (71), Arthritis Impact Measurement Scale 2 in RA and PMM, and Bath and Dougados Functional Indices in Spondylitis (72). These functional assessment tools singly and in combination are valuable tools in measuring both physical and psychosocial health parameters (**Tables 32-9** and **32-10**).

Functional assessment tools are also used in combination with traditional measures of disease state, including tender and swollen joint counts and biochemical markers of disease state such as the acute-phase reactants. The combination of these tools into core set outcome measures is used to define clinically significant improvement in diseases such as RA. The American College of Rheumatology (ACR) has chosen the definition of 20% improvement in tender and swollen joint counts and improvement in three of the five following ACR core set measures: patient assessment, physician global assessment of disease severity, pain, disability, and acute phase reactants (73). This is commonly referred to as the ACR-20. Clinical improvement in the preceding core set measures constitutes improvement of 50% and 70% (ACR-50 and ACR-70) and are often referred to in randomized control trials. The Outcome Measures

TABLE 32-9	**Assessments Measuring Physical Health Parameters**				
	Mobility	**Self-Care Roles**	**Communication**	**Pain**
American College of Rheumatology (ACR)	Global	Global	0	0
Stanford Health Assessment Questionnaire (HAQ)	++	+++	0	+
Arthritis Impact Measurement Scale (AIMS II)	+++	++	+	++
Sickness Impact Profile (SIP)	+++	+++	+	0
Short Form 36 ver. 2 (SF36)	++	+	0	+

Key: 0, No questions in this area; +, few questions in this area; ++, moderate number of questions in this area; +++, many questions in this area.
From Hicks JE, Joe JO, Shah JP, et al. Rehabilitation management of rheumatic diseases. In: O'Young BJ, Youn MA, Stiens SA, eds. *Physical Medicine and Rehabilitation Secrets*. 2nd ed. Philadelphia, PA: Hanley Belfus; 2002.

TABLE 32-10	Assessments Measuring Psychosocial Health Parameters		
	Mobility	**Self-Care Roles**	**Communication**
American College of Rheumatology (ACR)	0	0	0
Stanford Health Assessment Questionnaire (HAQ)	+	0	0
Arthritis Impact Measurement Scale (AIMS II)	++	++	++
Sickness Impact Profile (SIP)	++	++	+
Short Form 36 ver. 2 (SF36)	+	0	+

Key: 0, No questions in this area; +, few questions in this area; ++, moderate number of questions in this area; +++, many questions in this area.
From Hicks JE, Joe JO, Shah JP, et al. Rehabilitation management of rheumatic diseases. In: O'Young BJ, Young MA, Stiens SA, eds. *Physical Medicine and Rehabilitation Secrets*. 2nd ed. Philadelphia, PA: Hanley Belfus; 2002.

in Rheumatology Clinical Trials (OMERACT) group has reached consensus on the required core set measures of use in OA (74) and AS (75). Core set outcome measures in other populations, such as those with polymyositis/dermatomyositis, are currently in development. Although these tools are easily administered, results are often not immediately available for use because of scoring schemes. Some of these tools (e.g., HAQ) also have limited use because of ceiling effects and often miss subtle changes in the patient's disease process reflected in level of function; others may have significant flooring effects.

In the clinical setting of RA, a combination of factors including specific clinical and laboratory values is used to produce a Disease Activity Score (DAS28). The DAS28 is derived from the number of tender and swollen joints, patient assessment of disease activity via visual analog scale, ESR, and CRP (76).

Compliance

Rheumatic diseases are characterized by chronic relapsing and remitting symptoms and disease activity. It is a challenge for patients to adhere to complicated medication schedules and treatments to maintain strength and activity and control pain. It has long been recognized that a number of factors may influence adherence of patients with treatment in general. These include demographic features, natural history, types of treatment regimens, settings, patient-doctor relationships, support networks, and economic and educational levels.

Compliance depends on individual health beliefs, including the importance to the patient of the treatment goal, how likely the treatment is to achieve the goal and benefit the patient, and how likely the treatment is to lessen the disability and the physical, psychological, and functional barriers to treatment. In our clinical experience, patients who have pain are more likely to be compliant with medication, modalities, and techniques that relieve the pain. Education significantly increases adherence to drug regimens (77). Group education enhances self-management strategies (78,79). One study of adolescents with chronic diseases (including JRA) indicated good motivation was likely to result in better treatment compliance. Support from parents, physicians, and friends also predicted good compliance with regimens (80).

Compliance with unsupervised exercise programs tends to be low. In one study, two out of three patients with some form of arthritis management information used some technical orders and rested daily, and 50% used exercise and heat (one half on a daily basis) (81). Compliance at the 1-year level in patients on a home exercise program was predicted by self-efficacy for exercise, regular ROM before study intervention, and single

marital status (81). Perceived benefit of exercise was a significant predictor of participation in an aerobic exercise program. Those who reported exercising in their youth perceived more benefits. Subjects with less formal education, longer arthritis duration, and higher impact of arthritis scores perceived fewer exercise benefits (82).

Strategies to improve compliance with exercise can be seen in 📶 eTable 32-1. 📶 eTable 32-2 lists strategies for improving compliance with orthotics and gait aids.

TREATMENT

Pharmacologic Management

Pharmacologic management of rheumatic diseases often requires the use of one or more of a variety of medications. These may influence physical and psychological functioning. The well-known "treatment pyramid" approach to the management of rheumatic diseases was based on the view that RA was a benign disease and treatment should begin with the least toxic medications before advancing to those with more significant toxicity. It suggested that management begin with rest, patient education, joint protection, and nonsteroidal anti-inflammatory drugs (NSAIDs) with progression to steroids and sequential monotherapy and use of DMARDs later in the course of these diseases. There has been an inversion of the pyramid to encourage early use of DMARDs in order to stop progression as quickly as possible especially because DMARD toxicity profiles are not greater than other medications (83,84) (Fig. 32-3). At the onset of disease symptoms and diagnosis, the patient would begin early rehabilitation interventions: exercise, education, orthotics, physical modalities, joint protection, energy conservation, and strengthening, along with NSAIDs and low-dose steroid therapy in some cases. As we ascend the pyramid, introduction of DMARDs used singly or in combination and earlier use of biologic agents are noted. Patients are generally reevaluated every 3 months for drug response and either undergo dose escalation, addition of second or third agent, or switch to another medication altogether. The theme of "treat early and aggressively" with titration of medications after several months of remission has been shown to prevent joint damage and limitations, which is the goal in therapy (85).

Aspirin

Aspirin, or acetylsalicylic acid (ASA), has been the foundation of management of rheumatic conditions in the past and the symptoms of pain, fever, and inflammation. It has been shown to block the synthesis of PG in the anterior hypothalamus,

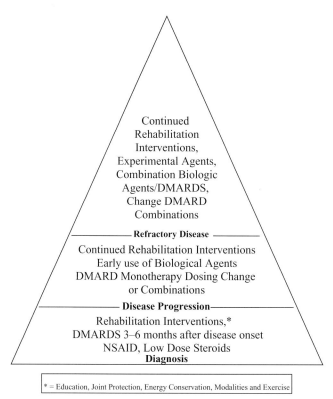

Continued
Rehabilitation
Interventions,
Experimental Agents,
Combination Biologic
Agents/DMARDS,
Change DMARD
Combinations

—————— **Refractory Disease** ——————

Continued Rehabilitation Interventions
Early use of Biological Agents
DMARD Monotherapy Dosing Change
or Combinations

———— **Disease Progression** ————

Rehabilitation Interventions,*
DMARDS 3–6 months after disease onset
NSAID, Low Dose Steroids
Diagnosis

* = Education, Joint Protection, Energy Conservation, Modalities and Exercise

FIGURE 32-3. Pyramid of the medical and rehabilitation treatment approach to inflammatory arthritis.

which is responsible for the antipyretic effect. The analgesic effect of ASA is not entirely understood. Musculoskeletal pain may be mediated by bradykinin, a synthesizer of PG, which sensitizes nerves to painful stimuli. Aspirin blocks PG synthesis. At doses higher than those used for analgesia (e.g., 5.3 g/d), ASA reduces joint inflammation and swelling. The mechanisms for this action are multifactorial. Aspirin affects leukocyte migration and vascular permeability, both of which may be influenced by PG synthesis. The toxicities of ASA include allergy, tinnitus and hearing loss, GI blood loss, ulcer, chemical hepatitis, and reduced glomerular filtration rate. For patients who have clinically significant GI symptoms, enteric-coated preparations are usually well tolerated. Other forms of salicylate can be used that are often less GI toxic (e.g., choline salicylate). However, given ASA does not change the disease course of inflammatory arthritides and now with the introduction of newer disease-modifying and biologic agents, ASA is not commonly used at this time, except for symptom management (86).

Nonsteroidal Anti-Inflammatory Drugs

The agents in use that form the group of drugs called NSAIDs, which include the cyclo-oxygenase-2 inhibitors (COX-2), continue to be used in part as first-line agents in management of the rheumatic diseases. These drugs also suppress inflammation through the inhibition of synthesis of PG. They inhibit the cyclooxygenase effect on platelets and effects on leukocyte migration. Toxicities include GI bleeding, pancreatitis, hepatotoxicity, decreased renal blood flow, hypertension, peripheral edema, and allergic interstitial nephritis. Some have more GI toxicity than others and cause more sodium retention. A review of the comparative NSAID toxicities is available (87).

Nonsteroidal anti-inflammatory drugs were widely used as first-line drugs in the treatment of RA, JIA, OA, and the spondyloarthropathies but have more recently been replaced by the early use of DMARDs in most cases. Only tolmetin sulfate, choline magnesium trisalicylate, ibuprofen, and naproxen sodium have been approved for use in children by the U.S. Food and Drug Administration.

Aspirin and NSAIDs are likely to provide some analgesic benefit for patients with OA, but not independently for the inflammatory arthropathies. The newest group of NSAIDs, the COX-2 inhibitors, has found more recent favor. They differ from traditional NSAIDs that do not inhibit COX-1 at normal therapeutic levels, thus likely avoiding some of the detrimental GI effects of other NSAIDs. These selective COX-2 inhibitors have been shown to increase risk of cardiovascular thrombotic events, acute myocardial infarction, and stroke. Hence, rofecoxib and valdecoxib have been removed from the market (88). Celecoxib remains on the market, with a warning. Dosing should be less than 200 mg/d (89).

Glucocorticoids

Glucocorticoids and therapeutics for rheumatic diseases are inseparable and probably have been tried in every rheumatic disease either systemically or locally. Exogenous glucocorticoids influence leukocyte movement, leukocyte function, and humoral factors; inhibit recruitment of neutrophils and monocytes into inflammatory sites; cause lymphocytopenia by inducing margination or redistribution of lymphocytes out of the circulation; modify the increased capillary and membrane permeability that occurs at an inflammatory site, reducing edema and antagonizing histamine-induced vasodilation; and inhibit PG synthesis.

Daily high-dose steroid use stimulates Cushing's syndrome, in which hypertension, hirsutism, acne, striae, obesity, psychiatric symptoms, and wound-healing problems occur. With exogenous doses above 12.5 mg/d, there is an increased incidence of glaucoma, cataracts, avascular necrosis, osteoporosis, and pancreatitis. The side effects are, in part, dependent on the particular glucocorticoid used and the dose. Alternate-day steroids are associated with fewer untoward effects. Current recommendations to reduce bone loss in patients receiving a prednisone equivalent of more than 5 mg/d include (a) use of supplemental calcium and vitamin D or activated form of vitamin D, (b) use of the bisphosphonates or calcitonin as a second-line agent for those with contraindications or intolerance of the bisphosphonates, and (c) hormone replacement therapy in those found to be hormone deficient (90). The oral route is usually selected for ease of administration, but glucocorticoids can safely be given intramuscularly, intravenously, or intra-articularly.

Glucocorticoids are used to treat several rheumatic diseases. In 2002, a consensus conference made the following recommendations for a standardized nomenclature for glucocorticoid dosing: dose of less than 7.5 mg is a low dose, 7.5 to 30 mg/d a medium dose, 30 to 100 mg a high dose, and greater than 100 mg/d a very high dose. Pulse-dosed therapies are greater than 250 mg/d (91). Higher doses are used in treating patients with SLE, vasculitis, and DM-PM (up to 100 mg prednisone every day) (92). The use of steroid therapy in RA, AS, and rarely in PSA (as can flare the psoriasis) is usually reserved for bridge therapy and/or to control acute flares of disease.

Similarly, for acute crystalline attacks, oral or intra-articular steroids are often the drug of choice, especially in patients with renal disease who are not candidates for NSAIDs/colchicine. In PSS, steroids are commonly avoided due to their increased risk in causing renal crisis in this population. However, in PSS patients that have severe ILD, inflammatory arthritis, or myositis, steroids are often used early and eventually replaced with DMARDs.

Disease-Modifying Antirheumatic Drugs

Methotrexate

This cytotoxic agent has become one of the first-line agents in the treatment of moderate to severe RA. It is a structural analog of folic acid and causes the deficiency of intracellular folate by inhibition of dihydrofolate reductase, an enzyme required for DNA synthesis. This may not be the true mechanism of action that makes methotrexate an effective anti-inflammatory agent. Methotrexate also may act to promote the extracellular adenosine release, which promotes the down-regulation of inflammatory pathways by binding surface receptors on lymphocytes, monocytes, and neutrophils and inhibiting interleukin (IL) production.

Methotrexate has been shown to be effective in RA, JIA, SLE, inflammatory myositis, and PSA (93,94) and is effective in combination with corticosteroids in the management of several vasculitides. It can be given in an oral form once per week at average doses of 7.5 to 15 mg/wk. Maximum doses of 25 mg/wk may be given. Weekly subcutaneous or intramuscular injections are well tolerated and less GI side effects are noted. Side effects include increased liver transaminases, myelosuppression, hypersensitivity pneumonitis, and cirrhosis. Methotrexate is highly teratogenic and contraindicated in pregnancy. It increases risk of infection. Patients on methotrexate must limit the use of alcohol.

Hydroxychloroquine

Antimalarials, such as hydroxychloroquine (HCQ), are one of the mainstay agents for SLE patients. They not only can control mild arthritis and skin lesions but also can reduce risk of SLE flares and renal or other internal organ involvement (95,96). They are also used as monotherapy in mild RA patients or in combination with moderate RA. Patients with RA improved in joint count, grip strength, walk time, and sedimentation rate. The antimalarials are slow-acting, taking 4 to 6 weeks before a therapeutic effect is observed. They are as effective as some of the other DMARDs, but a lower toxicity profile makes them one of the agents of choice in combination therapy (97,98).

The mechanism of action of these drugs is varied. They have been shown to impair enzymatic reactions, including phospholipase, cholinesterase-hyaluronidase, and proliferation of lymphocytes. They seem to block depolymerization by DNase and interfere with DNA replication. The incidence of side effects and toxicities varies widely. GI disturbance is quite common, and retinopathy is infrequent but of greatest concern; it rarely occurs before a cumulative dose of 300 mg is reached, specifically in chloroquine, but routine ophthalmologic examinations should be performed. The antimalarial agents are most often used in the treatment of RA, Sjögren's, and SLE.

Sulfasalazine

Sulfasalazine (SSA) is an agent that combines the antibiotic sulfapyridine with the anti-inflammatory agent 5-aminosalicylic. Its proposed mechanisms of action include inhibition of folate-dependent enzymes similar to methotrexate, immunomodulatory functions that decrease immunoglobulin and RF production, and several anti-inflammatory properties (98). SSA has been shown effective in treating mild RA, JIA, AS, and PSA with peripheral disease but not with axial involvement (99,100).

Leflunomide

Leflunomide is an immunosuppressive drug that inhibits *de novo* pyrimidine synthesis and impairs T-cell proliferation. In the treatment of RA, this drug has been shown to be as effective as methotrexate (101). This agent has been shown not only to be effective as monotherapy but to be even more effective when used in combination with methotrexate; however, concerns remain over the toxicity profile (102). Leflunomide is shown to be effective in the treatment of RA, SLE, and PSA (103,104). Monitoring while on this medication includes (a) liver function tests for toxicity and (b) platelet count for signs of thrombocytopenia.

Immunoregulatory Agents

Immunoregulatory drugs have been used in the management of rheumatic diseases in an attempt to restore a balanced immune response by eliminating certain cell subsets. None of these drugs has cured patients with rheumatic diseases, but they have produced control and long-term remissions (105). Commonly used agents are the alkylating agents (cyclophosphamide and chlorambucil), purine analogs (azathioprine and mercaptopurine), cyclosporine, tacrolimus, sirolimus, mycophenolate mofetil, dapsone, and thalidomide.

Cyclophosphamide and Chlorambucil

Cyclophosphamide and chlorambucil are alkylating agents, which form active metabolites that cross-link DNA, preventing replication and reducing DNA synthesis. Immunoregulatory effects are through the decrease of both T- and B-lymphocyte proliferation, antibody production, and suppression of delayed hypersensitivity reactions to new antigens. Cyclophosphamide has been shown to be effective in treating more severe SLE and vasculitis while chlorambucil is recommended for more severe RA (106). These agents have toxicity profiles that include myelosuppression, increased risk of infection, and risk of malignancy (105), which has led to less use of these medications.

Azathioprine and Mercaptopurine

The purine analogs, azathioprine and mercaptopurine, are converted to thiopurine, metabolized and incorporated into cellular DNA, which inhibits nucleic acid synthesis. It is believed that these agents function to decrease circulating lymphocyte count, suppress lymphocyte proliferation, and inhibit antibody production, monocyte activity, and cell-mediated and humoral immunity (105). These agents have been used as steroid-sparing agents to treat RA, inflammatory myopathies, and SLE. Increasingly, they are used for ILD often associated with RA or other CTDs. They are well tolerated. Most common side effects include GI symptoms, myelosuppression, and slight increased risk of infection (107).

Cyclosporine, Tacrolimus, Sirolimus, Mycophenolate Mofetil, Dapsone, and Thalidomide

Cyclosporine exerts its effects by inhibiting the production of IL-2 and other cytokines leading to reduction in T-cell activation and lymphocyte proliferation. It has been used in the treatment of RA and PSA. Toxicities include GI upset, hypertension, nephrotoxicity, and increased risk of lymphoma and skin cancer. Tacrolimus, a macrolide, functions by binding to an intracellular binding protein (FK-binding protein) and in association with calcineurin suppresses transcription of cytokines and inhibits the early steps of T-lymphocyte activation (108). Sirolimus also binds to the FK-binding protein but functions through blocking the progression of the cell cycle inhibiting cell signal transduction (109). Mycophenolate mofetil is converted to mycophenolate acid and reversibly inhibits inosine monophosphate dehydrogenase, an enzyme

required for the synthesis of purines, thus inhibiting T- and B-cell lymphocyte proliferation. It has been used in the treatment of SLE and associated nephritis, CTD-associated ILD, and inflammatory myopathies.

Thalidomide, a derivative of glutamic acid, is believed to exert its immunosuppressive effects through the inhibition of angiogenesis and tumor necrosis factor (TNF)-alpha. Its most notable toxicity is as a potent teratogen but is also associated with peripheral neuropathy. Currently only approved for the treatment of erythema nodosum, studies are evaluating its efficacy in RA, SLE, Sjögren's syndrome, and AS (110). Dapsone, an antimicrobial agent, is believed to inhibit neutrophil function by decreasing recruitment and chemotaxis (111). These drugs all cause marrow suppression and GI intolerance. A review of the therapeutic application of these drugs is presented in **Table 32-11**.

TABLE 32-11	Therapeutic Application of Drugs in Rheumatic Diseases		
Diseases	**Recommended Medications**	**Probable Mechanisms**	**Precautions**
RA	ASA, NSAIDs	Inhibition of cyclo-oxygenase (COX) enzyme needed for prostaglandin synthesis	Bleeding diathesis (platelet dysfunction)
	Antimalarials		Upper GI toxicity
	Gold	Block lysosomal enzymes	Renal toxicity
	D-Penicillamine	Inhibits phagocytic activity of macrophages	Retinal toxicity, psoriasis
	Steroids		Nephritis, rash, marrow suppression
	Azathioprine	Unknown	Nephritis, SLE, PM
	Methotrexate	Interfere with lymphocytic migration; decreases intra-articular membrane permeability	Lymphoid tumors
	Cyclophosphamide		Not used with allopurinol
	Cyclosporine		Cirrhosis, leukopenia
		Inhibits DNA synthesis	Marrow suppression, liver toxicity, lung fibrosis
	Infliximab/etanercept/adalumimab/ golimubab, certolizumab	Causes intracellular folate deficiency	
	Leflunomide	Prevents DNA replication	Ovarian cystitis
	Sulfasalazine	Inhibits IL-2 production	Nephrotoxicity, hypertension, ↑ infection risk
	Minocycline	Inhibits TNF	
	Rituximab	Inhibits pyrimidine synthesis, cellactivation and adhesion	Injection site rxn, ↑ infection risk
	Tocilizumab		Alopecia, stomatitis, abdominal pain, ↑ LFTs, hypertension
	Anakinra/canakinumab/ rilonacept	Suppress lymphocyte and leukocyte fxn	
	Abatacept	Up-regulation of IL-10 (anti-inflammatory cytokine)	Hepatitis, marrow suppression, rash diarrhea
		Inhibits B cells	GI toxicity, rash
		Inhibits IL-6	↑infection risk, infusion reaction
		Inhibits Il-1	↑infection risk, ↑ LFTs, ↑ lipids
		Inhibits costimulation of T cells	↑infection risk, Injection site rxn
			↑infection risk
Spondyloarthritis	ASA, NSAID	As above	As above
	Gold	As above	As above
	Methotrexate	As above	As above
	Sulfasalazine	As above	As above
	Infliximab/etanercept/adalumimab/ golimubab, certolizumab	As above	As above
	Ustekinumab	Inhibits Il-12	↑infections

Continued

TABLE 32.11	Therapeutic Application of Drugs in Rheumatic Diseases *(Continued)*		
Diseases	**Recommended Medications**	**Probable Mechanisms**	**Precautions**
Gout	NSAID	As above	As above
	Uricosurics (probenecid and Lesinurad)	Increases excretion of uric acid	Often need to alkalinize urine
	Allopurinol	Inhibits xanthine oxidase	Do not use with azathioprine
	Febuxostat	Inhibits xanthine oxidase	
	Colchicine	Inhibits microtubular assembly and inhibits	
	Canakinumab	lysosomal enzyme release	
	Pegloticase	Inhibits IL-1	↑infections
		Converts uric acid to allantoin	Antibody development/infusion reaction
SLE	NSAID	As above	As above
	Steroids	As above	As above
	Antimalarials	As above	As above
	Azathioprine	As above	As above
	Mycophenolate mofetil		
	Tacrolimus		
	Cyclophosphamide	As above	As above
	Rituximab		
PSS	ᴅ-Penicillamine	Unknown	As above
	Colchicine	As above	As above
DM-PM	Steroids	As above	As above
	Azathioprine	As above	As above
Primary vasculitis	Methotrexate	As above	As above
	Mycophenolate mofetil	As above	As above
	Rituximab	As above	As above
	Steroids	As above	As above
	Cyclophosphamide	As above	As above
	Rituximab	As above	As above
	Azathioprine	As above	As above
	Methotrexate	As above	As above

GI, gastrointestinal; DNA, dioxyribonucleic acid; TNF, tumor necrosis factor; SLE, systemic lupus erythematosus; PM, polymyositis; LFTs, liver function tests.

Antihyperuricemic Agents

Pain and inflammation of crystal-induced arthritis are frequently adequately controlled with NSAIDs. Although these drugs are effective in controlling symptoms, they do not alter the metabolism of the substances forming crystals, nor do they influence their excretion. Uricosuric agents like probenecid and recently FDA-approved medication, lesinurad, compete with the tubular transport mechanism for uric acid, reduce the reabsorption of uric acid, and hence increase its excretion (112). Their use is widespread, and their toxicities are well known, including nephrolithiasis, which is preventable if the urine is alkalinized and fluids are increased. Acute gout can be precipitated as the uric acid levels are lowered and GI symptoms are not infrequently seen. A second approach toward controlling serum urate levels is that of regulating production of uric acid by inhibiting xanthine oxidase. This is done by using allopurinol or febuxostat analogs of hypoxanthine. They too can precipitate an acute attack of gout and can cause xanthine renal stones. Side effects include rash and, rarely, blood dyscrasia. Febuxostat has recently been reported to be associated with increased cardiovascular events (113). Allopurinol should not be used with azathioprine. Allopurinol is an inhibitor of the principal pathway for the detoxification of azathioprine. In patients who develop a severe hypersensitivity rash to allopurinol, febuxostat is the next drug of choice.

Anticytokine Therapies

Due to the advances in molecular biology, immunology, and pharmacologic development since the early 1990s, newer treatment approaches for autoimmune diseases are now available. Biologic agents are a class of immunosuppressant medications that target or interfere with cytokine function and/or production, deplete B cells, or inhibit T-cell activation. These agents are further subdivided below based upon their specific cell or cytokine target.

TNF-Alpha Inhibitors

Etanercept (administered subcutaneously), infliximab (administered intravenously), adalimumab (administered subcutaneously), golimumab, and certolizumab function to inhibit TNF and have gained increasing popularity, as studies have shown these to be as effective, if not more effective, in preventing joint damage than methotrexate (114). Infliximab, adalimumab, golimumab, and certolizumab are monoclonal antibodies and bind to TNF-alpha. Etanercept binds to both TNF-alpha and lymphotoxin alpha, neutralizing their biologic activity. It is administered in doses of 25 mg twice weekly or 50 mg once weekly. It has been shown to be effective in RA (115), AS (116), and PSA (117). The most significant side effects include injection site reactions and infections and, to a lesser extent, development of autoantibodies. There is also some risk of lymphoproliferative disorders and, more rarely, lupus-like reactions and demyelinating disorders as well as other malignancies (118).

IL-1 Inhibitors

Anakinra (administered subcutaneously), canakinumab, and rilonacept are all inhibitors of the cytokine IL-1 through its effects on the inflammasome. These agents are approved for the treatment of autoinflammatory conditions such as cryopyrin-associated periodic syndrome (CAPS), TNF receptor-1–associated periodic fever (TRAPS), and familial Mediterranean fever, as well as second line for acute gout flares.

Anakinra is a recombinant human IL-1 receptor antagonist currently approved for the treatment of RA and autoinflammatory syndromes. Doses of 1 and 2 mg/kg were shown to make improvements in joint counts, pain scores, morning stiffness, and physician assessment of disease activity (119). Canakinumab, an anti–IL-1 beta monoclonal antibody with a longer half-life than anakinra, is approved for treatment of autoinflammatory syndromes and as a second-line treatment for acute gout flares. Rilonacept, a dimeric fusion protein, also known as IL-1 Trap, is approved for autoinflammatory conditions.

B-Cell Depletion and Inhibition

Rituximab and belimumab are two B-cell inhibitor agents. Rituximab is a monoclonal antibody directed against the extracellular domain of the CD20 antigen on B cell and initiates complement-mediated B-cell lysis. This medication has gained more popularity recently as its use has not been limited to RA alone but in refractory SLE patients, SVV, and inflammatory myopathies (120). Belimumab is an anti–B-lymphocyte stimulator (BLyS), which binds to soluble BLyS, preventing its binding and therefore stimulation of B cells. Its current use has been limited to SLE patients and is undergoing studies with other conditions like Sjögren's syndrome.

T-Cell Costimulation Inhibition

Abatacept binds to CD80/CD86 on the surface of antigen-presenting cells and inhibits T-cell activation. This agent continues to be studied, but it has shown significant promise when used in combination with methotrexate (121) for the treatment of RA and JIA.

IL-6 Inhibition

Tocilizumab is a human monoclonal antibody, which competes for both the membrane-bound and soluble forms of human IL-6 receptor, interfering with the cytokine's effects. IL-6 has both proinflammatory and anti-inflammatory effects and has been used successfully in the treatment of RA (122). Tocilizumab has recently been shown to have some benefit in Takayasu's and GCA (123).

Other Cytokine Inhibition

There are other cytokine inhibitors that have been approved in the treatment of PSA, including secukinumab (Il-17 inhibitor) and ustekinumab (Il-12/23 inhibitor) (123).

Combination Therapies

In the classic treatment paradigm for rheumatic diseases, the use of DMARDs earlier in the course of diseases has become increasingly common as has the use of these agents in combination. The benefits of using some of these combination therapies include additional therapeutic effects of drugs that may not have been fully effective as monotherapy and possible improvement in the toxicity profile as lower doses of these potentially toxic agents are needed. Traditional DMARDs can be combined with biologic agents; however, two or more biologic agents are not combined due to increased immunosuppression and increased risk for infection. Methotrexate is commonly used in combination with other DMARDs or with biologics. Often-used combinations include the following:

1. Cyclosporine and methotrexate have shown to be very safe and useful for the treatment of severe RA (124).
2. Methotrexate, HCQ, and sulfasalazine (SSF) combination therapy has shown some promise with moderate efficacy and no noted increased toxicity when compared with MTX alone or SSZ/Hcq in combination (125).
3. MTX and TNF-alpha blocking agent infliximab in a 2-year study showed good overall drug tolerance and sustained efficacy over a 2-year period (126).
4. MTX and leflunomide as a combination has shown some associated drug toxicity but good overall efficacy (102).
5. MTX with anti-TNF agent in combination with improved efficacy in RA (127).

Many other combinations of these agents have been evaluated. Some have shown promise but others have been marred by intolerable side effects.

Alternative and Complementary Medicine

The National Institutes of Health defines alternative and complementary medicine (CAM) as encompassing those treatments and health care practices that are not widely taught in medical schools, not generally used in hospitals, and not usually reimbursed by medical insurance companies. These therapies are sometimes called *unconventional therapies*, since they are outside the "mainstream of Western medicine." Often, these therapies have not undergone rigorous scientific analysis in randomized controlled trials (RCTs) (128–131). More medical schools have now introduced CAM into their curriculum (132). The term *alternative* alone has been used to refer to practices used in place of mainstream Western medicine, such as exclusive use of herbs instead of prescription drugs.

The Arthritis Foundation (AF) prefers the term *complementary medicine* for the use of unconventional therapies in arthritis that are used to support mainstream Western medicine.

There has been increasing use of CAM in the general population to treat disease. One recent study evaluated the potential economic benefit of complementary and integrative medicine (CIM) approaches to patients with rheumatic diseases (133). They found that of the 56 high-quality studies, 16 (29%) show a health improvement with cost savings for the CIM therapy versus usual care.

A 1998 review of surveys indicates use by 30% to 100% of arthritis patients (134). A 2004 study shows 90% of primary care clinic patients with arthritis use CAM, and RA patients used an average of 4.4 CAM therapies (135). A 2004 study reveals 33% of JAI patients use CAM as parents sought it for pain relief for their children (101). However, only 38% to 55% of patients reveal their use of CAM to their physicians (136). Physicians should ask patients about their use of CAM, as some treatments are contraindicated when used with conventional therapies (137). Arthritis patients and physicians have different perceptions about the usefulness of CAM. Arthritis patients generally perceive its usefulness (138). In a group of mixed arthritis patients in a 2005 review, homeopathy and acupuncture were the most used CAM types (44% and 41%). Significantly higher self-perceived efficacy scores were seen for CAM use in patients with spondyloarthropathies and OA. The lowest scores were among RA and connective tissue diseases (139). Some rheumatologists do not recommend them (140) and others do (141). The general trend is toward more approval by health care providers.

A number of practitioners and treatments are included under CAM (📶 **eTable 32-3**). The main categories are alternative healing systems; mind, body, and spirit treatments; prayer and spirituality; moving medicine; massage and touch; herbs and supplements; and miscellaneous treatments. In one study, RA patients most commonly used relaxation, glucosemine medication, and vitamin C. There was less common use of fish oil and gamma linolenic acid containing supplements. Patients used therapies to relieve pain, to prevent disease progression, and to feel better (138).

The benefit of some CAM therapies has been researched, and others have little research. Much of the older research consists of nonrandomized, noncontrolled trials. The issue of efficacy of popular CAM therapies (acupuncture, herbs of homeopathy) used by the general population has been explored in recent meta-analysis reviews of controlled trials (142–144).

There continues to be a growing interest in the use of herbal therapies in RA. A systemic review of RCTs in this area resulted in 14 such trials. There was moderate support for gamma linolenic acid (GLA) for reducing pain, tender joint count, and stiffness. Further research is needed to examine the safety and efficacy of herbal remedies (145).

A 2005 review summarizes the efficacy and toxicities of herbal remedies used in CAM therapies for rheumatic diseases. It elucidated the immune pathways through which they have anti-inflammatory and/or immunomodulatory activity, which may provide a scientific basis for efficacy. For instance, gamma linolenic acid acts as a competitive inhibitor of prostaglandin E_2 and leukotrienes (LTS). It appears to be efficacious in RA (146).

Proven benefits in noninflammatory arthritis include the following: (a) glucosamine/chondroitin decreases knee pain in OA, low level of evidence (147); (b) massage decreases insomnia, pain, fatigue, anxiety, and depression in FM, moderate level of evidence (148); and (c) acupuncture significantly decreases knee pain in OA and neck and low back pain, moderate level of evidence (149).

One study enrolled 662 participants with moderate-to-severe knee OA (147). They were randomly assigned either glucosamine (500 mg three times daily), chondroitin sulfate (400 mg three times daily), glucosamine and chondroitin sulfate combined (same doses), celecoxib (Celebrex, 200 mg once daily), or placebo. The primary outcome measure was a 20% reduction in pain scores (using the WOMAC pain scale). Function was a secondary outcome. All treatment groups improved in pain and function over the 2-year period. Clinical changes were identified as early as 24 weeks in all groups. There were no statistically significant differences among the four treatment groups, and none had a statistically significant improvement when compared with placebo.

Analysis of 17 acupuncture trials in 1997 (148) failed to show benefits of acupuncture in RA, SLE, AS, and PSS. A 2005 systematic review of studies on acupuncture and electroacupuncture for RA up to May 2005 concluded that although electroacupuncture showed significant knee pain reduction 24-hour and 4-month post treatment, the poor quality of the trials, including small sample sizes, precluded its recommendation. They further conclude, from the studies reviewed, that acupuncture has no significant effect on ESR, CPR, pain, patient global assessment, number of tender joints, general health, disease activity, and reduction of pain medications (149). A recent pilot study of two treatment groups of SLE patients (acupuncture or minimal needling) versus usual care revealed a greater than 30% improvement in pain measures in the acupuncture and minimal needling groups with no improvement in the control-usual care group (150). Low-level laser treatment decreases pain in RA in a Dutch study (151).

A cognitive-behavioral intervention (biofeedback) results in a decreased number of clinic visits and hospital days and medical costs in RA (152).

A yoga program based on upper body posture flexibility; correct hand, wrist, arm, and shoulder alignment; and stretching provided significant reduction in pain and increased grip strength in carpal tunnel syndrome (CTS), a common problem in RA (153). An NIH consensus conference in 1998 concluded that acupuncture was useful for Raynaud's (a common problem in SLE, MCTD, PSS) (154). A study by Yocum indicates biofeedback increased fingertip temperature in Raynaud's in SLE and PSS (155). Tai chi is safe in RA but benefits are not proven. A 2007 systematic review of 45 studies of tai chi for RA, up to January 2007, found only two RCTs and three nonrandomized case control trials (CCTs) meeting the Jadad score for methodologic quality. The RCTs demonstrated some positive findings for tai chi on disability index quality of life, depression, and mood but not on pain reduction. It was concluded by the author that collectively, at the current time, evidence is not convincing enough to suggest tai chi is an effective treatment for RA (156). A 1997 study indicates massage decreases pain and joint stiffness in JRA (157).

In general, diet can influence gout (158). However, there are no convincing data that diet is an effective treatment for inflammatory arthritis and no definitive evidence that diet can cure arthritis. There is some suggestive evidence that a decrease of omega fatty acids and substituting omega-3 oils may decrease pain and inflammation. Sources of omega-3 oils include cold-water oily fish, sardines, green soybeans, tofu, canola, and olive oils (130).

Most CAM therapies are low risk, but some do involve risks (130). Herbs can interfere with prescription medication. The following increase sensitivity to anticoagulants: bromelain, chondroitin, fish oil, GLA, garlic, ginkgo, ginger, ginseng, and primrose oil. Folic acid interferes with methotrexate. Ginger can increase NSAID effects. Ginseng may increase the effects of glucocorticoids and estrogens and should not be used in diabetes or with monoamine oxidase (MAO) inhibitors. Kava kava increases the effects of alcohol, sedatives, and tranquilizers. Magnesium may interfere with blood pressure medication. St. John's wort enhances the effects of narcotics, alcohol, and antidepressants and increases the risk of sunburn and can interfere with iron absorption. Valerian increases sedative effects. Zinc interferes with glucocorticoid and immunosuppressive drugs (130).

Caution should be noted in patients with inflammatory arthritis and manipulation therapy. These patients often have deranged joints that can sublux (RA, JRA) and ligamentous laxity (SLE). Patients with significant AS have rigid spines and can fracture. Those with moderate to severe osteoporosis from disease and steroids can also fracture. Spinal fractures can result in neurologic compromise. Patients with RA have C1-2 laxity or instability and can sublux with neurologic compromise.

Precautionary advice in CAM administration includes use of only sterile disposable needles and proscription of pulse electromagnetic field therapy in pregnant or cancer patients and magnets in those with implanted electronic devices or electric blankets.

Surgery: Soft Tissue and Reconstructive Procedures

Indications for surgeries in the rheumatic diseases include the restoration or preservation of joint mechanics and function and relief of pain. In general, pain relief is a more predictable outcome in arthritis surgery than is functional restoration. Contributors to functional outcome include motor strength, pain relief, postoperative complications, and participation in rehabilitation, all of which are highly variable (159).

The decision to operate on a patient with rheumatic disease requires a thorough preoperative evaluation. This must include the overall health status of the individual and identification of the medications that might increase the risk of surgical complications. This population is likely to be more than 55 years of age, have an altered immune system, and be receiving medication that could influence healing and postoperative infection control (159). Examples of these medications include steroids, nonsteroidal anti-inflammatory medications, methotrexate, and the newer cytokine inhibitors. Information about disease status and medication will help illuminate any additional risks for surgery.

Equally important is to perform a comprehensive physical examination and review of x-rays. The decision about which procedure to perform depends on properly identifying the cause of symptoms and the ability to determine whether they are likely to be correctable by the proposed procedure. Efforts to realign joints or soft tissue, although important, should be considered within the context of functional needs and symptom control. For example, pain is usually the result of joint deformity and its sequelae, but nerve entrapment, referred pain, and myopathy might need to be ruled out before surgery.

Proper identification of potential risk factors for the anesthesia, surgery, or postop course is also important. For example, C1-2 subluxation poses a significant risk for intubation. Carious teeth may increase the likelihood of developing postoperative infection. Obesity may make rehabilitation difficult and compromise the long-term outcome of surgery. These problems would need to be treated or accommodated before surgery.

Timing of surgery may be critical to outcome. For example, shoulder replacement in a patient who has had long-standing ROM deficits, in whom rotator cuff function is limited or absent, will have a poorer functional outcome than someone whose cuff is still working (159). When possible, surgery should be considered before development of significant joint contracture, muscle atrophy, and instability.

The surgical procedures relevant for joint and soft tissue management include synovectomy and joint debridement, tendon repair and realignment, osteotomy, arthrodesis, and arthroplasty. Each procedure has specific indications. Much has been written about the success of these procedures, their life expectancy, and long- and short-term complications. Rehabilitation professionals can assist in preparing patients for optimal outcomes by assisting patients to achieve a higher preoperative level of fitness, helping set realistic expectations, and educating them about health- and function-promoting behaviors (160). Data show benefits for improved postoperative strength and gait characteristics and shorter length of stay for both knee and hip arthroplasty (160,161).

Synovectomies

Synovectomies were first performed by Volkmann in 1877 for tuberculosis of the knee. Today, they are occasionally performed on patients with RA, most commonly to relieve pain and inflammation associated with chronic swelling uncontrolled by medication; to retard the progression of joint destruction, which is a controversial issue; and to prevent and retard tendon rupture. Other indications include the alleviation of decreased ROM caused by very hypertrophied synovial tissue and denervation effect (162).

Synovectomies are usually performed on the knee and wrist and may be performed by arthrotomy or arthroscopy. They are most frequently done in hemophilic arthropathy, for pigmented villonodular synovitis, or early RA. Synovectomy using radioactive intra-articular Yttrium-90 is therapeutic in a substantial proportion of patients with osteoarthritic knee pain and synovial inflammation. Clinical improvement is inversely related to radiographic knee damage (163).

Tenosynovectomy is most frequently performed for the extensor tendons of the hand. Regrowth of synovium commonly occurs postoperatively, so the procedure is not a curative one. Often local management using intra-articular injections of long-acting corticosteroids is tried, along with splinting of the joint when feasible and education to help develop alternative strategies for overuse (162).

Tendon Surgery

Tendon surgery is common in inflammatory disease. Frequent indications for surgery include repair of ruptured extensor tendons, realignment of tendons of the hand, synovectomies for tendons with severe tenosynovitis, and reanastomosis following tendon ruptures (Achilles and patellar tendons), and tendon releases for intrinsic tightness (164).

Arthrodesis

Arthrodesis is performed less often today than in the past because of the popularity and success of joint replacement. It may still be the best procedure to eradicate resistant infection that has destroyed significant bone. The stability provided by an arthrodesis should be permanent. Adolescents and young adults with many more years of activity might well be considered for an arthrodesis in selected instances rather than a joint replacement, which often does not stand the stress placed on it by a young, vigorous patient. Arthrodesis for patients with arthritis is usually limited to the wrist, interphalangeal (IP) joints of the hand, first metacarpal phalangeal (MCP) joint, subtalar joints, and vertebral bodies (165).

The triple arthrodesis remains one of the best procedures for reconstructing the hindfoot and restoring a pain-free, functional foot (166). Postoperative rehabilitation for this procedure requires 6 to 12 weeks of non–weight bearing, for which a roll-about can be prescribed for mobility (167). The roll-about is an ambulation aid, similar to a scooter, mounted 22 in. above the floor on four small wheels. It has a handle, a hand brake, and a padded shelf on which the leg is placed at 90 degrees of knee flexion. It is propelled by the nonoperative lower extremity and permits a reasonably rapid ambulation speed. The next level of independence is the cast boot and then a shoe with a custom insert and a rocker sole that assist in push-off. Somewhat more controversial is knee arthrodesis, a procedure that is rarely done but is occasionally suggested for the very young and highly mobile patient.

Common indications for arthrodesis of a joint are to relieve persistent pain, to provide stability where there is mechanical destruction of a joint, and to halt progress of the disease (e.g., infection, RA). Joints should be fused in optimal functional position (165,166). Contraindications for arthrodesis include significant bilateral joint disease. Joint replacement is indicated more in this instance and arthrodesis of the same joint on the contralateral side.

JOINT REPLACEMENTS

There have been several important trends recently in joint replacement. The first is that arthroplasty is being used successfully in younger patients. Additionally, postoperative length of stay has dropped dramatically, with immediate weight bearing for total hip arthroplasty (THA) and early rehabilitation.

Upper Extremity

Upper extremity joint replacements have become more common today (168). Patients with RA, JRA, OA, and AN in SLE may require joint replacement. Common indications for replacement are persistent pain despite adequate medical and rehabilitative management, loss of critical motion in the involved joint, and loss of functional status. The main contraindications for joint replacement are inadequate bone stock and periarticular support, serious medical risk factors, and presence of significant infection. Other contraindications include lack of patient motivation to cooperate in a postoperative rehabilitation program and inability of the procedure to increase the patient's total functional level (169).

Wrist arthroplasty is recommended for those with adequate bone stock, who have relatively low use requirements. Loosening over time is common (170). MCP arthroplasty is the procedure of choice, despite the relative frequency of subluxation and dislocation. Surgery performed before MCP dislocation usually has a better outcome (171).

Elbow surgery is usually restricted to radial head excision and arthroscopic synovectomy. Results from these procedures deteriorate over time (172). Elbow replacements have been shown to be effective in reducing pain and in improving ROM in pronation/supination, though improvement in flexion/extension is modest (173). Total elbow replacement has been recently used for patients with inflammatory arthritis with good success. Patients have noted substantial reduction in pain

and improved functional ROM (174). Excision of the radial head, however, remains one of the best procedures for pain reduction and improvement in elbow ROM.

Shoulder arthroplasty has been shown to be beneficial in relieving pain. Older patients have better function and longer-lasting results than younger patients. Those with rotator cuff tears have 33% to 50% return of ROM following surgery, which is half of what those without significant tears have (175). Shoulder replacement arthroplasty has been an excellent operation for pain relief. Long-term reports suggest it is also associated with good functional outcome when rotator cuff function is intact (176). The shoulder is stiff, but flexion and abduction can be performed (<50 degrees) using scapulothoracic movement. The best predictor of postoperative motion is preoperative motion (177). Significant observation of respiratory status postoperatively is critical (178).

Indication for fusion of the cervical spine in patients with RA remains somewhat controversial. There is agreement that pain unresponsive to nonsurgical treatment, cord compression, and peripheral sensory and/or motor loss are indications for cervical spine stabilization and/or cord decompression. Some studies suggest that early intervention is associated with better neurologic outcome. Instability of more than 10 mm at the atlantoaxial joint, or greater than 4 mm of basilar invagination, suggests the need for spinal stabilization (178).

Lower Extremity

Total hip replacement surgery has been performed in the United States for more than 30 years. More than 120,000 hip replacements are done annually, and function remains good 25 years after surgery (179). Hip surgeries are no longer limited to patients more than 60 years of age. Infection rates have been dramatically reduced to less than 1% (141). Loosening of the prosthesis is the reason for long-term failure. The acetabular component is more likely to loosen than the femoral, even in younger patients (180).

Total hip arthroplasty offers patients with RA, SLE (avascular necrosis), and AS pain relief and improved function. The decision about whether to offer a cemented or cementless prosthesis is usually based on the age and the functional requirements of the population to be treated. The older (more than 70 years of age) patients most frequently receive a cemented prosthesis, which provides good, immediate stability. The cementless prosthesis is associated with better preservation of bone but may be accompanied with persistent thigh pain.

There has been a significant change in technique for THA toward a direct anterior approach (DA), as compared with a posterolateral approach. A prospective, randomized study examined the very early outcome of THA performed through DA versus a posterolateral approach. Patients receiving DA had significantly higher functional scores at days 1 and 2, week 6, week 12, and 6 months. The difference in functional scores leveled out at 6 months (181).

One study reports a comparison of costs and postoperative care utilization between the anterior surgical approach and the more traditional posterolateral approach. The difference between the two groups is explained by a variety of factors including the following: "physician-led patient-focused care pathways, care coordination, rapid rehabilitation protocols, perioperative pain management protocols, and patient education are integral for effective patient care" (182).

Patients are given prophylactic antibiotics before surgery and low-molecular-weight heparin the night of surgery and for the duration of the hospital stay. Antibiotic prophylaxis is recommended for dental work. A good discussion by Sledge of the operative and postoperative course is recommended to the reader (182).

Total knee replacement surgery is commonly used for patients with bi- and unicompartmental joint space destruction, persistent pain from poor joint mechanics, and functional loss. Long-term complications tend to result from uneven patellar surface wear and loosening. Total knee arthroplasty has provided excellent pain relief and good functional outcomes for arthritics. Studies report prosthetic longevity with sustained, excellent function for more than 12 years (183). Problems with the patellar components are the most significant cause of knee joint replacement failure.

Ankle replacement arthroplasties have not been demonstrated to be effective over time. Loosening remains the most serious complication (184). Those patients with very limited mobility and functional requirements may be reasonable candidates for this procedure. Forefoot arthroplasty with total resection of the metatarsal heads is an excellent pain-relieving procedure. This enables patients to walk on a pain-free foot, although the toes become floppy, the foot size is smaller, and the mechanics of push-off, which are usually improved from the painful state, are not returned to normal. Use of a roller sole helps correct the dynamic abnormality (185).

Preoperative Rehabilitation Management

To maximize postoperative gains, preoperative rehabilitation interventions are desirable. These interventions include teaching the patient crutch walking with the appropriate type of crutch, weight reduction for the obese patient, and strengthening of the quadriceps before knee replacement and the hip abductors before hip surgery. Orienting patients to the types of pain they may experience postoperatively—such as acute, incisional, muscle strain or fatigue, and nerve root irritation—may help allay fears about the stability of the hip. Descriptions of the usual course of recovery may also prepare them for what to expect (160).

Postoperative Rehabilitation Management

The rehabilitation management goals of a total joint replacement program are to relieve pain, to redevelop comfortable musculoskeletal function, and to use joint protection techniques to avoid overstressing the prosthetic joint.

The postoperative management of hip replacement is unique to individual orthopedic surgeons and the needs of the patient. There are many published guidelines for postoperative management; however, the program usually includes the following (186). Bed mobility and ROM are started immediately with ankle pumps and isometric exercise to the quadriceps. The patients are usually stood by the bedside with full weight bearing and crutches if the hip is cemented or partial weight bearing if it is uncemented. Patients are placed in an abduction sling and told to restrict hip flexion to less than 90 degrees and to limit adduction and internal rotation (IR). While in bed, they are to sleep in a supine position with a pillow between their knees for a month. They need to be carefully monitored for signs of deep venous thrombosis and fever, excessive wound drainage, and/or infection. Patients should be instructed to use an elevated toilet seat and a high chair to minimize hip flexion. Discharge from the hospital is usually on the fifth day, provided they can get in and out of bed independently, walk independently with crutches or walker, and manage stairs. Key exercises include quadriceps, hip abductor, and hip flexor strengthening. Patients should expect to use a cane until hip abductor strength is in the four range and there is no Trendelenburg's sign. Many orthopedists permit return to full activity, including recreational tennis, cycling, and gardening (187).

There are many referenced guidelines for the postoperative management of knee replacement. Recommendations from the Cleveland Clinic include the following procedures (188): begin knee ROM immediately postoperatively, often with the aid of a continuous passive motion machine. Total weight bearing (to tolerance) with crutches and ad-lib ambulation are started on the first postoperative day using crutches or a walker. Active-assistive flexion is the cornerstone of management and usually needs to be done under supervision of the physical therapist. Knee replacement patients, unlike those undergoing hip replacement, frequently need some additional rehabilitation requiring admission to a rehabilitation hospital or step-down facility.

The extent of rotator cuff repair and function in part dictates the nature of the rehabilitation program, but the postoperative management of total shoulder replacement usually includes the following: immobilization of the shoulder for 2 to 8 weeks in an airplane splint with the shoulder in 80 degrees of flexion, 70 degrees of abduction, and 5 degrees of IR. Passive motion through range in excess of where the limb is in the splint is performed in the supine position. At the eighth to tenth postoperative day, active-assistive shoulder exercise is begun in the sitting position to 110 degrees of flexion and 20 degrees of external rotation (ER). At 6 weeks after surgery, active, unrestricted ROM is permitted, sometimes using an overhead pulley for assistance to end range. Lifting up to 10 lb is permitted (189).

GENERAL REHABILITATION INTERVENTIONS

Rehabilitation treatment plans must be individualized for the patient's needs; they should be practical, economical, and valued by the patient to enhance compliance. Treatment should begin early in the disease process to help prevent impairment and functional decline and so that the patient identifies this as part of the overall management plan. There is scientific and clinical rationale for the use of some specific rehabilitation treatments; others are based on clinical judgment. Rehabilitative rheumatology treatments and techniques must be monitored carefully, and periodic reevaluation of the patient with adjustments in treatment should be made.

Rest

Three forms of rest have been used by persons with arthritis: complete bed rest, local rest of a joint or joints with splints or casts, and short rest periods of 15 to 30 minutes dispersed throughout the day.

In the 1960s and 1970s, the literature revealed studies supporting bed rest for up to 4 weeks for persons with RA to decrease the number of inflamed joints, joint stiffness, and disease activity (83). However, systemic rest has many adverse effects, including muscle weakness and bone loss. Currently, the approach to the management of RA has changed. Much more adequate pharmacologic management of disease activity exists, such as early treatment with DMARDs. In addition, the literature clearly supports mobilizing and exercising patients with inactive and subacute inflammatory arthritis and encouraging them to be proactive in being active, maintaining fitness and healthy lifestyle behaviors through exercise and symptom control throughout the disease course (83). However, a Cochrane review suggests that there is little convincing evidence that physical activity and exercise for chronic pain is effective. This is largely due to small sample sizes and potentially underpowered studies. A number of studies had adequately long interventions, but planned follow-up was limited to less than 1 year in all but six reviews. There were some favorable effects in reduction in pain severity and improved physical function, though the findings were inconsistent among the studies and were usually for small number of patients (190).

Local rest of acutely or subacutely inflamed joints at night with nonfunctional resting splints and during the day with functional splints reduces inflammation and pain and may help prevent contracture. Immobilization of the wrist for painful periarticular syndromes (e.g., de Quervain's syndrome and CTS) is useful to relieve pain. One ROM exercise daily for joints during rest of 2 weeks' duration is not noted to cause an adverse effect. In terms of muscle effect, 4 weeks of knee immobilization in normal subjects causes a 21% decrease in muscle mass determined by computerized tomography and biopsy (191). Generally, it is recommended that short rest periods during the day of 20 to 30 minutes along with appropriate local splinting are the appropriate way to manage patients with inflammatory arthritis to help control joint inflammation and fatigue. Some workplace sites now provide rest areas for persons complete with cots. Negotiation with employers may also result in a person with an office being allowed to keep a small cot or sofa for napping.

Exercise

Arthritis commonly produces decreased biomechanical integrity of joints and their surrounding structures, which results in decreased joint motion, muscle atrophy, weakness, joint effusion, pain, instability, energy-inefficient gait patterns, and altered joint-loading responses (192,193).

Arthritis patients may lose muscle strength and bulk because of inactivity. A muscle can lose 30% of its bulk in a week and up to 5% of its strength a day when maintained at strict bed rest (194). Other factors contributing to loss of strength are myositis, myopathy secondary to steroids (195), inhibition of muscle contraction due to joint effusion (196), and direct effects of the disease itself on muscle. For example, in RA, some destruction of muscle fibers occurs as well as intermuscular and perimuscular adhesions, which may impair blood flow. Muscle fascicles adhere to one another, and the entire muscle may adhere to the intermuscular septum and perimuscular fascia, causing inhibition of muscle contraction and normal movement (192) with RA, PM, SLE, and PSS and resulting in weak, painful, and easily fatigable muscle. Reduced strength as determined by isometric testing has been documented in the quadriceps even in mild RA (197,198), PM (199), and JRA (200). Isokinetic strength testing has shown deficits in

the quadriceps in patients with RA (197) and DM-PM (201). Patients with RA, AS, SLE, JRA, DM, and JDM have been found to have decreased aerobic capacity (202–206).

The biomechanical advantage of joints is compromised by weak muscles. Normally, muscles function to provide postural stability and distribute forces of impact and stress across joints during activity. Normal joint function requires that muscles contract and relax synchronously. Atrophic muscles around joints do not coordinate well and are deficient in both static endurance and strength. There is decreased tone and increased spasm in muscle surrounding arthritic joints, resulting in less coordinated motion of the joint (204).

Exercise programs for patients with arthritis (🛜 eTable 32-4) have been shown to produce a variety of benefits, mainly in improving strength and function without convincing evidence about its impact on disease activity (207) (see Chapter 49). Some of these benefits have not yet reached a level of evidence to support their effectiveness and hence are areas for future research if these recommendations are to be supported as part of the development of formal guidelines. Nonetheless, they remain commonly used especially in people with RA. These include re-educating muscle to strengthen and enable improved static and dynamic muscle endurance (208–212) and utilizing overall conditioning exercise to improve functional activity and leisure (such as dance) (213–216). Some data suggest that exercise is associated with a reduction in joint inflammation (217,218) and possibly immune status (219,220). General benefits of exercise following both aerobic and strength training, in patients with rheumatic diseases, include increases in overall aerobic capacity and strength (221), assistance with weight reduction (222), improvement in metabolic status, and anabolic effects on muscle (223).

Exercise prescriptions should be designed to improve function that patients value. Once these goals are set, limits need to be established that preserve joint function and do not unduly fatigue inflamed muscle and joint structures. Exercise should be performed with proper joint support, after reduction of joint effusion is accomplished, and attention should be given to level of aerobic capacity (204). Patients with collagen diseases often have cardiac abnormalities (224), which should be evaluated before initiating an exercise program and regularly. Exercise programs for arthritis patients should specify whether exercise is aerobic, strengthening, or aimed at building muscle endurance. Prescriptions should specify the muscles that need strengthening; the type, intensity, duration, and frequency of exercise to be used; and the specific precautions (204). It is helpful and generally felt to improve compliance if the patient is provided with a written exercise program and verbal directions if the program is to be performed at home. Patients who exercise as part of a group or with a partner are more likely to adhere to a given program. The patient or family, or both, should be told the purpose of the exercises.

An exercise program should be progressive. It should start with relieving pain of the involved joints with appropriate modalities and/or pain medications. Once comfortable, a combination of stretching, strengthening, and fitness training should be initiated in a progressive manner. A program that shows results in terms of functional activity is best. Isometric exercise is usually the initial approach, with the addition of an isotonic exercise program for muscle endurance and for strengthening if joints permit. Isotonic low-resistive and low-weight progressive resistive exercise, as well as low-force isokinetic exercise, can be used without joint damage. Incorporating exercise into recreational activities may be the treatment of choice for the patient because of its inherent appeal and the fact that it is done outside of a medical setting. Depending on joint integrity (i.e., gardening, swimming, mall walking, low-impact dancing, table tennis), a variety of options are safe and effective for those with rheumatic diseases (204).

Passive Exercise

Passive exercise is beneficial for patients with severe muscle weakness due to PM or neuropathic disease associated with stroke, peripheral neuropathy, and vasculitis. Patients with acute joint flares should passively or actively move the acute joint through the range once or twice a day, to prevent motion loss. Passive exercise may also increase intra-articular pressure in the presence of joint effusion and has been associated with rupture of the joint capsule with large effusions (204).

Active Exercise

Active resistive exercise uses three types of muscle contraction:
1. Isometric or static contraction, which is highly suited for arthritis patients with mechanically deranged joints
2. Isotonic or dynamic contraction, which is most suited for patients without acutely inflamed or biomechanically deranged joints because it stresses the joint throughout its ROM
3. Isokinetic dynamic contraction, which in most cases is not recommended for arthritis patients

Strengthening Exercise

Strengthening of a muscle in arthritis patients may be achieved via isometric, isotonic, or isokinetic exercise. The degree of inflammation and disease stage should be evaluated before making an exercise choice.

Isometric (i.e., static) exercise is ideally suited for restoring and maintaining strength in patients with muscle atrophy from rheumatic diseases and steroids and for the recovery phase of DM-PM and for patients with significant biomechanically compromised joints. Machover and Sapecky demonstrated a significant increase (27%) in quadriceps strength in patients with RA on an isometric strengthening program (225). This program consisted of three daily maximal contractions held for 6 seconds, with 20 seconds of rest between each. The knee was in 90 degrees of flexion. The opposite quadriceps had a crossover effect with a 17% increase in strength. A similar program for a PM patient increased strength (199). To decrease force across a joint, a less than maximal contraction should be used. To affect strengthening, this should not be less than two thirds of the maximal contraction. The patient should be instructed how to do this.

An advantage of isometrics is that muscle tension can be generated with minimal joint stress. Pain has been reported with maximal contraction. One study of adults by Gnootveld and associates indicates that isometric quadriceps exercise of inflamed knee joints in RA yields increased oxidative damage to hyaluronate and glucose, determined by analyzing synovial fluid 1 hour following exercise (226). Therefore, isometric exercise in an inflamed joint is not recommended.

With isometric exercise, muscle strength is only achieved at the angle at which the muscle is trained. With isotonic exercise, resistance is constant throughout the range, hence strengthens.

In addition, strength increases with isometric training are not fully transferable to isotonic tasks. Therefore, the addition of isotonic exercise to the arthritic program is warranted where appropriate. DeLorme progressive resistive exercises with high loads and low repetitions build strength but put considerable stress across joints. A low-load resistive muscle training program in functional class II and III RA (12-week circuit weight bearing with light loads/high repetitions three times a week) resulted in significant improvement in self-reported joint count (number of tender and inflamed joints), the HAQ, grip strength, and knee extension strength. A 6-week high-intensity, progressive resistive strength training program in well-controlled RA patients resulted in significant improvements in strength, pain, and fatigue without exacerbating disease activity or joint pain (227). A recent study of moderate dynamic resistive exercise (with loads of 50% to 70% of repetition maximum) twice a week along with recreational activities showed a significant improvement in strength, disease activity (HAQ), and walking speed. Bone mineral density (BMD) of the spine was not significantly increased (212).

A comparison study of high-intensity aerobic bike exercise (70% to 85% of age-predicted heart rate) combined with full-weight-bearing exercises versus three combined low-intensity strengthening programs (group, individual, or home-based ROM and isometric) resulted in significant increases in aerobic capacity, muscle strength, and ROM that differed significantly from these changes in the other three groups (211). Strength increases were seen in PM patients on an isotonic resistive machine program (205,221,228).

Dynamic isotonic high-resistive exercise has the potential of exacerbating inflammation in general, which can increase muscle fatigue and joint pain, and secondarily decreases joint ROM. Progressive resistive high-intensity isotonic exercise and isokinetic exercise are not recommended for those with arthritis. Moderate-intensity isotonic programs can be used in selected cases. Joints should be nonactive and biomechanically intact. Strength gains with isokinetic exercise do not exceed those obtained with low-weight, isotonic strengthening programs, and equipment is expensive and only available in a clinic (229).

Isokinetic testing of strength has been done in a 1990 study of RA patients with mild joint disease (197) and in PM patients (201,230) without deleterious effects. An isokinetic strengthening program used in RA patients increased strength. Complications included several joint flares and a ruptured Baker cyst (231). A 1994 study on a small group of RA patients showed that isokinetic strength training at four speeds for 3 weeks significantly increased strength without joint flares (232). A 1999 study revealed increased knee flexion torques at 60 and 90 degrees per second in RA patients on a knee flexion/extensor training program. The patients had nonacute RA (233). An isokinetic program with medium (120 degrees/s) velocity is most likely used in RA patients. Low velocities (30 to 90 degrees/s) produce high torque around joints and are best avoided. Isokinetic exercise should not be used in arthritic patients with joint effusion, Baker cyst, ligamentous laxity, acute joints, or joint replacements. A study of isokinetic exercise in six PM-DM patients demonstrated a significant increase in strength without significant creatine phosphokinase (CPK) increases (234). See ᯤ eTable 32-4 and Table 32-12 for specific exercise regimens.

TABLE 32-12   Exercise Type Recommendations for Specific Joint Conditions and Functional Level

Joint Activity	Condition Exercise Type											
	ROM		Stretch		Isometric		Isotonic		Isokinetic		Aerobic	
	Full	Partial	Gentle	Full	Sub Max	Max	Low R	Moderate R	Low R	Moderate R	Low I	Moderate I
Acute	+	−	−	−	−	−	−	−	−	−	−	−
Subacute	+	−	+	−	+	−	+	−	−	−	+	−
Chronic (inactive)	+	−	−	+	−	+	−	+	+	+	+	+
Functional level												
I	+	−	+	−	+	+	+	+	+	+	+	+
II	+	−	−	+	+	+	+	+	+	+	+	+
III	+	+	+	+	+	−	−	−	−	−	+	−
IV		+	+	−	+	−	−	−	−	−	−	−
Biomechanical level joint												
Normal	+	−	−	+	+	+	+	+	+	+	+	+
Mild	+	−	−	+	+	+	+	−	+	−	+	+
Moderate	+	+	+	−	+		Gravity	−	−	−	Pool	−
Severe	−	+	−	−	+		−	−	−	−	−	−
Joint effusion												
0	+	−	+	−	+	+	+	+	+	+	+	+ (Pool)
Mild	+	−	+	−	+	+	+	−	−	−	(Bike)	+ (Pool)
Moderate	−	+	−	−	+	−	−	−	−	−	−	−
Severe	−	+	−	−	+	−	−	−	−	−	−	−
Joint replacement												
	−	+	+	−	+	−	←Check with orthopedic→	−	−	+	Pool	
Osteoporosis												
Mild	+	−	−	+	+	+	+	+	+	+	+	+
Moderate	+	−	+	−	+	−	+	−	−	−	+	−
Severe	−	+	−	−	+	−	−	−	−	−	Pool	−

ROM, range of motion; R, resistance; I, intensity.

Endurance

Patients with systemic rheumatic disease have overall limited endurance, and their ability to continue static or dynamic tasks is often impaired. Endurance exercise can lead to an increased functional level in RA patients (235,236).

In 1981, Nordemar described RA patients who were trained 4 to 8 years on a bicycle ergometer at home and a self-directed exercise program consisting of jogging, skiing, swimming, and cycling (237). He found improved ADL performance in the exercised group as well as less progression of x-ray changes in arthritis, more improvement in hamstring strength, and less sick leave (238). Harkcom and colleagues (239) also reported benefit from aerobic exercise in RA patients. Minor and colleagues showed that aerobic exercises increase aerobic capacity in both RA and OA patients. Decreased joint counts for pain and swelling also have been associated with aerobic programs for RA patients (216,218,235). Exercise programs using different combinations of ROM and strengthening and aerobic exercises on land and in the pool have been beneficial in RA (193).

Van den Ende in a 2000 Cochrane database study reviewed dynamic aerobic training and its effect on improving joint mobility, muscle strength, aerobic capacity, and function in RA patients. Negative effects such as increased pain, disease activity, and radiologic progression were also assessed. Selection criteria included randomized control trials on the effect of dynamic exercise therapy, an exercise program of at least 60% maximal heart rate for 20 minutes at least two times a week for 6 weeks. Only 6 of 30 controlled trials met the criteria. It was concluded that dynamic exercise has a positive effect on physical capacity as measured by aerobic capacity and strength. Further research is needed on the positive effect on functional ability and radiologic progression (240). A RCT of dynamic training revealed RA women on low-dose steroid on a dynamic weight-bearing program showed positive effects on physical function and fitness level and BMD with no disease exacerbation (241). Another trial reports the effect of intensive exercise in patients with active RA (208). A 2008 Cochrane database review summarizes dynamic exercise effect in RA (242).

A well-accepted, positive effect of aerobic exercise is the improvement in cardiovascular health. Mortality risk for patients with inflammatory rheumatic diseases has been associated with cardiovascular disease, which now adds an additional benefit for exercise in this population (243).

Recent studies have demonstrated that aerobic exercise has been associated with reduction in inflammatory biomarkers in the population with obesity, which may be of significance in the rheumatic disease population with obesity (244). High-intensity interval training (HIIT) has recently been introduced into fitness training for a variety of people in various diagnostic groups. Recent reports suggest it is a safe and effective treatment for people with RA and adult-onset juvenile arthritis (245).

Wiesinger reported improved physical fitness and muscle strength with short-term 6-week and long-term aerobic programs in DM-PM (230). Children with JRA can improve their aerobic endurance with a weight-bearing fitness program without disease exacerbation (246). SLE patients have been shown to increase their aerobic capacity by 20% on a bike aerobic program (162). A 12-week three times per week multimodal exercise program (aerobic stretching and pulmonary exercises vs. a medication-only control group) shared significant improvement in spinal mobility, work capacity, and chest expansion (247).

Bone mineralization is thought to be partially dependent on muscle contraction. Exercise has been shown to have a positive effect on bone mineralization in postmenopausal women (248). Patients with rheumatic disease develop osteopenia from disuse, medication, and calcium and collagen metabolism abnormalities. Most studies that support the positive effects of exercise in these areas cite the use of isotonic and some resistive exercises (211,212). Sinaki and Grubbs showed in a study that back extensor exercise can increase spinal bone density in postmenopausal women (249). This type of exercise may be useful for rheumatic disease patients.

Stretching Exercises

Stretching may be used to prevent contractures and maintain or restore ROM by breaking capsular adhesions (250). These exercises must be graded according to the degree of inflammation, pain present, and pain tolerance of the patient. Heat may be used to increase collagen extensibility and cold to decrease pain before stretching exercises. Stretching to preserve or increase ROM should not be performed if there is acute inflammation, because it may increase it.

Active-assistive stretching can be used for maintaining or increasing ROM when the problem is subacute and pain is decreased (251). The patient initiates muscle contraction, and the therapist or an assistive device serves as an aide. Forceful stretching should be avoided in the presence of a large joint effusion because capsular rupture may occur.

Active stretching is performed in the absence of pain and inflammation to maintain ROM. It may be facilitated by the use of pulleys. Devices may be needed to facilitate stretching for hip flexion contractures in JRA or knee flexion contractures in RA. Passive stretching has been found useful in increasing hip and shoulder motion in AS patients (252).

Aquatic Therapy

The benefits of performing exercise in a pool include elimination of gravity and the positive effect of water buoyancy, which may result in decreased joint compression and pain (see Chapter 50). Active stretching exercises in a pool are excellent (253,254). This may further result in increased muscle relaxation. In addition, a greater level of aerobic exercise may be tolerated in the water than on land. Therefore, therapeutic pool therapy may be most useful for those with moderate to severe arthritis, with recent joint replacement, with AS, and with any cardiopulmonary compromise.

Specifically, Danneskiold-Samsoe and colleagues have shown in a study on RA patients that isometric and isokinetic quadriceps strength can be increased by 38% and 16%, respectively, by adhering to a 2-month pool exercise program when compared with pretreatment values. A significant increase in aerobic

capacity also can be obtained in RA patients on a pool program (255). AS patients with low vital capacity (700, 1,500 cm^3) have been shown capable of undergoing pool therapy programs without untoward effect (217). In a RCT, it was demonstrated that combined spa-exercise therapy is effective in patients with AS (256). Exercise tolerance appears related to pulmonary function in these patients (257).

Recreational Exercise

Patients with rheumatic diseases often want to participate in recreational exercise programs (216). Care must be taken to advise the patient which activities or programs would be beneficial for him or her and to relate the use of recreational exercise to the condition of the joints (i.e., inflamed, subacute, chronic mechanical derangement problems). In exercise gyms, the use of preset rate-limited devices at high torque speeds of muscle contraction against high resistive forces on machines should be avoided. Light weights (3 lb or less) and minimal repetitions (10 or less) on isotonic machines are permitted for patients with RA with no inflammation, minimal x-ray changes, and no ligamentous laxity. If isotonic weight lifting is performed, it generally should be with light weights (1 to 3 lb) and 10 repetitions. A short arc of motion can be used to decrease joint pain. Swimming is an excellent form of isotonic exercise for arthritis patients because gravity is eliminated and ROM of the joints is less painful. ROM and stretching exercises and pool jogging or walking are good. Local chapters of the AF have aquatic courses for arthritic patients and often make heated pools available. The YMCA also has special pool exercise programs. Adaptive devices and special handgrips are available to help patients in specific sports (e.g., table tennis, golf, gardening, bowling).

Dance

Dance has become a popular recreational activity for patients with arthritis. It can help increase joint motion, muscle strength, and aerobic capacity. Van Deusen and Harlowe describe the efficacy of a ROM dance program for adults with RA (258). Other, more formal and therapeutic dance programs, such as Educize, have shown increased strength, flexibility, and aerobic capacity along with decreased joint pain and depression (236). Formal dance-based aerobic programs for RA have shown positive effects: (a) changes in fatigue, tension, and aerobic capacity; (b) positive changes in fatigue, depression, and anxiety with increased aerobic capacity in some patients with class III disease; and (c) significantly improved locomotor ability by gait test in class III RA (213,215,258,259).

Jogging

Dry land jogging, which involves repetitive joint motion and offers little chance for increase in strength, is not recommended if arthritis of the knee or hip or ankle is present. Data supporting running or jogging as a cause of OA or even a contributor to progression are not uniformly consistent. There are several recent reviews addressing this issue, all concluding there is need for more data (260–262).

It is a good rule that a patient should be made as strong as possible by isometrics, and strength and local muscle endurance increased by light isotonic exercises, before recreational exercise is begun. Indications of excess therapeutic and recreational exercise include postexercise pain at 2 or more hours, undue fatigue, increased weakness, decreased ROM, and joint swelling. If these occur, the program should be adjusted (262).

Treatment with Heath and Cold Modalities

Therapeutic heat can be applied with a number of devices and techniques (see Chapter 51). The effect on the tissue, location, surface area, depth of the tissue, and acuteness or chronicity of the arthritis must be considered in the selection of modalities.

Most investigations on the use of superficial and deep heat and cold modalities have produced conflicting data. Recent formal literature reviews utilizing the Cochrane databases and specific study selection criteria have been done for treating RA with thermotherapy (heat and cold) (263), balneotherapy (264), and therapeutic ultrasound (265). Only RCTs were selected for data analysis. Problems with poor methodologic quality and inadequate statistical analysis and outcome measures often hindered pooling data and made conclusions about treatment efficacy difficult. The general conclusions from the thermotherapy reviews indicate no effect on objective measures of disease activity (inflammation, pain, x-ray–measured joint destruction) of either ice versus control or heat versus control. Ninety-four percent of patients reported they preferred heat therapy to no therapy. There was no difference in patient preference for heat or cold, and no harmful side effects were noted.

The balneotherapy review indicates 10 studies report positive benefits, but the findings should be viewed with caution because of methodologic flaws. The review suggested that ultrasound (US) alone on the hand increases grip strength. It did not conclude that the combination of US with exercise, faradic current, or wax therapy was beneficial.

Heat

Superficial heat has been used for hundreds of years for pain relief in patients with arthritis. Patients report that warm baths, heated pools, hot packs, and warm mineral springs provide relief of joint pain and stiffness. Studies (266) indicate that superficial heat applied to patients with arthritis increases both skin and joint temperature in inflammatory arthritis. Painful stimuli, apprehension, alarm, or smoking lowers skin temperature and elevates knee joint temperature, as do active and passive exercise.

When joint temperature is increased from 30.5°C to 36°C, as it is in active RA, collagenase found in rheumatoid synovium is four times as active, resulting in lysis of cartilage (267). Increasing joint temperatures increases the metabolic rate and may increase inflammation and joint destruction (267). Mainardi and associates (268) found no increase and no decrease in joint destruction and inflammatory activity in the hand in RA with the use of superficial heat.

Heat affects the viscoelastic properties of collagen. As tension is applied, stretch is affected and an increase of creep (i.e., the plastic stretch of ligamentous structures placed under tension) occurs. Heat may enhance the efficacy of stretching if applied to appropriately chosen joints.

Both superficial and deep heat can raise the threshold for pain, producing sedation and analgesia by acting on free nerve endings of both peripheral nerves and gamma fibers of muscle spindles (269,270).

Cold

Cold modalities such as air or ice decrease skin, muscle, and joint temperature in arthritis patients (266). The application of cold to rheumatoid joints may therefore inhibit collagenase activity in the synovium. Some clinical studies have shown greater and more prolonged relief of pain with ice than deep or superficial heat in patients with RA (271). Other investigations found the increase of knee joint ROM to be the same with either ice or superficial heat applied daily for 5 days, with a 9-day interval between the two treatments (272).

Cold decreases muscle spasticity by direct action on the muscle spindle activity (273) and raises the pain threshold. Cold should not be used in patients with Raynaud's phenomenon, cold hypersensitivity, cryoglobulinemia, or paroxysmal cold hemoglobinuria. The abrupt application of cold causes discomfort and produces a stressful response.

In treating the acutely inflamed or subacute joint, the goal is pain relief. One is careful not to use interventions that may increase the metabolic rate and secondarily increase inflammation. The use of cold seems most logical because it can decrease the pain threshold, can relax surrounding spastic muscles, and is associated with decreased joint temperature, collagenase, and cell count in the joint fluid (274).

Later in the subacute period, when inflammatory pain is subsiding and stiffness is present, and the patient may have lost some ROM, either cold or superficial heat is appropriate and the patient should decide based on what is most convenient, economical, and effective.

Orthotics

Splints and orthotics are used to unweight joints, stabilize joints, decrease joint motion, support joints in a position of maximal function, and increase joint motion (i.e., dynamic splint) (see also Chapter 57). Splints may be prefabricated but are best when molded to fit the individual patient.

Upper Extremities

Orthotics for the upper extremities are mainly confined to the wrist and hand and include resting splints, functional wrist splints, thumb post splints, ring splints, and dynamic splints. Both level 1 and 2 evidence supports their use for pain reduction and improved prehension. In particular, thumb post splints are among the most effective (275–277).

Resting splints immobilize the hand and wrist and are used at night for patients with active RA, CTS, or extensor tendinitis. The role of splints in preventing deformity in RA has not yet been scientifically proven. Usual practice combines both resting and functional splints in early RA. In JRA, they probably help in delaying ulnar deviation and in reducing pain, synovitis, and edema. Functional wrist splints extend to the midpalmar crease, permit finger function, block wrist flexion, and are used for activities during periods of inflammation. They provide wrist and ligament support. A 2008 study using prefabricated working wrist splints revealed a 32% decrease in wrist pain (control group had a 17% increase in pain) (278). A functional thumb post splint may be used to relieve CMC and IP pain associated with OA. The same type of splint with a longer wrist extension is useful for de Quervain extensor tendinitis of the thumb. A functional wrist cock-up splint can help relieve pain in CTS.

Small ring splints (e.g., Bunnell orthoses, boutonniere orthoses) can reduce swan neck or boutonniere deformity. Cosmetic splints constructed of silver or gold and highlighted with semiprecious stones are available.

For patients who have had MCP replacements or who have a radial nerve neuropraxia, a dynamic outrigger splint pulls the fingers into extension, from which patients must actively work to pull into flexion. They provide gentle stretch through limited range while supporting the wrist and MTPs. Splints that realign digits to help reduce ulnar deviation are also available.

Elbow orthotics are rarely used. They may be useful in children with JRA and PM. Resting night splints may help to contain the advancement of an elbow flexion contracture. Braces with dial locks are used to increase extension during the day.

Lower Extremities

Foot and ankle orthoses are commonly used for people with rheumatic diseases (277). Those for the knee have been less successful, and there are none generally used for the hip. The advances in lighter materials for orthotics reduce energy and consumption with their use (277).

Foot/Ankle. Excess pronation at the subtalar joint, loss of the medial arch, and subtalar movement commonly seen in RA can cause pain, contribute to tarsal tunnel syndrome, and cause strain on the knee and hip. Control of pronation by bringing the calcaneus perpendicular to the floor often relieves pain and helps to balance the weight-bearing column. The first step toward control is to fit the patient with a shoe with a good heel counter and a soft or rigid orthotic insert lined with Spenco (AliMed, Dedham, MA). The sole should not be too soft. This will minimize the flotation effect on heel-strike and stance during gait and decrease stress, hypermobility, or instability at the ankle or a higher joint level. If pronation is not controlled by a shoe, a hindfoot orthotic has been shown to improve gait and reduce pain (**Fig. 32-4**). A beveled heel that makes a 20-degree angle with the floor can decrease ankle

motion and pain. For the very painful or arthritically involved RA ankle, a short-leg patellar tendon–bearing orthosis that shifts weight away from the ankle to the patellar tendon is useful. Plantar fasciitis may be relieved with a cup insert or an insert with a depression in the area of the tender fascia (279).

Appropriate wide-toe-box shoes should be used to accommodate a wide forefoot, cocked toes, and hallux valgus seen in RA or JRA, as well as the hallux valgus deformity seen in OA. A soft insert is added, as are metatarsal reliefs, whether in the form of a cookie inside the shoe or an external bar on the sole of the shoe. We prefer the former because we believe it to be safer. A rocker bottom shoe can facilitate rollover in the presence of a painful ankle. Sometimes, it is best coupled with a stirrup-type brace to provide subtalar support.

Knee. Bracing for the knee may be for pain, instability caused by ligamentous laxity, significant quadriceps weakness, or excess recurvatum. Evidence for its effectiveness is level 3, and in surveys, only 10% of practicing clinicians use them (280). A useful brace for quadriceps weakness is a double upright Klenzak (Pel Supply, Cleveland, OH) set at 5-degree plantar flexion at the ankle to put the knee in extension during heel-strike and stance. The Klenzak can be used for a unilateral problem or for the weaker side when the problem is bilateral, as in PM. Success also can be achieved with a plastic-molded AFO cast in 5-degree plantar flexion with a small added 3/8-in. heel incorporated into the orthosis, provided the patient is not overweight. A Lenox Hill orthosis (3-M, Long Island, NY) may be used to control mediolateral or rotational instability. These braces are rarely used in RA but are used for younger athletic individuals.

In our practice, we have used a knee, ankle, foot orthosis (KAFO) with ischial weight bearing and dial lock at the knee, which can be used to reduce knee pressure and may be adjusted to relieve medial or lateral compartmental stresses in OA or RA. This orthosis is difficult to fit with severe valgus deformities and in the obese patient. Compliance in the use of KAFOs is poor.

Smaller knee orthoses, such as hinged orthoses, the Swedish knee cage, or Lehrman orthoses (Pel Supply, Cleveland, OH), may be used to help control sagittal and frontal knee plane motion. A knee orthosis to help prevent dislocation of the patella is available and often effective. A shoe with a beveled heel at 20 degrees also decreases knee flexion and promotes a more stable extended knee. Orthoses with a dial lock turned 1 or 2 degrees daily can be used to reduce knee flexion contracture. Elasticized knee supports may help control swelling and often provide patients with a sense of control of the quadriceps.

Spinal Orthoses

Spinal orthoses are used primarily to relieve pain, limit motion, or support an unstable spine. A lumbar spinal orthosis or thoracic orthosis with mold and form insert will often relieve a painful back due to compression fracture or disk disease. This type of orthosis may reduce lordosis, reinforce abdominal muscles, and unload the spine. For thoracic compression fractures prone to gibbous deformity or an unstable lumbar or thoracic spine, a Jewett orthosis (Florida Brace, Winter Park, FL) or a molded polypropylene body jacket is required.

A lumbosacral corset does not limit motion but provides some abdominal support and relieves painful lower lumbar musculature.

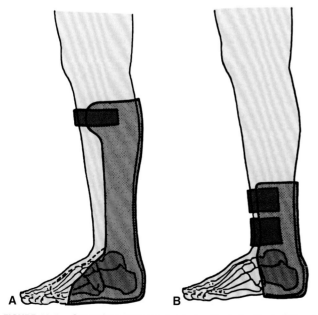

FIGURE 32-4. Comparison between standard ankle foot orthosis **(A)** and hindfoot orthosis **(B)** designed to control subtalar motion.

The cervical spine is involved in RA, OA, JRA, and spondyloarthropathies. Various collars provide different levels of support. A soft cervical collar only minimally limits motion but may provide pain relief. A Philadelphia collar (Pel Supply, Cleveland, OH) offers slightly more support and some limitation of extension. A two-poster, four-poster, or sterno-occipital mandibular immobilizer collar substantially limits flexion and extension, particularly at C1 and at C2 but also at C4 and C6. A halo is needed to completely control C1-2 instability.

ASSISTIVE DEVICES AND ADAPTIVE AIDS

It is not uncommon for clinicians to empirically select assistive devices and adaptive aids to compensate for limited ROM and pain, help promote independence, and reduce impairment and disability for arthritic patients (see Chapter 55). Systematic evaluation with publication of the effectiveness of these devices is rare (274). To help ensure patient acceptance, the appliance should be affordable and easy to use and improve patient function.

Ambulation and transfer skills are extremely important for persons with arthritis, and gait aids and devices may be needed.

Gait Aids

If joint pain is a problem, secondary to loss of cartilage, effusion, or active synovitis, the painful joint needs to be unloaded. Weight reduction is encouraged, because a 1-kg weight loss results in a 3- to 4-kg decrease in load across the hip joint. A straight cane when used properly unloads the limb by 25% (2), which is good for balance but not very efficient in unloading the limb, although a forearm crutch is. The elbow should be in 30 degrees of flexion when such a device is in use.

Custom handgrip pieces can be made by making a mold of the patient's hand in a functional position of weight bearing, or commercially made handpieces on canes can be used. Platform crutches distribute weight on the forearm, reducing the need for wrist extension and eliminating weight-bearing forces through the wrist and hand. Forearm attachments for walkers and wheelchairs are available.

For significant loss of strength as in DM-PM, or endurance, a small, lightweight wheelchair is recommended. There are also small motorized scooters, such as the sporty Amigo Chair (Amego Mobility Intl. Inc., Bridgeport, MI).

Adaptive Devices for Transfer

Chronic hip or knee pain, limited motion, and proximal muscle weakness make transfers from low-level chairs, toilets, and beds difficult. Upper extremities may be needed for push-off, but when these are incapacitated by RA, such simple motion becomes impossible. Independence in making transfers can be restored by elevating the seat with a cushion or using a levered seat or placing 3- or 4-in. blocks under each leg of chairs, tables, and beds. Chairs with elevating motorized seats, elevated toilet seats, and clamp-on tub seats are helpful.

Transfers in and out of the car are facilitated by the use of an extra-thick seat cushion, levered seat, or twist-about plastic disk and a mounted grab bar to increase leverage. In the car, use of the side, rearview, and wide-angle mirrors for patients with limited cervical ROM as a result of spondyloarthropathies becomes essential. A spinner bar for the steering wheel and a large-handled door opener and ignition piece are adaptations for the patient with significant hand problems. Patients with back pain benefit from a firm seat and back cushion, such as a PCP Champion Sacro cushion (OTC Professional Appliances, Ripley, OH). Those with neck pain need adjustable neck supports or pillows.

SELF-CARE

Dressing, undressing, and other daily self-care activities can be time- and energy-consuming tasks for those with RA, SLE, and PM (see Chapter 7). Adaptive and self-care aids such as long-handled reachers, shoehorns, elastic shoelaces, long-handled sponges, brushes and toothbrushes, Stirex scissors (North Coast Medical, San Jose, CA), button hooks, zipper hooks, toilet paper holders, and large-handled items are all helpful devices that also conserve energy. Clothing made with elastic and Velcro is easier to don than that with buttons and hooks. Wrinkle-resistant fabrics that do not require ironing and lightweight fabrics and wools (e.g., mohair, alpaca) are useful. Large buttons and partial zippering before putting on the garment may facilitate dressing, as will stretch straps and waists, garments with large raglan sleeves, and those with smooth linings. Capes, ponchos, and down jackets are easy to put on, warm, and lightweight.

Devices in the Kitchen

Useful kitchen devices include food processors, long-handled reachers, built-up handles on utensils, electric knives and vegetable peelers, mounted wedge-shaped jar openers, and lightweight aluminum pans. Lining pans with aluminum foil saves scrubbing. Bringing together items involved in a work area (e.g., kitchen stove, work area, sink, refrigerator) is helpful. A microwave oven cuts down on food preparation time. A kitchen cart loaded with often-used utensils cuts down on walking.

Environmental Design

Slopes, stairs with deep steps, high curbs, and buses or cars may be difficult to negotiate for someone with disease of the hips and knees (see Chapter 15). Appropriate placement of steps, lowered curbs, suitably graded inclines, and ramps are helpful. Buses that kneel to accept passengers are available in many communities. Indoors, thick carpets increase friction and are difficult to walk on or negotiate in a wheelchair. In the bathroom, guard rails are best for safety. The bathtub should have nonskid strips or an entire nonskid surface. A wheeling shower with a wall seat is excellent for wheelchair use. Door openings should be wide enough to accept a wheelchair. Chest-high storage cabinets and waist-high work surfaces are best; special door handles are available. For those patients in wheelchairs, proper positioning of doorknobs, light switches, and kitchen equipment is necessary. Large-handled pencils and eating utensils are helpful. Devices to help with spray cans are available. The AF provides a catalog of available assistive devices (www.arthritis.org).

EDUCATION

One of the most important aspects of care for patients with inflammatory disease, and perhaps all chronic illness, is a good rapport between physician and patient. This begins with clear communication between patient and health care providers so that patients can be assisted in habilitation or adjustment to the chronic disease process. In addition, educational groups consisting of arthritis patients who gather to hear experts in the field and talk about aspects of medical and rehabilitative management are very informational and supportive. They also provide a social context for coping with medical and psychosocial problems. Local hospitals, the YMCA, and the AF and other disease foundations and local interest groups offer such group activities.

It has been thought that patients with RA, and chronic disease in general, have had significant disability based on inactivity and lack of motivation. Approaches to solving this problem and promoting better patient function have included techniques to empower patients and to promote self-efficacy, thereby overcoming learned helplessness (281).

Educational intervention, using disease self-management programs, has been employed in the treatment of RA, SLE, AS, and fibromyalgia. These have reduced pain, improved function, and delayed the onset of disability. They are also underused (282–284). Studies show that information is helpful in empowering patients, and it often helps to relieve anxiety. However, educational interventions that only promote increased knowledge have little impact on disease activity and behavior. Educational models that establish approaches to problem solving, support groups, and healthy lifestyle/fitness behaviors are usually more effective in promoting improved function (281–284).

Patient education should include a discussion about the natural history of the disease and the likely impact that it will have on lifestyle, job, and leisure activities. Many systemic rheumatic diseases are chronic and have periods of remission and exacerbation that affect function. Planning activities so that they are done at the optimal time of day, or are broken up into smaller intervals for sustained activity, may permit completion of important activities without undue fatigue.

A full discussion of the impact that medication may have will help alert patients to medication-related problems. For example, corticosteroids may cause muscle atrophy, upset sleep patterns, and alter appearance. These changes may have profound effects on mood, energy, and strength, all of which may influence function.

Joint Protection

It is well known since the observations of Cordery that arthritic patients change their lifestyle and habits to protect their joints and use adaptive strategies and devices that make work easier rather than persist with activity that causes pain (285). However, patients need formal education in this area to learn techniques to reduce force across their joints. Principles of this program include the following: promoting good sitting posture; using adequate back contact, arm rests, and proper height such that the feet touch the floor; and changing position frequently to avoid gel phenomenon.

Use the largest possible joints to support activity, unweight painful lower extremity joints, avoid overuse by interrupting sustained activity with rest periods, use adaptive equipment and strategies for efficient use of joints, and use splints when limbs need to be supported in functional positions.

Energy Conservation

Rheumatic disease is most often accompanied by fatigue, so conserving energy to maximize function is an important part of the arthritic patient's lifestyle. Some of the mechanisms for conserving energy include the proper orthotics and assistive devices to affect energy-efficient ambulation and hand function, appropriate adaptive aids and clothing, proper environmental design and rest periods throughout the day, maintenance of ROM and strength, and maintenance of proper posture.

Good body posture, whether sitting or standing, balances the weight of the head and limbs on the body framework so that gravity helps to maintain joint position with minimal muscle activity. Significant changes in posture cause muscles to exert more energy to pull against the force of gravity. For example, standing takes 25% more energy than sitting to perform activities. Ideal posture cannot be maintained unless care is taken to preserve ROM and strength of muscles around the joints.

Psychosocial Interventions

Rheumatic disease has a major impact on the patient's mobility, ADLs, general lifestyle, self-image, family life, sexuality, and work (see Chapter 12). Stress and depression play major roles in influencing rheumatic disease (RD) patients' reporting of their symptoms and illness.

Two forms of stress play a role in RD: major life events, such as death of a spouse, and persistent negative events (286), such as conflicts with people. The latter stresses can influence immune function and increase global ratings of disease activity in RA (287), increase psychological distress in SLE (288), and increase symptoms in JRA (289).

These studies support the association between stress and symptom flares and indicate that interventions to help coping may be useful. Major patient reactions ranging from denial and repression to depression occur, as do other components of chronic illness, such as anger, bargaining, and acceptance.

Depression is common in RD. It has been reported that 37% of patients with RA have depression (290). Predictors of depression include scores in HAQ, pain intensity (291), and, in women, loss of valued activities. A history of depression in RA makes patients vulnerable to higher levels of pain, fatigue, and disability, even if they are not currently depressed but just in a dysphoric mood (292). The belief that there is a particular personality type prone to developing RA has been dropped. However, premorbid personality is an important determinant of the patient's reaction to illness. Patients with arthritis, in addition to coping with pain, may have to deal with losses in function and physical attractiveness because of the disease and side effects of medication, and they have to deal with the reactions of friends, spouse, and family. Some families adjust well, maintaining good communication, support, and flexibility in family routines. Other families are not able to reorganize and adjust to the needs of a person with arthritis.

The unpredictability of systemic disease complicates the coping process. Patients with RD often experience learned helplessness, believing no solutions exist to reduce stressful events, which leads to anxiety, depression, increased pain, decreased activities, and decreased ability to adapt to distress and disability (286). High levels of helplessness are associated with increased pain, depression, and functional impairment in RA and poorer physical health in SLE (293). Self-efficacy in patients with RD may vary for different actions to achieve health-related goals. High self-efficacy for pain is correlated with low frequency of pain behavior in RA and is related to physical and mental health in SLE (294,295). Coping strategies involve motor and cognitive actions to control the impact of stresses. Passive coping strategies are associated with high pain levels, disability, and poor illness adaptation (286). Psychosocial interventions help improve pain, affect, and function (152,295,296). They may also increase self-efficacy and health status. RA patients who use stress management programs increase self-efficacy and improve ratings of depression, pain, and walking speed (297). Treatment offered through telephone-based interventions has been associated with psychological improvement in SLE. Audiotapes and videos used at home yield improvements in physical function, pain, joint count, and global scores in RA (286). In summary, psychological and behavioral approaches are very useful in RD (298,299).

Sexual Adjustment

Many normal, well-educated, financially successful, and maritally stable US adults admit to sexual dysfunction or difficulties. However, arthritis may impose additional limitations or alterations that influence the sexual life as they do other ADLs (300).

Particular sexual problems in the arthritic patient arise as a result of mechanical problems associated with decreased ROM, pain, and stiffness; depression, with decreased self-image and interest; drug therapy resulting in decreased libido; psychosocial problems in the family unit related to the patient's arthritis; and fatigue. Studies indicate impairments occur in various indices of sexual function in a number of autoimmune diseases. In PSS, vaginal dryness, ulcers, and dyspareunia are significantly more common after disease onset in comparison with SLE and RA controls (301). Dyspareunia is also common in Sjögren's (302). There is a 50% decrease in the number and intensity of orgasms. Sexual satisfaction index is impaired in all three groups. Skin tightness, reflex, heartburn, and muscle weakness adversely affect sexual relations, more in PSS than in SLE and RA (301). Impotence occurs in males as a result of neurovascular problems in PSS and related syndromes (303). Arthritic involvement of the hips, knees, lumbar spine, hands, and shoulders commonly causes joint stiffness and painful mechanical problems that interfere with sexual performance. Hip involvement commonly causes mechanical problems. Analgesics and warm baths before intercourse may help. In women with more advanced disease, a posterior approach by the man for intercourse may be successful. With severe limitation of motion, either unilateral or bilateral hip replacements may be requisite to achieve intercourse. After hip surgery, intercourse should not be resumed at all for 6 weeks, and hip flexion of more than 90 degrees should be avoided. Attention to sexual adjustments after joint replacement is important (304). Neither pain nor stiffness nor limitation of motion of the knees should mechanically limit intercourse, but a change in position may be required for more comfort. For those patients with back pain (e.g., spondyloarthropathies, disk disease), a lateral position for both the man and the woman is preferable. Patients with significant muscle weakness, as in DM-PM, may need to assume a more passive sexual role. Significant problems in the joints of the hands and arms, as in RA, are more restrictive for the man than for the woman; a side-lying position may alleviate this. In both men and women, arthritis of these joints may interfere with the early stages of lovemaking involving caressing and manual stimulation.

Often, arthritic patients experience a decrease in self-image, a feeling of helplessness, and ultimately depression, which in turn is associated with decreased libido. Chronic pain may reduce a woman's efforts to make herself more attractive for her partner, and it is difficult to reassure the woman who has significant joint deformities that she is still physically attractive. A man may abstain from sexual relations rather than cause his arthritic spouse pain, and the spontaneity is reduced. In comparison to RA patients with a low degree of morning stiffness, RA patients with a high degree of morning stiffness worried more about self-image and reported significantly more problems in sexuality (305). Appropriate counseling may help alleviate these problems.

Certain medications are associated with decreased libido. High-dose steroids used in SLE and DM-PM may affect physical appearance and contribute to decreased self-image or acceptance by one's spouse. Immunosuppressive medications may interfere with conception. Reports have been made about gynecomastia and sexual impotence associated with methotrexate (306). The RDs as well as medications may cause significant fatigue. Education about energy conservation and the practice of aerobic exercise may be generally useful in managing this symptom.

Psychosocial problems in the family unit may lead to decreased sexual relationships between husband and wife. Such problems include inability to work, inadequate finances, limited acceptance by friends, and limited participation in social or recreational events. Misunderstanding and anxieties of the children about the chronic disease of the parents also contribute to tension and adversely influence sexual relationships.

Patients with JRA had similar attitudes toward sexual activity, conception, wish for children, age at first child, and duration of lactation. However, fecundity is significantly decreased, and an increased miscarriage rate has been reported. Males had greater problems than did females establishing relationships (307).

In our opinion, successful treatment of musculoskeletal disease does not necessarily serve as a sexual restorative; rather, understanding, counseling, alterations in sexual positions, and appropriate joint replacements are necessary.

Vocational Aspects

A vocational assessment should be part of the workup for rheumatic disease patients and should cover educational level, work history and achievements, physical functional level, and social and psychological adjustment (see Chapter 14). The capacity of individuals with RD to work is decreased when compared with those without RD (308,309), and those with RA are particularly impacted. Three years after diagnosis with SLE, patients are no longer working (310). For those patients who work as homemakers, the rheumatic disease has a negative impact on family activities and function (311).

Determinants of work disability exist at societal and individual levels (309). Societal factors include economic conditions, attitudinal and architectural barriers, types of jobs available, employers' practices, and types of disability pension plans available (308,309). Individual determinants include disease, social factors, and ability to maintain locus of control and anatomy on the job (309,311). Functional status is the most important determinant of household work performance (312,313).

A recent study indicates that women have higher degrees of work disability in RA (314). Remaining in the work force or being a homemaker is an important goal for the person with arthritis, and rehabilitative care and the support of the family help ensure success. The first step in vocational counseling is to see if adjustments can be made in the job or home setting so that the patient can continue working. If changes cannot be made, then the patient may have to receive formal vocational rehabilitation or training for another vocation.

REHABILITATION INTERVENTIONS FOR SPECIFIC DISEASES

Rheumatoid Arthritis

Rheumatoid arthritis is a systemic rheumatic disease characterized by an acute inflammatory response. It has different patterns of onset and can be divided into different types (315).

Depending on the severity of the progression of the disease, the pathologic process of RA has impact on joints, their surrounding structures, and other major organ systems. This process can produce a number of physical (anatomic and physiologic) and psychological (mental and emotional) impairments. These impairments cause functional problems that can result in disability. 📶 **eTable 32-5** lists the potential variables that can influence the extent of impairment, functional decline, and disability.

Course and Disease Outcome

Fewer than 25% of RA patients have a true remission in 5 years (315) as measured by ACR criteria. Most have progressive disease of varying degrees. The rate of progression to joint destruction and disability is proportional to the intensity of the inflammation, proliferative reaction in the joints, and persistence of disease over time. Low-grade attacks of synovitis, separated in time, are less likely to cause joint deformity than continuous active synovitis. Radiographic progression is highest in the first few years of the disease but can progress over decades. Once the synovium begins to destroy and invade cartilage, it is at risk for irreversible damage even if disease activity decreases (315,316).

In the 1980s, studies indicated RA patients had a progressive decline in functional capacity and ability to work and increase in mortality rate of 5 to 20 years (315). Work disability after 5 years is 60% to 70% in RA patients under 65 years of age (317). Other studies have developed models using baseline indices to predict outcomes in RA (318,319). This information has been useful to clinicians in planning treatment. One study predicted increased disability by both disease factors and nondisease variables. Disease-related factors explained 33% of total disability, and nondisease factors (depression, education, psychological status) explained 26%. Unexplained were 41% (319). Similarly, disease mortality has been predicted, and 5-year survival has been reported as 85% to 95% in patients who had favorable baseline variables (BLV) versus those who had unfavorable baseline variables (UBLV) and who had a mortality rate of 45% to 55% (320).

Treatment of RA

Early aggressive pharmacologic treatment by rheumatologists has been shown to be associated with improved function in early RA (4). Early functional assessment and rehabilitation treatment are also clinically indicated. Many treatments have proven of benefit in improving function. Team management is effective (321).

RA is associated with a high degree of disability, the causes of which have been frequently attributed to impairments and the biology of the disease. Recent literature suggests that the radiologic appearance in those with RA correlates highly with measures of functional ability (e.g., HAQ, Arthritis Impact Measurement Scale) (322). Critical to the management of RA should be treatment aimed at preventing disability and preserving or improving function. Usually, these include muscle strengthening while protecting joint integrity (isometric exercise may be preferred), aerobic conditioning using low-impact methods, and encouragement of leisure activity that promotes socialization and well-being (323,324).

Impairments in RA and Treatments

See **Table 32-13** for a listing of rehabilitative treatments and functional deficits and disabilities in RA.

Bone Health. All patients with inflammatory arthropathies are at risk for osteoporosis (OP). The location of bone changes may be (a) focal and affect subchondral bone and bone at the joint margins, (b) periarticular osteopenia, and (c) generalized osteoporosis involving the axial and appendicular skeleton (325).

Explanations for this include inactivity, medication and the inflammatory process, and up-regulation of IL-1α and IL-1β, TNF-α, macrophage colony-stimulating factor, IL-6, and IL-11. Also increased are parathyroid hormone–related peptide and the newly described T-cell–derived cytokine IL-17. Treatments for this include good disease management and possibly the use of intermittent low-dose parathyroid hormone to treat corticosteroid-induced osteoporosis (326).

Pain. Among patients with RA, 70% seek help for pain (327). Pain in RA is caused by active synovitis, stretch of the joint capsule by effusion, mechanical joint destruction, and moving and loading joints. Pain is complex and has physiologic and subjective components. It contributes significantly to functional disability in early RA (328). Treatment includes education, exercise, stress management, medication, physical modalities, orthotics, assistive devices, and joint protection.

Fatigue. Fatigue is one of the most common impairments in RA. Evidence is accumulating that this ubiquitous symptom is frequently associated with elevation of inflammatory cytokine (IL-6) interferon species. Characteristics of fatigue are varied and may include inability to sustain daily routines or leisure activities, sleepiness, inability to wake up refreshed, depression, and muscle weakness. For example, this may be a reflection of disease activity. Treatment is targeted at the most likely organ system contributing to the symptom. Fatigue in rheumatic diseases may be associated with thyroid abnormalities or the anemia of chronic illness. Lack of refreshing sleep is often associated with rheumatic diseases.

Disrupted sleep may best be treated with medication. Muscle weakness, on the other hand, is best treated with a strengthening program, and endurance problems are likely to respond to aerobic conditioning. Interrupting activity with periodic rest (20-minute) naps during the day has been shown to be effective in increasing physical activity levels (329). Also to be included are energy conservation techniques and depression management.

Decreased Aerobic Capacity. Deconditioning contributes to decreased aerobic capacity. Patients tend to limit activities because of joint pain fatigue and decreased motivation. Cardiovascular problems due to RA or other diseases may

	Deficit	Treatment
TABLE 32-13		**Rehabilitative Treatment of Impairment, Functional Deficits, and Disabilities in RA**
Impairment	Pain	Medication, education (self-efficacy), stress control joint protection, orthotics, assistive devices, in modalities, exercise
	Fatigue	Energy conservation, depression management, exercise (strengthening/aerobic) short rests
	Joint swelling (Acute inflammation) (Subacute/chronic)	Cold pack, ROM, heat, exercise (strengthening/aerobic)
	Weakness	Exercise (isometric/isotonic/isokinetic)
	Deconditioning	Aerobic exercise, energy conservation, short rests
	Joint Effusion (mod-lg)	Remove before exercise program
	Limited joint motion	ROM/strengthening (if biomechanically stable, not ankylosed and 0 to mild effusion), modalities
	Depression/anxiety/stress	Medication, counseling, relaxation techniques, coping, strategies
	Sleep disturbance	Medication, modalities before sleep, naps, stress reduction, mattress, and pillow changes
	Sexual dysfunction	Education, counseling, address course
Functional	Mobility	Gait aides, scooter
	ADL	Assistive devices, joint protection, education environmental strategies
	Gait	Assess cause of deviation, gait aids, appropriate shoes, and orthotics
	Homemaking	Environmental adjustments, adaptive devices, energy conservation joint protection
Disability	Can't work	
	Can't do housework	Vocational assessment; possible retraining, environmental adjustments
	Can't care for self	Home assistance, scooter/wheelchair, environmental changes

contribute. A 2006 Internet-based physical activity program for RA with individualized guidance (IT) in general information (GT) showed the IT program was more effective with respect to the number of patients who report meeting physical activity recommendations than the GT program. This program is inexpensive and readily accessible and should be useful for RA patients who have limited activity levels (330).

Aerobic capacity in RA is commonly evaluated by submaximal aerobic testing. A recent 2008 study identified that the HAP (Human Activity Profile) is useful in estimating fitness levels when aerobic standard testing is not feasible (331). Aerobic training has proven to be of benefit for class I through class III RA. It is generally of low intensity in class III or of moderate intensity in classes I and II (⎈ eTable 32-4). Appropriate forms include cycle ergometer, land (low-impact dance or aerobic routines), or pool. The latter is appropriate for class III deranged joints or joint replacements. Aerobic exercise can improve function, increase aerobic capacity, and improve cardiovascular health without increasing inflammation if chosen appropriately. In fact, it may reduce inflammation (332–334).

Sleep Disorder. Several different types of sleep disorders exist in RA: (a) fragmented with nocturnal clonus, (b) frequent prolonged wakefulness after sleep onset, and (c) sleep apnea. Insomnia or early AM awaking is not common.

In practice, treatment consists of modalities and appropriate pain medication before bedtime and provision of a good mattress or pillow. Medications such as clonazepam, L-dopa, short-acting benzodiazepines, and zolpidem can be used to improve sleep quality and quantity.

Depression. Depression can often accompany RA but is no more common in RA than in other chronic disorders (335). Depression and its subtypes in RA are correlated with health status measurements. Stress and anxiety are common.

Appropriate treatment for depression includes treating the underlying cause and medication. Depression, stress, and anxiety may benefit from stress management, relaxation techniques, and coping strategies.

Decreased Strength. Strength deficits occur very early in RA and are due to atrophy around painful joints, reflex inhibition by pain and joint effusion, inactivity, and myositis, which may be associated with RA.

Muscles around key joints (particularly the knee, hip, shoulder) should be strengthened. The literature provides evidence that isometric, isotonic, and low- and moderate-resistance exercise (210,242) and isokinetic exercise all strengthen muscles in RA. In addition, exercise as part of aerobic and aquatic programs also yields strength gains. Isotonic resistive exercise yields more gains than isometric exercise. The types of exercise, the intensity, and the frequency depend on ACR functional class, presence or absence of joint effusion, biomechanical joint integrity, inflammation stage, presence of moderate to severe OP, and presence of joint replacements (see **Table 32-12**). In general, keep the exercise simple, meet needed patient goals, and follow exercise guidelines for compliance (see ⎈ eTable 32-4). RA is a chronic disease that needs continued physical exercise with sufficient intensity to prevent muscle strength and function loss (336).

Decreased Range of Motion. In early RA, it is important to prevent contracture. In later stages, contractures may be present. Patients should be on a basic ROM program daily for all affected joints. In patients with limited ROM, due to contracture, ROM exercise should be in the available arc of motion.

Functional Problems. Such problems as decreased mobility, compromised ADL, and impaired gait are common in RA. Determining the impairments that produce these problems is necessary. The impairments should be managed appropriately. This will help reduce the functional limitation. Education on use of gait aids and assistive devices, orthotics, and environmental strategies is needed.

Disability. Although past studies indicate a significant number of persons with RA experience work and household disability, newer pharmacologic agents and early rheumatologic and rehabilitative care have resulted in improved function and less disability (337).

Management includes investigating the impairment and functional problem contributors to disability. Recently, subclinical disability, a need to modify task performance, or frequency without reported difficulty with the task has been identified as part of the disability continuum. Seventy-five percent of a group of 50% RA patients identified difficulties with valued life activities (VLA's)—subclinical disability. They were significantly more likely to experience functional limitations over a 2-year period. Subclinical disability may be a valuable marker for those in a disability transition phase where intervention may help maintenance of function (338). Intervention by vocational rehabilitation with patient interview and workplace assessment is essential. Ergonomic assessment may help people with arthritis maintain employment. An ergonomic assessment tool was developed and was shown to be feasible and comprehensive in identifying job issues that need accommodation strategies (339). All factors influencing disability need to be addressed, since workplace accommodations alone may not be associated with improvement in employment rate (340).

Specific Joints. RA may cause a variety of specific joint impairments that primarily affect the synovial lining of diarthrodial joints. It can affect almost any and all the peripheral joints, with relative sparing of the axial spine, except for the upper cervical (i.e., atlantoaxial) joints. However, degenerative change frequently accompanies it and involves C4-5 and C5-6 and the hands, knee, hips, and MTP joints. The end results of the process are joint pain, swelling, and malfunction. The muscles that surround the swollen, inflamed joints or biomechanically compromised joints are painful and are often atrophied or myositic. Ankylosis may occur, but subluxation is more common. Malalignment and pain result in increased problems with ADLs, mobility, and energy expenditure. Pain and deformity may cause problems with self-image and sexual activity (315).

Joint-Specific Problems

Shoulder. Shoulder RA affects the glenohumeral joint, distal third of the clavicle and surrounding bursae, capsule, and ligaments. Arthritis is associated with pain in the shoulder girdle, which is referred to the neck, back, and upper arm. Decreased motion of the joint, soft tissue contracture, and muscle atrophy follow. Because the capsule lies deep under the rotator cuff, effusion is difficult to detect on physical examination. Static and dynamic rotator cuff exercises in mild RA decrease arm pain, help swollen joints, and improve Sickness Impact Profile scores (341).

Pain causes decreased ROM. Limitation of IR is seen early. Proximal subluxation of the humeral head occurs late in the disease. Weakness of the rotator cuff may cause superior subluxation in about 33% of RA patients; about 21% of patients develop rotator cuff tears; and an additional 24% have fraying of the tendons (315). The insertion of the rotator cuff tendon into the greater tuberosity makes it vulnerable to erosion

by synovitis. Adhesive capsulitis, with anterolateral shoulder swelling, subacromial and subdeltoid bursitis, and bicipital tendinitis are associated problems. Anterolateral soft tissue shoulder swelling can indicate subacromial bursitis.

Adhesive capsulitis with motion loss can occur quickly. Pain is worse at night, when sleep movements stretch the capsule. Full motion is not needed for most daily activities, so pain may be less during the day. In addition to pain control with heat and cold, stretching and local steroid injection into the specific affected area is often useful (250,251). An ROM program to increase and prevent loss of mobility is crucial. For functional activities, the shoulder must have 30 to 45 degrees of flexion and 10 degrees of IR. Care must be taken to assess the degree of radiographic involvement and joint stability when prescribing mobilization so as not to injure a compromised joint. When pain and inflammation subside, Codman exercises and the use of a cane or wand can increase flexion and IR and ER. Wall walking is good for chronic capsulitis. In the presence of adhesive capsulitis, a technique of abduction-ER-flexion traction for 1 hour a day in conjunction with TENS has been successful in decreasing pain and increasing ROM (193). Isometric strengthening should first focus on the deltoid with the shoulder adducted, then wrist-restricted isometrics in IR and ER; finally, triceps and biceps isometrics are added.

Instruction in joint protection is essential to avoid overusing the shoulder. Arthroplasty should be considered before end-stage erosion and soft tissue contraction occur.

Elbow. Elbow involvement is common in RA (20% to 65%), depending on disease severity, with loss of full extension being an early problem. Loss of lateral stability can cause significant impairment. Preservation of flexion is needed for ADLs. In severe disease, lateral stability may be lost, which may cause significant pain and disability in ADL function. Olecranon bursitis and accumulation of RA nodules that may break down easily are annoying to the patient (315).

Bursitis may be caused by *Staphylococcus* infection, and care must be taken not to inject the bursae of the elbow with steroid before a culture is performed. Wearing a padded Heelbo (Heelbo, Niles, IL) is useful to relieve pressure.

Lateral and medial epicondylitis is common. Acute epicondylitis is managed with cold modalities. Steroid injection may be necessary. Stretching exercise should not be forceful because articular damage is often present in the arthritic elbow.

Hand and Wrist. The hand and wrist function as a unit. With weakness of the extensor carpi ulnaris, the carpal bones rotate (i.e., the proximal row in an ulnar direction and the distal ones radially), resulting in ulnar deviation of the MCPs. A power grasp and weakened intrinsic muscles contribute to these problems.

Synovial proliferation increases pressures in the wrist joint, so that ligaments, tendons, and cartilage may begin to be destroyed. When the ulnar collateral ligament is stretched or ruptures, the ulnar head rises dorsally and floats. In advanced disease, the carpus becomes significantly compacted. CTS may occur bilaterally. Progressive wrist disease results in decreased motion or ankylosis if the disease is severe and of long duration.

In the hand, muscle weakness and contraction occur and grip strength decreases. One study of male and female RA patients (average disease duration of 7.5 years) followed for 5 years showed at the 5-year mark that grip strengths, Keitel function tests, and HAQ scores were significantly worse in women. One fourth of patients in both groups needed more ADL assistance (342).

Swan neck deformity flexion of the distal interphalangeal joint (DIP) and hyperextension of the proximal interphalangeal joint (PIP) occur, as does Boutonniere deformity when the extensor hood of the PIP is stretched, causing flexion of the PIP and hyperextension of the IP. With incomplete profundus contraction, limitation of full flexion occurs at the DIP joints. Similarly, tight intrinsic muscles prevent full flexion of the PIP joints with the MCPs in extension.

Three types of deformity occur at the thumb: type I, a Boutonniere-type deformity at the IP joint (i.e., Nalebuff); type II, volar subluxation at the CMC joint during contraction of the adductor pollicis; and type III, in severe disease, exaggerated adduction of the first carpometacarpal joint and flexion at the MCP and hyperextension at the DIP joint. Flexor tenosynovitis and de Quervain thumb extensor synovitis are common (315).

Rehabilitative hand care involves stretching of tight intrinsic muscles, education about proper alignment, and support for functional activity and exercise. A controlled study of hand exercises versus no exercise for 48 months in female RA patients showed a significant increase in grip strength and pincer grip strength in the exercise group. The control group showed a significant decline in these parameters (343). A 3-week randomized control trial of combined ice massage and wax treatment and thermal and faradic baths with exercise revealed significantly improved Ritchie articular index, hand pain, ADL score and grip strength, and ROM in the treatment group. All parameters slightly declined in the control group (344). Use of functional wrist splints and finger ring–type splints to help reduce hyperextension or fixed flexion deformities, joint protection techniques, and postoperative care are important. These splints may help decrease synovitis, relieve pain and edema, and, when worn, reduce deformity and possibly retard its progression. A study of 273 RA patients indicated that in those with disease of less than 5 years, 269 needed help from a person with ADLs. The highest amount of disability resulted from impaired wrists. This indicates that early attention should be paid to treatment and stabilization of the wrist (345).

Hip. About 50% of patients with RA have radiographic hip involvement (315). Since this is a deep joint, early inflammation is not apparent. Palpation of effusion is difficult. Synovitis of the hip can cause pain radiating to the groin, whereas trochanteric bursitis causes pain radiating over the lateral thigh but can be in the buttock, anterior thigh, low back, and knee. Collapse of the femoral head and remodeling of the acetabulum, which is pushed medially (i.e., protrusio), occur in 5% of RA patients. Reduction in IR is an early finding with hip involvement. Synovial cysts can develop around the hip joint and communicate with the trochanteric bursae. Hip effusion can inhibit contraction of the gluteus medius muscle (346).

ROM exercises are important first to maintain at least the crucial 30 degrees of hip flexion. A tight tensor fascia lata should be stretched. Stretching in abduction helps to relieve pain. Stretching of the internal and external rotators, extensors, and abductors should be followed by isometric strengthening exercise for the hip abductors and extensors.

Ultrasound is best avoided in RA of the hip because it is somewhat difficult to assess the state of the inflammatory process in this deep joint. Because ultrasound increases joint temperature, it may aggravate an existing acute or subacute process.

Knee. The knees are commonly involved in RA, and synovial inflammation and proliferation and effusion are easily seen. Quadriceps atrophy occurs within weeks of the onset of the disease and leads to increased forces through the patella to the femoral surface. Loss of full knee extension also occurs early, and fixed contractions may ensue. Patients with lower limb involvement have been found to have quadriceps sensorimotor dysfunction that was associated with lower limb disability. A clinically applicable rehabilitation program increased quadriceps sensorimotor function and decreased lower limb disability without exacerbating pain or disease activity in well-controlled RA (347).

One study describes kinematic gait analysis differences in two groups of patients with (a) knee joint involvement and severe inflammation without progressive destruction and (b) knee joint involvement with progressive destruction. This analysis, which showed limitation in knee angle changes in swing and stance phases as well as a shortened swing phase duration in inflamed knee joints, can provide practical information about functional joint integrity in RA that could aid in therapeutic decision-making (348).

In the presence of moderate joint effusion, knee flexion in excess of 20 degrees is associated with significant increased articular pressure in the presence of moderate to large joint effusion, and caution must be observed in performing ROM exercises on a knee with significant fluid, as outpouching of the posterior joint space may occur, creating a popliteal or Baker cyst. Fluid from this popliteal portion does not readily return to the anterior joint space but rather adds increased pressure to the popliteal space. Forceful ROM may also cause rupture of the capsule. There may be uncomfortable fullness or pain in the popliteal space, and rupture into the calf may simulate thrombophlebitis. Ultrasound can define a cyst. If rupture occurs, a hematoma may be seen below the malleoli. Observe the patient from the rear while he or she is standing to check for a popliteal cyst.

Meniscal cartilage and cruciate ligaments can be easily destroyed by proliferative synovitis. Collateral ligaments become stretched, causing valgus and varus deformity. Tests for knee stability are always indicated in an examination. X-rays should be taken in the standing position to assess the cartilage and joint space.

Treatment is directed to the particular focal intra- or periarticular problem. The patient should be instructed in early ROM exercise to preserve knee extension and flexion. Ninety degrees of knee flexion is needed to kneel, and 100 degrees is needed to climb stairs. A pillow under the knee at night is to be avoided because this will encourage a knee flexion contracture. Stretching of the hamstrings is important. Strengthening of the quadriceps mechanism in nonacute joints by isometrics and in nonacute or subacute joints by low- and moderate-intensity isotonics in 30 degrees of flexion, if performed early in the disease process, helps to maintain the biomechanical advantage of the knee. Higher-intensity isotonic exercise should follow for the noninflamed joint.

Moderate to large effusions that inhibit contraction of the quadriceps and contribute to knee pain are best removed. Unweighting the knee is indicated with acute flares. Bracing the knee for instability is possible (see section on Orthotics), but patient compliance is low with bulky braces.

Inflamed periarticular or articular structures respond favorably to ice massage. When the joint is subacute or chronic, moist hot packs and TENS can be used.

Ankle and Foot. Arthritis affects the MTP, talonavicular, and tibiotalar joints in descending order. Ankles are less frequently involved than knees. Ankle damage is usually present in severe or progressive RA. Synovial involvement can be prominent and is seen anterior and posterior to the malleoli. The tarsal tunnel, posterior and inferior to the medial malleolus, contains the posterior tibial nerve, which is often painfully compressed by synovitis. In acute disease, stretching and erosion of collateral ligaments around the ankle occur, resulting in flattening of the arch and eversion of the calcaneus. This often results in an apropulsive gait. It also may promote knee valgus. Subtalar joint involvement is common, and patients experience more pain walking on uneven ground. About 85% of patients with RA have forefoot problems, such as widening at the metatarsal area, prominent MTP joints caused by subluxed metatarsal heads, hammer toe deformities, and hallux valgus of the great toe. Areas of skin breakdown are common on the dorsum of the toes (i.e., hammer toes), and callus is seen under the MTP heads. Plantar fasciitis and sub-Achilles bursitis may occur. Gait is typically flat-footed with little heel-strike or toe-off and a shuffling gait. Pronation of the hindfoot can be prominent. Appropriate footwear is extremely important. RA of this hindfoot and ankle can produce considerable dysfunction. A variety of nonoperative treatments may slow the progression of deformities, improve function, and provide symptomatic relief (349).

POLYMYOSITIS AND INFLAMMATORY MYOPATHIES

Polymyositis/dermatomyositis (DM-PM), IBM, and their subsets are systemic rheumatic diseases that affect skeletal muscle (see also Chapter 25). The mechanisms include autoimmune abnormalities as well as dysregulation of mitochondrial energy pathways. In fact, there seem to be metabolic defects in muscle metabolism, as well (350).

The clinical picture is predominantly one of profound weakness of the shoulder and hip girdle muscle, as well as of the neck and pharynx. In severe cases, the diaphragm and intercostal and abdominal muscles are involved. Twenty percent of patients also have some distal muscle weakness, and 50% of IBM patients have distal weakness. Some have weakness of the respiratory muscles. The muscle weakness is often compounded by steroid myopathy. A fair amount of muscle pain may be experienced when the inflammation is active. There may be complete remission of the disease, but chronic weakness is more common. Episodic periods of remission and exacerbation, which are often unpredictable, pose problems with functional activities and maintaining work status.

There are six types of inflammatory myopathy (351).

Type I (polymyositis): insidious onset, beginning in the pelvic girdle and later progressing to the shoulder girdle and neck muscles. Weakened posterior pharyngeal and laryngeal muscles result in dysphagia and dysphonia. Remission and exacerbations are quite common. Moderate to severe arthritis as well as Raynaud's phenomenon may be present. The skin over the knuckles and elbows is often atrophic.

Type II (dermatomyositis): acute onset. Proximal muscle weakness and an erythematous heliotropic rash on the skin of the eyelids and the dorsum of the hands are seen. Muscle tenderness is encountered in 25% of cases; subacute joint findings are common, as are systemic manifestations of malaise, fever, and weight loss.

Type III (cancer-associated myositis): associated with malignancy and most common in men more than 40 years of age. Often, muscle weakness precedes the diagnosis of malignancy by 1 to 2 years. The muscle weakness is usually progressive and does not respond well to steroids. Dysphagia and respiratory muscle weakness are common events. The mortality rate is high, and death is often the result of respiratory failure and pneumonia.

Type IV (juvenile dermatomyositis [JDM]): involves children. The muscle weakness is rapidly progressive, and problems with dysphagia, dysphonia, and respiratory weakness are quite common. It is important to remember that late exacerbations occur after 7 years of remission. The propensity for the development of severe joint contractures and muscle atrophy is high. Skin problems in the form of calcinosis universalis (i.e., cutaneous and muscle calcification), particularly over bony prominences, contribute to skin breakdown, draining lesions, and joint contracture (351).

Type V (myositis associated with other collagen vascular diseases): namely, RA, SLE, and PSS. The functional problems associated with the individual collagen disease often dominate the clinical picture.

Type VI (inclusion body myositis): most commonly involves men more than 40 years of age and has a slowly progressive course of muscle weakness. The quadriceps, hip, and shoulder girdle muscles often develop profound atrophy. In addition to proximal weakness, 50% of patients have significant distal weakness.

Each subtype has specific problems and impairments. Rehabilitation of the patients with DM-PM is influenced by the specific subtypes. However, there are some common impairments in the subgroups on which rehabilitation goals and treatment can be formulated (351–354).

Existing clinical subsets and 5-year survival rate include cancer-associated myositis (55%), dermatomyositis (80%), IBM (95%), and connective tissue–related myositis (85%). Autoantibody subsets include anti-SRP (30%), antisynthetase group (65%), and anti-M2 (95%). These subsets also predict response to treatment. Subtypes based on autoantibody status present with a different set of problems (94). Antisynthetase syndrome consists of ILDs, fever, arthritis, Raynaud's phenomenon, and mechanic's hands. The disease often has a rapid onset and aggressive course. The arthritis can affect the hands, knees, elbows, and shoulders and be chronic and deforming. The lung disease can be severe and can substantially limit ADLs and mobility.

Anti-SRP syndrome is associated with initial severe muscle weakness, myalgias, and cardiac involvement that significantly impact function. Anti-M2 presents with the rash of dermatomyositis and cuticle overgrowth and responds well to treatment.

Rehabilitation intervention must be tailored to suit the needs of each patient, depending on the disease type and associated impairments, functional problems, and disability present. Patients with type V PM and associated collagen vascular disease (e.g., PSS, RA, SLE) have muscle weakness plus the added problems of the additional disease, which needs to be addressed from a rehabilitation standpoint.

Survival and Prognosis

Much has been learned about medical management and the efficacy of rehabilitation for patients with DM-PM in the past 10 years. We have clearly advanced in our thinking from the view that that exercise is harmful and rest is needed to decrease inflammation (355). This is in part because medicine has generally recognized the value of physical activity and fitness for overall health and its importance in reducing all-cause mortality. The reluctance to provide patients with DM-PM with aerobic and resistive exercise programs has been, in part, due to concerns with the safety profile and risks of exacerbation. Recent studies have indicated that these types of exercises can safely be performed in this group of patients (228,356).

General factors associated with poor survival are listed as follows: older age, malignancy, delayed initiation of corticosteroid therapy, myocardial involvement, pharyngeal dysphagia with aspiration pneumonia, steroid and immunosuppressive drug complications, and GI vasculitis (children).

Adults with type I and II diseases can recover completely or be left with residual muscle weakness and fatigue, which can respond to rehabilitation management. The initial disease onset may be acute and require acute care hospitalization for significant weakness with respiratory and swallowing difficulty. Rehabilitation must be provided from day one in a progressive manner. Transfer to a rehabilitation unit after acute care management is appropriate (356). Patients with PM and associated incurable malignancy are not expected to recover from the disease. The rehabilitation goals are short term. Ambulation mobility and self-care functions progressively decline. Preserving ROM and strength will aid in keeping the person functional for as long as possible. Not being able to continue in the workforce for long is difficult for a middle-aged person to accept. Disability support payments and community support efforts need to be mobilized early on. Psychological support in coping with a chronic illness is needed. Good medical backup to contend with the problems of respiratory compromise and infection will be needed. Children with type IV disease need to be watched carefully for contractures.

Patients with type IV IBM have a slow, progressive course of proximal and distal weakness. Significant atrophy of the deltoid and quadriceps muscles is seen. Patients often have frequent falls resulting in fractures. The ability to increase the strength of significantly atrophied muscle has been shown to be poor (199). Lower extremity bracing to support a weak quadriceps mechanism is often needed.

Problems and Interventions

Scientifically proven impairments in isometric (199), isokinetic strength (201) and endurance exist. Also, studies document decreased aerobic capacity in DM-PM adults (205) and children (206). The functional problems that arise depend on the muscle groups involved and the extent of the weakness. For example, weakness of the pelvic girdle muscles is associated with difficulty in rising from a chair or a prone position, difficulty going up stairs, difficulty getting in and out of a bathtub, frequent falls with difficulty returning to the standing position, waddling gait, and toe walking caused by heel cord

tightness, which is common in children. Shoulder girdle weakness causes functional problems with dressing (e.g., difficulty pulling on shirt, hooking a bra) and grooming (e.g., combing hair, showering, shaving, brushing teeth), difficulty picking up heavy objects on a shelf, and difficulty eating. Neck weakness causes difficulty lifting and holding the head off a pillow and holding the head up while in a sitting position. Respiratory muscle weakness (e.g., intercostal muscles, diaphragm) results in difficulty with respiration, causing shallow and sometimes inefficient respiration. Distal muscle weakness (seen in 10% to 50%) may cause foot drop and related ambulation problems and difficulties with hand function and activities (353).

Rehabilitation goals in the acute phase consist of maintaining ROM of the joints and preventing joint contractures (357). In the recovery phase, the goals are to increase and regain muscle strength, maintain ROM, return to functional ADL and ambulatory activities, and restore previous lifestyle activities as much as possible.

UE ROM deficits are common in patients who have less than antigravity strength. The shoulder is most often involved in this case. Often, knee flexion contracture occurs because of overpull of the stronger hamstrings in PM over the weaker quadriceps. Elbow, knee, and plantar flexion contractures are common in children, particularly those with skin/muscle calcinosis.

Patients with DM-PM/JDM should be on a basic ROM/stretching exercise program. These may have to be adjusted in patients with active calcinosis, as stretching could increase muscle inflammation and calcinosis. In JDM patients without acute calcinosis or rash, stretching exercise, casting, or Dynasplints and aquatic exercise are appropriate. A text on the rehabilitation of persons with juvenile idiopathic inflammatory myopathy gives an excellent comprehensive overview of management of this patient group (358).

Isometric exercise is appropriate for DM-PM with inactive, mildly, and moderately active disease. Rest periods between contractions should be increased (20 seconds is appropriate) (199). Patients with significant atrophy are less likely to benefit. Therefore, early intervention is important. Clinically, low-weight concentric isotonic exercise is appropriate after a ROM, and isometric program is in place in inactive and mildly active disease (220). (Both short- and long-term aerobic exercises are appropriate for inactive and mildly active myositis (221,359).) The efficacy of programs to increase muscle strength by isometric (199), isotonic (229), and isokinetic exercise (234) without exacerbation of muscle inflammation, as determined by CPK, has been documented. The ability to increase aerobic capacity by short-term (6-week) and long-term (6-month) aerobic programs (221) has been documented. CPK should be monitored during exercise programs.

Patients with significant quadriceps weakness often trip and fall. A study of an IBM patient yielded some reasons for this (360). Clinically bracing a patient with significant isolated quadriceps weakness on one side can help stabilize the gait pattern, make it safer, and reduce falls. The appropriate bracing in this instance is a short leg brace—either polypropylene or Klenzac—positioned in 5-degree plantar flexion to create a hyperextension moment at the knee that will stabilize the limb. In patients with bilateral quadriceps weakness, it is appropriate to brace the weakest knee. Both knees cannot be braced in this manner, as the center of gravity would be shifted posteriorly and compromise the patient's balance. In the DM-PM patient who has both significant proximal and distal weakness, use of a 90-degree brace at the ankle or with a 10-degree dorsiflexion assist increases knee buckling. A 5-degree plantar flexion brace would stabilize the knee and basically correct the ankle foot drop. For those patients (less common) with only significant foot drop, a 90-degree or a 10-degree dorsiflexion brace is appropriate.

If pharyngeal and laryngeal weakness is present, referral to a speech pathologist to teach the patient techniques to avoid aspiration of food and prevent respiratory infection is needed (309). Neck flexor muscle weakness has been shown to correlate directly with swallowing dysfunction in patients with DM-PM, and its presence may cue the clinician to obtain a speech and language consultation (361). If respiratory muscle weakness is present, chest physical therapy breathing techniques, proper positioning, suctioning, postural drainage, and breathing exercises, if the patient is not in the acute stage, are indicated. Tidal volume should be checked daily with a bedside spirometer. A collar may be provided to support the neck when neck flexor or extensor weakness is present.

Most patients with polymyositis do not have arthritis. Polymyositis associated with anti–JO-1 antibody is characterized by arthritis that may become chronic and deforming without bone erosions. It occurs in the wrists, hands, elbows, knees, and shoulders. DM-PM with associated rheumatic disease (e.g., RA, SLE, PSS) is frequently associated with arthritis, which can be deforming; therefore, the use of modalities, splints, and joint conservation techniques is needed.

Iatrogenic steroid problems cause vertebral compression fractures in the thoracic and lumbar spine, resulting in back pain and muscle spasm. Osteoporosis is also common in the long bones and joints. Interventions include a corset to decrease spinal mobility, heat modalities to relieve pain, and a long-handled reacher and shoehorn. If avascular necrosis of the femoral head causes pain in the hip and groin on weight bearing, unweighting the hip is indicated. Deep heat (i.e., ultrasound) to the hip may relieve pain. Isotonic and isokinetic strength exercise should be available with moderate or severe OP. The therapeutic benefit of using superficial or deep heat and cold is frequently mentioned in textbooks, but their utility is primarily empirical.

Steroid myopathy presents with atrophy of muscle and increased muscle weakness. Repeated enzyme tests, electromyography (EMG), and muscle biopsy should be performed. If the enzymes have remained normal, the EMG will show no increased acute activity and the biopsy no increased active inflammation. The steroid should be reduced and the exercise program continued.

A number of problems can occur with the respiratory system. In addition to respiratory insufficiency, aspiration pneumonia may result because of weak pharyngeal and laryngeal muscles. Patients with the myositis-specific antibodies (MAS) anti–JO-1 commonly have ILD. Primary interstitial fibrosis in JO-1 patients with PM associated with SLE, RA, and PSS may have lung disease associated with these diseases. Pulmonary rehabilitation may be indicated.

Cardiovascular complications with DM-PM include congestive heart failure (3.3%), cardiomyopathy (1.3%), cor pulmonale (0.7%), and electrocardiogram abnormalities (50%) (16). They are most common in type I and type V diseases.

Rehabilitation includes cardiac precautions, energy conservation techniques, and an endurance program.

Dermatologic problems include pressure sores over bony prominences (e.g., sacrum, elbows, heels). Extensive calcinosis seen in childhood DM-PM causes breakdown of the skin over bony prominences of joints with drainage of calcium oxalate. Vasculitis with ulcerations of the fingertips and toes may occur in the overlap syndromes. Preventive measures include proper positioning, good nutrition with adequate protein intake, use of an egg crate mattress pad or waterbed, and padded support over elbows, knees, and heels. Restoration measures include appropriate treatment if deep pressure sores are present.

Raynaud's syndrome precipitated by cold and stress is usually mild when it occurs, unless associated with collagen vascular disease. Symptoms include painful cold fingers and color changes from white to blue. Wearing gloves and using biofeedback have been useful.

SYSTEMIC LUPUS ERYTHEMATOSUS

SLE is a chronic, autoimmune inflammatory disease that can affect any organ in the body. The most frequently involved sites are the skin, joints, pleuropericardium, kidneys, and central nervous system. Its course is varied in severity and duration.

People with SLE are universally fatigued. The causes of fatigue are multifactorial and may result from deconditioning resulting from decreased activity and release of inflammatory cytokines known to cause muscle atrophy and joint inflammation. These inflammatory cytokines may also influence mood and behavior. Interferon, TNF, and IL-2 are associated with fatigue and lack of motivation. Medication used in treating SLE, such as prednisone, is known to cause type 2 muscle fiber atrophy, which may be associated with muscle weakness. Several studies have shown that fatigue is more prevalent in those with SLE than in those without and that, characteristically, it is least on awakening and steadily increases as the day progresses (362,363). This pattern is clearly different from morning stiffness, characteristic of RA, and may be a result of deconditioning rather than an inflammatory process. Physical findings in this patient group include muscle weakness, disruption of sleep/wake cycle, cognitive difficulty, and psychomotor slowing (364). Depression is reported in about 30% of patients with SLE (365).

Fatigue is the best predictor of disease activity (364). Patients with SLE have reduced peak VO_2 and exercise duration. They also have reduced muscle strength and reduced forced expiratory volume (FEV) (366). A pilot study of 15 SLE patients aged 12 to 19 showed moderate impairment in aerobic fitness compared to referenced controls. Sixty-seven percent reported significant fatigue by questionnaire. There was no significant correlation between fitness and fatigue. Neither fitness nor fatigue is correlated with disease activity or damage or quality of life (367).

The symptoms prevalent in the SLE population (fatigue, deconditioning, and disability) respond to rehabilitation interventions. Central nervous system manifestations, such as poor concentration and memory impairment, do not. Isometric and aerobic conditioning programs are feasible in this population and effective in increasing fitness, strength, and functional capacity. Patients with SLE have been shown to have decreased aerobic capacity (364,366). An aerobic exercise program has been shown to increase endurance by 20% (368). A RCT of adult SLE patients showed significant improvement in exercise tolerance and aerobic capacity, quality of life, and depression after a supervised cardiovascular training program when compared to nonexercising controls (369). Treatment may include an energy conservation training program teaching that physical activity is interrupted by rest. Naps are taken during the day, and sleep can be promoted by the use of relaxation tapes.

Pain is common in the small joints of the hands and feet because of arthralgias and arthritis. Joint pain also can result from avascular necrosis of bone. Joint deformity is also seen. Control of joint pain has been successful with acupuncture and acupressure techniques, heat, cold, and TENS (370). These techniques are more effective in treating arthralgias than in treating avascular necrosis, which requires unweighting of the lower extremity. When unsuccessful, joint replacement to control symptoms may be required but should be undertaken with great caution because of the high degree of joint laxity (Jaccoud's arthropathy), which is often difficult to correct surgically.

The rashes of lupus are usually not responsive to nonpharmacologic treatments, but the skin ulceration that can occur as a result of active Raynaud's syndrome responds to hand-warming techniques (371). Temperature biofeedback has been used to relieve vasospastic disease.

One of the major challenges to the rehabilitation team is the request to evaluate and treat patients with central nervous system involvement. Stroke, psychosis, depression, and memory deficits all have a significant impact on function. Treatment is aimed at the underlying problem. An uncommon but well-described problem is transverse myelitis. Management may require mobility aids, including a wheelchair. Reeducation in self-care skills and exercise to help promote stamina is needed. Spasticity may be controlled with Baclofen or diazepam or local motor point blocks. Treatment of flaccidity with braces or adaptive equipment should be offered. Speech therapy can provide strategies to enhance memory with the use of lists and cues.

In a study of hand function in 109 SLE patients of the impact of hand function on daily activities, 73% of them reported interference with ADLs. Reduced grip strength, fumbling, and pain most commonly interfered with productivity (372).

The patient with SLE has to overcome major obstacles to successfully cope with this multifaceted illness. Support groups and family have been shown to be helpful in increasing compliance and are an essential component in the rehabilitation process.

SYSTEMIC SCLEROSIS

Management of progressive systemic sclerosis (SS) presents a significant challenge for rehabilitation specialists. The primary organ affected is the skin, but the pathogenesis is microvascular damage that can affect the kidney, the lung, and occasionally the heart (373). Whereas internal organ involvement usually requires pharmacologic treatment (blood pressure control, possible treatment of pulmonary fibrosis), musculoskeletal involvement leads to soft tissue contractures and loss of ROM for which rehabilitation interventions may be effective.

The skin in those with SS is often shiny and bound down and is associated with loss of soft tissue. This is most obvious with the hands, where fibrosis of the skin (with or without calcinosis) causes contractures, depigmentation, telangiectasias, ulceration, and loss of prehension. Raynaud's phenomenon often accompanies these findings.

The rehabilitation approaches include use of heat modalities. Care needs to be taken to avoid overheating relatively underperfused soft tissue that results from the microvascular damage. Paraffin and moist heat are usually best tolerated. Treatment of Raynaud's includes topical creams, such as nitroglycerine paste, and temperature biofeedback, as well as electric mittens. In general, heat and stretch programs are recommended, but few data are available to establish efficacy.

Several studies have reported beneficial effects of transcutaneous electrical nerve stimulation (TENS) and acupuncture. Both techniques are thought to increase skin block flow through increased vascularization (TENS) or activation of vasoactive peptides (acupuncture) (374).

Joint contracture is a frequent result of skin thickening and contraction at the joint. Disuse leads to muscle atrophy. Muscle may also be involved from an inflammatory process that begins as a cellular muscle infiltrate causing myositis and may lead to fibrotic change in muscle. This may be painful and may result in weakness accompanied by a rise in CPK and other muscle enzymes.

Physical medicine and rehabilitative treatment rely on a heat and stretch program of active or active-assistive ROM. Active contraction of muscle is usually needed to restore or preserve functional ROM. Usually, isometric exercise has been employed, but isotonic and isokinetic exercises appear to be well tolerated in many with rheumatic disease. Slow-rate isokinetic exercise (<60 degrees/s) may be very stressful on inflamed joints.

Adjunctively, splinting of the hand or wrist can be added to the heat and stretch program. Dynamic splinting appears to be ineffective and poorly tolerated (375).

The peripheral nervous system is commonly involved in SS, with a motor-sensory neuropathy (376), and occasionally autonomic dysfunction (377). CTS is most commonly seen, although weakness of the long flexors may be seen as well (377). Proper joint positioning, avoidance of compression at bony prominences, and short-term functional splinting may be useful.

The impact of SS on function is often profound and may reduce work capacity. Job modification, protection from cold, toxic exposures (urea formaldehyde, benzene, silica, etc.) and worksite modification may help preserve function and reduce risk of exacerbation. Adjustment to illness often depends on psychosocial support and preservation of function (378,379). Provision of treatment improves disease outcome (380).

A review of clinical management is available for the reader (380).

SPONDYLOARTHROPATHIES

Ankylosing spondylitis and other related diseases (e.g., PSA, reactive arthritis, and IBD–related arthritis) constitute a group of disorders involving the axial skeleton, enthesopathy, and extra-articular manifestations (e.g., skin rashes/psoriasis, uveitis, and aortitis). They are known as spondyloarthropathies.

The disability resulting from these diseases is usually attributable to the loss of spinal mobility and reduced pulmonary function. The impairments include pain at the enthesis, which is often worst at night and makes sitting difficult, and intervertebral fusion, producing substantial postural change.

Treatment for spondyloarthritis had typically consisted of NSAIDs, corticosteroids, and x-ray therapy, the latter two contributed to the development of osteoporosis. More recently, methotrexate, sulfasalazine, and now TNF blockers such as etanercept have been used successfully, and evidence supports the efficacy and safety of secukinumab, the first drug targeting the IL-17 pathway (381).

Rehabilitation therapies have been aimed at reducing pain, preserving joint alignment and posture, and promoting independence in functional activities. Fitness training is essential to maintain independent function.

At disease onset, the patient should be educated about maintaining mobility and preserving alignment. An ROM program designed to reduce hip flexor contractures and kyphosis should be initiated. Prone lying and sleeping without a pillow are encouraged. Some degree of muscle strengthening and especially abdominal breathing should be instituted (382–385). Often, therapies are suggested in conjunction with therapeutic pool/spa treatment, which seem to provide some symptomatic relief (386).

One report describes the use of a Jewett spinal orthotic as an effective treatment for increasing spinal mobility and reinstating the lumbar curve (387).

The most convincing data are presented for treatment efficacy of an intensive 3-week inpatient hospitalization (385). Using the Bath AS global assessment, diseases activity index, and visual analog scale for stiffness, improvements were demonstrated that were significantly better than those not treated for a similar 3-week period.

Patients with AS must be counseled about potential risk of cervical spine fractures that may result in tetraplegia. Cervical fracture is much more common than thoracic or lumbar. The likelihood of spinal cord injury is 11.4 times higher in this group than in those without AS (388). The cause of injury was usually slipping (53% of cases). Patients must be educated about self-protection to try to minimize injury, especially in the house; and to avoid contact sports, drinking, and driving; and to keep homes well lit in order to prevent injury. More recent RCTs have looked at the benefits of various combined exercise programs (combined flexibility, strengthening, breathing, and posture) and the latter further combined with aerobic exercise in supervised outpatient versus home settings. Control groups had received the same exercise, conventional, or no exercise. Results in the nonaerobic studies have indicated significant benefits in the areas of flexibility and function in both settings. In the aerobic incorporated study, only the supervised outpatient group had significant improvement when compared to the home group during similar exercises (389–395).

A recent 2008 Cochrane database review of 11 AS trials summarizes the scientific evidence on the effectiveness of physiotherapy interventions (individualized home exercise vs. supervised no intervention, supervised group therapy vs. individualized home exercise, initial inpatient Spa exercise followed by outpatient group therapy vs. outpatient group therapy and experimental exercise vs. conventional exercise). The author concludes that an individualized home-based or supervised program is better than no intervention; supervised group physiotherapy is better than home exercise, and combined inpatient Spa exercise followed by outpatient group exercise is better than group exercise alone (396).

Evaluation of occupational status and conditions is important in AS patients. A study of 397 AS patients showed that those with jobs that required dynamic flexibility had more functional limitations than those without this requirement (BASFI 48.3 vs. 38.1). A significantly increased BASRI and radiographic damage score was seen with dynamic flexibility and exposure to whole-body vibration jobs (397). Reviews of treatment for AS are available (389,398).

JUVENILE IDIOPATHIC ARTHRITIS

Juvenile idiopathic arthritis (JIA) is an umbrella term now used to refer to a heterogeneous group of disorders of childhood onset that have in common chronic arthritis. The term JIA now replaces the older classification for JRA and juvenile chronic arthritis. JIA is defined by an onset before age 16 with arthritis affecting one or more joints for more than 6 weeks with no other known etiology (399). There are eight subtypes of JIA: systemic onset, oligoarticular persistent, oligoarticular extended, RF-negative polyarthritis, RF-positive polyarthritis, PSA, enthesitis-related, and undifferentiated (399).

In general, the classification criteria for JIA are based on clinically presenting symptoms but also include exclusion criteria in defining each disease process. These are the following: (a) psoriasis or history of psoriasis in the patient or a first-degree family member; (b) arthritis in an HLA-B27–positive male beginning after the 6th birthday; (c) AS, enthesitis-related arthritis, sacroiliitis with IBD, Reiter's syndrome, an acute anterior uveitis, or a history of one of these disorders in a first-degree relative; (d) the presence of IgM RF on at least two occasions in at least 3 months; and (e) the presence of systemic JIA in the patient. Each of these subtypes has an adult counterpart, which may differ somewhat in presentation. JIA is more often manifested in large joints such as the ankles, knees, or wrists unlike adult forms. Rheumatoid or subcutaneous nodules and RF are less likely seen in this population as well.

Early identification of the disease, advances in drug therapy, appropriate and well-timed surgical intervention, and early active ongoing team rehabilitation programs have contributed to better quality of life and functional outcome (400–402). Many patients who in the past were wheelchair bound are now functionally ambulatory with early diagnosis and intervention (403). A recent 2008 study of 106 JIA patients showed 66% have low physical activity (PA) levels (not meeting public health standards for moderate to vigorous exercise) and are at risk for further loss in PA benefits. Low PA was not related to disease activity. These patients should be urged to increase PA (404). A 2008 review of exercise in pediatric rheumatic diseases reveals exercise capacity is significantly decreased in a large number of JIA patients and is most common with active inflammation especially in girls with RF-positive polyarticular JIA. Low levels of weight-bearing activity contribute to reduced bone mass, strength, and function. Increased levels of moderate to vigorous physical activity may improve exercise capacity, function, and general quality of life (405). Adults who have had JIA have significantly lower rates of employment and exercise tolerance than age-matched unaffected controls (405).

JIA Categories

Systemic onset JIA is defined as arthritis in one or more joints with or preceded by fever of at least 2-week duration with at least 3 days of daily documented temps greater than 39°C, evanescent rash, generalized lymphadenopathy, hepatosplenomegaly or splenomegaly or both, and serositis. In 50% of cases, five or more joints may be involved during some phase of the disease. This group comprises 2% to 17% of children with JIA and has a male/female ratio of 1:1 with peak onset during 1 to 6 years of age. They often have growth delays, osteopenia, anemia, leukocytosis, thrombocytosis, and elevated acute-phase reactants, while RF positivity is rare. In milder cases, patients will respond well to NSAIDs, but more involved cases will require initial intravenous steroids followed by tapering of oral regimens; DMARD therapy with cyclosporine and methotrexate is often given. The newer biologic agents such as anakinra that are being studied may show more usefulness in systemic onset JIA (406). The long-term prognosis is better for those with less severe arthritis. Patients who have systemic features that had lasted more than 6 months, polyarthritis with hip involvement, and thrombocytosis have a poorer overall outcome, and more of these children have long-term disability (407).

Oligoarticular JIA presents in two ways: (a) persistent oligoarthritis affecting 1 to 4 joints during the first 6 months of the disease affecting and (b) extended oligoarticular arthritis affecting greater than 4 joints in the first 6 months. Females are affected at a 4:1 ratio to males, with peak age onset around 6 years of age. It is the most common of the JIA subtypes affecting 50% to 60% of all children with JIA (408). The knee is the most commonly involved joint, followed by the ankle. Oligoarticular JIA may also involve the small joints of the hand and TMJ. Chronic anterior uveitis is seen in 20% to 30% of those with oligoarticular JIA. ANA positivity is seen in 50% to 70% of these children and has a high degree of association with chronic anterior uveitis. Treatment algorithms for these patients may begin with NSAIDs, but due to a low level of responders in this group, intra-articular steroid injections are more commonly used. Those with little or no response in these cases are treated with disease-modifying regimens such as methotrexate or antitumor necrosis antibody agents. Most patients respond to pharmacological therapies, with as many as 68% of those with the persistent type showing improvement and up to 70% of those in the extended oligoarticular group treated with methotrexate (409). Those who have not responded are eligible for TNF-alpha inhibition therapy or anakinra therapy. Level of evidence is moderate for effectiveness (410).

Polyarticular JIA is divided into two subgroups which include (a) JIA RF positive and (b) JIA RF negative. Both of these processes present with five or more joints involved during the first 6 months of the disease. The first of these groups differ with the presence of a positive immunoglobulin-M RF on at least two occasions at least 3 months apart. Female predominance is seen with ratios of 9:1 and 10% of total JIA cases. It is usually more aggressive in the patients affecting symmetrically small joints of the hands and wrists and some larger joints similar to the adult form of the disease. Ten percent of those affected may have rheumatoid nodules. RF-negative polyarticular JIA has the greatest risk for chronic, severe arthritis. It accounts for 30% of all cases of polyarticular JIA, with a 3:1 female preponderance. Early treatment is required with methotrexate. The joint distribution can be symmetric or asymmetric affecting large and small joints, which may include TMJ and cervical spine. Positive ANA may be seen in up to 40% of cases and a higher risk for anterior uveitis.

In both types of polyarticular JIA, early treatment with methotrexate is recommended. In RF-positive patients with signs of progressive disease, methotrexate in combination with anti-TNF antibody agents is recommended as this may play a role in preventing bony erosions (411).

Psoriatic JIA is a combination of arthritis and psoriasis and accounts for about 10% of the total JIA cases with a 2:1 female predominance. Diagnostic criteria include (a) dactylitis, (b) nail pitting and onycholysis, and (c) psoriasis in a first-degree relative. The arthritis typically involves peripheral, asymmetric joints of the hands, feet, knees, and ankles. When joint involvement is limited, NSAIDs and intra-articular injections can be used initially. Methotrexate is effective in treating skin involvement, and anti-TNF antibody therapy is useful when the disease is most aggressive.

Enthesopathic JIA represents about 10% of all and is characterized by arthritis, enthesitis, or both in addition to any two of the following: (a) sacroiliac joint tenderness and/or inflammatory lumbosacral pain, (b) positive HLA-B27 antigen, (c) acute symptomatic anterior uveitis, (d) onset of arthritis or enthesitis in a male greater than 6 years old, or (e) physician-diagnosed HLA-B27–associated disease in first- or second-degree relative. The lower limbs and axial skeleton are most often affected. Other clinical manifestations include anterior uveitis, IBD, and a reactive arthritis. Treatment with NSAIDs for symptomatic relief of enthesitis is often initially given. Those with specific articular involvement may be treated with intra-articular corticosteroids but may require DMARD therapy. Methotrexate, sulfasalazine, and more recently anti–TNF-alpha agents have been used as well.

Unclassified JIA are those subjects who do not fulfill any of the ILAR classification categories. This group constitutes, on average, 10% of all cases (402).

Special problem areas and impairments exist that deserve the attention of the rehabilitation specialist. Growth retardation, in general, may limit full stature. Abnormalities in growth related to specific joints result in a number of physical problems, cause impairment, and impact on function: short toes and fingers, leg length discrepancies, and micrognathia (i.e., small mandible). These abnormalities are due to premature closure of epiphyseal plates caused by intra-articular inflammation disturbing the development of the growth plate. Iritis and blindness are other major physical problems. It is important to remember that impairments of joint contractures and loss of ROM and muscle strength occur rapidly in JIA and must be managed quickly and efficiently. Impaired aerobic capacity is also present early in the course of the disease (412–414). Treatment goals and treatments should be initiated early in the disease course.

Specific Problems

An excellent review article has been published that addresses some of the generally accepted approaches to specific problems in JIA (415).

Upper Limbs. The wrist is often involved in JIA, and wrist flexion contracture can occur rapidly. A cock-up resting splint should be used at night. If the wrist is inflamed or forearm muscles are weak, contributing to wrist flexion, a functional splint should be used for activities. If a wrist flexion contracture is present, serial casting may be needed.

If there is PIP involvement, the resting splint should include the hand as well as the wrist. With interphalangeal (IP) joint contractures, a dynamic outrigger splint should be used during the day.

If the elbow is acute, an adjustable hinge splint can be used. ROM exercises to maintain extension, pronation, and supination are important. If a contracture exists, serial casting can be performed.

Neck. Every effort should be made to avoid flexion contracture at the neck. Proper positioning at night with the use of a single thin pillow, like a pediatric contour pillow, is recommended. When there is acute pain, a soft cervical collar is worn. Sometimes torticollis becomes a problem, and a firmer Plastazote collar may help. A collar is recommended for desk work. A desk with a tilt top may reduce pain and help maintain more ideal spinal posture.

Lower Limbs. Knee involvement should be managed promptly. If the joint is acute, a posterior resting splint should be used at night to prevent flexion contracture. If contracture already exists, a posterior splint may increase the danger of tibial subluxation and should not be used. Rather, the contracture should be reduced with a skin traction device or by serial casting. Occasionally soft tissue release is necessary.

Valgus deformity frequently occurs, and a supracondylar osteotomy may be needed to achieve realignment if conservative measures fail. A hip flexion deformity contributes to knee flexion problems and care must be taken to maintain hip extension. In severe disease, knee joint replacement can be considered if pain management and function cannot be achieved by medical and rehabilitative means.

An acute hip joint is most often associated with acute muscle spasm and rapid formation of a flexion contracture. Often, skin traction is used during acute hip pain to prevent contracture, with the patient lying supine in bed; 1 kg of weight for each 10 kg of body weight is used. In the child with a tendency toward knee flexion contracture, use of light hip traction during the night reduces the chance of the formation of hip and knee contractures. There should be periods of lying prone during the day to encourage maintenance of hip extension. A prone lying board also may be used in bed. If hip contracture is not responsive to conservative treatment, a soft tissue release may be needed. Joint replacement may be needed in severe disease and is usually performed before 16 years of age.

Ankle/Foot. Particular attention should be directed to management of the foot. Use of the proper shoe type and orthoses, as well as ROM exercise, is important. Leg length discrepancy should be corrected with a shoe insert or built-up shoe if a greater than 3/8-in. correction is needed.

Spine. Significant loss of motion, particularly in extension, can occur. The use of a small contour pillow while the child is supine provides suboccipital support while maintaining the neutral position limiting neck flexion. Cervical spine involvement in the systemic type and the polyarticular RF-negative form of JIA is common and requires careful attention to maintain alignment.

Compliance. Both the parents and the child should understand treatment regimens to ensure compliance. Many treatments are performed at home with parents supervising.

Exercise. Since patients with JIA have been demonstrated to have decreased ROM, muscle strength, and aerobic capacity, exercise in the form of ROM stretching and isometric, isotonic, and aerobic exercise are recommended early in the treatment program. Since most children lose strength rapidly around inflamed joints (particularly the knee), a few isometric contractions daily are recommended even with an inflamed joint (416).

Aquatic exercise has been shown to significantly improve hip motion (417). An 8-week weight-bearing conditioning program has been shown to increase aerobic capacity in polyarticular JIA without disease exacerbation or increased pain (217). A RCT of 80 JIA children consisted of a low to moderate (as tolerated) aerobic experimental group and a Qigong control group both exercising three times a week for 12 weeks. Both groups showed significant improvement in CHAQ but not in aerobic capacity. Adherence was higher in the Qigong group (418). Children with JIA often have osteoporosis resulting from glucocorticoids, and weight-bearing activity has a positive influence on bone density (BMD) (419).

A 2008 Cochrane review assessed RCTs on the effects of exercise on function, QOL, and aerobic capacity in JIA. Three out of 16 identified studies met selection criteria. Data were pooled for 212 JIA patients. The outcome measure favored a positive exercise effect but none was significant. Exercise in the excluded and included studies did not exacerbate arthritis. The author concludes that more "silver level" studies are needed to ascertain the short- and long-term effects of exercise for JIA patients (420).

Psychosocial Factors. The disease has an impact on the child's self-image, socialization, sexuality, and integration into school activities. Efforts should be made to keep acute admissions to hospitals at a minimum, so the child can participate as fully as possible in school, family, and social activities. Home schooling is not advocated. It is best to keep the child active in school. He or she should be allowed to participate as much as desired but should be given clear guidelines about limitations. Particular advice should be given in regard to sports activities. Body contact and high-impact sports are to be avoided (football, soccer, running, and ballet jumps). Cycling and swimming are to be encouraged. Guidance and support are needed during adolescence to deal with issues of vocation and sexuality.

Both children and parents should be educated in the disease and the benefits of treatment. One study shows parents in an education program improved significantly concerning their self-reported competencies on medical, exercise, pain, and social support issues (421).

GERIATRIC ARTHRITIDES

Care of the aged patient with arthritis is a challenge (422). Older people value the preservation of function and independence. They are often retired or working less than full time, so that they may enjoy family, travel, and more leisure and recreational activities.

As we age, the body experiences physiologic changes of normal aging. These changes include decreased proprioception and spatial orientation, difficulty in balancing and righting oneself, which may lead to falls. Other changes include muscle atrophy and decreased muscle power. The ability to sustain maximal muscle contraction is also reduced. Some older adults become less active and deconditioned (422).

In addition to normal aging changes, many older adults have comorbid conditions (i.e., congestive heart failure, OA, stroke, diabetes, hypertension, peripheral neuropathy, and emphysema). This necessitates the use of many medications. They have psychosocial challenges as a result of retirement income, and death of family members and friends, all of which may lead to some isolation and loneliness (423).

The elderly also may have chronic RA, which had its onset earlier in life. In addition, patients 60 years or older can present with elderly-onset RA (EORA). This tends to have more equal gender distribution, higher frequency of acute systemic onset with involvement of the shoulder, a higher disease activity, and in the later stages more radiographic damage and functional decline. Efficacy and tolerability of second-line drugs is similar in both age groups, but in the elderly, caution is needed with NSAIDs and prednisone (424,425).

The elderly with arthritis tend to be less physically active. Their diets may be poorly suited to their needs. Rehabilitation treatment goals in the elderly with arthritis are to reduce impairment, functional problems, and disability by relieving pain, fatigue, and psychological stress and by improving joint motion, muscle strength, and aerobic capacity. Achieving these goals will enhance safe mobility and ADLs and help prevent disability.

Treatments, both pharmacologic and rehabilitative, need to be altered in the elderly to accommodate for physiologic aging changes in body mechanics and pharmacokinetics, the effects of comorbid diseases, and the increased presence of biomechanically deranged joints and psychosocial issues attendant to the group (426,427).

In general, exercises tend to be ROM, isometric, low-resistance isotonic, and low-intensity aerobic. Isometrics are best if ligamentous laxity and effusion are present. Precautions need to be taken with joint replacements, which are common in the elderly. Comorbid cardiac and neurologic disease also limits exercise intensity and duration. Several RCTs show that regular exercise does not increase joint pain or accelerate disease progression. These studies suggest that exercise training may increase physiologic reserve and decrease dependency in older adults with joint disease (428). A program of progressive interval training with bicycles and step climbing in fragile elderly RA patients for 45 minutes twice a week increased work capacity 76% without increasing disease activity and has been shown to be effective (429). Heat/cold before exercise, deweighting painful lower extremity joints, and cognitive-behavioral strategies often diminish pain and improve function. Removing moderate to large joint effusions and carefully injecting any inflamed bursae or tendon sheaths also contribute to pain relief. Very painful biomechanically compromised joints that cause increased functional loss should be considered for joint replacement.

Correlates of fatigue in this population are pain severity, functional status, sleep quality, female gender, comorbid conditions, and disease duration (228). Treatment designed to decrease pain and improve sleep using short rest periods and energy conservation techniques may help reduce fatigue.

Foot problems are very common in the arthritic patient and even more common in the elderly. Proper footwear should provide a crepe sole to provide absorption of the ground reaction force, a wide base of support to promote balance, good fit with adequate depth to clear tops of toes and accommodate the width of the forefoot, and softness to relieve metatarsalgia. Foot hygiene and prompt care of skin breakdown are essential to prevent infection in a patient with possible vascular compromise of the lower extremity.

Management of patients with rheumatic diseases is very challenging and requires coordinated care among a variety of care professionals. These diseases are chronic and complex because of medications required, likelihood of medical comorbidities, and functional impact of disease and disabilities. Aging with chronic illness must be assessed in terms of multiorgan/multisystem and coordination of services from multiple professional groups, family, and the social and economic environment in which the patient resides.

REFERENCES

1. Elders MT. The increasing impact of arthritis on public health. *J Rheumatol.* 2000;60(suppl):6–8.
2. World Health Organization. The burden of musculoskeletal conditions at the start of the new millennium. *World Health Organ Tech Rep Ser.* 2003;919:i–x.
3. Barbour KE, Helmick CG, Theis KA, et al. Prevalence of doctor-diagnosed arthritis and arthritis-attributable activity limitation: United States, 2010–2012. *MMWR Morb Mortal Wkly Rep.* 2013;62:869–873.
4. Trogdon JG, Murphy LB, Khavjou OA, et al. Costs of chronic diseases at the state level: the chronic disease cost calculator. *Prev Chronic Dis.* 2015;12:E140.
5. Furner SE, Hootman JM, Helmick CG, et al. Health-related quality of life of US adults with arthritis: analysis of data from the Behavioral Risk Factor Surveillance System, 2003, 2005, and 2007. *Arthritis Care Res (Hoboken).* 2011;63:788–799.
6. Murphy L, Bolen J, Helmick CG, et al., eds. Comorbidities are very common among people with arthritis. *Proceedings of the 20th National Conference on Chronic Disease Prevention and Control; 2009 Feb 23–25.* Atlanta, GA: Centers for Disease Control and Prevention; 2009.
7. Murphy LB, Sacks JJ, Brady TJ, et al. Anxiety and depression among US adults with arthritis: prevalence and correlates. *Arthritis Care Res (Hoboken).* 2012;64: 968–976.
8. Fries, JF, Williams CA, Morfeld D, et al. Reduction in long-term disability in patients with rheumatoid arthritis by disease-modifying antirheumatic drug-based treatment strategies. *Arthritis Rheum.* 1996;39(4):616–622.
9. Vergara F, Rosa J, Orozco C, et al. Evaluation of learned helplessness, self-efficacy and disease activity, functional capacity and pain in Argentinian patients with rheumatoid arthritis. *Scand J Rheumatol.* 2017;46:17–21.
10. Lettre G, Rioux JD. Autoimmune diseases: insights from genome-wide association studies. *Hum Mol Genet.* 2008;17(R2):R116–R121.
11. Berdal G, Sand-Svartrud AL, Bo I, et al. Aiming for a healthier life: a qualitative content analysis of rehabilitation goals in patients with rheumatic diseases. *Disabil Rehabil.* 2018;40:1–17.
12. Clarke AK. Effectiveness of rehabilitation in arthritis. *Clin Rehabil.* 1999;13(suppl):51–62.
13. van Onna M, Boonen A. The challenging interplay between rheumatoid arthritis, ageing and comorbidities. *BMC Musculoskelet Disord.* 2016;17:184.
14. Kirwan J, Heiberg T, Hewlett S, et al. Outcomes from the patient perspective workshop at OMERACT 6. *J Rheumatol.* 2003;30(4):868–872.
15. Golbus J. Monoarticular arthritis. In: Firestein GS, Budd RC, Sergent JS, et al., eds. *Kelley's Textbook of Rheumatology.* 8th ed. Philadelphia, PA: WB Saunders; 2009:533–544.
16. Sergent J, Fuchs H. Polyarticular arthritis. In: Firestein GS, Budd RC, Sergent JS, et al. eds. *Kelley's Textbook of Rheumatology.* 8th ed. Philadelphia, PA: WB Saunders; 2009:545–555.
17. Klippel JH, Stone JH, Crofford LJ, et al. Appendix I. Criteria for the classification and diagnosis of the rheumatic diseases. In: Klippel JH, Stone JH, Crofford LJ, et al., eds. *Primer on the Rheumatic Diseases.* 13th ed. Atlanta, GA: Springer; 2008:669–682.
18. Jordan JM. Principles of epidemiology of the rheumatic diseases. In: Firestein GS, Budd RC, Sergent JS, et al., eds. *Kelley's Textbook of Rheumatology.* 8th ed. Philadelphia, PA: WB Saunders; 2009:433–439.
19. Firestein GS. Etiology and pathogenesis of rheumatoid arthritis. In: Firestein GS, Budd RC, Srgent JS, et al. *Kelley's Textbook of Rheumatology.* 8th ed. Philadelphia, PA: WB Saunders; 2009:1035–1087.
20. McInnes IB, Schett G. The pathogenesis of rheumatoid arthritis. *N Engl J Med.* 2011;365:2205.
21. Nielen MM, van Schaardenburg D, Reesink HW, et al. Specific autoantibodies precede the symptoms of rheumatoid arthritis: a study of serial measurements in blood donors. *Arthritis Rheum.* 2004;50(2):380–386.
22. Walderburg J-M, Firestein GS. Rheumatoid arthritis: epidemiology, pathology and pathogenesis. In: Klippel JH, Stone JH, Crofford LJ, et al., eds. *Primer on the Rheumatic Diseases.* 13th ed. Atlanta, GA: Springer; 2008:122–132.
23. Feldman M, Brennan FM, Maini RN. Rheumatoid arthritis. *Cell.* 1996;85: 307–310.

24. Brennan FM, Maini RN, Feldman M. Role of pro-inflammatory cytokines in rheumatoid arthritis. *Springer Semin Immunopathol.* 1998;20:133–147.

25. Goldring SR, Gravallese EM. Pathogenesis of bone erosions in rheumatoid arthritis. *Curr Opin Rheumatol.* 2000;12:195–199.

26. Koetz K, Bryl E, Spickschen K, et al. T cell homeostasis in patients with rheumatoid arthritis. *Proc Natl Acad Sci U S A.* 2000;97:9203–9208.

27. Abolghasemi S, Gitipour A, Morteza A. The sensitivity, specificity and accuracy of anti-citrulline antibody test in diagnosis of rheumatoid arthritis. *Rheumatol Int.* 2013;33(4):1027–1030.

28. Hannahs-Hahn B, Tsao BP. Pathogenesis of SLE. In: Firestein GS, Budd RC, Sergent JS, et al., eds. *Kelley's Textbook of Rheumatology.* 8th ed. Philadelphia, PA: WB Saunders; 2009:1233–1262.

29. Varga J, Denton CP. Systemic sclerosis and the scleroderma-spectrum disorders. In: Firestein GS, Budd RC, Sergent JS, et al., eds. *Kelley's Textbook of Rheumatology.* 8th ed. Philadelphia, PA: WB Saunders; 2009:1311–1352.

30. Dalakas MC. Inflammatory muscle diseases. *N Engl J Med.* 2015;372:1734–1747.

31. Nagaraju K, Lundberg IE. Inflammatory diseases of the muscle and other myopathies. In: Firestein GS, Budd RC, Sergent JS, et al., eds. *Kelley's Textbook of Rheumatology.* 8th ed. Philadelphia, PA: WB Saunders; 2009:1353–1380.

32. Kumar Y, Bhatia A, Minz RW. Antinuclear antibodies and their detection methods in diagnosis of connective tissue diseases: a journey revisited. *Diagn Pathol.* 2009;4:1.

33. Terkeltaub R. Diseases associated with articular deposition of calcium pyrophosphate dehydrate and basic calcium phosphate crystals. In: Firestein GS, Budd RC, Sergent JS, et al., eds. *Kelley's Textbook of Rheumatology.* 8th ed. Philadelphia, PA: WB Saunders; 2009:1507–1524.

34. Healy PJ. Classification of the spondyloarthropathies. *Curr Opin Rheumatol.* 2005;17(4):395.

35. Van der Heijde D. Ankylosing spondylitis: clinical features. In: Klippel JH, Stone JH, Crofford LJ, et al., eds. *Primer on the Rheumatic Diseases.* 13th ed. Atlanta, GA: Springer; 2008:193–199.

36. Paronen I. Reiter's disease: a study of 344 cases observed in Finland. *Acts Med Scand.* 1948;131(suppl 212):1.

37. Granfors K, Jalkanen S, von Essen R, et al. Yersinia antigens in synovial-fluid cells from patients with reactive arthritis. *N Engl J Med.* 1989;320(4):216–221.

38. Telfer NR, Chalmers RJ, Whale K, et al. The role of streptococcal infection in the initiation of guttate psoriasis. *Arch Dermatol.* 1992;128(1):39–42.

39. Denison HJ, Curtis EM, Clynes MA, et al. The incidence of sexually acquired reactive arthritis: a systematic literature review. *Clin Rheumatol.* 2016;35(11):2639–2648.

40. Braun J. Ankylosing spondylitis: pathology and pathogenesis. In: Klippel JH, Stone JH, Crofford LJ, et al., eds. *Primer on the Rheumatic Diseases.* 13th ed. Atlanta, GA: Springer; 2008:200–208.

41. Tung CH, Lai NS, Li CY, et al. Risk of rheumatoid arthritis in patients with hepatitis C virus infection receiving interferon-based therapy: a retrospective cohort study using the Taiwanese national claims database. *BMJ Open.* 2018;8(7):e021747.

42. Jennette JC, Falk RJ, Bacon PA, et al. 2012 revised International Chapel Hill Consensus Conference Nomenclature of Vasculitides. *Arthritis Rheum.* 2013;65:1.

43. Jennette JC, Falk RJ. Pathogenesis of antineutrophil cytoplasmic autoantibody-mediated disease. *Nat Rev Rheumatol.* 2014;10:463.

44. Olson SW, Arbogast CB, Baker TP, et al. Asymptomatic autoantibodies associate with future anti-glomerular basement membrane disease. *J Am Soc Nephrol.* 2011;22:1946.

45. Weyand CM. Medium- and large-vessel vasculitis. *N Engl J Med.* 2003;349(2):160.

46. Lie JT. Aortic and extracranial large vessel giant cell arteritis: a review of 72 cases with histopathologic documentation. *Semin Arthritis Rheum.* 1995;24(6):422.

47. Piggott K, et al. Vascular damage in giant cell arteritis. *Autoimmunity.* 2009;42(7):596–604.

48. Fries JF. Assessment of the patients with rheumatic disease. In: Ruddy S, Harris ED, Sledge CB, et al., eds. *Kelley's Textbook of Rheumatology.* 3rd ed. Philadelphia, PA: WB Saunders; 1989:361–365.

49. Robinson DB, El-Gabalawy HS. Evaluation of the patient: history and physical examination. In: Klippel JH, Stone JH, Crofford LJ, et al., eds. *Primer on the Rheumatic Diseases.* 13th ed. Atlanta, GA: Springer; 2008:6–14.

50. Siegel KL, Kepple TM, O'Connell P, et al. A technique to evaluate foot function during the stance phase of gait. *Foot Ankle.* 1995;16:764–770.

51. Platto MS, O'Connell PG, Hicks JE, et al. The relationship of pain and deformity of the rheumatoid foot to gait and an index of functional ambulation. *J Rheumatol.* 1991;18:38–44.

52. Khan S, Alvi A, Holding S, et al. The clinical significance of antinucleolar antibodies. *J Clin Pathol.* 2008;61:283.

53. Eyre S, Orozco G, Worthington J. The genetic revolution in rheumatology: large scale genomic arrays and genetic mapping. *Nat Rev Rheumatol.* 2017;13(7):421–432.

54. Alparslan L, Weissman BN. Imaging modalities of rheumatic disease. In: Firestein GS, Budd RC, Sergent JS, et al., eds. *Kelley's Textbook of Rheumatology.* 8th ed. Philadelphia, PA: WB Saunders; 2009:777–832.

55. Prasad A, Fessell DP, Vanderschueren GM, et al. Ultrasound of the ankle: technique, anatomy, and diagnosis of pathologic conditions. *Radiographics.* 1998;18:325–334.

56. Amato AA, Barohn RJ. Evaluation and treatment of inflammatory myopathies. *J Neurol Neurosurg Psychiatry.* 2009;80(10):1060.

57. Hauer HA, Bajema IM, van Houwelingen HC, et al. Renal histology in ANCA-associated vasculitis: differences between diagnostic and serologic subgroups. *Kidney Int.* 2002;61(1):80–89.

58. Descombes E, Gardiol D, Leuenberger P. Transbronchial lung biopsy: an analysis of 530 cases with reference to the number of samples. *Monaldi Arch Chest Dis.* 1997;52(4):324.

59. Kendall FP. Lower extremity strength tests. In: Kendall FP, Kendall EM, Provance PG, eds. *Muscles: Testing Function.* 4th ed. Baltimore, MD: Lippincott Williams & Wilkins; 1993:179–191.

60. Merritt JL, McLean TJ, Erickson RP, et al. Measurement of trunk flexibility in normal subjects: reproducibility of three clinical methods. *Mayo Clin Proc.* 1986;61:192–197.

61. Huskisson EC, Jones J, Scott PJ. Application of visual analog scales to the measurement of functional capacity. *Rheumatol Rehabil.* 1976;15:185–187.

62. Belza BL, Henke CJ, Yelin EH, et al. Correlates of fatigue in older adults with rheumatoid arthritis. *Nurs Res.* 1993;42:93–99.

63. Krupp LB, Larocca NG, Muirnash J, et al. The Fatigue Severity Scale: application to patients with multiple sclerosis and systemic lupus erythematosus. *Arch Neurol.* 1989;46:1121–1123.

64. Fix AJ, Daughton DM. *Human Activity Profile Professional Manual.* Odessa, FL: Psychological Assessment Resources, Inc.; 1988.

65. Hochberg MC, Chang RW, Dwosh I, et al. The American College of Rheumatology 1991 revised criteria for the classification of global functional status in rheumatoid arthritis. *Arthritis Rheum.* 1992;35(5):498–502.

66. Meenan RF, Gertman PM, Mason JH. Measuring health status in arthritis: the arthritis impact measurement scales. *Arthritis Rheum.* 1980;23:146–152.

67. Duffy CM, Tucker L, Burgos-Vargas R. Update on functional assessment tools. *J Rheumatol.* 2000;27(suppl 58):11–14.

68. Bombardier C, Tugwell P, Sinclair A, et al. Preference for end point measures in clinical trials: results of structured workshops. *J Rheumatol.* 1982;9:798.

69. Bergner M, Bobbitt RA, Pollard WE, et al. The Sickness Impact Profile: validation of a health status measure. *Med Care.* 1976;14(1):57–67.

70. Ramey DR, Raynauld J-P, Fries JF. The Health Assessment Questionnaire 1992: Status and review. *Arthritis Care Res.* 1992;5(3):119–129.

71. Mchorney CA, Ware JE, Lu JFR, et al. The MOS 36-item Short-Form Health Survey (SF-36): III. Tests of data quality, scaling assumptions, and reliability across diverse patient groups. *Med Care.* 1994;32(1):40–66.

72. Ruof J, Stucki G. Comparison of the duogados functional index and the bath ankylosing spondylitis functional index: a literature review. *J Rheumatol.* 1999;26:955–960.

73. Felsen DT, Anderson JJ, Boers M, et al. American College of Rheumatology preliminary core set of disease activity measured in rheumatoid arthritis clinical trials. *Arthritis Rheum.* 1993;30:729–740.

74. Bellamy N, Kirwan J, Boers M, et al. Recommendations for a core set of outcome measures for future phase 3 clinical trials in knee, hip and hand: Consensus development in OMERACT III. *J Rheumatol.* 1997;24:799–802.

75. van der Heijde D, Calin A, Dougados M, et al. Selection of instruments in the core set for DC-ART, SMARD, physical therapy, and clinical record keeping in ankylosing spondylitis: Progress report of the ASAS Working Group. Assessments in Ankylosing Spondylitis. *J Rheumatol.* 1999;26(4):951–954.

76. Oliver AM, St. Clair EW. Rheumatoid arthritis: treatment and assessment. In: Klippel JH, Stone JH, Crofford LJ, et al., eds. *Primer on the Rheumatic Diseases.* 13th ed. Atlanta, GA: Springer; 2008:133–141.

77. Hammond A. The use of self-management strategies by people with rheumatoid arthritis. *Clin Rehabil.* 1998;12:81–87.

78. Hell J, Bird H, Johnson S. Effect of patient education on adherence to drug treatment for rheumatoid arthritis: a randomized controlled trial. *Ann Rheum Dis.* 2001;60:869–875.

79. Taal E, Riemsma RP, Brus HL, et al. Group education for patients with rheumatoid arthritis. *Patient Educ Couns.* 1993;20:177–187.

80. Kyngas H, Rissanen M. Support as a crucial prediction of good compliance of adolescents with chronic disease. *J Clin Nurs.* 2001;10:767–774.

81. Stenstrom CH, Arge B, Sundbom A. Home exercise and compliance in inflammatory rheumatic disease—a prospective clinical trial. *J Rheumatol.* 1997;24:470–476.

82. Neuberger GB, Kasal S, Smith KV, et al. Determinants of exercise and aerobic fitness on outpatients with arthritis. *Nurs Res.* 1994;43:11–17.

83. Fries JF. Current treatment paradigms in rheumatoid arthritis. *Rheumatology (Oxford).* 2000;39(suppl 1):30–35.

84. Wolfe F, Rehman V, Lane NE, et al. Starting a disease modifying antirheumatic drug or a biologic agent in rheumatoid arthritis: standards of practice for RA treatment. *J Rheumatol.* 2001;28:1704–1711.

85. Smolen JS, Aletaha D, Bijlsma JW, et al. Treating rheumatoid arthritis to target: recommendations of an international task force. *Ann Rheum Dis.* 2010;69:631.

86. Silverstein FE, Faich G, Goldstein JL, et al. Gastrointestinal toxicity with celecoxib vs nonsteroidal anti-inflammatory drugs for osteoarthritis and rheumatoid arthritis: the CLASS study: a randomized controlled trial. Celecoxib Long-term Arthritis Safety Study. *JAMA.* 2000;284:1247.

87. Ballou LR, Wang BEW. Non-steroidal anti-inflammatory drugs. In: Firestein GS, Budd RC, Sergent JS, et al., eds. *Kelley's Textbook of Rheumatology.* 8th ed. Philadelphia, PA: WB Saunders; 2009:833–862.

88. Farkouh ME, Greenberg BP. An evidence-based review of the cardiovascular risks of nonsteroidal anti-inflammatory drugs. *Am J Cardiol.* 2009;103(9):1227–1237.

89. Lane JM. Advances in therapeutics and diagnostics. Anti-inflammatory medications: selective COX-2 inhibitors. *J Am Acad Orthop Surg.* 2002;10:75–78.

90. Recommendations for the prevention and treatment of glucocorticoid-induced osteoporosis: ACR 2001 Update. American College of Rheumatology Ad Hoc Committee on Glucocorticoid-Induced Osteoporosis. *Arthritis Rheum.* 2001;44(7):1496–1503.

91. Buttgereit F, daSilva JA, Boers M, et al. Standardised nomenclature for glucocorticoid dosages and glucocorticoid treatment regimens: current questions and tentative answers in rheumatology. *Ann Rheum Dis.* 2002;61(8):718–722.

92. Catoggio LJ. Inflammatory muscle disease: management. In: Klippel JH, Dieppe PA, eds. *Rheumatology*. 2nd ed. London: CV Mosby; 1998:15.1–15.5.
93. Choi HK, Hernán MA, Seeger JD, et al. Methotrexate and mortality in patients with rheumatoid arthritis: a prospective study. *Lancet*. 2002;359(9313):1173.
94. Joffe MM, Love LA, Leff RL, et al. Drug therapy of the idiopathic inflammatory myopathies: predictors of response to prednisone, azathioprine, and methotrexate and a comparison of their efficacy. *Am J Med*. 1993;94(4):379.
95. Ruiz-Irastorza G, Ramos-Casals M, Brito-Zeron P, et al. Clinical efficacy and side effects of antimalarials in systemic lupus erythematosus: a systematic review. *Ann Rheum Dis*. 2010;69:20.
96. A randomized trial of hydroxychloroquine in early rheumatoid arthritis: The HERA Study. *Am J Med*. 1995;98:156.
97. Case JP. Old and new drugs used in rheumatic arthritis: a historical perspective. Part 2: the newer drugs and drug strategies. *Am J Ther*. 2001;8(3):163–179.
98. Smedegard G, Bjork J. Sulphasalazine: mechanism of action in rheumatoid arthritis. *Br J Rheumatol*. 1995;34(suppl 2):7–15.
99. Sulfasalazine in early rheumatoid arthritis. The Australian Multicentre Clinical Trial Group. *J Rheumatol*. 1992;19(11):1672–1677.
100. Clegg DO, Reda DJ, Abdellatif M. Comparison of sulfasalazine and placebo for the treatment of axial and peripheral articular manifestations of the seronegative spondyloarthropathies: a Department of Veterans Affairs cooperative study. *Arthritis Rheum*. 1999;42(11):2325–2329.
101. Emery P, Breedveld FC, Lemmel EM, et al. A comparison of the efficacy and safety of leflunomide and methotrexate for the treatment of rheumatoid arthritis. *Rheumatology*. 2000;39:655–665.
102. Weinblatt ME, Kremer JM, Coblyn JS, et al. Pharmacokinetics, safety and efficacy of combination treatment with methotrexate and leflunomide in patients with active rheumatoid arthritis. *Arthritis Rheum*. 1999;42:1322–1328.
103. Scott DL, Smolen JS, Kalden JR, et al. Treatment of active rheumatoid arthritis with leflunomide: two year follow up of a double blind, placebo controlled trial versus sulfasalazine. *Ann Rheum Dis*. 2001;60(10):913–923.
104. Haibel H, Rudwaleit M, Braun J, et al. Six months open label trial of leflunomide in active ankylosing spondylitis. *Ann Rheum Dis*. 2005;64(1):124–126.
105. Stein CM, Taylor HG. Immunoregulatory drugs. In: Firestein GS, Budd RC, Sergent JS, et al., eds. *Kelley's Textbook of Rheumatology*. 8th ed. Philadelphia, PA: WB Saunders; 2009:909–927.
106. Hahn BH, McMahon MA, Wilkinson A, et al. American College of Rheumatology guidelines for screening, treatment, and management of lupus nephritis. *Arthritis Care Res (Hoboken)*. 2012;64(6):797–808.
107. Dheda K, Lalloo UG, Cassim B, et al. Experience with azathioprine in systemic sclerosis associated with interstitial lung disease. *Clin Rheumatol*. 2004;23(4):306.
108. Sehgal SN. Rapamune (RAPA, rapamycin, sirolimus): mechanism of action immunosuppressive effect results from blockade of signal transduction and inhibition of cell cycle progression. *Clin Biochem*. 1998;31(5):335–340.
109. Denton MD, Magee CC, Sayegh MH. Immunosuppressive strategies in transplantation. *Lancet*. 1999;353:1083–1091.
110. Matthews SJ, McCoy C. Thalidomide: a review of approved and investigational uses. *Clin Ther*. 2003;25:342–395.
111. Debol SM, Herron MJ, Nelson RD. Anti-inflammatory action of dapsone: inhibition of neutrophil adherence is associated with inhibition of chemo-attractant induced signal transduction. *J Leukoc Boil*. 1997;62:827–836.
112. Emmerson BT. The management of gout. *N Engl J Med*. 1996;334:445–451.
113. White WB, Saag KG, Becker MA, et al. Cardiovascular safety of febuxostat or allopurinol in patients with gout. *N Engl J Med*. 2018;378(13):1200–1210.
114. Bathon JM. A comparison of etanercept and methotrexate in patients with early rheumatoid arthritis. *N Engl J Med*. 2000;343:1586–1593.
115. Moreland LW, Schiff MH, Baumgartner SW, et al. Etanercept therapy in rheumatoid arthritis: a randomized controlled trial. *Ann Intern Med*. 1999;130:478–486.
116. Davis JC, Van der Heijde D, Braun J, et al. Recombinant tumor necrosis factor (etanercept) for treating ankylosing spondylitis: a randomized, controlled trial. *Arthritis Rheum*. 2003;48:3230–3236.
117. Mease PJ, Goffe BS, Metz J, et al. Etanercept in treatment of psoriatic arthritis and psoriasis: a randomized trial. *Lancet*. 2000;356:385–390.
118. Corinne RM, Duogados M. Tumor necrosis factor-alpha blockers in rheumatoid arthritis: review of clinical experiences. *BioDrugs*. 2001;15:251–259.
119. Bresnihan B, Alvaro-Garcia JM, Cobby M, et al. Treatment of rheumatoid arthritis with recombinant human interleukin-1 receptor antagonist. *Arthritis Rheum*. 1998;41:2196–2204.
120. Edwards JC, Szczepanski L, Szechinski J, et al. Efficacy of B-cell targeted therapy with rituximab patients with rheumatoid arthritis. *N Engl J Med*. 2004;350:2572–2581.
121. Kremer JM, Genant HK, Moreland LW, et al. Effects of abatacept in patients with methotrexate resistant active rheumatoid arthritis: a randomized trial. *Ann Intern Med*. 2006;144:865–876.
122. Scott LJ. Tocilizumab: a review in rheumatoid arthritis. *Drugs*. 2017;77(17):1865–1879.
123. Siebert S, Tsoukas A, Robertson J, et al. Cytokines as therapeutic targets in rheumatoid arthritis and other inflammatory diseases. *Pharmacol Rev*. 2015;67(2):280–309.
124. Stein CM, Pincus T, Yocum D, et al. Combination treatment of severe RA with cyclosporine and MTX for forty-eight weeks: an open label extension study. The Methotrexate-Cyclosporine Combination Study Group. *Arthritis Rheum*. 1997;40(10):1843–1851.
125. O'Dell JR, Leff R, Paulsen G, et al. Treatment of rheumatoid arthritis with methotrexate and hydroxychloroquine, methotrexate and sulfasalazine, or a combination of the three medications—Results of a two-year, randomized, double-blind, placebo-controlled trial. *Arthritis Rheum*. 2002;46:1164–1170.
126. Lipsky PE, van der Heijde DMFM, St. Clair EW, et al. Infliximab and MTX in the treatment of rheumatoid arthritis: Anti-tumor necrosis factor trial in rheumatoid arthritis with concomitant study group. *N Engl J Med*. 2000;343:1594–1602.
127. Seymour HE, Worsely A, Smith JM, et al. Anti-TNF agents for rheumatoid arthritis. *Br J Clin Pharmacol*. 2001;51(3):201–208.
128. Arnold WJ, ed. *Arthritis Foundation's Guide to Alternative Therapies*. Atlanta, GA: Arthritis Foundation; 1999:1–285.
129. Yang L, Sibbritt D, Adams J. A critical review of complementary and alternative medicine use among people with arthritis: a focus upon prevalence, cost, user profiles, motivation, decision-making, perceived benefits and communication. *Rheumatol Int*. 2017;37(3):337–351.
130. Arnold EA, Arnold WJ. Complementary and alternative therapies. In: Klippel JH, Stone JH, Crofford LJ, et al., eds. *Primer on the Rheumatic Diseases*. 13th ed. Atlanta, GA: Springer; 2008:664–668.
131. Cameron M, Gagnier JJ, Chrubasik S. Herbal therapy for treating rheumatoid arthritis. *Cochrane Database Syst Rev*. 2011;(2):CD002948.
132. Wetzel MS, Eisenberg DM, Kaptchuk TJ. Courses involving complimentary and alternative medicine at US medical schools. *JAMA*. 1998;280:784.
133. Herman PM, Poindexter BL, Witt CM, et al. Are complementary therapies and integrative care cost-effective? A systematic review of economic evaluations. *BMJ Open*. 2012;2(5).
134. Eisenberg DM, Davis RB, Ettner SL, et al. Trends in alternative medicine use in the United States. Results of a following national survey. *JAMA*. 1998;280:1569.
135. Herman CJ, Allen P, Hunt WC, et al. Use of complementary therapies among primary care clinic patients with arthritis. *Prev Chronic Dis*. 2004;1(4):A12.
136. Feldman DE, Duffy C, DeCivta M, et al. Factors associated with the use of complementary and alternative medicine in juvenile idiopathic arthritis. *Arthritis Rheum*. 2004;51(4):527–532.
137. Sugarman J, Burk L. Physicians ethical obligations regarding alternative medicine. *JAMA*. 1998;280:1623–1625.
138. Kanning M. Why I would want to use complimentary and alternative therapy: a patient's perspective. *Rheum Dis Clin North Am*. 1999;25(4):823–831.
139. Breuer GS, Orbach H, Elkayam O, et al. Perceived efficacy among patients of various methods of complementary alternative medicine for rheumatologic diseases. *Rheumatology*. 2005;23(5):693–696.
140. Kramer N. Why I would not recommend complimentary or alternative therapies: a physician's perspective. *Rheum Dis Clin North Am*. 1999;25(4):833–843.
141. Neims AH. Why I would recommend complimentary or alternative therapies: a physician's perspective. *Rheum Dis Clin North Am*. 1999;25(4):845–853.
142. Linde K, Vickers A, Hondras M, et al. Systematic reviews of complementary therapies—An annotated bibliography Part I: acupuncture. *BMC Complement Altern Med*. 2001;1:3.
143. Linde K, Riet G, Hondras M. Systematic reviews of complementary therapies—An annotated bibliography. Part II: herbal medicine. *BMC Complement Altern Med*. 2001;1:5.
144. Linde K, Hondras M, Vickers A, et al. Systematic reviews of complementary therapies—An annotated bibliography. Part III: homeopathy. *BMC Complement Altern Med*. 2001;1:4.
145. Soeken KL, Mill SA, Ernst E. Herbal medicine for the treatment of rheumatoid arthritis: a systematic review. *Rheumatology (Oxford)*. 2003;42(5):652–659.
146. Setty AR, Sigal LH. Herbal medications commonly used in the practice of rheumatology: mechanisms of action, efficacy and side effects. *Semin Arthritis Rheum*. 2005;34(6):773–784.
147. Sawitzke AD, Shi H, Finco MF, et al. Clinical efficacy and safety of glucosamine, chondroitin sulphate, their combination, celecoxib or placebo taken to treat osteoarthritis of the knee: 2-year results from GAIT. *Ann Rheum Dis*. 2010;69(8):1459–1464.
148. Lautenschlagen J. Acupuncture in the treatment of rheumatic diseases. *Z Rheumatol*. 1997;56(1):8–20.
149. Casmirol L, Burnsley L, Brosseau L, et al. Acupuncture and electroacupuncture for the treatment of rheumatoid arthritis. *Cochrane Database Syst Rev*. 2005;(4):CD0033788.
150. Greco CM, Kao AH, Maksimowicz-McKinnnon K, et al. Acupuncture for systemic lupus erythematosus; a pilot RCT feasibility and safety study. *Lupus*. 2008;17(12):1108–1116.
151. Beckeman H, de Bie RA, Bouter LM, et al. The efficacy of laser therapy for musculoskeletal and skin disorders: a criteria based meta-analysis of randomized controlled trials. *Phys Ther*. 1992;72:483–491.
152. Young LD, Bradley LA, Turner RA. Decreases in health care resource utilization in patients with rheumatoid arthritis following a cognitive behavioral intervention. *Biofeedback Self Regul*. 1995;20:259–268.
153. Garfinkel MS, Singhol A, Katz WA, et al. Yoga-based intervention for carpal tunnel syndrome: a randomized trial. *JAMA*. 1998;280:1601–1603.
154. NIH Consensus Conference. Acupuncture. *JAMA*. 1998;280(17):1518–1524.
155. Yocum DE, Hodes R, Sundstrom WR, et al. Use of biofeedback training in the treatment of Raynaud's disease and phenomenon. *J Rheumatol*. 1985;12:90–93.
156. Lee MS, Pittler MH, Ernst E. Tai Chi for rheumatoid arthritis: systematic review. *Rheumatology (Oxford)*. 2007;46(11):1648–1651.
157. Field T, Hernandez-Reif M, Seligman S, et al. Juvenile rheumatoid arthritis: Benefits from massage therapy. *J Pediatr Psychol*. 1997;22(5):607–617.

158. Beyl RN Jr, Hughes L, Morgan S. Update on importance of diet in gout. *Am J Med.* 2016;129(11):1153–1158.

159. Goodman SM, Figgie MA. Arthroplasty in patients with established rheumatoid arthritis (RA): mitigating risks and optimizing outcomes. *Best Pract Res Clin Rheumatol.* 2015;29(4-5):628–642.

160. Moyer R, Ikert K, Long K, et al. The value of preoperative exercise and education for patients undergoing total hip and knee arthroplasty: a systematic review and meta-analysis. *JBJS Rev.* 2017;5(12):e2.

161. Gerber LH, Hicks JE. Surgical and rehabilitation options in the treatment of the rheumatoid arthritis patient resistant to pharmacologic agents. *Rheum Dis Clin North Am.* 1995;21(1):19–39.

162. Whipple T, Duval MJ. Synovectomy. In: Ruddy S, Harris ED, Sledge CB, et al., eds. *Kelley's Textbook of Rheumatology.* 6th ed. Philadelphia, PA: WB Saunders; 2001:685–693.

163. Chatzopoulos D, Moralidis E, Markou P, et al. Yttrium-90 radiation synovectomy in knee osteoarthritis: a prospective assessment at 6 and 12 months. *Nucl Med Commun.* 2009;30(6):472–479.

164. Stern PT. Tendinitis, overuse syndromes, and tendon injuries. *Hand Clin.* 1990;6:467–475.

165. Sledge CB. The hand and wrist. In: Ruddy S, Harris ED, Sledge CB, et al., eds. *Kelley's Textbook of Rheumatology.* 6th ed. Philadelphia, PA: WB Saunders; 2001:1699–1718.

166. Christian CA, Donley, BG. Ankle arthritis. In: Crenshaw AH, ed. *Campbell's Operative Orthopaedics.* 9th ed. St. Louis, MO: CV Mosby; 1998:143–180.

167. Knupp M, Stufkens S, Hintermann B. Triple arthrodesis. *Foot Ankle Clin.* 2011;16(1):61–67.

168. Azar FM. Shoulder, elbow and wrist. In: Crenshaw AH, ed. *Campbell's Operative Orthopaedics.* 9th ed. St. Louis, MO: CV Mosby; 1998:188–208.

169. Christie A, Dagfinrud H, Engen Matre K, et al. Surgical interventions for the rheumatoid shoulder. *Cochrane Database Syst Rev.* 2010;(1):CD006188.

170. Carlson JR, Simmons BP. Total wrist arthroplasty. *J Am Acad Orthop Surg.* 1998;6:308.

171. Rothwell AG, Cragg KJ, O'Neill B. Hand function following silastic arthroplasty of the MCP joints in RA. *J Hand Surg Br.* 1997;22:90–93.

172. Lonner JH, Stuchin SA. Synovectomy, radial head excision, and anterior capsular releases in stage III inflammatory arthritis of the elbow. *J Hand Surg Am.* 1997;22A:279–285.

173. Gill DRJ, Morrey BE. The Conrad-Morrey total elbow arthroplasty in patients who have rheumatoid arthritis: a ten-to-fifteen-year follow-up study. *J Bone Joint Surg Am.* 1998;80A:1327–1335.

174. Kraay MJ, Figgie MP, Inglis AE, et al. Primary semi-constrained total elbow arthroplasty. Survival analysis of 113 consecutive cases. *J Bone Joint Surg.* 1994;76B:636–640.

175. Stewart MPM, Kelly IG. Total shoulder replacement in rheumatoid disease. 7-13 year follow-up of 37 joints. *J Bone Joint Surg Br.* 1997;79B:68–72.

176. Levy JC, Ashukem MT, Formaini NT. Factors predicting postoperative range of motion for anatomic total shoulder arthroplasty. *J Shoulder Elbow Surg.* 2016;25(1):55–60.

177. Bostrom LA, Wallensten R, Olsson E, et al. The Kessel prosthesis in total shoulder arthroplasty. A five-year experience. *Clin Orthop.* 1992;277:155–160.

178. Yoshihara H, Yoneoka D, Margalit A. National trends and in-hospital outcomes in patients with rheumatoid arthritis undergoing elective atlantoaxial spinal fusion surgery. *Clin Exp Rheumatol.* 2016;34(6):1045–1050.

179. Callaghan JJ, Albright JC, Goetz DD, et al. Charnley total hip arthroplasty minimum 25 year follow-up. *J Bone Joint Surg.* 2000;82A:487–497.

180. Fitzgerald RH. Total hip arthroplasty sepsis: prevention and diagnosis. *Orthop Clin North Am.* 1992;23:259–264.

181. Zhao HY, Kang PD, Xia YY, et al. Comparison of early functional recovery after total hip arthroplasty using a direct anterior or posterolateral approach: a randomized controlled trial. *J Arthroplasty.* 2017;32(11):3421–3428.

182. Sledge C. Principles of reconstructive surgery: the hip. In: Ruddy S, Harris ED, Sledge C, et al., eds. *Kelley's Textbook of Rheumatology.* 6th ed. Philadelphia, PA: WB Saunders; 2001:1743–1759.

183. Rand JA, Ilstrip DM. Survivorship analysis of total knee arthroplasty. Cumulative rates of survival of 920 total knee arthroplasties. *J Bone Joint Surg.* 1991;73:397–409.

184. Lachewicz PF. Rheumatoid arthritis of the ankle: the role of total ankle arthroplasty. *Semin Arthroplasty.* 1995;6:187–192.

185. Clayton ML, Leidholt JD, Clark W. Arthroplasty of rheumatoid metatarsophalangeal joint. An outcome study. *Clin Orthop.* 1997;340:48–57.

186. Health Quality Ontario. Physiotherapy rehabilitation after total knee or hip replacement: an evidenced-based analysis. *Ont Health Technol Assess Ser.* 2005;5(8):1–91

187. Kuster MS. Exercise recommendations after total joint replacement. *Sports Med.* 2002;32:433–445.

188. The Cleveland Clinic Foundation. *A Patient's Guide to Total Joint Replacement and Complete Care.* Available from: https://my.clevelandclinic.org/ccf/media/Files/Ortho/patient-education/total-joint-replacement-patient-guide.pdf?la=en. Accessed December 14, 2018.

189. Sledge CB. The shoulder. In: Ruddy S, Harris ED, Sledge CB, et al., eds. *Kelley's Textbook of Rheumatology.* 6th ed. Philadelphia, PA: WB Saunders; 2001:1728–1736.

190. Geneen LJ, Moore RA, Clarke C, et al. Physical activity and exercise for chronic pain in adults: an overview of Cochrane reviews. *Cochrane Database Syst Rev.* 2017;1:CD011279.

191. Veldhuizen JW, Verstappen FT, Vroemen JP, et al. Functional and morphological adaptations following four weeks of knee immobilization. *Int J Sports Med.* 1993;14:283–287.

192. Hicks JE. Rehabilitation and biomechanics. *Curr Opin Rheumatol.* 1990;2:320–326.

193. Hicks JE. Exercise in patients with inflammatory arthritis and connective tissue disease. *Rheum Dis Clin North Am.* 1990;16(4):845–870.

194. Kottke F. The effects of limitation of activity upon the human body. *JAMA.* 1966;196:825–830.

195. Danneskjold-Samsoe B, Grimby G. The relationship between the leg muscle strength and physical capacity in patients with rheumatoid arthritis, with reference to the influence of corticosteroids. *Clin Rheumatol.* 1986;5:468–474.

196. Fahrer H, Rentsch HU, Gerber NJ, et al. Knee effusion and reflex inhibition of the quadriceps. A bar to effective retraining. *J Bone Joint Surg Br.* 1988;70(4):635–638.

197. Hsieh LF, Didenko B, Schumacher HR. Isokinetic and isometric testing of knee musculature in patients with rheumatoid arthritis with mild knee involvement. *Arch Phys Med Rehabil.* 1987;68:294–297.

198. Nordemar L, Nordgren B, Wigren A, et al. Isometric strength and endurance in patients with severe rheumatoid arthritis or osteoarthritis in the knee joints. *Scand J Rheumatol.* 1983;12:152–156.

199. Hicks JE, Miller F, Plotz P, et al. Isometric exercise increases strength and does not produce sustained creatinine phosphokinase increases in a patient with polymyositis. *J Rheumatol.* 1993;20(8):1399–1401.

200. Lindehammar H, Backman E. Muscle function in juvenile chronic arthritis. *J Rheumatol.* 1995;22:1159–1165.

201. Hicks JE, Fromherz W, Miller F, et al. Cybex II strength and endurance testing in normal and polymyositis patients. *Arch Phys Med Rehabil.* 1987;68:637.

202. Nicholson CR, Daltroy L, Easton BSN, et al. Effects of aerobic conditioning in lupus fatigue: a pilot study. *Br J Rheumatol.* 1989;28:500–505.

203. Gerber L, Furst G, Drinkard B, et al. Assessment of fatigue in patients with rheumatoid arthritis, polymyositis and chronic fatigue syndrome. *Arthritis Rheum.* 1996;39(suppl):176.

204. Hicks JE. Rehabilitation strategies for patients with rheumatoid arthritis, Part I: the role of exercise. *J Musculoskelet Med.* 2000;17:191–204.

205. Wiesinger GF, Quittan M, Nuhr M, et al. Aerobic capacity in adult dermatomyositis/polymyositis patients and healthy controls. *Arch Phys Med Rehabil.* 2000;81:1–5.

206. Hicks JE, Drinkard B, Summers RM, et al. Decreased aerobic capacity in children with juvenile dermatomyositis. *Arthritis Rheum.* 2002;47(2):118–123.

207. Combe B, Landewe R, Lukas C, et al. EULAR recommendations for the management of early arthritis: report of a task force of the European Standing Committee for International Clinical Studies Including Therapeutics (ESCISIT). *Ann Rheum Dis.* 2007;66:34–25.

208. Van den Ende CH, Breedveld FC, le Cessie S, et al. Effects of intensive exercise in patients with active rheumatoid arthritis. *Ann Rheum Dis.* 2000;59:615–621.

209. Van den Ende CH, Hazes JM, le Cessie S, et al. Comparison of high and low intensity training in well controlled rheumatoid arthritis. Results of a randomized clinical trial. *Ann Rheum Dis.* 1996;55:798–805.

210. Komatiredely GR, Leitch RW, Cell K, et al. Efficacy of low load resistive muscle training in patients with rheumatoid arthritis functional class II, III. *J Rheumatol.* 1997;24:1531–1539.

211. Hakkinen A, Sokka T, Kontaniemi A. Dynamic strength training in patients with early rheumatoid arthritis increases muscle strength but not bone mineral density. *J Rheumatol.* 1999;26:1257–1263.

212. Hakkinen A, Sokka T, Kotaniemi A, et al. A randomized two year study of the effects of dynamic strength training on muscle strength, disease activity, functional capacity, and bone mineral density in early rheumatoid arthritis. *Arthritis Rheum.* 2001;44(3):515–522.

213. Moffet H, Noreau L, Parent E, et al. Feasibility of an eight-week dance-based exercise program and its effects on locomotor ability of persons with functional class III rheumatoid arthritis. *Arthritis Care Res.* 2000;13(2):100–111.

214. Minor M, Hewett J, Webel R, et al. Efficacy of physical conditioning exercise in patients with RA and OA. *Arthritis Rheum.* 1989;32:1396.

215. Novreau L, Martineau H, Roy L, et al. Effects of a modified dance based exercise on cardiorespiratory fitness, psychological state and health status of persons with rheumatoid arthritis. *Am J Phys Med Rehabil.* 1995;74:19–27.

216. Minor MA, Lane NE. Recreational exercise in arthritis. *Rheum Dis Clin North Am.* 1996;22:563.

217. Klepper SE. Effects of an eight-week physical conditioning program on disease signs and symptoms in children with chronic arthritis. *Arthritis Care Res.* 1999;12:52–60.

218. Lyngberg K, Danneskjold-Samsoe B, Halskov O. The effect of physical training on patients with rheumatoid arthritis: changes in disease activity, muscle strength and aerobic capacity: clinically controlled minimized cross-over study. *Clin Exp Rheumatol.* 1988;6:253–260.

219. Rall LC, Roubenoff R, Cannon JG, et al. Effects of progressive resistance training on immune response in aging and chronic inflammation. *Med Sci Sports Exerc.* 1996;28:1356–1365.

220. Shepard RJ, Shek PN. Autoimmune disorders, physical activity and training with particular reference to rheumatoid arthritis. *Exerc Immunol Rev.* 1997;3:53–67.

221. Wiesinger GF, Quittan M, Garinger M, et al. Improvement in physical fitness and muscle strength in polymyositis/dermatomyositis patients by a training program. *Br J Rheumatol.* 1998;37:196–200.

222. Engelhark M, Kondrup J, Hoie LH, et al. Weight reduction in obese patients with rheumatoid arthritis, with preservation of body cell mass and improvement in physical fitness. *Clin Exp Rheumatol.* 1996;14(3):289–293.

223. Rall LC, Rosen CJ, Dolnkowski G, et al. Protein metabolism in rheumatoid arthritis and aging effects of muscle strength, training and tumor necrosis factor alpha. *Arthritis Rheum.* 1996;39:1115–1124.

224. Toumanidis ST, Papamichael CM, Antomcades LG, et al. Cardiac involvement in collagen diseases. *Eur Heart J.* 1995;16:257–262.

225. Machover S, Sapecky AJ. Effect of isometric exercise on the quadriceps muscle in patients with rheumatoid arthritis. *Arch Phys Med Rehabil.* 1966;47:737–741.

226. Gnootveld M, Henderson EB, Farrell A, et al. Oxidative damage to hyaluronate and glucose in synovial fluid during exercise of the inflamed rheumatoid joint. *Biochem J.* 1991;273:459–467.

227. Rall LC, Maydone SN, Kahaylas JJ, et al. The effect of progressive resistance training in rheumatoid arthritis increased strength without changes in energy balance or body composition. *Arthritis Rheum.* 1996;39:415–426.

228. Alexanderson H, Stenstrom CH, Jenner G, et al. The safety of a restrictive home exercise program in patients with recent onset active polymyositis. *Scand J Rheumatol.* 2000;29(5):295–301.

229. Hicks JE. Exercise in rheumatoid arthritis. *Phys Med Rehabil Clin N Am.* 1994;5:701–708.

230. Wiesinger GF, Quittan M, Graninger M, et al. Benefit of 6 months' long-term training on polymyositis/dermatomyositis patients. *Br J Rheumatol.* 1998;37: 1338–1342.

231. Leventhal L, Ganjei A, Hirsch D, et al. Isokinetic strength training in patients with rheumatoid arthritis. *Arthritis Rheum.* 1990;33(suppl):123.

232. Lynberg KK, Ramsing BU, Nawrocke A. Safe and effective isokinetic knee extension training in rheumatoid arthritis. *Arthritis Rheum.* 1994;37:623–629.

233. McMeeken J, Stillman B, Story I, et al. The effects of knee extensors and flexion muscle training on the timed-up-and-go test in individuals with rheumatoid arthritis. *Physiother Res Int.* 1999;4:55–67.

234. Escalante A, Miller L, Beardmore TD. Resistive exercise in the rehabilitation of polymyositis/dermatomyositis. *J Rheumatol.* 1993;20:1340–1344.

235. Ekblom B, Lovgren O, Alderin M, et al. Effect of short-term physical training on patients with rheumatoid arthritis. *Scand J Rheumatol.* 1975;4(2):87–91.

236. Perlman SG, Connell KJ, Clark A, et al. Dance based aerobic exercise for rheumatoid arthritis. *Arthritis Care Res.* 1990;3:29–35.

237. Nordemar R, Berg U, Ekblom B, et al. Changes in muscle fiber size after physical performance in patients with rheumatoid arthritis after 7 months' physical training. *Scand J Rheumatol.* 1976;5:233–238.

238. Nordemar R. Physical training in rheumatoid arthritis: a controlled long term study: II. Functional capacity and general attitudes. *Scand J Rheumatol.* 1981;10(1):25–30.

239. Harkcom TM, Lampman RM, Banwell BF, et al. Therapeutic value of graded aerobic exercise training in rheumatoid arthritis. *Arthritis Rheum.* 1985;28:32–39.

240. Van den Ende CH, Vliet Vlieland TP, Munneke M, et al. Dynamic exercise therapy for rheumatoid arthritis. *Cochrane Database Syst Rev.* 2000;(2):CD000322.

241. Westby MD, Wade JP, Rangns KK. A randomized controlled trial to evaluate the effectiveness of an exercise program in women with rheumatoid arthritis taking low dose prednisone. *J Rheumatol.* 2000;27:1674–1680.

242. Van den Ende CH, Vliet Vlieland TP, Munneke M et al. Dynamic exercise therapy for treating rheumatoid arthritis. *Cochrane Database Syst Rev.* 2008;(1): CD000322.

243. Stavropoulos-Kalinoglou A, Metsios GS, Veldhuijzen van Zanten JJ, et al. Individualised aerobic and resistance exercise training improves cardiorespiratory fitness and reduces cardiovascular risk in patients with rheumatoid arthritis. *Ann Rheum Dis.* 2013;72(11):1819–1825.

244. Barry JC, Simtchouk S, Durrer C, et al. Short-term exercise training alters leukocyte chemokine receptors in obese adults. *Med Sci Sports Exerc.* 2017;49:1631–1640.

245. Sandstad J, Stensvold D, Hoff M, et al. The effects of high intensity interval training in women with rheumatic disease: a pilot study. *Eur J Appl Physiol.* 2015;115(10):2081–2089.

246. Klepper SE. Exercise in pediatric rheumatic diseases. *Curr Opin Rheumatol.* 2008;20(5):619–624.

247. Ince G, Sarpel I, Durgan B, et al. Effects of a multimodal exercise program for people with ankylosing spondylitis. *Phys Ther.* 2006;86(7):924–935.

248. Aloia JF, Cohn SH, Ostuni JA, et al. Prevention of involutional bone loss by exercise. *Ann Intern Med.* 1978;89:356–358.

249. Sinaki M, Grubbs N. Back strengthening exercises: quantitative evaluation of their efficacy in women aged 40 to 60 years. *Arch Phys Med Rehabil.* 1989;70:16–20.

250. Neviaser AS, Neviaser RJ. Adhesive capsulitis of the shoulder. *J Am Acad Orthop Surg.* 2011;19(9):536–542.

251. Park SW, Lee HS, Kim JH. The effectiveness of intensive mobilization techniques combined with capsular distension for adhesive capsulitis of the shoulder. *J Phys Ther Sci.* 2014;26(11):1767–1770.

252. Bulstrode SJ, Barefoot J, Harrison RA, et al. The role of passive stretching in the treatment of ankylosing spondylitis. *Br J Rheumatol.* 1987;26:40–42.

253. McNeal RL. Aquatic therapy for patients with rheumatic disease. *Rheum Dis Clin North Am.* 1990;16:915–929.

254. Bartels EM, Lund H, Danneskiold-Samsoe B. Pool exercise in therapy of rheumatoid arthritis. *Ugeskr Laeger.* 2000;163:5507–5513.

255. Danneskiold-Samsoe B, Lyngberg K, Risum T, et al. The effect of water exercise therapy given to patients with rheumatoid arthritis. *Scand J Rehabil Med.* 1987;19:31–35.

256. Harrison RA. Tolerance of pool therapy by ankylosing spondylitis patients with low vital capacities. *Physiotherapy.* 1981;67:296–297.

257. Van Tubergen A, Landewe RL, Van der Heijde D, et al. Combined spa-exercise therapy is effective in patients with ankylosing spondylitis: a randomized controlled trial. *Arthritis Rheum.* 2001;45:430–438.

258. Van Deusen J, Harlowe D. The efficacy of the ROM dance program for adults with rheumatoid arthritis. *Am J Occup Ther.* 1987;41:90.

259. Novreau L, Moffet H, Drolet M. Dance-based exercise program in rheumatoid arthritis. Feasibility in individuals with American College of Rheumatology class III disease. *Am J Phys Med Rehabil.* 1997;76:109–113.

260. Alentorn-Geli E, Samuelsson K, Musahi V, et al. The association of recreational and competitive running with hip and knee osteoarthritis: a systematic review and meta-analysis. *J Orthop Sports Phys Ther.* 2017;47(6):373–390.

261. Timmins KA, Leech RD, Batt ME, et al. Running and knee osteoarthritis: a systematic review and meta-analysis. *Am J Sports Med.* 2017;45(6):1447–1457.

262. Lefèvre-Colau MM, Nguyen C, Haddad R, et al. Is physical activity, practiced as recommended for health benefit, a risk factor for OA? *Ann Phys Rehabil Med.* 2016;59(3):196–206.

263. Brosseau WV, Shea B, McGowan J. Thermotherapy for treating rheumatoid arthritis. *Cochrane Database Syst Rev.* 2001;(2):CD002826.

264. Verhagen AP, Vet HC, de Bie RA, et al. Balneotherapy for rheumatoid arthritis and osteoarthritis. *Cochrane Database Syst Rev.* 2000;(2):CD000518.

265. Casimero L, Brosseau L, Robinson V, et al. Therapeutic ultrasound for the treatment of rheumatoid arthritis. *Cochrane Database Syst Rev.* 2002;(3):CD003787.

266. Oosterveld FG, Rasker JJ. Effects of local heat and cold treatment on the surface articular temperature of arthritic knees. *Arthritis Rheum.* 1994;37:1578–1582.

267. Osterveld FGJ, Rasker J, Jacobs JWG. The effect of local heat and cold therapy on the intraarticular and skin surface temperature of the knee. *Arthritis Rheum.* 1992;35:146–151.

268. Mainardi CL, Walter CM, Spiegel PK, et al. Rheumatoid arthritis: Failure of daily heat to affect its progression. *Arch Phys Med Rehabil.* 1979;60:390–393.

269. Warren CG, Lehmann JF, Koblanski JN. Heat and stretch procedures: an evaluation using rat tail tendon. *Arch Phys Med Rehabil.* 1976;57(3):122–126.

270. Petrofsky JS, Laymon M, Lee H. Effect of heat and cold on tendon flexibility and force to flex the human knee. *Med Sci Monit.* 2013;19:661–667.

271. Curkovi B, Vituli V, Nagle D, et al. The influence of heat and cold on the pain threshold in rheumatoid arthritis. *Z Rheumatol.* 1993;52:289–291.

272. Kirk JA, Kersley GD. Heat and cold in the physical treatment of rheumatoid arthritis of the knee: a controlled clinical trial. *Arch Phys Med.* 1968;9:270–274.

273. Price R, Lehmann JE, Boswell-Besette S, et al. Influence of cryotherapy on spasticity at the human ankle. *Arch Phys Med Rehabil.* 1993;74:300.

274. Hicks J. Modalities and devices for rheumatoid arthritis. *J Musculoskelet Med.* 2000;17:385–398.

275. Roll SC, Hardison ME. Effectiveness of occupational therapy interventions for adults with musculoskeletal conditions of the forearm, wrist, and hand: a systematic review. *Am J Occup Ther.* 2017;71(1):7101180010p1–7101180010p12.

276. Ramsey L, Winder RJ, McVeigh JG. The effectiveness of working wrist splints in adults with rheumatoid arthritis: a mixed methods systematic review. *J Rehabil Med.* 2014;46(6):481–492.

277. Frecklington M, Dalbeth N, McNair P, et al. Footwear interventions for foot pain, function, impairment and disability for people with foot and ankle arthritis: a literature review. *Semin Arthritis Rheum.* 2018;47(6):814–824.

278. Veehof MM, Taal E, Heijnsdjik-Rouwenhorst LM, et al. Efficacy of wrist working splints in patients with rheumatoid arthritis: a randomized controlled study. *Arthritis Rheum.* 2008;59(12):1698–1704.

279. Hennessy K, Woodburn J, Steultjens MP. Custom foot orthoses for rheumatoid arthritis: a systematic review. *Arthritis Care Res (Hoboken).* 2012;64(3):311–320.

280. Beaudreuil J. Orthoses for osteoarthritis: a narrative review. *Ann Phys Rehabil Med.* 2017;60(2):102–106.

281. Lorig KR, Ritter P, Stewart AL, et al. Chronic disease self-management program 2-year health status and health care utilization outcomes. *Med Care.* 2001;39: 1217–1223.

282. Hootman JM, Sniezek JE, Helmick CG. Women and arthritis: Burden, impact and prevention programs. *J Women's Health Gend Based Med.* 2002;11:407–416.

283. Ramos-Remus C, Salcedo-Rocha AL, Prieto-Parra RE, et al. How important is patient education? *Best Pract Res Clin Rheumatol.* 2000;14:689–703.

284. Lorig KR. Patient education: essential to good health care for patients with chronic arthritis. *Arthritis Rheum.* 1997;40:171–173.

285. Cordery JC. Joint protection: a responsibility of the occupational therapist. *Am J Occup Ther.* 1965;19:283–294.

286. Bradley LA, McKendra-Smith NL. Psychosocial factors. In: Klippel JH, ed. *Primer on the Rheumatic Diseases.* 12th ed. Atlanta, GA: Arthritis Foundation; 2001:563–567.

287. Harrington L, Affleck G, Arrows S, et al. Temporal covariation of soluble interleukin-2 receptor levels, daily stress and disease activity in rheumatoid arthritis. *Arthritis Rheum.* 1993;36:199–203.

288. Dacosta D, Dobkin PL, Pinard L, et al. The role of stress in functional disability among women with systemic lupus erythematosus: a prospective study. *Arthritis Care Res.* 1999;12:112–119.

289. Schanberg LE, Sandstrom MJ, Starr K, et al. The relationship of daily mood and stressful events to symptoms in juvenile rheumatic disease. *Arthritis Care Res.* 2000;13(1):33–41.

290. Hawley DJ, Wolfe F. Depression is not more common in rheumatoid arthritis: a 10 year longitudinal study of 6,153 patients with rheumatoid disease. *J Rheumatol.* 1993;20:2025–2031.

291. Wolf F, Hawley DJ. The relationship between clinical activity and depression in rheumatoid arthritis. *J Rheumatol.* 1993;20:2032–2037.
292. Fufield J, Tennen H, Reisine S, et al. Depression and long term risk of pain, fatigue, and disability in patients with rheumatoid arthritis. *Arthritis Rheum.* 1998;41:1851–1857.
293. Thumbo J, Fong KY, Chan SP, et al. A prospective study of factors affecting quality of life in systemic lupus erythematosus. *J Rheumatol.* 2000;27:1414–1420.
294. Lefebvre JC, Keefe FJ, Affleck G, et al. The relationship of arthritis self-efficacy to daily pain, daily mood, and daily pain coping in rheumatoid arthritis patients. *Pain.* 1999;80(1–2):425–435.
295. Karlson EW, Daltroy LH, Lew RA, et al. The relationship of socioeconomic status, race and modifiable risk factors to outcomes in patients with systemic lupus erythematosus. *Arthritis Rheum.* 1997;40:47–56.
296. Keefe FJ, Van Horn Y. Cognitive-behavioral treatment of rheumatoid arthritis pain: maintaining treatment gains. *Arthritis Care Res.* 1993;6(4):213–222.
297. Smarr KL, Parker JC, Wright GE, et al. The importance of enhancing self-efficacy in rheumatoid arthritis. *Arthritis Care Res.* 1997;10(1):18–26.
298. Bradley LA, Alberts KR. Psychological and behavioral approaches to pain management for patients with rheumatic disease. *Rheum Dis Clin North Am.* 1999;25:215–232.
299. Malseak R, Austin JS, West SG, et al. The effect of person centered counseling on the psychological status of persons with systemic lupus erythematosus or rheumatoid arthritis: a randomized, controlled trial. *Arthritis Care Res.* 1996;9:60–66.
300. Panush RS, Mihaelescu GD, Gomisiewicz MT, et al. Sex and arthritis. *Bull Rheum Dis.* 2000;49:1–4.
301. Bhadauria S, Moser DK, Clements PJ, et al. Genital tract abnormalities and female sexual function impairment in systemic sclerosis. *Am J Obstet Gynecol.* 1995;172:580–587.
302. Mulhern DM, Sheeran TP, Kumararatne DS, et al. Sjögren's syndrome in women presenting with chronic dyspareunia. *Br J Obstet Gynaecol.* 1997;104:1019–1023.
303. Clements PJ. Systemic sclerosis and related syndromes. In: Klippel JH, ed. *Primer on the Rheumatic Diseases.* 12th ed. Atlanta, GA: Arthritis Foundation; 2001:362.
304. Spica MM, Schwab MD. Sexual expression after total joint replacement. *Orthop Nurs.* 1996;15:41–44.
305. Gutweniger S, Kopp M, Mur E, et al. Body image of women with rheumatoid arthritis. *Clin Exp Rheumatol.* 1999;17(4):413–417.
306. Aguirre MA, Velez A, Romero M. Gynecomastia and sexual impotence associated with methotrexate treatment. *J Rheumatol.* 2002;29:1793–1794.
307. Oostensem M, Almberg K, Koksvik HS. Sex reproduction and gynecological disease in young adults with a history of juvenile chronic arthritis. *J Rheumatol.* 2000;27:1783–1787.
308. Callahan LF. Impact of rheumatic disease on society. In: Wegner ST, Belza BL, Gall EP, eds. *Clinical Care in the Rheumatic Diseases.* Atlanta, GA: American College of Rheumatology; 1996:209–213.
309. Allaire SH. Work disability. In: Wegner ST, Belza BL, Gall EP, eds. *Clinical Care in the Rheumatic Diseases.* Atlanta, GA: American College of Rheumatology; 1996:141–145.
310. Pastridge AJ, Karlson EW, Daltroy LH, et al. Risk factors for early work disability in systemic lupus erythematosis: results from a multicenter study. *Arthritis Rheum.* 1997;40:2199–2206.
311. Yellin EH. Work disability and rheumatoid arthritis. In: Wolf F, Pincus T, eds. *Rheumatoid Arthritis: Pathogenesis, Assessment, Outcome and Treatment.* New York: Marcel Dekker; 1994:261–271.
312. Reisine ST. Arthritis and the family. *Arthritis Care Res.* 1995;8:265–271.
313. Callahan LF, Yellin EH. The social and economic consequences of rheumatic disease. In: Klippel JH, ed. *Primer on the Rheumatic Diseases.* 12th ed. Atlanta, GA: Arthritis Foundation; 2001:1–4.
314. DeRoos AJ, Callahan LF. Difference by sex in correlates of work status in rheumatoid arthritis patients. *Arthritis Care Res.* 1999;12:381–391.
315. Harris ED, Firestein GS. Clinical features of rheumatoid arthritis. In: Firestein GS, Budd RC, Sergent JS, et al., eds. *Kelley's Textbook of Rheumatology.* 8th ed. Philadelphia, PA: WB Saunders; 2009:1087–1118.
316. Tehlirian CV, Bathon JM. Rheumatoid arthritis: clinical and laboratory manifestations. In: Klippel JH, Stone JH, Crofford LJ, et al., eds. *Primer on the Rheumatic Diseases.* 13th ed. Atlanta, GA: Springer; 2008:114–121.
317. Pincus T. Rheumatoid arthritis in clinical care in rheumatic disease. In: Wegner ST, Belza BL, Gall EP, eds. *Clinical Care in the Rheumatic Diseases.* Atlanta, GA: American College of Rheumatology; 1996:147–155.
318. Escalante A, Del Rincon I. How much disability in rheumatoid arthritis is explained by rheumatoid arthritis. *Arthritis Rheum.* 1999;42:1712–1721.
319. Drossaers-Bakker KW, Zwinderman AH, Vliet Vlieland TP, et al. Long term outcome in rheumatoid arthritis: a simple algorithm of baseline parameters can predict radiographic damage, disability and disease course at 12-year follow-up. *Arthritis Care Res.* 2002;47:383–390.
320. Pincus T, Brooks RH, Callahan LF. Prediction of long term mortality in patients with rheumatoid arthritis according to simple questionnaire and joint count measure. *Ann Intern Med.* 1994;120:26–34.
321. Scholten C, Brodowicz SC, Graninger W, et al. Persistent functional and social benefit 5 years after a multidisciplinary arthritis training program. *Arch Phys Med Rehabil.* 1999;80:1282–1287.
322. Hakala M, Nieminen P, Manelius J. Joint impairment is strongly correlated with disability measured by self report questionnaires. *J Rheumatol.* 1993;21:64–69.
323. Wiles NJ, Dunn G, Barrett EM, et al. One year follow-up variables predict disability five years after presentation with inflammatory polyarthritis with greater accuracy than at baseline. *J Rheumatol.* 2000;27:2360–2366.

324. Holm MB, Rogers JC, Kwoh CK. Predictors of functional disability in patients with rheumatoid arthritis. *Arthritis Care Res.* 1998;11:346–355.
325. Goldring SR, Gravallese EM. Mechanisms of bone loss in inflammatory arthritis: diagnosis and therapeutic implications. *Arthritis Res.* 1999;2:33.
326. Lane NE, Sanchez S, Modin GW, et al. Parathyroid hormone treatment can reverse corticosteroid-induced osteoporosis. Results of a randomized controlled clinical trial. *J Clin Invest.* 1998;102(8):1627–1633.
327. Heiberg T, Kvien TK. Preferences for improved health examined in 1,024 patients with rheumatoid arthritis: pain has highest priority. *Arthritis Care Res.* 2002;47(4):391–397.
328. Sarz I, Puttini P, Fiorini T, et al. Correlation of the score for subjective pain with physical disability, clinical and radiographic scores in recent onset rheumatoid arthritis. *BMC Muscloskelet Disord.* 2002;2:18.
329. Neuberger GB, Press AN, Lindsley HB, et al. Effects of exercise on fatigue, aerobic fitness and disease activity measures in persons with rheumatoid arthritis. *Res Nurs Health.* 1997;20:195–204.
330. Van den Berg MH, Ronday HK, Petters AJ, et al. Using internet technology to deliver a home based activity intervention for patients with rheumatoid arthritis. *Arthritis Rheum.* 2006;55(6):935–945.
331. Bilek LD, Venema DM, Willett GM, et al. Use of the Human Activity Profile for estimating fitness in persons with arthritis. *Arthritis Care Res.* 2008;59(5):659–664.
332. Beavers KM, Brinkley TE, Nicklas BJ. Effect of exercise training on chronic inflammation. *Clin Chim Acta.* 2010;411(11–12):785–793.
333. Stenström CH, Minor MA. Evidence for the benefit of aerobic and strengthening exercise in rheumatoid arthritis. *Arthritis Rheum.* 2003;49(3):428–434.
334. Lundberg IE, Nader GA. Molecular effects of exercise in patients with inflammatory rheumatic disease. *Nat Clin Pract Rheumatol.* 2008;4(11):597–604.
335. Smarr KL, Parker JC, Kosciulek JF. Implications of depression in rheumatoid arthritis: Do subtypes really matter. *Arthritis Care Res.* 2000;13:23–32.
336. Hakkinen A, Hakkinen ME, Laitenen L, et al. Effects of detraining subsequent to strength training on neuromuscular function in patients with inflammatory arthritis. *Br J Rheumatol.* 1997;36:1075–1081.
337. Escalante A, Del Rincón I. The disablement process in rheumatoid arthritis. *Arthritis Care Res.* 2002;47(3):333–342.
338. Katz P, Morris A, Yellin E. Subclinical disability in valued life activities among individuals with rheumatoid arthritis. *Arthritis Rheum.* 2008;59(10):1416–1423.
339. Backman CL, Village J, Lacaille D. The ergonomic assessment tool for arthritis: development and pilot testing. *Arthritis Rheum.* 2008;59(10):1495–1503.
340. Yelin E, Sonneborn D, Trupin L. The prevalence and impact of accommodations on the employment of persons 51-61 years of age with musculoskeletal conditions. *Arthritis Care Res.* 2000;13:168–176.
341. Bostrom C, Harms-Ringdahl K, Karreskog H, et al. Effects of static and dynamic shoulder rotator cuff exercise on women with rheumatoid arthritis: a randomized comparison of impairment, disability handicap and health. *Scand J Rheumatol.* 1998;27:281–290.
342. Dellhog B, Anders B. A five year follow-up of hand function and activities of daily living in the rheumatoid arthritis patients. *Arthritis Care Res.* 1999;12:33–41.
343. Brighton SW, Lubbe JE, Van der Merive CA. The effect of a long term exercise programme on the rheumatoid hand. *Br J Rheumatol.* 1993;32:392–395.
344. Baljima AI, Taljomavic MS, Audic DM, et al. Physical and exercise therapy for treatment of the rheumatoid hand. *Arthritis Rheum.* 2001;45:392–397.
345. Westhoff G, Listing J, Zink A. Loss of physical independence in rheumatoid arthritis: interview data from a representative sample of patients in rheumatologic care. *Arthritis Care Res.* 2000;13(1):11–22.
346. Buckwalter JA, Ballard WT. Operative treatment of arthritis. In: Klippel JH, Stone JH, Crofford LJ, et al., eds. *Primer on the Rheumatic Diseases.* 13th ed. Atlanta, GA: Springer; 2008:651–663.
347. Bearne LM, Scott DL, Harley MV. Sensorimotor function and decreased lower limb disability. *Rheumatology (Oxford).* 2002;41:157–166.
348. Sakauchi M, Narushuma K, Sone H, et al. Kinematic approach to gait analysis in patients with rheumatoid arthritis involving the knee joint. *Arthritis Rheum.* 2001;45:35–41.
349. Cumino WG, O'Malley MJ. Rheumatoid arthritis of the ankle and hindfoot. *Rheum Dis Clin North Am.* 1998;24:157–165.
350. Rayavarapu S, Coley W, Kinder TB, et al. Idiopathic inflammatory myopathies: pathogenic mechanisms of muscle weakness. *Skelet Muscle.* 2013;3:13.
351. Rennebohm R. Juvenile dermatomyositis. *Pediatr Ann.* 2002;31:426–433.
352. Hicks J. Rehabilitation of inflammatory myopathy. *J Musculoskelet Med.* 1995;12:41–54.
353. Hicks J. Role of rehabilitation in the management of myopathies. *Curr Opin Rheumatol.* 1998;10:548–555.
354. Sonies BC. Evaluation and treatment of speech and swallowing disorders associated with myopathies. *Curr Opin Rheumatol.* 1997;9:486–495.
355. Alexanderson H, Lundberg IE. Exercise as a therapeutic modality in patients with idiopathic inflammatory myopathies. *Curr Opin Rheumatol.* 2012;24(2):201–207.
356. Habers GE, Takken T. Safety and efficacy of exercise training in patients with an idiopathic inflammatory myopathy—a systematic review. *Rheumatology (Oxford).* 2011;50(11):2113–2124.
357. Hicks J. Rehabilitation of patients with myositis. In: Klippel JH, Deppe PA, eds. *Rheumatology.* 2nd ed. London: CV Mosby; 1998.
358. Rider LG, Pachman LM, Miller FW, et al. eds. *Myositis and You: A Guide to Juvenile Dermatomyositis for Patients, Families, and Healthcare Providers.* Alexandria, VA: The Myositis Association; 2007.

359. Daltroy LH, Robb-Nicholson C, Inverson MD, et al. Effectiveness of minimally supervised home aerobic training in patients with rheumatic disease. *Br J Rheumatol*. 1995;34(11):1064–1069.

360. Leff RL, Buczek FL, Hicks J, et al. A study of falling-slips and trips in a patient with muscle weakness due to myositis. *Arthritis Rheum*. 1992;35(suppl):S291.

361. Hicks J, Richardson D, Sonies B. Correlation of neck flexion weakness and swallowing dysfunction in polymyositis patients. *Arthritis Rheum*. 1990;33(suppl):123.

362. Godaert GL, Hartkamp K, Geenen R, et al. Fatigue in daily life in patients with primary Sjögren's syndrome and systemic lupus erythematosus. *Ann N Y Acad Sci*. 2002;966:320–326.

363. Trench CM, McCurdie I, White PD, et al. The prevalence and associations of fatigue in systemic lupus erythematosus. *Rheumatology*. 2000;39:1249–1254.

364. Tayer WG, Nicassio PM, Weisman MH, et al. Disease status predicts fatigue in systemic lupus erythematosus. *J Rheumatol*. 2001;28:1999–2007.

365. Iverson GL. Screening for depression in systemic lupus erythematosus with the British Columbia Major Depression Inventory. *Psychol Rep*. 2002;90:1091–1096.

366. Tench C, Bentley D, Vleck V, et al. Aerobic fitness, fatigue, and physical disability in systemic lupus erythematosus. *J Rheumatol*. 2002;29:474–481.

367. Houghton KM, Tucker LB, Potts JE, et al. Fitness, fatigue disease activity and quality of life in pediatric lupus. *Arthritis Rheum*. 2008;59(4):537–545.

368. Robb-Nicholson LC, Daltroy L, Eaton H, et al. Effects of aerobic conditioning in lupus fatigue: a pilot study. *Br J Rheumatol*. 1989;28(6):500–505.

369. Carvalho MR, Sato EI, Tebexreni AS, et al. Effects of supervised cardiovascular training program on exercise tolerance, aerobic capacity and quality of life in patients with systemic lupus erythematosis. *Arthritis Rheum*. 2005;53(6):838–844.

370. Mann SC, Buragar FD. Preliminary study of acupuncture in rheumatoid arthritis. *J Rheumatol*. 1974;1:126.

371. Gerber LH, Smith C, Novick A, et al. Autogenic training in the treatment of Raynaud's phenomenon. *Arch Phys Med Rehabil*. 1978;59:522.

372. Johnson PM, Sandqvist G, Bengtsson A, et al. Hand function and performance of daily activities in systemic lupus erythematosis. *Arthritis Rheum*. 2008;59(10):1432–1438.

373. Matucci-Cerinic M, Kahaleh BM, LeRoy EC. The vascular involvement in systemic sclerosis. In: Furst D, Clements P, eds. *The Pathogenesis of Systemic Sclerosis*. Baltimore, MD: Lippincott Williams & Wilkins; 1995:200–221.

374. Jansen G, Lundeberg T, Kjartansson J, et al. Acupuncture and sensory neuropeptides increase cutaneous blood flow in rats. *Neurosci Lett*. 1989;97:305–309.

375. Seeger MW, Furst DE. Effects of splinting in the treatment of hand contractures in progressive systemic sclerosis. *Am J Occup Ther*. 1987;41:118–121.

376. Cerinic MM, Generini S, Pignone A, et al. The nervous system in systemic sclerosis (scleroderma). Clinical features and pathogenetical mechanisms. *Rheum Dis Clin North Am*. 1996;24(4):879–892.

377. Lori S, Matucci-Cerinic M, Casale R, et al. Peripheral nervous system involvement in systemic sclerosis: the median nerve as target structure. *Clin Exp Rheumatol*. 1996;14(6):601–605.

378. Malcarne VL, Greenbergs HL. Psychological adjustment to systemic sclerosis. *Arthritis Care Res*. 1996;9(1):51–59.

379. Moser DK, Clements PJ, Brecht ML, et al. Predictors of psychosocial adjustment in systemic sclerosis. The influence of formal education level, functional ability, hardiness, uncertainty and social support. *Arthritis Rheum*. 1993;36:1398–1405.

380. Casale R, Buonocore M, Matucci-Cerinic M. Systemic sclerosis: an integrated challenge in rehabilitation. *Arch Phys Med Rehabil*. 1997;78:767–773.

381. van der Heijde D, Ramiro S, Landewé R, et al. 2016 update of the ASAS-EULAR management recommendations for axial spondyloarthritis. *Ann Rheum Dis*. 2017;76(6):978–991.

382. Hidding A, van der Linden S, Boers M, et al. Is group physical therapy superior to individualized therapy in ankylosing spondylitis? A randomized controlled trial. *Arthritis Care Res*. 1993;6(3):117–125.

383. Vitanen JV, Suni J, Kantiainen H, et al. Effect of physiotherapy on spinal mobility in ankylosing spondylitis. *Scand J Rheumatol*. 1992;21:38–41.

384. Vitanen JV, Lehtinen K, Suni J, et al. Fifteen months' follow-up of intensive inpatient physiotherapy and exercise in ankylosing spondylitis. *Clin Rheumatol*. 1995;14:413–419.

385. Vitanen JV, Heikkila S. Functional changes in patients with spondyloarthropathy. A controlled trial of the effects of short-term rehabilitation and 3-year follow-up. *Rheumatol Int*. 2001;20:211–214.

386. Tishier M, Brotovskyi Y, Yaron M. Effect of spa therapy on patients with ankylosing spondylitis. *Clin Rheumatol*. 1995;14:21–25.

387. Revel M, Rondier J, Amor B. Intérêt d'une orthése de courbure lombaire dans le traitement de la pelvis spondylite thumatismale. In: Simon L, Hérisson C, eds. *La Spondylarthrite Ankylosante: Actualités Nosologiques et Thérapeutiques*. Paris: Masson; 1988:155–159.

388. Alaranta H, Luoto S, Kontinnen YT. Traumatic spinal cord injury as a complication of ankylosing spondylitis. An extended report. *Clin Exp Rheumatol*. 2002;20:66–68.

389. Dougados M, Revel M, Khan MA. Spondyloarthropathy treatment: progress in medical treatment, physical therapy and rehabilitation. *Baillieres Clin Rheumatol*. 1998;12:717–736.

390. Karapolat H, Akkoc Y, Sari I, et al. Comparison of group-based exercise versus home-based exercise in patients with ankylosing spondylitis: effects on Bath Ankylosing Spondylitis Indices, quality of life and depression. *Clin Rheumatol*. 2008;27(6):695–700.

391. Analay Y, Ozcan E, Karne A, et al. The effectiveness of intensive group exercise on patients with ankylosing spondylitis. *Clin Rehabil*. 2003;17(6):631–636.

392. Durmus D, Alayli G, Cil E, et al. Effects of a home-based exercise program on quality of life, fatigue, and depression in patients with ankylosing spondylitis. *Rheumatol Int*. 2009;29(6):673–677.

393. Lim HJ, Moon YI, Lee MS. Effects of home-based daily exercise therapy on joint mobility, daily activity, pain, and depression in patients with ankylosing spondylitis. *Rheumatol Int*. 2005;25(3):255–259.

394. Fernández-de-Las-Peñas C, Alonso-Blanco C, Morales-Cabezas M, et al. Two exercise interventions for the management of patients with ankylosing spondylitis: a randomized controlled trial. *Am J Phys Med Rehabil*. 2005;84(6):407–419.

395. Fernández-de-Las-Peñas C, Alonso-Blanco C, Alguacil-Diego IM, et al. One-year follow-up of two exercise interventions for the management of patients with ankylosing spondylitis: a randomized controlled trial. *Am J Phys Med Rehabil*. 2006;85(7):559–567.

396. Dagfinrud H, Kvien TK, Hagen KB. Physiotherapy interventions in ankylosing spondylitis. *Cochrane Database Syst Rev*. 2008;(1):CD002822.

397. Ward MM, Reveille JD, Learch TJ. Occupational physical activities and long term functional and radiographic outcomes in patients with ankylosing spondylitis. *Arthritis Rheumatol*. 2008;59(6):822–832.

398. Stucki G, Kroeling P. Physical therapy and rehabilitation in the management of rheumatic disorders. *Best Pract Res Clin Rheumatol*. 2000;14:751–771.

399. Petty RE, Southwood TR, Manners P, et al. International League of Associations for Rheumatology classification of juvenile idiopathic arthritis: second revision, Edmonton, 2001. *J Rheumatol*. 2004;31(2):390–392.

400. Takei S, Hokonohara M. Quality of life and daily management of children with rheumatic disease. *Acta Paediatr Jpn*. 1993;35:454–456.

401. Hackett J, Johnson B, Parkin A, et al. Physiotherapy and occupational therapy for juvenile chronic arthritis: custom and practice in five centers in UK, USA and Canada. *Br J Rheumatol*. 1996;35:695–699.

402. Nistala K, Woo P, Wedderburn L. Juvenile idiopathic arthritis. In: Firestein GS, Budd RC, Sergent JS, et al., eds. *Kelley's Textbook of Rheumatology*. 8th ed. Philadelphia, PA: WB Saunders; 2009:1657–1676.

403. Lelieveld OT, Wineke A, Miek A. Physical activity in adolescents with juvenile idiopathic arthritis. *Arthritis Rheum*. 2008;59(10):1379–1384.

404. Giannnin SE. Exercise in pediatric rheumatic diseases. *Curr Opin Rheumatol*. 2008;20(50):619–624.

405. Peterson LS, Mason T, Nelson AM, et al. Psychosocial outcomes and health status of adults who had juvenile rheumatoid arthritis: a controlled population based study. *Arthritis Rheum*. 1997;40:2235–2240.

406. Lequerre T, Quartier P, Roselli D, et al. Interleukin-1 receptor antagonist (anakinra) treatment in patients with systemic-onset juvenile idiopathic arthritis or adult onset Stills' disease: preliminary experience in France. *Ann Rheum Dis*. 2008;67(3):302–308.

407. Lomater C, Gerloni V, Gattinara M, et al. Systemic onset juvenile idiopathic arthritis: a retrospective of 80 consecutive patient followed for 10 years. *J Rheumatol*. 2000;27:491–496.

408. Saurennman RK, Levin AV, Feldman BM, et al. Prevalence, risk factors, and outcome of uveitis in juvenile idiopathic arthritis: along-term followup study. *Arthritis Rheum*. 2007;56(2):647–657.

409. Woo P, Soutwood TR, Prieur AM, et al. Randomized, placebo controlled crossover trial of low dose oral methotrexate in children with extended oligoarticular or systemic arthritis. *Arthritis Rheum*. 2000;43:1849–1857.

410. Beukelman T, Patkar NM, Saag KG, et al. 2011 American College of Rheumatology recommendations for the treatment of juvenile idiopathic arthritis: initiation and safety monitoring of therapeutic agents for the treatment of arthritis and systemic features. *Arthritis Care Res (Hoboken)*. 2011;63(4):465–482.

411. van der Heijde D, Klareskog L, Rodriguez-Valerde V, et al. Comparison of etanercept and methotrexate, alone and combined, in the treatment of rheumatoid arthritis: two-year clinical and radiographic results from the TEMPO study, a double-blind, randomized trial. *Arthritis Rheum*. 2006;54(4):1063–1074.

412. Flatø B, Aasland A, Vinje O, et al. Outcome and predictive factors in juvenile rheumatoid arthritis and juvenile spondyloarthropathy. *J Rheumatol*. 1998;25(2):366–375.

413. Giannini MJ, Protas EJ. Comparison of peak isometric knee extension torque in children with and without juvenile rheumatoid arthritis. *Arthritis Care Res*. 1993;6:82–88.

414. Giannini MJ, Protas EJ. Aerobic capacity in juvenile rheumatoid arthritis. *Arthritis Care Res*. 1991;4:131–135.

415. Ravelli A. *Handbook of Juvenile Idiopathic Arthritis*. 1st ed. Switzerland: ADIS; 2016.

416. Klepper SE, Giannini MJ. Physical conditioning in children with arthritis: assessment and guidelines for exercise prescription. *Arthritis Care Res*. 1994;7:226–236.

417. Bacon MC, Nicholson C, Binder H, et al. Juvenile rheumatoid arthritis. Aquatic exercise and lower-extremity function. *Arthritis Care Res*. 1991;4(2):102–105.

418. Singh-Grewal D, Schneiderman-Walker J, Wright V, et al. The effects of vigorous exercise training on physical function in children with arthritis: a randomized, controlled, single-blinded trial. *Arthritis Rheum*. 2007;57(7):1202–1210.

419. Kotaniemi A, Savolainen A, Kroger H, et al. Weight-bearing physical activity, calcium intake, systemic glucocorticoids, chronic inflammation and body constitution as determinants of lumbar and femoral bone mineral in juvenile chronic arthritis. *Scand J Rheumatol*. 1999;28:19–26.

420. Takken T, Van Brussel M, Englebert RH. Exercise therapy in juvenile idiopathic arthritis: a Cochrane Review. *Eur J Phys Rehabil Med*. 2008;44(3):287–297.

421. André M, Hagelberg S, Stenström CH. Education in the management of juvenile chronic arthritis. Changes in self-reported competencies among adolescents and parents of young children. *Scand J Rheumatol*. 2001;30(6):323–327.

422. Ettinger WH. Physical activity, arthritis and disability in older people. *Clin Geriatr Med*. 1998;14:633–640.

423. Calkins E. Geriatrics and the rheumatic diseases. In: Ruddy S, Harris ED, Sledge CB, et al., eds. *Kelley's Textbook of Rheumatology*. 6th ed. Philadelphia, PA: WB Saunders; 2001:735–738.

424. van Schaardenburg D. Rheumatoid arthritis in the elderly. Prevalence and optimal management. *Drugs Aging*. 1995;7(1):30–37.

425. Sewell KL. Rheumatoid arthritis in older adults. *Clin Geriatr Med*. 1998;14:475–494.

426. Nesher G, Moore TL. Rheumatoid arthritis in the aged: Incidence and optimal management. *Drugs Aging*. 1993;3:487–501.

427. Daly MP, Berman BM. Rehabilitation of the elderly patient with arthritis. *Clin Geriatr Med*. 1993;9:783–801.

428. O'Grady M, Fletcher J, Ortiz S. Therapeutic and physical fitness exercise prescription for older adults with joint disease: an evidence-based approach. *Rheum Dis Clin North Am*. 2000;26:617–646.

429. Lyngberg KK, Harrebg M, Bentzen H, et al. Elderly rheumatoid arthritis patients on steroid treatment tolerate physical training without an increase in disease activity. *Arch Phys Med Rehabil*. 1994;75:1189–1195.

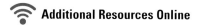 **Additional Resources Online**

CHAPTER **33**

Carmen M. Terzic
Jose R. Medina-Inojosa

Cardiac Rehabilitation

Cardiac rehabilitation (CR) is a comprehensive and multidisciplinary intervention offered to patients with cardiovascular diseases (CVDs), which incorporates components of health education, advice on cardiovascular risk reduction, physical activity/exercise, and stress management. Strong evidence confirms that CR reduces cardiovascular comorbidities, unplanned hospital admissions, and total and cardiovascular mortality (1–3), in addition to improvements in exercise capacity (1,4), quality of life, psychological well-being (4), and adherence to medications. CR is strongly recommended in all CVD prevention guidelines (5–7). This chapter provides an overview of heart anatomy, physiology, and diseases and focuses on CR program components, goals, performance measures, and benefits on CVDs control and secondary prevention.

OVERVIEW OF HEART ANATOMY AND PHYSIOLOGY

The heart is a muscular organ composed of three different layers known as epicardium, myocardium, and endocardium. A fourth layer of connective fibrous tissue or pericardium encompasses the entire heart and the roots of great vessels, functioning as a stabilizer of the heart within the mediastinum and preventing cardiac overload. The epicardium contains the coronary blood vessels and is in continuation with the myocardium internally and with the serous layer of the pericardium externally. It is composed largely of connective tissue, providing an additional layer of protection from trauma or friction. The myocardium, located between the epicardium and endocardium, consists mainly of cardiac cells or cardiomyocytes responsible for the contraction and relaxation of the cardiac walls. The endocardium (inner layer) is a lining of simple squamous epithelium, and it is continuous with the endothelium of the vein and arteries of the heart.

The heart is divided into four chambers, two upper atria and two lower ventricles that are separated by the atrioventricular septum and interventricular septum, respectively. Two valves, composed of collagenous fiber, elastic fibers, and endothelium, separate the right atria and the right ventricle (tricuspid valve) and the left atria and the left ventricle (mitral valve). Other two valves, pulmonary and aortic valves, are located at the base of the pulmonary artery and the aorta, respectively. Overall, the heart valves ensure blood flow in the correct direction through the heart and prevent blood return (**Fig. 33-1A**). The cardiac skeleton is made of connective tissue that forms the atrioventricular septum, which separates the atria from the ventricle, and the fibrous ring, which serves as a base and attachment for the heart valves.

There are two types of cardiac muscle cells: cardiomyocytes and pacemaker cells. The cardiomyocytes, or contractile cells, make up to 90% of all the cells in the atria and ventricle and are connected by intercalated disks. These disks allow a rapid response to an action potential, allowing these cells to enable the contraction that pumps blood through the heart into the major arteries.

The pacemaker cells make up around 1% of the cardiac cells of the heart. They are modified cardiomyocytes located at the sinoatrial node, responsible for generating regular and spontaneous action potentials, that will ultimately trigger the contraction of the entire heart. This autorhythmicity is modulated by the endocrine and nervous system. The electrical signal generated by the pacemaker cells travels through the right and left atrium via Bachmann's bundle, allowing both atria to contract together. The signal then travels throughout the atrioventricular node into the atrioventricular septum and into the ventricles through the left and right bundle branches of the bundle of His. In the ventricles, the signal is carried by specialized tissue called the Purkinje fibers, which then transmit the electric charge to the cardiomyocytes, allowing ventricular contraction (**Fig. 33-1A**).

Heart contractility and rate are controlled by the two branches of the autonomic nervous system: sympathetic trunk and parasympathetic system. The sympathetic trunk regulates heart rate acceleration, venous capacitance, and vasoconstriction. The parasympathetic nervous system is mainly involved in slowing heart rate through vagal impulses.

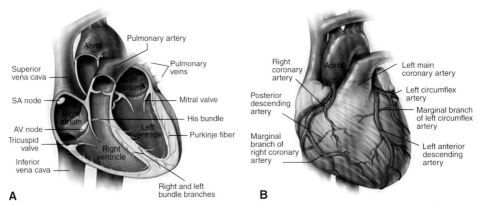

FIGURE 33-1. Heart anatomy and coronary artery circulation. **A:** Four-chamber view of the heart displaying the atria, ventricles, heart valves, and pacemaker system. **B:** Coronary artery circulation; right and left main coronary arteries and branches throughout the heart. (Courtesy of Jose R. Medina-Inojosa and Carmen M. Terzic. Used with permission of Mayo Foundation for Medical Education and Research. All rights reserved.)

Two major systemic veins, the superior and inferior vena cava, return deoxygenated blood from the body into the right atrium and from there into the right ventricle. Contraction of the right ventricle ejects the deoxygenated blood into the pulmonary arteries that carry it to each lung. After an exchange in the pulmonary capillaries of the lung, blood high in oxygen returns to the left atrium via pulmonary veins and from the atrium into the left ventricle. The blood is then pumped from the left ventricle into the circulatory system through the aorta. The coronary arteries emerge from the aorta and branch throughout the heart walls to form the coronary circulation that supply oxygen-rich blood to the heart (8) (**Fig. 33-1B**).

CARDIOVASCULAR DISEASES

CVDs are the world's largest cause of mortality (9). There are around 17.5 million cases a year, responsible for 31% of global deaths. CVD is particularly prevalent given our aging population (10) and creates a significant burden in health care with around 1.9 billion US dollars in overall costs (10). The majority of cardiovascular deaths, roughly 7.4 million, are due to coronary artery disease (CAD) (10). The most common manifestation of CAD is an acute coronary syndrome, caused by a flow-limiting lesion or plaque due to arteriosclerosis. It can manifest as chest pain or angina, dyspnea during exertion, or no symptoms at all. Besides atherosclerosis, less common causes of coronary artery obstruction include abnormal growth inside the artery and local or diffuse inflammatory process (11). Depending on the coronary artery involved and degree of ischemia, an electrocardiogram (ECG) may confirm the presence of an ST elevation myocardial infarction (STEMI), when a plaque completely or nearly completely blocks a major coronary artery resulting in extensive heart damage, or a non–ST elevation myocardial infarction (NSTEMI) when the blockage either occurs in a minor coronary artery or causes partial obstruction in a major coronary artery; see **Figure 33-1** and **Table 33-1**.

Not all CAD is obstructive in nature. Coronary arteries may display an impaired endothelium-dependent response to stress, where there is a reduction in coronary artery dilation and a compromised microvascular coronary flow reserve, limiting the flow of blood to the myocardium (12).

A second common cardiac condition is heart failure (HF) (13). HF is a complex clinical syndrome defined as the inability of the heart to pump enough blood to meet the needs of the body (13). HF could be classified as (a) systolic dysfunction, in which there is a decrease of the left ventricular ejection fraction, or (b) diastolic dysfunction, in which there is an impaired ventricular filling, meaning there is increased left ventricular and left atrial pressure (13). The pathophysiology of HF includes cardiac remodeling, in which the heart becomes hypertrophic initially and then dilated with an enlargement of the chambers; renin-angiotensin system activation with subsequent vasoconstriction and increased blood volume; and sympathetic nervous system stimulation to provide inotropic support to the failing heart. Another contributor to the pathophysiology of HF is the peripheral muscles that became myopathic due to reduction of vasodilation, decrease of mitochondrial metabolic capacity, reduction of aerobic motor units, and increasing numbers of anaerobic motor units (13).

Patients with HF typically exhibit reduced exercise capacity, early fatigue with physical activity, dyspnea with exertion, and edema (13). The most common causes of HF worldwide are ischemic heart disease, hypertension, valvular heart disease, arrhythmias, and cardiomyopathies such as Chagas' disease (American trypanosomiasis) (13). However, HF induced by ischemia is the major driver of late morbidity, mortality, and increase in health care cost (10).

Myocardial ischemia and HF create a heterogeneously distributed remodeled tissue that can promote the initiation and maintenance of electrical instability and generation

TABLE 33-1	Distribution of Myocardial Infarction According to Coronary Artery Involvement	
Coronary Artery	**Area of Damage**	**Affected ECG Leads**
Left anterior descending	Anterior heart wall	V_1–V_6
Left anterior descending distal		V_1–V_4
Left circumflex	Lateral heart wall	I, aVL, V_5, V_6
Right coronary artery	Inferior heart wall Right ventricle	II, III, aVF
Posterior descending artery	Posterior heart wall	V_7, V_8, V_9 (right leads)

ECG, electrocardiogram; MI, myocardial infarction.

of arrhythmias. Heart rhythm disorders or arrhythmias are responsible for considerable morbidity and mortality in patients with CVD (10). Cardiac arrest due to ventricular arrhythmias is the leading cause of death in the industrialized world, particularly among patients with prior MI (14).

CURRENT MANAGEMENT OPTIONS FOR CARDIOVASCULAR DISEASES

Risk factors for CVD include smoking, overweight, inactivity, high cholesterol, high blood pressure, and diabetes. In addition to lifestyle modification, current guidelines indicate pharmacologic therapy as the next line of intervention to control cardiovascular risk factors and disease progression (5–7). Initial antihypertensive treatment should include thiazide diuretics and calcium channel blockers, together with angiotensin-converting enzyme (ACE) inhibitors or angiotensin receptor blockers (ARBs) (15). Although in general beta-blockers are not considered the first line for treatment of high blood pressure, in patients with CAD, there are well-established benefits of the use of beta-blockers to decrease mortality and recurrence of cardiovascular events (16).

Aspirin, clopidogrel, and ticagrelor are antiplatelet aggregators indicated to prevent thrombus formation and restenosis, especially after percutaneous coronary intervention (PCI) or angioplasty. Drugs that affect blood coagulation like warfarin (vitamin K inhibitor), dabigatran (thrombin inhibitor), and rivaroxaban, apixaban, or edoxaban (factor Xa inhibitor) also prevent thrombus formation and embolism in patients with low ejection fraction, atrial fibrillation (AF), valvular heart disease, and artificial valves (17). The American College of Cardiology and the American Heart Association (ACC/AHA) recommend the use of high-intensity statins (HMG-CoA reductase inhibitors) in most high-risk patients (18). In this regard, simvastatin (20 to 40 mg/d), pravastatin (40 to 80 mg/d), atorvastatin (40 to 80 mg/d), or rosuvastatin (20 to 40 mg/d) is recommended (18). Myalgias and/or myopathy and liver failure are serious side effects of high intensive statin therapy (19). Liver function tests and markers of muscle damage are monitored if indicated. Other pharmacologic intervention for hyperlipidemia includes niacin, fibrates, cholesterol absorption inhibitors, omega-3 acid ethyl esters, and more recently lipoprotein convertase subtilisin/kexin type 9 (PCSK9) inhibitors (20).

ACE inhibitor or ARBs, beta-blockers, and calcium channel blockers also help to control blood pressure while improving the pumping ability of the heart. In addition, the inotropic agents dobutamine and digoxin, and the new angiotensin receptor blocker neprilysin inhibitors (ARNIs), are recommended in patients with HF to improve the overall muscle contractility and function of the heart (15). Oral hypoglycemics and insulin are used to control glucose and HbA1c levels in patients with diabetes (15).

Procedural interventions to control CVDs, such as PCI, in which a stent is placed in the coronary artery to open the artery and increase the blood flow to the heart muscle have improved early survival after MI (21). Surgical revascularization with coronary artery bypass graft (CABG) has been shown to improve mortality, symptomatic angina, and quality of life (22).

Although heart transplant remains the gold standard for the treatment of severe HF refractory to all the above interventions, durable mechanical assist devices have become an appealing option in light of the limited availability of heart donors. In this regard, new-generation, continuous-flow left ventricular assist devices (LVADs) have been used not only as a bridge to transplantation but also as destination therapy (23). Cardiac resynchronization therapy (CRT) has had a favorable impact on the care of patients with symptomatic HF, left ventricular ejection fraction less than 35%, and enlarged QRS (23). Catheter ablation is an effective treatment for a variety of arrhythmias. Pacemakers and defibrillators with a new generation of leadless pacing systems are essential tools to control arrhythmias and prevent sudden death (24). Finally, stem cell–based therapies delivered to the diseased myocardium after a coronary event, or in the setting of HF, have been shown to be safe and feasible with promising signals of efficacy (25). However, before the potential of biologic-based interventions can be translated into clinical benefits and services, appropriate research to define mechanisms of action and clinical applications, as well as the need to set regulatory mechanisms, must be outlined (26).

CARDIAC REHABILITATION PROGRAMS

Exercise as a medical intervention was perceived as a risk to patients with CVD, and mandatory bed rest period was commonly prescribed after an acute cardiac event. It was not until 1953 that the role of activity in lowering risk of CAD and associated mortality started to be recognized, after a pivotal study showing that bus, tram, and trolley conductors, who climbed an average of 500 to 750 steps per working day, had a decrease of CAD and cardiovascular mortality when compared with drivers who sat for over 90% during their work (27). In 1997, during the first International Congress on CR, the needs for early mobilization in patients with CVD were established, and since then, exercise as an intervention was gradually implemented (28). In 1993, The World Health Organization (WHO) stressed the importance of CR in the management of patients with CVD and set the definition as "the sum of the activities required to favorably influence both the subjacent cause of the disease and the physical, mental and social conditions of the patient, allowing patients to preserve or reassume their role in the community as soon as possible" (29).

Today, CR is considered the "gold standard of care" for patients after a cardiac event or procedure (5–7). CR programs consist of multiple supervised sessions that comprehensively address risk factors through education about cardiac diseases and medication use, exercise training, smoking cessation, adequate nutrition, and control of comorbidities such as diabetes, hypertension, obesity and sleep apnea, and psychosocial stressors. The multidisciplinary team is led by an experienced clinician and includes nurses, exercise physiologists, cardiologists, physiatrists, physical therapists, occupational therapists, dietitians, psychologists, and endocrinologists (5–7). The ultimate goal of a CR program is to control CVD risk factors and maximize physical function and return to work. CR program outcomes are outlined in **Table 33-2**.

CR programs are traditionally divided into phases: (a) hospital-based stage (inpatient setting, also known as phase I), (b) early outpatient supervised and monitored exercise sessions (or phase II), (c) late outpatient supervised CR to develop exercises with more intensity (or phase III), and (d) home-based exercise program (known as phase IV) (5–7).

TABLE 33-2	Cardiac Rehabilitation Program Outcomes
Maximizing the Medical Management of Risk Factors	• Smoking cessation • Lipid management (50% reduction of LDL-c to below 70 mg/dL) • Blood pressure control (<140/90 mm Hg for nondiabetics and <130/80 in people with diabetes) • Glucose control (<7% HbA1c) • Optimal weight and central obesity management (BMI 18.5–25 kg/m² and waist circumference <102 cm in men, <89 cm in women) • Diet modification • Obstructive sleep apnea management
Improving Quality of Life	• Increased exercise tolerance • Symptom control • Psychological well-being/stress management • Return to work

LDL-c, low-density lipoprotein; mg, milligrams; mm Hg, millimeters of mercury; Hb, hemoglobin; BMI, body mass index.

Hospital-Based CR (Phase I)

Hospital CR has grown in importance and is currently considered to be the most significant phase of the program. Hospital-based CR starts within 24 to 48 hours after admission (if patient is medically stable) and lasts until discharge. The team involved in this program includes nurses, physical and occupational therapists, and cardiologists. This phase focuses on clinical status assessment, education, physical function, patient mobilization and activities, family and social support, as well as a comprehensive discharge plan including follow-up options for transitional care and outpatient rehabilitation (5–7).

To set individualized interventions, a comprehensive assessment of clinical and functional status includes heart rate, ECG, blood pressure, oxygen saturation, upper and lower extremity strength and range of motion (ROM), mobility, activities of daily living, and tests such as Timed Up and Go (TUG) (30) and/or 6-Minute Walk Test (6-MWT) (31). One of the key elements in this phase is education, with a strong focus on understanding risk factors for CVD, medication use and effects, self-monitoring of heart rate and/or exertion level, and general wound precautions if postsurgery.

During hospital-based CR, the clinical team will ensure that patients can perform bed mobilization and safely transfer from bed to a chair. As patients progress in CR, more advanced activities are added including sitting to standing to ambulation (5 to 10 minutes, 2 to 4 times per day), stair climbing, and upper body exercises while monitoring heart rate, ECG changes, blood pressure, and oxygen levels (32). The ultimate goal is to reduce patient anxiety, increase independence and confidence, reduce deconditioning, and prepare the patient for outpatient CR. Finally, during the hospitalization, the team set comprehensive discharge plans that include follow-up options for transitional care and referral to outpatient CR.

Recommendations for the prescription of exercises in phase I CR are outlined in **Table 33-3**.

TABLE 33-3	Recommended Prescription of Exercises in Phase I of Cardiac Rehabilitation
Intensity	Rate of perceived effort below 13 Surgical patients: HR increase no >20 bpm above resting HR
Duration	Short burst of 3–5 min in duration, with 1–2 min resting time in between
Frequency	Two to three sessions per day
Progression	Increase duration first and then intensity. Should be individualized

Bpm, beats per minute; HR, heart rate.
Derived from Pescatello LS, American College of Sports Medicine. *ACSM's Guidelines for Exercise Testing and Prescription.* 7th ed. Philadelphia, PA: Wolters Kluwer Health/Lippincott Williams & Wilkins; 2013, Ref. (77).

Outpatient Cardiac Rehabilitation (Phase II to III to IV)

All patients hospitalized with a diagnosis of chronic stable angina, MI, CABG, PCI, cardiac transplantation, cardiac valve surgery, HF, and, more recently, peripheral arterial disease (PAD) should be referred to an outpatient CR (6,33). Outpatient CR is divided in early (phase II), late (phase III), and outpatient home-based program (phase IV) (5,6).

As in hospital-based programs, a comprehensive clinical evaluation is required prior to starting an outpatient CR program. Physicians perform a thorough physical examination searching for signs of complication after the cardiac event or surgical procedure. Findings of congestive heart failure or fluid overload (dyspnea at rest, rales, edema, and jugular distention) are evaluated. Surgical patients are carefully examined for proper wound healing. Past medical history, family and social history, and medication list are reviewed. Assessment of risk factors for disease progression is performed at the beginning and the end of the CR program. An ECG and cardiopulmonary stress tests are necessary to document work capacity and cardiopulmonary function (34). The 6-MWT is performed in patients deconditioned or with already known decreased functional capacity (not able to give maximal effort in stress test) (6,31).

Early outpatient CR programs (phase II) start 1 to 2 weeks postevent. During this phase, all exercise sessions are closely monitored with ECG to detect dysrhythmias or changes associated with ischemia, to follow intensity of exercise, and to increase patient self-confidence for independent activity. If patients are asymptomatic, have stable disease, and have excellent functional capacity, they may not require ECG monitoring during subsequent exercise sessions (late outpatient CR or phase III). However, ECG monitoring during aerobic exercise is recommended to continue later in the program for those patients with low ejection fraction, history of arrhythmias, abnormal blood pressure response to exercise, and ECG ST-segment depression during low level of exercise (5,6,35).

Upon completion of the 36 sessions of the phase II to III program, patients are ready to start a home-based program (phase IV) (6). This phase aims to continue exercising and preserve all behavioral changes and risk factor modifications learned during the previous phases of CR. A team member follows the patient on a regular basis to review cardiovascular symptoms, blood pressure, appropriate laboratory test (lipid profile, glycemia, liver function tests, creatinine, electrolytes), current exercise program and nutrition plan, weight control, and medications (5–7,35).

Intensive Cardiac Rehabilitation

Intensive cardiac rehabilitation (ICR) is also a comprehensive multidisciplinary physician-supervised program, and the main difference from traditional CR is that ICR is provided more frequently and in a more rigorous manner. ICR programs include up to 72 sessions lasting up to 18 weeks. A minimum of one session per week is required with a maximum of 6 sessions per day allowed. Patients must participate in aerobic exercise every day, and although exercise is not needed in every session, patients should participate in more than one session per day (36). Similar to traditional CR programs, indications for ICR include patients with chronic stable angina, MI, CABG, PCI, cardiac transplantation, cardiac valve surgery, HF, and PAD. Although ICR is becoming more popular, there is no scientific evidence showing that patients participating in ICR have better outcomes when compared to patients enrolled in traditional CR programs.

BENEFITS OF CARDIOVASCULAR REHABILITATION PROGRAMS

Control of Risk Factors

The specific beneficial effects of a structured exercise program on cardiovascular risk factors, exercise capacity, depression and stress, recurrence of cardiovascular events, and mortality have been fully established and will be described below (1,2,35, 37–43). It is recognized and proven that CR programs effectively manage lifestyle and provide optimal targets for intervention that address all modifiable CVD risk factors **(Box 33-1)** (38,44–47).

Tobacco

Smoking is directly associated with mortality and is considered the leading cause of preventable diseases and deaths in the United States, causing one of every three deaths from CVD according to the 2014 Surgeon General's Report (48,49). Smoking cessation is considered an essential outcome in all CR programs, and counseling on nicotine use together with pharmacologic therapy is mandatory. It has been clearly demonstrated that the strongest predictor of smoking cessation at 6 months after an acute cardiac event was participation in CR programs (50).

BOX 33-1

Modifiable Cardiovascular Risk Factors

- Smoking
- Diabetes
- Dyslipidemia
- Hypertension
- Overweight/abdominal obesity
- Sedentary lifestyle

Dyslipidemia

Strong evidence supports the benefits of managing dyslipidemias in patients with CVD (18). Reductions in CVD mortality, hospitalizations, and progression of atherosclerotic disease have been demonstrated with aggressive low-density lipoprotein (LDL) lowering (46). Participation in CR programs has been shown to improve lipid profile by reducing LDL (−11 mg/dL) and triglycerides (−5%) and increasing high-density lipoprotein (HDL) by 13% to 16% in patients with low levels of HDL (38).

Cholesterol levels are reviewed at the moment of the admission to the program and/or either 4 to 6 weeks post cardiac event or surgical intervention (6). The overall lipid control goals for patients participating in CR program are a 50% reduction in LDL-c to an LDL-c below 70 mg/dL and non-HDL cholesterol less than 100 mg/dL (18).

Hyperglycemia and Diabetes

Evidence suggests that hyperglycemia is a key risk factor not only for the development of diabetes but also for CVD (51,52). In addition, diabetes is currently considered a CVD equivalent, and patients with diabetes have premature mortality and morbidity related to CVD (51). It has been shown that an increase of 1 unit (%) of hemoglobin A1c is associated with roughly 18% increment of cardiovascular mortality (52).

Participation in CR programs has been associated with a clinically significant reduction of the hemoglobin A1c to levels that have been shown to reduce cardiac and diabetic complications (51,52). CR program motivates compliance with medications, diet, and exercise, important interventions to control hyperglycemia and diabetes.

The aim for patients participating in CR program is to maintain glucose levels less than 100 for nondiabetic patients and a hemoglobin A1c less than 7.0% for diabetic patients. The CR team must work closely with the primary medical provider to optimize management of diabetes and achieve desired targets.

Hypertension

Hypertension is an independent risk factor for stroke and the most common risk factor for MI and HF (53,54). Hypertension is highly prevalent in patients enrolled in CR (54,55). It has been demonstrated that patients participating in CR program have a significant reduction in systolic and diastolic blood pressure (55). Therefore, an important task for the CR team is to manage blood pressure and adjust medications as needed to achieve goal values of less than 140/90 mm Hg in nondiabetes and less than 130/80 mm Hg if diabetes is present (6,54).

Overweight and Obesity

The prevalence of obesity in the United States has risen remarkably over the past four decades, increasing from around 13% in the 1960s to 37.7% in 2014, according to the National Health and Nutrition Examination Survey (NHANES) (10). Obesity is an independent risk factor for CVD, and excess in adiposity also predisposes individuals to risk factors such as hypertension, diabetes, and dyslipidemia (10). Around 80% of patients enrolled in CR are overweight (56).

All patients entering CR program have weight, body mass index (BMI calculated as weight in kilograms divided by squared height in meters [kg/m^2]), and waist circumference recorded. Overweight by BMI measurements is defined as having a BMI between 25 and 29.0 kg/m^2, while a BMI greater than 30 kg/m^2 indicates the presence of obesity (56,57). Recently, dual-energy x-ray absorptiometry (DEXA) scan is used to have a more accurate diagnosis of obesity (58). Obesity by body adiposity is defined as a total body fat percentage over 25% for men and 35% for women (57). Patients with normal weight but high body fat content (defined as normal weight obesity) will have increased risk for CV mortality, especially women (59). Therefore, the determination of adiposity has significant health implications.

Changes in dietary patterns and increase in exercise and physical activities are the main components of the weight reduction program. Nutritional counseling and dietitian evaluation are indispensable to assist in weight management. Mediterranean style diet is highly recommended as it is rich in fish, complex carbohydrates, vegetables, fruits, olive oil, nuts, low salt, and saturated fat (6).

Prospective studies showed the beneficial effect of multidisciplinary lifestyle interventions, such as CR, on body weight and waist circumference (2). The goal is to achieve an optimal BMI of 18.5 to 24.9 and waist circumference less than 102 cm for men and less than 89 cm for women and decrease total body fat percentage to desired values.

Obstructive Sleep Apnea

Screening for obstructive sleep apnea (OSA) is another important assessment during the CR program, as OSA is an independent risk factor for ischemic heart disease and all-cause mortality (60). This evaluation can be performed using explorative tools designed to identify patients with OSA, such as Berlin questionnaire, or by measurements of O$_2$ saturation with an overnight oximetry (61,62). Advanced sleep studies such as polysomnography are performed if OSA screening tests were abnormal.

Psychological Well-Being

Depression is associated with an increased risk of death or rehospitalization in patients with HF, CAD, and stroke (63–66). Recently, the AHA recommended elevating depression to the status of a risk factor for adverse medical outcomes in patients with an acute coronary syndrome (67).

The PHQ-9 (68) and State-Trait Anxiety Inventory (69) are tools employed to assess depression and anxiety in the CR setting, as both provide useful information to guide intervention. Improvements in stress, anxiety, depression, and quality of life, regardless of patient age, have been reported after participation in CR programs (39,41).

Cardiovascular Outcomes

Extensive data in the literature support the impact of CR program participation on mortality, readmissions, and CVD progression. Several reasons explain this outstanding effect. CR is known to have a favorable impact on CVD risk factors and improves functional status as described in the previous section of this chapter (43). In addition, the nature of CR program offers a unique opportunity for continued assessment, communication, education, and counseling of patients after acute CVD events. Furthermore, CR improves adherence to guideline-recommended medications over time, with a favorable 3-year use of statins, beta-blockers, and ACE inhibitors (45).

Hospital Readmissions

Participation in CR programs has been shown to reduce hospital admissions and use of medical resources in participants regardless of their primary cardiovascular event (70). In a well-defined community cohort of patients with MI, CR participation was associated with a 25% reduction in long-term cardiovascular and noncardiovascular readmission (43). Other studies have shown an even higher reduction in the risk of hospital admission, which ranged from 30.7% to 26.1%, with a number needed to treat (NNT) of 22 (71). For HF patients, exercise-based CR reduces the risk of all-cause hospitalization (relative risk 0.75 [0.62 to 0.92], ARR 7.1%, NNT 15) and hospitalization for HF (relative risk 0.61 [0.46 to 0.80], ARR 5.8%, NNT 18) (72). In the case of heart transplant patients, participation in CR was associated with a 29% lower 1-year readmission risk (95% CI 13% to 42%) (73).

Mortality

It has been clearly established that CR participation decreases total and cardiovascular mortality for men and women, older and younger patients, and patients undergoing elective or nonelective cardiac interventions (3,40,42–44,47,74). Meta-analyses of randomized controlled trials and observational studies have demonstrated a reduction in mortality as high as 42%, after MI, an effect that is maintained over an average of 7.6 years post-CR participation (74). Also, CR attendance after CABG is associated with a significant reduction of 40% in 10 years of all-cause mortality rate (40,42,47). Similar impact on mortality was found in patients post PCI, CABG, and valve surgery (39,44). A meta-analysis of 10,794 patients with stable CAD also showed a reduction in total mortality and cardiovascular mortality (74).

A summary of all benefits of CR program is presented in **Table 33-4**.

EXERCISE TESTING IN THE CARDIAC REHABILITATION SETTING

Exercise tests are an objective tool to evaluate cardiorespiratory fitness, hemodynamic responses to exercise, and signs and symptoms associated with exertion. It gives the opportunity to not only follow clinical and functional improvement during patient participation in CR programs but also to define future interventions. The safety and low-risk rate of adverse events during exercise testing is well documented to be 1 to 5 per 100,000 tests with a rate of death less than 0.5 per 100,000 tests (75,76). However, appropriate risk stratification must be performed before beginning any exercise test, and an emergency workable plan and equipment must be set and readily available to the personnel in the program and exercise testing center (77). Absolute and relative contraindications to exercise testing are outlined in **Table 33-5**.

Exercise testing can have submaximal or symptom-limited endpoints. Submaximal exercise testing has a predetermined endpoint (percent predicted heart rate at 70%, an arbitrary metabolic equivalent [MET] [1 MET = 3.5 mL/kg/min]) or rating of perceived exertion (RPE) on the visual analogue Borg scale (**Table 33-6**) (78). Submaximal exercise testing is applied to higher-risk patients and provides satisfactory data for evaluating the patient's capacity to engage in daily activities and may serve as a guide for exercise prescription.

TABLE 33-4	Benefits of Cardiac Rehabilitation Programs
Improved Symptoms	• Dyspnea • Fatigue • Claudication • Stress • Depression
Autonomic Function	• Increased vagal activity • Attenuated sympathetic hyperactivity • Increased heart rate variability • Reduced resting pulse • Increased heart rate recovery • Decrease in blood pressure
Circulatory Function	• Antithrombotic effect • Peripheral adaptation of skeletal muscles • Decreased arterial stiffness • Enhance endothelium-dependent vasodilation
Cardiorespiratory Fitness	• Improve aerobic capacity • Increase metabolic equivalents
Metabolic Components	• Decrease in total and low-density lipoprotein (LDL) cholesterol and triglycerides • Increase in high-density lipoprotein (HDL) cholesterol • Improves insulin sensitivity • Improves metabolic syndrome • Total body fat reduction • Decrease inflammatory markers
Cardiovascular Outcomes	• Decrease all-cause hospital readmissions • Reduction in all-cause mortality rates • Diminution in cardiovascular mortality • Improved adherence with preventive medication

PCI, percutaneous coronary intervention; MI, myocardial infarction; CABG, coronary artery bypass graft; HF, heart failure.

TABLE 33-5	Absolute and Relative Contraindications to Exercise Testing
Absolute Contraindications	• Acute myocardial infarction (within 2 days) • High-risk unstable angina • Uncontrolled cardiac dysrhythmias causing symptoms or hemodynamic compromise • Active endocarditis • Severe symptomatic aortic stenosis • Decompensated symptomatic heart failure • Acute pulmonary embolus or pulmonary infarction • Acute noncardiac disorder that may affect exercise performance or be aggravated by exercise (e.g., infection, renal failure, thyrotoxicosis) • Acute myocarditis or pericarditis • Physical disability that would preclude safe and adequate test performance • Inability to obtain consent
Relative Contraindications[a]	• Left main coronary stenosis or equivalent • Moderate stenotic valvular heart disease • Electrolyte abnormalities • Tachyarrhythmias or bradyarrhythmias • Atrial fibrillation with rapid ventricular rate (>150 bpm) • Hypertrophic cardiomyopathy • Mental impairment leading to inability to cooperate with testing • High-degree atrioventricular block • Severe resting arterial hypertension (systolic BP > 200 mm Hg and diastolic BP > 110 mm Hg)

[a]Contraindications can be superseded if benefits outweigh risk of exercise.
Bpm, beats per minute; mm Hg, millimeters of mercury; BP, blood pressure.
Adapted from Gibbons RJ, Balady GJ, Bricker JT, et al. ACC/AHA 2002 guideline update for exercise testing: summary article. A report of the American College of Cardiology/American Heart Association Task Force on Practice Guidelines (Committee to Update the 1997 Exercise Testing Guidelines). *J Am Coll Cardiol.* 2002;40(8):1531–1540.

Symptom-limited protocols are indicated in lower-risk patients and are designed to be terminated when the protocol is completed or patients perceive any of the symptoms outlined in **Table 33-7**.

Treadmills and cycle ergometers are used to carry out exercise testing protocols. Treadmill tests provide a more physiologic testing context (comparable to walking), while ergometers are preferred for those with limited ability to walk or bear weight during exercise.

Testing protocols can also be ramped or staged. Ramp protocols are ideal for high-risk patients, as they provide less intense increments with stages no greater than 1 minute, aimed to have the patient achieve maximal effort in 8 to 12 minutes. In staged protocols, work increments can vary from 1 to 2.5 METs. The most used staged protocols are the Bruce, modified Bruce, Naughton, and modified Naughton (77).

Table 33-8 shows the most common protocols and the estimated metabolic requirements for each (79).

Exercise Testing Modalities

Different exercise testing modalities have different diagnostic, prognostic, and therapeutic applications, and the selection should be specific to each patient. Results should be interpreted in the context of the patient's clinical presentation and history of CVD. The following section will outline available exercise testing modalities and their indications.

TABLE 33-6	Borg Scale
15-Grade Scale	**Perceived Exertion**
6	No exertion at all
7	Extremely light
8	
9	Very light
10	
11	Fairly light
12	
13	Somewhat hard
14	
15	Hard (heavy)
16	
17	Very hard
18	
19	Extremely hard
20	Maximal exertion

Adapted with permission from Borg GA, Noble BJ. Perceived exertion. *Exerc Sport Sci Rev.* 1974;2(1):131–153, Ref. (78).

TABLE 33-7	Indications for Terminating Exercise Testing
Absolute Indications	• ST elevation on ECG (>1.0 mm) in leads without Q waves (other than V_1 or V_8) • Drop systolic blood pressure of >10 mm Hg (persistently bellow baseline) despite an increase in workload, when accompanied by evidence of ischemia • Moderated to severe angina • Central nervous system symptoms (e.g., ataxia, dizziness, or near-syncope) • Signs of poor perfusion (cyanosis or pallor) • Sustained ventricular tachycardia • Technical difficulties monitoring the ECG or SBP • Patient request to stop • Development of bundle branch block that cannot be distinguished from ventricular tachycardia
Relative Indications	• ST or QRS changes on ECG such as excessive ST displacement (horizontal or downsloping of >2 mm) or marked axis shift • Drop in systolic blood pressure of >10 mm Hg (persistently below baseline) despite an increase in workload, in the absence of other evidence of ischemia • Increasing chest pain • Fatigue, shortness of breath, wheezing, leg cramps, or severe claudication • Dysrhythmias other than sustained ventricular tachycardia, including frequent multifocal ectopic beats including ventricular pairs, supraventricular tachycardia, heart block, or bradyarrhythmias

ECG, electrocardiogram; SBP, systolic blood pressure; mm Hg, millimeters of mercury.
Adapted from Gibbons RJ, Balady GJ, Bricker JT, et al. ACC/AHA 2002 guideline update for exercise testing: summary article. A report of the American College of Cardiology/American Heart Association Task Force on Practice Guidelines (Committee to Update the 1997 Exercise Testing Guidelines). *J Am Coll Cardiol.* 2002;40(8):1531–1540.

Exercise ECG Testing

Exercise ECG testing is indicated in those patients who can exercise and provides useful information regarding exercise capacity, BP response to exercise, HR recovery (normal defined as an HR drop >13 bpm in the first minute of recovery), maximal predicted HR, and presence of ventricular ectopy while in the first minute of recovery, all predictors of future cardiovascular events including fatal MI (34,80). Exercise ECG testing should not be used as a single diagnostic tool as it cannot identify the distribution or extent of myocardial ischemia, which can significantly influence patient management decisions. In addition, its utility is limited in patients with resting ECG abnormalities (ST segment depression, left ventricular hypertrophy, left bundle branch block [LBBB], ventricular paced rhythms), valvular heart disease, and previous revascularization and those taking digoxin.

Cardiopulmonary Exercise Testing

Cardiopulmonary exercise testing (CPX) provides a dynamic summary of both submaximal and peak exercise responses involving the pulmonary, cardiovascular, neuropsychological, hematopoietic, and skeletal muscle systems (6,34,77). CPX is increasingly being used in a wide spectrum of clinical

applications and is most valuable in patients with ECG abnormalities that limit the evaluation of heart rate response to exercise and when evaluating patients with exercise intolerance. In the CR setting, CPX is considered the standard of care to define functional capacity and exercise impairment (81).

In addition to ECG recording and pulse oximetry (to determine arterial O_2 saturation), the global cardiorespiratory capacity is assessed through respiratory and ventilatory measures obtained during the CPX, including:

1. *Oxygen uptake (VO₂)*: represents the amount of oxygen (O_2) consumed during exercised and is a noninvasive analog for cardiac output (CO). VO_2 equals CO (stroke volume × HR) times the arterial minus mixed venous oxygen content:

$$VO_2 = CO \times (Cao_2 - Cvo_2)$$

2. *VO₂max*: defined as the maximal amount of oxygen that the body can use during maximal exercise and expressed in terms of mL of O_2 per kilogram of body weight per minute (mL/kg/min) (81). VO_{2max} is an indication of cardiac function, and it is considered a reliable and objective measurement of functional aerobic capacity in those that can achieve maximal effort. The VO_{2max} response to exercise is linear until maximal VO_2 is achieved. VO_2 plateau occurs at near maximal exercise and has traditionally been used as the best evidence of VO_{2max}. However, in clinical testing, a clear plateau may not be achieved before symptom limitation of exercise. Consequently, peak VO_2 (PVO_2) is often used as an estimate of VO_{2max} (81).

3. *Carbon dioxide output (VCO₂)*: represents the amount of carbon dioxide (CO_2) produced during respiration metabolism. VCO_2 is used to calculate the following:

   a. *Respiratory exchange ratio (RER)*: is the ratio of carbon dioxide production to oxygen consumption (VCO_2/VO_2) and expresses the source of substrates being used by the cells for the production of ATP. A normal range for RER at rest and during low-intensity exercise is 0.7 to 1.0 (82). Empirically, it has been determined that exercising to an RER greater than 1.15 is necessary for achievement of VO_{2max} during CPX (82).

   b. *Ventilatory efficiency to VCO₂ ratio (VE/VCO₂)*: is the relation between minute ventilation and the rate of CO_2 production, which provides useful diagnostic and prognostic superiority over VO_{2max} when patients are not able to achieve a maximal effort during CPX (83). A value of less than 35 is considered normal for adults without heart or lung disease. However, restrictive lung disease will increase the VE/VCO₂ ratio (83).

Interpretation of the CPX can be complex, but analysis of CPX data combined with patient clinical presentation allows for the evaluation and identification of causes for decreased exercise capacity (i.e., pulmonary abnormalities, poor effort, poor fitness, or poor cardiac function) (77,81). **Table 33-9** is a guide to the interpretation of exercise parameters obtained from CPX.

Exercise Stress Echocardiography

Exercise stress echocardiography is indicated to augment or supplement conventional exercise testing when ECG abnormalities are present at baseline. For this test, patients are required to lie down on their left side upon completion of an exercise

TABLE 33-8 Summary of Common Exercise Testing Protocols

METS	Cycle Ergometer For 70 kg Body Weight 1 Watt = 6.1 kpm/min	Ramp per 30 s		Modified Bruce 3-min Stages		Bruce 3-min Stages		Naughton 2-min Stages		Modified Naughton 2-min Stages	
		MPH	%GR	MPH	%GR	MPH	%GR	MPH	%GR	MPH	%GR
21											
20				6.0	22	6.0	22				
19											
18				5.5	20	5.5	20				
17											
16				5.0	18	5.0	18				
15										3.0	25
14	1,500										
13										3.0	22.5
	1,350										
		3.0	25.0	4.2	16	4.2	16			3.0	20
		3.0	24.0								
12		3.0	23.0								
		3.0	22.0							3.0	17.5
11	1,200	3.0	21.0								
		3.0	20.0								
		3.0	19.0	3.4	14	3.4	14			3.0	15
10	1,050	3.0	18.0								
9		3.0	17.0					2	17.5		
		3.0	16.0							3.0	12.5
	900	3.0	15.0					2	14.0		
8		3.0	14.0								
		3.0	13.0							3.0	10
	750	3.0	12.0	2.5	12	2.5	12				
7		3.0	11.0								
		3.0	10.0							3.0	7.5
	600	3.0	9.0								
6		3.0	8.0								
		3.0	7.0	1.7	10	1.7	10			2.0	10.5
5	450	3.0	6.0					2	10.5		
4	300	3.0	5.0					2	7.3		
		3.0	4.0							2.0	7.0
3		3.0	3.0	1.7	5			2	3.5		
	150	3.0	2.0	1.7	0			2	0		
		3.0	1.0							2.0	3.5
2		3.0	0					1	0		
		2.5	0								
		2.0	0							1.5	0
		1.5	0							1.0	0
		0.5	0								
1											

Common treadmill and stationary cycle ergometer protocols used in symptom-limited exercise testing with exercise workload and metabolic demand.

MET, metabolic equivalent; MPH, miles per hour; %GR, percent grade; kpm/min, kilopond meter/minute; kg, kilogram.

Adapted with permission from Fletcher GF, Ades PA, Kligfield P, et al. Exercise standards for testing and training: a scientific statement from the American Heart Association. *Circulation.* 2013;128(8):873–934.

test, by either treadmill or cycle ergometer. Echocardiography is then performed, and information on the possible distribution and extent of myocardial ischemia, chamber size, global and regional function, valvular integrity, and ejection fraction is obtained. Test interpretation is restricted when regional wall motion abnormalities exist at rest. Body habitus and pulmonary disease limit image query as well.

Exercise Myocardial Perfusion Imaging

Exercise myocardial perfusion imaging test employed isotopes, such as technetium (Tc)-99m or (thallium) chloride-20, that are delivered to the myocardium proportionally to the coronary blood flow (84). These tests evaluate the severity of myocardial ischemia, global ventricular size, function, and regional wall motion abnormalities. Exercise myocardial perfusion

TABLE 33-9	**Interpretation of the Cardiopulmonary Exercise Test According to Selected Exercise Parameters**				
	Normal	**Cardiac Limited**	**Lung Limited**	**Poor Fitness**	**Poor Effort**
O$_2$ saturation	>90%	Normal or Reduced	<90%	>90%	>90%
RER	>1.15	>1.15	<1.15	>1.15	<1.15
VO$_{2max}$	Normal	Low	Low	Low	Low
	Rise	Flat	Rise	Rise	Rise
VE/VCO$_2$	<35	Normal or high	High	Normal	Normal

O$_2$, oxygen; RER, respiratory exchange ratio; VO$_{2max}$, maximal oxygen uptake; VE/VCO$_2$, slope of ventilatory efficiency to carbon dioxide output.

imaging is indicated in those with an abnormal baseline ECG and resting wall motion abnormalities. It has been validated for both the detection and assessment of prognosis of CAD, with widely reproducible results (84).

Pharmacologic Stress Testing

The vasodilators adenosine, dipyridamole, regadenoson, and dobutamine are used to induce pharmacologic stress on the heart by increasing coronary vasodilation that results in increased flow in normal vessels with limited response in stenotic arteries, resulting in perfusion defects that are evident in nuclear scans. Pharmacologic stress tests are indicated in patients with CAD that are unable to exercise and/or those with LBBB or ventricular paced rhythms (84).

Alternate Measures of Physical Status Assessment

The 6-MWT is a simple, effective, and valid submaximal exercise test used to quantify the functional exercise capacity and exercise tolerance in patients deconditioned or with already known decreased functional capacity who are unable to give maximal effort in stress tests (such as patients with HF). Additionally, clinical questionnaires (i.e., the Duke Activity Status Index) (85) can be used to obtain rough estimates of exercise tolerance using MET activity tables (86).

PHYSICAL ACTIVITY AND EXERCISE PRESCRIPTION (SEE CHAPTER 49)

Of all the established risk factors, low aerobic exercise capacity appears to be the strongest predictor of mortality (87). Based on the cumulative body of evidence, it is clear that the relationship of CVDs and levels of physical activity are inverse, graded, and, most importantly, modifiable (87,88). It has been shown that for each MET increase in aerobic capacity, there is a reduction in cardiovascular events of up to 20% to 25% (87). Therefore, increased levels of physical activity, exercise training, and overall cardiorespiratory fitness have positive effect on primary and secondary prevention of CAD (88).

A baseline assessment is obtained to effectively dose the exercise prescription as well as to identify contraindications or potential limitations to exercise training. The International Physical Activity Questionnaire (IPAQ) is a suitable tool to standardize physical activity assessment (89). This tool quantifies duration, frequency, and intensity of the activity and also provides information regarding total sitting time (89).

For patients participating in early/late outpatient CR programs, exercise activities are closely monitored (heart rate, blood pressure, and ECG), and the exercise modality, intensity, and duration are set based on individual aerobic capacity and comorbidities.

A complete exercise program includes aerobic conditioning, activities to increase muscular health and endurance, flexibility exercises, and balance training.

Cardiorespiratory Endurance Training Exercises

Cardiorespiratory endurance training (aerobic conditioning exercises) is the foundation of all exercise routine for patients with CVD. The elements of an exercise prescription for endurance training include exercise modality, intensity, frequency, and duration. Initial exercise selection should be based on the individual fitness level, personal goals, and preferences (must be fun!), as well as pre-existing medical conditions, for example, musculoskeletal disorders (90). Jogging and running are very effective in increasing fitness and decreasing overall cardiovascular risk in patients with high fitness levels. On the other hand, walking represents a moderate-intensity exercise more appropriate for the elderly patients with low fitness levels and those who did not previously exercise. Other common modes of aerobic conditioning include cycling, swimming, rowing, stair climbing, elliptical, and treadmill use.

Intensity. Results of several studies have shown that exercise intensity is more important than duration to prevent CVD and mortality (91). Many approaches can be used to set the aerobic exercise intensity, but the accurate ones use data obtained from cardiopulmonary stress testing.

Heart rate reserve (HRR) uses the resting and peak heart rate obtained during the cardiopulmonary stress test to prescribe intensity of aerobic conditioning (target heart rate). In this method, HHR is obtained by subtracting resting heart rate from the maximal heart rate obtained during the stress. A percent of HRR (between 45% and 80%) is calculated and added to the resting heart rate to finally obtain the target heart rate.

Example:
1. If peak heart rate is 150 and resting heart rate is 70:
   HRR = 150 − 70 = **80**
2. A target of 60% of HHR is defined:
   80 × 0.6 = 48
3. Add resting heart rate to provide target heart rate:
   48 + 70 = 118
   TARGET HEART RATE = 118
   The above calculation can be summarized in the Karvonen formula (92):
   (HRR × % desired target) + resting heart rate = target heart rate

The visual analogue Borg scale rates of perceived exertion are another widely used method to prescribe intensity of the exercise when the stress test is not available, as it has been shown to display a linear correlation with heart rate and oxygen consumption (78). Borg scale indicates the self-assessed level of exertion and takes into account all sensations of exertion, physical stress, and fatigue (**Table 33-7**) (78). A level of 12 to 14 (somewhat difficult to reach) is recommended as a target (5,6). For patients taking beta-blockers, Borg scale rates of perceived exertion are a good method for heart rate monitoring, as the heart rate response is somehow blunted (78).

Frequency and duration. Twenty to thirty continuous minutes of exercise per CR session is commonly recommended when starting the program. Regardless of the total duration of the aerobic exercise, each session should include a 5-minute warm-up period of light exercise to decrease the risk of musculoskeletal or cardiovascular complications, followed by conditioning exercise at the desired intensity level, and finishing with a cooldown period of approximately 5 minutes to return heart rate and blood pressure to near pre-exercise values and to allow heat dissipation and removal of lactic acid. Depending on the individual aerobic capacity and comorbidities, the duration of exercise can vary. For severely deconditioned individuals that cannot tolerate 20 to 30 minutes of continuous exercise, accumulated multiple bouts of activities as short as 10 minutes in duration can produce similar benefits (5,6).

In CR programs, moderate-intensity continuous training (MCT) has been the gold standard for patients with cardiac disease. Recently, high-intensity interval training (HIIT) has emerged as an alternative, more effective exercise training (93). HIIT is defined as an exercise program that alternates brief periods of high-intensity aerobic exercise (near maximal capacity, e.g., >85% VO_{2max}) followed by intervals of low-intensity exercise (or rest period). Different HIIT protocols (intensity, stage duration, nature of the recovery, number of intervals) have been tested and used for CVD patients. HIIT can be introduced in CR programs when the patient is able to perform at least 20 minutes of continuous exercise at the target intensity. In general, three different categories of HIIT have been described in patients participating in CR programs including (a) short intervals of 10 seconds to 1 minute at 100% to 120% VO_{2max}, (b) medium intervals of 1 to 3 minutes at 95% to 100% VO_{2max}, and (c) long intervals of 3 to 15 minutes at 85% to 90% VO_{2max} (94). In general, the recommendations are for patients to start with 2 to 3 intervals of 30 to 60 seconds at RPE 15 to 17 interspersed with 1 to 5 minutes of moderate-intensity RPE 11 to 12 and then progress to 5 intervals of 1 to 2 minutes at RPE 15 to 17 during 30 to 45 minutes of training. HIIT can be performed with different exercise modes such as cycling, running, walking with inclination, rowing, swimming, or other activities (94). HIIT should be performed only during CR supervised sessions (94). HIIT in this setting elicits a greater training stimulus and results in greater improvements when compared with moderate exercise alone (93,94).

All recommended components for cardiorespiratory endurance exercises are summarized in **Table 33-10**.

Resistance/Strengthening Exercises

For appropriately screened patients, resistance training should be incorporated into the exercise program. Increases in subendocardial perfusion and attenuation of ischemic responses, as well as lower myocardial demand, are observed

TABLE 33-10	Components of the Exercise Prescription for Cardiorespiratory Endurance
Component	**Recommendation**
Intensity	• 40%–80% of HRR or VO_{2max} if maximal exercise data are available • RPE of 11–16 as adjunct to objective measure of HR • 10 bpm below HR associated with any of the following criteria: 　◦ The onset of angina or other symptoms of cardiovascular insufficiency 　◦ Plateau or ↓SBP; SBP > 240 mm Hg: DBP > 110 mm Hg 　◦ >2 mm ST depression, horizontal or downsloping 　◦ Radionuclide evidence of reversible myocardial ischemia or echocardiographic evidence of moderate to severe wall motion abnormalities during exertion 　◦ ↑ frequency of ventricular dysrhythmias 　◦ Other significant ECG disturbances (e.g., second- or third-degree AVB, atrial fibrillation, SVT, complex ventricular ectopy) 　◦ Other signs or symptoms of exertional intolerance
Duration	• 20–60 min per session • Longer durations of multiple sessions accumulating throughout the day are recommended to enhance total energy expenditure for weight reduction
Frequency	• Ideally, most days of the week (4–7 days/week)
Type	• Rhythmic, larger muscle group activities (i.e., walking, cycling, stair climbing, elliptical trainers, and other arm or leg ergometers that allow controlled movement and consistent intensity)

HRR, heart rate reserve; VO_{2max}, maximal oxygen uptake; RPE, rating of perceived exertion; SBP, systolic blood pressure; DBP, diastolic blood pressure, ECG, electrocardiogram; AVB, atrioventricular block; SVT, supraventricular tachycardia. Derived from Pescatello LS, American College of Sports Medicine. *ACSM's Guidelines for Exercise Testing and Prescription.* 9th ed. Philadelphia, PA: Wolters Kluwer Health/Lippincott Williams & Wilkins; 2013.

in patients performing resistance exercise training (95). Other established benefits include preservation of muscle mass, muscle strength, and endurance; improved bone density; increase in lean body mass and basal metabolism; improved glucose tolerance and insulin sensitivity as well as lipid profile; attenuated loss of skeletal muscle mass (size/number) present in aging (sarcopenia); decreased insomnia and depression; improved balance, coordination, and agility; and decrease in falls and prolonged functional independence in older patients (95).

The intensity of resistance exercise is prescribed relative to the one repetition performed at maximal weight (1 RM). Thirty to sixty percent of 1 RM can be used for initial training (94). Precautions to avoid uncontrolled elevations of blood pressure due to Valsalva are necessary. Patients already participating in an exercise routine can start with a 1 RM of 50%. If 1 RM data are not available, at perceived exertion (Borg scale), 11 to 13 is used (78). Patients with low performance or older patients should start with a 1 RM of less than 30% (95,96). If 1 RM is not available, light weight should be used with a gradual increase of load over time. General recommendations include 1 to 3 sets of 8 to 15 slow repetitions to result in volitional fatigue of the major muscle groups in the upper and lower extremities. Exercises are performed with a frequency of 2 to 3 times a week with at least 48 hours of resting time between sessions to allow muscle recovery (96). Precautions include avoiding isometric exercises in hypertensive patients and upper extremity exercises involving chest wall muscles in surgical patients. Heart failure patient's class I-II can perform resistance exercises with close supervision. Absolute contraindications for resistance training include Marfan syndrome and severe symptomatic aortic stenosis (95,96).

A summary of all elements of a strengthening exercise prescription is given in **Table 33-11**.

Flexibility/Stretching Exercises

The optimal musculoskeletal function requires that a patient maintain an adequate ROM in all joints. Therefore, a preventive and rehabilitative exercise program should include activities that promote the maintenance of flexibility. Stretching exercises help to improve circulation and relaxation, relieve stress, improve posture and coordination, and reduce the risk of musculoskeletal injuries (97). Flexibility/stretching exercises could

be performed during warm-up or cooldown period on a daily basis. Stretching should be held (pain-free) for at least 30 seconds and up to a minute. A minimum of three repetitions for each muscle group is recommended. As with endurance and strengthening exercises, the prescriptive elements of a flexibility program are individualized to the needs and goals of the patient.

Components of an exercise prescription for flexibility are summarized in **Table 33-12**.

Balance Exercises

Balance is dependent on sensory input (touch and pressure sensation on the plantar surface, joint position sense, visual acuity, visual edge detection, and vestibular input), central processing (brain, cerebellum), motor control, and muscle strength, all of which are affected by aging (97). Frailty, a geriatric syndrome that includes abnormalities in multiple areas, such as cognition, nutrition, mobility, motor processing, strength, endurance, physical activity, and balance, has been a causative and prognostic factor in patients with CVD (96,98). Poor balance in frail patients is associated with increased risk of falls (98), which may lead to bodily injury, loss of independence, chronic illness, and early mortality (99).

Significant improvements in balance have been previously reported after exercise interventions (99). All patients with CVD can benefit from balance exercises including single stance (hard surface, pillows, foam, wobble board, or shifting weight to 1 foot), tandem gait, walking on toes and heels, walking backward, walking sideways, and walking making a figure-of-8 pattern (99).

Tai chi is an effective intervention to improve balance, as it has been shown to be safe for all ages and fitness condition and, more important, has a positive effect on many cardiovascular risk factors, including stress, blood pressure, anxiety, and depression (100). Tai chi improves strength of muscles, balance, flexibility, coordination, energy, stamina, and agility, reducing risk for falls and improving physical functioning, feelings of well-being, and quality of life (99,100).

Once the initial exercise prescription has been established, patients should progress gradually toward predefined goals based on their CVD risk profile, training goals, and comorbidities. More structured programs are often designed with a frequency of three to four sessions per week; therefore, patients will need to engage in physical activity outside the structured

TABLE 33-11	Components of an Exercise Prescription for Muscular Strength and Endurance
Component	**Recommendation**
Intensity	• Resistance that allows approximately 10–15 repetitions
	• REP of 11–13 on Borg 6–20 scale
	• Complete movement through a full range of motion as possible, avoiding breath holding and Valsalva's maneuvers, by exhaling during the exertion phase of the motion and inhaling during the recovery phase
	• Maintaining a secure but no overly tight grip on the weight handles or bar to prevent an excessive BP response
	• RPP should not exceed that identified as threshold for CRE exercise
Volume	• Minimum of one set per exercise
	• May increase to two or three sets one accustomed to the regimen and, if greater gains are desired, approximately 8–10 different exercises using all major muscle groups of the upper and lower body; chest press, shoulder press, triceps extension, bicep curls, lat pulldown, lower back extension, abdominal crunch or curl up, quadriceps extension, leg curls (hamstrings), and calf raise
Frequency	• 2 or 3 nonconsecutive days/week
Type	• Variable: free weights, weight machines, resistance bands, pulley weights, dumbbells, light wrist or ankle weights
	• Select equipment that is safe, effective, and accessible
Progression	• Training loads may be increased approximately 5% when the patient can comfortably achieve the upper limit of the prescribed repetition range

RPE, rating of perceived exertion; BP, blood pressure; RPP, heart rate times systolic blood pressure product; CRE, cardiorespiratory endurance.
Derived from Pescatello LS, American College of Sports Medicine. *ACSM's Guidelines for Exercise Testing and Prescription.* 9th ed. Philadelphia, PA: Wolters Kluwer Health/Lippincott Williams & Wilkins; 2013, Ref. (77).

TABLE 33-12	Components of an Exercise Prescription for Musculoskeletal Flexibility
Component	**Recommendation**
Intensity	• Hold to a position of mild discomfort (not pain)
	• Exercises should be performed in a slow, controlled manner, with a gradual progression to greater ranges of motion
Duration	• Gradually increase to 30 seconds, then as tolerable to 90 seconds for each stretch, breathing normally
	• Three to five repetitions for each exercise
Frequency	• 2 or 3 nonconsecutive days/week
Type	• Static, with a major emphasis on the lower back and thigh regions

Derived from Pescatello LS, American College of Sports Medicine. *ACSM's Guidelines for Exercise Testing and Prescription.* 9th ed. Philadelphia, PA: Wolters Kluwer Health/Lippincott Williams & Wilkins; 2013, Ref. (77).

CR program to achieve the optimal/desired levels of activity. The overall goal is to exercise more than 150 min/wk of moderate activity or 75 min/wk of vigorous activity.

Figure 33-2 provides an example of a comprehensive exercise prescription.

PRACTICE CONSIDERATIONS IN SPECIAL POPULATIONS

CR delivers individualized programs of exercise and risk factor control according to the problems and needs that each cardiac patient brings to the rehabilitation program. In order to maximize patient safety and outcomes, it is imperative to recognize in unique populations and individuals specific medical and psychosocial issues that could potentially affect participation and effective deliverance of CR programs. For example, in women, symptoms of myocardial ischemia are more atypical, and CAD risk factors are more prevalent than in men (101). In addition, women are twice as likely as men to have poor outcomes after CABG and MI (101).

Elderly

In older patients, high disability rates due to multiple factors beyond the CAD, such as COPD, frailty, diabetes, arthritis, depression, and cognitive impairments, are markedly present (102). Therefore, the baseline evaluation of these patients prior to entering the program includes cognitive status assessment, gait, balance, mobility, activities of daily living, hearing, and sight (5–7,102). Severely deconditioned older patients that are unable to perform exercise stress test may need submaximal evaluations such as 6-MWT to assess their functional status. Other important physiologic and epidemiologic issues are important to consider.

Revascularization and Valve Repair/Replacement

Traditional CABG and valve surgery need sternotomy. Therefore, precaution for upper extremity exercise and sternal healing are considered and CR team should assess for wound healing on a periodic basis. Postsurgical patients should not be engaged in upper extremity resistance exercise for 5 weeks following the surgery. Moreover, resistance exercise should be

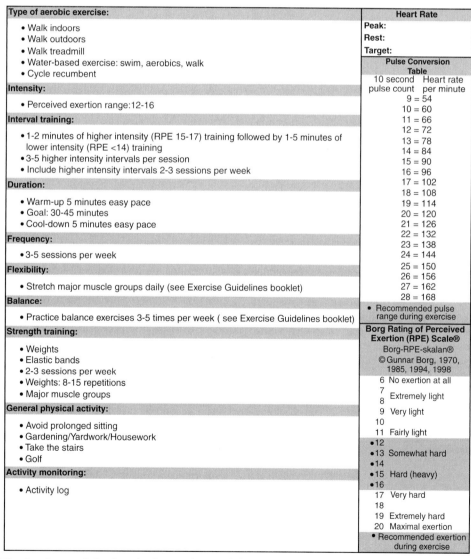

FIGURE 33-2. Exercise prescription. Example of an exercise prescription for aerobic, strengthening, flexibility, and balance exercise, including the recommended intensity, duration, and frequency of all exercise components.

preceded by at least 4 weeks of regular participation in the CR program (5–7,97).

Dysrhythmias, including atrial fibrillation, are not uncommon within the first several days after open heart surgery. Pleural and pericardial effusion related to postoperative inflammation may occur during outpatient CR and can be detected by evidence of decreasing exercise capacity, chest discomfort, and increasing dyspnea (72). It is important to know whether the revascularization was complete or incomplete. Complete revascularization (patent CABG of all significant atherosclerotic lesions) should alleviate all associated sign and symptoms of ischemia, while partial revascularization increases the likelihood of postsurgical signs and symptoms of residual myocardial ischemia during exercise (5–7).

The exercise prescription and training of patient following valve surgery are similar to those for CABG patients. However, some patients may have low functional capacity as they have been inactive for a long period of time prior to surgery. Therefore, they need to start and progress more slowly during the early stages of CR program (5–7). Valve surgery can also be performed either through a catheter-based procedure, and in this case, patients may be able to progress more rapidly during the program. Management of postsurgical anticoagulation is also important in patients with prosthetic valves (5–7).

Dysrhythmias, Pacemakers, Implantable Cardioverter-Defibrillators

Although cardiac dysrhythmias are not uncommon in CR participants, the majority of them are not life threatening. The most common benign ones are premature atrial complexes, premature ventricular complexes, atrial fibrillation or flutter, paroxysmal supraventricular tachycardia, mild bradycardia, first-degree AV block, and asymptomatic type I second-degree AV block (5–7). Potentially malignant dysrhythmias include atrial fibrillation or flutter with rapid response, symptomatic or severe bradycardia, symptomatic AV block, ventricular tachycardia, and ventricular fibrillation (10). Factors that can be associated with dysrhythmias are exercise intensity, autonomic nervous system variability, medications, electrolyte imbalance, and dehydration (24).

The physiologic response to exercise for patients with pacemakers can be essentially the same as for other patients. Evidence suggests that exercise training in patients with implantable cardioverter-defibrillator (ICD) and pacemakers is safe (24). However, patients with ICD often required more formal and prolonged ECG-supervised exercise programs. Details about pacemaker or ICD, rates, detection parameters, and algorithms should be obtained prior to participation in CR. Exercise testing is useful to perform in these patients to guide the adjustment of the pacemaker settings to ensure appropriated rate responses.

Heart Failure

Early initiation of exercise therapy in patients with compensated HF has been reported to improve exercise capacity, functional status, and quality of life (103). Individually tailored and medically guided program with low-level intensity training programs should be advocated as part of their lifestyle (103). The largest randomized controlled trial in HF (HF-ACTION) (104) demonstrated that exercise was safe for patients with advanced HF (ejection fraction [EF] <25%) and patients who were randomized to supervised exercise sessions exhibited a moderate reduction in cardiac and overall mortality, with significant improvements in the cardiopulmonary stress test, functional capacity, and quality of life (104). As patients with HF are at high risk for arrhythmias and decompensation, ECG monitoring during the entire CR program is strongly recommended.

In HF patients, continuous aerobic training is performed by using either a cycle or treadmill. Intensity as low as 40% of VO_{2max} has been effective in improving exercise capacity in patients with HF, and intensities of 50% to 60% of VO_{2max} have been shown to be safe (105). Aerobic sessions of short duration, 15 minutes, for example, are recommended at the beginning of the training program, specifically in patients with lower exercise capacity and who are deconditioned. Duration of exercise should be progressed according to a patient's tolerance, with the goal to reach duration of at least 30 minutes (105). For monitoring exercise intensity, the target heart rate may be used as well. However, if patients have severely reduced exercise capacity, chronotropic incompetence, or atrial fibrillation or are taking medications that affect heart rate, the Borg scale is more appropriate (see **Table 33-7**). Interval training has recently been studied in patients with HF and was also shown to be safe and beneficial (106).

Muscular atrophy is the hallmark of patients with CHF (107), and, although limited, there is growing evidence of the positive effects of resistance training related to the improvement of muscle function and quality of life in patients with HF (95). No adverse events have been reported in patients with New York Heart Association class I-II-III HF, and partial data exist regarding patients with New York Heart Association class IV (103). General recommendations include the use of small free weights (0.5 to 3 kg, 8 to 10 repetitions) or elastic bands and avoiding isometric high-resistance exercises.

Left Ventricular Assist Devices

As the need for donors increased, LVAD has become a standard therapeutic option for patients with severe HF, either as a bridge to transplant or as a destination therapy for those who are poor transplant candidates (103–105). LVAD provides hemodynamic support to organs and reverses the pathophysiologic sequelae of HF by helping the left ventricle with its pumping function. In appropriately selected advanced HF patients, treatment with LVAD is associated with significant improvements in physical function and quality of life (108).

Exercise training for LVAD patient as part of a CR program is effective and safe (108). Recent studies have demonstrated that CR following LVAD implantation is associated with no risk and greater improvement in functional capacity (109,110).

Although general considerations for LVAD patients participating in CR are similar to those of HF, some issues are important to consider. LVAD rate can increase automatically as the device senses the volume of blood in the pump chamber. Exercise is contraindicated if mean arterial pressure is less than 70 mm Hg, if the device alarm is activated, or if the patient exhibit intolerance to the workload. Due to the pulsatile flow of blood in the newer LVAD models, it will be difficult to assess blood pressure during the exercise sessions, requiring measuring it *via* Doppler ultrasound (5,6).

As in HF patients, peripheral factors might continue to limit physical function in LVAD recipients. Skeletal muscle weakness, as a marker of frailty, has been associated with an increased risk of poor clinical outcomes following LVAD implantation (111). Although the safety and efficacy of resistance training in LVAD patients have not been fully studied, recent studies have shown that resistance training is safe and is recommended (95).

Heart Transplant

Patients with heart transplants do not have intact pericardium, and they present with diastolic dysfunction, endothelial dysfunction with subsequent impaired peripheral, coronary vasodilatory capacity, and mildly elevated blood pressure (112). In addition, patients post heart transplant have decreased exercise capacity due to deconditioning, abnormal skeletal muscle structure and function, and muscle weakness (103,113). Exercises initiated as early as possible at an intensity of 50% of VO_{2max} or preferably by using an RPE (level of 12), for 20 to 30 min/d, have been shown to be beneficial for patients with heart transplant, increasing their exercise capacity between 18% and 30% (114).

The patient's transplanted heart loses parasympathetic innervation; therefore, the response to acute exercise is unique and needs to be carefully considered. First, the resting heart rate is elevated to 95 to 115 beats/min and does not increase during the first several minutes of exercise (115). Second, peak heart rate is lower than normal, and the highest exercise rate is achieved during the first few minutes of recovery from exercising and may remain high for a few minutes before returning to resting level (112). Due to the abnormal heart responses, the RPE is more useful when prescribing exercise intensity in patients with a heart transplant (115). Some patients can demonstrate partial reinnervation several months after transplantation (115). Although graded exercise testing is helpful in determining exercise capacity and prescribing exercise, it is best to wait 6 to 8 weeks after transplantation before performing a maximal exercise test.

Most patients may present with muscle atrophy, myopathies, osteopenia, or osteoporosis due to immunosuppression. Strengthening exercises partially reverse these adverse effects by improving muscle strength and positively change bone density (113). For the first week after surgery, bilateral arm lifting is restricted to avoid sternal dehiscence. After 6 to 8 weeks, patients may start a moderate resistance, 1 to 3 sets of exercises, 10 to 20 repetitions per set, 2 to 3 times per week by using the major muscle groups. The intensity of 50% 1 RM or with RPE of 12 to 14 is recommended (115).

ACCESS TO CARDIAC REHABILITATION

Despite solid evidence demonstrating the benefits of CR program, (40,42–44,47,74) participation remains low, ranging from 20% to 50% worldwide (35,116). Only 14% to 35% of eligible MI survivors and 31% of patients after coronary bypass surgery participate in a CR program (117). It is lowest for the elderly, African Americans, Hispanics, and women (118). The utilization rate for eligible Medicare beneficiaries is even lower at 12% (102).

Several barriers have been identified for CR participation, including lack of provider's awareness and enthusiasm to refer patients, lack of resources and space, and program availability (119,120). Adherence to CR programs is also affected by factors such as psychological well-being, geographical location, access to transport, limited health insurance coverage, and conflict with work and home responsibilities (121,122). Regrettably, the biggest predictor of participation and adherence is clinician promotion and referral (123).

The Centers for Medicare and Medicaid Services (CMS) guidelines cover standard CR and ICR (under current CMS decision memo for CR programs). Patients with a diagnosis of chronic stable angina, MI, CABG, PCI, cardiac transplantation, cardiac valve surgery, stable HF, and peripheral vascular disease (PAD) are eligible for CR referral and reimbursement. Under standard or traditional CR, CMS covers 2 to 3 sessions per week for 12 to 18 weeks up to a total of 36 sessions (6,33). Coverage for ICR is limited to 72 1-hour sessions (up to 6 sessions per week) for up to 18 weeks (124). Only three types of ICR have been approved by CMS: Dr. Dean Ornish's Program for Reversing Heart Disease, Pritikin ICR program, and Benson-Henry Institute for Cardiac Wellness Program (36). These programs are not commonly available. However, locations can be found by searching program websites (36).

To be eligible for coverage, both programs must include physician-prescribed exercise, cardiac risk factor modification, a psychosocial assessment, an outcome assessment, and individualized treatment plan reviewed and signed by a physician every 30 days. CMS may approve additional sessions, based on patient's medical necessity (6,33). Reimbursement under private insurer is also covered and varies significantly across policy and payers. The American Association for Cardiovascular and Pulmonary Rehabilitation (AACVPR) has made available an extensive array of toolkits for national and international medical professionals and administrators. These resources cover a variety of subjects including clinical management tools (with an updated section on PAD management in CR), practice guidelines, reimbursement resources, current legislative actions, marketing strategies, and others (125).

Home-based and tele-cardiac rehabilitation programs are options to overcome patient access limitations such as geographic, work schedule constraints, and transportation. These two models have been shown to provide comparable benefit to classic deliverable models (126–128). Outpatient CR program using virtual world technology may provide an effective alternative to conventional CR programs. However, these programs currently do not receive coverage by CMS guidelines.

SUMMARY

CR is a multidisciplinary and comprehensive program, considered the gold standard of care for patients after a cardiac event or cardiac procedure. It is the best and most well-established intervention for primary and secondary prevention and implementation of healthy lifestyle in the current health care model. CR after MI, CABG, PCI, cardiac transplantation, valve repair or replacement, and HF have reduced symptoms of dyspnea, slowed progression of CAD, decreased the number of recurrent events and hospitalization, reduced mortality, and improved risk factors (35). Patient referral and subsequent completion carry out several positive benefits that support the adoption and promotion of CR practice worldwide.

REFERENCES

1. Lavie CJ, Milani RV. Effects of cardiac rehabilitation, exercise training, and weight reduction on exercise capacity, coronary risk factors, behavioral characteristics, and quality of life in obese coronary patients. *Am J Cardiol*. 1997;79(4):397–401.

2. Rodriguez-Escudero JP, Somers VK, Heath AL, et al. Effect of a lifestyle therapy program using cardiac rehabilitation resources on metabolic syndrome components. *J Cardiopulm Rehabil Prev*. 2013;33(6):360–370.

3. Anderson L, Oldridge N, Thompson DR, et al. Exercise-based cardiac rehabilitation for coronary heart disease: cochrane systematic review and meta-analysis. *J Am Coll Cardiol*. 2016;67(1):1–12.

4. Gomadam PS, Douglas CJ, Sacrinty MT, et al. Degree and direction of change of body weight in cardiac rehabilitation and impact on exercise capacity and cardiac risk factors. *Am J Cardiol*. 2016;117(4):580–584.

5. Balady GJ, Williams MA, Ades PA, et al. Core components of cardiac rehabilitation/secondary prevention programs: 2007 update: a scientific statement from the American Heart Association Exercise, Cardiac Rehabilitation, and Prevention Committee, the Council on Clinical Cardiology; the Councils on Cardiovascular Nursing, Epidemiology and Prevention, and Nutrition, Physical Activity, and Metabolism; and the American Association of Cardiovascular and Pulmonary Rehabilitation. *Circulation*. 2007;115(20):2675–2682.

6. AACVPR. *Guidelines for Cardiac Rehabilitation and Secondary Prevention Programs*. 5th ed. Champaign, IL: Human Kinetics; 2013.

7. European Guidelines on cardiovascular disease prevention in clinical practice (version 2012): the Fifth Joint Task Force of the European Society of Cardiology and Other Societies on Cardiovascular Disease Prevention in Clinical Practice (constituted by representatives of nine societies and by invited experts). *Eur J Prev Cardiol*. 2012;19(4):585–667.

8. Moore KL. *Clinically Oriented Anatomy*. 7th ed. Baltimore, MD: Lippincott Williams & Wilkins; 2014.

9. Roth GA, Huffman MD, Moran AE, et al. Global and regional patterns in cardiovascular mortality from 1990 to 2013. *Circulation*. 2015;132(17):1667–1678.

10. Benjamin EJ, Blaha MJ, Chiuve SE, et al. Heart disease and stroke statistics—2017 update: a report from the American Heart Association. *Circulation*. 2017;135:e146–e603.

11. Eisen A, Giugliano RP, Braunwald E. Updates on acute coronary syndrome: a review. *JAMA Cardiol*. 2016;1(6):718–730.

12. Sharkey SW, Windenburg DC, Lesser JR, et al. Natural history and expansive clinical profile of stress (tako-tsubo) cardiomyopathy. *J Am Coll Cardiol*. 2010;55(4):333–341.

13. Bui AL, Horwich TB, Fonarow GC. Epidemiology and risk profile of heart failure. *Nat Rev Cardiol*. 2011;8(1):30–41.

14. Stecker EC, Reinier K, Marijon E, et al. Public health burden of sudden cardiac death in the United States. *Circ Arrhythm Electrophysiol*. 2014;7(2):212–217.

15. Smith SC, Benjamin EJ, Bonow RO, et al. AHA/ACCF secondary prevention and risk reduction therapy for patients with coronary and other atherosclerotic vascular disease: 2011 update: a guideline from the American Heart Association and American College of Cardiology Foundation. *Circulation*. 2011;124(22):2458–2473.

16. Bangalore S, Steg G, Deedwania P, et al. β-Blocker use and clinical outcomes in stable outpatients with and without coronary artery disease. *JAMA*. 2012;308(13):1340–1349.

17. Barnes GD, Kurtz B. Direct oral anticoagulants: unique properties and practical approaches to management. *Heart*. 2016;102(20):1620–1626.

18. Stone NJ, Robinson JG, Lichtenstein AH, et al. 2013 ACC/AHA guideline on the treatment of blood cholesterol to reduce atherosclerotic cardiovascular risk in adults: a report of the American College of Cardiology/American Heart Association Task Force on Practice Guidelines. *Circulation*. 2014;129(25 suppl 2):S1–S45.

19. Rosenson RS, Baker SK, Jacobson TA, et al. An assessment for the Statin Muscle Safety Task Force: 2014 update. *J Clin Lipidol*. 2014;8(3):S58–S71.

20. Everett BM, Smith RJ, Hiatt WR. Reducing LDL with PCSK9 inhibitors—the clinical benefit of lipid drugs. *N Engl J Med*. 2015;373(17):1588–1591.

21. Keeley EC, Hillis LD. Primary PCI for myocardial infarction with ST-segment elevation. *N Engl J Med*. 2007;356(1):47–54.

22. Yusuf S, Zucker D, Passamani E, et al. Effect of coronary artery bypass graft surgery on survival: overview of 10-year results from randomised trials by the Coronary Artery Bypass Graft Surgery Trialists Collaboration. *Lancet*. 1994;344(8922):563–570.

23. McMurray JJ, Adamopoulos S, Anker SD, et al. ESC guidelines for the diagnosis and treatment of acute and chronic heart failure 2012. *Eur J Heart Fail*. 2012;14(8):803–869.

24. Tracy CM, Epstein AE, Darbar D, et al. 2012 ACCF/AHA/HRS focused update incorporated into the ACCF/AHA/HRS 2008 guidelines for device-based therapy of cardiac rhythm abnormalities: a report of the American College of Cardiology Foundation/American Heart Association Task Force on Practice Guidelines and the Heart Rhythm Society. *J Am Coll Cardiol*. 2013;61(3):e6–e75.

25. Behfar A, Terzic A, Perez-Terzic CM. Regenerative principles enrich cardiac rehabilitation practice. *Am J Phys Med Rehabil*. 2014;93(11 suppl 3):S169–S175.

26. Fernandez-Aviles F, Sanz-Ruiz R, Climent AM, et al. Global position paper on cardiovascular regenerative medicine: scientific statement of the transnational alliance for regenerative therapies in cardiovascular syndromes (TACTICS) international group for the comprehensive cardiovascular application of regenerative medicinal products. *Eur Heart J*. 2017;38:2532–2546.

27. Morris JN, Crawford MD. Coronary heart disease and physical activity of work. *Br Med J*. 1958;2(5111):1485–1496.

28. Bethell HJ. Cardiac rehabilitation: from Hellerstein to the millennium. *Int J Clin Pract*. 2000;54(2):92–97.

29. Rehabilitation after cardiovascular diseases, with special emphasis on developing countries. Report of a WHO expert committee. *World Health Organ Tech Rep Ser*. 1993;831:1–122.

30. Shumway-Cook A, Brauer S, Woollacott M. Predicting the probability for falls in community-dwelling older adults using the Timed Up & Go Test. *Phys Ther*. 2000;80(9):896–903.

31. ATS Committee on Proficiency Standards for Clinical Pulmonary Function Laboratories. ATS statement: guidelines for the six-minute walk test. *Am J Respir Crit Care Med*. 2002;166(1):111–117.

32. de Macedo RM, Faria-Neto JR, Costantini CO, et al. Phase I of cardiac rehabilitation: a new challenge for evidence based physiotherapy. *World J Cardiol*. 2011;3(7):248–255.

33. Decision Memo for Supervised Exercise Therapy (SET) for Symptomatic Peripheral Artery Disease. Available from: https://www.cms.gov/medicare-coverage-database/details/nca-decision-memo.aspx?NCAId=287&NcaName=Supervised+Exercise+Therapy+%28SET%29+for+Symptomatic+Peripheral+Artery+Disease+%28PAD%29&ExpandComments=y&CommentPeriod=0&bc=gCAAAAAACAAAAA%3D%3D. Accessed 08/01/2017.

34. Gibbons RJ, Balady GJ, Bricker JT, et al. ACC/AHA 2002 guideline update for exercise testing: summary article: a report of the American College of Cardiology/American Heart Association Task Force on Practice Guidelines (Committee to Update the 1997 Exercise Testing Guidelines). *J Am Coll Cardiol*. 2002;40(8):1531–1540.

35. Dalal HM, Doherty P, Taylor RS. Cardiac rehabilitation. *BMJ*. 2015;351:h5000.

36. Centers for Medicare & Medicaid Services. Intensive Cardiac Rehabilitation (ICR) Programs. Available from: https://www.cms.gov/Medicare/Medicare-General-Information/MedicareApprovedFacilitie/ICR.html

37. Lavie CJ, Milani RV. Benefits of cardiac rehabilitation and exercise training. *Chest*. 2000;117(1):5–7.

38. Sadeghi M, Salehi-Abargouei A, Kasaei Z, et al. Effect of cardiac rehabilitation on metabolic syndrome and its components: a systematic review and meta-analysis. *J Res Med Sci*. 2016;21:18.

39. Lavie CJ, Arena R, Swift DL, et al. Exercise and the cardiovascular system. *Clin Sci Cardiovasc Outcomes*. 2015;117(2):207–219.

40. Goel K, Lennon RJ, Tilbury RT, et al. Impact of cardiac rehabilitation on mortality and cardiovascular events after percutaneous coronary intervention in the community. *Circulation*. 2011;123(21):2344–2352.

41. Milani RV, Lavie CJ, Mehra MR, et al. Impact of exercise training and depression on survival in heart failure due to coronary heart disease. *Am J Cardiol*. 2011;107(1):64–68.

42. Pack QR, Goel K, Lahr BD, et al. Participation in cardiac rehabilitation and survival following coronary artery bypass graft surgery: a community based study. *Circulation*. 2013;128:590–597.

43. Dunlay SM, Pack QR, Thomas RJ, et al. Participation in cardiac rehabilitation, readmissions and death after acute myocardial infarction. *Am J Med*. 2014;127(6):538–546.

44. Witt BJ, Jacobsen SJ, Weston SA, et al. Cardiac rehabilitation after myocardial infarction in the community. *J Am Coll Cardiol*. 2004;44(5):988–996.

45. Shah ND, Dunlay SM, Ting HH, et al. Long-term medication adherence after myocardial infarction: experience of a community. *Am J Med*. 2009;122(10):961.e7–961.e13.

46. Jarcho JA, Keaney JFJ. Proof that lower is better—LDL cholesterol and IMPROVE-IT. *N Engl J Med*. 2015;372(25):2448–2450.

47. Goel K, Pack QR, Lahr B, et al. Cardiac rehabilitation is associated with reduced long-term mortality in patients undergoing combined heart valve and CABG surgery. *Eur J Prev Cardiol*. 2013;22(2):159–168.

48. Critchley JA, Capewell S. Mortality risk reduction associated with smoking cessation in patients with coronary heart disease: a systematic review. *JAMA*. 2003;290(1):86–97.

49. 2014 Surgeon General's Report: The Health Consequences of Smoking—50 Years of Progress. Available from: https://www.cdc.gov/tobacco/data_statistics/sgr/50th-anniversary/index.htm

50. Sochor O, Lennon RJ, Rodriguez-Escudero JP, et al. Trends and predictors of smoking cessation after percutaneous coronary intervention (from Olmsted County, Minnesota, 1999 to 2010). *Am J Cardiol*. 2015;115(4):405–410.

51. Sarwar N, Gao P, Seshasai SR, et al. Diabetes mellitus, fasting blood glucose concentration, and risk of vascular disease: a collaborative meta-analysis of 102 prospective studies. *Lancet*. 2010;375(9733):2215–2222.

52. Selvin E, Marinopoulos S, Berkenblit G, et al. Meta-analysis: glycosylated hemoglobin and cardiovascular disease in diabetes mellitus. *Ann Intern Med*. 2004;141(6):421–431.

53. Rapsomaniki E, Timmis A, George J, et al. Blood pressure and incidence of twelve cardiovascular diseases: lifetime risks, healthy life-years lost, and age-specific associations in 1.25 million people. *Lancet*. 2014;383(9932):1899–1911.

54. Babu AS, Grace SL. Cardiac rehabilitation for hypertension assessment and control: report from the International Council of Cardiovascular Prevention and Rehabilitation. *J Clin Hypertens*. 2015;17(11):831–836.

55. Soja AM, Zwisler AD, Frederiksen M, et al. Use of intensified comprehensive cardiac rehabilitation to improve risk factor control in patients with type 2 diabetes mellitus or impaired glucose tolerance—the randomized DANish StUdy of impaired glucose metabolism in the settings of cardiac rehabilitation (DANSUK) study. *Am Heart J*. 2007;153(4):621–628.

56. Ades PA, Savage PD, Harvey-Berino J. The treatment of obesity in cardiac rehabilitation. *J Cardiopulm Rehabil Prev.* 2010;30(5):289–298.

57. Okorodudu DO, Jumean MF, Montori VM, et al. Diagnostic performance of body mass index to identify obesity as defined by body adiposity: a systematic review and meta-analysis. *Int J Obes (Lond).* 2010;34(5):791–799.

58. Palmieri GM, Bertorini TE, Griffin JW, et al. Assessment of whole body composition with dual energy x-ray absorptiometry in Duchenne muscular dystrophy: correlation of lean body mass with muscle function. *Muscle Nerve.* 1996;19(6):777–779.

59. Sahakyan KR, Somers VK, Rodriguez-Escudero JP, et al. Normal-weight central obesity: implications for total and cardiovascular mortality. *Ann Intern Med.* 2015;163(11):827–835.

60. Dong JY, Zhang YH, Qin LQ. Obstructive sleep apnea and cardiovascular risk: meta-analysis of prospective cohort studies. *Atherosclerosis.* 2013;229(2):489–495.

61. Netzer NC, Stoohs RA, Netzer CM, et al. Using the Berlin Questionnaire to identify patients at risk for the sleep apnea syndrome. *Ann Intern Med.* 1999;131(7):485–491.

62. Chung F, Yegneswaran B, Liao P, et al. STOP questionnaire: a tool to screen patients for obstructive sleep apnea. *Anesthesiology.* 2008;108(5):812–821.

63. Stenman M, Holzmann MJ, Sartipy U. Relation of major depression to survival after coronary artery bypass grafting. *Am J Cardiol.* 2014;114(5):698–703.

64. Dong J-Y, Zhang Y-H, Tong J, et al. Depression and risk of stroke: a meta-analysis of prospective studies. *Stroke.* 2012;43(1):32–37.

65. Rutledge T, Reis VA, Linke SE, et al. Depression in heart failure. *J Am Coll Cardiol.* 2006;48(8):1527–1537.

66. Barth J, Schumacher M, Herrmann-Lingen C. Depression as a risk factor for mortality in patients with coronary heart disease: a meta-analysis. *Psychosom Med.* 2004;66(6):802–813.

67. Lichtman JH, Froelicher ES, Blumenthal JA, et al. Depression as a risk factor for poor prognosis among patients with acute coronary syndrome: systematic review and recommendations: a scientific statement from the American Heart Association. *Circulation.* 2014;129:1350–1369.

68. Kroenke K, Spitzer RL, Williams JB. The PHQ-9: validity of a brief depression severity measure. *J Gen Intern Med.* 2001;16(9):606–613.

69. Tluczek A, Henriques JB, Brown RL. Support for the reliability and validity of a six-item state anxiety scale derived from the state-trait anxiety inventory. *J Nurs Meas.* 2009;17(1):19–28.

70. Stephens MB. Cardiac rehabilitation. *Am Fam Physician.* 2009;80(9):955–959; hand-out 960.

71. Anderson L, Thompson DR, Oldridge N, et al. Exercise-based cardiac rehabilitation for coronary heart disease. *Cochrane Database Syst Rev.* 2016;(1):CD001800.

72. Sagar VA, Davies EJ, Briscoe S, et al. Exercise-based rehabilitation for heart failure: systematic review and meta-analysis. *Open Heart.* 2015;2(1):e000163.

73. Bachmann JM, Shah AS, Duncan MS, et al. Cardiac rehabilitation and readmissions after heart transplantation. *J Heart Lung Transplant.* 2018;37:467–476.

74. Heran BS, Chen JM, Ebrahim S, et al. Exercise-based cardiac rehabilitation for coronary heart disease. *Cochrane Database Syst Rev.* 2011;(7):CD001800.

75. Balady GJ, Arena R, Sietsema K, et al. Clinician's guide to cardiopulmonary exercise testing in adults: a scientific statement from the American Heart Association. *Circulation.* 2010;122(2):191–225.

76. Keteyian SJ, Isaac D, Thadani U, et al. Safety of symptom-limited cardiopulmonary exercise testing in patients with chronic heart failure due to severe left ventricular systolic dysfunction. *Am Heart J.* 2009;158(4 suppl):S72–S77.

77. Pescatello LS; American College of Sports Medicine. *ACSM's Guidelines for Exercise Testing and Prescription.* Philadelphia, PA: Wolters Kluwer/Lippincott Williams & Wilkins Health; 2014.

78. Borg GA. Perceived exertion. *Exerc Sport Sci Rev.* 1974;2:131–153.

79. Fletcher GF, Ades PA, Kligfield P, et al. Exercise standards for testing and training: a scientific statement from the American Heart Association. *Circulation.* 2013;128(8):873–934.

80. Morshedi-Meibodi A, Larson MG, Levy D, et al. Heart rate recovery after treadmill exercise testing and risk of cardiovascular disease events (The Framingham Heart Study). *Am J Cardiol.* 2002;90(8):848–852.

81. Albouaini K, Egred M, Alahmar A. Cardiopulmonary exercise testing and its application. *Postgrad Med J.* 2007;83(985):675–682.

82. Goedecke JH, Gibson ASC, Grobler L, et al. Determinants of the variability in respiratory exchange ratio at rest and during exercise in trained athletes. *Am J Physiol Endocrinol Metab.* 2000;279(6):E1325–E1334.

83. Tabet J-Y, Beauvais F, Thabut G, et al. A critical appraisal of the prognostic value of the VE/VCO$_2$ slope in chronic heart failure. *Eur J Cardiovasc Prev Rehabil.* 2003;10(4):267–272.

84. Cheitlin MD, Armstrong WF, Aurigemma GP, et al. ACC/AHA/ASE 2003 guideline update for the clinical application of echocardiography: summary article. A report of the American College of Cardiology/American Heart Association Task Force on Practice Guidelines (ACC/AHA/ASE Committee to Update the 1997 guidelines for the clinical application of echocardiography). *Circulation.* 2003;108(9):1146–1162.

85. Hlatky MA, Boineau RE, Higginbotham MB, et al. A brief self-administered questionnaire to determine functional capacity (the Duke Activity Status Index). *Am J Cardiol.* 1989;64(10):651–654.

86. Pereira MA, FitzerGerald SJ, Gregg EW, et al. A collection of Physical Activity Questionnaires for health-related research. *Med Sci Sports Exerc.* 1997;29(6 suppl):S1–S205.

87. Ross R, Blair SN, Arena R, et al. Importance of assessing cardiorespiratory fitness in clinical practice: a case for fitness as a clinical vital sign: a scientific statement from the American Heart Association. *Circulation.* 2016;134(24):e653–e699.

88. Blair SN, Kohl HW III, Paffenbarger RS Jr, et al. Physical fitness and all-cause mortality. A prospective study of healthy men and women. *JAMA.* 1989;262(17):2395–2401.

89. Bassett DR Jr. International physical activity questionnaire: 12-country reliability and validity. *Med Sci Sports Exerc.* 2003;35(8):1396.

90. Goel K, Shen J, Wolter AD, et al. Prevalence of musculoskeletal and balance disorders in patients enrolled in phase II cardiac rehabilitation. *J Cardiopulm Rehabil Prev.* 2010;30(4):235–239.

91. Warburton DER, Nicol CW, Bredin SSD. Health benefits of physical activity: the evidence. *CMAJ.* 2006;174(6):801–809.

92. Karvonen MJ, Kentala E, Mustala O. The effects of training on heart rate; a longitudinal study. *Ann Med Exp Biol Fenn.* 1957;35(3):307–315.

93. Ito S, Mizoguchi T, Saeki T. Review of high-intensity interval training in cardiac rehabilitation. *Intern Med.* 2016;55(17):2329–2336.

94. Ribeiro PA, Boidin M, Juneau M, et al. High-intensity interval training in patients with coronary heart disease: prescription models and perspectives. *Ann Phys Rehabil Med.* 2017;60(1):50–57.

95. Williams MA, Haskell WL, Ades PA, et al. Resistance exercise in individuals with and without cardiovascular disease: 2007 update: a scientific statement from the American Heart Association Council on Clinical Cardiology and Council on Nutrition, Physical Activity, and Metabolism. *Circulation.* 2007;116(5):572–584.

96. Perez-Terzic CM. Exercise in cardiovascular diseases. *PM R.* 2012;4(11):867–873.

97. Nashner LM. *Practical Biomechanics and Physiology of Balance.* San Diego, CA: Singular Publishing; 1997.

98. Afilalo J, Karanananthan S, Eisenberg MJ, et al. Role of frailty in patients with cardiovascular disease. *Am J Cardiol.* 2009;103(11):1616–1621.

99. Gillespie LD, Robertson MC, Gillespie WJ, et al. Interventions for preventing falls in older people living in the community. *Cochrane Database Syst Rev.* 2012;(9):CD007146.

100. Dalusung-Angosta A. The impact of Tai Chi exercise on coronary heart disease: a systematic review. *J Am Acad Nurse Pract.* 2011;23(7):376–381.

101. Garcia M, Miller VM, Gulati M, et al. Focused cardiovascular care for women: the need and role in clinical practice. *Mayo Clin Proc.* 2016;91(2):226–240.

102. Hammill BG, Curtis LH, Schulman KA, et al. Relationship between cardiac rehabilitation and long-term risks of death and myocardial infarction among elderly Medicare beneficiaries. *Circulation.* 2010;121(1):63–70.

103. Vanhees L, Rauch B, Piepoli M, et al. Importance of characteristics and modalities of physical activity and exercise in the management of cardiovascular health in individuals with cardiovascular disease (Part III). *Eur J Prevent Cardiol.* 2012;19(6):1333–1356.

104. Flynn KE, Pina IL, Whellan DJ, et al. Effects of exercise training on health status in patients with chronic heart failure: HF-ACTION randomized controlled trial. *JAMA.* 2009;301(14):1451–1459.

105. Davies EJ, Moxham T, Rees K, et al. Exercise training for systolic heart failure: cochrane systematic review and meta-analysis. *Eur J Heart Fail.* 2010;12(7):706–715.

106. Wisloff U, Stoylen A, Loennechen JP, et al. Superior cardiovascular effect of aerobic interval training versus moderate continuous training in heart failure patients: a randomized study. *Circulation.* 2007;115(24):3086–3094.

107. Martinez PF, Okoshi K, Zornoff LA, et al. Chronic heart failure-induced skeletal muscle atrophy, necrosis, and changes in myogenic regulatory factors. *Med Sci Monit.* 2010;16(12):BR374–BR383.

108. Rogers JG, Aaronson KD, Boyle AJ, et al. Continuous flow left ventricular assist device improves functional capacity and quality of life of advanced heart failure patients. *J Am Coll Cardiol.* 2010;55(17):1826–1834.

109. Mahfood Haddad T, Saurav A, Smer A, et al. Cardiac rehabilitation in patients with left ventricular assist device: a systematic review and meta-analysis. *J Cardiopulm Rehabil Prev.* 2017;37:390–396.

110. Kerrigan DJ, Williams CT, Ehrman JK, et al. Cardiac rehabilitation improves functional capacity and patient-reported health status in patients with continuous-flow left ventricular assist devices: the Rehab-VAD randomized controlled trial. *JACC Heart Fail.* 2014;2(6):653–659.

111. Chung CJ, Wu C, Jones M, et al. Reduced handgrip strength as a marker of frailty predicts clinical outcomes in patients with heart failure undergoing ventricular assist device placement. *J Cardiac Fail.* 2014;20(5):310–315.

112. Squires RW. Cardiac rehabilitation issues for heart transplantation patients. *J Cardiopulm Rehabil Prevent.* 1990;10(5):159–168.

113. Braith RW, Mills RM, Welsch MA, et al. Resistance exercise training restores bone mineral density in heart transplant recipients. *J Am Coll Cardiol.* 1996;28(6):1471–1477.

114. Rosenbaum AN, Kremers WK, Schirger JA, et al. Association between early cardiac rehabilitation and long-term survival in cardiac transplant recipients. *Mayo Clin Proc.* 2016;91(2):149–156.

115. Squires RW. Exercise therapy for cardiac transplant recipients. *Prog Cardiovasc Dis.* 2011;53(6):429–436.

116. Anchique Santos CV, Lopez-Jimenez F, Benaim B, et al. Cardiac rehabilitation in Latin America. *Prog Cardiovasc Dis.* 2014;57(3):268–275.

117. Suaya JA, Shepard DS, Normand S-LT, et al. Use of cardiac rehabilitation by medicare beneficiaries after myocardial infarction or coronary bypass surgery. *Circulation.* 2007;116(15):1653–1662.

118. Supervia M, Medina-Inojosa JR, Yeung C, et al. Cardiac rehabilitation for women: a systematic review of barriers and solutions. *Mayo Clin Proc.* 2017;pii: S0025-6196(17)30026-5. doi: 10.1016/j.mayocp.2017.01.002. [Epub ahead of print].

119. Grace SL, Shanmugasegaram S, Gravely-Witte S, et al. Barriers to cardiac rehabilitation: does age make a difference? *J Cardiopulm Rehabil Prevent.* 2009;29(3):183–187.

120. Evenson KR, Fleury J. Barriers to outpatient cardiac rehabilitation participation and adherence. *J Cardiopulm Rehabil Prevent.* 2000;20(4):241–246.
121. Daly J, Sindone AP, Thompson DR, et al. Barriers to participation in and adherence to cardiac rehabilitation programs: a critical literature review. *Prog Cardiovasc Nurs.* 2002;17(1):8–17.
122. Balady GJ, Ades PA, Bittner VA, et al. Referral, enrollment, and delivery of cardiac rehabilitation/secondary prevention programs at clinical centers and beyond: a presidential advisory from the American Heart Association. *Circulation.* 2011;124(25): 2951–2960.
123. Ghisi GLM, Polyzotis P, Oh P, et al. Physician factors affecting cardiac rehabilitation referral and patient enrollment: a systematic review. *Clin Cardiol.* 2013;36(6):323–335.
124. Code of Federal Regulations. Title 42—public health. §410.49—cardiac rehabilitation program and intensive cardiac rehabilitation program: conditions of coverage.

2011. Available from: http://www.gpo.gov/fdsys/pkg/CFR-2011-title42-vol2/xml/CFR-2011-title42-vol2-sec410-49.xml
125. AACVPR. Resources for Cardiovascular & Pulmonary Rehabilitation Professionals. Available from: https://www.aacvpr.org/Resources/Resources-for-Professionals
126. Clark RA, Conway A, Poulsen V, et al. Alternative models of cardiac rehabilitation: a systematic review. *Eur J Prevent Cardiol.* 2015;22(1):35–74.
127. Jolly K, Lip GY, Taylor RS, et al. The Birmingham Rehabilitation Uptake Maximisation study (BRUM): a randomised controlled trial comparing home-based with centre-based cardiac rehabilitation. *Heart.* 2009;95(1):36–42.
128. Dalal HM, Evans PH, Campbell JL, et al. Home-based versus hospital-based rehabilitation after myocardial infarction: a randomized trial with preference arms-Cornwall Heart Attack Rehabilitation Management Study (CHARMS). *Int J Cardiol.* 2007;119(2):202–211.

Rehabilitation of the Patient with Respiratory Dysfunction

The beginning of wisdom is to call things by their right names.
Ancient Chinese Proverb

The names that are attached to clinical phenomena determine in part how they are managed. For example, "ventilator-associated pneumonia (VAP)" is responsible for over 60,000 excess hospital-related deaths annually. However, it is not the ventilator but the invasive interface that causes pneumonia. Similarly, since noninvasive ventilation doesn't cause pulmonary rehabilitation (PR), a more appropriate terminology might shift the emphasis of ventilatory support more to noninvasive management. Likewise, respiratory acidosis due to ventilatory pump failure results in "ventilatory" not "respiratory" failure, so assisted ventilation rather than conventional oxygen therapy is warranted. For primary pulmonary disability, many patients require "habilitation" rather than "rehabilitation." This brings us to the definition of "pulmonary rehabilitation."

As defined in the latest statement from a joint American Thoracic Society European Respiratory Society task force:

Pulmonary rehabilitation is a comprehensive intervention based on a thorough patient assessment followed by patient tailored therapies that include, but are not limited to, exercise training, education, and behavior change, designed to improve the physical and psychological condition of people with chronic respiratory disease and to promote the long-term adherence to health-enhancing behaviors (1).

REHABILITATION OF PATIENTS WITH OBSTRUCTIVE LUNG DISEASE

Thirty-two sources of chronic obstructive pulmonary disease (COPD) prevalence from 17 countries reveal a COPD prevalence from 0.23% to 18.3%. In Europe and North America, rates are between 4% and 10% (2). COPD is the most common pulmonary disease and second most common noninfectious disease in the world. It causes 2.75 million deaths annually with global mortality predicted to double by 2030. It is the fourth largest cause of major activity limitation (3). Thirty percent of COPD patients with forced expiratory volume in 1 second (FEV_1) less than 750 milliliters (mL) and 35% following an acute exacerbation die within 1 year (4) and 50% within 3 years (5).

By the GOLD recommendations, any patient with grade 2 to 4 COPD should have a PR program (6). Indeed, any motivated COPD patient who has respiratory symptoms that limit activities of daily living (ADL) and who has adequate medical, neuromusculoskeletal, financial, and psychosocial status to permit active participation is a candidate for PR. Active patients who are still able to walk several blocks but who have noted yearly decreases in exercise tolerance or who have recently begun to require ongoing medical attention for pulmonary symptoms or complications are ideal candidates. For patients with primary pulmonary disease, it is essential to consider PR for all conditions.

PATIENT EVALUATION

In addition to the elements of the patient evaluation noted in **Box 34-1**, medical, physical, financial, or psychological factors that could interfere with rehabilitation need to be addressed (5). Commonly overlooked is the fact that 13% of COPD patients are anemic. This may indicate erythropoietin resistance and be associated with increased serum inflammatory proteins (7).

Various dyspnea assessment surveys can be used to objectify the extent of dyspnea and the effects of rehabilitation (8–11). In addition, the presence of coughing, wheezing, chest pains, neurologic or psychological disturbances, allergies, previous communicable diseases, injuries, and nutritional imbalance is evaluated. A full nutritional assessment including total iron binding capacity, cholesterol, and serum vitamin levels, especially of vitamins A, C, and E, is important because COPD patients frequently have vitamin deficiencies. Hypophosphatemia, hypomagnesemia, hypocalcemia, and hypokalemia can cause or exacerbate respiratory muscle weakness, which is reversible with treatment (12). Complete social, educational, and vocational histories and relevant environmental factors are explored.

Besides spirometry, patients with interstitial disease also benefit from assessment of oxygenation and diffusion capacity for carbon monoxide. In COPD, exertional dyspnea tends to occur when the FEV_1 is less than 1,500 mL, and it decreases by 45 to 75 mL/y (5), a rate up to three times normal. Arterial oxygen tensions may be significantly decreased with the patient supine (13), and oxyhemoglobin desaturation may be episodically severe during sleep (14).

Because spirometry does not predict functional impairment, clinical exercise testing is recommended, before initiation of

BOX 34-1

Patient Evaluation

- Family history of pulmonary diseases
- Symptom progression and impact on function
- Exacerbation and hospitalization history
- Appetite, nutritional status, and weight changes
- Medications, substance abuse
- Physical examination for hyperresonant chest, poor breath, and cardiac sounds
- Hemoglobin/hematocrit, sedimentation rate, C-reactive protein, white cell count
- Radiographic assessment of (low, flattened) diaphragm, (long, narrow) heart shadow, retrosternal translucency, narrowing of peripheral pulmonary vessels
- $PaCO_2$ and PaO_2 and diffusion capacities (decreased in emphysema, normal in bronchitis)
- Pulmonary function tests for air and mucus trapping
- Low-maximum midexpiratory flow rates and increased midexpiratory times, normal or increased lung compliance and increased flow work, increased residual volume and total lung capacity
- Clinical exercise testing
- A 3-, 6-, or 12-minute walk
- Assessment of the VAT and maximum exercise tolerance for a precise exercise regimen

PR. Field and laboratory exercise tests complement each other. For severe patients, Cardiopulmonary Exercise Test (CPET) is recommended, whereas for those with milder impairments, a 6-minute walk test or shuttle walk test (SWT) may be appropriate (15). The CPET permits the clinician to determine whether the primary disability is pulmonary, cardiac, or related to exercise-induced bronchospasm (16) and can also be useful for documenting response to rehabilitation. The CPET can be done using a treadmill, stationary bicycle, or upper extremity ergometer. Monitoring typically includes vital signs, electrocardiography, oxygen consumption, carbon dioxide production, respiratory quotient, ventilatory equivalent, minute ventilation, and metabolic rate. The respiratory quotient is the ratio of the carbon dioxide produced divided by the oxygen consumed. The ventilatory equivalent is equal to the volume of air breathed for 1 L of oxygen consumed. Exercise is often reported in metabolic equivalents (METs), which is defined as 1 MET = 3.5 mL O_2/kg/min. One MET is the amount of energy an average person produces at rest. Another useful measure for noninvasively assessing cardiac function includes the oxygen pulse, which is the mL of oxygen consumed per heart beat (16). Maximum CPET is achieved when oxygen consumption fails to increase with increasing workload, peak heart rate is achieved (220—age in years), respiratory exchange ratio is >1.10, or for electrocardiographic changes, chest pain, O2 saturation below 80%, blood pressure exceeding parameters, severe dyspnea, or intolerable fatigue occurs. To assess ventilatory reserve, peak ventilation is compared to the maximum voluntary ventilation (MVV), which can be estimated as $37.5 \times FEV_1$ (17). Arterial blood gases may be normal at rest but are often abnormal during exercise in patients with pulmonary disease. During PR, supplemental oxygen should be provided to keep SpO_2 greater than 90% (18). It has been shown that supplemental oxygen benefits patients with COPD with moderate-to-severe airflow obstruction and mild hypoxemia at rest by improving exercise tolerance and reducing pulmonary hypertension during exercise (19).

When CPET is not available, maximum exercise tolerance can be estimated from field tests such as the 6MWT and SWT or using pulmonary function data (20). The patient is instructed to gradually increase walking speed and duration on subsequent walking tests (21).

Organization of a Comprehensive Rehabilitation Program

A comprehensive PR program involves an interdisciplinary team that includes a supervising physician, exercise physiologists, respiratory therapists, and nurses to administer therapeutic exercise, nutritional, social, and psychological support, and occupational therapy. This combination can create an environment of integrated care to support the many complex needs of these patients in both inpatient and outpatient settings. In many ways, PR is similar to cardiac rehabilitation, and often the resources for treating the patients can be shared. Although regulatory requirements require that these programs be separated, staff and facilities often overlap.

The most well-established evidence and most commonly offered programs for PR are for patients with COPD. Evidence of beneficial outcomes is very strong for COPD patients. Other than perhaps for smoking cessation (22,23), there is no evidence that inpatient programs are more effective than outpatient PR programs (22–25); so inpatient PR should be reserved for severely debilitated patients (26), for tracheostomy tube removal, or for optimizing the ventilatory support while initiating other aspects of comprehensive rehabilitation (27). Table 34-1 is a sample therapeutic prescription for an ambulatory, moderately affected COPD patient.

Recent evidence points to a variety of exercise programs and interventions having efficacy. Recent advances include a focus on home-based interventions, uses of telemedicine and other technologies, and interventions to improve self-efficacy. Outcomes and recommendations for exercise training will be reviewed.

Therapeutic Interventions

Medications

The patient's medical regimen is optimized prior to reconditioning exercise or a PR program. Inhaler bronchodilator administration is reviewed to avoid the deposition of medication on the tongue. Patient education also includes training in the use of "spacers" and nebulizers (28). One half to two thirds of 33 double-blinded, randomized, placebo-controlled studies demonstrated significant improvements in exercise tolerance with the use of anticholinergics and short-acting β-2 mimetics, especially salbutamol.

Early medical attention is important during intercurrent respiratory tract infections (29). Antibiotics, glucocorticoids, and adjustment of bronchodilators and mucolytic agents may be indicated. N-acetylcysteine at 1,200 mg/d was demonstrated in a randomized, double-blind, placebo-controlled study to normalize C-reactive protein levels, lung function, and symptoms during acute exacerbations and possibly preventing exacerbations (30).

TABLE 34-1	**A Sample Therapeutic Prescription for a Patient with COPD**
Diagnosis	Chronic obstructive pulmonary disease in 75-year-olds with no known CAD
Prognosis	Favorable, patient on stable self-medication program
Goals	• Improve endurance and efficiency
	• Optimize oxygen needs and control of secretions
	• Increase independence in ambulation and self-care activities
	• Reduce anxiety and improve self-esteem through enhanced body awareness
	• Home exercise program and independent exercise monitoring
	• Ease sleep-disordered breathing and rest inspiratory muscles
Precautions	• Supplemental oxygen as needed during exercise, up to 6 L via nasal cannula, Rest oxygen at 2 L via NC
	• Maintain oxygen saturation >90%
	• Systolic blood pressure >100, <180; diastolic BP > 60, <110 mm Hg
	• Heart rate <140 bpm, target HR for conditioning 120 bpm (from 6MWT)
	• Respiratory rate <24
	• Discontinue and notify physician if patient becomes severely dyspneic or develops chest pain with exercise
Respiratory therapy	• Monitor with pulse oximetry at rest and during exercise to determine portable oxygen flow rate needed to maintain oxygen saturation higher than 90%
	• Instruct patient in diaphragmatic and pursed-lip breathing
	• Instruct patient and family in postural drainage techniques
	• Instruct patient and family in portable oxygen use
	• Instruct in use of metered-dose inhaler before exercise, assure dosing prior to exercise sessions
	• Education in self-monitoring with oximetry and Borg scale for exertion and dyspnea
	• Instruct in use of nocturnal BiPAP
Physical therapy	• Assess baseline endurance, using 6-min walk test
	• 3 sessions a week for 12 weeks
	• Begin with 5-min warm-up and cooldown for each session, aim to improve tolerance to 20 min at target intensity, start with 5-min intervals
	• Review proper body mechanics and coordinate with breathing patterns, using diaphragmatic and pursed-lip breathing when appropriate
Occupational therapy	• Assess upper extremity mobility, strength, and endurance
	• Upper body ergometry: start with 5-min unloaded warm-up and cooldown and 5 Watts resistance. Build up to 20 min at targeted intensity
	• Evaluate basic and advanced self-care activities, and provide adaptive aids to improve independence with dressing, hygiene, bathing, cooking, and other chores
	• Train the patient in energy conservation and work simplification techniques
	• Evaluate home environment and make recommendations for workspace modifications and equipment to improve safety, efficiency, and independence
	• Provide relaxation exercise training with visual imagery techniques

Counseling and General Medical Care

Dyspnea can cause fear and panic. This may worsen tachypnea while increasing dead-space ventilation, the work of breathing, hyperinflation, and air trapping. Relaxation exercises, such as Jacobson exercises and biofeedback (31,32), yoga, and diaphragmatic and pursed-lip breathing, can decrease tension and anxiety. People with COPD have diminished quality of life with depression in up to 50% of patients and severe reduction in social interaction (33). Integrating psychosocial support with multimodal PR optimizes outcomes (34) and can help address loss of employment and independence.

Since COPD patients tend to overuse medications during periods of respiratory distress and underuse them otherwise, self-efficacy can be used to improve adherence to prescribed medication regimens (35). Patients are also counseled to avoid atmospheric or vocational pollutants and other aggravating factors such as pollen, aerosols, excessive humidity, stress, and respiratory tract pathogens. Yearly flu vaccinations along with pneumococcal vaccine administration every 5 to 10 years are warranted. For high-altitude travel, patients usually require an additional 0.5 L/min of supplemental oxygen administration and are taught to self-monitor their O_2 sat. For hypoxic patients, portable oxygen concentrators allow for greater ease of travel. For those with no resting hypoxemia, O_2 therapy is not generally needed for short flights (36). Good hydration should always be maintained.

Nutrition

Significant weight loss occurs in 19% to 71% of COPD patients (12). In a study of 255 stable COPD PR patients, depletion of body weight, fat-free mass, and muscle mass were noted in 40% to 50% of patients with chronic hypoxemia and in normoxemic patients with FEV_1 less than 35% (37). In one study, 30 of 50 consecutive COPD patients presenting with acute respiratory failure (ARF) were significantly undernourished, and impaired nutritional status was more prevalent in those patients requiring mechanical ventilation (74% vs. 43%) (38). Undernutrition is associated with increased susceptibility to infection due to impaired cell-mediated immunity, reduced secretory immunoglobulin A, depressed pulmonary alveolar macrophage function, and increased colonization and adherence of bacteria in the upper and lower airways. Patients with significant nutritional impairment are more frequently colonized by *Pseudomonas* species (39,40). In addition, malnutrition adversely affects lung repair, surfactant synthesis, control of ventilation and response to hypoxia, respiratory muscle function and lung mechanics (41), and water homeostasis. It can cause respiratory muscle atrophy and decreased exercise capacity, cor pulmonale, increased rate of respiratory hospitalizations, hypercapnic respiratory failure, and difficulty in ventilator weaning (38,42,43). Likewise, inappropriate nutrition, such as increasing carbohydrate intake, can exacerbate hypercapnia.

Short-term refeeding of malnourished patients can improve respiratory muscle endurance and increase respiratory muscle strength in the absence of demonstrable changes in skeletal muscle function (44). Because of bloating due to a low-riding diaphragm, patients are advised to take small mouthfuls of food, eat slowly, and take smaller and more frequent meals. O_2 saturation can be evaluated while eating. If desaturation occurs, supplemental O_2 is used or increased. For those with hypercapnia, a dietary regimen high in calories derived from fat can decrease hypercapnia. Although short-term refeeding can be beneficial, refeeding programs lasting more than 2 weeks have not consistently resulted in increases in body weight. Growth hormone has not been shown to be useful. Possible beneficial effects of anabolic steroids as adjuncts to nutritional support and exercise have been reported to increase lean body mass and promote weight gain (45–47).

Breathing Retraining

Shallow, rapid breathing is commonly seen in anxious, dyspneic patients. This increases dead-space ventilation and airflow through narrowed airways, increasing the flow work of breathing. Patients with chronic airflow obstruction also have an altered pattern of ventilatory muscle recruitment in which the most effective pressures generated for ventilating the lungs are generated by the rib-cage inspiratory muscles rather than by the diaphragm, with significant contribution by primarily expiratory muscles (48). Diaphragmatic breathing and pursed-lip exhalation (DPLB) can help to reverse these tendencies. These techniques are usually initiated in the supine or 15% to 25% head-down position. Diaphragmatic breathing is guided by having the patient place one hand over the abdomen and the other on the thorax just below the clavicle. Breathing deeply through the nose, the abdomen is distended forward as appreciated by movement of the hand on the abdomen. Movement of the rib cage and, thus, the hand on the thorax should be kept to a minimum. Small weights can be placed on the abdomen to provide some resistance training (RT) and enhance the patient's focus. During exhalation, the abdominal muscles and the hand on the abdomen compress the abdominal contents, and exhalation is via pursed lips (49). Classically, a lighted candle is put several feet in front of the patient, and the patient flickers the flame while exhaling. This equalizes pleural and bronchial pressures, preventing collapse of smaller bronchi and decreasing air trapping. The use of DPLB decreases respiratory rate, coordinates the breathing pattern, and can improve blood gases (50). It is used during routine ADL and exercise and can improve exercise performance by relaxing accessory muscles and improving breathing efficiency.

Air-shifting techniques may be useful to decrease microatelectasis. Air shifting involves taking a deep inspiration that is held with the glottis closed for 5 seconds, during which time the air shifts to lesser-ventilated areas of the lung. Expiration is via pursed lips. This technique may be most beneficial when performed several times per hour.

Airway Secretion Elimination

Airway secretion clearance is crucial because exacerbations of COPD can be caused by trapping of airway secretions in the peripheral airways. Often cough in COPD is weak and ineffective as a result obstructed airflow, and frequent bouts of coughing are fatiguing. The high expulsive pressures generated during coughing can exacerbate both air trapping and secretion retention. "Huffing," or frequent short expulsive bursts following a deep breath, is often an effective and more comfortable alternative to coughing. Chest percussion and postural drainage can be useful for patients with chronic bronchitis or others with greater than 30 mL of sputum production per day (51), although caution must be taken to increase oxygen delivery as necessary during treatment. Autogenic drainage involves breathing with low tidal volumes between the functional residual capacity and the residual volume to mobilize secretions in small airways. This is followed by taking increasingly larger tidal volumes and forced expirations to transport mucus to the mouth (52).

Application of positive expiratory pressure (PEP) breathing is based on the theory that mucus in small airways is more effectively mobilized by coughing or forced expirations if alveolar pressure and volume behind mucous plugs are increased. The PEP is applied by breathing through a face mask or a mouthpiece with an inspiratory tube containing a one-way valve and an expiratory tube having variable expiratory resistance. Expiratory pressures of 10 to 20 cmH$_2$O are maintained throughout expiration. The PEP increases functional residual capacity, reducing resistance to airflow in collateral and small airways (53,54), but studies on benefits of PEP breathing have been inconclusive for both cystic fibrosis (CF) and COPD (55–63).

Flutter breathing is a combination of PEP and oscillation applied at the mouth. The patient expires through a small pipe. A small stainless steel ball rests on the expiratory end of the pipe; it is pushed upward during expiration, producing PEP, and falls downward again, interrupting flow. The mucus-mobilizing effect is thought to be due to widening of the airways because of the increased expiratory pressure and airflow oscillations due to the oscillating ball (64). For this too, however, the results of clinical trials have been conflicting (65–69).

With currently available technology, mechanical vibration or oscillation can be mechanically applied to the thorax or directly to the airway to facilitate airway secretion elimination. Vibration is possible at frequencies up to 170 Hz applied under a soft plastic shell to the thorax and abdomen (the Hayek Oscillator, Breasy Medical Equipment Inc., Stamford, CT). Another device delivers rapid burst airflows at up to 25 Hz under a vest covering the chest and upper abdomen (THAIRapy System, The Vest System, Model 105—Home Care—Hill-Rom). The effects of mechanical chest percussion and vibration appear to be frequency dependent (70–72). In most animal studies, frequencies between 10 and 15 Hz appear best to facilitate mucous transport (70,72,73), especially the transport of a thicker mucous layer (74). Warwick and Hansen found long-term increases in forced vital capacity (FVC) and forced expiratory flows for CF patients treated with high-frequency chest-wall compression as compared with manual chest percussion alone (75). Others have reported improvement in pulmonary function and in gas exchange during high-frequency oscillation (76–80), and Sibuya et al. found that chest-wall vibration decreased dyspnea (79). Most studies on COPD and CF patients, however, have failed to demonstrate objective clinical benefits from percussion or vibration on mucous transport (80–83). Side effects of percussion and vibration can include increasing obstruction to airflow (84,85). In an animal model, the application of vibration and percussion was also associated with the development of atelectasis (86). Despite conflicting studies, the THAIRapy Vest has become popular for CF and familial dysautonomia patients, and there are claims of decreased hospitalization rates with its daily use (70). Patients with daily airways secretion encumbrance usually feel that it is beneficial.

The Percussionaire IPV-2C Lung Recruiter Model (Percussionaire Corp., Sandpoint, ID) can deliver aerosolized medications while providing high-flow percussive minibursts of air directly to the airways at rates of 2.5 to 5 Hz. This intrapulmonary percussive ventilation (IPV) has been reported to be more effective than chest percussion and postural drainage in the treatment of postoperative atelectasis and secretion mobilization in COPD patients (87,88). The majority of such patients feel that it is helpful (89,90).

Patterson et al. found in a 10-year study that good CF patient compliance with airway secretion mobilization methods was associated with a slower rate of loss of pulmonary function (91). Patient compliance is usually poor, however (92–94). There is greater patient compliance for simple methods that can be used independently. Little has been documented concerning long-term safety and efficacy of any of these. Because expensive devices have not been shown to be more effective than simple handheld percussors costing about $400 (Jeanie Rub Percussor, Morgan Inc., Mishawaka, IN or G5 NeoCussor, General Physiotherapy Inc., St. Louis, MO), the latter should be favored for routine use.

Inspiratory Resistive Exercises

Inspiratory resistive exercises, including maximum sustained ventilation, inspiratory resistive loading, and inspiratory threshold loading, can improve the endurance of respiratory muscles (95–97). Typically, patients breathe through these devices for a total of 30 minutes daily for 8 to 10 weeks. The settings of the devices are adjusted to increase difficulty as patients improve and the program advances.

Levine et al. conducted an evaluation of the isocapnic hyperpnea method and determined that no more benefits could be derived from it than could be achieved using periodic intermittent positive pressure breathing treatments, a regimen that was considered equivalent to placebo (98). However, Ries and Moser randomly assigned 18 patients to either a home isocapnic hyperventilation training program or a walking program and found that the former led to improvements in ventilatory muscle endurance and exercise performance and significant improvements in the maximum rate of O_2 consumption (VO_{2max}), whereas walking exercises improved lower limb exercise endurance but not ventilatory muscle endurance (99).

Twenty-one controlled studies of inspiratory resistive loading involving 259 COPD patients reported improvements in inspiratory muscle strength and endurance (100). The mean

increase in maximum inspiratory pressure was 19%. However, the subjects using inspiratory RT reduced their inspiratory flow rates and lengthened their inspiratory time to reduce the severity of the imposed loads. Thus, "targeted" or threshold inspiratory muscle training was and continues to be recommended over flow-resistive training to assure adequate intensity of inspiratory muscle activity.

With targeted training, the subject is provided feedback regarding the inspiratory flow rates through the resistor or the inspiratory pressure generated by flow through the resistor; with threshold training, the subject is unable to generate flow through the device until a predetermined pressure is achieved. Six of the nine controlled studies of the use of targeted or threshold resistor devices in COPD reported significantly greater improvements in inspiratory muscle function in the subjects than in the controls (100). In three of the six studies in which it was assessed, exercise tolerance was greater for trained subjects than for controls. In one controlled study comparing exercise reconditioning plus threshold inspiratory muscle training with exercise reconditioning alone, the former resulted in significantly greater increases in inspiratory muscle strength and endurance and in exercise tolerance (93). Exercise tolerance seemed to be improved particularly for those with electromyographic changes indicating inspiratory muscle fatigue with exercise (101). One controlled, well-designed, but small study of threshold inspiratory exercise for CF patients demonstrated significant improvements in inspiratory muscle strength, FVC, total lung capacity, and exercise tolerance in the experimental group (102). In another controlled study of patients taking corticosteroids, inspiratory muscle training appeared to prevent the muscle weakness that would have otherwise resulted from the steroid use (103). The combination of inspiratory muscle training along with bronchodilator therapy and reconditioning exercise was demonstrated to very significantly reduce dyspnea by comparison to the use of bronchodilators and general exercise without inspiratory muscle training (104). Benefits for incorporating inspiratory muscle training into PR programs have been reported (105) with targeted training preferred (106).

Respiratory Muscle Rest

Relatively minor changes in the pattern of breathing or respiratory muscle loading can trigger acute respiratory muscle fatigue and failure. Interspersing periods of exercise and muscle rest is a basic principle of rehabilitation. Hypercapnia is an indication of limited reserve before the appearance of overt fatigue and may indicate the need for periods of respiratory muscle assistance or rest before considering strengthening exercises (107). Diaphragm rest can be achieved by assisted ventilation using either body ventilators, mouth piece, or nasal noninvasive positive pressure ventilation (NIV), which is typically administered as bilevel positive airway pressure (PAP). Despite high ventilation rates in COPD, ventilatory response to both hypercapnia and hypoxia may be reduced. This is often exacerbated during sleep. The increase in pulmonary vascular resistance that occurs in the presence of pulmonary tissue hypoxia is exacerbated by acidosis. When this situation becomes severe, it may lead to right ventricular failure. The use of O_2 therapy alone can exacerbate CO_2 retention and acidosis.

Two groups of patients appear to be suited to home NIV administration during sleep. The first and smaller group includes those who need ventilatory assistance around the clock but who are medically and psychologically stable. They can use tracheostomy or noninvasive ventilatory support (NVS) where the ventilators are used at full ventilatory support settings. Ventilator-dependent patients require more frequent hospital readmission and have a poorer prognosis than did non–ventilator users. Tracheostomized patients are candidates for decannulation to NVS.

A second group of patients can benefit from nocturnal nasal NIV alone. While both nocturnal negative pressure body ventilator use and NIV can normalize arterial blood gases, improve sleep quality, and increase quality of life, 12-minute walk distance, respiratory muscle endurance, and decrease dyspnea (108), the former methods cause obstructive apneas during sleep and have fallen out of favor (109,110). The NIV methods, provided by portable ventilators and bilevel PAP devices, rest inspiratory muscles, assist ventilation, and splint, open the airway to prevent sleep apneas and airway collapse (111).

Belman et al. reported greater diaphragm relaxation by nasal NIV ventilation than by body ventilator use (112). Marino demonstrated reversal of nocturnal ventilatory insufficiency for COPD patients using nasal NIV (113), and others have used assisted ventilation via oral-nasal interfaces as an alternative to intubation and tracheostomy for COPD patients in acute exacerbation (114). Nasal bilevel PAP has the additional benefit of the expiratory PAP countering auto–positive end-expiratory pressure (PEEP) in these patients who trap air. This decreases their work of breathing. A number of studies have reported long-term improvements in daytime blood gases with the use of nocturnal nasal NIV for hypercapnic COPD patients (108,115,116), and they suggest that nocturnal ventilator use can also decrease dyspnea and improve quality of life (117) and survival (115). Nocturnal nasal bilevel PAP was also reported to improve sleep efficiency and total sleep time in hypercapnic COPD patients (118). In another study of 49 hypercapnic patients with COPD, while hospitalization rates were decreased by both long-term oxygen therapy (LTOT) and by LTOT with nocturnal nasal bilevel PAP, only the latter group had a significant decrease in intensive-care admissions and a significant improvement in 6-minute walk distance (119). However, a systematic review (69) of nocturnal bilevel PAP use for at least 3 months duration in stable hypercapnic COPD patients did not find a consistent statistically significant effect on lung function, gas exchange, respiratory muscle strength, sleep efficiency, or exercise tolerance although the studies included few subjects. Although it is widely considered appropriate to offer nocturnal bilevel PAP for hypercapnic COPD patients, little or no benefit has been reported with its use for nonhypercapnic patients (120).

Use of proportional assist ventilation and pressure support during exercise has been reported to facilitate high-intensity exercise training in severe COPD (121–123). Patients benefiting from proportional assist ventilation were reported to achieve 15% higher exercise levels at 6 weeks than those exercising without it. Users had a significant reduction in plasma lactate concentration at equivalent workloads after training.

Supplemental Oxygen Therapy

Supplemental O_2 therapy is indicated for patients with pO_2 continuously less than 55 to 60 mm Hg (124). Home O_2 therapy can decrease pulmonary arterial hypertension (PAH), polycythemia, and perception of effort during exercise, and it can prolong life (124,125). Patients with COPD have also been shown to have increased sympathetic modulation and reduced baroreflex sensitivity. Supplemental O_2 has been shown to significantly and favorably alter autonomic modulation and decrease blood pressure and pulse (126). In addition, cognitive function can be improved, or at least, better maintained, and hospital needs reduced. An international consensus on the current status and indications for LTOT suggested that the prescription be based on (127):

1. An appropriately documented diagnosis
2. Concurrent optimal use of other rehabilitative approaches, such as pharmacotherapy, smoking abstinence, and exercise training
3. Properly documented chronic hypoxemia

Oxygen therapy should be given with caution to hypercapnic patients whether or not they use NIV (128).

Supplemental O_2 can also improve exercise tolerance. Many patients exhibit exercise hypoxemia. Decreases in O_2 saturation are typically noted at physical activity levels comparable to those necessary to perform ADL. Often, the decrease in O_2 saturation occurs within the first minute after which O_2 saturation stabilizes, but occasionally, there is a progressive decline in O_2 saturation with exercise. In a study of 38 subjects in whom the mean resting O_2 saturation was 93% ± 3%, a decrease of 4.7% ± 3.6% (range: 1% to 18%) was observed during submaximal exercise (129). In patients with primary pulmonary disease, it is safe and effective to give as much O_2 as needed with activity to maintain their O_2 saturation above 90%. Even in patients with obstructive disease, this can be safe as long as the supplemental O_2 is returned to resting level supplementation at the end of exercise (130).

In a crossover study of 12 subjects with severe COPD (131), four patients more than doubled their duration of exercise while receiving 40% oxygen, but in only two of these were desaturation observed in the absence of oxygen. Bradley et al. reported that in subjects with mild hypoxemia and exercise desaturation, supplemental O_2 by nasal prongs did not influence maximum work rate but did influence endurance (132). Davidson et al. noted that O_2 increased mean walking endurance time by 59% and 6-minute walk distance by 17%. Moreover, submaximal cycle time at a constant workload was increased by 51% at a flow rate of 2 L/min and by 88% at 4 L/min, suggesting a dose-response curve (133). The exercise response to O_2 could not be predicted from the degree of desaturation, resting pulmonary function tests, echocardiographic measurements of right ventricular systolic pressure, or other clinical parameters (131). In fact, in nonhypoxemic COPD patients performing moderate exercise, O_2 supplementation decreased ventilatory requirement by its direct effect on chemoreceptor inhibition (134). Thus, exercise tolerance can be increased by O_2 therapy without improving O_2 consumption or utilization. A recent study found that supplemental O_2 during exercise prevented exercise-induced oxidative stress (135). Marcus et al. also reported significantly greater exercise tolerance in CF patients receiving O_2 (136). Improved exercise tolerance in CF patients in the Dead Sea basin compared with at sea level was also reported (137). This was thought to be due to the increased oxygen tension below sea level.

The most widely accepted guideline for prescribing O_2 use during exercise is that of exercise-induced O_2 saturation below

90%. However, it seems reasonable to recommend that measurements of dyspnea and exercise tolerance be undertaken with and without supplemental O_2 to determine which individuals are less short of breath or walk further (have greater exercise tolerance) when given it (138). Certainly, exercise-induced decreases in O_2 saturation below 90% when combined with increased exercise tolerance with O_2 therapy warrant its prescription for exercise. Patients with mild-to-moderate daytime hypoxemia often have marked nocturnal desaturation. Home overnight oximetry can be used to diagnose nocturnal oxyhemoglobin desaturation and assist in the O_2 prescription although guidelines for sleep supplemental O_2 have not been established (139).

Inspiratory phase or pulsed O_2 therapy, especially when delivered transtracheally, avoids waste and decreases discomfort and drying of mucous membranes. Oxygen flow delivery is 0.25 to 0.4 L/min compared to 2 to 4 L/min when delivered via nasal cannula or face mask (140,141). Oxygen therapy is used along with mechanical ventilation for patients with concomitant CO_2 retention.

Exercise

The hallmark of PR programs is exercise training to improve function. Although exercise is often limited by dyspnea, it is essential to improve the patient's ventilatory efficiency in order to permit increased functional capacity within the ventilatory limitations. The goal of PR exercise is not cure but to permit the person to do more with the ventilatory and gas exchange capacity they have, achieving "more steps per breath." Benefits of exercise training in COPD, the best studied primary pulmonary disease, include improving muscle function as well as improvements in exercise capacity (142–148). An added benefit of improved muscle function is the reduction of ventilatory requirement for a submaximal workload, leading to reduced dyspnea and increased endurance. In COPD, this also can reduce hyperinflation and ameliorate dyspnea even more (149). Other benefits include improved mood, improved cardiovascular function, and reduced symptom burden (1).

Exercise limitations in COPD results from any combination of ventilatory constraints, pulmonary gas exchange abnormalities, peripheral muscle dysfunction, cardiac dysfunction, anxiety, depression, poor motivation, and deconditioning (1). Ventilatory limitation, either from restrictive or obstructive pathophysiology, can be the major limitation for patients along with impaired gas exchange. Hypoxemia can be relieved using supplemental O_2, whereas approaches to ventilatory dysfunction center on appropriate use of medications and avoidance or reversal of deconditioning. Muscle dysfunction includes both inspiratory and skeletal muscles. Fortunately, exercise programs have been shown to ameliorate both forms of muscle weakness (150,151).

Exercise abnormalities in patients with COPD, as for patients with primary pulmonary disease, manifest an abnormally high ventilatory requirement and tachypnea with inability to adequately increase tidal volumes during exercise. In COPD, the maximal exercise ventilation (VE_{max}) can be close to or exceeds MVV. While cardiac output rises normally with exercise, peak cardiac output and heart rate are often limited because of the ventilatory limitations. Hypoxia—and in severely limited patients hypercapnia—can occur with exercise (152). Thus, many moderate to severely affected patients cannot attain the classical target of 60% to 70% of maximum heart rate for cardiac or aerobic exercise training. Because of this, there are modifications, which will be described below for exercise prescription in pulmonary disease.

The benefits of PR in COPD are clear, even at lower intensities. Independent of long-term O_2 therapy PR may prolong survival for COPD patients (153,154). For 149 patients (mean age 69, 89% of whom had COPD), age, sex, body mass index, and primary diagnosis were not related to survival after completion of a PR program. However, a higher postrehabilitation functional activities score, a longer postrehabilitation 6-minute walk distance, and being married were strongly associated with increased survival (155). Gerardi et al. also demonstrated that postrehabilitation 12-minute walk was a strong predictor of survival and much better than arterial partial pressure of oxygen (PaO_2), partial pressure of carbon dioxide ($PaCO_2$), FEV_1, and/or nutritional status (156). Thus, exercise tolerance is extremely important for predicting survival.

Exercise training programs have evolved from simple endurance training to now incorporating multiple exercise modalities. Endurance training is still the mainstay of most PR programs along with continuous aerobic training (CAT), which is based upon doing increasingly longer periods of progressively intensive exercise in order to achieve muscle training and endurance (142). For patients with profound dyspnea, there is potential to improve endurance using low-intensity CAT or to use interval training (IT). Although the benefits of low-intensity CAT may not be as robust, they still make a difference for COPD patients (157), and IT is now showing that it may actually be even more beneficial than CAT for many patients (158). For postexercise training maintenance, a new approach has been to encourage patients to maintain a minimum number of steps per day (159). Walking on a treadmill or in the community and cycle ergometry are two of the most common CAT modalities. Increases in leisure and community walking for patients with pulmonary disease translate into ongoing benefits that may be superior to cycle ergometry. At 6 and 9 months after a 3-month PR program, there were more benefits from walking than from cycle ergometry (160). When a patient has a higher level of function, more traditional techniques of exercise prescription can be used, basing the intensity of the CAT program on a cardiopulmonary exercise test (CPET) and using the ventilatory anaerobic threshold (VAT) for a target intensity. The ventilatory threshold is the point at which there is a respiratory compensation for the onset of lactic acidosis and in healthy individuals is a good target exercise intensity. In patients with severe lung disease who cannot reach VAT, exercise intensity is often closer to their peak capacity but still results in benefit. Indeed, a target intensity set at 60% to 70% of one's peak intensity can be effective. Thus, moderate to severely affected COPD patients perform exercise training successfully at intensity levels that represent higher percentages of their maximum physiologic capacities than typically recommended for unaffected individuals (161). For example, exercise performed at a heart rate target set at ventilation levels of 37.5 times the FEV_1 (16) can increase exercise ventilation and sustain it at a high percentage of MVV. With training, patients can exceed the levels attained during initial exercise testing (99). For example, 34 patients in one study got to walk at a work level of 86% of their baseline maximum for a mean duration of 22 minutes (99). Carter et al. also trained patients at near their ventilatory limits and reported mean peak exercise ventilation of 94% to 100% of measured MVV (162). Training above the VAT leads to a reduced ventilatory requirement during exercise and, therefore, improved maximum exercise tolerance (162). At home walking programs can be based on a program with a 5-minute warm-up and cooldown around 20 to 40 minutes of exercise at target intensities (142). Use of the Borg rating of perceived exertion, heart rate, and walking speed have all been used to monitor intensity and progress.

Innovation in exercise in PR has started to include IT, which has been shown to be more effective than CAT over the same time period when used by athletes. Benefits of IT have also been reported in COPD on quality of life, dyspnea, exercise capacity, and skeletal muscle adaptation to exercise. However, most studies have not included high-intensity interval training (HIIT) for patient populations (163,164). If programs of HIIT were to be applied to patients with pulmonary conditions, they might also achieve the greater benefits than with CAT as has been seen in heart failure populations (165).

RT is another important component of PR programs. Just as it helps frail patients with other conditions, RT appears to be beneficial for patients with COPD and other lung conditions as well (166). An issue with CAT is that there is usually little increase in muscle mass. The addition of RT to the exercise program of patients with pulmonary disease can increase muscle mass in this vulnerable, deconditioned, and inactive population, which in addition may be receiving long-term glucocorticoid therapy (167,168). Since the optimal dosage of resistance exercise for patients with COPD and other lung disease is not clear, the usual practice is to use the recommendation of the American Academy of Sports Medicine, which suggests 1 to 3 sets of 8 to 12 repetitions undertaken 2 to 3 days each week (169). Initial loads in RT are at 60% to 70% of a one repetition maximum and can be gradually increased as the patient strengthens. The addition of RT to CAT for patients with COPD has been demonstrated to increased muscle mass and strength but not add additional endurance capacity. However, the additional strength can assist patients with ADL including stair and hill climbing with decreased fatigue (170).

Upper limb training is an important component of PR programs since so many patients have upper limb weakness combined with deconditioning and dyspnea that lead to severe disability (171). Upper limb training includes a combination of CAT using upper body ergometry (UBE) and RT. The muscle groups that are focused on include the biceps, triceps, deltoids, latissimus dorsi, and pectorals. These training programs improve arm function and strength (172). Unsupported upper extremity activities range from typing, lifting, reaching, and carrying to athletic activities and personal daily care (eating, grooming, cleaning). Unsupported arm exercise shifts work to the diaphragm, leading to earlier fatigue (173). In a randomized controlled trial comparing supported arm exercise with unsupported arm exercise within a general rehabilitation program for COPD patients, the group performing the unsupported upper extremity exercise demonstrated significantly greater improvements and reduced O_2 consumption during upper extremity exercise than the supported upper extremity exercise group (174). Other studies have substantiated the greater benefits to be derived from unsupported exercise (173–177).

Another component of the PR exercise program is the inclusion of flexibility training. There are no clear studies demonstrating functional improvement from it; however, there may be some benefit in increasing pulmonary compliance and vital capacity (178). Flexibility training may also help to lessen the risk of musculoskeletal injuries in this sedentary population that has often been on corticosteroids and thus may be at increased risk of musculotendinous injuries.

For very disabled patients with COPD, there may be a benefit to the use of neuromuscular electrical stimulation (NMES) as it can provide training that does not increase dyspnea and may preserve and increase muscular function (179). NMES can increase limb muscle strength, exercise capacity, and decrease dyspnea for patients with severe COPD and can be done even during acute exacerbations (180). NMES can also be used in addition to traditional mobilization and CAT for additional benefits in mobility (181,182) and may decrease the risk of critical illness myopathy for critical care patients (183). For patients with severe debility, in a hospital setting or with severe limitations, NMES may prove beneficial in addition to traditional exercise modalities. It is unclear if there are any additional benefits for more mobile or only moderately impaired individuals (1).

PR has been studied to a lesser extent for conditions other than COPD but has been reported to be beneficial. This is likely due to the fact that most patients with a primary pulmonary disease labor under similar limitations and can benefit in similar fashion to PR. In interstitial lung disease (ILD), exercise intolerance is a hallmark of the condition with marked hypoxemia and dyspnea on exertion. The exercise limitations result from altered ventilatory mechanics as well as impaired gas exchange and pulmonary arterial hypertension (PAH) (184). There is also a prevalence of peripheral muscle dysfunction (185) as well as fatigue from chronic severe hypoxemia (186). Recent studies have shown short-term improvements in exercise tolerance, dyspnea, and quality of life in ILD (187,188). Similarly, CF patients have been reported to benefit from PR including demonstrating improved pulmonary toilet and secretion management. In CF, higher levels of physical activity, exercise capacity, and quality of life correlated with improved long-term outcomes (189) and participation in exercise (190).

For PAH, the role of PR has increased as the survival of patients has improved with the advent of vasodilator therapy. The primary limitation to exercise in patients with PAH is pulmonary vascular resistance and right heart failure. Patients also develop peripheral muscle dysfunction as well as deconditioning (191). Recent studies have demonstrated that patients with PAH can benefit from PR programs with increases in exercise capacity and symptom relief (192). The optimal dosage for training programs is not yet established, but avoidance of high level RT and IT with the use of CAT seems to be the most common strategy at this point (193).

PR is also an integral component of the preparation of patients for lung volume reduction surgery (LVRS) or lung transplantation as noted from outcomes of the National Emphysema Treatment Trial (NETT) (194). PR was shown to be safe and effective in improving exercise tolerance, quality of life, and dyspnea for this population of severely impaired COPD patients (195). The program for rehabilitation prior to LVRS is similar to a classical PR program for COPD with a focus on endurance and strength training as well as education geared toward the LVRS surgery. After LVRS, PR is targeted at restoration of function and improving exercise capacity since the mechanics of breathing were improved (196). For lung transplantation, there is a similar benefit from PR (197). A key additional component of PR for lung transplantation is the education of patients in posttransplant medication and lifestyle changes. An additional role in the pretransplant patient is in maintaining muscle strength and function in order for the patient to be strong enough to undergo the transplant as there is often a long wait for an acceptable donor organ (198). At the time of transplantation, an aggressive perioperative mobilization program and PR after discharge can help to improve function and alleviate muscle weakness due to transplant medications (199). Thus, PR can benefit patients before and after lung transplantation (200).

Role for Behavioral Management in Pulmonary Rehabilitation

Although it is beyond the scope of this chapter to go into too much detail regarding the full range of behavioral modifications that can be used for patients with pulmonary disease, it is an important component of PR to address psychosocial issues, self-efficacy, and lifestyle changes. In particular, smoking cessation is an essential component for any PR program. A favorite quote from a colleague was that "treating a patient with COPD who continued to smoke was like bailing water on the Titanic." In addition to controlling adverse behaviors, it is also important to establish better health behaviors and to facilitate patients regaining control over their condition and disease management (201). The focus of education in the PR program includes learning about their disease, medications, and health behaviors and also adaptive techniques and collaborative self-management. The program has four components: (a) changing cognitions, (b) enhancement of self-efficacy, (c) addressing motivational issues, and (d) collaborative self-management. Changing cognitions requires the patient to learn to control emotional responses to their disease by improving understanding of it. For example, dyspnea during exercise may trigger an emotional response to "suffocating." This occurs because the sensation of dyspnea with exertion is similar to the experience of dyspnea during a severe intercurrent exacerbation. By learning that not all dyspnea is the same, they can cognitively control the anxiety response to the sensation of dyspnea with exercise so that panic does not occur (202,203).

For enhancement of self-efficacy, it is essential for the patient to learn that they play the most important role for optimizing and maintaining their health. When they assume this control, they are more effective at adapting new health behaviors. Essentially, this is converting the patient from a passive bystander to an active agent in their own disease management. The strategies to help implement this include the use of mastery experiences, explicit experiences from other patients (in peer support groups), social persuasion, and positive mood. The peer support group is essential here as it allows patients to transfer their experiences and support other patients (204,205). Addressing motivational issues is also essential since the enrollment in PR requires a patient commitment. Determining goals that are meaningful can help tremendously and can keep a patient participating through an exacerbation or other challenge (204).

Finally, collaborative self-management is essentially training the patient in self-management with the support of the entire PR rehabilitation team. The key components of successful self-management programs include goal setting, problem solving, decision-making, and developing action plans. Collaborative self-management plans are custom tailored to each patient and their needs while taking into account available support systems and clinical resources. The benefits of self-efficacy can be seen in reduced health care utilization (206) and decreased hospitalizations (207).

Physical Aids

Wheelchairs and other assistive equipment are covered elsewhere in this text (see Chapters 55 and 58). However, certain aids like motorized scooters and rolling walkers (rollators with seats) can greatly improve function and quality of life for COPD patients. Rollators were reported to be effective in improving functional exercise capacity by reducing dyspnea and permitting rest periods for stable individuals with severe COPD (208,209). Those who walked less than 300 m and those who required a rest during an unaided 6-minute walk benefited the most by reduced dyspnea, reduced rest time, and improved distance walked. Hospital beds with an overhead trapeze, reachers, elevated toilet seats, and strategically placed hand rails at home can also be very useful.

The Results of Pulmonary Rehabilitation

When evaluating the efficacy of PR for patients with primary pulmonary disease, it is essential to keep the focus on patient-centered outcomes as well as outcomes on survival and exercise capacity. PR clearly benefits symptoms, quality of life, and exercise performance (142,210). The most important benefits are demonstrated by a minimally clinical important difference (MCID) when compared to before PR and that can be maintained long term (1). There are many questionnaires and scales that are currently used and are either generic (e.g., 36-item Short Form Health Survey [SF-36]) or more specific (e.g., Chronic Respiratory Questionnaire) that allow for comparison of the efficacy of treatments and interventions. We will review the specific benefits of PR in both patient-centered and classical realms.

Quality of life is definitively improved for patients with COPD and in other conditions. The most commonly used questionnaires are the St. George's Respiratory Questionnaire (SGRQ) (211) and the Chronic Respiratory Questionnaire (CRQ) (212,213). Dyspnea is also measured by several specific instruments and can be assessed in either the short term (Borg scale) or in situational measures (Baseline Dyspnea Index [BDI]) or impact measures (Chronic Respiratory Questionnaire [CRQ]). Depression and anxiety are also assessed in commonly employed instruments (e.g., components of the SGRQ).

Functional assessment is usually done with self-rating or by observing function while performing every day activities. Examples of these functional measures include the Manchester Respiratory Activities of Daily Living Scale (214) and the pulmonary Functional Status and Dyspnea Questionnaire (215). These instruments include direct assessment of physical capacity and performance. A most common measure is the 6-minute walk test (6MWT) (216) as well as the Cardiopulmonary Exercise Test (CPET) (1,217). Field tests such as the 6MWT are very useful in population-based assessments because they are inexpensive and easily applied. For more advanced evaluations the CPET may be more helpful, especially in more complex patients or for studies including physiologic parameters. Overall physical activity is also an important indicator of physical recovery and can be assessed with either subjective reporting, measures of energy expenditure, or through activity monitors (218). Finally, self-efficacy, or the ability to manage their condition, is a patient-centered outcome that assesses the effectiveness of the educational and psychological portions of the PR program. Other validated tools for these assessments include the Lung Information Needs Questionnaire (LINQ) (219). In an attempt to have an assessment that includes several measures in a simple and comprehensive assessment, the latest trend has been the creation of composite indices. The best known of these is the BODE Index for COPD (220). The benefits of the composite index are the combination of reported self-function, airflow obstruction, body mass index, and the functional measure in the form of the 6MWT. It has been shown to have predictive validity both for clinical outcomes and for mortality.

In a review of 48 PR studies that included exercise reconditioning, exercise tolerance improved significantly in all 48, including in 14 controlled studies (22). Exercise capacity improved significantly (proportionally) in patients with mild or advanced (hypercapnic) disease (221) with consistent decreases in the ventilatory equivalent, increases in work efficiency, exercise tolerance, ambulation capacity, general well-being, and dyspnea tolerance. The patients developed better performance strategies and greater confidence in performing the tests. Blood lactate levels were also observed to decrease in combination with higher VO_{2max}, implying a physiologic training effect as well as improved motivation and effort. Exercise dose was important with better results from higher intensity programs and for proportionally longer periods (142,210,222). Twenty-session outpatient programs had better outcomes than did 10-session programs (223). Even minimally supervised home exercise programs can result in improved health status (224).

In general, peak performance appeared to be reached in 26 to 51 weeks and lasted for as long as 5 years (210,222,225–227). Quality-of-life measures (22,228–230), hospitalization rates, postoperative pulmonary complications (231), and physical functioning were reported to be significantly improved in the majority of both the controlled and the repetitive measure studies (22). Outcomes were equivalent for inpatient and outpatient programs with many of the outpatient programs predominantly home based. Pulmonary function parameters, such as FEV_1, did not significantly improve in 31 of 35 studies (22).

Thus, virtually all studies indicate that PR with exercise training results in significant increases in ambulation capacity and exercise endurance for COPD and other lung disease patients (232). The often-reported decreased resting O_2 consumption and CO_2 production may, at least in part, account for the significant decrease in perception of dyspnea, the general increase in functional performance, and in the often-found improved sense of well-being. Indeed, a recent Cochrane meta-analysis of PR in COPD (233) concluded that "Rehabilitation relieves dyspnea and fatigue, improves emotional function, and enhances patients' control over their condition. These improvements are moderately large and clinically significant. Rehabilitation forms an important component of the management of COPD." Thus, hypercapnia is not a contraindication

to intensive rehabilitation as it can actually improve with exercise, and the use of rigorous reconditioning exercise does not precipitate respiratory muscle fatigue in this population (221). PR is even beneficial for bedridden ventilator-dependent COPD patients.

Although mortality risk is not altered, the majority of surviving patients can be successfully weaned from mechanical ventilation (27) with better 6MWT distances and mean inspiratory pressures.

Following the acute rehabilitation period, continued surveillance and attention to abstinence from smoking, bronchial hygiene, breathing retraining, physical reconditioning, O_2 therapy, and airway secretion mobilization have been shown to reduce hospital admissions, the length of hospital stays, and cost (234). As noted, the benefits of PR on exercise performance and quality of life can persist for up to 5 years (210,222,225,226,235–238). Pulmonary function parameters, dyspnea, exercise tolerance, and quality of life are not further improved long term by yearly repeated 2-month outpatient PR interventions, but rates of hospitalizations and acute exacerbations are further decreased by repeated interventions (239). The principles of PR for COPD are being increasingly applied to patients with asthma with similar outcomes (240), and PR is now recommended for other pulmonary conditions as well (1).

REFERENCES

1. ATS/ERS Task Force on Pulmonary Rehabilitation. An official American Thoracic Society/European Respiratory Society Statement: key concepts and advances in pulmonary rehabilitation. *Am J Respir Crit Care Med.* 2013;188(8):e13–e64.
2. Halbert RJ, Isonaka S, George D, et al. Interpreting COPD prevalence estimates: what is the true burden of disease. *Chest.* 2003;123:1684–1692.
3. Higgins ITT. Epidemiology of bronchitis and emphysema. In: Fishman AP, ed. *Pulmonary Diseases and Disorders.* 2nd ed. New York: McGraw-Hill; 1988:70–90.
4. Groenewegen KH, Schols AMWJ, Wouters EFM. Mortality and mortality-related factors after hospitalization for acute exacerbation of COPD. *Chest.* 2003;124:459–467.
5. Burrows B. An overview of obstructive lung diseases. *Med Clin N Am.* 1981;65:455–471.
6. Rabe KF, Hurd S, Anzueto A, et al. Global Initiative for Chronic Obstructive Lung Disease. Global strategy for the diagnosis, management, and prevention of chronic obstructive pulmonary disease: GOLD executive summary. *Am J Respir Crit Care Med.* 2007;176:532–555.
7. John M, Hoernig S, Dochner W, et al. Anemia and inflammation in COPD. *Chest.* 2005;127:825–829.
8. Holden DA, Stelmach KD, Curtis PS, et al. The impact of a rehabilitation program on functional status of patients with chronic lung disease. *Respir Care.* 1990;35:332–341.
9. Mahler DA, Weinberg DH, Wells CK, et al. The measurement of dyspnea: contents, interobserver agreement, and physiologic correlates of two new clinical indexes. *Chest.* 1984;85:751–758.
10. Moser K, Bokinsky G, Savage R, et al. Results of a comprehensive rehabilitation program: physiologic and functional effects on patients with chronic obstructive pulmonary disease. *Arch Intern Med.* 1980;140:1596–1601.
11. Stoller JK, Ferranti R, Feinstein AR. Further specification and evaluation of a new clinical index for dyspnea. *Am Rev Respir Dis.* 1986;134:1129–1134.
12. Lewis MI. Nutrition and chronic obstructive pulmonary disease: a clinical overview. In: Bach JR, ed. *Pulmonary Rehabilitation: The Obstructive and Paralytic Conditions.* Philadelphia, PA: Hanley & Belfus; 1996:156–172.
13. Stokes DC, Wohl MEB, Khaw KT, et al. Postural hypoxemia in cystic fibrosis. *Chest.* 1985;87:785–791.
14. Flick MR, Block AJ. Continuous in-vivo monitoring of arterial oxygenation in chronic obstructive lung disease. *Ann Intern Med.* 1977;86:725–730.
15. Jones NL. Current concepts: new tests to assess lung function. *N Engl J Med.* 1975;293:541–544.
16. Jones NL, Campbell EJM. *Clinical Exercise Testing.* 2nd ed. Philadelphia, PA: W.B. Saunders; 1982:158.
17. Reina-Rosenbaum R, Bach JR, Penek J. The cost/benefits of outpatient based pulmonary rehabilitation. *Arch Phys Med Rehabil.* 1997;78:240–244.
18. Goldstein RS. Supplemental oxygen in chronic respiratory disease. In: Bach JR, ed. *Pulmonary Rehabilitation: The Obstructive and Paralytic Conditions.* Philadelphia, PA: Hanley & Belfus; 1996:55–84.

19. Fujimoto K, Matsuzawa Y, Yamaguchi S, et al. Benefits of oxygen on exercise performance and pulmonary hemodynamics in patients with COPD with mild hypoxemia. *Chest.* 2002;122:457–463.

20. Carlson DJ, Ries AL, Kaplan RM. Prediction of maximum exercise tolerance in patients with COPD. *Chest.* 1991;100:307–311.

21. Guyatt GH, Thompson PJ, Berman LB, et al. How should we measure function in patients with chronic heart and lung disease? *J Chronic Dis.* 1985;38:517–524.

22. Bach JR. *The Effectiveness of Pulmonary Rehabilitation.* Washington, DC: Report to the Office of Civilian Health and Medical Programs for the Uniform Services; 1995.

23. Guilmette TJ, Motta SI, Shadel WG, et al. Promoting smoking cessation in the rehabilitation setting. *Am J Phys Med Rehabil.* 2001;80:560–562.

24. Hernandez MTE, Rubio TM, Ruiz FO, et al. Results of a home-based training program for patients with COPD. *Chest.* 2000;118:106–114.

25. Finnerty JP, Keeping I, Bullough I, et al. The effectiveness of outpatient pulmonary rehabilitation in chronic lung disease: a randomized controlled trial. *Chest.* 2001;119:1705–1710.

26. Votto J, Bowen J, Scalise P, et al. Short-stay comprehensive inpatient pulmonary rehabilitation for advanced chronic obstructive pulmonary disease. *Arch Phys Med Rehabil.* 1996;77:1115–1118.

27. Nava S. Rehabilitation of patients admitted to a respirator intensive care unit. *Arch Phys Med Rehabil.* 1998;79:849–854.

28. De Blaquiere P, Christensen DB, Carter WB, et al. Use and misuse of metered-dose inhalers by patients with chronic lung disease. *Am Rev Respir Dis.* 1989;140:910–916.

29. Nicotra MB, Rivera M, Awe RJ. Antibiotic therapy of acute exacerbations of chronic bronchitis: a controlled study using tetracycline. *Ann Intern Med.* 1982;97:18–21.

30. Zuin R, Palamidese A, et al. High-dose N-acetylcysteine in patients with exacerbations of chronic obstructive pulmonary disease. *Clin Drug Investig.* 2005;25:401–408.

31. Haas A, Pineda H, Haas F, et al. *Pulmonary Therapy and Rehabilitation: Principles and Practice.* Baltimore, MD: Williams & Wilkins; 1979;124–125.

32. Kahn AU. Effectiveness of biofeedback and counter conditioning in the treatment of bronchial asthma. *J Psychosom Res.* 1977;21:97–104.

33. Light RW, Marrill EJ, Despars JA, et al. Prevalence of depression and anxiety in patients with COPD: relationships to functional capacity. *Chest.* 1985;87:35–38.

34. Dudley DL, Glaser EM, Jorgenson BN, et al. Psychosocial concomitants in chronic obstructive pulmonary disease II: psychosocial treatment. *Chest.* 1980;77:544–551.

35. Dolce JJ, Crisp C, Manzella B, et al. Medication adherence patterns in chronic obstructive pulmonary disease. *Chest.* 1991;99:837–841.

36. Stoller JK. Travel for the technology-dependent individual. *Respir Care.* 1994;39:347–362.

37. Annemie M, Schols WJ, Soeters PB, et al. Prevalence and characteristics of nutritional depletion in patients with stable COPD eligible for pulmonary rehabilitation. *Am Rev Respir Dis.* 1993;147:1151–1156.

38. Laaban J-P, Kouchakji B, Dore M-F, et al. Nutritional status of patients with chronic obstructive pulmonary disease and acute respiratory failure. *Chest.* 1993;103:1362–1368.

39. Mohsenin V, Ferranti R, Loke JS. Nutrition for the respiratory insufficient patient. *Eur Respir J.* 1989;2:663s–665s.

40. Niederman MS, Merrill WW, Ferranti RD, et al. Nutritional status and bacterial binding in the lower respiratory tract in patients with chronic tracheostomy. *Ann Intern Med.* 1984;100:795–800.

41. Frankfort JD, Fischer CE, Stansbury DW, et al. Effects of high- and low-carbohydrate meals on maximum exercise performance in chronic airflow obstruction. *Chest.* 1991;100:792–795.

42. Memsic L, Silberman AW, Silberman H. Malnutrition and respiratory distress: who's at risk. *J Respir Dis.* 1990;11:529–535.

43. Juan G, Calverley P, Talamo C. Effect of carbon dioxide on diaphragmatic function in human beings. *N Engl J Med.* 1984;310:874–877.

44. Whittaker JS, Ryan CR, Buckley PA, et al. The effects of refeeding on peripheral and respiratory muscle function in malnourished chronic obstructive pulmonary disease patients. *Am Rev Respir Dis.* 1990;142:283–288.

45. Ferreira IM, Brooks D, Lacasse Y, et al. Nutritional intervention in COPD: a systematic overview. *Chest.* 2001;119:353–363.

46. Yeh SS, DeGuzman B, Kramer T, et al. Reversal of COPD-associated weight loss using the anabolic agent oxandrolone. *Chest.* 2002;122:421–428.

47. Creutzberg EC, Wouters EFM, Mostert R, et al. A role for anabolic steroids in the rehabilitation of patients with COPD? A double-blind, placebo-controlled, randomized trial. *Chest.* 2003;124:1733–1742.

48. Fartinez FJ, Couser JI, Celli BR. Factors influencing ventilatory muscle recruitment in patients with chronic airflow obstruction. *Am Rev Respir Dis.* 1990;142:276–282.

49. Haas A, Pineda H, Haas F, et al. *Pulmonary Therapy and Rehabilitation: Principles and Practice.* Baltimore, MD: Williams & Wilkins; 1979;128–131.

50. Mueller RE, Petty TL, Filley GE. Ventilation and arterial blood gas changes induced by pursed-lip breathing. *J Appl Physiol.* 1970;28:784–789.

51. Kirilloff LH, Owens GR, Rogers RM, et al. Does chest physical therapy work? *Chest.* 1985;88:436–444.

52. Schoi MH. Autogenic drainage: a modern approach to physiotherapy in cystic fibrosis. *J R Soc Med.* 1989;82(suppl 16):32–37.

53. Menkes HA, Traystman RJ. State of the art: collateral ventilation. *Am Rev Respir Dis.* 1977;116:287–309.

54. Peters RM. Pulmonary physiologic studies of the perioperative period. *Chest.* 1979;76:576–584.

55. Falk M, Kelstrup M, Andersen JB, et al. Improving the ketchup bottle method with positive expiratory pressure, PEP: a controlled study in patients with cystic fibrosis. *Eur J Respir Dis.* 1984;65:57–66.

56. Hofmeyer JL, Webber BA, Hodson ME. Evaluation of positive expiratory pressure as an adjunct to chest physiotherapy in the treatment of cystic fibrosis. *Thorax.* 1986;41:951–954.

57. Mortensen J, Falk M, Groth S, et al. The effects of postural drainage and positive expiratory pressure physiotherapy on tracheobronchial clearance in cystic fibrosis. *Chest.* 1991;100:1350–1357.

58. Tyrrell JC, Hiller EJ, Martin J. Face mask physiotherapy in cystic fibrosis. *Arch Dis Child.* 1986;61:598–611.

59. van Asperen PP, Jackson L, Hennessy P, et al. Comparison of positive expiratory pressure (PEP) mask with postural drainage in patients with cystic fibrosis. *Aust Paediatr J.* 1987;23:283–284.

60. van der Schans CP, van der Mark TW, de Vries G, et al. Effect of positive expiratory pressure breathing in patients with cystic fibrosis. *Thorax.* 1991;46:252–256.

61. Lagerkvist AL, Sten GM, Redfors SB, et al. Immediate changes in blood-gas tensions during chest physiotherapy with positive expiratory pressure and oscillating positive expiratory pressure in patients with cystic fibrosis. *Respir Care.* 2006;51:1154–1161.

62. Placidi G, Cornacchia M, Polese G, et al. Chest physiotherapy with positive airway pressure: a pilot study of short-term effects on sputum clearance in patients with cystic fibrosis and severe airway obstruction. *Respir Care.* 2006;51:1145–1153.

63. Olsni L, Midgren B, Honblad Y, et al. Chest physiotherapy in chronic obstructive pulmonary disease: forced expiratory technique combined with either postural drainage or positive expiratory pressure breathing. *Respir Med.* 1994;88:435–440.

64. Schibler A, Casaulta C, Kraemer R. Rational of oscillatory breathing in patients with cystic fibrosis. *Paediatr Pulmonol.* 1992;8:301S.

65. Konstan MW, Stern RC, Doershuk CF. Efficacy of the Flutter device for airway mucus clearance in patients with cystic fibrosis. *J Pediatr.* 1994;124:689–693.

66. Pryor JA, Webber BA, Hodson ME, et al. The Flutter VRP1 as an adjunct to chest physiotherapy in cystic fibrosis. *Respir Med.* 1994;88:677–681.

67. Bellone A, Lascioli R, Raschi S, et al. Chest physical therapy in patients with acute exacerbation of chronic bronchitis: effectiveness of three methods. *Arch Phys Med Rehabil.* 2000;81:558–560.

68. Wolkove N, Kamel H, Rotaple M, et al. Use of a mucus clearance device enhances the bronchodilator response in patients with stable COPD. *Chest.* 2002;121:702–707.

69. Wijkstra PJ, Lacasse Y, Guyatt GH, et al. Nocturnal non-invasive positive pressure ventilation for stable chronic obstructive pulmonary disease. *Cochrane Database Syst Rev.* 2002;(3):CD002878.

70. King M, Phillips DM, Gross D, et al. Enhanced tracheal mucus clearance with high frequency chest wall compression. *Am Rev Respir Dis.* 1983;128:511–515.

71. Radford R, Barutt J, Billingsley JG, et al. A rational basis for percussion augmented mucociliary clearance. *Respir Care.* 1982;27:556–563.

72. Rubin EM, Scantlen GE, Chapman GA, et al. Effect of chest wall oscillation on mucus clearance: comparison of two vibrators. *Pediatr Pulmonol.* 1989;6:123–127.

73. Flower KA, Eden RI, Lomax L, et al. New mechanical aid to physiotherapy in cystic fibrosis. *BMJ.* 1979;2:630–631.

74. Chang HK, Weber ME, King M. Mucus transport by high frequency nonsymmetrical airflow. *J Appl Physiol.* 1988;65:1203–1209.

75. Warwick WJ, Hansen LG. The long-term effect of high-frequency chest compression therapy on pulmonary complications of cystic fibrosis. *Pediatr Pulmonol.* 1991;11:265–271.

76. Christensen EF, Nedergaard T, Dahl R. Long-term treatment of chronic bronchitis with positive expiratory pressure mask and chest physiotherapy. *Chest.* 1990;97:645–650.

77. Holody B, Goldberg HS. The effect of mechanical vibration physiotherapy on arterial oxygenation in acutely ill patients with atelectasis or pneumonia. *Am Rev Respir Dis.* 1981;124:372–375.

78. Piquet J, Brochard L, Isabey D, et al. High frequency chest wall oscillation in patients with chronic air-flow obstruction. *Am Rev Respir Dis.* 1987;136:1355–1359.

79. Sibuya M, Yamada M, Kanamaru A, et al. Effect of chest wall vibration on dyspnea in patients with chronic respiratory disease. *Am J Respir Crit Care Med.* 1994;149:1235–1240.

80. Pryor JA, Parker RA, Webber BA. A comparison of mechanical and manual percussion as adjuncts to postural drainage in the treatment of cystic fibrosis in adolescents and adults. *Physiotherapy.* 1981;6:140–141.

81. Sutton PP, Parker RA, Webber BA, et al. Assessment of the forced expiration technique, postural drainage and directed coughing in chest physiotherapy. *Eur J Respir Dis.* 1983;64:62–68.

82. van Hengstum M, Festen J, Beurskens C, et al. No effect of oral high frequency oscillation combined with forced expiration maneuvers on tracheobronchial clearance in chronic bronchitis. *Eur Respir J.* 1990;3:14–18.

83. van der Schans CP, Piers DA, Postma DS. Effect of manual percussion on tracheobronchial clearance in patients with chronic airflow obstruction and excessive tracheobronchial secretions. *Thorax.* 1986;41:448–452.

84. Campbell AH, O'Connell JM, Wilson F. The effect of chest physiotherapy upon the FEV_1 in chronic bronchitis. *Med J Aust.* 1975;1:33–35.

85. Zapletal A, Stefanova J, Horak J, et al. Chest physiotherapy and airway obstruction in patients with cystic fibrosis—a negative report. *Eur J Respir Dis.* 1983;64:426–433.

86. Zidulka A, Chrome JF, Wight DW, et al. Clapping or percussion causes atelectasis in dogs and influences gas exchange. *J Appl Physiol.* 1989;66:2833–2838.

87. Toussaint M, De Win H, Steens M, et al. A new technique in secretion clearance by the percussionaire for patients with neuromuscular disease. In: Robert D, Leger P, eds. *Programme des journées internationales de ventilation à domicile*. Lyon, France: Hopital de la Croix Rousse; 1993:27(abst).

88. Thangathuria D, Holm AP, Mikhail M, et al. HFV in management of a patient with severe bronchorrhea. *Respir Manage*. 1988;1:31–33.

89. McInturff SL, Shaw LI, Hodgkin JE, et al. Intrapulmonary percussive ventilation in the treatment of COPD. *Respir Care*. 1985;30:885.

90. Toussaint M, Steens M, Wasteels G, et al. Diurnal ventilation via mouthpiece: survival in end-stage Duchenne patients. *Eur Respir J*. 2006;28:549.

91. Patterson JM, Budd J, Goetz D, et al. Family correlates of a 10-year pulmonary health trend in cystic fibrosis. *Pediatrics*. 1993;91:383–389.

92. Currie DC, Munro C, Gaskell D, et al. Practice, problems and compliance with postural drainage: a survey of chronic sputum producers. *Br J Dis Chest*. 1986;80:249–253.

93. Passero MA, Remor B, Salomon J. Patient-reported compliance with cystic fibrosis therapy. *Clin Pediatr (Phila)*. 1981;20:264–268.

94. Fong SL, Dales RE, Tierney MG. Compliance among adults with cystic fibrosis. *DICP*. 1990;24:689–692.

95. Pardy RL, Reid WD, Belman MJ. Respiratory muscle training. *Clin Chest Med*. 1989;9:287–295.

96. Belman MJ. Exercise in chronic obstructive pulmonary disease. *Clin Chest Med*. 1986;7:585–597.

97. Nield MA. Inspiratory muscle training protocol using a pressure threshold device: effect on dyspnea in chronic obstructive pulmonary disease. *Arch Phys Med Rehabil*. 1999;80:100–102.

98. Levine S, Weiser P, Gillen J. Evaluation of a ventilatory muscle endurance training program in the rehabilitation of patients with chronic obstructive pulmonary disease. *Am Rev Respir Dis*. 1986;133:400–406.

99. Ries AL, Moser KM. Comparison of isocapnic hyperventilation and walking exercise training at home in pulmonary rehabilitation. *Chest*. 1986;90:285–289.

100. Aldrich TK. Inspiratory muscle training in COPD. In: Bach JR, ed. *Pulmonary Rehabilitation: The Obstructive and Paralytic Conditions*. Philadelphia, PA: Hanley & Belfus; 1996:285–301.

101. Pardy RL, Rivington RM, Despas PJ, et al. Effects of inspiratory muscle training on exercise performance in chronic airflow limitation. *Am Rev Respir Dis*. 1981;123:426–433.

102. Sawyer EH, Clanton TL. Improved pulmonary function and exercise tolerance with inspiratory muscle conditioning in children with cystic fibrosis. *Chest*. 1993;104:490–497.

103. Weiner P, Azgad Y, Weiner M. Inspiratory muscle training during treatment with corticosteroids in humans. *Chest*. 1995;107:1041–1044.

104. Weiner P, Magadle R, Berar-Yanay N, et al. The cumulative effect of long-acting bronchodilators, exercise, and inspiratory muscle training on the perception of dyspnea in patients with advanced COPD. *Chest*. 2000;118:672–678.

105. Magadle R, McConnell AK, Beckerman M, et al. Inspiratory muscle training in pulmonary rehabilitation program in COPD patients. *Respir Med*. 2007;101:1500–1505.

106. Weiner P, Azgad Y, Ganam R, et al. Inspiratory muscle training in patients with bronchial asthma. *Chest*. 1992;102:1357–1361.

107. Braun NMT, Faulkner J, Hughes RL, et al. When should respiratory muscles be exercised? *Chest*. 1983;84:76–83.

108. Hill NS. Home noninvasive ventilation in patients with lung disease. In: Bach JR, ed. *Noninvasive Mechanical Ventilation*. Philadelphia, PA: Hanley & Belfus; 2002:241–258.

109. Bach JR, Penek J. Obstructive sleep apnea complicating negative pressure ventilatory support in patients with chronic paralytic/restrictive ventilatory dysfunction. *Chest*. 1991;99:1386–1393.

110. Levy RD, Bradley TD, Newman SL, et al. Negative pressure ventilation: effects on ventilation during sleep in normal subjects. *Chest*. 1989;65:95–99.

111. Elliott MW. Noninvasive ventilation: mechanisms of action. In: Bach JR, ed. *Noninvasive Mechanical Ventilation*. Philadelphia, PA: Hanley & Belfus; 2002:73–82.

112. Belman MJ, Soo Hoo GW, Kuei JH, et al. Efficacy of positive vs negative pressure ventilation in unloading the respiratory muscles. *Chest*. 1990;98:850–856.

113. Marino W. Intermittent volume cycled mechanical ventilation via nasal mask in patients with respiratory failure due to COPD. *Chest*. 1991;99:681–684.

114. Meduri GU, Abou-Shala N, Fox RC, et al. Noninvasive face mask mechanical ventilation in patients with acute hypercapnic respiratory failure. *Chest*. 1991;100:445–454.

115. Sivasothy P, Smith IE, Shneerson JM. Mask intermittent positive pressure ventilation in chronic hypercapnic respiratory failure due to chronic obstructive pulmonary disease. *Eur Respir J*. 1998;11:34–40.

116. Anton A, Guell R. Home mechanical ventilation: do we know when and how to use it? *Chest*. 2000;118:1525–1526.

117. Janssens JP, de Muralt B, Titelion V. Management of dyspnea in severe chronic obstructive pulmonary disease. *J Pain Symptom Manage*. 2000;19:378–392.

118. Krachman SL, Quaranta AJ, Berger TJ, et al. Effects of noninvasive positive pressure ventilation on gas exchange and sleep in COPD patients. *Chest*. 1997;112:623–628.

119. Sturani EC, Porta R, Scarduelli C, et al. Outcome of COPD patients performing nocturnal non-invasive mechanical ventilation. *Respir Med*. 1998;92:1215–1222.

120. Casanova C, Celli BR, Tost L, et al. Long-term controlled trial of nocturnal nasal positive pressure ventilation in patients with severe COPD. *Chest*. 2000;118:1582–1590.

121. Hawkins P, Johnson LC, Nikoletou D, et al. Proportional assist ventilation as an aid to exercise training in severe chronic obstructive pulmonary disease. *Thorax*. 2002;57:853–859.

122. Bianchi L, Foglio K, Pagani M, et al. Effects of proportional assist ventilation on exercise tolerance in COPD patients with chronic hypercapnia. *Eur Respir J*. 1998;11:422–427.

123. Maltais F, Reissmann H, Gottfried SB. Pressure support reduces inspiratory effort and dyspnea during exercise in chronic airflow obstruction. *Am J Respir Crit Care Med*. 1995;151:1027–1033.

124. Anthonisen NR. Home oxygen therapy in chronic obstructive pulmonary disease. *Clin Chest Med*. 1986;7:673–677.

125. Nixon PA, Orenstein DM, Curtis SE, et al. Oxygen supplementation during exercise in cystic fibrosis. *Am Rev Respir Dis*. 1990;142:807–811.

126. Bartels MN, Gonzalez JM, Kim W, et al. Oxygen supplementation and cardiac-autonomic modulation in COPD. *Chest*. 2000;118:691–696.

127. Pierson DJ. Current status of home oxygen in the U.S.A. In: Kira S, Petty TL, eds. *Progress in Domiciliary Respiratory Care—Current Status and Perspective*. New York: Elsevier Science BV; 1994:93–98.

128. Sassoon CSH, Hassell KT, Mahutte CK. Hyperoxic-induced hypercapnia in stable chronic obstructive pulmonary disease. *Am Rev Respir Dis*. 1987;135:907–911.

129. D'Urzo AD, Mateika J, Bradley TD, et al. Correlates of arterial oxygenation during exercise in severe chronic obstructive pulmonary disease. *Chest*. 1989;95:13–17.

130. Dyer F, Callaghan J, Cheema K, et al. Ambulatory oxygen improves the effectiveness of pulmonary rehabilitation in selected patients with chronic obstructive pulmonary disease. *Chron Respir Dis*. 2012;9:83–91.

131. Dean NC, Brown JK, Himelman RB, et al. Oxygen may improve dyspnea and endurance in patients with chronic obstructive pulmonary disease and only mild hypoxemia. *Am Rev Respir Dis*. 1992;146:941–945.

132. Bradley BL, Garner AE, Billiu D, et al. Oxygen assisted exercise in chronic obstructive lung disease: the effect on exercise capacity and arterial blood gas tensions. *Am Rev Respir Dis*. 1978;118:239–243.

133. Davidson AC, Leach R, George RID, et al. Supplemental oxygen and exercise ability in chronic obstructive airways disease. *Thorax*. 1988;43:965–971.

134. Somfay A, Porszdsz J, Sang-Moo L, et al. Effect of hyperoxia on gas exchange and lactate kinetics following exercise onset in nonhypoxemic COPD patients. *Chest*. 2002;121:393–400.

135. van Helvoort HA, Heijdra YF, Heunks LM, et al. Supplemental oxygen prevents exercise-induced oxidative stress in muscle-wasted patients with chronic obstructive pulmonary disease. *Am J Respir Crit Care Med*. 2006;173:1122–1129.

136. Marcus CL, Bader D, Stabile MW, et al. Supplemental oxygen and exercise performance in patients with cystic fibrosis with severe pulmonary disease. *Chest*. 1992;101:52–57.

137. Falk B, Nini A, Zigel L, et al. Effect of low altitude at the Dead Sea on exercise capacity and cardiopulmonary response to exercise in cystic fibrosis patients with moderate to severe lung disease. *Pediatr Pulmonol*. 2006;41:234–241.

138. Jolly EC, DiBoscio V, Aguirre L, et al. Effects of supplemental oxygen during activity in patients with advanced COPD without severe resting hypoxemia. *Chest*. 2001;120:437–443.

139. Lewis CA, Eaton TE, Fergusson W, et al. Home overnight pulse oximetry in patients with COPD: more than one recording may be needed. *Chest*. 2003;123:1127–1133.

140. O'Donohue WJ. The future of home oxygen therapy. *Respir Care*. 1988;33:1125–1130.

141. Tiep BL, Christopher KL, Spofford BT, et al. Pulsed nasal and transtracheal oxygen delivery. *Chest*. 1990;97:364–368.

142. Gimenez M, Servera E, Vergara P, et al. Endurance training in patients with chronic obstructive pulmonary disease: a comparison of high versus moderate intensity. *Arch Phys Med Rehabil*. 2000;81:102–109.

143. Sala E, Roca J, Marrades RM, et al. Effects of endurance training on skeletal muscle bioenergetics in chronic obstructive pulmonary disease. *Am J Respir Crit Care Med*. 1999;159:1726–1734.

144. Bernard S, Whittom F, Leblanc P, et al. Aerobic and strength training in patients with chronic obstructive pulmonary disease. *Am J Respir Crit Care Med*. 1999;159:896–901.

145. Maltais F, LeBlanc P, Simard C, et al. Skeletal muscle adaptation to endurance training in patients with chronic obstructive pulmonary disease. *Am J Respir Crit Care Med*. 1996;154:442–447.

146. Griffiths TL, Burr ML, Campbell IA, et al. Results at 1 year of outpatient multidisciplinary pulmonary rehabilitation: a randomised controlled trial. *Lancet*. 2000;355:362–368.

147. Franssen FM, Broekhuizen R, Janssen PP, et al. Effects of whole-body exercise training on body composition and functional capacity in normal-weight patients with COPD. *Chest*. 2004;125:2021–2028.

148. Spruit MA, Gosselink R, Troosters T, et al. Resistance versus endurance training in patients with COPD and peripheral muscle weakness. *Eur Respir J*. 2002;19:1072–1078.

149. Porszasz J, Emtner M, Goto S, et al. Exercise training decreases ventilatory requirements and exercise induced hyperinflation at submaximal intensities in patients with COPD. *Chest*. 2005;128:2025–2034.

150. Maltais F, Simard AA, Simard C, et al. Oxidative capacity of the skeletal muscle and lactic acid kinetics during exercise in normal subjects and in patients with COPD. *Am J Respir Crit Care Med*. 1996;153:288–293.

151. Rochester DF, Braun NM. Determinants of maximal inspiratory pressure in chronic obstructive pulmonary disease. *Am Rev Respir Dis*. 1985;132:42–47.

152. Dantzker DR, D'Alonzo GE. The effect of exercise on pulmonary gas exchange in patients with severe chronic obstructive pulmonary disease. *Am Rev Respir Dis.* 1986;134:1135–1139.

153. Niederman MS, Clemente PH, Fein AM, et al. Benefits of a multidisciplinary pulmonary rehabilitation program: improvements are independent of lung function. *Chest.* 1991;99:798–804.

154. Make BJ, Glenn K. Outcomes of pulmonary rehabilitation. In: Bach JR, ed. *Pulmonary Rehabilitation: the Obstructive and Paralytic/Restrictive Pulmonary Syndromes.* Philadelphia, PA: Hanley & Belfus; 1996:173–191.

155. Brown JB, Votto JJ, Thrall RS, et al. Functional status and survival following pulmonary rehabilitation. *Chest.* 2000;118:697–703.

156. Gerardi DA, Lovett L, Benoit-Connors ML, et al. Variables related to increased mortality following out-patient pulmonary rehabilitation. *Eur Respir J.* 1996;9:431–435.

157. Jenkins S, Hill K, Cecins NM. State of the art: how to set up a pulmonary rehabilitation program. *Respirology.* 2010;15:1157–1173.

158. Vogiatzis I, Nanas S, Roussos C. Interval training as an alternative modality to continuous exercise in patients with COPD. *Eur Respir J.* 2002;20:12–19.

159. de Blok BM, de Greef MH, ten Hacken NH, et al. The effects of a lifestyle physical activity counseling program with feedback of a pedometer during pulmonary rehabilitation in patients with COPD: a pilot study. *Patient Educ Couns.* 2006;61:48–55.

160. Leung RW, Alison JA, McKeough ZJ, et al. Ground walk training improves functional exercise capacity more than cycle training in people with chronic obstructive pulmonary disease (COPD): a randomised trial. *J Physiother.* 2010;56:105–112.

161. Punzal PA, Ries AL, Kaplan RM, et al. Maximum intensity exercise training in patients with chronic obstructive pulmonary disease. *Chest.* 1991;100:618–623.

162. Carter R, Nicotra B, Clark L, et al. Exercise conditioning in the rehabilitation of patients with chronic obstructive pulmonary disease. *Arch Phys Med Rehabil.* 1988;69:118–122.

163. Beauchamp MK, Nonoyama M, Goldstein RS, et al. Interval versus continuous training in individuals with chronic obstructive pulmonary disease—a systematic review. *Thorax.* 2010;65:157–164.

164. Zainuldin R, Mackey MG, Alison JA. Optimal intensity and type of leg exercise training for people with chronic obstructive pulmonary disease. *Cochrane Database Syst Rev.* 2011;(11):CD008008.

165. Wisløff U, Støylen A, Loennechen JP, et al. Superior cardiovascular effect of aerobic interval training versus moderate continuous training in heart failure patients: a randomized study. *Circulation.* 2007;115:3086–3094.

166. Simpson K, Killian K, McCartney N, et al. Randomised controlled trial of weight-lifting exercise in patients with chronic airflow limitation. *Thorax.* 1992;47:70–75.

167. Ortega F, Toral J, Cejudo P, et al. Comparison of effects of strength and endurance training in patients with chronic obstructive pulmonary disease. *Am J Respir Crit Care Med.* 2002;166:669–674.

168. Mador MJ, Bozkanat E, Aggarwal A, et al. Endurance and strength training in patients with COPD. *Chest.* 2004;125:2036–2045.

169. American College of Sports Medicine. American College of Sports Medicine position stand: progression models in resistance training for healthy adults. *Med Sci Sports Exerc.* 2009;41:687–708.

170. O'Shea SD, Taylor NF, Paratz JD. Progressive resistance exercise improves muscle strength and may improve elements of performance of daily activities for people with COPD: a systematic review. *Chest.* 2009;136:1269–1283.

171. Annegarn J, Meijer K, Passos VL, et al. Problematic activities of daily life are weakly associated with clinical characteristics in COPD. *J Am Med Dir Assoc.* 2012;13:284–290.

172. Janaudis-Ferreira T, Hill K, Goldstein R, et al. Arm exercise training in patients with chronic obstructive pulmonary disease: a systematic review. *J Cardiopulm Rehabil Prev.* 2009;29:277–283.

173. Celli B, Gotlief S. Biofeedback and upper extremity exercise in COPD. In: Bach JR, ed. *Pulmonary Rehabilitation: The Obstructive and Paralytic/Restrictive Pulmonary Syndromes.* Philadelphia, PA: Hanley & Belfus; 1996:285–301.

174. Martinez FJ, Vogel PD, Dupont DN, et al. Supported arm exercise vs unsupported arm exercise in the rehabilitation of patients with severe chronic airflow obstruction. *Chest.* 1993;103:1397–1402.

175. Couser J, Martinez F, Celli, BR. Pulmonary rehabilitation that includes arm exercise reduces metabolic and ventilatory requirements for simple arm elevation. *Chest.* 1993;103:37–41.

176. Lake FR, Hierndersen K, Briffa T. Upper limb and lower limb exercise training in patients with chronic airflow obstruction. *Chest.* 1990;97:1077–1082.

177. Holland AE, Hill CJ, Nehez E, et al. Does unsupported upper limb exercise training improve symptoms and quality of life for patients with chronic obstructive pulmonary disease? *J Cardiopulm Rehabil.* 2004;24:422–427.

178. Mathur S, Hornblower E, Levy RD. Exercise training before and after lung transplantation. *Phys Sportsmed.* 2009;37:78–87.

179. Vivodtzev I, Lacasse Y, Maltais F. Neuromuscular electrical stimulation of the lower limbs in patients with chronic obstructive pulmonary disease. *J Cardiopulm Rehabil Prev.* 2008;28:79–91.

180. Ngai SP, Jones AY, Hui-Chan CW, et al. Effect of 4 weeks of Acu-TENS on functional capacity and b-endorphin level in subjects with chronic obstructive pulmonary disease: a randomized controlled trial. *Respir Physiol Neurobiol.* 2010;173:29–36.

181. Zanotti E, Felicetti G, Maini M, et al. Peripheral muscle strength training in bedbound patients with COPD receiving mechanical ventilation: effect of electrical stimulation. *Chest.* 2003;124:292–296.

182. Gerovasili V, Stefanidis K, Vitzilaios K, et al. Electrical muscle stimulation preserves the muscle mass of critically ill patients: a randomized study. *Crit Care.* 2009;13:R161.

183. Routsi C, Gerovasili V, Vasileiadis I, et al. Electrical muscle stimulation prevents critical illness polyneuromyopathy: a randomized parallel intervention trial. *Crit Care.* 2010;14:R74.

184. Holland AE. Exercise limitation in interstitial lung disease—mechanisms, significance and therapeutic options. *Chron Respir Dis.* 2010;7:101–111.

185. Spruit MA, Thomeer MJ, Gosselink R, et al. Skeletal muscle weakness in patients with sarcoidosis and its relationship with exercise intolerance and reduced health status. *Thorax.* 2005;60:32–38.

186. Korenromp IH, Heijnen CJ, Vogels OJ, et al. Characterization of chronic fatigue in patients with sarcoidosis in clinical remission. *Chest.* 2011;140:441–447.

187. Holland AE, Hill CJ, Conron M, et al. Short term improvement in exercise capacity and symptoms following exercise training in interstitial lung disease. *Thorax.* 2008;63:549–554.

188. Nishiyama O, Kondoh Y, Kimura T, et al. Effects of pulmonary rehabilitation in patients with idiopathic pulmonary fibrosis. *Respirology.* 2008;13:394–399.

189. Yankaskas JR, Marshall BC, Sufian B, et al. Cystic fibrosis adult care: consensus conference report. *Chest.* 2004;125(suppl 1):1S–39S.

190. Bradley J, Moran F. Physical training for cystic fibrosis. *Cochrane Database Syst Rev.* 2008;(1):CD002768.

191. Mainguy V, Maltais F, Saey D, et al. Peripheral muscle dysfunction in idiopathic pulmonary arterial hypertension. *Thorax.* 2010;65:113–117.

192. Grünig E, Ehlken N, Ghofrani A, et al. Effect of exercise and respiratory training on clinical progression and survival in patients with severe chronic pulmonary hypertension. *Respiration.* 2011;81:394–401.

193. Desai SA, Channick RN. Exercise in patients with pulmonary arterial hypertension. *J Cardiopulm Rehabil Prev.* 2008;28:12–16.

194. Fishman A, Martinez F, Naunheim K, et al. A randomized trial comparing lung-volume reduction surgery with medical therapy for severe emphysema. *N Engl J Med.* 2003;348:2059–2073.

195. Ries AL, Make BJ, Lee SM, et al. The effects of pulmonary rehabilitation in the National Emphysema Treatment Trial. *Chest.* 2005;128:3799–3809.

196. Bartels MN. Rehabilitation management of lung volume reduction surgery. In: Ginsburg M, ed. *Lung Volume reduction Surgery.* St. Louis, MO: Mosby-Year Book, Inc.; 2001:97–124.

197. Rochester CL. Pulmonary rehabilitation for patients who undergo lung-volume-reduction surgery or lung transplantation. *Respir Care.* 2008;53:1196–1202.

198. Jastrzebski D, Ochman M, Ziora D, et al. Pulmonary rehabilitation in patients referred for lung transplantation. *Adv Exp Med Biol.* 2013;755:19–25.

199. Maury G, Langer D, Verleden G, et al. Skeletal muscle force and functional exercise tolerance before and after lung transplantation: a cohort study. *Am J Transplant.* 2008;8:1275–1281.

200. Wickerson L, Mathur S, Brooks D. Exercise training after lung transplantation: a systematic review. *J Heart Lung Transplant.* 2010;29:497–503.

201. Effing TW, Bourbeau J, Vercoulen J, et al. Self-management programmes for COPD: moving forward. *Chron Respir Dis.* 2012;9:27–35.

202. Neuringer A. Operant variability: evidence, functions, and theory. *Psychon Bull Rev.* 2002;9:672–705.

203. Bandura A. Social learning of moral judgments. *J Pers Soc Psychol.* 1969;11:275–279.

204. Bandura A. Self-efficacy: toward a unifying theory of behavioral change. *Psychol Rev.* 1977;84:191–215.

205. Lorig K, Holman H. Arthritis self-management studies: a twelve-year review. *Health Educ Q.* 1993;20:17–28.

206. Adams SG, Smith PK, Allan PF, et al. Systematic review of the chronic care model in chronic obstructive pulmonary disease prevention and management. *Arch Intern Med.* 2007;167:551–561.

207. Effing T, Monninkhof EM, van der Valk PD, et al. Self management education for patients with chronic obstructive pulmonary disease. *Cochrane Database Syst Rev.* 2007;4:CD002990.

208. Solway S, Brooks D, Lau L, et al. The short-term effect of a Rollator on functional exercise capacity among individuals with severe COPD. *Chest.* 2002;122:56–65.

209. Probst VS, Troosters T, Coosemans I, et al. Mechanisms of improvement in exercise capacity using a rollator in patients with COPD. *Chest.* 2004;126:1102–1107.

210. Ries AL, Kaplan RM, Limberg TM, et al. Effects of pulmonary rehabilitation on physiologic and psychosocial outcomes in patients with chronic obstructive pulmonary disease. *Ann Intern Med.* 1995;122:823–832.

211. Jones PW, Quirk FH, Baveystock CM, et al. A self-complete measure of health status for chronic airflow limitation: the St. George's Respiratory Questionnaire. *Am Rev Respir Dis.* 1992;145:1321–1327.

212. Guyatt GH, Berman LB, Townsend M, et al. A measure of quality of life for clinical trials in chronic lung disease. *Thorax.* 1987;42:773–778.

213. Williams JE, Singh SJ, Sewell L, et al. Health status measurement: sensitivity of the self-reported Chronic Respiratory Questionnaire (CRQ-SR) in pulmonary rehabilitation. *Thorax.* 2003;58:515–518.

214. Yohannes AM, Roomi J, Winn S, et al. The Manchester Respiratory Activities of Daily Living Questionnaire: development, American Thoracic Society Documents e59 reliability, validity, and responsiveness to pulmonary rehabilitation. *J Am Geriatr Soc.* 2000;48:1496–1500.

215. Lareau SC, Carrieri-Kohlman V, Janson-Bjerklie S, et al. Development and testing of the Pulmonary Functional Status and Dyspnea Questionnaire (PFSDQ). *Heart Lung.* 1994;23:242–250.

216. Spruit MA, Polkey MI, Celli B, et al. Evaluation of COPD Longitudinally to Identify Predictive Surrogate Endpoints (ECLIPSE) study investigators. Predicting outcomes from 6-minute walk distance in chronic obstructive pulmonary disease. *J Am Med Dir Assoc.* 2012;13:291–297.

217. Sava F, Laviolette L, Bernard S, et al. The impact of obesity on walking and cycling performance and response to pulmonary rehabilitation in COPD. *BMC Pulm Med.* 2010;10:55.

218. Pitta F, Troosters T, Probst VS, et al. Quantifying physical activity in daily life with questionnaires and motion sensors in COPD. *Eur Respir J.* 2006;27:1040–1055.

219. Hyland ME, Jones RC, Hanney KE. The Lung Information Needs Questionnaire: development, preliminary validation and findings. *Respir Med.* 2006;100:1807–1816.

220. Celli BR, Cote CG, Marin JM, et al. The body-mass index, airflow obstruction, dyspnea, and exercise capacity index in chronic obstructive pulmonary disease. *N Engl J Med.* 2004;350:1005–1012.

221. Foster S, Lopez D, Thomas HM. Pulmonary rehabilitation in COPD patients with elevated pCO_2. *Am Rev Respir Dis.* 1988;138:1519–1523.

222. Casaburi R, Patessio A, Ioli F, et al. Reductions in exercise lactic acidosis and ventilation as a result of exercise training in patients with obstructive lung disease. *Am Rev Respir Dis.* 1991;143:9–18.

223. Rossi G, Florini F, Romagnoli M, et al. Length and clinical effectiveness of pulmonary rehabilitation in outpatients with chronic airway obstruction. *Chest.* 2005;127:105–109.

224. Ferrari M, Vangelista A, Vedovi E, et al. Minimally supervised home rehabilitation improves exercise capacity and health status in patients with COPD. *Am J Phys Med Rehabil.* 2004;83:337–343.

225. Wijkstra PJ, TenVergert EM, van der Mark TW, et al. Relation of lung function, maximum inspiratory pressure, dyspnoea, and quality of life with exercise, capacity in patients with chronic obstructive pulmonary disease. *Thorax.* 1994;49(5):468–472.

226. Tydeman DE, Chandler AR, Graveling BM, et al. An investigation into the effects of exercise tolerance training of patients with chronic airways obstruction. *Physiotherapy.* 1984;70:261–264.

227. Oga T, Nishimura K, Tsukino M, et al. Exercise capacity deterioration in patients with COPD: longitudinal evaluation over 5 years. *Chest.* 2005;128:62–69.

228. Tu SP, McDonell MB, Spertus JA, et al. A new self-administered questionnaire to monitor health-related quality of life in patients with COPD. *Chest.* 1997;112:614–622.

229. Fuchs-Climent D, LeGallais D, Varray A, et al. Factor analysis of quality of life, dyspnea, and physiologic variables in patients with chronic obstructive pulmonary disease before and after rehabilitation. *Am J Phys Med Rehabil.* 2001;80:113–120.

230. Boueri FMV, Bucher-Bartelson BL, Glenn KA, et al. Quality of life measured with a generic instrument improves following pulmonary rehabilitation in patients with COPD. *Chest.* 2001;119:77–84.

231. Chumillas S, Ponce JL, Delgado F, et al. Prevention of postoperative pulmonary complications through respiratory rehabilitation: a controlled clinical study. *Arch Phys Med Rehabil.* 1998;79:5–9.

232. de Jong W, Grevink RG, Roorda RJ, et al. Effect of a home exercise training program in patients with cystic fibrosis. *Chest.* 1994;105:463–468.

233. Lacasse Y, Martin S, Lasserson TJ, et al. Meta-analysis of respiratory rehabilitation in chronic obstructive pulmonary disease: a Cochrane systematic review. *Eura Medicophys.* 2007;43:475–485.

234. Roselle S, D'Amico FJ. The effect of home respiratory therapy on hospital readmission rates of patients with chronic obstructive pulmonary disease. *Respir Care.* 1990;35:1208–1213.

235. Holle RHO, Williams DV, Vandree JC, et al. Increased muscle efficiency and sustained benefits in an outpatient community hospital-based pulmonary rehabilitation program. *Chest.* 1988;94:1161–1168.

236. Ilowite JS, Niederman M, Fein A, et al. Can benefits seen in pulmonary rehabilitation be sustained long term? *Chest.* 1991;100:182.

237. Mall RW, Medieros M. Objective evaluation of results of a pulmonary rehabilitation program in a community hospital. *Chest.* 1988;94:1156–1160.

238. Vale F, Reardon J, ZuWallack R. Is improvement sustained following pulmonary rehabilitation? *Chest.* 1991;100:56s.

239. Foglio K, Bianchi L, Ambrosino N. Is it really useful to repeat outpatient pulmonary rehabilitation programs in patients with chronic airway obstruction? A 2-year controlled study. *Chest.* 2001;119:1696–1704.

240. Cambach W, Wagenaar RC, Koelman TW, et al. The long-term effects of pulmonary rehabilitation in patients with asthma and chronic obstructive pulmonary disease: a research synthesis. *Arch Phys Med Rehabil.* 1999;80:103–111.

Burns

Burn injuries pose complex physical and psychological rehabilitation challenges. The incidence of burns has decreased dramatically in the past 50 years as a result of public education as well as home and work safety efforts. Additionally, survival after burn injury has increased significantly in the same time period (1). Advances in the field that have contributed to survival include the formation of specialized burn centers, early excision and grafting, improved resuscitation and intensive care, and the development of topical and systemic antibiotics (1,2). With dramatic improvements in survival, the focus of burn care is increasingly shifting toward rehabilitation and quality of life. Burn survivors have complicated rehabilitation needs including scarring, pruritus, chronic wounds, bone complications, metabolic abnormalities, contractures, pain, amputations, neurologic injuries, psychological problems, sleep disorders, and community integration issues. The period of rehabilitation may last from months to many years after injury. The physiatrist is an integral member of the burn care team from the time of injury to long-term follow-up.

EPIDEMIOLOGY

It is estimated that 1.25 million people experience burn injuries each year. Of those, approximately 500,000 receive some form of medical treatment and 40,000 are hospitalized, with 30,000 being at hospital burn centers (3). Burns predominantly affect young men (mode age, 20 to 40; male, 68%). Two thirds of burn injuries affect adults and one third affect children. Most burns occur by fire/flame (41%) or scald injuries (33%) (📶 **eFig. 35-1**). Other etiologies that constitute the minority of burns include electrical, contact, chemical, tar, radiation, and grease injuries as well as skin diseases. Approximately one third of burn injuries are associated with concomitant alcohol or drug use. The majority of burns are less than 20% total body surface area (TBSA) (4). A large majority of burn survivors have less than or equal to a high-school education (82%). About 73% of burns occur at home (3), while a minority of burn injuries (13%) occur at work.

Approximately 5% of burn injuries are the result of child abuse or adult assault or abuse. Among children less than 2 years old, burn injuries represent the most common cause of accidental death; most of these deaths are a result of abuse. Overall, the survival rate is approximately 95%. The risk of death is increased for those at the extremes of age, with inhalation injury and with larger burns (4–6). The most common in-hospital complications of burn injury for individuals less than 60 years old include urinary tract infection, pneumonia, and cellulitis (4).

PATHOPHYSIOLOGY

Normal Skin

The skin is the largest organ of the body. It serves multiple functions; it acts as a protective barrier to the external environment, regulates temperature and fluid homeostasis, plays a key role in sensation, is an active site of vitamin D synthesis, and contributes to our sense of identity and communication. The skin is a complex organ composed of two layers, the epidermis and dermis (**Fig. 35-1**).

The outermost epidermis consists of stratified squamous epithelium. This layer contains no blood vessels, and the cells are nourished by diffusion from capillaries in the upper layers of the dermis. Cells are formed through mitosis at the basal layer (stratum basale) that migrate toward the surface as they differentiate (7). In addition to forming the bottom layer of the epidermis, the stratum basale lines the hair follicles and sweat glands. (Hair follicles and sweat glands are a source of epidermal cells that enable partial-thickness burn injuries to heal spontaneously.) The mitotic daughter cells migrate toward the surface changing shape and composition as they die due to isolation from their blood source. The cytoplasm is released and the protein keratin is inserted. They eventually reach the outer layer and desquamate. This process is called keratinization and takes approximately 30 days. This keratinized layer of skin (stratum corneum) is responsible for keeping water in the body and keeping harmful chemicals and pathogens outside the body, making the skin a natural protective barrier.

The dermis resides beneath the epidermis and consists of a vascular connective tissue that supports and provides nutrition to the epidermis and skin appendages. The dermis contains nerve endings, capillaries, lymphatic vessels, as well as appendages that include hair follicles, sweat glands, and sebaceous glands. The eccrine sweat glands release heat from the body's surface though sweat, thereby contributing to thermoregulation. The sebaceous glands secrete an oily substance called sebum that protects the skin and hair and moisturizes the skin.

Classification of Burn Injury

One of the most common classification systems uses depth of injury to categorize the severity of the burn. Previously, burn injuries were labeled first, second, or third degree. Within the past decade, researchers and clinicians have transitioned to categorizing burns with descriptive terms (8). Superficial injuries, previously termed first-degree burns, solely affect the epidermis. The category of second-degree burns is now divided into superficial and deep partial-thickness burns. The former interrupt the epidermis and superficial dermis and present with

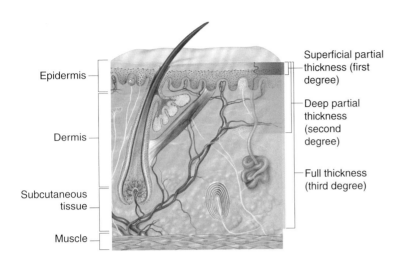

FIGURE 35-1. Diagram of normal skin histology with depth of burn injury indicated. Note the layers, epidermis and dermis, and skin appendages. (Courtesy of Anatomical Chart Company.)

blistering, moist, and painful skin that blanches with pressure. The latter involve the epidermis and deep dermis, including skin appendages, affecting some degree of sensory and sweat gland function. Deep partial-thickness burns present with a dry or waxy appearance and are less painful than more superficial burns. Full-thickness burns, formerly third-degree burns, affect the entire epidermal and dermal layers and result in complete loss of skin appendages. They present as white waxy to leathery gray to charred black appearance, are insensate to pain due to destruction of sensory nerves, and do not blanch to pressure. Deep injuries may affect muscle, tendon, and bone. Such deep injuries are not part of the newer classification system but were previously classified as fourth-degree burns (see **Fig. 35-1**; **Table 35-1**).

Burn injuries are also classified by size. Lund and Browder (9) diagrams provide a systematic method for calculating TBSA burned for both adults and children. In contrast to an adult, a child's head represents proportionally more and their legs represent proportionally less of their body surface area (**Fig. 35-2**). The rule of nines is used clinically as a quick estimate of TBSA (**Fig. 35-3**).

Many burn injuries are best treated in specialized burn centers. The American Burn Association in consultation with the American College of Surgeons has developed clinical criteria for referral to a burn center (10) (**Box 35-1**).

Effects of Thermal Injury

In thermal injury, the extent of tissue damage is related to the location, duration, and intensity (temperature) of heat exposure. Also of significance, those at the extremes of age have fewer protective layers of epithelium; therefore, the same location, duration, and intensity of heat will produce a more serious burn injury in children and elderly than in other adults.

After burn injury, a cascade of physiologic processes affect the thermal injury's ultimate impact. There is a complex interplay of local and circulating mediators, including histamine, prostaglandins, thromboxane, kinins, serotonin, catecholamines, oxygen free radicals, platelet aggregation factors, angiotensin II, and vasopressin. Initially, there is vasoconstriction at the site of injury mediated by these mediators. A few hours after injury, vasoconstriction turns to vasodilation, increased capillary permeability, and leakage of plasma into the extravascular space. Histamine is released, which contributes to edema. Damaged cells swell. Fluid shifts result in increased extravascular edema and intravascular hypovolemia. Platelets and leukocytes aggregate, leading to thrombotic ischemia (11). In severe burn injuries, inflammatory mediators are released and compromise cardiovascular function. Burn shock ensues, resulting in decreased intravascular volume, increased systemic vascular resistance, decreased cardiac output, end-organ ischemia, and metabolic acidosis. Resuscitation treatment helps

TABLE 35-1	Burn Severity Classifications		
Old Classification	**New Classification**	**Appearance/Symptoms**	**Course/Treatment**
First degree (epidermis)	Superficial thickness	Erythematous, dry, mildly swollen, blanches with pressure, painful	Exfoliation, heals spontaneously in 1 wk, no scarring
Second degree (dermis)	Superficial partial thickness	Blistering, moist, weeping, blanches with pressure, painful	Reepithelialization in 7–20 d
	Deep partial thickness	No blisters, wet or waxy dry, variable color, less painful, at risk for conversion to full thickness because of marginal blood supply	Reepithelialization in weeks to months. Skin grafting may speed recovery. Associated with scarring
Third degree (all of dermis and epidermis)	Full thickness	White waxy to leathery gray to charred black, insensate to pain, does not blanch to pressure	Reepithelialization does not occur, requires skin grafting, associated with scarring
Fourth degree (extends to muscle, bone, tendon)	N/A	Black (eschar), exposed bones, ligaments, tendons	May require amputation or extensive deep debridement

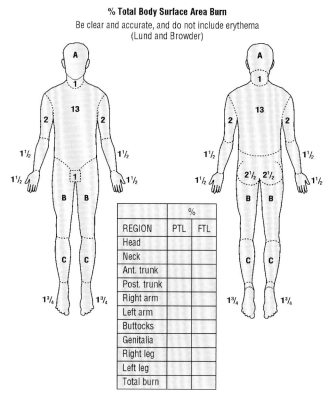

% Total Body Surface Area Burn
Be clear and accurate, and do not include erythema
(Lund and Browder)

	%	
REGION	PTL	FTL
Head		
Neck		
Ant. trunk		
Post. trunk		
Right arm		
Left arm		
Buttocks		
Genitalia		
Right leg		
Left leg		
Total burn		

AREA	Age 0	1	5	10	15	Adult
A = ½ OF HEAD	9½	8½	6½	5½	4½	3½
B = ½ OF ONE THIGH	2¾	3¼	4	4½	4½	4¾
C = ½ OF ONE LOWER LEG	2½	2½	2¾	3	3¼	3½

FIGURE 35-2. Lund and Browder diagram. (Adapted from Lund CC, Browder NC. The Estimation of Areas of Burns. *Surg Gynecol Obstet.* 1944; 79: 352–358. In: Wolfson AB, et al. Harwood-Nuss' Clinical Practice of Emergency Medicine. 6th ed. Philadelphia, PA: Wolters Kluwer; 2014. Copyright © 1944 Elsevier. With permission.)

reverse this potentially deadly cascade. When resuscitation is delayed or subpar, the kidneys and gastrointestinal tract are most at risk for ischemia.

Damaged skin results in impairment in most major functions of the integumentary system. In areas of burn injury, the skin loses its ability to act as a protective barrier and homeostatic regulator. This may lead to significant losses of body fluid, impaired thermoregulation, and increased susceptibility to infection. In large burns, loss of fluid by evaporation contributes to the development of hypovolemia and shock.

Release of catecholamines plays a key role in the development of a catabolic state after burn injury. Tachycardia, increased nutritional demand, and weight loss typically ensue. Gastric dilation and gastrointestinal ileus are common in the first few days after burn injury. Also, immune function is impaired. The arachidonic acid and cytokine cascades alter the function of lymphocytes, macrophages, and neutrophils. As a result, patients are at increased risk of infection. Inhalation injury is commonly associated with fire injuries. Noxious gaseous components of smoke directly damage the respiratory tract. Patients are at risk for carbon monoxide intoxication, upper airway edema and obstruction, pneumonia, and dependence on mechanical ventilation (11,12).

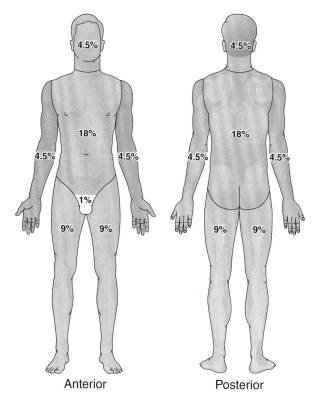

Anterior   Posterior

FIGURE 35-3. The rule of nines is used to estimate the percent of body surface area burned. (Reprinted with permission from Cohen BJ, DePetris A. *Medical Terminology.* 7th ed. Philadelphia, PA: Wolters Kluwer Health/ Lippincott Williams & Wilkins; 2013.)

Skin Regeneration and Scarring

Spontaneous reepithelialization is impossible with a full-thickness burn injury because of destruction of the dermal appendages; therefore, there are no stem cells for regeneration. Full-thickness burns result in hair loss, sensory impairment, loss of normal skin lubrication, and heat intolerance because of destruction of sweat glands.

BOX 35-1

American Burn Association Criteria for Referral to a Burn Center

- Partial-thickness burn greater than 10% TBSA
- Burns that involve the face, hands, feet, genitalia, perineum, or major joints
- Any full-thickness burn
- Electrical burns, including lightning injury
- Chemical burns
- Inhalation injury
- Burn injury in patients with preexisting medical disorders that could complicate management, prolong recovery, or affect mortality
- Any patient with burn injury and concomitant trauma in which the burn injury poses the greatest risk of morbidity and mortality
- Burned children in hospital without qualified personnel or equipment for the care of children
- Burn injury in patients who will require special social, emotional, or rehabilitative intervention

Healing and regeneration of skin in partial-thickness burns arise from the epithelial linings of the hair follicles and sweat glands (stratum basale). Depending on the depth, healing is completed within 14 to 21 days. The new skin again functions as a temperature regulator and a protective barrier against bacteria. After epithelialization, there is continued healing with regeneration of the peripheral nerves, sometimes associated with symptoms of neuropathic pain and itching. Although epithelium covers the wound, dermal scarring occurs in the burn wound on a continuous basis for several months after injury. The healing process is ongoing from 6 months to 2 years until the skin is mature. By that point, the vascularity of the wound has returned to near normal, and there is no further collagen deposition in the wound.

ACUTE MEDICAL MANAGEMENT

Acute Care of Burn Wounds

While the long-term goals of burn wound care are to restore skin integrity, function, and appearance, the immediate goals post resuscitation are to prevent infection, decrease pain, prepare wounds for grafting, prevent contracture and scarring, and maintain strength and function.

Debridement, the removal of eschar and necrotic tissue, prepares a viable base for wound healing and grafting. Eschar is a composite of coagulum and other tissue debris. Like necrotic tissue, eschar provides an excellent environment for bacterial growth. Since eschar has no microcirculation, bacterial invasion cannot be resolved with systemic antibiotics.

Debridement is performed by several methods, including mechanical debridement, enzymatic debridement, and surgical debridement. Water immersion, pulsed lavage, and wet to dry dressing are examples of mechanical debridement. Commercially available topical enzymes are available for debridement and include substances such as sutilains, trypsin, and streptokinase-streptodornase that induce proteolysis, fibrinolysis, and collagenolysis (13).

There are different types of surgical debridement. Sequential, also called tangential, debridement is the process of removing thin slices of necrotic tissue. Tissue is removed until a viable tissue bed is reached. Fascial debridement surgically removes tissue down to fascia. In this type, a viable wound bed is assured but a significant soft tissue defect results. Circumferential fascial debridement places patients at high risk for chronic edema.

Deep skin burns are inelastic, and the injured skin does not accommodate to the massive edema associated with acute burn injury. In a circumferential burn, the inelastic tissue acts as a tourniquet. The tourniquet effect can lead to a compartment syndrome, defined as compartment pressure of at least 40 mm Hg. If this occurs, escharotomy is indicated. Escharotomy, surgical decompression of the compartment, is urgently performed to avoid necrosis of the underlying tissues that results from sustained elevated pressure leading to ischemia. This procedure is critical in situations involving full-thickness circumferential injuries of the chest, arms, or legs. If escharotomy does not successfully reduce the elevated pressure, a fasciotomy is indicated.

Grafting

The introduction of early excision and grafting in the last 40 years has contributed significantly to decreased length of hospitalization as well as improved survival rates, cosmesis, and functional outcome.

Homografts, tissue taken from one's own species, include cadaveric tissue and human fetal membranes. Heterografts, also known as xenografts, are tissues taken from nonhuman species that are used as human grafts. These biologic tissues, most commonly porcine tissues, provide wound closure, modulate metabolic needs, and reduce evaporative fluid. These temporary grafts also act as a mechanical barrier to infection and aid in pain relief. Temporary grafts are useful as "test grafts" to determine if the wound bed will accept an autograft. Typically, homografts and heterografts are removed or replaced after several days because the patient's immune system rejects them. It is not routine to use immunosuppressant therapy in conjunction with grafting.

Synthetic wound dressings are available, including polyvinylchloride, polyurethanes, and other plastic membranes. They are vapor and gas permeable. Such grafts are employed until autografting is feasible or the wound heals. Bilaminate analogs composed of thin sheets of Silastic as well as epidermal and dermal components are available. Biobrane and Integra (bovine collagen and chondroitin 6-sulfate) are the two most common biosynthetic dressings.

In the world of skin substitutes and biologic dressings, autografts are the gold standard. The bioengineered substitutes can be used as a temporary covering prior to autografting or as a neodermal base on which the autograft is placed. Tissue-engineered skin substitutes are generally used to increase the rate of epithelialization and improve the long-term cosmetic outcomes and function (14). Artificial skin substitutes are either epidermal or dermal. Dermal substitutes generally require an overlying split-thickness autograft as an epidermal layer.

Debels et al., in a critical review of dermal matrices and bioengineered skin substitutes, concluded that there is no benefit of Biobrane over DuoDERM, which is lower in cost (15).

An evidence-based literature review of bioengineered skin substitutes concluded that Biobrane, TransCyte, Dermagraft, and allogeneic cultured skin are at least as safe and effective as other wound dressings or allografts for partial-thickness wounds. The authors concluded that Integra is best used for smaller burns; evidence suggests that burns of 45% or greater experienced higher infection rates. TransCyte provides good coverage in areas of high contour such as the face (16).

Autografts are harvested from the patient's own skin. In this process, skin is surgically removed from one's own body and is relocated to another site (grafted) (📶 **eFigs. 35-2** and **35-3**). Autografts are placed on a wound bed clean of any nonvital tissue or debris and without evidence of infection.

Split-thickness grafts are applied in sheets or may be meshed prior to application. Cutting small regularly staggered parallel slits in the sheet of harvested skin creates a meshed skin graft. This expands the size of the graft to several times its original surface area. Meshed grafts are less cosmetic than are full-thickness grafts. Meshed grafts heal quickly, and the epithelialization that occurs in the interstices creates a meshlike appearance to the healed skin (**Fig. 35-4**).

Full-thickness skin grafts are not meshed and result in a more cosmetic appearance. They are typically applied to cosmetically critical areas such as the face, neck, and hands. In addition, full-thickness grafts are used almost exclusively in reconstructive surgery.

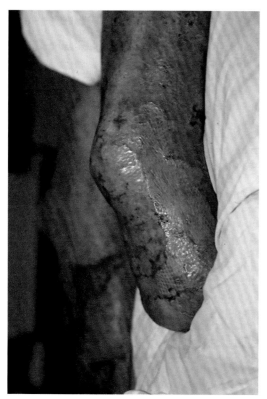

FIGURE 35-4. Split-thickness skin grafts used to close wounds of residual limb after amputation.

Dysphagia

Dysphagia is a common problem with large burn injuries and complicates the delivery of adequate nutrition for healing and recovery (see Chapter 13). Burn-induced hypermetabolism increases the caloric needs of the patient. Weakness, inhalation injury, tracheostomy, medication, oral motor dysfunction, and multiple other factors contribute to the development of dysphagia. Tracheostomy is associated with aspiration, pneumonia, and the development of tracheoesophageal fistulae. Vocal cord paresis is associated with inhalation injury and endotracheal intubation.

Vigilant monitoring is required to recognize dysphagia early and prevent aspiration and associated morbidity. Edelman et al. (17) demonstrated the importance of evaluating patients' swallowing function. In this study, dysphagia was initially assessed by bedside swallowing evaluation and, if abnormal, followed by modified barium swallow examination. They found that oral phase dysphagia is usually due to impaired range of motion (ROM), weak mastication, and impaired oral seal from burn wounds or scar formation. Esophageal dysfunction is a secondary complication of intubation or tracheostomy. Pharyngeal phase dysphagia is usually a result of inhalation injury, complications of tracheostomy, intubation, or burn scar. Pharyngeal dysphagia is associated with the highest risk of aspiration.

Interventions include evaluating endotracheal tube position, size, and location. Selection of appropriate food consistency and positioning, including head and neck positioning, are successful measures to reduce the risk of aspiration.

REHABILITATION

Restoration of independent function is the ultimate goal of rehabilitation. Functional restoration includes all aspects of the human life such as strength, ROM, mobility and self-care, reintegration into family and community, adaptive psychosocial responses, and self-determination.

Rehabilitation after a severe burn injury is a multistage process that may take years. Acute rehabilitation goals include interventions to facilitate wound healing, achieve pain control, prevent joint contracture and weakness, and promote independent mobility and activities of daily living (ADLs). Details of the injury, age, premorbid functional level, and health are determinants of an individual's rehabilitation plan. Therapy is individualized according to burn location, depth, and size as well as other associated injuries or complications. Successful rehabilitation involves multiple disciplines working collaboratively with the patient to achieve the highest level of functioning possible.

Positioning

Contractures are a common complication of deep partial- and full-thickness burn injuries. One review by Schouten et al. in 2012 found 5% to 40% of individuals with burn injuries develop contractures (18). Another study performed by Schneider et al. found that approximately one third of patients had a major joint contracture at discharge from rehabilitation (19). Proper positioning is a basic tenet of contracture prevention. Proper positioning also helps prevent other complications such as pressure ulcers and compression neuropathies (Fig. 35-5; 🛜 eTable 35-1).

Contracture prevention is based on the principle of tissue elongation. Patients often prefer to position injured tissue in a shortened, nonstretched state for comfort, which leads to contracture. Typically, this is a position of flexion and adduction.

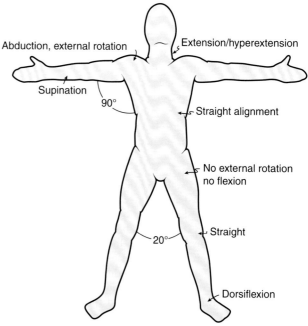

FIGURE 35-5. Therapeutic positioning to prevent contracture formation. (Reprinted from Helm PA, Kevorkian CG, Lushbaugh M, et al. Burn injury: rehabilitation management in 1982. *Arch Phys Med Rehabil.* 1982;63(1):6–16. Copyright © 1982 Elsevier. With permission.)

Positions of extension and abduction are usually indicated to counter the position of comfort. One must prescribe positioning in accord with the location of the injury and direction of the contracture. Joints with overlying deep burns are placed in a position of tissue elongation.

Contractures are not limited to joints. Other areas, such as the soft tissue of the lips and mouth, require stretching, exercise, and therapeutic devices to maintain tissue length and function. Contractures are more common in the upper extremities, particularly the elbow and shoulder. They are also more common in men, black race, Hispanic ethnicity, and individuals with neuropathy and medical problems (20). A system of cutaneous functional units (CFUs) was developed by Richard et al. to identify fields of skin that functionally contribute to joint ROM. Areas both proximal and distal to joints were found to affect joint motion. CFUs may be used to predict patients at risk for contracture and therefore allow for early prevention with range-of-motion exercises and splinting (21).

Splinting

Splints are commonly employed for burn injuries (see Chapter 57). These devices provide multiple functions including facilitating proper positioning, preventing joint contractures, protecting skin grafts or fragile wounds, or assisting desired motion. Splints are commonly needed in deep partial-thickness and full-thickness burns and less often in superficial partial-thickness burns due to rapid reepithelialization.

There are three types of splints used in burn rehabilitation. There are static splints, static progressive splints, and dynamic splints. Static splints are typically used for prevention of contracture, while static progressive and dynamic splints are used for the treatment of contracture. Classically, static progressive splints have been used for restrictive tissue shortening and dynamic splints used for more malleable tissues (22). The effects of splinting at the cellular level have mostly been studied *in vitro* and *in vivo* in animals. Some studies have assessed the effect of mechanical loading by splinting therapy on myofibroblast activity. There are conflicting results, including a concern for overactivation of myofibroblasts by mechanical tension, which may further exacerbate the contracture (18). Furthermore, Schouten et al. concluded that there is no strong scientific evidence to support the effectiveness of static splinting for burn contracture prevention. This may indicate that more rigorous studies need to be conducted.

Splints are fabricated from many materials, with low-temperature thermoplastic orthotics being the most common. Low-temperature plastics have several advantages including the ability to be warmed at the bedside in heated water and fitted to the patient immediately. These plastics are conformable at low temperatures and therefore can be readily remodeled and adjusted as needed in the clinic or at bedside.

Custom splints can be designed for virtually all parts of the body. Hand injuries commonly require custom splints. Custom splints are advantageous for difficult to fit areas and for sites that require unique design or built-in features.

Commercially available prefabricated splints may be cost-effective; however, these splints often require modification to fit properly or to achieve the intended purpose. Some clinicians believe that the commercially available prefabricated splints are best used for positioning the knee and ankle. Splints that are simple and straightforward in design and function are "user friendly" and more likely to be applied correctly and compliantly. Patient and family teaching is imperative for proper splint application. An incorrectly applied splint can lead to further injury, including nerve damage, loss of skin graft, and other skin traumas.

The basic rule of splinting is to splint the body part in a position opposite of the expected deformity. Factors to consider when prescribing a splint include burn size, burn location, burn type, functional goals, patient's cognition, and patient activity level.

The wearing schedule for splints is individualized. In the case of the comatose, vegetative, or minimally conscious patient, splints should be worn for 2 to 4 hours and then removed for a similar length of time and then reapplied. The wearing schedule can be modified as the patient's level of participation is increased. Splints may be worn to maintain the gains made in therapy.

If normal ROM of a joint is preserved, a splint is not indicated unless a joint or tendon is exposed or the patient is noncompliant with positioning. Common splints include the knee extension splint to prevent knee flexion contracture and posterior foot drop splint to maintain neutral ankle positioning.

The upper extremity is the most common site for contractures. For axillary burns, an "airplane" splint is used to prevent shoulder adduction contracture. An "airplane" splint holds the upper extremity in approximately 15 degrees of horizontal adduction and 90 degrees of abduction. This splint prevents shortening of the anterior and posterior axillary folds (**Fig. 35-6**). In injuries of other upper extremity joints, splints are fabricated to meet the specific positioning demands of the elbow, forearm, and wrist.

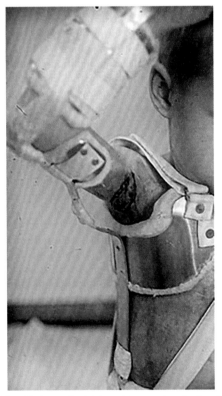

FIGURE 35-6. Airplane splint fabricated to prevent contracture development of the shoulder.

To correct a contracture, various static progressive splints or dynamic splints or orthoses are designed to provide a slow progressive sustained stretch. The literature documents success using serial casting to achieve contracture correction as well. Staley and Serghiou (23) summarized serial casting use in burn injury: long duration of stretch with minimal force, protection of exposed tendons, mechanical forces to remodel scar, cost-effective, treatment useful in children and noncompliant patients, and treatment option when an open wound is present.

Splints are also valuable in the postacute period to prevent contractures until the tissue length is stabilized, after surgical release of a contracture, or after skin grafting. Splints are useful in all stages of healing, because burn scar contractures begin with wound healing and continue through maturation of the scar around 2 years (22).

Hands

Hands require special attention. When evaluating the burned hand, individual joint motion should be assessed. Limitations in ROM result from decreased tendon sliding, decreased muscle strength, tendon shortening, skin/muscle/ligament/tendon tightness, joint restriction, or a combination of these processes.

During the acute phase, the hands are positioned and splinted to prevent shortening of the joint capsules, collateral ligaments, and muscle tendons. Edema can complicate care as it accentuates metacarpophalangeal (MCP) joint extension and interphalangeal (IP) joint flexion. The resulting combination of MCP hyperextension and IP joint flexion produces the intrinsic minus deformity of the hand, also called claw hand.

The hand is splinted with the wrist in slight extension, the MCP joints in 70 to 80 degrees flexion, IP joints in extension, and the thumb abducted from the palm (intrinsic plus position). Fingers are positioned in abduction (**Fig. 35-7**). If the burns are limited to the palmar aspect, then the MCP and IP joints are positioned in extension, fingers abducted, and the thumb abducted from the palm. Elastic wraps are applied in a figure of eight formation to avoid circumferential constriction. Straps should be soft and applied in a crisscross orientation.

Circumferential hand burns often damage the web spaces of the hand. Preservation of the web spaces is important for hand rehabilitation. For example, loss or shortening of the first web impairs thumb opposition and abduction and interferes

with grasp (24). Early intervention is critical. In order to maintain thumb and finger abduction there is focus on exercise to all digits, as well as applying dressings, soft inserts, or straps in the web spaces. Also, thermoplastic inserts may be customized and fitted in these areas. Compression gloves may be used in conjunction with the splints for positioning and edema control (eFig. 35-4). In mild cases, compression gloves may be sufficient to preserve web spaces and function. Passive exercise and scar suppression are also employed to assure restoration and maintenance of normal ROM.

Exposed tendons require splinting in a slack position. The tendon should be kept moist to avoid desiccation and denaturation. With time, the tendon may revascularize and become functional. If the exposed extensor hood of the fingers is not kept slack, the central slip can fail and lead to a boutonniere deformity. In cases of extensor hood rupture, the finger is positioned in extension. In approximately 6 weeks, scar tissue may form to bridge the extensor surface and act as a functional substitute. After that time, active ROM can be initiated (25).

Exercise

In burn rehabilitation, one of the earliest goals of exercise is to maintain or achieve normal ROM. For the obtunded or comatose patient, passive ROM exercises emphasizing the end ROM is appropriate. Alert and cooperative patients can participate in active and active-assisted exercise. With children, developmentally appropriate exercise and play activities are indicated to achieve the therapy goals.

Surgical anesthesia can provide an opportunity to perform ROM exercises and determine objective measurements of range while eliminating pain. The opportunity to assess ROM under anesthesia is valuable in the case of a child or an uncooperative patient or if pain is inhibiting ROM exercise.

The biomechanics of skin and muscle are different; therefore, the two tissues are stretched differently. Stretching of injured skin or scar tissue requires a slow sustained mechanical stretch to enhance elongation of collagen and underlying fibers. When a prolonged stretch is performed, the stretch is maintained until the tissue blanches. Blanching indicates that the tissue is near its yield point, the point at which the skin is at risk of tearing (26).

After burn injury, muscular weakness, fatigue, and deconditioning are serious problems. These sequelae interfere with function, such as ambulation, ADL skills, and endurance. Loss of muscle mass and, in children, the additional loss of bone mass interfere with the restoration of function and return to work or school (27,28).

The literature indicates that a structured exercise program, composed of aerobic and resistance training, leads to increased function as measured by increased muscle mass, strength, and cardiovascular endurance (29). Suman and Herndon (30) demonstrated the efficacy of a supervised exercise program for children, ages 7 to 18 years, which included resistance and aerobic exercise. The participants of a supervised resistance and aerobic program required significantly fewer surgical releases up to 2 years after the intervention (31). Suman et al. (32) also demonstrated that children had increased lean body mass and muscle strength with structured exercise and the concurrent administration of the anabolic steroid, oxandrolone, for 1 year after injury. Anabolic agents, such as oxandrolone and

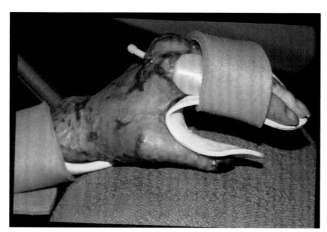

FIGURE 35-7. Resting hand splint.

human growth hormone, have been demonstrated to reduce the effects of hypermetabolism while also increasing muscle mass and strength and decreasing resting energy expenditure in children and adults (33–35). de Lateur et al. (36) reported that a structured aerobic exercise program, consisting of three times a week aerobic treadmill training for 12 weeks combined with a standard burn therapy program, achieved improved aerobic capacity. Clayton et al. in 2016 further found that at least 6 weeks of a rehabilitative exercise program was sufficient to improve muscle strength, cardiopulmonary fitness, and body composition in children with greater than 30% TBSA burns (37). This literature suggests that regular exercise after burn injury, like in other adults, results in improved flexibility, endurance, balance, and strength. Such gains are important for returning to full independence and function, reduced anxiety, and an improved sense of well-being (38).

Practice guidelines for cardiovascular fitness and strengthening exercises after burn injury were developed in 2016. Recommendations include exercise programs that may begin immediately after acute care discharge and should last 6 to 12 weeks for adults and up to 12 weeks for children. It is unclear whether longer programs are beneficial, due to lack of studies (39).

Gait

Independent walking may be the single most important factor in determining discharge disposition after severe burn injury. Farrell et al. (40) found that independent ambulation predicted discharge from the acute burn unit to home. As soon as the patient's condition permits, ambulation should begin. In addition to reducing the risk for contractures, deconditioning, and deep venous thromboses, early gait training maintains balance, lower extremity ROM, strength, and endurance. Physical therapists use a tilt table to perform graduated upright positioning and monitor for orthostasis. The literature indicates that muscles of the lower extremities, particularly the gastrocsoleus and quadriceps, are the first muscles to lose strength with bed rest. These same muscles experience a greater proportional loss of muscular torque when compared to other skeletal muscles (41). The physical therapist can initiate gait training and determine appropriate assistive devices; however, physical therapy sessions should not be the only time the patient walks. Nurses, family, and others can learn how to assist and provide needed support during walking. Walking reduces the effects of bed rest and improves aerobic conditioning.

Many consider new autografts to the lower extremities a contraindication to ambulation. Typically, ambulation is not initiated until the surgeon is confident that the graft will tolerate a dependent position. At 5 to 7 days after grafting, patients are instructed to begin lower extremity–dependent positioning. Dangling the lower extremities is a preambulation exercise that helps determine if the graft tolerates the dependent position. The application of elastic wraps or other elastic devices is used to minimize venous pooling and decrease the risk of graft loss. The typical protocol for dangling begins for 5 minutes two to three times per day. If inspection of the graft after dangling shows no signs of intolerance, the duration is progressively increased. Once the graft shows tolerance for dependency, ambulation is initiated. Like dangling, the time spent walking is methodically increased as the graft tolerates.

Patients excluded from early ambulation protocol include those with associated fractures, wounds greater than 300 cm^2, overriding social or psychiatric conditions, poor medical status, or plantar surface grafts. Bracing should be done if the burn crosses the ankle or knee joint. Currently, there are no formal recommendations for larger skin grafts to the lower extremities (42).

Gait deviations are common after burn injury. Some are transient, while others persist. Early correction of abnormal stance and gait reduces the risk that the deviation will be long-standing. Deviations result from pain, location of injury, deconditioning, weakness, contractures, and sensory and central nervous system dysfunction. Gait devices are commonly used to protect injured areas, reduce pain, assist with weight bearing, or to correct/prevent poor posture and gait deviations.

During times that the patient is unable to ambulate, wheelchairs provide mobility and are easily adapted to the patient's specific needs. Adaptations include attaching splints or wedges to elevate the arm or adding lower extremity positioning devices.

SURGICAL RECONSTRUCTION

The surgical goal is to minimize surgery and maximize results. If multiple areas are involved, an overall plan and timetable are developed that prioritize the fewest number of surgeries with the maximal functional benefit to the patient.

In terms of treating contractures, the timing of surgical release varies. Some surgeons believe that surgery should wait 6 to 12 months after injury. Others advocate waiting 2 years for full scar maturation prior to surgical intervention (43). However, there is limited evidence to support this recommendation. Other literature supports early intervention (44,45). There is evidence that early release does not worsen outcome, and surgery is indicated with the development of secondary deformities (46). Tendon and ligament injury impacts the completeness of the release that can be performed. Age, severity of the deformity, and time since injury impact surgical outcome (47).

Many reconstructive procedures are utilized in the burn-injured patient. Listed in the order of complexity are Z-plasty, skin graft, local skin flaps, local muscle flaps, fasciocutaneous flaps, free flaps, and cross-limb flaps. Full-thickness skin grafts are generally preferred to prevent recurrent contracture development (43).

Simple excision is indicated for scars that are limited in size and location. Z-plasties are employed to limit or correct joint contractures caused by hypertrophic scarring or for linear contractures that disrupt appearance. For example, this technique is employed to correct hypertrophic scarring over the chin that prevents adequate mouth closure (48). Release and skin grafting typically involve a fish-mouth incision and graft placement. Scar pressure therapy and silicone application are often combined with surgery to maximize outcome.

Severe axillary contractures are difficult to treat (📶 **eFig. 35-5**). If conservative treatment with passive ROM and splinting does not prevent axillary contracture after 6 to 12 months, then surgical release should be considered (43). For tight bands formed near unburned skin, five-flap releases are used (49). Local flaps are often used if anterior or posterior axillary fold contractures are present.

Contractures that are broader and involve the entire axilla require fasciocutaneous or similar flap procedures (50). Flaps generally heal faster than do skin grafts, which allows earlier mobilization (43).

Contractures at the elbow are often complicated by heterotopic ossification (HO), and this is taken into consideration during the surgical plan (51). A Z-plasty or five-flap release is used to treat a thin band of scarring (50). Surgical intervention for hand contractures requires expertise and experience. Full-thickness grafts are commonly used. Correction of flexion contracture of the MCP joint has a higher success rate than an extension deformity. Kirschner wires (K wires) are placed for 2 to 4 weeks after surgery for joint stabilization (52). Like the MCP joint, extension contractures of the thumb exhibit poor outcomes. Contractures associated with dislocated or subluxed joints have the worst results (50).

In recent years, face transplantation has garnered significant interest in the lay press. The first reported human face transplantation was performed in 2005 in France (53). To date, there have been more than 30 face transplants worldwide (53,54). These investigators utilize a cadaveric facial allograft that requires lifelong immunosuppressive treatment. There are unresolved questions regarding ethical, immunologic, and psychological issues. Does the improvement in quality of life justify the long-term risks of immunosuppression, including cancer, infection, and renal toxicity? Will the recipient experience graft rejection? What are the psychological consequences of a transplanted face? These and other issues are beginning to be addressed in the literature (55–57).

COMPLICATIONS

Burn survivors experience a wide range of complications that include neurologic, orthopedic, dermatologic, metabolic, pain, and psychosocial problems. These complications may develop in a few months to years after injury. The physiatrist plays an instrumental role in managing these problems, both on the wards and in the clinic.

NEUROLOGIC INJURIES

Localized Neuropathies

Peripheral mononeuropathies and plexopathies are common in severely burned patients (see Chapters 3 and 24). However, this complication is underreported in the literature, as the diagnosis is often delayed or missed entirely. The neurologic assessment is complicated by the complexity of medical problems and impaired consciousness of the critically ill patient. The reported incidence of peripheral neuropathy ranges from 15% to 37%. Kowalske et al. (58) examined 572 burn survivors and found that electrical injury, history of alcohol abuse, and length of intensive care unit stay were significant risk factors for the development of mononeuropathies. Polyneuropathies are more common than mononeuropathies after burn injury. It is also felt that elderly and diabetic patients are predisposed to peripheral nerve compromise (59,60). Compression and stretch of peripheral nerves place them at risk for injury. Bulky dressings can cause compression to superficial peripheral nerves. Improper and prolonged positioning is also a risk factor. Clinical pearls of specific mononeuropathies and brachial plexopathy are reviewed below (**Table 35-2**) (60,61).

Several bed and intraoperative positions may put the brachial plexus at risk for injury. To prevent compression or stretch injury to the brachial plexus, it is recommended to position the patient supine with 30 degrees of shoulder horizontal adduction (60).

In the lower extremity, mononeuropathies may include the peroneal and femoral nerves. Peroneal nerve injuries are relatively common. Windowing of dressings over the fibular head helps relieve pressure. Femoral nerve injury is uncommon (62).

Peripheral Polyneuropathy

Generalized peripheral polyneuropathy is a similarly common neurologic disorder in burn injury. The incidence ranges from 15% to 30% (59,63,64). Kowalske et al. (58) found that age and length of intensive care unit stay are risk factors for developing polyneuropathy. Polyneuropathy is more commonly seen in those with greater than 20% TBSA burns and electrical injuries (65). The etiology of peripheral neuropathies is uncertain; however, metabolic complications and neurotoxic drugs have been implicated. Electrophysiologic evidence of polyneuropathy is seen within 1 week of severe burn injury (66). The patient may have symptoms of paresthesia and signs of mild-to-moderate weakness in the muscles of the distal extremities. On manual muscle testing, most patients eventually recover their strength, although they may complain of easy fatigability for years after the burn (59,64). Critical illness polyneuropathy is understudied in the burn population. Risk factors include full-thickness burns, electrical burns, greater than 20% TBSA burns, multiorgan failure, and sepsis (67).

Mononeuritis Multiplex

Mononeuritis multiplex is an asymmetric sensory and motor peripheral neuropathy that involves two or more isolated peripheral nerves. The pathophysiology is not well understood but is thought to result from a combination of circulating neurotoxins, metabolic factors, and mechanical compression. Mononeuritis multiplex has been identified as the most common diagnosis in burn patients with a neuropathy, up to 69% (68). At 1 year after injury, lower extremity nerve lesions demonstrated better functional recovery than did upper extremity nerve lesions (69).

TABLE 35-2	Localized Neuropathies and Associated Risk Factors
Neuropathy	**Risk Factors**
Brachial plexus	Shoulder abduction >90, external rotation Axilla/lateral chest wall grafting position
Ulnar nerve	Elbow flexion 90 degrees, pronation, tourniquet paralysis
Radial nerve	At spiral groove: resting on side rails, hanging over the edge of the operating table, tourniquet paralysis At wrist: wrist restraints
Median nerve	Edema, prolonged or repeated wrist hyperextension, tourniquet paralysis
Peroneal nerve	Frog leg position, lateral decubitus position, metal stirrups, leg straps, bulky dressings
Femoral nerve	Hematoma at femoral triangle, retroperitoneal bleed

Pruritus

Itch is a significant symptom for many patients that may last up to several years in some cases (70). The prevalence of pruritus is as high as 93% at discharge, 86% at 6 months, 83% at 12 months, and 73% at 24 months after injury (70–72). A similar trend in pruritus after burn injury has been found in the pediatric population, with 93% reporting pruritus at discharge, 87% at 6 months, 78% at 12 months, and 64% at 24 months after injury (73). Intensity of pruritus is often greatest during the proliferative phase of wound healing as well as the remodeling phase. Risk factors for postburn pruritus include larger burn size, longer duration of time to wound closure, deep dermal injury, and early posttraumatic stress symptoms (72,74). Partial-thickness burn wounds are correlated with the most postburn itch (75). The mechanism of pruritus is not fully understood but is likely linked to histamine release from mast cells and induced by various inflammatory substances including prostaglandins, substance P, and kinins. Histamine receptors then activate unmyelinated C nerve fibers. Some investigators believe that it is related to axonal sprouting in the dermis. Various treatment regimens have demonstrated a decrease in reported itch symptoms; however, such interventions lack strong empirical evidence. Nonetheless, there exist multiple clinical treatment options. Topical moisturizers (75) and scar massage (76) are used in clinical practice on healed burn wounds. Topical medications include antihistamines and prudoxin, a tricyclic antidepressant. Oral medication options also include antihistamines (77) and prudoxin (DPT Laboratories, San Antonio, TX). There are reports of the use of transcutaneous electrical nerve stimulation (TENS), which works based on the Gate Theory (78). For those with severe itching, often a combination of interventions is needed to control symptoms. Gabapentin and pregabalin are some of the newest agents being investigated for postburn pruritus. Gabapentin works both centrally and peripherally and has been shown to control itch when given in doses of 300 to 900 mg/d (75). Recent studies show that gabapentin works better than do antihistamines and that antihistamines have limited efficacy (79–81).

BONE AND JOINT CHANGES

Contractures

Contractures are defined as an inability to perform full ROM of a joint. They result from a combination of possible factors—limb positioning, duration of immobilization, and muscle, soft tissue, and bony pathology. Postburn contractures are a combination of wound contracture and scar contracture secondary to the activity of fibroblasts and myofibroblasts, respectively (20). Individuals with burn injuries are at risk for developing contractures. Burn patients are often immobilized, both globally, as a result of critical illness in the severely burned, and focally, as a result of the burn itself due to pain, splinting, and positioning. Burns, by definition, damage the skin and may also involve damage to the underlying soft tissue, muscle, and bone. All of these factors contribute to contracture formation in burn injury.

Contractures place patients at risk for additional medical problems and functional deficits. Contractures interfere with skin and graft healing. Functionally, contractures of the lower extremities interfere with transfers, seating, weight-bearing activities, and ambulation. Contractures of the upper extremities may affect ADLs, such as grooming, dressing, eating, and bathing, as well as fine motor tasks.

Approximately 30% to 40% of hospitalized burn patients develop contractures, and on average, patients have three contractures per person (20). The shoulder, elbow, and hand/wrist are the most commonly involved joints (**Fig. 35-8**). Those with more extensive burns, amputations, and inhalation injuries are more likely to develop severe contractures (19). Positioning and ROM exercises are the mainstays of contracture prevention (25). Positions of comfort often include joint flexion and adduction, which often lead to contracture formation. For the bedbound burn patient, the ideal position to prevent contractures involves neck extension, shoulder abduction and external rotation, elbow extension and supination, hip abduction, and ankle dorsiflexion (see **Fig. 35-5**). Such positioning is coupled with regular ROM exercises. Once a patient has developed a contracture, treatment usually begins with conservative measures, including splinting (82–85) and serial casting (23,86). Richard et al. studied 52 patients with burn contractures, comparing treatment with a multimodal approach (massage, exercise, pressure) to a progressive approach (splinting and serial casting). Contractures are corrected in less than half the time in the progressive compared to the multimodal treatment group (83). Some investigators have reported success using ultrasound (87) and silicone gel (88) in treating contractures. Surgical correction of contractures (46,89) is reserved for contractures that significantly impact one's function and are not improved by conservative measures.

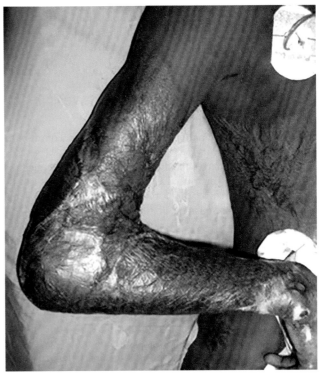

FIGURE 35-8. Burn contracture of the elbow.

Bone Growth

Significant growth delays occur in children after a severe burn injury (90). Growth disturbances in pediatric burns survivors may result from premature fusion of the epiphyseal plate of affected long bones. Bone growth issues should be considered in growing children with burn scars that cross a joint and with joint contractures. Partial epiphyseal plate fusion may cause bone deviation and deformity (91). In addition, case reports document that pressure garments for the treatment of facial burn injury in children alter facial bone growth. It is recommended to monitor closely facial development during and after pressure garment use in children for the development of normal dental and facial proportions (92,93). Children with burns greater than 15% TBSA exhibit decreased bone mineral density early (at 8 weeks) after injury and the loss is sustained (5 years after injury) (28). The mechanism for loss of bone mass is still being investigated; however, recent research demonstrates causal roles for multiple factors including increase in endogenous glucocorticoids, resorptive cytokines from the systemic inflammatory response and vitamin D deficiency, and disruption of calcium metabolism. Reduced bone density places children at risk for long bone fractures (94,95). Mayes et al. examined 104 burned children with greater than 40% TBSA and found a 5.8% incidence of fracture (96). Investigators have studied the use of recombinant human growth hormone without proven effect on bone formation (97). Studies have demonstrated improved bone mineral density with bisphosphonate therapy. Klein et al. performed a randomized controlled trial of 43 children with greater than 40% TBSA and examined the effects of acute administration (within 10 days of injury) of intravenous pamidronate. Subjects receiving pamidronate demonstrated higher whole-body and lumbar spine bone mineral content at discharge, 6 months, and 2 years compared to controls (98,99).

Osteophytes

Evans reports that osteophytes are the most frequently observed skeletal alteration in adult burn patients. They are most often seen at the elbow and occur along the articular margins of the olecranon or coronoid process (100).

Heterotopic Ossification

HO is the abnormal formation of bone in soft tissue. The incidence of HO is estimated at 1% to 4% of hospitalized burn patients (101). Only those with symptomatic joints, impaired ROM, joint pain, or other symptoms underwent radiographic examination. Therefore, reports in the literature reflect the incidence of clinically significant HO, not the true incidence. The etiology of this process is unknown. The elbow is the most frequent joint affected, constituting greater than 90% of cases in a 21-year review (101). Risk factors associated with the development of HO include size of burn (increased risk with >30% TBSA), ventilator support, sepsis, longer time to active movement, inhalation injury, intensive care unit stay, prolonged wound closure, wound infection, graft loss, number of trips to the operating room, and arm burns (101–104).

HO may occur as early as 5 weeks but usually develops at around 3 months after injury. One of the earliest signs of HO is loss of joint ROM. Other clinical findings may include swelling, erythema, pain, and peripheral nerve injury. Symptoms

may precede radiologic findings. A bone scan is the most sensitive diagnostic imaging test and may demonstrate positive findings up to 3 weeks prior to positive radiographic findings. Schneider et al. recently developed a scoring system to predict HO early after burn injuries (105).

Treatment of HO begins with conservative measures, including positioning and ROM to prevent worsening of joint motion. There is no evidence in the literature to support HO prophylaxis for burn patients. Timely surgical intervention is indicated when HO results in nerve entrapment. Surgical treatment is also indicated for HO that causes significant functional deficits, including impairments in upper and lower extremity function and impaired mobility and ADL. In these cases, it is common practice for surgeons to wait until the bone is mature to operate, which can take 12 to 18 months. One can follow the HO with serial radiographs every few months to monitor for bone stabilization. Surgical excision of HO at the elbow results in improvement in ROM and function (106,107). Tsionos et al. performed surgery on HO in 28 subjects and 35 elbows at a mean of 12 months after injury. At a mean follow-up of 21 months, the flexion/extension improved from 22 degrees preoperatively to 123 degrees postoperatively (106). Various postoperative treatments have been investigated to prevent recurrence of HO, including radiation, ROM, and anti-inflammatory medications (108).

Bony Changes in Electrical Burns

New bone formation is found at residual limb long bones in electrical burn survivors with amputation. Bony changes in the electrical burn include bone splitting, bony necrosis, bone swelling, lucent holes in bone, and periosteal new bone formation (109). Helm et al. reviewed 61 amputation sites in 43 burn survivors with electrical injuries. Twenty-three of twenty-eight patients with long bone amputations developed new bone formation at the amputation site. The etiology of new bone formation in the electrical amputee is unknown (110).

Scoliosis and Kyphosis

Asymmetric burns of the trunk, hips, and shoulder girdle can cause the patient to favor the affected side (see Chapter 28). In the growing child, the contracture of burn scars and resultant postural change can result in structural scoliosis. Moulton et al. performed a retrospective review that identified 40 pediatric burn patients with scoliosis and 1 with kyphosis. Average age at follow-up was 11 years 10 months. They identified that extensive burns at a young age can cause severe spine curves with risk factors including young age, large TBSA burn, deeper burn, and burn scar traversing the entire length of the trunk (111).

Similarly, childhood burns on the anterior neck, shoulders, and chest wall may produce a rounding of the shoulders and sunken chest. Likewise, burn scar shortening and protective posturing can result in kyphosis. Both scoliosis and kyphosis are amenable to bracing and surgical interventions. An orthopedic surgeon should follow such survivors.

Septic Arthritis

Septic arthritis is challenging to diagnose in the severely burned patient. The characteristic signs and symptoms are often absent or masked by the overlying burn wound. Joint pain, swelling, color change, and tenderness are common symptoms at the site of burn injury or grafting and therefore are difficult to distinguish from septic arthritis.

The two major causes of a septic joint are penetrating burns into a joint and hematogenous seeding in cases of bacteremia. Burn patients are at risk for infection because of their impaired immune system and concurrent illness. Septic arthritis may cause gross dislocation because of capsular laxity or cartilage and bone destruction (112), or it may result in severe restriction of movement or ankylosis. It occurs most frequently in the joints of the hands, hips, knees, and wrists.

Subluxations and Dislocations

Joint subluxation of the hands and feet is common after burn injury. Burns of the dorsal surface may contract resulting in joint hyperextension. With prolonged hyperextension, the joint can sublux. This is most commonly seen in the MCP and metatarsophalangeal (MTP) joints. Ulnar neuropathy places the patient at additional risk for subluxation of the fourth and fifth digits. For dorsal hand burns, prevention of subluxation is achieved with a combination of splinting and ROM exercises. Similarly, the MTP joints may become subluxed after contracture of healed wounds, especially in children. Application of surgical high-top shoes with a metatarsal bar keeps the toes in an antideformity position.

Posterior hip dislocation can be a problem in children. Hips maintained in an adducted and flexed position are at risk for dislocation. Anterior shoulder dislocations occur in positions of abduction and extension. Shoulder dislocations may result from positioning in the operating room (113).

PAIN COMPLICATIONS

Pain management is integral to the care of the burn survivor. Managing pain allows for greater participation in therapies after the acute period. In the acute stage after partial-thickness burn, some nerve endings in the dermis remain intact resulting in significant pain at the site of injury. In contrast, after full-thickness burn, the nerve endings are completely destroyed and the burned area is less painful or painless. Treatment of burns with daily dressing changes that debride necrotic tissue causes significant procedural pain. Patients may report unbearable levels of pain (114). It is important to manage the constant background pain of the burn injury itself as well as the intermittent procedural pain.

It is well documented that hospitalized burn patients' experience of pain varies among patients and across patients over time (115,116). Therefore, it is important to tailor the pain management plan for each individual. A few guiding principles are accepted as good clinical practice. Background pain can be treated with a continuous infusion of opioids, a long-acting oral opioid, or patient-controlled analgesia. Procedural pain is well managed with short-acting opioid medications scheduled prior to the procedure (117,118). In a randomized controlled trial of 79 hospitalized burn survivors, Patterson et al. (119) found that adding lorazepam to the standard opioid pain medication significantly reduced pain levels during procedures such as dressing changes for those with high baseline pain.

Nonpharmacologic interventions are important adjunctive interventions to standard pain medication regimens. This is an area of increasing interest in recent years. Simple environmental modifications and consistency are helpful. The goal is to create a calm atmosphere that incorporates as much patient autonomy as possible. Patients should be encouraged to direct their own dressing care. Some find the presence of family members and music helpful. The treatment team should provide consistent timing, staff, and routine of procedures. Investigators have found some success in the use of hypnosis to decrease procedural pain in burn injury (120,121). Virtual reality has demonstrated success as a distraction technique to help assuage pain during wound care (122,123). Morris et al. performed a systematic review on the effects of virtual reality on postburn pain and anxiety and found that it does reduce pain and anxiety during dressing changes and therapies (124). Other nonpharmacologic interventions that are validated in the literature include massage therapy for both acute and chronic pain in burn patients (76,125).

Neuropathic pain after burn injury is not well categorized in the literature. Neuropathic pain is defined as pain initiated or caused by a primary lesion or dysfunction in the peripheral or central nervous system. Neuropathic pain symptoms consisting of pins and needles, burning, stabbing, shooting, or electric sensations are common complaints of burn patients following healing of their open wounds. In two studies examining a total of 534 burn patients at least 1 year after injury, 71% and 82% reported paresthetic sensations in their burn scar, respectively. These sensations were associated with burn size and skin grafting (126,127). Schneider et al. retrospectively reviewed 72 patients with complaints of neuropathic pain and characterized their clinical course. Neuropathic pain symptoms first occurred at a mean of 4 months and persisted until 13 months after injury. Documented initial pain severity score was 7 out of 10. Typical exacerbating factors included temperature change, dependent position, light touch, and weight-bearing activities. Common alleviating factors included rest, massage, compression garment use, and elevation (128). Common treatment regimens include gabapentin, opioids, and steroid injections into areas of symptomatic hypertrophic scar.

SKIN COMPLICATIONS

Hypertrophic Scarring

Hypertrophic scarring can result from deep partial- and full-thickness burns. The scarring first presents as a firm, red area of healed burn scar. It progresses over weeks to become raised, erythematous, and rigid (**Fig. 35-9**). Scars can contract and, if present over a joint, can contribute to contracture formation. Over time, scars mature, taking on a pale, more pliable, and less thick appearance. This process may take up to 2 years. Scars may also be painful. Scarring can result in significant impairments in function. In addition to physical impairments, hypertrophic scarring may lead to psychosocial consequences. Scarring can impact self-esteem, social isolation, body image, and community reintegration (129,130). It is one of the most significant long-term complications of burn injury that impairs quality of life.

Histologically, scars demonstrate a whorled collage pattern, in contrast to the parallel array of collagen fibers in a normal skin. Scar tissue exhibits a proliferation of fibroblasts and capillaries, thickened epidermis, and a lack of rete pegs. Endothelial cell proliferation results in occlusion of the microvasculature

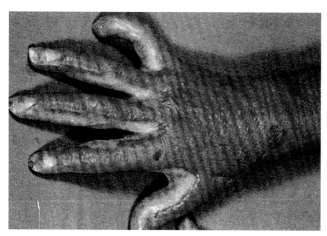

FIGURE 35-9. Hypertrophic scarring of the hand. Note the raised and rigid appearance of the scar.

leading to a local hypoxia. With maturation, the microvasculature degenerates and capillaries are reabsorbed (131–133). There exists a broad range of clinical presentations of scars that include varied thickness, color, rigidity, and corresponding symptoms. The prevalence of hypertrophic scarring is estimated at greater than 60% of white and greater than 75% of nonwhite survivors with severe burns (132). Interestingly, scarring is not documented in neonatal, elderly, and morbidly obese burn survivors. Prevalence data are confounded by lack of a standardized objective measure of hypertrophic scarring. The Vancouver Scar Scale and Observer Scar Assessment Scale are the most common methods of measurement; however, they are composed of subjective ratings of pigmentation, vascularity, and pliability and as a result have a relatively low interrater reliability (133,134). Risk factors for the development of hypertrophic scarring include open wounds for greater than 2 to 3 weeks, burns that require grafting, and heavily pigmented individuals (135). The etiology of hypertrophic scarring is largely unknown.

There exists little evidence in the literature to support specific treatment strategies for hypertrophic scarring. Current study limitations include sample size, randomization, adequate follow-up, and objective outcome measures. Given the seriousness of the problem, investigators are actively pursuing research in this area (136). Meanwhile, providers rely on clinically derived treatment approaches. Early excision of burns has been shown to reduce scarring (134). Management begins with early identification of hypertrophic scarring and those at risk of scarring. Initial conservative treatment measures include splinting, scar massage, compression garments, laser therapy, intense pulsed light, steroids, exercise, and positioning. Pressure therapy constitutes the main treatment intervention. It is postulated that pressure (at least 25 mm Hg) inhibits capillary blood flow resulting in local ischemia. A decrement in tissue metabolism leads to impaired fibroblastic activity and enhanced collagenase activity. Apoptosis ensues with release of proteases and liposomal contents (48).

The goal of therapy is to arrest scar development and flatten existing scars. Initially, pressure wrappings are applied around the affected areas using plastic elastic (ACE), cotton elastic (Tubigrip), or adhesive elastic (Coban) bandages. As edema resolves, the scarred area assumes a more stable shape and custom-made pressure garments are fit. It is recommended

to wear compression garments 23 hours of the day until the scar matures, which can be up to 2 years (137). Compliance with this regimen is difficult. The garments are warm, socially awkward, and difficult to don. They stretch and shift with wear, and replacement garments are recommended every 3 months. Concave areas are poorly compressed. To improve fit or pressure over areas with challenging contour features, such as the digital web space, silicone sheets or gels, sponges, or conformed pieces of plastic are used to improve the delivery of pressure and limit shear over the new and fragile epithelium (48,138,139).

Randomized controlled trials have been done to assess pressure garment therapy for hypertrophic scarring treatment, and no significant differences were seen in scar outcome (140,141). Both studies utilized subjective outcome measures to determine the number of days to scar maturation or the number of days for pressure therapy. In contrast, a meta-analysis of compression therapy showed a reduction in scar height (142). The efficacy of pressure therapy is unknown; however, there are no major treatment alternatives. Future research into the optimal pressure and duration of pressure therapy will greatly advance the care of burn survivors.

In addition, pressure therapy may have detrimental effects. Obstructive sleep apnea is an adverse effect that may occur with facial pressure therapy (143). In children, hypertrophic scarring of the head and neck and pressure garment treatment have been reported to cause deformities. Knowledge of such potential complications helps inform treatment decisions. Scar contractures of the mandible may lead to dental occlusion and difficulty with lip closure and subsequent drooling. Pressure garments at the mandible may cause mandibular hypoplasia. Severe neck scarring and resultant contractures may elongate the mandible. Mouth burns are associated with dental changes, including crossbite, crowding, and bite retrusion. Pressure garments may affect facial growth and development of normal contours (144).

Other treatments, silicone gel and massage, have been examined in the literature as well. Newer studies have also shown efficacy in gels and gel sheets for treatment of immature hypertrophic scars though most studies were superiority trials and did not include placebo treatments. Also, the number of studies and quality of evidence for burn survivor hypertrophic scar and keloid treatments were limited in burn-only populations. Studies to date have shown no difference in outcomes for gels versus gel sheets or nonsilicone versus silicone (145). Ahn et al. investigated the efficacy of an 8-week course of topical silicone gel in 10 adults with hypertrophic scars. Each subject acted as his or her own control; mirror-image or adjacent scars were untreated controls. Based on elastometry, skin biopsy, texture, color, thickness, durability, and itching, the silicone-treated areas demonstrated greater improvements than control scars at 4, 8, and 12 weeks (146). Most patients tolerate these products well, though adverse effects include pruritus, skin breakdown, and dermatitis. The suggested maximum wear time is 12 hours per day (146).

A study of 30 pediatric burn patients examined the use of frictional massage 30 minutes a day over a 3-month period. No significant effects were demonstrated with regard to the vascularity, pliability, and height of the hypertrophic scar (147). If conservative treatments fail, one may consider surgical resection with or without skin grafting.

Blisters

Blisters are a common complication of partial-thickness burns. Blisters result from inflammatory changes after injury that increases capillary permeability, thereby permitting fluid accumulation between the epidermis and dermis. Management of blisters remains a controversial topic in burn care. Sargent performed an extensive literature review on the topic, examining issues related to the care of blisters, including infection, healing, function, aesthetics, patient comfort, dressing care, and cost-effectiveness. The author issued clinical practice guidelines for management of blisters in partial-thickness burns. Small blisters (<6 mm) may be left intact, as they are unlikely to rupture spontaneously, damage underlying tissue, or impede healing. Large blisters (>6 mm) should be debrided and dressed. Thick-walled blisters on the palms and soles of the feet need not be debrided as they are less likely to become infected, and debridement may cause patient discomfort and impaired mobility. Debridement of blisters is associated with faster wound healing and decreased scarring. Decreased scarring is also associated with use of temporary skin substitutes to cover the debrided site (148,149).

UV Sensitivity and Skin Pigmentation

Sun protection is essential for burn survivors. The area of burn injury is susceptible to further damage from the sun's ultraviolet radiation. It is recommended that burn survivors of deep partial- and full-thickness burns avoid and protect against sun exposure for the first few years after injury. Especially after burn injury, people of all different skin pigmentations are at risk for sunburn from ultraviolet radiation. Avoiding direct sun exposure, especially during midday hours when ultraviolet exposure is highest, minimizes risk of sunburn. Covering sites of burn injury with clothing for at least the first year after injury is recommended. In addition, sunscreen with a sun protection factor of 15 or greater should be applied to healed burn sites prior to any sun exposure (150).

Pigmentation changes are common after burn injury. Hyperpigmentation correlates with premorbid skin color, age, sun exposure, and time after injury (151,152). Deep partial- and full-thickness burn injuries may result in hypopigmentation or depigmentation. Dyspigmentation after burn injury can be treated surgically. Al-Qattan reported treating 15 subjects with hyperpigmented skin grafts with surgical excision and split-thickness skin grafts. He also treated eight subjects with hypopigmented burn sites with dermabrasion and thin split-thickness skin grafts. The hyperpigmentation group exhibited color and texture match, while the hypopigmentation group demonstrated slight hyperpigmentation of the graft site (153). Other investigators demonstrated good results by treating depigmented burn scar using a carbon dioxide laser for dermabrasion followed by split-thickness skin grafting (154).

Malignancy

Development of malignant tumors in chronic burn wounds or scars is extremely rare but is a reported complication. Most tumors are squamous cell carcinoma; basal cell carcinoma and malignant melanoma are less common. Diagnosis ranges from 20 to 30 years after burn injury. Two large cohort studies followed 16,903 and 37,095 burn survivors, respectively, for a mean of 16 years. There was no increased risk for squamous cell carcinoma, basal cell carcinoma, or malignant melanoma in the burn survivors compared to the general population. In addition, subgroup analysis of those with more severe burns and longer follow-up exhibited no increased risk for skin cancer (155,156).

METABOLIC COMPLICATIONS

Catabolic State

Patients with burns greater than 30% to 40% TBSA experience a hypermetabolic response for at least 1 year or more after injury. Catabolism contributes significantly to morbidity and mortality. Patients with TBSA greater than 40% may experience 180% of the basal metabolic rate during acute admission, 150% at full healing, 140% at 6 months from injury, 120% at 9 months from injury, and 110% at 1 year from injury (157). The catabolic state in burn injury is associated with impaired wound healing, increased infection risk, loss of lean body mass, slowed rehabilitation, and delayed community reintegration. Increases in catecholamines, glucagon, glucocorticoids, and dopamine initiate the hypermetabolic response (158). Pharmacologic and nonpharmacologic strategies are implemented to help reverse the effects of catabolism. Nonpharmacologic interventions include early burn wound excision and closure; aggressive treatment of sepsis; maintenance of thermal neutrality by elevation of the ambient temperature; high-carbohydrate, high-protein diet; and early institution of resistive exercises. Pharmacologic interventions may include the use of recombinant human growth hormone, low-dose insulin infusion, synthetic testosterone analog (oxandrolone), and β-blockade (97,159,160).

The benefits of oxandrolone on hypermetabolism in burn injury are well supported by multiple well-designed studies in recent years. Jeschke et al. performed a prospective randomized controlled trial of 235 burned children with greater than 40% TBSA. Subjects receiving oxandrolone for at least 7 days during acute hospitalization exhibited shorter length of intensive care unit stay and higher lean body mass than controls (161). When oxandrolone was given to children for 1 year after severe burn, subjects demonstrated continued improved lean body mass, bone mineral content, muscle strength, height, and weight compared to controls (162). Cochran et al. found that administration of oxandrolone in individuals with TBSA 20% to 60% had shorter length of stay (163).

Temperature Regulation

Full-thickness burns damage the sweat glands of the dermis. Despite treatment with skin grafting, the sweat glands are not replaced or regenerated. Impaired sweating may affect thermoregulation (164), particularly with those with larger TBSA burns. Patients with large burn injuries often report overheating and exaggerated sweating response in areas of unburned skin with exercise and heat. Such complaints may interfere with burn survivors' exercise tolerance, overall fitness, and health, as well as occupational reintegration (165,166).

PSYCHOSOCIAL ISSUES

Psychosocial complications after burn injury are common and present major obstacles to burn survivors' rehabilitation and community integration. Burns are traumatic, functionally impairing, excruciatingly painful, and disfiguring. All of these factors contribute to the prevalence of psychosocial complications after burns. In addition, premorbid psychiatric history is higher in burn patients than in the general population. Approximately one third of burn injuries are associated with concomitant alcohol or drug use (5). Preinjury psychiatric problems, including anxiety, depression, and other problems, are more common in burn patients than in the general population and have been documented at 28% to 75% (167). Common psychosocial issues after burn injury include posttraumatic stress, depression, anxiety, sleep disorders, and difficulties with community integration. The research community has excelled in identifying and describing these important psychosocial issues after burn injury. An important aspect of community reintegration is return to work. One study reported 90% of individuals with burn injury return to work by 2 years (168). Future investigation in this area is needed.

Posttraumatic Stress and Acute Stress Disorder

Posttraumatic stress and/or acute stress disorder (ASD) occurs after one experiences a traumatic event with the threat of injury or death to self or others. Three types of symptoms characterize posttraumatic stress disorder (PTSD): reexperiencing the event, avoidance of reminders of the event, and an increased state of arousal. For the diagnosis of PTSD, symptoms must be present for greater than 1 month and for ASD symptoms must be present for greater than 2 days during the first 4 weeks after the event. Prevalence of ASD ranges from 6% to 33%, while PTSD prevalence is higher, with rates of 24% to 40% at 6 months and 15% to 45% at 12 months postinjury (169). Commonly reported symptoms include sleep disturbance, recurrent and intrusive recollections of the injury, avoidance of thoughts or feelings associated with the burn, and distress at reminders of the burn. Overall, posttraumatic stress symptoms decrease over time. It is common for burn survivors to endorse some posttraumatic stress symptoms but not fulfill the diagnostic criteria for posttraumatic stress and ASDs (170). Risk factors for the development of PTSD after burn injury include posttraumatic stress symptoms at earlier time points, female gender, social support, and the size and location of burn injury (171). Treatment interventions for posttraumatic stress have not been validated in the literature. Only a few small studies have been conducted. Screening for posttraumatic stress symptoms and referral for pharmacologic and nonpharmacologic treatment interventions are recommended.

Depression

Depression is a similarly common psychiatric problem after burn injury. Reported rates of depression vary based on the metric used, but some studies have reported 4% at discharge to 10% to 23% 1 year postinjury with increasing rates throughout the first year (172). Premorbid psychiatric problems, head or neck burns, length of hospital stay, and female gender are risk factors associated with depression (173,174). Edwards et al. followed 128 burn survivors and found that one third of subjects reported some form of suicidal ideation during the first year after injury. Pain severity at discharge was the only significant predictor of suicidal ideation (175). The frequency of suicidal ideation highlights the importance of early identification of symptoms in suicide prevention. Furthermore, psychosocial outcomes are complex and multifaceted. Pain management may impact depression and other psychiatric complications. Clinicians should identify those at risk for

depression and those with depressive symptoms and provide appropriate treatment options.

Sleep Disturbances

Sleep disturbances may be related to a psychiatric problem, medical issue, or a direct consequence of the burn injury. As many as 74% of burn survivors reported sleep problems at 1 week after discharge from the hospital. Common problems include nighttime awakenings, daytime napping, nighttime pain, and difficulty with sleep onset (176). Sleep problems, such as insomnia and nightmares, persist at 1 year after injury (170). Gottschlich et al. examined polysomnography in 11 severely burned inpatient children over forty-three 24-hour sessions. Deep sleep (stages III and IV) and rapid eye movement were completely missing in 40% and 19% of recordings, respectively. This demonstrates altered sleep architecture in the acute period after burn injury (177). High levels of pain and analgesic intake during the day were associated with poor sleep the following night in one study (178). Masoodi et al. studied 818 adults after burn injury at 1 year using the Pittsburgh Sleep Quality Index Questionnaire and discovered that 61% of burn-injured adults had poor sleep, while 39% of noninjured adults had poor sleep (179). A recent study by Lee et al. assessed risk factors for long-term sleep disturbances after burn injury in young adults ages 19 to 30 using the Young Adult Burn Outcome Questionnaire database. They concluded that 50% of subjects reported sleep dissatisfaction and some of the risk factors for long-term sleep disturbances include larger burn size, pain, itch, and lack of physical activity, though some of these factors are bidirectional (180).

It is important to ask burn patients about their sleep. Since other psychiatric problems can contribute to sleep problems, clinicians should consider these issues as well when treating sleep disorders in burn injury. Treatment of pain, pruritus, depression, and posttraumatic stress and anxiety may improve burn survivors' sleep.

Community Integration

The one main goal of rehabilitation is reintegration into society, including a return to one's work, school, and recreational and community activities. The various physical and psychological complications of burn injury detailed above may result in significant impairments that hinder community integration. In a study of 463 burn survivors who completed the Community Integration Questionnaire, researchers found significant problems in home integration, social integration, and productivity. Home integration was best predicted by gender and living situation; social integration was best predicted by marital status; productivity was best predicted by burn severity, age, and preburn job satisfaction (181). Return to work after burn injury has gained increased attention among researchers over the past several years.

Factors associated with unemployment after burn include severity of injury, length of hospital stay, older age, extremity burns, premorbid psychiatric history, and premorbid unemployment (130,182,183). Esselman et al. examined barriers to return to work in 154 burn survivors using a survey administered 16 times over 1 year. At 1 year, significant barriers included physical abilities, psychosocial factors (nightmares, flashbacks, body image), and working conditions (humidity, temperature, safety) (165).

Some burn survivors experience permanent impairment as a result of their injury. The American Medical Association publishes guidelines for determining the extent of impairment. Impairment is graded as a percentage of whole-body impairment. In the sixth edition of the guidelines, impairment in burn injury is primarily dependent upon the following factors: the severity of the skin condition; the frequency, intensity, and complexity of symptoms and the treatment regimen; and the ability to perform ADL. This impairment rating may be modified by objective physical examination findings, facial disfigurement, and related impairments of other organ systems including musculoskeletal, respiratory, cardiovascular, endocrine, and gastrointestinal. It is important to remember that these guidelines are intended for evaluation of patients with permanent impairments, those who have attained maximal recovery (184).

SPECIAL CONSIDERATIONS

Pediatric Burns

The physiologic and anatomic differences between adults and children need to be considered during acute and long-term medical management after burn injury (see Chapter 45). There are major differences in the anatomy and physiology of children and adults. Anatomically, the pediatric trachea is shorter, the glottis is more anterior, and the diameter of the airway is smaller compared to an adult. These anatomic differences are important during intubation and in the presence of facial burns, upper airway damage, inhalation injuries, or edema. Children have an increased risk of bronchospasm (185). The smaller airways make them more susceptible to occlusion if there is pulmonary debris, such as after an inhalation injury.

After a significant burn injury, children often demonstrate impaired cardiac function. This is particularly relevant if the child is less than 1 year of age, has underlying cardiac anomalies, or sustained an inhalation injury (186).

Pediatric Exercise

The goals of exercise are similar to adults, but the methods are different. Exercises are designed to be compatible with the child's level of development and incorporate play. Toys should be developmentally appropriate for the child. For instance, nesting blocks for the child less than 2 years old are used to enhance hand function. In an older child, wheelbarrow walking or crab walking stretches the shoulder muscles and strengthens the shoulder girdle. Bicycling and soccer ball kicking are appropriate for lower extremity stretching, strengthening, and endurance training in older children. A wide variety of products, such as TheraBand and therapy putty can provide resistance and facilitate strengthening. Handheld computer games are valuable for fine motor function of the hand. Interactive computer games, such as the Wii, utilize visual monitors and encourage gross motor participation.

Splints for Children

The skin of infants and children differs from that of adults. Because the skin of children is thinner, full-thickness wounds are more likely to occur (187). Stretching techniques, splint fabrication, and pressure garments (🛜 eTable 35-2) are designed to accommodate the thinner and more fragile skin of children. Therefore, the treatment of contractures in children is similar to that of adults, with a few modifications.

It is often difficult for parents to stretch a child's joints. Aggressive stretching of contracted joints is often difficult for children to tolerate. Stretching under anesthesia and pain medication administration prior to therapy may be indicated.

When using splints in the pediatric population, one must take into consideration the smaller size of body parts and the quality of the skin. Extra padding or foam may be needed. Compared to adults, children have hypermobile joints. Splints in children require frequent evaluation by caregivers because of normal growth.

Many suggest that splints for infants are applied when the child is sleeping and allow active use of the extremity during wakeful periods. If this is insufficient, wearing time is increased during the daytime and splints are removed for exercise or therapeutic activities. Children often tolerate prolonged joint immobilization and do not develop joint contractures like adults.

Dynamic splints are an option for adolescents but are generally not tolerated by infants or small children because they are too difficult to keep in place. Small children are better with static splints or serial casting. By age 3 or 4, children may use adjustable three-point splints at the knee or elbow. Dynamic ankle splints work in this older group as well.

For young children, hand and ankle splints are made with longer proximal extensions to secure the splint from sliding out of position. For instance, a hand splint may extend to the wrist and forearm. Soft straps that cross the volar aspect of the wrist and forearm secure the device. Splints may need to be covered with a garment, such as a sock, to prevent the child from removing the device. The hand of a young child or infant is typically splinted flat with the wrist in extension, fingers extended and abducted, and the thumb in extension and abducted radially. Sandwich splints lined with foam with a dorsal and ventral component are useful.

Pediatric Reconstructive Surgery

Children often require surgery to restore function. In addition, surgery may be indicated to correct deformities and functional impairments that develop as a result of growth. Scar tissue and some grafts do not elongate with growth and consequently reconstructive surgery is required. If ROM is normal as the child grows, surgery is not indicated. The neck and axillae require close monitoring. Reconstructive surgery is performed approximately 1 year after menarche for girls with significant scarring of the anterior chest.

Geriatric Burns

In the geriatric population, preexisting physical limitations or medical problems have a greater impact on rehabilitation than in younger survivors (see Chapter 47). Premorbid functional level and health are particularly important in establishing a geriatric rehabilitation plan. Older adults often have cardiovascular disease. In the face of a serious burn injury, an older patient may develop worsening cardiac function or myocardial infarction (188). There is a baseline decrease in pulmonary function that is associated with aging. Also, many older individuals have underlying pulmonary or cardiac disease that negatively impacts respiratory reserve and function. A burn injury coupled with inhalation injury markedly increases the risk of mortality and morbidity. Principles of cardiopulmonary rehabilitation are included in the exercise plan for these individuals.

Skin and Wound Healing

The atrophic skin of the elderly is characterized by the absence of rete pegs, a thinner dermis, and a reduced number of skin appendages. As a consequence, the elderly sustain more severe burns than do younger adults from the same injury (189). Additionally, the cellularity of the skin decreases with age, leading to a reduced number of macrophages and fibroblasts, thereby prolonging healing time. The skin of the elderly exhibits less turgor than that of younger people and is due in part to a decrease in glycosaminoglycans. The redundant tissue can be harvested for use as full-thickness grafts and improved functional outcome.

Early excision and grafting is a well-established approach to burn injury in children and adults; however, the risk-to-benefit ratio is not as clear in the elderly (190,191). The burn wound and donor site are additive, effectively increasing the surface area of open wounds resulting in increased rates of morbidity and mortality.

Exercise

During normal aging, one experiences sarcopenia or muscle mass loss as well as loss of strength (190). Strength declines at a rate of 15% per decade after age 50 and 30% after age 70. There is evidence that resistance training can reduce and reverse some of the muscle changes and strength loss of aging (191). However, sarcopenia, and the associated weakness, is aggravated by disuse or bed rest. As a result, elderly are at greater risk for loss of function after burn injury.

A geriatric burn exercise program takes into account one's preexisting musculoskeletal and neuromuscular conditions that influence the exercise prescription. One must determine if passive, active-assistive, or active exercise therapy is appropriate. An exercise regimen includes ROM, stretching, and strengthening.

Stretching principles are similar to those of any adult. Each joint is stretched individually. This progresses to stretching of an entire limb. With redundant tissue present in some body regions, scarring and contracture development are less frequent than in other adults.

ROM exercise is modified in the presence of underlying joint disease, such as degenerative osteoarthritis. A burn injury involving a chronically arthritic shoulder is treated differently than a nonarthritic joint. One may need to modify goals to achieve a functional range rather than full ROM.

Strength training starts slowly and gradually increases in intensity. It is important to closely monitor cardiopulmonary status. As in other age groups, strengthening usually begins with muscles that oppose scar contracture formation. Exercise should advance judiciously beginning with nonresistance exercises and progressing to resistance bands and light weights. Maximal exercise capacity and oxygen consumption decrease with age; however, there is evidence that aerobic capacity can increase with endurance training in the elderly.

FACIAL BURNS

Skin contractures and scars of the face are challenging to prevent. Facial tissue is highly mobile and has few points of fixation. Common facial deformities include ectropion of the lower eyelid and microstomia of the mouth. The development of ectropion prevents eyelid closing leading to eye irritation that may result in corneal ulcers. Microstomia is a contracture of the mouth that impairs mouth function.

Current review of the literature indicates that rehabilitation interventions for face burns lack general agreement. No generally accepted medical or rehabilitation protocols exist. Common treatment methodologies include positioning, splinting, exercise, stretching, and pressure therapy (192). A recent small study of 12 patients with full-thickness orofacial burns treated conservatively with exercise revealed improved vertical and horizontal mouth opening ranges though still in the lower limits of normal function compared to controls. The duration of rehabilitation was noted to be significant with 50% requiring more than 2 years (193).

During the acute phase, many begin treatment with splints for the neck, mouth, nose, and ears. Active ROM of the face, including the eyes and mouth, is initiated as soon as the patient can participate. For ear injuries, pillows are used to prevent chondritis and tissue adhering to the bed linens. Devices are fabricated to relieve pressure for an injured pinna.

Microstomia is a contracture of the oral aperture of the face (**Fig. 35-10**). It is associated with impaired oral hygiene, eating, and speech. In addition, microstomia may disrupt muscular and dental development in children (194). The contracture may involve the skin of the mouth or involve the perioral musculature that creates the sphincter of the mouth. The orbicularis oris muscle is separated from the surface by a thin subcutaneous layer and from the mucosa below by a thin submucosal layer.

Oral stretching splints are used to maintain the normal dimension of the mouth for those at risk of developing microstomia. These splints are often custom made and tailored to maximize comfort and benefit. Commercial devices are also available. Splint designs vary by direction of force (horizontal, vertical, or circumoral stretch) and orientation (intraoral or extraoral). Monitoring is required for skin irritation and breakdown. Factors to consider in prescribing a microstomia splint include age, dentition, stage of dental development in children, and location and depth of injury. Devices should be comfortable to wear, insert, and clean. Compliance is often challenging. To maximize success and achieve optimal patient compliance, a graduated wearing schedule is advised and more than one device is indicated (195,196).

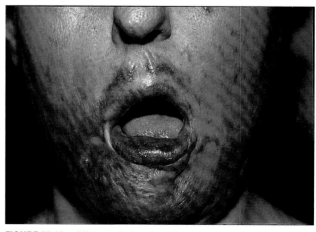

FIGURE 35-10. Microstomia from facial burns.

The timing of initiating pressure therapy in clinical practice for facial burns is variable (197). Pressure is an accepted treatment for facial burn scarring and deformity. Face masks or pressure garments fitted to the face are widely used. In 1979, Rivers et al. (198) first described the fabrication of a transparent face mask for application of pressure to prevent scarring. The transparent rigid face mask is the most common (192) facial pressure device ($\widehat{\mathbin{\widehat{\mathbb{\circ}}}}$ **eFig. 35-6**). There is better patient compliance and social acceptance of a transparent face mask than a fabric face garment (199,200). Accuracy of fit is critical to successful scar suppression. The transparent face mask allows for better fit, as one can easily monitor for scar blanching (198). Allely et al. described the use of laser Doppler imaging for mask fabrication. This technique holds the potential for increased precision and efficiency in fabricating transparent face masks (201).

There exists concern that pressure will alter the dental, maxillary, and mandibular features of a child. Some recommend the involvement of an orthodontist in all children with facial burns (202,203). Literature review reveals limited support for the effects of pressure therapy on preservation of craniofacial features after facial burns. A systematic review by Rappoport et al. in 2008 concluded that there is a lack of studies on dento-maxillofacial effects from pressure garment treatment of facial burns (204). One study met inclusion criteria and included six children, three with total face masks and three with partial face masks of the lower face. Those with the lower face mask exhibited anterior protrusion of the teeth and little reduction in the inferior growth of the mandible. These changes persisted after pressure therapy was discontinued. For subjects with full face masks, maxillary horizontal growth was more affected than vertical growth. Radiographs in both groups after pressure therapy was discontinued demonstrated resolution in the bony abnormalities (93,205).

CONCLUSION

With more patients surviving burn injuries, care is increasingly focused on the complications, rehabilitation, and long-term outcomes of burn survivors. Burn injuries may present as major catastrophic injuries, with a complex array of problems that include contractures, hypertrophic scarring, pain, neuropathy, and psychosocial problems. Physiatry is an integral component of the specialized multidisciplinary burn care team throughout the continuum of care. Rehabilitation interventions begin immediately after injury in the intensive care unit aimed at preventing long-term complications of burns. Splinting, positioning, and exercise are hallmarks of early rehabilitation. Burn care may continue for years after hospital discharge, managing physical and psychosocial impairments after burn injury and ultimately promoting maximal reintegration into the community.

REFERENCES

1. Ryan CM, Schoenfeld DA, Thorpe WP, et al. Objective estimates of the probability of death from burn injuries. *N Engl J Med*. 1998;338:362–366.
2. Pruitt BA Jr, Goodwin CW, Mason AD Jr. Epidemiological, demographic and outcome characteristics of burn injury. In: Herndon DN, ed. *Total Burn Care*. 2nd ed. New York, NY: Saunders; 2002:16–30.
3. *American Burn Association: Burn Incidence and Treatment in the US: 2016 Fact Sheet*. Available from: www.ameriburn.org/resources_factsheet.php
4. *National Burn Repository 2016 Report*. Available from: www.ameriburn.org/2016%20 ABA%20Full.pdf
5. *NIDRR Model Systems for Burn Injury Rehabilitation Adult Facts, Figures, and Selected Outcomes*. Available from: http://bms-dcc.uchsc.edu/. Accessed February 2017.
6. *NIDRR Model Systems for Burn Injury Rehabilitation Adult Facts, Figures, and Selected Outcomes*. Available from: http://bms-dcc.uchsc.edu/. Accessed March 2017.
7. Ojeh N, Pastar I, Tomic-Canic M, et al. Stem cells in skin regeneration, wound healing, and their clinical applications. *Int J Mol Sci*. 2015;16(10):25476–25501.
8. Kearns RD, Holmes JH, Cairns BA. Burn injury: what's in a name? Labels used for burn injury classification: a review of the data from 2000–2012. *Ann Burns Fire Disasters*. 2013;26(3):115–120.
9. Lund CC, Browder NC. Estimation of areas of burns. *Surg Gynecol Obstet*. 1944; 79:352–358.
10. Anderson JA, Coscia RL, Cryer HG. Guidelines for the operation of burn centers. In: Rotondo M, Cribari C, Smith RS, eds. *Resources for the Optimal Care of the Injured Patient*. Chicago, IL: American College of Surgeons Committee on Trauma; 2006:79–86.
11. Johnson C. Pathologic manifestations of burn injury. In: Richard R, Staley M, eds. *Burn Care and Rehabilitation: Principles and Practice*. Philadelphia, PA: F.A. Davis; 1994:29–48.
12. Munster A. The immunological response and strategies for intervention. In: Herndon DN, ed. *Total Burn Care*. London, UK: W.B. Saunders; 1997:279–292.
13. McCallon S, Weir D, Lantis JC. Optimizing wound bed preparation with collagenase enzymatic debridement. *J Am Coll Clin Wound Spec*. 2014;6:14–23.
14. Chua A, Khoo Y, Tan B, et al. Skin tissue engineering advances in severe burns: review and therapeutic applications. *Burns & Trauma*. 2016;4:3. DOI 10.1186/s41038-016-0027-y.
15. Debels H, Hamdi M, Abberton K, et al. Dermal matrices and bioengineered skin substitutes: a critical review of current options. *Plast Reconstr Surg Glob Open*. 2015;3(1):e284.
16. Pham C, Greenwood J, Cleland H, et al. Bioengineered skin substitutes for the management of burns: a systematic review. *Burns*. 2007;33:946–957.
17. Edelman DA, Sheehy-Deardorff DA, White MT. Bedside assessment of swallowing is predictive of an abnormal barium swallow examination. *J Burn Care Res*. 2008;29:89–96.
18. Schouten HJ, Nieuwenhuis MK, van Zuijlen PPM. A review on static splinting therapy to prevent burn scar contracture: do clinical and experimental data warrant its clinical application? *Burns*. 2012;38(1):19–25.
19. Schneider JC, Holavanahalli R, Helm P, et al. Contractures in burn injury: defining the problem. *J Burn Care Res*. 2006;27(4):508–514.
20. Goverman J, Mathews K, Goldstein R, et al. Adult contractures in burn injury: a burn model system national database study. *J Burn Care Res*. 2017;38(1):328–336.
21. Richard RL, et al. Identification of cutaneous functional units related to burn scar contracture development. *J Burn Care Res*. 2009;30(4):625–631.
22. Dewey W, Richard R, Parry I. Positioning, splinting, and contracture management. *Phys Med Rehabil Clin N Am*. 2011;22(2):229–247.
23. Staley M, Serghiou M. Casting guidelines, tips, and techniques: proceedings from the 1997 American Burn Association PT/OT Casting Workshop. *J Burn Care Rehabil*. 1998;19:254–260; discussion 253.
24. Torres-Gray D, Greene S. Rehabilitation of the burned hand. *Tech Hand Up Extrem Surg*. 1998;2:284–292.
25. Helm PA, Kevorkian CG, Lushbaugh M, et al. Burn injury: rehabilitation management in 1982. *Arch Phys Med Rehabil*. 1982;63:6–16.
26. Jensen LL, Parshley PH. Postburn scar contractures: histology and effects of pressure treatment. *J Burn Care Rehabil*. 1984;5:119–123.
27. Hart DW, Wolf SE, Chinkes DL, et al. Determinants of skeletal muscle catabolism after severe burn. *Ann Surg*. 2000;232:455–465.
28. Klein GL, Herndon DN, Langman CB, et al. Long-term reduction in bone mass after severe burn injury in children. *J Pediatr*. 1995;126:252–256.
29. Sakurai Y, Aarsland A, Herndon DN, et al. Stimulation of muscle protein synthesis by long-term insulin infusion in severely burned patients. *Ann Surg*. 1995;222:283–294, 294–297.
30. Suman OE, Herndon DN. Effects of cessation of a structured and supervised exercise conditioning program on lean mass and muscle strength in severely burned children. *Arch Phys Med Rehabil*. 2007;88:S24–S29.
31. Celis MM, Suman OE, Huang TT, et al. Effect of a supervised exercise and physiotherapy program on surgical interventions in children with thermal injury. *J Burn Care Rehabil*. 2003;24:57–61; discussion 56.
32. Suman OE, Henrdon DN, Przkora R. The effects of oxandrolone and exercise on muscle mass and function in severely burned children. *Burns*. 2006;10:269.
33. Przkora R, Herndon DN, Suman OE, et al. Beneficial effects of extended growth hormone treatment after hospital discharge in pediatric burn patients. *Ann Surg*. 2006;243:796–801; discussion 801–803.
34. Murphy KD, Thomas S, Mlcak RP, et al. Effects of long-term oxandrolone administration in severely burned children. *Surgery*. 2004;136:219–224.
35. Suman OE, Thomas SJ, Wilkins JP, et al. Effect of exogenous growth hormone and exercise on lean mass and muscle function in children with burns. *J Appl Physiol*. 2003;94:2273–2281.
36. de Lateur BJ, Magyar-Russell G, Bresnick MG, et al. Augmented exercise in the treatment of deconditioning from major burn injury. *Arch Phys Med Rehabil*. 2007;88:S18–S23.
37. Clayton RP, Wurzer P, Andersen CR, et al. Effects of different duration exercise programs in children with severe burns. *Burns*. 2017;43:796–803.
38. Pate RR, Pratt M, Blair SN, et al. Physical activity and public health. A recommendation from the Centers for Disease Control and Prevention and the American College of Sports Medicine. *JAMA*. 1995;273:402–407.
39. Nedelec B, Parry I, Acharya H, et al. Practice guidelines for cardiovascular fitness and strengthening exercise prescription after burn injury. *J Burn Care Res*. 2016;37(6):539–558.

40. Farrell RT, Gamelli RL, Sinacore J. Analysis of functional outcomes in patients discharged from an acute burn center. *J Burn Care Res.* 2006;27:189–194.

41. LeBlanc AD, Schneider VS, Evans HJ, et al. Regional changes in muscle mass following 17 weeks of bed rest. *J Appl Physiol.* 1992;73:2172–2178.

42. Nedelec B, Serghiou M, Niszczak J, et al. Practice guidelines for early ambulation of burn survivors after lower extremity grafts. *J Burn Care Res.* 2012;33(3):319–329.

43. Cartotto R, Cicuto BJ, Kiwanuka HN, et al. Postburn deformities and their management. *Surg Clin N Am.* 2014;94(4):817–837.

44. Kucan JO, Bash D. Reconstruction of the burned foot. *Clin Plast Surg.* 1992;19:705–719.

45. Kurtzman LC, Stern PJ. Upper extremity burn contractures. *Hand Clin.* 1990;6:261–279.

46. Greenhalgh DG, Gaboury T, Warden GD. The early release of axillary contractures in pediatric patients with burns. *J Burn Care Rehabil.* 1993;14:39–42.

47. Stern PJ, Law EJ, Benedict FE, et al. Surgical treatment of elbow contractures in postburn children. *Plast Reconstr Surg.* 1985;76:441–446.

48. Sherris DA, Larrabee WF Jr, Murakami CS. Management of scar contractures, hypertrophic scars, and keloids. *Otolaryngol Clin North Am.* 1995;28:1057–1068.

49. Hirshowitz B, Karev A. Axillary reconstruction: five-skin flap. In: Strauch B, Vasconez L, Findlay EH, eds. *Grabbs Encyclopedia of Flaps.* Toronto, ON: Little Brown and Company; 1990:1228–1289.

50. Schwarz RJ. Management of postburn contractures of the upper extremity. *J Burn Care Res.* 2007;28:212–219.

51. Ring D, Jupiter JB. Operative release of complete ankylosis of the elbow due to heterotopic bone in patients without severe injury of the central nervous system. *J Bone Joint Surg Am.* 2003;85-A:849–857.

52. Watson S. Hand burns. *Repair Reconstr.* 2001;2:2–4.

53. Devauchelle B, Badet L, Lengele B, et al. First human face allograft: early report. *Lancet.* 2006;368:203.

54. Giatsidis G, Sinha I, Pomaha B. Reflections on a decade of face transplantation. *Ann Surg.* 2017;265(3):439–500.

55. Morris P, Bradley A, Doyal A, et al. Face transplantation: a review of the technical, immunological, psychological and clinical issues with recommendations for good practice. *Transplantation.* 2007;83:109.

56. Wiggins P, Barker JH, Serge M, et al. On the ethics of facial transplantation research. *Am J Bioeth.* 2004;4:1.

57. Pomahac B, Aflaki P, Chandraker A, et al. Facial transplantation and immuno-suppressed patients: a new frontier in reconstructive surgery. *Transplantation.* 2008;85:1693–1697.

58. Kowalske K, Holavanahalli R, Helm P. Neuropathy after burn injury. *J Burn Care Rehabil.* 2001;22:353–357; discussion 352.

59. Helm P, Pandian G, Heck E. Peripheral neurological problems in the acute burn patient. *Burns.* 1977;3:123–125.

60. Helm PA, Pandian G, Heck E. Neuromuscular problems in the burn patient: cause and prevention. *Arch Phys Med Rehabil.* 1985;66:451–453.

61. Jackson L, Keats AS. Mechanism of brachial plexus palsy following anesthesia. *Anesthesiology.* 1965;26:190–194.

62. Reinstein L, Alevizatos AC, Twardzik FG, et al. Femoral nerve dysfunction after retroperitoneal hemorrhage: pathophysiology revealed by computed tomography. *Arch Phys Med Rehabil.* 1984;65:37–40.

63. Henderson B, Koepke GH, Feller I. Peripheral polyneuropathy among patients with burns. *Arch Phys Med Rehabil.* 1971;52:149–151.

64. Grube BJ, Heimbach DM, Engrav LH, et al. Neurologic consequences of electrical burns. *J Trauma.* 1990;30:254–258.

65. Khedr EM, Khedr T, el-Oteify MA, et al. Peripheral neuropathy in burn patients. *Burns.* 1997;23:579–583.

66. Chan Q, Ng K, Vandervord J. Critical illness polyneuropathy in patients with major burn injuries. *Eplasty.* 2010;10.

67. Lee MY, Liu G, Kowlowitz V, et al. Causative factors affecting peripheral neuropathy in burn patients. *Burns.* 2009;35(3):412–416.

68. Dagum AB, Peters WJ, Neligan PC, et al. Severe multiple mononeuropathy in patients with major thermal burns. *J Burn Care Rehabil.* 1993;14:440–445.

69. Carrougher GJ, Martinez EM, Mcmullen KS, et al. Pruritus in adult burn survivors: postburn prevalence and risk factors associated with increased intensity. *J Burn Care Res.* 2013;34(1):94–101.

70. Willebrand M, Low A, Dyster-Aas J, et al. Pruritus, personality traits and coping in long-term follow-up of burn-injured patients. *Acta Derm Venereol.* 2004;84:375–380.

71. Van Loey NE, Bremer M, Faber AW, et al. Itching following burns: epidemiology and predictors. *Br J Dermatol.* 2008;158:95–100.

72. Schneider JC, Nadler DL, Herndon DN, et al. Pruritus in pediatric burn survivors: defining the clinical course. *J Burn Care Res.* 2015;36(1):151–158.

73. Vitale M, Fields-Blache C, Luterman A. Severe itching in the patient with burns. *J Burn Care Rehabil.* 1991;12:330–333.

74. Zachariah J, Rao A, Prabha R, et al. Post burn pruritus—a review of current treatment options. *Burns J.* 2012;38(5):621–629.

75. Matheson JD, Clayton J, Muller MJ. The reduction of itch during burn wound healing. *J Burn Care Rehabil.* 2001;22:76–81; discussion 75.

76. Field T, Peck M, Hernandez-Reif M, et al. Postburn itching, pain, and psychological symptoms are reduced with massage therapy. *J Burn Care Rehabil.* 2000;21:189–193.

77. Baker RA, Zeller RA, Klein RL, et al. Burn wound itch control using H1 and H2 antagonists. *J Burn Care Rehabil.* 2001;22:263–268.

78. Hettrick HH, OBrien K, Laznick H, et al. Effect of transcutaneous electrical nerve stimulation for the management of burn pruritus: a pilot study. *J Burn Care Rehabil.* 2004;25:236–240.

79. Richardson C, Upton D, Rippon M. Treatment for wound pruritus following burns. *J Wound Care.* 2014;23(5):227–233.

80. Ahuja RB, Gupta R, Gupta G, et al. A comparative analysis of cetirizine, gabapentin and their combination in the relief of post-burn pruritus. *Burns.* 2011;37:203–207.

81. Ahuja RB, Gupta GK. A four arm, double blind, randomized and placebo controlled study of pregabalin in the management of post-burn pruritus. *Burns.* 2013;39(1):24–29.

82. Serghiou MA, McLaughlin A, Herndon DN. Alternative splinting methods for the prevention and correction of burn scar torticollis. *J Burn Care Rehabil.* 2003;24:336–340; discussion 322.

83. Richard R, Miller S, Staley M, et al. Multimodal versus progressive treatment techniques to correct burn scar contractures. *J Burn Care Rehabil.* 2000;21:506–512.

84. Manigandan C, Gupta AK, Venugopal K, et al. A multi-purpose, self-adjustable aeroplane splint for the splinting of axillary burns. *Burns.* 2003;29:276–279.

85. Van Straten O, Sagi A. "Supersplint": a new dynamic combination splint for the burned hand. *J Burn Care Rehabil.* 2000;21:71–73; discussion 70.

86. Johnson J, Silverberg R. Serial casting of the lower extremity to correct contractures during the acute phase of burn care. *Phys Ther.* 1995;75:262–266.

87. Ward RS, Hayes-Lundy C, Reddy R, et al. Evaluation of topical therapeutic ultrasound to improve response to physical therapy and lessen scar contracture after burn injury. *J Burn Care Rehabil.* 1994;15:74–79.

88. Wessling N, Ehleben CM, Chapman V, et al. Evidence that use of a silicone gel sheet increases range of motion over burn wound contractures. *J Burn Care Rehabil.* 1985;6:503–505.

89. Iwuagwu FC, Wilson D, Bailie F. The use of skin grafts in postburn contracture release: a 10-year review. *Plast Reconstr Surg.* 1999;103:1198–1204.

90. Prelack K, Dwyer J, Dallal GE, et al. Growth deceleration and restoration after serious burn injury. *J Burn Care Res.* 2007;28:262–268.

91. Mooney WR, Reed MH. Growth disturbances in the hands following thermal injuries in children. 1. Flame burns. *Can Assoc Radiol J.* 1988;39:91–94.

92. Leung KS, Cheng JC, Ma GF, et al. Complications of pressure therapy for postburn hypertrophic scars. Biomechanical analysis based on 5 patients. *Burns Incl Therm Inj.* 1984;10:434–438.

93. Fricke NB, Omnell ML, Dutcher KA, et al. Skeletal and dental disturbances in children after facial burns and pressure garment use: a 4-year follow-up. *J Burn Care Rehabil.* 1999;20:239–249.

94. Klein GL, Bi LX, Sherrard DJ, et al. Evidence supporting a role of glucocorticoids in short-term bone loss in burned children. *Osteoporos Int.* 2004;15:468–474.

95. Klein GL, Langman CB, Herndon DN. Vitamin D depletion following burn injury in children: a possible factor in post-burn osteopenia. *J Trauma.* 2002;52:346–350.

96. Mayes T, Gottschlich M, Scanlon J, et al. Four-year review of burns as an etiologic factor in the development of long bone fractures in pediatric patients. *J Burn Care Rehabil.* 2003;24:279–284.

97. Klein GL, Wolf SE, Langman CB, et al. Effects of therapy with recombinant human growth hormone on insulin-like growth factor system components and serum levels of biochemical markers of bone formation in children after severe burn injury. *J Clin Endocrinol Metab.* 1998;83:21–24.

98. Klein GL, Wimalawansa SJ, Kulkarni G, et al. The efficacy of acute administration of pamidronate on the conservation of bone mass following severe burn injury in children: a double-blind, randomized, controlled study. *Osteoporos Int.* 2005;16:631–635.

99. Przkora R, Herndon DN, Sherrard DJ, et al. Pamidronate preserves bone mass for at least 2 years following acute administration for pediatric burn injury. *Bone.* 2007;41:297–302.

100. Evans EB. Bone and joint changes secondary to burns. In: Lewis SR, ed. *Symposium on the Treatment of Burns.* St. Louis, MO: CV Mosby; 1973:76–78.

101. Hunt JL, Arnoldo BD, Kowalske K, et al. Heterotopic ossification revisited: a 21-year surgical experience. *J Burn Care Res.* 2006;27:535–540.

102. Klein MB, Logsetty S, Costa B, et al. Extended time to wound closure is associated with increased risk of heterotopic ossification of the elbow. *J Burn Care Res.* 2007;28:447–450.

103. Orchard GR, Paratz JD, Blot S, et al. Risk factors in hospitalized patients with burn injuries for developing heterotopic ossification—a retrospective analysis. *J Burn Care Res.* 2015;36(4):465–470.

104. Levi B, Jayakumar P, Giladi A, et al. Risk factors for the development of heterotopic ossification in seriously burned adults: a National Institute on Disability, Independent Living and Rehabilitation Research burn model system database analysis. *J Trauma Acute Care Surg.* 2015;79(5):870–876.

105. Schneider JC, Simko LC, Goldstein R, et al. Predicting heterotopic ossification early after burn injuries: a risk scoring system. *Ann Surg.* 2017;266(1):179–184.

106. Tsionos I, Leclercq C, Rochet JM. Heterotopic ossification of the elbow in patients with burns. Results after early excision. *J Bone Joint Surg Br.* 2004;86:396–403.

107. Gaur A, Sinclair M, Caruso E, et al. Heterotopic ossification around the elbow following burns in children: results after excision. *J Bone Joint Surg Am.* 2003;85-A:1538–1543.

108. Maender C, Sahajpal D, Wright T. Treatment of heterotopic ossification of the elbow following burn injury: recommendations for surgical excision and perioperative prophylaxis using radiation therapy. *J Shoulder Elbow Surg.* 2010;19(8):1269–1275.

109. Vrabec R, Kolar J. Bone changes caused by electrical current. Transactions of the Fourth International Congress of Plastic and Reconstructive Surgery, Rome. Amsterdam, The Netherlands: Excerpta Medica; 1969:215–217.

110. Helm PA, Walker SC. New bone formation at amputation sites in electrically burn-injured patients. *Arch Phys Med Rehabil.* 1987;68:284–286.

111. Moulton DL, Yngve DA, Evans EB. Spinal deformities in pediatric burn patients. *Spine Deform.* 2016;4(2):149–155.

112. Kim A, Palmieri TL, Greenhalgh DG, et al. Septic hip presenting with dislocation as a source of occult infection in a burn patient. *J Burn Care Res.* 2006;27:749–752.

113. Hinton AE, King D. Anterior shoulder dislocation as a complication of surgery for burns. *Burns.* 1989;15:248–249.

114. Carrougher GJ, Ptacek JT, Sharar SR, et al. Comparison of patient satisfaction and self-reports of pain in adult burn-injured patients. *J Burn Care Rehabil.* 2003; 24:1–8.

115. Ptacek JT, Patterson DR, Doctor J. Describing and predicting the nature of procedural pain after thermal injuries: implications for research. *J Burn Care Rehabil.* 2000;21:318–326.

116. Weinberg K, Birdsall C, Vail D, et al. Pain and anxiety with burn dressing changes: patient self-report. *J Burn Care Rehabil.* 2000;21:155–156; discussion 157–161.

117. Linneman PK, Terry BE, Burd RS. The efficacy and safety of fentanyl for the management of severe procedural pain in patients with burn injuries. *J Burn Care Rehabil.* 2000;21:519–522.

118. Robert R, Brack A, Blakeney P, et al. A double-blind study of the analgesic efficacy of oral transmucosal fentanyl citrate and oral morphine in pediatric patients undergoing burn dressing change and tubbing. *J Burn Care Rehabil.* 2003;24:351–355.

119. Patterson DR, Ptacek JT, Carrougher GJ, et al. Lorazepam as an adjunct to opioid analgesics in the treatment of burn pain. *Pain.* 1997;72:367–374.

120. Patterson DR, Ptacek JT. Baseline pain as a moderator of hypnotic analgesia for burn injury treatment. *J Consult Clin Psychol.* 1997;65:60–67.

121. Frenay MC, Faymonville ME, Devlieger S, et al. Psychological approaches during dressing changes of burned patients: a prospective randomised study comparing hypnosis against stress reducing strategy. *Burns.* 2001;27:793–799.

122. Hoffman HG, Patterson DR, Carrougher GJ, et al. Effectiveness of virtual reality-based pain control with multiple treatments. *Clin J Pain.* 2001;17:229–235.

123. Sharar SR, Carrougher GJ, Nakamura D, et al. Factors influencing the efficacy of virtual reality distraction analgesia during postburn physical therapy: preliminary results from 3 ongoing studies. *Arch Phys Med Rehabil.* 2007;88:S43–S49.

124. Morris L, Louw Q, Grimmer-Somers K. The effectiveness of virtual reality on reducing pain and anxiety in burn injury patients: a systematic review. *Clin J Pain.* 2009;25(9):815–826.

125. Field T, Peck M, Krugman S, et al. Burn injuries benefit from massage therapy. *J Burn Care Rehabil.* 1998;19:241–244.

126. Malenfant A, Forget R, Papillon J, et al. Prevalence and characteristics of chronic sensory problems in burn patients. *Pain.* 1996;67:493–500.

127. Choiniere M, Melzack R, Papillon J. Pain and paresthesia in patients with healed burns: an exploratory study. *J Pain Symptom Manage.* 1991;6:437–444.

128. Schneider JC, Harris NL, El Shami A, et al. A descriptive review of neuropathic-like pain after burn injury. *J Burn Care Res.* 2006;27:524–528.

129. Fauerbach JA, Heinberg LJ, Lawrence JW, et al. Effect of early body image dissatisfaction on subsequent psychological and physical adjustment after disfiguring injury. *Psychosom Med.* 2000;62:576–582.

130. Brych SB, Engrav LH, Rivara FP, et al. Time off work and return to work rates after burns: systematic review of the literature and a large two-center series. *J Burn Care Rehabil.* 2001;22:401–405.

131. Kischer CW. The microvessels in hypertrophic scars, keloids and related lesions: a review. *J Submicrosc Cytol Pathol.* 1992;24:281–296.

132. Bombaro KM, Engrav LH, Carrougher GJ, et al. What is the prevalence of hypertrophic scarring following burns? *Burns.* 2003;29:299–302.

133. Baryza MJ, Baryza GA. The Vancouver Scar Scale: an administration tool and its interrater reliability. *J Burn Care Rehabil.* 1995;16:535–538.

134. Finnerty CC, Jeschke MG, Branski LK, et al. Hypertrophic scarring: the greatest unmet challenge after burn injury. *Lancet.* 2016;388:1427–1436.

135. Deitch EA, Wheelahan TM, Rose MP, et al. Hypertrophic burn scars: analysis of variables. *J Trauma.* 1983;23:895–898.

136. Engrav LH, Garner WL, Tredget EE. Hypertrophic scar, wound contraction and hyper-hypopigmentation. *J Burn Care Res.* 2007;28:593–597.

137. Su CW, Alizadeh K, Boddie A, et al. The problem scar. *Clin Plast Surg.* 1998;25:451–465.

138. Carr-Collins JA. Pressure techniques for the prevention of hypertrophic scar. *Clin Plast Surg.* 1992;19:733–743.

139. Sawada Y. Alterations in pressure under elastic bandages: experimental and clinical evaluation. *J Dermatol.* 1993;20:767–772.

140. Chang P, Laubenthal KN, Lewis RW II, et al. Prospective, randomized study of the efficacy of pressure garment therapy in patients with burns. *J Burn Care Rehabil.* 1995;16:473–475.

141. Kealey GP, Jensen KL, Laubenthal KN, et al. Prospective randomized comparison of two types of pressure therapy garments. *J Burn Care Rehabil.* 1990;11:334–336.

142. Anzarut A, Olson J, Singh P, et al. The effectiveness of pressure garment therapy for the prevention of abnormal scarring after burn injury: a meta-analysis. *J Plast Reconstr Aesthet Surg.* 2009;62(1):77–84.

143. Hubbard M, Masters IB, Williams GR, et al. Severe obstructive sleep apnoea secondary to pressure garments used in the treatment of hypertrophic burn scars. *Eur Respir J.* 2000;16:1205–1207.

144. Staley M, Richard R, Billmire D, et al. Head/face/neck burns: therapist considerations for the pediatric patient. *J Burn Care Rehabil.* 1997;18:164–171.

145. Nedelec B, Carter A, Forbes L, et al. Practice guidelines for the application of nonsilicone or silicone gels and gel sheets after burn injury. *J Burn Care Res.* 2015;36(3):345–374.

146. Ahn ST, Monafo WW, Mustoe TA. Topical silicone gel: a new treatment for hypertrophic scars. *Surgery.* 1989;106:781–786; discussion 786–787.

147. Patino O, Novick C, Merlo A, et al. Massage in hypertrophic scars. *J Burn Care Rehabil.* 1999;20:268–271; discussion 267.

148. Sargent RL. Management of blisters in the partial-thickness burn: an integrative research review. *J Burn Care Res.* 2006;27:66–81.

149. Murphy F, Amblum J. Treatment of burn blisters debride or leave intact? Faye Murphy and Jeshi Amblum discuss the results of a systematic literature review on the categorization and management of minor burn injuries. *Emerg Nurse.* 2014;22(2):24.

150. Poh-Fitzpatrick MB. Skin care of the healed burned patient. *Clin Plast Surg.* 1992;19:745–751.

151. de Chalain TM, Tang C, Thomson HG. Burn area color changes after superficial burns in childhood: can they be predicted? *J Burn Care Rehabil.* 1998;19:39–49.

152. Carvalho Ddo A, Mariani U, Gomez Dde S, et al. A study of the post-burned restored skin. *Burns.* 1999;25:385–394.

153. Al-Qattan MM. Surgical management of post-burn skin dyspigmentation of the upper limb. *Burns.* 2000;26:581–586.

154. Acikel C, Ulkur E, Guler MM. Treatment of burn scar depigmentation by carbon dioxide laser-assisted dermabrasion and thin skin grafting. *Plast Reconstr Surg.* 2000;105:1973–1978.

155. Mellemkjaer L, Holmich LR, Gridley G, et al. Risks for skin and other cancers up to 25 years after burn injuries. *Epidemiology.* 2006;17:668–673.

156. Lindelof B, Krynitz B, Granath F, et al. Burn injuries and skin cancer: a population-based cohort study. *Acta Derm Venereol.* 2008;88:20–22.

157. Hart DW, Wolf SE, Mlcak R, et al. Persistence of muscle catabolism after severe burn. *Surgery.* 2000;128:312–319.

158. Jeschke MG, Gauglitz GG, Kulp GA, et al. Long-term persistence of the pathophysiologic response to severe burn injury. *PLoS One.* 2011;6(7):e21245.

159. Herndon DN, Tompkins RG. Support of the metabolic response to burn injury. *Lancet.* 2004;363:1895–1902.

160. Pereira CT, Herndon DN. The pharmacologic modulation of the hypermetabolic response to burns. *Adv Surg.* 2005;39:245–261.

161. Jeschke MG, Finnerty CC, Suman OE, et al. The effect of oxandrolone on the endocrinologic, inflammatory, and hypermetabolic responses during the acute phase postburn. *Ann Surg.* 2007;246:351–360; discussion 360–362.

162. Przkora R, Jeschke MG, Barrow RE, et al. Metabolic and hormonal changes of severely burned children receiving long-term oxandrolone treatment. *Ann Surg.* 2005;242:384–389; discussion 390–391.

163. Cochran A, Thuet W, Holt B, et al. The impact of oxandrolone on length of stay following major burn injury: a clinical practice evaluation. *Burns.* 2013;39(7): 1374–1379.

164. Davis SL, Shibasaki M, Low DA, et al. Impaired cutaneous vasodilation and sweating in grafted skin during whole-body heating. *J Burn Care Res.* 2007;28:427–434.

165. Esselman PC, Askay SW, Carrougher GJ, et al. Barriers to return to work after burn injuries. *Arch Phys Med Rehabil.* 2007;88:S50–S56.

166. Austin KG, Hansbrough JF, Dore C, et al. Thermoregulation in burn patients during exercise. *J Burn Care Rehabil.* 2003;24:9–14.

167. Patterson DR, Finch CP, Wiechman SA, et al. Premorbid mental health status of adult burn patients: comparison with a normative sample. *J Burn Care Rehabil.* 2003;24:347–350.

168. Mason S, Esselman P, Fraser R, et al. Return to work after burn injury: a systematic review. *J Burn Care Res.* 2012;33(1):101–109.

169. Corry NH, Klick B, Fauerbach JA. Posttraumatic stress disorder and pain impact functioning and disability after major burn injury. *J Burn Care Res.* 2010;31:13–15.

170. Ehde DM, Patterson DR, Wiechman SA, et al. Post-traumatic stress symptoms and distress 1 year after burn injury. *J Burn Care Rehabil.* 2000;21:105–111.

171. Van Loey NE, Maas CJ, Faber AW, et al. Predictors of chronic posttraumatic stress symptoms following burn injury: results of a longitudinal study. *J Trauma Stress.* 2003;16:361–369.

172. Tedstone JE, Tarrier N. An investigation of the prevalence of psychological morbidity in burn-injured patients. *Burns.* 1997;23:550–554.

173. Wiechman SA, Ptacek JT, Patterson DR, et al. Rates, trends, and severity of depression after burn injuries. *J Burn Care Rehabil.* 2001;22:417–424.

174. Fauerbach JA, Lawrence J, Haythornthwaite J, et al. Preburn psychiatric history affects posttrauma morbidity. *Psychosomatics.* 1997;38:374–385.

175. Edwards RR, Magyar-Russell G, Thombs B, et al. Acute pain at discharge from hospitalization is a prospective predictor of long-term suicidal ideation after burn injury. *Arch Phys Med Rehabil.* 2007;88:S36–S42.

176. Boeve SA, Aaron LA, Martin-Herz SP, et al. Sleep disturbance after burn injury. *J Burn Care Rehabil.* 2002;23:32–38.

177. Gottschlich MM, Jenkins ME, Mayes T, et al. The 1994 Clinical Research Award. A prospective clinical study of the polysomnographic stages of sleep after burn injury. *J Burn Care Rehabil.* 1994;15:486–492.

178. Raymond I, Ancoli-Israel S, Choiniere M. Sleep disturbances, pain and analgesia in adults hospitalized for burn injuries. *Sleep Med.* 2004;5:551–559.

179. Masoodi A, Ahmad I, Khurram F, et al. Changes in sleep architecture after burn injury: 'waking up' to this unaddressed aspect of postburn rehabilitation in the developing world. *Can J Plast Surg.* 2013;21(4):234–238.

180. Lee A, Ryan C, Schneider J, et al. Quantifying risk factors for long-term sleep problems after burn injury in young adults. *J Burn Care Res.* 2017;38(2):e510–e520.

181. Esselman PC, Ptacek JT, Kowalske K, et al. Community integration after burn injuries. *J Burn Care Rehabil.* 2001;22:221–227.

182. Fauerbach JA, Lawrence J, Stevens S, et al. Work status and attrition from longitudinal studies are influenced by psychiatric disorder. *J Burn Care Rehabil.* 1998; 19:247–252.

183. Wrigley M, Trotman BK, Dimick A, et al. Factors relating to return to work after burn injury. *J Burn Care Rehabil.* 1995;16:445–450; discussion 444.

184. Rondonelli RD, Genovese E, Katz RJ, et al., eds. *Guides to the Evaluation of Permanent Impairment.* 6th ed. Chicago, IL: American Medical Association; 2008.

185. McNiece WL, Dierdorf SF. The pediatric airway. *Semin Pediatr Surg.* 2004;13: 152–165.

186. Sheridan RL, Schnitzer JJ. Management of the high-risk pediatric burn patient. *J Pediatr Surg.* 2001;36:1308–1312.

187. Sheridan R, Remensnyder J, Prelack K, et al. Treatment of the seriously burned infant. *J Burn Care Rehabil.* 1998;19:115–118.

188. Meyers DG, Hoestje SM, Korentager RA. Incidence of cardiac events in burned patients. *Burns.* 2003;29:367–368.

189. Rao K, Ali SN, Moiemen NS. Etiology and outcome of burns in the elderly. *Burns.* 2006;32:802–805.

190. Pereira CT, Barrow RE, Sterns AM, et al. Age-dependent differences in survival after severe burns: a unicentric review of 1,674 patients and 179 autopsies over 15 years. *J Am Coll Surg.* 2006;202:536–548.

191. Evans WJ. What is sarcopenia? *J Gerontol A Biol Sci Med Sci.* 1995;50(spec no.): 5–8.

192. Poluri A, Mores J, Cook DB, et al. Fatigue in the elderly population. *Phys Med Rehabil Clin N Am.* 2005;16:91–108.

193. Serghiou MA, Holmes CL, McCauley RL. A survey of current rehabilitation trends for burn injuries to the head and neck. *J Burn Care Rehabil.* 2004;25:514–518.

194. Clayton NA, Ward EC, Maitz PKM. Full thickness facial burns: outcomes following orofacial rehabilitation. *Burns.* 2015;41(7):1599–1606.

195. Dougherty ME, Warden GD. A thirty-year review of oral appliances used to manage microstomia, 1972 to 2002. *J Burn Care Rehabil.* 2003;24:418–431; discussion 410.

196. Silverglade D, Ruberg RL. Nonsurgical management of burns to the lips and commissures. *Clin Plast Surg.* 1986;13:87–94.

197. Daughtry MB, Carr-Collins JA. Splinting techniques for the burn patient. In: Richard R, Staley M, eds. *Burn Care and Rehabilitation: Principles and Practice.* Philadelphia, PA: F.A. Davis; 1994:254.

198. Rivers EA, Strate RG, Solem LD. The transparent face mask. *Am J Occup Ther.* 1979;33:108–113.

199. Esselman PC, Thombs BD, Magyar-Russell G, et al. Burn rehabilitation: state of the science. *Am J Phys Med Rehabil.* 2006;85:383–413.

200. Groce A, Meyers-Paal R, Herndon DN, et al. Are your thoughts of facial pressure transparent? *J Burn Care Rehabil.* 1999;20:478–481.

201. Shons AR, Rivers EA, Solem LD. A rigid transparent face mask for control of scar hypertrophy. *Ann Plast Surg.* 1981;6:245–248.

202. Allely RR, Van-Buendia LB, Jeng JC, et al. Laser Doppler imaging of cutaneous blood flow through transparent face masks: a necessary preamble to computer-controlled rapid prototyping fabrication with submillimeter precision. *J Burn Care Res.* 2008;29:42–48.

203. Fricke NB, Omnell ML, Dutcher KD, et al. Skeletal and dental disturbances after facial burns and pressure garments. *J Burn Care Rehabil.* 1996;17:338–345.

204. Rappoport K, Muller R, Flores-Mir C. Dental and skeletal changes during pressure garment use in facial burns: a systematic review. *Burns.* 2008;34:18–23.

205. Silfen R, Amir A, Hauben DJ, et al. Effect of facial pressure garments for burn injury in adult patients after orthodontic treatment. *Burns.* 2001;27:409–412.

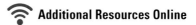 **Additional Resources Online**

CHAPTER 36

Julie K. Silver
Vishwa S. Raj
Sasha E. Knowlton
Lisa Marie Ruppert
Diana M. Molinares

Rehabilitation for Patients with Cancer Diagnoses

GENERAL ASPECTS OF REHABILITATION FOR CANCER PATIENTS

Basic Anatomy and Physiology

Cancers are classified in several different ways, based on the tissue of origin, the stage of histologic differentiation, and the anatomical location. Cancer nomenclature indicates the tissue of origin. For example, carcinomas refer to those types of cancers formed by epithelial cells; adenocarcinoma and squamous cell carcinoma being the most common in this category (1). Sarcomas are cancers of the bone (osteosarcomas), soft tissue (chondrosarcomas, liposarcomas, and synovial sarcomas), and blood and lymph vessels (angiosarcomas). Leukemia refers to the cancer of leukocyte precursors in the bone marrow and lymphoma to the cancers that originate in the lymphocytes. Multiple myeloma is the cancer of the plasma cells, and melanoma is the cancer of the melanocytes. The tumors of the central nervous system (CNS) will adopt the name of the cell from which they originate (e.g., astrocytoma, meningioma, glioma). Furthermore, cancers are histologically classified based on the similarity of the cancer cell to its progenitor; referred to as grade (2). This classification progresses from 1 to 4, with Grade 1 being well differentiated and Grade 4 being undifferentiated. Grades 2 and 3 refer to moderately and poorly differentiated, respectively. The higher the grade the more likely that there will be fewer similarities between the cancer cell and the normal cell and that the cancer will be more aggressive.

Once cancer cells have ensured their survival and have become a growing, self-sufficient tumor, the invasive process to other organs, known as metastasis, can begin. Staging, one of the most important components of cancer classification, refers to the anatomical location of the cancer cells that ultimately resulted in metastatic disease and patient mortality. Worldwide, the American Joint Committee on Cancer Tumor/Node/Metastasis (TNM) System is the most frequently used method to describe the extension of the cancer cells into adjacent or distant organs (3). The T stands for tumor and refers to the size of the primary tumor, N refers to the involvement of regional lymph nodes, and M to the presence of metastases. Classifications TX, NX, and MX denote that the size of the tumor, the involvement of lymph nodes, or metastatic disease, respectively, cannot be measured or determined. When the primary tumor cannot be found, it is classified as a T0. T corresponds to carcinoma *in situ*, while T1 to T4 refer to the extension of the primary tumor, with T1 indicating the smallest and T4 indicating the largest or most extensive. In terms of lymph node involvement, N0 indicates no lymph node involvement and N1 to N3 with N3 signifying the greatest lymph node involvement. Metastases are only classified as M0 or M1, based on the absence or presence of metastatic disease, respectively. Combination of the TNM classifications allows assignment of a final five-level overall stage ranked from 0 to IV; with 0 indicating *in situ*, I indicating early Stage, II and III indicating local-regionally advanced, and IV indicating the presence of metastatic disease.

The affinity of cancer cells for specific tissues is not completely understood; however, multiple studies point to the presence of a favorable microenvironment in these organs and the release of factors that promote the growth of organ-specific metastasis. Even though cancer cells have the ability to metastasize to any part of the body, this affinity increases the likelihood of different cancers to invade specific organs (**Table 36-1**) (2). The symptoms suggestive of the presence of metastasis are intrinsically related to the organs involved. Lung, bone, brain, and liver are the most common tissues hosting metastatic cells, and therefore, it is common to observe pain, fractures, ascites, jaundice, dyspnea, headaches, and neurologic deficits relative to organ involvement (2,4,5). Despite the fact that most cells that enter the circulatory system during the metastatic process do not survive, about 90% of the deaths related to cancer are due to complications related to metastatic disease (2).

Epidemiology

Patients with many cancer diagnoses are living longer because of a combination of early detection, a broader selection of cancer treatment options, and better, more-accessible general medical management. After the peak of cancer-related deaths observed in 1991, a drop of 25% mortality was observed in the following decades, going from 215 to 161 deaths per 100,000 persons between 1991 and 2014 (5). Despite this decline in mortality rate, cancer continues to be the second-leading cause of death in the United States (US) behind cardiovascular disease. It is responsible for one in every four deaths, with cancers of the lung and bronchus estimated to account for more than 25% of all cancer-related deaths in the US in 2017 (**Fig. 36-1**) (5,6). Although the age-standardized death rates from many types of cancer have decreased, the overall number of cancer deaths has increased (7). Changes in the demographics of the US are mainly responsible for these statistics, as the population is getting older, life expectancy is increasing, and estimates suggest that, though a 10% increase in the overall population of the US is expected between 2010 and 2020, the proportion of

TABLE 36-1	Primary Metastatic Sites of Common Cancers
Cancer Type	**Primary Sites of Metastasis**
Bladder	Bone, liver, lung
Breast	Bone, brain, liver, lung
Colon	Liver, lung, peritoneum
Kidney	Adrenal gland, bone, brain, liver, lung
Lung	Adrenal gland, bone, brain, liver, other lung
Melanoma	Bone, brain, liver, lung, skin, muscle
Ovary	Liver, lung, peritoneum
Pancreas	Liver, lung, peritoneum
Prostate	Adrenal gland, bone, liver, lung
Rectal	Liver, lung, peritoneum
Stomach	Liver, lung, peritoneum
Thyroid	Bone, liver, lung
Uterus	Bone, liver, lung, peritoneum, vagina

the mortality rates have decreased by almost 40% from 1998 to 2014 among both groups (5). In the interim, prostate cancer remains the most frequent cancer diagnosed in males, constituting 19% of all cancers in this group (1,2,4,5). Prostate cancer affects black males more frequently (74% higher risk); however, its mortality has decreased in all ethnicities. Even though prostate cancer is the most common cancer diagnosed in men, it is only the third leading cause of cancer death in males, with a steady 3% death rate decline since 1999 (📶 eFigs. **36-1** and **36-2**) (5,6). The leading cause of cancer death continues to be lung and bronchus cancer in both genders. It is the second most diagnosed cancer and is responsible for 27% and 25% of cancer mortalities in males and females, respectively (5). The overall incidence of lung and bronchus cancer has decreased over the last 30 years, which is associated with the increasing rates of smoking cessation (1,4,5). However, advanced stage at the time of the diagnosis is related to a 5-year survival rate of only 15% for males and 21% for females (5).

An increase in the incidence of cancer along with a decrease in the overall risk of mortality has resulted in a growing population of cancer survivors. At the beginning of 2016, an estimated 15.5 million people with a history of cancer were living in the US (5). In 2020, this number is projected to reach 18 million (7). While the treatment of cancer has moved toward less invasive and more preservation-oriented techniques, there remains a high incidence of disability in individuals with and surviving cancer (9–11). Cancer has become the second most common cause of new disability claims, following only musculoskeletal/connective tissue disease; and is fourth among ongoing claims (12).

Rehabilitation professionals should aim to examine the needs of survivors across the care continuum and throughout long-term survivorship. Of particular interest are the more

the population over 65 years of age is expected to increase from 13% to 16% (8). Currently, patients 50 years and older account for approximately 87% of the patients with new cancer diagnosis, and probability data demonstrates that the risk of cancer increases with age (**Fig. 36-2**) (5). Overall, risk of developing cancer in the US is 41% in males and 38% in females (6). By 2020, the incidence is predicted to reach 1.9 million people per year, an increase of more than 20% since 2010 (8).

Breast cancer continues to be the most common cancer among females, representing 30% of all cancers in this population (📶 eFig. **36-1**) (1,2,4–6). During the last 10 years, the incidence has slightly increased in black females (0.5% per year), while it has remained stable in white females; however,

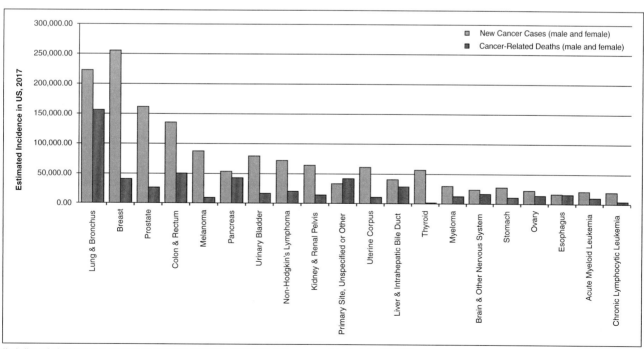

*Including only the 20 cancers with the highest combined estimated incidence of new cases and deaths in the US, 2017.

FIGURE 36-1. Total estimated incidence of new cancer cases and cancer-related deaths in the US, 2017. (*Data from American Cancer Society. *Cancer Facts & Figures 2017.* American Cancer Society website. Available from: https://www.cancer.org/research/cancer-facts-statistics/all-cancer-facts-figures/cancer-facts-figures-2017.html. Accessed December 18, 2018.)

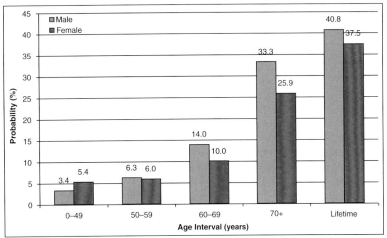

FIGURE 36-2. Probability of developing new invasive cancer in the US, 2011–2013. (*Data from American Cancer Society. *Cancer Facts & Figures 2017.* American Cancer Society website. Available from: https://www.cancer.org/research/cancer-facts-statistics/all-cancer-facts-figures/cancer-facts-figures-2017.html. Accessed December 18, 2018.)

*All sites, excluding basal and squamous cell skin cancers and *in situ* cancers except urinary bladder.

common cancers with large survivorship populations, such as breast and prostate cancer (5) and cancers known to have a high incidence of disabling complications (13). Since cancer is more common in older age groups, the impact of cancer within the geriatric population is receiving increasing attention. In general, cancer in the elderly may not be more disabling than other common medical conditions such as diabetes or congestive heart failure (14), but more severe symptoms or extensive treatment is associated with greater loss of function (15).

Functional Evaluation

A thorough history and physical examination may reveal issues at the symptom, impairment, and function levels. Visual analog scales have been described for pain, fatigue, appetite, mood, and sleep (16). Tests to assess impairments and basic function include manual muscle testing, grip dynamometry, range of motion, limb girths, up and go test (17), timed walking, single foot balance, tandem walking (18), modified sit-and-reach test (for flexibility), and stand and sit test (for strength) (19). Karnofsky Performance Status (**Table 36-2**) and Eastern Cooperative Oncology Group (ECOG) Scales measure performance status for cancer-directed treatment decision-making. Some questionnaire-based tools developed for oncology patients incorporate both functional and quality-of-life measures. Examples include the Functional Assessment of Cancer Therapy (FACT), European Organization for Research and Treatment of Cancer Quality of Life Questionnaire (EORTCQ), Cancer Rehabilitation Evaluation System (CARES), and Functional Living Index-Cancer (FLIC). The 36-Item Short Form Health Survey (SF-36), a health status instrument, has also been applied to the cancer population (20–22). Functional Independence Measure (FIM) scores can be used to monitor for functional gains or changes in functional status during rehabilitation efforts in this population.

Return to Work after Cancer

Cancer survivors' ability to return to work is an important area of study and often requires a multidisciplinary rehabilitation team approach (23) (see also Chapter 14). One large study exploring employment status of cancer survivors who had been working at the time of diagnosis found that 20% reported disabilities and that about 13% had stopped working for cancer-related

reasons, mostly after the 1st year (24). Diagnoses most likely to affect long-term employment status include CNS tumors, head and neck cancers, and advanced hematologic malignancies (24). Data from the Childhood Cancer Survivor Study found a 19.6% incidence of performance limitations for survivors, with 7.9% unable to attend work or school for health reasons (risk ratio 5.9) when compared to sibling controls (25).

Cancer survivors may be hampered by symptoms and also experience insurability concerns (especially affordability). One study of 253 long-term cancer survivors, many of whom were approaching retirement age, found 67% were actively working 5 to 7 years later, although some individuals reported that the cancer interfered with performing physical tasks (18%); lifting heavy loads (26%); stooping, kneeling or crouching (14%); prolonged mental concentration (12%); analyzing data (11%); keeping pace with others (22%); and learning new things (14%) (26). Given requirements of ongoing oncologic treatments, individuals may require extended or intermittent leave from work and/or flexible work schedules.

TABLE 36-2	Karnofsky Performance Status Scale

Able to carry on normal activity; no special care is needed.

10 Normal; no complaints, no evidence of disease

9 Able to carry on normal activity; minor signs or symptoms of disease

8 Normal activity with effort; some signs or symptoms of disease

Unable to work; able to live at home; cares for most personal needs; varying amounts of assistance is needed.

7 Cares for self; unable to carry on normal activity or do active work

6 Requires occasional assistance but is able to care for most of own needs

5 Requires considerable assistance and frequent medical care

Unable to care for self; requires equivalent of institutional or hospital care; disease maybe progressing rapidly.

4 Disabled; requires special care and assistance

3 Severely disabled; hospitalization is indicated, although death is not imminent

2 Very sick; hospitalization necessary; active supportive treatment necessary

1 Moribund, fatal process progressing rapidly

0 Dead

CANCER REHABILITATION SERVICE DELIVERY

"Cancer rehabilitation is medical care that should be integrated throughout the oncology care continuum and delivered by trained rehabilitation professionals who have it within their scope of practice to diagnose and treat patients' physical, psychological and cognitive impairments in an effort to maintain or restore function, reduce symptom burden, maximize independence and improve quality of life in this medically complex population" (27). The opportunity for care delivery is expansive and can occur from the time of diagnosis to the end of life.

Initial assessments identified that 54% of individuals with cancer had physical medicine problems (13), with very high incidence (70% or greater) among those with CNS, breast, lung, or head and neck tumors. However, despite the high prevalence rate for cancer-related disablement, treatment rates have remained relatively low and are as low as 1% to 2% in certain studies (28).

Because of the heterogeneity of rehabilitation needs across the cancer spectrum, as well as the complexity of care in individual cases, screening and surveillance tools should be employed which are both systematic and clinically practical. Settings in which to deliver this care include postacute and home care, acute care hospitalization, and outpatient ambulatory care (29).

Postacute Care

Inpatient rehabilitation facilities (IRF) are an often underutilized postacute care service. Patients with neoplastic spinal cord injury (SCI) (30) and brain tumors (31,32) have been shown to have shorter rehabilitation lengths of stay but similar discharge rates to home when compared to age-matched controls. Reasons may include higher initial FIM score, fewer behavioral sequelae, better social support, and expedited discharge planning due to poor long-term prognosis (33). Functional improvements made during acute rehabilitation have been maintained 3 months after discharge (34). Chemotherapy, radiation therapy, and specific tumor type have not been shown to adversely affect rehabilitation outcome (35,36).

The incidence of transfer back to acute care from rehabilitation is higher for cancer than noncancer patients in most (35,37,38) but not all (36) series. One study found that infection was more common in cancer patients than in controls (38). Low albumin, elevated creatinine, and use of a feeding tube or indwelling bladder catheter have been reported to be risk factors for transfer (39). For select populations, such as multiple myeloma, male gender and thrombocytopenia may also affect rate for transfer to acute care (40). Similarly, risk factors for transfer in lymphoma patients may include male gender, hematopoietic stem cell transplantation, and creatinine level ≥1.3 mg/dL (41). Prognosis and the patient's general tolerance of rehabilitation therapies must be weighed in the decision regarding inpatient rehabilitation.

However, poor expected long-term survival is not a contraindication if substantial patient benefit is expected in the short or intermediate term (e.g., family/caregiver training that will allow terminally ill patients to remain home with hospice services).

Postacute care can be delivered in other settings, such as skilled nursing facilities (SNF), long-term care hospitals (LTCH), and home health care (HH). Variation exists from a regulatory perspective regarding the cost per episode of care, medical requirements for participation, and rehabilitation services that can be provided (42). In addition, continuous care for patients after acute rehabilitation have not been well described (43). Further research is necessary to understand how each facility may benefit the oncology patient and what outcomes are relevant to substantiate the service.

Consultation during Acute Care

In the acute care setting, consultation is frequently requested for evaluation and treatment of mobility and self-care needs, as well as for the assessment of cognitive status, communication, and swallowing. Services for pain control or the provision of orthotic/prosthetic devices may also be indicated. One study administering the FIM instrument to acute oncology inpatients found that 87% of patients had rehabilitation needs on admission and 84% still had needs upon discharge (18). Another study applying organized interdisciplinary rehabilitation care to oncology inpatients reported significant functional improvement per Barthel Mobility Index and Karnofsky Performance Status Scale (44). Opportunities exist to triage patients through the spectrum of rehabilitation care based on needs while in the acute care hospital setting.

Outpatient Rehabilitation

Outpatient care typically addresses specific musculoskeletal or soft tissue problems, such as lymphedema, contracture, and pain, as well as mobility and self-care issues. Often there is need for surveillance of symptoms and function, both at critical points in care (e.g., in association with surgery) and over an extended period of time. One study of individuals with advanced breast cancer and remediable disabling impairments found that outpatients were markedly less likely than inpatients to receive rehabilitation services (45). However, models have been proposed to address this gap. In a prospective surveillance model for women with breast cancer, a three-staged approach was recommended to evaluate and educate patients preoperatively, reassess and implement an exercise program for early postoperative rehabilitation, and continue surveillance throughout the survivor plan of care (**Fig. 36-3**) (46). The costs of this models have been considered, though it is not clear whether it is cost-effective (47).

As the healthcare environment evolves, other novel approaches are being considered to provide appropriate rehabilitation services. For example, prehabilitation has been explored to improve performance status prior to oncologic intervention. "Prehabilitation is a process on the cancer continuum of care that occurs between the time of cancer diagnosis and the beginning of acute treatment and includes physical and psychological assessments that establish a baseline functional level, identify impairments, and provide interventions that promote physical and psychological health to reduce the incidence and/or severity of future impairments" (48).

Components of a prehabilitation program may include exercise prescription, nutrition, psychological stress reduction, and smoking cessation, and several of these components may factor into enhanced recovery strategies for surgical intervention

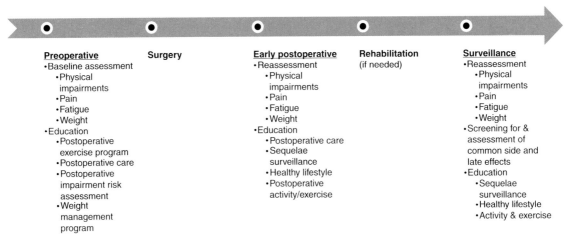

FIGURE 36-3.   Illustrated example of application of the prospective surveillance model for rehabilitation in surgical patients with cancer.

to improve stress reactions and recovery (**Fig. 36-4**). Models are currently being explored in the lung, colorectal, and breast populations (49). Similarly, rehabilitation can be provided to address symptomatic issues for cancer survivors, such as pain management, nausea, and bowel irregularity (50). Close collaboration of rehabilitation with palliative care specialists may allow for a unified approach to addressing cancer treatment–related side effects, health-related quality of life, and caregiver burden throughout the continuum of cancer care as well as through the end of life (27).

Precautions

Several absolute and relative contraindications exist for patients participating in a cancer rehabilitation program. Several of these recommendations have been compiled from multiple studies (**Table 36-3**); however, exceptions are often made based on medical condition and patient presentation. Specific considerations for treatment may include bedside interventions for significant thrombocytopenia and avoidance of

public areas such as therapy gyms until white blood cell count returns to a safe level ($\geq 500/mm^3$) (51). The physiatrist should perform routine follow-up as oncologic treatments may have an impact on the ability of the patient to safely tolerate some rehabilitation services, such as exercise or therapeutic heat.

CANCER-RELATED PAIN

General Approach to Assessment and Treatment

An estimated 60% of patients with cancer experience pain, with 25% to 30% having severe pain (52) (see also Chapter 39). Visceral pain is typically poorly localized, cramping, or deep aching. Somatic pain is well localized to discrete anatomic areas, often sharp or stabbing, whereas neuropathic pain has a burning, tingling, or throbbing quality. Presence of pain, as well as other symptoms such as fatigue and insomnia, is associated with a decrease in functional status, particularly in elderly cancer patients (15).

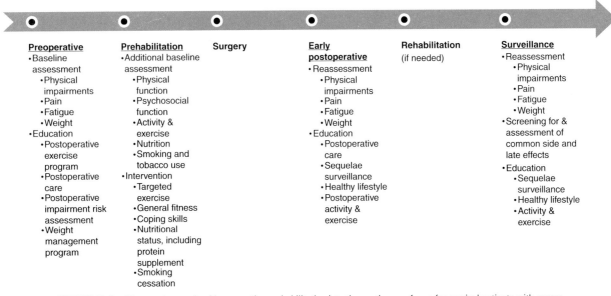

FIGURE 36-4.   Illustrated example of incorporating prehabilitation into the continuum of care for surgical patients with cancer.

TABLE 36-3	**Common Precautions and Contraindications for Patients Participating in Cancer Rehabilitation**

- Hematologic profile
  - Hemoglobin <7.5 g
  - Platelets <20,000
  - White blood cell count <3,000
- Metastatic bone disease
- Compression of a hollow viscous (bowel, bladder, or ureter), vessel, or spinal cord
- Fluid accumulation in the pleura, pericardium, abdomen, or retroperitoneum associated with persistent pain, dyspnea, or problems with mobility
- CNS depression or coma, or increased intracranial pressure
- Hypokalemia/hyperkalemia, hyponatremia, or hypocalcemia/hypercalcemia
- Orthostatic hypotension
- Heart rate in excess of 110 beats/min or ventricular arrhythmia
- Fever >101°F

The World Health Organization (WHO) analgesic ladder, which has been validated and is considered the cornerstone of cancer pain management, matches treatment to pain intensity. The first line of treatment is the nonopioid analgesics (e.g., aspirin, acetaminophen, and nonsteroidal anti-inflammatory drugs). If insufficient, an opioid (e.g., codeine, oxycodone, morphine, fentanyl, and methadone) should be added. In addition to intensity, one must consider multiple other factors including, but not limited to, acuity (acute, crescendo, chronic), pathophysiology (somatic, visceral, neuropathic), and temporal characteristics (continuous, intermittent, breakthrough) (52,53). While the WHO ladder remains fundamental, increasing attention is being paid to other treatments, such as early use of interventional procedures when clinical assessment suggests a high chance of success. In addition, there is growing support for the use of cannabinoids such as nabilone, dronabinol, and nabiximols. Although some evidence supports the use of medical marijuana for chronic neuropathic pain, further research with rigorous methodology is necessary to determine the role of cannabinoids in the treatment of cancer pain (54).

Medication regimens should be tailored to the pathophysiology of the pain generator. For example, when pain is due to direct tumor spread, antitumor therapy is most likely to be effective. Edema or antibody-mediated neurologic compromise is often managed with corticosteroids; inflammatory pain with nonsteroidal anti-inflammatory medication or corticosteroids; and neuropathic pain with antidepressants, anticonvulsants, and topical preparations (53). There is increasing recognition that in most cases, 33% to 50% pain reduction is clinically meaningful (55). Factors associated with difficulty attaining adequate pain control include neuropathic quality, psychological distress, history of addiction, and impaired cognition (52). Patient wishes should be included in the treatment plan, and use of a pain diary can assist in optimizing treatment (55). Technologic innovations such as an interactive computer program for education about pain and other symptoms have also been developed (56).

Opioid and Other Pharmacologic Strategies

Opioid agents that are commonly prescribed for cancer include oxycodone, morphine, hydromorphone, and fentanyl (**Table 36-4**) (see also Chapter 52). Meperidine should be avoided due to toxic metabolites that can lead to seizures or cardiac arrhythmias, especially in the case of dehydration or renal dysfunction (53). Methadone may be desirable in the case of renal failure; however, because of its high potential for interaction with other medications and marked individual variation in pharmacokinetics, it should only be prescribed by physicians highly experienced with this drug (52). While oral administration predominates in most physiatric settings, additional options have become available including parenteral routes such as transdermal, epidural, and intrathecal administration (57). In general, dosing is advanced to the level at which pain is controlled or at which toxicities preclude higher dosing. Daily effective dose can be established with short-acting preparations and then converted to longer-acting forms. Additional dosing should be available for breakthrough, intermittent, or incident pain (including that associated with rehabilitation therapies) consisting of the equivalent of a patient's 4-hour dosing needs, 25% to 50% of that dose, or 5% to 10% of the total daily opioid dose (52).

Management of opioid-related side effects is crucial. An effective bowel program, including stool softeners and laxatives should be prescribed. Sedation is often transient, but if it persists more than 1 week, measures such as caffeine intake or use of a stimulant such as methylphenidate can be helpful (53). However, in the case of delirium, a neuroleptic may be necessary after other metabolic causes have been excluded. Myoclonus related to opioid use may respond to baclofen, benzodiazepines, dantrolene, or valproate (52). While tolerance to a particular opioid may develop, reduced cross-tolerance between different agents allows rotation of opioid drugs to be an effective method of avoiding escalating dosage requirements and the resulting side effects (52).

Nonpharmacologic Pain Management Approaches

Physical modalities such as cryotherapy, biofeedback, iontophoresis, transcutaneous electrical nerve stimulation, and massage are well tolerated and believed to be safe; though traditionally, the latter two are not performed directly over areas with known tumors because of concerns about vasodilation and the possibility of tumor seeding (57). Similarly, deep heat such as ultrasound is contraindicated directly over an area with tumors. However, consideration for clinical stage and patient need may allow for exceptions in some cases, as the risk of tumor propagation could be mitigated via several variables (e.g., concurrent chemotherapeutic intervention). Routine physiatric procedures such as trigger point injections may be helpful. Psychological techniques including imagery, distraction training, relaxation techniques, and coping strategies are encouraged (53). Interventional options can include nerve blocks, vertebroplasty, spinal analgesia (including long-term catheter systems), dorsal column stimulators, and neuroablative procedures (e.g., neurectomy, rhizotomy, and cordotomy). Complementary and alternative medicine strategies are widely used, with increasing acceptance of massage and acupuncture, especially when other modalities have failed to achieve adequate pain relief (57) (see also Chapter 59).

TABLE 36-4   **Pharmacologic Management of Pain**

Analgesic	Route	Duration of Analgesic	Dosage	Side Effects
Aspirin	Oral	4–6 h	650 mg every 4 h	Gastritis, tinnitus
Acetaminophen	Oral	4–6 h	650 mg every 4 h	Hepatotoxicity
NSAIDs[a]	Oral	Varies by agent	Varies by agent	Gastritis
Tramadol	Oral	6–8 h	50–100 mg every 6 h	Sedation, nausea, constipation
Morphine[b]	Intravenous	1.5–2 h	2–10 mg	Sedation, respiratory depression, constipation, confusion, pruritus
	Epidural/intrathecal	Up to 24 h	5 mg	
	Oral	2–4 h	15–60 mg	
Delayed release MS Contin, Roxanol	Oral	8–12 h	15–60 mg	Sedation, respiratory depression, constipation, confusion, pruritus
Methadone	Oral	24 h	Varies	Sedation, respiratory depression, constipation, confusion; variable dosing efficacy
Oxycodone	Oral	3–6 h (standard) 12 h (sustained release)	5–10 mg every 4–6 h	Sedation, respiratory depression, constipation, confusion
Hydromorphone	Oral	2–4 h	7.5 mg	Sedation, respiratory depression, constipation, confusion
	Parenteral	2–4 h	1.5 mg	
	Rectal	6–8 h	3 mg	
Hydrocodone	Oral	3–5 h	30 mg	Sedation, respiratory depression, constipation (often more severe than with other opioids), confusion
Fentanyl	Transdermal	72 h	50 μg/h	Sedation, respiratory depression, constipation, confusion. Use transmucosal form only in opioid tolerant patients, for breakthrough; only for cancer patients
	Transmucosal (buccal)	4 h (variable)	200 μg	

[a]NSAIDs, nonsteroidal anti-inflammatory drugs. Numerous options, including COX-2 inhibitors (celecoxib) with reduced incidence of gastritis.
[b]Dosing of this agent and other opioids will be highly variable, depending on degree of opioid tolerance. Dosing can be advanced.

BONY METASTATIC DISEASE

Metastatic disease to the skeleton is one of the most problematic situations for clinicians managing musculoskeletal disorders. The skeleton is the third most common location for systemic metastatic disease (**Fig. 36-5**) (58). Breast, lung, prostate, kidney, and thyroid cancers account for 80% of malignancies to bone (59). Bone metastases are osteolytic, osteoblastic, or mixed (60). Lymphoma, multiple myeloma, thyroid, and renal cell malignancies have the highest rates of osteoclastic activity and therefore high levels of structural damage to bone and fracture risk. However, even in conditions where osteoblastic changes predominate, such as prostate cancer, pathologic fractures can occur. Early and aggressive management is imperative in maintaining function (61).

Pain is the most common clinical presentation of bone metastases (62). The pain is insidious, unrelenting, not associated with trauma or activity, and may be present or intensify at rest (63). The pain is frequently located in less common locations such as the thoracic spine or femoral shaft. Although pain is a common presentation, more than 25% of bone metastases are asymptomatic and found on routine imaging. Classic findings on physical examination include weight loss, exquisite point tenderness over the involved bone, and possibly neurologic impairment. Failure to respond to initial treatment and progressive symptoms are "red flags" that require further scrutiny (64).

The assessment of patients with suspected bone metastasis requires an efficient structured approach, including a detailed history and physical examination. Functional assessment and social history are imperative for establishing rehabilitation goals and the need for family support. Initial laboratory evaluation should include a complete blood count, serum protein electrophoresis, urinalysis, C-reactive protein, and a

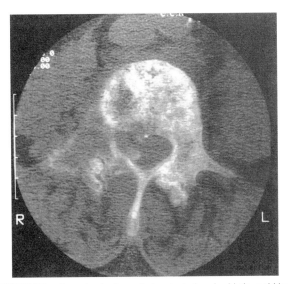

FIGURE 36-5. Extensive lumbar spinal metastasis, mixed lytic, and blastic lesions.

comprehensive metabolic panel including calcium and alkaline phosphatase. Plain radiographs, though inexpensive and easily accessible, have limited utility in identifying metastatic bone disease because greater than 50% of the cortex needs to be involved before metastatic disease will be identifiable (64). The most sensitive imaging study for the identification of bone metastases is the triple phase bone scan, as only 5% to 10% of cortical involvement is required to identify abnormalities (65). Bone scans identify osteoblastic activity in bone and therefore may produce normal results in patients with primarily osteolytic diseases such as myeloma or lymphoma. In addition, bone scans have poor specificity. For those patients with localized bone pain, equivocal bone scans, or neurologic impairment, magnetic resonance imaging (MRI) with gadolinium is the most appropriate test, particularly for suspected spinal lesions (66). The recent advent of PET scanning has helped to detect tumor activity in cases when the above imaging studies are equivocal or when the primary lesion is osteolytic (67). In some cases, biopsy may be indicated to guide treatment (63).

The median survival for patients with isolated bone disease from cancer of the breast, prostate, or from multiple myeloma is 21 to 33 months (68). During this time, the appropriate use of supportive measures to decrease morbidity and pain and improve function should be employed. Systemic management options, usually prescribed by a medical oncologist, include chemotherapy, hormonal therapy, monoclonal antibodies, and anti-angiogenesis agents. The administration of bisphosphonates is usually initiated when bone metastases are first detected, although in some cases, they may be administered prophylactically. Intravenous bisphosphonates decrease skeletal morbidity, fracture rate, and pain through the inhibition of osteoclastic activity and suspected modulation of local tumor activity (69,70). Radiation therapy, including direct beam and radiopharmaceutical options, frequently can be effective in decreasing local tumor burden and controlling pain (71). Nonsteroidal anti-inflammatory agents are employed to decrease periosteal bone reaction, and opioids are used for general pain control (65). In some cases, more aggressive interventional measures may be necessary.

Stabilization of the skeleton is imperative for pain control and function. Generally, the greater the amount of cortex involved with metastatic disease, the greater the risk of fracture (72).

Criteria for pathologic fracture risk in lower limb long bones include lesions measuring more than 2.5 cm, involvement of more than 50% of the bony cortex, and the Mirels' Score Incorporating pain, size, location, and radiographic appearance (**Table 36-5**) (66). A recent study comparing various methods found only axial cortical involvement of greater than 30 mm and circumferential cortical involvement predictive of fracture; the former having the advantage of being accessible with x-rays alone (73). Apart from radiographic assessment, pain that increases with weight bearing may be an indication of an unstable bony structure (63); warranting early surgical assessment. Fracture risk may actually increase during the first 6 to 8 weeks after radiation as a result of tumor necrosis and softening of bone. Therefore, surgical stabilization is typically done prior to radiation of unstable lesions.

In the spine, the stability of the bone and the presence of neurologic impairment guide the assessment in Harrington's

TABLE 36-5	Fracture Risk (>8 Point High Risk)		
	Points Assigned		
	1	**2**	**3**
Anatomic site	Upper extremity	Lower extremity	Trochanter
Lesion type	Blastic	Blastic/lytic	Lytic
Lesion size	<1/3 diameter	>1/3, <2/3 diameter	>2/3 diameter
Intensity of pain	Mild	Moderate	Severe

classification of vertebral metastases: (I) No significant neurologic involvement, (II) Involvement of bone without collapse or instability, (III) Major neurologic impairment without significant bone involvement, (IV) Vertebral collapse without neurologic impairment, and (V) Vertebral collapse with neurologic impairment. For class III to V involvement, surgical intervention is warranted (71). Surgical management of the unstable skeleton is effective in reducing pain and increasing function. Good or excellent pain relief was observed in 96% of long bone and 88% of spinal fractures, and improved function was seen in 82% of spine stabilization cases (74). A recent advance has been implementation of the NOMS algorithm, incorporating neurologic (cord compression), oncologic (radiosensitive or not), mechanical (movement-related pain; fracture/subluxation >5 mm, or angulation >11 degrees with subluxation >3.5 mm), and systemic (medical risks of surgery) factors into decision-making for surgery (75). In refractory cases or nonsurgical candidates, bracing can be considered, but wearing tolerance remains a significant barrier.

The rehabilitation of patients with bone metastasis is based on protection, pain control, energy conservation, and maintenance of function. Protection and pain control can be obtained through the use of bracing, mobility aids, and activity precautions. Some patients with exclusively lower extremity disease may be able to maintain mobility with the use of a cane or walker. Those with more diffuse (including upper limb) or bilateral disease may require a wheelchair or power mobility. Neutral spine techniques, which maintain spine physiologic curvatures while avoiding significant motion (flexion, extension, or rotation), preserve function and minimize pain in patients with spinal metastases. It is essential to assess the weight-bearing status of all limbs when prescribing assistive devices for patients with known or suspected bone metastases as they usually occur at multiple sites, with 20% of metastases present in the upper limbs, especially the humerus (66). Exercise prescriptions should focus on increasing strength, endurance, and function with minimal loading or torsion of the affected bone. A typical exercise program may include aquatic therapy, non–weight-bearing exercise such as cycling, and isometric exercise for strength maintenance. Compensatory techniques can decrease the biomechanical load on affected bones and maximize function. These include the use of reachers for activities of daily living, neutral spine techniques, and a step-to-gait pattern when climbing stairs. When metastatic disease limits independence, family training and education are beneficial in reducing the risk of injury to both caregiver and patient and to identifying needs for durable medical equipment.

CANCER-RELATED FATIGUE

Fatigue is a normal physiologic response to exertion. It becomes pathologic when it persists, occurs during routine activities, and does not respond to rest (76,77). Stringent clinical studies routinely find that the majority of cancer patients will meet criteria for cancer-related fatigue (CRF) at more than one-time during their disease continuum (78). High prevalence, negative impact on function and quality of life, and increased caregiver burden make the assessment and treatment of CRF a central goal of almost every cancer rehabilitation program (79,80).

Numerous fatigue assessment tools have been validated for oncology patients (81). Busy clinicians, however, may find it easiest to screen their patients using a mild/moderate/severe designation based on a 0 to 10 Likert-type scale. Patients reporting fatigue intensity of 1 to 3 are considered to have CRF that is mild, 4 to 6 moderate, and 7 to 10 severe. The National Comprehensive Cancer Network (NCCN) recommends screening for fatigue at the time of diagnosis, consistently during treatment, and as part of long-term follow-up care (82), even after the completion of successful oncologic treatment.

Clinical studies have identified specific factors that are consistently associated with CRF and are therefore thought to precipitate or intensify its impact. The most common associated factors are medication/side effects/drug interactions, pain, emotional distress, sleep disturbance, anemia, nutritional deficiencies, deconditioning, and medical comorbidities (**Table 36-6**) (82). Identification of lead factors guides the treatment process.

Successful management of CRF requires the coordinated collaboration between clinicians who can address etiologic factors affecting a specific patient. The NCCN guidelines recommend four types of treatment interventions: (a) education and counseling, (b) general strategies, (c) nonpharmacologic, and (d) pharmacologic. Since CRF affects patients throughout the cancer continuum, the NCCN provides guidelines for three types of patients: (a) patients in active treatment, (b) patients under long-term follow-up care, and (c) patients at the end of life (82).

General education about the nature and management of CRF provides reassurance and leads to earlier recognition and mitigation of its effects. General strategies, as opposed to cause-specific interventions, are intended to minimize the impact and intensity of existing CRF after reversible causes have been addressed. Energy conservation strategies developed for cardiac and pulmonary patients are equally effective for patients with CRF (83). Beneficial interventions include strengthening and endurance programs, psychosocial interventions, nutritional management, and sleep optimization.

The prevalence of disrupted sleep among persons with cancer diagnoses makes it one of the most common and intuitively obvious factors contributing to CRF. Many cognitive and behavioral strategies exist for promoting restorative night time sleep and minimizing daytime sleepiness (84). Addressing underlying anxiety and depression often improves sleep as does increasing physical activity. Sleep can also be addressed with judicious use of pharmacologic agents.

Anemia is a common cause of CRF that responds to medical management. Blood transfusions may be useful for more rapid correction of profound anemia, particularly after tumor resection or myeloablative chemotherapy. Several large-scale studies demonstrated the utility of erythropoietin for both increasing hemoglobin and reducing fatigue scores in patients with anemia associated with chemotherapy (85). However, the use of erythropoietin in cancer patients was reassessed in light of data concerning increased risk of thrombotic events in dialysis patients receiving erythropoietin (86). Some studies have also shown a decreased survival rate in cancer patients treated with erythropoietin that was not associated with thrombotic events (87). Recent data suggest that target hemoglobin levels of 12 g/dL can confer symptomatic benefit without increasing risk (88). However, consideration for transfusion must be balanced with institutional standards and recommendations given that evidence suggests across a range of clinical specialties that transfusions with allogeneic red blood cells can be avoided in most patients with hemoglobin thresholds above 7 to 8 g/dL (89).

In addition to medical management of factors contributing to CRF, physicians may use a range of prescription medications to treat CRF directly. Psychostimulants such as methylphenidate and modafinil have been used to treat CRF, but their efficacy has not been definitively established (90–93). Corticosteroids are used for numerous purposes in cancer patients and may modulate CRF (94). Numerous studies have explored the safety and efficacy of exercise interventions for patients with CRF. A meta-analysis identified the greatest statistically significant impact in studies limited to a specific disease population, such as breast cancer, with less effect demonstrated when patients with heterogeneous diagnoses were recruited (95). Even when exercise interventions do not directly reduce fatigue scores, they play an important role in the management of CRF by stemming the cycle of deconditioning that occurs as patients with CRF reduce their activity. Clinical literature supports the use of therapeutic exercise

TABLE 36-6	Interventions for Fatigue
Strategy	**Examples**
Restore energy balance	Correct anemia
	Nutritional and vitamin supplementation
	Correct endocrine dysfunction (thyroid)
Medications	Stimulants (methylphenidate, D-amphetamine)
	Analgesics
	Antidepressants (bupropion, SSRIs, TCAs)
	Regulate sleep/wake
	Glucocorticoids
	Investigational—cytokine-targeted therapy (including NSAIDs)
Exercise	Aerobic exercise is best-studied form
	Individualized
	Attention to precautions
	Cachectic patients may not tolerate
Energy conservation	Education
	Adaptive equipment
Psychological/coping	Recreational activities
	Relaxation techniques
	Support groups
	Spiritual supports, participation

for CRF in patients with Stage I to III disease. However, fewer guidelines exist for patients with advanced disease, particularly bony metastases. Walking has been the most frequently used mode of exercise in studies assessing the effect of physical activity on CRF, but a recent investigation studied the effect of higher intensity training utilizing cycle ergometry (96). None of the studies reviewed reported any serious adverse events related to the prescribed exercise program.

Strength training has been less well studied than aerobic exercise in oncology populations. Overall, moderate intensity aerobic exercise can help ameliorate CRF during and after treatment as well as minimize its effect on overall function and quality of life. Strength training is also beginning to show positive effects for fatigue management, although there are fewer studies supporting its role (97). It is best if cancer patients are screened prior to prescription of a moderate exercise program administered by clinicians who have experience with oncologic patients and are familiar with relevant precautions and contraindications.

Effective management of CRF requires a holistic approach that is best achieved through an integrated, interdisciplinary team including physicians, oncology nurses, physical therapists, occupational therapists, speech language therapists, nutritionists, and psychologists. A dedicated fatigue clinic has demonstrated high rates of patient satisfaction as well as some clinical improvement (79). Less formal CRF programs have been established elsewhere and are easily integrated into physiatric practices with established access to interdisciplinary team members who have oncologic experience.

COGNITIVE IMPAIRMENT IN THE PATIENT WITH CANCER

Cancer and its treatment can impair cognitive function and impairment occurs in a clinically relevant percentage of cancer patients and cannot be explained exclusively by depression or anxiety (98). Analysis in a national cross-sectional study showed that 14% of individuals with an identified cancer diagnosis self-reported memory problems, as compared to 8% of individuals without a cancer diagnosis, and that having cancer was independently associated with self-reported memory impairment (99). Associations have been noted for chemotherapy-induced cognitive deficits in the breast and prostate cancer populations (100).

Neuropsychological testing showed that breast and lymphoma survivors who received systemic chemotherapy, compared to local therapy, scored lower in psychomotor functioning and verbal memory (101). Women with breast cancer who received chemotherapy and tamoxifen were also noted to have deterioration on measures of visual memory and verbal working memory (102). Deficits were also noted in visuospatial ability compared to noncancer controls (103). Although mild cognitive impairments may occur in 10% to 40% of breast cancer survivors, they may take several years to resolve (104). Similarly, for men with extraprostatic prostate cancer receiving luteinizing hormone–releasing hormone analogues, cognitive testing showed deficits in memory and attention (105). Men who received combined androgen blockade showed a decline on spatial rotation ability after 9 months of treatment (106).

TABLE 36-7	Common Signs and Symptoms of Delirium

Acute (Hours to Days) Onset of

- Attention deficits
- Cognitive disturbance
- Dehydration
- Delusions
- Disorientation
- Disturbed consciousness
- Emotional lability
- Falls
- Impaired decision-making (confusion)
- Impaired judgment
- Impaired memory
- Incontinence (bowel and bladder)
- Perceptual disturbance
- Personality changes
- Psychomotor agitation
- Reduced clarity

Delirium is a confused mental state that can occur in patients with cancer, and many of the symptoms can be confused with either CRF or mild cognitive impairment from cancer and its treatment. Identified problems may include several symptoms (**Table 36-7**) (107,108). Types of delirium may include hypoactive (patients are not active and seem sleepy, tired, or depressed), hyperactive (patients are restless or agitated), or mixed (patients fluctuate between hypoactive and hyperactive states) (107). The incidence of delirium in patients with advanced cancer may range from 6% to 68%, depending on the health care setting, diagnostic tools, and the disease status of the patient (109). Although causes for delirium are multifactorial, often the symptoms are reversible and may be addressed through evaluating the medication regimen (e.g., opioids, benzodiazepines, corticosteroid, and anticholinergics), checking for electrolyte abnormalities, or diagnosing infection. Pharmacologic management may include antipsychotics such as haloperidol, and psychostimulants such as methylphenidate for the hypoactive population. Environmental strategies, with appropriate orientation and communication strategies, may also be beneficial (110).

EXERCISE FOR THE PATIENT WITH CANCER

General Aspects

Exercise studies performed in the cancer population have consistently substantiated gains in numerous parameters, including cardiopulmonary fitness, quality of life, depression, and anxiety (111–113) (see also Chapter 49). There may also be benefits of exercise on immune function, such as improved natural killer cell activity, monocyte function, proportion of circulating granulocytes, and duration of neutropenia; however, the implications of these effects are not well delineated on a clinical level, and not all studies have shown immune effects as a result of exercise (114).

Physical activity appears to exert a protective effect against the development of some types of cancers, most notably colon and breast cancers (115). Obesity has been associated with increased risk of death from cancer in both men and women. One large prospective study estimated the effect of overweight and obese status as accounting for 14% of cancer deaths in men and 20% of cancer deaths in women, with the strongest associations seen in gastrointestinal, kidney, breast, prostate, gynecologic, and some hematologic malignancies (116). Cancer prevention recommendations developed by the American Cancer Society include at least 150 minutes of moderately vigorous physical activity each week (e.g., 30 minutes or more on 5 or more days of the week for adults and at least 60 minutes each day for at least 3 days each week for children and adolescents) (117). Physician recommendation to exercise has been shown to improve self-reported total exercise among newly diagnosed cancer survivors (118).

While exercise studies overall have best explored use of aerobic forms of exercise in breast cancer, wider evidence is beginning to emerge, among a range of cancer types, with favorable outcomes (19,119,120). Cycle ergometry is often favored, with its advantages of positioning options and relative ease of use by individuals with balance or coordination deficits (121).

Patients often express interest in home or fitness center–based exercise, especially walking. However, at least one study suggests that a supervised program may be more likely to yield measurable gains in physical performance (122). Many perceive better readiness to start an exercise program after treatment (123,124).

Most hematologic-based restrictions for exercise are empiric. The concern with exercise in the thrombocytopenic state lies in the potential for (a) increased blood pressure, which occurs most dramatically with isometric exercise, to result in intracranial hemorrhage, (b) high-impact activities to result in muscular or intra-articular hemorrhage, and (c) falls. The risk of hemorrhage correlates with the platelet count but is mitigated by other systemic factors. In a study of acute leukemia patients (125), grossly visible hemorrhage was rare with a platelet count greater than 20,000, and no intracranial hemorrhage occurred with a platelet count greater than 10,000. In general, unrestricted exercise can be pursued with platelet counts greater than about 30,000 to 50,000. Aerobic, but not resistive, activities can be considered with platelet counts greater than 10,000 to 20,000. Active therapy is not advocated with platelet counts less than 10,000.

Exercise for Patients Undergoing Chemotherapy or Postchemotherapy

Cancer patients treated with cardiotoxic agents such as anthracyclines can sustain permanent cardiac damage that affects physical performance. Patients treated with significant doses of these agents (>100 mg/m²) can have reduced exercise time, reduced maximal oxygen uptake, abnormal heart rate response, ST-wave and T-wave changes, and exercise-induced hypotension. However, exercise time, peak oxygen uptake, and ventilatory anaerobic threshold can still improve with an exercise program due to peripheral adaptation, despite the fact that cardiac parameters, such as maximal heart rate and stroke volume, do not increase (126). A controlled study of patients undergoing aerobic exercise (supervised daily, supine bicycle ergometry) during treatment found multiple benefits in the exercise group, including less decrement in performance per treadmill testing, less pain, decreased duration of neutropenia, and shorter hospitalization (127). A study of home-based unsupervised exercise among early-stage breast cancer patients who had completed treatment (about half with treatment including chemotherapy) found higher self-reported physical activity and 1-mile walk test performance than controls but no difference in accelerometry or anthropomorphic measures (128). Use of a supervised program among breast cancer patients before and during treatment, focusing on both strength and aerobic training at 40% to 60% maximal twice weekly for 21 weeks, did result in improved lean body mass, reduced body fat, and improved strength per submaximal muscle endurance protocol (129). Another supervised program among breast cancer patients that had completed treatment, focusing on aerobic

training three times a week for 15 weeks, found improved peak oxygen consumption in the exercise group but no significant anthropomorphic differences (130).

Exercise for Patients Undergoing Bone Marrow Transplantation

Exercise programs have been developed for bone marrow transplant recipients to counteract the debility occurring with medical morbidity and prolonged hospitalization, as well as to address other factors such as depression and social isolation. Supine or sitting exercise is generally well tolerated, but standing exercise should be attempted at least for brief periods to minimize gastrocnemius soleus tightness. Supine exercise may be most comfortably performed with the head of the bed slightly elevated. Exercise programs emphasize range of motion, aerobic activity (e.g., walking or cycle ergometry), light resistive activities (e.g., bridging core exercises and light weights), and deep breathing to prevent atelectasis and pneumonia. In 1 program, referral to physical therapy is placed when the patient is isolated to the room or when unable to ambulate approximately 200 ft three times a day. For those in isolation, use of a sanitized bedside stationary bicycle or in-bed pedo cycle facilitates activity (131). In those with graft versus host disease (GVHD), skin erythema and rash may occur. Protective padding can prevent pain and skin irritation during exercise, especially over the soles of the feet. Attention should be paid to strengthening, due to risk of steroid myopathy. Medications such as quinine, carbamazepine, or baclofen may be useful for cramping symptoms of GVHD (132). One study of treadmill training (interval pattern) 30 minutes daily for 6 weeks in bone marrow transplant recipients with stabilized platelet counts and clinical condition resulted in improved physical performance, measured by distance of treadmill walking (133). Another controlled study of stretching and treadmill training found improved preservation of strength, measured by dynamometer in multiple muscle groups among the exercise group at 6 weeks posttransplant (134).

Cachexia

Endogenous tumor necrosis factor (TNF), or that administered exogenously as antineoplastic therapy, can reduce skeletal muscle protein stores. A low-to-moderate intensity of exercise that relies mainly on type I muscle fibers, which are fatigue resistant, should be encouraged. Another strategy may involve reducing activity at the onset of fatigue. While empirical evidence is limited in individuals with marked cachexia, rehabilitation efforts should focus on energy conservation and methods other than strenuous exercise to achieve functional goals.

NEUROLOGIC COMPLICATIONS OF CANCER

Neurologic impairments have been identified in 30% to 46% of cancer patients (135). Neurologic complications follow admission for routine chemotherapy as the second most common reason for admission to the hospital (136). Patients present most commonly with low back pain, limb weakness, headaches, and mental status changes (135). Because a high rate of associated disability and the vulnerability of the nervous system can lead to reversible and irreversible damage, early identification and treatment can prolong life and diminish disability.

Metastatic Brain Disease

Brain metastases are the most common catastrophic neurologic impairment in the cancer population. In CNS cancers, primary brain tumors are less common than metastatic brain tumors.

In fact, the incidence of metastatic disease to the brain is 10 times greater than the incidence of primary tumors (137). Brain metastases occur most frequently with lung, breast, colorectal, melanoma, and genitourinary cancers (135), with lung and breast malignancies accounting for 60% of all lesions. Approximately 85% of brain metastatic lesions are found in the cerebrum and 15% are found in the cerebellum. The most common presenting complaint is a progressive headache, often worse when recumbent. Hemiparesis, seizures, and mental status changes occur frequently. Evaluation includes a complete neurologic and clinical examination to exclude other etiologies such as stroke and CNS infection, and gadolinium-enhanced MRI is the gold standard assessment. Management includes early treatment with corticosteroids to decrease brain edema and anticonvulsants to decrease seizure risk. Excision of brain metastasis may be indicated, especially if the metastasis is single, the cancer is otherwise well controlled, and the lesion(s) appears to be the major factor limiting survival or quality of life. Clinical trials have shown that in certain patients, a combination of surgery and radiation therapy is superior to either treatment alone (138). Whole-brain radiation, with standard doses of 3,000 cGy given over 10 treatment sessions, as well as adjuvant chemotherapy are important components of treatment. Intrathecal methotrexate administered through a reservoir secured beneath the scalp has been used to treat CNS and leptomeningeal disease (LMD) with mixed results but does avoid some of the more toxic side effects of systemic methotrexate. Prognosis for solitary brain lesions and those able to maintain ambulatory function is good. Prognosis is poorer for those with persistent headache, visual dysfunction, or ongoing mental status changes (139).

LMD is a result of the spread of malignancy to cerebrospinal fluid (CSF). It is most commonly associated with breast cancer, small cell lung cancer, and melanoma (138). Some 75% to 80% of cases involve the spine, 50% of cases involve cranial nerves and greater than 50% of cases involve the brain (140). LMD causes back pain, radiculopathies, cranial nerve dysfunction, and mental status changes. The diagnosis is made by MRI with gadolinium and/or CSF analysis. Treatment includes intrathecal chemotherapy or radiation. The prognosis is uniformly poor.

Spinal Cord Involvement

Spinal cord compression due to metastatic disease occurs in 5% to 14% of all cancer patients (141). Notably, 25% of patients with neoplastic spinal cord compression do not have a previous diagnosis of cancer (135). The most common sources of metastases are primary prostate, breast, lung, and kidney cancers as well as multiple myeloma (142). The thoracic spine (70%) is the most frequent site of metastases followed by the lumbar (20%) and cervical (10%) regions.

Metastases to the spine characteristically present as progressive, insidious back pain that is worse when recumbent along with associated neurologic impairment (135,142). On average, patients have low back pain for 60 days before diagnosis (143). Clues to metastatic disease include a history

of cancer, constitutional symptoms, thoracic level pain, and bowel or bladder dysfunction. Signs and symptoms on physical examination may include point tenderness, paraparesis, sensory level, and upper motor neuron findings (141). Motor abnormalities often precede sensory changes as a result of epidural extension preferentially affecting the anterior spinal cord, with recovery in the reverse order. Early diagnosis is key, and patients presenting without paresis have longer survival than those presenting with paresis (144). Corticosteroids (usually dexamethasone) are administered with up to 100-mg loading dose, followed by 4 mg every 6 hours. Palliative radiation is indicated in those with metastatic disease and stable spinal structures. When disease renders the spine unstable, surgical decompression and stabilization may be pursued for patients who are operative candidates.

Paraneoplastic Neuromuscular Disorders

Paraneoplastic neuromuscular disorders (PND) are a remote effect of cancer caused by antibody formation by the primary tumor (145). Neuromuscular disorders can precede the diagnosis of cancer by years. These disorders are rare, seen in only 0.01% of cancer patients. The most common tumor associated with PND is small cell lung cancer, accounting for 50% to 75% of cases (146). Several forms of PND exist, including cerebellar degeneration, organic dementia, metabolic encephalopathy from electrolyte disturbance, proximal myopathies (as from carcinoid), and orthostasis from autonomic instability. In particular, Lambert-Eaton myasthenic syndrome (LEMS) is found in 3% of patients with small cell lung cancer. The disorder results from presynaptic inhibition of calcium release at the neuromuscular junction. Proximal weakness, autonomic dysfunction, and improvement with exercise are common clinical findings. Diagnosis is established by electromyography and nerve conduction (EMG/NCS) studies.

Myasthenia gravis (MG) is a postsynaptic neuromuscular junction disorder that is a result of autoimmune degradation of the postsynaptic membrane. MG is found in 15% of patients with a diagnosis of thymoma (146). The hallmarks of MG are ptosis, disconjugate gaze, fatigue on upward gaze, and proximal weakness worsened by activity. Electrodiagnostic studies, antibody analysis, and an anticholinesterase challenge are used to confirm diagnosis. Paraneoplastic subacute neuropathies include sensory, sensorimotor, and demyelinating forms (145). The clinical presentation is that of rapid (days to weeks) onset of peripheral neuropathy affecting various fiber types. The sensory and sensorimotor involvement is most commonly associated with small cell lung cancer, whereas demyelinating processes are associated with lymphoma. Monoclonal paraproteins create neuropathies in multiple myeloma, osteosclerotic myeloma, Waldenström's macroglobulinemia, amyloidosis, and γ heavy chain disease. Typically, the neuropathy is distal, mixed sensory, and motor, with axonal loss and segmental demyelination. The management of PND includes treatment of the primary tumor and immune mediation (146).

Polyneuropathy

Polyneuropathy can result from numerous factors in the cancer patient, including nutritional deficiencies, paraneoplastic disorders, and medical comorbidities. However, the most common cause is chemotherapy-induced peripheral neuropathy (CIPN). Dose-dependent toxicity occurs in peripheral

TABLE 36-8	Chemotherapy-Associated Polyneuropathies		
Tumor	**Agents**	**Trade Name**	**Nerve Fibers**
Breast	Taxanes	Taxol/taxotere	Sensory > motor
Lung	Taxanes	Taxol	Sensory > motor
	Platinum	Carboplatin	Pure sensory
		Cisplatin	Pure sensory
Ovarian	Platinum	Carboplatin	Pure sensory
		Cisplatin	Pure sensory
	Taxanes	Taxol	Sensory > motor
Myeloma	Thalidomide	Thalomid	Sensory > motor
Lymphoma	Vinca alkaloids	Vincristine	Motor = sensory
Colon	Platinum	Oxaliplatin	Pure sensory

TABLE 36-9	Radiation Therapy Side Effects	
Acute		**Delayed**
Fatigue		Soft tissue fibrosis
Nausea		Skin atrophy
Vomiting		Auditory changes
Anorexia		Pulmonary fibrosis
Skin erythema		GI stricture
Desquamation		Thyroid dysfunction
Mucositis		Brain necrosis
Xerostomia		Myelitis
Taste loss		Plexopathy
Proctitis		Lymphedema
Cystitis		Secondary malignancies
Decreased libido		Osteonecrosis
Sterility		
Amenorrhea		
Hematologic changes		

nerves and is commonly associated with a handful of agents (**Table 36-8**). The pathophysiology of CIPN includes disruption of axoplasmic microtubule transport, axonal "dying back," and direct effects to the dorsal root ganglion (147). The sensory nerves are typically more affected because of the smaller fibers and the location of the dorsal root ganglion outside the blood-brain barrier. The onset of neuropathy coincides with the administration of chemotherapy and symptoms and symptoms should not progress after treatment has stopped.

Symptoms of dysesthesias, sensory loss, and allodynia typically begin in the foot and ascend. Motor weakness and autonomic dysfunction are delayed findings and may be a sign of significant toxicity. The differential diagnosis of CIPN includes nutritional deficiencies, paraneoplastic disorders, mononeuropathies, radiculopathy, myelopathy, and brain disorders. Definitive diagnosis can be obtained through the use of electrodiagnostic studies. An accurate diagnosis of CIPN is required to avoid unnecessary discontinuation of chemotherapy as the management of CIPN includes alteration of dosing and symptom management with medications. Several agents have been evaluated as potential chemoprotective agents, but none have proven beneficial (148). Rehabilitation principles include education, safety awareness, gait and proprioceptive training, and prescription of orthoses and assistive devices for those with motor as well as sensory deficits.

RADIATION-INDUCED TISSUE DAMAGE

The local effects of RT can lead to many complications (**Table 36-9**) (149). Soft tissue injury, swallowing dysfunction, and neurologic impairments are some of the more commonly encountered issues for rehabilitation physicians. Soft tissue fibrosis as a direct result of RT results in dermal fibrosis, musculotendinous contraction, and joint restriction with resulting loss of range of motion and function. The most commonly affected joints are the glenohumeral joint after axillary RT for breast cancer, the femoroacetabular joint after RT for cutaneous malignancies, and the neck after treatment for head and neck cancer. The loss of range of motion may start with guarding from painful, irradiated skin and is followed by contraction of the musculotendinous unit and joint fibrosis. Prevention through meticulous skin care, soft tissue mobilization, and range of motion techniques is the primary means of management. The use of pentoxifylline may be beneficial to restore microvascular supply to the soft tissue structures and

thus help preserve mobility (150). The importance of delayed effects of RT and the need to maintain a stretching regimen for life should be emphasized for patients. Patients with radiation-induced skin damage should wash gently with warm water and mild soap and avoid sun exposure, rubbing (e.g., straps, belts, and collars), or chemical irritants (e.g., perfumes and deodorants) to the affected site. Mild cases may improve with emollients (e.g., baby oil) or other alcohol-free topical preparations (e.g., aloe or Aquaphor), whereas more severe cases might require a topical corticosteroid or specialized wound care preparations. Skin care recommendations should be made in conjunction with the practice of the radiation oncology team, especially during the period of ongoing radiation.

Neurologic complications of radiation therapy include myelopathy, plexopathy, peripheral nerve injury, and encephalopathy. Long-term neuropsychological sequelae have been reported even after low dose whole brain RT, especially in children. Restrictive dosing regimens and hyperfractionation have significantly decreased the rates of neurologic impairment secondary to RT. Myelopathy is typically seen with cumulative doses greater than 5,000 Gy. The symptoms consist of sensory abnormalities, Brown-Séquard syndrome, followed by ascending weakness to the site of RT. The onset is greater than 12 months after completion of RT, and the work-up should exclude possible reversible causes of myelopathy (149). Treatment is primarily supportive. Radiation-induced plexopathy is usually seen in the upper trunk of the brachial plexus and in the lumbosacral plexus. The clinical presentation is that of painless weakness with insidious progression that may even result in pan-plexopathy (151). Although brachial plexopathy is rarely seen today secondary to smaller fractions and lower cumulative doses, it was highly associated with breast cancer patients receiving fractions of greater than 2.2 Gy and cumulative doses greater than 44 Gy (152). Plexopathy is usually diagnosed via MRI, revealing fibrosis of the plexus, and electrodiagnostic studies may reveal the pathognomonic myokymic potentials.

Peripheral nerve injury secondary to RT is a rare occurrence, primarily occurring with cumulative doses greater than 6,000 Gy. Focal nerve injury results in painless weakness and may also be associated with myokymic discharges on electrodiagnostic studies (149).

Unwanted side effects of intracranial radiation are conventionally divided into acute (1 to 3 months), early-delayed (3 to 12 months), and late-delayed. There is limited risk of acute injury using contemporary protocols, but coadministration of methotrexate or anticonvulsants may precipitate acute encephalopathies or toxic epidermal necrolysis that mandate inpatient hospitalization. Acute radiation encephalopathy is typically seen with single doses greater than 300 Gy, is related to increased intracranial pressure, and is self-limiting. In addition to acute effects, early delayed effects after whole brain RT include neurologic deterioration with somnolence, headaches, and worsening of focal symptoms that may resolve over the following months. Comprehensive imaging, clinical, and laboratory evaluation are needed to distinguish this condition from tumor recurrence or infection. The mechanisms of the late delayed effects of radiation, specifically radiation necrosis and cerebral atrophy, are poorly understood. Necrosis is often difficult to distinguish from recurrence and may require evaluation by PET scan or surgical biopsy. Late radiation necrosis occurs in 3% to 5% of patients receiving greater than 5,000 Gy and usually begins 1 to 2 years after completion of RT (149). Management is with corticosteroids or resection. Late radiation changes secondary to atrophy present with ataxia, dementia, and incontinence usually 1 year or more after whole brain irradiation of greater than 3,000 cGy. Treatment is supportive.

LYMPHEDEMA

Lymphedema is an irregular painless accumulation of fluid, typically in an extremity, that may also involve the face, thorax, or abdomen, secondary to a disorder of the lymphatic system. The most common malignancies associated with lymphedema include breast, melanoma, gynecologic malignancies, and lymphoma. In breast cancer, a full axillary dissection typically involves removal of lymph nodes below the axillary vein, whereas in melanoma, all regional lymph nodes below the clavicle are removed (153). Sentinel lymph node dissection, which includes sampling of lymph nodes that drain directly from the site of the tumor, leads to smaller numbers of lymph nodes being removed and reduces, but does not eliminate, risk of lymphedema (154,155). Associated risk factors include axillary lymph node dissection (ALND), metastatic involvement of lymph nodes, radiation therapy, obesity, and increasing age (156).

Lymphedema usually presents gradually, however for patients presenting with rapid onset of swelling with pain or erythema, one must exclude metastatic seeding (malignant lymphedema), infection, and thromboembolic disease. Two types of presentation are usually seen in patients with lymphedema. The first type has a gradual onset of fluid accumulation after lymph node removal secondary to overload of the lymphatic system with normal daily fluid production (normal output lymphedema). The second presentation consists of an acute increase in lymphatic fluid that overwhelms the compromised system (high output lymphedema). Common causes of high output lymphedema include cellulitis, lymphangitis, trauma, thermal burns, and increased metabolism in the at-risk limb (**Table 36-10**). Lymphedema progresses in stages. Stage 1 is a primarily fluid stage in which arm volumes diminish

TABLE 36-10	Factors Promoting Increased Lymphatic Fluid Production and Prevention Strategies	
Factor	**Example**	**Prevention**
Infection	Cellulitis, lymphangitis	Prevent breaks in skin
		Avoid venipuncture
		Gloves during high-risk activities
Lymphatic constriction	Tourniquets	Avoid blood pressure cuffs
	Tight clothes	Blood draws in opposite arm
	Scar tissue	Scar tissue mobilization
Increased metabolism	Burns/extremes of heat	Avoid hot tubs/sauna Sun screen
Anaerobic metabolism	Excessive exercise	Avoid fatigue and soreness with exercise; build exercise routine gradually
Trauma	Fractures, surgery	Protection, compression garment
Air travel	Low ambient air pressure	Compression garment

with elevation and use of external compression. As lymphatic fluid accumulates in the extremity, an inflammatory reaction ensues which results in subcutaneous fibrosis and hardening of tissue. This is considered the hallmark for Stage 2 lymphedema. Stage 2 lymphedema does not resolve with elevation and compression garments. Stage 3 lymphedema is identified by cutaneous fibrosis and verrucous hyperplastic changes of the skin and is rarely seen in the upper extremity (153). As lymphedema progresses, pain may develop secondary to constriction of underlying soft tissue structures and overload of the supporting structures such as the shoulder (157).

The clinical evaluation of lymphedema should include a history of the primary malignancy and the aspects of treatment that have impacted the lymphatic system. The onset, duration, and progression of lymphatic swelling should be identified. In addition, identifying attempted management methods is important. Functional restrictions related to lymphedema (loss of shoulder or hand function) should be identified. Full musculoskeletal and neurologic examination is needed to identify any underlying deficits. The skin examination should include general skin and soft tissue characteristics, with a specific focus on surgical and irradiated sites. In addition, identification of cellulitis or lymphangitis is paramount to halt processes that may lead to worsening lymphedema. The lymphatic evaluation includes palpation of all lymphatic territories. Examination should include limb girth measurements, usually performed via tape measure or volumetric displacement of the affected and contralateral extremities (158).

Suspicion for recurrent malignant disease, while often unlikely to occur, should be part of care. In addition, evaluation of new onset suspected lymphedema should involve ruling out deep vein thrombosis (DVT), infection, and malignancy (e.g., cancer recurrence).

The management of lymphedema is performed to reduce symptoms, preserve cosmesis, maintain function, and decrease risk of infection. Complex decongestive therapy (CDT) is the most effective treatment (159). One component of CDT consists of manual lymphatic drainage, which is a massage technique promoting proximal lymph decongestion by fluid mobilization toward unaffected lymphatic territories. Skin care to reduce risk of infection is important and should be combined with stretching and soft tissue mobilization techniques to the proximal limb, helping to reduce stasis of the lymphatic system. Wrapping the extremity with short stretch bandages to promote lymphatic flow out of the limb is the next phase and can be augmented by use of high tensile foam to break up fibrosis. The foam use in lymphedema cases is usually a moderately rigid open-cell material applied over boney prominences or fibrotic areas that require more pressure to mobilize the fluid and to soften the tissue. The final phase uses exercises with gentle compressive wrapping in order to use the physiologic muscle pump to propel fluid to the proximal lymphatics. CDT is typically divided into a (a) decongestive phase that consists of 24 hours/day compression usually under the guidance of a trained physical or occupational therapist and (b) maintenance phase that consists of wrapping at night (performed by the patient or caregiver) and compressive garments during the day. In the maintenance phase, regular surveillance by a physician should be performed to assure volume reduction is maintained. Pneumatic pumps are also available but are controversial. They may be helpful in situations where the above treatments are not clinically feasible or response is poor. Pneumatic pump use requires a time-consuming daily routine, and clinical response may be modest (158,159). Although individuals with secondary lymphedema can safely participate in progressive and regular exercise, there was no effect of exercise on lymphedema or associated symptoms (160). However, a slowly progressive weight lifting program did not result in increased lymphedema for breast cancer survivors, which indicates resistance-based exercise programs may be appropriate for lymphedema patients (161). Evidence confirming the importance of early detection and intervention is emerging. A recent case series employing preoperative and postoperative volumetric measurements via optoelectronic perometry demonstrated subclinical lymphedema in 49% of ALND patients. Early treatment with provision of a 30/20 mm Hg compression sleeve and gauntlet was effective in reducing limb volume to near baseline levels (162,163).

Malignant lymphedema, resulting from spread of cancer into remaining lymphatics, presents with rapid swelling and a mottled appearance of the skin in the affected limb. Clinical examination may also reveal lymph node fullness. Evaluation should include exclusion of DVT and imaging of the regional lymphatics with computed tomography (CT) or MRI. Identifying locoregional recurrence is imperative to initiate early treatment to reduce functional loss and maximize life expectancy. The primary treatment is management of the occluding tumor.

IMPACT OF CANCER AND ONCOLOGY-DIRECTED TREATMENTS ON NUTRITION

Nutrition is an essential variable for all rehabilitation outcomes, but specific concerns apply to cancer patients at different points during the disease continuum. Many cancers as well as oncologic treatments affect nutritional status resulting in delayed wound healing, longer hospital stays, diminished

quality of life, lower survival rates, and reduced functional performance (164,165). One study noted a 50% prevalence of below normal prealbumin (<18 mg/dL) in cancer patients admitted to an inpatient rehabilitation unit (166). Older studies found that close to two thirds of cancer patients developed inanition during the course of their disease, demonstrating severe risk in the absence of systematic intervention (167). Multiple anthropometric and laboratory measures can be used to elegantly characterize malnutrition in individual cancer patients, but serum albumin below 3 g/dL and loss of 10% or more of stable preillness body weight continue to be the most reliable indicators of malnutrition in clinical practice. Laboratory and radiographic studies are necessary for identifying and responding to reversible components of malnutrition in cancer patients. Folate or B_{12} deficiencies may precipitate symptomatic anemia while hypercalcemia may induce anorexia and nausea. The Bristol-Myers Anorexia/Cachexia Instrument and the Functional Assessment of Anorexia/Cachexia Therapy provide validated means for assessing the impact of malnutrition on patients and can be used sequentially to track the effects of prescribed interventions (168).

Weight loss and malnutrition in cancer patients occur as the result of primary and secondary processes. Secondary processes that interfere with intake and absorption are common and more easily reversible. Nausea and anorexia may be associated with specific chemotherapy regimens as well as with malignancies involving the gastrointestinal system. Depression may be a cause of reduced intake. Patients with head and neck cancers and other diagnoses frequently present with or develop significant dysphagia. Others develop mucositis as the result of treatment regimens. Radiation enteritis can cause malabsorption, intestinal obstruction, and even fistulas that may require total bowel rest and parenteral nutrition. Secondary causes of malnutrition in cancer patients should be identified proactively, and tailored treatment plans should be introduced as early as possible. Mucositis can be treated with ice chips and oral analgesics although these may decrease enjoyment of food. Avoiding anticholinergic medication and adding oral rinses or pilocarpine to promote salivary flow can limit the effect of dry mouth on oral intake. Oral supplements may be more easily tolerated and appreciated than solid foods. Modifications can be made to minimize the effect of acquired aversions such as the use of plastic utensils by patients complaining of a metallic taste or the elimination of odors that affect odor-sensitive patients. Antiemetics such as ondansetron, prochlorperazine, and trimethobenzamide can be used to mitigate nausea while prokinetic agents such as metoclopramide can reduce early satiety from gastric stasis. Appetite stimulants including megestrol acetate and dronabinol are widely used and have been shown to increase intake and promote weight gain (169). It remains unclear, however, whether these gains reflect the actual increase in fat-free mass (FFM) needed for improved function. Concern over the prothrombotic effect of megestrol acetate has led to successful trials with lower dosages (170). Anabolic steroids such as oxandrolone may be used to promote lean body mass in patients with androgen receptor–negative malignancies (171). Extreme weight loss, specifically the loss of lean body mass, may be a primary disease–related process. Cancer cachexia was previously thought to result from direct tumor effect, but more recent investigations have suggested that cytokine-mediated processes alter the overall metabolic balance in cancer patients and animal models. TNF, proteolysis-inducing factor (PIF), and interleukin 6–dependent mechanisms shift metabolic processes; increasing lipolysis, protein consumption, and energy expenditure (172). Timely nutritional assessment and intervention are essential to effective cancer rehabilitation. The American Dietetic Association has published standards of practice and professional performance for specialty accreditation in the area of nutritional management of oncology patients (173). In addition to early assessment and monitoring the impact of nutritional interventions, nutritionists in many cancer programs serve as a de facto clearing house for patient use of complementary medicine and nutraceuticals—topics that patients are often uncomfortable discussing with their physicians. A growing body of literature endorses the addition of immunomodulating nutrients, specifically *n*-3 polyunsaturated fatty acids (eicosapentaenoic acid, docosahexaenoic acid), arginine, and nucleotides (174). Nutritionists often work one-to-one with patients and their families, but they can also contribute through organized support groups, addressing shared concerns such as weight gain during and after treatment for breast cancer, care provider responses to dysphagia, or healthy eating habits for long-term survivors.

CANCER-RELATED SEXUAL DYSFUNCTION

Sexual dysfunction may occur as a primary effect of malignancy but more commonly occurs as a side effect of treatment. Sexual function can be affected by disturbance at many levels, including psychological, central or peripheral nervous system, endocrine, pelvic, vascular, and local effects on gonadal structures. Physical changes may interfere with the patient's concept of his or her sexual attractiveness. Depression may result in low sexual drive. Sexual dysfunction in cancer patients may persist long after treatment is completed, and it is important for the practitioner to inquire about this during follow-up visits (175).

In men, chemotherapy can have adverse effects on spermatogenesis and also on testosterone production. Neuropathies, including dysautonomia, can interfere with the emission phase of male orgasm. Endocrine effects occur in men with prostate cancer treated with orchiectomy or with hormonal regimens to reduce serum testosterone. Radiation therapy to the prostate or testicles can produce erectile dysfunction, possibly as a result of acceleration of preexisting atherosclerosis from postradiation fibrotic changes. After prostate surgery, reports of erectile dysfunction have varied widely from 9% to 86%, probably related both to the extent of surgery (and other therapies) and assessment techniques (176). More rarely, urinary incontinence occurs. Similar problems may occur after radical cystectomy and abdominoperineal resection of gastrointestinal tumors. First-line therapies for erectile dysfunction include education and counseling, oral medications (e.g., sildenafil, vardenafil, or tadalafil), and the use of a vacuum device. Second-line therapies include use of intraurethral agents such as alprostadil and intracavernous injection therapy (as with papaverine), while the third-line option is surgery for penile prosthesis. Following retropubic prostatectomy, higher doses of sildenafil may increase smooth muscle content, with potential benefit of maintaining the proerectile ultrastructure during the recovery process (176).

In women, gonadal toxicity can occur with chemotherapy, especially alkylating agents, and permanent menopause may

occur with combination chemotherapy. Among breast cancer survivors, chemotherapy has been associated with greater reported sexual problems (177). Hormonal therapies, especially tamoxifen, may also produce side effects such as menstrual changes, vasomotor symptoms (hot flashes, headaches), and vaginal dryness (175). Radiation therapy to the pelvis produces premature menopause. A radiation dose of as low as 600 to 1,000 rad permanently destroys ovarian function. Radiation also produces damage to the vaginal epithelium, and the fibrotic process can continue over years. The result can be dyspareunia, postcoital bleeding, and even vaginal ulcers. After local radiation therapy for cervical cancer, stenosis of the upper vagina can occur. Among women presenting to a sexual medicine clinic at a large cancer hospital, the most common problems were dyspareunia (72%) and vulvovaginal atrophy (65%). The most common interventions included vaginal moisturizers and water-based lubricants (89%), psychosexual counseling (46%), and local, estradiol vaginal tablets (35%), with 70% of those attending follow-up sessions reporting improvement (178). In general, greasy lubricants, such as petroleum jelly, should be avoided because they may block the urethral opening. Counseling is usually short term and optimally includes both partners. Disease-specific or treatment-specific effects on sexual function should be discussed with the patient, including the use of diagrams when appropriate. For women who have undergone resection of pelvic tumors, vaginal dilators or pelvic floor exercises may also be indicated. Preservation of fertility is an increasing focus in many programs.

THE IMPACT OF CANCER ON MENTAL HEALTH

Psychological comorbidity has been described as a major source of distress in cancer patients (see also Chapter 12). Factors that may affect the mental health of cancer survivors include grief about current and anticipated losses, fear of death, concerns about loved ones, effects of chemotherapy on mood, and the biology of malignancy. This psychological distress in turn can lead to amplified pain, increased desire for hastened death, disability, difficulty participating in end-of-life planning, and psychosocial dysfunction of caregivers (179).

Behavior symptoms are a common side effect of breast cancer diagnosis and treatment and include disturbances in energy, sleep, cognition, and mood. Disturbances in mood may include depression and have been treated with intervention and pharmacotherapy using antidepressants (180). Intrusive thoughts were greater at baseline and at 12 months post treatment. They influenced the trajectory of pain, depressive symptoms, negative affect, and physical functioning over time (181). Cancer-related posttraumatic stress disorder (PTSD) has also been noted in a minority of patients and their families and has been correlated with distress, reduced quality of life, preexisting psychiatric conditions, and poor social support (182). Meta-analysis estimated an odds ratio of 1.66 for PTSD after cancer diagnosis in adults compared to controls (183). Cancer survivors, when compared to adults without cancer, were significantly more likely to report taking medication for anxiety (16.8% vs. 8.6%), depression (14.1% vs. 7.8%), and one or both of these conditions combined (19.1% vs. 10.4%) (184). Elderly individuals (≥66 years) with incident cases of breast, colorectal, or prostate cancer were followed for

6 months after a new diagnosis of depression, and two thirds of patients did receive intervention for the depression (antidepressants only 46%, combined therapy 18%, and psychotherapy only 9%) (185). Impact of cancer and its treatment on the mood of survivors and family should remain an important consideration in treatment given potential effects for recovery and quality of life.

SPECIFIC CANCERS AND THEIR REHABILITATION NEEDS

Breast Cancer

Breast cancer is the most common malignancy in women. Approximately 3 million women are living in the US with this diagnosis (186) and over 250,000 women were estimated to be newly diagnosed with breast cancer in 2017 (6). Breast cancer diagnosed in men correspond to only 0.5% to 1% of all breast cancers (187). Breast cancer can be treated with breast-conserving surgery, mastectomy, radiation, chemotherapy, and antihormonal therapy (188). Sentinel lymph node biopsy or ALND may occur with surgical intervention. The overall 5-year survival rate for breast cancer is approximately 90% as a result of improved treatment and earlier diagnosis through improved screening protocols (186).

Specific impairments may be related to the cancer or to the treatment, and it is therefore essential to know the potential side effects of the oncology-directed therapy. For example, cardiomyopathy may occur with trastuzumab, and CIPN may occur with taxane-based chemotherapy (48). Lymphedema is one of the most well-known impairments associated with breast cancer as a result of surgical intervention, lymph node dissection, and radiation therapy (186). Approximately 20% of women with breast cancer will develop lymphedema, with a higher incidence in those that underwent axillary compared to sentinel lymph node dissection (189). Cording, otherwise known as axillary web syndrome, occurs in approximately 30% of patients as a result of treatment and contributes to functional impairment of the upper extremity (190).

Pain is very common in breast cancer and can last a year or longer after treatment (191).

Postsurgical pain, often referred to as postmastectomy pain syndrome, occurs in over 40% of women (192). Postsurgical pain syndromes include phantom breast pain (193), incisional allodynia, neuroma formation, pectoralis muscle pain, and intercostobrachial neuropathy (194). Incisional allodynia is related to the dense cutaneous innervation of the breast, resulting in hypersensitivity approximating the incision. Neuroma formation typically occurs at the end of the incision and results in a focal area of pain and sometimes a small palpable mass. The pectoralis muscle may be impacted mechanically from surgery and presents with diffuse chest wall pain, that is worse with shoulder flexion and external rotation (195). The intercostobrachial nerve, which traverses across the chest wall, enters the axilla and provides sensation to the lateral chest wall and posteromedial portion of the arm, which is frequently sacrificed during axillary dissection, resulting in sensory impairment and occasionally allodynia.

In addition to lymphedema and pain, patients can experience adhesive capsulitis, pectoralis tightness, myofascial pain syndromes, and rotator cuff dysfunction (196). The etiologies

of these symptoms are multifactorial and can be related to immobilization, muscle weakness, atrophy, mechanical alterations in the shoulder girdle musculature, radiation therapy, and neurologic impairment. Cervical radiculopathy and brachial plexopathy (especially of the lower trunk) can result from breast cancer extension or metastases (197).

Treatment of breast cancer with aromatase inhibitors such as anastrozole has been well documented to result in carpal tunnel syndrome, trigger finger, decreased grip strength, morning stiffness, and generalized arthralgia in addition to bone loss (198,199).

The assessment of pain, lymphedema, and shoulder dysfunction begins with a history including descriptions of symptoms, postoperative complications, durations of immobilizations, functional restrictions, weaknesses, and sensory disturbances. The history should also identify red flags for recurrence such as constitutional symptoms, progressive pain complaints, concurrent plexopathy, or unusual presentations of lymphedema. The physical examination should identify atrophy; assess restriction in regional musculature, scapulohumeral and glenohumeral mobility, and regional muscle strength; and include a comprehensive neurologic exam.

Management is multimodal and dependent on symptoms. The primary management of pain consists of self-applied techniques including cutaneous desensitization, soft tissue mobilization, stretching of regional muscle groups, and shoulder range of motion exercises. These techniques usually can be commenced once the surgical incision is healed. For those with persistent pain, severe loss of function, or sleep loss, additional care, including a more extended course of physical or occupational therapy, pharmaceutical management, and even interventional procedures may be warranted (195). Thermal modalities should be used with caution secondary to concern about provoking lymphedema. The management of shoulder impairment ideally begins preoperatively with a home stretching regimen to maximize shoulder mobility. After surgery, pendulum exercises and range of motion exercises below 90 degrees of shoulder abduction and flexion are advocated until postsurgical drains are removed (200). Once drains are removed, aggressive pain management and daily shoulder stretching, targeting the pectoralis complex and latissimus dorsi, are initiated. Once full range is obtained, strengthening of the scapular stabilizers, rotator cuff, and deltoid musculature should begin. For those with persistent or progressive shoulder dysfunction, advanced imaging with MRI and referral to a skilled therapist who understands cancer principles is warranted. Management of intercostobrachial neuropathy and axillary web syndrome (cording) includes scar tissue mobilization and shoulder range of motion exercises.

Head and Neck Cancer

Approximately 600,000 new cases of head and neck cancer occur worldwide each year (201). In the US, 3% of all cancers are due to those in the head and neck, which includes cancers of the nasal cavity, sinus, oral cavity, salivary glands, tongue, pharynx, and larynx (202). Men are twice as likely as women to be diagnosed with head and neck cancer, and the incidence increases after the age of 45 (202). Head and neck cancer presents with a variety of symptoms depending upon the location of the tumor, including hoarseness, stridor, dysphonia, dysphagia, or cranial nerve palsy (203).

Head and neck cancer and its treatment result in a number of impairments. Pain is very common at the time of diagnosis, during treatment, and after completion of treatment (204). Dysphagia, like pain, can be a presenting symptom of head and neck cancer but can also result from surgical and radiation treatment; causing patients to lose weight, become malnourished and fatigued, and be at higher risk for infection and other complications resulting from aspiration (205,206). Mucositis and xerostomia result in pain and sticky saliva and have a high prevalence after chemotherapy and radiation and contribute to dysphagia as well as poor oral hygiene and increased risk for fungal infections and dental caries (205,207). Reduced mouth opening, otherwise known as trismus, results in dysphagia, poor oral hygiene, and poor speech production and can also predispose patients to weight loss and malnutrition (208,209). Communication difficulties in head and neck cancer include dysarthria, dysphonia, and aphonia resulting from tongue, vocal cord, or other dysfunction caused by the tumor or treatment (205,206,210). Lymphedema can result from damage to the lymphatic system as the result of surgical excision (208). Dysfunction and pain of the neck and shoulders can result from surgery, such as radical neck dissection which involves removal of muscles such as the sternocleidomastoid in addition to the spinal accessory nerve, via trapezius dysfunction and biomechanical imbalances of the upper trunk, shoulder and neck (208).

Assessment of these symptoms requires a thorough history of cancer diagnosis, oncologic management, treatment complications, functional impairments, and quality of life. Clinical examination should focus on the oral mucosa, dentition, posture, cervical and shoulder range of motion, and a thorough neurologic examination.

Rehabilitation management should aim to address symptoms and functional deficits. The primary management for mucositis includes topical agents for pain control, oral hygiene, and artificial lubrication. For severe oral pain, opioids may be utilized to maintain oral intake. Treatment of xerostomia consists of strict oral hygiene including sodium fluoride gel; rinses with saline, salt and baking soda (one teaspoon of each in a quart of water) or diluted peroxide; artificial lubricants or use of a spray mister; and salivary gland stimulating agents such as pilocarpine or sugarless gum or lozenges. Diet should emphasize fluids, moist foods, and high-calorie supplements. Patients with trismus may benefit from rehabilitation efforts focusing on intraoral skills (mastication, mouth opening, swallowing, phonation), scar tissue mobilization, strengthening of the masticatory muscles, and consideration of a TheraBite or Dynasplint System to provide prolonged passive stretch. Of note, patients should be evaluated and cleared by their dentist prior to initiation of any intraoral therapy or stretching. When dysphagia is present, a speech and language pathologist should be incorporated into the plan of care. Management of dysphagia should begin with a swallowing study, performed bedside or via a modified barium swallow to identify aspiration. Therapy then focuses on airway protection techniques, such as breath holding during the swallow, throat clearing afterward, chin tuck, and dietary modification. Communication difficulties can be quite devastating for patients with head and neck cancers, and basic management strategies include use of good eye contact, appropriate gestures, oral exercises, tongue mobilization for articulation, and modification of pitch, loudness, and voice quality (211). Aphonia is one of the most feared complications

in cancer treatment and is usually a result of total laryngectomy (210). Communication after total laryngectomy occurs through esophageal speech (propelling air into the esophagus and expelling it, making sound), an electrolarynx (handheld device to the larynx, making sound), or tracheoesophageal puncture (also known as TEP, tracheoesophageal prosthesis, or fistula and includes placement of a valve that allows for speech production, such as a Passy-Muir valve) (212). Management of facial and cervical lymphedema includes manual lymphatic drainage in combination with compression garments to reduce fluid accumulation in the face when recumbent (213). In cases of severe acute swelling, thrombosis of the superior vena cava or jugular veins should be excluded. For patients with pain and neurologic impairments, efforts should include manual desensitization, scar tissue mobilization, neuromuscular reeducation, postural correction, range of motion exercises, compensatory strategies, and muscle strengthening. Education on injury prevention especially for those with axillary nerve injuries should be provided. If needed, topical anesthetics and neuropathic pain medications can be initiated.

Hematologic Malignancies

Hematologic malignancies include lymphomas, leukemias, and myelomas, and they were estimated to be over 135,000 new cases of hematologic malignancies diagnosed in the US in 2016 (214). The average age of onset for each of these malignancies varies by tumor type.

For example, acute lymphocytic leukemia is usually diagnosed around age 14 while acute myelocytic leukemia is usually diagnosed around 67 years of age (186). Similarly, the majority of non-Hodgkin's lymphoma cases are diagnosed after the age of 50, whereas Hodgkin's lymphoma is usually diagnosed before age 50 (186). In general, the survival of patients with hematologic malignancies has improved over the years, though prognosis depends on the particular type of tumor (186,214,215).

Hematologic malignancies are associated with a number of signs and symptoms as a result of cancer and treatment. Alterations in blood cell count at time of diagnosis and throughout the disease course result in fatigue, increased episodes of bleeding, and increased risk of infection. Cardiopulmonary dysfunction resulting in reduced endurance and increased fatigue can occur with chemotherapy or radiation use (186). Weakness, reduced ambulation, reduced range of motion, and peripheral neuropathy as a result of chemotherapy, radiation, or disease can occur during or after diagnosis and treatment (216). Balance can also be impaired (216). Bony tumor involvement can result in biologic pain, while fractures can occur in the case of treatment-induced osteopenia or bony tumor involvement (217). In the multiple myeloma population, compression of nerve roots such as carpal tunnel syndrome or compression of the spinal cord may occur from relapsing disease (217). Side effects of chemotherapy and radiation may also include dysphagia, difficulty speaking, and memory impairments (217–220). Steroids can cause steroid-induced myopathy and avascular necrosis of the femoral or humeral heads while mantle field radiation can cause dropped head syndrome (221–223). Individuals undergoing autologous or allogeneic transplantation may experience chemotherapy-related or steroid-induced myopathy, deconditioning, fatigue, and peripheral neuropathy (224).

Complications of allogeneic stem cell transplantation include acute or chronic graft versus host disease. In chronic graft-versus-host disease, cutaneous skin changes commonly occur and can involve the dermis and fascia resulting in edema, reduced range of motion, and joint contracture with skin breakdown and, ultimately, destruction of involved joints (221,225,226). Inflammatory myositis, inflammatory neuropathy, and avascular necrosis may be manifestations of chronic graft versus host disease (225,227).

Rehabilitation efforts in this population focus on symptoms and functional impairments. These efforts may include walking to maintain endurance during treatment, strengthening exercises particularly for proximal muscles, sensory and balance training, range of motion, and activities of daily living. Blood counts and vital signs must be closely monitored during activity to ensure no adverse events.

Lung Cancer

Lung cancer is one of the most commonly occurring cancers with over 200,000 new cases estimated in the US in 2017 (6). Lung cancer is more common in men, and the average age of diagnosis is 70 (186,228). Lung cancer is the most common cause of cancer-related mortality among men and women in developed countries, and survival is reported to be better for non–small cell lung cancer than for small cell lung cancer cases (186,228). In recent years, studies have demonstrated the benefit of low-dose CT screening for reducing lung cancer mortality, and the U.S. Preventive Services Task Force currently recommends annual screening for lung cancer in adults aged 55 to 80 years old who have a 30–pack-year smoking history and either currently smoke or have stopped within the past 15 years (229,230).

Lung CT screening for high-risk patients means that more cancers will be picked up at earlier stages, and thus, an increase in the number of patients who will have surgery is anticipated. As such, this population may be ideal for prehabilitation (49). Treatment of either small cell or non–small cell lung cancer can include chemotherapy, radiation therapy, surgical intervention, or targeted drug therapy (186).

Fatigue, pain, dyspnea, decreased physical activity, and reduced function are commonly reported symptoms and clinical findings at the time of diagnosis (231,232). Similarly, after treatment, patients with lung cancer have impaired lung function, exercise capacity, and quality of life (233). Initiating a pulmonary rehabilitation program at time of diagnosis with continuation throughout the continuum of care has been shown to improve respiratory function (234,235). In this population, other cancer-related impairments include myasthenic syndromes, plexopathies, and radiculopathies from tumor invasion while treatment-related impairments can include postthoracotomy pain, peripheral neuropathy, and cognitive impairments (236). Similar to other cancer types, patients with lung cancer should undergo a thorough history and clinical evaluation. Electrodiagnostic testing can be incorporated to evaluate neuropathies, radiculopathies, and myasthenic syndromes. Physical therapy focused on chest wall mobilization, endurance training, muscle strengthening, desensitization, and scar tissue mobilization as well as occupational therapy focused on activities of daily living play an important role in the management of this population.

Gastrointestinal Malignancies

Gastrointestinal malignancies include colorectal, stomach, liver, esophageal, small intestine, and pancreatic cancers. Screening with routine colonoscopy has reduced the incidence of colorectal cancer as has improved diet and treatment (16,17). However, the incidence rates for some types of gastrointestinal malignancy such as liver cancer have increased (18). The survival rate for a number of gastrointestinal cancers, including colorectal and esophageal cancer, has increased as a result of improved prevention, screening, and treatment, while the survival rate for pancreatic and liver cancer has not improved as significantly (186,237,238).

Impairments commonly experienced by the colorectal and gastrointestinal cancer populations include bowel and bladder dysfunction from surgery or radiation. Some patients may have an ostomy placed for bowel management (186). Pelvic floor therapy can improve bowel dysfunction in addition to bladder incontinence (239,240). Depending on the extent of intervention, patients may have absent anal sphincters and present similar to a lower motor neuron pattern of injury requiring increased fiber and hydration in addition to timed toileting and/or manual removal to promote continence and emptying (239). Bladder dysfunction can include incontinence or difficulty emptying resulting from detrusor dysfunction from neurologic injury or scar tissue formation (241). Patients may also experience sexual dysfunction (241). In the general gastrointestinal cancer population, patients may experience dysphagia, odynophagia, pain, fatigue, CIPN, increased fracture risk, and lymphedema (242). These impairments should be symptomatically managed with speech, physical, occupational, or lymphedema therapies.

Brain Tumors

Brain tumors account for 85% to 90% of all primary CNS tumors, and there are more than 125 types of brain tumors officially recognized by the WHO (243). The majority of brain tumors are located in meninges (34%) followed by the frontal, temporal, parietal, and occipital lobes of the brain (22%). Meningiomas represent 34% of all primary tumors and are the most common benign tumor of the brain. Gliomas represent 30% of all tumors and 80% of all malignant brain tumors. Glioblastomas account for the majority of all gliomas. Other histologies include astrocytomas, pituitary tumors, lymphomas, oligodendrogliomas, and medulloblastomas (243).

Brain metastases are the most common nonterminal neurologic event in individuals with cancer. Each year approximately 100,000 individuals are diagnosed with brain metastases (244–246). In adults, most metastatic lesions arise from lung and breast cancers and cutaneous melanomas. Renal cell carcinoma, colon cancer, and gynecologic malignancies are also known to metastasize to the brain. In individuals under the age of 21, sarcomas including osteogenic sarcoma, rhabdomyosarcoma, Ewing sarcoma, and germ cell tumors are the most common sources of metastases (244–246). Brain metastases tend to occur at the junction of the grey-white matter, a pattern characteristic of an embolic event, and are associated with severe peritumoral edema. The distribution of metastases roughly correlates with cerebral blood flow and volume; with approximately 80% of metastatic lesions occurring in the cerebral hemispheres, 15% in the cerebellum, and 5% in the brain stem. Metastases are multiple in approximately 50% of patients (244).

Neurologic impairments from primary brain tumors and metastases are the result of destruction or displacement of normal brain tissue by the growing lesion and its associated edema.

Hydrocephalus, increased intracranial pressure, and vascular injury may also ensue and play a role in development of impairments (244,247). Typically, patients have a subacute to chronic progression of symptoms; however, symptoms may also appear rapidly and episodically from associated hemorrhage, nonconvulsive seizures, or by cerebral ischemia/infarction from embolic or compressive occlusion of blood vessels (245,246). The clinical presentation of neurologic impairments related to primary and metastatic brain tumors is often similar to that seen in stroke or traumatic brain injury. The neuroanatomical location of the tumor determines the presenting signs and symptoms (31,248). Survival factors including age, extent of systemic disease, neurologic status at time of diagnosis, and extent of metastatic disease are considered when determining optimal treatment for individuals with primary and metastatic brain tumors (246).

Surgical intervention is a standard treatment option in individuals with accessible single lesions, good functional performance status, and controlled or absent extracranial disease, as it provides tissue for definitive diagnosis and immediate relief of neurologic symptoms due to mass effect (244). Postoperatively, individuals may experience residual neurologic deficits from subtotal tumor resection or new deficits related to postoperative edema and resection of functional brain tissue along with the tumor (249). Postoperative neurologic deficits may present with generalized signs and symptoms such as headache, seizures, and personality changes, or focal deficits such as weakness, sensory impairments, gait abnormalities, language dysfunction, cognitive impairments, visual perceptual deficits, and dysphagia.

Radiation therapy is a mainstay in the treatment of both primary and metastatic tumors in the brain (250). The goal of radiation therapy is to achieve maximal effect to the tumor with minimal toxicity to normal brain tissue (249). The very young (age <10) and the elderly (age >70) appear to be most vulnerable to the adverse effects of radiation exposure (250). Three clinical phases of adverse effects from radiation therapy have been identified: acute, subacute, and delayed effects (250). Adverse effects occurring during radiation therapy are usually temporary but can be disturbing enough to warrant symptom-based therapy. Common acute phase symptoms include headache, nausea, vomiting, fever, and new or progressive focal neurologic deficits. Individuals experiencing acute effects should be assured that they are temporary (250). Subacute effects develop within the first 6 months of receiving radiation therapy and are usually temporary. They can however persist longer and be more severe than acute adverse effects. During the subacute period, individuals may experience increased fatigue/lethargy, impaired cognition, and new or worsening focal neurologic deficits (250).

Delayed phase adverse effects occur several months to years post treatment and are attributed to microvasculature damage resulting in tissue hypoxia. These adverse effects are the most feared complications, because they are generally considered irreversible and can be disabling.

Classically described delayed effects include cerebral radiation necrosis, leukoencephalopathy, and vascular abnormalities (250,251).

Chemotherapy plays a role in the treatment of both intracranial and extracranial malignancies and has contributed to significant improvements in clinical outcomes (252). Neurologic involvement after treatment with chemotherapeutic agents can range from cognitive impairments and visual changes to encephalopathy, leukoencephalopathy, cerebrovascular complications, and cerebellar syndromes. Factors contributing to the development of neurologic involvement include total dose received, route of administration, presence of structural brain lesions, exposure to concomitant radiation therapy, and medication interactions (252). Functional gains are possible for many patients with brain tumors; however, rehabilitation services for patients with steadily worsening neurologic status should focus on caregiver training for palliative goals. Rehabilitation outcomes for patients with brain tumors compare favorably to gains made by patients with other types of brain disorders such as traumatic brain injury or stroke, and standard rehabilitation strategies for those diagnoses can be effectively used for brain tumor patients. Brain tumor patients participating in comprehensive inpatient rehabilitation programs have been shown to achieve meaningful gains in FIM scores with characteristically shorter lengths of stay than patients with traumatic brain injuries and some strokes (32,33). Concurrent radiotherapy treatment does not significantly alter these gains (35). Most studies show a higher than average rate of transfer back to an acute medical setting, with the majority (69%) of these patients returning to meet their rehabilitation goals prior to discharge to a private home/community setting (33,35). Patients with primary brain tumors and metastatic disease show similar functional gains (253,254), though gains are better during the initial presentation to rehabilitation than with recurrence (255). Depression and anxiety can be a barrier to rehabilitation efforts, and care should be taken when initiating medication management as it may further affect cognition. Data collected from patients with gliomas have documented improvements in function with 10 mg twice daily methylphenidate and have led to the recommendation of this agent as an adjuvant in the treatment of brain tumors (255).

Radiation treatments may produce fatigue, limiting participation in therapy sessions. If possible, treatments should be scheduled later in the day after rehabilitation therapies have completed (33) Continuation of oral corticosteroids is needed during radiation treatment, as edema due to radiation can precipitate or intensify neurologic and cognitive symptoms. Corticosteroid regimens ranging from 2 to 24 mg/d in divided doses of oral dexamethasone or equivalent agent are typically given. Treating clinicians should be aware of potential side effects including steroid psychosis, gastrointestinal bleeding, avascular necrosis, and proximal myopathy. Anticonvulsant therapy appears to be justified in patients with a history of seizure and possibly for short-term use perioperatively, but efficacy of long-term prophylaxis for patients without history of seizure has not been established (256). Incidence of DVT in brain tumor patients is high, and prophylaxis such as intermittent pneumatic compression with or without low-dose heparin is warranted. Incidence of postoperative deep venous thrombosis in malignant glioma was found to range from 3% to 60% (257).

Anticoagulation must be judiciously restarted in collaboration with the treating neurosurgeon following any kind of intracranial tumor resection.

Spinal Tumors

Spinal tumors can be primary or secondary to metastatic disease and can occur in any region of the spinal column or spinal cord. They are classically grouped into three categories: extradural, intradural extramedullary, and intradural intramedullary tumors. Primary and metastatic lesions may be osteolytic, osteoblastic, or mixed in nature. Osteolytic lesions are more common with breast, lung, and thyroid cancers. Osteoblastic lesions typically occur with prostate and bladder cancers and carcinoid tumors. Mixed lesions can be seen with lung, breast, cervical, and ovarian cancers (258). Both osteolytic and osteoblastic lesions alter normal bone architecture resulting in deformity or collapse of the affected vertebral body. This deformity can lead to spinal instability by increasing strain on the support elements of the spine including muscles, tendons, ligaments, and joint capsules (259). It can also result in retropulsion of fractured bone fragments into the epidural space causing spinal cord compression (260).

Extradural lesions may grow into the epidural space resulting in spinal cord compression. Epidural spinal cord compression (ESCC) results in mechanical injury to axons and myelin. ESCC may also result in vascular compromise of the spinal arteries and epidural venous plexus, leading to spinal cord ischemia and/or infarction. Depending on the underlying malignancy, 2% to 5% of patients will develop clinical signs and symptoms of ESCC during the course of their disease (261). ESCC is most commonly diagnosed in thoracic lesions; though cadaveric studies have shown that the most common site of tumor burden in the spine is the lumbar region (260). Extramedullary metastases, or LMD, are a relatively common complication of cancer, occurring in 3% to 8% of all patients (258).

Pain is the most common initial symptom in patients with ESCC (83% to 95%) and may precede the development of other neurologic symptoms by weeks to months (262). Moreover, pain related to spinal metastases is the initial manifestation of systemic disease in 10% of cancer patients (263). Motor weakness is the next most common symptom of ESCC and is present in 35% to 85% of patients with metastatic disease at time of initial presentation. This weakness may be upper motor neuron, lower motor neuron, or a combination of both depending on the area of the cord involved. Patients with cervical involvement may have a lower motor neuron pattern of weakness in the upper extremities and an upper motor neuron pattern in the lower extremities. Thoracic lesions may result in upper motor neuron findings in the lower extremities, with flexor musculature weaker than extensor. Lumbosacral involvement often presents with a lower motor neuron pattern secondary to injury at the level of the cauda equina (259). Sensory symptoms or impairments are usually present at time of diagnosis with ESCC (60%) but are rarely the initial symptom. The pattern of sensory impairments corresponds to the location of nerve injury. Involvement of the spinal thalamic tracts at the level of the spinal cord results in sensory level disturbances to pin prick and temperature tests. Dorsal column injuries commonly produce ascending tingling and an encircling sensation of tightness about the trunk or limb. Sensory ataxia from dorsal column involvement is also common. Lhermitte's phenomenon is frequently noted by patients with cord compression in the cervical and upper thoracic levels and reflects compression injury to the dorsal columns. Root compression results in a dermatomal distribution of paresthesia

(261). Autonomic symptoms including bowel, bladder, and sexual dysfunction; loss of sweating below the lesion; and orthostatic hypotension are unusual as an initial symptom but are often present at the time of diagnosis. Autonomic symptoms usually correlate with the degree of motor involvement (259,261). Gait and truncal ataxia mimicking cerebellar involvement may be seen.

Primary extradural tumors and metastases present in a similar fashion to ESCC but with a higher incidence of neurologic impairments. Approximately 70% to 90% of individuals will have pain as an initial symptom, and more than 60% of individuals undergoing surgical resection will have some degree of weakness. Motor deficits may manifest in the absence of pain. Almost all patients will have some degree of sensory involvement. Given predilection for cauda equine involvement, bowel, bladder, and sexual dysfunction have been noted; usually as an early finding. LMD may present with radiculopathy, neuropathy or in a Brown-Séquard, conus medullaris, or cauda equina pattern (264,265). Intramedullary tumors may also present with clinical manifestations similar to epidural tumors. Pain, the most common initial symptom, is present in 30% to 85% of patients (258,265).

Séquard, central cord, conus medullaris, and cauda equina syndrome (261,264,266). Benefits of rehabilitation in traumatic SCI are well established. Studies in neoplastic spinal cord injuries have shown that conventional rehabilitation approaches including medical management, initiation of bowel and bladder programs, physical and occupational therapies, bracing, and adaptive equipment can be utilized to relieve symptoms, prevent further complications, enhance functional independence, and improve quality of life in this patient population (265).

Sarcomas of Bone and Soft Tissue

Sarcomas are mesenchymal tumors that develop in bone and soft tissue, represent approximately 1% of cancer cases, yet present as over 50 different subtypes (267). The incidence of soft tissue sarcomas generally increases with older age, while bone sarcomas are more common at ages 15 to 24 and over the age of 65 (268). Treatment of sarcomas is dependent on tumor type and location and can include chemotherapy, radiation, and surgery (269,270).

Comprehensive sarcoma clinics, involving specialists who have experience in caring for this population, can be beneficial in addressing the multiple needs of these patients (271). Because both soft tissue and bone sarcomas often involve the extremities, impairments reported are related to mobility and activities of daily living. Pain is extremely common and may include postoperative pain, neuropathic pain, or phantom limb pain (269,272). Limb-sparing surgery and amputation are the methods of choice for treatment. Multiple factors influence the surgical decision between the two, including activity level, cosmesis, and prior level of function (269). Limb-sparing surgery can require multiple reconstruction and resection surgeries and can result in significant functional impairment (269,272). Amputation requires preprosthetic management that includes diligence, care for limb shaping, and skin preservation that is followed by prosthetic training (269,272). In some cases, a rotationplasty to replace a knee joint may be performed in young patients (269). Both limb-sparing and amputation rehabilitation should focus on range of motion, strength, endurance training, and wound healing as indicated by the individual's weight-bearing status (269,272). Sarcoma patients can be approached therapeutically in ways similar to the non-oncologic amputee population.

Prostate Cancer

Prostate cancer is the most commonly diagnosed cancer in men over the age of 50 years in the US, with an estimated 220,800 cases diagnosed in 2016 (273), and was the third leading cause of cancer death in males in 2017 (6). Prostate cancer has a distinct tropism for bone, making it the most common and frequently the only site of metastatic disease (274).

Spinal bone represents the most common site of skeletal involvement (275). Treatment options for localized disease include intensity-modulated radiation therapy to the intact prostate bed (IMRT), low dose rate brachytherapy, radical prostatectomy (RP) with or without postoperative radiation therapy, and active surveillance (273,276). For many men with prostate cancer, the treatment decision is based on the potential toxicity and anticipated impact on quality of life, as prostate cure rates are roughly equivalent across modalities (273).

Obstructive urinary symptoms with or without incontinence, and sexual dysfunction can occur as a result of prostate cancer and worsen as a result of treatment. Postoperative stress urinary incontinence and erectile dysfunction related to external sphincter insufficiency and possible nerve injury are the most common complications after RP and have a significant impact on quality of life (276). The standard first-line treatment for advanced disease is androgen deprivation therapy (ADT), and as of 2014, roughly 1/3 of the 3 million men diagnosed with prostate cancer in the US had or were scheduled to receive ADT (277). The initiation of ADT results in tumor regression but at the same time may result in sexual dysfunction, gynecomastia, hot flashes, osteoporosis, cognitive deficits, reduced muscle mass, increased fat mass, fatigue, and increased incidence of both cardiovascular disease and type 2 diabetes (277). More recently, systemic therapeutic approaches for metastatic disease have targeted the osteoclastic/osteoblastic pathway with the goal of reducing existing bone-related symptoms, prolonging the time to onset of a new bone-related insult, increasing patient survival, and improving quality of life (274).

Perioperative education regarding bladder and sexual dysfunction plays an important role in patient satisfaction. Included in this education should be the role of rehabilitation efforts. Rehabilitation efforts in this population should include pelvic floor therapy for scar tissue mobilization, muscle coordination, and biofeedback, as well as physical therapy with resistance training, core strengthening, spine stabilization, and aerobic exercise. These efforts should be considered from time of diagnosis throughout the continuum of care.

Gynecologic Cancers

Endometrial cancer is the most common gynecologic malignancy in the US, with 61,380 new cases diagnosed in 2017 (6). Cancer of the endometrium accounts for 6% of all cancers in women. Treatment options include hysterectomy with bilateral salpingo-oophorectomy and possible pelvic and paraaortic lymph node dissection, vaginal brachytherapy, radiation therapy alone or as an adjuvant treatment postoperatively, chemotherapy, and hormonal therapy. Treatment is based on extent of disease (278).

Vulvar cancer affects approximately 6,000 women in the US each year (6). The most common histology is squamous cell carcinoma. Treatment of localized vulvar cancer involves surgical resection, with adjuvant radiation therapy reserved for those with high-risk factors.

Locally advanced disease is treated with a combination of radical surgery and adjuvant chemoradiation. Surgical intervention may also include sentinel lymph node biopsies or inguinofemoral lymphadenectomy. For advanced and metastatic disease, palliation with chemotherapy and/or radiation therapy is recommended (279).

As of 2017, cervical cancer affected over 12,000 women in the US and accounted for more than 4,200 deaths annually (280). Treatment options include surgical intervention with/without sentinel lymph node biopsy or lymphadenectomy, radiation therapy, brachytherapy, and chemotherapy.

Ovarian cancer is the second most common gynecologic malignancy and the most common cause of gynecologic cancer death in the US (6). Standard treatment recommendations for patients with ovarian cancer include surgical debulking followed by adjuvant chemotherapy. Similar to other gynecologic cancers, lymph node resection may be performed during surgical intervention.

Pelvic surgery and radiation therapy as treatment for gynecologic cancers can result in changes to the pelvic floor, scar tissue formation, and injury to the autonomic and somatic nerves in the pelvis. These injuries can result in bladder, bowel, and sexual dysfunction. In the gynecologic literature, postoperative bladder dysfunction has been reported to occur in 70% to 85% of patients who underwent radical hysterectomy (281). In addition, pelvic radiation can result in vaginal erythema, moist desquamation, and confluent mucositis of the vagina in the acute phases of treatment. In some patients, these changes can progress to epithelial sloughing, ulcer formation, and necrosis leading to vaginal wall thinning, adhesions, atrophy, and fibrosis followed by vaginal stenosis. These anatomical changes can result in sexual dysfunction and pain (282).

Sexual dysfunction can occur from dryness, scarring, narrowing of the vaginal entrance, shortening of the canal, and pain. Similar effects are observed in the bladder and rectum resulting in late effects such as urgency, hemorrhagic cystitis, tenesmus, and incontinence (282,283). Rehabilitation interventions should address scar tissue mobilization, tissue health, neuromuscular reeducation, sensory and muscle training, biofeedback, and dilator therapy. Bowel and bladder programs should be initiated to promote emptying. Lower extremity lymphedema is one of the most disabling side effects of surgical and radiation therapy.

Lymphedema presents as swelling in the lower extremities within the first 12 months post treatment and results in pain, heaviness, difficulty with mobility, and impaired quality of life (284). When present, lymphedema therapy should focus on manual lymphatic drainage, compression wrapping and/or use of compression garments, education on self-drainage, and skin hygiene.

ACKNOWLEDGMENTS

The authors wish to acknowledge the authors of the original version of this chapter: Mary M. Vargo, Justin C. Riutta, and Deborah J. Franklin. The authors would like to thank Julie A. Poorman, Ph.D., for her help with manuscript preparation.

REFERENCES

1. Howlader N, Noone AM, Krapcho M, et al. *SEER Cancer Statistics Review (CSR) 1975–2013.* Bethesda, MD: National Cancer Institute; 2016.
2. Niederhuber JE, Armitage JO, Doroshow JH, et al. *Abeloff's Clinical Oncology.* Electronic version/5th ed. Philadelphia, PA: Saunders; 2014.
3. What is cancer staging? American Joint Committee on Cancer; 2017. Available from: https://cancerstaging.org/references-tools/Pages/What-is-Cancer-Staging.aspx. Accessed February 24, 2017.
4. DeVita VT. *DeVita, Hellman, and Rosenberg's Cancer: Principles & Practice of Oncology.* Electronic version/10th ed. Philadelphia, PA: Wolters Kluwer; 2015.
5. *Cancer Facts & Figures 2016.* Atlanta, GA: American Cancer Society; 2016.
6. American Cancer Society. *Cancer Facts & Figures 2017.* Atlanta, GA: American Cancer Society; 2017.
7. Weir HK, Thompson TD, Soman A, et al. Meeting the healthy people 2020 objectives to reduce cancer mortality. *Prev Chronic Dis.* 2015;12:E104.
8. Weir HK, Thompson TD, Soman A, et al. The past, present, and future of cancer incidence in the United States: 1975 through 2020. *Cancer.* 2015;121(11):1827–1837.
9. Hewitt M, Rowland JH, Yancik R. Cancer survivors in the United States: age, health, and disability. *J Gerontol A Biol Sci Med Sci.* 2003;58(1):82–91.
10. Ness KK, Gurney JG, Zeltzer LK, et al. The impact of limitations in physical, executive, and emotional function on health-related quality of life among adult survivors of childhood cancer: a report from the Childhood Cancer Survivor Study. *Arch Phys Med Rehabil.* 2008;89(1):128–136.
11. Sweeney C, Schmitz KH, Lazovich D, et al. Functional limitations in elderly female cancer survivors. *J Natl Cancer Inst.* 2006;98(8):521–529.
12. *The 2014 Council for Disability Awareness: Long Term Disability Claims Review.* Portland, ME: Council for Disability Awareness; 2014.
13. Lehmann JF, DeLisa JA, Warren CG, et al. Cancer rehabilitation: assessment of need, development, and evaluation of a model of care. *Arch Phys Med Rehabil.* 1978;59(9):410–419.
14. Corsonello A, Pedone C, Carosella L, et al. Health status in older hospitalized patients with cancer or non-neoplastic chronic diseases. *BMC Geriatr.* 2005;5:10.
15. Given B, Given C, Azzouz F, et al. Physical functioning of elderly cancer patients prior to diagnosis and following initial treatment. *Nurs Res.* 2001;50(4):222–232.
16. Guo Y, Young BL, Hainley S, et al. Evaluation and pharmacologic management of symptoms in cancer patients undergoing acute rehabilitation in a comprehensive cancer center. *Arch Phys Med Rehabil.* 2007;88(7):891–895.
17. Hurria A, Gupta S, Zauderer M, et al. Developing a cancer-specific geriatric assessment: a feasibility study. *Cancer.* 2005;104(9):1998–2005.
18. Movsas SB, Chang VT, Tunkel RS, et al. Rehabilitation needs of an inpatient medical oncology unit. *Arch Phys Med Rehabil.* 2003;84(11):1642–1646.
19. Monga U, Garber SL, Thornby J, et al. Exercise prevents fatigue and improves quality of life in prostate cancer patients undergoing radiotherapy. *Arch Phys Med Rehabil.* 2007;88(11):1416–1422.
20. Ware JE, Jr, Sherbourne CD. The MOS 36-item short-form health survey (SF-36). I. Conceptual framework and item selection. *Med Care.* 1992;30(6):473–483.
21. Schag CA, Ganz PA, Heinrich RL. CAncer Rehabilitation Evaluation System—short form (CARES-SF). A cancer specific rehabilitation and quality of life instrument. *Cancer.* 1991;68(6):1406–1413.
22. Zebrack BJ, Ganz PA, Bernaards CA, et al. Assessing the impact of cancer: development of a new instrument for long-term survivors. *Psychooncology.* 2006;15(5):407–421.
23. Silver JK, Baima J, Newman R, et al. Cancer rehabilitation may improve function in survivors and decrease the economic burden of cancer to individuals and society. *Work.* 2013;46(4):455–472.
24. Short PF, Vargo MM. Responding to employment concerns of cancer survivors. *J Clin Oncol.* 2006;24(32):5138–5141.
25. Ness KK, Mertens AC, Hudson MM, et al. Limitations on physical performance and daily activities among long-term survivors of childhood cancer. *Ann Intern Med.* 2005;143(9):639–647.
26. Bradley CJ, Bednarek HL. Employment patterns of long-term cancer survivors. *Psychooncology.* 2002;11(3):188–198.
27. Silver JK, Raj VS, Fu JB, et al. Cancer rehabilitation and palliative care: critical components in the delivery of high-quality oncology services. *Support Care Cancer.* 2015;23(12):3633–3643.
28. Cheville AL, Mustian K, Winters-Stone K, et al. Cancer rehabilitation: an overview of current need, delivery models, and levels of care. *Phys Med Rehabil Clin N Am.* 2017;28(1):1–17.
29. Stout NL, Silver JK, Raj VS, et al. Toward a National Initiative in Cancer Rehabilitation: recommendations from a subject matter expert group. *Arch Phys Med Rehabil.* 2016;97(11):2006–2015.
30. McKinley WO, Huang ME, Brunsvold KT. Neoplastic versus traumatic spinal cord injury: an outcome comparison after inpatient rehabilitation. *Arch Phys Med Rehabil.* 1999;80(10):1253–1257.
31. Huang ME, Cifu DX, Keyser-Marcus L. Functional outcome after brain tumor and acute stroke: a comparative analysis. *Arch Phys Med Rehabil.* 1998;79(11):1386–1390.
32. O'Dell MW, Barr K, Spanier D, et al. Functional outcome of inpatient rehabilitation in persons with brain tumors. *Arch Phys Med Rehabil.* 1998;79(12):1530–1534.
33. Kirshblum S, O'Dell MW, Ho C, et al. Rehabilitation of persons with central nervous system tumors. *Cancer.* 2001;92(4 suppl):1029–1038.
34. McKinley WO, Conti-Wyneken AR, Vokac CW, et al. Rehabilitative functional outcome of patients with neoplastic spinal cord compressions. *Arch Phys Med Rehabil.* 1996;77(9):892–895.
35. Marciniak CM, Sliwa JA, Spill G, et al. Functional outcome following rehabilitation of the cancer patient. *Arch Phys Med Rehabil.* 1996;77(1):54–57.
36. Cole RP, Scialla SJ, Bednarz L. Functional recovery in cancer rehabilitation. *Arch Phys Med Rehabil.* 2000;81(5):623–627.
37. O'Toole DM, Golden AM. Evaluating cancer patients for rehabilitation potential. *West J Med.* 1991;155(4):384–387.
38. Alam E, Wilson RD, Vargo MM. Inpatient cancer rehabilitation: a retrospective comparison of transfer back to acute care between patients with neoplasm and other rehabilitation patients. *Arch Phys Med Rehabil.* 2008;89(7):1284–1289.
39. Guo Y, Persyn L, Palmer JL, et al. Incidence of and risk factors for transferring cancer patients from rehabilitation to acute care units. *Am J Phys Med Rehabil.* 2008;87(8):647–653.
40. Fu JB, Lee J, Shin BC, et al. Return to the primary acute care service among patients with multiple myeloma on an acute inpatient rehabilitation unit. *PM R.* 2017;9(6):571–578.
41. Fu JB, Lee J, Smith DW, et al. Frequency and reasons for return to the primary acute care service among patients with lymphoma undergoing inpatient rehabilitation. *PM R.* 2014;6(7):629–634.
42. Buntin MB, Colla CH, Escarce JJ. Effects of payment changes on trends in postacute care. *Health Serv Res.* 2009;44(4):1188–1210.
43. Guo Y, Fu JB, Guo H, et al. Postacute care in cancer rehabilitation. *Phys Med Rehabil Clin N Am.* 2017;28(1):19–34.
44. Sabers SR, Kokal JE, Girardi JC, et al. Evaluation of consultation-based rehabilitation for hospitalized cancer patients with functional impairment. *Mayo Clin Proc.* 1999;74(9):855–861.
45. Cheville AL, Troxel AB, Basford JR, et al. Prevalence and treatment patterns of physical impairments in patients with metastatic breast cancer. *J Clin Oncol.* 2008;26(16):2621–2629.
46. Stout NL, Binkley JM, Schmitz KH, et al. A prospective surveillance model for rehabilitation for women with breast cancer. *Cancer.* 2012;118(8 suppl):2191–2200.
47. Cheville AL, Nyman JA, Pruthi S, et al. Cos consideration regarding the prospective surveillance model. *Cancer.* 118(8):2325–2329.
48. Silver JK, Baima J, Mayer RS. Impairment-driven cancer rehabilitation: an essential component of quality care and survivorship. *CA Cancer J Clin.* 2013;63(5):295–317.
49. Carli F, Silver JK, Feldman LS, et al. Surgical prehabilitation in patients with cancer: state-of-the-science and recommendations for future research from a panel of subject matter experts. *Phys Med Rehabil Clin N Am.* 2017;28(1):49–64.
50. Raj VS, Silver JK, Pugh TM, et al. Palliative care and physiatry in the oncology care spectrum: an opportunity for distinct and collaborative approaches. *Phys Med Rehabil Clin N Am.* 2017;28(1):35–47.
51. Rajarajeswaran P, Vishnupriya R. Exercise in cancer. *Indian J Med Paediatr Oncol.* 2009;30(2):61–70.
52. Davis MP, Lasheen W, Gamier P. Practical guide to opioids and their complications in managing cancer pain. What oncologists need to know. *Oncology (Williston Park).* 2007;21(10):1229–1238; discussion 1238–1246, 1249.
53. Swarm R, Anghelescu DL, Benedetti C, et al. Adult cancer pain. *J Natl Compr Canc Netw.* 2007;5(8):726–751.
54. Maida V, Daeninck PJ. A user's guide to cannabinoid therapies in oncology. *Curr Oncol.* 2016;23(6):398–406.
55. Gordon DB, Dahl JL, Miaskowski C, et al. American pain society recommendations for improving the quality of acute and cancer pain management: American Pain Society Quality of Care Task Force. *Arch Intern Med.* 2005;165(14):1574–1580.
56. Wilkie DJ, Huang HY, Berry DL, et al. Cancer symptom control: feasibility of a tailored, interactive computerized program for patients. *Fam Community Health.* 2001;24(3):48–62.
57. Silver J, Mayer RS. Barriers to pain management in the rehabilitation of the surgical oncology patient. *J Surg Oncol.* 2007;95(5):427–435.
58. Hage WD, Aboulafia AJ, Aboulafia DM. Incidence, location, and diagnostic evaluation of metastatic bone disease. *Orthop Clin North Am.* 2000;31(4):515–528, vii.
59. Buckwalter JA, Brandser EA. Metastatic disease of the skeleton. *Am Fam Physician.* 1997;55(5):1761–1768.
60. Roodman GD. Mechanisms of bone metastasis. *N Engl J Med.* 2004;350(16):1655–1664.
61. Coleman RE, Smith P, Rubens RD. Clinical course and prognostic factors following bone recurrence from breast cancer. *Br J Cancer.* 1998;77(2):336–340.
62. Mercadante S. Malignant bone pain: pathophysiology and treatment. *Pain.* 1997;69(1–2):1–18.
63. Riccio AI, Wodajo FM, Malawer M. Metastatic carcinoma of the long bones. *Am Fam Physician.* 2007;76(10):1489–1494.
64. Selvaggi G, Scagliotti GV. Management of bone metastases in cancer: a review. *Crit Rev Oncol Hematol.* 2005;56(3):365–378.
65. Mercadante S, Fulfaro F. Management of painful bone metastases. *Curr Opin Oncol.* 2007;19(4):308–314.
66. Weber KL, Lewis VO, Randall RL, et al. An approach to the management of the patient with metastatic bone disease. *Instr Course Lect.* 2004;53:663–676.
67. Schirrmeister H. Detection of bone metastases in breast cancer by positron emission tomography. *Radiol Clin North Am.* 2007;45(4):669–676, vi.
68. Saad F, Lipton A, Cook R, et al. Pathologic fractures correlate with reduced survival in patients with malignant bone disease. *Cancer.* 2007;110(8):1860–1867.
69. Ross JR, Saunders Y, Edmonds PM, et al. Systematic review of role of bisphosphonates on skeletal morbidity in metastatic cancer. *BMJ.* 2003;327(7413):469.

70. Higano CS. Understanding treatments for bone loss and bone metastases in patients with prostate cancer: a practical review and guide for the clinician. *Urol Clin North Am.* 2004;31(2):331–352.

71. van der Linden YM, Dijkstra SP, Vonk EJ, et al. Prediction of survival in patients with metastases in the spinal column: results based on a randomized trial of radiotherapy. *Cancer.* 2005;103(2):320–328.

72. Mirels H. Metastatic disease in long bones. A proposed scoring system for diagnosing impending pathologic fractures. *Clin Orthop Relat Res.* 1989(249):256–264.

73. Van der Linden YM, Dijkstra PD, Kroon HM, et al. Comparative analysis of risk factors for pathological fracture with femoral metastases. *J Bone Joint Surg Br.* 2004;86(4):566–573.

74. Harrington KD. Orthopedic surgical management of skeletal complications of malignancy. *Cancer.* 1997;80(8 suppl):1614–1627.

75. Bilsky MH. New therapeutics in spine metastases. *Expert Rev Neurother.* 2005;5(6):831–840.

76. Dimeo FC. Effects of exercise on cancer-related fatigue. *Cancer.* 2001;92(6 suppl): 1689–1693.

77. Fukuda K, Straus SE, Hickie I, et al. The chronic fatigue syndrome: a comprehensive approach to its definition and study. International Chronic Fatigue Syndrome Study Group. *Ann Intern Med.* 1994;121(12):953–959.

78. Vogelzang NJ, Breitbart W, Cella D, et al. Patient, caregiver, and oncologist perceptions of cancer-related fatigue: results of a tripart assessment survey. The Fatigue Coalition. *Semin Hematol.* 1997;34(3 suppl 2):4–12.

79. Escalante CP, Grover T, Johnson BA, et al. A fatigue clinic in a comprehensive cancer center: design and experiences. *Cancer.* 2001;92(6 suppl):1708–1713.

80. Schneider CM, Dennehy CA, Carter SD. *Exercise and Cancer Recovery.* Champaign, IL: Human Kinetics; 2003.

81. Franklin DJ, Packel L. Cancer-related fatigue. *Arch Phys Med Rehabil.* 2006;87(3 suppl 1):S91–S93; quiz S94–S95.

82. Berger AM, Mooney K, Banerjee C, et al. *NCCN Clinical Practice Guidelines in Oncology: Cancer-Related Fatigue, Version 1.2017.* Fort Washington, PA: National Comprehensive Cancer Network, Inc.; 2016.

83. Barsevick AM, Dudley W, Beck S, et al. A randomized clinical trial of energy conservation for patients with cancer-related fatigue. *Cancer.* 2004;100(6):1302–1310.

84. Lee K, Cho M, Miaskowski C, et al. Impaired sleep and rhythms in persons with cancer. *Sleep Med Rev.* 2004;8(3):199–212.

85. Itri L. Epoetin alpha intervention for anemia-related fatigue in cancer patients. In: Marty M, Pecorelli S, eds. *Fatigue and Cancer.* New York: Elsevier Science; 2001:129–144.

86. Lenzer J. Safety of anaemia drug erythropoietin is to be reviewed. *BMJ.* 2007;334:495.

87. Leyland-Jones B, Semiglazov V, Pawlicki M, et al. Maintaining normal hemoglobin levels with epoetin alfa in mainly nonanemic patients with metastatic breast cancer receiving first-line chemotherapy: a survival study. *J Clin Oncol.* 2005;23(25):5960–5972.

88. Jacobsen PB, Garland LL, Booth-Jones M, et al. Relationship of hemoglobin levels to fatigue and cognitive functioning among cancer patients receiving chemotherapy. *J Pain Symptom Manage.* 2004;28(1):7–18.

89. Carson JL, Stanworth SJ, Roubinian N, et al. Transfusion thresholds and other strategies for guiding allogeneic red blood cell transfusion. *Cochrane Database Syst Rev.* 2016;10:CD002042.

90. Bruera E, Driver L, Barnes EA, et al. Patient-controlled methylphenidate for the management of fatigue in patients with advanced cancer: a preliminary report. *J Clin Oncol.* 2003;21(23):4439–4443.

91. Morrow GR, Shelke AR, Roscoe JA, et al. Management of cancer-related fatigue. *Cancer Invest.* 2005;23(3):229–239.

92. Hanna A, Sledge G, Mayer ML, et al. A phase II study of methylphenidate for the treatment of fatigue. *Support Care Cancer.* 2006;14(3):210–215.

93. Bruera E, Valero V, Driver L, et al. Patient-controlled methylphenidate for cancer fatigue: a double-blind, randomized, placebo-controlled trial. *J Clin Oncol.* 2006;24(13):2073–2078.

94. Lundstrom SH, Furst CJ. The use of corticosteroids in Swedish palliative care. *Acta Oncol.* 2006;45(4):430–437.

95. Stevinson C, Lawlor DA, Fox KR. Exercise interventions for cancer patients: systematic review of controlled trials. *Cancer Causes Control.* 2004;15(10):1035–1056.

96. Andersen C, Adamsen L, Moeller T, et al. The effect of a multidimensional exercise programme on symptoms and side-effects in cancer patients undergoing chemotherapy—the use of semi-structured diaries. *Eur J Oncol Nurs.* 2006;10(4):247–262.

97. Segal RJ, Reid RD, Courneya KS, et al. Resistance exercise in men receiving androgen deprivation therapy for prostate cancer. *J Clin Oncol.* 2003;21(9):1653–1659.

98. Poppelreuter M, Weis J, Kulz AK, et al. Cognitive dysfunction and subjective complaints of cancer patients. A cross-sectional study in a cancer rehabilitation centre. *Eur J Cancer.* 2004;40(1):43–49.

99. Jean-Pierre P, Winters PC, Ahles TA, et al. Prevalence of self-reported memory problems in adult cancer survivors: a national cross-sectional study. *J Oncol Pract.* 2012;8(1):30–34.

100. McDougall GJ Jr, Oliver JS, Scogin F. Memory and cancer: a review of the literature. *Arch Psychiatr Nurs.* 2014;28(3):180–186.

101. Ahles TA, Saykin AJ, Furstenberg CT, et al. Neuropsychologic impact of standard-dose systemic chemotherapy in long-term survivors of breast cancer and lymphoma. *J Clin Oncol.* 2002;20(2):485–493.

102. Bender CM, Sereika SM, Berga SL, et al. Cognitive impairment associated with adjuvant therapy in breast cancer. *Psychooncology.* 2006;15(5):422–430.

103. Jim HS, Phillips KM, Chait S, et al. Meta-analysis of cognitive functioning in breast cancer survivors previously treated with standard-dose chemotherapy. *J Clin Oncol.* 2012;30(29):3578–3587.

104. Matsuda T, Takayama T, Tashiro M, et al. Mild cognitive impairment after adjuvant chemotherapy in breast cancer patients—evaluation of appropriate research design and methodology to measure symptoms. *Breast Cancer.* 2005;12(4):279–287.

105. Green HJ, Pakenham KI, Headley BC, et al. Altered cognitive function in men treated for prostate cancer with luteinizing hormone-releasing hormone analogues and cyproterone acetate: a randomized controlled trial. *BJU Int.* 2002;90(4):427–432.

106. Cherrier MM, Rose AL, Higano C. The effects of combined androgen blockade on cognitive function during the first cycle of intermittent androgen suppression in patients with prostate cancer. *J Urol.* 2003;170(5):1808–1811.

107. Delirium (PDQ®)—Patient Version. National Cancer Institute; 2016. Available from: https://www.cancer.gov/about-cancer/treatment/side-effects/memory/delirium-pdq. Accessed February 17, 2017.

108. Delirium (PDQ®)—Health Professional Version. National Cancer Institute; 2016. Available from: https://www.cancer.gov/about-cancer/treatment/side-effects/memory/delirium-hp-pdq. Accessed February 27, 2017.

109. Kang JH, Shin SH, Bruera E. Comprehensive approaches to managing delirium in patients with advanced cancer. *Cancer Treat Rev.* 2013;39(1):105–112.

110. Bush SH, Kanji S, Pereira JL, et al. Treating an established episode of delirium in palliative care: expert opinion and review of the current evidence base with recommendations for future development. *J Pain Symptom Manage.* 2014;48(2):231–248.

111. Holtzman J, Schmitz K, Babes G, et al. *Effectiveness of Behavioral Interventions to Modify Physical Activity Behaviors in General Populations and Cancer Patients and Survivors. Summary, Evidence Report/Technology Assessment: Number 102.* Rockville, MD: Agency for Healthcare Research and Quality; 2004.

112. Knols R, Aaronson NK, Uebelhart D, et al. Physical exercise in cancer patients during and after medical treatment: a systematic review of randomized and controlled clinical trials. *J Clin Oncol.* 2005;23(16):3830–3842.

113. Galvao DA, Newton RU. Review of exercise intervention studies in cancer patients. *J Clin Oncol.* 2005;23(4):899–909.

114. Fairey AS, Courneya KS, Field CJ, et al. Physical exercise and immune system function in cancer survivors: a comprehensive review and future directions. *Cancer.* 2002;94(2):539–551.

115. Thune I, Furberg AS. Physical activity and cancer risk: dose-response and cancer, all sites and site-specific. *Med Sci Sports Exerc.* 2001;33(6 suppl):S530–S550; discussion S609–S510.

116. Calle EE, Rodriguez C, Walker-Thurmond K, et al. Overweight, obesity, and mortality from cancer in a prospectively studied cohort of U.S. adults. *N Engl J Med.* 2003;348(17):1625–1638.

117. Kushi LH, Doyle C, McCullough M, et al. American Cancer Society Guidelines on nutrition and physical activity for cancer prevention: reducing the risk of cancer with healthy food choices and physical activity. *CA Cancer J Clin.* 2012;62(1):30–67.

118. Jones LW, Courneya KS, Fairey AS, et al. Effects of an oncologist's recommendation to exercise on self-reported exercise behavior in newly diagnosed breast cancer survivors: a single-blind, randomized controlled trial. *Ann Behav Med.* 2004;28(2):105–113.

119. Coleman EA, Coon S, Hall-Barrow J, et al. Feasibility of exercise during treatment for multiple myeloma. *Cancer Nurs.* 2003;26(5):410–419.

120. Courneya KS, Friedenreich CM, Quinney HA, et al. A randomized trial of exercise and quality of life in colorectal cancer survivors. *Eur J Cancer Care (Engl).* 2003;12(4):347–357.

121. Courneya KS, Mackey JR, McKenzie DC. Exercise for breast cancer survivors: research evidence and clinical guidelines. *Phys Sportsmed.* 2002;30(8):33–42.

122. Segal R, Evans W, Johnson D, et al. Structured exercise improves physical functioning in women with stages I and II breast cancer: results of a randomized controlled trial. *J Clin Oncol.* 2001;19(3):657–665.

123. Jones LW, Guill B, Keir ST, et al. Exercise interest and preferences among patients diagnosed with primary brain cancer. *Support Care Cancer.* 2007;15(1):47–55.

124. Vallance JK, Courneya KS, Jones LW, et al. Exercise preferences among a population-based sample of non-Hodgkin's lymphoma survivors. *Eur J Cancer Care (Engl).* 2006;15(1):34–43.

125. Gaydos LA, Freireich EJ, Mantel N. The quantitative relation between platelet count and hemorrhage in patients with acute leukemia. *N Engl J Med.* 1962;266:905–909.

126. Sharkey AM, Carey AB, Heise CT, et al. Cardiac rehabilitation after cancer therapy in children and young adults. *Am J Cardiol.* 1993;71(16):1488–1490.

127. Dimeo F, Fetscher S, Lange W, et al. Effects of aerobic exercise on the physical performance and incidence of treatment-related complications after high-dose chemotherapy. *Blood.* 1997;90(9):3390–3394.

128. Pinto BM, Frierson GM, Rabin C, et al. Home-based physical activity intervention for breast cancer patients. *J Clin Oncol.* 2005;23(15):3577–3587.

129. Battaglini C, Bottaro M, Dennehy C, et al. The effects of an individualized exercise intervention on body composition in breast cancer patients undergoing treatment. *Sao Paulo Med J.* 2007;125(1):22–28.

130. Courneya KS, Mackey JR, Bell GJ, et al. Randomized controlled trial of exercise training in postmenopausal breast cancer survivors: cardiopulmonary and quality of life outcomes. *J Clin Oncol.* 2003;21(9):1660–1668.

131. Gillis TA, Donovan ES. Rehabilitation following bone marrow transplantation. *Cancer.* 2001;92(4 suppl):998–1007.

132. Trovato MK, Pidcock FS, Christensen JR, et al. Chronic graft versus host disease in children: a review of function and rehabilitative needs. Poster presented at: 60th Annual Assembly of the American Academy of Physical Medicine and Rehabilitation; 1998; Seattle, WA.

133. Dimeo F, Bertz H, Finke J, et al. An aerobic exercise program for patients with haematological malignancies after bone marrow transplantation. *Bone Marrow Transplant*. 1996;18(6):1157–1160.

134. Mello M, Tanaka C, Dulley FL. Effects of an exercise program on muscle performance in patients undergoing allogeneic bone marrow transplantation. *Bone Marrow Transplant*. 2003;32(7):723–728.

135. Newton HB. Neurologic complications of systemic cancer. *Am Fam Physician*. 1999;59(4):878–886.

136. Clouston PD, DeAngelis LM, Posner JB. The spectrum of neurological disease in patients with systemic cancer. *Ann Neurol*. 1992;31(3):268–273.

137. Newton HB. Primary brain tumors: review of etiology, diagnosis and treatment. *Am Fam Physician*. 1994;49(4):787–797.

138. Buckner JC, Brown PD, O'Neill BP, et al. Central nervous system tumors. *Mayo Clin Proc*. 2007;82(10):1271–1286.

139. Zimm S, Wampler GL, Stablein D, et al. Intracerebral metastases in solid-tumor patients: natural history and results of treatment. *Cancer*. 1981;48(2):384–394.

140. Wasserstrom WR, Glass JP, Posner JB. Diagnosis and treatment of leptomeningeal metastases from solid tumors: experience with 90 patients. *Cancer*. 1982;49(4):759–772.

141. Sioutos PJ, Arbit E, Meshulam CF, et al. Spinal metastases from solid tumors. Analysis of factors affecting survival. *Cancer*. 1995;76(8):1453–1459.

142. Byrne TN. Spinal cord compression from epidural metastases. *N Engl J Med*. 1992;327(9):614–619.

143. Tazi H, Manunta A, Rodriguez A, et al. Spinal cord compression in metastatic prostate cancer. *Eur Urol*. 2003;44(5):527–532.

144. Hosono N, Ueda T, Tamura D, et al. Prognostic relevance of clinical symptoms in patients with spinal metastases. *Clin Orthop Relat Res*. 2005;(436):196–201.

145. Spies JM, McLeod JG. Paraneoplastic neuropathy. In: Dyck PJ, Thomas PK, eds. *Peripheral Neuropathy*. 4th ed. Philadelphia, PA: Saunders; 2005:2471–2485.

146. Darnell RB, Posner JB. Paraneoplastic syndromes involving the nervous system. *N Engl J Med*. 2003;349(16):1543–1554.

147. Hausheer FH, Schilsky RL, Bain S, et al. Diagnosis, management, and evaluation of chemotherapy-induced peripheral neuropathy. *Semin Oncol*. 2006;33(1):15–49.

148. Gandara DR, Perez EA, Weibe V, et al. Cisplatin chemoprotection and rescue: pharmacologic modulation of toxicity. *Semin Oncol*. 1991;18(1 suppl 3):49–55.

149. Casciato DA, Lowitz BB. *Manual of Clinical Oncology*. 4th ed. Philadelphia, PA: Lippincott Williams & Wilkins; 2000.

150. Okunieff P, Augustine E, Hicks JE, et al. Pentoxifylline in the treatment of radiation-induced fibrosis. *J Clin Oncol*. 2004;22(11):2207–2213.

151. Posner JB. *Neurological Complications of Cancer. Contemporary Neurology Series*. Vol 45. Philadelphia, PA: F. A. Davis Company; 1995.

152. Johansson S. Radiation induced brachial plexopathies. *Acta Oncol*. 2006;45(3):253–257.

153. Morrell RM, Halyard MY, Schild SE, et al. Breast cancer-related lymphedema. *Mayo Clin Proc*. 2005;80(11):1480–1484.

154. Langer I, Guller U, Berclaz G, et al. Morbidity of sentinel lymph node biopsy (SLN) alone versus SLN and completion axillary lymph node dissection after breast cancer surgery: a prospective Swiss multicenter study on 659 patients. *Ann Surg*. 2007;245(3):452–461.

155. Schulze T, Mucke J, Markwardt J, et al. Long-term morbidity of patients with early breast cancer after sentinel lymph node biopsy compared to axillary lymph node dissection. *J Surg Oncol*. 2006;93(2):109–119.

156. Herd-Smith A, Russo A, Muraca MG, et al. Prognostic factors for lymphedema after primary treatment of breast carcinoma. *Cancer*. 2001;92(7):1783–1787.

157. Herrera JE, Stubblefield MD. Rotator cuff tendonitis in lymphedema: a retrospective case series. *Arch Phys Med Rehabil*. 2004;85(12):1939–1942.

158. Petrek JA, Pressman PI, Smith RA. Lymphedema: current issues in research and management. *CA Cancer J Clin*. 2000;50(5):292–307; quiz 308–311.

159. Erickson VS, Pearson ML, Ganz PA, et al. Arm edema in breast cancer patients. *J Natl Cancer Inst*. 2001;93(2):96–111.

160. Singh B, Disipio T, Peake J, et al. Systematic review and meta-analysis of the effects of exercise for those with cancer-related lymphedema. *Arch Phys Med Rehabil*. 2016;97(2):302–315.e313.

161. Schmitz KH, Ahmed RL, Troxel AB, et al. Weight lifting for women at risk for breast cancer-related lymphedema: a randomized trial. *JAMA*. 2010;304(24):2699–2705.

162. Stout Gergich NL, Pfalzer LA, McGarvey C, et al. Preoperative assessment enables the early diagnosis and successful treatment of lymphedema. *Cancer*. 2008;112(12):2809–2819.

163. Yang EJ, Ahn S, Kim EK, et al. Use of a prospective surveillance model to prevent breast cancer treatment-related lymphedema: a single-center experience. *Breast Cancer Res Treat*. 2016;160(2):269–276.

164. Ravasco P, Monteiro-Grillo I, Vidal PM, et al. Cancer: disease and nutrition are key determinants of patients' quality of life. *Support Care Cancer*. 2004;12(4):246–252.

165. Bauer JD, Capra S. Nutrition intervention improves outcomes in patients with cancer cachexia receiving chemotherapy—a pilot study. *Support Care Cancer*. 2005;13(4):270–274.

166. Guo Y, Palmer JL, Kaur G, et al. Nutritional status of cancer patients and its relationship to function in an inpatient rehabilitation setting. *Support Care Cancer*. 2005;13(3):169–175.

167. Dewys WD, Begg C, Lavin PT, et al. Prognostic effect of weight loss prior to chemotherapy in cancer patients. Eastern Cooperative Oncology Group. *Am J Med*. 1980;69(4):491–497.

168. Ribaudo JM, Cella D, Hahn EA, et al. Re-validation and shortening of the Functional Assessment of Anorexia/Cachexia Therapy (FAACT) questionnaire. *Qual Life Res*. 2000;9(10):1137–1146.

169. Maltoni M, Nanni O, Scarpi E, et al. High-dose progestins for the treatment of cancer anorexia-cachexia syndrome: a systematic review of randomised clinical trials. *Ann Oncol*. 2001;12(3):289–300.

170. Bruera E, Ernst S, Hagen N, et al. Effectiveness of megestrol acetate in patients with advanced cancer: a randomized, double-blind, crossover study. *Cancer Prev Control*. 1998;2(2):74–78.

171. Couch M, Lai V, Cannon T, et al. Cancer cachexia syndrome in head and neck cancer patients: part I. Diagnosis, impact on quality of life and survival, and treatment. *Head Neck*. 2007;29(4):401–411.

172. Skipworth RJ, Fearon KC. The scientific rationale for optimizing nutritional support in cancer. *Eur J Gastroenterol Hepatol*. 2007;19(5):371–377.

173. Robien K, Levin R, Pritchett E, et al. American Dietetic Association: standards of practice and standards of professional performance for registered dietitians (generalist, specialty, and advanced) in oncology nutrition care. *J Am Diet Assoc*. 2006;106(6):946–951.

174. Marin Caro MM, Laviano A, Pichard C. Nutritional intervention and quality of life in adult oncology patients. *Clin Nutr*. 2007;26(3):289–301.

175. Pelusi J. Sexuality and body image. Research on breast cancer survivors documents altered body image and sexuality. *Am J Nurs*. 2006;106(3 suppl):32–38.

176. Miranda-Sousa AJ, Davila HH, Lockhart JL, et al. Sexual function after surgery for prostate or bladder cancer. *Cancer Control*. 2006;13(3):179–187.

177. Ganz PA, Desmond KA, Belin TR, et al. Predictors of sexual health in women after a breast cancer diagnosis. *J Clin Oncol*. 1999;17(8):2371–2380.

178. Krychman ML. Sexual rehabilitation medicine in a female oncology setting. *Gynecol Oncol*. 2006;101(3):380–384.

179. Kadan-Lottick NS, Vanderwerker LC, Block SD, et al. Psychiatric disorders and mental health service use in patients with advanced cancer: a report from the coping with cancer study. *Cancer*. 2005;104(12):2872–2881.

180. Bower JE. Behavioral symptoms in patients with breast cancer and survivors. *J Clin Oncol*. 2008;26(5):768–777.

181. Dupont A, Bower JE, Stanton AL, et al. Cancer-related intrusive thoughts predict behavioral symptoms following breast cancer treatment. *Health Psychol*. 2014;33(2):155–163.

182. Cordova MJ, Riba MB, Spiegel D. Post-traumatic stress disorder and cancer. *Lancet Psychiatry*. 2017;4(4):330–338.

183. Swartzman S, Booth JN, Munro A, et al. Posttraumatic stress disorder after cancer diagnosis in adults: a meta-analysis. *Depress Anxiety*. 2016;34(4):327–339.

184. Hawkins NA, Soman A, Buchanan Lunsford N, et al. Use of medications for treating anxiety and depression in cancer survivors in the United States. *J Clin Oncol*. 2017;35(1):78–85.

185. Alwhaibi M, Madhavan S, Bias T, et al. Depression treatment among elderly medicare beneficiaries with incident cases of cancer and newly diagnosed depression. *Psychiatr Serv*. 2017;68(5):482–489.

186. DeSantis CE, Lin CC, Mariotto AB, et al. Cancer treatment and survivorship statistics, 2014. *CA Cancer J Clin*. 2014;64(4):252–271.

187. Ruddy KJ, Winer EP. Male breast cancer: risk factors, biology, diagnosis, treatment, and survivorship. *Ann Oncol*. 2013;24(9):1434–1443.

188. Senkus E, Kyriakides S, Ohno S, et al. Primary breast cancer: ESMO clinical practice guidelines for diagnosis, treatment and follow-up. *Ann Oncol*. 2015;26(suppl 5):v8–v30.

189. DiSipio T, Rye S, Newman B, et al. Incidence of unilateral arm lymphoedema after breast cancer: a systematic review and meta-analysis. *Lancet Oncol*. 2013;14(6):500–515.

190. O'Toole J, Miller CL, Specht MC, et al. Cording following treatment for breast cancer. *Breast Cancer Res Treat*. 2013;140(1):105–111.

191. Meretoja TJ, Leidenius MH, Tasmuth T, et al. Pain at 12 months after surgery for breast cancer. *JAMA*. 2014;311(1):90–92.

192. Couceiro TC, Valenca MM, Raposo MC, et al. Prevalence of post-mastectomy pain syndrome and associated risk factors: a cross-sectional cohort study. *Pain Manag Nurs*. 2014;15(4):731–737.

193. Rothemund Y, Grusser SM, Liebeskind U, et al. Phantom phenomena in mastectomized patients and their relation to chronic and acute pre-mastectomy pain. *Pain*. 2004;107(1–2):140–146.

194. Jung BF, Ahrendt GM, Oaklander AL, et al. Neuropathic pain following breast cancer surgery: proposed classification and research update. *Pain*. 2003;104(1–2):1–13.

195. Cheville AL, Tchou J. Barriers to rehabilitation following surgery for primary breast cancer. *J Surg Oncol*. 2007;95(5):409–418.

196. Yang EJ, Park WB, Seo KS, et al. Longitudinal change of treatment-related upper limb dysfunction and its impact on late dysfunction in breast cancer survivors: a prospective cohort study. *J Surg Oncol*. 2010;101(1):84–91.

197. Custodio CM. Electrodiagnosis in cancer rehabilitation. *Phys Med Rehabil Clin N Am*. 2017;28(1):193–203.

198. Gaillard S, Stearns V. Aromatase inhibitor-associated bone and musculoskeletal effects: new evidence defining etiology and strategies for management. *Breast Cancer Res*. 2011;13(2):205.

199. Niravath P. Aromatase inhibitor-induced arthralgia: a review. *Ann Oncol*. 2013;24(6):1443–1449.

200. Gerber LH AE, McGarvey CL, et al. *Preserving and Restoring Function Breast Cancer Survivors.* 3rd ed. Philadelphia, PA: Lippincott Williams and Wilkins; 2004.

201. Ferlay J, Shin HR, Bray F, et al. Estimates of worldwide burden of cancer in 2008: GLOBOCAN 2008. *Int J Cancer.* 2010;127(12):2893–2917.

202. Pulte D, Brenner H. Changes in survival in head and neck cancers in the late 20th and early 21st century: a period analysis. *Oncologist.* 2010;15(9):994–1001.

203. Mehanna H, Paleri V, West CM, et al. Head and neck cancer—part 1: epidemiology, presentation, and preservation. *Clin Otolaryngol.* 2011;36(1):65–68.

204. Macfarlane TV, Wirth T, Ranasinghe S, et al. Head and neck cancer pain: systematic review of prevalence and associated factors. *J Oral Maxillofac Res.* 2012;3(1):e1.

205. List MA, Bilir SP. Functional outcomes in head and neck cancer. *Semin Radiat Oncol.* 2004;14(2):178–189.

206. Lokker ME, Offerman MP, van der Velden LA, et al. Symptoms of patients within curable head and neck cancer: prevalence and impact on daily functioning. *Head Neck.* 2013;35(6):868–876.

207. Dirix P, Nuyts S, Van den Bogaert W. Radiation-induced xerostomia in patients with head and neck cancer: a literature review. *Cancer.* 2006;107(11):2525–2534.

208. Guru K, Manoor UK, Supe SS. A comprehensive review of head and neck cancer rehabilitation: physical therapy perspectives. *Indian J Palliat Care.* 2012;18(2):87–97.

209. Pauli N, Fagerberg-Mohlin B, Andrell P, et al. Exercise intervention for the treatment of trismus in head and neck cancer. *Acta Oncol.* 2014;53(4):502–509.

210. American Society of Clinical Oncology; Pfister DG, Laurie SA, et al. American Society of Clinical Oncology clinical practice guideline for the use of larynx-preservation strategies in the treatment of laryngeal cancer. *J Clin Oncol.* 2006;24(22):3693–3704.

211. Rinkel RN, Verdonck-de Leeuw IM, Doornaert P, et al. Prevalence of swallowing and speech problems in daily life after chemoradiation for head and neck cancer based on cut-off scores of the patient-reported outcome measures SWAL-QOL and SHI. *Eur Arch Otorhinolaryngol.* 2016;273:1849–1855. 281.

212. Levendag PC, Teguh DN, Voet P, et al. Dysphagia disorders in patients with cancer of the oropharynx are significantly affected by the radiation therapy dose to the superior and middle constrictor muscle: a dose-effect relationship. *Radiother Oncol.* 2007;85(1):64–73.

213. Piso DU, Eckardt A, Liebermann A, et al. Early rehabilitation of head-neck edema after curative surgery for orofacial tumors. *Am J Phys Med Rehabil.* 2001;80(4):261–269.

214. Teras LR, DeSantis CE, Cerhan JR, et al. 2016 US lymphoid malignancy statistics by World Health Organization subtypes. *CA Cancer J Clin.* 2016;66(6):443–459.

215. Pulte D, Gondos A, Brenner H. Improvement in survival of older adults with multiple myeloma: results of an updated period analysis of SEER data. *Oncologist.* 2011;16(11):1600–1603.

216. Ness KK, Hudson MM, Pui CH, et al. Neuromuscular impairments in adult survivors of childhood acute lymphoblastic leukemia: associations with physical performance and chemotherapy doses. *Cancer.* 2012;118(3):828–838.

217. Snowden JA, Greenfield DM, Bird JM, et al. Guidelines for screening and management of late and long-term consequences of myeloma and its treatment. *Br J Haematol.* 2017;176(6):888–907.

218. Krull KR, Brinkman TM, Li C, et al. Neurocognitive outcomes decades after treatment for childhood acute lymphoblastic leukemia: a report from the St Jude lifetime cohort study. *J Clin Oncol.* 2013;31(35):4407–4415.

219. Armstrong GT, Reddick WE, Petersen RC, et al. Evaluation of memory impairment in aging adult survivors of childhood acute lymphoblastic leukemia treated with cranial radiotherapy. *J Natl Cancer Inst.* 2013;105(12):899–907.

220. Wouters H, Baars JW, Schagen SB. Neurocognitive function of lymphoma patients after treatment with chemotherapy. *Acta Oncol.* 2016;55(9–10):1121–1125.

221. Smith SR, Asher A. Rehabilitation in chronic graft-versus-host disease. *Phys Med Rehabil Clin N Am.* 2017;28(1):143–151.

222. Talamo G, Angtuaco E, Walker RC, et al. Avascular necrosis of femoral and/or humeral heads in multiple myeloma: results of a prospective study of patients treated with dexamethasone-based regimens and high-dose chemotherapy. *J Clin Oncol.* 2005;23(22):5217–5223.

223. Rowin J, Cheng G, Lewis SL, et al. Late appearance of dropped head syndrome after radiotherapy for Hodgkin's disease. *Muscle Nerve.* 2006;34(5):666–669.

224. Steinberg A, Asher A, Bailey C, et al. The role of physical rehabilitation in stem cell transplantation patients. *Support Care Cancer.* 2015;23(8):2447–2460.

225. Smith SR, Haig AJ, Couriel DR. Musculoskeletal, neurologic, and cardiopulmonary aspects of physical rehabilitation in patients with chronic graft-versus-host disease. *Biol Blood Marrow Transplant.* 2015;21(5):799–808.

226. Janin A, Socie G, Devergie A, et al. Fasciitis in chronic graft-versus-host disease. A clinicopathologic study of 14 cases. *Ann Intern Med.* 1994;120(12):993–998.

227. Stevens AM, Sullivan KM, Nelson JL. Polymyositis as a manifestation of chronic graft-versus-host disease. *Rheumatology (Oxford).* 2003;42(1):34–39.

228. Torre LA, Bray F, Siegel RL, et al. Global cancer statistics, 2012. *CA Cancer J Clin.* 2015;65(2):87–108.

229. Moyer VA, Force USPST. Screening for lung cancer: U.S. Preventive Services Task Force recommendation statement. *Ann Intern Med.* 2014;160(5):330–338.

230. Humphrey LL, Deffebach M, Pappas M, et al. Screening for lung cancer with low-dose computed tomography: a systematic review to update the US Preventive Services Task Force recommendation. *Ann Intern Med.* 2013;159(6):411–420.

231. Bayly JL, Lloyd-Williams M. Identifying functional impairment and rehabilitation needs in patients newly diagnosed with inoperable lung cancer: a structured literature review. *Support Care Cancer.* 2016;24(5):2359–2379.

232. Granger CL, McDonald CF, Irving L, et al. Low physical activity levels and functional decline in individuals with lung cancer. *Lung Cancer.* 2014;83(2):292–299.

233. Cavalheri V, Jenkins S, Cecins N, et al. Impairments after curative intent treatment for non-small cell lung cancer: a comparison with age and gender-matched healthy controls. *Respir Med.* 2015;109(10):1332–1339.

234. Tarumi S, Yokomise H, Gotoh M, et al. Pulmonary rehabilitation during induction chemoradiotherapy for lung cancer improves pulmonary function. *J Thorac Cardiovasc Surg.* 2015;149(2):569–573.

235. Glattki GP, Manika K, Sichletidis L, et al. Pulmonary rehabilitation in non-small cell lung cancer patients after completion of treatment. *Am J Clin Oncol.* 2012;35(2):120–125.

236. Vijayvergia N, Shah PC, Denlinger CS. Survivorship in non-small cell lung cancer: challenges faced and steps forward. *J Natl Compr Canc Netw.* 2015;13(9):1151–1161.

237. Siegel RL, Miller KD, Jemal A. Cancer statistics, 2015. *CA Cancer J Clin.* 2015;65(1):5–29.

238. Castro C, Bosetti C, Malvezzi M, et al. Patterns and trends in esophageal cancer mortality and incidence in Europe (1980–2011) and predictions to 2015. *Ann Oncol.* 2014;25(1):283–290.

239. Laforest A, Bretagnol F, Mouazan AS, et al. Functional disorders after rectal cancer resection: does a rehabilitation programme improve anal continence and quality of life? *Colorectal Dis.* 2012;14(10):1231–1237.

240. Visser WS, Te Riele WW, Boerma D, et al. Pelvic floor rehabilitation to improve functional outcome after a low anterior resection: a systematic review. *Ann Coloproctol.* 2014;30(3):109–114.

241. Fish D, Temple LK. Functional consequences of colorectal cancer management. *Surg Oncol Clin N Am.* 2014;23(1):127–149.

242. Numico G, Longo V, Courthod G, et al. Cancer survivorship: long-term side-effects of anticancer treatments of gastrointestinal cancer. *Curr Opin Oncol.* 2015;27(4):351–357.

243. Ostrom QT, Gittleman H, Liao P, et al. CBTRUS statistical report: primary brain and central nervous system tumors diagnosed in the United States in 2007–2011. *Neuro Oncol.* 2014;16(suppl 4):iv1–iv63.

244. Lu-Emerson C, Eichler AF. Brain metastases. *Continuum (Minneap Minn).* 2012;18(2):295–311.

245. O'Neill BP, Buckner JC, Coffey RJ, et al. Brain metastatic lesions. *Mayo Clin Proc.* 1994;69(11):1062–1068.

246. Patchell RA. The treatment of brain metastases. *Cancer Invest.* 1996;14(2):169–177.

247. Ruppert LMM G, Stubblefield M. *Cancer Survivorship.* New York: Springer; 2017.

248. Stubblefield MD, O'Dell MW, eds. *Cancer Rehabilitation.* New York: Demos Medical; 2009.

249. Giordana MT, Clara E. Functional rehabilitation and brain tumour patients. A review of outcome. *Neurol Sci.* 2006;27(4):240–244.

250. Rogers LR. Neurologic complications of radiation. *Continuum (Minneap Minn).* 2012;18(2):343–354.

251. Correa DD, DeAngelis LM, Shi W, et al. Cognitive functions in survivors of primary central nervous system lymphoma. *Neurology.* 2004;62(4):548–555.

252. Newton HB. Neurological complications of chemotherapy to the central nervous system. *Handb Clin Neurol.* 2012;105:903–916.

253. Mukand JA, Blackinton DD, Crincoli MG, et al. Incidence of neurologic deficits and rehabilitation of patients with brain tumors. *Am J Phys Med Rehabil.* 2001;80(5):346–350.

254. Marciniak CM, Sliwa JA, Heinemann AW, et al. Functional outcomes of persons with brain tumors after inpatient rehabilitation. *Arch Phys Med Rehabil.* 2001;82(4):457–463.

255. Meyers CA, Weitzner MA, Valentine AD, et al. Methylphenidate therapy improves cognition, mood, and function of brain tumor patients. *J Clin Oncol.* 1998;16(7):2522–2527.

256. Bell K, Barr K, et al. Rehabilitation of the patient with brain tumor. *Arch Phys Med Rehabil.* 1998;79:S37–S46.

257. Marras LC, Geerts WH, Perry JR. The risk of venous thromboembolism is increased throughout the course of malignant glioma: an evidence-based review. *Cancer.* 2000;89(3):640–6282.

258. Kim DHCU, Kim S, Bilsky M, ed. *Tumor of the Spine.* Philadelphia, PA: Saunders Elsevier; 2008.

259. Sciubba DM, Gokaslan ZL. Diagnosis and management of metastatic spine disease. *Surg Oncol.* 2006;15(3):141–151.

260. Raj VS, Lofton L. Rehabilitation and treatment of spinal cord tumors. *J Spinal Cord Med.* 2013;36(1):4–11.

261. Hammack JE. Spinal cord disease in patients with cancer. *Continuum (Minneap Minn).* 2012;18(2):312–327.

262. Cole JS, Patchell RA. Metastatic epidural spinal cord compression. *Lancet Neurol.* 2008;7(5):459–466. 283.

263. Sciubba DM, Petteys RJ, Dekutoski MB, et al. Diagnosis and management of metastatic spine disease. A review. *J Neurosurg Spine.* 2010;13(1):94–108.

264. Lin W, ed. *Spinal Cord Medicine Principles and Practice.* 2nd ed. New York: Demos; 2010.

265. Ruppert LM. Malignant spinal cord compression: adapting conventional rehabilitation approaches. *Phys Med Rehabil Clin N Am.* 2017;28(1):101–114.

266. Sawaya R, Zuccarello M, Elkalliny M, et al. Postoperative venous thromboembolism and brain tumors: part I. Clinical profile. *J Neurooncol.* 1992;14(2):119–125.

267. Lahat G, Lazar A, Lev D. Sarcoma epidemiology and etiology: potential environmental and genetic factors. *Surg Clin North Am.* 2008;88(3):451–481, v.

268. Stiller CA, Trama A, Serraino D, et al. Descriptive epidemiology of sarcomas in Europe: report from the RARECARE project. *Eur J Cancer*. 2013;49(3):684–695.

269. Smith SR. Rehabilitation strategies and outcomes of the sarcoma patient. *Phys Med Rehabil Clin N Am*. 2017;28(1):171–180.

270. Harwood JL, Alexander JH, Mayerson JL, et al. Targeted chemotherapy in bone and soft-tissue sarcoma. *Orthop Clin North Am*. 2015;46(4):587–608.

271. Bobowski NP, Baker LH. The University of Michigan Sarcoma Survivorship Clinic: preventing, diagnosing, and treating chronic illness for improved survival and long-term health. *J Adolesc Young Adult Oncol*. 2016;5(3):211–214.

272. Tobias K, Gillis T. Rehabilitation of the sarcoma patient-enhancing the recovery and functioning of patients undergoing management for extremity soft tissue sarcomas. *J Surg Oncol*. 2015;111(5):615–621.

273. Johnson ME, Zaorsky NG, Martin JM, et al. Patient reported outcomes among treatment modalities for prostate cancer. *Can J Urol*. 2016;23(6):8535–8545.

274. Autio KA, Scher HI, Morris MJ. Therapeutic strategies for bone metastases and their clinical sequelae in prostate cancer. *Curr Treat Options Oncol*. 2012;13(2):174–188.

275. Rief H, Petersen LC, Omlor G, et al. The effect of resistance training during radiotherapy on spinal bone metastases in cancer patients—a randomized trial. *Radiother Oncol*. 2014;112(1):133–139.

276. Kretschmer A, Buchner A, Grabbert M, et al. Perioperative patient education improves long-term satisfaction rates of low-risk prostate cancer patients after radical prostatectomy. *World J Urol*. 2017;35(8):1205–1212.

277. Moyad MA, Newton RU, Tunn UW, et al. Integrating diet and exercise into care of prostate cancer patients on androgen deprivation therapy. *Res Rep Urol*. 2016;8:133–143.

278. Endometrial Cancer Treatment (PDQ®): Health Professional Version. *PDQ Cancer Information Summaries*. Bethesda, MD: National Cancer Institute; 2002.

279. Dellinger TH, Hakim AA, Lee SJ, et al. Surgical management of vulvar cancer. *J Natl Compr Canc Netw*. 2017;15(1):121–128.

280. Mayadev J, Viswanathan A, Liu Y, et al. American Brachytherapy Task Group Report: a pooled analysis of clinical outcomes for high-dose-rate brachytherapy for cervical cancer. *Brachytherapy*. 2017;16(1):22–43.

281. Kato K, Tate S, Nishikimi K, et al. Bladder function after modified posterior exenteration for primary gynecological cancer. *Gynecol Oncol*. 2013;129(1):229–233.

282. Jensen PT, Froeding LP. Pelvic radiotherapy and sexual function in women. *Transl Androl Urol*. 2015;4(2):186–205.

283. Dunberger G, Lind H, Steineck G, et al. Fecal incontinence affecting quality of life and social functioning among long-term gynecological cancer survivors. *Int J Gynecol Cancer*. 2010;20(3):449–460.

284. Beesley V, Janda M, Eakin E, et al. Lymphedema after gynecological cancer treatment: prevalence, correlates, and supportive care needs. *Cancer*. 2007;109(12):2607–2614.

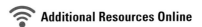 **Additional Resources Online**

CHAPTER 37

Karen L. Andrews
Mary E. Matsumoto

Matthew T. Houdek
Melissa J. Neisen

Amputations and Vascular Diseases

The term *vascular disease* encompasses a variety of acute and chronic pathophysiologic syndromes caused by congenital and acquired disorders affecting the arterial, venous, and lymphatic systems. *Arterial diseases* include those acute or chronic disorders that result in partial or complete and functional or anatomic occlusion or aneurysmal dilation of the arteries. An example of functional occlusion is abnormal vascular reactivity of the arteries supplying a given tissue such as vasospasm. *Venous disease* includes acute or chronic occlusion of the systemic venous or pulmonary arterial system, usually as a result of thromboembolism. Chronic venous disease is a spectrum of diseases and disorders of the limbs, with spider veins and varicosities on one end of the spectrum and edema, skin changes such as venous hyperpigmentation, and ulceration on the other. The cause is either primary valvular incompetence or previous deep vein thrombosis (DVT, postphlebitic/postthrombotic syndrome). Lymphatic diseases are discussed in Chapter 36.

The rehabilitation professional is often asked to evaluate the patient with a painful, swollen, or ulcerated limb and determine if amputation will be necessary. A thorough understanding of the pathophysiology, available diagnostic testing, and clinical evaluation will help the practitioner to choose the appropriate vascular diagnosis and treatment regimen.

In this chapter, we (a) review evaluation and management of acute and chronic arterial occlusive disease including the most frequent vasospastic and vasculitic disorders; (b) discuss arterial diagnostic testing; (c) discuss limb salvage, amputation, amputation surgery, and levels of amputation; (d) discuss early management and rehabilitation strategies following amputation; (e) review evaluation and management of venous obstruction and venous insufficiency; and (f) discuss selected venous diagnostic testing.

ARTERIAL DISEASES

Acute Arterial Occlusion
Most cases of acute arterial occlusion can be attributed to one of three causes: thrombosis, dissection, and embolism.

Thrombosis
Thrombosis usually occurs at the site of an underlying vascular abnormality such as an atherosclerotic lesion or an aneurysm.

Dissection
A dissection is a tear in the inner lining of the artery, which allows blood to travel between the layers of the wall, leading to stenosis or occlusion. Dissections are associated with hypertension, atherosclerosis, connective tissue disorders, trauma, and iatrogenic causes (related to invasive diagnostic and therapeutic cardiovascular interventions) (1).

Embolism
Embolization occurs when material, usually a clot, is created in one location and travels to another where it creates an obstruction. Emboli sizeable enough to occlude relatively large arteries typically have a cardiac source. The most common abnormalities causing cardiac-derived emboli include ventricular mural thrombi, valvular diseases, and atrial disorders such as chronic or paroxysmal atrial fibrillation. An unusual cause of arterial embolus includes a paradoxical embolus (a DVT that passes through an atrial septal defect, ventricular septal defect, or patent foramen ovale and enters the arterial system). In about 5% to 10% of cases, no source of embolism is found. Emboli tend to be multiple and recurrent. Certain hypercoagulable states, such as protein C and S deficiency, the presence of antiphospholipid antibody, and malignancy have been associated with peripheral embolism.

Clinical Presentation
The clinical presentation of acute arterial occlusion is described as "six Ps": pain, pallor, paresthesias, paralysis, pulselessness, and poikilothermia. Some or all of these findings may be present. The limb is at risk if blood flow is not restored quickly. Once the tissues become ischemic, cells compensate for the lack of oxygen by converting to anaerobic metabolism. Lactic and pyruvic acids are produced and released into the circulation. If the ischemia persists, cellular adenosine triphosphate stores are depleted, and the cells swell due to their inability to maintain the sodium/potassium pump. Tissue swelling eventually overcomes the capillary filling pressure; this produces ischemia. Clinically, this phase is characterized by pain, muscular rigidity, nonpitting edema of the extremities, and metabolic acidosis. If the ischemia persists, cell membrane disruption occurs with release into the circulation of large amounts of potassium, lactic acid, myoglobin, creatinine phosphokinase, lactic dehydrogenase, serum glutamic-oxaloacetic transaminase, and glutamic-pyruvic transaminase. These findings can also be seen with reperfusion following delayed revascularization.

Chronic Arterial Disease
There are many causes of arterial occlusive disease, the most common of which is atherosclerosis obliterans (ASO). Other disease processes include thromboangiitis obliterans (TAO) (Buerger disease), Mönckeberg medial calcific sclerosis, vasospastic disorders (Raynaud's phenomenon, livedo reticularis, and acrocyanosis), and vasculitis.

Clinical Presentation

The presentation of arterial occlusive disease varies with the course of progression, the presence and extent of collateral vessels, comorbidities, and activity of the patient. Patients with peripheral arterial occlusive disease commonly present with symptoms of intermittent claudication or critical leg ischemia. If the patient is active, intermittent claudication is the typical presenting complaint. If the patient is inactive, rest pain, ulceration, dependent rubor, or gangrene may be the presenting finding (**Fig. 37-1**). In general, symptoms occur distal to the level of stenosis.

Intermittent claudication indicates an inadequate supply of arterial blood to contracting muscles. It occurs primarily in chronic arterial occlusive disease or severe arteriospastic disease. Intermittent claudication is brought on by continuous exercise and is relieved promptly by rest without change of position of the affected limb. Patients describe claudication as leg numbness, weakness, buckling, aching, cramping, or pain. It may change in character as the causative lesions progress. Claudication occurs at a predictable distance or time. When the workload is increased (rapid pace, walking up hills, or walking over rough terrain), the time to claudication decreases. Claudication may worsen over a period of inactivity (e.g., following hospitalization) but usually returns to baseline with reconditioning. When claudication abruptly increases, thrombosis *in situ* or an embolic event should be considered. Claudication at the arch of the foot suggests occlusion at or above the ankle; claudication at the calf suggests occlusion at or above this region. Claudication is less frequent above the knee (likely due to the rich collateral circulation in the thigh); occlusion of the iliac arteries or aorta may cause thigh, lumbar, and buttock claudication (2).

Recognition of the broad differential diagnosis of lower extremity arterial disease is important to optimize management. Although many other disorders can cause the symptoms of lower extremity arterial insufficiency (TAO, arterial thromboemboli), these conditions account for only a small percentage of lower extremity arterial disease. Progression of lower extremity arterial occlusive disease may be slow. In patients presenting with intermittent claudication, symptomatic worsening occurs in 15% to 30% over 5 to 10 years following the initial diagnosis. Tissue necrosis or progression to rest pain requiring vascular surgery occurs in 2.7% to 5% of limbs with claudication annually. Amputation is required in 1% of patients per year (3).

Critical Limb Ischemia

Critical limb ischemia (CLI) is a clinical syndrome in which patients with arterial occlusive disease experienced chronic ischemic rest pain, ulcer, or gangrene (4). CLI is a severe form of peripheral arterial disease (PAD) and is associated with grave prognoses with 1-year mortality exceeding 25% and 30% to 50% major limb amputation at 1 year from diagnosis (4). The number of patients with PAD having CLI is estimated at 1% to 3%, and the annual number is estimated to be around 160,000 in the United States (5).

Patients with CLI are at risk of limb loss. Revascularization is not always an option. Occlusion of the crural and pedal vessels in 14% to 20% of patients with CLI makes them unsuitable for surgical revascularization (6).

ARTERIAL DIAGNOSTIC TESTING

Arterial diagnostic testing is typically performed to confirm a clinical diagnosis and document the severity of disease. Other indications for arterial testing include monitoring disease progression, assessing outcome after an intervention, and localizing lesions to specific segments of the limb. Vascular diagnostic studies are generally classified as noninvasive (ankle-brachial index, segmental pressure measurements, pulse volume recording, continuous wave Doppler, transcutaneous oximetry, duplex scanning, CT angiography, and MR angiography) or invasive (catheter angiography).

Ankle-Brachial Index

The ABI provides objective data about arterial perfusion of the lower limbs (**Table 37-1**). Pressures are obtained using blood pressure cuffs placed around the patient's lower calves or ankles. A handheld Doppler detects systolic blood movement

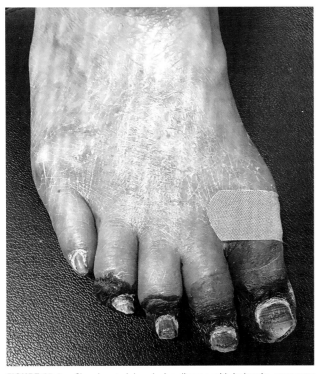

FIGURE 37-1. Chronic arterial occlusive disease with ischemia, cutaneous ulcerations, and gangrene.

TABLE 37-1	ABI Criteria to Assess Perfusion of the Lower Extremities	
Category	**Index (ABI)**
Noncompressible	≥1.4
Normal	1.0–1.39
Borderline	0.9–0.99
Mild	0.8–0.89
Moderate	0.5–0.79
Severe	<0.50
	Index (TBI)
Normal	>0.7

in the dorsalis pedis and the posterior tibial arteries. The brachial (arm) pressure is measured in the standard fashion. In normal individuals, there should be no interarm systolic pressure gradient, or this pressure difference should be minimal (<12 mm Hg). If the arm blood pressures are not equal, a subclavian or axillary arterial stenosis is present in the arm with the lower pressure. The higher of the two blood pressures is then used for subsequent blood pressure ratio (ABI) calculations. In a healthy individual, due to peripheral amplification of the pulse pressure, the ankle pressure should be higher than the brachial arterial systolic pressure; the normal ankle-to-arm systolic blood pressure ratio is, therefore, greater than 1.0. ABI values are considered to be low-normal when they are less than 1.0 and more than 0.90, mildly diminished when they are less than 0.90 and more than or equal to 0.80, moderately diminished between 0.50 and 0.79, and severely decreased when less than 0.50. An ABI identifies individuals who are at risk for developing rest pain, ischemic ulcerations, or gangrene, and it is a marker of generalized atherosclerosis (7). The risk for death, usually from a cardiovascular event, increases dramatically as the ABI decreases. The 5-year mortality rate in patients with an ABI less than 0.85 is 10%; when the ABI is less than 0.40, the 5-year mortality rate approaches 50% (8,9).

The ABI is not accurate when the systolic blood pressure cannot be abolished using a blood pressure cuff. The incidence of noncompressible (artifactually high), calcified conduit arteries is highest in diabetic, elderly, and chronic renal failure patients. Despite high recorded systolic pressure, these individuals may have severe disease. Patients with severely stenotic or occluded iliofemoral arteries may also have a normal ankle pressure if sufficient collateral circulation is present. If such patients have symptomatic evidence of arterial disease, the test should be repeated after exercise.

Segmental Pressure Measurements

Arterial pressures can be measured using blood pressure cuffs placed at various levels (upper thigh, lower thigh, upper calf, and lower calf above the ankle) sequentially along the limb. Systolic blood pressures obtained in this manner can be indexed relative to the brachial artery pressure in a manner analogous to the ABI. Segmental pressure analysis is often used to determine the location of arterial stenoses. The presence of a significant systolic pressure gradient (>10 to 15 mm Hg) between the brachial artery pressure and the upper thigh systolic pressure usually signifies the presence of aortoiliac obstruction. A pressure gradient located between the upper and lower thigh cuff signifies obstruction in the superficial femoral artery. A gradient between the lower thigh and upper calf cuff indicates distal superficial femoral or popliteal artery obstruction. A gradient between the upper and lower calf cuffs identifies infrapopliteal disease. Gradients of 10 to 15 mm Hg between adjacent sites may represent physiologically important obstruction. Segmental pressure measurements may be artifactually elevated or unpredictable in patients with calcified or noncompressible vessels (as described with ABI). In such individuals, Doppler waveform analysis, arterial duplex studies, or transcutaneous oximetry studies may be of benefit.

Pulse Volume Recording

Pulse volume recording (PVR) is used to assess the arterial pulsatility of the limb (10). An external pneumatic cuff is filled to a low pressure (typically 40 to 60 mm Hg). The pneumatic cuff is connected by a flexible hose to a pressure transducer. The blood ejected from the left ventricle during cardiac systole causes a transient distention of the limb, which in turn produces a transient rise in cuff pressure. The cyclic changes in cuff pressure with each heartbeat provide an index of arterial pulsatility. Measurements are typically made at multiple levels along the limb (as described with segmental pressures). The tracings are analyzed to determine whether the waveform changes shape or pulse dampening occurs at a particular level (11). When an altered pulse volume waveform is present, it can be inferred that there is a hemodynamically significant lesion proximal to the site of the cuff.

Continuous Wave Doppler

Waveform analysis can provide important information that may confirm arterial patency or identify occlusive lesions (📶 eFig. 37-1). In many circumstances, a change in blood velocity or pulse waveform such as a change from a triphasic to monophasic waveform provides reasonable, accurate information about the location and extent of specific lower extremity lesions. Doppler waveform analyses are reliable even in highly calcified vessels that are not amenable to pressure determinations.

Transcutaneous Oximetry

Transcutaneous oximetry ($TcPO_2$) determinations provide a very sensitive means to assess skin perfusion (**Table 37-2**) and the potential for cutaneous healing at a specific site (12). $TcPO_2$ measurements are relatively simple and reproducible. Surface oxygen-sensing electrodes calibrated to 45°C are attached to the skin and allowed to equilibrate before recording the $TcPO_2$ value. The feet are then elevated to 30 degrees for 3 minutes, and the $TcPO_2$ values are again recorded. Normal $TcPO_2$ values are greater than 50 to 60 mm Hg. $TcPO_2$ values less than 20 to 30 mm Hg suggest severe local ischemia and bode poorly for future wound healing (13). A decrease in the $TcPO_2$ value of 10 mm Hg with elevation is significant (12) and suggests tenuous perfusion.

Duplex Scanning

Duplex scanning using B-mode imaging combined with directional Doppler can visualize and assess vessel diameter and patency and detect flow velocity changes at sites of localized stenosis or occlusion. Duplex studies can assess plaque morphology and surgical graft patency and establish the presence of arteriovenous fistulae. This technique requires a technically proficient examiner, may require extensive time for a complete examination, and is significantly more expensive than most physiologic noninvasive testing methods. Duplex scanning is particularly helpful in assessing proximal iliofemoral stenosis that may be amenable to angioplasty, providing follow-up data

TABLE 37-2	Transcutaneous Oximetry ($TcPO_2$) Values Assess Skin Perfusion	
Category	**$TcPO_2$ (mm Hg)**
Normal	>45
Mild	40–45
Moderate	20–39
Severe	<20

to assess continued patency of both venous and prosthetic arterial grafts, and evaluating the patency of prior angioplasty sites or intravascular stents.

Axial Imaging Techniques

Technologic advances are enabling computed tomography angiography (CTA) and magnetic resonance angiography (MRA) to replace catheter angiography as a means of identifying arterial stenoses and occlusions.

CT Angiography

During the past decade, CTA has become a standard noninvasive imaging modality for vascular anatomy and pathology. With continued improvement in spatial resolution, CTA is now the mainstay for preoperative imaging of abdominal aortic aneurysms.

CT with three-dimensional reconstruction provides a global view of the chest, abdomen, pelvis, and associated large vessels (**Fig. 37-2**). The accuracy is less operator dependent when compared to ultrasound and is especially useful in patients with a large body habitus. CTA requires radiation exposure and contrast administration for image acquisition.

Magnetic Resonance Angiography

MRA can be used to determine the morphology of blood vessels, assess blood flow velocity, evaluate the lumen for the presence of thrombosis, and evaluate for the presence of hemorrhage, infection, or the status of the end organ. MRA has been found to have a sensitivity of 99.6%, a specificity of 100%, a positive predictive value of 100%, and a negative predictive value of 98.5% for detecting patent segments, occluded

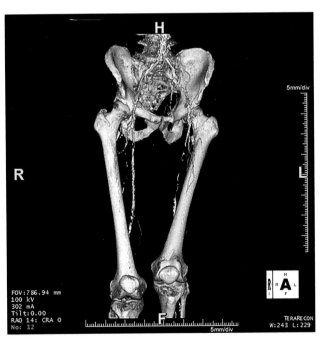

FIGURE 37-2. CTA of the abdominal aortic artery with runoff showing diffuse moderate to severe disease of the common, external, and iliac arteries bilaterally. On the right, the common femoral artery is severely diseased and occludes near its bifurcation; the superficial femoral artery is severely diseased and segmentally occluded. On the left, the common femoral artery is critically stenosed or occluded with heavy calcification just above the profunda origin; the superficial femoral artery is chronically occluded.

segments, and hemodynamically significant stenosis in the aorta, iliac, and femoral vessels (14). Unlike ultrasound, MRA is not compromised by overlying bone, bowel gas, or calcification. When MRA is compared with conventional contrast angiography in preoperative studies of the aorta, iliac artery, and femoral artery, the two imaging modalities are concordant in almost all cases (14). MRA is relatively expensive and its use limited in situations in which metallic instrumentation may be required. MRA is the optimum imaging alternative in pregnant women and those with severe iodinated contrast allergy.

Magnetic resonance studies using gadolinium have a long safety record with little nephrotoxicity at the doses used. Reports that gadolinium may play a role in inducing nephrogenic systemic fibrosis (NSF) are a concern. Although rare, NSF can be catastrophic. Caution is recommended with reduced glomerular filtration rate (GFR) (definitely a GFR < 30, possibly <60) (15). There are new techniques available to allow for angiographic imaging without the use of contrast (16).

Catheter Angiography

Catheter angiography remains the traditional "gold standard" for lower extremity arterial evaluation, remaining the definitive approach for preprocedural evaluation in patients requiring open revascularization if noninvasive axial imaging is inconclusive or for intraprocedural planning for endovascular repair. Angiography is especially helpful for evaluation of the tibial and pedal arteries, which are more difficult to assess on axial imaging.

Catheter angiography is associated with an overall minor and major complication rate of about 8%. Most of the complications result from the side effects of the iodinated contrast material and access site complications. Patients with preexisting renal insufficiency, diabetes, or dehydration are at greatest risk for contrast-induced renal failure. To minimize the risk of nephrotoxicity, bicarbonate hydration and oral acetylcysteine can be used starting the day prior to the procedure. The risk for contrast reaction, which may include hives, worsening of renal function, laryngeal edema, anaphylaxis, or death, varies from 0.04% to 0.22% (17,18). The arterial puncture necessary for the study may be associated with bleeding, hematoma, pseudoaneurysm, and pain at the site.

Treatment of Acute Arterial Occlusion

Ideally, all acute occlusion warrants immediate repair, although the urgency is governed by the degree of ischemia. If a patient presents with symptoms consistent with the "six Ps," a medical-surgical emergency exists. Immediate evaluation and intervention must be performed. Severe ischemia is suggested by pallor at rest, profound coolness, tender or hard muscles, and loss of motor and sensory functions. When severe ischemia is present, repair must occur within hours to salvage the limb. Immediate measures are needed to open the vessel lumen and restore the blood flow. The most common site of embolization is the femoral bifurcation. Ideal treatment consists of expeditious diagnosis of acute arterial ischemia, recognition of any embolic source, rapid systemic anticoagulation, percutaneous thrombolysis with an infusion catheter placed into the vessel, or surgical embolectomy. Heparin is given to prevent thrombus propagation and treat any embolic source. Angiography may be required to plan a repair when there is preexisting occlusive or aneurysmal disease or when the etiology is uncertain.

Balloon embolectomy is performed without angiography when the embolic source is certain and the vessel was previously normal. In acute arterial thrombosis, lysis of acute occlusion can be effective (19). If a thrombolytic strategy is elected, one must ensure that the infusion catheter can be positioned within the substance of the thrombus. An open operative approach is necessary when access to the thrombus cannot be achieved. Successful thrombolysis should be followed by endovascular or open surgical revision of any lesion unmasked after dissolution of the thrombus. Endovascular modalities such as balloon angioplasty with or without stenting can be performed at the conclusion of thrombolysis (usually through the same access site used for the infusion).

Historically, it has been thought that 4 to 6 hours (following the onset of symptoms) is the maximal length of tolerable ischemia. Patients with prior chronic limb ischemia tend to tolerate longer period of acute ischemia. The physiologic state of the limb, determined mainly by a balance between metabolic supply and demand, rather than the elapsed time from the onset of occlusion, is actually the best predictor of limb salvage.

Treatment of Chronic Arterial Disease

Medical

The management of patients with intermittent claudication has traditionally focused on relief of symptoms. The goals of medical care should be to reduce cardiovascular risk and alleviate symptoms of intermittent claudication. Medical therapies can both effectively modify the natural history of atherosclerotic lower extremity arterial occlusive disease and significantly reduce the morbidity of this disorder.

Screening for elevated homocysteine should be considered in young patients with PAD. An elevated plasma homocysteine level is recognized as an independent predictor of PAD (20). An increased plasma total homocysteine level confers an independent risk for vascular disease similar to that of smoking or hyperlipidemia. It further increases the risk associated with smoking and hypertension (21). Elevated homocysteine levels can be lowered by folic acid and other vitamin supplementation; however, no studies to date have examined how this treatment affects atherosclerosis or intermittent claudication symptoms (22).

Among apparently healthy men, elevated baseline levels of C-reactive protein (CRP), a marker for systemic inflammation, may predict future risk for developing symptomatic peripheral arterial occlusive disease. CRP may serve as a molecular marker for underlying systemic atherosclerosis (23).

Risk factor management. All patients presenting for treatment of peripheral arterial occlusive disease should have their risk factors rigorously assessed (24). On average, an age-matched control group has an all-cause mortality rate of 1.6% per year. This rate increases to 4.8% per year for patients with PAD. Cardiovascular mortality rates are similarly affected, with an overall event rate of 0.5% per year in controls and 2.5% per year in patients with PAD. The presence of PAD is an independent risk factor for mortality even when other known risk factors are controlled (25–28). The increased cardiac event rate in patients with PAD underscores the importance of intensive medical management to reduce the risks for cardiovascular morbidity and mortality.

Treatment needs to focus on both the effects of atherosclerosis in the peripheral circulation and the systemic nature of the disease. Appropriate therapy should be instituted to decrease the risk for both peripheral progression and cardiovascular mortality. Patients with known PAD should be treated aggressively with a combination of a HMG-CoA reductase inhibitor (statin), an angiotensin-converting enzyme (ACE) inhibitor, an antiplatelet agent, and a beta-blocker (if there is a history of coronary disease). They should also control their blood pressure and blood sugar level. Smokers should be encouraged to stop smoking (25). Smokers are 2.3 times more likely to develop symptomatic PAD than nonsmokers. For heavy smokers, the incidence of PAD is 9.8%.

Diabetic management. Diabetes is an independent risk factor for complications and amputations in patients with CLI. Hemoglobin A1C should be less than 7% (29). Optimal diabetic management is presumed to improve the rate of lower extremity disease progression and to decrease the incidence of wound infection, gangrene, and amputation (30).

Nicotine cessation. Cigarette smoking is an exceptionally positive risk factor for lower extremity PAD. It is two to three times more likely to cause lower extremity PAD than coronary artery disease (1). Cigarette smoking nearly doubles the risk for progression of peripheral arterial occlusive disease, independent of other associated risk factors (24). Patients should be informed that continued tobacco use is likely to accelerate disease progression and cause progressive symptomatic worsening. Eighteen percent of patients with claudication who continue to smoke cigarettes develop rest pain over the subsequent 5 years of observation (31). In contrast, in those patients who stop smoking, the development of rest pain is exceedingly rare. The 5-year mortality rate for patients with claudication who continue to smoke may be as high as 40% to 50%.

Lipid management. Effective lipid management should be considered a mandatory component of the medical therapy of patients with objective evidence of atherosclerotic peripheral arterial occlusive disease. ACC/AHA PAD recommendations are for LDL less than 100 mg/dL in the general population and less than 70 mg/dL for patients at very high risk for significant cardiovascular events such as patients with CLI (32). Statins may also have a positive effect on intermittent claudication and survival in severe PAD (29).

Health care providers should increase statin therapy in a graduated fashion to adequately determine the patient's response and tolerance. Since statins are cleared hepatically, it is recommended that liver enzymes be tested before initiating the medication, 12 weeks following imitation of therapy, upon any elevation of the medication dose, and every 6 months. Other side effects of HMG-CoA reductase inhibitors include myopathy and rhabdomyolysis with acute renal failure secondary to myoglobinuria. Therefore, statins should be prescribed with caution in patients with predisposing factors for myopathy and discontinued if markedly elevated creatinine kinase doubles or myopathy is noted. Statins have favorable effects on multiple interrelated aspects of vascular biology important in atherosclerosis. In particular, they have beneficial effects on inflammation, plaque stabilization, endothelial dysfunction, and thrombosis. Statins have also been shown to be beneficial in acute vascular events. Unless contraindicated, all patients with PAD should be on a statin medication especially patients presenting with CLI.

Hypertension management. Fifty-five percent of patients with PAD also have hypertension. The goal of treated hypertension in patients with PAD should be similar to that in patients who have other cardiovascular diseases. Antihypertensive therapies should be administered to hypertensive patients with lower extremity PAD to achieve a goal of less than 140 mm Hg systolic/90 mm Hg diastolic (nondiabetics) or less than 130 mm Hg systolic/80 mm Hg diastolic (diabetics and individuals with chronic renal disease) to reduce the risk of MI, stroke, congestive heart failure, and cardiovascular death (1,30).

ACE inhibitors. ACE inhibitors have been shown to reduce cardiovascular morbidity and mortality rates in patients with PAD by 25% regardless of the presence or absence of hypertension (21). The overall treatment effect achieved by ace inhibitors is more than that of other therapeutic agents for intermittent claudication such as cilostazol and pentoxifylline but less than that of a supervised exercise program (33).

Antiplatelet therapy. Antiplatelet therapy may decrease the rate of atherosclerotic disease progression, decrease the incidence of thrombotic events in the limbs, and decrease the rate of adverse coronary and cerebral vascular ischemic events (30).

Aspirin in doses of 75 to 325 mg is recommended as safe and effective antiplatelet therapy to reduce the risk of MI, stroke, or vascular death in individuals with atherosclerotic lower extremity PAD (30). Patients with documented arterial occlusive disease may benefit from antiplatelet therapy unless otherwise contraindicated.

Vasodilator drugs. In general, vasodilator drugs do not improve symptoms in patients with arterial claudication. Direct-acting vasodilators have minimal effect at the focal atherosclerotic site. Vasodilator drugs do not vasodilate lower extremity collateral vessels. In addition, this class of medications may elicit a fall in blood pressure and limb perfusion pressure if a preferential vasodilatory effect occurs in other nondiseased circulation (34).

Beta-blockers. Although beta-blockers were previously believed to have detrimental clinical effects in patients with claudication, clinical trials have demonstrated a symptom-neutral effect for these agents in most patients (35). Because beta-blocker therapy may be efficacious for the treatment of associated coronary artery disease or myocardial infarction, these drugs do not need to be empirically withdrawn from the patient with claudication.

Agents for intermittent claudication. Cilostazol inhibits the action of phosphodiesterase and increases the amount of intracellular cyclic adenosine monophosphate. This results in significant platelet and vasodilatory activity as well as antiproliferative properties. Since antiplatelet and vasodilatory drugs have been shown to have no positive effect on claudication-limiting walking distance, the mechanism by which cilostazol achieves improvement in PAD patients remains speculative (36). Cilostazol (100 mg orally two times per day) is indicated as an effective therapy to improve symptoms and increase walking distances in patients with lower extremity PAD and intermittent claudication (in the absence of heart failure) (30). This medication is contraindicated in patients with congestive heart failure.

Pentoxifylline has received variable reports of success in patients with arterial occlusive disease (37). Minimal efficacy and caffeine-like side effects limit use of this medication.

In summary, although there are few widely accepted pharmacologic interventions for PAD, current recommendations are that all PAD patients should receive antiplatelet therapy, stop smoking, exercise, and be screened and treated for hyperlipidemia, hypertension, diabetes, and hypercoagulability in accordance with national guidelines and community standards (38).

Revascularization

The angiosome concept, which has been successfully used in plastic surgery for years, has recently been the topic of discussion in the field of vascular and endovascular surgery. In 2006, Attinger et al. described six angiosomal regions in the foot and ankle, each supplied by one of the crural arteries and its terminal branches (39,40). Based on this knowledge, several consecutive studies have been carried out applying the angiosome concept to the treatment of CLI. Although the angiosome concept is anatomic rather than physiologic, all efforts should be made when selecting the target artery to consider the specific angiosome vessel.

Previously, surgical revascularization was considered for patients with rest pain, impending tissue loss, or significant limitations of lifestyle who failed medical treatment. The Bypass Versus Angioplasty in Severe Ischaemia of the Leg (BASIL) trial reported that 50% of patients who had a diagnostic angiogram were unsuitable for revascularization (41,42). Recent advances in endovascular revascularization have changed the rates of limb salvage and potentially the prognosis of patients with CLI with a shift in the treatment (43–45).

Among CLI patients who are poor surgical candidates, the simultaneous combination of antegrade and distal retrograde access improves the overall success of endovascular therapies (46). Endovascular intervention coupled with aggressive proactive medical management is replacing previous conventional paradigms (38).

Endovascular. Endovascular therapy is a broad term that encompasses several treatment modalities: percutaneous transluminal angioplasty (PTA) with plain or drug-eluting balloons; stenting with bare-metal, covered, or drug-eluting stents; atherectomy; cryoplasty; and cutting-balloon angioplasty. The updated TASC II guidelines suggest best practices for percutaneous intervention versus surgical intervention for arterial occlusive disease above and below the inguinal ligament (47).

As a controlled injury to the vessel wall, PTA is indicated for focal stenosis or short segmental occlusions in which the adjacent vessels are relatively free of disease (38). Smooth muscle cell proliferation within the media (normal <1%) increases to more than 20% within 48 hours after angioplasty. After balloon angioplasty, there are thrombosis formation, intimal hyperplasia development, elastic recoil, and remodeling.

Endovascular stents were introduced to help resolve the problems of residual stenosis, elastic recoil, and flow-limiting arterial dissection and to improve patency rates after balloon angioplasty. After stent placement, elastic recoil and remodeling are eliminated, and thrombosis followed by intimal hyperplasia is the main contributor to in-stent restenosis (38). The response of a vessel to a stent is dependent on the stent design, length, composition, delivery system, and deployment technique (38). Stents may be bare-metal or covered and plain or drug-eluting. In a recent meta-analysis of the endovascular treatment of the superficial femoral artery, drug-eluting stents appear to have the best primary patency of any stents. Plain balloon angioplasty was found to have the lowest rate of primary patency (48). Lesion length and location play a role in device and treatment selection. The biology of in-stent restenosis is different than that seen after balloon angioplasty. In a retrospective study, nitinol stents significantly demonstrated improved primary patency rates in femoropopliteal arteries compared with stainless steel stents (49). In the intermediate term, a randomized controlled study has shown superior results with nitinol stents compared to PTA with the option of secondary stenting (50). The policy of routine primary stenting versus angioplasty for femoropopliteal lesions with stenting reserved for angioplasty failure remains controversial.

The potential role of ionizing radiation to inhibit cellular proliferation and prevent restenosis has been evaluated. Endovascular brachytherapy has shown a delay but not an inhibition of restenosis when compared to PTA alone (51). This technology is rarely used.

Cryoplasty combines conventional balloon angioplasty with application of cryotherapy. While the hope was that cryoplasty would allow more accurate angioplasty and reduce dissection and recoil (38), in practice, this has not been shown to be an effective stand-alone treatment. Further study is needed to determine the effectiveness of cryoplasty in combination with other therapies, such as stents (48).

There is decreasing long-term effectiveness of stenting and angioplasty in below-knee vessels because of the reduction in both artery size and flow rate. It is reasonable to consider distal angioplasty for limb salvage in patients at high risk for limb loss who are not surgical candidates. Although the rate of long-term clinical success appears to be less than that for conventional surgical reconstruction, the benefits in terms of decreased morbidity and probable cost savings may well justify the use of PTA in these circumstances.

Subintimal recanalization. Subintimal recanalization of infrainguinal occlusions is a minimally invasive percutaneous endovascular technique that allows revascularization of occluded infrainguinal arteries by creating a new lumen between the intima and the adventitia of the arterial wall. Unlike conventional PTA, subintimal angioplasty displaces the atheromatous and calcified intima and media to one side of the vessel lumen, thereby producing a relatively smooth neolumen. The catheter and wire are redirected to the true arterial lumen distal to the area of occlusion. Subintimal recanalization can be used in patients with CLI (52). These patients frequently have multiple comorbidities and consequently long-term survival is poor, irrespective of the technique used to revascularize the ischemic limb. The success rate of subintimal recanalization has been reported to be 78% to 90% depending on the length of the occluded arterial segment treated. Treatment may involve use of a plain or drug-eluting balloon and stent. Patency rates are approximately 50% at 1-year follow-up, with higher (70% to 80%) limb salvage rate. The most common complications include peripheral embolization, inadvertent ruptures, and bleeding. Other alternative endovascular modalities in patients with long-segment disease include percutaneous directional, orbital, rotational, or laser atherectomy devices, which remove the atherosclerotic plaque from the artery (53).

Surgical. Ischemic rest pain and tissue necrosis, including ischemic ulceration or gangrene, are well accepted as indicators of advanced ischemia and threatened limb loss. Without treatment, most limbs with these symptoms experience disease progression and require major amputation. These symptoms represent an unequivocal indication for arterial revascularization, if anatomically feasible. Large vessel bypass surgery with synthetic graft material is well established and durable. Aortobifemoral grafting continues to be regarded as the gold standard for the treatment of aortoiliac occlusive disease (54). If early and long-term patency is to be achieved, it is important that the site for vascular reconstruction has a relatively unobstructed inflow and a patent distal runoff.

The purpose of profundoplasty is to relieve a significant stenosis or an occlusion of the proximal portion of the profunda femoris artery in order to restore its function. The procedure is employed as an adjunct to an inflow procedure or when patients present with an occluded limb of an aortobifemoral bypass. The profunda femoris artery is often the only major outflow vessel in the groin. In this case, a profundoplasty ensures continued patency of the aortofemoral limb. In addition, profundoplasty can be performed to optimize healing after transtibial amputation.

Judicious selection of the appropriate method of infrainguinal reconstruction for a given patient requires an appreciation of the results obtained with all available approaches. Although PTA may be appropriate for some patients with short-segment lesions, and profundoplasty may be effective in others, many patients with an ischemic limb require conventional surgical bypass. Most claudicants achieve sustained relief, and 80% to 90% of limbs threatened with critical ischemia are salvaged with vascular reconstruction. Of variables influencing the ultimate outcome, the choice of conduit is most important. For optimal results, every effort must be made to use autogenous vein for infrainguinal reconstruction (55,56).

Inframalleolar revascularization (pedal bypass grafting) has become an accepted treatment for patients with severe distal disease, limb-threatening ischemia, and tissue loss, regardless of age or diabetic status (57,58). *In situ* distal bypass using reverse or intact saphenous vein has shown promising long-term patency. Patient mortality rate following revascularization averages about 5%. Patient survival rates range from 30% to 70% at 3 years (annual mortality rate following recovery from operation is between 10% and 20%) (59). If the arterial anatomy of the foot permits, autologous vein bypass should be offered to all patients with severe limb ischemia before a major amputation is considered. Pedal bypass grafting has low perioperative mortality and morbidity. Postoperative surveillance with duplex ultrasonography is warranted to detect hemodynamically significant abnormalities within the graft that can be corrected before thrombosis occurs. With this, failing grafts can be salvaged, secondary patency can be improved, and the rate of late amputations can be diminished (60). Once thrombosis occurs, attempts to restore long-term patency are unlikely, and only modest limb salvage rates will be achieved. Patients with chronic renal insufficiency have been shown to have a poor outcome following reintervention. Data suggest that reintervention should not be considered when these patients present with failed grafts following an initial pedal bypass procedure (61,62).

Attempts at revascularization should be avoided in the presence of life-threatening sepsis, chronic flexion contracture, or paralysis and in patients with markedly reduced life expectancy. A multicenter randomized trial showed that coronary artery revascularization before elective vascular surgery does not alter long-term survival (63). Revascularization should be delayed in most individuals with a significant acute comorbidity (recent myocardial infarction) unless the limb is eminently threatened and a higher perioperative morbidity is acceptable (64).

Rehabilitation

General self-care measures. Patients with PAD should be instructed to wear protective footwear at all times (never walk barefoot or in socks) and monitor their extremities carefully for redness or skin breakdown. Extremes of temperature should be avoided. The feet should be washed carefully with mild soap and warm water. Drying is best performed by blotting or patting with a soft clean towel (rubbing should be avoided because it may injure the skin). The skin between the toes should be carefully dried to avoid maceration. Emollients without preservative or perfume should be used (avoid between the toes) to prevent cracking of the skin. Proper footwear, which accommodates the foot without areas of point pressure, should be used. Whenever new shoes are purchased, the patient should gradually (over a period of a week) wear-in the shoes to make sure there are no areas of point pressure. Warm outer footwear should be used in the winter to protect against cold injury.

Decreased activity due to symptomatic lower extremity arterial occlusive disease can result in deconditioning and further disease impairment. Deconditioning may also be "iatrogenic" as a result of a prolonged period of limited mobility to avoid trauma to ischemic wounds.

Exercise. Regular exercise training produces a reduction in the inflammatory markers associated with endothelial damage (1). Evidence suggests that following an exercise regimen improves both claudication distance and cardiovascular risk profiles (38). Exercise training may lead to improvements in maximal walking time of 25% to 200% (65). Exercise training is thought to augment limb flow, improve blood viscosity, improve the efficiency of gait, and alter the ischemic pain threshold or tolerance. Multiple studies have demonstrated the effectiveness of supervised exercise therapy (SET) for symptomatic PAD. Unfortunately, many patients have limitations (such as fear of walking, unsafe walking paths, or weather conditions not conducive to walking) that limit self-directed programs. To optimize the benefits of an exercise program, patients should receive a structured claudication exercise rehabilitation program for at least 3 sessions weekly over a period of 12 weeks (65–69). Improvement can be seen over 24 weeks of training. Strength training, whether sequential or concomitant, does not augment the response to a walking exercise program (70). The optimal exercise program for improving claudication pain distances in patients with PAD is intermittent walking to near maximal pain during a program of at least 6 months. Such a program should be a part of the standard medical care for patients with intermittent claudication (71). Patients should be instructed to walk until claudication occurs, rest until it subsides, and continue repeating the cycle for 1 hour each day. Improved walking performance has also been demonstrated through upper limb aerobic exercise training in patients with PAD (72). Patients with advanced CLI may not be able to participate in a supervised exercise training program (29).

Intermittent Pneumatic Compression

Every effort should be made to identify alternative therapies that would benefit patients who are not candidates for revascularization. Conservative management of lower extremity nonhealing wounds in selected patients with PAD is successful in over two thirds of the patients. The failure of conservative management does not increase morality or amputation rates (73).

Sequential pneumatic compression has been proposed as an adjunct to best medical care, aimed at preventing amputation, relieving pain, and promoting wound healing by increasing arterial blood flow in distal limbs (74). Intermittent pneumatic compression has been shown to achieve wound healing and limb salvage in patients with severe infrapopliteal disease and limb-threatening ischemia who are not suitable for revascularization (75,76,77).

In a study of 707 patients with CLI, 518 underwent intervention, and 189 were not suitable for intervention; a total of 171 patients used an impulse pump for 3 months. The impulse pump was a cost-effective, clinically efficacious solution in CLI patients with no option for revascularization (78).

Intermittent pneumatic foot and calf compression has also been shown to improve walking distance comparable with supervised exercise (79).

External compression briefly raises the tissue pressure, emptying the underlying veins and transiently reducing the venous pressure without occluding arterial blood flow. The proposed mechanism to explain the increased flow is analogous to the pumping action of the calf muscle during walking (80). The transient inflation imitates the effects of normal gait by generating vigorous hemodynamic impulses throughout the veins each time the lower extremity is compressed. The pneumatic impulse enhances the venous return and causes venous pressure to decrease transiently until veins are refilled by forward flow from the arteries. An increase in the hydrostatic pressure gradient during this brief period is thought to be a major mechanism for the enhancement of arterial leg inflow. The altered flow and shear forces generated by the inflation of the pneumatic cuff may mediate the release of endothelial and humoral factors having local and systemic effects (80). A direct reduction in peripheral resistance is also postulated via release of nitric oxide secondary to shear stress across the vessel wall (81). This may be a useful device in rehabilitation centers involved in wound management after providers are properly trained in its use. Skin blood flow, as reflected by $TcPO_2$, can be augmented acutely in ischemic limbs by intermittent venous occlusion with an externally applied inflatable cuff (82).

Spinal Cord Stimulation

Spinal cord stimulation was evaluated in inoperable patients with CLI with some efficacy concerning pain relief and reduced amputation rate (29).

Gene Therapy

Molecular therapies that result in increased levels of vascular endothelial growth factor, fibroblast growth factor, and hepatocyte growth factor have been used in claudication populations. The Regional Angiogenesis with Vascular Endothelial growth factor (RAVE) in PAD trial concluded that a single IM administration of adenoviral vascular endothelial growth factor was not associated with improved treadmill exercise performance or quality of life over placebo (83).

Chelation Therapy

Given its lack of efficacy and important safety concerns, EDTA should not be used to treat patients with intermittent claudication (30).

AMPUTATIONS AND VASCULAR DISEASES

Amputations due to vascular disease, commonly referred to as dysvascular amputations, encompass pathology related to PAD and diabetic vascular disease. Amputation is a significant cause of disability, as it profoundly affects a patient's life, including functional mobility, independence, self-image, vocational, and avocational activities. Over the years, advances in prosthetic rehabilitation have included improved preoperative management, surgical techniques, postoperative management, and advances in prosthetic technology (discussed in Chapter 56). The role of the rehabilitation team is to optimize care at each stage to reduce morbidity and mortality and maximize functional outcome and quality of life for the person with amputation.

Epidemiology

Amputation due to vascular disease is an important cause of morbidity. In 2005, there were 1.6 million people living with limb loss in the United States, 54% due to vascular disease. This number is predicted to increase to 3.6 million by 2050, driven by increasing number of dysvascular amputations (84). This increase in prevalence is attributed to the aging population, the obesity epidemic, and high rates of diabetes and vascular disease in older and obese adults. With the changes in population demographics, the number of individuals older than 65 years continues to increase, and the absolute number of patients with vascular amputations will remain large (85,86).

Vascular disease is by far the most common cause of amputation, accounting for 82% of all amputations (87). Moreover, while the incidence of amputations due to trauma and cancer has decreased (87,88), amputations due to vascular disease continue to increase. There are an estimated 150,000 amputations per year in the United States due to PAD (89). This rate increased by 27% between the years 1988 and 1996 (87). Ninety-seven percent of amputations due to vascular disease are in the lower extremity (87). Moreover, patients who undergo one dysvascular lower extremity amputation are at high risk of reamputation, with 25% undergoing reamputation within 1 year (89).

In comparing trends among levels of amputation, recent studies looking at the incidence of lower limb amputations in Australia and England have found that while the incidence of amputation above the ankle, commonly referred to as major amputation, was decreasing, the incidence of amputation below the ankle or minor amputation was increasing (90,91). Fifty-five to seventy-five percent of lower extremity amputations are now performed below the ankle (90,91). Studies suggest that the rate of major amputations has decreased as a result of the increased use of surgical and endovascular revascularization procedures, such as balloon angioplasty and peripheral arterial bypass grafting (4,92–95).

Several risk factors have been identified for amputation due to vascular disease. Diabetes greatly increases the risk of amputation, with studies showing a 6- to 15-fold greater risk of amputation in this population (91,96,97). Moreover, in studies in Europe and the United States, approximately half to two thirds of all lower extremity amputations occur in persons with diabetes (91,97–99). This rate may vary between 25% and 90% depending on the geographic location (100). End-stage renal disease also carries an extremely high risk of amputation of 6.2 per 100 persons in this population (101).

Another risk factor is age. The incidence of major amputation rises steeply with age (87,100), with the highest rates in those over 70 years old (88). Seventy-five percent of all lower extremity amputations occur in people aged 65 or older (102). Arteriosclerotic vascular disease is a significant risk factor and is the cause of 90% of the amputations in the elderly population (103).

Male gender also increases the risk for vascular limb loss. Men have twice the risk of amputation compared to women (91). This is even higher at the transfemoral level where they have 70% greater rate of amputation than women (104).

Minority populations in the United States also have an increased risk of amputation. African Americans have a two to four times greater risk of amputation (87,88). Native American and Mexican Americans also have increased risk of diabetes-related amputation compared to white Americans (88,100).

Preoperative Consultation

When amputation is considered for a person with vascular disease, careful consideration should be given to level of amputation. Ideally, this should be a collaborative decision with input from the surgeon, the physiatrist, and the patient. A physiatrist can assess the functional implications of different levels of amputation, given medical comorbidities, life expectancy, preoperative functional status, postoperative functional goals, and risk of nonhealing or reamputation. In general, more distal surgery provides a better functional outcome but has increased risk of nonhealing, reulceration, and reamputation. The physiatrist can also use their knowledge of prosthetic rehabilitation to make recommendations regarding residual limb length and if prosthetic management should be considered.

Levels of Amputation

The benefit of a partial foot amputation (**Fig. 37-3A**) (toe, ray, transmetatarsal, Lisfranc [tarsometatarsal], and Chopart [transtarsal]) is that it preserves a full weight-bearing surface, allowing standing and short distance walking without a prosthesis. The drawback of a partial foot amputation in persons with vascular disease is the high rate of nonhealing and reamputation. Studies report healing rates of transmetatarsal amputations (TMAs) of 40% to 70% and rates of revision to above ankle amputation of about 30% to 40% (105–108). The wound may fail to heal after amputation or may heal initially with subsequent reulceration of the residual foot. The loss of the normal architecture of the foot after partial foot amputation can lead to increased and abnormal pressures in the residual foot, placing it at high risk of reulceration. In Chopart or Lisfranc amputations, the residual foot is prone to equinovarus deformity due to the loss of muscular attachments. Surgeons may perform an Achilles tendon lengthening procedure at the time of amputation to avoid an equinovarus deformity.

The next amputation level (**Fig. 37-3B**) is a Syme amputation or ankle disarticulation. Because this is a disarticulation procedure, the bony integrity is not disrupted, which can decrease the risk of osteomyelitis in cases of soft tissue infection. Other

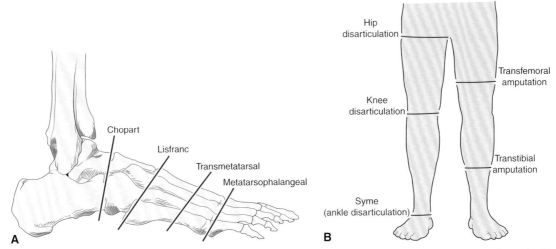

advantages of the Syme level amputation are the long lever arm, greater proprioception, and ability to end weight bearing on the residual limb. The disadvantages are poor cosmesis due to the bulbous shape of the residual limb and limited prosthetic foot options due to limited build height at this level.

The transtibial level is the most common major lower extremity amputation (90,109). Compared to a partial foot amputation, the benefit of transtibial amputation is low risk of reamputation. Conversion to a higher level is reported in 9% to 19% of transtibial amputations (4,89,109–112). The drawback is that the patient must use a prosthesis for weight bearing through their residual limb.

Comparing partial foot to transtibial level amputation, the partial foot amputation has traditionally been thought to allow a more energy-efficient gait by preserving a functional ankle joint. This has been called into question by recent research comparing these levels, which show similar functional outcomes (113), similar energy expenditure of walking (114), and similar quality of life (115).

Knee disarticulation is a relatively rare level of amputation compared to transtibial and transfemoral levels. Like the ankle disarticulation amputation, the benefits of this level include no disruption of the bony cortex, greater proprioception, greater end weight-bearing ability, and long lever arm of the residual limb. The drawbacks are again poor cosmesis due to the bulbous shape of the limb and less room for knee componentry. The leg lengths of the prosthetic and sound thigh can also appear uneven at this level, especially in sitting. For persons with vascular disease, the more common proximal amputation level is the transfemoral amputation. This is not a preferred level from a functional point of view due to the loss of the knee joint and the increased metabolic cost of ambulation. It is considered when more distal levels are not an option due to inadequate tissue or poor perfusion.

Comparing transtibial to knee disarticulation and transfemoral levels, a transtibial amputation is always preferred, as long as attachment of the patellar tendon to the tibial tubercle is intact, preserving a functional knee joint. The metabolic cost of prosthetic ambulation is higher in transfemoral compared to transtibial amputees (116,117). Patients undergoing transfemoral amputation are less likely to be fit with a prosthesis (103,118,119) and, if fit, have reduced functional outcome

and ambulation (110,120–123) compared to those with transtibial amputation. In many persons with vascular disease, comorbidities and the increased energy expenditure associated with the use of a transfemoral prosthesis make prosthetic fitting untenable (124).

Recognition of the functional advantages associated with preservation of the knee and advances in surgical techniques have brought about a change in surgical policy (125,126). As a result, the ratio of transtibial amputations to transfemoral amputations has increased over the years (92,93). Studies from the 1980s (102) and 1990s (112) report that two thirds of all amputations due to PAD were below the knee. A more recent study reports an even higher ratio of 2.8:1 transtibial compared to transfemoral amputations (109).

Proximal to the transfemoral level are the hip disarticulation and hemipelvectomy level amputation, which are relatively uncommon. These are only performed if no more distal amputation is possible.

Predicting Prosthetic Use

The perioperative consultation by the physiatrist should address the likelihood of successful prosthetic fitting and use. This can assist the team to determine the optimal level of amputation. If a patient is not a prosthetic candidate, they may be better served with a transfemoral level amputation to optimize healing, avoid dependent edema, and avoid a knee flexion contracture with risk of excess pressure at the distal residual limb. This information is also important to discuss with the patient and their family to allow shared decision-making and help set realistic expectations as they prepare for life after amputation.

Predicting whether a patient will use a prosthesis is a clinical judgment taking many factors (physical, medical, psychological, and social) into account (**Table 37-3**). Several studies have looked at preoperative factors to predict successful prosthetic use. Preoperative factors associated with not using a prosthesis postoperatively include being nonambulatory or only ambulating in the household before amputation, age greater than 70 years, dementia, end-stage renal disease, and coronary artery disease (127). Age, number of medical problems, presence of coronary artery disease, or presence of diabetes mellitus were associated with worse postoperative mobility following transtibial amputation (128).

TABLE 37-3	Factors Affecting Prosthetic Use		
Physical	**Medical**	**Psychosocial**	**Function**
Level of amputation	Cognition	Motivation to use a prosthesis	Preoperative level of function
Length of residual limb	Renal insufficiency/end-stage renal disease	Anxiety/depression	Support after amputation
Strength and range of motion	Coronary artery disease	Level of education	
Soft tissue coverage	Diabetes	Social support/marital status	
Age	COPD	Alcohol use disorder	
	Hypertension		

From Smith DG, Michael JW, Bowker J. *Atlas of Amputations and Limb Deficiencies—Surgical, Prosthetic, and Rehabilitation Principles.* 3rd ed. Rosemont, IL: American Academy of Orthopedic Surgeons; 2004.

Amputation Surgery

The decision to attempt limb salvage or proceed with amputation is complex. Amputation should not be viewed as an ablative procedure but as a reconstructive procedure. The basic principle of all amputations is to restore patient function, control disease, and optimize surgical wound management. Adherent scarred distal tissues or redundant soft tissue should be avoided.

Each level of amputation in the lower extremity has its own nuances, which are important considerations for postoperative function; however, the general principles of each level are similar.

Skin and soft tissue. Preoperatively, the integrity of the skin and soft tissues plays an important role in determining the level of amputation and is more important than the osseous integrity to determine the length of the residual limb and amputation level. In the lower extremity, the skin and soft tissue envelope need to be robust in order to tolerate the sheer forces associated with prosthetic rehabilitation. Adequate blood flow to the skin is assessed preoperatively through a combination of various factors including $TcPO_2$ levels (>20 to 30 mm), hair growth, presence of warm skin, and bleeding of the skin at the time of surgery. If there is no bleeding of the skin or muscle at the time of surgery, the level of amputation should be changed to a more proximal level.

Intraoperatively, meticulous handling of the skin and soft tissues is critical as traumatic handling can lead to postoperative wound necrosis and further complications. Skin incisions should be made under tourniquet control and in a layered fashion: first only going through the skin, then through the subcutaneous tissues, fascia, and deeper layers. This allows for a layered closure and obtaining full-thickness soft tissue flaps (eFig. 37-2). An incision straight through the skin, subcutaneous tissue, and fascia is not advised as this makes it difficult to obtain a robust layered closure. The wound is typically closed from the periphery moving central in order to avoid dog-ears; however, if dog-ears are present, they should not be trimmed as

this could lead to flap failure. As a tenant of closure, the wound should be closed without tension (eFig. 37-3).

Skin flap design varies based on the level of amputation. For toe amputations, equal fish-mouth style incisions are planned, either with a long plantar flap or with a side-to-side flap depending on wound location. For partial foot/transmetatarsal amputations, a fish-mouth incision is used with a longer planter flap, as the integrity of the distal plantar skin makes it critical to determine the level of amputation. If this is not the case, a transtibial amputation should be performed. If the plantar skin is not conducive for TMA, a Syme level amputation can be performed as long as the patient has a palpable posterior tibial artery; however, this is unreliable in the setting of peripheral arterial disease. If this is not the case, a transtibial amputation should be performed.

For a transtibial amputation, the skin and soft tissue flap is based on the posterior tissues. Even if the more distal skin near the ankle is intact, an amputation at this level is not advised due to the subcutaneous location of the tibia and fibula and lack of posterior tissue for a flap. The anterior incision for the transtibial amputation is placed at a level approximately a loose handsbreadth from the tibial tubercle (typically 8 to 10 cm) as this will allow for sufficient length for prosthetic rehabilitation. The skin incision should be made approximately 1.5 cm distal to the planned bone cut level in order to allow for adequate closure. The anterior incision is then carried 2/3 of the way medial and lateral, and at this point, the posterior flap is designed. The flap should be rounded distally; however, the transition from the anterior to the posterior incision should be sharp 90 degrees perpendicular to the anterior incision and not rounded. The flap length is typically the same length or a little longer than the length of anterior incision. A contraindication to a transtibial amputation in the setting of arterial disease is proximal skin necrosis near the knee joint as this is typically associated with an acute, thrombotic, or embolic occlusion of the femoral artery.

Flap design for a through knee amputation is different from other distal leg amputations since the main flap relies on the anterior skin and soft tissue. A fish-mouth incision with a flap that is twice as long anteriorly as it is posteriorly is used. This is to allow for adequate mobilization of the patella tendon.

In the setting of a transfemoral amputation, flap design is based on the medial and lateral soft tissues. Similar to other amputations, a fish-mouth–designed flap is used, with a medial flap that is longer than the lateral flap. This is to allow for mobilization of the adductor muscle group and perform a myodesis. The ideal length of a transfemoral residual limb is 5 to 7 cm proximal to the knee joint (7 cm allows adequate space for a rotation unit).

Although not commonly performed in the setting of vascular disease, hip disarticulations and hindquarter amputations are indicated in select situations. Since these procedures are most commonly performed in the setting of a failed vascular graft, it is critical to assess the patency of the iliac arteries in order to ensure adequate flap perfusion. The traditional hip disarticulation is based on a gluteal flap, as the patency of the internal iliac and gluteal vessels is essential. For this flap, a buttock incision, which allows for mobilization of the gluteus maximus, is used. The classic hindquarter amputation involved ligation of the common iliac artery, as there was a high incidence of wound complications. Due to this, modified hindquarter amputations have been developed based on either the internal or external iliac vessels. Depending on the patency of the vascular supply, a large soft tissue flap based on the external iliac system and superficial femoral artery, which includes the quadriceps musculature, can be mobilized. This provides a large myocutaneous flap of essentially the entire anterior thigh. Similar to hip disarticulation, a posterior flap based on the internal iliac and gluteal vessels can also be used allowing for mobilization of the gluteus maximus when there is an occluded external iliac system (129,130).

Unlike upper extremity amputations where a split-thickness skin graft (STSG) can be used to provide durable coverage of skin defects and maximize residual limb length with little complications, there is debate on their use in the lower extremity. This in part is due to the high shear forces across the STSG, which can potentially lead to wound complications, especially when used on the terminal surface of the residual limb. In the setting of traumatic amputation, Polfer et al. noted that, although there were increased complications and reoperations, a STSG can be used to maintain residual limb length and adequate coverage (131). Likewise, other studies have shown similar results, including a series by Kent et al. (132) that included patients with PAD, diabetes, and gangrene. In the setting of a terminal bearing STSG, it is essential that the graft has completely healed prior to starting prosthetic rehabilitation to reduce early wound complications.

Nerves and blood vessels. At all levels of lower extremity and hindquarter amputations, nerves are encountered that require transection. For larger nerves such as the sciatic and femoral nerves, the nerves should be suture ligated prior to transection since they are accompanied by a large vasa nervorum. All nerves should be transected sharply under tension (📶 **eFig. 37-4**). Prior to allowing the nerve to retract, they can be infiltrated with local anesthetic in order to provide postoperative pain control. The transected nerve is then allowed to retract into the adjacent soft tissues, permitting the nerves to move away from the amputation site and away from the areas where it could become adherent and a source of pressure irritation from the socket.

Meticulous hemostasis is mandatory to avoid postoperative hematoma formation. It is essential that all larger blood vessels are suture ligated and, when indicated, oversewn. All wounds are drained for at least 48 hours postoperatively. It is not uncommon to have drains in place longer for more proximal level amputations. Incisional negative pressure wound dressings can also be used for hip disarticulations and hindquarter amputations to reduce wound drainage.

Bone. In all lower extremity amputations, the bone is typically transected proximal to any soft tissue flap wound edge to allow for adequate closure. All bone edges should be rounded to prevent bony prominences and assist with closure (📶 **eFig. 37-5**). Prior to the osteotomy, the periosteum of the bone should be stripped and pushed proximal allowing for a clean cut.

For TMAs, the metatarsals should be osteotomized at the same level. This is in contrast to the transtibial amputation where the tibia and fibula are osteotomized at different levels. The fibula is typically cut 1.5 cm proximal to the planned tibial cut and then a further 5 cm more proximal. The portion of the fibula is then removed allowing for visualization of the posterior compartment of the leg.

In transfemoral amputations, the femur is typically transected 12 cm proximal to the knee joint. This allows for the adductor magnus to be used as a dynamic stabilizer of the residual limb. As the amputation is taken more proximal, there is a reduction in the strength of the adductors and less stabilization.

There are different levels of hindquarter amputation based on the amount of residual ilium and sacrum. The traditional hindquarter amputation involves disarticulation of the sacroiliac joint, while an extended procedure transects the sacrum and a modified procedure preserves the sacroiliac joint. If a portion of the ilium is preserved, the patient is able to wear a suspension belt to assist prosthetic management.

Muscle stabilization. If able, a myodesis of the remaining muscle provides excellent residual limb control and patient function and is essential for a balanced limb. Whenever possible, an attempt to mitigate opposing muscle forces should be done. This will reduce the risk of joint contracture. In certain situations, such as burns, paralytic disease, and scarred tissue, and in elderly patients with severe vascular disease, stabilization procedures cannot be performed.

Unlike other lower extremity amputations, a transfemoral amputation requires stabilization of the muscle and firm fixation to the remaining bone. If opposing muscles are only sewn to each other over the bone or joint, a bursa can form due to the creation of a "sling-like" effect. The formation of the bursa reduces the muscle strength and can be painful. Myodesis of the residual muscle groups should be performed using transosseous sutures passed through drill holes. An attempt to preserve the adductor magnus should be made since this muscle belly has the largest cross-sectional area with a moment arm that provides the greatest mechanical advantage.

Postamputation Management

After amputation surgery, the patient begins postoperative or preprosthetic rehabilitation. Goals of this period are to protect the residual limb, to promote wound healing, to control edema, to promote residual limb shaping to prepare for possible prosthetic use, to prevent contractures, to desensitize the residual limb and prevent adhesions, to control pain, and to facilitate early weight bearing. Many of these goals are the same whether or not the patient will go on to eventual prosthetic use.

Wound Healing

Wound healing is of primary importance after amputation due to the morbidity associated with prolonged wound healing and reamputation. Wound care, edema management, diabetic control, smoking cessation, and adequate nutrition are all important factors. Optimally, wound healing takes 6 to 8 weeks after amputation. However, amputations due to vascular disease may have a more prolonged course. Healing for TMA due to vascular disease ranged from 3 to 20 months with a mean of 7 months (133). Healing at 100 and 200 days was 55% and 83% for transtibial and 76% and 85% for transfemoral amputations, respectively (110).

Postoperative Dressings

There are different types of dressings that can be applied to the residual limb in the postoperative period to help achieve these goals. For transtibial amputations, either a rigid or a soft dressing can be used (**Fig. 37-4**). Following transfemoral amputation, typically soft dressings are used. The benefits of the soft

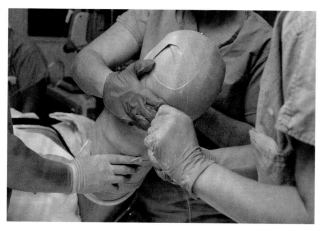

FIGURE 37-4. A postoperative splint applied in the immediate postoperative period.

dressing are ease of application, low cost, and easy access to wound. The drawbacks are that they tend to become loose and fall off easily, they do not prevent joint contracture, and there is a risk of choking of the distal residual limb if too much compression is applied proximally. Different kinds of soft, compressive dressings include self-adherent compressive bandage, figure-of-8 compressive dressing, and postoperative sock with a garter suspension.

Rigid dressings are either a plaster cast or a rigid removable dressing. The benefits of a nonremovable rigid dressing are that they help to control edema, protect the limb from trauma, prevent knee flexion contracture, reduce pain, and increase tolerance to weight bearing. The drawbacks of a plaster cast are that it requires weekly application by a skilled professional, prevents monitoring of the wound, and is heavier and more costly than a soft dressing. A rigid removable dressing can be taken off to monitor the wound and is less heavy and costly than a nonremovable rigid dressing. Studies of rigid dressings show that they decrease time to prosthetic fitting compared to other management (134,135).

The plaster cast also allows for the attachment of an immediate postoperative prosthesis (IPOP), which includes a connector, pylon, and foot. The IPOP has been purported to allow patients with transtibial amputations the opportunity for early ambulation without increased complication rates compared with other postoperative dressings (136,137). The impact of this early weight bearing on wound healing is unclear. Despite IPOP dressings, patients were mostly sedentary and had a low quality of life in the first 6 weeks after transtibial amputation (138). Potential complications include tissue necrosis if incorrectly wrapped and mechanical tissue trauma inside the cast (139). At the transfemoral level, a locking knee is used in the IPOP to avoid excess motion and shearing along the surgical incision.

Preprosthetic Rehabilitation

Goals of preprosthetic rehabilitation include flexibility and contracture prevention, muscle strength and endurance, cardiovascular conditioning, and balance (140). The patient should also be taught techniques for skin desensitization, scar, and soft tissue mobilization.

Patients should be educated about stretching and positioning to avoid joint contracture. To prevent hip flexion

contractures, patients are educated to spend time prone with a pillow or towel under the anterior thigh (if tolerated). Knee flexion contractures can be prevented by using an elevated leg rest on the wheelchair, by using a residual limb support, and by educating the patient about proper positioning (avoid lying with a pillow under the knee). Although the focus is usually on the amputated side, attention should also be paid to the contralateral side, as patients are at risk of joint contractures on that side as well due to immobility after surgery.

The rehabilitation program should include strengthening of upper extremities, core, and lower extremities. Upper extremity and core strength is important for transfers, sitting balance, bed mobility, propelling a wheelchair, and ambulating with a walker or crutches. Residual limb strength is important for eventual control of the prosthesis during prosthetic ambulation. Contralateral limb strength is important because it will allow the patient to stand and ambulate in the parallel bars or with assistive devices in the preprosthetic period.

A focus of rehabilitation should be to develop standing balance on the intact limb and to progress to hopping in the parallel bars and then with an assistive device. This will prevent contractures in the intact limb, build muscle strength and endurance, and increase cardiovascular fitness. Cardiovascular conditioning is also important to prepare the patient for the greater energy demands of unipedal and prosthetic ambulation.

Contralateral Limb Protection

It is essential to evaluate the contralateral foot in the perioperative period, postoperative period, and lifelong. Patients with amputations due to vascular disease are at a very high risk of contralateral amputation. Following major lower extremity amputation due to vascular disease, 53% to 67% will undergo contralateral amputation within 5 years (98,141). If a patient has wounds on the contralateral side, this should be addressed with vascular evaluation and wound care. If the patient lacks protective sensation, accommodative footwear, foot orthoses, and follow-up with a podiatrist for routine foot care should be recommended.

Determination of Discharge Setting

Another important perioperative rehabilitation team goal is to ensure that the patient can adequately function in their home with or without a prosthesis after discharge. This should include evaluation for adaptive and durable medical equipment needs. If the patient cannot safely function in their home environment after amputation, discharge to a rehabilitation setting is necessary. One study looking at the effect of post-acute discharge setting on mortality and morbidity in patients with limb loss due to vascular disease found that patients who discharged to inpatient rehabilitation had an improved 1-year survival, increased likelihood of being prescribed a prosthesis, decreased hospital readmissions for non-amputation–related causes, and decreased risk of additional amputation compared to those discharged home. In addition, improved 1-year survival and increased likelihood of receiving a prosthetic prescription compared to those discharged to subacute rehabilitation were noted as well. Those discharged to subacute rehabilitation had improved 1-year survival and improved likelihood of receiving a prosthetic prescription compared to those discharged to home (142).

Psychosocial Adjustment

Patients are noted to have higher rates of depression and anxiety in the first 2 years after amputation (143). They may also experience body image disturbance and social discomfort. If persistent, these can contribute to decreased physical functioning, quality of life, and self-esteem, as well as social isolation after amputation. The rehabilitation consultant can play an important role in helping the patient during this period of adjustment by discussing feelings of loss, grief, or anger, providing information on the rehabilitation process after amputation, discussing realistic functional expectations as an amputee, and directing their rehabilitation care to ensure they get needed services. They can also connect the patient with supportive services, such as psychology, peer visitors, or amputee support groups, that can assist with adjustment.

Prosthetic Management

Prosthetic rehabilitation begins when the wound is healed. The rehabilitation process is best accomplished with a comprehensive, multidisciplinary, specialized treatment team including a physiatrist, prosthetist, and physical therapist. The team may also include a rehabilitation psychologist, occupational therapist, recreational therapist, and vocational therapist. The goal of the team is to prevent morbidity and mortality and maximize function following amputation.

After amputation, many patients are focused on the goal of getting a prosthetic leg. They frequently have unrealistic expectations that a prosthesis will simply replace their lost extremity. The rehabilitation team can help them to understand that prosthetic use is one tool to improve function after amputation but that it may not be the best tool for everyone. Other options for mobility include a manual wheelchair or powered mobility. Taking into account the patient's premorbid functional status and their lifestyle and future goals, the rehabilitation team can work with the patient to find the best mobility option to safely achieve these functional goals. It is important to discuss realistic expectations early on. For some patients, the risks and burden of care associated with prosthetic use are not worth the benefit. For others, prosthetic use allows them to regain or improve their preoperative level of function.

Lower extremity muscle strength, particularly of the hip extensors and abductors, and joint range of motion are important to prosthetic ambulation. Joint contractures at the knee or hip increase the challenge of prosthetic fitting and ambulation. Presence of joint contracture has been shown to reduce success of prosthetic ambulation (144).

Musculoskeletal and neurologic evaluation of the remaining extremities is also important. Many patients have comorbid diabetic peripheral neuropathy affecting their intact limbs, which may affect their balance, proprioception, and ability to don and doff a prosthesis. Degenerative joint disease is another common comorbidity that may be a barrier to prosthetic ambulation or, in the upper extremities, to the use of some walking aids.

Cognitive function should be assessed to determine if the patient has the capability to learn how to don and doff a prosthesis, manage sock ply, monitor their residual limb for complications, and relearn how to transfer and walk. Impaired cognition has been shown to correlate with poor functional outcomes following amputation (145,146).

The metabolic cost of prosthetic ambulation is another important consideration. The metabolic cost of ambulation, which is a measure of the economy of ambulation, is greater in persons with limb loss than controls at any speed. These measures are higher in persons with vascular compared to traumatic amputation and in transfemoral compared to transtibial level amputation (116,117). Persons with limb loss walk at slower self-selected walking speed to normalize their metabolic energy expenditure and relative metabolic load. The exception is persons with vascular transfemoral amputation who experience higher metabolic costs of ambulation even at their self-selected walking speed (116,117,147). In patients with vascular amputations who often have comorbid coronary artery disease, it is important to consider whether they will be able to tolerate the increased cardiac work of prosthetic ambulation.

The patient's postoperative level of function is also an important consideration. Studies have shown that one-legged balance after amputation is a strong predictor of successful prosthetic ambulation (145,148). An important part of the evaluation to determine whether a patient is a prosthetic candidate includes having them stand on their sound leg in the parallel bars and hop several lengths of the parallel bars if they can tolerate it. This evaluation assesses lower extremity strength, balance, and cardiovascular endurance. If a patient becomes excessively fatigued or experiences shortness of breath or chest pain, they may not be able to tolerate prosthetic ambulation or may need further medical evaluation.

Taking all of these factors into consideration, every patient with a transtibial level amputation who is motivated to use a prosthesis, can transfer independently, and walk short distances without a prosthesis should be given the opportunity to use a prosthesis, recognizing that it is ultimately the person's choice whether a prosthesis becomes part of his or her daily life. At the transtibial level, even if a patient will not be a prosthetic ambulator, they may benefit from using the prosthesis to transfer. This has the additional benefit of decreasing stress on the contralateral foot. In the person with a vascular transfemoral amputation, the decision of whether or not to prescribe a prosthesis is a matter of clinical judgment, on which even experienced physiatrists may disagree (86). In contrast to the transtibial prosthesis, the transfemoral prosthesis provides no benefit for transfers. Additionally, as previously discussed, the person with a vascular transfemoral amputation experiences increased metabolic cost of prosthetic ambulation.

Knowing the likelihood of successful prosthetic fitting is important in decision-making and counseling of the patient. We examined the medical charts of geriatric amputee residents of Olmsted County, MN, to define better the characteristics and predictors of successful prosthetic fitting in this population (103). Overall, only 71 (36%) of all unilateral geriatric vascular amputee patients were successfully fitted with a prosthesis. Transtibial amputees were more likely to be fitted than transfemoral amputees (47.2% vs. 14.5%, $p < 0.001$). The success rate was much greater in the subgroup of patients who were referred to the amputee clinic with 60 patients (74.1%) being fitted (77.6% of transtibial, 57.1% of transfemoral). However, only 11 (9.3%) of those patients not seen in the clinic were fitted (19.1% of transtibial, 2.9% of transfemoral). These patients were referred by a physician directly to their local prosthetists. Nine (20%) bilateral amputee patients were fitted with both prostheses: 8 of 23 with bilateral transtibial (35%), 1 of 6 with transtibial/transfemoral (17%), and none of 14 bilateral transfemoral (0%). Persons with bilateral amputations who were referred to the amputee clinic were significantly more likely to be successfully fitted (38% vs. 4%, $p = 0.007$). Other population-based studies in Denmark and Finland report similar results with 40% to 50% of lower extremity amputees successfully fit with a prosthesis and increased success among transtibial compared to transfemoral amputees (62% to 66% transtibial vs. 27% to 49% transfemoral) (118,119).

Univariate predictors of successful fit were presence of family member at home ($p = 0.03$), marriage ($p = 0.04$), and diabetes with peripheral neuropathy ($p < 0.001$). Negative predictors of fit on univariate analysis were increased age ($p < 0.001$), CVD ($p = 0.001$), dementia ($p < 0.001$), and transfemoral level ($p < 0.001$). Age greater than 85 ($p < 0.001$), CVD ($p < 0.001$), dementia ($p = 0.002$), and transfemoral level ($p < 0.001$) were negatively associated with prosthetic fit (103).

Whether or not a patient receives a prosthesis, the rehabilitation team will ideally maintain lifelong follow-up. In addition to prosthetic management, the rehabilitation team also manages postamputation complications including dermatologic issues, bone issues, and pain. If a prosthesis is not provided, the rehabilitation team can manage the patient's functional and mobility needs, durable medical equipment, assistive devices, and therapy needs. They also should address any issues on the contralateral foot to prevent further amputation.

Prosthetic Rehabilitation

If the decision is made to prescribe a prosthesis, details of the prosthetic prescription including socket design, suspension, interface, pylon, knee, and foot components are decided upon with input from the prosthetist and the patient. A plan for prosthetic training should be made at this time. Options include outpatient physical therapy, subacute rehabilitation, and inpatient rehabilitation. Once the prosthesis is fabricated, the physiatrist will often evaluate the fit and quality of the limb before or during prosthetic training. A well-fitting prosthesis with appropriate components, supervised training, and ongoing follow-up optimizes prosthetic use and function.

A patient must understand that successful prosthetic and physical rehabilitation is a prerequisite for optimal performance. A state-of-the-art prosthesis will not provide optimal performance to a user who is not physically capable of taking advantage of its features. Conversely, optimal performance will not be achieved with a prosthesis that does not provide a level of technical sophistication that matches or challenges the user's physical capabilities.

Functional Outcomes

Functional outcomes after amputation are highly variable and are often related to age, premorbid function, and medical comorbidities. At 1-year postamputation, functional prosthetic use is reported in 47% to 70% of persons with limb loss (110,112,121,122,127,145). Persons with transtibial level limb loss were more likely to be prosthetic ambulators (60% to 70%) than those with transfemoral level amputation (40% to 50%) (122,127). In one study following postamputation patients for 5 years, the number of prosthetic ambulators had decreased to 17% (112).

Increased age is associated with poor functional outcomes after amputation (122,145,149). Schoppen reported a very

low functional level in amputees over 60 years old (145). Those over 75 years old rarely used a prosthesis or were ambulatory (110).

Premorbid level of function is also predictive of postamputation level of function (128). Patients who are nonambulatory prior to amputation are unlikely to resume ambulation after amputation (110).

Postamputation function is also influenced by the patient's medical and social condition. The number of medical comorbidities is associated with poorer function (128). In particular, chronic obstructive pulmonary disease, end-stage renal disease requiring hemodialysis, diabetes, hypertension, alcohol use disorder, and history of treatment for anxiety or depression are all associated with worse functional outcomes (122,149). On the contrary, white race, being married, and having at least a high school education are associated with better outcomes (122).

A subset of patients experienced improvements in their functional mobility after amputation. Norvell reported that 37% of amputee patients returned to or exceeded their premorbid level of function at 1-year postamputation (149). Johnson also reported that many persons with unilateral transtibial amputation are able to maintain or improve their function after amputation (128). Because patients undergoing vascular lower extremity amputation have often been functionally limited by PAD, foot ulcers, infections, and weight-bearing restrictions sometimes for years prior to amputation, definitive management with amputation surgery can sometimes improve their function.

It has been suggested that persons with amputations comprise two distinct groups: the fit (often traumatic amputation) and the older, medically unfit patient who has vascular disease and a poor prognosis (120). Among this latter group, however, there is a great variation in functional outcome dependent on age, medical status, and other factors. The ability to predict which among these patients are better prosthetic candidates may reduce the costs and burden of care resulting from unsuccessful attempts at prosthetic fitting in this population and allow for earlier focus on other interventions that will increase the patient's independence and quality of life.

Interestingly, when prosthetic fitting patterns were examined over 40 years, no marked changes in the rate of fitting or in wear patterns occurred, despite technologic developments, advances in revascularization procedures, and provision of rehabilitation services. This suggests that a physiologic limit to successful prosthetic fitting may exist in the geriatric patient due to advanced age and comorbidity. This will have implications on health care allocation in the future, as the number of major lower extremity amputations due to dysvascular disease increases (85).

Mortality

Mortality after amputation is very high in the dysvascular population. Thirty-day mortality after amputation is 8% to 10% (109,110,150). 1-Year survival is 60% to 70% and 5-year survival is 35% overall after vascular amputation (109,142).

Certain comorbid conditions also increase risk. Perioperative systemic sepsis, congestive heart failure, renal failure, and liver disease were associated with higher mortality in hospital, at 30 days and at 1 year (109,151). 1-Year and 5-year survival was found to be comparable in patients with diabetes (69.4% and 30.9% survival at 1 and 5 years) but much worse in patients with either end-stage renal disease (51.9% and 14.4% survival at 1 and 5 years) or renal insufficiency (55.9% and 19.4% at 1 and 5 years) (109). Patients with renal insufficiency were also more likely to undergo repeat amputation within 30 days (152).

Higher level of amputation is also associated with increased mortality. Mortality from inhospital to 5 years is higher for those with transfemoral compared to transtibial amputation (109,151). One-year survival was 75% in persons with transtibial compared to 50% with transfemoral amputation. Five-year survival was 38% in persons with transtibial level amputation compared to 23% in persons with transfemoral amputation (109).

Given the high mortality after vascular amputation, it is important to identify appropriate interventions and rehabilitation goals early on to improve mobility, functional independence, and quality of life in the first months and years after amputation. Delayed wound healing will mean more time spent in the hospital, more medical appointments, and greater burden of care over many months. It is important to discuss prognosis and realistic goals with the patient and their family so that they do not spend a prolonged time trying to heal a distal amputation level or attempt prosthetic rehabilitation if they are unlikely to be a functional prosthetic user and may be better served by a more proximal amputation, healing, and wheelchair mobility.

Other Arterial Diseases

Upper Extremity Ischemia

Symptomatic vascular diseases involving the upper extremity are rare in comparison with those involving the lower extremity. However, ischemia caused by vasospasm is much more common in the upper extremities than in the lower extremities. Upper extremity arterial occlusive disease is less common, but more varied in etiology, than disease of the lower extremity; associated vasospastic and microcirculatory disorders are more common. Coolness and color changes are the most common presenting symptoms in upper extremity ischemia (**Fig. 37-5**). Ischemia may be constant or intermittent; may be a manifestation of a fixed arterial obstruction, vasospasm, or both; and may reflect involvement of large proximal arteries, small distal arteries, or the microvasculature. Impairment of the arterial circulation to the upper extremities may result in a variety of symptoms including weakness, intermittent vasospasm, or irreversible tissue loss with digital ulcers, skin necrosis, and gangrene.

The manifestation of acute arterial occlusion of the upper extremity depends on the location and extent of the clot, the pre-existing status of the vascular bed, and the collateral flow. Occlusion of the ulnar artery may be asymptomatic if the radial and palmar arch circulation is intact. In contrast, occlusion of the axillary artery (before the bifurcation of the brachial and profunda brachial artery) will typically result in severe ischemia. Raynaud's phenomenon, connective tissue disease, vasculitis, TAO (Buerger disease), erythromelalgia, acrocyanosis, livedo reticularis, pernio, frost bite, and occupational trauma may result in microvascular disease of the upper extremity (1). Arteriolar constriction is usually well-tolerated. When arteriolar constriction is super imposed on fixed arterial obstruction, previously viable fingers may become ischemic.

Establishing the underlying etiology is essential for both definitive treatment and prognosis. Upper extremity ischemia may cause a significant impairment due to decreased hand function.

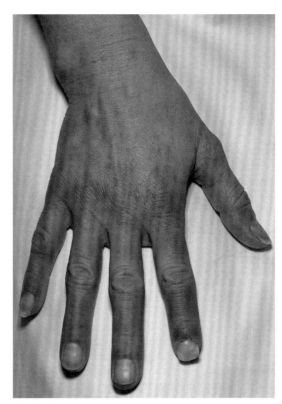

FIGURE 37-5. Upper extremity ischemia in a person with fixed arterial obstruction and vasospasm.

Raynaud Syndrome

Raynaud syndrome is characterized by episodic attacks of vasospasm in response to cold or emotional stress. The fingers and hands are most often affected. In certain cases, the toes and feet may be involved. Classic episodes of vasospasm cause an intense pallor of the distal extremity followed in sequence by cyanosis and rubor on rewarming. Most people with Raynaud syndrome do not experience the complete triple color response. Typically, only pallor or cyanosis is noted during attacks. Generally, the attacks are over within 30 to 60 minutes. Episodes are usually bilateral. Attacks may occur infrequently (some may only have symptoms during the winter), but others may have a significant impairment/disability with multiple daily episodes. Digital ulcerations are rare but may occur. Females are affected more commonly than males. The symptoms may be related to abnormalities in adrenergic function, blood viscosity, or endothelial disorders (153). The normal regulation of blood flow to the fingers is affected by a number of different factors acting by local, humeral, and nervous mechanisms. Disturbance of any of these may predispose to vasospastic attacks. The exact mechanism of digital artery vasospasm remains unknown; however, it is felt to be due to an exaggeration of the normal thermoregulatory system. In clinical practice, it is helpful to differentiate patients with Raynaud syndrome as having either vasospasm or obstructive disease.

Raynaud disease refers to a primary vasospastic disorder where there is no identifiable underlying cause. Raynaud's phenomenon refers to vasospasm, secondary to another underlying condition or disease. Predisposing factors include atherosclerosis, arteritis, cancer, collagen vascular disease, thoracic outlet syndrome, embolic occlusion, occupational disease, and certain medications (153). Secondary Raynaud's phenomenon is occasionally unilateral and may produce skin breakdown. The distinction between Raynaud disease and Raynaud's phenomenon has important clinical utility as it underscores the different pathologic mechanisms, treatment options, and outcomes of these two groups.

Treatment

Treatment of primary Raynaud syndrome may be difficult. Fortunately, the majority of patients with Raynaud disease have only mild-to-moderate symptoms that respond well to conservative measures. Dressing warmly, using mittens rather than gloves, heat conservation, and avoiding unnecessary cold exposure may substantially improve symptoms. Nicotine and drugs with a potential for vasoconstriction should be avoided. Biofeedback is effective in certain cases. If a secondary cause of vasospasm is not identified, often reassurance and patient education are all that is necessary. Occasionally, it is necessary for a patient to move to a warmer climate to achieve complete relief.

Pharmacologic therapy is indicated for patients with severe symptoms whose activities of daily living are affected or those who are at risk of ischemic tissue damage. A number of vasodilator medications have shown to be beneficial for patients with Raynaud syndrome. Calcium channel blockers are the most commonly prescribed medications for vasospasm associated with Raynaud syndrome. Multiple studies have shown dihydropyridines, such as nifedipine, to be effective in reducing the frequency and severity of vasospastic attacks. Alpha-1 blockers such as doxazosin and terazosin may also be of benefit in reducing the frequency and severity of attacks. Angiotensin converting inhibitors and angiotensin-II receptor antagonists may be of benefit in both primary and secondary Raynaud's (153).

Novel therapies for Raynaud syndrome with upper extremity ischemia refractory to standard therapy include (a) prostacyclin, (b) a potent endothelial-derived endothelin blocker bosentan, and (c) an intermittent pneumatic compression (154). Interruption of the sympathetic innervation, either through ganglionic injection or surgical sympathectomy, is reserved for patients with severe symptoms.

Vasculitic Syndrome

Vasculitis, or angiitis, is an inflammatory disease of blood vessels. It often causes damage to the vessel wall, stenosis or occlusion of the vessel lumen by thrombosis, and progressive intimal proliferation. Vasculitic symptoms reflect systemic inflammation and the ischemic consequences of vascular occlusion. The distribution of vascular lesions and the size of the blood vessels involved vary considerably in different vasculitic syndromes and in different patients with the same syndrome. Vasculitis can be transient, chronic, self-limited, or progressive. It can be the primary abnormality or secondary to another systemic process. Histopathologic classification does not distinguish local from systemic illness or secondary from primary insult.

Rheumatoid Vasculitis

Rheumatoid vasculitis usually occurs in patients who have severe deforming arthritis and a high titer of rheumatoid factor (155). The vasculitis is mediated by the deposition of circulating immune complexes on the blood vessel wall with activation of compliment. Proliferation of the vascular intima and media causes an obliterative endarteropathy. Leukocytoclastic, or small vessel vasculitis, produces palpable purpura or cutaneous ulceration. A systemic necrotizing vasculitis, histopathologically indistinguishable from polyarteritis nodosa (PAN), complicates some cases of seropositive rheumatoid arteritis. Rheumatoid arthritis–associated polyarteritis is three times as common as primary polyarteritis. Type II cryoglobulin and vasculitis may complicate many different connective tissue diseases. Cryoglobulin should be assayed in any patient with an autoimmune disease that develops vasculitis (155).

Cryoglobulinemia

Cryoglobulins are immunoglobulins that reversibly precipitate at reduced temperatures. Type I cryoglobulins are aggregates of a single monoclonal immunoglobulin. Patients with type I cryoglobulinemia are often asymptomatic. Type II cryoglobulins are frequently associated with chronic infection (hepatitis C) and immune disorders. The typical presentation of type II cryoglobulinemia is that of a nonsystemic small vessel vasculitis with palpable purpura, urticaria, and cutaneous ulceration. Peripheral neuropathy, arthralgias, and arthritis are common.

Polyarteritis

Polyarteritis occurs by itself (PAN) or in association with another disease (secondary polyarteritis). PAN is an acute necrotizing vasculitis that affects primarily medium-sized and small arteries. It is a systemic disorder that may involve the kidneys, joints, skin, nerves, and various other tissues. Biopsy typically shows necrotizing changes and disruption of the blood vessels (156). If untreated, the systemic form of PAN is associated with a less than 15% survival rate at 5 years. With steroid therapy, the 5-year survival rate increases to more than 50% (156).

Other Vasculitides

A wide variety of other vasculitides may affect small- and medium-size vessels. These include allergic angiitis (Churg-Strauss syndrome), Henoch-Schönlein purpura, various forms of hypersensitivity vasculitis, and numerous nonspecific necrotizing and nonnecrotizing vasculitides. Knowledge of the etiology of an underlying vasculitis is critical for rehabilitation professionals involved in the management of ischemic wounds.

Treatment

General measures should be performed as outlined for patients with PAD. In addition, because vasculitic processes typically involve small vessels (arterioles, venules), gentle compression with a low-stretch wrap or graduated compression stockings (20 to 30 mm Hg) may decrease associated venous congestion and enhance skin perfusion.

Giant Cell Arteritis

Giant cell arteritis often involves the arch, thoracic, and abdominal aorta as well as proximal branch arteries.

Temporal Arteritis

Temporal arteritis primarily affects older individuals (>50 years) and involves branches of the external carotid, brachial, and femoral arteries (157). In an elderly person with a new onset of mild-to-moderate temporal headache, temporal arteritis should be considered. Only about 50% of persons with temporal arteritis have headache or tender temporal arteries. Common symptoms include low-grade fever, jaw claudication, weight loss, anorexia, and other systemic symptoms (157). The erythrocyte sedimentation rate is usually elevated.

Treatment

With vision loss, emergent therapy with corticosteroids is needed. In those with no vision loss, prednisone should be initiated immediately after the diagnosis is made. Temporal biopsy is used to confirm the diagnosis before prescribing long-term prednisone therapy. If the biopsy cannot be performed immediately, prednisone therapy may be initiated until biopsy results are available. High-dose prednisone (40 to 60 mg/daily initially) is usually instituted for 3 to 6 weeks or until the sedimentation rate has stabilized in the normal range. Biopsy results remain accurate, if the biopsy is performed within several days after starting treatment with corticosteroids. Immune-modifying agents may decrease the complications of prolonged steroid suppression. The rate of steroid taper should be modified according to the sedimentation rate and the clinical picture. When surgical correction is necessary, efforts should be made to hold off until the disease has been adequately treated or preferably until it has "burned out." Although angiography can be used to make the diagnosis, biopsy is much more commonly used due to accessibility of the temporal artery. Advances in noninvasive imaging (CT and MR angiography) have increased their diagnostic accuracy and provide a marker to follow disease progression.

Vibration Syndrome

Vibratory tools such as chain saws, grinders, and jackhammers can induce hand dysesthesias and Raynaud's phenomenon when used for several years. Symptoms initially occur during use of the instrument. Subsequently, dysesthesias and cold sensitivity persist when the vibratory tool is not being used. After several years, a late stage can be seen with frank digital artery occlusion, cyanosis, ulceration, and gangrene. Ischemia is a rare and late occurrence (158). The exact mechanism of injury is unknown. Repetitive trauma from the vibration of tools is obviously the main cause of the problem. Both the frequency and the intensity of the vibration affect the extent of damage to the endothelium (159).

Treatment

The treatment of vibration injuries include simple measures and medications outlined for the treatment of Raynaud's phenomenon. In addition, vibration gloves and modifications to decrease vibratory trauma may be of benefit.

Hypothenar Hammer Syndrome

Occlusive disease in the hands can result from trauma to the hypothenar area caused by using the palm of the hand as a hammer in an activity that involves pushing, pounding, or twisting. This results in intimal injury to the ulnar artery as it crosses the hamate bone. When this area is repeatedly traumatized, ulnar or digital arterial spasm, aneurysm, occlusion, or a combination of these lesions can result. This may result in Raynaud's phenomenon and digital ischemia as the artery either becomes aneurysmal and embolizes or occludes (160).

External Iliac Syndrome in Cyclists

Cyclists with high-level training/competition over several years may report claudication (typically, buttock and thigh) followed by heaviness or numbness of the limb. The symptoms often occur under maximal stress (hill climbing or sprinting) with quick relief as the pace is reduced. Pulse and ankle systolic pressures are normal at rest but drop when symptoms are reproduced by strenuous ergometric cycling. The history and clinical findings are compatible with subclinical stenosis that becomes hemodynamically significant with maximal stress. Surgical repair includes segmental resection to shorten the artery, endarterectomy, and ligation of a prominent psoas arterial branch (that may enhance arterial lengthening) when present (161).

VENOUS AND ARTERIAL DISEASE

Thromboangiitis Obliterans (Buerger Disease)

TAO is a segmental disease of the small-to-medium arteries and veins, usually involving more than one extremity. The first manifestation of TAO may be superficial thrombophlebitis. TAO occurs predominantly in young adult male smokers. Few, if any, cases occur in the absence of tobacco use.

There are two distinguishing features of TAO compared with other forms of vasculitis: (a) pathologically, the thrombus is highly cellular with relative sparing (less intense cellular activity) in the wall of the blood vessel; (b) the disease usually affects the small distal arteries first and progresses proximally if smoking continues (162). In addition, the usual immunologic markers (sedimentation rate and CRP, circulating immune complexes, antinuclear antibody, rheumatoid factor, and compliment) are usually normal or negative. It is not known whether the vascular lesions of TAO are primarily thrombotic or inflammatory. In either case, the intense inflammatory infiltration and cellular proliferation seen in the acute-stage lesions are distinctive, especially when the veins are involved. TAO is segmental with angiographic "skip lesions" and histopathologic areas of normal vessel adjacent to diseased segments, often with variable intensity of periadventitial reaction within different segments of the same vessel (163).

Treatment

Cessation of smoking is an absolute necessity. If smoking is discontinued, the disease process is frequently arrested. Other treatments such as antiplatelet therapy and sympathectomy are of variable benefit.

Thoracic Outlet Syndrome

Thoracic outlet syndrome occurs when the brachial plexus, subclavian artery, or subclavian vein becomes compressed in the region of the thoracic outlet. Symptoms are thought to result from nerve compression in 90% to 95% of cases (164). The second most common presentation is venous compression. Repetitive trauma to the artery can lead to intimal damage, embolization, aneurysm formation, or acute thrombosis. Although only a small number of cases of thoracic outlet syndrome are clearly due to arterial compression, thoracic outlet syndrome is the most common cause of acute arterial occlusion in the upper extremity of adults younger than 40 years old and the most common cause of acute upper extremity venous occlusion in the young adult. The cause of arterial thoracic outlet syndrome is often a cervical or rudimentary first rib. Primary venous thoracic outlet syndrome is generally due to the costoclavicular ligament and subclavius muscle compressing the subclavian vein. Arterial involvement is suggested by obliteration of the radial or brachial pulse during provocative maneuvers of the arm (this finding may also be a normal variant). Duplex ultrasound or arteriography can be used to document the presence of a functional hemodynamic change with thoracic outlet maneuvers.

Treatment

Nonsurgical measures, including stretching (scalenes, pectorals, and trapezius muscle) without recreating symptoms, positioning, and avoidance of aggravating factors may be of benefit. If nonsurgical measures fail and symptoms warrant, surgical resection of the first rib is frequently curative. In those with significant arterial involvement (such as intimal damage or aneurysmal formation), the involved section of an artery should be replaced with a graft. Advances in the management of arterial and venous complications include thrombolysis, mechanical thrombectomy, and endovascular stenting. Patients with recent venous thrombosis can have the thrombus cleared with thrombolytic therapy before rib resection. Stenting, if needed, is performed after removal of the first rib and should not be applied if the first rib has not been resected.

VENOUS DISEASE

Venous Thromboembolism

DVT is a serious medical condition that continues to plague immobilized patients and those rehabilitation professionals who care for them. The incidence of venous thromboembolism (VTE) exceeds 1 per 1,000 (165). Of all VTE patients, when including pulmonary embolism, 30% die within 30 days (166). When a patient presents with the possibility of a DVT, predisposing risk factors such as prolonged immobilization during car or plane trips, use of estrogen, prior DVT, or family history of thrombosis should be elicited. Hypercoagulable states such as those associated with cancer or inherited coagulopathies and those caused by vessel wall injury from surgery or local trauma are major predisposing factors for thrombosis. About 30% of surviving patients develop recurrent VTE within 10 years. Independent predictors for recurrence include increasing age, obesity, malignant neoplasm, and extremity paresis. About 28% of patients develop postthrombotic syndrome within 20 years. To reduce VTE incidence, improve survival, and prevent recurrence and complications, patients with these characteristics should receive appropriate prophylaxis (167).

As initially postulated by Virchow, three factors are of primary importance in the development of venous thrombosis: (a) abnormalities of blood flow (especially reduced flow, or *stasis*), (b) abnormalities of blood, and (c) vessel wall injury.

The normal hemostatic response requires interactions among the vessel wall, endothelium, platelets, and the coagulation cascade responsible for thrombin generation. Early phases of thrombosis are marked by increases in permeability followed by leukocyte adhesion, migration, and endothelial disruption (168). Stasis may facilitate endothelial leukocyte adhesion and cause endothelial hypoxia leading to a procoagulant state. In addition, stasis allows the accumulation of activated coagulation factors in areas prone to thrombosis.

Although the hemostatic system is continuously active, thrombus formation is generally confined to sites of local injury by a precise balance between activators and inhibitors of coagulation and fibrinolysis. A prothrombotic state may result from imbalances in the regulatory and inhibitory system or from activation exceeding antithrombotic capacity (169).

Thrombosis may occur anywhere but most commonly involves the deep veins of the lower extremity. Once a thrombus forms, several events may occur: (a) the thrombus may propagate, (b) it may embolize, (c) it may be removed by fibrinolytic activity, or (d) it may undergo organization (including recanalization and retraction). An initial inflammatory response leads to fibroblast and capillary ingrowth, which helps to stabilize the thrombus. Organization occurs over weeks to months as the thrombus becomes incorporated into the vessel wall. Once luminal flow is disturbed, antegrade and retrograde propagation of the thrombus may also be promoted by hemodynamic factors. The competing processes of recanalization and recurrent thrombosis determine the extent of acute DVT and its sequelae. Venous thrombi rarely lyse completely unless they are subjected to pharmacologic lysis.

The natural history and clinical consequences of a lower extremity venous thrombosis depend on the site of thrombus. Because the tibial and peroneal veins run in parallel, a thrombosis confined to one of these veins is unlikely to cause significant obstruction to the outflow of blood. Small calf vein thrombi frequently occur, especially in postoperative patients. A calf thrombosis may remain asymptomatic; half lyse spontaneously without sequelae by natural fibrinolysis (170). Five to twenty percent of calf vein thrombi propagate centrally. If extension occurs into the popliteal or more central veins, the chance of pulmonary embolism increases from less than 5% to about 50% (171). Thrombus isolated to the calf is less dangerous than thrombus in the thigh, but greater than 20% of such thrombi can extend proximally, and 10% embolize. Surveillance of lesions is required if anticoagulants are not used (172). Thrombi involving the central femoral through iliac veins may not undergo spontaneous recanalization even with heparin therapy. A large prospective study evaluating the use of thrombolysis for large central DVT (ATTRACT trial) (173) suggests that patients with iliac vein involvement and those presenting with severe symptoms who received pharmacomechanical catheter-directed thrombolysis in addition to anticoagulation showed decreased incidence of moderate to severe postthrombotic syndrome than those receiving anticoagulation alone.

Phlegmasia Cerulea Dolens

Phlegmasia cerulea dolens is a rare complication of DVT, characterized by rapid and massive lower extremity edema, severe pain, and cyanosis (171). Distal cyanosis may indicate extensive blockage to venous return. Phlegmasia cerulea dolens most commonly occurs with central, iliofemoral obstruction with extensive distal thrombus of deep and superficial veins. The arterial pulses may not be palpable, although anatomically the arteries are patent. In severe cases, gangrene, which may necessitate amputation, occurs (171). Urgent treatment, including placement of a caval filter, heparinization, and surgical thrombectomy or thrombolysis if possible, is essential to minimize loss of life or limb.

Chronic Venous Insufficiency

Chronic venous disease is an important cause of discomfort and disability and is present in a significant percentage of the population worldwide. A clinical score of Clinical-Etiologic-Anatomic-Pathophysiologic has been developed as a standard for reporting venous disease (174).

Many factors can result in the development of venous insufficiency, including heredity, local trauma, thrombosis, and intrinsic defects in the veins or valves themselves. Venous flow is based on a force that pushes the blood proximally, an adequate outflow, and the presence of competent valves limiting reflux. Any disruption of these components results in chronic venous hypertension (175). Normally, the pressure in the leg veins is equal to the hydrostatic pressure from a vertical column of blood extending to the right atrium of the heart. At the ankle level, the hydrostatic pressure is about 90 mm Hg (176). The pumping action of the calf muscles during exercise reduces this venous pressure by two thirds. Even slight muscular movements during normal standing will lower the pressure (176). Patients with venous insufficiency might fail to reduce ankle pressure or show a rapid return of venous pressure to resting levels at the end of exercise. The time required for the ankle vein pressure to return to resting levels after exercise is an indicator of the degree of reflux in the limb. Elevated ambulatory venous pressure is associated with an increased incidence of ulceration (177). When ambulatory venous ankle pressure is below 30 mm Hg, the incidence of ulceration is close to 0%. The incidence of ulceration increases linearly, reaching 100% when the ambulatory venous pressure is greater than 90 mm Hg (177). The superficial leg veins normally carry 10% to 15% of the venous return. Incompetent valves in the superficial veins rarely cause serious venous hypertension, although 10% of patients with venous ulcers have superficial venous incompetence alone.

Postthrombotic syndrome (venous occlusion or valve destruction after thrombosis) develops in 67% to 80% of patients after DVT, although ulcers form in less than 5% of the patients (178). Venous insufficiency may present up to 5 to 10 years after the resolution of the acute episode of thrombosis. Postthrombotic damage in the deep veins is an important cause of chronic venous insufficiency. Advanced venous insufficiency develops only when the valves in the perforator or deep veins are also incompetent. Ultimately, venous hypertension is the result of valve damage and retrograde venous blood flow to the superficial veins. The true mechanism by which venous hypertension leads to induration and fibrosis of the skin (lipodermatosclerosis) and ulceration (**Fig. 37-6**) remains unclear (179).

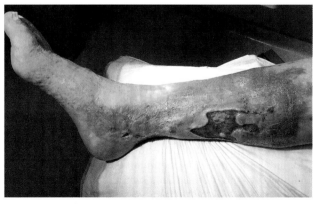

FIGURE 37-6. Chronic venous insufficiency with edema, increased pigmentation, induration, dermatitis, and ulceration.

May-Thurner Syndrome and Pelvic Venous Occlusion

May-Thurner syndrome (iliac vein compression syndrome) is defined as isolated left lower extremity symptoms similar to those seen in venous insufficiency but due to compression of the left iliac vein by the right common iliac artery. Treatment of May-Thurner syndrome has historically involved anticoagulation therapy. Advances in interventional management have allowed relief of the associated mechanical compression by open surgical or endovascular repair. Endovascular stents are the most common treatment. Similarly, chronic occlusion of the common femoral through iliac veins and inferior vena cava can be recanalized percutaneously and stented. Surgical bypass is also an option for chronic iliocaval occlusion.

VENOUS DIAGNOSTIC TESTING

Continuous Wave Doppler

Continuous wave Doppler (described previously) is also used clinically to test the integrity of the venous system. This method can identify the presence of venous obstruction or incompetence, quantify severity of the venous disease, and roughly localize these abnormalities to a particular segment of the limb. The venous flow signal is obtained at several sites in the limb. Normal venous flow is spontaneous and phasic with respiration. With continuous wave Doppler, the patency, spontaneous flow, phasicity, augmentation, competency, and pulsatility of the venous flow are determined and graded. Obstruction of a vein is characterized by either the absence of normal spontaneous venous flow or by the loss of phasic variation with respiration. If the Doppler probe is placed directly over an area of obstruction, there is absence of spontaneous flow. If the probe is placed below the site of obstruction, there is a loss of phasic change in the venous flow with respiration (a monophasic low-frequency signal). Several maneuvers (deep breathing, Valsalva, and distal compression of the calf or forearm) can produce augmentation of venous flow. Because continuous wave Doppler provides subjective information, if positive for obstruction, findings should be followed by an objective test.

Venous Plethysmography

Plethysmography is a noninvasive method of detecting blood volume changes in an extremity (🛜 **eFig. 37-6**). Plethysmographic techniques have been developed to measure the changes in limb volume that occur when venous return is enhanced (venous insufficiency) or impeded (venous obstruction). With normal venous outflow, positional change (leg elevation) or release of an externally inflated cuff results in rapid emptying of the leg veins. If the valves are competent, refilling occurs in an antegrade fashion through the arteries and capillaries. In normal individuals, this takes a minute or more.

With venous incompetence, the leg volume returns to baseline more rapidly than normal. If the incompetence is primarily superficial, tourniquets placed around the leg or using a finger to compress an incompetent superficial vein will normalize the refilling time. In venous obstruction, the peripheral venous pressure and baseline venous volume are elevated (increased venous outflow resistance). In this case, leg elevation or a rapid release of the cuff results in slower emptying of the leg veins.

Segmental plethysmography uses a sleeve to demonstrate changes in limb volume. Sequential timed inflation and deflation of a proximal cuff produces changes in limb volume, which are measured to determine the venous capacitance and maximal venous outflow. The presence of a proximal lower extremity DVT causes (a) minimal change in the limb volume with cuff inflation and (b) a decreased change in limb volume when the cuff is released.

Duplex Ultrasound

Duplex ultrasound (a) directly visualizes and locates intraluminal obstruction, (b) assesses the characteristics of venous flow distal to the inguinal ligament, (c) identifies the presence of collateral veins around an obstructed venous segment, (d) permits direct detection of valvular reflux, (e) allows visualization of specific venous valves and valve leaflet motion, (f) quantitates the degree of incompetence, (g) locates and assesses veins before harvest for bypass procedures, (h) evaluates venous perforator incompetence, and (i) evaluates conditions that may mimic venous disease. Duplex scanning has become the method of choice for testing individual veins of the superficial, deep, and perforating systems.

Contrast Venography

Lower extremity contrast venography remains a powerful, but decreasingly used, tool in the evaluation of both acute and chronic DVT. With advances in duplex ultrasonography, venography has been largely replaced by duplex scanning to evaluate patients with suspected deep venous obstruction or incompetence. In chronic venous disease, ascending venography demonstrates the location and extent of postthrombotic disease, as manifested by occlusion, venous recanalization, collateral channels, and superficial varicosities. Ascending venography may also help with planning of endovascular and open surgical procedures such as iliac and inferior vena cava (IVC) recanalizations and venous bypass grafts. Ascending contrast venography is performed primarily in patients with significant chronic deep venous occlusive disease who are candidates for endovascular treatment with stents, surgical venous bypass, venous valve repair, or valve transplantation.

CT Venous Imaging

The two advantages of CT in venous imaging are the speed and resolution of image acquisition. The disadvantages include radiation exposure and the necessity for administration of iodinated contrast material. Patients with a significant allergic reaction to iodinated contrast material or decreased renal function should be evaluated with alternate imaging techniques.

Magnetic Resonance Imaging

The effectiveness of MRI for detection of DVT has been compared with that of contrast venography in a number of trials. Sensitivity and specificity values as high as 100% have been reported (180). MRI can also be used to distinguish acute from chronic DVT. Because MRI is more expensive than a duplex scan, it is rarely used to diagnose DVT.

TREATMENT OF ACUTE DVT

Standard therapy of acute DVT consists of anticoagulation, elevation, and compression. Of primary importance is the prevention of thrombosis, with recognition of high-risk groups and effective prophylaxis of thromboembolic disease.

Anticoagulants

Anticoagulants remain the main form of treatment for thromboembolic disease. The two goals of anticoagulation are to prevent death from pulmonary embolism and to limit venous damage and subsequent postthrombotic syndrome. Prophylactic anticoagulation is warranted in patients with prior VTE or known clotting disorders that have trauma or undergo medical or surgical treatments with prolonged bed rest. If anticoagulation must be interrupted, consideration could be given to placement of an optionally retrievable IVC filter.

Vena Cava Filters

Vena cava filters are indicated to prevent pulmonary embolism in patients with VTE who have a contraindication to anticoagulation, failed anticoagulation, VTE during pregnancy, preoperative prophylaxis, bariatric surgery, multitrauma and neurosurgery, or orthopedic surgery with a recent DVT (1 month). Anticoagulation should be considered when the temporary contraindication to anticoagulation therapy is no longer present. If a removable filter is used, it can be removed when the thrombosis risk is over or when anticoagulation can be initiated.

TREATMENT FOR CHRONIC VENOUS INSUFFICIENCY

Surgery/Endovenous Management

Treatment of superficial venous reflux is performed via thermal ablation (laser or radiofrequency) or nonthermal ablation (chemical or mechanochemical ablation or sclerotherapy), microphlebectomy, or, uncommonly today, vein stripping or subfascial endoscopic perforator surgery (SEPS).

Thermal ablation. Thermal ablation imparts heat to the refluxing vessel of the superficial system or the refluxing perforator vein, to close the vein. This is performed via a small catheter inserted into the target vein.

Nonthermal ablation. Sclerotherapy (which uses the injection of an irritant substance into the vein) can be used to obliterate incompetent veins in certain settings (175,181). Sclerotherapy is used for the treatment of spider veins, small distal varicose veins, and venous insufficiency resulting from superficial and perforator incompetence. Ultrasound-guided sclerotherapy has been used successfully to treat incompetent perforator veins (182). Complications are rare and usually minor and include skin discoloration, thrombophlebitis, and hematoma formation. The temporary use of elastic compression is suggested after treatment.

Regarding perforating veins, the currently accepted standard is to treat perforating veins (outward flow of greater than 500-ms duration with a diameter of greater than 3.5 mm located beneath a healed or open venous ulcer) with either ultrasound-guided sclerotherapy or endovenous thermal ablation with radiofrequency or laser rather than open ligation or SEPS. In the setting of wounds, it is acceptable to treat the saphenous vein incompetence first with close reevaluation of the incompetent perforators and then a staged approach to the incompetent perforator veins if they remain pathologic (183).

Subfascial endoscopic perforator vein surgery. SEPS is a minimally invasive technique performed in patients with advanced chronic venous insufficiency. The objective of the operation is to interrupt incompetent medial calf perforating veins to decrease venous reflux and reduce ambulatory venous hypertension in critical areas above the ankle where venous ulcers most frequently develop.

Deep vein reconstruction. Surgical bypass may need to be considered in patients with iliac or iliofemoral venous occlusion. Deep vein valve repair or valve transplantation can be attempted in patients with valvular incompetence and venous ulcers. Stenting of the iliofemoral veins and inferior vena cava has emerged as the preferred treatment of venous outflow obstruction. Severe (>50%) in-stent recurrent stenosis of iliofemoral venous stents is uncommon over the short term (184).

Rehabilitation

Because venous hypertension in the upright position and during ambulation is the physiologic cause of the damage in chronic venous insufficiency, the first step of treatment should be to reduce the ambulatory venous pressure. Compression therapy is the mainstay of treatment for chronic venous insufficiency.

Compression. To prevent postthrombotic syndrome, compression stockings should be used routinely following diagnosis of a proximal DVT and continued for a minimum of 1 year (185). Compressive dressings aid venous return by compressing the leg and increasing the interstitial tension. Compression of dilated, engorged, superficial, and intramuscular veins indirectly increases the efficiency of the calf pump mechanism (176).

Patients with severe obstruction of the iliocaval venous outflow track are recalcitrant to compression therapy due to venous claudication resulting in poor healing rates with compression therapy. Stenting of the venous outflow improves the ability of compression to eliminate edema, reduces venous hypertension, and decreases pain and other symptoms in patients with severe chronic venous insufficiency. Patients not responding to compression and/or other treatments should undergo ultrasound or other imaging to evaluate for this condition (183).

With no history of congestive heart failure and no evidence of venous obstruction (on noninvasive studies), lower extremity volume can be stabilized with an intermittent pneumatic compression pump (40 to 50 mm Hg). Compression wraps should be used between pumping sessions. After the volume stabilizes, the patient can be measured for stockings. Elastic stockings should provide graduated compression, exerting most pressure at the ankle, less at the calf, and least at the thigh. Typically, knee-length graduated compression stockings with a pressure of 30 to 40 mm Hg (at the ankles) are prescribed.

When elevation is used for edema control, the extremity is typically elevated above the level of the heart. The patient should lie on a sofa or sit in a recliner to elevate the legs appropriately. The correct duration and frequency of leg elevation should be tailored to the severity of disease. The leg should be elevated whenever possible and long periods of standing or sitting should be avoided. In patients with concomitant arterial disease, modified elevation is used to avoid further compromise of arterial inflow.

Venous ulceration results from an elevated ambulatory venous pressure (venous hypertension). The use of a class III compression is strongly recommended in the treatment of venous ulcers. Compression can be applied successfully using many methods including multilayered elastic compression, inelastic compression, Unna boot, compression stockings, and others. Although these modalities are similar in effectiveness, they can differ significantly in comfort and cost. Patients who use compression stockings regularly had a lower rate of wound recurrence if they used higher level of compression, but significantly fewer patients were able to use the higher level of compression regularly (186). Because venous hypertension is an ongoing condition, a degree of compression therapy should be continued constantly and forever in patients with a history of wounds (183).

The degree of compression must be modified when mixed venous/arterial disease is confirmed during the diagnostic workup (187). Application of moderate amounts of compression may be successful in healing venous leg ulcers in patients with mild-to-moderate arterial insufficiency (188). Intermittent pressure stimulates venous return and can be utilized when constant compression is not tolerated (189).

Exercise. Exercise to increase calf muscle pump function has been demonstrated to be helpful in long-term maintenance of venous ulcer prevention (190). Exercises involving the leg musculature, such as walking, bicycling, or swimming, promote muscle tone in the calf and enhance venous return. Exercise produces variable reductions in venous hypertension. Patients with chronic venous stasis due to incompetent deep vein valves generally do not obtain as much reduction in venous pressure as do those in which the primary defect is due to incompetent perforator valves (191).

SUMMARY

The patient with vascular disease poses a significant challenge to the rehabilitation professional. Arterial or venous dysfunction may be the primary issue or a critical comorbidity in many patients who present to rehabilitation. These diseases may also be present in patients who present for presumably unrelated problems. A detailed vascular history, examination, and selected diagnostic tests should be inherent in the rehabilitation evaluation. When identified early by the rehabilitation professional, interventions including exercise, appropriate compression, modalities, positioning, protection, and proper footwear may help to avoid limb loss.

REFERENCES

1. Hirsh AT, Haskal ZJ, Hertzer NR, et al. ACC/AHA Guidelines for the Management of Patients with Peripheral Arterial Disease (lower extremity, renal, mesenteric, and abdominal aortic): a collaborative report from the American Associations for Vascular Surgery/Society for Vascular Surgery, Society for Cardiovascular Angiography and Interventions, Society for Vascular Medicine and Biology, Society of Interventional Radiology, and the ACC/AHA Task Force on Practice Guidelines. *J Vasc Interventional Radiol.* 2006;17:1383–1397.
2. Allen EV, Barker NW, Hines EA. *Peripheral Vascular Diseases.* 3rd ed. Philadelphia, PA: WB Saunders; 1962.
3. McDaniel MD, Cronenwett JL. Basic data related to the natural history of intermittent claudication. *Ann Vasc Surg.* 1989;3:273–277.
4. Nogren L, Haitt WR, Dormandy JA, et al. Inter-society consensus for the management of peripheral arterial disease (TASC II). *J Vasc Surg.* 2007;45:S5–S67.
5. Becker F, Robert-Ebadi H, Ricco JB, et al. Chapter I: Definitions, epidemiology, clinical presentation and prognosis. *Eur J Vasc Endovasc Surg.* 2011;42:S4–S12.
6. Jacob S, Nassef A, Belli AM, et al. Vascular surgical society of Great Britain and Ireland: distal venous arterialization for non-reconstructable arterial disease. *Br J Surg.* 1999;86:694.
7. Yao ST. Haemodynamic studies in peripheral arterial disease. *Br J Surg.* 1970; 57:761–766.

8. Criqui MH, Denenberg JO. The generalized nature of atherosclerosis: how peripheral arterial disease may predict adverse events from coronary artery disease. *Vasc Med.* 1998;3(3):241–245.
9. McKenna M, Wolfson S, Kuller L. The ratio of ankle and arm arterial pressure as an independent predictor of mortality. *Atherosclerosis.* 1991;87:119–128.
10. Darling RC, Raines JK, Brener BJ, et al. Quantitative segmental pulse volume recorder: a clinical tool. *Surgery.* 1972;72:873–877.
11. Symes JF, Graham AM, Mousseau M. Doppler waveform analysis versus segmental pressure and pulse-volume recording: assessment of occlusive disease in the lower extremity. *Can J Surg.* 1984;27:345–347.
12. Bacharach JM, Rooke TW, Osmundson PJ, et al. Predictive value of transcutaneous oxygen pressure and amputation success by use of supine and elevation measurements. *J Vasc Surg.* 1992;15:558–563.
13. Kram HB, Appel PL, Shoemaker WC. Multisensor transcutaneous oximetric mapping to predict below-knee amputation wound healing: use of a critical Po2. *J Vasc Surg.* 1989;9:796–800.
14. Carpenter JP, Owen RS, Holland GA, et al. Magnetic resonance angiography of the aorta, iliac, and femoral arteries. *Surgery.* 1994;1116:17–23.
15. Thomsen HS, Marckmann P, Logager VB. Enhanced computed tomography or magnetic resonance imaging: a choice between contrast medium-induced nephropathy and nephrogenic system fibrosis? *Acta Radiol.* 2007;48:593–596.
16. Peak AS, Sheller A. Risk factors for developing gadolinium-induced nephrogenic systemic fibrosis. *Ann Pharmacother.* 2007;41:1481–1485.
17. D'Elia JA, Gleason RE, Alday M, et al. Nephrotoxicity from angiographic contrast material: a prospective study. *Am J Med.* 1982;72:719–775.
18. Waugh JR, Sacharias N. Arteriographic complications in the DSA era. *Radiology.* 1992;182:243–246.
19. Ouriel K, Veith FJ, Sasahara AA. Thrombolysis or peripheral arterial surgery: phase I results. TOPAS Investigators. *J Vasc Surg.* 1996;23:64–73.
20. Clarke R, Daly L, Robinson K, et al. Hyperhomocystinemia: an independent risk factor for vascular disease. *N Engl J Med.* 1991;324:1149–1155.
21. Graham IM, Daly LE, Refsum HM, et al. Plasma homocysteine as a risk factor for vascular disease: the European Concerted Action Project. *JAMA.* 1997;277:1775–1781.
22. Ostergren J, Sleight P, Dagenais G, et al. HOPE study investigators: impact of ramipril in patients with evidence of clinical or subclinical peripheral arterial disease. *Eur Heart J.* 2004;25:17–24.
23. Ridker PM, Cushman M, Stampfer MJ, et al. Plasma concentration of C-reactive protein and risk of developing peripheral vascular disease. *Circulation.* 1998;97:425–428.
24. Holm J, Schersten T. Anticoagulant treatment during and after embolectomy. *Acta Chir Scand.* 1972;138:683–687.
25. Rice TW, Lumsden AB. Optimal medical management of peripheral arterial disease. *Vasc Endovascular Surg.* 2006;40:312–327.
26. Criqui MH, Langer RD, Fronek A, et al. Mortality over a period of 10 years in patients with peripheral arterial disease. *N Engl J Med.* 1992;326:381–386.
27. Leng GC, Fowkes FG, Lee AJ, et al. Use of ankle brachial pressure index to predict cardiovascular events and death: a cohort study. *BMJ.* 1996;313:1440–1444.
28. Leng GC, Lee AJ, Fowkes FG, et al. Incidence, natural history and cardiovascular events in symptomatic and asymptomatic peripheral arterial disease in the general population. *Int J Epidemiol.* 1996;25:1172–1181.
29. Ubbink DT, Vermeulen H, Spincemaille GH, et al. Systematic review and meta-analysis of controlled trials assessing spinal cord stimulation for inoperable critical leg ischaemia. *Br J Surg.* 2004;91:948–955.
30. Marso SP, Hiatt WR. Peripheral arterial disease in patients with diabetes. *J Am Coll Cardiol.* 2006;47:921–929.
31. Jonason T, Bergstrom R. Cessation of smoking in patients with intermittent claudication: effects on the risk of peripheral vascular complications, myocardial infarction and mortality. *Acta Med Scand.* 1987;221:253–260.
32. Rooke TW, Hirsch AT, Misra S, et al. 2011 ACCF/AHA focused updated of the guideline for the management of patients with peripheral artery disease (updating the 2005 guideline): a report of the American College of Cardiology Foundation/American Heart Association Task Force on Practice Guidelines. *Circulation.* 2011;124:2020–2045.
33. Shahin Y, Barnes R, Barakat H, et al. Meta-analysis of angiotensin converting enzyme inhibitors effect on walking ability and ankle brachial pressure index in patients with intermittent claudication. *Atherosclerosis.* 2013;231:283–290.
34. Coffman JD. Drug therapy: vasodilator drugs in peripheral vascular disease. *N Engl J Med.* 1979;300:713–717.
35. Radack K, Deck C. Beta-adrenergic blocker therapy does not worsen intermittent claudication in subjects with peripheral arterial disease: a meta-analysis of randomized controlled trials. *Arch Intern Med.* 1991;151:1769–1776.
36. Kim CK, Schmalfuss CM, Schofield RS, et al. Pharmacological treatment of patients with peripheral arterial disease. *Drugs.* 2003;63:637–647.
37. Hood SC, Moher D, Barber GG. Management of intermittent claudication with pentoxifylline: meta-analysis of randomized controlled trials. *CMAJ.* 1996;155:1053–1056.
38. Davies MG, Waldman DL, Pearson TA. Comprehensive endovascular therapy for femoropopliteal arterial atherosclerotic occlusive disease. *J Am Coll Surg.* 2005;201:275–296.
39. Taylor GI, Palmer JH. The vascular territories (angiosomes) of the body: experimental study and clinical applications. *Br J Plast Surg.* 1987;40:113–141.
40. Attinger CE, Evans KK, Bulan E, et al. Angiosomes of the foot and ankle and clinical implications for limb salvage: reconstruction, incisions, and revascularization. *Plast Reconstr Surg.* 2006;117:261S–293S.
41. Adam DJ, Beard JD, Cleveland T, et al. Bypass versus angioplasty in severe ischaemia of the Leg (BASIL): multicentre, randomized, controlled trial. *Lancet.* 2005;366:1925–1934.
42. Bradbury AW, Adam DJ, Bell J, et al. Bypass versus angioplasty in severe ischaemia of the leg (BASIL) trial: a description of the severity and extent of disease using the Bollinger angiogram scoring method and the TransAtlantic Inter-Society Consensus II classification. *J Vasc Surg.* 2010;51:32S–42S.
43. Egorova NN, Guillerme S, Gelijn A, et al. An analysis of the outcomes of a decade of experience with lower extremity revascularization including limb salvage, lengths of stay, and safety. *J Vasc Surg.* 2010;51:878–885.
44. Fernandez N, McEnaney R, Marone LK, et al. Multilevel versus isolated endovascular tibial interventions for critical limb ischemia. *J Vasc Surg.* 2011;54:722–729.
45. Sachs T, Pomposelli F, Hamdan A, et al. Trends in the national outcomes and costs for claudication in limb threatening ischemia: angioplasty versus bypass graft. *J Vasc Surg.* 2011;54:1021–1031.
46. Venkatachalam S, Bunte M, Monteleone P, et al. Combined antegrade-retrograde intervention to improve chronic total occlusion recanalization in high-risk critical limb ischemia. *Ann Vasc Surg.* 2014;28:1439–1448.
47. TASC Steering Committee; Jaff MR, White CJ, et al. An update on methods for revascularization and expansion of the TASC lesion classification to include below-the-knee arteries: a supplement to the inter-society consensus for the management of peripheral arterial disease (TASC II). *Vasc Med.* 2015;20:465–478.
48. Antonopoulos CN, Mylonas SN, Konstantinos G, et al. A network meta-analysis of randomized controlled trials comparing treatment modalities for de novo superficial femoral artery occlusive lesions. *J Vasc Surg.* 2017;65:234–245.
49. Sabeti S, Schillinger M, Amighi J, et al. Primary patency of femoropopliteal arteries treated with nitinol versus stainless steel self-expanding stents: propensity score-adjusted analysis. *Radiology.* 2004;232:516–521.
50. Schillinger M, Sabeti S, Loewe C, et al. Balloon angioplasty versus implantation of nitinol stents in the superficial femoral artery. *N Engl J Med.* 2006;2006:1879–1888.
51. Wolfram RM, Budinsky AC, Pokrajac B, et al. Endovascular brachytherapy for prophylaxis of restenosis after femoropopliteal angioplasty: five-year follow-up—prospective randomized study. *Radiology.* 2006;240:878–884.
52. Yilmaz S, Sindel T, Luleci E. Subintimal versus intraluminal recanalization of chronic iliac occlusions. *J Endovasc Ther.* 2004;11:107–118.
53. Akkus NI, Abdulbaki A, Jimenez E, et al. Atherectomy devices: technology update. *Med Devices (Auckl).* 2014;8:1–10.
54. Brewster DC. Current controversies in the management of aortoiliac occlusive disease. *J Vasc Surg.* 1997;25:365–379.
55. Belkin M, Conte MS, Donaldson MC, et al. The impact of gender on the results of arterial bypass with in situ greater saphenous vein. *Am J Surg.* 1995;170:97–102.
56. Shah DM, Darling RC III, Chang BB, et al. Long-term results of in situ saphenous vein bypass: analysis of 2058 cases. *Ann Surg.* 1995;222:438–446.
57. Gloviczki P, Bower TC, Toomey BJ, et al. Microscope-aided pedal bypass is an effective and low-risk operation to salvage the ischemic foot. *Am J Surg.* 1994;168:76–84.
58. Panneton JM, Gloviczki P, Bower TC, et al. Pedal bypass for limb salvage: impact of diabetes on long-term outcome. *Ann Vasc Surg.* 2000;14:640–647.
59. McDaniel MD, Macdonald PD, Haver RA, et al. Published results of surgery for aortoiliac occlusive disease. *Ann Vasc Surg.* 1997;11:425–441.
60. Mills JL, Harris EJ, Taylor LM Jr, et al. The importance of routine surveillance of distal bypass grafts with duplex scanning: a study of 379 reversed vein grafts. *J Vasc Surg.* 1990;12:378–386.
61. Gloviczki P, Kalra MS, Bower TC. Limits of distal revascularization of limbs with critical ischemia: are multiple procedures in high-risk patients justified? *Cardiovasc Surg.* 2001;9:12.
62. Rhodes JM, Gloviczki P, Bower TC, et al. The benefits of secondary interventions in patients with failing or failed pedal bypass grafts. *Am J Surg.* 1999;178:151–155.
63. McFalls EO, Ward HB, Moritz TE, et al. Coronary-artery revascularization before elective major vascular surgery. *N Engl J Med.* 2004;351:2795–2804.
64. Rivers SP, Scher LA, Gupta SK, et al. Safety of peripheral vascular surgery after recent acute myocardial infarction. *J Vasc Surg.* 1990;11:70–75.
65. Hiatt WR, Regensteiner JG, Hargarten ME, et al. Benefit of exercise conditioning for patients with peripheral arterial disease. *Circulation.* 1990;81:602–609.
66. Hiatt WR, Regensteiner JG. Exercise rehabilitation in the treatment of patients with peripheral arterial disease. *J Vasc Med Biol.* 1990;2:163.
67. Regensteiner JG, Wolfel EE, Brass EP, et al. Chronic changes in skeletal muscle histology and function in peripheral arterial disease. *Circulation.* 1993;87:413–421.
68. Dahllof AG, Holm J, Schersten T, et al. Peripheral arterial insufficiency, effect of physical training on walking tolerance, calf blood flow, and blood flow resistance. *Scand J Rehabil Med.* 1976;8:18.
69. Larsen OA, Lassen NA. Effect of daily muscular exercise in patients with intermittent claudication. *Lancet.* 1996;2:1093–1096.
70. Hiatt WR, Wolfel EE, Meier RH, et al. Superiority of treadmill walking exercise versus strength training for patients with peripheral arterial disease: implications for the mechanism of the training response. *Circulation.* 1994;90:1866–1874.
71. Gardner AW, Poehlman ET. Exercise rehabilitation programs for the treatment of claudication pain: a meta-analysis. *JAMA.* 1995;274:975–980.
72. Zwierska I, Walker RD, Choksy SA, et al. Upper- vs lower-limb aerobic exercise rehabilitation in patients with symptomatic peripheral arterial disease: a randomized control trial. *J Vasc Surg.* 2005;42:1122–1130.
73. Chiriano J, Bianchi C, Teruya TH, et al. Management of lower extremity wounds in patients with peripheral arterial disease: a stratified conservative approach. *Ann Vasc Surg.* 2010;24:1110–1116.

74. Moran PS, Teljeur C, Harrington P, et al. A systematic review of intermittent pneumatic compression for critical limb ischemia. *Vasc Med.* 2005;20(1):41–50.

75. van Bemmelen PS, Gitlitz DB, Faruqi RM, et al. Limb salvage using high pressure intermittent compression arterial assist device in cases unsuitable for surgical revascularization. *Arch Surg.* 2001;136:1280–1285.

76. Louridas G, Saadia R, Spelay J, et al. The art-assist device in chronic lower extremity ischemia: a pilot study. *Int Angiol.* 2002;21(1):28–35.

77. Montori VM, Kavros SJ, Walsh EE, et al. Intermittent compression pump for non-healing wounds in patients with limb ischemia. The Mayo Clinic experience (1998–2000). *Int Angiol.* 2002;24:360–366.

78. Sultan S, Hamada N, Sylou E, et al. Sequential compression biomechanical device in patients with critical limb ischemia and nonreconstructible peripheral vascular disease. *J Vasc Surg.* 2011;54:440–447.

79. Kakkos SK, Geroulakos G, Nicolaides AN. Improvement of the walking ability in intermittent claudication due to superficial femoral artery occlusion with supervised exercise and pneumatic foot and calf compression: a randomized control trial. *Eur J Vasc Endovasc Surg.* 2005;30:164–175.

80. Koch CA. External leg compression in the treatment of vascular disease. *Angiology.* 1997;48:S3–S15.

81. Delis KT, Nicolaides AN. Effect of intermittent pneumatic compression of foot and calf, on walking distance, hemodynamics, and quality of life in patients with arterial claudication: a prospective randomized controlled study with 1-year follow up. *Ann Surg.* 2005;241:431–441.

82. Rooke TW, Osmundson PJ. Effect of intermittent venous occlusion on transcutaneous oxygen tension in lower limbs with severe arterial occlusive disease. *Int J Cardiol.* 1988;21:76–78.

83. Rajagopalan S, Mohler E, Lederman RJ, et al. Regional angiogenesis with vascular endothelial growth factor trial. Regional angiogenesis with vascular endothelial growth factor (VEGF) in peripheral arterial disease: design of the RAVE trial. *Am Heart J.* 2003;145:1114–1118.

84. Ziegler-Graham K, MacKenzie EJ, Ephraim PL, et al. Estimating the prevalence of limb loss in the United States: 2005 to 2050. *Arch Phys Med Rehabil.* 2008;89:422–429.

85. Fletcher DD, Andrews KL, Hallett JW Jr, et al. Trends in rehabilitation after amputation for geriatric patients with vascular disease: implications for future health resource allocation. *Arch Phys Med Rehabil.* 2002;83:1389–1393.

86. Frieden RA, Brar AK, Esquenazi A, et al. Fitting an older patient with medical comorbidities with a lower-limb prosthesis. *PM R.* 2012;4:56–64.

87. Dillingham TR, Pezzin LE, MacKenzie EJ. Limb amputation and limb deficiency: epidemiology and recent trends in the United States. *South Med J.* 2002;95:875–883.

88. Ephraim PL, Dillingham TR, Sector M, et al. Epidemiology of limb loss and congenital limb deficiency: a review of the literature. *Arch Phys Med Rehabil.* 2003;84:747–761.

89. Dillingham TR, Pezzin LE, Shore AD. Reamputation, mortality, and health care costs among persons with dysvascular lower-limb amputations. *Arch Phys Med Rehabil.* 2005;86:480–486.

90. Dillon MP, Kohler F, Peeva V. Incidence of lower limb amputation in Australian hospitals from 2000 to 2010. *Prosthet Orthot Int.* 2014;38:122–132.

91. Ahmad N, Thomas GN, Gill P, et al. The prevalence of major lower limb amputation in the diabetic and non-diabetic population of England 2003-2013. *Diab Vasc Dis Res.* 2016;13:348–353.

92. Hallett JW Jr, Byrne J, Gayari MM, et al. Impact of arterial surgery and balloon angioplasty on amputation: a population-based study of 1155 procedures between 1973 and 1992. *J Vasc Surg.* 1997;25:29–38.

93. Lindholt JS, Bovling S, Fasting H, et al. Vascular surgery reduces the frequency of lower limb major amputations. *Eur J Vasc Surg.* 1994;8:31–35.

94. Mayfield JA, Reiber GE, Maynard C, et al. Trends in lower limb amputation in the Veterans Health Administration, 1989–1998. *J Rehabil Res Dev.* 2000;37:23–30.

95. Luther M. The influence of arterial reconstructive surgery on the outcome of critical leg ischaemia. *Eur J Vasc Surg.* 1994;8:682–689.

96. Most RS, Sinnock P. The epidemiology of lower extremity amputations in diabetic individuals. *Diabetes Care.* 1983;6:87–91.

97. Siitonen OI, Niskanen LK, Laakso M, et al. Lower-extremity amputations in diabetic and nondiabetic patients. A population-based study in eastern Finland. *Diabetes Care.* 1993;16(1):16–20.

98. Shah SK, Bena JF, Allemang MT, et al. Lower extremity amputations: factors associated with mortality or contralateral amputation. *Vasc Endovascular Surg.* 2013;47:608–613.

99. Icks A, Haastert B, Trautner C, et al. Incidence of lower-limb amputations in the diabetic compared to the non-diabetic population. findings from nationwide insurance data, Germany, 2005–2007. *Exp Clin Endocrinol Diabetes.* 2009;117:500–504.

100. Global Lower Extremity Amputation Study Group. Epidemiology of lower extremity amputation in centres in Europe, North America and East Asia. The Global Lower Extremity Amputation Study Group. *Br J Surg.* 2000;87:328–337.

101. Eggers PW, Gohdes D, Pugh J. Nontraumatic lower extremity amputations in the Medicare end-stage renal disease population. *Kidney Int.* 1999;56:1524–1533.

102. Clark SC, Blue B, Bearer JB. Rehabilitation of the elderly amputee. *J Am Geriatr Soc.* 1983;31:439–448.

103. Fletcher DD, Andrews KL, Butters MA, et al. Rehabilitation of the geriatric vascular amputee patient: a population-based study. *Arch Phys Med Rehabil.* 2001;82:776–779.

104. Feinglass J, Brown A, LoSasso MW, et al. Rates of lower-extremity amputation and arterial reconstruction in the United States, 1979 to 1996. *Am J Public Health.* 1999;89:1222–1227.

105. Pollard J, Hamilton GA, Rush SM, et al. Mortality and morbidity after transmetatarsal amputation: retrospective review of 101 cases. *J Foot Ankle Surg.* 2006;45:91–97.

106. Nguyen TH, Gordon IL, Whalen D, et al. Transmetatarsal amputation: predictors of healing. *Am Surg.* 2006;72:973–977.

107. Landry GJ, Silverman DA, Liem TK, et al. Predictors of healing and functional outcome following transmetatarsal amputations. *Arch Surg.* 2001;146:1005–1009.

108. Mueller M, Allen BT, Sinacore DR. Incidence of skin breakdown and higher amputation after transmetatarsal amputation: implications for rehabilitation. *Arch Phys Med Rehabil.* 1995;76:50–54.

109. Aulivola B, Hile CN, Hamdan AD, et al. Major lower extremity amputation: outcome of a modern series. *Arch Surg.* 2004;139:395–399; discussion 9.

110. Nehler MR, Coll JR, Hiatt JG, et al. Functional outcome in a contemporary series of major lower extremity amputations. *J Vasc Surg.* 2003;38:7–14.

111. Barber GG, McPhail NV, Scobie TK, et al. A prospective study of lower limb amputations. *Can J Surg.* 1983;26:339–341.

112. McWhinnie DL, Gordon AC, Collin J, et al. Rehabilitation outcome 5 years after 100 lower-limb amputations. *Br J Surg.* 1994;81:1596–1599.

113. Dillon MP, Fatone S. Deliberations about the functional benefits and complications of partial foot amputation: do we pay heed to the purported benefits at the expense of minimizing complications? *Arch Phys Med Rehabil.* 2013;94:1429–1435.

114. Goktepe AS, Cakir B, Yilmaz B, et al. Energy expenditure of walking with prostheses: comparison of three amputation levels. *Prosthet Orthot Int.* 2010;34:31–36.

115. Quigley M, Dillon MP, Duke EJ. Comparison of quality of life in people with partial foot and transtibial amputation: a pilot study. *Prosthet Orthot Int.* 2016;40:467–474.

116. Waters RL, Perry J, Antonelli D, et al. Energy cost of walking of amputees: the influence of level of amputation. *J Bone Joint Surg Am.* 1976;58:42–46.

117. Wezenberg D, van der Woude LH, Faber WX, et al. Relation between aerobic capacity and walking ability in older adults with a lower-limb amputation. *Arch Phys Med Rehabil.* 2013;94:1714–1720.

118. Pohjolainen T, Alaranta H, Wikstrom J. Primary survival and prosthetic fitting of lower limb amputees. *Prosthet Orthot Int.* 1989;13:63–69.

119. Christensen S. Lower extremity amputations in the county of Aalborg 1961–1971. Population study and follow-up. *Acta Orthop Scand.* 1976;47:329–334.

120. Houghton AD, Taylor PR, Thurlow S, et al. Success rates for rehabilitation of vascular amputees: implications for preoperative assessment and amputation level. *Br J Surg.* 1992;79:753–755.

121. Pohjolainen T, Alaranta H, Karkkainen M. Prosthetic use and functional and social outcome following major lower limb amputation. *Prosthet Orthot Int.* 1990;14:75–79.

122. Czerniecki JM, Turner AP, Wiliams RM, et al. The development and validation of the AMPREDICT model for predicting mobility outcome after dysvascular lower extremity amputation. *J Vasc Surg.* 2017;65:162–171.

123. Siriwardena GJ, Bertrand PV. Factors influencing rehabilitation of arteriosclerotic lower limb amputees. *J Rehabil Res Dev.* 1991;28:35–44.

124. Davis WC, Blanchard RS, Jackson FC. Rehabilitation of the geriatric amputee: a plea for moderation. *Arch Phys Med Rehabil.* 1967;48:31–36.

125. Andrews KL. Rehabilitation in limb deficiency 3. The geriatric amputee. *Arch Phys Med Rehabil.* 1996;77:S14–S17.

126. Kihn RB, Warren R, Beebe GW. The "geriatric" amputee. *Ann Surg.* 1972;176:305–314.

127. Taylor SM, Kalbaugh CA, Blackhurst DW, et al. Preoperative clinical factors predict postoperative functional outcomes after major lower limb amputation: an analysis of 553 consecutive patients. *J Vasc Surg.* 2005;42:227–235.

128. Johnson VJ, Kondziela S, Gottschalk F. Pre and post-amputation mobility of transtibial amputees: correlation to medical problems, age and mortality. *Prosthet Orthot Int.* 1995;19:159–164.

129. Karakousis CP, Emrich LJ, Driscoll DL. Variants of hemipelvectomy and their complications. *Am J Surg.* 1989;158:404–408.

130. Senchenkov A, Moran SL, Petty PM, et al. Soft-tissue reconstruction of external hemipelvectomy defects. *Plast Reconstr Surg.* 2009;124:144–155.

131. Polfer EM, Tintle SM, Forsberg JA, et al. Skin grafts for residual limb coverage and preservation of amputation length. *Plast Reconstr Surg.* 2015;136:603–609.

132. Kent T, Yi C, Livermore M, et al. Skin grafts provide durable end-bearing coverage for lower-extremity amputations with critical soft tissue loss. *Orthopedics.* 2013;36:132–135.

133. Thomas SR, Perkins JM, Magee TR, et al. Transmetatarsal amputation: an 8-year experience. *Ann R Coll Surg Engl.* 2001;83:164–166.

134. Churilov I, Churilov L, Murphy D. Do rigid dressings reduce the time from amputation to prosthetic fitting? A systematic review and meta-analysis. *Ann Vasc Surg.* 2014;28:1801–1808.

135. Sumpio B, Shine SR, Mahler D, et al. A comparison of immediate postoperative rigid and soft dressings for below-knee amputations. *Ann Vasc Surg.* 2013;27:774–780.

136. Mazari FA, Mockford K, Barnett C, et al. Hull early walking aid for rehabilitation of transtibial amputees—randomized controlled trial (HEART). *J Vasc Surg.* 2010;52:1564–1571.

137. Ali MM, Loretz L, Shea A, et al. A contemporary comparative analysis of immediate postoperative prosthesis placement following below-knee amputation. *Ann Vasc Surg.* 2013;27:1146–1153.

138. Samuelsen BT, Andrews KL, Houdek MT, et al. The impact of immediate postoperative prosthesis on patient mobility and quality of life after transtibial amputation. *Am J Phys Med Rehabil.* 2017;96(2):116–119.

139. Smith DG, McFarland LV, Sangeorzan BJ, et al. Postoperative dressing and management strategies for transtibial amputations: a critical review. *J Rehabil Res Dev.* 2003;40:213–224.

140. Esquenazi A, DiGiacomo R. Rehabilitation after amputation. *J Am Podiatr Med Assoc.* 2001;91:13–22.

141. Izumi Y, Satterfield K, Lee S, et al. Risk of reamputation in diabetic patients stratified by limb and level of amputation: a 10-year observation. *Diabetes Care.* 2006;29:566–570.

142. Dillingham TR, Pezzin LE. Rehabilitation setting and associated mortality and medical stability among persons with amputations. *Arch Phys Med Rehabil.* 2008;89:1038–1045.

143. Horgan O, MacLachlan M. Psychosocial adjustment to lower-limb amputation: a review. *Disabil Rehabil.* 2004;26:837–850.

144. Munin MC, Espejo-De Guzman MC, Boninger ML, et al. Predictive factors for successful early prosthetic ambulation among lower-limb amputees. *J Rehabil Res Dev.* 2001;38:379–384.

145. Schoppen T, Boonstra A, Groothoff JW, et al. Physical, mental, and social predictors of functional outcome in unilateral lower-limb amputees. *Arch Phys Med Rehabil.* 2003;84:803–811.

146. Williams R, Turner AP, Green M, et al. Relationship between cognition and functional outcomes after dysvascular lower extremity amputation: a prospective study. *Am J Phys Med Rehabil.* 2015;94:707–717.

147. Czerniecki JM, Morgenroth DC. Metabolic energy expenditure of ambulation in lower extremity amputees: what have we learned and what are the next steps? *Disabil Rehabil.* 2017;39:143–151.

148. Chin T, Sawamura S, Fujita H, et al. %VO2max as an indicator of prosthetic rehabilitation outcome after dysvascular amputation. *Prosthet Orthot Int.* 2002;26:44–49.

149. Norvell DC, Turner AP, Williams RM, et al. Defining successful mobility after lower extremity amputation for complications of peripheral vascular disease and diabetes. *J Vasc Surg.* 2011;54:412–419.

150. Collins TC, Johnson M, Daley J, et al. Preoperative risk factors for 30-day mortality after elective surgery for vascular disease in Department of Veterans Affairs hospitals: is race important? *J Vasc Surg.* 2001;34:634–640.

151. Bates B, Stineman MG, Reker DM, et al. Risk factors associated with mortality in veteran population following transtibial or transfemoral amputation. *J Rehabil Res Dev.* 2006;43:917–928.

152. O'Hare AM, Feinglass J, Reiber GE, et al. Postoperative mortality after nontraumatic lower extremity amputation in patients with renal insufficiency. *J Am Soc Nephrol.* 2004;15:427–434.

153. Shepherd RF, Shepherd JT. Raynaud's phenomenon. *Int Angiol.* 1992;11:41–45.

154. Pfizenmaier DH, Kavros SJ, Liedl DA, et al. Use of intermittent pneumatic compression for treatment of upper extremity vascular ulcers. *Angiology.* 2005;56:417–422.

155. Scott DG, Bacon PA, Tribe CR. Systemic rheumatoid vasculitis: a clinical and laboratory study of 50 cases. *Medicine (Baltimore).* 1981;60:288–297.

156. Cohen RD, Conn DL, Ilstrup DM. Clinical features, prognosis, and response to treatment in polyarteritis. *Mayo Clin Proc.* 1980;55:146–155.

157. Huston KA, Hunder GG, Lie JT, et al. Temporal arteritis: a 25-year epidemiologic, clinical, and pathologic study. *Ann Intern Med.* 1978;88:162–167.

158. National Institute of Occupational Safety and Health. *Vibration Syndrome: Current Intelligence Bulletin 38.* Washington, DC; 1982. Available from: https://www.cdc.gov/niosh/docs/83-110/default.html

159. Nerem RM. Vibration-induced arterial shear stress: the relationship to Raynaud's phenomenon. *Arch Environ Health.* 1973;26:105–110.

160. Conn J Jr, Bergan JJ, Bell JL. Hypothenar hammer syndrome: posttraumatic digital ischemia. *Surgery.* 1970;68:1122–1128.

161. Rousselet MC, Saint-Andre JP, L'Hoste P, et al. Stenotic intimal thickening of the external iliac artery in competition cyclists. *Hum Pathol.* 1990;21:524–529.

162. Papa M, Bass A, Adar R, et al. Autoimmune mechanisms in thromboangiitis obliterans (Buerger's disease): the role of tobacco antigen and the major histocompatibility complex. *Surgery.* 1992;111:527–531.

163. Olin JW, Young JR, Graor RA, et al. The changing clinical spectrum of thromboangiitis obliterans (Buerger's disease). *Circulation.* 1990;82:IV3–IV8.

164. Machleder HI. *Vascular Disorders of the Upper Extremity.* New York: Futura; 1983.

165. Rosendaal FR. Risk factors for venous thrombosis: prevalence, risk, and interaction. *Semin Hematol.* 1997;34:171–187.

166. Anderson FA Jr, Wheeler HB, Goldberg RJ, et al. The Worcester DVT Study. A population-based perspective of the hospital incidence and case-fatality rates of deep vein thrombosis and pulmonary embolism. *Arch Intern Med.* 1991;151:933–938.

167. Heit JA, Silverstein MD, Mohr DN, et al. The epidemiology of venous thromboembolism in the community. *Thromb Haemost.* 2001;86:452–463.

168. Stewart GJ. Neutrophils and deep venous thrombosis. *Haemostasis.* 1993;23(suppl 1):127–140.

169. Amiral J, Fareed J. Thromboembolic diseases: biochemical mechanisms and new possibilities of biological diagnosis. *Semin Thromb Hemost.* 1996;2:41–48.

170. Kakkar VV, Howe CT, Flanc C, et al. Natural history of postoperative deep-vein thrombosis. *Lancet.* 1969;2:230–232.

171. Shephard RF. Acute deep vein thrombosis. *Cardiovasc Clin.* 1992;22:47–66.

172. Ridker PM, Hennekens CH, Lindpaintner K, et al. Mutation in the gene coding for coagulation factor V and the risk of myocardial infarction, stroke, and venous thrombosis in apparently healthy men. *N Engl J Med.* 1995;332:912–917.

173. Vedantham S, Goldhaber SZ, Julian JA, et al. Pharmacomechanical catheter-directed thrombolysis for deep-vein thrombosis. *N Engl J Med.* 2017;377(23):2240–2252.

174. Beebe HG, Bergan JJ, Bergqvist D, et al. Classification and grading of chronic venous disease in the lower limbs. A consensus statement. *Eur J Vasc Endovasc Surg.* 1996;12:487–491.

175. Jamieson WG. State of the art of venous investigation and treatment. *Can J Surg.* 1993;36:119–128.

176. Lofgren KA. Surgical management of chronic venous insufficiency. *Acta Chir Scand Suppl.* 1988;544:62–68.

177. Nicolaides AN, Hussein MK, Szendro G, et al. The relation of venous ulceration with ambulatory venous pressure measurements. *J Vasc Surg.* 1993;17:414–419.

178. Cronan JJ. Venous thromboembolic disease: the role of US. *Radiology.* 1993;186:619–630.

179. Coleridge-Smith PD. Pathogenesis of chronic venous insufficiency and possible effects of compression and pentoxifylline. *Yale J Biol Med.* 1993;66:47–59.

180. Tapson VF, Carroll BA, Davidson BL, et al. The diagnostic approach to acute venous thromboembolism: clinical practice guideline. *Am J Respir Crit Care Med.* 1999;160:1043–1066.

181. Puggioni A, Kalra M, Gloviczki P. Superficial vein surgery and SEPS for chronic venous insufficiency. *Semin Vasc Surg.* 2005;18:41–48.

182. Masuda EM, Kessler DM, Lurie F, et al. The effect of ultrasound-guided sclerotherapy of incompetent perforator veins on venous clinical severity and disability scores. *J Vasc Surg.* 2006;43:551–557.

183. Marston W, Tang J, Kirschner RS. Wound Healing Society 2015 update on guidelines for venous ulcers. *Wound Repair Regen.* 2016;24:136–144.

184. Neglen P, Raju S. In-stent recurrent stenosis in stents placed in the lower extremity venous outflow tract. *J Vasc Surg.* 2004;39:181–187.

185. Snow V, Qaseem A, Barry P, et al. Management of venous thromboembolism: a clinical practice guideline from the American College of Physicians and the American Academy of Family Physicians. *Ann Fam Med.* 2007;5:74–80.

186. Nelson EA, Bell-Syer SE. Compression for preventing recurrence of venous ulcers. *Cochrane Database Syst Rev.* 2012;(9):CD002303.

187. O'Meara S, Cullum N, Nelson EA, et al. Compression for venous ulcers. *Cochrane Database Syst Rev.* 2012;(11):CD000265.

188. Mosti G, Iabichella ML, Partsch H. Compression therapy in mixed venous ulcers increases venous output and arterial perfusion. *J Vasc Surg.* 2012;55:122–128.

189. Nelson EA, Mani R, Thomas K, et al. Intermittent pneumatic compression for treating venous leg ulcers. *Cochrane Database Syst Rev.* 2011;(2):CD001899.

190. Heinen MM, van der Vleuten C, de Rooij MJ, et al. Physical activity and adherence to compression therapy in patients with venous leg ulcers.. *Arch Dermatol.* 2007;143(10):1283–1288.

191. Fitzpatrick JE. Stasis ulcers: update on a common geriatric problem. *Geriatrics.* 1989;44:19–21, 5–36, 31.

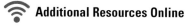 **Additional Resources Online**

CHAPTER

38

Patrick Kortebein

Physical Inactivity: Physiologic Impairments and Related Clinical Conditions

Lack of activity destroys the good condition of every human being, while movement and methodical physical exercise save it and preserve it

Plato (1)

Your love of repose will lead, in its progress, to a suspension of healthy exercise, …an indifference to everything around you, and finally to a debility of body…

Thomas Jefferson (2)

While physical activity and exercise are generally well-accepted concepts in healthy persons, the consequences of inactivity (including bed rest) tend to be less well recognized by clinicians and the general public. The deleterious effects of immobility and physical inactivity are quite broad and impact multiple organ systems; the insidiousness of these effects may minimize the awareness of these dangers and their timely prevention and treatment. This chapter reviews the myriad effects of inactivity beginning with a discussion of the most extreme example of reduced physical activity, bed rest. Subsequently, relevant information is discussed regarding the clinical populations in which reduced physical activity may have a substantial impact on function, namely hospitalized patients and, in particular, patients requiring treatment in an intensive care unit (ICU). Not infrequently, rehabilitation clinicians may have the opportunity to care for these patient populations and should be prepared to address their functional deficits. Finally, information regarding the public health consequences of physical inactivity is presented.

"Rest," in the form of reduced physical activity to allow the body to recover from illness or injury, has most certainly been a common sense form of medical "therapy" throughout history. However, the concept of complete inactivity, as in bed rest, as a therapeutic intervention is a relatively recent phenomenon in the history of medicine. In the mid-19th century, several advocates of bed rest came to prominence, including the surgeons Hugh Owen Thomas and John Hilton (3). With time, bed rest was advocated more broadly for a variety of medical conditions. It was generally assumed that rest fostered healing and recovery of the body. However, it was not appreciated that immobility and inactivity could also be potentially harmful to the body. It was not until the 1940s that the adverse effects of prolonged bed rest became more well recognized (4–7). More recently, it has been further argued that bed rest is in fact not an effective treatment for many medical conditions (8).

Over the past decades, numerous bed rest studies have been completed with normal subjects most typically as a paradigm to extrapolate the effects of microgravity in preparation for space travel. More recently, similar studies have been completed in an effort to differentiate the specific impact of bed rest inactivity from the effects of illness or injury (9). The cumulative knowledge from these studies indicates that inactivity/immobility may adversely impact virtually every human organ system (see **Table 38-1**). In clinical rehabilitation medicine, all of these complications may be need to be considered and addressed while evaluating patients in the acute care hospital setting, and many remain relevant while managing these patients in a post–acute care (PAC) setting as well. Fortunately, the recent evolution of the health care systems has, for instance, resulted in reduced acute hospital lengths of stay and thus a lower incidence of many of these sequelae (e.g., kidney stones, joint contractures). Nonetheless, rehabilitation clinicians should remain vigilant in surveilling for, and initiating prevention and/or management of, the sequelae of inactivity. Rehabilitation clinicians managing patients in the outpatient setting also have an opportunity to positively

TABLE 38-1	Adverse Effects of Immobility and Inactivity
System	**Effect(s)**
Musculoskeletal	Skeletal muscle atrophy, decreased muscle protein synthesis, decreased muscle strength and endurance (LExt > UExt, Extensors > Flexors)
	Joint contractures (Hip/knee flexion)
	Osteoporosis
	Impaired balance/fall risk
Cardiovascular	Decreased aerobic/cardiopulmonary function (e.g., VO_{2max}) due to decreased cardiac output from reduced venous return and stroke volume
	Orthostatic hypotension (secondary to reduced blood volume and increased venous compliance of lower extremities)
	Venous thromboembolism
Pulmonary	Atelectasis
	Hypostatic pneumonia
Gastrointestinal	Decreased appetite
	Constipation
Genitourinary	Urinary stasis, stones, and infection
Metabolic/endocrine	Glucose intolerance
Dermatological	Pressure ulcers
Psychological/behavioral	Sensory deprivation
	Disorientation/confusion
	Depression/anxiety

Reprinted with permission from Kortebein P. Rehabilitation for hospital associated deconditioning. *Am J Phys Med Rehabil.* 2009;88(1):66–77.
LExt, lower extremities; UExt, upper extremities; VO_{2max}, maximal aerobic capacity.

address the public health consequences of physical inactivity as discussed at the end of this chapter.

The following sections review the effects of physical inactivity on each of the major organ systems with the majority of this information acquired from bed rest studies.

MUSCLE EFFECTS

Skeletal muscle, in concert with our nervous and skeletal systems, is the "engine" of physical function. Physical inactivity can rather rapidly impact muscle function, and this tends to be most readily identifiable in the acute hospital setting, and particularly in more susceptible individuals such as older adults. If not recognized and addressed early on in an individual's hospital course, these patients may experience more long-term functional compromise, including reduced ambulatory function and impairment of an individual's ability to perform basic activities of daily living.

Bed rest studies ranging in duration from only a few days to over 10 weeks have been completed in the preceding decades, and a majority of these studies have focused on the impact on skeletal muscle (6,10,11). On average, the reported rate of muscle loss from these studies is 0.5% to 0.6% of total muscle mass per day, although this value can vary depending upon the method of measurement (e.g., MRI, DEXA) (10). The majority of muscle loss with bed rest is from the lower extremities (9,10,12), and predominantly of the antigravity extensor muscle groups with the ankle plantar flexors most affected. For example, a 20-day bed rest study utilizing MRI revealed that the muscle volume of the gastrocnemius and soleus muscles (–9.4% and –10.3%, respectively) were reduced to a greater extent than that of the knee extensors and flexors (–5.1% and –8.0%, respectively) (13). In another study with MRI, Trappe et al. reported declines of 21% and 29% of the quadriceps and triceps surae muscle volume, respectively, after 60 days

of bed rest in younger women (14). The latter study also highlights the fact that there appears to be a more pronounced loss of muscle within the first several days of bed rest with a slower, more consistent loss thereafter (10). Age appears to be a relevant factor as well. Although a majority of bed rest studies have been completed in young adults, older individuals appear to be more sensitive to the effects of inactivity (9,12). In the first study of bed rest in older adults, 10 days of bed rest resulted in the loss of almost 1 kg of muscle from the lower extremities, while younger adults from a 14-day study only lost slightly more than 600 g of lower extremity muscle (9,15). A subsequent study by Drummond et al. with older adults noted an even more substantial loss of whole body lean tissue (1.6 kg) with only 7 days of bed rest (12). Subsequently, in studies directly comparing old and young subjects, Tanner et al. found a 4% reduction in lower extremity mass with 5 days of bed rest in older individuals as compared to no change in their younger counterparts, and Pisot et al. reported an 8% loss of quadriceps muscle volume (by MRI) in their older subjects after 14 days of bed rest with only a 6% decline in the young subjects (16,17). Not all of these data are necessarily consistent, though, as Suetta et al. noted a more pronounced loss of quadriceps muscle volume (by MRI) in young as compared to older subjects (9% vs. 5%) in a study with 2 weeks of lower extremity cast immobilization (18). Gender does not appear to be a factor, as multiple bed rest studies have not found any significant difference in muscle loss in women as compared to men (14). It should however be noted that all of these studies were completed with healthy individuals and not with the typical patient seen in an acute care hospital or outpatient clinical practice.

The specific mechanism of muscle loss due to inactivity has been evaluated with multiple distinct methods of analysis with much of this work focused on muscle protein synthesis and breakdown. From these studies, the primary mechanism of muscle loss appears to be a decrease in muscle protein synthesis, both in the rested/basal state where reductions of 30% to 50% are noted as well as in the postprandial state (10,19); the latter has been termed "anabolic resistance" as protein synthesis should increase after meal ingestion. As muscle loss is greater within the first several days of bed rest, it has been hypothesized that there is a concomitant spike in muscle degradation that then returns to basal levels (10), and subsequent muscle loss is more gradual due to a sustained reduction in muscle protein synthesis. However, as measures of muscle protein degradation are more technically challenging, less data are available for interpretation. However, one recent study with young and older participants only noted increased markers of muscle proteolysis in the older subjects after short-term bed rest (16). It should also be noted that these alterations in protein synthesis occur despite the provision of the recommended daily allowance of protein (0.8 to 1 g/kg/d) in all these bed rest studies and that older subjects have been found to be in negative nitrogen balance even at the onset of bed rest (9).

Not surprisingly, in concert with the loss of muscle mass, there is an associated decline in muscle strength with bed rest inactivity, although the reduction in strength is generally more pronounced than that for muscle mass. Specifically, muscle strength decreases approximately 1% per day although there is again some variability depending upon the method of measurement (e.g., isometric vs. isotonic). In addition, as with muscle atrophy, there tend to be less pronounced declines with more prolonged periods of bed rest (10,11) and the antigravity extensors are typically most adversely affected. For instance, knee extensor strength reductions of 13% to 16% have been reported in young and older adults with bed rest studies of 10 to 14 days' duration (9,17,20) while a 43% decline was noted in younger subjects after 84 days of bed rest (11). These reductions in strength appear to be consistent regardless of age or gender, although Tanner et al. reported a 16% reduction in knee extensor isometric strength in older subjects as compared to only a 6% decline in younger individuals after 5 days of bed rest (16). Also, while measurement of extensor and flexor muscle strength is not that common, Kortebein et al. found nearly identical declines in both knee extensor and flexor strength in older men and women after 10 days of bed rest (9). Although not consistently measured, muscle power declines to about the same degree as does strength with bed rest in both young and older participants (11,21).

Since strength changes with bed rest are not fully commensurate with muscle loss, other factors including altered neural drive, changes in motor unit recruitment, and/or intrinsic properties of muscle (e.g., excitation-contraction mechanisms, calcium sensitivity) have been hypothesized to explain this difference (11,16,22). In addition, analysis of single muscle fibers has been reported in multiple bed rest studies. Consistently, these studies have found that slow/type I fibers are more adversely impacted by inactivity as compared with fast/type II fibers, and that there is also an overall shift in fiber type to fast/type II fibers (10,11). Another potential contributor may be the transforming growth factor–beta protein myostatin as it inhibits muscle protein synthesis and has been noted to increase during bed rest (23). Zachwieja et al. reported that total lean body mass declined by an average of 2.2 kg after 25 days of bed rest, and plasma myostatin-immunoreactive protein levels increased by 12% (24). In contrast, performing resistance exercise throughout a period of prolonged bed rest was able to maintain myostatin levels in younger individuals

(23). In immobilized patients, changes in muscle length can contribute to decreased strength as well; when muscle is held in a fixed shortened position (e.g., hamstring muscles with knee flexion), the number of sarcomeres in series is reduced as a result of diminished chronic stretch and muscle adaptation to the new resting length.

Despite the rather pronounced impact of bed rest inactivity on muscle function, no studies to date have documented a substantial detrimental impact on whole body function even in older adult subjects. For instance, after 10 days of bed rest, healthy older subjects had no significant change in a valid reliable measure of whole body physical function (Short Physical Performance Battery), and were able to return home with no assistive device or gait aid, and suffered no other adverse sequelae (21). These findings would indicate that bed rest in and of itself is typically not sufficient to induce substantial functional compromise in previously healthy individuals.

A number of studies have examined interventions to ameliorate the loss of muscle mass and strength associated with bed rest. Of these, the most robust method of prevention reported has been resistance exercise. Ferrando et al. found that high-intensity resistance exercise (80% maximum) performed every other day during 14 days of bed rest was able to maintain premorbid muscle protein synthesis as well as strength (15). Subsequently, Trappe et al. completed a study in which male subjects completed a high-intensity squat regimen with a gravity-independent inertial ergometer every 3rd day during 84 days of bed rest; the exercise group had no decrement in knee extensor muscle mass or strength at the completion of the study while the control group experienced declines of 17% and 40% in mass and strength, respectively (11). More recently, a high-intensity jumping program during 60 days of bed rest was reported to maintain muscle mass and power in young adult subjects (25). Whole body vibration has been noted to improve muscle mass, and a recent bed rest study found this intervention had no additional benefit in ameliorating lower extremity muscle loss when combined with resistance exercise in young men during 60 days of bed rest (26). Nutritional interventions to augment muscle protein synthesis have also been evaluated with a primary emphasis on essential amino acid supplementation. Paddon-Jones et al. noted that muscle protein synthesis and lower extremity muscle mass were maintained during 28 days of bed rest with a daily essential amino acid/sucrose supplement, while knee extensor strength declined only half that of the control subjects (–9% vs. –18%) (27). In a 14-day bed rest study with leucine supplementation, there was partial preservation of muscle protein synthesis (–10% leucine group [L] vs. –30% control [C]), knee extensor strength (–7% L vs. –15% C), and muscle mass (–2% L vs. –3% C) (20). A direct comparison of exercise (resistance and aerobic) and protein supplementation was evaluated in women in a 60-day bed rest study; similar to other resistance exercise interventions, knee extensor muscle size and strength, as well as ankle plantar flexor strength, at the end of the study remained unchanged in the resistance exercise group while plantar flexor size declined only slightly (–8%). In contrast to the aforementioned dietary studies, the female subjects receiving the protein supplement (1.6 g/kg/d; 60% more than control subjects) in this study experienced similar declines in muscle mass and strength of the knee extensors and plantar flexors as did the control group (–19% to –46%) (14).

The time course of recovery of muscle mass and strength after bed rest has only been evaluated in a limited number of studies. Tanner et al. had young and older subjects complete an 8-week high intensity eccentric resistance exercise program in conjunction with postexercise protein supplementation after 5 days of bed rest; knee extensor strength increased substantially (+10% to 15%) in both groups as compared to pre–bed rest values, while lower extremity lean mass returned to premorbid levels in older subjects and exceeded pre–bed rest levels in the younger participants (16). In a 10-day bed rest study with older subjects, lower extremity muscle strength returned to pre–bed rest values within 30 days after bed rest with a combined high-intensity (70% to 80% maximum) resistance and moderate-intensity (60% to 70% maximum) aerobic exercise regimen (unpublished data, 9). Pisot et al. investigated recovery after 14 days bed rest in young and older men; they found that young subjects recovered quadriceps muscle mass and strength/power after a 14-day combined resistance and aerobic exercise rehabilitation program while the older men recovered knee extensor strength but had continued deficits of muscle mass and power (17). These findings would indicate that the time required for full recovery of muscle function in healthy individuals, just from the effects of bed rest, and utilizing a high-intensity rehabilitative exercise program, may be two to three times longer than the duration of the immobility, particularly for older individuals. This information is relevant for rehabilitation clinicians caring for patients recovering from an illness or injury that necessitated acute care hospitalization (and/or prolonged bed rest). Full recovery of function in these patients can understandably be quite prolonged as high-intensity exercise is often not feasible during postacute rehabilitation. As such, these patients often remain functionally impaired for substantial periods of time after completion of a formal rehabilitation program.

To summarize, bed rest inactivity has a rather stereotypic effect on skeletal muscle. Muscle atrophy and weakness most typically affects the lower extremities more than the upper extremities and extensor muscle groups more than the flexors with atrophy primarily attributable to declines in muscle protein synthesis. These changes begin within a few days of initiation of bed rest, and the majority of the declines in muscle mass and strength occur within the first one to 2 weeks with less pronounced declines thereafter. Lastly, older adults are more susceptible to the effects of bed rest inactivity, which is relevant clinically as older individuals represent the majority of hospitalized patients in the United States (28).

Muscle-Tendon Effects

Stretching to maintain optimal resting muscle length as well as muscle-tendon viscoelastic properties is considered important for maintaining normal muscle function. Animal studies indicate that passive stretching of striated muscle is associated with muscle hypertrophy, including an increase in muscle fiber area and number of sarcomeres (29). However, some element of muscle contraction is required as well, and this appears primarily related to the associated elevation of cytoplasmic calcium levels with contraction (29). Undifferentiated, quiescent myoblasts (satellite cells) residing on the sarcolemma of muscle fibers are activated and believed to be responsible for this stretch-induced muscle hypertrophy (30).

Muscle stiffness is felt to occur due to structural changes in the muscle, such as altered muscle fiber angulation, reduction of sarcomeres in series, and rearrangement of collagen fibers and their cross-links. Even a relative increase in muscle connective tissue may lead to muscle stiffness and potentially a reduction of joint motion. Muscles that cross two joints such as the hip flexors and hamstrings are particularly prone to stiffness. Stiffness and subsequent muscle shortening of two-joint muscles, for example, can interfere with functional walking. For instance, a hip-flexion contracture of 35 degrees as a result of hip flexor muscle tightness can result in up to a 60% increase in energy consumption during ambulation (31). In immobilized persons, however, this process can be accelerated because of the absence of activity-induced stretch; thus, it is typically recommended to initiate a prophylactic range of motion and passive stretching program for the major joints and muscle groups of the limbs to prevent stiffness. Intuitively, this seems reasonable; however, there is limited scientific evidence to support these interventions. A recent Cochrane review of stretching for the prevention of contractures in individuals at risk for, or with, joint contractures (including those with or without neurologic conditions) concluded that stretching, when performed for up to 7 months, has no clinically relevant effect on joint mobility (32). In addition, a prior Cochrane review evaluating stretching for the prevention or abolition of post exercise muscle soreness also found no supportive evidence (33). Despite the limited literature demonstrating efficacy of benefit, stretching and range of motion exercises are low-risk activities and are the best options currently available to prevent joint stiffness and the development of contractures in at-risk patients. The optimal frequency and duration of a range of motion and stretching regimen is not known; however, it appears most judicious to perform these at least daily, and perhaps even two or three times per day, for individuals on prolonged bed rest, or restricted to a wheelchair, for instance. Stretching should be performed just to the point of mild discomfort and held in that position for approximately 30 seconds continuously. Of note, in older (>65 years old) community-dwelling adults, recent guidelines recommend that these individuals perform flexibility exercises of the major muscle groups thrice weekly (each stretch for 20 to 30 seconds) as part of a regular physical activity program (34).

CARDIOVASCULAR EFFECTS

Numerous studies have evaluated the impact of bed rest on cardiovascular function, and Saltin et al. published one of the seminal investigations in this area in 1968 (35). In that study, young males completed 20 days of bed rest followed by approximately 8 weeks of exercise training. Subjects experienced a 26% decline, on average, in their maximal oxygen consumption (VO_{2max}) after bed rest. Subsequent studies in young and older individuals have similarly found an approximate 1% per day decline in VO_{2max} (17,20,21,36). However, similar to the effects on skeletal muscle, the rate of decline in VO_{2max} slows with longer periods of bed rest. For instance, 60 days of bed rest in younger women resulted in only a 21% decline in maximal oxygen consumption (37). As with the diet and exercise interventions evaluating muscle, this study also noted no benefit with a nutritional supplement (26% decline) but a near complete preservation of aerobic capacity (3% decline) with a combined moderate-intensity aerobic and resistance exercise regimen during bed rest.

The mechanism for the decrease in VO_{2max} with bed rest has been identified definitively as due to a reduction in cardiac output secondary to a commensurate decline in stroke volume (35,38). Several factors have been identified to explain the reduced stroke volume including decreased plasma volume, reduced venous return, and increased venous capacitance (36). The combination of these factors also results in orthostatic hypotension, which is a relatively common phenomenon after prolonged bed rest. Heart rate, both at rest and with maximal exertion, does increase slightly after extended bed rest, and, as anticipated with the reduced stroke volume, submaximal heart rate is increased at a given workload as compared to pre–bed rest values (36). Similar to findings from detraining studies, oxidative enzyme activity and content as well as the number and size of mitochondria are all reduced as a result of immobility (23,35). Also, in conjunction with the shift to fast/type II glycolytic muscle fibers, there is decreased fatty acid utilization. A recent analysis of muscle metabolic changes with 84 days of bed rest found that oxidative enzyme activity and gene expression declined while those for anaerobic/glycolytic metabolism remained unchanged (23).

Hemodynamic Effects

During periods of bed rest, there is a prompt decline in blood volume, with the maximum reduction occurring within the first 1 to 2 weeks (39). This decrease is due to increased diuresis as result of decreased antidiuretic hormone secretion. Plasma volume typically decreases to a greater extent than does red-cell mass, leading to increased blood viscosity and, possibly, an increased propensity for thromboembolism. The loss of plasma volume after 24 hours is approximately 5%, while after 6 and 14 days, the loss can be up to 10% and 20%, respectively, of the pre–bed rest level (40). Exercise can ameliorate the reduction of plasma volume with isotonic exercises almost twice as effective as isometric (39,41). In addition to plasma volume change, a reduction of plasma proteins is noted after prolonged bed rest. A short period of intensive exercise produces smaller losses of plasma proteins, whereas sustained submaximal exercise actually induces a net gain in plasma protein, which can contribute to maintenance of plasma volume (41).

Due to reduced blood volume, orthostatic hypotension is a common complication of prolonged bed rest. Early mobilization is the most effective means of counteracting orthostatic intolerance and should include trials of partial or fully upright posture, passive and active range of motion (ROM) exercises of the lower extremities in particular, and progression to ambulation. In the hospital setting, initial partial upright posture may be completed in bed, and progress to sitting in a chair and then standing; infrequently, a tilt table may be necessary. Isotonic or even isometric exercises, as well as elevation, of the lower extremities can address venous stasis and pooling, while abdominal strengthening is beneficial for trunk stability. Support garments, such as elastic bandages and thigh-high elastic stockings, in addition to abdominal binders may also be used to prevent orthostasis. If there are no clinical contraindications (e.g., severe renal disease), maintenance of adequate

salt and fluid intake can also ameliorate hypotension secondary to blood volume contraction (42). Intravenous infusions may infrequently be indicated when fluid volume and dehydration cannot be corrected by these other interventions (43).

Venous Thromboembolism

Immobility exposes the patient to two of the three risk factors from Virchow's triad: venous stasis and increased blood coagulability. The increased coagulability appears related to reduce plasma volume and increased blood viscosity. There is a direct relationship between the frequency of venous thromboembolism (VTE) and the duration of bed rest (44). However, during bed rest studies with healthy human subjects, VTE prophylaxis and surveillance is typically instituted, and, fortunately, there have been no reported instances of VTE or pulmonary embolism (PE) in any of these studies. Nonetheless, given the substantial morbidity and mortality related to VTE and PE, prophylaxis and/or active surveillance should be a consideration in any individual exposed to prolonged immobility.

In the outpatient clinical setting, patients with classic symptoms of VTE (lower extremity swelling, pain, and erythema) should be evaluated for the multiple known risk factors for VTE including the following: recent bed rest/immobility or surgery or lower extremity trauma/paralysis/casting, obesity, prior VTE, prior stroke, use of oral contraceptives or hormone replacement therapy, pregnant/postpartum, or malignancy. For patients in an acute care hospital, bed rest/immobility is, of course, often a key risk factor, and consideration for deep vein thrombosis (DVT) prophylaxis should be evaluated in every patient. Several risk scoring systems that include historical elements and examination findings have been developed for predicting the probability of a DVT (44–46); a low clinical probability score in conjunction with negative D-dimer testing has been found to have an excellent negative predictive value thus obviating the need for further evaluation/testing. However, if further diagnostic testing is warranted based on the scoring system and/or D-dimer results, or purely by clinical suspicion, venous compression ultrasonography is the test of choice. Contrast venography is usually only performed when ultrasonography cannot be performed or results are equivocal.

For patients with clinical suspicion of PE (e.g., new-onset dyspnea, pleuritic chest pain), clinical prediction criteria are also available (47,48). The modified Wells criteria include the following key elements: clinical symptoms of DVT, other diagnoses less likely than PE, tachycardia, immobilization ≥3 days or surgery in preceding month, prior DVT/PE, hemoptysis, and malignancy (47). If scoring from one of the prediction criteria is positive, or if there is strong clinical suspicion (including hemodynamic instability), computed tomography pulmonary angiography is the preferred definitive diagnostic test with ventilation perfusion scanning or other modalities as secondary alternatives. It is beyond the scope of this article to discuss specific management options for VTE or PE as management guidelines frequently change; however, this information may be obtained from any of a number of sources including the frequently updated guidelines from the American College of Chest Physicians (49) or from an electronic clinical decision support resource (e.g., UpToDate). It should also be noted that while bed rest was previously recommended as part of the management of VTE, recent analysis indicates that there is no increased risk of PE, or worsening of DVT with mobilization/ambulation; as such, patients with VTE may be promptly mobilized (50,51).

CONNECTIVE TISSUE EFFECTS

Multiple factors play a role in the development of joint contractures including reduction of sarcomeres in series, changes in the angulation of muscle fibers with respect to their origin and insertion, and increases in collagen content of connective tissues of muscle, joints, and soft tissue, as well as aberrant organization of muscle extracellular matrix (52,53).

Mechanical Properties of Connective Tissues

Connective tissue can be subdivided into five major groups: (a) loose connective tissue, (b) dense connective tissue (e.g., tendon, ligament), (c) cartilage, (d) bone, and (e) blood vessels. It is not always well appreciated that connective tissues are living, malleable tissues that can adapt their structure and composition to a change in mechanical stress in particular. Both loose and dense connective tissues are composed of cells (fibroblasts) and intercellular macromolecules surrounded by polysaccharide gel (i.e., extracellular matrix). The primary components of the extracellular matrix include proteins (e.g., collagen, elastin) and glycoproteins (e.g., proteoglycans, fibronectin). The extracellular matrix affects the mechanical properties of the tissue, whereas cells are important for homeostasis, adaptation, and repair functions (54).

Collagen

Fibers in tendons, ligaments, joint capsules, and muscle (e.g., endomysium, perimysium) are predominantly of the collagen type, while there is also a significant proportion of elastic fibers in tendons. This is consistent with their function in that tendons have excellent tensile strength and some elasticity, while ligaments are relatively inelastic and composed primarily of collagen fibers. Collagen is the most abundant protein in the body and accounts for more than 20% of total body protein; at least 28 different collagen types have been well characterized (55,56).

All collagen molecules have a triple helix conformation, a result of three constituent polypeptide chains of the collagen molecule coiled together. The precise amino acid sequence differs between the different types of collagens and accounts for their tissue-specific properties.

In tendons and ligaments, type I collagen predominates, although types III, IV, and VI are also present. Important variations in collagen diameter have been found in association with location, age, and activity level. Investigations in both animal and human models have demonstrated that changes in collagen diameter, density, and orientation follow Wolff's law; that is, connective tissues orient themselves in form and mass to best resist extrinsic forces. This has been established in response to physiologic conditions (e.g., immobilization or exercise) as well as in response to injury. These factors shift the dynamic equilibrium toward synthesis or degradation (57). If extrinsic factors, such as stretch or weight bearing, are limited, or if a joint is immobilized in a foreshortened position, then collagen fiber density and mass will be readjusted to the new position or the new load, reducing ROM of the joint and potentially the failure point of ligaments and tendons (58).

Disuse Changes in Connective Tissue

The synthesis of collagen tissue in muscle is strongly influenced by the tension produced by muscular contraction, stretch, and weight bearing. Hence, muscle collagen synthesis is greater during activity and reduced during immobility. Immobilization for 1 week has been found to result in substantial decreases in collagen synthetic activity in both untrained and trained experimental animals (59). The declines in connective tissue synthesis during immobility are nearly proportionally to that of muscle protein synthesis, though both can be reversed by exercise (60).

Joint Contractures

While joint contractures can be associated with primary joint pathology, more frequently this is a multifactorial process including a lack of joint motion. The specific pathophysiology of joint contractures is not fully understood, although there are believed to be a variety of contributing factors; tissues that may be involved in contracture development include muscle, joint capsule, tendon, ligament, cartilage, bone, and skin (61). Limited joint motion may stem from joint pain, arthropathies, paralysis, capsular or periarticular tissue fibrosis, or muscletendon injury/trauma. Regardless, the common factor that contributes to the occurrence of fixed contractures is a lack of joint mobilization through its full allowable range. For instance, prolonged elbow immobilization in a flexed position will cause reduction of elbow flexor resting muscle length and capsular or soft tissue tightness with a resultant fixed joint contracture.

The rate of contracture development is affected by other factors, including limb position, duration of immobilization, and preexisting joint pathology. Edema, ischemia, bleeding, and other alterations to the microenvironment of muscle and periarticular tissue can precipitate the development of fibrosis. Advanced age is also a factor as both muscle fiber loss and a relative increase in the proportion of structural connective tissue occur with aging (62). Contractures that are precipitated by pathologic changes in the joints or muscles may be classified into three groups (see **Table 38-2**): arthrogenic, myogenic, and soft tissue related. It is important to note that all tissues surrounding a joint are likely to eventually become affected by contracture regardless of the initiating/perpetuating process.

Myogenic Contracture

Myogenic contracture is a shortening of resting muscle length that is due to intrinsic or extrinsic factors, limiting full ROM and causing abnormal positioning of the limbs or body. Intrinsic factors are structural and may be associated with inflammatory, degenerative, or traumatic processes. Extrinsic muscle contracture is secondary to neurologic conditions or mechanical factors (see **Table 38-2**).

Chronic progressive muscle weakness as with a muscular dystrophy can, for example, result in contracture due to the replacement of functional muscle fibers with collagen and fatty tissue in concert with a chronically shortened muscle (63). Curiously, however, sarcomere length in cerebral palsy patients with muscle contracture has been found to be increased as compared with normal (53).

Among the processes that may also cause intrinsic muscle shortening is heterotopic ossification (HO) wherein lamellar bone forms in nonosseous tissue. This is most commonly

TABLE 38-2	**Anatomical Classification of Contractures**		
Type	**Primary Cause**		**Secondary Cause**
Myogenic			
Intrinsic (structural)	Traumatic (e.g., bleeding, edema)		Immobility
	Inflammatory (e.g., myositis, polymyositis)		Fibrosis
	Degenerative (e.g., muscular dystrophy)		
	Ischemic (e.g., diabetes, peripheral vascular disease, compartment syndrome)		Immobility
Extrinsic	Spasticity (e.g., stroke, multiple sclerosis, spinal cord injury)		Lack of stretch
	Flaccid paralysis (e.g., muscle imbalance)		Aberrant joint position
	Mechanical (e.g., aberrant joint position)		Immobility
	Immobilization		Reduced/absent stretch
Arthrogenic	Cartilage damage, congenital deformities, infection, trauma, degenerative joint disease		Immobility
	Synovial and fibrofatty tissue proliferation (e.g., inflammation, effusion)		Immobility
	Capsular fibrosis (e.g., trauma, inflammation)		Reduced/absent ROM
	Immobilization		Mechanical position
Soft tissue	Periarticular soft tissue (e.g., trauma, inflammation)		Immobility
	Skin, subcutaneous tissue (e.g., trauma, burns, infection, systemic sclerosis)		
	Tendons and ligaments (e.g., tendinopathy, bursitis, ligamentous tear, and fibrosis)		Immobility
Mixed	Combination of arthrogenic, soft tissue, and contractures		

noted after trauma (especially elbow and acetabular fractures), spinal cord injury (SCI—see Chapter 22), or other central nervous system injury (e.g., traumatic brain injury—see Chapter 19). The actual initiating mechanism for HO is unknown, although there is a prolonged or increased inflammatory response in tissues prone to HO, and muscle mesenchymal stem cells are felt to be the primary osteogenic cell population (64).

Extrinsic myogenic contracture is most common after neurologic insult but may also occur in chronically sedentary individuals. In planning a therapeutic approach, it is useful to identify the cause of the extrinsic contracture (e.g., paralysis, spasticity). A simple example is the shortened triceps surae muscle group in patients with chronic fibular nerve palsy. Stretch of the stronger triceps surae muscle is essential to prevent contracture, although strengthening of the weak muscle, if possible, and proper positioning may be effective as well. Similarly, in spasticity, a dynamic muscle imbalance exists across one or more joints. The spastic muscle is shortened and precipitates a functional, or fixed, contracture (see 📶 **eFig. 38-1**).

Arthrogenic Contracture

Pathologic processes involving joint components, such as cartilage degeneration, congenitally incongruent joints, or synovial inflammation and effusion, may each limit joint mobility chronically secondary to pain, for instance, and this may result in arthrogenic contractures. In experimental chronic arthritis, joint immobilization for several weeks results in increased destruction of joint cartilage as compared to ad libitum mobilization (65). In contrast, short-term immobilization can be beneficial for acute inflammatory arthritis. Studies indicate that even passive ROM with acute inflammatory arthritis may increase the release of interleukin-1 into synovial fluid, and inhibition of production of protective proteoglycans (65). However, a study by van den Ende et al. demonstrated that intensive dynamic exercise in addition to ordinary physical activity in active rheumatoid arthritis patients did not induce worsening of the disease process, but

rather, induced significant gains in physical functioning (66). Thus, regular aerobic and resistance exercise training is now considered an essential aspect of care for patients with rheumatoid arthritis (67).

Soft Tissue Contracture

Cutaneous, subcutaneous, and loose connective tissue around the joint may also become contracted during immobility. An extreme example of soft tissue contracture is that due to severe thermal injury. During recovery, burns that cross any joint must be ranged diligently, via active and passive ROM exercises, and positioned to oppose the shortening forces of the scarred tissue; compression garments can be beneficial as well.

Functional Limitations Due to Contracture

Contractures can interfere with mobility, basic activities of daily living (ADL) function, and nursing care. Lower extremity contractures may alter the gait pattern and, in extreme cases, can prevent ambulation. Hip-flexion contracture, for example, reduces hip extension, shortens stride length, and may require the patient to walk with a plantar flexed ankle and increased lumbar lordosis; these alterations result in increased energy consumption. If not addressed, patients with hip flexion contractures may also develop knee and ankle joint contractures. Individuals with multiple lower extremity joint contractures may even have difficulties with bed positioning/mobility and perineal hygiene. Joint contractures may also result in an increased risk of pressure ulcers if positioning is problematic.

Management of Contractures

The basic approach to treatment of contractures starts with a careful determination of predisposing factors, as well as an evaluation of the specific affected joint components or tissues. An observant neuromuscular examination emphasizing active and passive ROM and joint stability is essential. Particular attention should be directed to two joint muscles and to the application of special maneuvers to detect shortening (e.g., Thomas test for hip flexion contracture). Of course, the best treatment is prevention, so a careful analysis of abnormal joint positioning and factors limiting ROM should be undertaken.

Flexibility and ROM Exercises

Once a contracture has developed, the sine qua non for treatment is active and passive ROM exercises combined with a sustained terminal stretch on a daily basis (see **Table 38-3**). For mild contractures, sustained or intermittent stretching for 5 to 10 minutes daily may be effective. Prolonged stretches (e.g., >10 minutes) combined with subsequent appropriate joint positioning and splinting may be effective for more severe contractures. This is generally more successful when used in combination with the application of deep heat at the musculotendinous junction or joint capsule, for instance. Ultrasound may increase tissue temperature to 40–43°C (see Chapter 51, Therapeutic Physical Agents), and maximize the effect of a stretching program.

Serial casting may gradually improve joint ROM. Typically, a cast is applied immediately after the use of heat and manual stretching to obtain maximal ROM. The cast can then be reapplied weekly. Dynamic splinting provides tension in the desired direction with the use of springs or elastic bands. This type of splinting is often used in the hand and arm because it allows a measure of function while improving flexibility.

To achieve optimal joint position, it sometimes is necessary to lengthen tendons via surgical intervention; evaluation by a surgical team with significant experience in these procedures is prudent.

Prevention of Contractures

Prevention of contracture in an immobilized patient, for instance, starts with proper bed positioning, and a bed-mobility training program. Patients should be mobilized as soon as their medical condition allows; the initiation of an early mobility program in critically ill patients is discussed below. When

TABLE 38-3   Basic Principles in the Prevention and Treatment of Contractures

Prevention	*In healthy individuals with sedentary lifestyle (e.g., older adults):* • Flexibility exercises—stretch all major muscle groups, yoga *In individual with preexisting condition(s) or predisposition:* • Range of motion (active or passive) with terminal stretch • Proper positioning (e.g., in bed, wheelchair), splinting, casting • Early mobilization and standing/ambulation (weight bearing) • CPM (continuous passive motion) • Active ROM/resistance exercise of muscle antagonist
Treatment	• Passive range of motion with terminal stretch • Prolonged stretch using low passive tension and heat (e.g., ultrasound) • Progressive (e.g., dynamic) splinting, casting

bed rest is unavoidable, then positioning and bed-mobility/transfer training are incorporated into the patient's nursing and physical therapy management program. For the patient with immobility due to paralysis or compromised extremity function, a variety of assistive devices/orthoses may be used to maintain a functional joint posture. Active and/or passive ROM exercises and stretching are, again, mainstays of management. Rehabilitative therapy including the use of early and progressive ambulation and ADL training helps to maintain joint motion and, ideally, functional mobility. Ambulation and weight bearing provide a physiologic stretch, and are important components in the prevention and treatment of contractures.

BONE EFFECTS

Maintenance of skeletal mass depends largely on mechanical loading applied to the bone by muscle contraction and bone loading/weight bearing, and it has been long recognized that bone adapts to an imposed demand (i.e., Wolff's law). Bone mass will increase with repeated loading and will decrease with the absence of muscle activity or with actual or simulated microgravity (68,69). Healthy adults on bed rest lose bone at a rate that exceeds the rate of new bone formation, leading to osteopenia (70,71). Mean bone losses range from 1% to 3% per month of bed rest and are similar for men and women; these findings are true for whole body as well as site specific measurements (e.g., lumbar spine, hip). For instance, non–weight bearing over several weeks can cause trabecular and endosteal (and later cortical) mineral bone loss in the tibia, which may require one to one and a half years to return to baseline levels with normal activity (72). As would be anticipated, bone resorption markers increase substantially during bed rest, while markers of bone formation are unchanged or increase only slightly (71). In immobilized healthy persons, urinary calcium excretion increases above normal levels within 2 weeks of initiation of bed rest and, in general, remains consistently elevated up to 90 days although other studies have reported that maximum loss occurs during the 4th or 5th week of immobility (71,73). As with muscle loss, declines are greater in the weight-bearing lower extremities as compared with the upper extremities (74). This decrease in total calcium continues even after resumption of physical activity, and negative calcium balance can last for months and even years (70).

Regional bone loss can occur with even relatively minor muscle dysfunction; for instance, persons with rotator cuff ruptures have been shown to have significantly decreased bone mineral density of the affected arm (as compared with controls) that is proportional to their remaining shoulder function (75).

Recovery of bone mass can be rather protracted. It has been documented that with longer duration immobility, an extended time period is required to restore bone density to the preimmobility level. Full body recumbency for 3 weeks in animals resulted in a loss of both trabecular and compact bones, which remained below baseline even 2 months after returning to normal activity (76). In human bed rest studies, similar findings have been noted, with full restoration of bone mass requiring more than a threefold greater time period than the original bed rest (77).

Prevention and Treatment

Physical inactivity is a significant contributing factor to osteoporosis, and loss of bone density and frequency of subsequent fractures may be reduced by optimizing bone development early in life; weight-bearing exercise and physical activity, as well as sufficient calcium and vitamin D, are key components of bone growth as well as the maintenance of bone density through the life span (69). Regular exercise participation through the life span can result in a lower risk of fracture in older age (78).

In adults, the importance of exercise in preventing inactivity-induced osteopenia should not be underestimated whether for otherwise healthy or disabled individuals. Disuse osteoporosis can be prevented by regular performance of resistance exercise, particularly weight-bearing and functional exercise training. There is a great deal of evidence that resistance exercise in particular can increase bone mass in humans. These studies also demonstrate a significant correlation between muscle strength and bone mineral density. For example, paraspinal muscle strength correlates well with bone mineral density of the lumbar spine (79). In contrast, reduced back extensor muscle strength is associated with a higher incidence of vertebral fractures, indicating that inactivity plays an important role in the development of osteoporosis in women. Back extensor strengthening exercises can improve low bone mineral density of the spine (80). In addition, avoiding flexed spine activities, including lifting, is recommended for those with known osteoporosis or those at risk for vertebral fractures. Weight-bearing activities and resistance exercise are particularly important in preventing progression of bone loss. In the elderly, exercise targeted at strengthening lower extremity muscles and improving balance will lessen progression of bone loss as well as fall risk (80). Sufficient calcium and vitamin D, in conjunction with physical activity, are essential in maintaining healthy bones (81). Please see Chapter 31 for detailed information regarding the evaluation and management of osteoporosis.

PULMONARY EFFECTS

With supine positioning, initial pulmonary alterations result from restricted movement of the chest and gravity-induced changes in the perfusion of blood through the dependent portions of the lung. As such, the balance between perfusion and ventilation is altered during recumbency (82). Regional changes in the ventilationperfusion ratio in dependent areas occur when ventilation is reduced and perfusion increased. This may lead to significant arteriovenous shunting with lowered arterial oxygenation. Studies in normal subjects have found that a change of position from upright to supine results in a 2% reduction in vital capacity, a 7% reduction in total lung capacity, a 19% reduction in residual volume, and a 30% reduction in functional residual capacity (83). After prolonged bed rest, vital capacity and functional reserve capacity may be reduced by 25% to 50%. Mechanisms responsible for this may include diminished diaphragmatic movement in the supine position, decreased chest excursion, progressive decrease in costovertebral and costochondral joint range of motion, and reduced tidal volume with a concomitant increase in respiratory rate. Clearance of secretions is also more difficult in a recumbent position. The dependent (i.e., usually posterior) lobes accumulate more secretions, whereas the upper lung regions (i.e., anterior) become less humidified, rendering the ciliary lining ineffective for clearing secretions and secretions to thus pool in the lower bronchial tree. The effectiveness of coughing is impaired because of ciliary malfunction and abdominal muscle weakness. The intercostal and axillary respiratory muscles also tend to lose strength and endurance with prolonged bed rest. Atelectasis and hypostatic pneumonia may develop due to these numerous alterations of the pulmonary system.

Prevention involves early mobilization, frequent respiratory toilet, and position changes. At-risk hospitalized patients should perform regular pulmonary toilet, including deep breathing and coughing exercises, and also maintain adequate hydration. An incentive spirometer, chest percussion, and postural drainage with oropharyngeal suctioning, if needed, can prevent aspiration and atelectasis. Management of pre-existing pulmonary disease is, of course, also essential (see Chapter 34).

GENITOURINARY EFFECTS

Prolonged bed rest contributes to an increased risk of renal stones and urinary tract infections. Contributing factors for stone formation in immobilized individuals includes hypercalciuria, an altered ratio of citric acid to calcium, and decreased urine volume (71); phosphorus excretion does not change during bed rest, although oxalate and magnesium excretion are increased in men only. In the supine position, urine must flow against gravity from the renal collecting systems through the ureters. Patients often find it difficult to initiate voiding while supine, a situation that is often exacerbated by reduced intra-abdominal pressure from weakened abdominal muscles. Studies have demonstrated that less complete voiding occurs in immobilized animals, leading to urinary retention and infection (84).

If there is incomplete bladder emptying, patients are at greater risk for bladder stone formation. The most common types of stones are struvite and carbonate apatite. Bladder stones may allow bacterial growth and decrease the efficacy of standard antimicrobial treatment. Irritation and trauma to the bladder mucosa by stones can also encourage bacterial overgrowth and infection. Urea-splitting bacteria increase urine pH, leading to further precipitation of calcium and magnesium (84).

Treatment of these problems lies first in prevention, which includes adequate fluid intake to increase urine production and more frequent micturition thereby reducing bacterial colonization, as well as voiding in a side-lying or upright posture if able. Other therapeutic approaches might include acidification of the urine with vitamin C, and, in those populations at highest risk for stone formation, a urease inhibitor. Treatment of stones after they have formed may require surgical removal or the use of ultrasonic lithotripsy. If a urinary tract infection develops, appropriate antibiotic selection is based on results of urine culture and sensitivity testing. If retention is suspected, postvoid residual volumes should be measured and regular catheterization initiated if persistently elevated. In all hospitalized patients, Foley catheters should be removed as promptly as possible to reduce the risk of infection.

GASTROINTESTINAL EFFECTS

Gastrointestinal alterations induced by immobility may be overlooked, but can contribute to functional compromise. Reduced appetite and a slower rate of absorption may lead to nutritional compromise including hypoproteinemia. Overall gastrointestinal transit is slowed in the supine position, while upright posture increases the velocity of esophageal waves and shortens the relaxation time of the lower esophagus (85). Few studies have evaluated motility; results are inconsistent as an older study noted slowed gastric transit, while a more recent evaluation found no change in gastric emptying during bed rest but increased small and large intestine motility (86,87). Eating in an elevated or upright posture during bed rest may improve gastric transit. Sleeping on two or three pillows with the trunk elevated in bed may have therapeutic implications in preventing gastroesophageal reflux.

Constipation is a common complication that results from the interaction of multiple factors. In addition to probable slowed transit time, immobility causes increased adrenergic activity, which inhibits peristalsis and causes sphincter contraction (88). The loss of plasma volume and dehydration also aggravate constipation. In addition, the use of a bedpan for fecal elimination places the patient in a nonphysiologic position. The result can be fecal impaction, which may require pharmacologic agents (including enemas) or manual disimpaction.

The basic tenets of constipation prevention include a fiber-rich diet, (including raw fruits and vegetables, if possible), intake of liberal amounts of fluid, and regular activity/mobilization. Stool softeners and bulk-forming agents may also be helpful in maintaining intestinal function. The use of opioids or other medications that slow peristalsis should be avoided whenever possible. Glycerin or peristalsis-stimulating suppositories, or other pharmacologic agents (e.g., oral polyethylene glycol), may also be utilized to assist in regulating bowel function (89).

SKIN EFFECTS

Pressure injury (ulcers) is a well-recognized risk of immobility and bed rest (90,91). These lesions develop in areas of unrelieved pressure; quite frequently, this is over a bony prominence. Key risk factors include older age, male sex, moisture, friction, shear, immobility, altered cognition, and nutritional compromise (90,91). It is relevant to note that there have not been any reports of pressure ulcers in the numerous bed rest studies completed to date in healthy adults, both young and old. In general, older adults are at most at risk and pressure wounds are most common in the acute hospital and nursing home settings. Several specific patient populations are also at high risk of pressure injury including several core rehabilitation populations (e.g., SCI, stroke, severe traumatic brain injury) (90,91). Staging of pressure injury is most typically completed with the National Pressure Ulcer Advisory Panel Staging System (see www.npuap.org/resources/educational-and-clinical-resources/npuap-pressure-injury-stages/); this staging system was most recently updated in 2016. The fundamental components of pressure injury management include pressure relief, wound cleansing (including debridement of necrotic tissue if present), reducing bacterial growth, and wound dressings (90). Nutritional optimization is typically recommended, although there is no convincing evidence of its efficacy (90). More detailed information regarding the evaluation and management of pressure injury may be found in Chapter 22.

METABOLIC EFFECTS

Daily human energy needs include basal metabolic activity, thermogenesis of food, and that required for ADL and mobility/locomotion. It has not been definitively determined whether basal metabolism changes during bed rest, but it appears that it remains stable or perhaps declines slightly. As previously discussed, most bed rest studies note that lean body mass decreases, while there is a concomitant equivalent gain in body fat with no overall change in body weight (71,92). However, a recent study reporting on a compilation of five bed rest studies (14 to 90 days duration) noted that caloric intake declined approximately 10% despite a weight maintenance diet over the course of the investigations (71). The previously discussed decline in lean body mass with bed rest does result in overall decreased metabolic activity from muscle, a shift to more glycolytic metabolism secondary to the transition to fast/type II muscle, and insulin resistance (93).

Effects on Electrolyte Balance

Prolonged immobility, especially if associated with posttraumatic electrolyte changes, can alter the balance of sodium, sulfur, phosphorus, and potassium. A mild decrease in total body sodium occurs in tandem with the diuresis seen early during bed rest (71). However, serum sodium levels do not correlate well with the degree of orthostatic intolerance. Potassium levels may also decrease to a mild degree during the early weeks of bed rest (94). Immobility alone rarely causes serious electrolyte disturbances, although in long-term critically ill patients hypercalcemia and other electrolyte disturbances may occur (95).

Endocrine Effects

Although not clinically evident during short term immobility, numerous changes have been demonstrated to occur in the endocrine system. The most relevant change is that of insulin resistance, noted to occur as early as the 3rd day of immobility; peripheral insulin resistance may increase over 50% with 1 to 2 weeks of bed rest (93,96,97). Typically, the duration of immobility correlates proportionally with the degree of glucose intolerance. Insulin resistance induced by bed rest can be ameliorated by exercise including resistance exercise of the lower extremity muscle groups (97,98).

Several other hormonal effects occur, including an increase in serum parathyroid hormone, which is thought to be related to hypercalcemia from immobility, although its precise mechanism is unknown (95). Triiodothyronine (T3) blood levels are either slightly elevated or unchanged during immobility (99,100). In a 54-day bed rest study, growth hormone levels were noted to decrease after 10 days of bed rest, increase after 20 days, and then decline thereafter (101). In men, testosterone levels have been found to remain unchanged during long-duration bed rest (102). Serum cortisol levels do not change with short-term bed rest (<14 days) but are mildly increased with longer duration immobility, and these latter studies have noted an associated increase in urinary cortisol excretion (103,104).

Free Radicals and Oxidative Stress

Free radicals are highly reactive compounds that cause oxidation of a number of molecules in the body. Antioxidants, conversely, are enzymes, vitamins, or other types of compounds that are capable of reducing or preventing the harmful effects of free radicals. Vitamins E, C, and A, and nonvitamin compounds like glutathione peroxidase and superoxide dismutase are important antioxidants that are reduced in older adults and, possibly, with chronic immobility. Whether free radicals interfere with metabolic processes in muscle, including contractility, causing functional limitation in mobility and ADL, is not entirely known. It has been theorized that increased free radicals in elderly subjects may indeed contribute to decreased functional mobility with aging (104). However, there are no studies to definitively prove that free radicals contribute to muscle disuse atrophy or reduced function in bed rest subjects.

IMMUNE SYSTEM EFFECTS

There are no known effects of short term bed rest on immune system function. However, chronic inactivity and associated conditions such as cardiovascular disease, diabetes, and obesity are associated with a low-level chronic inflammatory state, while regular physical activity/exercise has a demonstrable anti-inflammatory effect (105,106). The anti-inflammatory effect of exercise is thought to be due to reduced visceral fat, and the release of anti-inflammatory cytokines (i.e., myokines) from muscle although other factors are likely involved as well (105). However, excessive training as with high-level athletes can adversely impact immune function and put these individuals at an increased risk of infection, particularly of the respiratory system; in these individuals, factors such as psychological stress and sleep dysfunction are also felt to contribute (105). Collectively, the relationship between physical activity and immune function/illness is best characterized by a J-shaped curve with the greatest adverse impact on immunity, and thus increased risk of infection, at the extremes of physical activity, although recent information indicates a relatively lower incidence of illness in ultra high-level athletes (107).

NERVOUS SYSTEM EFFECTS

During prolonged bed rest studies, exposure to social and chronological cues, such as time of day and movement through space, may be reduced causing emotional, cognitive, and intellectual declines (108). Social isolation alone with preserved mobility can cause emotional lability and anxiety but does not appear to cause any intellectual alterations; while a variety of tests of cognitive function have been reported from numerous bed rest studies, no consistent identifiable change has been identified (109). Balance, gait, and coordination are mildly impaired after prolonged immobility, and while not fully understood, this effect appears related to muscle atrophy and perhaps alterations of the central nervous system; exercise can ameliorate the gait and balance dysfunction of prolonged bed rest (110).

In hospitalized patients, an important strategy in the prevention and treatment of these complications is to apply appropriate physical and psychosocial stimulation early in the course of illness. Options for the treatment of these effects include attention to socialization, encouraging family interaction, and, in the PAC rehabilitation setting, group therapy sessions with identification of avocational pursuits to be pursued upon discharge, as well as continued participation in a regular physical activity/exercise program. According to a recent meta-analysis, there is strong evidence from multiple studies that physical activity/exercise, especially aerobic and resistance exercise of at least moderate intensity and of 45 to 60 minutes duration per session, results in improved cognitive function of individuals

over 50 years of age; this is concordant with the physical activity guidelines for all adults (34).

CLINICAL POPULATIONS AND BED REST/IMMOBILITY

In the realm of clinical medicine, hospitalized patients, and critically ill patients in particular, are at greatest risk of the adverse sequelae of bed rest inactivity. Rehabilitation clinicians need to be familiar with these risks as well as the optimal methods for their prevention and management as we are frequently asked to evaluate these patients in the acute hospital setting, and often continue to manage their care in a PAC setting (e.g., inpatient or subacute rehabilitation facility). In addition, as discussed below, rehabilitation, including early mobility, has more recently come to the fore in the ICU, and rehabilitation clinicians may also be asked to provide their expertise for patients in this setting

Hospitalization and Deconditioning

The cumulative effects of inactivity are often termed "deconditioning." However, while this term certainly applies to and encompasses the deleterious impact on muscular and cardiovascular function in the recreational or elite athlete upon cessation of training, in the sphere of clinical rehabilitation medicine this term is most appropriately applied to patients suffering from functional compromise related to the effects of a prolonged acute care hospitalization. More specifically, this condition has been termed "hospital-associated deconditioning" (HAD) and may be defined as the functional decline that occurs during acute hospitalization due to illness, injury, or both, and is unrelated to a specific neurologic or orthopedic insult (111,112). It is also worthwhile to note that the related term "posthospital syndrome" has been coined to characterize the clinical population of patients (usually older adults with limited functional reserve) at increased risk for readmission after acute hospital discharge (113).

Approximately one third of patients experience some element of functional decline during an acute hospitalization, and these individuals are at increased risk of rehospitalization, institutionalization, and death (114). While these patients may be considered to have some element of HAD, functional decline that is sufficient to prevent a patient from returning to their premorbid independent living setting may be considered to have "clinically relevant" HAD. It also needs to be kept in mind, however, that a number of factors aside from functional ability (e.g., social support, financial resources) may impact one's ability to return home after hospitalization; these issues will be discussed below. Given that there are no distinct diagnostic criteria, nor a diagnostic billing code for HAD, it is not possible at this time to determine the specific incidence and prevalence of this condition (112). Older adults are most frequently affected, although any patient may experience functional compromise during a sufficiently severe or protracted hospitalization. Critically ill patients are at increased risk, and this will be discussed separately (see Critical Illness and Rehabilitation below). One relatively straightforward means of identifying patients at risk for poor outcomes is a simple measure of function, namely, gait speed. In the community setting, gait speed has been demonstrated to predict hospitalization, institutionalization, and mortality, while more recently, low gait speed at hospital admission was found to be strongly predictive of longer hospital stays and a lower likelihood of discharge to home (115–117).

The etiology of HAD is multifactorial, and is due to more than just the effects of bed rest inactivity alone (112). As noted previously, bed rest studies in older adults have reported substantial declines in muscle mass and strength with no significant impact on whole body function (16,21). While muscle mass and strength changes have not been formally evaluated in hospitalized patients, a recent analysis of a cohort of older adults did find that hospitalization in the preceding year was associated with a more substantial loss of muscle mass and strength as compared to adults not hospitalized, and this was most pronounced in those individuals hospitalized for a total of 8 days or more in the prior year (118). In addition to bed rest/immobility, other factors contributing to the development of HAD include the following: prehospitalization functional capacity/reserve, specific medical/surgical condition necessitating hospitalization, comorbid medical conditions, inflammation (illness associated), nutritional compromise (calories and protein), pain, sleep dysfunction/insomnia, fatigue, anemia, and depression.

Several different interventions have been evaluated to address the functional compromise associated with hospitalization. As older adults are most at risk, specialized hospital units specifically focused on the needs of these patients have been developed (e.g., Acute Care for Elders), and have generally reported positive results (119–121). Prompt mobilization, polypharmacy reduction, delirium surveillance/prevention, restful sleep, and nutritional optimization are key elements of these geriatric units. Numerous studies have also examined formal rehabilitative exercise training initiated in the acute care hospital setting. A recent review of these studies, found that, in general, rehabilitation initiated in the acute care hospital setting is safe and does result in functional benefit (122). Subsequently, Hastings et al. found that hospitalized older adults participating in a supervised walking program had shorter lengths of stay and were more likely to be discharged to home (123). Another more recent study examined the feasibility of a specific physical therapist directed sit-stand exercise program in at-risk older hospitalized patients, and as a result of their positive findings, a larger scale trial has been initiated (124,125). These efforts are of substantial relevance as improving mobility during hospitalization is associated with lower mortality 2 years after an index hospitalization, while declining mobility is even more strongly associated with higher mortality (126).

Rehabilitation clinicians most frequently encounter patients with HAD during an acute care consultation, or upon admission to an inpatient rehabilitation facility (IRF). In the acute care setting, physiatrists are frequently consulted to determine a patient's suitability for transfer to an IRF or other PAC setting. Key criteria to be considered when evaluating whether a particular patient is appropriate for admission to an IRF are listed in **Box 38-1**; of note, these criteria have not been formally evaluated to determine if they are predictive of subsequent relevant outcomes (e.g., functional improvement, discharge to community). In the United States, HAD (i.e., debility) patients are the fifth largest IRF patient population at nearly 11% (127). For patients not transferred to an IRF, other PAC options include subacute rehabilitation (typically as part of a skilled nursing facility), home health or outpatient therapy services (e.g., physical therapy), or less commonly long-term acute care facilities. While the percentage of HAD patients

---

BOX 38-1

Evaluation Criteria for Post–Acute Care Rehabilitation

- Prehospitalization functional status/ability
- Prehospitalization living setting (e.g., house/apartment, stairs)
- Family/social support
- Current/active medical problems
- Current participation/tolerance with physical and/or occupational therapy
- Cognition/ability to learn
- Anticipated potential/time frame for functional recovery
- Patient/family preference (e.g., specific facility, location)
- Financial (e.g., patient/family resources, insurance coverage, CMS 60% rule)
- Ultimate discharge location identified and appropriate (e.g., home with adequate family/social support)

---

discharged to an IRF versus other PAC settings is not known, the overwhelming majority of patients requiring PAC rehabilitation services receive their care in a skilled nursing facility (aka, subacute rehabilitation facility) (127).

As with other rehabilitation populations, the goal of rehabilitation training for patients with HAD is to maximize functional recovery and independence in a safe, cost-effective manner (112). Physical and occupational therapy are the cornerstones of rehabilitation, and the key components of these therapy programs are outlined in **Table 38-4**. While HAD patients often receive low-intensity general conditioning–type exercises during IRF rehabilitation, higher intensity exercise with an emphasis on functional resistance exercise and gait/balance training may be more effective (112,128). The physical and occupational therapy programs for HAD patients receiving rehabilitation in a subacute rehabilitation or home

---

TABLE 38-4 Rehabilitative Therapy for Hospital-Associated Deconditioning

Physical therapy
- Bed mobility/transfers
- Gait and balance training
- Ambulatory endurance with/without gait aid/stair climbing
- Muscle strength and endurance training—hip and knee extensors primarily
- Range of motion and muscle flexibility/stretching of major joints and muscle groups of the lower extremities

Occupational therapy
- Activities of daily living (ADL) training, including fine motor skills and adaptive equipment needs
- Instrumental ADL/homemaking/community survival skills
- Cognitive and safety awareness assessment and remediation, if needed
- Range of motion and muscle flexibility/stretching of major muscle groups of the upper extremities to facilitate ADL training
- Energy conservation and joint protection principles, if needed
- Muscle strength and endurance training—shoulder abductors/adductors, elbow flexors/extensors, and finger flexors/grip strength

Reprinted with permission from Kortebein P. Rehabilitation for hospital associated deconditioning. *Am J Phys Med Rehabil.* 2009;88(1):66–77.

health care setting should be very similar to that of the IRF program, although the therapy sessions are necessarily less frequent. In contrast to the required 3 hours of daily therapy mandated in an IRF (i.e., 15 hours per week) the time allotted for therapy in subacute rehabilitation settings is generally only 3 to 5 hours per week, and similar or even less frequent with home health therapy. Tolerance for higher intensity exercise is a potential concern with HAD patients regardless of PAC setting, and contraindications to participation in a therapeutic exercise program are listed in **Box 38-2**. These contraindications are applicable to all HAD patients regardless of the rehabilitation setting. In addition to rehabilitation therapy, nutritional optimization with an emphasis on total calories and protein intake, ideally with the assistance of a dietician, is strongly encouraged as nutrition is frequently compromised in HAD patients. Bed rest studies have noted improved muscle protein synthesis with essential amino acids (leucine and lysine in particular), and the nutritional supplement creatine has been found to increase muscle power as well; if not contraindicated, a trial of one of these could be initiated in HAD patients during rehabilitation (27,129). Pharmacologic agents for improving muscle mass/strength and function would also be of benefit for this population; however, none are approved for HAD or any other similar clinical population. Short-term (3 to 6 months) use of testosterone might be considered in HAD patients with no contraindications (e.g., prostate cancer); a small pilot study examining testosterone supplementation in older deconditioned men did note greater functional gains with testosterone (130). Other myoanabolic agents, including myostatin inhibitors and selective androgen receptor modulators, are being investigated for muscle wasting conditions and may be available in the future for these patients (131).

Outcomes after IRF treatment are available for HAD-type patients (i.e., debility) while no similar data exist for these patients after admission to a subacute rehabilitation facility or for those receiving rehabilitative therapy via home health services. In a large retrospective analysis of 10 years of IRF data including more than 250,000 patients, Galloway et al. found that debility patients are rather stereotypic of an HAD patient in that they are older (mean age 74 years), had been admitted from an acute care hospital (93%), and had previously been living in the community (94%) (132). With regard to outcomes, these debility patients were quite comparable to other more traditional IRF patient populations including mean length of stay (12.6 days), rate of discharge to the community (75%), and Functional Independence Measure improvement (23), although their rate of discharge to the acute care setting was higher (12%). In a follow-up study, these investigators noted that debility patients have the highest acute hospital readmission rate (19% at 30 days after IRF discharge) among the six most common IRF patient populations, while their readmission rate climbs to 34% up to 90 days after discharge (133,134). The latter study also found that debility patients with higher motor function at IRF discharge were less likely to be readmitted within 60 days; this is perhaps not surprising since other studies have also noted that lower extremity function is highly predictive of important health outcomes (116). While HAD/debility patients are more medically fragile both during and after IRF care, the findings from this large database indicate that this patient population does in fact derive tangible functional benefits during an IRF stay. Future investigations might evaluate proactive methods for identifying those debility/HAD patients at greatest risk for acute medical problems, and, ideally, initiating interventions to avoid discharge to acute care setting and/or early readmission after discharge. In addition, as IRF care is typically more expensive than subacute rehabilitation or home health therapy, it would be worthwhile to determine which debility/HAD patients are most appropriate for and most likely to benefit from (e.g., functional gains) IRF care as opposed to one of these other PAC programs.

Critical Illness and Rehabilitation

Individuals experiencing critical illness are the clinical population at greatest risk for the multiple adverse consequences attendant with bed rest inactivity. Muscle weakness, in particular, has been one of the most recognizable consequences of critical illness and has been termed ICU–acquired weakness (ICUAW) due to its significance in this population (135). ICUAW is defined as a syndrome of generalized clinically detectable limb weakness that develops in ICU patients and for which there is no alternative explanation other than the critical illness itself (136,137). Approximately 25% to 30% of patients requiring prolonged mechanical ventilation develop ICUAW, and while the specific etiology is not clear there is overlap with critical illness myopathy (CIM) and critical illness polyneuropathy (CIP), though patients may not necessarily have either of these discrete conditions (135,137); more recent analysis indicates impaired muscle regenerative capacity manifest by factors including decreased muscle satellite cell content (138). Similar to the HAD population, bed rest is certainly a contributing factor in ICUAW although systemic inflammation and nutritional compromise are likely more consequential in critically ill patients (139). There are a number of additional pathophysiologic factors felt to be contributing to the development of ICUAW though many questions remain unanswered (140). Risk factors for ICUAW include duration of mechanical ventilation, ICU length of stay, severity of illness/sepsis, serum glucose, hyperosmolality, and parenteral

---

BOX 38-2

Contraindications to Therapeutic Exercise/ Rehabilitation

Unstable angina or severe left main coronarydisease
End-stage congestive heart failure
Severe valvular heart disease
Malignant or unstable arrhythmias
Elevated resting blood pressure (systolic, >200 mm Hg; diastolic, >110 mm Hg)
Large or expanding aortic aneurysm
Known cerebral aneurysm or recent intracranial bleed
Uncontrolled or end-stage systemic disease
Acute retinal hemorrhage or recent ophthalmologic surgery
Acute or unstable musculoskeletal injury
Acute illness with systemic features, (e.g., pneumonia)
Severe dementia or behavioral disturbance

Reprinted from Kortebein P. Rehabilitation for hospital associated deconditioning. *Am J Phys Med Rehabil.* 2009;88(1):66–77. Copyright © 2009 Elsevier. With permission.

nutrition, while early mobilization has been associated with a reduced risk (139,141). Corticosteroids and neuromuscular blocking agents have been implicated as well though not consistently (139); of note, in healthy bed rest subjects, the addition of corticosteroids has been found to result in increased muscle protein breakdown as compared with bed rest alone (142). The diagnosis of ICUAW is most typically made based on a standardized examination of muscle strength, as electrodiagnostic testing (or muscle biopsy) is often not feasible or available (135). Manual muscle strength testing of three muscle groups each of the bilateral upper (shoulder abduction, elbow flexion, wrist extension) and lower (hip flexion, knee extension, ankle dorsiflexion) extremities is performed using the Medical Research Council scale (0 to 5 with 0 being no visible/palpable muscle contraction and 5 normal strength); a score of less than 48 of 60 is deemed clinically relevant (137,141). While prolonged mechanical ventilation and hospitalization are the immediate effects of ICUAW, the long-term consequences include persistent functional compromise for up to several years after an ICU stay as well as increased one-year mortality (137,143). These adverse sequelae initially gained widespread clinical recognition in survivors of acute respiratory distress syndrome (144,145).

In addition to the immediate and long-term consequences of ICUAW, it has relatively recently been recognized that ICU survivors suffer long-term cognitive and psychological impairments (e.g., depression, posttraumatic stress) (144,145). These more global effects of critical illness have been termed the post–intensive care syndrome, and result in compromised quality of life not only for the patient but for their family/caregivers as well (146,147). As more individuals survive critical illness, this has become an increasingly prevalent problem for medical teams caring for these patients and their families.

In recognition of the long-term deleterious consequences of critical illness, there has been a rather dramatic shift in critical care patient management (137,148). Harkening back to the early days of intensive care management, efforts are once again focused on limiting sedation and increasing mobilization in concert with treatment of an individual's critical illness (148). This revised construct of critical care management to proactively address the post–intensive care syndrome is termed the ABCDEF bundle (148). The "A" indicates "Assessment, Prevention, and Management of Pain"; "B" stands for "Both spontaneous awakening and breathing trials"; "C" indicates "Choice of sedation and analgesia"; "D" stands for "Delirium Assessment, Prevention, and Management"; and "E" emphasizes "Early mobility and exercise." Utilization of this bundle in randomized clinical trials has demonstrated that patients receiving this comprehensive program have significantly reduced days of mechanical ventilation and in the ICU, as well as improved mobility and survival (148). Some bundles also include an "F" for "Family engagement and empowerment" as early and ongoing family interaction has been found to be important as well. More detailed information regarding how to operationalize the ABCDE bundle may be obtained from the Society of Critical Care Medicine ICU liberation Web site (www.iculiberation.org).

Interventions more specifically focused on early mobilization have also demonstrated positive outcomes. In one of the initial randomized trials with early mobility, Schweickert et al.

found that patients receiving early physical and occupational therapy (initiated 1.5 days after intubation vs. 7.4 days after intubation in control group) were significantly more likely to have a shorter duration of mechanical ventilation (3.4 days vs. 6.1 days), to have fewer days with delirium (2 days vs. 4 days), and to return to independent physical functioning at hospital discharge (59% vs. 35%) (149). Subsequent studies have typically demonstrated similar positive findings although a recent meta-analysis of early mobility in the ICU reported improved walking ability but no association with improved functional status, muscle strength, health care utilization, or quality of life (150). Additional studies to determine the optimal timing of early mobility as well as the most efficacious frequency, intensity, and duration of early mobility training are needed. The safety of mobilizing this high-risk population has, of course, been a concern, though the reported incidence of safety issues has been very low even in patients intubated or with other invasive devices (137). Specific screening criteria are used to reduce the safety risks associated with mobilization, and a report from one institution noted potential safety events in only 0.6% of over 5,000 physical therapy sessions; most events were mild changes in blood pressure or oxygen saturation, and no medical intervention was necessary (137). However, despite the increasing literature demonstrating the potential benefits of early mobility, the prevalence of early physical and occupational therapy within ICUs is still rather low with one recent study noting that only 32% of respiratory failure patients across 42 ICUs received therapist mobilization, and for patients on mechanical ventilation, out-of-bed mobility occurred only 16% of the time (151). In addition, as not all critically ill patients may be safely mobilized out of bed, alternative methods to augment muscle function have been utilized including cycle ergometry (with or without functional electrical stimulation) and neuromuscular stimulation (137). Additional clinical literature and educational information related to ICU mobilization may be found at www.mobilization-network.org.

As with the HAD population, rehabilitation clinicians may only initially become involved in the care of critically ill patients during an acute care consultation or on admission to an IRF. However, some rehabilitation clinicians are now collaborating with ICU teams to initiate mobilization and rehabilitation efforts in the intensive care with the goal of then providing continuing rehabilitation interventions through the acute and PAC settings. Therapy interventions for this patient population would be the same as those for the HAD population (see **Table 38-4**) with a primary emphasis on functional recovery of muscle strength and ambulation. No studies have specifically evaluated the functional outcomes of critically ill patients receiving rehabilitation in an IRF or other PAC system, although an indeterminate percentage of debility/HAD patients are likely ICU survivors. A recent Cochrane review has, however, reported that exercise rehabilitation had no significant effect on functional exercise capacity or health-related quality of life in patients surviving critical illness, although there were only a limited number of studies to analyze and there was substantial variability across the studies (152). As with HAD patients, nutritional optimization, with an emphasis on protein intake, is also warranted to improve muscle protein synthesis; a trial of essential amino acids or creatine could be initiated, if there are no contraindications. Also, as there are no pharmacologic agents approved to treat ICUAW or its long-term sequelae, testosterone or other anabolic steroids (e.g., oxandrolone) may be considered during PAC rehabilitation with continued treatment through the short term after rehabilitation discharge.

Physical Inactivity and Public Health

It has been known for at least the past several decades that physical inactivity is a major public health problem due to its well-established association with multiple adverse health consequences including cardiovascular disease, diabetes mellitus, obesity, and some cancers (breast and colon), as well as increased all-cause mortality (153,154). In contrast, physical activity results in positive effects on numerous parameters associated with chronic disease (e.g., reduced blood pressure, increased insulin sensitivity, improved lipid profile), and there is an inverse relationship between cardiorespiratory fitness and all-cause mortality (155). Participation in a regular physical activity program is also associated with lower rates of dementia and depression. Despite this information, approximately 30% of the US population is not engaged in any regular physical activity, with older adults most likely to be inactive, and only 21% achieve the recommended minimum amount of physical activity (156). Individuals who are the least physically active are at the highest risk of adverse consequences, and yet they have the most to gain since a majority of risk reduction is attained merely by engaging in just some degree of physical activity (155). To address this public health problem, physical activity recommendations for the general public have been published and public health education campaigns have been initiated (153,156). Full details are available from these publications (156, 157; see also Chapter 49); however, the key components for adults are aerobic exercise and resistance training. Specifically, all adults should perform a minimum of 150 minutes per week (30 minutes 5 days per week) of moderate-intensity (5 to 6 on 0 to 10 scale) or 75 minutes (25 minutes 3 days per week) of vigorous-intensity (7 to 8 on 0 to 10 scale) aerobic exercise, as well as resistance exercise of the major muscle groups of the upper and lower extremities at least twice per week (8 to 10 exercises total, 1 to 3 sets of 8 to 12 repetitions at moderate to vigorous intensity). In addition, to the previously noted guidelines, more specific guidance regarding exercise interventions for adults may be found in Chapter 49 and from the American College of Sports Medicine (157, www.acsm.org). Rehabilitation clinicians/physicians are also encouraged to address physical inactivity in the clinical setting as part of the Exercise is Medicine initiative (www.exerciseismedicine.org).

Separate physical activity recommendations have also been published for older adults (>65 years old) (see also Chapter 47). The recommendations regarding aerobic and resistance exercise are the same as described above for adults, and, in addition, these individuals are advised to include balance and flexibility exercises as part of their physical activity program (34). Older adults are also advised to develop an individualized physical activity plan that addresses all of these recommended elements, and this may be completed in conjunction with a physician visit, for instance. Specific evidence of the positive effects of physical activity in older individuals can be found in a recent large randomized trial examining a structured physical activity program in older adults at risk for disability; while the effects were rather modest, a physical activity intervention was found to be more effective than a health education program at reducing further progression of mobility dysfunction (158).

Low physical activity is also a significant risk factor for impaired mobility in community-dwelling older adults (159). As impaired mobility, manifest as slow gait speed (critical value <0.8 m/s), is associated with falls and increased mortality, and as the older adult population worldwide is anticipated to double by 2030, this will most certainly be a public health problem in the coming decades (116,160). In addition to lifelong low physical activity, a number of other risk factors for mobility disability have been identified, including obesity, strength or balance impairments, and the chronic medical conditions diabetes and arthritis (159,161). The three-item Short Physical Performance Battery test (repetitive chair rises, 4 m gait speed and balance) is a more global measure of lower extremity function and is strongly predictive of subsequent morbidity and mortality in older adults (162). In addition to measures of lower extremity strength and function, a more recent investigation reported that the novel parameters of slow leg velocity and lower trunk extensor muscle endurance are also predictive of future functional decline (163). The related condition, sarcopenia (age-related loss of muscle mass and function) will be discussed separately (see Chapter 47) although an excellent summary of progress in this field was recently published, and includes the first evidence-based cut-points for clinically relevant muscle mass and weakness (164).

Interventions to improve mobility disability have primarily focused on exercise interventions including lower extremity resistance exercise and gait/balance training including ambulatory endurance (158,165), although a novel resistance exercise program utilizing a weighted vest during functional activities resulted in more substantial, and clinically meaningful, gains in lower extremity power and leg velocity as compared with a traditional resistance exercise program (166).

CONCLUSION

Physical inactivity results in deleterious sequelae of almost every organ system though the musculoskeletal and cardiopulmonary systems are typically the most compromised. In clinical medicine, patients in the acute hospital setting, including those requiring intensive care, are most at risk of these sequelae although functionally immobile individuals living in the community may develop these complications as well. Rehabilitation clinicians often participate in the care of hospitalized patients, either as a consultant or as the lead physician during postacute rehabilitation, for instance, and thus we must be vigilant in surveilling for these sequelae and proactively initiating prevention and treatment as well as coordinating the rehabilitation of these patients. As with other areas of rehabilitation medicine, treatment for patients impacted by physical inactivity, regardless of setting, is focused on functional recovery with the primary modality being therapeutic exercise.

REFERENCES

1. Izquotes. Available from: http://izquotes.com/author/plato/?q=physical+activity&x=0&y=0. Accessed March 23, 2017.
2. https://www.monticello.org/site/research-and-collections/exercise. Accessed March 23, 2017.
3. Ghormley RK. The abuse of rest in bed in orthopedic surgery. *JAMA.* 1944;125(16):1085–1087.

4. Dock W. The evil sequelae of complete bed rest. *JAMA*. 1944;125(16):1083–1085.
5. Asher RAJ. The dangers of going to bed. *Br Med J*. 1947;2:967–968.
6. Deitrick JE, Whedon GD, Shorr E. Effect of immobilization upon various metabolic and physiologic functions of normal men. *Am J Med*. 1948;4(1):3–36.
7. Taylor HL, Henschel A, Brozek J, et al. Effects of bed rest on cardiovascular function and work performance. *J Appl Physiol*. 1949;2(5):223–239.
8. Allen C, Glasziou P, Del Mar C. Bed rest: a potentially harmful treatment needing more careful evaluation. *Lancet*. 1999;354(9186):1229–1233.
9. Kortebein P, Ferrando A, Lombeida J, et al. Effect of ten days of bed rest on skeletal muscle in healthy older adults. *JAMA*. 2007;297(16):1772–1774.
10. Wall BT, Dirks ML, van Loon LJC. Skeletal muscle atrophy during short term disuse: implications for age-related sarcopenia. *Ageing Res Rev*. 2013;12:898–906.
11. Trappe S, Trappe T, Gallagher P, et al. Human single muscle fibre function with 84 day bed-rest and resistance exercise. *J Physiol*. 2004;557(2):501–513.
12. Drummond MJ, Timmerman KL, Markofski MM, et al. Short term bed rest increases TLR4 and IL-6 expression in skeletal muscle of older adults. *Am J Physiol Regul Integr Comp Physiol*. 2013;305:R216–R223.
13. Akima H, Kuno S, Suzuki Y, et al. Effects of 20 days of bed rest on physiological cross-sectional area of human thigh and leg muscles evaluated by magnetic resonance imaging. *J Gravit Physiol*. 1997;4(1):S15–S21.
14. Trappe TA, Burd NA, Louis ES, et al. Influence of concurrent exercise or nutrition countermeasures on thigh and calf muscle size and function during 60 days of bed rest in women. *Acta Physiol (Oxf)*. 2007;191:147–159.
15. Ferrando AA, Tipton KD, Bamman MM, et al. Resistance exercise maintains skeletal muscle protein synthesis during bed rest. *J Appl Physiol*. 1997;82:807–810.
16. Tanner RE, Brunker LB, Agergaard J, et al. Age-related differences in lean mass, protein synthesis and skeletal muscle markers of proteolysis after bed rest and exercise rehabilitation. *J Physiol*. 2015;593(18):4259–4273.
17. Pisot R, Marusic U, Biolo G, et al. Greater loss in muscle mass and function but smaller metabolic alterations in older compared with younger men following 2 wk of bed rest and recovery. *J Appl Physiol*. 2016;120:922–929.
18. Suetta C, Hvid LG, Justesen L, et al. *J Appl Physiol*. 2009;107:1172–1180.
19. Rudrappa SS, Wilkinson DJ, Greenhaff PL, et al. Human skeletal muscle disuse atrophy: effects on muscle protein synthesis, breakdown, and insulin resistance—a qualitative review. *Front Physiol*. 2016;7(361):1–10.
20. English KL, Mettler JA, Ellison JB, et al. Leucine partially protects muscle mass and function during bed rest in middle-aged adults. *Am J Clin Nutr*. 2016;103:465–473.
21. Kortebein P, Symons TB, Ferrando A, et al. Functional impact of 10 days of bed rest in healthy older adults. *J Gerontol A Biol Sci Med Sci*. 2008;63A(10):1076–1081.
22. Hvid LG, Suetta C, Aagaard P, et al. Four days of muscle disuse impairs single fiber contractile function in young and old healthy men. *Exp Gerontol*. 2013;48:154–161.
23. Irimia JM, Guerrero M, Rodriguez-Miguelez P, et al. Metabolic adaptations in skeletal muscle after 84 days of bed rest with and without concurrent flywheel resistance exercise. *J Appl Physiol*. 2017;122:96–103.
24. Zachwieja JJ, Smith SR, Sinha-Hikim I, et al. Plasma myostatin-immunoreactive protein is increased after prolonged bed rest with low-dose T3 administration. *J Gravit Physiol*. 1999;6(2):11–15.
25. Kramer A, Kummel J, Mulder E, et al. High-intensity jump training in tolerated during 60 days of bed rest and is very effective in preserving leg power and lean body mass: an overview of the Cologne RSL study. *PLoS One*. 2017;12:e0169793.
26. Miokovic T, Armbrecht G, Gast U, et al. Muscle atrophy, pain, and damage in bed rest reduced by resistive (vibration) exercise. *Med Sci Sports Exerc*. 2014;46:1506–1516.
27. Paddon-Jones D, Sheffield-Moore M, Urban RJ, et al. Essential amino acid and carbohydrate supplementation ameliorates muscle protein loss in humans during 28 days bedrest. *J Clin Endocrinol Metab*. 2004;89:4351–4358.
28. McDermott KJ, Elixhauser A, Sun R. *Trends in Hospital Inpatient Stays in the United States, 2005-2014. HCUP Statistical Brief #225*. Rockville, MD: Agency for Healthcare Research and Quality; 2017.
29. Riley DA, Van Dyke JM. The effects of active and passive stretching on muscle length. *Phys Med Rehabil Clin N Am*. 2012;23:51–57.
30. Berg HE, Dudley GA, Haggmark T, et al. Effects of lower limb unloading on skeletal muscle mass and function in humans. *J Appl Physiol*. 1991;70(4):1882–1885.
31. Kottke FJ. The effects of limitation of activity upon the human body. *JAMA*. 1966;196(10):825–830.
32. Harvey LA, Katalinic OM, Herbert RD, et al. Stretch for the treatment and prevention of contractures. *Cochrane Database Syst Rev*. 2017;(1):CD007455.
33. Herbert RD, de Noronha M, Kamper SJ. Stretching to prevent or reduce muscle soreness after exercise. *Cochrane Database Syst Rev*. 2011;(7):CD004577.
34. Nelson ME, Rejeski WJ, Blair SN, et al. Physical activity and public health in older adults: recommendation from the American College of Sports Medicine and the American Heart Association. *Med Sci Sports Exerc*. 2007;39:1435–1445.
35. Saltin B, Blomqvist G, Mitchell JH, et al. Response to exercise after bed rest and after training. *Circulation*. 1968;38(5 suppl):VII 1–VII 78.
36. Convertino VA. Cardiovascular consequences of bed rest: effect on maximal oxygen uptake. *Med Sci Sports Exerc*. 1997;29:191–196.
37. Schneider SM, Lee SMC, Macias BR, et al. WISE-2005: exercise and nutrition countermeasures for upright VO2pk during bed rest. *Med Sci Sports Exerc*. 2009;41:2165–2176.
38. Wagner PD. A re-analysis of the 1968 Saltin et al 'Bedrest' paper. *Scand J Med Sci Sports*. 2015;25(suppl 4):83–87.
39. Convertino VA. Blood volume response to physical activity and inactivity. *Am J Med Sci*. 2007;334:72–79.
40. Van Beaumont W, Greenleaf JE, Juhos L. Disproportional changes in hematocrit, plasma volume, and proteins during exercise and bed rest. *J Appl Physiol*. 1972;33(1):55–61.
41. Greenleaf JE, Stinnett HO, Davis GL, et al. Fluid and electrolyte shifts in women during +Gz acceleration after 15 days' bed rest. *J Appl Physiol*. 1977;42(1):67–73.
42. Greenleaf JE, Wade CE, Leftheriotis G. Orthostatic responses following 30-day bed rest deconditioning with isotonic and isokinetic exercise training. *Aviat Space Environ Med*. 1989;60(6):537–542.
43. Haruna Y, Takenaka K, Suzuki Y, et al. Effect of acute saline infusion on the cardiovascular deconditioning after 20-days head-down tilt bedrest. *J Gravit Physiol*. 1998;5(1):P45–P46.
44. Wells PS, Forgie MA, Rodger MA. Treatment of venous thromboembolism. *JAMA*. 2014;311:717–728.
45. Subramaniam RM, Snyder B, Heath R, et al. Diagnosis of lower limb deep venous thrombosis in emergency department patients: performance of Hamilton and modified Wells scores. *Ann Emerg Med*. 2006;48:678–685.
46. Wells PS, Anderson DR, Rodger M, et al. Evaluation of D-dimer in the diagnosis of suspected deep-vein thrombosis. *N Engl J Med*. 2003;349:1227–1235.
47. Van Belle A, Buller HR, Huisman MV, et al.; Christopher Study Investigators. Effectiveness of managing suspected pulmonary embolism using an algorithm combining clinical probability, D-dimer testing, and computed tomography. *JAMA*. 2006;295:172–179.
48. Lucassen W, Geersing GJ, Erkens PM, et al. Clinical decision rules for excluding pulmonary embolism: a meta-analysis. *Ann Intern Med*. 2011;155:448–460.
49. Kearon C, Akl EA, Omelas J, et al. Antithrombotic therapy for VTE disease: CHEST guideline and expert panel report. *Chest*. 2016;149:315–352.
50. Aissaoui N, Martins E, Mouly S, et al. A meta-analysis of bed rest versus early ambulation in the management of pulmonary embolism, deep vein thrombosis, or both. *Int J Cardiol*. 2009;137:37–41.
51. Anderson CM, Overend TJ, Godwin J, et al. Ambulation after deep vein thrombosis: a systematic review. *Physiother Can*. 2009;61:133–140.
52. Williams PE. Use of intermittent stretch in the prevention of serial sarcomere loss in immobilised muscle. *Ann Rheum Dis*. 1990;49(5):316–317.
53. Mathewson MA, Lieber RL. Pathophysiology of muscle contractures in cerebral palsy. *Phys Med Rehabil Clin N Am*. 2015;26:57–67.
54. Alberts B, Bray D, Lewis J, et al. *Molecular Biology of the Cell*. New York: Garland Science; 1983:673–715.
55. Kjaer M, Langberg H, Miller BF, et al. Metabolic activity and collagen turnover in human tendon in response to physical activity. *J Musculoskelet Neuronal Interact*. 2005;5:41–52.
56. Mouw JK, Guanqing O, Weaver VM. Extracellular matrix assembly: a multiscale deconstruction. *Nat Rev Mol Cell Biol*. 2014;15:771–785.
57. Harper J, Amiel D, Harper E. Collagenases from periarticular ligaments and tendon: enzyme levels during the development of joint contracture. *Matrix*. 1989;9(3):200–205.
58. Saamanen AM, Tammi M, Jurvelin J, et al. Proteoglycan alterations following immobilization and remobilization in the articular cartilage of young canine knee (stifle) joint. *J Orthop Res*. 1990;8(6):863–873.
59. Karpakka J, Vaananen K, Orava S, et al. The effects of preimmobilization training and immobilization on collagen synthesis in rat skeletal muscle. *Int J Sports Med*. 1990;11(6):484–488.
60. Kjaer M, Jorgenson NR, Heinemeier K, et al. Exercise and regulation of bone and collagen tissue biology. *Prog Mol Biol Transl Sci*. 2015;135:259–291.
61. Wong K, Trudel G, Laneuville O. Noninflammatory joint contractures arising from immobility: animal models to future treatments. *Biomed Res Int*. 2015; 2015:8484290.
62. Garcia-Bunuel L, Garcia-Bunuel VM. Connective tissue metabolism in normal and atrophic skeletal muscle. *J Neurol Sci*. 1980;47(1):69–77.
63. Johnson EW. Pathokinesiology of Duchenne muscular dystrophy: implications for management. *Arch Phys Med Rehabil*. 1977;54:4–7.
64. Ranganathan K, Loder S, Agarwal S, et al. Heterotopic ossification: basic science principles and clinical correlates. *J Bone Joint Surg Am*. 2015;97:1101–1111.
65. van Lent PL, van den Bersselaar L, van de Putte LB, et al. Immobilization aggravates cartilage damage during antigen-induced arthritis in mice. Attachment of polymorphonuclear leukocytes to articular cartilage. *Am J Pathol*. 1990;136(6):1407–1416.
66. van den Ende CH, Breedveld FC, le Cessie S, et al. Effect of intensive exercise on patients with active rheumatoid arthritis: a randomised clinical trial. *Ann Rheum Dis*. 2000;59(8):615–621.
67. Hurkmans E, van der Giesen FJ, Vliet Vlieland TP, et al. Dynamic exercise programs (aerobic capacity and/or muscle strength training) in patients with rheumatoid arthritis. *Cochrane Database Syst Rev*. 2009;(4):CD006853.
68. Van Loon JJ, Bervoets DJ, Burger EH, et al. Decreased mineralization and increased calcium release in isolated fetal mouse long bones under near weightlessness. *J Bone Miner Res*. 1995;10(4):550–557.
69. Stagi S, Cavalli L, Iurato C, et al. Bone metabolism in children and adolescents: main characteristics of the determinants of peak bone mass. *Clin Cases Miner Bone Metab*. 2013;10:172–179.
70. Leblanc AD, Schneider VS, Evans HJ, et al. Bone mineral loss and recovery after 17 weeks of bed rest. *J Bone Miner Res*. 1990;5(8):843–850.
71. Morgan JL, Heer M, Hargens AR, et al. Sex-specific responses of bone metabolism and renal stone risk during bed rest. *Physiol Rep*. 2014;2:e12119.
72. Ito M, Matsumoto T, Enomoto H, et al. Effect of nonweight bearing on tibial bone density measured by QCT in patients with hip surgery. *J Bone Miner Metab*. 1999;17(1):45–50.
73. Schneider VS, McDonald J. Skeletal calcium homeostasis and countermeasures to prevent disuse osteoporosis. *Calcif Tissue Int*. 1984;36(suppl 1):S151-154.
74. LeBlanc AD, Spector ER, Evans HJ, et al. Skeletal responses to space flight and the bed rest analog: a review. *J Musculoskelet Neuronal Interact*. 2007;7:33–47.

75. Kannus P, Leppala J, Lehto M, et al. A rotator cuff rupture produces permanent osteoporosis in the affected extremity, but not in those with whom shoulder function has returned to normal. *J Bone Miner Res.* 1995;10(8):1263–1271.

76. Cann CE, Genant HK, Young DR. Comparison of vertebral and peripheral mineral losses in disuse osteoporosis in monkeys. *Radiology.* 1980;134(2):525–529.

77. Belavy DL, Beller G, Ritter Z, et al. Bone structure and density via HR-pQCT in 60d bed-rest, 2-years recovery with and without countermeasures. *J Musculoskelet Neuronal Interact.* 2011;11:215–226.

78. Warden SJ, Fuchs RK, Castillo AB, et al. Exercise when young provides lifelong benefits to bone structure and strength. *J Bone Miner Res.* 2007;22(2):251–259.

79. Sinaki M, Wahner HW, Bergstralh EJ, et al. Three-year controlled, randomized trial of the effect of dose-specified loading and strengthening exercises on bone mineral density of spine and femur in nonathletic, physically active women. *Bone.* 1996;19(3):233–244.

80. Sinaki M, Pfeifer M, Preisinger E, et al. The role of exercise in the treatment of osteoporosis. *Curr Osteoporos Rep.* 2010;8:138–144.

81. Khosla S, Hofbauer LC. Osteoporosis treatment: recent developments and ongoing challenges. *Lancet Diabetes Endocrinol.* 2017;5(11):898–907. doi: 10.1016/S2213-8587(17)30188-2.

82. Svanberg L. Influence of posture on the lung volumes, ventilation and circulation in normals; a spirometric-bronchospirometric investigation. *Scand J Clin Lab Invest.* 1957;9(suppl 25):1–195.

83. West JB. *Ventilation/Blood Flow and Gas Exchange.* 4th ed. Oxford, UK: Blackwell Scientific; 1985.

84. Anderson RL, Lefever FR, Francis WR, et al. Urinary and bladder responses to immobilization in male rats. *Food Chem Toxicol.* 1990;28(8):543–545.

85. Dooley CP, Schlossmacher B, Valenzuela JE. Modulation of esophageal peristalsis by alterations of body position. Effect of bolus viscosity. *Dig Dis Sci.* 1989;34(11):1662–1667.

86. Moore JG, Datz FL, Christian PE, et al. Effect of body posture on radionuclide measurements of gastric emptying. *Dig Dis Sci.* 1988;33:1592–1595.

87. Prakash M, Fried R, Gotze O, et al. Microgravity simulated by the 6° head-down tilt bed rest test increases intestinal motility but fails to induce gastrointestinal symptoms of space motion sickness. *Dig Dis Sci.* 2015;60:3053–3061.

88. LeBlanc A, Schneider V, Specter E, et al. Calcium absorption, endogenous excretion, and endocrine changes during and after long-term bed rest. *Bone.* 1995;16(4):S301–S304.

89. Wald A. Constipation: advances in diagnosis and treatment. *JAMA.* 2016;315:185–191.

90. Bluestein D, Javaheri A. Pressure ulcers: prevention, evaluation, and management. *Am Fam Physician.* 2008;78:1186–1194.

91. Cushing CA, Phillips LG. Evidence based medicine: pressure sores. *Plast Reconstr Surg.* 2013;132:1720–1732.

92. Krebs JM, Schneider VS, Evans H, et al. Energy absorption, lean body mass, and total body fat changes during 5 weeks of continuous bed rest. *Aviat Space Environ Med.* 1990;61(4):314–318.

93. Stuart CA, Shangraw RE, Prince MJ, et al. Bed-rest-induced insulin resistance occurs primarily in muscle. *Metabolism.* 1988;37(8):802–806.

94. Zorbas YG, Merkov AB, Nobahar AN. Nutritional status of men under hypokinesia. *J Environ Pathol Toxicol Oncol.* 1989;9(4):333–342.

95. Mechanick JI, Brett EM. Endocrine and metabolic issues in the management of the chronically critically ill patient. *Crit Care Clin.* 2002;18:619–641.

96. Hamburg, NM, McMackin CJ, Huang AL, et al. Physical inactivity rapidly induces insulin resistance and microvascular dysfunction in healthy volunteers. *Arterioscler Thromb Vasc Biol.* 2007;27:2650–2656.

97. Bergouignan A, Rudwill F, Simon C, et al. Physical inactivity as the culprit of metabolic inflexibility: evidence from bed-rest studies. *J Appl Physiol.* 111:1201–1210.

98. Dolkas CB, Greenleaf JE. Insulin and glucose responses during bed rest with isotonic and isometric exercise. *J Appl Physiol.* 1977;43(6):1033–1038.

99. Balsam A, Leppo LE. Assessment of the degradation of thyroid hormones in man during bed rest. *J Appl Physiol.* 1975;38(2):216–219.

100. Smith SR, Lovejoy JC, Bray GA, et al. Triiodothyronine increases calcium loss in a bed rest antigravity model for space flight. *Metabolism.* 2008;57:1696–1703.

101. Vernikos-Danellis J, Leach CS, Winget CM, et al. Changes in glucose, insulin, and growth hormone levels associated with bedrest. *Aviat Space Environ Med.* 1976;47:583–587.

102. Smith SM, Heer M, Wang Z, et al. Long-duration space flight and bed rest effects on testosterone and other steroids. *J Clin Endocrinol Metab.* 2012;97:270–278.

103. Ferrando AF. Effects of inactivity and hormonal mediators on skeletal muscle during recovery from trauma. *Curr Opin Clin Nutr Metab Care.* 2000;3:171–175.

104. Geffken DF, Cushman M, Burke GL, et al. Association between physical activity and markers of inflammation in a healthy elderly population. *Am J Epidemiol.* 2001;153(3):242–250.

105. Gleeson M, Bishop NC, Stensel DJ, et al. The anti-inflammatory effects of exercise: mechanisms and implications for the prevention and treatment of disease. *Nat Rev Immunol.* 2011;11:607–615.

106. Beavers KM, Brinkley TE, Nicklas BJ. Effect of exercise training on chronic inflammation. *Clin Chim Acta.* 2010;411:785–793.

107. Schwellnus M, Soligard T, Alonso JM, et al. How much is too much? (Part 2) International Olympic Committee consensus statement on load in sport and risk of illness. *Br J Sports Med.* 2016;50:1043–1052.

108. Ryback RS, Lewis OF, Lessard CS. Psychobiologic effects of prolonged bed rest (weightless) in young, healthy volunteers (Study II). *Aerosp Med.* 1971;42(5):529–535.

109. Lipnicki DM, Gunga HC. Physical inactivity and cognitive functioning: results from bed rest studies. *Eur J Appl Physiol.* 2009;105:27–35.

110. Koppelmans V, Mulavara AP, Yuan P, et al. Exercise as potential countermeasure for the effects of 70 days of bed rest on cognitive and sensorimotor performance. *Front Syst Neurosci.* 2015;9:121.

111. Hoenig HM, Rubenstein LZ. Hospital-associated deconditioning and dysfunction. *J Am Geriatr Soc.* 1991;39(2):220–222.

112. Kortebein P. Rehabilitation for hospital-associated deconditioning. *Am J Phys Med Rehabil.* 2009;88:66–77.

113. Krumholz HM. Post-hospital syndrome- an acquired, transient condition of generalized risk. *N Engl J Med.* 2013;368:100–102.

114. Covinsky KE, Pierluissi E, Johnston CB. Hospitalization-associated disability: "She was probably able to ambulate but I'm not sure." *JAMA.* 2011;306:1782–1793.

115. Abellan van Kan G, Rolland Y, Andrieu S, et al. Gait speed at usual pace as a predictor of adverse outcomes in community-dwelling older people an International Academy on Nutrition and Aging (IANA) Task Force. *J Nutr Health Aging.* 2009;13:881–889.

116. Studenski S, Perera S, Patel K, et al. Gait speed and survival in older adults. *JAMA.* 2011;305:50–58.

117. Ostir GV, Berges I, Kup YF, et al. Assessing gait speed in acutely ill older adults admitted to an acute care for elders hospital unit. *Arch Intern Med.* 2012;172:353–358.

118. Alley DE, Koster A, Mackey D, et al. Hospitalization and change in body composition and strength in a population-based cohort of older persons. *J Am Geriatr Soc.* 2010;58:2085–2091.

119. Rubenstein LZ, Wieland D, English P, et al. The Sepulveda VA Geriatric Evaluation Unit: data on four-year outcomes and predictors of improved patient outcomes. *J Am Geriatr Soc.* 1984;32:503–512.

120. Applegate WB, Miller ST, Graney MJ, et al. A randomized, controlled trial of a geriatric assessment unit in a community rehabilitation hospital. *N Engl J Med.* 1990;322:1572–1578.

121. Landefeld CS, Palmer RM, Kresevic DM, et al. A randomized trial of care in a hospital medical unit especially designed to improve functional outcomes of acutely ill older patients. *N Engl J Med.* 1995;332:1338–1344.

122. Kosse NM, Dutmer AL, Dasenbrock L, et al. Effectiveness and feasibility of early physical rehabilitation programs for geriatric hospitalized patients: a systematic review. *BMC Geriatr.* 2013;13:107.

123. Hastings SN, Sloane R, Morey MC, et al. Assisted early mobility for hospitalized older veterans: preliminary data from the STRIDE program. *J Am Geriatr Soc.* 2014;62:2180–2184.

124. Pedersen MM, Petersen J, Bean JF, et al. Feasibility of progressive sit-to-stand training among older hospitalized patients. *Peer J.* 2015;3:e1500.

125. Pedersen MM, Petersen J, Beyer N, et al. Supervised progrssive cross-continuum strength training compared with usual care in older medical patients: study protocol for a randomized controlled trial (the STAND-Cph trial). *Trials.* 2016;17:176.

126. Ostir GV, Berges IM, Kuo YF, et al. Mobility activity and its value as a prognostic indicator of survival in hospitalized older adults. *J Am Geriatr Soc.* 2013;61:551–557.

127. *A Data Book: Health Care Spending and the Medicare Program.* Medicare Payment Advisory Commission; 2017.

128. Falvey JR, Mangione KK, Stevens-Lapsley JE. Rethinking hospital-associated deconditioning: proposed paradigm shift. *Phys Ther.* 2015;95:1307–1315.

129. Ferrando A, Paddon-Jones D, Hays NP, et al. EAA supplementation to increase nitrogen intake improves muscle function during bed rest in the elderly. *Clin Nutr.* 2010;29:18–23.

130. Bakhshi V, Elliott M, Gentili A, et al. Testosterone improves rehabilitation outcomes in ill older men. *J Am Geriatr Soc.* 2000;48:550–553.

131. Meriggioli MN, Roubenoff R. Prospect for pharmacological therapies to treat skeletal muscle dysfunction. *Calcif Tissue Int.* 2015;96:234–242.

132. Galloway RV, Granger CV, Karmarkar AM, et al. The Uniform Data System for Medical Rehabilitation: report of patients with debility discharged from inpatient rehabilitation programs in 2000–2010. *Am J Phys Med Rehabil.* 2013;92:14–27.

133. Ottenbacher KJ, Karmarkar A, Graham JE, et al. Thirty-day hospital readmission following discharge from postacute rehabilitation in fee-for-service Medicare patients. *JAMA.* 2014;311:604–614.

134. Galloway RV, Karmarkar AM, Graham JE, et al. Hospital readmission following discharge from inpatient rehabilitation for older adults with debility. *Phys Ther.* 2016;96:241–251.

135. Fan E, Cheek F, Chlan L, et al. An official American Thoracic Society Clinical Practice guideline: the diagnosis of intensive care unit-acquired weakness in adults. *Am J Respir Crit Care Med.* 2014;190:1437–1446.

136. Stevens RD, Marshall SA, Cornblath DR, et al. A framework for diagnosing and classifying intensive care unit-acquired weakness. *Crit Care Med.* 2009;37(suppl 10): S299–S308.

137. Hashem MD, Nelliot A, Needham DM. Early mobilization and rehabilitation in the ICU: moving back to the future. *Respir Care.* 2016;61:971–979.

138. Dos Santos C, et al. Mechanisms of chronic muscle wasting and dysfunction after intensive care unit stay. A pilot study. *Am J Respir Crit Care Med.* 2016;194:821–830.

139. Truong AD, Fan E, Brower RG, et al. Bench-to-bedside review: mobilizing patients in the intensive care unit—from pathophysiology to clinical trials. *Crit Care.* 2009;13:216.

140. Batt J, dos Santos CC, Cameron JI, et al. Intensive care unit-acquired weakness: clinical phenotypes and molecular mechanisms. *Am J Respir Crit Care Med.* 2013;187:238–246.

141. Hermans G, Van den Berghe G. Clinical review: intensive care unit-acquired weakness. *Crit Care.* 2015;19:274.

142. Ferrando AA, Stuart CA, Sheffield-Moore M, et al. Inactivity amplifies the catabolic response of skeletal muscle to cortisol. *J Clin Endocrinol Metab.* 1999;84:3515–3521.

143. Hermans G, Van Mechelen H, Clerckx B, et al. Acute outcomes and 1-year mortality of intensive care unit-acquired weakness. A cohort study and propensity matched analysis. *Am J Respir Crit Care Med.* 2014;190:410–420.

144. Herridge MS, Cheung AM, Tansey CM, et al. One-year outcomes in survivors of the acute respiratory distress syndrome. *N Engl J Med.* 2003;348:683–693.

145. Herridge MS, Tansey CM, Matte A, et al. Functional disability 5 years after acute respiratory distress syndrome. *N Engl J Med.* 2011;364:1293–1304.

146. Needham DM, Kamdar BB, Stevenson JE. Rehabilitation of mind and body after intensive care unit discharge: a step closer to recovery. *Crit Care Med.* 2012;40:1340–1341.

147. Jutte JE, Erb CT, Jackson JC. Physical, cognitive and psychological disability following critical illness: what is the risk? *Semin Respir Crit Care Med.* 2015;36:943–958.

148. Ely EW. The ABCDEF bundle: science and philosophy of how ICU liberation serves patients and families. *Crit Care Med.* 2017;45:321–330.

149. Schweickert WD, Pohlman MC, Pohlman AS, et al. Early physical and occupational therapy in mechanically ventilated, critically ill patients: a randomized controlled trial. *Lancet.* 2009;373:1874–1882.

150. Castro-Avila AC, Seron P, Fan E, et al. Effect of early rehabilitation during intensive care unit stay on functional status: systematic review and meta-analysis. *PLoS One.* 2015;10:e0130722.

151. Jolley SE, Moss M, Needham DM, et al. Point prevalence study of mobilization practices for acute respiratory failure patients in the United States. *Crit Care Med.* 2017;45:205–215.

152. Connolly B, Salisbury L, O'Neill B, et al. Exercise rehabilitation following intensive care unit discharge for recovery from critical illness. *Cochrane Database Syst Rev.* 2015;(6):CD008632.

153. Haskell WL, Blair SN, Hill JO. Physical activity: health outcomes and importance for public health policy. *Prev Med.* 2009;49:280–282.

154. Kohl HW III, Craig CL, Lambert EV, et al. The pandemic of physical inactivity: global action for public health. *Lancet.* 2012;380:294–305.

155. Ross R, Blair SN, Arena R, et al. Importance of assessing cardiorespiratory fitness in clinical practice: a case for fitness as a clinical vital sign: a scientific statement from the American Heart Association. *Circulation.* 2016;134:e653–e699.

156. Centers for Disease Control and Prevention. *Physical Activity Data and Statistics.* Available from: www.cdc.gov/physicalactivity/data/facts.htm. Accessed July 25, 2017.

157. Garber CE, Blissmer B, Deschenes MR, et al. American College of Sports Medicine position stand. Quantity and quality of exercise for developing and maintaining cardiorespiratory, musculoskeletal, and neuromotor fitness in apparently healthy adults: guidance for prescribing exercise. *Med Sci Sports Exerc.* 2011;43:1334–1359.

158. Pahor M, Guralnik JM, Ambrosius WT, et al. Effect of structured physical activity on prevention of major mobility disability in older adults. The LIFE study randomized clinical trial. *JAMA.* 2014;311:2387–2396.

159. Brown CJ, Flood KL. Mobility limitation in the older patient: a clinical review. *JAMA.* 2013;310:1168–1177.

160. United Nations, Department of Economic and Social Affairs, Population Division. World Population Prospects: the 2012 revision, highlights and advance tables. Working Paper No. ESA/P/WP.228; 2013.

161. Stenholm S, Koster A, Valkeinen H, et al. Association of physical activity history with physical function and mortality in old age. *J Gerontol A Biol Sci Med Sci.* 2016;71:496–501.

162. Guralnik JM, Ferrucci L, Pieper CF, et al. Lower extremity function and subsequent disability: consistency across studies, predictive models, and value of gait speed alone compared with the short physical performance battery. *J Gerontol A Biol Sci Med Sci.* 2000;55:M221–M231.

163. Ward RE, Beauchamp MK, Latham NK, et al. Neuromuscular impairments contributing to persistently poor and declining lower-extremity mobility among older adults: new findings informing geriatric rehabilitation. *Arch Phys Med Rehabil.* 2016;97:1316–1322.

164. Studenski SA, Peters KW, Alley DE, et al. The FNIH Sarcopenia Project: rationale, study description, conference recommendations and final estimates. *J Gerontol A Biol Sci Med Sci.* 2014;69:547–558.

165. Brown LG, Ni M, Schmidt CT, et al. Evaluation of an outpatient rehabilitative program to address mobility limitations among older adults. *Am J Phys Med Rehabil.* 2017;96:600–606.

166. Bean JF, Beauchamp MK, Ni M. Targeted exercise training to optimize leg power, leg speed, and mobility in older adults. *J Am Geriatr Soc.* 2016;64:2608–2609.

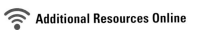 **Additional Resources Online**

CHAPTER 39

Andrea Dompieri Furlan
Nimish Mittal
Dinesh Kumbhare
Mario Giraldo-Prieto
Angela Mailis-Gagnon

Chronic Pain

Chronic pain is a complex clinical phenomenon that poses a challenge for treating clinicians since it can affect the physical, emotional, cognitive, and functional aspects of a patient. This chapter provides an up-to-date resource that outlines the mechanisms, epidemiology, and socioeconomic factors of chronic pain as well as the impact upon an individual who suffers from chronic pain. The chapter also provides a review of the anatomy and physiology of pain, the clinical evaluation, and diagnostic procedures that can be utilized. This is followed by a brief review of conditions that are commonly associated with chronic pain. The chapter also reviews the clinical management including nonpharmacologic, pharmacologic, interventional, and surgical management strategies.

DEFINITIONS

Pain is purely subjective, difficult to define, and often hard to characterize or interpret. It is currently defined as an unpleasant sensory and emotional response to a stimulus associated with actual or potential tissue damage or described in terms of such damage (1–3). Pain is a complex biologic phenomenon modulated by descending endogenous excitatory and inhibitory pain modulation mechanisms (4). However, pain has never been shown to be a simple function of the amount of physical injury; it is extensively influenced by anxiety, depression, expectation, and other psychological and physiologic variables. It is a multifaceted experience, an interweaving of the physical characteristics of the stimulus with the individual's motivational, affective, and cognitive functions. The pain experience is in part behavior based on an interpretation of the event, influenced by present and past experiences.

Acute pain is a biologic symptom of an apparent nociceptive stimulus, such as tissue damage that is due to disease or trauma that persists only as long as the tissue pathology itself persists. The pain may be highly localized or may radiate. Acute somatic pain may be well localized, aching, and sharp, whereas acute visceral pain may be burning, cramping, and radiating. It is usually associated with up-regulated sympathetic activity, tachycardia, hypertension, tachypnea, increased metabolic rate, and hypercoagulability. Acute pain is generally self-limiting, and as the nociceptive stimulus lessens, the pain decreases. Acute pain usually lasts a few days to a few weeks (2). If it is not effectively treated, it may progress to a chronic form.

Chronic pain is a disease process in which the pain is a persistent symptom of an autonomous disorder with neurologic, psychological, and physiologic components. Differing significantly from acute pain, it is defined as pain lasting longer than anticipated (>3 months) within the context of the usual course of an acute disease or injury. The pain may be associated with continued pathology, that is, when there is still an active pathology such as inflammatory arthritis or neuroma, or the pain may persist beyond the usual time of healing after recovery from a disease or injury, such as when there is peripheral or central sensitization or when psychoemotional or pain disability arises. Due to the complex nature of chronic pain, many other definitions have been proposed. Some include factors such as the persistence of pain despite extraordinary measures in a nonacute setting or pain that is without apparent biologic value (5). Operational definitions include aspects such as pain sensation, pain behavior, functional status, emotion, and somatic preoccupation. As with acute pain, treatable chronic pain that is due to organic disease is managed by effectively treating the underlying disorder; however, in many cases, no such identifiable organic disease may be evident. Chronic pain can mimic the qualities of acute pain except that associated signs of autonomic nervous system response may be absent, and the patient may appear exhausted, listless, depressed, and withdrawn. Chronic pain can have exacerbations that are triggered by progression of organic pathology, physiologic stress, or worsening emotional, social, and psychiatric problems. As these problems subside, the patient's general well-being may improve, but there might still be some residual sensations of pain. The pain sensations may also be highly persistent and reported as severe for years without remission.

ANATOMY AND PHYSIOLOGY OF PAIN

Pain is a central perception of multiple primary sensory modalities. This interpretive function is complex, involving psychological, neuroanatomic, neurochemical, and neurophysiologic factors of both the pain stimulus and the memory of past pain experiences. The peripheral mechanisms for sensing and modulating pain have been extensively studied during the past 40 years. The pathways for pain sensation, from the initial stimulus of the nociceptors to the central nervous system (CNS), are summarized in **Figure 39-1** (6–10). There appear to be several descending systems that play a role in the control of the ascending pain pathways, which are summarized in **Figure 39-2** (7,10–14).

Polymodal nociceptors respond to stimuli that damage tissue. This stimulation results in impulses ascending in the A-delta or C fibers to the marginal layers of the dorsal horn of the spinal cord. The A-delta fibers primarily synapse in laminae I and V, whereas C fibers synapse primarily in lamina II. Deeper regions of the dorsal horn may be polysynaptically

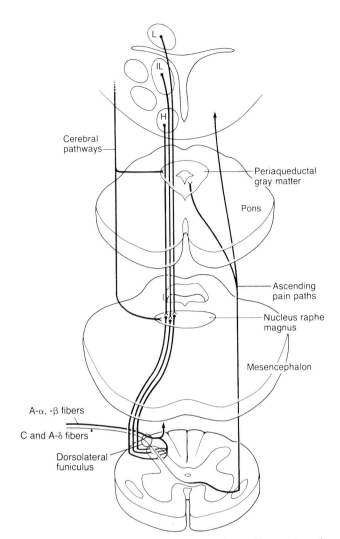

FIGURE 39-1. Central nervous system structures that modify ascending pain pathways. H, hypothalamus; IL, intralaminar thalamic nuclei; L, limbic system.

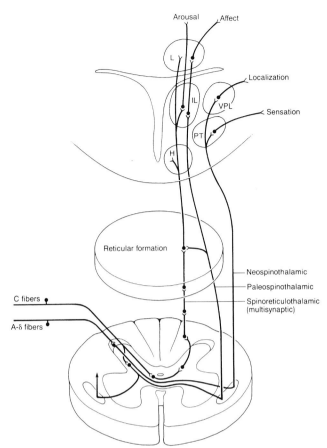

FIGURE 39-2. Ascending pathways for pain sensation from nociceptors to the central nervous system. H, hypothalamus; IL, intralaminar thalamic nuclei; L, limbic system; PT, posterior thalamic nuclei; VPL, ventral posterolateral thalamic nuclei.

involved in the processing of noxious stimuli. Before synapsing, these entering roots of the spinal cord arrange themselves as a longitudinal white matter small bunch of axons, also called the Lissauer's tract or the dorsolateral fasciculus (funiculus), that ascends or descends one or two levels just adjacent to the dorsal horn; after synapsing the new fibers decussate throughout the spinal white commisure, which gives origin to the spinothalamic tracts (15).

The major *ascending nociceptive pathways* are the spinothalamic and spinoreticular tracts, which involve both oligosynaptic and polysynaptic neurons. The oligosynaptic pathways are fast conducting, with discrete somatotopic organization resulting in rapid transmission of nociceptive information regarding site, intensity, and duration of stimulus. Further, the oligosynaptic tracts provide somatic information by way of the posterior ventral nuclei of the thalamus to the postcentral cortex. The sensory discriminatory characteristics are delineated from the neospinothalamic portion of the lateral spinothalamic tract and the nonproprioceptive portion of the dorsal columns. The polysynaptic pathways are slow conducting, with a lack of somatotopic organization resulting in poor localization as well as dull aching and burning sensations. The nociceptive

impulses transmitted through the polysynaptic pathway system result in suprasegmental reflex responses related to ventilation, circulation, and endocrine function. Pathways contributing to this slow-conducting system are the paleospinothalamic tract, spinoreticular, spinocollicular, and the dorsal intercornual, as well as the spinomesencephalic tracts. The polysynaptic tracts form the brainstem reticular activating system with projections to the medial and interlaminar (IL) nuclei of the thalamus. From these nuclei, diffuse radiation occurs to the cerebral cortex, limbic system, and basal ganglia.

There are multiple levels of processing and convergence of nociceptive information in its ascending transmission to the cerebral cortex. In addition, there appear to be several *descending pain control systems* that play a role in the control and modification of the ascending pain pathways. The periaqueductal gray (PAG) region of the midbrain plays an interconnecting role among ascending and descending pathways of pain (16). There is an increased functional connectivity (FC) of the PAG with the amygdala and insula under painful conditions that seems to regulate the behavioral components of emotion and memory associated with pain; on the contrary, the FC with the ventromedial prefrontal cortex (MPFC) seems to be decreased during painful stimulation (17). The decreased activity of the prefrontal cortex is even lower in patients with depressive disorder when compared with healthy controls, while the activation in the areas associated with memory of pain and emotion, such as the right anterior insular region, the dorsal anterior cingulate cortex, and the right amygdala, is higher during anticipation of painful stimuli; moreover, the increased activity in the right amygdala is associated with greater levels of perceived helplessness (18).

Stimulation of the PAG neurons and the subsequent descending impulses result in the release of endogenous opioids at the nucleus locus ceruleus (NLC) in the midbrain and nucleus raphe magnus (NRM) that extends from the midbrain to the pons and medulla oblongata. Endogenous opioids activate the serotonergic cells in the NRM and norepinergic neurons in the NLC. These monoamines activate opioid-secreting interneurons. The morphine-like transmitter released may vary, depending on what type of receptor in the periphery has been activated. Both A-delta and C afferent fibers are inhibited by descending influences in the dorsal horn. The opioid inhibitory interneurons may be influenced by intersegmental and descending pathways, but the intersegmental and segmental mechanisms have not been established. These interneurons may function either by presynaptic inhibition on the terminals with the primary nociceptive afferents preventing the release of substance P or by postsynaptic inhibition on second-order neurons. Cells in the raphe magnus are activated by ascending sensory pathways transmitted to the reticular formation as well as by descending input from cells in the PAG region. The descending modulatory pathways involve not only opioid systems but also antiopioid cholecystokinin systems (19); serotonergic, noradrenergic, dopaminergic systems (20); and endocannabinoid systems (21). Other descending monoamine systems include the locus ceruleus to the dorsal horn interneurons, the nucleus reticularis, the magnocellularis to the dorsal horn interneurons, and the mesencephalic lateral reticular formation to the dorsal horn interneurons (4).

EPIDEMIOLOGY OF CHRONIC PAIN

It is challenging to calculate the prevalence of chronic pain for many reasons. First, pain is a subjective experience that cannot be measured "objectively." Second, there is no consensus on a definition of what constitutes chronic pain, for example, does it have to be constant 24-hour pain or intermittent daily or weekly episodes? When defining chronic pain, some studies only include certain types of chronic pain, and therefore, the prevalence is skewed or underestimated for all types of chronic pains. Third, the populations and settings in which prevalence estimates of chronic pain are obtained vary from study to study, for example, surveys of community samples, in the general population, among patients attending a primary care practice or hospital. Last, the methods to collect and analyze data differ from study to study, making it difficult to compare results.

For the abovementioned reasons, the estimated prevalence of the chronic pain ranges from 8% to nearly 60% and more (22–29). The majority of the reported literature on the chronic pain is represented from cross-sectional studies with a limited number of longitudinal studies. According to the U.S. Institute of Medicine report published in 2010, pain was reported as a significant health problem with an estimated prevalence of chronic pain in America as 40% affecting around 100 million Americans (30). The health care costs and productivity losses

amount to 560 to 635 billion (2010 data) to the society, with annual per capita costs as high as $2,000 (30). Recent data from the Centers for Disease Control and Prevention (CDC) and National Center for Health Statistics (NCHS) suggest substantial rates of pain from the various causes and that most people in chronic pain have multiple sites of pain. The most common causes of pain reported by the U.S. adults include low back pain (LBP) (28.1%), severe headache or migraine (15.3%), and neck pain (14.6%) (31). The data from national health and nutritional examination survey suggested that the prevalence of the chronic LBP increased with age with a maximum likelihood in the fifth and sixth decades of life (32). Adults with LBP reported worse physical and mental health and are four times more likely to report psychological issues as compared to people without LBP.

Chronic widespread pain is a subset of chronic pain conditions and is characterized by long-standing diffuse musculoskeletal pain and presence of one or more other physical symptoms like fatigue, psychological distress, and concentration. According to a recent comprehensive review, females are more affected than males in all age groups with the female-to-male prevalence ratios ranging from 1.06:4.80 (33). There is little evidence to suggest the existence of geographic variation and the effects of sociocultural issues on the pain prevalence (33). The variations seem to be related to lack of standard definition and risk of bias in the studies conducted to date (34).

PERIPHERAL AND CENTRAL SENSITIZATION

Peripheral sensitization is defined when there are increased responsiveness and reduced threshold of nociceptive neurons in the periphery to the stimulation of their receptive field (4). In the presence of tissue damage and peripheral nerve injury, there are ectopic discharges from the proximal neuron in the dorsal root ganglion, which leads to antidromic stimulation of afferent C fibers and the release of mediators in the periphery (neurogenic inflammation) (4).

Central sensitization occurs when peripheral nociceptor hyperactivity induces changes in the spinal cord dorsal horn neurons, basically by increased excitability and enhanced synaptic efficacy. Clinically, central sensitization manifests as secondary hyperalgesia (pain sensitivity beyond the site of tissue damage or inflammation) and dynamic mechanical allodynia (light touch and hair movement generating sensations of pain or tenderness) (4).

Peripheral and central sensitizations are indicative of maladaptive neuronal response to an acute painful phenomenon. However, other structures are also involved in the chronification of pain: oligodendrocytes, immune system, and glial cells. Glial cells are more common in the CNS than in neurons. They are microglia, astrocytes, and Schwann cells. Initially, it was thought that glial cells were only supportive to the function of the neurons, but it is now known that they have important modulating function in the CNS and in the control of ascending and descending pain pathways (35).

Psychological factors such as depression, anxiety, and positive expectations also interact with the descending pain pathways in the development, persistency, and treatment of pain, which contribute to the central sensitization phenomenon (4).

EFFECTS OF CHRONIC PAIN ON THE INDIVIDUAL

Chronic pain is not merely a physical sensation. In the affective component of chronic pain, most patients show a degree of depression, and many show anger and anxiety. For many individuals, depression is the primary factor in the perception or experience of pain. Fifty to seventy percent of patients with chronic pain have either a primary depression or depression secondary to their pain. Chronic pain, with accompanying depression, often leads to extensive periods of reduced productivity as well as inactivity. Prolonged inactivity alters cardiovascular function, impairs musculoskeletal flexibility, and causes abnormal joint function (36,37). Prevention involves the encouragement of patient activity as soon as it is reasonable.

The motivational component of chronic pain is concerned with the vocational, economic, and interpersonal reinforcement contingencies that contribute to the learning of pain behaviors and the maintenance of chronic pain. More than 75% of patients with chronic pain display adverse behavioral characteristics, including problems with job or housework, leisure activities, sexual function, and vocational endeavors (38). Sleep disturbances and depression are highly associated with chronic pain. The patient also may have significant functional limitations as a result of multiple previous surgeries with little success and prolonged convalescence, disuse/physical deconditioning syndrome, or opioid medication (39).

Chronic pain's cognitive component involves how patients think and the part that pain plays in their belief system and view of self. The more the patient perceives pain as a threat signal, requiring a reduction of activity and protection of the affected part, the more difficult it is for the rehabilitation team to achieve compliance with exercise, stretching, and other elements of the treatment program. The memories of pain from acute pain episodes may significantly hinder a patient's recovery and contribute to chronic pain syndrome (40–42). Pain is often the result of sensory input, affective state, cognition, motivational, and memory factors, which require a multidimensional evaluation process, including treatment interventions directed at those components most responsible for the pain experience (43–45).

PROGNOSIS OF ACUTE AND CHRONIC PAIN

Acute pain is frequently the result of tissue damage in which the initial pain leads to an increase in anxiety, which magnifies the pain experience. The amount of anxiety generated and possibly the level of pain seem to be more influenced by the setting in which the pain develops rather than personality variables. With the healing process comes a reduction or termination of the anxiety and acute pain perception. When acute pain (which functions as a warning signal) fails to respond to treatment with conventional medical therapies, illness behavior and chronic pain develop. The anxiety characteristic of acute pain is replaced by depression with hopelessness, helplessness, and despair. When the expected pain relief is not attained, physical activities decrease and suffering and depression increase.

Acute pain usually resolves when the source of nociception is removed or cured and subsides quickly with application of appropriate pharmacologic or regional analgesic therapy. The cause of acute pain can be documented by physical examination findings and diagnostic procedures. A short course (i.e., a few days) of analgesic medication usually controls postoperative pain, and a return to full, painless functional state can be anticipated in a matter of weeks. Acute pain control requires the administration of an efficacious analgesic dosage of nonopioid analgesics, anti-inflammatories, or muscle relaxants. Opioids should not be considered first-line treatment for acute pain, unless when the other options are contraindicated. Too little analgesia promotes suffering and anxiety, thus defeating the purpose of prescribing medications. Fear of opioid tolerance, abuse, and addiction contribute to the underutilization of opioid medications (46). Addiction in the acute pain situation occurs in a small proportion, but it can reach much higher incidence in individuals with risk factors such as previous history of substance use disorder, current mood or anxiety disorder, history of psychological trauma, or family history of substance use disorder (47). Higher risk of opioid use disorder is correlated with the physician being more liberal in prescribing opioids for acute pain (48).

Unfortunately, a significant minority of acute pain patients continues to experience pain, which may progress into a more complex disease entity. The transition to chronic pain may be related to the brain's emotional learning circuitry (49). Except in cases where there is presence of a definable substantial biomedical disorder that persists, chronic pain is a symptom of physiologic malfunction and now becomes the disease itself. The latter is chronic pain in the absence of a structural pathology, and it is associated with a major pain-related disability; in this case, chronic pain represents a complex interaction of physical, psychological, and social factors in which the pain complaint is a socially acceptable manifestation of the disease (50,51).

The optimal intervention for chronic pain is prevention. Once the disease state of chronic pain commences, perpetuating factors such as monetary compensation, presence of job-related problems, manipulation of the environment to satisfy unmet needs, and retirement from the competitive world may obstruct complete disease resolution. Therapies designed for acute pain are often ineffective for chronic pain.

Prevention of chronic pain requires identifying contributing factors and resolving them early in the acute stage. Physicians should set a reasonable time frame for the resolution of the acute pain process. Patients should be advised when the pain medication will no longer be needed and that those medications that are no longer effective will not be continued. The patient's attention should be directed to a gradual return of full activity on a prescribed schedule. Follow-up appointments should be planned at specified intervals to enable a proper rehabilitation plan, which includes leisure, school, or work reintegration.

GENETICS OF CHRONIC PAIN

With the advance in techniques in this field, there is a great interest in explaining interindividual variability related to pain sensitivity and response to analgesic therapies. Over the last decades, at least 23 genes have been identified with the potential association with experimental pain, clinical pain, or analgesia in human and animal studies (52).

The genetic determinants have been evaluated in humans with pain associated with clinical conditions (52,53). The variability in pain syndromes has been partially associated with inherited genetic factors in back pain (54), fibromyalgia (FM) (55), menstrual pain (56), and migraine (57). Family and twin heritability estimates indicate genetic as well as significant environmental factors modulating pain (58,59). Polymorphic pain genes have been associated with congenital insensitivity to pain (60), drug metabolism due to cytochrome P-450 (61), familial hemiplegic migraine (58,62), FM (63), and reflex sympathetic dystrophy (64,65).

Gene therapy and other advances in molecular medicine may offer a means of enhancing antinociceptive receptors (cannabinoid, 1 and 2; acetylcholine, m and n; opioid, μ and κ; adrenergic, α_2) or blocking pronociceptive receptors (neurokinin, 1-α-amino-3-hydroxy-5-methyl-4-isoazolepropionate [AMPA]; N-methyl-D-aspartate [NMDA]), acting directly on the calcium channels of pain fibers, or acting directly on membrane receptors, protein C-GAMA, or other areas of the CNS involved in the transmission of pain (66,67). Definitive applications of gene intervention in pain control remain to be developed.

SOCIOECONOMIC FACTORS IN CHRONIC PAIN

Socioeconomic status likely plays an important role in the prevalence and risks of developing chronic pain. Persons with low socioeconomic status have an increased incidence of a variety of musculoskeletal pains including LBP, as well as increased incidence of psychological problems. In a large cohort study of over 9,000 adults, lowest adult socioeconomic status (defined as having a "nonskilled" manual profession) was associated with a nearly threefold relative risk of chronic widespread pain and at least a 1.5-fold relative risk for regional pain problems (68). Conversely, higher socioeconomic status (e.g., professional, managerial, and technical careers) was associated with a higher incidence of forearm pain (68).

LITIGATION AND COMPENSATION FACTORS

Disability, along with pain and suffering, greatly determines the amount of compensation awarded in worker's compensation cases and in personal injuries. The patient/client's pain behavior may be reinforced, maximized, and groomed with the hope of a large cash settlement. As a result of this reinforcement, the pain behavior develops into a learned response. The pain also becomes the disability for which the patient/client is seeking compensation. Therefore, a learned behavior becomes a determining factor in the amount of compensation awarded (69).

Alteration of the disability and/or compensation laws could decrease the number of acute pain patients who develop the behavioral disease of chronic pain. The relationship between compensation systems and pain following an acute trauma is complex, especially when superimposed by secondary mental health problems. There is some evidence that clients seeking or receiving financial compensation following a motor vehicle accident may have poor outcomes of recovery and worse pain (70). Changes that might discourage the development of chronic pain include allowing an injured worker to continue working at a job he or she is physically able to accomplish during the recuperation period,

rapid adjudication of disability and compensation claims, and physicians restricting the patient's use of addicting and depressant medication to less than 1 month. The extensive use of conservative intervention to include physical therapy and stress management early in treatment also could prevent the emergence of chronic pain (71). For additional information on disability determination and medical-legal aspects, the reader is referred to Chapter 8.

EVALUATION OF A PATIENT WITH CHRONIC PAIN

The goals of comprehensive assessment in a chronic pain patient should focus on measurement of the severity of disease, magnitude of the functional limitations, and impact of psychological factors affecting the medical condition. The failure of the biomedical approach to pain due in part to inadequate treatment outcomes has resulted in the evolution of a newer biopsychosocial model of pain. The complex interrelationships among biologic changes, psychological status, and the sociocultural context need evaluation for better understanding of a person's perception, nature, severity, persistence of pain and disability, and response to pain and illness. Moreover, interdisciplinary care has shown more promise in terms of cost efficacy and outcomes of all the available chronic pain management approaches (1–3). Hence, objective measurement and longitudinal tracking of these measurements should be more widely used to guide diagnosis and treatment and used to assess treatment outcomes. This is accomplished by a thorough pain evaluation, including a detailed history, comprehensive physical examination and clinical interview, standardized objective assessment instruments, and review of appropriate diagnostic tests.

History

A detailed history of the pain report identifies the pain in terms of its origin, radiation, quality, severity, and time intensity attributes, as well as mode of onset, duration, time of occurrence, and factors that aggravate and relieve it. Previous treatments for pain should be noted, including comments regarding usefulness in the reduction of pain. Medications currently being taken, as well as those used in the past, should be recorded, along with the patient's perceptions as to the results achieved by each. The details of physical therapy, including types of modalities, exercise (passive and active), and effectiveness of regimes, should be recorded. An inquiry as to the patient's attempts at biofeedback, relaxation, and hypnosis is also helpful. Information regarding associated findings including sensory deficits, muscle weakness, and altered body function should be obtained. It should be determined whether compensation is involved and if the patient is working; if not, the employment history should be obtained.

Physical Examination

The general goals of physical examination should be focused to (a) assess if the patient's clinical findings can explain the severity of symptoms and functional limitations, (b) assess need for additional diagnostic evaluation, and (c) formulate the treatment objectives and plan appropriate management focused on symptom alleviation and better functional status.

Physical examination always includes examination of related spine and musculoskeletal components, as well as a neurologic evaluation (see Chapter 1). Painful regions need to be compared with normal areas on the contralateral side of the patient for sensation, temperature, and sensitivity to palpation (72). Functional evaluation measures the appropriateness of the patient's functional capabilities for the level of impairment. Objective, quantitative measurements give a baseline with which to evaluate progress and long-term outcome.

Many medically unexplained pains have now been attributed to complex interplay of peripheral and central neuropsychologic mechanisms. The most commonly assessed aspect of pain is its sensory severity. Patients' response to different thermal and electrochemical sensory modalities (light touch, pinprick, hot, cold, etc.) can help to differentiate between primary and secondary hyperalgesia patterns (72,73). Further, the distribution of sensory symptoms in the body quadrants can help assess and understand possible peripheral and central pain mechanisms (72). Special attention should be given to rule out hyperalgesia patterns in chronic opioid drug overuse, possibility of neurologic sensory symptoms due to involvement of small nerve fibers not amenable to assessment in routine electrodiagnostic testing, and chronic myofascial muscle pains.

Objective Measures of Pain, Function, and Mental Health

Most pain patients present a complex array of physical, motivational, cognitive, and affective manifestations and therefore require detailed psychological and social evaluations. Objective measures of pain intensity and interference should be used to track the pain intensity and interference with function and assess response to the interventions. At least 50% of the patients suffering from chronic pain suffer from coexisting depression and anxiety (4).

Brief Pain Inventory (BPI) is a widely accepted and commonly used objective tool for clinical pain assessment (5). It allows the patient to rate the severity of the pain on a 10-point numeric rating scale (NRS) system and also allows for characterization of pain interference with feeling and function. Simple and easy self-reported questionnaires such as Patient Health Questionnaire-4 (PHQ-4) (6) and Pain Catastrophizing Scale (PCS) (7) allow a physician to quickly assess patient psychological distress by measuring depression and anxiety and serve as possible predictors to tailor appropriate treatment approaches (74).

Providers should also assess for special patient population groups with traumatic past experiences and posttraumatic stress disorder (PTSD) like sexual abuse, military veterans, etc., as these subgroups have higher abnormal pain perception and risk of opioid dependence (8). Given the well-known estimates of co-occurrence of chronic pain and addiction, there are several simple objective tools, such as the "Opioid Risk Tool" (9), that can be utilized to assess the risk for addiction. Due care should be taken to list other potentially risky medications as benzodiazepines and sedative hypnotics.

Diagnostic Procedures

Laboratory Testing

Until recently, laboratory findings in acute and chronic pain had been shown to have no features distinct from those found in patients with a primary disease. However, drug screening tests of the blood and urine may provide valuable information as to the variety and type of pain medications being used. Serum drug level testing provides data to determine the bioavailability of medications being taken by the patient.

Recently, altered milieu of inflammatory biomarkers has been shown to exist in acute and chronic myofascial pain conditions (75). However, the association of these systematic biomarkers and clinical findings is not yet established and remains more of research value at the moment. Epidemiologic studies have linked low levels of vitamin D to chronic pain (76). Still, its role as causative or confounding factor has not been fully elucidated. Recent systematic reviews and meta-analysis have shown inconclusive evidence but promising treatment outcomes with vitamin D supplementation in patients with chronic pain (77).

Drug infusions like sodium amobarbital and pentobarbital can be used in conjunction with the psychological interview and may be helpful in differentiating patients with significant somatic/peripheral pain from mood disorders, somatoform disorders, factitious disorders, and conscience exaggerators (78–81). However, their criticism of cognitive effects masking real pain experience has precluded their widespread use.

Imaging

The recently published consensus statement from the presidential task force of the International Association for the Study of Pain (IASP) emphasized that the use of brain imaging in the diagnosis of chronic pain has the potential to increase our understanding of the neural underpinnings of chronic pain, inform the development of therapeutic agents, and predict treatment outcomes for use in personalized pain management. However, the task force does not recommend brain imaging measures as suitable for clinical or legal purposes, especially as it is not an effective method as a pain lie detector (82).

Since the early 1990s, neuroimaging studies have allowed an access to the human brain function and *in vivo* analysis of pain-associated responses in the CNS. The positron emission tomography (PET) localizes a specified radionuclide that works as a tracer, which is concentrated within a brain area with high metabolic activity. The functional magnetic resonance imaging (fMRI) detects a blood-oxygen-level–dependent signal (BOLD) (83). The diffusion tensor imaging provides insights about brain connectivity by providing information about anisotropy and white matter orientation (84). The neuroimaging techniques are reconstructed after a defined sensory stimulus or a cognitive task, so higher pain-related brain functions can be mapped, such as the anticipation to a pain stimuli, the emotional response, the memory associated with pain, and the conditioning. Most of the methodologic designs of imaging studies are cross-sectional studies. Although the costs, the limited methodologic design of research studies, the heterogeneous responses among individuals, and the diverse spatial resolution of imaging studies are barriers to obtain strong high-quality evidence and to draw definite recommendations for diagnostic or therapeutic purposes, there are some insights about the pain-related functional neuroanatomy (85,86).

Radiography, computed tomography (CT), and magnetic resonance imaging (MRI) demonstrate anatomic or structural disorders, which account for a low percentage of functional abnormalities. However, CT, myelography, and MRI are well established in the diagnosis of disk herniation though they provide significant false-positive results in subjects with no history of back pain (87). The recent interest in high-frequency musculoskeletal ultrasound has given some possible diagnostic insights into the structural and mechanical properties of muscles in chronic myofascial pains (88).

Recent advances in functional brain imaging have shown evidence of changes in brain structure and function in patients with chronic pain (86,89). Although the neural mechanisms that contribute to these pain-related changes in brain structure and function remain largely unknown, the evidence reflects its potential use in the future for mechanism-related pains. Given the current cost and the emerging nature of findings, these brain imaging methods are not yet ready for clinical implementation. The clinical usage of diagnostic tests requires a careful correlation between clinical signs, symptoms, and test results. For additional information on imaging studies, the reader is referred to Chapter 5.

Electrodiagnosis

Electrodiagnosis is an objective neurophysiologic extension of the physical examination. It typically includes the determination of nerve conduction velocities and needle electromyographic (EMG) studies of individual muscles. In addition, somatosensory-evoked potentials have expanded the armamentarium of the electromyographer in evaluating the peripheral and CNS (90). For additional information on electrodiagnostic evaluation, the reader is referred to Chapter 3. EMG and evoked potential studies demonstrate the neurophysiologic changes that the clinician should associate with structural abnormalities as demonstrated by imaging techniques such as MRI and CT scanning. The diagnosis of conditions such as radiculopathy, plexopathy, peripheral entrapment neuropathy, and polyneuropathy is important consideration for the clinical management of chronic pain patients. Careful clinical correlation is essential when interpreting all tests related to chronic pain (91).

CONDITIONS COMMONLY ASSOCIATED WITH CHRONIC PAIN

Low Back Pain and Sciatica

Chronic low-LBP is a serious problem, especially affecting adults of working age (see Chapter 27). Although most individuals recover from an acute episode of LBP, those who remain in pain after 12 weeks have a slower and uncertain recovery. It is estimated that 60% recover within 6 weeks and 90% within 12 weeks, but in those individuals who have been disabled for 2 years, the rate of return to work is almost close to zero (92). It is estimated that the 10% of workers who develop chronic LBP (remaining off work for 3 months or longer) are responsible for 80% of the costs, in terms of lost wages, compensation, medical expenses, etc. (93). The prevalence of LBP is higher in older adults (94). Strategies to prevent acute LBP from progressing to chronic LBP include using conservative interventions, returning to work as soon as possible, or continuing working at a modified job the worker is physically able to accomplish during the recuperation period and rapid adjudication of disabilities/compensation claims (95).

An extensive review of randomized, controlled trials in chronic LBP over the past 20 years has repeatedly shown methodologic limitations including high risk of selection, performance, measurement, attrition, and reporting biases (96,97). Despite the limitations in clinical trial design and conduct, it is good clinical practice to recommend behavioral treatments to reduce disability through modification of maladaptive pain behaviors and cognitive processes (98). Nonsteroidal anti-inflammatory drugs (NSAIDs) are effective and the most commonly used medications for back pain symptoms and must be consumed preferably for short courses or in anticipation of pain aggravation with functional activities, given their side effects of bleeding and unestablished safety profile in hypertensive states and cardiovascular disease risks (99). Low-dose opioids for a short duration of 3 to 7 days may be considered only as a last resource after exhausting all nonpharmacologic and nonopioid pharmacologic options (see Chapter 52). Long-term opioid use for the treatment of chronic LBP has shown minimal functional improvement with significant increase in the risk for the adverse effects of opioid use including CNS depression, constipation, development of tolerance, and aberrant behavior (100).

Adjunctive treatment options include therapeutic rehabilitative physical therapy regimes and physical treatment modalities (heat, ice, soft tissue mobilization, and transcutaneous electrical nerve stimulation [TENS]) (see Chapter 51) (101). Alternative treatment options may include spinal manipulation, as well as acupuncture, yoga, and other exercise-based therapy programs (102–104). Many alternative therapies lack conclusive scientific evidence supporting their efficacy in the treatment of chronic back pain (see Chapter 59). Physical therapy or exercise-based programs tend to focus on core muscle strengthening and aerobic conditioning. No differences have been found when comparing the effectiveness of supervised with home-based exercise programs for chronic LBP. It seems that muscle energy technique is not effective for LBP (105). Pilates has been reported to be a little superior than other forms of exercises, but the decision should be based on patient's or care provider's preferences and costs (106). Motor control exercise seems to be effective for chronic but not for acute LBP (107,108).

Spinal injections have a limited role in the treatment of chronic, mechanical LBP (109–111). Specific subset of patients may receive short periods of benefit from facet injections or epidural steroid injections after exhaustion of other conservative treatment options (see Chapter 53). Treatment goals for chronic LBP should shift from "disease cure" to address symptom alleviation and achievement of better functional status. For additional information on rehabilitation of the patient with spinal pain, the reader is referred to Chapter 27.

Neck Pain and Whiplash Syndrome

Chronic neck pain is a complex disorder that consists of biologic, psychological, and social factors and presents as a combination of physical and psychological symptoms (112) and signs with decreased health-related quality of life, daily activity limitations, increased health care utilization, and decreased work productivity (113) (see Chapter 26). In the United States, neck pain contributes to approximately 10.2 million annual visits to physicians and hospital outpatient clinics (114).

Injury severity is classified in five categories of whiplash-associated disorder (WAD), ranging from 0 (no symptoms) to IV (fracture or dislocation of the neck) (112). More recently, the 2000–2010 Bone and Joint Decade Task Force has proposed the classification of neck pain and associated disorders (NAD) (115) as follows:

I. No signs or symptoms suggestive of structural pathology and/or minor interference with activities of daily living

II. No signs or symptoms suggestive of structural pathology, with major interference with activities of daily living

III. No signs or symptoms suggestive of structural pathology but presence of neurologic signs such as decreased deep tendon reflexes, weakness, or sensory deficits

IV. Signs or symptoms suggestive of structural pathology

About 30% to 50% of patients report chronic symptoms (116). The development of chronicity is thought to occur because of peripheral and central sensitization. This is an area of active research, and the risk factors for the development of chronicity are still under investigation. Many neurotrophins (e.g., nerve growth factor) and tachykinins (e.g., substance P) have been shown to enhance the sensitivity of nociceptors and modify the expression of cytokines (IL-1ra, IL-8, IL-6) that are implicated in increased nociceptive sensitivity and sympathetic nervous system activation (117–119). Neuroimaging studies have demonstrated that mechanical stimulation can cause abnormal (or enhanced) pain processing at higher cortical levels such as anterior cingulate cortex and prefrontal areas (120,121). In addition, the chronic pain experience has been associated with a spatial pattern of brain activity (122). The existence of a persistent high-intensity nociceptive input can cause neuroplastic changes in the CNS with expansion of receptive fields, and more widespread symptoms have research support (123).

There is some evidence that provides the clinician with clues as to which patient may become chronic (124). These clues include higher than expected pain complaints (125,126), high levels of catastrophization (121), and comorbid pain syndromes such as irritable bowel syndrome (IBS), irritable bladder syndrome, restless leg syndrome, and/or migraine headaches (127). Furthermore, women are overrepresented among the chronic widespread pain group (128). In addition, the coexistence of depression and/or anxiety may also cause more disability in the chronic pain patient (129). There is also an association with positive family history of chronic widespread pain and history of abuse (126). We encourage the astute clinician to keep these factors in mind when assessing their patients.

Extensive literature review suggests the following management plan (113):

1. Major structural pathology should be ruled out.
2. Assess for prognostic factors for delayed recovery.
3. Education with regard to pathophysiology of WAD/NAD.
4. Importance of maintenance of activity.
5. Physical therapies with emphasis on range of motion, strengthening exercises, manipulation, or mobilization.
6. Pharmacotherapy using NSAIDs and muscle relaxants.
7. There is little to no evidence for massage therapy, laser, short wave diathermy, electroacupuncture and Botox injections, and cervical collar or cervical traction.

Myofascial Pain Syndrome

Myofascial pain syndrome (MPS) is a common, nonarticular musculoskeletal disorder, characterized by myofascial trigger points (MTrPs). MTrPs have been defined as hard, palpable, discrete, localized nodules located within taut bands of skeletal muscle that are painful on compression (130). Travell and Simons (131,132) originally described the criteria for identification of trigger points by clinical assessment as palpation of a taut band, local tenderness, a pain recognition, a referred pain, a local twitch response, and the "jump sign."

It has been estimated that some 44 million Americans have pain that is associated with MTrPs (133). Another study reported that myofascial pain affects up to 85% of the general internal medicine clinic (134,135). This study reported results of lower back pain only and so it would be expected that the prevalence is much higher. Thus, MPS is very common, and its diagnosis primarily rests upon the presence of MTrPs since they are thought to be the most important aspect of the diagnostic criteria. An extensive literature search was conducted investigating the epidemiology of MPS, and very limited information is available.

MTrPs have been detected in the shoulder girdle musculature in nearly half of a group of young, asymptomatic military personnel (136) and with a similar prevalence in the masticatory muscles of a group of unselected student nurses (137). Active MTrPs, defined as those causing spontaneous pain, have been diagnosed as the primary source of pain in 74% of 96 patients with complaints of musculoskeletal pain seen by a neurologist in a community pain medical center (134) and in 85% of 283 consecutive admissions to a comprehensive pain center (138). Of 164 patients referred to a dental clinic for chronic head and neck pain, 55% were found to have active MTrPs as the cause of their pain (139), as were 30% of those presenting with pain to a university primary care internal medicine group practice from a consecutive series of 172 patients (133). A study of musculoskeletal disorders in villagers from rural Thailand has demonstrated myofascial pain as the primary diagnosis in 36% of 431 subjects with pain during the previous 7 days (140). There is evidence of an increasing awareness that active MTrPs often play a role in the symptoms of patients with tension headaches (141), LBP (142), neck pain (141), temporomandibular pain (143), forearm and hand pain (144), postural pain (145), and pelvic/urogenital pain syndromes (146–149).

For the majority of the history of MPS, identification of the trigger points has been primarily based on manual palpation described initially by Simons et al. (131). According to a systematic review by Tough et al. (150), the originally proposed criteria are utilized inconsistently in research with many studies including only subsets of the criteria. An attempt to standardize diagnostic criteria has been made by surveying practicing clinicians concerning the importance of purported diagnostic criteria for MPS. Surveys conducted on physician opinion agreed that point tenderness and reproduction of pain are key to diagnosis, while autonomic symptoms are unnecessary (151,152). Rivers et al. (152) utilized their survey results and proposed the following diagnostic criteria based on clinician consensus:

1. A tender spot is found with palpation, with or without referral of pain ("trigger point").
2. Recognition of symptoms by patient during palpation of tender spot.

3. At least three of the following:
   a. Muscle stiffness or spasm
   b. Limited range of motion of an associated joint
   c. Pain worsens with stress
   d. Palpation of taut band and/or nodule associated with tender spot

Unfortunately, palpation has come into question as an effective method of diagnosing and locating trigger points. Previously published reviews (150,153,154) on the reliability of manual palpation for MTrPs generally report poor clinician agreement and reliability. Using meta-analysis, Rathbone et al. have found unacceptably poor interrater reliability (kappa = 0.474) of the clinician's ability to detect an MTrP (155). Unfortunately, palpation of a nodule in a taut band, the target of injection-based therapies, was significantly less reliable with a kappa of 0.336.

The lack of interrater reliability may be related to the small size of MTrPs. A recent ultrasound study of MTrPs in the ankle and foot region found that MTrPs ranged in size from 0.05 to 0.21 cm², with a mean of 0.09 cm² (156). Moreover, Sikdar et al. also previously attempted to use ultrasound imaging to visualize and characterize trigger points within the trapezius muscle. They observed that MTrPs appear as discrete, focal, hypoechoic regions of elliptical shape, with a size of approximately 0.16 ± 0.11 cm² (157). These small sizes of the MTrPs identified on ultrasound imaging would present difficulty in identification through palpation. One study that examined intrarater reliability of trigger point localization in the upper trapezius found a 0.15-cm test-retest mean difference in localization between exams (158). Therefore, even before accounting for the difficulty of palpating while injecting, we suggest that the mean difference in localization is approximately the average size of a trigger point, which would contribute to a large susceptibility of mistakenly missing the trigger point on injection. Given this information, we suggest that successful injection will not be possible without ultrasound imaging guidance. The poor detection accuracy of the trigger points may be why previous studies have failed to clearly identify benefits from trigger point injections. Therefore, we believe that the use of an imaging modality is necessary to improve the MTrP detection rate, reliability, and diagnostic objectivity.

MTrPs are a common therapeutic target for the management of chronic pain caused by MPS, including dry needling (102,130), injections, and manual therapies.

In addition, there is considerable overlap with FM since MTrPs are very prevalent in FM. Furthermore, MTrPs are thought to represent important pain generators (159). Therefore, the clinician should consider the presence of MPS and FM carefully. This can be especially confusing during the evolution of either disorders; the clinical picture has not fully evolved to the point where the criteria of each have been fulfilled. This is important since the treatment recommendations can be quite different depending upon the diagnosis that becomes established.

MPS can appear to be a different syndrome and have different clinical presentations based upon the muscle(s) and region involved. Therefore, the clinician is encouraged to have an excellent working knowledge of pertinent regional anatomy and the "Trigger Point Manual" (131,132). Other conditions within the differential diagnosis should be ruled out; some of the important diagnoses to consider include radiculopathy and complex regional pain syndrome (CRPS).

Important considerations for the comprehensive management of MPS include:
1. Education to provide the patient with:
   a. Pathophysiology of MPS
   b. The importance of a multifaceted management program
   c. Recognizing that underlying psychological factors can impact MPS
   d. Importance of proper sleep, cardiovascular fitness, and biomechanics
2. Physical therapies including *s*trengthening, *s*tretching, *a*erobics, and *r*elaxation exercises, or S.S.A.R. for short form (see Chapter 49).
3. Pharmacologic management using NSAIDs (topical or oral), muscle relaxants, antidepressants (tricyclics or SNRIs), or lidocaine patches (see Chapter 52).
4. Trigger point injections—many different agents have been used, but there is no convincing evidence to suggest one is better than another, and there has been no universal acceptance of any one practice.
5. Psychological interventions.

Fibromyalgia

Fibromyalgia syndrome (FMS) is a common chronic condition of unknown etiology. It is characterized by chronic widespread pain, fatigue, cognitive dysfunction (memory and attention deficits), psychological distress, sleep disturbance, and other functional symptoms. The global prevalence of FM is estimated to be 2.7% but was based on the old American College of Rheumatology (ACR)-established diagnostic criteria (1990) (160). A recent study based on the newer provisional 2010 criteria estimated the prevalence to be 7.7%, with a female-to-male ratio of 1.6:1 (161), alike as in chronic pain conditions (162).

The pathogenesis of FMS is unknown, and there is an ongoing debate whether it is a rheumatologic, somatoform, or neuroendocrine disorder. However, there is general consensus about the heterogeneous nature of FMS with variable sensory symptoms and comorbidities (163). Further, it is believed that different subgroups may exist that have different pathophysiology with different treatment response characteristics (164). FMS is thought to develop from aberrant sensory and pain processing with contributions from peripheral, central, and autonomic nervous systems. Unlike the known causes of pain related to an identifiable tissue or nerve damage, several hypothetical mechanisms have been suggested on the pathogenesis of FMS. Some researchers argue that FMS is predominantly characterized by neurochemical alterations in the CNS that lead to an augmentation of pain perception, most commonly including allodynia and hyperalgesia (165). CNS influences involving several mechanisms, including central sensitization and reduction of descending inhibition, may play the major role in FMS in a similar fashion with other common chronic pain conditions. Further, contributions from peripheral and autonomic mechanisms encompassing neurogenic and neuroendocrine inflammation may also play a role in the pathogenesis. Recently, there have been many studies debating the peripheral neuropathic component in FMS and its association with peripheral small fiber neuropathy (166). Moreover, psychoemotional contributory factors as poor stress response mechanisms, vulnerable psychological status, low social support, and previous life adverse events further add susceptibility for FMS (167). Irrespective of the proposed several pathogenesis models, health researchers still lack a consensus to fit FMS relative to other peripheral and central pain disorders.

FMS shall be considered in the differential diagnosis if the patient presents with multifocal or diffuse pain. The original ACR criteria of 1990 were developed for research purposes and were not widely used due to the inconsistencies in symptom recognition and low awareness of the guidelines resulting in late diagnosis and ineffective treatment outcomes. A recent modification of the original 1990 ACR criteria was provisionally released in 2011 and utilized a patient–self-reported survey to determine the pain locations (widespread pain index) and presence/severity of other associated symptoms instead of physician-reported tender point examination in the old 1990 criteria. However, the 2011 criteria came under severe criticism due to the blurring of the distinction between FMS and more localized functional pain syndromes by dropping generalized pain as a criterion (168). Hence, a revision to the original 2010/2011 criteria was published in 2016 and combines physician assessment, questionnaire criteria, as well as emphasizing a widespread pain state, thus minimizing misclassification of regional pain syndromes (169).

The self-reported version of criteria yet remains to be validated. FMS does not cause joint pathology but may occur in the presence of other rheumatologic and pain disorders. However, basic tests such as blood counts, serum chemistries, and thyroid function tests can be helpful for disease assessment. FM is no longer considered a diagnosis of exclusion, and the diagnosis can be established by assessment of patient's symptoms and if they meet the diagnostic criteria. However, physicians must be mindful of the illness validation–seeking behavior of FMS individuals for compensation purposes, preventing them from the motivation to get well (170). The treatment should be initiated immediately. However, due to the lack of consensus on the causative pathogenesis, minimal research has been done on the disease-modifying treatments. Patient education is a critical part of disease management and starts with patient understanding, setting the expectations, and self-management. A multidisciplinary approach to treatment and an individualized treatment plan are important for better outcomes. Pharmacologic management includes FDA-approved medications as pregabalin, duloxetine, and milnacipran, which work through central pain modulation mechanisms (171). The dose should be gradually titrated for effective patient response. Several other non–FDA-approved medications as amitriptyline and cyclobenzaprine have fair evidence of efficacy. The choice of pharmacologic agent or combination therapy shall be tailored according to patient factors and comorbid symptoms.

Nonpharmacologic interventions include low- to moderate-intensity aerobic exercises with a goal to reach 30 minutes of activity two to three times per week (172). Referrals for cognitive behavioral therapy (CBT) and sleep hygiene should be considered, if required, as they have shown to be effective as patient management strategies. The goal of treatment is to maintain everyday activities and enhance quality of life. The best results are obtained using a combination of pharmacologic and nonpharmacologic therapies.

Complex Regional Pain Syndrome

The International Association for the Study of Pain (IASP)-accepted criteria for CRPS are the "Budapest Criteria" (173). CRPS is defined as a syndrome with continuing (spontaneous and/or evoked) regional pain that is seemingly disproportionate in time or degree to the usual course of pain after trauma or other lesion. The pain must be regionally distributed, but not in a specific nerve territory or dermatome. Usually, there is distal predominance of abnormal sensory, motor, sudomotor, vasomotor edema, and/or trophic findings.

The clinical diagnostic criteria for CRPS are as follows:

A. Continuing pain, disproportionate to any inciting event

B. Must report at least one *symptom* in three of the four categories:
1. Sensory: hyperalgesia and/or allodynia
2. Vasomotor: temperature asymmetry and/or skin color changes and/or skin color asymmetry
3. Sudomotor/edema: edema and/or sweating changes and/or sweating asymmetry
4. Motor/trophic: decreased range of motion and/or motor dysfunction (weakness, tremor, dystonia) and/or trophic changes (hair, nails, or skin)

C. Must display at least one *sign* at time of evaluation in two or more of the following categories:
1. Sensory: evidence of hyperalgesia (to pinprick) and/or allodynia (to light touch and/or deep somatic pressure and/or joint movement)
2. Vasomotor: evidence of temperature asymmetry and/or skin color changes and/or asymmetry
3. Sudomotor/edema: evidence of edema and/or sweating changes and/or sweating asymmetry
4. Motor/trophic: evidence of decreased range of motion and/or motor dysfunction (weakness, tremor, dystonia) and/or trophic changes (hair, nails, skin)

D. There is no other diagnosis that better explains the signs and symptoms.

It is very important to perform a good differential diagnosis for local pathology such as nonunion of a fracture, compartment syndrome, traumatic vasospasm, regional vascular disease, cellulitis, regional infection, Raynaud's disease, thromboangiitis obliterans, thrombosis, specific neuropathy, erythromelalgia, specific regional motor disease, or a regional autoimmune process.

There are two types of CRPS with similar signs and symptoms but different etiologies: CRPS type I (previously known as reflex sympathetic dystrophy) develops after any type of trauma, most commonly fracture or a soft tissue lesion (e.g., crush injury), but may also occur after immobilization. It may also be related to visceral disease such as angina or a central neurologic disease such as stroke. CRPS II (previously known as causalgia) occurs with electrodiagnostic or physical evidence of a major nerve damage. In type II, the initial symptoms and signs correspond to a single peripheral nerve distribution but may become more diffuse over time. The median and sciatic nerves are the most affected in the vast majority of cases (174).

The concept of "sympathetically maintained pain" has lost its previous significance as CRPS-related mechanisms may shift and change over time (175). The response to sympathetic blocks should not be used to make the diagnosis.

The mainstay of the diagnosis of CRPS is a detailed history and physical examination. Investigations are not necessary to make the diagnosis, but only to exclude other causes that could explain the symptoms and signs. In the past, three-phase bone scan was considered important to help in the diagnosis of CRPS, especially if it was done within 12-month postinitiation of the symptoms. The typical findings of periarticular uptake in the delayed phase are not equivalent to having CRPS, because it may also be observed in other conditions such as immobility, after sympathectomy, in asymptomatic persons, or even in factitious disorders (175). Besides, the three-phase bone scan has a low sensitivity for CRPS, so it should not be used for screening purposes, because it may result in false-negative results and therefore a delayed treatment (176). Plain radiographs of the affected body part and contrast-enhanced MRI have low sensitivity and high specificity to make the diagnosis of CRPS and do not need to be used routinely (177). Other tests such as galvanic reflex tests, thermography, quantitative sudomotor axon reflex test, and resting sweat output have been suggested to document the sympathetic nervous system hyperactivity, but their low diagnostic accuracy does not suggest routine use and is restricted to research studies (178).

The incidence of CRPS ranges from 5.5 to 26.2 per 100,000 person-years at risk (179,180).

There is a paucity of preventive measures for CRPS. The only evidence-based strategy is the use of low-dose vitamin C (200 mg/d) in patients who had a wrist fracture (181).

The management of patients with CRPS should focus on function restoration. The pharmacologic and nonpharmacologic modalities serve primarily to facilitate the restoration of normal function (182). Early mobilization of the involved limb is essential to avoid central and peripheral nerve system sensitization. For patients with refractory pain, an interdisciplinary pain rehabilitation team may be required to provide specific exercises, reconditioning, biofeedback, relaxation, psychotherapy, and education.

Historically, pharmacologic treatments have included NSAIDs, steroidal anti-inflammatories, sodium channel blockers (intravenous [IV] lidocaine), N-methyl-D-aspartate (NMDA) receptor blockers (ketamine, dextromethorphan, memantine), calcium-regulating drugs (calcitonin, clodronate, alendronate), free radical scavengers (transdermal dimethyl sulfoxide [DMSO], oral N-acetylcysteine [NAC]), α_2-adrenoceptor agonist (clonidine), and oral phenoxybenzamine (183). The use of corticosteroids in CRPS is reported since the early 1980s (184), but it is not possible to establish a well-defined protocol yet. Oral prednisone (185), intramuscular metilprednisone (186), intravenous systemic (187), or regional dexamethasone (188) is reported in trials with diverse methodologies. The duration of treatment is reported from one session of a regional IV block (188) to a daily oral regimen of around 4 months (189), but many trials reported a poor strategy to detect or record side effects. Given the heterogeneity of treatments, there are no clear guidelines (190) on the type of patient, the underlying condition, the type of medication, the dosage, the route of administration, and the safest protocol with the least risk of adverse events. In general, these trials report a significant improvement of swelling, pain, range of motion, and grip strength, but a clear guideline in CRPS is yet lacking. There is a very-low-quality evidence that oral corticosteroids do not improve pain and that the corticosteroid IV block is not effective (191).

The use of opioids may be indicated in the early phases to allow mobilization and functional restoration (FR). The evidence base is scarce and there is no supporting literature on how to safely use the opioids for CRPS. A randomized trial found no differences between a sustained-released dose of morphine and placebo (192). Clinicians need to be careful not to escalate the dose without a clear assessment of baseline risk and goals or without safety measures and patient education. This could lead to increased risks of overdose, misuse, diversion, or complications of long-term opioid therapy such as opioid-induced constipation, hypogonadism, hyperalgesia, or sleep apnea (193,194).

There are very few trials of anticonvulsants in CRPS type I, including carbamazepine 600 mg/d, with better results than placebo (192). Although the reports on gabapentin 600 to 1,800 mg/d resulted in a modest improvement in a randomized controlled trial (RCT) study (195), a Cochrane systematic review concluded that there is no improvement of pain with gabapentin and it induces a higher frequency of adverse events (191).

Intranasal or subcutaneous calcitonin has been used for CRPS. The evidence is conflicting (196), and there is some suggestion that its analgesic effect is not superior than paracetamol (acetaminophen) (191).

Bisphosphonates are widely used for CRPS due to a significant relief of pain reported in individual studies and a meta-analysis at the short (<2 months) and long term (>2 months). They also reduce the swelling and improve range of motion. In patients with symptom duration less than a year, the trials with alendronate 7.5 mg/d IV for 3 days (197) and clodronate 300 mg/d IV for 10 days (198) reported significant relief of pain in the short term; another study with oral alendronate 40 mg/d for 56 days found a relief even at 84 days of follow-up (199). In patients with a longer duration of the CPRS type I, pamidronate 60 mg in an IV single infusion reported symptom relief at 90 days (200). The long use of bisphosphonates increases the risk of pathologic fractures, jaw osteonecrosis (201), and prolonged union times of distal radius fractures (202).

Topical preparations have the advantage of reducing or avoiding systemic side effects, but there are not enough clinical trials to form a solid evidence base. Topical cream with 10% ketamine has been used in CRPS with relief of allodynia and hyperalgesia (203,204). A 5% lidocaine-impregnated patch and capsaicin has been used for other kinds of neuropathic pain; capsaicin may be limited by the patient acceptance due to a painful burning sensation until it causes dying-back denervation of nociceptive nerve endings (193).

Other pharmacologic treatments have very limited or no evidence of efficacy, and they are not currently recommended for CRPS. These include muscle relaxants, baclofen, botulinum toxin, mannitol, phenytoin, antidepressants, benzodiazepines, or calcium channel blockers (178,193,201,205,206).

There is evidence that spinal cord stimulators reduce pain and improve health-related quality of life in carefully selected patients with chronic CRPS type I (207); however, the pain-alleviating effects diminished over time, as compared with the control group of physiotherapy, and were no longer significant after 3 years of follow-up (208).

When treating a patient with long-standing pain that is due to CRPS, it is important to consider the psychological aspects.

PTSD is also a common but unidentified psychological problem in CPRS patients. Appropriate psychological and psychiatric consultation for relaxation training and biofeedback, in addition to other treatment modalities, is important. The prognosis is poorer when there is anxiety and pain-related fear; therefore, these could be considered target for early intervention (209). Psychological factors must be adequately treated; otherwise, the patient is unlikely to improve regardless of other interventions.

Painful Peripheral Neuropathy

Pain is a common feature of peripheral neuropathy that is due to diabetes, amyloidosis, alcoholism, polyarteritis, Guillain-Barré syndrome, brachial neuritis, acquired immune deficiency syndrome (AIDS), porphyria, and riboflavin deficiency. The pain sensations may vary depending on the type of neuropathy but can be of either a constant or an intermittent nature and are often described as burning, aching, or lancinating. It may occur with or without signs of sensory loss, muscle weakness, atrophy, or reflex loss (210). The pain can disturb sleep as it is often bothersome at night. For specific recommendations regarding diagnosis and management of painful neuropathies, read Chapter 24.

Spinal Cord Injury

Pain related to spinal cord injury (SCI) is often complex and multifactorial. SCI pain may be broadly classified into nociceptive pain (musculoskeletal and visceral) and neuropathic pain located above level, at level, and below level of the spinal injury (**Table 39-1**). Studies indicate that 66% of all patients with SCI have pain that is mild to moderate in severity. Pain after SCI is common, poorly understood, complex, and often difficult to treat. Also note that 50% of patients with cauda equina syndrome report severe pain.

The reported prevalence of chronic pain in the population with SCI is variable with an average of 65%; approximately one third rate the pain as severe (211).

Many of the nociceptive types of pain are variations of those found in patients without SCI and are treated in a similar fashion with adaptation to the underlying injury. However, patients with SCI are more susceptible to mechanical instability of the spine that is due to trauma of the musculoskeletal system, muscle spasm pain that is due to trauma to the neurologic system, as well as both overuse and nerve compression syndromes primarily involving the upper extremities.

Mechanical instability of the spine is usually best treated with NSAIDs and opiates (as needed), as well as immobilization using orthosis or surgical fusion. These are effective treatments in most patients. Pain that is due to muscle spasm is best treated with antispasmodics, motor point blocks, or botulism toxin to decrease spasticity. Secondary overuse syndromes are often relieved by rest and NSAIDs, with significant adaptation by the patient and modification of environmental factors. Nerve compression syndromes are often relieved through the use of orthotics or surgical decompression. Visceral nociceptive pain is often due to afferent input from the sympathetic nervous system and may be due to underlying pathology. A headache that is due to autonomic dysreflexia is a medical emergency and should be treated appropriately.

With neuropathic pain, evidence suggests that trauma and neural alterations of the pain pathways are primarily involved

TABLE 39-1	**Classification and Causes of Pain Related to Spinal Cord Injury**

Nociceptive Pain
Musculoskeletal (often dull, aching, worse with movement, decreased with immobilization, responsive to NSAIDs and opioids)
Secondary overuse syndromes
Bone, joint, muscle trauma, or inflammation
Mechanical instability
Bone, joint, muscle trauma, or inflammation
Scar infection
Muscle spasm
Visceral structures (often dull, cramping, burning, and constant but fluctuating pain in the abdomen with preserved innervation)
Regional calculus
Bowel or sphincter dysfunction
Headache associated with autonomic dysreflexia
Neuropathic (often sharp, shooting, burning, electrical sensation [hyperalgesia, hyperesthesia])
Above level (located in the region of sensory preservation)
Compressive mononeuropathies
Complex regional pain syndromes
Routinely treated as neuropathic pain of peripheral nerve origin
At level (located in segmental pattern of level of injury)
Nerve-root compression (including cauda equina)
Syringomyelia, spinal cord trauma/ischemia (transitional zone, etc.)
Presents with an ascending neurologic deficit often with alterations in pain/temperature
Dual-level cord and root trauma and double-lesion syndrome
Below level (located diffusely below level of injury)
Spinal cord trauma/ischemia (central dysesthesia syndrome, etc.)
Phantom sensations

(211,212). Neuropathic pain following SCI is associated with significant differences in regional brain anatomy located in pain-related regions as well as regions of the classic reward circuitry, that is, the nucleus accumbens and orbitofrontal, dorsolateral prefrontal, and posterior parietal cortices (213). The precise etiology underlying pain in spinal cord injuries is not known, but evidence suggests that trauma-induced alterations of the pain pathways are primarily involved (212). Hypersensitivity of the structures in the ascending pathway may play a role (213). Patients describe their pain as having one or more of the following components: burning in body parts below the injury; a deep, aching sensation over and around the site of injury; and radicular with lancinating characteristics. Burning pain in spinal cord–injured patients may be a variation of deafferentation pain occurring as a result of loss of inhibitory or augmentation of excitatory influences. The most effective treatments of this type of pain include gabapentin, tricyclic antidepressants (TCAs) and SNRIs, and neuroaugmentative techniques (214,215).

Patients describe their pain as having one or more of the following components at the level of injury: lancinating, burning, or stabbing pain in a radicular distribution. This pain may also be related to spinal instability or nerve-root entrapment. Pain is typically relieved by opioids, neuropathic pain medications, and spinal decompression, if necessary. Pain from cauda equina injury is usually neuropathic of peripheral nerve origin that has a burning sensation routinely affecting the groin and bilateral lower extremities. Segmental deafferentation pain often occurs at the border of sensory loss. Transitional zone pain is often associated with allodynia and hyperalgesia and may respond to neuropathic pain medications, epidural or somatic root blocks, dorsal root entry zone (DREZ) procedures, or spinal cord stimulation (SCS). The combination of spinal cord and root trauma often results in severe burning pain over a region that is otherwise denervated. Pain with root evulsion may be responsive to neuropathic pain medications, DREZ procedures, or SCS. DREZ procedure was shown to be more effective for segmental pain than for diffuse pain after SCI (214). The segmental deafferentation pain may be secondary to spinal cord trauma or ischemia. Neuropathic pain below the level of entry is often referred to as deafferentation or central dysesthesia syndrome, commonly described as burning, tingling, numb, aching, or throbbing. Pain is usually constant and unrelenting. Pain may be relieved by neuropathic pain-relieving medication, intrathecal opioids, and clonidine and occasionally by dorsal column stimulator. Pharmacologic and nonpharmacologic treatments for pain in patients with SCI have a minimal number of subjects per treatment approach, and only a limited number of studies have been subjected to randomized, controlled trials.

Spinal fracture site pain results from an alteration of body mechanics causing pain-sensitive structures to be stretched or compressed. This mechanical pain may be the result of vertebral endplate fractures, annulus fibrous tears, or internal disk herniation after a spinal fracture. Fracture site pain or mechanical pain is often exacerbated by activity. NSAIDs, trigger point injections, TENS, cognitive/behavioral techniques, and adjuvant medication may be used, but the evidence from randomized trials is scarce or weak (216). Orthotics also may be used to decrease the mechanical stress and alleviate the underlying etiology. Radicular pain in these patients may be secondary to compression of nerve roots by a herniated nucleus pulposus, fracture fragment, dislocated vertebra, or the results of traumatic arachnoiditis.

New therapies have emerged in the past 10 years, including transcranial direct current stimulation (tDCS), high-definition tDCS (HD-tDCS), repetitive transcranial magnetic stimulation (rTMS), cranial electrotherapy stimulation (CES), TENS, SCS, and motor cortex stimulation (MCS). The results show a great variability in the mean improvement in chronic pain after SCI (217).

For additional information on SCI, the reader is referred to Chapter 22.

Stroke and Brain Injury

Chronic pain after stroke (see Chapter 18) is common and affects nearly 50% of the affected population (218). It is an underreported phenomenon, which is poorly identified and inadequately treated (219). Pain after a cerebral vascular accident may be secondary to multiple etiologies, including central poststroke pain, CRPS, pain due to spasticity, and pain from dysfunction of the affected extremities (220).

Central poststroke pain is a neuropathic pain due to a lesion or dysfunction of the CNS, develops usually within 1 to 3 months after the stroke, and is often characterized as an agonizing, burning pain on the side contralateral to that of the lesion. Dejerine-Roussy syndrome is a specific condition developed after a thalamic stroke. It is important to exclude other causes of pain like obvious nociceptive, psychogenic, or peripheral pain (221).

The diagnostic criteria for central poststroke pain have been revised in 2009 (222):

Mandatory criteria:

- Pain within an area of the body corresponding to the lesion of the central nerve system.
- History suggestive of a stroke and onset of pain at or after stroke onset.
- Confirmation of a central nerve system lesion by imaging or negative or positive sensory signs confined to the area of the body corresponding to the lesion.
- Other causes of pain, such as nociceptive or peripheral neuropathic pain, are excluded or considered highly unlikely.

Supportive criteria:

- No primary relation to movement, inflammation, or other local tissue damage
- Descriptors such as burning, painful cold, electric shocks, aching, pressing, stinging, and pins and needles, although all pain descriptors can apply
- Allodynia or dysesthesia to touch or cold

The reported prevalence of central poststroke pain is variable and depends on the site of the infarct, study design, and sample cohorts, ranging from 2% to 25% (223,224). CNS lesions producing central pain can be extremely small, especially if located in central pathways. Almost 100% of central pain patients are affected by change in temperature perception. Pain is constant in 85% of the patients and intermittent but daily in 15%. Pain is primarily burning, aching, prickling, and lancinating. Patients make the point that central pain is not truly pain but an unpleasant sensation that drastically affects their quality of life. Multiple factors including peripheral and central, psychological, and autonomic mechanisms contribute to the central poststroke pain. Neuronal reorganization of the CNS architecture is most likely the cause of central pain. The plasticity of the CNS may result in changes in receptor structure and function that are likely to be delayed in onset. CNS neurons are responsible for nociceptive perception and can exhibit long-lasting changes and responsiveness after transient or permanent damage in input. Either excitatory or inhibitory mechanisms can be affected, and as this responsiveness changes, so does modulation of the signals. Central poststroke pain that is due to thalamic infarction is often characterized as an agonizing, burning pain on the side contralateral to that of the lesion. Pain to minimal cutaneous stimulation and aggravation by emotional stress and fatigue are characteristic findings. Sensory alteration is variable in these patients, with minimal findings of motor weakness. Central pain that is due to lesions involving central thalamic spinal tracts may be manifest in pain distributed to the level of the tract involved. This results in loss of pain and temperature perception on the contralateral side at the level below the injury. Central pain of tract origin is similar to pain of thalamic origin but is usually less intense. This pain may be described as burning, pulling, or swelling. Information on central pain syndromes is scarce, with treatments limited in efficacy.

Resolution of the central poststroke pain is rarely obtained; therefore, it is important to manage patient's expectations with treatment. As it is the case with all types of chronic pain, it is recommended to manage chronic poststroke pain in an interdisciplinary setting to provide optimal pharmacologic, physical, and psychological support (221). Initial pharmacologic treatment includes TCAs (amitriptyline nortriptyline, trazodone), anticonvulsants (lamotrigine, gabapentin, pregabalin), and selective serotonin reuptake inhibitors (SSRIs) (fluvoxamine). The last option for pharmacologic treatment is opioids (morphine, tramadol, tapentadol, oxycodone, methadone, or buprenorphine) because of the potential for adverse complications such as opioid-induced hyperalgesia, sleep apnea, and hypogonadism (221,225). Other pharmacologic options that have been used for central poststroke pain include carbamazepine, phenytoin, ketamine, intrathecal baclofen, subanesthetic infusions of thiamylal/thiopental, and subhypnotic doses of propofol.

Physical modalities and exercises have been shown to improve the well-being and function in patients with central poststroke pain. These include TENS, desensitization techniques, and mirror therapy (226).

There are other therapies that have shown little effect on pain and function or contradictory results (227). These include dorsal column stimulators, DREZ, thalamic stimulation, and deep brain stimulation. Electrical stimulation such as deep brain stimulation and rTMS seems to be effective in certain cases (228).

Chronic pain after stroke that is due to dysfunction of the affected extremities is most often manifest in the upper extremity. This pain may be the result of shoulder subluxation, decreased range of motion because of adhesive capsulitis, or brachial plexus injury (229). Spasticity secondary to stroke may result in pain. This may be treated with medication or nerve blocks. Other factors of affected limb dysfunction include bicipital tendonitis, arthritis, fracture, heterotopic ossification, and knee/ankle instability. Appropriate use of modalities, as well as orthotics and assistive devices, is indicated in the resolution if some of these problems are contributing to the patient's pain (230).

Amputations

After an amputation, the patients may develop phantom limb pain or residual limb pain. The residual limb pain is classified as neuropathic and somatic. The neuropathic pain may be due to a painful neuroma, a complex regional pain syndrome (CRPS) or other neuropathic conditions. Somatic pain refers to pain in either the scar, soft tissue, muscle or bone of the amputated limb (231,232).

Phantom Limb Pain

Phantom limb pain involves an amputated portion of the body. The etiology of phantom pain appears to be related to peripheral, spinal, and central factors. Peripheral components of phantom limb pain appear to be the result of loss of previously present peripheral nerve activity triggering changes in the CNS. Development of abnormal activity in a neuroma or dorsal root ganglion results in pain fiber transmission and an alteration in ion channel activity at site of injury resulting in pain fiber activation. Spinal-level factors involved in phantom limb pain include

deafferentation of neurons and their spontaneous and evoked hyperexcitability resulting from the loss of large A-afferent nerve fiber input in the dorsal horn cells with an unopposed C fiber input. Cortical reorganization has been observed in the primary motor and somatosensory cortex in humans after amputation. These reorganizational changes appear to be a significant factor in the occurrence and intensity of phantom limb pain. The remapping of regions of the brain receiving touch, pain, and temperature input from the amputated limb to other parts of the brain appears to be an etiology of phantom limb pain. Pain may be continuous, in character with intermittent exacerbations. It is often reported by patients as cramping, aching, or burning, with occasional superimposed electric-like components. Reported incidence of phantom limb pain is highly variable often due to the setting and circumstances in which the data were collected. Prospective research suggests approximately 82% of patients experience phantom pain following amputation. It is estimated that 65% experience phantom pain at 6 months and 59% experience phantom pain 2 years after amputation. Severe disabling phantom limb pain incidence is reported at 10% after several years. Of note are reports that severe pain occurs more often with proximal amputations (41,233–235).

There is some indication that psychological factors may predict poor prognosis in patients with amputations and phantom pain. Catastrophizing thoughts, poor social supports, solicitous responses from family members, and high reliance on resting as a coping response are poor predictors (236).

Multiple modalities, adjuvant medications, and anesthetic and surgical procedures have been used in the treatment of phantom limb pain with varying long-term success. Although more than 70 methods of treating phantom limb pain have been identified, successful treatment of persistent types of pain is not commonly reported (234,235,237–243). Transcutaneous nerve stimulation, TCAs, anticonvulsants, calcitonin, lidocaine, mexiletine, and mirror therapy have been used with varying success. Chemical sympathectomy or neurosurgical procedures also have had variable success, but there is a high incidence of complications (242,243). Treatments yielding a temporary decrease in pain include analgesics, anesthetic procedures, stump desensitization, physical modalities, and sedative/hypnotic medication. Studies of various therapeutic regimens have reported up to a 70% efficacy in the treatment of phantom limb pain, but reviews of most with long-term follow-up suggest a limited response to any intervention.

Underlying mechanisms for phantom limb pain include reorganization that appears to occur at the dorsal horn of the spinal cord, in the thalamus, and in the cortex. *Residual limb pain* is pain at the site of the limb amputation. Residual limb pain is common, with approximately 57% of patients experiencing residual limb pain following amputation, 22% at six months and 10% two years after amputation. Residual limb pain may be rated as more severe than the patient's phantom limb pain and its incidence is close to 5% after several years. (235). Residual limb pain was rated as the worst problem by 33% of the patients, phantom limb pain by 24%, back pain by 17%, and sites other than the involved limb by 26%.

Neuroma

Injury to the nerve with a resulting neuroma or entrapment of the branches of the nerve in the scar tissue can produce disabling pain. The pain caused by a neuroma is sharp, often jabbing, pain in the stump and is usually aggravated by pressure or by infection in the residual limb. Pain is often elicited by tapping over a neuroma in a transected nerve. The increased sensitivity of sprouts from cut peripheral nerves to noradrenaline and adrenaline may partially explain why adrenergic-influenced emotional states (i.e., stress or anxiety) occasionally provoke attacks of phantom limb pain.

Neuromas are suspected when numbness appears in the distribution of a particular nerve and when pain is produced by palpation of the neuroma. It has been shown that the nerve fibers in the neuroma develop α-receptors, which respond to catecholamines with spontaneous firing and pain production. Painful neuromas are difficult to treat; many patients continue to have pain despite multiple attempts at surgical excision of the neuroma. Suspected scar pain can be evaluated by picking up the scar from the deeper tissues with two fingers and palpating. If this does not reproduce the patient's pain, the pain is probably not originating in the scar tissue. Pain that is due to neuroma or scar tissue can be associated with CRPS. Diagnosis can be established by infiltration of the scar or the neuroma with a local anesthetic agent, resulting in complete pain relief (246). Repeated injection of a local anesthetic agent has proven to be an extremely useful technique. This should be followed by appropriate physical therapy to the scar; stretching or deep massage of the scar are proposed, although the evidence is scarce. When the local anesthetics, with or without steroids, do not provide prolonged relief, other methods, such as Neurolytic techniques or surgical revision should be considered. Neurolytic techniques should be used only after repeated injections of local anesthetics produce consistent pain relief proportional to the duration of action of the local anesthetic agent. Although surgical revision of the scar is often considered, it is not very successful when the scar cannot be stretched out and there is significant nerve entrapment.

Somatic Pain

The somatic pain may have multiple aetiologies including chronic swelling in patients with predisposing conditions, such as diabetes, renal, cardiac or venous insufficiency, residual ischemia in arterial vascular disease, wound dehiscence, osteomyelitis, bone spur, hematoma, or infection. The soft tissue damage may result from poor stump qualities, such as insufficient myoplasty covering, aggressive bone edge, heterotopic ossification, redundant tissue, thin stump, or direct trauma from a poorly unfitted prosthesis with non-well distributed pressure or shearing-related wound due to telescoping or pistoning (247,248). Causes of painful stump after intense or repetitive trauma include bursitis in the weight bearing area, soft tissue inflammation without fluid collection or bone bruise (247). Diabetes, older age, smoking, arterial ischemia, infection and malignancy are predisposing factors of wound dehiscence (249–252). Skin problems in the stump include acroangiodermatitis, allergic contact dermatitis, bullous diseases, epidermal hyperplasia, hyperhidrosis, infections, malignancies and ulcerations (253). Skin complications in the stump may appear even decades after the amputation; a report of veterans with combat-related amputations found complaints of skin problems in 48.2% of cases during the preceding year in more than 50% of the time; it caused pain or discomfort in the stump in 61.5% of them and prevented the prosthesis use in 55.6% (254). Myodesis for patients with traumatic or

ischemic amputation is recommended by experts instead of myoplasty. It offers a better stability of the stump, decreases the pain and facilitates the use of the prosthesis (255).

Chronic Pain After Cancer Treatment

Cancer pain can be viewed as pain associated with advanced cancer (palliative or end-of-life care) or chronic pain in cancer survivors. Despite all advances in cancer treatment, there is still an estimated 40% of survivors who continue to experience pain as a result of treatment (256). Unbearable pain is one of the greatest fears and a major source of morbidity for patients with cancer. Clinical experience suggests that patients with cancer pain (palliative or survivors) are treated most effectively with a multidisciplinary approach, including multiple modalities, appropriate analgesic drugs, neurosurgical and anesthetic procedures, psychological intervention, and supportive care (257,258). The goals of pain therapy for palliative cancer patients are a significant relief of pain to maintain the functional status of their choice, a reasonable quality of life, and a death relatively free of pain. The goals of pain therapy for cancer survivors are improved quality of life, return to function or meaningful activities with minimal side effects from treatment modalities, and self-management strategies. For additional information on cancer rehabilitation, the reader is referred to Chapter 36.

There are multiple invasive measures to control cancer pain. The most common is the surgical removal of all or part of the tumor with the hope of relieving pain and obtaining a cure. Radiotherapy or chemotherapy also may relieve pain by shrinking the tumor. Common invasive anesthetic procedures include trigger point injections and nerve blocks. MPSs are often the result of inactivity and disuse and are commonly found in the cancer patient. Neuropathic pain may result from direct tumor invasion or as a side effect of chemotherapy. Patients who have side effects with large doses of opioids may derive long-term benefit with a chronically implanted epidural catheter or an intrathecal catheter and pump to administer opioids and/or other pharmacologic agents. Multiple neurosurgical procedures have been used for the control of cancer pain.

The American Society of Clinical Oncology released a new guideline on chronic pain management in adult cancer survivors (259). The highlights of this guideline are as follows:

- Clinicians should screen for pain at each encounter.
- Recurrent disease, second malignancy, or late onset treatment effects in any patient who reports new-onset pain should be evaluated, treated, and monitored.
- Clinicians should determine the need for other health professionals to provide comprehensive pain management care in patients with complex needs.
- Systemic nonopioid analgesics and adjuvant analgesics may be prescribed to relieve chronic pain and/or to improve function.
- Clinicians may prescribe a trial of opioids in carefully selected patients with cancer who do not respond to more conservative management and who continue to experience distress or functional impairments.
- Risks of adverse effects of opioids should be assessed.
- Clinicians should clearly understand terminology such as tolerance, dependence, abuse, and addiction as it relates to the use of opioids and should incorporate universal precautions to minimize abuse, addiction, and adverse consequences.

The nonpharmacologic interventions recommended for the management of chronic pain in cancer survivors are exercises, orthotics, ultrasound, heat/cold, massage, acupuncture, and music therapy. Interventional therapies include nerve blocks, neuraxial infusions, vertebroplasty, or kyphoplasty. The psychological approaches recommended include CBT, distraction, mindfulness meditation, and guided imagery. The neurostimulation interventions include TENS, SCS, peripheral nerve stimulation (PNS), and transcranial stimulation (259).

Pain Associated with Multiple Sclerosis

Multiple sclerosis (MS) is a chronic, remitting, and relapsing disease characterized by multiple foci of demyelination that are randomly distributed in the white matter of the CNS. Patients with MS often have symptoms of psychiatric distress, sleep problems, chronic pain, and sexual dysfunction that affect their quality of life and function (260).

A recent meta-analysis of 28 articles (7,101 subjects) describing overall pain or pain syndromes in MS showed that the overall prevalence of pain was 63%. Marked heterogeneity in this estimate was not significantly explained by selected study design variables (outpatient sample, time frame prior to study over which pain was assessed) or sample demographic variables (disability, disease duration, sex, and proportion with progressive MS). The prevalence of headache was 43%, neuropathic extremity pain 26%, back pain 20%, painful spasms 15%, Lhermitte's sign 16%, and trigeminal neuralgia 3.8% (261).

Patients often present initially with paroxysmal lancinating and intense burning pain that primarily affects the face, shoulder region, or pelvic girdle. In MS, the central pain usually involves the bilateral lower extremities. Treatment of pain resulting from MS has been limited. Pharmacologic interventions that showed some efficacy for chronic pain in MS include antidepressants, anticonvulsants, dextromethorphan/quinidine, cannabinoids, and opioids/opioid antagonists (262). If the patients have intrathecal baclofen pumps, neuropathic pain adjuvant medications can be added to the infusion. For additional information on MS, the reader is referred to Chapter 20.

Postherpetic Neuralgia

Herpes zoster (shingles) is a reactivation of the varicella (chicken pox) virus, which has remained latent. The viral inflammation of the dorsal nerve root and ganglion causes vesicle formation and severe burning, aching, and lancinating pain in a radicular distribution. During the acute stage, a course of antiviral medication, along with NSAIDs and/or steroids, provides good pain relief (263). Most patients recover from the acute episode in approximately 2 weeks without sequelae. However, some patients develop postherpetic neuralgia secondary to deafferentation from neuronal cell death with and without allodynia. Postherpetic neuralgia is uncommon in patients younger than 40 years of age but occurs in more than 50% of patients older than 60 years of age after an episode of herpes zoster. Varicella-zoster virus vaccine is effective to prevent episodes of herpes zoster. Varicella-zoster immunoglobulin is useful to modify the course of zoster in patients who are immunocompromised. Pharmacologic treatment of postherpetic neuralgia includes topical or systemic analgesics. Topical agents are lidocaine and capsaicin. Systemic agents include anticonvulsants, TCAs, and opioid analgesics (264). Peripheral nerve blocks and destructive neurosurgical procedures have not proved useful in treating established postherpetic neuralgia.

Functional Pain Disorders

Functional abdominal pain syndrome is defined as frequent or continuous abdominal pain associated with some loss of daily activity, where there is no identifiable structural, biochemical, or immunologic abnormality (4). It is important to differentiate from IBS as there are no changes in bowel habits, eating, or other gut-related symptoms (265). Prevalence has been estimated to be 0.5% to 1.7% and tends to show a female predominance (265). It is likely that injury or inflammation in a psychologically predisposed individual may lead to the peripheral sensitization of visceral afferents, thus augmenting the ascending input of nociceptive information to the spinal dorsal horn leading to central sensitization. The physical exam of a patient with functional abdominal pain must exclude any abnormality that can explain the symptoms. The Carnett's test is useful to differentiate between myofascial pain of the abdominal wall and intra-abdominal origin of the pain: the painful area is palpated before and after the patient raises the head and tenses the abdominal wall. If there is pain on palpation, then the most likely cause is myofascial pain because usually intra-abdominal pain improves with tension of the abdominal musculature. Treatment of patients with IBS involves good patient-physician relationship, education, general measures, and pharmacologic (antidepressants) and psychological interventions (CBT, hypnosis). Opioids should be avoided because they are implicated in opioid-induced hyperalgesia and narcotic bowel syndrome (266).

CLINICAL MANAGEMENT

The primary goals of treating a patient with pain are alleviating the pain and enhancing the patient's quality of life and functional capabilities. The biomedical model of chronic pain management is outdated because it implies a biologic pathway for cure and elimination of the pain, and it has been replaced by a biopsychosocial approach that describes the complex and dynamic interactions among physiological, psychological, and social factors that perpetuate or worsen one another, resulting in the complex phenomenon of chronic pain syndromes (267).

Multidisciplinary and Interdisciplinary Pain Teams

The treatment of pain with physical modalities is as ancient as the history of humanity, but the use of interdisciplinary rehabilitation techniques has gained acceptance only within the past few decades. The chronic pain problem is clearly multifaceted. No single physician has the resources to care comprehensively for the complex psychological, social, legal, medical, and physical problems involved in chronic pain. Therefore, the multidisciplinary team approach is necessary. The American Pain Society in its recent white paper on the interdisciplinary care of pain emphasized on the difference between multidisciplinary and interdisciplinary care. Multidisciplinary care usually involves several disciplines in parallel with an independent approach and may not necessarily be coordinated. In a multidisciplinary pain management approach, there are several health care providers, but there is limited communication and collaboration among them, as they may not even be located in the same facility (268). Using an interdisciplinary team approach does not mean the patient is referred from one specialist to another, because this tends to result in conflicting and overlapping treatment and a loss of hope of treatment in the patient. Ideally, the team should have complimentary roles and discrete skill sets and work in a coordinated manner to provide a unified explanation of the illness. The interdisciplinary team usually assesses the patient together, although this is not mandatory. Comprehensive treatment program enhancing patient care is the hallmark of an interdisciplinary approach/interdisciplinary pain service and has the advantage of offering a variety of coherent treatment approaches to the patient. This type of program recognizes that a multifaceted problem requires a multifaceted approach, as well as continuity of care in which the patient is an active participant (269). The main characteristic of an interprofessional approach is the common philosophy of rehabilitation, constant communication, and active patient involvement (268).

The International Association for the Study of Pain (IASP) task force recommended that multidisciplinary/interdisciplinary pain centers offer a diversity of health care providers with sufficient professional breadth to comprehensively address the biopsychosocial model of pain (270). They suggest the core group to include at least two medical doctors as well as a clinical psychologist, a physical therapist, and additional health care providers (if needed) to address the particular needs of specific pain populations. This group may vary considerably according to local needs, resources, and available expertise. The physiatrist has advantages over other medical specialties as the medical doctor because of the training in working with multidisciplinary/interdisciplinary teams, pharmacologic approaches, and physical and psychosocial management of various chronic conditions. Other medical specialities are well suited for the team such as neurology, psychiatry, and anesthesia. However, the team must have the knowledge to manage the pharmacologic, physical, psychological, and social problems with optimal evidence-based treatments. They must also have a thorough understanding of physical treatments and the rehabilitation process. Our clinical experience demonstrates that nurses, nurse practitioners, pharmacists, occupational therapists, social workers, chiropractors, acupuncturists, massage therapists, and sex therapists may also play important role in the assessment, management, and education of patients with chronic pain.

The referral to a multidisciplinary/interdisciplinary pain team should be as early as possible to restore the person to society and avoid the high costs of chronic pain investigations, which usually occur in the first year (271).

The multidisciplinary/interdisciplinary pain approach begins with a complete clinical evaluation. Comprehensive medical and psychosocial evaluations with emphasis on functional capabilities and behavioral responses to pain are essential. The somatic, affective, cognitive, and emotional components of the chronic pain experience are explored. All previous medical records are needed to avoid repeating appropriately performed studies and unsuccessful treatment approaches. The psychosocial evaluation focuses on the behavioral response to pain, adjustments to the physical impairment, and degree of motivation (272).

Patient education with setting the expectations right and agreement for a common goal based on functional improvement with manageable pains, if not curable, as the main focus helps avoid potential conflicts and shall be the mainstay of treatment. The multidisciplinary/interdisciplinary team functions at several levels within the treatment process. It attempts to identify and resolve documentable organic problems when present and

to improve the patient's ability to cope with the pain through medication, manual/physical therapy, psychological interventions, and patient education. In addition, considerable effort is devoted to exercise rehabilitation in order to improve the patient's functional outcome as measured by increased activity time, improved activities of daily living, increased distance walked, and increased tolerance for specific homemaking or vocational activities (101,273,274). To accomplish these objectives, the multidisciplinary/interdisciplinary team must use many skills. Selective use of interventions (e.g., injections in soft tissues, joints, nerves, or the spine) in appropriate time at an appropriate stage of disease process can help them effectively manage the pain levels serving as enabler to participate and engage in other pain interventions including physical therapy and psychological interventions. In many cases, the patient with chronic pain is so entrenched in pain behavior that a behavior modification approach is essential. These patients are often characterized by low levels of activities of daily living, high demand for medication accompanied by physical and psychological dependency, high verbalization of pain, and the inability to work. The American Pain Society evidence-based guidelines also support the use of interdisciplinary treatments in patients with ongoing axial back pain and associated disability before proceeding with surgical interventions (275).

Pain Clinics or Pain Treatment Centers

The organization and operation of the multidisciplinary pain clinic has been discussed by multiple authors (276,277). Many behavior modification programs use the Fordyce model (278,279). This approach uses the general principles of interruption of the pain behavior reinforcement cycle; reward of healthy behavior; appropriate goals that the patient must achieve; measurement of improvement by functional assessment, as well as pain level; and psychosocial adjustment. Particular emphasis is placed on detoxification and medication reduction, pain reduction, increased activity, and modification of pain behavior. FR started as a program for pain rehabilitation in 1988 by Mayer and Gatchel (280). Multiple studies in various jurisdictions have shown the benefits of FR approach, including the US military (268). The U.S. Department of Defense started a Functional Occupational Restoration Treatment (FORT) program in 2003 with the goals to improve the management of chronic pain, increase functioning, and retain military members on active duty using an interprofessional approach. This program was able to achieve all goals over 1 year in a randomized trial design (281).

The patient with chronic pain usually exhibits a decreased activity level, which results in a disuse syndrome. The exercise programs are based on the initial specific and general exercise that the individual can perform. The exercise regimen is progressive, with the goals rising along with the patient's ability. Rewards for accomplishing tasks are a mainstay of this program with no reinforcement given for pain behavior. The achievable goals provide success and confidence and allow for frequent reinforcement when they are met. Cooperation by all staff members is essential; they must consistently ignore reports of pain and encourage improved function. Psychological intervention is used as indicated. The chronic pain behavior modification programs report short-term success rates in medication reduction, increased activity, and more productive behavior patterns (282). Statistics suggest improvement of 60% to 80% in patients with chronic pain without major psychosocial components, 30% to 50% in patients with significant psychosocial components, and approximately 20% in patients with major psychiatric components or secondary gains (283–285).

Multidisciplinary chronic pain treatment is a focused, unified approach to the chronic pain syndrome. In the United States, pain treatment centers differ widely in organization and emphasis. They are generally multidisciplinary centers that use some combination of physiatrists, anesthesiologists, clinical psychologists, dentists, neurologists, orthopedists, pharmacists, and psychiatrists. The goals of these centers are to provide holistic treatments to help diminish, if not eliminate, chronic pain, increase the patient's functional capabilities to allow for a more active life, and decrease the patient's dependence on drugs for pain control.

However, an important criticism of multidisciplinary/interdisciplinary care has been failure to consider costs and other concerns important to involved stakeholders including third-party payers. In view of same, due attention must be paid to assessment of measurable outcomes to assess treatment effects.

Pharmacologic Interventions for Chronic Pain

Pharmacologic treatments commonly follow the World Health Organization pain relief three-step ladder that was developed for cancer pain and can be adapted to chronic noncancer pain. The *first step* consists of nonopioid analgesics (**Table 39-2**), with or without adjuvants. The *second step* consists of mild opioids such as codeine, with or

TABLE 39-2	**Step 1: Nonopioid Analgesics and Anti-inflammatories**		
Drug	**Usual Dose (mg)**[a]	**Maximum Recommended Dose (mg/d)**[b]	**Comments**
Analgesic/Antipyretic			
Acetaminophen	650 q4–6h	4,000 for acute use 3,000 for chronic use	Less effect on gastric mucosa, platelet aggregation, or anti-inflammatory response. Hepatotoxic >4 g/d
Salicylates			
Acetylsalicylic acid	325–1,000 q4–6h	4,000	Standard of comparison for nonopioids, irreversible effect on platelet aggregation
Diflunisal	500 q12h	1,500	Less effect on platelet aggregation with <1 g/d, decreased GI toxicity
Choline magnesium trisalicylate	1,000–1,500 q12h	3,000	Less effect on platelet aggregation Lower GI toxicity
Salsalate	1,000 q8h	4,000	Less effect on platelet aggregation Lower GI toxicity
Nonsteroidal Anti-inflammatory Drugs (NSAIDs)			
Diclofenac	50–75 q12h	150	Lower GI toxicity than indomethacin
Indomethacin	25–50 q8h	200	Not routinely used because of greater incidence of GI toxicity and CNS side effects
Ibuprofen	400–800 q8h	2,400	Rapid onset of action. Side effects include nephrotoxicity, tinnitus, CNS, and cardiovascular problems
Flurbiprofen	50 q4–6h	300	Less effect on platelet aggregation. Decreased GI toxicity <20%
Naproxen	250–500 q12h	1,500	Available in liquid suspension
Piroxicam	20 q24h	40	Not recommended with liver or kidney dysfunction. Higher incidence of side effects at a dosage of 40 mg qd over 3 wk
Meloxicam	5–7.5 once daily	15	Avoid in >65 years of age
Sulindac	150 q12h	400	Lower renal toxicity
Nabumetone	500 q12h	2,000	Near placebo level GI side effects
COX-2 Inhibitors			
Celecoxib	200 q12h	800	Lower GI toxicity
Atypical Analgesic			
Tramadol	37.5–50 q6h	300 or 400	Atypical central-acting analgesic.[c] Risk of seizure, serotonin syndrome, mu opioid agonist, lower GI toxicity

CNS, central nervous system; GI, gastrointestinal; NSAIDs, nonsteroidal anti-inflammatory drugs; q12h, every 12 hours, etc. The authors will not assume liability for this table. No medication should be given until the complete prescribing recommendations, drug use indications, and potential side effects that are listed in the package insert with the product or contained in a drug reference manual are reviewed and understood thoroughly by the physician and patient.

[a]Dosage should be adjusted in the elderly and patients on multiple medications and patients with renal insufficiency or hepatic failure. Doses may be increased at weekly intervals if pain relief is inadequate and dosage is tolerated. Doses and intervals titrated to effect.

[b]The patient should be evaluated routinely for hepatic toxicity. Patients receiving NSAIDs also should be evaluated for renal function and fecal blood loss that is due to gastrointestinal irritation. It is recommended that patients who develop visual symptoms during treatment undergo ophthalmic evaluation. Gastrointestinal disturbance may be reduced if taken with milk, on a full stomach, with antacids, or with a gastroprotective agent such as proton pump inhibitor.

[c]Combined action as an opioid agonist and monoaminergic drug with potential abuse potential. Nausea and vomiting side effects at same rate as opioid medications. Classified by the World Health Organization as weak opioid, however, classified in the United States as nonopioid medication. Serious potential consequences of overdose are central nervous system depression, respiratory depression, and death.

TABLE 39-3 Step 2: Opioid Analgesics for Moderate Pain

Drug	Equivalent to 90 mg Oral Morphine	Usual Initial Oral Dose (mg)	Usual Oral Dose Limits (mg)	Comments
Codeine IR or CR	600 mg	IR: 15–30 mg q12h CR: 50 mg q12h	IR: 600 mg/d CR: 300 q12h	Weak opioid, as dose increases, nausea, vomiting, and constipation occur more frequently
Hydrocodone	90 mg	2.5–10 mg q4–6h	Limited by maximum acetaminophen or NSAID	Only available combined with NSAIDs
Pentazocine	450 mg	50 mg q4h	600 mg/d	Partial opioid agonist
Buprenorphine transdermal	30–40 µg/h patch	5 µg/h q7d	Varies by country	Partial opioid agonist
Meperidine	Oral administration is not recommended for treatment of acute or chronic pain. IV, IM, or subcutaneous administration does not indicate for chronic pain. If use in acute pain (in patients without renal or CNS disease) cannot be avoided, treatment should be limited to ≤48 h and doses should not exceed 600 mg/24 h			
Propoxyphene	Discontinued in many countries due to increased risk of serious abnormal heart rhythms			

CR, controlled release; IM, intramuscularly; IR, immediate release; IV, intravenous; NSAIDs, nonsteroidal anti-inflammatory drugs; q4h, every 4 hours; etc. The authors will not assume liability for this table. No medication should be given until the complete prescribing recommendations, drug use indications, and potential side effects that are listed in the package insert with the product or contained in a drug reference manual are reviewed and understood thoroughly by the physician and patient. The dosage should be adjusted in elderly patients and patients with impaired ventilation, increased intracranial pressure, liver failure, or bronchial asthma.

without nonopioid analgesics or adjuvants (**Table 39-3**), and the *third step* includes strong opioids such as morphine (**Table 39-4**), with or without nonopioid analgesics or adjuvants. Opioid analgesics are used on time-limited regimes to minimize the development of complications such as opioid-induced hyperalgesia, hypogonadism, sleep apnea, addiction, or overdose.

Pharmacologic intervention is the most common means of treatment for all forms of chronic pain; however, the physiatrist has knowledge and access to other modalities that could be employed to reduce the polypharmacy and to improve the patients' well-being. Pharmacologic substances may be divided into the following classes: analgesics (acetaminophen), anti-inflammatories (nonsteroidal and steroidal), muscle relaxants (nonbenzodiazepines and benzodiazepines), opioids, cannabinoids, and adjuvant drugs (antidepressants and anticonvulsants).

Nonopioid Analgesics and Anti-inflammatories

Nonopioid analgesics are primarily acetaminophen and NSAIDs (see **Table 39-2**). These drugs are centrally and peripherally active analgesics that do not inhibit nociception or alter the perception of the pain input. They are best considered remittent agents that alter the pathologic processes that generate pain. Salicylates and other NSAIDs reduce pain by interfering with prostaglandin sensitization of nociceptors and inhibiting the synthesis of prostaglandins. Additional NSAID actions include inhibition of tissue reaction to bradykinin, suppressed release of histamine, and decreased vascular permeability. This improves the environment of the nociceptor, increasing pain control by decreasing sensitivity. NSAIDs are mostly used for the treatment of inflammatory pain; however, given their properties to block COX-2 activity in the spinal cord, they are also useful to prevent the development of central

TABLE 39-4 Step 3: Opioid Analgesics for Severe Pain

Drug	Equivalent to 90 mg Oral Morphine	Usual Initial Oral Dose (mg)	Usual Oral Dose Limits (mg)	Comments
Morphine IR, CR, and ER (12 or 24 h release)	90 mg	IR: 5–10 mg q4h 12-h capsules: 10 mg q12h 24-h capsules: 10 mg q24h	N/A	Standard of comparison for opioid equianalgesic doses
Oxycodone IR or CR	60 mg	IR: 5–10 mg q6h CR: 10 mg q12h	N/A	Immediate release available in combination with acetaminophen or NSAIDs
Hydromorphone IR, CR (12 h), and PR (24 h)	18 mg	IR: 1–2 mg q4–6h CR: 3 mg q12h PR: 4 mg q24h	N/A	Long-acting available for twice-a-day or once-a-day doses
Levorphanol	6 mg	1–2 mg q6–8h	N/A	Increased sedation with repeated doses
Methadone	Dose equivalence is unreliable	N/A	N/A	Avoid in patients with significant respiratory, hepatic, cardiac, or renal failure
Fentanyl transdermal patch	25 µg/h patch	Not recommended for opioid naïve patients	N/A	Recommend a patch-for-patch return to the pharmacy (286)

CR, controlled release; ER, extended release; IR, immediate release; N/A, not available; PR, prolonged release. The authors will not assume liability for this table. No medication should be given until the complete prescribing recommendations, drug use indications, and potential side effects that are listed in the package insert with the product or contained in a drug reference manual are reviewed and understood thoroughly by the physician and patient.
The dosage should be adjusted in elderly patients and patients with impaired ventilation, increased intracranial pressure, liver failure, or bronchial asthma.

sensitization and chronic pain syndrome (4). NSAIDs also possess anti-inflammatory effects that reduce local heat, swelling, and stiffness. These drugs are used to treat patients with acute and chronic pain of low to moderate severity. NSAIDs are preferred over opioids because they cause no constipation, very little sedation, no psychological or physical dependence, and no development of tolerance. All NSAIDs have ceiling effects, but the ceilings for some of these drugs are higher than that of acetyl salicylic acid (238).

Although acetyl salicylic acid, acetaminophen, and other NSAID compounds are available over the counter, they all have potential side effects. The most common complication, involving the gastrointestinal (GI) tract, is seen in 5% to 10% of patients. These drugs produce in varying degrees gastrointestinal, hematologic, renal, and hepatic toxicities. It is important to note that some patients demonstrate difficulty with compliance because of the gastrointestinal side effects; in these cases, it is recommended to prescribe a gastroprotective drug to reduce the symptoms and protect from upper GI bleeding (287). NSAIDs are associated with an increased risk of adverse cardiovascular thrombotic events, including myocardial infarction (288). For additional information on NSAID medications, the reader is referred to Chapter 52.

Opioid Analgesics

The use of opioids for chronic noncancer pain is controversial. The benefits are small in terms of improvement in pain and function when compared to placebo, but the effects are not different from NSAIDs, antidepressants, and anticonvulsants (229,289–291). However, there are serious risks and complications that have sparkled some jurisdictions to declare a public health crisis due to the number of fatal and nonfatal opioid-related overdoses and number of people who are addicted to opioids (292–295). Among patients without history of substance use disorder, the rate of addiction to prescription opioids prescribed for chronic noncancer pain is 5.5%, the rate of nonfatal overdose is 0.1%, and the rate of fatal of overdose is 0.2%. These risks increase in people with active substance use disorder to 8.9% for addiction, 0.9% for nonfatal overdose, and 0.5% for fatal overdose (296). See **Table 39-5** for glossary.

Patient selection is very important. Opioid medications should be avoided in patients who exhibit signs of central sensitization because opioids activate the abnormal NMDA receptors in the spinal cord, thus potentiating the painful stimulus and therefore participating in the transition from acute to chronic pain (127,297). Opioid-induced hyperalgesia has been demonstrated in experimental and clinical studies (297–301). Long-term use of opioid drugs often produces behavioral complications that are more difficult to manage than the pain problem itself. Deficits of cognition and motor function, as well as the masking of psychological disorders, are common with opioids (302). Opioids are also implicated in higher incidence of road trauma (303), immunosuppression, hormonal axis suppression, and increased risk of falls and fractures (304,305). For workers who perform safety-sensitive tasks, it is better not to initiate opioids as the patient will have difficulty to perform tasks safely under the cognitive side effects of the opioids (306). Opioids should be avoided in women who are planning pregnancy because of the high risk of neonatal

TABLE 39-5	**Definitions Related to the Use of Opioids**

Opioid Use Disorder (OUD)—OUD, previously referred as "addiction," is a primary chronic neurobiologic disease with genetic psychosocial and environmental factors influencing its development and manifestations (http://www.asam.org, 2001). The DSM-5 diagnostic criteria classifies mild OUD when there are two to three symptoms, moderate for four to five, and severe, when there are six or more symptoms.

Physical dependence—Physical dependence is an adaptation that is manifested by a drug class–specific withdrawal syndrome that can be produced by abrupt sensation, rapid dose reduction, decreasing blood level of the drug, and/or administration of an antagonist.

Tolerance—Tolerance is a state of adaptation in which exposure to a drug induces change that results in a diminution of one or more of the drug's effects over time.

Diversion—Diversion is the illegal use or inappropriate use of medications. Diversion of controlled substances should be the concern of every health professional, but efforts to stop diversion should not interfere with prescribing opioids for pain management. Attention to patterns of prescription requests and prescribing of opioids is part of an ongoing relationship between a patient and health care provider that can decrease the risk of diversion.

abstinence syndrome (307,308). Opioids are not considered safe in persons with current or past substance use disorder or patients with an active psychiatric disorder (296).

The most common immediate adverse effects are nausea, vomiting, constipation, dry mouth, drowsiness, fatigue, confusion, pruritus, and headache (229). These complications compromise a patient's main goal of maintaining a normal lifestyle. It is often necessary to educate the patient and family regarding the appropriate use of opioids for pain. In high-risk patients, it has been demonstrated that coprescribing of naloxone reduces the proportions of opioid-related overdoses and deaths (309,310).

Morphine is the opiate drug prototype and commonly prescribed by many clinicians. Pain relief is often obtained by titrating the dose to the patient's needs. At equianalgesic doses, there is no significant pharmacologic evidence to suggest the efficacy of one opioid over another, but there are significant differences in their action times, adverse events profile, and parenteral/oral ratio (see **Tables 39-4** and **39-5**). Inappropriate drug dosing often occurs because of a lack of knowledge or attention to equianalgesic doses, resulting in inadequate pain relief.

When introducing opioid medications for the first time or changing a patient's chronic dosage, it is imperative to counsel them about precautions regarding increased sedation, driving impairment, risk of falls, and risk of respiratory depression over the next days to weeks until the patient becomes acclimated.

It is good clinical practice to document the physician's and patient's responsibilities in an opioid agreement. Both patient and physicians should retain a copy for future consultation and follow-up if necessary. The document should outline the consequences of breaking the agreement. A typical treatment agreement includes name of the only physician responsible for writing the prescriptions, name of the dispensing pharmacy, no early refills are allowed, patient will provide urine samples for drug screens when requested, patient will not give opioids to others and will not receive opioids from other sources, patient will comply with scheduled follow-up visits, etc.

Oral administration of medication is preferred in the treatment of all chronic pain. A time-contingent, round-the-clock schedule for pain medications is superior to an as-needed schedule for patients with chronic pain. This form of administration minimizes variations in plasma levels and provides optimal pain control. The schedule should be based on such variables as potency, duration of the analgesic effect, and efficacy of the analgesic medication. A regularly scheduled dosage optimizes the reduction of pain by minimizing the peaks and valleys of pain intensity. The as-needed, or "prn," schedule does not have a place in the control of chronic constant pain but may be employed in acute or chronic exacerbations or activity-related pain. However, prn schedule may result in operant conditioning, craving, a sense of dependence, and anxiety about the drug wearing off. Short-acting opioids may be used in the initial prescriptions to adjust the dose until optimal dose is achieved. In chronic pain management, the drugs with longer duration of action are usually preferred. There is considerable patient-to-patient variation with respect to effective analgesic dosage; therefore, it is important to individualize the medication regime for each patient. Titration of opioids is generally accomplished by increasing or decreasing the next dose by one fourth or one half of the previous dose. During titration, patients are often provided with medication for breakthrough pain. Short-acting opioids of approximately 10% of the individual's baseline opioid equianalgesic dose may be given every 2 to 3 hours as needed.

The optimal (or stable) opioid dose should be achieved in a few weeks. After this period of dose adjustment, the patient should be monitored very closely for the development of opioid-related complications. The optimal dose should not be excessive. In doses above 90 mg of morphine equivalents per day, there are increased chances of opioid-related overdoses, all-cause mortality, motor vehicle accidents, opioid-induced hyperalgesia, sleep apnea, hypogonadism, and development of addiction (290).

Once the patient is on long-term opioid therapy for chronic pain, there is a need for close monitoring and reassessments. Urine drug screening is a valuable tool to monitor compliance with medication and detection of other substances that are not known to the prescriber (311). It is important to monitor for aberrant behaviors suggestive of opioid use disorder and increased risk of overdose.

In patients who are willing to stop chronic opioid therapy or in patients who have developed complications or are being harmed by opioids, it is useful to consider tapering and stopping the opioids completely. This can be achieved by slowly tapering the dose 10% every 2 weeks during the first few weeks, then 5% every 4 weeks until the opioid is completely stopped (311). The physician can help the patient to manage withdrawal symptoms using nonpharmacologic or pharmacologic interventions. For pregnant women, it is recommended to taper opioids to avoid neonatal abstinence syndrome; however, the tapering has to be careful and slow to avoid miscarriage or premature labor.

Opioid rotation, or opioid switching, is useful when the patient still has persistent pain with the opioid or intolerable adverse effects. There are various methods to switch opioids, with no evidence that one method is superior than the others. The most straightforward method is to discount 25% to 50% of the total daily dose and switch to a new opioid equivalent dose.

The discount is important because the patient is usually not tolerant to the new opioid and could have an overdose if they switched to 100% of the previous dose. Withdrawal symptoms are unpleasant, but not life threatening. Buprenorphine is a partial agonist opioid that can be administered in transdermal patch or sublingual tablets combined with naloxone. Buprenorphine is indicated for substitution treatment in patients with problematic opioid drug dependence. It is also used to taper opioids because it causes very little withdrawal symptoms.

Adjuvant Analgesics (Antidepressants and Anticonvulsants) and Muscle Relaxants

The adjuvant analgesic drugs produce or potentiate analgesia by mechanisms not directly mediated through the opiate receptor system. This group includes a wide variety of compounds with no inherent specific analgesic properties: antidepressants and anticonvulsants (**Table 39-6**).

TCAs, such as amitriptyline, nortriptyline, doxepin, and imipramine, have been used in the treatment of chronic pain syndromes. One of the primary mechanisms of tricyclic compounds is to block the reuptake of the neurotransmitter serotonin in the CNS. This enhances pain inhibition by way of the dorsolateral pathway (11,312). In addition, amitriptyline is a potent sedative drug, which may be used as a sleeping medication in patients with chronic pain; however, there is not enough evidence to suggest antidepressants are indicated for mechanical LBP (313). The combination of antidepressant effect, enhanced cortical serotonergic mechanism, and improved sleep contributes to these medications being one of the most commonly used groups of psychotropic agents in pain management (225,314). The evidence base for the use of TCAs in chronic pain is not so strong as the evidence for duloxetine or pregabalin, but they continue to be used for a variety of chronic pain conditions such as neuropathic pain and FM (225,315–319) (**Table 39-7**).

Gabapentin, pregabalin, and other antiepileptic drugs are used in the management of pain syndromes affecting the CNS. Their applications include trigeminal neuralgia, postherpetic neuralgia, CRPS, phantom pain syndromes, painful diabetic neuropathy, and FM (327–330). Although the mechanism is unclear, they appear to have a stabilizing effect on excitable cell membranes, which decreases afferent and deafferent second-order neuron activity (331).

Alternative anticonvulsants used for pain control are valproic acid and clonazepam. They increase the effectiveness of GABA-induced inhibition in the pre- and postsynaptic systems. These drugs appear to be most effective in the treatment of neuralgias and neuropathies (329,332).

In addition to these medications, a number of other adjuvant medications have been used. Steroids such as prednisone and dexamethasone are thought to interfere with prostaglandin sensitization of nociceptors. Serotonin antagonists such as ergot alkaloids, the β-blocking agents such as propranolol, and the antihistamines such as hydroxyzine all function by antagonizing transmitters that directly activate nociceptors. These medications have been used extensively in the treatment of migraine and cluster headaches.

Benzodiazepines and barbiturates are two groups that have little or no place as adjuvant drugs in chronic pain management. Long-term use of these medications may result in psychological and physical dependence as well as in interference with cognition

TABLE 39-6   **Adjuvant Analgesic Medications**

Drug Class	Drug	Indication	Usual Dose[a]	Maximum Dose (mg/d)	Comments
Antidepressants	Amitriptyline	For neuropathic deafferentation and somatic pain complicated by insomnia or depression	25–75 mg qhs or divided dose	300 mg/d	Tertiary amines—sedative, if morning somnolence is a problem, give dose earlier in the evening
	Doxepin			50 mg/d	
	Imipramine		25 mg tid–qid	300 mg/d	
	Clomipramine		50–200 mg qd	375 mg/d	
	Nortriptyline		37.5 mg bid	60 mg/d	Secondary amines—less sedative
	Desipramine		20 mg qam		80 mg/d
	Venlafaxine		20 mg qam	200 mg/d	Selective serotonin and norepinephrine reuptake inhibitor (SSNRI)
	Duloxetine		30–60 mg qam	120 mg/d	
Anticonvulsants	Pregabalin	Intermittent lancinating and continuous neuropathic pain	50 mg tid	450 mg/d	Few side effects, few drug-drug interactions
	Gabapentin		300 mg qid	3,600 mg/d	
	Topiramate		50 mg bid	1,800 mg/d	Risk of leucopenia
	Phenytoin	Lancinating pain	100 mg tid	600 mg/d	
	Lamotrigine		50 mg bid	400 mg/d	
	Carbamazepine		200 mg bid	1,200 mg/d	
Local anesthetics	Lidocaine	Burning neuropathic pain	50–100 mg IV	300 mg/h	2–50 mg/min q5min
Neuroleptics	Fluphenazine	Refractory pain	2.5 mg tid	40 mg/d	Used with pain complicated by nausea or delirium
Corticosteroids	Dexamethasone	Refractory bone and nerve pain	16 mg/d	96 mg/d	Used for malignant lesions, multiple side effects
	Prednisone		10 mg/d	60 mg/d	
Bisphosphonates	Pamidronate	Metastatic bone pain	90 mg IV	90 mg q4wk	Inhibit bone resorption
	Alendronate		10 mg qd	70 mg qwk	
Neurostimulants	Dextroamphetamine	Somatic and visceral pain	5 mg bid	40 mg/d	Reduce sedative effects of opioids
	Methylphenidate		10–20 mg tid	60 mg/d	
	Caffeine		65 mg/d	200 mg/d	
Topical agents	Lidocaine	Peripheral neuropathy	q12h		Transdermal patch
	Capsaicin		3–4 times/d		Causes burning sensation
α_2-Adrenergic agonist	Clonidine	Neuropathic pain, withdrawal from opioids	25–50 mg	150 mg/d	Epidural injection (significant hypotension may occur)
NDMA antagonists	Ketamine	Neuropathic pain	12.5–25 mg IV 50 mg PO	150 mg IV test 250 mg/d	Possible hallucinations and nightmares
Miscellaneous	Calcitonin	Bone pain	200 IU qd	200 IU/d	Intranasal
	Baclofen	Muscle pain associated with spasticity	5 mg tid	80 mg/d	GABA agonist
	Diazepam	Muscle relaxant	5 mg tid	40 mg/d	Benzodiazepine
	Tizanidine	Muscle relaxant	8 mg tid	36 mg/d	α_2-Adrenergic agonist

The authors will not assume liability for this table. No medication should be given until the complete prescribing recommendations, drug use indications, and potential side effects that are listed in the package insert with the product or contained in a drug reference manual are reviewed and understood thoroughly by the physician and patient. Drug dosages may need to be modified for the elderly.

[a]Dosage should be adjusted in elderly patients, patients on multiple medications, and patients with renal insufficiency or hepatic failure. Doses may be increased at varied intervals if pain relief is inadequate and dosage is tolerated. Doses and intervals are titrated to effect.

bid, twice a day; IU, international unit; PO, by mouth; q12h, every 12 h; q4wk, every 4 week; qam, every morning; qd, every day; qhs, at bedtime; qid, four times a day; tid, three times a day.

and motor function. Historically, benzodiazepines, because of their claimed muscle relaxant properties, are often prescribed to patients with pain. However, their role as muscle relaxants is questionable in clinical studies (333). In addition to the adverse effects of dependency, it has been suggested that these medications adversely affect the serotonin system. These medications are depressants that, with long-term use, lower pain tolerance, increase hostility, and tend to induce clinical depression as well as psychological and physical dependence. Because of their sedative effects, depressants often act as potent reinforcers of pain in drug-seeking behaviors. Chronic use of these medications may result in physical and mental incapacitation, emotional

instability, and the inability to deal with initial physiologic or psychological problems. Benzodiazepines deplete serotonin, alter sleep patterns, and increase pain perception. It is recommended that these two groups of medications should not be part of the long-term management of chronic pain. The only possible indication for these sedatives, or for antianxiety agents, is the short-term (<1 month) treatment of a self-limited crisis unrelated to the particular pain problem or as an adjunct when detoxifying a patient from opioid medication.

Muscle relaxants (cyclobenzaprine) have little effect in chronic pain caused by MPS (334) or FM. Their effects seem to be more related to sedation and improved sleep.

Many of the medications used in pharmacologic intervention in pain may produce dependence, and some may lead to addiction in susceptible individuals. These medications include anxiolytics, cannabinoids, muscle relaxants, opioids, sedatives, stimulants, and steroids. The clinical implications in management of physical dependence, tolerance, addiction, and diversion of medications are discrete and different phenomena (see glossary in **Table 39-5**). Behavior suggestive of addiction may include inability to take medication according to agreed-upon schedule, taking multiple doses together, frequent reports of lost or stolen prescriptions, doctor shopping, isolation from family and friends, and use of nonprescription psychoactive drugs in addition to prescribed medications. Other behaviors that may raise concerns are the use of analgesic medications for other than analgesic affects (such as sedation), an increase in energy, a decrease in anxiety, intoxication, noncompliance with recommended nonopioid treatments or evaluations, insistent on rapid-onset formulation or routes of administration, and all reports of no relief whatsoever from any nonopioid treatments (291,335).

Cannabinoids

The use of cannabis (marijuana) for chronic noncancer pain is controversial. There are a growing number of clinical trials showing that cannabinoids have some effects in a range of pain disorders. Dronabinol and nabilone are synthetic cannabinoids with analgesic potential, and the herbal extract nabiximols are approved in many countries for neuropathic pain associated with MS and in advanced cancer. Smoked or inhaled cannabis has analgesic properties in neuropathic pain associated with HIV/AIDS, trauma, and MS (225). Cannabinoids are considered third-line treatment in the consensus of the Canadian Pain Society for the treatment of neuropathic pain (225). There is some suggestion from preclinical studies that coadministration of cannabinoids to opioids is useful to reduce the dose of opioid (sparing effect) (336).

The cannabis phenotypes are classified dependent on the content of delta-9-tetrahydrocannabinol (delta-9-THC) and cannabidiol (CBD). CB1 receptors are present in brain structures related to the psychoactive effects of cannabis, gastrointestinal tract, adipocytes, the liver, and skeletal muscles. The brain has a small number of CB2 receptors, which are mainly expressed in macrophages, microglia, osteoclasts, and osteoblast. Both CB1 and CB2 signal through the transducing G proteins, Gi and Go, and their activation by delta-9-THC or other agonists causes the inhibition of adenylyl cyclase activity, the closing of voltage-gated calcium channels, the opening of inwardly rectifying potassium channels, and the stimulation of mitogen-activated protein kinases such as extracellular signal-regulated kinases (ERK) and focal adhesion kinases (FAKs) (337).

The safety concerns with cannabinoids are related to the boundaries between recreational and medicinal use, in addition to the potential for early-onset psychosis, myocardial infarction, stroke, and driving impairment (338). The effects of short-term heavy use of marijuana include short-term memory impairment, impaired motor coordination, paranoia, and psychosis (in high doses). The effects of long-term heavy use include addiction, altered brain development, poor educational outcomes, cognitive impairment, poor life achievements, chronic bronchitis, and increase risk of chronic psychosis (338). Cannabis dependency is well recognized, and these patients need to be referred to substance use specialists

for evaluation and possible treatment (339). Cannabis and cannabinoids are contraindicated in pregnant and breastfeeding women, in patients with severe liver or kidney diseases, and in persons younger than 25 or elderly individuals.

Combination of Multiple Drugs

In some circumstances, the combination of two drugs with different mechanisms of action may be synergistic and achieve better effects with less adverse events. Unfortunately, there are not many well-conducted studies to draw any firm conclusion about which combination is better than the isolated drugs for chronic pain. It is important to remember that polypharmacy is also a serious problem, especially when the various drugs have similar action or adverse effects, such as respiratory depression (340).

Physical Modalities and Exercises

Prior to the prescription of physical modalities for the chronic pain patient, the clinician is encouraged to perform a thorough evaluation in order to determine the presence of an impairment that requires such treatments. Physical modalities are valuable adjuncts in the successful management of chronic pain. In general, their application should be minimized since to overarch management strategy would be to "demedicalize" and return to function. Another important aspect is to educate the patient on self-management of their symptoms. Within this context, the patient should be educated when it is appropriate to use physical modalities as well as what impairment they are used to treat. This goal aims at improving the patient's functional independence and less reliance on the medical system.

Physical modalities should be used with caution and to a limited extent. Passive treatment programs such as hot packs, massage, and ultrasound may be appropriate for a short period of time; however, an active treatment program should be implemented as early as possible. The patient should be transitioned to a home program involving exercise, stretching, and self-applied modalities as early as possible.

For additional information on physical agents, the reader is referred to Chapter 51.

Cryotherapy

In addition to acute musculoskeletal injuries, cryotherapy has been shown to benefit some chronic painful conditions. Pain may be alleviated by direct or indirect mechanisms. Direct cold application serves to decrease temperature in the affected area. Reduced pain sensation is presumed to result through an indirect effect on the nerve fibers and sensory end organs. Additionally, the lowered temperature reduces muscle spindle firing rate and decreases the painful muscle tone (341).

The direct application of ice massage has shown modest benefits in some clinical trials (342). The application of cold as a vapocoolant spray was popularized by Travell in treating MPSs (132). A counterirritant effect is presumed to provide the mechanism of muscle spasm relief and pain alleviation. The combination of vapocoolant spray, stretching, and trigger point injection has been reported to provide significant pain relief in MPSs (131).

Heat Therapy

Heat application is a common form of chronic pain treatment. It is generally accepted that therapeutic heat is best tolerated in the subacute and chronic phases of a disease process.

The physiologic responses produced by heat are increased collagen extensibility, increased blood flow and metabolic rate, and inflammation resolution. Decreased joint stiffness, muscle spasm, and pain are also beneficial effects of heat.

Therapeutic heat is believed to have direct and indirect effects on the muscle spindle. Local elevated temperatures have been shown to directly decrease the spindle sensitivity, and superficial heating of the skin has been demonstrated to indirectly reduce spindle excitability (343).

Pain associated with numerous conditions has been successfully treated with therapeutic heat application (344). Musculoskeletal contractures respond well to deep heat used in association with prolonged stretch. Joint stiffness associated with chronic inflammatory diseases, particularly those affecting the limbs, responds to superficial heating with decreased pain and increased range of motion and function. Subacute and chronic bursitis, tenosynovitis, and epicondylitis also may respond to heat with decreased pain and symptom resolution (342).

Therapeutic Exercise

Therapeutic exercise has been well documented as an essential component of treatment for the patient with chronic pain with beneficial effects upon pain, sleep, mood, and cognitive and physical functioning (345–349). It is important to note that the exercise programs described in most studies with chronic pain patients do not meet the CDC or ACSM guidelines (350). There is low-quality evidence of benefit with low- to moderate-intensity water or land-based exercise performed two to four times per week for at least 4 weeks (350,351). There is evidence that females (352) with FM can safely perform a resistance exercise program (348). However, hyperalgesic effects have been demonstrated in FM patients with strenuous bouts of aerobic or isometric exercise that is performed (353,354). The clinician should also be aware of the patient's fear-avoidance beliefs and behaviors as this may present a significant barrier to and detrimentally impact the patient's ability to exercise (355–357).

In the chronic phase of pain, the optimal treatment methodology combines graded stretching movements, strengthening exercises, heat or cold, and massage. The patient is also educated regarding proper body mechanics and the need to continue the prescribed therapeutic exercise regimen outside of formal therapy sessions.

Therapeutic exercise, prescribed to correct a specific abnormal condition, is often used to treat chronic painful conditions. The primary goal is to aid the patient in achieving pain control. This may be accomplished through the restoration of normal muscle tone, length, strength, and optimal joint range of motion (358). Finally, the patient is urged to continue a home program after formal therapy sessions have ceased.

Therapeutic exercise consists of passive movements, active-assistive exercises, active exercises, stretching, and relaxing exercises. Each may be used alone or in combination to achieve the desired effect. In the case of LBP, there has been disagreement as to which exercise program is most effective in the treatment of chronic LBP. A recent meta-analysis of randomized, controlled trials in patients with LBP showed a positive effect in function both immediately and at follow-up (359). While this study highlighted the variety of programs that are incorporated under the umbrella of "exercise," the majority (12 out of 16) incorporated an element of strengthening.

There is an emerging school of thought that the maintenance of lumbar spinal stability over time can limit the pain associated with degenerative disk disease and spondylosis. This stability is thought to be secondary to three components: the bones and ligaments of the spine, the muscles, and the nerves that coordinate muscle activation (360). The muscles are the major stabilizers, specifically the multifidi, the transversus abdominis, the pelvic floor muscles, and the diaphragm (361). Without the assistance of the muscles and their nerves, a cadaver spine with bones and ligaments intact will buckle and collapse under a load of 20 lb (362,363).

The multifidi are rich in muscle spindles; therefore, they act both to stabilize individual segments of the spine and to provide proprioceptive feedback of spinal movement. The other muscles, including the transversus abdominis, form a muscular cylinder that increases intra-abdominal pressure, also effectively stabilizing the spine. The transversus abdominis is one of the first muscles to be activated to stabilize the spine; however, studies have suggested that its activation may be delayed in patients with back pain (364).

Several small studies have shown a promising effect of lumbar stabilization programs targeted at strengthening the above, deep muscles in treating a number of painful and potentially destabilizing spinal conditions. Of note, O'sullivan and colleagues reported a significant improvement in pain and function of a group of patients with spondylolysis and spondylolisthesis treated with lumbar stabilization compared to patients treated with general exercise (365). Various outcome studies have demonstrated the effectiveness of therapeutic exercise for chronic back pain patients. Unfortunately, there remains limited consensus regarding the most effective exercise programs for patients with LBP. Motor control exercises (107), Pilates (106), and yoga (104) have shown benefits for patients with chronic LBP. Passive forms of therapeutic exercise (mobilization, manipulation, muscle energy technique, and massage) have not been shown to be superior to other routine treatments (general practitioner care, analgesics, home exercises, or back school) in the management of neck and back pain (105,366,367). Aerobic exercise has proven to be an effective treatment option for individuals with depressive symptoms. A review by Blumenthal et al. highlights several studies that have undertaken the task of investigating the association, and many have found positive associations in regard to aerobic exercise on depression. Since depression, at times, presents itself along with pain, aerobic exercise also seems like a viable option for the treatment of pain (349). For additional information on therapeutic exercise, the reader is referred to Chapter 49.

Transcutaneous Electrical Nerve Stimulation Therapy

The use of electrical currents dates back to the Greeks, who applied torpedo fish to individuals suffering from pain (184,368). The exact physiologic basis by which TENS produces pain control remains unknown. TENS also has been used extensively to manage chronic pain. The results have been less promising and more variable than those in acute pain trials. Rigorous controlled trials suggest that TENS is no better than placebo in the management of chronic LBP (369,370). Patients with CRPS, phantom limb pain, and peripheral nerve injury have demonstrated pain control with TENS (371). Treatment comparisons of TENS and sham TENS concluded that TENS had a positive effect on chronic pain at one point or another

(372). This review did not find evidence to support the use of TENS alone in chronic pain management. One should remember that the lack of evidence of effect is clearly different from evidence of lack of effect. Further research that elucidates the effects of TENS in chronic pain is clearly required.

Acupuncture

Acupuncture (originating from the Latin *acus* or "sharp point" and *punctura*, "to puncture") is an ancient Chinese therapy practiced for more than 2,500 years to cure disease or relieve pain. Thin, solid metal needles are inserted into specific body sites and slowly twisted manually or stimulated electrically. Various sensations may be produced, ranging from a dull ache or warmth to that of a pinprick. Researchers have considered acupuncture to be a form of neuromodulation. Two theories have been proposed for its use in pain control. First, acupuncture may stimulate large sensory afferent fibers and suppress pain perception as explained by the gate control theory of pain. Second, the needle insertion may act as a noxious stimulus and induce endogenous production of opioid-like substances to effect pain control (371).

It has been demonstrated that there is a significant overlap between traditional acupuncture sites, MTrPs, and muscular motor points (373). The sensation induced by the application of an acupuncture needle is very similar to the dull ache often experienced by the patient when a trigger point is injected. The insertion of a needle, regardless of the substance injected, appears to produce the beneficial pain relief and is termed the *needle effect*. The injection of trigger points may share not only similar areas of needle insertion but also associated mechanisms of pain control.

Acupuncture has been used in a wide variety of painful conditions (374). The insertion of a needle is considered an invasive procedure, and many states require a physician to perform or supervise the treatment. Uniform agreement does not yet exist as to the preferred time necessary for an adequate trial of acupuncture. There is limited evidence to suggest that acupuncture is more effective than placebo or sham acupuncture for chronic LBP in the short term only (102). There is no evidence that acupuncture is more effective than other treatments such as NSAIDs. While acupuncture may be a useful adjunctive treatment in pain management, more high-quality studies are needed to confirm its efficacy and guide its use. A recent meta-analysis of acupuncture treatments was conducted for the following chronic pain conditions: neck/back pain, osteoarthritis, and chronic headache (374). Within these groups, they demonstrated pain scores were 0.23, 0.16, and 0.15 standard deviations better that sham and 0.55, 0.57, and 0.42 standard deviations better when compared to no acupuncture controls. In clinical terms, they suggest that the improvement in pain ratings corresponded to approximately 50%.

Low-Level Laser Therapy

The physiologic mechanisms responsible for low-level laser therapy (LLLT) are variable and are not well understood (375–377). However, several studies have shown mixed results and suggest that LLLT may have short-term analgesic effects. A systematic review and meta-analysis in 2009 suggested that LLLT may be beneficial to reduce pain in acute neck pains and up to 22 weeks post in chronic neck pains (375). Till date, there is no standard of care with variable dosing, frequency, and wavelength options limiting the possibility to derive conclusions.

Traction

In regard to traction therapy, a Cochrane systematic review with 2,206 patients concluded that traction, either alone or in combination with other treatments, is not effective to improve pain intensity, functional status, global improvement, and return to work among people with LBP (378). Another systematic review does not support the use of traction for neck pain (379).

Behavioral Treatment Modalities

Among the treatment goals of pain management are the decrease in illness behavior (reduced drug use and visits to physicians) and the increase in well behavior (increased physical activities, mobility, and return to gainful employment). This may be accomplished by blocking noxious sensory input, decreasing tension and depression, rearranging reinforcement contingencies, or assisting in the learning of new behaviors (380). Examples of modalities that can assist in the treatment of certain types of chronic pain include biofeedback, cognitive behavior modification, acceptance and commitment therapy (ACT), operant approaches, hypnosis, and relaxation training (191,216,227,241,337,381,382).

An alternative approach is ACT, which aims to increase valued action in the presence of pain. The principles of ACT are that the person will accept that pain, grief, disappointment, illness, and anxiety are inevitable parts of being a human being and they will adapt to these challenges by developing resilience and flexibility rather than denying and attempting to eliminate or suppress those undesirable experiences. The therapy is achieved by them committing to pursuit of valued life areas and directions even when the natural desire is to escape or avoid those painful experiences, emotions, or thoughts (383). ACT does not reduce pain intensity, but there is evidence that it improves pain acceptance, psychological well-being, functioning, anxiety, and mood (384).

Biofeedback has found use in the treatment of some types of chronic pain (381). Typically, biofeedback teaches muscle relaxation (through surface EMG) or temperature control. The instrumentation is reported to be somewhat useful, although clinical experience suggests that relaxation without instrumentation is of equal value. Through biofeedback training, the patient learns self-regulation of pain. A meta-analysis of 21 studies showed that biofeedback, either as a stand-alone or as an adjunctive intervention, reduced pain intensity with a small-to-medium effect size up to a follow-up of 8 months. It also reduced depression, disability, muscle tension, and improved cognitive coping (381).

CBT helps the patient learn self-coping statements and problem-solving cognitions in order to alter the cognitive structures (schemata, beliefs) and cognitive process (automatic thoughts, images, and internal dialogue) associated with the pain experience (43,345,385). Cognitive strategies of imaginative inattention, imaginative transformation of pain, focused attention, and somatization in a dissociation manner have been found helpful. There are mainly three distinct concepts of CBT: operant, cognitive, and respondent treatment. A recent review of 35 studies of CBT for a variety of chronic pain conditions found that either online or in-person delivery methods were comparable to provide pain intensity reduction in 43% of the included trials (386). CBT has also the potential to prevent chronic LBP, especially the graded activity, an operant treatment approach (387).

TABLE 39-7	**Nutritional Advice for Patients with Chronic Pain (230,320–326)**
Increase	**Reduce**
Vitamins D, B$_6$ (chronic pain, fibromyalgia)	Glutamate, MSG (fibromyalgia, headache, migraine)
Vitamin B$_{12}$ (pain, insomnia, and fatigue)	Aspartate (fibromyalgia, depression)
Probiotics (irritable bowel syndrome, abdominal pain)	Omega-6 fatty acids (complex regional pain syndrome)
Magnesium (postoperative pain, chronic neuropathic pain, fibromyalgia, muscle cramps, myofascial trigger points, and muscle spasms)	Caffeine (insomnia)
Zinc (fibromyalgia)	
Careful: Too much zinc intake cause impairment of the microbiome	
Omega-3 polyunsaturated fatty acids (inflammatory arthritis, dysmenorrhea, IBS, headaches, and neuropathic pain)	
Caffeine (fatigue)	

The operant approach involves the identification of behaviors to be produced, increased, maintained, or eliminated. Reinforcement is then regulated to achieve the desired outcome. Activity and walking programs are followed to the prescribed level, not to discomfort. All medication is prescribed by schedule. Family and friends are instructed to avoid reinforcing all pain behavior.

Relaxation methods to reduce tension may include deep muscle relaxation, deep diaphragmatic breathing, meditation, yoga, and autogenic training (388). Patients also may be taught self-hypnosis (216,241,388–390). Hypnosis has the advantage of providing pain relief without unpleasant side effects, no reduction in normal function, and no development of tolerance. Hypnotic strategies can suggest analgesia or anesthesia, substitute another feeling for pain, move the pain perception to a smaller or less vulnerable area, alter the meaning of pain, increase tolerance to pain, or, in some individuals, dissociate the perception of the body from the patient's awareness.

Lifestyle Modifications

Self-Management Programs

Self-management programs (SMPs) are a form of structured program to help patients learn to better manage their own chronic disease, and they have been shown to reduce pain intensity and disability in patients with chronic LBP (391).

The Stanford Chronic Disease Self-Management Program (CDSMP) has been shown to produce moderate, short-term improvements in pain, disability, fatigue, depressive symptoms, health distress, self-rated health, and health-related quality of life (392). The program has been evaluated in a RCT, and it has been shown effective for patients with chronic pain (393).

The Stanford CDSMP is a community-based self-management support program based on Bandura's self-efficacy theory that states that successful behavior change requires confidence in one's ability to carry out an action (i.e., self-efficacy) and the expectation that a specific goal will be achieved (i.e., outcome expectancy) (394). The CDSMP usually involves group sessions of 10 to 15 participants that meet for about 3 hours on a weekly basis for six sessions. The meetings are usually held at community settings such as libraries, churches, hospitals, and community centers. Each session is facilitated by laypersons who are trained in the methodology. The group follows a range of topics such as exercises, stress, pain reduction techniques, positive thinking, and progressive muscle relaxation. There is also discussion about the use of mediations, community resources, communication with others (health care professionals, relatives, family), and problem-solving and decision-making. There is a book that participants receive with activities to do between the sessions (395). The Stanford CDSMP has been modified and translated to various languages. There are a license fee and required training in order to implement the Stanford CDSMP.

Mindful-Based Meditation

Mindfulness-based interventions have been used in the management of chronic pain since 1982. It has been shown to be safe for substance use disorder and insomnia, which occur frequently with chronic pain conditions (396).

Diet and Nutrition

An important aspect of chronic pain management is to understand how nutrition and diet may affect the symptoms of pain, fatigue, and sleep quality. It is important to take a detailed history of intake of proteins, carbohydrates, fat, vitamins, micronutrients, glutamate, aspartate, alcohol, and caffeine. There is no strong evidence that special diets may be better than a regular well-balanced diet. There has been suggestion that an anti-inflammatory diet such as the Mediterranean diet (which is rich in vegetables, legumes, fruits, whole grains, fish, and healthy oils but low in meat) may provide benefits in reducing inflammation (230,397). An anti-inflammatory diet can reduce the prevalence of many of the chronic diseases that are associated with pain: diabetes, cardiovascular disease, and obesity. A diet of processed foods tends to be high in calories with an abundance of unhealthy fat, refined carbohydrates, salt, and chemicals such as pesticides, stabilizers, antibiotics, and preservatives. Such a diet is poor in fiber, micronutrients, and antioxidants and is proinflammatory (230). Chronic inflammation is associated with medical and psychiatric disorders, including cardiovascular diseases, metabolic syndrome, cancer, autoimmune diseases, schizophrenia, and depression, all of which adversely affect health and life expectancy and can exacerbate pain (398).

Vitamins

The prevalence of vitamin D deficiency is higher in geographical areas with low exposure to sunlight (320). Severe deficiency of vitamin D during childhood may lead to rickets; however, moderate chronic deficiency may lead to osteoporosis and muscle pain (321). Regular monitoring of blood levels of vitamin D is not necessary in areas where it is well known that the prevalence of deficiency is high; therefore, it is acceptable that the majority of the population should receive supplements of vitamin D on a daily basis. However, in areas where the sunlight exposure might be adequate, a measurement of blood levels might be necessary to detect deficiency and monitor therapy with supplements. A recent review of randomized trials demonstrated that in patients with chronic pain, vitamin D supplementation significantly reduced pain scores compared to placebo suggesting that supplementation has a role in the management of chronic pain (77).

Vitamin B_6 is a cofactor for the enzyme glutamate decarboxylase, which converts glutamate (excitatory neurotransmitter) into GABA (inhibitory neurotransmitter) (397). Vitamin B_{12} is needed to make healthy blood cells and for optimal bone density. It is well known that neurologic dysfunction and chronic pain are consequences of deficiencies of vitamin B_{12} (230). A dose of 1,000 mg/d taken sublingually may produce improved symptoms of pain, insomnia, and fatigue. The sublingual route avoids the need for injections while still bypassing any impairment in gastrointestinal tract absorption.

Vitamin B_{12} and folate deficiencies predispose to painful peripheral neuropathies. Patients who use proton pump inhibitors (PPIs) on a regular basis are more susceptible to deficiency of vitamin B_{12}, magnesium, and iron and dysbiosis in the gut (322). Metformin causes vitamin B_{12} malabsorption, which may increase the risk of developing vitamin B_{12} deficiency (399).

Excitotoxicity leads to oxidative stress in the CNS. Two main vitamins have antioxidant effects: vitamin C (a water-soluble antioxidant) and vitamin E (a fat-soluble antioxidant). Other chemicals found in fruits and vegetables also have sown important antioxidant abilities such as resveratrol in grapes and polyphenols in green tea.

Magnesium and Zinc

Magnesium is known for its analgesic properties in acute (postoperative pain) and chronic (neuropathic) pain. The physiologic mechanism is the antagonist effect of the N-methyl-D-aspartate (NMDA) receptor ion channel, and that NMDA receptor is implicated in the development of central sensitization. In addition, magnesium also blocks calcium channels, modulates potassium channels, and activates the nitric oxide (NO) pathway, which is an important role in the antinociception effects of systemic magnesium sulfate in the somatic, but not in visceral, models of inflammatory pain (323).

Zinc plays an important role in the normal neuronal functioning and in regulating specially the NMDA receptor, which is the main glutamate receptor implicated in excitotoxicity. Magnesium blocks the NMDA receptor, and zinc is coreleased with glutamate to negatively modulate the excitatory response (352). Magnesium is a muscle relaxant; therefore, it is useful for MTrPs, muscle cramps, and tightness. Magnesium supplementation is better absorbed using magnesium glycinate, malate, and citrate (230).

Prebiotics, Probiotics, and Synbiotics

The microbiome is the group of microorganisms that inhabit the guts and can affect the absorption of nutrients, function of the immune system, and dysbiosis, which may cause some forms of abdominal pain, such as IBSs. Certain substances like antibiotics, NSAIDs, steroids, PPIs, and hormones may affect the microbiome (230). IBS and chronic idiopathic constipation (CIC) are considered functional bowel disorders that may be associated with disturbance in the gastrointestinal microbiota (324). Probiotics are beneficial for global symptoms in IBS, abdominal pain, bloating, and flatulence. Data for prebiotics and symbiotic in IBS are sparse.

Omega-3 Fatty Acids

Omega-3 polyunsaturated fatty acids (PUFAs) increase the fluidity of the cell membrane, which could potentially modulate the expression of glutamate transporters, therefore clearing the excess of glutamate from the synapses and reducing excitotoxicity (352). Omega-3 fatty acids have a regulatory role against inflammatory pain associated with rheumatoid arthritis, dysmenorrhea, and inflammatory bowel disease (IBS) (325). Omega-3 fatty acids also block the activity of mitogen-activated protein kinase, which is involved in the modulation of central sensitization induced by inflammation and neuropathic pain. Omega-3 fatty acids are alpha-linolenic acid (found in flax seeds), eicosapentaenoic acid (EPA), and docosahexaenoic acid (DHA) found in fish, eggs, and grass-fed beef.

The two types of omega-6 fatty acids are linoleic acid and arachidonic acid. The North American diet is generally too high in omega-6 PUFAs and deficient in omega-3 PUFAs. Linoleic acid is the predominant omega-6 PUFA that promotes inflammation (400). Arachidonic acid may be converted to prostaglandins, thromboxane, and leukotrienes, which are pronociceptive; however, it may also be converted to 14,15-epoxyeicosanoic acid, which has antinociceptive properties (325). An analysis of patients with CRPS demonstrated an increase in levels of omega-6 fatty acids in comparison with omega-3 levels.

Coffee, Tea, Wine, and Dark Chocolate

Willett, MD of Harvard, in his book *Eat, Drink, and be Healthy*, provides an alternative food pyramid to that of the U.S. Department of Agriculture. He explains that moderate use of coffee, tea, wine, and dark chocolate is recommended under the antioxidant banner (326).

Interventional and Surgical Pain Management

Nearly 50% of the patients suffering from common chronic pain diseases continue to suffer as a result of inadequate pain relief with the available conservative pain measures. Advanced interventional pain measures can be chosen judiciously for some, if not all for better pain management and reduction of their lifelong suffering. Further, a vast majority of chronic pain patients are treated with chronic opioid therapy with a potential risk of addiction and life-threatening complications. Hence, interventional options may be considered to ameliorate suffering in complex chronic pain diseases. Interventional pain management options should be considered as only one of the therapeutic modalities used in the multidisciplinary pain clinic. Other factors, such as psychological problems and associated muscle tightness and weakness, should be treated by using other appropriate modalities. Interventional pain treatment options may include basic interventions as trigger point injections and epidural steroids for temporary pain relief to more permanent options as neuromodulation including SCS and advanced intrathecal drug delivery systems.

Trigger Point Injections

Trigger point injections are one of the most common and basic interventions for chronic pain management. A common practice is to inject a drug mixture at the point of maximum tenderness, felt on palpation, for pain alleviation. Several techniques and injectate mixtures are used with varied results, efficacy, duration of effect, and outcomes (401,402). Recently, ultrasound visualization of trigger points has been debated for better objectivity in diagnosis and needle guidance in terms of accuracy (157,403).

Neurolysis and Neural Blockade

Blocking the nerve with a local anesthetic agent is one of the most common procedures in the management of chronic pain. Nerve blocks are useful in delineating the pain mechanisms and in blocking the pain when the patients are required to take part in physical therapy to mobilize the muscles and joints. Patients who have a nerve block followed by appropriate physical therapy usually have excellent results. There are various nerve block techniques used in pain clinics; the most common and useful include epidural use of a local anesthetic with or without steroid and peripheral nerve block (404). Further, intra-articular facet joint injections and medial branch blocks have been employed in the treatment of axial back pain as an alternative to more invasive interventions. The steroids are injected into the epidural space close to the involved root and can be performed at any level, including cervical, thoracic, or lumbar. Differences in injection route, region, injectate mixture, frequency, number of injections, and patient pathology determine the patient outcomes. Epidural steroid injections may be administered via the three common techniques of transforaminal (TF), IL, and caudal routes. The general consensus among practitioners is that TF approach is superior to IL or caudal technique (405–407).

Steroid preparations commonly used are methylprednisolone (40 to 80 mg), betamethasone (3 to 6 mg), dexamethasone (6 to 15 mg), and triamcinolone (10 to 40 mg). Although steroid preparations may be used to produce anti-inflammatory action, many of the steroid preparations contain various preservatives, such as benzyl alcohol, which may produce serious side effects, including paralysis. Agents with preservatives that are designated for articular injections should not be used as epidural agents. Only preservative-free steroid preparations have been extensively used in the epidural space without producing significant neurologic damage. However, any particulate-based steroid can cause embolic spinal cord infarction if injected into the spinal arterial supply. In comparing nonparticulate and particulate steroids, recent systematic reviews have demonstrated nonstatistically significant superiority of particulate steroids over nonparticulate steroids in the short- and long-term treatment of lumbar radicular pain (408). The preferred procedure is to administer one injection and wait 2 weeks in order to assess the patient's response. If the patient is significantly pain-free, no further injections are administered. If there is minimal or limited response, then further injections are administered. If the patient does not respond to two or three epidural steroid injections or the patient receives only short-term/subtherapeutic pain relief, then steroid injections are discontinued. Frequent injections of epidural steroid can produce problems related to chronic steroid administration as well as a remote possibility of infection. Epidural steroid injection is also a useful technique in patients who have neural irritation. In addition, steroids may be injected into the subarachnoid space, especially in patients who have had multiple surgeries and in whom the epidural space has been obliterated. These patients, especially those with arachnoiditis, show significant pain relief. For more information on injection techniques, the reader is referred to Chapter 53.

The facet joint is supplied by two medial branches of the spinal nerve root, one from the same level and one from the level above in case of a lumbar facet. Diagnostic facet joint medial branch blocks and procedures like radiofrequency ablation of the sensory nerves can be done under radiologic fluoroscopy guidance in chronic complex axial LBPs for diagnostic and short-term therapeutic benefits.

Neuromodulation

Advanced interventions like neuromodulation therapies have shown promise of effective pain alleviation in refractory chronic pain conditions (233,409–412). The most common forms of therapies include SCS, PNS, and brain stimulation by electric impulses. The electrical signals affect pain by the principles of gate control theory and various mechanisms including neurotransmitter release, modulation of action potential, and sympathetic nervous system alteration. The earliest clinical trials for the use of neuromodulation in chronic pain started in the late 1960s and early 1970s. Since then, the appropriate indications for use of both PNS and SCS have been expanding due to improving technology and efforts by clinicians to explore new and novel uses of these modalities.

Despite an incomplete understanding of mechanism of pain modulation, both PNS and SCS have become popular with proven efficacy in neuropathic pains (413). The current research-based indications of PNS include greater occipital nerve stimulation to manage intractable headache, sacral plexus stimulation for pelvic pains, brachial plexus stimulation for neuropathic pains, and peripheral neuropathic, visceral, cardiac, abdominal, low back, and facial pain. Further, the use of PNS in modulating organ function in conditions such as epilepsy, incontinence, and obesity with vagal, tibial, and gastric stimulation is under investigation.

The current available SCS systems include conventional SCS (Con-SCS) (frequency ranges from 35 to 80 Hz) and the newer high-frequency SCS systems (HF-SCS, 500 to 10,000 Hz) (414). The mechanism of pain relief in the Con-SCS systems is thought to be spinal modulation of the inhibitory GABA system and the segmental spinal dorsal column. The HF-SCS (10,000 Hz) delivers subthreshold stimulation of A-beta fibers due to low charge per pulse resulting in the absence of paresthesia. However, the technique of implantation varies slightly as compared to Con-SCS. The burst variant of HF-SCS delivers 500-Hz stimulation in groups of five pulses with 1-ms pulse width, with bursts repeated 40 times per second. Generally, this technique limits the paresthesia experienced in the Con-SCS systems and has shown more effects on the dorsal anterior cingulate gyrus resulting in effect on the patients' focus on pain and reduction in the attention to pain and pain changes (415).

The current chronic pain indications of SCS include radicular pain in failed back surgery syndrome, CRPS I, and diabetic neuropathy (411). The effectiveness in chronic intractable angina pectoris and peripheral vascular disease still remains debatable with multiple conflicting trials (416). However, a cost-effectiveness analysis comparing SCS added to conventional medical management showed that SCS is cost-effective compared to conventional medical management alone for failed back surgery syndrome, CRPS, peripheral arterial disease, and refractory angina pectoris (417).

The SCS implantation is a two-stage process beginning with the trial evaluation period, of approximately 3 to 7 days. Percutaneous leads are used to place electrodes in the epidural space under local anesthesia and connected to an external pulse generator that delivers the stimulation. This is followed by the surgical implant of the permanent system approximately 4 to 8 weeks after the completion of a successful trial. Common complications include device-related (lead migration, hardware malfunction, fracture electrode, and battery replacement), tissue-related (superficial and deep infection, localized implant site pain, seroma, hematoma), and the neuraxial complications (epidural hematoma, abscess, fibrosis, and nerve injury). The trends in complication rates related to SCS have shown severe reductions with the technologic and hardware improvements in the last few years (418).

Several other novel and promising invasive pain modalities have evolved over the period of time. These include deep brain stimulation, tDCS, and intrathecal delivery systems. However, till date, their use has been confounded by the technical difficulties and mixed results of large trials with reported variable therapeutic utility.

REFERENCES

1. Deyo RA, Walsh NE, Martin DC, et al. A controlled trial of transcutaneous electrical nerve stimulation (TENS) and exercise for chronic low back pain. *N Engl J Med.* 1990;322(23):1627–1634.
2. Merskey HE. Classification of chronic pain: descriptions of chronic pain syndromes and definitions of pain terms. *Pain.* 1986;3(suppl):1–225.
3. Merskey HE, Bogduk N. *Classification of Chronic Pain—Descriptions of Chronic Pain Syndromes and Definitions of Pain Terms.* 2nd ed. Seattle: IASP Press; 1994.
4. Peng P. The basic science of pain; 2016. Available from: https://itunes.apple.com/ca/book/the-basic-science-of-pain/id1174147456?mt=11
5. Geertzen JH, Van Wilgen CP, Schrier E, et al. Chronic pain in rehabilitation medicine. *Disabil Rehabil.* 2006;28(6):363–367.
6. Bishop B. Pain: its physiology and rationale for management. Part I. Neuroanatomical substrate of pain. *Phys Ther.* 1980;60(1):13–20.
7. Terman GW, Bonica JJ. Spinal mechanisms and their modulation. In: Loeser JD, ed. *Bonica's Management of Pain.* 3rd ed. Philadelphia, PA: Lippincott, Williams & Wilkins; 2001:73–152.
8. Edmeads J. The physiology of pain: a review. *Prog Neuropsychopharmacol Biol Psychiatry.* 1983;7(4–6):413–419.
9. Zimmerman M. The somatovisceral sensory system. In: Schmidt RF, Thews G, eds. *Human Physiology.* 3rd ed. New York: Springer-Verlag; 1989:224–233.
10. Schmidt RE. Nociception and pain. In: Schmidt RF, Thews G, eds. *Human Physiology.* 3rd ed. New York: Springer-Verlag; 1989:223–236.
11. Basbaum AI, Fields HL. Endogenous pain control systems: brainstem spinal pathways and endorphin circuitry. *Annu Rev Neurosci.* 1984;7:309–338.
12. Kruger L, Mantyh P. Changing concepts in the anatomy of pain. *Semin Anesth.* 1985;4:209–217.
13. Liebeskind JC, Sherman JE, Cannon T. Neural and neurochemical mechanisms of pain inhibition. *Anaesth Intensive Care.* 1982;10(2):139–143.
14. Snyder SH. Opiate receptors and internal opiates. *Sci Am.* 1977;236(3):44–56.
15. Traub RJ, Sedivec MJ, Mendell LM. The rostral projection of small diameter primary afferents in Lissauer's tract. *Brain Res.* 1986;399(1):185–189.
16. Linnman C, Moulton EA, Barmettler G, et al. Neuroimaging of the periaqueductal gray: state of the field. *Neuroimage.* 2012;60(1):505–522.
17. Hemington KS, Coulombe MA. The periaqueductal gray and descending pain modulation: why should we study them and what role do they play in chronic pain? *J Neurophysiol.* 2015;114(4):2080–2083.
18. Strigo IA, Simmons AN, Matthews SC, et al. Association of major depressive disorder with altered functional brain response during anticipation and processing of heat pain. *Arch Gen Psychiatry.* 2008;65(11):1275–1284.
19. Benedetti F, Amanzio M, Thoen W. Disruption of opioid-induced placebo responses by activation of cholecystokinin type-2 receptors. *Psychopharmacology (Berl).* 2011;213(4):791–797.
20. Potvin S, Grignon S, Marchand S. Human evidence of a supra-spinal modulating role of dopamine on pain perception. *Synapse.* 2009;63(5):390–402.
21. Benedetti F, Amanzio M, Rosato R, et al. Nonopioid placebo analgesia is mediated by CB1 cannabinoid receptors. *Nat Med.* 2011;17(10):1228–1230.
22. Blyth FM, March LM, Brnabic AJ, et al. Chronic pain in Australia: a prevalence study. *Pain.* 2001;89(2–3):127–134.
23. Perquin CW, Hazebroek-Kampschreur AA, Hunfeld JA, et al. Pain in children and adolescents: a common experience. *Pain.* 2000;87(1):51–58.
24. Elliott AM, Smith BH, Penny KI, et al. The epidemiology of chronic pain in the community. *Lancet.* 1999;354(9186):1248–1252.
25. Crook J, Rideout E, Browne G. The prevalence of pain complaints in a general population. *Pain.* 1984;18(3):299–314.
26. Woolf AD, Pfleger B. Burden of major musculoskeletal conditions. *Bull World Health Organ.* 2003;81(9):646–656.
27. Tsang A, Von Korff M, Lee S, et al. Common chronic pain conditions in developed and developing countries: gender and age differences and comorbidity with depression-anxiety disorders. *J Pain.* 2008;9(10):883–891.
28. Fayaz A, Croft P, Langford RM, et al. Prevalence of chronic pain in the UK: a systematic review and meta-analysis of population studies. *BMJ Open.* 2016;6(6):e010364.
29. Dureja GP, Jain PN, Shetty N, et al. Prevalence of chronic pain, impact on daily life, and treatment practices in India. *Pain Pract.* 2014;14(2):E51–E62.
30. The National Academies Collection: Reports funded by National Institutes of Health. *Relieving Pain in America: A Blueprint for Transforming Prevention, Care, Education, and Research.* Washington, DC: National Academies Press (US); 2011.
31. CDC. Health status and determinants 2015. Available from: https://www.cdc.gov/nchs/data/hus/2015/041.pdf
32. Shmagel A, Foley R, Ibrahim H. Epidemiology of chronic low back pain in US adults: data from the 2009-2010 National Health and Nutrition Examination Survey. *Arthritis Care Res (Hoboken).* 2016;68(11):1688–1694.
33. Mansfield KE, Sim J, Jordan JL, et al. A systematic review and meta-analysis of the prevalence of chronic widespread pain in the general population. *Pain.* 2016;157(1):55–64.
34. Hoy D, Bain C, Williams G, et al. A systematic review of the global prevalence of low back pain. *Arthritis Rheum.* 2012;64(6):2028–2037.
35. Salter MW, Beggs S. Sublime microglia: expanding roles for the guardians of the CNS. *Cell.* 2014;158(1):15–24.
36. Baldwin KM, Haddad F. Effects of different activity and inactivity paradigms on myosin heavy chain gene expression in striated muscle. *J Appl Physiol (1985).* 2001;90(1):345–357.
37. Bogdanis GC. Effects of physical activity and inactivity on muscle fatigue. *Front Physiol.* 2012;3:142.
38. Snow BR, Pinter I, Gusmorino P, et al. Incidence of physical and psychosocial disabilities in chronic pain patients: initial report. *Bull Hosp Jt Dis Orthop Inst.* 1986;46(1):22–30.
39. Guck TP, Meilman PW, Skultety FM, et al. Prediction of long-term outcome of multidisciplinary pain treatment. *Arch Phys Med Rehabil.* 1986;67(5):293–296.
40. Arnstein PM. The neuroplastic phenomenon: a physiologic link between chronic pain and learning. *J Neurosci Nurs.* 1997;29(3):179–186.
41. Wilkins KL, McGrath PJ, Finley GA, et al. Phantom limb sensations and phantom limb pain in child and adolescent amputees. *Pain.* 1998;78(1):7–12.
42. Kalso E. Memory for pain. *Acta Anaesthesiol Scand Suppl.* 1997;110:129–130.
43. Villemure C, Bushnell MC. Cognitive modulation of pain: how do attention and emotion influence pain processing? *Pain.* 2002;95(3):195–199.
44. Tasmuth T, Estlanderb AM, Kalso E. Effect of present pain and mood on the memory of past postoperative pain in women treated surgically for breast cancer. *Pain.* 1996;68(2–3):343–347.
45. Chaplin ER. Chronic pain: a sociobiological problem. *Phys Med Rehabil Stars.* 1991;5:1–48.
46. Allen MJ, Asbridge MM, Macdougall PC, et al. Self-reported practices in opioid management of chronic noncancer pain: a survey of Canadian family physicians. *Pain Res Manag.* 2013;18(4):177–184.
47. Webster LR, Webster RM. Predicting aberrant behaviors in opioid-treated patients: preliminary validation of the opioid risk tool. *Pain Med.* 2005;6(6):432–442.
48. Barnett ML, Olenski AR, Jena AB. Opioid-prescribing patterns of emergency physicians and risk of long-term use. *N Engl J Med.* 2017;376(7):663–673.
49. Apkarian AV, Baliki MN, Farmer MA. Predicting transition to chronic pain. *Curr Opin Neurol.* 2013;26(4):360–367.
50. Mailis-Gagnon A, Nicholson K, Yegneswaran B, et al. Pain characteristics of adults 65 years of age and older referred to a tertiary care pain clinic. *Pain Res Manag.* 2008;13(5):389–394.
51. Mailis-Gagnon A, Yegneswaran B, Lakha SF, et al. Pain characteristics and demographics of patients attending a university-affiliated pain clinic in Toronto, *Pain Res Manag.* 2007;12(2):93–99.
52. Lacroix-Fralish ML, Mogil JS. Progress in genetic studies of pain and analgesia. *Annu Rev Pharmacol Toxicol.* 2009;49:97–121.
53. Mogil JS, Yu L, Basbaum AI. Pain genes?: natural variation and transgenic mutants. *Annu Rev Neurosci.* 2000;23:777–811.
54. Bengtsson B, Thorson J. Back pain: a study of twins. *Acta Genet Med Gemellol (Roma).* 1991;40(1):83–90.
55. Buskila D, Neumann L, Hazanov I, et al. Familial aggregation in the fibromyalgia syndrome. *Semin Arthritis Rheum.* 1996;26(3):605–611.
56. Treloar SA, Martin NG, Heath AC. Longitudinal genetic analysis of menstrual flow, pain, and limitation in a sample of Australian twins. *Behav Genet.* 1998;28(2):107–116.
57. Peroutka SJ. Genetic basis of migraine. *Clin Neurosci.* 1998;5(1):34–37.
58. Mogil JS. The genetic mediation of individual differences in sensitivity to pain and its inhibition. *Proc Natl Acad Sci U S A.* 1999;96(14):7744–7751.
59. Turk DC, Flor H, Rudy TE. Pain and families. I. Etiology, maintenance, and psychosocial impact. *Pain.* 1987;30(1):3–27.
60. Indo Y, Tsuruta M, Hayashida Y, et al. Mutations in the TRKA/NGF receptor gene in patients with congenital insensitivity to pain with anhidrosis. *Nat Genet.* 1996;13(4):485–488.

61. Meyer UA. The molecular basis of genetic polymorphisms of drug metabolism. *J Pharm Pharmacol.* 1994;46(suppl 1):409–415.

62. Ophoff RA, Terwindt GM, Vergouwe MN, et al. Familial hemiplegic migraine and episodic ataxia type-2 are caused by mutations in the Ca2+ channel gene CACNL1A4. *Cell.* 1996;87(3):543–552.

63. Offenbaecher M, Bondy B, de Jonge S, et al. Possible association of fibromyalgia with a polymorphism in the serotonin transporter gene regulatory region. *Arthritis Rheum.* 1999;42(11):2482–2488.

64. Kemler MA, van de Vusse AC, van den Berg-Loonen EM, et al. HLA-DQ1 associated with reflex sympathetic dystrophy. *Neurology.* 1999;53(6):1350–1351.

65. Mailis A, Wade J. Profile of Caucasian women with possible genetic predisposition to reflex sympathetic dystrophy: a pilot study. *Clin J Pain.* 1994;10(3):210–217.

66. Lazorthes Y, Sagen J, Sallerin B, et al. Human chromaffin cell graft into the CSF for cancer pain management: a prospective phase II clinical study. *Pain.* 2000;87(1):19–32.

67. Finegold AA, Mannes AJ, Iadarola MJ. A paracrine paradigm for in vivo gene therapy in the central nervous system: treatment of chronic pain. *Hum Gene Ther.* 1999;10(7):1251–1257.

68. Macfarlane GJ, Norrie G, Atherton K, et al. The influence of socioeconomic status on the reporting of regional and widespread musculoskeletal pain: results from the 1958 British Birth Cohort Study. *Ann Rheum Dis.* 2009;68(10):1591–1595.

69. Mendelson G. Chronic pain and compensation: a review. *J Pain Symptom Manage.* 1986;1(3):135–144.

70. Giummarra MJ, Ioannou L, Ponsford J, et al. Chronic pain following motor vehicle collision: a systematic review of outcomes associated with seeking or receiving compensation. *Clin J Pain.* 2016;32(9):817–827.

71. Rohling ML, Binder LM, Langhinrichsen-Rohling J. Money matters: a meta-analytic review of the association between financial compensation and the experience and treatment of chronic pain. *Health Psychol.* 1995;14(6):537–547.

72. Mailis-Gagnon A, Nicholson K. On the nature of nondermatomal somatosensory deficits. *Clin J Pain.* 2011;27(1):76–84.

73. Meyer RA, Ringkamp M, Campbell JN, et al. Neural mechanisms of hyperalgesia after tissue injury *Johns Hopkins APL Tech Dig.* 2005;26:56–66.

74. Nelli JM, Nicholson K, Fatima Lakha S, et al. Use of a modified Comprehensive Pain Evaluation Questionnaire (CPEQ): characteristics and functional status of patients on entry to a tertiary care pain clinic. *Pain Res Manag.* 2012;17(2):75–82.

75. Shah JP, Danoff JV, Desai MJ, et al. Biochemicals associated with pain and inflammation are elevated in sites near to and remote from active myofascial trigger points. *Arch Phys Med Rehabil.* 2008;89(1):16–23.

76. Straube S, Andrew Moore R, Derry S, et al. Vitamin D and chronic pain. *Pain.* 2009;141(1–2):10–13.

77. Wu Z, Malihi Z, Stewart AW, et al. Effect of vitamin D supplementation on pain: a systematic review and meta-analysis. *Pain Physician.* 2016;19(7):415–427.

78. Russo MB, Brooks FR, Fontenot JP, et al. Sodium pentothal hypnosis: a procedure for evaluating medical patients with suspected psychiatric co-morbidity. *Mil Med.* 1997;162(3):215–218.

79. Simon EP, Dahl LF. The sodium pentothal hypnosis interview with follow-up treatment for complex regional pain syndrome. *J Pain Symptom Manage.* 1999;18(2):132–136.

80. Ellis JS, Schoenfeld LS, Ramamurthy S. Nonsomatic pain. *Phys Med Rehabil Stars.* 1991;5:103–132.

81. Mailis A, Amani N, Umana M, et al. Effect of intravenous sodium amytal on cutaneous sensory abnormalities, spontaneous pain and algometric pain pressure thresholds in neuropathic pain patients: a placebo-controlled study. *Pain.* 1997;70(1):69–81.

82. Davis KD, Flor H, Greely HT, et al. Brain imaging tests for chronic pain: medical, legal and ethical issues and recommendations. *Nat Rev Neurol.* 2017;13(10):624–638.

83. Peyron R, Faillenot I. [Functional brain mapping of pain perception]. *Med Sci (Paris).* 2011;27(1):82–87.

84. Alexander AL, Lee JE, Lazar M, et al. Diffusion tensor imaging of the brain. *Neurotherapeutics.* 2007;4(3):316–329.

85. Kolesar TA, Fiest KM, Smith SD, et al. Assessing nociception by fMRI of the human spinal cord: a systematic review. *Magn Reson Insights.* 2015;8(suppl 1):31–39.

86. Apkarian AV. Human brain imaging studies of chronic pain: translational opportunities. In: Kruger L, Light AR, eds. *Translational Pain Research: From Mouse to Man.* Boca Raton, FL: Frontiers in Neuroscience; 2010.

87. Ferrari R. Imaging studies in patients with spinal pain: practice audit evaluation of Choosing Wisely Canada recommendations. *Can Fam Physician.* 2016;62(3):e129–e137.

88. Kumbhare DA, Elzibak AH, Noseworthy MD. Assessment of myofascial trigger points using ultrasound. *Am J Phys Med Rehabil.* 2016;95(1):72–80.

89. Davis KD, Moayedi M. Central mechanisms of pain revealed through functional and structural MRI. *J Neuroimmune Pharmacol.* 2013;8(3):518–534.

90. Dumitru D, Zwartz MJ, Amato AA. *Electrodiagnostic Medicine.* 2nd ed. Philadelphia, PA: Hanley & Belfus; 2001.

91. Dumitru D. Electrophysiologic evaluation of the pain patient. *Phys Med Rehabil Stars.* 1991;5:187–208.

92. Petit A, Fouquet N, Roquelaure Y. Chronic low back pain, chronic disability at work, chronic management issues. *Scand J Work Environ Health.* 2015;41(2):107–110.

93. Andersson GBJ, Pope MH, Frymoyer JW, et al. Epidemiology and cost. In: Pope MH, Andersson GBJ, Frymoyer JW, et al., eds. *Occupational Low Back Pain: Assessment, Treatment and Prevention.* St. Louis, MO: CV Mosby; 1991:95–113.

94. Leopoldino AA, Diz JB, Martins VT, et al. Prevalence of low back pain in older Brazilians: a systematic review with meta-analysis. *Rev Bras Reumatol Engl Ed.* 2016;56(3):258–269.

95. Aronoff GM, Dupuy DN. Evaluation and management of back pain: preventing disability. In: Aronoff GM, ed. *Evaluation and Treatment of Chronic Pain.* 3rd ed. Baltimore, MD: Williams & Wilkins; 1998:247–257.

96. Furlan AD, Malmivaara A, Chou R, et al. 2015 updated method guideline for systematic reviews in the cochrane back and neck group. *Spine (Phila Pa 1976).* 2015;40(21):1660–1673.

97. van Tulder M, Koes B. Low back pain. In: McMahon SB, Koltzenburg M, eds. *Wall and Melzack's Textbook of Pain.* 5th ed. Philadelphia, PA: Elsevier Churchill Livingstone; 2006:699–708.

98. Henschke N, Ostelo RW, van Tulder MW, et al. Behavioural treatment for chronic low-back pain. *Cochrane Database Syst Rev.* 2010;(7):CD002014.

99. Enthoven WT, Roelofs PD, Deyo RA, et al. Non-steroidal anti-inflammatory drugs for chronic low back pain. *Cochrane Database Syst Rev.* 2016;(2):CD012087.

100. Deshpande A, Furlan A, Mailis-Gagnon A, et al. Opioids for chronic low-back pain. *Cochrane Database Syst Rev.* 2007;(3):CD004959.

101. Karjalainen K, Malmivaara A, van Tulder M, et al. Multidisciplinary biopsychosocial rehabilitation for subacute low back pain among working age adults. *Cochrane Database Syst Rev.* 2003;(2):CD002193.

102. Furlan AD, van Tulder MW, Cherkin DC, et al. Acupuncture and dry-needling for low back pain. *Cochrane Database Syst Rev.* 2005;(1):CD001351.

103. Furlan AD, Yazdi F, Tsertsvadze A, et al. Complementary and alternative therapies for back pain II. *Evid Rep Technol Assess (Full Rep).* 2010;(194):1–764.

104. Wieland LS, Skoetz N, Pilkington K, et al. Yoga treatment for chronic non-specific low back pain. *Cochrane Database Syst Rev.* 2017;(1):CD010671.

105. Franke H, Fryer G, Ostelo RW, et al. Muscle energy technique for non-specific low-back pain. *Cochrane Database Syst Rev.* 2015;(2):CD009852.

106. Yamato TP, Maher CG, Saragiotto BT, et al. Pilates for low back pain. *Cochrane Database Syst Rev.* 2015;(7):CD010265.

107. Saragiotto BT, Maher CG, Yamato TP, et al. Motor control exercise for nonspecific low back pain: a cochrane review. *Spine (Phila Pa 1976).* 2016;41(16):1284–1295.

108. Macedo LG, Saragiotto BT, Yamato TP, et al. Motor control exercise for acute non-specific low back pain. *Cochrane Database Syst Rev.* 2016;(2):CD012085.

109. Waseem Z, Boulias C, Gordon A, et al. Botulinum toxin injections for low-back pain and sciatica. *Cochrane Database Syst Rev.* 2011;(1):CD008257.

110. Dagenais S, Yelland MJ, Del Mar C, et al. Prolotherapy injections for chronic low-back pain. *Cochrane Database Syst Rev.* 2007;(2):CD004059.

111. Nelemans PJ, de Bie RA, de Vet HC, et al. Injection therapy for subacute and chronic benign low back pain. *Cochrane Database Syst Rev.* 2000;(2):CD001824.

112. Spitzer WO, Skovron ML, Salmi LR, et al. Scientific monograph of the Quebec Task Force on Whiplash-Associated Disorders: redefining "whiplash" and its management. *Spine (Phila Pa 1976).* 1995;20(8 suppl):1S–73S.

113. Cote P, Wong JJ, Sutton D, et al. Management of neck pain and associated disorders: a clinical practice guideline from the Ontario Protocol for Traffic Injury Management (OPTIMa) Collaboration. *Eur Spine J.* 2016;25(7):2000–2022.

114. Riddle DL, Schappert SM. Volume and characteristics of inpatient and ambulatory medical care for neck pain in the United States: data from three national surveys. *Spine (Phila Pa 1976).* 2007;32(1):132–140; discussion 41.

115. Guzman J, Hurwitz EL, Carroll LJ, et al. A new conceptual model of neck pain: linking onset, course, and care: the Bone and Joint Decade 2000–2010 Task Force on Neck Pain and Its Associated Disorders. *Spine (Phila Pa 1976).* 2008;33(4 suppl):S14–S23.

116. Carroll LJ, Hogg-Johnson S, van der Velde G, et al. Course and prognostic factors for neck pain in the general population: results of the Bone and Joint Decade 2000–2010 Task Force on Neck Pain and Its Associated Disorders. *Spine (Phila Pa 1976).* 2008;33(4 suppl):S75–S82.

117. Seidel MF, Herguijuela M, Forkert R, et al. Nerve growth factor in rheumatic diseases. *Semin Arthritis Rheum.* 2010;40(2):109–126.

118. Sarchielli P, Alberti A, Candeliere A, et al. Glial cell line-derived neurotrophic factor and somatostatin levels in cerebrospinal fluid of patients affected by chronic migraine and fibromyalgia. *Cephalalgia.* 2006;26(4):409–415.

119. Bazzichi L, Rossi A, Massimetti G, et al. Cytokine patterns in fibromyalgia and their correlation with clinical manifestations. *Clin Exp Rheumatol.* 2007;25(2):225–230.

120. Grant MA, Farrell MJ, Kumar R, et al. fMRI evaluation of pain intensity coding in fibromyalgia patients and controls. *Arthritis Rheum.* 2001;44 [abstract].

121. Gracely RH, Geisser ME, Giesecke T, et al. Pain catastrophizing and neural responses to pain among persons with fibromyalgia. *Brain.* 2004;127(Pt 4):835–843.

122. Kucyi A, Davis KD. The neural code for pain: from single-cell electrophysiology to the dynamic pain connectome. *Neuroscientist.* 2016;23(4):397–414.

123. Vardeh D, Mannion RJ, Woolf CJ. Toward a mechanism-based approach to pain diagnosis. *J Pain.* 2016;17(9 suppl):T50–T69.

124. Holm LW, Carroll LJ, Cassidy JD, et al. Widespread pain following whiplash-associated disorders: incidence, course, and risk factors. *J Rheumatol.* 2007;34(1):193–200.

125. Bergman S, Herrstrom P, Jacobsson LT, et al. Chronic widespread pain: a three year follow-up of pain distribution and risk factors. *J Rheumatol.* 2002;29(4):818–825.

126. Kindler LL, Jones KD, Perrin N, et al. Risk factors predicting the development of widespread pain from chronic back or neck pain. *J Pain.* 2010;11(12):1320–1328.

127. Sarzi-Puttini P, Atzeni F, Mease PJ. Chronic widespread pain: from peripheral to central evolution. *Best Pract Res Clin Rheumatol.* 2011;25(2):133–139.

128. Stisi S, Cazzola M, Buskila D, et al. Etiopathogenetic mechanisms of fibromyalgia syndrome. *Reumatismo.* 2008;60(suppl 1):25–35.

129. Buskila D, Cohen H. Comorbidity of fibromyalgia and psychiatric disorders. *Curr Pain Headache Rep.* 2007;11(5):333–338.

130. Tekin L, Akarsu S, Durmus O, et al. The effect of dry needling in the treatment of myofascial pain syndrome: a randomized double-blinded placebo-controlled trial. *Clin Rheumatol.* 2013;32(3):309–315.

131. Simons DG, Travell JG, Simms LS. *Myofascial Pain and Dysfunction. The Trigger Point Manual. Upper Half of the Body Extremities.* 2nd ed. Baltimore, MD: Williams & Wilkins; 1998.

132. Travell JG, Simons DG. *Myofascial Pain and Dysfunction. The Trigger Point Manual. Lower Extremities.* Baltimore, MD: Williams & Wilkins; 1998.

133. Skootsky SA, Jaeger B, Oye RK. Prevalence of myofascial pain in general internal medicine practice. *West J Med.* 1989;151(2):157–160.

134. Gerwin RD. A study of 96 subjects examined both for fibromyalgia and myofascial pain. *J Musculoskelet Pain.* 1995;3(suppl 1):121.

135. Kaergaard A, Andersen JH. Musculoskeletal disorders of the neck and shoulders in female sewing machine operators: prevalence, incidence, and prognosis. *Occup Environ Med.* 2000;57(8):528–534.

136. Sola AE, Rodenberger ML, Gettys BB. Incidence of hypersensitive areas in posterior shoulder muscles; a survey of two hundred young adults. *Am J Phys Med.* 1955;34(6):585–590.

137. Schiffman EL, Fricton JR, Haley DP, et al. The prevalence and treatment needs of subjects with temporomandibular disorders. *J Am Dent Assoc.* 1990;120(3):295–303.

138. Fishbain DA, Goldberg M, Meagher BR, et al. Male and female chronic pain patients categorized by DSM-III psychiatric diagnostic criteria. *Pain.* 1986;26(2):181–197.

139. Fricton JR, Kroening R, Haley D, et al. Myofascial pain syndrome of the head and neck: a review of clinical characteristics of 164 patients. *Oral Surg Oral Med Oral Pathol.* 1985;60(6):615–623.

140. Chaiamnuay P, Darmawan J, Muirden KD, et al. Epidemiology of rheumatic disease in rural Thailand: a WHO-ILAR COPCORD study. Community Oriented Programme for the Control of Rheumatic Disease. *J Rheumatol.* 1998;25(7):1382–1387.

141. Fernandez-de-las-Penas C, Alonso-Blanco C, Miangolarra JC. Myofascial trigger points in subjects presenting with mechanical neck pain: a blinded, controlled study. *Man Ther.* 2007;12(1):29–33.

142. Borg-Stein J, Wilkins A. Soft tissue determinants of low back pain. *Curr Pain Headache Rep.* 2006;10(5):339–344.

143. Fernandez-de-Las-Penas C, Alonso-Blanco C, Cuadrado ML, et al. Myofascial trigger points and their relationship to headache clinical parameters in chronic tension-type headache. *Headache.* 2006;46(8):1264–1272.

144. Hwang M, Kang YK, Kim DH. Referred pain pattern of the pronator quadratus muscle. *Pain.* 2005;116(3):238–242.

145. Treaster D, Marras WS, Burr D, et al. Myofascial trigger point development from visual and postural stressors during computer work. *J Electromyogr Kinesiol.* 2006;16(2):115–124.

146. Jarrell J. Myofascial dysfunction in the pelvis. *Curr Pain Headache Rep.* 2004;8(6):452–456.

147. Doggweiler-Wiygul R. Urologic myofascial pain syndromes. *Curr Pain Headache Rep.* 2004;8(6):445–451.

148. Anderson RU, Wise D, Sawyer T, et al. Sexual dysfunction in men with chronic prostatitis/chronic pelvic pain syndrome: improvement after trigger point release and paradoxical relaxation training. *J Urol.* 2006;176(4 Pt 1):1534–1538; discussion 8–9.

149. Simons DG. Clinical and etiological update of myofascial pain from trigger points. *J Musculoskelet Pain.* 1996;4(1–2):93–122.

150. Tough EA, White AR, Richards S, et al. Variability of criteria used to diagnose myofascial trigger point pain syndrome—evidence from a review of the literature. *Clin J Pain.* 2007;23(3):278–286.

151. Grosman-Rimon L, Clarke H, Mills PB, et al. Clinicians' perspective of the current diagnostic criteria for myofascial pain syndrome. *J Back Musculoskelet Rehabil.* 2017;30(3):509–514.

152. Rivers WE, Garrigues D, Graciosa J, et al. Signs and symptoms of myofascial pain: an international survey of pain management providers and proposed preliminary set of diagnostic criteria. *Pain Med.* 2015;16(9):1794–1805.

153. Hsieh CY, Hong CZ, Adams AH, et al. Interexaminer reliability of the palpation of trigger points in the trunk and lower limb muscles. *Arch Phys Med Rehabil.* 2000;81(3):258–264.

154. Gerwin RD. Myofascial pain and fibromyalgia: diagnosis and treatment. *J Back Musculoskelet Rehabil.* 1998;11(3):175–181.

155. Rathbone A, Grosman-Rimon L, Kumbhare D. Inter-rater agreement of manual palpation for identification of myofascial trigger points: a systematic review and meta-analysis. *Clin J Pain.* 2017;33(8):715–729.

156. Zale KE, Klatt M, Volz KR, et al. A mixed-method approach to evaluating the association between myofascial trigger points and ankle/foot pain using handheld sonography equipment. *J Diagn Med Sonogr.* 2015;31(4):210–220.

157. Sikdar S, Shah JP, Gebreab T, et al. Novel applications of ultrasound technology to visualize and characterize myofascial trigger points and surrounding soft tissue. *Arch Phys Med Rehabil.* 2009;90(11):1829–1838.

158. Barbero M, Bertoli P, Cescon C, et al. Intra-rater reliability of an experienced physiotherapist in locating myofascial trigger points in upper trapezius muscle. *J Man Manip Ther.* 2012;20(4):171–177.

159. Ge HY. Prevalence of myofascial trigger points in fibromyalgia: the overlap of two common problems. *Curr Pain Headache Rep.* 2010;14(5):339–345.

160. Queiroz LP. Worldwide epidemiology of fibromyalgia. *Curr Pain Headache Rep.* 2013;17(8):356.

161. Wolfe F, Clauw DJ, Fitzcharles MA, et al. Fibromyalgia criteria and severity scales for clinical and epidemiological studies: a modification of the ACR preliminary diagnostic criteria for fibromyalgia. *J Rheumatol.* 2011;38(6):1113–1122.

162. Clauw DJ. Fibromyalgia: a clinical review. *JAMA.* 2014;311(15):1547–1555.

163. Rehm SE, Koroschetz J, Gockel U, et al. A cross-sectional survey of 3035 patients with fibromyalgia: subgroups of patients with typical comorbidities and sensory symptom profiles. *Rheumatology (Oxford).* 2010;49(6):1146–1152.

164. Turk DC, Okifuji A, Sinclair JD, et al. Differential responses by psychosocial subgroups of fibromyalgia syndrome patients to an interdisciplinary treatment. *Arthritis Care Res.* 1998;11(5):397–404.

165. Clauw DJ, Arnold LM, McCarberg BH, FibroCollaborative. The science of fibromyalgia. *Mayo Clin Proc.* 2011;86(9):907–911.

166. Serra J, Collado A, Sola R, et al. Hyperexcitable C nociceptors in fibromyalgia. *Ann Neurol.* 2014;75(2):196–208.

167. McBeth J, Silman AJ, Gupta A, et al. Moderation of psychosocial risk factors through dysfunction of the hypothalamic-pituitary-adrenal stress axis in the onset of chronic widespread musculoskeletal pain: findings of a population-based prospective cohort study. *Arthritis Rheum.* 2007;56(1):360–371.

168. Egloff N, von Kanel R, Muller V, et al. Implications of proposed fibromyalgia criteria across other functional pain syndromes. *Scand J Rheumatol.* 2015;44(5):416–424.

169. Wolfe F, Clauw DJ, Fitzcharles MA, et al. 2016 revisions to the 2010/2011 fibromyalgia diagnostic criteria. *Semin Arthritis Rheum.* 2016;46(3):319–329.

170. Fitzcharles MA, Ste-Marie PA, Mailis A, et al. Adjudication of fibromyalgia syndrome: challenges in the medicolegal arena. *Pain Res Manag.* 2014;19(6):287–292.

171. Arnold LM, Gebke KB, Choy EH. Fibromyalgia: management strategies for primary care providers. *Int J Clin Pract.* 2016;70(2):99–112.

172. Arnold LM. Biology and therapy of fibromyalgia. New therapies in fibromyalgia. *Arthritis Res Ther.* 2006;8(4):212.

173. Harden RN, Bruehl S, Perez RS, et al. Validation of proposed diagnostic criteria (the "Budapest Criteria") for complex regional pain syndrome. *Pain.* 2010;150(2):268–274.

174. Hassantash SA, Afrakhteh M, Maier RV. Causalgia: a meta-analysis of the literature. *Arch Surg.* 2003;138(11):1226–1231.

175. Mailis-Gagnon A, Chaparro LE. Diagnosis and management of complex regional pain syndrome. *J Musculoskelet Med.* 2008;25:464–469, 490.

176. Ringer R, Wertli M, Bachmann LM, et al. Concordance of qualitative bone scintigraphy results with presence of clinical complex regional pain syndrome 1: meta-analysis of test accuracy studies. *Eur J Pain.* 2012;16(10):1347–1356.

177. Held U, Brunner F, Steurer J, et al. Bayesian meta-analysis of test accuracy in the absence of a perfect reference test applied to bone scintigraphy for the diagnosis of complex regional pain syndrome. *Biom J.* 2015;57(6):1020–1037.

178. Geertzen JHB, Perez RSGM, Dijkstra PU, et al. *Guidelines Complex Regional Pain Syndrome Type I.* Netherlands Society of Anesthesiologists and Netherlands Society of Rehabiltiation Specialties; 2006.

179. de Mos M, de Bruijn AG, Huygen FJ, et al. The incidence of complex regional pain syndrome: a population-based study. *Pain.* 2007;129(1–2):12–20.

180. Sandroni P, Benrud-Larson LM, McClelland RL, et al. Complex regional pain syndrome type I: incidence and prevalence in Olmsted county, a population-based study. *Pain.* 2003;103(1–2):199–207.

181. Zollinger PE, Tuinebreijer WE, Breederveld RS, et al. Can vitamin C prevent complex regional pain syndrome in patients with wrist fractures? A randomized, controlled, multicenter dose-response study. *J Bone Joint Surg Am.* 2007;89(7):1424–1431.

182. Burton AW, Bruehl S, Harden RN. Current diagnosis and therapy of complex regional pain syndrome: refining diagnostic criteria and therapeutic options. *Expert Rev Neurother.* 2005;5(5):643–651.

183. Baron R. Complex regional pain syndromes. In: McMahon SB, Koltzenburg M, eds. *Wall and Melzack's Textbook of Pain.* 5th ed. Philadelphia, PA: Elsevier Churchill Livingstone; 2006:1011–1027.

184. Kozin F, Ryan LM, Carerra GF, et al. The reflex sympathetic dystrophy syndrome (RSDS). III. Scintigraphic studies, further evidence for the therapeutic efficacy of systemic corticosteroids, and proposed diagnostic criteria. *Am J Med.* 1981;70(1):23–30.

185. Christensen K, Jensen EM, Noer I. The reflex dystrophy syndrome response to treatment with systemic corticosteroids. *Acta Chir Scand.* 1982;148(8):653–655.

186. Grundberg AB. Reflex sympathetic dystrophy: treatment with long-acting intramuscular corticosteroids. *J Hand Surg Am.* 1996;21(4):667–670.

187. Zyluk A, Puchalski P. Treatment of early complex regional pain syndrome type 1 by a combination of mannitol and dexamethasone. *J Hand Surg Eur Vol.* 2008;33(2):130–136.

188. Taskaynatan MA, Ozgul A, Tan AK, et al. Bier block with methylprednisolone and lidocaine in CRPS type I: a randomized, double-blinded, placebo-controlled study. *Reg Anesth Pain Med.* 2004;29(5):408–412.

189. Lukovic TZ, Ilic KP, Jevtic M, et al. Corticosteroids and physical agents in treatment of complex regional pain syndrome type I. *Medicus.* 2006;7:70–72.

190. Borchers AT, Gershwin ME. Complex regional pain syndrome: a comprehensive and critical review. *Autoimmun Rev.* 2014;13(3):242–265.

191. O'Connell NE, Wand BM, McAuley J, et al. Interventions for treating pain and disability in adults with complex regional pain syndrome. *Cochrane Database Syst Rev.* 2013;(4):CD009416.

192. Harke H, Gretenkort P, Ladleif HU, et al. The response of neuropathic pain and pain in complex regional pain syndrome I to carbamazepine and sustained-release morphine in patients pretreated with spinal cord stimulation: a double-blinded randomized study. *Anesth Analg.* 2001;92(2):488–495.

193. Harden RN, Oaklander AL, Burton AW, et al. Complex regional pain syndrome: practical diagnostic and treatment guidelines, 4th edition. *Pain Med.* 2013;14(2):180–229.

194. Furlan AD, Reardon R, Weppler C, et al. Opioids for chronic noncancer pain: a new Canadian practice guideline. *CMAJ.* 2010;182(9):923–930.

195. Serpell MG; Neuropathic Pain Study Group. Gabapentin in neuropathic pain syndromes: a randomised, double-blind, placebo-controlled trial. *Pain.* 2002;99(3):557–566.

196. Benzon HT, Liu SS, Buvanendran A. Evolving definitions and pharmacologic management of complex regional pain syndrome. *Anesth Analg.* 2016;122(3):601–604.

197. Adami S, Fossaluzza V, Gatti D, et al. Bisphosphonate therapy of reflex sympathetic dystrophy syndrome. *Ann Rheum Dis.* 1997;56(3):201–204.

198. Varenna M, Zucchi F, Ghiringhelli D, et al. Intravenous clodronate in the treatment of reflex sympathetic dystrophy syndrome. A randomized, double blind, placebo controlled study. *J Rheumatol.* 2000;27(6):1477–1483.

199. Manicourt DH, Brasseur JP, Boutsen Y, et al. Role of alendronate in therapy for posttraumatic complex regional pain syndrome type I of the lower extremity. *Arthritis Rheum.* 2004;50(11):3690–3697.

200. Robinson JN, Sandom J, Chapman PT. Efficacy of pamidronate in complex regional pain syndrome type I. *Pain Med.* 2004;5(3):276–280.

201. Goh EL, Chidambaram S, Ma D. Complex regional pain syndrome: a recent update. *Burns Trauma.* 2017;5(2):1–11.

202. Molvik H, Khan W. Bisphosphonates and their influence on fracture healing: a systematic review. *Osteoporos Int.* 2015;26(4):1251–1260.

203. Finch PM, Knudsen L, Drummond PD. Reduction of allodynia in patients with complex regional pain syndrome: a double-blind placebo-controlled trial of topical ketamine. *Pain.* 2009;146(1–2):18–25.

204. Gammaitoni A, Gallagher RM, Welz-Bosna M. Topical ketamine gel: possible role in treating neuropathic pain. *Pain Med.* 2000;1(1):97–100.

205. Wertli M, Bachmann LM, Weiner SS, et al. Prognostic factors in complex regional pain syndrome 1: a systematic review. *J Rehabil Med.* 2013;45(3):225–231.

206. Perez RS, Zollinger PE, Dijkstra PU, et al. Evidence based guidelines for complex regional pain syndrome type 1. *BMC Neurol.* 2010;10:20.

207. Kemler MA, Barendse GA, van Kleef M, et al. Spinal cord stimulation in patients with chronic reflex sympathetic dystrophy. *N Engl J Med.* 2000;343(9):618–624.

208. Kemler MA, de Vet HC, Barendse GA, et al. Spinal cord stimulation for chronic reflex sympathetic dystrophy—five-year follow-up. *N Engl J Med.* 2006;354(22):2394–2396.

209. Bean DJ, Johnson MH, Heiss-Dunlop W, et al. Do psychological factors influence recovery from complex regional pain syndrome type 1? A prospective study. *Pain.* 2015;156(11):2310–2318.

210. Galer BS, Gianas A, Jensen MP. Painful diabetic polyneuropathy: epidemiology, pain description, and quality of life. *Diabetes Res Clin Pract.* 2000;47(2):123–128.

211. Siddall PJ. Pain following spinal cord injury. In: McMahon SB, Koltzenburg M, eds. *Wall and Melzack's Textbook of Pain.* 5th ed. Philadelphia, PA: Elsevier Churchill Livingstone; 2006:1043–1055.

212. Boivie J. Central pain. In: McMahon SB, Koltzenburg M, eds. *Wall and Melzack's Textbook of Pain.* 5th ed. Philadelphia, PA: Elsevier Churchill Livingstone; 2006:1057–1074.

213. Gustin SM, Wrigley PJ, Siddall PJ, et al. Brain anatomy changes associated with persistent neuropathic pain following spinal cord injury. *Cereb Cortex.* 2010;20(6):1409–1419.

214. Mehta S, Orenczuk K, McIntyre A, et al. Neuropathic pain post spinal cord injury part 2: systematic review of dorsal root entry zone procedure. *Top Spinal Cord Inj Rehabil.* 2013;19(1):78–86.

215. Mehta S, Orenczuk K, McIntyre A, et al. Neuropathic pain post spinal cord injury part 1: systematic review of physical and behavioral treatment. *Top Spinal Cord Inj Rehabil.* 2013;19(1):61–77.

216. Boldt I, Eriks-Hoogland I, Brinkhof MW, et al. Non-pharmacological interventions for chronic pain in people with spinal cord injury. *Cochrane Database Syst Rev.* 2014;(11):CD009177.

217. Moreno-Duarte I, Morse LR, Alam M, et al. Targeted therapies using electrical and magnetic neural stimulation for the treatment of chronic pain in spinal cord injury. *Neuroimage.* 2014;85(Pt 3):1003–1013.

218. Naess H, Lunde L, Brogger J. The effects of fatigue, pain, and depression on quality of life in ischemic stroke patients: the Bergen Stroke Study. *Vasc Health Risk Manag.* 2012;8:407–413.

219. Langhorne P, Stott DJ, Robertson L, et al. Medical complications after stroke: a multicenter study. *Stroke.* 2000;31(6):1223–1229.

220. Widar M, Samuelsson L, Karlsson-Tivenius S, et al. Long-term pain conditions after a stroke. *J Rehabil Med.* 2002;34(4):165–170.

221. Harvey RL, Macko RF, Stein J, et al. *Stroke Recovery and Rehabilitation.* Demos Medical Publishing, Springer Publishing Company; 2008.

222. Klit H, Finnerup NB, Jensen TS. Central post-stroke pain: clinical characteristics, pathophysiology, and management. *Lancet Neurol.* 2009;8(9):857–868.

223. O'Donnell MJ, Diener HC, Sacco RL, et al. Chronic pain syndromes after ischemic stroke: PRoFESS trial. *Stroke.* 2013;44(5):1238–1243.

224. MacGowan DJ, Janal MN, Clark WC, et al. Central poststroke pain and Wallenberg's lateral medullary infarction: frequency, character, and determinants in 63 patients. *Neurology.* 1997;49(1):120–125.

225. Moulin D, Boulanger A, Clark AJ, et al. Pharmacological management of chronic neuropathic pain: revised consensus statement from the Canadian Pain Society. *Pain Res Manag.* 2014;19(6):328–335.

226. Hebert D, Lindsay MP, McIntyre A, et al. Canadian stroke best practice recommendations: stroke rehabilitation practice guidelines, update 2015. *Int J Stroke.* 2016;11(4):459–484.

227. Mulla SM, Wang L, Khokhar R, et al. Management of central poststroke pain: systematic review of randomized controlled trials. *Stroke.* 2015;46(10):2853–2860.

228. Akyuz G, Kuru P. Systematic review of central post stroke pain: what is happening in the central nervous system? *Am J Phys Med Rehabil.* 2016;95(8):618–627.

229. Furlan A, Chaparro LE, Irvin E, et al. A comparison between enriched and nonenriched enrollment randomized withdrawal trials of opioids for chronic noncancer pain. *Pain Res Manag.* 2011;16(5):337–351.

230. Tick H. Nutrition and pain. *Phys Med Rehabil Clin N Am.* 2015;26(2):309–320.

231. Buchheit T, Van de Ven T, Hsia HL, et al. Pain phenotypes and associated clinical risk factors following traumatic amputation: results from veterans integrated pain evaluation research (VIPER). *Pain Med.* 2016;17:149–161.

232. Clarke C, Lindsay DR, Pyati S, et al. Residual limb pain is not a diagnosis: a proposed algorithm to classify postamputation pain. *Clin J Pain.* 2013;29:551–562.

233. Aiyer R, Barkin RL, Bhatia A, et al. A systematic review on the treatment of phantom limb pain with spinal cord stimulation. *Pain Manag.* 2017;7(1):59–69.

234. Ehde DM, Czerniecki JM, Smith DG, et al. Chronic phantom sensations, phantom pain, residual limb pain, and other regional pain after lower limb amputation. *Arch Phys Med Rehabil.* 2000;81(8):1039–1044.

235. Nikolajsen L, Jensen TS. Phantom limb pain. *Br J Anaesth.* 2001;87(1):107–116.

236. Jensen MP, Ehde DM, Hoffman AJ, et al. Cognitions, coping and social environment predict adjustment to phantom limb pain. *Pain.* 2002;95(1–2):133–142.

237. Challapalli V, Tremont-Lukats IW, McNicol ED, et al. Systemic administration of local anesthetic agents to relieve neuropathic pain. *Cochrane Database Syst Rev.* 2005;(4):CD003345.

238. Gold MS, Chessell I, Devor M, et al. Peripheral nervous system targets: rapporteur report. In: Campbell JN, Bausbaum AI, Dray A, et al., eds. *Emerging Strategies for the Treatment of Neuropathic Pain.* Seattle: IASP Press; 2006:3–36.

239. Alviar MJ, Hale T, Dungca M. Pharmacologic interventions for treating phantom limb pain. *Cochrane Database Syst Rev.* 2016;(10):CD006380.

240. Barbin J, Seetha V, Casillas JM, et al. The effects of mirror therapy on pain and motor control of phantom limb in amputees: a systematic review. *Ann Phys Rehabil Med.* 2016;59S:e149.

241. Batsford S, Ryan CG, Martin DJ. Non-pharmacological conservative therapy for phantom limb pain: a systematic review of randomized controlled trials. *Physiother Theory Pract.* 2017;33(3):173–183.

242. Flor H. Phantom-limb pain: characteristics, causes, and treatment. *Lancet Neurol.* 2002;1(3):182–189.

243. McCormick Z, Chang-Chien G, Marshall B, et al. Phantom limb pain: a systematic neuroanatomical-based review of pharmacologic treatment. *Pain Med.* 2014;15(2):292–305.

244. Furlan AD, Lui PW, Mailis A. Chemical sympathectomy for neuropathic pain: does it work? Case report and systematic literature review. *Clin J Pain.* 2001;17(4):327–336.

245. Furlan AD, Mailis A, Papagapiou M. Are we paying a high price for surgical sympathectomy? A systematic literature review of late complications. *J Pain.* 2000;1(4):245–257.

246. Winnie AP, Candido KD. Differential neural blockade in the diagnosis of pain mechanisms. In: Raj PP, ed. *Practical Management of Pain.* 3rd ed. St. Louis, MO: Mosby; 2000:427–438.

247. Henrot P, Stines J, Walter F, et al. Imaging of the Painful Lower Limb Stump. *RadioGraphics.* 2000;20:S219–S235.

248. Neil MJE. Pain after amputation. *BJA Educ.* 2016;16:107–112.

249. Dunkel N, Belaieff W, Assal M, et al. Wound dehiscence and stump infection after lower limb amputation: risk factors and association with antibiotic use. *J Orthop Sci.* 2012;17:588–594.

250. Vanross ER, Johnson S, Abbott CA. Effects of early mobilization on unhealed dysvascular transtibial amputation stumps: a clinical trial. *Arch Phys Med Rehabil.* 2009;90:610–617.

251. Rubin JR, Yao JS, Thompson RG, et al. Management of infection of major amputation stumps after failed femorodistal grafts. *Surgery.* 1985;98:810–815.

252. Buikema KE, Meyerle JH. Amputation stump: Privileged harbor for infections, tumors, and immune disorders. *Clin Dermatol.* 2014;32:670–677.

253. Meulenbelt HE, Geertzen JH, Dijkstra PU, et al. Skin problems in lower limb amputees: an overview by case reports. *J Eur Acad Dermatol Venereol.* 2007;21:147–155.

254. Yang NB, Garza LA, Foote CE, et al. High prevalence of stump dermatoses 38 years or more after amputation. *Arch Dermatol.* 2012;148:1283–1286.

255. Lugo L, Plata J, Salinas F, et al. Guía de Práctica Clínica para el diagnóstico y tratamiento preoperatorio, intraoperatorio y postoperatorio de la persona amputada, la prescripción de la prótesis y la rehabilitación integral [Internet]. Guía de Práctica Clínica. Ministerio de Salud y Seguridad Social. 2015. Available from: http://gpc.minsalud.gov.co/gpc_sites/Repositorio/Conv_637/GPC_amputacion/GPC_AMP_compl

256. Haumann J, Joosten EB, Everdingen MH. Pain prevalence in cancer patients: status quo or opportunities for improvement? *Curr Opin Support Palliat Care.* 2017;11(2):99–104.

257. Fitzgibbon DR, Chapman CR. Cancer pain: assessment and diagnosis. In: Loeser JD, ed. *Bonica's Management of Pain.* 3rd ed. Philadelphia, PA: Lippincott, Williams & Wilkins; 2001:623–658.

258. Foley KM. The treatment of cancer pain. *N Engl J Med.* 1985;313(2):84–95.

259. Paice JA, Portenoy R, Lacchetti C, et al. Management of chronic pain in survivors of adult cancers: American Society of Clinical Oncology Clinical Practice Guideline. *J Clin Oncol.* 2016;34(27):3325–3345.

260. Gromisch ES, Schairer LC, Pasternak E, et al. Assessment and treatment of psychiatric distress, sexual dysfunction, sleep disturbances, and pain in multiple sclerosis: a survey of members of the consortium of multiple sclerosis centers. *Int J MS Care*. 2016;18(6):291–297.

261. Foley PL, Vesterinen HM, Laird BJ, et al. Prevalence and natural history of pain in adults with multiple sclerosis: systematic review and meta-analysis. *Pain*. 2013;154(5):632–642.

262. Jawahar R, Oh U, Yang S, et al. A systematic review of pharmacological pain management in multiple sclerosis. *Drugs*. 2013;73(15):1711–1722.

263. Dworkin RH, Johnson RW, Breuer J, et al. Recommendations for the management of herpes zoster. *Clin Infect Dis*. 2007;44(suppl 1):S1–S26.

264. Gan EY, Tian EAL, Tey HL. Management of herpes zoster and post-herpetic neuralgia. *Am J Clin Dermatol*. 2013;14(2):77–85.

265. Sperber AD, Drossman DA. Review article: the functional abdominal pain syndrome. *Aliment Pharmacol Ther*. 2011;33(5):514–524.

266. Farmer AD, Ferdinand E, Aziz Q. Opioids and the gastrointestinal tract—a case of narcotic bowel syndrome and literature review. *J Neurogastroenterol Motil*. 2013;19(1):94–98.

267. Gatchel RJ, Peng YB, Peters ML, et al. The biopsychosocial approach to chronic pain: scientific advances and future directions. *Psychol Bull*. 2007;133(4):581–624.

268. Gatchel RJ, McGeary DD, McGeary CA, et al. Interdisciplinary chronic pain management: past, present, and future. *Am Psychol*. 2014;69(2):119–130.

269. Loeser JD. Multidisciplinary pain programs. In: Loeser JD, ed. *Bonica's Management of Pain*. 3rd ed. Philadelphia, PA: Lippincott, Williams & Wilkins; 2001:255–264.

270. Loeser J, Boureau F, Brooks P. *Desirable Characteristics for Pain Treatment Facilities and Standards for Physician Fellowship in Pain Management*. Seattle: IASP; 1990.

271. Kronborg C, Handberg G, Axelsen F. Health care costs, work productivity and activity impairment in non-malignant chronic pain patients. *Eur J Health Econ*. 2009;10(1):5–13.

272. King JC, Kelleher WJ. The chronic pain syndrome: the in-patient interdisciplinary rehabilitative behavioral modification approach. *Phys Med Rehabil Stars*. 1991;5:165–186.

273. Karjalainen K, Malmivaara A, van Tulder M, et al. Biopsychosocial rehabilitation for upper limb repetitive strain injuries in working age adults. *Cochrane Database Syst Rev*. 2000;(3):CD002269.

274. Karjalainen K, Malmivaara A, van Tulder M, et al. Multidisciplinary rehabilitation for fibromyalgia and musculoskeletal pain in working age adults. *Cochrane Database Syst Rev*. 2000;(2):CD001984.

275. Turk DC, Stanos SP, Palermo TM, et al. *Interdisciplinary Pain Management*. APS Position Statement; 2010. Available from: http://www.ampainsoc.org/advocacy/downloads/2010%20Interdisciplinary%20White

276. Grabois M. Pain clinics: role in the rehabilitation of patients with chronic pain. *Ann Acad Med Singapore*. 1983;12(3):428–433.

277. Loeser JD, Turk DC. Multidisciplinary pain management. In: Loeser JD, ed. *Bonica's Management of Pain*. 3rd ed. Philadelphia, PA: Lippincott, Williams & Wilkins; 2001:2069–2079.

278. Fordyce WE. Learned pain: pain as a behavior. In: Loeser JD, ed. *Bonica's Management of Pain*. 3rd ed. Philadelphia, PA: Lippincott, Williams & Wilkins; 2001:478–482.

279. Fordyce WE. *Behavioral Methods for Chronic Pain and Illness*. St. Louis, MO: CV Mosby; 1976:41–221.

280. Mayer TG, Gatchel RJ. *Functional Restoration for Spinal Disorders: Sports Medicine Approach*. Philadelphia, PA: Lea and Febiger; 1988.

281. Gatchel RJ, McGeary DD, Peterson A, et al. Preliminary findings of a randomized controlled trial of an interdisciplinary military pain program. *Mil Med*. 2009;174(3):270–277.

282. Deardorff WW, Rubin HS, Scott DW. Comprehensive multidisciplinary treatment of chronic pain: a follow-up study of treated and non-treated groups. *Pain*. 1991;45(1):35–43.

283. Maruta T, Swanson DW, McHardy MJ. Three year follow-up of patients with chronic pain who were treated in a multidisciplinary pain management center. *Pain*. 1990;41(1):47–53.

284. Peters JL, Large RG. A randomised control trial evaluating in- and outpatient pain management programmes. *Pain*. 1990;41(3):283–293.

285. Bendix AF, Bendix T, Lund C, et al. Comparison of three intensive programs for chronic low back pain patients: a prospective, randomized, observer-blinded study with one-year follow-up. *Scand J Rehabil Med*. 1997;29(2):81–89.

286. RxFiles. Opioid Patch Exchange Disposal Tool. Available from: http://www.rxfiles.ca/rxfiles/uploads/documents/Opioid-Patch-Exchange-Disposal-Tool.pdf

287. Saarto T, Wiffen PJ. Antidepressants for neuropathic pain. *Cochrane Database Syst Rev*. 2007;(4):CD005454.

288. Bally M, Dendukuri N, Rich B, et al. Risk of acute myocardial infarction with NSAIDs in real world use: Bayesian meta-analysis of individual patient data. *BMJ*. 2017;357:j1909.

289. Finestone HM, Juurlink DN, Power B, et al. Opioid prescribing is a surrogate for inadequate pain management resources. *Can Fam Physician*. 2016;62(6):465–468.

290. Dowell D, Haegerich TM, Chou R. CDC guideline for prescribing opioids for chronic pain—United States, 2016. *JAMA*. 2016;315(15):1624–1645.

291. Manchikanti L, Helm S II, Fellows B, et al. Opioid epidemic in the United States. *Pain Physician*. 2012;15(3 suppl):ES9–ES38.

292. Volkow ND, Collins FS. The role of science in addressing the opioid crisis. *N Engl J Med*. 2017;377(4):391–394.

293. Brown RE Jr, Sloan PA. The opioid crisis in the united states: chronic pain physicians are the answer, not the cause. *Anesth Analg*. 2017;125(5):1432–1434.

294. Soelberg CD, Brown RE Jr, Du Vivier D, et al. The US opioid crisis: current federal and state legal issues. *Anesth Analg*. 2017;125(5):1675–1681.

295. Makary MA, Overton HN, Wang P. Overprescribing is major contributor to opioid crisis. *BMJ*. 2017;359:j4792.

296. Busse JW, Craigie S, Juurlink DN, et al. Guideline for opioid therapy and chronic noncancer pain. *CMAJ*. 2017;189(18):E659–E666.

297. Stoicea N, Russell D, Weidner G, et al. Opioid-induced hyperalgesia in chronic pain patients and the mitigating effects of gabapentin. *Front Pharmacol*. 2015;6:104.

298. Roeckel LA, Le Coz GM, Gaveriaux-Ruff C, et al. Opioid-induced hyperalgesia: cellular and molecular mechanisms. *Neuroscience*. 2016;338:160–182.

299. Mauermann E, Filitz J, Dolder P, et al. Does fentanyl lead to opioid-induced hyperalgesia in healthy volunteers?: a double-blind, randomized, crossover trial. *Anesthesiology*. 2016;124(2):453–463.

300. Yi P, Pryzbylkowski P. Opioid Induced Hyperalgesia. *Pain Med*. 2015;16(suppl 1):S32–S36.

301. Hooten WM, Lamer TJ, Twyner C. Opioid-induced hyperalgesia in community-dwelling adults with chronic pain. *Pain*. 2015;156(6):1145–1152.

302. Mailis-Gagnon A, Lakha SF, Furlan A, et al. Systematic review of the quality and generalizability of studies on the effects of opioids on driving and cognitive/psychomotor performance. *Clin J Pain*. 2012;28(6):542–555.

303. Gomes T, Redelmeier DA, Juurlink DN, et al. Opioid dose and risk of road trauma in Canada: a population-based study. *JAMA Intern Med*. 2013;173(3):196–201.

304. Soderberg KC, Laflamme L, Moller J. Newly initiated opioid treatment and the risk of fall-related injuries. A nationwide, register-based, case-crossover study in Sweden. *CNS Drugs*. 2013;27(2):155–161.

305. Li L, Setoguchi S, Cabral H, et al. Opioid use for noncancer pain and risk of fracture in adults: a nested case-control study using the general practice research database. *Am J Epidemiol*. 2013;178(4):559–569.

306. Mai J, Franklin G, Tauben D. Guideline for prescribing opioids to treat pain in injured workers. *Phys Med Rehabil Clin N Am*. 2015;26(3):453–465.

307. Juurlink DN, Gomes T, Guttmann A, et al. Postpartum maternal codeine therapy and the risk of adverse neonatal outcomes: a retrospective cohort study. *Clin Toxicol (Phila)*. 2012;50(5):390–395.

308. Turner SD, Gomes T, Camacho X, et al. Neonatal opioid withdrawal and antenatal opioid prescribing. *CMAJ Open*. 2015;3(1):E55–E61.

309. Delaney W, Huff J, Mini S, et al. Coprescribing naloxone for patients on chronic opioid therapy: les-sons learned from a patient-safety initiative in primary care training sites. *J Opioid Manag*. 2016;12(5):360–366.

310. Bird SM, McAuley A, Perry S, et al. Effectiveness of Scotland's National Naloxone Programme for reducing opioid-related deaths: a before (2006–10) versus after (2011–13) comparison. *Addiction*. 2016;111(5):883–891.

311. Furlan AD, Reardon R, Salach L. The opioid manager: a point-of-care tool to facilitate the use of the Canadian Opioid Guideline. *J Opioid Manag*. 2012;8(1):57–61.

312. Walsh TD. Antidepressants in chronic pain. *Clin Neuropharmacol*. 1983;6(4):271–295.

313. Urquhart DM, Hoving JL, Assendelft WW, et al. Antidepressants for non-specific low back pain. *Cochrane Database Syst Rev*. 2008;(1):CD001703.

314. Arnold LM, Keck PE Jr, Welge JA. Antidepressant treatment of fibromyalgia. A meta-analysis and review. *Psychosomatics*. 2000;41(2):104–113.

315. Dworkin RH, O'Connor AB, Backonja M, et al. Pharmacologic management of neuropathic pain: evidence-based recommendations. *Pain*. 2007;132(3):237–251.

316. Moore RA, Derry S, Aldington D, et al. Amitriptyline for neuropathic pain in adults. *Cochrane Database Syst Rev*. 2015;(7):CD008242.

317. Derry S, Wiffen PJ, Aldington D, et al. Nortriptyline for neuropathic pain in adults. *Cochrane Database Syst Rev*. 2015;(1):CD011209.

318. Hearn L, Moore RA, Derry S, et al. Desipramine for neuropathic pain in adults. *Cochrane Database Syst Rev*. 2014;(9):CD011003.

319. Hearn L, Derry S, Phillips T, et al. Imipramine for neuropathic pain in adults. *Cochrane Database Syst Rev*. 2014;(5):CD010769.

320. Holick MF. Vitamin D deficiency. *N Engl J Med*. 2007;357(3):266–281.

321. Plotnikoff GA, Quigley JM. Prevalence of severe hypovitaminosis D in patients with persistent, nonspecific musculoskeletal pain. *Mayo Clin Proc*. 2003;78(12):1463–1470.

322. Ito T, Jensen RT. Association of long-term proton pump inhibitor therapy with bone fractures and effects on absorption of calcium, vitamin B_{12}, iron, and magnesium. *Curr Gastroenterol Rep*. 2010;12(6):448–457.

323. Srebro D, Vuckovic S, Milovanovic A, et al. Magnesium in pain research: state of the art. *Curr Med Chem*. 2016 Dec 12. [Epub ahead of print] PubMed PMID: 27978803.

324. Ford AC, Quigley EM, Lacy BE, et al. Efficacy of prebiotics, probiotics, and synbiotics in irritable bowel syndrome and chronic idiopathic constipation: systematic review and meta-analysis. *Am J Gastroenterol*. 2014;109(10):1547–1561; quiz 1546, 1562.

325. Tokuyama S, Nakamoto K. Unsaturated fatty acids and pain. *Biol Pharm Bull*. 2011;34(8):1174–1178.

326. Willett W. *Eat, Drink, and Be Healthy: The Harvard Medical School Guide to Healthy Eating: Simon and Schuster*. 2011. Simon & Schuster Source. A division of Simon & Schuster Rockefeller Centre; Copyright 2001 by the President and Fellows of Harvard College.

327. Derry S, Cording M, Wiffen PJ, et al. Pregabalin for pain in fibromyalgia in adults. *Cochrane Database Syst Rev*. 2016;9:CD011790.

328. Moore RA, Wiffen PJ, Derry S, et al. Gabapentin for chronic neuropathic pain and fibromyalgia in adults. *Cochrane Database Syst Rev*. 2014;(4):CD007938.

329. Wiffen PJ, Derry S, Moore RA, et al. Antiepileptic drugs for neuropathic pain and fibromyalgia—an overview of Cochrane reviews. *Cochrane Database Syst Rev.* 2013;(11):CD010567.

330. Wiffen PJ, Derry S, Lunn MP, et al. Topiramate for neuropathic pain and fibromyalgia in adults. *Cochrane Database Syst Rev.* 2013;(8):CD008314.

331. Moshe SL. Mechanisms of action of anticonvulsant agents. *Neurology.* 2000;55(5 suppl 1):S32–S40; discussion S54–S58.

332. Corrigan R, Derry S, Wiffen PJ, et al. Clonazepam for neuropathic pain and fibromyalgia in adults. *Cochrane Database Syst Rev.* 2012;(5):CD009486.

333. van Tulder MW, Touray T, Furlan AD, et al. Muscle relaxants for non-specific low back pain. *Cochrane Database Syst Rev.* 2003;(2):CD004252.

334. Leite FM, Atallah AN, El Dib R, et al. Cyclobenzaprine for the treatment of myofascial pain in adults. *Cochrane Database Syst Rev.* 2009;(3):CD006830.

335. Lakha SF, Louffat AF, Nicholson K, et al. Characteristics of chronic noncancer pain patients assessed with the opioid risk tool in a Canadian tertiary care pain clinic. *Pain Med.* 2014;15(10):1743–1749.

336. Nielsen S, Sabioni P, Trigo JM, et al. Opioid-sparing effect of cannabinoids: a systematic review and meta-analysis. *Neuropsychopharmacology.* 2017;42(9):1752–1765.

337. Mackie K. Cannabinoid receptors as therapeutic targets. *Annu Rev Pharmacol Toxicol.* 2006;46:101–122.

338. Volkow ND, Baler RD, Compton WM, et al. Adverse health effects of marijuana use. *N Engl J Med.* 2014;370(23):2219–2227.

339. Hazekamp A, Heerdink ER. The prevalence and incidence of medicinal cannabis on prescription in The Netherlands. *Eur J Clin Pharmacol.* 2013;69(8):1575–1580.

340. Chaparro LE, Wiffen PJ, Moore RA, et al. Combination pharmacotherapy for the treatment of neuropathic pain in adults. *Cochrane Database Syst Rev.* 2012;(7):CD008943.

341. Lehmann JF, DeLateur BJ. Therapeutic heat. *Therapeutic heat and Cold.* 1990:2. Copyright © 2016 by F. A. Davis Company.

342. French SD, Cameron M, Walker BF, et al. Superficial heat or cold for low back pain. *Cochrane Database Syst Rev.* 2006;(1):CD004750.

343. Taylor BF, Waring CA, Brashear TA. The effects of therapeutic application of heat or cold followed by static stretch on hamstring muscle length. *J Orthop Sports Phys Ther.* 1995;21(5):283–286.

344. Nadler SF, Steiner DJ, Erasala GN, et al. Continuous low-level heat wrap therapy provides more efficacy than Ibuprofen and acetaminophen for acute low back pain. *Spine (Phila Pa 1976).* 2002;27(10):1012–1017.

345. Hassett AL, Williams DA. Non-pharmacological treatment of chronic widespread musculoskeletal pain. *Best Pract Res Clin Rheumatol.* 2011;25(2):299–309.

346. Langhorst J, Klose P, Dobos GJ, et al. Efficacy and safety of meditative movement therapies in fibromyalgia syndrome: a systematic review and meta-analysis of randomized controlled trials. *Rheumatol Int.* 2013;33(1):193–207.

347. Tang NK, Sanborn AN. Better quality sleep promotes daytime physical activity in patients with chronic pain? A multilevel analysis of the within-person relationship. *PLoS One.* 2014;9(3):e92158.

348. Busch AJ, Webber SC, Richards RS, et al. Resistance exercise training for fibromyalgia. *Cochrane Database Syst Rev.* 2013;(12):CD010884.

349. Blumenthal JA, Smith PJ, Hoffman BM. Is exercise a viable treatment for depression? *ACSMs Health Fit J.* 2012;16(4):14–21.

350. Jones KD, Adams D, Winters-Stone K, et al. A comprehensive review of 46 exercise treatment studies in fibromyalgia (1988-2005). *Health Qual Life Outcomes.* 2006;4:67.

351. Hauser W, Klose P, Langhorst J, et al. Efficacy of different types of aerobic exercise in fibromyalgia syndrome: a systematic review and meta-analysis of randomised controlled trials. *Arthritis Res Ther.* 2010;12(3):R79.

352. Holton K. The role of diet in the treatment of fibromyalgia. *Pain Manag.* 2016;6(4):317–320.

353. Staud R, Robinson ME, Price DD. Isometric exercise has opposite effects on central pain mechanisms in fibromyalgia patients compared to normal controls. *Pain.* 2005;118(1–2):176–184.

354. Vierck CJ Jr, Staud R, Price DD, et al. The effect of maximal exercise on temporal summation of second pain (windup) in patients with fibromyalgia syndrome. *J Pain.* 2001;2(6):334–344.

355. Nijs J, Kosek E, Van Oosterwijck J, et al. Dysfunctional endogenous analgesia during exercise in patients with chronic pain: to exercise or not to exercise? *Pain Physician.* 2012;15(3 suppl):ES205–ES213.

356. Nijs J, Roussel N, Van Oosterwijck J, et al. Fear of movement and avoidance behaviour toward physical activity in chronic-fatigue syndrome and fibromyalgia: state of the art and implications for clinical practice. *Clin Rheumatol.* 2013;32(8):1121–1129.

357. Stubbs B, Patchay S, Soundy A, et al. The avoidance of activities due to fear of falling contributes to sedentary behavior among community-dwelling older adults with chronic musculoskeletal pain: a multisite observational study. *Pain Med.* 2014;15(11):1861–1871.

358. Mannion AF, Taimela S, Muntener M, et al. Active therapy for chronic low back pain part 1. Effects on back muscle activation, fatigability, and strength. *Spine (Phila Pa 1976).* 2001;26(8):897–908.

359. Hayden JA, van Tulder MW, Malmivaara A, et al. Exercise therapy for treatment of non-specific low back pain. *Cochrane Database Syst Rev.* 2005;(3):CD000335.

360. Panjabi MM. The stabilizing system of the spine. Part I. Function, dysfunction, adaptation, and enhancement. *J Spinal Disord.* 1992;5(4):383–389; discussion 97.

361. Barr KP, Griggs M, Cadby T. Lumbar stabilization: core concepts and current literature, Part 1. *Am J Phys Med Rehabil.* 2005;84(6):473–480.

362. Crisco JJ III, Panjabi MM. Euler stability of the human ligamentous lumbar spine. Part I: Theory. *Clin Biomech (Bristol, Avon).* 1992;7(1):19–26.

363. Crisco JJ, Panjabi MM, Yamamoto I, et al. Euler stability of the human ligamentous lumbar spine. Part II: Experiment. *Clin Biomech (Bristol, Avon).* 1992;7(1):27–32.

364. Ferreira PH, Ferreira ML, Hodges PW. Changes in recruitment of the abdominal muscles in people with low back pain: ultrasound measurement of muscle activity. *Spine (Phila Pa 1976).* 2004;29(22):2560–2566.

365. O'Sullivan PB, Phyty GD, Twomey LT, et al. Evaluation of specific stabilizing exercise in the treatment of chronic low back pain with radiologic diagnosis of spondylolysis or spondylolisthesis. *Spine (Phila Pa 1976).* 1997;22(24):2959–2967.

366. Furlan AD, Giraldo M, Baskwill A, et al. Massage for low-back pain. *Cochrane Database Syst Rev.* 2015;(9):CD001929.

367. Furlan AD, Yazdi F, Tsertsvadze A, et al. A systematic review and meta-analysis of efficacy, cost-effectiveness, and safety of selected complementary and alternative medicine for neck and low-back pain. *Evid Based Complement Alternat Med.* 2012;2012:953139.

368. Taub A, Kane A, eds. History of local electrical analgesia in abstracts. First World Congress on Pain; 1975.

369. Brosseau L, Milne S, Robinson V, et al. Efficacy of the transcutaneous electrical nerve stimulation for the treatment of chronic low back pain: a meta-analysis. *Spine (Phila Pa 1976).* 2002;27(6):596–603.

370. Khadilkar A, Odebiyi DO, Brosseau L, et al. Transcutaneous electrical nerve stimulation (TENS) versus placebo for chronic low-back pain. *Cochrane Database Syst Rev.* 2008;(4):CD003008.

371. Hansson P, Lundeberg T. Transcutaneous electrical nerve stimulation and acupuncture. In: McMahon SB, Koltzenburg M, eds. *Wall and Melzack's Textbook of Pain.* 5th ed. Philadelphia, PA: Elsevier Churchill Livingstone; 2006:583–590.

372. Nnoaham KE, Kumbang J. Transcutaneous electrical nerve stimulation (TENS) for chronic pain. *Cochrane Database Syst Rev.* 2008;(3):CD003222.

373. Melzack R, Stillwell DM, Fox EJ. Trigger points and acupuncture points for pain: correlations and implications. *Pain.* 1977;3(1):3–23.

374. Vickers AJ, Linde K. Acupuncture for chronic pain. *JAMA.* 2014;311(9):955–956.

375. Chow RT, David MA, Armati PJ. 830 nm laser irradiation induces varicosity formation, reduces mitochondrial membrane potential and blocks fast axonal flow in small and medium diameter rat dorsal root ganglion neurons: implications for the analgesic effects of 830 nm laser. *J Peripher Nerv Syst.* 2007;12(1):28–39.

376. Moriyama Y, Nguyen J, Akens M, et al. In vivo effects of low level laser therapy on inducible nitric oxide synthase. *Lasers Surg Med.* 2009;41(3):227–231.

377. Cidral-Filho FJ, Mazzardo-Martins L, Martins DF, et al. Light-emitting diode therapy induces analgesia in a mouse model of postoperative pain through activation of peripheral opioid receptors and the L-arginine/nitric oxide pathway. *Lasers Med Sci.* 2014;29(2):695–702.

378. Wegner I, Widyahening IS, van Tulder MW, et al. Traction for low-back pain with or without sciatica. *Cochrane Database Syst Rev.* 2013;(8):CD003010.

379. Damgaard P, Bartels EM, Ris I, et al. Evidence of physiotherapy interventions for patients with chronic neck pain: a systematic review of randomised controlled trials. *ISRN Pain.* 2013;2013:567175.

380. Fulton WM. Psychological strategies and techniques in pain management. *Semin Anesth.* 1985;4:247–254.

381. Sielski R, Rief W, Glombiewski JA. Efficacy of biofeedback in chronic back pain: a meta-analysis. *Int J Behav Med.* 2017;24(1):25–41.

382. Heymans MW, van Tulder MW, Esmail R, et al. Back schools for non-specific low-back pain. *Cochrane Database Syst Rev.* 2004;(4):CD000261.

383. Dindo L, Van Liew JR, Arch JJ. Acceptance and commitment therapy: a transdiagnostic behavioral intervention for mental health and medical conditions. *Neurotherapeutics.* 2017;14(3):546–553.

384. Hughes LS, Clark J, Colclough JA, et al. Acceptance and commitment therapy (ACT) for chronic pain: a systematic review and meta-analyses. *Clin J Pain.* 2016;33(6):552–568.

385. Gatchel RJ, Turk DC. *Psychological Approaches to Pain Management: A Practitioner's Guide.* New York: The Guilford Press; 1996.

386. Knoerl R, Lavoie Smith EM, Weisberg J. Chronic pain and cognitive behavioral therapy: an integrative review. *West J Nurs Res.* 2016;38(5):596–628.

387. Brunner E, De Herdt A, Minguet P, et al. Can cognitive behavioural therapy based strategies be integrated into physiotherapy for the prevention of chronic low back pain? A systematic review. *Disabil Rehabil.* 2013;35(1):1–10.

388. Edmonston W, William E, Sanders SJ. Hypnosis and relaxation: modern verification of an old equation. *Am J Clin Hypn.* 1981;24(1):65–66.

389. Eimer BN. Clinical applications of hypnosis for brief and efficient pain management psychotherapy. *Am J Clin Hypn.* 2000;43(1):17–40.

390. Turner JA, Chapman CR. Psychological interventions for chronic pain: a critical review. II. Operant conditioning, hypnosis, and cognitive-behavioral therapy. *Pain.* 1982;12(1):23–46.

391. Du S, Hu L, Dong J, et al. Self-management program for chronic low back pain: a systematic review and meta-analysis. *Patient Educ Couns.* 2017;100(1):37–49.

392. Franek J. Self-management support interventions for persons with chronic disease: an evidence-based analysis. *Ont Health Technol Assess Ser.* 2013;13(9):1–60.

393. LeFort SM, Gray-Donald K, Rowat KM, et al. Randomized controlled trial of a community-based psychoeducation program for the self-management of chronic pain. *Pain.* 1998;74(2–3):297–306.

394. Lorig KR, Sobel DS, Stewart AL, et al. Evidence suggesting that a chronic disease self-management program can improve health status while reducing hospitalization: a randomized trial. *Med Care.* 1999;37(1):5–14.

395. Lorig K, Holman H, Sobel D, et al. *Living a Healthy Life with Chronic Conditions: Self-Management of Heart Disease, Arthritis, Diabetes, Depression, Asthma, Bronchitis, Emphysema & Other Physical & Mental Health Conditions.* 4th ed. Boulder, CO: Bull Publishing; 2012.

396. Khusid MA, Vythilingam M. The emerging role of mindfulness meditation as effective self-management strategy, Part 2: Clinical implications for chronic pain, substance misuse, and insomnia. *Mil Med.* 2016;181(9):969–975.

397. Tick H. Integrative pain medicine: a holistic model of care. *Pain Clin Updates.* 2014;22(2):1–6.

398. Barclay AW, Petocz P, McMillan-Price J, et al. Glycemic index, glycemic load, and chronic disease risk—a meta-analysis of observational studies. *Am J Clin Nutr.* 2008;87(3):627–637.

399. Mazokopakis EE, Starakis IK. Recommendations for diagnosis and management of metformin-induced vitamin B_{12} (Cbl) deficiency. *Diabetes Res Clin Pract.* 2012;97(3):359–367.

400. Ramsden CE, Mann JD, Faurot KR, et al. Low omega-6 vs. low omega-6 plus high omega-3 dietary intervention for chronic daily headache: protocol for a randomized clinical trial. *Trials.* 2011;12:97.

401. Criscuolo CM. Interventional approaches to the management of myofascial pain syndrome. *Curr Pain Headache Rep.* 2001;5(5):407–411.

402. Scott NA, Guo B, Barton PM, et al. Trigger point injections for chronic non-malignant musculoskeletal pain: a systematic review. *Pain Med.* 2009;10(1):54–69.

403. Botwin KP, Sharma K, Saliba R, et al. Ultrasound-guided trigger point injections in the cervicothoracic musculature: a new and unreported technique. *Pain Physician.* 2008;11(6):885–889.

404. Breivik H. Local anaesthetic blocks and epidurals. In: McMahon SB, Koltzenburg M, eds. *Wall and Melzack's Textbook of Pain.* 5th ed. Philadelphia, PA: Elsevier Churchill Livingstone; 2006:507–519.

405. Candido KD, Raghavendra MS, Chinthagada M, et al. A prospective evaluation of iodinated contrast flow patterns with fluoroscopically guided lumbar epidural steroid injections: the lateral parasagittal interlaminar epidural approach versus the transforaminal epidural approach. *Anesth Analg.* 2008;106(2):638–644.

406. Lee JH, Moon J, Lee SH. Comparison of effectiveness according to different approaches of epidural steroid injection in lumbosacral herniated disk and spinal stenosis. *J Back Musculoskelet Rehabil.* 2009;22(2):83–89.

407. Manchikanti L, Pakanati R, Pampati V. Comparison of three routes of epidural steroid injections in low back pain. *Pain Digest.* 1999;9:277–285.

408. Mehta P, Syrop I, Singh JR, et al. Systematic review of the efficacy of particulate versus nonparticulate corticosteroids in epidural injections. *PM R.* 2017;9(5):502–512.

409. Deer TR, Krames E, Mekhail N, et al. The appropriate use of neurostimulation: new and evolving neurostimulation therapies and applicable treatment for chronic pain and selected disease states. Neuromodulation Appropriateness Consensus Committee. *Neuromodulation.* 2014;17(6):599–615; discussion 615.

410. Deer TR, Mekhail N, Petersen E, et al. The appropriate use of neurostimulation: stimulation of the intracranial and extracranial space and head for chronic pain. Neuromodulation Appropriateness Consensus Committee. *Neuromodulation.* 2014;17(6):551–570; discussion 570.

411. Deer TR, Mekhail N, Provenzano D, et al. The appropriate use of neurostimulation of the spinal cord and peripheral nervous system for the treatment of chronic pain and ischemic diseases: the Neuromodulation Appropriateness Consensus Committee. *Neuromodulation.* 2014;17(6):515–550; discussion 550.

412. Deer TR, Mekhail N, Provenzano D, et al. The appropriate use of neurostimulation: avoidance and treatment of complications of neurostimulation therapies for the treatment of chronic pain. Neuromodulation Appropriateness Consensus Committee. *Neuromodulation.* 2014;17(6):571–597; discussion 597–598.

413. Moir L. Managing chronic neuropathic pain: the role of spinal cord stimulation. *Br J Community Nurs.* 2009;14(5):207–209.

414. Miller JP, Eldabe S, Buchser E, et al. Parameters of spinal cord stimulation and their role in electrical charge delivery: a review. *Neuromodulation.* 2016;19(4):373–384.

415. De Ridder D, Perera S, Vanneste S. Are 10 kHz stimulation and burst stimulation fundamentally the same? *Neuromodulation.* 2017;20(7):650–653.

416. Ubbink DT, Vermeulen H. Spinal cord stimulation for non-reconstructable chronic critical leg ischaemia. *Cochrane Database Syst Rev.* 2013;(2):CD004001.

417. Kumar K, Rizvi S. Cost-effectiveness of spinal cord stimulation therapy in management of chronic pain. *Pain Med.* 2013;14(11):1631–1649.

418. Eldabe S, Buchser E, Duarte RV. Complications of spinal cord stimulation and peripheral nerve stimulation techniques: a review of the literature. *Pain Med.* 2016;17(2):325–336.

CHAPTER 40

Amanda L. Harrington
Michael A. Kryger
Jessica B. Berry

Spasticity

Muscle spasticity is a common problem in patients with neurologic injury and can lead to drastic changes in function and quality of life (1,2). Fortunately, there are effective treatments available to reduce the impact of spasticity. An in-depth understanding of spasticity management can allow the provider to offer effective counseling and treatment to a patient. This requires knowledge of several different areas related to the motor system, including normal motor function, the pathophysiology of spasticity, as well as evaluation and treatment options.

The normal physiologic function of the motor system is governed by a complex system of inhibitory and excitatory control signals. When this communication system is compromised by a lesion proximal to anterior horn cells, such as in the spinal cord, brainstem, or brain, it may result in an upper motor neuron syndrome (UMNS). The UMNS is characterized by positive signs of spasticity, hypertonicity, exaggerated reflexes, clonus, and primitive reflexes (3). Patients often present with multiple positive signs simultaneously, which can build up clinical suspicion of a UMNS. For the purposes of this chapter, the term spasticity is used to describe the collective positive signs of the UMNS.

Spasticity is defined as a velocity-dependent increase in muscle tone (4) and will worsen with quick passive movements of the affected muscles. Severe cases may present as rigidity or contracture. An individual's function and health may be considerably compromised by spasticity. Depending on the pattern of spasticity, patients may present with gait dysfunction, hand or fine motor dysfunction, spontaneous muscle contractions, difficulty with hygiene, or pain. While treatment can be challenging, these potential consequences make spasticity an important problem to manage. The goal of treatment is to reduce problematic spasticity with the fewest side effects in order to improve function and reduce pain.

EPIDEMIOLOGY OF SPASTICITY

The reported incidence and prevalence of spasticity vary across studies and between different etiologic diagnoses. After spinal cord injury (SCI), spasticity has been reported to affect between 40% and 78% of persons (5–8) (see Chapter 21). Up to 85% of individuals with multiple sclerosis (MS) report spasticity (2,9)(see Chapter 20). Studies performed at varying time frames after stroke have reported 19% to 42% of persons develop spasticity between 3 and 12 months after the neurologic insult (10–12) (see Chapter 18). In a recent study of noncommunicative disorders of consciousness patients, up to 89% demonstrated signs of spasticity (13) (see Chapter 19 on Traumatic Brain Injury). Spasticity is also known to be common in children and adults with cerebral palsy. Clearly, spasticity can be a significant problem in people with neurologic disease.

NORMAL MOTOR FUNCTION

There are several components of the motor system pathway that allow for effective control of muscles (14). Cortical signals related to motor control are generated in the brain, primarily in the motor cortex and premotor planning areas, then travel to the internal capsule, decussate in the medullary pyramids, and descend down the corticospinal tracts of the spinal cord. These signals travel via upper motor neurons and synapse via interneurons with lower motor neurons in the spinal cord. α-motor neurons and γ-motor neurons are both types of lower motor neurons that originate in the ventral horn of the spinal cord. Signals from the α-motor neuron exit the spinal cord and continue through a peripheral nerve to the synapse at the neuromuscular junction, resulting in muscle contraction. Gamma motor neurons, on the other hand, project to intrafusal muscle fibers within muscle spindles (Fig. 40-1).

Simultaneously, multiple peripheral sensory signals are providing feedback to the spinal cord. These signals include not only traditional senses, such as light touch and pain, but also muscle velocity, muscle tension, and joint position. This information travels back up the spinal cord to the brain and also circles back as a reflex arc. To function effectively, the motor system must be able to integrate sensory feedback, control reflex activity, and coordinate volitional movement.

The Motor Unit

The motor unit refers to the collective system that comprises an α-motor neuron, its axon, and all of the muscle fibers that it innervates. Individual motor units can differ in recruitment patterns and firing rates, depending on each unit's demands and functions. When working properly, motor units fire with coordination of agonist and antagonist systems, in normal patterns of recruitment and decruitment (15). Coordination is accomplished using a sensory feedback loop that integrates muscle length, velocity, muscle tension, and joint position. This integration is mediated by a combination of immediate monosynaptic reflexes and more complex higher-level control involving spinal and supraspinal polysynaptic activity. The sum total of inhibitory versus excitatory signals results in coordinated muscle contraction and cocontraction.

Muscle Spindle and Golgi Tendon Organs

Muscle stretch receptors play a critical role in carrying sensory information regarding muscle length, tension, position, and velocity to the central nervous system (CNS). This afferent information relayed via reflexes allows for quick adjustments to motor activity and is carried to the CNS via various types of nerve fibers (14). Muscle spindles provide afferent information

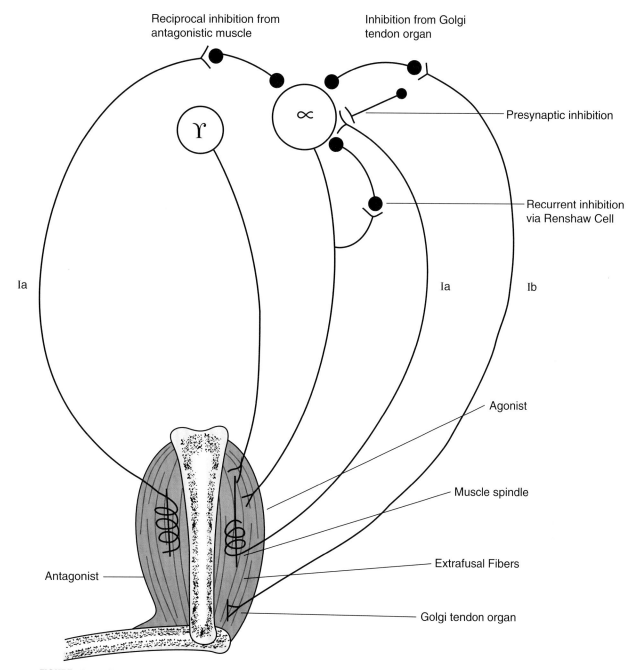

FIGURE 40-1. Normal reflex physiology combines supraspinal input with peripheral sensory signals from muscle spindles and Golgi tendon organs. Balancing excitatory and inhibitory sensory input via multiple mechanisms allows for controlled movement. (Copyright © 2010 Mukherjee and Chakravarty. In: Mukherjee A, Chakravarty A. Spasticity Mechanisms – for the Clinician. *Front Neurol.* 2010; 1:149.)

via group Ia and group II nerve fibers. Muscle spindles are innervated by γ-motor neurons, are composed of intrafusal fibers, and are attached in parallel to the extrafusal fibers of the muscle. Therefore, muscle spindles relay information related to muscle lengthening but are not activated by shortening. Golgi tendon organs are located in series with extrafusal muscle fibers and relay afferent information via group Ib nerve fibers. Golgi tendon organs are receptors for muscle tension and are activated by both lengthening and shortening of the muscle. Thus,

passive stretch of a muscle causes afferent firing from both the muscle spindle and the Golgi tendon organs, but active muscle contraction only activates Golgi tendon organs.

Spinal Interneurons

Spinal interneurons play a crucial role in motor control, providing an integration point for sensory and supraspinal inputs to influence motor neurons. There are a number of important pathways in which the complex interneuron system normally results in the net inhibition of reflexes at rest (3,14). Ia afferent fibers have excitatory connections to both the α-motor neurons from which they originate and to the α-motor neurons of synergistic muscles. At the same time, Ia afferent fibers have excitatory connections to inhibitory interneurons of antagonist muscles. Thus, the concept of *Ia reciprocal inhibition* refers to the innate inhibition of antagonist muscles when an agonist muscle is stretched. Facilitation of agonist activity while simultaneously inhibiting antagonist muscles prevents futile cocontraction. *Presynaptic Ia inhibition* results when inhibitory interneurons reduce Ia firing to the α-motor neurons from which they originate. At baseline, this helps to maintain inhibitory control over the monosynaptic reflex arc. *Ib nonreciprocal inhibition* describes Ib firing from Golgi tendon organs, which, via interneuron activation of α-motor neurons, results in inhibition of agonist muscles and facilitation of antagonist muscles. This negative feedback loop from the Golgi tendon organ serves to impose a ceiling effect on muscle contraction and prevent musculotendinous injury (16). The Renshaw cell is a specific type of inhibitory interneuron that can suppress both α- and γ-motor neurons via a negative feedback loop known as *recurrent inhibition*. Similar to other suppressive pathways, the Renshaw cell limits Ia reflexes to reduce agonist activity and facilitate antagonist function (17).

PATHOPHYSIOLOGY OF SPASTICITY

An in-depth discussion of all possible causes of spasticity is beyond the scope of this text. However, a brief mention of more common pathways is warranted. Although the exact pathology of spasticity is unknown, the loss of supraspinal influence on baseline interneuron inhibition is thought to exaggerate normal reflexes. Cocontraction of muscles and muscles firing out of phase may result in the loss of the normal recruitment and decruitment patterns and may play a key role in spasticity (18). At the level of the spinal interneurons, a number of pathways are thought to play a role in the development of spasticity, either independently or in combination (3,14). First, there is likely to be impairment in normal reciprocal inhibition; thus, when agonist muscle groups are activated, antagonists are not suppressed and cocontraction occurs. Second, a decrease in presynaptic Ia inhibition results in increased firing of α-motor neurons, resulting in increased excitability of α-motor neurons. Next, there is thought to be a reduction in Ib nonreciprocal inhibition from Golgi tendon organs, which results in the loss of the protective negative feedback loop. Finally, a counterintuitive increase in Renshaw cell inhibition may play a role in the development of spasticity by contributing to the reduction of reciprocal inhibition (3).

EVALUATION OF SPASTICITY

There are multiple methods a clinician can employ to assess spasticity. A focused physical exam utilizing range of motion (ROM) and reflex testing serves as the basis of the clinical evaluation. Many scales and assessment tools have been described, which may help to standardize exams among clinicians and allow for temporal comparison of the physical exam in clinical documentation. An important component of spasticity evaluation rests with patient or caregiver self-report of response to treatment and impact of spasticity on daily life. Several mechanical and electrophysiologic tools have also been described, which can more objectively measure spasticity.

Clinical Assessment Scales

A number of assessment scales are commonly used to evaluate spasticity in the clinical setting. While it is beyond the scope of this text to detail each instrument, several of the most widely used and novel assessment tools will be highlighted. The Ashworth Scale was first described in a 1964 study that evaluated medication effectiveness in MS (19). In utilizing the Ashworth Scale, the level of resistance of limb passive ROM is measured on an ordinal scale. The scale was later expanded as the Modified Ashworth Scale (MAS) **(Table 40-1)**, which is more commonly used in clinical practice (20). Despite being one of the most widely used scales, the MAS has not demonstrated good intra- or interrater reliability for spasticity assessment (21,22).

Because the reliability of the MAS has been questioned, a Modified Modified Ashworth Scale (MMAS) was developed, which eliminates the 1+ grade and adjusts the definition of grade 2 to attempt to create a more ordinal relationship (21). The updated grade 2 is described as a marked increase in tone with a catch in the middle of the ROM and resistance throughout the remainder of the movement. The MMAS has demonstrated possible improvements in interrater reliability compared to the MAS (23,24). Similarly, the Tardieu Scale and the Modified Tardieu Scale have demonstrated varying degrees of reliability to measure passive resistance to stretch at varying velocities on an ordinal scale (25–29). A number of multi-item scales have been created to combine facets of clinical exams into more useful qualitative date. Examples of multi-item scales include the Spinal Cord Assessment Tool for Spastic Reflexes (SCATS) for SCI (30) and the Triple Spasticity Scale (TSS) for use in persons with spasticity secondary to stroke (31). The SCATS, which is evaluated in the lower limb, grades severity of clonus, degree of flexor spasms after noxious stimuli, and degree of extensor spasm after movement from a flexed position. The TSS grades resistance at different speeds, duration of clonus, and dynamic muscle length, which is calculated via goniometer measurements.

Patient-Reported Assessment Scales

Although physicians should use their own examination to measure spasticity, often, a patient's subjective report is invaluable, particularly when assessing response to treatment. A number of self-reported scales have been created to further help to quantify spasticity. The Penn Spasm Frequency Scale grades the frequency of spasms over a 1-hour period in persons with

TABLE 40-1	Modified Ashworth Scale
0	No increase in tone
1	Slight increase in tone with a catch or minimal resistance at the end of the ROM
1+	Slight increase in tone with a catch followed by minimal resistance through the remainder of the ROM
2	Moderate increase in tone through most of the ROM but limb easily moved
3	Considerable increase in tone with passive movement difficult
4	Limb rigid or contracted

ROM, range of motion.
Adapted from Bohannon RW, Smith MB. Interrater reliability of a Modified Ashworth Scale of muscle spasticity. *Phys Ther.* 1987;67(2):206–207.

spasticity of spinal origin (32), whereas its modified version, the Modified Penn Spasm Frequency Scale, ranks spasticity based on severity (33). The Patient-Reported Impact of Spasticity Measure (PRISM) evaluates both positive and negative effects of spasticity on various life experiences over a 7-day period (34). A similar scale, the Spinal Cord Injury Spasticity Evaluation Tool (SCI-SET), is specific for persons with SCI (35). A self-reported scale of spasticity has also been developed for patients with stroke (36). In general, the use of a combination of assessment measures is thought to be most appropriate in clinical evaluations.

Quantitative Assessments

Mechanical assessments are most often utilized in research settings in order to obtain objective measures of the resistance to joint passive ROM. One of the more basic techniques was first described by Wartenberg in the 1950s, in which the time and quality of leg pendulum swing were measured in a seated position (37). The classic pendulum assessment has been enhanced over time to include measurements of resistive torque of the joint, tachometer measurements of joint velocity, and electrogoniometer recordings of joint angles (38–40). In more recent years, devices such as the NeuroFlexor and the Electric Spastic Ankle Measure (E-SAM) have been created to provide quantification of spasticity components in both arm (41,42) and leg tone (43). EMG response can be recorded during limb ROM at varying velocities (44,45). H-reflex, H/M ratios, and F-wave amplitudes have also been measured as means to quantify response to spasticity treatment (46). Although mechanical and EMG measures of spasticity may provide accurate data, use in clinical practice is limited by the need for equipment, specialized training, and time (47).

MANAGEMENT OF SPASTICITY AND THE UMNS

Not all persons with spasticity require treatment. Those with minimal spasticity may not want treatment due to side effect risks. Some people use spasticity to their advantage, as it can occasionally help with activities of daily living, transfers, standing, or ambulation (6,34,48). The decision to treat spasticity should be made by weighing possible adverse effects against potential benefits.

Treatment of spasticity can be divided into two core goals: managing passive function and improving functional activities (49). Improving passive function may help to reduce pain, improve positioning and hygiene, facilitate splint wearing, and prevent contracture. Common functional activities that are targeted by spasticity treatment include transfers, ambulation, and activities of daily living. To accomplish treatment goals, several interventions are frequently utilized, often in combination (**Table 40-2**). Selection of management techniques is made based on potential benefits as well as possible disadvantages.

There are several aspects to consider when identifying treatments. One important consideration is the timing of intervention in relation to the neurologic insult. As a general rule, spasticity interventions and medications that may impair recovery should be used later in the course of an event. For example, low-functioning patients with traumatic brain injury (TBI) are less likely to be prescribed sedating antispasticity agents. Similarly, phenol neurolysis is rarely used early in recovery, as the scarring of muscle and nerve and long duration of action may be undesirable in a recovering patient. Orthopedic interventions are almost never offered early on, as there needs to be stabilization of the neuromuscular structures before permanent surgical intervention. Although intrathecal baclofen (ITB) pumps were traditionally selected for treatment after spasticity had stabilized, earlier placement has become more common in severe spasticity (50).

The overall medical condition of the patient and their location of spasticity must be considered. Patients with hypotension, syncope, balance disturbances, or ataxia may be unable to tolerate the side effect profile of certain agents. If there are focal areas of spasticity, then chemodenervation may be considered, whereas if the target condition is more systemic, more global treatment will be necessary.

Cost may also be a consideration during treatment selection. ITB and botulinum toxin injections are quite expensive. Paying out of pocket for some modalities is not realistic, and the physician, patient, and family have to utilize third-party payers to make treatment affordable. Some insurance companies require trials with less expensive agents such as oral

TABLE 40-2	Comparisons of Different Treatment Modalities for Spasticity		
Spasticity Treatment	**Indications**	**Advantages**	**Disadvantages**
Therapeutic modalities	Used by therapist for early management and facilitation of chemodenervation	Minimal side effects	Short duration of effect
Oral medications	Generalized tone, spasms	Systemic administration. Can treat large area of spasticity	Systemic side effects such as sedation, metabolic load
Botulinum toxins	Focal area of spasticity	Can treat spastic area without systemic side effects	Expensive, requires repeat injections to maintain effectiveness
Phenol	Focal area of spasticity	Can treat spastic area without systemic side effects. Much cheaper than botulinum toxins and longer duration	Requires considerable skill of injector, risk of dysesthesias, painful procedure
Orthopedic procedure	Potential improvement in passive or active ADLs	Long-term repair	Surgical risk, loss of motor strength
Intrathecal baclofen	Significant tone not adequately treated by other modalities	Minimal systemic side effects	Surgical risk, pump requires replacement at end of battery life, requires office visits for refills

antispasticity medications before approving toxin injections. Clinicians are often required to justify their decisions and recommendations in order to gain approval.

Providers should consider each individual patient when making management decisions. Disease etiology, medical comorbidities, type of spasticity, and cost will all factor into the treatment plan. To maximize quality of life improvements for patients undergoing spasticity management, the entire treatment team must monitor the efficacy and adverse effects of spasticity interventions and adjust treatment accordingly.

Nonpharmacologic Treatment Options

Reduction of Noxious Stimulation

The first step in any program to manage spasticity is the reduction of noxious stimulation, which has been shown to increase spasticity (51). The term *noxious stimulation* encompasses a wide variety of conditions. More common causes include pressure ulcers, ingrown toenails, contractures, kinked catheters, urolithiasis, urinary tract infections, deep venous thrombosis (DVT), heterotopic ossification, fecal impaction, sepsis, and fractures. Addressing these conditions should generally be the first approach in spasticity management.

Positioning

Proper positioning is an important component of spasticity management. Poor positioning can result in an increase in spasticity, a decreased ROM, contractures, noxious stimulation, pain, and exacerbation of a vicious cycle that can lead to worsening spasticity (52). Postures that should be avoided include a leg scissoring posture (bilateral hip extension, adduction, and internal rotation), windswept position (hip flexion, abduction, and external rotation on one side and relative hip extension, adduction, and internal rotation on the other), and frog-leg position (bilateral hip external rotation). Positioning is also important in the wheelchair. Tone can be minimized by placing the patient with the hips and knees at 90 degrees and by using adequate seating support to maintain neutral upright torso position (52).

Stretch and Casting

Immobilization of paralyzed muscles in shortened positions results in a decrease in longitudinal tension (muscle unloading) and can predispose to contracture. Stretching is a focal treatment that can prevent muscle shortening (53). Schmit et al. have demonstrated the benefit of a relatively brief stretch in the management of spasticity (54). However, the benefit is short-lived, as the tone returns after a single contraction (55). Therefore, stretch needs to be applied for a longer period of time to have potential functional benefit. Stretch has been shown to be useful in volitional movement in both agonist (56) and antagonist muscles (57).

Chronic stretch via casting or splints changes reflexive activity and reduces the stretch reflex (58–60). Splints and orthotics are often utilized to facilitate prolonged stretch, particularly overnight. Serial casting is defined as the use of successive casts to treat increased tone and contractures. It is not definitively known how often to change serial casts; however, when casts are changed more frequently (every 1 to 4 days), there are fewer complications compared to longer intervals of cast changes (5 to 7 days) (61). Using casting to facilitate the

action of chemical denervation has been shown to increase the treatment effect in the stroke (62) and cerebral palsy populations (63).

Physical Modalities

Physical modalities can play a role in the management of spasticity. Like stretching, they have the benefit of being benign interventions with localized treatment benefits. Cooling of muscles is beneficial in the management of spasticity (64,65). It both inhibits the monosynaptic stretch reflexes and lowers receptor sensitivity after it is removed (66,67). Cooling can be used in different ways. The quick icing technique, with ice applied with a light striking movement, results in facilitation of α- and γ-motor neurons and is used to facilitate antagonist function (68). Another method of cooling delivery includes the use of an evaporating spray, such as ethyl chloride (69). Because of their short duration of action, the cooling modalities may have their greatest utility by therapists to reduce muscle overactivity to allow other therapeutic interventions.

Heat is another modality that can be applied in various forms, including ultrasound, paraffin, fluidotherapy, superficial heat, and whirlpool. Heat has a short duration of action (70), and like cold, its application should be followed immediately by stretching and exercise. The major effect of heat on spasticity appears to be related to an increase in elasticity that may assist in stretching activities (71).

Electrical Stimulation

Electrical stimulation is another modality that may be an adjunct to spasticity management. Transcutaneous electrical nerve stimulation (TENS) units reduce pain via a nociceptive action that may also reduce spasticity by decreasing the flexor reflex afferents that are facilitated by nociceptive stimulation (72). Improved outcomes have been noted when TENS is used in combination with active therapy for the management of limb spasticity (73). Although electrical stimulation devices are predominantly used to facilitate motor recovery secondary to CNS pathology, they may also result in reduction of spasticity. A number of studies have demonstrated improvements in spasticity after functional electrical stimulation in patients with stroke (74–77), SCI (78–80), and MS (81).

Other Nonpharmacologic Treatments

Although less traditional, a number of other interventions have been investigated as tools to manage spasticity. Whole-body vibration (WBV), which is a modality often utilized by elite athletes, has been shown to reduce lower limb spasticity in adults and children with cerebral palsy (82,83). WBV as well as focal vibration may also reduce spasticity for short periods of time in persons with SCI (84) and may be beneficial in treating poststroke spasticity (85,86). Traditional Chinese acupuncture has been trialed in multiple studies as an intervention to reduce spasticity. Although results of acupuncture studies are varied and many studies are of poor quality, some suggest effectiveness in treating spasticity after stroke and brain injury (87–90). In a number of studies, transcranial magnetic stimulation and repetitive magnetic stimulation have been used to reduce limb spasticity in persons with stroke, SCI, and MS (91–94). More recently, extracorporeal shock wave therapy has been utilized with beneficial results in persons with both stroke and cerebral palsy (95–97).

Pharmacologic Treatments

Oral and Transdermal Medications

Oral and transdermal medications are commonly used in the treatment of spasticity. **Table 40-3** summarizes the usage of these medications. Considering the pathology of spasticity is thought to be a loss of baseline inhibition of the spinal reflex interneuron system; most oral medications work by up-regulating inhibitory neurotransmitters or by activating their receptors.

Benzodiazepines

The benzodiazepines were the first agents used in the management of spasticity. Of this class, diazepam is most commonly used. Their mechanism of action is central in origin, acting on the brainstem reticular formation and spinal polysynaptic pathways (98). They demonstrate their effect via GABA$_A$ (γ-aminobutyric acid), which opens membrane Cl$^-$ channels with resultant hyperpolarization. The net effect is a reduction of monosynaptic and polysynaptic reflexes and an increase in presynaptic inhibition (99).

Diazepam is generally dosed from 2 to 10 mg, three or four times daily (100). Benzodiazepines are well absorbed after enteral administration and peak at 1 hour. There is a relatively long half-life for benzodiazepines when accounting for their active metabolites, which ranges between 20 and 80 hours. The side effect profile can be quite problematic, including issues with addiction and withdrawal, ataxia, weakness, cognitive impairment, hypotension, respiratory depression, poor coordination, fatigue, and CNS depression that can be potentiated by alcohol. Research with diazepam has demonstrated improvements in painful spasms, hyperreflexia, and passive ROM. Evidence concerning functional improvement is limited.

The greatest benefit for diazepam has been demonstrated in persons with SCI (101) and MS (102–104). Benzodiazepines are rarely used in the acquired brain injury (ABI) population because of their potential for cognitive side effects as well as their potential to compromise motor recovery (105).

Baclofen

Baclofen also mediates its activity through the GABA system, acting as a GABA$_B$ receptor agonist, which inhibits both monosynaptic and polysynaptic reflexes. It is FDA approved for management of spasticity in cerebral palsy, SCI, and MS (100). Baclofen is eliminated via the kidney, and its half-life is roughly 5 hours (100). When initiating treatment, 5 mg twice or three times daily is recommended, and this can be increased by 5 to 10 mg/d each week. The suggested maximum dose per day is 80 mg, but while not routinely recommended, doses as high as 300 mg/d have been used safely (99). Possible side effects of baclofen include sedation, hypotension, fatigue, weakness, nausea, dizziness, paresthesias, hallucinations, and a lowering of the seizure threshold. The patient is at greatest risk when the agent is abruptly discontinued, as hallucinations and withdrawal seizures have been reported (106). Since baclofen primarily undergoes renal clearance, dosing may need to be adjusted with renal impairment (107).

Baclofen is effective in reducing systemic spasticity and painful flexor spasms in both persons with SCI and MS (107–116). It is generally avoided in ABI and stroke due to sedation (117); however, positive effects have been noted (114,118,119).

Dantrolene Sodium

Unlike many other agents, dantrolene acts peripherally, at the level of the muscle itself. Its mechanism of action is to inhibit calcium release from the sarcoplasmic reticulum during muscle contraction. Rather than dampening neuronal activation, it reduces the strength of contraction. In addition to its action on the muscle extrafusal fibers, dantrolene reduces muscle spindles' sensitivity by acting on the γ-motor neuron (120). Starting dose is 25 mg by mouth once or twice daily and can be increased weekly by 25 to 50 mg to a maximum of 400 mg/d (100,121). The most well-known side effect of dantrolene is potential liver toxicity. However, overall, this is a rare occurrence, with a rate of only 1.8% (122) when administered for more than 60 days. Even when discovered, it is usually reversible. It is found most commonly in women over the age of 40, especially if they have been on doses greater than 300 mg/d for a long period of time (123). Fatal liver failure has been reported in 0.3% of those who received the medication. Therefore, it is critical for clinicians to follow liver function tests (LFT) when prescribing dantrolene. In addition to liver toxicity, other more common side effects of dantrolene include weakness, flushing, paresthesias, nausea, and diarrhea (99,100).

Although dantrolene can be effective in controlling spasticity and improving ROM after SCI and MS (124,125), it

TABLE 40-3	Commonly Used Oral Medications		
Medication	**Common Dosing**	**Mechanism of Action**	**Comments**
Baclofen	5–40 mg q6-8h	GABA$_B$ agonist. Presynaptic inhibition of GABA$_B$ receptors	Risk of withdrawal seizures and hallucinations. Dose must be adjusted with renal disease. Sedating
Diazepam	2–10 mg q6-8h	Facilitates postsynaptic effects of GABA$_A$ by opening chloride channels in membranes resulting in increased presynaptic inhibition	Can have very long half-life. Sedating
Dantrolene	25–100 mg q6-12h	Interferes with calcium release from sarcoplasmic reticulum	Only truly peripherally acting oral agent. LFTs must be watched carefully
Clonidine	0.05–0.3 mg PO q12h or 1–6 patch/wk	α_2-Agonist. Decreases tonic facilitation via locus coeruleus and in spinal cord enhances presynaptic inhibition	Primary use in SCI population. Theoretical limitation to use in ABI secondary to interference with recovery
Tizanidine	2–8 mg q6-8h	α_2-Agonist. Blocks release of excitatory neurotransmitters and facilitates inhibitory neurotransmitters	Slow titration reduces sedation side effect that is a major limiting factor

is associated with greater weakness (126–128). Because dantrolene does not cause significant sedation, it is often the agent of choice after ABI (106). After stroke, dantrolene has been noted to improve ROM, deep tendon reflexes, and upper limb function (129).

Clonidine

Clonidine is an imidazoline derivative that is primarily used as an antihypertensive agent. It is a central acting α_2-adrenergic agonist that has been shown to demonstrate some efficacy in spasticity management, primarily in SCI. It peaks in 3 to 5 hours when taken orally and has a usual half-life of 5 to 19 hours or up to 40 hours in persons with renal impairment. Clonidine's clearance is primarily renal, with half of it first metabolized by the liver. Clonidine has two distinct mechanisms of action. First, it acts directly on the locus coeruleus and decreases tonic facilitation (99). Second, it also has a spinal mechanism, acting to enhance α_2-mediated presynaptic inhibition (130–132). Clonidine doses as low as 0.1 mg orally are often effective in treating spasticity (131). A transdermal system that allows for more uniform blood levels and easier administration is also available. Side effects reported with clonidine include bradycardia, depression, lethargy, syncope, and hypotension (131,133). Although clonidine has been shown to be effective in treating spasticity after SCI (134,135), blood pressure effects may limit use (130). Clonidine can impair motor recovery after ABI (105), thus making its use in these patients somewhat controversial.

Tizanidine

Like clonidine, tizanidine is an imidazoline derivative with α_2-agonist effects and is a widely used antispasticity agent. Tizanidine increases presynaptic inhibition of γ-motor neurons and decreases excitatory amino acids (100). Its onset is rapid, and it has a very short 2.5-hour half-life, which may require frequent dosing. It is cleared via liver metabolism and then is excreted by the kidneys.

The side effects of tizanidine can be quite troubling, with close to 15% of clinical trial participants discontinuing the medication due to side effects (136). Drowsiness has been reported in up to 50% of patients (136–138). Other major side effects are dry mouth, fatigue, dizziness, hypotension, muscle weakness, nausea, and vomiting (136–139). There is also a potential for liver damage, and LFT should be evaluated periodically. Initial dosing begins at 2 to 4 mg before bedtime and can be increased to a maximum of 36 mg/d (99).

Tizanidine has been well studied in patients with SCI (140,141) and has demonstrated a significant reduction in spasticity and an early reduction in spasm frequency. Several studies have demonstrated the efficacy of tizanidine in patients with MS, demonstrating an improvement in clonus, spasms, and deep tendon reflexes (136,138,142–144). In those with ABI, significant decreases in their upper and lower extremity Ashworth scores and lower extremity spasm scores have been seen with the use of tizanidine. Additional benefits, including reduction of clonus and walking distance on flat ground, have also been described (137). While it can be effective for spasticity treatment, a concern that needs to be highlighted is that tizanidine, like clonidine, is a member of the imidazoline family. Therefore, it also has the potential to impair neurologic recovery after ABI (105).

Cannabinoids

While cannabinoids have traditionally been used recreationally for psychological relaxation, there is developing evidence that they may provide relief of spasticity in persons with MS or SCI. As the legalization of cannabinoids in certain parts of the United States has made medical use more common, more patients are likely to request treatment in the future. Pharmacokinetics vary based on route of administration. Smoked cannabis has been found to reduce both pain and spasticity in persons with MS (145). In Europe, a tetrahydrocannabinol (THC)/cannabidiol (CBD) oromucosal spray under the trade name Sativex has been used to treat spasticity in treatment-resistant MS (146). The mechanism of action is thought to be twofold: reduction of both intracortical and spinal excitability by acting as a partial cannabinoid receptor agonist, which can modulate the effects of both excitatory and inhibitory neurotransmitters (147). Thus far, the treatment has demonstrated symptomatic relief of spasticity with fairly good tolerability. There appears to be no effect on mood or cognition, suggesting side effects of recreational cannabis use may be avoided using THC/CBD oromucosal spray (148). The long-term adverse effects of cannabinoids are not well studied.

Chemical Denervation

Clinical Considerations

Chemical deinnervation is a procedure by which localized injections are used to decrease neural signal transmission through the neuromuscular junction or peripheral nerve. While ethanol and phenol have historically been common injectable agents, the advent of purified botulinum toxin proteins has resulted in a significant change in practice over the past 30 years. Botulinum toxin injections have become a standard of care for many patients with spasticity (149,150). The use of chemical deinnervation injections is best suited for those with localized spasticity in which a specific goal can be identified that would be achievable by reducing tone in the focal muscle group. For example, if a patient's tight hip adductors are limiting access to perform perineal hygiene, localized injections to the hip adductors may make hygiene more easily accomplishable. However, should a patient have global spasticity in all limbs, the use of injections as a primary means of management becomes impractical.

Prior to initiation of injections, it is best to identify specific goals of treatment. In addition to outlining functional goals for injections, it is important to remind patients that injections do not restore strength and may make the muscle slightly weaker. Given the temporary response to injections, patients should be aware that repeated injections are usually necessary. While there is variable evidence on the impact of rehabilitation in combination with botulinum toxin treatment, initiation of a rehabilitation program to achieve functional or passive goals may be recommended when the toxin reaches peak effect (151). Therefore, it is important that the patient can comply with such a program. Botulinum toxins may be avoided as a first-line treatment due to the high cost of the medication, as insurance companies in the United States may require that a patient try and fail other antispasticity medications first, even if the spasticity is localized. However, given the minimal systemic side effects of botulinum toxins when appropriately administered, these medications may still be preferable to oral agents.

Botulinum Toxin

Mechanism of Action. Botulinum toxin acts primarily at the neuromuscular junction. The toxin protein, which consists of a heavy chain and light chain, effects the presynaptic nerve terminal. In normal physiology, synaptic vesicles filled with acetylcholine (ACh) molecules attach to soluble NSF attachment protein receptors (SNARE) proteins, enabling exocytosis of the vesicle and release of ACh into the neuromuscular junction. However, once botulinum toxin enters the presynaptic nerve terminal, the light chain detaches and cleaves a portion of the SNARE proteins, thus preventing the release of ACh (**Fig. 40-2**). Without a substantial release of ACh, the neuromuscular junction will not cause as significant of a muscle contraction, thereby reducing spasticity in the target muscle.

Interestingly, it has been found that botulinum toxin may also act more proximally in the motor unit and CNS to reduce spasticity via retrograde axonal transport of the toxin proteins.

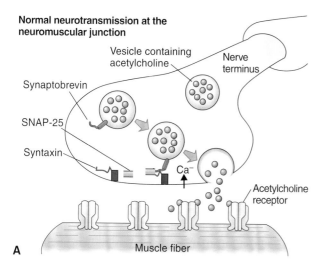

Normal neurotransmission at the neuromuscular junction

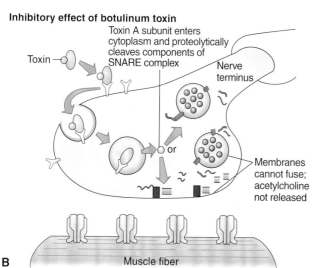

Inhibitory effect of botulinum toxin

FIGURE 40-2. **A:** Normal neuromuscular junction transmission. Fusion of ACh vesicles with the cell membrane with release of ACh into the neuromuscular junction. **B:** Mechanism of action of botulinum toxins. Cleavage of the SNARE complex prevents fusion of ACh vesicles with the cell membrane. (Reprinted from Engleberg NC, Dermody T, DiRita V. *Schaechter's Mechanisms of Microbial Disease.* 5th ed. Baltimore, MD: Lippincott Williams & Wilkins; 2012, with permission.)

Studies have shown that injection of botulinum toxin can result in depression of recurrent inhibition (152). It was theorized that the toxin blocks ACh releases between Renshaw cells and motor neuron recurrent collaterals. In stroke patients, the use of botulinum toxin causes changes in cortical excitability in the unaffected hemisphere, suggesting that maladaptive cortical reorganization may also contribute to spasticity and may improve with peripheral botulinum toxin injection (153).

Immunogenicity of Botulinum Toxins. When commercial botulinum toxins were first released, it was found that in some patients, injections that had previously produced positive results later lost efficacy. This subset of patients became known as "secondary nonresponders." Studies demonstrate that antibodies to the toxins can develop, and this immunogenicity has been theorized to be a cause of secondary nonresponse to botulinum toxins. In a study examining over 500 secondary nonresponders between 1995 and 2000, 44.5% of secondary nonresponders were positive for toxin antibodies (154). Since the early 2000s, the makers of the various toxins have begun manufacturing much more pure forms of the toxins with fewer superfluous proteins. As a result, the incidence of secondary nonresponse has become increasingly uncommon (154–156). However, due to past experience, it is still recommended to minimize the chances of developing immunogenicity by using the smallest effective dose and to wait at least 3 months between injections (157).

Types of Botulinum Toxin. There are several different serotypes of botulinum toxins, lettered A through G. Each subtype has a different target in the SNARE protein complex, all resulting in decreased synaptic vesicle exocytosis. Only two subtypes of toxin are currently used in clinical practice: A and B.

Botulinum toxin A targets the synaptosomal-associated protein (SNAP)-25 on the SNARE complex. There are currently three A-toxins that are used in clinical practice: onabotulinumtoxinA (trade name BOTOX), abobotulinumtoxinA (trade name Dysport), and incobotulinumtoxinA (trade name Xeomin). All formulations have been found to be effective for use in focal upper and lower limb spasticity and have FDA indications for upper extremity spasticity and cervical dystonia (158–160). In addition, onabotulinumtoxinA has been approved for treatment of lower limb spasticity and bladder spasticity (158). AbobotulinumtoxinA is also approved for pediatric lower limb spasticity (159). The choice of one formulation over the other may depend on insurance and physician preference. However, should a patient be primarily or secondarily nonresponsive to one formulation, a second agent may be trialed.

Each formulation has different ranges of dosages, and there is no equivalence conversion between the various units. OnabotulinumtoxinA should not exceed 400 to 600 units based on safety data, though higher cumulative doses have been observed (157,158). Maximum recommended abobotulinumtoxinA dosage is 1,000 units (159), and incobotulinumtoxinA should not exceed 400 units (160). All of these formulations do not recommend injecting more frequently than every 12 weeks.

Botulinum toxin B targets the vesicle-associated membrane protein, or synaptobrevin portion of the SNARE protein complex. There is one clinically used toxin in this class: rimabotulinumtoxinB (trade name Myobloc in the United States and

NeuroBloc in Europe). This formulation is only approved for use in cervical dystonia. Doses in a single session range from 2,500 to 10,000 units (161). Immunogenicity has been found to be much higher with rimabotulinumtoxinB (162,163).

Side Effects. Side effects associated with botulinum toxin injections often depend on the site of injection. Local injection-related side effects, which are often transient, may include bleeding, erythema, and pain (164). Transient weakness has also been reported (165). At higher doses, limb edema and more prolonged weakness have been reported (166,167). There is a small risk of infection, which can be mitigated with aseptic technique. There is a concern for remote spread of the toxin particularly when used for cervical dystonia. This may result in dysphagia or symptoms similar to upper respiratory infections (168). The most common systemic effects tend to be headache, flulike symptoms, fatigue, and nausea and are benign with no long-term sequelae (169). There are also case reports of iatrogenic botulism resulting in respiratory depression, dysphagia, generalized weakness, dysarthria, ptosis, and dry mouth (170–174).

Injection Guidance. Once the target spastic muscle groups have been selected via history and physical exam, one must ensure accurate localization of these muscles for toxin injection. Comparison of needle guidance techniques has been investigated in several studies in order to better establish a standard of care for this procedure. Using anatomic localization or palpation alone has been found to be inferior to using other guidance techniques. In one study comparing anatomic localization to muscle stimulation, experienced injectors missed the gastrocnemius-soleus complex 22% of the time and the biceps brachii 38% of the time when using anatomy alone (175). Success rates decline even more in smaller muscle groups such as forearm muscles (176). While anatomical localization may be helpful for initial needle placement, ultimately further guidance can result in more accurate delivery of toxin.

Neurophysiologic data are often used for additional needle guidance, in the form of electromyography (EMG) or muscle stimulation. Using a monopolar needle electrode with a bore for toxin delivery, EMG may be used to identify areas of nonvolitional motor unit action potentials (MUAPs) suggestive of spasticity, isolate motor endplates that theoretically should be the target of injection (177), and detect which MUAPs activate with volitional movement of the target muscle. A muscle stimulator may also be used for guidance as it will cause repeated contractions of the target muscle once it is isolated. Both neurophysiologic approaches will provide similar localization for toxin injection (178); however, due to increased discomfort, these methods are not always used (149).

Ultrasound guidance for toxin injection allows for visualization of the target muscle and direct observation of the toxin entering the muscle. This visualization also allows one to avoid nerves or blood vessels that are often close in proximity to a target muscle (179). Spasticity may eventually lead to changes in the muscle architecture that could impact toxin effectiveness (180); thus, ultrasound can allow the injector to avoid areas of the muscle with high echogenicity suggestive of fibrosis (181). Given that ultrasound offers real-time, direct visualization of the needle and tissue, it may become a more commonly used method for botulinum toxin guidance, although comparisons between techniques have not shown conclusively improved clinical measures of spasticity (182). Additional training and cost of ultrasound machines may be barriers for clinical use in many settings.

Phenol and Ethanol

Phenol and ethanol injections have been used for over a century for the treatment of focal spasticity (183,184). Several methods have been proposed for injecting these agents for the purpose of reducing spasticity, including intramuscularly, intraspinally, and perineurally (185). Both are nonselective agents that effectively destroy tissue via protein denaturing. While helpful when injected intramuscularly, the resulting tissue necrosis can cause muscle weakness, particularly with ethanol. As a result, perineural phenol is a preferred method of injection as it appears to reduce spasticity without significant loss of muscle strength. Additionally, perineural phenol has been shown to have a more complete and longer-lasting effect than ethanol (150). Perineural phenol achieves peripheral nerve blockade via demyelination and axonal degeneration (186). Because phenol can damage both motor and sensory fibers, dysesthesias are common side effects of these injections (150,185,186). Common targets for perineural injection include the musculocutaneous nerve to treat elbow flexor spasticity, the obturator nerve for hip adductor spasticity, the sciatic nerve for hamstring spasticity, and the tibial nerve for plantar flexion spasticity.

Given the minimal side effect profile of botulinum toxins, the use of phenol and ethanol has fallen out of favor in recent years (150). However, phenol may be appropriate in certain clinical situations and recalcitrant cases. Advantages to phenol include the ability to target several muscles by injection around a single peripheral nerve, generally longer effect than botulinum toxin (185), and lower cost. Given that a peripheral nerve is a much smaller target than a muscle, injections require skill and patience. Traditionally, electrical stimulation has been used to confirm proximity to the nerve; however, stimulation in combination with ultrasound may allow for visualization of perineural delivery of the phenol.

Intrathecal Medications

Intrathecal Baclofen

ITB can be a safe and effective treatment of spasticity. ITB was initially demonstrated by Penn et al. (32) to have clear benefits versus placebo in severe spasticity in patients with MS and SCI and was later demonstrated to have efficacy for spasticity related to cerebral palsy (187), TBI (188), anoxia (189), and stroke (190–194). ITB therapy for the management of severe spasticity of cerebral origin was approved by the U.S. FDA in 1996.

The ITB system delivers a continuous supply of baclofen through a catheter that terminates in the subarachnoid space. This allows for placement of medication in close proximity to the targeted $GABA_B$ receptors, resulting in reduction in spasticity at doses substantially lower than required via oral administration (195–197). Clinically efficacious intrathecal doses have been reported at approximately 1% of doses needed for oral administration (198). Given this lower dose of medication, the CNS side effects of baclofen are greatly reduced with intrathecal delivery; thus, ITB can be an effective option for those who see some improvement in spasticity with oral antispasticity agents but are unable to tolerate increases in dosage due to side effects (199,200). In addition to a reduction in side effects, patients often benefit from improved control of spasticity, with decreased frequency and severity of spasms (201).

Although these benefits make ITB a good therapeutic choice, consideration should be given to the requirements of an ITB system and potential adverse effects. Placement of an ITB device requires a commitment to a surgical procedure, strict compliance for follow-up visits for reservoir refills, attention to pump alarms, and replacement of the device every 7 years. Adverse effects are rare but can be serious, including infection (202), CSF leak (203), pump dysfunction, and kinking or disconnection of catheter tubing resulting in baclofen overdose or withdrawal and associated seizures (204–207). Some studies reveal concern for rapid progression of scoliosis with long-term use (208–210), potentially increased risk of seizures (211,212), and variable effects on respiratory function and aspiration risk (213–216).

Clinically, patient selection for ITB therapy involves the assessment of the severity of spasticity, response and tolerance to less invasive methods of spasticity management, and factors affecting patient compliance. The severity of spasticity may include objective measures by the clinician as well as subjective input from the patient regarding the effect of spasticity on pain, function, and quality of life (217). Historically, ITB therapy was considered for patients after failure of multiple conservative therapies and/or only after a defined time period from upper motor neuron injury. However, further studies have challenged these ideas, demonstrating potential benefits of intrathecal therapy earlier after injury (50,218,219) and in conjunction with, rather than after failure of, conservative measures (217). Factors that may preclude use of ITB therapy for a patient include history of noncompliance, lack of family/caregiver support, financial burden or geographic challenges impeding access to care, history of hypersensitivity or allergy to baclofen, or active infection.

Potential candidates for ITB undergo screening for tolerance and efficacy with a trial of ITB. A trial is most commonly performed using a lumbar puncture to deliver an intrathecal bolus of 50 µg of baclofen. Spasticity is evaluated at baseline and following the bolus; if there is substantial improvement in spasticity, the screen is considered successful. If improvement is not demonstrated, the bolus is repeated with an escalation of dose, up to a maximum bolus of 100 µg. If any of the trials proves successful, the patient is offered the ITB system, with a starting dose typically set at twice the effective bolus dose per 24 hours.

A trial of continuous infusion with an external pump connected to an intrathecal catheter may also be used. This trial method may be useful for patients with additional considerations beyond reduction in spasticity, such as effect of treatment on ambulatory function. Continuous infusion allows for assessment of the patient's ambulation while on ITB and possibly for closer titration of starting dose for pump placement. Studies on the use of continuous infusion ITB trials have also reported associated adverse effects (220), including CSF leak and chemical meningitis, though are generally positive regarding the procedure's overall safety and efficacy (221).

Implanted pumps are programmable to deliver ITB at a constant or variable rate, with options for periodic bolus delivery or change in the rate of delivery at certain times. The options for dosing and delivery of ITB allow treatment to be individualized for each patient (193,222,223). Continuous dosing minimizes high peak and low trough medication levels. Use of periodic bolus delivery or rate changes may accommodate patients who experience variation in spasticity through the day or desire different levels of spasticity control for functional activities such as ADLs (222,224,225). Use of periodic bolus dosing has also been suggested to enhance ITB effects on upper limb spasticity or to enhance distribution of the drug in the CSF (193,222,225–227), though there remains a lack of clear guidance in the literature regarding choice of dosing method.

The level of catheter placement may also affect the distribution of baclofen in the CSF and influence upper limb spasticity. While originally the most cephalad placement of the catheter was between the levels of T8 and T10 (228), higher placement has been shown to be safe and effective for treating spasticity in both the upper and lower limbs (188,229–232).

Other Intrathecal Medications

Pharmacologic agents other than baclofen have been administered intrathecally for spasticity management, either alone or in combination with baclofen. These agents include morphine, clonidine, midazolam, lidocaine, and fentanyl (233–237).

Intrathecal Morphine. Morphine has also been used intrathecally in the management of spasticity, with reduction in tone noted with boluses of 1 to 2 mg (238) and doses of 2 to 4 mg administered daily in the treatment of SCI-induced spasticity (239). Intrathecal morphine has been used successfully in combination with ITB to control spasticity and pain in patients with MS (240) and in patients with SCI (241). Case report evidence also supports using intrathecal morphine to control spasticity as a temporary agent for a "drug holiday" from ITB in cases of ITB resistance (242) or as replacement therapy when ITB tolerance develops (243). The significant side effect profile of intrathecal morphine limits its use, including development of tolerance; itching; GI disturbances, including delayed gastric emptying (244); hypotension; urinary retention (99); and respiratory depression (245). As a result, the role of intrathecal morphine in the management of spasticity is uncertain (99).

Intrathecal Clonidine. Intrathecal clonidine has also been used in the management of spasticity (233), especially in SCI patients (234). In the incomplete SCI population, intrathecal clonidine has shown potential benefit in improvement of spasticity control and gait velocity, though overall functional results are mixed (234,246). Another potential benefit of intrathecal clonidine is its ability to reduce detrusor hyperreflexia in the SCI population (247,248). The hemodynamic side effects of intrathecal clonidine, including hypotension, bradycardia, and decreased blood flow, may be its most limiting factor (99,234,249). Other common side effects include dry mouth and sedation.

Other Agents. Fentanyl has been shown to be effective in cases of developed resistance to ITB (235). Midazolam has been used intrathecally for the management of spasticity. Animal studies have shown that the agent functions as a CNS depressant, analgesic, anticonvulsive, and myorelaxant (99); however, some studies report neurotoxicity, including potential toxicity to the blood-brain barrier, neurons, and the myelin sheath (250,251). As a result, its use in humans is controversial. Midazolam use for spasticity management is also limited by its sedating properties.

Surgical Procedures

In addition to intrathecal administration of pharmacologic agents, other surgical procedures are available for the management of spasticity. In general, surgical interventions are only considered when other treatments have failed. As all surgeries carry risk of anesthesia, bleeding, and infection, the potential benefits must be worth the surgical risk. Traditionally, neurosurgical procedures were performed for pain; however, there may be some benefit in management of spasticity. Selective dorsal rhizotomy has been described in children with cerebral palsy and in persons with MS and SCI (252–259). Initially, rhizotomy did not selectively ablate motor and sensory roots. The technique of interrupting a limited number of the most pathologic sensory rootlets and sparing the remainder was an innovation derived later in the history of the rhizotomy procedure. This method reduces the propensity of anesthesia due to sensory nerve root ablations and leaves the motor system intact. Numerous complications have been reported as a result of selective dorsal root rhizotomy, but they are often transient. Complications include bronchospasm, aspiration pneumonia, urinary retention, ileus, sensory loss, hypotonia, and bowel dysfunction (260–262).

Other more aggressive neurosurgical interventions such as myelotomy or cordotomy are available. These procedures are generally reserved for intractable cancer pain, and most studies describing myelotomy or cordotomy involve pain management (263–265). Some have advocated the use of myelotomy or cordotomy in severely spastic patients; however, these more aggressive interventions are controversial because they may cause dysfunction of the bowel and bladder (266).

There is an additional role for orthopedic interventions in complex spasticity cases. Osteotomy, capsulotomy, myotomy, and tendon lengthening may be utilized to restore ROM in a contractured joint (267). A common operation is the split anterior tibial tendon transfer procedure, which is used to reduce spasticity of the tibialis anterior when there is excessive inversion of the foot during swing phase. During the surgery, the tendon's distal attachment is anchored into the medial and lateral aspect of the foot, reducing the inversion moment with limited loss of dorsiflexor strength (268). Knee flexion contractures may be treated with a release of the hamstrings to improve positioning and function (269). Achilles lengthening is beneficial to reduce plantar flexion contractures, but there may be some loss of strength at the ankle joint as a result. If there is a hip flexor contracture of greater than 20 degrees, an iliopsoas tenotomy may be necessary after failure of more conservative measures (269). In patients with severe spasticity from MS or CP, the problem of hip subluxation may be encountered. This can be treated with adductor myotomies or, if not successful, femoral osteotomy (266). The decision to consult orthopedic surgery for surgical consideration is generally made when restoration of ROM is desired and other interventions have failed.

REFERENCES

1. Westerkam S, Sunders LL, Krause JS. Association of spasticity and life satisfaction after spinal cord injury. *Spinal Cord.* 2011;49(9):990–994.
2. Milinis K, Tennant A, Young CA, et al. Spasticity in multiple sclerosis: associations with impairments and overall quality of life. *Mult Scler Relat Disord.* 2016;5:34–39.
3. Young RR. Spasticity: a review. *Neurology.* 1994;44(suppl 9):S12–S20.
4. Lance JW. Symposium synopsis. In: Feldman RG, Youg RR, Koela WP, eds. *Spasticity: Disordered Motor Control.* Chicago, IL: Year Book Medical; 1980:487–489.
5. Maynard FM, Karunas RS, Waring WP III. Epidemiology of spasticity following traumatic spinal cord injury. *Arch Phys Med Rehabil.* 1990;71(8):566–569.
6. Sköld C, Levi R, Seiger Å. Spasticity after traumatic spinal cord injury: nature, severity and location. *Arch Phys Med Rehabil.* 1999;80:1548–1557.
7. Noreau L, Proulx P, Gagnon L, et al. Secondary impairments after spinal cord injury: a population-based study. *Am J Phys Med Rehabil.* 2000;79(6):526–535.
8. Walter JS, Sacks J, Othman R, et al. A database of self-reported secondary medical problems among VA spinal cord injury patients: its role in clinical care and management. *J Rehabil Res Dev.* 2002;39(1):53–61.
9. Rizzo MA, Hadjimichael OC, Preiningerova J, et al. Prevalence and treatment of spasticity reported by multiple sclerosis patients. *Mult Scler.* 2004;10(5):589–595.
10. Sommerfeld DK, Eek EU, Svensson AK, et al. Spasticity after stroke: its occurrence and association with motor impairments and activity limitations. *Stroke.* 2004;35(1):134–139.
11. Watkins CL, Leathley MJ, Gregson JM, et al. Prevalence of spasticity post stroke. *Clin Rehabil.* 2002;16(5):515–522.
12. Urban PP, Wolf T, Uebele M, et al. Occurrence and clinical predictors of spasticity after ischemic stroke. *Stroke.* 2010;41(9):2016–2020.
13. Thibaut FA, Chatelle C, Wannez S, et al. Spasticity in disorders of consciousness: a behavioral study. *Eur J Phys Rehabil Med.* 2015;51(4):389–397.
14. Sehgal N, McGuire JR. Beyond Ashworth: electrophysiologic quantification of spasticity. *Phys Med Rehabil Clin N Am.* 1998;9(4):949–979.
15. American Academy of Physical Medicine and Rehabilitation, ed. *Spasticity Management in the Patient with Brain Injury.* Orlando, FL: American Academy of Physical Medicine and Rehabilitation; 1995.
16. Moore JC. The Golgi tendon organ: a review and update. *Am J Occup Ther.* 1984;38:227–236.
17. Brooks VB. *The Neural Basis of Motor Control.* New York: Oxford University Press; 1986.
18. Katz R, Pierrot-Deseilligny E. Recurrent inhibition of alpha-motor neurons in patients with upper motor neuron lesions. *Brain.* 1982;105(pt 1):103–124.
19. Ashworth B. Preliminary trial of carisoprodol in multiple sclerosis. *Practitioner.* 1964;192:540–542.
20. Bohannon RW, Smith MB. Interrater reliability of a modified Ashworth scale of muscle spasticity. *Phys Ther.* 1987;67(2):206–207.
21. Ansari NN, Naghdi S, Moammeri H, et al. Ashworth scales are unreliable for the assessment of muscle spasticity. *Physiother Theory Pract.* 2006;22(3):119–125.
22. Craven BC, Morris AR. Modified Ashworth scale reliability for measurement of lower extremity spasticity among patients with SCI. *Spinal Cord.* 2010;48(3):207–213.
23. Ansari NN, Naghdi S, Mashayekhi M, et al. Intra-rater reliability of the Modified Modified Ashworth Scale (MMAS) in the assessment of upper-limb muscle spasticity. *NeuroRehabilitation.* 2012;31(2):215–222.
24. Ghotbi N, Ansari NN, Naghdi S, et al. Measurement of lower-limb muscle spasticity: intrarater reliability of Modified Modified Ashworth Scale. *J Rehabil Res Dev.* 2011;48(1):83–88.
25. Tardieu G, Shentoub S, Delarue R. A la recherché d'une technique de mesure de la spasticite. *Rev Neurol (Paris).* 1954;91:143–144.
26. Haugh AB, Pandyan AD, Johnson GR. A systematic review of the Tardieu scale for the measurement of spasticity. *Disabil Rehabil.* 2006;28(15):899–907.
27. Naghdi S, Ansari NN, Abolhasani H, et al. Electrophysiological evaluation of the Modified Tardieu Scale (MTS) in assessing poststroke wrist flexor spasticity. *NeuroRehabilitation.* 2014;34(1):177–184.
28. Ansari NN, Naghdi S, Hasson S, et al. Clinical assessment of ankle plantarflexor spasticity in adult patients after stroke: inter- and intra-rater reliability of the Modified Tardieu Scale. *Brain Inj.* 2013;29(5):605–612.
29. Ben-Shabat E, Palit M, Fini NA, et al. Intra- and interrater reliability of the Modified Tardieu Scale for the assessment of lower limb spasticity in adults with neurologic injuries. *Arch Phys Med Rehabil.* 2013;94(12):2494–2501.
30. Benz EN, Hornby TG, Bode RK, et al. A physiologically based clinical measure for spastic reflexes in spinal cord injury. *Arch Phys Med Rehabil.* 2005;86:52–59.
31. Li F, Wu Y, Xiong L. Reliability of a new scale for measurement of spasticity in stroke patients. *J Rehabil Med.* 2014;46(8):746–753.
32. Penn RD, Savoy SM, Corcos D, et al. Intrathecal baclofen for severe spinal spasticity. *N Engl J Med.* 1989;320:1517–1521.
33. Priebe MM, Sherwood AM, Thornby JI, et al. Clinical assessment of spasticity in spinal cord injury: a multidimensional problem. *Arch Phys Med Rehabil.* 1996;77:713–716.
34. Cook KF, Teal CR, Engebretson JC, et al. Development and validation of Patient Reported Impact of Spasticity Measure (PRISM). *J Rehabil Res Dev.* 2007;44:363–372.
35. Adams MM, Martin Ginis KA, Hicks AL. The spinal cord injury spasticity evaluation tool: development and evaluation. *Arch Phys Med Rehabil.* 2007;88:1185–1192.
36. Barker S, Horton M, Kent RM, et al. Development of a self-report scale of spasticity. *Top Stroke Rehabil.* 2013;20(6):485–492.
37. Wartenberg R. Pendulousness of the legs as a diagnostic test. *Neurology.* 1951;1:18–24.
38. Bajd T, Vodovnik L. Pendulum testing of spasticity. *J Biomed Eng.* 1984;6:9–16.
39. Firoozbakhsh KK, Kunkel CF, Scremin AME, et al. Isokinetic dynamometric technique for spasticity assessment. *Am J Phys Med Rehabil.* 1993;72:379–385.
40. Lamontagne A, Malouin F, Richards CL, et al. Evaluation of reflex- and nonreflex-induced muscle resistance to stretch in adults with spinal cord injury using hand-held and isokinetic dynamometry. *Phys Ther.* 1998;78(9):964–978.
41. Pennati GV, Plantin J, Borg J, et al. Normative NeuroFlexor data for detection of spasticity after stroke: a cross-sectional study. *J Neuroeng Rehabil.* 2016;13:30.

42. Gäverth J, Sandgren M, Lindberg PG, et al. Test-retest and inter-rater reliability of a method to measure wrist and finger spasticity. *J Rehabil Med.* 2013;45(7):630–636.

43. Chino N, Muraoka Y, Ishihama H, et al. Measurement of ankle plantar flexor spasticity following stroke: assessment of a new quantitative tool. *J Rehabil Med.* 2015;47(8):753–755.

44. Penn RD. Intrathecal baclofen for severe spasticity. *Ann N Y Acad Sci.* 1988;531: 157–166.

45. van der Salm A, Veltink PH, Hermens HJ, et al. Development of a new method for objective assessment of spasticity using full range passive movements. *Arch Phys Med Rehabil.* 2005;86:1991–1997.

46. Yablon SA, Stokic DS. Neurophysiologic evaluation of spastic hypertonia: implications for management of the patient with the intrathecal baclofen pump. *Am J Phys Med Rehabil.* 2004;83(suppl):S10–S18.

47. Burridge JH, Wood DE, Hermens HJ, et al. Theoretical and methodological considerations in the measurement of spasticity. *Disabil Rehabil.* 2005;27:69–80.

48. Little JW, Micklesen P, Umlauf R, et al. Lower extremity manifestations of spasticity in chronic spinal cord injury. *Am J Phys Med Rehabil.* 1989;68(1):32–36.

49. Gans BM, Glenn MB. Introduction. In: Glenn MB, Whyte J, eds. *The Practical Management of Spasticity in Children and Adults.* Philadelphia, PA: Lea & Febiger; 1990:1–7.

50. Francois B, Vacher P, Roustan J, et al. Intrathecal baclofen after traumatic brain injury: early treatment using a new technique to prevent spasticity. *J Trauma.* 2001;50(1):158–161.

51. Gracies JM, Elovic E, McGuire J, et al. Traditional pharmacological treatments for spasticity. Part I: local treatments. In: Mayer NH, Simpson DM, eds. *Spasticity: Etiology, Evaluation, Management and the Role of Botulinum Toxin.* New York, NY: We Move; 2002:44–64.

52. Zafonte RD, Elovic E. Spasticity and abnormalities of muscle tone. In: Grabois M, Garrison SJ, Hart KA, et al., eds. *Physical Medicine & Rehabilitation: The Complete Approach.* Malden, MA: Blackwell Science; 2000:848–858.

53. Gracies JM. Pathophysiology of impairment in patients with spasticity and use of stretch as a treatment of spastic hypertonia. *Phys Med Rehabil Clin N Am.* 2001;12(4):747–768.

54. Schmit BD, Dewald JP, Rymer WZ. Stretch reflex adaptation in elbow flexors during repeated passive movements in unilateral brain-injured patients. *Arch Phys Med Rehabil.* 2000;81(3):269–278.

55. Wilson LR, Gracies JM, Burke D, et al. Evidence for fusimotor drive in stroke patients based on muscle spindle thixotropy. *Neurosci Lett.* 1999;264(1–3):109–112.

56. Tremblay F, Malouin F, Richards CL, et al. Effects of prolonged muscle stretch on reflex and voluntary muscle activations in children with spastic cerebral palsy. *Scand J Rehabil Med.* 1990;22(4):171–180.

57. Carey JR. Manual stretch: effect on finger movement control and force control in stroke subjects with spastic extrinsic finger flexor muscles. *Arch Phys Med Rehabil.* 1990;71(11):888–894.

58. Brouwer B, Davidson LK, Olney SJ. Serial casting in idiopathic toe-walkers and children with spastic cerebral palsy. *J Pediatr Orthop.* 2000;20(2):221–225.

59. Hill J. The effects of casting on upper extremity motor disorders after brain injury. *Am J Occup Ther.* 1994;48(3):219–224.

60. Otis JC, Root L, Kroll MA. Measurement of plantar flexor spasticity during treatment with tone-reducing casts. *J Pediatr Orthop.* 1985;5(6):682–686.

61. Pohl M, Ruckriem S, Mehrholz J, et al. Effectiveness of serial casting in patients with severe cerebral spasticity: a comparison study. *Arch Phys Med Rehabil.* 2002;83(6):784–790.

62. Farina S, Migliorini C, Gandolfi M, et al. Combined effects of botulinum toxin and casting treatments on lower limb spasticity after stroke. *Funct Neurol.* 2008;23(2):87–91.

63. Ackman JD, Russman BS, Thomas SS, et al. Comparing botulinum toxin A with casting for treatment of dynamic equinus in children with cerebral palsy. *Dev Med Child Neurol.* 2005;47(9):620–627.

64. Lightfoot E, Verrier M. Neurophysiological effects of prolonged cooling of the calf in patients with complete spinal cord transection. *Physiotherapy.* 1976;62(4):114–117.

65. Weiss M, Duma-Drzewinska A. Cooling as a method of reducing spasticity. *Neurol Neurochir Pol.* 1976;10(3):335–343.

66. Knutsson E. On effects of local cooling upon motor functions in spastic paresis. *Prog Phys Ther.* 1970;1(2):124–131.

67. Knutsson E. Topical cryotherapy in spasticity. *Scand J Rehabil Med.* 1970;2(4): 159–163.

68. Gracies JM. Physical modalities other than stretch in spastic hypertonia. *Phys Med Rehabil Clin N Am.* 2001;12(4):769–792.

69. Travell J. Ethyl chloride spray for painful muscle spasm. *Arch Phys Med Rehabil.* 1952;33(5):291–298.

70. Lehmann JF, deLateur BJ. Diathermy and superficial heat and cold therapy. In: Krusen F, ed. *Handbook of Physical Medicine.* Philadelphia, PA: WB Saunders; 1996.

71. Warren CG, Lehmann JF, Koblanski JN. Heat and stretch procedures: an evaluation using rat tail tendon. *Arch Phys Med Rehabil.* 1976;57(3):122–126.

72. Lund S, Lundberg A, Vyklicky L. Inhibitory action from the flexor reflex afferents on transmission to Ia afferents. *Acta Physiol Scand.* 1965;64(4):345–355.

73. Mills PB, Dossa F. Transcutaneous electrical nerve stimulation for management of limb spasticity: a systematic review. *Am J Phys Med Rehabil.* 2016;95(4):309–318.

74. Yan T, Hui-Chan CW, Li LS. Functional electrical stimulation improves motor recovery of the lower extremity and walking ability of subjects with first acute stroke: a randomized placebo-controlled trial. *Stroke.* 2005;36(1):80–85.

75. Chen SC, Chen YL, Chen CJ, et al. Effects of surface electrical stimulation on the muscle-tendon junction of spastic gastrocnemius in stroke patients. *Disabil Rehabil.* 2005;27(3):105–110.

76. Aydin G, Tomruk S, Keles I, et al. Transcutaneous electrical nerve stimulation versus baclofen in spasticity: clinical and electrophysiologic comparison. *Am J Phys Med Rehabil.* 2005;84(8):584–592.

77. Bakhtiary AH, Fatemy E. Does electrical stimulation reduce spasticity after stroke? A randomized controlled study. *Clin Rehabil.* 2008;22(5):418–425.

78. Granat MH, Ferguson ACB, Andrews BJ, et al. The role of functional electrical stimulation in the rehabilitation of patients with incomplete spinal cord injury—observed benefits during gait studies. *Paraplegia.* 1993;31:207–215.

79. Mirbagheri MM, Ladouceur M, Barbeau H, et al. The effects of long-term FES-assisted walking on intrinsic and reflex dynamic stiffness in spastic spinal-cord-injured subjects. *IEEE Trans Neural Syst Rehabil Eng.* 2002;10(4):280–288.

80. Agarwal S, Triolo RJ, Kobetic R, et al. Long-term over perceptions of an implanted neuroprosthesis for exercise, standing, and transfers after spinal cord injury. *J Rehabil Res Dev.* 2003;40(3):241–252.

81. Krause P, Szecsi J, Straube A. FES cycling reduces spastic muscle tone in a patient with multiple sclerosis. *NeuroRehabilitation.* 2007;22(4):335–337.

82. Ahlborg L, Andersson C, Julin P. Whole-body vibration training compared with resistance training: effect on spasticity, muscle strength, and motor performance in adults with cerebral palsy. *J Rehabil Med.* 2006;38(5):302308.

83. Cheng HY, Yu Y, Wong AM, et al. Effects of an eight-week whole body vibration on lower extremity muscle tone and function in children with cerebral palsy. *Res Dev Disabil.* 2015;38:256–261.

84. Sadeghi M, Sawatzky B. Effects of vibration on spasticity in individuals with spinal cord injury: a scoping systematic review. *Am J Phys Med Rehabil.* 2014;93(11): 995–1007.

85. Miyara K, Matsumoto S, Uema T, et al. Feasibility of using while body vibration as a means for controlling spasticity in post-stroke patients: a pilot study. *Complement Ther Clin Pract.* 2014;20(1):70–73.

86. Caliandro P, Celletti C, Padua L, et al. Focal muscle vibration in the treatment of upper limb spasticity: a pilot randomized controlled trial in patients with chronic stroke. *Arch Phys Med Rehabil.* 2012;93(9):1656–1661.

87. Fink M, Rollnik JD, Bijak M, et al. Needle acupuncture in chronic poststroke leg spasticity. *Arch Phys Med Rehabil.* 2004;85:667–672.

88. Moon SK, Whang YK, Park SU, et al. Antispastic effect of electroacupuncture and moxibustion in stroke patients. *Am J Chin Med.* 2003;31(3):467–474.

89. Mukherjee M, McPeak LK, Redford JB, et al. The effect of electro-acupuncture on spasticity of the wrist joint in chronic stroke survivors. *Arch Phys Med Rehabil.* 2007;88:159–166.

90. Zhao W, Wang C, Li Z, et al. Efficacy and safety of transcutaneous electrical acupoint stimulation to treat muscle spasticity following brain injury: a double-blinded, multicenter, randomized controlled trial. *PLoS One.* 2015;19(2):e0116976.

91. Krause P, Straube A. Repetitive magnetic and functional electrical stimulation reduce spastic tone increase in patients with spinal cord injury. *Suppl Clin Neurophysiol.* 2003;56:220–225.

92. Centonze D, Koch G, Versace V. Repetitive transcranial magnetic stimulation of the motor cortex ameliorates spasticity in multiple sclerosis. *Neurology.* 2007;68: 1045–1050.

93. Mälly J, Dinya E. Recovery of motor disability and spasticity in post-stroke after repetitive transcranial magnetic stimulation (rTMS). *Brain Res Bull.* 2008;76: 388–395.

94. Naghdi S, Ansari NN, Rastgoo M, et al. A pilot study on the effects if low frequency repetitive transcranial magnetic stimulation on lower extremity spasticity and motor neuron excitability in patients after stroke. *J Bodyw Mov Ther.* 2015;19(4):616–623.

95. Daliri SS, Forogh B, Emami Razavi SZ, et al. A single blind, clinical trial to investigate the effects if a single session extracorporeal shock wave therapy on wrist flexor spasticity after stroke. *NeuroRehabilitation.* 2015;36(1):67–72.

96. El-Shamy SM, Eid MA, El-Banna MF. Effect of extracorporeal shock wave therapy on gait pattern in hemiplegic cerebral palsy: a randomized controlled trial. *Am J Phys Med Rehabil.* 2014;93(12):1065–1072.

97. Santamato A, Micello MF, Panza F, et al. Extracorporeal shock wave therapy for the treatment of poststroke plantar-flexor muscles spasticity: a prospective open-label study. *Top Stroke Rehabil.* 2014;21(suppl 1):S17–S24.

98. Tseng TC, Wang SC. Locus of action of centrally acting muscle relaxants, diazepam and tybamate. *J Pharmacol Exp Ther.* 1971;178(2):350–360.

99. Gracies JM, Elovic E, McGuire J, et al. Traditional pharmacological treatments for spasticity. Part II. General and regional treatments. In: Mayer NH, Simpson DM, eds. *Spasticity: Etiology, Evaluation, Management and the Role of Botulinum Toxin.* New York: We Move; 2002:65–93.

100. Truven Health Analytics. *Micromedex® Solutions.* Available from: http://www.micromedexsolutions.com/micromedex2/librarian/. Accessed March 19, 2017.

101. Corbett M, Frankel HL, Michaelis L. A double blind, cross-over trial of Valium in the treatment of spasticity. *Paraplegia.* 1972;10(1):19–22.

102. Cartlidge NE, Hudson P, Weightman D. A comparison of baclofen and diazepam in the treatment of spasticity. *J Neurol Sci.* 1974;23(1):17–24.

103. From A, Heltberg A. A double-blind trial with baclofen (Lioresal) and diazepam in spasticity due to multiple sclerosis. *Acta Neurol Scand.* 1975;51(2):158–166.

104. Roussan M, Terrence C, Fromm G. Baclofen versus diazepam for the treatment of spasticity and long-term follow-up of baclofen therapy. *Pharmatherapeutica.* 1985;4(5):278–284.

105. Goldstein LB; The Sygen in Acute Stroke Study Investigators. Common drugs may influence motor recovery after stroke. *Neurology.* 1995;45(5):865–871.

106. Whyte J, Robinson KM. Pharmacologic management. In: Glenn MB, Whyte J, eds. *The Practical Management of Spasticity in Children and Adults.* Malvern, PA: Lea & Febiger; 1990:201–226.

107. Basmajian JV. Lioresal (baclofen) treatment of spasticity in multiple sclerosis. *Am J Phys Med.* 1975;54(4):175–177.

108. Duncan GW, Shahani BT, Young RR. An evaluation of baclofen treatment for certain symptoms in patients with spinal cord lesions. A double-blind, cross-over study. *Neurology.* 1976;26(5):441–446.

109. Hudgson P, Weightman D. Baclofen in the treatment of spasticity. *Br Med J.* 1971;4(778):15–17.

110. Nance PW. A comparison of clonidine, cyproheptadine and baclofen in spastic spinal cord injured patients. *J Am Paraplegia Soc.* 1994;17(3):150–156.

111. Feldman RG, Kelly-Hayes M, Conomy JP, et al. Baclofen for spasticity in multiple sclerosis. Double-blind crossover and three-year study. *Neurology.* 1978;28(11):1094–1098.

112. Hedley DW, Maroun JA, Espir ML. Evaluation of baclofen (Lioresal) for spasticity in multiple sclerosis. *Postgrad Med J.* 1975;51(599):615–618.

113. Basmajian JV, Yucel V. Effects of a GABA—derivative (BA-34647) on spasticity. Preliminary report of a double-blind cross-over study. *Am J Phys Med.* 1974;53(5):223–228.

114. Jones RF, Lance JW. Baclofen (Lioresal) in the long-term management of spasticity. *Med J Aust.* 1976;1(18):654–657.

115. Pedersen E, Arlien-Soborg P, Grynderup V, et al. GABA derivative in spasticity. (Beta-(4-chlorophenyl)-gamma-aminobutyric acid, Ciba 34.647-Ba). *Acta Neurol Scand.* 1970;46(3):257–266.

116. Ashby P, White DG. "Presynaptic" inhibition in spasticity and the effect of beta (4-chlorophenyl)GABA. *J Neurol Sci.* 1973;20(3):329–338.

117. Hulme A, MacLennan WJ, Ritchie RT, et al. Baclofen in the elderly stroke patient its side-effects and pharmacokinetics. *Eur J Clin Pharmacol.* 1985;29(4):467–469.

118. Pedersen E. Clinical assessment and pharmacologic therapy of spasticity. *Arch Phys Med Rehabil.* 1974;55(8):344–354.

119. Pinto OS, Polikar M, Debono G. Results of international clinical trials with Lioresal. *Postgrad Med J.* 1972;48(suppl 25):18–25.

120. Elovic E. Principles of pharmaceutical management of spastic hypertonia. *Phys Med Rehabil Clin N Am.* 2001;12(4):793–816.

121. Katz RT, Campagnolo DI. Pharmacologic management of spasticity. In: Katz RT, ed. *Spasticity: State of the Arts Review.* Philadelphia, PA: Hanley & Belfus; 1994:473–480.

122. Utili R, Boitnott JK, Zimmerman HJ. Dantrolene associated hepatic injury: incidence and character. *Gastroenterology.* 1977;72:610.

123. Zafonte R, Lombard L, Elovic E. Antispasticity medications: uses and limitations of enteral therapy. *Am J Phys Med Rehabil.* 2004;83(10 suppl):S50–S58.

124. Weiser R, Terenty T, Hudgson P, et al. Dantrolene sodium in the treatment of spasticity in chronic spinal cord disease. *Practitioner.* 1978;221(1321):123–127.

125. Monster AW. Spasticity and the effect of dantrolene sodium. *Arch Phys Med Rehabil.* 1974;55(8):373–383.

126. Glass A, Hannah A. A comparison of dantrolene sodium and diazepam in the treatment of spasticity. *Paraplegia.* 1974;12(3):170–174.

127. Gelenberg AJ, Poskanzer DC. The effect of dantrolene sodium on spasticity in multiple sclerosis. *Neurology.* 1973;23(12):1313–1315.

128. Tolosa ES, Soll RW, Loewenson RB. Letter: treatment of spasticity in multiple sclerosis with dantrolene. *JAMA.* 1975;233(10):1046.

129. Chyatte SB, Birdsong JH, Bergman BA. The effects of dantrolene sodium on spasticity and motor performance in hemiplegia. *South Med J.* 1971;64(2):180–185.

130. Donovan WH, Carter RE, Rossi CD, et al. Clonidine effect on spasticity: a clinical trial. *Arch Phys Med Rehabil.* 1988;69(3 pt 1):193–194.

131. Nance PW, Shears AH, Nance DM. Clonidine in spinal cord injury. *Can Med Assoc J.* 1985;133(1):41–42.

132. Nance PW, Shears AH, Nance DM. Reflex changes induced by clonidine in spinal cord injured patients. *Paraplegia.* 1989;27(4):296–301.

133. Rosenblum D. Clonidine-induced bradycardia in patients with spinal cord injury. *Arch Phys Med Rehabil.* 1993;74(11):1206–1207.

134. Weingarden SI, Belen JG. Clonidine transdermal system for treatment of spasticity in spinal cord injury. *Arch Phys Med Rehabil.* 1992;73(9):876–877.

135. Yablon SA, Sipski ML. Effect of transdermal clonidine on spinal spasticity. A case series. *Am J Phys Med Rehabil.* 1993;72(3):154–157.

136. Bass B, Weinshenker B, Rice GP, et al. Tizanidine versus baclofen in the treatment of spasticity in patients with multiple sclerosis. *Can J Neurol Sci.* 1988;15(1):15–19.

137. Bes A, Eyssette M, Pierrot-Deseilligny E, et al. A multi-centre, double-blind trial of tizanidine, a new antispastic agent, in spasticity associated with hemiplegia. *Curr Med Res Opin.* 1988;10(10):709–718.

138. Lapierre Y, Bouchard S, Tansey C, et al. Treatment of spasticity with tizanidine in multiple sclerosis. *Can J Neurol Sci.* 1987;14(3 suppl):513–517.

139. Johnson TR, Tobias JD. Hypotension following the initiation of tizanidine in a patient treated with an angiotensin converting enzyme inhibitor for chronic hypertension. *J Child Neurol.* 2000;15(12):818–819.

140. Nance PW, Bugaresti J, Shellenberger K, et al. Efficacy and safety of tizanidine in the treatment of spasticity in patients with spinal cord injury. North American Tizanidine Study Group. *Neurology.* 1994;44(11 suppl 9):S44–S51.

141. Mathias CJ, Luckitt J, Desai P, et al. Pharmacodynamics and pharmacokinetics of the oral antispastic agent tizanidine in patients with spinal cord injury. *J Rehabil Res Dev.* 1989;26(4):9–16.

142. Smith C, Birnbaum G, Carter JL, et al. Tizanidine treatment of spasticity caused by multiple sclerosis: results of a double-blind, placebo-controlled trial. US Tizanidine Study Group. *Neurology.* 1994;44(11 suppl 9):S34–S42.

143. Eyssette M, Rohmer F, Serratrice G, et al. Multi-centre, double-blind trial of a novel antispastic agent, tizanidine, in spasticity associated with multiple sclerosis. *Curr Med Res Opin.* 1988;10(10):699–708.

144. United Kingdom Tizanidine Trial Group. A double-blind, placebo-controlled trial of tizanidine in the treatment of spasticity caused by multiple sclerosis. *Neurology.* 1994;44(11 suppl 9):S70–S78.

145. Corey-Bloom J, Wolfson T, Gamst A, et al. Smoked cannabis for spasticity management in multiple sclerosis: a randomized, placebo-controlled trial. *CMAJ.* 2012;184(10):1143–1150.

146. Trojano M, Vila C. Effectiveness and tolerability of the THC/CBD oromucosal spray for multiple sclerosis spasticity in Italy: first data from a large observational study. *Eur Neurol.* 2015;74(3–4):178–185.

147. Russo M, Calabrò RS, Naro A, et al. Sativex in the management of multiple sclerosis-related spasticity: role of the corticospinal modulation. *Neural Plast.* 2015;2015:656582. doi: 10.1155/2015/656582.

148. Fernandez O. Advances in the management of multiple sclerosis spasticity: recent clinical trials. *Eur Neurol.* 2014;72(suppl 1):9–11.

149. Wissel J, Ward AB, Erztgaard P, et al. European consensus table on the use of botulinum toxin type A in adult spasticity. *J Rehabil Med.* 2009;41:13–25.

150. Lapeyre E, Kuks J, Meijler WJ. Spasticity: revisiting the role and the individual value of several pharmacological treatments. *NeuroRehabilitation.* 2010;27:193–200.

151. Kinnear BZ, Lannin NA, Cusick A, et al. Rehabilitation therapies after botulinum toxin-A injection to manage limb spasticity: a systematic review. *Phys Ther.* 2014;94:1569.

152. Marchand-Pauvert V, Aymard C, Giboin L-S, et al. Beyond muscular effects: depression of spinal recurrent inhibition after botulinum neurotoxin A. *J Physiol.* 2013;591:1017–1029.

153. Huynh W, Krishnan AV, Lin CS-Y, et al. Botulinum toxin modulates cortical maladaptation in post-stroke spasticity. *Muscle Nerve.* 2013;48:93–99.

154. Lange O, Bigalke H, Dengler R, et al. Neutralizing antibodies and secondary therapy failure after treatment with botulinum toxin type A: much ado about nothing? *Clin Neuropharmacol.* 2009;32:213–218.

155. Coleman C, Hubble J, Schwab J, et al. Immunoresistance in cervical dystonia patients after treatment with abobotulinumtoxinA. *Int J Neurosci.* 2012;122:358–362.

156. Brin MF, Comella CL, Jankovic J, et al. Long-term treatment with botulinum toxin type A in cervical dystonia has low immunogenicity by mouse protection assay. *Mov Disord.* 2008;23:1353–1360.

157. Francisco GE. Botulinum toxin: dosing and dilution. *Am J Phys Med Rehabil.* 2004;83:S30–S37.

158. Allergan, Inc. BOTOX (onabotulinumtoxinA) for injection, for intramuscular, intradetrusor, or intradermal use. Available from: https://www.allergan.com/assets/pdf/botox_pi.pdf. Accessed February 1, 2017.

159. Ipsen Biopharm Ltd. DYSPORT® (abobotulinumtoxinA) for injection, for intramuscular use. Available from: https://www.allergan.com/assets/pdf/botox_pi.pdf. Accessed February 1, 2017.

160. Merz Pharmaceuticals, LLC. XEOMIN (incobotulinumtoxinA) for injection, for intramuscular use. Available from: http://www.xeomin.com/wp-content/uploads/xeomin-full-prescribing-information.pdf. Accessed February 1, 2017.

161. Solstice Neurosciences, Inc. Myobloc® (rimabotulinumtoxinB) Injection. Available from: http://www.myobloc.com/hp_about/PI_5-19-10.pdf. Accessed February 1, 2017.

162. Jankovic J, Hunter C, Dolimbek BZ, et al. Clinico-immunologic aspects of botulinum toxin type B treatment of cervical dystonia. *Neurology.* 2006;67:2233–2235.

163. Callaway JE. Botulinum toxin type B (Myobloc®): pharmacology and biochemistry. *Clin Dermatol.* 2004;22:23–28.

164. Cheng CM, Chen JS, Patel RP. Unlabeled uses of botulinum toxins: a review, part 1. *Am J Health Syst Pharm.* 2006;63(2):145–152.

165. Mancini F, Sandrini G, Moglia A, et al. A randomized, double-blind, dose-ranging study to evaluate efficacy and safety of three doses of botulinum toxin type A (Botox) for the treatment of spastic foot. *Neurol Sci.* 2005;26:26–31.

166. Nuanthaisong U, Abraham N, Goldman HB. Incidence of adverse events after high doses of onabotulinumtoxinA for multiple indications. *Urology.* 2014;84:1044–1048.

167. Baricich A, Grana E, Carda S, et al. High doses of onabotulinumtoxinA in post-stroke spasticity: a retrospective analysis. *J Neural Transm.* 2015;122:1283–1287.

168. Ramirez-Castaneda J, Jankovic J, Comella C, et al. Diffusion, spread, and migration of botulinum toxin. *Mov Disord.* 2013;28:1775–1783.

169. Yablon SA, Agana BT, Ivanhoe CB, et al. Botulinum toxin in severe upper extremity spasticity among patients with traumatic brain injury: an open-labeled trial. *Neurology.* 1996;47(4):939–944.

170. Maan Z, Al-Singary W, Shergill I, et al. Alternative use of botulinum toxin in urology. *Expert Opin Pharmacother.* 2004;5(5):1015–1021.

171. Chang H. Botulism toxin: use in disorders of the temporomandibular joint. *Dent Today.* 2005;24(12):48, 50–51.

172. Clark GT. The management of oromandibular motor disorders and facial spasms with injections of botulinum toxin. *Phys Med Rehabil Clin N Am.* 2003;14(4):727–748.

173. Crowner BE, Brunstrom JE, Racette BA. Iatrogenic botulism due to therapeutic botulinum toxin a injection in a pediatric patient. *Clin Neuropharmacol.* 2007;30(5):310–313.

174. Rossi RP, Strax TE, Di RA. Severe dysphagia after botulinum toxin B injection to the lower limbs and lumbar paraspinal muscles. *Am J Phys Med Rehabil.* 2006;85(12):1011–1013.

175. Chin TYP, Nattrass GR, Selber P, et al. Accuracy of intramuscular injection of botulinum toxin A in juvenile cerebral palsy: a comparison between manual needle placement and placement guided by electrical stimulation. *J Pediatr Orthop.* 2005;25:286–291.

176. Molloy FM, Shill HA, Kaelin-Lang A, et al. Accuracy of muscle localization without EMG: implications for treatment of limb dystonia. *Neurology*. 2002;58:805–807.

177. Lapatki BG, Van Dijk JP, Van de Warrenburg BPC, et al. Botulinum toxin has an increased effect when targeted toward the muscle's endplate zone: a high-density surface EMG guided study. *Clin Neurophysiol*. 2011;122:1611–1616.

178. Geenen C, Consky E, Ashby P. Localizing muscles for botulinum toxin treatment of focal hand dystonia. *Can J Neurol Sci*. 1996;23:194–197.

179. Henzel MK, Munin MC, Niyonkuru C, et al. Comparison of surface and ultrasound localization to identify forearm flexor muscles for botulinum toxin injections. *PM R*. 2010;2:642–646.

180. Picelli A, Bonetti P, Fontana C, et al. Is spastic muscle echo intensity related to the response to botulinum toxin type A in patients with stroke? A cohort study. *Arch Phy Med Rehabil*. 2012;93:1253–1258.

181. Picelli A, Tamburin S, Cavazza S, et al. Relationship between ultrasonographic, electromyographic, and clinical parameters in adult stroke patients with spastic equinus: an observational study. *Arch Phy Med Rehabil*. 2014;95:1564–1570.

182. Kwon J-Y, Hwang JH, Kim J-S. Botulinum toxin A injection into calf muscles for treatment of spastic equinus in cerebral palsy: a controlled trial comparing sonography and electric stimulation-guided injection techniques: a preliminary report. *Am J Phys Med Rehabil*. 2010;89:279–286.

183. May O. The functional and histological effects of intraneural and intraganglionic injections of alcohol. *Br Med J*. 1912;2:465.

184. Khalili AA, Betts HB. Peripheral nerve block with phenol in the management of spasticity: indications and complications. *JAMA*. 1967;200:1155–1157.

185. Zafonte RD, Munin MC. Phenol and alcohol blocks for the treatment of spasticity. *Phys Med Rehabil Clin N Am*. 2001;12:817–832.

186. Van Kuijk AA, Geurts ACH, Bevaart BJW, et al. Treatment of upper extremity spasticity in stroke patients by focal neuronal or neuromuscular blockade: a systematic review of the literature. *J Rehabil Med*. 2002;34:51–61.

187. Albright AL, Barron WB, Fasick MP, et al. Continuous intrathecal baclofen infusion for spasticity of cerebral origin. *JAMA*. 1993;270(20):2475–2477.

188. Meythaler JM, Guin-Renfroe S, Grabb P, et al. Long-term continuously infused intrathecal baclofen for spastic—dystonic hypertonia in traumatic brain injury: 1-year experience. *Arch Phys Med Rehabil*. 1999;80(1):13–19.

189. Becker R, Alberti O, Bauer BL. Continuous intrathecal baclofen infusion in severe spasticity after traumatic or hypoxic brain injury. *J Neurol*. 1997;244(3):160–166.

190. Gwartz BL. Intrathecal baclofen for spasticity caused by thrombotic stroke. *Am J Phys Med Rehabil*. 2001;80(5):383–387.

191. Meythaler JM, Guin-Renfroe S, Brunner RC, et al. Intrathecal baclofen for spastic hypertonia from stroke. *Stroke*. 2001;32(9):2099–2109.

192. Ivanhoe CB, Francisco GE, McGuire JR, et al. Intrathecal baclofen management of poststroke spastic hypertonia: implications for function and quality of life. *Arch Phys Med Rehabil*. 2006;87(11):1509–1515.

193. Francisco GE, Yablon SA, Schiess MC, et al. Consensus panel guidelines for the use of intrathecal baclofen therapy in poststroke spastic hypertonia. *Top Stroke Rehabil*. 2006;13(4):74–85.

194. Guillaume D, Van HA, Vloeberghs M, et al. A clinical study of intrathecal baclofen using a programmable pump for intractable spasticity. *Arch Phys Med Rehabil*. 2005;86(11):2165–2171.

195. Passat R, Perrouin Verbe B, Menei P, et al. Treatment of spasticity with intrathecal baclofen administration: long term follow-up, review of 40 patients. *Spinal Cord*. 2004;42:686–693.

196. Detrembleur C, Plaghki L. Quantitative assessment of intrathecally administered baclofen in spasticity. *Arch Phys Med Rehabil*. 2000;81:279–284.

197. Albright AL, Thompson Carlos S, Minnigh MB. Cerebrospinal fluid baclofen concentrations in patients undergoing continuous intrathecal baclofen therapy. *Dev Med Child Neurol*. 2007;49:423–425.

198. Dralle D, Muller H, Zierski J, et al. Intrathecal baclofen for spasticity [letter]. *Lancet*. 1985;2(8462):1003.

199. Coffey RJ, Cahill D, Steers W, et al. Intrathecal baclofen for intractable spasticity of spinal origin: results of a long-term multicenter study. *J Neurosurg*. 1993;78:226–232.

200. Avellino AM, Loeser JD. Intrathecal baclofen for treatment of intractable spasticity of spine or brain etiology. *Neuromodulation*. 2000;3:75–81.

201. McCormick ZL, Chu SK, Binler D, et al. Intrathecal versus oral baclofen: a matched cohort study of spasticity, pain, sleep, fatigue and quality of life. *PM R*. 2016;8:553–562.

202. Teddy P, Jamous A, Gardner B, et al. Complications of intrathecal baclofen delivery. *Br J Neurosurg*. 1992;6(2):115–118.

203. Albright AL, Ferson SS. Intrathecal baclofen therapy in children. *Neurosurg Focus*. 2006;21(2):e3.

204. Kofler M, Kronenberg MF, Rifici C, et al. Epileptic seizures associated with intrathecal baclofen application. *Neurology*. 1994;44(1):25–27.

205. Green LB, Nelson VS. Death after acute withdrawal of intrathecal baclofen: case report and literature review. *Arch Phys Med Rehabil*. 1999;80(12):1600–1604.

206. Reeves RK, Stolp-Smith KA, Christopherson MW. Hyperthermia, rhabdomyolysis, and disseminated intravascular coagulation associated with baclofen pump catheter failure. *Arch Phys Med Rehabil*. 1998;79(3):353–356.

207. Coffey RJ, Edgar TS, Francisco GE, et al. Abrupt withdrawal from intrathecal baclofen: recognition and management of a potentially life-threatening syndrome. *Arch Phys Med Rehabil*. 2002;83:735–741.

208. Ginsburg GM, Lauder AJ. Progression of scoliosis in patients with spastic quadriplegia after the insertion of an intrathecal baclofen pump. *Spine*. 2007;32(24):2745–2750.

209. Sansone JM, Mann D, Noonan K, et al. Rapid progression of scoliosis following insertion of intrathecal baclofen pump. *J Pediatr Orthop*. 2006;26(1):125–128.

210. Senaran H, Shah SA, Presedo A, et al. The risk of progression of scoliosis in cerebral palsy patients after intrathecal baclofen therapy. *Spine*. 2007;32(21):2348–2354.

211. Buonaguro V, Scelsa B, Curci D, et al. Epilepsy and intrathecal baclofen in children with cerebral palsy. *Pediatr Neurol*. 2005;33:110–113.

212. Scheule SU, Kellinghuas C, Shook SJ, et al. Incidence of seizures in patients with multiple sclerosis treated with intrathecal baclofen. *Neurology*. 2005;64:1086–1087.

213. Tasseel Ponche S, Ferrapie A-L, Chenet A, et al. Intrathecal baclofen in cerebral palsy: a retrospective study of 25 wheelchair-assisted adults. *Ann Phys Rehabil Med*. 2010;53:483–498.

214. Kishima H, Yanagisawa T, Goto Y, et al. Respiratory function under intrathecal baclofen therapy in patients with spastic tetraplegia. *Neuromodulation*. 2016;19:650–654.

215. Bensmail D, Quera Salva MA, Roche N, et al. Effect of intrathecal baclofen on sleep and respiratory function on patients with spasticity. *Neurology*. 2006;67:1432–1436.

216. Bensmail D, Marquer A, Roche N, et al. Pilot study assessing the impact of intrathecal baclofen administration mode on sleep-related respiratory parameters. *Arch Phys Med Rehabil*. 2012;93:96–99.

217. Saulino M, Ivanhoe CB, McGuire JR, et al. Best practices for intrathecal baclofen therapy: patient selection. *Neuromodulation*. 2016;19:607–615.

218. Francisco GE, Hu MM, Boake C, et al. Efficacy of early use of intrathecal baclofen therapy for treating spastic hypertonia due to acquired brain injury. *Brain Inj*. 2005;19(5):359–364.

219. Turner MS. Early use of intrathecal baclofen in brain injury in pediatric patients. *Acta Neurochir*. 2003;87:81–83.

220. Phillips MM, Miljkovic N, Ramos-Lamboy M, et al. Clinical experience with continuous intrathecal baclofen pump trials prior to pump implantation. *PM R*. 2015;7(10):1052–1058.

221. Bleyenheuft C, Filipetti P, Caldas C, et al. Experience with external pump trial prior to implantation for intrathecal baclofen in ambulatory patients with spastic cerebral palsy. *Neurophysiol Clin*. 2007;37(1):23–28.

222. Krach LE, Kriel RL, Nugent AC. Complex dosing schedules for continuous intrathecal baclofen infusion. *Pediatr Neurol*. 2007;37(5):354–359.

223. Saval A, Chiodo AE. Intrathecal baclofen for spasticity management: a comparative analysis of spasticity of spinal vs cortical origin. *J Spinal Cord Med*. 2010;33(1):16–21.

224. Schiess MC, Oh IJ, Stimming EF, et al. Prospective 12-month study of intrathecal baclofen therapy for poststroke spastic upper and lower extremity motor control and functional improvement. *Neuromodulation*. 2011;14:38–45.

225. Rawlins PK. Intrathecal baclofen therapy over 10 years. *J Neurosci Nurs*. 2004;36(6):322–327.

226. Stokic DS, Yablon SA. Effect of concentration and mode of intrathecal baclofen administration on soleus H-reflex in patients with muscle hypertonia. *Clin Neurophysiol*. 2012;123:2200–2204.

227. Saval A, Chiodo AE. Effect of intrathecal baclofen concentration on spasticity control: case series. *J Spinal Cord Med*. 2008;31:394–397.

228. Ivanhoe CB, Tilton AH, Francisco GE. Intrathecal baclofen therapy for spastic hypertonia. *Phys Med Rehabil Clin N Am*. 2001;12(4):923–938.

229. Grabb PA, Guin-Renfroe S, Meythaler JM. Midthoracic catheter tip placement for intrathecal baclofen administration in children with quadriparetic spasticity. *Neurosurgery*. 1999;45(4):833–836.

230. McCall TD, MacDonald JD. Cervical catheter tip placement for intrathecal baclofen administration. *Neurosurgery*. 2006;59(3):634–640.

231. Burns AS, Meythaler JM. Intrathecal baclofen in tetraplegia of spinal origin: efficacy for upper extremity hypertonia. *Spinal Cord*. 2001;39:413–419.

232. Chappuis DM, Boortz-Marx RL, Stuckey MW, et al. Safety of continuously infused intrathecal baclofen in the cervical and high thoracic areas for patients with spasticity, dystonia, and movement disorders. *Arch Phys Med Rehabil*. 2002;83:1676.

233. Middleton JW, Siddall PJ, Walker S, et al. Intrathecal clonidine and baclofen in the management of spasticity and neuropathic pain following spinal cord injury: a case study. *Arch Phys Med Rehabil*. 1996;77(8):824–826.

234. Remy-Neris O, Denys P, Bussel B. Intrathecal clonidine for controlling spastic hypertonia. *Phys Med Rehabil Clin N Am*. 2001;12(4):939–951.

235. Chabal C, Jacobson L, Terman G. Intrathecal fentanyl alleviates spasticity in the presence of tolerance to intrathecal baclofen. *Anesthesiology*. 1992;76(2):312–314.

236. Chabal C, Jacobson L, Schwid HA. An objective comparison of intrathecal lidocaine versus fentanyl for the treatment of lower extremity spasticity. *Anesthesiology*. 1991;74(4):643–646.

237. Muller H, Gerlach H, Boldt J, et al. Spasticity treatment with spinal morphine or midazolam. In vitro experiments, animal studies and clinical studies on compatibility and effectiveness. *Anaesthesist*. 1986;35(5):306–316.

238. Erickson DL, Lo J, Michaelson M. Control of intractable spasticity with intrathecal morphine sulfate. *Neurosurgery*. 1989;24(2):236–238.

239. Erickson DL, Blacklock JB, Michaelson M, et al. Control of spasticity by implantable continuous flow morphine pump. *Neurosurgery*. 1985;16(2):215–217.

240. Sadiq SA, Poopatana CA. Intrathecal baclofen and morphine in multiple sclerosis patients with severe pain and spasticity. *J Neurol*. 2007;254(10):1464–1465.

241. Saulino M. Simultaneous treatment of intractable pain and spasticity: observations of combined intrathecal baclofen-morphine therapy over a 10-year clinical experience. *Eur J Phys Rehabil Med*. 2012;48(1):39–45.

242. Vidal J, Gregori P, Guevara D, et al. Efficacy of intrathecal morphine in the treatment of baclofen tolerance in a patient on intrathecal baclofen therapy (ITB). *Spinal Cord*. 2004;42(1):50–51.

243. Soni BM, Mani RM, Oo T, et al. Treatment of spasticity in a spinal cord-injured patient with intrathecal morphine due to intrathecal baclofen tolerance—a case report and review of literature. *Spinal Cord*. 2003;41:586–589.

244. Lydon AM, Cooke T, Duggan F, et al. Delayed postoperative gastric emptying following intrathecal morphine and intrathecal bupivacaine. *Can J Anaesth*. 1999;46(6):544–549.

245. Glass PS. Respiratory depression following only 0.4 mg of intrathecal morphine. *Anesthesiology*. 1984;60(3):256–257.

246. Remy-Neris O, Barbeau H, Daniel O, et al. Effects of intrathecal clonidine injection on spinal reflexes and human locomotion in incomplete paraplegic subjects. *Exp Brain Res*. 1999;129(3):433–440.

247. Chartier-Kastler E, Azouvi P, Yakovleff A, et al. Intrathecal catheter with subcutaneous port for clonidine test bolus injection. A new route and type of treatment for detrusor hyperreflexia in spinal cord-injured patients. *Eur Urol*. 2000;37(1):14–17.

248. Denys P, Chartier-Kastler E, Azouvi P, et al. Intrathecal clonidine for refractory detrusor hyperreflexia in spinal cord injured patients: a preliminary report. *J Urol*. 1998;160(6 pt 1):2137–2138.

249. Kroin JS, McCarthy RJ, Penn RD, et al. Intrathecal clonidine and tizanidine in conscious dogs: comparison of analgesic and hemodynamic effects. *Anesth Analg*. 1996;82(3):627–635.

250. Malinovsky JM, Cozian A, Lepage JY, et al. Ketamine and midazolam neurotoxicity in the rabbit. *Anesthesiology*. 1991;75(1):91–97.

251. Erdine S, Yucel A, Ozyalcin S, et al. Neurotoxicity of midazolam in the rabbit. *Pain*. 1999;80(1–2):419–423.

252. Boscarino LF, Ounpuu S, Davis RB III, et al. Effects of selective dorsal rhizotomy on gait in children with cerebral palsy. *J Pediatr Orthop*. 1993;13(2):174–179.

253. Gul SM, Steinbok P, McLeod K. Long-term outcome after selective posterior rhizotomy in children with spastic cerebral palsy. *Pediatr Neurosurg*. 1999;31(2):84–95.

254. Hodgkinson I, Berard C, Jindrich ML, et al. Selective dorsal rhizotomy in children with cerebral palsy. Results in 18 cases at one year postoperatively. *Stereotact Funct Neurosurg*. 1997;69(1–4 pt 2):259–267.

255. Wright FV, Sheil EM, Drake JM, et al. Evaluation of selective dorsal rhizotomy for the reduction of spasticity in cerebral palsy: a randomized controlled trial. *Dev Med Child Neurol*. 1998;40(4):239–247.

256. Morrison G, Yashon D, White RJ. Relief of pain and spasticity by anterior dorsolumbar rhizotomy in multiple sclerosis. *Ohio State Med J*. 1969;65(6):588–591.

257. Sindou M, Millet MF, Mortamais J, et al. Results of selective posterior rhizotomy in the treatment of painful and spastic paraplegia secondary to multiple sclerosis. *Appl Neurophysiol*. 1982;45(3):335–340.

258. Barolat G. Surgical management of spasticity and spasms in spinal cord injury: an overview. *J Am Paraplegia Soc*. 1998;11(1):9–13.

259. Smyth MD, Peacock WJ. The surgical treatment of spasticity. *Muscle Nerve*. 2000;23:153–163.

260. Abbott R. Complications with selective posterior rhizotomy. *Pediatr Neurosurg*. 1992;18(1):43–47.

261. Kim DS, Choi JU, Yang KH, et al. Selective posterior rhizotomy in children with cerebral palsy: a 10-year experience. *Childs Nerv Syst*. 2001;17(9):556–562.

262. Steinbok P, Schrag C. Complications after selective posterior rhizotomy for spasticity in children with cerebral palsy. *Pediatr Neurosurg*. 1998;28(6):300–313.

263. Crul BJ, Blok LM, van EJ, et al. The present role of percutaneous cervical cordotomy for the treatment of cancer pain. *J Headache Pain*. 2005;6(1):24–29.

264. Gildenberg PL. Evolution of spinal cord surgery for pain. *Clin Neurosurg*. 2006;53:11–17.

265. Hong D, Andre-Sandberg A. Punctate midline myelotomy: a minimally invasive procedure for the treatment of pain in inextirpable abdominal and pelvic cancer. *J Pain Symptom Manage*. 2007;33(1):99–109.

266. Elovic E, Zafonte RD. Spasticity management in traumatic brain injury. *Phys Med Rehabil State Art Rev*. 2001;15(2):327–348.

267. Eltorai I, Montroy R. Muscle release in the management of spasticity after spinal cord injury. *Paraplegia*. 1990;28:433–440.

268. Keenan MA. Surgical decision making for residual limb deformities following traumatic brain injury. *Orthop Rev*. 1988;17(12):1185–1192.

269. Keenan MA, Ure K, Smith CW, et al. Hamstring release for knee flexion contracture in spastic adults. *Clin Orthop Relat Res*. 1988;236:221–226.

CHAPTER 41

William Micheo   Luis Baerga-Varela
Gerardo Miranda-Comas   Gerard A. Malanga

Sports Medicine

Sports medicine is an interdisciplinary medical specialty concerned with physical fitness and the diagnosis, treatment, and rehabilitation of injuries sustained in sports activities. An expanded definition and scope of Sports and Exercise Medicine has been proposed by McCrory and includes management of medical problems of exercising individual at all ages and all levels of participation, the physiology, biomechanics, and optimization of human performance, the use of exercise in the promotion of health and the prevention and treatment of disease or injury at a population level (1). In the United States, sports medicine is a subspecialty of Physical Medicine and Rehabilitation (PM&R), Family Medicine, Internal Medicine, Pediatrics and Emergency Medicine or a subspecialty of Orthopedic Surgery, while in many countries around the world, Sports and Exercise Medicine is considered a primary specialty.

Sports medicine is an important area of practice for many PM&R specialists. The PM&R model applies well to sports medicine since the majority of injuries related to sports and exercise participation do not require surgical management, are treated with aggressive conservative care, and are delivered with an interdisciplinary team approach.

Physiatric involvement in the field of sports medicine has greatly increased over the past two decades. The development of sports medicine fellowships with PM&R as the core specialty and subspecialty board certification has played a major role in increasing involvement in the field. Many PM&R specialists are serving as team physicians at the high school, collegiate, Olympic/Paralympics, and professional levels. In addition, there has been increased involvement in professional societies such as American College of Sports Medicine (ACSM) and American Medical Society for Sports Medicine (AMSSM) as members, leaders, and presenters at scientific meetings. Physiatrists are conducting research, publishing book chapters, and scientific articles related to sports medicine and exercise sciences, thus increasing PM&R's contribution to the scientific literature.

Validation of the effectiveness of nonoperative treatment, rehabilitation programs, interventional procedures and preventive strategies of various sports injuries will highlight the role of physiatrists as leaders in sports medicine.

The purpose of this chapter is to present selected concepts pertaining to the evaluation, treatment, rehabilitation, and prevention of sports injuries as well as recent advances in the specialty.

BASIC CONCEPTS OF SPORTS INJURY

Epidemiology of Injury

Understanding the incidence and prevalence of injuries based on variables such as type and nature of the injury, age group, type of sports, sex, and time since the onset of symptoms, among others, has contributed to the development of programs aimed at prevention, treatment, and rehabilitation of sports injuries (2). Athletic injuries occur from acute or chronic overload on the muscles, nerves, tendons, bones, or joints. The knee, shoulder, foot, and ankle are common sites of injury in athletes, and frequent diagnoses include tendinopathies, ligament sprains, and patellofemoral pain (3).

The location, type, and specific diagnoses of injuries seen in athletes are influenced by the particular sport involved. Overhead sports such as baseball, tennis, or volleyball often lead to injuries in the shoulder and elbow that include rotator cuff tendinopathy, shoulder instability, and suprascapular neuropathy. Sports that require trunk rotation, flexion, and extension such as gymnastics, diving, judo, and wrestling lead to trunk and spine injuries such as spondylolysis, disc disease, and facet joint syndrome. Running and jumping sports result in injuries to the knee and ankle, like ankle sprains, patellofemoral pain, and anterior cruciate ligament (ACL) tears of the knee.

The age and sex of the individual also influences the type of athletic injury (2,3). Young and female athletes present with injuries as a result of overuse and ligamentous laxity while older individuals present with degenerative conditions exacerbated by athletic activity.

Physiatrists working as team physicians or traveling with sports teams to different competitions should be prepared to deal with general medical problems in addition to musculoskeletal injuries. Reports on the utilization of health services during international sports competitions have shown that although the most common reason for medical evaluation was musculoskeletal injury (39.1%), many individuals presented with medical problems, including respiratory (17.2%), gastrointestinal (12.2%), and skin (5.8%) complaints (4).

Identification of Risk Factors

Athletic injury can be caused by extrinsic and intrinsic factors, which can be divided into modifiable and nonmodifiable (Table 41-1). Modifiable extrinsic factors include volume of activity, inappropriate equipment, and surfaces in which training and competition occur. Training errors have been reported to account for the majority of running injuries. Running more than 40 to 45 miles per week, excessive running of hills, and doing interval training significantly increase the rate of injury (5).

Intrinsic factors can be modifiable (poor flexibility, muscle weakness, and body mass index) or nonmodifiable (sex, height, ligamentous laxity, and anatomic malalignment) (6–8).

Classification of Injury

A sports injury can be defined as a physical complaint or tissue damage that occurs during an athletic activity, regardless of whether it received medical attention or resulted in time loss from competition or training (6). Sports injuries are usually divided into two basic types: those that result from macrotrauma and those associated with overuse and repetitive microtrauma.

Athletic injury can be classified by mode of onset, mechanism of injury, diagnosis (type of injury), involved body part, severity depending of time loss from competition or training, and using the classification of acute, subacute, chronic, or an acute exacerbation of a chronic injury (6).

Patient Evaluation

Pertinent information that should be obtained in the history includes the type of sport, the mechanism of injury, the severity of the injury, and prior treatment strategies (if any). Information regarding growth and development, menstrual history, previous history of similar or related injuries, training and competition history, and associated medical problems should be obtained. Psychological issues include anxiety associated with competition, parental involvement in sports, abnormal attitude toward eating, and fear of recurrent injury.

TABLE 41-1	Sport Injury Risk Factors
Intrinsic Factors	**Extrinsic Factors**
• Age[a] 　• Skeletal immaturity • Gender[a] • BMI 　• Weight 　• Height[a] • Previous injury[a] • Anatomic misalignment[a] • Muscle fatigue and weakness • Inadequate flexibility 　• Extreme joint laxity 　• Soft tissue tightness	• Biomechanical and physical sports-specific demands • Early sport specialization • Nutritional state • Training equipment and environment

[a]Nonmodifiable.

TABLE 41-2	Framework for Sports-Related Injuries	
Musculoskeletal injuries	Clinical symptoms	Pain Instability Dysfunction
	Anatomic alterations	Tissue injury Tissue overload
	Functional alterations	Biomechanical deficits Subclinical adaptations

The physical exam should identify postural asymmetry, lack of flexibility, muscle weakness and imbalance, neurologic as well as proprioceptive deficits, and ligamentous laxity. It is also important to evaluate core trunk and pelvic muscle strength, dynamic flexibility, and sports-specific techniques.

The treating physician also has the responsibility of ordering and interpreting the appropriate diagnostic studies. These include laboratory tests, x-rays, musculoskeletal ultrasound (US), bone scan, computerized tomography (CT), and magnetic resonance imaging (MRI) (see Chapter 5, Imaging Techniques). Complete diagnosis of athletic injury can be established using a modification of the musculoskeletal injury complex model (7). This model identifies the anatomic site of injuries, the clinical symptoms, and the functional deficits (Table 41-2).

The clinical symptom complex addresses the main complaints of the injured athlete, which include pain, swelling, feeling unstable, numbness, weakness, or change in performance. The anatomic alteration complex identifies the site of the primary injury causing patients the symptoms and associated areas of tissue overload. The functional alteration complex addresses the biomechanical deficits that result from an athletic injury, adaptations used by the athletes who continue to participate in sports and changes in sports and exercise performance.

Principles of Sports Rehabilitation

Rehabilitation of the injured athlete can be divided into acute, recovery, and functional phases. Each phase has specific goals and criteria for progression (Table 41-3). Rehabilitation should start early in the postinjury period to reduce the deleterious effects of inactivity, immobilization, and to reduce the overall level of physical impairment (8).

The acute phase addresses the clinical symptoms and should focus on treating tissue injury. This phase correlates with the

TABLE 41-3	Rehabilitation Goals of Sports-Related Injuries
Acute phase	Treat symptom complex Protect anatomic injury site
Recovery phase	Correct biomechanical deficits Improve muscle control and balance Retrain proprioception Start sports-specific activity
Functional phase	Increase power endurance Improve neuromuscular control Work on entire kinematic chain Return to competition

inflammatory stage of injury in that primary tissue damage is followed by secondary injury, resulting from hypoxia and inflammatory enzymatic activity. The goal at this stage should be to reduce pain and inflammation and promote tissue healing. Reestablishment of nonpainful range of motion (ROM), prevention of muscle atrophy, and maintenance of general fitness should be addressed.

Therapeutic strategies used in this phase include ice, electrical stimulation, static exercise, and protected ROM exercise. Cryotherapy, transcutaneous nerve or high-voltage galvanic electrical stimulation, and analgesics or a short course of nonsteroidal anti-inflammatory drugs (NSAIDs) medication should be used early in the rehabilitation process to reduce pain, inflammation, and muscle inhibition. In addition, orthotic equipment can be used to protect the injured part.

Static muscle contractions are used to maintain muscle strength if dynamic exercise is detrimental to injured tissue. Static contractions should be performed at multiple joint angles, using a maximal voluntary effort, with repetitions lasting 5 to 10 seconds. If pain or swelling inhibits voluntary muscle contraction, low-voltage electrical stimulation used in combination with static exercise can facilitate muscle recruitment (9). Active exercise should be started as soon as the patient can tolerate minimal external load through pain-free ROM. Pain and swelling control should be accomplished prior to progressing to the next rehabilitation phase.

The recovery phase correlates with the fibroblastic repair stage, in which inflammatory changes at the site of the injury are replaced by granulation tissue. This phase should focus on obtaining normal passive and active range of motion (PROM and AROM), improving muscle control, achieving normal muscle balance, and working on proprioception. Loading of injured tissues should be done in a progressive manner since the tensile strength of affected tissue may be reduced. Biomechanical and functional deficits including lack of flexibility and inability to run or jump should be addressed in this phase (see Chapter 49, Exercise).

Therapeutic strategies used include superficial heat, ultrasound, soft tissue laser and electrical stimulation, as well as flexibility and strengthening exercises. In addition, proprioceptive retraining for the upper and lower extremities should be undertaken.

Flexibility training includes both static and dynamic techniques (10). Muscles that cross two joints such as the hamstrings are prone to shorten as a result of injury and require static stretching. Improvement in flexibility could result from static stretching, and stretching is recommended for 30 seconds, at least three times a day for a total of three repetitions. Changes in muscle length can be expected after 7 days, and the benefits of daily stretching can last to up to 21 days (9,11). Proprioceptive neuromuscular facilitation techniques that include contract-relax and contract-relax-antagonist-contract methods can be used with individual repetitions lasting 10 seconds (12).

Dynamic flexibility in which training is performed in the sagittal, frontal, and transverse planes of motion combining eccentric, static, and concentric muscle actions in a functional manner can be incorporated in this stage of rehabilitation.

Dynamic strengthening exercises are very important during the recovery phase of rehabilitation. Open kinetic chain (OKC) exercises allow joint isolation and train both the concentric and eccentric phases of muscle contraction. Eccentric muscle contractions generate the greatest muscle force and consequent adaptation, important in the rehabilitation of tendinopathy but have to be used judiciously since this type of exercise can result in muscle damage (8). Loading the muscle gradually allows recovery of tissue tensile strength and reduces the pain and swelling associated with delayed onset muscle soreness. Resistive exercises that attempt to reproduce sports-specific actions should be added to the rehabilitation program when isolated single-joint exercises can be performed through a full ROM.

Closed kinetic chain (CKC) exercises that involve multiple joints and muscle cocontraction are also used. These exercises emphasize sequential movement of functionally related joints, control joint centers of motion, and transfer of applied loads (10,13). In addition, these exercises can reduce strain, translation loads, and shear in injured or operated knee ligaments and allow the transition to functional activities of the lower limb following injury (14). In patients with shoulder instability, closed chain exercises that result in scapular and rotator cuff muscle coactivation are beneficial to emphasize proximal stability (15).

Core muscle strengthening is incorporated into functional rehabilitation. Strengthening of abdominal, gluteal, hip girdle, paraspinal, and pelvic floor muscles is important since these stabilize the spine, allow a stable platform for sports activity, act as force generators, and transfer links in the kinetic chain and decelerators. The dynamic spine stabilization program has been used as a base for the development of progressive functional core exercise (16,17).

Proprioceptive training is also an important component of this phase. Proprioception can be defined in the clinical context as a complex neuromuscular process that involves afferent input and efferent responses and allows the body to maintain stability during static and dynamic activities. Proprioception has been found to be trainable, and improvement in function can be expected despite changes in joint laxity following injury (18). Exercises to retrain proprioception and balance typically progress from standing on both legs on a stable supported surface to single limb exercises with eyes open and closed.

Sports-specific training should be initiated in this stage. Progression of the training without recurrence of symptoms is necessary prior to advancing to the functional stage.

The functional phase correlates with the maturation and remodeling stage of tissue healing, in which the tensile strength of the granulation tissue increases and the collagen fibers are realigned. This phase should focus on increasing strength, power, and endurance while improving neuromuscular control. Emphasis is placed on working on the entire kinematic chain addressing specific functional deficits. This program should be continuous with the ultimate goal of prevention of recurrent injury.

Therapeutic strategies used in this stage typically include plyometric exercises, progressive overload whole body vibration, and increased complexity of sports-specific tasks. Plyometrics combine eccentric muscle activity prior to a concentric contraction and are used to gain power and in sports-specific training to improve technique (9).

Return to Play Considerations

Once the athlete completes a rehabilitation program, the decision to clear the individual to practice his/her sport and finally to participate in competition must be made. This decision should be based on clinical evaluation, results of objective tests, and psychologic readiness and not solely on the absence of symptoms and time elapsed from injury or surgery.

Factors to consider include the type of sport and position played, the treatment or surgery offered to the patient, absence of symptoms at rest and with sports activity, normal flexibility, strength and neuromuscular control based on clinical evaluation, isokinetic dynamometry, and functional tests. Patient satisfaction with the treatment offered, sense of confidence with sports activity and psychologic readiness to participate in sports need to be addressed prior to returning to play and may require the use of validated questionnaires (19,20).

Prevention of Sports Injury

For the athlete who returns to practice and competition, prevention of recurrent injury is very important. Prevention programs have been developed for athletes who have not been injured (primary prevention) and for those who have been injured (secondary prevention). Prehabilitation is defined as conditioning strategies for athletes susceptible to injury because of sports-specific demands, and in formerly injured athletes, to prepare them for the stresses and demands of their sport. Prevention programs focus on education about the injury and modifiable intrinsic and extrinsic risk factors (see **Table 41-1**) (19).

Components of a prehabilitation program include stretching, strengthening, proprioception, and plyometric exercises. Thacker reported that while stretching has been found to improve flexibility (especially static flexibility), it has not been conclusively shown to reduce the risk of injury and in the immediate poststretching period, loss of strength has adverse effects on jump and running performance (10). Conditioning strategies and appropriate warm-up using sports-specific dynamic movements can be better alternatives to reduce injury risk.

Strengthening exercises are known to reduce the risk of injury. Eccentric exercise, in particular, has been found to reduce the risk of hamstring strains in elite athletes and should be included as part of the training and prehabilitation program for the running athlete (21). Balance training, learning how to fall from a jump, modifying cutting techniques, and plyometric exercises that activate the hamstrings have been found to reduce the risk of ACL injuries in athletes and should be integrated into injury prevention programs (21,22).

MANAGEMENT OF UPPER LIMB INJURIES (SEE CHAPTER 29, DISORDERS OF THE UPPER LIMBS)

Shoulder Injuries

The glenohumeral joint has a high degree of mobility at the expense of stability. Static and dynamic restraints maintain the shoulder in place with overhead activity. Muscle action, particularly of the rotator cuff and scapular stabilizers, is important in maintaining joint congruity in midranges of motion. Static stabilizers such as the glenohumeral ligaments, joint capsule, and glenoid labrum are important for stability in the extremes of motion (23).

Acute Injuries

Glenohumeral Dislocation

Anterior dislocation of the glenohumeral joint usually results from a fall on an outstretched externally rotated and abducted arm. A blow to the posterior aspect of the shoulder can also result in anterior dislocation. Posterior dislocation usually results from a fall on the forward flexed and adducted arm or by direct blow in the posterior direction when the arm is above the shoulder. An acutely dislocated shoulder can usually be recognized by the position of the arm. In anterior dislocation, the arm is held in external rotation while the humeral head can be palpated anterior to the glenoid. Posterior dislocations present with internal rotation and posterior fullness of the shoulder (24).

In acute anterior dislocation, the injured individual presents with pain, decreased active motion, and deformity. If the injury was observed, the mechanism of injury is clear, and no evidence of neurologic or vascular damage is evident on the clinical exam, reduction can be attempted (24). There are multiple techniques that have been described for reduction of an anterior shoulder dislocation. Classic maneuvers include the Stimson and Milch techniques, but more recently, the Spaso technique and the Fast, Reliable, and Safe (FARES) method have been described with good outcomes (25). If there is a suspicion of fracture or posterior dislocation, the patient should undergo radiologic evaluation prior to attempting a reduction. The x-rays should be repeated after the reduction.

There is some controversy regarding the treatment of first-time anterior dislocations. Although some clinicians have recommended immobilization for as long as 6 weeks, it appears that the time of immobilization is not related to improved outcome. Many advocate functional rehabilitation following a period of immobilization until the patient is pain free and able to progress in the treatment program.

Age is a very important factor in management since younger patients have a higher rate of recurrence (26). The young athlete returning to competition after shoulder dislocation should be advised about the possibility of recurrence and the future need for surgical intervention. In the case of the older adolescent and adult overhead athlete with a traumatic dislocation of the throwing arm, early surgical intervention is recommended (27).

Acromioclavicular Dislocation

Dislocations of the acromioclavicular (AC) joint are caused by a direct blow on the posterior aspect of the acromion and spine of the scapula such as when a player falls on the tip of his shoulder. They are classified from type 1 to type 6 based on the anatomic relationship between the acromion and the clavicle following the injury. Type 1 AC dislocations represent complete tears of the capsule with no major break in continuity between the acromion and clavicle. Type 2 dislocations involve a complete tear of the capsule and sprain of the coracoclavicular ligaments. Point tenderness is associated with this ligamentous disruption, and on visual examination the distal end of the clavicle is prominent. Type 3 lesions involve a complete disruption of both the joint capsule and coracoclavicular ligaments. Type 4 injury results in posterior dislocation of the clavicle relative to the acromion, type 5 shows superior displacement of the clavicle through the trapezius with more than 100% of clavicle displacement, and type 6 shows inferior displacement of the clavicle (28).

Physical examination reveals an obvious depression of the scapula with elevation of the clavicle, localized tenderness to palpation, and limited active shoulder motion. Radiographic examination should be performed to assess degree of injury.

Nonoperative treatment is used for type 1 and type 2 injuries. A sling is used to support the upper limb at rest until the athlete is pain free. Heavy lifting and contact sports should be avoided until full ROM, scapular control, and normal strength are restored, with no pain on joint palpation. In type 1 injuries, this process usually takes 2 weeks but can take up to 6 weeks in type 2 injuries.

The treatment of a type 3 AC dislocation is somewhat controversial. Some clinicians recommend surgical intervention, while others prefer conservative treatment and rehabilitation after a period of immobilization. Type 4 to type 6 injuries require surgical treatment (29).

Overuse Injuries

Rotator Cuff Injury

Overload of the rotator cuff can occur with recurrent overhead sports activity. The resulting symptoms of reduced motion, muscle weakness, and pain can interfere with activity. In the young patient, rotator cuff overload is often associated with shoulder instability (15). The repeated stress of throwing places great demands on the dynamic and static stabilizers of the glenohumeral joint, including the rotator cuff, ligaments, capsule, and glenoid labrum. These biomechanical stress leads to increased translation of the humeral head and to pain associated with external subacromial or secondary impingement of the rotator cuff. The individual reports that the shoulder slips out of the joint or that the arm goes "dead." Weakness with overhead activity is also a frequent complaint. Some patients present with symptoms associated with internal impingement. In these cases, the rotator cuff tendon is compressed against the superoposterior aspect of the glenoid labrum with repeated abduction and external rotation particularly in the early phases of the throwing motion (15).

Older athletes can present with primary impingement associated with a curved or hooked acromion, osteophytes of the AC joint, or thickened coracoacromial ligament. These can cause rotator cuff symptoms with abduction of the arm. Symptoms of pain at rest, particularly at night in the older athlete, can be due to a rotator cuff tear.

The physical examination should start with inspection for the presence of deformity, atrophy of muscle, asymmetry, and scapular dyskinesia. Palpation of soft tissue and bone should be systematic and includes the rotator cuff, biceps tendon, subacromial and AC regions, and the glenohumeral joint.

Passive and active range of shoulder motion should be evaluated. Differences between passive and active motion can be secondary to pain, weakness, or neurologic damage. Repeated overhead activity in baseball can lead to an increase in external rotation accompanied by a reduction in internal rotation (30). Participation in tennis can result in an internal rotation deficit with less of an increase in external rotation. Strength testing should be performed to identify weakness of specific muscles of the rotator cuff and the scapular stabilizers, in particular the infraspinatus, lower trapezius, and serratus anterior. The supraspinatus muscle can be tested in the scapular plane with internal rotation or the so-called "empty can" position. The external rotators can be tested with the arm at the side of the body, and the subscapularis muscle can be tested by using the "lift-off test" in which the palm of the hand is lifted away from the lower back. The scapular stabilizers such as the serratus anterior and lower trapezius muscle by doing standing pushups against a wall. Sensory and motor exam of the shoulder girdle should always be performed to rule out nerve injuries (31).

Rotator cuff external impingement can be assessed by testing the shoulder in 90 degrees of forward flexion with internal rotation, or extreme forward flexion with the forearm pronated. Glenohumeral translation testing looking for laxity (asymptomatic) or instability (associated with symptoms) should be documented. Apprehension testing can be performed with the patient sitting, standing, or in the supine position. The shoulder joint is stressed in abduction and external rotation, looking for reproduction of the feeling of instability in the patient. A relocation maneuver that reduces the symptoms also aids in the diagnosis (31). The individual with internal impingement presents with posterior shoulder pain rather than apprehension in this position of shoulder abduction and external rotation.

Other tests include the load and shift maneuver to document humeral head translation in anterior or posterior directions, the sulcus sign to document inferior humeral head laxity, and the active compression test. This test involves a downward force applied to the forward flexed, adducted, and internally rotated shoulder looking for reproduction of pain associated with labral tears or AC joint pathology (32). The across chest adduction maneuver can also be used to reproduce AC symptomatology.

The goals of nonsurgical management of rotator cuff injury include reducing pain, restoring full motion, correction of muscle strength deficits, achieving muscle balance, and returning to full activity free of symptoms (33–35). Static and closed chain exercises to the rotator cuff and scapular stabilizers and pain-free ROM of the shoulder as well as strengthening of the trunk and lower extremities should be started as early as possible. Biomechanical and functional deficits such as glenohumeral internal rotation deficits and throwing motion abnormalities should be addressed. Functional activities should be started, including squats, lunges, and rotational exercises to improve core and lower extremities muscle strength. Sports-specific training should also be incorporated into the treatment program (33–35). A supervised throwing program is required prior to returning to sports participation.

Shoulder Instability

The spectrum of shoulder instability ranges from acute traumatic dislocation (which is usually unidirectional) to recurrent subluxation not related to trauma. Patients with recurrent instability can have a history of recurrent dislocations, but more commonly that of subluxation or pain associated with repeated overhead activity (36). The patient can complain of weakness, locking, transient giving way of the shoulder, or having a "dead arm." Some patients present with impingement symptoms of the rotator cuff secondary to failure of the capsuloligamentous structures that stabilize the shoulder at the extremes of ROM (23).

The key to diagnosing recurrent shoulder instability is the demonstration of asymmetry of glenohumeral translation from side to side. This is particularly important in the patient with evidence of generalized ligamentous laxity, who might also exhibit laxity of other joints as demonstrated by hyperextension of the elbow and knee. The shoulder exam should emphasize maneuvers for instability or labral injury.

The initial treatment of patients with multidirectional or microtraumatic shoulder instability is nonoperative. Symptom reduction is the first goal. This is followed by rehabilitation addressing weakness of the scapular stabilizers and rotator cuff muscles. Emphasis should be placed on working the scapular and rotator cuff muscles in "closed chain" cocontraction methods which emphasizes joint stability (33,34).

In patients with failed rehabilitation, recurrent episodes of instability or those who suffered injury to the dominant extremity and participate in overhead sports surgical reconstructive surgery should be considered. Open versus arthroscopic repair techniques can be considered, based on factors such as age and the cause of the instability (previous shoulder dislocations or generalized ligamentous laxity) (37–39).

ELBOW INJURIES

Elbow injuries resulting from repetitive overuse can be seen often in overhead sports. In other sports such as gymnastics, judo, and basketball, elbow injuries are less common but can occur from repeated upper limb activity or trauma such as falling on an outstretched arm. Forces that can damage the elbow include valgus stress to the medial structures, compression of the lateral structures, and extension overload of the posterior structures. Because of a stable joint structure, single traumatic events require substantial forces to result in fracture or dislocation.

Acute Injuries

Elbow Fractures and Dislocations

Single-event injuries are most often a result of collision of an outstretched hand with the ground. If the elbow is somewhat flexed, posterolateral dislocation can occur. If the elbow is fully extended, transmission of force up the radius can result in a fracture of the radial head or capitellum. Varus/valgus shear forces at the time of impact can result in fracture of the condylar and supracondylar structures. Direct impact on the elbow is another mechanism of injury that can result in fractures about the elbow, usually to the olecranon (40).

The basics of treatment of fractures of the elbow region include early reduction, management of associated injuries, ongoing assessment of the neurovascular status, and early protected ROM to minimize the risk of contracture. In most cases, complete immobilization should not exceed 2 weeks. Use of a removable splint that permits active elbow ROM including flexion-extension and supination-pronation can be used early in the rehabilitation process. By 10 to 14 days, if the fracture or dislocation is stable, the splint should be discontinued and full elbow flexibility and strengthening begun (41). On return to play, the elbow can be braced or taped to limit elbow hyperextension and for protection from valgus forces.

Overuse Injuries

Epicondylopathy, Ligament, and Nerve Injuries

Injuries to soft tissue include lateral or medial epicondylopathy, ulnar collateral ligament (UCL) sprain, and ulnar neuropathy (42).

The patient with lateral epicondylopathy complains of pain anterior and distal to the lateral elbow associated with gripping and excessive use of the wrist extensor musculature, usually the extensor carpi radialis brevis (42). The pain is increased on resisted wrist extension with the elbow extended and the forearm pronated. The examination typically shows localized tenderness anterior to the lateral epicondyle over the forearm extensors origin, weakness of wrist extension due to pain inhibition of function, and loss of passive wrist flexion in chronic cases.

Management includes relative rest, icing, and therapeutic modalities as well as NSAIDs. Stretching of the wrist extensors is initially performed with the elbow bent and progressed to stretching with extended elbow and pronated forearm. This should be combined with eccentric strengthening in different wrist positions (43). A local corticosteroid injection may provide adequate short-term relief of symptoms to patients who present with pain at rest or cannot tolerate rehabilitation interventions, but regenerative techniques, such as platelet-rich plasma (PRP) may be more beneficial in the long term (44). The use of a counterforce brace to reduce the load on the extensor muscles has been advocated when athletes return to practice or competition (45). Evaluation of appropriate sports-specific technique is important prior to allowing return to sports.

Athletes with medial epicondylopathy typically have injury to the forearm flexor and pronator muscle groups associated with tensile overload. Pain occurs distal to the medial epicondyle at the origin of the flexor/pronator group and increases with resisted forearm pronation or wrist flexion (42). Weakness of shoulder girdle and trunk muscles is also present in many individuals with this condition.

Management includes symptom control combined with stretching and strengthening of the flexor/pronator muscle group. The program should also include strengthening of the shoulder girdle, trunk, and lower limb muscles. In severe cases, local injection with corticosteroids, or regenerative techniques such as PRP and counterforce bracing, may be used as previously described for lateral epicondylopathy (44,45).

Some patients with chronic medial elbow region symptoms have injury to the capsule and ligamentous structures, or of the ulnar nerve. The symptoms are related to repeated activity in which valgus and extension forces are applied to the elbow. The throwing athlete typically complains of medial elbow pain during the late cocking and acceleration phases of throwing. As a result, there is loss of throwing velocity and control. Physical examination shows tenderness over the medial side of the elbow joint. Stability testing with the elbow in 20 to 30 degrees of flexion can reproduce pain symptoms in UCL injury (42). Patients with ulnar neuropathy can present with pain or paresthesias in the distribution of the nerve. In many instances, sensory symptoms might not be present at rest and are only reproduced following activity.

Management of medial injury to the UCL includes avoiding activities with valgus stress, strengthening of the whole upper limb kinetic chain, and improvement of sports-specific technique such as leading with the elbow when pitching. Surgical reconstruction is needed in some cases, but only after failure of an appropriate rehabilitation program of 3 to 6 months' duration (46).

Ulnar neuropathy typically occurs in the cubital tunnel and can be treated with an elbow pad to avoid direct pressure over the nerve. In severe cases, it might be necessary to use an elbow orthosis that holds the elbow in 45 degrees of flexion. In the early stages of recovery, the orthosis should be worn during most of the day. As the patient's symptoms improve, it should be used only at night. Appropriate stretching, strengthening of the whole kinetic chain, and sports biomechanics should also be addressed (43).

WRIST AND HAND INJURIES

Hand and upper limb injuries are among the most common injuries sustained by athletes, comprising 3% to 9% of sports injuries. Unfortunately, there is a tendency to minimize their severity as the hand does not bear weight and the injuries rarely render the athlete unable to compete. Although soft tissue injuries are more common, fractures are also seen quite frequently, more common in adolescents than in adults due to epiphyseal trauma (47).

Acute Injuries

Wrist and Hand Fractures

The scaphoid (navicular) is the most commonly fractured carpal bone. The mechanism of injury is usually a fall on the outstretched hand causing hyperextension of the wrist.

The patient presents with complaints of wrist pain localized to the anatomic snuffbox and x-rays including ulnar deviation views should be obtained. If the x-rays are negative, but there is a strong clinical suspicion of fracture, a thumb spica splint could be applied for 2 weeks and the x-rays repeated after 14 days. A bone scan or MRI can be performed, particularly in the elite athlete, to rule out a fracture when the x-rays are negative. Early diagnosis is important to avoid postfracture avascular necrosis (47).

The treatment of a nondisplaced scaphoid fracture consists of a thumb spica cast for approximately 6 to 8 weeks until the fracture is clinically and radiographically healed. The more proximal the fracture of the scaphoid, the longer it will take to heal, due to compromise of its blood supply. Early open reduction and internal fixation are recommended as the treatment of choice if the scaphoid fracture is proximal or displaced. An open reduction and internal fixation is frequently used in the elite competitive athlete to shorten the recovery time. The athlete usually returns to sports within 3 to 4 months after an open reduction (47).

Fractures due to athletic trauma are typically stable because of the low energy involved as a cause of the injury. Phalangeal fractures constitute more than half of all hand fractures and are associated with crush injury or a direct blow to the hand. In basketball, the most common fracture is in the distal phalanx of the middle finger. These fractures are usually stabilized by the nail plate dorsally and the pulp septa volarly, and when nondisplaced treated with an extension splint for 3 weeks. Displaced distal phalanx fractures require referral for possible surgical treatment (47).

Middle and proximal phalanx fractures usually occur as a result of a direct blow to the finger. Fractures having no malrotation and minimal angulation can be treated with splinting or "buddy taping" to the next finger. The athletes can return to competition as soon as there is no tenderness over the fracture site. Closed reduction and percutaneous pin fixation might

be required if the alignment is unacceptable or the fracture is displaced. Special attention is required when dealing with adolescents because the physeal plate at the base of the phalanx can be involved (48).

Metacarpal fractures are very common and represent up to 36% of all hand injuries. Metacarpal fractures that involve the middle and ring fingers are usually more stable than those of the index and small fingers. This is due to the support provided by the transverse metacarpal ligament. The treatment of metacarpal fractures is closed reduction and splinting for 3 to 4 weeks followed by active ROM. Fractures through the diaphysis of the metacarpals tend to shorten or rotate as well as angulate, and surgery is necessary in some cases (48).

The thumb is frequently traumatized because of its unprotected position. Thumb fractures are usually caused by impact to the radial side of the thumb and typically occur at the proximal one third of the thumb metacarpal. Fracture angulation is usually in adduction and volar flexion. Closed treatment can be used if there is only minimal angulation. Fractures to moderate degrees of angulation or malrotation usually require open reduction and internal fixation.

Hand Dislocations

Dorsal dislocation of the PIP joint is a common dislocation in sports. For a dorsal dislocation to occur, the volar plate must be torn, leading to a dorsal displacement of the middle phalanx of the finger.

The treatment of this dislocation is immediate reduction on the field, followed by buddy taping for 3 to 6 weeks. The player can return to competition immediately after a reduction using buddy taping, but when not playing, the athlete should have the joint immobilized with a dorsal splint in 30 degrees of flexion to promote the healing of the volar plate (48). Inadequately treated dorsal dislocations can develop a pseudo-boutonnière deformity.

Hand Tendon Injuries

Injuries to the flexor or extensor tendons of the hand are often believed to be minor and go untreated. However, if these are not diagnosed and treated early in the course of injury, permanent deformity can result.

The most common of the closed tendon injuries of the hand is the mallet finger. It is caused by direct impact against an extended distal interphalangeal joint (DIP). The patient presents with pain, swelling on the dorsum of the joint, and an inability to extend the joint. This injury usually involves the terminal extensor tendon, but it can also be associated with an avulsion fracture of the dorsal aspect of the distal phalanx at the DIP joint. Treatment of injury to the substance of the extensor tendon consists of applying a dorsal splint in extension. The splint is used continuously for 6 weeks, followed by an additional 4 weeks of dorsal night splinting to prevent the recurrence of the deformity. It is important that the athlete wears a protective splint maintaining the DIP in extension for approximately 2 months to protect the joint during competition. It should be noted that good results can be obtained with treatment 3 to 4 months after the injury (48).

An avulsion fracture of the dorsal aspect of the DIP joint that does not involve the articular surface can be treated with dorsal splinting, but surgery may be required if the fracture involves more than a third of the articular surface.

A traumatically induced boutonnière deformity occurs as a result of an injury to the central slip of the extensor tendon at or near its insertion into the base of middle phalanx. The cause is usually a blow to the dorsal aspect of the middle phalanx that forces the digit into flexion while the athlete is actively extending the PIP joint. It can also be caused by unrecognized palmar dislocation of the PIP joint that spontaneously reduced or reduced on the field by the athlete.

The clinical presentation of the boutonnière deformity is weakness of PIP extension or an extensor deficit, accompanied by swelling, pain, and tenderness at the dorsal aspect of the joint. The classic deformity of flexion of the PIP and hyperextension of the DIP joints is rarely seen acutely. If the injury goes untreated, the central slip retracts, the triangular ligament becomes stretched, and the lateral bands fall palmar to the axis of rotation flex the PIP joint and hyperextend the DIP joint.

The treatment of choice of an acute boutonnière deformity is the use of a volar splint as early as possible after the injury. This palmar splint holds the metacarpophalangeal (MP) and PIP joint in extension, while allowing active and passive flexion of the DIP joint. DIP flexion is important because it helps the lateral bands maintain the anatomic position at the PIP joint. The splint should be worn continuously for 5 to 6 weeks, an additional 2 weeks as a night splint. After 5 weeks of splinting, gentle active and passive ROM exercises are begun at the PIP joint. In the event that the boutonnière deformity has developed, surgical release with reconstruction might be necessary.

Avulsion of the flexor digitorum profundus (FDP) tendon, also known as "Jersey" finger, is a relatively common injury seen in many sports. It is most common in American football, usually occurs in the ring finger, with the mechanism of injury being forceful extension of the finger during maximum contraction of the FDP. The athlete presents acutely with swelling and pain of the palmar aspect of the hand, and inability to actively flex the DIP joint of the involved finger.

This injury is classified into three types: type 1 in which the FDP tendon retracts into the palm of the hand and the patient presents with pain and swelling at the level of the lumbrical muscles; type 2 in which the FDP tendon retracts back to the level of the PIP joint and is held there by the intact long vinculum; type 3 when the avulsion of the profundus tendon is associated with a large bony fragment that is held in place by the A-4 pulley. Radiographs of the hand usually show a bony fragment just proximal to the DIP joint. The treatment for this injury is usually surgical, and type 1 requires early intervention because the tendon retracted to the palm may have compromised blood supply (48).

Hand Ligamentous Injuries

Skier's or Gamekeeper's thumb is the most common soft tissue injury of the thumb and is due to rupture of the UCL. This injury occurs from a fall on the hand or from trauma associated with excessive thumb abduction and hyperextension. The ligaments can be partially or completely torn. Failure to diagnose this injury can lead to chronic instability. First- and second-degree tears can be treated with immobilization with a short-arm thumb spica cast for 4 weeks. After 2 weeks, the cast can be changed, and if the patient is pain free, a removable splint can be used and ROM exercises started (47).

Stress radiographs or dynamic evaluation with ultrasound can help make the diagnosis when the UCL is completely torn. The radiographs are also helpful in detecting an avulsion fracture. A nondisplaced avulsion fracture can be treated with a cast for 4 to 6 weeks. Operative treatment should be considered if the avulsion fracture is greater than 10% to 15% of the articular surface, displacement is more than 2 to 3 mm or if angulation is present (47).

The most common wrist ligament injury is scapholunate dissociation, which usually results from a fall on an outstretched hand with excessive wrist extension and ulnar deviation. The patient presents with pain and swelling in the dorsal aspect of the wrist. The scaphoid shift maneuver (also known as Watson's test) can be performed by applying dorsal stress to the scaphoid as the wrist is moved from ulnar to radial deviation. Reproduction of the pain and/or hearing a pop constitutes a positive test (49).

In a severe injury, a separation of 2 to 3 mm between the scaphoid and the lunate can be seen on posteroanterior radiographs. Less severe injuries with dynamic partial scapholunate dissociations can sometimes be demonstrated on clenched fist or radial-ulnar deviation views (49).

Treatment of acute static scapholunate ligament dissociation is surgical, with closed reduction and pinning, or with open reduction and repair of the ligament. Acute partial ligament injuries without any of the collapse deformities are best treated in a short-arm thumb spica cast for at least 6 weeks (49).

Overuse Injuries

Wrist Impingement

Dorsal wrist impingement syndromes are common in all sports where repetitive dorsiflexion of the wrist occurs during axial loading. Gymnasts have a high incidence of wrist pain that can be associated with dorsal wrist capsulitis, dorsiflexion impaction syndrome, and distal radius stress reaction or fractures. In addition, ulnar impaction syndrome and triangular fibrocartilage complex damage can occur with repeated pronation and ulnar deviation on the weight-bearing forearm (50). The patient presents with swelling and tenderness of the distal wrist and has limited wrist extension and pain with motion. Management includes splinting, rest from weight-bearing activities, NSAIDs, and in some instances local injection with corticosteroids.

Wrist and Hand Tenosynovitis

De Quervain's syndrome is a tenosynovitis of the first dorsal compartment of the wrist (abductor pollicis longus and the extensor pollicis brevis tendon) that occurs in activities requiring forceful grasp, coupled with radial and ulnar deviation, as well as repetitive use of the thumb. Pain over the radial aspect of the wrist is the most common presenting symptom. The physical examination shows tenderness of the first dorsal compartment of the wrist and reproduction of symptoms with the Finkelstein's test. This test is done by having the patient place the thumb inside a fist and radially deviating the wrist, with reproduction of the patient's pain. The initial treatment for this condition is rest, immobilization and NSAIDs. Physical therapy modalities such as ultrasound and electrical stimulation can also be helpful. If the patient does not improve, an ultrasound-guided steroid injection in the first dorsal compartment of the wrist can be of benefit. In the rare case in which conservative measures fail, a surgical release of the first dorsal compartment is indicated (50).

The extensor carpi ulnaris (ECU) is the second most common site for tenosynovitis in the wrist. It presents as pain and swelling along the dorsal ulnar aspect of the wrist. It commonly occurs in tennis players due to repetitive twisting and ulnar deviation of the wrist. The initial treatment is NSAIDs and splinting. If this fails, an ultrasound-guided injection with a corticosteroid into the area of the tendon sheath is usually effective. In rare recalcitrant cases, surgical release of the tendon sheath along with repair might have to be performed (50). Technical factors such as extreme ulnar deviation with the forehand stroke in tennis players needs to be addressed.

Trigger finger or stenosing tenosynovitis of the flexor digitorum tendon is an overuse syndrome of the hand that can be associated with racquet sports because of repeated grasping. Repetitive impact at the level of the metacarpophalangeal joint can cause thickening of the A-1 pulley, resulting in swelling and pressure over the flexor tendon sheath. Initial treatment includes relative rest and NSAIDs. It usually responds to an ultrasound-guided steroid injection of the flexor tendon sheath under the A-1 pulley. Surgical release of the A-1 pulley is needed in some cases.

MANAGEMENT OF LOWER LIMB INJURY (SEE CHAPTER 30, DISORDERS OF THE LOWER LIMBS)

Hip Injuries

The hip can be injured in a variety of sports, from either direct trauma or musculotendinous overload. In either case, the athlete is often greatly impaired in sport participation as a result of significant alterations in gait. It is important to determine the etiology of the problem, allow for a period of rest, and maintain strength and flexibility as these injuries heal.

Acute Injuries

The "hip pointer" injury or hip contusion is a direct blow to the pelvic brim or hip region, which results in a contusion to the soft tissues and often the underlying bone. It is relatively common in collision sports. Common areas include the greater trochanter and iliac crest. The injury can result in hematoma formation, but often there is little visible swelling or ecchymosis. There is, however, a significant amount of pain and focal tenderness that is due to bony contusion and periosteal irritation. The athlete has difficulty with quick bursts of running and with any contact to the area.

The diagnosis is made by the above history or on field observation. On examination, it is important to note full ROM of the hip and the knee. If there is pain with passive hip ROM, then x-rays should be obtained to rule out any significant bony pathology. For most injuries, further imaging studies are not necessary.

Treatment includes frequent and repeated icing, a short course of NSAIDs, active ROM, and a period of rest until the gait can be normalized. Crutches with weight bearing as tolerated may be necessary to unload the hip. Once an athlete has no pain at rest, with sports activities and minimal pain on palpation, he or she can return to play with protective padding. Most of these injuries do not result in long-term sequelae.

Hip flexor strains are commonly seen in sprinting as well as in other sports, such as soccer, baseball, and football.

They occur as a result of an eccentric overload of the psoas muscle or as the athlete attempts to flex the fully extended hip, such as in hurdling. The examination reveals tenderness to palpation over the area and pain with resisted hip flexion and passive hip extension. The majority of these injuries require plain x-rays of the hip (usually an anteroposterior and frog-leg lateral view) to exclude bony injury. This is particularly important in the adolescent or skeletally immature athlete, as avulsion fracture of the apophysis can occur. These avulsion fractures, whether in the adult or adolescent athlete, can be treated nonoperatively unless significant displacement occurs.

Treatment of hip flexor strains and/or avulsions consists of protected weight bearing, icing, and gentle active ROM as soon as tolerated. Strengthening exercises of the lower extremities should be avoided until the gait is nonantalgic and ROM is full and pain free. Then the athlete should be progressed through a strengthening program consisting of both open and closed kinetic exercises. Eccentric and plyometric training should be added when the athlete tolerates functional activities and can be of benefit in preventing recurrence of injury.

Hamstring injuries are very common in athletes. Acute hamstring strains can occur with high-speed running or with excessive lengthening of the hamstrings, commonly affecting the biceps femoris and semimembranosus muscles, respectively. The patient can present with a palpable muscle gap, ecchymosis, and tenderness to palpation over the injured area. Evaluation with MRI can be used to classify the severity of the injury, although imaging findings generally have not been shown to correlate with the prognosis of return to play (51). Treatment includes a progressive rehabilitation protocol, which involves a gradual increase in intensity, ROM, and eccentric resistance leading to more sports-specific and neuromuscular control exercises. The type of injury, especially the lengthening injury mechanism correlates with more delayed time to return to play (51).

Overuse Injuries

Greater trochanteric pain syndrome can be associated with various etiologies that may involve the gluteus medius and minimus muscle-tendon complex, subgluteus maximus (trochanteric) bursa, iliotibial band (ITB), and hip external rotator muscles (52). Trochanteric bursitis can occur secondary to repeated irritation of the bursa, or less commonly from direct trauma. Traumatic inflammation of the bursa is seen in collision sports, such as football and hockey, and at times in soccer and baseball after sliding hard into a base or hitting the ground after diving for a ball. Irritation can be associated to other biomechanical abnormalities such as a tight ITB and/or weakness of the hip abductors. The athlete reports an aching pain along the lateral aspect of the hip that is worse with running and jumping and any contact on the area, including laying on the affected side at night. Physical examination will demonstrate weakness of the hip abductors on the affected side, a tight ITB, and significant pain with direct palpation over the trochanter. Rather than a true "bursitis," greater trochanteric pain syndrome represents an insertional tendinopathy of the gluteus medius and/or gluteus minimus tendons. Treatment should be directed at strengthening these muscles both concentrically and eccentrically as well as stretching-associated muscle/tendons such as the ITB and the hip internal and external rotators. Ultrasound can be helpful in delineating the pathology and guiding directed treatment.

In refractory cases, regenerative techniques could be tried. Corticosteroids should be avoided in these cases.

Femoroacetabular impingement (FAI) is associated with the presence of aberrant morphology involving the proximal femur and acetabulum that results in abnormal contact between the femoral neck and the acetabular rim during the movements of the hip (53). Two main types have been described: cam and pincer, although a mixed type is common. Symptoms include slow-onset groin pain exacerbated by excessive demands on the hip during athletic activities or with prolonged sitting or walking. Physical exam can reveal limited ROM, especially internal rotation and adduction. The impingement test is usually positive, described as pain on adduction and internal rotation, when the hip is at 90 degrees of flexion (54). Plain radiographs may reveal coxa profunda and acetabular retroversion in the anteroposterior view and the presence of bony prominence at the anterolateral head and neck junction in the lateral view. MR arthrography is the modality of choice to quantify the reduced femoral waist and to evaluate the cartilage and labrum.

Initial treatment is nonsurgical and includes activity modification and NSAIDs. If a trial of conservative treatment fails or there is evidence of labral tear, then surgery is recommended (53,54).

Pain over the proximal posterior thigh may be secondary to a chronic proximal hamstring tendinopathy. This injury often occurs without an inciting event with the patient presenting progressive discomfort and pain in the posterior thigh, especially with maximal knee extension with the hip in flexion, and forceful hamstring contraction during physical activity. The patient will present with tenderness to palpation over the proximal hamstring at the ischium, which may be associated with ischial bursitis. Diagnostic modalities include MRI and ultrasound to evaluate for hamstring tendinosis, partial tears, bursitis, and the latter is useful in dynamic evaluation. A rehabilitation protocol with focus on eccentric strengthening exercises is used for management. Other potential interventions when traditional management fails may include ultrasound-guided corticosteroid injections to the ischial bursa, extracorporeal shockwave therapy (ESWT), PRP injection with or without tenotomy, published studies have shown mixed therapeutic results (55).

KNEE INJURIES

Athletes participating in sports activities involving running, jumping, or changing directions often present with traumatic or overuse injuries to the knee. Acute knee injury can result from direct contact that induces a valgus stress such as a tackle in football, noncontact deceleration and change of direction resulting from a cut in basketball, and forced flexion associated with a squat. Overuse injuries can result from repeated activity such as running downhill, jumping, or lifting weights.

Acute Injuries

ACL Tears
ACL injury is very common in sports. It is commonly injured in female athletes participating in high-demand sports such as soccer, downhill skiing, and basketball (56). The ACL is a static stabilizer of the knee with a primary function of resisting hyperextension and anterior tibial translation in flexion

and providing rotatory control. It is also a secondary restraint to valgus and varus forces. Biomechanical studies of the ACL have shown that forces in the ligament are the highest in the last 30 degrees of extension and in hyperextension. ACL forces are also high during anterior tibial translation, internal rotation, and varus (57).

ACL injury usually presents with pain, immediate swelling, and limited ROM associated with a noncontact mechanism. The injury usually results from sudden deceleration during a high-velocity movement and requires a forceful contraction of the quadriceps muscle. Injury has also been described as a result of a valgus stress, hyperextension, and external rotation, such as when landing from a jump. It can also occur with severe internal rotation of the knee, or hyperextension with internal rotation. Traumatic injury to the ligament can occur with valgus stress to the knee in combination with injury to the medial collateral ligament and the medial meniscus (58).

Some patients present with a history of recurrent episodes of knee instability, associated with swelling and limited motion. These patients often give a history of a remote injury to the knee that was rested, immobilized but not rehabilitated (58).

The physical examination is sensitive and specific in the diagnosis of ACL tears. The examiner should observe for asymmetry, palpate for areas of tenderness, measure active and passive ROM, and document muscle atrophy. Special maneuvers such as the apprehension test to rule out patellar subluxation, collateral ligament testing, and flexion-rotation tests such as the McMurray's for meniscal injury should be done to rule out associated injuries. Testing for the integrity of the ACL in the patient with an acute injury should include a Lachman's test. This is done by applying an anterior force to the tibia with the knee in 30 degrees of flexion. Another important test in the acute setting is the lateral pivot shift in which the examiner attempts to reproduce anterolateral rotatory instability by internally rotating the leg and applying a valgus stress to the knee as it is flexed. In the patient with chronic ACL insufficiency, the anterior drawer test in which an anterior force is applied to the tibia with the knee flexed to 90 degrees can also be used.

Protection of secondary structures is of paramount importance in the acutely injured knee. The rate of progression of rehabilitation depends on the extent of damage to other knee structures. The individual with a recurrently unstable knee frequently benefits from a trial of rehabilitation. This involves correction of muscle weakness, proprioceptive deficits, and functional retraining in combination with activity modification. This can often reduce the episodes of instability (58).

Recurrent anterolateral instability is a functionally unacceptable outcome in the adolescent and competitive athlete as well as active adults who participate in activities that involve pivoting and jumping. Athletes with chronic ACL deficiency typically have an increased incidence of meniscal injuries that can lead to early osteoarthritis. Reconstruction of the ligament using the central portion of the patellar tendon or semitendinosus/gracilis tendon grafts has become the treatment of choice for this athletic population (59,60). The choice of graft depends on several factors, including a history of patellofemoral pain and the preference of the surgeon.

Rehabilitation should begin after reconstructive surgery on the first postoperative day. The early use of cryotherapy, compression, and elevation has been shown to reduce swelling postoperatively. It is very important to achieve full passive extension and to initiate early active flexion in the first days post surgery. Partial weight bearing with crutches is usually started immediately after the operation.

Rapid progression of the rehabilitation program has reduced complications usually associated with ACL surgery such as stiffness, muscle weakness and atrophy, and patellofemoral pain (61). Early in the rehabilitation, it is important to avoid the excessive strain of the reconstructed ligament with terminal (0 to 30 degrees) extension OKC–resisted quadriceps exercises. OKC exercises can be safely used in the 90 to 45 degrees range at this stage. Use of CKC exercises such as minisquats, steps, and lunges results in quadriceps strengthening with tolerable shear forces to the graft. Aquatic exercises that allow progressive weight bearing can be started as soon as the sutures are removed (58).

Specific factors to consider in the return to play decision include timing and type of surgery, patient symptoms, physical examination, results from isokinetic and functional testing, and information from validated questionnaires that assess subjective factors such as patient satisfaction and psychological readiness for return to sports (62,63). Although some programs have reported very early return to activity following reconstruction, delaying return to activity to 9 months and achieving symmetric quadriceps strength after ACL reconstruction significantly reduces the risk of reinjury (64).

Prevention of ACL injury has become very important for athletes participating in basketball, handball, and soccer. Neuromuscular training has been shown to reduce the incidence of ACL injury in male and female athletes and has been incorporated as a prehabilitation strategy in this population (62).

Meniscal Tears

The menisci serve as shock absorbers, decrease load concentration, and help guide normal knee kinematics. As much as 50% of the compressive load across the knee is transmitted through the menisci, and this increases during flexion. Injury to the menisci reduces the weight contact area of the knee, placing the articular cartilage at risk for failure or degenerative changes (65). Common causes of injury include acute macrotrauma following hyperflexion or twisting, and chronic microtrauma due to running or jumping. The meniscus is affected by the aging process and can tear by shear failure in the older runner without acute trauma.

Symptoms of meniscal tears include pain with activity or mechanical symptoms of catching, grinding, locking, and slight swelling. Clinical signs include joint line tenderness, and pain upon hyperflexion or hyperextension. Physical exam maneuvers like McMurray's test, Thessaly, and the Apley grind test have been described to aid in the diagnosis of meniscal injury. These maneuvers have shown high specificity, but limited sensitivity (66).

A trial of rehabilitation for 3 to 6 months that includes ice, NSAIDs, reductions of weight-bearing activity, and strengthening exercises is the first line of treatment in most patients, especially those with degenerative meniscus injury or an arthritic knee (67). Surgical consultation is recommended in athletes with acute meniscal tears and refractory cases, if the patient continues to have mechanical symptoms and swelling with sports activity. The surgical options include meniscal repair of a peripheral tear, or partial meniscectomy. In the young athlete, repair of the meniscus is the preferred option if clinically possible. Meniscectomy and debridement is often the only alternative in the older athlete (65).

Rehabilitation after meniscal surgery has progressed in recent years. Accelerated rehabilitation programs that allow early weight bearing and progressive ROM have replaced more conservative protocols in which the patient was maintained non–weight bearing and limited in ROM post surgery (68). Special precautions, however, should be taken with extreme flexion and rotation and axial loading in the postoperative period. The patient with meniscal repair and an ACL-deficient knee needs to be counseled about the possibility of recurrent instability and failure of the meniscal repair.

Overuse Injuries

Patellofemoral Pain Syndrome

The athlete with patellofemoral pain syndrome usually presents with pain associated with activity such as running down hills, descending stairs, or jumping. Female and young athletes with patellar instability may present with pain associated to abnormal tracking.

Anterior knee pain is very common in runners and jumpers and can be secondary to more than one pathologic process. The pain generators in extensor mechanism disorders include the subchondral bone of the patella, synovial capsular and retinacular soft tissues, and tendon insertion on the patella. The resulting pain can be associated with stimulation of free nerve endings, secretion of inflammatory mediators, and abnormal transmission of forces through the cartilage to the subchondral bone (69).

Modifiable intrinsic factors for injury include muscle weakness (hip abductors, external rotators, and knee extensors); inflexibility of the ITB, quadriceps, hamstring, and gastrocsoleus tendons; vastus medialis dysfunction; and increased joint reactive forces with heel strike. Nonmodifiable intrinsic risk factors include patella alta, pes planus, age, gender, and race. Extrinsic factors include rapid increase in training intensity, inappropriate running shoes, uphill running, and hard playing surfaces. Preventive strategies include identification and correction of modifiable risk factors (70).

Symptoms include dull, aching retropatellar or peripatellar pain of insidious onset. It typically worsens with activities in knee flexion such as squatting, sitting for prolonged periods (theater sign), descending stairs, or running hills. The physical examination usually shows patellar crepitus, pain with patellar compression or quadriceps contraction, and quadriceps muscle atrophy. Tightness of the hip flexors and hamstrings is also frequently found. In the patients with coexisting patellar instability, apprehension can be identified in addition to pain over the superior lateral facet. Proximal muscle weakness can also be present, as evidenced by the patient having difficulty with single leg stance, step-down, and eccentric muscle control.

Acute treatment of patellofemoral pain syndrome includes modified rest, ice, and NSAIDs. Stretching the ITB and strengthening the quadriceps with both open and closed chain exercises should be instituted early, in combination with cross-training strategies. In some patients, closed chain exercises are the preferred mode of strength training because of reduced patellofemoral joint stress. Other important considerations include gluteal strengthening to reduce femoral internal rotation with weight-bearing activities; and strengthening the ankle muscles in combination with heel cord stretching to manage hyperpronation (70).

Patellar taping that forces the patella to track medially can be used in the early stages of training (71). Other interventions include neoprene knee sleeves or other patellofemoral orthoses that attempt to control patellar laxity. Shoe orthoses to control hyperpronation can also be helpful.

Arthroscopic surgery is rarely indicated in the patient with patellofemoral pain and should be used judiciously when approaching this problem. In patients with lateral pressure syndrome, an arthroscopic lateral release can relieve patellar tilt (72).

LEG, ANKLE, AND FOOT INJURIES

Leg and foot injuries are common occurrences, especially in athletes who participate in sports that emphasize repetitive lower limb activity, such as track and field, jogging, basketball, and soccer.

Acute Injuries

Ankle Sprains

Acute ankle sprains are a very common cause of lost playing time and disability among athletes. Although they are considered to be benign injuries, many athletes present with recurrent sprains, functional instability, and inability to return to their sport at the previous level of performance (73,74).

Stability of the ankle depends on its bony architecture, static effects of the ligaments, and dynamic function of muscles. The lateral ligamentous complex consists of the anterior talofibular ligament (ATFL), calcaneofibular ligament (CFL), posterior talofibular ligament (PTFL), and lateral talocalcaneal ligament (LTCL). The ATFL is the weakest of the lateral ankle ligaments and the one most commonly injured. The CFL is the second weakest ligament and crosses both the tibiotalar and subtalar joints, both of which can be involved in an acute ankle sprain (75).

The most common mechanism of injury to the lateral ankle ligaments occurs from a forced plantar flexion and inversion of the ankle. The sequence of ligament tears in an inversion injury is the ATFL, followed by the anterolateral capsule, and finally the distal tibiofibular ligament. Progressive inversion forces also result in a CFL tear (75).

The patient complains of acute lateral ankle pain that is usually accompanied by swelling, difficulty with weight bearing, and ecchymosis. The physical examination shows diffuse swelling, tenderness over the lateral ligament complex, pain with inversion, and in many instances fibular (peroneal) muscle weakness. Palpation of bony structures such as the posterior malleoli, fifth metatarsal, and the navicular should be performed to rule out associated fractures. The anterior drawer test stresses the ATFL and should be performed to document ligamentous laxity. The talar tilt test evaluates the CFL in inversion but can be somewhat limited in the acute stage by pain.

Early management emphasizes reduction of ankle effusion and pain as well as protection of the lateral ligament complex. Ice, NSAIDs, elevation, taping, physical modalities or wrapping with lateral felt pads can be useful in early recovery. Physical therapy emphasizing movement in pain-free ROM can be combined with the use of functional stirrup braces and early weight bearing. Followed by static and dynamic exercises for strengthening, while avoiding inversion stress to the ankle. Gentle stretching of the Achilles tendon is done to avoid a plantar flexion contracture. Proprioceptive training instituted early in the rehabilitation process reduces the risk of functional instability following the injury (76).

The timing of return to activity varies depending on the severity of the sprain. Athletes with grade I sprains usually return to play in 1 to 2 weeks, but those with grade II sprains can be out of competition for up to 6 weeks. Athletes with grade III sprains can take several months to return to their sports. The use of ankle bracing during athletic activity should be considered for up to 6 months following an injury to the ankle (77).

Achilles Rupture

Degenerative changes in the Achilles tendon associated with poor tendon vascularity can lead to an Achilles tendon rupture. The mechanisms of rupture include forefoot push off with the knee in extension, sudden unexpected dorsiflexion of the ankle, and arising following violent dorsiflexion of the plantarflexed foot when falling from a jump (78). Clinically, the patient presents with pain and a history of hearing an audible snap when falling from a jump or starting to sprint. In many instances, the patients are unable to walk or bear weight.

On physical examination, there is a palpable defect proximal to the tendon insertion. Significant swelling can be present, making the exam difficult. The patient may be able to plantarflex the foot but cannot perform a calf raise. The Thompson's test that evaluates the integrity of the tendon can be performed by squeezing the posterior calf in the prone position and observing passive plantarflexion. This test can be falsely negative because the intact plantaris muscle can plantar flex the ankle when the calf is squeezed.

In the cases of complete or partial tears, nonsurgical management with casting and functional bracing can be used. This treatment, however, carries a higher risk of rerupture, mainly after complete tears, and should be reserved for patients who are not interested in high levels of activity. Open surgical repair of the Achilles tendon can restore the anatomy and allow transition to early rehabilitation. Recently, shorter immobilization periods and the use of functional bracing have gained popularity, with an earlier recovery of ROM (78).

Midfoot Sprain

It is important for the sports medicine physician to be aware of midfoot sprains as they can be confused with ankle injury. The injury occurs with landing of the forefoot, usually in inversion. On careful examination, the tenderness to palpation is localized to the dorsal-medial midfoot, swelling and ecchymosis in the area, and pain can be elicited with a varus stress to the foot. Most of these athletes are unable to walk without an antalgic gait pattern. It is important to get plain x-rays of the foot and note any widening between the first and second metatarsal rays. Widening of greater than 5 mm is associated to unstable injury and requires surgical fixation. If there is no significant widening on x-rays, 4 to 6 weeks of immobilization in plantar flexion and supination will allow for healing (79).

Metatarsophalangeal Sprain ("Turf Toe")

Great toe metatarsophalangeal joint hyperextension injury occurs in sports such as football and soccer. It has been named "turf toe" because trauma occurs on stiff synthetic surfaces. In addition to hyperextension, there are often added forces, such as other players falling on the injured athlete. This is associated with localized pain at the metatarsophalangeal joint with weight bearing and especially during push off in running. The examination can demonstrate localized tenderness, swelling, and decreased ROM. In recurrent injuries, loss of motion and degenerative changes about the joint may occur. The treatment consists of the protection, rest, ice, compression, and elevation, with taping to limit motion of the joint. A long rigid shoe orthotic may assist in decreasing force across the joint to facilitate return to play. This can be a very disabling injury, requiring several weeks of rest before return can be accomplished. Occasionally, a corticosteroid injection is necessary to control pain and inflammation of the joint and to facilitate a progressive rehabilitation program.

Overuse Injuries

Medial Tibial Stress Syndrome

Medial tibial stress syndrome (MTSS), also known as shin splints, is a common injury seen in running sports. Although runners are most commonly afflicted, individuals involved in jumping sports can also develop MTSS. Although the exact anatomic changes that cause MTSS have been debated, most experts agree that there is an inflammatory process at the periosteum of the tibia caused by overuse and by biomechanical abnormalities. Recent studies point to the fascial insertion of the medial fibers of the soleus muscles into the tibia as the possible cause of the pain symptoms. Biomechanical factors that can be associated with the syndrome include excessive foot pronation, loss of leg flexibility, limited ankle ROM, and abnormal running technique (80).

The clinical presentation is pain associated with activity that initially improves with warm-up but recurs at the end of the workout. Commonly, symptoms arise when athletes are beginning a training program or when abruptly increasing the intensity of their training. The physical examination shows diffuse tenderness over the posteromedial aspect of the distal third of the tibia with occasional localized edema in the region. Initial x-rays are usually negative, and the diagnosis can be confirmed with an MRI or bone scan. MRI offers the advantages of multiplanar capability, high sensitivity for pathology, ability to precisely define the location and extent of bony injury, lack of exposure to ionizing radiation, and significantly less imaging time than a 3-phase bone scan, which may reveal patchy areas of increased uptake along the medial border of the tibia (81). In chronic cases, there can be periosteal thickening on plain radiographs.

The initial treatment of this condition includes relative rest, ice, NSAIDs, active rest, and gentle stretching of the gastrocnemius and soleus. Other therapeutic modalities such as iontophoresis and ultrasound can be useful adjuncts in the rehabilitation (80). As symptoms begin to subside a gradual return to activities is recommended, but with a decrease in training intensity, and running on soft, flat surfaces. Running technique should be assessed, and emphasis on midfoot strike can be implemented to decrease the ground reaction forces to the lower limbs (80). Additional measures include flexibility exercises for the entire lower limb, strengthening of the whole kinetic chain, and cross-training activities to maintain cardiovascular conditioning. Management of foot pronation might include the use of stability shoes, and the prescription of shoe orthoses.

Stress Fractures

Stress fractures are very common injuries, and the location varies from sport to sport. In a series of 196 stress fractures, Iwamoto found that basketball players predominantly sustained stress fractures of the tibial shaft, medial malleolus, and metatarsal bones (82). Tennis and volleyball players predominately had fractures of the tibial shaft. Stress fractures are overuse injuries to bone which occur when bone breakdown exceeds bone remodeling. Stress to bone can range from stress reaction with edema, to a stress fracture that can progress to a complete fracture. The diagnosis and treatment of these fractures depends on their location and potential for spontaneous healing. Fractures that are low risk with good potential for healing include the posteromedial tibial cortex, fibula, and metatarsal shaft. High-risk fractures with a lower potential for healing include the anterior cortex of the tibia, the base of the fifth metatarsal, and the tarsal navicular (80).

Clinically, this injury presents with a gradual increase in activity-related pain that is aggravated by repetitive loading of the lower limb and improved by rest. Physical exam shows localized tenderness that reproduces the symptoms of pain. Minimal soft tissue swelling is often present as well. Maneuvers that reproduce the pain symptoms such as hopping on one leg or jumping can also aid in making the diagnoses.

X-rays are usually negative for the first 2 to 4 weeks following the stress fracture. If the clinical picture is highly suspicious for stress fracture, then a bone scan or MRI should be considered. Bone scan and MRI are both sensitive and specific examinations for the diagnosis of stress fractures. MRI provides anatomic information about the surrounding structures and can be superior to bone scan for following up the healing fracture (81,82).

Treatment during the acute phases consists of relative rest, ice, and NSAIDs. High-risk stress fractures such as the fifth metatarsal or navicular require non–weight bearing, casting, and in some instances surgery. Low-risk stress fractures such as the medial tibial and metatarsals can be treated with functional activity progression. When the patient is asymptomatic at rest, a program of progressive return to running should be instituted. Initially, runs are allowed on even soft surfaces, and progression is allowed weekly provided that no symptoms recur with proper running technique (80).

Achilles Tendinopathy

The Achilles tendon is the largest and strongest tendon in the body, and during sports activities, it is under large tensile loads that can result in degeneration and injury. Achilles tendon disorders are very common in sports, particularly in running sports, with a 7% to 9% annual incidence reported in elite runners (78).

The term tendinopathy should be used in the majority of individuals to describe the Achilles tendon injury, since the most common pathologic findings is tendinosis with intratendinous degeneration without inflammation. In the athlete with acute symptoms, the Achilles tendon develops acute edema and inflammation in the paratenon. Chronic Achilles tendon symptomatology usually includes thickening of the tendon and localized tenderness to palpation.

Achilles tendon injuries frequently affect mature male athletes who are active in running and jumping activities. The typical history is one of gradual onset of pain that worsens with activity, associated with changes in intensity of the exercise, running surfaces, or footwear. Physical exam shows tenderness to palpation of the Achilles tendon 2 to 6 cm from its insertion, inflexibility of the ankle dorsiflexors, and weakness of the ankle plantar flexors.

Conservative treatment for Achilles tendinopathy includes relative rest, as well as physical modalities and exercises that address the biomechanical deficits. Exercise prescription for tendinopathy should include eccentric programs for stretching and strengthening the gastrocnemius muscle (83,84). One exercise that is very important in the rehabilitation of these disorders is the heel drop. This exercise is performed standing on a bench, and the individual allows the heel to drop eccentrically with the knee extended and subsequently returns the foot to a neutral position. As symptoms improve, the rehabilitation program should progress to include fast eccentric exercises. A gradual running and jumping program can be started when the patient is asymptomatic at rest. A heel lift used in the initial stages can relieve pain by reducing tensile load.

Plantar Fasciopathy

Plantar fasciopathy is the most common cause of heel pain and affects 15% to 20% of runners (5). The plantar fascia is a tough fibrous, aponeurotic structure arising from the medial calcaneal tubercle and inserting into the plantar plates of the metatarsophalangeal joints, the bases of the proximal phalanges of the toes, and the flexor tendon sheaths. It provides shape and support to the longitudinal arch and acts as a shock absorber on foot impact.

Plantar fasciopathy is an overload injury usually associated with tight plantar flexors and short foot flexor muscles, weakness of posterior calf muscles, and increased pronation. Other biomechanical abnormalities of the lower limb such as hip abductor weakness, external rotation of the leg, and supinated high-arch feet can also be factors (85).

Patients usually complain of heel pain upon arising in the morning that decreases during the day and then worsens with increased activity. Commonly, this is not associated with trauma and presents insidiously. It can be diffuse initially, but over time it localizes to the medial calcaneus. Patients often relate the onset of symptoms to a rapid increase in distance, speed, intensity, or frequency of running. Other factors can include changing to a flexible shoe having minimal rearfoot control.

The diagnosis is based mainly on the history and physical examination. The patient presents with tenderness to palpation over the medial calcaneal tubercle and, in more advanced cases, over the proximal medial longitudinal arch. Slight swelling in the area and Achilles tendon tightness is present in most patients. Other findings on the exam can include pronated and everted foot, tightness of the hamstrings, and weakness of the leg and intrinsic foot muscles.

Treatment is initially directed to relieve pain and includes NSAIDs and icing to the affected area. Heel pads and arch supports to maintain the longitudinal arch during ambulation can aid in symptom management.

Rehabilitation includes an exercise program to correct the biomechanical deficits. Stretching of plantar flexors, hamstrings, and plantar fascia should be combined with strengthening of short foot flexors and plantar flexors.

Localized steroid and anesthetic injection can provide initial pain relief, but superficial injections that cause fat pad atrophy should be avoided. The use of night splints or, in severe cases, casting can reduce pain. Emerging regenerative techniques, such as ESWT is recommended in treating refractory cases (86,87). Surgery should be considered only if the pain has not responded to appropriate conservative treatment for 6 to 12 months. The athlete can return to activity when pain is absent and the biomechanical deficits have been corrected.

MANAGEMENT OF HEAD AND CERVICAL SPINE INJURIES

The physician covering athletic events, particularly contact sports, needs to be prepared to deal with the athlete who presents with head or neck injuries. These injuries can result in significant morbidity, and rarely even in mortality. Proper management requires an emergency action plan (EAP) established by the sports medicine team prior to the event.

Head and neck injuries comprise about 11.9% of all severe injuries in college athletes (88). Head injuries alone occur at a rate of 132 to 367 cases per 100,000 people per year, with sports activities accounting for approximately 14% of these injuries (89). It has been estimated that 8.9% of the 12,000 cervical injuries occurring in the United States every year result from sports activity (90). The sports having the highest risk of cervical injuries include American football, wrestling, and gymnastics (88). During the 10-year period from 2005 to 2014, a total of 28 deaths (2.8 deaths per year) from traumatic brain and spinal cord injuries occurred among high school and college football players combined (91).

Sport-Related Concussion (Also See Chapter 19 on Traumatic Brain Injury)

Sport-related concussion (SRC) is defined as a traumatic brain injury induced by biomechanical forces that may be caused by either a direct blow to the head, face, neck, or elsewhere in the body. It typically results in the rapid onset of short-lived impairments associated with altered neural function that may or may not involve loss of consciousness, disturbance of vision, or equilibrium (92,93). The incidence of sport-related concussions is as high as 3.8 million per year, although as many as 50% of episodes are not documented (92). Contact sports, female gender, individual aggressive play, and history of concussion are factors that may increase the risk of suffering a concussion. Other factors that affect prognosis and recovery include a greater number, severity, and duration of symptoms, younger age, catastrophic injury, preinjury mood disorders, learning disorders, attention deficit disorders, and migraine headaches.

In assessing an athlete with a head injury who is conscious, the level of alertness is the most sensitive criteria for establishing the nature of the head injury and subsequently treating the athlete. Initial evaluation of concussion should be guided

TABLE 41-4	Sideline Cognitive Evaluation (94,95)
Recent memory (only for sideline diagnosis)	Location, half/period/quarter, who scored last, last opponent, who won the last game
Orientation	Month, date, day of the week, year, time
Immediate memory	Recall five words
Concentration	Numerate digits backward, months in reverse
Delayed recall	Recall five words

by a symptom checklist, which may include amnesia, headache, dizziness, blurred vision, attention deficit, and nausea. There are also a wide variety of other complaints that can be encountered in concussed athletes. These include descriptions of vacant stare, irritability, emotional liability, impaired coordination, sleep disturbance, noise/light intolerance, lethargy, behavioral disturbance, and altered sense of taste/smell. Cognitive evaluation (**Table 41-4**), balance tests, and further neurologic physical examination are required. There are several assessment tools that have been proposed to guide serial evaluations to follow symptoms, but their validity has received limited attention (94–97).

When an individual shows any signs of SRC, he/she must be removed from competition or practice and should not be allowed to return to play the same day. Some patients may need to be referred to an emergency facility if they present worsening headache, severe drowsiness, develops nausea or vomiting, unusual behavior and disorientation, seizures, weakness, slurred speech, or gait unsteadiness.

The return to play after the diagnosis of a concussion is a controversial topic. The young athlete poses a unique challenge in which cognitive rest and academic accommodation should be implemented, along with physical rest, although the exact amount is not well defined (92). While scientifically validated return-to-play guidelines do not yet exist, the consensus of experts in this field suggests that complete resolution of concussion symptoms (both at rest and during exercise) is mandatory prior to the resumption of training or playing (**Table 41-5**) (92). The use of neuropsychologic testing can also be considered in the return to play decision-making, particularly in the case where baseline test values were established prior to the injury.

Sequelae to concussion include irreversible cognitive deficits and depression as seen in chronic traumatic encephalopathy,

TABLE 41-5	Concussion Return to Play Protocol (92)
Rehabilitation Stage	**Goal of Stage**
No activity	Recovery
Light aerobic exercise	Increase heart rate
Sports-specific exercise	Add movement
Noncontact training drills	Exercise, coordination, and cognitive load
Full-contact practice	Restore the athlete's confidence and coaching staff assess functional skills
Return to play	

or death due to second impact syndrome. Postconcussion syndrome is a less serious, yet potentially debilitating result of a concussion. It involves prolonged, disabling, and sometimes permanent symptoms such as headache, dizziness, nausea, tinnitus, depression, irritability, slowed mental processing, impaired attention, and deficits in memory. Rare but severe brain injury associated with sports includes second impact syndrome or malignant brain edema, hematomas, and intracranial hemorrhages. The second impact syndrome occurs when an athlete is still symptomatic from an initial head injury and sustains a second head injury. Usually within seconds to minutes of the second impact, the initially conscious but stunned athlete precipitously collapses, with rapidly dilating pupils, loss of eye movement, and evidence of respiratory failure. The management of severe brain injury in an athlete who has collapsed includes protection of the cervical spine, cardiopulmonary resuscitation, and prompt transportation to a medical facility that has the capability of performing computer tomography or MRI of the brain, and neurosurgical consultation.

There are no evidence-based guidelines for disqualifying or retiring an athlete from sport after a concussion. The recommendation should be individualized, but disqualification from the sport may be suggested if there is structural abnormality on neuroimaging, history of multiple concussions, diminished academic or workplace performance, persistent postconcussive symptoms, prolonged recovery course, or a perceived reduced threshold of sustaining recurrent concussions (92).

Injury prevention may be possible with modification and enforcement of the rules and fair play. Equipment modifications like helmets have shown to decrease the incidence of fractures and laceration, but not concussions. Secondary prevention can be achieved by raising awareness and through legislation to promote safe play, rule changes, proper training to health care providers, as well as the presence of trained health professionals in sporting events.

Cervical Spine Injuries (See Also Chapter 26 on Disorders of the Cervical Spine)

Cervical spine injuries result when the accelerating head and neck strike a stationary object and associated with axial loading of the flexed cervical spine. Cervical injury can range in severity from sprain or strain to cervical spinal cord injury with resultant tetraplegia.

The sports medicine team should be prepared to deal with a cervical spine emergency during practice or competition. This includes practice on how to manage a player who is injured while wearing a helmet. Protective athletic equipment should be removed *prior* to transport to an emergency facility for an athlete with suspected cervical spine instability. Helmet removal should be performed by at least three trained and experienced rescuers to protect the cervical spine (98).

Sports-related tetraplegia is the most dreaded complication that can result from spinal cord injury. Incorrect tackling techniques in which the head is used as a spear to make initial contact with the opponent can lead to this injury. A reduction of spinal cord injury in American football has resulted from a prohibition of this tackling method, and educating coaches and athletes on the consequences of tackling the opponent with a flexed cervical spine. Management of tetraplegia includes assessment of the airway, breathing, and circulation as well as protection from further damage to the spinal cord. The athlete should be transported to the hospital for radiologic evaluation and emergency management.

Athletes with cervical cord neuropraxia and temporary loss of strength or sensation merit special attention. The decision regarding returning to play following a reversible spinal injury is a challenging and controversial one. Athletes with a history of transient cervical cord neuropraxia, who have a normal neurologic examination, normal imaging studies as well as normal cervical strength and ROM, are permitted by some clinicians to return to sports. Others counsel the athletes against returning to sports following this injury (99,100). The athlete with spinal stenosis documented by MRI or spear tackler's spine in which there is loss of cervical lordosis and degenerative changes documented by x-rays should be advised about the possibility of irreversible neurologic injury when returning to contact sports and should be excluded from participation.

A stinger is a transient neurologic event characterized by pain and paresthesia in a single upper limb following a blow to the neck or shoulder. The players present with tingling or burning sensations, and numbness of the involved limb. One mechanism of injury seen in young American football players is depression of the shoulder accompanied by lateral flexion of the neck in the opposite direction. This causes traction to the upper branches of the brachial plexus. The other mechanism is rotation and extension of the neck toward the ipsilateral shoulder affecting the cervical roots by compression in the neural foramina. Stingers are usually reversible, but some athletes have recurrent symptoms that require protective equipment, improvement in technique, and cervical muscle strength. Return to play should be permitted when the athlete has a normal examination, including ROM and strength of the upper limb and cervical spine (101).

The athlete with a soft tissue injury to the cervical region should be evaluated to rule out neurologic injury. Once a neurologic injury has been ruled out, the management includes NSAIDs, therapeutic modalities, and a stretching and strengthening program to the shoulder girdle and cervical muscles. Postural abnormalities that need to be corrected typically include forward head with tight pectoral muscles, increased thoracic kyphosis, scapular protraction, and hypermobility of the cervical spine (101).

MANAGEMENT OF LUMBAR SPINE INJURIES

The patterns of back injury differ in child and adolescent athletes and adults (102). Young athletes involved in sports that require trunk rotation and hyperextension usually present with posterior elements injury. Repeated stresses associated with gymnastics, diving, and wrestling places the athlete at increased risk of pars interarticularis injury such as spondylolysis (103). These athletes can present with acute or gradual onset of pain and limited motion that restricts activity.

Older athletes who participate in sports like golf, tennis, gymnastics, football, wrestling, dance, and hockey can present with injuries to the anterior elements of the spine including the vertebral endplate and the intervertebral discs (104). These individuals usually present with symptoms associated with trunk flexion and rotation. They can present with episodes of axial back pain and limited motion followed by episodes of radiculopathy.

Repeated exposure to rotational activities can lead to progressive degenerative disc and facet joint disease associated with spinal stenosis. These athletes can present with leg pain, weakness, or numbness associated with activity that improves with sitting or trunk flexion.

The physical examination may show limited back motion a lateral trunk tilt that can be associated with an annulus fibrosus tear or with muscle-ligament injury. Flexibility testing of the hip rotators, flexors, and hamstring muscles should be performed. Neurologic examination should address areas of sensory loss, abnormal muscle stretch reflexes, and focal muscle weakness. Special tests to identify abnormal neural tension and reproduce leg symptoms such as the straight leg raising maneuver, the slump test (in which the sitting patients knee is extended after flexion of the cervical spine), or the femoral stress test in which the hip is extended while flexing the knee should be performed.

The direction of motion that worsens the patient's pain should be identified. Increased pain with flexion and rotation is usually associated with discogenic injury, while pain with extension and rotation is usually associated with posterior element injury. A useful test in the patient with suspected spondylosis is the one-legged hyperextension maneuver in which the patient extends the lumbar spine while standing in one leg and reproducing the patient's ipsilateral symptoms. The other factors that should be identified include inflexibility of the hip and hamstrings muscles, weakness of the core muscles, as well as abnormalities in balance. Rehabilitation of the athlete with a back injury should focus on reducing pain, protecting injured tissue, limited bed rest, and early mobilization (105).

In the initial phase of treatment, modalities such as ice and electrical stimulation can be used in combination with static exercises to train proper muscle firing. Identification of the neutral spine position of comfort and education about proper spine biomechanics should be done at this stage. Light aerobic exercise, muscle relaxants, and NSAIDs that facilitate participation in the rehabilitation program should also be used.

In the recovery phase of treatment, flexion- or extension-biased exercise should be used, depending on the direction that exacerbates the symptoms. Patients with radicular pain secondary to discogenic disease can benefit from extension exercises, while patients with facet syndrome or spondylolysis benefit from flexion exercises (106). Back stabilization exercises in the neutral spine position are used to strengthen the back and pelvic core musculature. The muscles that are targeted for exercise training include the multifidi, quadratus lumborum, abdominals, and hip muscles (13,14). Dynamic flexibility training in sagittal, frontal, and transverse planes of motion should be started gradually as the core strength improves. As the patient's pain improves, specific inflexibilities of the hip flexors, rotators, and hamstrings, as well as muscle imbalances are addressed.

In the functional treatment phase, the progression of trunk strengthening is emphasized. Exercises with gym balls, rotational patterns, and eccentric loading of the spine are done. Normal spine mechanics for sports activities and progression of sports-specific training are required prior to allowing the athlete to return to competition.

Considerations should be given to the use of spinal bracing in patients with spondylolysis who do not respond to treatment. The use of epidural steroid injections can be considered in patients who have a radiculopathy that inhibits participation in the rehabilitation program, and other spinal injection techniques such as medial branch blocks or intra-articular facet steroid injections can be considered for facet-mediated pain.

Surgery can be required in the rare case of failure of conservative treatment for discogenic pain. Return to play after surgical treatment is variable, but aggressive rehabilitation frequently allows a rapid return to competition. Patients with percutaneous discectomy or microdiscectomy can return to sports activities several months after their injury; however, patients having a surgical spinal fusion typically take up to a year to return to noncontact sports (107).

Prevention of low back pain is very important for the athlete, since a history of previous symptoms statistically predispose to recurrent injury (108). Hip muscle imbalance has been considered as one of the predisposing factors for back pain and core strengthening programs for the correction of these imbalances show promise as a prehabilitation strategy (109).

SPECIFIC POPULATIONS IN SPORTS MEDICINE

Older Athlete (See Also Chapter 47 on Geriatric Rehabilitation)

With improvement in medical care, there has been a significant increase in the aging population that is participating in exercise and competitive sports. This trend is accelerating, and by 2030, approximately 20% of Americans will be elderly. Structured physical activity in the form of regular exercise appears to have a significant role in preventing and reversing some of the changes typically associated with age. Regular exercise benefits older adults through improved overall health and physical fitness, increased opportunities for social contacts, gains in cerebral function, lower rates of mortality, and fewer years of disability in later life. Walking and to some extent running, as well as strength training are forms of regular exercise that can be performed throughout life and result in physiologic as well as functional benefits, that in turn improve the quality of life of the elderly (110).

An important issue in the older athlete is the relationship of exercise and osteoarthritis (OA). Available information about the effects of sports on the synovial joint and the development of OA is not conclusive and sometimes contradictory. Exercise therapy benefits pain control, self-reported disability, walking performance, and patient's global assessment in this population (111). The existing literature fails to support an association or causal relationship between low- and moderate-distance running and osteoarthritis. Increasing age, previous joint injury, and greater body mass index have consistently been associated with an increased risk of developing osteoarthritis. There is evidence that high-volume running may be associated to the development of osteoarthritis, but the definition of high-volume running is not clear (112,113).

Many of the patients with OA eventually benefit from arthroplasty to improve function, decrease pain symptoms, and allow the return to sports after joint replacements. The majority of patients are permitted to return to low-impact sports like golf, hiking, dancing, cycling, and bowling (111). Patients who did not participate in sports preoperatively are less likely to begin sports after surgery. There is still debate about the long-term effect of sports activity on prosthesis wear, loosening, and revision rates. It appears that light exercise has no deleterious effect on replaced hips, and some authors have found the risk of loosening to be lower in patients who returned to sports (111).

Female Athlete

Female athletes participating in competitive sports, particularly the ones involving weight categories and scoring systems that can be affected by physical appearance, are under intense pressure to have a low percentage of body fat because of perceived benefits on performance. This can lead to abnormal eating behavior and the development of the female athlete triad. The triad includes low energy availability with or without disordered eating, menstrual dysfunction, and low bone mineral density (114).

Physicians treating female athletes should have a high index of suspicion for this condition, particularly in the athlete who presents with a stress fracture. Management of the female athlete triad involves adequate nutrition to achieve a positive energy balance, supplementation with calcium and vitamin D, weight-bearing exercise that is not excessive, and in some instances medications that can include oral contraceptives. Education of athletes aimed at preventing this condition is key in the young female athlete because bone health and reduced risk of osteoporosis in later life depends on achieving normal peak bone mass in early adulthood.

Osteoporosis is another condition more prevalent in the female athlete, especially postmenopausal females. Risk factors for developing osteoporosis, in addition to excessive exercise and menstrual dysfunction, include sedentary lifestyle. Weight-bearing exercise is an important part of the prevention and treatment of the disease. Exercisers who report lifelong, strenuous, or moderate exercise have a higher bone mass density of the hip than those who report using mild exercises. Postmenopausal women who receive exercise plus calcium supplementation have less bone loss than those who receive calcium supplementation alone.

High-intensity strength training is effective in maintaining femoral neck bone mass density as well as improving muscle mass, strength, and balance in postmenopausal women when compared to unexercised controls (111). Resistance training should take place at least two nonconsecutive days per week and include 2 to 3 sets of 8 to 12 repetitions for each muscle, with short rests between sets to allow for an intensity that can approach muscular fatigue. The amount of weight that is lifted should increase as strength builds, keeping resistance to approximately 60% to 80% of one repetition maximum. Sessions of exercise lasting 20 to 30 minutes are recommended, since sessions lasting 60 minutes or more lead to reduced compliance.

Another issue in the female athlete is the susceptibility to specific musculoskeletal injuries such as ACL tears, patellofemoral pain, and stress fractures. Multiple factors have been identified as possible causes of these injuries in women, including ligamentous laxity, hormonal influences, anatomical variants, muscle strength, and muscle recruitment deficits. Factors that play a role in ACL injury include weakness of proximal muscles, and dynamic movement patterns such as landing on a single limb, with an extended knee that falls into a valgus position (62).

Young Athlete

Sports injuries in children and adolescents are the most common cause of musculoskeletal injury that requires emergency treatment. The most common diagnoses that present to the emergency department are sprains, contusions, and fractures.

The risk of developing sports injuries in the young athlete is associated with nonmodifiable intrinsic factors such as sex, age, and history of previous injury, and modifiable intrinsic and extrinsic factors such as lack of preseason conditioning and poor endurance (see **Table 41-1**) (115). Biomechanical considerations related to overuse injuries include timing of the adolescent growth spurt, quality of movement control, and imbalances between flexibility and muscle strength. Injuries in the young athlete that are related to these biomechanical factors include tibial tubercle and calcaneal apophysitis, patellofemoral pain, and rotator cuff impingement associated with shoulder instability. Early sport specialization may increase rates of overuse injury and sport burnout (116).

Identification of these injury risk factors is very important for planning the medical care of the pediatric athlete. The structured preparticipation examination (PPE) is a valuable tool for the physician practicing sports medicine and possibly the only encounter that the young athlete has with a physician. It has the objectives of identifying medical and orthopedic conditions that would make sports participation unsafe, screens for underlying medical illness and facilitates the development of preventive conditioning programs. Components of the PPE include a brief medical and family history, a general medical examination, and a clinical evaluation of the major joints. The scheduling of the PPE should be one that allows sufficient time to address the treatment and the rehabilitation issues identified prior to the competitive season, typically at least 6 to 8 weeks prior to the beginning of the season.

The benefits of strength training for the pediatric age athlete have been debated over the last several years. It appears that strength training in this population can have health-related benefits that include an increase in bone mass and loss of body fat as well as fitness-related benefits such as increase in power and strength. Strength training can also lead to a reduction in sports injuries. Strength training programs also appear to be safe when they are structured appropriately and emph size light weights lifted with correct technique for 10 to 15 repetitions. The program should combine single-joint, open chain exercises with multijoint, closed chain exercises (117).

Physically Challenged Athletes (See Also Chapter 42 on Paralympic Athlete and Chapter 43 on Physical Activity for People with Disabilities)

The opportunity to participate in sports competition has increased for physically challenged athletes in recent years. It has been estimated that over 2 million disabled athletes participate in sports competition in the United States. In addition, many athletes have had the opportunity to represent their country in international competitions and participate at an elite level. In the 2016 Rio Summer Paralympic Games, 4,350 athletes participated, compared to 400 athletes in the 1960 Games.

The type of physical impairment of the athlete and the sports in which they participate typically determines the type of injury that the competitor is most likely to suffer. Wheelchair athletes who compete in track and field or basketball usually present with soft tissue injuries of the upper limb, particularly the shoulder. While ambulating, athletes suffered injuries that involve the lower limbs (118).

Medical issues that need to be addressed in physically challenged athletes include respiratory illnesses, skin integrity, gastrointestinal issues, and coexisting diseases (119). The proper fit of adaptive equipment, wheelchairs, prostheses, and orthoses should be carefully assessed. Other factors that can affect exercise performance include venous pooling of the lower extremities in the sitting athlete, poor trunk muscle control that affects upper limb function, and muscle imbalances secondary to neurologic injury.

Medical Issues in Sports Medicine

The team physician should be prepared to deal with medical issues that arise in the care of their athletes. These issues can include identification of cardiac risk factors for sudden death, management of respiratory problems such as exercise-induced asthma, gastrointestinal problems like gastroenteritis, and fluid and electrolytes balance. Other issues that also need to be addressed include inappropriate weight loss behavior, the use of ergogenic aids, and doping rules in sports competition.

Cardiovascular Issues in Sports

An integral part of the preparticipation physical examination for athletes is the cardiovascular evaluation. The goal of this evaluation is to identify athletes who are at risk for sudden cardiac death during vigorous physical activity. By applying elements of the personal history, the family history, and the physical exam, the most important signs and symptoms of the most common cardiac reasons for sudden death can be obtained. These include hypertrophic cardiomyopathy (HCM), selected arrhythmias, coronary artery anomalies, and ruptured aortic aneurysms (120). In particular, HCM has received much attention in the press and in the literature as it has taken the lives of several high-profile athletes. It is the primary cause of sudden atraumatic death in athletes, responsible for nearly 35% of those deaths (121).

General Cardiac Evaluations

The guideline recommendations for preparticipation athletic screening of the cardiovascular system include a thorough evaluation of the family history, the personal and present medical history, and the physical evaluation (121).

Importantly, one should ask if there is a history of premature or sudden cardiac death, or if there have been any deaths of unknown etiologies in young family members under the age of 50. As mentioned earlier, HCM is a familial disease, as is Marfan's syndrome, which can lead to ruptured aortic aneurysms. There are also elements of the personal history that are crucial to the cardiovascular evaluation of any athlete. Questions regarding medical history of heart murmurs, systemic hypertension, and exertional symptoms are important (121).

The physical exam is key to identifying possible at-risk athletes. Auscultation of a murmur warrants further evaluation and requires employment of tactics like Valsalva, squatting, standing, to be able to demonstrate the qualities of the murmur, and to possibly define pathology. Abnormal pulse and heart rhythm abnormalities need to be evaluated further.

Lateral and inferior migration of the point of maximal impact (PMI) of the heart on the chest wall may also be a sign of left ventricular hypertrophy. If any of the abovementioned scenarios are uncovered, the athlete must be precluded from exercise until further workup has occurred with electrocardiogram (EKG), echocardiogram, and possibly a Holter monitor.

Corrado et al. performed a multiyear study in Italy, analyzing the efficacy of a nationally implemented standardized preparticipation cardiovascular evaluation for the detection of at-risk athletes for sudden death (122). They included EKG in addition to a standard history and physical exam. This multiyear study concluded that there was decreased incidence of sudden cardiac deaths since the initiation of the national screening program secondary to better detection of the at-risk athletes and precluding them from participation. However, there have been questions raised regarding cost-effectiveness and the risk of false-positive diagnoses with the use of EKG as a part of the routine screening cardiac evaluation (121).

Needless to say, a focused cardiac preparticipation evaluation must be an essential part of the armamentarium of the sports medicine physician. The physician must also serve as an educator to coaches, players, and parents about the warning signs of dangerous cardiac scenarios.

Doping Considerations

Physicians who treat athletes and cover teams that participate at the college, professional, and Olympic level need to understand local, national, and international doping regulations that may affect eligibility to participate in sports. The list of prohibited substances and methods is the international standard that determines what is prohibited in sports and out of competition and is produced by the World Anti-Doping Agency (WADA) (123). Other governing organizations such as the National Collegiate Athletic Association (NCAA) have drug-testing programs to deter athletes from using performance-enhancing drugs that may impact eligibility to participate, affect their health, and provide an unfair advantage in competition (124).

The use of anabolic steroids, stimulants, and other ergogenic substances has become widespread in sports as athletes look to develop an advantage on their competitors. Anabolic agents are commonly used and have been shown to contribute to an increase in body weight, lean body mass, and muscle strength in the athlete who uses them in combination with high-intensity exercise and adequate nutrition. The side effects of these agents are multiple, particularly when used in very high doses, and include decreased testicular size, infertility, increased cholesterol, elevated blood pressure, and aggressive behavior (125).

The sports medicine physician and the members of the health care team need to be aware of the risks associated with the use of these agents, counsel athletes, and instill in the athlete the importance of fair play and competition.

ADVANCES IN SPORTS MEDICINE

Sports Ultrasound (see Chapter 6 on Diagnostic Ultrasound)

The use of ultrasound in sports medicine has increased in the past decade (126). Improvements in technology, reduced cost, and widespread availability of training have made this tool available to nonradiologists. Because of its many advantages, such as, high-resolution soft tissue imaging, real-time and dynamic examination, patient interaction, portability, lack of radiation, and low cost, it has become a very attractive diagnostic and procedure guidance tool. Nevertheless, it is not free of limitations, including inability to see through bone, limited penetration, limited field of view, and significant operator dependence (127).

This technology is very appealing to the sports physician for its diagnostic and interventional capabilities. The use of ultrasound to diagnose musculoskeletal injuries including fascia, muscle, tendon, ligament, bone, and articular pathologies has been well described in the literature (127–130). It has been shown to increase the accuracy of infiltration or aspiration of joints, bursae, muscles, tendon sheaths, and nerves, (131) in addition to guide interventions such as tenotomies, releases, hydrodissection, percutaneous needle scraping among others (131,132).

Because ultrasound's indications extend well beyond the realm of musculoskeletal medicine, it has been suggested that the term "sport ultrasound" can be used as a more accurate term for the broad applications of ultrasound in sports medicine. Nonmusculoskeletal uses of ultrasound include the extended Focused Assessment with Sonography for Trauma (eFAST), limited preparticipation echocardiographic screening, assessment of glycogen stores, optic nerve sheath diameter in athletes with increased intracranial pressure, and vocal cord dysfunction in athletes (133).

Regenerative Medicine

Regenerative medicine has provided the sports medicine physicians with new tools to provide better patient care using minimally invasive procedures. Understanding of pathology in overuse and degenerative injuries has changed with the knowledge that not all injuries have an inflammatory etiology but are associated with chronic degeneration and an impaired healing response (134). Treatments that have traditionally been used in sports medicine, such as NSAIDs and corticosteroids, have been questioned in the treatment of overuse and degenerative injuries. NSAIDs provide effective short-term relief in acute injuries, including ankle sprains, and acute tendon injuries, in part due to its analgesic properties. However, the inhibition of prostaglandins caused by NSAIDs reduces the inflammatory response. This could lead to impaired tendon healing by reducing fibroblast proliferation and affect fracture healing by preventing callus formation (134). Corticosteroids provide adequate short-term relief, which in turn helps patients participate in a comprehensive rehabilitation program. However, evidence suggests that corticosteroids may affect tendon and cartilage structural properties. Its use in recurrent injuries or when evidence of tendon or cartilage degeneration is present might be limited unless there is a clear rationale of achieving short-term pain relief in order to meet other rehabilitation goals (135).

Regenerative medicine treatments include prolotherapy, PRP, and mesenchymal stem cells. Several studies on the effectiveness of PRP in the treatment of chronic tendinopathies have been published (136–140). There is also some evidence for the use of PRP and mesenchymal stem cells in osteoarthritis (141–146). The exact mechanism by which regenerative treatments work is not yet clear, but basic science seems to support the theory of enhancing the local environment and up-regulating the healing factors of local tissues (147).

Despite the great promise of regenerative medicine, there is still a long way to go before treatments and protocols are standardized. Currently, there is variability in the preparations and techniques utilized for PRP, including the role of leukocytes, number of platelets, activation, and the timeframe before another intervention is attempted. Similarly, there is variability in the harvesting and preparation of mesenchymal stem cell, including the tissue to be harvested, bone marrow or adipose tissue, the method of extraction, and whether the stem cells need to be concentrated, processed, or expanded. Choosing the appropriate treatment protocol can be a challenge with the variability of pathologies and different stages of disease seen in our athletes (148).

Finally, the appropriate postprocedure and rehabilitation protocols need to be further defined in order to potentiate the healing effects of the treatments. When and how much to load ligaments and joints after different regenerative procedures in each specific condition needs to be delineated. In the meantime, general concepts of postprocedure rehabilitation include protected weight bearing in the first days after treatment, avoiding NSAIDs 1 week before and 2 to 4 weeks after procedure, and gentle ROM after initial joint protection. Two weeks after the injection, the patient may begin stretching and concentric strengthening. During the collagen-strengthening phase (approximately 4 to 6 weeks after injection), the patient may begin eccentric training. Finally, sports-specific and functional training can be instituted in the final stages of the rehabilitation regimen (149).

TRAINING AND CERTIFICATION IN SPORTS MEDICINE

In the United States, sports medicine fellowship training programs are accredited by the Accreditation Council for Graduate Medical Education (ACGME) and are sponsored by core specialties such as PM&R and Family Medicine. The sports medicine subspecialty programs are of 1-year duration and fellowship training requirements are similar for programs sponsored by PM&R, Family Medicine, Emergency Medicine, Pediatrics, and Internal Medicine.

Fellows should have a clinical and academic curriculum which includes lectures; journal clubs; training experiences in sports medicine clinics; primary care of the athlete; and event and team coverage including management of emergencies in the field of play. Training in musculoskeletal ultrasound has become an integral part of sports medicine training, and experience in this area is mandatory for all fellows (150).

At present, there are 19 sports medicine fellowship programs in the United States sponsored by core PM&R programs accredited by ACGME, but PM&R residents can apply to sports medicine programs sponsored by the other core specialties that offer subspecialty training.

Subspecialty certification in sports medicine granted by the American Board of Physical Medicine and Rehabilitation (ABPMR) started in 2006, initial candidates qualifying for the examination through a clinical pathway. At this time, only individuals who train in ACGME-accredited fellowships qualify for the board exam and subspecialty certification.

REFERENCES

1. McCrory P. What is sports and exercise medicine? *Br J Sports Med*. 2006;40(12): 955–957.
2. Frontera WR. Epidemiology of sports injuries: implications for rehabilitation. In: Frontera WR, ed. *Rehabilitation of Sports Injuries: Scientific Basis*. Malden, MA: Blackwell; 2003:3–9.
3. Frontera WR, Micheo WF, Amy E, et al. Patterns of injuries in athletes evaluated in an interdisciplinary clinic. *P R Health Sci J*. 1994;13(3):165–170.
4. Frontera WR, Micheo WF, Aguirre G, et al. Patterns of disease and utilization of health services during international sports competitions. *Arch Med Dep*. 1997;14:479–484.
5. Fredericson M. Common injuries in runners. Diagnosis, rehabilitation and prevention. *Sports Med*. 1996;21(1):49–72.
6. Timpka T, Alonso JM, Jacobsson J, et al. Injury and illness definitions and data collection procedures for use in epidemiological studies in Athletics (track and field): consensus statement. *Br J Sports Med*. 2014;48(7):483–490.
7. Kibler WB. A framework for sports medicine: evaluation and treatment. *Phys Med Rehabil Clin N Am*. 1994;5:1–8.
8. Dale B. Principles of rehabilitation. In: Andrews J, Harrelson G, Wilk K, eds. *Physical Rehabilitation of the Injured Athlete*. 4th ed. Philadelphia, PA: Elsevier/Saunders; 2012:41–66.
9. Frontera WR. Exercise and musculoskeletal rehabilitation: restoring optimal form and function. *Phys Sportsmed*. 2003;31:39–45.
10. Micheo W, Baerga L, Miranda G. Basic principles regarding strength, flexibility, and stability exercises. *PM R*. 2012;4(11):805–811.
11. Schwellnus M. Flexibility and joint range of motion. In: Frontera WR, ed. *Rehabilitation of Sports Injuries: Scientific Basis*. Malden, MA: Blackwell; 2003:232–257.
12. Krivickas L. Training flexibility. In: Frontera W, Dawson D, Slovik S, eds. *Exercise in Rehabilitation Medicine*. Champaign, IL: Human Kinetics; 1999:83–102.
13. Kibler WB. Closed kinetic chain rehabilitation for sports injuries. *Phys Med Rehabil Clin N Am*. 2000;11(2):369–384.
14. Escamilla RF, Fleisig GS, Zheng N, et al. Biomechanics of the knee during closed kinetic chain and open kinetic chain exercises. *Med Sci Sports Exerc*. 1998;30(4):556–569.
15. Kibler WB, Wilkes T, Sciascia A. Mechanics and pathomechanics in the overhead athlete. *Clin Sports Med*. 2013;32:637–651.
16. Akuthota V, Ferreiro A, Moore T, et al. Core stability exercise principles. *Curr Sports Med Rep*. 2008;7:39–44.
17. McGill S. Building better rehabilitation programs for low back injuries. In: McGill S, ed. *Low Back Disorders: Evidence-based Prevention and Rehabilitation*. Champaign, IL: Human Kinetics; 2002:205–222.
18. Laskowski ER, Newcomer-Aney K, Smith J. Proprioception. *Phys Med Rehabil Clin N Am*. 2000;11(2):323–340.
19. Kibler W, Chandler T. Functional rehabilitation and return to training and competition. In: Frontera W, ed. *Rehabilitation of Sports Injuries: Scientific Basis*. Malden, MA: Blackwell; 2003:288–300.
20. Creighton DW, Shrier I, Shultz R, et al. Return-to-play in sport: a decision-based model. *Clin J Sport Med*. 2010;20:379–385.
21. Brockett CL, Morgan DL, Proske U. Predicting hamstring strain injury in elite athletes. *Med Sci Sports Exerc*. 2004;36(3):379–387.
22. Gilchrist J, Mandelbaum BR, Melancon H, et al. A randomized controlled trial to prevent noncontact anterior cruciate ligament injury in female collegiate soccer players. *Am J Sports Med*. 2008;36(8):1476–1483.
23. Kibler WB, Kuhn JE, Wilk K, et al. The disabled throwing shoulder: spectrum of pathology-10-year update. *Arthroscopy*. 2013;29:141.e26–161.e26.
24. Bahr R, Craig EV, Engebretsen L. The clinical presentation of shoulder instability including on field management. *Clin Sports Med*. 1995;14(4):761–776.
25. Ufberg JW, Vilke GM, Chan TC, et al. Anterior shoulder dislocations: beyond traction-countertraction. *J Emerg Med*. 2004;27:301–306.
26. Zaremski JL, Galloza J, Sepulveda F, et al. Recurrence and return to play after shoulder instability events in young and adolescent athletes: a systematic review and meta-analysis. *Br J Sports Med*. 2017;51:177–184.
27. Harris JD, Romeo AA. Arthroscopic management of the contact athlete with instability. *Clin Sports Med*. 2013;32:709–730.
28. Wolin P. Shoulders injuries. In: Kibler WB, ed. *ACSM's Handbook for the Team Physician*. Baltimore, MD: Lippincott Williams & Wilkins; 1996:253–271.
29. Bradley JP, Elkousy H. Decision making: operative versus nonoperative treatment of acromioclavicular joint injuries. *Clin Sports Med*. 2003;22:277–290.
30. Wilk KE, MacRina LC, Fleisig GS, et al. Correlation of glenohumeral internal rotation deficit and total rotational motion to shoulder injuries in professional baseball pitchers. *Am J Sports Med*. 2011;39(2):329–335.
31. Manske R, Ellenbecker T. Current concepts in shoulder examination of the overhead athlete. *Int J Sports Phys Ther*. 2013;8(5):545–567.
32. O'Brien SJ, Pagnani MJ, Fealy S, et al. The active compression test: a new and effective test for diagnosing labral tears and acromioclavicular joint abnormality. *Am J Sports Med*. 1998;26(5):610–613.
33. Sciascia A, Thigpen C, Namdari S, et al. Kinetic chain abnormalities in the athletic shoulder. *Sports Med Arthrosc Rev*. 2012;20:16–21.
34. Wilk KE, Meister K, Andrews JR. Current concepts in the rehabilitation of the overhead throwing athlete. *Am J Sports Med*. 2002;30(1):136–151.
35. Krabak BJ, Sugar R, McFarland EG. Practical nonoperative management of rotator cuff injuries. *Clin J Sports Med*. 2003;12:102–105.

36. Micheo W, Rivera A, Miranda G. Glenohumeral instability. In: Frontera WR, Silver J, eds. *Essentials of Physical Medicine and Rehabilitation*. 3rd ed. Philadelphia, PA: Hanley & Belfus; 2014:76–89.

37. Zhang AL, Montgomery SR, Ngo SS, et al. Arthroscopic versus open shoulder stabilization: current practice patterns in the United States. *Arthroscopy*. 2014;30(4):436–443.

38. Freedman KB, Smith AP, Romeo AA, et al. Open Bankart repair versus arthroscopic repair with transglenoid sutures or bioabsorbable tacks for recurrent anterior instability of the shoulder: a meta-analysis. *Am J Sports Med*. 2004;32(6):1520–1527.

39. Ticker JB, Warner JJP. Selective capsular shift technique for anterior and anterior-inferior glenohumeral instability. *Clin Sports Med*. 2000;19:1–17.

40. McGuire DT, Bain GI. Management of dislocations of the elbow in the athlete. *Sports Med Arthrosc Rev*. 2014;22:188–193.

41. Plancher KD, Lucas TS. Fracture dislocations of the elbow in athletes. *Clin Sports Med*. 2001;20:59–76.

42. Akuthota V, Chou LH, Drake DF, et al. Sports and performing arts medicine. 2. Shoulder and elbow overuse injuries in sports. *Arch Phys Med Rehabil*. 2004; 85(3 suppl 1):S52–S58.

43. Wilk KE, Macrina LC, Cain EL, et al. Rehabilitation of the overhead athlete's elbow. *Sports Health*. 2012;4(5):404–414.

44. Nguyen RT, Borg-Stein J, McInnis K. Applications of platelet-rich plasma in musculoskeletal and sports medicine: an evidence-based approach. *PM R*. 2011;3(3):226–250.

45. Micheo W, Esquenazi A. Orthoses in the prevention and rehabilitation of injuries. In: Frontera W, ed. *Rehabilitation of Sports Injuries: Scientific Basis*. Malden, MA: Blackwell; 2003:301–315.

46. Naylor M. Elbow injury in the throwing athlete. *Curr Sports Med Rep*. 2016;15: 309–310.

47. Brunton L, Graham T, Atkinson R. Hand injuries. In: Miller M, Thompson S, DeLee J, et al., eds. *DeLee & Drez's Orthopedic Sports Medicine Principles and Practice*. Philadelphia, PA: Saunders; 2015:884–907.

48. Rettig AC. Athletic injuries of the wrist and hand. Part I: traumatic injuries of the wrist. *Am J Sports Med*. 2003;31(6):1038–1048.

49. Lewis DM, Lee Osterman A. Scapholunate instability in athletes. *Clin Sports Med*. 2001;20:131–140.

50. Rettig AC. Athletic injuries of the wrist and hand: part II: overuse injuries of the wrist and traumatic injuries to the hand. *Am J Sports Med*. 2004;32(6):262–273.

51. Chu SK, Rho ME. Hamstring injuries in the athlete: diagnosis, treatment, and return to play. *Curr Sports Med Rep*. 2016;15(3):184–190.

52. Mallow M, Nazarian LN. Greater trochanteric pain syndrome diagnosis and treatment. *Phys Med Rehabil Clin N Am*. 2014;25:279–289.

53. Jagtap P, Shetty G, Mane P, et al. Emerging intra-articular causes of groin pain in athletes. *Eur J Orthop Surg Traumatol*. 2014;24:1331–1339.

54. Byrd JWT. Femoroacetabular impingement in athletes: current concepts. *Am J Sports Med*. 2014;42(3):737–751.

55. Beatty NR, Félix I, Hettler J, et al. Rehabilitation and prevention of proximal hamstring tendinopathy. *Curr Sports Med Rep*. 2017;16:162–171.

56. Arendt E, Dick R. Knee injury patterns among men and women in collegiate basketball and soccer. *Am J Sports Med*. 1995;23(6):694–701.

57. Woo SL, Debski RE, Withrow JD, et al. Biomechanics of knee ligaments. *Am J Sports Med*. 1999;27(4):533–543.

58. Micheo W, Hernández L, Seda C. Evaluation, management, rehabilitation, and prevention of anterior cruciate ligament injury: current concepts. *PM R*. 2010;2(10):935–944.

59. Fu FH, Bennett CH, Lattermann C, et al. Current trends in anterior cruciate ligament reconstruction. Part 1: biology and biomechanics of reconstruction. *Am J Sports Med*. 1999;27(6):821–830.

60. Fu FH, Bennett CH, Ma CB, et al. Current concepts current trends in anterior cruciate ligament reconstruction part II. Operative procedures and clinical correlations. *Sports Med*. 2000;28(1):124–130.

61. Arnold T, Shelbourne KD. A perioperative rehabilitation program for anterior cruciate ligament surgery. *Phys Sportsmed*. 2000;28(1):31–44.

62. Acevedo RJ, Rivera-Vega A, Miranda G, et al. Anterior cruciate ligament injury: Identification of risk factors and prevention strategies. *Curr Sports Med Rep*. 2014;13(3):186–191.

63. Sepúlveda F, Sánchez L, Amy E, et al. Anterior cruciate ligament injury: return to play, function and long-term considerations. *Curr Sports Med Rep*. 2017;16(3):172–178.

64. Grindem H, Snyder-Mackler L, Moksnes H, et al. Simple decision rules can reduce reinjury risk by 84% after ACL reconstruction: The Delaware-Oslo ACL cohort study. *Br J Sports Med*. 2016;50(13):804–808.

65. Cox CL, Deangelis JP, Magnussen RA, et al. Meniscal tears in athletes. *J Surg Orthop Adv*. 2009;18(1):2–8.

66. Beutler A, O'Connor F. Physical examination of the knee. In: Malanga G, Mautner K, eds. *Musculoskeletal Physical Examination*. 2nd ed. Philadelphia, PA: Elsevier; 2016:173–198.

67. Katz JN, Brophy RH, Chaisson CE, et al. Surgery versus physical therapy for a meniscal tear and osteoarthritis. *N Engl J Med*. 2013;368(18):1675–1684.

68. Kozlowski EJ, Barcia AM, Tokish JM. Meniscus repair: the role of accelerated rehabilitation in return to sport. *Sports Med Arthrosc Rev*. 2012;20:121–126.

69. Witvrouw E, Callaghan MJ, Stefanik JJ, et al. Patellofemoral pain: consensus statement from the 3rd International Patellofemoral Pain Research Retreat held in Vancouver, September 2013. *Br J Sports Med*. 2014;48(6):411–414.

70. Dutton RA, Khadavi MJ, Fredericson M. Update on rehabilitation of patellofemoral pain. *Curr Sports Med Rep*. 2014;13(3):172–178.

71. McConnell J. The physical therapist's approach to patellofemoral disorders. *Clin Sports Med*. 2002;21:363–387.

72. Pidoriano AJ, Fulkerson JP. Arthroscopy of the patellofemoral joint. *Clin Sports Med*. 1997;16:17–28.

73. Kaminski TW, Hertel J, Amendola N, et al. National athletic trainers' association position statement: conservative management and prevention of ankle sprains in athletes. *J Athl Train*. 2013;48(4):528–545.

74. DiGiovanni BF, Partal G, Baumhauer JF. Acute ankle injury and chronic lateral instability in the athlete. *Clin Sports Med*. 2004;23:1–19.

75. Safran MR, Benedetti RS, Bartolozzi AR, et al. Lateral ankle sprains: a comprehensive review: part 1: etiology, pathoanatomy, histopathogenesis, and diagnosis. *Med Sci Sports Exerc*. 1999;31(7 suppl):S429–S437.

76. Verhagen E. The effect of a proprioceptive balance board training program for the prevention of ankle sprains: a prospective controlled trial. *Am J Sports Med*. 2004;32(6):1385–1393.

77. Gross MT, Liu H-Y. The role of ankle bracing for prevention of ankle sprain injuries. *J Orthop Sports Phys Ther*. 2003;33(10):572–577.

78. Egger AC, Berkowitz MJ. Achilles tendon injuries. *Curr Rev Musculoskelet Med*. 2017;10:72–80.

79. Molloy A, Selvan D. Ligamentous injuries of the foot and ankle. In: Miller M, Thompson SR, DeLee J, et al., eds. *DeLee & Drez's Orthopedic Sports Medicine Principles and Practice*. Philadelphia, PA: Saunders; 2015:1392–1407.

80. Tenforde AS, Kraus E, Fredericson M. Bone stress injuries in runners. *Phys Med Rehabil Clin N Am*. 2016;27:139–149.

81. Fredericson M, Jennings F, Beaulieu C, et al. Stress fractures in athletes. *Top Magn Reson Imaging*. 2006;17:309–325.

82. Iwamoto J, Takeda T. Stress fractures in athletes: review of 196 cases. *J Orthop Sci*. 2003;8:273–278.

83. Barr KP, Harrast MA. Evidence-based treatment of foot and ankle injuries in runners. *Phys Med Rehabil Clin N Am*. 2005;16:779–799.

84. Sorosky B, Press J, Plastaras C, et al. The practical management of achilles tendinopathy. *Clin J Sport Med*. 2004;14(1):40–44.

85. Simons SM. Foot injuries in the runner. In: O'Connor FG, Wilder RP, eds. *Textbook of Running Medicine*. New York: McGraw-Hill; 2001:213–226.

86. Berbrayer D, Fredericson M. Update on evidence-based treatments for plantar fasciopathy. *PM R*. 2014;6:159–169.

87. Lou J, Wang S, Liu S, et al. Effectiveness of extracorporeal shock wave therapy without local anesthesia in patients with recalcitrant plantar fasciitis. *Am J Phys Med Rehabil*. 2017;96(8):529–534.

88. Kay MC, Register-Mihalik JK, Gray AD, et al. The epidemiology of severe injuries sustained by National Collegiate Athletic Association student-athletes, 2009–2010 through 2014–2015. *J Athl Train*. 2017;52(2):117–128.

89. Ghiselli G, Schaadt G, McAllister DR. On-the-field evaluation of an athlete with a head or neck injury. *Clin Sports Med*. 2003;22:445–465.

90. Spinal Cord Injury (SCI) facts and figures at a glance. *J Spinal Cord Med*. 2016;39(2):243–244.

91. Kucera KL, Yau RK, Register-Mihalik J, et al. Traumatic brain and spinal cord fatalities among high school and college football players—United States, 2005–2014. *MMWR Morb Mortal Wkly Rep*. 2017;65(52):1465–1469.

92. McCrory P, Meeuwisse W, Dvorak J, et al. Consensus statement on concussion in sport- the 5th international conference on concussion in sport held in Berlin, October 2016. *Br J Sports Med*. 2017;13(2):53–65.

93. Heads up to Brain Injury Awareness. Centers for Disease Control and Prevention. https://www.cdc.gov/headsup/index.html. Updated June 22, 2017. Accessed: November 24, 2018.

94. Maddocks DL, Dicker GD, Saling MM. The assessment of orientation following concussion in athletes. *Clin J Sport Med*. 1995;5:32–35.

95. McCrea M. Standardized mental status testing on the sideline after sport-related concussion. *J Athl Train*. 2001;36(3):274–279.

96. Echemendia RJ, Meeuwisse W, McCrory P, et al. The sport concussion assessment tool 5th edition (SCAT5): background and rationale. *Br J Sports Med*. 2017;51:848–850.

97. Davis GA, Purcell L, Schneider KJ, et al. The child sport concussion assessment tool 5th edition (Child SCAT5): background and rationale. *Br J Sports Med*. 2017;51(11):859–861.

98. Appropriate Care of the Spine Injured Athlete. The National Athletic Trainers' Association (NATA) and the Inter-Association Task Force. https://www.nata.org/sites/default/files/Executive-Summary-Spine-Injury.pdf. Updated 2015. Accessed: November 24, 2018.

99. Morganti C. Recommendations for return to sports following cervical spine injuries. *Sports Med*. 2003;33(8):563–573.

100. Fagan K. Transient quadriplegia and return-to-play criteria. *Clin Sports Med*. 2004;23:409–419.

101. Weinstein SM. Assessment and rehabilitation of the athlete with a "stinger." *Clin Sports Med*. 1998;17:127–135.

102. Friedly J, Standaert C, Chan L. Epidemiology of spine care: the back pain dilemma. *Phys Med Rehabil Clin N Am*. 2010;21:659–677.

103. Stracciolini A, Casciano R, Levey Friedman H, et al. Pediatric sports injuries: an age comparison of children versus adolescents. *Am J Sports Med*. 2013;41(8):1922–1929.

104. Borg-Stein J, Elson L, Brand E. The aging spine in sports. *Clin Sports Med*. 2012;31(3):473–486.

105. Dahm KT, Jamtvedt G, Hagen KB, et al. Advice to rest in bed versus advice to stay active for acute low-back pain and sciatica. *Cochrane Database Syst Rev*. 2010;(6):CD007612.

106. Donelson R. The McKenzie approach to evaluating and treating low back pain. *Orthop Rev*. 1990;19(8):681–686.

107. Eck JC, Riley LH. Return to play after lumbar spine conditions and surgeries. *Clin Sports Med.* 2004;23:367–379.
108. Greene HS, Cholewicki J, Galloway MT, et al. A history of low back injury is a risk factor for recurrent back injuries in varsity athletes. *Am J Sports Med.* 2001;29(6):795–800.
109. Nadler SF, Malanga GA, Bartoli LA, et al. Hip muscle imbalance and low back pain in athletes: influence of core strengthening. *Med Sci Sports Exerc.* 2002;34(1):9–16.
110. Chodzko-Zajko WJ, Proctor DN, Fiatarone Singh MA, et al. Exercise and physical activity for older adults. *Med Sci Sports Exerc.* 2009;41:1510–1530.
111. Concannon LG, Grierson MJ, Harrast MA. Exercise in the older adult: from the sedentary elderly to the masters athlete. *PM R.* 2012;4(11):833–839.
112. Hansen P, English M, Willick SE. Does running cause osteoarthritis in the hip or knee? *PM R.* 2012;4(5 suppl):S117–S121.
113. Straker JS, Vannatta CN, Waldron K. Treatment strategies for the master athlete with known arthritis of the hip and knee. *Top Geriatr Rehabil.* 2016;32:39–54.
114. De Souza MJ, Nattiv A, Joy E, et al. 2014 female athlete triad coalition consensus statement on treatment and return to play of the female athlete triad: 1st international conference held in San Francisco, CA, May 2012, and 2nd international conference held in Indianapolis, IN, May 2013. *Clin J Sport Med.* 2014;24(2):96–119.
115. Emery CA. Risk factors for injury in child and adolescent sport: a systematic review of the literature. *Clin J Sport Med.* 2003;13(4):256–268.
116. Difiori JP, Benjamin HJ, Brenner JS, et al. Overuse injuries and burnout in youth sports: a position statement from the American Medical Society for Sports Medicine. *Br J Sports Med.* 2014;48(4):287–288.
117. McCambridge TM, Stricker PR. Strength training by children and adolescents. *Pediatrics.* 2008;121(4):835–840.
118. Webborn N, Emery C. Descriptive epidemiology of paralympic sports injuries. *PM R.* 2014;6(8 suppl):S18–S22.
119. Simon LM, Ward DC. Preparing for events for physically challenged athletes. *Curr Sports Med Rep.* 2014;13(3):163–168.
120. Gregory A, Kerr Z, Parsons J. Selected issues in injury and illness prevention and the team physician: a consensus statement. *Curr Sports Med Rep.* 2016;15(1):48–59.
121. Drezner JA, O'Connor FG, Harmon KG, et al. AMSSM position statement on cardiovascular preparticipation screening in athletes: current evidence, knowledge gaps, recommendations and future directions. *Br J Sports Med.* 2017;51(3):153–167.
122. Corrado D, Basso C, Pavei A, et al. Trends in sudden cardiovascular death in young competitive athletes after implementation of a preparticipation screening program. *J Am Med Assoc.* 2006;296(13):1593–1601.
123. Available from: https://www.wada-ama.org. [cited 2018 Feb 20]
124. Available from: http://www.ncaa.org/sport-science-institute/doping-and-substance-abuse. [cited 2018 Feb 20].
125. Sturmi JE, Diorio DJ. Anabolic agents. *Clin Sports Med.* 1998;17:261–282.
126. Primack SJ. Past, present, and future considerations for musculoskeletal ultrasound. *Phys Med Rehabil Clin N Am.* 2016;27:749–752.
127. Smith J, Finnoff JT. Diagnostic and interventional musculoskeletal ultrasound: part 1. Fundamentals. *PM R.* 2009;1(1):64–75.
128. Smith J, Finnoff JT. Diagnostic and interventional musculoskeletal ultrasound: part 2. Clinical applications. *PM R.* 2009;1(2):162–177.
129. Lesniak BP, Loveland D, Jose J, et al. Use of ultrasonography as a diagnostic and therapeutic tool in sports medicine. *Arthroscopy.* 2014;30(2):260–270.
130. Tok F, Özçakar L, De Muynck M, et al. Musculoskeletal ultrasound for sports injuries. *Eur J Phys Rehabil Med.* 2012;48:651–663.
131. Finnoff JT, Hall MM, Adams E, et al. American Medical Society for Sports Medicine (AMSSM) position statement: interventional musculoskeletal ultrasound in sports medicine. *PM R.* 2015;7(2):151–168.
132. Peck E, Jelsing E, Onishi K. Advanced ultrasound-guided interventions for tendinopathy. *Phys Med Rehabil Clin N Am.* 2016;27:733–748.
133. Finnoff JT, Ray J, Corrado G, et al. Sports ultrasound: applications beyond the musculoskeletal system. *Sports Health.* 2016;8(5):412–417.
134. Chen MR, Dragoo JL. The effect of nonsteroidal anti-inflammatory drugs on tissue healing. *Knee Surg Sports Traumatol Arthrosc.* 2013;21:540–549.
135. Nichols AW. Complications associated with the use of corticosteroids in the treatment of athletic injuries. *Clin J Sport Med.* 2005;15(5):370–375.
136. Mishra A, Pavelko T. Treatment of chronic elbow tendinosis with buffered platelet-rich plasma. *Am J Sports Med.* 2006;34(11):1774–1778.
137. Mautner K, Colberg RE, Malanga G, et al. Outcomes after ultrasound-guided platelet-rich plasma injections for chronic tendinopathy: a multicenter, retrospective review. *PM R.* 2013;5(3):169–175.
138. Finnoff JT, Fowler SP, Lai JK, et al. Treatment of chronic tendinopathy with ultrasound-guided needle tenotomy and platelet-rich plasma injection. *PM R.* 2011;3(10):900–911.
139. Gosens T, Peerbooms JC, van Laar W, et al. Ongoing positive effect of platelet-rich plasma versus corticosteroid injection in lateral epicondylitis: a double-blind randomized controlled trial with 2-year follow-up. *Am J Sports Med.* 2011;39(6):1200–1208.
140. Peerbooms JC, Sluimer J, Bruijn DJ, et al. Positive effect of an autologous platelet concentrate in lateral epicondylitis in a double-blind randomized controlled trial: platelet-rich plasma versus corticosteroid injection with a 1-year follow-up. *Am J Sports Med.* 2010;38(2):255–262.
141. Filardo G, Kon E, Roffi A, et al. Platelet-rich plasma: why intra-articular? A systematic review of preclinical studies and clinical evidence on PRP for joint degeneration. *Knee Surg Sports Traumatol Arthrosc.* 2015;23:2459–2474.
142. Emadedin M, Aghdami N, Taghiyar L, et al. Intra-articular injection of autologous mesenchymal stem cells in six patients with knee osteoarthritis. *Arch Iran Med.* 2012;15(7):422–428.
143. Koh YG, Jo SB, Kwon OR, et al. Mesenchymal stem cell injections improve symptoms of knee osteoarthritis. *Arthroscopy.* 2013;29(4):748–755.
144. Koh YG, Choi YJ, Kwon OR, et al. Second-look arthroscopic evaluation of cartilage lesions after mesenchymal stem cell implantation in osteoarthritic knees. *Am J Sports Med.* 2014;42(7):1628–1637.
145. Jo C, Lee Y, Shin W. Intra-articular injection of mesenchymal stem cells for the treatment of osteoarthritis of the knee: a proof-of-concept clinical trial. *Stem Cells.* 2014;32:1254–1266.
146. Orozco L, Munar A, Soler R, et al. Treatment of knee osteoarthritis with autologous mesenchymal stem cells. *Transplant J.* 2013;95(12):1535–1541.
147. Malanga GA. Regenerative treatments for orthopedic conditions. *PM R.* 2015;7(4):S1–S3.
148. Sepúlveda F, Baerga L, Micheo W. The role of physiatry in regenerative medicine: the past, the present, and future challenges. *PM R.* 2015;7(4):S76–S80.
149. Mautner K, Malanga G, Colberg R. Optimization of ingredients, procedures and rehabilitation for platelet-rich plasma injections for chronic tendinopathy. *Pain Manag.* 2011;1(6):523–532.
150. Fredericson M. On the horizon: defining the future of sports medicine and the role of the physiatrist. *PM R.* 2012;4(10):707–710.

Paralympic Sports

...and yet a true creator is necessity, which is the mother of our invention.

Plato, The Republic Book II, 369c

Four values underpin the Paralympic Movement: determination, equality, inspiration, and courage (1). This concise set of universal principles weaves its way through the stories of individual Paralympic athletes, the history of the Paralympic Movement, and international sport itself. Interestingly, the historical context that gave rise to the Paralympic Movement is shared by the field of physical medicine and rehabilitation. Both movements began against the backdrop of the two great world wars; both were created, among other things, as a response to the need for progressive medical services for war-wounded citizens with an impairment; both aspire to make for a more inclusive society for people with an impairment; and both continue to require determination and courage to emphasize hope, possibility, and equality despite differences. In this chapter, we will first contextualize the modern Paralympic Movement by reviewing its history and describing its 31 sports. Then, we will review a cornerstone feature of Paralympic sport, athlete classification. This concept may be new to some but should resonate with clinicians who practice a function-focused physical exam in diverse clinical settings. The chapter will then explore issues of ergonomics and physiology in Paralympic sport and review common illnesses and injuries among Para athletes. We conclude by discussing the public health impact of Paralympic sport, and reviewing a few of the interconnected initiatives for health, equality, and inclusion that the Paralympic Movement touches.

HISTORY OF THE PARALYMPIC MOVEMENT

Historical Context

Lasting innovation in physical medicine arose during and after the two great world wars. Physical medicine and rehabilitation (physiatry) and Paralympic sport share this common foundation. Both began as targeted, clinical efforts to restore war-wounded citizens to full physical, mental, emotional, and social health (2,3), and this history continues to influence the values and aims of the contemporary Paralympic Movement.

Origins of Sport for Athletes with Impairment

The origins of international sport for athletes with impairment predate the Paralympic Games. In 1888, the inaugural Sports Club for the Deaf was established in Berlin, Germany (4). As neighboring European countries increasingly followed suit, a community of hearing-impaired athletes and activists grew in size, scope, and ability throughout Europe, culminating in the 1924 International Silent Games, held in Paris, France. These were the first-ever international games for athletes with an impairment and featured just under 150 athletes (5). Every 4 years, the Deaflympics, previously called the World Games for the Deaf, continues to dazzle spectators (4).

Sir Ludwig Guttmann and the Stoke Mandeville Hospital

In 1939, World War II began. In the same year, Dr. Frank Krusen coined the term "physiatrist" (6), and a skilled Jewish neurosurgeon, Dr. (later Sir) Ludwig Guttmann, arrived with his family in Oxford, England (7). Guttmann was a refugee fleeing Nazi Germany, and his early professional work in the United Kingdom comprised clinical research at the prestigious Oxford University and the Wingfield-Morris Orthopedic Hospital (5). In 1943, anticipating a significant uptick in the number of injured servicemen and women returning home during and after the war's second front, the British government asked Sir Guttmann to run a spinal injuries unit at the Stoke Mandeville Hospital. Guttmann agreed under the condition that he would have complete creative autonomy. The 26-bed national spinal injuries unit at the Ministry of Pensions Hospital, Stoke Mandeville, opened on February 1, 1944, in Aylesbury, Buckinghamshire. Its primary mission was to care for servicemen and women returning home with paraplegia and tetraplegia.

Attitudes Toward Spinal Cord–Injured Patients

Prior to the advent of sulfa antibiotics near the conclusion of World War II, even the most progressive clinicians viewed severe spinal injuries as fatal due to the severe attendant secondary complications such as septicemia, renal failure, major depression, and others. Approximately 80% of British and American spinally injured World War I veterans did not survive (3), and those who did "dragged out their lives as useless and hopeless cripples, unemployable and unwanted...with no incentive or encouragement to return to a useful life" (8). Thus, clinicians generally regarded this patient group as unappealing. Guttmann's "[colleagues] could not understand how [he] could leave Oxford University to be engulfed in the hopeless and depressing task of looking after traumatic spinal paraplegics" (9).

As he'd seen in the 1930s Germany (9), Guttmann found a clinical culture characterized by pessimism and resignation in his new spinal unit: morale among clinical staff was low, functional expectations of patients were minimal, and there was great difficulty identifying and recruiting sub–specialty-trained therapists (5). At the time, expectations surrounding the clinical and social outcomes of spinal cord–injured patients were decidedly unambitious. Guttmann famously commented that paraplegia was the "most depressing and neglected [subject] in medicine and society" (10). Medicine and society had essentially excluded an entire class of patients—an entire group of people, from full and complete social inclusion because no satisfactory treatment and rehabilitation protocols seemed to be available.

Guttmann's Revolutionary Rehabilitation Program

Perhaps, his personal experience with the downside of human discrimination and social exclusions enabled Guttmann to immediately recognize this paradigm and to see medicine's "most depressing and neglected" (10) subjects with "one of the most devastating calamities in human life" (8) as equal and respected members of the human community worthy of full lives. Perhaps, his time as a student-fencer (3) gave him a deep personal understanding of the joy of athletic effort informed his professional path. With a pioneering spirit, Guttmann revolutionized the way that veterans with paraplegia and tetraplegia were rehabilitated and understood. Challenging the idea that spinal cord injury (SCI) inevitably portended a short life with little meaning and predictably fatal illness, Guttmann created an intensive, dynamic clinical rehabilitation program (9,11). Patients were led through the initial phases of recovery to community reentry using practical nursing care, a systems-based approach to health maintenance and therapeutic modalities (5,7,9). Multidisciplinary care teams turned patients every 2 hours to help prevent deep tissue injuries, implemented a rigorous genitourinary hygiene program, regularly took patients' limbs through permissible ranges of motion, engaged patients in community recreation, and established pre-vocational work programs, helping to facilitate health, happiness, confidence, and independence (12,13).

Uniquely, Guttmann's program incorporated competitive sport, one of the most social and spirited therapeutic modalities. Taking a holistic view of health and well-being, Guttmann recognized the biopsychosocial value of sport in the inpatient setting (14–16). He described sport as "the most natural form of remedial exercise" and saw it as a powerful tool to restore physical strength, cardiorespiratory fitness, and coordination while also repairing psychological health (13). Using long-held sporting values in the service of rehabilitation, Guttmann's program emphasized competitive sport as a tool to enable self-worth, connection, and meaning, even among those with severe physical impairments. A fitting foundation to the Paralympic Movement, Guttmann's inpatient rehabilitation program was characterized by determination, equality, inspiration, and courage (**Fig. 42-1**).

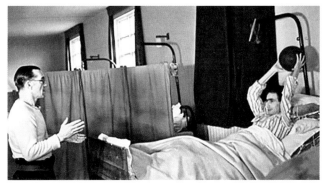

FIGURE 42-1. "Q" Hill, Remedial Gymnast, using a medicine ball to strengthen a patient's upper body at Stoke Mandeville Hospital. (© International Wheelchair & Amputee Sports (IWAS) – www.iwasf.com)

Early Vision, Values, and Aims of the Games

Guttmann's aim was to "not only give hope and a sense of self-worth to the patients, but to change the attitudes of society towards the spinally injured by demonstrating to them that they could not only continue to be useful members of society, but could take part in activities and complete tasks most of the non-disabled society would struggle with" (7). From the outset, Guttmann expressed interest in exploring the therapeutic value of sport, but also in using sport to test the limits of human performance and change societal perceptions of persons with impairment:

> These experiments were the beginning of a systematic development of competitive sport for the paralysed as an essential part of their medical rehabilitation and social re-integration in the community of a country like Great Britain where sport in one form or another plays such an essential part in the lives of so many people (17).

Indeed, Guttmann would take patients into nondisabled community archery clubs, engaging nondisabled persons in competitions with Stoke Mandeville teams, further eroding barriers between the community and paraplegic persons (7).

Guttmann and his staff "started [the sports program] modestly and cautiously with darts, snooker, punch-ball and skittles." Wheelchair polo was then introduced but quickly changed to wheelchair netball (later wheelchair basketball). Archery was started next and was "of immense value in strengthening, in a very natural way, just those muscles of the upper limbs, shoulders and trunk, on which the paraplegic's well-balanced, upright position depends" (**Fig. 42-2**) (17). Like darts, archery also offered impaired athletes an opportunity to compete with their able-bodied counterparts on equal footing (7).

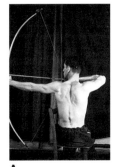
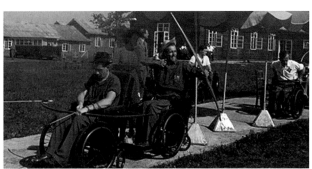

A   **B**

FIGURE 42-2. Archery. In Image B, Roy Jennings (Stoke Mandeville team) releases his *arrow* watched by his fiancée, Effie Wright. "Old Bill," the specially adapted bus, can be seen in the background. (© International Wheelchair & Amputee Sports (IWAS) – www.iwasf.com)

Early Editions of the Stoke Mandeville Games (1948–1959)

In 1948, Guttmann organized a small archery competition among 16 paralyzed British war veterans from two hospitals, the Stoke Mandeville Games (later the "International Stoke Mandeville Games") (18). Two teams of eight archers each competed over distances of 50, 40, and 30 yards; the day included an informal lunch and the presentation of a specially adapted, accessible bus on behalf of the British Legion and London Transport (3,5,7). What started as a modest contest between Stoke Mandeville and the Star and Garter Home for Injured War Veterans evolved in name and scope over the next 12 years, featuring an increasing number of sports, athletes, and nations every year (🛜 **eTable 42-1**).

Fiscal support for the Games came from organizations like the War Veterans Federation and British Paraplegic Fund. They were promoted in three primary ways: word of mouth, often initiated by former Stoke Mandeville patients and staff; media attention, often attracted by the presence of invited celebrity guests; and Guttmann's individual effort in promoting the Games at international conferences and meetings. Guttmann's intentional alignment of the Stoke Mandeville Games with the Olympic Games (18) also helped generate publicity. Indeed, the first archery competition at Stoke Mandeville took place on July 29, 1948, the same day the opening ceremony of the

14th Olympiad took place in London, England. During the 1952 Games' opening remarks, Guttmann reminded the audience that the Helsinki Olympic Games were getting underway at the same time, and he shared his hope that "one day the paraplegic games would be as international and as widely known in its own sphere as the Olympics" (**Fig. 42-3**) (17). As he later described, "like the Olympic Games, which were started by a small group of people who believed in sport as a great medium for furthering true sportsmanship and understanding among human beings, our Stoke Mandeville Games will, we believe, unite paralysed men and women of different nations to take their rightful place in the field of sport" (17).

Growth and Development of the Games After Rome (1960–2016)

By 1960, the International Stoke Mandeville Games had evolved into the first large international Para sport festival, held in Rome, Italy, and using the same venue as the Rome Olympic Games (3). The event featured 400 athletes, all of whom were spinally injured, representing 23 countries. As Guttmann explained, "the vast majority of competitors and escorts have fully understood the meaning of the Rome Games as a new pattern of re-integration of the paralysed into society, as well as the world of sport" (3).

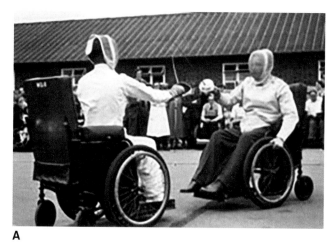

A

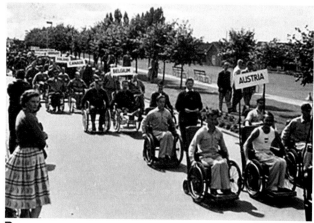

B

FIGURE 42-3.   **(A)** Wheelchair fencing, **(B)** early "Parade of Nations," and **(C)** Dr. Ludwig Guttmann with Dr. Kenneth More. (© International Wheelchair & Amputee Sports (IWAS) – www.iwasf.com)

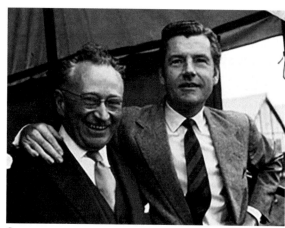

C

The contemporary Paralympic Movement is currently enjoying unprecedented growth in both size and exposure. In 2016, the 15th meeting of the Paralympic Games was contested in Rio de Janeiro, Brazil. It featured more than 4,300 athletes representing 160 countries including a team of independent Paralympic athletes, competing in 23 sports (1). Media coverage of the Paralympic Games has experienced similar rates of expansion. In 2014, NBC and NBCSN combined to air 50 hours of television coverage for the Sochi 2014 Winter Paralympic Games including coverage of the opening and closing ceremonies and daily coverage of all five Paralympic sports in the Sochi program. In 2016, NBCUniversal showed 66 hours of television coverage for the Rio de Janeiro 2016 Summer Paralympic Games, an increase of 60.5 hours from the coverage of the London 2012 Summer Games. NBCUniversal aimed to build on the success of London 2012, which were broadcast to a global cumulated audience of 3.8 billion in 115 countries, via numerous global television networks. The Rio 2016 Summer Games achieved a cumulative global audience of 4.1 billion (1).

The Paralympic Games has an ever-increasing presence in social media as well, which is important given modern modes of information sharing. During the 2016 contest, Paralympic Games gained 14k followers on Twitter, 125k fans on Facebook, and 13k followers on Instagram (almost 50% growth). Paralympic Games subscriber based on YouTube gained 14,672 during the Games, which was a 22% increase, and a single Snapchat Live Story about football 5-a-side, goalball, and athletics attracted 5 million views from outside of the United States. In the United States, thanks to a partnership with NBC, 2.5 million people, bringing the grand total to 7.5 million, viewed the Live Story. All told, 386 million people were reached via Twitter during the Games, a cumulative total of 3,137,837 visited the Games' Web site (1).

Moreover, the International Paralympic Committee (IPC) celebrated its quarter-century anniversary in 2014, a momentous achievement for the largest international sport organization dedicated to the core values of courage, determination, inspiration, and equality through sport.

Historical Overview

In many ways, the great world wars accelerated innovation in physical medicine, and enabled a pioneering physician to see a clear and pressing need to respond against the prevailing view held by medicine and society: that SCI was akin to invalidism. Using sport, among other therapeutic modalities, Sir Guttmann laid a firm foundation for the Paralympic Movement.

Guttmann's personal history of discrimination and competitive sport may have contributed to his tenacity in transforming a dilapidated spinal injuries unit, his determination in establishing the International Stoke Mandeville Games, and his grand aspirations for competitive Para sport. Out of this spirit, the Paralympic Movement has steadily become one of the most successful sporting initiatives in history. What started as a grassroots effort to restore war-wounded citizens to physical, mental, and social health has evolved into a global campaign for unification and empowerment through sport (19). True to Guttmann's vision, as contemporary Para athletes continue to push the envelope of human performance forward, societal perceptions of people who are differently abled are rocked.

PARALYMPIC SPORTS

"Para athlete(s)" is the IPC's term for all sportspersons with impairment, at all levels of competition (1). "Paralympic athletes" and "Paralympians," in contrast, refer only to athletes who have competed at the Paralympic Games (1). Similarly, "Para sport" refers to sports for persons with impairment at all competitive levels, which "Paralympic sport" indicates sports contested at the Paralympic Games, only (1). Thirty-one sports are currently recognized by the IPC, although not all are included in the Paralympic program (1). Twenty-seven sports were contested at the most recent editions of the Paralympic Games: the Rio 2016 Summer Paralympic Games (22 sports) and the Sochi 2014 Winter Paralympic Games (5 sports). A summary of each sport is found in **Table 42-1**. The Paralympic Movement offers sporting opportunities to athletes who fall into one or more of 10 different eligible impairment categories, outlined here and described throughout Section 2.0 of the chapter. As shown in **Table 42-2**, the first eight categories constitute physical impairments; one is visual impairment and the final category is intellectual impairment.

Athlete Classification in Para Sport

Classification is a process in which a single group of things, or units, are ordered into a number of smaller groups, or classes, based on perceptible properties (3,21). Classification has an integral function in science, health and functioning, and in sports, including Para sport. The unique systems of classification used by Para sport carry out two very important functions to uphold the achievement of the Paralympic Movement's vision:

1. Defines who is eligible to compete in Para sport and as a result has the opportunity to reach the goal of becoming a Paralympic athlete
2. Groups athletes into sport classes, which intend to make sure that the impact of impairment is minimized and sporting excellence decides which athlete or team is victorious in the end

The individuals who carry out athlete classification in Para sport are known as classifiers. The essence of classifiers' work determines "who is in and who is out" of Para sport and, equally as important, authenticates success in Para sport (22). Classifiers conduct the evaluation of Para athletes as a member of a classification group, known as a classification panel, to determine if an athlete has an eligible impairment and to assign the athlete a sport class in which to compete (23–25). The sport class is determined on the basis of the severity of the impairment and its impact on performing fundamental activities of a specific sport (25). Of note, physiatrists have the necessary education and practical experience in the evaluation of impairments eligible for Para sport to become trained and certified as classifiers.

To understand why classification is so critical to Para sport and to appreciate the vital role classifiers play in partnership with Para athletes, it is important to understand the classification definitions, the historical foundations of classification in Para sport, the evolution of classification systems in Para sport, and the conceptual models that have shaped classification in Para sport in the past, present, and into the future.

TABLE 42-1	Sports of the Paralympic Movement				
	Summer Sport	Eligible Impairment Category	Features of the Sport	Number of Competitors in the Rio 2016 Games	Governing Body
	Wheelchair Basketball	Impaired muscle power Athetosis Impaired passive ROM Hypertonia Limb deficiency Ataxia Leg length difference	Same ball, court dimensions, playing time, and scoring system as the able-bodied game. Total classification points cannot exceed 14 per team on court during play. Travel violation occurs when a player in possession of the ball pushes his/her wheelchair greater than twice without dribbling	263	International Wheelchair Basketball Federation
	Para Canoe	Impaired muscle power Impaired passive ROM Limb deficiency	Debuted at the 2016 Games. Exactly the same as canoeing for able-bodied athletes, allowing those with physical impairments at all levels to enjoy this inclusive sport	60	International Canoe Federation
	Para Cycling	Impaired muscle power Athetosis Impaired passive ROM Hypertonia Limb deficiency Ataxia Leg length difference Visual impairment	Originally developed for athletes with visual impairments. Athletes race on bicycles, tricycles, tandem, or handcycles based on their impairment. Individuals and teams compete in sprints, individual pursuits, 1,000-m time trials, road races, and road time trials	235	International Cycling Union
	Para Athletics	All	Open to male and female athletes from all impairment groups. Those who are visually impaired receive guidance from a sighted guide who trains and competes alongside the Para athlete	1,140	International Paralympic Committee
	Rowing	Impaired muscle power Athetosis Impaired passive ROM Hypertonia Limb deficiency Ataxia Visual impairment	Debuted at the 2008 Games. There are four boat classes, and in all four events, races are 2,000 m. The equipment (boat, etc.) is adapted to the athletes	96	World Rowing
	Para Table Tennis	Impaired muscle power Athetosis Impaired passive ROM Hypertonia Limb deficiency Ataxia Leg length difference Short stature Intellectual impairment	Sitting or standing athletes compete in individual, doubles, or team events. Matches consist of 5 sets of 11 points each and are played in a best-of-five format	269	International Table Tennis Federation
	Wheelchair Tennis	Impaired muscle power Athetosis Impaired passive ROM Hypertonia Limb deficiency Ataxia Leg length difference	Same rules as the able-bodied game, with one exception: the ball is allowed to bounce twice. Competitors must have a permanent or substantial loss of function in one or both legs and matches are played in a best-of-three sets format	100	International Tennis Federation

Continued

	Summer Sport	Eligible Impairment Category	Features of the Sport	Number of Competitors in the Rio 2016 Games	Governing Body
TABLE 42-1		**Sports of the Paralympic Movement** *(Continued)*			
	Boccia	Impaired muscle power Athetosis Impaired passive ROM Hypertonia Limb deficiency Ataxia	One of the two Paralympic sports with no Olympic counterpart. Originally designed for athletes with cerebral palsy. Players throw or roll colored balls as close as possible to a white target ball, the "jack." The player, pair, or team with the most balls near the jack wins.	106	Boccia International Sports Federation
	Wheelchair Fencing	Impaired muscle power Athetosis Impaired passive ROM Hypertonia Limb deficiency Ataxia Leg length difference	Males and females with amputations, spinal cord injuries, and cerebral palsy are eligible to compete in foil epee (both genders) and saber (men only) events. Wheelchairs are fastened to the floor during competition.	89	International Wheelchair and Amputee Sports Federation
	Football 5-a-side	Visual impairment	Similar to able-bodied football, except: five players per team, smaller field, 50-minute games, no offside rulings, bells inside the ball help orient players, and all players except goalies wear blindfolds for fairness. Goalies may be sighted and verbally guide athletes during the game.	64	International Blind Sports Federation
	Football 7-a-side	Athetosis Hypertonia Ataxia	Similar to able-bodied football, except: seven players per team, smaller field, 60-minute games, no offside rulings, and throw-ins may be made with one hand. Designed for athletes with cerebral palsy.	112	International Federation of Cerebral Palsy Football
	Goalball	Visual impairment	One of two Paralympic sports with no Olympic counterpart. Two 12-minute halves; athletes wear blindfolds for fairness and the object is to roll the ball into the opposite goal. Opponents block the ball with their bodies. Silence is required in the venue.	119	International Blind Sports Federation
	Para Archery	Impaired muscle power Athetosis Impaired passive ROM Hypertonia Limb deficiency Ataxia Leg length difference Visual impairment[a]	Para archery has three different classifications. Athletes compete as individuals or teams in wheelchair or standing competitions.	137	World Archery Federation
	Shooting Para Sport	Impaired muscle power Athetosis Impaired passive ROM Hypertonia Limb deficiency Ataxia	There are 12 Paralympic shooting events. Athletes compete over 10 m, 25 m, and 50 m in single-sex events and there are both rifle and pistol events.	147	International Paralympic Committee

	TABLE 42-1	Sports of the Paralympic Movement *(Continued)*			
	Summer Sport	**Eligible Impairment Category**	**Features of the Sport**	**Number of Competitors in the Rio 2016 Games**	**Governing Body**
	Wheelchair Rugby	Impaired muscle power Athetosis Impaired passive ROM Hypertonia Limb deficiency Ataxia	Originally developed by athletes with tetraplegia in Canada; two teams with at least four players compete for four periods of 8 minutes each. Total classification points cannot exceed 8 per team on court during play.	96	International Wheelchair Rugby Federation
	Para Powerlifting	Impaired muscle power Athetosis Impaired passive ROM Hypertonia Limb deficiency Ataxia Leg length difference Short stature	Open to male and female athletes, bench press is the only discipline. There are 10 weight categories and each athlete has three attempts at each weight. Athletes lower the bar to their chest, hold it motionless, and then press it up with elbows locked at the end. The winner lifts the most.	179	International Paralympic Committee
	Para Equestrian	Impaired muscle power Athetosis Impaired passive ROM Hypertonia Limb deficiency Ataxia Leg length difference Short stature Visual impairment	Introduced at the 1996 Games. Individual athletes compete in dressage events including a championship test with set movements and a freestyle test to music. Teams comprised of 3–4 members also compete in team events.	76	International Equestrian Federation
	Para Taekwondo[a]	Impaired muscle power Athetosis Impaired passive ROM Hypertonia Limb deficiency Ataxia Leg length difference Short stature	At the Paralympic Games, athletes currently compete in the kyorugi (sparring) discipline. A major difference between Para Taekwondo and Taekwondo is that no kicks to the head are allowed in Para Taekwondo.	n/a	World Taekwondo
	Sitting Volleyball	Impaired muscle power Athetosis Impaired passive ROM Hypertonia Limb deficiency Ataxia Leg length difference	Six players on each side play in a best-of-five set format; the first to reach 25 points with a 2-point lead wins. Smaller court, lower net, and considerably faster pace than the able-bodied game. At all times, an athlete's pelvis must touch the ground.	187	World ParaVolley
	Para Dance Sport[b]	Impaired muscle power Athetosis Impaired passive ROM Hypertonia Limb deficiency Ataxia Leg length difference	Combi style (dancing with a standing able-bodied partner), or duo dance (two wheelchair users); group dance, or single-dance events showcase standard, Latin American, or freestyle dances.	n/a	International Paralympic Committee
	Judo	Visual impairment	Added to the Games in 1988; women's weight categories were added in 2004. Contests last 5 minutes and the athlete who scores the higher number of points wins.	129	International Blind Sports Federation

Continued

	TABLE 42-1 **Sports of the Paralympic Movement** *(Continued)*				
	Summer Sport	**Eligible Impairment Category**	**Features of the Sport**	**Number of Competitors in the Rio 2016 Games**	**Governing Body**
	Para Swimming	All	Freestyle, backstroke, butterfly, breaststroke, and medley events. Optional starting platforms and in-water starts are available for some athletes. Signals or "tappers" can be used for the visual impaired. No prostheses/assistive devices are permitted in the pool.	593	International Paralympic Committee
	Para Badminton[a]	Impaired muscle power Athetosis Impaired passive ROM Hypertonia Limb deficiency Ataxia Leg length difference Short stature	Will be debuted at the 2020 Games. Athletes compete in six different classes.	n/a	Badminton World Federation
	Sailing	Impaired muscle power Athetosis Impaired passive ROM Hypertonia Limb deficiency Ataxia Visual impairment Short stature	Athletes compete in different events, which are not specified by gender. Different boats are available in different configurations, either one- or two-person boats.	80	World Sailing
	Para Triathlon	Impaired muscle power Athetosis Impaired passive ROM Hypertonia Limb deficiency Ataxia Visual impairment	Debuted at the 2016 Games. Athletes swim 750 m, then bike 20 km, and finally run 5 km. Athletes may use handcycle, tandem bicycle, or bicycle in the cycling portion and either ambulate the course or use a racing wheelchair for the last segment.	60	International Triathlon Union
	Winter Sport	**Eligible Impairment Category**	**Features of the Sport**	**Number of Competitors in the Sochi 2014 Games**	**Governing Body**
	Para Snowboard[a]	Impaired muscle power Athetosis Impaired passive ROM Hypertonia Limb deficiency Ataxia Leg length difference	Four disciplines are contested: snowboard cross head to head, banked slalom, snowboard cross time trial, and giant slalom. There are specific equipment rules/adaptations based on athletes' impairment.	n/a	International Paralympic Committee
	Para Alpine Skiing	Impaired muscle power Athetosis Impaired passive ROM Hypertonia Limb deficiency Ataxia Leg length difference Visual impairment	There are 14 sport classes in Para alpine skiing based on athletes' impairment, including both seated and standing categories. Athletes with visual impairment ski with a guide in front of them. The guide verbally gives directions to the athlete.	214	International Paralympic Committee
	Para Biathlon	Impaired muscle power Athetosis Impaired passive ROM Hypertonia Limb deficiency Ataxia Leg length difference	Skiers in cross-country and biathlon compete in 15 different sport classes based on impairment. A guide may be optional or mandatory based on severity of visual impairment.	95	International Paralympic Committee

TABLE 42-1	Sports of the Paralympic Movement *(Continued)*				
	Summer Sport	**Eligible Impairment Category**	**Features of the Sport**	**Number of Competitors in the Rio 2016 Games**	**Governing Body**
	Para Cross Country Skiing	Impaired muscle power Athetosis Impaired passive ROM Hypertonia Limb deficiency Ataxia Leg length difference	Skiers in cross-country and biathlon compete in 15 different sport classes based on impairment. A guide may be optional or mandatory based on severity of visual impairment.	147	International Paralympic Committee
	Para Ice Hockey	Impaired muscle power Athetosis Impaired passive ROM Hypertonia Limb deficiency Ataxia Leg length difference	Originally developed in Sweden, Para ice hockey follows the rules of able-bodied hockey except the only rule unique to Para ice hockey: it is illegal to T-charge an opponent using any part of the front radius of the sled.	128	International Paralympic Committee
	Wheelchair Curling	Impaired muscle power Impaired passive ROM Hypertonia Limb deficiency Ataxia	Debuted at the Games in 2006. Teams are comprised of both men and women who have a lower body impairment.	50	World Curling Federation

[a]Did not participate in winter 2014 or summer 2016 Paralympic Games.
[b]Not included in the Paralympic program.
Images © Yetsa A. Tuakli-Wosornu, M.D., M.P.H.
From *International Paralympic Committee*. 2017. Available from: www.paralympic.org. Accessed February 1, 2017, ref. (20).

History of Classification

Since the early beginnings of Para sport in the 1940s (26), several conceptual models have supported the development and subsequent progression of Para sport classification: (a) *medical*, (b) *functional* sport-specific, and (c) *evidence-based* sport-specific.

Medical Model: Para Sport as Rehabilitation

Rehabilitation was the most important early driver for development in Para sport. Classification initially appeared in the mid-1950s, as a way to divide competitors with SCI participating in wheelchair basketball into two classes—one for higher and one for lower–SCI lesions to make the competitions "more fair"

TABLE 42-2	Eligible Impairment Categories
Physical impairment	• **Impaired muscle power:** Reduced force generated by muscles or muscle groups, such as muscles of one limb or the lower half of the body, as caused, for example, by spinal cord injuries, spina bifida, or polio • **Impaired passive ROM:** ROM in one or more joints is reduced permanently, for example, due to arthrogryposis. Hypermobility of joints, joint instability, and acute conditions, such as arthritis, are not considered eligible impairments • **Limb deficiency:** Total or partial absence of bones or joints as a consequence of trauma (e.g., car accident), illness (e.g., bone cancer), or congenital limb deficiency (e.g., dysmelia) • **Leg length difference:** Bone shortening in one leg due to congenital deficiency or trauma • **Short stature:** Reduced standing height due to abnormal dimensions of bones of upper and lower limbs or trunk, for example, due to achondroplasia or growth hormone dysfunction • **Hypertonia:** Abnormal increase in muscle tension and a reduced ability of a muscle to stretch, due to a neurologic condition, such as cerebral palsy, brain injury, or multiple sclerosis • **Ataxia:** Lack of coordination of muscle movements due to a neurologic condition, such as cerebral palsy, brain injury, or multiple sclerosis • **Athetosis:** Generally characterized by unbalanced, involuntary movements and a difficulty in maintaining a symmetrical posture, due to a neurologic condition, such as cerebral palsy, brain injury, or multiple sclerosis
Visual impairment	Vision is impacted by either an impairment of the eye structure, optical nerves or optical pathways, or the visual cortex
Intellectual impairment	A limitation in intellectual functioning and adaptive behavior as expressed in conceptual, social, and practical adaptive skills, which originates before the age of 18

(27). The influence of impairment, such as impaired motor power, and how this affected wheelchair propulsion was not yet a part of classification systems.

During these early decades, classification was medically based, and the medical diagnosis was the only factor used to determine in which sport class the athlete competed. Athletes received a single sport class based on a doctor's medical diagnosis, and they competed in that class for all sports that existed at the time (26).

Although the conceptual model of medically based classification is widely used to describe early classification, a transition occurred where athletes with SCI, poliomyelitis, and spina bifida competed together despite having three separate medical conditions. These conditions resulted in a common impairment in strength. The focus was thus beginning to shift away from medical diagnosis toward how much impairments impacted sport performance (26).

Functional and Sport-Specific Models: Para Sport as Sport

As the Paralympic Movement matured, classification rapidly became more sport focused, driving the development of classification from a medical model to functional and sport-specific models (28,29). The 1988 Seoul Paralympic Games signified the shift from sport as rehabilitation and recreation to elite sport, while the 1992 Barcelona Paralympic Games advanced the use of sport-specific functional classification systems (30).

Decisions for fewer classes, supported by functional classification, were popular with event organizers and accelerated the transition to functional and sport-specific systems, although the science to support an objective, reliable, and valid classification system was immature. Classifiers made decisions based on their professional medical experience and clinical judgment. In most cases, the expert classifier made credible and valid decisions based on the comparable effect on performance of sport-specific activities. At times, these decisions made sense. Sometimes, however, these decisions were not clearly understood by athletes, coaches, media, spectators, or even other classifiers.

Classifiers, mostly medically trained clinical experts who learned about sport as part of rehabilitation, worked individually in the developing and administering of classification rules for specific sports. Classification systems were not published or publicly available, and classifiers from different sports were not in contact with each other and rarely if ever exchanged ideas, skills, or techniques. This group of dedicated advocates of sport developed clinical expertise in Para sport that served the Paralympic Movement well (30). Yet, even more was needed to keep pace with the explosive growth of Para sport.

There was considerable variability across the increasing number of Para sports on essential issues such as a consistent approach to classification. Para sport classification was viewed as "too complicated to be understood." What was needed for better understanding was a standardized language, an unambiguous purpose, and a transparent structure for decisions on who was eligible for Para sport and who was not. A conceptual model was looked for to guide classification forward (26).

With each major event following the successful 2000 Sydney Paralympic Games, and in the context of growing global popularity of the Games, the fundamental importance of classification to Para sport started to be widely recognized. The next step for Para sport was to define the eligible impairments for which it could provide sporting opportunities, delineate the level of impairment that would be required to participate in specific sports along with the impact of the impairment on the sport-specific activities (31), and harmonize classification issues across the Paralympic Movement (30).

Evidence-Based Model: Para Sport Classification and Science

The evolution of standardized Para sport classification systems was guided by three primary documents: the 2003 IPC Classification Strategy, the 2007 IPC Classification Code, and the 2009 IPC Position Stand on Background and Scientific Principles of Classification (22,32). The latter two are discussed.

The Paralympic Movement approved the IPC Classification Code in November 2007. The purpose of this code was to uphold confidence in classification and promote participation by a wide range of athletes by specifying policies and procedures common across all Para sports and by setting principles to be applied by all Para sports (32). The 2007 Code adopted the use of a universal language, the International Classification of Functioning, Disability and Health (ICF), to interconnect with sport. Each sport governance body was to determine which eligible impairment types would be included in their sport. The presence of a permanent, verifiable impairment, and an underlying health condition was mandated. Sport class decisions were to be based on how the resulting impairment caused activity limitation in the fundamental activities of the sport (32).

The 2007 Code did not make the scientific background and conceptual basis for Paralympic Classification available. Tweedy and Vanlandewijck filled in the gap with the 2009 IPC Position Stand on Background and Scientific Principles of Classification. The authors of this foundational document offered a theoretically grounded description of the scientific principles underpinning classification in Para sport, defined the term evidence-based classification, and provided guidelines for how this may be achieved through a unique application of taxonomy, ICF language, and selective classification (22).

Taxonomy, the science of how to classify, includes principles, procedures, and rules and is well recognized in scientific fields as the method to develop systems of naming and ordering to make possible clear communication, understanding, and recognition of how things interrelate (3,21). The ICF is the most widely accepted classification for health and functioning and uses terminology recognized around the world (33).

The intersection of classification in Para sport and in health and functioning was explained, and the key ICF relationship with Para sport classification was established as impairment and its impact on sport-specific activity (31,34). This intersection is represented by 🛜 **eFigure 42-1**. The unit of classification in Para sport was clearly described as impairment in body functions and body structures together with the impact of the impairment on the fundamental activities of each specific Para sport (22).

Taken together, the 2007 Code and the 2009 Position Statement on Classification provided the assertion of the unique role of classification in Paralympic Sport and gave a clear and cohesive position on classification across all Para sports. The foundation was set to build the scientific body of evidence to advance just how classification would support the values of the Paralympic Movement (1).

Contemporary Principles and Practice

Prior to the IPC Classification Code, there were ambiguous purposes for classification, that is, to make sport fair and to enable all to participate equally. The Code provided a clearly stated and unambiguous purpose for classification—to define who competes in Para sport and to ensure that the impact of eligible impairment in each event is minimized.

Evidence-Based Classification

The evidence-based model, using a taxonomy perspective, defined the unit of classification as impairment and aligned classification in Para sports with other selective classification systems used in sport, such as age, body mass, and sex. Each sport is required to identify the eligible impairments in that sport, to describe the severity of impairment permitted, known as minimum impairment criteria (MIC), to classify the impairments according to the extent of resulting sport-specific activity limitation, and to develop the evidence to support that the methods used for assigning a sport class achieved the defined purpose of Para classification (22).

Currently, the Paralympic Movement offers sport opportunities for athletes who have an impairment that belongs to one of the ten eligible impairment types identified in the IPC International Standard for Eligible Impairments (23). **Table 42-2** lists all 10 eligible impairments in Para sport, briefly described in the first section of this chapter. Even if the athlete has one of the eligible impairments made available in that specific sport, an athlete may still not be eligible to participate if the athlete does not meet the MIC demonstrating the impairment is severe enough to affect how the athlete does the fundamental activities for the sport (25).

Of note, Para sports are not required to include all 10 eligible impairments. Some Paralympic sports are only designed for athletes with one impairment. Goalball, for example, is open only for athletes with visual impairment, while athletics and swimming are open to athletes with any of the 10 eligible impairments. The Classification Code requires the impairment to be permanent, meaning the impairment will not resolve in the foreseeable future regardless of physical training or any other therapeutic intervention. Classification systems are developed, administered, and regulated by the International Federations (IFs) governing the sport, which decide which impairments will be included in their sport and what will be the MIC for the sport.

Because fundamental sport activities are different, MIC are sport-specific. As a consequence, an athlete may meet MIC in one sport, but not meet the MIC in another. If an athlete does not meet the MIC and is consequently not eligible to compete in that sport, this does not question the presence of a genuine impairment. It is a sport ruling specific for that sport only. Examples of MIC could be a level of amputation for athletes with limb deficiency or a maximum height for athletes with short stature (32).

MIC should be explained on the basis of scientific research, which assesses the extent of impairment and the impact of impairment on the fundamental activities for that specific sport in a valid and reliable way. Through scientific research evidence, it can be determined how much an impairment impacts on carrying out the fundamental activities in a certain sport. Although this evidence did not exist at the time of the 2007 Code, this body of research is now starting to develop and opportunities to contribute to this growing body of knowledge abound.

Current Best Practices for Classifiers

The sport class an athlete is placed in for competition has a significant effect on the possibility of successful performance, but the research to develop new evidence-based methods of classifying is still lacking. Using current best practices, classification panels should always consider three questions when evaluating a Para athlete: (a) does the athlete have an eligible impairment for this sport; (b) does the athlete's eligible impairment meet the MIC of the sport; and (c) which sport class describes the athlete's activity limitation most accurately?

Tweedy recommends four sources of information to assist all classification experts in making decisions, several of which are already part of athlete evaluation processes in many sports and documented in classification recording forms (35): (a) *impairment(s)*, (b) *novel activities*, (c) *practiced activities*, and (d) *training history* and other factors.

To measure impairment, classifiers should have simple, readily available, affordable, objective, valid, and reliable tests such as manual muscle testing to measure impairment in motor power (35). Novel activities, which are new and unpracticed by the athlete but relevant to sport activity, help relate impairment test results. Practiced activities incorporate elements of strength, coordination, and range of motion trained by the athlete in sport preparation. For example, in wheelchair rugby, athletes would perform wheelchair propulsion drills with stops, starts, and turns (36). And lastly, taking a training history includes questions about frequency; duration; intensity; and periodization of training, quality, and level of coaching; and other personal or environmental factors, such as age and gender (37).

Classifiers can reliably assess activity limitation by defining key components of sport-specific activity to examine and then look at novel and practice tasks to filter out training-sensitive measures and training responsiveness of impairment measures. Performance on novel tasks should be consistent with impairments across all athletes in the sport. In contrast, performance on practiced tasks is likely to vary. For example, a well-trained athlete may do better on practiced tasks than on novel tasks, where an untrained or novice athlete is not likely to display much difference in athletic performance of a novel or practiced task. Without this crucial step, there is a risk of classifying performance rather than impairment, and compromising the value of Para sport classification in that a Para athlete should not change class based on his or her training status (37).

Factors Not Considered in Para Classification

A number of other factors should not affect an athlete's class in any sport, including body size or type such as height, arm length or hand size, gender, and equipment that allows enhanced technique. In most individual sports, men and women compete in separate competitions because of the impact of gender on maximum performance. However, because of the low number of female athletes in wheelchair rugby, this sport is coed, with sport rule adjustments to encourage female participation (38).

Also, selective rather than performance classification is ideal. That is, an athlete should not be penalized for training and/or good equipment use. Equally, an athlete should not be rewarded for not training and for poorly fitting equipment. The competition rules of each sport should specify which equipment types and designs are allowed, such as wheelchair or cycle configuration, prosthetic design, gloves, or strapping (25).

Classifier Qualifications

Classifiers are experts in impairment type and in specific sports. International classifiers are trained for one specific impairment category, for a physical, visual, or intellectual impairment. This specialization is necessary because classifiers must have qualifications appropriate for the impairments they evaluate (24).

The following qualifications are most typical:
1. Physical impairment: medical doctors, physiotherapists, physical therapists, occupational therapists, and experts in sport and biomechanics
2. Visual impairment: ophthalmologists and optometrists
3. Intellectual impairment: psychologists and experts in sport and biomechanics

National-level involvement in classification is a good way to be introduced to classification. International classifiers are trained and certified by the specific sport IFs. For international classifier courses, the IF of the sport one is most interested in is the best contact. The National Paralympic Committees (NPCs) can also help. As of January 1, 2017, the IPC listed on its website IF and NPC contacts to learn more about classifier training (1).

Future of Para Sport Classification

Classification is moving toward a sport-specific evidence-based model, driven by the sports, classification, and scientific communities. All stakeholders acknowledge that collaboration as essential for Para sport classification to achieve the vision of the Paralympic Movement in a way that is clear, consistent, and properly understood.

2015 Code and International Standards

At the beginning of 2013, the IPC launched a consultation process to revise the 2007 Classification Code. This revised Code is expected to further develop sport-specific evidence-based classification in all sports. In November 2015, the Paralympic Movement approved the revised Athlete Classification Code, with compliance by all Para sports by January 1, 2018. In September 2016, the IPC published a series of documents to accompany the Code, providing specific operational guidance for key areas in classification consisting of international standards for (a) *eligible impairments*, (b) *athlete evaluation*, (c) *protest and appeals*, (d) *classifier personnel and training*, and (e) *data protection* (23–25,39,40).

Future Challenges and Opportunities

Para sport classification continues to have significant challenges. First, there is a critical need for research to improve current systems. In a few sports, such as Para athletics and wheelchair rugby, a growing body of research is rapidly emerging (41–50). Identifying intentional misrepresentation poses another challenge to classification (22). Intentional misrepresentation is "a deliberate attempt to mislead a classification panel regarding the existence or extent of skills and/or abilities

relevant to a Para sport and/or the degree or nature of eligible impairment during athlete classification or at any point after the allocation of a sport class" (51). The goal is to obtain the most favorable outcomes from testing, and classification is essentially used as a tactic for an athlete to compete in a sport class with less impairment than is allowable. Anecdotal evidence suggests that some athletes, whether on their own initiative or with advice from others, may not cooperate with full effort during testing or attempt to exaggerate the severity of their impairments. Better tools for detecting intentional misrepresentation are needed, and preliminary research is underway (50).

To take on these challenges, expertise and resources from Para athletes, classification experts, and scientists are needed (52). These challenges represent opportunities for various groups to engage with the Paralympic Movement. By honoring all past and present contributors, maintaining strong links between medical communities, and engaging scientific and research communities, athlete classification will advance to be the strong cornerstone of the Paralympic Movement into the future.

BIOMECHANICS, ERGONOMICS, AND PHYSIOLOGY IN PARA SPORT

A specific feature that distinguishes a Para athlete from a non-disabled athlete is the use of individually adapted assistive technology. Two areas are specifically in focus: wheelchairs for athletes with mobility limitations and prosthetics for amputees.

Kinematics and Kinetics of Wheelchair Sports

Research in wheelchair design ergonomics has led to an increased awareness of overuse problems in spinal cord–injured athletes (53) (see Chapter 58). The "power balance model" describes the interaction between the athlete's energy input and power output. When an athlete in a wheelchair moves at a certain speed, there are three factors that act as resistive forces: rolling resistance, air resistance, and gravitational effects going up or down a slope (54). Rolling resistance relates to the actual surface, wheels, and tires, where the tire pressure, profile, wheel diameter, and wheel alignment all contribute to the resistance. The seating position together with seat height also contributes; the athlete should not be tipping forward or backward in the chair (55). Air resistance, which is most important at high speeds, is the second important factor. The size of the frontal area, that is, the athlete's body, should therefore be kept at a minimum to reduce the force that the air gives. This, in turn, is related to the athlete's position during an event and the athlete's body composition. Finally, going up or down a slope contributes to acceleration/deceleration during a race. By choosing a wheelchair in light-weight material, the mass is reduced, which thereby improves power output.

To improve power output, the design of the wheelchair is also important. Here, the size of the wheel matters, as larger wheels positively affect rolling resistance (56). Secondly, the force applied to the rim through the hand is important (57), and athletes use gloves to get maximum grip. Thirdly, cambered rear wheels affect power output. Practically, all sport wheelchairs have cambered wheels. This gives the athlete greater stability and makes it easier to handle the wheelchair. Field studies have found that an 18-degree camber is the best for both sprint and maneuverability skills (58,59). Different models of wheelchairs used for different sports have been developed. In Para athletics and wheelchair racing, historically, athletes competed in more or less daily-use wheelchairs. Today, three-wheeled racing chairs are of high-tech design and individually customized, enabling athletes to reach speeds up to 10 m/s. These chairs are made of lightweight material, with small hand rims, high-pressure tubular tires, and up to 15 degrees of camber.

Sport wheelchairs more closely resemble daily-use wheelchairs, are of lightweight material, and have larger hand rims compared to racing wheelchairs, in order to maximize the turning moment (46). In rugby, there is significant chair contact. Chairs are designed to allow for hitting and blocking. Rugby players, who are always affected in both their upper and lower extremities, generally choose a low-seat height for maximum balance. In basketball, players select a seat height based on impairment and role on the court.

Prosthetics and Running

With the development of modern prosthetics, amputee running has seen tremendous growth (60,61) (see Chapter 56). A functionally designed prosthesis for highly active amputees, the carbon fiber flex foot, was originally launched in 1996. It has helped enable Para athletes to compete in disability-specific and able-bodied sports, transcending stereotypes, and perceived societal limitations. Most recently, a German long jumper and single below-knee amputee, Markus Rehm, garnered international recognition. At the 2015 Doha IPC Athletics World Championships, Rehm jumped a length of 8.40 m, making him the new IPC world record holder. This same jump would have earned a gold medalist at the London 2012 Olympic Games. In his attempt to compete in able-bodied track and field, Rehm has undergone biomechanics testing at a German Sport University. The results were inconclusive on whether he has an advantage over his able-bodied counterparts. However, the International Association of Athletics Federations rules require him to prove that he has no advantage, so he remains barred from able-bodied competition until further evidence is brought to the fore.

Physiology

For a majority of Paralympic athletes, the responses to physical activity and training are similar to those of nondisabled athletes (see Chapter 49). Much of our knowledge of the underlying physiologic principles from research in nondisabled athletes can be used when designing Paralympic training programs. Still, there are some differences that have to be considered, the majority of which are seen in athletes who have a SCI (62).

Athletic performance is closely linked to the volume of blood transported by the central circulation and the perfusion of the contracting muscle. Cardiac output, as a function of heart stroke volume and heart rate, is considerably altered in athletes with a SCI (63). This results from the reduced sympathetic input, which is closely related to the level and severity of lesion. In particular, athletes with a lesion above thoracic level 6 (T6) have a reduced maximal heart rate compared to nondisabled athletes.

Considering maximum oxygen uptake, a well-established predictor of athletic performance, Paralympic athletes can reach values similar to nondisabled elite athletes (64). Para athletes with reduced muscle mass have maximum oxygen uptake proportional to their mass. Athletes with a SCI, however, have lower values, as a result of both reduced muscle mass and changes in the autonomic nervous system.

Athletes with a SCI above T6 also have impaired blood pressure control, causing low resting blood pressure and orthostatic hypotension (65). This can cause dizziness and nausea with position changes and during intense exercise. Compression socks and adequate hydration can alleviate some of these symptoms.

Both aerobic and anaerobic performances in athletes with a SCI are closely linked to the level and severity of the lesion. As a general rule, the lower the lesion, the better the athletic performance. As an example, high-performance athletes with paraplegia competing in wheelchair racing or handcycling can reach peak oxygen uptakes well above 50 mL/kg/min during an exercise test, whereas wheelchair rugby players or wheelchair tennis players with quadriplegia, both examples of athletes with high-level SCI, have significantly lower values, closer to 20 mL/kg/min (66).

Autonomic Dysreflexia

A physiologic reaction that can occur in persons who are spinally injured above level T6 is autonomic dysreflexia (AD) (67) (see Chapter 22). This can be a life-threatening condition and requires immediate treatment. AD is acute uncontrolled sympathetic activity leading to rapid onset of high blood pressure, headache, flushing, sweating above the level of the lesion, nasal congestion, and anxiety. AD is caused by a stimulus below the lesion level, usually a full bladder or bowel, or some other noxious stimuli such as pain. The rise in blood pressure can lead to intracranial hemorrhages, retinal bleedings, seizures, cardiac failure and asystole, and pulmonary edema. Treatment involves both nonpharmacologic and pharmacologic interventions. A person with AD should be placed in an upright position to produce an orthostatic decrease in blood pressure and restrictive clothing should be removed. Usually, the bladder is emptied by catheterization, as is the bowel by gently inserting a gloved finger. If blood pressure remains high, above 150 mm Hg, it can be treated by oral nifedipine, a calcium antagonist.

AD also has specific implications for Paralympic athletes and relates to what is named "boosting" (68). Boosting is the intentional induction of AD for unfair performance enhancement by athletes. In elite wheelchair sports, athletes have been known to fill their bladders to induce AD. The higher sympathetic activation leads to increases in blood pressure, stroke volume, peak heart rate, and an overall performance enhancement of around 10%. For decades, the practice of "boosting" has been under scrutiny in Paralympic sport, and it is strictly prohibited by the IPC due to its inherent health risks (69). Since 2008, the IPC has implemented a testing program for boosting in major Paralympic competition (70). Systolic blood pressure has been used as a marker for boosting. Athletes are being tested just before competition, and a blood pressure of above 180 mm Hg is considered a "positive" test. From 2008 to 2015, a total of 159 tests have been conducted, none of which were positive. It has also been noted that athletes could be dysreflexic with blood pressure levels much less than 180 mm Hg. Using historic data of precompetition baseline blood pressure in athletes with SCI, the IPC Governing Board (on recommendation of the IPC Medical Committee) has amended its rules to lower this threshold for a "positive" test to 160 mm Hg.

The effect on the autonomic and somatic nervous system in persons with a SCI also reduces the capacity to regulate heat (62). This decreased thermoregulatory capacity compared to nondisabled persons leads to a disturbed skin blood flow below the lesion level and thereby a reduced ability to sweat and consequently increased body core temperatures during exercise. Sweat rates can be reduced by up to 30% compared to nondisabled athletes, which consequently can lead to reduced performance. Athletes with a higher lesion level and those with complete lesions are most affected. Athletes with a SCI are therefore advised to develop a clear rehydration plan during competition (71). An alternative way to drinking excessive fluid is to cool the body with wet and cold towels during exercise.

PARALYMPIC SPORT MEDICINE

In parallel with the growth of the Paralympic Movement, the field of Paralympic sport medicine has emerged as an exciting new frontier of clinical care and scientific exploration (72) (see Chapter 41). Additionally, optimizing athlete health in Para athletes is important for both sport performance as well as long-term functional outcomes. When considering the issues unique to Paralympic sport medicine, it is important to note that the majority of clinical needs encountered by Para athletes are the same as those pertaining to the general athlete population. For those considerations that are unique to Paralympic sport, further information will be provided here.

Sports-Related Injury Epidemiology and Prevention

It is generally accepted that participation in sport and physical activity leads to improvements in health, yet it is often inevitable that athletes may incur sports-related injury. Such injuries have the risk of causing detriments to performance, an early end to one's sport career, and/or musculoskeletal symptoms into the future. These relative risks require even greater emphasis in Para sport given that sport injuries, incurred at a young age, may result in functional decline later in life. For example, a wheelchair basketball player with SCI may develop a rotator cuff tear during a game, with immediate onset of symptoms. If left untreated, this tear may progress and ultimately lead to rotator cuff tear arthropathy later in life. Given that the athlete uses his/her shoulder for both sports and functional tasks such as wheelchair transfers and propulsion, this has the potential to cause significant morbidity. Thus, injury prevention in this population is of utmost importance.

The field of sport injury epidemiology in the Para athlete is a growing field of sport medicine research (73). Earnest attempts to better understand injury patterns in multisport events began in 2002 when the Paralympic Injury Surveillance System was implemented at the Winter Paralympic Games (74,75). Following on this success, an advanced online injury and illness surveillance system was initiated for the London 2012 Paralympic Summer Games—the first to comprehensively capture injury patterns across a wide range of summer Para sports as well as enabling the monitoring of both injury

and illness (76). Currently, many countries and sport federations are striving to implement similar systems to enable prospective data collection.

In summer Paralympic sport, the five sports with the highest rates of injury are football 5-a-side, powerlifting, goalball, wheelchair fencing, and wheelchair rugby (77). The upper extremity is most frequently injured, particularly involving the shoulder, elbow, and wrist/hand. This pattern varies in comparison to similar data from an Olympic athlete population, for whom the lower limb is more commonly injured. Older athletes and athletes with SCI are at increased risk for upper limb injuries (78). Additionally, across all athletes, males and females have similar rates of injury (77).

Recent sport-specific subanalysis have enabled a more detailed analysis of injury, noting that in the sport of track and field, wheelchair/seated athletes are at higher risk of upper limb injury, which is seen most commonly in the throw events (shot put, discus, and javelin) (79). Additionally, among ambulant track athletes, those with cerebral palsy are at decreased risk of lower extremity injury when compared to amputees and athletes with visual impairment (79). This may be due to increased lower extremity muscle tone in athletes with cerebral palsy, which may in fact be protective against injury given the lack of full, forceful eccentric muscle contraction during sprints and distance running events. In the sport of Paralympic football, visually impaired athletes in football 5-a-side experience a high incidence of acute injury, particularly to the head/neck and lower limb (80). Of interest, greater than 60% of these injuries are reported as being attributable to foul play. In Paralympic powerlifting, chronic/overuse injuries are very common, accounting for greater than 60% of all injuries (81). Of these, the shoulder/clavicle was most commonly involved, and athletes in heavier weight classes were more likely to experience injury.

In Paralympic winter sport, Para ice hockey and Para alpine skiing/snowboarding demonstrate a high incidence of injury, while Para cross-country skiing/biathlon and wheelchair curling have relatively low injury rates (82). Of interest, sports such as Nordic skiing may be somewhat protective against upper limb injury, given that the nature of propulsion heavily involves scapular retraction, unlike wheelchair court sports, which predominantly rely on activation of the anterior chest resulting in overuse injuries, particularly to the rotator cuff. Additionally, concussions, fractures, and contusions are more common in winter Paralympic sport, likely due to the high-speed, high-impact nature of these events (82).

Sports-Related Illness Epidemiology and Prevention

Similar to patterns of injury, sports-related illnesses in Para athletes also show unique features when compared to the general athlete population. Indeed, the incidence of illness is higher at the Paralympic Games when compared to the Olympic Games (83,84). The respiratory, integumentary, and digestive systems are most impacted by sports-related illness, in the order of decreasing frequency (83). Additionally, the genitourinary system is disproportionately involved, a pattern unique to Para athletes. Across all systems, most illnesses are due to infections, particularly urinary tract infections (82% of all genitourinary illnesses) (85). This is likely due to the fact that a large proportion of Paralympic athletes are individuals with central neurologic injury (e.g., SCI, brain injury) with resultant neurogenic bladder and use of catheterization.

Skin and subcutaneous tissue infections are also common among athletes with SCI, amputation/limb deficiency, and cerebral palsy (85). This may be attributable to reduced sensation resulting in risk for skin breakdown, as well as complications at the stump-socket interface in amputee athletes using sport prosthesis.

Of great interest is the fact that Para athletes typically delay the reporting of symptoms after onset of illness in comparison to their able-bodied counterparts, a phenomenon described as "transcendence of injury" in the literature (86). Further educational initiatives are needed to encourage athletes to report symptoms at the time of onset, thus leading to optimization of care and reduced detrimental impact on performance.

Antidoping and Therapeutic Use Exemptions

For the Para athlete engaged in national and international competition, issues related to the antidoping program are of paramount importance. Similar to Olympic sport, Paralympic sport must conform to the World Anti-Doping Agency (WADA) Code as well as the IPC Anti-Doping Code (87,88). For athletes, this typically includes being subject to both in and out of competition testing via urine and/or blood samples. Additionally, according to the WADA prohibited list, certain categories of medications, as well as certain methods, are prohibited given their potential for abuse (89). It is extremely important for sport medicine practitioners to be aware of what agents are or are not allowable under this program, to avoid providing the athlete with a medication that may lead to a positive test. Of note, several classes of medication that are commonly used by individuals with disabilities, such as oral antispasticity agents and medications for neurogenic bowel and bladder, are not prohibited. Please see 📶 **eTable 42-2** for further details.

In certain instances, athletes may require a medication that is prohibited, however is required for a valid medical indication. In these cases, the athlete and his or her physician may apply a Therapeutic Use Exemption (TUE) via a rigorous process, subject to approval by a TUE committee with jurisdiction over the event. Guidelines for the granting of TUEs are subject to the International Standard for Therapeutic Exemption, which denotes that, among other factors, the athlete must have exhausted all potential treatments involving nonprohibited substances (90).

Pain Management in the Para Athlete

Athletes may experience pain for a number of reasons, inclusive of symptoms attributable to sports-related injury or illness. In Para athletes, this phenomenon may be complicated by pre-existing pain that is directly related to his or her disability. For example, an athlete with history of neurologic injury may experience significant neuropathic pain that worsens in stressful, competitive settings, or an athlete with history of rheumatoid arthritis may experience nociceptive joint pain, exacerbated by sport competition. In all circumstances, safe and effective pain management is critical to protect the health of Para athletes.

Treatment strategies for pain in any competitive athlete involve the optimization of conservative, nonpharmacologic

strategies prior to the initiation of pharmacologic intervention. When medications are used via any route (oral, topical, intravenous, ophthalmic), specific care must be taken to avoid the use of substances and/or methods prohibited by the WADA (89), as noted above.

Although the full management of painful conditions is beyond the scope of this chapter and also described in other portions of this text, we will choose to focus this discussion on the treatment of neuropathic pain, given that it is of significant, specific concern to the Para athlete population and has the distinct potential to impact quality of life, as well as sport performance, in athletes with neurologic injury (91). By definition, neuropathic pain is noted to arise from a lesion or other pathology involving the somatosensory system, resulting in discomfort often described as numbness, tingling, burning, shooting, or electrical (92). In a Para athlete population, the athletes most commonly affected are those with SCI, brain injury, stroke, burns, and/or any type of peripheral nerve injury. A full history and physical (inclusive of a neurologic exam with motor/sensory testing) is required for diagnosis. At times, additional tests such as electromyography (EMG) with nerve conduction studies (NCS) may be helpful in determining a diagnosis, particularly in cases of peripheral nerve entrapment or peripheral neuropathy.

In all cases, initial conservative treatment should include nonpharmacologic management. This may include tools such as heat/cold application, compression wraps, soft tissue massage for desensitization, and acupuncture. If pharmacologic treatment is warranted, initial trials of nonprohibited substances such as the oral agents gabapentin, pregabalin, or duloxetine may be of benefit (92). Additionally, topical agents such as lidocaine ointment/patch and topical capsaicin may be of helpful as either monotherapy or in combination with oral medications. Two additional agents often used in the treatment of neuropathic pain—opiates and cannabis—should be strictly avoided in an athlete population, if possible, given that they are prohibited substances. If use of these medications is required, the athlete may apply for a TUE, noting that approval is only granted if all other nonprohibited treatments have been exhausted. Additionally, for international-level athletes, consideration must be given to domestic laws for import when competitions take place in countries where these substances are deemed to be illegal.

PUBLIC HEALTH IMPACT OF PARALYMPIC SPORT

It is well known that individuals with disabilities are more likely to experience the effects of sedentary lifestyle such as cardiovascular disease, diabetes, and obesity when compared to the general population (see Chapter 43). Multiple barriers likely contribute to these disparities, including those related to structural, socioeconomic, and attitudinal factors that reduce participation in physical activity and organized sport. In this context, the Paralympic Movement may provide a platform for the reframing of societal expectations around the engagement of people with disabilities in physical activity and sport while also catalyzing the development of programs to meet the needs of this population (93).

Disability and Health Disparities Related to Sedentary Lifestyles

Similar to trends noted in the general population, population health studies have reliably shown the impact of chronic disease and detrimental health behavior on the lives of people with disabilities. Once thought to impact only a small minority, it is now known that these trends affect a large sector of the United States (USA) and global population, given that an estimated 56.7 million civilian, noninstitutionalized Americans, or 18.7% of the population, are individuals with self-reported disability (94). This figures grows to an estimated one billion people worldwide (95). Additionally, it is important to note that disability is heterogeneous, accounting for impairments in mobility, sensory difficulties (e.g., vision and/or hearing deficits), mental and emotional health concerns, and cognitive impairments, all of which may impact an individual's ability to engage in routine physical activity.

In the United States, data from the National Health Interview Survey report a higher prevalence of obesity in individuals with disabilities as compared to those without disabilities, for example, 28.4% compared to 17.8% for ages 18 to 44 (96). Adults with severe lower extremity mobility impairment are at particularly high risk for obesity and also less likely to receive physician counseling regarding the importance of exercise (97). Adults with intellectual disability are more likely to be obese or morbidly obese, regardless or whether one lives in independent or supervised settings (98). Cardiovascular health, including hypertension, hyperlipidemia, and coronary artery disease, also present an important concern, given that they are known to disproportionately impact individuals with disabilities. There is likely a compounded effect of obesity and reduced mobility that place individuals with physical disability at particularly high risk (99). For example, as life expectancies increase, cardiovascular disease is now a leading cause of morbidity and mortality following SCI (100).

Several additional factors are likely to exacerbate the prevalence of chronic disease in this population. First, people with disabilities are more likely to be vulnerable in engaging in detrimental health behaviors such as tobacco smoking when compared to the general population (96). Additionally, adults with disabilities are more likely to report not engaging in "leisure time physical activity"—a marker of meaningful engagement in physical activity and sport (96). This negative trend is noted already in youth. For example, a study commissioned by the Women's Sports Foundation notes that girls with disabilities in grades 9 to 12 report obtaining the recommended 60 minutes of physical activity per day only 3.1 days/week, compared to 4.5 days/week for their able-bodied peers (101). Second, people with disabilities are more likely to be unemployed and to report living below the poverty line when compared to their able-bodied peers (94). Previous literature has noted that reduced financial resources often limit the ability of persons with disabilities to participate in sports and exercise (102,103).

Increasing Physical Activity: The Intersection of Public Health, Policy, and Sport

Although it is clear that health disparities exist, further research is needed to fully understand the impact of various interventions that may be effective in reducing the impact of sedentary lifestyles on people with disabilities. To more fully promote the participation of people with disabilities in physical activity and sport, a multipronged strategy may be the most effective in capitalizing on the intersection of public health programming, policy change, and sport-specific opportunities. Here, we present concepts regarding how each of these broad categories may be able to create impact.

Public Health Measures and Policy Change

Across populations, the rising rate of obesity and chronic disease has catalyzed the formation of numerous public health initiatives (104) aimed at increasing population engagement in physical activity. In the United States, several federal agencies have the stated priority of ensuring that all programming is inclusive of people with disabilities (105), although it remains unclear to what extent this is implemented. An excellent example of disability-specific programming is the National Center on Health, Physical Activity and Disability (NCHPAD), which collaborates with leading disability and health advocacy organizations to promote inclusion in physical activity and sport (106). Into the future, it is recommended that organizations seek a "twin track" approach through which disability-specific programming is supplemented by the concomitant inclusion of people with disabilities in all public health programs and services, even those that do not have a specific disability focus (93).

Public health initiatives exist against a backdrop of laws and policies enhancing equal access for people with disabilities to myriad public and private services. Many of these laws have both direct and indirect implications for participation in sport and physical activity at the grassroots and community level. Additionally, programming for elite Para athletes, such as US-based Paralympic programming, must conform to US laws. For example, an athlete who may be training for an upcoming Paralympics will require access to his or her local fitness facility for strength and conditioning training.

The majority of civil rights law in the United States pertaining to the rights of people with disabilities focus on establishing equal access to the same programs, services, and venues enjoyed by members of the general community. The first such legislation was Section 504 of the Rehabilitation Act of 1973, which applies to federal programs and private programs and settings receiving federal funds—for example, public schools and national parks (107). Several years later, in 1990, the Americans with Disabilities Act (ADA) extended these guarantees to also include private settings—for example, private gyms and health clubs (108). Although not retroactive, under the ADA, newly constructed fitness facilities must meet basic accessibility requirements to meet the needs of individuals with disabilities.

More recently, in 2013, the Department of Education issued a Federal Guidance notification confirming that the tenets of the Rehabilitation Act of 1973 also apply to extracurricular athletics, to include club and interscholastic sports in schools receiving federal funding and at all educational levels, including collegiate (109). This Guidance was prompted by findings of a U.S. Government Accountability Office (GAO) report noting that students with disabilities were being broadly excluded from extracurricular sports in public schools—for example, in a sample of 11 schools, 6% to 25% of students with disabilities were involved in sports, compared to 18% to 73% of students with no disability (110).

At the state level, local advocacy by athletes and their families has led to the passage of legislation ensuring access to school-based sports in several regions. In 2005, wheelchair racer Tatyana McFadden sued the Maryland Public Schools Athletics Association for discrimination that prevented her from being a full, point-scoring member of her high school track and field team (111). This successful fight led to the passage of the 2008 Maryland Fitness and Athletics Equity for Students with Disabilities Act, ensuring access to public school interscholastic athletic programs (112).

Sport-Specific Programming

Given their profile and societal reach, sport organizations have an opportunity to promote physical activity and sport participation for health. The Paralympic Movement is specifically poised to promote these concepts. Little hard data link Paralympic sport to public health outcomes such as increased levels of leisure time physical activity, but a more compelling argument is that of legacy, that is, the long-term outcomes enjoyed by a city and/or country after hosting a Paralympic event. The Paralympic Movement may thus have an impact related to structural change, removal of barriers, and shifting of attitudes, all of which may contribute to expanded opportunities for engagement in sport and physical activity for the broad population of people with disabilities.

One such example is the enhancement of the built environment in cities that host the Summer and Winter Paralympic Games every 2 years. Often, preparation for the Games creates a proactive deadline for the infrastructure-based projects that promote accessibility and universal design. Given the "one bid, one city" model of the Olympic and Paralympic Movement, all enhancements are required to be accessible to people with disabilities. For example, after hosting the 2008 Summer Olympic and Paralympic Games, the city of Beijing now has 2,834 low-floor accessible busses, and several bus and train stations now include ramps, accessible signage, and raised tile walkways to increase the independence of visually impaired travelers (113).

Additionally, the international Paralympic Movement has continued to state its commitment to be a change agent for the promotion of health and disability rights. For example, the IPC 2015–2018 strategic plan notes an aspiration "to make for a more inclusive society for people with an impairment through Para sport" (114). Additionally, in 2012, the IPC Agitos Foundation was launched as a vehicle to build the capacity of international Paralympic programming. Additionally, an innovative partnership between the IPC and an international nongovernmental organization called Motivation U.K. has led to the development of low-cost sport wheelchairs, serving to lower the financial barriers to entry that are experienced by many athletes. Into the future, it is expected that capacity building will remain a high priority of the organization, serving to increase awareness and resources available to the movement as a whole.

SUMMARY

Although physical activity is a mainstay of health promotion and chronic disease prevention, people with disabilities are too often excluded from accessing opportunities for physical activity and sports due to myriad barriers such as poor physical access, negative attitudes, and low financial resources, among others. Efforts to improve the health of this broad population can be enhanced by more uniform inclusion in public health initiatives, enforcement of policy, and proactive partnership with the Paralympic sport community. The Paralympic Movement has the capacity to enhance public awareness regarding the capabilities of individuals with disabilities both on and off the field of play, thus increasing societal expectations regarding physical activity and sport participation as a key component of health promotion.

REFERENCES

1. International Paralympic Committee. Available from: https://www.paralympic.org/the-ipc/about-us. Accessed February 1, 2017.
2. Verville RE, et al. Physical education, exercise, fitness and sports: early PM&R leaders build a strong foundation. *PM R*. 2015;7(9):905–912.
3. Bailey S. *Athlete First: A History of the Paralympic Movement*. West Sussex, UK: John Wiley & Sons, Ltd.; 2008.
4. Deaflympics. 2017. Available from: www.deaflympics.com. Accessed February 1, 2017.
5. Gold JR, Gold MM. Access for all: the rise of the Paralympic Games. *J R Soc Promot Health*. 2007;127(3):133–141.
6. Kinney CL, DePompolo R. "Rehabilitation ... a key word in medicine": the legacy of Dr. Frank H. Krusen. *PM R*. 2013;5(3):163–168.
7. Brittain I. *From Stoke Mandeville to Stratford: A History of the Summer Paralympic Games*. Champaign, IL: Common Ground Publishing, LLC; 2012.
8. Guttmann L. *Spinal Cord Injuries: Comprehensive Management and Research*. Oxford, UK: Blackwell Scientific Publications; 1973.
9. Goodman S. *Spirit of Stoke Mandeville: The Story of Sir Ludwig Guttmann*. London, UK: Harper Collins Publishing LLC; 1986.
10. Guttmann L. Looking back on a decade. *The Cord*. 1954;6(4):9–23.
11. Guttmann L. History of the National Spinal Injuries Centre, Stoke Mandeville Hospital, Aylesbury. *Paraplegia*. 1967;5:115–126.
12. Gallagher M. *Athletics*. Aylesbury, UK: British Sports Association for the Disabled; 1982.
13. Guttmann L. *Textbook of Sport for the Disabled*. Aylesbury, UK: HM & M Publishers; 1976.
14. McCann C. Sports for the disabled: the evolution from rehabilitation to competitive sport. *Br J Sports Med*. 1996;30(4):279–280.
15. Guttmann L. Reflections on sport for the physically handicapped. *Physiotherapy*. 1965;51:252–253.
16. Guttmann L. Sport and recreation for the mentally and physically handicapped. *R Soc Health J*. 1973;93(4):208–212.
17. Guttmann L. On the way to an International sports movement for the Paralysed. *The Cord*. 1952;5(3):7–23.
18. Guttmann L. The annual stoke mandeville games. *The Cord*. 1949;3:24.
19. Tuakli-Wosornu Y. "And Thereby Hangs a Tale": current medical and scientific controversies in Paralympic Sport. *Palaestra*. 2016;30(3):9–13.
20. International Paralympic Committee. 2017. Available from: https://www.paralympic.org/paralympic-games. Accessed February 1, 2017.
21. Fleishman E, Quaintance M. *Taxonomies of Human Performance*. Orlando, FL: Harcourt Brace Jovanovich. Inc.; 1983.
22. Tweedy SM, Vanlandewijck YC. International Paralympic Committee position stand—background and scientific principles of classification in Paralympic sport. *Br J Sports Med*. 2011;45(4):259–269.
23. International Paralympic Committee. *International Standard for Eligible Impairments*. Bonn, Germany: International Paralympic Committee. Available frpm: https://www.paralympic.org/the-ipc/handbook. Accessed December 24, 2018.
24. International Paralympic Committee. *International Standard for Classifier Personnel and Training*. Bonn, Germany: International Paralympic Committee.
25. International Paralympic Committee. *International Standard for Athlete Evaluation*. Bonn, Germany: International Paralympic Committee.
26. Tweedy S, David HP. Introduction to the Paralympic Movement. In: Thompson W, Vanlandewijck Y, eds. *The Paralympic Athlete*. West Sussex, UK: Wiley Blackwell; 2011.
27. Van de Vliet P. Paralympic athlete's health. *Br J Sports Med*. 2012;46(7):458–459.
28. Strohkendl H. *Junktionelle Klassifizierung für den Rollstuhlsport [Functional Classification in Wheelchair Sport]*. Berlin, Germany: Springer-Verlag; 1978.
29. Strohkendl H. Player classification. In: Thiboutot A, ed. *The 50th Anniversary of Wheelchair Basketball: A History by Horst Strohkendl*. 1st ed. Waxmann Publishing: Munster/Ne; 1996:47–53.
30. Hart A. Classification: conceptual models. In: *International Convention on Science, Education and Medicine in Sport (ICSEMIS)*. ICSSPE/CIEPSS: Berlin, Germany; 2012.
31. Tweedy SM. Biomechanical consequences of impairment: a taxonomically valid basis for classification in a unified disability athletics system. *Res Q Exerc Sport*. 2003;74(1):9–16.
32. International Paralympic Committee. *IPC Classification Code and International Standards*. Bonn, Germany: International Paralympic Committee; 2007.

33. World Health Organization. *International Classification of Functioning, Disability, and Health*. Geneva, Switzerland: World Health Organization; 2001.

34. Tweedy SM. Taxonomic theory and the ICF: foundations for a unified disability athletics classification. *Adapt Phys Activ Q*. 2002;19(2):220–237.

35. Tweedy S, Williams G, Bourke J. Selecting and modifying methods of manual muscle testing for classification in Paralympic sport. *Eur J Adapt Activ*. 2010;3(2):7–16.

36. Yilla A, Sherrill C. Validating the beck battery of quad rugby skills. *Adapt Phys Activ Q*. 1998;15:155–167.

37. Tweedy S. Assessing extent of activity limitation resulting from impairment. In: Bourke J, Tweedy S, eds. *IPC Athletics Classification Project for Physical Impairments: Final Report—Stage 1*. Bonn, Germany: International Paralympic Committee; 2009:74–76.

38. International Wheelchair Rugby Federation. *IWRF Classification Manual*. 3rd ed. 2015. Available from: http://www.iwrf.com/?page=classification. Accessed December 24, 2018.

39. International Paralympic Committee. *International Standard for Protest and Appeals*. Bonn, Germany: International Paralympic Committee; 2016.

40. International Paralympic Committee. *International Standard for Data Protection*. Bonn, Germany: International Paralympic Committee; 2016.

41. Altmann VC, et al. Reliability of the revised wheelchair rugby trunk impairment classification system. *Spinal Cord*. 2013;51(12):913–918.

42. Altmann VC, et al. Improvement of the classification system for wheelchair rugby: athlete priorities. *Adapt Phys Activ Q*. 2014;31(4):377–389.

43. Altmann VC, et al. The impact of trunk impairment on performance of wheelchair activities with a focus on wheelchair court sports: a systematic review. *Sports Med Open*. 2015;1(1):6.

44. Altmann VC, et al. The impact of trunk impairment on performance-determining activities in wheelchair rugby. *Scand J Med Sci Sports*. 2017;27:1005–1014.

45. Altmann VC, et al. Construct validity of the trunk impairment classification system in relation to objective measures of trunk impairment. *Arch Phys Med Rehabil*. 2016;97(3):437–444.

46. Vanlandewijck Y, Theisen D, Daly D. Wheelchair propulsion biomechanics: implications for wheelchair sports. *Sports Med*. 2001;31(5):339–367.

47. Vanlandewijck YC, Verellen J, Tweedy S. Towards evidence-based classification in wheelchair sports: impact of seating position on wheelchair acceleration. *J Sports Sci*. 2011;29(10):1089–1096.

48. Vanlandewijck YC, et al. Trunk strength effect on track wheelchair start: implications for classification. *Med Sci Sports Exerc*. 2011;43(12):2344–2351.

49. Connick M, Beckman E, Deuble R, et al. Developing tests of impaired coordination for Paralympic classification: normative values and test-retest reliability. *Sports Eng*. 2016;19:147–154.

50. Deuble RL, et al. Using Fitts' Law to detect intentional misrepresentation. *J Mot Behav*. 2016;48(2):164–171.

51. International Paralympic Committee. *Athlete Classification Code*. Bonn, Germany: International Paralympic Committee; 2015.

52. Malone L, Morgulec-Adamowicz N, Orr K. Contribution of sport science to performance: wheelchair rugby. In: Thompson W, Vanlandewijck Y, eds. *The Paralympic Athlete*. West Sussex, UK: Wiley Blackwell; 2011:249–263.

53. Mason BS, van der Woude LH, Goosey-Tolfrey VL. The ergonomics of wheelchair configuration for optimal performance in the wheelchair court sports. *Sports Med*. 2013;43(1):23–38.

54. Churton E, Keogh JW. Constraints influencing sports wheelchair propulsion performance and injury risk. *BMC Sports Sci Med Rehabil*. 2013;5:3.

55. Kotajarvi BR, et al. The effect of seat position on wheelchair propulsion biomechanics. *J Rehabil Res Dev*. 2004;41(3b):403–414.

56. van der Woude LH, et al. Wheelchair racing: effects of rim diameter and speed on physiology and technique. *Med Sci Sports Exerc*. 1988;20(5):492–500.

57. van der Linden ML, et al. The effect of wheelchair handrim tube diameter on propulsion efficiency and force application (tube diameter and efficiency in wheelchairs). *IEEE Trans Rehabil Eng*. 1996;4(3):123–132.

58. Mason B, et al. The effects of rear-wheel camber on maximal effort mobility performance in wheelchair athletes. *Int J Sports Med*. 2012;33(3):199–204.

59. Mason B, et al. Effects of camber on the ergonomics of propulsion in wheelchair athletes. *Med Sci Sports Exerc*. 2011;43(2):319–326.

60. Matthews D, Sukeik M, Haddad F. Return to sport following amputation. *J Sports Med Phys Fitness*. 2014;54(4):481–486.

61. Buckley JG. Sprint kinematics of athletes with lower-limb amputations. *Arch Phys Med Rehabil*. 1999;80(5):501–508.

62. Bhambhani Y. Physiology of wheelchair racing in athletes with spinal cord injury. *Sports Med*. 2002;32(1):23–51.

63. Schmid A, et al. Physical performance and cardiovascular and metabolic adaptation of elite female wheelchair basketball players in wheelchair ergometry and in competition. *Am J Phys Med Rehabil*. 1998;77(6):527–533.

64. Katch V, McArdle WD, Katch F. *Essentials of Exercise Physiology*. 4th ed. Philadelphia, PA: Lippincott Williams & Wilkins; 2010:1–699.

65. Ravensbergen HJ, et al. Cardiovascular function after spinal cord injury: prevalence and progression of dysfunction during inpatient rehabilitation and 5 years following discharge. *Neurorehabil Neural Repair*. 2013;28(3):219–229.

66. Perret C, et al. Correlation of heart rate at lactate minimum and maximal lactate steady state in wheelchair-racing athletes. *Spinal Cord*. 2012;50(1):33–36.

67. Sharif H, Hou S. Autonomic dysreflexia: a cardiovascular disorder following spinal cord injury. *Neural Regen Res*. 2017;12(9):1390–1400.

68. Gee CM, West CR, Krassioukov AV. Boosting in elite athletes with spinal cord injury: a critical review of physiology and testing procedures. *Sports Med*. 2015;45(8):1133–1142.

69. Bhambhani Y, et al. Boosting in athletes with high-level spinal cord injury: knowledge, incidence and attitudes of athletes in paralympic sport. *Disabil Rehabil*. 2010;32(26):2172–2190.

70. Blauwet CA, et al. Testing for boosting at the Paralympic games: policies, results and future directions. *Br J Sports Med*. 2013;47(13):832–837.

71. Griggs KE, Price MJ, Goosey-Tolfrey VL. Cooling athletes with a spinal cord injury. *Sports Med*. 2015;45(1):9–21.

72. Blauwet C, Lexell J, Derman W. Paralympic sports medicine. In: Thompson W, Vanlandewijck Y, eds. *IOC Handbook of Sports Medicine and Science: Training and Coaching the Paralympic Athlete*. England: Wiley Blackwell; 2016:75–95.

73. Ferrara MS, et al. A longitudinal study of injuries to athletes with disabilities. *Int J Sports Med*. 2000;21(3):221–224.

74. Webborn N, Willick S, Emery CA. The injury experience at the 2010 winter paralympic games. *Clin J Sport Med*. 2012;22(1):3–9.

75. Webborn N, Willick S, Reeser JC. Injuries among disabled athletes during the 2002 Winter Paralympic Games. *Med Sci Sports Exerc*. 2006;38(5):811–815.

76. Derman W, et al. Illness and injury in athletes during the competition period at the London 2012 Paralympic Games: development and implementation of a web-based surveillance system (WEB-IISS) for team medical staff. *Br J Sports Med*. 2013;47(7):420–425.

77. Willick SE, et al. The epidemiology of injuries at the London 2012 Paralympic Games. *Br J Sports Med*. 2013;47(7):426–432.

78. Roussot M. *Upper Limb Injuries in Athletes Participating at the London 2012 Paralympic Games*. 2014. A dissertation prepared by Mark Roussot (RSSMAR024) in partial fulfillment of the requirements for the Master of Philosophy degree in Sport and Exercise Medicine (MPhil Sport and Exercise Medicine) from the University of Cape Town, South Africa.

79. Blauwet CA, et al. Risk of injuries in Paralympic track and field differs by impairment and event discipline: a prospective cohort study at the London 2012 Paralympic games. *Am J Sports Med*. 2016;44(6):1455–1462.

80. Webborn N, et al. The epidemiology of injuries in Football at the London 2012 Paralympic Games. *PM R*. 2016;8(6):545–552.

81. Willick SE, et al. The epidemiology of injuries in powerlifting at the London 2012 Paralympic Games: an analysis of 1411 athlete-days. *Scand J Med Sci Sports*. 2016;26(10):1233–1238.

82. Derman W, et al. High incidence of injury at the Sochi 2014 Winter Paralympic Games: a prospective cohort study of 6564 athlete days. *Br J Sports Med*. 2016;50(17):1069–1074.

83. Schwellnus M, et al. Factors associated with illness in athletes participating in the London 2012 Paralympic Games: a prospective cohort study involving 49,910 athlete-days. *Br J Sports Med*. 2013;47(7):433–440.

84. Derman W, et al. The incidence and patterns of illness at the Sochi 2014 Winter Paralympic Games: a prospective cohort study of 6564 athlete days. *Br J Sports Med*. 2016;50(17):1064–1068.

85. Derman W, Schwellnus M, Jordaan E. Clinical characteristics of 385 illnesses of athletes with impairment reported on the WEB-IISS system during the London 2012 Paralympic Games. *PM R*. 2014;6(8 suppl):S23–S30.

86. Derman W, Ferreria S, Subban K, et al. Transcendence of musculoskeletal injury in athletes with disabilities during major competition. *S Afr J Sports Med*. 2011;23: 95–97.

87. World Anti-Doping Agency Code. 2015. Available from: https://www.wada-ama.org/en/what-we-do/the-code. Accessed March 4, 2017.

88. International Paralympic Committee Anti-Doping Code. 2015. Available from: https://www.paralympic.org/antidoping. Accessed March 4, 2017.

89. World Anti-Doping Agency Prohibited List. 2017. Available from: https://www.wada-ama.org/en/prohibited-list. Accessed March 4, 2017.

90. World Anti-Doping Agency International Standard for Therapeutic Use Exemptions. 2015. Available from: https://www.wada-ama.org/en/resources/therapeutic-use-exemption-tue/international-standard-for-therapeutic-use-exemptions-istue. Accessed March 4, 2017.

91. Burke D, et al. Neuropathic pain prevalence following spinal cord injury: a systematic review and meta-analysis. *Eur J Pain*. 2017;21(1):29–44.

92. Watson JC, Sandroni P. Central neuropathic pain syndromes. *Mayo Clin Proc*. 2016;91(3):372–385.

93. Blauwet CA, Iezzoni LI. From the Paralympics to public health: increasing physical activity through legislative and policy initiatives. *PM R*. 2014;6(8 suppl):S4–S10.

94. Brault MW. Americans with disabilities: 2010. Household economic studies. In: *Current Population Reports*. Washington, DC: United States Census Bureau; 2012:70–131.

95. *World Report on Disability*. Geneva, Switzerland: World Health Organization and the World Bank; 2011.

96. Altman B, Bernstein A. *Disability and Health in the United States, 2001–2005*. Hyattsville, MD: National Center for Health Statistics; 2008.

97. Weil E, et al. Obesity among adults with disabling conditions. *JAMA*. 2002; 288(10):1265–1268.

98. Hsieh K, Rimmer JH, Heller T. Obesity and associated factors in adults with intellectual disability. *J Intellect Disabil Res*. 2014;58(9):851–863.

99. Froehlich-Grobe K, Lee J, Washburn RA. Disparities in obesity and related conditions among Americans with disabilities. *Am J Prev Med*. 2013;45(1):83–90.

100. Garshick E, et al. A prospective assessment of mortality in chronic spinal cord injury. *Spinal Cord*. 2005;43(7):408–416.

101. Sabo D, Veliz P. *Go Out and Play: Youth Sports in America*. East Meadow, NY: Women's Sports Foundation; 2008.

102. Rimmer JH, Wang E, Smith D. Barriers associated with exercise and community access for individuals with stroke. *J Rehabil Res Dev*. 2008;45(2):315–322.

103. Scelza WM, et al. Perceived barriers to exercise in people with spinal cord injury. *Am J Phys Med Rehabil.* 2005;84(8):576–583.

104. Healthy People 2020: Disability and Health. 2014. Available from: http://www. healthypeople.gov/2020/topicsobjectives2020/overview.aspx?topicid=9. Accessed March 23, 2017.

105. Boyle CA. *Message from the Director.* National Center on Birth Defects and Developmental Disabilities; 2014. Available from: http://www.cdc.gov/ncbddd/ aboutus/director.html. Accessed March 23, 2017.

106. National Center on Health, Physical Activity and Disability. 2017. Available from: http://www.ncpad.org/Aboutus. Accessed March 23, 2017.

107. A Guide to Disability Rights Laws: The Rehabilitation Act. 2017. Available from: http://www.ada.gov/cguide.htm#anchor65610. Accessed March 23, 2017.

108. A Guide to Disability Rights Laws: The Americans with Disabilities Act. 2017. Available from: http://www.ada.gov/cguide.htm#anchor62335. Accessed March 23, 2017.

109. Students with Disabilities in Extracurricular Athletics. 2017. Available from: http://www2.ed.gov/about/offices/list/ocr/docs/dcl-factsheet-201301-504.pdf. Accessed March 23, 2017.

110. Students with Disabilities: More Information and Guidance Could Improve Opportunities in Physical Education and Athletics. Washington, DC: U.S. Government Accountability Office; 2010.

111. Gallo J, Otto M. Wheelchair athlete wins right to race alongside runners. *Washington Post.* 2006.

112. Fitness and Athletics Equity for Students with Disabilities Act. 2015. Available from: http://mlis.state.md.us. Accessed March 23, 2017.

113. Shuhan S, Le Clair J. Legacies and tensions after the 2008 Beijing Paralympic Games. In: Gilbert K, Legg D, eds. *Paralympic Legacies.* Champaign, IL: Common Ground Publishing; 2011:111–129.

114. *The International Paralympic Committee Strategic Plan 2015 to 2018.* Bonn, Germany: International Paralympic Committee; 2015.

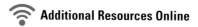 **Additional Resources Online**

CHAPTER 43

Byron W. Lai
James H. Rimmer

Physical Activity for People with Disabilities

Studies have reported that people with disabilities are more likely to be inactive or sedentary (1,2) compared to the general adult population. National prevalence data from 2009 to 2012 has demonstrated that people with disabilities in the United States are nearly twice as likely to be inactive (47% vs. 26% with no reported disability) (3). Inactive lifestyles, combined with tendencies for non-use and worsening health conditions, place people with disabilities at risk for rapid deconditioning. Together, these issues increase the likelihood that, as people with disabilities age, they will have greater difficulty maintaining their ability to work, participating in recreational activities, performing self-care activities (4,5), and engaging in various activities in their community (6).

Regular engagement in physical activity (see Chapter 49) is generally acknowledged for its ability to improve health and function for people with disabilities (7). Growing evidence indicates that active people with disabilities have a lower prevalence of chronic health conditions (e.g., cardiovascular disease, diabetes, and stroke) (3), as well as secondary health conditions (e.g., limited mobility, fatigue, depression, and anxiety) (8); experience greater levels of participation in all aspects of society, including work, leisure, and recreation (9,10); and achieve a higher satisfaction with life (11). These benefits stress the importance of promoting physical activity among people with disabilities. An important first step in this process is for clinicians and health professionals to find effective ways to identify and remove the many challenges that people with disabilities encounter to participate in physical activity.

A generally accepted explanation for low levels of physical activity is that people with disabilities experience substantially more barriers to participation (12). Fortunately, with correct adaptations/modifications, physical activity can be made accessible to people with a range of disabling conditions by overcoming many of the barriers reported in the literature. Examples of these barriers may include lack of accessible and usable equipment, knowledge, affordable programs, or barriers that are directly related to the built or natural environment (e.g., lack of accessible fitness facilities, parks, sidewalks, or public transportation) (13). In addition to these physical impediments, promoters of physical activity should also pay careful attention to a variety of personal factors such as the needs and preferences of the individual who is interested in starting a new program.

The focus of this chapter is to guide health care professionals in their efforts to increase physical activity in people with disabilities, by providing suggestions that overcome barriers and enhance the personalization of physical activity programs. The first section discusses how community-based physical activity programs can be used as a mechanism for transitioning people in rehabilitation to self-maintenance of health and function across the life span. This section includes a framework to assist this transition or transformation. The second section provides a model for systematically prescribing tailored physical activity programs to people with disabilities, which is complemented by general recommendations for exercise training. The final section focuses on specific types of recreation, fitness, and sports activities that individuals with disabilities can engage in and identifies appropriate community-based resources.

TRANSITIONING FROM REHABILITATION TO COMMUNITY-BASED PHYSICAL ACTIVITY

Inpatient or outpatient rehabilitation can lead to substantial gains in health and function for individuals who aim to improve their functional independence or recover from a serious injury or accident. However, for these gains to be maintained after rehabilitation is completed, health professionals should prescribe home- or community-based physical activity programs to maintain or further improve health and function. As evident from summative reviews of the literature, participation in research trials of physical activity or exercise (a subset of physical activity) can improve several indicators of fitness, health, and function (7,14,15). Yet, despite these benefits, the majority of people with disabilities do not meet the recommended guidelines necessary to elicit such benefits (3). This information implies that there is a gap between participation in rehabilitation services and lifelong physical activity behavior. To explain this gap, **Figure 43-1** provides a conceptual illustration of what may occur after an injury, accident, or onset of a new health condition that, without regular participation in physical activity, can potentially lead to a progressive decline in health and function.

Most rehabilitation is limited to the subacute period and is designed to restore or improve the most critical functional skills needed to assist the person in performing BADL (basic activities of daily living) and/or IADL (instrumental activities of daily living). Typically, after therapy is completed and clients are discharged, rehabilitation professionals will prescribe clients a therapeutic exercise plan to continue within their community. Unfortunately, people with disabilities are often impeded from community physical activity by numerous intrapersonal barriers (e.g., lack of energy/motivation, outcome

FIGURE 43-1. Getting beyond rehabilitation and transitioning people with disabilities into community-based physical activity.

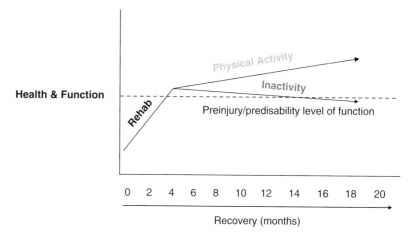

expectations, and time), and perhaps, more importantly, environmental or organizational barriers to exercise. Barriers within the community range from those that are structural in nature, such as access, usability of equipment, and transportation to those that prevent activity at the organizational level, such as policies or laws (12). Therefore, after people are discharged to the home to what is often a considerable alteration in health, function, and lifestyle, numerous barriers prevent them from living a healthy and active lifestyle. In theory, these barriers may contribute to reports of low levels of participation in physical activity after rehabilitation discharge (16,17), along with declines in health and function that are associated with inactivity or sedentary behavior during this period (18).

Transforming Rehabilitation *Patients* into *Participants* in Physical Activity

To prevent deconditioning that occurs after rehabilitation discharge, ideally, *patients* should undergo a structured transition to becoming *participants* in community-based physical activity. However, there is no general consensus for how this process might occur. Exercise professionals have access to a wide variety of strategies to promote physical activity, with limited empirical evidence to support choosing one approach versus another. To address this issue, we discuss this transformation along a theoretical continuum of four focus areas: (a) Rehabilitation, (b) Condition-Specific Exercise, (c) Physical Fitness, and (d) Lifetime Physical Activity. The continuum is referred to as

the Transformative Exercise (TE) Framework and (**Fig. 43-2**) (19), and suggests that before patients are transitioned into Lifetime Physical Activity, they may require a gradual transition through intermediary areas that focus on different aspects of training and rehabilitation.

The end goal of TE is to transition people from exercises focused on restoration of function in Rehabilitation to exercise as a means of prevention in lifelong Physical Activity. Activities within the Physical Activity focus area consist of those that aim to promote or sustain long-term activity behavior. Examples may include recreation, sports, and group activities that promote social, enjoyable, and meaningful experiences. The latter section of this chapter discusses physical activity options and modifications in more detail.

The challenge engaging in physical activities immediately after rehabilitation, is that, aside from the environmental barriers to participation, physical activities often involve more dynamic movements that are performed for higher intensities or durations than conventional exercises. For example, wheelchair users travel approximately 2.5 km in a single wheelchair basketball or rugby game (20). This value not only exceeds the average distance of 1.6 km that manual wheelchair users travel throughout a given day (21), but the distance traveled during a game is also accumulated within a shorter length of time (i.e., one basketball game amounted to 2.6 km distance traveled, whereas 90 separate bouts of mobility throughout an entire day amounted to a distance of 1.6 km). This physiologic demand

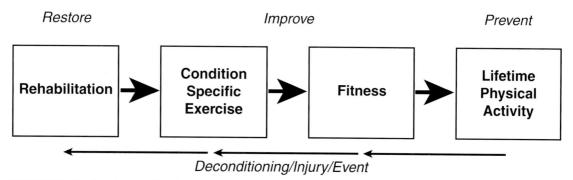

FIGURE 43-2. The Transformative Exercise Framework portrays a continuum from Rehabilitation focused on recovery, to exercises focused on improvement that are Condition-Specific and Fitness-related, and finally to prevention in lifelong Physical Activity participation. (Modified and reprinted from Rimmer J, Lai B. Framing new pathways in transformative exercise for individuals with existing and newly acquired disability. *Disabil Rehabil.* 2015;39(2):173–180.)

likely explains why evidence demonstrates that an individual's physical capacity is linked with their physical activity participation. A study by Janssen and colleagues (22) found that weekly sport participation in people with spinal cord injury is associated with common measures of physical capacity, specifically maximal power output and peak oxygen consumption. In other words, people with spinal cord injury who had a higher physical capacity participated in greater durations of physical activity in a given week, whereas individuals with a lower physical capacity performed less physical activity. These findings are further supported and expanded upon by evidence-based conceptual models demonstrating that physical deconditioning (e.g., decreases in strength, power, and aerobic capacity) results in increased difficulty with performing tasks (e.g., increased fatigability, risk of falls, and mobility issues), which makes individuals less likely to perform physical activity (23,24).

In addition to considering the physical demand of physical activity, health professionals should also consider incorporating behavioral change techniques to enhance physical activity participation (25). Strong evidence demonstrates that exercise confidence (i.e., self-efficacy) and goal-setting contribute heavily towards an individual's decision to start and maintain a behavior (26,27), including physical activity or exercise. In fact, self-efficacy is often a predominant construct that is incorporated in many prevalent theories/models of health behavior (28). In summary, physical activity participation depends on physical and psychosocial factors, which may be difficult for people with disabilities who are discharged from rehabilitation and face a myriad of lifestyle changes to which they must begin to adapt (29–31). Due to these issues, we suggest that there be a gradual progression through a Condition-Specific Exercise and Fitness focus area, in order to bridge the gap between Rehabilitation and Physical Activity.

Therapeutic exercise programs after rehabilitation discharge should focus on modalities that manage health conditions: exercises that are Condition-Specific. As defined by the Institute of Medicine Report (*Disability in America*, 1991) (32), secondary health conditions are "causally related to a primary disabling condition and include pressure ulcers, contractures, physical deconditioning, cardiopulmonary conditions, and depression." These conditions can affect the individual physically (e.g., severe muscle weakness from prolonged bed rest, pressure ulcers due to inadequate blood flow, and abnormal blood pressure) or psychosocially (e.g., depression, anxiety, and isolation) (8). To exercise through the impact of these conditions, the individual with a disability will likely require exercises that are carefully tailored towards their conditions with assistance from an exercise professional, who has knowledge of the disability. We recommend that these professionals prescribe Condition-Specific exercises in a two-step process: (a) identify secondary conditions that prevent the individual from progressing to Fitness or Physical Activity, and (b) prescribe evidence-based exercises that alleviate or reduce the signs or symptoms of the condition.

To prescribe Condition-Specific exercise, exercise professionals will first have to identify and understand that secondary conditions vary among different populations of people with disabilities. For example, people who use a wheelchair as a primary means of mobility might experience conditions that arise from poor blood flow due to prolonged sitting or severe muscle atrophy of the lower extremities. In contrast, people post-stroke may experience abnormally high blood pressure

throughout the day, which places significant strain on internal organs and places them at risk for cardiovascular events, including a recurrent stroke. Four of the most common secondary conditions reported in people with disabilities include, mobility problems, fatigue, deconditioning, and chronic pain (8). Psychosocial conditions include perceived difficulties with access, sleep problems, depression, and isolation (8).

After identifying relevant conditions, the last step for Condition-Specific exercise is to prescribe activities that alleviate, improve, or prevent against the worsening of secondary conditions. This task will prove challenging, as a summative review of the literature published for the 2008 Physical Activity Guidelines for Americans report (US Department of Health and Human Services) by the Advisory Committee found insufficient evidence to support the prescription of specific exercise doses (e.g., frequency, intensity, time, and type) that might best affect health conditions for people with disabilities (15). Nevertheless, the US Department of Health and Human Services has established general national physical activity guidelines of 150 minutes of moderate aerobic exercise and 2 days per week of muscular strengthening exercises (33). For Condition-Specific exercise, we recommend that health professionals target bodily systems (e.g., musculoskeletal, cardiovascular/circulatory, respiratory, sensory, and nervous system) that underlie the condition experienced by the individual with a disability.

Therefore, Condition-Specific exercises should target secondary conditions with evidence-based activities that emphasize exercises and equipment that are tailored for the specific functional needs and identified secondary conditions of the participant. For example, an individual who uses a wheelchair and has impaired function of their lower extremities may aim to improve the circulatory system to prevent or reduce the risk of pressure ulcers. In this case, the individual could use an arm-crank ergometer as the modality of exercise, and perform the activity in the standing position with a device that alleviates weight (e.g., body weight supported system; shown in **Fig. 43-3**) or

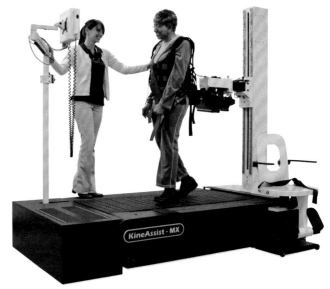

FIGURE 43-3. An individual using a robotic body-weight-support system (the KineAssist): a safe, yet challenging, method for mobility and balance training for individuals with limited levels of strength, balance, and coordination. (Courtesy of HDT Expeditionary Systems, Inc.)

assists the individual into a standing position (e.g., a standing tilt-table or wheelchair) to reduce seated pressure. Moreover, an individual with multiple sclerosis who aims to improve his/her gait and has high symptoms of fatigue and heat sensitivity could perform aquatic exercise in a pool with cool water temperatures. The aquatic environment provides buoyancy and reduces body-weight and core temperature. Additionally, evidence suggests that walking in a pool at slower speeds requires less energy expenditure than overground walking (34,35), which may be beneficial for people who experience high levels of fatigue.

Ideally, exercise professionals should first target secondary conditions that are most severe in nature (e.g., extreme weakness, fatigue, pain, falls risk), before transitioning to the remaining two focus areas—Fitness and Lifetime Physical Activity. Due to the complexity of this task, exercise professionals and people with disabilities will likely require the guidance or consultation of a physical therapist or disability exercise specialist (certifications discussed later under "General Exercise Programming").

Once significant secondary health conditions are better managed and the participant is able to move to a higher level of training, the main focus area is Fitness. The Fitness stage focuses primarily on five types of health: cardiorespiratory, musculoskeletal, functional, metabolic and mental health and prepares individuals to work from improvement towards prevention. Training components could include cardiovascular, balance, flexibility, and musculoskeletal strength or endurance exercise. Typical modalities of Fitness consist of those generally associated with exercise such as walking, jogging, lifting weights, and cycling. Some of the same activities may be modified for people with disabilities, which could include, arm cycling, recumbent cycling, accessible weight machines, and pool walking.

Fitness activities could help certain individuals increase their sports performance. For example, someone who wants to play wheelchair basketball will require sufficient strength to pass or shoot the ball and push and maneuver their wheelchair; have enough sitting balance to maintain their posture during activity and perturbations; and have adequate aerobic power to maintain performance for the entire game. In contrast to Condition-Specific exercise, individuals performing exercise as Fitness will typically need little to no supervision. Theoretically, they will have or be close to obtaining the functional ability to perform many exercises independently. Exercise professionals should still pay careful attention to safety during Fitness (more detail provided in section three of this chapter). The naturally high intensity of these exercises may present some potential health risks for people with disabilities starting a fitness program until they become accustomed and comfortable with the training routine (e.g., transfers onto weight machines, knowing the signs and symptoms of overexertion, reducing risk of overuse injuries).

In summary, after Rehabilitation, clients should undergo Condition-Specific Exercise and then focus on increasing their Fitness to a sufficient level to participate in Lifetime Physical Activity that they enjoy and can sustain over the long-term. This transition might not always proceed in a linear, stepwise fashion, which is why we refer to the four TE domains as "focus areas" versus "steps" or "phases." When considering progression, it is possible that an individual has a high enough level of function after rehabilitation and can skip one or more focus areas and proceed directly to participation in Fitness or Lifetime Physical Activity. In contrast, people can also return to a previous focus area. If they experience an exacerbation of an existing condition or experience a new injury/event, Rehabilitation or more carefully prescribed exercises that reflect their current health status (Condition Specific) may be required. Finally, individuals may remain in one focus area indefinitely. Some individuals may not be able to restore function to the point where they can exercise independently. Likewise, a single exercise program could consist of all focus areas of the TE Framework. Although there is a handful of evidence to show that transitioning people into physical activity after rehabilitation is beneficial for long-term participation (36), further investigations are needed to validate the TE framework. In summary, TE provides an overarching foundation for exercise professionals to prescribe and design general exercise plans and goals for people with disabilities after rehabilitation discharge. The next section (below) discusses how to design programs that are tailored towards the needs of the individual.

TAILORING PHYSICAL ACTIVITY

Tailoring physical activity programs that recognize the unique circumstances surrounding each individual is an important aspect of prescribing physical activity programs that have a greater likelihood of successful initiation and adherence (37). For example, research on physical activity for people post-stroke indicates that generic programs not targeted to the needs of any particular end user are far less likely to result in long-term maintenance of health-promoting behaviors (38). By assessing a combination of factors, including the person's motivational level (i.e., readiness to change), physical activity profile, health and mobility limitations, and barriers to participation, a program can be developed that meets each person's specific needs, interests, and circumstances. Thus, physical activity recommendations for people with disabilities may be more effective if they are individually and culturally appealing and are implemented in a setting of the individual's own choosing. This includes establishing realistic, achievable goals to meet the person's needs and build self-efficacy, while also finding solutions for the barriers to participation that frustrate even the most enthusiastic participant. Furthermore, programs should be dynamic (i.e., interesting, enjoyable) and provide the flexibility to change frequently to accommodate changes in the life of the participant (e.g., boredom, getting a new job, experiencing some pain performing certain types of exercises, etc.). So many programs fail because the individuals' health or personal interests change, making the program either too challenging or uninteresting, or the environment changes and individuals no longer have access to the same resources needed to participate in the program or activity.

PEP Intervention Model

One method that can assist rehabilitation professionals in providing more tailored physical activity recommendations to their clients as they transition from in-patient rehabilitation to community-based activities is the Personalized Exercise Program (PEP). The *PEP* intervention model (shown in **Fig. 43-4**) begins with problem identification accomplished through a detailed assessment of the individual's needs, interests, activity

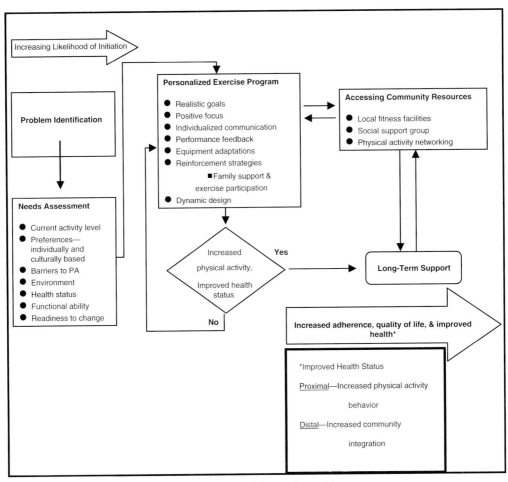

FIGURE 43-4. PEP intervention model.

level, health status, functional ability, and readiness to change. This assessment of individual health, lifestyle behaviors, and function, in conjunction with an evaluation of the individual's family support, community resources, and environmental barriers, allows a personalized physical activity program to be tailored for the individual. Jointly, individual-, family-, and community-level *strengths* and *resources* are harnessed to help the individual overcome barriers to physical activity.

While implementation of the resulting *PEP* intervention in the context of long-term support is expected to result in increased physical activity and improved health outcomes, more research needs to be conducted to determine the effectiveness of this model. Establishment and maintenance of social support networks are an important component of maintaining physical activity behaviors in people with disabilities. The individualized assessment, in conjunction with an evaluation of community resources (e.g., community swim programs, accessible fitness centers), allows for a personalized physical activity program that is based on customized information. Both individual and community-level *strengths* and *resources* are utilized to help the client overcome barriers to participating in a sport or other type of physical activity at home or in the community. Establishment and maintenance of social support networks that include building community friendships with other people, in addition to parental and/or caregiver support, are important components for maintaining participation over

an extended period until health benefits are achieved. These networks may include personal contacts with family members or caregivers or may involve friendships formed through exercise classes or nutritional cooking classes offered as part of a community-based program.

The dynamic design of the *PEP* intervention model and its *person-centered* approach allow the rehabilitation professional to revise and modify the program at any time until the recommendations are *calibrated* or *recalibrated* (as in the case with an illness or new secondary health condition) to the user's needs and interest level. In **Figure 43-4**, the first step of the *PEP* intervention model is illustrated in the left column, *comprehensive needs assessment*, which includes the following components: (a) physical activity profile and activity preferences, (b) barriers to participation, (c) health status and mobility limitations, and (d) motivational level (readiness to change). Each of these components is described below.

Components of the *PEP* Intervention Model

Physical Activity Profile

Understanding the clients' physical activity participation history in sports, recreation, and/or fitness before (when possible) and after the onset of a disability is critical for designing an effective program. An assessment of a client's specific disability and functional level, along with personal activity preferences, can help determine potential activities. For example, if a person with a spinal cord injury was an enthusiastic softball or basketball player before his or her disability, finding links to participating in wheelchair softball or basketball and establishing relevant goals, whenever possible, may be more appealing and increase the individual's participation. Any recreation, fitness, and sport activity can be adapted for an individual with a disability (discussed in the final section of this chapter), and there are multiple opportunities for offering individuals meaningful, enjoyable, and sustainable physical activities.

Barriers to Physical Activity

As discussed previously, personal and environmental barriers can impose substantial limitations in maintaining a physically active lifestyle (see Chapter 15). Among people with disabilities, some of the more common barriers are pain, lack of transportation, insufficient financial resources to pay for a health club membership, lack of awareness of community-based programs, and not knowing how to perform certain types of exercises or recreational activities. Usually, more specification is required in developing exercise programs for people with disabilities because certain impairments and activity limitations can limit an individual's access to a program or activity.

One of the major concerns associated with increasing physical activity participation among people with disabilities is the lack of access to many community sports, recreation, and fitness programs (12). People with disabilities can often encounter enormous barriers in the built and natural environment. Indoor and outdoor structures have a major effect on participation in physical activity among people with disabilities (39). Structures such as gyms, fitness centers, outdoor trails, parks, and swimming pools often have poor signage, lack detail on how to use the equipment or participate in a program, or provide poor access routes to and from the facility or program.

Indoor environments of many fitness and recreation facilities also need to become more accessible. Another major barrier to exercise is inaccessible exercise equipment (12). Most manufacturers do not consider in their design specifications how to make their equipment accessible to people with physical, cognitive, and sensory disabilities. Typically, commercial cardiovascular exercise equipment requires propulsion by using the musculature of the lower extremities (e.g., treadmills, stationary bikes, elliptical cross-trainers, and steppers), thereby restricting use among people with lower-extremity disabilities (e.g., paralysis, limb loss). While a few fitness facilities may be able to purchase a commercial quality arm cycle or wheelchair ergometer, the vast majority of fitness centers either cannot afford this equipment or do not find it cost-effective to purchase one for a small percentage of their clientele. Aside from access, people with disabilities also have difficulty with using exercise equipment. For example, people with visual or cognitive disabilities might find that display panels are often difficult to read or understand, or getting on and off the equipment presents some risk of falling (40). Likewise, people with low strength levels often find that exercise machines at even the lowest settings are hard to propel or lift.

Programmatic issues are also barriers for people with disabilities. Fitness and recreation classes such as aerobic dance, yoga, and tai chi are often taught by instructors who have minimal knowledge of how to adapt their program for someone with a disability. Therefore, class activities or even spoken directions may not be suitable for people with disabilities. Professionals aimed at promoting physical activity must have a good understanding of how to overcome certain barriers in order to ensure that the participant can successfully engage in various types of community-based programs.

Health Status and Other Conditions

In line with Condition Specific exercise, the exercise professional must understand the health and mobility limitations that prevent a client from engaging in certain types of physical activities and prescribe the appropriate set of exercises to address these deficits. Examples of mobility limitations include difficulty walking, climbing steps, and transferring from a wheelchair. Other limiting factors include loss of balance, low vision, hearing difficulty, pain, fatigue, decreased cognition and paralysis.

Motivational Level

For successful participation in any form of physical activity, the rehabilitation/exercise professional must find innovative ways to encourage participants to obtain regular physical activity. One behavioral theory that resembles an individual's progression towards adoption of physical activity is the Stages of Change model (41,42). This model includes five stages: precontemplation—no intention to change a behavior in the foreseeable future; contemplation—individual is aware of the needs for physical activity but has not yet made a commitment to take action; preparation—intending to take action in the next month but has unsuccessfully taken action in the past year; action—interested in modifying behavior to increase physical activity; and maintenance—individual is engaging in physical activity. The stage of change that a client is experiencing is dependent on a variety of factors, which can include intrapersonal, interpersonal, and environmental barriers, as well as exercise self-efficacy (mentioned previously). Therefore, assistance in identifying and addressing these factors will be critical towards improving physical activity participation.

General Exercise Programming for People with Disabilities

After prescribing a tailored exercise program, careful attention will be required to ensure that movements are performed comfortably and safely. Exercise guidelines for the general adult population are often suitable for people with disabilities, assuming appropriate modifications/adaptations are made where necessary.

This section provides a series of general recommendations for three primary components of exercise, namely, cardiorespiratory endurance, muscular strength and endurance, and flexibility. Cardiorespiratory endurance or aerobic capacity refers to the ability of the heart (cardio) and lungs (respiratory) to provide sufficient blood flow to working muscles for sustained physical activity. Muscular endurance is defined as the muscle's ability to exert force for a sustained period of time, and muscular strength refers to the ability to generate force one time. Both contribute to improved balance, mobility and stability. Flexibility is the movement capability (i.e., range of motion) of muscle groups around a joint and can help to reduce injury, improve posture, and perform ADL and IADL (43,44). Note that the recommendations below may not apply to leisure and competitive sports and activities (the Physical Activity focus are of the TE Framework), which are less likely to be closely monitored for safety and specific conditioning effects.

Starting an Exercise Program

Before beginning an exercise program, a client's physician should be informed so that adequate precautions, if necessary, can be taken, and possible side effects of medications considered (**Box 43-1**). The American College of Sports Medicine (ACSM) (45) recommends that individuals with certain risk factors for exercise have a graded exercise test to determine how the heart responds to stress and whether there is adequate blood flow to the heart during increasing levels of activity. However, maximal graded exercise testing in some subgroups of people with disabilities (e.g., stroke, high lesion-level spinal cord injury) must be carefully supervised to avoid cardiovascular events. Likewise, participant's functional limitations may limit the ability to achieve a true maximal test of exertion. Standardized exercise tests often require treadmills and stationary cycles, which must reach high enough intensity levels to obtain a true measure of maximal effort. Therefore, we recommend performing submaximal exercise tests using validated and reliable methods on equipment that is suitable for certain populations (e.g., recumbent cycle or an arm ergometer).

In order to locate an exercise professional who has adequate education and experience, seek out recommendations from health professionals or national disability organizations. Though there are no national standards or educational requirements necessary to be an exercise professional, the ACSM, the American Council on Exercise (ACE), and the National Strength and Conditioning Association (NSCA) all issue certifications recognized nationally by exercise professionals. For example, exercise professionals can become certified disability exercise specialists through the Certified Inclusive Fitness Trainer provided by the ACSM and the National Center on Health, Physical Activity and Disability. Other important considerations of the exercise professional include the personality, gender, and flexibility to conduct training in the home or fitness facility (**Box 43-2**).

In choosing an exercise facility, similar considerations apply. Depending on the client's disability and functional level, accessibility of both the center and the equipment is

---

BOX 43-1

Considerations Prior to Involvement in Exercise Training

- Inform physician of intentions to engage in physical activity if you are uncertain the patient/client is safe to participate in higher intensity levels of exercise.
- Determine side effects of medication on exercise.
- Consult a trained exercise professional to design an exercise prescription or identify resources for exercise programming for people with disabilities through the ACSM website (www.acsm.org).
- A graded exercise test may be warranted for some patients/clients if there is any concern about safely performing moderate- to vigorous-intensity exercise.

BOX 43-2

Parameters for Choosing an Exercise Professional and Fitness Center

- Education and experience
- Personal preferences
- Training frequency
- Location
- Cost
- Social skills

---

critical. Exercise equipment using universal equipment design is preferable, as it is accessible for people with and without disabilities. Moreover, other factors to consider are availability of staff on site, location, transportation options, and cost. The last section of this chapter provides an online resource with a national database of local exercise centers and programs for people with disabilities.

During Exercise

Safety

A variety of guidelines should be followed to help ensure the safety and general effectiveness of a physical activity program or sport (**Table 43-1**). The client must be aware of how his or her body is responding to the activity, so that appropriate adjustments can be made. Ideally, an exercise program should include a variety of movements based on the TE focus area and the target systems (e.g., cardiorespiratory, musculoskeletal). One particular issue that must be addressed is avoidance of overuse injuries. For wheelchair users, certain muscle

---

TABLE 43-1	**Safety Guidelines and Reducing Injury**
Reducing injury in people with disabilities	• Stop exercise if pain, discomfort, nausea, dizziness, light-headedness, chest pain, irregular heartbeat, shortness of breath, or clammy hands are experienced.
	• Adequate fluid intake is necessary.
	• Appropriate clothing can help to avoid overheating.
	• Realistic short-term and long-term goals must be established.
	• The exercise program must meet the patient/client's goals.
	• Overuse injuries can be avoided by varying exercise routine (e.g., cross-training) and using proper equipment.
	• Pain and fatigue levels must be monitored closely.
	• Balance must be assessed prior to engaging in standing activities (e.g., weight routine, aerobic dance class).
Reducing injury in wheelchair users	• Workout gloves with adequate padding can help avoid hand injury.
	• Push rims should be padded.
	• The angle of push rims to the seat must be optimally positioned to provide the most comfortable and efficient push angle.
	• Legs should be securely strapped.
	• Adequate stretching is necessary prior to the workout.

groups in the shoulder region are often overused due to the effort required to push a wheelchair. Thus, exercise professionals could prescribe exercises that focus on the back musculature. Standing and seated balance should also be assessed to determine readiness for various activities. With all activities, a disability exercise specialist should be primarily concerned with helping their clients avoid and prevent falls.

Various indicators of exertion should be monitored during exercise programming so that the individual stays within an optimal and safe training zone. Rating of perceived exertion (RPE) should be monitored by using the Borg RPE scale, which measures intensity of exercise on a scale from 6 to 20, or the conversation rule, in which one is able to converse while exercising. Heart rate must be gauged by finding the pulse and comparing this to the target heart rate. In some cases, blood pressure should also be checked by an exercise professional during exercise or sport. For some individuals with physical disabilities, hypertension (e.g., stroke), hypotension, and autonomic dysreflexia (e.g., spinal cord injury) are common health conditions that should be carefully monitored. Once the individual adjusts to the program without wide fluctuations in blood pressure, it can be measured before and after until the person is comfortable enough to exercise independently without supervision.

Although we provide general safety guidelines, an individual's exercise plan can be affected by a multitude of health factors and conditions, which extends beyond the capacity of this chapter. For more detailed suggestions, we recommend consulting a disability exercise specialist (discussed later).

Cardiorespiratory Endurance (Often Referred to as Aerobic Exercise)

General suggestions for cardiorespiratory endurance are shown in **Box 43-3**. Though a wide range of activities and sports are available to obtain a cardiovascular workout, including walking, wheelchair rolling, cycling, and swimming, as well as recreational and competitive sports (discussed later), specific types of cardiovascular exercise equipment can assist wheelchair users and individuals with lower-extremity impairments in obtaining a cardiovascular workout (**Box 43-4**).

BOX 43-3

Cardiorespiratory Exercise Suggestions

- An exercise prescription for individuals with neurologic conditions should include the same four elements that are used with the general population: frequency, intensity, duration, and type. Check the ACSM website (www.acsm.org) for resources on developing exercise prescription guidelines.
- Any activity that increases energy expenditure above rest safely and effectively can be used to improve cardiorespiratory fitness.
- Patients taking β-blockers and those with autonomic dysfunction can have a blunted heart rate response. In these instances, consider using the RPE scale.
- Monitor RPE, heart rate, and blood pressure during early stages of activity and new programs.
- Teach proper breathing techniques (i.e., deeper vs. shallow breaths and "think tall" to maintain good posture) to avoid dyspnea (breathlessness).
- Vary workout to maintain interest.

BOX 43-4

Sample Cardiovascular Exercise Equipment for People with Disabilities Who Are Unable to Use Their Legs to Exercise

- Upper arm ergometer
- Wheelchair ergometer
- NuStep recumbent stepper
- BioStep Semi-Recumbent Elliptical

An ergometer is an upper and/or lower body–driven exercise device that is powered from a stationary position and provides an aerobic workout. The common stationary exercise bike represents one type/mode. Other variations exist for individuals with physical disabilities. Most ergometers use some form of hand or foot pedal for the basic motion, and some models allow for wheelchair access. Ergometers come in upper-arm, lower-leg, and dual-extremity models and are often the primary mode of aerobic exercise for people who use wheelchairs as a primary means of mobility (**Fig. 43-5**). Some arm ergometers also come with removable or rotating seats to allow access to both people who use and do not use wheelchairs. When necessary, hand grips or foot straps can be used to be provide better attachment to the exercise device. Additionally, wheelchair ergometers allow for upper-body workouts and propulsion mechanics training through wheelchair propulsion on a stationary-supported mount.

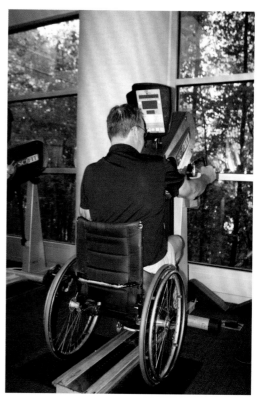

FIGURE 43-5. An individual using a Scifit upper-body ergometer. (Courtesy of Lakeshore Foundation [www.lakeshore.org] and the National Center on Health, Physical Activity and Disability [www.nchpad.org].)

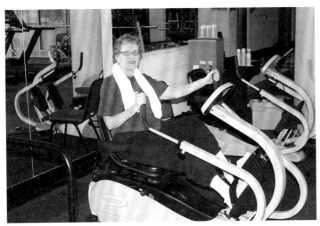

FIGURE 43-6. An individual using the NuStep recumbent stepper, with a reclining back rest and a swivel seat, allows for an upper- and/or lower-body workout. (Courtesy of Lakeshore Foundation [www.lakeshore.org] and the National Center on Health, Physical Activity and Disability [www.nchpad.org].)

Another type of cycle/ergometer that can be powered by upper, lower, and dual extremities is the NuStep recumbent stepper (**Fig. 43-6**). The NuStep includes a reclining back rest and a swivel seat, which simultaneously allows the arms and legs to move in a smooth motion. Design features allow for either the lower and/or upper body to power the stepper, depending on the individual's disability and strength capacity.

Muscular Strength and Endurance

Strength training prescriptions for people with disabilities are based largely on disability severity, functional muscle mass, and health status (**Box 43-5**). Some individuals can train at very high intensity levels, while others will only be able to perform at minimal levels of resistance (i.e., lifting a body part against gravity). The training load (number of sets and

---

BOX 43-5

Strength Training Guidelines

- Strength training prescription and training load are determined by disability severity, functional muscle mass, and health status.
- Resistance goals must be clarified to determine strength training schedule.
- Proper breathing techniques and a complete range of motion must be followed.
- Blood pressure should be monitored periodically during strength training.
- Adaptations may be necessary for individuals with hand dysfunction and asymmetrical weakness.
- Focus on stability, coordination, ROM, and timing.
- Wide benches, low seats, and trunk and pelvic strapping will help support and protect the person from injury during the exercise routine.
- Avoid "hiking" the body on the weak side.
- Avoid person holding breath while lifting weight (i.e., Valsalva maneuver).
- Use straps whenever necessary to keep body part in contact or alignment while lifting weight.

---

repetitions, frequency, rest interval between sets) also varies by disability type, health status, and functional muscle mass. With respect to disability type, individuals who do not have a progressive disorder (e.g., spinal cord injury, cerebral palsy) may work at higher intensity levels than persons at later stages of progressive disorders (e.g., multiple sclerosis, Parkinson disease).

The amount of functional muscle mass also affects training volume. Persons with paralysis, hemiplegia, impaired motor control, or limited joint mobility have less functional muscle mass and will therefore require a lower training volume. For individuals who cannot lift the minimal weight on certain resistance machines, resistance bands or cuff weights or even the person's own body weight can be used as the resistance.

Modes of resistance exercise consist of three general categories: free weights, portable equipment (e.g., elastic bands, tubing), and machines. While free weights may be preferable because they resemble functional daily activity, they require good trunk stability and may be difficult to perform for individuals with severe limitations in motor control and coordination. For individuals with very low strength levels, gravity-resistance exercise may be all that the person is capable of doing, and active-assistive exercise may be required for certain muscle groups that are too weak (paresis) or tight (spasticity) to be moved independently.

Precautions for assisting people with disabilities with strength training include avoiding fatigue and exacerbations, assisting with asymmetrical weakness and hand dysfunction, and periodically checking blood pressure. Fatigue and delayed-onset muscle soreness in individuals with physical disabilities should be avoided, though this is common in new resistance training programs. Exercise should be stopped temporarily if soreness in certain muscle groups prevents the person from performing routine daily activities. Similarly, individuals with asymmetrical weakness may tend to hike their body disproportionately in resistance training and must be encouraged to use proper form.

For individuals with hand dysfunction who have difficulty grasping barbells or handles on different strength machines, a variety of specially designed gloves allow the person's hand(s) to maintain contact with the resistance equipment. Gloves will also protect the hand(s) from injury while performing resistance training routines. Individuals who do not have good grip strength can use wrist cuffs or leather mitts with velcro and buckles to secure their hands to dumbbells or weight equipment (**Fig. 43-7**). Blood pressure should also be monitored during the early stages of the program. Hypertension or hypotension can be a common problem for some disabilities.

Finally, safe and effective strength training must include proper breathing techniques and extend through a complete range of motion. Breath should not be held during strength training, and the client should be taught to exhale or breathe out while pushing the weight up or out and inhale or breathe in while letting the weight down or in. Proper posture facilitates effective breathing techniques.

Flexibility

Flexibility exercises help to improve range of motion, balance, and coordination, as well as the ability to carry out

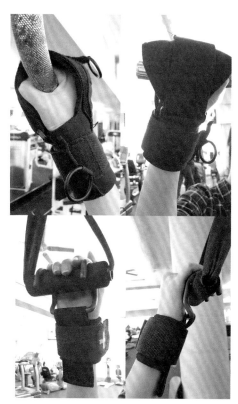

FIGURE 43-7. Activity mitts or gloves can assist a person with hand dysfunction to grip equipment handles. (Courtesy of Lakeshore Foundation and the National Center on Health, Physical Activity and Disability [www. nchpad.org].)

regular activities of daily living. They can be performed daily, before or after a cardiovascular and strength workout. In some cases, stretching prior to exercise may increase an individual's range of motion to a sufficient level that allows successful completion of a movement. However, if the joint has been in a "fixed" position for many years (i.e., contracture), it may not be possible to fully extend the joint. An exercise professional should consult with a physical therapist, physician, or appropriate medical professional to determine how to stretch the muscle appropriately without causing injury.

In summary, we recommend that stretches should be held and progressed slowly for major muscle groups, with careful precaution taken to avoid spasticity and pain. Exercise specialists should be familiar with normal ranges of motion for each body joint, be aware of conditions that might contraindicate the performance of flexibility exercises, and seek consultation when necessary. Flexibility training can often be combined with more enjoyable forms of activities, which can easily be adapted for people with disabilities, such as yoga, Tai-Chi, and Pilates.

PHYSICAL ACTIVITY TYPES AND RESOURCES

One of the most important elements of this chapter is to provide rehabilitation and health professionals with a one-stop resource for identifying physical activity materials that can be used to facilitate/promote/prescribe participation among people with disabilities.

Resources for Fitness and Leisure Physical Activities

While textbooks provide a framework for guiding professionals in planning and developing rehabilitation programs, when it comes to physical activity, the Internet is extremely important for identifying key resources that can be passed on to the client. Resources should include specific information on how physical activity can improve certain conditions or symptoms associated with a disability; resources on how to exercise or use an exercise facility, and, most importantly, video clips demonstrating various types of exercises or physical activities that are easier to visualize than explain. The National Center on Health, Physical and Disability (NCHPAD, nchpad.org) has been funded by the Centers for Disease Control and Prevention (CDC) since 1999 to promote physical activity among people with disabilities. This resource center acts as a central hub for public health professionals, health care providers, educators, fitness professionals, and individuals with disabilities to access a variety of disability-related information, including physical activity, nutrition, and lifestyle weight management.

For health professionals interested in physical activity promotion, this 'one-stop' can assist exercise professionals in identifying, developing, and prescribing disability-specific options for physical activity. NCHPAD has actively promoted the importance of physical activity in attaining and maintaining optimal health for people with disabilities through a variety of promotional resources and outreach activities in partnership with advocacy organizations, service providers, and individual consumers.

NCHPAD's information is centralized on its website (www.nchpad.org), which provides a range of resources on physical activity and disability: information on physical activity and disability, networking opportunities, searchable databases, assessment tools, and research. NCHPAD Expert Information Specialists are available at 800-900-8086 or email@nchpad. org to answer questions, about appropriate exercise for individuals with a specific disability, available adaptive equipment, the location of accessible fitness programs and sport team opportunities, and more. NCHPAD serves as a central repository of information, actively collecting information from research, best professional practices, information on public and private recreation and fitness facilities serving people with disabilities, and businesses that provide equipment and services supporting physical activity participation by people with disabilities. Rehabilitation professionals can use NCHPAD resources when designing discharge programs for clients ending rehabilitation.

As has been discussed in the previous sections, participation in physical activity, including all stages of the TE framework is more likely to succeed if programming is tailored to the participant's abilities and interest levels, while simultaneously addressing the barriers that these individuals may encounter for participating in such activities. NCHPAD addresses these problems by making sports and physical activity programs more accessible to people with disabilities. For example, the NCHPAD *14 Week Program to a Healthier You* (www.nchpad.org/14weeks/) gives Internet users access to a free web-based physical activity and nutrition program developed by trained their disability-specialists. Information specialists offer personalized exercises and nutritional advice and prescribe online resources (e.g., instructional videos, newsletters, research articles, and local physical activity options) that are suitable to the varying functional levels and preferences of individuals with disabilities.

Searchable Databases of Local Physical Activity Resources

NCHPAD's online searchable databases can assist professionals in locating appropriate resources for people with disabilities within their community. Databases (located at www.nchpad.org/directories/) are searchable by city and state within the United States. Resources include information on community-based physical activity programs and organizations, adaptive equipment and devices, accessible parks, and opportunities for youth with disabilities.

Assessment Tools

NCHPAD and its related projects include assessment instruments and resources on accessibility for people with disabilities to participate in fitness and recreation programs and facilities. One example is NCHPAD's AIMFREE (*Accessibility Instruments Measuring Fitness and Recreation Environments*) assessment manuals, which are a validated series of questionnaire measures that can be used by people with mobility limitations and professionals (i.e., fitness and recreation center staff, rehabilitation professionals, owners/managers of fitness centers) to assess the accessibility of recreation and fitness facilities, including fitness centers and swimming pools. The Community Health Inclusion Index (CHII) also helps communities identify and assess the inclusivity of physical activity and nutrition resources within their community (http://www.nchpad.org/1273/6358/Commu). Additional resources are available to assist professionals who are developing evidence-based programs, applying for grants, or designing a research study.

Involvement of People with Disabilities in the Transformative Exercise Framework's Lifetime Physical Activities

In this section, types of leisure/recreational and competitive physical activities are provided, along with direct resources that the professional can use in connecting the client with community programs and resources. **Figure 43-8** identifies some activities falling into Lifetime Physical Activity. Lifetime Physical Activity can be categorized on a spectrum from those associated with leisure/recreation to competitive activities. Provided below are resources that can be pursued in further detail on the nchpad.org website (see Chapter 42 for information related to paralympic athletes and sports).

Gardening

Gardening is considered an excellent leisure activity for increasing energy expenditure and for using various muscle groups that are not typically used in general activities. Bending, reaching, twisting, digging, etc., are all aspects of gardening that are helpful for performing functional activities throughout the day. A garden can be adapted for access in a variety of ways, starting with appropriate grades and paving,

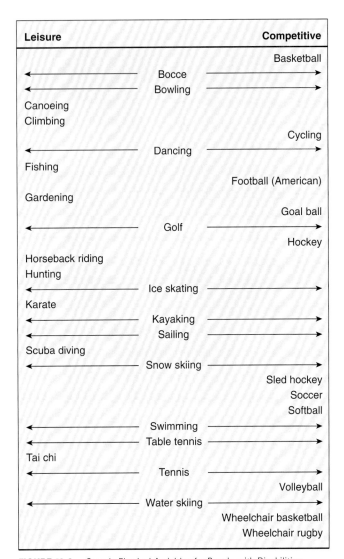

FIGURE 43-8. Sample Physical Activities for People with Disabilities.

then careful selection and placement of planters, vertical gardening techniques such as hanging baskets, and, where possible, larger raised beds. These are all used to position soil and plants safely and comfortably within reach. A barrier-free or enabling garden can be as simple as an easily-reached window box hung from a balcony railing at waist height or an entire home landscape designed to be accessible and maintained by a wheelchair user.

All physical activities described in this section require careful attention to adaptations/modifications, which are often made to prevent injury and provide a rewarding experience for the individual. For example, gardening tools and equipment enable the individual to reduce effort, maximize abilities, and encourage independence while working in the garden. Long-handled tools decrease the need to extend or bend the body to work areas beyond the gardener's reach. Comfort and gripping ability can be improved by modifying handles with soft padding. Knee pads or kneelers can be useful for tasks close to the ground. Such tools help protect muscles and joints from fatigue and injury.

- For additional information, refer to the gardening articles on the NCHPAD website as well as: American Horticultural Therapy Association: http://www.ahta.org, which can help identify a nearby horticultural therapist who is adept at working with people with disabilities. The association also provides referrals to local health care agencies and public gardens with horticultural therapy programs, educational opportunities, and publications.
- Chicago Botanic Garden's Horticultural Therapy Services program: http://www.chicagobotanic.org/therapy provides demonstrations on enabling gardening, an extensive adaptive tool collection, publications, and educational programming.

Bowling

Bowling is a popular recreational and competitive activity that can be enjoyed by individuals with disabilities through minimal equipment adaptations. Adapted equipment is available for individuals of all ability levels to participate and compete in bowling. These include ball ramps, assisting those unable to throw a bowling ball; ball pushers or bowling sticks, which provide the participant with increased control over the force of the throw and the angle at which the ball travels down the lane; and aids for persons with visual impairments.

Organized bowling opportunities for people with disabilities include groups associated with Special Olympics International (SOI), the United States Deaf Bowling Federation (USADBF) the American Wheelchair Bowling Association (AWBA), and the American Blind Bowling Association (ABBA). Refer to the following websites for additional resources:

- SOI: http://www.specialolympics.org
- AWBA: http://www.awba.org
- ABBA: http://www.abba1951.org
- USADBF: http://www.usdeafsports.org

Dance

Dance is a recreational or competitive activity for individuals with varying abilities. It involves creativity and expression while promoting movement, flexibility, and endurance. Dance can decrease stress and increase muscle tone, physical endurance, and self-confidence. It may also increase brain activity and stimulate memory through the use of choreography and help prevent or lessen the effects of secondary conditions such as depression and social isolation.

The basic rules of wheelchair dance include the pairing of a male and female partner, one of which must be a wheelchair user with at least a minimal disability that involves nonambulation (**Fig. 43-9**). Although competitive dance typically involves people with lower extremity disability (e.g., amputation, paralysis, cerebral palsy, and shortened limb (at least 7 cm), dance forms (e.g., hip hop, waltz, jazz, quickstep) can be adapted for other disability groups including people with intellectual/developmental disabilities.

Social or recreational dance opportunities for people with disabilities can be located through accessible dance troupes and

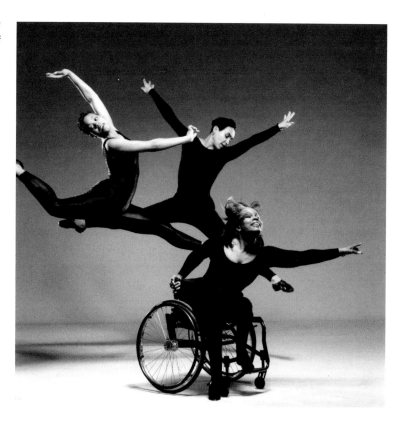

FIGURE 43-9. Diverse-ability dance troupe, "Dance Detour," comprised of artists with and without disabilities. (Courtesy of William Frederking, Dance Detour, Chicago, IL.)

organizations. Refer to the following websites for additional resources:

- Axis Dance Company: http://www.axisdance.org
- Dancing Wheels: http://www.dancingwheels.org
- Gallaudet Dance Company: https://www.gallaudet.edu/department-of-art-communication-and-theatre/gallaudet-dance-company

Swimming

Swimming is an excellent recreational, competitive, and therapeutic activity that can be enjoyed indoors or outdoors. To increase access, stair systems, pool lifts, and all-terrain wheelchairs can be used to reach natural bodies of water. Adaptations could include different prosthetic devices to reduce resistance in the water, or flotation devices to help stabilize individuals.

For competitive swimming, a sport classification ensures that swimmers compete against others with similar functional abilities. Swimmers with disabilities are encouraged to train under the supervision of a qualified coach who understands stroke mechanics and can recommend special stroke adaptations. Swimmers are expected to perform strokes according to the rules of nondisabled swimming, and rulebooks are available from USA Swimming. USA Swimming teams (http://www.usaswimming.org) are an excellent place to find a coach. The most elite swimmers compete in the Paralympic Games every 4 years. Refer to the following websites for additional resources:

- United States of America Deaf Sports Federation (USADSF): http://www.usdeafsports.org/
- Dwarf Athletic Association of America (DAAA): http://www.daaa.org)
- Disabled Sports USA (DSUSA): http://www.disabledsportsusa.org/

- United States Association of Blind Athletes (USABA): http://www.usaba.org/

Sailing

Sailing for people with disabilities can be practiced in both leisure and competitive contexts. It made its debut as a demonstration event in the 1996 Atlanta, GA, Paralympics, and became a full medal sport at the 2000 Sydney Paralympic Games. Using the International Association for Disabled Sailing (IFDS) Functional Classification System, Paralympic sailors with disabilities are classified according to their ability and can compete on a relatively equal basis.

With some adaptations, many standard boats are suitable for competition by people with disabilities. Types of adaptations include accessible and stable seats, transfer benches, and steering assists. Seats and transfer benches can consist of low-tech furniture, such as lawn chairs or coolers, and specifically-designed equipment, such as a translating seat. Steering systems can also be adapted for the user. Bars and handles are secured throughout the boat for sailor stability and safety. For additional resources, please access the IFDS website.[1]

Water Skiing

Water skiing is a recreational and competitive warm-weather activity that can be easily adapted for individuals with disabilities (**Fig. 43-10**). A ski harness assists skiers who have difficulty holding onto the towrope. Outriggers can be attached to the sit ski to help skiers who have difficulty with balance. Skiers with disabilities may also use a board (ski) that is similar

---

[1]Additional sailing resources are available at: http://www.sailing.org/disabled

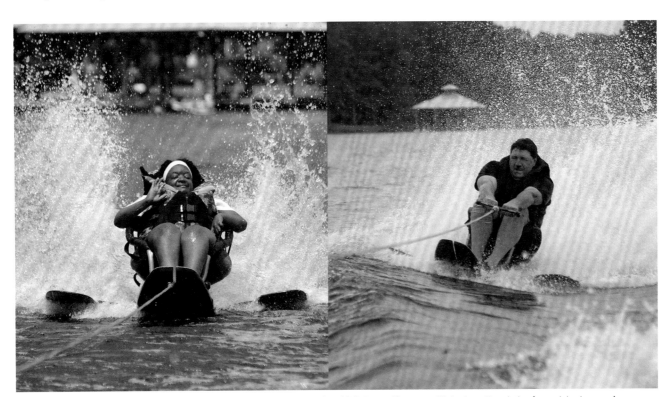

FIGURE 43-10.   A man and woman skiing, with outriggers to assist with balance. (Courtesy of Lakeshore Foundation [www.lakeshore.org] and the National Center on Health, Physical Activity and Disability [www.nchpad.org].)

to a surfboard with a seat (cage) attached to the top. The cage, typically made of padded metal tubes, is deep so that the skier can sit securely.

Competitive water skiing includes three events—slalom, trick skiing, and jumping—and six broad category divisions for the disability water skiing events. The sit skier division includes individuals with spinal cord injuries (paraplegia, tetraplegia), bilateral leg amputations, or other conditions that affect the lower limbs. The vision impairment division includes people with complete and partial vision impairment. The leg division is for skiers who have an amputation above or below the knee, in which skiers can ski with or without their prosthesis. The arm division includes skiers with either an arm amputation or an impairment of one arm, and the arm and leg division for skiers with an impairment of both upper and lower limbs. Refer to the following websites for additional resources:

- USA Water Ski: http://www.usawaterski.org/, a national governing body for water skiing, which works through the Water Skiers with Disabilities Association to serve individuals with disabilities.
- U Can Ski 2: http://www.ucanski2.com, dedicated to providing public awareness and outreach opportunities for individuals with disabilities.

Snow Skiing

Snow skiing is a competitive and recreational winter activity in which individuals use skis to maneuver downhill or cross-country. Skiing can be readily adapted for people with disabilities and offers opportunity for competition or recreating with friends. Various organizations offer skiing events to encourage individuals of all abilities to participate. Information on adaptive equipment, teaching techniques, workshops, and certification clinics can be obtained from the Professional Ski Instructors of America (http://www.psia.org). Competitive alpine events include slalom, giant slalom, super giant slalom, and downhill. Cross-country events include men's 10K and 30K and women's 5K, 10K, and 4 × 10K relay races.

Skiing adaptations for people with disabilities include adapted skis and prosthetics, as well as adequate communication and instruction for the individual with the disability. The monoski consists of a bucket-style seat attached to a single ski, with outriggers (crutches with skis at the end) to maintain stability (**Fig. 43-11**). A biski has a bucket-style seat attached to two skis and outriggers attached to the sled, three track skiing requires one ski and two hand held outriggers, and four track skiing requires two skis and two hand held outriggers. Skiing for persons with visual impairments involves good communication between the visually impaired skier and a sighted guide providing the ski instructions. Disabled Sports USA (http://www.disabledsportsusa.org/sport/down hill-skiing) offers individuals who are interested in participating in adapted sports, including skiing, with a variety of references and nearby locations to get started. Additionally, the U.S. Deaf Ski & Snowboard Association (http://www.ussa.org), affiliated with USADSF (http://www.usdeafsports.org), sponsors various championships, selects U.S. Deaf Ski and Snowboard Teams, and can provide information on skiing with a hearing impairment. Refer to the following websites for additional resources:

- United States Ski and Snowboard Association: http://www.ussa.org
- Ski for Light, Inc.: http://www.sfl.org
- Outdoors For All Foundation: http://www.outdoorsforall.org
- United States Deaf Ski and Snowboard Association: http://www.usdssa.org
- United States Deaf Sports Federation: http://www.usdeafsports.org

Tennis

Tennis is a competitive recreational activity that has become increasingly popular among individuals with disabilities (**Fig. 43-12**). The two versions of tennis within disability sport include ambulatory tennis and wheelchair tennis. Ambulatory tennis is governed by two disability sport organizations, the United States Deaf Sports Federation and Special Olympics. Wheelchair tennis was developed in 1976 and is currently governed by the International Tennis Federation (ITF, http://www.itftennis.com) and Wheelchair

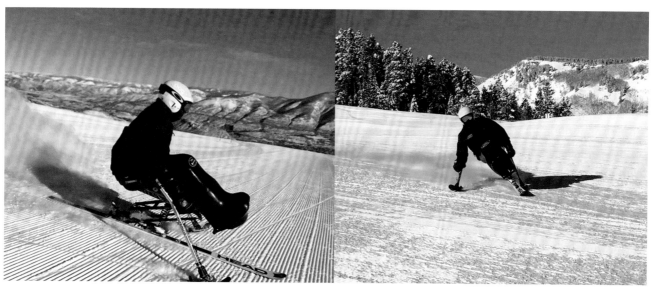

FIGURE 43-11. Use of the monoski with outriggers. (Courtesy of Jimmy Soliz.)

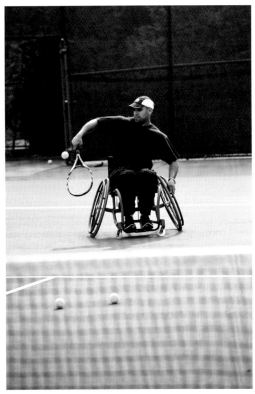

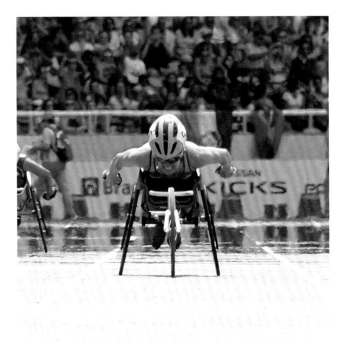

FIGURE 43-13. Kerri Morgan using a racing wheelchair to speed towards the finish line at the Rio 2016 Paralympics. (Courtesy of Peggy Turner.)

FIGURE 43-12. A wheelchair tennis player. (Courtesy of Lakeshore Foundation [www.lakeshore.org] and the National Center on Health, Physical Activity and Disability [www.nchpad.org].)

Tennis Committee, with advisement by the International Wheelchair Tennis Association (IWTA). Wheelchair tennis follows the same rules as able-bodied tennis as endorsed by the ITF, with several key exceptions, the most significant of these being the "two-bounce rule," where the wheelchair tennis player is allowed two bounces before the ball must be returned across court.

- Wheelchair tennis requires only a few pieces of equipment, a tennis racquet, ball, and a wheelchair, and is played on the same courts and surfaces as able-bodied tennis. Players use a sports wheelchair that is lighter than everyday chairs to allow for ample flexibility, and the wheelchair is considered part of the player so that general rules of contact apply. To keep the player stable on the chair, a positioning strap across the waist and/or thighs is used. If necessary, grip devices can allow players who do not have the grip strength to hold a racquet. Refer to the following websites for additional resources: ITF: http://www.itftennis.com
- United States Tennis Association: http://www.usta.com

Cycling

Cycling is a recreational and competitive sport (**Fig. 43-13**), which can involve the upper or lower extremities. It is an official sport of DSUSA, SOI, USABA, and the USADSF. Competitive hand cycling is governed by the United States Handcycling Federation (USHF). Each of these disability sports organizations work cooperatively with USA Cycling to develop cycling opportunities throughout the United States. Events range from 400-m junior races to 40-km road races. A wide variety of adapted cycles exist, including handbikes, arm-driven cycles, dual-recumbent cycles, and tandem cycles. Refer to the following websites for additional resources:

- DSUSA: http://www.disabledsportsusa.org
- United States Deaf Cycling Association: http://www.usdeafcycling.org
- USADSF: http://www.usdeafsports.org
- USA Cycling: http://www.usacycling.org
- USHF: http://www.ushf.org

Basketball

Basketball is a team sport that can be played by individuals with a variety of disabilities. Though numerous variations exist, the two major versions of basketball popular within disability sport are ambulatory and wheelchair basketball. Benefits of playing basketball include the development of aerobic capacity and strength, as well as the opportunity to participate in different roles and positions on a team.

In wheelchair basketball, the wheelchair is considered part of the player, and therefore, general rules of contact apply (**Fig. 43-14**). The National Wheelchair Basketball Association (NWBA) has an extensive list of rules, and rule modifications can also be found for other disability organizations (SOI, DAAA). Basketball variations include bankshot basketball, which relies entirely on shooting skill and no running, dribbling, jumping, or body contact, and twin basketball, which is set up for athletes with cervical-level spinal cord injuries, with players surrounding a free throw circle. Refer to the following websites for additional resources:

- NWBA: http://www.nwba.org
- USADSF: http://www.usdeafsports.org
- International Wheelchair Basketball Federation: http://www.iwbf.org

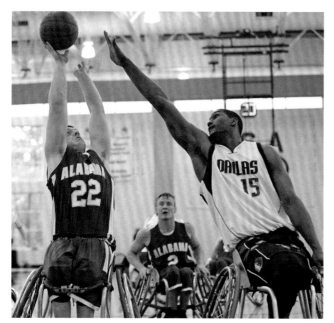

FIGURE 43-14. A competitive wheelchair basketball game. (Courtesy of Lakeshore Foundation [www.lakeshore.org] and the National Center on Health, Physical Activity and Disability [www.nchpad.org].)

Softball

The game of softball can be easily adapted for individuals with disabilities and played within competitive or recreational contexts. Variations to the game include wheelchair softball and beep baseball. Batting and fielding equipment are available for individuals with upper-extremity amputations. Competition is offered by the USADSF, the DAAA (http://www.daaa.org), SOI, the National Wheelchair Softball Association (NWSA), and the National Beep Baseball Association (NBBA). Rule modifications for competitive play and general information are available from the NWSA.

Beep baseball is an adaption for individuals with visual impairment and blindness. The game consists of 4-ft-high padded cylinders with speakers and a sighted pitcher and catcher. Beeping tones are emitted as the pitcher places the ball, and after the ball is hit, the base operator activates a buzzing sound for the batter to identify and run to the base prior to the defense fielding the ball. For more information, contact the NBBA.

For additional softball and Beep baseball resources refer to the following websites:

- USADSF: http://www.usdeafsports.org
- National Wheelchair Softball Association (NWSA): http://www.wheelchairsoftball.org
- National Softball Association: http://www.playnsa.com
- National Beep Baseball Association (NBBA): http://www.nbba.org
- DAAA: http://www.daaa.org

Volleyball

The game of volleyball can be played by people of different ability levels in recreational or competitive settings (**Fig. 43-15**). While standing and sitting volleyball are the two main forms of this activity, adapted versions of volleyball include wallyball and water volleyball.

Adaptations on the game allow for greater participation by people with disabilities. Players with amputations can participate with or without prostheses in standing volleyball (see **Fig. 43-15**). Sitting volleyball is played with six players per

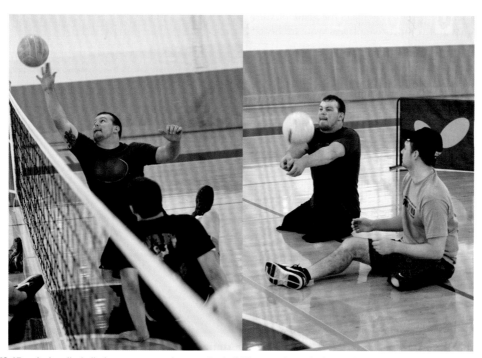

FIGURE 43-15. A sit volleyball player returns and serves the ball. The use of prosthetic or orthopedic devices is not allowed in the sit volleyball competition. (Courtesy of Lakeshore Foundation [www.lakeshore.org] and the National Center on Health, Physical Activity and Disability [www.nchpad.org].)

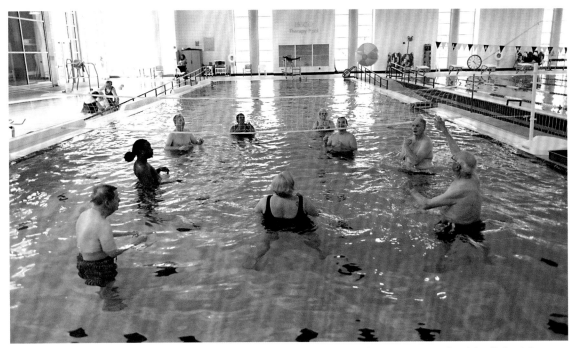

FIGURE 43-16. A group aquatic volleyball class. (Courtesy of Lakeshore Foundation [www.lakeshore.org] and the National Center on Health, Physical Activity and Disability [www.nchpad.org].)

team on a smaller court with a lowered net. This version of volleyball enables double-leg amputees and individuals with spinal cord injuries, polio, and various other lower-extremity disabilities to participate. Volleyball can also be played in the aquatic setting to accommodate individuals who may not have the functional ability to play on land (**Fig. 43-16**). The United States Deaf Volleyball Association (USDVA) and the American Deaf Volleyball Association (ADVA) manage the game of volleyball for recreational and competitive players who are hearing impaired.

- For additional volleyball resources refer to the following websites: World Para Volley: http://www.worldparavolley.org
- DSUSA: http://www.disabledsportsusa.org

Wheelchair Rugby

Developed in 1977, wheelchair rugby is a competitive game in which two teams of four players in wheelchairs attempt to maneuver the game ball over their opponent's goal line while in possession of the ball. The game is played primarily by individuals who have paraplegia or tetraplegia, as well as people with other disabling conditions (e.g., limb loss). There are seven classification divisions that range from 0.5 to 3.5 points based on functional ability. Most rugby chairs have metal guards on the front, sides, and/or back of the chair to prevent opponents from hooking the chair during play. In addition, the wheels are attached at an angle (camber) for greater stability. Trunk, waist, leg, and foot strappings are allowed, depending on individual needs. Gloves and the use of taping at the forearms can protect against skin abrasions.

The game moves at a fast pace with aggressive players that utilize a variety of offensive and defensive techniques (**Fig. 43-17**). A goal is scored when a player carrying a ball

crosses over the opponents' goal line with two wheels. For more detailed information about quad rugby rules, consult the United States Quad Rugby Association website.

- For additional rugby resources refer to the following websites: United States Quad Rugby Association: http://www.usqra.org
- WSUSA: http://www.wsusa.org

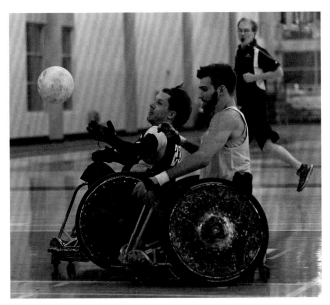

FIGURE 43-17. Wheelchair rugby players illustrating the intensity of competition. (Courtesy of Lakeshore Foundation [www.lakeshore.org] and the National Center on Health, Physical Activity and Disability [www.nchpad.org].)

SUMMARY

The transition from rehabilitation to community-based physical activity is a critical one. There is a small window of opportunity for rehabilitation and health professionals to establish effective community-based Lifetime Physical Activity recommendations that are more likely to be adhered to if the program is tailored to the needs of the individual, readily accessible, and has an element of social engagement.

Most individuals recovering from an injury or health condition will appreciate the benefits of rehabilitation during the subacute period, but once the person returns home and stops performing certain rehabilitative exercises and increases his or her sedentary behavior, these gains are often lost or diminished and the risk of health complications increases. Considering that generic exercise programming is far less likely to result in long-term maintenance of health-promoting behaviors, a tailored approach is necessary for maintaining good adherence. First, the individual's current goals and need should be considered along a continuum, such as the one we describe in this chapter (TE Framework). This will provide a more specific set of recommendations that will more precisely meet the person's health and functional needs and interest level. The *PEP* model combines key factors including a person's motivational level (readiness to change), physical activity profile, health and mobility limitations, and barriers to participation, so that the rehabilitation and health professional can prescribe a program that meets each person's specific needs, interests, and circumstances.

This chapter provides rehabilitation professionals with a variety of resources that they can use to assist their patients in becoming more physically active. The importance of physical activity in preventing secondary health conditions cannot be underestimated. It is one of the most important protective behaviors that can be engaged in to prevent a various of secondary health conditions.

ACKNOWLEDGMENT

This work was supported by the National Institute on Disability, Independent Living, and Rehabilitation Research (NIDILRR); Rehabilitation Engineering Center on Exercise and Recreational Technologies for People with Disabilities, Grant #90REGE0002. NIDILRR is a Center within the Administration for Community Living (ACL), Department of Health and Human Services (HHS). The contents of this chapter do not necessarily represent the policy of NIDILRR, ACL, or HHS and you should not assume endorsement by the Federal Government.

REFERENCES

1. Centers for Disease Control and Prevention (CDC). Physical activity among adults with a disability–United States, 2005. *MMWR Morb Mortal Wkly Rep.* 2007;56:1021–1024.
2. McGuire LC, Strine TW, Okoro CA, et al. Healthy lifestyle behaviors among older U.S. adults with and without disabilities, Behavioral Risk Factor Surveillance System, 2003. *Prev Chron Dis.* 2007;4:A09
3. Carroll DD, Courtney-Long EA, Stevens AC, et al. Vital signs: disability and physical activity—United States, 2009–2012. *MMWR Morb Mortal Wkly Rep.* 2014;63(18):407–413.
4. Rimmer J. Exercise and physical activity in persons aging with a physical disability. *Phys Med Rehabil Clin N Am.* 2005;16(1):41–56.
5. Martin Ginis K, Hicks A. Considerations for the development of a physical activity guide for Canadians with physical disabilities. *Appl Physiol Nutr Metab.* 2007;32:S135–S147.
6. Corr S, Bayer A. Poor functional status of stroke patients after hospital discharge: scope for intervention. *Br J Occup Ther.* 1992;55:383–385.
7. Rimmer J, Chen M-D, McCubbin JA, et al. Exercise intervention research on persons with disabilities. What we know and where we need to go. *Am J Phys Med Rehabil.* 2010;89:249–263.
8. Rimmer JH, Chen MD, Hsieh K. A conceptual model for identifying, preventing, and managing secondary conditions in people with disabilities. *Phys Ther.* 2011;91(12):1728–1739.
9. Lord E, Patterson I. The benefits of physically active leisure for people with disabilities: an Australian perspective. *Ann Leis Res.* 2008;11(1–2):123–144.
10. Crawford A, Hollingsworth HH, Morgan K, et al. People with mobility impairments: physical activity and quality of participation. *Disabil Health J.* 2008;1:7–13.
11. Tasiemski T, Kennedy P, Gardner B, et al. The association of sports and physical recreation with life satisfaction in a community sample of people with spinal cord injuries. *NeuroRehabilitation.* 2005;20:253–265.
12. Martin Ginis KA, Ma JK, Latimer-Cheung AE, et al. A systematic review of review articles addressing factors related to physical activity participation among children and adults with physical disabilities. *Health Psychol Rev.* 2016;10(4):478–494.
13. Rimmer JH, Riley B, Wang E, et al. Physical activity participation among persons with disabilities: barriers and facilitators. *Am J Prev Med.* 2004;26(5):419–425.
14. Lai B, Young HJ, Bickel CS, et al. Current trends in exercise intervention research, technology, and behavioral change strategies for people with disabilities: a scoping review. *Am J Phys Med Rehabil.* 2017;96(10):748–761.
15. Physical Activity Guidelines Advisory Committee. *Physical Activity Guidelines Advisory Committee Report.* Washington, DC: U.S. Department of Health and Human Services; 2008. Available from: https://health.gov/paguidelines/report/pdf/CommitteeReport.pdf
16. van den Berg-Emons RJ, Bussmann JB, Haisma JA, et al. A prospective study on physical activity levels after spinal cord injury during inpatient rehabilitation and the year after discharge. *Arch Phys Med Rehabil.* 2008;89(11):2094–2101.
17. Forkan R, Pumper B, Smyth N, et al. Exercise adherence following physical therapy intervention in older adults with impaired balance. *Phys Ther.* 2006;86(3):401–410.
18. Askim T, Bernhardt J, Churilov L, et al. Changes in physical activity and related functional and disability levels in the first six months after stroke: a longitudinal follow-up study. *J Rehabil Med.* 2013;45(5):423–428.
19. Rimmer J, Lai B. Framing new pathways in transformative exercise for individuals with existing and newly acquired disability. *Disabil Rehabil.* 2015;39(2):173–180.
20. Sporner ML, Grindle GG, Kelleher A, et al. Quantification of activity during wheelchair basketball and rugby at the National Veterans Wheelchair Games: a pilot study. *Prosthet Orthot Int.* 2009;33(3):210–217.
21. Sonenblum SE, Sprigle S, Lopez RA. Manual wheelchair use: bouts of mobility in everyday life. *Rehabil Res Pract.* 2012;2012:753165.
22. Janssen TW, Dallmeijer AJ, van der Woude LH, et al. Normative values and determinants of physical capacity in individuals with spinal cord injury. *J Rehabil Res Dev.* 2002;39:29–39.
23. Hunter GR, McCarthy JP, Bamman MM. Effects of resistance training on older adults. *Sports Med.* 2004;34(5):329–348.
24. Rimmer JH, Schiller W, Chen MD. Effects of disability-associated low energy expenditure deconditioning syndrome. *Exerc Sport Sci Rev.* 2012;40(1):22–29.
25. Michie S, Richardson M, Johnston M, et al. The behavior change technique taxonomy (v1) of 93 hierarchically clustered techniques: building an international consensus for the reporting of behavior change interventions. *Ann Behav Med.* 2013;46(1):81–95.
26. Ma JK, Ginis KA. A meta-analysis of physical activity interventions in people with physical disabilities: Content, characteristics, and effects on behaviour. *Psychol Sport Exerc.* 2018;37:262–273.
27. Kroll T, Kratz A, Kehn M, et al. Perceived exercise self-efficacy as a predictor of exercise behavior in individuals aging with spinal cord injury. *Am J Phys Med Rehabil.* 2012;91(8):640–651.
28. Glanz K, Rimer BK, Viswanath K. *Health Behavior and Health Education Theory, Research, and Practice.* San Francisco, CA: Jossey-Bass; 2015.
29. Vissers M, Van den Berg-Emons R, Sluis T, et al. Barriers to and facilitators of everyday physical activity in persons with a spinal cord injury after discharge from the rehabilitation centre. *J Rehabil Med.* 2008;40(6):461–467.
30. Levins SM, Redenbach DM, Dyck I. Individual and societal influences on participation in physical activity following spinal cord injury: a qualitative study. *Phys Ther.* 2004;84(6):496–509.
31. Morris J, Oliver T, Kroll T, et al. The importance of psychological and social factors in influencing the uptake and maintenance of physical activity after stroke: a structured review of the empirical literature. *Stroke Res Treat.* 2012;2012:1–20.
32. Institute of Medicine. *Disability in America: Toward a National Agenda for Prevention.* Washington, DC: The National Academies Press; 1991. Available from: https://doi.org/10.17226/1579
33. United States Department of Health and Human Services. *2018 Physical Activity Guidelines for Americans.* Washington, DC; 2018. Available from: https://health.gov/paguidelines/second-edition/report/pdf/PAG_Advisory_Committee_Report.pdf
34. Hall J, Grant J, Blake D, et al. Cardiorespiratory responses to aquatic treadmill walking in patients with rheumatoid arthritis. *Physiother Res Int.* 2004;9:59–73.
35. Jung T, Ozaki Y, Lai B, et al. Comparison of energy expenditure between aquatic and overground treadmill walking in people post-stroke. *Physiother Res Int.* 2014;19:55–64.

36. Pelletier CA, Latimer-Cheung AE, Warburton DE, et al. Direct referral and physical activity counselling upon discharge from spinal cord injury rehabilitation. *Spinal Cord*. 2014;52(5):392–395.

37. Bulger DW, Smith AB. Message tailoring: an essential component for disease management. *Dis Manag Health Outcomes*. 1999;5:127–134.

38. Morris JH, MacGillivray S, Mcfarlane S. Interventions to promote long-term participation in physical activity after stroke: a systematic review of the literature. *Arch Phys Med Rehabil*. 2014;95(5):956–967.

39. Rimmer JH, Rowland JL. Health promotion for people with disabilities: implications for empowering the person and promoting disability-friendly environments. *Am J Life Med*. 2008;2(22):409–420.

40. Rimmer JH. Building inclusive physical activity communities for people with vision loss. *J Vis Impair Blind*. 2006;100(suppl):863–865.

41. Prochaska JO, Redding CA, Evers KE. The transtheoretical model and stages of change. In: Glanz K, Lewis FM, Rimer BK, eds. *Health Behavior and Health Education*. 2nd ed. San Francisco, CA: Jossey-Bass; 1997.

42. Prochaska JO, DiClemente CC, Norcross JC. In search of how people change: applications to addictive behaviors. *Am Psychol*. 1992;47(9):1102–1114.

43. Wilmore JH, Costill DL. *Physiology of Sport and Exercise*. Champaign, IL: Human Kinetics; 1994.

44. U.S. Department of Health and Human Services. *Physical Activity and Health: A Report of the Surgeon General*. Atlanta, GA: U.S. Department of Health and Human Services, Centers for Disease Control and Prevention (CDC), National Center for Chronic Disease Prevention and Health Promotion; 1996.

45. Durstine JL, Moore GE. *ACSM's Exercise Management for Persons with Chronic Diseases and Disabilities*. 2nd ed. Illinois: Human Kinetics; 2003.

CHAPTER 44

Sonya Rissmiller
Lauren A. Chambers
Katie Weatherhogg

Performing Arts Medicine

The body says what words cannot.
Martha Graham, Dancer and Choreographer, 1894–1991

Performing arts medicine is a branch of physical medicine and rehabilitation devoted to the care of musicians and dancers. A key concept of performing arts medicine is the ability to prevent, recognize, treat, and rehabilitate musculoskeletal injuries as related to each student, amateur, and professional performing artist. This chapter discusses in further detail common injuries found in musicians and dancers, including injury diagnosis, management, and rehabilitation (see also Chapters 29, 30, and 41). The injuries primarily focus on the upper limbs for musicians and the lower limbs for dancers. Practitioners of performing arts medicine should have a solid understanding of musculoskeletal medicine and an appreciation for the physical effort and specific movement required to perform in each of the various arts. Performing artists are performing athletes.

DANCE MEDICINE

Most current dance-related medical literature focuses on ballet (1–4). Research must therefore be extrapolated to treat other types of dance. The majority of this chapter focuses on the injuries associated with ballet, understanding that the performing arts practitioner treats all types of dance including modern, jazz, tap, folk, ethnic, ballroom, and hip hop, all of which can lead to medical problems (5,6). Each style places demands on the body and may vary with respect to footwear, dance surfaces, training, and alignment.

Dance Training

Ballet training typically begins for female dancers by 5 or 6 years of age. Young dancers often begin training daily for 2 to 6 hours at a time with annual or semiannual performances by age 11 or 12. In order to pursue ballet professionally, preteen and teenage students with high-level ability and skills attend intensive summer programs, and those with the greatest ability and potential move to preprofessional ballet schools for year-round training. These exceptional students may participate in work study programs with school in the morning, blended with class and rehearsals in the afternoon and evening. Some dancers obtain their general education degree early to join professional companies, while others continue to dance through college and join companies later. A large component of a dancer's early career involves auditions. These tryouts can be critical to obtaining roles in performances and in the development of a professional career. Performing arts physicians need to acknowledge the high importance of auditions and should

inquire about upcoming dates. This knowledge may aid in the decision to tolerate a higher risk of reinjury than under normal circumstances.

Terminology and Positions

Knowledge about the technical requirements for dance is important. Performing arts medicine practitioners excel at understanding the biomechanical demands placed on dancers and the maladaptations many dancers use to compensate for inadequate anatomy, conditioning, or biomechanics. Dancers should be evaluated for onset of symptoms and triggers, in addition to demonstrating the movements or positions that reproduce the symptoms (7). Common dance terms are

Plié—heel remains on the floor with the knee in flexion **Fig. 44-1**
Grand plié—heels lift off the floor with deep knee flexion
Pointe—dancing on the tips of the toes, ankle in maximal plantar flexion (**Fig. 44-2**)
Demipointe—weight bearing on the metatarsal joints, ankle plantar flexion, and metatarsal joint extension (**Fig. 44-3**)
Barre work—dance classes are divided into three stages: *barre*, center, and movement from the corners across the floor. *Barre* work involves holding on to a bar during warm-up exercises and conditioning.
Center floor work—the second stage of a dance class performed in the middle of the studio involves balancing, jumps, and short sequences of movement.

Causes of Injury and Risk Factors

Extrinsic

There are many common extrinsic and intrinsic causes of injury and risk factors in dance. One extrinsic factor is the type of dance floor. The presence of adequate shock absorption and the degree of surface friction can lead to injuries of the knee, foot, and ankle if there is too much surface resistance. Likewise, a floor that is too firm leads to fatigue and injuries such as tendonitis of the leg and foot (8).

Footwear can also influence injuries. Most ballet dancers wear either slippers, composed of only fabric or leather and no structural support, or *pointe shoes*, which are made of a solid toe box, metal or wood shank, and fabric. Theoretically, *pointe shoes* act as an additional stabilizer of the foot as demonstrated by cadaveric studies (9). However, these shoes are not designed to provide adequate stability or shock absorption and have changed very little since the 1600s (4,8). Furthermore, principal dancers may wear out one to three pairs of pointe shoes per performance because if the shoe becomes too soft, it can often lead to injury, such as tendonitis and stress fractures (9).

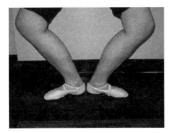

FIGURE 44-1. *Plié*—ankle dorsiflexion and knee flexion, performed in any of the basic positions.

Intrinsic

Intrinsic causes of injury or risk factors include, but are not limited to, malalignment of the lower limbs, muscle imbalance, and inappropriate training (7,8,10,11). Proper alignment in ballet is based on turnout (the maximal amount of external rotation at the hips), which will ideally enable a dancer to stand with the feet placed at 180 degrees in *first position*. Although dancers may appear to be able to achieve 160 to 190 degrees of turnout at the feet, they may not have the corresponding degree of external rotation at the hip (12,13). When the lower extremity is properly aligned in *first position* (14,15), the knee flexes directly over the foot. Many students will not be able to attain this ideal position and will compensate by forcing their turnout. "Rolling in" forces the feet into a position with a valgus heel and forefoot pronation (**Fig. 44-4**), leading to subsequent collapse of the medial arch and thereby increasing the torque on the ankle and knee (**Fig. 44-5**) (7,9,11). Young dancers, both female and male, will sometimes increase their lumbar lordosis in order to tip the pelvis anteriorly and thus obtain increased hip rotation. In addition to potentially leading to low back pain, other complaints may arise from the increased torque placed on the lower limb (7,11).

Muscle imbalance is often due to inadequate strength or altered flexibility. Ballet emphasizes hip flexion, external rotation, and abduction, which can lead to weakening of the antagonist muscles (8). Deficits in strength and endurance at the hip may lead to injuries of the foot, ankle, and knee (16–18). Focusing the treatment on the injured joint without addressing any underlying hip muscle imbalances may frustrate both dancers and physicians alike as pain and dysfunction are likely to recur. By nature, dancing *en pointe* involves loading the ankle joint in maximal plantar flexion with accompanying distal pressure placed on the first and second toes. Significant ankle flexibility and intrinsic foot strength are required to maintain the position (9). Elite and professional dancers usually display appropriate alignment as malalignment problems

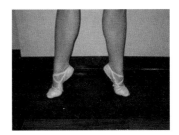

FIGURE 44-3. Demipointe—dancing on the metatarsals in either slippers or pointe shoes.

typically extinguish careers prior to this level. Generally speaking, at the professional level, limb injuries more often result from overuse rather than from issues of alignment. In young dancers, immature skeletal formation may contribute to musculoskeletal injury. Similarly, growth spurts may further lead to muscle imbalances, where a gain of 1 to 3 in. in growth might overwhelm the muscular strength required to move and change positions. As a result, young dancers can develop muscle tightness relative to bone length and/or inadequate strength, particularly in the hip rotators (19).

The effects of inappropriate training are often related to factors such as excessive duration and intensity (7,10). As in other aesthetic sports that place a large degree of importance on the appearance of the performer such as diving and figure skating, dancers often have delayed menarche due to caloric restriction coupled with large amounts of exercise (20). As dancers are often subjectively judged on their appearance, eating disorders are common in preprofessional dance schools with some reports estimating up to 30% of the students being affected (21–23). Such behavior can often place dancers at increased risk of developing the "female athlete triad": disordered eating, amenorrhea, and osteoporosis (7,10).

Incidence of Dance Injuries

In 2005, a United Kingdom (UK) national survey reported that 80% of 1,056 professional dancers sustained at least one injury per year (24). Further UK national survey studies demonstrated that 36% of retired professional dancers stopped due to musculoskeletal injury by age 29; the most common causes were hip and back (25). In similar studies, 66% to 90% of injuries occurred in the lower extremity and two thirds were classified as overuse injuries (26,27). A systematic review of the literature from 1984 to 2014 of 1,365 amateur and 900 professional dancers found the incidence of injury among amateur dancers at 1.09 injuries per 1,000 dance hours with 75% due to overuse and 1.46 injuries per 1,000 dance hours in female

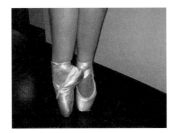

FIGURE 44-2. *Sur les pointes*, dancing on the tips of the toes in pointe shoes.

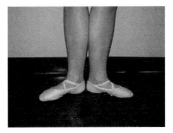

FIGURE 44-4. "Rolling in" of the feet, demonstrating collapse of the medial arch.

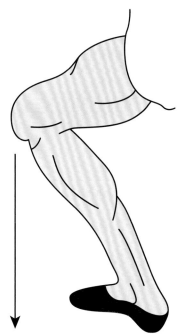

FIGURE 44-5. "Rolling in" at the knee, with tracking medial to the foot. This often occurs with insufficient hip external rotation strength and forcing of the physiologic barrier.

professional dancers with 64% due to overuse; rates were slightly lower in males (27). Of all the disciplines in dance, classical ballet necessitates the longest training, places the most physical demands on the musculoskeletal system, and studies indicate that 67% of all dance injuries occur from the practice of classical ballet (4).

Common Dance Injuries

Spine Injuries

Dancers routinely suffer spine injuries similar to many other athletes, including but not limited to fractures of the pars interarticularis and sacroiliac dysfunction. Back injuries are often associated with high preseason training, a history of low back pain, low body weight, scoliosis, young age, and hypermobile hip external rotation (28) (see also Chapter 27). Delay in the treatment of pars fractures may progress to fibrous unions that will not calcify and potentially result in spondylolisthesis. If underlying biomechanical issues are corrected within an appropriate time frame, dancers may continue dancing with spondylolisthesis. However, dancers should restrict activity with relative rest in the event of a new pars fracture and may require either an antilordotic-modified Boston brace or a nonspecific conventional lumbar corset (29).

Sacroiliac pain occurs frequently and is often difficult to resolve (7,30). Jumping and leg extension on the affected side may incite pain in dancers experiencing sacroiliac dysfunction. Special physical examination maneuvers such as sacroiliac joint compression and Gillet's test are useful in diagnosis. Treatment of sacroiliac dysfunction may include mobilization of the joint and pelvic stabilization exercises.

Repetitive microtrauma from hyperextension may result in damage to posterior elements, such as the pars interarticularis, facets, pedicles, and spinous processes (31). Poor technique

may cause painful injuries to the periosteum during hyperextension. Although this injury is painful, it requires no special treatment other than correction of technique unless it proceeds to pars fracture.

Hip Injuries

"Snapping hip" accounts for 50% of hip problems in dancers, occurring either medially or laterally with or without pain (4). When it occurs laterally, the iliotibial band or tensor fascia lata snaps anteriorly and posteriorly over the greater trochanter when landing from a jump in poor turnout and with excessive anterior pelvic tilt (7) or as the thigh moves between the anterior and posterior positions. "Snapping hip" may also occur medially and is sometimes referred to as "iliopsoas syndrome" (32). This phenomenon occurs when a hypertrophied iliopsoas crosses the femoral neck when bringing the hip into extension during a semicircular motion known as *rond de jambe* (7) (**Fig. 44-6**). A dancer with this injury will experience intense anterior groin pain during this arcing movement, particularly as the iliopsoas stretches over the femoral head from medial to lateral; it is also typically more painful while in the air than with the foot on the floor (33) (📶 **eFig. 44-1**). "Snapping hip" rarely causes significant disability and responds well to focused stretching, hip strengthening (especially the external rotators, adductors, and internal rotators), pelvic mobilization, and modification of technique with a concentration on conservative care rather than surgery or corticosteroid injection (11,33,34). Other hip injuries such as acetabular dysplasias, femoral-acetabular impingement associated with hyperlaxity, labral tears, osteoarthritis, stress fractures of the femoral neck, hip avulsion injuries, and femoral neuropraxia have been described in the medical literature as well (7,35).

Knee Injuries

Knee problems are often attributed to insufficient hip strength in external rotation or forcing greater foot turnout than physiologically possible (as noted previously). Hip weakness

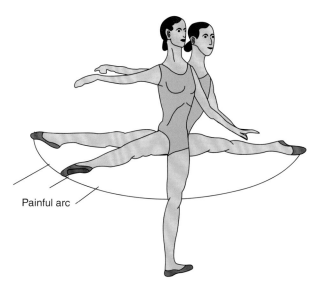

Painful arc

Rond de jambe en l'air

FIGURE 44-6. Rond de jambe en l'air. For a dancer with iliopsoas syndrome, circling the leg with the foot in the air is more painful than *rond de jambe, with* the foot on the floor.

or alignment problems are the usual causes of knee pain. The typical sports-related knee injuries also occur in dancers, including anterior and medial collateral ligament sprains, patellar subluxation, and patellofemoral syndrome (36,37). Tears and injuries often result from slips, twisting falls, and improper landings from jumps. Diagnosis and rehabilitation of such injuries follow standard sports medicine guidelines.

Acute Ankle Injuries

Ankle sprains are the most common acute dance-related injury (7). These sprains commonly occur when a dancer loses balance while landing from a jump while the foot is in plantar flexion. They can also occur from rolling over the lateral aspect of the foot while on *demipointe* (9). Interestingly, in full *pointe*, the ankle is relatively stable as the posterior lip of the tibia locks on the calcaneous, and thus, the subtalar joint locks in varus. It should be noted, however, that slight dorsiflexion relaxes the chain and may predispose the ankle to injury (10). As noted with other sports, the anterior talofibular ligament is the weakest ankle ligament and most susceptible to injury (9,10). The Ottawa ankle rules recommend ankle radiographs if a patient is unable to walk three steps or if there is tenderness over either malleoli (10). Ultrasound is helpful for evaluating soft tissues, tendons, and ligaments in the foot and ankle and can also be used therapeutically to guide interventions and for dynamic assessment (38). Specific rehabilitation of acute ankle injuries includes pool therapy, plantar flexion exercises, proprioceptive retraining, and peroneal strengthening with an emphasis on resuming full mobility of the talar, subtalar, and transverse tarsal joints (7,9).

Overuse Ankle Injuries

Anterior Ankle Impingement

In anterior ankle impingement, the anterior distal tibia and the talus pinch the bony or soft tissue during ankle dorsiflexion, particularly during *grand plié* (7) (**Fig. 44-7**). The medical history is often notable for chronic anterior or anterolateral ankle pain on jump landings or a limited *demi-plié* (9). Other mechanisms and the source of pathology of ankle impingements are found in **Table 44-1**.

Physical examination might include an effusion, audible click, palpable tenderness, and limited dorsiflexion when compared to the contralateral side. Pain is also present with passive

TABLE 44-1	Anterior Ankle Impingement Etiology	
Site	**Pathologic Change**	**Mechanism**
Anterior talofibular ligament	Hypertrophic scar	Inversion ankle sprains
Soft tissue	Synovitis, tears	Plantar flexion
Anterior tibia	Osteophytes, traction spurs	Repetitive forced dorsiflexion
Distal tibia	Avulsion fracture	Rapid plantar flexion
Talar neck	Loose bodies	Rapid plantar flexion
Capsule	Calcium deposits	Forced plantar flexion

Modified from Valencia KM. Dance-related injury. *Phys Med Rehabil Clin N Am.* 2006;17(3):708. Copyright © 2006 Elsevier. With permission.

dorsiflexion when the knee is bent (9). This is primarily a clinical diagnosis. Treatment includes restricting *pointe* and center floor work, encouraging exercises at the *barre*, nonsteroidal anti-inflammatory drugs (NSAIDs), local injections, modalities, and in refractory cases, arthroscopic surgery (7). Return to a *full plié* position may take 3 to 4 months (9).

Posterior Ankle Impingement

Posterior ankle impingement is caused by the posterior tibia and calcaneous compressing the posterior talus and surrounding structures. This impingement may frequently be caused by a symptomatic os trigonum (7,9). The os trigonum is an accessory ossicle posterior to the talus, which is often asymptomatic (11) (📶 **eFig. 44-2**). When a dancer positions herself in extreme plantar flexion, the os trigonum is pinched between the tibia and calcaneous. Patients will present with posterior ankle pain, worsened with plantar flexion (11), and the pain and inflammation may limit the dancer's ability to perform *pointe*, as well as the movement from flat foot to *demipointe*. Os trigonum syndrome will also cause pain with both active and passive plantar flexion (7). This pain is usually posterolateral, behind the peroneal tendons and often with associated ankle stiffness (9). Diagnosis is again primarily clinical; however, a standard lateral view ankle x-ray can demonstrate the presence of an os trigonum (7). Magnetic resonance imaging (MRI) may also show bony edema of the distal tibia and inflammatory changes surrounding soft tissue (7). Treatment of posterior impingement syndrome includes dance training modifications including limiting *pointe work*, NSAIDs, physical therapy modalities, and exercises, with the refractory case leading to surgical excision (7). Changing *pointe* shoe wear to a half or three-quarter shank to more easily facilitate *pointe work* may also provide some relief (9).

Achilles Tendinosis

Achilles tendinosis is classically seen in *pointe* overuse, excessive pronation and "forced turnout" during *plié*, or the wearing of too tight *pointe shoe* ribbons (10,11). Pain is localized to the zone of avascularity of the distal tendon, approximately 2 to 8 cm proximal to the insertion, and is often aggravated during landing from jumps (7). Physical exam is often notable for palpable tendon nodules, swelling, and crepitus (10). MRI and ultrasound are useful tools for demonstrating tendon degeneration. Treatment includes gastrocnemius stretching, concentric to eccentric muscle strengthening, with approximately 25% of cases proceeding to surgical intervention to excise and debride

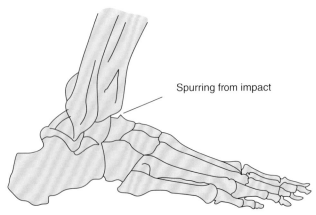

FIGURE 44-7. Anterior ankle impingement during *plié* due to spurring.

Spurring from impact

the focal area of tendon degeneration (10). Stretch boxes strategically placed in the studio and theatre have been shown to provide some degree of prevention for some dance companies (9).

Acute Foot Injuries

Subluxation

Cuboid subluxation may result in acute or chronic lateral midfoot pain (7). It is often associated with lateral ankle sprain injury (10) or is sustained during landing from a jump onto *demipointe* with the lower limb in external rotation (4). The medial border of the cuboid subluxes inferiorly, with dorsal displacement of the fourth metatarsal base, and plantar displacement of the metatarsal head (9,10). Physical exam is notable for tenderness over the cuboid bone, decreased mobility in passive supination/pronation, and a step-off of the fourth metatarsal head (10). A dancer may walk on the lateral edge of the injured foot as extreme supination is the most rigid position. Early diagnosis and treatment are key to preventing progress toward chronic injury. The cuboid should be immediately realigned using manipulation techniques (9).

Subtalar subluxation is caused by ankle hyperflexion, external rotation, and slight inversion, often occurs when performing *grand plié en pointe*, or landing from a jump on *demipointe* (39). Dancers may experience a sudden sharp talonavicular pain and a sensation of forward displacement of the foot, interfering with ambulation (7,39). Physical exam shows tenderness to palpation of the talonavicular ligament, anterior talofibular ligament, anterior tibiotalar ligament, posterior joint, and hypomobility of the subtalar joint (39). Imaging has not shown to be useful due to anatomic variation (4). Treatment includes manual reduction, taping, and relative rest for 6 weeks. Dancing may be started in a pool after the initial 2 weeks. Proprioceptive training may begin after 3 to 4 weeks followed by continued close observation (7,39).

Metatarsal Fractures

Metatarsal fractures generally occur at the fifth metatarsal bone. These fractures are usually caused by missed landings and rolling over the lateral border of the foot on *demipointe* (9). Dancers present with tenderness, swelling, and ecchymoses over the fifth metatarsal bone and lateral foot pain particularly with weight bearing (9,10). The most common proximal fifth metatarsal fracture is an avulsion fracture, which is commonly caused by an inversion injury (10). A "Jones fracture" involves the metaphyseal-diaphyseal junction and often leads to nonunion due to the poor blood supply. "Dancer's fractures" are oblique or spiral fractures of the mid-distal fifth metatarsal associated with twisting and inversion (10). Surgical intervention is needed for high-level dancers to avoid prolonged immobilization for Jones fractures and diaphyseal fractures (9,10). Avulsion fractures and Dancer's fractures can typically be treated conservatively and symptomatically with immobilization with a removable cast boot (9,10). Once fractures have healed adequately, rehabilitation goals return to strengthening the intrinsic foot musculature, retraining proprioception, initiating aquatic therapy, and gently returning to dance.

Lisfranc's Joint Dysfunction

Midfoot sprains most commonly involve injury to Lisfranc's joint, where the second metatarsal articulates with the intermediate cuneiform. The Lisfranc's joint is crucial to midfoot stability and the longitudinal and midfoot arches of the foot (9,10). This type of injury is typically caused by a loss of balance on *pointe*, or spinning and landing jumps, which subsequently result in an inability to roll through *demipointe* or full *pointe* (9,10). Physical examination is significant for midfoot swelling, ecchymosis, and tenderness to palpation and pain with both passive pronation and supination (9,10). Imaging may reveal avulsion fragments or diastasis between the first and second metatarsal bases (9). Treatment depends on the severity of the injury, from non–weight-bearing cast immobilization to operative fixation if diastasis is present (10). However, a simple strain without evidence of instability should be treated nonsurgically (9).

Second metatarsal stress fractures at Lisfranc's joint are almost exclusive to women practicing *pointe work* (32). Ballerinas with long second toes are particularly vulnerable to Lisfranc's fracture (40), as the load through the foot is carried mostly on the first two toes with partial weight bearing of the third toe. Studies implicate that the fully plantar flexed or hyperflexed forefoot places the highest risk of injury due to the anatomy of the Lisfranc's joint (33), and increased load on a long second toe can thus lead to fracture at the base of the second metatarsal head or middle cuneiform bone (41–43).

Overuse Foot Injuries

Metatarsal Stress Fractures

Most stress fractures in dancers occur in the metatarsal bones (9). Multiple risk factors have been identified in placing dancers at risk for stress fracture including, but not limited to, long duration of practice hours per day, female athlete triad, and a pronated "overpointed" foot with excessive strain on the capsule and ligaments on the dorsum of the foot (9,44). Early diagnosis improves outcomes and may avoid delayed return to dance (7,44). Dancers typically present with poorly localized midfoot pain initially after dance but progressing to pain during activity and at night. Bone scans and MRI will reveal bone marrow edema and microfractures. Diaphyseal stress fractures are often seen with repetitive adduction, movements that involve cutting and pivoting. These fractures have poor healing potential due to their poor blood supply in the metaphyseal-diaphyseal region (9,10). Treatment of stress fractures involves immobilization or use of a removable cast boot with custom molded footplate for 6 to 12 weeks and consideration of external shock wave therapy (44). The contralateral shoe may need to be modified, as a cast boot or footplate may cause a leg length discrepancy leading to sacroiliac dysfunction, and adjusting the height of the opposite shoe may help prevent imbalance and pain. Weight bearing is progressed as tolerated and aquatic therapy or Pilates starting as soon as possible is recommended for approximately 6 weeks and until the fracture has healed. A padding system or toe cap for the second metatarsal and properly fitted *pointe* shoes may subsequently support the Lisfranc region, enabling a more balanced weight distribution (7).

Flexor Hallucis Longus Tendon Dysfunction

Flexor hallucis longus (FHL) tendon dysfunction is also known as "dancer's tendonitis" (45). This condition often occurs with symptomatic os trigonum. The FHL is used as an accessory push-off muscle for *plié*, transitioning from flat foot to *demipointe*, and during jumps (33). These repetitive movements from full plantar flexion to dorsiflexion cause the FHL to become compressed within the fibro-osseous tunnel postero-medial to the talus with subsequent inflammation (9). Dancers present with pain when jumping and dancing on *pointe* and may have crepitus and triggering, or locking of the big toe in a flexed position much like a trigger finger of the flexor tendons of the hand (10). Physical examination may further reveal tenderness to palpation along the course of the tendon with painful passive extension of the big toe (7). Conservative treatment includes limiting *pointe work* and jumps, correcting malalignments related to forced turnout, NSAIDs, physical therapy, and aquatic *barre* exercises (4,7,9).

Sesamoid Disorders

Sesamoid injuries occur in dancers due to the increased load on the sesamoid bones when rolling through *demipointe*, forcing turnout, out-toeing gait, and during abrupt landings (7). Sesamoids are located both in the tendon of the flexor hallucis brevis (FHB) and on the plantar surface of the proximal first metatarsal-phalangeal joint (MTP) and increase the mechanical advantage of the FHB. Dancers typically present with pain on the plantar aspect of the first MTP joint (10). Physical examination demonstrates tenderness to palpation of the sesamoid, pain with resisted MTP flexion, and restricted passive dorsiflexion (10). Injecting a small amount of local anesthetic can confirm the diagnosis (9). MRI can help differentiate bipartite sesamoids with smooth edges versus acute sesamoid fractures (9). Treatment is to correct alignment problems including avoiding excessive turnout, restricting *demipointe*, using sesamoid pads, wearing a stiff-soled shoe outside of class, physical therapy for mobilization of the joint, restoration of range of motion, balance/proprioceptive retraining and intrinsic foot strengthening, and occasionally corticosteroid injections (9,10).

Hallux Rigidus

Hallux rigidus presents as arthritic changes of the first MTP joint. Dancers experience pain at the first MTP joint with dorsiflexion, particularly on *demipointe*, which causes the dancer to roll onto the lateral metatarsals. Physical examination demonstrates tenderness to palpation of the first MTP and decreased passive dorsiflexion. Imaging may reveal osteophytes, joint space narrowing, or subchondral sclerosis (9,10). Early treatment is usually conservative, including avoidance of *demipointe* and strengthening of the intrinsic foot muscles (9). While surgery may be an option, it may not lead to full restoration of movement, and some of these dancers may need to retire (9).

Hallux Valgus

Hallux valgus is a painful bunion on the medial border first MTP and is commonly exacerbated with *pointe work*. Dancing in *pointe shoes* does not cause bunion deformities (9); however, the condition can be exacerbated by poor technique, inadequate shoe inserts, flat first MTP surface, and long second toe (4). Treatment includes orthotics for regular walking shoes, NSAIDs, modalities, and foot strengthening of FHL, adductor hallucis, and flexor digitorum longus with the use of exercise bands to simulate relevé, pushing the foot from demipointe to pointe, and progressing to weight-bearing exercises (7), with surgery reserved for retiring professionals as intervention may lead to loss of range of motion (9).

Dance-Specific Rehabilitation

Prevention remains the key in dance rehabilitation. Dance screening clinics may provide screening for adequacy of training, physical conditioning, malalignment, poor technique, prior injuries, and other medical problems (7). Ideally, dancers should be assessed in functional foot movements of plantar flexion, dorsiflexion, pronation, supination as well as *plié*, *demipointe*, parallel position, and at the individual affected joint (10). Much of dance rehabilitation is similar to sports medicine management including pain management, restoration of range of motion, muscle strengthening, and balance and proprioceptive retraining. Studies also indicate that supplementary physical conditioning or cross-training can both improve fitness and decrease injuries in dancers (46). Modification of dance activities may include strengthening initially in neutral position where the feet are in parallel position and not turned out and then progressing from *barre* exercises to the center floor (10). Pilates-based exercises are often very effective for promoting balance and coordination (7) and enable injured dancers to remain relatively fit while recovering from injury. While acknowledging that improper technique may increase the likelihood of injury recurrence, rehabilitation should emphasize biomechanical reeducation, possibly with a transitional dance class supervised by both a specialized physical therapist and dance coach (7) or supervision with both a dance-medicine–trained practitioner and dance instructor (33). Additional intervention may include psychological care for stress management, anxiety and coping with limitations, identifying proper shoes, nutritional assessment to screen for eating disorders, and advocating for general health improvement including smoking cessation (7).

The benefit of dance rehabilitation is cited in several studies (47,48). One study demonstrated savings in one ballet company of $1.2 million over a 5-year period as well as a decrease in annual incidence of injury with the provision of in-house medical and therapy services (47). A second retrospective cohort study conducted with the Alvin Ailey Dance Company revealed that comprehensive management inclusive of prevention, intervention, and case management, over a 5-year period, significantly decreased the number of worker's compensation cases from 81% to 17% and decreased the number of lost workdays by 60% (48).

MUSCULOSKELETAL PROBLEMS IN THE MUSICIAN

Musicians of all ages and playing levels are susceptible to musculoskeletal pain and injury due to repetitive and unique biomechanical movement required to play an instrument. An interesting study in 2013 demonstrated that the odds ratio of developing an injury over 12 months was 2.33 in music academy students versus medical students (49). A study of professional orchestra musicians in Puerto Rico published in 2007 revealed increased risk in younger musicians (ages 22 to 29) and older musicians (ages 50 to 61). Risk was also higher for females, increased playing time, and technical difficulty (50).

Most of the injuries observed in musicians are similar to musculoskeletal injuries seen in the nonmusicians. It is imperative, however, to understand the biomechanics involved in developing these injuries in order to treat this population. In many cases, an isolated musculoskeletal injury can be career ending or life altering. The incidence of specific injuries depends on the instrument played (📶 eTable 44-1). The remainder of this chapter reviews common musculoskeletal disorders in the musician organized primarily by body part. The emphasis is on risk factors and treatment unique to musicians.

For those not familiar with instruments and terminology, below is a brief overview (51):

Woodwind instrument—produces sound when the player blows against the edge of or opening in the instrument, causing air to vibrate within a resonator. These include the flute, piccolo, clarinet, bassoon, saxophone, and oboe.

Brass instrument—tone is produced by vibration of the lips, as the player blows into a tubular resonator. These include the trombone, trumpet, tuba, and the French horn.

String instrument—produces sound by means of vibrating strings. These include the violin, viola, cello, bass, electric guitar, bass guitar, acoustic guitar, harp, and banjo. The violin is the smallest of all the strings and the most common orchestral instrument.

Percussion instrument—any object which produces a sound by any action, which causes it to vibrate and produce sound. These include the snare and bass drums, cymbals, and in some references, the piano.

Keyboards such as the piano, organ, and accordion are sometimes classified in the percussion group and sometimes in the strings. For the purpose of this chapter, the term keyboards or the specific instrument is used.

Embouchure—position of the lips and tension of the face to produce a good tone on a brass or woodwind instrument.

Disorders of the Head and Face

The temporomandibular joints (TMJs) connect the temporal bone to the mandible. TMJ disorder occurs when the surrounding muscles become hyperactive causing malocclusion or when the meniscus of the joint becomes displaced causing poor articulation (52). TMJ occurs in violin and viola players due to pressure on the mandible, clenching mastication muscles, and from vibrations transmitted from the instrument. It may occur in trumpet, trombone, and tuba players due to displacement of the mandible. Treatment includes modifying the shoulder rest, use of occlusal splints, and physical therapy. The goal of physical therapy is to increase joint flexibility and decrease muscle tightness. Modalities include ultrasound, transcutaneous electrical nerve stimulation (TENS), massage, biofeedback, and myofascial spray and stretch (53).

Embouchure overuse syndrome is the most common performance injury suffered by brass players. Symptoms include lip pain, swelling, embouchure weakness, and lack of endurance. Chin bunching indicates embouchure fatigue or evidence of a problem in technique (📶 eFig. 44-3A and B). Rest is essential to recover from these symptoms. Once they improve, working with an appropriately trained music instructor to optimize technique and avoid excess strain can prevent further injury or even rupture (53). Louis Armstrong suffered a rupture of the orbicularis oris from repeated straining to play the trumpet. Surgical intervention is required if rupture occurs. A useful Web site for patients and clinicians is www.embouchures.com.

Disorders of the Neck and Shoulder

Playing an instrument involves dynamic and static positions that can cause discomfort in the neck. Violin and viola players support the instrument between their left shoulder and left side of the neck and mandible. This prolonged static position can lead to myofascial pain and eventually, degenerative changes in the cervical spine. Cervical radiculopathy is more common on the left in violinists due to prolonged neck rotation and flexion (54) (see also Chapter 26). Support devices such as shoulder rests and chin rests can be used to optimize position. A properly fitted violin allows the player to turn his/her head and tilt it slightly to stabilize the violin. The hand is not required to support the instrument distally and the neck should not strain to hold it (**Fig. 44-8**). Neck pain can occur as the artist clamps the chin down on the chin rest to hold a poorly balanced instrument. The chin and shoulder rests are often placed too low, causing the musician to raise his or her shoulder or thrust the head forward to compensate (54).

Keyboard players may develop neck pain from looking down at their hands, especially on the right side. Cervical radiculopathy is more common on the right side in pianists (55). Orchestra partners must keep their head turned to one side to read the music on the stand. The flute player is also at risk for cervical degenerative changes due to static position of the tilted and rotated head. There is a mouthpiece available that has a 30-degree obtuse angle just past the lip plate. This allows for a near neutral position.

Shoulder injury is included in this section because many of the positions that contribute to neck pain also contribute to shoulder pain. Myofascial pain in the shoulder is common on the same side of the neck from positions described above. Rotator cuff impingement is likely in musicians that must keep their arms in a raised position with elbow pointing outward or forward. Instruments that require this position include the violin, viola, cello, and bassoon. In flute players, the right shoulder is more commonly affected than the left because it is abducted and externally rotated (**Fig. 44-9A** and **B**).

The physician who treats musculoskeletal injuries is sure to see numerous patients with neck and shoulder pain. Current literature does not suggest that these problems are more common in musicians than in the general population, but when

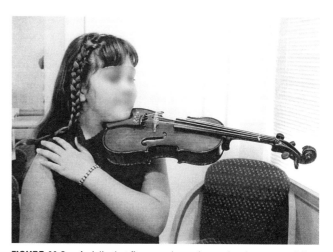

FIGURE 44-8. A violin that fits properly requires no hand support and does not strain the neck.

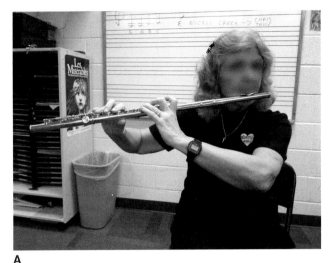
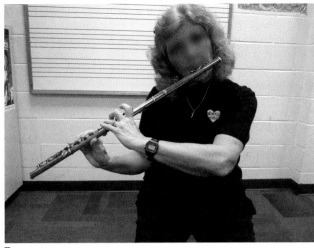

A   **B**

FIGURE 44-9.   **A:** Shoulder abduction and external rotation required to play the flute may lead to impingement and shoulder fatigue. **B:** The flautist may drop the shoulder to avoid discomfort, which strains the neck.

a musician presents with neck and shoulder discomfort, the instrument is usually the cause as it requires repetitive motion and unnatural positions. A study published in 2004 (56) in Sweden compared the risk of musculoskeletal injury in actors and orchestra musicians. The neck and shoulders were the most frequently injured anatomical areas and the prevalence of 25% was similar in both groups. The orchestra musicians, however, had a threefold to fivefold increased risk for pain affecting their performance capacity (56). Upper body strengthening and stretching to compensate for these postural asymmetries is helpful in these patients.

Thoracic Outlet Syndrome

Thoracic outlet syndrome (TOS) is a condition that may result in compression of the brachial plexus or subclavian vessels. This may cause paresthesias of the digits, vascular changes, and/or weakness of the hand. Musicians can be particularly susceptible owing to their need to maintain shoulder abduction or extension for prolonged periods of time (**Fig. 44-10**) (57). Musicians commonly have tight pectoralis and scalene

muscles, which can cause compression of the neurovascular bundle. Irregular breathing patterns and breath-holding may be a risk factor in woodwind and brass instrumentalists (58). The presence of a cervical rib and the first rib are known contributors to TOS. It is imperative to stretch the tight anterior muscles and to strengthen the posterior scapular stabilizing muscles to treat this condition.

TOS has been reported to be more common on the left side in violin, viola, and guitar players, and bilaterally in flute and piano players. In one study, there was a 12% prevalence of TOS among musicians, most prevalent in pianists, string, and wind players (59). In an earlier study, the same author found that physical therapy to correct postural errors and range of motion was successful in 76% of 17 musicians with TOS (59).

Disorders of the Arm and Hand

Entrapment of the ulnar nerve may occur between the two heads of the flexor carpi ulnaris in the cubital tunnel or in the bony sulcus between the medial epicondyle and the ulnar olecranon process. As in ulnar neuropathy of nonmusicians, excessive elbow flexion is the most significant risk factor. It is more likely to occur in the left arm of viola, violin, and guitar players, due to continuous elbow flexion. Treatment consists of position awareness and limiting elbow flexion. This is not usually feasible while playing, but needs to be emphasized during other activities, and sleep.

Medial epicondylitis occurs with repetitive wrist flexion, finger flexion, or pronation of the forearm. Medial epicondylitis occurs in the harpist on the left side. Lateral epicondylitis is due to repeated wrist extension, finger extension, or supination. It is more likely seen in clarinet players bilaterally and in oboe and trombone players on the right side. Percussionists and keyboard players are at risk for bilateral medial and lateral epicondylitis. Proper bench height is important to maximize a neutral wrist and elbow position. Forearms should be parallel to the floor when touching the keyboards (**Fig. 44-11A–C**).

Repetitive wrist flexion with ulnar deviation leads to de Quervain tenosynovitis. This is an inflammation of the extensor pollicis brevis and adductor pollicis longus muscles on the radial side of the wrist. The clarinet, oboe, flute, keyboard,

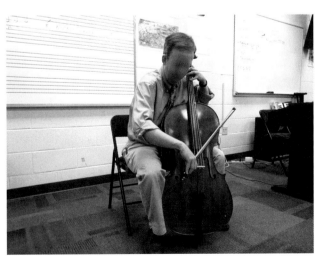

FIGURE 44-10.   Playing an instrument in a slumped position contributes to tight anterior muscles such as the pectoralis muscles and scalenes.

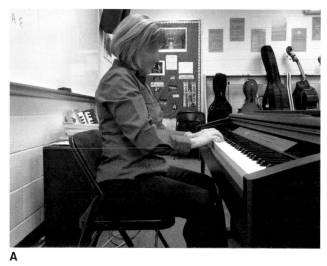

A

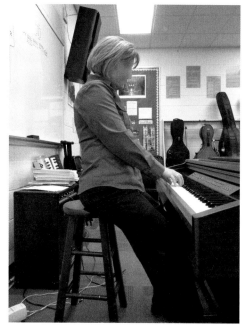

B

FIGURE 44-11. **A:** A low bench causes the wrists to be maintained in extension. Also with a low bench, a pianist may shrug shoulders to maintain neutral wrists, which strain the trapezius, neck, and shoulders. **B:** A high bench causes the wrists to be in flexion and adds stress to the fingers. **C:** Proper bench height allows neutral position of the shoulders, elbows, and wrists.

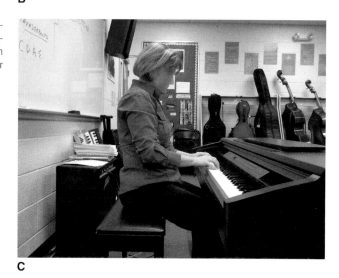

C

percussion, violin, and viola are the primary culprits. Use of a spica splint to immobilize the thumb as much as possible is helpful. A localized steroid injection provides relief in 81% of patients at 6 weeks (60). Ergonomics can be improved by repositioning the proximal arm so the left hand does not have to twist so radically to perform fingering work (**Fig. 44-12**).

Carpal tunnel syndrome (CTS), entrapment of the median nerve at the wrist, is the most common entrapment neuropathy in musicians (61). As in nonmusicians, the primary risk factor is repetitive wrist flexion. Because CTS is such a prevalent disorder among the general population, causality from instrument playing is less clear than in other musculoskeletal disorders. Dawson studied 98 musicians with CTS and reported that only 18.4% had no risk factors for CTS other than playing music (62). Among right-handed musicians, the left hand in violin, viola, and guitar players is more likely to develop CTS. Treatment includes rest with splinting, icing, physical

therapy, and especially, technique modification. Fortunately, for musicians with CTS, over 90% have complete recovery with surgical and nonsurgical treatment (62).

The actual manipulation of keys, valves, and strings is performed mostly by the small intrinsic muscles of the hands (63). The intrinsics include the thenar, hypothenar, interossei, and lumbrical muscles. Involvement of these small muscles is less studied and referenced in the literature. Dawson, however, addressed this problem in a retrospective chart review of 1,354 instrumentalists with hand and upper extremity injuries, 51 of whom had strains of hand intrinsic muscles. Risk factors included playing keyboards, string instruments, female sex, and higher-level musicians. It is hypothesized that females are more affected due to smaller, and therefore, weaker hand muscles (63). Treatment includes relative rest, modification of technique, analgesics, and occupational therapy, which can address ergonomics of playing.

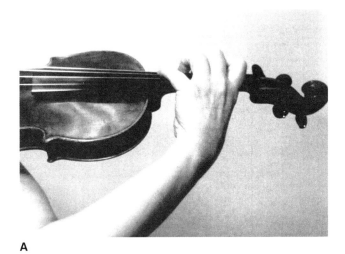

A

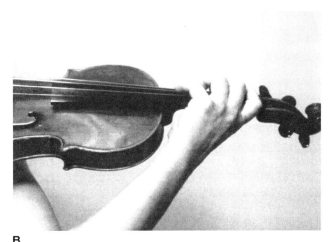

B

FIGURE 44-12. **A:** Poor glenohumeral joint motion restricts arm position and generates poor wrist ergonomics. **B:** By increasing glenohumeral motion, the hand is positioned with less wrist deviation.

Disorders Related to Joint Laxity

Many authors have described joint laxity as a risk factor for injury among musicians. Brandfonbrener found that 34% of 128 musicians presenting with arm and hand pain had hyperlaxity, which appeared to play a role in the etiology of pain (64). Many joints can have hyperextensibility. Having more than 10 degrees beyond 180 degrees of proximal interphalangeal joint extension and/or 10 degrees or more beyond 90 degrees of metacarpophalangeal joint extension seems to put musicians at most risk (65). More women than men have joint laxity. Smaller hands are also a risk factor for hand injury in musicians; thus, the clinician should be especially vigilant when dealing with hand pain in women musicians (65). Awareness, education, supportive splints or taping, and joint protection are the cornerstones of treatment (**Fig. 44-13**).

Disorders Related to Focal Dystonia

Focal dystonia is characterized by involuntary muscle contractions that selectively interfere with the execution of specific motor tasks such as writing or playing a musical instrument (66). Similar to writer's cramp, a focal dystonia of the hand, dystonia may affect the fingers of instrumentalists and more

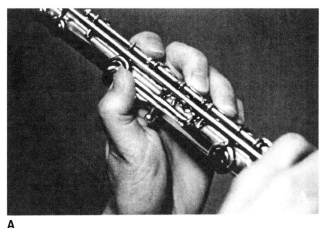

A

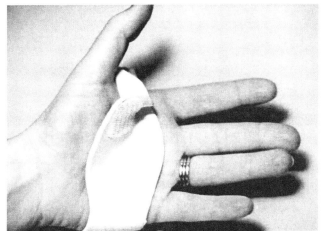

B

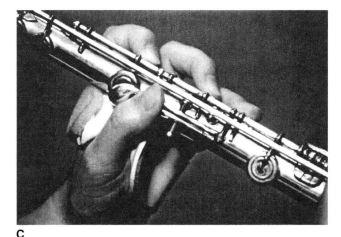

C

FIGURE 44-13. **A:** Postpregnancy hyperlaxity at metacarpophalangeal (MCP) joint. **B:** Orthosis fabricated to prevent abnormal MCP joint motion. **C:** Functional hand orthosis preserves hand movement but limits hyperlaxity.

rarely, the embouchure in wind instrumentalists (67). The dystonia causes the finger or lip to contract when it should not, or otherwise move involuntarily (eFig. 44-4). Lederman found a pattern of involvement of the left hand in string players and the right hand in keyboard and wind players (68). Keyboard players appear to be the most commonly affected of all instrumentalists, usually involving the fourth and fifth digits of the right hand, which plays melody more than the left hand (69). Dystonia of the fourth and fifth digits may be more common in patients who have developed ulnar neuropathy (69).

A study of patients with focal hand dystonia suggested that these patients have alterations in the cortical somatosensory representation of the digits. The representation of the fingers spans outside the area normally occupied in persons without focal dystonia. This may affect sensorimotor feedback and cause involuntary cocontraction of other muscles (70). The onset is insidious and usually painless (71). It should be considered when a musician begins to experience difficulties with speed and precision of playing and when he or she has to work harder to play. It is helpful for the examiner to observe the musician playing and watch for subtle signs of slow, hesitant, or abnormal movements of fingers or lips (72).

Treatment of focal dystonia is challenging. An evidence-based review by the American Academy of Neurology in 2008 concluded that botulinum toxin is potentially effective in the treatment of focal upper limb dystonia (73). Priori et al. found that immobilization of the forearm and hand for 4 to 5 weeks resulted in improved function (66). The hypothesis is that immobilization leads to plastic changes at the motor cortical level, reducing excitability. A treatment known as the sensory trick has shown promise in some individuals. Application of a sensory stimulus may disrupt the habituated somatosensory cortex. One study showed that 19% of pianists who played with a latex glove had statistically significant improvement in motor control (74). This may also help some guitarists. Oral medications cited in the literature include levodopa, lioresal, clonazepam, gabapentin, and trihexyphenidyl. Unfortunately, treatments are not always successful, and in more than half of the musicians with dystonia, it is career ending (75).

Myofascial Upper Back Pain

Myofascial pain commonly occurs in the trapezius, levator scapulae, and periscapular muscles. As in the general population, it is caused by maintaining a static position, poor posture, and muscle fatigue. The tendency toward counterclockwise rotation of the guitarist's spine facilitates right shoulder protraction and placement of the strumming hand. Widening of the strap can help decrease tension on the left trapezius and periscapular muscles (76). The physician may offer trigger point injections or make a referral to physical therapy for myofascial release and neuromuscular therapy, but restoring postural symmetry, strength, and flexibility is again the crux of treatment. Dry needling of myofascial trigger points has emerged as popular technique by many physical therapists. Most studies have demonstrated short-term benefits. A study published in 2017 showed sustained relief 6 weeks after completion of three dry needling sessions in the upper trapezius muscles of patients who had pain over 3 months before treatment (77).

Low Back Pain

An important risk factor for muscular strain in the low back is maintenance of a position in which the weight of the spine is not well balanced (78). This is a likely scenario in many musicians. A discogenic etiology of pain is more likely with lumbar flexion. Musicians who play leaning forward, especially while seated, are likely more at risk for disc bulging and degenerative disk disease. Lifting and carrying heavy instruments is also a risk factor for muscular strain and discogenic pain. The clinician should recommend wheeled carts to transport heavier instruments, for instance, the harp, drums, and bass (79).

The practitioner and music instructor should focus on the posture of the musician while playing. Paull and Harrison, authors of "The Athletic Musician," recommend a chair designed specifically for musicians with the front end sloped and the rear horizontal (80). This puts about one third of the body weight through the feet, taking the weight off the spine (80). Similarly, a wedge cushion can be added to a standard chair. If using a standard chair, it is best to have the legs parallel to the ground and the back straight (📶 **eFig. 44-5**). It is helpful for guitarists to have a footstool so that he/she can rest the guitar on the elevated thigh. A string player with low back pain may improve symptoms by playing standing up, though the technique is different. A strap can be added to support the guitar while standing.

General Guidelines for the Treatment of the Injured Musician

Novice musicians should gradually increase their practice time and rest at appropriate intervals to avoid muscle fatigue. There are several suggested guidelines such as 5 minutes of rest for every 20 minutes of playing, 10 minutes of rest for 50 minutes of playing, and 10 to 15 minutes of rest for 30 minutes of playing (58). During rest, the musician should stretch and change positions. An abrupt increase in practice time is the most important risk factor for playing-related musculoskeletal disorders (81).

Communication with the music instructor and musician is essential to optimize performance. Together, they can assure proper instrument size, adjustment pads, benches, straps, and harnesses. Most of the problems discussed can be prevented with education regarding posture, technique, and instrument-specific conditioning.

Important Medical Considerations and Barriers to Care in the Performance Athlete

Performance athletes participate in events year-round. In addition to injury prevention, management, and recommendations for performance enhancement, this population also needs medical oversight for other health care needs and overall wellness (82). When providing care for performance athletes, it is important to address fundamental principles of wellness such as the benefits of a well-balanced diet and participation in appropriate levels of physical activity so as to reap health benefits. Some evidence shows that general nutrition knowledge and understanding of the health benefits of exercise are lacking in dance students (83). Despite regular participation in dance or long hours playing an instrument, performance athletes may not be reaching the recommended level of exercise required to gain health benefits. Education should be provided about guidelines for diet and exercise with specific recommendations tailored to the individual needs of each patient. A unique consideration to keep in mind for the touring musician is lack of readily available healthy eating options on the road (84). Dancers have several unique considerations, one of which includes the concept of changing nutritional needs based on periodization of the training schedule, and this is further complicated by the fact that nutritional demands in this population are not well studied.

Also, the ideal body type for a dancer is lean with low weight and low body fat composition, yet this population tends to rely on nutritional advice from peers instead of trained healthcare professionals (85,86). This may put dancers at risk for health disparities. Providers should be sensitive to the fact that dancers demonstrate a low level of trust in physicians and should try to build a rapport with their patients to help facilitate stronger provider-patient relationships (87). Also, since few dancers receive preventive care from physicians (87), it is important that the patient is established with a primary care provider and not only receiving intermittent care for isolated injuries.

Providers should also be aware that musicians are at risk for noise-induced hearing loss and music performance anxiety (MPA). In addition to physical and mental health effects, both can limit the musician's ability to perform or maintain their livelihood. Musicians should receive regular audiometric examinations along with education about the risks of noise exposure including methods to protect hearing (88). Audiology referral can be helpful to address these issues. Many musicians experience MPA regardless of demographic factors, time spent practicing, or professional experience, and MPA may prevent some music students from pursuing a music career (89). A full discussion of evaluation and treatment is outside the scope of this chapter, but providers can consider referral to psychiatry or psychology.

It is important to understand that barriers to care often include lack of medical insurance or financial coverage. Worker's compensation is usually only found in large dance companies or in the university setting for dancers. Similarly, worker's compensation and health insurance are often unobtainable for musicians. The median hourly wage for musicians and singers in 2015 was $24.20, and they may have periods of unemployment between jobs because of the part-time or intermittent nature of their work. The median hourly wage for dancers and choreographers in 2015 was $16.85, and schedules can vary depending on the nature of their employment (90). Physical therapy, occupational therapy, physician visits, medications, and durable medical equipment may be unaffordable. It is necessary to prescribe rest at times, which in many cases, results in lost income. There is often pressure from parents or managers of dancers and musicians to continue through the discomfort. More seasoned musicians may choose to perform injured during their busy seasons and audition periods when they are in the most need of treatment and rest.

CONCLUSION

Musicians and dancers are a wonderfully unique group of people. Knowledge of the body mechanics is required to play an instrument and dance, and the accompanying lifestyle is vital to optimize the outcome of musculoskeletal problems. Organizations such as the Performing Arts Medicine Association (PAMA) and National Association of Schools of Music (NASM) are excellent resources for the performing athlete and those who care for them.

ACKNOWLEDGMENTS

We would like to acknowledge the following individuals for their help with this chapter: Konrad Weatherhogg, PT, for assistance with rehabilitation techniques; Stephanie Levi, PT, for sharing her library of arts medicine articles; the music department at Charlotte Christian School—Don Humphries, Kelly Goley, and Jane Mendlik for being our musician models, and Laura Goodyear and Terry Efird, Charlotte Christian School for facilitating our photography session.

REFERENCES

1. Evans RW, Evans RI, Carvajal S. Surveys of injuries among West end performers. *Occup Environ Med.* 1998;55(9):585–593.
2. Nilsson C, Leanderson J, Wykman A, et al. The injury panorama in a Swedish professional ballet company. *Knee Surg Sports Traumatol Arthrosc.* 2002;9(4):242–246.
3. Khan K, Brown J, Way S, et al. Overuse injuries in classical ballet. *Sports Med.* 1995;19(5):341–357.
4. Stretanski M, Weber GJ. Medical and rehabilitation issues in classical ballet: literature review. *Am J Phys Med Rehabil.* 2002;81(5):383–391.
5. Tuffery AR. The nature and incidence of injuries in morris dancers. *Br J Sports Med.* 1989;23(3):155–160.
6. Evans RW, Evans RI, Carvajal S, et al. A survey of injuries among Broadway performers. *Am J Public Health.* 1996;86(1):77–80.
7. Motta-Valencia K. Dance-related injury. *Phys Med Rehabil Clin N Am.* 2006;17:697–723.
8. Milan K. Injury in ballet: a review of relevant topics for the physical therapist. *J Orthop Sports Phys Ther.* 1994;19(2):121–129.
9. Kadel N. Foot and ankle injuries in dance. *Phys Med Rehabil Clin N Am.* 2006;17:813–826.
10. Macintyre J, Joy E. Foot and ankle injuries in dance. *Clin Sports Med.* 2000;19(2):351–368.
11. Toledo S, Akuthota V, Drake D, et al. Sports and performing arts medicine. 6. Issues relating to dancers. *Arch Phys Med Rehabil.* 2004;85(suppl 1):S75–S78.
12. Garrick JG, Requa RK. Tournout and training in ballet. *Med Probl Perform Art.* 1994;9(2):43–49.
13. Watkins A, Woodhull-McNeal AP, Clarkson PM, et al. Lower extremity alignment and injury in young, preprofessional, college and professional ballet dancers: turnout and knee-foot alignment. *Med Probl Perform Art.* 1989;4(4):148–153.
14. Trepman E, Gellman RE, Solomon R, et al. Electromyographic analysis of standing posture and demi-plie in ballet and modern dancers. *Med Sci Sports Exerc.* 1994;26(6):771–782.
15. Trepman E, Gellman RE, Micheli LJ, et al. Electromyographic analysis of grand-plie in ballet and modern dancers. *Med Sci Sports Exerc.* 1998;30(12):1708–1720.
16. Luke AC, Kinney SA, D'Hemecourt PA, et al. Determinants of injuries in young dancers. *Med Probl Perform Art.* 2002;17(3):105–112.
17. Macintyre J. Kinetic chain dysfunction in ballet injuries. *Med Probl Perform Art.* 1994;9(2):39–42.
18. DiTullio M, Wilczek L, Paulus D, et al. Comparison of hip rotation in classical ballet dancers versus female nondancers. *Med Probl Perform Art.* 1989;4(4):154–158.
19. Micheli LJ, Gillespie WJ, Walaszek A. Physiologic profiles of female professional ballerinas. *Clin Sports Med.* 1984;3(1):199–209.
20. Brooks-Gunn J, Warren MP, Hamilton LH. The relation of eating problems and amenorrhea in ballet dancers. *Med Sci Sports Exerc.* 1987;19(1):41–44.
21. Hamilton LH, Brooks-Gunn J, Warren MP, et al. The impact of thinness and dieting on the professional ballet dancer. *Med Probl Perform Art.* 1987;2(4):117–123.
22. Schnitt JN, Scnitt D. Eating disorders in dancers. *Med Probl Perform Art.* 1986;1(2):39–44.
23. Hamilton LH, Brooks-Gunn J, Warren MP, et al. The role of selectivity in the pathogenesis of eating problems in ballet dancers. *Med Sci Sports Exerc.* 1988;20(6):560–565.
24. Dobson R. Eight in 10 dancers have an injury each year, survey shows. *BMJ.* 2005;331:594.
25. Smith T, et al. National survey to evaluate musculoskeletal health in retired professional ballet dancers in the United Kingdom. *Phys Ther Sport.* 2017;23:82–85.
26. Denton J. Overuse foot and ankle injuries in ballet. *Clin Podiatr Med Surg.* 1997;14(3):525–532.
27. Smith P, et al. Incidence and prevalence of musculoskeletal injury in ballet: a systematic review. *Orthop J Sports Med.* 2015;3(7):2325967115592621.
28. Steinburg N, et al. Injuries in female dancers aged 8 to 16 years. *J Athl Train.* 2013;48(1):118–123.
29. Stadaert C, Herring S. Spondylolysis: a critical review. *Br J Sports Med.* 2000;34:415–422.
30. DeMann LE Jr. Sacroiliac dysfunction in dancers with low back pain. *Man Ther.* 1997;2(1):2–10.
31. Sammarco GJ. The hip in dancers. *Med Probl Perform Art.* 1987;2(1):5–14.
32. Sammarco GJ. The dancer's hip. In: Ryan AJ, Septhens RE, eds. *Dance Medicine: A Comprehensive Guide.* Chicago, IL: Pluribus Press; 1987:220–242.
33. Solomon R, Brown T, Gerbino P, et al. The young dancer. *Clin Sports Med.* 2000;19(4):717–736.
34. Laible C, et al. Iliopsoas syndrome in dancers. *Orthop J Sports Med.* 2013;1(3):2325967113500638.
35. Weber A, et al. The hyperflexible hip. *Sports Health.* 2015;7(4):346–358.
36. Meuffels D, Verhaar J. Anterior cruciate ligament injury in professional dancers. *Acta Orthop.* 2008;79(4):515–518.

37. Ostwald P, Baron B, Byl N, et al. Performing arts medicine. *West J Med.* 1994;160:48–52.

38. Rehmani R et al. Lower extremity injury patterns in elite ballet dancers: ultrasound/MRI imaging features and an institutional overview of therapeutic ultrasound guided percutaneous interventions. *HSS J.* 2015;11(3):258–277.

39. Menetrey J, Fritschy D. Subtalar subluxation in ballet dancers. *Am J Sports Med.* 1999;27(2):143–149.

40. Ogilvie-Harris DJ, Car MM, Fleming PJ. The foot in ballet dancers: the importance of second toe length. *Foot Ankle Int.* 1995;16(3):144–147.

41. Micheli LJ, Solomon R. Stress fractures of the second metatarsal involving Lisfranc's joint in ballet dancers: a new overuse injury of the foot. *J Bone Joint Surg Am.* 1985;67(9):1372–1375.

42. O'Malley MJ, Hamilton WG, Munyak J, et al. Stress fractures at the base of the second metatarsal in ballet dancers. *Foot Ankle Int.* 1996;17(2):89–94.

43. Harrington T, Crichton KJ, Anderson IF. Overuse ballet injury of the base of the second metatarsal: a diagnostic problem. *Am J Sports Med.* 1993;21(4):591–598.

44. Albisetti W, et al. Stress fractures of the base of the metatarsal bones in young trainee ballet dancers. *Int Orthop.* 2010;34(1):51–55.

45. Peterson W, Pufe T, Zantop T, et al. Blood supply of the flexor hallucis longus tendon with regard to dancer's tendonitis: injection and immunohistochemical studies of cadaver tendons. *Foot Ankle Int.* 2003;24(8):591.

46. Koutedakis Y, Jaumurtas A. The dancer as a performing athlete: physiological considerations. *Sports Med.* 2004;34(10):651–661.

47. Solomon R, Solomon J, Micheli LJ, et al. The "cost" of injuries in a professional ballet company: a five year study. *Med Probl Perform Art.* 1999;164–169.

48. Bronner S, Ojofeitimi S, Rose D. Injuries in a modern dance company: effect of comprehensive management on injury incidence and time loss. *Am J Sports Med.* 2003;31(3):365–373.

49. Kok L, Vlieland T, et al. A comparative study on the prevalence of musculoskeletal complaints among musicians and non-musicians. *BMC Musculoskelet Disord.* 2013;14:9.

50. Abreu-Ramos AM, Micheo WF. Lifetime prevalence of upper-body musculoskeletal problems in a professional-level symphony orchestra. *Med Probl Perform Art.* 2007;22:97–104.

51. Wikipedia. Musical instruments. Available from: http://en.wikipedia.org/wiki/musical_instrument. Accessed November 20, 2008.

52. Berman SA, Chadhary A, Appelbaum J. Temporomandibular disorders. *E-Medicine.* June 30, 2006.

53. Bejjani FJ, Kaye GM, Benham M. Musculoskeletal and neuromuscular conditions of instrumental musicians. *Arch Phys Med Rehabil.* 1996;77:406–413.

54. Levy CE, Lee WA, Brandfonbrener AG, et al. Electromyographic analysis of muscular activity in the upper extremity generated by supporting a violin with and without a shoulder rest. *Med Probl Perform Art.* 1992;7(4):103–109.

55. Lederman RJ. Peripheral nerve disorders in instrumentalists. *Ann Neurol.* 1989;26:640–646.

56. Engquist K, Orbaek P, Jakobsson K. Musculoskeletal pain and impact on performance in orchestra musicians and actors. *Med Probl Perform Art.* 2004;19:55–61.

57. Clearman RR. Arts medicine. In: Delisa A, ed. *Physical Medicine and Rehabilitation.* 4th ed. Philadelphia, PA: Lippincott Williams & Wilkins; 2005:595–613.

58. Robinson D, Zander J. *Preventing Musculoskeletal Injuries for Musicians and Dancers: A Resource Guide.* Vancouver, BC: Safety and Health in Arts Production and Entertainment; 2002.

59. Lederman RJ. Thoracic outlet syndromes: review of the controversies and report of 17 instrumental musicians. *Med Probl Perform Art.* 1987;2:87–91.

60. Anderson BC, Manthey R, Brouns MC. Treatment of DeQuervain's tenosynovitis with corticosteroids: a prospective study of the response to local injection. *Arthritis Rheum.* 1991;34(7):793–798.

61. Lederman RJ. Entrapment neuropathies in instrumental musicians. *Med Probl Perform Art.* 1993;8:35–39.

62. Dawson WJ. Carpal tunnel syndrome in instrumentalists: a review of 15 years' clinical experience. *Med Probl Perform Art.* 1999;14:25–29.

63. Dawson WJ. Intrinsic muscle strain in the instrumentalist. *Med Probl Perform Art.* 2005;20:66–69.

64. Fishbein M, Middlestadt SE. Medical problems among ICSOM musicians: overview of a national survey. *Med Probl Perform Art.* 1998;3:1–8.

65. Brandfonbrener AG. Joint laxity and arm pain in musicians. *Med Probl Perform Art.* 2000;15:22–24.

66. Priori A, Pesenti A, Cappellari A, et al. Limb immobilization for the treatment of focal occupational dystonia. *Neurology.* 2001;57:405–409.

67. Lederman RJ. Embouchure problems in brass instrumentalists. *Med Probl Perform Art.* 2001;16:53–57.

68. Lederman RJ. Focal dystonia in instrumentalists: clinical features. *Med Probl Perform Art.* 1991;6:110–115.

69. Charness ME, Ross MH, Shefner JM. Ulnar neuropathy and dystonic flexion of the fourth and fifth digits: clinical correlation in musicians. *Muscle Nerve.* 1996;19:431–437.

70. McKenzie AL, Nagarajan SS, Roberts TPL, et al. Somatosensory representation of the digits and clinical performance in patients with focal hand dystonia. *Am J Phys Med Rehabil.* 2003;82:737–749.

71. Newmark J. Musicians' dystonia: the case of Gary Graffman. *Semin Neurol.* 1999;19(suppl 1):41–45.

72. Brandfonbrener AG. Musicians with focal dystonia: a report of 58 cases seen during a ten-year period at a performing arts medicine clinic. *Med Probl Perform Art.* 1995;10(4):121–127.

73. Simpson DR, Blitzer A, Brashear A, et al. Assessment: botulinum toxin for the treatment of movement disorders (an evidence-based review): report of the Therapeutics and Technology Assessment Subcommittee of the American Academy of Neurology. *Neurology.* 2008;70:1699.

74. Paulig J, Jabusch HC, et al. Sensory trick phenomenon improves motor control in pianists with dystonia: prognostic value of glove-effect. *Front Psychol.* 2014;5:1012.

75. Scheuele S, Lederman R. Focal dystonia in woodwind instrumentalists: long term outcome. *Med Probl Perform Art.* 2003;18:15–20.

76. Storm SA. Assessing the instrumentalist's interface: modifications, ergonomics, and maintenance of play. *Phys Med Rehabil Clin N Am.* 2006;17:893–903.

77. Gerber LH, Sikdar S, et al. Beneficial effects of dry needling for treatment of chronic myofascial pain persist for 6 weeks after treatment completion. *PM R.* 2017;9(2):105–112.

78. Jenkins DB. *Hollinshead's Functional Anatomy of the Limbs and Back.* Philadelphia, PA: W.B. Saunders Company; 1998.

79. Brandfonbrener AG. Musculoskeletal problems of instrumental musicians. *Hand Clin.* 2003;19:231–239.

80. Paull B, Harrison C. *The Athletic Musician.* Lanham, MD: The Rowman and Littlefield Publishing Group, Inc.; 1997.

81. Hoppman RA. Instrumental musicians' hazards. *Occup Med.* 2001;16(4):619–621.

82. Dick RW. The arts and athletes—the role of sports medicine in the performing arts. *Curr Sports Med Rep.* 2013;12(6):397–403.

83. Hanna K, Hanley A, Huddy A, et al. Physical activity participation and nutrition and physical activity knowledge in university dance students. *Med Probl Perform Art.* 2017;32(1):1–7.

84. Cizek E, Kelly P, Kress K, et al. Factors affecting healthful eating among touring popular musicians and singers. *Med Probl Perform Art.* 2016;31(2):63–68.

85. Sousa M, Carvalho P, Moreira P, et al. Nutrition and nutritional issues for dancers. *Med Probl Perform Art.* 2013;28(3):119–123.

86. Brown D, Wyon M. An international study on dietary supplementation use in dancers. *Med Probl Perform Art.* 2014;29(4):229–234.

87. Alimena S, Air ME. Trust, satisfaction, and confidence in health care providers among student and professional dancers in France. *Med Probl Perform Art.* 2016;31(3):166–173.

88. McIlvaine D, Stewart M, Anderson R. Noise exposure levels for musicians during rehearsal and performance times. *Med Probl Perform Art.* 2012;27(1):31–36.

89. Brugués AO. Music performance anxiety—part 1. A review of its epidemiology. *Med Probl Perform Art.* 2011;26(2):102–105.

90. Bureau of Labor Statistics. *Occupational Outlook Handbook.* 2015. Available from: www.bls.gov/ooh/. Accessed April 11, 2017.

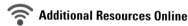 **Additional Resources Online**

CHAPTER 45

Tobias J. Tsai
Kelly L. D. Pham

Rehabilitation of Children with Disabilities and Adults with Childhood-Onset Disabling Conditions

The rehabilitation of children differs in several ways from that of adults. Children have many differences in physiology that predispose them to different patterns of injury and recovery and a variety of conditions not seen in the adult population. Throughout childhood, growth and development create different therapeutic challenges that require unique approaches that differ from the adult patient. This chapter provides an overview of the context of care in which pediatric rehabilitation services are provided, a discussion of childhood growth and development, a review of common pediatric clinical conditions and treatments that may be seen by members of the rehabilitation team, and considerations for the management of adults with two of the most common pediatric-onset conditions: cerebral palsy (CP) and spina bifida.

THE CONTEXT OF CARE AND THE MEDICAL HOME

According to 2010 US nationwide census data, approximately 8% of children under the age of 15 have a disability (1). The current standard of care for children is a medical home model. This is particularly important for children with disabilities, for whom utilization of health care services may be increased and, in many cases, spread among multiple providers. The concept of a medical home refers to an approach to care that is accessible, patient and family centered, continuous, comprehensive, coordinated, compassionate, and culturally effective (2). However, many children with special health care needs do not receive care provided by a medical home (3,4). Furthermore, though care coordination has been associated with positive outcomes such as increased satisfaction and decreased unplanned hospitalizations, repeated surveys have shown that less than half of children with special health care needs report receiving care coordination (5).

The medical home concept is supported in part by grants provided by Title V of the Social Security Act. Many states use Title V funds to support care coordination and screening services with the goal of identifying children with special health care needs.

An important part of the medical home for the child with a disability includes early intervention (EI) services. These services, funded through grants to states authorized by Part C of the Individuals with Disabilities Education Act (IDEA), are available to children age 0 up until the age of 3, who have certain conditions known to have a high risk of developmental delay or who have developmental delay in the areas of cognitive development, physical development, communication development, social or emotional development, or adaptive development. The definition of "developmental delay" varies by state.

EVALUATION OF THE PEDIATRIC PATIENT

In the pediatric evaluation, a careful review of the pregnancy, birth history, and developmental history as well as the family history is essential. In children with acquired disabilities, detailed information about the illness or injury that produced the disability should be obtained. Most parents will have a good idea of how their child with developmental delay compares to a typical child; asking "what age does your child act like?" can be a quick way to get a sense of a child's overall functional level.

PEDIATRIC GROWTH AND DEVELOPMENT

Knowledge of the patterns of growth and development is key to understanding, anticipating, and managing the difficulties that children with disabilities may experience. In the child's early years, head circumference, weight, and height are important parameters to monitor. Specialized growth charts for various conditions (e.g., CP, Down's syndrome) are available (6). Motor and cognitive milestones are achieved in a predictable pattern and when they are not should prompt a provider to do further investigation (Table 45-1).

PRIMITIVE REFLEXES

Many reflex behaviors are age and development dependent. For example, the asymmetric tonic neck reflex (ATNR) (📶 eFig. 45-1) is a normal behavior when elicited before 6 months of age but is pathognomonic for neurologic dysfunction if it persists after that time or emerges at a later time.

Because they are more commonly observed in children with neurologic conditions, major primitive reflex patterns that

TABLE 45-1	**Examples of Gross Motor Milestones**		
Age	**Gross Motor**	**Fine Motor**	**Social**
2 mo	Head in midline	Increasing opening of hands	Smiles
3 mo		Hands to midline	
4 mo	Rolls prone to supine		Social smile
5 mo	Rolls supine to prone		
6 mo	Sits	Transfers hand to hand, raking grasp	Raises arms to be picked up
9 mo	Crawls ("creeps") Note: Some children may skip this milestone	Pincer grasp	
10 mo	Pulls to stand		Waves bye, peekaboo
12–15 mo	Walks	Stacks two blocks	Shows toy, approximately two words
21–24 mo	Up and down stairs, hands on rail		Two-word phrases
3 y	Pedals tricycle, up stairs reciprocally, runs	Copies circle	
4 y	Hops	Copies cross	Cooperative play
5 y	Skips	Copies square, writes name	

may either interfere with or facilitate skilled motor actions should be well understood. The times of appearance and disappearance of these reflexes in the developmental sequence are summarized in **Table 45-2**.

EVALUATION BY THE PHYSICIAN

The pediatric physical examination may be challenging depending on the ability of the child to participate and may reflect the child's age or developmental level. Observational evaluations provide important data that can inform the clinician and assist with the diagnosis and treatment plans. Frequently, significant information such as head and trunk control, other motor skills such as crawling and walking, and communication skills are obtained through observation before the formal examination begins. Strategies for examination of the young patient may include removing a white coat before entering the room, having the child sit on the parent's lap, demonstrating the exam on the parent or doll first, using small toys to assist in the exam, showing instruments such as a reflex hammer first, and starting with the least invasive or threatening portion of the exam first.

Manual muscle testing is usually not possible in a child less than 5 years old. Observation of the young child's spontaneous movements as well during play provides the examiner with information about antigravity muscle strength.

TABLE 45-2	**Normal Acquisition and Regression of Primitive Reflex Behaviors**	
Reflex	**Age of Onset**	**Age Reflex Disappears**
Moro	Birth	6 mo
Palmar grasp	Birth	6 mo
Plantar grasp	Birth	9–10 mo
Adductor spread of patellar reflex	Birth	7 mo
Tonic neck	2 mo	5 mo
Landau	3 mo	24 mo
Parachute response	8–9 mo	Persists

Reprinted with permission from Swaiman KF, Jacobson RI. Developmental abnormalities of the central nervous system. In: Baker AB, Joynl RJ, eds. *Clinical Neurology*. Philadelphia, PA: Harper & Row; 1984.

Sensory testing is limited in the infant, but response to noxious stimuli such as pinprick can be assessed. Regarding vision assessment in the pediatric patient, assessment for red reflex is typically done before the newborn leaves the hospital. The American Academy of Ophthalmology recommends that if strabismus, amblyopia, or refractive errors are suspected, an infant or preschool-aged child should be referred to an ophthalmologist. Hearing screening is typically done before the newborn leaves the hospital; if the infant does not pass that initial screen, he or she should follow up with an audiologist.

At different ages, standardized assessment tools are utilized to evaluate specific functional domains including gross and fine motor abilities, cognition and communication, and adaptive and social skills. Knowledge of the tools, the age ranges encompassed by these tools, and the interpretation of the results can be assisted by the interdisciplinary team members. Commonly used tests are described in **Table 45-3**.

SPECIFIC CLINICAL CONDITIONS

Cerebral Palsy

CP is defined as "a group of permanent disorders of the development of movement and posture, causing activity limitation, that are attributed to nonprogressive disturbances that occurred in the developing fetal or infant brain" (7). It is the most common motor disability of childhood with an overall prevalence of approximately 2 to 3 per 1,000 live births, which has remained stable over recent years (8–10). Low birth weight is associated with a higher prevalence of CP (59.2 per 1,000 live births if <1,500 g compared to 1.33 per 1,000 live births if >2,500 g) as is prematurity (111.8 per 1,000 live births if <28 weeks compared to 1.35 per 1,000 live births if >36 weeks (8)).

General risk factors for CP can be found in 🛜 **eBox 45-1** (11,12). Birth-related asphyxia is a rare cause occurring in only roughly 6% of children born with CP (11). Though CP is not as common in term infants, risk factors include placental abnormalities, birth defects, low birth weight, meconium aspiration, emergency cesarean section, birth asphyxia, neonatal seizures, respiratory distress syndrome, hypoglycemia, and neonatal infection (13). Postnatal risk factors for CP include infection (meningitis), trauma (nonaccidental trauma, falls,

TABLE 45-3	Commonly Used Developmental Assessments	
Test	**Age**	**Domains Tested**
Bayley Scales of Infant and Toddler Development	1–42 mo	Gross motor, fine motor
Bayley Infant Neurodevelopmental Screener (BINS)	3–24 mo	Basic neurologic functions, expressive functions, receptive functions, cognitive functions
Test of Infant Motor Performance (TIMP)	32 wk post gestation to 4 mo	Gross motor
Denver Developmental Screening Test-II	1 mo to 6 y	Gross motor, fine motor, personal-social, language
Ages & Stages Questionnaire	4–60 mo	Gross motor, fine motor, communication, personal-social, problem solving

motor vehicle accidents), cerebrovascular events (arteriovenous malformations, sickle cell disease, congenital heart disease), and anoxic injury (submersion, cardiac arrest) (14).

Classification

CP can be classified by topography, type of movement disorder, and functional level. Approximately 40% of children with CP are hemiplegic with impairment of one side of the body, another 35% with diplegia involving bilateral lower extremities, and the remaining 23% with quadriplegia involving all four extremities (15). Triplegia and monoplegia, three- and one-extremity involvement, respectively, are less common. The type of movement disorder is characterized as spastic, dyskinetic, hypotonic, ataxic, and mixed. Epidemiology studies suggest that the spastic subtype represents 75% to 85% of children with CP, dyskinetic 7% to 14% and ataxic 4% to 11% (9,16). The topographical organization and movement disorder often correlate with the functional level of the child, which is delineated for gross motor, fine motor, and communication skills.

The Gross Motor Function Classification System (GMFCS) was developed as a means of classifying children with CP based on their self-initiated gross motor movements in their typical environments (i.e., home, school, and community) (17). Levels are defined as follows: level I a child who is totally independent; level II a child who may need modified independence with stairs and uneven surfaces and may use a wheelchair for longer distances as he or she ages; level III a child who requires an assistive device to ambulate but is independent in a manual wheelchair, which becomes the primary means of mobility with age; level IV a child who is able to ambulate with assistance and an assistive device but is independent with power mobility; and level V a child who is totally dependent for all functional mobility (🛜 eFig. 45-2) (18). Classification of GMFCS level varies depending on age and is outlined for children age less than 2 years, 2 to 4 years, 4 to 6 years, 6 to 12 years, and 12 to 18 years of age, which accounts for developmental level (19). Approximately 75% of children with quadriplegic CP function at a GMFCS level IV or V with the remaining 25% at a GMFCS level I to III. Ninety-eight percent of children with diplegia and 99% of those with hemiplegia function at a GMFCS level I to III (20). One large observational study has outlined the motor development curves illustrating the prognosis of gross motor function based on GMFCS level in children with CP, which is useful in predicting gross motor function over time including a child's ability to ambulate (21).

Like the GMFCS, the Manual Ability Classification System (MACS) was developed as a means of classifying children with CP based on their ability to handle objects in everyday activities such as self-care skills and play (22). It ranges from level I denoting easy manipulation of objects to level V denoting limited ability to perform simple actions. Likewise, the Communication Function Classification System (CFCS) is a means of classifying everyday communication performance of a child with CP. It too ranges from I, the most effective level of communication, to level V, the most ineffective (23). These scales provide a means for clinicians to describe children with CP across disciplines and are used both clinically and in research.

Initial Evaluation

Children with CP are typically identified by their families and/or pediatricians to have delays in their motor milestones such as rolling, sitting, crawling, and walking. Others may be identified by abnormal motor patterns such as spasticity, dystonia, athetosis, or choreoathetosis. This may manifest as "early" milestones such as early head control due to spasticity of the neck muscles, early rolling related to posturing, or early development of handedness, which is typical in children with hemiplegia. CP may also be suspected in the presence of associated conditions (see below). The diagnosis is typically made by approximately 2 years of age based on birth history, developmental history, physical examination, and imaging (24). The American Academy of Neurology (AAN) recommends initial imaging with magnetic resonance imaging (MRI) of the brain as opposed to computed tomography (CT) scan of the head (25).

The European CP study demonstrates that MRI findings include white matter disease of prematurity, most commonly periventricular leukomalacia (PVL) in 43%, basal ganglia lesions in 13%, cortical/subcortical lesions in 9%, brain malformations in 9%, focal infarcts in 7%, and 12% of children with normal MRI (26). Children with normal MRI results tend to have milder functional impairments and warrant further evaluation for metabolic or neurodegenerative disorders, though often testing fails to clarify the etiology (27). In this case, the AAN recommends further testing only if the history or physical examination is atypical for CP in the setting of normal MRI of the brain (25).

Differential diagnosis includes, but is not limited to, idiopathic toe walking, dopa-responsive dystonia, hereditary spastic paraplegia, Friedreich's ataxia, tethered cord, a leukodystrophy, or a metabolic disorder (25,28).

Associated Conditions (24,29)

Population-based studies have identified a multitude of medical comorbidities associated with CP. Intellectual disability is present in approximately 30% of all children with CP. Speech impairment ranges from impaired yet understandable in 10% to severely impaired or nonverbal in 22% to 28%. Cortical blindness or severe impairment of vision is found in 5% to 10% of children with CP. Severe hearing impairment is seen in only 4% and does not correlate with topographical involvement or GMFCS level. Presence of epilepsy is seen in 17% to 28% of children with CP and more commonly in those with bilateral versus unilateral involvement. Feeding via gastrostomy tube is observed in 8% due to dysphagia. Children with oromotor dysfunction resulting in dysphagia may also have sialorrhea. Five times the number of medical comorbidities is seen in children with ataxic-hypotonic, spastic quadriplegic, and dyskinetic CP compared to those with spastic diplegia or hemiplegia. There are 10 times more comorbidities in those children functioning at a GMFCS level V compared to those who function at a GMFCS level I.

Hypertonicity and Movement Disorders

Hypertonicity is an increase in tone, or resistance to passive range of motion, and typically is thought to include spasticity, rigidity, and posturing. Movement disorders in CP include dystonia, choreoathetosis, and rarely ataxia. Many children with CP have truncal hypotonia with hypertonia of the extremities, though there are rare cases of hypotonic CP characterized by low tone throughout. The Hypertonia Assessment Tool (HAT) is a means of categorizing a child's hypertonicity as spasticity, dystonia, or rigidity, which may guide management by the treating clinician (30). Spasticity scales commonly used include the Modified Ashworth Scale and the Tardieu Scale, both of which are described in the spasticity chapter of this book (see Chapter 40). Hypertonicity can affect a child's function including their ability to ambulate, manipulate objects, care for themselves, and communicate.

Gait is affected by hypertonicity or presence of a movement disorder as well as by weakness and impaired motor control. Those gait patterns commonly seen in ambulatory children with spastic diplegic and hemiplegic CP are well defined by Rodda et al. (📶 **eFig. 45-3**) (31).

True equinus, seen in the young child with CP, is characterized by ankle plantar flexion spasticity with extension at the knees and hips resulting in a shortened step and stride length due to loss of the three rockers of gait. One may also see genu recurvatum due to the anterior to posterior ground reaction force on the knee. A jump knee pattern is characterized by ankle plantar flexion with flexion at the knee and the hip. This is often due to spasticity or contracture of the hamstrings and hips flexors in addition to weakness resulting in inability to maintain an upright posture. A stiff knee pattern, also seen in jump gait, appears as lack of movement at the knee in the swing phase and is attributed to rectus femoris spasticity and contraction that is out of phase. Apparent equinus, typically seen as a child gets older, is similarly characterized by hip and knee flexion but with the ankle in neutral and not plantar flexed, though it appears to be plantar flexed due to the knee and hip flexion. Crouch gait, which typically happens later in adolescence or after isolated tendo-Achilles lengthening, is illustrated by ankle dorsiflexion oftentimes at the expense of the foot with planovalgus deformity due to gastrocnemius/soleus contracture and weakness of the plantar flexors. The knees and hips are flexed due to contracture and weakness.

In children with hemiplegia, five patterns of gait are common (31). Type I hemiplegia involves footdrop with lack of ankle dorsiflexion through swing phase resulting in a compensatory steppage pattern. Type 2A, or true equinus, consists of ankle plantar flexion spasticity with knee and hip extension. Type 2B furthermore includes genu recurvatum of the knee. Type 3 is a jump knee pattern like that in bilateral CP gait. Type 4 hemiplegia involves an equinus foot/ankle with a jump knee and pelvic rotation, hip flexion, adduction, and internal rotation. Clinical observation in both the frontal and sagittal planes is necessary to fully characterize the different gait patterns.

Hypertonicity can also affect a child's ability to perform fine motor skills such as manipulating toys, writing, typing, feeding, dressing, and bathing. It can affect a parent's ability to provide care if severe enough, making tasks such as bathing, dressing, and diapering difficult. It can be painful for the child but can also result in difficulty with positioning. These may be reasons for treatment, though not all hypertonicity and movement disorder is dysfunctional and requires treatment. Some children use their hypertonicity functionally for things such as standing, transfers, and even ambulation.

Musculoskeletal

The most common musculoskeletal abnormalities of the foot include equinus, planovalgus, and equinovarus, which result from a combination of muscle imbalance, hypertonicity, dystonia, and impaired motor control (32). Equinus is due to spasticity of the gastrocnemius and soleus muscles resulting in ankle plantar flexion. Equinovarus consists of ankle plantar flexion with inversion of the foot (varus) due to spasticity or dystonia in the tibialis posterior. Over time, with contracture of the ankle plantar flexors and eventual weakness of the plantar flexors, children may develop planovalgus deformity. This involves valgus deformity of the hindfoot, midfoot pronation, and forefoot abduction.

Contractures, the result of hypertonicity, muscle imbalance, and positioning, occur in any joint but most commonly in those muscles that cross two joints such as the gastrocnemius, medial hamstrings, and hip adductors. A typical pattern of contractures is hip adduction, hip flexion, knee flexion, and ankle plantar flexion (equinus). Patella alta, also due to spasticity, more specifically of the rectus femoris muscle is very common in CP and can result in knee pain especially in children who are ambulatory.

Rotational deformities can occur at the level of the femur and the tibia. Femoral anteversion is due to a lack of derotation of the femur throughout development due to muscle imbalance and spastic or dystonic hip muscles including the hip flexors, adductors, and medial hamstrings. Often, the history includes "W-sitting" and on physical examination in-toeing, excessive internal rotation, and limited external rotation range of motion of the hip. Tibial torsion, either internal or external, results from a similar lack of typical rotation during development.

In addition to rotational deformities of the hip, children with CP are at a high risk for hip subluxation or dislocation over time due to hypertonicity and muscle imbalance. On physical examination, range of motion of the hips in abduction is measured as well as special tests such and the Thomas test looking for hip flexor tightness, the Phelps test looking at gracilis tightness, and the Galeazzi test looking for evidence of hip subluxation or dislocation. Hip surveillance protocols have been developed and revised in the last 10 years giving guidance to clinicians regarding frequency and timing of hip x-ray based on GMFCS level (33,34). Approximately 25% of children with CP have hip displacement at the time of initial x-ray, which includes both subluxation and dislocation (35). Ninety-nine percent of children who function at a GMFCS level I have normal hips in contrast to 28% of children who function at a GMFCS level V. Children with hemiplegia and ataxic CP are less likely to have hip displacement, while those with quadriplegia are the most likely.

Like the lower extremities, children with CP can develop contractures in the upper extremities due to muscle imbalance, spasticity, and dystonia. Common patterns of contracture include shoulder adduction and internal rotation, elbow flexion, forearm pronation, wrist flexion, finger flexion, and thumb in palm deformity (36).

Scoliosis is common in CP, and in one population-based study looking at all children with any type of CP, 17% of children had mild scoliosis and 11% moderate to severe. It was most common in the thoracolumbar spine. Children with higher GMFCS levels (III to V) were most likely to have moderate to severe scoliosis with those functioning at a GMFCS level IV to V most likely to require surgical intervention. Children with hemiplegia were unlikely to have scoliosis, and those most likely to have moderate to severe scoliosis and require surgical correction were those with spastic bilateral CP and dyskinetic CP (37).

Treatment

There are many interventions geared toward the treatment of motor dysfunction, hypertonicity, and associated conditions in CP, but few aimed at lessening mortality and disability in the neonate born with encephalopathy. Therapeutic hypothermia, now the standard of care in the treatment of neonatal encephalopathy, has demonstrated significant reductions in mortality and in neurodevelopmental disability in term and late preterm neonates with moderate to severe encephalopathy due to intrapartum asphyxia (38).

Therapy

Therapies generally start when a child is discovered to have developmental delays and is initially through the EI (birth to 3) Program, which is a federally funded program that provides therapy services to children under the age of 3. These therapies typically will begin with a motor therapist and a speech therapist if needed. As the child ages, the physical and occupational therapists treat separately to focus on discipline-specific areas. Depending on a child's level of function, the therapists are typically focusing on developmental skills such as functional mobility, fine motor skills, feeding, and eventually dressing and bathing, as it becomes age appropriate. Once a child turns 3 and still requires therapy services, the family develops an Individualized Education Plan (IEP) with the school district, which provides them with access to a developmental preschool class and ongoing therapies including physical therapy (PT), occupational therapy (OT), speech and language pathology (SLP), and if needed vision therapy. School-based therapies tend to focus on access to a child's education, which changes as they age. In addition to school-based therapies, many children receive private outpatient therapies to supplement either throughout the year or as a boost of therapies over the summer while out of school. There are numerous methods of therapeutic intervention, a few of which will be described in the section that follows.

Goal-directed training/functional training involves repetitive gross or fine motor actions used to obtain a goal that is meaningful to the child; this has good evidence in the literature (39). Context-focused therapy is similar though it involves compensatory measures and environmental modifications to promote success in an activity. Partial body weight–supported treadmill training involves ambulation on a treadmill with variable amounts of support, allowing a child to focus on the quality of the movements with many repetitions (40).

Therapies focused on upper extremity function include constraint-induced movement therapy, which is used in children with hemiplegic CP and involves constraint of the unaffected arm followed by repetitive activity of the affected arm to promote its use (41). This as well as bimanual therapy are well supported in the literature. Bimanual therapy involves a structured program of repetitive activities using both hands together to promote bimanual use (42).

Orthoses (see Chapter 57)

Lower extremity orthoses can be helpful with providing stability to a joint, maintaining range of motion, and providing a prolonged stretch and may even be effective in improving gait dysfunction (43). In children with CP, one frequently used low-profile brace for children with hyperpronation is a supramalleolar orthosis (SMO), which extends the length of the foot and up just above the medial and lateral malleoli. It is used to provide medial-lateral support about the hindfoot. This is typically only used in a child who is just starting to stand and does not have excessive ankle plantar flexion tone or ankle dorsiflexor weakness. More commonly used is an ankle-foot orthosis (AFO), which extends the length of the foot and proximally to just below the knee. There are many variations, though the most commonly used AFOs include the posterior leaf spring (PLS), hinged AFO, solid ankle AFO, and ground reaction AFO (GRAFO). The PLS, a low-profile brace posteriorly, does not provide a great deal of medial-lateral support of the foot. It is generally used to provide support during the swing phase of gait for a child with footdrop and little plantar flexor tone. A solid AFO wraps around the ankle and the leg providing medial-lateral support of the hindfoot, preventing footdrop or plantar flexor spasticity, and providing stability to the knee in a patient with genu recurvatum (knee hyperextension). A hinged AFO is like a solid ankle AFO with the addition of a hinge allowing ankle dorsiflexion, but typically limiting the amount of plantar flexion. It is used in a child who needs medial-lateral support, who has ankle dorsiflexion range of motion, and who has the strength to maintain an upright position (strong enough ankle plantar flexors, knee extensors, and hip extensors). A GRAFO is like a solid ankle AFO except that the proximal portion wraps anteriorly around the leg resulting in an anterior to posterior moment about the knee preventing further knee flexion. It is used for children who are in crouch and have enough range of motion at their knees to tolerate its use. One study looking at the efficacy of various types of AFOs in the gait of children with CP demonstrated improved step length but otherwise no change in gait parameters (44).

The most commonly used upper extremity orthoses include both functional and nonfunctional splints. Nonfunctional splints are those worn at night for stretching purposes as they render the hand and wrist unable to perform functional tasks. This includes nighttime resting hand splints, which support the wrist and fingers into slight extension providing a prolonged stretch. Elbow splints are typically used for a prolonged stretch at nighttime, as they are not functional. There is some evidence to suggest that nonfunctional hand splints result in improved functional upper extremity measures (45). There are many types of functional hand and wrist splints, which are used to position the hand such that it can be used functionally such as a neoprene hand splint that maintains the thumb in an abducted position or the wrist and fingers in a neutral position. Some neoprene and nonneoprene splints provide wrist extension to place the fingers in a more functional position to support finger flexion or tenodesis.

Equipment

There is a variety of equipment that is used by children with CP depending on their functional level and care needs. Some of the most commonly used include assistive devices such as Lofstrand crutches, which provide a widened base of support for a higher functioning child who is ambulatory. A posterior walker is used in children who need more support in their ambulation but who have good trunk control. Those who have less trunk control in standing benefit from the use of a gait trainer. This provides support with a harness system allowing the child to be in an upright position to continue working on gait. In children who are not ambulatory, they may start with an off-the-shelf stroller and as they grow out of this can benefit from an adaptive stroller or, when age appropriate (age 2 or older), a wheelchair. For those children who have good truncal stability and upper extremity function, a lightweight manual wheelchair is the best option. For those children who are GMFCS level IV with impaired upper extremity function, a power wheelchair provides them with the most independence. Children also benefit from bath equipment for safe bathing. This can range from a tub bench for a child who has good trunk support to a shower commode chair with a tilt mechanism for a child who is a GMFCS level V and dependent for all cares. Car seats for younger children are important for safe transportation. As children age and grow, often a wheelchair-accessible vehicle is helpful for transportation in their wheelchair.

Hypertonicity and Movement Disorder Management

Hypertonicity and movement disorders are best treated initially with conservative measures such as therapy, stretching, range of motion, and bracing. Reasons for treatment with medication include impairment of a child's function, pain, or difficulty with cares such as diapering, dressing, bathing, or transfers. Despite its presumed negative impact, some children use their hypertonicity or dystonia in a functional way such as to maintain upright positioning for transfers in children with equinus. If conservative measures fail, then enteral medications can be useful in the treatment of generalized hypertonicity. Other treatments for generalized hypertonicity include intrathecal baclofen (ITB) and selective dorsal rhizotomy (SDR), which will be discussed below. Focal management of spasticity or dystonia targeting specific muscles is with chemodenervation or chemoneurolysis.

Enteral Medications

Enteral medications are initiated when the spasticity or dystonia is generalized, as an enteral medication has systemic effects on the child. Baclofen, a GABA-B agonist, is targeted to the spinal cord and results in a decrease in excitatory neurotransmitters. Side effects include sedation, constipation, and a theoretical lowering of the seizure threshold, though this has not been demonstrated in the literature. Studies of efficacy are conflicting and it has not clearly demonstrated improvements in spasticity or function in children with CP (46). Diazepam, also commonly used to treat spasticity, dystonia, and choreoathetosis, is a GABA-A agonist that functions by inhibition of mono- and polysynaptic reflexes as well as increasing presynaptic inhibition. Side effects include sedation, weakness, and constipation. Another consideration is that a child with epilepsy may not respond as well to seizure rescue with a benzodiazepine medication if they are on a scheduled dose of a similar medication due to tolerance. Studies of efficacy have demonstrated improvement in spasticity and range of motion and an increase in spontaneous movements but without demonstration of functional gains (46).

Commonly used medications for predominantly dystonia include trihexyphenidyl and carbidopa/levodopa. Trihexyphenidyl is an acetylcholine receptor antagonist; common side effects include constipation, dry mouth, urinary retention, and behavior changes. Carbidopa/levodopa is a combination medication in which the levodopa increases the dopamine release in the brain while the carbidopa decreases the peripheral dopamine decarboxylation, resulting in fewer side effects from peripheral action of the medication. Common side effects include gastrointestinal upset, dyskinesia, bradykinesia, and confusion.

Less commonly used medications, typically reserved for second- or third-line treatment of hypertonicity and dystonia, include dantrolene, clonidine, and tizanidine.

Chemodenervation and Chemoneurolysis

Chemodenervation and chemoneurolysis are both means of focal tone management used when there are target areas that don't necessitate an enteral medication with systemic effects. Chemodenervation is the process by which a botulinum toxin denervates the muscle into which it is injected. It is used, as is chemoneurolysis, for focal treatment of spasticity and dystonia. Botulinum toxins include onabotulinum toxin A, abobotulinum toxin A, incobotulinum toxin A, and rimabotulinum toxin B. These injectable medications act presynaptically blocking the release of acetylcholine into the neuromuscular junction. The onset is typically about 3 days with peak effect at about 3 weeks after injection. In children, often the results of the injection are seen anywhere from 3 to 6 months after the injection when paired with therapies, stretching, and bracing (46). Botulinum toxin is effective in improving the ease of care and comfort in nonambulatory children with CP (47). In children who are higher functioning, it is effective in improving upper extremity function when paired with OT and improving ambulation with PT when compared to PT alone (48,49). There is a theoretical risk that the botulinum toxin can spread to distant muscle groups resulting in weakness of respiratory muscles and dysphagia. This is described in case reports and thought to be related to either high doses of the botulinum toxin or other sedating medications that patients were receiving in combination with botulinum toxin (50–52).

Chemoneurolysis is the process by which phenol or alcohol causes nonselective axonal degeneration of peripheral nerve fascicles subsequently disrupting the reflex arc that causes hypertonicity. Injections are directed either at the nerve in a purely motor nerve (or almost purely motor nerve) such as the obturator nerve or at the endplate for mixed motor and sensory nerves such as the tibial division of the sciatic nerve. These injections are technically more challenging and require the use of anatomical localization as well as electrical stimulation to ensure that the medication is injected at the nerve or endplate. Phenol injections have been found to reduce spasticity and improve range of motion and function (53,54). The results of chemoneurolysis are thought to be immediate and lasting 6 months or longer in the majority of patients (55). One potential side effect is painful dysesthesias with sensory nerve involvement, which can be treated with gabapentin. There is also a risk of arrhythmia at higher doses of phenol and the risks associated with anesthesia given that phenol injections are done in children under general anesthesia in the operating room.

Intrathecal Baclofen Pump

An intrathecal baclofen (ITB) pump is a means of delivering baclofen directly into the intrathecal space via a programmable pump implanted subfascially into the abdomen and connected to a catheter that is threaded into the intrathecal space. This allows the delivery of baclofen directly into the cerebrospinal fluid (CSF) where it in turn reduces spasticity and dystonia at doses that are considerably lower and therefore with fewer side effects than enteral baclofen. Changes in the dose as well as mode of delivery (simple continuous, bolus dosing, etc.) can be made with a telemetry unit placed on the skin overlying the pump. ITB has been shown to be effective in the treatment of spasticity with improvements in comfort, ease of care, and quality of life in children with CP (56). Theoretically with a higher catheter tip placement, there can be more effect on the upper extremities, but there is no consensus on the appropriate level and how this affects outcomes. Complications of the ITB pump include CSF seroma, catheter kinking or dislodgement, infection, pump failure, and pump flip. Baclofen withdrawal is a medical emergency and typically presents with pruritus, increase in spasticity or dystonia, hyperthermia, tachycardia, hypertension, and seizures. Baclofen overdose is also a medical emergency presenting with decreased tone, decreased respiratory drive, altered mental status, hypothermia, hypotension, and seizures.

Selective Dorsal Rhizotomy

Selective dorsal rhizotomy (SDR) is a neurosurgical procedure for the treatment of spasticity in children. A lumbar laminectomy is performed to access the lumbosacral nerve roots. The ventral roots are isolated for specific target muscles with the use of neuromonitoring. Once isolated, a portion of the target dorsal roots are cut, in effect decreasing the sensory input that results in spasticity. The most successful candidate for SDR is a child who has spastic diplegic CP who functions at a GMFCS level II to III and is typically 3 to 8 years old. Given the effect on spasticity, postoperative course generally includes intensive rehabilitation for neuromuscular reeducation and eventual gait retraining. There is typically an initial decline in function followed by a slow improvement over time. Short-term effects include improved spasticity and improved

functional outcomes with SDR and PT compared to PT alone (57). Long-term outcomes have demonstrated improvements in lower limb muscle tone, gross motor function, and performance of activities of daily living (ADLs) at 1, 5, 10, and 15 years postoperatively (58).

Management of Musculoskeletal Conditions

Musculoskeletal deformities are common in CP and often require surgical intervention. The type of surgery, timing of surgery, and rehabilitation postoperatively are important in promoting ambulation in an ambulatory child or ease of care, positioning, and pain control in a nonambulatory child.

There are a number of approaches to lower extremity surgical intervention in children with CP. For many years, single-level or staged multilevel procedures were used, but resulted in numerous hospitalizations and periods of recovery often referred to as "birthday syndrome." This has led to the development and wide acceptance of a single-event multilevel surgery (SEMLS) in which multiple levels of orthopedic deformity are corrected in a single surgery and recovery period. This typically involves soft tissue tendon lengthening, muscle transfer, correction of bony deformity of the foot, and correction of rotational deformity and dislocation of the hip. SEMLS has been found to improve gait, though its long-term effects remain unclear at this time (59).

In the upper extremity, spasticity, dystonia, and muscle imbalance typically result in a position of shoulder internal rotation and adduction, elbow flexion, forearm pronation, wrist and finger flexion, and thumb in palm deformity. If these deformities are affecting function, causing difficulty with cares or hygiene, or resulting in skin breakdown, treatment is warranted. Typically, this is approached with stretching, range of motion, bracing, OT, and tone management. Should these conservative measures fail, surgical intervention is considered and includes tendon lengthening, tendon transfer, arthrodesis, or capsulodesis (36).

Scoliosis is monitored in children with CP, especially those who function at a GMFCS level IV or V given the higher incidence in that population. Bracing with a thoracolumbar-sacral orthosis (TLSO) is not thought to be effective in preventing progression of scoliosis, but can be used to improve sitting balance. It is difficult for most children to tolerate and therefore is used uncommonly. When a scoliotic curve progresses to a Cobb angle of greater than 40 to 50 degrees, surgical intervention is considered. In a child who has not reached skeletal maturity, growing rods that can be expanded as the child grows are used to prevent crankshaft deformity in which the anterior spine grows, as the posterior aspect is fused and unable to grow. Advances in this technology have resulted in the use of vertical expandable prosthetic titanium rods (VEPTR) and now magnetic expansion control (MAGEC) rods that do not require surgery to adjust for growth. Older children can undergo definitive spinal fusion surgery for treatment of scoliosis. This has been found to improve quality of life especially as it relates to pain in children who function at a GMFCS level IV or V (60).

Hypotonia

The differential diagnosis of hypotonia in the young patient—sometimes colloquially referred to as the "floppy infant"—is broad. Early on, CP may present with hypotonia. Prader-Willi syndrome and Angelman syndrome, both disorders of genomic imprinting involving chromosome 15, are marked by hypotonia. Prader-Willi syndrome is characterized by early failure to thrive and then hyperphagia; patients with Angelman syndrome are at risk for seizure and tend to have a happy demeanor. Beckwith-Wiedemann syndrome is also caused by an imprinting error, but involves chromosome 11. It is characterized by macroglossia and risk for certain childhood cancers, particularly Wilms tumor. Rett syndrome is an X-linked dominant disorder marked by developmental regression, seizures, and stereotyped movements, particularly hand flapping. Hypotonia is also a feature of trisomy 21 (Down syndrome), and the facies characteristic of this condition may aid in diagnosis. If the hypotonia is paroxysmal, alternating hemiplegia of childhood should be considered. Peripheral causes of hypotonia include Dejerine-Sottas syndrome. Botulism is an important acquired cause of infantile hypotonia. Other common causes of hypotonia are discussed in more detail below, but an exhaustive list is beyond the scope of this chapter. Referral to a geneticist should be strongly considered for all patients with hypotonia, particularly those without an established diagnosis.

Neuromuscular Disease

Over the past decade, the diagnosis of neuromuscular diseases, historically accomplished electrodiagnostically and by muscle biopsy, is increasingly accomplished by genetic testing (see Chapters 23 and 25). Furthermore, the availability of genetic therapies for some diseases has the potential to change the natural history of conditions for which few treatments were originally available.

Approach to Diagnosis

In the history and physical examination, one should look for evidence of hypotonia with weakness, disproportionately delayed motor milestones compared to other developmental areas, and hyporeflexia or areflexia. Serum creatine kinase (CK) is a useful laboratory test for possible primary muscle disease, although consistent elevations are seen in dystrophinopathies and inflammatory muscle disease only. Serum electrolytes (particularly potassium), organic acids (lactate, pyruvate), and amino acids (carnitine) may also be useful. Genetic testing has revolutionized our collective understanding of many neuromuscular disorders, but even in the era of increased availability of genetic testing, electrodiagnostic studies may be helpful in guiding further workup and avoiding more costly tests and procedures. A list (not exhaustive) of genetic loci of selected pediatric diseases is given in 🛜 **eTable 45-1**.

ANTERIOR HORN CELL DISEASES

Spinal Muscular Atrophy

Spinal muscular atrophy (SMA) is classified into multiple types based on severity of muscle weakness. Cognition is spared. The traditional natural history of SMA will be reviewed here, although the expected clinical course may now be quite different with the recent availability of genetic therapy, as noted later in this section. Guidelines for care of patients with SMA were published in 2007 (61).

SMA is an autosomal recessive disorder. The cause is a mutation of a gene on chromosome 5q13, SMN1, which codes for the SMN (survival motor neuron) protein. There is a

paralogous gene, SMN2, of which individuals have a variable number of copies. SMN2 also codes for SMN, but the majority of the protein coded for by SMN2 rapidly degrades, with only a small percentage being functional. SMN2 copy number is related to severity of phenotype.

Infantile SMA, or SMA I, also known as Werdnig-Hoffman disease, is seen in 1/15,000 to 25,000 live births. The onset of hypotonia (🛜 **eFig. 45-4**) and global weakness with facial muscle sparing within the first weeks of life is typical. Weakness is typically so profound that children with SMA I never sit independently. Tongue fasciculations are a hallmark and, if seen, may aid in diagnosis. Stretch reflexes are absent, but sensation is normal. Electrodiagnosis reveals normal motor conduction velocities but markedly decreased compound muscle action potential (CMAP) amplitudes. Sensory latencies and amplitudes are normal. EMG may demonstrate "chronic neuropathic" changes, although fibrillations may also be seen. Muscle biopsy shows rounded fibers, with areas of atrophy and compensatory hypertrophy. The clinical course, historically, was marked by death by age 2, although improvement in respiratory management and availability of genetic therapy now make longer survival more likely. Rehabilitative efforts should focus on provision of appropriately supportive adaptive seating and assistive technology for mobility and ADLs.

SMA II, sometimes known as intermediate SMA, has the onset of progressive weakness and areflexia later in infancy. Typically, patients with SMA II sit but do not walk. A few patients become limited household ambulators during childhood with the assistance of bracing and walkers. Fasciculations, including at the tongue, are more common and minipolymyoclonus is seen. In addition to the nerve conduction abnormalities seen in type I SMA, large-amplitude motor units are more frequent on needle EMG. A tremulous baseline in the EKG represents cardiac muscle fasciculations and is almost pathognomonic for this disease. The clinical course is one of gradual progression with long-term complications, including scoliosis, contractures, and respiratory insufficiency, typically leading to death in early adulthood (🛜 **eFig. 45-5**).

SMA III (Kugelberg-Welander disease) presents with proximal weakness during early childhood to young adulthood. Ambulation may be maintained into later years. EMG shows a chronic neuropathic pattern (minimal fibrillations and positive sharp waves with large-amplitude polyphasic motor unit action potentials and diminished recruitment).

In 2016, the FDA approved Spinraza (nusinersen), an antisense oligonucleotide therapy directed at SMN2, delivered intrathecally. Though adult data are lacking, the therapy is approved for all patients with SMA. Early studies indicate that improvement in achievement of motor milestones, as well as decreased dependence on ventilatory support, is possible with this therapy (62,63).

Acute Flaccid Myelitis

In the past decade, clusters of acute flaccid myelitis, some cases correlating with exposure to enterovirus D68, have been noted throughout the United States and worldwide (64). The disease process appears to affect the anterior horn cell. Limb and trunk weakness, often more notable proximally than distally, is a hallmark. Diaphragmatic paralysis is possible. To date, treatment with steroids, intravenous immunoglobulin, or plasmapheresis has not been shown to be beneficial. Prognosis is poor, with most children making no significant recovery in strength at 1-year follow-up (65). However, some functional gains were apparent as children learned compensatory mechanisms, suggesting the importance of rehabilitation for this disorder.

Congenital Myopathies of Infancy

Congenital myotonic dystrophies are autosomal dominant disorders transmitted from an affected mother. Type 1, often called DM1, is marked by typical features including severe hypotonia at birth with respiratory distress often requiring prolonged ventilator support (66). Facial diplegia with a characteristic triangular-shaped mouth, equinovarus contractures, and mental retardation are also seen (📶 **eFig. 45-6**). Clinical myotonia may not appear until 3 to 4 years of age, while electrical myotonia is rarely seen at birth and may be absent until 2 to 3 years old. Clinical diagnosis is confirmed genetically. An abnormal genetic locus on the long arm of chromosome 19 (19q13.3), involving the DMPK gene, results in a trinucleotide repeating sequence (CTG) (67). The number of repetitions, normally between 5 and 35, may be as high as 2,000 and is directly correlated with severity of disease, including cardiomyopathy (68). The genetic and clinical abnormalities tend to increase in severity with successive generations (termed genetic *anticipation*). The clinical course is one of gradual improvement with hypotonia no longer clinically significant by 4 years. All will eventually become at least household ambulators, although soft tissue surgeries and bracing may be required. Mild to moderate intellectual disability, exacerbated by oromotor immobility affecting expressive language skills more than receptive skills, is common. Multisystem disease consists of frontal baldness, cataracts, testicular atrophy in males, and smooth muscle and cardiac muscle dysfunction. Typically, life span is shortened, with death most commonly due to cardiac dysrhythmias.

Type 2, often called DM2, was previously known as proximal myotonic myopathy and is due to a mutation on the long arm of chromosome 3 (3q21), related to expansion of a CCTG repeat. The onset is typically in the third decade of life. Myotonia, muscle pain, and muscular weakness are hallmarks, but the clinical course tends to be milder than that of DM1.

The Myotonic Dystrophy Association has published guidelines for PT in individuals with myotonic dystrophy (69).

Note that these conditions are distinct from *myotonia congenita*, a channelopathy caused by a mutation in the CLCN1 gene.

Congenital muscular dystrophies (CMD) refer to a heterogeneous group of conditions, usually transmitted in an autosomal recessive pattern (📶 **eFig. 45-7**). They include structural protein (laminin, collagen) deficiencies (this category includes the disorders previously named Ullrich muscular dystrophy and Bethlem myopathy), dystroglycogenopathies (which previously included several named syndromes such as Walker-Warburg syndrome and Fukuyama muscular dystrophy), and Emery-Dreifuss muscular dystrophy. Impact on function, including cognition, ranges from mild to severe depending on the specific genetic disorder. In 2015, the AAN published evidence-based guidelines for the evaluation, diagnosis, and management of CMD (70).

Other myopathies are named after histologic changes seen in biopsy specimens treated with special staining techniques. Examples include nemaline myopathies, central core disease, centronuclear (myotubular) myopathy, and fiber-type disproportion (71). With improvements in genetic analysis, more is becoming known about the genetic basis of these histopathologic findings (72).

Myasthenic Syndromes

Transient neonatal myasthenia is due to maternal antibodies that cross the placenta. A weak cry and weak suck are typically noted, and the infant may need respiratory support. The syndrome is self-limited, once the maternal antibodies leave the infant's circulation.

Congenital myasthenic syndromes, by contrast, represent a group of genetic disorders. Most are inherited in an autosomal recessive pattern, though some forms are autosomal dominant. Serum acetylcholine receptor antibodies are absent. Diagnosis can and should be made genetically, since medical treatment depends on subtype. The onset is early in life, typically by the age of 2—some forms can present later. In the neonatal period, respiratory insufficiency is common, and joint contractures have been reported. Weakness worsens with repeated activity. Facial weakness is common. Cognition is usually normal. Rehabilitation interventions include PT, OT, and SLP and provision of orthoses and equipment to assist mobility.

Autoimmune MG occurs with a prevalence of 5 to 10/100,000 population and is four times as frequent in females. Clinically, abnormal fatigue occurs after activity and improves with rest. The onset is usually insidious although it may present precipitously after a febrile illness, allergic reaction, or emotional upset. The most common presenting sign is ptosis (ocular MG) that increases with reading and is accompanied by compensatory forehead wrinkling. Facial weakness may also be seen, presenting as a slack jaw, slurred speech or difficulty swallowing, and limb weakness, proximal more than distal with a positive Gower sign and Trendelenburg gait. Tensilon, a short-acting AChE, given intravenously, reverses weakness within 30 to 60 seconds and lasts 5 to 10 minutes. Electrodiagnostic testing reveals a decrement of more than 10% on 2 to 3 Hz stimulation, while single-fiber EMG (SFEMG) shows abnormal jitter but is difficult to perform in children. Finally, antibodies to ACh receptors (anti-AChR Abs) can be measured and are elevated in 85% to 90% of patients with generalized MG, but only 50% in ocular MG. Treatment is based on either improving NMJ transmission with AChEs or decreasing the lytic effect of anti-AChR Abs by steroids, immunosuppressive therapy, or thymectomy. Commonly used AChEs include Prostigmin (neostigmine) or Mestinon (pyridostigmine). IV gamma globulin or plasma exchange is sometimes employed during crisis. The role of thymectomy is still somewhat controversial, but a recent randomized controlled trial found that patients who underwent thymectomy had improved time-weighted average Quantitative Myasthenia Gravis scores over a 3-year period and improved outcomes, including decreased requirement for immunosuppression and fewer hospitalizations for exacerbations (73).

MUSCULAR DYSTROPHY

Duchenne Muscular Dystrophy

Duchenne muscular dystrophy (DMD), an X-linked recessive disorder, is seen in 1 to 3/10,000 male births. The gene coding for dystrophin, on the short arm of the X chromosome (Xp21), is the largest gene in the human body. The dystrophin protein links the extracellular matrix to the actin cytoskeleton, stabilizing the sarcolemma (74). Deficiency of dystrophin leads to collapse of the muscle cell membrane and fatty infiltration of the muscle. Many different mutations may affect this gene. Mutations that cause a loss of the reading frame most often lead to DMD and a more severe phenotype, whereas mutations that maintain the reading frame result in a truncated but still somewhat functional protein and the less severe phenotype of *Becker muscular dystrophy* (BMD).

The first sign of weakness is typically noted at the neck flexors. Gait deviations present after 2 years of age eventually lead to a Trendelenburg gait, pathognomonic of hip abductor weakness. Patients come to stand through the Gower maneuver, pathognomonic of proximal pelvic girdle weakness. Gradually, a characteristic posture of tight heel cords, calf pseudohypertrophy (sometimes also deltoid hypertrophy), a widely abducted stance, and hyperlordosis develops. Intellectual disability is seen in about one third. CK is markedly elevated, maximally in the preclinical stage, with values greater than 10,000 not unusual. A "myopathic" EMG (brief, small-amplitude, abundant polyphasic potentials, early recruitment) is seen. Biopsy shows variation in fiber size, fiber splitting, central nuclei, fibrous/fatty replacement, and absence of type 2B fibers.

Therapeutically, ongoing drug trials continue. In 2016, Exondys 51 (eteplirsen) received accelerated approval from U.S. FDA as an exon-skipping therapy for patients with a known mutation in dystrophin amenable to exon-51 skipping. Because some but not all individuals with DMD may be candidates for available genetic therapies, diagnosis of DMD should always be made genetically. Many different therapeutic targets have been identified, involving different potential strategies for treatment of the disease (including but not limited to gene replacement, anti-inflammatories, and antifibrotics). The status of clinical trials is rapidly changing—refer to https://clinicaltrials.gov for a recent list. As of this writing, https://www.duchenne-connect.org also provides a list of trials, with family-friendly summaries provided as well.

The clinical course is variable, with loss of ambulation typically in the first part of the second decade. Steroids can prolong ambulation somewhat; prednisone or deflazacort is used, with the latter (under the trade name Emflaza) recently gaining FDA approval in the United States. The age at loss of ambulation occurs may depend in part on the underlying mutation (75).

Care of the Patient with DMD

Multidisciplinary care guidelines for the diagnosis and management of DMD were published in 2010 (76,77). In an effort to improve adherence to these guidelines, streamlined "imperatives" were introduced in 2015 (78).

Functional Considerations

For fitness, submaximal exercise has been recommended (79). Patients are taught to "listen to their body," and if there is muscle pain, activity should be modified to avoid this. Stretching and range of motion are important to minimize risk for contracture. AFOs are used in the nighttime for this purpose, but typically avoided in the daytime since patients with DMD tend to use a plantar flexion moment at the ankle to stabilize the knee. Knee-ankle-foot orthoses (KAFOs) are sometimes used in the late ambulatory phase to prolong ambulation. An ultralightweight manual wheelchair with solid seat is often considered during this phase. As lower extremity strength and mobility decline, power mobility is offered; with decline in upper extremity strength, access to environmental controls should be provided.

Pulmonary

Respiratory disease is a major cause of morbidity and mortality in DMD. Assisted ventilation has had a profound effect on the natural history. In addition to recommendations published in the multidisciplinary guidelines mentioned above, guidelines for management have also been published by the American Thoracic Society (ATS) (80).

Patients of all ages should have access to a pulmonologist and routine immunizations, including pneumococcal vaccine and yearly influenza vaccine. In the ambulatory patient, annual assessment of sitting forced vital capacity (FVC) is recommended. ATS guidelines recommend evaluation by a physician specializing in respiratory care at least once between the ages of 4 and 6 for assessment including baseline pulmonary function tests (PFTs), as well as anticipatory guidance.

Once the patient is nonambulatory, the 2010 guidelines by Bushby et al. recommend that routine evaluations should include oxyhemoglobin saturation, sitting FVC, and peak cough flow, at least every 6 months. The ATS guidelines add spirometric measurements of FEV1, maximal midexpiratory flow rate, and maximum inspiratory and expiratory pressures. The ATS guidelines also recommend assessment of CO_2 (optimally by capnography) at least yearly, as well as annual CBC, serum bicarbonate concentration, and chest radiograph. The patient should be assessed for sleep-disordered breathing and, if available, should have annual polysomnography.

There are a multitude of techniques for management of the respiratory status of the individual with DMD, and these generally proceed in a stepwise fashion as the disease progresses (eBox 45-2).

Cardiac

In DMD, the heart is almost always affected by progressive cardiomyopathy, and patients are also at risk for ventricular arrhythmias. With improvement in respiratory management, cardiac causes have become the leading cause of death in DMD (80). Traditionally, EKG and echocardiograms formed the mainstay of evaluation; more recently, the value of cardiovascular MRI for the evaluation of asymptomatic patients has been acknowledged (81). Dilated cardiomyopathy primarily involves the left ventricle, and treating this before the patient becomes symptomatic is recommended. Angiotensin-Converting Enzyme (ACE) inhibitors or angiotensin-receptor blockers often constitute first-line therapy; the use of a beta-blocker with an ACE inhibitor improves survival in presymptomatic patients with left ventricular dysfunction (82). Right ventricle failure can result from respiratory failure and pulmonary hypertension.

Recommendations call for echocardiogram at diagnosis or age 6, then every 2 years until age 10, and annually thereafter (76). EKG should be done at each cardiology visit. Monitoring for hypertension is important when the patient is on steroids.

Gastrointestinal and Nutrition

Both undernutrition and obesity are potential concerns for the child with DMD over the course of the life span. Steroids are associated with weight gain (83). Some, but not all (84), studies suggest that deflazacort may lead to less weight gain than prednisone. Weight should be monitored routinely, and patients should be referred for a nutritional assessment at diagnosis, at initiation of steroids, or if concern for weight, if planning major surgery, if there is suspicion for dysphagia, or if there is chronic constipation (76). Constipation is managed with stool softeners and other laxatives, as well as by attention to adequate fluid intake. Gastroesophageal reflux may develop and is treated with medications typical for this condition. Videofluoroscopic swallowing study should be considered once there is concern for dysphagia. If swallowing dysfunction is severe or weight cannot be maintained, gastrostomy tube placement is considered.

Conditions Affecting Bone

Patients with DMD are at risk for scoliosis, though use of steroids appears to ameliorate this risk somewhat (85). However, with steroids, risk of fracture is increased. Spinal radiographs are done around the time of transition to a wheelchair, unless scoliosis is noted earlier. Guidelines suggest this should be done annually for curves of 15 to 20 degrees and every 6 months for curves greater than 20 degrees, until spinal maturity (76). Evidence suggests posterior spinal fusion improves quality of life, but there is some debate regarding its effect on respiratory function in patients with DMD (⌃ **eFig. 45-8**) (86).

Fractures are common, and guidelines suggest assessment of markers of bone health, including calcium, phosphate, alkaline phosphatase, and vitamin D level (76). Baseline DEXA scan should be obtained, and this should also be assessed at the start of steroid therapy; for those at high risk, this should be repeated annually (76). For patients who do experience fracture, bisphosphonates are sometimes used, but controversy remains (87). Case reports suggest that patients with DMD who experience fracture may be at particular risk for development of fat embolism syndrome (88).

Psychosocial Concerns

All patients with DMD should have at least an informal emotional status assessment at every visit. Assessment by a social worker or other social services professional should be offered. Because there may be a higher risk for neuropsychiatric disorders in children with DMD, referral to speech-language pathology should be initiated if there are concerns for speech or language delays; referral to a specialist should be initiated if there is concern for autism spectrum disorder (89). For children at least 5 years old, neuropsychological assessment is recommended at or near diagnosis, and prior to the start of schooling, with comprehensive developmental assessment made available for younger children (76).

End-of-Life Planning

Advance care planning is important in the care of the individual with DMD. Though medical professionals acknowledge that end-of-life directives are a critical part of anticipatory care, studies indicate that many families may be reluctant to discuss end-of-life issues during times of stability, and it is not unusual for families to rescind decisions that they made earlier (90). Education about ventilatory and palliative options should be discussed prior to ventilatory failure (80). However, though anticipatory guidance is recommended, this issue is further complicated because there is evidence that health care

professionals underestimate the quality of life of ventilator-dependent people with DMD (91). Before the end of life, palliative care should be offered, as well as hospice care when appropriate.

Other Muscular Dystrophies

The presentation of *facioscapulohumeral muscular dystrophy* (FSHD) is often in adolescent or early adult years. Facial weakness often precedes shoulder girdle weakness. In later years, there may be progression to abdominal and pelvic girdle muscles. Associated abnormalities include high- (and rarely low-) frequency hearing loss and retinal abnormalities (telangiectasia, microaneurysms) in up to 75%. There are no cardiac abnormalities and cognition is preserved. CK elevation and muscle biopsy changes may be minimal. An abnormal genetic locus has been found at the 4q35 site.

Limb-girdle muscular dystrophies refer to a group of genetic disorders marked by proximal muscle wasting. Age of onset is variable, though many present in childhood; muscles at the pelvic girdle are frequently the first affected. Some of the limb-girdle muscular dystrophies are autosomal dominant, while others are autosomal recessive. Guidelines for treatment and management of LGMD were published in 2010 (92).

Neonatal Brachial Plexus Palsy

Neonatal brachial plexus palsy (NBPP) is an injury to the brachial plexus, including cervical nerves, C5-8 and thoracic, T1, often due to complications of birth. The reported incidence of NBPP in the United States is 1.5 per 1,000 live births (93). The mechanism of injury is traction of the brachial plexus during delivery resulting in neurapraxia, axonotmesis, neurotmesis, or avulsion of the nerve roots, which translates into a spectrum of clinical presentation and recovery. Risk factors include shoulder dystocia, large for gestational age (>4.5 kg), forceps delivery, vacuum extraction, and breech delivery (93).

Presentation depends on the portion of the brachial plexus involved. An upper trunk palsy, or Erb's palsy, involves C5 and C6 presenting with a "waiter's tip" with the shoulder internally rotated and adducted, elbow extended, and forearm pronated (⌃ **eFig. 45-9**). This is due to weakness in shoulder abduction, external rotation, elbow flexion, and forearm supination. An extended Erb's palsy, involving C5, C6, and C7, additionally presents with impaired finger extension, wrist extension, and elbow extension. A lower trunk palsy, otherwise known as Klumpke's palsy, involves C8 and T1, presenting with weakness in the intrinsic muscles of the hand, finger flexors and wrist flexors (⌃ **eFig. 45-10**), though this is quite rare. A pan plexus injury involving the brachial plexus in its entirety presents with a flail arm with flaccid paralysis. Additionally, Horner's syndrome (ptosis, miosis, and anhydrosis) can be present with avulsion of the lower nerve roots from the spinal cord and resulting from disconnection of the sympathetic chain. Other portions of the birth history that may be reported include clavicle fracture, humeral fracture, cervical spine fracture (though less common), and respiratory distress secondary to diaphragm dysfunction (innervated by cervical roots C3-5).

Many neonates present with deficits that resolve fully, with estimates upward of 90%, though more conservative studies report 20% to 30% with residual deficits (94). Some studies report lower residual deficit (14% without complete recovery) with C5-6 injuries compared to more persistent deficits in those with more extensive injuries involving C7 (62% without complete recovery) (95). Those with ongoing deficits should be monitored for recovery while receiving PT.

The focus of PT in the neonate with brachial plexus palsy is typically on a stretching program to maintain range of motion and prevent contracture as well as working on age-appropriate developmental skills. These children are at risk for developing contractures, especially in shoulder internal rotation, elbow flexion, and forearm pronation. Other therapeutic interventions include constraint-induced movement therapy, which involves constraining the unaffected arm to promote recovery of the affected arm. There is little literature to support this, most in the form of case reports and case series (96,97). Electrical stimulation is another intervention with limited evidence, though with some support for use in shoulder function and bone mineralization in children with NBPP (98).

While engaging in therapies, monitoring continues in the first years of life and is done with the use of the active movement scale (AMS), which is a common measure used to grade strength and subsequently to guide decision-making for intervention in the treatment of NBPP. Other commonly used scales include the Toronto Score Grading System and the Modified Mallet, among others. These can be useful in determining if a brachial plexus exploration and reconstruction surgery would be beneficial. The presence of antigravity elbow flexion, for example, is often used as a guide at 3 months and for some providers up to 9 to 12 months to predict need for or benefit from nerve reconstruction surgery (99). This is undertaken by a plastic surgeon or a neurosurgeon trained in peripheral nerve surgery. It can involve neurotization, neurolysis, nerve transfer and excision, and grafting of donor peripheral nerves. A meta-analysis by Coroneos and colleagues has demonstrated that nerve repair reduces functional impairments in neonates with obstetric-related brachial plexus palsy (100).

In addition to monitoring of neurologic recovery, it is also important to monitor the development of the glenohumeral joint due to the risk of glenohumeral dysplasia (GHD). This is thought to be due to muscle imbalance with strong shoulder internal rotators and weak or absent external rotators resulting in glenoid abnormality and humeral head subluxation posteriorly. Studies demonstrate that GHD can present as early as 3 months and should be followed closely with serial examinations and shoulder ultrasound (101). In addition to conventional PT including stretching and range of motion, there are emerging studies on the use of passive bracing of the forearm into supination and the shoulder into external rotation, using a Sup-ER splint, which has been found to improve function in NBPP (102). Botulinum toxins can also be used in some instances to weaken the tight internal rotators to prevent shoulder subluxation and allow external rotator recovery. It can also be used to weaken the triceps when there is cocontraction of the triceps and biceps to allow for further recovery of the biceps. Onabotulinum toxin A has been demonstrated to be effective in management of muscle imbalance in NBPP (103).

Despite early monitoring and treatment, both surgical and nonsurgical, a portion of these neonates go on to have impairments into childhood and adulthood. Their affected limb is often smaller in size with tightness or contracture in the shoulder internal rotators, elbow flexors, and forearm pronators, which can limit function. Surgical intervention in childhood in the form of tendon transfers and nerve transfers is a

possibility depending on age and function of potential donor muscles or nerves.

Childhood Torticollis

Torticollis may be congenital or acquired. Congenital muscular torticollis, common in infants, is associated with a nontender, soft enlargement in the sternocleidomastoid (SCM) muscle, the so-called olive sign, which may be seen within the first 6 weeks (104). It is mobile within the belly of the muscle, gradually decreases in size, and is usually gone within 4 to 6 months. Secondary deformities including flattening of the ipsilateral face and orbital asymmetry can be seen (105). Plagiocephaly is a common comorbidity (106). Acquired torticollis has a broad differential diagnosis, including tumor, ocular disorders, and vertebral abnormalities (107).

The treatment of congenital torticollis should be based first on correcting identified etiologic factors. PT may hasten improvement in range of motion (108); conservative therapy should include stretching of the tight neck muscles as well as functional strengthening of contralateral neck muscles by use of lateral and anterior head righting reactions. Directing the gaze toward the ipsilateral superior direction should also be encouraged. The use of skull-shaping orthoses has been advocated as an additional cosmetic corrective measure although much controversy exists (109). Surgical intervention is sometimes considered when other methods have failed, but here, too, controversy exists as to the optimal timing of the procedure; it has been suggested that the patient's ability to adhere to a postoperative rehabilitation regimen is an important factor in this regard (110).

SPINAL CORD DYSFUNCTION (SEE ALSO CHAPTER 22)

There are multiple etiologies of pediatric spinal cord dysfunction including congenital (e.g., spinal dysraphism), acquired traumatic spinal cord injury, vascular causes such as AVM or spinal cord infarction, infectious or autoimmune disorders, and tumors. In addition to presenting key distinctions between pediatric and adult traumatic spinal cord injury (see Chapter 22), this chapter provides an overview of the management of spina bifida, the most common spinal dysraphism (111).

Traumatic Spinal Cord Injury

The reported incidence of pediatric traumatic spinal cord injury varies among studies, but is much lower than in the adult population. Cervical injury, and therefore quadriplegia, is comparatively more common. This is in part because young children have proportionally larger heads compared to their body size. Therefore, the fulcrum of injury is higher resulting in higher cervical injuries than in adults (112).

Anatomical differences between the child and the adult patient predispose the child to spinal cord injury without radiographic abnormalities (SCIWORA). This condition, first defined by Pang in 1982 (113), originally referred to clinical evidence of myelopathy without radiographic evidence on radiographs or CT. (With the advent of MRI, some authors/clinicians have raised the issue that term should be used only if no MRI findings are present, but they also indicate further discussion on this issue is warranted.) (114) The pediatric spinal column is more elastic than that of an adult and so may stretch more than the spinal cord can tolerate (115). SCIWORA typically occurs in the cervical region and is more common in younger children than in older children.

Another pattern of injury seen in the pediatric population is spinal cord injury resulting from an improperly placed lap belt. The classic triad is that of abdominal wall bruising, intra-abdominal injury, and spinal fracture—in a series studied by Achildi et al., vertebral fractures were associated with spinal cord injury in 11% (116).

Examination of the Patient with Pediatric SCI

The exam of the pediatric patient is often limited by the child's ability to cooperate. Because of this, it may not be possible in many cases to designate the injury as complete or incomplete or to assign an ASIA Impairment Scale grade. At approximately age 5, depending on the cognitive abilities of the child, accurate manual muscle testing can be performed. It is important to remember that when assessing the pediatric patient, the resistance during manual muscle testing is not the same as exhibited by an adult. In children who cannot participate in manual muscle testing, observational motor exam is recommended. For children younger than age 6, sensory level should be estimated. Grading the sensory exam in infants is virtually impossible and only an estimate of the sensory level can be obtained. Intrarater agreement for the anorectal exam has been characterized as poor for children (and even adolescents) (117). The child's response to anorectal (grimace, cry) can be documented for the child who is preverbal or who had not yet been toilet-trained.

Neurogenic Bowel and Bladder

In infants and very young children who had not yet achieved continence prior to their injury, initiation of a bowel program is sometimes delayed and then introduced later to promote social continence as appropriate. Intermittent catheterization to manage neurogenic bladder is typically introduced in the early postacute phase once an indwelling catheter is removed (118). As the practitioner monitors bladder volumes, bladder capacity in the child can be estimated by adding two to the child's age in years, which gives the capacity in ounces (1 oz is equal to 30 mm) (119) Surveillance of the urinary tract with regular renal ultrasound and with urodynamics is important to monitor urinary tract health and function (120).

There are limited data on venous thromboembolism (VTE) in the pediatric patients with spinal cord injury. The incidence seems to be less than in the adult population. Schottler et al. found an incidence of 2.2% in a study of 159 patients (121). Leeper et al., in a retrospective review of 753 pediatric trauma patients, reported an incidence of 8.9% (122). For the immature adolescent and child, the issue of VTE prophylaxis is not clear-cut and further investigation is warranted (123).

Spinal Dysraphism

The spectrum of spinal dysraphism includes both open and closed defects. The most common open defect is myelomeningocele (also called meningomyelocele and sometimes abbreviated MMC), which involves the significant disruption of all elements of the bony spine, typically with an open malformed neural tube covered by a membranous sac. If only the meninges herniate into the sac, this is termed meningocele. In anencephaly, there is failure of neural tube closure in the cranial region. Prenatal detection of these defects, originally enabled by assessment of alpha-fetoprotein, now is also done by fetal ultrasound (124). Closed spinal dysraphism is sometimes known as spina bifida occulta. Prevalence is quite high, over 20% in some series (125), and the defect may occur with or without subcutaneous lipoma. Visible stigmata may include a dimple or tuft of hair in the sacral region, though there may be no obvious clinical signs (126). Sometimes, the condition may come to attention because of urologic concerns or back pain.

Demographics

In the United States, it is estimated that about 1,500 infants are born each year with spina bifida (127), and individuals of Hispanic origin have a higher risk for neural tube defects, whereas the risk is lowest among African Americans (128). The incidence is decreasing worldwide, particularly in countries that mandate folic acid fortification of foods (see below (129)).

Etiology

The specific etiology of neural tube defects has not been elicited. However, the etiology seems to be multifactorial, involving genetic and nongenetic factors. Evidence for the former includes studies that show a 2% to 5% risk that a future sibling of an individual with myelomeningocele will also be affected (129,130), with a 10% risk if a woman has had two affected pregnancies. If one parent has spina bifida, the risk that the child will also have spina bifida has been estimated at 4% (131). A variation (C677T) in a gene coding for methylenetetrahydrofolate reductase (MTHFR) has also been found to be associated with neural tube defects. Evidence that nongenetic factors play a role includes the implication of hot tub or sauna use during early pregnancy as a risk factor, as well as studies indicating that maternal use of valproic acid or carbamazepine increases risk (132). Studies also indicate that maternal diabetes and maternal obesity raise the risk for neural tube defects (133).

The risk of recurrence can be reduced by up to 70% with periconceptual use of folic acid (134). The Centers for Disease Control and Prevention (CDC) recommends that all women of childbearing age consume 0.4 mg/d of folic acid. Multiple organizations, including the American College of Obstetricians and Gynecologists and the CDC, believe that higher doses such as 4 mg/d should be used if the woman has already had a child with a neural tube defect (135). The exact mechanism of folic acid in prevention has not yet been determined, though it has been proposed that it is involved in methylation of septin2, a regulator of cilium structure and function (136).

Surgical Closure

Sac closure is usually performed within the first 24 to 48 hours to reduce the risk of infection. Microsurgical closure with reapproximation of the neural tube and construction of a fluid-filled pouch to "bathe" the cord has reduced the incidence of early tethering of the spinal cord.

Newer neurosurgical techniques now involve in utero repair. Patients undergoing fetal myelomeningocele repair have been shown to have a reduction in need for ventriculoperitoneal (VP) shunt placement at 1 year of life, an improvement in neuromotor function at 30 months of age including an improvement in ambulation, and less hindbrain herniation. However, risks include premature birth (137).

ASSOCIATED NEUROLOGIC ABNORMALITIES

Chiari Malformation Type II and Hydrocephalus

The Chiari malformation type II, associated with a small posterior fossa and common in myelomeningocele, is defined as downward displacement of the inferior portion of the cerebellar vermis, the medulla, lower pons, and an elongated ("slit-like") fourth ventricle through the foramen magnum. Other abnormalities seen include a beaked tectum and an associated kinking of the medulla.

The brainstem abnormalities lead to swallowing difficulty, stridor, and apnea, which can sometimes be fatal. Hydrocephalus occurs in a significant percentage of patients with spina bifida. Rintoul et al. have suggested that the need for a shunt may be dependent on the level of the lesion; in their series, while 100% of infants with a thoracic-level lesion received a shunt, only 68% of those with a sacral-level lesion received one (138). More recently, endoscopic third ventriculostomy has shown promise as a possible alternative to shunt placement (139).

Tethered Cord

While descriptions of the phenomenon of cord tethering were published earlier (140), the 1976 description of "tethered spinal cord" by Hoffman et al. referred to patients with a low-lying conus medullaris in which the cord was fixed by a thickened terminal filum (141). More recently, others have chosen to define the tethered cord syndrome as a "stretch-induced functional disorder of the spinal cord with its caudal part anchored by an inelastic structure" (142).

A tethered spinal cord may be due to a lipoma, scarring at the closure site, or diastematomyelia (i.e., split-cord syndrome). Presenting symptoms may include deterioration in bladder and bowel function, loss of strength or sensation, spasticity (or, occasionally, decreased tone,) low back pain or radicular pain, and/or rapidly progressive scoliosis. However, the imaging diagnosis is distinct from the clinical syndrome—that is, not all patients with imaging findings of a low-lying conus or a thick filum will have symptoms. A tethered cord is present in almost all patients with meningomyelocele though it may be asymptomatic (143).

The issue of when and whether to perform surgery is the subject of some controversy. Though there is consensus that surgical detethering is indicated for the symptomatic patient with a thickened filum, opinions differ on the management of the asymptomatic patient (144,145). Even after surgery, retethering can occur.

Syringomyelia

Syringomyelia refers to central canal dilation extending across multiple segments. The term is sometimes used interchangeably with hydromyelia, where CSF dilates the central canal. Multiple etiologic theories have been proposed, but the cause remains unknown. Presenting symptoms include deterioration of neurologic function, loss of sensory and motor function in the upper limbs, and spasticity. Scoliosis is an early sign. Patients with syringomyelia may also be asymptomatic. Shunting is often done for patients whose symptoms interfere with function.

Cognition

Many individuals with spina bifida have intellectual disability. On neuropsychological profiling, verbal ability may be a relative strength compared to nonverbal abilities (146). A study by Swartwout et al. found that lower socioeconomic status is associated with lower verbal IQ in Hispanic children with spina bifida. Deficits in attention and executive function are common (147). Baseline neuropsychological assessment will be helpful around the age that the child starts school, and this testing should be updated as the child ages.

ORTHOPEDIC ISSUES

Lower Extremity

Imbalance of muscular forces around the hip places the patient with spina bifida at risk for subluxation/dislocation as well as contracture. The child with L3-level myelomeningocele is particularly at risk for hip dislocation, due to unopposed hip flexion and adduction (148). However, it appears that the patient's neurologic level, rather than the reduction of the hip, most influences the ability to ambulate (149,150). Contracture release appears to have a role in improving gait symmetry (151).

Depending on neurologic level, the knees may be at risk for flexion contracture or extension contracture. In the ambulatory patient, releases for knee flexion contracture can improve gait. In the nonambulatory patient, it may only be necessary to consider releases if contractures interfere with seating/positioning. The initial management of knee extension contractures is often by serial casting, with surgery considered if this fails (152). Knee pain is common, due to stresses on the knee as a result of weakness and muscular imbalance, and when available, gait analysis is helpful to evaluate which factors are contributing to this. Femoral and tibial torsion may be seen, with tibial torsion being more common. As above, gait analysis may be helpful as osteotomy is considered.

Abnormalities of the foot/ankle affect almost all individuals with spina bifida. Patterns seen include clubfoot (often corrected by the Ponseti method early in life), equinus, calcaneal deformity, hindfoot deformity, and vertical talus. Though surgery to achieve a plantigrade foot is regarded as helpful for ambulators, patients undergoing such surgery still remain at risk for pressure ulcers and, potentially later, amputations (153).

Spine (see also Chapter 28)

Spinal deformity is common in patients with spina bifida. Kyphosis may be present in the thoracic or lumbar region. Congenital kyphosis is seen in up to 20%, but the condition may also be acquired (154). With lumbar kyphosis, a compensatory thoracic lordosis is seen. With progression of the kyphosis (despite use of bracing), skin ulcers can occur at the apex of the curvature.

Scoliosis is common as well, and the prevalence of this condition, but not its severity, is correlated with the patient's motor level (155). Whether or not to undertake spinal surgery to correct the scoliosis is a matter of debate. Studies suggest that, if performed, a combined anterior and posterior approach has better rates of curve correction and lower rates of nonunion (150). However, relatively few studies have investigated functional outcomes after surgery. Wright, in a 2011 review of the evidence, found that the clinical relevance of a possible small improvement in pulmonary function is not clear, and though there may be some improvement with sitting/positioning, some studies indicate that ambulation may decline after surgery (150).

Genitourinary

The majority of patients with spina bifida have a neurogenic bladder. In addition, there are associated genitourinary abnormalities seen in up to 20% of patients including horseshoe kidneys, hypoplastic kidneys, or renal agenesis, as well as ureteral duplications and posterior urethral valves.

A renal ultrasound should be performed early in infancy to delineate the anatomy. A voiding cystourethrogram (VCUG) can define bladder contour and determine the presence of ureteral reflux. Since the physiology can change over the first year of life, serial ultrasounds should be performed regularly to monitor the status of the kidneys and detect any changes that would necessitate further intervention. Most patients will be managed with clean intermittent catheterization (CIC). The age at which this should begin is still controversial, with some practitioners advocating "expectant" management and other practitioners choosing a proactive approach (156). While the caregiver will manage catheterization initially, children with good fine motor skills and good cognition can be taught self-catheterization at approximately age 5.

The long-term goals of bladder management are to prevent renal damage by preventing infection (though the use of prophylactic antibiotics remains controversial), by preventing reflux, and also to prevent wetness between catheterizations. As the patient ages, routine renal-bladder ultrasounds should be performed every 6 to 12 months in order to properly monitor the urologic system. Pharmacologic intervention may be needed based on the results of urodynamics and the patient's clinical status with anticholinergic medication such as oxybutynin being used for spastic bladders.

Surgical procedures include bladder augmentation for small-capacity bladders, urethral implantation for patients with reflux, and suprapubic vesicostomy to allow for an alternative method of drainage. The Mitrofanoff procedure, in which a catheterizable conduit is created between the bladder and the surface of the skin, can be helpful for patients in order to promote independence (157). The artificial sphincter is an implantable device used to help achieve urinary continence. In the past decade, procedures for neural reconstruction have shown promise, though authors investigating the application of these techniques for spina bifida indicate further studies are needed (158).

Bowel

Training in timed bowel regulation may be started by 2 to 3 years of developmental age. Every effort should be made to achieve at least social continence, to limit stigmatization and the impact on socialization.

Since peristalsis and the gastrocolic reflex are still intact, evacuations after meals are usually more successful. Diet is an important component of the bowel program. Adequate fluid intake is important as well as knowing which foods soften or harden the stools. Bulk additives, stimulant suppositories, and enemas may be needed. Transanal colonic irrigation can be helpful for some patients (159). For patients with uncontrollable incontinence, the Malone antegrade continence enema (ACE) provides a surgical alternative, with a conduit using either the cecum or the appendix between the intestine and the abdominal wall. This is a catheterizable conduit that can be used to deliver tap water or saline enemas and allow for evacuation through the rectum. Another alternative is a Chait cecostomy, in which a tube is placed in the cecum that remains in place. An adapter can then be hooked to this tube for delivery of an anterograde enema.

Skin

Patients with spina bifida are at risk for decubitus sores due to impaired mobility and impaired sensation. Occipital decubiti are more common in younger children that are immobile due to the large head size. Lower extremities are a common site for ulcers due to poorly fitting orthotics and improper biomechanics created by muscle imbalance and associated foot deformities, but bare feet are also a risk factor (160). Those dependent on wheelchair mobility are susceptible to pressure in the ischial and sacral areas. Frequent pressure relief and an appropriate cushion are imperative, and pressure mapping may be necessary for more complex cases. Meticulous skin care is important with weight shifts being done routinely by the family/caregivers and ultimately the child once they are older. However, a recent study by Psihogios et al. showed that increasing a child's responsibility to manage his or her own skin checks was related to greater nonadherence to checking the skin, suggesting the importance of continued parental involvement even as the child ages (161). For advanced wounds, surgical closure or even amputation may ultimately be necessary.

Latex

Latex protein allergy should be considered in every child with meningomyelocele. Historically, it was estimated that 18% to 40% of children with meningomyelocele were latex sensitive (162). Previous reports indicated that atopic disposition, number of operations, and presence of a shunt increase the risk of becoming not only sensitized but also allergic to latex (163), but more recent data call this into question (164). Certain catheters are also a potential source of latex exposure. In recent years in the United States, the avoidance of latex in hospital settings seems to be correlated with a decrease in the number of cases of latex sensitivity and latex allergy in patients with spina bifida (165).

Awareness that certain foods have cross-reactivity with latex, including banana, avocado, chestnuts, and kiwi, is also important. A longitudinal study has suggested that the sensitization to fruit develops after the sensitivity to latex (166).

Rehabilitation

The rehabilitation program for children with meningomyelocele begins in the newborn period. A careful examination in the newborn period, often by observation of the position of the infant, can help discern the functional level of the patient that result from imbalance of muscular forces around major pivots. Therefore, as the child grows, he or she should be monitored closely for the development of contractures.

Referral should be made to early intervention services, and the child's development should be followed closely, ideally in a multidisciplinary clinic if one is available. Though there exists little literature on whether care provided in a multidisciplinary clinic improves outcomes for individuals with spina bifida, Kaufman et al. report that 46% to 66% of patients with myelomeningocele failed to go for regular medical and specialty care after a previously available multidisciplinary clinic disbanded (167).

As the child reaches school age, the rehabilitation team should ensure that the child is receiving appropriate accommodations in school. Since many individuals with spina bifida have some degree of intellectual disability, the most appropriate mechanism for the provision of these accommodations may be as part of an IEP.

Mobility

Rehabilitation specialists are uniquely qualified to help patients with myelomeningocele achieve mobility. For the infant, proper seating with appropriate relief for deformities allows the infant to sit upright and view the environment. At about 1 year of age, standing devices can be considered.

Ambulation is likely to be delayed in children with spina bifida, regardless of the level of the lesion (168). There are multiple factors that affect ambulation. Data from the National Spinal Bifida Patient Registry indicates, as would be expected, that individuals with midlumbar (knee extension) or low lumbar/sacral (ankle dorsi-/plantar flexion) motor levels were more likely to be community ambulators. Factors having an inverse relationship to ambulation included history of shunting and history of hip or knee contracture release.

Charney and Melchionni, in a retrospective study, evaluated high lumbar– and thoracic-level patients and found that the significant factors determining ambulation were the degree of intellectual disability, whether the child received PT for ambulation, and parental involvement (169).

In the younger patient with a higher motor level, a parapodium is sometimes used. The parapodium can be used as a stander or for ambulation. In standing, the advantage of a parapodium over crutches is that it allows the child the ability to have their arms free for other activities. One disadvantage compared to crutches is that that the child will need assistance to don/doff the device. The parapodium can also be used with crutches for ambulation. However, the device does not allow a reciprocal gait pattern. The ORLAU (Orthotic Research and Locomotor Assessment Unit) swivel walker is similar to a parapodium except that the baseplate is attached to swiveling footplates, which pivot as the child shifts weight from side to side. This allows ambulation without crutches. Eventually, the parapodium can be replaced by hip-knee-ankle-foot orthoses (HKAFOs) with the use of a walker or Lofstrand crutches, depending on the child's abilities. The reciprocating gait orthosis (RGO) allows for an upright, reciprocal (or, alternatively, swing-through) gait pattern. The isocentric RGO uses a bar with a central pivot (eFig. 45-11). The quality of gait is improved if the patient can assist with active hip flexion. However, obesity, age, lack of patient/family motivation, scoliosis, and spasticity are factors that contribute to many patients' decision to cease using this device over the long term (170).

High–lumbar-level patients may receive bracing as early as 10 to 12 months, usually with HKAFOs. For lower-level patients, the residual motor movements will dictate the type of orthosis needed.

Although ambulation in childhood, even in high-motor-level patients, is a reasonable goal, eventually wheelchair mobility may be required as a result of the energy demands of upright ambulation (168). Wheeled mobility can be achieved by 18 to 24 months, and steering a power wheelchair can be achieved before 3 (in some cases, potentially before 2) years of age.

As the child becomes an adolescent and reaches driving age, consideration should be given to whether he or she may need hand controls or a specialized driving evaluation by an occupational therapist.

TRANSITION TO ADULT CARE

As young adults with disabilities transition to more independence, physicians need to educate patients and their families about potential age-related changes and medical issues.

In addition to acknowledging common medical conditions and quality of life issues encountered as a person ages, the pediatric rehabilitation practitioner can help with transitioning a young person to adult services by viewing transition as a process that occurs over time. Well before (and several times before) the individual with a disability reaches the age of 18, the practitioner should assess that individual's autonomy and child and family readiness with conversations beginning as early as 12 years of age (171). Some groups, such as the Spina Bifida Association, argue that preparing for the transition to adult self-care begins at birth (172). Establishing strong relationships with adult providers is also essential in ensuring the young person will be successful in the adult system of care.

Management of Adults with Specific Pediatric-Onset Conditions

Adults with Cerebral Palsy

Although CP is a nonprogressive disorder, adults face a unique set of medical and social problems compared to their younger cohorts. It is helpful to consider this population in the context of the International Classification of Functioning, Disability and Health (ICF) defined by the World Health Organization (173) (see also Chapter 9). This provides a means of demonstrating the interaction between body function and structure, health conditions, participation, personal factors, environment, and activities. Many of these factors in the ICF evolve with age and can result in changes in function both physically and socially. However, many adults with CP live and work independently in the community and lead full, productive lives (174).

Functional Changes

Adults with CP, similar to those without disability, become more sedentary with age. This is thought to be related to secondary conditions that affect motor function. It has been shown that the GMFCS level observed around age 12 is highly predictive of adult motor function (175). By age 25, improvement in ambulation is unlikely and decline more likely (176). In a population of 101 adults living with CP in California, about 75% stopped ambulating by the age of 25 due to fatigue and increased efficiency of wheelchair mobility compared to ambulation (177). For those persons who are ambulatory when they reach adulthood, there is a significant decline in ambulation, especially in late adulthood, and few of the 60-year-olds who walk well maintain this skill over the following 15 years (178). Older persons often lose the ability to dress themselves as well. Speech, self-feeding, and the ability to order meals in public are often preserved in those who are still alive at age 60. These functional changes often affect a person's ability to care for themselves and may result in less independent living. Most young adults live in their families' home or in small private group homes, while only 18% of the 60-year-olds live independently or semi-independently, and 41% reside in medical care facilities (178).

Pain

Pain has been recognized as a serious secondary problem in adults with CP. Chronic pain has been reported in 30% to 67% of adults, with low back, hips, legs, and feet being the most commonly affected (179–181). Adults with dyskinetic CP tend to report more cervical pain (182). Fifty percent of adults report pain in more than one body part (174). It is thought that irregular biomechanical forces due to spasticity, contractures, and physical stress could lead to overuse injuries, but this has not been widely studied in CP (182). Spasticity has been shown to play a significant role in the development of chronic pain in persons with CP. Spasticity can result in muscular and joint pain and often increases in response to pain. It has been found to be associated with higher rates of osteoarthritis, joint dislocation, pain, and pressure ulcers (183).

Tone management including enteral medications such as baclofen, chemodenervation with botulinum toxin, chemoneurolysis with phenol, and ITB can be used to treat spasticity and therefore potentially for treatment of pain. In a study of adults with spasticity, including CP, botulinum toxin combined with therapy improved function and ADLs in up to 91%, while pain was improved in 90% (184). Treatment of pain is challenging, and it has been described that the majority of adults with CP and chronic pain do not seek help from health care providers for pain management. Treatments most commonly used and found to be moderately effective include physical interventions such as PT, strengthening and range of motion, over-the-counter and opioid medications, as well as heat or ice (181). One study demonstrated no significant change in pain intensity over 2 years despite an increased use of varied pain treatments (185). Often, once an adult develops chronic pain, there may be few treatments that will be effective (186). Multidisciplinary and cognitive behavioral therapies have proven beneficial for patients with CP-related chronic pain. Coping in this population has been shown to improve when the training is focused on teaching and encouraging patients to learn to maintain their daily tasks despite pain (186).

Several studies have documented the impact of chronic pain on the lives of adults with CP. Many adults experience limitations in their activities, social withdrawal, decreased self-esteem, depression, loss of roles, relationship strain, and emotional distress that leads to a cycle of despair and hopelessness (186,187).

Musculoskeletal

It has been suggested that adults with CP may show musculoskeletal or functional changes typical of advanced aging earlier than their nondisabled peers (182). Lifetime disabilities, such as CP, can result in excessive wear and tear on the muscular, skeletal, and other body systems.

Contractures are common in adults with CP and may contribute to joint pain, joint deformity, positioning difficulty, impaired ambulation and transfers, and pressure sores. Eighty percent of adults report contractures with 33% of these occurring in 2 to 3 joints (174). Hip adduction contracture, hip flexion contracture, and windswept deformity of the hips

are associated with hip pain and difficulty with perineal care (183). The presence of a unilateral hip dislocation can create a pelvic obliquity that has the potential to result in sitting imbalance, hip pain, and pressure ulcers. The reported incidence of hip pain in adults with varied severity of CP is 18% to 50% (183,188,189). Some studies report pain correlating with hip migration, whereas in other studies, hip subluxation or dislocation has been found to be associated with osteoarthritis on imaging, but not with hip pain (183,190). By adulthood, extent of deformity can preclude many interventions that may have been suitable early on (188). If a dislocated hip becomes painful in adulthood or contractures interfere with ADLs or positioning, a salvage procedure can be considered. Proximal femoral resection arthroplasty (PFRA), subtrochanteric valgus osteotomy (SVO) with femoral head resection, and proximal femur prosthetic interposition arthroplasty (PFIA) have demonstrated good results in 67%, 67%, and 73% of patients, respectively, in a study comparing outcomes of the three procedures (191).

Scoliosis is a significant problem for many youth and adults with CP. Severe curves can be associated with pelvic obliquity, pressure sores, and functional decline (192). Few studies have evaluated the natural history of scoliosis in adults with CP, and it has been shown that there is a high risk of progression with curves of 40 degrees at skeletal maturity (192,193). Average progression rate has been shown to range from 3 to 4.4 degrees per year, depending on function (192). Cardiopulmonary compromise can also occur and is associated with severity of curve and age (194). Surgical correction in these adults may improve respiratory function, but outcomes are variable (195). Close surveillance of pulmonary function is needed, and it is important to continually monitor seating, skin integrity, and comfort.

Cervical myelopathy is a potentially devastating secondary condition in adults with athetoid and dystonic CP. Presenting symptoms can be difficult to discern given baseline neurologic dysfunction and difficulty in performing neurologic examination in the presence of athetosis or dystonia. The most common presenting symptoms are hand clumsiness, lower limb weakness, gait impairment or falls, hyperreflexia, upper limb weakness, spasticity, and neck pain (196). The main risk factors for cervical myelopathy in a population of adults with dystonic CP include increased age, more severe dystonia, and longer duration of dystonia (196). Imaging commonly demonstrates disk herniation, spinal stenosis, and spine instability (197). Treatment involves surgical decompression and spinal fusion with or without botulinum toxin injections to manage the patient's movement disorder postoperatively. Postoperative stabilization is with a variety of bracing from the least restrictive Philadelphia collar to the most restrictive halo immobilization. In one long-term follow-up study of individuals with athetoid CP who underwent spinal decompression and fusion, eight of ten patients had late neurologic deterioration, five of whom had a poor outcome and three of whom required a repeat operation (198).

Life Expectancy

Life expectancy in persons with CP can be quite good in those with milder functional impairment. Mortality is not common in childhood, but more concentrated in infancy, often attributed to severe brain injury, as well as in adulthood (199).

Studies demonstrate higher mortality with increased severity of CP, implying lower gross motor functional level. One study out of California, for example, reports in a population greater than 60 years old with severe CP a mortality of 99% compared to 44% in those with milder CP. In 30- to 45-year-olds, those with severe CP had a mortality rate of 32% compared with only 6% in those with milder forms (200). Another study out of the UK demonstrates higher mortality in any age group with severe impairments in motor, fine motor, cognitive, and visual functions (201).

Adults with Spina Bifida

Health management for adults with spina bifida has gathered increasing attention. The Spina Bifida Association of America has led an effort toward better education of patients and health care providers working with this patient population. Improved management of neurogenic bladder dysfunction and hydrocephalus has increased the survival into early adulthood to 75% (202).

Incontinence

The majority of adults with spina bifida require some type of bladder management program. Most young adults in one study reported urinary incontinence regardless of the type of management used (203). Patients without hydrocephalus were more likely to perceive incontinence as a problem. Management options include intermittent catheterization (used by the majority of patients), indwelling catheters, urinary diversion, and artificial sphincters. Medication is often used, and first-line treatment tends to be with anticholinergic medication. Another option for some patients includes therapeutic botulinum toxin injections to the bladder.

Optimization of medical health is not the only reason to attend to incontinence—it can easily affect socialization as well. Studies have shown that for individuals with spina bifida, continence is correlated with the likelihood of being sexually active (204).

Urinary tract infections were found in one study to be the most common reason for inpatient admission in adults with spina bifida (205), while renal failure is the leading cause of death for adults with spina bifida (204,206). The rate of renal failure in adults with spina bifida has declined significantly due to appropriate intermittent catheterization techniques. Risk factors include chronic urinary tract infections and nephrolithiasis. Peritoneal dialysis can be complicated by VP shunts or urinary stomata, but studies have shown that having a shunt is not an absolute contraindication (207). Renal transplantation has been shown to have good outcomes (208). Adults with spina bifida and neurogenic bladder have an increased risk of bladder cancer, and this may be influenced by bladder augmentation (156) or use of a chronic indwelling catheter (209). Careful surveillance is required.

Annual renal function tests, blood pressure, and ultrasound are important tools to monitor urologic function (210). Quan et al. showed that when serum creatinine is greater than 0.5, it is not an accurate marker of renal function, suggesting instead a radioisotope clearance study (211). Newer literature suggests determining Glomerular Filtration Rate (GFR) from cystatin C is more sensitive than GFR calculated on the basis of the serum creatinine (212). Any change in bladder function should be thoroughly evaluated in the adult patient, as a change could also indicate a neurologic abnormality.

While most adults with spina bifida have some degree of bowel dysfunction, management of the neurogenic bowel in the adult follows similar principles to those outlined in this chapter's earlier discussion of management of the bowel for children with spina bifida. One study found that individuals with spina bifida over 18 years old were more likely than younger individuals with spina bifida to report bowel incontinence (213). As adults with spina bifida age, bowel patterns may change—in some, this may mean more of a tendency toward looser stools, while others may experience more of a tendency toward constipation (214). In adults, the issue of bowel incontinence is especially important as it may present a barrier to employment (215).

Skin

While most common during adolescence, wounds remain common in adults with spina bifida (160). Studies have shown that complications from wounds represent the reason for a significant percentage of hospital admissions for adults with spina bifida, creating a substantial economic burden (216). Furthermore, a study over a 10-year period showed that individuals with skin ulcers had significantly increased mortality compared to those without ulcers (217).

Neurologic

Individuals with shunts, including those with spina bifida, should be followed indefinitely. Though the need for shunt revision tends to be higher in early life, a recent study by Dupepe et al. suggested that there was also a high incidence of shunt failure in patients over the age of 30 (218). Symptoms of failure can be subtle, presenting as only mild cognitive decline, or severe (death) (206).

Spinal cord tethering may occur at any age. Adults who have had prior repair of myelomeningocele may have worse outcomes compared to individuals with spina bifida occulta (219). In addition, postsurgical outcomes may be worse for individuals who again undergo surgical detethering after a prior detethering procedure (220).

Chronic headaches are also common in adults with spina bifida. There are many possible causes. The most serious possible causes, for example, shunt malfunction, should be ruled out. Several studies have shown a high prevalence of the Chiari/hydrosyringomyelia complex in adults with spina bifida with symptoms including headaches, upper limb weakness, sensory changes, ataxia, and lower cranial nerve palsies (221). One study found that 10% of adults with spina bifida and hydrocephalus, for whom no definitive cause of the headache was found, required specialist pain management (222).

Musculoskeletal

Those children with spina bifida who are still ambulatory as teenagers tend to remain so into their adult years (202). It is described that deterioration of ambulation can occur in adults due to change in the neurologic level of lesion, spasticity, knee and hip flexion contractures, low back pain, lack of motivation, as well as major events such as stroke (223). Adults often develop improper biomechanics created by muscular imbalance that can result in pain. Ultimately, this may lead to degenerative changes—some have argued that onset of these changes may be delayed or prevented by orthopedic surgery, for example, derotational osteotomy (224). Charcot arthropathy can also develop due to these imbalances and impaired sensation. The most common location is the foot/ankle (206). An appropriate brace such as a patellar-tendon-bearing AFO may be helpful.

Somewhat counterintuitively, Sawatzky et al. demonstrated adults with spina bifida who were wheelchair users from childhood seemed to have less shoulder pain than adults with acquired traumatic spinal cord injury (225). The reasons for this are unclear but may include a decreased expectation of independence in early childhood for children with spina bifida or the possibility that the immature shoulder may remodel in such a way as to better accommodate the forces seen during wheelchair use.

Osteoporosis is common among adults with spina bifida (226). Individuals are at increased risk for fracture, particularly those who are nonambulatory, but adults with spina bifida appear to have a lower risk of fracture than children with spina bifida (227). Treatment includes appropriate calcium and vitamin D supplementation. Data on bisphosphonates are lacking.

Scoliosis is common, seen in almost half of adults with spina bifida. Typically, by the time the patient with spina bifida is an adult, the scoliotic curve is static. Bracing may nonetheless be useful to help with positioning (206).

Nutrition

A study by Buffart et al. characterized 39% of studied individuals with spina bifida as inactive and 37% as extremely inactive; 19% of males and 52% of females were obese (228). Maintaining an ideal body weight is of critical importance in adults with spina bifida when considering prevention of long-term effects of obesity. Complications of obesity include hypertension, diabetes, cardiovascular disease (one study identified cardiac disease as the second leading cause of death for individuals with spina bifida, behind renal dysfunction (229)), hyperlipidemia, obstructive sleep apnea, and osteoarthritis. One study found a 30% prevalence of metabolic syndrome in adolescents/young adults with spina bifida (the prevalence increased to 45% in those with obesity.) Nutritional counseling should not only include dietary recommendations but also include information on physical activity.

Sexuality

The majority of young adults with spina bifida report being sexually active. However, studies have shown that many individuals with spina bifida felt they needed more information on sexuality/fertility (230,231). Counseling regarding the increased risk of neural tube defects in the children of those with spina bifida is important. When considering contraception, it is important to give information about the risk of latex in many condoms and the risk of thromboembolism associated with oral contraceptive pills.

Infertility issues such as erectile or ejaculatory dysfunction need to be addressed by physicians. Erectile dysfunction in spina bifida has been well studied and largely depends on neurologic level. Twenty-five percent of men with thoracic/high lumbar spina bifida achieve erections, while about 75% of those with spina bifida at L3 or lower are able to do so (206). Sildenafil has been shown to improve erectile function in 80% of men with spina bifida (232). Ejaculation is more common in those with sacral-level lesions. Azoospermia is more prevalent among those with a lesion above T10 (233).

Compared to studies of men, there are fewer studies of sexual function in women who have spina bifida. One study of 35 women with spina bifida found that over 80% had vulvar sensation and 37% experienced orgasm (234).

Women with spina bifida are able to carry pregnancies to term. Particular risks may include UTI and exacerbation of pressure ulcers if mobility decreases. One series of 70 shunt-dependent women (138 pregnancies) found that 4 of the women required shunt revisions during pregnancy and 13 required revision within 6 months of delivery (235).

SUMMARY

Pediatric rehabilitation specialists recognize the many issues that may be faced by children with disabilities. While many of these issues are similar to those seen in adults, ongoing growth, development, family considerations, and the interplay of the child's condition with the educational setting create a unique milieu in which interventions can be offered. Using a team approach will help ensure that the different stakeholders in the child's care have an understanding of the goals and effects of these interventions, so that care can be optimized throughout childhood.

REFERENCES

1. Brault MW. *Americans With Disabilities: 2010.* 2012. Available from: https://www2.census.gov/library/publications/2012/demo/p70-131.pdf. Accessed October 23, 2017.
2. Medical Home Initiatives for Children With Special Needs Project Advisory Committee (American Academy of Pediatrics). The medical home. *Pediatrics.* 2002;110(1 Pt 1):184–186.
3. Houtrow AJ, et al. Profiling health and health-related services for children with special health care needs with and without disabilities. *Acad Pediatr.* 2011;11(6):508–516.
4. Bethell CD, et al. Using existing population-based data sets to measure the American Academy of Pediatrics definition of medical home for all children and children with special health care needs. *Pediatrics.* 2004;113(5 suppl):1529–1537.
5. Council on Children with Disabilities and Medical Home Implementation Project Advisory Committee. Patient- and family-centered care coordination: a framework for integrating care for children and youth across multiple systems. *Pediatrics.* 2014;133(5): e1451–e1460.
6. Brooks J, et al. Low weight, morbidity, and mortality in children with cerebral palsy: new clinical growth charts. *Pediatrics.* 2011;128(2):e299–e307.
7. Rosenbaum P, et al. A report: the definition and classification of cerebral palsy April 2006. *Dev Med Child Neurol Suppl.* 2007;109:8–14.
8. Oskoui M, et al. An update on the prevalence of cerebral palsy: a systematic review and meta-analysis. *Dev Med Child Neurol.* 2013;55(6):509–519.
9. Nordmark E, Hagglund G, Lagergren J. Cerebral palsy in southern Sweden I. Prevalence and clinical features. *Acta Paediatr.* 2001;90(11):1271–1276.
10. Christensen D, et al. Prevalence of cerebral palsy, co-occurring autism spectrum disorders, and motor functioning—Autism and Developmental Disabilities Monitoring Network, USA, 2008. *Dev Med Child Neurol.* 2014;56(1):59–65.
11. Nelson KB. Causative factors in cerebral palsy. *Clin Obstet Gynecol.* 2008;51(4): 749–762.
12. Nelson KB, Grether JK. Causes of cerebral palsy. *Curr Opin Pediatr.* 1999;11(6): 487–491.
13. McIntyre S, et al. A systematic review of risk factors for cerebral palsy in children born at term in developed countries. *Dev Med Child Neurol.* 2013;55(6):499–508.
14. Sewell MD, Eastwood DM, Wimalasundera N. Managing common symptoms of cerebral palsy in children. *BMJ.* 2014;349:g5474.
15. ACPR Group. Australian Cerebral Palsy Register Report. 2016.
16. Prevalence and characteristics of children with cerebral palsy in Europe. *Dev Med Child Neurol.* 2002;44(9):633–640.
17. Palisano R, et al. Development and reliability of a system to classify gross motor function in children with cerebral palsy. *Dev Med Child Neurol.* 1997;39(4):214–223.
18. Reid B, et al. The Royal Children's Hospital Melbourne. Available from: https://canchild.ca/system/tenon/assets/attachments/000/002/114/original/GMFCS_English_Illustrations_V2.pdf
19. Palisano R, Rosenbaum P, Bartlett D, et al. *Gross Motor Function Classification System—Expanded & Revised.* 2007.
20. Shevell MI, et al. The relationship of cerebral palsy subtype and functional motor impairment: a population-based study. *Dev Med Child Neurol.* 2009;51(11):872–877.
21. Rosenbaum PL, et al. Prognosis for gross motor function in cerebral palsy: creation of motor development curves. *JAMA.* 2002;288(11):1357–1363.
22. Eliasson AC, et al. The Manual Ability Classification System (MACS) for children with cerebral palsy: scale development and evidence of validity and reliability. *Dev Med Child Neurol.* 2006;48(7):549–554.
23. Hidecker MJ, et al. Developing and validating the Communication Function Classification System for individuals with cerebral palsy. *Dev Med Child Neurol.* 2011;53(8):704–710.

24. Andersen GL, et al. Cerebral palsy in Norway: prevalence, subtypes and severity. *Eur J Paediatr Neurol.* 2008;12(1):4–13.

25. Ashwal S, et al. Practice parameter: diagnostic assessment of the child with cerebral palsy: report of the Quality Standards Subcommittee of the American Academy of Neurology and the Practice Committee of the Child Neurology Society. *Neurology.* 2004;62(6):851–863.

26. Bax M, Tydeman C, Flodmark O. Clinical and MRI correlates of cerebral palsy: the European Cerebral Palsy Study. *JAMA.* 2006;296(13):1602–1608.

27. Leonard JM, et al. Should children with cerebral palsy and normal imaging undergo testing for inherited metabolic disorders? *Dev Med Child Neurol.* 2011;53(3):226–232.

28. Huntsman R, et al. The differential diagnosis of spastic diplegia. *Arch Dis Child.* 2015;100(5):500–504.

29. Shevell MI, et al. Comorbidities in cerebral palsy and their relationship to neurologic subtype and GMFCS level. *Neurology.* 2009;72(24):2090–2096.

30. Jethwa A, et al. Development of the Hypertonia Assessment Tool (HAT): a discriminative tool for hypertonia in children. *Dev Med Child Neurol.* 2010;52(5):e83–e87.

31. Rodda J, Graham HK. Classification of gait patterns in spastic hemiplegia and spastic diplegia: a basis for a management algorithm. *Eur J Neurol.* 2001;8(suppl 5):98–108.

32. Kedem P, Scher DM. Foot deformities in children with cerebral palsy. *Curr Opin Pediatr.* 2015;27(1):67–74.

33. Wynter M, et al. The consensus statement on hip surveillance for children with cerebral palsy: Australian standards of care. *J Pediatr Rehabil Med.* 2011;4(3):183–195.

34. Wynter M, et al. Australian hip surveillance guidelines for children with cerebral palsy: 5-year review. *Dev Med Child Neurol.* 2015;57(9):808–820.

35. Terjesen T. The natural history of hip development in cerebral palsy. *Dev Med Child Neurol.* 2012;54(10):951–957.

36. Lomita C, Ezaki M, Oishi S. Upper extremity surgery in children with cerebral palsy. *J Am Acad Orthop Surg.* 2010;18(3):160–168.

37. Persson-Bunke M, et al. Scoliosis in a total population of children with cerebral palsy. *Spine (Phila Pa 1976).* 2012;37(12):E708–E713.

38. Jacobs SE, et al. Cooling for newborns with hypoxic ischaemic encephalopathy. *Cochrane Database Syst Rev.* 2013;(1):CD003311.

39. Novak I, et al. A systematic review of interventions for children with cerebral palsy: state of the evidence. *Dev Med Child Neurol.* 2013;55(10):885–910.

40. Mattern-Baxter K. Effects of partial body weight supported treadmill training on children with cerebral palsy. *Pediatr Phys Ther.* 2009;21(1):12–22.

41. Chen YP, et al. Effectiveness of constraint-induced movement therapy on upper-extremity function in children with cerebral palsy: a systematic review and meta-analysis of randomized controlled trials. *Clin Rehabil.* 2014;28(10):939–953.

42. Novak I. Evidence-based diagnosis, health care, and rehabilitation for children with cerebral palsy. *J Child Neurol.* 2014;29(8):1141–1156.

43. Davids JR, Rowan F, Davis RB. Indications for orthoses to improve gait in children with cerebral palsy. *J Am Acad Orthop Surg.* 2007;15(3):178–188.

44. Ries AJ, Novacheck TF, Schwartz MH. The efficacy of ankle-foot orthoses on improving the gait of children with diplegic cerebral palsy: a multiple outcome analysis. *PM R.* 2015;7(9):922–929.

45. Jackman M, Novak I, Lannin N. Effectiveness of hand splints in children with cerebral palsy: a systematic review with meta-analysis. *Dev Med Child Neurol.* 2014;56(2):138–147.

46. Quality Standards Subcommittee of the American Academy of Neurology and the Practice Committee of the Child Neurology Society, et al. Practice parameter: pharmacologic treatment of spasticity in children and adolescents with cerebral palsy (an evidence-based review): report of the Quality Standards Subcommittee of the American Academy of Neurology and the Practice Committee of the Child Neurology Society. *Neurology.* 2010;74(4):336–343.

47. Copeland L, et al. Botulinum toxin A for nonambulatory children with cerebral palsy: a double blind randomized controlled trial. *J Pediatr.* 2014;165(1):140.e4–146.e4.

48. Hoare BJ, et al. Botulinum toxin A as an adjunct to treatment in the management of the upper limb in children with spastic cerebral palsy (UPDATE). *Cochrane Database Syst Rev.* 2010;(1):CD003469.

49. Ryll U, et al. Effects of leg muscle botulinum toxin A injections on walking in children with spasticity-related cerebral palsy: a systematic review. *Dev Med Child Neurol.* 2011;53(3):210–216.

50. Howell K, et al. Botulinum neurotoxin A: an unusual systemic effect. *J Paediatr Child Health.* 2007;43(6):499–501.

51. Crowner BE, Brunstrom JE, Racette BA. Iatrogenic botulism due to therapeutic botulinum toxin a injection in a pediatric patient. *Clin Neuropharmacol.* 2007;30(5):310–313.

52. Partikian A, Mitchell WG. Iatrogenic botulism in a child with spastic quadriparesis. *J Child Neurol.* 2007;22(10):1235–1237.

53. Khalili AA, Betts HB. Peripheral nerve block with phenol in the management of spasticity. Indications and complications. *JAMA.* 1967;200(13):1155–1157.

54. Spira R. Management of spasticity in cerebral palsied children by peripheral nerve block with phenol. *Dev Med Child Neurol.* 1971;13(2):164–173.

55. Halpern D, Meelhuysen FE. Duration of relaxation after intramuscular neurolysis with phenol. *JAMA.* 1967;200(13):1152–1154.

56. Hasnat MJ, Rice JE. Intrathecal baclofen for treating spasticity in children with cerebral palsy. *Cochrane Database Syst Rev.* 2015;(11):CD004552.

57. McLaughlin J, et al. Selective dorsal rhizotomy: meta-analysis of three randomized controlled trials. *Dev Med Child Neurol.* 2002;44(1):17–25.

58. Dudley RW, et al. Long-term functional benefits of selective dorsal rhizotomy for spastic cerebral palsy. *J Neurosurg Pediatr.* 2013;12(2):142–150.

59. Narayanan UG. Management of children with ambulatory cerebral palsy: an evidence-based review. *J Pediatr Orthop.* 2012;32(suppl 2):S172–S181.

60. Sewell MD, et al. A preliminary study to assess whether spinal fusion for scoliosis improves carer-assessed quality of life for children with GMFCS level IV or V cerebral palsy. *J Pediatr Orthop.* 2016;36(3):299–304.

61. Wang CH, et al. Consensus statement for standard of care in spinal muscular atrophy. *J Child Neurol.* 2007;22(8):1027–1049.

62. Finkel RS, et al. Treatment of infantile-onset spinal muscular atrophy with nusinersen: a phase 2, open-label, dose-escalation study. *Lancet.* 2016;388(10063):3017–3026.

63. Chiriboga CA, et al. Results from a phase 1 study of nusinersen (ISIS-SMN(Rx)) in children with spinal muscular atrophy. *Neurology.* 2016;86(10):890–897.

64. Sejvar JJ, et al. Acute flaccid myelitis in the United States, August-December 2014: results of Nationwide Surveillance. *Clin Infect Dis.* 2016;63(6):737–745.

65. Martin JA, et al. Outcomes of Colorado children with acute flaccid myelitis at 1 year. *Neurology.* 2017;89(2):129–137.

66. Keller C, et al. Congenital myotonic dystrophy requiring prolonged endotracheal and noninvasive assisted ventilation: not a uniformly fatal condition. *Pediatrics.* 1998;101(4 Pt 1):704–706.

67. Lieberman AP, Fischbeck KH. Triplet repeat expansion in neuromuscular disease. *Muscle Nerve.* 2000;23(6):843–850.

68. Igarashi H, et al. Hypertrophic cardiomyopathy in congenital myotonic dystrophy. *Pediatr Neurol.* 1998;18(4):366–369.

69. Pandya S, Eichinger K. *Role of Physical Therapy In the Assessment and Management of Individuals with Myotonic Dystrophy.* Available from: https://www.myotonic.org/sites/default/files/Physical%20Therapy%20FINAL.pdf

70. Kang PB, et al. Evidence-based guideline summary: evaluation, diagnosis, and management of congenital muscular dystrophy: report of the guideline development subcommittee of the American Academy of Neurology and the Practice Issues Review Panel of the American Association of Neuromuscular & Electrodiagnostic Medicine. *Neurology.* 2015;84(13):1369–1378.

71. Bodensteiner JB. Congenital myopathies. *Muscle Nerve.* 1994;17(2):131–144.

72. North KN, et al. Approach to the diagnosis of congenital myopathies. *Neuromuscul Disord.* 2014;24(2):97–116.

73. Randomized trial of thymectomy in myasthenia gravis. *N Engl J Med.* 2017;376(21):2097.

74. Ervasti JM, Campbell KP. Membrane organization of the dystrophin-glycoprotein complex. *Cell.* 1991;66(6):1121–1131.

75. Bello L, et al. DMD genotypes and loss of ambulation in the CINRG Duchenne Natural History Study. *Neurology.* 2016;87(4):401–409.

76. Bushby K, et al. Diagnosis and management of Duchenne muscular dystrophy, part 2: implementation of multidisciplinary care. *Lancet Neurol.* 2010;9(2):177–189.

77. Bushby K, et al. Diagnosis and management of Duchenne muscular dystrophy, part 1: diagnosis, and pharmacological and psychosocial management. *Lancet Neurol.* 2010;9(1):77–93.

78. Kinnett K, et al. Imperatives for DUCHENNE MD: a simplified guide to comprehensive care for duchenne muscular dystrophy. *PLoS Curr.* 2015;7.

79. Fowler WM Jr, Taylor M. Rehabilitation management of muscular dystrophy and related disorders: I. The role of exercise. *Arch Phys Med Rehabil.* 1982;63(7):319–321.

80. Finder JD, et al. Respiratory care of the patient with Duchenne muscular dystrophy: ATS consensus statement. *Am J Respir Crit Care Med.* 2004;170(4):456–465.

81. D'Amario D, et al. A current approach to heart failure in Duchenne muscular dystrophy. *Heart.* 2017;103:1770–1779.

82. Ogata H, et al. Beneficial effects of beta-blockers and angiotensin-converting enzyme inhibitors in Duchenne muscular dystrophy. *J Cardiol.* 2009;53(1):72–78.

83. Bonifati MD, et al. A multicenter, double-blind, randomized trial of deflazacort versus prednisone in Duchenne muscular dystrophy. *Muscle Nerve.* 2000;23(9):1344–1347.

84. McAdam LC, et al. The Canadian experience with long-term deflazacort treatment in Duchenne muscular dystrophy. *Acta Myol.* 2012;31(1):16–20.

85. Alman BA, Raza SN, Biggar WD. Steroid treatment and the development of scoliosis in males with duchenne muscular dystrophy. *J Bone Joint Surg Am.* 2004;86-A(3):519–524.

86. Alexander WM, et al. The effect of posterior spinal fusion on respiratory function in Duchenne muscular dystrophy. *Eur Spine J.* 2013;22(2):411–416.

87. Bell JM, et al. Interventions to prevent and treat corticosteroid-induced osteoporosis and prevent osteoporotic fractures in Duchenne muscular dystrophy. *Cochrane Database Syst Rev.* 2017;(1):CD010899.

88. Medeiros MO, et al. Fat embolism syndrome in patients with Duchenne muscular dystrophy. *Neurology.* 2013;80(14):1350–1352.

89. Hendriksen JG, Vles JS. Neuropsychiatric disorders in males with duchenne muscular dystrophy: frequency rate of attention-deficit hyperactivity disorder (ADHD), autism spectrum disorder, and obsessive—compulsive disorder. *J Child Neurol.* 2008;23(5):477–481.

90. Edwards JD, et al. End-of-life discussions and advance care planning for children on long-term assisted ventilation with life-limiting conditions. *J Palliat Care.* 2012;28(1):21–27.

91. Kohler M, et al. Quality of life, physical disability, and respiratory impairment in Duchenne muscular dystrophy. *Am J Respir Crit Care Med.* 2005;172(8):1032–1036.

92. Narayanaswami P, et al. Evidence-based guideline summary: diagnosis and treatment of limb-girdle and distal dystrophies: report of the guideline development subcommittee of the American Academy of Neurology and the practice issues review panel of the American Association of Neuromuscular & Electrodiagnostic Medicine. *Neurology.* 2014;83(16):1453–1463.

93. Foad SL, Mehlman CT, Ying J. The epidemiology of neonatal brachial plexus palsy in the United States. *J Bone Joint Surg Am.* 2008;90(6):1258–1264.

94. Pondaag W, et al. Natural history of obstetric brachial plexus palsy: a systematic review. *Dev Med Child Neurol.* 2004;46(2):138–144.

95. Lindqvist PG, et al. Characteristics and outcome of brachial plexus birth palsy in neonates. *Acta Paediatr.* 2012;101(6):579–582.

96. Berggren J, Baker LL. Therapeutic application of electrical stimulation and constraint induced movement therapy in perinatal brachial plexus injury: a case report. *J Hand Ther.* 2015;28(2):217–220; quiz 221.

97. Buesch FE, et al. Constraint-induced movement therapy for children with obstetric brachial plexus palsy: two single-case series. *Int J Rehabil Res.* 2010;33(2):187–192.

98. Elnaggar RK. Shoulder function and bone mineralization in children with obstetric brachial plexus injury after neuromuscular electrical stimulation during weight-bearing exercises. *Am J Phys Med Rehabil.* 2016;95(4):239–247.

99. Fisher DM, et al. Evaluation of elbow flexion as a predictor of outcome in obstetrical brachial plexus palsy. *Plast Reconstr Surg.* 2007;120(6):1585–1590.

100. Coroneos CJ, et al. Primary nerve repair for obstetrical brachial plexus injury: a meta-analysis. *Plast Reconstr Surg.* 2015;136(4):765–779.

101. Iorio ML, et al. Glenohumeral dysplasia following neonatal brachial plexus palsy: presentation and predictive features during infancy. *J Hand Surg.* 2015;40(12):2345.e1–2351.e1.

102. Verchere C, et al. An early shoulder repositioning program in birth-related brachial plexus injury: a pilot study of the Sup-ER protocol. *Hand (N Y).* 2014;9(2):187–195.

103. Michaud LJ, et al. Use of botulinum toxin type A in the management of neonatal brachial plexus palsy. *PM R.* 2014;6(12):1107–1119.

104. Cheng JC, Tang SP, Chen TM. Sternocleidomastoid pseudotumor and congenital muscular torticollis in infants: a prospective study of 510 cases. *J Pediatr.* 1999;134(6):712–716.

105. Golden KA, et al. Sternocleidomastoid imbalance versus congenital muscular torticollis: their relationship to positional plagiocephaly. *Cleft Palate Craniofac J.* 1999;36(3):256–261.

106. Kuo AA, Tritasavit S, Graham JM Jr. Congenital muscular torticollis and positional plagiocephaly. *Pediatr Rev.* 2014;35(2):79–87; quiz 87.

107. Gupta AK, et al. Torticollis secondary to posterior fossa tumors. *J Pediatr Orthop.* 1996;16(4):505–507.

108. Kaplan SL, Coulter C, Fetters L. Physical therapy management of congenital muscular torticollis: an evidence-based clinical practice guideline: from the Section on Pediatrics of the American Physical Therapy Association. *Pediatr Phys Ther.* 2013;25(4):348–394.

109. van Vlimmeren LA, et al. Torticollis and plagiocephaly in infancy: therapeutic strategies. *Pediatr Rehabil.* 2006;9(1):40–46.

110. Shim JS, Jang HP. Operative treatment of congenital torticollis. *J Bone Joint Surg Br.* 2008;90(7):934–939.

111. Dias M, Partington M; Section on Neurologic Surgery. Congenital brain and spinal cord malformations and their associated cutaneous markers. *Pediatrics.* 2015;136(4):e1105–e1119.

112. Eleraky MA, et al. Pediatric cervical spine injuries: report of 102 cases and review of the literature. *J Neurosurg.* 2000;92(1 suppl):12–17.

113. Pang D, Wilberger JE Jr. Spinal cord injury without radiographic abnormalities in children. *J Neurosurg.* 1982;57(1):114–129.

114. Yucesoy K, Yuksel KZ. SCIWORA in MRI era. *Clin Neurol Neurosurg.* 2008;110(5):429–433.

115. Knox J. Epidemiology of spinal cord injury without radiographic abnormality in children: a nationwide perspective. *J Child Orthop.* 2016;10(3):255–260.

116. Achildi O, Betz RR, Grewal H. Lapbelt injuries and the seatbelt syndrome in pediatric spinal cord injury. *J Spinal Cord Med.* 2007;30(suppl 1):S21–S24.

117. Vogel L, et al. Intra-rater agreement of the anorectal exam and classification of injury severity in children with spinal cord injury. *Spinal Cord.* 2009;47(9):687–691.

118. Bauer SB. Neurogenic bladder: etiology and assessment. *Pediatr Nephrol.* 2008;23(4):541–551.

119. Kaefer M, et al. Estimating normal bladder capacity in children. *J Urol.* 1997;158(6):2261–2264.

120. Chao R, Mayo ME. Long-term urodynamic follow up in pediatric spinal cord injury. *Paraplegia.* 1994;32(12):806–809.

121. Schottler J, Vogel LC, Sturm P. Spinal cord injuries in young children: a review of children injured at 5 years of age and younger. *Dev Med Child Neurol.* 2012;54(12):1138–1143.

122. Leeper CM, et al. Venous thromboembolism in pediatric trauma patients: ten-year experience and long-term follow-up in a tertiary care center. *Pediatr Blood Cancer.* 2017;64(8).

123. Radecki RT, Gaebler-Spira D. Deep vein thrombosis in the disabled pediatric population. *Arch Phys Med Rehabil.* 1994;75(3):248–250.

124. Coleman BG, Langer JE, Horii SC. The diagnostic features of spina bifida: the role of ultrasound. *Fetal Diagn Ther.* 2015;37(3):179–196.

125. Fidas A, et al. Prevalence and patterns of spina bifida occulta in 2707 normal adults. *Clin Radiol.* 1987;38(5):537–542.

126. Fletcher JM, Brei TJ. Introduction: Spina bifida—a multidisciplinary perspective. *Dev Disabil Res Rev.* 2010;16(1):1–5.

127. Parker SE, et al. Updated National Birth Prevalence estimates for selected birth defects in the United States, 2004–2006. *Birth Defects Res A Clin Mol Teratol.* 2010;88(12):1008–1016.

128. Frey L, Hauser WA. Epidemiology of neural tube defects. *Epilepsia.* 2003;44(suppl 3):4–13.

129. Atta CA, et al. Global birth prevalence of spina bifida by folic acid fortification status: a systematic review and meta-analysis. *Am J Public Health.* 2016;106(1):e24–e34.

130. Sebold CD, et al. Recurrence risks for neural tube defects in siblings of patients with lipomyelomeningocele. *Genet Med.* 2005;7(1):64–67.

131. Cheschier N; ACOG Committee on Practice Bulletins-Obstetrics. ACOG practice bulletin. Neural tube defects. Number 44, July 2003. (Replaces committee opinion number 252, March 2001). *Int J Gynaecol Obstet.* 2003;83(1):123–133.

132. Mitchell LE. Epidemiology of neural tube defects. *Am J Med Genet C Semin Med Genet.* 2005;135C(1):88–94.

133. Salbaum JM, Kappen C. Neural tube defect genes and maternal diabetes during pregnancy. *Birth Defects Res A Clin Mol Teratol.* 2010;88(8):601–611.

134. Cavalli P. Prevention of Neural Tube Defects and proper folate periconceptional supplementation. *J Prenat Med.* 2008;2(4):40–41.

135. U.S. Preventive Services Task Force, et al. Folic acid supplementation for the prevention of neural tube defects: US preventive services task force recommendation statement. *JAMA.* 2017;317(2):183–189.

136. Toriyama M, et al. Folate-dependent methylation of septins governs ciliogenesis during neural tube closure. *FASEB J.* 2017;31(8):3622–3635.

137. Copp AJ, et al. Spina bifida. *Nat Rev Dis Primers.* 2015;1:15007.

138. Rintoul NE, et al. A new look at myelomeningoceles: functional level, vertebral level, shunting, and the implications for fetal intervention. *Pediatrics.* 2002;109(3):409–413.

139. Elbabaa SK, et al. First 60 fetal in-utero myelomeningocele repairs at Saint Louis Fetal Care Institute in the post-MOMS trial era: hydrocephalus treatment outcomes (endoscopic third ventriculostomy versus ventriculo-peritoneal shunt). *Childs Nerv Syst.* 2017;33(7):1157–1168.

140. Garceau GJ. The filum terminale syndrome (the cord-traction syndrome). *J Bone Joint Surg Am.* 1953;35-A(3):711–716.

141. Hoffman HJ, Hendrick EB, Humphreys RP. The tethered spinal cord: its protean manifestations, diagnosis and surgical correction. *Childs Brain.* 1976;2(3):145–155.

142. Yamada S, Won DJ. What is the true tethered cord syndrome? *Childs Nerv Syst.* 2007;23(4):371–375.

143. McEnery G, et al. The spinal cord in neurologically stable spina bifida: a clinical and MRI study. *Dev Med Child Neurol.* 1992;34(4):342–347.

144. Tuite GF, et al. Evaluation and management of tethered cord syndrome in occult spinal dysraphism: recommendations from the international children's continence society. *Neurourol Urodyn.* 2018;37:890–903.

145. Bui CJ, Tubbs RS, Oakes WJ. Tethered cord syndrome in children: a review. *Neurosurg Focus.* 2007;23(2):E2.

146. Fletcher JM, et al. Verbal and nonverbal skill discrepancies in hydrocephalic children. *J Clin Exp Neuropsychol.* 1992;14(4):593–609.

147. Dennis M, Barnes MA. The cognitive phenotype of spina bifida meningomyelocele. *Dev Disabil Res Rev.* 2010;16(1):31–39.

148. Broughton NS, et al. The natural history of hip deformity in myelomeningocele. *J Bone Joint Surg Br.* 1993;75(5):760–763.

149. Sherk HH, et al. Treatment versus non-treatment of hip dislocations in ambulatory patients with myelomeningocele. *Dev Med Child Neurol.* 1991;33(6):491–494.

150. Wright JG. Hip and spine surgery is of questionable value in spina bifida: an evidence-based review. *Clin Orthop Relat Res.* 2011;469(5):1258–1264.

151. Gabrieli AP, et al. Gait analysis in low lumbar myelomeningocele patients with unilateral hip dislocation or subluxation. *J Pediatr Orthop.* 2003;23(3):330–334.

152. Swaroop VT, Dias L. Orthopedic management of spina bifida. Part I: hip, knee, and rotational deformities. *J Child Orthop.* 2009;3(6):441–449.

153. Roach JW, Short BF, Saltzman HM. Adult consequences of spina bifida: a cohort study. *Clin Orthop Relat Res.* 2011;469(5):1246–1252.

154. Lalonde F, Jarvis J. Congenital kyphosis in myelomeningocele. The effect of cordotomy on bladder function. *J Bone Joint Surg Br.* 1999;81(2):245–249.

155. Mummareddy N, et al. Scoliosis in myelomeningocele: epidemiology, management, and functional outcome. *J Neurosurg Pediatr.* 2017;20(1):99–108.

156. Snow-Lisy DC, Yerkes EB, Cheng EY. Update on urological management of spina bifida from prenatal diagnosis to adulthood. *J Urol.* 2015;194(2):288–296.

157. Reddy MN, et al. Laparoscopic Mitrofanoff continent catheterisable stoma in children with spina bifida. *Afr J Paediatr Surg.* 2015;12(2):126–130.

158. Peters KM, et al. Outcomes of lumbar to sacral nerve rerouting for spina bifida. *J Urol.* 2010;184(2):702–707.

159. Pacilli M, et al. Use of Peristeen(R) transanal colonic irrigation for bowel management in children: a single-center experience. *J Pediatr Surg.* 2014;49(2):269–272; discussion 272.

160. Ottolini K, et al. Wound care challenges in children and adults with spina bifida: an open-cohort study. *J Pediatr Rehabil Med.* 2013;6(1):1–10.

161. Psihogios AM, Kolbuck V, Holmbeck GN. Condition self-management in pediatric spina bifida: a longitudinal investigation of medical adherence, responsibility-sharing, and independence skills. *J Pediatr Psychol.* 2015;40(8):790–803.

162. Meeropol E, et al. Latex allergy in children with myelodysplasia: a survey of Shriners hospitals. *J Pediatr Orthop.* 1993;13(1):1–4.

163. Niggemann B, et al. Latex provocation tests in patients with spina bifida: who is at risk of becoming symptomatic? *J Allergy Clin Immunol.* 1998;102(4 Pt 1):665–670.

164. Eiwegger T, et al. Early exposure to latex products mediates latex sensitization in spina bifida but not in other diseases with comparable latex exposure rates. *Clin Exp Allergy.* 2006;36(10):1242–1246.

165. Blumchen K, et al. Effects of latex avoidance on latex sensitization, atopy and allergic diseases in patients with spina bifida. *Allergy*. 2010;65(12):1585–1593.

166. Cremer R, Mennicken O. Longitudinal study on specific IgE against natural rubber latex, banana and kiwi in patients with spina bifida. *Klin Padiatr*. 2011;223(6):352–355.

167. Kaufman BA, et al. Disbanding a multidisciplinary clinic: effects on the health care of myelomeningocele patients. *Pediatr Neurosurg*. 1994;21(1):36–44.

168. Williams EN, Broughton NS, Menelaus MB. Age-related walking in children with spina bifida. *Dev Med Child Neurol*. 1999;41(7):446–449.

169. Charney EB, Melchionni JB, Smith DR. Community ambulation by children with myelomeningocele and high-level paralysis. *J Pediatr Orthop*. 1991;11(5): 579–582.

170. Guidera KJ, et al. Use of the reciprocating gait orthosis in myelodysplasia. *J Pediatr Orthop*. 1993;13(3):341–348.

171. American Academy of Pediatrics; American Academy of Family Physicians; American College of Physicians; Transitions Clinical Report Authoring Group; Cooley WC, Sagerman PJ. Supporting the health care transition from adolescence to adulthood in the medical home. *Pediatrics*. 2011;128(1):182–200.

172. Spina Bifida Association. Available from: http://spinabifidaassociation.org/wp-content/uploads/2015/07/HOW-SB-LESIONS-IMPACT-DAILY-FUNCTION1.pdf. Accessed October 23, 2017.

173. World Health Organization. International classification of functioning, disability and health. 2001. Available from: http://www.who.int/classifications/icf/en/. Accessed October 15, 2017.

174. Andersson C, Mattsson E. Adults with cerebral palsy: a survey describing problems, needs, and resources, with special emphasis on locomotion. *Dev Med Child Neurol*. 2001;43(2):76–82.

175. McCormick A, et al. Stability of the gross motor function classification system in adults with cerebral palsy. *Dev Med Child Neurol*. 2007;49(4):265–269.

176. Day SM, et al. Change in ambulatory ability of adolescents and young adults with cerebral palsy. *Dev Med Child Neurol*. 2007;49(9):647–653.

177. Murphy KP, Molnar GE, Lankasky K. Employment and social issues in adults with cerebral palsy. *Arch Phys Med Rehabil*. 2000;81(6):807–811.

178. Strauss D, et al. Decline in function and life expectancy of older persons with cerebral palsy. *NeuroRehabilitation*. 2004;19(1):69–78.

179. Schwartz L, Engel JM, Jensen MP. Pain in persons with cerebral palsy. *Arch Phys Med Rehabil*. 1999;80(10):1243–1246.

180. Jahnsen R, et al. Musculoskeletal pain in adults with cerebral palsy compared with the general population. *J Rehabil Med*. 2004;36(2):78–84.

181. Hirsh AT, et al. Survey results of pain treatments in adults with cerebral palsy. *Am J Phys Med Rehabil*. 2011;90(3):207–216.

182. Murphy KP, Molnar GE, Lankasky K. Medical and functional status of adults with cerebral palsy. *Dev Med Child Neurol*. 1995;37(12):1075–1084.

183. Noonan KJ, et al. Hip function in adults with severe cerebral palsy. *J Bone Joint Surg Am*. 2004;86-A(12):2607–2613.

184. Bergfeldt U, et al. Focal spasticity therapy with botulinum toxin: effects on function, activities of daily living and pain in 100 adult patients. *J Rehabil Med*. 2006;38(3):166–171.

185. Jensen MP, et al. Natural history of chronic pain and pain treatment in adults with cerebral palsy. *Am J Phys Med Rehabil*. 2004;83(6):439–445.

186. Jensen MP, Engel JM, Schwartz L. Coping with cerebral palsy pain: a preliminary longitudinal study. *Pain Med*. 2006;7(1):30–37.

187. Castle K, Imms C, Howie L. Being in pain: a phenomenological study of young people with cerebral palsy. *Dev Med Child Neurol*. 2007;49(6):445–449.

188. Knapp DR Jr, Cortes H. Untreated hip dislocation in cerebral palsy. *J Pediatr Orthop*. 2002;22(5):668–671.

189. Cooperman DR, et al. Hip dislocation in spastic cerebral palsy: long-term consequences. *J Pediatr Orthop*. 1987;7(3):268–276.

190. Boldingh EJ, et al. Determinants of hip pain in adult patients with severe cerebral palsy. *J Pediatr Orthop B*. 2005;14(2):120–125.

191. Wright PB, et al. Outcomes after salvage procedures for the painful dislocated hip in cerebral palsy. *J Pediatr Orthop*. 2013;33(5):505–510.

192. Majd ME, Muldowny DS, Holt RT. Natural history of scoliosis in the institutionalized adult cerebral palsy population. *Spine (Phila Pa 1976)*. 1997;22(13): 1461–1466.

193. Saito N, et al. Natural history of scoliosis in spastic cerebral palsy. *Lancet*. 1998; 351(9117):1687–1692.

194. Lin MC, et al. Pulmonary function and spinal characteristics: their relationships in persons with idiopathic and postpoliomyelitic scoliosis. *Arch Phys Med Rehabil*. 2001;82(3):335–341.

195. Rizzi PE, et al. Adult spinal deformity and respiratory failure. Surgical results in 35 patients. *Spine (Phila Pa 1976)*. 1997;22(21):2517–2530; discussion 2531.

196. Guettard E, et al. Risk factors for spinal cord lesions in dystonic cerebral palsy and generalised dystonia. *J Neurol Neurosurg Psychiatry*. 2012;83(2):159–163.

197. Jameson R, Rech C, Garreau de Loubresse C. Cervical myelopathy in athetoid and dystonic cerebral palsy: retrospective study and literature review. *Eur Spine J*. 2010; 19(5):706–712.

198. Azuma S, et al. Long-term results of operative treatment for cervical spondylotic myelopathy in patients with athetoid cerebral palsy: an over 10-year follow-up study. *Spine (Phila Pa 1976)*. 2002;27(9):943–948; discussion 948.

199. Haak P, et al. Cerebral palsy and aging. *Dev Med Child Neurol*. 2009;51(suppl 4): 16–23.

200. Strauss D, et al. Survival in cerebral palsy in the last 20 years: signs of improvement? *Dev Med Child Neurol*. 2007;49(2):86–92.

201. Hutton JL, Pharoah PO. Life expectancy in severe cerebral palsy. *Arch Dis Child*. 2006;91(3):254–258.

202. Bowman RM, et al. Spina bifida outcome: a 25-year prospective. *Pediatr Neurosurg*. 2001;34(3):114–120.

203. Verhoef M, et al. High prevalence of incontinence among young adults with spina bifida: description, prediction and problem perception. *Spinal Cord*. 2005;43(6): 331–340.

204. Smith K, et al. Urinary continence across the life course. *Pediatr Clin North Am*. 2010;57(4):997–1011.

205. Dicianno BE, Wilson R. Hospitalizations of adults with spina bifida and congenital spinal cord anomalies. *Arch Phys Med Rehabil*. 2010;91(4):529–535.

206. Dicianno BE, et al. Rehabilitation and medical management of the adult with spina bifida. *Am J Phys Med Rehabil*. 2008;87(12):1027–1050.

207. Grunberg J, et al. Comparison of chronic peritoneal dialysis outcomes in children with and without spina bifida. *Pediatr Nephrol*. 2007;22(4):573–577.

208. Muller T, Arbeiter K, Aufricht C. Renal function in meningomyelocele: risk factors, chronic renal failure, renal replacement therapy and transplantation. *Curr Opin Urol*. 2002;12(6):479–484.

209. Ho CH, et al. Chronic indwelling urinary catheter increase the risk of bladder cancer, even in patients without spinal cord injury. *Medicine (Baltimore)*. 2015; 94(43):e1736.

210. Ahmad I, Granitsiotis P. Urological follow-up of adult spina bifida patients. *Neurourol Urodyn*. 2007;26(7):978–980.

211. Quan A, et al. Serum creatinine is a poor marker of glomerular filtration rate in patients with spina bifida. *Dev Med Child Neurol*. 1997;39(12):808–810.

212. Fox JA, et al. Cystatin C as a marker of early renal insufficiency in children with congenital neuropathic bladder. *J Urol*. 2014;191(5 suppl):1602–1607.

213. Schechter MS, et al. Sociodemographic attributes and spina bifida outcomes. *Pediatrics*. 2015;135(4):e957–e964.

214. Johnsen V, et al. Problematic aspects of faecal incontinence according to the experience of adults with spina bifida. *J Rehabil Med*. 2009;41(7):506–511.

215. Leibold S, Ekmark E, Adams RC. Decision-making for a successful bowel continence program. *Eur J Pediatr Surg*. 2000;10(suppl 1):26–30.

216. Kinsman SL, Doehring MC. The cost of preventable conditions in adults with spina bifida. *Eur J Pediatr Surg*. 1996;6(suppl 1):17–20.

217. Cai B, et al. Skin ulcers and mortality among adolescents and young adults with spina bifida in South Carolina during 2000–2010. *J Child Neurol*. 2016;31(3): 370–377.

218. Dupepe EB, et al. Rate of shunt revision as a function of age in patients with shunted hydrocephalus due to myelomeningocele. *Neurosurg Focus*. 2016;41(5):E6.

219. George TM, Fagan LH. Adult tethered cord syndrome in patients with postrepair myelomeningocele: an evidence-based outcome study. *J Neurosurg*. 2005;102 (2 suppl):150–156.

220. Lee GY, et al. Surgical management of tethered cord syndrome in adults: indications, techniques, and long-term outcomes in 60 patients. *J Neurosurg Spine*. 2006; 4(2):123–131.

221. McDonnell GV, McCann JP. Issues of medical management in adults with spina bifida. *Childs Nerv Syst*. 2000;16(4):222–227.

222. Edwards RJ, Witchell C, Pople IK. Chronic headaches in adults with spina bifida and associated hydrocephalus. *Eur J Pediatr Surg*. 2003;13(suppl 1):S13–S17.

223. Bartonek A, et al. Ambulation in patients with myelomeningocele: a 12-year follow-up. *J Pediatr Orthop*. 1999;19(2):202–206.

224. Dunteman RC, Vankoski SJ, Dias LS. Internal derotation osteotomy of the tibia: pre- and postoperative gait analysis in persons with high sacral myelomeningocele. *J Pediatr Orthop*. 2000;20(5):623–628.

225. Sawatzky BJ, et al. Prevalence of shoulder pain in adult- versus childhood-onset wheelchair users: a pilot study. *J Rehabil Res Dev*. 2005;42(3 suppl 1):1–8.

226. Valtonen KM, et al. Osteoporosis in adults with meningomyelocele: an unrecognized problem at rehabilitation clinics. *Arch Phys Med Rehabil*. 2006;87(3): 376–382.

227. Trinh A, et al. Fractures in spina bifida from childhood to young adulthood. *Osteoporos Int*. 2017;28(1):399–406.

228. Buffart LM, et al. Triad of physical activity, aerobic fitness and obesity in adolescents and young adults with myelomeningocele. *J Rehabil Med*. 2008;40(1): 70–75.

229. Singhal B, Mathew KM. Factors affecting mortality and morbidity in adult spina bifida. *Eur J Pediatr Surg*. 1999;9(suppl 1):31–32.

230. Akre C, et al. What young people with spina bifida want to know about sex and are not being told. *Child Care Health Dev*. 2015;41(6):963–969.

231. Sawyer SM, Roberts KV. Sexual and reproductive health in young people with spina bifida. *Dev Med Child Neurol*. 1999;41(10):671–675.

232. Palmer JS, Kaplan WE, Firlit CF. Erectile dysfunction in patients with spina bifida is a treatable condition. *J Urol*. 2000;164(3 Pt 2):958–961.

233. Bong GW, Rovner ES. Sexual health in adult men with spina bifida. *ScientificWorldJournal*. 2007;7:1466–1469.

234. Cass AS, Bloom BA, Luxenberg M. Sexual function in adults with myelomeningocele. *J Urol*. 1986;136(2):425–426.

235. Liakos AM, et al. Hydrocephalus and the reproductive health of women: the medical implications of maternal shunt dependency in 70 women and 138 pregnancies. *Neurol Res*. 2000;22(1):69–88.

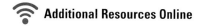 **Additional Resources Online**

Amie Brown (Jackson) McLain
Marcalee S. Alexander

CHAPTER 46

Health for Women with Disabilities

Recognizing that the American people should be encouraged to achieve healthier lifestyles, the Department of Health and Human Services (DHHS) began an initiative in 1990 known as *Healthy People 2000: National Health Promotion and Disease Prevention Objectives* (1,2). This resource focused on improving the health of all people in the United States by developing processes to strategically identify, investigate, and manage wellness activities while at the same time preventing unhealthy behaviors. The federal government with state, community, private, and public entities continues to support *Healthy People* by defining health improvement priorities in specific populations. Guidelines are determined, and progress is subsequently monitored via science-based, standard benchmarks. For nearly four decades, this initiative has continued to build a strategy for implementing 1,200 detailed, health-related objectives linked to larger, more general goals to promote outcomes for longer, healthier lives (3). The overarching goals of *Healthy People 2020* give emphasis to (a) *General Health Status*, (b) *Disparities and Inequity*, (c) *Social Determinants of Health*, and (d) *Health-Related Quality of Life and Well-Being* (4). Achievement of these goals is measured by demonstrating improvement of 26 associated "Leading Health Indicators (LHIs)," which include determinants of health, such as health service access, clinical preventive services, injury and violence consequences, maternal-fetal well-being, reproductive and sexual health, and socioeconomic factors.

Healthy People has always had an overarching goal focused on reducing and eliminating health disparities. Health *equity* is the "attainment of the highest level of health for all people." This "requires valuing everyone equally with focused and ongoing societal efforts to address avoidable inequalities, historical and contemporary injustices, and the elimination of health and health care disparities" (3). Health *disparity* is "a particular type of health difference that is closely linked with social, economic, and/or environmental disadvantage. Health disparities adversely affect groups of people who have systematically experienced greater obstacles to health based on their racial or ethnic group; religion; socioeconomic status; gender; age; mental health; cognitive, sensory, or physical disability; sexual orientation or gender identity; geographic location; or other characteristics historically linked to discrimination or exclusion" (5). Individuals with disabilities are a vulnerable population at high risk for disparities in health care delivery due to lack of equitable practices. When the individual with a disability is also of female gender, further attention is required to ensure that her medical complexities are understood. Lack of comprehensive knowledge regarding the health and wellness of women with disabilities predisposes them to receiving inequities and disparity of care.

The World Health Organization (WHO) defines *disability* by the International Classification of Functioning, Disability and Health (ICF) as "an umbrella term for impairments, activity limitations and participation restrictions" (6). *Disability* is determined by an individual's health characteristics interacting with his/her functioning environment. The U.S. Census Bureau has defined *disability* as having a "difficulty" with hearing, vision, cognition, ambulation, self-care, or independent living (7). Based on the U.S. Census Bureau data, the Cornell University Yang-Tan Institute developed the American Community Survey (ACS), which is a population-based sampling of self-reported disabling conditions. In 2016, extrapolation from the sample size utilized in the analysis revealed a base population for the United States of approximately 162 million people, 50.9% of which were female. Sub-analysis of the gender cohorts showed that 12.7% of all females responding to the ACS claimed to have one or more types of disabilities. Further stratification revealed 8.0%, 6.5%, and 3.0% of all women reported a disability related to "difficulties" with ambulation, independent living, and self-care, respectively (8). Thus, it is important to fully understand those specific disabilities that can uniquely impact the woman's reproductive health.

In recent years, studies have confirmed that the incidence and/or prevalence of some disabling disorders are greater in females compared to males. The awareness that previous medical studies included predominantly male cohorts when examining diagnosis and treatment of disease states led to a consumer outcry for inclusive gender-specific research. The unequal representation of women in health care research launched the Women's Health Initiative of the National Institutes of Health in 1991 (9). This was a major effort to address the deficiencies during a 15-year commitment of funding for large multicenter studies on topics such as breast and colon cancer, osteoporosis, and heart disease. Unfortunately, women with disabilities were not identified as a subpopulation for study; thus, despite the richness of the information, it did not help answer particular questions about the similarities or distinctions of these health issues in the context of disability.

We are just beginning to understand how disabling disorders have adverse repercussions on a woman's reproductive health and pregnancy. For example, the physiologic changes a woman experiences due to her acquired or congenital disability often exhibit neurologic and/or musculoskeletal consequences that impact gynecologic and obstetrical outcomes. On the other hand, the usual neuroendocrine fluctuations of a woman's reproductive system can affect expression or exacerbation of secondary conditions resulting from the disability. Thus, the interrelationship of gender and disability must be evaluated

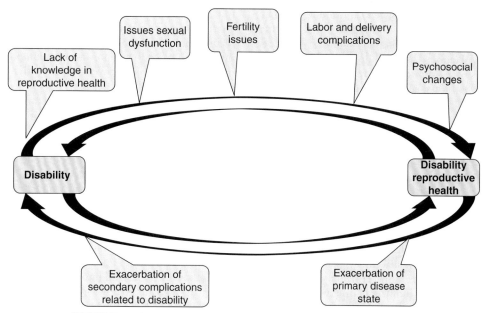

FIGURE 46-1. Interrelationship of women's reproductive health and her disabilities.

together in order to guarantee the highest quality of health care for women (**Fig. 46-1**).

This chapter will discuss several specific conditions that affect functional and reproductive health outcomes of women. It will then focus on the biologic, physiologic, and psychosocial aspects of women who have disabilities and face challenges in terms of their reproductive health and underlying disease/disorder. Specifically, unique concerns regarding *fertility, sexual function, reproductive endocrine expression, menstrual management, contraception, and obstetrical outcomes* will be addressed. The chapter will also include a discussion of the distinctive *psychosocial issues* such as violence and abuse that women with disabilities encounter but are often missed by health care providers (HCPs). Any practitioner involved in the health care of women—for any reason—has a responsibility to understand conditions that may require preventive counseling, integrative management, or specialty referral. It is only through improved access, education, and empowerment that all women will reach their maximum health status.

GENERAL CONSIDERATIONS FOR ALL WOMEN

Women's health care includes preventive as well as diagnostic and management approaches to developmental, sexual, psychosocial, and disease-specific conditions. Recognition of "normal" health status, in addition to "unhealthy" risk factors, should be part of an assessment for any practitioner or health care team. The practitioner has an obligation to assess and educate the female patient regardless of the health care environment in which she presents. Not all patients will be under the care of a primary care physician/provider or obstetrical and gynecologic specialist. In fact, a recent study supported the need for integrated care models with improved coordination among women's health specialists and primary, mental health, and other types of care providers so that all HCPs

accept responsibility for ensuring comprehensive care (10). Counseling patients about preventive care and referring to appropriate services lessen morbidity and mortality (11).

Information should be provided that directs a woman to the preventive health care for appropriate age screening of cervical, uterine, anogenital, and breast cancer. An extensive set of endorsements for age-appropriate preventive health actions for women (and men) has been published by the U.S. Preventive Services Task Force (USPSTF) (12). The USPSTF Web site gives many links that recommend preventive health care practices for providers and patients (i.e., specific disease/disorder screening, resources for counseling, preventive medication and vaccination information) and appropriate time and frequency these procedures should be completed. For example, the *Electronic Preventive Services Selector (ePSS) Tool* (13) is a link where recommendations are personalized based on age, gender, pregnancy status, tobacco use, and whether the individual is sexually active. The *Guide to Clinical Preventive Services* (14) provides a complete list of preventive health service recommendations that are reviewed and updated annually. Guidelines for screening and counseling for specific reproductive cancers found in women can also be found on the *Center for Disease Control, CDC 24/7: Saving Lives, Protecting People* Web site on the link *Inside Knowledge: Get the Facts About Gynecologic Cancer* (15).

This educational information can be downloaded and printed for patients. Expanding knowledge of practitioners, as well as promoting advocacy of the female patient for responsibility to her own health care, will contribute to improved health outcomes. Prompt recognition of conditions that may carry higher morbidity and disability allows for timely intervention and effective management that lessen impairment and mortality.

Many effective preventive initiatives for young women (and men) unfortunately continue to be underutilized despite the proven increased survival rates for those individuals who participate in these practices. For example, appropriate populations receiving vaccination to deter infection by human papillomavirus (HPV) are disappointingly low. The Center for Disease Control (CDC) reports that about 27% of U.S. women aged 14 to 59 (almost 24.9 million women) have tested positive for HPV (16). Despite the proven efficacy of HPV vaccines, only 41.9% of age-appropriate girls (and 28.1% of age-appropriate males) have received the recommended number of doses (17). Counseling from *any* HCP on the benefits and safety of HPV vaccination for females aged 9 to 26 years (and boys aged 9 to 12 years old) significantly increases utilization of the vaccine and reduces the incidence of anogenital cancer and genital warts.

Some disabling conditions develop more commonly in women and should be part of the practitioner's surveillance. HCPs should routinely screen for those risk factors indicating possible development of metabolic syndrome and other chronic illnesses. Studies have shown that two out of three women die from heart disease, cerebral vascular accidents (CVAs), diabetes, and chronic respiratory diseases (18). Permanent impairments may result as a consequence of intimate partner violence (IPV) (19). Women, more than men, have significantly greater and more severe injuries related to IPV. Furthermore, survivors of IPV have a high rate of disability, and women with disabilities are more commonly targets of IPV. Thus, the need for screening questions for IPV is vital. **Figure 46-2** was developed by McFarlane et al., as a valid, short screening tool specifically for abuse assessment in women with disabilities (20).

Osteoporosis is a very disabling condition for women. Although many factors contribute to the development and severity of osteoporosis, it generally peaks around menopausal age. Some risk factors include genetic predisposition, nutrition/vitamin and calcium intake, tobacco and caffeine consumption, immobility or lack of activity/exercise, and some medications. For women with disabilities, the neurogenic and immobility-related osteoporosis only compounds an underlying state. This topic is covered in extensive detail in another chapter of this book (see Chapter 31), but it is mentioned here as an example of a systemic process that women may develop under normal aging but also as a comorbid consequence of a disabling pathologic state.

From prevalence studies, it has been shown that women have chronic pain more frequently than do men. Furthermore, they are less likely to receive appropriate treatment. Recent investigations have shown that women respond differently to opioid medications and other types of treatment used for chronic pain management (21). This may be due to the unique relationship of pain perception, sex-related hormonal influences, and gender variability (22). It is known that estrogen receptors are present in the dorsal root ganglion and small fiber afferent nerves (23). In addition, estrogen can direct regulation (either up-regulate or down-regulate) neighboring ganglionic receptors involved in primary afferent sensitization or development of pain. Animal studies have shown that estrogen and its metabolites contribute to the sprouting and growing of small pain fibers in the dorsal spinal cord. Its action increases the affinity of nerve growth factor (NGF) for the trkA receptors, which in turn produces messenger ribonucleic acid (mRNA) expression to up-regulate nociceptive sensitivity (24,25). More recent studies with functional magnetic resonance imaging (fMRI) have looked at how estrogen, progesterone, and testosterone interact with multiple endogenous pain modulatory systems and the central nervous system (CNS). Sex hormone

---

CROWD Abuse Assessment Screen – Disability (AASD)

1. Within the last year, have you been hit, slapped, kicked, pushed, shoved, or otherwise physically hurt by someone? YES _____ NO _____
    If YES, who? (circle all that apply)
    Intimate partner   Care provider   Health professional   Family member   Other
    Please describe:

2. Within the last year, has anyone forced you to have sexual activities? YES _____ NO _____
    If YES, who? (circle all that apply)
    Intimate partner   Care provider   Health professional   Family member   Other
    Please describe:

3. Within the last year, has anyone prevented you from using a wheelchair, cane, respirator, or other assistive devices? YES _____ NO _____
    If YES, who? (circle all that apply)
    Intimate partner   Care provider   Health professional   Family member   Other
    Please describe:

4. Within the last year, has anyone you depend on refused to help you with an important personal need, such as taking your medicine, getting to the bathroom, getting out of bed, bathing, getting dressed, or getting food or drink? YES _____ NO _____
    If YES, who? (circle all that apply)
    Intimate partner   Care provider   Health professional   Family member   Other
    Please describe:

FIGURE 46-2. Screening tool to assess (confidentially) the likelihood of a woman with a disability experiencing physical, emotional, and sexual abuse. (From McFarlane J, Hughes RB, Nosek MA, et al. Abuse assessment screen-disability (AAS-D): measuring frequency, type and perpetrator of abuse towards women with physical disabilities. *J Womens Health Gend Based Med.* 2001;10(9):861–866. The publisher for this copyrighted material is Mary Ann Liebert, Inc. publishers.)

activity was assessed either by corresponding menstrual cycle levels to endogenous hormone levels or by exogenously manipulating serum levels. Functional imaging of brain activation patterns suggests that during high-estradiol states, the μ-opioid system is "turned on" to diminish effects of a sustained painful stimulus (26–29). Increased activation was seen in the thalamus, anterior hypothalamus, nucleus accumbens, and amygdala. Animal studies have provided evidence that many more interactions exist between sex hormones and the attenuation or amplification of other non-μ-opioid, pain modulatory systems that utilize many neurotransmitters such as noradrenalin, serotonin, dopamine, and γ-aminobutyric acid (GABA). Investigation (30,31) continues with other reproductive hormone such as opioids with testosterone, progesterone with GABA, and dopamine with testosterone. These studies are encouraging in understanding that pain management should be gender specific; however, much more research is needed.

WOMEN WITH DISABILITIES

In 1988, the first women's clinic for the disabled was established at the University of Alabama at Birmingham in response to women with spinal cord injury (SCI) who expressed frustration about their special needs and concerns not being met in the community. It became apparent that women with disabilities faced many barriers that prevented them from getting reproductive health care. Furthermore, it was evident that practitioners had a scarcity of specific information about these women's unique bodies in order to treat them appropriately (32). Since that time, attention slowly evolved to provide the full scope of health and wellness for women with disabilities. With wisdom and resilience born out of years of hardship, exclusion, and prejudice, women with disabilities began finding their voices and reshaping the medical care delivery system (33). In parallel with the national directive for gender-specific research, clinical investigators began looking at the demands and problems of these women through a new health care paradigm. Pioneer investigators such as Welner and Nosek elucidated what women with disabilities deemed important in obtaining health care (34,35). Overwhelmingly, women prioritized *barriers* as being the front-line encumbrance to accessing care.

Barriers to Health Care

Many types of barriers exist that have been recognized as impediments to accessing health care for people with disabilities (**Table 46-1**). Due to these efforts, *physical barriers* have been

TABLE 46-1	**Access Barriers Impacting Women's Health Care**

Physical
   Environmental
   Equipment
   Adaptive assistance
Service
Communication
Programmatic
Financial/Economics
Attitudinal
Medical Provider Knowledge

initially targeted for removal. The most overt physical barriers are stairs, narrow doorways, curbs, and inaccessible bathrooms (36,37). Curb cuts, accessible transportation, communication systems, and greater access to public spaces have been lacking in the past. Another type of physical barrier is inaccessible medical equipment, such as examination tables, bariatric scales, and mammogram machines (38). *Service barriers*, however, have not changed as much for women with disabilities who require a large range of reproductive health care services. Availability of "wellness" and "illness" resources, critical in the lives of many people with disabilities, has been the slowest domain to adapt (39–41). *Communication barriers* include shortage of sign language interpreters, materials in Braille, or large print. Other types of communication shortfalls comprise unawareness of asking and discussing concerns central to the reproductive health of individuals with disabilities. It is important for the HCP to not just prescribe a treatment or procedure, but she/he must also enquire about the ability of the woman to access the management plan. *Programmatic barriers* encompass lack of trained physical assistance to safely transfer, position, and then perform appropriate physical examinations or diagnostic testing (42). The absence of informed health care professionals and staff who understand disability-related issues may impede examination and care, especially for women who have limited hand/upper extremity function, neurogenic bowel and bladder issues, mobility pain, and fragile joints, skin, and bones. Inflexible scheduling and transportation difficulties keep women from opportunities to see providers, accept specialty referrals, obtain tests, or receive treatments (43,44). *Economic barriers* also play a significant role in preventing people with disabilities from accessing health care community services (45). The most insidious barriers, however, are erected by *ignorance and negative social attitudes* about life with disability (46). Women with disabilities, in particular, are disproportionately affected by discriminatory practices in obtaining preventive health care screening employment, education, vocational services, economic programs, access to benefits and services, health care, and parenting activities (47–49). With the passage of civil rights laws such as the Americans with Disabilities Act (ADA) in 1990, and expanding clinical services targeting the needs of women with disabilities, this situation is beginning to improve (50,51) (see Chapter 15). We are a long way, though, from full integration, where a woman with a disability can go to a community health center with the expectation that it will be fully accessible with wheelchair-adapted equipment and knowledgeable staff trained to assist women with a variety of disabilities in a manner respectful of their womanhood.

Preventive Reproductive Health Care

Women with disabilities often report difficulties obtaining balanced information about reproductive health care issues concerning menstruation management, birth control and fertility methods, pregnancy outcomes and risks, labor and delivery practices, and information about sexual functioning, dating, lesbian and gay issues, and gender identity (52,53). Basic preventive health and gynecologic screening for women with disabilities is often overshadowed by more obvious or neurologic problems, which may require more immediate focus (54). Thus, screening for diabetes, hypertension, hyperlipidemia, and thyroid imbalance, all of which are common concerns for women, may be neglected in women with disabilities (55).

Many women avoid gynecologic and subspecialty care because of difficulty in obtaining an accessible, comfortable, and dignified examination (41,53). Consequently, treatable early-stage problems may escalate and become much more difficult to manage. These concerns include Papanicolaou (Pap) smear screening as well as breast cancer evaluation. Performance of the pelvic examination must be tailored to a woman's physical impairments often using creative positioning techniques (38,56,57). An accessible examination table that lowers to wheelchair height and has security features, such as handrails, boots, and straps, can be indispensable. Leg adjustments should be performed slowly and gradually to minimize pain and spasticity yet discourage pressure points that cause skin breakdown. Liberal application of lidocaine gel to the perineal area can be helpful in minimizing spasticity or in preventing episodes of autonomic hyperreflexia (AH) in some spinal cord–injured women with high lesions (above T6) (58); however, care must be exercised to avoid contact with cervical and vaginal sampling due to possible interference with accuracy of test results.

In 2013 (the most recent data available before the publication of this chapter), 230,815 women and 2,109 men in the United States were diagnosed with breast cancer, and 40,860 women and 464 men in the United States died from this disease (59). Excluding some types of skin cancer, breast cancer in the United States is "the most common cancer in all women, independent of race or ethnicity" (see Chapter 36). Furthermore, it is "most common cause of death from cancer among Hispanic women, the second most common cause of death from cancer among white, black, and Asian/Pacific Islander women, and the third most common cause of death from cancer among American Indian/Alaska Native women." Currently, it is estimated that one in eight women will develop breast cancer. As a screening tool, mammography detects 80% to 90% of breast cancers. Mammography as a screening precaution (60) should consider the age of the woman, known presence of genetic mutation, history of chest radiation, or known family history of breast cancer. For women aged 40 to 49 years, the screening schedule should be individualized based on the woman's "circumstances" and "values." Also, the HCP must consider the likelihood for false-positive results and unnecessary need for a surgical biopsy at a time of life when women have fewer occurrences of breast cancer findings. However, "Women with a parent, sibling, or child with breast cancer are at higher risk for breast cancer and thus may benefit more than average-risk women from beginning screening in their 40s." If without risk factors, it is generally recommended for women aged 50 to 70 years old to begin screening at least every 2 years. Of note, of all the age groups, "women aged 60 to 69 years are most likely to avoid breast cancer death through mammography screening." Unfortunately, many facilities do not have equipment that easily accommodates mobility-impaired women (42). Though universal design mammography equipment is available, not all mammography centers or technicians are knowledgeable about how to accommodate women with disabilities. There are ongoing efforts to educate breast health providers how to accommodate women with disabilities (38,61,62). Women with disabilities should ask their HCP for the names of facilities in their area best able to accommodate their disability and should contact the center in advance to notify them of any special needs they might have.

Although many authorities dispute the value of the breast self-examination, the consensus from the 2013 USPSTF recommendations (63) concludes that "the evidence is insufficient to recommend for or against teaching or performing routine breast self-examination." Being aware of the changes in one's body remains important for all preventive health measures, so monthly self-breast examinations may be performed at the same time as other skin checks such as examination for skin cancer (especially melanoma), pressure sores, or infections. Women with disabilities, particularly those lacking manual sensation or dexterity, might need to rely on a partner or personal attendant or adaptive aids such as mirrors to assist with this examination.

In a longitudinal study of medical expenditure survey data (64), disabled women were less likely to receive Pap smears, mammography, and other cancer screening services but more likely to receive influenza immunization and colorectal and cholesterol screening. Another study (65) of young adults reported similar results in regard to cervical cancer screening. Even when controlled for sexual activity, females with physical disabilities aged 18 to 26 years old were significantly less likely to report receiving a Pap smear in the past year compared to able-bodied females. Interestingly, there was no statistical difference in their reporting having received a "gynecologic" examination. The investigators infer that "provider attitudes" may have factored into the young women seeing an HCP for reproductive health issues and yet not having a Pap smear performed. Another study analyzed the 2000 and 2005 National Health Interview Surveys of 20,907 women, aged 21 to 64, who were interviewed about receiving preventive health care. Encouraging results revealed only a small (not statistically significant) gap in the percentage of women with disabilities receiving less preventive health recommendations than their able-bodied counterparts (66). Unfortunately, the study could not explain why women with disabilities were statistically less likely to follow recommendations and receive a Pap smear even when there were no differences between the groups for being insured. Other researchers examined health care access using eight measures, including sources of care, insurance status, satisfaction, Pap test utilization, and breast examination. They conclude that "although the women with disabilities had similar or better potential health care access than nondisabled women, they generally had worse realized health care." (67) More specifically, women with disabilities were more likely to postpone evaluations and medications and were less satisfied with their medical care than women without disabilities, although they had higher rates of a "usual source of health care." The authors conclude that disability is a barrier to preventive clinical services and "a key issue for improving women's health care is to identify those who are at risk for specific measures of preventive care and also recognize subgroup disparities in care." (64) Interventions have been developed to promote self-advocacy and improved practices to receive preventive health care for women with disabilities, but these have not been routinely employed in today's health care environment (48).

There is growing evidence of similar health discrepancies in the treatment phase of an illness and not just in health care screenings. In a retrospective observational study of women with stage I to IIIA breast cancer, those with disabilities were much less likely to receive radiotherapy following breast-conserving surgery than nondisabled women (68). Many reasons are posited for such disparities, ranging from absent or inadequate health insurance, patient preferences, lack of physical access or transportation resources, and attitudinal bias (69,70). Further research is needed to uncover the causes for these health disparities in preventive care.

Menstruation Management and Contraception

Menarche is a symbolic moment in most women's lives, marking the transition from "girlhood" to "womanhood," with the attendant procreative possibilities. For young girls growing up with their disabilities, it can also bring a host of stresses—from the practicalities of managing menstrual hygiene to the parental anxieties and concerns raised by menstruation (71,72). Parental discomfort can encompass a wide range of issues: the need to assist with menstrual hygiene; concerns about menstrual cramps and painful periods (particularly for those daughters with intellectual or communicative disabilities); maturation and secondary sexual characteristics of their daughters with awareness of vulnerabilities for sexual abuse; interest in dating and sexuality; and potential pregnancy. For women with acquired disabilities who are still menstruating, management of menstrual flow becomes a practical issue shortly after the onset of disability, and often as a part of a rehabilitation program. Women may be able to work with a nurse or occupational therapist to develop a system for managing menstrual hygiene, which may include wheelchair modifications. Other women may find that switching to sanitary pads if they had previously used tampons may be all that is needed. Still other women may elect to work with a personal assistant to manage their menstrual hygiene. Those with more extensive physical disabilities may find these options impractical and choose to look for pharmacologic or surgical alternatives to regulate or discontinue menstruation (73–77). While there are a number of options used by women in general, there are few data on the usage, satisfaction and safety, and of these treatments in women with disabilities. Unfortunately, some physical disabilities and chronic disease states are inherently associated with menstrual irregularities, leading exactly to the unpredictable menses that is so unwelcome.

The topic of *menstrual manipulation* can imply several aspects of patient care. In the past menstrual manipulation invigorated much societal passion and concern due to a history of misuse, misunderstanding and at times, misguided objectives when utilized for women with mental and/or physical disabilities. For this reason, communication regarding the short- and long-term goals of menstrual cycle regulation is critical for the woman or female adolescent and the HCP. As explained above, curtailing or stopping menstruation is often sought by women with disabilities in order to *improve their quality of life.* Another reason includes the woman's personal desire for *contraception* during a time in her reproductive years. When *permanent contraception (i.e., sterilization)* is desired, menstrual manipulation usually involves a procedural intervention. Unfortunately, events have come to light—not too many decades ago—exposing egregious abuse and wrongful enforcement of surgical sterilization in children, adolescents, and women with physical and/or mental disabilities (78). Therefore deciding on which course of menstrual manipulation to use should only be considered with total respect for the

female and her "reproductive autonomy" without any "coercion toward forcible sterilization practices" (79).

With the development of safer, reversible hormonal interventions, menstrual suppression becomes a reasonable choice for adolescents and women with disabilities who wish contraception or reduction/cessation of menstruation (77). Studies have shown that long-acting reversible contraception (LARC) and continuous hormone contraception (CHC) are tolerated well and provide effective management for women with many types of disabilities. Menstrual suppression before menarche, however, is not recommended by American College of Obstetricians and Gynecologists (80) or the Canadian Paediatric and Adolescent Gynaecology and Obstetricians. Kirkham et al. (77) summarizes some of the available hormonal regimens and some of their risks and benefits. These interventions, however, must be considered in light of the underlying disability and its associated sequelae or required treatment. Considerations of disability-related issues should be explored before initiating hormonal therapies that may interact to exacerbate disability symptoms. After review of the individualized advantages and disadvantages to a woman's desires and disability, a gynecologic consultation/examination is recommended.

It should not be assumed that women with disabilities have no interest in permanent contraception or sterility. In fact, one study (81) of an online survey of 520 women aged 14 to 45 years old with a sampling to ensure inclusion of women of non-Caucasian races and women with disabilities reported that women with disabilities were significantly more interested in female sterilization than all subgroups analyzed. Furthermore, many of the women with disabilities responded that they currently used LARCs or had interest in using LARCs. Contraceptive coercion was not a significant concern. As a general group, 8.1% of women aged 15 to 49 years living in developing countries use some type of sterilization strictly for contraception (82). Currently, permanent sterilization includes other options than hysterectomy. While the complication and/or failure of hysteroscopic sterilization or various types of laparoscopic methods of tubal ligation have not been studied in women with disabilities, these methods may be options for permanent contraception in carefully selected women (83). Reported complications include occurrence of high-risk pregnancies in addition to abdominal infections, severe pain, and fistula formation. Performing an endometrial ablation without tubal obliteration is not an accepted contraceptive method (84).

Menstrual Irregularity and Other Gynecologic Issues

For most women with physical disabilities, fertility potential is preserved, and menses resemble the patterns of women without disabilities (85). In some cases, though, menstrual irregularity and fertility problems can occur (**Table 46-2**). Any type of abnormal uterine bleeding should be explored, and the primary etiology corrected if treatment benefits outweigh risks. When menses becomes too unpredictable and impacts the woman's function, mobility, and independence, interventions to stop menstruation are appropriate. Some of these methods were described above and include contraception. Often, abnormal uterine bleeding results in other comorbid

TABLE 46-2	Some Menstrual Problems That Impact Reproductive Health	

Menstrual Cycle Abnormalities

Condition	Types	Definition
Abnormal Uterine Bleeding	Dysfunctional uterine bleeding (DUB)	*Excessive* menstrual blood flow (MBF), usually of endocrine etiology
	Menometrorrhagia	*Prolonged* uterine bleeding at *irregular* intervals
	Menorrhagia	*Prolonged* heavy uterine bleeding at *regular* intervals
	Metrorrhagia	*Frequent irregular* menses
Dysmenorrhea	Primary	Painful abdominal cramping occurring just before or during menstruation, often associated with other somatic symptoms such as nausea vomiting, headache, and diaphoresis AND occurs at the time of menarche but not related to pelvic pathologic conditions
	Secondary	Same condition and symptoms as primary BUT occurrence is due to pathologic pelvic condition and after menarche has been established
Amenorrhea	Primary	Failure to undergo menarche before 16.5 years of age
	Secondary	Cessation of menstruation for at least 3–12 months after a woman has had a previous pattern of spontaneous menstruation

problems such as anemia, pain, and worsening spasticity/tone. Treatment options may include placement of levonorgestrel-releasing intrauterine system, or performing surgical procedures such as hysterectomy or endometrial ablation (84,86).

The most common hormonal imbalances found in women are disorders of prolactin secretion or thyroid function. Disorders of neuroendocrine function are not uncommon after traumatic brain injury (TBI) (see Chapter 19), though there are no clear data on the frequency with which it affects the menstrual cycle or fertility (87). Furthermore, recent scrutiny gives evidence that the prevalence of hypopituitarism is overreported and dependent on the acuity of TBI and testing methodology. Only cases of clinical suspicion of adrenal and antidiuretic hormone insufficiency should warrant further standardized testing (88). On the other hand, women—especially of reproductive age—who have sustained a TBI are recognized as a subpopulation who require closer endocrine monitoring.

For women with SCI (see Chapter 22), almost all women will resume their normal cycle within the first 3 to 6 months post injury (55) about 25% of one population of women studied report increased autonomic symptoms (sweating, headaches, flushing, gooseflesh) around menstruation (89). Occasionally, medications can also cause menstrual irregularities. Phenytoin and corticosteroids may affect thyroid function and ovulation; tricyclic antidepressants, antipsychotic medications, and some antihypertensive medications may also cause menstrual irregularities by affecting the hypothalamus creating labile prolactin levels (85,90,91). Treatment of menstrual irregularities varies with age and medical condition. Pregnancy should always be considered in evaluating menstrual irregularity. Thyroid and parathyroid function tests and prolactin, estradiol, follicle-stimulating hormone (FSH), luteinizing hormone (LH) and testosterone assays can be helpful in evaluating women with irregular or abnormal menstrual periods (92,93). For women who sometime during their life may have required placement of a ventriculoperitoneal (VP) shunt for increased intracranial pressure, hormonal and menstrual changes may be presenting signs of shunt malfunction or blockage (94). Correcting hormonal causes of menstrual irregularities can often regulate the menstrual cycle successfully and improve fertility.

In summary, for women who desire to conceive and are having difficulties, they need to undergo an evaluation identical to those without disabilities (94). Special consideration should be directed toward documenting normal menstrual physiology. Some research (95) hypothesizes that autonomic dysfunction or imbalance during the menstrual phases may be a cause for infertility. Evidence exists for sympathetic dominance during the luteal phase, which results in an immunologic environment that favors implantation and gestation. This may be a key problem for those women with autonomic nervous system dysfunction. Finally, the male partner needs to be involved in the process by providing a semen specimen for analysis, as about 40% of all couples who present with infertility problems will have a male factor (96).

Abnormal bleeding can also occur with structural problems such as uterine or endocervical polyps, fibroids, cervical pathology, and vulvovaginal lesions (97). Some of these problems may more frequently be associated with congenital disabilities. Menstrual irregularities become more common as women approach menopause. Careful gynecologic evaluation is required to determine an appropriate course of treatment.

It is not known if the occurrence of abnormal menstrual cycles from other causes is more common in women with some types of disability. They are at least as prevalent as that found in able-bodied women. Gynecologic referral is appropriate for evaluation; however, some of these conditions may exacerbate conditions such as bladder spasms, muscle spasms, autonomic dysfunction, and hyperirritable or constipated bowels. Understanding the relationship between the female's reproductive cycle and disability-related systemic reactions enables the HCPs to explain these symptoms and treat as management of the primary etiology.

Sexual Function

Sexuality is an important issue for people, yet it can also be problematic. In a general sample of 1,480 women seeking gynecologic care of 65% who responded to a questionnaire, 98.8% reported some types of sexual concern (98). Based on the National Health and Social Life Survey, 43% of women in the United States complain of sexual dysfunction (99). When one adds disability to the issues that a woman must tackle, the rate of sexual concerns only increases. Despite the decreases in sexual satisfaction, frequency, and desire that are known to occur after neurologic and rheumatologic disorders, the use of a systematic approach to educating and treating the sexual concerns of women with disabilities can assist in helping to improve their sexual responsiveness. The foundation for this approach comes from the "Guidelines to Promote Sexual Sustainability after SCI," a recommendation for treatment of the concerns of persons with SCIs (100); however, the framework is easily modifiable to address the concerns of persons with general disabilities; thus, it will be used here.

The first step when addressing the sexual concerns of a woman with a disability is to communicate with her in a nonjudgmental fashion assuring the woman that it is safe and it is appropriate to discuss sexual issues with you. For women with an acquired disability, once this baseline level of trust is achieved, it is then important to take a good sexual history and determine whether there were any preexisting sexual concerns prior to their disability. Among other things, these issues could include a history of childhood or partner sexual abuse; baseline sexual dysfunction including desire, arousal, orgasm or sexual pain problems; issues related to gender dysphoria or sexual orientation; depression and other preexisting psychiatric disorders; and medical problems such as diabetes, hypertension, cardiac or pulmonary disease; or gynecologic or urologic dysfunction, which could negatively impact sexual response. For women with a history of preexisting, long-standing sexual concerns, it is highly recommended that the clinician suggest referral to a physician or psychologist with special expertise in treating sexual dysfunction.

Along with the medical and sexual history, it is important to address partner issues that women with disabilities may have. Although not often addressed in research, in clinical practice, it is common to find that the spouses of persons with disabilities choose to refrain from sexual activity once their partner becomes ill. This can result in negative feelings in the person with disability and is an issue that is important to address first with the patient and then, if the patient desires and partner is willing to participate in the discussion, to add them. Moreover, it may be appropriate at this point to recommend masturbation to the woman as a source for relief of sexual tension and rediscovery of the potential for her body to respond sexually as the confidence obtained through masturbation may allow her to successfully pursue renewed sexual activity with her partner.

Cultural and religious issues are also important to consider when working to improve the sexual function of women with disabilities. For women from Africa, Asia, and the Middle East, the clinician needs to be aware of the practice of female cutting, otherwise known as circumcision or genital mutilation. Moreover, for women of the Muslim faith, many will choose not to see male physicians and if married, only to do so in the presence of their husband. Therefore, it is best in these situations to have any discussions related to sexual concerns first approached by a female. For women of the Catholic faith, the issue of premarital sex and opposition to birth control may also be a concern, and physicians must also be aware of these beliefs during their discussions.

In addition to cultural and religious issues, psychological concerns are prevalent in women with disabilities. Depression is a common issue after illness or injury that can independently cause sexual dysfunction. Anxiety and fear about the future can impact a woman's interest in sex. Altered body image and insecurity can hinder a woman's ability to seek out and engage in sexual activity, and posttraumatic stress can cause flashbacks and negative images that can impact on a woman's ability to relax during sexual activity. If these issues are found in women, it is recommended that you refer them for psychological support.

It is important to perform a detailed neurologic assessment when considering the sexual concerns of women with disabilities. Cranial nerve dysfunction can result in problems with communication, vision, or oral motor control. These issues can negatively impact the woman's ability to communicate with her partner and to participate in face-to-face activities that are very important to women, such as kissing or performing oral sex. Altered motor control and spasticity can make performance of previous sexual activities difficult and can result in a need for the woman to rethink positioning for sexual activities, require assistance to get into bed or result in the need for special care and attention from her partner in order to access body parts. Cerebellar function is important to assess and then to clarify for women ways to deal with ataxia, dysmetria, or tremor associated with sexual activity. Moreover, Positron Emission Tomography (PET) studies have showed increased activity in the left deep cerebellar nuclei in association with orgasm (101). Finally, evaluation of sensation is important to highlight insensate or dysesthetic areas for women with disabilities and educate women about them. If a woman is insensate, there is the risk of friction burns, shearing, or pressure ulcers during sexual activities that she needs to be aware of. Furthermore, detailed assessment of preservation of sensation can be helpful in women with spinal cord disorders to determine the potential impact of their injury on sexual response.

The neurologic examination of women with SCI (see Chapter 22) and disorders deserves special attention because of the association of specific patterns and degrees of injury with loss of specific aspects of arousal and orgasm. Moreover, recent studies (102,103) have shown evidence of the location for the spinal ejaculator in women. Based upon postmortem data, galanininergic neurons were found in the L2-5 spinal segments in both women and men, but at a lower density in women. These findings correspond to the dimorphic nature of ejaculation and orgasm and the levels of the spinal injury, which result in failure of response to electroejaculation. In order to assess women with SCI/D with regard to their sexual potential, it is important to perform the International Standards for the Neurologic Classification of SCI Assessment. Using the International Standards, it has been documented that the maintenance of psychogenic female arousal is related to the degree of preservation of light touch and pinprick sensation in the T11-L2 dermatomes (104). The greater the preservation of sensation in these dermatomes, the greater likelihood there is that women with SCI/Ds will be able to achieve psychogenic genital vasocongestion. The reason for this is the location of the sympathetic cell bodies at this level of the spinal cord. These dermatomes roughly correspond to the area between the umbilicus and the pockets; thus, a useful technique is to tell patients that the more they can feel in this area, the more importance there is to maximizing the romantic or psychologic sex to achieve lubrication. Another area that is important to assess in women with SCI/Ds is that of anal reflexes and sensation. With regard to reflex lubrication, although it has not been conclusively proven (105), it is generally accepted that preservation of reflex sacral function is necessary for women to have reflex lubrication. Based upon laboratory-based analyses, it has been shown in women (105) and separately in men (106), that without preservation of the bulbocavernosus reflex and anal wink reflexes, voluntary anal contraction or S3-5 sensation, individuals are unlikely to achieve genital orgasm. Whereas about 50% of women with SCIs report the ability to achieve orgasm, only 1 of 10 men and women with complete lower motor neuron injuries affecting their lower sacral cord who were studied in a laboratory reported orgasm; thus, this population should be directed toward attempting to achieve orgasm through nongenital means. Additionally for women with SCIs, the International Standards to Assess Autonomic Function (107) are available as a guideline to document the impact of level and degree of injury on sexual responses, and the Female Sexual and Reproduction Function Basic Data Sets (108) are available to document whether the woman with SCI also complains of sexual dysfunction.

Other important aspects of the physical examination include assessment of the mouth for dryness; evaluation of the joints for range of motion, tenderness, and swelling; and evaluation of the urethrogenital region for evidence of infection, lesions, urethral or vaginal prolapse, or vulvar atrophy in women who are postmenopausal or with a history of receipt of chemotherapy, regional surgery, or radiation. Additionally, the anorectal examination will provide evidence of incontinence, fissure, hemorrhoids, or other lesions that may impact on sexual activity.

Once a thorough physical examination has been performed, it is important to educate the patient regarding the impact of her disability on sexual function. Explaining the physical and psychological effects of the injury on sexuality and sexual response and educating the patient on what can be practically done to ameliorate these issues can be all that is necessary to relieve a patient's distress. Additionally, providing basic information regarding sexuality and sexual response may be necessary for some patients and can be done at the same time. Depending on the patient's age and relationship status, it may or may not be appropriate to include the patient's significant other in this discussion. As part of the educational process, it is important to broach the topic of masturbation with the patient. Many women may feel uncomfortable speaking about the topic, and bringing it up with them validates it as an area they can feel safe exploring. Furthermore, the use of masturbation is an excellent way for women without and with partners to "relearn" their bodies after illness, neurologic injury, or surgical procedures that may affect their genital responses. By becoming comfortable in achieving orgasm without a partner, it may also facilitate a woman feeling comfortable enough to achieve orgasm with a partner.

After the initial encounter with a patient who has questions about her sexual function, it is recommended that the clinician encourage the patient to go home and participate in sexual activities alone or with a partner. By giving the patient this type of "assignment," it is stressing the importance of sexuality to the patient and letting her know that you are willing and able to follow up regarding her needs. At the first visit, it is also beneficial to tell patients that use of aids like KY jelly and vibrators is commonplace among the able-bodied and that they should also feel free to explore use of these assists, which may make it easier for patients to achieve sexual satisfaction.

At the follow-up appointment, it is recommended that the practitioner review the events of the previous appointment, asking the patient, in a nonjudgmental fashion whether she had "practiced" the suggestions and whether the couple's sexual issues are resolved or if they have persistent or other concerns. At this time, it may also be necessary to review problems that were addressed at the last appointment with patients in order to ensure the patient accurately recalls the recommendations. If there are persistent concerns, it is recommended that the practitioner move to discuss confounding and iatrogenic issues that may be related to sexuality.

Confounding issues related to the impact of disability on sexuality include concomitant medical problems. Women with both type I and type II diabetes have increased sexual dysfunction (109), which can be associated with peripheral or autonomic neuropathy. Additionally, increased clitoral vascular resistance, thought to be a measure of sexual function in women, has been noted in conjunction with the metabolic syndrome (110). For women with cardiovascular disease and myocardial infarction, decreased desire, arousal, orgasm, and lubrication as compared to able-bodied controls (111) has been documented. Moreover, exercise and cardiac rehab are reported to be effective in reducing the risk of cardiovascular, sexually related complications associated with ischemic heart disease (112) (see Chapter 33). Bronchial asthma (113) and obstructive sleep apnea have been associated with increased sexual dysfunction in women (114); thus, maximizing treatment of these conditions would be beneficial. Morbid obesity has also been reported to be associated with increase sexual concerns in women (115).

Bladder and bowel dysfunction are also common confounders to sexual activity. Fear of urinary incontinence has been associated with sexual dysfunction in women (116), and the use of extended-release tolterodine (117) has been associated with improved desire, arousal, lubrication, orgasm, satisfaction, and pain in women. Pelvic organ prolapse has been associated with increased sexual problems, and randomized controlled trials have provided evidence that pelvic muscle training and/or (later) surgical correction can improve sexual function in women with prolapse (118,119). Fecal incontinence has been associated with worse sexual function in women (120,121), although the benefit of reversal of incontinence on sexual function has not been documented.

Aside from concomitant medical issues, iatrogenic concerns often impact the sexual function of women with disabilities. Many of the medications routinely used in rehabilitation have sexual side effects that can cause or compound the sexual problems of a woman with a disability. Antidepressants are commonly used in rehabilitation. In fact, according to a recent review (122), one in six women in the United States are taking antidepressants; thus, before initiating antidepressants, the clinician should be attuned to the issue of the women's sexual function, and during therapy, they should consider various means such as dose reduction, discontinuation, or changing to a different antidepressant if sexual concerns increase. Antihypertensive medications are also known to cause sexual dysfunctions. Other medications that are commonly used in rehabilitation and are associated with sexual dysfunction include pregabalin, gabapentin (123), and baclofen (124). Additionally, opiate use is associated with sexual dysfunction in women (125); thus, in addition to the adverse effects of dependence and constipation, practitioners should make certain to inform their patients about this potential if they are considering use of chronic opioids for pain management. Other iatrogenic causes of sexual dysfunction include surgeries that affect the genital neuroanatomy, radiation, or certain forms of chemotherapy.

After the clinician has reviewed the concerns regarding any impact of a disabling injury on sexual responses and has worked to alleviate concomitant medical concerns, it is recommended that the woman return home again to continue to explore her sexual potential. As sexual concerns are generally not an emergency, it is recommended that a slow approach be used so that the woman knows this is a lifelong issue. The practitioner can also remind the patient at this time of other techniques such as timing of sexual activity and using lubrication and vibratory stimulation to assist in improving her sexual responsiveness.

For some patients, these actions will resolve their sexual concerns, whereas others will still have concerns. In this case, the clinician may concern other therapies to treat sexual dysfunction. For women who complain of dyspareunia associated with vulvar atrophy, ospemifene (126) has been shown to be an effective treatment. Flibanserin was approved in 2015 to treat of hypoactive sexual desire disorder in women (127); however, its limitations include requirement for complete cessation of alcohol consumption, risk of symptomatic hypotension, and high expense and lack of third-party payment. Testosterone (128) has been shown to improve desire, arousal, and satisfaction in women; however, although it is used in the United States to treat female desire and orgasm dysfunction, it is on an off-label basis and it has not received FDA approval. For arousal dysfunction, the use of off-label PDE5 inhibitors such as sildenafil may be attempted; however, the practitioner must be aware that although sildenafil was shown to improve psychological female sexual arousal after SCI in a laboratory setting (129), it did not show improved sexual responsiveness in a multicenter trial (130). Additionally, the use of a clitoral vacuum stimulation device has been shown effective in treating orgasmic dysfunction in able-bodied women (131) and women with multiple sclerosis (MS) (132).

Once you have prescribed a treatment for sexual dysfunction, again it is worthwhile to refer the woman home for practice and evaluation of the new therapy. Reviewing the progress makes sense again at a follow-up visit. Moreover, if the woman fails to respond to any of the measures above, it may be useful to take a step back and determine whether general psychotherapy or referral to a more specialized practitioner would be beneficial. Additionally, couples therapy should definitely be considered if there is any interest on the part of the woman and her partner.

Fertility

We know that women with disabilities have neurologic, physical, physiologic, or psychosocial secondary conditions that can directly influence the pregnancy continuum. Whether a woman is able to conceive has contingencies depending on the type and expression of a disabling disease/disorder and other "non–disability"-related factors. Thus, when a woman with a disability wishes to become pregnant, planning may involve fertility assessment. Depending on the disability, studies have shown (133) that women with disabilities tend

to be older than able-bodied counterparts and those who choose to become pregnant have less functional impairments than do the women with disabilities who do not report pregnancies. Although interrelated, two spheres of influence for determining pregnancy outcomes appear to be evident: (a) disability-specific influences and (b) age-induced conditions. Disability-related factors include physical/physiologic and psychosocial consequences that encompass the woman's ability to conceive due to her underlying disability and the degree of functioning and psychological adjustment she considers before deciding to become pregnant. Age-related factors from women waiting longer to enter motherhood may impact fertility rates for the same medical reasons that are found in the able-bodied population. Regardless of those factors of concern, prenatal counseling is recommended with a health care team that may include a physiatrist, high-risk obstetrician, anesthesiologist, neurologist, neonatologist, physical and occupational therapist, lactation nurse, or others who will ensure an informed pregnancy process. It should not be assumed that a woman with a disability is asexual and not desiring motherhood. In fact, one study (134) utilized a qualitative interpretative phenomenology analysis (IPA) technique for interviewing women with spinal cord disabilities to explore their feelings and understanding of childbirth and parenting. The results concluded that (a) "childbirth is perceived by women with SCI as unique and positive"; (b) "person-centered care and control are critical"; and (c) "there is a need to recognize the biopsychosocial framework with women in this setting."

Obstetrical Issues of Pregnancy

Often women with physical disabilities are erroneously assumed to have little interest or ability to perform sexual activity and therefore have no desire to conceive children. Unfortunately, public prejudices promote negative perceptions against these women's abilities to be mothers (135). Some HCPs counsel against pregnancy due to inaccurate presumptions regarding the ability of these women to take care of their children or misconceptions that "harm" will always result to either the mother or infant (136,137). Advances in medical science have improved overall morbidity and mortality of many disabling disorders such that more women with disabilities are reaching childbearing years and having children (**Fig. 46-3**) (35,138). Unless rendered physiologically infertile by their disorder or its treatment, many women have proven capable of becoming pregnant, delivering healthy babies, and successfully accomplishing motherhood (see **Fig. 46-3**).

However, evidence from population-based surveys show that women with disabilities have significantly greater comorbid health conditions that negatively impact pregnancy outcomes. Furthermore, lack of social opportunity, economic support, and knowledge of reproductive health seem to lengthen the time for pregnancy decisions. Therefore, these women tend to be older than their able-bodied counterparts when they have their first or postinjury pregnancy.

Only in recent years have studies focused on the unique fertility and obstetrical challenges of women with disabilities. Accumulative information supports that full reproductive management of these women requires comprehension of the association between the underlying disabling disease and its impact on the pregnancy and postpartum state (135). While some disorders affect fertility, women with disabilities may also

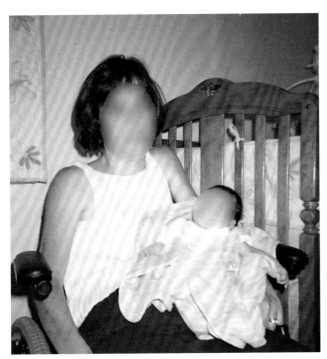

FIGURE 46-3. Early postpartum for mother with right C6, left C7 complete tetraplegia holding her 1-month infant.

have other secondary conditions that directly influence the pregnancy outcome. Conversely, during pregnancy, the adapting female reproductive system may produce direct or indirect control on the expression of the neurologic or musculoskeletal disorder. For example, in disorders such as systemic lupus erythematosus, MS, and rheumatoid arthritis, pregnancy and/or the postpartum period may improve or exacerbate the progression or symptomatology of the disease course (136–139).

Many women with disabilities have a neurogenic bladder, which is associated with a higher risk of impaired kidney function and altered urologic structures. Today, urologic management provides many options to prevent or delay the genitourinary (GU) symptoms and complications experienced by woman with neurologic disabilities such as SCI, spina bifida, MS, and transverse myelitis. Many of these women have undergone various urinary diversion procedures as a child or sometime before becoming pregnant (140). Challenges present when permanent anatomical modifications exist from a previously performed ureterosigmoidostomy, ileal or colonic conduit, abdominal or pelvic pouch, augmentation cystoplasty, or neobladder construction. The growing fetus may impair the altered GU functioning, and delivery may damage the GU diversion. Hautmann (140) and Thomas (141) performed a thorough review of published delivery outcomes of women with urinary diversions and concluded that due to the risks of complications, the diversion type should dictate the delivery method. Recommendations stated that vaginal delivery should be contraindicated for women with a narrow bony pelvis, artificial sphincter (with or without electrical stimulation), bladder neck reconstruction, or contracted hips. It should only be allowed with careful attention in women with ureterosigmoidostomy, malpresentation, or cervical prolapse. Cesarean sections are generally not contraindicated but should be performed very cautiously in women with pouches,

enterocystoplasty, or neobladders. Of course, the situation and parturient's health should always take priority before deciding any procedure.

During pregnancy, women with disabilities may experience changes to their baseline bladder function. Pressure from the growing fetus, hormonal fluctuations, increase in urinary bladder detrusor tone and spasms (seen in reflexive upper motor neuron disorders), or exacerbation of incompetence from her flaccid pelvic floor musculature (seen in areflexive, lower motor neuron disorders) can promote unusual urine leakage. For some women a modification in how she manages her bladder during pregnancy may be advisable. Placing an indwelling catheter may be considered if incontinence is significant. However, this must be evaluated in light of increasing GU infections and possibly commencement of autonomic dysreflexia (AD).

Urinary tract infections (UTIs) are very common in women with disabilities, and years of treatment predispose the woman to antibiotic resistance. Pregnancy is also associated with an increased incidence of UTIs so that the woman with a disability must be monitored more closely for these complications. Few studies have examined the issue of how to prevent or treat UTIs in these women. Two controlled studies (142,143) showed that checking cultures frequently and prescribing trimester-appropriate antibiotics for prophylaxis or treatment significantly decreased the frequency of UTIs seen in women with spinal cord injuries. The important point of the study was that specific, targeted treatment was more efficacious than indiscriminate prophylaxis.

Respiratory function may be compromised in women with disabilities. This may be from the underlying disorder or a developed abnormal adaptation such as a spinal curve deformity. If a spinal curve deformity (discussed further below) exists, the rostral-caudal dimensions of the chest wall are much less, which compromise lung volume measurements. In able-bodied women (144,145), a normal respiratory adjustment in the second half of pregnancy results in elevation of the diaphragm and anatomical rearrangement of the chest components. This situation also creates a relative physiologic alkalosis and hypoxemia with a 20% decrease in functional residual capacity (FRC) and a 15% increase in oxygen consumption. For women who have developed spinal curve deformities, or intrinsic pulmonary dysfunction, their diminished baseline function worsens when pregnancy advances (146,147). Furthermore, the expanding gravid uterus promotes diminished force vital capacity (FVC) and FRC due to restriction of lung expansion. Even in the early trimesters, pneumonia, atelectasis, gastric reflux, and significant sleep apnea may be problematic. Obtaining pulse oxygen saturations at the initial and subsequent intrapartum clinic examinations warns the clinician when asymptomatic hypoxemic conditions present. Interventions may require supplemental oxygen, use of incentive spirometry, or intermittent continuous positive airway pressure (CPAP). On occasion, portable ventilatory assistance—either intermittently or continuously—may be required during pregnancy, labor, or delivery.

Neurogenic bowel dysfunction is common in women with neurologic disabilities. Regardless of whether women have lower (areflexive) or upper (reflexive) motor neuron deficits, bowel evacuation and incontinence during pregnancy is often a primary concern. A minority of women will have bowel-specific diversions, and many will have had bowel used for a urinary diversion. Common bowel surgeries are colostomies and Malone antegrade continence enema (MACE) procedures. In 1990, Malone (148) adapted the Mitrofanoff principle (149) for fecal incontinence by creating a cutaneous appendicocecostomy whereby the lumen of the conduit closes via a physiologic valve to promote continence. The individual evacuates the bowel by introducing a catheter for installation of an enema. This procedure has been successfully used in women with SCI (150) and spina bifida (151). One report (152) even recounts successful pregnancy after surgical placement of the MACE. Understanding the changes in anatomy from these procedures is especially important when C-sections are required for delivery.

Regardless of bowel management method, problems may develop during pregnancy, especially when the consequences of neurogenic bowel are superimposed on the gastrointestinal (GI) changes that occur in a normal pregnancy. Development of hemorrhoids is common. Women undergo physiologic GI adaptations, such as decreased gastric pH and motility, and slowing of gastroesophageal sphincter activity. As the intra-abdominal pressure increases, there is a predisposition for gastroesophageal reflux and aspiration. For a woman with a neurogenic bowel, serious complications may develop such as severe constipation, chronic impactions, persistent diarrhea, paralytic ileus, abdominal pain, persistent nausea and vomiting, AD, bowel compression with necrosis, and bowel obstruction. Prenatal vitamins usually combine iron supplementation, which potentiates constipation predisposing to impactions. Programs utilizing high fiber, liberal fluids, natural laxatives, and suppositories are only partially effective. Caution should be utilized when using any medication during pregnancy and lactation due to maternal-fetal adverse effects. Although no study has been published on the safety during pregnancy of the transanal irrigation (TI) system (also called pulsatile irrigation enema [PIE]) (153), it may be an option if the woman has trunk balance and hand dexterity to introduce the rectal catheter. This becomes more difficult with abdominal enlargement. It should be prescribed cautiously, however, as one complication of this type of bowel management method is bowel perforation.

Muscle and bone often adapts to the influences of disabling neurologic and rheumatologic disorders. Musculotendinous contractures arise from increases in muscle tone, unequal muscle strengths around a joint, disuse or lack of voluntary muscle activity, or intrinsic fibrotic shortening of the connective tissue. Women with neurologic disabilities such as SCI, spina bifida, MS, cerebral palsy (CP), amyotrophic lateral sclerosis (ALS) as well as those disabilities with muscle deterioration and atrophy such as muscular dystrophies (MDs), myopathies, and arthritides are especially prone to extremity and trunk contractures. The malaligned deformity is an impediment to joint movement and body positioning (**Fig. 46-4A**).

Other bony alterations include types of osseous fusion around joints. Heterotopic ossification (H.O.), a condition that may occur following events such as SCI, TBI, burns, joint arthroplasty, and CVAs, may develop (154). Ectopic bone forms from a central neural deregulation whereby progenitor cells within the soft tissue converts to osteogenic precursor cells. These osteogenic cells transform into osteoblasts within the muscle and produce osteoid-like material around the joint. Calcium deposits form and fuse the joint. The most common

sites of H.O. formation are dependent on the primary disorder but often affect the hips followed by the knees, elbows, and shoulders. H.O. occurs within the first few months after CNS injury, but it has been reported to develop long after the initial CNS injury when that individual develops an acute inflammatory illness, sustains a long bone fracture, or undergoes a surgical procedure (155). Joint fusion may be intentional from orthopedic procedures such as ankle bone fusions with or without tendon lengthening to promote ambulation in children with congenital disabilities such as CP and spina bifida (156). Abnormal hip bone and joint development may create malformations that inhibit normal joint movement. Even without structural limitations, lower extremity limitations may occur in CNS disabilities when significant spasticity, hypertonicity, dystonia, or other uncontrolled bodily movements exist. For the pregnant woman with a disability, these problems impede safe body shifting, transferring, and positioning. For the parturient (i.e., the woman about to give birth), lower extremity joint restriction and contractures adversely impact pelvic examinations and vaginal and cesarean deliveries.

Any woman with a physical disability who has had paralysis and been non–weight bearing will develop immobility osteoporosis. Studies looking at the first year after an acquired neurologic injury reported an increase in the rate of bone loss. A potential decrease of 50% in bone mass may develop resulting in a twofold increase of fracture risk (157,158). Women of reproductive age with long-standing, immobility osteoporosis may sustain fractures with minimal tension on the bone from repositioning or ranging of the extremities. Femur fractures have even been shown to occur during sexual intercourse from the external rotation and flexion of the woman's osteoporotic bone. Similarly, sacral, pelvic, and femur bones have been reported to fracture during labor and delivery in women with disabilities. Women who have disabilities from inflammatory arthropathies may have osteoporosis from periarticular demineralization (159). Concomitant bone loss also develops when medications such as steroids and other disease-modulating therapies are used for slowing the primary disease processes or when some hormone-containing medications are taken earlier for birth control.

The progressive spine deformities, with/without spinal corrective surgery, present in females with disabilities may interfere with progression of pregnancy (**Fig. 46-4B**). These spinal changes may be congenital, idiopathic, or acquired. Progressive spinal scoliosis with or without excessive lordosis or kyphosis severely impacts the positioning of the gravid uterus during pregnancy and delivery. In women whose disability predisposes them to congenital axial skeletal abnormalities, the developing kyphoscoliosis accompanies compensatory pelvic bone deformities and hip/femoral obliquity. The tortuous vasculature around these areas encourages hemodynamic instability—especially during pregnancy. In fact, superior mesenteric artery syndrome has been reported to occur from vascular compression in a pregnant woman with severe spinal curvature distortion. Compromise of the mesenteric arteries of the duodenum from the growing fetus and enlarging uterus produced bowel ischemia and ultimately fetal distress (160,161). It is important to know about the anatomical and structural "rearrangement" of the skeletal-vascular systems so that the health care team can appropriately instruct the woman about proper positioning while in the bed or wheelchair.

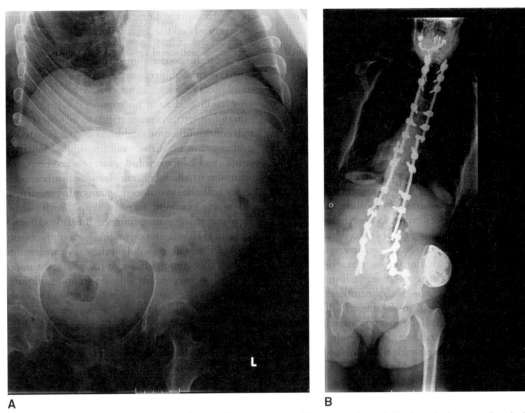

A   **B**

FIGURE 46-4. Spine and pelvic malalignment that may impact pregnancy, labor and delivery. **A:** Radiograph demonstrating significant spine and pelvic alignment changes that may impact pregnancy continuum in young woman with spina bifida contemplating pregnancy. **B:** Radiograph demonstrating limitations resulting from spinal instrumentation. Also note baclofen pump is present.

In some cases, pregnancy may initiate or exacerbate new spinal curve formation from axial-spine calcium/bone loss due to fetal requirements. Biomechanical stability of the spine becomes challenged from the added effects of altered tension on the spinal column and pregnancy-related ligamentous laxity. The literature reports an increased risk for thoracolumbar vertebral disc herniation (162), spondylolisthesis (163) during pregnancy, and sacral stress fractures during labor (164). Neural compromise may ensue creating back and leg pain, loss of lower extremity strength and sensation, and new bowel or bladder dysfunction. Unfortunately, these conditions are often missed due to the assumption that these symptoms are commonly seen in "normal" pregnancy. Progression of these conditions, however, can result in neurologic decline. Spinal scoliosis/kyphosis leading to functional deterioration, before or during pregnancy, often requires surgical reconstruction and placement of intervertebral rods, pedicle screws, or other metallic devices (165,166). Therefore, knowledge of the woman's baseline neurologic and spine status is important to document early in the pregnancy and closely observed throughout the pregnancy continuum. The woman's obstetric health care record should document all events of spine stabilization or correction for consideration of delivery method (i.e., cesarean section) and decision of general or spinal anesthesia (167–170).

Other issues of immobility are of concern for the pregnant woman with a disability. Even finding a practitioner to manage their pregnancy may be difficult. One study (43) looked at this issue by exploring the difficulty for mobility-impaired women to obtain physician appointments. The investigators

"created" a prototypical patient who was female, obese, physically disabled, and unable to self-transfer from chair to examination table. Using a specialty-determined script, the investigator "patient" called 256 medical practices in four U.S. cities and attempted to arrange a first-time appointment. Eight subspecialties were identified and stratified into two groups. One hundred and sixty practices would require transfer of the woman to a table for her to have standard, adequate evaluation, and 96 practices included specialties where the woman could be examined from her wheelchair (e.g., physiatry and ophthalmology). Of the "transfer required" group, only 14% of these practices reported having use of height-adjustable tables or a lift for transfer (and thus agreed to schedule the woman). Among the subspecialties that required transfer of the woman, gynecology had the highest rate (44% of all OB/GYN practices) of declining the woman due to inaccessibility.

Lack of height-adjustable examination tables and wheelchair weight scales impede quality management. Those who require wheelchairs and other assistive devices will need assistance with transfers, placement, and positioning on an examination or delivery table. They will be unable to place their legs in stirrups, much less maintain that position. Extra personnel may be required to hold her legs. Limitations to receiving satisfactory care may contribute to women being noncompliance with prenatal visits and testing (135). Paralysis and lack of sensation predispose any woman to a pressure sore if she is left in one position too long. Many reports exist of women who developed pressure sores during labor and delivery (170). The added weight with pregnancy may require the woman with the disability, who was once independent, to call for assistance with all activity and mobility. It is helpful for the clinical care team to review the techniques and precautions of transferring the woman on and off the examination table as well as positioning her while on the table.

Pain may or may not be associated with a disabling disorder. To date, no studies have addressed the effects of pregnancy in women with disabilities who have concomitant chronic pain syndrome(s). Chronic pain can be from many etiologies, and how the woman with a disability and chronic pain will respond to the changes from pregnancy, labor, and delivery is unique for each woman. Central, neuropathic pain, often described as burning or throbbing, can become more intense as a result of neuroendocrine adaptations. Weight gain and new mobility restrictions may strain preexisting, painful musculoskeletal problems. Pain management for pregnant women with disabilities can be challenging to manage for the practitioner who must examine the physical and functional benefits of all pain medications and the associated risks of neonatal addiction and withdrawal and fetal teratogenicity. Unfortunately, few studies have looked at treatment for these types of pregnancy-related pain. Evidence exists that safe modalities such as auricular (171) or conventional acupuncture, (172) diadynamic current applications and transcutaneous electrical neural stimulation (TENS) may confer some relief during pregnancy, especially if the pain pathology is related to spinal disorders (173,174). Studies using these modalities for relief of pain in labor have not shown effectiveness (175). Other treatments that may have palliative properties during pregnancy are prolonged (176) or short-course (177) epidural analgesia and osteopathic manipulation (178). Maternity support belts (179) lack substantiating evidence for their use, and risk of skin breakdown from the pressure is a concern for the woman with minimal or no sensation in the pelvic/abdominal dermatomes.

An intervention specific for neuropathic pain studied in women with disabilities is a spinal cord stimulator. This is a device that is implanted usually in the pelvis. Its wires connect the stimulator to the epidural space over the dorsum of the spinal cord. Electrical activation over single or multiple channel electrodes are controlled by preset frequencies. The literature (180) does not support placement of this device during pregnancy, but a case study demonstrated maternal and fetal safety for a woman who had a spinal cord stimulator placed prior to her pregnancies. Following the birth of her third child, she reexperienced the onset of her severe pain. Removal of the device revealed that one of the wires from the stimulator was broken in two places. Women with specific types of disabilities often require medications that target the primary disability or the secondary physiologic consequences from the disability. As for all women who are pregnant, or are considering pregnancy, clinical care mandates careful evaluation of their prescribed or over-the-counter medications and supplements.

Labor and Delivery

By far the most critical complication of labor and delivery occurs specifically with women with SCI or disorders. Sixty to eighty percent (181–183) of women with SCI with lesions at T6, and above, and a small percentage below T6, (183) will experience AD during uterine contractions during labor and delivery. AD (described in more detail in Chapter 22) occurs when there is a noxious stimulus or pain below the level of

injury in the spinal cord. It is an alarm system of visceral disturbances and also has been reported to occur during breast-feeding (184). It develops when cerebral control of the sympathetic-parasympathetic balance is blocked and uncontainable mass autonomic reflexes occur. If the stimulus is not found and alleviated, AD becomes a medical emergency.

When the "stimulus" is uterine contraction in labor or descent of the baby in delivery, management must be directed toward arresting maternal and fetal problems. Maternal complications may arise including cardiac arrest; hypertensive cerebral or cerebellar vascular accident or encephalopathy; intraventricular or retinal hemorrhage; coma; seizures; and death. Fetal complications involve uteroplacental vasoconstriction, fetal hypoxia, and fetal bradycardia. Treatment is regional epidural or general anesthesia and prompt delivery of the baby and placenta. Occasionally, parenteral antihypertensives are required (185). Due to the similarity of the cardiovascular symptoms of AD to those of preeclampsia/eclampsia, it is important to distinguish the difference between these very different syndromes and their treatments (186). Preeclampsia occurs with the same frequency in both able-bodied women and women with disabilities (**Fig. 46-5**). The hypertension, tachycardia, and proteinuria of eclampsia occur throughout labor, whereas AD is concomitant with uterine contractions.

Preparation for labor and delivery is an important consideration for the woman with a disability; however, depending on her disability, the traditional childbirth classes may not be adequate for her and her partner (187). Information to assist the woman in proper recognition of labor involves understanding expected signs and symptoms in the context of her particular disability (186). For example, a woman with extensive sensory impairments may not be able to sense pain from uterine contractions but have to rely on manual or electronic detection of the contractions. If she has high paraplegia or tetraplegia, periodic headaches from recurring AD due to uterine contractions, may be the first symptom she recognizes. It is important that the pregnant woman be instructed on the early signs of labor, including recognition of amniotic fluid leakage, and know when to seek immediate care. Frequent regular checkups with her practitioner are recommended with closer monitoring in the last 2 months. Finally, a discussion of anesthesia before labor and delivery is important in establishing a care plan.

Mothering with a Disability

Although mothers with disabilities share the same basic needs and concerns as nondisabled mothers, their capabilities to function aptly in a parenting role are greatly enhanced with the use of adaptive equipment and techniques. Also vital is having regular access to peer support and knowledgeable HCPs (188,189). Mothers with disabilities now have more possibilities for support and resources such as the Internet, specialized resource centers, and rehabilitation specialists. Yet, many women with disabilities live in fear of their children being taken away from them if they do not live up to other people's expectations and thus feel that they have to go to great lengths to present themselves and their children as managing "normally" in order to be accepted as "ordinary" mothers (190). This is a realistic fear, as historically the lay public and HCPs have questioned the capacity of women with disabilities to be care providers, based upon the perception and presumption that those who receive care (e.g., Personal Assistants) could not

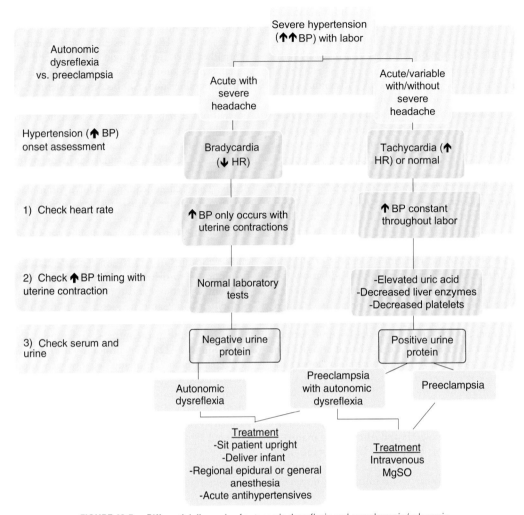

FIGURE 46-5. Differential diagnosis of autonomic dysreflexia and preeclampsia/eclampsia.

then provide care to others (190). Findings from a national study of parents with disabilities confirm the prevalence of discrimination that mothers with disabilities face regarding their rights to bear and raise children (191–195). Of the more than 1,000 parents with physical, sensory, and/or cognitive disabilities surveyed, 15% reported that others attempted to remove their children (191).

SUMMARY

The reproductive health care of women with disabilities requires understanding of the interdynamics of the disabling condition as well as risk management. Not all of these women will be predestined to significant complications, but consideration of their unique systems will require close observation so that difficulties can be recognized early and treated or accommodated. As this population grows, a collaborative approach must develop among physical medicine and rehabilitation (PM&R) specialists, obstetricians, gynecologists, urologist, GI physicians, family practitioners, nurses, physical and occupational therapist, and any other health care delivery practitioner participating in the woman's care. Finally, it is imperative that the medical team listens closely to the woman with a disability

as she is usually the most knowledgeable about her body and the changes that occur.

ACKNOWLEDGMENT

The authors would like to acknowledge Kristi L Kirschner MD, who generously allowed use of the section content from the 2nd edition chapter "Empowering Women with Disabilities to be Self-Determining in their Health Care" to be updated and serve as templates for some parts of this chapter. Dr Kirschner and her co-authors, Judy Panko Reis MA MS, Debjani Mukherjee PhD, and Cassing Hammond MD are credited with establishing valuable information that remains pertinent today. While we cannot list all of those who have also taken part in the evolution of this chapter we would like to acknowledge the following contributors of past (and present) editions: Megan Kirshbaum PhD, Judi Rogers OTR/L, Christi Tuleja MS, OTR/L, Rosemary Hughes PhD, Carol J Gill PhD, and the late Sandra Welner MD. These authors and advocates, and many others, have provided "influence, passion, and wisdom" for promoting reproductive healthcare for all women with disabilities. Finally, we thank Barrett B Jackson MA, and Elizabeth Cooper for much needed technical assistance.

REFERENCES

1. National Center for Health Statistics. *Healthy People 2000. Public Health Service: Final Review.* Hyattsville Maryland: Public Health Service, 2001.
2. Sullivan LW. Sounding board: healthy people 2000. *N Engl J Med.* 1990;323:1065–1068.
3. U.S. Department of Health and Human Services, Office of Minority Health. National Partnership for Action to End Health Disparities. *The National Plan for Action Draft as of February 17, 2010 [Internet]. Chapter 1: Introduction.* Available from: http://panko.minorityhealth.hhs.gov/npa/templates/browse.aspx?&lvl=2&lvlid=34.
4. CDC/National Center for Health Statistics Healthy People 2000 priority areas. 2009 (last updated) 2016 (last reviewed) accessed January 16, 2016 https://www.cdc.gov/nchs/healthy_people/hp2000/hp2000_priority_areas.htm
5. U.S. Department of Health and Human Services, The Secretary's Advisory Committee on National Health Promotion and Disease Prevention Objectives for 2020. *Phase I Report: Recommendations for the Framework and Format of Healthy People.* 2010. Available from: http://www.healthypeople.gov/sites//default/files/Phase1_0.pdf. Accessed April, 2017.
6. World Health Organization Factsheet on Disability and Health. 2016. Available from: http://who.int//mediacentre/factsheets/fs352/en/. Accessed April, 2017.
7. Erickson W, Lee C, von Schrader S. *Disability Statistics from the American Community Survey.* Available from: http://www.disabilitystatistics.org. Accessed April, 2017.
8. Brault MW. *Americans with Disabilities: 2010 [Brief]. Current Populations Report.* 2012. Available from: http://census.g-131.pdf. Accessed November, 2015.
9. Rossouw JE, Finnegan LP, Harlan WR, et al. The evolution of the women's health initiative: perspectives from the NIH. *J Am Med Womens Assoc.* 1995;50(2):50–55.
10. Hall KS, Patton EW, Crissman H. A population-based study on U.S. women's preferred versus usual sources of reproductive health care. *Am J Obstet Gynecol.* 2015;213(23):352.e1–352.e14.
11. The American College of Obstetricians and Gynecologists. Women's Health Care Physicians. *Well Woman's Visit: Committee Opinion No. 534.* 2012 (Reaffirmed 2016) ACOG-pub, Committee on Gynecologic Practice.
12. U.S. Preventive Task Force. Information for Health Professionals. Available from: http://uspreventiveservicetaskforce.org/Page/Name/tools-and-resources-for-better-preventive-care. Accessed April, 2017.
13. U.S. Preventive Task Force. Available from: https://epss.ahrq.gov/PDA/index.jsp; https://ahrq.gov/sites/all/themes/ahrgtheme/images/ahrg-logo.png. Accessed September 22, 2017.
14. Guide to Clinical Preventive Services. *U.S. Department of Health and Human Services Agency for Healthcare Research and Quality.* Available from: www.ahrq.gov. AHRQ Pub No. 14-05158 May, 2014. Accessed September 22, 2017.
15. Center for Disease Control. *Inside Facts: Get the Facts About Gynecological Cancer.* Available from: https://cdc.gov/2017. Accessed April, 2017. Available from: https://www.cdc.gov/cancer/knowledge/pdf/cdc_gynecologiccomprehensivebrochure_brochure.pdf
16. Dunne EF, Naleway A, Smith N, et al. Reduction in human papillomavirus vaccine type prevalence among young women screened for cervical cancer in an integrated US healthcare delivery system in 2007 and 2012-2013. *J Infect Dis.* 2015;212(12):1970–1975.
17. The American College of Obstetricians and Gynecologists Women's Health Care Physicians. *The Human Papillomavirus Vaccination: Committee Opinion No 704.* 2017. The Committee on Adolescent Health Care. ACOG.
18. Bonita R, Beaglehole R. Gender and health. Women in NCD's: overcoming the neglect. *Glob Health Action.* Available from: http://dox.doi.org/10.3402/gha/v.7.23742. Accessed April, 2017.
19. Zolotor AJ, Denham AC, Weil A. Intimate partner violence. *Obstet Gynecol Clin North Am.* 2009;36:847–860.
20. McFarlane J, Hughes RB, Nosek MA, et al. Abuse assessment screen-disability (AAS-D): measuring frequency, type and perpetrator of abuse towards women with physical disabilities. *J Womens Health Gend Based Med.* 2001;10(9):861–866.
21. Bartley EJ, Fillingim RB. Sex differences in pain: a brief review of clinical and experimental findings. *Br J Anaesth.* 2013;111(1):52–58.
22. Fillingim RB, King CD, et al. Sex, gender, and pain: a review of recent clinical and experimental findings. *J Pain.* 2009;10:447–485.
23. Aloisi AM, Bonifazi M. Sex hormones, central nervous system and pain. *Horm Behav.* 2006;50:1–7.
24. Sohrabji F, Miranda RC, Toran-Allerand CD. Estrogen differentially regulates estrogen and nerve growth factor receptor mRNAs in adult sensory neurons. *J Neurosci.* 1994;14:459–471.
25. Liuzzi FJ, Scoville SA, Bufton SM. Long-term estrogen replacement coordinately decreases trkA and beta-PPT mRNA levels in dorsal root ganglion neurons. *Exp Neurol.* 1999;155:260–267.
26. Vincent K, Tracey I. Sex hormones and pain: the evidence from functional imaging. *Curr Pain Headache Rep.* 2010;14:396–403.
27. Choi JC, Park SK, Kim YH, et al. Different brain activation patterns to pain and pain-related unpleasantness during the menstrual cycle. *Anesthesiology.* 2006;105:120–127.
28. De Leeuw R, Albuquerque RJ, Andersen AH, et al. Influence of estrogen on brain activation during stimulation with painful heat. *J Oral Maxillofac Surg.* 2006;64:158–166.
29. Smith YR, Stohler CS, Nichols TE, et al. Pronociceptive and antinociceptive effects of estradiol through endogenous opioid neurotransmission in women. *J Neurosci.* 2006;26:5777–5785.
30. Fields HL, Basbaum AI. Central nervous system mechanisms of pain modulation. In: MacMahan SB, Kolzenburg M, eds. *Wall and Melzack's Textbook of Pain.* 5th ed. London: Churchill Livingstone; 2005:125–142.
31. Craft RM. Modulation of pain by estrogens. *Pain.* 2007;132(suppl 1):S3–S12.
32. Becker H, Stuifbergen A, Tinkle M. Reproductive health care experiences of women with physical disabilities: a qualitative study. *Arch Phys Med Rehabil.* 1997;78:S26–S33.
33. Panko R, Breslin ML, Iezzoni LI, et al. *It Takes More Than Ramps to Solve the Crisis of Healthcare for People with Disabilities.* Chicago, IL: Rehabilitation Institute of Chicago; 2004. Available from: http://www.ric.org/community/RIC_whitepaperfinal82704.pdf. Accessed October 8, 2008.
34. Welner SL, Hammond C. Gynecological and obstetric issues facing women with disabilities. In: *Gynecology and Obstetrics.* Philadelphia, PA: Lippincott Williams & Wilkins; 1999.
35. Nosek MA, Howland CA, Rintala DH, et al. National study of women with disabilities: final report. *Sex Disabil.* 2001;19(1):5–39.
36. Gill CJ, Kirschner KL. *Learning to Act in Partnership: Women with Disabilities Speak to Health Care Professionals [Educational Video].* Chicago, IL: Health Resource Center for Women with Disabilities at the Rehabilitation Institute of Chicago; 2002.
37. *Educational DVD and Training Curriculum. Access to Medical Care.* World Institute on Disability; 2005. Available from: www.wid.org/programs/health-access-and-long-term-services. Accessed January 31, 2009.
38. Poulos A, Balandin S, Llewellyn G, et al. Women with physical disability and the mammogram; an observation study to identify barriers and facilitators. *Radiology.* 2011;11:14–19.
39. Iezzoni L, O'Day R. *More than Ramps: A Guide to Improving Health Care Quality and Access for People with Disabilities.* New York: Oxford University Press; 2006.
40. U.S. Department of Health and Human Services, Office of the Surgeon General. *The Surgeon General's Call To Action To Improve the Health and Wellness of Persons with Disabilities.* Washington, DC: U.S. Department of Health and Human Services; 2005. Available from: http://www.surgeongeneral.gov/library/disabilities/calltoaction/calltoaction.pdf. Accessed October 8, 2008.
41. Gill CJ. Becoming visible: personal health experiences of women with disabilities. In: Krotoski DM, Nosek MA, Turk MA, eds. *Women with Physical Disabilities.* Baltimore, MD: PH Brookes Publishing Co.; 1996:5–16.
42. Mayeda-Letourneau J. Safe patient handling and movement: a literature review. *Rehabil Nurs.* 2014;39:123–129.
43. Lagu T, Hannon NS, Rothberg MB, et al. Access to subspecialty care of patients with mobility impairment. *Ann Intern Med.* 2013;(1585):441–446.
44. Caban M, Nosek M, Graves D, et al. Breast carcinoma treatment received by women with disabilities compared with women without disabilities. *Cancer.* 2002;94(5):1391–1396.
45. Blanchard JC, Hosek HD. *Financing Healthcare for Women with Disabilities.* Santa Monica, CA: Rand; 2003. Available from: http://www.rand.org/pubs/white_papers/WP139/. Accessed October 8, 2008.
46. Albrecht GA, Seelman KD, Bury M, eds. *Handbook of Disability Studies.* Thousand Oaks, CA: Sage Publications; 2001.
47. Coyle CP, Santiago MC. Healthcare utilization among women with physical disabilities. *Medscape Womens Health.* 2002;7(4):2.
48. Suzuki R, Peterson JJ, Weatherby AV, et al. Using intervention mapping to promote the receipt of clinical preventive services among women with physical disabilities. *Health Promot Pract.* 2012;13:106–115.
49. Tate DG, Roller S, Riley B. Quality of life for women with physical disabilities. In: Cardenas D, special ed. *Women's Issues, Physical Medicine and Rehabilitation Clinics of North America.* Vol 12. Philadelphia, PA: WB Saunders; 2001:23–37.
50. Grabois E, Nosek MA. The Americans with Disabilities Act and medical providers for women—ten years after passage of the act. *Policy Stud J.* 2001;29(4):682–689.
51. Grabois E. Guide to getting reproductive health care services for women with disabilities under the Americans with Disabilities Act of 1990. *Sex Disabil.* 2001;19(3):191–208.
52. Jackson AB. Pregnancy and delivery. In: Krotoski DM, Nosek MA, Turk MA, eds. *Women with Physical Disabilities: Achieving and Maintaining Health and Well-Being.* Baltimore, MD: Paul H. Brookes; 1996:91–99.
53. Nosek MA, Rintala DH, Young M, et al. Sexual functioning among women with physical disabilities. *Arch Phys Med Rehabil.* 1996;77:107–115.
54. Piotrowski K, Snell K. Health needs of women with disabilities across the lifespan. *J Obstet Gynecol Neonatal Nurs.* 2007;36:79–87.
55. Burns AS, Jackson AB. Gynecological and reproductive issues in women with spinal cord injury. *Phys Med Rehabil Clin N Am.* 2001;12(1):183–199.
56. Welner S, Temple B. General health concerns and the physical examination. In: Welner S, Haseltine F, eds. *Welner's Guide to the Care of Women with Disabilities.* Philadelphia, PA: Lippincott Williams & Wilkins; 2004:95–108 [Chapter 9].
57. Bates CK, Carroll N, Potter J. The challenging pelvic examination. *J Gen Intern Med.* 2011;26(6):651–657.
58. Colachis SC III. Autonomic hyperreflexia with spinal cord injury. *J Am Paraplegia Soc.* 1992;15:171–186.
59. U.S. Cancer Statistics Working Group. *United States Cancer Statistics: 1999-2013 Incidence of Mortality Web-based Report.* Dept of Health and Human Services, Centers for Disease Control and prevention and National Cancer Institute; 2016. Available from: https://www.cdc.gov/cancer/breast/statistics/. Accessed May, 2017.

60. U.S. Preventive Task Force 2016. *First Annual Report to Congress on High-Priority Evidence Gaps for Clinical Preventive Services—Appendix C.* Accessed April, 2017. Available from: http://uspreventiveservicestaskforce.org/Page/Name/first-annual-report-to-congress-on-high-priority-evidence-gaps-for-clinical-preventive-services

61. Toveg F. *Breast Health and Beyond: A Provider's Guide to the Examination and Screening of Women with Disabilities.* 2nd ed. Berkeley, CA: Breast Health Access for Women with Disabilities (BHAWD); 2007.

62. Llewellyn G, Balandin S, Poulos A. Disability and mammography screening: intangible barriers to participation. *Disabil Rehabil.* 2011;33(19–20):1755–1767.

63. U.S. Preventive Services Task Force 2013. *First Annual Report to Congress on High-Priority Evidence Gaps for Clinical Preventive Services—Appendix C.* 2013. Available from: https://www.uspreventiveservicestaskforce.org/Page/Name/first-annual-report-to-congress-on-high-priority-evidence-gaps. Accessed April, 2017.

64. Wei W, Findley PA, Sambamoorthi U. Disability and receipt of clinical preventive services amongst women. *Womens Health Issues.* 2006;16(6):286–296.

65. McRee AL, Haydon AA, Halpern CT. Reproductive health of young adults with physical disabilities in the U.S. *Prev Med.* 2010;51:502–504.

66. Rivera Drew JA, Short SE. Disability and pap smear receipt among U.S. Women, 2000 and 2005. *Perspect Sex Reprod Health.* 2010;42(4):258–266.

67. Parish SL, Huh J. Health care for women with disabilities: population-based evidence of disparities. *Health Soc Work.* 2006;31(1):7–15.

68. McCarthy EP, Ngo LH, Roetzheim RD, et al. Disparities in breast cancer treatment and survival for women with disabilities. *Ann Intern Med.* 2006;145:637–645.

69. Iezzoni LI, Kilbridge K, Park ER. Physical access barriers to care for diagnosis and treatment of breast cancer among women with mobility impairments. *Oncol Nurs Forum.* 2010;37(6):711–717.

70. Iezzoni LI, Frakt AB, Pizer SD. Uninsured persons with disability confront substantial barriers to health care services. *Disabil Health J.* 2011;4(4):238–244.

71. Stainton MA. Piece of my mind. Raising a woman. *JAMA.* 2006;296(12):1445–1446.

72. Gunther DF, Diekema DS. Attenuating growth in children with profound developmental disability: a new approach to an old dilemma. *Arch Pediatr Adolesc Med.* 2006;160(10):1013–1017.

73. Kiley J, Hammond C. Combined oral contraceptives: a comprehensive review. *Clin Obstet Gynecol.* 2007;50(4):868–877.

74. Jensen JT, Speroff L. Health benefits of oral contraceptives. *Obstet Gynecol Clin North Am.* 2000;27:705–721.

75. Istre O, Trolle B. Treatment of menorrhagia with the levonorgestrel intrauterine system versus endometrial resection. *Fertil Steril.* 2001;76:304–309.

76. Dizon C, Allen LM, Ornstein MP. Menstrual and contraceptive issues among young women with developmental disabilities. Review of cases at the Hospital for Sick Children, Toronto. *J Pediatr Adolesc Gynecol.* 2005;18:157–162.

77. Kirkham YA, Allen L, Kives S, et al. Trends in menstrual concerns and suppression in adolescents with developmental disabilities. *J Adolesc Health.* 2013;53(3):407–412.

78. Largent MA. *Breeding Contempt: The History of Coerced Sterilization in the United States.* New Brunswick, NB: Rutgers University Press; 2008.

79. Committee on Ethics. American College of Obstetricians and Gynecologists. Committee Opinion No 695. Sterilization of women: ethical issues and considerations. *Obstet Gynecol.* 2017;129:e109–e116.

80. Committee on Adolescent Health Care. American College of Obstetricians and Gynecologists. Committee opinion No 668. Menstrual manipulation for adolescents with physical and developmental disabilities. *Obstet Gynecol.* 2016;128:e20–e25.

81. Burns B, Grindlay K, Dennis A. Women's awareness of, interest in, and experiences with long-acting reversible and permanent contraception. *Womens Health Issues.* 2015;25(3):224–231.

82. Lawrie TA, Nardin JM, Kulier R, et al. Techniques for the interruption of tubal patency for female sterilisation. *Cochrane Database Syst Rev.* 2011;(2):CD003034.

83. La Chapelle CF, Veersema S, Brolmann HA, et al. Effectiveness and feasibility of hysteroscopic sterilization techniques: a systematic review and meta-analysis. *Fertil Steril.* 2015;103(6):1516–1525.

84. Cleary TP, Tepper NK, Cwiak C, et al. Pregnancies after hysteroscopic sterilization: a systematic review. *Contraception.* 2013;87(5):539–548.

85. Roche NE, Weiss G. Infertility diagnosis and treatment for the disabled woman. In: Welner S, Haseltine F, eds. *Welner's Guide to the Care of Women with Disabilities.* Philadelphia, PA: Lippincott Williams & Wilkins; 2004:185–194.

86. Bonafede MM, Miller JD, Lukes A, et al. Comparison of direct and indirect costs of abnormal uterine bleeding treatment with global endometrial ablation and hysterectomy. *J Comp Eff Res.* 2015;4(2):115–122.

87. Sandel ME, Delmonico R, Kotch MJ. Sexuality, reproduction, and neuroendocrine disorders following TBI. In: Zasler ND, Katz DI, Zafonte RD, eds. *Brain Injury Medicine: Principles and Practice.* New York: Demos Medical Publishing; 2007.

88. Klose M, Feldt-Rasmussen U. Chronic endocrine consequences of traumatic brain injury—what is the evidence? *Nat Rev Endocrinol.* 2018;14(1):57–62.

89. Jackson AB, Wadley V. A multicenter study of women's self reported reproductive health after spinal cord injury. *Arch Phys Med Rehabil.* 1990;80:1420–1428.

90. Smith PJ, Surks MI. Multiple effects of 5,5-diphenylhydantoin on the thyroid hormone systems. *Endocr Rev.* 1984;5:514–524.

91. Kletzky OA, Davajan V. Hyperprolactinemia. In: Mishell DR, Davajan V, Lobo RA, eds. *Infertility, Contraception, and Reproductive Endocrinology.* Boston, MA: Blackwell Scientific Publications; 1991:809–851.

92. Wathen PI, Hendersen MC, Witz CA. Abnormal uterine bleeding. *Med Clin North Am.* 1995;2:329–344.

93. Ratchev E, Dokumov S. Premenopausal bleeding associated with hyperprolactinaemia. *Maturitas.* 1995;3:197–200.

94. Bedaiwy MA, Fathalla MM, Shaaban OM, et al. Reproductive implications of endoscopic third ventriculostomy for the treatment of hydrocephalus. *Eur J Obstet Gynecol Reprod Biol.* 2008;140(1):55–60.

95. Lee PY, Bazar LA, Yun AJ. Menstrual variation of autonomic balance may be a factor in exacerbations of certain diseases during the menstrual cycle. *Med Hypotheses.* 2004;63(1):163–167.

96. Smith S, Pfeifer SM, Collins JA. Diagnosis and management of female infertility. *JAMA.* 2003;290(13):1767–1770.

97. Severino M. Endocrinology, infertility, and genetics. *Gynecol Obstet.* 1995;5:2.

98. Bachman GA, Avei D. Evaluation and management of female sexual dysfunction. *Endocrinologist.* 2004;14:337–345.

99. Lauman EP, Paik A, Rosen RC. Sexual dysfunction in the United States: prevalence and predictors. *JAMA.* 1999;281(6):537–544.

100. Alexander M, Courtois F, Elliott S, et al. Improving sexual satisfaction in persons with SCIs: collective wisdom. *Top Spinal Cord Inj Rehabil.* 2017;23(1):57–70.

101. Georgiadis JR, Kortekaas R, Kuipers R, et al. Regional cerebral blood flow changes associated with clitorally induced orgasm in healthy women. *Eur J Neurosci.* 2006;24(110):3305–3316.

102. Chehensse C, Facchinetti P, Bahrami S, et al. Human spinal ejaculation generator. *Ann Neurol.* 2017;81:35–45.

103. Alexander, MS, Kozyrev N, Bosma RL, et al. fMRI localization of spinal cord processing underlying female sexual arousal. *J Sex Marital Ther.* 2016;42:36–47.

104. Sipski ML, Alexander CJ, Rosen RC. Sexual arousal and orgasm in women: effects of spinal cord injury. *Ann Neurol.* 2001;49(1):35–44.

105. Sipski ML, Alexander CJ, Gomez-Marin O, et al. Effects of vibratory stimulation on sexual response in women with spinal cord injury. *J Rehabil Res Dev.* 2005;42(5):609–616.

106. Sipski M, Alexander CJ, Gomez-Marin O. Effects of level and degree of spinal cord injury on male orgasm. *Spinal Cord.* 2006;44:798–804.

107. Alexander MS, Biering-Sorensen F, Bodner D, et al. International standards to document remaining autonomic function after spinal cord injury. *Spinal Cord.* 2009;47:36–43.

108. Alexander MS, Biering-Sorensen F, Elliott S, et al. International spinal cord injury female sexual function basic data set. *Spinal Cord.* 2011;49:787–790.

109. Pontiroli AE, Cortelazzi D, Morabito A. Female sexual dysfunction and diabetes: a systematic review and meta-analysis. *J Sex Med.* 2013;10(4):1044–1051.

110. Maseroli E, Fanni E, Cipriani S, et al. Cardiometabolic risk and female sexuality: focus on clitoral vascular resistance. *J Sex Med.* 2016;13(11):1651–1661.

111. Oskay U, Can G, Camci G. Effect of myocardial infarction on female sexual function in women. *Arch Gynecol Obstet.* 2015;291(5):1127–1133.

112. Lange R, Levine G. Sexual activity and ischemic heart disease. *Curr Cardiol Rep.* 2014;16:445.

113. Skrzypulec V, Drosdzol A, Nowosielski K. The influence of bronchial asthma on the quality of life and sexual functioning of women. *J Physiol Pharmacol.* 2007;58 suppl 5(Pt 2):647–655.

114. Liu L, Kang R, Zhao S, et al. Sexual dysfunction in patients with obstructive sleep apnea: a systematic review and meta-analysis. *J Sex Med.* 2015;12(10):1992–2003.

115. Steffen KJ, King WC, White GE, et al. Sexual functioning of men and women with severe obesity before bariatric surgery. *Surg Obes Relat Dis.* 2017;13(2):334–343.

116. Çayan S, Yaman Ö, Orhan İ, et al. Prevalence of sexual dysfunction and urinary incontinence and associated risk factors in Turkish women. *Eur J Obstet Gynecol Reprod Biol.* 2016;203:303–308.

117. Zachariou A, Filiponi M. The effect of extended release tolterodine used for overactive bladder treatment on female sexual function. *Int Braz J Urol.* 2017;43(4):713–720.

118. Braekken IH, Majida M, Ellström Engh M, et al. Can pelvic floor muscle training improve sexual function in women with pelvic organ prolapse? A randomized controlled trial. *J Sex Med.* 2015;12(2):470–480.

119. Uçar MG, İlhan TT, Şanlıkan F, et al. Sexual functioning before and after vaginal hysterectomy to treat pelvic organ prolapse and the effects of vaginal cuff closure techniques: a prospective randomised study. *Eur J Obstet Gynecol Reprod Biol.* 2016;206:1–5.

120. Cichowski SB, Yuko M, Komesu, GC, et al. The association between fecal incontinence and sexual activity and function in women attending a tertiary referral center. *Int Urogynecol J.* 2013;24(9):1489–1494.

121. Pauls RN, Rogers RG, Parekh M, et al. Sexual function in women with anal incontinence using a new instrument: the PISQ-IR. *Int Urogynecol J.* 2015;26(5):657–663.

122. Lorenz T, Rullo J, Faubion S. Antidepressant-induced female sexual dysfunction. *Mayo Clin Proc.* 2016;91(9):1280–1286.

123. Yang Y, Wang X. Sexual dysfunction related to antiepileptic drugs in patients with epilepsy. *Expert Opin Drug Saf.* 2016;15(1):31–42.

124. Saval A, Chiodo A. Sexual dysfunction associated with intrathecal baclofen use: a report of two cases. *J Spinal Cord Med.* 2008;31(1):103–105.

125. Ajo R, Segura A, Inda MD, et al. Opioids increase sexual dysfunction in patients with non-cancer pain. *J Sex Med.* 2016;13(9):1377–1386.

126. Wurz GT, Kao CJ, DeGregorio MW. Safety and efficacy of ospemifene for the treatment of dyspareunia associated with vulvar and vaginal atrophy due to menopause. *Clin Interv Aging.* 2014;9:1939–1950.

127. Gelman F, Atrio J. Flibanserin for hypoactive sexual desire disorder: place in therapy. *Ther Adv Chronic Dis.* 2017;8(1):16–25.

128. Khera M. Testosterone therapy for female sexual dysfunction. *Sex Med Rev.* 2015;3(3):137–144.

129. Sipski ML, Alexander CJ, Rosen RC, et al. Sildenafil effects on sexual and cardiovascular responses in women with spinal cord injury. *Urology.* 2000;55:812–815.

130. Alexander MS, Rosen RC, Steinberg S, et al. Sildenafil in women with sexual arousal disorder following spinal cord injury. *Spinal Cord.* 2011;49(2):273–279.

131. Josefson D. FDA approves device for female sexual dysfunction. *BMJ.* 2000;320(7247):1427.

132. Alexander M, Bashir K, Alexander C, et al. Randomized Trial of Clitoral Vacuum Suction Versus Vibratory Stimulation in Neurogenic Female Orgasmic Dysfunction. *Arch Phys Med Rehabil.* 2018 Feb;99(2):299–305. doi: 10.1016/j.apmr.2017.09.001. Epub 2017 Sep 9.

133. Iezzoni LI, Chen Y, McLain AB. Current pregnancy among women with spinal cord injury findings from the US national spinal cord injury database. *Spinal Cord.* 2015;53(111):821–826.

134. Tebbett M, Kennedy P. The experience of childbirth for women with spinal cord injuries: an interpretative phenomenology analysis study. *Disabil Rehabil.* 2012;34(9):726–769.

135. Iezzoni LI, Wint AJ, Smeltzer SC, et al. Effects of disability on pregnancy experiences among women with impaired mobility. *Acta Obstet Gynecol Scand.* 2015;94(2):133–140.

136. Mitra M, Smith LD, Smeltzer SC, et al. Barriers to providing maternity care to women with physical disabilities: perspectives from health care practitioners. *Disabil Health J.* 2017;10(3):445–450.

137. Long-Bellil L, Mitra M, Iezzoni LI, et al. The impact of physical disability on pregnancy and childbirth. *J Womens Health (Larchmt).* 2017;26(8):878–885.

138. Iezzoni LI, Yu J, Wint AJ, et al. Prevalence of current pregnancy among US women with and without chronic physical disabilities. *Med Care.* 2013;51(6):555–562.

139. Silver RM, Branch DW. Autoimmune disease in pregnancy. *Clin Perinatol.* 1997;21:291–319.

140. Hautmann RE, Volkmer BG. Pregnancy and urinary diversion. *Urol Clin North Am* 2007;34(1):71–88.

141. Thomas JC, Adams MC. Female sexual function and pregnancy after genitourinary reconstruction. *J Urol.* 2009;182(6):2578–2584.

142. Salomon J, Schnitzler A, Ville Y, et al. Prevention of urinary tract infection in six spinal cord-injured pregnant women who gave birth to seven children under a weekly oral cyclic antibiotic program. *Int J Infect Dis.* 2009;13(3):399–402.

143. Michau A, Dinh A, Denys P, et al. Control cross-sectional study evaluating an antibiotic prevention strategy in 30 pregnancies under clean intermittent self-catheterization and review of literature. *Urology.* 2016;91:58–63.

144. Madorsky JG. Influence of disability on pregnancy and motherhood. *West J Med.* 1995;162:153–154.

145. Norwitz ER, Repke JT. Obstetric issues in women with neurologic disabilities. In: Kaplan PW, ed. *Neurologic Disease in Women.* New York: Demos; 2005:151–167.

146. Winslow C, Rozovsky J. Effect of spinal cord injury on the respiratory system. *Am J Phys Med Rehabil.* 2003;82(10):803–815.

147. Nash CL, Kevins K. A literal look at pulmonary function in scoliosis. In proceedings of the Scoliosis Research Society. *J Bone Joint Surg.* 1974;46A:440.

148. Malone PS, Ransley PG, Kiely EM. Preliminary report: the antegrade continence enema. *Lancet.* 1990;336:1217–1218.

149. Adams MC, Joseph DB. Urinary tract reconstruction in children. In: Wein AJ, ed. *Campbell-Walsh Urology.* 10th ed. Philadelphia, PA: Saunders; 2007:3458–3502.

150. Teichman JMH, Barber DB, Rogenes VJ, et al. Malone antegrade continence enemas for autonomic dysreflexia secondary to neurogenic bowel. *J Spinal Cord Med.* 1998;21:245–247.

151. Squire R, Kiely EM, Carr B, et al. The clinical application of the Malone antegrade colonic enema. *J Pediatr Surg.* 1993;28:1012–1015.

152. Macdonald MC, Garner JP, Selby KF, et al. Successful pregnancy and delivery following a Malone antegrade continence enema procedure. *Tech Coloproctol.* 2009;13:337–339.

153. Krassioukov A, Eng JJ, Claxton G, et al. Neurogenic bowel management after spinal cord injury: a systematic review of the evidence. *Spinal Cord.* 2010;48(10):718–733.

154. Ranganathan K, Loder S, Agarwal A, et al. Heterotopic ossification: basic-science principles and clinical correlates. *J Bone Joint Surg.* 2015;97(13):1101–1111.

155. Sullivan MP, Torres SJ, Mehta S, et al. Instructional review, trauma: heterotopic ossification after central nervous system trauma. *Bone Joint Res.* 2013;2(3):51–57.

156. Sarwark JF. Common orthopedic problems II. *Pediatr Clin North Am.* 1996;43(5):1151–1158.

157. Maimoun L, Fattal C, Sultan C. Bone remodeling and calcium homeostasis in patients with spinal cord injury: a review. *Metabolism.* 2011;60(12):1655–1663.

158. Sarikaya S, Ozdolap S, Acikgoz G, et al. Pregnancy-associated osteoporosis with vertebral fractures and scoliosis. *Joint Bone Spine.* 2004;71(1):84–85.

159. Sarikaya S, Basaran A, Tekin Y, et al. Is osteoporosis generalized or localized to central skeleton in ankylosing spondylitis? *J Clin Rheumatol.* 2007;13(1):20–24.

160. Elmadag M, Guzel Y, Uzer G, et al. Superior mesenteric artery syndrome due to a vertebral hemangioma and postpartum osteoporosis following treatment. *Orthopedics.* 2010;33(7):519.

161. Marecek GS, Barsness KA, Sarwark JF. Relief of superior mesenteric artery syndrome with correction of multiplanar spinal deformity by posterior spinal fusion. *Orthopedics.* 2010;33(7):519.

162. Brown MD, Levi AD. Surgery for lumbar disc herniation during pregnancy. *Spine.* 2001;26(4):440–443.

163. Russell R, Reynolds F, Editorial. Back pain, pregnancy, and childbirth: postpartum pain is most likely to be a continuation of antepartum pain. *BMJ.* 1997;314:106.

164. Thein R, Burstein G, Shabshin N. Labor-related sacral stress fracture presenting as lower limb radicular pain. *Orthopedics.* 2009;32:447–452.

165. Nossek E, Ekstein M, Rimon E, et al. Neurosurgery and pregnancy. *Acta Neurochir.* 2011;153(9):1727–1735.

166. Hedequist DJ. Instrumentation and fusion for congenital spine deformities. *Spine.* 2009;34(17):1783–1790.

167. Kuczkowski KM. Planning for labor (and labor analgesia) in a parturient with spinal cord injury: a need for multidisciplinary approach. *Spine J.* 2004;4(3):370–377.

168. Bansal N, Gupta S. Anaesthetic management of a parturient with severe Kyphoscoliosis. *Kathmandu Univ Med J (KUMJ).* 2008;6(23):379–382.

169. Lavelle WF, Demers E, Fuchs A, et al. Pregnancy after anterior spinal surgery: fertility, cesarean-section rate, and use of neuraxial anesthesia. *Spine J.* 2009;(4):271–274.

170. Darney BG, Biel FM, Quigley BP, et al. Primary cesarean delivery patterns among women with physical, sensory, or intellectual disabilities. *Womens Health Issues.* 2017;27(3):336–344.

171. Wang SM, Dezinno P, Lin EC, et al. Auricular acupuncture as a treatment for pregnant women who have low back and posterior pelvic pain: a pilot study. *Am J Obstet Gynecol.* 2009;201(3):271.e1–271.e9.

172. Ernst E, Lee MS, Choi TY. Acupuncture in obstetrics and gynecology: an overview of systematic review. *Am J Chin Med.* 2011;39(3):423–431.

173. Ratajczak B, Hawrylak A, Demidas A, et al. Effectiveness of diadynamic currents and transcutaneous electrical nerve stimulation in disc disease lumbar part of spine. *J Back Musculoskelet Rehabil.* 2011;24(3):155–159.

174. Han IH. Pregnancy and spinal problems. *Curr Opin Obstet Gynecol.* 2010;22(6):477–481.

175. Dowswell T, Bedwell C, Lavender T, et al. Transcutaneous electrical nerve stimulation (TENS) for pain relief in labour. *Cochrane Database Syst Rev.* 2009;(2):CD007214.

176. Khan M, Mahmood T. Prolonged epidural analgesia for intractable lumbo-sacral pain in pregnancy. *J Obstet Gynaecol.* 2008;28(3):350–351.

177. Winder AD, Johnson S, Murphy J, et al. Epidural analgesia for treatment of a sickle cell crisis during pregnancy. *Obstet Gynecol.* 2011;118(2 Pt 2):495–497.

178. Licciardone JC, Buchanan S, Hensel KL, et al. Osteopathic manipulative treatment of back pain and related symptoms during pregnancy: a randomized controlled trial. *Am J Obstet Gynecol.* 2010:202(1):43–48.

179. Ho SS, Yu WW, Lao TT, et al. Effectiveness of maternity support belts in reducing low back pain during pregnancy: a review. *J Clin Nurs.* 2009;18(11):1523–1532.

180. Takeshima N, Okuda K, Takatanin J, et al. Trial spinal cord stimulator reimplantation following lead breakage after third birth. *Pain Physician.* 2010;13(6):523–526.

181. Guttman L, Paeslack V. Cardiac irregularities during labor in paraplegic women. *Paraplegia.* 1965;3:144–147.

182. Wanner MB, Rageth CJ, Zach OA. Pregnancy and autonomic hyperreflexia in patients with spinal cord lesions. *Paraplegia.* 1986;6:482–490.

183. Gimovsky ML, Ojeda A, Otaki R, et al. Management of autonomic hyperreflexia associated with a low thoracic spinal cord lesion. *Am J Obstet Gynecol.* 1985;153(2):223–224.

184. Dakhil-Jerew F. Autonomic dysreflexia triggered by breastfeeding in a tetraplegic mother. *J Rehabil Med.* 2008;40:780–782.

185. Kuczkowski KM. Labor analgesia for the parturient with spinal cord injury: what does an obstetrician need to know? *Arch Gynecol Obstet.* 2006;274:108–112.

186. Baker ER, Cardena DI, Benedetti TJ. Risks associated with pregnancy in spinal cord injury women. *Obstet Gynecol.* 1992;80(3):425–428.

187. Rogers J. *The Disabled Woman's Guide to Pregnancy and Birth.* New York: Demos Medical Publishing; 2006.

188. Kopala B, Young M. *Mothers with Disabilities: An Introduction.* Loyola University Niehoff School of Nursing; 1992 (Available through Judy Panko-Reis, MA,MS, UIC College of Nursing, 312-996-1866).

189. Filax G, Taylor D, eds. *Disabled Mothers: Stories and Scholarship By and About Mothers with Disabilities.* Bradford, Ontario, Canada: Demeter Press; 2014.

190. Grue K, Laerum T. "Doing Motherhood": some experiences of mothers with physical disabilities. *Disabil Soc.* 2002;17(6):671–683.

191. Toms-Barker L, Maralani V. *Challenges and Strategies of Disabled Parents: Findings From a National Survey of Parents with Disabilities. Final Report.* Available from: http://www.berkeleypolicyassociates.com/photo/20030608_223938/488-1_Final_Report.pdf. Accessed January 31, 2009.

192. Kirshbaum M. Disability cultural perspective on early intervention with parents with physical or cognitive disabilities and their infants. *Infants Young Child.* 2000;23(2):9–20.

193. Kirshbaum M, Olkin R. Parents with physical systemic or visual disabilities. *Sex Disabil.* 2002;20(1):65–80.

194. Buck F, Hohmann G. Personality behavior, values and family relations of children of fathers with spinal cord injury. *Arch Phys Med Rehabil.* 1981;62:432–438.

195. Greene BF, Norman R, Searle M, et al. Child abuse and neglect by parents with disabilities: a tale if two families. *J Appl Behav Anal.* 1995;28(4):417–434.

Geriatric Rehabilitation

Aging is the stage of life in which maximum functioning gradually declines. Many factors contribute to this, and traditionally physiologic deterioration has been seen as the primary driver of decline. Multiple chronic illnesses are almost inevitable in advanced older age. However, it is increasingly recognized that social and environmental factors also contribute. Rehabilitation for older people aims to reduce disability through enhancing and maintaining optimal functioning in the context of an older person's usual environment.

Until recently, rehabilitation involving older people has developed mainly in the context of disabilities related to specific health conditions, for example, stroke and hip fracture. However, increasingly, it is now recognized as a broader health strategy to assist older people improve functioning, particularly in the areas of mobility and self-care. Similarly, its setting has traditionally been institutional (principally hospital based), but increasingly, its application in community settings is recognized and promoted.

The World Health Organization recognizes that access to rehabilitation influences older people's ability to recover physical capacity and regain and sustain independence (1) **Figure 47-1**.

It also recognizes that there is great diversity in the capacities and health needs of older people, which has its origins in events throughout the person's life, and thus, an understanding of aging is relevant to rehabilitation medicine for younger people (1). The life course approach recognizes that a number of events and processes that are determinants of health in older age can be modified (1).

The goals of this chapter are to:
- Review epidemiology and theories of aging
- Discuss common syndromes and health conditions associated with aging
- Examine the impact of contextual factors (personal and environmental) on functioning in older adults
- Review studies of functioning in older adults
- Introduce principles and methods of assessing limitations of functioning as a basis for formulation of rehabilitation interventions
- Detail appropriate rehabilitation interventions for a number of disabling health conditions and syndromes with high prevalence in older adults

AGING—EPIDEMIOLOGY AND THEORIES OF AGING

Demography and Epidemiology of Aging

Demographic Imperative

The context for the increasing interest, and concern, about health care needs of older adults is found in demographic projections of an expanding population of older people in the United States and other developed countries.

At the turn of the 20th century, 1 of every 25 Americans (4%) was 65 years of age or older. By 2015, this population had increased to 1 of every 7 Americans (14.9%), or 47.8 million (2). Current projections indicate that 88.0 million, or 1 of every 5 Americans (22.1%), will be 65 years of age or older by the year 2050 (2). By 2029, all "baby boomers" (Americans born post–WW II, between 1946 and 1964) will be 65 years or over. However, the rate of aging of the population and the absolute percentage of older people in the United States are less than most other developed countries, particularly Europe and Japan (3). In addition, life expectancy in the United States is expected to increase less than in most other countries (4).

Distribution of the older people is uneven across the United States, with 50% living in just nine states. While California has the greatest number of citizens over the age of 65, Florida has the highest proportion of older people (18.6%) (5). There are also ethnic aging trends, with projections that by 2050 the proportion of older White individuals will have decreased, with corresponding increases of older Hispanic and Black American citizens (2).

There is increasing recognition of differences in health care needs and issues among subgroups of older people. Of particular significance from a health care standpoint is the rapidly expanding relative proportions of the population aging 65 years and older who are 75 to 85 years of age (old-old) and 85 years of age or older (oldest-old). These groups include many of the so-called frail older people, with a disproportionately high prevalence of disabilities and consumption of health services (6). Another related dynamic is recognition of increasing racial and ethnic health disparities among older Americans, as the relative proportions of racial and ethnic minorities increase.

Compression of Morbidity and Disability

Older people are also living longer, and this increase in life expectancy is projected to continue. Between 2010 and 2030, estimated longevity at 65 years of age is projected to increase by approximately 2 years for women and 3 years for men in the United States (4). Contributing factors to these increases in longevity include improved access to health care, advances in medical care, overall healthier lifestyles, as well as better health prior to age 65 (7). The increasingly delayed occurrence of death at all ages appears in part to be due to reduced lethality of such diseases as stroke, cancer, and myocardial infarction, resulting from risk factor reduction as well as improved health care interventions (8). Increasingly, people are surviving their initial encounter with these previously fatal diseases,

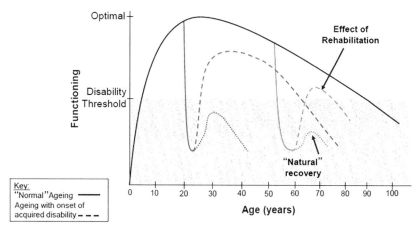

FIGURE 47-1. Theoretical impact of rehabilitation on functioning at different ages.

resulting instead in chronic illness. This trend has been termed the fourth stage of epidemiologic transition (i.e., the postponement of death from degenerative diseases) (9). These significant reductions in mortality are associated with an increasing risk for development of various chronic diseases.

Certainly, the incidence and prevalence of many potentially disabling chronic illnesses increase substantially among older adults, including arthritis, osteoporosis with associated fractures, stroke, amputation, and various neurodegenerative disorders (e.g., Alzheimer's disease, Parkinson's disease) (6,10–12).

This demographic imperative has far-reaching implications for increasingly limited U.S. health care resources and dollars: 84% of U.S. health care spending is for people with chronic health conditions (13). In 2012, the average annual health care expenses were $18,988 for the 65+ population, compared to $6,632 for the working age population (14). The old-old and oldest-old groups consume the greatest proportion of resources, and a disproportionate amount of these health care costs represent nursing home and other institutional care (6). While the overall proportion of older individuals residing in nursing homes decreased from 6.8% in 1982 to 4.2% in 1999, these rates vary dramatically by age (15). Only 1% of young-old (65- to 74-year-olds) reside in nursing homes, contrasted with 20% of the oldest-old (85 years of age or older) (8). In fact, the latter group constitutes 45% of all older nursing home residents.

It appears that much of the increased health care cost associated with aging (across all health care settings) is significantly related to activity limitation, rather than chronic disease (13,16). There is some evidence that disability among older individuals may be decreasing, but this may vary from country to country, and there may be a differential reduction in restriction of basic activities of daily living (ADLs) rather than instrumental activities of daily living (IADLs) (1). **Figure 47-2** shows the prevalence of ADL disability over time in one population group. Obesity does not seem to be the cause of this in the United States, and it may relate to self-reporting differences or other factors (17).

These findings could lend credence to the concept advanced by Fries in 1980 of "compression of morbidity," in which he predicted that if the age of onset of disability

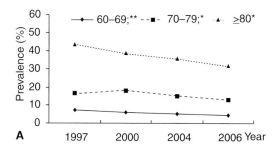

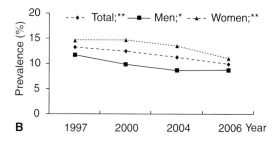

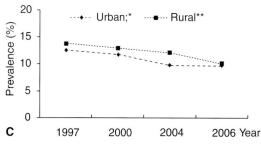

FIGURE 47-2. Prevalence of ADL disability over time in Chinese older people. Prevalence of disability in basic activities of daily living over time in 1997, 2000, 2004, and 2006, by age groups **(A)**, sex **(B)**, and living regions **(C)**. $*p_{trend} < 0.05$; $**p_{trend} < 0.01$. The prevalence of disability in basic activities of daily living significantly decreased from 1997 to 2006: $p_{trend} < 0.01$ for the total sample, for people aged 60 to 69 years, for women, and for rural residents; $p_{trend} \leq 0.05$ for people aged 70 to 79 years and ≥ 80 years, for men, and for urban residents. (From Liang Y, Song A, Du S, et al. Trends in disability in activities of daily living among Chinese older adults, 1997–2006: the China Health and Nutrition Survey. *J Gerontol A Biol Sci Med Sci.* 2015;70(6):739–745. Reproduced by permission of The Gerontological Society of America.)

could be significantly delayed (e.g., with regular exercise, healthier diets, elimination of smoking, improved health care interventions) in the context of a relatively "fixed" life span, then terminal predeath disability could be compressed into a shorter interval (18). He postulated that health care needs for older people would decrease because they would be relatively healthy and functional until shortly before their death. A related prediction was that this anticipated short duration of predeath morbidity, and accompanying disability, would be expected and accepted with acknowledged futility of medical intervention. There is consistent evidence of increased health care costs associated with aging, with one study documenting nearly one half of lifetime health care costs occurring after age 65 (19). Interestingly, although a number of reports have documented dramatically increasing health care costs near the end of life, it should be noted that these are costs generated close to death, not of living longer *per se* (20). Further, there is evidence suggesting that the incremental costs associated with extending life may actually plateau or even decrease (21–23). These findings are of critical significance in the context of increasing focus on cost containment and debate over the feasibility and appropriateness of rationing of health care (24). Twenty years after his initial predictions, Fries (and others) cites increasing evidence in support of the trend of compression of morbidity, even though the mechanisms are not clear (25,26). He reiterates the importance of a research agenda focused on delineation of the epidemiology of disability, determination of the fundamental basis of age-associated chronic conditions, and identification of effective interventions for preventing or delaying resulting disability (25). This call to action has been echoed by others as well (12,19,27). On the other hand, Kane raises disturbing questions regarding potentially adverse economic, cultural, and individual consequences of successfully overcoming the aging (and dying) process and urges ongoing dialogue to further explore these ethical questions (28).

Active Life Expectancy

A derivative of research into longevity and epidemiology of aging relates to issues of quality of life, given the increased incidence of frequently disabling chronic disorders such as degenerative neurologic diseases (e.g., Alzheimer's disease, Parkinson's disease), degenerative musculoskeletal conditions (e.g., osteoporosis, osteoarthritis), and multisensory losses (e.g., cataracts, presbycusis). One concept that attempts to delineate quality of life for older individuals has been termed "active life expectancy," referring to the proportion of remaining life span characterized by functional independence (29). This concept, also referred to as "disability-free life expectancy," has been expanded to consider both physical and cognitive impairments, as well as their interrelationships (26,30). A significant sex difference in active life expectancy with aging has been identified. As can be seen in **Table 47-1**, older men have a greater proportionate active life expectancy at all ages. However, due to greater longevity, older women enjoy longer actual durations of active life expectancy than older men, until age 85 (31,32). A longitudinal British study confirmed a sex difference, with men aged 65 showing 79% active life expectancy (12.1 of 15.3 years) and women aged 65 showing 57% active life expectancy (11.0 of 19.4 years) (26). Further investigation into dynamics impacting active life expectancy reveals the deleterious effects of diabetes (decreased total life expectancy and active life expectancy at all ages, with a 25% reduction in active life expectancy in 85-year-olds) and depression (reduction of active life expectancy by 6.5 years in 70-year-old males and by 4.2 years in 70-year-old women) (33,34).

Comorbidity, Frailty, and Disability

Although the increasing incidence and prevalence of (often multiple) chronic diseases with aging are well documented, there is no one-to-one correlation between either disease and illness (35) or disease and disability (36). A significant proportion of older people are limited in the amount or kind of

TABLE 47-1	Active Life Expectancy (Remaining Years of Functional Independence, Compared to Projected Longevity) by Gender and Age Cohort[a]			
	Males		**Females**	
	1990 Period Estimates	**Completed-Cohort Estimates**	**1990 Period Estimates**	**Complete-Cohort Estimates**
At Age 65				
Total	15.1	15.7	18.9	22.2
Active	7.4	13.7	9.8	15.7
Disabled in community	7.0	1.7	7.5	5.0
Institutionalized	0.6	0.4	1.5	1.6
At Age 85				
Total	5.2	6.4	6.4	9.3
Active	1.6	4.2	1.6	3.1
Disabled in community	2.7	1.5	3.0	4.2
Institutionalized	0.9	0.7	1.8	1.9

[a]Sum of life expectancies in states may not add to total expectation of life because of rounding.

Adapted by permission from Springer: Manton KG, Land KC. Active life expectancy estimates for the U.S. elderly population: a multidimensional continuous-mixture model of functional change applied to completed cohorts, 1982–1996. *Demography.* 2000;37(3):253–265. Copyright © 2000 Population Association of America.

their usual activity or mobility secondary to chronic impairments: over 60% of adults with functional impairments due to chronic health problems are 65 years of age or older (10).

However, disability in this older population can also be very dynamic, with frequent transitions between periods of independence and disability and levels of disability (37,38). Also, the overall health of progressive cohorts of older persons has been changing. Although there have been predictions that future generations may well be healthier than current generations, due in part to higher levels of education and health awareness (38), there are disturbing trends of increasing obesity and diabetes in older adults, with significant associated morbidity and mortality (11).

Fried et al. have helped to clarify the dynamics of interrelationships among comorbidity, frailty, and disability—terms frequently used interchangeably—by providing discrete definitions of each entity and describing the synergistic impact of each on the other(s) (39). As seen in **Figure 47-5**, disability accordingly is defined as "difficulty or dependency in carrying out activities essential to independent living" (such as ADLs, mobility, IADLs), while frailty is "a physiologic state of increased vulnerability to stressors that results from decreased physiologic reserves, and even dysregulation, of multiple physiologic systems." Frailty appears to represent an aggregate expression of risk resulting from age- or disease-associated physiologic accumulation of subthreshold decrements affecting multiple physiologic systems (39). Fried cites evidence in support of a phenotype of the clinically frail older adult, characterized by the presence of a critical mass of three or more "core elements" of frailty (weakness, poor endurance, weight loss, low physical

activity, and slow gait speed) (40). Comorbidity is commonly defined as the concurrent presence of two or more disease processes in the same individual. Fried suggests that comorbidity is the aggregation of clinically manifested diseases present in an individual, while frailty is the aggregate of subclinical losses of reserve across multiple physiologic systems (39).

Fried further documents the interrelationships between frailty, comorbidity, and disability (**Fig. 47-3**), noting that frailty and comorbidity each predict disability, while disability appears to exacerbate frailty and comorbidity (39). While medical care for each of these entities is typically complex, particularly when they coexist, Fried specifically notes that rehabilitation interventions for disabled older adults to regain function and/or prevent further functional decline need to factor in recognition and treatment of frailty and comorbidity to maximize likelihood of success. She cites growing evidence to suggest that frailty, comorbidity, and disability may be preventable but with different intervention strategies (39). The importance of prevention is reinforced by the clear association of each entity, especially when concurrent, with higher health care costs and poorer survival (39,41). Recent research is further differentiating between various subtypes of disability in older individuals (transient, short term, long term, recurrent, and unstable) and their relative clinical significance (42).

In summary, an increasing proportion of older people are living longer and are at increased risk of developing varying (and changing) degrees of comorbidity, frailty, and functional losses with disability. The challenge for health care providers, accordingly, is to try to prevent the onset/progression of these entities with early and effective medical and rehabilitation interventions and to reverse or at least minimize their deleterious effects on health and function.

Active Aging and Healthy Aging

Distinctions have been made between aging processes representing "primary aging" (i.e., apparently universal changes that occur with aging, independent of disease and environmental effects) and "secondary aging," which includes lifestyle and environmental consequences and disease associated with aging (43,44). A number of tenets associated with aging research are being re-examined, particularly with the observation that a pathologic process may exaggerate an aging process believed to be normal, even before the disease is detected clinically (43). There is increasing evidence that the nonpathologic processes of aging are distinct from, but not necessarily independent of, the pathologic processes of disease (39,45).

Most studies of normal aging have focused on the physiologic and biochemical changes occurring with aging, with explicit exclusion of disease. However, it is increasingly apparent that such factors as personal habits (e.g., diet, exercise, nutrition), environmental exposures, and body composition may have significant impact on observed aging changes (44). Rowe has proposed a conceptual distinction between "successful aging" and "usual aging" (46). He suggests that "successful aging" could be characterized by minimal or no physiologic losses in a particular organ system and would comprise a relatively small subset of the total "normal" (i.e., nonpathologic) aging population. The remaining majority of "normal" older adults demonstrate "usual aging," with gradually progressive but significant declines in various physiologic functions.

The significance of this concept lies in the implications for modifiability of usual aging by virtue of addressing such

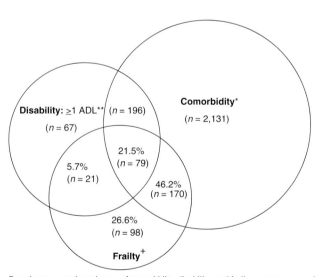

Prevalences—and overlaps—of comorbidity, disability, and frailty among community-dwelling men and women 65 years and older participating in the Cardiovascular Health Study. Percents listed indicate the proportion among those who were frail (n = 368), who had comorbidity and/or disability, or neither. Total represented: 2,762 participants who had comorbidity and/or disability and/or frailty.⁺n = 368 frail participants overall. *n = 2,576 overall with 2 or more of the following 9 diseases: myocardial infarction, angina, congestive heart failure, claudication, arthritis, cancer, diabetes, hypertension, chronic obstructive pulmonary disease. Of these, 249, total were frail. **n = 363 overall with an activity of daily living disability; of these, 100 (total) were also frail.

FIGURE 47-3. Overlap of frailty, comorbidity, disability. (From Fried LP, Ferrucci L, Darer J, et al. Untangling the concepts of disability, frailty, and comorbidity: implications for improved targeting and care. *J Gerontol A Biol Sci Med Sci.* 2004;59(3):M255–M263. Reproduced by permission of The Gerontological Society of America.

variables as level of physical activity, diet and nutrition, and environmental exposures (25,44,45). This principle is demonstrated in studies documenting the effects of exercise, diet, and drugs on the usual aging observations of carbohydrate intolerance. Rowe proposes that geriatric research into health promotion initiatives concentrates on increasing the proportion of older adults who "successfully age" by identifying and modifying extrinsic risk factors contributing to "usual aging" and decreasing the manifestations of "pathologic aging" by preventing or minimizing adverse effects of acquired disease processes (46). This would reinforce the previously described concept of compression of morbidity, with greater active life expectancy. Indeed, studies are helping to determine which factors distinguish high-functioning older adults from other populations of older adults (26,33,44,47).

The World Health Organization has more recently defined and discussed "active aging" with emphasis on the importance of activity, particularly physical activity (1), and Active and Healthy Aging, which is a broad concept and particularly acknowledges environmental influences on aging well (1). **Figure 47-4** shows factors associated with healthy aging.

Theories of Aging

With continuing research, it appears likely that there is no single cause of aging (45,48). The current concepts of aging characterize the process as extremely complex and multifactorial and suggest that various theories of aging should be viewed not as mutually exclusive but rather complementary (48). From this perspective, hypotheses based on passive (i.e., random) and/or active processes

of genetic programming could be considered in conjunction with superimposed nongenetic mechanisms (e.g., environment, lifestyle), producing varying individual vulnerability (43,45,46,49). Certainly, this would help explain the well-documented phenomenon of differential aging, whereby individuals of the same species appear to age at different rates (45,47). Multiple levels of research suggest that rates of aging are affected to varying extents by heredity, lifestyle, environment, occurrence of disease, and psychological coping abilities (31,43,47,50).

Active investigation continues in the areas of neuroendocrine pacemakers, telomere shortening, and attenuation of inducible stress responses (49,51–53). A number of studies have also focused on the phenomena of apoptosis and autophagy, related to cell death of proliferating and postmitotic cells, respectively, as well as mitochondrial degradation in long-living cells (54,55). There is some evidence suggesting that pathologic stimulation of apoptosis may result in a number of degenerative disorders commonly associated with aging, whereas inhibition appears to be associated with a variety of forms of cancer (54). For example, osteoporosis may be related to accelerated cell death, while failure of apoptosis appears to be an important mechanism in cancer, particularly metastatic cancer.

Physiology of Normal Aging

The normal aging process involves gradual decreases in body system capabilities and homeostatic controls that are relatively benign (i.e., asymptomatic or subclinical) in the absence of disease or stress (35). Although the older person progressively adapts to these changes without need (or desire) for outside

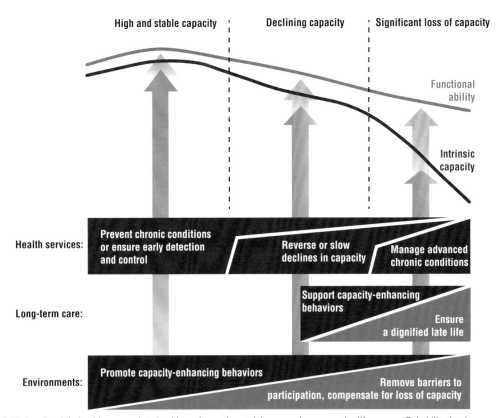

FIGURE 47-4. A public health approach to healthy aging and sustaining capacity across the life course. Rehabilitation has a major role in both the situations of "declining capacity" and "significant loss of capacity." It is a health service, but it can influence functioning in the long-term care setting and also advocate for environmental adaptations. (Reprinted with permission from World Health Organization. *World Report on Aging and Health.* Geneva 2015.)

intervention, the steady decreases of physiologic reserves make older adults potentially vulnerable to functional decline as a result of acute and/or chronic illnesses (43,56). One way of understanding these processes is via the "disposable soma" theory, which attributes aging to the buildup of accumulated deficits due to random molecular damage that is influenced by both genetic and environmental factors (57). Characteristics of aging include the following:

- Decreased reserve capacity of body systems, which is typically apparent only during periods of exertion or stress
- Decreased homeostatic control (e.g., decreased ability to remain upright with perturbations, decline in baroreceptor sensitivity)
- Decreased ability to adapt in response to different environments (e.g., vulnerability to falls in response to uneven or slippery surfaces, risk of hypothermia and hyperthermia with changing temperatures)
- Decreased capacity to respond to stress (e.g., exertion, fever, anemia) (35)

The end result of these age-related declines is an increased risk of disease and injury or frailty (39).

Problems in Study Design

Inherent with studying physiologic changes in aging adults are several potentially confounding variables, which are unique to this population. Awareness of these dynamics will facilitate more accurate interpretations of clinical studies of older adults, with particular reference to generalizability.

Definition of Normal

A significant concern, in view of the heterogeneity of the aging population, is what is truly normal. As noted, there is great variability in rates of aging among healthy older people and wide variations in individual performance (31,35). More than 80% of the population over 65 years has at least one chronic disease and 50% two or more disorders (30). One question is whether the relative minority of older people who have escaped serious illness should be considered "normal" for the purpose of studies of aging and whether the results of such studies can be generalized to the rest (majority) of the older population. Another area of uncertainty is that multimorbidity is not coincident with disability or frailty.

On the other hand, it is important clinically to be able to differentiate the physiologic and functional consequences of aging (i.e., normal aging) from those of accompanying disease (i.e., pathologic aging) (58). Because detection of disease depends on determination that a patient is other than normal, it is critical to define appropriate age-adjusted criteria for clinically relevant variables in older people (59). Although many laboratory values do change gradually with aging, abnormalities should not be a priori attributed to old age. In fact, a number of age-related changes may resemble the changes associated with a specific disease (45). For example, an age-related decline in glucose tolerance is well documented. So dramatic is this change that most people over 60 years of age would be diagnosed as diabetic if traditional criteria, based on studies of primarily younger patients, were applied (60).

Methodology Limitations

A number of methodologic problems are associated with the study of aging. Well recognized is the tendency for very old people to report an age that is greater than their actual chronologic age (61). This is coupled with difficulties in verifying reported ages, due in part to lost or nonexistent birth records.

Another major problem in the design and evaluation of aging studies is the relative validity of both cross-sectional and longitudinal studies. Cross-sectional studies, although easier and less costly (in time and money) to perform, often overemphasize (but may also underestimate) age-related changes (62,63). This can result from a cohort bias, due to significant differences in educational, nutritional, health, and social experiences of people born in different decades.

Contributing further to this distortion is the high proportion of older people in the United States who were foreign born, with relatively less schooling. This has implications in particular for studies of psychological and cognitive changes with aging (36). A further issue to consider is a period effect in which there is a change in the rate of a health condition affecting the entire population at a given point in time.

On the other hand, longitudinal studies tend to underestimate changes due to aging, primarily as a result of withdrawal and survivor biases with high dropout rates (47,56,62). Some studies have experienced as much as a 50% dropout rate over just a 10-year period, leading to questions of self-selection for relative preservation of function (and again, the issue of "supernormals").

Subtle changes in methodology over time may introduce laboratory drifts that are difficult to differentiate from true age-related changes (5). A further concern with serial measurements is the potential for distortion due to learning effects.

Mean Versus Maximal Performance

Another issue in the characterization of aging is that a focus on "average" or "mean" changes in various parameters can hide remarkable individual variation, particularly regarding peak performance (18). Consider marathon running, which tends to attract a very select ("supernormal") population and, thus, individuals with a higher maximal aerobic capacity. For example, a 50-year-old male with a marathon time of 3.5 hours is in the 99th percentile for his age group, yet this same time would not be an age group record until over 80 years of age.

Although there also is a slow linear decline in maximal aerobic performance with aging based on world age group records, this is only on the order of about 1% per year between the ages of 30 and 70 years (18). This linear decline appears to accelerate after 70 years of age (64).

Effects of Age on Organ System Performance

There are several general principles regarding aging effects on the performance of various organ systems (65).

Wide Individual Differences in the Rate of Aging

Linear regressions show average changes with aging, but variation between subjects is so great that it is not always possible to determine accurately if age decrements are linear over the entire age span or whether the rate of decline accelerates in later years (66). However, Fleg et al. recently reported that VO_{2max} declines more precipitously after the age of 70, especially in men, irrespective of habitual physical activity (64) and long-distance world records for endurance running support this.

Different Organ Systems Age at Different Rates

There is great individual variation in the rate of decline for various organ system functions (35). For instance, there is up to a 60% decline in maximal breathing capacity with aging but only a 15% decline in nerve conduction velocity and basal metabolic rate during the same time interval. Another demonstration of this principle is the localized cellular growth, aging, and death that occur continuously in some tissues and organs (e.g., hematopoietic system, skin, and mucosa).

Furthermore, a significant decline in function of one organ system (e.g., kidney) does not necessarily entail a similar decline in other organ systems (65).

Age Changes with Complex Performances

Complex performances (e.g., running) will show greater changes with aging because of the need to coordinate and integrate multiple organ system functions (e.g., rate, degree and sequence of muscle contraction, balance, proprioception, vision, cardiovascular response), as opposed to simple performances involving a single system (e.g., renal glomerular filtration) (65).

Age Changes in Adaptive Responses

Adaptive responses (e.g., to temperature change or change in position) are most affected by aging due to a decline in the effectiveness of physiologic control mechanisms (e.g., sensory feedback), which is magnified during stressful situations (e.g., disease, sudden changes in environment) (35,65).

Prevention and Reversibility of Physiologic Decline

There is little question that biologic systems, regardless of the direct effects of aging, can be profoundly influenced by environment and lifestyle (31,35,44). Obvious examples include a sedentary versus active lifestyle and the deleterious effects of smoking (67,68).

The modifiability or plasticity of aging is demonstrated by studies in which performance can be improved despite age, within relatively broad ranges (18,69). Physical training can improve or even reverse age-related declines in aerobic power and muscle strength (70–72). These gains have been demonstrated to translate to improvements in functional skills (73,74).

Functional Implications of Body System Aging

The clinician must be aware of specific age-related physiologic changes to properly understand disease in older people because these changes significantly influence not only the presentation of disease but also the response to treatment and potential complications that may ensue. Similarly, such knowledge is essential to understand the underlying mechanisms of functional deterioration secondary to disease and to formulate effective rehabilitation approaches (58). The following is a summary of clinically significant physiologic changes that occur with aging.

Geriatric Syndromes

Providing health care to older people involves frequent encounters with syndromes that have high prevalence in older people. These occur as a consequence of disease and age-related changes in body systems. These "geriatric giants" were recognized by British geriatricians last century and are characterized by the "Is": immobility and instability, incontinence, and impaired intellect (75). "Impaired intellect" may be due to dementia, delirium, a combination of both conditions, or, less commonly, psychiatric disorders. These syndromes are discussed in more detail later in this chapter.

Sensory System

Deterioration of vision is one of the most recognized sensory changes occurring with aging. The most common visual change with increasing age is a gradual loss of the ability to increase

thickness and curvature of the lens to focus on near objects (i.e., presbyopia) and physiologic miosis (60). Cataract formation, with opacification of the lens, occurs to some degree in 95% of the 65 years or older population. Older people are also at significantly higher risk for further disease-related visual decrements (e.g., glaucoma, macular degeneration, diabetic retinopathy) (76). The result of these various changes is a loss of visual acuity, decrease in lateral fields of vision, decline in both dark adaptation ability and speed of adaptation, and higher minimal threshold for light perception. These changes have obvious implications in relation to the higher incidence of falls in older people, particularly at night (77,78).

Gradual decline in hearing acuity (i.e., presbycusis) also is characteristic of aging, although again a number of treatable disorders can cause superimposed hearing loss (e.g., wax occluding the outer canal, cholesteatomas, acoustic neuromas). Older people most commonly manifest a conductive hearing loss, possibly due to increased stiffness of the basilar membrane or distortion of perceived sound with increase in threshold sensitivity, narrower range of audibility, abnormal loudness, and difficulty discriminating complex sounds (79). Continuing advances in hearing aid technology make remediation of such hearing deficits increasingly feasible (80). Early recognition and treatment of hearing impairments are particularly critical in the presence of cognitive deficits to avoid adverse sequelae of social isolation and development of paranoid ideations or frank psychiatric reactions (77).

Neurologic System

Numerous changes in the functioning of the neurologic system have been noted with aging (81). Important areas of dysfunction accompanying normal aging include loss of speed of motor activities (with slowing in the rate of central information processing) and changes in posture, proprioception, and gait (60).

The major controversy over neurologic changes with aging concerns cognitive functioning. A significant proportion of the observed decline in fluid intelligence with aging appears to be related to a decrease in the rate of central information processing (82–84). There is progressive deterioration in performance after age 20 on timed motor or cognitive tasks, including abstraction tests (e.g., digit symbol substitution test), reaction time tasks, and other tests requiring speed in processing of new information. Although there are declines with aging in motor and sensory nerve conduction velocities and rate of muscle contraction, they account for only a fraction of these slowed responses (83).

Many aspects of learning and memory remain relatively intact during normal aging, including immediate or primary memory as measured by digit span recall, retrieval from long-term storage, storage and retrieval of overlearned material, and semantic memory (85). However, age-related impairments have been documented consistently in tasks involving episodic short-term memory and incidental learning (86). Examples include difficulties with free recall of long (i.e., supraspan) lists of digits or words and paired-associate and serial rate learning, for both visually and verbally presented material. What these investigations indicate is that older adults are capable of new learning but at a slower rate (85).

Because much of rehabilitation involves learning, these findings have major implications for rehabilitation programming for older people with disabilities. This is particularly true in the context of superimposed cognitive deficits, given that intellectual ability is an important determinant of the effectiveness of a standard geriatric rehabilitation program (87).

A final area of neurologic age-related physiologic changes involves posture, proprioception, and gait (88). Older people in general are noted to demonstrate progressive declines in coordination and balance, related in part to impaired proprioception (89). This may have significant implications for degree of mobility and stability, although there are a number of common, potentially concomitant, pathologic changes that may contribute further to gait problems in older people (e.g., vertebral compression fractures with kyphosis, arthritis, sarcopenia, degenerative cerebral changes, cerebral infarcts) (78,90).

Musculoskeletal System

There is a well-documented progressive loss of muscle strength with aging from the fourth decade, in the order of 14% to 16% per decade (men and women) for lower extremity muscles and 2% (women) to 12% (men) per decade for upper extremity muscles (47). A major contributing factor to this observed decline in strength appears to be an overall decrease in muscle cross-sectional area and mass with age (91). However, there may be significant contributions of cellular, neural, or metabolic factors to changes in strength, as loss of strength was observed even without loss of muscle mass (47). Significant gains in muscle strength, as well as functional mobility, have been demonstrated in older individuals with a structured, high-intensity resistance exercise program, even in frail nursing home residents up to 96 years of age (71).

Sarcopenia, meaning a loss of skeletal muscle tissue with aging, has been recognized for many decades. More recently, its implications on functioning of older people have been better understood as having the underlying multifactorial processes that contribute to its development (92). For a long period, the study of sarcopenia was hampered by the lack of an accepted definition. This has now been remedied. It is generally accepted that sarcopenia involves both a reduction of muscle mass and also deterioration in muscle strength or body function. The European consensus definition of sarcopenia is best known and accepted (93).

Treatment is through adequate nutrition and targeted exercise (92). The increasing understanding of sarcopenia is of considerable importance to rehabilitation programs as many rehabilitation patients have sarcopenia, and this should be a target for therapeutic interventions. The essential treatment is an exercise program.

Sarcopenic obesity is, as the name suggests, the combination of these two conditions. The combination is clinically important because of the metabolic and functional changes associated with this syndrome. The combination of excess energy intake, physical inactivity, low-grade inflammation, insulin resistance, and other hormonal changes leads to both obesity and reduced muscle mass. This is associated with reductions in functioning. Reviews have pointed out that there are detrimental changes in muscle composition and quality rather than reduced muscle mass *per se* (94). The approach to treatment is to achieve weight loss through nutritional intervention and also to increase physical activity, generally with an exercise program. It has been suggested that these two approaches act synergistically and hence both should be used (95).

In both sarcopenia and sarcopenic obesity, there are clinical trials of pharmacologic therapies being conducted. Currently, it has not been established that a pharmacologic approach to treatment is associated with improvements in functioning except with reference to use of anabolic steroids. Exercise and nutritional approaches, however, are effective (96).

The high prevalence of both osteoporosis and degenerative joint disease (i.e., osteoarthritis) in older people again raises the question about normal physiologic changes versus ubiquitous pathologic processes (46,97). The physiologic changes and sequelae associated with osteoporosis are discussed further in Chapter 31.

Distinction of the "disease" of osteoarthritis from the normal or usual aging changes that occur in weight-bearing joints can be made on a biochemical basis: with osteoarthritis, there are increases in the water content of cartilage and the ratio of chondroitin-4-sulfate to chondroitin-6-sulfate, with decreases in keratin sulfate and hyaluronic acid content (the opposite of what occurs in aging) (97). There is a strong relationship between aging and osteoarthritis: Degenerative joint changes in weight-bearing joints are essentially a universal occurrence in both genders by 60 years of age (98). These changes include biochemical alteration of cartilage, especially the proteoglycan component, with reduced ability to bear weight without fissuring, focal fibrillation and ulceration of cartilage, and eventual exposure of the subchondral bone (97). The wear and tear hypothesis of osteoarthritis suggests that this process is the result of the cumulative stresses of a lifetime of joint use. Accordingly, "primary" osteoarthritis results from the stress of repetitive weight loading (e.g., spine, knees) or strain (e.g., distal interphalangeal joints), whereas "secondary" osteoarthritis may be related to occupational factors or congenital factors with unusual patterns of stress (e.g., congenital hip dysplasia). There appear to be other factors operating, however, because there are specific differences in distribution and prevalence between genders and races, and other explanatory models have been proposed (98–100). Obesity appears to be a risk factor for knee osteoarthritis in particular, although it is not clear whether this is due to a mechanical or a metabolic etiology. Further details regarding arthritis can be found in Chapters 27 to 30.

Osteoporosis as a defined entity has been long recognized as a risk factor for fracture (and fracture-related disability). Treatment for it was advanced in the 1990s when the World Health Organization defined it based on a measurement of bone mineral density (BMD) that lies 2.5 standard deviations or more below the average value for young healthy women (a T-score of <–2.5 SD) (101). More recently, the emphasis has shifted to preventing fragility fractures and their negative consequences, rather than on treating low BMD *per se*. Low BMD is viewed as only one of the several risk factors for fracture of which fall risk is the most important in frail older people. Treatment of osteoporosis is now based on absolute risk of fracture and a number of online calculators are available for this purpose. The FRAX calculator is best known (102). Pharmacologic treatment of osteoporosis when there is a high absolute risk of future fracture is clearly effective and the risk reduction is approximately 50% (103). However, in older patients who are participants in rehabilitation programs, fall risk should be addressed through appropriate interventions, particularly exercise programs (104). Further information about osteoporosis is provided in Chapter 31.

Renal System

There are a number of age-related anatomic and physiologic changes in the kidney, including decreases in renal mass, number and functioning of glomeruli and tubules, renal blood flow, and glomerular filtration rate (105–107). These reductions in renal function have major implications for drug excretion, with prolonged half-lives for those drugs cleared primarily by glomerular filtration (e.g., aminoglycosides, digoxin, lithium, penicillin, chlorpropamide) (108).

Studies show a mean age-related decrease in renal function of about 1% per year from approximately 40 years of age, with a decrease in creatinine clearance of 7.5 to 10 mL per decade. However, there is wide variability, with up to third of older individuals showing no significant decline (107). Because of a corresponding decline in daily urinary creatinine excretion (reflecting decreases in muscle mass), there is no significant change in serum creatinine level with aging. As a result, neither serum blood urea nitrogen (BUN) (which is dependent on dietary intake and metabolic function) nor creatinine is valid for accurately gauging renal function in older people (108).

Other common physiologic changes with aging include impaired ability to concentrate and dilute urine, impaired sodium conservation, reduction of urine acidification, and decreased ability to excrete an acid load (105). This erosion of reserve capacity allows maintenance of fluid and electrolyte homeostasis under normal conditions, but not with sudden changes in volume, acid load, or electrolyte balance. As a result, older people are more vulnerable to hyponatremia, hyperkalemia, dehydration, and, perhaps most seriously, water intoxication (60,109).

Because of difficulty in concentrating urine in conjunction with a blunted thirst mechanism, a hypernatremic state with attendant mental confusion can result if an older person is stressed by higher than usual insensible losses (e.g., high or prolonged fever, heat exposure, exercise) with poor fluid intake (109).

Just as older patients are prone to volume depletion when deprived of salt, acute volume expansion from an elevated sodium load caused by inappropriate intravenous fluids, dietary indiscretion, or intravenous radiographic contrast dye can result in congestive heart failure, even in older people without preexisting myocardial disease (108,110). A further potential complication of the use of radiocontrast materials in older people is the risk of acute renal failure, which is exacerbated by the presence of preprocedure dehydration (105). Because renin and aldosterone plasma concentrations are decreased by 30% to 50% in older people, with increased susceptibility to hyperkalemia, potassium-sparing diuretics (e.g., spironolactone, triamterene) should be used with great caution (111).

Hyponatremia due to water intoxication may be the most serious electrolyte disorder of older adults (60,109). Most frequently complicating an acute illness, the clinical picture includes nonspecific signs of depression, confusion, lethargy, anorexia, and weakness. Serum sodium concentrations below 110 mEq/L may result in seizures and stupor (112). The syndrome of inappropriate antidiuretic hormone secretion (SIADH), with water retention and hyponatremia, can occur with infections (e.g., pneumonia, meningitis), strokes, various drugs (e.g., diuretics), brain injury, or the stress of anesthesia and surgery (107).

Pulmonary System

Although progressive declines in pulmonary function are observed with aging, in the absence of significant pulmonary, cardiovascular, or neuromuscular disease, these declines are reflected primarily as a loss of reserve capacity without major functional limitations at rest (113) (see Chapter 34). However, impaired pulmonary function on spirometric testing does indicate increased risk for subsequent disability and several common causes of death in older people, including cardiovascular disease and chronic obstructive pulmonary disease (COPD) (114,115). Changes in pulmonary function observed with aging reflect effects of aging *per se* (in the pulmonary as well as cardiovascular and neuromuscular systems) together with the cumulative effects of inhaled noxious agents (especially cigarette smoke and air pollutants) and infectious processes (113). The latter typically have a far greater impact on pulmonary function.

Progressive decline in a number of pulmonary function tests has been documented with aging, including vital capacity, maximum voluntary ventilation, expiratory flow rate, and forced expiratory ventilation (113). These declines reflect aging changes in the pulmonary system combined with those in related organ systems, which are collectively stressed by the maximum volitional inspiration and expiration required to complete the tests. Examples include stiffening of the rib cage from degenerative calcification of costochondral cartilage (i.e., decreased compliance), weakening of intercostal and abdominal muscles, and increased airflow resistance from small airway narrowing due to decreased elasticity (114). Residual volume and functional residual capacity increase, related to the loss of elastic recoil (increased compliance), although total lung capacity remains unchanged.

Normal gas exchange requires both uniform ventilation of alveoli and adequate blood flow through the pulmonary capillary bed. With increasing age, there is a progressive ventilation-perfusion imbalance due to collapse of small peripheral airways with decreased ventilation of alveoli, resulting in a linear decline in pO_2 with aging ($pO_2 = 110 - [0.4 \times \text{age}]$) (113). Due to altered thoracic mechanics, pO_2 in older individuals is lower in the supine position than with sitting or standing. No changes occur in pCO_2 or pH, and oxygen saturation is typically normal or only slightly reduced.

This reduction in arterial oxygen tension is clinically relevant because it represents an additional loss of reserve. Older people patients are more vulnerable to significant hypoxia from a relatively minor insult (e.g., anemia, congestive heart failure, respiratory infection) or the stress of physical inactivity because they are closer to the steep slope of the oxygen-hemoglobin dissociation curve (113). Blunting of central and peripheral chemoreceptor responsiveness exacerbates this vulnerability further: both hypercapnic and hypoxic ventilatory responses markedly diminish with aging, independent of lung mechanics. There is a significant increase in sleep-related breathing disorders with aging, and this appears to be related to this phenomenon (60).

Maximal oxygen consumption (VO_{2max}), an overall measure of exercise capacity and cardiopulmonary fitness, depends on pulmonary ventilation, cardiac output, peripheral circulatory control (i.e., ability to shunt blood to exercising muscles), and muscle oxidative capacity (i.e., oxygen extraction from the blood). Although a progressive decline in VO_{2max} is observed with aging, this does not appear to be on a pulmonary basis (114,116). In fact, it appears that decreases in VO_{2max} in older adults with mild-to-moderate COPD are due primarily to cardiac and peripheral muscle deconditioning resulting from limited activity levels (114). Regular exercise to maintain or improve fitness is critical with aging because it is possible to improve fitness with training at any age, and this is associated with a reduced vulnerability to stress or disease (and thereby increased active life expectancy) (68,69,72,73,117). The tendency of physicians and society to tolerate (or even encourage) decreased activity among older people, in conjunction with trends toward obesity and increased recumbency, probably contributes more to poor pulmonary function than aging alone (114,118).

Although most attention regarding the high incidence of pneumonia in older people is focused on immunologic declines, there appear to be contributing factors, direct or indirect, relating to the pulmonary system itself. Because many pneumonias result from aspiration of the infecting organism, impaired mucociliary function and decreased chest wall compliance with weaker cough (resulting in impaired ability to clear aspirated material or secretions) likely play a role (113,114). Other nonimmunologic contributing factors may include dysphagia, disruption of lower esophageal sphincter integrity, various esophageal disorders, and reduced levels of consciousness, as well as the presence of diabetes or cardiovascular disease (119).

Cardiovascular System

A number of established tenets about the aging cardiovascular system have been revised, based on continuing research using more rigorous methodologies to exclude occult disease and controlling for degree of habitual physical activity (see Chapter 33). As a result, it now appears that cardiac output at rest and during graded exercise is relatively unaffected by age directly (60,116,120).

Although resting heart rate does not change with aging, maximal heart rate with exercise does decrease progressively, related to decreased chronotropic responsiveness to adrenergic stimuli. The clinical formula reflecting this decline in maximal heart rate involves subtracting the age from 220 for men and ($0.8 \times$ age) from 190 for women (117,120). Decreased inotropic responsiveness to adrenergic stimulus results in decreased myocardial contractility, with decreased ejection fraction and increased risk of congestive heart failure (121). Maintenance of cardiac output at rest and with modest exercise is accomplished by early involvement of the Frank-Starling mechanism, with increased stroke volume via higher left ventricular end-diastolic volumes (60,120).

Another age-associated change is a decrease in the rate of early diastolic filling, with a much greater dependency on late filling through atrial contraction (120). As a result, older people are more vulnerable to deleterious effects of atrial tachycardia or fibrillation, including congestive heart failure (116,121).

Both cross-sectional and longitudinal studies demonstrate decreases in maximal oxygen consumption with aging, regardless of habitual activity levels (64,67,116). However, physically active people retain significantly greater maximal aerobic capacity with aging compared to their sedentary counterparts (69). In fact, trained older subjects may have greater maximal oxygen consumption than sedentary subjects who are much younger (70). Furthermore, endurance training, even when

begun in old age, can significantly improve exercise capacity (69,117). Of clinical relevance is that the energy of walking represents an increasing percentage of the total aerobic capacity with advancing age, such that walking becomes a very effective physical conditioning activity (122).

A final age-related physiologic change in the cardiovascular system with important clinical applications is decreased baroreceptor sensitivity (122,123). This results in a diminished reflex tachycardia on rising from a recumbent position and accounts in part (possibly along with blunted plasma renin activity and reduced angiotensin II and vasopressin levels) for the increased incidence of symptomatic orthostatic hypotension in older people, as well as cough and micturition syncope syndromes (120,124).

Immunologic System

Significant alterations in immunocompetence occur with aging, involving both cellular and humoral immune functions (125,126). Although the total number of lymphocytes decreases by about 15% in older adults, this does not appear to contribute significantly to the marked decline in immunocompetence (116). There is a decline in lymphocyte proliferation in response to antigen stimulation in older adults, as well as a higher incidence of energy (125). Age-related shifts have been observed in the regulatory activities of T cells (i.e., fewer T cells with suppressor or helper activity) and monocytes or macrophages.

Changes in humoral immunity with aging include increases in circulating autoantibodies and immune complexes, with decreased antibody production (125). The latter is characterized by an attenuated response to immunization, with difficulty maintaining specific serum antibody levels.

The increased susceptibility of older people to infection is a function of both these age-related changes in immune function and the frequency of concomitant factors that further impair host defenses (e.g., diabetes, malignancy, vascular disease, malnutrition, and stress) (125). Altered local barriers to infection, such as skin breakdown or an indwelling urinary catheter, often compromise resistance to infection further. Common infectious processes in older people include influenza, pneumonia, urinary tract infection, sepsis, herpes zoster, and postoperative wound infections.

Of particular clinical relevance is the fact that older people react differently to infections than do their younger counterparts. There is a less active leukocytosis in response to inflammation, and the total white blood cell count often is not increased (although usually there is still a shift of the differential count to the left) (116). The older patient may have less pain or other symptomatologies and frequently absent, or only low-grade, fever (127).

Endocrine System

The endocrine system also undergoes significant changes as we grow older. There is a gradual decrease in glucose tolerance with aging, although the fasting blood sugar level remains relatively unchanged (60). Accordingly, age-adjusted criteria for diabetes mellitus have been developed. This age-related decline in glucose tolerance is due to reduced sensitivity of tissues to the metabolic effects of insulin or insulin resistance (128,129). Compounding these aging changes are secondary conditions that further reduce tissue sensitivity to insulin, including lifestyle changes (e.g., obesity, diet changes, stress, sedentary lifestyle), other diseases (e.g., chronic infections, prolonged immobilization), and effects of medications (46,130). Older adults with diabetes are also at increased risk for common geriatric syndromes (e.g., depression, falls) (131).

Of clinical importance is the risk for untreated hyperglycemia, osmotic diuresis, and dehydration, potentially leading to hyperosmolar nonketotic coma or ketoacidosis (130). Certain drugs can cause or potentiate hyperglycemia (e.g., thiazide diuretics, glucocorticoids, tricyclic antidepressants, phenothiazines, phenytoin) (132). Control of serum glucose in older diabetics with oral sulfonylureas or insulin can be fragile, with significant risk for hypoglycemia.

However, even borderline hyperglycemia appears to result in accelerated atherosclerosis and multiple end-organ involvement (60). On the other hand, data indicate that extremely tight glycemic control in type 2 diabetics may also be harmful (133). Of interest are the contributions of obesity and physical inactivity to the increased incidence of diabetes in older adults and the benefits of weight loss and regular exercise in improving control (46).

There are multiple other endocrine changes associated with aging. The primary clinical impact of altered thyroid physiology with aging is the need to maintain a high index of suspicion for unusual presentation of thyroid disease (134). Presenting signs and symptoms of the older thyrotoxic patient may include palpitations, congestive heart failure, angina, atrial fibrillation, major weight loss associated with anorexia, and either diarrhea or constipation (135). Goiter and serious ophthalmopathy frequently are absent. Apathetic hyperthyroidism may not be recognized until late in the course of the illness: patients appear depressed and withdrawn, with clinical clues of muscle weakness, dramatic weight loss, and cardiac dysfunction (130). Signs and symptoms of hypothyroidism essentially are unchanged with aging, but the diagnosis still may be delayed because of the many similarities between the stereotype of senescence and the hypothyroid state (e.g., psychomotor retardation, depression, constipation, cold intolerance).

The relationships between the hypothalamus, pituitary, and adrenal cortex remain unchanged with age, with preserved diurnal rhythm and stress response (130). However, in older women, serum cortisol concentrations vary more over the course of a day, and mean daily cortisol and ACTH (adrenocorticotropic hormone)-stimulated serum cortisol levels are higher (136,137). Primary adrenocortical disease is uncommon in the older people. Significant hyponatremia or hyperkalemia, suggestive of adrenocortical insufficiency, is not uncommon in older people but more often is secondary to drugs (e.g., thiazide diuretics, chlorpropamide, carbamazepine) (111).

Age-related changes in gonadal function are well documented. There are variable and gradual declines in serum testosterone levels in healthy men with aging, likely due to partial testicular failure; however, there is no indication for routine androgen replacement (60,138).

Postmenopausal declines in estrogen levels are well documented, with clinical expression variably including vasomotor instability syndrome (i.e., hot flashes), atrophic vaginitis, and osteoporosis (44,139). Controversy continues over prophylaxis and treatment of the latter, particularly with regard to potential benefits of dietary supplements and exercise (44,46,140). The reader is referred to Chapter 31 for further details.

Thermoregulatory System

Older people have an impaired temperature regulation system due to a combination of diminished sensitivity to temperature change and abnormal autonomic vasomotor control (141). As a result, they have a reduced ability to maintain body temperature with changes in environmental temperature and are vulnerable to both hypothermia and hyperthermia (60,109). The risk of hypothermia is compounded further by impaired thermogenesis (i.e., inefficient shivering), with potential aggravation by a variety of conditions (e.g., hypothyroidism, hypoglycemia, malnutrition) or medications (e.g., ethanol, barbiturates, phenothiazines, benzodiazepines, narcotics) (109). Conversely, diminished sweating (due to higher body temperature to initiate sweating and decreased sweat production) is a major contributing factor in heat exhaustion and heat stroke in hot conditions. Hypohidrosis is aggravated by anticholinergics, phenothiazines, and antidepressants (111). Two thirds of deaths from heat stroke occur in people over 60 years of age, reflecting this impairment in regulatory systems. This has implications for rehabilitation exercise programs, particularly when combined with a tendency for dehydration (69).

Genitourinary System

Benign prostatic hyperplasia is common in men older than 60 years of age and develops under hormonal rather than neoplastic influence (142). Accordingly, after ruling out other etiologies (e.g., anticholinergic or diuretic medication side effects), cystoscopy should be considered in patients with persisting obstructive symptomatology but minimal prostatic tissue on rectal examination to detect median lobe hypertrophy (143). Usual indications for surgical intervention (e.g., prostatectomy) include increasing obstructive symptoms, recurrent/persistent gross hematuria, bladder calculi, recurrent infections, and postvoid residual volumes greater than 100 mL (142,144).

Incontinence in older people, although increasingly prevalent with advancing age, should be regarded as a symptom of underlying disease; it does not result from the natural aging process (145). Normal aging typically results in decreases in bladder capacity, ability to postpone voiding, detrusor contractility, and urinary flow rate (146). Postvoid residual volumes are typically increased, with a tendency for increased urine output later in the day, as well as propensity for uninhibited detrusor contractions. Each of these changes predisposes older adults to incontinence, but none alone precipitates it.

The primary clinical significance of these aging changes is that the new onset, or exacerbation, of incontinence in an older person is likely to be due to a precipitating factor outside the urinary tract (145). Usually, remedial intervention can restore continence.

Contrary to stereotypes, although there is a decrease in sexual functioning with aging, most older people retain sexual interest and desire and, to a variable extent, capability (147–149).

Older men experience a decrease in the ability to have psychogenic erections and require more intense physical stimulation for erection; erections may be partial, and orgasm with ejaculation may occur without full engorgement (150). The force of ejaculation is less, along with a less intense sensation of orgasm. Impotence may be caused by a variety of diseases (e.g., atherosclerosis, diabetes, hypothyroidism) and medications (e.g., antihypertensives, phenytoin, cimetidine). Treatment of erectile dysfunction in older men has been revolutionized with availability of such medications as sildenafil, tadalafil, and vardenafil (151,152).

Older women experience postmenopausal changes, including increased fragility of the vaginal wall and attenuation of the excitement phase (e.g., decreased vaginal lubrication) (149).

Common sexual difficulties identified included partner's impotence, anorgasmia, decreased libido, and insufficient opportunities for sexual encounters. Despite these changes, most women maintain the ability to engage in sexual intercourse throughout the life cycle (99).

Hematologic System

Although anemia (i.e., hemoglobin <13 g/dL in men and <12 g/dL in women) (153) occurs with increasing prevalence with aging, there is convincing evidence that it is not a normal consequence of aging and should be investigated, especially if hemoglobin is less than 10.5 g/dL (154–156). Anemia in older people appears to be due most commonly to iron deficiency (typically from gastrointestinal [GI] blood loss) or chronic disease (such as infection, polymyalgia rheumatica, or cancer) (156). Other potential causes include hemolysis (e.g., secondary to lymphoma, leukemia, or medication effect), B12 deficiency (pernicious anemia, diet), or folate deficiency (diet). Of note, D-dimer levels have been shown to double with aging, with even more dramatic increases among African Americans and functionally impaired older individuals (157). Increases in the erythrocyte sedimentation rate and C-reactive protein levels also have been noted with aging (158,159).

The functional consequences of anemia can be significant because of further reduction of reserve capacity, such that previously subclinical disease states may become symptomatic (e.g., orthostatic blood pressure changes, change in anginal pattern with lower exercise tolerance) (155,160). This has obvious implications with regard to tolerance of relatively intensive and sustained rehabilitation exercise programs. There is also evidence of correlation of even relatively mild anemia with impaired mobility (161,162). A very anemic older patient may present with nonspecific fatigue and confusion, with the potential for misdiagnosis and mistreatment (154).

There are several related hematologic changes with aging that can affect pharmacokinetics, particularly drug distribution. Decreased drug binding for highly protein-bound drugs (e.g., warfarin, tolbutamide) may result in a higher unbound, or free, drug concentration with correspondingly magnified actions (108). This effect is even more significant for patients taking multiple drugs because of competition for fewer binding sites.

The volume of distribution is also altered in older adults due to a reduction in total body water and lean body mass, with a relative increase in body fat (163). As a result, water-soluble drugs (e.g., digoxin) tend to have a smaller volume of distribution, with higher plasma concentrations and greater pharmacologic effect (164). Conversely, fat-soluble drugs (e.g., diazepam, phenobarbital) usually have a larger volume of distribution because of relatively greater storage in fatty tissue. This may result in delayed therapeutic effects, with the potential for unexpected late toxicity. By the same token, prolonged drug effects are seen after dosage change or discontinuation because of the amount of drug stored in adipose tissue (108).

Gastrointestinal System

There are multiple changes in esophageal function commonly observed with aging, such as delayed esophageal emptying, incomplete sphincter relaxation, and decreased amplitude of peristaltic contractions. Only the latter appears to be a direct result of aging, but it is not clinically significant; the other changes are related to associated disease processes and may have significant clinical ramifications (165). Most importantly, there is an increased risk of aspiration with aging due to less coordinated swallowing.

Age-related changes occur throughout the GI system although the more distal portion is most affected (166). Alterations in colon function include slightly decreased force and coordination of smooth muscle contraction resulting in slower transit time, as well as impaired rectal perception of feces (167). The high incidence of constipation in older people accordingly is thought to be related to multiple additional factors, such as low dietary fiber and fluid intake, sedentary habits, and various associated diseases interfering with intrinsic bowel function (e.g., Parkinson's disease, stroke) (168). A variety of medications are potentially constipating as well, including minerals (e.g., aluminum antacids, iron, calcium), opioids, nonsteroidal anti-inflammatory drugs (NSAIDs), antihypertensives (e.g., calcium channel blockers, clonidine), anticholinergics (e.g., tricyclic antidepressants, neuroleptics, antispasmodics), and sympathomimetics (e.g., pseudoephedrine, isoproterenol, terbutaline) (111). Prolonged use of stimulant laxatives or enemas can also impair bowel contractility and result in constipation or obstipation (168). Older adults often report straining and hard bowel movements along with their constipation (169). Straining may indicate rectal dyschezia (i.e., impaired rectal sensation and contractility).

Fecal incontinence in older people is due most commonly to overflow incontinence secondary to fecal impaction but can also occur as a result of decreased sphincter tone, cognitive impairment (e.g., from drugs, dementia), diarrhea, or dyschezia (168,169). Diarrhea among older patients is most frequently caused by fecal impaction, intestinal infection, or drugs (e.g., broad-spectrum antibiotics, digoxin toxicity) but also can be due to chronic laxative abuse (170). More appropriate interventions for bowel regulation include increasing diet fiber, using bulk agents or stool softeners, and avoiding frequent use of enemas or laxatives.

Despite these physiologic changes with aging, little effect is seen on absorption of most orally administered drugs (164). Drug absorption in general is more significantly affected by concomitant administration of multiple drugs; in particular, antacids and laxatives bind to or reduce dissolution of other medications (108).

Hepatic System

The primary changes in the hepatic system with aging involve a gradual progressive decline in liver size (5% to 15%) and hepatic blood flow, as well as slowing of hepatic biotransformation, specifically and most consistently microsomal oxidation and hydrolysis (164,167). This can have major implications on the circulating concentration of certain drugs and their metabolites, depending on the mode of metabolism and clearance. Drugs with high first-pass clearance (e.g., propranolol, major tranquilizers, tricyclic antidepressants, antiarrhythmic drugs) are cleared less effectively owing to reduced hepatic blood flow, resulting in greater bioavailability (108). Comorbid processes such as congestive heart failure can exacerbate these effects.

Drugs metabolized by means of phase I biotransformation (i.e., oxidation, reduction, hydrolysis) tend to have prolonged elimination in older people (e.g., diazepam, chlordiazepoxide, prazepam), whereas those undergoing phase II metabolism (i.e., glucuronidation, acetylation, sulfation) generally are not affected by aging changes (e.g., oxazepam, lorazepam, triazolam) (108,111).

It is important to note that studies of drug elimination with aging demonstrate significant interindividual variability that is likely to be due to genetic variation as well as the effects of such factors as smoking, alcohol, caffeine intake, diet, and concurrent use of other medications (164). As a result, caution should be exercised when using age-based guidelines for dosage determination (66).

IMPACT OF THE ENVIRONMENT ON THE HEALTH OF OLDER ADULTS

Psychological and Social Issues in Aging

Ageism and Myths of Aging

Butler coined the term "ageism" (or agism) to describe negatively biased perceptions of older people by the younger population in today's youth-oriented culture, as well as perceptions of old age by older individuals themselves (171). There are many adverse sequelae of ageism, including devaluation of older people (by themselves, as well as others both younger and older), diversion of health care professional focus from the real health problems of older patients, the dearth of physicians interested and trained in geriatric medicine, and lack of curriculum time in medical schools regarding geriatrics (172–174). There is evidence of a negative impact of perceived discrimination on mortality in older adults (175). According to Rowe et al., it is time to "discard the many derogatory myths about older people, who are often seen as sick, senile, silly, sexless, and sedentary, as well as inflexible, irritable, non-contributing, and too old for preventive interventions" (176). The evidence is clear: the majority of older people are cognitively intact, live independently in the community, and are fully independent in ADL (36,50).

Cumulative Changes

There is increasing awareness of the critical interrelationships, particularly for older people, of physical health, mental health, and life circumstances. The emotional and life stress associated with major losses are well documented, and older people may be exposed progressively to multiple significant losses: job, income, health, functional ability and independence, parents, spouse, siblings, children, friends, social roles and status, and self-esteem (177). There are in fact few norms or defined role expectations regarding appropriate behavior or activities in old age (178,179). Bereavement, isolation, poverty, illness, and physical disability all are associated with a higher incidence of depression in older adults (180), which in turn is associated with decreased physical and cognitive functioning, disability, and increased mortality (34,181–183).

Social Support Networks

Social support networks include a wide variety of sources that can be categorized as informal (family), semiformal (church, clubs, family doctor, local pharmacist), and formal (health care system, social service agencies, insurance companies, etc.) (184,185). Older persons often use supports from a combination of these networks (10). There is mounting evidence of the positive impact of social support networks on the cognitive, health, and functional statuses of older individuals (185–187).

Older people with children sometimes live near them and may visit frequently or at least maintain regular telephone contact (188). Older people without children tend to maintain closer ties with young relatives or with siblings (189). It is important to consider the extended family, including cousins, in-laws, and others, with regard to support networks, rather than just immediate household members (178,185,190).

Institutionalization of an impaired older person usually is the last resort for families, used only when all other efforts fail; in fact, 64% of individuals over the age of 85 who are dependent in self-care or homemaking still live in the community (191). Families, rather than the formal system of government and agencies, provide the bulk (up to 90%) of personalized long-term care for their disabled older relatives (13). This includes home health and nursing care, personal care, household maintenance, transportation, cooking, and shopping. With advancing age, however, older adults tend to have increasingly limited and relatively fragile support systems. Dependency in aging parents can result in significant physical, emotional, and financial stresses on their family network (188). An alternative support system may evolve gradually over a period of time as the older person loses family support (e.g., death of spouse and siblings, children moving away and unable to actively assist). Such a system might include friends and neighbors in an extended network to assist with shopping, cooking, cleaning, and self-care (185,192).

With whatever combination of support systems, a significant additional insult (e.g., onset of a new disease or complication) may overtax an already marginal arrangement. It is commonly observed that as the patient's dependence on the formal network of the health care system increases, the informal or family network support decreases (187). Furthermore, if the older person is hospitalized for a prolonged period, the network(s) may dissipate and may be difficult or impossible to reassemble (193). The critical importance of maintaining the integrity of support networks is illustrated by the observation that for every aged impaired person in a nursing home, there are two equally impaired older people living in the community (58). The difference is the role played by the latter's informal support systems, providing most of their long-term care.

Increasingly, issues concerning family functioning with aging are being studied. Even when family members are seemingly available to assist older relatives, their support cannot always be counted on unless they too receive help. Fortunately, there is evidence that patients' families can benefit from educational interventions to help prevent weakening in this crucial source of patient support. Caregivers of older patients with cancer and chronic pain are often frustrated, fearful, and anxious. Patient care improved when caregivers were provided with guidelines on what they could do within the home to help the patient (187). Similarly, caregivers of stroke survivors had less depression and better outcomes with more formal training (194). Nursing home placement has been delayed by specific family interventions for patients with Alzheimer's disease (195).

Caregiver burden is another dynamic receiving increasing attention (196). Increased caregiver burden can be associated with increased mortality after controlling for known risk factors (197). Adding to the physical stress of providing personal care aid may be the unpleasantness of incontinence or exhaustion due to a relative's sleep disorder. Behavioral problems, such as agitation or impulsivity with poor safety awareness, create proportionately greater caregiver burden than the demands of providing physical assistance (196). Physical and emotional health problems among caregivers have been documented, including depression and immunosuppression. Physical aggression to a caregiver by a patient is not uncommon and may lead to reciprocal abuse (198). Potential intervention strategies include encouraging the use of other support systems to augment care provided by family members, as well as the use of respite programs (199,200). Education, information, counseling, and support, as well as aids and equipment, are also effective. Service provision, including respite, should ideally be provided on an ongoing basis (201). Elder abuse is present in all societies and, on occasions, will be recognized by rehabilitation services for older people. Elder abuse is strongly associated with disability in an older person (1). Financial abuse may require legal interventions. Interventions to address caregiver burden will be beneficial for the older people having significant disability, but, in this situation, it may be necessary to separate the abuser and the victim with the victim moving to a residential care facility.

Functional Impact

Physically impaired older people tend to become socially isolated, which can result in exacerbation of medical problems, functional deficits, and mental health problems (particularly depression) (34,181) (see Chapter 7 and 15). Other factors contributing to a vicious cycle of depression, withdrawal, and functional decline may include the stress of multiple losses, malnutrition, chronic ill health, pain, and adverse drug effects that aggravate depression (183). Unfortunately, the environment too often fosters dependency. A classic illustration is the acute hospital setting, where the focus is on routinely providing care and assistance, rather than encouraging self-care (202,203).

Additional psychosocial barriers can interfere with maintaining or improving functional ability in older people. Handicapping sequelae of ageism include devaluation of older people who have disabilities (by themselves as well as others), lack of interest (actual and/or perceived) among health care professionals in their problems, and limited opportunity for access to appropriate rehabilitation services (172,176). Further attitudinal obstacles encountered among disabled older people include the "right of dependency," perceived as earned by virtue of longevity, and the "apathy of fatigue," both physical and emotional, associated with multiple illnesses and hospitalizations (204).

Increasingly, physical environments are being recognized as either preventing or contributing to disability (205). While full discussion is beyond the scope of this chapter, the development of a requirement for some housing to meet visitability criteria (one entrance without stairs, bathroom on the first floor, and wide bathroom doorway to accommodate a wheelchair) is encouraging (206). Housing adapted in this manner may more easily accommodate older adults as they age and facilitate social visits to or from friends by minimizing physical barriers. Visitability is less than full accessibility and universal design (207,208). Full accessibility provides enough additional features to support continuing use by people with mobility limitations, and universal design provides a wide array of other features that improve usability, safety, and health for a diverse group of people with varying abilities.

The obvious conclusion, and why rehabilitation plays a key role in restoring function in older people living with disabilities, is the importance of awareness and intervention regarding significant psychosocial factors affecting their health. Many of these factors can be anticipated and prevented or at least minimized in terms of their adverse effects.

Cumulative Functional Sequelae of Disease

Older adults can experience acute onset of disability just as in younger people, from such conditions as stroke, traumatic brain injury, spinal cord injury (SCI), and amputation. However, many experience a gradual progression of difficulties in function. The effects of multiple and chronic illnesses usually are gradual over time with cumulative erosion of organ reserves, leaving the older person reasonably functional with various adaptations, such as walking more slowly or taking more frequent rests (25,35,46). As functional problems develop, it can be hard to determine if the disability can be treated generically (i.e., regardless of the contributing diseases and other factors) or it is due to a reversible underlying disease process that needs to be treated. Also, an older individual may be only marginally functional with little or no reserve capacity, so that even a relatively minor superimposed acute complication or disease process (e.g., influenza) may result in functional decompensation (58,209). Of even greater concern is that this significant functional decompensation may be difficult to reverse even though the intercurrent acute illness is appropriately treated and resolves (209–212). This can be seen as a manifestation of frailty, particularly when conceptualized using an accumulated deficit model (213).

Underreporting of Illness

Older people as a group are more vulnerable to functional sequelae of diseases for a variety of reasons, including ageism. The latter commonly results in underreporting of symptomatology related to illness (35,171). Health care providers may not be trained adequately to evaluate and treat symptoms and signs of functional disability in older patients and may as a result not recognize the significance of vague and inconsistent symptoms. Older people themselves may think that such vague symptoms are a natural result of aging (212). As a result, the underlying disease process may become quite advanced before care is sought, making treatment that much more difficult.

From the older person's viewpoint, the available system of care may seem unresponsive (35). Physician's offices can be perceived as inconveniently located, with inadequate parking and limited access for the physically impaired. A typically brief physician encounter may not allow for development of rapport and full elaboration of symptoms. Busy office staff may appear to be uninterested or discourteous.

Other issues may contribute further to underreporting of illness. There may be denial of disease coupled with fear of consequences, especially financial (171). Depression is common among older people and may result in the attitude "What have I got to gain?" (35,181). Increasing isolation, with fewer opportunities for others to observe and react to changes in appearance or behavior, is an additional barrier. Finally, older people may not recognize significant symptoms or seek medical attention because of cognitive impairments, which not infrequently may be secondary to or aggravated by an underlying and potentially reversible disease process (83).

Altered Response to Illness

There is often an altered response to illness in older people, which contributes to a delayed, or incorrect, initial diagnosis (35). Many specific diseases present with atypical signs and symptoms. For example, the presentation of myocardial infarction in an older person is less likely to include classic retrosternal chest pain; more often, it will involve nausea, dizziness, syncope, or congestive heart failure with decreased activity tolerance (160). Furthermore, a wide variety of diseases may present with similar nonspecific symptoms, including confusion, weakness, weight loss, and general "failure to thrive" (35,214). Accordingly, the differential diagnosis of possible disease processes is much broader in older patients.

Variable Patterns of Disease

Further confounding accurate elucidation of the underlying illness are the frequent changes in disease patterns and distribution (35). Abnormalities in one organ system may be accompanied by secondary abnormalities in other organ systems. Traditional medical training focuses on disease recognition and treatment in a relatively young population, with emphasis on synthesizing multiple signs and symptoms into a single unifying diagnosis (35,215). Older people typically have concurrent symptomatology, relating to multiple diseases. Although accurate diagnosis is important, the functional impact of each disease, particularly the cumulative and additive impact of multiple diseases, must be determined (58).

Atypical Responses to Treatment

There is an increased frequency of many chronic diseases in this population, including osteoarthritis, osteoporosis, cardiovascular disease, malignancy, anemia, and malnutrition. Palliation and prevention of secondary complications, and setting appropriate and realistic goals, are more important than cure of the primary condition (35,215). There often are atypical (and potentially confusing) behaviors and responses to treatment, however, due to coexisting diseases and decreased functional reserves of multiple organ systems (e.g., affecting drug metabolism and distribution) (35).

Older people also are more prone to a wide variety of concomitant and complicating diseases, which may further cloud diagnosis and treatment decisions. Examples include thrombophlebitis, dehydration, fluid and electrolyte disturbances, adverse drug interactions or toxicity, pressure ulcers, pneumonia, and general deleterious effects of deconditioning due to inactivity, which occurs earlier and with greater severity in older adults (216,217).

Frailty

Frailty as a concept refers to more than just older individuals who experience functional loss; it represents a state of vulnerability resulting from the balance and interplay of medical and social factors (39,40,218). Characteristics of frail older institutionalized persons included female gender, being unmarried, absence of a caregiver, presence of cognitive deficit, functional impairment, and medical condition (e.g., diabetes mellitus, stroke, Parkinson's disease) (219).

"Frailty" is becoming better characterized as a biologic syndrome of older adults associated with decreased reserve and resistance to stressors (39,40). Contributing factors are the multiple decrements in physiologic systems, as previously discussed. Clinical characteristics have been defined as unintentional weight loss (10 lb [4.5 kg] in prior year), self-reported exhaustion, weakness (decreased grip strength), slow walking speed, and decreased physical activity. Using these criteria, if three or more of these characteristics are present, the individual may be classified as frail (39,40). An alternative conceptualization of frailty is the accumulated deficit model in which a frailty index, which relates deficit accumulation to the individual risk of death, is used (213).

Effects of Acute Hospitalization

There is increasing recognition of the multiple deleterious effects of acute hospitalization on older people, separate and distinct from sequelae due primarily to their presenting illness (210,220). Disorientation due to the foreign hospital environment and relatively infrequent and brief interactions with unfamiliar health care personnel may contribute to delirium and agitation (181,202,221). Contributing to this may be enforced bed rest, and relative sensory and social isolation with few familiar environmental cues or social interactions, especially if the patient is confined to a private room or intensive care setting. Moreover, there are atypical routines and schedules (e.g., blood drawing, vital sign checks at odd hours), which, coupled with unusual noises (e.g., overhead paging, machines, other patients), may contribute to insomnia. A patient with insomnia typically is treated with a sedative medication, which may begin a cycle (or cascade) of drug side effects and interactions that may adversely affect the patient's health (210,220).

Increased incidence of medical and iatrogenic complications in older adults is well documented (35,215). Drug side effects, complications, and toxicity, together with adverse interactions related to polypharmacy, make up a large proportion of such morbidity (35,108). There also is a greater frequency of diagnostic and therapeutic misadventures in this age group, related in part to decreased organ reserve with resultant increased vulnerability (220).

There also are a variety of emotional sequelae of hospitalization that may affect health and functional statuses. Anxiety and confusion relating to the underlying illness and prognosis, or just to hospitalization itself, may interfere with cooperation with medical treatment or therapy programs (222–224). Depression from similar origins may result in dependency and poor motivation to cooperate or improve function (181,182). Functional dependency frequently is reinforced during acute hospitalizations, both by the older patients who expect hospital staff to assist and by hospital staff who tend routinely to perform self-care tasks without taking the extra time to supervise the patient in performing his or her own self-care (204,210). Documented functional decline after hospitalization for acute medical illnesses also may result from other, as yet unexplained, factors (220). Deconditioning from inadequate activity during the hospital stay may contribute to poorer functional outcomes, and older adults are more sensitive to the deleterious effects of bed rest as compared to younger individuals (225). Preliminary results are mixed as to whether exercise during hospitalization can help improve functional outcomes (226,227).

In addition to significant implications for health care in the hospital setting, these sequelae related to acute hospitalization often affect social support systems and discharge disposition

(193,210). The older patient may experience loss of confidence or motivation as a result of multiple insults and complications, coupled with erosion of functional abilities from deconditioning (216,217). This by itself will put greater stress on often relatively fragile social support systems, making it more difficult for older patients to return home to their prior living situation (193).

To try to address these problems, several randomized trials have investigated alternative models attempting to change the organization of care (and outcomes) for older persons during hospitalization. Use of a geriatric consultation team approach did not yield improved outcomes (228). In another randomized clinical trial of 651 patients 70 years of age and older, the experimental patients received care on a special unit (Acute Care of the Elderly [ACE] Unit), which had the additional components of daily team conferences, active discharge planning, and use of therapy staff for functional training—the core components of an acute rehabilitation unit. Patients in the experimental group were discharged at higher functional levels, and fewer were discharged to skilled nursing facilities (14% vs. 22%). Neither cost of hospitalization nor length of stay was increased (229). In a Veterans Administration study, older patients, after stabilization, were randomized to usual care or to a geriatric rehabilitation unit (230). At hospital discharge, patients receiving the geriatric unit care had greater improvements in scores for four of the eight SF-36 subscales, ADL, and physical performance. These studies suggest potential strategies to improve acute hospital care for older persons, with less functional sequelae. Unfortunately, similar programs have not been routinely implemented despite their demonstrated benefit (231).

Effects of Deconditioning

Deconditioning can be defined as the multiple changes in physiology and anatomy induced by physical inactivity and reversed through physical activity (217), and it can be coded using the International Classification of Diseases as "debility, unspecified" (232). This topic is covered in detail in Chapter 38 but will be discussed here relative to unique aspects relating to aging.

Older adults' (75 to 120 years old) physical functioning and associated physical activities have been classified by Spirduso into five categories: physically elite, physically fit, physically independent, physically frail, and physically dependent (233). Deconditioning can be one component, in addition to disease, that may contribute to a patient's lower level of function. In addition, low fitness is an important predictor of cardiovascular and all-cause mortality in older adults (234).

As noted before, older adults have a more substantial loss of muscle mass than younger adults with bed rest inactivity (225). However, the associated declines in lower extremity strength and maximal aerobic capacity in these older subjects were similar to that reported in younger adults exposed to similar periods of bed rest. Reversal of the deleterious effects of deconditioning has been amply demonstrated through focused muscle-strengthening programs as well as comprehensive exercise programs in both nursing homes and the community (71,235–237). These programs variably included exercises for flexibility, muscle strength, and aerobic endurance.

The functional consequences of deconditioning in older people may be of major clinical significance and may be confused with changes intrinsic to aging or changes from diseases (217). In addition to deconditioning, sarcopenia is another process that can affect overall function in older individuals (238). Deconditioning *per se* may result in functional losses when certain threshold values for physical performance are crossed (239). Quadriceps weakness may progress to the point of dependency in getting in and out of a car solely from progressive deconditioning, not related to intrinsic aging or new onset of disease (216). Multiple factors associated with falls may originate from deconditioning or be exacerbated by deconditioning (240,241). For people living in the community, factors associated with falls include impairments in static balance, leg strength, and hip and ankle flexibility (242,243). In nursing home patients, falls are associated with decreased muscle strength at the knees and ankles (244,245). Weakened muscles also may contribute to other injuries and pain syndromes by allowing abnormal forces to act on bone, joints, ligaments, and tendons. In addition, lack of exercise is being viewed increasingly as a risk factor not only for functional loss but also for onset of various disease processes, including cardiovascular disease and diabetes, among others (246).

Deconditioning affecting older people can be differentiated into acute inactivity secondary to bed rest (such as during acute illness) and chronic inactivity from sedentary lifestyles (often more difficult to reverse) (217). A variety of types and combinations of exercises are available to treat deconditioning in older individuals; a precise prescription of a therapeutic exercise and activity program, including appropriate precautions and instruction, is suggested (69,72,122,247).

Psychological issues in maintaining exercise habits are being studied increasingly (237). Currently, health professionals can help older persons increase their physical activity levels by discussing the issue openly and then helping the patient decide what approach may be most appropriate (118). One option may be group classes, which offer the benefits of social interaction and support, and perhaps even friendly competition. Exercising on their own at home may be preferable for some, especially if they are self-conscious about their own abilities (248).

Care Transitions

Care transitions have been recognized as hazardous, particularly for older people. These have been defined as events in which there are transfers between health care locations (249). Hazards occur due to inadequate transfer of information about medications and support requirements. Risks for older people are noted specifically when an older person is transferred to post–acute care facilities (250). This may include both admission to and discharge from rehabilitation facilities. Evidence-informed interventions are available and the benefit of the broader concept of discharge planning has been established (251).

Disability Prevention in Older Adults

The future impact of increased disability as the population ages is of major concern to clinicians, health care administrators, insurers, and policy-makers. Increasingly, prevention strategies are being proposed both to improve the number of disability-free years of life and to contain health care costs (15,26,30,34,36,38,39). Some of the themes around prevention can be organized according to the concepts of primary, secondary, and tertiary prevention. Primary prevention involves preventing the onset of a disease (e.g., annual influenza vaccine), whereas secondary prevention involves the diagnosis and treatment of asymptomatic diseases to prevent the development of symptoms (e.g., treatment of hypertension to prevent stroke or myocardial infarction). Tertiary prevention involves treatment once a disease becomes symptomatic to avoid complications (e.g., deep venous thrombosis prophylaxis and appropriate mobilization to prevent skin breakdown in poststroke patients). However, as previously discussed, what becomes increasingly important in older persons with chronic disease (comorbidity) is focused attention to preventing or minimizing frailty and, therefore, decreasing risk of development of disability (39).

Another model that may help in the development of prevention strategies has been proposed by Lawrence and Jette (252). They have studied the application of a model for the disablement process in 1,048 community-residing adults (mean age 74 years) without functional limitations or disabilities over a 6-year period. The model hypothesized a process in which risk factors (age, gender, education, body mass, and physical activity measured as frequency of walking 1 mi.) would lead to functional limitations with or without the presence of pathology or impairments.

Over time, the functional limitations (e.g., inability to walk well) would lead to subsequent disability such as inability to go shopping. Guralnik et al. likewise found that among nondisabled persons living in the community, impairments in the lower extremity were highly predictive of later disability (253). Fried et al. characterized a functional level of "preclinical disability" (task modification but no difficulty by self-report) in a study of women 70 to 80 years old (254).

Measurement of their physical function was intermediate between women with high function (no modifications) and disability (difficulty with tasks). The potential role of interventions involving increased physical activity and exercise as types of primary prevention of disability for older persons is supported by studies documenting the dynamic nature of functional loss and impact on both morbidity and mortality (37,39,41).

There may in fact be significant overlap of risk factors for multiple problems in older persons. For instance, the risk factors associated with falls, incontinence, and functional dependence are similar—slowed chair stand, decreased arm strength, decreased vision and hearing, and either a high anxiety or depression score (255).

From these types of models, successful prevention strategies are being tested, often entailing multiple interventions covering multiple domains. For instance, incidence of falls can be reduced by a combination of medication adjustments, exercise, safety training, and environmental modifications. A comprehensive nurse-practitioner evaluation program for community-residing seniors resulted in a delay in onset of disability and decreased nursing home admission (256).

Another study demonstrated that higher self-efficacy was associated with lesser functional decline in persons with diminished physical capacity (257). Research also suggests that self-efficacy (i.e., a person's confidence or belief that he or she can achieve a specific behavior or cognitive state) may be modifiable and therefore help guide preventive strategies (258). Research continues to identify which targeted intervention for which specific risk factor in which specific patient at what specific point in time will be most efficacious in preventing or minimizing disability (39).

PRINCIPLES OF ASSESSMENT AND REHABILITATIVE MANAGEMENT OF OLDER ADULTS WITH DISABILITY

Assessment of the Older Patient

Rehabilitation medicine and geriatric medicine share common principles and have complementary approaches (174). This is seen in patient assessments and initial medical assessment is relevant for both disciplines (259). **Box 47-1** provides further

---

BOX 47-1

Essential Elements of a Brief Assessment of an Older Patient

History
- Ensure patient has spectacles and hearing aids in place if appropriate. Use a headphone amplification device if the patient is not able to hear you speaking.
- Introduce yourself and explain the purpose of your visit.
- Seal yourself at the level of the patient and speak slowly and clearly.
- Ask the patient what is troubling them (presenting symptoms) and the history of these symptoms.
- Ask about other medical conditions including recent illnesses, doctor and hospital visits, and falls.
- Check what medication the patient is taking (a current list is preferred), any known allergies, alcohol intake, and smoking status.
- Ask about function in activities of daily living, including continence, before the current admission.
- Ask about the patient's home situation, whether they live alone or with someone, if that person provides care to them, or if there are services in place to assist them.
- Ask whether they have completed an advance care directive or appointed a proxy health care decision-maker.
- When the patient has significant cognitive impairment, information will need to be obtained from a carer or family member.

Physical Examination
- Assess general appearance, personal hygiene, nutrition, and hydration. Check vision, hearing, and dentition. Assess swallowing with a small amount of water (20 to 30 mL).
- Perform a brief cognitive screening test to assess orientation, attention, memory, and language. Check ability to follow a two-step command. Briefly assess mood.
- Check pulse and blood pressure in both sitting-lying and standing positions.
- Assess movement of all limbs, including a brief assessment of tone and power, muscle wasting, and active range of motion at major joints.
- While checking limb movement, assess peripheral pulses and presence of edema, skin integrity, and pressure ulceration (particularly heels and sacrum).
- Where possible, stand the patient up to check ability to transfer and standing balance, and ask the patient to walk several steps (ensure walking aid is available and provide standby assistance).
- Examine the cardiovascular and respiratory systems and abdomen, including bladder palpation (and rectal examination if indicated).

Reproduced from Kurrle SE, Cameron ID, Geeves RG. A quick ward assessment of older patients by junior doctors. *BMJ*. 2015;350:h607. With permission from BMJ Publishing Group Ltd.

details. Rehabilitation of older adults requires attention to multiple areas. Benefits of organized, comprehensive assessments and care have been documented for acute-onset disabilities like stroke and are described elsewhere in this textbook. Assessments of older patients with more insidious onset of multiple disabilities are evolving. They are collectively referred to as comprehensive geriatric assessment (CGA). Pioneering work by Dr. Marjorie Warren in Britain laid the foundation for CGA while evaluating many institutionalized older adults (260). The process was formally defined in the United States in a National Institutes of Health Consensus Development Conference in 1988 (261). CGA is "a multidisciplinary evaluation in which the multiple problems of older persons are uncovered, described, and explained, if possible, and in which the resources and strengths of the person are catalogued, need for services is assessed, and a coordinated care plan is developed to focus interventions of the person's problems" (261).

Since that time, numerous studies have evaluated CGA programs in different sites of care. While the majority focuses on the general medical geriatric population, a growing literature examines benefits in specific areas like oncology. CGA programs vary depending on the clinical setting and program design. A general conclusion from this work is that there can be benefits depending on patients targeted and the nature of the program. Targeting aims to identify older adults who are not terminally ill and who have multiple conditions. These patients also have associated disabilities amenable to known multifactorial interventions. Usually, beneficial programs include actual control of care provided rather than consultation alone.

Benefits for some, but not all, inpatient programs have included shorter lengths of stay, better management of specific syndromes, delays in functional decline, decreased bodily pain at 1 year, decreased need for home health care services, and higher likelihood of living at home in 6 months (230,260,262). In some recent studies, mortality at 1 year has not been changed.

Some, but not all, outpatient CGA programs have shown delays in functional decline, improved mental health at 1 year, and earlier diagnosis of common health problems like cognitive impairment, depression and anxiety, and incontinence (230,263–265).

CGA topics are similar to what needs to be assessed during comprehensive rehabilitation. Issues include sensory, cognitive, emotional, functional, social, financial, legal, and home issues. Other commonalities are screening and evaluation of syndromes like incontinence and falls. These syndromes are common entities that result from multiple diseases and multiple risk factors (255,266).

A standardized framework for assessing older patients, and managing care, can facilitate both rehabilitation and follow-up care by other providers. With so many types of issues requiring assessment, and follow-up, a practical standard framework would help avoid oversight of relevant factors. Communication among team members would be easier. This is especially important because older adults receive care from multiple providers in multiple settings. One estimate suggests Medicare patients should receive annually, on average, care from five specialists and two primary care providers in four different practice sites (267). Another estimate for stroke survivors is that they can receive care from up to 89 providers distributed among 8 different health care teams in 7 different locations (268).

There are a number of frameworks for organizing rehabilitation programs for older people. These can relate to domains, for example, medical, psychological, social, and functional (269,270), or can be organized with reference to the World Health Organization's International Classification of Functioning, Disability and Health (ICF) (205). Steiner and colleagues in an extensively cited paper (271) set out a "Rehabilitation Problem-Solving Form." This form is based on the ICF and includes both patient and family perspectives and the views of rehabilitation health professionals. It defines domains but these are expressed with an emphasis on functioning and personal and environmental influences on functioning, in addition to the health conditions experienced by the patient. This model explicitly recognizes the potential for both positive and negative interactions between domains and incorporates a biopsychosocial model. The classification system of the ICF can be used but that is not essential. The form is used as part of a Rehab-Cycle. This involves identifying the issues from the patient's perspective ("problems"), relating these to relevant person, environment, and health condition factors, defining rehabilitation goals, planning and implementing interventions, and assessing their effects (271). This Rehab-Cycle is consistent with the usual rehabilitation goal setting and review processes as discussed below.

Rehabilitation Goal Setting

Increasingly, there is recognition that health care and rehabilitation goals may not be uniformly shared by patients and their caregivers (272,273). For example, patients may want to return home after rehabilitation, while rehabilitation staff may strongly disagree, at times, out of undue fear of what may occur (274). Our focus as health care providers is typically on general health and well-being, as well as functional independence. Our tacit assumption is that these goals are necessarily shared by our patients and their caregivers and perhaps that these are the only goals they value. However, there is evidence of differing goals, and priorities of goals, between health care providers, case managers, patients, and their caregivers (272,273,275). Alternative goals also valued by patients and their caregivers included such areas as education and referrals, social/family relations, emotional issues, and caregiver burden. Of significance is that patients and family caregivers often focus on process goals and shorter time frames, as opposed to typical health care providers' emphasis on specific outcomes and longer-range time frames (273). While goal setting is seen as intrinsic to rehabilitation programs, the evidence base for its specific patient outcome-related benefits is not strong (276).

Prescription of Rehabilitation Programs

An appropriate therapeutic prescription is critical to the success of a rehabilitation program. The process for achieving this will vary with the country and health system in which the practitioner is working. It must be based on a careful analysis of the patient's current functional limitations, with realistic goal setting in the context of premorbid functioning and anticipated improvement in medical status (277). Specific therapy techniques will be used based on physical status (e.g., neurologic, musculoskeletal, cardiovascular systems) and medical stability. Social and cultural barriers to certain exercises or activities also must be taken into account. The patient should participate in goal setting, such that the rehabilitation plan is relevant to his or her own goals.

Without a strong therapeutic alliance between all health professional team members and the patient (and family), progress will be slow and/or limited. Functional training approaches usually are well accepted by most older individuals because they can clearly see the relevance and importance. Many therapeutic goals can be achieved by incorporating formal therapy techniques into the context of functional tasks. Examples of this approach include the following techniques:

- Repeated sit to stand to improve strength and balance
- Participation in bathing and dressing to practice basic activities
- Feeding using modified food or utensils to remediate perceptual problems and to practice basic activities
- Participation in group-based activities to assist social skills and to encourage engagement with others
- Participation in daily activities with supervision or assistance of family members to increase practice and to educate family members

Prescription of the rehabilitation program must be tailored to the person to accommodate limitations imposed by comorbid medical problems (69,117,122). Cardiovascular (e.g., blood pressure/pulse response, cardiac symptomatology) and pulmonary (e.g., use of oxygen) restrictions should be established as appropriate. In patients with limited exercise tolerance, it may be necessary to use flexibility with therapy scheduling and duration of treatment, with frequent rest periods. A number of authors have suggested practical rehabilitation guidelines that summarize these recommendations (122,278–280). Weight-bearing limits can be accommodated by means of assistive devices or aquatic therapy but should not be commonly imposed in hip fracture (408).

Resnick proposes a seven-step model to help motivate older individuals to exercise, including education, goal setting, role modeling, and verbal encouragement/rewards (281).

Realistic goal setting is complex in any rehabilitation setting but may be complicated further in older patients in two unique respects. First, older adults frequently have potential caregivers (e.g., spouse, siblings, and children) who also are aging and have medical problems of their own. Thus, the fitness and capability of the proposed caregiver after discharge must be considered in the discharge planning process (189,190,193). The second problem relates to the limited remaining life expectancy of the older disabled patient. For example, diabetic amputees over 65 years of age have average survival of approximately a year (282). In view of their potentially limited longevity, an expedited rehabilitation program to facilitate return home with family would be most appropriate. This would also apply to people with conditions that are progressively disabling and require increasingly frequent episodes of hospitalization and/or skilled nursing care.

A number of potentially negative or counterproductive team dynamics can develop in rehabilitation settings that may interfere with or limit a patient's progress (283,284). Patients and families tend to trust their health care providers as the experts who will know and do what is best for them. It is critical that the rehabilitation team maintain vigilance for and strive to counter such negative attitudes as paternalism (e.g., overriding patient goals judged by the team to be unrealistic or inappropriate), arrogance (e.g., presumptive familiarity by addressing patients by their first name without requesting permission or preference), and self-fulfilling prophecies (e.g., patients judged not to have potential for improvement and not receiving as much attention or effort as patients felt to have a good prognosis). Other team

issues that can impact effectiveness include relative team member roles (e.g., lack of clarity or excess rigidity), communication barriers, or decision-making conflicts (283). The ongoing challenge for rehabilitation teams is to foster an individual and collective philosophy of respect for and empowerment of the individuals they treat, facilitating functional independence.

Significance of Functional Status in Residential Placement Issues

Reference already has been made to the critical nature of functional status with regard to the ability to live independently in the community. Older people often live alone and must perform their own self-care and other daily activities, including homemaking. Issues of safety in this home environment frequently are raised, particularly after an acute adverse event or illness (e.g., a fall with hip fracture). A patient who achieves a level of mobility (i.e., ambulation or transfers) requiring only close supervision or contact guard assistance because of an occasional loss of balance may not be able to safely return home alone. Home-based supervision by an aide, unless paid privately, typically is available only a few hours a day, 5 days a week, for relatively limited intervals. In this instance, return to a community setting may only be possible if a relative is available to live with this individual. If not, he or she may not even qualify for a group home or intermediate care/assisted living facility; most intermediate care facility admission criteria include independent safe locomotion. This patient accordingly may require a skilled nursing facility (SNF, or nursing home) admission as the only source of 24-hour/day supervision available. Unfortunately, alternatives are limited for more homelike settings with other residents of similar functional level. These same issues apply worldwide, although the structure of home support and residential aged care facilities can vary substantially between countries (285). However, there is a clear trend toward increasing home support for older people.

Health Care Policy Issues

These issues have substantial impacts on older people. Internationally, there is support for an "aging in place" philosophy because older people generally prefer to live in their own homes and the cost of support in the person's own home is less than in an institutional setting until paid support twice daily is needed (1,285). While greater income inequality in society is strongly established as being bad for health, the relative situation of older people varies substantially by country, and there is some evidence that younger people are currently experiencing greater income inequality than older people (286).

In the American context, it is not clear what changes will occur to Medicare, Medicaid, and other programs as a result of changes in health care policy (287). However, these could have substantial effects on systems of support for older people with disabilities.

REHABILITATION APPROACHES TO COMORBIDITY AND GERIATRIC SYNDROMES

Medical Issues

Reassessment of Medical Status

Transfer of a patient from an acute medical or surgical service to a rehabilitation unit has been identified as an opportunity for a fresh and objective reassessment of medical status (288). Such an appraisal is even more critical in geriatric rehabilitation and should include confirming the accuracy of referral diagnoses, evaluating for previously unrecognized conditions, and reviewing medications for continuing appropriateness (215). Often, an older patient's physiologic status has improved or stabilized by the time of transfer, warranting consideration of altering dosage or discontinuing certain medications. Creating and using tools like a patient care notebook with medication lists is one process that can help clarify medication use (289). Patients can be encouraged to take these notebooks to all health care appointments.

Avoiding Adverse Drug Effects

The incidence of adverse drug reactions approaches 25% in people older than 80 years of age (35). Adverse drug reactions account for 11% to 20% of hospitalizations in people older than 65 years of age and are a frequent cause of mental deterioration (290–292). The reasons for drug problems in older adults revolve around five key interrelated areas:

1. Polypharmacy
2. Medications not taken as prescribed
3. Increased susceptibility to adverse reactions
4. Altered pharmacokinetics
5. Altered receptor sensitivity

Polypharmacy

Polypharmacy is frequent in older people and often compounded by the frequent use of nonprescription drugs, resulting in preventable adverse drug reactions and unnecessary financial costs (293,294). Physicians all too often contribute to this problem; one study found that one in five older patients received a prescription for a potentially inappropriate medication (295).

Frequently, known risk factors are not taken into account when prescribing a particular medication and dosage (296,297). Medication histories obtained by physicians often are inaccurate in both inpatient and outpatient settings (298,299), related in part to lack of questioning and underreporting of over-the-counter (OTC) medications, which are used almost as frequently as prescription medications by older adults (300,301). Over 50% of OTC medications are oral analgesics, with the remainder consisting of cough-and-cold preparations, vitamins, antacids, and laxatives (299,301).

The hospital setting is an excellent opportunity to discontinue drugs of questionable value because careful monitoring is possible. Accordingly, all medications should be reviewed carefully on admission to a rehabilitation unit and regularly thereafter. In addition to OTC medications, special attention should be directed to psychotropic medication, NSAIDs, and digitalis preparations (302). The Modified Beers Criteria provide an excellent basis for a medication review (303).

In addition to unawareness of concurrent medications, other factors have been identified as potentially influencing prescribing habits and contributing to polypharmacy in older people. These include pharmaceutical advertising (particularly involving new drugs inadequately tested in older people) and patient and family expectations (or even demands) for treatment, usually in the form of a prescription (304). In one nursing home study, treatments (i.e., medication prescriptions) occurred more often if a patient's problem produced ongoing discomfort for the staff (e.g., agitation); conditions tended to be undertreated if symptoms were intermittent or had less impact on staff (e.g., arthritis) (305).

Medications Not Taken as Prescribed

Patients do not take medications as prescribed in one third to one half of all cases (306). Patients over 75 years of age who live alone are especially likely to not take medications as prescribed (299,301). Reasons given by patients in one study for not taking medications included "feeling the prescribed dosage was too high" and experiencing problematic side effects (307). These patient choices can cause postdischarge deterioration; patient education prior to discharge is critical to avoid such problems. Allowing patients to self-medicate in the hospital with flexible administration times may be a useful way to monitor their understanding and an opportunity to reinforce the need for medications (308). This strategy also may help to decrease the frequency of incorrect drug frequency or dosage, omitted medications, and use of expired medications (309). However, challenges remain in determining the best methods for enhancing patient adherence to medication prescriptions (310).

Drug toxicity can result when a patient is admitted to the hospital and given all the drugs (in the "correct" dosages and frequency) that have been previously prescribed but were not being taken at home. Such a problem should be suspected when a patient shows a decline in cognitive or functional status 5 to 10 days after admission and other medical workup are unrevealing (311).

Increased Susceptibility to Adverse Reactions

Adverse drug reactions appear to be more common in older patients, even when medications are given in the proper dosages (312). This may be related to a relative lack of resiliency in their homeostatic mechanisms (35,302). Although not all adverse drug reactions are avoidable, some investigators suggest that 70% to 90% could be anticipated and prevented (293,305,306).

That some patients choose not to adhere to prescriptions given by physicians may in fact help decrease the frequency of adverse drug reactions (307). Serious side effects can occur secondary to OTC medications, especially from antihistamines with anticholinergic side effects, leading to fatigue and confusion even in middle-aged adults (300).

Altered Pharmacokinetics

There are a number of age-related changes in pharmacokinetics (see Chapter 52) with significant implications for drug dosing, timing of dosage changes, and potential for unexpected toxicity or interactions. The reader is referred to the previous discussion of organ system aging for hematologic, GI, hepatic, and renal systems.

Altered Receptor Sensitivity

Age-related changes in receptor sensitivity to drug effects are an additional reason for untoward drug effects in older people. There is evidence, for example, that benzodiazepines and warfarin have a greater effect at similar concentrations in the young compared with older people (304,312). Such changes are difficult to evaluate separately from the pharmacokinetic changes related to aging (313).

The common philosophy of "start low, go slow" is a sound advice when prescribing drugs for older people. Evaluation of response to drug therapy is critical, and elimination of unnecessary medication is essential for improving function. Patient and family education as to the indications, contraindications, and adverse effects of drugs is even more important in older individuals to try to improve adherence and avoid adverse reactions (308,309).

Hypotension

Symptomatic orthostatic hypotension can occur in many older patients after even relatively short periods of bed rest (123,217). Orthostatic hypotension is defined as a decline of 20 mm Hg or more in systolic blood pressure when rising from supine to standing, and after standing for 3 minutes, usually accompanied by symptoms of dizziness or light-headedness (314). It is accordingly a frequent problem during early remobilization of older people patients in rehabilitation settings. Symptoms can persist if there are underlying problems with blood pressure maintenance related to drug therapy, salt restriction, or autonomic dysfunction (160).

Evaluation of the orthostatic patient should include a review of medications (particularly nitrates, antihypertensives, levodopa, diuretics, phenothiazines, and tricyclic antidepressants), examination for autonomic dysfunction (e.g., pupillary response, abnormal sweating) or recent fluid loss, and laboratory tests to rule out abnormalities in aldosterone and cortisol levels (215,314,315). Treatment for symptomatic orthostasis includes discontinuing any prescribed or OTC medication that could be contributing to the hypotension. The patient should be instructed to exercise (i.e., ankle dorsiflexion/plantar flexion) before arising, to sit up initially, and then to stand up slowly while holding onto a support. Thigh-high elastic stockings or an abdominal binder may help minimize lower extremity blood pooling (314). High-sodium diet and fludrocortisone acetate, a synthetic mineralocorticoid, are useful for plasma expansion in the absence of congestive heart failure. Other medications to consider include NSAIDs (inhibit prostaglandin synthesis), clonidine or midodrine (α2-adrenergic agonists), propranolol (blocks β-2 vasodilatory receptors), pindolol (a β-adrenergic antagonist with intrinsic sympathomimetic activity), or phenylpropanolamine (a sympathomimetic) (316).

Significance of Mental and Emotional Status

Depression

Depressed mood is a significant problem in older persons and is often missed. Given the importance of improving recognition of depression, a recent review has covered the topic in detail (317) (see Chapter 12). Rates of major depression vary from 16% to 30% for the older clinical populations, and prevalence rates in community-dwelling older persons range from 2% to 5%. The risk of depression has been estimated to be three-fold greater for older persons with disability, compared to their functionally independent counterparts (182,318). The reverse appears to also be true: depression in older adults is associated with significant reductions in active life expectancy (34). Essential is the distinction, sometimes hard to make, between depressed mood that will respond to supportive counseling and more severe depression requiring more aggressive intervention (e.g., psychotherapy, medication, electroconvulsive therapy) (319). Symptoms can include depressed mood, poor motivation, fatigue, and suicidal ideation. The rehabilitation team

should maintain a high index of suspicion for the presence of depression that may require aggressive treatment. Vegetative signs suggestive of more severe depression may include the following:
- Sleep disturbance
- Loss of appetite
- Constipation
- Impaired concentration
- Poor memory
- Psychomotor retardation (181)

Other less specific complaints include other somatic symptoms such as pain and ill-characterized dyspnea (180). Depressed patients may appear as if they have cognitive impairment.

In many patients with mild reactive depression, the activity and milieu of the rehabilitation unit will alleviate the depression. Progress in therapy and the support of peers and staff often are therapeutic. When the depression is more profound, antidepressants may prove helpful; however, medical contraindications may limit or preclude their use. Medications such as the selective serotonin reuptake inhibitors (SSRIs), for example, citalopram or sertraline, have low anticholinergic activity and should be considered in preference to the tricyclic antidepressants. If these are not effective, consultation with a geriatric psychiatrist is suggested.

Evidence-based psychotherapy is recommended for older persons. Depressed outpatient volunteers in generally good health have shown benefits with cognitive behavior, interpersonal relationships, and short-term psychodynamic therapies. Clinically, interventions like these are potentially beneficial and require more evaluation, especially because medication alone cannot address such associated issues as altered life role (especially with disabilities), chronic medical illness, and losses of a spouse and/or close friends (181,320).

Anxiety

Anxiety syndromes are another frequent problem during rehabilitation (321). Symptoms can manifest in multiple body systems, as in depression. Careful differential diagnosis is required to distinguish between primary anxiety disorders and those secondary to medical illness or medication. A detailed interview and chronology of onset are needed, and assistance from psychiatry is sometimes needed. Diagnostic categories include adjustment disorder with anxious mood, generalized anxiety disorder, posttraumatic stress disorder, and panic attacks (322,323). When feasible, nonpharmacologic interventions, such as behavioral management techniques, physical therapy for muscle relaxation, or psychotherapy, should be used first (324).

Nonetheless, judicious and appropriate medication use is frequently necessary to control anxiety symptoms and facilitate participation in the rehabilitation process. Commonly used options include lorazepam, buspirone, imipramine, and SSRIs (322,324).

A baseline anxiety disorder may be exacerbated by hospitalization, leading to agitation with nonpurposeful excessive motor activity. Depression, as well as preexisting psychoses, can also present with agitation (321). The former usually responds to the more sedating tricyclic antidepressants (e.g., doxepin). Paraphrenia is an example of a psychosis occurring in older people that often presents with agitation (324). This paranoid psychosis, with onset typically late in life, is characterized by bizarre paranoid delusions in a socially isolated person.

Antipsychotics may assist in the management of this problem, coupled with therapeutic alliance with a geriatric psychiatrist and an attempt to redevelop social contacts for the patient. A history of preexisting psychiatric disorders should always be investigated in the agitated patient.

Schizophrenia can continue into old age, although exacerbations respond well to antipsychotics (321).

Delirium

Delirium, a syndrome characterized by the acute onset of fluctuating cognitive deficits in conjunction with attention disorder and disorganized thought, can cause sleep disturbances, hallucinations, and agitation (221,325). It occurs more often in patients with prior cognitive impairments and can coexist with a dementia, making accurate diagnosis very difficult (326). Any acute medical illness can present in the older person with delirium without the classic signs of the underlying acute illness (215). Infections, dehydration, stroke, hypothermia, uremia, heart or liver failure, and pulmonary emboli are the most common examples of this phenomenon (327). Drug toxicity is another frequent cause of delirium in the older people, with common offenders including neuroleptics and narcotics (326,327). There are evolving data on factors associated with postoperative delirium states (328). Delirium is still present in 16% of admissions to postacute facilities, presenting diagnostic and management challenges in the SNF setting (329). Delirium represents a medical emergency, with significant independent morbidity (330); identifying the cause is critical to its resolution. Detailed clinical guidelines with reference to prevention, diagnosis, and management are now available (331).

Dementia

Dementia occurs in about 5% of individuals over 65 years of age and in about 22% of those over 80 years of age (332,333). It is found in more than half of nursing home residents and is the most common precipitating cause of admission (332). Women appear to be affected more frequently than men. Insidious onset of memory loss, loss of abstract reasoning and problem-solving ability, impairment of judgment and orientation, and personality changes with relatively intact alertness and awareness are all hallmarks of the disease (334). A patient with early dementia, premorbidly not interfering with daily activities, can become severely disoriented during an acute hospitalization with the development of a delirium (203,215,335). This agitated confusion may resolve without any specific therapy in 1 to 2 weeks. Appreciation of this possibility is important with regard to evaluating and working with this population in the rehabilitation setting.

Fifty to sixty percent of dementias represent dementia of the Alzheimer type, and another 20% are vascular in origin (333). The current terminology is vascular dementia, rather than the older term multi-infarct dementia. Dementia with Lewy bodies and frontotemporal dementia are seen in 10% to 15% of cases of dementia, and the remaining causes include alcohol-related brain damage and traumatic brain injury and Parkinson's disease with dementia. There are a very small number of reversible causes of dementia, and it is stressed that in unselected series of older people presenting with gradual onset cognitive impairment, these are uncommon:

- Subdural hematoma, brain tumor
- Occult (normal pressure) hydrocephalus, sleep apnea
- Hypothyroidism or hyperthyroidism, hypercalcemia
- Vitamin B_{12} deficiency, niacin deficiency, drug toxicity, depression
- Cardiac, renal, or hepatic failure (334)

Limited diagnostic evaluation should be performed to rule out these possible causes. Even if one of these potentially treatable etiologies is established, however, reversibility of the dementia may be limited because of permanent damage from the condition (336). Although there are differing guidelines for recommended laboratory tests for evaluating dementia (334), a standard dementia workup, in addition to detailed history and physical examination with cognitive screening, should include at least a complete blood count (CBC), blood chemistry profiles (including electrolytes, calcium, glucose, liver function and creatinine, BUN), erythrocyte sedimentation rate, thyroid function studies, and serum B12 and folate levels.

Imaging of the brain (e.g., CT [computed tomography], MRI [magnetic resonance imaging]) should be undertaken as it may clarify the etiology, such as vascular dementia versus Alzheimer's disease (337). While the cause of Alzheimer's disease remains unknown, there are symptomatic treatments available. These are the cholinesterase inhibitors and include donepezil, rivastigmine, and galantamine, and they have all been shown to have similar modest efficacy (337). Symptomatic treatment of depression may also be indicated (214,338).

Patients with moderate or severe dementia can be limited in their ability to learn in the rehabilitation setting because their ability to form new memory is poor. Day-to-day carryover may be limited and makes certain types of therapeutic gains difficult to achieve (339). A rehabilitation trial may still be justified in such situations to clarify learning abilities and to train the family in appropriate care of a patient with a new disability. For instance, the patient may show the ability for procedural learning (learning by performing the activity) even if declarative learning (learning from verbal instruction) is impaired (195,224). Care should be taken not to unreasonably discriminate against older people with dementia in assessment for rehabilitation programs.

When evaluating the older patient for admission to a rehabilitation program, it is critical to determine the mental status before onset of the new disability by talking to family or others who have observed the patient. Too often, the mental status as seen in the acute hospital setting underestimates the patient's cognitive function when healthier and in a more supportive and stimulating environment (340).

Discharge planning for patients with dementia needs to include family education as to the nature of the patient's cognitive strengths and weaknesses and how to handle potential behavioral problems (195). Community resources for adult day care and respite care programs may be very helpful for families, as well as educational materials such as those available from the Alzheimer's Association Web site.

Pharmacologic treatment of older patients with severe dementia, particularly with behavioral and psychological disturbances, is controversial and confusing. In 1995, the Food and Drug Administration (FDA) issued "black box" warnings for atypical (second-generation) antipsychotic medications in older patients, due to multiple clinical trials documenting greater mortality risk (341,342), which has been shown to occur in both the first- and second-generation antipsychotics. These medications should be used carefully and for as short a period as clinically indicated. Current treatment guidelines emphasize shared decision-making with caregivers, thorough documentation, and frequent monitoring (337).

Common Geriatric Syndromes

Incontinence

An all too common complication, devastating to patient self-esteem and family commitment to patient care, is urinary incontinence. For diagnostic classification and evaluation procedures, the reader is referred to Chapter 23. Several recent reviews cover this topic thoroughly (343–346). Treatment for incontinence in the older patient hinges on proper diagnosis, which usually is possible with a complete history of the problem combined with careful neurologic, pelvic, rectal, and mental status examinations.

Laboratory studies should include urinalysis, culture and sensitivity, serum creatinine and BUN, and a postvoid residual urine volume (344,347). A voiding diary often is helpful in determining the nature of the problem, and cystometrics/urodynamics might also be indicated (348).

Treatment is directed at the cause of the incontinence. Unfortunately, many of the etiologies have no uniformly successful therapy, and there may even be multiple causes. A timed voiding program is useful in many patients, offering toileting opportunities at regular intervals to try to maintain continence (344). Initially, the intervals are very short (e.g., every 15 to 20 minutes), with a progressive increase as indicated. Modifications of this technique include patterned urge-response toileting (PURT) (349) and functional incidental training (FIT) (350), with reports of excellent success in nursing home settings.

Surgical procedures may be useful in the treatment of prostatic hypertrophy and sphincteric incompetence (343,348). Anticholinergics (e.g., tolterodine, solifenacin, trospium) may be useful in the management of detrusor instability but with the potential risk of retention (351). Other pharmacologic approaches include direct smooth muscle relaxants (e.g., oxybutynin) and imipramine (343,344). However, great caution should be used with the use of anticholinergics with older people due to the strong associations with delirium and cognitive impairment (303). Overflow incontinence due to detrusor decompensation (from overstretching) may require long-term indwelling catheterization, although frequent intermittent catheterization and cholinergic drugs to stimulate detrusor contraction may be helpful (352).

Where detrusor decompensation has occurred gradually, it may be possible to monitor the patient over an extended period of time so that it can be established whether intervention is likely to benefit the patient. Excellent patient and health care professional educational materials are available (353,354).

Bowel incontinence may imply severe bilateral brain disease (most frequently moderate to severe dementia) or loss of sensory input from the rectal ampulla (355). Biofeedback has been shown to be helpful in managing sensory bowel incontinence (356,357), but the management of incontinence secondary to diffuse brain disease usually requires a behavioral approach with bowel movements induced by suppositories at regular intervals (355).

Sleep Disorders

Sleep disorders and daytime fatigue are related problems common in the hospitalized older people as well as those living in the community (216,220,358). The hospital environment alone can disrupt the sleep cycle, an effect further compounded by foreign routines (vital sign checks and medication administration at odd hours), unfamiliar noises (from machines, overhead paging, and neighboring patients), and the depression often associated with the onset of new major chronic illness (220). Sleep deprivation at night leads to fatigue during the day. Napping during the day further disrupts nocturnal sleep patterns, and a vicious cycle can ensue (359).

It is important to document whether insufficient sleep is actually occurring because patients can complain of sleep difficulties when no problem is documented and they remain alert throughout the day. Simple reassurance in such cases is warranted. In cases of documented sleep disorder, contributing factors such as delirium, medication toxicities, depression, anxiety, restless leg syndrome, chronic pain syndrome, or nighttime medical problems (e.g., congestive heart failure, angina) should be considered (215,220). It is also important to differentiate acute insomnia from chronic insomnia. Acute insomnia (present for <1 month) is often related to a stressor (e.g., bereavement) and is treated with support and short-term, intermittent medication. Chronic insomnia (persisting for >1 month) should be viewed more as a symptom of another illness (359). Hypnotics should be used judiciously and only if other interventions, such as improved sleep hygiene, and treatment of the underlying illness, are unsuccessful.

After addressing these issues, good sleep hygiene practices may help. These include a regular sleep schedule, keeping the patient out of the bed and bedroom until bedtime, a snack before bedtime, daily exercise, relaxing activities in the evening before bedtime, and instruction in mental imagery or deep breathing relaxation techniques to be used as needed in bed at night (360). In addition, patients should not watch clocks during the night. Naps during the day should be avoided unless absolutely needed, briefly after lunch.

Only if these interventions fail should a sleep medication be considered. Selected antidepressants can be used in low doses at night to take advantage of sedative side effects while minimizing anticholinergic activity (e.g., trazodone) (361). If a benzodiazepine-type hypnotic is used, the choice should be one with a very short half-life (e.g., zaleplon, zolpidem, temazepam) to avoid accumulation with hangover effects (347,362). In general, diphenhydramine should be avoided because of anticholinergic effects (302,304). In the patient who remains persistently fatigued without clear organic cause, occult depression should be suspected (214,315). Additional nonmedication treatments that appear promising in older adults include behavioral treatments (e.g., stimulus control to induce good sleep hygiene behaviors) and increased exposure to light (363,364). Recent research indicates melatonin can be a useful adjunct in the management of sleep disorders in the older people (365,366).

Primary sleep disorders in older adults increase in prevalence substantially with increasing age. Common are periodic limb movements during sleep, insomnia, obstructive sleep apnea (OSA), and restless leg syndrome (358).

Pain

Pain is very common in older people, and studies are increasingly focused on this subject (367–369); prevalence estimates range from 25% to 50% of community-dwelling older people to 45% to 80% of nursing home residents (369,370). The consequences of pain are significant and include depression, decreased socialization, sleep disturbance, impaired ambulation, and increased health care use and costs (368). The pain experienced and reported by older people is no less threatening than that experienced by younger people and, similarly, must be addressed promptly (369).

Special considerations in managing pain (see Chapters 39 and 52) in older persons include difficulty in assessment secondary to patient fears, the higher incidence of comorbid illnesses compared with younger persons, complications in reporting pain in patients with memory and other cognitive impairments, validity difficulties with proxy reporting, and the importance of assessing functional implications of the pain (369,371). Furthermore, physicians understandably tend to attribute new pain to prior conditions (e.g., osteoarthritis). Cognitive impairment does not mask pain at the time of patient questioning, but accurate reporting of past pain is not necessarily reliable (372). Patients may be able to respond appropriately to pain intensity scales concerning current pain, with visual cueing as needed and taking short attention spans into account (373). Special functional considerations include the recognition that instrumental ADLs may be more sensitive to changes in pain.

Common etiologies of pain in older people include osteoarthritis, cancer, herpes zoster, temporal arteritis, polymyalgia rheumatica, and atherosclerotic peripheral vascular disease (370).

Approaches to pain management are similar across age groups and include use of physical modalities (e.g., heat, cold, massage), transcutaneous electrical nerve stimulation (TENS), biofeedback, hypnosis, and distractive techniques and other cognitive strategies (368).

Concurrent depression with pain may occur as in younger persons, requiring direct assessment for depression and intervention if required (374). Of note, older patients with depression are more likely to report pain as a somatic expression of their mood disturbance (372).

Medications for pain should be prescribed judiciously and in conjunction with nonpharmacologic approaches (368). Acetaminophen remains one of the best initial medications to be used routinely in patients with pain (375,376). Nonsteroidal anti-inflammatory medications are problematic in this population, given the limited study of patients over age 65 (377) and the known fourfold higher risk of peptic ulcer disease (378). Long-term use of opioid analgesics is appropriate for pain due to malignancy and probably in some cases of nonmalignant chronic disabling pain unresponsive to other medications. Tricyclic antidepressants or anticonvulsants may be useful in treating neuropathic pain (368). Physical mobility and activities should be encouraged as much as possible. All these treatments are best administered as part of a multidisciplinary team approach, regardless of the setting (e.g., home, SNF, or outpatient department) (369).

A particularly challenging clinical population includes older adults who experience chronic pain, often with repeated failures to respond to traditional medical or surgical treatments.

The cognitive-behavioral model of therapy, developed with younger persons, is useful in these patients (379,380). This therapy is safer, more effective, and probably lower in cost than a long-term analgesic regimen, especially if applied early in the course of an evolving pain syndrome.

This model divides contributory factors to the pain experience into biomedical variables, psychological variables (e.g., pain coping strategies, depression, personality), and socioenvironmental variables (e.g., social support, spousal criticism). Behavior therapy encourages wellness behaviors, and cognitive therapy helps patients reassess how they view themselves and their pain experience. This model also highlights the importance of assessing family behaviors in the presence of pain. Specific interventions for family coping can be beneficial (381,382).

Family and caregiver training, as well as semiformal social supports in the community, may be especially important in the setting of chronic pain in older persons (369). For example, chronic back pain sufferers (typically with associated depression) tend to exhaust their social support (383). Preventing the resulting social isolation would likely improve efficacy of treatment intervention and avoid a cascade of complications (211).

Falls

Many of the age-related physiologic declines in multiple organ systems combine to increase dramatically the incidence of falls in older people, including visuoperceptual difficulty, postural instability, impaired mobility, orthostatic hypotension, lower extremity weakness, and vertigo due to degenerative or vascular changes in the vestibular apparatus (240,241,384). Other factors contribute to increase the risk of falling, including environmental hazards, adverse effects of medications, concomitant acute or chronic disease states, depression, apathy, or confusion (333,385–387). A model attempting to identify the degree of risk for recurrent falls stratified patients into high and low risk depending on sitting and standing balance, walking ability, and stair climbing (388). In addition, attitudes toward risk were measured, as were social supports and environmental status. Recurrent falls were associated with impaired mobility, risk-taking behavior, and environmental score.

Prevention of these injurious falls is more problematic. A prospective study of 9,516 community-residing white women (average follow-up 4.1 years) found that the likelihood of hip fracture increased in the presence of multiple risk factors and low bone density (389). Suggested possible interventions to decrease risk include maintaining body weight, walking for exercise, avoiding long-acting benzodiazepines, minimizing caffeine intake, and treating impaired visual function. Tai chi reduced risk of multiple falls by 48% in a randomized control trial in community-residing persons 70 years of age and older without chronic illness, many of whom had fallen in the prior year (390). Whether this intervention would work for older persons with chronic illnesses needs to be assessed. In another study of community-dwelling older people with at least one risk factor for falls, a multifactorial intervention (medication adjustments, behavioral instruction, and exercise) reduced falls from 47% in the control group to 35% in the intervention group (391).

What multiple studies appear to consistently substantiate is that exercise is an important component of any fall prevention strategy (104,392,393).

Fear of falling resulting in decreased mobility is also a clinical problem in many older adults (394,395). Patient training in fall recovery techniques and education regarding adaptive and preventive strategies are being evaluated as methods to help prevent activity restriction from the fear of falling (396).

Assessment and intervention for falls in older people are complex due to the large number of potentially contributing factors. This task is aided by an algorithm that has been developed as a component of falls prevention and management guidelines (392). See **Figure 47-5**.

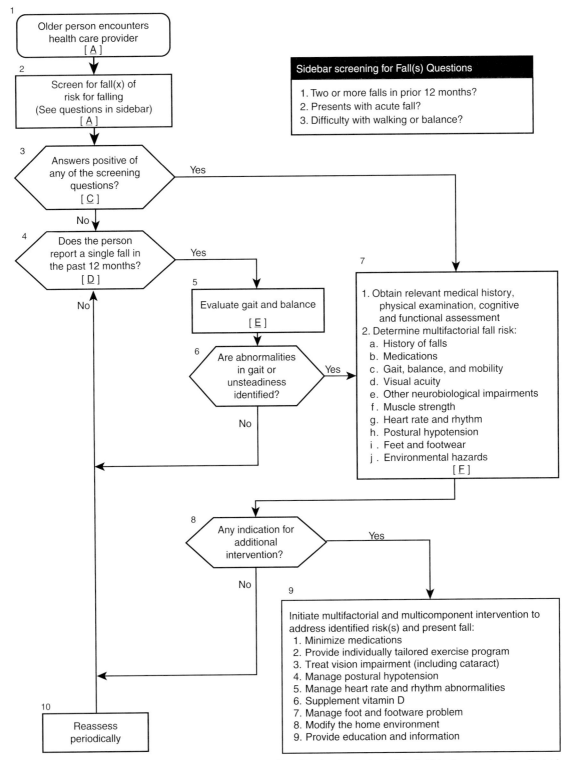

FIGURE 47-5. Algorithm for prevention of falls in older persons. (From Panel on Prevention of Falls in Older Persons, American Geriatrics Society and British Geriatrics Society. Summary of the Updated American Geriatrics Society/British Geriatrics Society clinical practice guideline for prevention of falls in older persons. *J Am Geriatr Soc.* 2011;46(1):148–157. Reprinted by permission of John Wiley & Sons, Inc.)

REHABILITATION INTERVENTIONS FOR COMMON DISABLING CONDITIONS IN OLDER ADULTS

Hip Fracture

Although 95% of falls in older persons fortunately do not result in serious injury (397), hip fractures continue to be one of the most serious sequelae (398). Strategies considered for intervention to prevent hip fracture have included both public health initiatives (e.g., emphasizing weight-bearing exercise) and individualized approaches focused on high-risk patients (78,90,399). The most effective approaches have yet to be worked out. In situations involving rehabilitation of an older patient after repair of hip fracture, it is critical to evaluate, and treat, the cause of the incident fall to prevent future recurrence.

A number of controversies involve proper care of the older patient after hip fracture. The literature is increasingly evaluating factors affecting outcomes from hip fractures and potential cost-effective changes in practice (400–404).

Issues relating to preoperative decisions include how long to wait for medical stabilization. One guideline suggests that hip fracture patients who have two or fewer comorbidities should have the operation within 2 days of admission but that a longer delay is beneficial for patients with three or more comorbidities (405). Another study found that a delay of greater than 4 days, or delay due to the management of acute medical problems, resulted in increased mortality (406).

Several factors affect the decision to operate and selection of the most appropriate type of surgery. A tendency to treat hip fractures conservatively (i.e., nonsurgically) in older patients with dementia is countered by findings of better function with less morbidity and mortality with surgical management (407). For patients with severe cardiovascular disease that contraindicates general anesthesia, percutaneous pinning with Ender rods under local anesthesia can be performed. Femoral neck fractures can be treated either by resection of the femoral head with endoprosthesis with immediate postoperative weight bearing or by internal fixation with multiple pins. Although intertrochanteric fractures have in the past been managed by internal fixation with nail or compression screw with delayed weight bearing, guidelines now suggest mobilization soon after (408).

The postoperative period can be divided into the acute hospital period and posthospital (or postacute) care. The urgency of early mobilization after repair of hip fracture is twofold: the vulnerability to many postoperative complications (e.g., pulmonary problems, thromboembolism, genitourinary sequelae, delirium) and the risk of secondary complications from bed rest or relative inactivity (400,404). Also, early initiation of physical therapy has been found to be beneficial for improving mobility in the first 2 months after hip fracture (409).

By far, the majority of hip fracture patients in the United States receive postacute hospital care in other facilities—either acute rehabilitation hospitals/units or skilled nursing facilities. These settings are increasingly necessary as hospital length of stay continues to dramatically decline.

Which setting is best for which patient is still not clear, although a recent prospective evaluation found that hip fracture patients had greater functional recovery at 12 weeks with treatment in an acute rehabilitation setting as compared to an SNF (410). What is necessary during the recuperative phase from hip fracture, regardless of setting, is close attention to the multiple medical problems that can arise (400,403). Optimal length of stay in these settings likewise is not yet clear and also continues to decline.

Arthritis and Joint Replacements

Management of arthritic conditions in older people, just as in a younger population, must be individualized with close monitoring of benefits (407,411). Treatment principles are comparable, although the balance between rest and activity is much more delicate because of the adverse sequelae of inactivity in the older people. There is evidence that older people with arthritis may respond better to therapeutic programs and often are more patient and compliant with long-term exercise and activity programs (412,413). Treatment goals include relief from fear, fatigue, stiffness, and pain, suppression of the inflammatory process, prevention or correction of deformity, and maximizing function (376,412). This is accomplished via a combination of psychological, pharmacologic, physical, and surgical measures.

Important psychological approaches have been developed through the Arthritis Self-Help Course. The multifaceted interventions include education and exercise (414). Part of the benefit may derive from facilitating the patient's ability to manage his or her own chronic condition.

Successful exercise interventions include programs of focused muscle strengthening (e.g., quadriceps strengthening for osteoarthritis of the knee), general conditioning, and aerobic activities (415–417).

Patients can be educated about the beneficial results of using various assistive devices to maintain independent community living, such as a firm chair of appropriate height with armrests, utensils with built-up handles, elevated toilet seat with grab bars, or ambulation aids (e.g., cane, walker). As with any patient care equipment, having patients try to use various devices before purchase will help ensure actual functional use (376).

Pharmacologic interventions for pain control should start with acetaminophen (up to 2 to 3 g/d) (375,376). Opioids (tramadol or codeine) can provide additional analgesia for breakthrough pain. Topical capsaicin cream may be helpful for persistent knee or finger pain, although usage may be limited by cost, need for frequent application, and initial burning sensation with application. NSAIDs may be needed for control of pain and inflammation but with great care and close monitoring given the increased risk of acute renal impairments and GI bleeding (375). In older patients with a history of gastritis or ulcers who require use of NSAIDs, concurrent administration of misoprostol or other cytoprotective agents should be considered (376,418). The use of the nutraceuticals glucosamine and chondroitin sulfate is not recommended as initial therapy for hip or knee osteoarthritis (419).

A limited number of intra-articular steroid injections can be considered (generally no more than 2 to 3 per year for any joint) but with anticipation of only short-term benefit (376). The FDA has approved another type of intra-articular injection (hyaluronan, a glycosaminoglycan) for patients who have failed other forms of therapy (376).

Age should not be a primary factor in considering potential benefits of surgical intervention in the older arthritic patient

(375,420). Significant functional gains may be realized with an appropriately timed procedure (e.g., ligament or tendon repair, osteotomy, arthroplasty, prosthetic joint replacement) to improve stability and range or to decrease pain (412). Attention to preoperative and postoperative therapy programs and early mobilization are critical to maximize functional gains and minimize secondary complications from inactivity. Further details of rehabilitation management, including principles for prescription of medication and therapeutic modalities, can be found in Chapters 30, 32, and 52.

Stroke

Studies to date suggest that age may have a negative or no effect on functional outcomes, that older stroke patients may require longer lengths of stay to achieve the same functional gains as younger patients, and that functional outcomes may be similar in differing rehabilitation settings (421–431). The most significant aspect of rehabilitating older stroke patients relates to the severity of their neurologic and functional deficits, medical stability and impact of their frequent multiple comorbid conditions on endurance, and their ability to understand, cooperate, and learn in therapy sessions. Severe language or cognitive deficits, significant neglect or apraxia, poor balance or endurance, or recurrent medical complications/instability may negatively impact the feasibility and goals of a rehabilitation program. Clinical practice guidelines for stroke rehabilitation that incorporate these and other variables have been published (432). It is clear that depression, a common complication after stroke at any age, is particularly problematic in older patients due to the deleterious effect on cognitive functioning (433). There is evidence of potential to enhance neural plasticity after stroke, even in older individuals, with improved functional recovery (434). Research continues in an effort to clarify the most appropriate (and cost-effective) role, timing, methods, setting, intensity, and duration of rehabilitation services for older people after stroke (421,435). Chapter 18 reviews concepts of stroke rehabilitation in detail, with reference to older patients.

Amputation

Although a detailed review of rehabilitation of patients with dysvascular amputation can be found in Chapter 37, several aspects require emphasis here. An ageist bias may result in the belief that a patient's age should be a factor in determining whether or not to prescribe a prosthesis. Other comorbidities rather than age *per se* are the relevant determinants for prosthetic fitting (421,436,437). A number of studies have documented the successful outcomes of rehabilitation programs for older amputees, including bilateral amputees and amputees with concurrent hemiplegia (437–441). Even in the face of severe medical comorbidity (e.g., cardiovascular disease), a prosthesis still may be both therapeutic and functional, even if only from the standpoint of standing, transfers, or cosmesis (436). For bilateral amputees, although energy costs are significantly higher and ambulation training is more difficult, prosthetic fitting still may be useful to allow periodic standing during the day and for walking short distances in the home, which are therapeutic from both an aerobic exercise and psychological standpoint (438). Wheelchair locomotion will usually be a preferable alternative for longer distance travel in view of significantly lower energy costs and ability to stop and rest. The former criterion of successful crutch ambulation to justify prosthetic prescription is not appropriate (436,437).

Spinal Cord Injury

Although SCI usually is considered a disability occurring primarily in the younger population, there is increasing recognition of its significance for older people. The mean age at injury has increased from 29 years in the 1970s to 42 years currently. However, in the United States for people with SCI, there has been no definite increase in the remaining years of life since the 1980s (442).

Epidemiology of SCI with older age at onset differs from that of younger populations. The etiology of injury is much more likely to be falls (60% in the 75 and older age group), followed by motor vehicle accidents (32% in the 75 and older group) (443–445). SCI from metastatic disease and cervical myelopathy occurs primarily in older adults. There is a marked increase in proportionate incidence of tetraplegia (TC) and tetraparesis (TI) in older people (67% in the 61- to 75-year-old age group, 88% in the 75 and older group), as opposed to the more nearly equal distribution between paraplegia (PC) and paraparesis (PI) and TC and TI in younger age groups (438). Older SCI patients are much more likely to have TI as opposed to TC (444).

There is a progressive disparity in 10-year survival rates between SCI and non-SCI populations with advancing age at injury (445). For those 70 to 98 years of age, the grouped SCI 10-year survival rate is 32%, compared with 48% for their non-SCI counterparts. Life expectancies reported for SCI patients differ depending on whether patients who die before discharge from rehabilitation programs—usually within the first year post injury—are included in the analysis. If such first-year fatalities are included, life expectancy for SCI patients injured at 60 years of age is 6.5 years for PI, 5.9 years for PC, 4.2 years for TI, and 1.9 years for TC, compared with 20.0 years for the non-SCI population (445). Two-year life expectancy is 46% for SCI patients between 61 and 86 years of age, compared to 95% for their younger counterparts (446,447).

Older patients with SCI were more likely than their younger counterparts to develop various medical complications, such as pneumonia, GI hemorrhage, pulmonary emboli, or renal stones (448,449). Although overall survival post-SCI is reduced for older adults, with increased morbidity, there does not appear to be a direct relationship between age and functional outcome (450,451).

These significant life expectancies, and potential for functional gains, make rehabilitation efforts appropriate for all patients following SCI, regardless of age (448,451). Rehabilitation goals should be comparable with those for a younger SCI population (see Chapter 22), except as impacted by comorbidity (e.g., arthritis with limitation of hand function, deconditioning, etc.). Personal care assistance becomes more critical with regard to ability to return to the community to live.

Traumatic Brain Injury

Although the concerns regarding falls in older persons are focused primarily on the risk of hip or other skeletal fractures, there is evidence of a significant incidence of traumatic brain injury as well (452,453). Similarly to older individuals after stroke, the rehabilitation interventions after brain injury must factor in premorbid and current cognitive status, severity of neurologic and functional deficits, and comorbidity issues. Experience with the federally designated Traumatic Brain Injury Model Systems project reveals that older brain-injured patients are capable of significant functional improvement but more often at a slower pace (with longer lengths of stay and higher costs) (452,453). However, increasing age is significantly associated with greater long-term disability in severe traumatic brain injury (454).

Chapter 19 provides detailed rehabilitation approaches to traumatic brain injury.

GERIATRIC REHABILITATION PERSPECTIVES

Geriatric Rehabilitation Settings

Older people with disabling medical conditions may have difficulty tolerating and participating in an intensive inpatient rehabilitation program, owing to such factors as severity of deficits, medical comorbidity, and deconditioning (455,456). Combined with the quest for least costly health care alternatives, the ideal system of inpatient rehabilitative care would provide for varying levels of intensity and settings (277). Indeed, in the United States, there is evolving interest in the role and effectiveness of various levels of postacute rehabilitative care, encompassing hospital-based comprehensive or "acute rehabilitation," SNF, or nursing home- based "subacute rehabilitation," long-term acute care hospitals (LTACHs), or outpatient clinic-based therapies. Each of these settings offers varying degrees and frequency of physician involvement in medical care and supervision and varying frequency and intensity of rehabilitation therapy treatments. Outcome studies continue to address the question of which older patients, with what underlying disability, will benefit most cost-effectively from which level(s) of care and at what time post onset of disability (425,426,455,456).

Another nontraditional setting for rehabilitation is the day hospital, which provides comprehensive, relatively intensive, and structured rehabilitation therapies designed to reverse disability and train family members to facilitate maintenance of the patient at home (457,458). This provides a greater intensity of therapy, with a wider array of equipment, under closer medical supervision, than usually is feasible in a home-based treatment program. Day hospitals may allow earlier transition from inpatient rehabilitation hospitals/units to the more familiar and comfortable home setting, with lower health care costs (457). However, there is little recent evaluative literature on this topic.

There is also an increasing interest and program development in augmented home care services, including rehabilitative care (459,460). New and innovative programs to provide intensive rehabilitation services in the home are being developed and tested (461). A randomized controlled trial of an occupational therapy preventive assessment and treatment program for older people living in the community showed improvements across various health, function, and quality of life domains (462). Such community-based programs may prove cost-effective and feasible and help resolve accessibility problems in both urban and rural settings.

These alternative levels and settings of rehabilitation services for older adults provide the potential for a continuum of care, facilitating individually tailored rehabilitative care that can be modified to meet an individual patient's changing needs over time. It is also important to utilize effective therapies across a range of different settings (463). Further research is required to document the cost-effectiveness and benefits of these varied rehabilitation programs, particularly among subsets of different disability and age groups.

Critical Issues Relating to Outcomes

The rehabilitation approach to care of older individuals with disability, like geriatric care in general, must be longitudinal in perspective and coordinated with other aspects of the individual's health care, not episodic and in isolation (464). The team work background and training of the physiatrist are ideal bases to accomplish this critical goal of geriatric care.

There are a number of critical issues impacting the quality, cost-effectiveness, and outcomes of rehabilitation interventions. Determining the appropriate treatment setting, timing, and duration of care is of obvious importance. Coupled with this is the need for individualized, realistic, functional, and relevant goal setting, which includes engagement by the older patient during formulation. Facilitating access to needed services is critical, whether referencing insurance coverage or physical transportation to the care setting. In keeping with the longitudinal perspective, periodic re-evaluation is necessary, with review and revision of therapeutic goals as warranted.

Even though "maintenance" treatment or activity is typically unfunded (as opposed to "restorative" care), the concept nonetheless is appropriate. By "maintaining" an older individual's functional status, he or she can stay in the community at far lower costs than if institutionalized. Waiting for a patient to deteriorate from lack of "maintenance" care risks initiating a cascade of complications with concomitant decreased prospects of regaining premorbid function. It is also important to remember the potential benefits of group therapy/activities (e.g., peer support and encouragement, even friendly competition), as opposed to individual treatment.

The need for patient and family education and training, perhaps on multiple occasions or even continually, should be recognized with respect to compliance and follow-through with health care recommendations and treatment (465). Finally, the longitudinal perspective mandates long-term follow-up to monitor for complications, recidivism, or underlying disease progression (with prompt intervention, if necessary), as well as to assess counseling or respite needs.

Role of the Physiatrist in Geriatrics

Physicians from various specialties traditionally have had differing perspectives on their respective roles in geriatrics (451). Physiatrists may serve a variety of roles relating to geriatrics, depending on the practice setting. These contributions range from providing primary care in a rehabilitation inpatient hospital setting or subacute (SNF-based) setting (288,339) to consulting in various health care settings (e.g., acute care hospital, SNF, day hospital, or home health care) to outpatient care (339,401,457). In the latter settings, the physiatrist assesses functional and medical statuses, works closely with therapy staff, helps formulate appropriate rehabilitation goals, helps coordinate interdisciplinary team care if needed, and monitors the efficacy of therapy.

Hoenig provides an interesting analysis of rehabilitation providers, noting that physicians of whatever specialty typically act at the disease or impairment level (e.g., prescription of medication, surgical procedure, etc.), may function as rehabilitation team leaders, and are often designated as gatekeepers in facilitating access to rehabilitation services (via prescription of therapies, insurance authorization, etc.) (466). She points out that there is a great deal of overlap and variability in the roles played by various rehabilitation providers, with a need to network, communicate, and coordinate to best serve the needs of older patients. She also provides perspectives on aging and rehabilitation from a geriatric medicine background (http://www.uptodate.com/contents/overview-of-geriatric-rehabilitation-patient-assessment-and-common-indications-for-rehabilitation?source=see_link).

Further progress in this regard is demonstrated by an interdisciplinary interaction and consensus process among ten medical and surgical specialties, spearheaded and funded by the American Geriatrics Society and John A. Hartford Foundation, respectively (467). As part of this process, Strasser et al. articulate the overlapping principles and complementary treatment approaches of geriatrics and physiatry and the importance of improving the consistency and level of expertise of all physiatrists regarding geriatric rehabilitation, to facilitate improved health care and functional outcomes for our older patients (174).

ACKNOWLEDGMENT

The contributions of Dr. Gary S Clarke and Dr. Hilary C Siebens to the previous version of this chapter is acknowledged.

REFERENCES

1. World Health Organization. *World Report on Aging and Health*. Geneva: World Health Organization; 2015. Available from: http://apps.who.int/iris/bitstream/10665/67215/1/WHO_NMH_NPH_02.8.pdf. Accessed April 10, 2018.
2. National Center for Health Statistics. *Health, United States 2015. With Special Feature on Racial and Ethnic Health Disparities*. Hyattsville, MD: National Center for Health Statistics (US); 2016.
3. United Nations, Department of Economic and Social Affairs, Population Division. *World Population Aging 2015*. Available from: http://www.un.org/en/development/desa/population/publications/pdf/ageing/WPA2015_Report.pdf. Accessed April 10, 2018.
4. Kontis V, Bennett JE, Mathers CD, et al. Future life expectancy in 35 industrialised countries: projections with a Bayesian model ensemble. *Lancet*. 2017;389(10076): 1323–1335.
5. Hobbs FB, Damon BL. Sixty-five plus in America. In: *Current Population Reports, Special Studies*. Washington, DC: US Department of Commerce, Economics, and Statistics Administration, Bureau of the Census; 1996:P23–P190.
6. Schneider EL, Guralnik JM. The aging of America. Impact on health care costs. *JAMA*. 1990;263(17):2335–2340.
7. Fried LP. Epidemiology of aging. *Epidemiol Rev*. 2000;22(1):95–106.
8. National Center for Health Statistics. *Health, United States. With Health and Aging Chartbook*. Hyattsville, MD: US Department of Health and Human Services, National Center for Health Statistics; 1999. DHHS Publication No. (PHS) 99–1232.
9. Olshansky SJ, Ault AB. The fourth stage of the epidemiologic transition: the age of delayed degenerative diseases. *Milbank Q*. 1986;64(3):355–391.
10. The Institute for Health and Aging. *Chronic Care in America: A 21st Century Challenge*. Princeton, NJ: Robert Wood Johnson Foundation Publications; 1996.
11. National Center for Health Statistics. *Health, United States. With Chartbook on Trends in the Health of Americans*. Hyattsville, MD: National Center for Health Statistics; 2007.
12. Lee LW, Siebens HC. Geriatric rehabilitation. In: LoCicero JI, Rosenthal RA, Katlic MR, et al., eds. *A Supplement to New Frontiers in Geriatric Research-An Agenda for Surgical and Related Medicine Specialties*. New York: American Geriatrics Society; 2007:301–345.
13. Anderson G. *Chronic Care—Making the Case for Ongoing Care*. Robert Johnson Foundation. 2010. Available from: http://www.rwjf.org/en/library/research/2010/01/chronic-care.html. Accessed April 10, 2018.
14. Centres for Medicare and Medicaid Services. *National Health Expenditures 2015*. Available from: www.cms.gov/research-statistics-data-and-systems/statistics-trends-and-reports/nationalhealthexpenddata/nhe-fact-sheet.html. Accessed April 10, 2018.
15. Manton KG, Gu X. Changes in the prevalence of chronic disability in the United States black and nonblack population above age 65 from 1982 to 1999. *Proc Natl Acad Sci U S A*. 2001;98(11):6354–6359.
16. Chan L, Beaver S, Maclehose RF, et al. Disability and health care costs in the Medicare population. *Arch Phys Med Rehabil*. 2002;83(9):1196–1201.
17. Lin SF, Beck AN, Finch BK, et al. Trends in US older adult disability: exploring age, period, and cohort effects. *Am J Public Health*. 2012;102(11):2157–2163.
18. Fries JF. Aging, natural death, and the compression of morbidity. *N Engl J Med*. 1980;303(3):130–135.
19. Alemayehu B, Warner KE. The lifetime distribution of health care costs. *Health Serv Res*. 2004;39(3):627–642.
20. Experton B, Ozminkowski RJ, Branch LG, et al. A comparison by payor/provider type of the cost of dying among frail older adults. *J Am Geriatr Soc*. 1996;44(9):1098–1107.
21. Lubitz J, Beebe J, Baker C. Longevity and Medicare expenditures. *N Engl J Med*. 1995;332(15):999–1003.
22. Payne G, Laporte A, Deber R, et al. Counting backward to health care's future: using time-to-death modeling to identify changes in end-of-life morbidity and the impact of aging on health care expenditures. *Milbank Q*. 2007;85(2):213–257.
23. Seshamani M, Gray A. Time to death and health expenditure: an improved model for the impact of demographic change on health care costs. *Age Ageing*. 2004;33(6):556–561.
24. Fisher ES, Welch HG, Wennberg JE. Prioritizing Oregon's hospital resources. An example based on variations in discretionary medical utilization. *JAMA*. 1992;267(14): 1925–1931.
25. Fries JF. Reducing disability in older age. *JAMA*. 2002;288(24):3164–3166.
26. Jagger C, Matthews R, Matthews F, et al. The burden of diseases on disability-free life expectancy in later life. *J Gerontol A Biol Sci Med Sci*. 2007;62(4):408–414.
27. Hoenig H, Siebens H. Geriatric rehabilitation. In: Solomon DH, LoCicero JI, Rosenthal RA, eds. *New Frontiers in Geriatrics Research: An Agenda for Surgical and Related Medical Specialties*. New York: American Geriatrics Society; 2004:339–367.
28. Kane RS. The defeat of aging versus the importance of death. *J Am Geriatr Soc*. 1996;44(3):321–325.
29. Katz S, Branch LG, Branson MH, et al. Active life expectancy. *N Engl J Med*. 1983;309(20):1218–1224.
30. Manton KG, Stallard E. Cross-sectional estimates of active life expectancy for the U.S. elderly and oldest-old populations. *J Gerontol*. 1991;46(3):S170–S182.
31. Crimmins EM, Hayward MD, Saito Y. Differentials in active life expectancy in the older population of the United States. *J Gerontol B Psychol Sci Soc Sci*. 1996;51(3): S111–S120.
32. Manton KG, Land KC. Active life expectancy estimates for the U.S. elderly population: a multidimensional continuous-mixture model of functional change applied to completed cohorts, 1982–1996. *Demography*. 2000;37(3):253–265.
33. Jagger C, Goyder E, Clarke M, et al. Active life expectancy in people with and without diabetes. *J Public Health Med*. 2003;25(1):42–46.
34. Reynolds SL, Haley WE, Kozlenko N. The impact of depressive symptoms and chronic diseases on active life expectancy in older Americans. *Am J Geriatr Psychiatry*. 2008;16(5):425–432.
35. Williams ME, Hadler NM; Sounding Board. The illness as the focus of geriatric medicine. *N Engl J Med*. 1983;308(22):1357–1360.
36. Freedman VA, Martin LG, Schoeni RF. Recent trends in disability and functioning among older adults in the United States: a systematic review. *JAMA*. 2002;288(24):3137–3146.
37. Gill TM, Allore HG, Hardy SE, et al. The dynamic nature of mobility disability in older persons. *J Am Geriatr Soc*. 2006;54(2):248–254.
38. Manton KG, Stallard E, Liu K. Forecasts of active life expectancy: policy and fiscal implications. *J Gerontol*. 1993;48(Spec No):11–26.
39. Fried LP, Ferrucci L, Darer J, et al. Untangling the concepts of disability, frailty, and comorbidity: implications for improved targeting and care. *J Gerontol A Biol Sci Med Sci*. 2004;59(3):255–263.
40. Fried LP, Tangen CM, Walston J, et al. Frailty in older adults: evidence for a phenotype. *J Gerontol A Biol Sci Med Sci*. 2001;56(3):M146–M156.
41. Klein BE, Klein R, Knudtson MD, et al. Frailty, morbidity and survival. *Arch Gerontol Geriatr*. 2005;41(2):141–149.
42. Gill TM, Guo Z, Allore HG. Subtypes of disability in older persons over the course of nearly 8 years. *J Am Geriatr Soc*. 2008;56(3):436–443.
43. Fozard JL, Metter EJ, Brant LJ. Next steps in describing aging and disease in longitudinal studies. *J Gerontol*. 1990;45(4):P116–P127.
44. Holloszy JO. The biology of aging. *Mayo Clin Proc*. 2000;75(suppl):S3–S8; discussion S8–S9.
45. Vijg J, Wei JY. Understanding the biology of aging: the key to prevention and therapy. *J Am Geriatr Soc*. 1995;43(4):426–434.
46. Rowe JW. Toward successful aging: limitation of the morbidity associated with "normal aging". In: Hazzard WR, Andres R, Bierman EL, eds. *Principles of Geriatric Medicine and Gerontology*. 2nd ed. New York: McGraw-Hill; 1990:138–141.
47. Seeman TE, Charpentier PA, Berkman LF, et al. Predicting changes in physical performance in a high-functioning elderly cohort: MacArthur studies of successful aging. *J Gerontol*. 1994;49(3):M97–M108.
48. Tosato M, Zamboni V, Ferrini A, et al. The aging process and potential interventions to extend life expectancy. *Clin Interv Aging*. 2007;2(3):401–412.
49. Johnson FB, Sinclair DA, Guarente L. Molecular biology of aging. *Cell*. 1999;96(2): 291–302.
50. Fries JF. The sunny side of aging. *JAMA*. 1990;263(17):2354–2355.
51. Lipsitz LA, Goldberger AL. Loss of "complexity" and aging. Potential applications of fractals and chaos theory to senescence. *JAMA*. 1992;267(13):1806–1809.
52. Martin GR, Danner DB, Holbrook NJ. Aging—causes and defenses. *Annu Rev Med*. 1993;44:419–429.
53. Aubert G, Lansdorp PM. Telomeres and aging. *Physiol Rev*. 2008;88(2):557–579.

54. Thompson CB. Apoptosis in the pathogenesis and treatment of disease. *Science.* 1995;267(5203):1456–1462.

55. Salvioli S, Capri M, Tieri P, et al. Different types of cell death in organismal aging and longevity: state of the art and possible systems biology approach. *Curr Pharm Des.* 2008;14(3):226–236.

56. Manton KG, Vaupel JW. Survival after the age of 80 in the United States, Sweden, France, England, and Japan. *N Engl J Med.* 1995;333(18):1232–1235.

57. Kirkwood TB. Understanding the odd science of aging. *Cell.* 2005;120(4):437–447.

58. Fried LP, Guralnik JM. Disability in older adults: evidence regarding significance, etiology, and risk. *J Am Geriatr Soc.* 1997;45(1):92–100.

59. Robbins J, Wahl P, Savage P, et al. Hematological and biochemical laboratory values in older Cardiovascular Health Study participants. *J Am Geriatr Soc.* 1995;43(8):855–859.

60. Abrass IB. The biology and physiology of aging. *West J Med.* 1990;153(6):641–645.

61. Sorlie PD, Rogot E, Johnson NJ. Validity of demographic characteristics on the death certificate. *Epidemiology.* 1992;3(2):181–184.

62. Desrosiers J, Hebert R, Bravo G, et al. Comparison of cross-sectional and longitudinal designs in the study of aging of upper extremity performance. *J Gerontol A Biol Sci Med Sci.* 1998;53(5):B362–B368.

63. Hughes VA, Frontera WR, Wood M, et al. Longitudinal muscle strength changes in older adults: influence of muscle mass, physical activity, and health. *J Gerontol A Biol Sci Med Sci.* 2001;56(5):B209–B217.

64. Fleg JL, Morrell CH, Bos AG, et al. Accelerated longitudinal decline of aerobic capacity in healthy older adults. *Circulation.* 2005;112(5):674–682.

65. Shock NW. Aging of regulatory systems. In: Cape RDT, Coe RM, Rossman I, eds. *Fundamentals of Geriatric Medicine.* New York: Raven; 1983:51–62.

66. Rochon PA, Gurwitz JH. Drug therapy. *Lancet.* 1995;346(8966):32–36.

67. McGuire DK, Levine BD, Williamson JW, et al. A 30-year follow-up of the Dallas Bedrest and Training Study: I. Effect of age on the cardiovascular response to exercise. *Circulation.* 2001;104(12):1350–1357.

68. Nelson ME, Rejeski WJ, Blair SN, et al. Physical activity and public health in older adults: recommendation from the American College of Sports Medicine and the American Heart Association. *Med Sci Sports Exerc.* 2007;39(8):1435–1445.

69. Christmas C, Andersen RA. Exercise and older patients: guidelines for the clinician. *J Am Geriatr Soc.* 2000;48(3):318–324.

70. McGuire DK, Levine BD, Williamson JW, et al. A 30-year follow-up of the Dallas Bedrest and Training Study: II. Effect of age on cardiovascular adaptation to exercise training. *Circulation.* 2001;104(12):1358–1366.

71. Fiatarone MA, Marks EC, Ryan ND, et al. High-intensity strength training in nonagenarians. Effects on skeletal muscle. *JAMA.* 1990;263(22):3029–3034.

72. Singh MA. Exercise and aging. *Clin Geriatr Med.* 2004;20(2):201–221.

73. Gill TM, Baker DI, Gottschalk M, et al. A program to prevent functional decline in physically frail, elderly persons who live at home. *N Engl J Med.* 2002;347(14):1068–1074.

74. Coleman EA, Fox PD. Translating evidence-based geriatric care into practice: lessons from Managed Care Organizations—Part I: introduction and physical inactivity. *Ann Long Term Care Clin Care Aging.* 2002;10:42–48.

75. Isaacs B. *An Introduction to Geriatrics.* London: Baillière, Tindall & Cassell; 1965.

76. Fine SL, Berger JW, Maguire MG, et al. Age-related macular degeneration. *N Engl J Med.* 2000;342(7):483–492.

77. Keller BK, Morton JL, Thomas VS, et al. The effect of visual and hearing impairments on functional status. *J Am Geriatr Soc.* 1999;47(11):1319–1325.

78. American Geriatrics Society, British Geriatrics Society, and American Academy of Orthopaedic Surgeons Panel on Falls Prevention. Guideline for the prevention of falls in older persons. *J Am Geriatr Soc.* 2001;49(5):664–672.

79. Cohn ES. Hearing loss with aging: presbycusis. *Clin Geriatr Med.* 1999;15(1):145–161, viii.

80. Mansour-Shousher R, Mansour WN. Nonsurgical management of hearing loss. *Clin Geriatr Med.* 1999;15(1):163–177, viii.

81. Rossini PM, Rossi S, Babiloni C, et al. Clinical neurophysiology of aging brain: from normal aging to neurodegeneration. *Prog Neurobiol.* 2007;83(6):375–400.

82. Rubichi S, Neri M, Nicoletti R. Age-related slowing of control processes: evidence from a response coordination task. *Cortex.* 1999;35(4):573–582.

83. Keefover RW. Aging and cognition. *Neurol Clin.* 1998;16(3):635–648.

84. Small SA, Stern Y, Tang M, et al. Selective decline in memory function among healthy elderly. *Neurology.* 1999;52(7):1392–1396.

85. Corey-Bloom J, Wiederholt WC, Edelstein S, et al. Cognitive and functional status of the oldest old. *J Am Geriatr Soc.* 1996;44(6):671–674.

86. Petersen RC, Doody R, Kurz A, et al. Current concepts in mild cognitive impairment. *Arch Neurol.* 2001;58(12):1985–1992.

87. Hoenig H, Nusbaum N, Brummel-Smith K. Geriatric rehabilitation: state of the art. *J Am Geriatr Soc.* 1997;45(11):1371–1381.

88. Wolfson L. Gait and balance dysfunction: a model of the interaction of age and disease. *Neuroscientist.* 2001;7(2):178–183.

89. Wolfson L, Whipple R, Derby C, et al. Balance and strength training in older adults: intervention gains and Tai Chi maintenance. *J Am Geriatr Soc.* 1996;44(5):498–506.

90. Rubinstein TC, Alexander NB, Hausdorff JM. Evaluating fall risk in older adults: steps and missteps. *Clin Geriatr.* 2003;11(1):52–60.

91. Frontera WR, Hughes VA, Fielding RA, et al. Aging of skeletal muscle: a 12-yr longitudinal study. *J Appl Physiol (1985).* 2000;88(4):1321–1326.

92. Walston JD. Sarcopenia in older adults. *Curr Opin Rheumatol.* 2012;24(6):623–627.

93. Cruz-Jentoft AJ, Baeyens JP, Bauer JM, et al. Sarcopenia: European consensus on definition and diagnosis: report of the European Working Group on Sarcopenia in Older People. *Age Ageing.* 2010;39(4):412–423.

94. Stenholm S, Harris TB, Rantanen T, et al. Sarcopenic obesity: definition, cause and consequences. *Curr Opin Clin Nutr Metab Care.* 2008;11(6):693–700.

95. Bouchonville MF, Villareal DT. Sarcopenic obesity: how do we treat it? *Curr Opin Endocrinol Diabetes Obes.* 2013;20(5):412–419.

96. Morley JE. Sarcopenia: diagnosis and treatment. *J Nutr Health Aging.* 2008;12(7):452–456.

97. Creamer P, Hochberg MC. Management of osteoarthritis. In: Hazzard WR, Blass JP, Ettinger WHJ, eds. *Principles of Geriatric Medicine and Gerontology.* 4th ed. New York: McGraw-Hill; 1999:1155–1162.

98. Lawrence RC, Helmick CG, Arnett FC, et al. Estimates of the prevalence of arthritis and selected musculoskeletal disorders in the United States. *Arthritis Rheum.* 1998;41(5):778–799.

99. Martin JA, Brown TD, Heiner AD, et al. Chondrocyte senescence, joint loading and osteoarthritis. *Clin Orthop Relat Res.* 2004;(427 suppl):S96–S103.

100. DeGroot J, Verzijl N, Wenting-van Wijk MJ, et al. Accumulation of advanced glycation end products as a molecular mechanism for aging as a risk factor in osteoarthritis. *Arthritis Rheum.* 2004;50(4):1207–1215.

101. Kanis JA, Melton LJ III, Christiansen C, et al. The diagnosis of osteoporosis. *J Bone Miner Res.* 1994;9(8):1137–1141.

102. Centre for Metabolic Bone Diseases, University Of Sheffield, UK. *FRAX® Fracture Risk Assessment Tool 2008.* Available from: https://www.shef.ac.uk/FRAX/. Accessed April 20, 2018.

103. Papaioannou A, Morin S, Cheung AM, et al. 2010 clinical practice guidelines for the diagnosis and management of osteoporosis in Canada: summary. *CMAJ.* 2010;182(17):1864–1873.

104. Gillespie LD, Robertson MC, Gillespie WJ, et al. Interventions for preventing falls in older people living in the community. *Cochrane Database Syst Rev.* 2012;(9):CD007146.

105. Roy AT, Johnson LE, Lee DB, et al. Renal failure in older people. *J Am Geriatr Soc.* 1990;38(3):239–253.

106. Martin JE, Sheaff MT. Renal ageing. *J Pathol.* 2007;211(2):198–205.

107. Lindeman RD, Tobin J, Shock NW. Longitudinal studies on the rate of decline in renal function with age. *J Am Geriatr Soc.* 1985;33(4):278–285.

108. Podrazik PM, Schwartz JB. Cardiovascular pharmacology of aging. *Cardiol Clin.* 1999;17(1):17–34.

109. Pandolf KB. Aging and human heat tolerance. *Exp Aging Res.* 1997;23(1):69–105.

110. Luchi RJ, Taffet GE, Teasdale TA. Congestive heart failure in the elderly. *J Am Geriatr Soc.* 1991;39(8):810–825.

111. Beers MH. Explicit criteria for determining potentially inappropriate medication use by the elderly. An update. *Arch Intern Med.* 1997;157(14):1531–1536.

112. Halawa I, Andersson T, Tomson T. Hyponatremia and risk of seizures: a retrospective cross-sectional study. *Epilepsia.* 2011;52(2):410–413.

113. Chan ED, Welsh CH. Geriatric respiratory medicine. *Chest.* 1998;114(6):1704–1733.

114. Enright PL. Aging of the respiratory system. In: Hazzard WR, Blass JP, Ettinger WH, et al., eds. *Principles of Geriatric Medicine and Gerontology.* 4th ed. New York: McGraw-Hill; 1999:721–728.

115. Fragoso CA, Gahbauer EA, Van Ness PH, et al. Peak expiratory flow as a predictor of subsequent disability and death in community-living older persons. *J Am Geriatr Soc.* 2008;56(6):1014–1020.

116. Geokas MC, Lakatta EG, Makinodan T, et al. The aging process. *Ann Intern Med.* 1990;113(6):455–466.

117. Evans WJ. Exercise training guidelines for the elderly. *Med Sci Sports Exerc.* 1999;31(1):12–17.

118. Damush TM, Stewart AL, Mills KM, et al. Prevalence and correlates of physician recommendations to exercise among older adults. *J Gerontol A Biol Sci Med Sci.* 1999;54(8):M423–M427.

119. Yende S, Angus DC, Ali IS, et al. Influence of comorbid conditions on long-term mortality after pneumonia in older people. *J Am Geriatr Soc.* 2007;55(4):518–525.

120. McLaughlin MA. The aging heart. State-of-the-art prevention and management of cardiac disease. *Geriatrics.* 2001;56(6):45–49; quiz 50.

121. Tresch DD, McGough MF. Heart failure with normal systolic function: a common disorder in older people. *J Am Geriatr Soc.* 1995;43(9):1035–1042.

122. Heath JM, Stuart MR. Prescribing exercise for frail elders. *J Am Board Fam Pract.* 2002;15(3):218–228.

123. Gupta V, Lipsitz LA. Orthostatic hypotension in the elderly: diagnosis and treatment. *Am J Med.* 2007;120(10):841–847.

124. Linzer M, Yang EH, Estes NA III, et al. Diagnosing syncope. Part 2: Unexplained syncope. Clinical efficacy assessment project of the American College of Physicians. *Ann Intern Med.* 1997;127(1):76–86.

125. Burns EA, Goodwin JS. Immunology and infectious disease. In: Cassel CK, Reisenberg DE, Sorenson LB, et al., eds. *Geriatric Medicine.* 2nd ed. New York: Springer-Verlag; 1990:312–329.

126. Gruver AL, Hudson LL, Sempowski GD. Immunosenescence of ageing. *J Pathol.* 2007;211(2):144–156.

127. Mouton CP, Bazaldua OV, Pierce B, et al. Common infections in older adults. *Am Fam Physician.* 2001;63(2):257–268.

128. Halter JB. Diabetes Mellitus. In: Hazzard WR, Blass JP, Ettinger WH, et al., eds. *Principles of Geriatric Medicine and Gerontology.* 4th ed. New York: McGraw-Hill; 1999:991–1012.

129. Scheen AJ. Diabetes mellitus in the elderly: insulin resistance and/or impaired insulin secretion? *Diabetes Metab.* 2005;31(Spec No 2):5S27–5S34.

130. Gruenewald DA, Matsumoto AM. Aging of the endocrine system. In: Hazzard WR, Blass JP, Ettinger WH, et al., eds. *Principles of Geriatric Medicine and Gerontology.* 4th ed. New York: McGraw-Hill; 1999:949–966.

131. Brown AF, Mangione CM, Saliba D, et al. Guidelines for improving the care of the older person with diabetes mellitus. *J Am Geriatr Soc.* 2003;51(5 suppl Guidelines):S265–S280.

132. Miller M. Fluid and electrolyte homeostasis in the elderly: physiological changes of ageing and clinical consequences. *Baillieres Clin Endocrinol Metab.* 1997;11(2):367–387.

133. Gerstein HC, Miller ME, Byington RP, et al. Effects of intensive glucose lowering in type 2 diabetes. *N Engl J Med.* 2008;358(24):2545–2559.

134. Ladenson PW, Singer PA, Ain KB, et al. American Thyroid Association guidelines for detection of thyroid dysfunction. *Arch Intern Med.* 2000;160(11):1573–1575.

135. Chiovato L, Mariotti S, Pinchera A. Thyroid diseases in the elderly. *Baillieres Clin Endocrinol Metab.* 1997;11(2):251–270.

136. Van Cauter E, Leproult R, Kupfer DJ. Effects of gender and age on the levels and circadian rhythmicity of plasma cortisol. *J Clin Endocrinol Metab.* 1996;81(7):2468–2473.

137. Parker CR Jr, Slayden SM, Azziz R, et al. Effects of aging on adrenal function in the human: responsiveness and sensitivity of adrenal androgens and cortisol to adrenocorticotropin in premenopausal and postmenopausal women. *J Clin Endocrinol Metab.* 2000;85(1):48–54.

138. Harman SM, Metter EJ, Tobin JD, et al. Longitudinal effects of aging on serum total and free testosterone levels in healthy men. Baltimore Longitudinal Study of Aging. *J Clin Endocrinol Metab.* 2001;86(2):724–731.

139. Casper RF, Yen SS. Neuroendocrinology of menopausal flushes: an hypothesis of flush mechanism. *Clin Endocrinol (Oxf).* 1985;22(3):293–312.

140. Rosen CJ. Clinical practice. Postmenopausal osteoporosis. *N Engl J Med.* 2005;353(6):595–603.

141. Kenney WL, Munce TA. Invited review: aging and human temperature regulation. *J Appl Physiol (1985).* 2003;95(6):2598–2603.

142. Medina JJ, Parra RO, Moore RG. Benign prostatic hyperplasia (the aging prostate). *Med Clin North Am.* 1999;83(5):1213–1229.

143. Krahn MD, Mahoney JE, Eckman MH, et al. Screening for prostate cancer. A decision analytic view. *JAMA.* 1994;272(10):773–780.

144. Beckman TJ, Mynderse LA. Evaluation and medical management of benign prostatic hyperplasia. *Mayo Clin Proc.* 2005;80(10):1356–1362.

145. Fantl JA, Newman DK, Colling J. *Urinary Incontinence in Adults: Acute and Chronic Management.* Clinical Practice Guideline No. 2, 1996 Update. Rockville, MD: U.S. Department of Health and Human Services. Public Health Service, Agency for Health Care Policy and Research. AHCPR Publication No. 96–0682. March 1996.

146. Ouslander JG. Aging and the lower urinary tract. *Am J Med Sci.* 1997;314(4):214–218.

147. Duffy LM. Lovers, loners, and lifers: sexuality and the older adult. *Geriatrics.* 1998;53(suppl 1):S66–S69.

148. Lindau ST, Schumm LP, Laumann EO, et al. A study of sexuality and health among older adults in the United States. *N Engl J Med.* 2007;357(8):762–774.

149. Meston CM. Aging and sexuality. *West J Med.* 1997;167(4):285–290.

150. Kaiser FE. Sexuality in the elderly. *Urol Clin North Am.* 1996;23(1):99–109.

151. Kaiser FE. Erectile dysfunction in the aging man. *Med Clin North Am.* 1999;83(5):1267–1278.

152. Montorsi F, Salonia A, Deho F, et al. The ageing male and erectile dysfunction. *World J Urol.* 2002;20(1):28–35.

153. WHO/UNICEF/UNU. *Iron Deficiency Anaemia: Assessment, Prevention, and Control.* Geneva: World Health Organization; 2001. Available from: http://www.who.int/iris/bitstream/10665/66914/1/WHO_NHD_01.3.pdf?ua=1. Accessed April 10, 2018.

154. Aapro MS, Cella D, Zagari M. Age, anemia, and fatigue. *Semin Oncol.* 2002;29(3 suppl 8):55–59.

155. Lipschitz D. Medical and functional consequences of anemia in the elderly. *J Am Geriatr Soc.* 2003;51(3 suppl):S10–S13.

156. Smith DL. Anemia in the elderly. *Am Fam Physician.* 2000;62(7):1565–1572.

157. Pieper CF, Rao KM, Currie MS, et al. Age, functional status, and racial differences in plasma D-dimer levels in community-dwelling elderly persons. *J Gerontol A Biol Sci Med Sci.* 2000;55(11):M649–M657.

158. Piva E, Sanzari MC, Servidio G, et al. Length of sedimentation reaction in undiluted blood (erythrocyte sedimentation rate): variations with sex and age and reference limits. *Clin Chem Lab Med.* 2001;39(5):451–454.

159. Osei-Bimpong A, Meek JH, Lewis SM. ESR or CRP? A comparison of their clinical utility. *Hematology.* 2007;12(4):353–357.

160. Stern N, Tuck ML. Homeostatic fragility in the elderly. *Cardiol Clin.* 1986;4(2):201–211.

161. Chaves PH, Ashar B, Guralnik JM, et al. Looking at the relationship between hemoglobin concentration and prevalent mobility difficulty in older women. Should the criteria currently used to define anemia in older people be reevaluated? *J Am Geriatr Soc.* 2002;50(7):1257–1264.

162. Maraldi C, Ble A, Zuliani G, et al. Association between anemia and physical disability in older patients: role of comorbidity. *Aging Clin Exp Res.* 2006;18(6):485–492.

163. Schwartz JB. The current state of knowledge on age, sex, and their interactions on clinical pharmacology. *Clin Pharmacol Ther.* 2007;82(1):87–96.

164. Parker BM, Cusack BJ, Vestal RE. Pharmacokinetic optimisation of drug therapy in elderly patients. *Drugs Aging.* 1995;7(1):10–18.

165. Altman DF. Changes in gastrointestinal, pancreatic, biliary, and hepatic function with aging. *Gastroenterol Clin North Am.* 1990;19(2):227–234.

166. Camilleri M, Cowen T, Koch TR. Enteric neurodegeneration in ageing. *Neurogastroenterol Motil.* 2008;20(3):185–196.

167. Shamburek RD, Farrar JT. Disorders of the digestive system in the elderly. *N Engl J Med.* 1990;322(7):438–443.

168. De Lillo AR, Rose S. Functional bowel disorders in the geriatric patient: constipation, fecal impaction, and fecal incontinence. *Am J Gastroenterol.* 2000;95(4):901–905.

169. Harari D, Gurwitz JH, Avorn J, et al. How do older persons define constipation? Implications for therapeutic management. *J Gen Intern Med.* 1997;12(1):63–66.

170. Holt PR. Diarrhea and malabsorption in the elderly. *Gastroenterol Clin North Am.* 2001;30(2):427–444.

171. Butler RN. Age-ism: another form of bigotry. *Gerontologist.* 1969;9(4):243–246.

172. Hummert ML. Age and typicality judgments of stereotypes of the elderly: perceptions of elderly vs. young adults. *Int J Aging Hum Dev.* 1993;37(3):217–226.

173. Salzman B. Myths and realities of aging. *Care Manag J.* 2006;7(3):141–150.

174. Strasser DC, Solomon DH, Burton JR. Geriatrics and physical medicine and rehabilitation: common principles, complementary approaches, and 21st century demographics. *Arch Phys Med Rehabil.* 2002;83(9):1323–1324.

175. Barnes LL, de Leon CF, Lewis TT, et al. Perceived discrimination and mortality in a population-based study of older adults. *Am J Public Health.* 2008;98(7):1241–1247.

176. Rowe JW, Kahn RL. *Successful Aging: The MacArthur Foundation Study.* New York: Pantheon Books; 1998:11–35.

177. Solomon R. Coping with stress: a physician's guide to mental health in aging. *Geriatrics.* 1996;51(7):46–48, 50–1; quiz 2.

178. Medalie JH. The elderly and their families. In: Reichel WR, ed. *Clinical Aspects of Aging.* 3rd ed. Baltimore, MD: Lippincott Williams & Wilkins; 1989:477–486.

179. Fried LP, Freedman M, Endres TE, et al. Building communities that promote successful aging. *West J Med.* 1997;167(4):216–219.

180. Kennedy GJ, Kelman HR, Thomas C, et al. Hierarchy of characteristics associated with depressive symptoms in an urban elderly sample. *Am J Psychiatry.* 1989;146(2):220–225.

181. Covinsky KE, Fortinsky RH, Palmer RM, et al. Relation between symptoms of depression and health status outcomes in acutely ill hospitalized older persons. *Ann Intern Med.* 1997;126(6):417–425.

182. Harris RE, Mion LC, Patterson MB, et al. Severe illness in older patients: the association between depressive disorders and functional dependency during the recovery phase. *J Am Geriatr Soc.* 1988;36(10):890–896.

183. Penninx BW, Leveille S, Ferrucci L, et al. Exploring the effect of depression on physical disability: longitudinal evidence from the established populations for epidemiologic studies of the elderly. *Am J Public Health.* 1999;89(9):1346–1352.

184. Roy R, Thomas M, Cook A. Social context of elderly chronic pain patients. In: Ferrell BR, Ferrell BA, eds. *Pain in the Elderly.* Seattle, WA: IASP Press; 1996:111–117.

185. Fiori KL, Smith J, Antonucci TC. Social network types among older adults: a multidimensional approach. *J Gerontol B Psychol Sci Soc Sci.* 2007;62(6):P322–P330.

186. Crooks VC, Lubben J, Petitti DB, et al. Social network, cognitive function, and dementia incidence among elderly women. *Am J Public Health.* 2008;98(7):1221–1227.

187. Mavandadi S, Rook KS, Newsom JT. Positive and negative social exchanges and disability in later life: an investigation of trajectories of change. *J Gerontol B Psychol Sci Soc Sci.* 2007;62(6):S361–S370.

188. Lang FR, Carstensen LL. Close emotional relationships in late life: further support for proactive aging in the social domain. *Psychol Aging.* 1994;9(2):315–324.

189. Connidis IA. Sibling support in older age. *J Gerontol.* 1994;49(6):S309–S317.

190. Mendes de Leon CF, Gold DT, Glass TA, et al. Disability as a function of social networks and support in elderly African Americans and Whites: the Duke EPESE 1986–1992. *J Gerontol B Psychol Sci Soc Sci.* 2001;56(3):S179–S190.

191. Hing E, Bloom B. Long-term care for the functionally dependent elderly. *Am J Public Health.* 1991;81(2):223–225.

192. Unger JB, McAvay G, Bruce ML, et al. Variation in the impact of social network characteristics on physical functioning in elderly persons: MacArthur Studies of Successful Aging. *J Gerontol B Psychol Sci Soc Sci.* 1999;54(5):S245–S251.

193. Brody EM. Informal support systems in the rehabilitation of the disabled elderly. In: Brody SJ, Ruff GE, eds. *Aging and Rehabilitation: Advances in the State of the Art.* New York: Springer-Verlag; 1986:87–103.

194. McCullagh E, Brigstocke G, Donaldson N, et al. Determinants of caregiving burden and quality of life in caregivers of stroke patients. *Stroke.* 2005;36(10):2181–2186.

195. Mittelman MS, Ferris SH, Shulman E, et al. A family intervention to delay nursing home placement of patients with Alzheimer disease. A randomized controlled trial. *JAMA.* 1996;276(21):1725–1731.

196. Tsuji I, Whalen S, Finucane TE. Predictors of nursing home placement in community-based long-term care. *J Am Geriatr Soc.* 1995;43(7):761–766.

197. Schulz R, Beach SR. Caregiving as a risk factor for mortality: the Caregiver Health Effects Study. *JAMA.* 1999;282(23):2215–2219.

198. Lachs MS, Berkman L, Fulmer T, et al. A prospective community-based pilot study of risk factors for the investigation of elder mistreatment. *J Am Geriatr Soc.* 1994;42(2):169–173.

199. Von Korff M, Gruman J, Schaefer J, et al. Collaborative management of chronic illness. *Ann Intern Med.* 1997;127(12):1097–1102.

200. Levine C. The loneliness of the long-term care giver. *N Engl J Med.* 1999;340(20):1587–1590.

201. Cameron ID, Aggar C, Robinson AL, et al. Assessing and helping carers of older people. *BMJ.* 2011;343:d5202.

202. Creditor MC. Hazards of hospitalization of the elderly. *Ann Intern Med.* 1993;118(3):219–223.

203. Volpato S, Onder G, Cavalieri M, et al. Characteristics of nondisabled older patients developing new disability associated with medical illnesses and hospitalization. *J Gen Intern Med.* 2007;22(5):668–674.

204. Hesse KA, Campion EW, Karamouz N. Attitudinal stumbling blocks to geriatric rehabilitation. *J Am Geriatr Soc.* 1984;32(10):747–750.

205. *International Classification of Functioning, Disability, and Health*. Geneva: World Health Organization; 2001. Available from: http://www.who.int/classifications/icf/en/. Accessed April 10, 2018.

206. Maisel JL, Ranahan M. *Visitability*. Center for Inclusive Design & Environmental Access (IDeA). Washington DC: National Institute of Building Sciences. 2017. Available from: https://www.wbdg.org/resources/visitability. Accessed April 20, 2018.

207. World Health Organization. *World Report on Disability*. Geneva: World Health Organization; 2011. Available from: http://whqlibdoc.who.int/publications/2011/9789240685215_eng.pdf. Accessed April 10, 2018.

208. WBDG Accessible Committee; Maisel JL, Ranahan M. *Beyond Accessibility to Universal Design*. Washington DC: Center for Inclusive Design & Environmental Access (IDeA). Available from: https://www.wbdg.org/design-objectives/accessible/beyond-accessibility-universal-design. Accessed April 10, 2018.

209. Gill TM, Allore H, Guo Z. The deleterious effects of bed rest among community-living older persons. *J Gerontol A Biol Sci Med Sci*. 2004;59(7):755–761.

210. Hirsch CH, Sommers L, Olsen A, et al. The natural history of functional morbidity in hospitalized older patients. *J Am Geriatr Soc*. 1990;38(12):1296–1303.

211. Mold JW, Stein HF. The cascade effect in the clinical care of patients. *N Engl J Med*. 1986;314(8):512–514.

212. Williamson JD, Fried LP. Characterization of older adults who attribute functional decrements to "old age". *J Am Geriatr Soc*. 1996;44(12):1429–1434.

213. Searle SD, Mitnitski A, Gahbauer EA, et al. A standard procedure for creating a frailty index. *BMC Geriatr*. 2008;8:24.

214. Sarkisian CA, Lachs MS. "Failure to thrive" in older adults. *Ann Intern Med*. 1996;124(12):1072–1078.

215. Fried LP, Storer DJ, King DE, et al. Diagnosis of illness presentation in the elderly. *J Am Geriatr Soc*. 1991;39(2):117–123.

216. Hoenig HM, Rubenstein LZ. Hospital-associated deconditioning and dysfunction. *J Am Geriatr Soc*. 1991;39(2):220–222.

217. Siebens H. Deconditioning. In: Kemp B, Brummel-Smith K, Ramsdell JW, eds. *Geriatric Rehabilitation*. Boston, MA: Little, Brown; 1990:177–192.

218. Rockwood K, Fox RA, Stolee P, et al. Frailty in elderly people: an evolving concept. *CMAJ*. 1994;150(4):489–495.

219. Rockwood K, Stolee P, McDowell I. Factors associated with institutionalization of older people in Canada: testing a multifactorial definition of frailty. *J Am Geriatr Soc*. 1996;44(5):578–582.

220. Sager MA, Franke T, Inouye SK, et al. Functional outcomes of acute medical illness and hospitalization in older persons. *Arch Intern Med*. 1996;156(6):645–652.

221. Inouye SK. Delirium in older persons. *N Engl J Med*. 2006;354(11):1157–1165.

222. Inouye SK. Delirium in hospitalized older patients: recognition and risk factors. *J Geriatr Psychiatry Neurol*. 1998;11(3):118–125; discussion 57–58.

223. Marcantonio ER, Flacker JM, Michaels M, et al. Delirium is independently associated with poor functional recovery after hip fracture. *J Am Geriatr Soc*. 2000;48(6):618–624.

224. Kemp B. Psychosocial and mental health issues in rehabilitation of older persons. In: Brody SJ, Ruff GE, eds. *Aging and Rehabilitation: Advances in the State of the Art*. New York: Springer-Verlag; 1986:122–158.

225. Kortebein P, Ferrando A, Lombeida J, et al. Effect of 10 days of bed rest on skeletal muscle in healthy older adults. *JAMA*. 2007;297(16):1772–1774.

226. de Morton NA, Keating JL, Jeffs K. Exercise for acutely hospitalised older medical patients. *Cochrane Database Syst Rev*. 2007;(1):CD005955.

227. Siebens H, Aronow H, Edwards D, et al. A randomized controlled trial of exercise to improve outcomes of acute hospitalization in older adults. *J Am Geriatr Soc*. 2000;48(12):1545–1552.

228. Reuben DB, Borok GM, Wolde-Tsadik G, et al. A randomized trial of comprehensive geriatric assessment in the care of hospitalized patients. *N Engl J Med*. 1995;332(20):1345–1350.

229. Landefeld CS, Palmer RM, Kresevic DM, et al. A randomized trial of care in a hospital medical unit especially designed to improve the functional outcomes of acutely ill older patients. *N Engl J Med*. 1995;332(20):1338–1344.

230. Cohen HJ, Feussner JR, Weinberger M, et al. A controlled trial of inpatient and outpatient geriatric evaluation and management. *N Engl J Med*. 2002;346(12):905–912.

231. Landefeld CS. Care of hospitalized older patients: opportunities for hospital-based physicians. *J Hosp Med*. 2006;1(1):42–47.

232. ICD9Data.com. 2012. Available from: http://www.icd9data.com/2012/Volume1/780-799/797-799/799/799.3.htm. Accessed April 20, 2018.

233. Spirduso WW. *Physical Dimensions of Aging*. Champaign, IL: Human Kinetics; 1995.

234. Sui X, Laditka JN, Hardin JW, et al. Estimated functional capacity predicts mortality in older adults. *J Am Geriatr Soc*. 2007;55(12):1940–1947.

235. Frontera WR, Meredith CN, O'Reilly KP, et al. Strength training and determinants of VO$_{2max}$ in older men. *J Appl Physiol (1985)*. 1990;68(1):329–333.

236. Morey MC, Pieper CF, Sullivan RJ Jr, et al. Five-year performance trends for older exercisers: a hierarchical model of endurance, strength, and flexibility. *J Am Geriatr Soc*. 1996;44(10):1226–1231.

237. American College of Sports Medicine. *ACSM's Resource Manual for Guidelines for Exercise Testing and Prescription*. Philadelphia, PA: Lea & Febiger; 1993.

238. Doherty TJ. Invited review: aging and sarcopenia. *J Appl Physiol (1985)*. 2003;95(4):1717–1727.

239. Young A. Exercise physiology in geriatric practice. *Acta Med Scand Suppl*. 1986;711:227–232.

240. Lach HW, Reed AT, Arfken CL, et al. Falls in the elderly: reliability of a classification system. *J Am Geriatr Soc*. 1991;39(2):197–202.

241. Robbins AS, Rubenstein LZ, Josephson KR, et al. Predictors of falls among elderly people. Results of two population-based studies. *Arch Intern Med*. 1989;149(7):1628–1633.

242. Gehlsen GM, Whaley MH. Falls in the elderly: Part I, Gait. *Arch Phys Med Rehabil*. 1990;71(10):735–738.

243. Gehlsen GM, Whaley MH. Falls in the elderly: Part II, Balance, strength, and flexibility. *Arch Phys Med Rehabil*. 1990;71(10):739–741.

244. Tinetti ME. Factors associated with serious injury during falls by ambulatory nursing home residents. *J Am Geriatr Soc*. 1987;35(7):644–648.

245. Whipple RH, Wolfson LI, Amerman PM. The relationship of knee and ankle weakness to falls in nursing home residents: an isokinetic study. *J Am Geriatr Soc*. 1987;35(1):13–20.

246. Fentem PH. Exercise in prevention of disease. *Br Med Bull*. 1992;48(3):630–650.

247. Edwards D. *Prime Moves: An Exercise Program for Mature Adults*. New York: Avery; 1990.

248. Mills KM, Stewart AL, Sepsis PG, et al. Consideration of older adults' preferences for format of physical activity. *J Aging Phys Act*. 1997;5(1):50–58.

249. Coleman EA, Berenson RA. Lost in transition: challenges and opportunities for improving the quality of transitional care. *Ann Intern Med*. 2004;141(7):533–536.

250. Farris G, Sircar M, Bortinger J, et al. Extension for community healthcare outcomes-care transitions: enhancing geriatric care transitions through a multidisciplinary videoconference. *J Am Geriatr Soc*. 2017;65(3):598–602.

251. Goncalves-Bradley DC, Lannin NA, Clemson LM, et al. Discharge planning from hospital. *Cochrane Database Syst Rev*. 2016;(1):CD000313.

252. Lawrence RH, Jette AM. Disentangling the disablement process. *J Gerontol B Psychol Sci Soc Sci*. 1996;51(4):S173–S182.

253. Guralnik JM, Ferrucci L, Simonsick EM, et al. Lower-extremity function in persons over the age of 70 years as a predictor of subsequent disability. *N Engl J Med*. 1995;332(9):556–561.

254. Fried LP, Young Y, Rubin G, et al. Self-reported preclinical disability identifies older women with early declines in performance and early disease. *J Clin Epidemiol*. 2001;54(9):889–901.

255. Tinetti ME, Inouye SK, Gill TM, et al. Shared risk factors for falls, incontinence, and functional dependence. Unifying the approach to geriatric syndromes. *JAMA*. 1995;273(17):1348–1353.

256. Evans LK, Yurkow J, Siegler EL. The CARE Program: a nurse-managed collaborative outpatient program to improve function of frail older people. Collaborative Assessment and Rehabilitation for Elders. *J Am Geriatr Soc*. 1995;43(10):1155–1160.

257. Mendes de Leon CF, Seeman TE, Baker DI, et al. Self-efficacy, physical decline, and change in functioning in community-living elders: a prospective study. *J Gerontol B Psychol Sci Soc Sci*. 1996;51(4):S183–S190.

258. Tinetti ME, Powell L. Fear of falling and low self-efficacy: a case of dependence in elderly persons. *J Gerontol*. 1993;48(Spec No):35–38.

259. Kurrle SE, Cameron ID, Geeves RB. A quick ward assessment of older patients by junior doctors. *BMJ*. 2015;350:h607.

260. Ellis G, Langhorne P. Comprehensive geriatric assessment for older hospital patients. *Br Med Bull*. 2004;71:45–59.

261. National Institutes of Health Consensus Development Conference Statement: geriatric assessment methods for clinical decision-making. *J Am Geriatr Soc*. 1988;36(4):342–347.

262. Harari D, Martin FC, Buttery A, et al. The older persons' assessment and liaison team "OPAL": evaluation of comprehensive geriatric assessment in acute medical inpatients. *Age Ageing*. 2007;36(6):670–675.

263. Boult C, Boult LB, Morishita L, et al. A randomized clinical trial of outpatient geriatric evaluation and management. *J Am Geriatr Soc*. 2001;49(4):351–359.

264. Silverman M, Musa D, Martin DC, et al. Evaluation of outpatient geriatric assessment: a randomized multi-site trial. *J Am Geriatr Soc*. 1995;43(7):733–740.

265. Toseland RW, O'Donnell JC, Engelhardt JB, et al. Outpatient geriatric evaluation and management. Results of a randomized trial. *Med Care*. 1996;34(6):624–640.

266. Olde Rikkert MG, Rigaud AS, van Hoeyweghen RJ, et al. Geriatric syndromes: medical misnomer or progress in geriatrics? *Neth J Med*. 2003;61(3):83–87.

267. Pham HH, Schrag D, O'Malley AS, et al. Care patterns in Medicare and their implications for pay for performance. *N Engl J Med*. 2007;356(11):1130–1139.

268. Black-Schaffer RM. Communication among levels of care for stroke patients. *Top Stroke Rehabil*. 2002;9(3):26–38.

269. Siebens H. Applying the domain management model in treating patients with chronic diseases. *Jt Comm J Qual Improv*. 2001;27(6):302–314.

270. Aronow H, Siebens H. Community assessment. In: Capezuti SE, Siegler EL, Mezey MD, eds. *The Encyclopedia of Elder Care—The Comprehensive Resource on Geriatric and Social Care*. 2nd ed. New York: Springer Publishing Company; 2008:153–156.

271. Steiner WA, Ryser L, Huber E, et al. Use of the ICF model as a clinical problem-solving tool in physical therapy and rehabilitation medicine. *Phys Ther*. 2002;82(11):1098–1107.

272. Bogardus ST Jr, Bradley EH, Tinetti ME. A taxonomy for goal setting in the care of persons with dementia. *J Gen Intern Med*. 1998;13(10):675–680.

273. Bradley EH, Bogardus ST Jr, van Doorn C, et al. Goals in geriatric assessment: are we measuring the right outcomes? *Gerontologist*. 2000;40(2):191–196.

274. Frost FS. Rehabilitation and fear: what happens if the house catches on fire? *Am J Phys Med Rehabil*. 2001;80(12):942–944.

275. Stineman MG, Maislin G, Nosek M, et al. Comparing consumer and clinician values for alternative functional states: application of a new feature trade-off consensus building tool. *Arch Phys Med Rehabil*. 1998;79(12):1522–1529.

276. Levack WM, Weatherall M, Hay-Smith EJ, et al. Goal setting and strategies to enhance goal pursuit for adults with acquired disability participating in rehabilitation. *Cochrane Database Syst Rev.* 2015;(7):CD009727.

277. Clark GS, Bray GP. Development of a rehabilitation plan. In: Williams TF, ed. *Rehabilitation in the Aging.* New York: Raven; 1984:125–143.

278. Hunt TE. Homeostatic malfunctions in the aged. *Br C Med J.* 1980;22:379–381.

279. Bean JF, Vora A, Frontera WR. Benefits of exercise for community-dwelling older adults. *Arch Phys Med Rehabil.* 2004;85(7 suppl 3):S31–S42; quiz S3–S4.

280. Karani R, McLaughlin MA, Cassel CK. Exercise in the healthy older adult. *Am J Geriatr Cardiol.* 2001;10(5):269–273.

281. Resnick B. Testing a model of exercise behavior in older adults. *Res Nurs Health.* 2001;24(2):83–92.

282. Bodily KC, Burgess EM. Contralateral limb and patient survival after leg amputation. *Am J Surg.* 1983;146(2):280–282.

283. Clark GS. Rehabilitation team: process and roles. In: Felsenthal G, Garrison SJ, Steinberg FU, eds. *Rehabilitation of the Aging and Elderly Patient.* Baltimore, MD: Lippincott Williams & Wilkins; 1994:439–448.

284. Strasser DC, Falconer JA. Rehabilitation team process. *Top Stroke Rehabil.* 1997;4(2):34–39.

285. OECD. *Ensuring Quality Long-term Care for Older.* Policy Brief. 2005. Available from: www.oecd.org/els/health-systems/Ensuring-quality-long-term-care-for-older-people.pdf. Accessed April 10, 2018.

286. OECD. *Income Equality Update—Youth and Poor Fall Further Behind.* 2014. Available from: https://www.oecd.org/social/OECD2014-Income-Inequality-Update.pdf. Accessed April 10, 2018.

287. Kane RL, Saliba D, Hollmann P. The evolving health policy landscape and suggested geriatric tenets to guide future responses. *J Am Geriatr Soc.* 2017;65(3):462–465.

288. Felsenthal G, Cohen BS, Hilton EB, et al. The physiatrist as primary physician for patients on an inpatient rehabilitation unit. *Arch Phys Med Rehabil.* 1984;65(7):375–378.

289. Siebens H, Weston H, Parry D, et al. The Patient Care Notebook: quality improvement on a rehabilitation unit. *Jt Comm J Qual Improv.* 2001;27(10):555–567.

290. Beers MH, Dang J, Hasegawa J, et al. Influence of hospitalization on drug therapy in the elderly. *J Am Geriatr Soc.* 1989;37(8):679–683.

291. Colt HG, Shapiro AP. Drug-induced illness as a cause for admission to a community hospital. *J Am Geriatr Soc.* 1989;37(4):323–326.

292. Sinoff GD, Kohn D. Prevalence of adverse drug reactions. *J Am Geriatr Soc.* 1990;38(6):722.

293. Willcox SM, Himmelstein DU, Woolhandler S. Inappropriate drug prescribing for the community-dwelling elderly. *JAMA.* 1994;272(4):292–296.

294. Brook RH, Kamberg CJ, Mayer-Oakes A, et al. Appropriateness of acute medical care for the elderly: an analysis of the literature. *Health Policy.* 1990;14(3):225–242.

295. Zhan C, Sangl J, Bierman AS, et al. Potentially inappropriate medication use in the community-dwelling elderly: findings from the 1996 Medical Expenditure Panel Survey. *JAMA.* 2001;286(22):2823–2829.

296. Doucet J, Jego A, Noel D, et al. Preventable and non-preventable risk factors for adverse drug events related to hospital admission in the elderly. *Clin Drug Investig.* 2002;22(6):385–392.

297. Juurlink DN, Mamdani M, Kopp A, et al. Drug-drug interactions among elderly patients hospitalized for drug toxicity. *JAMA.* 2003;289(13):1652–1658.

298. Beers MH, Munekata M, Storrie M. The accuracy of medication histories in the hospital medical records of elderly persons. *J Am Geriatr Soc.* 1990;38(11):1183–1187.

299. Spagnoli A, Ostino G, Borga AD, et al. Drug compliance and unreported drugs in the elderly. *J Am Geriatr Soc.* 1989;37(7):619–624.

300. Abrams RC, Alexopoulos GS. Substance abuse in the elderly: over-the-counter and illegal drugs. *Hosp Community Psychiatry.* 1988;39(8):822–823, 9.

301. Stoehr GP, Ganguli M, Seaberg EC, et al. Over-the-counter medication use in an older rural community: the MoVIES Project. *J Am Geriatr Soc.* 1997;45(2):158–165.

302. Goldberg PB, Roberts J. Pharmacologic basis for developing rational drug regimens for elderly patients. *Med Clin North Am.* 1983;67(2):315–331.

303. American Geriatrics Society. Updated beers criteria for potentially inappropriate medication use in older adults. *J Am Geriatr Soc.* 2015;63(11):2227–2246.

304. Beers MH, Ouslander JG. Risk factors in geriatric drug prescribing. A practical guide to avoiding problems. *Drugs.* 1989;37(1):105–112.

305. Rozzini R, Bianchetti A, Zanetti O, et al. Are too many drugs prescribed for the elderly after all? *J Am Geriatr Soc.* 1989;37(1):89–90.

306. Morrow D, Leirer V, Sheikh J. Adherence and medication instructions. Review and recommendations. *J Am Geriatr Soc.* 1988;36(12):1147–1160.

307. Cooper JK, Love DW, Raffoul PR. Intentional prescription nonadherence (noncompliance) by the elderly. *J Am Geriatr Soc.* 1982;30(5):329–333.

308. Pereles L, Romonko L, Murzyn T, et al. Evaluation of a self-medication program. *J Am Geriatr Soc.* 1996;44(2):161–165.

309. Hsia Der E, Rubenstein LZ, Choy GS. The benefits of in-home pharmacy evaluation for older persons. *J Am Geriatr Soc.* 1997;45(2):211–214.

310. McDonald HP, Garg AX, Haynes RB. Interventions to enhance patient adherence to medication prescriptions: scientific review. *JAMA.* 2002;288(22):2868–2879.

311. Larson EB, Kukull WA, Buchner D, et al. Adverse drug reactions associated with global cognitive impairment in elderly persons. *Ann Intern Med.* 1987;107(2):169–173.

312. Nolan L, O'Malley K. Prescribing for the elderly: Part II. Prescribing patterns: differences due to age. *J Am Geriatr Soc.* 1988;36(3):245–254.

313. Mangoni AA, Jackson SH. Age-related changes in pharmacokinetics and pharmacodynamics: basic principles and practical applications. *Br J Clin Pharmacol.* 2004;57(1):6–14.

314. Lipsitz LA. Orthostatic hypotension in the elderly. *N Engl J Med.* 1989;321(14):952–957.

315. Samiy AH. Clinical manifestations of disease in the elderly. *Med Clin North Am.* 1983;67(2):333–344.

316. Figueroa JJ, Basford JR, Low PA. Preventing and treating orthostatic hypotension: As easy as A, B, C. *Cleve Clin J Med.* 2010;77(5):298–306.

317. National Guideline Clearinghouse (NGC). Guideline summary: Diagnosis and treatment of depression in adults: 2012 clinical practice guideline. In: *National Guideline Clearinghouse (NGC)* [Web site]. Rockville, MD: Agency for Healthcare Research and Quality (AHRQ); 2012 Jun 01. Available from: https://www.guideline.gov. Accessed April 10, 2018.

318. Gurland BJ, Wilder DE, Berkman C. Depression and disability in the elderly: reciprocal relations and changes with age. *Int J Geriatr Psychiatry.* 1988;3(3):163–179.

319. Rapp SR, Davis KM. Geriatric depression: physicians' knowledge, perceptions, and diagnostic practices. *Gerontologist.* 1989;29(2):252–257.

320. Hirschfeld RM, Keller MB, Panico S, et al. The National Depressive and Manic-Depressive Association consensus statement on the undertreatment of depression. *JAMA.* 1997;277(4):333–340.

321. Flint AJ. Epidemiology and comorbidity of anxiety disorders in the elderly. *Am J Psychiatry.* 1994;151(5):640–649.

322. Alwahhabi F. Anxiety symptoms and generalized anxiety disorder in the elderly: a review. *Harv Rev Psychiatry.* 2003;11(4):180–193.

323. Brown CS, Rakel RE, Wells BG, et al. A practical update on anxiety disorders and their pharmacologic treatment. *Arch Intern Med.* 1991;151(5):873–884.

324. Martin LM, Fleming KC, Evans JM. Recognition and management of anxiety and depression in elderly patients. *Mayo Clin Proc.* 1995;70(10):999–1006.

325. Francis J, Martin D, Kapoor WN. A prospective study of delirium in hospitalized elderly. *JAMA.* 1990;263(8):1097–1101.

326. Schor JD, Levkoff SE, Lipsitz LA, et al. Risk factors for delirium in hospitalized elderly. *JAMA.* 1992;267(6):827–831.

327. Inouye SK, Charpentier PA. Precipitating factors for delirium in hospitalized elderly persons. Predictive model and interrelationship with baseline vulnerability. *JAMA.* 1996;275(11):852–857.

328. Marcantonio ER, Goldman L, Mangione CM, et al. A clinical prediction rule for delirium after elective noncardiac surgery. *JAMA.* 1994;271(2):134–139.

329. Kiely DK, Bergmann MA, Murphy KM, et al. Delirium among newly admitted postacute facility patients: prevalence, symptoms, and severity. *J Gerontol A Biol Sci Med Sci.* 2003;58(5):M441–M445.

330. O'Keeffe S, Lavan J. The prognostic significance of delirium in older hospital patients. *J Am Geriatr Soc.* 1997;45(2):174–178.

331. National Institute for Health and Care Excellence. *Delirium: Prevention, Diagnosis and Treatment.* Clinical Guideline 103, London. 2008. Available from: http://nice.org.uk/guidance/cg103. Accessed April 10, 2018.

332. Rowe JW. Health care of the elderly. *N Engl J Med.* 1985;312(13):827–835.

333. Wolfson LI, Katzman R. The neurologic consultation at age 80. In: Katzman R, Terry RD, eds. *The Neurology of Aging.* Philadelphia, PA: FA Davis; 1983:221–244.

334. Fleming KC, Adams AC, Petersen RC. Dementia: diagnosis and evaluation. *Mayo Clin Proc.* 1995;70(11):1093–1107.

335. Warshaw GA, Moore JT, Friedman SW, et al. Functional disability in the hospitalized elderly. *JAMA.* 1982;248(7):847–850.

336. Clarfield AM. The reversible dementias: do they reverse? *Ann Intern Med.* 1988;109(6):476–486.

337. National Institute for Health and Care Excellence. Supporting people with dementia and their carers in health and social care. Clinical Guideline 42, London 2006 revised 2016. Available from: http://nice.org.uk/guidance/cg42. Accessed April 10, 2018.

338. McKhann G, Drachman D, Folstein M, et al. Clinical diagnosis of Alzheimer's disease: report of the NINCDS-ADRDA Work Group under the auspices of Department of Health and Human Services Task Force on Alzheimer's Disease. *Neurology.* 1984;34(7):939–944.

339. Schuman JE, Beattie EJ, Steed DA, et al. Geriatric patients with and without intellectual dysfunction: effectiveness of a standard rehabilitation program. *Arch Phys Med Rehabil.* 1981;62(12):612–618.

340. Beck JC, Benson DF, Scheibel AB, et al. Dementia in the elderly: the silent epidemic. *Ann Intern Med.* 1982;97(2):231–241.

341. Jeste DV, Blazer D, Casey D, et al. ACNP White Paper: update on use of antipsychotic drugs in elderly persons with dementia. *Neuropsychopharmacology.* 2008;33(5):957–970.

342. Recupero PR, Rainey SE. Managing risk when considering the use of atypical antipsychotics for elderly patients with dementia-related psychosis. *J Psychiatry Pract.* 2007;13(3):143–152.

343. Ham RJ, Lekan-Rutledge DA. Incontinence. In: Ham RJ, Sloane PD, eds. *Primary Care Geriatrics.* St. Louis, MO: CV Mosby; 1997:321–349.

344. Resnick NM. An 89-year-old woman with urinary incontinence. *JAMA.* 1996;276(22):1832–1840.

345. Holroyd-Leduc JM, Straus SE. Management of urinary incontinence in women: scientific review. *JAMA.* 2004;291(8):986–995.

346. Tannenbaum C, Perrin L, DuBeau CE, et al. Diagnosis and management of urinary incontinence in the older patient. *Arch Phys Med Rehabil.* 2001;82(1):134–138.

347. National Institutes of Health Consensus Development Conference on Urinary Incontinence in Adults. Bethesda, Maryland, October 3–5, 1988. Proceedings. *J Am Geriatr Soc.* 1990;38(3):263–386.

348. Resnick NM, Yalla SV. Management of urinary incontinence in the elderly. *N Engl J Med.* 1985;313(13):800–805.

349. Colling J, Ouslander J, Hadley BJ, et al. The effects of patterned urge-response toileting (PURT) on urinary incontinence among nursing home residents. *J Am Geriatr Soc.* 1992;40(2):135–141.

350. Schnelle JF, MacRae PG, Ouslander JG, et al. Functional Incidental Training, mobility performance, and incontinence care with nursing home residents. *J Am Geriatr Soc.* 1995;43(12):1356–1362.

351. Germain CB, Gitterman A. The life model approach to social work practice revisited. In: Turner F, ed. *Social Work Treatment.* New York: Free Press; 1986:618–643.

352. Williams ME, Pannill FC III. Urinary incontinence in the elderly: physiology, pathophysiology, diagnosis, and treatment. *Ann Intern Med.* 1982;97(6):895–907.

353. Burgio KC, Pearce KL, Lucco AJ. *Staying Dry: A Practical Guide to Bladder Control.* Baltimore, MD: Johns Hopkins University Press; 1989.

354. Urinary Incontinence Guideline Panel. *Urinary Incontinence in Adults: Clinical Practice Guideline.* AHCPR Publication No. 92–0038. Rockville, MD: Agency for Health Care Policy and Research, Public Health Service, United States Department of Health and Human Services; 1992.

355. Ouslander JG, Schnelle JF. Incontinence in the nursing home. *Ann Intern Med.* 1995;122(6):438–449.

356. Marzuk PM. Biofeedback for gastrointestinal disorders: a review of the literature. *Ann Intern Med.* 1985;103(2):240–244.

357. Wald A. Biofeedback therapy for fecal incontinence. *Ann Intern Med.* 1981;95(2):146–149.

358. Bloom HG, Ahmed I, Alessi CA, et al. Evidence-based recommendations for the assessment and management of sleep disorders in older persons. *J Am Geriatr Soc.* 2009;57(5):761–789.

359. Gottlieb GL. Sleep disorders and their management. Special considerations in the elderly. *Am J Med.* 1990;88(3a):29S–35S.

360. King AC, Oman RF, Brassington GS, et al. Moderate-intensity exercise and self-rated quality of sleep in older adults. A randomized controlled trial. *JAMA.* 1997;277(1):32–37.

361. Ancoli-Israel S. Insomnia in the elderly: a review for the primary care practitioner. *Sleep.* 2000;23(suppl 1):S23–S30; discussion S6–S8.

362. Folks DG, Burke WJ. Psychotherapeutic agents in older adults. Sedative hypnotics and sleep. *Clin Geriatr Med.* 1998;14(1):67–86.

363. Campbell SS, Dawson D, Anderson MW. Alleviation of sleep maintenance insomnia with timed exposure to bright light. *J Am Geriatr Soc.* 1993;41(8):829–836.

364. Morin CM, Azrin NH. Behavioral and cognitive treatments of geriatric insomnia. *J Consult Clin Psychol.* 1988;56(5):748–753.

365. Garfinkel D, Laudon M, Nof D, et al. Improvement of sleep quality in elderly people by controlled-release melatonin. *Lancet.* 1995;346(8974):541–544.

366. Olde Rikkert MG, Rigaud AS. Melatonin in elderly patients with insomnia. A systematic review. *Z Gerontol Geriatr.* 2001;34(6):491–497.

367. AGS Panel on Chronic Pain in Older Persons, American Geriatrics Society. The management of chronic pain in older persons. *J Am Geriatr Soc.* 1998;46(5):635–651.

368. Ferrell BA. Pain management in elderly people. *J Am Geriatr Soc.* 1991;39(1):64–73.

369. Ferrell BR, Ferrell BA. *Pain in the Elderly. A Report of the Task Force on Pain in the Elderly of the International Association for the Study of Pain.* Seattle, WA: IASP Press; 1996.

370. Ferrell BA, Ferrell BR, Osterweil D. Pain in the nursing home. *J Am Geriatr Soc.* 1990;38(4):409–414.

371. Nishikawa ST, Ferrell BA. Pain assessment in the elderly. *Clin Geriatr Long Term Care.* 1993;1:15–28.

372. Parmelee PA, Smith B, Katz IR. Pain complaints and cognitive status among elderly institution residents. *J Am Geriatr Soc.* 1993;41(5):517–522.

373. Ferrell BA, Ferrell BR, Rivera L. Pain in cognitively impaired nursing home patients. *J Pain Symptom Manage.* 1995;10(8):591–598.

374. Rothschild AJ. The diagnosis and treatment of late-life depression. *J Clin Psychiatry.* 1996;57(suppl 5):5–11.

375. Michet CJ Jr, Evans JM, Fleming KC, et al. Common rheumatologic diseases in elderly patients. *Mayo Clin Proc.* 1995;70(12):1205–1214.

376. Recommendations for the medical management of osteoarthritis of the hip and knee: 2000 update. American College of Rheumatology Subcommittee on Osteoarthritis Guidelines. *Arthritis Rheum.* 2000;43(9):1905–1915.

377. Rochon PA, Fortin PR, Dear KB, et al. Reporting of age data in clinical trials of arthritis. Deficiencies and solutions. *Arch Intern Med.* 1993;153(2):243–248.

378. Griffin MR, Piper JM, Daugherty JR, et al. Nonsteroidal anti-inflammatory drug use and increased risk for peptic ulcer disease in elderly persons. *Ann Intern Med.* 1991;114(4):257–263.

379. AGS Panel on Persistent Pain in Older Persons. The management of persistent pain in older persons. *J Am Geriatr Soc.* 2002;50(6 suppl):S205–S224.

380. Nicholas MK, Asghari A, Blyth FM, et al. Long-term outcomes from training in self-management of chronic pain in an elderly population: a randomized controlled trial. *Pain.* 2017;158(1):86–95.

381. Evans RL, Matlock AL, Bishop DS, et al. Family intervention after stroke: does counseling or education help? *Stroke.* 1988;19(10):1243–1249.

382. Ferrell B, Rivera L. Cancer pain: impact on elderly patients and their family caregivers. In: Roy R, ed. *Chronic Pain in Old Age: An Integrated Biopsychosocial Perspective.* Toronto, ON: University of Toronto Press; 1995.

383. Billings AG, Moos RH. The role of coping responses and social resources in attenuating the stress of life events. *J Behav Med.* 1981;4(2):139–157.

384. Thurman DJ, Stevens JA, Rao JK. Practice parameter: assessing patients in a neurology practice for risk of falls (an evidence-based review): report of the Quality Standards Subcommittee of the American Academy of Neurology. *Neurology.* 2008;70(6):473–479.

385. King MB, Tinetti ME. Falls in community-dwelling older persons. *J Am Geriatr Soc.* 1995;43(10):1146–1154.

386. Lipsitz LA. An 85-year-old woman with a history of falls. *JAMA.* 1996;276(1):59–66.

387. Tinetti ME. Performance-oriented assessment of mobility problems in elderly patients. *J Am Geriatr Soc.* 1986;34(2):119–126.

388. Studenski S, Duncan PW, Chandler J, et al. Predicting falls: the role of mobility and nonphysical factors. *J Am Geriatr Soc.* 1994;42(3):297–302.

389. Cummings SR, Nevitt MC, Browner WS, et al. Risk factors for hip fracture in white women. Study of Osteoporotic Fractures Research Group. *N Engl J Med.* 1995;332(12):767–773.

390. Wolf SL, Barnhart HX, Kutner NG, et al. Reducing frailty and falls in older persons: an investigation of Tai Chi and computerized balance training. Atlanta FICSIT Group. Frailty and Injuries: Cooperative Studies of Intervention Techniques. *J Am Geriatr Soc.* 1996;44(5):489–497.

391. Tinetti ME, Baker DI, McAvay G, et al. A multifactorial intervention to reduce the risk of falling among elderly people living in the community. *N Engl J Med.* 1994;331(13):821–827.

392. Panel on Prevention of Falls in Older Persons, American Geriatrics Society and British Geriatrics Society. Summary of the Updated American Geriatrics Society/British Geriatrics Society clinical practice guideline for prevention of falls in older persons. *J Am Geriatr Soc.* 2011;59(1):148–157.

393. Oakley A, Dawson MF, Holland J, et al. Preventing falls and subsequent injury in older people. *Qual Health Care.* 1996;5(4):243–249.

394. Lawrence RH, Tennstedt SL, Kasten LE, et al. Intensity and correlates of fear of falling and hurting oneself in the next year: baseline findings from a Roybal Center fear of falling intervention. *J Aging Health.* 1998;10(3):267–286.

395. Tinetti ME, Richman D, Powell L. Falls efficacy as a measure of fear of falling. *J Gerontol.* 1990;45(6):P239–P243.

396. Zijlstra GA, van Haastregt JC, van Rossum E, et al. Interventions to reduce fear of falling in community-living older people: a systematic review. *J Am Geriatr Soc.* 2007;55(4):603–615.

397. Bezon J, Echevarria KH, Smith GB. Nursing outcome indicator: preventing falls for elderly people. *Outcomes Manag Nurs Pract.* 1999;3(3):112–116; quiz 6–7.

398. Gardner MM, Robertson MC, Campbell AJ. Exercise in preventing falls and fall related injuries in older people: a review of randomised controlled trials. *Br J Sports Med.* 2000;34(1):7–17.

399. Jarvinen TL, Sievanen H, Khan KM, et al. Shifting the focus in fracture prevention from osteoporosis to falls. *BMJ.* 2008;336(7636):124–126.

400. Bernardini B, Meinecke C, Pagani M, et al. Comorbidity and adverse clinical events in the rehabilitation of older adults after hip fracture. *J Am Geriatr Soc.* 1995;43(8):894–898.

401. Cameron ID, Lyle DM, Quine S. Cost effectiveness of accelerated rehabilitation after proximal femoral fracture. *J Clin Epidemiol.* 1994;47(11):1307–1313.

402. Guccione AA, Fagerson TL, Anderson JJ. Regaining functional independence in the acute care setting following hip fracture. *Phys Ther.* 1996;76(8):818–826.

403. Kiel DP, Eichorn A, Intrator O, et al. The outcomes of patients newly admitted to nursing homes after hip fracture. *Am J Public Health.* 1994;84(8):1281–1286.

404. Koval KJ, Zuckerman JD. Functional recovery after fracture of the hip. *J Bone Joint Surg Am.* 1994;76(5):751–758.

405. Zuckerman JD, Skovron ML, Koval KJ, et al. Postoperative complications and mortality associated with operative delay in older patients who have a fracture of the hip. *J Bone Joint Surg Am.* 1995;77(10):1551–1556.

406. Moran CG, Wenn RT, Sikand M, et al. Early mortality after hip fracture: is delay before surgery important? *J Bone Joint Surg Am.* 2005;87(3):483–489.

407. Hochberg MC, Altman RD, Brandt KD, et al. Guidelines for the medical management of osteoarthritis. Part I. Osteoarthritis of the hip. American College of Rheumatology. *Arthritis Rheum.* 1995;38(11):1535–1540.

408. National Institute for Health and Care Excellence. Hip fracture: management. Clinical Guideline 124, London 2011 revised 2014. Available from: http://nice.org.uk/guidance/cg124. Accessed April 10, 2018.

409. Penrod JD, Boockvar KS, Litke A, et al. Physical therapy and mobility 2 and 6 months after hip fracture. *J Am Geriatr Soc.* 2004;52(7):1114–1120.

410. Munin MC, Seligman K, Dew MA, et al. Effect of rehabilitation site on functional recovery after hip fracture. *Arch Phys Med Rehabil.* 2005;86(3):367–372.

411. Hochberg MC, Altman RD, Brandt KD, et al. Guidelines for the medical management of osteoarthritis. Part II. Osteoarthritis of the knee. American College of Rheumatology. *Arthritis Rheum.* 1995;38(11):1541–1546.

412. Nesher G, Moore TL, Zuckner J. Rheumatoid arthritis in the elderly. *J Am Geriatr Soc.* 1991;39(3):284–294.

413. van Baar ME, Assendelft WJ, Dekker J, et al. Effectiveness of exercise therapy in patients with osteoarthritis of the hip or knee: a systematic review of randomized clinical trials. *Arthritis Rheum.* 1999;42(7):1361–1369.

414. Lorig KR, Mazonson PD, Holman HR. Evidence suggesting that health education for self-management in patients with chronic arthritis has sustained health benefits while reducing health care costs. *Arthritis Rheum.* 1993;36(4):439–446.

415. Ettinger WH Jr, Burns R, Messier SP, et al. A randomized trial comparing aerobic exercise and resistance exercise with a health education program in older adults with knee osteoarthritis. The Fitness Arthritis and Seniors Trial (FAST). *JAMA.* 1997;277(1):25–31.

416. Minor MA. Exercise in the management of osteoarthritis of the knee and hip. *Arthritis Care Res*. 1994;7(4):198–204.

417. Puett DW, Griffin MR. Published trials of nonmedicinal and noninvasive therapies for hip and knee osteoarthritis. *Ann Intern Med*. 1994;121(2):133–140.

418. Silverstein FE, Faich G, Goldstein JL, et al. Gastrointestinal toxicity with celecoxib vs nonsteroidal anti-inflammatory drugs for osteoarthritis and rheumatoid arthritis: the CLASS study: a randomized controlled trial Celecoxib Long-term Arthritis Safety Study. *JAMA*. 2000;284(10):1247–1255.

419. Hochberg MC, Altman RD, April KT, et al. American College of Rheumatology 2012 recommendations for the use of nonpharmacologic and pharmacologic therapies in osteoarthritis of the hand, hip, and knee. *Arthritis Care Res*. 2012;64(4):465–474.

420. Felson DT, Lawrence RC, Hochberg MC, et al. Osteoarthritis: new insights. Part 2: treatment approaches. *Ann Intern Med*. 2000;133(9):726–737.

421. Cruise CM, Sasson N, Lee MH. Rehabilitation outcomes in the older adult. *Clin Geriatr Med*. 2006;22(2):257–267; viii.

422. Granger CV, Clark GS. Functional status and outcomes of stroke rehabilitation. *Top Geriatr Rehabil*. 1994;9(3):72–84.

423. Granger CV, Hamilton BB, Gresham GE. The stroke rehabilitation outcome study—Part I: general description. *Arch Phys Med Rehabil*. 1988;69(7):506–509.

424. Granger CV, Hamilton BB, Gresham GE, et al. The stroke rehabilitation outcome study: Part II. Relative merits of the total Barthel index score and a four-item subscore in predicting patient outcomes. *Arch Phys Med Rehabil*. 1989;70(2):100–103.

425. Keith RA, Wilson DB, Gutierrez P. Acute and subacute rehabilitation for stroke: a comparison. *Arch Phys Med Rehabil*. 1995;76(6):495–500.

426. Kramer AM, Steiner JF, Schlenker RE, et al. Outcomes and costs after hip fracture and stroke. A comparison of rehabilitation settings. *JAMA*. 1997;277(5):396–404.

427. Lindmark B. Evaluation of functional capacity after stroke with special emphasis on motor function and activities of daily living. *Scand J Rehabil Med Suppl*. 1988;21:1–40.

428. Osberg JS, DeJong G, Haley SM, et al. Predicting long-term outcome among post-rehabilitation stroke patients. *Am J Phys Med Rehabil*. 1988;67(3):94–103.

429. Scmidt EV, Smirnov VE, Ryabova VS. Results of the seven-year prospective study of stroke patients. *Stroke*. 1988;19(8):942–949.

430. Shah S, Vanclay F, Cooper B. Efficiency, effectiveness, and duration of stroke rehabilitation. *Stroke*. 1990;21(2):241–246.

431. Wade DT, Langton-Hewer R, Wood VA. Stroke: the influence of age upon outcome. *Age Ageing*. 1984;13(6):357–362.

432. Duncan PW, Zorowitz R, Bates B, et al. Management of adult stroke rehabilitation care: a clinical practice guideline. *Stroke*. 2005;36(9):e100–e143.

433. Kimura M, Robinson RG, Kosier JT. Treatment of cognitive impairment after post-stroke depression: a double-blind treatment trial. *Stroke*. 2000;31(7):1482–1486.

434. Liepert J, Bauder H, Wolfgang HR, et al. Treatment-induced cortical reorganization after stroke in humans. *Stroke*. 2000;31(6):1210–1216.

435. Cifu DX, Stewart DG. Factors affecting functional outcome after stroke: a critical review of rehabilitation interventions. *Arch Phys Med Rehabil*. 1999;80(5 suppl 1):S35–S39.

436. Clark GS, Blue B, Bearer JB. Rehabilitation of the elderly amputee. *J Am Geriatr Soc*. 1983;31(7):439–448.

437. Cutson TM, Bongiorni DR. Rehabilitation of the older lower limb amputee: a brief review. *J Am Geriatr Soc*. 1996;44(11):1388–1393.

438. DuBow LL, Witt PL, Kadaba MP, et al. Oxygen consumption of elderly persons with bilateral below knee amputations: ambulation vs wheelchair propulsion. *Arch Phys Med Rehabil*. 1983;64(6):255–259.

439. Frieden RA. The geriatric amputee. *Phys Med Rehabil Clin N Am*. 2005;16(1):179–195.

440. O'Connell PG, Gnatz S. Hemiplegia and amputation: rehabilitation in the dual disability. *Arch Phys Med Rehabil*. 1989;70(6):451–454.

441. Wolf E, Lilling M, Ferber I, et al. Prosthetic rehabilitation of elderly bilateral amputees. *Int J Rehabil Res*. 1989;12(3):271–278.

442. National Spinal Cord Injury Statistical Centre. *Spinal Cord Injury Facts and Figures at a Glance: 2016 Datasheet*. Birmingham, AL: National Spinal Cord Injury Statistical Centre; 2016. Available from: www.nscisc.uab.edu/Public/Facts%202016.pdf. Accessed April 10, 2018.

443. McGlinchey-Berroth R, Morrow L, Ahlquist M, et al. Late-life spinal cord injury and aging with a long term injury: characteristics of two emerging populations. *J Spinal Cord Med*. 1995;18(3):183–193.

444. Roth EJ, Lovell L, Heinemann AW, et al. The older adult with a spinal cord injury. *Paraplegia*. 1992;30(7):520–526.

445. Stover SL, Fine PR. *Spinal Cord Injury: The Facts and Figures*. Birmingham, AL: University of Alabama; 1986.

446. DeVivo MJ, Fine PR, Maetz HM, et al. Prevalence of spinal cord injury: a reestimation employing life table techniques. *Arch Neurol*. 1980;37(11):707–708.

447. DeVivo MJ, Stover SL, Black KJ. Prognostic factors for 12-year survival after spinal cord injury. *Arch Phys Med Rehabil*. 1992;73(2):156–162.

448. Capoor J, Stein AB. Aging with spinal cord injury. *Phys Med Rehabil Clin N Am*. 2005;16(1):129–161.

449. DeVivo MJ, Kartus PL, Rutt RD, et al. The influence of age at time of spinal cord injury on rehabilitation outcome. *Arch Neurol*. 1990;47(6):687–691.

450. Adkins RH. Research and interpretation perspectives on aging related physical morbidity with spinal cord injury and brief review of systems. *NeuroRehabilitation*. 2004;19(1):3–13.

451. Yarkony GM, Roth EJ, Heinemann AW, et al. Spinal cord injury rehabilitation outcome: the impact of age. *J Clin Epidemiol*. 1988;41(2):173–177.

452. Cifu DX, Kreutzer JS, Marwitz JH, et al. Functional outcomes of older adults with traumatic brain injury: a prospective, multicenter analysis. *Arch Phys Med Rehabil*. 1996;77(9):883–888.

453. Testa JA, Malec JF, Moessner AM, et al. Outcome after traumatic brain injury: effects of aging on recovery. *Arch Phys Med Rehabil*. 2005;86(9):1815–1823.

454. Steyerberg EW, Mushkudiani N, Perel P, et al. Predicting outcome after traumatic brain injury: development and international validation of prognostic scores based on admission characteristics. *PLoS Med*. 2008;5(8):e165; discussion e165.

455. Good DC. Overview of stroke rehabilitation. In: *Timing, Intensity, and Duration of Rehabilitation for Hip Fracture and Stroke: Report of a Workshop*. National Center for Medical Rehabilitation Research (NCMRR); 2001:3–9. Available from: http://www.nichd.nih.gov/ncmrr/StrokeWorkshopReport.pdf. Accessed April 20, 2018.

456. Worsowicz GM, Stewart DG, Phillips EM, et al. Geriatric rehabilitation. 1. Social and economic implications of aging. *Arch Phys Med Rehabil*. 2004;85(7 suppl 3):S3–S6; quiz S27–S30.

457. Cummings V, Kerner JF, Arones S, et al. Day hospital service in rehabilitation medicine: an evaluation. *Arch Phys Med Rehabil*. 1985;66(2):86–91.

458. Fisk AA. Comprehensive health care for the elderly. *JAMA*. 1983;249(2):230–236.

459. Council on Scientific Affairs. Home care in the 1990s. *JAMA*. 1990;263(9):1241–1244.

460. Grieco AJ. Physician's guide to managing home care of older patients. *Geriatrics*. 1991;46(5):49–55, 9–60.

461. Frank JC, Miller LS. Community-based rehabilitation for the elderly. In: Felsenthal G, Garrison SJ, Steinberg FU, eds. *Rehabilitation of the Aging and Elderly Patient*. Baltimore, MD: Lippincott Williams & Wilkins; 1994:477–485.

462. Clark F, Azen SP, Zemke R, et al. Occupational therapy for independent-living older adults. A randomized controlled trial. *JAMA*. 1997;278(16):1321–1326.

463. Legg LA, Drummond AE, Langhorne P. Occupational therapy for patients with problems in activities of daily living after stroke. *Cochrane Database Syst Rev*. 2006;(4):CD003585.

464. Cameron ID, Kurrle SE. 1: Rehabilitation and older people. *Med J Aust*. 2002;177(7):387–391.

465. Marcus C. Strategies for improving the quality of verbal patient and family education: a review of the literature and creation of the EDUCATE model. *Health Psychol Behav Med*. 2014;2(1):482–495.

466. Hoenig HM. Rehabilitation. In: Duthie EH, Katz PR, eds. *Practice of Geriatrics*. 3rd ed. Philadelphia, PA: WB Saunders Company; 1998:146–172.

467. American Geriatrics Society; John A. Hartford Foundation. A statement of principles: toward improved care of older patients in surgical and medical specialties. *Arch Phys Med Rehabil*. 2002;83(9):1317–1319.

The Role of PM&R in Disaster Relief

You could hear the shrieks of women, the wailing of infants, and the shouting of men; some were calling their parents, others their children or their wives, trying to recognize them by their voices. People bewailed their own fate or that of their relatives, and there were some who prayed for death in their terror of dying.

Pliny the Younger, survivor of the Mount Vesuvius
eruption in 79 A.D. (1)

There has been no more constant a source of disability, whether due to injury or to chronic illness, than war, one of the oldest of human practices… In contrast to disabled veterans, the bystander is not easily assimilated into the romanticized and heroic depictions of warriors.

Encyclopedia of Disability (2)

A disaster is defined as an event that overwhelms the ability of local resources to respond. War, terrorism, building collapse, nuclear or chemical leak can overwhelm local resources. So can earthquake, tsunami, mudslide, flooding and other natural events. Experts often separate disasters into natural and man-made disasters. Yet, from a rehabilitation standpoint, it is fair to say that almost all of the overwhelming is the consequence of human factors. This is an optimistic statement—it implies that we have an opportunity to profoundly affect the consequences of disaster. This chapter reviews the issue of disaster as it relates to disability, outlines the rehabilitation responses, and provides concrete direction for those who hope to help in the face of a human tragedy.

DISASTERS ARE NO SURPRISE

The reality of disasters is that they are predictable—mostly. We know with 100% certainty that there will be another earthquake, tsunami, flood, hurricane, tornado, and volcano eruption. We just do not know exactly when and where. As this chapter is being written someone is being tortured, another has just been blown up by a bomb, and still others are lying wounded by shrapnel, poison gas, or landmines. There is only a little less certainty about nuclear leaks, the form and timing of bioterrorism and epidemics, and the nature of industrial errors.

Each of these overwhelming incidents is measured by the World Health Organization (WHO) as a Major Emergency. The WHO report on Major Emergencies for January to October 2016 is daunting (3). It lists response to Major Emergencies in 47 countries, including 31 acute and 19 protracted emergencies. The scope of emergencies ranges from war and civil strife to earthquakes and floods, to Ebola, Zika, and other infectious disease crises. The cost in resources and lives is

gigantic. The size, incidence, and cost of disasters are increasing, too (4). The Centre for Research on the Epidemiology of Disasters relates this to increasing populations, increasing concentration of populations in urban centers, and global warming's effect on weather patterns.

When a colleague with experience in Haiti heard of the massive earthquake in 2010, she commented, "What disaster? Haiti's already a disaster." The scope of this particular disaster was epic, and far beyond her initial understanding. Still, the earthquake disaster in this poorest country in the Western hemisphere had as much to do with lack of food, water, sanitation, and government competency as with the collapse of cheaply built buildings.

For rehabilitation experts, the daunting part of the WHO's 17-page Major Emergency summary is the absence of the word "disability." "Rehabilitation" is only mentioned once and only in the context of the Syrian civil war: "The long-term rehabilitation of severely wounded patients remains a challenge." Even in Syria the document neglects any analysis of the "challenge," with no discussion of needs or plans, successes or failures. It is as if the only meaningful intervention was heroic rescue and the only outcomes from disaster were death or cure.

Indeed, until recently the WHO and most governments did only measure death and cure as metrics for health care system adequacy. In the last decades a concept called "Disability-Adjusted Life Years" or DALY evolved, portending to represent the cost of disability (5). In fact, DALY is not useful for rehabilitation purposes. With DALY, once a person crosses the threshold from "ability" to "disability," there is no change in value of a human life. An amputation is an amputation, whether a prosthetic leg is provided or not. Employment, schooling, child rearing, and participation in society and government—all of the functions that add value to a community are not valued. So the value of rehabilitation towards these goals is counted as zero in the DALY model. WHO and most national policymakers have no way of understanding the missed opportunity to rehabilitate. Yet the crisis and opportunity is clear.

Even when there is a company or person at fault for the disaster, they often do not contribute to recovery. The Bhopal chemical spill in India killed thousands and disabled many more. The companies involved successfully spent enormous money and political energy to avoid liability (6).

War is the more common example. In many countries, the largest medical rehabilitation resources are provided for soldiers and veterans. The moral imperative to care for those who serve the country is unquestioned, and the political strength of the military and veterans is huge. On the absolute opposite end of the spectrum of resources are the innocent victims of war. Foreign forces go home, local governments are strapped for resources, and few have the insight or political will to invest in long-term individual independence, even where dependent people cost the economy so much. In cases of civil war, political retribution often takes the form of withholding of resources. Especially when it comes to refugee camps, international aid organizations may be paralyzed by perceptions that their response favors one side or the other. The civilian victims live in a war zone, and wars often do not stop completely after a disabling incident. There is real danger to foreign aid workers, and the ability to build the kind of sustained programs needed for successful rehabilitation is heavily compromised.

Terrorism is defined as acts of violence targeting civilian or innocent persons for political purpose. The rehabilitation response to terrorism always comes from whatever local infrastructure already exists. So, victims of terrorism in industrialized countries do receive rehabilitation, and many, such as the Boston bombing victims, are lauded as heroes. However, the vast majority of terrorism occurs in low-resource or conflict areas where the rehabilitation infrastructure is poor. Aid organizations often do not respond to terror acts because the number of injured victims is relatively small and the acute event is over before they can meaningfully mobilize. So, the opportunity to build rehabilitation in response to a terror disaster is minimal, even where the need is substantial.

Nuclear disaster has been a reality since the atomic bombs hit Hiroshima and Nagasaki in Japan in World War II. It has continued with contamination events such as the Chernobyl and Fukushima power plant leaks. Terrorist threats of "dirty bombs" mean that nuclear disaster can occur almost anywhere.

The spectrum of human-made disasters is large. Chemical leaks, radiation leaks, building collapses, dam breaks, release of infectious agents, and other calamities result in highly varied medical problems and require different rehabilitation responses. **Table 48-1** provides a framework for the nature of rehabilitation response one might anticipate after a man-made disaster.

Despite the apparent increased risk of man-made disasters in the future, a Medline review finds very little specific about the science of rehabilitation response to such events. There certainly are experts who have lived through these disasters; however, their expertise needs to be more public. Even more important, national and international organizations must be convinced by this information that a special rehabilitation response is appropriate after humans cause disability in other humans.

HUMANITARIAN RESPONSE TO DISASTER

Rehabilitation providers who have not been personally involved in disaster response often see one end of the humanitarian response when a disaster hits. Their colleagues, hospital, or local service organizations raise funds and send workers into the crisis. This valuable effort is not the core of disaster response. Local professional and well-prepared volunteer teams coordinated by local or international government are almost always the core of humanitarian response.

Numerous organizations with substantial experience and resources have created policies and procedures, have evolved resources, and are on the ground within hours of any major disaster. Most countries (85% according to a World Health Organization survey [7]) (and in the United States, each state and city) have an extensive disaster response plan. The World Health Organization and numerous nongovernmental organizations such as the Red Cross/Red Crescent, Doctors Without Borders, Handicap International, and others have professionals whose careers revolve around preparing for the inevitable next disaster.

The volume and predictability of disasters mean that international emergency medical teams are increasingly composed of, or led by, professionals trained specifically in this area (8), and core competencies have been spelled out (9,10). These include integration of rehabilitation efforts into the response (11–13). Rehabilitation professionals or teams that hope to respond to an international disaster must follow the plans of the government and nongovernment organizations that are leading the response to any particular incident.

Politics between aid organizations should be recognized but should not dissuade responders from joining in. Responders on the ground are almost uniformly heroic and collaborative, dedicated to saving lives while respecting the people and improving the community they are responding to. However some of the best aid organizations are also competitive multimillion dollar businesses run by salaried administrators who are rewarded for raising funds and visibility and who are climbing their professional career ladder (14). As in all areas of medicine, some of the clinical leaders have conflicting professional views on how things should be done on the ground. Some of the worst organizations show up for a photo shoot to raise funds and feed egos. They create chaos and confusion, and then get back on the plane home leaving only a small percentage of their money with the victims. These unsavory aspects of

TABLE 48-1	Rehabilitation Issues of Survivors of Man-Made Disasters[a]				
	War	**Explosion**	**Radiation Exposure**	**Chemical Event**	**Biologic Event**
Spinal cord injury	Frequent	Occasional	Uncommon	Uncommon	Uncommon
Brain injury	Frequent	Frequent	Uncommon	Uncommon	Uncommon
Amputation	Frequent	Frequent	Uncommon	Uncommon	Uncommon
Burns	Frequent	Frequent	Occasional	Occasional	Occasional
Multiple fractures	Frequent	Frequent	Uncommon	Uncommon	Uncommon
Nerve disease	Occasional	Uncommon	Frequent	Frequent	Frequent
Cardiopulmonary	Uncommon	Occasional	Occasional	Occasional	Occasional

[a]Theoretical distribution of rehabilitation issues among persons cared for after various man-made disasters. Brain injury includes hypoxic toxic infectious or metabolic brain injury. Burns include exfoliative skin disorders.

disaster response need to be seen for what they are, but do not diminish the good done by volunteer teams who join up with major aid organizations.

The precise plans for acute medical and surgical response are varied based on location, disaster, and organization in charge. So they are beyond the scope of this chapter. What is important is that rehabilitation responders seek out the leaders and follow their acute plans, adding rehabilitation expertise ahead of time if possible, or tactfully in the moment when they see gaps related to people with disability (PWD).

EVOLUTION OF THE FIELD OF DISASTER REHABILITATION

No doubt there have been rehabilitation efforts after disasters going back for millennia. However, professional and scientific efforts by rehabilitation medicine specialist physicians to understand and respond have been surprisingly recent.

Perhaps the first scientific description of rehabilitation medicine in disaster relief came from American physiatrist George Kevorkian, M.D., and colleagues who responded to the earthquake in Kevorkian's ancestral home of Armenia (15). Burke described the development of a spinal cord injury unit after this disaster (16). Many decades later, the prosthetic center Kevorkian established remains a national resource.

Occasional papers have described the disabling results of disaster since. The first scientific meeting on the subject of PM&R intervention was decades later at the 2009 meeting of a grassroots group called International Rehabilitation Forum in Kayseri, Turkey. At that meeting colleagues who had responded to earthquakes in Pakistan and China and to the New Orleans flood presented their experience. Presciently, the future leaders of responses to the 2010 Haiti earthquake and the 2015 Nepal disaster were also involved in the small group. Almost a decade later, this group has published dozens of studies and position papers (including those by Rathore, Gosney, Li, Haig, and others within this chapter) responded to a number of global disasters, and remains the core leadership of the International Society for Physical and Rehabilitation Medicine (ISPRM) Disaster Rehabilitation Committee.

A vast country under central control, China has provided us with one of the best laboratories for rehabilitation response to disaster. It was some time after a first earthquake in the Sichuan province before Jianan Li was allowed to bring his well-organized rehabilitation teams to the region. Their work was seen as so impressive and necessary that when another earthquake hit a few years later, rehabilitation was called in among the very first responding teams. The difficulty in serving a large disaster region also resulted in a natural experiment where some areas got rehabilitation services early and others did not. The Chinese team has now established a scientific research team that studies disaster rehabilitation, and in his tenure as ISPRM president Dr. Li has led the organization towards taking more responsibility for disaster response.

A number of important policy papers and reviews evolved (17,18). Rathore described the need for a response (19). Gosney reviewed the role of these important organizations in creating adequate response (20,21). Perhaps Reinhardt's detailed review provides the best sense of the need for rehabilitation and the trends (22). He found that the survival rate ("injury:death ratio") from earthquakes has increased since 1970, implying that disability is a more frequent consequence, and that various rehabilitation interventions seemed to show positive outcomes.

THE ROLE OF MEDICAL REHABILITATION

The Nature of Disability after Disaster

The types and number of disabling injuries and complications after a disaster are the result of many complex factors, including the type of disaster, the time of day, the physical infrastructure, cultural factors, and the nature of the response. Table 48-2 presents the spectrum of disabling conditions that occur after various natural disasters.

While an earthquake results in spinal cord injuries, amputations, and crush injuries, we know that a daytime earthquake in a farming community may spare men working in the fields and disproportionately affect women and children who may be at home or at school in poorly built facilities. The opposite proportion might happen in an urban setting where men typically would be working in construction and other higher risk occupations (23). If spinal cord injuries are evacuated by helicopter or other stable transportation, there may be some patients with tetraplegia; otherwise, they mostly die in the field (24,25).

Tsunamis are waves of physical energy that travel through oceans after an earthquake. Close to shore, they turn into physical waves that can grow rapidly and travel at very high speed, ruining everything in front of them and leaving injured victims drowning in the floodwaters.

TABLE 48-2	Rehabilitation Issues of Survivors of Natural Disasters[a]					
	Earthquake	**Wind Storms**	**Floods**	**Volcano**	**Tsunami**	**Fire**
Spinal cord injury	Frequent	Frequent	Occasional	Moderate	Frequent	Moderate
Brain injury	Frequent	Frequent	Moderate	Moderate	Frequent	Moderate
Amputation	Frequent	Frequent	Moderate	Frequent	Moderate	Moderate
Burns	Moderate	Moderate	Moderate	Frequent	Uncommon	Frequent
Multiple fractures	Frequent	Frequent	Occasional	Moderate	Moderate	Moderate
Nerve disease	Uncommon	Uncommon	Uncommon	Uncommon	Uncommon	Moderate
Cardiopulmonary	Uncommon	Uncommon	Uncommon	Moderate	Uncommon	Frequent

[a]Theoretical distribution of rehabilitation issues among persons cared for after various natural disasters. Brain injury includes hypoxic toxic infectious or metabolic brain injury.

Floods cause varying injuries and illnesses related to the cause of flooding (river overflow, hurricane tide surges, dam bursting) and the location (cold, tropical, widespread regional vs. local). Unique concerns are wound infections and animal bites (26). Hurricanes result in wind damage, wave damage, and flooding. Evacuation of PWD and large and small new injuries of varying sorts can result (27–29).

Much has been written about the steps that must be taken in order to be ready for rehabilitation after disaster (30,31). Rehabilitation nurses play critical roles in planning, especially where the facilities they work may be involved (32,33). Media planning is an important early step. As noted below, a very first step involves educating first responders including the lay public about management. Pamphlets and other communications can be designed and translated into appropriate language and media long before a disaster occurs (34–36).

An earthquake caused tsunami and radiation leak from the Fukushima power plant in Japan. E-mails and calls of assistance flooded the Japanese Association of Rehabilitation Medicine. Their responses were gracious. However, it was clear that Japan had the expertise, resources, and organization to respond to the rehabilitation part of the disaster. The last thing they needed was to host foreigners. In this case a humanitarian disaster was not technically a rehabilitation disaster because it did not overwhelm the local country's outstanding ability to respond.

People with Preexisting Disability

The failure of disaster planners to take into account the fact that 15% or more of the population already has a significant physical disability has been tragic. Lives were lost and ethics were severely compromised in the poorly designed evacuation of PWD from the New Orleans hurricane and flood (27,28,37,38).

Researchers have described problems and solutions relating to people with previous disabilities in general (39–42).

Some have commented on the needs of specific populations. Evacuation of people with previous spinal cord injuries presents a special challenge due to risk of pressure sores, interrupted bladder and bowel programs, spasticity drug management, and separation from assistive devices and caregivers (43). People with rheumatoid arthritis may have difficulty with fine motor activities as well as mobility, and pain control may be a challenge (44). Because hearing and vision are not classically part of PM&R training curricula, people with these impairments may be overlooked in planning. Yet evacuation and care should take into account the needs of these people (45,46). People with seizure disorders are often left without medication (47), and pain patients on narcotics can go into serious withdrawal (48).

The frailty associated with aging results in special requirements related to care of premorbid illnesses, cognitive impairment, emotional inflexibility and disorientation, and physical limitations related to age, sedentary lifestyle, and specific disabling conditions. Evacuation considerations (43,49) must be followed by accommodations in acute care, rehabilitation, and discharge planning (50,51,52).

Box 48-1 shows Handicap International's schema for educating acute responders on the needs of PWD. These steps largely focus on trusting that the person with disability and his or her family usually know what is needed.

BOX 48-1

Handicap International Instructions for Rescue Workers' Response to People with Disability (PWD)

- **Respect the dignity and wishes of PWDs.**
- **Be patient with psychosocially and intellectually impaired persons.**
- **Ask the person with disability for advice.**
- **Find the regular caregiver or family members.**
- **Do not separate a person with disability from his or her assistive aids/devices.**
- **Follow up on other specific needs of a PWD.**

(Derived from LeBourgeois B, Sherrer V, eds. *How to Include Disability Issues in Disaster Management Following Floods 2004 in Bangladesh.* Dhaka, Bangladesh: Handicap International Bangladesh; 2005.)

The Rehabilitation Team

The first author teaches, "Surgeons use knives, internists use pills, and physiatrists use teams." It is obvious, yet still needs to be emphasized, that the response to a disaster must include the team of experts that PM&R physicians typically work with. Back in 1956, Lee pointed out the need for physical and occupational therapists as well as dieticians (53). Over the years, each of the rehabilitation specialty areas has focused on its role in disaster.

As far back as 1960, McDaniel (54) pointed out that occupational therapists have an important role in responding to disaster. Scaffa et al. (55) expanded on this with a delineation of the many different skills and tasks involving occupational therapy. They range from basic functioning of evacuated persons with disability to support of patients with posttraumatic stress disorder to vocational planning and testing early after recovery. Edgar et al. (56) in response to the Bali bombing disaster pointed out the challenges in providing top-quality physiotherapy.

Social work issues are more important than one might think. Shortly after the Haiti earthquake, the US Navy's hospital was filled with people who did not need inpatient care but could not/would not leave. This was a simple failure to follow the rehabilitation mantra, "discharge planning begins on admission." There were not enough crutches for patients to walk home, and there was little effort to identify and train family members. The family may also be in shock and disarray, with destroyed housing. Without food, water, clothing and shelter for themselves, the family cannot take the patient home.

Psychology is critical for many issues. They include premorbid psychological problems. Posttraumatic stress disorder is frequent and relates to other adjustment issues such as hopelessness and social support (57–60). Management of acute grief reaction, treatment of reactive depression, and more classical rehabilitation psychology problems such as adjustment to disability are important (61). Counselors provide education and support to patient caregivers (62). Therapy dogs have been successfully deployed (63). The role of psychologists and other counselors goes beyond the victims to support of the responding team. Acute and rehabilitation providers are typically wholly unprepared for the tragedy they experience.

Rehabilitation technology and engineering are important. Accessibility of the environment is always a challenge, but the hospital itself and the patient's home must be made accessible, or discharge and independence will be impossible. Wheelchairs and other mobility devices are important; however, in developing regions, donated high-tech devices such as battery-powered prostheses or titanium-based wheelchairs are often left in the ditch, because they are not rugged enough and impossible to fix.

Farooq Rathore was a physician in the Pakistan Army's Physical Medicine and Rehabilitation residency—the only training program in the country—when a huge earthquake hit. He and fellow trainees, with leadership from their faculty, commandeered a women's hospital and other facilities, eventually admitting over 300 spinal cord–injured patients within just a few days. They not only cared for the patients but also screened for venous thrombosis, measured function, and followed outcomes. The outcome was zero deaths, two babies, and an impressive database that lead to a number of publications that help us understand the nature of disability after earthquake and the appropriate management of victims. Dr. Rathore and his colleagues have gone on to be internationally respected in the field, and the increased attention to rehabilitation has helped build rehabilitation on the civilian side.

Rehabilitation Triage

As much as possible, specific diagnostics and treatment should emulate the standards presented throughout the rest of this textbook. So most of the important knowledge presented here relating to disaster rehabilitation is organizational in nature. Still there are some clinical differences that require special skills.

Rapid admission of dozens or hundreds of patients means that complete rehabilitation intake assessment and orders may need to be compromised. The goal should be to prioritize and revisit, rather than abandon details. First priority is missed life-, limb-, and nerve-threatening problems. The rushed and tired acute team is more likely to miss these things. There is also a need to prophylax for important dangerous problems. Venous thrombosis, GI ulcers, bladder problems, and seizure disorders may need attention. Second is detection of causes for disability that can be prevented with action, such as contracture or pressure sore. Next is maintenance of prior or stable medical problems that may include bowel, bladder, diabetes, and hypertension. Then comes detection of disabling problems that will need to be rehabilitated but do not require acute medical or surgical evaluation. Mild brain injury, minor fractures, and musculoskeletal disorders are commonly found and will affect life if not managed during the initial interaction with the health care system.

Crush injuries and urgent evacuation by less trained persons result in poorly planned or difficult-to-treat amputations. The acute surgical team may also feel rushed and may not be expert in amputation, so it is critical that PM&R review every potential amputation (64). Especially in low-resource regions, immediate postoperative fitting such as Yeongchi

Wu's old but effective removable rigid dressing process should be considered (65).

Injuries and evacuation may also cause rhabdomyolysis leading to renal failure, hypothermia, electrolyte abnormalities, and pressure sores. Acute or sometimes chronic malnutrition may need to be treated.

Urgent bladder management may not follow standards of a typical rehabilitation program. Clean intermittent catheterization may be optimal, but with limited human resources a Foley catheter may be needed at first (66). Chang followed 74 spinal cord patients who learned the Credé maneuver for voiding over 20 years after an earthquake (67). The complications including pyuria, stones, and ureteral dilatation were quite high, making this technique not desirable.

Usually the functional, psychological, and social factors so critical to success in the long term can wait for a more calm and measured evaluation a few days after admission.

RESPONDING TO DISASTER

Physical Medicine and Rehabilitation specialists may be called upon or volunteer to help after natural disaster in their home country or overseas. Rapid PM&R response is critical, but a few hours of thoughtful planning can ensure that the response is safe, meaningful, and lasting. Leadership, organization, and logistics are the key skill sets, especially since many PM&R responders are bringing teams or working with teams that have not worked together and will not be in the community long term. Leadership issues come before individual response issues.

The first question is, to go or not to go. A natural reaction to disaster may be to rush in to help. However, there are many instances of rehabilitation responders adding to the burden, being ineffective, interfering with established plans, and ignoring local expertise and leadership. They can cause harm to patients and put themselves and others at risk. So any potential responder must first convince themselves that they are personally the right person and that they are in a position to truly contribute.

Figure 48-1 provides a summary checklist of the issues to consider in deciding whether to participate in a disaster response. Careful consideration about everything from finances to logistics to role within the disaster response before departure can make the response safe and effective.

Responders

Responders with expert skill are not experts at disaster. So they must partner with the experts. Each nation, the World Health Organization, and many nongovernmental organizations have professionals whose lives are dedicated to disaster preparedness. They have detailed plans, stockpiled supplies, and equipment. Increasingly these groups have sophisticated rehabilitation plans as well. No individual or team should travel without aligning with and coordinating with one of these organizations.

The World Health Organization has well-established regional disaster plans and teams. Read the appropriate plan including designated lead organizations for PWD and

☐ You have approval from the destination country

☐ You have checked on safety

☐ You have established contact with an organization already on the grounds

☐ You have funding

☐ You have resources (food, water, medications, generators, shelter, etc.)

☐ You have transportation in the country

☐ You know where you are going and who to report to when you arrive

☐ You are medically healthy (medications for chronic illnesses) and emotionally stable

☐ You have clearance from your employer (responsibilities at your job, your patients at home)

FIGURE 48-1. *Go–no go checklist.*

for medical rehabilitation. Nongovernmental organizations involved in acute response include the following:

- Doctors Without Borders
- Red Cross/Red Crescent
- Handicap International
- International Spinal Injury Society
- International Society for Prosthetics and Orthotics

Response to the request of a local hospital or group is not advised until it is reviewed or approved by a lead disaster group.

Visas and Requirements

Before leaving, the responders have a lot of work to do. They should obtain a visa by visiting their country's embassy Web site and search for visa requirements to the destination country. In the United States, the U.S. Department of State—Bureau of Consular Affairs Web site is a helpful resource.[1] Partnering with a major aid agency can help expedite your visa in many cases. Responders need to check local licensing requirements and the rules for any waiver of licensure.

Immunizations

Responders should obtain appropriate immunizations and medications. In the United States, an excellent resource is the Centers for Disease Control and Prevention Web site.[2] Note that certain malaria regimes require travelers to start days before travel. The responders need to be sure that prescriptions for their usual medications are sufficient for the trip.

Travel Plans

Flights, local transportation, security, housing, food, and water must be arranged. The financial support must be sorted out. The responders need to bring appropriate cash with them. They should also make arrangements for fundraising, transfer of funds to them while away, and safekeeping of money on site.

Life at home will be substantially disrupted, and the responders must organize things for their absence and their return. Important plans include the following:

- Permission for work leave
- Any employer or institutional travel permission forms
- Discussion of plans with family
- Plans for care of home, pets, children, and personal finances
- Ensure that the traveler's will, living will, and health insurance are updated and known by others

Protection and Safety Concerns

Protection from the disaster must be planned. Disaster sites are not pretty. Late damage can occur. Panicked or angry people can become uncontrollable. The typical health and hygiene infrastructure is often broken down and was sometimes poor before the disaster. Responders can crash from emotional and physical exhaustion. Rehabilitation professionals must plan to avoid becoming part of the disaster instead of part of the relief.

One aspect of safety has to do with the disaster environment. There can be aftershocks, flooding, or more storms. Especially after an earthquake, the living and working facilities must be shown to be structurally intact. Fire, gas leaks, toxic chemicals, radiation, and isolation from food and water can occur. The local environment can have problems including stray pets, unstable trees, landslides, displaced snakes and venomous animals, and sewage.

Workers themselves can get sick or injured. So, the team must prepare for infections such as cholera, AIDS, malaria, or rabies. They need to get their shots and pills and have treatments readily available in the case of an incident. Hard work in tough environments can lead to a number of exposure problems including dehydration, heat exhaustion, hypothermia, and starvation. So the team must have plans for food, water and water purification, appropriate clothing, and interpersonal monitoring for symptoms.

The work, stress, and environment create risk for musculoskeletal injuries and lacerations. So pain medications, splints, cleaning materials, bandages, and access or transportation to more advanced care for more serious injuries must be available.

The social environment after a disaster is often horrific, and cultural norms for responders may be different from local expectations. Responders may run into prison outbreaks, looting, gang activity, mass riots, political upheaval that targets travelers, chaos in accessing care, and harassment related to gender. Important protections include an established relationship with military and police, hired security for transport, guarding of facilities, guarding of supplies, and contact with locals or members of the diaspora who know how to get around before traveling. Assigned daily check on the local radio news and rumor mill. Responders are encouraged to not bring valuables, stay in groups, stay away from political gatherings or crowd gatherings, set an alarm system to notify all and contact help rapidly, and set meeting points, hiding places, and evacuation plans.

For well over a decade before the Haiti earthquake, Jeff Randle's Healing Hands for Haiti was a model of sustainable and locally respectful rehabilitation in the country. A wide spectrum of rehabilitation "help" flooded the country. Some did excellent

---

[1] https://travel.state.gov/content/travel.html
[2] http://wwwnc.cdc.gov/travel/

work, but some appeared to stay for only a week or so and take photos, and others arrived without resources, requiring help themselves. International aid organizations largely did not seek the expertise of this local resource. So Colleen O'Connell of Healing Hands joined with other high-functioning rehabilitation response teams to coordinate care, provide daily updates to each other and the support systems, and reach out to improve care in the acute settings.

The Healing Hands facility was severely damaged, and many of the local staff lost family and home. So the Healing Hands leadership focused as much on funding long-term resources as on the emergency itself. As a result Healing Hands has opened a new and improved facility and has expanded its mission of training local persons in rehabilitation careers.

Most disaster responders arrive back home physically safe. Yet many are scarred for life by the experience. Even experienced responders can get serious psychological problems. Concrete plans must be made specifically for this eventual consequence. Individuals need to know their own mental health frailties, and team leaders must be able to restrict or reject volunteers who may pose a harm to themselves or others when under stress. Teams should have at least one team meeting before leaving to discuss coping with burnout. They might read and watch the news before leaving, watch videos of disasters and aftermath, listen to testimonies from experienced colleagues, and openly discuss the limits of their ability to help. Good teams have on-site debriefing at the end of each day, during which they might talk about the realistic limits of

their efforts or learn deep breathing or biofeedback exercises. Leaders need to watch for silent members, try to establish ways for members to contact family, and establish a mental health source for the team. It is good policy for the team to take time to recovery after return home, meet a week or so after reentry, and insist that struggling team members seek help.

Equipment, Supplies, and Preparations

Actual equipment and supplies vary according to the disaster, location, and larger response organizations.

Figure 48-2 is a list of supplies to consider. Each person must bring supplies for their own survival and personal needs. Team leaders need to consider food, shelter, medical supplies, group safety, means of communication with other professionals, and patient teaching resources.

Rehabilitation supplies depend on these variables as well as the expertise and duties of the team. **Figure 48-3** is a simple list. General medical equipment, medications, and supplies are augmented by rehabilitation-specific items for acute response, while a more advanced or prolonged plan will include technology like EMG machines.

Finally, distant responders need to know and appreciate the environment to which they are traveling. They need to know the country and the medical infrastructure. The United States Central Intelligence Agency Fact Book or another document on the destination country can be accessed. Respondents might keep a card with 11 basic words in the local language: hello, goodbye, please, thank you, no, yes, go away, help, bathroom,

---

Individuals should consider:

- Survival supplies: Be prepared to be fully autonomous for up to five days
  - ☐ Food, water, water purification, shelter (mosquito net?), basic medical supplies, electricity/generator, clothing, gas/fuel if permitted

- Personal clothing:
  - ☐ Dress appropriately for your role and the job you must do
  - ☐ Respect local cultural norms
  - ☐ Easy drying clothes
  - ☐ Clothing for weather, for bug and sun protection

- Personal needs:
  - ☐ Toiletries, soap including laundry soap
  - ☐ Medications and personal first aid, sun block, bug spray
  - ☐ Documentation of medical history and meds. Family and medical contacts
  - ☐ Glasses, sunglasses, hat, camera, paper, pens, possibly computer, phone, pocket knife
  - ☐ Reading material, deck of cards, or other avocational stuff
  - ☐ Maybe small gifts

- Personal logistics:
  - ☐ Money including enough money to buy supplies
  - ☐ Valid passport
  - ☐ Uniforms, name tags
  - ☐ Copy of license and business cards

Teams should consider:

- ☐ Food, water, shelter, basic medical supplies, electricity/generator, clothing, gas/fuel for five days
- ☐ Communication: cell phones, satellite communication, walkie talkies
- ☐ Recommendations: freezer for food or medications, electricity
- ☐ Interpreters and/or language guides
- ☐ Print-outs from the team's own training modules
- ☐ Paper copies of important documents
- ☐ A written plan for evacuation and repacking, escape to safety
- ☐ Uniforms/t-shirts to identify team members

FIGURE 48-2. Packing list for response to a distant rehabilitation disaster.

Seriously consider:

☐ Reference books: rehab medicine, family medicine, emergency med, electromyography

☐ Instructions for allied health professionals and families of patients in appropriate language

☐ Basic medical needs (needles, syringes, bandages, suture material, anesthetics, gloves (sterile and protective), betadine (PVPI), various tapes, masks, minor surgery kits): pressure relief and pressure sore dressings, bladder catheterization (straight and Foley), bowel program, stretching protocols

☐ Equipment: stethoscope, otoscope, goniometer, reflex hammer, light pen, thermometers, sphygmomanometer, monofilament

☐ Medical term translation list or book

Maybe

☐ Meds, e.g., injectable steroids and anesthetics, phenol for blocks, Pain meds (check to see if opiates can be imported), seizure meds (specify by checking with other experts; ex: phenobarbital), spasticity meds?

    ○ Antibiotics, antidepressants, anticoagulants

☐ Casting materials (plaster and fiberglass cast material, stockinette, padding, manual and electric cast saw, cast wedge opener), splinting materials

☐ Removable rigid dressing for amputees: White athletic tube socks, velcro M/F strips w/ adhesive on back, heat moldable plastic

☐ Supplies to measure function and outcome (L.I.F.E., survey instruments, etc.?)

Advanced or long term

☐ EMG machine (electrodes, needles, tape measure, tape, normal references, gel) and supplies?

☐ Portable ultrasound (gel, textbook)

☐ Medical record keeping: computer, paper forms, clipboards, pens, folders, wristbands with permanent marker

☐ Off the shelf orthotics, crutches, canes

FIGURE 48-3. Rehabilitation supplies to consider in response to a distant disaster.

hungry, thirsty. They should understand the culture: general manners, gender roles (especially in health care), hospitality, corruption, education level, government, political hot topics, and locals' perception of their country. The socioeconomic status of the country should be appreciated, including means of employment, education, housing architecture, government roles, and resources. Often, the natural environment is quite different for the travelers, so extended forecast, terrain, flora, and fauna should be sought.

The predisaster hospitals, medical schools, and NGO involvement need to be known. The rehabilitation infrastructure and rehabilitation leaders might be explored through Web sites and contact with national leaders or organizations through the International Society for Physical and Rehabilitation Medicine. Even the most resource-poor regions have a disability culture and disabled persons' organizations that can ensure that the efforts of outsiders are respectful and sustainable.

The real job of visiting responders is to create a sustainable response. Successful lifesaving results in a population of PWD who will need medical, physical, and psychosocial adaptation for a lifetime. However, investment in the long term is not in the interest of most acute care response organizations and often beyond the understanding of the local health care system. Donor fatigue means that support for long-term sustainable care must occur early in the disaster, too. Even where there is local expertise, these experts are often in shock, exhausted, and critically needed on the ground. This creates a compelling need for expert responder groups to aggressively advocate for the long-term support of the PWD in the region.

Fortunately, most of the work of creating sustainability can fall on volunteers who are not busy on site, or on volunteers whose skills are not medical care. Tasks include liaison and planning with other like-minded organizations; developing and executing fundraising and media strategies; gathering data on the nature and extent of disabling injuries and presenting this information to aid organizations and policymakers; sorting out the resources and gaps within the local health care system and educational system; and looking at support options including long-term volunteers, telemedicine consultation, and capital for local entrepreneurs to build sustainable rehabilitation businesses. The volunteers may be able to influence payment policies that can sustain rehabilitation programs beyond the acute phase, such as increased government payment for outpatient therapies, assistive devices, and vocational rehabilitation.

Often first-responding rehabilitation professionals feel a real commitment to the place and people they have served. With efforts to organize things, this can be converted into a long-term beneficial relationship in which distant partners provide advice, become visiting teachers, act as advocates or board members for local organizations, and return again and again to help in a place where they have developed cultural expertise and friendship.

Work on the Ground

The response to disaster should be well planned and well organized ahead of time. And it often is, except that rehabilitation is often an afterthought. So rehabilitation responders need to understand the overall schema in order to insert themselves into the process effectively. Where does a rehabilitation professional and team plug into the disaster response? **Table 48-3** summarizes general goals.

TABLE 48-3	**Timeline for Rehabilitation Goals after a Disaster**
Days 1–7	• Get the word out to first responders about appropriate evacuation (e.g., stabilize spinal cord; transport to specialized center via helicopter) • Consult on potential amputees • Identify and tag probable rehab candidates: persons whose disease would likely lead to rehab admission
Week 2	• Second look: Reassess all persons still in hospital for potential rehab • Begin to manage musculoskeletal and pain cases • Begin appropriate therapy and education on patients

Week 3	• Establish a "real" inpatient rehab ward:
	  ◦ Specialized team of rehab nurses along with PT, OT, SLP, psych
	  ◦ Weekly team meeting: Record goals, time frames, discharge planning, discharge location, family patient teaching, equipment, medication, barriers
	  ◦ Therapy equipment
	• Begin long-term rehab needs assessment

Many rehabilitation physicians, rehabilitation nurses, and perhaps therapists also have competency in acute medicine and surgery. They may take on these roles while maintaining a rehabilitation presence in the first days. Otherwise, in the first week, the rehabilitation team needs to advise first responders and emergency workers and get out of the way.

Urgent radio broadcasts, pamphlet drops, etc., about spinal precautions, pressure without tourniquets to control bleeding, and watching for progression of minor brain injuries should be considered. The team might brief professional evacuators on spinal cord injury issues including helicopter evacuation, pressure relief, and use of indwelling catheters. They might set a policy that surgeons should contact a PM&R doctor before an amputation. Attention may need to be drawn to the need to help evacuate people with preexisting disability.

The United States is widely viewed as a wealthy country with sophisticated and well-organized government functions and one of the top medical systems in the world. Yet when a hurricane and flood hit the southern city of New Orleans, the emergency response was seen as pathetic (68). There was looting in the streets. People were trapped in the roofs of their houses; food, water, and shelter were lacking; and a general consensus across the country was that the government had let the people down. From a rehabilitation standpoint, there was chaos in the beginning. Rescue of people with disability was delayed and poorly executed. Individuals were separated from their caregivers, equipment, and important medications and supplies. One postacute facility was accused of abandoning or euthanizing some of its most disabled residents. Once identified and rescued, patients were rapidly evacuated to world-class rehabilitation facilities in nearby areas.

In the chaotic environment of a disaster response, an important task for the rehabilitation team is to systematically and repeatedly identify rehabilitation patients. Early on, it seems obvious that some patients with spinal cord injury, amputation, and severe brain injury are in need of rehabilitation. A few days later, the patients who were bypassed need to be screened again. Fractures are frequently missed in the context of multisystem injury (69). Some who appeared to be dying will be saved, while others with apparent minor trauma will

be found to have neurologic deficits, failed salvage of a limb, or preexisting disability that complicates discharge. "Minor" disabilities such as back pain, single focal nerve injury, or mild brain injury may not be a priority in week 1, but can cause a lifetime of pain and disability if left undetected and untreated.

Regardless of disaster or diagnosis, a number of common issues arise. Pain management, especially in the field, is important both from a humanitarian standpoint and to prevent long-term pain issues. The psychological response to disaster can include posttraumatic stress disorder and grieving, and the epidemiology of mental health disorders tells us that many PWD will have premorbid complex and serious mental health problems.

THE IMPACT OF DISASTER REHABILITATION

While it seems intuitive that rehabilitation is important, scientific evidence is important if rehabilitation is to be included in the larger sphere of disaster policy and resource allocation.

Very little prospective research has been done. However, Zhang et al. found that the administrative constraints on their response resulted in a natural experiment after an earthquake in China (70). Two hundred ninety-eight people who received institutional-based rehabilitation with community-based follow-up were compared to 101 people who received delayed rehabilitation services and 111 who never received rehabilitation services. Rehabilitation showed significant improvement on the Barthel Index of function, although the differences between early and late rehabilitation were not large.

Long-term follow-up has shown continued challenges. After earthquakes, Li's team (71,72) found improvement in wheelchair skills and activities of daily living in over 50 spinal cord patients who underwent rehabilitation. Positive outcome related to early evacuation and early rehabilitation.

Lessons learned from earthquakes have set the stage for future research on evacuation and management of people who suffer from spinal cord injuries as a result (73). Reviewers of the Haiti earthquake thought in retrospect that the weakness of the local rehabilitation infrastructure had a lot to do with failure, yet the building of support afterwards made the international response a positive lesson for future disasters (74,75).

Child survivors of disaster have different medical and social needs. Gamulin found over 1,000 pediatric admissions after the Haiti earthquake, about half of whom were treated by surgeons and half by medical specialists (76). The acute phase in which a lot of surgery was done was approximately 11 days after the earthquake.

Rasco and North (77) and Tomata et al. (78) studied employment among survivors of disaster. Tomata's review of a national disability database showed that persons from the tsunami region had double the disability rate (14%) compared to other regions of the country (78). In contrast, Rasco looked at 3-year follow-up of survivors of seven major disasters, and found little change in employment.

The consequences of man-made disaster have been studied in a number of situations. In addition to the physical impairments, psychological trauma is common (60). After the 9/11 terrorist attack, Perlman et al. (79) found that risk factors for posttraumatic stress disorder in the population included "proximity to the site on 9/11, living or working in lower Manhattan, rescue or recovery work at the World Trade Center site, event-related loss of spouse, and low social support."

SUMMARY

Certainly humans can be blamed for war, terrorism, and failure of infrastructure. Yet, even when the "disaster" is due to the forces of nature, the need for rehabilitation relates to human factors. One can contrast Japan's tsunami and Haiti's earthquake. Local infrastructure determined the number and nature of injuries. Local acute response determined the type of rehabilitation needed. The resiliency of local rehabilitation resources determined the need for outside help. Human factors predominate in rehabilitation after man-made or natural disasters.

A small minority of readers of this chapter will be responsible for prospective design of rehabilitation response for their community. Most of us will be strangers hoping to help. Our technical and medical expertise is invaluable, but we must be aware of the need to follow leaders rather than strike out on our own. We must ensure that our teams are safe, sane, and effective in the context of the local environment. Finally, as visitors who care, we have a unique opportunity to focus on building the long-term infrastructure that is so often neglected after the acute teams pack their bags for home.

ACKNOWLEDGMENTS

Much of the research and infrastructure of this paper come from work of the Disaster Acute Rehabilitation Team project of the ISPRM, funded by the University of Michigan's Center for Global Health and led by the author and Prof. Jianan Li of Nanjing University (80–84). Josh Verson, Lars Johnson Huacon (Wendy) Wen and Yih-Chieh Chen were the key leaders of this project. All tables and figures (with the exception of **Box 48-1**) were created by Andrew J. Haig, MD, 2013.

The educational modules of the DART team are not officially recognized by the ISPRM, but may be of use to disaster rehabilitation leaders and teams.

REFERENCES

1. Pliny the Younger. The Destruction of Pompeii, 79 AD. Translation by EyeWitness to History; 1999. Available from: www.eyewitnesstohistory.com. Accessed March 13, 2017.
2. Gerber DA. War. In: Albrecht GL, ed. *Encyclopedia of Disability*. Thousand Oaks, CA: SAGE Publications, Inc.; 2006:1629.
3. World Health Organization. Health Emergencies. WHO Response in Severe Large Scale Emergencies. EB140/7, 140th Session; 2016. Available from: http://www.who.int/hac/crises/en/. Accessed March 15, 2017.
4. Vos F, Rodriguez J, Below R, et al. *Annual Disaster Statistical Review 2009: The Numbers and Trends*. Brussels: Centre for Research on the Epidemiology of Disasters (CRED); 2010.
5. Anand S. Disability-adjusted life years: a critical review. *J Health Econ.* 1997;16(6):685–702.
6. Sarangi S. Compensation to Bhopal gas victims: will justice ever be done? *Indian J Med Ethics.* 2012;9(2):118–120.
7. World Health Organization. Global Assessment of National Health Sector Emergency Preparedness and Response; 2008. Available from: http://www.who.int/hac/about/Global_survey_inside.pdf. Accessed October 15, 2018.
8. Burkle FM Jr. The development of multidisciplinary core competencies: the first step in the professionalization of disaster medicine and public health preparedness on a global scale. *Disaster Med Public Health Prep.* 2012;6:10–12.
9. World Health Organization. Classification and Minimum Standards for Foreign Medical Teams in Sudden Onset Disasters; 2017. Available from: https://extranet.who.int/emt/page/home. Accessed March 26, 2017.
10. Chackungal S, Nickerson JW, Knowlton LM, et al. Best practice guidelines on surgical response in disasters and humanitarian emergencies: report of the 2011 Humanitarian Action Summit Working Group on Surgical Issues within the Humanitarian Space. *Prehosp Disaster Med.* 2011;26(06):429–437.
11. World Health Organization. *Emergency Medical Teams: Minimum Technical Standards and Recommendations for Rehabilitation*. Licence: CC BY-NC-SA 3.0 IGO. Geneva, Switzerland: WHO; 2016.
12. Mills J-A, Durham J, Packirisamy V. Rehabilitation services in disaster response. *Bull World Health Organ.* 2017;95(2):162–164. Available from: http://www.who.int/bulletin/volumes/95/2/15-157024.pdf. Accessed March 26, 2017.
13. Knowlton LM, Gosney JE, Chackungal S, et al. Consensus statements regarding the multidisciplinary care of limb amputation patients in disasters or humanitarian emergencies: report of the 2011 Humanitarian Action Summit Surgical Working Group on amputations following disasters or conflict. *Prehosp Disaster Med.* 2011;26(6):438–448.
14. Smith A. The Aid Racket. Socialist Worker; 2010. Available from: https://socialistworker.org/2010/02/24/the-aid-racket. Accessed October 15, 2018.
15. Gellert GA, Walsh W Jr, Petrosian L, et al. Role of voluntarism and nongovernmental organizations in internationalizing rehabilitation medicine. *Am J Phys Med Rehabil.* 1995;74(6):460–463.
16. Burke DC, Brown D, Hill V, et al. The development of a spinal injuries unit in Armenia. *Paraplegia.* 1993;31(3):168–171.
17. Smith J, Roberts B, Knight A, et al. A systematic literature review of the quality of evidence for injury and rehabilitation interventions in humanitarian crises. *Int J Public Health.* 2015;60(7):865–872.
18. Khan F, Amatya B, Gosney J, et al. Medical rehabilitation in natural disasters: a review. *Arch Phys Med Rehabil.* 2015;96(9):1709–1727.
19. Rathore FA, Gosney JE, Reinhardt JD, et al. Medical rehabilitation after natural disasters: why, when, and how?. *Arch Phys Med Rehabil.* 2012;93(10):1875–1881.
20. Gosney JE Jr. Physical medicine and rehabilitation: critical role in disaster response. *Disaster Med Public Health Prep.* 2010;4(2):110–112.
21. Gosney J, Reinhardt JD, Haig AJ, et al. Developing post-disaster physical rehabilitation: role of the World Health Organization Liaison Sub-Committee on Rehabilitation Disaster Relief of the International Society of Physical and Rehabilitation Medicine. *J Rehabil Med.* 2011;43(11):965–968.
22. Reinhardt JD, Li J, Gosney J, et al. Disability and health-related rehabilitation in international disaster relief. *Glob Health Action.* 2011;4:7191.
23. Shapira S, Novack L, Bar-Dayan Y, et al. An integrated and interdisciplinary model for predicting the risk of injury and death in future earthquakes. *PLoS One.* 2016;11(3):e0151111.
24. Rathore MF, Rashid P, Butt AW, et al. Epidemiology of spinal cord injuries in the 2005 Pakistan earthquake. *Spinal Cord.* 2007;45(10):658–663.
25. Burns AS, O'Connell C, Rathore F. Meeting the challenges of spinal cord injury care following sudden onset disaster: lessons learned. *J Rehabil Med.* 2012;44(5):414–420.
26. Du W, FitzGerald GJ, Clark M, et al. Health impacts of floods. *Prehosp Disaster Med.* 2010;25(3):265–272.
27. Bloodworth DM, Kevorkian CG, Rumbaut E, et al. Impairment and disability in the Astrodome after hurricane Katrina: lessons learned about the needs of the disabled after large population movements. *Am J Phys Med Rehabil.* 2007;86(9):770–775.
28. Chiou-Tan FY, Bloodworth DM, Kass JS, et al. Physical medicine and rehabilitation conditions in the Astrodome clinic after hurricane Katrina. *Am J Phys Med Rehabil.* 2007;86(9):762–769.
29. LeBourgeois B, Sherrer V, eds. *How to Include Disability Issues in Disaster Management Following Floods 2004 in Bangladesh*. Dhaka, Bangladesh: Handicap International Bangladesh; 2005.
30. Snyder AP. The role of the physical therapist in disaster planning. *Phys Ther Rev.* 1958;38(9):593–598.
31. Eldar R. Preparedness for medical rehabilitation of casualties in disaster situations. *Disabil Rehabil.* 1997;19(12):547–551.
32. Miller ET, Farra S. Disaster preparedness, a rehabilitation nursing priority. *Rehabil Nurs.* 2012;37(3):95–96.
33. Brown LM, Hickling EJ, Frahm K. Emergencies, disasters, and catastrophic events: the role of rehabilitation nurses in preparedness, response, and recovery. *Rehabil Nurs.* 2010;35(6):236–241.
34. Wolf-Fordham SB, Twyman JS, Hamad CD. Educating first responders to provide emergency services to individuals with disabilities. *Disaster Med Public Health Prep.* 2014;8(6):533–540.
35. Motoki E, Mori K, Kaji H, et al. Development of disaster pamphlets based on health needs of patients with chronic illnesses. *Prehosp Disaster Med.* 2010;25(4):354–360.
36. Morris JT, Mueller JL, Jones ML. Use of social media during public emergencies by people with disabilities. *West J Emerg Med.* 2014;15(5):567–574.
37. Jenkins JL, McCarthy M, Kelen G, et al. Changes needed in the care for sheltered persons: a multistate analysis from hurricane Katrina. *Am J Disaster Med.* 2009;4(2):101–106.
38. Dosa D, Feng Z, Hyer K, et al. Effects of hurricane Katrina on nursing facility resident mortality, hospitalization, and functional decline. *Disaster Med Public Health Prep.* 2010;4(suppl 1):S28–S32.
39. Zakour MJ. Effects of support on evacuation preparedness of persons with disabilities. *J Soc Work Disabil Rehabil.* 2015;14(1):1–22.
40. McDermott S, Martin K, Gardner JD. Disaster response for people with disability. *Disabil Health J.* 2016;9(2):183–185.
41. Sinclair K. Global policy and local actions for vulnerable populations affected by disaster and displacement. *Aust Occup Ther J.* 2014;61(1):1–5.
42. Bethel JW, Foreman AN, Burke SC. Disaster preparedness among medically vulnerable populations. *Am J Prev Med.* 2011;40(2):139–143.
43. McClure LA, Boninger ML, Oyster ML, et al. Emergency evacuation readiness of full-time wheelchair users with spinal cord injury. *Arch Phys Med Rehabil.* 2011;92(3):491–498.

44. Tomio J, Sato H, Mizumura H. Impact of natural disasters on the functional and health status of patients with rheumatoid arthritis. *Mod Rheumatol.* 2011;21(4): 381–390.

45. Gee CJ, Bonkowske J, Kurup SK. Visual disability in selected acts of terror, warfare, and natural disasters of the last 25 years: a concise narrative review. *Am J Disaster Med.* 2008;3(1):25–30.

46. Cripps JH, Cooper SB, Austin EN. Emergency preparedness with people who sign: toward the whole community approach. *J Emerg Manag.* 2016;14(2):101–111.

47. Kobayashi S, Endo W, Inui T, et al. The lack of antiepileptic drugs and worsening of seizures among physically handicapped patients with epilepsy during the Great East Japan Earthquake. *Brain Dev.* 2016;38(7):623–627.

48. Tofighi B, Grossman E, Williams AR, et al. Outcomes among buprenorphine-naloxone primary care patients after hurricane Sandy. *Addict Sci Clin Pract.* 2014;9:3.

49. McGuire LC, Ford ES, Okoro CA. Natural disasters and older US adults with disabilities: implications for evacuation. *Disasters.* 2007;31(1):49–56.

50. Bhalla MC, Burgess A, Frey J, et al. Geriatric disaster preparedness. *Prehosp Disaster Med.* 2015;30(5):443–446.

51. Goldstraw P, Strivens E, Kennett C, et al. The care of older people during and after disasters: a review of the recent experiences in Queensland, Australia and Christchurch, New Zealand. *Australas J Ageing.* 2012;31(2):69–71.

52. Tomata Y, Kakizaki M, Suzuki Y, et al. Impact of the 2011 Great East Japan Earthquake and Tsunami on functional disability among older people: a longitudinal comparison of disability prevalence among Japanese municipalities. *J Epidemiol Community Health.* 2014;68:530–533.

53. Lee HS. The role of dietitians, physical and occupational therapists in the management of mass casualties. *Mil Med.* 1956;118(4):396–398.

54. McDaniel ML. The role of the occupational therapist in natural disaster situations. *Am J Occup Ther.* 1960;14:195–198.

55. Scaffa ME, Gerardi S, Herzberg G, et al. The role of occupational therapy in disaster preparedness, response, and recovery. *Am J Occup Ther.* 2006;60(6):642–649.

56. Edgar D, Wood F, Goodwin-Walters A. Maintaining physical therapy standards in an emergency situation: solutions after the Bali bombing disaster. *Burns.* 2005;31(5):555–557.

57. Rajkumar AP, Mohan TS, Tharyan P. Lessons from the 2004 Asian tsunami: nature, prevalence and determinants of prolonged grief disorder among tsunami survivors in South Indian coastal villages. *Int J Soc Psychiatry.* 2015;61(7):645–652.

58. Zhou X, Song H, Hu M, et al. Risk factors of severity of post-traumatic stress disorder among survivors with physical disabilities one year after the Wenchuan earthquake. *Psychiatry Res.* 2015;228(3):468–474.

59. Ozdemir O, Boysan M, Guzel Ozdemir P, et al. Relationships between posttraumatic stress disorder (PTSD), dissociation, quality of life, hopelessness, and suicidal ideation among earthquake survivors. *Psychiatry Res.* 2015;228(3):598–605.

60. Miller L. Psychological interventions for terroristic trauma: prevention, crisis management, and clinical treatment strategies. *Int J Emerg Ment Health.* 2011;13(2): 95–120.

61. Takahashi A, Watanabe K, Oshima M, et al. The effect of the disaster caused by the great Hanshin earthquake on people with intellectual disability. *J Intellect Disabil Res.* 1997;41(Pt 2):193–196.

62. Sawa M, Osaki Y, Koishikawa H. Delayed recovery of caregivers from social dysfunction and psychological distress after the Great East Japan Earthquake. *J Affect Disord.* 2013;148(2–3):413–417.

63. Shubert J. Therapy dogs and stress management assistance during disasters. *US Army Med Dep J.* Apr-June, 2012:74–78.

64. Kelly JD. Haitian amputees—lessons learned from Sierra Leone. *N Engl J Med.* 2010;362(11):e42.

65. Wu Y, Keagy RD, Krick HJ, et al. An innovative removable rigid dressing technique for below-the-knee-amputation. *J Bone Joint Surg Am.* 1979;61A:724–729.

66. Hoshii T, Nishiyama T, Takahashi K. Influence of the great earthquake in the Chuetsu district on patients managing urination with clean intermittent self-urethral catheterization. *Int J Urol.* 2007;14(9):875–878.

67. Chang SM, Hou CL, Dong DQ, et al. Urologic status of 74 spinal cord injury patients from the 1976 Tangshan earthquake, and managed for over 20 years using the Crede maneuver. *Spinal Cord.* 2000;38(9):552–554.

68. The Economist. *When Government Fails: The Pathetic Official Response to Katrina Has Shocked the World How Will It Change American*; 2005. Accessed October 15, 2018.

69. Born CT, Ross SE, Iannacone WM, et al. Delayed identification of skeletal injury in multisystem trauma: the 'missed' fracture. *J Trauma.* 1989;29(12):1643–1646.

70. Zhang X, Reinhardt JD, Gosney JE, et al. The NHV rehabilitation services program improves long-term physical functioning in survivors of the 2008 Sichuan earthquake: a longitudinal quasi experiment. *PLoS One.* 2013;8(1):e53995.

71. Li Y, Reinhardt JD, Gosney JE, et al. Evaluation of functional outcomes of physical rehabilitation and medical complications in spinal cord injury victims of the Sichuan earthquake. *J Rehabil Med.* 2012;44(7):534–540.

72. Hu X, Zhang X, Gosney JE, et al. Analysis of functional status, quality of life and community integration in earthquake survivors with spinal cord injury at hospital discharge and one-year follow-up in the community. *J Rehabil Med.* 2012;44(3): 200–205.

73. Gosney JE, Reinhardt JD, von Groote PM, et al. Medical rehabilitation of spinal cord injury following earthquakes in rehabilitation resource-scarce settings: implications for disaster research. *Spinal Cord.* 2013;51(8):603–609.

74. Wolbring G. Disability, displacement and public health: a vision for Haiti. *Can J Public Health.* 2011;102(2):157–159.

75. Iezzoni LI, Ronan LJ. Disability legacy of the Haitian earthquake. *Ann Intern Med.* 2010;152(12):812–814.

76. Gamulin A, Armenter-Duran J, Assal M, et al. Conditions found among pediatric survivors during the early response to natural disaster: a prospective case study. *J Pediatr Orthop.* 2012;32(4):327–333.

77. Rasco SS, North CS. An empirical study of employment and disability over three years among survivors of major disasters. *J Am Acad Psychiatry Law.* 2010;38(1):80–86.

78. Tomata Y, Suzuki Y, Kawado M, et al. Long-term impact of the 2011 Great East Japan Earthquake and tsunami on functional disability among older people: a 3-year longitudinal comparison of disability prevalence among Japanese municipalities. *Soc Sci Med.* 2015;147:296–299.

79. Perlman SE, Friedman S, Galea S, et al. Short-term and medium-term health effects of 9/11. *Lancet.* 2011;378(9794):925–934.

80. Verson J, Haig AJ. Building the ISRPM Disaster Acute Rehabilitation Team Program. Consortium of Universities for Global Health (CUGH), Boston, MA, March 26–28, 2015.

81. Verson J, Haig AJ, Wen H, et al. Building the ISPRM Disaster Acute Rehabilitation Team. ISPRM, Beijing, June 14–20, 2013.

82. Verson J, Haig A, Wen H, et al. Rehabilitation Planning: The Michigan Center for Global Health and the ISPRM Disaster Acute Rehabilitation Team. ISPRM, Beijing, June 14–20, 2013.

83. Johnson L, Haig AJ, Verson J, et al. Comparative Rehabilitation Consequences of Tsunamis and Floods. ISPRM, Beijing, June 14–20, 2013.

84. Wen H, Haig AJ, Johnson L, et al. A Comparison of Rehabilitation Management after Natural Disasters in Different Countries. ISPRM, Beijing, June 14–20, 2013.

CHAPTER **49**

Frank E. Lorch
Lee Stoner
Jesse A. Lieberman

Alicia H. Lazeski
Michael Masi

Exercise

The term *exercise* traditionally refers to regular and structured physical activity for the sake of training or improvement of health and fitness. Regular physical activity reduces the risk of many adverse health outcomes, and it is known that any amount of physical activity confers some health benefits (1). It is also well known that the risks of remaining inactive are substantial (2,3). Additionally, the use of exercise in the treatment of injuries is not a new concept. Hippocrates (460 to 370 B.C.) reportedly advocated exercise as an important factor in the healing of injured ligaments, and the Hindus and Chinese used therapeutic exercise in the treatment of athletic injuries as early as 1,000 B.C.

Exercise as a concept encompasses a vast range of activities and methods, ultimately to be applied toward the goal of improving function and health. Function itself can be conceptualized as the interrelated performance of balance/postural control, cardiopulmonary fitness/endurance, flexibility/mobility, muscle performance, neuromuscular control/coordination, and stability (4). As a subset of function, physical fitness, that is, cardiopulmonary fitness, muscular fitness (strength, endurance, and power), body composition, flexibility, and neuromotor fitness, is known to confer health benefits (5). Exercise can be used therapeutically to address all these areas for the prevention, treatment, and rehabilitation of illness and disabling conditions.

This chapter focuses on the use of activities requiring physical exertion to improve fitness and health. The pertinent exercises considered in this chapter include those to develop aerobic and muscular fitness, flexibility, and neuromotor (balance, coordination, proprioception) control. A portion of this chapter is devoted to information that provides the physiologic foundation for the clinical use of exercise.

MUSCLE PHYSIOLOGY FUNDAMENTALS

The movement of limbs, and therefore physical activity, results from the generation of force by activated skeletal muscle(s). The following section will focus on the structure and function of skeletal muscle (see also Chapter 2), prior to discussing how the energy for fueling skeletal muscle force is produced.

Structure and Function of Muscle

Morphology

The human body is composed of over 650 skeletal muscles. As displayed in **Figure 49-1**, each skeletal muscle is composed of structural subunits, including fascicles and muscle fibers (muscle cells) (6). Each structural unit is surrounded by connective tissue, which is continuous with the skeletal muscle and connects from tendon to bone. Force generated by a skeletal muscle acts on the tendons through the connective tissue.

More precisely, the force, which acts on the tendons, is developed by sarcomeres. Sarcomeres, which are contained within a muscle fiber, are aligned end to end to form a myofibril. The force developed by sarcomeres results from the action of two basic protein filaments, a thicker one, called *myosin*, and a thinner one, called *actin*. These proteins are arranged in such a way as to give skeletal muscle its *striated* appearance.

Sliding Filament Theory

As mentioned above, the primary function of skeletal muscle is to develop force. The sliding filament theory (**Fig. 49-2**) (7) provides an explanation of how muscle fibers shorten and so develop force.

Muscle shortening requires an adequate supply of calcium and adenosine triphosphate (ATP). Under resting conditions, a protein called tropomyosin blocks the site at which myosin attaches to actin. To expose the actin site, an action potential must reach the sarcoplasmic reticulum, where calcium ions are stored. Once released, these calcium ions attach to troponin and induce a conformational change that pulls tropomyosin away from the actin site. Subsequently, the myosin head attaches to actin, forming a *cross-bridge* and permitting a *power stroke* to occur. During a power stroke, the angle of the myosin heads changes, causing actin filaments to be pulled over the myosin filaments and narrowing the distance between Z lines

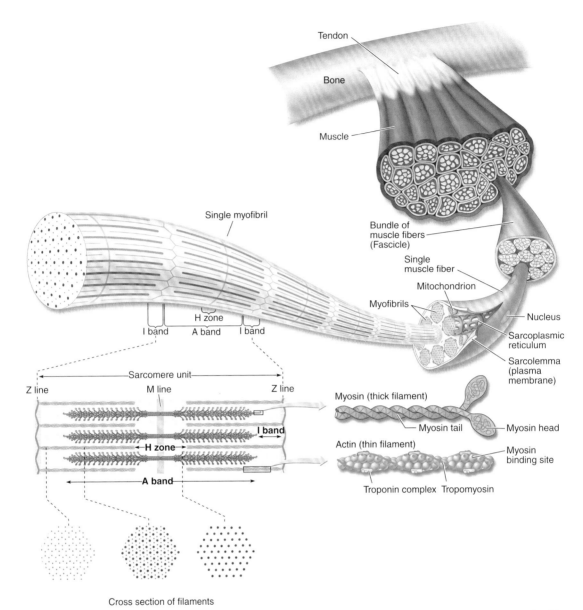

FIGURE 49-1. Structural and functional subunits of skeletal muscle. (Reprinted with permission from Moorcroft C. *Myology and Kinesiology for Massage Therapists.* Philadelphia, PA: Wolters Kluwer Health/Lippincott Williams & Wilkins, 2011: 22.)

(see **Fig. 49-1**). For more shortening to occur, the actin-myosin bond must be broken, allowing binding of myosin to another actin site closer to the Z line. Energy, in the form of ATP, is required for both the cocking (power stroke) and detachment of myosin. For repetitive contractions to occur, that is, subsequent cross-bridge cycles, ATP must be replenished.

Mechanical Model

Figure 49-3 shows a useful model to understand the mechanical properties of muscles (8). This model consists of the contractile element with both parallel and series elastic elements. The contractile element, which represents the sarcomere, generates force through the cross-bridge cycle. The elastic elements are purely passive components acting as mechanical springs. The parallel elastic element represents the connective tissue surrounding the various subunits of the muscle, and the series elastic element represents the tendinous insertions of muscle. Force generated by contractile elements acts on the series elastic element through the parallel elastic element.

Force-Velocity Relationship

The maximum force a muscle can exert depends on the speed at which it is contracting. The maximal static (isometric) force of a muscle is always greater than the force that can be exerted during shortening, and the maximal force exerted during lengthening is always greater than that exerted during static contraction. This relationship is displayed in **Figure 49-4**.

It is thought that the shape of the force-velocity curve is explained on the basis of the sliding filament theory of muscle contraction (9).

Muscle Fiber Types

Skeletal muscles contain a mixture of muscle fiber types that can be distinguished by their physical and biochemical characteristics (see Chapter 2). These physiologic and biochemical characteristics have been used to coin the skeletal muscle nomenclature outlined in **Table 49-1**. An understanding of the origins of physical and biochemical characterization, and subsequent nomenclature, is important for the following discussion

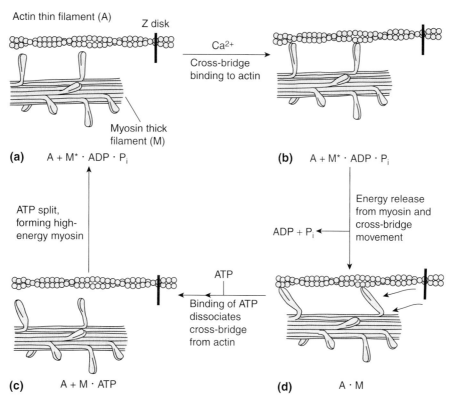

FIGURE 49-2. The cyclic process of muscle contraction and relaxation. In the resting state **(a)**, actin (A) and energized myosin (M*·ADP·P$_i$) cannot interact because the binding site is blocked by tropomyosin. Upon release of calcium (Ca^{2+}) from the sarcoplasmic reticulum, M*·ADP·P$_i$ binds to A **(b)**. Tension is developed, and movement occurs with the release of ADP and Pi **(c)**. Dissociation of actin and myosin requires the presence of ATP to bind to myosin and to pump Ca^{2+} in to the SR **(d)**. Myosin is energized upon return to resting state **(a)**. (Republished with permission of McGraw-Hill Education from Vander A, Sherman JH, Luciano DS. *Human Physiology.* 3rd ed. New York: McGraw-Hill, 1980:218; permission conveyed through Copyright Clearance Center, Inc.)

In figure (a): A + M* · ADP · P$_i$, with labels "Actin thin filament (A)", "Z disk", "Myosin thick filament (M)"

Between (a) and (b): Ca^{2+} Cross-bridge binding to actin

In figure (b): A + M* · ADP · P$_i$

Between (b) and (d): Energy release from myosin and cross-bridge movement, ADP + P$_i$

Between (a) and (c): ATP split, forming high-energy myosin

In figure (c): A + M · ATP

Between (c) and (d): ATP, Binding of ATP dissociates cross-bridge from actin

In figure (d): A · M

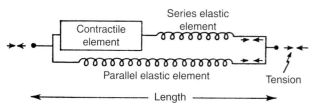

FIGURE 49-3. Mechanical model of muscle consisting of a contractile element and two elastic elements. (Reprinted from Roberts TDM. *Neurophysiology of Postural Mechanics.* 2nd ed. London: Butterworth; 1978. Copyright © 1978 Elsevier. With permission.)

Labels in figure: Contractile element, Series elastic element, Parallel elastic element, Tension, Length

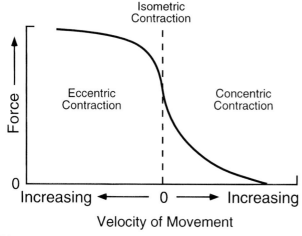

FIGURE 49-4. Schematic relationship between maximal muscular force and velocity of movement.

Labels in figure: Force, Isometric Contraction, Eccentric Contraction, Concentric Contraction, Increasing ← 0 → Increasing, Velocity of Movement

of muscle physiology. A common approach for characterizing muscle is to assay the enzyme myosin ATPase (mATPase). This enzyme is located on the myosin head, hydrolyzes ATP, and enables the cross-bridge cycle. Fibers with high mATPase activity are able to hydrolyze ATP quickly and are able to contract "fast." There are also muscle fibers that express more than one type of myosin heavy chain isoform simultaneously and are known as hybrid fibers (e.g., I/IIa, IIa/IIx, I/IIa/IIx). These hybrid muscles lie on a continuum and variably express qualities of both slow and fast fibers. An alternative approach is to assess the oxidative metabolic characteristics of muscle by assaying, for example, succinate dehydrogenase (SDHase). Finally, the type of myosin heavy chain can be identified using electrophoresis. Based on these histochemically and biochemically determined classifications, a continuum (**Table 49-1**) of muscle types has been identified: (a) type I, slow-oxidative (SO);

TABLE 49-1	Muscle Fiber Type Continuum Using the Myosin ATPase Classification and Succinate Dehydrogenase Systems		
	Type I	**IIa**	**Type IIx**
Contractile speed	Low/"slow twitch"	High	Highest/"fast twitch"
Oxidative capacity	High	Intermediate	Low
Endurance capacity	High	Intermediate	Low
Force capacity	Low	High	Highest
Mitochondrial density	High	Intermediate	Low
Appearance	Intermediate	Red	White

(b) type IIa, fast-oxidative glycolytic (FOG); and (c) type IIx, fast-glycolytic (FG). The discussion below outlines how and why these fiber types are utilized during exercise.

Motor Units

Each muscle fiber is attached to a *motor unit*. A motor unit consists of a cell body, an α motor neuron, and all the fibers innervated by the motor neuron. While the fibers attached to a given motor unit are distributed across a single muscle, all the fibers within a given motor unit have nearly identical physical and biochemical characteristics. Two main categories of motor units can be distinguished—fast units and slow units. Fast units, which are attached to type II fibers, are larger than slow units, achieve peak tension and relaxation more rapidly, and achieve greater peak tension, but have a higher recruitment threshold and fatigue more rapidly. Conversely, slow units, which are attached to type I fibers, are smaller, have a lower recruitment threshold and are fatigue resistant, achieve peak tension and relaxation more slowly, and achieve a lower peak tension.

According to Henneman's size principle (10), those units with smaller cell bodies (slow motor units) will be recruited first and more frequently. Further, recruitment patterns are additive, meaning that slow motor units will be recruited when walking a normal speed or lifting a light load. When one breaks into a sprint or lifts heavy weight, slow units will still be recruited, but so too will fast motor units in order to generate the necessary force. This basic principle is an important consideration when prescribing exercise for patients experiencing sarcopenia, such as the elderly or those with type II diabetes mellitus. Sarcopenia results in selective loss of motor units that are infrequently used, that is, fast motor units. Higher-intensity exercise, including resistance training, is necessary to engage the fast motor units (11).

METABOLIC FUNDAMENTALS

The first law of thermodynamics states that "energy cannot be created or destroyed but, instead, is transformed from one form to another." Therefore, the body does not produce, consume, or use up energy; instead, it transforms it from one state into another as physiologic systems undergo continual change. This is true for generating the energy required for muscular contraction. During the cross-bridge cycle, energy, in the form of ATP, is required. A limited supply of ATP is available inside the muscle cell, which can fuel muscle contractions for a few seconds (12). However, for cellular activity to continue, ATP

must be generated. For this to occur, fuel stored in the body must be converted to ATP using the basic energy systems.

Substrate Storage

The three fuels that may be used to generate ATP for muscular contraction are carbohydrate, fat, and protein (**Table 49-2**). Because fat serves as the primary form of stored energy in the body, it is fortunate that it has a caloric density that is much higher than carbohydrate (9.3 kcal/g, compared with 4.1 kcal/g). Amino acids can also be metabolized to produce energy for muscular actions, although this contribution is generally 10% or less.

The fuel used during exercise is predominantly influenced by exercise intensity and duration. As the intensity of the exercise is increased, the predominant fuel source shifts toward carbohydrate. This is partly because ATP production shifts toward anaerobic metabolism during high-intensity exercise and the only fuel available for anaerobic glycolysis is carbohydrate. Carbohydrates are made available to the contracting muscle through mobilization of muscle and liver glycogen stores as well as through ingested carbohydrates that are circulating in the bloodstream. Exercise duration also has an effect on the fuel utilization pattern. During long bouts of exercise, fat usage in the form of free fatty acids gradually increases. Free fatty acids are made available to the contracting muscle through lipolysis of triglycerides within extramuscular (e.g., adipose) and intramuscular stores.

Considering fat is stored in abundance (**Table 49-2**), whereas carbohydrate stores are limited, there is been much interest in the use of low-carbohydrate (<25% energy), high-fat (>60% energy) diets to increase muscle fat utilization (13,14). The evidence does indicate that such diets can enhance muscle fat-burning capacity in as little as 5 days (14). However, studies have failed to detect clear performance benefits during endurance/ultra-endurance protocols. The lack of translation to performance may be explained by the following: (a) low-carbohydrate diets limit the capacity to train at high intensities; (b) impaired glycogenolysis and energy flux limit ATP production; and (c) for endurance events lasting up to 3 hours, carbohydrates are the predominant fuel for the working muscles, and therefore carbohydrate availability becomes rate limiting for performance (13).

The Basic Energy Systems and Continuum

Three energy systems interplay to replenish ATP during exercise: (a) the adenosine triphosphate–creatine phosphate (ATP-CP) system, (b) the anaerobic glycolysis system, and (c) the aerobic system (**Table 49-2**). The anaerobic system can only use

TABLE 49-2	**Power and Capacity of Energetics Processes**			
	Moles ATP Available	**Max Power mmol ATP kg⁻¹ d·wt·s⁻¹**	**Relative Exercise Intensity Supported**	**Exercise Time**
ATP stores	0.02	11.2	Very high	5–10 s
PC stores	0.34	8.6	Very high	30 s
Anaerobic glycolysis	5.2	5.2	High	7 min
Aerobic oxidation				
Carbohydrate	70	2.7	Moderate-high	90 min
Lipid	8,000	1.4	Low	350 h

ATP, adenosine triphosphate; PC, phosphocreatine.

*Assuming a male subject of 70 kg body weight, 15% body fat, and a $\dot{V}O_{2max}$ of 4.0 L/min.

Adapted from Sahlin K, Tonkonogi M, Söderlund K. Energy supply and muscle fatigue in humans. *Acta Physiol Scand.* 1998;162(3):261–266. Reprinted by permission of John Wiley & Sons, Inc.

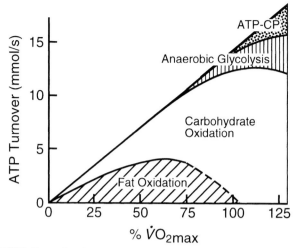

FIGURE 49-5. Relative importance of the different metabolic systems as a function of exercise intensity. (Adapted from Sahlin K. Metabolic changes limiting muscle performance. In: Saltin B, ed. *Biochemistry of Exercise VI.* Champaign, IL: Human Kinetics; 1986:323–343.)

carbohydrate to produce ATP, whereas the aerobic system can use carbohydrates, fat, and to a limited extent protein.

All three energy systems supply a portion of energy to the body at all times. However, one energy system may predominate during a particular activity. Which energy system is predominant during a given activity depends on the rate of energy (power) requirement during the activity (**Fig. 49-5**) (15). In activities performed at maximal intensity for only a few seconds (e.g., 100-m sprint), most of the ATP is supplied by the ATP-CP system. Activities of lower intensity, such as those at a maximal effort that can be sustained for 1 to 2 minutes (e.g., 400- to 800-m sprint), primarily rely on the anaerobic glycolysis system.

Longer-duration, lower-intensity activities that may last several minutes (e.g., 1,600 m) or hours (e.g., marathon) are supplied almost entirely through aerobic metabolism. However, aerobic metabolism is dependent on oxygen delivery, including the ability of the lungs to extract oxygen from the environment, the capacity of the heart to pump blood (cardiac output), and the blood flow to the active muscle fibers. Understanding these three systems, including the advantages and limitations of each system, is important for optimally conditioning an individual for participation in a particular activity or sport.

Anaerobic Metabolism

Anaerobic metabolism refers to a series of chemical reactions that do not require the presence of oxygen. Two of the systems that supply energy for muscular contraction are anaerobic.

The ATP-CP System

ATP and CP are high-energy phosphagen compounds stored within the muscle and ready for immediate use. The breakdown of ATP produces adenosine diphosphate (ADP), inorganic phosphate, and energy used in muscular contraction. The phosphate (P) can be cleaved from CP and phosphorylate ADP to ATP. This system provides an immediate source of energy for the muscle and has a large power capacity. In other words, a large amount of energy per unit time can be

supplied through this system. However, because of the small stores of ATP and CP, the total capacity for exercise with the ATP-CP system is limited. In fact, the energy resources from the ATP-CP system will be exhausted in 30 seconds or less during an all-out bout of exercise (12).

Anaerobic Glycolysis System

Glycolysis refers to a series of reactions resulting in the breakdown of carbohydrate. Anaerobic glycolysis means that this breakdown of carbohydrate is performed in the absence of oxygen. While carbohydrates can be utilized by either anaerobic or aerobic metabolism, the by-product of aerobic metabolism is pyruvate, whereas during anaerobic metabolism, pyruvate is converted to lactate.

During maximal exercise lasting 1 to 2 minutes, lactate produced by the skeletal muscles accumulates in the muscles and blood. This is accompanied by an increase in proton release causing acidosis. When the concentration of lactate is high enough, nerve endings are stimulated, resulting in the sensation of pain. In addition, the lactate within the muscle cell inhibits the production of more ATP and the binding of calcium to troponin, thereby inhibiting the cross-bridge cycle (16). As such, the amount of energy obtained from the anaerobic glycolysis system is limited. Nevertheless, the anaerobic glycolysis system is extremely important because it can provide a rapid supply of energy.

Aerobic Metabolism

In the presence of oxygen, glycolysis produces pyruvate, which is further metabolized through the tricarboxylic acid (TCA) cycle (also known as the *Krebs* or *citric acid cycle*) and electron transport system to yield carbon dioxide, water, and energy. Relative to anaerobic glycolysis, the energy produced from a given amount of carbohydrate is about 13 times greater through aerobic metabolism. Furthermore, there are no fatiguing or painful by-products through aerobic metabolism, and fat may be metabolized in addition to carbohydrates. Although the ability to metabolize fat means that this system provides a virtually unlimited source of energy, aerobic metabolism, particularly when utilizing fats, provides energy at the slowest rate of the three energy systems.

ACUTE PHYSIOLOGIC RESPONSES TO EXERCISE

During dynamic exercise, various physiologic systems must be coordinated to enable and maintain force production. In the case of short, explosive activities, neuromuscular recruitment and anaerobic metabolism are particularly important. However, in the case of more prolonged activities, the maximal ability to deliver and consume oxygen, that is, maximal oxygen uptake ($\dot{V}O_{2max}$), is crucial. The relationship between oxygen delivery and consumption can be explained by the Fick principle, developed by Adolf Fick in the 1870s. According to this principle, $\dot{V}O_{2max}$ is equal to the product of cardiac output and the arteriovenous difference [(a-v)O_2], whereby the (a-v) O_2 difference reflects oxygen being extracted by active muscle fibers. However, while $\dot{V}O_{2max}$ governs the upper limit to aerobic metabolism, the maximal lactate steady state (MLSS) governs the proportion of $\dot{V}O_{2max}$ that can be maintained for a prolonged period. Lastly, the ability to sustain a given $\dot{V}O_2$ is also dependent on the endocrine system to mobilize nutrients and preserve body fluids and the thermoregulatory system to dissipate heat.

Pulmonary

During exercise, ventilation increases from a resting value of approximately 6 to 10 L/min up to 100 to 125 L/min in untrained participants and 150 to 200 L/min in well-trained athletes (17). Accompanying the changes in ventilation, there are increases in mean pulmonary arterial pressure, increases in pulmonary blood flow, and improvements in the ventilation-perfusion ratio. The pulmonary system does not tend to be a limiting factor for exercise performance in persons without pulmonary disorders at sea level (17).

Cardiovascular

Once oxygen has been inspired into the lungs, it diffuses from the alveoli to the capillaries surrounding the alveoli and is bound to the protein hemoglobin. The oxygenated hemoglobin is transported to the left atrium by way of the pulmonary veins and then into the left ventricle prior to being pumped into the systematic circulation. From here, adequate oxygen delivery is dependent on two factors: (a) the amount of blood pumped out of the left ventricle per minute, or cardiac output, and (b) the ability of the autonomic nervous system to direct the blood. These factors can limit exercise performance.

Cardiac output, which is the product of heart rate and stroke volume, can increase from approximately 5 L/min at rest up to 20 L/min in untrained participants and 40 L/min or more in well-trained athletes (18). To achieve this increase in cardiac output, heart rate increases in direct proportion to exercise rate, or $\dot{V}O_2$, and stroke volume increases until somewhere between 40% and 60% of $\dot{V}O_{2\,max}$ (18,19). The rise in heart rate is controlled by the autonomic nervous system, including parasympathetic withdrawal and increased sympathetic nerve activity. The rise in stroke volume is a function of increased contractility, also resulting from increased sympathetic activity, and increased myocardial preload. Increased preload, which can be defined as the initial stretching of the cardiac myocytes prior to contraction, increases as a function of enhanced venous return. Venous return is enhanced through muscle contraction (muscle pump) and venoconstriction. Collectively, the increased left ventricular end-diastolic volume (preload), coupled with the more complete emptying of the left ventricle (contractility), leads to a great volume of blood being pumped each contraction cycle. However, the upper limit for stroke volume tends to plateau between 40% and 60% of $\dot{V}O_{2\,max}$ when the contraction cycle (heart rate) becomes too fast, and there is inadequate time to fill the left ventricle prior to contraction (preload). Any subsequent increase in cardiac output is attributed to heart rate.

Up to 80% of cardiac output can be distributed to the active muscles at maximal effort, compared with only about 20% of cardiac output being distributed to the muscles at rest and other organs (20). Marked blood flow redistribution is accomplished by arterial vasodilation in the active muscles and arterial vasoconstriction in other vascular regions (e.g., splanchnic, inactive muscle, renal) (20). Although muscle

sympathetic nerve activity appears to increase in the active muscles, metabolic by-products override this vasoconstriction effect to produce vasodilation. Control of the autonomic nervous system during exercise originates from both central and peripheral receptors located in the motor cortex, ergoreceptors, and arterial and cardiopulmonary baroreceptors (21).

Lactate Threshold and Maximal Lactate Steady State

The aerobic lactate threshold refers to the intensity of exercise at which blood lactate begins to rise above resting values, whereas MLSS (also referred to as the anaerobic lactate or ventilatory threshold) refers to the intensity of exercise at which a continuous increase in blood lactate is unavoidable (22). Although the precise mechanism(s) for MLSS is unresolved, a number of factors may explain the continuous increase in blood lactate, including (a) insufficient lactate removal by the heart, liver, and kidneys; (b) increased activation of the sympathetic nervous system, resulting in increased glycogenosis and decreased blood flow to the liver and kidneys; (c) insufficient supply of oxygen to active mitochondria; (d) imbalance between glycolysis and mitochondrial respiration; and (e) recruitment of FG muscle fibers (**Table 49-1**), which produce lactate whether or not oxygen is available (17). As discussed above, high concentrations of lactate result in the sensation of pain, inhibit the production of ATP, and interfere with cross-bridge recycling (16).

While $\dot{V}O_{2\,max}$ governs the upper limit to aerobic metabolism, the MLSS governs the proportion of $\dot{V}O_{2\,max}$ that can be maintained for a prolonged period. This concept is of particular importance to elite endurance athletes, including long-distance runners (**Fig. 49-6**). In elite runners, $\dot{V}O_{2\,max}$ demonstrates limited improvements with training, whereas the running velocity at which MLSS occurs is highly trainable and correlates well with improved running performance (19,23).

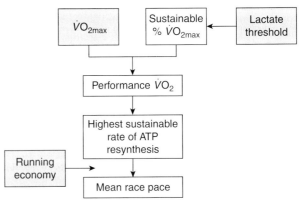

FIGURE 49-6. Flow diagram showing that long-distance running performance is predominantly determined by maximal oxygen uptake ($\dot{V}O_2$), the lactate threshold (determines the fraction of $\dot{V}O_{2\,max}$ that can be sustained), and running economy. Performance oxygen uptake ($\dot{V}O_2$) represents the highest mean $\dot{V}O_2$ that can be sustained during the race. Running economy refers to how efficient the runner is at converting available energy into running speed. ATP, adenosine triphosphate. (Reprinted by permission from Springer: Midgley AW, McNaughton LR, Jones AM. Training to enhance the physiologic determinants of long-distance running performance: can valid recommendations be given to runners and coaches based on current scientific knowledge? *Sports Med.* 2007;37(10):857–880. Copyright © 2007 Adis Data Information BV.)

Endocrine

Hormones released from the endocrine system are essential for mobilizing fuels and maintaining fuel homeostasis. The levels of several hormones including catecholamines (epinephrine and norepinephrine), growth hormone, cortisol, and glucagon increase during exercise, while insulin decreases (24). Collectively, these changes promote the breakdown of muscle glycogen, increase blood glucose, and increase lipolysis and mobilization of free fatty acids (25). In addition, activation of the renin-angiotensin-aldosterone and release of antidiuretic hormone assist in maintaining blood volume by retaining sodium and water, respectively. The release of the aforementioned hormones plays a crucial role during sustained exercise.

Thermoregulation

The final product of metabolism is heat. Particularly during prolonged exercise, this heat production can lead to marked increases in core temperature and subsequent heat illness if not managed. The heat produced following cellular activity is transported to cutaneous vascular beds via the cardiovascular system, where it is dissipated predominantly by evaporation. This increased blood flow is accomplished in part by blood flow redistribution away from splanchnic and renal arterial vascular beds.

Sustained levels of high work intensity, especially when performed in combination with heat stress, can lead to high rates of sweat loss, reaching 2 to 3 L/h. These rates of sweating can lead to dehydration and decreased total blood volume. The loss of blood volume, coupled with increased cutaneous blood flow, can lead to *cardiovascular drift*. Cardiovascular drift refers to the increase in heart rate during prolonged exercise with little or no change in exercise rate. Heart rate increases to compensate for decreased stroke volume, which occurs due to decreased preload as a function of decreased venous return. To avoid excessive fluid/electrolyte during prolonged exercise, the ideal hydration practice is to consume fluid at a rate and composition approximate to that of sweat loss (26).

Static (Isometric) Exercise

The hemodynamic responses to static (isometric) exercise are related to the percentage of maximal voluntary contraction (MVC) and the amount of muscle mass involved in the contraction (27). Increases in $\dot{V}O_2$, cardiac output, and heart rate are typically modest during static exercise compared with dynamic exercise (**Fig. 49-7**) (28). Additionally, total peripheral vascular resistance does not decrease, and stroke volume typically fails to rise as occurs with dynamic exercise. However, blood pressure, especially mean and diastolic blood pressure, can significantly increase. The rise in blood pressure can be attributed to a pressor response, which occurs due to mechanical and metabolic activation of skeletal muscle afferent nerve fibers (29). The metabolic activation of afferent nerve fibers can be attributed to the effects of static exercise on blood flow.

Blood flow through the active muscle is dependent on a balance between metabolically induced vasodilation and mechanical restriction of flow associated with contraction of the surrounding muscle. At high static efforts, blood flow through the active muscle is restricted and may be completely occluded. Reduced muscle blood flow relative to metabolic

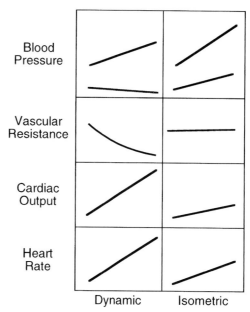

FIGURE 49-7. Schematic comparison of hemodynamic responses to dynamic and isometric exercise. (Adapted from Hanson P, Rueckert P. Hypertension. In: Pollock ML, Schmidt DH, eds. *Heart Disease and Rehabilitation.* 3rd ed. Champaign, IL: Human Kinetics; 1995:343–356.)

demands results in greater reliance on anaerobic metabolism, greater metabolic waste, and earlier onset of fatigue than occurs with dynamic exercise (19,29).

THE PRESCRIPTION OF EXERCISE

General Considerations

Despite the well-known benefits of physical activity and regular exercise, physical inactivity remains a global pandemic (30). There is an ever-growing recognition of the vital importance of the medical community in the promotion of physical activity. *Exercise is Medicine* is one such program based on the concept that it is both the role and the responsibility of the clinician to prescribe exercise to patients who would benefit from it (31). The Foundation for PM&R has also begun an initiative called *Rx for Exercise* emphasizing the importance of doctor-recommended exercises (www.foundationforpmr.org/ADF).

Although the specific goals of an exercise program depend on the individual, basic exercise goals include counteracting the detrimental effects of sedentary living or reduced activity, for example, from disease or injury, and optimizing functional capacity. Additionally, exercise training programs can provide valuable clinical information for the ongoing treatment of a patient. Using these basic goals as a foundation, an individual's specific health history, risk factors, behavioral characteristics, personal goals, and exercise preferences will shape and detail the exercise prescription.

Appropriate exercise prescriptions should systematically and individually recommend physical activity to develop fitness, maintain health, and/or treat specific conditions. The optimal exercise prescription should address the health-related physical fitness components of cardiorespiratory (aerobic) fitness; muscular strength, power, and endurance; flexibility; body composition; and neuromotor fitness (32). Also, due to the known health risks of long periods of sedentary activity

(33), it should include a plan to decrease periods of inactivity in addition to an increase in physical activity (34).

As a starting point for the prescription of exercise, it is important to familiarize oneself with established recommendations for activity for all individuals. Current physical activity guidelines from the American College of Sports Medicine (ACSM) and the American Heart Association (AHA) can be found in **Table 49-3**.

The 2018 Physical Activity Guidelines for Americans (1) report has similar recommendations but with a greater emphasis on acquired volume of exercise per week, an elimination of the requirement for adults to accrue exercise in bouts of at least 10 minutes, and new guidelines for preschool-aged children and children and adolescents. A summary of these guidelines can be seen in 🛜 **eTable 49-1**.

Adaptation and Adherence

It is important to remember that the prescription of exercise will not benefit patients without their acceptance and participation. However, if this were easily achieved, the numbers of individuals engaging in moderate-to-vigorous physical activity in the United States still would not be at low levels (35). No single approach for encouraging patients to become regular exercisers works for everyone. Indeed, there are at least six behavioral theories one can employ to understand exercise participation and the factors that may facilitative or impede physical activity (34). Motivation is the one common requirement necessary for exercise participation and adherence. For the most part, it must be inner-directed (36). Various evidence-based cognitive and behavioral strategies are presented in **Table 49-4** to aid the clinician in helping patients find their motivation to increase physical activity.

Brief counseling using the "five As" model is a promising area for helping patients resolve ambivalence and increase their motivation for change (37). With this technique, the clinician (a) **A**ssesses physical activity behavior, beliefs, knowledge, and readiness to change; (b) **A**dvises patients on the benefits of physical activity and the health risks of inactivity; (c) **A**grees collaboratively on physical activity goals based on patient's interests, confidence, ability, and readiness to change; (d)

TABLE 49-3	The ACSM-AHA Physical Activity Recommendations

- All healthy adults aged 18–65 years should participate in moderate-intensity aerobic physical activity for a minimum of 30 minutes on 5 days/week or vigorous-intensity aerobic physical activity for a minimum of 20 minutes on 3 days/week
- Combinations of moderate- and vigorous-intensity exercise can be performed to meet this recommendation
- Moderate-intensity aerobic activity can be accumulated to total the 30-minute minimum by performing bouts each lasting 10 minutes or more
- Every adult should perform activities that maintain or increase muscular strength and endurance for a minimum of 2 days/week
- Because of the dose-response relationships between physical activity and health, individuals who wish to further improve their fitness, reduce their risk for chronic disease and disabilities, and/or prevent unhealthy weight gain may benefit by exceeding the minimum recommended amounts of physical activity

Reprinted with permission from Pescatello LS, American College of Sports Medicine. *ACSM's Guidelines for Exercise Testing and Prescription.* 9th ed. Philadelphia, PA: Wolters Kluwer Health/Lippincott Williams & Wilkins; 2013.

TABLE 49-4	Cognitive and Behavioral Strategies for Increasing Physical Activity
Cognitive-Behavioral Strategy	**Description**
Enhancing self-efficacy	Increase individuals' confidence by ensuring realistic goals, watching others similar to them have positive experiences, offering encouragement, and helping them experience positive mood states
Goal setting	Help individuals establish specific, measurable, action-oriented, realistic, timely, and self-determined (SMARTS) short- and long-term goals
Reinforcement	Encourage individuals to reward themselves for meeting behavioral goals. Reinforcements can be external or internal
Social support	Encourage individuals to enlist social support for physical activity from family, friends, and coworkers
Self-monitoring	Encourage individuals to track their physical activity through a physical activity log, pedometer, smart watch, or other technology device
Problem solving	Help individuals find ways to overcome barriers to physical activity
Relapse prevention	Prepare individuals for lapses in physical activity and develop plans for overcoming them so that lapses do not become relapses

Derived from American College of Sports Medicine. In: Riebe D, Ehrman J, Liguori G, et al., eds. *ACSM's Guidelines for Exercise Testing and Prescription.* 10th ed. Philadelphia, PA: Wolters Kluwer; 2017.

Assists patients to identify and overcome barriers using problem-solving techniques and social and environmental support and resources; and (e) **A**rranges a specific plan for follow-up, feedback, assessment, and support (34). In general, the behavioral change process is facilitated when the patient becomes an active partner in the decision-making process, and the process is then codified by a written exercise prescription (38).

A key principle to improve the likelihood of adoption of a life-long habit of regular exercise is goal setting—a powerful tool that leads to positive changes in exercise behavior by mobilizing motivation (38,39). Using the SMARTS principle will help individuals establish effective goals: (a) **S**pecific—goals should be precise; an exercise prescription is invaluable here; (b) **M**easurable—goals should be quantifiable; (c) **A**ction-oriented—goals should indicate what needs to be done; (d) **R**ealistic—goals should be achievable; (e) **T**imely—goals should have a specific and realistic time frame; and (f) **S**elf-determined—goals should be developed primarily by the patient.

Another important factor in establishing regular exercise habits is prioritizing a time for exercise. Individuals should be encouraged to initially focus on finding the time to establish a regular pattern of exercise rather than on an amount (38). If a protected amount of time is not achievable, individuals should be encouraged to build physical activity into their normal routines and/or participate in more active recreational activities. Examples include using a walk-behind mower, taking the stairs, getting off the bus at an earlier stop, meeting for a walk instead of a coffee, and parking at the far end of the parking lot. Other useful strategies include beginning an exercise program in small increments with a gradual progression over weeks and emphasizing that some exercise or physical activity is better than none (38). An approach of gradual progression of intensity and volume will decrease the likelihood of overuse and other musculoskeletal injuries and thus cessation of the activity. Lastly, an appreciation of potential unique beliefs, cultural values, environments, and health conditions that may exist across diverse populations will help ensure proper tailoring of physical activity recommendations to promote adherence (34).

Components of the Exercise Prescription

An individually tailored exercise prescription to improve physical fitness and health can be developed for most patients using the FITT-VP principle: frequency, intensity, time (duration), type (mode), volume (quantity), and progression (advancement) (40). This formula can also be applied to patients with various health conditions and disabilities when appropriately screened as detailed later in this section. It is infinitely adaptable to an individual's circumstance, needs, and goals.

Frequency refers to the number of days per week dedicated to physical activity. In general, aerobic exercise should occur 3 to 5 days per week dependent upon intensity, resistance and flexibility training should occur 2 to 3 days per week, and neuromotor exercise training involving balance, agility, coordination, and gait is recommended at least 2 to 3 days per week (5,34).

Intensity refers to the rate at which the activity is being performed or the magnitude of the effort required to perform an activity or exercise. It can be thought of as "How hard a person works to perform the activity" (41). In regard to the overload principle, an individual should reach a minimum threshold of activity, which is a level of intensity at which the body is challenged enough to change physiologic parameters (34). This minimum threshold of intensity for benefit varies depending on an individual's level of fitness and other factors, and there is a positive dose response of health and fitness benefits that result from increasing intensity (5,34). Intensity can be measured and monitored in a number of practical ways, some more subjective than others. Examples include heart rate monitoring, the Borg Rating of Perceived Exertion (RPE) scale, the talk test, and motion sensors (42). Currently, there are no studies available comparing all exercise prescription intensity methods against each other, and thus the methods may not be equivalent. **Table 49-5** provides an overview of some of these measures.

In general, the more subjective, but simpler, "talk test" (43) and Borg RPE scale (44) will translate more easily from the exam room to real-world applicability. Also, relative measures of intensity (e.g., percent of heart rate reserve [HRR] or Borg RPE) are often more appropriate than absolute measures for individual exercise prescription, especially for older and deconditioned individuals (45–47). A more detailed explanation of intensity will follow in subsequent sections.

Time of exercise, or duration, refers to the amount of time physical activity is performed. As previously noted, it is recommended that most adults accumulate between 75 and 150 minutes per week of aerobic exercise and that moderate-intensity physical activity be accumulated in bouts of ≥ 10 minutes each (5,34). In sedentary individuals, continuous exercise sessions of less than 20 minutes per day or bouts less than 10 minutes at a time can be beneficial, but for weight management, longer durations of exercise along the lines of 60 to 90 minutes per day may be needed (34,48). High-intensity aerobic interval training done in bouts of less than 10 minutes may also yield favorable adaptations in deconditioned individuals, but further research is needed (5,49,50).

The type of physical activity chosen for the exercise prescription must take into consideration the patient's preferences, capabilities, goals, health status, environment, available equipment and facilities, and existing fitness level. Rhythmic aerobic-type exercises involving large muscle groups are recommended for improving cardiorespiratory fitness (5). Walking is a good example. It is available to most individuals and is an appropriate initial activity for sedentary patients. Other activities of various intensities are also appropriate when performed for the necessary time. 📶 **eTable 49-2** gives examples of activities with their associated intensities in metabolic equivalents of tasks (METs). Types of resistance exercise training can include machines, free weights, resistance bands, and even body weight. Multijoint exercises affecting more than one muscle group and targeting agonist and antagonist muscle groups are recommended for all adults, and single-joint exercises can also be included (34).

The volume, or quantity, of aerobic exercise is a product of frequency, intensity, and time and is a representation of energy expenditure (34). Energy expenditure can be expressed in a standardized manner as MET/min and kcal/min and will be discussed in greater detail later in the chapter. It has been established that there is a dose-response association between the volume of aerobic exercise and health outcomes, and it is known that an energy expenditure of approximately 1,000 kcal/wk, which equates to about 150 minutes per week of moderate-intensity physical activity, is associated with lower rates of cardiovascular disease (CVD) and premature mortality (5). As measures of energy expenditure, MET/min and kcal/min are

TABLE 49-5	Classification of Exercise Intensity					
Intensity	**Subjective/Relative Measures**		**Objective/Relative Measures**		**Absolute Measure**
	"Talk test"	**Perceived exertion (6–20 RPE scale)**	**% HRR or % $\dot{V}O_2R$**	**%HR_{max}**	**METs**
Light	Able to talk and/or sing	9–11	30–39	57–63	2.0–2.9
Moderate	Able to talk but not sing	12–13	40–59	64–76	3.0–5.9
Vigorous/hard	Difficulty talking	14–17	60–89	77–95	6.0–8.7

HR_{max}, maximal heart rate (HR); %HR_{max}, percent of maximal HR; HRR, HR reserve; $\dot{V}O_2R$, oxygen uptake reserve; METs, metabolic equivalent units (1 MET = an oxygen uptake of 3.5 [mL/kg/min]).
Derived from Pescatello LS, American College of Sports Medicine. *ACSM's Guidelines for Exercise Testing and Prescription.* 9th ed. Philadelphia, PA: Wolters Kluwer Health/Lippincott Williams & Wilkins; 2013.

often used to estimate exercise volume in research, but are seldom used for exercise prescription for individuals (5). Of note, lower volumes of exercise, for example, 300 to 500 kcal/wk, can result in fitness benefits, especially in inactive individuals (1). In resistance training, volume is the sum of the number of repetitions and sets performed multiplied by the resistance used and reflects the duration muscles are being stressed (51). This training variable will be discussed more thoroughly later in the chapter.

Progression of an aerobic exercise program occurs by increasing frequency, intensity, time (duration), or a combination of these components. In a resistance program, progression is accomplished by increasing the resistance lifted, the repetitions performed, and/or the frequency the muscle groups are trained (34). The rate of progression will depend upon the patient's health, fitness level, and goals. It should occur gradually to avoid injury, muscle soreness, and excessive fatigue and to promote long-term adherence. For an initial aerobic exercise program with a patient selecting a duration of exercise that can be accomplished three times a week at a low-to-moderate intensity, progression should begin with an increase in exercise time/duration of 5 to 10 minutes per session every 1 to 2 weeks over the first 4 to 6 weeks. After the patient has been exercising for a month or more, frequency, intensity, and time can be gradually progressed over 4 to 8 months (or longer for very deconditioned individuals) until the recommended guidelines are met (34). For more detailed models of progression in exercise prescription, the interested reader is referred to *ACSM's Exercise is Medicine* (38). To progressively overload muscle as they adapt to resistance training, muscle fatigue must occur. Muscles can be fatigued by increasing resistance, repetitions, and frequency, with the goal of increasing muscle mass and strength. Further details will be outlined in subsequent sections.

Risk Assessment

Previous recommendations from the ACSM for preparticipation health screening focused on reducing the likelihood of "at-risk" individuals experiencing serious exercise-related cardiovascular (CV) events (40). Individuals were stratified as low, moderate, and high risk for CV disease, and those at moderate risk were recommended to undergo a medical examination prior to starting a vigorous exercise program. While vigorous-intensity exercise has a small acute risk of CV disease complications, particularly in sedentary men and women with known or occult CV disease, the absolute and relative risks of a CV event during exercise are extremely low and the risk decreases with increasing volumes of regular exercise (2). Much of the risk associated with vigorous exercise can be mitigated by gradually increasing the duration, frequency, and intensity of exercise over 2 to 3 months (52,1). Because the benefits of exercise far outweigh the risks of remaining sedentary in most children and adults and studies have suggested that using the previous ACSM screening process can result in excessive physician referrals and possibly create a barrier to exercise participation, the ACSM updated the preparticipation process (2,34).

The new ACSM exercise preparticipation health screening algorithm (**Fig. 49-8**) is designed to identify individuals at risk for CV complications during, or immediately after, aerobic exercise. There is currently insufficient evidence on CV complications during resistance training to make formal prescreening recommendations (34). The new health screening process is based on (a) the individual's current level of physical activity; (b) presence of signs or symptoms and/or known cardiovascular, metabolic, or renal disease; and (c) desired exercise intensity, because these three factors have been identified as important risk modulators of exercise-related cardiovascular events (2).

Both healthy and asymptomatic physically active and inactive (i.e., not performing structured physical activity of at least 30 minutes at moderate intensity, at least 3 days per week for the last 3 months) individuals may continue moderate-to-vigorous, or begin light-to-moderate, exercise, respectively, without medical clearance (2). Asymptomatic physically active individuals with known CV, metabolic, or renal disease may begin moderate-intensity exercise without medical clearance, but all other categories should undergo medical clearance (2). An important point is that the type of medical clearance is left to the discretion of the provider to whom the participant is referred because there is no single, universally recommended screening test (34). In adults, the risk of exercise-induced CV events can be reduced with an exercise prescription that (a) addresses the FITT-VP principle of exercise prescription, (b) encourages appropriated warm-up and cool-down strategies, (c) promotes education of warning signs/symptoms (e.g., chest pain or pressure, light-headedness, heart palpitations/arrhythmias, unusual shortness of breath), (d) encourages sedentary individuals to engage in regular brisk walking, and (e) counsels physically inactive individuals to avoid unaccustomed vigorous- to near maximal-intensity physical activity (2).

Children and young adults rarely die during physical activity, but the infrequent deaths that occur generally relate to congenital and hereditary abnormalities including hypertrophic cardiomyopathy, coronary artery abnormalities, and aortic stenosis (34). Sudden cardiac death (SCD) is the leading cause of death during exercise for athletes younger than 35 years (53), with structural cardiac abnormalities responsible for 84% of SCDs among competitive athletes (54). The best screening protocol for detecting athletes at risk for SCD is still under debate. The AHA recommends the use of a 14-element history and physical examination (H&P) (54), whereas European standards call for a focused H&P and 12-lead electrocardiogram (ECG) (55). ECG screening in the United States has been repeatedly rejected because of the high rate of false-positive results and an abundance of evidence suggesting that it is a cost-ineffective tool for screening (56). However, in its recent position stand, the American Medical Society for Sports Medicine stated the absence of definitive outcome-based evidence precludes it from endorsing any single or universal cardiovascular screening strategy for all athletes (57). Point-of-care preparticipation screening echocardiography by a frontline physician is another method that is appealing in its ability to detect structural abnormalities and seems to offer promising reliability and feasibility (56).

Injury and Illness Precautions

All exercises carry some risk of injury, but individualizing the exercise prescription minimizes the chance of causing or exacerbating health problems. The intensity and type of exercise may be the most important factors related to the incidence of injury (5). Stretching, warm-up and cool-down periods, and

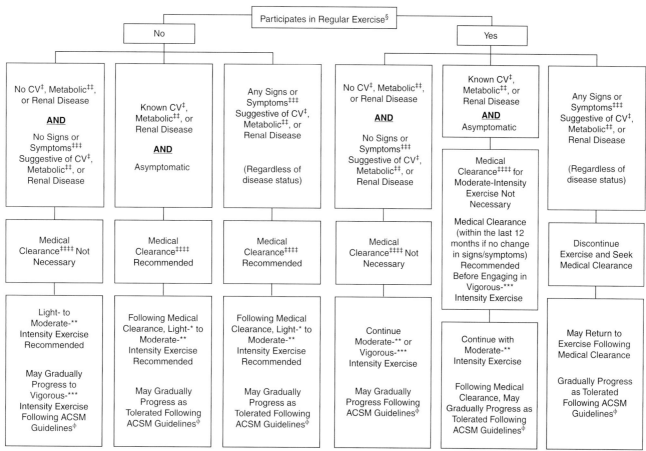

FIGURE 49-8. Exercise preparticipation health screening logic model for aerobic exercise participation. §Exercise participation, performing planned, structured physical activity at least 30 minutes at moderate intensity on at least 3 days/week for at least the last 3 months. *Light-intensity exercise, 30% to less than 40% HRR or $\dot{V}O_2R$, 2 to less than 3 METs, 9 to 11 RPE, an intensity that causes slight increases in HR and breathing. **Moderate-intensity exercise, 40% to less than 60% HRR or $\dot{V}O_2R$, 3 to less than 6 METs, 12 to 13 RPE, an intensity that causes noticeable increases in HR and breathing. ***Vigorous-intensity exercise, ≥60% HRR or $\dot{V}O_2R$, ≥6 METs, ≥14 RPE, an intensity that causes substantial increases in HR and breathing. ‡CVD, cardiac, peripheral vascular, or cerebrovascular disease. ‡‡Metabolic disease, type 1 and 2 diabetes mellitus. ‡‡‡Signs and symptoms, at rest or during activity; include pain and discomfort in the chest, neck, jaw, arms, or other areas that may result from ischemia; shortness of breath at rest or with mild exertion; dizziness or syncope; orthopnea or paroxysmal nocturnal dyspnea; ankle edema; palpitations or tachycardia; intermittent claudication; known heart murmur; or unusual fatigue or shortness of breath with usual activities. ‡‡‡‡Medical clearance, approval from a health care professional to engage in exercise. φACSM *Guidelines, see ACSM's Guidelines for Exercise Testing and Prescription,* 9th edition, 2014. (Reprinted with permission from Riebe D, Franklin BA, Thompson PD, et al. Updating ACSM's recommendations for exercise preparticipation health screening. *Med Sci Sports Exerc.* 2015;47(11):2473–2479.)

gradual progression of exercise intensity and volume are commonly used methods to reduce musculoskeletal injuries, but their effectiveness is unconfirmed (5).

Exercise also exerts a noticeable influence on immune function. Individual exercise bouts transiently alter immune status, but this acute response reverses with moderate chronic training; appropriately trained individuals demonstrate better immune function and decreased risk of infection compared to sedentary counterparts (58–60). The stress imposed by overtraining (i.e., an imbalance between training volume and recovery) will increase the incidence of infection and illness in athletes, but further studies are required to determine the individual contributions of intensive exercise versus recovery on the immune system (61,62). No studies have systematically determined the effects of repeated aerobic exercise bouts of different intensity and duration on immunosuppression, and there are also no data on the effects of repeated bouts of anaerobic or resistance/strength exercise or a combination of different types of exercise on the same day (62). Among the

various nutritional interventions and physical therapies (e.g., massage, vibration therapy, electrical stimulation, cold-water immersion, compression garments) that that have been studied to counteract immunodepression during exercise recovery, carbohydrate supplementation has been proven the most effective (62). How exercise affects the progression of existing infectious diseases is poorly understood, but there is no evidence to suggest regular participation in an exercise program of moderate intensity will suppress immune function of asymptomatic or symptomatic individuals with HIV (34). During an active viral infection manifest by fever, malaise, myalgia, and/or anorexia, individuals should avoid strenuous exercise as myocarditis can develop (63).

Environmental Factors

Hot and/or humid conditions increase the physiologic challenge and health risk associated with exercise. Combining exercise and environmental heat stress produces a competition for blood flow between active muscle (to deliver oxygen

TABLE 49-6	**Fluid Replacement Recommendations Before, During, and After Exercise**	
	Fluid	**Comments**
Before exercise	• Drink 5–7 mL/kg at least 4 h before exercise (12–17 oz for 154 lb individual)	• If urine is not produced or very dark, drink another 3–5 mL/kg before exercise • Sodium-containing beverages or salted snacks will help retain fluid
During exercise	• Monitor individual body weight changes during exercise to estimate sweat loss • Composition of fluid should include 20–30 mEq/L of sodium, 2–5 mEq/L of potassium, and 5%–10% of carbohydrate	• Prevent a >2% loss in body weight • Amount and rate of fluid replacement depend on individual sweating rate, environment, and exercise duration
After exercise	• Consumption of normal meals and beverages will restore euhydration • If rapid recovery is needed, drink 1.5 L/kg of body weight lost	• Goal is to fully replace fluid and electrolyte deficits • Consuming sodium will help recovery by stimulating thirst and fluid retention

Adapted from Sawka MN, Burke LM, Eichner ER, et al. American College of Sports Medicine position stand. Exercise and fluid replacement. *Med Sci Sports Exerc.* 2007;39(2):377–390; Armstrong LE, Casa DJ, Millard-Stafford M, et al. American College of Sports Medicine position stand. Exertional heat illness during training and competition. *Med Sci Sports Exerc.* 2007;39(3):556–572.

and nutrients) and cutaneous vascular beds (to dissipate heat), reducing exercise performance and/or thermoregulatory capacity (64). Decreases in total body water (i.e., hypohydration) exacerbate this situation by increasing core temperature, heart rate, and perceived exertion (65). To counteract dehydration, determining sweat rate by measuring body weight before and after exercise provides a fluid replacement guide. Active individuals should drink 0.5 L (1 pint) of fluid for each pound of body weight lost (66). **Table 49-6** provides recommendations for hydration prior to, during, and following exercise or physical activity (66,67).

Acclimatization allows for optimal performance in hot or humid weather through decreased core temperature, heart rate, RPE, and sweat salt and increased sweat rate and exercise tolerance time (68). Seasonal acclimatization will occur gradually through exposure to the heat, but this process can be facilitated through a structured moderate exercise program in the heat across 10 to 14 days (34). If an exercise prescription specifies a target heart rate, reducing the workload to maintain the same target heart rate in the heat will help reduce the risk of heat illness (e.g., heat exhaustion) during acclimatization (34). For further details, see the ACSM Position Stand describing heat illnesses during exercise (67).

In extremely cold environments, exercisers must protect against hypothermia and cold injuries to exposed skin (frostbite and nonfreezing cold injuries). Hypothermia develops when heat loss exceeds heat production and has an increased risk with immersion, rain, wet clothing, low body fat, age 60 and above, and hypoglycemia (69). Cold injuries occur less frequently than heat illnesses because exercise produces large metabolic heat loads, defending core temperature against all but the coldest temperatures. However, exercise-related cold stress may increase the risk of morbidity and mortality in at-risk populations such as those with CVD and asthmatic conditions (34). In most conditions, appropriately layered clothing and protection of sensitive areas (e.g., hands, feet, and face) allow exercise to continue comfortably. Shoveling snow, walking in snow, and swimming in water less than 25°C can pose a risk to individuals with CVD by substantially increasing pressure rate product or energy requirements or blunting angina symptoms, and therefore exercise intensity and/or duration should be reduced (34,69,70). After repeated exposures to

a cold environment, the body does exhibit adaptations that enhance heat production or minimize heat loss; however, cold acclimatization causes far less dramatic physiologic changes than does heat acclimatization (69).

Exposure to moderate (1,200 to 2,400 m) and high (>2,400 m) altitudes also challenges exercise. Altitude exposure reduces work capacity because the lower atmospheric pressure directly translates to less available oxygen. The body compensates by increasing ventilation and cardiac output, the latter usually through an increase in heart rate. Physical performance decreases with increasing altitude above 1,200 m (3,937 ft) for most people (34). Acclimatization consists of physiologic changes acquired during repeated or continuous exposures to moderate and high altitudes—changes that benefit exercise performance (primarily through increased blood oxygen–carrying capacity) and reduce the incidence of altitude-related illnesses (e.g., acute mountain sickness). Stays at moderate altitude of at least 3 days are necessary to reduce the incidence of altitude sickness, and 6 to 12 days are required to improve physical work performance (34). For an exercise prescription specifying a target heart rate, the individual should maintain the same heart rate at higher elevations (34). Available information suggests cardiac patients can safely exercise to at least moderate altitudes (71,72).

Air pollution detrimentally affects exercise performance. Several air pollutants (e.g., particulate matter, carbon monoxide, sulfur dioxide, nitrogen oxides, and ozone) negatively impact work tolerance or cardiovascular responses to exercise (73,74). Furthermore, increased pulmonary ventilation during exercise exposes the individual to increased doses of pollutants. As strong evidence now suggests a link between air pollution and CVD (75), individuals should avoid exercising in highly polluted areas or near traffic congestion and in environments where ozone reaches a critical threshold. These recommendations especially apply to those with coronary artery or pulmonary disease.

AEROBIC EXERCISE

Physiologic Adaptations to Aerobic Conditioning

As early as the 1960s and 1970s, investigators have sought to understand how patients were able to increase their overall aerobic capacity by engaging in aerobic conditioning. Aerobic exercise training produces many physiologic adaptations

TABLE 49-7	Physiologic Adaptations to Aerobic Exercise		
Respiratory	**Cardiovascular**	**Musculoskeletal**
↑O_2 exchange in lungs	↑ Cardiac output	↑ Capillarization
↑Blood flow through lungs	↑ Blood volume	↑ Mitochondrial size and density
↓Submax respiratory rate	↑ Blood flow to skeletal muscle	↑ Myoglobin concentration
↓Submax pulmonary ventilation	↓ Submax heart rate	↑ Enzyme concentration
	↑ Thermoregulation	↑ a-VO_2 diff

(Table 49-7). An important adaptation is increased exercise capacity, or $\dot{V}O_{2\,max}$. As previously noted, the $\dot{V}O_{2\,max}$ can be mathematically defined as the product of maximal cardiac output and maximal arteriovenous oxygen difference and assesses the integrated functioning of the pulmonary, cardiovascular, and muscle systems to uptake (diffusive O_2 transport at the lung and muscle microvasculature), transport (conductive O_2 transport), and utilize O_2 predominantly in the contracting muscle mitochondria (76). Most studies indicate that sedentary people within diverse populations (age, gender, income, ethnic background, health status) will experience ≥15% improvement in $\dot{V}O_{2\,max}$ within 3 months of starting aerobic training (17,77,78). This increase is caused about equally by central cardiovascular adaptations that raise maximal cardiac output and peripheral adaptations that enhance oxygen extraction from the circulating blood (17).

The rise in maximal cardiac output with aerobic conditioning resides in increased stroke volume. Maximal heart rate does not rise with aerobic conditioning and may even be lower in well-conditioned endurance athletes than in sedentary individuals. The mechanism by which maximal stroke volume increases appears to be related to an increase in cardiac preload, which in turn is related to the rise in total blood volume that occurs with aerobic training and which is likely the main mechanism for endurance-enhanced increases in maximal cardiac output (17,79). Enhanced myocardial contractility and relaxation as well as a reduced end-systolic volume may also play a role (80,81). As training progresses, a common finding among male endurance athletes is an increased heart size (athlete's heart) characterized by increased left ventricular end-diastolic volume and a proportional increase in left ventricular mass and normal wall tension (82,83). While highly trained women frequently show cardiac adaptations, they rarely demonstrate cardiac dimensional changes outside of normal limits (84). It is important to note that the enlarged heart of the athlete differs from the enlarged heart in hypertension and congestive heart failure where indices of left ventricular function are impaired (85). In the athlete, left ventricular hypertrophy is eccentric rather than concentric, and ventricular dilation is proportional to wall thickness.

Increased oxygen extraction with aerobic training stems from changes within the trained muscle, including increased capillary density, capillary-fiber ratio, and tissue myoglobin (17). Aerobic training will also increase the amount of retinaculum and respiratory enzyme capacity per mitochondrion, and recent research has determined that exercise volume may be important in increasing mitochondrial content whereas exercise intensity is important for increasing mitochondrial function (86,87). These muscular adaptations are believed to raise the anaerobic lactate threshold (or MLSS) through enhanced oxidative capacity and improve tolerance for sustained work.

Physiologic adaptations to aerobic training are not restricted to conditioning programs that focus on the legs. Arm training is more stressful than leg training as measured by a number of parameters and can result in improvements in peak oxygen uptake through increases in cardiac output and stroke volume (central) and arteriovenous oxygen differences (peripheral), especially in subjects who are initially unfit (88,89). However, specificity of training takes precedent, and there is limited transfer of training benefit from one set of limbs to the other, with improvements in exercise performance, to include $\dot{V}O_{2\,max}$, due primarily to peripheral adaptations in the trained muscles (90,91).

Assessment of Aerobic Capacity

The $\dot{V}O_{2\,max}$ provides a reliable and precise measure of cardiovascular fitness and the body's maximal use of oxygen. It can be thought of as a surrogate for intensity of effort and is generally considered the gold standard measurement of exercise performance. However, its determination requires spirometry techniques, a monitored clinical laboratory setting, and a generally healthy, young, and motivated subject to exercise to exhaustion. The $\dot{V}O_{2\,peak}$, another clinic measure used to determine the upper ceiling of the O_2 transport/utilization system, represents the highest $\dot{V}O_2$ reached on a given test and defines the limits of the cardiopulmonary system (92). It too cannot discriminate among subjects who cease exercise because of lack of motivation, perceived discomfort, or a plethora of other reasons (76). Many factors influence $\dot{V}O_{2\,max}$, including age, gender, chronic levels of exercise, genetics, and disease (17,93). With increasing age, $\dot{V}O_{2\,max}$ declines about 1% per year after peaking at age 25 (94). Men have a 10% to 20% greater $\dot{V}O_{2\,max}$ than women with the difference largely attributed to the smaller muscle mass, lower hemoglobin, and smaller stroke volume in women (95). The high levels of $\dot{V}O_{2\,max}$ observed in elite endurance athletes (e.g., 70 to 85 mL/kg/min) compared with average young men (e.g., 40 to 50 mL/kg/min) probably stem from prolonged intense training plus genetic factors that enhance responsiveness to training (93,96).

Determination of Intensity

A prescribed exercise intensity based on a percentage of the $\dot{V}O_{2\,max}$ or similarly derived measure (76) has limitations as noted above, can over- and underestimate intensity (5,97), and is more suited to performance and cardiopulmonary exercise testing (92). A number of surrogates for maximal oxygen consumption/uptake exist to include anaerobic lactate (ventilatory) threshold (or MLSS), maximum heart rate, respiratory exchange ratio, oxygen uptake reserve, and MET (22,76,92). These also have various limitations, either in terms of accurately measuring energy expenditure or in practicality in an office setting.

Intensity can be expressed in absolute or relative measures. 🛜 eTable 49-3 provides an overview of various measures of aerobic exercise intensity. A MET is a measure of the absolute energy expenditure for a given activity. It is the ratio of energy expended during an activity to the rate of energy expended at rest, and one MET is equal to an oxygen uptake of 3.5 mL/kg/min—the energy an average person spends seated at rest. The measure MET-minutes describes the minutes a patient spends over their resting rate of energy expenditure (1). For example, a 4 MET activity expends 4 times the energy used by the body at rest. If a person does a 4 MET activity for 30 minutes, they have done 4 x 30 = 120 MET-minutes of physical activity. While METs are standardized and resources listing MET equivalents for specific activities are widely available (📶 eTable 49-2), they can overestimate actual oxygen use and do not take into consideration physical fitness, body weight, or gender (34,98). As an example, a healthy, active 20-year-old would likely find doubles tennis (approximately 5 METs) to feel less intense than would a sedentary 65-year-old.

Relative measures of intensity can be subjective and objective (**Table 49-5**). The ACSM recommends measures of perceived effort (i.e., talk test and Borg RPE) in prescribing exercise intensity (34). In particular, the talk test (i.e., can you speak comfortably while exercising) has been validated as a surrogate of the ventilatory or lactate threshold and is a valid, reliable, practical, and inexpensive tool for prescribing and monitoring exercise intensity in competitive athletes, healthy active adults, and patients with CVD (43,99). Exercise testing is required to accurately determine the objective measure of percent of maximum heart rate and therefore not practical for most. Thus, estimating the maximum heart is often based on the formula $HR_{max} = 220 - age$ (100). While simple to use, it can under- or overestimate the measured HR_{max} (101–103). To base the prescribed intensity of effort on a target heart rate, the ACSM recommends the HRR because it more accurately reflects intensity than the percent of maximum heart rate and oxygen uptake (34). It is also a more accurate estimate of energy expenditure as it takes into account the range of working heart rate (92). The formula for prescribing exercise intensity using HRR is target $HR = [(HR_{max/peak} - HR_{rest}) \times \%$ intensity desired] + HR_{rest} where $HR_{max/peak}$ is the highest value obtained during maximal/peak exercise or it can be estimated by 220-age or some other predication equation.

Principles of Aerobic Exercise Prescription

As noted earlier, the ACMS recommends prescription of physical activity based on the FITT-VP principle, with the first three parameters being frequency, intensity, and time, which determine exercise volume (**Table 49-8**).

Exercise volume can thereby increase by varying any of those parameters. The recommendation for exercise volume is ≥500 to 1,000 MET-minutes per week, which equates to roughly 1,000 kcal/wk. To reach the recommended exercise volume, individuals can (a) maintain their physical activity intensity level, but increase frequency by performing that activity on more days of the week; (b) maintain a certain frequency, but increase the intensity of their activity (i.e., exchange a low MET activity for a mid to high MET activity); or (c) maintain frequency and intensity, but increase the time allotted to a particular activity.

As physical fitness levels increase, individuals will need to progress their physical activity to continue reaching the minimum threshold of intensity required to challenge the body. The optimal rate of progression depends on several factors, including the individual's current activity level, physiologic limitations, health, age, and exercise goals (5,34). Progression typically starts by increasing the time spent doing a given activity. For instance, the ACSM recommends an increase of exercise session time by 5 to 10 minutes every 1 to 2 weeks and to "start low and go slow" (34). Once a previously inactive individual has participated in an aerobic conditioning regimen for at least 4 to 6 weeks, he or she can start to adjust the FITT parameters gradually over the next 4 to 12 months, making sure to avoid large increases in any of the components. It is important that all progression is done gradually to avoid burnout, muscle soreness, overtraining, and/or overuse injuries (34).

In the past, if a more individualized exercise prescription based on current fitness levels was desirable, a target heart

TABLE 49-8	**Aerobic Exercise Evidence-Based Recommendations**
FITT-VP	**Evidence-Based Recommendation**
Frequency	• ≥5 days/week of moderate exercise, or ≥3 days/week of vigorous exercise, or a combination of moderate and vigorous exercise on ≥3–5 days/week
Intensity	• Moderate and/or vigorous intensity for most adults • Light-to-moderate intensity exercise may be beneficial in deconditioned individuals
Time	• 30–60 minutes/day of purposeful moderate exercise, or 20–60 minutes/day of vigorous exercise, or a combination of moderate and vigorous exercise for most adults • <20 minutes of exercise per day can be beneficial, especially in previously sedentary individuals
Type	• Regular, purposeful exercise that involves major muscle groups and is continuous and rhythmic in nature
Volume	• A target volume of ≥500–1,000 MET-minute/week • Increasing pedometer step counts by ≥2,000 steps per day to reach a daily step count ≥7,000 steps per day is beneficial • Exercising below these volumes may still be beneficial for individuals unable or unwilling to reach this amount
Pattern	• Exercise may be performed in one continuous session, in one interval session, or in multiple sessions ≥10 minutes to accumulate the desired duration and volume of exercise per day • Exercise bouts of <10 minutes may yield favorable adaptations in very deconditioned individuals
Progression	• A gradual progression of exercise volume by adjusting exercise duration, frequency, and/or intensity is reasonable until the desired exercise goal (maintenance) is attained • This approach of "start low and go slow" may enhance adherence and reduce risks of musculoskeletal injury and adverse cardiac events

Derived from American College of Sports Medicine. In: Riebe D, Ehrman J, Liguori G, et al., eds. *ACSM's Guidelines for Exercise Testing and Prescription.* 10th ed. Philadelphia, PA: Wolters Kluwer; 2017.

method was employed. As noted above, this requires an estimate of the maximal heart rate or formal exercise testing. It is known that the anaerobic lactate (ventilatory) threshold is highly trainable for all individuals whereas $\dot{V}O_{2\,max}$ is not (104). In high-level athletes, almost all improvements in running performance are due to training at the MLSS, and the person who wins is typically the one who can sustain their MLSS at the greatest relative proportion of their $\dot{V}O_{2\,max}$ (22). There is good evidence to show that the ventilatory threshold is reliable for normalizing exercise intensity and placing individuals into specific training zones (105). There is also good evidence that ratings of perceived exertion and the "talk test" are effective at determining training zones (106–109).

Methods of Aerobic Conditioning

Traditional endurance training refers to submaximal aerobic effort for a fixed period of time, which produces physiologic adaptations such as increased cardiac output, increased utilization of oxygen by the muscles, metabolic changes, and an improved exercise capacity (110,111). Endurance training is typically performed at a moderate intensity of about 65% to 75% of $\dot{V}O_{2\,max}$ and starts to induce positive central and metabolic adaptations in as little as 7 days (111). Activities may include running, cycling, swimming, or walking.

One of the drawbacks to aerobic training is the large amount of time required to meet the recommended guidelines. In fact, a cross-sectional study performed in 1994 reported that lack of time was the most commonly cited reason for not exercising (112). Interval training is a technique in which the level of intensity is varied at fixed intervals during a single session of exercise and can result in an equal or greater volume of exercise for a given time period. It has been shown to result in similar or greater improvements in cardiorespiratory fitness and cardiometabolic biomarkers in healthy adults and in those with metabolic, cardiac, or pulmonary disease compared to single-intensity exercise (5). High-intensity interval training (HIIT) relies on repeated short bursts of high-intensity exercise performed at 90% $\dot{V}O_{2\,max}$ (approximately 85% to 90% of max HR or vigorous-to-near maximal intensity) separated by brief periods of low-intensity exercise (approximately 65% max HR) to allow for partial recovery (113). With HIIT training, it is possible to get training effects while varying the mode (e.g., running, cycling, swimming), work, and recovery interval number, intensity, and duration and number of repetitions of the intervals (114–117). A popular HIIT technique known as Tabata training involves exercising at maximal effort for 20 seconds followed by resting for 10 seconds and then repeating the sequence for a total of 4 minutes (118). HIIT has been shown to have comparable, if not superior, physiologic improvements to traditional endurance training despite a 90% decrease in training duration (50,119,120).

Walking is a readily available form of exercise that can be used to meet the recommended amount of aerobic exercise per week. A relatively new measure to track walking volume is steps per day (5). Pedometers, which track number of steps, are popular, are easy to access, and have been shown to improve physical activity (121). However, the quality of the steps (i.e., speed and duration) cannot be determined via pedometers, and there is no consensus on recommended steps per day currently. Although 10,000 steps per day is regularly cited, studies suggest that 5,400 to 7,900 steps per day may provide health benefits (122–124). Higher step counts may be necessary for weight management (34). Walking 100 steps per minute provides a very rough approximation of moderate-intense exercise (121,122).

RESISTANCE EXERCISE

Importance of Resistance Training

Muscular fitness gained through resistance training is important for maintaining functional capacity, preventing and recovering from injuries, and improving sports performance (125). With the many physiologic conditions that promote catabolic breakdown of the muscle and connective tissues (e.g., aging, injury, disease), resistance training presents the only natural method to offset such wasting conditions. Furthermore, a small difference in the quantity of lean muscle mass could have a significant effect on energy balance, which has implications on treatment and prevention of metabolic syndromes and disease states (126). Enhanced muscular fitness is associated with improved cardiometabolic risk factors (127), lower all-cause mortality (128–130), fewer cardiovascular events (130,131), and lower risk of developing nonfatal disease and functional limitations (127,132,133). Variables such as speed, jumping ability, and other measures of motor performance may be enhanced by resistance training. The focus of this section is on exercise prescription and program design for general muscular fitness and health benefits. The reader interested in more advanced regimens designed to achieve maximum strength, power, and hypertrophy is referred to the ACSM Position Stand "Progression Models in Resistance Training for Healthy Adults" (134).

Concepts

Components of muscular fitness include strength, endurance, and power. Muscular strength refers to maximal force production with a single contraction and is related to, or influenced by, muscle fiber cross-sectional area and pennation, muscle length, joint angle, contraction velocity, and motor unit activation (135–137). Strength, as well as muscular endurance, is often the focus of a general training regimen. Endurance, or more precisely, local muscular endurance, is the ability of a muscle or group of muscles to maintain a submaximal resistance over time. Training of this type may lead to an enhanced ability to perform submaximal exercise and recreational activities (134). Muscular power is the optimal amount of work performed in a given time period, is the product of force generation and movement velocity, and is demonstrable as the highest power output attainable during a given movement (134). Total-body exercises (to be discussed later) are very effective for enhancing power (138). Muscular power is an important training objective and may particularly benefit older adults because this element of muscle fitness declines most rapidly with aging (139).

Muscle fibers can generate force whether they remain static, become shorter, or increase in length (140). Static (isometric) muscle action occurs when the muscles generate force without changing length, and there is no associated joint movement (141). Strength gains are limited to the angle at which the joint is exercised (142). Squeezing a crutch handle to avoid losing grip is an example. Dynamic muscle actions are divided into concentric, eccentric, and isokinetic actions. In dynamic concentric muscle action, the muscle shortens as it overcomes external resistance (e.g., the shortening phase of a biceps curl). Concentric actions accelerate joints and produce greater torque with slow contractions (142). During dynamic eccentric muscle action, the muscle lengthens as it works to slow joint movement, resulting in high force generation. Exercises that focus on this type of action are sometimes called *negatives*. The activation of the hamstrings during the terminal swing phase of gait to slow the forward movement of the leg is an example of an eccentric action. Dynamic isokinetic muscle actions are characterized by constant velocity concentric or eccentric movements, a condition that exists in the laboratory or clinic but not in nature (143). Isokinetic training requires computerized equipment to maximize resistance at each angle of a range of motion (ROM) and can simulate actual speeds of sport-specific activities (141).

Plyometric training, while technically not a form of resistance training (but often confused with ballistic resistance exercise), is a technique involving rapid stretching and contracting of muscles (e.g., jump squats, one-leg hops) to ultimately increase power. Body weight and a combination of eccentric and concentric muscle action are typically used with this type of training. The eccentric prestretch phase of plyometric activity involves a quick powerful movement to prestretch the muscle, thereby activating the muscle stretch reflex, which inhibits the agonist muscle(s) through the Golgi tendon organ. As such, this type of exercise could be considered a form of neuromuscular training. Attaining a prestretch of the muscle through an eccentric contraction that produces elastic energy, which is stored in the musculotendinous unit for later use in a subsequent concentric contraction, is referred to as the stretch-shortening cycle (SSC) (144). It is this eccentric-concentric coupling that forms the basis of the SSC and increases force development (145). The time spent between the end of the eccentric phase and the initiation of a concentric contraction (i.e., the concentric phase) is called the amortization phase. The longer the duration of this phase, the larger the risk of losing elastic energy as heat within the muscle (146). Plyometric training can decrease the length of the amortization phase and theoretically can increase average power and velocity, increase peak force and velocity of acceleration, and increase time for force development (147). From a practical standpoint, plyometric training has been well shown to increase maximal vertical jump height (148–151) and sprint speed or velocity (151–155) and play a role in anterior cruciate ligament (ACL) injury prevention (156,157).

Progression in resistance training is defined as "the act of moving forward or advancing toward a specific goal over time until the target goal has been achieved," and *progressive overload* is the gradual increase of stress placed upon the body during exercise training to increase muscle strength and mass (134). As trained muscles strengthen and enlarge (i.e., hypertrophy), the resistance training stimulus must be progressively increased (e.g., increasing the amount of resistance lifted) if additional gains are to be accrued (34). In addition to progressive overload, specificity and variation (or periodization) are also important for progression. The principle of specificity predicts that the closer the training routine is to the requirements of the desired outcome (i.e., a specific exercise task or performance criteria), the better will be the outcome—that is, to become better at a particular exercise or skill, you must perform that exercise or skill. Although there is some limited

carryover of resistance training effects to areas such as agility and balance, the most effective training programs are those that are designed to target specific training goals for that activity. Variation, or *periodization*, is the process of altering one or more program variable(s) over time. Because the human body adapts quickly to a resistance training program, at least some changes are needed for long-term progression to occur, and the systematic variation of volume and intensity has been found to be the most effective (134). There are three common models of periodization: classical, reverse, and undulating. The interested reader is referred to the relevant ACSM Position Stand for further details (134).

One repetition maximum (1 RM) is the greatest amount of weight that can be lifted for a single repetition; it is often used to guide the prescription of intensity (or loading) of resistance exercise. The ACSM has proposed guidelines for relative intensity based on the 1 RM (**Table 49-9**). In the prescription of resistance training, intensity is usually progressed by (a) increasing the load based on a percentage of 1 RM, (b) increasing the absolute load based on a targeted repetition number, or (c) increasing loading within a prescribed zone (e.g., 8 to 12 RM) (134).

A total-body workout regimen implies that all the major muscle groups (chest, shoulders, upper and lower back, hips, legs, abdomen, and arms) are to be exercised on the same day in the same session to meet the general guideline for resistance training of each major muscle group of 2 to 3 days a week (34). Alternatively, in a split-body routine, each session day may be divided into an upper/lower body routine (upper body musculature trained on one day and lower body on another) and/or a muscle group routine (individual muscles trained during a workout) (5,134). In the muscle group split, an individual muscle is trained with different techniques. For example, the triceps could be trained by a triceps extension exercise for one set and by push-ups with another set. This split training program requires four training sessions a week to train each muscle group twice a week. Further details about this regimen will be discussed later.

TABLE 49-9	Method of Estimating Intensity of Resistance Exercise	
Relative Intensity		
Intensity	**Perceived Exertion (on 6–20 RPE Scale)**	**% of One Repetition Maximum**
Very light	RPE < 9 (less than very light effort)	<30
Light	RPE 9–11 (very to fairly light effort)	30–49
Moderate	RPE 12–13 (fairly light to somewhat hard effort)	50–69
Vigorous	RPE 14–17 (somewhat hard to very hard effort)	70–84
Near-maximal to maximal	RPE ≥ 18 (greater than or equal to very hard effort)	≥85

Adapted with permission from Garber CE, Blissmer B, Deschenes MR, et al. Quantity and quality of exercise for developing and maintaining cardiorespiratory, musculoskeletal, and neuromotor fitness in apparently healthy adults: guidance for prescribing exercise. *Med Sci Sports Exerc*. 2011;43(7):1334–1359.

Physiologic Effects of Resistance Training

Nervous System Adaptations

Maximal force production from a muscle requires the maximal recruitment of all motor units (158). Part of the adaptation to resistance training is the development of the ability to recruit all motor units as well as increased synchronization of those units (158,159). Such neural adaptations are thought to be responsible for the acute increase in strength that precedes an increase in muscle size during the early phase of a resistance training program. Improvements in strength also may result from reduced inhibition from the central nervous system (CNS) (139).

Muscle Hypertrophy

During heavy-resistance training, motor units containing both type I and type II muscle fibers are recruited. As a result, resistance training typically induces increases in the cross-sectional area of both type I and type II muscle fibers and thus of the intact muscle. This hypertrophy can be observed after several weeks or months of training (160,161). Muscle fiber hypertrophy occurs through remodeling of protein within the cell and an increase in the size and number of myofibrils (162). Satellite cells are activated in the very early stages of training; their proliferation and later fusion with existing fibers appear to be intimately involved in the hypertrophy response (163). Increases in the number of actin and myosin filaments and myofilament density, along with sarcomere addition, also contribute to the increase in muscle fiber size (162,164).

It is hypothesized that three primary factors are responsible for initiating the hypertrophic response to resistance exercise: mechanical tension, metabolic stress, and muscle damage (165–168). Mechanically induced tension produced both by force generation and stretch is considered essential to muscle growth, and the combination of these stimuli appears to have a pronounced additive effect (168–170). Conversely, unloading muscle for a given time results in atrophy (171). Muscle atrophy also results from fiber denervation with loss of some fibers and atrophy of others, especially fast twitch, with aging and inactivity (172).

Metabolic stress from using anaerobic glycolysis to produce ATP may also play a large role in optimizing the hypertrophic response (167,173–175). Buildup of metabolites such as lactate, hydrogen ions, creatine, and inorganic phosphates has been implicated in signaling an anabolic response (176,177). Muscle ischemia also creates metabolic stress and may have an additive hypertrophic effect when combined with glycolytic training (178,179).

Lastly, local muscle damage can produce an anabolic cascade that extends beyond what is required for local repair resulting in muscle hypertrophy (166,180). Resistance training programs involving higher working volume have consistently proven superior over single-set protocols (181,182), though it is still unclear whether the hypertrophic superiority is the product of greater muscle damage, muscle tension, metabolic stress, or a combination of these factors (183).

Muscle Fiber Conversion

Transition within the muscle fiber subtypes from type IIx to type IIa and vice versa may occur with resistance training (184–186), and this conversion begins to occur within about 2 weeks of initiation of training (187). However, any transformation from type I to type II muscle fibers seems less probable (185,186).

Other Adaptations Within the Muscle

It is widely accepted that mitochondrial abundance, oxidative enzyme activities, and oxidative capacity increase in skeletal muscles from rodents to humans in response to exercise (160). However, the degree to which skeletal muscle mitochondria adapt to exercise probably depends on the mode of exercise, and whether resistance training consistently increases oxidative capacity is still unclear. Skeletal muscle mitochondrial function declines and oxidative stress increases with advancing age (188,189), and these changes have been implicated in the etiology of sarcopenia (190,191). Moreover, aged skeletal muscle from sedentary older adults exhibits reduced mitochondrial abundance, oxidative enzyme activities, and oxidative capacity (188,192,193). While it appears that low-volume resistance exercise does not increase skeletal muscle oxidative capacity or reduce reactive oxygen species production in older adults (194), a combination of endurance and resistance training was found to be better than either modality alone at significantly increasing oxidative capacity and expression of mitochondrial proteins and transcription factors independent of age (195).

Body Compositional Changes

Body compositional changes associated with resistance training are primarily associated with gains in lean muscle mass (196,197). These gains can accrue during short-term (6 to 24 weeks) resistance training programs (198,199). Increases in fat-free mass normally mirror increases in muscle tissue weight, but because of concomitant decreases in fat, total body weight generally increases little over short training periods. The largest gains in fat-free mass that can be expected are a little more than 3 kg (6.6 lb) in 10 weeks of training (125).

Endocrine System Adaptations

The endocrine system plays a major role in the adaptational responses of skeletal muscle to resistance training (200). Serum testosterone, growth hormone, and cortisol concentrations have been demonstrated to increase immediately after exercise (201). During the time that serum testosterone concentrations are elevated, significant changes in the type of muscle proteins (e.g., myosin ATPase hybrids or myosin proteins) occur. Resistance training is also well known to improve insulin sensitivity through an increase in the anabolic hormone insulin; it also increases insulin-like growth factor-1, which is critical to skeletal muscle growth (199,200,202).

Adaptations to Connective Tissue, Bone, and Cartilage

As muscles develop greater tension through the effects of resistance training, ligaments and tendons also gain in strength (203,204). It is now acknowledged that the dense fibrous tissues that make up tendons and ligaments are adaptable, and it is known that eccentric loading will induce tendon remodeling (205) and heavy-resistance training will increase tendon stiffness (206). Physical activity also causes increased metabolism, thickness, weight, and strength of ligaments (207,208). Damaged ligaments regain their strength at a faster rate if physical activity is performed after the injury (207,208).

The connective tissue sheaths that surround the entire muscle (epimysium), groups of muscle fibers (perimysium), and individual muscle fibers (endomysium) also adapt to resistance training. These sheaths are of major importance in the tensile strength and elastic properties of muscle, as they form the framework that supports an overload on the muscle. It has been found that muscle hypertrophy is accompanied by an increase in the absolute collagen content of these connective tissue sheaths (209,210), but the amount of connective tissue appears to increase at the same rate as the muscle tissue (162).

Bone adapts to resistance training, but much more slowly than muscle, requiring 6 to 12 months for adaptations to be observed (211). Bone is sensitive to compression and strain. Such forces are common in resistance training and are related to the type of exercise used, the intensity of the resistance, and the number of sets performed. Training characterized by high-power exercise movements, heavy resistances, and multiple sets appears to be most likely to produce changes in bone metabolism. A direct and positive relationship between the effects of resistance training and bone density exists, and in contrast to pharmacologic interventions, resistance training has the additive effect of mitigating multiple risk factors for osteoporosis (212).

Resistance training also has been found to increase the thickness of hyaline cartilage on the articular surfaces of bone (213). Hyaline cartilage acts as a shock absorber between the bony surfaces of a joint. Increasing the thickness of cartilage could facilitate the performance of this shock absorber function.

Principles of Resistance Exercise Prescription

The prescription and development of a resistance training regimen/program is dependent upon the development of appropriate and specific training goals and should be a highly individualized process. Appropriate equipment, program design, and exercise techniques are needed for safe and effective implementation (134). Training programs may be developed for rehabilitation from disease or injury, fitness (e.g., to make activities of daily living less physiologically stressful), prevention of chronic diseases or injury, sports, or other activities. Trainable characteristics include muscular strength, power, hypertrophy, and local muscular endurance. These characteristics can be effected by the manipulation of various program variables (i.e., frequency, intensity, choice and order of exercise, number of sets and repetitions, repetition speed, and rest periods). Over time, changes made in program variables will create the progressions, variations, and overloads needed to produce physiologic adaptations and improved functional abilities.

The initial resistance program should be viewed only as a starting point and must be progressed to meet the goals of the individual. Program design should be adjusted over time to optimize each person's physiologic potential for a particular training goal with the understanding that individual differences in development of adaptations to a resistance training program are what drive the need for individualized programs. With all the variables of a resistance training program, nearly an infinite number of programs can be designed. As noted earlier, the ACSM's FITT-VP principle (📶 **eTable 49-4**) provides a good framework for exercise prescription but should be tailored to the individual's goals (34).

The Needs Analysis

A needs analysis is a process that can be used to help design a resistance training program (214) and establish priorities for the many options available in the prescription of resistance training to attain goals related to health, fitness, and physical performance. The major questions to be addressed for the purposes of this chapter are:

1. What are the specific needs for muscle strength, endurance, and power?
2. What muscle groups need to be trained?
3. What type of muscle action(s) (e.g., isometric, eccentric) need to be trained?
4. What is the prior injury history and what are the primary sites of injury for the particular activities in which the individual participates?

Determination of the Need for Various Components of Muscular Fitness

Determination of the magnitude of improvement needed for muscle strength, power, and endurance is a very important step in the overall resistance training program design. This determination requires an understanding of the benefits each component of muscular fitness conveys and the goals of the individual. For example, as alluded to earlier, insufficient power in older adults has been associated with a greater risk of accidental falls (14,23). Training for local muscular endurance can facilitate prolonged participation in activities. Many sports require a high strength-to-mass or a high power-to-mass ratio. In such a case, resistance training programs should be designed to maximize strength and power while minimizing increases in body mass. Thus, the need for these components of muscular fitness must be evaluated so that proper resistance training partitioning may be used.

Biomechanical Analysis to Determine What Muscles Need to Be Trained

The second question requires an appreciation of which muscles, and their specific joint angles, need to be trained to accomplish a specific goal. This examination involves a basic analysis of the movements performed and muscles involved with an activity. Because of the principle of specificity, the greatest improvements are observed when resistance training programs are prescribed that are specific to the task or the activity (134). Understanding exactly what movement one is trying to mimic during resistance training is an important aspect of program design. Such analyses will allow the proper selection of exercises that use muscles and actions in a manner specific to the desired activity or outcome. The best way to select such exercises is to analyze the biomechanics of the activity and match it to exercises. However, an appreciation of the chosen exercises' impact on physiologic variables should also be taken into account. For example, when training for improved health and well-being, the training specificity will be related to picking the right exercises that can impact a given physiologic variable (e.g., bone mineral density [BMD]). The decisions made at this stage will help define the choice of exercises, a program variable to be discussed later.

Determination of What Type of Muscle Actions Should Be Used

After the basic biomechanical analysis described above has identified what muscles to train based on their involvement in an activity, the next step is to identify the type of muscle action to train. Decisions regarding the use of static (isometric), dynamic concentric, dynamic eccentric, and isokinetic forms of exercise are important in the preliminary stages of planning a resistance training program for sport, fitness, or rehabilitation. Most resistance training programs use several types of muscle actions, and indeed during most types of exercise, muscles alternate between static and dynamic muscle actions (141). For most exercise programs, resistance training will include dynamic concentric and eccentric muscle actions.

Whether a muscle action is performed concentrically, eccentrically, or isometrically has an influence on the adaptation to the resistance exercise. Greater force can be produced during eccentric muscle actions with the advantage of requiring less energy per unit of muscle force (215–217). It has been known for some time that there is a need for an eccentric component to optimize muscle hypertrophy (183,186,218,219). This is why techniques such as *heavy negatives*, *forced negatives*, and *slow negatives* have been used by individuals (e.g., bodybuilders) to maximize muscle hypertrophy. With pure eccentric resistance exercise, especially in untrained individuals, delayed-onset muscle soreness (DOMS) can be more prominent than with concentric actions (220). Eccentric training causes greater muscle fiber and connective tissue disruption, enzyme release, DOMS, and impaired neuromuscular function that limits force production and ROM (221). In addition, performing a high-intensity training session or performing new exercises at novel angles can result in greater muscle soreness when an eccentric action is involved. Nevertheless, dynamic strength improvements and hypertrophy are greatest when eccentric actions are combined with concentric actions in a repetition (219). Individuals adapt to eccentric actions and subsequently the muscle damage mentioned above becomes much lower after training.

Isometric muscle actions are less metabolically demanding and less conducive to hypertrophy than dynamic muscle actions (222,223). Static exercise may play a role in a resistance training program when working around a musculoskeletal injury or in the very deconditioned where the volume of exercise can be increased for a fraction of the metabolic fatigue experienced with dynamic training.

Assessment of the Primary Sites of Injury

Lastly, it is important to understand the injury profile of the individual and/or determine the primary sites for potential injury in work or sports activities. In addition to the rehabilitation of injuries, another goal of a resistance training program is to enhance the strength and function of tissue so that it better resists injury. The concept of *prehabilitation* refers to preventing initial injury by training the joints and muscles that are most susceptible to injury during an activity. The prevention of reinjury can also be an important goal of a resistance training program. Thus, understanding the typical sites of injury for the activity (e.g., knee joints in alpine skiing or low back in office workers) and the individual's prior history of injury can aid in the proper design of a resistance training program.

Program Prescription

After the needs analysis has been completed, a specific exercise program is prescribed that addresses the goals and needs of the individual, whether for rehabilitation, fitness, or performance. The program variables mentioned earlier (FITT-VP) serve as

the framework of a training session, and subsequent changes to these variables will make up the progression of a planned training period in the overall program. Understanding the influence and importance of each of the program variables in achieving a specific training goal is vital to creating the optimal exercise stimulus. Over long periods of training, the concepts of the SAID (Specific Adaptation to Imposed Demands) principle imply the need for variation, or *periodization*, of program variables to ensure progression (125,224). Although periodization usually implies manipulation of the volume and intensity variables of resistance exercises, in the rehabilitation setting, such variation may mean that focused strengthening exercises are shifted to more functional exercises emphasizing the development of muscular endurance.

Each program must be designed to meet the individual's needs and training goals with recognition of the individual's initial fitness level. It is important to remember that evaluation of a fitness level (e.g., 1 RM strength test) is typically not done until it is known that the individual can tolerate the test demands so that the data generated are meaningful (225). One of the most serious mistakes made in designing a resistance workout is placing too much stress on the individual before it can be tolerated.

Program Variables

Frequency (Number of Workouts per Week)

Optimal training frequency (number of workouts per week) depends on several factors, such as volume, intensity, exercise selection, level of conditioning and/or training status, recovery ability, nutrition, and training goals (134). Numerous resistance training studies have used frequencies of 2 or 3 alternating days per week in untrained subjects (219,226). This has been shown to be a very effective initial frequency. If the resistance training is not excessive, only moderate amounts of delayed muscular soreness should be experienced 1 day after the session. The ACSM recommends that novice individuals perform full-body workouts 2 to 3 days per week when training for muscular strength, hypertrophy, power, or endurance (134). A meta-analysis showed that strength gains in untrained individuals were highest with a frequency of 3 days per week (227). A reduced frequency is adequate for maintenance training; training 1 or 2 days per week is adequate for muscle mass, power, and strength retention (228). However, this appears effective for only short time periods, as such long-term maintenance training (i.e., reduced frequency and volume) may lead to detraining.

The progression from beginning to more aggressive training does not necessitate a change in frequency but may be more dependent on alterations in other acute variables, such as exercise selection, volume, and intensity (i.e., periodization). However, it is common to see three or four training sessions per week among those individuals who are training more aggressively. Increasing training frequency allows for greater specialization (i.e., greater exercise selection per muscle group and/or volume in accordance with more specific goals). To achieve a higher frequency of training, more detailed workouts should be developed, as simply performing the same exercises four times rather than three times per week is not the optimal approach to increasing frequency. Programs should use exercises that involve similar muscle groups but use different angles for particular movements (referred to as *split programming*) (125). For example, a 4-days-per-week routine that involves performing the bench press all 4 days would be better designed by having the individual perform a regular bench press on 2 days and an alternate type of bench press (e.g., incline bench press) on the other 2 days. Thus, split programming allows for more variety (progression) in the exercise choices, because of the increase in the number of training days available. In addition, total-body or split-body-part workouts have been used to allow more training variety. Both styles have been shown to produce improvements in muscle strength and size (229). However, it is recommended that similar muscle groups or exercises not be performed on consecutive days during split-routine workouts to allow adequate recovery and to minimize the risk of overtraining. The ASCM recommends using a training frequency of 3 to 4 days per week for muscular strength, hypertrophy, power, and endurance in intermediate and advanced individuals: 3 days a week for total-body workouts and 4 days a week for muscle group split routines (134).

Intensity (Loading, or Resistance Used)

The intensity of effort, reflected in the amount of resistance used for a specific exercise, is probably one of the key factors in any resistance training program (230). It is the major stimulus related to changes observed in measures of strength, power, and local muscular endurance. When implementing a resistance training program, a load for each exercise must be chosen. Either the maximum number of repetitions (RM) or the load that only allows a specific number of repetitions to be performed probably provides the easiest way to determine intensity. Typically, one uses a RM target (e.g., 10 RM) or target zone (a range such as 4 to 6 RM) to choose the load and thus the intensity of effort. Another method of determining load for an exercise involves using a percentage of the 1 RM (e.g., 80% of the 1 RM). If the patient's 1 RM for an exercise is 100 lb, 80% of the 1 RM would be 80 lb. This method requires that the maximal strength in various lifts used in the training program be evaluated regularly. If 1 RM testing is not done regularly (e.g., each week), the percentage of 1 RM used in training decreases and therefore the training intensity is reduced. From a practical perspective, determining percentage of 1 RM for many lifts may not be feasible because of the amount of testing time required. Use of an RM target or an RM target zone allows the individual to adjust resistances in response to an ability to perform greater repetitions to stay at the RM target or within the RM target zone. Also, the reader needs to appreciate that the load lifted per repetition is highly dependent on other variables, such as exercise order, volume, frequency, muscle action, repetition speed, and rest period length (231).

Classic studies have indicated that training with loads corresponding to 1 to 6 RM (mostly 5 to 6 RM) was most conducive to increasing maximal dynamic strength (232,233). A load of at least 45% to 50% of 1 RM is needed to increase dynamic muscular strength in beginners (234). However, greater loads are needed in more experienced subjects (235). Although significant strength increases have been reported using loads corresponding to 8 to 12 RM (187,236–238), and this load range appears most effective for increasing muscular hypertrophy (239), loads lighter than this (i.e., 12 to 15 RM and lighter) have only had small effects on maximal strength in

previously untrained individuals (240). However, these lighter loads have been shown to be very effective for increasing local muscular endurance (241).

Contrary to early studies in resistance training, it appears that training loads must be tailored to an individual's situation to most effectively increase their muscular fitness as opposed to performing all exercises with a 6 RM load (242). Neural adaptations precede hypertrophy during intense training periods, and it appears that a variety of loads is conducive to increasing both neural function (i.e., increased motor unit recruitment, firing rate, and synchronization) and hypertrophy. Therefore, periodized training in which great load variation is included appears most effective for long-term improvements in muscular fitness.

In general, a certain percentage of the 1 RM with free-weight exercises will allow fewer repetitions than the same percentage of 1 RM on a similar exercise performed on a machine. This is probably due to the need for greater balance and control in space when using free weights. The larger muscle group exercises appear to need much higher percentages of the 1 RM than smaller muscle groups to keep them in the RM target zone when using free weights but not necessarily exercise machines (243–245). Thus, using percentages of the 1 RM is dependent upon exercise equipment (free weights vs. machines) and exercise choice, and the RM zone should be checked to be sure the percentage is yielding the proper number of repetitions to meet training-related goals.

The ACSM recommends that novice to intermediate individuals train with loads corresponding to 60% to 70% of 1 RM (moderate-to-vigorous intensity) for 8 to 12 repetitions to maximize strength, with the concurrent addition of a power component consisting of light-to-moderate loading (i.e., 30% to 60% 1 RM for upper body exercises and 0% to 60% 1 RM for lower body) with the understanding that for progression to occur, heavy loading (i.e., 85% to 100% 1 RM) is necessary for increasing the force component of power, while light-to-moderate loading performed at an explosive velocity is necessary for increasing fast force production (134). For muscular endurance in novice and intermediate training, light loads of less than 50% 1 RM with higher repetitions of 10 to 15 (15 to 25 or more in advanced training) are recommended (34,134).

Type of Exercise (Choice of Exercise)

As described in the needs analysis, the choice and types of exercises selected for a resistance training program will be related to the biomechanical and functional characteristics of the identified goals for improvement. For example, if the needs analysis discovers that a lack of strength in the lower extremities is causing difficulty with chair transfers, exercise selection should facilitate sit-to-stand transfer movements. In this scenario, squat or glute bridge exercises might be appropriate. In addition to body weight exercises, various types of resistance training equipment can be used effectively to improve muscular fitness including free weights, machines, and resistance bands (34). Both free weights and machines are effective for increasing strength, and the choice should be based on the primary training objective, the level of training status, and familiarity with specific exercise movements (134). For general fitness, it is recommended that exercises target the major muscle groups of the chest, shoulders, back, hips, legs, trunk, and arms (134).

Exercises of choice can be structural (i.e., multiple-joint) or body part (i.e., single-joint), and both have been shown to be effective for increasing muscular strength in the targeted muscle groups (134). Structural or multijoint exercises require the coordinated action of multiple muscle groups through complex neural communications and have generally been regarded as more effective for increasing overall muscular strength because they enable a greater magnitude of weight to be lifted (246,247). Examples include power cleans, dead lifts, squats, bench press, military press, and latissimus pulldowns (📶 **eFig. 49-1**). It is especially important to include multiple-joint exercises in a program when whole-body-strength movements are required for a particular activity. Due to the necessity of full-body stabilization for many multijoint exercises, numerous muscles are trained that otherwise might not be. Exercises like dead lifts and squats engage almost all the muscles of the lower extremities, to include the distal muscles involved in ankle stabilization. They also require significant core stabilization through the abdominal and low back muscles, as well as the trapezius, rhomboids, and others (248). Most sports and functional activities in everyday life depend on structural multiple-joint movements.

Single-joint or body-part exercises focus on individual muscle groups such as the lumbar extensors, hamstrings, and triceps. Biceps curls, crunches, knee extensions, and knee curls are examples of isolated single-joint or body-part exercises (📶 **eFig. 49-2**). These exercises usually require less skill and technique and may be less intimidating for novices. All exercises should be executed using correct form and technique, including performing the repetitions deliberately and in a controlled manner, and using proper breathing techniques (i.e., exhalation during the concentric phase and inhalation during the eccentric phase; avoiding holding one's breath) (5).

A change in angle due to altering body posture, grip, and hand width or foot stance and position will affect which muscle tissue is activated. Using magnetic resonance imaging technology, investigators have shown that the type of resistance exercise (relative to joint angle and loading method) alters the activation pattern of the muscle (249). As a result, the number of possible angles and exercises is almost limitless. Including unilateral and bilateral training is another way to vary an exercise. Unilateral training may increase bilateral strength (in addition to unilateral strength) (250). Therefore, it is important to understand that if the muscle tissue is not activated by using the most appropriate resistance load (periodized loadings) or joint angles, the desired tissue may not be affected and therefore the optimal rehabilitation progression will not occur.

The ACSM recommends the use of unilateral and bilateral, multi- and single-joint exercises, with emphasis on multijoint, for maximizing strength and local muscle endurance (134). Exercises stressing multiple or large muscle groups stimulate metabolic adaptations within skeletal muscle necessary to improve endurance (251). For power enhancement, multijoint exercises, and in particular total-body explosive lifts (e.g., power clean, push press, jump squat), should be used predominantly (134).

Order of Exercise

In the sequencing of multi- and single-joint exercises, the more complex multiple-joint exercises are performed initially followed by the less complex single-joint exercises. The sequencing rationale is that the exercises performed in the beginning of the workout require the greatest amount of muscle mass and energy for optimal performance (252). Thus, this sequencing strategy focuses on attaining a greater training effect for the large muscle groups. If multijoint exercises are performed early in the workout, more resistance can be used due to a limited amount of fatigue. Additionally, the complex movements of multijoint exercises are easier and safer to learn before fatigue begins to inhibit motor skills. Single-joint exercises attempt to isolate functionally important muscle groups. Exercise focusing on these single muscle groups is added with the goal to eventually improve performance in the multijoint exercise.

To prevent muscular imbalances, training opposing muscle groups (i.e., agonists and antagonists), such as the chest and upper back, quadriceps and hamstrings, and the abdominal musculature and lumbar extensors, is important (5). Push/pull protocols, where a pushing exercise is followed by a pulling exercise (e.g., bench press followed by bent-over rows), are also utilized for the same purpose. It also may be advantageous to alter the order of the body parts exercised (e.g., arm followed by leg) to allow for some recovery of the muscles while another area is exercised.

Improper sequencing of exercises can compromise the lifter's ability to perform the desired number of repetitions with the desired load. Recommendations for sequencing exercises for novice, intermediate, and advanced strength training for total-body, upper/lower body split, and muscle group split workouts designed to improve strength, power, and hypertrophy are

- Rotation of agonist/antagonist exercises for total-body sessions
- Rotation of upper/lower body exercises for total-body sessions
- Large muscles before smaller ones
- Multijoint exercises performed before single-joint exercises
- Olympic lifts before basic strength and single-joint exercises
- Most intense exercises performed before least intense (particularly when performing several exercises consecutively for the same muscle group)

Volume (Number of Repetitions and Sets)

Resistance training volume represents the total number of repetitions performed (sets × repetitions) multiplied by the resistance (intensity) used and is reflective of the duration of which muscles are being exercised (51). To improve strength, a resistance that allows an individual to complete 8 to 12 repetitions per set should be selected. As noted earlier in the "Intensity" subsection, this number usually translates to a resistance that is approximately 60% to 80% of an individual's 1 RM. As resistance, and by association force, increases, fewer number of repetitions will need to be completed to improve strength. Each set should be performed to the point of muscle fatigue but not failure. For power training, three to six repetitions of light-to-moderate loading is recommended and fast or ballistic lifting velocities are needed to optimize power development (134).

The speed at which a repetition is conducted is important and has been shown to significantly affect neural (216,235), hypertrophy (253,254), and metabolic (251) adaptations. In general, force production is greatest at slower speeds and lowest during high-speed movements. This relationship is graphically represented by the force-velocity curve discussed earlier in this chapter. The implications of the force-velocity relationship are that training at slow velocities with maximal tension will be effective for strength training and training with high velocities will be effective for power/speed enhancement. Generally, moderate-to-rapid speeds (i.e., 1 to 2 seconds concentric, 1 to 2 seconds eccentric) are most effective for enhancing gains in strength and power. Thus, improving set performance (i.e., number of repetitions or load) may be best accomplished with use of moderate-to-fast speeds. Increasing the time under tension (with sufficient loading) can increase muscular fatigue, and fatigue is important in improving muscular endurance (51). Slower speeds will result in more fatigue than moderate-to-rapid speeds, but it is difficult to perform a large number of repetitions at slow speeds. Therefore, a higher number of repetitions (15 to 25 or more) should be conducted at moderate-to-fast speeds (227,236), while intentionally slow speeds should be used with a lower number of repetitions (10 to 15) to improve local muscular endurance (134).

Most individuals respond favorably to two to four sets of resistance exercises per muscle group for strength, power, and endurance training. However, even a single set of exercise may significantly improve muscle strength and size, particularly in untrained exercisers (5). Multiple studies have shown that multiset resistance training programs are superior for strength enhancement in untrained and trained individuals both for short and long training periods (182,227,255,256). While single-set training programs are effective in increasing strength in untrained to moderately trained individuals over short training periods (i.e., 6 to 12 weeks), multiset programs are necessary for long-term improvement (i.e., 17 to 40 weeks) (182,227,256). A relatively recent meta-analysis found that two to three sets produce 46% greater increases in strength than single-set programs in both trained and untrained subjects (255). Additional strength gains peak at a volume of four sets per muscle group at 60% of 1 RM, three times a week (227). For continued improvement, variation (periodization) is important, and this includes the use of lower-volume training programs for certain phases of the overall training cycle to provide rest and recovery periods. The key factor may be variation of training volume (and its interaction with intensity) rather than absolute number of sets (134). These findings have prompted the recommendation from the ACSM for periodized multiple-set programs when long-term progression (not maintenance) is the goal (134).

Pattern (Rest Periods Between Sets, Exercises, and Repetitions)

As noted earlier, strength gains are mediated by mechanical, metabolic, and hormonal factors, and rest intervals between sets are one of the most important variables that affects both the mechanical and metabolic acute effects of training. The amount of rest between sets and exercises influences the stress of the workout and thus training adaptations through the amount of resistance lifted. Rest periods determine the magnitude of ATP-CP energy source resynthesis and the concentrations of lactate in the blood. The length of the rest period significantly alters the metabolic, hormonal, and cardiovascular responses to an acute bout of resistance exercise, as well as performance of subsequent sets (237,257–260). Strength and power performances are highly dependent on anaerobic energy metabolism, primarily through the phosphagen system. It appears that the majority of phosphagen repletion occurs within 3 minutes (261,262). In addition, removal of lactate and other metabolites may require at least 4 minutes (263). Kraemer (237) reported differences in performance with 3- versus 1-minute rest periods. All subjects were able to perform 10 repetitions with 10 RM loads for three sets with 3-minute rest periods for the leg press and bench press. However, when rest periods were reduced to 1 minute, 10, 8, and 7 repetitions were performed, respectively. Other studies in recreational weight lifters (264) and resistance-trained men came to the same conclusions (265). For this reason, it may be prudent to rest longer when performing exercise of high complexity and rest less between less technical assistance exercises that isolate muscle groups. Current recommendations to improve strength and power by the ACSM suggest a 2- to 3-minute rest between core exercises utilizing heavier loads and a 1- to 2-minute rest between sets of complimentary assistance exercises (134).

Local muscular endurance is also affected by the duration of rest intervals between sets. Short rest periods between sets in a high-volume (e.g., loading of 70% to 100% 1 RM for 6 to 12 repetitions or more for three to six sets per exercise) program improves fatigue rate (257). Circuit training in which minimal rest is taken between exercise stations is also known to improve local muscle endurance (266,267). Training for local muscular endurance implies the individual (a) performs multiple repetitions (perhaps up to 15 to 25), (b) trains to and beyond the point of fatigue, and/or (c) minimizes recovery between sets (i.e., training in a semifatigued state). The ACSM recommends 1- to 2-minute rest periods for high-repetition sets (15 to 20 or more) and less than 1 minute for moderate (10 to 15 repetitions) sets (134).

The amount of rest taken between repetitions has variable training effects. With regard to strength, and in confirmation of the traditional continuous method, Rooney et al. found significantly greater improvements in a group performing consecutive repetitions than in a group utilizing 30-second rest periods between repetitions and suggested that fatigue contributes to the strength training stimulus (173). However, in power resistance training, it appears that avoiding excessive fatigue and failure is important, and rest intervals ranging from 20 to 100 seconds between repetitions improve maximum and total power output (268,269). The optimum rest interval needs further research, but if a high percentage of peak velocity or power is desired for each repetition in a workout, having longer rest periods of 50 to 100 seconds with fewer repetitions for several sets is prudent.

Progression

Progression of an exercise/training program implies that the individual desires to continue to increase muscular strength, power, mass, and local muscular endurance. As discussed above, this goal must be accomplished through progressive overload and most commonly by gradually increasing resistance, sets per muscle group, and/or frequency. If an individual is satisfied with his or her level of muscular fitness, he or she can take comfort in knowing that maintenance of strength, functional performance, and metabolic health can be achieved through training as little as 1 day a week (5,270–272). However, intensity of effort must remain at a moderate to hard level as it is an important component of maintaining the effects of resistance training (271).

Older and very deconditioned individuals should begin resistance training exercises with higher numbers of repetitions (i.e., 10 to 15) at 40% to 50% of 1 RM (i.e., a very light-to-light) intensity to reduce the chance of injury (34). Progression should be individualized and tailored to patient tolerance and preference. Completing three sets of 8 to 12 repetitions at a very light-to-moderate intensity (i.e., 20% to 50% of 1 RM) has been shown to effectively increase strength and power and improve balance in older persons (273,274). As adaptation and musculotendinous conditioning progress, older and frail persons can safely increase resistance and follow the guidelines for younger adults as detailed above (46). Given the important role of power in the older population, it bears repeating that healthy older adults should increase power by using single- and multijoint exercises (one to three sets) using light-to-moderate intensity (30% to 60% of 1 RM) for 6 to 10 high-velocity repetitions (34).

NEUROMOTOR EXERCISE

Importance and Challenges

The importance of neuromotor exercise in the pursuit of improved function can be appreciated by the number of independent but interrelated areas it encompasses: balance, coordination, postural control, stability, muscle strength/power, and agility. The objectives of neuromuscular training are to improve the nervous system's ability to generate a fast and optimal muscle firing pattern, to increase dynamic joint stability, to decrease joint forces, and to relearn movement patterns and skills (275). Neuromotor exercise programs are typically implemented with the aim of fall and injury prevention, rehabilitation from injury, and optimizing performance. However, research in this area is hampered by the large variety of exercises used in neuromuscular training programs. These can include balance and stabilization exercises as well as multi-intervention programs with a combination of balance, strength, plyometric, agility, and sport-specific exercises (276). Gait and flexibility training as well as Pilates, yoga, tai chi, qigong, and dance have been utilized in programs to improve functional balance and address fall and injury prevention and rehabilitation (4,277). Because there is no agreed-upon standard in the literature for training that incorporates balance exercise, various terms are used to include static and dynamic balance and neuromuscular, proprioceptive, sensorimotor, instability, and perturbation training. Contributing to the complexity of comparing and determining effectiveness of various training programs is the fact that essential factors for optimal neuromuscular functioning include reliable sensory information from the visual, vestibular, proprioceptive, and mechanoreceptive systems; a well-functioning CNS with feedback and feed forward loops able to withstand external and internal volitions; as well as adequate musculoskeletal strength and sufficient ROM in the joints for adequate movement (278). However, these mechanisms integral to neuromotor control are not consistently measured in most studies. The wide variety of distinct but interrelated exercise interventions, their often comingling during therapeutic intervention trials, and their often diverse populations have made it difficult to determine the distinct contributions of each exercise on various outcomes (279).

Despite these challenges, neuromotor exercise training is felt to be an important part of a comprehensive exercise program for older adults, especially to improve balance, agility, and muscle strength and reduce the risk of falls (34). Additionally, a number of recent meta-analyses and systematic reviews have shown that neuromotor exercise is effective in reducing fall and injury risk, enhancing performance after injury, and enhancing certain aspects of functional performance (276,280–283).

Neuromotor Function Programs and Outcomes

As noted above, there is a large variety of exercises used in neuromuscular training programs as well as a variety of techniques to assess outcome. Regarding programs, it is helpful to distinguish between balance-specific training and multimodal training ones. The former use postural exercises that typically incorporate static (i.e., maintaining a steady position in sitting and standing positions) and dynamic (i.e., maintaining a steady position during limb segment or whole-body movement) testing and training exercises. Dynamic balance can be further subdivided as proactive balance (i.e., anticipation of a predicted disturbance) and reactive balance (i.e., compensation for a perturbation) (284). Examples of static and dynamic exercises can include single-leg or tandem balancing exercises on stable or unstable platforms, with or without recurrent destabilization (e.g., star excursion, tiltboard, foam mat, wobble board, BOSU ball, ball throwing or catching on a trampoline, and elastic band kicks) (**Fig. 49-9** and 📶 **eFigs. 49-3** and **49-4**).

Multimodal training programs will usually include two or more components of strength, balance, plyometrics, proximal control, or flexibility exercises and often incorporate agility drills and sport-specific exercises. Plyometric exercises utilize

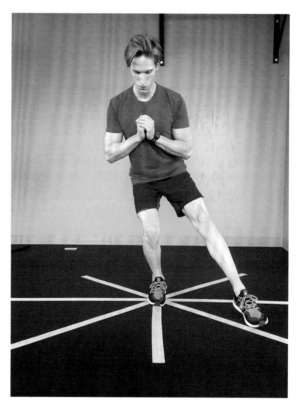

FIGURE 49-9. Balance training exercise using star excursion technique.

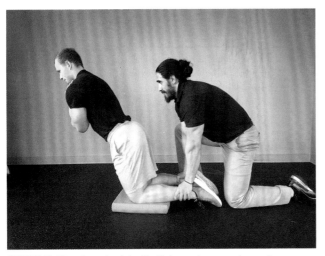

FIGURE 49-10. Example of the Nordic hamstring strength exercise.

ballistic movements containing both concentric and eccentric phases and often incorporate jumping forward and backward, jumping side to side, and tuck and scissors jumps (285). Strengthening exercises aim to promote greater muscular force development—a common exercise is the Nordic hamstring curl (**Fig. 49-10**). Proximal control exercises typically address trunk strengthening (and are thus sometimes categorized as strengthening exercises) and often use the plank, abdominal curls, push-ups, hyperextension, and upper body weight training including bench press, pullover, and pulldown (285). Yoga, Pilates, and tai chi are also considered multimodal programs. A representative multimodal training program determined to be effective for the prevention of ACL injuries is the Prevent injury and Enhance Performance (PEP) program (📶 **eTable 49-5**) (286).

Outcome measures of training interventions aimed at enhancing neuromuscular control and functional performance are varied and extensive. One systematic review counted 68 balance-specific tests in the literature (273). Balance exercises should be separated into different categories because it is thought that balance control is highly task specific as there appears to be only weak to moderate associations between each type (281). Neuromuscular training outcome measures generally fall into the following categories: static and dynamic balance during functional activities, balance test batteries, and computerized dynamic posturography. As noted above, static and dynamic balance tests have also been more narrowly defined as static/dynamic balance, proactive balance, and reactive balance. Examples of static measures would be center of pressure displacement during single-limb stance and the Romberg test. Dynamic measures (including proactive and reactive balance) include the five-times-sit-to-stand test, gait speed/time over 10 m, time to stabilize after single-leg jump landing, Functional Reach Test, and Push and Release Test. Functional measures involving balance can include the Timed Up and Go test and Berg Balance Scale. Other outcomes in the neuromotor literature include recurrence and prevention of injury; muscle strength, agility, gait, jump, and sprint performance; muscle reflex activity; rate of force development; and electromyography. A complete description of these outcomes is beyond the scope of this chapter, but the interested reader is referred to additional resources (4,280,281,287).

Neuromotor Training Guidelines

Many different neuromuscular exercises to improve balance and its related functional activities have been proposed over time and only recently have isolated components begun to be investigated. In a systematic review in 2008, Orr and colleagues found that the use of progressive resistance training in isolation did not improve balance in older adults (273). And a recent meta-analysis investigating correlations between balance and lower extremity muscle strength/power found only a small correlation between measures of maximal strength (which varied by age) and dynamic steady-state balance (e.g., 10-m walk test), leading the authors to conclude that these components are independent of each other (i.e., task specific) and should be tested and trained complementarily across the life span (287). Also, muscle power (force × velocity) may have more influence on balance than strength. Power declines more rapidly than strength with advancing age and is more strongly associated with performance in everyday activities (288). The implication for training is that programs should include task-specific balance, strength, and power components to increase balance and muscular strength/power (287).

The influence of trunk muscle strength on balance and the most effective techniques to improve core strength are coming to light. Anatomically, the core is defined as the axial skeleton and all soft tissues with a proximal attachment originating on the axial skeleton. Functionally, the core is a kinetic link that facilitates the transfer of torques and angular momentum between upper and lower extremities during the execution of whole-body movements as part of sports and occupational skills, fitness activities, and activities of daily living (248). Traditional core and Pilates strength training often utilize a number of trunk muscle exercises through variations on abdominal bracing, planks, bridges, partial sit-ups, lumbar extension, and trunk rotations (**Fig. 49-11**).

A recent systematic review found that compared to traditional strength training, core strength training resulted in more pronounced effects regarding balance and mobility in older adults; the addition of unstable elements (e.g., balance pads, Swiss balls) was recommended to contribute to progression of exercises (289). It is known that performing exercises on unstable bases appears to increase core activation (290).

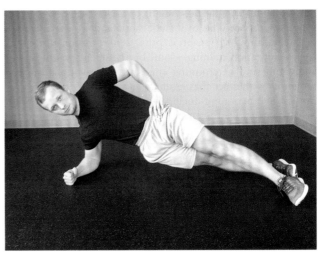

FIGURE 49-11. Participant performing a core strength exercise (side plank).

However, Behm and colleagues determined that ground-based free-weight exercises, such as Olympic lifts, squats, and dead lifts, can result in core activation similar to or higher than that achieved with traditional unstable core exercises (248). Also, a recent meta-analysis found that training programs utilizing proximal control and strength training demonstrated the greatest prophylactic effects on ACL injury (285). Thus, it appears that core strengthening and Pilates should be used as an adjunct, or even an alternative, to traditional balance and/or resistance training programs to develop more efficient use of the upper and lower extremities and thus improve balance, functional performance, and injury prevention (289).

For quite some time, the optimal frequency, intensity, time, type, volume, and progression of neuromotor exercise were not known (5,34,46). In a recently published meta-analysis of 25 studies, of which only 7 were classified as high quality, dose-response relationships for balance training parameters leading to balance improvements in young healthy adults with differing levels of athletic ability were proposed (280). Based on this analysis of primarily single mode balance training techniques (e.g., wobble board, biomechanical ankle platform system, single-leg balance), Lesinski and colleagues found that balance training appears to be most effective in improving measures of steady-state balance in elite athletes (280). They found that an effective training protocol that improves measures of steady-state and proactive balance is characterized by a training period of 11 to 12 weeks, a frequency of three to six training sessions per week, at least 16 to 19 training sessions, four exercises per training session, two sets per exercise, and a duration of 21 to 40 seconds for a single balance exercise (280) (**Table 49-10**). Due to the task-specific nature of balance training, it should include exercises that promote static/dynamic steady-state (e.g., single-leg balance), proactive (e.g., star excursion), and reactive (e.g., push-pull) balance, which should additionally be performed in a sport- or task-specific context (291,292).

Lesinski and colleagues were not able to determine the best time to perform balance training (i.e., before or after sport-specific training sessions). They also could not say whether the improvements in balance were protocol specific or whether other types of training regimens (e.g., plyometrics) might produce similar effects. This has implications in the design of multimodal training regimens. In addressing intensity, they noted that there is no methodologic approach available in the literature on how to properly assess intensity during balance training (280). Exercise progression is also necessary to persistently challenge postural control during the course of a training period in keeping with the overload principle of performing exercise at or near the limit of an individual's capability to induce a training effect. Progression can occur through increased task difficulty by narrowing the base of support and limiting the use of sensory information (i.e., from eyes open to closed and from standing on firm ground to standing on foam).

To address balance training program parameters in older adults, Lesinski et al. published another meta-analysis of 23 studies, of which only 6 were considered of high quality (281). Excluded in the analysis were studies that used a combined (i.e., multimodal) type of balance training (e.g., balance and resistance training) and only one specific type of balance training (e.g., tai chi and water-based training). They found that balance training utilizing static/dynamic steady-state, proactive, and reactive balance exercises on stable and unstable surfaces with eyes opened or closed leads to improvements in the respective proxies for each area (e.g., dynamic steady-state balance proxy = gait speed, proactive balance proxy = Functional Reach Test, reactive balance proxy = perturbation test), as well as in balance test batteries. To achieve improvements in balance in healthy older adults, they suggest a protocol involving a training period and frequency similar to that of young adults (i.e., 11 to 12 weeks, 3 sessions per week), but with a greater number of total training sessions (36 to 40 vs. 16 to 19), longer duration of a single training session (31 to 45 minutes vs. 11 to 15 minutes), and higher total duration of balance training per week (91 to 120 minutes vs. 33 to 90 minutes). Parameters for sets and/or repetitions per exercise and the duration of a single exercise could not be determined with the available data.

Injury and Fall Prevention

The key to the development of effective fall- and injury-preventive strategies is to address modifiable risk factors. Anatomic, hormonal, and genetic components are nonmodifiable, whereas biomechanical and neuromuscular components are modifiable (285). Deficits in balance and lower extremity muscle strength/power have been identified as important intrinsic risk factors for injury and falls in children, adolescents, adults, and seniors (293–296). In the elderly, the two most important intrinsic predictors for a fall are medication use and poor balance (297). Proxies of poor balance associated with a two- to threefold increased risk of falls are (a) a standing time of ≤ 19 seconds in the modified Romberg test, (b) a habitual gait speed of less than 1 m/s, and (c) a duration of ≥ 13.5 seconds to compete the Timed Up and Go test (281). A large body of evidence now documents the favorable effects of balance training on motor performance and injury prevention (281). Well-designed exercise programs targeting strength and balance, and sometimes walking, have been shown to prevent falls and injuries in community-dwelling elderly (297–300). Strength training alone does not transfer effectively to improvements in balance, activities of daily living, or fall risk (273). And as mentioned earlier, strength and dynamic steady-state balance (e.g., time/speed while walking) are independent of each other (i.e., task specific) and should therefore be tested

TABLE 49-10	Dose-Response Relationships in Balance Training in Young Healthy Adults
Training Modalities	**Results/Most Effective Dose**
Training period	11–12 wk
Training frequency	Three or six times per week
Number of training sessions	16–19 training sessions
Duration of a single training session	11–15 min
Number of exercises per training session	Four exercises
Number of sets per exercise	Two sets
Duration of a single balance training exercise	21–40 s

and trained in a complementary manner (287). Recently, Hafström et al. developed a multimodal home exercise program based on existing fall intervention programs but simplified to be used without devices and to include reweighting strategies as well as challenges to the vestibulo-ocular and the vestibulocervical systems to improve gaze stabilization (301). They found this balance-enhancing exercise program to be safe, efficient, and cost-effective (📶 eTable 49-6).

In their systematic review of core and Pilates training for balance, functional performance, and fall prevention, Granacher et al. were able to determine that (a) there is a significant relationship between trunk muscle strength and balance, functional performance, and falls in seniors; (b) core strength training is effective for the promotion of trunk muscle strength, balance/mobility, and functional performance; and (c) Pilates exercise training can have a positive impact on various measures of trunk muscle strength, balance, functional performance, and falls in older adults (289). The addition of unstable elements (e.g., Swiss ball, balance pad) further enhances balance performance and core strength but must be applied with proper supervision and progressed in a safe manner and with the correct prescription (i.e., frequency, intensity, number of exercises, sets, repetitions, duration, which is currently under investigation) (289). However, it appears that a longer-duration (i.e., 12 weeks) Pilates program is likely more effective than shorter ones at reducing the occurrence of falls (302). Whether a trunk muscle strengthening program alone has the ability to reduce fall rate in older individuals is currently unresolved.

Exercise-based prevention strategies are primarily developed and applied to modify parameters of proprioception, neuromuscular control, flexibility, jumping and landing skills, strength, and balance. In a systematic review, Hubscher et al. reported that balance training or the combination of balance training with plyometric, strengthening, sport-specific, and/or stretching exercises is effective in preventing knee and ankle injuries in young basketball, handball, soccer, volleyball, hockey, and floor ball players (283). In their meta-analysis of multimodal neuromuscular training programs, which implemented balance, strength, plyometric, and/or proximal control exercises for ACL injury prevention, Sugimoto et al. further elucidated that strength and proximal control training had the greatest prophylactic effect (285). Also, although not statistically significant, they found that those programs using plyometrics reduced ACL injury incidence and that balance training alone did not reduce ACL injuries. However, balance exercise in conjunction with other types of exercises appears to be effective (285). Therefore, a reasonable approach to prevention is to incorporate warm-up programs not requiring balance equipment but utilizing stretching, strengthening, sport-specific agility drills, and landing techniques (which can be considered a form a balance training if knee position is properly coached) applied for longer than 3 consecutive months (303). In a systematic review, it was determined that the "11+" prevention strategy significantly reduces overall and overuse lower limb injuries as well as knee injuries among young female footballers; the "Knee Injury Prevention Program" significantly reduced the risk of noncontact lower limb and overuse injuries in young amateur female football and basketball players; the "PEP program" strategy reduces the incidence of ACL injuries; the "HarmoKnee" program reduces the risk of knee injuries

in teenage female footballers; and the "Anterior Knee Pain Prevention Training Program" significantly reduces the incidence of anterior knee pain in military recruits (303).

Rehabilitation

Rehabilitation of neuromuscular function after surgery or injury aims to improve and optimize sensorimotor control. It is assumed that altered feedback mechanisms of mechanoreceptors after joint injury lead to CNS reorganization processes in sensorimotor integration (i.e., learning) and subsequently to alterations of motor responses (e.g., adaptations of neuromuscular control) (304). Neuromotor training is incorporated into rehabilitation programs to restore proprioception and neuromuscular function compromised by injury (282). A systematic review of 15 trials of relatively low methodologic quality found that there is moderate evidence that neuromotor training consisting of balance, perturbation, or plyometric exercises is effective for the prevention of further injuries and for the enhancement of joint functionality after ankle instability and ACL ruptures (282). Due to the large variety of exercises included in these programs, it is currently not possible to determine if one component may be more effective than another. Previously, Hess et al. determined that 4 weeks of agility training alone did not improve static single-leg balance in subjects with functionally unstable ankles (305). However, it seems possible that training periods of 6 weeks or longer are more effective for effecting physiologic adaptations responsible for recurrent injury prevention (282). Emery et al. investigated a home balance training program with a wobble board done daily for 6 weeks and then weekly for 6 months (306). It was found to be effective in preventing all self-reported athletic injury over 6 months, that it might reduce the risk of ankle sprain, and that the intervention was more effective for participants with a history of previous injury than for those without previous injury (306). In a study of basketball and soccer players utilizing single-leg stance and balance board exercises five times a week for 4 weeks before the start of the season and then three times a week throughout the season, the ankle sprain incidence among athletes with a history of a sprain was significantly reduced (307). Also, in a study of female collegiate soccer players, Gilchrist et al. found 12 weeks of multimodal neuromuscular training (i.e., the PEP program) to have a preventative effect on the risk of ACL injury, especially among athletes with a history of ACL injury (286).

Performance Improvement

Performance improvement or enhancement involves procedures or techniques enacted to achieve a greater level of success. The concept implies that an individual or athlete is presently functioning at a successful or steady-state level. It is now well known that balance training in its many forms improves measures of steady-state, proactive, and reactive balance and is effective in preventing and rehabilitating lower extremity injuries (276,280,283,285). Parameters for achieving improved balance have also been elucidated, as noted above. What remains unclear is whether improvement in these measures of postural and neuromuscular control translates into enhanced performance. The large variety of exercises included in neuromuscular training programs has made it difficult to determine which intervention, or combination, might be responsible for improved performance. The literature also is unspecific as to whether and how training-related balance improvements transfer to sport- or task-specific skill enhancement (280). As the importance of trunk strengthening on balance becomes realized, it is reasonable to assume improvements in core strength translate to improvements in performance. However, the best program to achieve this is not clear. While unstable conditions and ground-based free-weight resistance exercises are both techniques to improve core activation, the addition of unstable bases to resistance exercises can decrease force, power, velocity, and ROM and thus is not recommended as the primary training mode for athletic conditioning (248). Zech et al. also recommended the use of balance exercises for postural and neuromuscular control improvement but stated that to achieve optimal enhancements in sprint, jumping, or strength performance, other training programs (e.g., strength or plyometric training) are more effective (276).

FLEXIBILITY

Importance

Flexibility is the ability of a structure or segment of the body to move freely through an available ROM. Mobility is often used interchangeably with flexibility although, in the strictest sense, the former is a more complex construct. Active mobility requires neuromuscular activation to allow the occurrence of ROM for functional activities (4). Mobility also can be used to describe the quality of movement achieved. A closely related concept to flexibility and mobility is performance. If performance is the ability to accomplish a task, whether to rebound a basketball or squat down and pick an object up off the floor, flexibility can be a potential limiting factor to performance. The foundation for all performance starts with the underlying quality of movement. If that movement is compromised, performance will be suboptimal.

It is important to maintain a ROM adequate to perform one's desired activities. Even relatively small reductions in ROM may result in biomechanical accommodations that place abnormal stress on tissues elsewhere in the body and theoretically predispose an individual to injury. Severe restrictions in ROM may even produce complications such as skin breakdown. An injured body segment or joint can often present with restricted ROM. It is this correlation that drives specific professions, for example, physical and occupational therapists, to use various techniques to focus on restoring this motion with the goal of re-establishing the individual's prior level of function. When movement, and by association flexibility and mobility, is compromised, collaboration with the appropriate health care providers is paramount for optimal outcomes.

Although restoration and maintenance of a functional ROM are intuitively desirable, research has only recently confirmed that flexibility appears to be of greater benefit than cost in terms of performance, ROM, and injury outcomes (308). While pre-exercise static stretching (SS) less than 60 seconds can be performed without compromising maximal muscle performance to a substantial degree, and can enhance performance in activities performed at longer muscle lengths, detrimental effects of SS are mainly limited to durations greater than a minute (309). Proprioceptive neuromuscular facilitation (PNF) stretching appears to have a small negative impact on muscle performance if conducted within 5 minutes of an activity (308). Overall, dynamic stretching (DS) does not have

robust evidence to support performance enhancement but can produce small to moderate performance improvements when performed minutes before physical activity and utilizing faster, and/or more intense ballistic, stretches (308,310–313). All types of stretching improve ROM, with one technique not determined to be more effective than another (308). While SS and PNF have no clear effect on all-cause or overuse injuries, the current research indicates that preactivity stretching may be beneficial for injury prevention in sports with a sprint running component (308).

It has been demonstrated that running economy may be better among those who have some lower extremity tightness (314,315), but this still is not a settled topic (316) and may depend on individual variables of flexibility and stiffness (317). Also, most studies demonstrate that stretching prior to exercise is ineffective in reducing soreness (308).

Stretch-induced loss of force has been attributed to alterations in the muscle force-length relationship, stretch-induced muscle damage, reduced blood flow, diminished electromechanical coupling, and reduced central drive (308). Reduced central drive through cortical modulation of muscle spindle facilitation of the motor neuron (318) has the most consistent human evidence underpinning changes in muscular force production after stretching (308).

It is appropriate to include stretching in a preactivity routine that is preceded by a warm-up aerobic activity and followed by poststretching dynamic activities that replicate the forthcoming task or activity. Prolonged stretching is not recommended within 5 minutes of an activity. Where concerns of optimized strength and power take precedence over increased ROM and reduced muscle injury risk, it is prudent to perform flexibility exercises after these activities (34). However, dynamic stretching can induce performance enhancements when performed soon before an activity and can be utilized to replicate task-specific movements during the stretch and dynamic activity warm-up phases. Overall, stretching is recommended for reducing muscle injuries and increasing joint ROM with inconsequential effects on subsequent athletic performance (308).

Measuring Flexibility and Mobility

Flexibility and mobility may be assessed in various ways. Angle measurements can be made with a goniometer, electrogoniometer, or flexometer. Inclinometers are also popular tools and smartphone applications have been found to be convenient as well as reliable and valid (319–321). Flexibility for some movements is also commonly assessed through distance measurements between specific reproducible reference points. One example of this technique would be the assessment of temporomandibular joint motion through measurement of the distance between the upper and the lower incisors. Furthermore, landmarks may be utilized to assess flexibility within specific patterns of motion. For instance, when reaching behind the back, the practitioner can record the highest vertebrae the patient can reach to with that hand.

Each one of these techniques has a set of norms, sometimes in ranges, to be measured and applied quantitatively across and within individuals (322). However, it is often prudent to compare measurements bilaterally and assess for asymmetry that might otherwise fall within normal ranges. Another technique involves evaluating the quality of a person's movement or functional mobility. Movement assessments such as the Selective Functional Movement Assessment have been designed to categorize patients as either functional or dysfunctional by assessing the quality and quantity of a patient's movement using key indicators. For instance, when assessing multisegmental flexion (reaching and touching toes), the inability to evenly flex the spine, or keep the knees from flexing, may categorize this patient as dysfunctional (323).

Factors Affecting Range of Motion

Many factors can limit joint ROM, including tightness of soft tissue structures such as the muscle, tendon, ligament, neural tissue, and joint capsule. Involuntary muscle contraction in the form of spasm or trigger point formation can also restrict range. The bony contour of the joint is important in accessing full ROM. When there is abnormal bone growth around a joint, range can be restricted. In addition, intra-articular loose bodies (e.g., bone or cartilage) and excessive fluid may inconsistently restrict joint ROM.

Range of motion varies widely among individuals. Regular activities using a full ROM will help maintain range, but the maintenance of ROM is specific to the joints that are used. For instance, an individual can have normal range in one joint but severely restricted range in another. When connective tissue is not stretched, the collagen component gradually shortens. As a result, the periarticular collagen and the connective tissue of the muscle shorten. Furthermore, immobilization of a muscle in a shortened position also causes a decrease in the muscle length through a decrease in the number of sarcomeres in the muscle (324).

Age and sex also seem to affect ROM. Women tend to have greater ROM than do men, and young people usually have greater range than do the elderly. Tissue temperature is another factor affecting ROM, with warm tissue having greater distensibility than cool tissue (325).

Methods to Improve Range of Motion

Techniques

Identifying the primary limiting structure will ultimately guide the treatment approach or prescribed exercises. Neural tension is a common limiting factor and may present as limitations in specific combinations of movements depending on the neural structure involved. A solid understanding of neuroanatomy and musculoskeletal anatomy may help guide succeeding treatment by identifying common areas of neural encroachment. For instance, the pectoralis minor and anterior scalene muscles are common areas of compression of the brachial plexus (326). Improving the extensibility of these tissues may improve overall upper-quarter mobility in the presence of median nerve neural tension. Furthermore, flossing techniques, in which one end of the nerve is tensioned while the other is slackened, are commonly used to improve neurodynamics through the spine and involved extremity (327).

Tightness of ligaments and joint capsules is commonly seen after a trauma or immobilization and may accompany other tight structures. Joint mobilization is a method that can ameliorate these deficits. An understanding of the arthrokinematics of the affected joint is necessary to help restore ROM when these structures are suspected (319,328). A joint mobilization can be applied to stretch the particular area of a joint capsule over which the moving bone segment glides. For instance, to restore ankle dorsiflexion, the talus must move posteriorly on the tibia. Shearing the talus posteriorly with respect to the tibia would stretch the posterior aspect of the joint capsule of the ankle and can improve limited dorsiflexion ROM (329).

The most commonly implicated structures for limiting ROM are muscle and tendon. Because these are contractile units, neuromuscular states such as reflexive guarding and hypertonicity can be major contributing factors in acute and chronic conditions, respectively. In these instances, it may be prudent to address the neural system with stretching using the principals of PNF developed by Kabat (330). The two most common PNF stretching techniques are the contract-relax technique and the agonist contract-relax technique. With the former, the muscle is statically stretched, then contracted for 6 to 8 seconds, and then relaxed and passively stretched further to an increased pain-free range. This process is repeated three to six times. The agonist contract-relax technique is identical to the contract-relax technique except that the stretch is accompanied by a submaximal contraction of the opposing muscle to the one being stretched. This voluntary contraction of the opposing muscle theoretically results in reciprocal inhibition of the stretched muscle.

While it has been theorized that PNF works through autogenic and/or reciprocal inhibition and use of the stretch reflex, this concept is controversial (331). As PNF involves a component of SS, its efficacy at increasing ROM is likely shared with this technique. Stretch tolerance, that is, increases in the capacity to tolerate loading prior to stretch termination (332,333), reduced muscle stiffness, that is, changes in mechanical properties (334,335); and reduction in tendon stiffness (336) have been reported after SS and PNF stretching.

In most cases, muscles may become shortened or lengthened secondary to postural impairments, muscle imbalances, and/or simply not accessing specific ranges of motion over long periods of time. However, because multiple muscles with similar actions often cross each joint, it may be difficult to implicate which of the group is involved, and this may require a more in-depth analysis or movement assessment. Movement tests, such as the modified Thomas test, help identify which of the major hip flexors are involved by passively extending a leg into hip extension off the edge of a bed and examining the predilection of the limb to rest in a specific position (337) (🛜 **eFig. 49-5** and **Fig. 49-12**). This knowledge can help develop a more effective stretching protocol individualized to a patient's needs.

In addition to PNF stretching, static and dynamic stretching are techniques used to restore soft tissue extensibility and consequently flexibility. Static stretching involves a slowly applied stretch that is held for a prescribed length of time. Proponents of this technique believe that the muscle stretch reflex is minimized through a slow, progressive stretch (338). Static stretches can be active or passive (339). Active SS involves holding the stretched position using the strength of the agonist muscle. Passive SS involves assuming a position such that an external force is exerted upon the limb to move it into the new position (5). Passive stretching can be achieved with the use of a partner or devices such as stretch-out straps, yoga blocks, or elastic bands. Static stretching is generally easy to perform, has little associated risk of injury, and is also known to not increase the risk of injury (308). Holding a stretch for 10 to 30 seconds to the point of tightness seems prudent to enhance flexibility, and

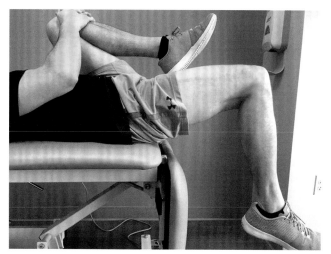

FIGURE 49-12. Subject performing a modified Thomas test with restricted hip flexor flexibility.

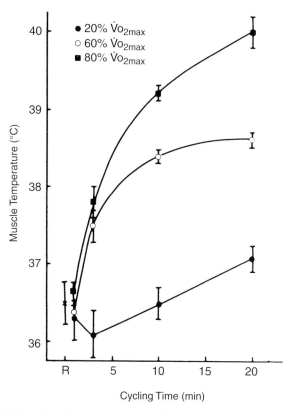

FIGURE 49-13. Effect of leg cycling at different intensities and durations on intramuscular temperature of the quadriceps at a depth of 3 cm. The mean resting value is represented at R. (Reprinted by permission from Springer: Hoffman MD, Williams CA, Lind AR. Changes in isometric function following rhythmic exercise. *Eur J Appl Physiol.* 1985;54(2):177–183. Copyright © 1985 Springer-Verlag.)

as noted above, it has been found there is clear dose-response effect in which longer stretch durations, for example, ≥60 seconds, likely elicit performance impairments (309,340). While this may have important implications for elite competitions, there is also evidence to suggest that longer-duration stretching interventions, for example greater than 5 minutes, may have a greater potential to decrease risk of injury (308). In older adults, stretching is recommended for 30 to 60 seconds as this may result in greater flexibility than shorter-duration techniques (5).

Dynamic stretching involves the performance of controlled movements through the ROM of the active joint(s) and can take the form of high- and low-frequency movements or ballistic stretching (stretching using momentum in an attempt to exceed the normal ROM, which can include bouncing) (311). DS is sometimes thought to be preferable to SS in preparation for physical activity because it can replicate the movement patterns of the activity to be performed, increase central drive, and elevate core temperature (308). However, as noted above, there currently is no robust evidence to support significantly improved performance after DS.

When able to participate, the patient can provide valuable feedback to ensure that appropriate positioning is used so that the desired tissues are being stretched. The patient should also understand that some discomfort may be required for adequate stretching, but prolonged poststretching pain is indicative of an overzealous approach. It also seems to be of considerable importance for the patient and the clinician to understand that the most rapid gains in ROM will be achieved through regular stretching. The ROM of a joint is improved immediately after all types of stretching and shows chronic improvement after about 3 to 4 weeks of regular stretching (34). Stretching exercises are most effective when performed daily, but improvements in flexibility can be seen by stretching 2 to 3 days per week. Stretching routines can be completed by most individuals in approximately 10 minutes if each stretching exercise is repeated two to four times as recommended (5).

Modalities

Some modalities may be used to enhance ROM. Because the distensibility of warm tissue is greater than that of cool tissue (325), heat is commonly used before stretching. Ultrasound

is the best therapeutic modality for heating deep-lying tissues (341) and can be used effectively as a prestretching treatment when there are no contraindications for its use. Exercise also increases tissue temperature. For example, the quadriceps intramuscular temperature can be elevated by 2°C after 10 minutes of cycling at a moderate intensity (**Fig. 49-13**) (342). One way in which DS is thought to produce benefits in ROM is through an elevation in core temperature (343). The use of passive modalities is becoming less popular as we understand the therapeutic effects of movement and the psychological benefits of becoming increasingly independent of the health care provider. Active interventions, rather than passive, will empower the patient to improve their condition and should be encouraged whenever possible.

EFFECTS OF EXERCISE TRAINING, PHYSICAL ACTIVITY, AND SEDENTARY BEHAVIOR

In the past two decades, there has been a substantial increase in the prevalence of obesity in the United States with an estimated 30% of the adult population over the age of 20 classified as obese (344). This trend is multifactorial and attributed to changes in diet and daily level of physical activity (344). Opportunities to burn calories have diminished as daily activities have become more automated, leisure activities have become more sedentary, and focus on physical activity in schools has lessened (344). The rise in obesity and sedentary behavior has large implications on the prevalence of chronic health conditions and risk of mortality. Not only are obesity and physical inactivity independent risk factors in the development of CVD, diabetes, and some cancers, they are also associated with other major risk factors such as hypertension, hyperlipidemia, and metabolic syndrome. Fortunately, the detrimental effects of obesity and sedentary behavior can be countered with regular physical activity with some health benefits starting immediately after exercise and others beginning with as little as 60 minutes a week (1). It is known that even short episodes of physical activity are beneficial and once the health benefits from physical activity begin to accumulate, additional amounts of activity provide additional benefits (1) (see 🛜 **eTable 49-7** for the major research findings of health benefits of physical activity).

All-Cause Mortality

The health benefits of physical activity are many (**Table 49-11**). Although the minimal and/or optimal intensity, frequency, and duration of physical activity remain under investigation, multiple studies have reported that there is a strong inverse relationship between level of physical activity and risk of all-cause and cardiovascular mortality (345). Additionally, this decrease in mortality risk appears to be independent of other risk factors, including cigarette smoking, hyperlipidemia, gender, and age (345,346). The largest reduction in mortality was observed in the most sedentary groups of subjects, indicating that even modest increases in

physical activity can have a large impact on all-cause mortality (345,347). Initial attempts to develop physical activity guidelines focused on results from a prospective long-term follow-up study following middle-aged male subjects that showed a 20% to 40% reduction in mortality associated with the beginning of a moderately vigorous sports activity (MET > 4.5) (346). Thus, major health organizations suggested subjects exercise at an intensity of 3 to 6 METs with an overall energy expenditure of at least 1,000 kcal/wk (345). The ACSM has developed more practical recommendations for physical activity guidelines based on minutes of moderate-intensity activity and minutes of vigorous-intensity activity, a concept easier to understand than the MET construct. In this system, the recommendation is for at least 150 minutes of moderate-intensity activity per week, which is equivalent to 500 MET-minutes, long held as the minimum requirement for exercise to decrease mortality risk.

Although multiple, large cohort studies have shown an increased mortality risk with sedentary behavior and, conversely, a lowered mortality risk in subjects with increased physical activity, it is also important to note that the exercise-related health benefits are only evident with consistent physical activity throughout a subject's lifetime. In the landmark study following Harvard Alumni, subjects who participated in college athletics but went on to be sedentary during adulthood had a much higher mortality risk than those subjects who maintained a physically active lifestyle (348).

TABLE 49-11	**The Health Benefits of Physical Activity**
Children and Adolescents	**Adults and Older Adults**

• Improved bone health (ages 3 through 17 y)
• Improved weight status (ages 3 through 17 y)
• Improved cardiorespiratory and muscular fitness (ages 6 through 17 y)
• Improved cardiometabolic health (ages 6 through 17 y)
• Reduced risk of depression (ages 6 to 17 y)
• Improved cognition (ages 6 to 13 y)
  • Includes performance on academic achievement tests, executive function, processing speed, and memory
	• Lower risk of all-cause mortality
	• Lower risk of cardiovascular disease mortality
	• Lower risk of cardiovascular disease (including heart disease and stroke)
	• Lower risk of hypertension
	• Lower risk of type 2 diabetes
	• Lower risk of adverse blood lipid profile
	• Lower risk of cancers of the bladder, breast, colon, endometrium, esophagus, kidney, lung, and stomach
	• Improved quality of life
	• Reduced anxiety
	• Reduced risk of depression
	• Improved sleep
	  • Includes increased sleep efficiency, sleep quality, deep sleep; reduced daytime sleepiness, and frequency of use of medication to aid sleep
	• Slowed or reduced weight gain
	• Weight loss, particularly when combined with reduced calorie intake
	• Prevention of weight regain following initial weight loss
	• Improved bone health
	• Improved physical function
	• Lower risk of falls (older adults)
	• Lower risk of fall-related injuries (older adults)
	• Reduced risk of dementia (including Alzheimer's disease)
	• Improved cognition
	  • Includes executive function, attention, memory, crystallized intelligence[a] and processing speed

Note: Only outcomes with strong or moderate evidence of effect of health benefits of physical activity are included in this table.

[a]Crystallized intelligence is the ability to retrieve and use information that has been acquired over time. It is different from fluid intelligence, which is the ability to store and manipulate new information.

Adapted from U.S. Department of Health and Human Services. *2018 Physical Activity Guidelines for Americans*. 2nd ed. Washington, DC: U.S. Department of Health and Human Services; 2018. Available from: https://health.gov/paguidelines/second-edition/

Cardiovascular Disease

According to the Centers for Disease Control, CVD is the leading cause of death in men and women with coronary artery disease predominating. The mechanism by which physical activity reduces the risk of CVD is not entirely clear but may in part be related to its positive impact on risk factors such as hypertension and hyperlipidemia (348). However, physical inactivity is also an independent risk factor for coronary artery disease after statistical adjustment for other risk factors (349).

Multiple well-controlled studies and subsequent review articles have consistently shown that physical activity can significantly reduce blood pressure (350–352). Aerobic exercise training lowers blood pressure in subjects with stage 1 hypertension on average 3.4 to 10 mm Hg for systolic blood pressure and 2.4 to 7.6 mm Hg for diastolic blood pressure. Similar reductions in blood pressure were also seen in subjects with stage 2 hypertension who engaged in an aerobic exercise regimen for up to 32 weeks (345). Furthermore, a meta-analysis investigating the role of resistance training on blood pressure found that progressive resistance training reduced systolic and diastolic blood pressures by 2% to 4% (353). This translates to an approximate 3 mm Hg decrease in systolic and diastolic blood pressure, which is admittedly less than the results achieved by aerobic activity. However, this data indicates that resistance training may be a useful adjunct to aerobic activity in the control of hypertension and, subsequently, CVD.

Although moderate-intensity aerobic activity has been shown to reduce blood pressure, there has been a resistance to recommending more intense activity (MET > 5) secondary to some studies suggesting an increased risk of left ventricular hypertrophy. However, it appears the effect of elevated blood pressure related to exercise on left ventricular mass may be modulated by level of fitness. For moderately fit to highly fit individuals, exercise blood pressure was routinely 10 mm Hg lower than that of their low-fitness counterparts. Additionally, for every 1 MET increased in workload achieved, there was a 42% reduction in risk for left ventricular hypertrophy (345).

The effect of physical activity on blood lipids is less clear than that seen with reduction in blood pressure. A meta-analysis looked at 51 studies, half of which were randomized controlled trials, that prescribed aerobic exercise of varying intensities for a duration of at least 12 weeks and then evaluated blood lipids and lipoproteins including total cholesterol, triglycerides, high-density lipoprotein (HDL), and low-density lipoprotein (LDL). The effect on blood lipids and lipoproteins was inconsistent across all of the studies. The most consistent result was an increase in HDL by a mean of 4.5% (354). Reductions in LDL reached up to 5.0%, with a potential greater reduction when combined with dietary intervention (354). These findings indicated that although physical activity appears to have a positive effect on blood lipids and lipoproteins, further investigation is required to determine a dose-dependent relationship and/or the optimal exercise prescription for lipid reduction.

Physical activity has also been linked to increased myocardial perfusion, although the exact mechanism remains unclear. One theory focuses on the correction of endothelial dysfunction noted in subjects with coronary artery disease (355). There have also been studies looking at the intima-media thickness of carotid and coronary arteries, which is used to quantify atherosclerosis. Studies have shown that physically inactive subjects have increased intima-media thickness, but there appears to be an inverse relationship between intima-media thickness of the carotid artery and aerobic exercise capacity. Additionally, sufficient exercise has been shown to actually decrease carotid and coronary stenosis (356).

In addition to coronary artery disease, a significant proportion of SCDs are related to arrhythmias with ventricular tachyarrhythmia predominating. Predisposition to cardiac arrhythmias appears to be related to cardiac autonomic control, particularly an increase in sympathetic activity. Physical activity modulates this risk by increasing the cardiac parasympathetic tone (357).

Physical activity is important for secondary prevention as well. In a meta-analysis reviewing 48 randomized controlled trials comparing standard medical care versus an exercise rehabilitation program in subjects following a cardiac event, all-cause mortality and cardiac mortality were reduced by 20% and 26%, respectively (358). As hospital stays become shorter and subjects present with more complicated clinical scenarios including multiple comorbidities, exercise rehabilitation may assume a large role in the secondary prevention of CVD. For additional information on secondary prevention of CVD, the reader is referred to Chapter 33.

Metabolic Syndrome

Several definitions for metabolic syndrome have been proposed, but common features include dyslipidemia, insulin resistance, hypertension, and obesity (359). Each of these factors is an independent risk factor in the promotion of atherosclerosis and CVD; however when present together, they confer an even greater risk for the development of CVD and premature mortality.

Research thus far mostly includes observational studies following diabetic subjects and their rate of CVD and mortality. Consistently, an inverse relationship between physical activity and risk of CVD and/or mortality has been found (359). Additionally, increased physical activity has been shown to decrease the risk of nondiabetic patients becoming diabetic as demonstrated in the Finnish Diabetes Prevention Study and Diabetes Prevention Program (360,361). Although research focusing on physical activity and metabolic syndrome is sparse, one epidemiologic study focusing on level of physical activity and development of metabolic syndrome revealed a dose-dependent relationship between leisure-time activity and reduction in prevalence of metabolic syndrome (362). Finally, a cross-sectional study surveyed over 1,400 subjects by obtaining detailed medical records, performing thorough physical exams, blood pressure measurements, and blood work in order to evaluate the association between prevalence of metabolic syndrome and level of physical activity. Results suggested that a high level of physical activity (i.e., walking >14 km/wk) was significantly associated with a lower prevalence of metabolic syndrome (363).

Obesity is a strong independent risk factor for CVD and mortality and is rapidly becoming more prevalent as lifestyles become more sedentary. Increased physical activity has been shown to result in modest weight reduction but, when combined with dietary intervention, may result in more substantial weight loss. Weight loss through physical activity is directly related to the amount of kilocalories expended, thus making duration of physical activity important (349). To combat obesity, the ACSM recommends moderate-intensity physical activity for 150 to 250 minutes per week to prevent weight gain and greater than 250 minutes per week to promote weight loss (48). Following weight loss, continued increased levels of physical activity at a moderate intensity for greater than 250 minutes per week may help prevent weight gain, but further studies are needed to investigate the best intervention to prevent weight gain (48). However, contrary to popular belief, weight reduction alone does not seem to appreciably modify risk of CVD and mortality. Large epidemiologic studies suggest that level of fitness may play a larger role in risk reduction than simply weight loss (345).

Improved Psychological Well-Being and Quality of Life

Mood state is improved immediately after aerobic exercise among regular exercisers (364). Furthermore, it is well recognized that regular physical activity improves general sense of well-being and quality of life (365–367). It is postulated that reduced psychological stress and improved tolerance for activities of daily living contribute to the perception of improved well-being and quality of life. In addition, regular exercise may help improve quality of life by protecting people from development of disabling diseases such as heart disease, diabetes, cancer, and cognitive decline as well as enabling people with diseases to regain functional work tolerance. Freedom from disease and ability to function independently into old age are important factors in quality of life. Shephard estimated that remaining physically active into old age could allow one to maintain functional independence for 10 to 20 years longer than if one is inactive (368).

Maintenance of Bone Density

Osteoporosis is an important health problem. It causes considerable societal disability among the elderly and is a major contributor to health care costs. Regular physical activity is recommended to slow the age-related decline in BMD, delay the onset of osteoporosis, and reduce fracture risk (369–372). Exercise habits during peak bone-forming years may impact on bone density years later (373). Intuitively, adequate nutrition should accompany exercise to achieve the most beneficial skeletal effects, but optimum amounts of dietary protein are still being determined (374). Additionally, a recent meta-analysis concluded that increasing calcium intake from dietary sources, as well as supplements, produces small, nonprogressive increases in BMD but was unlikely to translate into clinically meaningful reductions in fractures, and therefore, increasing calcium intake is unlikely to be beneficial (375). A positive interaction may exist between calcium supplementation and exercise in increasing BMD over that of exercise alone (376), but more research is needed in this area. The benefits of exercise on bone health are due primarily to increases in bone density, volume, and strength and to a parallel increase in muscle strength (34). Although the optimal duration and/or intensity of physical activity for bone health remains unclear, in general, weight-bearing aerobic exercise in combination with some form of high-impact, high-velocity, high-intensity resistance training is considered the best choice (34).

Decreased Inflammatory Biomarkers

Chronic low levels of inflammation, as measured by levels of CRP, IL-6, and TNF-α, are associated with CVD, obesity, chronic kidney disease, sarcopenia, and osteoarthritis and may contribute to risk of mortality and poor physical functioning. As delineated by Woods et al., multiple cohort studies and randomized controlled trials have reported an inverse, dose-response relationship between physical activity, weight loss, and inflammatory biomarkers, particularly CRP (377). The mechanism whereby inflammatory biomarkers are reduced through exercise is not entirely clear but may result from the loss of adipose tissue, which is known to store proinflammatory

macrophages (377). Additionally, acute exercise has been shown to up-regulate endogenous antioxidant defense systems and increase muscle production of IL-6, which has both inflammatory and anti-inflammatory properties resulting in the reduction of circulating TNF-α (377).

Improved Sleep

The prevalence of insomnia increases with age and has a negative impact on quality of life, mood, and cognition. Currently, treatment for sleep disorders is often pharmacologic. However, there is an increasing body of literature that may support exercise for better sleep. In 2002, a systematic review looked at randomized controlled trials studying the effect of physical activity on insomnia in individuals older than 60 years old and showed an increase in sleep latency, sleep duration, and sleep quality in patients who participated in an exercise program (378). Additionally, a randomized controlled trial of 17 sedentary adults older than 55 showed a statistically significant improvement in sleep quality, sleep latency, sleep duration, and sleep efficiency in the intervention group treated with exercise and sleep hygiene techniques versus the control group, which was treated with sleep hygiene techniques alone (379).

Cognitive Function

With regard to cognitive decline associated with advancing age and dementia, there appears to be a protective factor with physical activity (1). In 2008, a randomized controlled trial studied 170 middle-aged patients with self-reported memory deficits but without a diagnosis of dementia. The patients were randomized to either education plus standard care or a 24-week exercise program. At the beginning and end of the study, patients performed an Alzheimer Disease Assessment Scale—Cognitive Subscale. The study reported a significant increase in cognitive performance in the exercise group as compared to the control group, which actually showed a decline in cognitive functioning (380). There have also been multiple meta-analyses studying the effectiveness of exercise on improving cognitive function. In 2003, a meta-analysis reviewed the effect of aerobic fitness on the cognitive vitality of healthy, sedentary older patients and showed positive effects on overall cognitive functioning, but in particular on executive processing (381). Another meta-analysis performed in 2011 reported an improvement in overall cognitive functioning in both healthy and mildly cognitively impaired patients performing at least 6 weeks of exercise amounting to 60-minute sessions, three times per week (382). There are several theories as to how exercise modulates cognitive functioning. First, it is thought that exercise augments cerebral blood flow, increases the brain's utilization of oxygen and glucose, and may also enhance antioxidant enzyme activity, clearing oxidative free radicals in the brain more quickly (383). Second, it has been shown that exercise can increase the production of neurogrowth factors such as insulin-like growth factor and brain-derived neurotrophic factor, which helps stimulate neurogenesis and may enhance nerve message processing capacity (384). Finally, exercise can stimulate the release of calcium, dopamine, and acetylcholine, all of which are necessary to maintain normal nerve functioning and cognitive function (385).

Reduced Cancer Risk

A growing number of studies have shown that increased physical activity is moderately to strongly associated with a reduced risk of bladder, breast, colon, endometrium, esophagus, kidney, lung, and stomach cancer (1). Besides counteracting the effects of inactivity and improving psychological status (386), evidence suggests moderate exercise improves immune function (61). Other potential direct and/or indirect pathways by which exercise may be beneficial include reduced bowel lining exposure to mutagens via accelerated movement of food through the intestines, reduced breast tissue exposure to circulating estrogen, lowered circulating concentrations of blood insulin and growth factors, and improved body weight management. Exercise may also have positive effects on cancer survivors. A meta-analysis focusing on the effect of exercise on breast cancer patients and survivors reported that exercise promoted a statistically important increase in quality of life, physical functioning, and peak oxygen consumption (387).

EXERCISE PRESCRIPTION IN SPECIAL POPULATIONS

Considerations in Chronic Disease States

Exercise effectively assists in managing numerous medical and disabling conditions. Many individuals treated in the rehabilitation setting with exercise also suffer concomitant medical conditions or disabilities that affect the ability to perform and respond to specific exercises. Accordingly, effective program design requires special considerations for people with disease or disability. In general, the exercise program must not interfere with the standard medical treatment and must vary according to the presence or severity of disease. The following section discusses important considerations for medical conditions and disabilities commonly encountered in rehabilitation settings. Further recommendations for other disease states can be found in the relevant chapters of this book. As noted previously, the *ACSM's Guidelines for Exercise Testing and Prescription* uses the FITT-VP principle for exercise prescription (34). The following sections also will follow this model where the evidence exists in the literature.

Cardiac Disease

Cardiac disease occurs commonly among individuals in the rehabilitation setting. Although CVD generally does not preclude exercise, those prescribing exercise must recognize the presence and extent of disease to design and initiate a safe program. Risk stratification (discussed earlier) significantly assists this process.

It is recommended that cardiac rehabilitation (see Chapter 33) follow the acute hospitalization for a myocardial infarction. Once completed, a regular exercise program should commence (34). General guidelines for aerobic exercise apply to patients with stable cardiac disease. Patients with ischemic changes, angina, or arrhythmias during exercise should exercise at an intensity 10 to 15 beats per minute below the ischemic, angina, or dysrhythmic threshold (34). Individuals at high risk for exercise-induced cardiac emergencies (📶 eTable 49-8) require a more cautious application of exercise intensity and professional supervision, potentially including electrocardiographic and blood pressure monitoring. This population should complete gradual and prolonged cooldowns to reduce the risk of arrhythmias and postexercise hypotension.

Most low- to moderate-risk patients with stable cardiac disease can also safely perform and benefit from resistance

exercise (388,389). The ACSM has published exclusion criteria precluding resistance training for those with a history of cardiac disease, which include congestive heart failure, severe valvular disease, uncontrolled hypertension, uncontrolled dysrhythmias, and other unstable symptoms (34). When monitoring exercise intensity during resistance exercise, rate pressure product likely better indicates ischemic threshold than heart rate because resistance exercises frequently generate large blood pressures. Accurate determination of the rate pressure product requires the measurement of blood pressure during muscular actions, as blood pressure decreases rapidly during relaxation.

Stroke (See Also Chapter 18)

Recent studies, including several meta-analysis and systematic reviews, have shown that aerobic and resistance training, as well as combinations of them, can convey a wide variety of benefits to individuals with subacute and chronic strokes (390–393). A large systematic review demonstrated that progressive resistance training can improve strength and activity in individuals with an acute and chronic stroke without increasing spasticity (393). In one study of participants with subacute stroke, an exercise program consisting of aerobic, resistance, and balance training resulted in improved endurance, balance, and mobility and, subsequently, function and quality of life (394). In a similar study in the same patient population, depressive symptom were improved with aerobic and resistance training (395).

Currently, there are no guidelines for exercise in the subacute and chronic stroke population, but the American Heart Association/American Stroke Association has published recommendations for stroke survivors (396). The scientific statement recognizes that both aerobic and resistance training can improve functional capacity and quality of life. It states that exercise programs need to be customized to the tolerance of the individual with the stroke, their stage of recovery, specific impairments, social support, and physical activity preferences. They recommend low- to moderate-intensity aerobic activity, reduction of sedentary behavior, and resistance training. No other specific recommendations are given.

Arthritis

A variety of different types of exercise can be beneficial for individuals with both osteoarthritis and rheumatoid arthritis (397–400). A Cochrane review of exercise articles for knee osteoarthritis determined that there was high-quality evidence that exercise reduces pain and moderate-quality evidence that exercise can improve physical function (401). They concluded that the magnitude of the treatment effect from exercise was moderately small, but comparable with estimates reported for nonsteroidal anti-inflammatory drugs (401). A narrative review of aerobic and resistance training in individuals with rheumatoid arthritis determined that both water-based and land-based aerobic and resistance training can improve muscle strength and reduce activity limitations (402). Even high-intensity weight-bearing exercises do not appear to increase progression of radiologic joint damage of the hands and feet and may even be protective (403).

In general, the exercise prescription for those with arthritis is consistent with healthy adults. FITT recommendations consider the individual's stability, pain, and functional limitations.

Aerobic training is recommended 3 to 5 days per week. Resistance training is recommended 2 to 3 days per week, and flexibility/ROM exercises are recommended daily. For the most part, aerobic training should be done at a light-to-moderate intensity. Both high and low intensity have both shown improvements in pain, function, and strength in individuals with osteoarthritis and rheumatoid arthritis (397,404,405). However, exercise programs for individuals with arthritis, and especially rheumatoid arthritis, vary according to disease state; when disease activity peaks, minimizing activity might avoid tissue damage (406). For example, high-intensity exercise is contraindicated when there is acute inflammation (34). Programs for arthritis generally rely more heavily on shorter, more frequent exercise sessions, non–weight-bearing or low-impact activities (e.g., swimming and cycling), and flexibility exercises to motivate positive adaptations while concurrently minimizing joint stress (34,407). For resistance training, light-to-moderate intensity is typically recommended, such as 10 to 15 repetitions at a lower percentage of the individuals 1 RM (40% to 60% 1 RM).

For the time component of the exercise prescription for aerobic training, the goal should be the same as healthy adults, ≥150 minutes each week. However, long aerobic training sessions may be difficult for some with arthritis. These individuals can start with 10 minutes per session and gradually build up. The optimal time for resistance training in this population is not known, but it should be determined by pain levels (34).

The type of exercise chosen should be the least painful. Aerobic training with low joint stress, like walking, swimming, or cycling, is recommended. Some with arthritis will be able to use a treadmill for walking, but others may be better off only cycling, swimming, or participating in other nonimpact aerobic exercises. In the prescription of exercise, it is important to base progression of aerobic, flexibility, and resistance training on the individual's pain and other symptoms (34).

There are some special considerations that need to be made in the exercise prescription for those with arthritis. An adequate warm-up and cool-down period of movements through a joint's ROM for approximately 5 to 10 minutes is important. Patients should not exercise during an acute flare-up, but they should continue to do range-of-motion exercises. Exercise should be done at the time of day when pain is least severe. It is important patients understand that some level of pain after exercise is expected, but the pain level should come back to baseline within 2 hours of completing exercise. When exercising in the water, the temperature should be 83°F to 88°F. Functional exercises should be incorporated as often as possible. Finally, appropriate shoes that provide stability and shock absorption are important for this population, and some will benefit from a referral to an orthotist or shoe specialist (34).

Spinal Cord Injury

Spinal cord injury (SCI) affects exercise capacity by altering the amount of functional muscle mass, compromising autonomic nervous control of cardioacceleration, redistributing blood flow, and limiting thermoregulation (see also Chapter 22). Each issue affects exercise capacity, potential training adaptations, and safety during exercise. Despite these physiologic limitations, spinal cord–injured people safely participate in many activities (e.g., long-distance wheelchair propulsion, swimming, kayaking, and skiing) and commonly complete exercise programs of wheelchair propulsion or arm crank ergometry.

Depending on the characteristics of the lesion, a SCI can limit functional muscle mass to the upper body. SCI might severely limit the adaptive potential of central cardiovascular structure and function. As the most effective aerobic exercise rhythmically recruits large muscle groups, this reduction in available muscle mass limits training-induced aerobic demands and therefore alters potential adaptations. People with paraplegia can exercise intensely and adapt to exercise training (as demonstrated by the clearly positive effect of upper body endurance training on peak and work capacity during exercise), but most adaptations occur peripherally (91,408). SCI research suggests several techniques, including lower body compression (409–411), functional electrical stimulation of the paralyzed lower limbs (412,413), or supine body position concomitant with upper body exercise (326,414), might enhance venous return and cardiac output, thereby increasing the opportunity for central training adaptations.

Complete spinal cord lesions also affect the autonomic nervous system. Loss of sympathetic cardiac innervation from lesions above the sixth thoracic vertebra can limit maximal heart rate to 110 to 130 beats per minute (409). Lesions at the cervical and thoracic levels can impair control over regional blood flow during exercise, causing venous blood pooling in the legs and consequently reducing cardiac preload. As a result, stroke volume and cardiac output at a given oxygen uptake tend to decline in those with SCI (415,416). Furthermore, the loss of sympathetic nervous control over vasomotor and sudomotor responses of the insensate skin impairs thermoregulation (417).

Individuals with SCI should complete exercise testing before initiating an exercise program for two reasons in addition to screening for coronary artery disease. One, testing helps identify cardiovascular issues that might otherwise remain undetected because some people with tetraplegia lack classical symptoms of angina pectoris (as most cardiac visceral afferents enter the spinal cord at the upper thoracic levels). And two, exercise testing can identify and assist in the treatment of exercise-induced hypotension. Overall risk of serious problems from participating in appropriately structured exercise programs appears minimal for the spinal cord injured.

Some individuals with SCI should be encouraged to follow the ACSM physical activity guideline recommendations of 30 minutes of moderate physical activity five times a week for a total of 150 minutes per week (5). However, the able-bodied guidelines are not always appropriate for all individuals with a SCI. It is important not to subject the upper extremities to overuse in those who depend upon them for independent living. Others with tetraplegia may not be able to tolerate the standard physical activity guidelines. Therefore, in 2011, SCI physical activity guidelines were established (**Table 49-12**) (418). These guidelines call for aerobic activity two times per week for at least 20 minutes at a moderate to vigorous intensity. The guidelines also call for resistance training two times per week in the muscles that have voluntarily use. It is recommended that individuals gradually work up to three sets of 8 to 10 repetitions of each exercise with 1 to 2 minutes of rest between each set and each exercise (418).

TABLE 49-12 **Spinal Cord Injury Physical Activity Guidelines**

For important fitness benefits, adults with a spinal cord injury should engage in:
At least 20 minutes of moderate- to vigorous-intensity aerobic activity two times per week,
AND
Strength training exercises two times per week, consisting of 3 sets of 8–10 repetitions of each exercise for each major muscle group

How…?	Aerobic activity	Strength training activity
How often?	Two times per week	Two times per week
How much?	Gradually increase your activity so that you are doing at least 20 minutes of aerobic activity during each workout session.	Repetitions are the number of times you lift and lower a weight. Try to do 8–10 repetitions of each exercise. This counts as one set. Gradually work up to doing three sets of 8–10 repetitions of each exercise.
How hard?	These activities should be performed at a moderate to vigorous intensity. Moderate intensity: activities that feel somewhat hard, but you can keep doing them for a while without getting tired Vigorous intensity: activities that make you feel like you are working really hard, almost at your maximum, and you cannot do these activities for very long without getting tired	Pick a resistance (free weights, cable pulleys, bands, etc.) heavy enough that you can barely, but safely, finish 8–10 repetitions of the last set. Be sure to rest for 1–2 minutes between each set and exercise.
How to?	There are many ways to reach this goal, including: *Upper body exercises*: wheeling, arm cycling, sports *Lower body exercises*: Body weight–supported treadmill walking, cycling *Whole-body exercise*: recumbent stepper, water exercise	There are many ways to reach this goal, including: • Free weights • Elastic resistance bands • Cable pulleys • Weight machines • Functional electrical stimulation

Adapted from Ginis KAM, Hicks AL, Latimer AE, Warburton DER, Bourne C, Ditor DS, et al. The development of evidence-informed physical activity guidelines for adults with spinal cord injury. *Spinal Cord.* 2011;49:1088–1096.

Postpoliomyelitis Syndrome

Although once thought that those who suffered postpolio syndrome (PPS) might experience overuse-induced muscle weakness with exercise, most evidence suggests these individuals can safely exercise without adverse effects. Individuals with PPS generally respond to aerobic (419,420) and resistance (421,422) training like healthy adults. In a study of strength training in individuals with PPS and hand weakness, participants were able to improve their strength without any deleterious effect on motor units (421). A study consisting of flexibility and aerobic training conducted for approximately 1.5 hours per session, three times per week for 8 weeks resulted in improved fatigue and quality of life (423). However, another study utilizing aerobic and resistance training did not show a reduction in severe fatigue (424). Although physical training is generally regarded as safe in this population, it is still prudent to monitor each individual with assessment of symptoms in relation to function and with periodic muscle function measurements (419).

Multiple Sclerosis

Most concerns regarding exercise safety in persons with multiple sclerosis (MS) center around potential adverse effects from the autonomic dysfunction that frequently accompanies the disease and exacerbations of the disease via exercise-induced thermal stress. Studies have shown that aerobic and resistance training is safe and beneficial for individuals with MS who are mild to moderately impaired (425–427). Exercise can reduce fatigue (428) and improve walking speed (426). Aerobic training has been shown to improve quality of life (429) and cardiorespiratory fitness (427). Other studies using resistance training and aerobic training have shown improvements in quality of life (430), strength (431), balance (432), and functional capacity (433).

Individuals with MS can perform endurance exercise at intensities above the anaerobic threshold without developing significant neurologic symptoms (434) and can experience training-induced cardiovascular adaptations (435). Individuals with mild to moderate disability should perform aerobic training three to five times per week for 20 to 30 minutes if possible. Initially, it may be best to start with 10 minutes. The intensity should be 40% to 70% of $\dot{V}O_2R$ or maximum HR. Lower intensities and discontinuous bouts of aerobic training can be used in those with excessive fatigue (34).

The frequency of resistance training initially should be 2 days a week. The intensity should be 60% to 80% of the 1 RM. The sessions should consist of 1 to 2 exercises per body part for major muscle groups (legs, chest, back) and 1 exercise for the smaller muscle groups (shoulders, biceps, triceps, abdominals). Either two or three sets should be performed, with 8 to 15 repetitions per set. For those with excessive fatigue, the rest times between sets can be increased to 2 to 5 minutes (34).

To allow individuals with MS to exercise safely, certain precautions should be taken. Close supervision is recommended. Some people have their MS symptoms worsen when they are exposed to higher ambient temperatures. Precooling prior to the exercise session and/or interval training may be preferable for them. Fans, evaporative cooling garments, and cooling vests can also help with reducing the effects of the heat. During MS exacerbations, the FITT of the exercise prescription should be adapted to the level that the individual can tolerate (34).

Cancer

The medical community increasingly accepts exercise as an important component of rehabilitation for cancer patients (see also Chapter 36). Besides the disease itself, the treatments for cancer challenge exercise capacity and prescription. Cancer treatments can induce cytotoxicity, immunosuppression, bleeding disorders, and anemia. Further, direct or peripheral effects of cancer or its treatments inhibit exercise performance by causing (a) direct damage to cardiac and pulmonary tissue; (b) difficulty in maintaining adequate nutrition, hydration, and electrolyte balance; and (c) fatigue and infection.

Various types of exercise, including aerobic and resistance training, yoga, and tai chi, have been shown to improve a myriad of health issues associated with cancer and the treatment of cancer (436–440). These include sarcopenia (441–443), psychological status (444,445), fatigue (437,446–448), strength (441,449), cognitive decline (438), and, probably most importantly, quality of life (447,450,451).

In 2009, the ACSM convened an expert roundtable to review the literature on exercise in cancer survivors and develop guidelines for physical activity (452). These recommendations can be seen in 🛜 **eTable 49-9**. The guidelines recommend that those with active cancer and cancer survivors should start a regular exercise regimen at a relatively low frequency, duration, and intensity and gradually build up to the recommended 150 minutes of moderate-intensity aerobic training or 75 minutes of vigorous-intensity aerobic training. However, exercise prescriptions for this patient population should be individualized and based on the individuals' current function and fitness level, preferences, health status, treatment course, and disease trajectory. Symptom burden has been reduced and quality of life improved with as little as 10 minutes of moderate-intensity aerobic training and not more than 90 minutes a day three to seven times a week (439,453). Resistance training involving all of the major muscle groups should be done two to three times a week for at least 20 minutes. This can be increased as tolerated. Flexibility training can occur daily, even during treatment. Intensity will vary greatly depending upon disease severity and time of treatment. Intensity should be 60% to 70% of 1 RM. Cancer survivors may need slower progression. If fatigue or other adverse symptoms worsen as a result of the prescribed exercise, the FITT should be reduced to a level that can be tolerated better (34).

People with bone malignancies (particularly of the spine, pelvis, femur, and ribs) require non–weight-bearing modalities. Individuals suffering associated conditions that increase the risk of bruising, fractures, or falls should perform resistance exercise on machines rather than with free weights to minimize the risk of injury.

Osteoporosis

Both resistance and aerobic training can be beneficial in those with osteoporosis (454,455). Multiple trials in postmenopausal women have shown improvements in bone mineral density as a result of resistance training (456–458). They have also shown improvements in strength and muscle mass, which can help with functional activities (11,459,460). Aerobic training has also been shown to improve bone density (281,461).

A Delphi consensus process on physical activity and exercise recommendations for adults with osteoporosis and vertebral fractures determined that those without fractures are safe to follow the ACSM Exercise and Physical Activity Guidelines for Older Adults (462). These include 150 minutes of moderate-intensity (5 to 6 on a scale of 0 to 10) aerobic training per week or 75 minutes of vigorous-intensity (7 to 8 on a scale of 0 to 10) aerobic training per week. Balance exercises

are recommended at least 2 days per week for those who have balance deficits or fall frequently. Resistance training, with a focus on major muscle groups, should be performed at least two times per week. The resistance training program should be progressive, with the individual building up to 8 to 10 exercises involving the major muscle groups with 2 to 3 sets, with 10 to 12 repetitions each set (463).

REFERENCES

1. U.S. Department of Health and Human Services. 2008 Physical activity guidelines for Americans. 2nd ed. Washington, DC: U.S. Department of Health and Human Services; 2018.
2. Riebe D, Franklin BA, Thompson PD, et al. Updating ACSM's recommendations for exercise preparticipation health screening. *Med Sci Sports Exerc.* 2015;47(11):2473–2479.
3. Warburton DE, Charlesworth S, Ivey A, et al. A systematic review of the evidence for Canada's Physical Activity Guidelines for Adults. *Int J Behav Nutr Phys Act.* 2010;7(1):39.
4. Kisner C, Colby Lynn A. *Therapeutic Exercise, Foundations and Techniques.* 6th ed. Philadelphia, PA: FA Davis; 2012:1023.
5. Garber CE, Blissmer B, Deschenes MR, et al. Quantity and quality of exercise for developing and maintaining cardiorespiratory, musculoskeletal, and neuromotor fitness in apparently healthy adults: guidance for prescribing exercise. *Med Sci Sports Exerc.* 2011;43(7):1334–1359.
6. Lamb D. *Physiology of Exercise: Responses and Adaptations.* 2nd ed. New York: Macmillan; 1984.
7. Vander AJ, Sherman H, Lucian K. *Human Physiology.* 3rd ed. New York: McGraw-Hill; 1980:218.
8. Roberts TDM. *Neurophysiology of Postural Mechanisms.* London: Butterworths; 1978:415.
9. Rothwell J. *Control of Human Voluntary Movement.* Rockwell, MD: Aspen Publishers; 1987.
10. Henneman E, Clamann HP, Gillies JD, et al. Rank order of motoneurons within a pool: law of combination. *J Neurophysiol.* 1974;37(6):1338–1349.
11. Rogers MA, Evans WJ. Changes in skeletal muscle with aging: effects of exercise training. *Exerc Sport Sci Rev.* 1993;21:65–102.
12. Sahlin K, Tonkonogi M, Söderlund K. Energy supply and muscle fatigue in humans. *Acta Physiol Scand.* 1998;162(3):261–266.
13. Hawley JA, Leckey JJ. Carbohydrate dependence during prolonged, intense endurance exercise. *Sports Med.* 2015;45(S1):5–12.
14. Burke LM. Re-examining high-fat diets for sports performance: did we call the "Nail in the Coffin" Too Soon? *Sports Med.* 2015;45(suppl 1):S33–S49.
15. Sahlin K. Metabolic changes limiting muscle performance. In: Saltin B, ed. *Biochemistry of Exercise VI.* Champaign, IL: Human Kinetics; 1986:323–343.
16. Robergs RA, Ghiasvand F, Parker D. Biochemistry of exercise-induced metabolic acidosis. *Am J Physiol Regul Integr Comp Physiol.* 2004;287(3):R502–R516.
17. Brooks GA, Fahey TD, Baldwin KM. *Exercise Physiology: Human Bioenergetics and Its Applications.* 4th ed. New York: McGraw-Hill; 2005:283–291.
18. Montero D, Díaz-Cañestro C. Maximal cardiac output in athletes: influence of age. *Eur J Prev Cardiol.* 2015;22(12):1588–1600.
19. Midgley AW, McNaughton LR, Jones AM. Training to enhance the physiological determinants of long-distance running performance: can valid recommendations be given to runners and coaches based on current scientific knowledge? *Sports Med.* 2007;37(10):857–880.
20. Mitchell JH, Blomqvist G. Maximal oxygen uptake. *N Engl J Med.* 1971;284(18):1018–1022.
21. Mitchell JH. Neural control of the circulation during exercise: insights from the 1970–1971 Oxford studies. *Exp Physiol.* 2012;97(1):14–19.
22. Hall MM, Rajasekaran S, Thomsen TW, et al. Lactate: friend or foe. *PM R.* 2016;8(3):S8–S15.
23. Tanaka K, Watanabe H, Konishi Y, et al. Longitudinal associations between anaerobic threshold and distance running performance. *Eur J Appl Physiol Occup Physiol.* 1986;55(3):248–252.
24. Kjaer M, Kiens B, Hargreaves M, et al. Influence of active muscle mass on glucose homeostasis during exercise in humans. *J Appl Physiol.* 1991;71(2):552–557.
25. Kjaer M, Engfred K, Fernandes A, et al. Regulation of hepatic glucose production during exercise in humans: role of sympathoadrenergic activity. *Am J Physiol.* 1993;265(2 Pt 1):E275–E283.
26. Baker LB, Jeukendrup AE, Baker LB, et al. Optimal composition of fluid-replacement beverages. In: *Comprehensive Physiology.* Hoboken, NJ: John Wiley & Sons, Inc.; 2014:575–620.
27. Lewis SF, Snell PG, Taylor WF, et al. Role of muscle mass and mode of contraction in circulatory responses to exercise. *J Appl Physiol.* 1985;58(1):146–151.
28. Hanson P, Rueckert P. Schematic comparison of hemodynamic responses to dynamic and isometric exercise. *Heart Disease and Rehabilitation.* 3rd ed. Champaign, IL: Human Kinetics, 1995:343–356.
29. Williamson JW, Olesen HL, Pott F, et al. Central command increases cardiac output during static exercise in humans. *Acta Physiol Scand.* 1996;156(4):429–434.

30. Kohl HW, Craig CL, Lambert EV, et al. The pandemic of physical inactivity: global action for public health. *Lancet*. 2012;380(9838):294–305.

31. Rauworth A. F.I.T.T.: The Wonder Drug: Exercise is Medicine. National Center on Health, Physical Activity, and Disability. Available at: https://www.nchpad.org/548/2487/2008-04--The-Wonder-Drug--Exercise-is-Medicine--8482-

32. American College of Sports Medicine. *ACSM's Guidelines for Exercise Testing and Prescription*. Philadelphia, PA: Lippincott Williams & Wilkins; 2013.

33. Dunstan DW, Howard B, Healy GN, et al. Too much sitting—a health hazard. *Diabetes Res Clin Pract*. 2012;97(3):368–376.

34. American College of Sports Medicine. In: Riebe D, Ehrman J, Liguori G, et al., eds. *ACSM's Guidelines for Exercise Testing and Prescription*. 10th ed. Philadelphia, PA: Wolters Kluwer Health; 2017:472.

35. Metzger JS, Catellier DJ, Evenson KR, et al. Patterns of objectively measured physical activity in the United States. *Med Sci Sports Exerc*. 2008;40(1):630–638.

36. Curry SJ, Wagner EH, Grothaus LC. Evaluation of intrinsic and extrinsic motivation interventions with a self-help smoking cessation program. *J Consult Clin Psychol*. 1991;59(2):318–324.

37. Armit CM, Brown WJ, Marshall AL, et al. Randomized trial of three strategies to promote physical activity in general practice. *Prev Med*. 2009;48(2):156–163.

38. Jonas S, Phillips E. *ACSM's Exercise is Medicine: A Clinician's Guide to Exercise Prescription*. Philadelphia, PA: Lippincott Williams & Wilkins; 2012.

39. Artinian N, Fletcher G, Mozaffarian D, et al. Interventions to promote physical activity and dietary lifestyle changes for cardiovascular risk factor reduction in adults a scientific statement from the American Heart Association. *Circulation*. 2010;122(4):406–441.

40. Pescatello LS, Arena R, Deborah R, et al. *ACSM'S Guidelines for Exercise Testing and Prescription*. 9th ed. Philadelphia, PA: Lippincott Williams & Wilkins; 2014:482.

41. World Health Organization. *What is Moderate-intensity and Vigorous-intensity Physical Activity?* [Internet]. World Health Organization; 2017. Available from: http://www.who.int/dietphysicalactivity/physical_activity_intensity/en/ [cited February 3, 2017]

42. Reed JL, Pipe AL. Practical approaches to prescribing physical activity and monitoring exercise intensity. *Can J Cardiol*. 2016;32(4):514–522.

43. Persinger R, Foster C, Gibson M, et al. Consistency of the Talk Test for exercise prescription. *Med Sci Sports Exerc*. 2004;36(9):1632–1636.

44. Borg GA. Perceived exertion. *Exerc Sport Sci Rev*. 1974;2:131–153.

45. Howley ET. Type of activity: resistance, aerobic and leisure versus occupational physical activity. *Med Sci Sports Exerc*. 2001;33(suppl):S364–S369.

46. Nelson ME, Rejeski WJ, Blair SN, et al. Physical activity and public health in older adults: recommendation from the American College of Sports Medicine and the American Heart Association. *Med Sci Sports Exerc*. 2007;39(8):1435–1445.

47. Mezzani A, Hamm LF, Jones AM, et al. Aerobic exercise intensity assessment and prescription in cardiac rehabilitation: a joint position statement of the European Association for Cardiovascular Prevention and Rehabilitation, the American Association of Cardiovascular and Pulmonary Rehabilitation and the Canadian Association of Cardiac Rehabilitation. *Eur J Prev Cardiol*. 2013;20(3):442–467.

48. Donnelly JE, Blair SN, Jakicic JM, et al. Appropriate physical activity intervention strategies for weight loss and prevention of weight regain for adults. *Med Sci Sports Exerc*. 2009;41(2):459–471.

49. Sisson SB, Katzmarzyk PT, Earnest CP, et al. Volume of exercise and fitness non-response in sedentary, postmenopausal women. *Med Sci Sports Exerc*. 2009;41(3):539–545.

50. Burgomaster KA, Howarth KR, Phillips SM, et al. Similar metabolic adaptations during exercise after low volume sprint interval and traditional endurance training in humans. *J Physiol*. 2008;586(1):151–160.

51. Tran QT, Docherty D, Behm D. The effects of varying time under tension and volume load on acute neuromuscular responses. *Eur J Appl Physiol*. 2006;98(4):402–410.

52. Thompson PD, Arena R, Riebe D, et al. ACSM's new preparticipation health screening recommendations from ACSM's guidelines for exercise testing and prescription, ninth edition. *Curr Sports Med Rep*. 2013;12(4):215–217.

53. Harmon KG, Drezner JA, Wilson MG, et al. Incidence of sudden cardiac death in athletes: a state-of-the-art review. *Heart*. 2014;100(16):1227–1234.

54. Maron BJ, Thompson PD, Ackerman MJ, et al. Recommendations and considerations related to preparticipation screening for cardiovascular abnormalities in competitive athletes: 2007 update: a scientific statement from the American Heart Association Council on Nutrition, Physical Activity, and Metabol. *Circulation*. 2007;115(12):1643.

55. Corrado D, Basso C, Schiavon M, et al. Pre-participation screening of young competitive athletes for prevention of sudden cardiac death. *J Am Coll Cardiol*. 2008;52:1981–1989.

56. Kerkhof DL, Gleason CN, Basilico FC, et al. Is there a role for limited echocardiography during the preparticipation physical examination? *PM R* 2016;8:S36–S44.

57. Drezner JA, O'Connor FG, Harmon KG, et al. AMSSM position statement on cardiovascular preparticipation screening in Athletes: current evidence, knowledge gaps, recommendations and future directions. *Curr Sports Med Rep*. 2016;15(5):359–375.

58. Nieman DC, Pedersen BK. Exercise and immune function. Recent developments. *Sports Med*. 1999;27:73–80.

59. Mackinnon L. *Advances in Exercise Immunology*. Champaign, IL: Human Kinetics; 1999.

60. Gleeson M. Immune function in sport and exercise. *J Appl Physiol*. 2007;103(2):693–699.

61. Pedersen BK, Rohde T, Ostrowski K. Recovery of the immune system after exercise. *Acta Physiol Scand*. 1998;162:325–332.

62. Peake JM, Neubauer O, Walsh NP, et al. Recovery of the immune system after exercise. *J Appl Physiol*. 2017;122(5):1077–1087.

63. Friman G, Ilbäck NG. Acute infection: metabolic responses, effects on performance, interaction with exercise, and myocarditis. *Int J Sports Med*. 1998;19(suppl 3):S172–S182.

64. Gagge AP, Gonzalez RR. Mechanisms of heat exchange: biophysics and physiology. In: Fregly MJ, ed. *Handbook of Physiology/Section 4, Environmental Physiology*. Bethesda, MD: American Physiological Society; 1996:45–84.

65. Sawka MN, Young YJ. Physiological systems and their responses to conditions of heat and cold. *ACSM's Adv Exerc Physiol*. 2006;(April):535–563.

66. Sawka MN, Burke LM, Eichner ER, et al. American College of Sports Medicine position stand. Exercise and fluid replacement. *Med Sci Sports Exerc*. 2007;39(2):377–390.

67. Armstrong LE, Casa DJ, Millard-Stafford M, et al. American College of Sports Medicine position stand. Exertional heat illness during training and competition. *Med Sci Sports Exerc*. 2007;39(3):556–572.

68. Periard JD, Racinais S, Sawka MN. Adaptations and mechanisms of human heat acclimation: applications for competitive athletes and sports. *Scand J Med Sci Sports*. 2015;25:20–38.

69. Castellani J, Young A, Ducharme M, et al. American College of Sports Medicine position stand: prevention of cold injuries during exercise. *Med Sci Sports Exerc*. 2006;38(11):2012–2029.

70. Franklin BA, Hogan P, Bonzheim K, et al. Cardiac demands of heavy snow shoveling. *JAMA*. 1995;273:880–882.

71. Vona M, Mazzuero G, Lupi A, et al. Effects of altitude on effort tolerance in non-acclimatized patients with ischemic left ventricular dysfunction. *Eur J Cardiovasc Prev Rehabil*. 2006;13:617–624.

72. Schmid J-P, Noveanu M, Gaillet R, et al. Safety and exercise tolerance of acute high altitude exposure (3,454 m) among patients with coronary artery disease. *Heart*. 2006;92(7):921–925.

73. Gong H Jr, Bradley PW, Simmons MS, et al. Impaired exercise performance and pulmonary function in elite cyclists during low-level ozone exposure in a hot environment. *Am Rev Respir Dis*. 1986;134(4):726–733.

74. Oliveira RS, Barros Neto TL, Braga ALF, et al. Impact of acute exposure to air pollution on the cardiorespiratory performance of military firemen. *Braz J Med Biol Res*. 2006;39(12):1643–1649.

75. Sharman JE, Cockcroft JR, Coombes JS. Cardiovascular implications of exposure to traffic air pollution during exercise. *QJM*. 2004;97:637–643.

76. Poole DC, Jones AM. Measurement of the maximum oxygen uptake ($\dot{V}_{O_{2max}}$): $\dot{V}_{O_{2peak}}$ is no longer acceptable. *J Appl Physiol*. 2017;122:997–1002.

77. Sheldahl LM, Tristani FE, Hastings JE, et al. Comparison of adaptations and compliance to exercise training between middle-aged and older men. *J Am Geriatr Soc*. 1993;41(8):795–801.

78. National Institutes of Health. Physical activity and cardiovascular health. NIH Consensus Development Panel on Physical Activity and Cardiovascular Health. *JAMA*. 1996;276:241–246.

79. Bonne TC, Doucende G, Flück D, et al. Phlebotomy eliminates the maximal cardiac output response to six weeks of exercise training. *Am J Physiol Regul Integr Comp Physiol*. 2014;306(50):752–760.

80. Thomas SG, Paterson DH, Cunningham DA, et al. Cardiac output and left ventricular function in response to exercise in older men. *Can J Physiol Pharmacol*. 1993;71(2):136–144.

81. Schulman SP, Fleg JL, Goldberg AP, et al. Continuum of cardiovascular performance across a broad range of fitness levels in healthy older men. *Circulation*. 1996;94(3):359–367.

82. Maron BJ. Distinguishing hypertrophic cardiomyopathy from athlete's heart physiological remodelling: clinical significance, diagnostic strategies and implications for preparticipation screening. *Br J Sports Med*. 2009;43(9):649–656.

83. Buttrick PM, Scheuer J. Execise and the heart: acute hemodynamics, conditioning training, the athlete's heart, and sudden death. In: Schlant RC, Alexander RW, eds. *The Heart*. 8th ed. New York: McGraw-Hill; 1994:2057–2066.

84. Pelliccia A, Maron BJ, Culasso F, et al. Athlete's heart in women. Echocardiographic characterization of highly trained elite female athletes. *JAMA*. 1996;276(3):211–215.

85. Schannwell CM, Schneppenheim M, Plehn G, et al. Left ventricular diastolic function in physiologic and pathologic hypertrophy. *Am J Hypertens*. 2002;15(6):513–517.

86. Bishop DJ, Granata C, Eynon N. Can we optimise the exercise training prescription to maximise improvements in mitochondria function and content? *Biochim Biophys Acta*. 2014;1840(4):1266–1275.

87. Ljubicic V, Joseph AM, Saleem A, et al. Transcriptional and post-transcriptional regulation of mitochondrial biogenesis in skeletal muscle: effects of exercise and aging. *Biochim Biophys Acta*. 2010;1800(3):223–234.

88. Franklin BA. Aerobic exercise training programs for the upper body. *Med Sci Sports Exerc*. 1989;21:S141–S148.

89. Pendergast DR. Cardiovascular, respiratory, and metabolic responses to upper body exercise. *Med Sci Sports Exerc*. 1989;21(5 suppl):S121–S125.

90. Magel JR, McArdle WD, Toner M, et al. Metabolic and cardiovascular adjustment to arm training. *J Appl Physiol*. 1978;45(1):75–79.

91. Bhambhani YN, Eriksson P, Gomes PS. Transfer effects of endurance training with the arms and legs. *Med Sci Sports Exerc*. 1991;23(9):1035–1041.

92. Nelson N, Asplund CA. Exercise testing: who, when, and why? *PM R*. 2016;8(3):S16–S23.

93. Bouchard C, Rankinen T, Timmons JA. Genomics and genetics in the biology of adaptation to exercise. *Compr Physiol*. 2011;1(3):1603–1648.

94. Fleg JL, Pina IL, Balady GJ, et al. Assessment of functional capacity in clinical and research applications: an advisory from the committee on exercise, rehabilitation, and prevention, council on Clinical Cardiology, American Heart Association. *Circulation.* 2000;102(13):1591–1597.

95. Fletcher GF, Ades PA, Kligfield P, et al. Exercise standards for testing and training: a scientific statement from the American heart association. *Circulation.* 2013;128(8):873–934.

96. Joyner MJ, Coyle EF. Endurance exercise performance: the physiology of champions. *J Physiol.* 2008;586(1):35–44.

97. Swain DP. Energy cost calculations for exercise prescription: an update. *Sports Med.* 2000;30(1):17–22.

98. Forman DE, Myers J, Lavie CJ, et al. Cardiopulmonary exercise testing: relevant but underused. *Postgrad Med.* 2010;122(6):1941–9260.

99. Reed JL, Pipe AL. The talk test. *Curr Opin Cardiol.* 2014;29(5):475–480.

100. Fox S, Naughton J, Haskell W. Physical activity and the prevention of coronary heart disease. *Ann Clin Res.* 1971;3(6):404–432.

101. Gellis RL, Goslin BR, Oson RE, et al. Longitudinal modeling of the relationship between age and maximal heart rate. *Med Sci Sports Exerc.* 2007;822–829.

102. Tanaka H, Monahan KD, Seals DR. Age-predicted maximal heart rate revisited. *J Am Coll Cardiol.* 2001;37(1):153–156.

103. Zhu N, Suarez-Lopez JR, Sidney S, et al. Longitudinal examination of age-predicted symptom-limited exercise maximum HR. *Med Sci Sports Exerc.* 2010;42(8):1519–1527.

104. Londeree BR. Effect of training on lactate/ventilatory thresholds: a meta-analysis. *Med Sci Sports Exerc.* 1997;29(6):837–843.

105. Mann T, Lamberts RP, Lambert MI. Methods of prescribing relative exercise intensity: physiological and practical considerations. *Sports Med.* 2013;43::613–625.

106. Dantas JL, Doria C, Rossi H, et al. Determination of blood lactate training zone boundaries with rating of perceived exertion in runners. *J Strength Cond Res.* 2015;29(2):315–320.

107. Ballweg J, Foster C, Porcari J, et al. Reliability of the talk test as a surrogate of ventilatory and respiratory compensation thresholds. *J Sports Sci Med.* 2013;12:610–611.

108. Lyon E, Menke M, Foster C, et al. Translation of incremental talk test responses to steady-state exercise training intensity. *J Cardiopulm Rehabil Prev.* 2014;34(4):271–275.

109. Gillespie BD, McCormick JJ, Mermier CM, et al. Talk test as a practical method to estimate exercise intensity in highly trained competitive male cyclists. *J Strength Cond Res.* 2015;29(4):894–898.

110. Green HJ, Ball-Burnett M, Symon S, et al. Short-term training, muscle glycogen, and cycle endurance. *Can J Appl Physiol.* 1995;20(3):315–324.

111. Green HJ, Helyar R, Ball-Burnett M, et al. Metabolic adaptations to training precede changes in muscle mitochondrial capacity. *J Appl Physiol.* 1992;72(2):484–491.

112. Godin G, Desharnais R, Valois P, et al. Differences in perceived barriers to exercise between high and low intenders: observations among different populations. *Am J Health Promot.* 2012;8(4):279–385.

113. Laursen PB, Jenkins DG. The scientific basis for high-intensity interval training: optimising training programmes and maximising performance in highly trained endurance athletes. *Sports Med.* 2002;32(1):53–73.

114. Zadow E, Gordon N, Abbiss C, et al. Pacing, the missing piece of the puzzle to high-intensity interval training. *Int J Sports Med.* 2014;36(3):215–219.

115. Gillen JB, Gibala MJ. Is high-intensity interval training a time-efficient exercise strategy to improve health and fitness? *Appl Physiol Nutr Metab.* 2014;39(3):409–412.

116. Buchheit M, Laursen PB. High-intensity interval training, solutions to the programming puzzle: Part II: anaerobic energy, neuromuscular load and practical applications. *Sports Med.* 2013;43:927–954.

117. Buchheit M, Laursen PB. High-intensity interval training, solutions to the programming puzzle: Part I: cardiopulmonary emphasis. *Sports Med.* 2013;43:313–338.

118. Tabata I, Nishimura K, Kouzaki M, et al. Effects of moderate-intensity endurance and high-intensity intermittent training on anaerobic capacity and Vo_{2max}. *Med Sci Sports Exerc.* 1996;28(10):1327–1330.

119. Weston KS, Wisløff U, Coombes JS. High-intensity interval training in patients with lifestyle-induced cardiometabolic disease: a systematic review and meta-analysis. *Br J Sports Med.* 2014;48(16):1227–1234.

120. Gibala MJ, Little JP, Van Essen M, et al. Short-term sprint interval versus traditional endurance training: similar initial adaptations in human skeletal muscle and exercise performance. *J Physiol.* 2006;575(3):901–911.

121. Tudor-Locke C, Lutes L. Why do pedometers work?: a reflection upon the factors related to successfully increasing physical activity. *Sports Med.* 2009;39(12):981–993.

122. Kang M, Marshall SJ, Barreira TV, et al. Effect of pedometer-based physical activity interventions: a meta-analysis. *Res Q Exerc Sport.* 2009;80(3):648–655.

123. Jordan A, Jurca G, Locke C, et al. Ovid: pedometer indices for weekly physical activity recommendations in postmenopausal women. *Med Sci Sports Exerc.* 2005;37(9):1627–1632.

124. Bravata DM, Smith-Spangler C, Sundaram V, et al. Using pedometers to increase physical activity and improve health. *JAMA.* 2007;298(19):2296.

125. Fleck S, Kramer W. *Designing Resistance Training Programs.* 4th ed. Champaign, IL: Human Kinetics; 2014:520.

126. Wolfe RR. The underappreciated role of muscle in health and disease. *Am J Clin Nutr.* 2006;84:475–482.

127. Jurca R, Lamonte MJ, Barlow CE, et al. Association of muscular strength with incidence of metabolic syndrome in men. *Med Sci Sports Exerc.* 2005;37(11):1849–1855.

128. Newman AB, Kupelian V, Visser M, et al. Strength, but not muscle mass, is associated with mortality in the health, aging and body composition study cohort. *J Gerontol A Biol Sci Med Sci.* 2006;61(1):72–77.

129. Fitzgerald SJ, Barlow CE, Kampert JB, et al. Muscular fitness and all-cause mortality: prospective observations. *J Phys Act Heal.* 2004;1(1):7–18.

130. Gale CR, Martyn CN, Cooper C, et al. Grip strength, body composition, and mortality. *Int J Epidemiol.* 2007;36(1):228–235.

131. Tanasescu M, Leitzmann MF, Rimm EB, et al. Exercise type and intensity in relation to coronary heart disease in men. *JAMA.* 2002;288(16):1994–2000.

132. Manini TM, Everhart JE, Patel KV, et al. Daily activity energy expenditure and mortality among older adults. *JAMA.* 2006;296(2):171.

133. Brooks N, Layne JE, Gordon PL, et al. Strength training improves muscle quality and insulin sensitivity in Hispanic older adults with type 2 diabetes. *Int J Med Sci.* 2007;4(1):19–27.

134. American College of Sports Medicine. American College of Sports Medicine position stand. Progression models in resistance training for healthy adults. *Med Sci Sports Exerc.* 2009;41(3):687–708.

135. Finer JT, Simmons RM, Spudich JA. Single myosin molecule mechanics: piconewton forces and nanometre steps. *Nature.* 1994;368(6467):113–119.

136. Knapik JJ, Mawdsley RH, Ramos MU. Angular specificity and test mode specificity of isometric and isokinetic strength training. *J Orthop Sports Phys Ther.* 1983;5(2):58–65.

137. Gülch R. Force-velocity relations in human skeletal muscle. *Int J Sports Med.* 1994;15(suppl 1):S2–S10.

138. Tricoli V, Lamas L, Carnevale R, et al. Short-term effects on lower-body functional power development: weightlifting vs. vertical jump training programs. *J Strength Cond Res.* 2005;19(2):433.

139. Häkkinen K, Kraemer WJ, Newton RU, et al. Changes in electromyographic activity, muscle fibre and force production characteristics during heavy resistance/power strength training in middle-aged and older men and women. *Acta Physiol Scand.* 2001;171(1):51–62.

140. Behm DG. Neuromuscular implications and applications of resistance training. *J Strength Cond Res.* 1995;9(4):264–274.

141. Rivera-Brown AM, Frontera WR. Principles of exercise physiology: responses to acute exercise and long-term adaptations to training. *PM R.* 2012;4(11):797–804.

142. Micheo W, Baerga L, Miranda G. Basic principles regarding strength, flexibility, and stability exercises. *PM R.* 2012;4(11):805–811.

143. MacDougall J. *The Encyclopedia of Sports Medicine.* Oxford: Blackwell; 1992:20–38.

144. Bosco C, Vitasalo J, Komi P, et al. Potentiation during stretch-shortening cycle exercise. *Acta Physiol Scand.* 1982;(114):557–565.

145. Potach DH, Chu DA. Plyometric training. In: *Essentials of Strength Training and Conditioning.* Champaign, IL: Human Kinetics; 2000.

146. Wilk KE, Voight ML, Keirns MA, et al. Stretch-shortening drills for the upper extremities: theory and clinical application. *J Orthop Sports Phys Ther.* 1993;17(5):225–239.

147. Davies G, Riemann BL, Manske R. Current concepts of plyometric exercise. *Int J Sports Phys Ther.* 2015;10(6):760–786.

148. Fatouros IG, Jamurtas AZ, Leontisini D, et al. Evaluation of plyometric exercise training, weight training, and their combination on vertical jumping performance and leg strength. *J Strength Cond Res.* 2000;14(4):470–476.

149. Chimera NJ, Swanik KA, Swanik CB, et al. Effects of plyometric training on performance in female athletes. *J Athl Train.* 2004;39(1):24–31.

150. Adams K, O'Shea JP, O'Shea KL, et al. The effect of six weeks of squat, plyometric and squat-plyometric training on power production. *J Strength Cond Res.* 1992;6:36.

151. Chelly MS, Hermassi S, Shephard RJ. Effects of in-season short-term plyometric training program on sprint and jump performance of young male track athletes. *J Strength Cond Res.* 2015;29(8):2128–2136.

152. Ozbar N, Ates S, Agopyan A. The effect of 8-week plyometric training on leg power, jump and sprint performance in female soccer players. *J Strength Cond Res.* 2014;28(10):2888–2894.

153. Chelly MS, Ghenem MA, Abid K, et al. Effects of in-season short-term plyometric training program on leg power, jump- and sprint performance of soccer players. *J Strength Cond Res.* 2010;24(10):2670–2676.

154. Sáez de Villarreal E, Requena B, Cronin JB. The effects of plyometric training on sprint performance: a meta-analysis. *J Strength Cond Res.* 2012;26(2):575–584.

155. Markovic G, Jukic I, Milanovic D, et al. Effects of sprint and plyometric training on muscle function and athletic performance. *J Strength Cond Res.* 2007;21(2):543–549.

156. Griffin LY, Albohm MJ, Arendt EA, et al. Understanding and preventing noncontact anterior cruciate ligament injuries: a review of the Hunt Valley II meeting, January 2005. *Am J Sports Med.* 2006;34(9):1512–1532.

157. Myer G, Ford K, McLean S, et al. The effects of plyometric versus dynamic stabilization and balance training on lower extremity biomechanics. *Am J Sports Med.* 2006;34(3):445–455.

158. Sale DG. Neural adaptation to strength training. In: Komi PV, ed. *Strength and Power in Sports The Encyclopaedia of Sports Medicine.* Oxford: Blackwell; 1992:249–265.

159. Enoka RM. Muscle strength and its development. New perspectives. *Sports Med.* 1988;6:146–168.

160. Booth FW, Thomason DB. Molecular and cellular adaptation of muscle in response to exercise: perspectives of various models. *Physiol Rev.* 1991;71(2):541–585.

161. Billeter R, Hoppeler H. Muscular basis of strength. In: Komi PV, ed. *Strength and Power in Sports The Encyclopaedia of Sports Medicine.* Oxford: Blackwell; 1992:39–63.

162. Macdougall JD. Hypertrophy and hyperplasia. In: Komi PV, ed. *The Encyclopedia of Sports Medicine: Strength and Power in Sport.* 2nd ed. Oxford: Blackwell Science Ltd; 1992:252–264.

163. Folland JP, Williams AG. The adaptations to strength training. *Sports Med.* 2007;37(2):145–168.

164. Antonio J, Gonyea W. Muscle fiber splitting in stretch-enlarged avian muscle. *Med Sci Sports Exerc.* 1994;26(973–977):973–977.

165. Jones D, Rutherford O. Human muscle strength training: the effects of three different regimes and the nature of the resultant changes. *J Physiol.* 1987;391(1):1–11.

166. Evans WJ. Effects of exercise on senescent muscle. *Clin Orthop Relat Res.* 2002;(403 suppl):S211–S220.

167. Shinohara M, Kouzaki M, Yoshihisa T, et al. Efficacy of tourniquet ischemia for strength training with low resistance. *Eur J Appl Physiol Occup Physiol.* 1998; 77(1–2):189–191.

168. Vandenburgh HH. Motion into mass: how does tension stimulate muscle growth? *Med Sci Sports Exerc.* 1987;19(5 suppl):S142–S149.

169. Goldspink G. Gene expression in skeletal muscle. *Biochem Soc Trans.* 2002; 30(2):285–290.

170. Hornberger TA, Chien S. Mechanical stimuli and nutrients regulate rapamycin-sensitive signaling through distinct mechanisms in skeletal muscle. *J Cell Biochem.* 2006;97(6):1207–1216.

171. Goldberg AL, Etlinger JD, Goldspink DF, et al. Mechanism of work-induced hypertrophy of skeletal muscle. *Med Sci Sports Exerc.* 1975;7(3):185–198.

172. Brunner F, Schmid A, Sheikhzadeh A, et al. Effects of aging on type II muscle fibers: a systematic review of the literature. *J Aging Phys Act.* 2007;15(3):336–348.

173. Rooney KJ, Herbert RD, Balnave RJ. Fatigue contributes to the strength training stimulus. *Med Sci Sports Exerc.* 1994;26(9):1160–1164.

174. Schott J, McCully K, Rutherford OM. The role of metabolites in strength training - II. Short versus long isometric contractions. *Eur J Appl Physiol Occup Physiol.* 1995;71(4):337–341.

175. Carey Smith R, Rutherford OM. The role of metabolites in strength training—I. A comparison of eccentric and concentric contractions. *Eur J Appl Physiol Occup Physiol.* 1995;71(4):332–336.

176. Suga T, Okita K, Morita N, et al. Intramuscular metabolism during low-intensity resistance exercise with blood flow restriction. *J Appl Physiol.* 2009;106(4):1119–1124.

177. Tesch PA, Larsson L. Muscle hypertrophy in bodybuilders. *Eur J Appl Physiol Occup Physiol.* 1982;49(3):301–306.

178. Pierce JR, Clark BC, Ploutz-Snyder LL, et al. Growth hormone and muscle function responses to skeletal muscle ischemia. *J Appl Physiol.* 2006;101(6):1588–1595.

179. Toigo M, Boutellier U. New fundamental resistance exercise determinants of molecular and cellular muscle adaptations. *Eur J Appl Physiol.* 2006;97:643–663.

180. Hill M, Goldspink G. Expression and splicing of the insulin-like growth factor gene in rodent muscle is associated with muscle satellite (stem) cell activation following local tissue damage. *J Physiol.* 2003;549(Pt 2):409–418.

181. Krieger JW. Single vs. multiple sets of resistance exercise for muscle hypertrophy: a meta-analysis. *J Strength Cond Res.* 2010;24(4):1150–1159.

182. Wolfe BL, LeMura LM, Cole PJ. Quantitative analysis of single- vs. multiple set programs in resistance training. *J Strength Cond Res.* 2004;18(1):35–47.

183. Schoenfeld BJ. The mechanisms of muscle hypertrophy and their application to resistance training. *J Strength Cond Res.* 2010;24(10):2857–2872.

184. Kraemer WJ, Patton JF, Gordon SE, et al. Compatibility of high-intensity strength and endurance training on hormonal and skeletal muscle adaptations. *J Appl Physiol.* 1995;78(3):976–989.

185. Beardsley C. Muscle fiber type [Internet]. *Strength & Conditioning Research.* Available from: https://www.strengthandconditioningresearch.com/hypertrophy/muscle-fiber-type/ [cited July 8, 2017].

186. Hather BM, Tesch PA, Buchanan P, et al. Influence of eccentric actions on skeletal muscle adaptations to resistance training. *Acta Physiol Scand.* 1991;143(2):177–185.

187. Staron RS, Karapondo DL, Kraemer WJ, et al. Skeletal-muscle adaptations during early phase of heavy resistance training in men and women. *J Appl Physiol.* 1994;76(3):1247–1255.

188. Short KR, Bigelow ML, Kahl J, et al. Decline in skeletal muscle mitochondrial function with aging in humans. *Proc Natl Acad Sci U S A.* 2005;102(15):5618–5623.

189. Petersen KF, Morino K, Alves TC, et al. Effect of aging on muscle mitochondrial substrate utilization in humans. *Proc Natl Acad Sci.* 2015;112(36):11330–11334.

190. Cadenas E, Davies KJA. Mitochondrial free radical generation, oxidative stress, and aging. *Free Radic Biol Med.* 2000;29(3–4):222–230.

191. Joseph A-M, Adhihetty PJ, Leeuwenburgh C. Beneficial effects of exercise on age-related mitochondrial dysfunction and oxidative stress in skeletal muscle. *J Physiol.* 2015;0:1–45.

192. Petersen KF, Befroy D, Dufour S, et al. Mitochondrial dysfunction in the elderly: possible role in insulin resistance. *Science.* 2003;300(5622):1140–1142.

193. Joseph AM, Adhihetty PJ, Buford TW, et al. The impact of aging on mitochondrial function and biogenesis pathways in skeletal muscle of sedentary high- and low-functioning elderly individuals. *Aging Cell.* 2012;11(5):801–809.

194. Flack KD, Davy BM, DeBerardinis M, et al. Resistance exercise training and in vitro skeletal muscle oxidative capacity in older adults. *Physiol Rep.* 2016;4(13).

195. Irving BA, Lanza IR, Henderson GC, et al. Combined training enhances skeletal muscle mitochondrial oxidative capacity independent of age. *J Clin Endocrinol Metab.* 2015;100(4):1654–1663.

196. Hunter G, McCarthy J, Bamman M. Effects of resistance training on older adults. *Sports Med.* 2004;34(5):329–348.

197. Dietz P, Hoffmann S, Lachtermann E, et al. Influence of exclusive resistance training on body composition and cardiovascular risk factors in overweight or obese children: a systematic review. *Obes Facts.* 2012;5(4):546–560.

198. Sillanpaa E, Laaksonen DE, Hakkinen A, et al. Body composition, fitness, and metabolic health during strength and endurance training and their combination in middle-aged and older women. *Eur J Appl Physiol.* 2009;106(2):285–296.

199. Westcott WL. Resistance training is medicine: effects of strength training on health. *Curr Sports Med Rep.* 2012;11(4):209–216.

200. Kraemer WJ, Ratamess NA. Hormonal responses and adaptations to resistance exercise and training. *Sports Med.* 2005;35:339–361.

201. Shaner AA, Vingren JL, Hatfield DL, et al. The acute hormonal response to free weight and machine weight resistance exercise. *J Strength Cond Res.* 2014;28(4):1032–1040.

202. Klimcakova E, Polak J, Moro C, et al. Dynamic strength training improves insulin sensitivity without altering plasma levels and gene expression of adipokines in subcutaneous adipose tissue in obese men. *J Clin Endocrinol Metab.* 2006;91(12):5107–5112.

203. Stone M. Connective tissue and bone response to strength training. In: Komi PV, ed. *The Encyclopedia of Sports Medicine: Strength and Power in Sport.* 2nd ed. Oxford: Blackwell Science Ltd; 1992:279–290.

204. Zernicke RF, Loitz B. Exercise-related adaptations in connective tissue. *Strength Power Sport Encycl Sport Med.* 1992;77–95.

205. Alfredson H, Pietilä T, Jonsson P, et al. Heavy-load eccentric calf muscle training for the treatment of chronic Achilles tendinosis. *Am J Sports Med.* 1998;26(3):360–366.

206. Couppe C, Kongsgaard M, Aagaard P, et al. Habitual loading results in tendon hypertrophy and increased stiffness of the human patellar tendon. *J Appl Physiol.* 2008;105(3):805–810.

207. Tipton CM, Matthes RD, Maynard JA, et al. The influence of physical activity on ligaments and tendons. *Med Sci Sports.* 1975;7:165–175.

208. Staff PH. The effect of physical activity on joints, cartilage, tendons and ligaments. *Scand J Soc Med.* 1982;29(suppl):59–63.

209. Laurent GJ, Sparrow MP, Bates PC, et al., Collagen content and turnover in cardiac and skeletal muscles of the adult fowl and the changes during stretch-induced growth. *Biochem J.* 1978;176(2):419–427.

210. Turto H, Lindy S, Halme J. Protocollagen proline hydroxylase activity in work-induced hypertrophy of rat muscle. *Am J Physiol.* 1974;226:63–65.

211. Conroy BP, Kraemer WJ, Maresh CM, et al. Adaptive responses of bone to physical activity. *Med Exerc Nutr Health.* 1992;1:64–74.

212. Layne JE, Nelson ME. The effects of progressive resistance training on bone density: a review. *Med Sci Sports Exerc.* 1999;31(1):25–30.

213. Ingelmark BE, Ekholm R. A study on variations in the thickness of the articular cartilage in association with rest and periodical load. *Upsala Lakareforen Forh.* 1948;53:61–64.

214. Kraemer WJ. Detraining the "bulked-up" athlete: prospects for lifetime health and fitness. *Nat Strength Cond Assoc J.* 1983;5:10–12.

215. Komi PV, Kaneko M, Aura O. EMG activity of the leg extensor muscles with special reference to mechanical efficiency in concentric and eccentric exercise. *Int J Sports Med.* 1987;1:22–29.

216. Eloranta V, Komi P. Function of the quadriceps femoris muscle under maximal concentric and eccentric contraction. *Electromyogr Clin Neurophysiol.* 1980;20:159.

217. Bonde-Petersen F, Knuttgen HG, Henriksson J. Muscle metabolism during exercise with concentric and eccentric contractions. *J Appl Physiol.* 1972;33(6):792–795.

218. Schoenfeld BJ, Ogborn D, Vigotsky AD, et al. Hypertrophic effects of concentric versus eccentric muscle actions: a systematic review and meta-analysis. *J Strength Cond Res.* 2017;31:2599–2608.

219. Dudley GA, Tesch PA, Miller BJ, et al. Importance of eccentric actions in performance adaptations to resistance training. *Aviat Space Environ Med.* 1991;62(6):543–550.

220. Ebbeling CB, Clarkson PM. Exercise-induced muscle damage and adaptation. *Sports Med.* 1989;7(4):207–234.

221. Saxton JM, Clarkson PM, James R, et al. Neuromuscular dysfunction following eccentric exercise. *Med Sci Sports Exerc.* 1995;27:1185–1193.

222. Ikai M, Fukunaga T. A study on training effect on strength per unit cross-sectional area of muscle by means of ultrasonic measurement. *Int Z Angew Physiol.* 1970;28(3):173–180.

223. Ryschon TW, Fowler MD, Wysong RE, et al. Efficiency of human skeletal muscle in vivo: comparison of isometric, concentric, and eccentric muscle action. *J Appl Physiol (1985).* 1997;83:867–874.

224. Kraemer WJ, Fleck SJ. *Optimizing Strength Training: Designing Nonlinear Periodization Workouts.* Champaign, IL: Human Kinetics Publishers; 2007.

225. Kraemer W, Fry A. Strength testing: development and evaluation of methodology. In: Maud P, Foster C, eds. *Physiologic Assessment of Human Fitness.* Champaig, IL: Human Kinetics; 1995:115–138.

226. Hickson RC, Hidaka K, Foster C. Skeletal muscle fiber type, resistance training, and strength-related performance. *Med Sci Sports Exerc.* 1994;26(5):593–598.

227. Rhea MR, Alvar BA, Burkett LN, et al. A meta-analysis to determine the dose response for strength development. *Med Sci Sports Exerc.* 2003;35(3):456–464.

228. Rico-Sanz J, Jagim A, Baechle T, et al. Essentials of strength training and conditioning: National strength and conditioning association. *Am J Physiol Cell Physiol.* 2010;109:1490–1496.

229. Calder AW, Chilibeck PD, Webber CE, et al. Comparison of whole and split weight training routines in young women. *Can J Appl Physiol.* 1994;19(2):185–199.

230. Kramer JB, Stone MH, O'Bryant HS, et al. Effects of single vs. multiple sets of weight training: impact of volume, intensity, and variation. *J Strength Cond Res.* 1997;11(3):143–147.

231. Kraemer WJ, Ratamess NA. Physiology of resistance training: current issues. *Orthop Phys Ther Clin North Am.* 2000;9(4):467–513.

232. Berger R. Effect of varied weight training programs on strength. *Res Quarterly Am Assoc Heal Phys Educ Recreat.* 1962;33(2):168–181.

233. O'Shea P. Effects of selected weight training programs on the development of strength and muscle hypertrophy. *Res Q.* 1966;37(1):95–102.

234. Baechle T, Earle R, Wathen D. Resistance training. In: Baechle T, Earle R, eds. *Essentials of Strength Training and Conditioning.* 2nd ed. Champaig, IL: Human Kinetics; 2000:395–425.

235. Häkkinen K, Komi PV, Alén M. Effect of explosive type strength training on isometric force- and relaxation-time, electromyographic and muscle fibre characteristics of leg extensor muscles. *Acta Physiol Scand.* 1985;125(4):587–600.

236. Campos GER, Luecke TJ, Wendeln HK, et al. Muscular adaptations in response to three different resistance-training regimens: specificity of repetition maximum training zones. *Eur J Appl Physiol.* 2002;88(1–2):50–60.

237. Kraemer WJ. A series of studies—the physiological basis for strength training in american football: fact over philosophy. *J Strength Cond Res.* 1997;11(3):131.

238. DeLorme T, Watkins A. Technics of progressive resistance exercise. *Arch Phys Med Rehabil.* 1948;29:263–273.

239. Kraemer WJ, Fleck SJ, Evans WJ. Strength and power training: physiological mechanisms of adaptation. *Exerc Sport Sci Rev.* 1996;24:363–397.

240. Anderson T, Kearney JT. Effects of three resistance training programs on muscular strength and absolute and relative endurance. *Res Q Exerc Sport.* 1982;53(1):1–7.

241. Stone WJ, Coulter SP. Strength/endurance effects from three resistance training protocols with women. *J Strength Cond Res.* 1994;8(4):231–234.

242. Fleck SJ. Periodized strength training: a critical review. *J Strength Cond Res.* 1999;13(1):82–89.

243. Shimano T, Kraemer WJ, Spiering BA, et al. Relationship between the number of repetitions and selected percentages of one repetition maximum in free weight exercises in trained and untrained men. *J Strength Cond Res.* 2006;20(4):819–823.

244. Hoeger WW, Hopkins DR, Barette SL, et al. Relationship between repetitions and selected percentages. *J Strength Cond Res.* 1987;1(1):11–13.

245. Hoeger WW, Hopkins DR, Barette SL, et al. Relationship between repetitions and selected percentages of one repetition maximum: a comparison between untrained and trained males and females. *J Strength Cond Res.* 1990;4(2):47–54.

246. Chilibeck PD, Calder AW, Sale DG, et al. A comparison of strength and muscle mass increases during resistance training in young women. *Eur J Appl Physiol Occup Physiol.* 1998;77(1–2):170–175.

247. Stone ME, Plisk SS, Stone MH, et al. Athletic performance development: volume load—1 set vs. multiple sets, training velocity and training variation. *Strength Cond J.* 1998;20(6):22.

248. Behm DG, Drinkwater EJ, Willardson JM, et al. Canadian Society for Exercise Physiology position stand: the use of instability to train the core in athletic and nonathletic conditioning. *Appl Physiol Nutr Metab.* 2010;35(1):109–112.

249. Tesch PA, Dudley GA. *Muscle Meets Magnet.* Stockholm: Myuobio Technologies; 1994.

250. McCurdy KW, Langford GA, Doscher MW, et al. The effects of short-term unilateral and bilateral lower-body resistance training on measures of strength and power. *J Strength Cond Res.* 2005;19(1):9.

251. Ballor DL, Becque MD, Katch VL. Metabolic responses during hydraulic resistance exercise. *Med Sci Sports Exerc.* 1987;19:363–367.

252. Spreuwenberg LPB, Kraemer WJ, Spiering BA, et al. Influence of exercise order in a resistance-training exercise session. *J Strength Cond Res.* 2006;20(1):141–144.

253. Coyle EF, Feiring DC, Rotkis TC, et al. Specificity of power improvements through slow and fast isokinetic training. *J Appl Physiol.* 1981;51(6):1437–1442.

254. Housh DJ, Housh TJ, Johnson GO, et al. Hypertrophic response to unilateral concentric isokinetic resistance training. *J Appl Physiol.* 1992;73(1):65–70.

255. Krieger JW. Single versus multiple sets of resistance exercise: a meta-regression. *J Strength Cond Res.* 2009;23(6):1890–1901.

256. Rhea MR, Alvar BA, Burkett LN. Single versus multiple sets for strength: a meta-analysis to address the controversy. *Res Q Exerc Sport.* 2002;73(February 2015):485–488.

257. Kraemer WJ, Noble BJ, Clark MJ, et al. Physiologic responses to heavy-resistance exercise with very short rest periods. *Int J Sports Med.* 1987;8(4):247–252.

258. Kraemer W, Gordon S, Fleck S, et al. Endogenous anabolic hormonal and growth factor responses to heavy resistance exercise in males and females. *Int J Sports Med.* 1991;12(2):228–235.

259. Kraemer WJ, Marchitelli L, Gordon SE, et al. Hormonal and growth factor responses to heavy resistance exercise protocols. *J Appl Physiol.* 1990;69(4):1442–1450.

260. Kraemer WJ, Fleck SJ, Dziados JE, et al. Changes in hormonal concentrations after different heavy-resistance exercise protocols in women. *J Appl Physiol.* 1993;75(2):594–604.

261. Fleck S. Bridging the gap: interval training physiological basis. *NSCA J.* 1983;5:40:57–62.

262. Volek JS, Kraemer WJ. Creatine supplementation: its effect on human muscular performance and body composition. *J Strength Cond Res.* 1996;10(3):200–210.

263. Robinson JM, Stone MH, Johnson RL, et al. Effects of different weight training exercise/rest intervals on strength, power, and high intensity exercise endurance. *J Strength Cond Res.* 1995;9(4):216–221.

264. Richmond SR, Godard MP. The effects of varied rest periods between sets to failure using the bench press in recreationally trained men. *J Strength Cond Res.* 2004;18(4):846.

265. Schoenfeld BJ, Pope ZK, Benik FM, et al. Longer interset rest periods enhance muscle strength and hypertrophy in resistance-trained men. *J Strength Cond Res.* 2016;30(7):1805–1812.

266. Wilmore JH, Parr RB, Girandola RN, et al. Physiological alterations consequent to circuit weight training. *Med Sci Sports Exerc.* 1978;10:79–84.

267. Marcinik EJ, Hodgdon JA, Mittleman K, et al. Aerobic/calisthenic and aerobic/circuit weight training programs for Navy men: a comparative study. *Med Sci Sports Exerc.* 1985;17(4):482–487.

268. Lawton TW, Cronin JB, Lindsell RP. Effect of interrepetition rest intervals on weight training repetition power output. *J Strength Cond Res.* 2006;20(1):172.

269. Iglesias-Soler E, Carballeira E, Sánchez-Otero T, et al. Acute effects of distribution of rest between repetitions. *Int J Sports Med.* 2012;33(5):351–358.

270. Trappe S, Williamson D, Godard M. Maintenance of whole muscle strength and size following resistance training in older men. *J Gerontol A Biol Sci Med Sci.* 2002;57(4):B138–B143.

271. Fatouros IG, Kambas A, Katrabasas I, et al. Strength training and detraining effects on muscular strength, anaerobic power, and mobility of inactive older men are intensity dependent. *Br J Sports Med.* 2005;39(10):776–780.

272. Fatouros IG, Kambas A, Katrabasas I, et al. Resistance training and detraining effects on flexibility performance in the elderly are intensity-dependent. *J Strength Cond Res.* 2006;20(3):634–642.

273. Orr R, Raymond J, Fiatarone Singh M. Efficacy of progressive resistance training on balance performance in older adults: a systematic review of randomized controlled trials. *Sports Med.* 2008;38(4):317–343.

274. de Vos NJ, Singh NA, Ross DA, et al. Optimal load for increasing muscle power during explosive resistance training in older adults. *J Gerontol A Biol Sci Med Sci.* 2005;60(5):638–647.

275. Risberg M, Mørk M, Jenssen HK, et al. Design and implementation of a neuromuscular training program following anterior cruciate ligament reconstruction. *J Orthop Sports Phys Ther.* 2001;31(ll):620–631.

276. Zech A, Hübscher M, Vogt L, et al. Balance training for neuromuscular control and performance enhancement: a systematic review. *J Athl Train.* 2010;45(4):392–403.

277. Heyward V, Gibson A. *Advanced Fitness Assessment and Exercise Prescription.* 7th ed. Champaign, IL: Human Kinetics; 2014:552.

278. Horak FB. Postural orientation and equilibrium: what do we need to know about neural control of balance to prevent falls? *Age Ageing.* 2006;35(suppl 2):ii7–ii11.

279. Howe TE, Rochester L, Neil F, et al. Exercise for improving balance in older people (Review). *Cochrane Database Syst Rev.* 2011;(11):CD004963.

280. Lesinski M, Hortobágyi T, Muehlbauer T, et al. Dose-response relationships of balance training in healthy young adults: a systematic review and meta-analysis. *Sports Med.* 2015;45(4):557–576.

281. Lesinski M, Hortobagyi T, Muehlbauer T, et al. Effects of balance training on balance performance in healthy older adults: a systematic review and meta-analysis. *Sports Med.* 2015;45(12):1721–1738.

282. Zech A, Hübscher M, Vogt L, et al. Neuromuscular training for rehabilitation of sports injuries: a systematic review. *Med Sci Sports Exerc.* 2009;41(10):1831–1841.

283. Hübscher M, Zech A, Pfeifer K, et al. Neuromuscular training for sports injury prevention: a systematic review. *Med Sci Sports Exerc.* 2010;42(3):413–421.

284. Granacher U, Muehlbauer T, Zahner L, et al. Comparison of traditional and recent approaches in the promotion of balance and strength in older adults. *Sports Med.* 2011;41:377–400.

285. Sugimoto D, Myer GD, Barber Foss KD, et al. Specific exercise effects of preventive neuromuscular training intervention on anterior cruciate ligament injury risk reduction in young females: meta-analysis and subgroup analysis. *Br J Sports Med.* 2015;49:282–289.

286. Gilchrist J, Mandelbaum BR, Melancon H, et al. A randomized controlled trial to prevent noncontact anterior cruciate ligament injury in female collegiate soccer players. *Am J Sports Med.* 2008;36(8):1476–1483.

287. Muehlbauer T, Gollhofer A, Granacher U. Associations between measures of balance and lower-extremity muscle strength/power in healthy individuals across the lifespan: a systematic review and meta-analysis. *Sports Med.* 2015;45(12):1671–1692.

288. Granacher U, Muehlbauer T, Gruber M. A qualitative review of balance and strength performance in healthy older adults: impact for testing and training. *J Aging Res.* 2012;2012:708905.

289. Granacher U, Gollhofer A, Hortobagyi T, et al. The importance of trunk muscle strength for balance, functional performance, and fall prevention in seniors: a systematic review. *Sports Med.* 2013;43(7):627–641.

290. Anderson K, Behm DG. Trunk muscle activity increases with unstable squat movements. *Can J Appl Physiol.* 2005;30(1):33–45.

291. Gioftsidou P, Pafis G, Beneka A, et al. The effects of soccer training and timing of balance training on balance ability. *Eur J Appl Physiol.* 2006;96(6):659–664.

292. Zemková E. Sport-specific balance. *Sports Med.* 2014;44(5):579–590.

293. Razmus I, Wilson D, Smith R, et al. Falls in hospitalized children. *Pediatr Nurs.* 2006;32(6):568–572.

294. Wang HK, Chen CH, Shiang TY, et al. Risk-Factor analysis of high school basketball-player ankle injuries: a prospective controlled cohort study evaluating postural sway, ankle strength, and flexibility. *Arch Phys Med Rehabil.* 2006;87(6):821–825.

295. Fousekis K, Tsepis E, Poulmedis P, et al. Intrinsic risk factors of non-contact quadriceps and hamstring strains in soccer: a prospective study of 100 professional players. *Br J Sports Med.* 2011;45(9):709–714.

296. Rubenstein LZ. Falls in older people: epidemiology, risk factors and strategies for prevention. *Age Ageing.* 2006;35(suppl 2):ii37–ii41.

297. Gillespie LD, Robertson MC, Gillespie WJ, et al. Interventions for preventing falls in older people living in the community. *Cochrane Database Syst Rev.* 2012;9(9):CD007146.

298. El-Khoury F, Cassou B, Charles M-A, et al. The effect of fall prevention exercise programmes on fall induced injuries in community dwelling older adults: systematic review and meta-analysis of randomised controlled trials. *BMJ.* 2013;347 (suppl 2):f6234.

299. Campbell AJ, Robertson MC, Gardner MM, et al. Randomised controlled trial of a general practice programme of home based exercise to prevent falls in elderly women. *BMJ.* 1997;315(7115):1065–1069.

300. Sherrington C, Tiedemann A, Fairhall N, et al. Exercise to prevent falls in older adults: an updated meta-analysis and best practice recommendations. *N S W Public Health Bull.* 2011;22(3–4):78–83.

301. Hafström A, Malmström E-M, Terdèn J, et al. Improved balance confidence and stability for elderly after 6 weeks of a multimodal self-administered balance-enhancing exercise program: a randomized single arm crossover study. *Gerontol Geriatr Med.* 2016;2:2333721416644149.

302. Irez GB, Ozdemir RA, Evin R, et al. Integrating pilates exercise into an exercise program for 65+ year-old women to reduce falls. *J Sports Sci Med.* 2011;10(1):105–111.

303. Herman K, Barton C, Malliaras P, et al. The effectiveness of neuromuscular warm-up strategies, that require no additional equipment, for preventing lower limb injuries during sports participation: a systematic review. *BMC Med.* 2012;10(1):75.

304. Kapreli E, Athanasopoulos S, Gliatis J, et al. Anterior cruciate ligament deficiency causes brain plasticity: a functional MRI study. *Am J Sports Med.* 2009;37(12):2419–2426.

305. Hess DM, Joyce CJ, Arnold BL, et al. Effect of a 4-week agility-training program on postural sway in the functionally unstable ankle. *J Sport Rehabil.* 2001;10:24–35.

306. Emery CA, Cassidy JD, Klassen TP, et al. Effectiveness of a home-based balance-training program in reducing sports-related injuries among healthy adolescents: a cluster randomized controlled trial. *Can Med Assoc J.* 2005;172(6):749–754.

307. McGuine TA, Keene JS. The effect of a balance training program on the risk of ankle sprains in high school athletes. *Am J Sports Med.* 2006;34(7):1103–1111.

308. Behm DG, Blazevich AJ, Kay AD, et al. Acute effects of muscle stretching on physical performance, range of motion, and injury incidence in healthy active individuals: a systematic review. *Appl Physiol Nutr Metab.* 2016;41(1):1–11.

309. Kay AD, Blazevich AJ. Effect of acute static stretch on maximal muscle performance: a systematic review. *Med Sci Sports Exerc.* 2012;44(1):154–164.

310. Woolstenhulme MT, Griffiths CM, Woolstenhulme EM, et al. Ballistic stretching increases flexibility and acute vertical jump height when combined with basketball activity. *J Strength Cond Res.* 2006;20(4):799–803.

311. Fletcher IM. The effect of different dynamic stretch velocities on jump performance. *Eur J Appl Physiol.* 2010;109(3):491–498.

312. Hough PA, Ross EZ, Howatson G. Effects of dynamic and static stretching on vertical jump performance and electromyographic activity. *J Strength Cond Res.* 2009;23(2):507–512.

313. Sekir U, Arabaci R, Akova B, et al. Acute effects of static and dynamic stretching on leg flexor and extensor isokinetic strength in elite women athletes. *Scand J Med Sci Sports.* 2010;20(2):268–281.

314. Trehearn TL, Buresh RJ. Sit-and-Reach flexibility and running economy of men and women collegiate distance runners. *J Strength Cond Res.* 2009;23(1):158–162.

315. Hunter GR, Katsoulis K, McCarthy JP, et al. Tendon length and joint flexibility are related to running economy. *Med Sci Sports Exerc.* 2011;43(8):1492–1499.

316. Beaudoin CM, Blum JW. Flexibility and running economy in female collegiate track athletes. *J Sports Med Phys Fitness.* 2005;45(3):295–300.

317. Barnes KR, Kilding AE. Strategies to improve running economy. *Sports Med.* 2014;45:37–56.

318. Trajano GS, Seitz LB, Nosaka K, et al. Can passive stretch inhibit motoneuron facilitation in the human plantar flexors? *J Appl Physiol.* 2014;117(12):1486–1492.

319. Clarkson HM. *Musculoskeletal Assessment: Joint Range of Motion and Manual Muscle Strength.* Baltimore, MD: Lippincott Williams & Wilkins; 2000:158–160.

320. Ockendon M, Gilbert R. Validation of a novel smartphone accelerometer-based knee goniometer. *J Knee Surg.* 2012;25(4):341–346.

321. van de Pol RJ, van Trijffel E, Lucas C. Inter-rater reliability for measurement of passive physiological range of motion of upper extremity joints is better if instruments are used: a systematic review. *J Physiother.* 2010;56(1):7–17.

322. Swaim D. *ACSM's Resource Manual for Guidelines for Exercise Testing and Prescription.* 7th ed. Philadelphia, PA: Lippincott Williams & Wilkins; 2014.

323. Cook G. *Movement: Functional Movement Systems: Screening, Assessment, and Corrective Strategies.* Santa Cruz, CA: On Target Publications; 2010.

324. Herring SW, Grimm AF, Grimm BR. Regulation of sarcomere number in skeletal muscle: a comparison of hypotheses. *Muscle Nerve.* 1984;7(2):161–173.

325. Noonan TJ, Best TM, Seaber AV, et al. Thermal effects on skeletal muscle tensile behavior. *Am J Sports Med.* 1993;21(4):517–522.

326. Bottros MM, AuBuchon JD, McLaughlin LN, et al. Exercise-enhanced, ultrasound-guided anterior scalene muscle/pectoralis minor muscle blocks can facilitate the diagnosis of neurogenic thoracic outlet syndrome in the high-performance overhead athlete. *Am J Sports Med.* 2016;45(1):363546516665801.

327. Bonser RJ, Hancock CL, Hansberger BL, et al. Changes in hamstring range of motion following neurodynamic sciatic sliders: a critically appraised topic. *J Sport Rehabil.* 2017;26:311–315.

328. Palmer ML, Epler M. *Fundamentals of Musculoskeletal Assessment Techniques.* Philadelphia, PA: Lippincott-Raven; 1998.

329. Collins N, Teys P, Vicenzino B. The initial effects of a Mulligan's mobilization with movement technique on dorsiflexion and pain in subacute ankle sprains. *Man Ther.* 2004;9(2):77–82.

330. Kabat H. Studies on neuromuscular dysfunction. XV. The role of central facilitation in restoration of motor function in paralysis. *Arch Phys Med.* 1952;33(9):521–533.

331. Hindle KB, Whitcomb TJ, Briggs WO, et al. Proprioceptive Neuromuscular Facilitation (PNF): its mechanisms and effects on range of motion and muscular function. *J Hum Kinet.* 2012;31(March):105–113.

332. Magnusson SP, Simonsen EB, Aagaard P, et al. Mechanical and physical responses to stretching with and without preisometric contraction in human skeletal muscle. *Arch Phys Med Rehabil.* 1996;77(4):373–378.

333. Mitchell UH, Myrer JW, Hopkins JT, et al. Acute stretch perception alteration contributes to the success of the PNF "contract-relax" stretch. *J Sport Rehabil.* 2007;16:85–92.

334. Morse CI, Degens H, Seynnes OR, et al. The acute effect of stretching on the passive stiffness of the human gastrocnemius muscle tendon unit. *J Physiol.* 2008;586(1):97–106.

335. Magnusson SP, Simonsen EB, Aagaard P, et al. A mechanism for altered flexibility in human skeletal muscle. *J Physiol.* 1996;497(1):291–298.

336. Kay AD, Husbands-Beasley J, Blazevich AJ. Effects of contract-relax, static stretching, and isometric contractions on muscle-tendon mechanics. *Med Sci Sports Exerc.* 2015;47(10):2181–2190.

337. Harvey D. Assessment of the flexibility of elite athletes using the modified Thomas test. *Br J Sports Med.* 1998;32(1):68–70.

338. Anderson B, Burke ER. Scientific, medical, and practical aspects of stretching. *Clin Sports Med.* 1991;10(1):63–86.

339. Winters MV, Blake CG, Trost JS, et al. Passive versus active stretching of hip flexor muscles in subjects with limited hip extension: a randomized clinical trial. *Phys Ther.* 2004;84(9):800–807.

340. Behm DG, Chaouachi A. A review of the acute effects of static and dynamic stretching on performance. *Eur J Appl Physiol.* 2011;111:2633–2651.

341. Lehmann J, Warren C, Scham S. Therapeutic heat and cold. *Clin Orthop Relat Res.* 1974;99:207–245.

342. Hoffman MD, Williams CA, Lind AR. Changes in isometric function following rhythmic exercise. *Eur J Appl Physiol Occup Physiol.* 1985;54(2):177–183.

343. Fletcher IM, Jones B. The effect of different warm-up stretch protocols on 20 meter sprint performance in trained rugby union players. *J Strength Cond Res.* 2004;18(4):885–888.

344. National Center for Health Statistics, Centers for Disease Control and Prevention. *Health, United States, 2011: With Special Feature on Socioeconomic Status and Health.* Hyattsville, MD: CDC; 2012:1–583.

345. Kokkinos P, Myers J. Exercise and physical activity: clinical outcomes and applications. *Circulation.* 2010;122:1637–1648.

346. Paffenbarger RS, Hyde RT, Wing AL, et al. The association of changes in physical-activity level and other lifestyle characteristics with mortality among men. *N Engl J Med.* 1993;328(8):538–545.

347. Blair SN, Kohl HW III, Paffenbarger RS Jr, et al. Physical fitness and all cause mortality a prospective study of healthy men and women. *JAMA.* 1989;262(17):2395–2401.

348. Kokkinos P. Physical activity, health benefits, and mortality risk. *ISRN Cardiol.* 2012;2012:718789.

349. Kokkinos P, Sheriff H, Kheirbek R. Physical inactivity and mortality risk. *Cardiol Res Pract.* 2011;2011:924945.

350. Fagard RH. Exercise characteristics and the blood pressure response to dynamic physical training. *Med Sci Sports Exerc.* 2001;33(6):S484–S492.

351. Cornelissen VA, Fagard RH. Effects of endurance training on blood pressure, blood pressure-regulating mechanisms, and cardiovascular risk factors. *Hypertension.* 2005;46(4):667–675.

352. Kokkinos PF, Narayan P, Papademetriou V. Exercise as hypertension therapy. *Cardiol Clin.* 2001;19(3):507–516.

353. Kelley GA, Kelley KS. Progressive resistance exercise and resting blood pressure: a meta-analysis of randomized controlled trials. *Hypertension.* 2000;35(3):838–843.

354. Leon AS, Sanchez OA. Response of blood lipids to exercise training alone or combined with dietary intervention (dyslipidemias). *Med Sci Sports Exerc.* 2001;33(S2):S502–S515.

355. Ribeiro F, Alves AJ, Duarte JA, et al. Is exercise training an effective therapy targeting endothelial dysfunction and vascular wall inflammation? *Int J Cardiol.* 2010;141(3):214–221.

356. Szostak J, Laurant P. The forgotten face of regular physical exercise: a "natural" anti-atherogenic activity. *Clin Sci.* 2011;121(3):91–106.

357. Harper CM. Invited review. *Muscle Nerve.* 2004;(March):339–351.

358. Contractor AS. Cardiac rehabilitation after myocardial infarction. *J Assoc Physicians India.* 2011;59(suppl December):51–55.

359. Pitsavos C, Panagiotakos D, Weinem M, et al. Diet, exercise and the metabolic syndrome. *Rev Diabet Stud.* 2006;3(3):118–126.

360. Brouwer BG, van der Graaf Y, Soedamah-Muthu SS, et al. Prevention of type 2 diabetes mellitus by changes in lifestyle among subjects with impaired glucose tolerance. *Diabetes Res Clin Pract.* 2010;87(3):372–378.

361. Knowler W, Barrett-Connor E, Fowler S, et al. Reduction in the incidence of type 2 diabetes with lifestyle intervention or metformin. *N Engl J Med.* 2006;346(6):393–403.

362. Panagiotakos DB, Pitsavos C, Chrysohoou C, et al. Impact of lifestyle habits on the prevalence of the metabolic syndrome among Greek adults from the ATTICA study. *Am Heart J.* 2004;147(1):106–112.

363. Dai D-F, Hwang J-J, Chen C-L, et al. Effect of physical activity on the prevalence of metabolic syndrome and left ventricular hypertrophy in apparently healthy adults. *J Formos Med Assoc.* 2010;109(10):716–724.

364. Hoffman MD, Hoffman DR. Exercisers achieve greater acute exercise-induced mood enhancement than nonexercisers. *Arch Phys Med Rehabil.* 2008;89(2):358–363.

365. Hoffman MD, Hoffman DR. Does aerobic exercise improve pain perception and mood? A review of the evidence related to healthy and chronic pain subjects. *Curr Pain Headache Rep.* 2007;11:93–97.

366. Petruzzello SJ, Landers DM, Hatfield BD, et al. A meta-analysis on the anxiety-reducing effects of acute and chronic exercise. *Sports Med.* 1991;11(3):143–182.

367. Spirduso WW, Cronin DL. Exercise dose-response effects on quality of life and independent living in older adults. *Med Sci Sports Exerc.* 2001;33(6 suppl):S598–S610.

368. Shephard RJ. Exercise and aging: extending independence in older adults. *Geriatrics.* 1993;48(5):61–64.

369. Marques E, Wanderley F, Machado L, et al. Effects of resistance and aerobic exercise on physical function, bone mineral density, OPG and RANKL in older women. *Exp Gerontol.* 2011;46(7):524–532.

370. PolidoulisI I, Beyene J, Cheung AM. The effect of exercise on pQCT parameters of bone structure and strength in postmenopausal women—a systematic review and meta-analysis of randomized controlled trials. *Osteoporos Int.* 2012;23:39–51.

371. Bolam KA, van Uffelen JG, Taaffe DR. The effect of physical exercise on bone density in middle-aged and older men: a systematic review. *Osteoporos Int.* 2013;24(11):2749–2762.

372. Kemmler W, Haberle L, Von Stengel S. Effects of exercise on fracture reduction in older adults: a systematic review and meta-analysis. *Osteoporos Int.* 2013;24:1937–1950.

373. Karlsson MK, Nordqvist A, Karlsson C. Physical activity increases bone mass during growth. *Food Nutr Res.* 2008;52:1–10.

374. Shams-White MM, Chung M, Du M, et al. Dietary protein and bone health: a systematic review and meta-analysis from the National Osteoporosis Foundation. *Am J Clin Nutr.* 2017;105:1528–1543.

375. Tai V, Leung W, Grey A, et al. Calcium intake and bone mineral density: systematic review and meta-analysis. *BMJ.* 2015;351:h4183.

376. Arabameri E, Dehkhoda MR, Hemayattalab R. Bone mineral density changes after physical training and calcium intake in students with attention deficit and hyper activity disorders. *Res Dev Disabil.* 2012;33(2):594–599.

377. Woods JA, Wilund KR, Martin SA, et al. Exercise, inflammation and aging. *Aging Dis.* 2012;3(1):130–140.

378. Montgomery P, Dennis JA. Physical exercise for sleep problems in adults aged 60+. *Cochrane Database Syst Rev.* 2002;(4):CD003404.

379. Reid KJ, Baron KG, Lu B, et al. Aerobic exercise improves self-reported sleep and quality of life in older adults with insomnia. *Sleep Med.* 2010;11(9):934–940.

380. Lautenschlager NT, Cox KL, Flicker L, et al. Effect of physical activity on cognitive function in older adults at risk for alzheimer disease. *JAMA.* 2008;300(9):1027.

381. Colcombe S, Kramer AF. Fitness effects on the cognitive function of older adults: a meta-analytic study. *Psychol Sci.* 2003;14(2):125–130.

382. Tseng C, Gau B, Lou M. The effectiveness of exercise on improving cognitive function in older people: a systematic review. *J Nurs Res.* 2011;19(2):119–131.

383. Radák Z, Kaneko T, Tahara S, et al. Regular exercise improves cognitive function and decreases oxidative damage in rat brain. *Neurochem Int.* 2001;38(1):17–23.

384. Pereira AC, Huddleston DE, Brickman AM, et al. An in vivo correlate of exercise-induced neurogenesis in the adult dentate gyrus. *Proc Natl Acad Sci.* 2007;104(13):5638–5643.

385. Cotman CW, Berchtold NC. Exercise: a behavioral intervention to enhance brain health and plasticity. *Trends Neurosci.* 2002;25(6):295–301.

386. Friedenreich CM, Courneya KS. Exercise as rehabilitation for cancer patients. *Clin J Sport Med.* 1996;6(4):237–244.

387. McNeely ML, Campbell KL, Rowe BH, et al. Effects of exercise on breast cancer patients and survivors: a systematic review and meta-analysis. *Can Med Assoc J.* 2006;175(1):34–41.

388. McKelvie RS. Exercise training in patients with heart failure: clinical outcomes, safety, and indications. *Heart Fail Rev.* 2008;13:3–11.

389. Bjarnason-Wehrens B, Mayer-Berger W, Meister ER, et al. Recommendations for resistance exercise in cardiac rehabilitation. Recommendations of the German Federation for Cardiovascular Prevention and Rehabilitation. *Eur J Cardiovasc Prev Rehabil.* 2004;11(May):352–361.

390. Harris JE, Eng JJ. Strength training improves upper-limb function in individuals with stroke: a meta-analysis. *Stroke.* 2010;41(1):136–140.

391. Veerbeek JM, Koolstra M, Ket JCF, et al. Effects of augmented exercise therapy on outcome of gait and gait-related activities in the first 6 months after stroke: a meta-analysis. *Stroke.* 2011;42(11):3311–3315.

392. Marzolini S, Oh P, McIlroy W, et al. The effects of an aerobic and resistance exercise training program on cognition following stroke. *Neurorehabil Neural Repair.* 2013;27(5):392–402.

393. Ada L, Dorsch S, Canning CG. Strengthening interventions increase strength and improve activity after stroke: a systematic review. *Aust J Physiother.* 2006;52(4):241–248.

394. Duncan P, Studenski S, Richards L, et al. Randomized clinical trial of therapeutic exercise in subacute stroke. *Stroke.* 2003;34(9):2173–2180.

395. Lai SM, Studenski S, Richards L, et al. Therapeutic exercise and depressive symptoms after stroke. *J Am Geriatr Soc.* 2006;54(2):240–247.

396. Billinger SA, Arena R, Bernhardt J, et al. Physical activity and exercise recommendations for stroke survivors: a statement for healthcare professionals from the American Heart Association/American Stroke Association. *Stroke.* 2014;45(8):2532–2553.

397. Ettinger WHJ, Burns R, Messier SP, et al. A randomized trial comparing aerobic exercise and resistance exercise with a health education program in older adults with knee osteoarthritis. The Fitness Arthritis and Seniors Trial (FAST). *JAMA.* 1997;277(1):25–31.

398. Helmark IC, Mikkelsen UR, Børglum J, et al. Exercise increases interleukin-10 levels both intraarticularly and peri-synovially in patients with knee osteoarthritis: a randomized controlled trial. *Arthritis Res Ther.* 2010;12(4):R126.

399. Brorsson S, Hilliges M, Sollerman C, et al. A six-week hand exercise programme improves strength and hand function in patients with rheumatoid arthritis. *J Rehabil Med.* 2009;41(5):338–342.

400. Metsios GS, Stavropoulos-Kalinoglou A, Veldhuijzen van Zanten J, et al. Individualised exercise improves endothelial function in patients with rheumatoid arthritis. *Ann Rheum Dis.* 2014;73(4):748–751.

401. Fransen M, McConnell S, Harmer AR, et al. Exercise for osteoarthritis of the knee. In: Fransen M, ed. *Cochrane Database of Systematic Reviews.* Chichester, UK: John Wiley & Sons, Ltd; 2015.

402. Swärdh E, Brodin N. Effects of aerobic and muscle strengthening exercise in adults with rheumatoid arthritis: a narrative review summarising a chapter in physical activity in the prevention and treatment of disease (FYSS 2016). *Br J Sports Med.* 2016;50:1–7.

403. de Jong Z, Munneke M, Zwinderman AH, et al. Long term high intensity exercise and damage of small joints in rheumatoid arthritis. *Ann Rheum Dis.* 2004;63(11):1399–1405.

404. Jan MH, Lin JJ, Liau JJ, et al. Investigation of clinical effects of high- and low-resistance training for patients with knee osteoarthritis: a randomized controlled trial. *Phys Ther.* 2008;88(4):427–436.

405. Van Den Ende CH, Hazes JM, Le Cessie S, et al. Comparison of high and low intensity training in well controlled rheumatoid arthritis. Results of a randomised clinical trial. *Ann Rheum Dis.* 1996;55(11):798–805.

406. Finckh A, Iversen M, Liang MH. The exercise prescription in rheumatoid arthritis: primum non nocere. *Arthritis Rheum.* 2003;48(9):2393–2395.

407. Lundeberg N. Exercise prescription for older adults with osteoarthritis pain: consensus practice recommendations. *J Am Geriatr Soc.* 2001;49(6):808–823.

408. Clausen JP, Trap-Jensen J, Lassen NA. The effects of training on the heart rate during arm and leg exercise. *Scand J Clin Lab Invest.* 1970;26(3):295–301.

409. Hoffman MD. Cardiorespiratory fitness and training in quadriplegics and paraplegics. *Sports Med.* 1986;3:312–330.

410. Pitetti KH, Barrett PJ, Campbell KD, et al. The effect of lower body positive pressure on the exercise capacity of individuals with spinal cord injury. *Med Sci Sports Exerc.* 1994;26(4):463.

411. Hopman MT, Oeseburg B, Binkhorst RA. The effect of an anti-G suit on cardiovascular responses to exercise in persons with paraplegia. *Med Sci Sports Exerc.* 1992;24:984–990.

412. Davis GM, Servedio FJ, Glaser RM, et al. Cardiovascular responses to arm cranking and FNS-induced leg exercise in paraplegics. *J Appl Physiol.* 1990;69(2):671–677.

413. Hooker SP, Figoni SF, Rodgers MM, et al. Metabolic and hemodynamic responses to concurrent voluntary arm crank and electrical stimulation leg cycle exercise in quadriplegics. *J Rehabil Res Dev.* 1992;29(3):1–11.

414. McLean KP, Skinner JS. Effect of body training position on outcomes of an aerobic training study on individuals with quadriplegia. *Arch Phys Med Rehabil.* 1995;76(2):139–150.

415. Davis GM. Exercise capacity of individuals with paraplegia. *Med Sci Sports Exerc.* 1993;25(4):423–432.

416. Davis GM, Shephard RJ. Cardiorespiratory fitness in highly active versus inactive paraplegics. *Med Sci Sports Exerc.* 1988;20(5):463–468.

417. Hopman MT, Oeseburg B, Binkhorst RA. Cardiovascular responses in persons with paraplegia to prolonged arm exercise and thermal stress. *Med Sci Sports Exerc.* 1993;25(5):577–583.

418. Ginis KAM, Hicks AL, Latimer AE, Warburton DER, Bourne C, Ditor DS, et al. The development of evidence-informed physical activity guidelines for adults with spinal cord injury. *Spinal Cord.* 2011;49:1088–1096.

419. Ernstoff B, Wetterqvist H, Kvist H, et al. Endurance training effect on individuals with postpoliomyelitis. *Arch Phys Med Rehabil.* 1996;77(9):843–848.

420. Dean E, Ross J. Modified aerobic walking program: effect on patients with postpolio syndrome symptoms. *Arch Phys Med Rehabil.* 1988;69(12):1033–1038.

421. Chan KM, Amirjani N, Sumrain M, et al. Randomized controlled trial of strength training in post-polio patients. *Muscle Nerve.* 2003;27(3):332–338.

422. Einarsson G. Muscle conditioning in late poliomyelitis. *Arch Phys Med Rehabil.* 1991;72(1):11–14.

423. Oncu J, Durmaz B, Karapolat H. Short-term effects of aerobic exercise on functional capacity, fatigue, and quality of life in patients with post-polio syndrome. *Clin Rehabil.* 2009;23(2):155–163.

424. Koopman FS, Voorn EL, Beelen A, et al. No reduction in severe fatigue in patients with postpolio syndrome by exercise therapy or cognitive behavioral therapy: results of an RCT. *Neurorehabil Neural Repair.* 2016;30(5):402–410.

425. Rietberg MB, Brooks D, Uitdehaag BMJ, et al. Exercise therapy for multiple sclerosis. *Cochrane Database Syst Rev.* 2009;(4):CD003980.

426. Romberg A, Virtanen A, Ruutiainen J, et al. Effects of a 6-month exercise program on patients with multiple sclerosis: a randomized study. *Neurology.* 2004;63(11):2034–2038.

427. Bansi J, Bloch W, Gamper U, et al. Endurance training in MS: short-term immune responses and their relation to cardiorespiratory fitness, health-related quality of life, and fatigue. *J Neurol.* 2013;260(12):2993–3001.

428. Surakka J, Romberg A, Ruutiainen J, et al. Effects of aerobic and strength exercise on motor fatigue in men and women with multiple sclerosis: a randomized controlled trial. *Clin Rehabil.* 2004;18(7):737–746.

429. Sutherland G, Andersen MB, Stoové MA. Can aerobic exercise training affect health-related quality of life for people with multiple sclerosis? *J Sport Exerc Psychol.* 2001;23(2):122–135.

430. Motl RW, Gosney JL. Effect of exercise training on quality of life in multiple sclerosis: a meta-analysis. *Mult Scler.* 2008;14(1):129–135.

431. Dalgas U, Stenager E, Jakobsen J, et al. Resistance training improves muscle strength and functional capacity in multiple sclerosis. *Neurology.* 2009;73(18):1478–1484.

432. DeBolt LS, McCubbin JA. The effects of home-based resistance exercise on balance, power, and mobility in adults with multiple sclerosis. *Arch Phys Med Rehabil.* 2004;85(2):290–297.

433. White LJ, McCoy SC, Castellano V, et al. Resistance training improves strength and functional capacity in persons with multiple sclerosis. *Mult Scler.* 2004;10(6):668–674.

434. Kosich D, Molk B, Feeney J, et al. Cardiovascular testing and exercise prescription in multiple sclerosis patients. *Neurorehabil Neural Repair.* 1987;1(4):167–170.

435. Schapiro RT, Petajan JH, Kosich D, et al. Role of cardiovascular fitness in multiple sclerosis: a pilot study. *Neurorehabil Neural Repair.* 1988;2(2):43–49.

436. Janelsins MC, Peppone LJ, Heckler CE, et al. YOCAS©® yoga reduces self-reported memory difficulty in cancer survivors in a nationwide randomized clinical trial: investigating relationships between memory and sleep. *Integr Cancer Ther.* 2016;15(3):263–271.

437. Sprod LK, Fernandez ID, Janelsins MC, et al. Effects of yoga on cancer-related fatigue and global side-effect burden in older cancer survivors. *J Geriatr Oncol.* 2015;6(1):8–14.

438. Demark-Wahnefried W, Clipp EC, Morey MC, et al. Lifestyle intervention development study to improve physical function in older adults with cancer: outcomes from project LEAD. *J Clin Oncol.* 2006;24(21):3465–3473.

439. Courneya KS, Segal RJ, Mackey JR, et al. Effects of aerobic and resistance exercise in breast cancer patients receiving adjuvant chemotherapy: a multicenter randomized controlled trial. *J Clin Oncol.* 2007;25(28):4396–4404.

440. Sprod LK, Janelsins MC, Palesh OG, et al. Health-related quality of life and biomarkers in breast cancer survivors participating in tai chi chuan. *J Cancer Surviv.* 2012;6(2):146–154.

441. Stene GB, Helbostad JL, Balstad TR, et al. Effect of physical exercise on muscle mass and strength in cancer patients during treatment—a systematic review. *Crit Rev Oncol Hematol.* 2013;88:573–593.

442. Coleman EA, Coon S, Hall-Barrow J, et al. Feasibility of exercise during treatment for multiple myeloma. *Cancer Nurs.* 2003;26(5):410–419.

443. Battaglini C, Bottaro M, Dennehy C, et al. The effects of an individualized exercise intervention on body composition in breast cancer patients undergoing treatment. *Sao Paulo Med J.* 2007;125(1):22–28.

444. Kaltsatou A, Mameletzi D, Douka S. Physical and psychological benefits of a 24-week traditional dance program in breast cancer survivors. *J Bodyw Mov Ther.* 2011;15(2):162–167.

445. Pinto BM, Clark MM, Maruyama NC, et al. Psychological and fitness changes associated with exercise participation among women with breast cancer. *Psychooncology.* 2003;12(2):118–126.

446. Schwartz AL, Mori M, Gao R, et al. Exercise reduces daily fatigue in women with breast cancer receiving chemotherapy. *Med Sci Sports Exerc.* 2001;33(5):718–723.

447. Peddle CJ, Au HJ, Courneya KS. Associations between exercise, quality of life, and fatigue in colorectal cancer survivors. *Dis Colon Rectum.* 2008;51(8):1242–1248.

448. Tomlinson D, Diorio C, Beyene J, et al. Effect of exercise on cancer-related fatigue. *Am J Phys Med Rehabil.* 2014;93(8):675–686.

449. Winters-Stone KM, Dobek J, Bennett JA, et al. The effect of resistance training on muscle strength and physical function in older, postmenopausal breast cancer survivors: a randomized controlled trial. *J Cancer Surviv.* 2012;6(2):189–199.

450. Mustian KM, Peppone L, Darling TV, et al. A 4-week home-based aerobic and resistance exercise program during radiation therapy: a pilot randomized clinical trial. *J Support Oncol.* 2009;7(5):158–167.

451. Mock V, Pickett M, Ropka ME, et al. Fatigue and quality of life outcomes of exercise during cancer treatment. *Cancer Pract.* 2001;9(3):119–127.

452. Schmitz KH, Courneya KS, Matthews C, et al. American college of sports medicine roundtable on exercise guidelines for cancer survivors. *Med Sci Sports Exerc.* 2010;42(7):1409–1426.

453. Holmes MD, Chen WY, Feskanich D, et al. Physical activity and survival after breast cancer diagnosis. *JAMA.* 2005;293(20):2479.

454. Saarto T, Sievänen H, Kellokumpu-Lehtinen P, et al. Effect of supervised and home exercise training on bone mineral density among breast cancer patients. A 12-month randomised controlled trial. *Osteoporos Int.* 2012;23(5):1601–1612.

455. Shipp KM. Exercise for people with osteoporosis: translating the science into clinical practice. *Curr Osteoporos Rep.* 2006;4(4):129–133.

456. Iwamoto J, Takeda T, Ichimura S. Effect of exercise training and detraining on bone mineral density in postmenopausal women with osteoporosis. *J Orthop Sci.* 2001;6(2):128–132.

457. Martyn-St. James M, Carroll S. High-intensity resistance training and postmenopausal bone loss: a meta-analysis. *Osteoporos Int.* 2006;17(8):1225–1240.

458. Borba-Pinheiro CJ, Dantas EH, Vale RG, et al. Resistance training programs on bone related variables and functional independence of postmenopausal women in pharmacological treatment: a randomized controlled trial. *Arch Gerontol Geriatr.* 2016;65:36–44.

459. Mosti MP, Kaehler N, Stunes AK, et al. Maximal strength training in postmenopausal women with osteoporosis or osteopenia. *J Strength Cond Res.* 2013;27(10):2879–2886.

460. Watson SL, Weeks BK, Weis LJ, et al. Heavy resistance training is safe and improves bone, function, and stature in postmenopausal women with low to very low bone mass: novel early findings from the LIFTMOR trial. *Osteoporos Int.* 2015;26(12):2889–2894.

461. Alghadir AH, Gabr SA, Al-Eisa ES, et al. Correlation between bone mineral density and serum trace elements in response to supervised aerobic training in older adults. *Clin Interv Aging.* 2016;11:265–273.

462. Giangregorio LM, McGill S, Wark JD, et al. Too Fit To Fracture: outcomes of a Delphi consensus process on physical activity and exercise recommendations for adults with osteoporosis with or without vertebral fractures. *Osteoporos Int.* 2015;26(3):891–910.

463. Chodzko-Zajko WJ, Proctor DN, Fiatarone Singh MA, et al. American College of Sports Medicine position stand. Exercise and physical activity for older adults. *Med Sci Sports Exerc.* 2009;41(7):1510–1530.

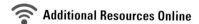 **Additional Resources Online**

CHAPTER 50

Bruce E. Becker

Aquatic Rehabilitation

INTRODUCTION AND BRIEF HISTORY

Historical Applications

Throughout all recorded history, the sick and suffering have resorted to springs, baths, and pools for their soothing, healing, and powerful effects. Healing water rituals appeared in the river valley civilizations of Mesopotamia, Egypt, India, China as well as in ancient Greek, Hebrew, Roman, Christian, and Islamic cultures (1). In Europe, the beginnings of formal resorts formed for the purposes of healing began to emerge, and these became the progenitors of the current group of European spas. A spa has been defined as a "place where mineral-containing waters flow from the ground naturally, or to which it is pumped or conducted, and is there used for therapeutic purposes" (2). This chapter will, however, deal not with spas in their historical context but with contemporary aquatic therapy practice. Simon Baruch established the American medical standards for hydrotherapy in *The Principles and Practice of Hydrotherapy*, and in 1921, shortly before he died, Baruch published his last book, *An Epitome of Hydrotherapy* (3,4). Baruch writes in the Preface to the second edition of *The Principles and Practice of Hydrotherapy*, "So flexible is this therapeutic agent that, unlike medicinal remedies, it may be utilized to meet indications which seem contradictory to the uninitiated" (3). This statement holds true today.

Although most writings concerned the internal and external curative benefits of the waters, baths, and pools, limited emphasis was placed on water exercise. In 1911, Charles Leroy Lowman began using therapeutic tubs to treat spastic patients and those with cerebral palsy. He visited the Spaulding School for Crippled Children in Chicago, where he observed paralyzed patients exercising in a wooden tank. Lowman had founded the Orthopedic Hospital in Los Angeles in 1913, later to become Rancho Los Amigos. On his return to California, he transformed the Orthopedic Hospital's lily pond into two therapeutic pools (5). In Warm Springs, Georgia, Leroy Hubbard developed his famous tank, and in 1924, Warm Springs received its most famous aquatic patient, Franklin D. Roosevelt. Roosevelt would go on to purchase Warm Springs in 1926 and expand it with residential and better therapeutic facilities, and it subsequently became the destination of choice for American polio survivors for rehabilitation (6).

At Saratoga Springs, New York, financier Bernard M. Baruch, Roosevelt's friend and the son of Dr. Simon Baruch, headed a special commission to plan a scientific American spa (7). The commission studied spa design, natural treatments, and efficient operations based on what was then felt to be the sound medical and scientific care for chronically ill patients, especially those suffering from cardiac, vascular, and circulatory ailments, and selected Dr. Walter S. McClellan to be the Medical Spa Director (8,9). At Northwestern University Medical School in Chicago, Dr. John S. Coulter presented lectures on physical therapy that he placed within the history of spa medicine (10). In 1933, the Simon Baruch Research Institute of Balneology at Saratoga Springs Spa was established, and the facility began the printing of their scientific bulletin, *The Publications of Saratoga Spa*. At Hot Springs, Arkansas, a warm swimming pool was installed for special underwater physical therapy exercises and pool therapy treatments with chronic arthritic patients (11). In 1937, Dr. Charles Leroy Lowman published his *Technique of Underwater Gymnastics: A Study in Practical Application,* in which he detailed pool therapy methods of specific underwater exercises that "carefully regulated dosage, character, frequency, and duration for remedying bodily deformities and restoring muscle function" (5). During the 1950s, the National Foundation for Infantile Paralysis supported the corrective swimming pools and hydrogymnastics of Dr. Lowman and the therapeutic use of pools and tanks for the treatment of poliomyelitis. With polio seen as a national epidemic, aquatic therapy became widely supported within rehabilitation medicine.

Current Trends and Uses

With the end of the polio epidemic and the rise of newer and more exciting technology in rehabilitative therapeutics, the use of the aquatic environment in rehabilitation waned. Fortunately, basic science research in the biologic effects of immersion accelerated during the late 1960s for two fortuitous reasons. Aquatic immersion was recognized as a wonderful surrogate for the weightlessness of space, and as we prepared to place humans outside gravity, it became essential to forecast the effects of space flight. At the same time, researchers realized that aquatic immersion was a benign means of simulating central volume expansion to better understand volume homeostasis (12,13). The end result of these research efforts and recent research has been that aquatic therapy now has a considerable foundation of high-quality basic science research (14).

THE PHYSICS OF WATER AND ITS RELATIONSHIP TO AQUATIC REHABILITATION

Because water is a substance with many physical properties, nearly all of which impact human physiology, the relevance of these physical properties cannot be readily understood without a brief discussion of the physics behind these properties.

Density and Specific Gravity

Density is defined as mass per unit volume. In addition to density, substances are defined by their specific gravity, the ratio of the density of that substance to the density of water. By definition, water has a specific gravity equal to 1.00 at 4°C. Although the human body is mostly water, the body's density is slightly less than that of water and averages a specific gravity of 0.974, with males averaging higher density than females. Lean body mass, which includes bone, muscle, connective tissue, and organs, has a typical density near 1.10, whereas fat mass, which includes both essential body fat plus fat in excess of essential needs, has a density of about 0.90 (15). Consequently, the human body displaces a volume of water weighing slightly more than the body, forcing the body upward by a force equal to the volume of the water displaced. The buoyancy differences between lean and fat body mass make aquatic activity particularly useful for severely obese individuals, for whom land-based exercise may produce joint pain.

Hydrostatic Pressure

Pressure is defined as force per unit area, and is measured in Newtons $(N)/m^2$, dynes/cm^2, kg/m^2, and pounds per square inch (PSI). Fluids have been experimentally found to exert pressure in all directions. The pressure exerted on a theoretical point surrounded by a fluid is equal from all directions. Obviously, if unequal pressure were being exerted, the point would move until the pressures were equalized on it. Pressure is directly proportional to both the liquid density and the immersion depth, when the fluid is incompressible, as water is at the depths used in therapeutic environments. Because pressure responds not only to the fluid depth but also to any force exerted on its surface, the pressure of the Earth's atmosphere is an important contributor to the total force from immersion. Water exerts a pressure of 22.4 mm Hg for every foot of water depth, which translates to 0.73 mm Hg/cm or slightly under 2 mm Hg per inch of H_2O depth. Thus, a body immersed to a depth of 48 inches is subjected to a distal pressure equal to 88.9 mm Hg, far greater than venous or lymphatic pressures. Even shallow water immersion increases hydrostatic pressure substantially more than air pressure plus gravity. This external compressive force significantly aids the resolution of edema in an injured body part or where postsurgical edema resolution is a therapeutic goal.

Buoyancy

Buoyancy causes immersed objects to have less apparent weight than the same object on land. Buoyancy, a force opposite to gravity, acts on the object with a force generated by the volume of H_2O displaced. This principle was discovered by Archimedes (287–212 B.C.) and is the reason that water can be used to advantage in the management of medical problems, such as arthritis or severe obesity requiring weight off-loading. A human with a specific gravity of 0.97 will reach floating equilibrium when 97% of his or her volume is submerged.

Because the force of buoyancy is an upward force, there are important consequences in the therapeutic aquatic environment. The center of gravity is a point at which all force moments are in equilibrium. For an average male adult human being standing in the "anatomic" position, this point is located slightly posterior to the mid-sagittal plane and at about the level of the second sacral vertebra, because the human body is nonuniform with respect to density and varies depending upon body build within a radius of 1.9 to 9 cm (16). The lungs obviously are less dense than the lower limbs, for example. The center of buoyancy is defined as the center of all buoyancy force moments summating on each body segment. Typically, the human center of buoyancy is in the mid-chest. The difference between the center of gravity (a downward force) and the center of buoyancy (an upward force) may generate rotational torque. This rotational torque may produce instability for some patients and should be carefully monitored, preferably by a therapist in the pool with the patient.

Water in Motion

Flow Characteristics

When water moves smoothly, in layers moving at the same speed, the water is defined as in laminar or streamline flow. When water moves more rapidly, even minor oscillations create uneven flow, and parallel paths are knocked out of alignment, resulting in turbulent flow. Within the mass of water, flow patterns arise that run dramatically out of parallel. These paths are called eddy currents. An example of the latter are the eddy currents that form in the blood stream behind artery walls encrusted with cholesterol plaque. Turbulent flow absorbs energy at a much greater rate than does streamline flow, and the internal friction within the fluid determines the rate of energy absorption. The major determinants of water motion are viscosity, turbulence, and speed. Flow rates decrease when turbulence occurs, largely due to the significant nonlinear increase in internal friction in the fluid. The onset of turbulent flow obviously is a function of fluid velocity, but it is also related to fluid density, viscosity, and enclosure radius. The transition from laminar flow to turbulent flow often occurs abruptly with increasing velocity.

Viscosity and Drag

Viscosity refers to the magnitude of internal friction specific to the fluid. As layers of fluid molecules are set into motion, molecular attraction creates resistance to movement and is detected as friction. Energy must be exerted to create movement, and as in the first law of thermodynamics, energy is never lost but rather is transformed and stored as potential or kinetic energy. Some energy is transformed into heat, some into kinetic energy, and some may be stored as potential energy by increasing surface tension. Fluids are in part defined by individual viscosity, expressed quantitatively as the coefficient of viscosity. The greater the coefficient, the more viscous the fluid and the greater the force required to create movement within the fluid. Water is intermediate in viscosity as liquids go, but it still presents much resistance to movement. Under turbulent flow conditions, this resistance increases as a log function of velocity. The greatest surface area drag on a swimming man is his head, although the negative pressure following the swimmer causes the greatest force resisting forward movement. There is turbulence produced by fast-moving body surface areas and a drag force produced by the turbulence behind. Viscosity, with all its attendant physical properties, is a quality that makes water a useful strengthening medium. Viscous resistance increases as more force is exerted against it, but resistance drops to zero almost immediately on cessation of force because there is only a small amount of inertia (viscosity effectively counteracts inertial momentum). Thus, when a rehabilitating person feels pain and stops movement, the force decreases precipitously, and water viscosity damps movement almost instantaneously. The combination of buoyancy and viscosity means that, unlike in thin air, gravity is taken out of the movement equation during active movement. This allows great control of strengthening activities within the envelope of patient movement comfort.

Specific Heat

Water is used therapeutically in all three of its thermal states: solid, liquid, and gas. A major reason for its usefulness lies in the physics of aquatic thermodynamics. All substances on earth possess energy stored as heat. A mass of water possesses a measurable amount of stored energy in the form of heat. Energy stored may be released through a change to a lower temperature, or additional energy may raise the water temperature. If the temperature of the water exceeds the temperature of a submersed body, the system equilibrates to a different level, with the submersed body warming through transference of heat energy from the water, and the water cooling through loss of heat energy to the body. By the first law of thermodynamics, the total heat (and thus energy) contents of the system remain the same. Energy applied to this system increases the kinetic energy of some of the molecules, and when high kinetic energy molecules collide with lower kinetic energy molecules, they transfer some of their energy, increasing and equilibrating the total energy of the system. Water is defined as having a specific heat capacity equal to 1.00. Air, in contrast, has a far lower specific heat capacity = 0.001. Thus, water retains heat 1,000 times more than does an equal volume of air.

Thermal Energy Transfer

The therapeutic utility of water is greatly dependent on both its ability to retain heat and its ability to transfer heat energy. Exchange of energy in the form of heat occurs in three ways: conduction, convection, and radiation. Conduction may be thought of as occurring through molecular collisions that take place over a small distance. For example, a hydrocollator pack transfers heat by conduction. Substances vary widely in their ability to conduct heat. Convection requires water molecules to move over a large distance. For example, a whirlpool bath transfers heat by convection. Heat transfer across a gradient is measured by the amount of heat in calories transferred per second across an imaginary membrane. Liquids and gases are generally poor conductors but good convectors. Water is an efficient conductor of heat and transfers heat 25 times faster than does air. Radiation transfers heat through the transmission of electromagnetic waves. For example, a heating lamp transfers heat by radiation. The thermal conductive property of water, in combination with water's high specific heat, makes its use in rehabilitation versatile, as it retains heat or cold while transferring it easily to the immersed body part.

BIOLOGIC ASPECTS OF AQUATIC REHABILITATION

Cardiovascular System Effects

Water begins to exert external pressure on the body immediately on immersion. Intrinsic pressure within the venous and lymphatic side of the circulation is much lower than pressure on the arterial side of the system. Consequently, venous and lymphatic return is sensitive to external pressure changes,

including compression from surrounding muscles and from external water pressure. During water immersion, hydrostatic pressure displaces blood upward through this one-way system, first into the thighs, then into the abdominal cavity vessels, and finally into the great vessels of the chest cavity and into the heart. Central venous pressure begins to increase with immersion to the xiphoid and increases until the body is completely immersed. Right atrial distension occurs, and pressure increases by 14 to 18 mm Hg during immersion to the neck, going from about −2 to −4 mm Hg to +14 to +17 mm Hg (17,18). The transmural pressure gradient of the right atrium increases significantly, measured by Arborelius, who was the first researcher to intensively study the impact of immersion on human physiology at 13 mm Hg, going from 2 to 15 mm Hg. Extra systoles may result, especially early into immersion (17).

Pulmonary blood flow increases with increased central blood volume and pressure. Mean pulmonary artery wedge pressure increases from 5 mm Hg on land to 22 mm Hg during immersion to the neck (18). Most of the increased pulmonary blood volume is distributed in the larger vessels of the pulmonary vascular bed and only a small percentage (5% or less) at the capillary level. This is validated by the fact that the diffusion capacity of the lungs changes very little.

Central blood volume increased by 0.7 L in Arborelius' classic study (17). This represents a 60% increase in central volume, with one third of this volume taken up by the heart and the remainder by the great vessels of the lungs. Cardiac volume increases 27% to 30% with immersion to the neck (19), but the heart is not a static receptacle. The healthy cardiac response to increased volume (stretch) is to increase the force of contraction. As the myocardium stretches, an improved actin/myosin filament relationship is produced, enhancing the myocardial efficiency (Starling's law) (20). Mean stroke volume increases 35% on average with immersion to the neck from a resting baseline of about 71 mL/beat to about 100 mL/beat, which is close to the exercise maximum for a sedentary, deconditioned individual on land (21,22). There is both an increase in end-diastolic volume and a decrease in end-systolic volume (17). Stroke volume is one of the major determinants of the increase in cardiac output seen with training because heart rate response ranges remain relatively fixed despite cardiovascular fitness levels, although the upper range decreases through the life span (21).

Most of the changes are temperature dependent, with cardiac output increasing progressively with increasing water temperatures. Weston found cardiac output to increase by 30% at 33°C rising to 121% at 39°C (19). There is considerable individual variance in the many studies assessing this phenomenon.

As cardiac filling and stroke volume increase with deeper immersion from symphysis to xiphoid, the heart rate typically decreases (18,23). This decrease is variable, with the amount of decrease dependent on water temperature. Typically, at average pool temperatures, the rate decreases by 12% to 15% (19). There is a significant relationship between water temperature and heart rate. At 25°C, the heart rate decreases by approximately 12 to 15 beats/min (19,24), whereas at thermoneutral temperatures, the rate of decrease is less than 15%, and in warm water, the rate generally increases significantly, contributing to the major increase in cardiac output at high temperatures. The reduction variability is believed to be related to decreased peripheral resistance at higher temperatures and increased vagal effects (25). Ongoing work in our lab has corroborated the heart rate effects, with both healthy college-aged students and middle-aged adults showing a reduction of heart rate in cool (30°C) water, an increase to about baseline in neutral (36°C), and elevation averaging about 10% in warm water (39°C) (26,27). At the same time, by monitoring autonomic nervous system activity, we found elevation of sympathetic activity in cool water, substantially reducing in warm water, with vagal power increasing through the cool to warm immersion sequence, the end result being an increase in sympathovagal balance. Earlier investigators found similar results (28).

Because the ultimate purpose of the heart as an organ is to pump blood, its ultimate measure of performance is the amount of blood pumped per unit time. Cardiac output is the product of stroke volume times pulse rate per unit time. The most efficient way for the heart to deliver more blood during exercise is to increase stroke volume. Maximal myocardial oxygen consumption efficiency (peak heart muscle efficiency) occurs when stroke volume increases because heart rate acceleration is a less efficient means of increasing output (20,29). Thus, as cardiovascular conditioning occurs, cardiac output increases are achieved through smaller increases in heart rate but greater stroke volumes per beat. This is the reason that conditioned athletes are able to maintain lower pulse rates for a given cardiac output than those who are deconditioned (20,30).

Submersion to the neck increases cardiac output by more than 30% (17). Output increases by about 1,500 mL/min, of which 50% is directed to increased muscle blood flow (17). Normal resting cardiac output is approximately 5 L/min. Maximum output in a conditioned athlete is about 40 L/min, which is equivalent to 205 mL/beat times 195 beats/min. Maximum output at exercise for a sedentary individual on land is approximately 20 L/min, equivalent to 105 mL/beat times 195 beats/min (30). Because immersion to the neck produces a cardiac stroke volume of about 100 mL/beat, a resting pulse of 86 beats/min produces a cardiac output of 8.6 L/min and is already producing increased cardiac work. The increase in cardiac output appears to be somewhat age dependent, with younger subjects demonstrating greater increases (59%) than older subjects (22%) (31). The increase is also highly temperature dependent, varying directly with temperature increase from 30% at 33°C to 121% at 39°C (19). Conditioned athletes demonstrate an even greater increase in cardiac output than do untrained control subjects during immersed exercise, and this increase seems sustained for longer periods than in an untrained control group (32). Therefore, the myth that water exercise is not aerobically efficient is faulty; it may be an ideal cardiovascular conditioning medium. There is an emerging body of research on water exercise–induced cardiac output, but significant work needs to be done to delineate the effects of age, gender, temperature, and conditioning, as well as to explain the significant individual response variations. The cascade of cardiovascular responses to immersion is shown in **Figure 50-1**.

FIGURE 50-1. Cardiovascular schematic.

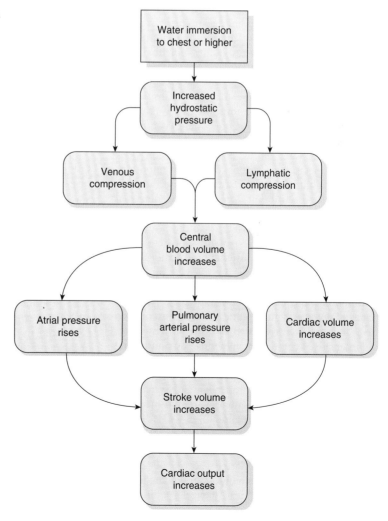

In 1989, Gleim and Nicholas found that oxygen consumption (VO_2) was three times greater at a given running speed (53 m/min) in water than on land (33). Therefore, during water walking and running, only one-half to one third the speed was required to achieve the same metabolic intensity as on land (33). It is important to note that the relationship of heart rate to VO_2 parallels the relationship during land-based exercise, even with accounting for the heart rate decrease in water. Consequently, metabolic intensity in water may be predicted as on land from monitoring heart rate.

During immersion to the neck in thermoneutral water, systemic vascular resistance decreases by 30% (17). Diminished sympathetic vasoconstriction produces this decrease, with peripheral venous tone decreasing by 30% from 17 to 12 mm Hg at thermoneutral temperatures (13). Total peripheral resistance decreases during the first hour of immersion and remains low for several hours thereafter. This decrease is related to temperature, with higher temperatures producing greater reductions. This resistance drop decreases end-diastolic pressures. Immersed systolic pressures increase with increasing workload, as they do on land, but these increases appear to be reduced in magnitude when compared with equivalent land-based work (33). Venous pressures also decrease during immersion because less vascular tone is required to support the system. This venous pressure drop may lead to light-headedness upon exiting warm or hot water.

Effects upon Blood Pressure

The effect of immersion on blood pressure has been quite extensively studied. A consistent finding has been the striking individual variation, but trends have emerged that are useful. Very short-term immersion (10 minutes) in thermoneutral temperatures has been found to slightly increase both systolic and diastolic pressures, perhaps as part of the thermal accommodation process (33). In contrast, a pilot study in our institution found that mean arterial pressures demonstrated a 15% to 25% decrease at 5 minutes of immersion. Other studies conducted in carefully controlled environments have found no effects or actual decreases in pressures during longer immersion periods more typical of therapeutic sessions (34). In an important study for aquatic rehabilitation, Coruzzi et al. found that longer immersion produced significant decreases in mean arterial pressure, with sodium-sensitive hypertensive patients showing even greater decreases (18 to 20 mm Hg) than did normotensive patients, and sodium-insensitive patients showing smaller decreases (5 to 14 mm Hg) (35). No studies have demonstrated consistent sustained increases in systolic pressure with prolonged immersion, although several have found no significant decrease. Based on a substantial body of research, therapy pool appears to be both a safe and potentially therapeutic environment for both normotensive and hypertensive patients, with both sodium-sensitive and insensitive hypertensive individuals demonstrating decreases in pressure during therapeutically customary periods of immersion (36). In summary, the preponderance of literature supports the safety of aquatic immersion and exercise for both healthy normals as well as individuals with mild-moderate hypertension and may even be therapeutic (27,37–41).

Cardiac Rehabilitation

Recent research has generally supported the use of aquatic environments in cardiovascular rehabilitation following infarct and ischemic cardiomyopathy (see also Chapter 33). Since the late 1980s, studies have validated the use of aquatic environments in cardiovascular rehabilitation after infarct and ischemic cardiomyopathy by actively rehabilitating heart patients in an aquatic environment (42,43).

Japanese investigators studied patients with severe congestive heart failure (mean ejection fractions 25 ± 9%) under the hypothesis that in this clinical problem, the essential pathology was the inability of the heart to overcome peripheral vascular resistance. They reasoned that since exposure to a warm environment causes peripheral vasodilatation, a reduction in vascular resistance and cardiac afterload might be therapeutic. During a series of studies, these researchers found that during a single 10-minute immersion in a hot-water bath (41°C), both pulmonary wedge pressure and right atrial pressure dropped by 25%, while cardiac output and stroke volume both increased. In a subsequent study of patients using warm-water immersion or sauna bath 1 to 2 times per day, 5 days a week for 4 weeks, they found improvement in ejection fractions of nearly 30% accompanied by reduction in left ventricular end-diastolic dimension, along with subjective improvement in quality of life, sleep quality, and general well-being (44–48). Recent work on the use of aquatic exercise in heart disease has shown significant benefit in both mild to moderate heart failure and general cardiac rehab (37,38,49–56). Clinical aquatic cardiac treatment programs are discussed extensively in a recent textbook chapter by Andrea Salzman, RPT (57). Severe congestive heart failure may still be a contraindication to aquatic exercise, however, and concerns should also be raised when the patient has bivalvular systolic failure (58,59). An algorithm for clinical decision-making in the use of aquatic therapy for rehabilitation of cardiac failure is found in **Figure 50-2** (60).

Pulmonary System Effects

The pulmonary system is profoundly affected by immersion of the body to the level of the thorax. Part of the effect is due to the shift of blood into the chest cavity, and part is due to compression of the chest wall itself by water. The combined effect is to alter pulmonary function, increase the work of breathing, and change respiratory dynamics (61).

Functional residual capacity reduces to about 54% of the normal value with immersion to the xiphoid (62). Most of this loss is due to reduction in expiratory reserve volume (ERV), which decreases by 75% at this level of immersion (22). The change in this volume may be readily experienced at poolside: while sitting on the edge of the pool, exhale normally, and then expel the rest of the reserve volume forcibly. Take a normal breath and then enter the water to neck level and perform the same experiment. The difference is very perceptible. Little air remains to exhale at the end point of relaxed exhalation. ERV is reduced to 11% of vital capacity, equal to breathing at a negative pressure of –20.5 cm H_2O (62,63). There is some loss of residual volume that decreases by 15% (62). Vital capacity decreases by about 6% to 9% when comparing neck submersion to controls submerged to the xiphoid (22,62). About 50% to 60% of this vital capacity reduction is due to increased thoracic blood volume, and 40% to 50% is due to hydrostatic forces counteracting the inspiratory musculature (22,62). Pressure on the rib cage shrinks the rib cage circumference by approximately 10% during submersion (22). Different immersion depths alter the effects upon the respiratory system, demonstrating hydrostatic pressure as the primary cause of

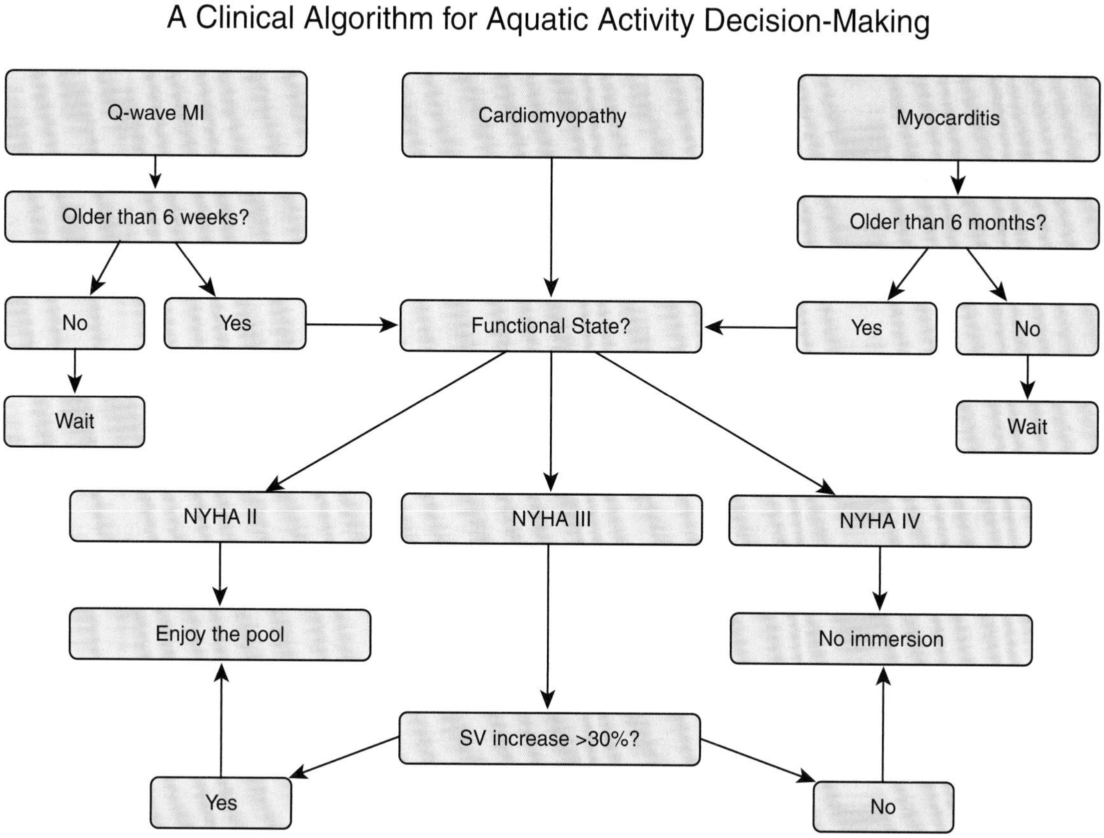

A Clinical Algorithm for Aquatic Activity Decision-Making

FIGURE 50-2. Aquatic activity algorithm for congestive heart failure. (Adapted with permission from Meyer K, Leblanc MC. Aquatic therapies in patients with compromised left ventricular function and heart failure. *Clin Invest Med.* 2008;31(2):E90–E97.)

these changes (61). The reduction in vital capacity does appear to fluctuate somewhat with temperature, with cooler water immersion (25°C) producing a greater reduction and warm-water immersion (40°C) a smaller reduction (64). **Figure 50-3** depicts the changes in pulmonary function during immersion.

The ability of the alveolar membrane to exchange gases is called diffusion capacity. Diffusion capacity of the lungs

is reduced slightly, as is partial pressure of oxygen (PO_2), as the lung beds become distended with blood shifted from the extremities and abdomen. Total intrapulmonary pressure shifts to the right by 16 cm H_2O (65). This causes airway resistance to the movement of air to increase by 58% or more, resulting from reduced lung volume (22). Expiratory flow rates are reduced, increasing the time to move air into and out of

FIGURE 50-3. Pulmonary effects schematic.

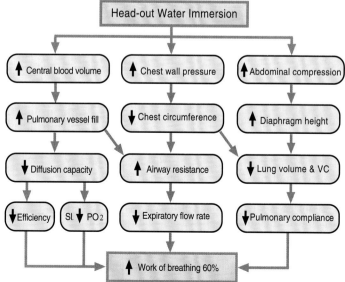

the lungs. Chest wall compliance is reduced as a result of the pressure of water on the chest wall, increasing pleural pressure from a -1 mm Hg to $+1$ mm Hg (66).

The combined effect of all these changes is to increase the total work of breathing. The total work of breathing for a tidal volume of 1 L increases by 60% during submersion to neck. Three quarters of this effort is attributable to an increase in elastic work (redistribution of blood from the thorax), and the rest is due to dynamic work (hydrostatic force on the thorax) (22,67,68). Because the preponderant force is blood flow return through pulmonary vasculature, this workload increase is defined by Poiseuille's equation in flow through a tube. An increase in the rate of breathing in turn produces a logarithmic increase in the work of breathing, as even with a constant vessel radius, the flow velocity is derivative of the fourth power of the radius.

Rehabilitation Applications

For an athlete accustomed to land-based conditioning exercises (see also Chapter 49), a program of water-based exercise results in a significant workload challenge to the respiratory apparatus. Because fluid dynamics enter into both the elastic workload component as well as the dynamic component of breathing effort, as respiratory rate increases, turbulence enters into the equation. Consequently, there is an exponential workload increase with more rapid breathing, as during high-level exercise with rapid respiratory rates. A 2016 Japanese study demonstrated that clavicle-depth immersion produced greater inspiratory muscle fatigue during inspiratory load breathing when compared to umbilicus and mid-chest depth immersion, supporting this concept (69). In the authors' experience, this challenge can raise the efficiency of the respiratory system and improve athletic performance if the time spent in water conditioning is sufficient to achieve respiratory musculature strength gains. When an athlete begins to experience respiratory fatigue, a cascade of physiologic changes follows. The production of metabolites, plus neurologic signaling through the sympathetic nervous system, sends a message to the peripheral arterial tree to shunt blood from the locomotor musculature through peripheral vasoconstriction (70–73). With a decline in perfusion of the muscles of locomotion, the rate of fatigue increases quite dramatically (72,74). Corroboration of this experience has been found in two studies done on elite cyclists following an inspiratory muscle-strengthening program (75,76). These studies found athletic performance improvement as well as measurable strength and endurance gains in respiratory function. Researchers investigating respiratory changes in competitive swimmers comparing the effects of inspiratory muscle specific training (IMT) in combination with routine swim training found no advantage to IMT in the combined training cohort compared to the sham IMT swim-trained cohort, suggesting that intense swim training achieves comparable benefits to IMT training (77–79). A series of studies on patients with emphysema found that a treatment program involving breathing out into water for 30 minutes/day, 5 days/week for 8 weeks, increased the FeV1 percentage of forced vital capacity, and PaO$_2$, and that clinical improvement followed these laboratory results (80–83). A 2013 Cochrane review of the literature on aquatic exercise in COPD found benefits in exercise capacity and quality of life for aquatic exercise–trained individuals when compared to controls and to land-based exercisers,

although no long-term effects had been studied at the time of that paper (84). Inspiratory muscle strengthening has also been shown to improve both ventilatory function and perceived difficulty of breathing in tetraplegia (85,86). Aquatic exercise has been used successfully in both young and old asthmatic patients (51,87–91).

In summary, the hydrostatic pressure of immersion can be used therapeutically to produce physiologic changes in the respiratory system useful in healthy competitive athletes as well as in clinical populations in need of rehabilitative efforts.

Musculoskeletal Effects

Joint Effects

As the body gradually immerses, water is displaced, creating a progressive off-loading of the immersed joints (**Figure 50-4**). With neck immersion, only about 15 pounds of compressive force (the approximate weight of the head) is exerted on the spine, hips, and knees. A person immersed to the symphysis pubis has effectively off-loaded 40% of body weight, and when further immersed to the umbilicus, approximately 50%. Xiphoid immersion produces 60% or more off-loading, depending on whether the arms are overhead or beside the trunk (92). A body suspended or floating in water essentially counterbalances the downward effects of gravity by the upward force of buoyancy. This effect may be of great therapeutic utility (93,94). For example, a fractured pelvis may not become mechanically stable under full-body loading for a period of many weeks, but with water immersion, gravitational forces may be partially or completely offset so that only muscle torque forces are present on the fracture site(s), allowing "active-assisted" range-of-motion activities, gentle strength building, and even gait training.

The effects of buoyancy and water resistance make possible high levels of energy expenditure with relatively little movement and strain on lower extremity joints (95). Off-loading occurs as a function of immersion, but the water depth chosen may be adjusted for the amount of loading desired.

Shallow-water vertical exercises generally approximate closed chain exercise, but with reduced joint loading because of the partial buoyancy counterforce. Deep-water exercises more generally approximate an open chain system, as do horizontal exercises such as swimming. Paddles and other resistive equipment tend to close the kinetic chain. Thus, the therapist can vary the amount of open versus closed chain joint loading by varying the activity and resistive equipment used.

The ground counteracts the force exerted against the floor by the walking body (see Chapter 4). This force is termed *ground reaction force* and may easily be measured through a force plate. It has been found to differ substantially during walking in chest-deep water. Force plate tracings of the pressure generated during a gait cycle on dry land compared with

Effective Loading Force

Neck depth = 10% Body Weight

Xiphoid depth = 20%

Waist depth = 50% Body Weight

Thigh depth = 75% Body Weight

FIGURE 50-4. Effective off-loading by buoyancy.

chest-deep water walking are substantially reduced in magnitude by more than 50% and are generated more slowly. Moreover, the forces are transmitted over a longer time interval during water walking (96). Clinically, this means that less joint compression is produced, and impact strain is diminished.

Water immersion causes significant effects on blood circulation through muscle tissue. These effects are caused by the compressive effects of immersion and by the increase in cardiac output as well as by the reflex regulation of blood vessel tone. During immersion, it is likely that much of the increased cardiac output is redistributed to skin and muscle rather than to the splanchnic beds (13). To resist blood pooling during dry land conditions, sympathetic vasoconstriction tightens the resistance vessels of skeletal muscle. Immersion pressure removes the biologic need for vasoconstriction, thus increasing muscle blood flow. Resting muscle blood flow has been found to be more than double during immersion to the neck, and with this increased perfusion, muscle tissue washout was found to increase 130% above dry land clearance (97,98). Thus, oxygen delivery is significantly increased during immersion, as is the removal of muscle metabolic waste products. Hydrostatic forces add an additional circulatory drive to remove edema, muscle lactate, and other metabolic end products.

Renal and Endocrine Effects

Because aquatic immersion produces central volume expansion in a pharmacologically and physiologically noninvasive manner, aquatic immersion serves as an excellent model for volume homeostasis. Aquatic immersion creates many effects on renal blood flow, on the renal regulatory systems, and on the endocrine systems. These effects have been studied extensively in both the American and international literatures. Murray Epstein, one of the most skilled and prolific early researchers in studying immersion effects on the human, published an exhaustive summary of these effects in 1992 (13). The flow of blood to the kidneys increases immediately on immersion. This causes an increase in creatinine clearance, a measure of renal efficiency, initially on immersion (13). Renal sympathetic nerve activity decreases because of the vagal response caused by left atrial distension, as discussed earlier in this chapter, and this decrease in sympathetic nerve activity increases renal tubular sodium transport (99). Calculated renal vascular resistance decreases by about one third (13). Renal venous pressure increases almost twofold (13). Sodium excretion increases tenfold in individuals with normal total-body sodium, and this sodium excretion is accompanied by free water, creating a major part of the diuretic effect of immersion. This increase in sodium excretion is a time-dependent phenomenon. Sodium excretion also increases as a function of depth, as a result of the shifting of circulating central blood volume (13). Potassium excretion also increases with immersion (34). The renal effects of immersion are shown in **Figure 50-5**.

Renal function is largely regulated by the hormones renin, aldosterone, and antidiuretic hormone (ADH), by the dopaminergic system, and by the atrial natriuretic peptide (ANP) system. All these hormones are greatly affected by immersion. Aldosterone controls Na^+ reabsorption in the distal renal tubule and accounts for most of the Na^+ loss with immersion (13). ADH release is significantly suppressed with immersion by 50% or more and is the other major contributor to diuresis. Another factor important in sodium regulation is ANP, which has both sodium excretion-facilitating and diuretic activity. ANP relaxes vascular smooth muscle and inhibits production

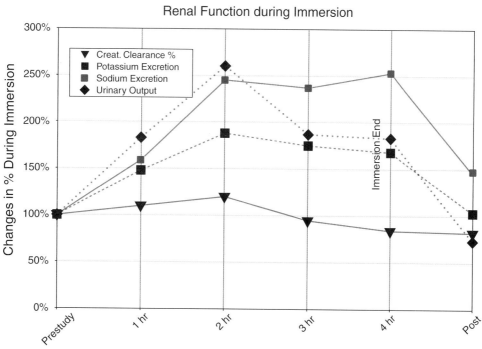

FIGURE 50-5. Renal function changes during immersion. (From Epstein M. Renal effects of head-out water immersion in humans: a 15-year update. *Physiol Rev.* 1992;72(3):563–621.)

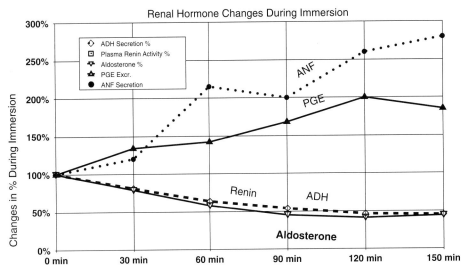

FIGURE 50-6. Renal hormone changes during immersion. (From Epstein M. Renal effects of head out immersion in humans: a 15-year update. *Physiol Rev.* 1992;72(3):563–621.)

of aldosterone. Immersion produces a prompt and continuing increase in ANP (34). Renal prostaglandin E secretion increases steadily through the first 2 hours of immersion and then decreases gently over the next 3 hours. Plasma renin activity is reduced by 33% to 50% at 2 hours of immersion to the neck (13) (**Fig. 50-6**). Overall, immersion-induced central volume expansion causes an increase in urinary output accompanied by significant sodium and potassium excretion, beginning almost immediately on immersion, steadily increasing over several hours of immersion. This may cause a decrease in blood pressure, and the resultant decrease may be sustained over a period of several to many hours. Immersion was historically one of the few effective ways of treating congestive heart failure noninvasively before the discovery of digitalis.

Accompanying the renal hormone effects are changes in the autonomic nervous system neurotransmitters, collectively called catecholamines, which act to regulate vascular resistance, cardiac rate, and force. The most important of these are epinephrine, norepinephrine, and dopamine. Catecholamine levels begin changing immediately on immersion (99,100) (**Fig. 50-7**).

REHABILITATIVE APPLICATIONS

Arthritis and Related Disorders

The value of the aquatic environment has a longer history in the management and scientific literature of arthritic diseases than in almost any other disease group. The losses that accompany chronic joint disease are many: loss of strength, loss of joint mobility and stability, and ultimately loss of functional capacity. It has been noted that rheumatoid patients as a group have lower than expected aerobic capacity and physical performance, with overall muscle strength 60% below that of age-matched control subjects. These deficits respond promptly to active rehabilitation, with well-tailored strengthening and endurance programs achieving gains in physical performance levels in as brief a time as 6 weeks (101). Long-term exercise regimens in rheumatoid patients over many years have been

well tolerated, with resultant improvement in functional and other outcome measures (102,103). A recent study of the cost-benefit in persons with osteoarthritis demonstrated that individuals enrolled in an Arthritis Foundation aquatics course significantly reduced perceived disability related to arthritis and improved perceived quality of life specific to physical health, although once all costs of participation were calculated, the program did not show dramatic cost-effectiveness over standard care (104). A number of recent systematic meta-analyses have demonstrated the value of aquatic exercise in reducing arthritis-related pain and other joint-related symptoms and increased physical functioning (105–107). With respect to knee and hip osteoarthritis specifically, a series of meta-analyses have shown short-term and medium-term benefits in managing pain, disability, and improving quality of life for individuals with functionally limiting symptoms (105,106,108–111). Recent work assessing MRI evidence on femoral cartilage has shown a reduction in T2 signaling following 16 weeks of aquatic resistance training, consistent with clinical findings over the study period (112).

Because patients with arthritis have been shown to have decreased endurance, these individuals should participate in some form of aerobic exercise to enhance their overall fitness. Studies have demonstrated the benefits of aerobic exercise for many conditions, including fibromyalgia pain (51,113–119), rheumatoid arthritis (51,102,103,120–124), lupus (125), and osteoarthritis (51,101,109,126–129). Low-impact exercise has been shown to be more efficacious than medications in the self-management of osteoarthritis (130). In a study of rheumatoid patients, Danneskiold-Samsoe et al. found markedly increased isometric and isokinetic muscle strength of the quadriceps after only moderate training in the pool. Other gains included an increase in aerobic capacity, freedom of movement, and a higher degree of independence in activities of daily living (121). Postural sway, a factor associated with fall risk, has been shown to decrease in patients undergoing a 6-week aquatic exercise intervention (101). Bunning et al. concluded that pool therapy was efficacious and achieved

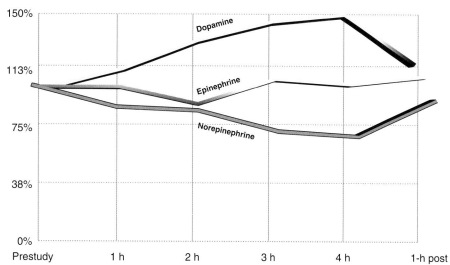

FIGURE 50-7. Sympathoadrenal hormone responses to immersion. (From Grossman E, Goldstein DS, Hoffman A, et al. Effects of water immersion on sympathoadrenal and dopa-dopamine systems in humans. *Am J Physiol.* 1992;262(6 Pt 2):R993–R999.)

high compliance for those with osteoarthritis and that aquatic exercise should be the cornerstone of active rehabilitation for severe arthritis (126). More recent studies have corroborated these results (51,101,102,106,108,109,113,115,116,121–123,127,131,132). The aquatic treadmill has been shown to produce quite specific gains in gait, knee angular velocities, and reductions in pain in individuals with knee osteoarthritis following aquatic treadmill training (133,134). Aquatic exercise has been shown to have benefit in individuals with ankylosing spondylitis, with improvements in pain, general health perceptions, general mental health (SF-36), and even social functioning (135).

Spine Rehabilitation

The spine is especially well protected during aquatic exercise programs, thus facilitating early rehabilitation (see Chapters 26 and 27). The combination of buoyancy off-loading of the spine combined with hydrostatic pressure on the abdomen and independent pain-reducing effects of immersion have been found to increase spinal height, with improved pain reduction when compared to land-based exercises (136–139). Accurate diagnosis of patients' spinal injuries and observation of their initial responses to land-based or aquatic stabilization programs helps determine further therapeutic exercise treatment. A transition from dry to wet exercise conditions minimizes certain dry land risks such as axial loading of the spine or falling onto a hard surface and limits the chance of rapid uncontrolled motion from occurring. It also establishes a supportive training environment due to reduction in axial loads, better control of spinal and peripheral joint motion and seems to improve the psychological framework in which spine pain patients function, providing a new therapeutic activity, decreasing the risk of peripheral joint injury, and allowing a return to prior activity. Moving from dry to wet environments also should be considered if patients cannot tolerate axial or gravitational loads, they require increased support in the presence of a

strength or proprioceptive deficit (140), or they are at risk of a compression fracture due to decreased bone density (141). Remaining in a water-supported environment is appropriate if a dry environment exacerbates symptoms or if patients prefer water. Transition from a wet to a dry environment should occur if patients are doing well in the water but must return to land to meet functional training needs efficiently and attain their ultimate competitive goals (142).

The aquatic rehabilitation programs that will be reviewed are based on dynamic lumbar, thoracic, and cervical stabilization techniques that have been previously described for land programs (143–146). Dynamic land-based stabilization training is also referred to as segmental or core stabilization exercise. This type of exercise program seeks to improve the neuromuscular control, strength, and endurance of muscles in the trunk, pelvic floor, thorax, and cervical spine, theoretically helping patients gain dynamic control of segmental spine forces, eliminate repetitive injury to motion segments (i.e., discs, zygapophyseal joints, and related structures), encourage healing of injured motion segments, and possibly alter the degenerative process. The underlying premise is that motion segments and supporting soft tissues react to minimize applied stresses and reduce risk of injury (143–145). There are, however, few prospective studies on patients with low back pain and less discussion of patient selection, dose-response, and long-term outcome with this type of rehabilitation construct, although aquatic exercise has been found to at least equal land-based exercise in most study metrics (138,146,147). The goals of aquatic stabilization exercise and swimming programs incorporate these elements but take into account the unique properties of water so that risk of spine injury is reduced. Aquatic stabilization programs help develop patients' flexibility, strength, and body mechanics so that a smooth transition to aquatic stabilization swimming programs or other spine-stabilized activities may occur. Such programs can help first-time swimmers or patients who previously swam (148–150).

Graded elimination of gravitational forces through buoyancy allows patients to train with decreased yet variable axial loads and shear forces. In essence, water increases the safety margin of patient postural error by decreasing the compressive and shear forces on the spine. Gravitational forces may be further attenuated by using aquatic traction techniques for lumbar, thoracic, and cervical spine dysfunction and pain (136,137,151,152). Velocity can be better controlled by water resistance, viscosity, buoyancy, and training devices. Buoyancy increases the range of training positions. The psychological outlook of athletes may be enhanced because rehabilitation occurs in their competitive environment. Many believe that pain attenuation takes place in the water because of the sensory overload generated by hydrostatic pressure, temperature, and turbulence (153).

Aquatic Spine Stabilization Techniques

Although the spine stabilization principles discussed for land programs also apply to aquatic programs, certain exercises that can be performed on land cannot be reproduced in water and vice versa. Aquatic programs can be designed for patients who cannot train on land or for those whose land training has reached a plateau. Richard Eagleston first described aquatic stabilization in 1989 (139).

Eight core aquatic stabilization exercises with four levels of difficulty have been developed to provide graded training of stabilization skills (139). **Figures 50-8 to 50-13** demonstrate progressive gravitational loading during spine stabilization exercises. Programs must be customized to meet the needs of each patient's unique spine pathology, related musculoskeletal dysfunctions, and comfort with the aquatic environment. Also, patients who have had joint replacements require particular

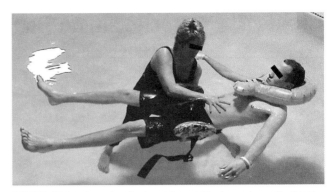

FIGURE 50-9. Assessing lumbopelvic mobility in supine with flotation devices.

care during positioning in the water because the replacements can change the center of buoyancy and may cause patients to sink due to high specific gravity (154). When a program is mastered, a more advanced program is provided. That said, there are numerous types of aquatic spine stabilization programs. All share at least one similar goal to enhance dynamic stabilization. The aquatic spine specialist must be aware of as many styles and types of aquatic stabilization programs as possible. They can then pick the most appropriate exercises from each program when creating an exercise regime that best meets their patient's needs.

Eventually, if a patient wants to incorporate a swimming program, a series of transitional aquatic stabilization exercises are initiated. These help to establish a spine-stabilized swimming style that minimizes the risk of further spine injury and helps maximize swimming performance (155).

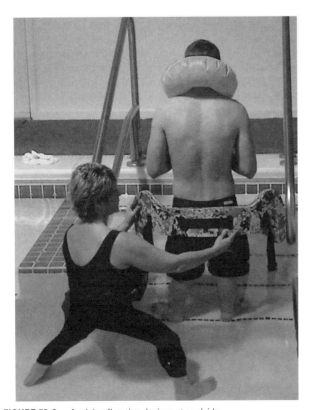

FIGURE 50-8. Applying flotation devices at poolside.

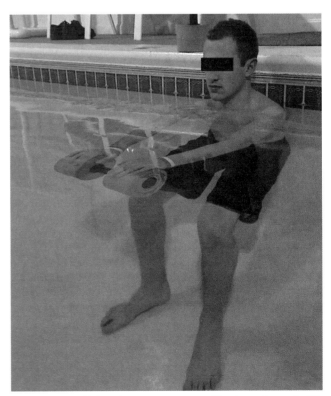

FIGURE 50-10. Maintaining core engagement with spine against wall while using foam barbells.

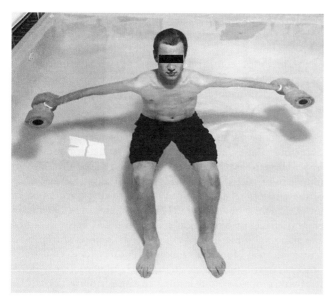

FIGURE 50-11. Progressing away from wall while maintaining core stability.

In summary, the aquatic environment provides numerous advantages to assist rehabilitation of patients with spine pain. A series of aquatic stabilization exercises has been designed that incorporates the intrinsic properties of water and enhance rehabilitative efforts. When these exercises are mastered, injured patients can soon advance to spine-safe swimming or other high-level aquatic training activities (156). Swimming programs, in particular, require that close attention be directed to proper swim-stroke biomechanics and to the effect that abnormal mechanics may have on the spine (157–159).

Neurologic Disorders

The advantages of the aquatic environment in the rehabilitation of neurologic disease have been noted for many centuries. Roosevelt's poliomyelitis rehabilitation at Warm Springs,

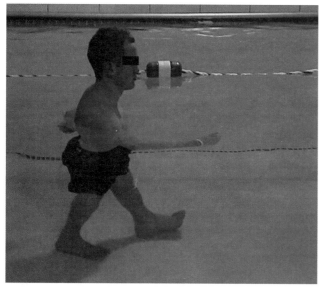

FIGURE 50-12. Beginning water walking in neutral spine position.

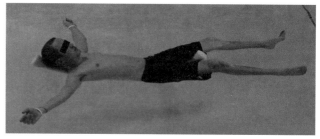

FIGURE 50-13. Supine flotation in neutral spine position using noodle for support is challenging.

Georgia, is common knowledge (6). The use of pool exercises for spinal cord injury rehabilitation is a mainstay at many rehabilitation centers, and Sir Ludwig Guttman built a central focus for aquatics in the Spinal Injury Unit at Stoke-Mandeville (see also Chapters 22 and 42). Throughout the United States, the Easter Seals organization has focused on the rehabilitation of children with cerebral palsy through pool-based programs. Programs have been designed for many neurologic diseases, and efficacy has been noted for multiple sclerosis (157–160), late poliomyelitis (161,162), and spinal cord injury (85,163,164). From a technical standpoint, there is little difference in the aquatic techniques used in neurologic rehabilitation, with some disease-specific exceptions (165,166).

Multiple Sclerosis

Patients with multiple sclerosis may benefit greatly from aquatic programs, in part because of the ability of water to prevent core temperature increase during exercise, but the pool temperature should be cool to start, below thermoneutral (see also Chapter 20). Studies have demonstrated improvements in gait speed, balance, timed up and go (TUG), reductions in pain, and improvements in fatigue scores 167–170. The authors have found ideal pool temperatures for patients with multiple sclerosis to be in the range of 25°C to 28°C (77°F to 82°F). There are literature reports of warmer temperatures being used with safety, but patient comfort should be an essential consideration (171).

Spinal Cord Injury

In contrast, spinal-injured patients lacking thermoregulatory capacity require much higher temperatures, in the range of 35°C to 37°C (95°F to 98°F). All neurologically impaired individuals obviously require close monitoring by poolside or in-water personnel. Patients with normal thermoregulatory ability and tolerance may be safely treated between 28°C and 35°C. Among the physiologic effects that aquatic exercise may produce are reduction in spasticity, improvement in strength particularly in incomplete SCI, and improvements in respiratory function for the reasons discussed earlier (164,172–176).

Parkinsonism

The combination of buoyancy in protecting from injurious falls during therapy plus recent research demonstrating improvements in cerebral blood flow make the aquatic environment particularly useful in treating individuals with parkinsonism (see also Chapter 21). Levels of exercise should seek to reach aerobic training levels to maximize benefits, but even programs such as Ai Chi, the aquatic version of Tai Chi, have shown gains in balance and postural stability, pain reduction, and gait speed (177–181).

Dementia and Stroke

Recent research has demonstrated an increase in cerebral blood flow during immersion and immersed exercise (182,183). These studies have potentially significant implications for individuals poststroke and with dementia. Improved cerebral blood flow and cerebral vasomotor reactivity has been demonstrated to correlate with improved cognition in stroke survivors (184,185). While research is still at case study–based publication in dementia, several remarkable reports have shown utility in improving mobility, cognitive function, and language in individuals with dementia using an aquatic therapy program (186–190). A therapeutic technique called Watsu, an aquatic adaptation of shiatsu massage, has shown some benefit in the management of spasticity in stroke (191).

Cerebral Palsy

The techniques developed at Bad Ragaz, Switzerland, and the methods developed by James McMillan, which have been called the Halliwick Method because of their initial development and use at the Halliwick School for Crippled Girls in England, have been used extensively in the management of cerebral palsy rehabilitation (see also Chapter 45). Their descriptions are beyond the limitations of this chapter, but these methods are described thoroughly elsewhere (192–194). Essentially, the techniques use the properties of buoyancy, warmth, and careful body positioning to achieve reduction in muscle tone. The patient is floated through the use of buoyant rings to support arms, legs, and head as clinically warranted. More active aquatic exercise programs have shown benefits in respiratory function, gross motor skills, and walking endurance with higher scores in physical activity enjoyment than in land-based exercise programs (195–200).

Pregnancy

Aquatic immersion during pregnancy has a lengthy history, but the benefits of aquatic exercise have only recently received scientific study (201). Aquatic exercise programs have been found to have a significant effect on preventing excessive maternal weight gain (202,203), gestational diabetes (202,204–207), positively impacting the quantity of the amniotic fluid seen on ultrasonography called the amniotic fluid index (AFI) (208,209), and reducing blood pressure during later stages of pregnancy (210). In addition, positive impacts have been found in improving sleep quality, reducing stress and increasing mental well-being, and reducing musculoskeletal complaints including low back pain (147,201,208,211). No studies have shown fetal risk from such programs, and some data exist showing increased fetal health following birth (212).

Sports Medicine

The aquatic environment has broad utility in sports medicine both for recovery from injury and rehabilitation as well as for cross-training using the properties of water for conditioning and protection from overuse injuries (93,213,214) (see Chapter 41). The aquatic environment has been used extensively throughout history, in both warm and cold temperatures as a result of the many physiologic effects of both the properties of water and the consequent physiologic changes brought about. Versey et al. have published an extensive review of the literature comparing effects of hot-water immersion, cold-water immersion, thermoneutral immersion, and contrast baths on performance following recovery from intense athletic activity (213).

In recent years, the use of chiller tanks has increased, particularly following intense exercise. Cold-water immersion in numerous studies has shown benefit in reducing muscle stiffness, delayed-onset muscle soreness, and some measures of muscle injury (213,215–219). It has been suggested that some of these effects relate to cold water producing a reduction in lower extremity blood flow (217). No significant difference in clinical effects or blood flow has been noted between seated and standing immersion (220). There are reports of improved return to play function following postexercise cold-water immersion with no suggestion that such immersion may interfere with proprioception leading to risk of injury (216,221). The ideal cold-water immersion temperatures and immersion times remain unresolved, although immersion temperatures in the 10°C to 15°C see most likely to assist recovery and 5 to 15 minutes duration as most tolerable (213).

The warm-water environment may be very useful for sedentary injury recovery but is not advisable for active exercise, as the increase in heart rate and core temperature gains produced during warm-water immersion preclude longer sessions of exercise (14). No currently published studies clearly demonstrate a role for hot-water immersion following exercise as a method of performance recovery in uninjured athletes (213). As a consequence, cross-training activities are better served by normal exercise pool temperatures. Contrast water immersion therapy has been shown in several studies to have a positive effect on postexercise recovery, although the literature has been inconsistent on immersion temperatures, cycle repetition times, and number of repetitions. The study most carefully assessing these variables used immersion in 38°C and 15°C cycling at 1 minute each for 6 to 12 minutes finding improved recovery from high-intensity running (222).

Both shallow water and deep water may be useful in these programs (223–228). Aquatic techniques for specific athletic injury rehabilitation have been comprehensively detailed elsewhere (229). Deep-water running may be successfully utilized even when weight bearing is contraindicated but also has been extensively studied as an effective means of cross-training (156,223,230,231). **Figures 50-14** and **50-15** depict commonly used devices for aquatic cross training using an underwater treadmill and a flotation device. In athletic training, the aquatic environment may provide a more protected opportunity for plyometric training, achieving comparable performance improvement with potential reduction in stress forces upon lower extremities (232–235).

Aquatic Therapy Precautions and Contraindications

Precautions require close supervision and assessment prior to initiation of aquatic therapy, as well as generally in-pool oversight. Contraindications generally preclude aquatic therapy as long as these conditions persist. If resolved, it is prudent to still view them as precautions (**Table 50-1**).

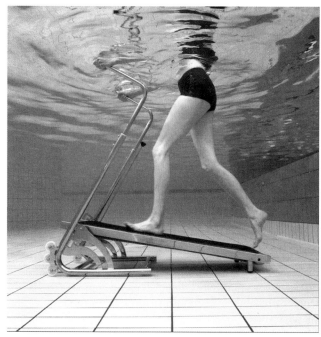

FIGURE 50-14. Underwater treadmill in use.

Health Facility Pools

Aquatic facilities located within health care facilities are generally warm-water pools, which usually cannot be adjusted for temperature, and are often shallow, rarely exceeding a depth of 4.5 ft. They are usually in-ground pools. They often offer ramp access or may use slings to gain access for disabled individuals. The pools are usually small, because of constraints imposed by expensive space and construction. Although warm water is more comfortable for low-level activities and acute rehabilitation, it is not ideal for patients with multiple sclerosis, and it makes high-level activities exhausting. Pool size limits high-level activities as well, and often group therapy must be done in small groups only. Staff is medically knowledgeable but often varies in aquatic skill. Facility-based pools are suitable for the acute rehabilitation of orthopedic populations, neurologic rehabilitation (with the exception of patients with multiple sclerosis), and arthritis rehabilitation. Common

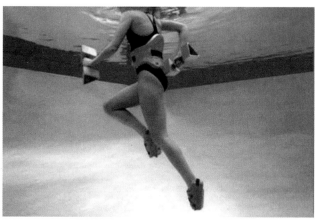

FIGURE 50-15. Foam waist belt and foot booties in deep-water use.

TABLE 50-1	Precautions and Contraindications
Precautions	**Contraindications**
Bowel incontinence—firm stool (manage with bowel program and plastic pants	Diarrhea, either active or within 4 days
Communicable disease (colds, flu, hepatitis)	Uncontrolled seizures
Autonomic dysreflexia	Unstable angina or cardiac arrhythmia
Sensitivity to halogens	Open wounds or bleeding
Abnormal heat tolerance (both warm or cold)	Tracheostomy prior to healing
Rashes, skin conditions	Serious active risk of aspiration
Severe orthostatic hypotension	Acute DVT without stable anticoagulation
Hydrophobia	Active fever >37°F
Combative or difficult populations	MRSA, VRSA
Ambulation dependency	
Controlled seizures	
Exercise-induced angina	
Open wounds with bio-occlusive dressings	
Immune system compromise	
On chemotherapy	
On dialysis	
Healed tracheostomy (must protect airway)	
History of aspiration	
Ostomy bags require occlusive dressings	
Skin at risk for maceration (diabetes, other)	
Severe respiratory compromise	

appropriate techniques include Bad Ragaz, Halliwick, aquatic spine stabilization, Red Cross arthritis, and low-level conditioning programs. Some health facilities also offer the Arthritis Foundation YMCA Aquatic Exercise Program, which has added adaptations for both deep-water and juvenile programs.

Community Pools

Community pools nearly always use cool water; vary in depth, often to 9 ft; usually offer stair or ladder access; and are in-ground designs. Varied depths make a wide range of programs possible, both horizontal and vertical, although the cool water precludes sedentary activities. Staff size is usually limited and without medical sophistication. These facilities are ideal for transitioning patients from the acute health facility pool, especially to group activities such as aquaerobics, low back classes, arthritis classes, or general conditioning. Because of access difficulty and cool water, they are often difficult for populations with severe physical limitations.

Hot Tubs and Spas

Hot tubs and spas usually feature hot water, are small and very shallow (rarely exceeding 3 ft in depth), and are most commonly above-ground designs. Most offer added turbulence through jets and temperature adjustability through a narrow range. Although the high temperature is useful for acute treatments, patients quickly elevate their core temperatures even when not exercising. Hot tubs and spas are suitable for acute joint rehabilitation and relaxation; movements are limited. Staff is varied in skill level but often does not have a therapy background.

Deep-Water Environments

Deep-water environments, including therapeutic tanks, may be deeper and cooler and facilitate suspended activities for avoidance of weight bearing. These environments are very adaptable, permitting even high-level conditioning, including aqua running, cross-country skiing, and ballet movements, if the temperature can be brought to an appropriate level. Tethering may be used to stabilize the immersed individual during exercise. Swimming skill is not required, although tank use usually requires flotation and always requires immediate supervision. Deep-water facilities are ideal for athletic rehabilitation, rehabilitation of early fractures when weight bearing is precluded, and high-level conditioning activities. Staff tends to come from an athletic training background.

Aquatic Techniques in Current Use

Treatment foundational techniques include Bad Ragaz (236,237), Halliwick (192), and Watsu (193,238,239). All these methods of aquatic therapy are techniques consisting of a developmental and progressive set of structured exercises. The first two are primarily intended for neurologic impairment, and the latter is an offshoot of shiatsu massage technique and was not originally developed for medical therapy, although more recently it has been found useful in the management of cerebral palsy (200,239). Many therapists will incorporate elements of each of these as well as other techniques into a program adapted to an individual patient.

Specialized Equipment

Flotation and Resistance Devices

A broad range of flotation devices have been developed for aquatic rehabilitation as seen in **Figures 50-8** and **50-9** for central trunk flotation. Neoprene vests and foam waist belts are the most commonly used. Bad Ragaz techniques use foam rings that are placed around arms and legs or under the head. Kick boards, leg floats, vinyl foam flexible buoys, and combinations of the preceding are all important pieces of the aquatic rehabilitation armamentarium if a broad base of patients is to be treated. **Figure 50-13** demonstrates a foam noodle in use for spine stabilization work. As strengthening proceeds, the natural resistance of the water may be augmented through devices to increase the surface area of the moving part. Finned dumbbells, finned boots, kick boards, and flotation devices all may be used to add resistance to movement.

Performance Measurement Tools

Water is a more challenging environment for the therapist wishing to quantify performance. Waterproof heart rate monitors and stop watches are useful, and as in the spine section, quantifying time, resistance, and movement freedom can add quantification (156,231).

SUMMARY

Aquatic use is growing, both publically and in medical rehabilitation. There may be no more broadly applicable therapeutic venue for the population in need of rehabilitation therapies than that of aquatics. It may be safely used in virtually all age groups, in both acute disease management as well as in chronic disabling conditions, and if used under supervision is virtually without side effects. That said, while many physiatrists and therapists today understand its potential benefits, there are too few aquatic facilities available and too few trained therapists with the skills and creativity to most fully realize this potential. In a time of scrutiny of health care expenditures, it becomes critical to find safe, inexpensive treatment modalities for common problems. We must find methods that are suitable for self-management regimens, ideally across a large variety of clinical concerns, and which may be easily learned and facilitate treatment adherence by the patient (240). The aquatic environment offers a significant step toward these goals. Aquatic therapy is a scientifically grounded, useful approach to a broad range of rehabilitative problems from acute to chronic, and patients usually find it helpful and pleasurable. Although specific aquatherapeutic approaches are plentiful, many problems lend themselves to creative aquatic-based solutions as well. Successful rehabilitation may occur with a high safety margin and at low cost, especially when community pools are used, and professional extender personnel may be used for group programs, further decreasing cost while increasing regimen adherence. With increasing understanding, knowledge of the scientific basis behind the value of immersion and immersed exercise, we should be hopeful for a better rehabilitative future for aquatic therapy.

REFERENCES

1. deVierville J. Aquatic rehabilitation: a historical perspective. In: Cole A, Becker B, eds. *Comprehensive Aquatic Rehabilitation*. 3rd ed. Pullman, WA: Washington State University Publishing; 2011:1–21.
2. Licht S, ed. *Medical Hydrology*. 1st ed. Baltimore, MD: Waverly; 1963. Licht E, ed. The Physical Medicine Library; No. 7.
3. Baruch S. *The Principles and Practice of Hydrotherapy. A Guide to the Application of Water in Disease for Students and Practitioners of Medicine*. 1st ed. London: Balliere, Tindall & Cox; 1900.
4. Baruch S. *An Epitome of Hydrotherapy for Physicians, Architects and Nurses. Illustrated*. 1st ed. Philadelphia, PA/London: W. B. Saunders Company; 1920.
5. Lowman CL. *Technique of Underwater Gymnastics: A Study in Practical Application*. 1st ed. Los Angeles, CA: American Publications; 1937.
6. Ditunno JF Jr, Becker BE, Herbison GJ. Franklin Delano Roosevelt: the diagnosis of poliomyelitis revisited. *PM R*. 2016;8(9):883–893.
7. Groedel F. *The Mineral Springs and Baths at Saratoga Springs*. Saratoga Springs, NY: Saratoga Springs Commission; 1932.
8. McClellan W. What is being done at New York State's great enterprise: Saratoga Springs. *J Am Med Hydrol*. 1932;1(27):30.
9. *Minutes of Working Committee*. French Lick, IN: The American Society of Medical Hydrology; December 4, 1931.
10. Coulter J. *Physical Therapy*. Vol 7. New York: P. B. Hoebner, Inc.; 1932.
11. Smith E. Hydrotherapy in arthritis: underwater therapy applied to chronic atrophic arthritis. Paper presented at: 14th Annual Session of the American Congress of Physical Therapy; September 11, 1935; Kansas City, MO.
12. Epstein M. Cardiovascular and renal effects of head-out water immersion in man: application of the model in the assessment of volume homeostasis. *Circ Res*. 1976;39(5):619–628.
13. Epstein M. Renal effects of head-out water immersion in humans: a 15-year update. *Physiol Rev*. 1992;72(3):563–621.
14. Becker BE. Aquatic therapy: scientific foundations and clinical rehabilitation applications. *PM R*. 2009;1(9):859–872.
15. Bloomfield J, Fricker PA, Fitch K. *Textbook of Science and Medicine in Sport*. Champaign, IL: Human Kinetics Books; 1992.
16. Duggar BC. The center of gravity of the human body. *Hum Factors*. 1962;4:131–148.

17. Arborelius M Jr, Balldin UI, Lilja B, et al. Hemodynamic changes in man during immersion with the head above water. *Aerosp Med.* 1972;43(6):592–598.

18. Risch WD, Koubenec HJ, Beckmann U, et al. The effect of graded immersion on heart volume, central venous pressure, pulmonary blood distribution, and heart rate in man. *Pflugers Arch.* 1978;374(2):115–118.

19. Weston CF, O'Hare JP, Evans JM, et al. Haemodynamic changes in man during immersion in water at different temperatures. *Clin Sci.* 1987;73(6):613–616.

20. Schlant RC, Sonnenblick E. Normal physiology of the cardiovascular system. In: Hurst J, ed. *The Heart.* 6th ed. New York: McGraw-Hill; 1986:51.

21. Dressendorfer RH, Morlock JF, Baker DG, et al. Effects of head-out water immersion on cardiorespiratory responses to maximal cycling exercise. *Undersea Biomed Res.* 1976;3(3):177–187.

22. Hong SK, Cerretelli P, Cruz JC, et al. Mechanics of respiration during submersion in water. *J Appl Physiol.* 1969;27(4):535–538.

23. Gabrielsen A, Johansen LB, Norsk P. Central cardiovascular pressures during graded water immersion in humans. *J Appl Physiol.* 1993;75(2):581–585.

24. Park KS, Choi JK, Park YS. Cardiovascular regulation during water immersion. *Appl Human Sci.* 1999;18(6):233–241.

25. Craig AB Jr, Dvorak M. Thermal regulation during water immersion. *J Appl Physiol.* 1966;21(5):1577–1585.

26. Becker BE, Hildenbrand K, Whitcomb RK, et al. Biophysiologic effects of warm water immersion. *Int J Aquatic Res Educ.* 2009;3(1):24–37.

27. Hildenbrand K, Becker B, Whitcomb R, et al. Age-dependent autonomic changes following immersion in cool, neutral, and warm water temperatures. *Int J Aquatic Res Educ.* 2010;4 (2):127–146.

28. Itoh M, Fukuoka Y, Kojima S, et al. Comparison of cardiovascular autonomic responses in elderly and young males during head-out water immersion. *J Cardiol.* 2007;49(5):241–250.

29. McArdle WD, Katch F, Katch VL. Functional capacity of the cardiovascular system. *Exercise Physiology.* 3rd ed. Malvern, PA: Lea & Febiger; 1991:330–331.

30. McArdle WD, Katch F, Katch VL. *Exercise Physiology, Nutrition and Human Performance.* 3rd ed. Malvern, PA: Lea & Febiger; 1991.

31. Tajima F, Sagawa S, Claybaugh JR, et al. Renal, endocrine, and cardiovascular responses during head-out water immersion in legless men. *Aviat Space Environ Med.* 1999;70(5):465–470.

32. Gehring MM, Keller BA, Brehm BA. Water running with and without a flotation vest in competitive and recreational runners. *Med Sci Sports Exerc.* 1997;29(10):1374–1378.

33. Gleim GW, Nicholas JA. Metabolic costs and heart rate responses to treadmill walking in water at different depths and temperatures. *Am J Sports Med.* 1989;17(2):248–252.

34. Epstein M, Lifschitz MD, Hoffman DS, et al. Relationship between renal prostaglandin E and renal sodium handling during water immersion in normal man. *Circ Res.* 1979;45(1):71–80.

35. Coruzzi P, Biggi A, Musiari L, et al. Renin-aldosterone system suppression during water immersion in renovascular hypertension. *Clin Sci (Colch).* 1985;68(5):609–612.

36. Coruzzi P, Musiari L, Mossini GL, et al. Water immersion and salt-sensitivity in essential hypertension. *Scand J Clin Lab Invest.* 1993;53(6):593–599.

37. Lazar JM, Khanna N, Chesler R, et al. Swimming and the heart. *Int J Cardiol.* 2013;168(1):19–26.

38. Schmid JP, Noveanu M, Morger C, et al. Influence of water immersion, water gymnastics and swimming on cardiac output in patients with heart failure. *Heart.* 2007;93(6):722–727.

39. Schega L, Claus G, Almeling M, et al. Cardiovascular responses during thermoneutral, head-out water immersion in patients with coronary artery disease. *J Cardiopulm Rehabil Prev.* 2007;27(2):76–80.

40. Ward EJ, McIntyre A, van Kessel G, et al. Immediate blood pressure changes and aquatic physiotherapy. *Hypertens Pregnancy.* 2005;24(2):93–102.

41. Shin TW, Wilson M, Wilson TW. Are hot tubs safe for people with treated hypertension? *CMAJ.* 2003;169(12):1265–1268.

42. McMurray RG, Fieselman C, Avery KE, et al. Exercise hemodynamics in water and on land in patients with coronary artery disease. *Cardiopulm Rehabil.* 1988;8:69.

43. Bucking J, Krey S. [Swimming after myocardial infarct. Oxygen saturation, pulmonary arterial and capillary pressure in underwater immersion and during swimming after myocardial infarct]. *Dtsch Med Wochenschr.* 1986;111(48):1838–1841.

44. Tei C, Horikiri Y, Park JC, et al. [Effects of hot water bath or sauna on patients with congestive heart failure: acute hemodynamic improvement by thermal vasodilation]. *J Cardiol.* 1994;24(3):175–183.

45. Tei C, Horikiri Y, Park JC, et al. Acute hemodynamic improvement by thermal vasodilation in congestive heart failure. *Circulation.* 1995;91(10):2582–2590.

46. Tei C, Tanaka N. [Treatment of chronic congestive heart failure to improve their quality of life—clinical study of thermal vasodilation therapy]. *Nippon Naika Gakkai Zasshi.* 1995;84(9):1475–1482.

47. Tei C, Tanaka N. Thermal vasodilation as a treatment of congestive heart failure: a novel approach. *J Cardiol.* 1996;27(1):29–30.

48. Tei C, Tanaka N. Comprehensive therapy for congestive heart failure: a novel approach incorporating thermal vasodilation. *Intern Med.* 1996;35(1):67–69.

49. Cider A, Svealv BG, Tang MS, et al. Immersion in warm water induces improvement in cardiac function in patients with chronic heart failure. *Eur J Heart Fail.* 2006;8(3):308–313.

50. Cider A, Carlsson S, Arvidsson C, et al. Reliability of clinical muscular endurance tests in patients with chronic heart failure. *Eur J Cardiovasc Nurs.* 2006;5(2):122–126.

51. Pedersen BK, Saltin B. Evidence for prescribing exercise as therapy in chronic disease. *Scand J Med Sci Sports.* 2006;16(suppl 1):3–63.

52. Gruner Svealv B, Cider A, Tang MS, et al. Benefit of warm water immersion on biventricular function in patients with chronic heart failure. *Cardiovasc Ultrasound.* 2009;7:33.

53. Mussivand T, Alshaer H, Haddad H, et al. Thermal therapy: a viable adjunct in the treatment of heart failure? *Congest Heart Fail.* 2008;14(4):180–186.

54. Choi JH, Kim BR, Joo SJ, et al. Comparison of cardiorespiratory responses during aquatic and land treadmill exercise in patients with coronary artery disease. *J Cardiopulm Rehabil Prev.* 2015;35(2):140–146.

55. Teffaha D, Mourot L, Vernochet P, et al. Relevance of water gymnastics in rehabilitation programs in patients with chronic heart failure or coronary artery disease with normal left ventricular function. *J Card Fail.* 2011;17(8):676–683.

56. Mourot L, Teffaha D, Bouhaddi M, et al. Exercise rehabilitation restores physiological cardiovascular responses to short-term head-out water immersion in patients with chronic heart failure. *J Cardiopulm Rehabil Prev.* 2010;30(1):22–27.

57. Salzman A. Aftercare and wellness group programming. In: Becker B, Cole A, eds. *Comprehensive Aquatic Therapy.* 3rd ed. Pullman, WA: Washington State University Publishing; 2011:385–406.

58. Meyer K. Left ventricular dysfunction and chronic heart failure: should aqua therapy and swimming be allowed? *Br J Sports Med.* 2006;40(10):817–818.

59. Svealv BG, Tang MS, Cider A. Is hydrotherapy an appropriate form of exercise for elderly patients with biventricular systolic heart failure? *J Geriatr Cardiol.* 2012;9(4):408–410.

60. Meyer K, Leblanc MC. Aquatic therapies in patients with compromised left ventricular function and heart failure. *Clin Invest Med.* 2008;31(2):E90–E97.

61. de Andrade AD, Junior JC, Lins de Barros Melo TL, et al. Influence of different levels of immersion in water on the pulmonary function and respiratory muscle pressure in healthy individuals: observational study. *Physiother Res Int.* 2014;19(3):140–146.

62. Agostoni E, Gurtner G, Torri G, et al. Respiratory mechanics during submersion and negative-pressure breathing. *J Appl Physiol.* 1966;21(1):251–258.

63. Taylor NA, Morrison JB. Static respiratory muscle work during immersion with positive and negative respiratory loading. *J Appl Physiol.* 1999;87(4):1397–1403.

64. Choukroun ML, Varene P. Adjustments in oxygen transport during head-out immersion in water at different temperatures. *J Appl Physiol.* 1990;68(4):1475–1480.

65. Derion T, Guy HJ, Tsukimoto K, et al. Ventilation-perfusion relationships in the lung during head-out water immersion. *J Appl Physiol.* 1992;72(1):64–72.

66. Arborelius M Jr, Balldin UI, Lila B, et al. Regional lung function in man during immersion with the head above water. *Aerosp Med.* 1972;43(7):701–707.

67. Taylor NA, Morrison JB. Static and dynamic pulmonary compliance during upright immersion. *Acta Physiol Scand.* 1993;149(4):413–417.

68. Morrison JB, Taylor NA. Measurement of static and dynamic pulmonary work during pressure breathing. *Undersea Biomed Res.* 1990;17(5):453–467.

69. Yamashina Y, Yokoyama H, Naghavi N, et al. Forced respiration during the deeper water immersion causes the greater inspiratory muscle fatigue in healthy young men. *J Phys Ther Sci.* 2016;28(2):412–418.

70. Dempsey JA, Amann M, Romer LM, et al. Respiratory system determinants of peripheral fatigue and endurance performance. *Med Sci Sports Exerc.* 2008;40(3):457–461.

71. Dempsey JA, Sheel AW, St Croix CM, et al. Respiratory influences on sympathetic vasomotor outflow in humans. *Respir Physiol Neurobiol.* 2002;130(1):3–20.

72. Sheel AW, Derchak PA, Morgan BJ, et al. Fatiguing inspiratory muscle work causes reflex reduction in resting leg blood flow in humans. *J Physiol.* 2001;537(Pt 1):277–289.

73. Sheel AW. Respiratory muscle training in healthy individuals: physiological rationale and implications for exercise performance. *Sports Med.* 2002;32(9):567–581.

74. Dempsey JA, Miller JD, Romer L, et al. Exercise-induced respiratory muscle work: effects on blood flow, fatigue and performance. *Adv Exp Med Biol.* 2008;605:209–212.

75. Romer LM, McConnell AK, Jones DA. Effects of inspiratory muscle training upon recovery time during high intensity, repetitive sprint activity. *Int J Sports Med.* 2002;23(5):353–360.

76. Romer LM, McConnell AK, Jones DA. Inspiratory muscle fatigue in trained cyclists: effects of inspiratory muscle training. *Med Sci Sports Exerc.* 2002;34(5):785–792.

77. Clanton TL, Dixon GF, Drake J, et al. Effects of swim training on lung volumes and inspiratory muscle conditioning. *J Appl Physiol.* 1987;62(1):39–46.

78. Mickleborough TD, Stager JM, Chatham K, et al. Pulmonary adaptations to swim and inspiratory muscle training. *Eur J Appl Physiol.* 2008;103(6):635–646.

79. Wells GD, Plyley M, Thomas S, et al. Effects of concurrent inspiratory and expiratory muscle training on respiratory and exercise performance in competitive swimmers. *Eur J Appl Physiol.* 2005;94(5–6):527–540.

80. Kurabayashi H, Kubota K, Machida I, et al. Effective physical therapy for chronic obstructive pulmonary disease. Pilot study of exercise in hot spring water. *Am J Phys Med Rehabil.* 1997;76(3):204–207.

81. Kurabayashi H, Machida I, Handa H, et al. Comparison of three protocols for breathing exercises during immersion in 38 degrees C water for chronic obstructive pulmonary disease. *Am J Phys Med Rehabil.* 1998;77(2):145–148.

82. Kurabayashi H, Machida I, Tamura K, et al. Breathing out into water during subtotal immersion: a therapy for chronic pulmonary emphysema. *Am J Phys Med Rehabil.* 2000;79(2):150–153.

83. Kurabayashi H, Machida I, Yoshida Y, et al. Clinical analysis of breathing exercise during immersion in 38 degrees C water for obstructive and constrictive pulmonary diseases. *J Med.* 1999;30(1–2):61–66.

84. McNamara RJ, McKeough ZJ, McKenzie DK, et al. Water-based exercise training for chronic obstructive pulmonary disease. *Cochrane Database Syst Rev.* 2013;(12):CD008290.

85. Liaw MY, Lin MC, Cheng PT, et al. Resistive inspiratory muscle training: its effectiveness in patients with acute complete cervical cord injury. *Arch Phys Med Rehabil.* 2000;81(6):752–756.

86. Pachalski A, Mekarski T. Effect of swimming on increasing of cardio-respiratory capacity in paraplegics. *Paraplegia.* 1980;18(3):190–196.

87. Ram FS, Wellington SR, Barnes NC. Inspiratory muscle training for asthma. *Cochrane Database Syst Rev.* 2003;(4):CD003792.

88. Rosimini C. Benefits of swim training for children and adolescents with asthma. *J Am Acad Nurse Pract.* 2003;15(6):247–252.

89. Weisgerber MC, Guill M, Weisgerber JM, et al. Benefits of swimming in asthma: effect of a session of swimming lessons on symptoms and PFTs with review of the literature. *J Asthma.* 2003;40(5):453–464.

90. Wicher IB, Ribeiro MA, Marmo DB, et al. Effects of swimming on spirometric parameters and bronchial hyperresponsiveness in children and adolescents with moderate persistent atopic asthma. *J Pediatr (Rio J).* 2010;86(5):384–390.

91. Wang JS, Hung WP. The effects of a swimming intervention for children with asthma. *Respirology.* 2009;14(6):838–842.

92. Harrison RA, Hillman M, Bulstrode S. Loading of the lower limb when walking partially immersed. *Physiotherapy.* 1992;78:165.

93. Torres-Ronda L, Del Alcazar XS. The properties of water and their applications for training. *J Hum Kinet.* 2014;44:237–248.

94. Aquatic physical therapy: running in water decreases stress on the body. *J Orthop Sports Phys Ther.* 2012;42(5):445.

95. Severin A, Burkett B, McKean M, et al. Biomechanical aspects of aquatic therapy: a literature review on application and methodological challenges. *J Fit Res.* 2016;5(1):48–62.

96. Nakazawa K, Yano H, Miyashita M. Ground reaction forces during walking in water. In: Mutoh Y, Miyashita M, Richardson AB, eds. *Medicine and Science in Aquatic Sports.* Vol 39. Basel: Karger AG; 1994:28.

97. Balldin UI, Lundgren CE. Effects of immersion with the head above water on tissue nitrogen elimination in man. *Aerosp Med.* 1972;43(10):1101–1108.

98. Balldin UI, Lundgren CE, Lundvall J, et al. Changes in the elimination of 133 xenon from the anterior tibial muscle in man induced by immersion in water and by shifts in body position. *Aerosp Med.* 1971;42(5):489–493.

99. Grossman E, Goldstein DS, Hoffman A, et al. Effects of water immersion on sympathoadrenal and dopa-dopamine systems in humans. *Am J Physiol.* 1992;262 (6 Pt 2):R993–R999.

100. Krishna GG, Danovitch GM, Sowers JR. Catecholamine responses to central volume expansion produced by head-out water immersion and saline infusion. *J Clin Endocrinol Metab.* 1983;56(5):998–1002.

101. Suomi R, Collier D. Effects of arthritis exercise programs on functional fitness and perceived activities of daily living measures in older adults with arthritis. *Arch Phys Med Rehabil.* 2003;84(11):1589–1594.

102. Stenstrom CH, Lindell B, Swanberg E, et al. Intensive dynamic training in water for rheumatoid arthritis functional class II—a long-term study of effects. *Scand J Rheumatol.* 1991;20(5):358–365.

103. Stenstrom CH. *Dynamic Therapeutic Exercise in Rheumatoid Arthritis* [Doctoral]. Stockholm: Rehabilitation and Physical Medicine, Karolinska Institutet; 1993.

104. Patrick DL, Ramsey SD, Spencer AC, et al. Economic evaluation of aquatic exercise for persons with osteoarthritis. *Med Care.* 2001;39(5):413–424.

105. Lu M, Su Y, Zhang Y, et al. Effectiveness of aquatic exercise for treatment of knee osteoarthritis: systematic review and meta-analysis. *Z Rheumatol.* 2015;74(6): 543–552.

106. Waller B, Ogonowska-Slodownik A, Vitor M, et al. Effect of therapeutic aquatic exercise on symptoms and function associated with lower limb osteoarthritis: a systematic review with meta-analysis. *Phys Ther.* 2014;94(10):1383–1395.

107. Al-Qubaeissy KY, Fatoye FA, Goodwin PC, et al. The effectiveness of hydrotherapy in the management of rheumatoid arthritis: a systematic review. *Musculoskeletal Care.* 2013;11(1):3–18.

108. Bartels EM, Juhl CB, Christensen R, et al. Aquatic exercise for the treatment of knee and hip osteoarthritis. *Cochrane Database Syst Rev.* 2016;3:CD005523.

109. Bartels EM, Lund H, Hagen KB, et al. Aquatic exercise for the treatment of knee and hip osteoarthritis. *Cochrane Database Syst Rev.* 2007;(4):CD005523.

110. Dannaway J, New CC, New CH, et al. Aquatic exercise for osteoarthritis of the knee or hip (PEDro synthesis). *Br J Sports Med.* 2017;51(16):1233–1234.

111. Gibson AJ, Shields N. Effects of aquatic therapy and land-based therapy versus land-based therapy alone on range of motion, edema, and function after hip or knee replacement: a systematic review and meta-analysis. *Physiother Can.* 2015;67(2): 133–141.

112. Waller B, Ogonowska-Slodownik A, Vitor M, et al. The effect of aquatic exercise on physical functioning in the older adult: a systematic review with meta-analysis. *Age Ageing.* 2016;45(5):593–601.

113. Assis MR, Silva LE, Alves AM, et al. A randomized controlled trial of deep water running: clinical effectiveness of aquatic exercise to treat fibromyalgia. *Arthritis Rheum.* 2006;55(1):57–65.

114. Busch A, Schachter CL, Peloso PM, et al. Exercise for treating fibromyalgia syndrome. *Cochrane Database Syst Rev.* 2002;(3):CD003786.

115. Gowans SE, deHueck A. Pool exercise for individuals with fibromyalgia. *Curr Opin Rheumatol.* 2007;19(2):168–173.

116. Gusi N, Tomas-Carus P, Hakkinen A, Hakkinen K, Ortega-Alonso A. Exercise in waist-high warm water decreases pain and improves health-related quality of life

117. Jentoft ES, Kvalvik AG, Mengshoel AM. Effects of pool-based and land-based aerobic exercise on women with fibromyalgia/chronic widespread muscle pain. *Arthritis Rheum.* 2001;45(1):42–47.

118. McCain GA. Role of physical fitness training in the fibrositis/fibromyalgia syndrome. *Am J Med.* 1986;81(3A):73–77.

119. Tomas-Carus P, Hakkinen A, Gusi N, et al. Aquatic training and detraining on fitness and quality of life in fibromyalgia. *Med Sci Sports Exerc.* 2007;39(7):1044–1050.

120. Bacon MC, Nicholson C, Binder H, et al. Juvenile rheumatoid arthritis. Aquatic exercise and lower-extremity function. *Arthritis Care Res.* 1991;4(2):102–105.

121. Danneskiold-Samsoe B, Lyngberg K, Risum T, et al. The effect of water exercise therapy given to patients with rheumatoid arthritis. *Scand J Rehabil Med.* 1987;19(1):31–35.

122. Hall J, Grant J, Blake D, et al. Cardiorespiratory responses to aquatic treadmill walking in patients with rheumatoid arthritis. *Physiother Res Int.* 2004;9(2):59–73.

123. Hall J, Skevington SM, Maddison PJ, et al. A randomized and controlled trial of hydrotherapy in rheumatoid arthritis. *Arthritis Care Res.* 1996;9(3):206–215.

124. Takken T, Van Der Net J, Kuis W, et al. Aquatic fitness training for children with juvenile idiopathic arthritis. *Rheumatology (Oxford).* 2003;42(11):1408–1414.

125. Robb-Nicholson LC, Daltroy L, Eaton H, et al. Effects of aerobic conditioning in lupus fatigue: a pilot study. *Br J Rheumatol.* 1989;28(6):500–505.

126. Bunning RD, Materson RS. A rational program of exercise for patients with osteoarthritis. *Semin Arthritis Rheum.* 1991;21(3 suppl 2):33–43.

127. Hinman RS, Heywood SE, Day AR. Aquatic physical therapy for hip and knee osteoarthritis: results of a single-blind randomized controlled trial. *Phys Ther.* 2007;87(1):32–43.

128. Wang TJ, Belza B, Elaine Thompson F, et al. Effects of aquatic exercise on flexibility, strength and aerobic fitness in adults with osteoarthritis of the hip or knee. *J Adv Nurs.* 2007;57(2):141–152.

129. Wyatt FB, Milam S, Manske RC, et al. The effects of aquatic and traditional exercise programs on persons with knee osteoarthritis. *J Strength Cond Res.* 2001;15(3):337–340.

130. Hampson SE, Glasgow RE, Zeiss AM, et al. Self-management of osteoarthritis. *Arthritis Care Res.* 1993;6(1):17–22.

131. Suomi R, Lindauer S. Effectiveness of arthritis foundation aquatic program on strength and range of motion in women with arthritis. *J Aging Phys Act.* 1997;5:341–351.

132. Mattos F, Leite N, Pitta A, et al. Effects of aquatic exercise on muscle strength and functional performance of individuals with osteoarthritis: a systematic review. *Rev Bras Reumatol Engl Ed.* 2016;56(6):530–542.

133. Roper JA, Bressel E, Tillman MD. Acute aquatic treadmill exercise improves gait and pain in people with knee osteoarthritis. *Arch Phys Med Rehabil.* 2013;94(3):419–425.

134. Bressel E, Wing JE, Miller AI, et al. High-intensity interval training on an aquatic treadmill in adults with osteoarthritis: effect on pain, balance, function, and mobility. *J Strength Cond Res.* 2014;28(8):2088–2096.

135. Dundar U, Solak O, Toktas H, et al. Effect of aquatic exercise on ankylosing spondylitis: a randomized controlled trial. *Rheumatol Int.* 2014;34(11):1505–1511.

136. Simmerman SM, Sizer PS, Dedrick GS, et al. Immediate changes in spinal height and pain after aquatic vertical traction in patients with persistent low back symptoms: a crossover clinical trial. *PM R.* 2011;3(5):447–457.

137. Kurutz M, Bender T. Weightbath hydrotraction treatment: application, biomechanics, and clinical effects. *J Multidiscip Healthc.* 2010;3:19–27.

138. Dundar U, Solak O, Yigit I, et al. Clinical effectiveness of aquatic exercise to treat chronic low back pain: a randomized controlled trial. *Spine (Phila Pa 1976).* 2009;34(14):1436–1440.

139. Cole AJ, Johnson J, Alford J, et al. Spine pain: aquatic rehabilitation strategies. In: Becker B, Cole A, eds. *Comprehensive Aquatic Therapy.* 3rd ed. Pullman, WA: Washington State University Publishing; 2011:219–244.

140. Minor MA, Hewett JE, Webel RR, et al. Efficacy of physical conditioning exercise in patients with rheumatoid arthritis and osteoarthritis. *Arthritis Rheum.* 1989;32(11):1396–1405.

141. Bravo G, Gauthier P, Roy PM, et al. A weight-bearing, water-based exercise program for osteopenic women: its impact on bone, functional fitness, and well-being. *Arch Phys Med Rehabil.* 1997;78(12):1375–1380.

142. LeFort SM, Hannah TE. Return to work following an aquafitness and muscle strengthening program for the low back injured. *Arch Phys Med Rehabil.* 1994;75(11):1247–1255.

143. Keane GP, Saal JA. The sports medicine approach to occupational low back pain. *West J Med.* 1991;154(5):525–527.

144. Saal JA. Dynamic muscular stabilization in the nonoperative treatment of lumbar pain syndromes. *Orthop Rev.* 1990;19(8):691–700.

145. Saal JA. The new back school prescription: stabilization training. Part II. *Occup Med.* 1992;7(1):33–42.

146. Standaert CJ, Herring SA. Expert opinion and controversies in musculoskeletal and sports medicine: core stabilization as a treatment for low back pain. *Arch Phys Med Rehabil.* 2007;88(12):1734–1736.

147. Waller B, Lambeck J, Daly D. Therapeutic aquatic exercise in the treatment of low back pain: a systematic review. *Clin Rehabil.* 2009;23(1):3–14.

148. Cole A. Getting backs in the swim. *Rehabil Mgmt.* 1992;5(62):71.

149. Cole A, Frederickson M, Johnson J, et al. Spine pain: aquatic rehabilitation strategies. In: Cole C, Becker B, eds. *Comprehensive Aquatic Therapy.* 2nd ed. Philadelphia, PA: Butterworth Heinemann; 2004:177–206.

150. Cole AJ, Moschetti M, Eagleston RA, et al. Spine pain: aquatic rehabilitation strategies. In: Becker BE, Cole AJ, ed. *Comprehensive Aquatic Therapy*. 1st ed. Boston, MA: Butterworth-Heinemann; 1997:73–101.

151. Kurutz M, Oroszvary L. Finite element analysis of weightbath hydrotraction treatment of degenerated lumbar spine segments in elastic phase. *J Biomech*. 2010;43(3):433–441.

152. Olah M, Molnar L, Dobai J, et al. The effects of weightbath traction hydrotherapy as a component of complex physical therapy in disorders of the cervical and lumbar spine: a controlled pilot study with follow-up. *Rheumatol Int*. 2008;28(8):749–756.

153. Constant F, Collin JF, Guillemin F, et al. Effectiveness of spa therapy in chronic low back pain: a randomized clinical trial. *J Rheumatol*. 1995;22(7):1315–1320.

154. Brewster NT, Howie CR. That sinking feeling. *BMJ*. 1992;305(6868):1579–1580.

155. Cole AJ, Moschetti ML, Eagleston RA. Swimming. In: White AH, ed. *Spine Care*. St. Louis, MO: CV Mosby; 1995:727–745.

156. Wilder RP, Brennan DK. Physiological responses to deep water running in athletes. *Sports Med*. 1993;16(6):374–380.

157. Gehlsen G, Beekman K, Assmann N, et al. Gait characteristics in multiple sclerosis: progressive changes and effects of exercise on parameters. *Arch Phys Med Rehabil*. 1986;67(8):536–539.

158. Gehlsen GM, Grigsby SA, Winant DM. Effects of an aquatic fitness program on the muscular strength and endurance of patients with multiple sclerosis. *Phys Ther*. 1984;64(5):653–657.

159. Zamparo P, Pagliaro P. The energy cost of level walking before and after hydro-kinesi therapy in patients with spastic paresis. *Scand J Med Sci Sports*. 1998;8(4):222–228.

160. Pagliaro P, Zamparo P. Quantitative evaluation of the stretch reflex before and after hydro kinesy therapy in patients affected by spastic paresis. *J Electromyogr Kinesiol*. 1999;9(2):141–148.

161. Jubelt B. Post-polio syndrome. *Curr Treat Options Neurol*. 2004;6(2):87–93.

162. Willen C, Sunnerhagen KS, Grimby G. Dynamic water exercise in individuals with late poliomyelitis. *Arch Phys Med Rehabil*. 2001;82(1):66–72.

163. Bosch PR, Wells CL. Effect of immersion on residual volume of able-bodied and spinal cord injured males. *Med Sci Sports Exerc*. 1991;23(3):384–388.

164. Kesiktas N, Paker N, Erdogan N, et al. The use of hydrotherapy for the management of spasticity. *Neurorehabil Neural Repair*. 2004;18(4):268–273.

165. Plecash AR, Leavitt BR. Aquatherapy for neurodegenerative disorders. *J Huntingtons Dis*. 2014;3(1):5–11.

166. Morris D. Aquatic rehabilitation for the treatment of neurologic disorders. In: Becker B, Cole AJ, eds. *Comprehensive Aquatic Therapy*. 3rd ed. Pullman, WA: Washington State University Publishing; 2011:193–218.

167. Bayraktar D, Guclu-Gunduz A, Yazici G, et al. Effects of Ai-Chi on balance, functional mobility, strength and fatigue in patients with multiple sclerosis: a pilot study. *NeuroRehabilitation*. 2013;33(3):431–437.

168. Kargarfard M, Etemadifar M, Baker P, et al. Effect of aquatic exercise training on fatigue and health-related quality of life in patients with multiple sclerosis. *Arch Phys Med Rehabil*. 2012;93(10):1701–1708.

169. Castro-Sanchez AM, Mataran-Penarrocha GA, Lara-Palomo I, et al. Hydrotherapy for the treatment of pain in people with multiple sclerosis: a randomized controlled trial. *J Evid Based Complementary Altern Med*. 2012;2012:473963.

170. Salem Y, Scott AH, Karpatkin H, et al. Community-based group aquatic programme for individuals with multiple sclerosis: a pilot study. *Disabil Rehabil*. 2011;33(9):720–728.

171. Peterson C. Exercise in 94 degrees F water for a patient with multiple sclerosis. *Phys Ther*. 2001;81(4):1049–1058.

172. Stevens SL, Caputo JL, Fuller DK, et al. Effects of underwater treadmill training on leg strength, balance, and walking performance in adults with incomplete spinal cord injury. *J Spinal Cord Med*. 2015;38(1):91–101.

173. West CR, Taylor BJ, Campbell IG, et al. Effects of inspiratory muscle training on exercise responses in Paralympic athletes with cervical spinal cord injury. *Scand J Med Sci Sports*. 2014;24(5):764–772.

174. Jung J, Chung E, Kim K, et al. The effects of aquatic exercise on pulmonary function in patients with spinal cord injury. *J Phys Ther Sci*. 2014;26(5):707–709.

175. Berlowitz DJ, Tamplin J. Respiratory muscle training for cervical spinal cord injury. *Cochrane Database Syst Rev*. 2013;(7):CD008507.

176. Verges S, Flore P, Nantermoz G, et al. Respiratory muscle training in athletes with spinal cord injury. *Int J Sports Med*. 2009;30(7):526–532.

177. Perez-de la Cruz S, Garcia Luengo AV, Lambeck J. Effects of an Ai Chi fall prevention programme for patients with Parkinson's disease. *Neurologia*. 2016;31(3):176–182.

178. Vivas J, Arias P, Cudeiro J. Aquatic therapy versus conventional land-based therapy for Parkinson's disease: an open-label pilot study. *Arch Phys Med Rehabil*. 2011;92(8):1202–1210.

179. Crizzle A, Newhouse I. Water exercise for individuals with Parkinson's disease: a pilot study. *Aquat Ther J*. 2007;8(2):22–26.

180. Murray DK, Sacheli MA, Eng JJ, et al. The effects of exercise on cognition in Parkinson's disease: a systematic review. *Transl Neurodegener*. 2014;3(1):5.

181. Petzinger GM, Fisher BE, McEwen S, et al. Exercise-enhanced neuroplasticity targeting motor and cognitive circuitry in Parkinson's disease. *Lancet Neurol*. 2013;12(7):716–726.

182. Pugh CJ, Sprung VS, Ono K, et al. The effect of water immersion during exercise on cerebral blood flow. *Med Sci Sports Exerc*. 2015;47(2):299–306.

183. Carter HH, Spence AL, Pugh CJ, et al. Cardiovascular responses to water immersion in humans: impact on cerebral perfusion. *Am J Physiol Regul Integr Comp Physiol*. 2014;306(9):R636–R640.

184. Ivey FM, Ryan AS, Hafer-Macko CE, et al. Improved cerebral vasomotor reactivity after exercise training in hemiparetic stroke survivors. *Stroke*. 2011;42(7):1994–2000.

185. Brown AD, McMorris CA, Longman RS, et al. Effects of cardiorespiratory fitness and cerebral blood flow on cognitive outcomes in older women. *Neurobiol Aging*. 2010;31(12):2047–2057.

186. Henwood T, Neville C, Baguley C, et al. Physical and functional implications of aquatic exercise for nursing home residents with dementia. *Geriatr Nurs*. 2015;36(1):35–39.

187. Neville C, Henwood T, Beattie E, et al. Exploring the effect of aquatic exercise on behaviour and psychological well-being in people with moderate to severe dementia: a pilot study of the Watermemories Swimming Club. *Australas J Ageing*. 2014;33(2):124–127.

188. Sherlock LA, Guyton Hornsby JW, Rye J. The physiological effects of aquatic exercise on cognitive function in the aging population. *Int J Aquatic Res Educ*. 2013;7(3):266–278.

189. Myers K, Capek D, Shill H, et al. Aquatic therapy and Alzheimer's disease. *Ann Long-Term Care Aging*. 2013;21(5):36–41.

190. Becker BE, Lynch S. Case report: aquatic therapy and end-stage dementia. *PM R*. 2018;10(4):437–441.

191. Chon SC, Oh DW, Shim JH. Watsu approach for improving spasticity and ambulatory function in hemiparetic patients with stroke. *Physiother Res Int*. 2009;14(2):128–136.

192. Cunningham J. Halliwick method. In: Ruoti RG, Morris DM, Cole AJ, eds. *Aquatic Rehabilitation*. Philadelphia, PA: Lippincott-Raven; 1996:331.

193. Lambeck J, Gamper U. The Bad Ragaz ring method. In: Becker BE, Cole AJ, eds. *Comprehensive Aquatic Therapy*. 3rd ed. Pullman, WA: Washington State University Publishing; 2011:109–136.

194. Lambeck J, Gampers U. The Halliwick concept. In: Becker BE, Cole AJ, eds. *Comprehensive Aquatic Therapy*. 3rd ed. Pullman, WA: Washington State University Publishers; 2011:77–107.

195. Lai CJ, Liu WY, Yang TF, et al. Pediatric aquatic therapy on motor function and enjoyment in children diagnosed with cerebral palsy of various motor severities. *J Child Neurol*. 2015;30(2):200–208.

196. Fragala-Pinkham MA, Smith HJ, Lombard KA, et al. Aquatic aerobic exercise for children with cerebral palsy: a pilot intervention study. *Physiother Theory Pract*. 2014;30(2):69–78.

197. Gorter JW, Currie SJ. Aquatic exercise programs for children and adolescents with cerebral palsy: what do we know and where do we go? *Int J Pediatr*. 2011;2011:712165.

198. Ballaz L, Plamondon S, Lemay M. Group aquatic training improves gait efficiency in adolescents with cerebral palsy. *Disabil Rehabil*. 2011;33(17–18):1616–1624.

199. Fragala-Pinkham M, Haley SM, O'Neil ME. Group aquatic aerobic exercise for children with disabilities. *Dev Med Child Neurol*. 2008;50(11):822–827.

200. Hutzler Y, Chacham A, Bergman U, et al. Effects of a movement and swimming program on vital capacity and water orientation skills of children with cerebral palsy. *Dev Med Child Neurol*. 1998;40(3):176–181.

201. Prather H, Spitznagle T, Hunt D. Benefits of exercise during pregnancy. *PM R*. 2012;4(11):845–850; quiz 850.

202. Barakat R, Perales M, Cordero Y, et al. Influence of land or water exercise in pregnancy on outcomes: a cross-sectional study. *Med Sci Sports Exerc*. 2017;49(7):1397–1403.

203. Bacchi M, Mottola MF, Perales M, et al. Aquatic activities during pregnancy prevent excessive maternal weight gain and preserve birth weight. *Am J Health Promot*. 2018;32(3):729–735.

204. Cordero Y, Mottola MF, Vargas J, et al. Exercise is associated with a reduction in gestational diabetes mellitus. *Med Sci Sports Exerc*. 2015;47(7):1328–1333.

205. Ruchat SM, Mottola MF. The important role of physical activity in the prevention and management of gestational diabetes mellitus. *Diabetes Metab Res Rev*. 2013;29(5):334–346.

206. da Silva JR Jr, Borges PS, Agra KF, et al. Effects of an aquatic physical exercise program on glycemic control and perinatal outcomes of gestational diabetes: study protocol for a randomized controlled trial. *Trials*. 2013;14:390.

207. Barakat R, Cordero Y, Coteron J, et al. Exercise during pregnancy improves maternal glucose screen at 24–28 weeks: a randomised controlled trial. *Br J Sports Med*. 2012;46(9):656–661.

208. Sechrist DM, Tiongco CG, Whisner SM, et al. Physiological effects of aquatic exercise in pregnant women on bed rest. *Occup Ther Health Care*. 2015;29(3):330–339.

209. San Juan Dertkigil M, Cecatti JG, Sarno MA, et al. Variation in the amniotic fluid index following moderate physical activity in water during pregnancy. *Acta Obstet Gynecol Scand*. 2007;86(5):547–552.

210. Vazquez-Lara JM, Ruiz-Frutos C, Rodriguez-Diaz L, et al. Effect of a physical activity programme in the aquatic environment on haemodynamic constants in pregnant women. *Enferm Clin*. 2018;28(5):316–325.

211. Rodriguez-Blanque R, Sanchez-Garcia JC, Sanchez-Lopez AM, et al. The influence of physical activity in water on sleep quality in pregnant women: a randomised trial. *Women Birth*. 2018;31(1):e51–e58.

212. Rodriguez-Blanque R, Sanchez-Garcia JC, Sanchez-Lopez AM, et al. [Influence of physical exercise during pregnancy on newborn weight: a randomized clinical trial]. *Nutr Hosp*. 2017;34(4):834–840.

213. Versey NG, Halson SL, Dawson BT. Water immersion recovery for athletes: effect on exercise performance and practical recommendations. *Sports Med*. 2013;43(11):1101–1130.

214. Wilcock IM, Cronin JB, Hing WA. Physiological response to water immersion: a method for sport recovery? *Sports Med*. 2006;36(9):747–765.

215. Fonseca LB, Brito CJ, Silva RJ, et al. Use of cold-water immersion to reduce muscle damage and delayed-onset muscle soreness and preserve muscle power in jiu-jitsu athletes. *J Athl Train*. 2016;51(7):540–549.

216. Pointon M, Duffield R. Cold water immersion recovery after simulated collision sport exercise. *Med Sci Sports Exerc*. 2012;44(2):206–216.

217. Gregson W, Black MA, Jones H, et al. Influence of cold water immersion on limb and cutaneous blood flow at rest. *Am J Sports Med*. 2011;39(6):1316–1323.

218. Bailey DM, Erith SJ, Griffin PJ, et al. Influence of cold-water immersion on indices of muscle damage following prolonged intermittent shuttle running. *J Sports Sci*. 2007;25(11):1163–1170.

219. Eston R, Peters D. Effects of cold water immersion on the symptoms of exercise-induced muscle damage. *J Sports Sci*. 1999;17(3):231–238.

220. Leeder JD, van Someren KA, Bell PG, et al. Effects of seated and standing cold water immersion on recovery from repeated sprinting. *J Sports Sci*. 2015;33(15):1544–1552.

221. Elias GP, Varley MC, Wyckelsma VL, et al. Effects of water immersion on post-training recovery in Australian footballers. *Int J Sports Physiol Perform*. 2012;7(4):357–366.

222. Versey NG, Halson SL, Dawson BT. Effect of contrast water therapy duration on recovery of running performance. *Int J Sports Physiol Perform*. 2012;7(2):130–140.

223. Killgore GL. Deep-water running: a practical review of the literature with an emphasis on biomechanics. *Phys Sportsmed*. 2012;40(1):116–126.

224. Wicker A. Sport-specific aquatic rehabilitation. *Curr Sports Med Rep*. 2011;10(2):62–63.

225. Kim E, Kim T, Kang H, et al. Aquatic versus land-based exercises as early functional rehabilitation for elite athletes with acute lower extremity ligament injury: a pilot study. *PM R*. 2010;2(8):703–712.

226. Becker BE, Lindle-Chewning JM, Huff K, et al. Aquatic cross training for athletes: Part 2. *Strength Cond J*. 2008;30(3):67–73.

227. Haff G, Becker BE, Lindle-Chewning JM, et al. Aquatic cross training for athletes: Part 1. *Strength Cond J*. 2008;30(2):18–26.

228. Haff GG, Becker BE, Lindle-Chewning JM, et al. Aquatic cross training for athletes: Part 2. *Strength Cond J*. 2009;30(3):7.

229. Alleva J, Biondi M, Hudgins T. Aquatic strategies in musculoskeletal pain. In: Becker B, Cole A, eds. *Comprehensive Aquatic Therapy*. 3rd ed. Pullman, WA: Washington State University Publishing; 2011:245–265.

230. Brennan D, Wilder R. Aqua running. In: Becker B, Cole A, eds. *Comprehensive Aquatic Therapy*. 3rd ed. Pullman, WA: Washington State University Publishing; 2011:155–169.

231. Wilder RP, Brennan D, Schotte DE. A standard measure for exercise prescription for aqua running. *Am J Sports Med*. 1993;21(1):45–48.

232. Donoghue OA, Shimojo H, Takagi H. Impact forces of plyometric exercises performed on land and in water. *Sports Health*. 2011;3(3):303–309.

233. Stemm JD, Jacobson BH. Comparison of land and aquatic-based plyometric training on vertical jump performance. *J Strength Cond Res*. 2007;21(2):568–571.

234. Gulick D, Libert C, O'Melia M, et al. Comparison of aquatic and land plyometric training on strength, power and agility. *J Aquatic Phys Ther*. 2007;15(1):11–18.

235. Martel GF, Harmer ML, Logan JM, et al. Aquatic plyometric training increases vertical jump in female volleyball players. *Med Sci Sports Exerc*. 2005;37(10):1814–1819.

236. Garrett G. Bad Ragaz ring method. In: Ruoti R, Morris D, Cole A, eds. *Aquatic Rehabilitation*. Philadelphia, PA: Lippincott; 1997:289–292.

237. Harrison RA, Allard LL. An attempt to quantify the resistances produced using the Bad Ragaz ring method. *Physiotherapy*. 1982;68(10):330–331.

238. Lutz ER. Watsu-aquatic bodywork. *Beginnings*. 1999;19(2):9, 11.

239. Schoedinger P. Watsu in aquatic rehabilitation. In: Becker BE, Cole A, eds. *Comprehensive Aquatic Therapy*. 3rd ed. Pullman, WA: Washington State University Publishing; 2011:137–153.

240. Becker B. Motivating adherence in the rehabilitation setting. *J Back Musculoskeletal Med*. 1991;1(37):48.

The Physical Agents

This chapter reviews the physical agents with an emphasis on their clinical use, scientific basis, and effectiveness. Although the properties of many agents overlap, discussion will begin with superficial heat and cold and progress to hydrotherapy, the diathermies, and the electrically based therapies. The chapter will conclude with an analysis of some of the newer and less established modalities.

HEAT AND COLD

The benefits of therapeutic heat and cold have been appreciated from the earliest of times. Each has potent effects on tissue. For example, temperatures above 42°C are painful, and prolonged exposure to those above 45°C may cause injury. Temperatures below 13°C are uncomfortable, and systemic temperatures below 28°C can cause death (1). In addition, metabolic and enzymatic processes are temperature dependent: an increase of 3°C increases collagenase activity several fold (2). Heating the hands to 45°C reduces metacarpophalangeal joint stiffness by a fifth, whereas cooling them to 18°C increases stiffness by a similar amount (3). Temperature changes of several degrees centigrade produce significant changes in nerve conduction velocity, blood flow (4–6), and collagen extensibility.

In practice, most clinical treatments attempt to warm tissues between 40°C and 45°C. As a point of reference, 20-minute immersions of the body in 22°C cold or 42°C warm baths result in core temperature changes of 0.3°C to 0.4°C (7). Cold therapy can produce intense localized effects; ice massage over an inflamed knee joint reduces skin temperatures by 16°C and intra-articular temperatures by 5°C or 6°C (8). Conversely, hot paraffin is reported to increase local skin temperature and knee intra-articular temperature by 7.5°C and 1.7°C, respectively (8). Although the heating modalities differ, most gain their effects by producing analgesia, hyperemia, changes in temperature, and reduced muscle tone. As a result, they share many of the indications and contraindications (**Boxes 51-1** and **51-2**) of heat in general. Cold's main effects are analgesia, reduced perfusion, and muscle tone reduction. As a result, heat and cold have indications (**Box 51-3**) and contraindications (**Box 51-4**) that are often surprisingly similar.

Tissue can be heated or cooled in one of three ways. The first, conduction, requires the physical contact of two or more objects at different temperatures such as a hot pack and the body. The second, convection, also involves the transfer of energy between objects at different temperatures. In this case (e.g., a whirlpool), however, one object, the medium, is moving relative to the other, which permits more intensive heating or cooling than would occur in a stationary setting. The last

approach, conversion, involves the transformation of one form of energy to another such as occurs when the radiant energy of heat lamp is used to heat tissue.

Superficial Heat

The physical properties of superficial heating and cooling modalities differ, but none is able to overcome the combination of skin tolerance, tissue thermal conductivity, and the patient's comfort to produce temperature changes of more than a few degrees at depths of a few centimeters (9). The following sections review the characteristics of the most common superficial agents.

Hot Packs

Hot packs typically consist of segmented cloth bags filled with a hydroscopic material that, when exposed to water, absorb many times their own weight. Packs are available in various sizes and are stored in water baths at temperatures of 70°C to 80°C. When needed, the packs are removed from the reservoirs and excess water is allowed to drain off. The packs are then wrapped or laid on layer of toweling and placed on the patient (**Fig. 51-1**).

Hot packs, due to their advantages of low cost and ease of use, have been one of the most commonly used heat modalities (10). While now increasingly rare in the clinic, home use is common and a number of options are available. Some, such as packs containing sodium acetate, are quiescent until activated by being placed in a microwave or boiling water. Once heated, and particularly when they are wrapped in an insulating material, they will cool slowly and may maintain a therapeutic temperature for 20 or 30 minutes.

These packs have heat-associated risks that are outlined in **Box 51-2**. In addition, scalding is possible, and it is important that excess water is drained off and an insulating layer provided before they are placed on (not under) the patient.

Electric heating pads, hot water bottles, and circulating water heating pads are alternatives to hot packs. Many of these do not cool spontaneously and not all have reliable timers or thermostats. Burns are possible, and the risk factors outlined in **Box 51-2** become particularly prominent for people with diminished sensation or those who may fall asleep during treatment.

Heat Lamps

Heat lamps, although now rarely used, remain an easy way to warm superficial tissue. Specialized infrared (IR) sources are available. However, incandescent light bulbs release almost all their energy as heat and can serve as an inexpensive alternative.

General Indications for Therapeutic Heat

Pain
Muscle spasm
Contracture
Tension myalgia
Production of hyperemia
Acceleration of metabolic processes
Hematoma resolution
Bursitis
Tenosynovitis
Fibrositis
Fibromyalgia
Superficial thrombophlebitis
Induction of reflex vasodilation
Collagen-vascular diseases

Skin temperatures are controlled by adjusting the distance between the lamp and the patient. Although the drop-off of a lamp's intensity depends on its geometry as well as the beam's angle with the patient, in practice, lamps are typically placed perpendicular to, and about 40 to 50 cm from, the patient.

Choice

The physiologic effects of the "dry" heat of a heat lamp differ little from those of the "moist" heat of a hot pack (11). As a result, the choice between agents depends on ease of use and patient/therapist preference.

Safety

The precautions in **Box 51-2** apply to these agents (12). In addition, chronic use of these modalities can produce a permanent reddish-brown skin discoloration known as erythema ab igne (literally "erythema from fire").

Effectiveness

As noted above, superficial heat and cold have clear and established physiologic effects. The translation of these effects, other than as a temporary amelioration of symptoms or as an adjunct to active treatment, into clear clinical benefit, however, has been difficult. As a result, while their use is declining, they

General Contraindications and Precautions for Therapeutic Heat

Acute inflammation, trauma, or hemorrhage
Bleeding disorders
Cutaneous insensitivity
Inability to communicate or respond to pain
Poor thermal regulation (e.g., from neuroleptics)
Malignancy
Edema
Ischemia
Atrophic skin
Scar tissue
Unstable angina or blood pressure
Decompensated heart failure within 6–8 weeks of a myocardial infarction

General Indications for Therapeutic Cold

Acute musculoskeletal trauma
   Edema
   Hemorrhage
   Analgesia
Pain
Spasticity
Adjunct in muscle reeducation
Reduction of local and systemic metabolic activity

continue to be utilized to lessen discomfort and, to a lesser extent, for the control of swelling and edema. Although they have a limited penetration (9), there is some support for their use as an adjunct to the treatment of a variety of musculoskeletal conditions (13–16).

Hydrotherapy

Hydrotherapy uses a fluid to transfer thermal energy and mechanical forces to tissue. Whirlpool baths, for example, use agitated water to produce convective heating and cooling, as well as massage and gentle debridement. Agitation, however, is not essential as sitz, paraffin, and contrast baths all use a stationary medium. Submersion itself has effects. Subjects immersed in warm water will display obvious changes such as an elevated heartrate, diaphoresis, and an increased core temperature. In addition, they will also show more subtle effects such as increased levels of atrial natriuretic protein and augmented venous return to the right atrium (17). This section discusses hydrotherapy as well as other alternatives, such as balneotherapy, misting, and fluidotherapy.

Whirlpool Baths

Hydrotherapy is traditionally associated with water-filled tanks ranging in size from more than a thousand liters to smaller units designed to treat a hand or foot. Contamination concerns and research findings have resulted in even these later devices often being replaced by alternative and potentially more effective approaches. However, some knowledge of the older approaches remains necessary as the larger tanks still have their uses and new findings could result in their increased use.

Temperature choice depends on the amount of the body immersed, treatment goals, and the patient's tolerance/medical condition. Neutral temperatures of 33°C to 36°C are usually well tolerated, although higher temperatures of 42°C to as

General Precautions and Contraindications for Therapeutic Cold

Ischemia
Cold intolerance
Raynaud's phenomenon or disease
Severe cold pressor responses
Cold allergy
Inability to communicate or respond to pain
Poor thermal regulation
Cutaneous insensitivity

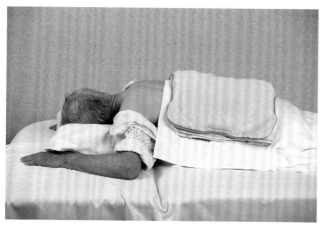

FIGURE 51-1. Hot pack treatment of the low back. Note that the patient is positioned in a comfortable position and that scalding is prevented by placing several layers of toweling between the pack and the patient.

much as 45°C or 46°C are possible on limited portions of the body. Since full-body immersion can increase systemic temperature, immersion tank temperatures are usually limited to 39°C. Temperature selection must take into account the fact that for any given temperature, turbulent water heats and cools more vigorously than its stationary counterpart.

Larger size whirlpools (e.g., Hubbard tanks) may still be used at times for large wounds and widespread dermatologic conditions for which gentle agitation, heat, and solvent action are needed. Neutral to somewhat warmer temperatures, depending on comfort, are chosen. Once the patient is immersed, agitation is gradually increased to provide gentle debridement and aid in dressing removal.

"Sterile" tanks should be specified for burns and wounds. Although true sterility is not possible, disinfecting protocols can make disease transmission unlikely. If a wound is large or if there is a significant exposure of internal tissue, sodium chloride may be added to the water (5 kg or more may be needed for the largest tanks) to improve comfort and lessen the risk of hemolysis or electrolyte imbalances. Agents such as potassium permanganate and gentle detergents raise cytotoxic concerns but may be added in particular situations.

Contrast Baths

Contrast baths are now rarely used but represent an interesting attempt to desensitize tissue, lessen pain, and improve autonomic regulation. The baths consist of two reservoirs, one typically at 38°C to 40°C and the other significantly cooler at about 13°C to 16°C. Treatment begins with the involved hand or foot being placed in the warm bath for about 10 minutes and then undergoing four cycles of alternating 1- to 4-minute cold and 4- to 6-minute warm soaks. If edema is an issue, a case can be made for ending with a cool, rather than a warm, soak.

In the past, contrast baths commonly featured in the treatment of rheumatoid arthritis and complex regional pain. Use has lessened due to the complexity of their use, a poor evidence base (18), and improvements in the medical care.

Sitz Baths

Warm sitz baths are enshrined in the treatment of hemorrhoids, anorectal fistulas, and postpartum pain. While there has been criticism about the limitations of our knowledge of

their effectiveness (19), they have some support. For example, sitting in warm water decreases sphincter tone and lessens rectal pain following anal surgery (20,21). Risks seem minimal and limited to that of any heat and water modality.

Edema

The ancient Greeks and 18th-century physicians treated edema with water immersion—a practice mimicked today with compressive sleeves. Research supports this intuitively reasonable treatment; immersion increases natriuretic proteins (17) and renal water and salt loss in normal subjects as well as those with the nephrotic syndrome and cirrhosis (22). Because warmth produces a reactive vasodilation, neutral temperatures appear to be the most effective.

Water-Based Exercise

Water-based exercise is a popular way to permit training in a limited weight-bearing setting (23) for which a 2016 Cochrane review found "moderate quality evidence" for a short-term but clinically significant benefit for people with hip and knee osteoarthritis (24). Its benefits over land-based alternatives remain unclear. For example, a number of studies have found that water-based programs provide little or no benefits over their land-based counterparts for patients with chronic obstructive pulmonary disease (25), stroke (26), rheumatoid arthritis, anterior cruciate rehabilitation (27,28), or fibromyalgia (29).

Balneotherapy

Balneotherapy (spa) therapy is little more than a curiosity in North America although its acceptance in Europe remains stronger (30). Treatments tend to be holistic and involve a combination of physical therapy, exercise, diet, hydrotherapy/mineral water baths, mud treatments, mineral water consumption, and education that may take place in a resort-like atmosphere. The fundamental tenet of the approach is the belief that water containing dissolved gases (such as nitrogen and carbon dioxide), elements (e.g., calcium, magnesium, zinc, and cobalt), and compounds (e.g., hydrogen sulfide) has therapeutic effects. It should be noted that while intact skin is relatively impervious, penetrance of these substances increases if skin integrity is impaired (31,32).

Overall, evidence of benefit is weak or lacking. Thus, while well-done systematic reviews may find no benefit (33), they, by necessity, group relatively disparate findings together and obscure isolated benefits reported for people with osteoarthritis (34,35), (inflammatory arthritides) (36), and fibromyalgia (37–40). In all, balneotherapy studies are often limited in their rigor, but their findings can be intriguing and an open, but questioning, mind seems warranted.

Fluidotherapy

Hydrotherapy uses water as the heat-exchanging medium, but substances such as pulverized corncobs and small beads "fluidized" by hot air jets may be substituted. Although these devices have been available since the 1970s, the benefits of this high-temperature, low–heat capacity approach over other approaches for improving joint mobility and sensory desensitization remain, as is true for many physical agents, controversial (41).

Safety

The general precautions of heat and cold apply to hydrotherapy. Although reports of their occurrence are minimal, drowning, cardiac disease, systemic hyperthermia, heat-associated seizures (42), and disease transmission are concerns.

Cardiac disease may not be an absolute contraindication to hyperthermia. For example, even though sauna baths (80°C to 100°C) elevate body temperatures by 1°C or 2°C (43,44), research indicates that at least at more moderate temperatures, they may improve the function and quality of life of individuals with severe congestive heart failure (CHF) (45). Furthermore, Finnish heart attack survivors return to sauna bathing without apparent increased risk, and 15-minute soaks in 40°C hot tubs do not create ischemic electrocardiogram changes or alter systolic and diastolic blood pressures more than cardiac rehabilitation–associated stationary bicycle exercises (43,44,46).

Hydrotherapy-associated infections seem to be rare. However, prolonged hyperthermia may reduce fertility (47) and it seems reasonable to limit exposure if this is a concern.

Paraffin Baths

Paraffin baths, while now rarer in the clinic, remain commercially available and deserve a brief discussion. These baths consist of a thermostatically controlled reservoir filled with a 1:7 mixture of mineral oil and paraffin. Bath temperatures (45°C to 54°C) are higher than in most hydrotherapy but are well tolerated because of the low heat capacity of the mixture and the tendency for an insulating layer of wax to build up on the surface of the treated area.

Two paraffin treatment approaches predominate. Dipping is the most common and consists of the patient submerging the treated extremity in the bath about 10 times, with pauses between dips to permit a layer of paraffin to solidify. The treated area is then covered with a plastic sheet and placed in an insulating cover for about 20 minutes (**Fig. 51-2**). The paraffin is then stripped off and returned to the container.

Dipping initially increases skin temperatures to about 47°C, but by the end of a 30-minute session, skin temperatures have fallen to within a few degrees of baseline. Subcutaneous temperatures may increase by 3°C and intramuscular/intra-articular temperatures by 1°C (48).

Continuous immersion is an alternative approach in which the treated extremity is kept immersed for 20 to 30 minutes following 6 to 10 dips in the bath. Heating, while more intense, is still well tolerated due to the presence of an insulating layer of solidified paraffin. Immersion produces the same initial maximum skin temperature as dipping; however, temperatures decrease less rapidly. At the end of a session, skin temperatures are about 41.5°C with subcutaneous and superficial intramuscular temperature increases (about 5°C and 3°C, respectively), which are higher than those of dipping (48). The dip-and-wrap method in conjunction with limb elevation is preferable for a patient at risk for edema.

Paraffin baths were often used to treat hand contractures associated with rheumatoid arthritis, scleroderma, burns, and injury. Dipping or immersion was the most common technique, but, at times, paraffin was brushed on difficult-to-treat areas. Reports in the literature are scant, but do report benefits in rheumatoid arthritis (49) and posttraumatic hand

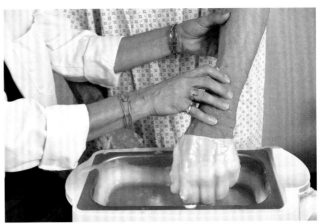

FIGURE 51-2. Paraffin bath treatment. Paraffin baths typically involve either dipping or immersion. In the dipping technique, the area to be treated is immersed in the bath, removed briefly to allow the wax to solidify, and redipped for a total of 10 repetitions. After the dipping, the treated area is wrapped in an insulating cover for about 20 minutes before the wax is removed. The immersion technique provides more vigorous heating and is similar to the dipping approach, except that after a number of dips, the extremity is kept immersed in the paraffin.

stiffness when combined with mobilization relative to the results of mobilization alone (8,50,51).

Safety

A thermometer should be kept in the reservoir, and paraffin temperature should be checked (typical values are about 48°C) before each use to ensure that the paraffin is at the correct temperature. (A film of solidified wax around a reservoir's margins suggests that temperatures are not dangerously elevated.) If the feet have poor circulation, a few insulating layers of paraffin may be brushed on before they are dipped or immersed.

Most avoid treating acutely inflamed joints and tissues vigorously given concerns that increases in intra-articular temperatures will increase enzymatic activity (2). Although there has been controversy about its benefits, warmth often improves comfort, and there seems to be little risk in using this agent in the subacute situation.

Diathermy

The diathermies, which encompass ultrasound, shortwave, and microwave, were once a mainstay of practice but have lessened in importance with time. Ultrasound remains the most commonly used of the three, but shortwave diathermy (SWD) is still in use not only as a heating agent but also as a pulsed relatively athermic variant. Microwave diathermy (MWD) no longer has a place in routine practice but continues to have specialized medical applications. All three will be reviewed but with an emphasis commensurate with their current use.

Ultrasound

Ultrasound (US) is sound that occurs at frequencies above the 17,000- to 20,000-Hz limit of human hearing. As such, it shares the characteristics of sound in general: it requires a medium for transmission; its waves consist of alternating compressions and rarefactions; it transmits energy; and it can be focused, refracted, and reflected. Although arguments are made for a variety of frequencies, most therapeutic units operate between 0.8 and 3 MHz due to the trade-offs between focusing and penetration.

Biophysics

US has both thermal and nonthermal effects. Heat production, with its goals of hyperemia, enhanced soft tissue extensibility, and lessened pain, is the best known. Nonthermal processes—which include cavitation, streaming, standing waves, and mechanical deformation—may also be sought because of their ability to alter cell membrane permeability and function (52). The first of these nonthermal processes, cavitation, occurs when high-intensity ultrasound passes through a liquid and produces small bubbles that may either rhythmically oscillate in size or grow and abruptly collapse. In either case, large temperature and pressure changes may occur (53) and produce localized tissue distortion and injury. Pressure asymmetries produced by the presence of an ultrasonic beam can generate shear forces that may lead to media movement (streaming), tissue damage, or accelerated metabolic processes (52,54). Standing waves produce fixed regions of high and low pressure at half-wavelength intervals (about 0.75 mm for 1-MHz ultrasound). Graphic effects are possible; exposure to static ultrasonic fields can result in standing wave patterns in multiple tissues such as the blood and brain (55).

Tissue penetration depends on frequency, orientation, and the tissue itself. Frequency is particularly important as the intensity of a beam decreases by a factor of 6 as the frequency increases from 0.3 to 3.3 MHz (56). Orientation is also critical. For example, about 50% of a 0.87-MHz ultrasound beam penetrates 7 cm in a direction parallel to muscle fibers, but only 2 cm in a transverse direction (56). Tissue type is also significant. Fifty percent of an ultrasound beam penetrates several centimeters in muscle, only a few tenths of a millimeter in the bone, and 7 to 8 cm in fat (56,57). In practice, 3-MHz US is used for the more superficial tissues, while lower frequencies are used when deeper penetration is desired. US treatments are frequently delivered to anisotropic tissue, and it should be remembered that localized areas of temperature elevations of 5°C or more may occur at sound absorption discontinuities such as those that occur at bone-soft tissue interfaces (56–58).

Equipment

US machines typically use ferromagnetic ceramics to convert electrical energy into sound. Machines are computerized, and in addition to indicating treatment, times, frequencies, and waveforms are often provided with predesigned treatment programs. Additional capabilities such as concurrent electrical stimulation are also common.

While the output parameters of ultrasound machines are relatively stable, they can vary both with age and during a treatment. Given this, they should be routinely calibrated and safety checked.

Technique

There are two philosophies of US therapy. The first is that its benefits are due to heating. This approach typically uses a continuous-wave (CW) or high-intensity pulsed beam with intensities of 0.5 to 2.5 W/cm². The second approach is designed to optimize ultrasound's nonthermal properties. In this case, the beam is modulated to deliver brief high-intensity pulses

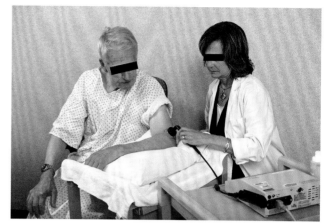

FIGURE 51-3. Direct-contact ultrasound treatment of the elbow. Note the use of a pillow to support the patient comfortably. Although not shown in the picture, a coupling agent is used to acoustically couple the applicator and the skin.

separated by no-power pauses. Heating is, thus, minimized and ultrasound's nonthermal effects are emphasized.

US is usually delivered by moving the applicator (**Fig. 51-3**) over the treated area in slow (a few cm/s), overlapping strokes. Treatments cover areas of about 100 cm² and last 5 to 10 minutes. Indirect US, while less common, is used to treat irregular surfaces such as the ankle. In these situations, the body part is placed in a container filled with degassed water (water that has been allowed to sit for several hours). The applicator is held a short distance away (0.5 to 3.0 cm) and moved without touching the skin. Power intensities may need to be higher due to transmission losses.

Safety and energy transmission require a good coupling between the applicator and the skin. The treatment area should be cleansed before treatment, and a coupling agent is necessary. Little practical difference exists between commercial gels and mineral oil for direct applications, but gels are often chosen due to convenience (59). Coupling agents should not be salt based (e.g., those used for EMG or ECG), as the salt may damage the applicator.

Phonophoresis is an US variant in which biologically active substances are combined with the coupling medium with the hope that the US will speed the movement of the active material into tissue. Although this technique has been in use since the 1960s, neither its effectiveness, penetration, optimal frequency, coupling mediums, nor amount of material lost to the subcutaneous circulation is well established. Although claims of increased cortisol concentrations at depths of several centimeters following corticosteroid phonophoresis have been made, evidence of deep penetration remains limited (60,61). Clinical reports are mixed. Thus, although some studies report phonophoresis with a variety of agents successful in terms of improved shoulder range of motion and pain following the treatment (62,63), others may find the approach no more effective than ultrasound alone (64,65).

Indications

Musculoskeletal Conditions. Research support is surprisingly limited (66). For example, a study of 63 patients with calcific shoulder tendonitis treated with pulsed ultrasound (0.89 MHz, 2.5 W/cm²) found that the treated patients had significantly larger improvements in their pain and decreases in calcium deposits relative to sham controls at the end of an intensive 6-week treatment program. However, this difference had disappeared at follow-up 9 months later (67). Although ultrasound may be more beneficial than corticosteroid injection in the treatment of shoulder pain, other studies and reviews find it no more effective than placebo or nonsteroidal anti-inflammatory medications for a variety of conditions ranging from subacromial bursitis and lateral epicondylitis (68) to heel pain (69). More tellingly, perhaps, an evidence-based practice guideline panel came to the conclusion that although ultrasound was effective in the treatment of calcific tendonitis of the shoulder, there was no compelling evidence of clinical benefits for other sources of musculoskeletal pain (70). Although these studies raise legitimate issues about its effectiveness, many remain convinced that ultrasound is useful for the treatment of at least some forms of musculoskeletal pain. In support of this, several reviews have found weak but supportive evidence of benefits in the form of increased motion and lessened stiffness from the cautious use of ultrasound in patients with rheumatoid arthritis (49,71,72).

Contractures. Ultrasound in conjunction with stretching is effective in increasing the range of motion of the heel cords, periarthritic shoulders, and contracted hips (73,74). In fact, due to its penetration and focusing capabilities, it is the only agent that can significantly heat (by 8°C to 10°C) the hip joint (58). Hand and Dupuytren's contractures also may benefit from ultrasound (75), although a small study of burns did not find treatment beneficial (76). Stretching is essential and should begin during heating and continue as the tissue cools and "sets."

Soft Tissue Wounds and Inflammation. The benefits of ultrasound in wound healing, regardless of whether delivered either via a conventional or pulsed high-frequency or by an increasingly accepted non-contact low-frequency "mist" technique, remain intriguing but controversial. As conventional high frequency treatment is discussed elsewhere in this section, we will focus here on the newer low-frequency approaches that typically operate at 0.1 to 0.8 W/cm² intensities and far lower (30 to 40 kHz) frequencies.

Treatment begins by covering the area surrounding the wound with clean towels and the operator using a sterile technique. Treatment is delivered in a continuous sweeping manner with the applicator's tip held 0.5 to 1.5 cm from the wound. The most common mediums are sterile saline and 0.25% acetic acid. Loosened debris and fluid runoff are collected by an absorbent towel. Treatments are usually delivered on a once a day, 3 to 5 times/week schedule with their durations (typically 3 to 5 minutes) depending on the size of the wound.

Treatment is well tolerated and associated with low pressure changes of about 13 to 22 kPa (1.9 to 3.2 psi) or less. Benefits are thought to result from an accelerated loosening of debris, metabolic stimulation, and enhanced antibiotic penetration. While widely used, the benefits of the approach remain controversial—a situation that was not helped by the fact that Food and Drug Administration (FDA) approval was obtained via a 510(k) process rather than the demands of a more far more scientifically rigorous full premarket approval (PMA) process. Given this, a brief review of the evidence is useful.

On one hand, a number of studies including RCTs of varying quality often find that pressure sores (77) as well as wounds such as those associated with diabetes, surgery, burns, venous stasis, and skin grafts heal more rapidly following treatment (e.g., at rates of 40% to 60% relative to the 13% to 25% rates of standard care) (78–83).

It may be that the UK's National Institute for Clinical Excellence (NICE) put it the most succinctly in 2011 when it concluded that while the approach "showed promise," an "overall low quality of evidence and uncertainty about its effectiveness" precluded its adoption for use (84). In summary, low-frequency, noncontact US is a potentially effective, but still arguable approach to wound treatment (85).

Trauma. Although ultrasound may aggravate tissue damage and swelling if used too soon after an injury, subacute hematomas (86) and postpartum perineal pain (87) may improve more rapidly with treatment. Ankle sprains are a common indication for treatment. Even here, benefits are unclear with a systematic review involving more than 570 patients concluding that current evidence, at best, supporting a limited benefit (88). A number of studies find evidence that ultrasound at intensities on the order of 1 W/cm² may provide at least short-term benefits in the treatment of symptomatic carpal tunnel syndrome (89,90). Although these reports are intriguing, benefits are not always evident and remain controversial (91).

Fractures. Although ultrasound is not typically used for this purpose, it has been approved by the FDA for the treatment of some fractures. For example, low-intensity pulsed US has been shown to accelerate the healing of fractures and nonunions (92).

Precautions and Contraindications

Ultrasound is capable of producing intense heating and, under some conditions, potentially destructive nonthermal effects such as cavitation and fluid streaming. The precautions for therapeutic heat (**Box 51-2**) are applicable. In addition, fluid-filled cavities such as the eyes and gravid uterus are avoided, and the heart, brain, cervical ganglia, tumors, acute hemorrhages/inflammation, ischemic areas, and pacemakers should not be treated for obvious heat, neurophysiologic, and mechanical reasons. The spine should not be exposed to high intensities, and laminectomy sites seem particularly problematic. Ultrasound is used in children with particular concern about the effects of excessive energy and heat on immature growth plates.

A common concern is that ultrasound treatment over metal implants in muscle or next to the bone will elevate tissue temperatures to a higher level than would occur in their absence (93,94). The concept is certainly valid and, although some studies found the effect smaller than might be expected, only a limited number of objects and geometries were studied. Although clear indications and contraindications do not exist, many simply avoid using ultrasound near metal.

Shortwave Diathermy

Shortwave diathermy heats tissue with a combination of induced electrical currents and the vibration that it imposes on the molecules of a tissue. Since SWD produces radio waves that can cause electrical interference, its use is restricted to 27.12, 13.56, and 40.68 MHz (wavelengths of 11, 22, and 7 m), respectively, with most therapeutic machines operating at 27.12 MHz. While the use of SWD has decreased over the years, it continues to be used and some review is warranted.

Biophysics

Penetration depends on the specifics of tissue as well as the frequency and characteristics of the applicator. Inductive applicators induce electrical ("eddy") currents in tissue and, as a rule, produce the highest temperatures in water-rich, highly conductive tissues such as muscle. Capacitively coupled applicators, on the other hand, emphasize electric field heating. Maximum temperatures tend to occur in water-poor substances, such as fat, ligaments, tendons, and joint capsules (95). Although heating depends on the dosage and application approach, SWD can increase subcutaneous fat temperatures by 15°C and 3- to 5-cm-deep intramuscular temperatures by 4°C to 6°C (9,96).

SWD machines may produce pulsed as well as continuous-wave (CW) output. CW is used when the treatment goal is heating. In contrast, pulsed approaches, often termed pulsed electromagnetic fields (PEMFs), alternate brief periods of high power with longer no power pauses. As is true for ultrasound, the pulsed approach may be chosen to emphasize nonthermal effects. Some investigators, for example, believe that certain pulse frequencies, even at low intensities, can increase blood flow and have resonant effects on cell function. Although nonthermal SWD phenomena have been observed, their clinical importance remains unclear.

Technique

A SWD machine is essentially a radio transmitter that automatically tunes itself to optimize coupling with the body. Two treatment approaches are possible. In the inductive approach, the SWD machine, as noted above, induces eddy currents, which are degraded into heat by the body's electrical resistance. In the capacitive approach, the tissue to be heated is placed between two plates that are connected to the SWD machine's output and serves as the dielectric of a capacitor. In this case, heating currents are produced as the radio wave polarity oscillates across the plates.

There are a variety of inductive applicators. Drum applicators consist of coils encased in rigid containers that may be positioned with hinges around the body (**Fig. 51-4**). Pad applicators and semiflexible mats are also available.

Research in SWD has been limited recently and shows, at best, variable support for the modality. Thus, while no additional benefit has been found for spinal pain over exercise and advice, others have reported that treatment produced significant reductions in knee pain (97–99).

Microwave Diathermy

Microwave diathermy is now a curiosity for most of us. However, as noted above, it still finds use in specialized applications and some discussion is warranted. The FCC-approved industrial, scientific, and medical frequencies for MWD are 915 and 2,456 MHz (33- and 12-cm wavelengths, respectively).

Biophysics

Microwaves, while highly focusable, do not penetrate tissue as deeply as shortwaves and ultrasound, but, like them, penetration decreases as frequency increases. Microwaves are absorbed by water and should theoretically preferentially heat muscle. However, fat usually overlies muscle and absorbs a significant portion of the beam. As an example, at 915 MHz,

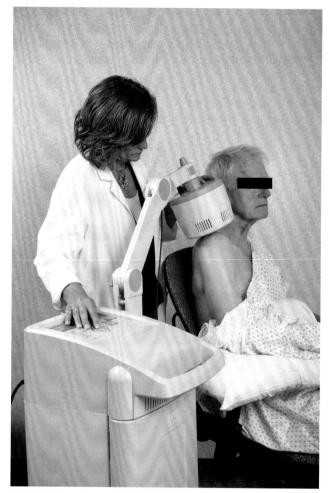

FIGURE 51-4. Shortwave diathermy treatment using a drum applicator. Careful positioning is necessary and the patient should wear no jewelry and be positioned on a nonconductive surface.

subcutaneous fat temperatures may increase by 10°C to 12°C, whereas 3- to 4-cm-deep muscles will be warmed by only 3°C to 4°C.

Precautions and Contraindications

While the general contraindications of heat listed in **Box 51-2** apply to short- and MWD, additional restrictions stem from their electromagnetic nature. For example, perspiration is conductive and, if present in a field, heats the skin. Metal produces localized heating; patients should not wear jewelry, and treatment takes place on a nonconductive surface. Pacemakers, stimulators, surgical implants, contact lenses, and the menstruating or pregnant uterus should not be exposed to these agents. Although many of these concerns seem almost academic, this is not always the case. For example, implanted devices are a particular concern with a report of an application of pulsed diathermy to the jaw leading to a persistent vegetative state in a man with a deep brain stimulator (100). Some believe that small, metallic surgical clips or metallic intrauterine devices do not produce significant localized temperature elevations. This may be correct, but at least one study found that 1-cm wires positioned to mimic a surgical site produced localized 3°C to 4°C temperature elevations (101). Many follow a rule of "no metal" when using any diathermy. Microwaves selectively heat

TABLE 51-1	Therapeutic and Environmental Magnetic Fields (T)[a]
Typical residential exposure	0.4
Earth's magnetic field	25–65
Automobile interior	2
Subway passenger compartment	16–64
Standard therapeutic magnet	250–5,000
Credit card erasure	5,000
Pulsed electromagnetic field devices	2,000–8,000
Bone growth stimulator	5,000
Exposure limits (continuous)	
Occupational	2×10^5
General public	4×10^4
MRI	$1.5+ \times 10^6$

[a]1 Tesla = 10 Gauss.

water, and treatment of edematous tissue, moist skin, the eyes, and fluid-filled cavities/blisters can produce unacceptable temperature elevations and cataracts.

Workplace safety has been addressed by the American National Standards Institute (ANSI) guidelines (102). Pregnant women may want to take particular precautions (103,104), but as fields fall rapidly with distance and therapists work only intermittently with these agents, their exposures seem to fall well within the ANSI limits (**Table 51-1** and **Box 51-5** display typical electromagnetic exposures and contraindications for use).

Cold (Cryotherapy)

Chilling a limited portion of the body produces local and distant physiologic effects. In the case of ice, skin temperatures initially decrease rapidly and then more slowly approach an equilibrium of about 12°C to 13°C in 10 minutes. Subcutaneous and deeper intramuscular temperatures fall more slowly by 3°C to 5°C at 10 minutes in the former case and by a degree or less in the latter (105). Chilling for longer periods generates more pronounced cooling with intramuscular forearm temperature decreases of 6°C to 16°C after 20 minutes to 3 hours of cooling (6,8) and intra-articular knee

temperatures decreases of 5°C to 6°C over a prolonged period of cooling with ice chips (8).

Cooling produces an initial period of vasoconstriction that may (106) or may not be followed by a reactive vasodilation (106–108). Vasoconstriction becomes evident within 5 minutes of cooling, and after 25 minutes of packing a knee in ice, soft tissue and bone blood flows are decreased by 30% and 20%, respectively (8). Superficial cold also decreases metabolic activity and with prolonged application lessens muscle tone, increases gastrointestinal motility (109), slows nerve conduction, and produces analgesia.

Technique

Ice has a high heat capacity and cools treated tissue more rapidly than alternatives such as gel packs (see below) (110). Treatments tend to last 10 to 20 minutes. Techniques are straightforward, but if ice packs are used, a slightly damp, thin towel is placed between the pack and the skin.

Iced whirlpools cool vigorously and usually are used for 10- to 20-minute periods. Although an athlete may be motivated to tolerate them, the average patient finds temperatures below 15°C uncomfortable. If the feet or hands are exposed to a cold bath, neoprene booties or woolen socks/gloves may increase tolerance.

Ice massage consists of rubbing a piece of ice (e.g., an ice cube or water frozen in a small cup) over the painful area (**Fig. 51-5**). Analgesia is often achieved in 3 to 5 minutes with patients typically reporting successive sensations of cold, burning, aching, and numbness. A moisture barrier should be present between ice and the skin, and ice should slide smoothly over the treated area. Although chemical and refrigerated agents may have temperatures below 0°C and can produce frostbite, ice treatments of healthy people for periods of less than 30 minutes do not seem to cause injury.

Vapocoolant and liquid nitrogen sprays can abruptly reduce skin temperature by 20°C (8) and are used for local skin analgesia and myofascial "spray-and-stretch" techniques. Prepackaged chemical ice packs often consist of two compartments (e.g., one filled with water, the other with ammonium nitrate) that, when mixed, produce a cooling reaction. Although these packs are convenient and pliable, they are

BOX 51-5
General Contraindications and Precautions for Electromagnetic Agents

Jewelry
Moist tissue
Ischemia
Acute hemorrhage/injury/inflammation
Neoplasm
Implants
   Metal
   Pacemakers
   Stimulators
   Pumps
   Small clips/IUDs
Eyes
Gonads
Growth plates
Infection (e.g., joint)

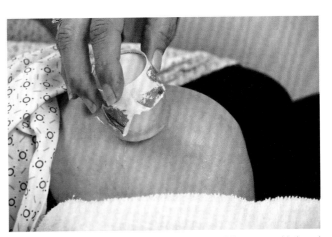

FIGURE 51-5. Ice is a mainstay of cryotherapy. While more sophisticated approaches are possible, ice massage using water frozen in a paper cup remains a common approach.

expensive and tend to cool rapidly (110). Alternatives such as commercially available cuffs that apply both chilled water and pressure to a joint such as the knee are also available. In many cases, plastic bags of frozen peas, which conform to the body once struck on a hard surface, serve as effective and inexpensive alternatives.

Indications

Trauma

Many studies have found that chilling limits hypoxic damage, lessens edema, speeds recovery, and reduces compartmental pressures after injury (111). Although there are concerns that cooling does not reduce posttraumatic swelling, it does lessen metabolic activity and blood flow (107).

Rest, ice, compression, and elevation (RICE) are the initial steps in treating many musculoskeletal injuries. For example, icing 20 minutes per half hour to 30 minutes every 2 hours, for the first 6 to 24 hours, is a common acute ankle sprain recommendation. Although ice is often the mainstay of acute soft tissue injury treatment, research indicates that the evidence supporting its use is more limited than might be thought (112–115).

After the first 48 to 72 hours, the choice between cryotherapy and heat is typically a matter of preference. Some prefer heat and will use it unless there is a worsening of edema or pain. Others prefer cooling and believe that a combination of icing for 10 to 20 minutes to reduce pain, along with active exercising, is the most effective way to speed recovery. In any event, heat and cold are only adjuncts to a mobilization and exercise program.

Chronic Pain

Research results are again mixed; while some investigators have found ice massage and transcutaneous electrical nerve stimulation (TENS) comparable for chronic low back pain, a subsequent Cochrane review found limited evidence of the effectiveness of cryotherapy in low back pain (14). Ultimately, patient tolerance will limit the applicability of ice therapy.

Spasticity

The effect of cooling on spasticity remains unclear although cooling muscles before therapy might be helpful; its utility must be balanced against discomfort and the time required. It is interesting that cooling via cold water baths and cooling vests has been reported to both improve and worsen the spasticity in patients with multiple sclerosis (116,117).

Whole-Body Cryotherapy

Whole-body cryotherapy has gained some prominence recently. In essence, the approach involves a patient entering into a chamber and being exposed to short, less than 3-minute durations of air that has been cooled to −100°C or so. Research support for the approach remains limited with a 2014 review (118) finding only 10 reports, primarily involving limited numbers of athletes. The authors concluded that (a) the exposures resulted in limited tissue cooling; (b) that there was only weak evidence that the exposures altered antioxidant, autonomic, or inflammatory responses in clinically meaningful manner; (c) that there was little objective evidence of accelerated musculoskeletal recovery; and (d) that conventional cold agents were cheaper than, and as likely, to be as beneficial.

Precautions and Contraindications

The precautions shown in **Box 51-4** should be heeded. Pressor responses aggravating cardiovascular disease should be considered, as well as the effects of direct and consensual vasoconstriction on ischemic limbs and in people with Raynaud's phenomenon. Cold hypersensitivity, urticaria, and even frostbite are possible. Patients with insensate areas and those who are unresponsive should not be treated with cryotherapy. Cryotherapy is uncomfortable, and it is important to explain its rationale before beginning treatment.

ULTRAVIOLET

Ultraviolet (UV) therapy, although a commonly used wound treatment in the 1980s, has now almost disappeared from the clinic. However, a brief discussion remains warranted due to its past importance and its continued use, in other medical areas.

The biomedical literature divides the UV spectrum into three parts: UV-A (0.315 to 0.4 µm), UV-B (0.29 to 0.315 µm), and UV-C (0.2 to 0.29 µm). UV-A penetrates most deeply but has the least biologic activity. UV-B produces sunburn and skin erythema. UV-C is bactericidal and also produces erythema.

Treatment

UV exposure is limited by the nature of the tissue treated, source strength, and the separation of the tissue from the applicator. Exposures are quantified in terms of the time required to produce a minimal erythema (i.e., one minimal erythemal dose [MED]) and are established by determining the time required to produce a minimal erythema on the volar forearm several hours later. For reference, 2.5 MEDs produce erythema and pain that persists for a few days, 5 MEDs edema and desquamation, and 10 MEDs blistering (119).

In general, UV treatments began with 1 or 2 MEDs and were kept to less than 5 MEDs to avoid tissue damage (119). Open wounds were treated directly with a lamp. Specially designed probes were used for fistulas, undermined wounds, or the oral cavity.

UV-C was once a common skin ulcer treatment as its bactericidal effects (on motile bacteria but not spores) are well recognized (120). UV may also accelerate wound healing and wound margin vascularization (121), but alternatives may be more effective, easier to use, and less likely to produce side effects. It may be that antibiotic-resistant bacteria will provide a reason for increased use in the future.

ELECTROTHERAPY

The ancient Greeks knew that that shocks from electric eels and fish could produce analgesia. This knowledge had little practical impact until the 18th and 19th centuries when rapid increases in the understanding of electricity caught the public's imagination. Early "medicinal" electrical applications were haphazard. Electrostatic baths, spark treatments, and galvanically induced limb movement all had momentary popularity. Unfortunately, their utility was minimal and scientific interest waned until the last half of the 20th century (122).

Today, electrical stimulation may be used to strengthen muscles, move paralyzed limbs, produce analgesia, deliver medications, and, at very low intensities, improve fracture healing (see also Chapter 54). Soft tissue wounds, osteoporosis, and musculoskeletal pain represent additional potentially important but still investigational electrical stimulation applications. This section discusses these agents.

Transcutaneous Electrical Nerve Stimulation

The gate theory of pain postulated in 1965 that cells in the spinal substantia gelatinosa serve as gates to pain perception by inhibiting the passage of nociceptive information to the brain if nonpainful sensory afferent signals are present (123). TENS provided sensory afferent signals and, after some successful trials, became widely accepted.

The mechanism of action of TENS remains controversial. Although research shows that stimulation reduces dorsal horn cell activity (124), the gate theory does not explain phenomena such as painless sensory neuropathy, analgesia persisting after stimulation, or a delayed onset of analgesia. As a result, explanations such as those involving frequency-dependent effects and central nervous system endorphins have been advanced by a number of investigators (125).

TENS units consist of a battery, one or more signal generators, and a set of electrodes. Units are small, are programmable, and generate a variety of stimuli with currents of less than 100 mA, pulse rates ranging from a few to 200 Hz, and pulse widths of 10 to a few hundred microseconds. Biphasic waveforms improve comfort and avoid the electrolytic and iontophoretic effects associated with unidirectional currents. Additional features such as "burst" modes and wave-train modulation are common but of unclear benefit.

Electrode positioning is more art than science. Placement over the painful area is usually the first choice, but locations over afferent nerves, nerve roots, and acupuncture and trigger points, as well as contralateral to the pain, are also possible. Parameter choice is also subjective. Many prefer to begin with low-amplitude, 40- to 80-Hz "conventional" settings and use the less comfortable high-intensity, 4- to 8-Hz alternative if the first trials are unsuccessful. Ideally, initial benefit is established in a few therapy sessions and a home trial. Response is difficult to predict, and parameter selection is ultimately based on trial and error. TENS can be quite expensive and, as benefits often wane with time, purchase should be considered only if benefits persist for at least a few months.

Indications

TENS studies range in quality from well-designed, prospective, randomized controlled trials to case reports. Success rates vary from placebo levels to 95% and may be affected by the choice of stimulating parameters, electrode placement, condition treated, chronicity, and length of follow-up. Even when studies are controlled, it is not clear whether the controls should be sham TENS or an alternative treatment.

Acute Pain

Surgical pain is a convenient model for acute pain. Benefits are not universally found and may be limited to specific conditions (126). Parameter choice appears important. Thus, two RCTs that used peri-incisional either low frequency (2 Hz), high frequency (100 Hz), or a combination of the two in large groups of women undergoing gynecologic surgery found that TENS resulted in a 30% to 50% reduction in the use of

analgesics with the combination approach appearing the most beneficial (126–128).

Musculoskeletal Pain

While the earlier reports were relatively encouraging, more recent research places a harsher light on TENS benefits. For example, a 2015 Cochrane review of 19 trials involving more than 1,300 subjects found at most "tentative evidence" that TENS reduces pain intensity more effectively than its sham counterpart for acute pain (129). Similarly, the authors of a number of recent Cochrane reviews have found little or no benefit in postsurgical stump pain (129), cancer-related pain (130), or in the treatment of rotator cuff disease (131). Findings for subacute low back pain may be more positive but are still equivocal (132).

It is intriguing that while the evidence of TENS effectiveness in spinal pain seems so limited, a stronger case appears possible for its use in osteoarthritis. For example, several reviews and panels find that TENS is beneficial in the treatment of osteoarthritis (particularly of the knee). There is also evidence that benefits require treatments of 40 minutes or more duration (133).

In summary, support for its use remains mixed and may depend on factors such as chronicity, parameter choice (134), and the condition treated (135).

Urologic and Gynecologic Issues

While musculoskeletal pain is the main focus for many TENS applications, a significant amount of attention has also been placed on other conditions such as gynecologic pain. Here again, the picture is mixed. While a number of RCTs support the benefits of TENS in labor, pregnancy-related low back pain, and dysmenorrhea (136,137), a 2009 Cochrane review involving almost 1,700 women found only weak support for the use of TENS during labor (138).

Other New and Potential Applications

Ischemia

TENS appears capable of altering cutaneous blood flow and skin temperatures in normal subjects (139–141). However, its ability to do so in a clinically significant manner in ischemic conditions such as angina and peripheral vascular disease remains more controversial (142). While there are suggestions that TENS may reduce cardiac ischemia perhaps by lessening sympathetic tone, concerns about the risk of precordial placement make more research in monitored settings essential before its use could be recommended for this application.

Spasticity

Spasticity reduction following TENS use has been reported for patients with stroke, spinal cord injury, and multiple sclerosis (143). Effects are controversial, with a 2007 study and a 2013 systematic review of nonpharmacologic treatment of spasticity in multiple sclerosis finding no benefit (144,145).

Precautions and Contraindications

Only a limited proportion of patients who try TENS benefit. Studies of long-term users find that about 75% of individuals who have purchased a unit may be still using it after 6 months to a year (146,147), with use continuing to decline to about 30% at 3 years (148). The best results seem to occur in musculoskeletal pain, neurogenic pain, and angina. People with psychogenic pain, central pain, autonomic dysfunction, and social distress may respond less well (148).

TENS has few common safety issues other than contact dermatitis and skin irritation, which usually respond to changes in electrode type and placement. High current densities, either due to the setting of the unit or to a partially detached electrode, are uncomfortable but are easily corrected. Cardiac pacemakers seem resistant to TENS (149), but even a small concern about the possibility of ectopically generated rhythms dictates avoidance over the pericardial area or in patients with pacemakers, electrical implants, and dysrhythmias. Treatment near the carotid sinus and epiglottis and over the low backs, abdomens, and lower extremities of pregnant women should be avoided.

Iontophoresis

Iontophoresis uses electrical fields to force electrically charged or polarized ions and molecules into tissue. Speed of movement is related to voltage and field strength, whereas the amount of material introduced into the tissue is proportional to the current. Penetration is dependent on a substance's size and polarity and may be particularly strong at sweat glands and areas of skin breakdown (150). It may not always be necessary to have an "active ingredient" as treatment with tap water at current intensities of 10 $\mu A/cm^2$ has been reported to increase both local skin temperatures and microcirculation (151).

An iontophoretic unit is simple and may be contained within a disposable skin patch. In general, it consists of a direct-current power source, two electrodes, and a pad moistened with a dilute solution of the desired (charged or polar) substance placed under the electrode of the same polarity. Currents are determined by multiplying the area of the active electrode by 0.1 to 0.5 mA/cm^2. The size of the inactive electrode is immaterial but is kept as large as convenient for patient comfort.

Indications

Although the first-line treatment of hyperthyrosis lies in the use of antiperspirants such as aluminum chloride hexahydrate, tap water iontophoresis has been reported to produce benefits in the majority of treated patients (150,152). The treatment approach varies with location. In the case of the distal limbs, the hands or feet may be placed in a container with both the anode and cathode, or with one extremity and one electrode in each of two containers. Currents vary with the approach but are often 10 to 30 mA. The mechanism of action is unclear but may result from the preferential flow of ions along the sweat ducts.

Iontophoresis has been found to improve delivery of a variety of antibiotics such as gentamicin, penicillin, and cefoxitin into the poorly vascularized tissues such as burns and cartilage (153,154). Iontophoretic treatment of postherpetic neuralgia with methylprednisolone and lidocaine as well as Achilles tendonitis with dexamethasone has been reported to produce prolonged benefits (155,156). There is, thus far, minimal evidence of benefit in neck pain (157) or patellar tendinopathy (158). Similarly, RCTs of steroidal iontophoresis in the treatment of plantar fasciitis and lateral epicondylitis, as well as acetic acid in shoulder tendinitis, found minimal to no benefits over conventional therapy or placebo (159–161).

Safety

Iontophoresis is a safe therapy. Complications tend to involve allergic reactions or to be similar to those of TENS.

Electric and Low-Intensity Electromagnetic Fields

Bone and soft tissue injuries produce electrical fields and currents that can alter cell orientation, proliferation, calcium concentrations, and motility (162). These fields have very low intensities (approximately 1 V/m rather than the 70,000 V/m [70 mV/m] associated with cell membrane potentials), and their mechanism of action may include a switch effect that alters cell permeability.

Wound Healing

Interest in electrically stimulated wound healing extends back to at least the early 1970s (163), but those early reports were marred by poor design and the approach was not widely accepted. More recent protocols are often similar to the earlier studies and use low-frequency (10 to 200 Hz) and low-intensity (10 $\mu A/cm^2$) electric currents and electromagnetic fields to speed the healing of soft tissue wounds. Benefits remain difficult to establish, but there is some experimental support for the approach in stem cell research (164), and the recognition of electrical stimulation's impact on nonhealing bony fractures (165) has served to maintain interest.

Wound studies are notoriously difficult to carry out, and this has proven true for those involving electrical stimulation as well. Thus, while TENS stimulation has been reported to improve healing and elevate distal limb temperatures in patients with diabetic neuropathy and scleroderma (166), research may or may not show accelerated healing. In fact, two updated Cochrane reviews concluded as recently as 2015 that the data remain too limited to permit an assessment of benefits of electromagnetic therapy in the healing of either venous or pressure ulcers (167).

Musculoskeletal Pain

Musculoskeletal pain has proven to be a focus of electrotherapeutic research with a particular emphasis on pulsed EMF (PEMF/PEME). The results are again intriguing but less than convincing. For example, while controlled studies have reported that low-intensity pulsed SWD produced clinically and statistically significant improvements in neck pain or ankle sprains (168,169), other investigations involving subacromial impingement failed to find benefit from the addition of PEMF to their rehabilitation program (170). Reviews provide a similarly mixed picture. For example, a 2013 Cochrane review encompassing more than 600 subjects concluded that while electromagnetic therapies may provide moderate amounts of pain relief for osteoarthritis, the clinical significance of the relief remained unclear (171).

Interferential Current

TENS units and muscle simulators are limited at times by the discomfort that strong stimulation at low (e.g., <80 Hz) frequencies produces in the skin. However, skin impedance decreases with frequency, and higher-frequency waves can penetrate to deeper tissues without discomfort. Interferential current (IFC) devices take advantage of this fact by having two high-frequency (e.g., 2,000 to 4,000 Hz) sine waves differing by 20 to 100 Hz overlap each other in tissue. Beat frequencies equal to the sum and differences of the sine waves are produced with the difference in frequency within the therapeutic 20- to 80-Hz range.

IFC is often used when TENS effects are desired. Immediate effects in terms of pain reduction and shoulder ROM may be found (172), but there is no clear demonstration of its superiority over TENS or other devices (173) for either musculoskeletal or neuropathic pain (174). IFC is used at times for the treatment of osteoarthritis and musculoskeletal injury. Here also, information is limited: while positive studies can be found, no conclusions of more than transient benefit can be drawn.

Safety

IFC devices operate at low powers and are used for limited periods. Although there has been a report of a burn arising from treatment (175), the devices appear safe, and the precautions necessary seem to be those outlined for TENS and electrical devices in general.

Epidemiologic studies have at times associated prolonged exposure to low-intensity EMFs (such as those associated with power lines, hairdryers, and cell phones) with increased rates of cancer and miscarriage (**Table 51-1**). These studies are of concern, but all have methodologic shortcomings. Public concern led to the formation of a number of national and international review panels that have consistently concluded that neither static magnetic nor ELF electric fields pose a known risk (176).

Alternative Therapies

Vibration

Vibration and tapping have a long history in neuromuscular rehabilitation as a way to facilitate muscle recruitment (177). Research is limited, but many clinicians believed that frequencies of about 150 Hz and amplitudes of 1.5 mm were particularly effective and might have some analgesic or wound healing effects (178).

More recently, attention has focused on the utility of whole-body vibration (WBV) in which the subject sits or stands on a vibrating platform. While findings remain mixed (179), there are suggestions that WBV may improve balance in cerebral palsy and the elderly (180), lessen knee pain and improve function in knee osteoarthritis (181), and improve strength (182). Adverse effects appear minimal and transient. More investigation seems warranted given mixed findings, variable study quality, as well as the plethora of frequencies, vibration amplitudes, and training regimens utilized.

Light and Laser Therapy

Laser and monochromatic light sources ("photobiomodulation") have been used since the late 1960s to lessen pain and speed the healing of a variety of neuropathic, inflammatory, and soft tissue conditions (183). Initially, treatment involved short exposures to a variety of ≤1- to 5-mW lasers. However, with time, therapy practices have coalesced, and now, most treatments are performed with 30- to 150-+mW IR diode lasers. Higher power sources, which have the advantage of being able to treat larger areas, may be utilized at times as well.

Photobiomodulation received its first impetus due to claims about its ability to heal chronic, nonhealing wounds (184),

which have been surprisingly difficult to substantiate at the clinical level. Thus, while the underlying mechanisms have been well researched (e.g., increased collagen production and altered DNA synthesis) (185,186), support for clinically significant benefits remains more limited than we would like.

Use of this approach lagged in the United States until the FDA reduced its requirements for acceptance in 2002 to that of single positive clinical study. Currently, however, it is widely available.

As is true for many modalities, confirmation of benefit is conflicting and confusing. Thus, several systematic reviews find evidence of variable benefits in the treatment of complex regional pain syndrome (CRPS) (174) and shoulder disorders such as impingement and adhesive capsulisites (187). Similarly, lateral epicondylitis (188) may benefit, while more generalized syndromes such as myofascial pain may be more resistant. Although several trials have indicated potential benefits in the treatment of fibromyalgia (189) and chronic low back pain (190), others have found conflicting support. Effectiveness seems to depend, at least in part, upon parameter choice. Dosage guidelines are now available (191) and may have some relevance in terms of clinical effectiveness (192). As seems true for almost all modalities, more research is needed, effectiveness does not arise from stand-alone treatment alone (193), and the benefits of this over other approaches are often unknown.

Safety

While medical laser devices are subject to strict regulation (e.g., use of safety goggles), based upon risk to the unprotected skin and eyes, safety does not seem to be a particularly worrisome issue at the lower-energy parameters typically employed in clinical practice.

Static Electric and Magnetic Fields

The potential health benefits of electric and magnetic fields have intrigued humans for thousands of years. Interest has fluctuated with time, but the magnetic devices advertised today differ little, other than in complexity, from the magnetic rings of the Greeks and therapies of 150 years ago.

Indications

Although enthusiasm flared up a decade or more ago, objective clinical support is limited. Thus, although a study may find magnetic fields beneficial in conditions such as rheumatoid arthritis, others may not (194).

Safety

Safety does not seem to be a particular issue. As noted earlier, a number of panels have concluded that neither static electric nor magnetic fields pose any known risk (195,196). As a point of reference, 1.5-, 3-T, and higher-strength MRI machines have long records of safety. For example, even hour-long exposures to 8-T field strengths, while producing temporary changes in ECG readings, do not alter heart or respiratory rates, blood pressure, or body temperature (197,198).

Extracorporeal Shock Wave Therapy

Although extracorporeal shock wave therapy (ESWT) gained prominence as a potential treatment of a variety of soft tissue disorders, its potential for benefits over conventional treatment remains unclear. Limited research is available with minimal benefits reported in nonspecific shoulder pain (199), but more significant results have been reported in a number of musculoskeletal conditions (200). As is true for other agents, treatment in combination with exercise appears more effective than its isolated counterpart (201). Thus, whether, and to what extent, ESWT has any unique benefits or is merely a new way to apply controlled trauma to reinitiate healing is yet to be established.

MODALITY CHOICE AND PRESCRIPTION

The physical agents are almost always more effective when prescribed as part of a program that may also include massage, exercise, and education. A well-written prescription involves the same elements that are common to all good writing: who (the patient), what (the agent), why (the diagnosis), where (the treatment area), when (the frequency and duration), and how (intensity, device settings). Consultation and discussion with an experienced therapist are appropriate if the prescriber is unsure of the specifics of a particular approach.

Modality choice depends on a balancing of the diagnosis, the characteristics of the agent, evidence of effectiveness, concurrent issues (e.g., patient preference, anticoagulation, etc.), and treatment goals. General rules do exist. For example, acute (<24 to 48 hours) musculoskeletal conditions are usually treated with cooling. Hot packs, cool packs, hydrotherapy, SWD, and some of the electrical therapies are commonly used to treat broader areas. More intense agents such as ice massage and ultrasound are restricted to smaller regions. The diathermies appear preferential for deeper tissues. In the end, choice involves blending an understanding of the agents, experience, and equipment availability. As research continues, our knowledge will grow. Choices common today will undoubtedly appear quaint in the future.

REFERENCES

1. Frachimont P, Juchmes J, Lecomite J. Hydrotherapy: mechanisms and indications. *Pharmacol Ther.* 1983;20:79–93.
2. Harris ED, McCroskery PA. The influence of temperature and fibril stability on degradation of cartilage collagen by rheumatoid synovial collagenase. *N Engl J Med.* 1974;290:1–6.
3. Wright V, Johns RJ. Quantitative and qualitative analysis of joint stiffness in normal subjects and in patients with connective tissue diseases. *Ann Rheum Dis.* 1961;20:36–46.
4. Knight KL. *Cryotherapy: Theory, Technique and Physiology.* 1st ed. Chattanooga, TN: Chattanooga Corporation; 1985:83–100.
5. Guyton AC. *Textbook of Medical Physiology.* 7th ed. Philadelphia, PA: W.B. Saunders; 1986:336–346.
6. Denys EH. AAEM minimonograph #14: the influence of temperature in clinical neurophysiology. *Muscle Nerve.* 1991;14:795–811.
7. Doering TJ, Aaslid R, Steuernagel B, et al. Cerebral autoregulation during whole-body hypothermia and hyperthermia. *Am J Phys Med Rehabil.* 1999;78:33–38.
8. Oosterveld FG, Rasker JJ. Effects of local heat and cold treatment of surface and articular temperature of arthritic knees. *Arthritis Rheum.* 1994;31:1578–1582.
9. Draper DO, Knight K, Fujiwara T, et al. Temperature change in human muscle during and after pulsed short-wave diathermy. *J Orthop Sports Phys Ther.* 1999;29: 13–18; discussion 9–22.
10. Lindsay DM, Dearness J, McGinley CC. Electrotherapy usage trends in private physiotherapy practice in Alberta. *Physiother Can.* 1995;47:30–34.
11. Poindexter RH, Wright EF, Murchison DF. Comparison of moist and dry heat penetration through orofacial tissues. *Cranio.* 2002;20:28–33.
12. Batavia M. Contraindications for superficial heat and therapeutic ultrasound: do sources agree? *Arch Phys Med Rehabil.* 2004;85:1006–1012.
13. Chou R, Huffman LH. Nonpharmacologic therapies for acute and chronic low back pain: a review of the evidence for an American Pain Society/American College of Physicians clinical practice guideline. *Ann Intern Med.* 2007;147:492–504.
14. French SD, Cameron M, Walker BF, et al. Superficial heat or cold for low back pain. *Cochrane Database Syst Rev.* 2006;(1):CD004750.
15. Lin YH. Effects of thermal therapy in improving the passive range of knee motion: comparison of cold and superficial heat applications. *Clin Rehabil.* 2003;17:618–623.
16. Brosseau L, Robinson V, Pelland L, et al. Efficacy of thermotherapy for rheumatoid arthritis: a meta-analysis. *Phy Ther Rev.* 2002;7:5–15.
17. Kurabayashi H, Tamura K, Tamura J, et al. The effects of hydraulic pressure on atrial natriuretic peptide during rehabilitative head-out water immersion. *Life Sci.* 2001;69:1017–1021.
18. Cochrane DJ. Alternating hot and cold water immersion for athlete recovery: a review. *Phys Ther Sport.* 2004;5:26–32.
19. Tejirian T, Abbas MA. Sitz bath: where is the evidence? Scientific basis of a common practice. *Dis Colon Rectum.* 2005;48:2336–2340.
20. Pinho M, Correa JCO, Furtado A, et al. Do hot baths promote anal sphincter relaxation? *Dis Colon Rectum.* 1993;36:273–274.
21. Gupta P, Gupta P. Randomized, controlled study comparing sitz-bath and no-sitz-bath treatments in patients with acute anal fissures. *ANZ J Surg.* 2006;76:718–721.
22. Adler AJ. Water immersion: lessons from antiquity to modern times. *Contrib Nephrol.* 1993;102:171–186.
23. Geytenbeek J. Evidence for effective hydrotherapy. *Physiotherapy (London).* 2002;88:514–529.
24. Bartels EM, Juhl CB, Christensen R, et al. Aquatic exercise for the treatment of knee and hip osteoarthritis. *Cochrane Database Syst Rev.* 2016;(3):CD005523.
25. McNamara RJ, McKeough ZJ, McKenzie DK, et al. Acceptability of the aquatic environment for exercise training by people with chronic obstructive pulmonary disease with physical comorbidities: additional results from a randomised controlled trial. *Physiotherapy.* 2015;101:187–192.
26. Mehrholz J, Kugler J, Pohl M. Water-based exercises for improving activities of daily living after stroke. *Cochrane Database Syst Rev.* 2011;(1):CD008186.
27. Epps H, Ginnelly L, Utley M, et al. Is hydrotherapy cost-effective? A randomised controlled trial of combined hydrotherapy programmes compared with physiotherapy land techniques in children with juvenile idiopathic arthritis. *Health Technol Assess.* 2005;9:iii–iv.
28. Foley A, Halbert J, Hewitt T, et al. Does hydrotherapy improve strength and physical function in patients with osteoarthritis—a randomised controlled trial comparing a gym based and a hydrotherapy based strengthening programme. *Ann Rheum Dis.* 2003;62:1162–1167.
29. Bidonde J, Busch AJ, Webber SC, et al. Aquatic exercise training for fibromyalgia. *Cochrane Database Syst Rev.* 2014;(10):CD011336.
30. Bender T, Balint PV, Balint GP. A brief history of spa therapy. *Ann Rheum Dis.* 2002;61:949–950.
31. Rishler M, Brostovski Y, Yaron M. Effect of Spa therapy in tiberias on patients with ankylosing spondylitis. *Clin Rheumatol.* 1995;14:21–25.
32. Sukenik S, Giryes H, Halevy S, et al. Treatment of psoriatic arthritis at the dead sea. *J Rheumatol.* 1994;21:1305–1309.
33. Verhagen AP, Bierma-Zeinstra SM, Cardoso JR, et al. Balneotherapy for rheumatoid arthritis. *Cochrane Database Syst Rev.* 2003;(4):CD000518.
34. Brosseau L, Macleay L, Robinson V, et al. Efficacy of balneotherapy for osteoarthritis of the knee: a systematic review. *Phy Ther Rev.* 2002;7:209–222.
35. Pascarelli NA, Cheleschi S, Bacaro G, et al. Effect of mud-bath therapy on serum biomarkers in patients with knee osteoarthritis: results from a randomized controlled trial. *Isr Med Assoc J.* 2016;18:232–237.
36. Altan L, Bingol U, Aslan M, et al. The effect of balneotherapy on patients with ankylosing spondylitis. *Scand J Rheumatol.* 2006;35:283–289.
37. Codish S, Dobrovinsky S, Abu Shakra M, et al. Spa therapy for ankylosing spondylitis at the Dead Sea. *Isr Med Assoc J.* 2005;7:443–446.
38. Yurtkuran M, Ay A, Karakoc Y. Improvement of the clinical outcome in Ankylosing spondylitis by balneotherapy. *Joint Bone Spine.* 2005;72:303–308.
39. Zijlstra TR, van de Laar MA, Bernelot Moens HJ, et al. Spa treatment for primary fibromyalgia syndrome: a combination of thalassotherapy, exercise and patient education improves symptoms and quality of life. *Rheumatology.* 2005;44:539–546.
40. Bagdatli AO, Donmez A, Eroksuz R, et al. Does addition of "mud-pack and hot pool treatment" to patient education make a difference in fibromyalgia patients? A randomized controlled single blind study. *Int J Biometeorol.* 2015;59:1905–1911.
41. Kelly R, Beehn C, Hansford A, et al. Effect of fluidotherapy on superficial radial nerve conduction and skin temperature. *J Orthop Sports Phys Ther.* 2005;35:16–23.
42. Bebek N, Gurses C, Gokyigit A, et al. Hot water epilepsy: clinical and electrophysiologic findings based on 21 cases. *Epilepsia.* 2001;42:1180–1184.
43. Hannuksela ML, Ellahham S. Benefits and risks of sauna bathing. *Am J Med.* 2001;110:118–126.
44. Keast ML, Adamo KB. The Finnish sauna bath and its use in patients with cardiovascular disease. *J Cardiopulm Rehabil.* 2000;20:225–230.
45. Basford JR, Oh JK, Allison TG, et al. Safety, acceptance, and physiologic effects of sauna bathing in people with chronic heart failure: a pilot report. *Arch Phys Med Rehabil.* 2009;90:173–177.
46. Allison TG, Miller TD, Squires RW, et al. Cardiovascular responses to immersion in a hot tub in comparison with exercise in male subjects with coronary artery disease. *Mayo Clin Proc.* 1993;68:19–25.
47. Dreier JW, Andersen AM, Berg-Beckhoff G. Systematic review and meta-analyses: fever in pregnancy and health impacts in the offspring. *Pediatrics.* 2014;133:e674–e688.
48. Abramson DI, Tuck S, Chu LSW, et al. Effect of paraffin bath and hot fomentations on local tissue temperatures. *Arch Phys Med Rehabil.* 1964;45:87–94.
49. Robinson V, Brosseau L, Casimiro L, et al. Thermotherapy for treating rheumatoid arthritis. *Cochrane Database Syst Rev.* 2002;(1):CD002826.
50. Sibtain F, Khan A, Shakil-Ur-Rehman S. Efficacy of paraffin wax bath with and without joint mobilization techniques in rehabilitation of post-traumatic stiff hand. *Pak J Med Sci.* 2013;29:647–650.

51. Sandqvist G, Akesson A, Eklund M. Evaluation of paraffin bath treatment in patients with systemic sclerosis. *Disabil Rehabil.* 2004;26:981–987.

52. Nyborg WL. Biological effects of ultrasound: development of safety guidelines. Part II: general review. *Ultrasound Med Biol.* 2001;27:301–333.

53. Flint EB, Suslick KS. The temperature of cavitation. *Science.* 1991;253:1397.

54. Dyson M. Non-thermal cellular effects of ultrasound. *Br J Cancer.* 1982;45: 165–171.

55. O'Reilly MA, Huang Y, Hynynen K. The impact of standing wave effects on transcranial focused ultrasound disruption of the blood-brain barrier in a rat model. *Phys Med Biol.* 2012;55:5251–5267.

56. Goldman DE, Heuter TF. Tabular data of the velocity and absorption of high-frequency sound in mammalian tissues. *J Acoust Soc Am.* 1956;28:35–37.

57. Lehmann JF, deLateur BJ, Stonebridge JB, et al. Therapeutic temperature distribution produced by ultrasound as modified by dosage and volume of tissue exposed. *Arch Phys Med Rehabil.* 1967;48:662–666.

58. Lehmann JF, deLateur BJ, Warren CG, et al. Heating of joint structures by ultrasound. *Arch Phys Med Rehabil.* 1968;49:28–30.

59. Poltawski L, Watson T, Poltawski L, et al. Relative transmissivity of ultrasound coupling agents commonly used by therapists in the UK. *Ultrasound Med Biol.* 2007;33:120–128.

60. Bare AC, McAnawa MB, Pritchard AE, et al. Phonophoretic delivery of 10% hydrocortisone through the epidermis of humans as determined by serum cortisol concentrations. *Phys Ther.* 1996;76:738–745, discussion;46–49.

61. Meidan VM, Walmsley AD, Docker MF, et al. Ultrasound-enhanced diffusion into coupling gel during phonophoresis of 5-fluorouracil. *Int J Pharm.* 1999;185: 205–213.

62. Vlak T. Comparative study of the efficacy of ultrasound and sonophoresis in the treatment of painful shoulder syndrome. *Reumatizam.* 1999;46:5–11.

63. Ebrahimi S, Abbasnia K, Motealleh A, et al. Effect of lidocaine phonophoresis on sensory blockade: pulsed or continuous mode of therapeutic ultrasound? *Physiotherapy.* 2012;98:57–63.

64. Klaiman MD, Shrader JA, Danoff JV, et al. Phonophoresis versus ultrasound in the treatment of common musculoskeletal conditions. *Med Sci Sports Exerc.* 1998;30:1349–1355.

65. Loew LM, Brosseau L, Tugwell P, et al. Deep transverse friction massage for treating lateral elbow or lateral knee tendinitis. *Cochrane Database Syst Rev.* 2014;(11):CD003528.

66. van der Windt DA, van der Heijden GJ, van den Berg S, et al. Ultrasound therapy for acute ankle sprains. *Cochrane Database Syst Rev.* 2002;(1):CD001250.

67. Ebenbichler GR, Erdogmus CB, Resch KL, et al. Ultrasound therapy for calcific tendinitis of the shoulder. *N Engl J Med.* 1999;340:1533–1538.

68. Lundeberg T, Abrahamsson P, Haker E. A comparative study of continuous ultrasound and rest in epicondylalgia. *Scand J Rehabil Med.* 1988;20:99–101.

69. Crawford F, Thomson C. Interventions for treating plantar heel pain. *Cochrane Database Syst Rev.* 2003;(3):CD000416.

70. Harris GR, Susman JL, Harris GR, et al. Managing musculoskeletal complaints with rehabilitation therapy: summary of the Philadelphia Panel evidence-based clinical practice guidelines on musculoskeletal rehabilitation interventions. *J Fam Pract.* 2002;51:1042–1046.

71. Casimiro L, Brosseau L, Robinson V, et al. Therapeutic ultrasound for the treatment of rheumatoid arthritis. *Cochrane Database Syst Rev.* 2002;(3):CD003787.

72. Ottawa P. Ottawa panel evidence-based clinical practice guidelines for electrotherapy and thermotherapy interventions in the management of rheumatoid arthritis in adults. *Phys Ther.* 2004;84:1016–1043.

73. Knight CA, Rutledge CR, Cox ME, et al. Effect of superficial heat, deep heat, and active exercise warm-up on the extensibility of the plantar flexors. *Phys Ther.* 2001;81:1206.

74. Lehmann JF, Fordyce WE, Rathbun LA, et al. Clinical evaluation of a new approach in the treatment of contracture associated with hip fracture after internal fixation. *Arch Phys Med Rehabil.* 1961;42:95.

75. Markham DE, Wood MR. Ultrasound for Dupuytren's contracture. *Physiotherapy.* 1980;66:55–58.

76. Ward RS, Hayes-Lundy C, Reddy R, et al. Evaluation of topical therapeutic ultrasound to improve response to physical therapy and lessen scar contracture after burn injury. *J Burn Care Rehabil.* 1994;15:74–79.

77. Polak A, Franek A, Blaszczak E, et al. A prospective, randomized, controlled, clinical study to evaluate the efficacy of high-frequency ultrasound in the treatment of Stage II and Stage III pressure ulcers in geriatric patients. *Ostomy Wound Manage.* 2014;60:16–28.

78. Kavros SJ, Liedl DA, Boon AJ, et al. Expedited wound healing with noncontact, low-frequency ultrasound therapy in chronic wounds: a retrospective analysis. *Adv Skin Wound Care.* 2008;21:416–423.

79. Gibbons GW, Orgill DP, Serena TE, et al. A prospective, randomized, controlled trial comparing the effects of noncontact, low-frequency ultrasound to standard care in healing venous leg ulcers. *Ostomy Wound Manage.* 2015;61:16–29.

80. Prather JL, Tummel EK, Patel AB, et al. Prospective randomized controlled trial comparing the effects of noncontact low-frequency ultrasound with standard care in healing split-thickness donor sites. *J Am Coll Surg.* 2015;221:309–318.

81. Driver VR, Yao M, Miller CJ. Noncontact low-frequency ultrasound therapy in the treatment of chronic wounds: a meta-analysis. *Wound Repair Regen.* 2011;19(4):475–480.

82. Thomas R. Acoustic pressure wound therapy in the treatment of stage II pressure ulcers. *Ostomy Wound Manage.* 2008;54:56–58.

83. Mojtaba Olyaie M, Rad FS, Elahifar MA, et al. High-frequency and noncontact low-frequency ultrasound therapy for venous leg ulcer treatment: a randomized, controlled study. *Ostomy Wound Manage.* 2013;59:14–20.

84. National Institute for Clinical Excellence. *The MIST Therapy System for the Promotion of Wound Healing.* London: NICE; July 2011. Available from: http://www.nice.org.uk/nicemedia/live/13548/55637/55637.pdf

85. Aetna. *Ultrasound Therapy for Wound Healing;* October 18, 2016. Available from: http://www.aetna.com/cpb/medical/data/700_799/0746.html

86. Oakley EM. Evidence for effectiveness of ultrasound treatment in physical medicine. *Br J Cancer.* 1982;45:233–237.

87. Foulkes J, Yeo B. The application of therapeutic pulsed ultrasound to the traumatised perineum. *Br J Clin Pract.* 1980;34:114–117.

88. van den Bekerom MP, van der Windt DA, Ter Riet G, et al. Therapeutic ultrasound for acute ankle sprains. *Eur J Phys Rehabil Med.* 2012;48:325–334.

89. Oztas O, Turan B, Bora I, et al. Ultrasound therapy effect in carpal tunnel syndrome. *Arch Phys Med Rehabil.* 1988;79:1540–1544.

90. Ebenbichler GR, Resch KL, Nicolakis P, et al. Ultrasound treatment for treating the carpal tunnel syndrome: randomised "sham" controlled trial. *BMJ.* 1998;316: 731–735.

91. Gerritsen AA, de Krom MC, Struijs MA, et al. Conservative treatment options for carpal tunnel syndrome: a systematic review of randomised controlled trials. *J Neurol.* 2002;249:272–280.

92. Padilla F, Puts R, Vico L, et al. Stimulation of bone repair with ultrasound. *Adv Exp Med Biol.* 2016;880:385–427.

93. Skoubo-Kristensen E, Sommer J. Ultrasound influence on internal fixation with a rigid plate in dogs. *Arch Phys Med Rehabil.* 1982;63:371–373.

94. Gersten JW. Effect of metallic objects on temperature rises produced in tissue by ultrasound. *Am J Phys Med.* 1958;37:75–82.

95. Kantor G. Evaluation and survey of microwave and radiofrequency applicators. *J Microw Power.* 1981;16:135–150.

96. Lehmann JF, deLateur BJ, Stonebridge JB. Selective heating by shortwave diathermy with a helical coil. *Arch Phys Med Rehabil.* 1969;50:117–123.

97. Dziedzic K, Hill J, Lewis M, et al. Effectiveness of manual therapy or pulsed shortwave diathermy in addition to advice and exercise for neck disorders: a pragmatic randomized controlled trial in physical therapy clinics. *Arthritis Care Res.* 2005;53:214–222.

98. Jan MH, Chai HM, Wang CL, et al. Effects of repetitive shortwave diathermy for reducing synovitis in patients with knee osteoarthritis: an ultrasonographic study. *Phys Ther.* 2006;86:236–244.

99. Atamaz FC, Durmaz B, Baydar M, et al. Comparison of the efficacy of transcutaneous electrical nerve stimulation, interferential currents, and shortwave diathermy in knee osteoarthritis: a double-blind, randomized, controlled, multicenter study. *Arch Phys Med Rehabil.* 2012;93:748–756.

100. Nutt JG, Anderson VC, Peacock JH, et al. DBS and diathermy interaction induces severe CNS damage. *Neurology.* 2001;56:1384–1386.

101. Lee ER, Sullivan DM, Kapp DS. Potential hazards of radiative electromagnetic hyperthermia in the presence of multiple metallic surgical clips. *Int J Hyperthermia.* 1992;8:809–817.

102. D'Andrea JA, Ziriax JM, Adair ER. Radio frequency electromagnetic fields: mild hyperthermia and safety standards. *Prog Brain Res.* 2007;162:107–135.

103. Ouellet-Hellstrom R, Stewart WF. Miscarriages among female physical therapists who report using radio-and microwave-frequency electromagnetic radiation. *Am J Epidemiol.* 1993;138:775–786.

104. Guberane E, Campana A, Faval P, et al. Gender ratio of offspring and exposure to short-wave radiation among female physiotherapists. *Scand J Work Environ Health.* 1994;20:345–348.

105. Lehmann JF, de Lateur BJ. Diathermy and superficial heat and cold therapy. In: Kottke FJ, Stillwell GK, Lehmann JF, eds. *Krusen's Handbook of Physical Medicine and Rehabilitation.* 3rd ed. Philadelphia, PA: W.B. Saunders; 1982:275–350.

106. Guyton AC, Hall JE. Body temperature, temperature regulation and fever. In: *Textbook of Medical Physiology.* 9th ed. Philadelphia, PA: W.B. Saunders; 1996:911–922.

107. Ho SS, Illgen RL, Meyer RW, et al. Comparison of various icing times in decreasing bone metabolism and blood flow in the knee. *Am J Sports Med.* 1995;23:74–76.

108. Taber C, Contryman K, Fahrenbruch J, et al. Measurement of reactive vasodilation during cold gel pack application to nontraumatized ankles. *Phys Ther.* 1992;72:294–299.

109. Bisgard JD, Nye D. The influence of hot and cold application upon gastric and intestinal motor activity. *Surg Gynecol Obstet.* 1940;71:172–180.

110. Kanlayanaphotporn R, Janwantanakul P, Kanlayanaphotporn R, et al. Comparison of skin surface temperature during the application of various cryotherapy modalities. *Arch Phys Med Rehabil.* 2005;86:1411–1415.

111. Bert JM, Stark JG, Maschka K, et al. The effect of cold therapy on morbidity subsequent to arthroscopic lateral retinacular release. *Orthop Rev.* 1991;20:755–758.

112. Bleakley C, McDonough S, Gardner E, et al. Cold-water immersion (cryotherapy) for preventing and treating muscle soreness after exercise. *Cochrane Database Syst Rev.* 2012;(2):CD008262.

113. Radkowski CA, Pietrobon R, Vail TP, et al. Cryotherapy temperature differences after total knee arthroplasty: a prospective randomized trial. *J Surg Orthop Adv.* 2007;16:67–72.

114. van der Westhuijzen AJ, Becker PJ, Morkel J, et al. A randomized observer blind comparison of bilateral facial ice pack therapy with no ice therapy following third molar surgery. *Int J Oral Maxillofac Surg.* 2005;34:281–286.

115. Kerkhoffs GM, van den Bekerom M, Elders LA, et al. Diagnosis, treatment and prevention of ankle sprains: an evidence-based clinical guideline. *Br J Sports Med.* 2012;46:854–860.

116. Ku YT, Montgomery LD, Lee HC, et al. Physiologic and functional responses of MS patients to body cooling. *Am J Phys Med Rehabil.* 2000;79:427–434.

117. Chiara T, Carlos J Jr, Martin D, et al. Cold effect on oxygen uptake, perceived exertion, and spasticity in patients with multiple sclerosis. *Arch Phys Med Rehabil.* 1998;75:523–528.

118. Bleakley CM, Bieuzen F, Davison GW, et al. Whole-body cryotherapy: empirical evidence and theoretical perspectives. *Open Access J Sports Med.* 2014;5:25–36.

119. Stillwell GK. Ultraviolet therapy. In: Krusen FH, Kottke FJ, Elwood PM, eds. *Handbook of Physical Medicine and Rehabilitation.* 2nd ed. Philadelphia, PA: W.B. Saunders; 1971:363–373.

120. Thai TP, Houghton PE, Campbell KE, et al. Ultraviolet light C in the treatment of chronic wounds with MRSA: a case study. *Ostomy Wound Manage.* 2002;48:52–60.

121. Nussbaum EL, Biemann I, Mustard B. Comparison of ultrasound/ultraviolet-C and laser for treatment of pressure ulcers in patients with spinal cord injury. *Phys Ther.* 1994;74:812–823.

122. Basford JR. A historical perspective of the popular use of electric and magnetic therapy. *Arch Phys Med Rehabil.* 2001;82:1261–1269.

123. Melzack R, Wall PD. Pain mechanisms: a new theory. *Science.* 1965;150:971–979.

124. Garrison DW, Foreman RD. Effects of transcutaneous electrical nerve stimulation (TENS) on spontaneous and noxiously evoked dorsal horn cell activity in cats with transected spinal cords. *Neurosci Lett.* 1996;216:125–128.

125. Sluka KA, Walsh D, Sluka KA, et al. Transcutaneous electrical nerve stimulation: basic science mechanisms and clinical effectiveness. *J Pain.* 2003;4:109–121.

126. Philadelphia Panel. Philadelphia panel evidence-based clinical practice guidelines on selected rehabilitation interventions for knee pain. *Phys Ther.* 2001;81:1675–1699.

127. Chen L, Tang J, White PF, et al. The effect of location of transcutaneous electrical nerve stimulation on postoperative opioid analgesic requirement: acupoint versus nonacupoint stimulation. *Anesth Analg.* 1998;87:1129–1134.

128. Hamza MA, White PF, Ahmed HE, et al. Effect of the frequency of transcutaneous electrical nerve stimulation on the postoperative opioid analgesic requirement and recovery profile. *Anesthesiology.* 1999;91:1232–1238.

129. Johnson MI, Mulvey MR, Bagnall AM. Transcutaneous electrical nerve stimulation (TENS) for phantom pain and stump pain following amputation in adults. *Cochrane Database Syst Rev.* 2015;(5):CD007264.

130. Hurlow A, Bennett MI, Robb KA, et al. Transcutaneous electric nerve stimulation (TENS) for cancer pain in adults. *Cochrane Database Syst Rev.* 2012;(3):CD006276.

131. Page MJ, Green S, Mrocki MA, et al. Electrotherapy modalities for rotator cuff disease. *Cochrane Database Syst Rev.* 2016;(6):CD012225.

132. Pengel HM, Maher CG, Refshauge KM, et al. Systematic review of conservative interventions for subacute low back pain. *Clin Rehabil.* 2002;16:811–820.

133. Cheing GL, Tsui AY, Lo SK, et al. Optimal stimulation duration of tens in the management of osteoarthritic knee pain. *J Rehabil Med.* 2003;35:62–68.

134. Chesterton LS, Foster NE, Wright CC, et al. Effects of TENS frequency, intensity and stimulation site parameter manipulation on pressure pain thresholds in healthy human subjects. *Pain.* 2003;106:73–80.

135. Carroll D, Moore RA, McQuay HJ, et al. Transcutaneous electrical nerve stimulation (TENS) for chronic pain. *Cochrane Database Syst Rev.* 2001;(3):CD003222.

136. Keskin EA, Onur O, Keskin HL, et al. Transcutaneous electrical nerve stimulation improves low back pain during pregnancy. *Gynecol Obstet Invest.* 2012;74:76–83.

137. Proctor ML, Smith CA, Farquhar CM, et al. Transcutaneous electrical nerve stimulation and acupuncture for primary dysmenorrhoea. *Cochrane Database Syst Rev.* 2002;(1):CD002123.

138. Carroll D, Tramer M, McQuay H, et al. Transcutaneous electrical nerve stimulation in labour pain: a systematic review. *Br J Obstet Gynaecol.* 1997;104:169–175.

139. Nolan MF, Hartsfield JK Jr, Witters DM, et al. Failure of transcutaneous electrical nerve stimulation in the conventional and burst modes to alter digital skin temperature. *Arch Phys Med Rehabil.* 1993;74:182–187.

140. Cramp FL, McCullough GR, Lowe AS, et al. Transcutaneous electric nerve stimulation: the effect of intensity on local and distal cutaneous blood flow and skin temperature in healthy subjects. *Arch Phys Med Rehabil.* 2002;83:5–9.

141. Hallén K, Hrafnkelsdóttir T, Jern S, et al. Transcutaneous electrical nerve stimulation induces vasodilation in healthy controls but not in refractory angina patients. *J Pain Symptom Manage.* 2010;40:95–101.

142. Hallén K, Hrafnkelsdóttir T, Jern S, et al. Transcutaneous electrical nerve stimulation induces vasodilation in healthy controls but not in refractory angina patients. *J Pain Symptom Manage.* 2012;40:95–101.

143. Miller L, Mattison P, Pasul L, et al. The effects of transcutaneous electrical nerve stimulation on spasticity. *Phys Ther Rev.* 2005;10:201–208.

144. Hsieh JT, Wolfe DL, Connolly S, et al. Spasticity after spinal cord injury: an evidence-based review of current interventions. *Top Spinal Cord Inj Rehabil.* 2007;13:81–97.

145. Amatya B, Khan F, La Mantia L, et al. Non pharmacological interventions for spasticity in multiple sclerosis. *Cochrane Database Syst Rev.* 2013;(2):CD009974.

146. Fishbain DA, Chabal C, Abbott A, et al. Transcutaneous electrical nerve stimulation (TENS) treatment outcome in long-term users. *Clin J Pain.* 1996;12:201–214.

147. Verdouw BC, Zuurmond WWA, De Lange JJ, et al. Long-term use and effectiveness of transcutaneous electrical nerve stimulation in treatment of chronic pain patients. *Pain Clin.* 1995;8:341–346.

148. Meyler WJ, de Jongste MJ, Rolf CA. Clinical evaluation of pain treatment with electrostimulation: a study on TENS in patients with different pain syndromes. *Clin J Pain.* 1994;10:22–27.

149. Rasmussen MJ, Hayes DL, Vlietstra RE, et al. Can transcutaneous electrical nerve stimulation be safely used in patients with permanent cardiac pacemakers? *Mayo Clin Proc.* 1988;63:443–445.

150. Hill AC, Baker GF, Jansen GT. Mechanisms of action of iontophoresis in the treatment of palmar hyperhidrosis. *Cutis.* 1981;28:69–70, 72.

151. Berliner MN. Skin microcirculation during tapwater iontophoresis in humans: cathode stimulates more than anode. *Microvasc Res.* 1997;54:74–80.

152. Peterson JL, Read SI, Rodman OG. A new device in the treatment of hyperhidrosis by iontophoresis. *Cutis.* 1982;29:82–83, 87–89.

153. Fishman PH, Jay WM, Rissing JP, et al. Iontophoresis of gentamicin into aphakic rabbit eyes. Sustained vitreal levels. *Invest Ophthalmol Vis Sci.* 1984;25:343–345.

154. Greminger RF, Elliott RA, Rapperport A. Antibiotic iontophoresis for the management of burned ear chondritis. *Plast Reconstr Surg.* 1980;66:356–360.

155. Neeter C, Thomee R, Silbernagel KG, et al. Iontophoresis with or without dexamethasone in the treatment of acute Achilles tendon pain. *Scand J Med Sci Sports.* 2003;13:376–382.

156. Ozawa A, Haruki Y, Iwashita K, et al. Follow-up of clinical efficacy of iontophoresis therapy for postherpetic neuralgia (PHN). *J Dermatol.* 1999;26:1–10.

157. Kroeling P, Gross A, Graham N, et al. Electrotherapy for neck pain. *Cochrane Database Syst Rev.* 2009;(4):CD004251.

158. Rigby JH, Mortensen BB, Draper DO. Wireless versus wired iontophoresis for treating patellar tendinopathy: a randomized clinical trial. *J Athl Train.* 2015;50:1165–1173.

159. Gudeman SD, Eisele SA, Heidt RS Jr, et al. Treatment of plantar fasciitis by iontophoresis of 0.4% dexamethasone. A randomized, double-blind, placebo-controlled study. *Am J Sports Med.* 1997;25:312–316.

160. Leduc BE, Caya J, Tremblay S, et al. Treatment of calcifying tendinitis of the shoulder by acetic acid iontophoresis: a double-blind randomized controlled trial. *Arch Phys Med Rehabil.* 2003;84:1523–1527.

161. Runeson L, Haker E, Runeson L, et al. Iontophoresis with cortisone in the treatment of lateral epicondylalgia (tennis elbow)—a double-blind study. *Scand J Med Sci Sports.* 2002;12:136–142.

162. Robinson KR. The responses of cells to electrical fields: a review. *J Cell Biol.* 1985;101:2023–2027.

163. Gault WR, Gatens PF Jr. Use of low intensity direct current in management of ischemic skin ulcers. *Phys Ther.* 1976;56:265–268.

164. Banks TA, Luckman PS, Frith JE, et al. Effects of electric fields on human mesenchymal stem cell behaviour and morphology using a novel multichannel device. *Integr Biol (Camb).* 2015;7:693–712.

165. Aaron RK, Ciombor DM, Simon BJ. Treatment of nonunions with electric and electromagnetic fields. *Clin Orthop Relat Res.* 2004;(419):21–29.

166. Kaada B. Vasodilatation induced by transcutaneous nerve stimulation in peripheral ischemia (Raynaud's phenomenon and diabetic neuropathy). *Eur Heart J.* 1982;3:303–341.

167. Aziz Z, Bell-Syer SE. Electromagnetic therapy for treating pressure ulcers. *Cochrane Database Syst Rev.* 2015;(9):CD002930.

168. Foley-Nolan D, Barry C, Coughlan RJ, et al. Pulsed high frequency (27MHz) electromagnetic therapy for persistent neck pain. A double blind, placebo controlled study of 20 patients. *Orthopedics.* 1990;13:445–451.

169. Foley-Nolan D, Moore K, Codd M, et al. Low energy high frequency pulsed electromagnetic therapy for acute whiplash injuries: a double blind randomized controlled study. *Scand J Rehabil Med.* 1992;24:51–59.

170. Aktas I, Akgun K, Cakmak B. Therapeutic effect of pulsed electromagnetic field in conservative treatment of subacromial impingement syndrome. *Clin Rheumatol.* 2007;26:1234–1239.

171. Li S, Yu B, Zhou D, et al. Electromagnetic fields for treating osteoarthritis. *Cochrane Database Syst Rev.* 2013;(12):CD003523.

172. Suriya-amarit D, Gaogasigam C, Siriphorn A, et al. Effect of interferential current stimulation in management of hemiplegic shoulder pain. *Arch Phys Med Rehabil.* 2014;95:1441–1446.

173. Grabianska E, Lesniewicz J, Pieszynski I, et al. [Comparison of the analgesic effect of interferential current (IFC) and TENS in patients with low back pain]. *Wiad Lek.* 2015;68:13–19.

174. Smart KM, Wand BM, O'Connell NE. Physiotherapy for pain and disability in adults with complex regional pain syndrome (CRPS) types I and II. *Cochrane Database Syst Rev.* 2016;(2):CD010853.

175. Ford KS, Shrader MW, Smith J, et al. Full-thickness burn formation after the use of electrical stimulation for rehabilitation of unicompartmental knee arthroplasty. *J Arthroplasty.* 2005;20:950–953.

176. World Health Organization. *What are Electromagnetic Fields?* Available from: http://www.who.int/peh-emf/about/WhatisEMF/en/index1.html

177. Gabriel DA, Basford JR, An K-N. Vibratory facilitation of strength in fatigued muscle. *Arch Phys Med Rehabil.* 2002;83:1202–1205.

178. Leduc A, Lievens P, Dewald J. The influence of multi-directional vibrations on wound healing and on regeneration of blood and lymph vessels. *Lymphology.* 1981;14:179–185.

179. Sitjà Rabert M, Rigau Comas D, Fort Vanmeerhaeghe A, et al. Whole-body vibration training for patients with neurodegenerative disease. *Cochrane Database Syst Rev.* 2012;(2):CD009097.

180. Sucuoglu H, Tuzun S, Akbaba YA, et al. Effect of whole-body vibration on balance using posturography and balance tests in postmenopausal women. *Am J Phys Med Rehabil.* 2015;94:499–507.

181. Zafar H, Alghadir A, Anwer S, et al. Therapeutic effects of whole-body vibration training in knee osteoarthritis: a systematic review and meta-analysis. *Arch Phys Med Rehabil.* 2015;96:1525–1532.

182. Santin-Medeiros F, Rey-López JP, Santos-Lozano A, et al. Effects of eight months of whole-body vibration training on the muscle mass and functional capacity of elderly women. *J Strength Cond Res.* 2015;29:1863–1869.

183. Anders JJ, Lanzafame RJ, Arany PR. Low-level light/laser therapy versus photobio-modulation therapy. *Photomed Laser Surg.* 2015;33:183–184.

184. Mester E, Spiry T, Szende B, et al. Effect of laser rays on wound healing. *Am J Surg.* 1971;122:532–535.

185. Peplow PV, Chung TY, Baxter GD. Laser photobiomodulation of wound healing: a review of experimental studies in mouse and rat animal models. *Photomed Laser Surg.* 2010;28:291–325.

186. Peplow PV, Chung TY, Ryan B, et al. Laser photobiomodulation of gene expression and release of growth factors and cytokines from cells in culture: a review of human and animal studies. *Photomed Laser Surg.* 2001;29:285–304.

187. Jain TK, Sharma NK. The effectiveness of physiotherapeutic interventions in treatment of frozen shoulder/adhesive capsulitis: a systematic review. *J Back Musculoskelet Rehabil.* 2014;27:247–273.

188. Dingemanse R, Randsdorp M, Koes BW, et al. Evidence for the effectiveness of electrophysical modalities for treatment of medial and lateral epicondylitis: a systematic review. *Br J Sports Med.* 2014;48:957–965.

189. Gur A. Physical therapy modalities in management of fibromyalgia. *Curr Pharm Des.* 2006;12:29–35.

190. Esmaeeli Djavid G, Mehrdad R, Ghasemi M, et al. In chronic low back pain, low level laser therapy combined with exercise is more beneficial than exercise alone in the long term: a randomised trial. *Aust J Physiother.* 2007;53:155–160.

191. Bjordal JM. Low level laser therapy (LLLT) and World Association for Laser Therapy (WALT) dosage recommendations. *Photomed Laser Surg.* 2012;30:61–62.

192. Tumilty S, Munn J, McDonough S, et al. Low level laser treatment of tendinopathy: a systematic review with meta-analysis. *Photomed Laser Surg.* 2010;28:3–16.

193. Manca A, Limonta E, Pilurzi G, et al. Ultrasound and laser as stand-alone therapies for myofascial trigger points: a randomized, double-blind, placebo-controlled study. *Physiother Res Int.* 2014;19:166–175.

194. Collacott EA, Zimmerman JT, White DW, et al. Bipolar permanent magnets for the treatment of chronic low back pain. A pilot study. *JAMA.* 2000;283:1322–1325.

195. Kaiser J. Panel finds EMFs post no threat. *Science.* 1996;274:910.

196. IARC classification of static and extremely low frequency electric and magnetic fields. *J Radiol Prot.* 2001;21:313–314.

197. Hartwig V. Engineering for safety assurance in MRI: analytical, numerical and experimental dosimetry. *Magn Reson Imaging.* 2015;33:681–689.

198. Kangarlu A, Burgess RE, Zhu H, et al. Cognitive, cardiac, and physiological safety studies in ultra high field magnetic resonance imaging. *Magn Reson Imaging.* 1999;17:1407–1416.

199. Goldgrub R, Côté P, Sutton D, et al. The effectiveness of multimodal care for the management of soft tissue injuries of the shoulder: a systematic review by the Ontario Protocol for Traffic Injury Management (OPTIMa) collaboration. *J Manipulative Physiol Ther.* 2016;39:121–139.

200. Saggini R, Di Stefano A, Saggini A, et al. Clinical application of shock wave therapy in musculoskeletal disorders: part II related to myofascial and nerve apparatus. *J Biol Regul Homeost Agents.* 2015;29:771–785.

201. Rompe JD, Furia J, Cacchio A, et al. Radial shock wave treatment alone is less efficient than radial shock wave treatment combined with tissue-specific plantar fascia-stretching in patients with chronic plantar heel pain. *Int J Surg.* 2015;24:135–142.

CHAPTER 52

Todd P. Stitik
Vivan P. Shah
Harmeet S. Dhani

Nourma Sajid
Shruti Amin
Patrick J. Bachoura

Pharmacotherapy of Disability

See 📶 **eTable 52-1** for abbreviations

ANALGESIC MEDICATIONS

Acetaminophen (Tylenol)

Relevance to Physiatry

Although acetaminophen is unsatisfactory as a single agent for patients requiring significant analgesic, it can be an effective primary or adjuvant medication for pain of mild to moderate intensity. In particular, it is considered to be the initial medication of choice for patients with osteoarthritis of the knee or hip who present without obvious signs of inflammation (1). Acetaminophen is also an alternative for some patients who experience gastrointestinal (GI) side effects with nonsteroidal anti-inflammatory drugs (NSAIDs) or celecoxib or who are at particular risk for renal toxicity associated with these agents. In addition, it is often used in combination with both opioid and nonopioid analgesics so as to decrease potential side effects (and thereby lessen interference with a rehabilitation program) by lowering the dose requirement of these other medications. In contrast to aspirin, it is often used in the pediatric rehabilitation setting due to the lack of an association with Reye's syndrome.

Other potential uses for acetaminophen include headaches for which it can be used as a single agent or as a combination product with various narcotic analgesics, as well as with butalbital and caffeine (i.e., Fioricet or Esgic). Acetaminophen is also the primary agent used to suppress fever in the inpatient rehabilitation setting.

Acetaminophen has negligible anti-inflammatory effects; it therefore cannot be substituted for anti-inflammatory agents when treating conditions associated with significant inflammation such as rheumatoid arthritis.

Due to the potential for chronic acetaminophen overdosage leading to hepatotoxicity, patients must be counseled to not exceed dosage limitations when taking scheduled doses of acetaminophen. Patients also might not realize that over-the-counter (OTC) headache or cold/flu remedies often contain acetaminophen and this can lead to inadvertent overdosage if they are also prescribed acetaminophen either in the form of Tylenol or in combination with analgesic medications.

Mechanism of Action and Pharmacokinetics

Despite clinical use of acetaminophen for over 120 years, its exact mechanism of action remains under investigation. Studies have confirmed a pathway whereby acetaminophen decreases production of prostaglandins by reducing prostaglandin H_2 synthase, a COX (2). This mechanism is notably distinct from NSAIDs, which physically block arachidonic acid from accessing COX enzyme's active site, and is hypothesized to explain its diminished action at anti-inflammatory sites—where the activated immune system produces oxidizing agents that can reverse the reduction step.

Acetaminophen is rapidly and almost completely absorbed from the upper GI tract. It is then uniformly distributed throughout the body, partly bound by plasma proteins, while the unbound portion exerts the therapeutic effects. Acetaminophen can penetrate both the placenta and blood-brain barrier (3). It is rapidly metabolized in the liver and excreted by the kidneys at its recommended dosage.

When ingesting subtherapeutic levels of acetaminophen, hepatic stores of glucuronide and sulfate are depleted, resulting in an increased formation of the toxic metabolite N-acetyl-para-benzoquinoneimine (NAPQI). NAPQI is normally detoxified by glutathione. Insufficient glutathione results in excess NAPQI, leading to cellular necrosis of the liver. Administration of N-acetylcysteine offers reduction in toxicity by regenerating glutathione stores. Acute overdose leading to hepatic toxicity is less common in young children than in older children and adults. This may be because there is either decreased metabolism of acetaminophen throughout the CYP450 system or an increased ability to synthesize glutathione (4,5).

Preparations and Dosing

Acetaminophen is administered orally, rectally, or intravenously. The brand name Tylenol is frequently used interchangeably with the generic term acetaminophen. There are three major oral Tylenol preparations, and they are shown in **Table 52-1**, which lists the dosing regimens that would provide a maximum dose of 2 g per 24 hours for those patients with normal hepatic function. For those with abnormal liver function, specific dosing information should be consulted prior to prescribing.

Relevant Side Effects and Drug Interactions

Acetaminophen has an extremely favorable side effect profile when used within recommended dosage limitations (6). In those with normal hepatic function, the maximum daily recommended dose is 2 g/d. Precaution must be taken when it is used:

1. Chronically in excess of the recommended dose
2. At more than approximately 2 g/d in patients who consume excessive amounts of alcohol (defined as more than 3 alcoholic drinks per day)
3. When taken as a single dose in excess of approximately 15 g.

Fatalities in children due to accidental overdose were reported, and OTC cold medicines in the United States were subsequently withdrawn for children under 2 years of age.

TABLE 52-1	Acetaminophen Preparations and Dosing for Adults	
Tylenol Formulation	**Acetaminophen Content**	**Dose (Maximum No. of Units)**
Tylenol	325 mg	1 tab q4h
Extra Strength Tylenol (ES-Tylenol)	500 mg	1 tab q6h or 1 tab q6h
Tylenol Arthritis	650 mg	1 tab PO q8h

Acetaminophen is metabolized into an intermediate, *N*-acetyl-benzoquinoneimine, that accumulates and may cause fatal hepatic necrosis (7). While the liver is the primary target of toxicity, chronic use of acetaminophen is also associated with renal failure (8). However, aside from cases of overdosage, acute nephrotoxic effects of acetaminophen are not common in the nonalcoholic population (9). The National Kidney Foundation, for this reason, has not amended its 1996 recommendation, making acetaminophen the drug of choice for analgesia in those with renal dysfunction (10).

Acetaminophen has a very favorable medication interaction profile. One potentially important exception, however, is warfarin as large acetaminophen doses can potentiate its effect by prolonging its half-life (11). Although this is believed to only be clinically significant in patients with a relatively high international normalized ratio (INR), the INR should be monitored in patients who are chronically taking acetaminophen while also on warfarin (12). To reduce the risk of liver damage and hypersensitivity reactions, the U.S. Food and Drug Administration (FDA) has recommended to discontinue prescribing combination prescription medications containing more than 325 mg of acetaminophen per dosage unit (5).

Antidepressants

Relevance to Physiatry

Because depression is a common consequence of illnesses and injuries, particularly if they are associated with functional loss, physiatrists should familiarize themselves with this medication class. Antidepressants are also used off-label to treat chronic nonmalignant pain syndromes and neuropathic pain (13–15). Not only do these agents treat the psychiatric component of chronic pain, but there is also evidence that they have independent analgesic effects (16,17). This chapter will specifically address their use as analgesics.

Analgesic action of tricyclic antidepressant (TCA) medications for neuropathic pain has been extensively studied. Secondary amine TCAs, nortriptyline and desipramine, are preferred over tertiary amine TCAs (e.g., amitriptyline) because they have been shown to be equally effective and have fewer side effects (e.g., drowsiness) (18,19). Another TCA, doxepin has shown some efficacy as a topical analgesic in managing chronic neuropathic pain (20).

The selective serotonin reuptake inhibitor (SSRI) class of antidepressants is hypothesized to affect brain stem pain-modulating systems. Initial interest in using this class of medication for analgesia developed from a few promising case reports. The evidence for the ability of SSRIs in the treatment of neuropathic pain is modest at best. Serotonin-norepinephrine reuptake inhibitors (SNRIs), such as venlafaxine and duloxetine,

have been shown to be efficient in the treatment of painful diabetic neuropathy and polyneuropathy. For the treatment of fibromyalgia, both SSRIs (fluoxetine and paroxetine) and SNRIs (duloxetine and milnacipran) have been shown to provide pain relief and improve quality of life (21).

The SNRIs have been replacing SSRIs for neuropathic pain conditions. Venlafaxine (Effexor) and duloxetine (Cymbalta) are two SNRIs that have been studied in the treatment of pain due to postherpetic neuralgia (PHN) and diabetic neuropathy. Duloxetine is currently approved for the treatment of pain due to diabetic neuropathy and chronic musculoskeletal pain such as osteoarthritic pain, while venlafaxine was found to be as effective as imipramine in the treatment of pain due to polyneuropathy (22,23).

The popularity of SNRIs is also vested in their cost-effectiveness and more favorable side effect profiles (24). However, there are reports of withdrawal associated with discontinuation of duloxetine (25).

The serotonin reuptake mechanism is not only present in neurons but also notable in cells such as platelets. SSRIs have a remarkable effect on homeostasis dependant on an inverse relationship of serotonin concentration. Abnormal activation of platelets may lead to a prothrombotic state, as may occur in patients with major depressive disorder, that is, up-regulation of the 5-HTT. However, down-regulation of the 5-HTT, as occurs in patients treated with SSRIs, has two clinical consequences. This is especially in the elderly as there is both an increased risk of bleeding and a potential benefit with the reduction of thrombosis. There is no study at the time of this writing in the peer-reviewed literature in relation to the risk of upper GI bleeding and dose or duration of therapy, after the first few weeks of treatment, suggesting that at therapeutic drug levels, the bleeding risk is greatest and persistent. There is an increased risk of bleeding, associated with concomitant use of SSRIs with NSAIDs or low-dose aspirin (26). Other antidepressants that have been studied as analgesics include those (i.e., trazodone, bupropion, mirtazapine, and nefazodone) that do not fall into any one particular chemical class. Both of these have received somewhat less attention than the previous three classes of antidepressants but deserve further comment. There is some literature on the use of trazodone and bupropion in the treatment of pain. Trazodone is chemically unrelated to other antidepressants. It is rarely used for depression but is more commonly used as a hypnotic. Although there is some literature on it as an analgesic, a review of 59 randomized placebo-controlled trials of antidepressants as analgesics concluded that trazodone is not effective (27,28). A placebo-controlled cross-over trial confirmed that bupropion SR (sustained release, 150 to 300 mg daily) is effective and well tolerated in treating neuropathic pain (29). In contrast, it was found to be ineffective in treating nonneuropathic, chronic pain (30).

Mechanism of Action and Pharmacokinetics

TCAs increase aminergic transmission by inhibiting serotonin and norepinephrine reuptake to different degrees at presynaptic nerve ending terminals. For example, amitriptyline primarily inhibits serotonin reuptake, whereas nortriptyline primarily inhibits norepinephrine reuptake. As a result, TCAs elevate pain thresholds in depressed and nondepressed patients. Analgesic doses are usually lower than those for primary depression.

TCAs are well absorbed in the GI tract. These agents are rapidly absorbed and bind avidly to plasma albumin. Metabolism first involves demethylation of tertiary amine to secondary amine, followed by hydroxylation, glucuronidation, and eventual renal excretion as inactive metabolites. They are metabolized in the liver by the cytochrome P450 system. The CYP2D6 isoenzyme is of particular importance, since around 7% of the population have reduced activity of CYP2D6, therefore resulting in increased plasma concentrations of medications, including TCAs. Concomitant administration of the TCAs with medications that inhibit cytochrome P450 can cause clinically significant interactions (31).

SSRIs selectively inhibit serotonin reuptake, with less of an effect on norepinephrine reuptake. This selectivity offers the advantage of a superior side effect profile. End results include prolonged decreased production of serotonin and down-regulation of pre- and postsynaptic receptors. Paroxetine and sertraline are the most frequently used agents in this class, and both have a chemical structure that is unique among the SSRIs as well as other antidepressants. As a whole, this class is well absorbed orally and then undergoes hepatic metabolism followed by renal excretion.

Bupropion's mechanism of action is still uncertain, but evidence suggests that it inhibits dopamine and norepinephrine reuptake; its effect is greater on the former than the latter (32). Bupropion is hepatically metabolized into an active metabolite, 4-hydroxybupropion, which is excreted in the urine.

Trazodone possibly acts via serotonin reuptake inhibition and mixed serotonin agonist-antagonist effects. Although extensively metabolized in the liver, it has variable clearance that may lead to accumulation in some patients.

SNRIs act as norepinephrine inhibitors via α_2-adrenergic receptor blockade, serotonin reuptake inhibitors, and it bind to opioid receptors. This combined mechanism of action is somewhat similar to that of tramadol.

Preparations and Dosing

Dosage, side effects, and miscellaneous information about the most commonly used antidepressants for neuropathic and chronic pain are shown in **Table 52-2**.

Relevant Side Effects and Drug Interactions

Antidepressants in general are associated with a high incidence of sexual dysfunction that is often underreported in product literature (33), and all FDA-regulated antidepressants are associated with an increased risk of suicidal ideation and worsening of mood (34). Antidepressants that inhibit serotonin reuptake (e.g., SSRIs, SNRIs, trazodone) can cause "serotonin syndrome," a hyperexcitable state of nervousness and insomnia.

TCA side effects are mainly anticholinergic and include dry mouth, blurred vision, tachycardia, constipation, exacerbation of glaucoma, and urinary retention. They also cause antihistaminergic side effects such as sedation (therefore, they are often prescribed as a single bedtime dose) and weight gain, related to an increased appetite for carbohydrates. TCAs also exert some quinidine-like cardiac effects, including atrioventricular conduction time prolongation. It may be beneficial, to acquire a baseline EKG, to screen for long QT syndrome, prior to starting a TCA. In addition, if the patient has a history of an increased propensity for developing arrhythmia,

consideration should be given for choosing a non-TCA medication (35). Cognitive/behavioral alterations (e.g., agitation and memory impairment) appear at plasma TCA concentrations greater than 0.450 µg/mL (36); many TCAs, notably dothiepin, are fatal at concentrations greater than 1 µg/mL (37). Nortriptyline is generally considered superior to all TCAs because it is more potent and has a comparatively wide therapeutic range (38). Elderly and otherwise medically fragile patients should probably be started on nortriptyline rather than amitriptyline for the above reason and because side effects such as orthostatic hypotension and significant morning sedation, which can potentially interfere with rehabilitation efforts in this patient population, are relatively less common.

SSRIs, including fluoxetine and paroxetine, inhibit CYP2D6 activity and can cause elevated serum concentrations of TCAs and therefore increase the risk for TCA–related side effects. Decreased serum concentrations of TCAs may be caused by cigarette smoking, lithium, ascorbic acid, and barbiturates. Oral contraceptives may increase the activity of hepatic enzymes and decrease TCA serum concentrations. TCAs may also block the activity of antihypertensives (31).

Since SSRIs have a relatively specific effect on serotonin reuptake without a significant effect on norepinephrine reuptake, their side effect profile is generally superior to TCAs—especially with respect to cardiovascular issues—and they are much safer in cases of overdose. However, abrupt cessation of SSRI has been reported to cause SSRI discontinuation syndrome in some individuals. This syndrome includes dizziness, light-headedness, insomnia, fatigue, anxiety/agitation, nausea, headache, and sensory disturbance.

Bupropion has caused seizures and interference with cardiac conduction (ventricular arrhythmias and third-degree heart block). Idiosyncratic reactions including Stevens-Johnson syndrome, rhabdomyolysis, and severe hepatotoxicity have also been reported (37,39,40). Bupropion is a cytochrome P450-2D6 (CYP2D6) inhibitor (41). The sustained-release (SR) bupropion is generally better tolerated than the immediate-release (IR) form.

Trazodone can be quite sedating and possesses other mild anticholinergic effects, but these are generally less than those from TCAs. It also exhibits α-adrenergic blocking properties, which can cause penile or clitoral priapism (42).

TCAs, SSRIs, and bupropion should not be used in patients taking monoamine oxidase inhibitors (MAOIs) and should be instituted cautiously in patients who have been off MAOIs for at least 2 weeks. The only exception to this rule is nortriptyline, which can be safely combined with MAOIs or sertraline (an SSRI) (38). Concomitant use of other TCAs or any of SSRIs and MAOIs can cause hyperpyretic crises, seizures, and death. TCAs should also be used cautiously in patients taking other anticholinergic medications, neuroleptics, or central nervous (CNS) depressants.

It is not known whether interactions occur between trazodone and MAOIs. Trazodone may increase serum digoxin and phenytoin levels and can cause either an increase or a decrease in prothrombin times in patients on warfarin (43).

Venlafaxine's most common side effects not only are from increased serotonin levels (irritability, insomnia, and sexual dysfunction) but also include constipation and nausea. There are several case reports of false-positive phencyclidine (PCP) results from ingesting high dosage of venlafaxine (44,45).

TABLE 52-2	Antidepressants Used in the Treatment of Neuropathic Pain	
Generic Name	**Dose (mg) Neuropathic Pain and (Depression)**	**Miscellaneous**
[TCAs]		
Amitriptyline Elavil/Saroten/ Endep/Vanatrip	10–100 at H/S (150–300/d); begin at 12.5–25 qH/S, and titrated as tolerated	Dry mouth and sedation very common, long QT syndrome Demethylated to nortriptyline
Nortriptyline (Aventyl, Pamelor)	10–30 at H/S (50–150/d)	First metabolite of amitriptyline; less side effects but not as potent
Doxepin (Sinequan) topical	Topical application of 3.3% doxepin, 0.025% capsa-icin, and 3.3% doxepin/0.025% capsaicin produces analgesia of similar magnitude. The combination produces more rapid analgesia. Cream: 50 mg/g	Minor side effects
Desipramine (Norpramin)	Start 25–100 PO once daily or in divided doses increase to effective dose of 100–200 mg/d, MAX 300 mg/d (111 mg) used in studies	• Cardiovascular: decreases of blood pressure on rising from a sitting or lying position, which may cause dizziness or fainting; increases of blood pressure, rapid heart rate, pounding heart, altered heart rhythm • Nervous system: sedation, confusion, nervousness, rest-lessness, sleep difficulties, numbness, tingling sensations, tremors, increased seizure tendency • Autonomic: blurred vision, dry mouth, decreased sweating, difficulty urinating, constipation • Skin: rashes, sensitivity to sunlight • Body as a whole: weight gain
Imipramine (Tofranil)	Start 75 mg PO qhs. Increase to 150 mg PO qhs or in divided doses	Dry mouth, constipation, urinary retention, increased heart rate, sedation, irritability, dizziness, and decreased coordination
[SSRIs]		All SSRIs are associated with an increased risk of bleeding at therapeutic doses, especially if used in conjunction with NSAIDs
Citalopram (Celexa)	20–40 QD (20–60 QD)	Relatively short half-life
Fluoxetine		Very popular when first released; blamed by the press as a contributing factor to several high-profile murders
(Prozac)	20 QD (20–80 QD)	
(Prozac Weekly)	90 Qw of Prozac Q wk	
(Sarafem)	20–40 QD (20–60 QD) throughout menstrual cycle or 14 d prior to menses	
Fluvoxamine (Luvox)	100 QD (50–150 BID)	Least studied of the SSRIs for pain
Paroxetine (Paxil) (Pexeva)	20–50 QD (20–50 QD)	Most selective of the SSRIs
(Paxil CR)	25 mg PO qam MAX 62.5 mg/d	
Sertraline (Zoloft)	50–150 QD (50–200 QD)	Tablets and oral concentrate; serotonin syndrome (hypersero-tonergic state) with tramadol coadministration; also used for obsessive-compulsive disorder (OCD) and posttraumatic stress disorder (PTSD)
[Other antidepressants]		
Bupropion SR (Wellbutrin SR)	150–300 QD (100–450 QD)	SR formulation has a better side effect profile vs. IR prepara-tion, esp. for sexual dysfunction and seizures; also used for smoking cessation (Zyban)
Wellbutrin, Zyban, Buproban	Start 100 mg PO BID immediate-release tab increase to TID	
Wellbutrin XL	150–300 QD (100–450 QD)	
Trazodone (Desyrel)	Start 50–150 mg/d PO in divided doses; H/S (200–300 BID), usual effective dose is 400–600 mg/d	Priapism that can be severe; less anticholinergic side effects vs. TCAs
Mirtazapine (Remeron)	Initiate at 7.5 mg/d at bedtime and rapidly adjust upward to 30–45 mg/d to avoid subtherapeutic dose-related side effects	Side effects are sleepiness and nausea. Other common side effects are dizziness, increased appetite, and weight gain. Less common adverse effects include weakness and muscle aches, flulike symptoms, low blood cell counts, high cholesterol, back pain, chest pain, rapid heartbeats, dry mouth, constipation, water retention, difficulty sleep-ing, nightmares, abnormal thoughts, vision disturbances, ringing in the ears, abnormal taste in the mouth, tremor, confusion, upset stomach, and increased urination

Continued

TABLE 52.2	Antidepressants Used in the Treatment of Neuropathic Pain *(Continued)*	
Generic Name	**Dose (mg) Neuropathic Pain and (Depression)**	**Miscellaneous**
Remeron SolTab		
Nefazodone (Serzone)	50-, 100-, 150-, 200-, and 250-mg tablets. Initial dose of nefazodone is 100 mg taken by mouth twice daily. The dose may be increased in 100- or 200-mg increments once a week. Most commonly, final dosages range between 300 and 600 mg taken by mouth each day	Side effects: dizziness, difficulty sleeping, weakness, or agitation. Other common adverse effects are sleepiness, dry mouth, nausea, constipation, blurred vision, and confusion
[Antidepressants] SNRIs		
Venlafaxine (Effexor)	18.75–75 QD, divided BID or TID (37.5–75 divided BID or TID) 75 mg/d divided BID–TID MAX 375 mg/d 25, 37.5, 50, 75,100	An extended-release form (Effexor XR) is used for depression but not studied yet for pain
(Effexor XR)	(37.5–75 mg PO daily) MAX 225 mg/d Tabs: 37.5, 75, 150	
Duloxetine (Cymbalta)	Total dose of 40 mg/d (given as 20 mg BID) to 60 mg/d (given either once a day or 30 mg BID), no evidence that doses >60 mg/d confer any additional benefits	Side effects: Impaired thinking or reactions. Be careful if you drive or do anything that requires you to be awake and alert

Corticosteroids

Relevance to Physiatry

Anti-inflammatory effects of corticosteroids are usually more important to the physiatrist than their mineralocorticoid and androgenic/estrogenic effects. Physiatrists today are using corticosteroids for a range of injection procedures, including fluoroscopic-guided spinal injection procedures and peripheral joint injection procedures. They are also prescribing them in either short, tapering oral courses (e.g., Medrol Dosepak) for patients with radiculopathy and other localized musculoskeletal conditions or chronically for systemic inflammatory diseases. Besides their oral and injectable forms, corticosteroids can additionally be delivered transdermally by iontophoresis or phonophoresis and via inhaled and topical applications.

Mechanism of Action and Pharmacokinetics

There are three general categories of corticosteroids: glucocorticoids, sex steroids, and mineralocorticoids. The main topic this section will focus on is the glucocorticoid class. Glucocorticoids diffuse passively across the cellular membrane and bind to the intracellular glucocorticoid receptor. Binding of the drug to this receptor creates a complex, which then translocates into the nucleus, where it can interact directly with specific DNA sequences (glucocorticoid-responsive elements [GREs]) and other transcription factors (46). At physiologic but not pharmacologic doses, glucocorticosteroid exerts anti-inflammatory and immunosuppressive effects via the following mechanisms:

1. Inhibition of prostaglandin and leukotriene synthesis, occurs by preventing arachidonic acid release from phospholipids. This contrasts with NSAIDs and COX-II inhibitors, both of which act at a later step in prostaglandin synthesis via inhibition of COX isoenzymes.
2. Inhibition of chemotactic factor release, leading to a diminished attraction of white blood cells (i.e., neutrophil migration) to sites of inflammation. This prevents the release of inflammatory cytokines such as IL-1 and TNF-alpha.

3. Decrease in circulating lymphocytes and monocytes. This major mechanism of immunosuppression occurs through inhibition of nuclear factor kappa-light-chain-enhancer of activated B cells (NF-κB).
4. Stabilization of lysosomal membranes, which subsequently prevents the release of inflammatory mediators (e.g., histamine, bradykinin).

Oral glucocorticoids are hepatically metabolized and renally excreted at a rate proportional to the particular agent's water solubility. Hence, longer-acting glucocorticoids are less water soluble.

Preparations and Dosing

The two most commonly used oral steroid preparations in many physiatric practices are prednisone and methylprednisolone. The latter is often prescribed as Medrol Dosepak of 4-mg tabs, which provides an initial 24 mg of Medrol (equivalent to 30 mg of prednisone) and tapers to 0 mg over 7 days. The popularity of Dosepak comes from the fact that patients' instructions are conveniently printed on the package, and it eliminates the need for patients to count out a different set of pills each day. Potential drawbacks to Medrol Dosepak are its higher expense compared to generic prednisone and a limited peak dose of merely 30 mg of prednisone. Some physicians overcome the low peak dose by prescribing two Medrol Dosepak to be taken simultaneously.

Corticosteroid selection can be made on the basis of equivalent cortisone dose, relative anti-inflammatory potency, relative mineralocorticoid potency, and onset and duration of action (47,48) (**Table 52-3**). For comparison, physiologic steroid doses are equivalent to 30 mg/d of hydrocortisone (7.5 mg/d of prednisone), whereas stress doses are equivalent to 300 mg/d of hydrocortisone (75 mg/d of prednisone). General dosing guidelines have also been developed (**Tables 52-3** and **52-4**), but recent popularity of injectable corticosteroids has raised concern that there is a lack of uniform guidelines for treating intra-articular joint conditions (49).

| TABLE 52-3 | Corticosteroid Preparations | | | | |

Corticosteroid Generic (Trade) Name	Route	Equivalent Oral Dose (mg)	Relative Potencies: Anti-inflammatory (Mineralocorticoid)	Relative Duration
Betamethasone (Celestone)	PO/IM	0.6–0.75	20–30 (0)	Long
Cortisone (Cortone)	PO	25	0.8 (2)	Short
Dexamethasone (Decadron)	PO/IM/IV	0.75	20–30 (0)	Long
Hydrocortisone (Cortef, Solu-Cortef)	PO/IM/IV	20	1 (2)	Short
Methylprednisolone (Medrol, Medrol Dosepak, Solu-Medrol)	PO/IM/IV	4	5 (0)	Intermediate
Prednisolone (Hydeltra)	PO/IM/IV	5	4 (1)	Intermediate
Prednisone (Deltasone, Orasone)	PO	5	4 (1)	Intermediate
Triamcinolone (Aristocort, Kenacort, Kenalog)	PO/IM	4	5 (0)	Intermediate

Relevant Side Effects and Drug Interactions

Most side effects occur after prolonged administration, and many are simply manifestations of Cushing's syndrome as shown in eTable 52-2. Among these conditions, steroid myopathy and avascular necrosis are particularly pertinent to physiatry. Firstly, osteonecrosis, particularly of the femoral or humeral head, is a potentially devastating event that can be seen with chronic use of steroids. Physiatrists who routinely perform electrodiagnostic studies are likely to be familiar with the need to "rule out steroid myopathy." It has been traditionally taught that the injection frequency for a "series of steroid injections" (e.g., up to a series of 3 weekly or biweekly [i.e., once every 2 weeks]), that is, epidural steroid injections, be limited to no less than 3- to 4-month intervals to reduce the chance of steroid-related side effects.

Skin depigmentation and subcutaneous atrophy are dermatologic complications that can occur with corticosteroid injections but can be minimized by adding local anesthetic or normal saline vehicle into the injectate and flushing the needle of residual corticosteroid with saline or local anesthetic injection before removal from the skin. Skin changes from chronic oral corticosteroids can lead to pressure ulcers and easy bruising.

Acceleration of corticosteroid metabolism occurs with medications that induce hepatic microsomal enzymes, especially phenobarbital, phenytoin, carbamazepine, and rifampin. In contrast, corticosteroid potency is increased by NSAIDs and exogenous estrogens (50). Clinicians should consider discontinuing NSAIDs or switching to a COX-II inhibitor if concomitant corticosteroid use is needed as corticosteroids are risk factors for NSAID-induced GI bleeding.

Lastly, although not a true side effect, a potential problem with corticosteroids is that they mask forewarning inflammation of various disorders. Thus, there is a tendency for patients to overvalue temporary relief and ignore the underlying disorder. An example is a patient who has received a subacromial steroid injection and soon resumes repetitive overhead activities that initially led to impingement.

| TABLE 52-4 | Corticosteroid Dosing Guidelines |

- Use these only after a less toxic therapy has been ineffective or is not an alternative
- Use the smallest corticosteroid amount that can control symptoms
- Administer the corticosteroid locally rather than systemically whenever possible

Short-term Use: Dosing QD (preferably in the AM) is more convenient and causes less adrenal suppression than QID dosing at ¼ the total dose

Chronic Use: Dosing QOD is less likely to suppress adrenal function

- Do not use the term "steroids" because of this word's negative connotations.
  - Although the terms cortisone and prednisone may also have negative connotations, explain that osteoporosis and truncal obesity only occur with chronic use
- Forewarn patients that oral steroids typically cause a metallic taste

Adrenal suppression is likely for dose, potency, and duration
- Doses >100 mg hydrocortisone (25 mg prednisone) daily × 3 d
- Doses >30 mg hydrocortisone (7.5 mg prednisone) daily × 30 d

- Wean patients off over weeks or months if taking steroids for more than several weeks
- If unsure that patient has become adrenally suppressed, refer to endocrinologist for metyrapone or insulin tolerance testing. Recovery of adrenal function is variable

Corticosteroid Injections
- Can decrease chance of corticosteroid arthropathy with limit of 3/y; 20/lifetime
- Never inject directly into a tendon and avoid weight-bearing peritendinous injections (e.g., Achilles, patellar, posterior tibial) or risk tendon rupture

Membrane-Stabilizing Medications: Antiarrhythmics

Relevance to Physiatry

There are three circumstances under which a physiatrist might prescribe antiarrhythmics: first, in the inpatient rehabilitation setting, for a patient who needs ongoing treatment for existing cardiac conditions; second, for a patient with neuropathic pain that responds to off-label use of type I antiarrhythmics (i.e., mexiletine, tocainide, lidocaine, and phenytoin); and third, for a patient with myotonia-associated pain from certain neuromuscular disorders. Intravenous (IV) lidocaine, as an analgesic agent, will not be discussed in detail in this chapter because it is infrequently used other than as a predictive test for mexiletine treatment in highly specialized pain management clinics (49). In contrast, the low diagnostic sensitivity of IV lidocaine infusion renders the test inappropriate for definitive diagnosis of neuropathic pain (51).

The literature pertaining to oral antiarrhythmics for neuropathic pain is still limited to mexiletine because other oral analogues (e.g., flecainide and tocainide) have some potentially lethal adverse effects (52). It is noteworthy that, prior to tocainide's withdrawal from the US market over safety concerns, there were successful reports on using the agent as treatment for myotonic pain in paramyotonia congenita and Thomsen-Becker myotonia (53).

Earlier case reports and prospective studies suggested that mexiletine is efficacious and safe in various neuropathic pain states including pain from traumatic peripheral nerve damage, diabetic neuropathy, alcoholic neuropathy, phantom limb pain, multiple sclerosis complicated by painful dysesthesias, and thalamic pain syndrome (52,54–59). A 2005 systematic review of local anesthetics found mexiletine (at a median dose of 600 mg daily) to be "superior to placebo in relieving neuropathic pain and as effective as other analgesics used for this condition" (60). However, most of these studies were of relatively short duration, and fewer than 400 patients had been studied altogether (61).

Mechanism of Action and Pharmacokinetics

Type I antiarrhythmics (e.g., lidocaine, mexiletine, and tocainide) block Na$^+$ channels in nerve and muscle cell membranes with a subsequent reduction in the number of abnormal ectopic impulse generated by dysfunctional peripheral nerves. Lidocaine and oral analogues differ, in that the latter have low first-pass metabolism, which enhances their oral bioavailability.

Preparations and Dosing

Mexiletine is available in 150-, 200-, and 250-mg caplets. Neuropathic pain doses are lower (150 to 300 mg TID) than those used for arrhythmias (200 to 400 mg TID). It can be initiated as a 150-mg/d regimen, titrated weekly.

Relevant Side Effects and Drug Interactions

Mexiletine's potential side effects are acute in onset and can involve the GI, neurologic, and cardiovascular systems. One mexiletine study of experimentally induced pain found that analgesic dosing caused side effects at an average of 993 mg/d, whereas another study found negligible side effects at doses up to 900 mg/d (62). GI side effects include nausea, anorexia, and gastric irritation in up to 40% of patients. Another 10% of patients experience neurologic side effects similar to those of other class I antiarrhythmics, including dizziness, visual disturbances, anxiety in patients with history of anxiety disorder, tremor, and altered coordination. Individuals with abnormal cardiac conduction are also at risk of mexiletine-induced exacerbation; mexiletine is absolutely contraindicated in second- and third-degree heart block uncontrolled by a pacemaker. Patients in fact should obtain an EKG prior to starting this medication.

Mexiletine's pharmacologic disposition is susceptible to multiple alterations. For example, opioid analgesics, atropine, and antacids slow its absorption, while metoclopramide enhances it. Phenytoin, rifampin, and smoking increase its metabolism. Mexiletine, in turn, may significantly reduce the clearance of theophylline and caffeine (63).

Membrane-Stabilizing Medications: Anticonvulsants

Relevance to Physiatry

When anticonvulsants are used to treat neuropathic pain, they are generally referred to as membrane-stabilizing medications. Their initial use as antineuralgic drugs in the 1960s was derived merely from positive clinical observations. Similarities between neuropathic pain and epilepsy pathophysiology models might explain the efficacy of anticonvulsants in treating both conditions (64). As supportive evidence continues to accumulate, anticonvulsants have marked a new era in the treatment of pain.

Various anticonvulsants have yielded good results thus far. Specific drugs will be discussed individually as there are some significant differences among them with respect to side effects and mechanisms of action (**Tables 52-5** and **52-6**).

Gabapentin (Neurontin)

Relevance to Physiatry

Gabapentin remains among the first-line treatments for neuropathic pain. It has been shown to be as effective as TCAs and carbamazepine and has a highly favorable side effect profile and minimal drug interactions (65). Although evidence is lacking for its efficacy in acute pain states (66), there is evidence supporting its efficacy in treating painful diabetic neuropathy (61,67–69). Gabapentin was approved by the FDA in December 1993 as an adjunct medicine for partial seizures and later was approved in May 2002 for the treatment of PHN (70); in April 2011, the FDA approved gabapentin enacarbil extended-release tablets for the management of PHN in adults (71).

Based on a recent Cochrane review, only two conditions can be effectively treated with gabapentin, postherpetic neuralgia, and diabetic neuropathy. Cochrane review concluded that gabapentin was effective in providing pain relief in comparison with administration of placebo after performing searches for clinical trials where gabapentin was used to treat neuropathic pain. The review found that 5,633 participants had been involved in 37 studies of acceptable quality, where gabapentin provided 3 to 4 people out of 10 by reducing their pain by at least 50%, while with the placebo only 2 out of 10 people had this outcome (72). It has also been investigated for spasticity reduction in SCI patients (73,74).

TABLE 52-5		Anticonvulsant Efficacy and Pharmacokinetics in Neuropathic Pain	
Efficacy	**Medication**	**Specific Neuropathic Pain Uses**	**Pharmacokinetics**
Efficacious			
	Gabapentin (Neurontin)	Especially diabetic neuropathy and postherpetic neuralgia (FDA approved)	Not protein bound or metabolized; renal excretion
	Carbamazepine (Tegretol)	Trigeminal neuralgia (FDA approved), glossopharyngeal neuralgia, painful diabetic neuropathy, and postherpetic neuralgia	Binds and prolongs inactivation of voltage-dependent sodium channels. The number of action potentials is consequently decreased. Highly plasma protein-bound, variable $t_{1/2}$ as it induces its own metabolism
	Pregabalin (Lyrica)	FDA approved in treating diabetic neuropathy pain, postherpetic neuralgia pain. Used off-label for other neuropathic pain conditions. There is mounting evidence that it can help to manage pain due to fibromyalgia	Does not bind to plasma proteins and nearly the entire dose is excreted unchanged in the urine, with elimination following first-order kinetics
Unclear			
	Clonazepam (Klonopin)	Some efficacy in trigeminal neuralgia	Good absorption; highly plasma protein bound, lipid soluble and hepatically metabolized
	Lamotrigine (Lamictal)	Primarily indicated in treatment for epilepsy and bipolar disorder. Provides minimal, if any, therapeutic effects in acute and chronic pain. Some efficacy in trigeminal neuralgia; peripheral neuropathy poststroke syndromes	Good oral absorption; hepatic conjugation; renal excretion
	Oxcarbazepine (Trileptal)	Efficacy in newly diagnosed and refractory trigeminal neuralgia and possible merit in areas of neuropathic pain and bipolar disorder and other neuropathic pain conditions	Hepatically metabolized to its active metabolite; renal excretion
	Phenobarbital (Solfoton)	No clinical studies in humans in peer-reviewed literature	Moderate protein binding; hepatic metabolism; pH-dependent renal excretion
	Phenytoin (Dilantin)	Conflicting results in trigeminal neuralgia and diabetic neuropathy	Metabolism saturable at high plasma levels, thus large concentration increases from additional small doses
	Tiagabine (Gabitril)	Two small trials showed beneficial outcome in painful sensory neuropathy	Highly protein bound; at least two metabolic pathways
	Topiramate (Topamax)	Conflicting results in studies of neuropathic pain and diabetic neuropathy. Some evidence in refractory intercostal neuralgia, trigeminal neuralgia, and trigeminal autonomic cephalgias	Rapidly absorbed orally, a third of the drug is metabolized by the hepatic CYP450 system into inactive metabolites, remainder excreted renally unchanged
	Valproate (valproic acid, Depakene)	Efficacy in neuropathic cancer pain but not paraplegia central pain. Mixed results in neuropathic pain, postherpetic neuralgia, and polyneuropathy	A lipid-soluble compound, rapidly absorbed, and becomes tightly protein bound. Metabolized in the liver through oxidation and glucuronidation pathways. Active metabolites and a small, unchanged portion are renally eliminated
	Zonisamide (Zonegran)	Studies in neuropathic pain are lacking	Renally excreted intact and as a glucuronide metabolite

Mechanism of Action and Pharmacokinetics

See **Tables 52-5** and **52-6**.

Gabapentin's mechanism of action is by which gabapentin exerts its anticonvulsant activity is not known; however, it does not seem to be related to its structure as a gamma-aminobutyric acid (GABA) analogue. Studies have shown that gabapentin does not act at GABA receptors. It was originally thought to inhibit GABA receptors because of its structural similarity to GABA, a major CNS excitatory neurotransmitter. Gabapentin acts on the α_2-δ subunit of the voltage-gated calcium channels, inhibiting calcium influx, which then indirectly reduces the release of substance P and glutamate and thereby reducing pain (75).

Gabapentin is transported from the GI tract into the bloodstream by the amino acid transport system. It does not bind to

TABLE 52-6	Proposed Mechanism of Action of Anticonvulsants in Neuropathic Pain
Proposed Mechanism	**Medications**
Na$^+$ channel blocker	Carbamazepine; lamotrigine; oxcarbazepine; phenytoin; valproate; zonisamide
Ca^{2+} channel blocker	Gabapentin; oxcarbazepine; zonisamide
GABA receptor activity	Barbiturates; benzodiazepines
GABA metabolism	Gabapentin; tiagabine; valproate
Glutamate receptor activity	Carbamazepine; lamotrigine; topiramate
Glutamate metabolism	Gabapentin

plasma protein, is not metabolized, and ultimately is excreted by the kidneys at the rate of creatinine clearance, which can mean that gabapentin has an elimination half-life of 5 to 7 hours (76).

Gabapentin enacarbil has a different metabolism in comparison with gabapentin (Neurontin). Gabapentin enacarbil is primarily absorbed in the intestine through numerous pathways, particularly through the monocarboxylate transporter type-1 (MCT-1). After absorption through the gut, gabapentin enacarbil is then metabolized to gabapentin. Gabapentin is a substrate to a transporter in the kidney, organic cation transporter type-2 (OCT); the drug is then excreted renally (77).

Preparations and Dosing

The reported dosage that provides adequate relief from neuropathic pain ranges from 900 to 2,400 mg/d, divided TID. When initiating therapy, a 300-mg dose given at bedtime on the 1st day, then BID dosing on the 2nd day, and TID dosing thereafter can be used as a way to help patients accommodate its CNS depressive effects. A maximum of 3,600-mg daily dose has been well-tolerated in some patients.

Relevant Side Effects and Drug Interactions

CNS depression (e.g., somnolence, dizziness, ataxia, and fatigue) is the main side effect. Nystagmus has also been reported. Side effects are generally transient with resolution in 2 weeks. There have been only rare reports of adverse events (e.g., rash, leukopenia, increased blood urea nitrogen (BUN), thrombocytopenia, and nonlethal ECG abnormalities) that required its discontinuation. Although larger studies are needed to provide substantiated evidence, the following are possible adverse effects of gabapentin: visual field defects, risks of misuse, myopathy, self-harm, and suicidal behavior. The risks of misuse of gabapentin have been associated with prison populations and simultaneous recreational drug use in various but limited studies, even though a strong correlation is present between concomitant opioid and gabapentin abuse (78).

Gabapentin may act synergistically with numerous medications. Frequent morphine administration with intrathecal injections along with gabapentin potentiates an antinociceptive response (79). With the same reasoning, gabapentin may also potentiate methadone and alleviate opioid withdrawal symptoms (78).

Cimetidine minimally decreases renal gabapentin excretion, since both drugs are substrates to OCT2. Gabapentin enacarbil if given with naproxen would increase gabapentin drug concentration by 8% on average. There is no need for dose adjustment with coadministration of naproxen or cimetidine with gabapentin enacarbil, due to the associated pharmacokinetics (77).

Carbamazepine (Tegretol)

Relevance to Physiatry

Carbamazepine was the first anticonvulsant to be studied in neuropathic pain clinical trials. Results from these trials confirmed its indication in treating trigeminal neuralgia (FDA approved), glossopharyngeal neuralgia, painful diabetic neuropathy, and PHN. It has not been as extensively studied in other neuropathic conditions. Traditional belief is that carbamazepine is especially effective for neuropathic pain that is acute and lancinating, as is often found in postamputation neuroma.

Its relative lack of CNS side effects compared to other anticonvulsants offers an obvious advantage with respect to functional activities. The unfortunate combination of potential hematologic toxicity, the need for periodic laboratory monitoring, baseline and periodic eye examinations, and numerous medication interactions limit carbamazepine's usefulness.

Mechanism of Action and Pharmacokinetics

See **Tables 52-5** and **52-6**.

Carbamazepine binds and prolongs inactivation of voltage-dependent sodium channels. The number of action potentials is consequently decreased.

Because of its high lipid solubility, it is slowly absorbed into the body following oral administration and becomes highly protein bound. It induces the hepatic CYP450 enzymes, and this increases the metabolism of multiple medications—including its own.

Preparations and Dosing

Carbamazepine is available in tablets, chewable tablets, extended-release capsules, syrup, suspensions, and rectal suppository preparations. Although there are no dosing guidelines for trigeminal neuralgia, it is commonly used to treat this condition with 100 mg BID initially, and then, the dose is gradually increased to a maximum of 400 mg TID. Given the potential for hematologic toxicity, the maintenance dose should be reduced to the minimum effective level. The extended-release form, Tegretol-XR can be given BID to achieve the same total daily doses as described above.

Relevant Side Effects and Drug Interactions

Severe toxicity can occur with carbamazepine including leukopenia and thrombocytopenia, aplastic anemia and agranulocytosis (rare), hepatotoxicity, skin reactions (e.g., Stevens-Johnson syndrome and toxic epidermal necrolysis), and (80), to a lesser degree, renal dysfunction. Prior to initiating carbamazepine, a complete blood count (CBC), liver function tests (LFTs), BUN and urinalysis, reticulocyte count, and serum iron levels are recommended. CBC and LFTs should be reviewed periodically, and if toxicity is suspected, consideration should be given for medication discontinuation.

Due to the pharmacokinetics described previously, carbamazepine interacts with many medications (eTable 52-3). In addition, it should neither be given to individuals with TCA hypersensitivity due to potential cross-reactivity, nor should it be used within 2 weeks of an MAOI.

Clonazepam (Klonopin)

Relevance to Physiatry

This benzodiazepine has been used to provide relief in neuropathic pain states (especially in patients with trigeminal neuralgia who are either intolerant to or have failed carbamazepine, baclofen, or phenytoin) and movement disorders (e.g., sleep-related nocturnal myoclonus, restless legs syndrome, tardive dyskinesia, phantom limb pain, and opioid-related myoclonic jerks).

Mechanism of Action and Pharmacokinetics

See **Tables 52-5** and **52-6**.

Clonazepam is avidly bound to plasma protein and highly lipid soluble. It is acetylated into nonactive metabolites in the liver and gradually excreted by the kidneys. Low level of metabolites is also excreted in breast milk. In spite of this, there have not been reports of adverse outcome in newborns; lactation is therefore not a contraindication (81).

Preparations and Dosing

Clonazepam is available as 0.5-, 1-, and 2-mg tablets. Brand name tablets distinguish themselves with a unique K-shaped perforation in the middle of the pill. For movement disorders, clonazepam is begun at either 0.5 mg at bedtime or 0.5 mg TID, and it can be titrated up to 2 mg TID. A daily dose of 0.5 to 1.0 mg is recommended to treat trigeminal neuralgia (82).

Relevant Side Effects and Drug Interactions

Ataxia and personality changes can develop early in the treatment course but may subside with long-term use. At the other end of the spectrum, withdrawal often causes a flulike syndrome, and abrupt discontinuation of a chronic, high-dose regimen can even lead to seizures. Moreover, common to all benzodiazepines, chronic clonazepam use can result in psychological addiction and physical tolerance. Caution should be exercised when clonazepam is given along with another CNS depressant.

Lamotrigine (Lamictal, Lamictal Cd)

Relevance to Physiatry

Lamotrigine is primarily indicated as a treatment for epilepsy and bipolar disorder. Multiple, well-designed clinical trials have investigated its efficacy in neuropathic pain, but a systematic review concluded that lamotrigine provides minimal, if any, therapeutic effects in acute and chronic pain (83). In addition, potentially fatal skin reactions including Stevens-Johnson syndrome and toxic epidermal necrolysis have been reported.

Oxcarbazepine (Trileptal)

Relevance to Physiatry

Oxcarbazepine is a structural analogue of carbamazepine. It has been used in the treatment of epilepsy since 1990. There is convincing evidence of its efficacy in newly diagnosed and refractory trigeminal neuralgia (84). In addition, it has emerging merit in areas of neuropathic pain and bipolar disorder (85).

Mechanism of Action and Pharmacokinetics

See **Tables 52-5** and **52-6**.

Liver microsomes metabolize oxcarbazepine into an active metabolite, 10-monohydroxy metabolite (MHD), which exerts the desired pharmacologic effects. This process minimally induces hepatic CYP450 enzymes. MHD is excreted by the kidneys.

Preparations and Dosing

Oxcarbazepine is available as 150-, 300-, and 600-mg scored tablets and as a 60 mg/mL suspension. Rapid titration (over 7 to 10 days) from the initial dose (ranging from 75 to 300 mg BID) to a maximum of 1,200 mg BID is recommended. Therapeutic range for trigeminal neuralgia extends from 600 to 1,800 mg/d.

Relevant Side Effects and Drug Interactions

Although a carbamazepine analogue, oxcarbazepine is not associated with serious hematologic toxicity. CNS and GI disturbances are instead reported; between 20% and 25% of patients discontinue oxcarbazepine due to its side effects.

The coadministration of felodipine/calcium channel blockers (CaCBs) and/or oral contraceptives should be avoided. The specific mechanism is undetermined, but the CaCB verapamil is known to decrease oxcarbazepine concentration by 20%, and oxcarbazepine, in turn, decreases CaCB felodipine concentration by 30%. As for contraceptives, oxcarbazepine stimulates their metabolism and, in effect, diminishes their efficacy (86). Antiepileptic drug (AED) coadministration, a regular practice in the setting of epilepsy but not neuropathic pain, also warrants caution because CYP450 enzyme inducers (e.g., carbamazepine, phenobarbital, and phenytoin) decrease mean plasma oxcarbazepine concentrations by 40%.

Phenobarbital (Luminal, Solfoton)

There is limited evidence for the effectiveness of phenobarbital in pain management (87). As is true of all barbiturates, human neuropathic pain studies are lacking, and sedative properties limit their usage. Phenobarbital thus has a very limited role in neuropathic pain management.

Phenytoin (Dilantin)

Relevance to Physiatry

Besides its well-known anticonvulsant use, phenytoin is also used off-label as a neuropathic pain agent. It was the first anticonvulsant used as an antinociceptive agent and was confirmed (via controlled clinical trials) to be effective in managing trigeminal neuralgia and diabetic neuropathy more than 25 years ago. Clinical trials have ironically shown conflicting evidence (88). In addition to this ambiguity, there is a significant potential for medication interactions. In contrast, phenytoin offers the advantage of relative low cost and once a day dosing.

Mechanism of Action and Pharmacokinetics

See **Tables 52-5** and **52-6**.

Oral absorption of phenytoin in the stomach is slow because it is weakly acidic. The drug is mainly bound to plasma proteins, and it readily traverses the blood-brain barrier. The liver hydroxylates phenytoin into nonactive metabolites, which are excreted by the kidneys; this metabolic pathway is progressively saturated as the concentration of phenytoin increases.

Preparations and Dosing

Phenytoin is available as tablets, extended-release capsules, chewable tablets, injectable solution, and oral suspension. Neuropathic pain doses are often less than those used for seizures, but a specific therapeutic range has not yet been defined. Given the complex pharmacokinetics, it is important to monitor serum phenytoin levels because small increases in the dose can produce unexpectedly large increase in plasma concentrations.

Relevant Side Effects and Drug Interactions

Side effects can be classified into three different categories: dose-related toxic effects, true side effects, and idiosyncratic reactions:

- *Dose-related toxic effects* generally occur between plasma levels of 20 and 40 µg/mL, but there is marked individual variation. The effects include sedation, ataxia, and nystagmus. Ingesting high doses over a prolonged period can result in painful peripheral neuropathy.

- *True side effects* from long-term use include hirsutism, osteomalacia and hypocalcemia (secondary to interference with vitamin D metabolism), megaloblastic anemia (secondary to interference with vitamin B12 metabolism), and gingival hyperplasia (secondary to interference with fibroblastic activity).
- *Idiosyncratic reactions* include blood dyscrasias and a rare clinical picture, which resembles malignant lymphoma.

Phenytoin should not be prescribed to pregnant women as there are conflicting reports on its teratogenic effects, including the fetal hydantoin syndrome. Cerebellar ataxia can occur at seizure management doses and may interfere with rehabilitation efforts.

Pregabalin (Lyrica)

Relevance to Physiatry

A second analogue of GABA, pregabalin, is FDA approved for use in treating diabetic neuropathic pain, PHN pain, partial seizures, fibromyalgia, and spinal cord injury–associated neuropathic pain. It is also being used off-label for other neuropathic pain conditions. Furthermore, there is mounting evidence that this potent "sibling" of gabapentin can help to manage anxiety symptoms of anxiety disorder (89–91).

Mechanism of Action and Pharmacokinetics

Based on its structure, pregabalin is expected to be a calcium channel blocker (92). However, it is also theorized to have other mechanisms of action, including modulating the release of various neurotransmitters (i.e., glutamate, noradrenaline, and substance P) (93) to produce its net inhibitory effect on neurons.

Pregabalin has an oral bioavailability of greater than 90%. Concomitant food intake reduces the absorption rate but the total amount absorbed remains constant. Pregabalin does not bind to plasma proteins, and nearly the entire dose is excreted unchanged in the urine, with elimination following first-order kinetics.

Preparations and Dosing

Pregabalin is available as capsules in the following strengths: 25, 50, 75, 100, 150, 200, 225, and 300 mg. For the treatment of painful diabetic neuropathy, it is generally started at 50 mg TID for 1 week and then increased to a maximum of 1,000 mg TID. Therapeutic level of pregabalin for PHN can be achieved with an initial dose of 75 mg BID or 50 mg TID and increased to 150 mg BID or 100 mg TID after 1 week; the maximum dose for this purpose is 600 mg/d.

Relevant Side Effects and Drug Interactions

Dizziness, somnolence, and dry mouth have been frequently reported (94). Complaints of headache, weight gain, edema, blurred vision, and difficulty in concentration are also sometimes reported. Pregabalin is classified as a Schedule V controlled substance because it leads to euphoria in selected individuals (95). As it is true for gabapentin, pregabalin has no known drug interactions.

Tiagabine (Gabitril)

Relevance to Physiatry

Tiagabine became available at the turn of the century. Although it demonstrated antihyperalgesic and antinociceptive activity for neuropathic pain in animal models, placebo-controlled trial data are lacking; there are only two small clinical trials to date

documenting its beneficial outcome (96–98). New research also proposes that tiagabine is indicated for Stiff man syndrome, bruxism, and tonic spasms in multiple sclerosis; however, more studies are needed to draw definite conclusions (99–101).

Mechanism of Action and Pharmacokinetics

See **Tables 52-5** and **52-6**.

Tiagabine is well absorbed orally; concomitant consumption of food decreases the absorption rate but the fraction absorbed remains constant. It is highly bound to plasma proteins. Metabolism of tiagabine involves oxidation and glucuronidation. Both pathways produce inactive metabolites, which are excreted by the biliary system (major) and the kidneys (minor).

Preparations and Dosing

Tiagabine is available in multiple strength tablets (2, 4, 12, 16, and 20 mg). Its neuropathic pain dosing schedule has not been established. The two published clinical trials investigated its efficacy in the range from 4 to 24 mg daily. When used as an anticonvulsant however, it should be initiated at 4 mg every day and then increased to 8 mg at the beginning of week 2 and increased by 4 to 8 mg at weekly intervals thereafter, until clinical response is achieved or up to 32 mg/d.

Relevant Side Effects and Drug Interactions

Side effects are mild. CNS and GI disturbances (e.g., tiredness, somnolence, nausea, and abdominal pain) are the primary reasons that participants withdraw from tiagabine-related clinical trials. Tiagabine is also free of significant drug interactions.

Topiramate (Topamax)

Relevance to Physiatry

Structurally derived from D-fructose, topiramate is FDA approved for seizure management and migraine prophylaxis but is also used off-label for neuropathic pain and myoclonic jerks (102). Despite that several small studies support its efficacy in neuropathic pain, including diabetic neuropathy, larger studies have been disappointing (103,104). Minor studies also found that topiramate provides pain relief in refractory intercostal neuralgia, trigeminal neuralgia, and trigeminal autonomic cephalgias; these findings will likely invite additional future research (105,106). Another possible indication applicable to physiatry is to promote weight loss. The phentermine/topiramate combination can result in significant weight loss and improvements in cardiometabolic risk factors in patients with obesity (71). A possible indication of less physiatric relevance includes bipolar disorder (107).

Mechanism of Action and Pharmacokinetics

See **Tables 52-5** and **52-6**.

Topiramate is rapidly absorbed into the body and does not bind well to plasma proteins (<20%). Only a third of the drug is metabolized by the hepatic CYP450 system into inactive metabolites. The remainder is excreted unchanged in the urine.

Preparations and Dosing

Topiramate is available as tablets (25, 50, 100, and 200 mg) and sprinkle capsules (15 and 25 mg). Its recommended daily dose as an adjunctive therapy for seizure prophylaxis is 200 mg BID, and gradual titration from an initial daily dose of 25 mg over 8 weeks can reduce adverse cognitive effects. There are no dosing guidelines in neuropathic pain, but topiramate has been used between 200 and 400 mg/d.

Relevant Side Effects and Drug Interactions

Topiramate causes two general CNS-related side effects: delayed psychomotor actions (e.g., difficulty concentrating and sluggish speech) and somnolence. Weight loss (secondary to appetite suppression) and paresthesia can develop with chronic intake. The reversible effects discussed above are generally more common at seizure prophylaxis doses (108). Occasional cases of acute myopia and angle-closure glaucoma have been associated with topiramate use as well (109). Finally, animal models suggest that it may be teratogenic.

Topiramate is a carbonic anhydrase inhibitor; concomitant use with another carbonic anhydrase inhibitor should be avoided to prevent increased risk of renal stone formation. It also has mild inductive effect on hepatic CYP450 enzymes and can hence increase metabolism of digoxin and oral contraceptive.

Valproate (Valproic Acid, Depakene)

Relevance to Physiatry

Valproate has been used as a third-line agent for epilepsy and migraine prophylaxis. It has also been studied for use in neuropathic pain including PHN and polyneuropathy (110–114). Similar to several other anticonvulsants though, evidence of its efficacy is weak. Previously, it was the subject of a small randomized clinical trial in paraplegic central pain and was not effective (115). It has yield variable results in experimentally induced central pain (116).

Mechanism of Action and Pharmacokinetics

See **Tables 52-5** and **52-6**.

Valproate, a lipid-soluble compound, is rapidly absorbed and becomes tightly protein bound. It is then metabolized in the liver through oxidation and glucuronidation pathways. Active metabolites and a small, unchanged portion are then renally eliminated.

Preparations and Dosing

Valproate is widely available in the following forms: caplet, sprinkle capsule, delayed-release tablet, extended-release tablet, syrup, and parental preparation. It is often initiated at 250 mg/d and then titrated to a maximum dose of 1,000 mg BID.

Side Effects and Drug Interactions

Nausea, tremors, drowsiness, and weight gain are commonly encountered in the clinical setting. More serious complications include hepatotoxicity among the children population, pancreatitis, and prolonged bleeding time. Frequent monitoring of the previous parameters is recommended. Rare instances of valproate-induced encephalopathy are presumed to be caused by inhibition of ammonia metabolism (117). However, there are recent reports of encephalopathy in the absence of hyperammonemia (118).

Valproate is an inhibitor of the oxidation and glucuronidation pathways; it inhibits the metabolism of phenytoin, carbamazepine, and lamotrigine. It also decreases the clearance of amitriptyline and nortriptyline.

Zonisamide (Zonegran)

Relevance to Physiatry

Zonisamide is FDA approved as an adjunctive therapy in partial seizures. A small, randomized clinical trial in 2005 concluded that it produces statistically insignificant effects when used in diabetic neuropathy (119,120). Another study, in 2015, found a lack of evidence suggesting that the medication may provide relief of neuropathic pain (121).

Mechanism of Action and Pharmacokinetics

See **Tables 52-5** and **52-6**.

Preparations and Dosing

Zonisamide 100-mg capsules are given daily for the first 2 weeks, after which the dose may be increased to 200 mg/d for at least 2 weeks. It can be increased to 300 and 400 mg/d, with the dose stable for at least 2 weeks to achieve steady state at each level. Evidence from controlled trials as an anticonvulsant suggests that 100 to 600 mg/d doses are effective, but there is no suggestion of increasing efficacy above 400 mg/d.

Relevant Side Effects and Drug Interactions

Zonisamide is contraindicated in sulfonamide allergy. Rare cases of aplastic anemia and agranulocytosis have been reported. It can also cause adverse psychiatric CNS events (depression and psychosis), psychomotor slowing (concentration difficulties and speech/language problems, especially word-finding difficulties), and somnolence and fatigue. Concomitant phenytoin or carbamazepine use increases zonisamide clearance.

Local Anesthetics-Injectable Anesthetics

Relevance to Physiatry

In the outpatient physiatric setting, injectable and sometimes topical anesthetics are frequently used to provide local anesthesia for a variety of procedures and as a diagnostic tool during intra-articular, soft tissue, nerve block, or hydrodissection procedures. They can also be combined with corticosteroids in intra-articular and soft tissue injections to attain immediate pain relief. Injectable anesthetics can also be used as a component of proliferant solutions used in prolotherapy.

Local anesthetics are classified as esters (e.g., procaine) or amides (e.g., bupivacaine, lidocaine, ropivacaine) based upon their chemical structure. Amide anesthetics are preferred over ester anesthetics because the latter are associated with a higher incidence of allergic reactions. Cross-sensitivity between the two classes does not occur (122). The amide class is further subdivided according to each drug's duration of action. Lidocaine, a short-acting injectable anesthetic, is commonly used in percutaneous infiltration anesthesia. Long-acting injectable anesthetics are often reserved for procedures in which a longer degree of postprocedure pain relief is desirable. Bupivacaine, an example of a long-acting injectable, is slowly released from its binding site resulting in a longer duration of action (123,124). For example, after a positive lidocaine diagnostic shoulder impingement test, bupivacaine can be added to the corticosteroid to provide longer pain relief to help bridge the time gap while the corticosteroid gradually takes effect. This section will examine the amide anesthetics in greater detail.

Bupivacaine (Marcaine, Sensorcaine)

Bupivacaine has been widely used for over half a century. Two comparable variants, levobupivacaine and ropivacaine, were subsequently introduced to circumvent the drawbacks of bupivacaine-related side effects; however, bupivacaine remains as a viable, inexpensive choice (125,126). Though spinal anesthesia for surgical procedures is considered to be the best indication for bupivacaine, a combination of bupivacaine and corticosteroid can also be injected as part of intra-articular, soft tissue, and some spinal injection procedures to provide longer-term relief; candidates for this procedure are typically individuals who responded to prior lidocaine injection (127). Bupivacaine is also used as part of a comparative local anesthetic medial branch block paradigm as a precursor to possible facet radio-frequency ablation.

Clinical and laboratory studies have shown that the local anesthetics bupivacaine, lidocaine, ropivacaine, mepivacaine, and levobupivacaine can be toxic to human chondrocytes and thus to the cartilage (128–130). Bupivacaine, ropivacaine, and mepivacaine are chondrotoxic in a time-dependent, concentration-dependent, and drug-dependent manner (130). In animal studies of rabbit joints, intra-articular bupivacaine 0.5% caused synovial membrane changes and articular cartilage inflammation, and another study showed after 48 hours of continuous intra-articular bupivacaine infusion with and without epinephrine resulted in chondrolysis after 1 week (131,132). Numerous clinical reports have shown that intra-articular pain pump catheter infusions with prolonged use of local anesthetics carry a high risk of chondrolysis and should be used with caution especially in compromised joints (128,129,133). While there is limited evidence that a single injection can cause chondrolysis, high concentration doses are best avoided (128,133,134). One *in vitro* study showed that buffering bupivacaine to a pH of 7.4 resulted in greater chondrolysis than bupivacaine alone and thus recommends against it (135). When bupivacaine is encapsulated in a liposome, a phospholipid bilayer with an aqueous core, it allows for slow release of the anesthetic, allowing for a longer duration of action and delay in peak plasma concentration. Liposomal bupivacaine is a new approved treatment for postoperative pain after bunionectomy and hemorrhoidectomy (136). It has predictable kinetics, an acceptable side effect profile without any opioid effects, and acceptable in patients with hepatic impairment (124,137,138).

Lidocaine (Xylocaine)

Lidocaine has been used as an anesthetic for over half a century. It has clearly replaced procaine, the first synthetic anesthetic, as the short-acting injectable anesthetic of choice because of its favorable side effect profile. Lidocaine is regularly used in outpatient physiatry for procedures such as regional anesthesia for musculoskeletal injections, nerve blocks, or tissue hydrodissection.

Mechanism of Action and Pharmacokinetics

All amide anesthetics are sodium channel blockers, which selectively inhibit tetrodotoxin-resistant sodium channels. These axonal structures are involved in generating nociceptive and temperature sensation. Local anesthetics cause a differential neural block—that is, sensory block with minimal loss of motor function (139,140). They are also shown to have a neuropathic anti-inflammatory effect attributed by the blockade of neural transmission at the site of tissue injury (141).

Many factors influence an injectable anesthetic's activity including lipid solubility, degree of ionization, molecular size, and vasodilatory capacity that are proportional to its potency, onset, and duration of action. Amides undergo extensive hepatic metabolization to become active metabolites—whereas esters are hydrolyzed by plasma enzymes to para-aminobenzoic acid (a potential allergen). Serum levels peak between 5 and 25 minutes postinjection, depending on the route of administration and rate of renal excretion.

Preparations and Dosing

Table 52-7 summarizes the dosing guidelines for using lidocaine and bupivacaine in percutaneous infiltration anesthesia. There are more concentrated preparations available (e.g., a 2% and 4% lidocaine solution) for use in procedures where minimal injectable volume is desirable, such as digital nerve blocks and small joint injections.

The smallest effective dose should always be used. Dosages should be adjusted for factors such as a patient's age and general health, because children, the elderly, debilitated, and acutely ill patients are at greater risk for anesthetic toxicity. Individuals with hepatic dysfunction or reduced hepatic blood flow (e.g., those taking β-blockers or those with congestive heart failure [CHF]) are at risk as well. Anesthetic doses should also be adjusted according to the systemic absorption rate at the site of injection. Highly vascular regions such as intercostal or epidural region result in a large, relatively quick increase in serum concentration, thereby warranting a lower effective dose. Conversely, subcutaneous tissues have lower perfusion and therefore do not lead to rapid increases in serum concentration nor require dosage adjustment.

Other Medications Sometimes Used in Conjunction with Local Anesthetics

Epinephrine

Coadministration of epinephrine counteracts the anesthetic-induced vasodilation, thereby slowing the systemic absorption rate from the injection site. The combined effect may potentiate and prolong the effective analgesic dose, as well as reduce the systemic toxicity of the anesthetic (142–144). Epinephrine is also used to dilute high-dose preparations to prevent anesthetics-associated systemic side effects. Concentrations between 2 and 10 μg/mL (i.e., ratio from 1:500,000 to 1:100,000) are generally used.

TABLE 52-7	**Commonly Used Local Anesthetics**				
Generic (Trade) Name	Applicable Preparations and Concentrations	Onset of Action (Duration)	Usual Dosage (mL): Bursal Injection (A); (IP); (Ish); (SA); (T)[a]	Usual Dosage (mL): Joint Injection Small (Large)	Dosage: Percutaneous Infiltration (Maximum Amount)
Bupivacaine (Marcaine, Sensorcaine)	0.25% or 0.5%	5 min (2–4 h)	(A) 2½–4½; (IP) 4–4½; (Ish) 2½–4; (SA) 4–6; (T) 4½–9	1–2 mL (2–4 mL)	Up to 70 mL
Lidocaine (Xylocaine)	0.5% or 1%	1/2–1 min (1½ h)	(A) 2½–4½; (IP) 4–4½; (Ish) 2½–4; (SA) 4–6; (T) 4½–9	1–2 mL (2–4 mL)	Up to 60 mL

[a]A, Anserine bursa; IP, Iliopectineal bursa; Ish, Ischial bursa; SA, Subacromial bursa; T, Trochanteric bursa.

Despite its benefits, epinephrine may expose patients to additional side effects such as wound infection, tachycardia, and hypertension (HTN). It is generally believed that tissue ischemia can occur when the mixture is injected into body regions, especially the digits, that have compromised or limited blood supply. The other concern is that epinephrine solutions contain sodium metabisulfite, which can serve as an allergen in certain individuals (145).

Overall, it is unlikely that epinephrine would be part of the injectate solution for typical physiatric injection procedures. The senior author, in fact, does not administer epinephrine for injection procedures.

7.5% Sodium Bicarbonate

Lidocaine causes a memorable burning sensation upon intradermal and subcutaneous injection because lidocaine solutions are acidic. This is especially true for multidose bottles due to the presence of a preservative. The addition of epinephrine worsens the burn by further decreasing the pH. This unpleasant feeling can be minimized by buffering a lidocaine solution with 7.5% sodium bicarbonate typically at a 9:1 ratio (e.g., 2 mL sodium bicarbonate added to 20 mL of 1% lidocaine) (120,146). The mixture should be administered within 24 hours to avoid risk of contamination due to the unclear effect upon the preservative when the solution has been buffered. The rate of anesthetic effect is also increased by buffering lidocaine. Local anesthetics are typically made as water-soluble hydrochloride salts (LAH+) to increase shelf life and stability and are thus acidic. As local anesthetic is diffused across the nerve sheath and membrane to receptor sites, only the uncharged base (LA) can penetrate the lipid membrane. Bicarbonate is added to increase the unionized fraction, quickening the onset of action of anesthesia (147).

Relevant Side Effects and Drug Interactions

Amide anesthetics have a wide therapeutic index. Although toxicity can occur and it is dose-related; when used alone, lidocaine and bupivacaine maximal recommended doses for a 70-kg person are 28 and 56 mL, respectively (148,149).

Calculation for a 70-kg person is shown below:
- lidocaine MAX dose 4 mg/kg × 70 kg = 280 mg
  280 mg/10 mg/mL = 28 mL MAX (lidocaine 1% bottles made as 10 mg/mL)
- bupivacaine MAX dose 2 mg/kg × 70 kg = 140 mg
  140 mg/2.5 mg/mL = 56 mL MAX (bupivacaine 0.25% bottles made as 2.5 mg/mL)

Spinal injections carry higher likelihood of significant toxicity from possible inadvertent intrathecal administration. Cervical spine injection procedures in particular can incur the risk of immediate systemic toxicity due to inadvertent vertebral artery injection. This explains why some injectionists even use the presence of early systemic toxicity during a "lidocaine test injection" as an indicator of inadvertent intravascular injection prior to injecting corticosteroid (even nonparticulate corticosteroids). Another potential local anesthetic side effect that is especially pertinent to spinal injection procedures pertains to ropivacaine. Specifically, ropivacaine combined with dexamethasone demonstrated rapid crystal formation large enough to act as emboli if inadvertent intravascular injection occurred during a targeted spinal injection. However, crystallization was not seen when dexamethasone was mixed with lidocaine or bupivacaine (150).

Systemic toxicity, albeit uncommon, unless there has been inadvertent intravascular injection or an excessive administered dose, can affect the CNS followed by the cardiovascular system (125). Bupivacaine is more CNS toxic and notably more arrhythmogenic than lidocaine and ropivacaine (148,151). The patient suffering from systemic local anesthetic injection toxicity may initially complain of drowsiness, tremors, and altered special senses (e.g., tinnitus and/or a metallic taste); however, as the serum level of the offending agent increases, an arrhythmia, seizure, and respiratory/cardiac arrest can develop (152). Lipid infusion can reportedly treat late-phase systemic toxicity (153,154). The results of one study suggest that lipid emulsion can counteract inhibition of mitochondrial function and abnormal mitochondrial calcium concentration in myocardiocytes induced by bupivacaine toxicity (153).

There are a few notable potential medication interactions pertinent to local anesthetics. Because local anesthetics are CNS depressants, they should not be combined with other CNS depressants. Anesthetics can enhance the action of neuromuscular blocking agents (155). Preparations containing epinephrine should not be given concomitantly with MAOIs or TCAs due to risk of severe HTN.

Local Anesthetics-Topical Anesthetics

In addition to injectable preparations, local anesthetics are available as a cream and as a transdermal patch that are sometimes employed for preprocedural soft tissue anesthesia. Topical lidocaine patch has also become a recommended first-line treatment for PHN and is becoming increasingly used off-label for various neuropathic and musculoskeletal pain conditions (156,157).

Eutectic Mixture of Local Anesthetics (EMLA Cream)

EMLA cream is an emulsion composed of 2.5% prilocaine and 2.5% lidocaine droplets. This topical compound has a lasting anesthetic effect for up to 4 hours (158). It can be applied to an intact skin an hour prior to painful outpatient procedures. EMLA is applied in a thick layer of 1 to 2 g/10 cm^2, up to a maximal dose of 20 g/200 cm^2, to an intact skin. The palms and soles have variable penetration (159). Numerous studies confirmed its efficacy over placebo cream, ethyl chloride, and lidocaine administrated subcutaneously or via iontophoresis (160). Although EMLA was deemed less effective than intradermal lidocaine, it is nonetheless preferred by patients (161).

Lidocaine Cream and Patch

Lidocaine cream (LMX) is regarded as an equivalent of EMLA but with faster onset of action (i.e., half an hour vs. 1 hour) (162). The patch form, with its dual mechanism of nociceptive sensation blockade and a mechanical barrier from friction against an injured skin, is FDA approved for treatment of PHN pain. There is also some evidence that lidocaine patches are effective for other neuropathic pain, low back pain, and osteoarthritic knee pain (156,163,164). Two small, uncontrolled studies reported significant pain relief in reflex sympathetic dystrophy (RSD)/complex regional pain syndrome (CRPS), stump neuroma pain, intercostal neuralgia, postthoracotomy pain, and meralgia paresthetica (117,165).

A 5% lidocaine-medicated plaster has been shown to be helpful in the treatment of pain due to PHN and diabetic polyneuropathy. Studies have shown that when compared to pregabalin, lidocaine plaster is more efficacious in treating PHN, has comparable efficacy for diabetic peripheral neuropathy, and has a more favorable safety profile and patient satisfaction for both indications (166,167).

The branded lidocaine patch, Lidoderm, contains 700 mg of 5% lidocaine. The recommended guideline to treat PHN is to apply a maximum of three simultaneous patches on an intact skin for 12 hours a day. Clothing may be worn over the application area. Weaker preparations of both the cream and patch can be found over the counter.

Lidocaine, Epinephrine, and Tetracaine (LET)

LET solution and gel are both formulated with 4% lidocaine, 0.1% epinephrine, and 0.5% tetracaine. The gel has obvious advantages over the liquid form and is widely used half an hour before suturing uncomplicated facial and scalp lacerations (168). In a randomized study of 221 children between the ages of 3 and 17 years, who underwent pretreatment of minor wounds with LET solution adhesive before tissue repair, they experienced decreased pain and increased amount of pain-free repairs (169). LET can also ameliorate pain from infiltrative anesthesia. Doses between 1 and 3 mL are effective in the aforementioned procedures. LET is not effective when used to anesthetize large wounds on the trunk or extremities at typical recommended doses.

Lidocaine-Tetracaine (LT) Patch (Synera)

The LT patch is a novel topical anesthetic with a built-in oxygen-activated heating element containing a eutectic 1:1 ratio of 7% lidocaine and 7% tetracaine. It has a more rapid onset than Lidoderm with effective anesthesia within 10 minutes of application (170). The LT patch has shown some benefit in patients with shoulder outlet impingement syndrome (171) and myofascial pain syndromes (172,173).

LT Peel (S-Caine Peel, Pliaglis)

A 7% lidocaine and 7% tetracaine cream dries within half an hour of application and is then peeled off. There is evidence that it is superior to EMLA yet with similar efficacy to LT patch in adults undergoing cutaneous procedures (174).

Relevant Side Effects and Drug Interactions

Topical agents are associated with potential side effects that are similar to their injectable counterparts. The transdermal mode of delivery has a predilection to cause local skin erythema and irritation. Eight trials reported erythema, burning, itching, and edema at the application site (174). Importantly, these local reactions are usually not due to anesthetic allergy. Overall, topical anesthetics are safe, as no serious adverse events have been observed in more than 120,000 patch-hours in patients who used the patch for up to 8.7 years (175). However, topical anesthetics should be used cautiously in patients who are taking class I antiarrhythmics (e.g., tocainide and mexiletine) as the toxic effects of both drugs are potentially synergistic (176).

Muscle Relaxants

Relevance to Physiatry

Skeletal muscle relaxants are often divided into two categories: antispasticity agents (such as baclofen and dantrolene when they are used for conditions such as multiple sclerosis or cerebral

palsy) and antispasmodic agents (carisoprodol, chlorzoxazone, cyclobenzaprine, metaxalone, orphenadrine, and methocarbamol) (177). Diazepam and tizanidine are considered under both categories (178). Muscle relaxants are intended for short-term use in musculoskeletal conditions where muscle "tightness" is one of the pain generators. Common conditions in which skeletal muscle relaxants are typically prescribed are low back and neck pain with a presumed significant muscular pain component, fibromyalgia, tension headache, and other myofascial pain syndromes (177,179,180). Although there are no published studies comparing the relative efficacy of NSAIDs and muscle relaxants, muscle relaxants appear to offer some benefits in patients with nonspecific back pain. In fact, 35% of patients with nonspecific low back pain are prescribed with muscle relaxants and 18.5% receive initial muscle relaxant therapy (178). Of note, concomitant use of muscle relaxants with analgesics may increase the efficacy of the muscle relaxant allowing for a reduced effective dose (155).

Muscle relaxants act by decreasing muscle excitability and thus diminishing muscle tension–induced pain. Unlike antispasticity agents, muscle relaxants offer the advantage of not compromising muscle strength. Unfortunately, sedation limits their application and sometimes obliges physicians to prescribe them for bedtime use only. Cyclobenzaprine, carisoprodol, dantrolene, diazepam, metaxalone, methocarbamol, and tizanidine are some of the most commonly prescribed muscle relaxants (181).

Mechanism of Action and Pharmacokinetics

Muscle relaxants are a unique group of medications as they have different mechanisms and pharmacokinetics (see **Table 52-8**). The only common denominator among them is that they all act in some manner on the CNS, rather than at the muscle fiber level, to interrupt nociceptive signals and therefore cause skeletal muscle relaxation. Dantrolene is the one exception to this as this medication acts at the level of muscle fibers.

Muscle Relaxant Preparations, Dosing, Relevant Side Effects, and Drug Interactions

See **Table 52-8**.

Muscle Relaxants and Antispastic Agents

Baclofen (Kemstro, Gablofen, Lioresal)

Baclofen is a centrally acting muscle relaxant that is primarily used to treat spasticity and improve mobility in disorders such as multiple sclerosis and cerebral palsy, as well as spinal cord injury. It is a direct agonist on GABA$_B$ receptors, which inhibits pre- and postsynaptic transmission on the spinal cord (182). Although it has been used off-label as a muscle relaxant for musculoskeletal conditions, there is little literature to support this (177,180,183). Despite this, some insurance companies are requiring that baclofen be used as the first-line muscle relaxant due to cost issues. Baclofen is often the first drug of choice for lower limb spasticity in multiple sclerosis and spinal cord injury; however, its efficacy in spasticity of cerebral origin is less well established (184–186). Regardless of severity or origin, oral baclofen is effective for reducing muscle tone and spasm frequency and is comparable with other oral antispasmodic agents. At first, the dose is 5 to 30 mg/d depending on the degree of spasticity. The MAX dose varies from

TABLE 52-8	**Muscle Relaxants**		

[Class] Generic (Trade) Name	Structural Analogue	Dose (mg)	Other Properties and Side Effects
[Single agents]			Sedation often occurs from muscle relaxants
Carisoprodol (Soma) (Rela)	Meprobamate (Equanil, Miltown)	250–350 mg TID and at bedtime; MAX: 1,400 mg QD	Unclear exact mechanism of action but centrally acting; sedation, tachycardia, shortness of breath, dizziness, drowsiness, headache, rare first dose idiosyncratic reactions (transient quadriplegia, loss of vision), contraindicated in acute intermittent porphyria; addictive; use lower initial dose and increase gradually as needed/tolerated for hepatic dysfunction
Cyclobenzaprine (Flexeril, Amrix)	Tricyclic antidepressants	IR: 5 mg 3 times QD MAX: 10 mg 3 times QD ER: 15 mg QD; MAX: 30 mg QD	Unclear exact mechanism of action but centrally acting; widely used; plasma levels vary widely; sedation and other anticholinergic side effects (avoid use in the elderly, cardiac disease); absolute contraindication for use with MAOIs
Diazepam (Valium)	Benzodiazepines	2–10 mg TID–QID QD	Enhances GABA effect by binding to benzodiazepine receptors; also used as an antispasticity agent; sedation, amnesia, dizziness, ataxia, high risk of tolerance, dependence, abuse, and withdrawal, delirium and falls in the elderly, overdose leads to respiratory failure and death
Metaxalone (Skelaxin)	None	800 PO TID–QID	Unclear exact mechanism of action but centrally acting; commonly drowsiness, dizziness, nervousness, nausea, vomiting, and headache, rarely CNS paradoxical excitation; hematologic toxicity, esp. hemolytic anemia or leukopenia; avoid if with hepatic or renal dysfunction
Methocarbamol (Robaxin)	Mephenesin (first muscle relaxant)	Initial: 1,500 mg QID for 2–3 d Maintenance: 750 mg q4h, 1,500 mg PO TID, or 1,000 mg QID; MAX: 4 g QD	Unclear exact mechanism of action but centrally acting; IM form inconvenient since you should inject into each buttock rather than entire dose into one; lowers seizure threshold; black, brown, or green urine; possible mental status impairment; and possible exacerbation of myasthenia gravis symptoms
Orphenadrine (Norflex)	Antihistamines	100 mg PO BID 60 mg IV/IM BID	Unclear exact mechanism of action but centrally acting; sedation, hallucinations, agitation, and euphoria, tachycardia (avoid in CHF and arrhythmias), anticholinergic effects (avoid in the elderly); rare cases of aplastic anemia, reports of anaphylaxis in some asthmatics with IM/IV dosing
Chlorzoxazone		250–750 mg TID–QID	Dizziness, light-headedness, malaise, red or orange urine, GI irritation, and rare GI bleeding
[Muscle relaxant/analgesic]			
Carisoprodol with aspirin (Soma Compound)		1–2 tabs PO QID; MAX duration: up to 2–3 wk	Contents (mg): carisoprodol 200/ASA 325; addictive, side effects same as carisoprodol with addition of salicylate toxicity
Soma Compound with codeine		1–2 tabs PO QID; MAX duration: up to 2–3 wk	Contents (mg): carisoprodol 200/ASA 325/codeine 16; potentially quite sedative; same as above with higher addiction potential
Methocarbamol and aspirin (Robaxisal)		2 tabs PO QID	Contents (mg): methocarbamol 400/ ASA325 side effects same as methocarbamol with addition of salicylate toxicity

20 to 120 mg/d depending on the presence of mild, moderate, or severe spasticity (184). One study of 16 subjects showed that the combination of baclofen and diazepam might inhibit the acquisition of motor skills by interrupting the neuroplastic changes that are involved in motor performance. Therefore, it is important to take caution in patients receiving concomitant physiotherapy (187). Intrathecal baclofen is a practical option for patients intolerant to oral baclofen from adverse effects or failure to respond to maximum oral dose in severe hypertonia of spinal and supraspinal origin (188–191). In patients with hereditary spastic paraplegia, intrathecal baclofen is an appropriate treatment to improve gait performance (192).

Dantrolene

Dantrolene, structurally similar to phenytoin (193), is a direct-acting skeletal muscle–relaxing agent which causes depression of excitation-contraction coupling in the skeletal muscle. Once bound to the ryanodine receptor, free intracellular and released calcium from the sarcoplasmic reticulum in the skeletal muscle is decreased, thereby depressing contraction (194). The first use of oral dantrolene was for spasticity treatment (195). Although this FDA-approved agent is well known for the treatment of malignant hyperthermia, it may also be used for management of neuroleptic malignant syndrome, ecstasy intoxication, and spasticity from upper neuronal disorders, including spinal cord injury, multiple sclerosis, and cerebral palsy (194,196). For spasticity, adults initially receive an oral capsule dose of 25 mg/d with the dose increased every 3 to 7 days. The maximum dose is no more than 100 mg four times a day. If there is no effect after 45 days, it is best to discontinue the drug. As it is metabolized by the liver (194), some adverse effects of dantrolene include generalized muscle weakness and hepatotoxicity (183,197). A retrospective study found 1 of 243 patients to have hepatic dysfunction after at least 4 weeks of low-dose oral dantrolene administration. Low-dose dantrolene may safely be used with close clinical and laboratory monitoring of hepatic function (197).

Carisoprodol (Soma)

Carisoprodol, a commonly prescribed muscle relaxant, primarily acts on the GABA_A receptor chloride channels (198). A common brand name, Soma Compound, also contains 325 mg of aspirin in addition to 200 mg of carisoprodol allowing for an added analgesic and antipyretic effect (199). The recommended adult dosage is 250 to 350 mg three times daily and at bedtime with a maximum duration of 2 to 3 weeks. One study comparing carisoprodol with cyclobenzaprine for muscle pain, spasms, tension, tenderness, or functional status showed no significant difference in therapy (177). Although not a controlled substance, concerns of carisoprodol abuse have been discussed over the past decade. Accordingly, numerous reviews have discussed its abuse potential (198,200–202). Carisoprodol is both structurally and pharmacologically similar to its psychoactive metabolite meprobamate, an approved anxiolytic (199). Meprobamate, a carbamate, likely accounts for the chronic effects observed from carisoprodol, tolerance and withdrawal (198,200–203). The barbiturate antagonist precipitated withdrawal demonstrated in one study suggests possible addiction potential similar to that of benzodiazepine or barbiturate compounds (198). Carisoprodol is metabolized by the liver and excreted by the kidney (199). Adverse effects include sedation, tachycardia, shortness of breath, dizziness, drowsiness, headache, and rare idiosyncratic reactions after the first dose such as transient quadriplegia and temporary loss of vision (178,204). Given the addition of aspirin, overdose of Soma Compound commonly produces salicylate toxicity as well (199). Physicians should be warned when administering carisoprodol to patients with reduced CYP2C19 activity or when coadministering drugs that inhibit or induce CYP2C19 (205). One study of 15 healthy nonabusing volunteers found that carisoprodol induced psychomotor effects minimally to none at therapeutic doses and significantly higher feelings of euphoria at supratherapeutic doses (206). Of note, 1 study of 10 subjects showed that when carisoprodol is prescribed alone, it is no different to placebo giving a "coasting, dreamy, drug liking feeling"; however, concomitant use with opioid in 3 of 10 patients produced liability-related abuse—"pleasant bodily sensations, drug liking, take again" feeling (207). One case report observed reports of euphoria and relaxation with concomitant use of carisoprodol and tramadol (208). Given these effects, it is particularly important to use caution in the elderly (177).

Cyclobenzaprine (Flexeril)

Cyclobenzaprine is perhaps the most commonly used muscle relaxant for nonspastic muscle pain. It can also be used for sleep disturbance in fibromyalgia (181). It is a centrally acting treatment, which acts at the level of the brain stem and spinal cord with an antagonistic effect on 5HT2 receptors in descending serotonergic neurons. It carries no direct peripheral action on the affected muscles (209). As a glucuronidated metabolite, this drug is extensively metabolized by the liver and excreted through the kidneys. It possesses a long half-life of approximately 18 hours and can continue to accrue for up to 4 days when given three times per day. For dosing, immediate release is 5- to 10-mg tablet three times a day, and extended release is 15- to 30-mg tablet daily. Of note, cyclobenzaprine is structurally similar to TCAs and has potent anticholinergic properties; thus, caution should be exercised when considering its use in the elderly or in patients with cardiac disease. Concomitant use with MAOIs is absolutely contraindicated because this combination can result in a fatal hyperpyretic crisis. The initial starting dose is 5 mg three times per day as needed and can be titrated up to 10 mg three times per day per therapeutic effect or side effect. In some patients who report therapeutic benefit but also report sedation, the senior author (TPS) instructs patients to either use 2.5-mg doses as long as this achieves benefit or to limit cyclobenzaprine to nighttime use. In patients with hepatic or renal impairment, cyclobenzaprine should initially be administered only once per day given its somewhat long half-life. In addition, one study showed equal efficacy of 5- and 10-mg doses, with the smaller dose showing a lower level of sedation (210). The most common adverse effects are drowsiness, fatigue, dry mouth, and headache, followed by less often occurring adverse effects of confusion, dizziness, abdominal pain, nausea, diarrhea, nervousness, and blurred vision (211,212).

Methocarbamol (Robaxin)

Methocarbamol is structurally related to the muscle relaxants chlorphenesin and mephenesin and expectorant guaifenesin. This muscle relaxant acts by centrally suppressing spinal polysynaptic reflexes having no direct effect on the skeletal muscle. It is largely metabolized by the liver and excreted by the kidneys and a minute amount excreted via feces (212). Recommended dosage includes 1,500 mg four times daily for the first 2 to 3 days, followed by 750 mg four times daily (177). The concomitant use of methocarbamol and paracetamol is a commonly used approach. A pharmacokinetic bioequivalence study demonstrated linearity in concentration with the combination of 500 mg of paracetamol and 400 mg of methocarbamol in healthy volunteers (213). Oral methocarbamol has shown to be a well-tolerated treatment option for patients with acute lower back pain and the typically associated restricted mobility (214). In a cohort study, methocarbamol did not improve pain control after acute injury from trauma during the first

3 days of hospitalization (215). Deep dry needling of trigger points in the lateral pterygoid muscle for myofascial pain and temporomandibular dysfunction was found to be more efficacious than methocarbamol/paracetamol treatment (216). Side effects of methocarbamol can include black, brown, or green urine, mental status impairment, and exacerbation of myasthenia gravis symptoms (177).

Diazepam (Valium)

Diazepam is a benzodiazepine that is both antispastic and antispasmodic. Diazepam is a broadly distributed, lipid-soluble CNS penetrant. Upon binding to the $GABA_A$ receptor, it produces an increase in chloride ion influx, which hyperpolarizes postsynaptic membranes augmenting CNS depression. Diazepam is a skeletal muscle relaxant approved for skeletal muscle spasms in addition to its anxiolytic, antiepileptic, and hypnotic effects (178,179,217–220). One study comparing diazepam with tizanidine for muscle pain, spasms, tension, tenderness, or functional status showed no significant difference in efficacy (177). The rapid onset of action and clinical efficacy attribute to its risk of tolerance, dependence, abuse, and withdrawal; hence, it is a Schedule IV controlled substance. Off-label uses include insomnia, restless leg syndrome, and pre-/postoperative sedation. Recommended adult dosages are 2 to 10 mg three to four times daily. Maximum dosage of diazepam in adults ranges up to 30 mg every 8 hours. This drug is metabolized by the liver CYP450 enzyme and glucuronidated for biphasic elimination with redistribution into the muscle and adipose tissue. Side effects from chronic diazepam use include amnesia, dizziness, ataxia, confusion, sedation, tachycardia, and depression. Patients with anxiety or seizure disorder may have increased frequency of anxiety or seizures, respectively. Serious adverse events are rare and often seen when combined with another drug such as opiates or alcohol. It is best to use it with caution in the elderly, as there is an increased risk of cognitive impairment, delirium, falls, and fractures. Overdose results in heavy sedation, motor function inhibition, cognitive delays, respiratory failure, coma, and sometimes even death (217–220).

Metaxalone (Skelaxin)

Metaxalone a centrally acting antispasmodic agent used for acute, painful musculoskeletal conditions such as back pain. Its exact mechanism of action is unknown. Adult dosing typically consists of 800 mg three to four times per day. It is not recommended in children younger than 12 years of age. It is metabolized by the liver and excreted via the kidneys in the form of metabolites. It is advised to monitor hepatic function after initiation of this agent. Common side effects include drowsiness, dizziness, nervousness, nausea, vomiting, and headache. The following are rare but serious adverse reactions that have been reported: hemolytic anemia, leukopenia, jaundice, and hypersensitivity reactions. Interestingly, metaxalone is an oxazolidinone structurally similar to reversible MAOIs; therefore, there is a potential risk of serotonin syndrome. There have been a few recent case reports of serotonin syndrome as a side effect with metaxalone overdose alone or with other proserotonergic medications (221,222). Rarely, patients may have paradoxical muscle cramping. This drug is contraindicated in severe renal or hepatic impairment (177,211,212).

Orphenadrine (Norflex)

Orphenadrine is a muscle relaxant used to treat muscle spasm associated with acute painful musculoskeletal conditions. One clinical study revealed some therapeutic efficacy for fibromyalgia (212,223). Its chemical structure is similar to diphenhydramine, in a manner that it possesses stronger anticholinergic and comparatively weaker sedation properties. Its precise mechanism of action is unknown; however, we know it has centrally acting anticholinergic effects without any direct effects on the skeletal muscle. It also has some euphorigenic and analgesic properties as well. This drug is mostly excreted via the kidneys. The typical recommended adult dose is 100 mg administered orally twice per day or 60 mg intravenous or intramuscular twice per day attributable to its fairly long half-life. Common adverse effects include drowsiness and dizziness, followed by other CNS effects such as hallucinations, agitation, and euphoria. Since patients may experience palpitations or tachycardia, it is important to avoid its use in CHF and patients with arrhythmia. Due to its anticholinergic properties, patients may experience dry mouth, nausea, constipation, urinary retention, tachycardia, blurred vision, and mental confusion; therefore, caution is advised in the elderly. Rare cases of aplastic anemia have also been reported (178,211,212).

Chlorzoxazone (Parafon Forte)

Chlorzoxazone, an approved centrally acting antispasmodic muscle relaxant, is used in acute, painful musculoskeletal conditions and discomfort relating to muscle spasms. This agent is a small potassium-type channel activator. Because of this targeted mechanism, chlorzoxazone may also be used to treat alcoholism (224). The brand name Parafon Forte is a combination of chlorzoxazone and acetaminophen. One study that compared tizanidine with chlorzoxazone (Parafon Forte) showed no significant difference in efficacy for outcomes of muscle pain, spasms, tenderness, and functional status (225). The usual dosage for adults is 250 to 750 mg three to four times daily. Adverse effects that patients may experience include dizziness, light-headedness, malaise, red or orange urine, GI irritation, and rare GI bleeding (177).

N-Methyl-D-Aspartate Receptor Antagonists

Relevance to Physiatry

Chronic pain such as neuropathic pain can result in grief and reduced quality of life. Tissue and nerve injury enhances the release of glutamate, which binds to glutamate N-methyl-D-aspartate (NMDA) receptors. Once bound to NMDA receptors in the spinal cord, especially in the dorsal horn, it triggers central sensitization and pain sensation. NMDA receptor antagonists (also known as NMDA glutamatergic antagonists), such as ketamine, dextromethorphan, or memantine, act to inhibit this pathway. Neuropathic pain remains a therapeutic challenge to treat since existing analgesic treatment may be ineffective or have serious side effects (226). NMDA receptor antagonists are prospective drugs for reducing persistent neuropathic pain in conditions such as PHN, painful diabetic peripheral neuropathy, multiple sclerosis–associated neuropathic pain, and neuropathic cancer pain (226–231). Shown in animal models, NMDA receptor antagonist can reduce hyperalgesia and allodynia related to nerve injury or diabetic peripheral neuropathy (226). Despite numerous laboratory studies demonstrating the efficacy of these agents for neuropathic pain, clinical studies show limited effects of NMDA antagonists for chronic neuropathic pain in a subpopulation of patients (226). According to a 2003 study, dosing guidelines for myofascial and neuropathic pain have not yet been established and are still considered off-label. However, there are a variety of off-label treatments for neuropathic myofascial pain including NMDA antagonists, gabapentin, and TCAs. Other potential applications include oral/epidural preemptive analgesia prior to surgery and coadministration with opioids to improve postoperative pain relief (232–235). In addition to their independent analgesic effect, NMDA receptor antagonists are also synergists with opioids and can prevent tolerance to opioids (236). Two opioids (i.e., methadone and dextropropoxyphene) also possess NMDA antagonistic properties. These agents are discussed in the opioid section of this chapter. Other NMDA receptor antagonists exist, but their use is significantly limited by side effects.

Several NMDA receptor antagonist clinical trials have been discontinued due to psychotomimetic adverse effects as well as ataxia and coordination impairment (237). This has led to the development of moderate affinity channel blockers (e.g., glycine B and NR2B selective antagonists), which selectively block peripheral NMDA receptors (238). This new generation of drugs has shown a more favorable side effect profile in animal models.

Ketamine (Ketalar)

Ketamine hydrochloride is a noncompetitive NMDA receptor antagonist that is primarily used in veterinary practices as a tranquilizer. Indications for ketamine include IV induction for intubation in sepsis patients, reactive airway disease, induction in children with poor health such as congenital heart disease, burns, and an adjunct to local or regional anesthesia procedures (239). Though with positive results, further studies are needed for its use. It causes a state of consciousness known as dissociative anesthesia. Ketamine may be used for a variety of applications given its neuroprotective, anti-inflammatory, and antitumor effects (239–241). It also interacts with opioid, monoamine, and cholinergic receptors (240). Ketamine produces numerous effects such as sedation, somatic analgesia, cataplexy, bronchodilation, and stimulation of the sympathetic nervous system (239). There are limited studies present on the clinical off-label use of ketamine administered topically or intravenously for the treatment of chronic pain conditions such as acute and chronic migraine, breakthrough noncancer pain, chemotherapy-induced neuropathy, CRPS, fibromyalgia, painful limb ischemia, traumatic peripheral nerve injury, phantom limb pain, PHN, spinal cord injury, temporomandibular pain, trigeminal neuropathic pain, and whiplash (239,242–245). Ketamine has been found to produce a strong analgesia in neuropathic pain states presumably via its antagonistic effect on NMDA receptors (239,246). A limited number of studies have demonstrated pain relief from chronic pain lasting for months after long-term IV infusion of ketamine (244). Though not officially indicated, there has been some mounting literature on its successful use in RSD/CRPS (242,247–250).

Ketamine can potentially relieve pain due to CRPS, generally without eliciting respiratory depression and/or prolonged sedation. Some studies have found that ketamine infusions are efficacious for the management of CRPS (247–249,251–255), and other studies have found it to exert an antidepressant effect. It has been generally found to be relatively safe.

Ketamine has been studied both in the outpatient setting using subanesthetic doses and two of a lesser extent, in the inpatient setting using anesthetic doses. A meta-analysis, however, of NMDA receptor antagonists for the treatment of neuropathic pain, which included a review of the effects of IV ketamine for CRPS, found that no significant effect on pain reduction could be demonstrated (256). It concluded that "no conclusions can yet be made about the efficacy of NMDA receptor antagonists on neuropathic pain. Additional randomized controlled trials (RCTs) in homogeneous groups of pain patients are needed to explore the therapeutic potential of NMDA receptor antagonists in neuropathic pain." A meta-analysis published in 2015 in a leading pain management journal also concluded that there is currently only weak evidence supporting the efficacy of ketamine for CRPS, yet there is clearly a rationale for definitive study (257).

There is no predetermined dosing guideline for its analgesic use, but a dose ranging from 6.5 to 13 mg/kg IM is administered for 12 to 25 minutes of surgical anesthesia. One study used 0.4 mg/kg IM doses to treat trigeminal neuralgia (258). Low-dose ketamine is recommended for pain management in the emergency department as an adjunct to morphine. The dosage for this includes a starting bolus of 0.2 to 0.3 mg/kg IV over 10 minutes with subsequent infusion of 0.1 to 0.3 mg/kg/h.

Ketamine is classified as a Schedule III controlled substance because its psychotomimetic effects are comparable to inhaling PCP. Furthermore, it has the potential to cause addiction (243).

Dextromethorphan

Dextromethorphan has shown to have anti-inflammatory effects *in vivo* (259). It attenuates acute pain at doses of 30 to 90 mg, divided every 4 to 6 hours (5 to 10 mg/mL), and reduces analgesic requirements in postoperative patients without major side effects, but it has a suboptimal analgesic effect in treatment of chronic pain (260). There is some preclinical evidence of neuroprotective properties in the setting of perioperative brain injury, amyotrophic lateral sclerosis, and methotrexate neurotoxicity (245,261,262). Dextromethorphan has been shown to be helpful in painful diabetic peripheral neuropathy and PHN (228). This agent has no effect on opioid requirement for control of acute pain in children admitted to the intensive care unit (263). The concomitant use of dextromethorphan and oxycodone may enhance the antiallodynia effects of oxycodone (264). There is no known antidote for dextromethorphan toxicity (261).

Amantadine

Amantadine is an antiviral agent with NMDA receptor antagonist properties. It is also used in Parkinson's disease and traumatic brain injury (TBI). Oral amantadine was unsuccessful as an agent used to prevent postmastectomy pain syndrome due to intolerable side effects and inadequate pain reduction for neuropathic pain (76,265). One study demonstrates that intravenous infusion of amantadine decreases the intensity of continuous postsurgical neuropathic pain in cancer patients (239).

Memantine

Memantine is a moderate affinity NMDA receptor antagonist. It is indicated for moderate Alzheimer's disease. There is some evidence from case reports and small, controlled trials on its application in neuropathic pain (228,266–271). For example, memantine has shown to reduce pain and possibly prevent phantom limb syndrome (268,269,271,272). One RCT study confirms that memantine could be a new prophylactic therapy given prior to mastectomy to counteract neuropathic pain development (227). Another recent study demonstrates that the therapeutic benefit of administering memantine prior to mastectomy can prevent the presence of postsurgery pain and chemotherapy-induced pain symptoms (273).

Nonsteroidal Anti-Inflammatory Drugs

Relevance to Physiatry

Oral NSAIDs are frequently used in the outpatient musculoskeletal medicine setting. At low doses, NSAIDs display primarily analgesic properties, while at high doses, it has both anti-inflammatory and analgesic properties, generally without causing sedation. All NSAIDs share the same mechanism of action and overall side effect profile, but they also have individual characteristics that distinguish them from each other. Not one NSAID has been demonstrated as being superior in terms of efficacy to others. Ideally, physiatrists should be familiar with at least one agent from each NSAID classes. This will allow the physician to comfortably switch a patient off an agent from one NSAID class to an agent from a different class. This strategy can be emplaced if they do not respond and/or have side effects with the use of an NSAID from one class.

Mechanism of Action and Pharmacokinetics

NSAIDs exert their primary effects by inhibiting the synthesis of prostaglandins and other related inflammatory compounds (e.g., thromboxanes and leukotrienes). The four primary properties of NSAIDs are analgesia for mild to moderate pain, anti-inflammatory effects, antipyretic effects, and reversible platelet inhibition. Anti-inflammatory effects also contribute to analgesia by preventing inflammatory-mediated sensitization of nociceptors.

Oral NSAIDs are absorbed in the upper GI tract. A large percent of the drug becomes bound to plasma protein, while the unbound portion exerts its pharmacologic effects. NSAIDs undergo hepatic metabolism and renal excretion. NSAIDs are available as short-acting and long-acting preparations with a half-life ranging from 30 to 50 hours at steady state. The consequence of accumulating long-acting agents (e.g., oxaprozin [Daypro] and piroxicam [Feldene]) in the human body is unclear, but to date, there are no reports of any additional significant adverse events beyond those typically seen with NSAIDs (274).

Preparations and Dosing

Table 52-9 shows a classification scheme of NSAIDs based on their chemical structure. Additional information on the individual classes is as follows:

- *Salicylates*: These include aspirin and three nonacetylated salicylates. Compared to other NSAIDs, nonacetylated salicylates are less potent but cause less GI complications and less platelet inhibition. It is unclear if any one particular nonacetylated salicylate in this category is more advantageous than the other two.
- *Propionic acids*: This is the most popular NSAID class due to the OTC availability of ibuprofen and naproxen and the direct marketing of the agent to the general public.

- *Acetic acids*: This class is the most potent and most potentially toxic of all NSAIDs. It includes drugs that can be administered via intramuscular and parental routes (e.g., ketorolac, indomethacin, diclofenac, etodolac).
  - This group of NSAIDs contains two subclasses, pyrrole acetic acids (indomethacin, sulindac, tolmetin, ketorolac, etodolac) and phenylacetic acids (diclofenac, bromfenac).
- *Fenamates*: Meclofenamate and mefenamic acid offer no advantage over other NSAIDs but can cause significant GI toxicity and dysmenorrhea pain, respectively.
- *Oxicams*: Only piroxicam and meloxicam are currently available in the United States. Piroxicam has convenient once-daily dosing but is associated with severe dermatologic reactions such as exfoliative dermatitis and pemphigus vulgaris. The risk of adverse effects is lower for meloxicam. It was FDA approved for treatment of pain due to osteoarthritis in 2004.
- *Naphthyl alkanones*: The only clinically available NSAID in this class is nabumetone. It is a prodrug, most noted for its nonacidic chemical structure, similar to naproxen but unlike that of other clinically used NSAIDs (275).

Relevant Side Effects and Drug Interactions

Individuals regularly using NSAIDs have up to five times the risk of developing GI complications (276). NSAIDs act directly to increase gastric acid secretion and indirectly to inhibit prostaglandin, which protects the GI tract lining. The direct effect varies among NSAIDs and only occurs with oral administration. The direct effect, on the contrary, remains constant regardless of the rate of administration. And all adverse events increase with higher doses of NSAIDs. The elderly and patients with a history of peptic ulcer disease are particularly vulnerable to epigastric discomfort and ulceration. Recent studies indicate that ketorolac, piroxicam, followed by indomethacin confer the highest GI risks at low dose and ibuprofen confers the least (277). The theory behind relative GI risks is that certain NSAIDs undergo extensive biliary excretion of their active metabolites and this, in turn, prolongs mucosal contact.

The most common adverse effects, GI bleeding and cardiovascular problems, begin almost immediately after starting a patient on NSAIDs, whether it is a short- or long-term course (278). It has been a general consensus that to reduce the risk of GI complications, one should include taking NSAIDs with meals and select enteric-coated preparations, when available. But a 2015 study in the British Journal of Pharmacology regarding NSAIDs instructions showed that the t_{max} (t_{max} is time to maximum concentration), when taken with meals, was longer than the fasting t_{max}. The study concludes that taking analgesics with food may make them less effective but acknowledges further studies need to be undertaken, as taking NSAIDs with food has not shown to worsen the GI risk (279). Prophylactic medications can be given if the patient has concomitant use of corticosteroids and warfarin or a history of GI bleeding or peptic ulcer disease (📶 **eTable 52-4**). The classes of available prophylactic medications include antacids, H_2 blockers, misoprostol, proton pump inhibitors (PPIs), and sucralfate (📶 **eTable 52-4**). Only misoprostol and PPIs are FDA approved for gastric ulcer prevention, and H_2 blocker has not been shown to be effective in chronic NSAID users (280).

TABLE 52-9	NSAIDs	
[Class] Generic (Trade) Name	**Dose (Oral in mg)**	**Other Properties and Side Effects**
[Salicylates: acetylated]		

Aspirin (Ecotrin, Empirin, Bayer, Entrophen)	325–650 q4–6h	Used esp. for antipyretic and cardioprotective effects
		Other formulations available:
		    800-mg controlled release (prescription)
		    975-mg enteric coated (prescription)
		    suppositories: 100, 200, 300, 600 mg
		    combined with narcotics and muscle relaxants
		Side effects: allergy esp. if triad of nasal polyps, hay fever, asthma; GI toxicity but enteric-coated and buffered forms exist; tinnitus; Reye's syndrome in children

[Salicylates: nonacetylated]		
Diflunisal (Dolobid)	500–1,000 load 250–500 q8–12h	Relatively weak anti-inflammatory effect; lacks antipyretic activity
Salsalate (Disalcid, Salflex)	3,000/d divided q8–12h	Relatively weak anti-inflammatory effect; no platelet inhibition
Salicylate combination (Trilisate)	1,500 BID	Relatively weak anti-inflammatory effect; no ASA allergic reactions may be present; liquid preparation available (500 mg/5 mL)
[Propionic Acids]		
Flurbiprofen (Ansaid)	200–300/d divided BID–QID	Available in ophthalmic solution (Ocufen); TD form available
Ibuprofen (Motrin)	600–800 TID–QID	Inexpensive and widely used; frequent dosing; [OTC]: Advil, Motrin IB; Nuprin, Rufen; TD form available
Ketoprofen (Orudis, Oruvail, Orafen)	50–75 TID 200 QD	Accumulates if poor renal function (OTC): Orudis-KT; Actron; TD form available
Naproxen (Naprosyn)	250–500 BID	High incidence of GI side effects; advantage of enteric-coated form may be present, although expensive; [OTC]: Aleve
(EC-Naprosyn)	375–500 BID	
Naproxen-Na (Naprelan)	750–1,000 QD	Naprelan has Intestinal Protective Drug Absorption System (IPDAS): immediate- and sustained-release components
(Anaprox)	275–550 BID	
Oxaprozin (Daypro)	600 BID; 1,200 QD	QD or BID dosing
[Acetic Acids]		
Diclofenac (Cataflam, Voltaren)	50 BID–TID	LFT monitoring if prolonged use; side effects in up to 20%
(Voltaren-XR)	50 BID–TID 100 QD	Arthrotec = diclofenac (50 or 75 mg) + misoprostol (200 μg)
Etodolac (Lodine)	200–400 BID–TID	Gastric-sparing properties may be present
(Lodine XL)	400–1,200 QD	
Indomethacin (Indocin)	25–50 TID	Most potent and toxic NSAID; PR preparation (Indotec); drug of choice in ankylosing spondylitis; indicated in other highly inflammatory conditions—e.g., acute gouty arthritis; prevents heterotopic ossification s/p THR and used for myositis ossificans; dose-related CNS/hematologic side effects, in up to 25%–50%; GI toxicity
(Indocin SR)	75 QD	
Ketorolac (Toradol)	10 QID (PO) 15–60 (IM) Lower doses if age >65 or renal dysfunction	FDA approved only for 5 consecutive days; GI bleeding at higher doses; rapid analgesia with IM form—decrease dose For age >65, renal dysfunction, weight <110; IV preparation also available
Sulindac (Clinoril)	150–200 BID	Prodrug; possibly renal-sparing because urinary excretion primarily as biologically inactive forms, may be more GI toxic
Tolmetin (Tolectin)	200–600 TID–QID	Frequent dosing; frequent GI toxicity
[Fenemates]		
Meclofenamate (Meclomen)	50–100 TID–QID	Frequent dosing; diarrhea common
Mefenamic acid (Ponstel)	500 × 1, then 250 QID	Frequent dosing; used for dysmenorrheic pain
[Oxicams]		
Piroxicam (Feldene)	20 QD or 10 BID	QD dosing; accumulation in the elderly possibly due to enterohepatic recirculation; dermatologic side effects and cases of serum sickness; PR form (Fexicam)
[Naphthyl alkanones]		
Nabumetone (Relafen)	500–1,000 BID	QD or BID dosing; nonacidic prodrug that undergoes hepatic biotransformation into active metabolite; preliminary studies suggest that unlike other NSAIDs, no evidence of enterohepatic recirculation of active metabolite—this may be an advantage

Misoprostol is recommended over PPIs in patients without active *H. pylori* infection (281). Ideally, the selected prophylactic medication should be taken for the duration of NSAID therapy in order to provide maximum protection.

Less common regions of GI side effects include the esophagus, the nonduodenal portion of the small bowel, colon, and liver. Esophageal side effects include esophagitis and benign esophageal strictures. Irritable bowel disease can be unmasked while the small bowel and colon can develop ulcers, erosions, and weblike strictures. NSAID enteropathy is not believed to occur via an acid mechanism and is therefore not prevented by antacids, H_2 blockers, or PPIs.

A large study in 2005 found that NSAIDs are the second main cause of drug-induced liver injury. Despite this, hepatotoxicity is rare except in individuals with a history of liver disease (282). Clinically significant hepatic enzyme elevation does occur with certain NSAIDs, particularly diclofenac. When employing these NSAIDs, LFTs are recommended throughout the course of treatment. There is however currently no established recommended schedule for liver function testing.

In large part due to studies of coxibs (see below), all NSAIDs now carry a black box warning that warns against potential cardiovascular and GI side effects. This will be discussed in more detail in the coxib section below.

The risk of kidney failure increases the longer NSAIDs are used. Individuals with preexisting kidney disease or comorbid medical conditions that impair renal blood flow (e.g., CHF and hypovolemia) are prone to acquire NSAID-induced renal toxicity. Acute renal failure, nephrotic syndrome, and interstitial nephritis are examples. It has been suggested but not proven that sulindac is somewhat renal-sparing compared to other NSAIDs (283).

There is less evidence that NSAIDs per se can cause tendinopathy. Many physicians still treat tendinopathy as though it is tendonitis, causing a potential issue. There is some animal evidence in rat studies which suggest NSAIDs reduce tendon healing, especially of the supraspinatus tendon. In addition, it was found that ibuprofen was the most correlated with the development of tendinopathy (284).

In light of all adverse effects discussed above, a significant amount of research has been dedicated to find an alternative to traditional NSAIDs. The effort yielded only one product, the COX-II inhibitor celecoxib, that is still available on the market, and it will be further explored in the following section. More options are currently under investigation. They include dual COX and 5-lipooxygenase (5-LOX) inhibitors, synthetic lipoxins, nitric oxide–releasing NSAIDs, and hydrogen sulfide–releasing NSAIDs (285). The mechanism of action for these drugs involves either combining current NSAIDs with a moiety (i.e., nitric oxide and hydrogen sulfide) that releases gastro-protective mediators or targeting new processes of the inflammatory process.

True NSAID allergic reactions occur in 1% of the population and range from simple skin rashes and rhinitis to anaphylaxis. NSAIDs should not be used in patients allergic to aspirin.

Cyclooxygenase-II Inhibitors

Relevance to Physiatry
In the late 1990s, the FDA approved COX-II inhibitors (also known as, coxibs) as an alternative to NSAIDs. Coxibs in general were generally thought to confer the advantage of less GI toxicity compared to traditional NSAIDs. This appeal led to them becoming the most frequently prescribed new medication within the first year of being introduced in 1999. Celecoxib, the only currently available coxib in the United States, is FDA approved for the treatment of pain associated with rheumatoid and osteoarthritis and acute pain. Celecoxib is especially used in those individuals who require oral anti-inflammatories but are on concomitant anticoagulation therapy, are at high risk for GI side effects, or are to undergo certain injection procedures such as fluoroscopic-guided spinal injection procedures or injection procedures into deep joint structures, where the risk of inadvertent bleeding makes the use of traditional NSAIDs potentially dangerous (286). There also continues to be interest in coxibs because COX-II expression is implicated in colon cancer and Alzheimer's disease (287).

Mechanism of Action and Pharmacokinetics
Coxibs reduce prostaglandin synthesis by selectively inhibiting one isoform of cyclooxygenase enzyme over another—namely, COX-II over COX-I. This mechanism contrasts with that of NSAIDs, which inhibit COX-II and COX-I equally. COX-I is constitutively expressed in all human tissues including the GI tract. Only a low level of COX-II is constitutively expressed in the brain, kidney, bone, and female reproductive tissues; however, the expression of COX-II can be induced at sites of inflammation. By sparing COX-I, coxibs achieve comparable anti-inflammatory and analgesic effects, with less adverse GI toxicity. The lack of effect on thromboxane synthesis explains the absence of antiplatelet effect.

Food has no significant effect on either peak plasma concentration or absorption at therapeutic doses. Higher doses ($\geq$400 mg BID) should, however, be taken with food to improve absorption.

Preparations and Dosing
Celecoxib is available as 100-, 200-, and 400-mg capsules. It is currently only approved for the indications as shown in 📶 **eTable 52-5**. The lowest effective dose should be used, especially in patients with HTN or CHF because coxibs may cause renal prostaglandin-mediated fluid retention. In patients with moderate hepatic impairment, doses should be decreased by approximately 50%.

Relevant Side Effects and Drug Interactions
Clinical trials found that coxibs caused less gastropathy than traditional NSAIDs; the most notable trials included the TARGET (Therapeutic Arthritis Research and Gastrointestinal Event Trial) and CLASS (Celebrex Long-term Arthritis Safety Study) studies (288–290). There is, however, growing evidence that coxibs impair healing of damaged gastric mucosa and may negatively affect both the small and large intestines (291–293). These findings have led to further questioning as to whether there really is an advantage of less GI toxicity from coxibs over traditional NSAIDs.

The FDA produced a black box warning for Celebrex, for its increased risk for cardiovascular events including myocardial infarction and stroke. Coxibs can cause a dose-dependent risk of adverse cardiovascular events, including myocardial infarction and stroke (294,295). Rofecoxib was withdrawn upon completion of the 3-year APPROVe study, which showed that daily intake of 25 mg of this coxib doubled the risk of thrombotic events (296). It was also shown that doubling the dose of celecoxib increased adverse cardiovascular events by (risk ratio 3.4; 95% confidence interval, 1.5 to 7.9) above that of the 200-mg QD Celebrex dose (2.6; 95% CI, 1.1 to 6.1) (177,297). The pathophysiology behind this effect is that coxibs inhibit vascular endothelium production of prostaglandin I$_2$, a lipid that counteracts thromboxane A$_2$, to prevent platelet aggregation leading to atherosclerosis and cause a similar blood pressure elevation as NSAIDs (298). It is not known if cardioprotective aspirin or low-salt diet can mitigate coxibs' cardiovascular risks (299).

This issue of increased cardiovascular risk led to a black box warning that is now part of the package inserts of celecoxib and all NSAIDs as follows:
- Cardiovascular Risk
  - NSAIDs and celecoxib may cause an increased risk of serious cardiovascular thrombotic events, myocardial infarction, and stroke, which can be fatal. This risk may increase with duration of use. Patients with cardiovascular disease or risk factors for cardiovascular disease may be at greater risk.
  - NSAIDs and celecoxib are contraindicated for the treatment of perioperative pain in the setting of coronary artery bypass graft (CABG) surgery.
- Gastrointestinal Risk
  - NSAIDs and celecoxib cause an increased risk of serious GI adverse events including bleeding, ulceration, and perforation of the stomach or intestines, which can be fatal. These events can occur at any time during use and without warning symptoms.
    - Elderly patients are at greater risk for serious GI events.

Traditional NSAIDs and coxibs have equal potential to cause renal toxicity (e.g., fluid retention leading to edema, renal HTN, interstitial nephritis, and papillary necrosis) (300,301). Elderly, patients with renal insufficiency or hepatic failure, and individuals at risk for renal failure should avoid coxibs (302).

Mean INR can increase up to 10% for a subset of patients receiving both warfarin and coxibs, and there have been infrequent reports of increased INR associated with bleeding events. This notion, however, was subsequently challenged by the results of a randomized, controlled crossover trial to assess the effect on INR of celecoxib in 15 patients who were receiving warfarin therapy (303). Nonetheless, patients on anticoagulation therapy should have their INRs monitored when a coxib is initiated or its dose changed.

There are case reports of celecoxib having induced serious skin reactions such as toxic epidermal necrolysis, erythema multiforme, and Stevens-Johnson syndrome (304,305). Celecoxib is contraindicated in sulfonamide allergy (approximately 3% of the general population) and in patients with a history of aspirin or NSAID allergy.

Prostaglandins are involved in bone metabolism, and animal models show that coxibs reduce bone, tendon, and ligament healing. Although clinical trials on humans have yet to be undertaken, many orthopedists and physiatrists avoid coxibs in patients with fractures (306,307).

The main potential drug interactions involving coxibs include those with angiotensin converting enzyme (ACE) inhibitors and diuretics. Specifically, celecoxib can interfere with the antihypertensive effects of those agents. Medications that alter celecoxib's serum concentration and whose concentrations are altered by celecoxib are summarized in 🛜 **eTable 52-6.**

Other Adjuvant Analgesics

Tizanidine (Zanaflex)

Relevance to Physiatry
Tizanidine, an antispastic and antispasmodic agent, is approved for use in spasticity due to multiple sclerosis or spinal cord injury. It has also been studied for acute low back pain accompanied by muscle "spasm" and neuropathic pain conditions, including trigeminal neuralgia and phantom pain syndrome (308–310). An open-label study in humans concluded that tizanidine may be an effective treatment for pain associated with idiopathic peripheral neuropathy, and another animal study showed that it relieved thermal hyperalgesia in rats with induced neuropathic pain (311,312). However, there are no large, randomized clinical trials to date on its use in neuropathic pain. In one study in Russia, tizanidine was shown to decrease spasticity, increase muscle strength, and improve pain syndrome intensity when combined with botulinum toxin A (313). Other indications that are not as applicable to physiatry include its use along with long-acting NSAIDs for detoxification of rebound headache, chronic tension headache, and narcotic withdrawal (314–317). Tizanidine 4 mg administered orally before laparoscopic cholecystectomy was shown in one study to reduce postoperative pain, opioid consumption, and recovery room stay (318).

Mechanism of Action and Pharmacokinetics
Tizanidine is a centrally acting agonist to α_2-adrenergic G protein–coupled receptor known to prevent the release of excitatory neurotransmitters by suppressing polysynaptic excitation of spinal cord interneurons (319). Furthermore, it presumably reduces spasticity by increasing presynaptic motor neuron inhibition. Following oral administration, 95% of the dose undergoes first-pass hepatic metabolism to inactive metabolites, and peak plasma level is reached in 1.5 hours. Concomitant food intake decreases peak plasma concentration and increases the time it takes to reach peak level (320).

Preparations and Dosing
Tizanidine is available in 2-, 4-, and 6-mg capsules or 4-mg tablets. Dosing for spasticity is accomplished by gradually increasing a starting dose of 4 mg by 2 to 4 mg until a daily maximum of 36 mg divided TID is reached; the desired therapeutic effect is achieved or dose-limiting side effects occur. Although the maximum total daily dose is generally denoted as 36 mg, clinical experience beyond 24 mg is limited (321).

Side Effects and Medication Interactions
Hypotension, dry mouth, CNS depression, and muscle weakness are commonly associated with α_2-adrenergic antagonism. Muscle weakness associated with tizanidine is comparatively less than other antispasticity agents (322). Tizanidine should be used with caution in patients with hepatic impairment, as hepatotoxicity is a rare but clinically significant side effect. In controlled clinical studies, 5% of participants had serum transaminase elevated three times that of normal (or twice if baseline levels were elevated); most cases resolved upon medication withdrawal, but some individuals developed nausea, vomiting, anorexia, and jaundice. Liver function testing is recommended during the first 6 months (i.e., baseline, 1, 3, and 6 months) of initiating tizanidine therapy and then periodically monitored. Tizanidine should be discontinued in patients

found experiencing hallucinations (3% in two controlled studies) or hypersensitivity reactions (321). CYP1A2 primarily metabolizes tizanidine; therefore, it is contraindicated to take potent CYP1A2 inhibitors such as fluvoxamine or ciprofloxacin when taking tizanidine (321,323–325). Oral contraceptives have shown to lower tizanidine clearance (326). However, if concomitant use is clinically necessary, start with a single 2-mg dose and increase in 2- to 4-mg increments daily based on patient response (321). One case report noted hypotension with the first dose of tizanidine in patients taking lisinopril (327).

Opioid Analgesics

Relevance to Physiatry

Narcotic analgesics are often referred to as opioid or opiate analgesics, as some are opium-derived. They are indicated for moderate to severe acute and ongoing malignant and nonmalignant pain, especially that which is of a nociceptive quality (i.e., generally dull or aching). In contrast, opiate analgesics are considered second-line treatments for various neuropathic pain syndromes such as phantom leg pain, diabetic neuropathy, and PHN (328–330). These indications are partly adapted from the World Health Organization (WHO) three-step ladder that guides analgesic treatment (331). The first step consists of nonopioid analgesics and adjuvants. Weak opioids (e.g., codeine) comprise the second step of pain management when the first-step options have failed. Step three consists of stronger opioids (e.g., morphine) plus or minus the first-step options.

CDC Guidelines for prescribing opioids for chronic pain in the United States were updated in 2016. Of note are the following recommendations to keep in mind as a clinician: (a) clinicians should establish treatment goals with all patients, including realistic goals for pain and function, and should consider how therapy will be discontinued; (b) when opioids are started, clinicians should prescribe the lowest effective dosage; (c) clinicians should review the patient's history of controlled substance prescriptions using state Prescription Drug Monitoring Program (PDMP) data to determine whether the patient is receiving opioid dosages or dangerous combinations that put him or her at high risk for overdose; (d) clinicians should use urine drug testing before starting opioid therapy and consider urine drug testing at least annually to assess for prescribed medications as well as other controlled prescription drugs and illicit drugs (332).

The lack of end-organ toxicity (especially GI, hepatic, and renal) with pure narcotic analgesics, other than meperidine, makes them an appealing choice for chronic therapy. However, the potential for serious adverse events (e.g., respiratory depression), abuse, and diversion represents drawbacks (333).

More common side effects associated with opioid analgesics include nausea, vomiting, constipation, sedation, euphoria, tolerance, and physical/psychological dependence. There may be minor variations to this side effect profile for individual agents (i.e., some have more pronounced side effects than others at equivalent doses) (334,335). Since all pure opioid agonists have equianalgesic doses with each other, selection of a specific agent is based upon the desired route of administration, duration of action, and desired side effect.

Other physiatric applications for opioids include diarrhea treatment and cough suppression; the latter is particularly pertinent for patients with nonproductive cough that is interfering with sleep and, thus, their rehabilitation. The recent discovery of opioid receptors beyond the CNS has led to much interest in "peripheral opioid analgesia"; there is now evidence that intramuscular, intra-articular, and intravenous injection of low-dosed opioid provides localized, peripheral analgesia and anti-inflammatory effects (336–340). Recent studies have implicated peripheral opioid analgesia in a cotreatment approach with other therapies, such as cytokine modulators or TNF-α antagonists in certain conditions, thereby providing an alternative for management of chronic inflammatory conditions (341).

Mechanism of Action and Pharmacokinetics

This class of medication mimics the action of opioids naturally produced by the body. Endorphins, enkephalins, and dynorphins are examples of these endogenous opioids. All opioids exert their effects by binding, with varying degrees of affinity, to three primary receptor types: mu (μ), kappa (κ), and delta (δ). Each receptor type has a unique CNS distribution and results in different physiologic responses, via variable biochemical pathways. Receptors have also been identified in immune cells, peripheral sensory nerves, and joints; these sites account for the peripheral analgesic and anti-inflammatory effects of opioids (342,343). The unifying property among all opioid receptors is that they are coupled to a G protein, which inhibits adenylyl cyclase. An activated receptor acts via its specific biochemical pathway to inhibit neuronal excitability and, thus, blocks pain impulse transmission.

Opioid analgesics can be categorized based on their affinity for a receptor and their intrinsic activity (i.e., amount of receptor stimulation they can produce). Morphine and methadone are designated as full agonists because they have high affinity for receptors and produce strong analgesia. Partial agonists, such as codeine, have lower affinity and are thus less potent than full agonists. Pentazocine is an example of a mixed agonist/antagonist that can activate unoccupied opioid receptors while blocking occupied ones. Antagonists (e.g., naloxone) are effective in reversing the effects of a full opioid agonist.

Slightly basic opioids are generally well absorbed in the small intestine. Short-acting agents demonstrate maximal effects between 30 and 60 minutes of administration and have durations of approximately 4 hours. Long-acting or sustained-release agents achieve peak effects within 2 to 24 hours and last for 12 to 72 hours—the first value correlates with oral administration and the second value correlates with transdermal application. Many opioids undergo first-pass metabolism in the liver. Hepatic conjugation is the primary route of metabolism for most opioids, but metabolism can also occur in the kidneys, lungs, and CNS. Active and inactive metabolites are excreted in urine and/or bile.

Preparations and Dosing

Opioid analgesics can be administered orally, intramuscularly, intravenously, subcutaneously, intraspinally, intranasally (e.g., naloxone), rectally (e.g., hydromorphone), transdermally (e.g., fentanyl patch), and transmucosally (e.g., fentanyl buccal tablet). The preferred route of administration and duration of action (i.e., long-acting vs. short-acting) will vary for a given patient. Short-acting agents can be used to manage acute pain syndromes and episodes of breakthrough pain. Long-acting agents are generally more convenient for patients with chronic conditions, and their sustained effects often help prevent pain-related nocturnal awakening.

Opioid preparations most relevant to physiatry, along with their usual dosage ranges and relative potencies, are shown in **Table 52-10**; although partial agonists and mixed agonist/

TABLE 52-10   Narcotic Analgesics

[Narcotic Class] Subclass Generic (Trade) Name	Usual Dosage Range (mg) (time = hours)	Relative Potency PO (IM) [Others]
[AGONISTS]		
Codeine	15–60 PO q4–6; 15–60 IM q4–6	200 (120)
Fentanyl transdermal (Duragesic patch)	1 patch q72	Refer PDR for table of equivalent doses
Hydromorphone (Dilaudid)	2–4 mg PO q4–6; 3 mg PR q6–8 0.5–2 mg IM/SC or slow IV q4–6	1.5
(Dilaudid-5)	5 mg/5 mL liquid PO q6	
Meperidine (Demerol)	1–1.8 mg/kg PO/IM/SC q3–4—MAX 150 mg Slow IV q3–4	300 (75)
Morphine sulfate		
Sustained-release tabs (MS Contin; Oramorph SR)	30 q8–12	60
Sustained-release caps (Kadian)	20 q12–24	
Oral solution (Roxanol)	Various concentrations: 10–30 q4	
Immediate release (MS IR)	10–30 q4	
Oxycodone		
Immediate-release tabs (OxyIR; Roxicodone)	5 q6	30
Immediate-release tabs (Percolone)	10–30 q4	
Oral concentrate solution (OxyFast)	5 mg q6 of a 20 mg/mL solution	
Sustained release (OxyContin)	10–40 q12	
Propoxyphene (Darvon Pulvules) (Darvon-N)	**[Removed from the US Market (2010)]**	
[PARTIAL AGONISTS]		
Buprenorphine (Buprenex)	Parenteral only	N/A
[MIXED AGONIST-ANTAGONISTS]		
Butorphanol tartrate nasal spray (Stadol NS)	1 mg (1 spray per nostril) q3–4	N/A
Pentazocine		
(Talwin)	1 tab PO q3–4	N/A
(Talwin NX){pentazocine, 50mg/naloxone, 0.5 mg}	1–2 tabs PO q3–4	
[ANALGESIC COMBINATIONS]		
Narcotic/acetaminophen		
Propoxyphene/acetaminophen (Darvocet) (*N* – 50 = 50/325; *N* – 100 = 100/650)	1–2 tabs PO q4	N/A
Hydrocodone/acetaminophen (Lortab) {2.5/500, 5/500, 7.5/500}	1–2 tabs PO q4–6	N/A
Anexsia (hydrocodone/acetaminophen) {5/500, 7.5/650, 10/660}	1 tab PO q4–6	
Hydrocodone/acetaminophen (Lorcet) {5/500}	1 tab PO q6	N/A
Oxycodone/acetaminophen (Percocet) {5/325}	1 tab PO q6	N/A
Pentazocine/acetaminophen (Talacen) {25/650}	1 caplet PO q4 (MAX. 6/24 h)	
APAP/codeine (Tylenol with codeine) {Tylenol #2, #3, #4 = 300/15; 300/30; 300/60}	1–2 tabs PO q4–6	N/A
Oxycodone/acetaminophen (Tylox) {5/500}	1 PO q6	
Hydrocodone/acetaminophen (Vicodin) {5/500}	1–2 tabs PO q4–6	N/A
Vicodin-ES {7.5/750}	1 tab PO q4–6	N/A
Narcotic/aspirin		
Propoxyphene/ASA/caffeine (Darvon Compound-65 Pulvules) {65/389/32.4}	1 tab PO q4	N/A
Oxycodone/aspirin (Percodan) {5/325}	1 tab PO q6	N/A
ASA/codeine (Empirin with Codeine #3) {325/30}		N/A
Empirin with Codeine # 4 (ASA/Codeine) {325/60}		
Pentazocine/ASA (Talwin compound) {12.5/325}	2 caplets PO q6–8	N/A

antagonist are listed in the table, they have limited application. Required oral doses are greater than parenteral ones because of first-pass metabolism effect following oral administration. The management of neuropathic pain usually requires higher doses than for nociceptive pain.

Patients requiring chronic opioid therapy are often initiated on a short-acting agent that is titrated over several weeks to achieve adequate analgesia and then converted to an equivalent dose of the long-acting agent (344). Doses can be titrated as high as necessary to relieve pain as long as they are tolerated well. Studies have shown that daily doses up to 120 mg of morphine equivalent can provide pain relief and improve sleep, without impairing cognitive function (330,344,345). Opioid rotation, which involves replacing one opioid with one that has incomplete cross-tolerance than the original, is a technique that is used in an attempt to avoid tolerance buildup and to overcome dose-limiting side effects (346,347). An individual is considered to be tolerant to opioid therapy when he/she is consuming greater than 60-mg oral morphine daily, greater than 25-μg transdermal fentanyl hourly, greater than 30-mg oxycodone daily, greater than 8-mg hydromorphone daily, or an equivalent dose of another opioid for greater than 1 week (348).

WHO recommends that all opioid therapies follow a fixed-interval dosing schedule, rather than being dispensed as needed (331). This strategy helps maintain a stable serum medication level and, in turn, minimizes side effects experienced at peak levels and breakthrough pain at trough levels. Another recommendation is for health care providers to recognize individual variability in opioid metabolism and pain tolerance. Therapy must therefore be individualized to maximize analgesia while minimizing side effects. Other guidelines within this document are designed to help optimize opioid analgesic use and minimize the side effects.

Opioid-Related Androgen Deficiency in Males

While opioids are prescribed widely for pain, the literature is lacking regarding some of the potential long-term risks associated with daily use of these drugs. For example, the issue of androgen deficiency in men with daily opioid use is in need of further study. This is particularly important because androgen deficiency has been linked to metabolic syndrome (i.e., obesity, HTN, hyperlipidemia, and glucose intolerance) (349).

Previous studies have elucidated the differences between long-acting and short-acting opioids with respect to structure, lipophilicity, and other factors affecting the hypothalamic-pituitary axis (HPA). These studies have concluded that long-acting opioids are associated with higher odds ratio of androgen deficiency than with equipotent doses of short-acting opioids. However, other studies have questioned these differences (349).

Rubinstein et al. further investigated the relationship between opioid use and androgen deficiency in males by conducting a retrospective cohort study. They hypothesized that certain prescribed opioids are associated with higher androgen deficiency when compared to hydrocodone. Morning serum testosterone levels were sampled for at least 90 days in 1,159 men (ages 18 to 80) on a single opioid for chronic noncancer pain. They concluded that men on transdermal fentanyl, methadone, and oxycodone were more likely to be androgen-deficient than men on hydrocodone. Of these, transdermal

fentanyl followed by methadone had the highest odds of androgen deficiency.

Altogether, these studies suggest that testosterone screening before opioid use may play an important role in order to identify both preexisting deficiency and perhaps those at greatest risk of developing androgen deficiency (349).

Individual Agents

Partial Agonists

Codeine

Codeine is a natural opioid present in opium that can be used as an analgesic, antitussive, or antidiarrheal agent. It possesses less than one seventh the analgesic potency of morphine and is often either combined with acetaminophen or used concomitantly with NSAIDs to manage mild to moderate pain (350). It has a relative lack of respiratory depression and a low abuse potential (due to its relative lack of euphoria). Codeine has high oral bioavailability because its phenyl ring shields the molecule from first-pass metabolism. Following administration, codeine is demethylated to morphine, an active metabolite, and, an inactive metabolite, norcodeine; these metabolites are then hepatically conjugated, and most are renally excreted. Individuals unable to convert codeine to morphine would experience negligible analgesic effects.

Potential adverse effects associated with codeine are typical of narcotic analgesics in general. Codeine is regulated under the Controlled Substances Act. Codeine is considered to be unsafe when consumed at high doses or for prolonged time during pregnancy. Some codeine-containing preparations may contain sodium metabisulfite, a potentially allergenic preservative. Sustained-release codeine, Codeine Contin, is available outside the United States for chronic pain management (351).

Propoxyphene (Darvon, Darvon Pulvules, Dolene)
This narcotic analgesic was removed from the US market in 2010 in response to an FDA recommendation because of its cardiotoxicity (prolongation of PR and QT intervals and QRS complex widening) at therapeutic doses (352).

Full Agonists

Fentanyl Transdermal (Duragesic), Fentanyl Transmucosal (Actiq, Fentora)
Fentanyl is a potent (i.e., >80 times that of morphine), short-acting opioid with therapeutic uses including analgesia, preprocedural anxiolysis, sedation, and supplemental anesthesia. It is available as an injectable preparation, a nebulized preparation, a transdermal patch, and a transmucosal lozenge/tablet. Management of terminally ill patients with dyspnea is an off-label use of nebulized fentanyl (342).

A transdermal delivery system for fentanyl is possible because it has a low molecular weight and is highly lipophilic, which enables the drug to be absorbed through the skin and subsequently distributed throughout the body. The fentanyl patch, with an average duration of 72 hours, is used to manage chronic pain that requires regular administration of narcotic analgesics. The advantages of transdermal fentanyl include lower incidences of constipation, nausea, and drowsiness (353). Cutaneous reactions are limited to localized dermatitis but systemic adverse effects may occur. The patch cannot be used in acute pain syndromes because initial absorption is delayed for 17 to 48 hours, and it should not be used in narcotic-naive patients due to the risk of significant hypoventilation. There is, however, a trend of employing a patient-controlled iontophoresis transdermal system, fentanyl HCl iontophoretic transdermal system (fentanyl ITS), to manage acute postoperative pain within inpatient settings (259,354,355). In clinical trials, fentanyl ITS was found to be superior to placebo and as effective as morphine IV PCA in patients with moderate to severe postoperative pain (356).

When initiating a fentanyl patch therapy for narcotic-naive patients, one should start with the lowest available dose (currently 12.5 µg/h). There is a wide variability of absorption among patients, and titration can be accomplished by combining various available patch strengths (e.g., 25, 50, 75, and 100 µg/h) (357). As for patients who are accustomed to opioid therapy, the initial dose is estimated from previous equianalgesic morphine doses. Fever, diaphoresis, cachexia, morbid obesity, and ascites can all affect the rate of transdermal absorption, and dosage should hence be adjusted accordingly (358). Physiatrists involved in pain management should also become familiar with dosage titration, discontinuation strategies, and drug interactions for the fentanyl patch.

With an average onset of action in 5 minutes, transmucosal delivery provides a rapid route of absorption into the bloodstream. The lozenge and buccal tablet are only FDA approved for treatment of breakthrough cancer pain in patients who are tolerant to their current opioid therapies, but various off-label uses have been reported (359–362). Dosing should be individualized to achieve adequate analgesia with tolerable side effects. If the pain is not relieved following transmucosal administration, a second dose of lozenge and buccal tablet can be administered 15 and 30 minutes after completion of the first, respectively (363). Patients should not exceed 4 units per day. Single doses between 100 and 800 µg are generally well-tolerated, causing mild to moderate opioid-associated side effects (364).

Hydromorphone (Dilaudid)

This semisynthetic opioid is derived from morphine. These two compounds have similar pharmacokinetic profiles, except that hydromorphone has a shorter duration of action but five times the analgesic efficacy. An open-labeled study found that hydromorphone causes less nausea, emesis, and constipation (365,366). Hydromorphone may be a valuable alternative for patients with "pseudoallergy" (i.e., flushing and itching due to histamine release) to morphine in managing moderate to severe chronic pain because it appears to induce minimal histamine release (367). It is also preferred for patients with renal failure because its metabolite is nontoxic (368). Finally, hydromorphone's superior water solubility allows high doses to be dissolved into solution and delivered to opioid-tolerant patients.

Several hydromorphone-containing products are FDA approved as antitussives, and a nebulized form is available for off-label use in terminally ill patients with dyspnea (369,370). Although Hydromorph Contin remains available in Canada, a similar extended-release formulation was withdrawn from the US market in 2005 due to a high risk of overdose when consumed with alcohol.

Meperidine (Demerol)

Once a popular fast-acting agent used for management of moderate to severe postoperative pain, meperidine is of limited use in physiatry for four major reasons. First, it has only one tenth of morphine's potency, yet the two have similar addiction and physical dependence risks (371). Second, its short duration of action necessitates frequent dosing, and this practice cycles through peaks and troughs in serum concentrations. Third, meperidine is metabolized to normeperidine, a toxic metabolite which causes CNS hyperexcitability that can manifest as seizure, anxiety, tremors, and myoclonus (371). Patients with impaired renal function are obviously susceptible to meperidine toxicity, but healthy individuals are also vulnerable because normeperidine accumulates with use greater than several days.

Methadone

Methadone is both an agonist to µ-receptors and a weak, noncompetitive antagonist to NMDA receptors. Discovery of this unique dual action has led to increased use of methadone for the treatment of neuropathic pain, including phantom limb pain, and burn pain in recent years (372–374). Methadone is also becoming increasingly used as a second-line agent in treating cancer pain unresponsive to conventional opioids (375). Traditional uses include management of severe, chronic pain and suppression of withdrawal symptoms from heroin and morphine. For the latter reason, there is social stigma associated with methadone.

This Schedule II controlled opioid has several advantages including its lack of active metabolites, its high lipid solubility, its excellent absorption after oral and rectal delivery, and its low cost (48). Despite these advantages, the conversion schedule (i.e., dose and time course) between methadone and other opioids remains indeterminate. Deaths have been reported in conversion to methadone from other opioid agonists and during initiation of methadone treatment of addiction. Therefore, particular vigilance is required during conversion and initiation. Confusion arises from the fact that parenteral methadone is proposed, but not proven to be equianalgesic to morphine, and traditional opioid conversion charts have underestimated the potency of methadone, leading to safety concerns (376). Another drawback of methadone is its long half-life because unpredictable drug accumulation at the beginning of a regimen carries a risk of respiratory depression. Myoclonus and electrocardiographic changes (e.g., QT prolongation and torsade de pointes) have been reported as well (377). Methadone is also increasingly being abused by recreational drug users and has been associated nationally with increases in overdose and death. Because it does not lead to quick onset or significant euphoria, its substance abuse potential had been considered as low. Unfortunately, it can be hours before a user feels any effect, which increases the risk that they may be alone at the time of overdose.

Oxycodone (OxyIR, OxyContin, Eth-Oxydose)

Oxycodone is a morphine derivative that is available as a generic short-acting form, a short-acting immediate-release form (OxyIR), a controlled-release form (OxyContin), as well as several combination analgesic products. Pure oxycodone products offer the advantage of not being limited by the potential for end-organ toxicity, in contrast to combination products due to the presence of aspirin and acetaminophen. Its efficacy in managing neuropathic and somatic pain has been established, but OxyContin is only approved for management of chronic, moderate to severe pain (378).

OxyContin has high oral availability due to minimal first-pass metabolism. Easy access has historically led to its widespread abuse in the United States (379). This in fact has led the FDA to place a black box warning on the product, categorize it as a Schedule II controlled substance, and order the discontinuation of the 160-mg tablets. Despite these problems with diversion, OxyContin is still a valuable medication with a fast onset and long duration of action—the apparent dichotomy of prompt yet sustained analgesia can be explained by the AcroContin delivery system, whereby oxycodone is released relatively quickly after ingestion and continues to be steadily released over the subsequent 12 hours. When dosed around the clock, it provides sustained serum levels through the night and potentially minimizes narcotic side effects often associated with peak serum drug levels. A relatively short half-life also allows OxyContin to reach steady state in a short time period, thereby achieving its full analgesic potential within a day or 2 of treatment initiation. An additional benefit is that, unlike MS Contin, its absorption is independent of pH; this allows patients to take this opioid with or without food.

The short-acting immediate-release form, OxyIR, can be used as premedication prior to physical therapy for patients whose pain level interferes with meaningful participation in therapeutic exercises. One fourth to one third of the 12-hour dose of OxyContin can also be prescribed to treat breakthrough pain. If greater than two rescue doses are needed during any 24-hour period, the OxyContin regimen should be titrated.

The liver extensively metabolizes oxycodone into oxymorphone, which has even greater analgesic potency, and noroxycodone, a weak analgesic. Neither metabolite causes end-organ toxicity. Efficacy and adverse events are believed to be similar for both OxyIR and OxyContin (380,381). Compared to morphine, they appear to cause less nausea and vomiting but more constipation (382).

Partial Agonists

Buprenorphine (Buprenex, Subutex, Suboxone)

Buprenorphine, a mild to moderate analgesic, has been available via parenteral administration for many years. This partial agonist, with agonistic activity at κ- and δ-receptors, became available to the United States in a sublingual form (Subutex) in 2002, and it was FDA approved for medication-assisted treatment of opioid addiction (383). A transdermal delivery system for this medication can also be found in European markets. A review of various clinical studies concluded that oral, intravenous, intrathecal, and transdermal buprenorphine are all efficacious in managing neuropathic pain. Further research is still required to develop guidelines for different pain syndromes (384). Intravenous and oral administrations, additionally, have sustained antihyperalgesia effect in inflammatory models (385).

Slow dissociation from the μ-receptor makes buprenorphine a long-acting agent. Fewer withdrawal signs occur because buprenorphine minimally affects GI motility and sphincter tone. It does not have an analgesic ceiling, but it can

cause respiratory depression at high doses and this cannot be readily reversed with naloxone (386,387).

Mixed Agonists-Antagonists

These analgesics are used for moderate to severe pain but do not offer any superiority over opioid agonists. They have a lower respiratory depression risk compared to traditional agonists, but this benefit is minimal given that all agonist users build tolerance to respiratory depression over time. There are several disadvantages inherent to class, including an analgesic ceiling and the potential to precipitate a withdrawal syndrome among previous opioid users. It is nonetheless important to be somewhat familiar with several key medications.

The synthetically prepared prototype agent, pentazocine (Talwin, Talacen), is an antagonist at μ-receptors and an agonist at κ- and δ-opioid receptors. It is approximately equianalgesic to codeine on a milligram-per-milligram basis. Several different pentazocine combinations are available as shown in **Table 52-10**. It is unclear how pentazocine-containing medications can be best used in pain management. A pentazocine-methylphenidate combination—known by various street terms including "crackers," "poor man's heroin," and "T's and rits"—is subject to illicit use because the compound produces an effect similar to that of heroin mixed with cocaine. Talwin NX blends pentazocine with naloxone to maintain analgesic effects but minimizes abuse.

Butorphanol tartrate (Stadol NS) is a mixed agonist-antagonist (i.e., agonist at κ-opioid receptors and a mixed agonist-antagonist at μ-opioid receptors) that offers the flexibility of intranasal administration. Of note, widespread abuse of the nasal spray led to its classification as a Schedule IV controlled substance in the late 1990s. Butorphanol has not been widely used by physiatrists, and there remains scant literature on its use in musculoskeletal pain (388,389). Instead, it has a niche in the general surgical setting, where it is used as a preoperative/postoperative sedative and analgesic, a supplement to balanced anesthesia, a conscious sedative, and a postanesthesia shaking suppressor. Additional applications include analgesia during labor, relief of moderate postpartum pain, and a treatment for migraine headache.

Relevant Side Effects and Drug Interactions

Before discussing opioid-related side effects, it is important to clarify three terms: tolerance, addiction, and dependence. *Tolerance* can be defined as a reduced reaction to a drug following its repeated administration. Tolerance can be a double-edged sword. It potentially negatively affects treatment when an increasing amount of a drug is needed to produce a given therapeutic effect. Tolerance to side effects (other than constipation), however, is of obvious benefit. *Dependence* is the onset of withdrawal symptoms when a drug is abruptly removed. *Addiction* is the habitual use of a substance to achieve a certain effect—usually euphoria—that the patient perceives as pleasurable. Confusion of these terms has led to bias against the use of narcotic analgesics, particularly for nonmalignant pain. Fear of patient addiction is also the main reason why physicians tend to underprescribe narcotics (390). There is controversy as to whether psychological addiction actually develops in patients with chronic pain without a past history of substance abuse (391–393).

Health care providers may need to explain the concept of tolerance to patients and their families to quell the anxiety associated with increased narcotic requirement that often occurs after approximately 1 month of treatment. Tolerance begins after the first dose but does not become clinically apparent until the 2nd or 3rd week and generally lasts for up to 2 weeks after the regimen concludes. Since there is incomplete cross-tolerance among the different narcotic agents, analgesia can often be sustained with a schedule of opioid rotation (394). Finally, there is a notion that tolerance can be avoided altogether if opioid doses are matched with the patient's needs, such that there is no excess medication to cause euphoria and then tolerance.

Abrupt cessation of opioid therapy in a physically dependent patient can lead to withdrawal symptoms, which can sometimes be subtle and manifest only as complaints of mild, nonspecific muscle aches. Onset and duration of the withdrawal process correlate with the half-life of the specific drug, but autonomic symptoms can be blunted with the use of oral or transdermal clonidine, at a dose of 0.1 to 0.2 mg/d. Similar to tolerance, there is a notion that if doses are matched with the patient's needs, then physical dependence will never develop. However, traditional teaching is that most patients who take opioids for more than 1 month will have some degree of physical dependence. In order to avert withdrawal symptoms in physically dependent patients, detailed guidelines have been developed for weaning patients off opioid treatment (395,396).

The overall side effect profile for narcotic analgesics is relatively favorable, especially in the elderly population. Constipation is the most common narcotic side effect, and it is also the only one to which tolerance will not develop over time. Since it can profoundly negatively affect patients' lives, the initiation of prophylactic bowel stimulants or osmotic agents should be strongly considered with opioid therapy. If constipation develops despite prophylaxis, it should be treated aggressively.

Another prevalent GI side effect includes nausea with or without vomiting. Prophylaxis against nausea is not routinely employed because patients usually build tolerance to nausea over time. Treatment of nausea depends upon its etiology. If it is due to constipation, then the latter should be treated; in contrast, if nausea is due to a primary effect of the medication (i.e., stimulation of the chemotrigger zone), then prochlorperazine is a first-line agent for treatment of this. If the patient remains nauseous after addressing the above and other possible etiologies, agents such as haloperidol could be considered. If the patient additionally develops agitation, chlorpromazine would be an appropriate second-line agent of choice. Metoclopramide can be employed if the suspected etiology is gastric outlet obstruction, secondary to the antimotility effect of opioids. Nonoral adjuvant analgesics (e.g., IV indomethacin or IM ketorolac) may be more appropriate for patients suffering from narcotic-related nausea.

Patients on opioid therapy can also experience significant non–gastrointestinal-related adverse events. Orthostatic hypotension, for example, can reach a degree where it limits rehabilitative transfer and ambulation training. Respiratory depression, manifested as reduced respiratory rate in the early stage, can also become severe enough to cause respiratory arrest. Habitual users are less likely than narcotic-naive patient to suffer the extremes of either event because of a phenomenon

known as tolerance, where patients adapt to a drug's effects over time. Evolving theories attribute receptor desensitization and receptor down-regulation to tolerance (397).

Opioids can induce a variety of additional side effects. For example, opioids can influence various hormones of the hypothalamus-pituitary-gonad system (398,399). Both acute administration and chronic use of opioids, in the absence of pain, can be immunosuppressive (400). Repeated administration may produce hyperalgesia (397,401,402). Potential CNS side effects include sedation and euphoria. Sedation can be countered using stimulants such as caffeine, dextroamphetamine, and methylphenidate. Euphoria is comparatively more problematic as it is the basis behind psychological addiction.

Tramadol HCL (Ultram), Tramadol HCL and Acetaminophen (Ultracet)

Relevance to Physiatry. Tramadol is a centrally acting, synthetic analgesic with FDA approval for management of moderate to severe pain. It is a unique drug because it was not initially classified as a controlled substance (though its μ-receptor binding affinity is similar to codeine) and it has an additional mechanism of action akin to many antidepressants. Given the dual mechanism, tramadol can be an effective analgesic for both nociceptive and neuropathic pain (403). However, the Federal Drug Enforcement Agency published its decision to schedule tramadol as a Schedule IV controlled substance in 2014. Randomized controlled trials have demonstrated its efficacy in treating PHN, phantom limb pain, diabetic neuropathy, and polyneuropathy of various etiologies (404–407). As for chronic nociceptive pain, the American College of Rheumatology (ACR) continues to recommend tramadol for osteoarthritis (OA) patients who have failed to achieve adequate benefit from nonnarcotic analgesic medications (408). Finally, this weak opioid agonist can also be used to treat migraine, moderately severe episodic breakthrough pain, and it has been studied in acute dental and surgical pain (409,410).

Ultracet contains 37.5 mg of tramadol and 325 mg of acetaminophen. Its exact role in pain management is still evolving. Its advantages, like any other combination analgesics, are synergistic analgesia and reduced dose-dependent side effects (411). Only a few randomized, placebo-controlled studies have been conducted to date using Ultracet, and they have overall shown that it is as effective as and better tolerated than acetaminophen with codeine (at 300/30 mg) for chronic, nonmalignant low back pain, OA pain, and fibromyalgia (412–414). Lee et al. conducted a multicenter, double-blind clinical trial to investigate Ultracet's efficacy in treating pain associated with rheumatoid arthritis. They found that Ultracet, as an add-on therapy in patients with symptomatic rheumatoid arthritis, was associated with a significant improvement in pain relief and a statistically significant reduction in pain intensity when compared with placebo. Lee et al. concluded that Ultracet may be a viable analgesic option when combined with conventional NSAIDs and disease-modifying antirheumatic drugs in patients with rheumatoid arthritis (415).

The extended-release form, Ultram ER, has a convenient once-daily dosing schedule for managing chronic pain conditions. It is shown to have similar tolerability and effectiveness at relieving moderate to severe OA pain as the original tramadol (416).

In summary, tramadol is potentially advantageous compared to NSAIDs and COX-II inhibitors because it does not cause GI bleeding nor exacerbation of HTN or CHF (417). There may also be decreased tolerance to tramadol's therapeutic effect with chronic use in treatment of pain due to knee and hip OA (418,419).

Mechanism of Action and Pharmacokinetics. Tramadol has two complementary analgesic mechanisms including weak activation of μ-receptors and pain impulse transmission modification, via weak inhibition of norepinephrine and serotonin reuptake. This compound can therefore be thought of as both a synthetic opioid and a TCA.

Tramadol has high bioavailability. Following oral administration, one fifth of the drug is protein bound and it undergoes extensive first-pass hepatic metabolism. Onset of analgesia is apparent within 1 hour, and a mean peak plasma concentration is reached within 1.5 to 2 hours. The liver demethylates and glucuronidates tramadol into several metabolites, only one of which have analgesic properties (420). All metabolites and the unchanged portion are renally excreted. Tramadol has a half-life of 6 hours and steady-state is achieved within 2 days when it is taken four times daily.

Preparations and Dosing. Tramadol is available in the United States as 50-mg immediate-release tablets. Extended-release tablets (Ultram ER in denominations of 100, 200, and 300 mg) are available in the United States. Intravenous, intramuscular, rectal, and subcutaneous preparations are available internationally.

The usual dosing range for immediate-release tramadol is between 50 and 100 mg, every 4 to 6 hours. The maximum recommended dose is 400 mg daily. Dosing adjustments are recommended for patients older than 75 years old (<300 mg/d), with a creatinine clearance less than 30 mL/min (administer every 12 hours, with a maximum daily dose of 200 mg), and with a history of hepatic dysfunction. Patients with nonacute pain are initiated on a starting dose of 50 mg every day, increased by one 50-mg dose every 3 days until the maximum daily dose is reached; this strategy minimizes side effects. Patients with acute pain can be treated with an initial 50-mg dose, followed by another 25- to 50-mg dose if adequate analgesia is not achieved within the first hour.

The starting dose for extended-release therapy is 100 mg daily, which can be increased at a rate of 100 mg/d for every 5 days. The recommended maximum dose is 300 mg/d, but a daily dose of 400 mg has been safely prescribed for patients under 75 years old (421,422).

Relevant Side Effects and Drug Interactions. Nausea, drowsiness, and constipation are the most common side effects (423). The frequency of both is notably less than traditional opioids. Vomiting, somnolence, abdominal pain, headache, dry mouth, dyspepsia, and vertigo have also been reported (411). Respiratory depression and pruritus are potential side effects associated with all opioids, but tramadol has a much lower risk of either (424). Serious, and rarely fatal, anaphylactoid reactions have occurred following the first tramadol dose; individuals with a history of anaphylactoid reactions to opioids may be at higher risk.

Seizure is a rare but significant potential side effect of tramadol. Caution should be exercised if tramadol is prescribed to patients with epilepsy, a seizure history, or seizure risk factors (e.g., TBI, metabolic disorders, alcohol/drug withdrawal, and

CNS infections). SSRIs or TCAs should not be prescribed with tramadol because they may further lower the seizure threshold. CNS depressants and MAOIs should be avoided as well because they pose risks of respiratory depression and hypertensive crisis, respectively. One should also be aware that carbamazepine markedly induces tramadol's metabolism, such that twice the usual tramadol dose might be needed. Additionally, the FDA has restricted the use of tramadol in children and recommended against use in breastfeeding women (425).

Tramadol is a Schedule IV opioid and but has limited abuse potential because it rarely produces euphoria. However, abrupt cessation of therapy can lead to opioid withdrawal symptoms—though they may not be as severe as with other opioids—and atypical withdrawal symptoms (e.g., hallucinations and paranoia) (426).

FDA's Role in Ensuring Safe Opioid Use

In 2014, approximately 3.8 million people aged 12 years or older reported nonmedical use of prescription opioid analgesics in the United States, making opioid abuse the second most commonly abused drug after marijuana (427). This opioid abuse epidemic has been linked to significant morbidity and mortality. From 1999 to 2014, the number of drug poisoning deaths involving opioid analgesics rose more than 4.5-fold from 4,030 to 18,893 (428).

In light of the rising prescription opioid abuse and subsequent overdoses, on August 31, 2016, the FDA created new boxed warnings on labels of all opioid analgesics, opioid-containing cough substances, and benzodiazepines. The FDA also has created the Opioid Action Plan, which aims to curb prescription opioid abuse, but still allow for patients with chronic pain to obtain access to clinically indicated pain management options. Some notable features of this plan are shown in 🛜 **eTable 52-7**.

Abuse-Deterrent Opioids

In addition to mandatory boxed warnings and the Opioid Action Plan (as outlined in 🛜 **eTable 52-7**), the FDA is encouraging the development of opioid formulations that have abuse-deterrent (AD) properties, which should make abuse more difficult. These formulations act to target the known or expected routes of abuse, such as snorting, crushing, or injecting, by creating physical or chemical barriers. Some products may contain substances that, when altered, release substances that cause unpleasant effect. The science of these AD opioids is a relatively new and evolving technology. In 2015, the FDA released a guidance document for the evaluation of abuse-deterrent opioids. In it, the FDA outlined four abuse-deterrent study categories: (a) lab-based *in vitro* manipulation and extraction studies, (b) *in vivo* pharmacokinetic studies assessing manipulated drugs, (c) human abuse potential studies, and (d) postmarketing studies (429).

Currently, 10 AD opioids have been approved by the FDA, many of which are extended-release (ER) formulations (see 🛜 **eTable 52-8**). To date, there are no intermediate-release AD opioids approved by the FDA. All of the companies with approved brand name AD opioids are required to conduct postmarket studies to determine the impact of AD technologies, including evidence from *in vitro* and *in vivo* studies. Additionally, all of the following FDA-approved drugs are Schedule II controlled substances indicated for the management of pain severe enough to require daily, around-the-clock, long-term opioid treatment and for which alternative treatment options are inadequate. Below outlines a brief description of each of the 10 FDA-approved AD opioid medications (see 📶 **eTable 52-8**).

Hysingla ER

Abuse-Deterrence Property
Hysingla ER contains water-soluble hydrocodone bitartrate, which exists as fine white crystals or a crystalline powder, and is affected by light. AD characteristics of Hysingla ER include forming a gelatinous hydrogel when exposed to aqueous environments (430).

Mechanism of Action and Pharmacokinetics
As compared to an immediate-release hydrocodone combination product, Hysingla ER results in similar bioavailability at the same daily dose. Steady-state plasma concentrations are approximated to be 72 hours with the mean terminal $t_{1/2}$ life of 7 hours (430).
(See *Codeine* section for mechanism of action.)

Preparations and Dosing
The Hysingla ER tablets are available in 20, 30, 40, 60, 80, 100, and 120 mg. For opioid-naive patients, initiate with 20-mg tablets orally every 24 hours (430).

Relevant Side Effects and Drug Interactions
See *Codeine* section.

Vantrela ER

Abuse-Deterrence Property
Vantrela ER contains hydrocodone bitartrate, a white to yellow-white crystalline powder. It resists crushing, breaking, and dissolution. Upon small volumes of extraction, it forms a viscous hydrogel when exposed to aqueous environments (431).

Mechanism of Action and Pharmacokinetics
Oral bioavailability of Vantrela ER is similar to the profile of hydrocodone bitartrate. Steady state of Vantrela is 24 hours, with a half-life between 11 and 12 hours (431).
(See *Codeine* section for mechanism of action.)

Preparations and Dosing
Vantrela ER tablets are available in 15, 30, 45, 60, and 90 mg. For opioid-naive and opioid nontolerant patients, 15-mg tablet orally every 12 hours is the suggested starting dose (431).

Relevant Side Effects and Drug Interactions
See *Codeine* section.

Arymo ER

Abuse-Deterrence Property
Similar to other AD opioids, Arymo ER tablets form a viscous hydrogel when exposed to liquid environment. This gelatinous mass is what produces the AD property of the substance, further making it more difficult for abuse via injection. Any manipulation of the tablet (cutting, breaking, chewing, crushing, and dissolving) will result in delivery of morphine that could lead to overdose and death (432).

Mechanism of Action and Pharmacokinetics
The oral bioavailability of morphine is approximately 20% to 40%, with a steady state of 24 hours, and half-life (after intravenous administration) is normally 2 to 4 hours (432).
(See *Morphine* section for mechanism of action.)

Preparations and Dosing
Arymo ER is available in doses of 15, 30, and 60 mg. Treatment with Arymo ER can be initiated with 15-mg tablets every 8 or 12 hours (432).

Relevant Side Effects and Drug Interactions
See *Morphine* section.

Embeda

Abuse-Deterrence Property
Embeda capsules contain pellets of morphine sulfate and sequestered naltrexone hydrochloride. When Embeda capsules are crushed, it results in the simultaneous release and rapid absorption of morphine sulfate and naltrexone hydrochloride (433).

Mechanism of Action and Pharmacokinetics
The bioavailability of oral Embeda is only 20% to 40%, while the steady-state plasma concentrations are approximated to be 24 to 36 hours. The terminal elimination half-life of morphine following single-dose Embeda administration is approximately 29 hours (433).
(See *Morphine* section for mechanism of action.)

Preparations and Dosing
Embeda is available in six dosage strengths, including 20/0.8, 30/1.2, 50/2, 60/2.4, 80/3.2, and 100/4 mg. It is administered once daily in opioid-naive patients or twice daily (every 12 hours, BID) in opioid nontolerant patients (433).

Relevant Side Effects and Drug Interactions
See *Morphine* section.

MorphaBond ER

Abuse-Deterrence Property
MorphaBond ER contains morphine sulfate and is formulated with inactive ingredients that make abuse via injection or insufflation more difficult while maintaining ER characteristics in spite of physical manipulation or chemical extraction; MorphaBond ER also forms gelatinous hydrogel when exposed to aqueous environments (434).

Mechanism of Action and Pharmacokinetics
The oral bioavailability of morphine is approximately 20% to 40%. When MorphaBond ER is given on a fixed dosing regimen, steady state is achieved in about 24 hours. Steady-state levels are also approximated to be 24 hours. Morphine has a 2- to 4-hour half-life after intravenous administration (434).
(See *Morphine* section for mechanism of action.)

Preparations and Dosing
MorphaBond ER tablets are available in 15-, 30-, 60-, and 100-mg dosing strengths. It is recommended to initiate treatment with 15-mg tablets orally every 12 hours (434).

Relevant Side Effects and Drug Interactions
See *Morphine* section.

OxyContin ER

Abuse-Deterrence Property
In 2010, FDA approved an AD form of OxyContin ER, and then in April 2013, it became the first opioid analgesic to receive labeled description of abuse-deterrent properties (435). OxyContin ER contains oxycodone, and when exposed to aqueous environments, OxyContin ER forms a gelatinous

hydrogel, which provides its AD properties, further making abuse via intravenous or intranasal routes more difficult (436).

Mechanism of Action and Pharmacokinetics

The oxycodone release is pH-independent, giving it an oral bioavailability of 60% to 87%. This high oral bioavailability is due to low presystemic and/or first-pass metabolism. Steady-state levels were achieved within 24 to 36 hours, and the apparent elimination half-life of oxycodone following the administration of OxyContin ER is 4.5 hours (436).

(See *Oxycodone* section for mechanism of action.)

Preparations and Dosing

OxyContin ER tablets are available in 10-, 15-, 20-, 30-, 40-, 60-, and 80-mg tablets for oral administration. For opioid-naive and opioid nontolerant patients, FDA recommends initiating treatment with 10-mg tablets orally every 12 hours (436).

Relevant Side Effects and Drug Interactions

See *Oxycodone* section.

Targiniq ER

Abuse-Deterrence Property

Targiniq ER contains a combination of oxycodone hydrochloride and naloxone hydrochloride. It can be crushed and dissolved in solution. However, according to the FDA drug fact sheet, complete separation or complete inactivation of naloxone from oxycodone was not achieved despite using various techniques and conditions. Based on *in vitro* study results, Targiniq ER tablets will lessen abuse via the intravenous and intranasal routes of administration by its inability to separate the two active components. Cutting, breaking, chewing, crushing, or dissolving Targiniq ER impairs the ER delivery mechanism and results in the rapid release and absorption of a potentially fatal dose of oxycodone (437).

Mechanism of Action and Pharmacokinetics

The oral bioavailability of oxycodone from Targiniq ER is 60% to 87%. Steady-state plasma concentrations are reached in approximately 48 hours. The oxycodone is rapidly eliminated from the body with a mean half-life of approximately 3.9 to 5.3 hours after a single oral dose administration of Targiniq ER in healthy subjects. Naloxone is eliminated from the body with mean $t_{1/2}$ ranging from 4.1 to 17.2 hours (437).

(See *Oxycodone* section for mechanism of action.)

Preparations and Dosing

Targiniq ER is available in 10/5, 20/10, and 40/20 mg. For opioid-naive and opioid nontolerant patients, it is recommended to initiate treatment of Targiniq ER with 10/5 mg tablets orally every 12 hours (437).

Relevant Side Effects and Drug Interactions

See *Oxycodone* section.

Troxyca ER

Abuse-Deterrence Property

Troxyca ER capsules contain pellets of oxycodone hydrochloride with sequestered naltrexone hydrochloride (an opioid antagonist). When taken as directed, the naltrexone remains sequestered and patients receive oxycodone in an extended-release manner. Crushing the pellets releases sequestered naltrexone, thereby counteracting the effects of oxycodone (438).

Mechanism of Action and Pharmacokinetics

Oral bioavailability of Troxyca ER is 60% to 87%, while steady state was reached within 48 hours with twice-daily dosing (12 hours apart). The apparent elimination half-life of oxycodone is approximately 7.2 hours (438).

(See *Oxycodone* section for mechanism of action.)

Preparations and Dosing

Troxyca ER is available in fixed dosage strengths of 10/1.2, 20/2.4, 30/3.6, 40/4.8, 60/7.2, and 80/9.6 mg. For opioid-naive and opioid nontolerant patients, initiate with 10/1.2 mg capsule every 12 hours (438).

Relevant Side Effects and Drug Interactions

See *Oxycodone* section.

RoxyBond

Abuse-Deterrence Property

RoxyBond contains oxycodone hydrochloride. It has an AD formulation that deters intranasal and IV abuse by forming a viscous hydrogel that resists passage through a needle when attempting to inject intravenously (439).

Mechanism of Action and Pharmacokinetics

RoxyBond has demonstrated comparable bioavailability to Roxicodone (60% to 87%). Steady-state plasma concentrations take 18 to 24 hours, with an apparent elimination half-life between 3.8 and 4.3 hours (439).

(See *Oxycodone* section for mechanism of action.)

Preparations and Dosing

Dosage strengths are same as Roxicodone, both of which are available in 5-, 15-, and 30-mg dosing regimens. Dosing can be initiated with a range of 5 to 15 mg every 4 to 6 hours as needed (439).

Relevant Side Effects and Drug Interactions

See *Oxycodone* section.

Xtampza ER

Abuse-Deterrence Property

Xtampza ER is an opioid analgesic containing a microsphere in-capsule formulation, with each individual microsphere acting as its own drug delivery system. Each microsphere consists of oxycodone homogeneously dispersed in a hydrophobic matrix of fatty acid and waxes. The small particle size and waxy, hydrophobic nature create the AD properties of Xtampza ER (440).

Modes of administration include oral via intact capsule, sprinkling directly into the mouth, or on soft foods and via enteral tubes such as nasogastric and gastrostomy tubes; these various routes of administration provide flexible dosing options for those who have difficulty swallowing. Additionally, characteristics of Xtampza ER are maintained if chewed or crushed, making it the only ER-formulated opioid without a boxed warning against crushing or chewing (440).

Mechanism of Action and Pharmacokinetics

Bioavailability of Xtampza ER is 114% in fed state when compared to 75% in fasted state. Steady-state levels were achieved within 24 to 36 hours, with a half-life of 5.6 hours in fed state (440).

(See *Oxycodone* section for mechanism of action.)

Preparations and Dosing

Xtampza ER is available in fix dosage strengths, including 9, 13.5, 18, 27, and 36 mg. For opioid-naive and opioid non-tolerant patients, initiate Xtampza ER treatment with 9-mg capsule orally, twice a day, every 12 hours with food. It is imperative that patients take Xtampza ER with food as the oral bioavailability is dependent on the food consumed (greatest after a high-fat and high-calorie meal) (440).

Relevant Side Effects and Drug Interactions

See *Oxycodone* section.

Investigational Drugs

Oliceridine (TRV130)

Oliceridine is the first μ-receptor G protein pathway selective modulator, or "μGPS." It is indicated for the management of moderate to severe acute pain where intravenous therapy is preferred. In February 2016, the FDA granted Breakthrough Therapy status to oliceridine with hopes to improve delivery of the pain-reducing potential of an opioid with fewer adverse effects. Oliceridine is available only in intravenous form and may provide benefit over IV morphine with less side effects (441).

Transdermal and Topical Analgesic Medications

The skin can be used to deliver medications locally, to an underlying target tissue, or systemically. Depending upon the medication, delivery can be via an exogenous, disposable transdermal (TD) delivery system or topical application of cream or ointment. While the terms "transdermal" and "topical" are often used interchangeably, TD delivery aims to achieve systemic therapeutic levels similar to that of oral administration and can be administered distal to the target site over an extended period of time. The fentanyl patch is an example of a true TD delivery system, while topical NSAIDs, the topical NSAIDs patch Flector (topical diclofenac epolamine), and the lidocaine patch are examples of topical application.

TD delivery and topical application have become increasingly popular as it circumvents the unpredictability of GI tract absorption and hepatic first-pass metabolism. Topical medications can also achieve higher therapeutic concentration at local sites than do systemically administered medications.

All TD delivery systems are comprised of three elements: a backing, the active drug, and the adhesive. First-generation reservoir systems release active drug via a rate-limiting membrane. Second-generation matrix systems have the active drug embedded in polymer layers and are directly applied to the skin. Both systems deliver the active drug at a constant rate and thereby maintain constant drug-plasma level. This feature, in turn, extends the therapeutic activity for drugs with short half-lives and improves patient compliance by increasing the dosing interval.

An increasing number of medications will likely be delivered via the skin in the future as new mechanical enhancements are developed to increase TD topical permeability and allow patient-controlled administration. Iontophoresis is a currently available enhancement mechanism, and various others (e.g., electroporation, sonophoresis, and microneedles) are being investigated (442–444).

Unfortunately, several factors limit TD and topical analgesic medication application. For one, significant contact dermatitis can occur among selected individuals. TD delivery and topical application are also not suitable for all medications. The efficacy of individual analgesic medications is further complicated by certain variables including humidity of the skin, ambient temperature, a drug's thermodynamic properties, and the target tissue's properties. The major disadvantage remains that most TD preparations (especially that of topical NSAIDs) have relatively short shelf lives, which makes mass production difficult.

The physiatrist should become familiar with TD delivery and topical application because they may encounter some of these medications in daily practice. A partial list of available TD medication classes includes analgesics, antibiotics, anticholinergics, antiemetics, and hormones. The aforementioned medications can also be delivered across mucous membranes using intranasal sprays, ophthalmologic solutions, and suppository.

Topical agents are widely available over the counter, but many TD medications are only available using a specialized pharmacy known as a compounding pharmacy.

Individual Agents

EMLA, LIDOCAINE, and FENTANYL patches have been discussed previously in this chapter.

Diclofenac Epolamine (Flector Patch)

Relevance to Physiatry

Although the international community has had significant experience with topical NSAIDs and they are reported to be well-tolerated, particularly with respect to their lack of associated GI side effects, as of early 2017, there are 3 approved topical NSAIDs in the United States, Flector patch, diclofenac sodium topical gel 1% (Voltaren gel), and diclofenac sodium topical solution 1.5%.

The active ingredient in Flector patch is 1.3% diclofenac epolamine. It is indicated for minor sprains, strains, and contusions. RCTs have also shown that it is effective in short-term treatment of symptomatic knee OA and epicondylitis (445,446).

Of these, both diclofenac sodium topical gel 1% and diclofenac sodium topical solution 1.5% are approved by the FDA for the management of OA (447).

An investigation of a combination preparation (heparin and lecithin with diclofenac epolamine) is underway, and preliminary results suggest that this combination has superior anti-inflammatory, hemorheologic, and antiedema effects for treating local trauma (448,449).

Mechanism of Action and Pharmacokinetics

The anti-inflammatory, analgesic, and antipyretic effects of diclofenac epolamine are similar to other NSAIDs. Flector patch reaches peak plasma level between 10 and 20 hours after application, and the half-life of each patch is approximately 12 hours (450). Diclofenac avidly binds to plasma protein, is metabolized by the liver, and is then excreted along with urine and bile.

Preparation and Dosing

Voltaren gel—Lower limb joints: Can be applied 4 g QID, MAX 16 g/joint/day, while in the upper limb joints, apply 2 g QID, MAX 8 g/day/joint.

Each Flector patch contains 180 mg of diclofenac epolamine in an aqueous base. The recommended dose is one Flector patch to the intact skin o the affected area BID.

Relevant Side Effects and Drug Interactions

The most common adverse effects of Flector patch are local skin reactions. Although diclofenac has similar side effect and drug interaction profiles as other NSAIDs, the minimal serum medication levels associated with use in patch formulation lead to a lower risk of GI side effects.

Capsaicin (Zostrix, Zostrix-HP)

Relevance to Physiatry

Capsaicin is a naturally occurring, reversible neurotoxin extracted from Solanaceae family plants (i.e., "hot" chili peppers) and is classified as a capsaicinoid. It is used by physiatrists to manage localized pain states (e.g., focal neuropathic pain) and joint arthralgias (e.g., knee and finger OA). Topical capsaicin is FDA approved for the treatment of diabetic neuropathy and PHN, along with pain due to OA and rheumatoid arthritis. Several studies found it to be beneficial for postoperative pain, trigeminal neuralgia, and cluster headache (451–456). There is also some scant literature on management of CRPS type I and traumatic amputee neurogenic residual limb pain (457,458).

Capsaicin has recognizable efficacy in managing chronic musculoskeletal and neuropathic pain but is generally considered as an adjuvant analgesic. Study outcomes on the combined use of capsaicin and other topical medications have generally been favorable. For example, the combination of capsaicin (0.25%) and topical 3.3% doxepin was found to produce synergistic effects in neuropathic pain (18). A 2004 systematic review declared that capsaicin might be useful as an adjunct or sole therapy for patients with refractory pain (459).

Less direct physiatric applications of capsaicin include painful urologic conditions, temporomandibular pain, oral mucositis, rhinitis, and psoriasis (17,180,460,461).

In addition to its clinical use, capsaicin has also become an integral part of pain management research (462,463). A human trigeminal sensitization pain model was developed to examine gender differences (464). In addition, basic science research suggests that an endogenous capsaicin-like substance is released in inflamed tissues and produces nociceptive neural impulses by acting on capsaicin receptors on sensory neurons (465).

Mechanism of Action and Pharmacokinetics

Analgesia is achieved by its binding to vanilloid receptor-1 (VR1), which leads to the depletion of and inhibited accumulation of substance P (SP) at the target site. SP is an endogenous neuropeptide produced by small-diameter, primary, sensory "pain" fibers; it is involved in the afferent transmission of pain impulse and stimulates immune cells (466,467). In addition to SP depletion, capsaicin also inhibits SP transport and *de novo* synthesis. The overall effect is a reversible sensory degeneration that leads to pain desensitization. Inflammation is also indirectly inhibited in the above process because inflammation has a neural component, which is referred to as neurogenic inflammation. The major proinflammatory players in this model are SP and related peptides (468). Capsaicin's biochemistry is still under investigation (469,470).

Preparations and Dosing

Capsaicin is available under various trade names including 0.025% (Zostrix) and 0.075% (Zostrix-HP) topical cream preparations that are to be applied three to four times daily.

It is also available as an 8% patch, which is applied as single application patches that last 60 minutes, as well as in a 0.25% to 0.75% stick form. Patients should be initiated on the lower-concentration preparation to minimize early, unfavorable effects.

Relevant Side Effects and Drug Interactions

Transient application site stinging and burning, caused by activation of C fibers, are experienced by up to 50% of patients at the onset of treatment, particularly with the higher potency formulation. Capsaicin studies have on average incurred 13% participant withdrawal rate due to intolerable burning. Capsaicin is not deemed appropriate for acute musculoskeletal pain for this reason though this side effect usually remits after the first few days (471). This phenomenon is attributed to the depletion of substance P with repeat application. Cough is another possible adverse effect. No adverse effect upon nerve function and no drug interactions have been documented to date (472).

Other NSAID Topicals

Ketoprofen is available in several forms including a 2.5% to 10% gel as well as a TD patch. It has shown promise with soft tissue injuries in the setting of reducing acute pain. Salicylates, including aspirin cream, have shown in a small sample size studies to significantly reduce pain in patients with acute herpetic neuralgia (473).

REFERENCES

1. Altman R, Hochberg M, Moskowitz R, et al. Recommendations for the medical management of osteoarthritis of the hip and knee: 2000 update. *Arthritis Rheum.* 2000;43(9):1905–1915.
2. Flower RJ, Vane JR. Inhibition of prostaglandin synthetase in brain explains the antipyretic action of paracetamol (4-acetamidophenol). *Nature.* 1972;240:410.
3. Batchlor EE, Paulus HE. Principles of drug therapy. In: Moskowitz RW, Howell DS, Goldberg VM, et al., eds. *Osteoarthritis: Diagnosis and Medical/Surgical Management.* Philadelphia, PA: WB Saunders; 1992.
4. Klopčič I, Poberžnik M, Mavri J, et al. A quantum chemical study of the reactivity of acetaminophen (paracetamol) toxic metabolite *N*-acetyl-*p*-benzoquinone imine with deoxyguanosine and glutathione. *Chem Biol Interact.* 2015;242:407–414. Available from: ScienceDirect, Ipswich, MA. Accessed May 16, 2017.
5. FDA reminds health care professionals to stop dispensing prescription combination drug products with more than 325 mg of acetaminophen. Fdagov. 2017. Available from: https://www.fda.gov/Drugs/DrugSafety/ucm394916.htm. Accessed May 16, 2017.
6. Benison H, Kaczynski J, Wallerstedt S. Paracetamol medication and alcohol abuse: a dangerous combination for the liver and the kidney. *Scand J Gastroenterol.* 1987;22:701–704.
7. Jones AF, Vale JA. Paracetamol poisoning and the kidney. *J Clin Pharm Ther.* 1993;18:5–8.
8. Henrich WL, Agodaoa LE, Barret B, et al. Analgesics and the kidney: summary and recommendations to the Scientific Advisory Board of the National Kidney Foundation from an Ad Hoc Committee of the National Kidney Foundation. *Am J Kidney Dis.* 1996;27:162–165.
9. Hylek EM, Heiman H, Skates SJ, et al. Acetaminophen and other risk factors for excessive warfarin anticoagulation. *JAMA.* 1998;279(9):657-662.
10. Fitzmaurice DA, Murray JA. Potentiation of anticoagulant effect of warfarin. *Postgrad Med J.* 1997;73:439–440.
11. Max MB. Thirteen consecutive well-designed randomized trials show that antidepressants reduce pain in diabetic neuropathy and postherpetic neuralgia. *Pain Forum.* 1995;4(4):248–253.
12. Onghena P, Van Houdenhove B. Antidepressant-induced analgesia in chronic non-malignant pain: a meta-analysis of 39 placebo-controlled studies. *Pain.* 1992;49:205–219.
13. McQuay HJ, Tramer M, Nye BA, et al. A systematic review of antidepressants in neuropathic pain. *Pain.* 1996;68:217–227.
14. Sullivan MJL, Reesor K, Mikail S, et al. The treatment of depression in chronic low back pain: review and recommendations. *Pain.* 1992;50:5.
15. McQuay HJ, Carroll D, Glynn CJ. Low dose amitriptyline in the treatment of chronic pain. *Anesthesia.* 1992;47:646.
16. Kishore-Kumar R, Max MB, Schafer SC, et al. Desipramine relieves post-herpetic neuralgia. *Clin Pharmacol Ther.* 1990;47:305–312.

17. Max MB, Lynch SA, Muir J, et al. Effects of desipramine, amitriptyline, and fluoxetine (prozac) on pain in diabetic neuropathy. *N Engl J Med.* 1992;326:1250–1256.

18. McCleane G. Topical application of doxepin hydrochloride, capsaicin and a combination of both produces analgesia in chronic human neuropathic pain: a randomized, double-blind, placebo-controlled study. *Br J Clin Pharmacol.* 2000;49(6):574–579.

19. Finestone DH, Ober SK. Fluoxetine and fibromyalgia. *JAMA.* 1990:264: 2869–2870.

20. Wolfe F, Cahtey MA, Hawley DJ. A double-blind placebo controlled trial of fluoxetine in fibromyalgia. *Scand J Rheumatol.* 1994:23:255–259.

21. Lee Y, Chen P. A review of SSRIs and SNRIs in neuropathic pain. *Expert Opin Pharmacother.* 2010;11(17):2813–2825. Available from: Science Citation Index, Ipswich, MA. Accessed May 22, 2017.

22. Sindrup SH, Gram LF, Bronsen K, et al. The selective serotonin reuptake inhibitor paroxetine is effective in the treatment of diabetic neuropathy symptoms. *Pain.* 1990;42:135–144.

23. Sindrup SH, Bjerre U, Dejgaard A, et al. The selective serotonin reuptake inhibitor citalopram relieves the symptoms of diabetic neuropathy. *Clin Pharmacol Ther.* 1992;52(5):547–552.

24. Goodnick PJ, Jimenez I, Kumar A. Sertraline in diabetic neuropathy: preliminary results. *Ann Clin Psychiatry.* 1997;9:255–257.

25. Hou YC, Lai CH. Long-term duloxetine withdrawal syndrome and management in a depressed patient. *J Neuropsychiatry Clin Neurosci.* 2014;26(1):E4.

26. Abajo F. Effects of selective serotonin reuptake inhibitors on platelet function. *Drugs Aging.* 2011;28(5):345–367. Available from: CINAHL with Full Text, Ipswich, MA. Accessed April 25, 2017.

27. Manna V, Bolino F, Di Cicco L. Chronic tension-type headache, mood depression and serotonin: therapeutic effects of fluvoxamine and mianserine. *Headache.* 1994;34(1):44–49.

28. Brannon GE, Stone KD. The use of mirtazapine in a patient with chronic pain. *J Pain Symptom Manage.* 1999;18(5):382–385.

29. Brannon GE, Stone KD. Potentiation of opioid analgesia by the antidepressant nefazodone. *Eur J Pharmacol.* 1992;211(3):375–381.

30. Lynch ME. Antidepressants as analgesics: a review of randomized controlled trials. *J Psychiatry Neurosci.* 2001;26(1):30–36.

31. Swaiman K. *Swaiman's Pediatric Neurology.* 5th ed. Edinburgh, UK: Elsevier Saunders; 2012:664–702.

32. Wilson RC. The use of low-dose Trazodone in the treatment of diabetic neuropathy. *J Am Podiatr Med Assoc.* 1999;89(9):468–471.

33. Sumpton JE, Moulin DE. Treatment of neuropathic pain with venlafaxine. *Ann Pharmacother.* 2001;35(5):557–559.

34. Friedman RA, Leon AC. Expanding the black box—depression, antidepressants, and the risk of suicide. *N Engl J Med.* 2007;356(23):2343–2346. doi:http://dx.doi.org.proxy.libraries.rutgers.edu/10.1056/NEJMp078015.

35. Wood AJJ, Roden DM. DRUG THERAPY: Drug-induced prolongation of the QT interval. *N Engl J Med.* 2004;350(10):1013–1022. Available from: https://search-proquest-com.proxy.libraries.rutgers.edu/docview/223946445?accountid=13626

36. Lithner F. Venlafaxine in treatment of severe painful peripheral diabetic neuropathy. *Diabetes Care.* 2000;23(11):1710–1711.

37. Pernia A, Mro JA, Calderon E, et al. Venlafaxine for the treatment of neuropathic pain. *J Pain Symptom Manage.* 2000;19(6):408–410.

38. Markowitz JS, Petrick KS. Venlafaxine-tramadol similarities. *Med Hypotheses.* 1998;51(2):167–168.

39. Kiayias JA, Vlachou ED, Lakka-Papadodima E. Venlafaxine HCl in the treatment of painful peripheral diabetic neuropathy. *Diabetes Care.* 2000;23:699.

40. Davis JL, Smith RL. Painful peripheral diabetic neuropathy treated with venlafaxine HCl extended release capsules. *Diabetes Care.* 1999;22 (11):1909–1910.

41. Coles R, Kharasch ED. Stereoselective metabolism of bupropion by cytochrome P4502B6 (CYP2B6) and human liver microsomes. *Pharm Res.* 2008;25(6):1405–1411.

42. Galer BS. Neuropathic pain of peripheral origin: advances in pharmacological treatment. *Neurology.* 1995;45(suppl 9):S17–S25.

43. Nutt D, Johnson FN. Potential applications of venlafaxine. *Rev Contemp Pharmacother.* 1998;9:321–331.

44. Semenchuk MR, Davis B. Double-blind, randomized trial of bupropion SR for the treatment of neuropathic pain. *Neurology.* 2001;57(9):1583–1588.

45. Clayton AH, Pradko JF, Croft HA, et al. Prevalence of sexual dysfunction among newer antidepressants. *J Clin Psychiatry.* 2002;63(4):357–366.

46. Chatham W. Glucocorticoid effects on the immune system. *UptoDate.* 2017.

47. Green SM, ed. *The 1997 Tarascon Pocket Pharmacopoeia.* Loma Linda, CA: Tarascon Publishing; 1997.

48. Lennard TA. *Physiatric Procedures in Clinical Practice.* Philadelphia, PA: Hanley & Belfus, Inc.; 1995.

49. American Medical Association Department of Drugs, Division of Drugs and Technology. *Drug Evaluations.* 6th ed. Chicago, IL: American Medical Association; 1986.

50. Skedros JG, Hunt KJ, et al. Variations in corticosteroid/anesthetic injections for painful shoulder conditions: comparisons among orthopedic surgeons, rheumatologists, and physical medicine and primary-care physicians. *BMC Musculoskelet Disord.* 2007;8:63.

51. Trentin L, Visentin M. The predictive lidocaine test in treatment of neuropathic pain. *Minerva Anestesiol.* 2000;66(3):157–161.

52. Galer BS, Dworkin RH. Pharmacologic treatment of neuropathic pain. In: Galer BS, Dworkin RH, eds. *A Clinical Guide to Neuropathic Pain.* Minneapolis, MN: The McGraw-Hill Companies; 2000:53–83.

53. Kalso E, Tramer MR, McQuay HJ, et al. Systemic local-anaesthetic-type drugs in chronic pain: a systematic review. *Eur J Pain.* 1998;2(1):3–14.

54. Chabal C, Jacobson L, Mariano A, et al. The use of oral mexiletine for the treatment of pain after peripheral nerve injury. *Anesthesiology.* 1992;76(4):513–517.

55. Stracke H, Meyer U, Schumacher H, et al. Mexiletine in treatment of painful diabetic neuropathy. *Med Klin.* 1994;89(3):124–131.

56. Oskarsson P, Ljunggren JG, Lins PE. Efficacy and safety of mexiletine in the treatment of painful diabetic neuropathy. The Mexiletine Study Group. *Diabetes Care.* 1997;20(10):1594–1597.

57. Stracke H, Meyer UE, Schumacher HE, et al. Mexiletine in the treatment of diabetic neuropathy. *Diabetes Care.* 1992;15(11):1550–1555.

58. Dejgard A, Petersen P, Kastrup J. Mexiletine for treatment of chronic painful diabetic neuropathy. *Lancet.* 1988;1(8575–8576):9–11.

59. Nishiyama K, Sakuta M. Mexiletine for painful alcoholic neuropathy. *Intern Med.* 1995;34(6):577–579.

60. Davis RW. Successful treatment for phantom pain. *Orthopedics.* 1993;16(6): 691–695.

61. Ando K, Wallace MS, Braun J, et al. Effect of oral mexiletine on capsaicin-induced allodynia and hyperalgesia: a double-blind, placebo-controlled, crossover study. *Reg Anesth Pain Med.* 2000;25(5):468–474.

62. Awerbuch GI, Sandyk R. Mexiletine for thalamic pain syndrome. *Int J Neurosci.* 1990;5(2–4):129–133.

63. Okada S, Kinoshita M, Fujioka T, et al. Two cases of multiple sclerosis with painful tonic seizures and dysesthesia ameliorated by the administration of mexiletine. *Jpn J Med.* 1991;30(4):373–375.

64. Kemper CA, Kent G, Burton S, et al. Mexiletine for HIV-infected patients with painful peripheral neuropathy: a double-blind, placebo-controlled, crossover treatment trial. *J Acquir Immune Defic Syndr Hum Retrovirol.* 1998;19(4):367–372.

65. Chio-Tan FY, Tuel SM, Johnson JC, et al. Effect of mexiletine on spinal cord injury dysesthetic pain. *Am J Phys Med Rehabil.* 1996;75(2):84–87.

66. Pascual J, Berciano J. Failure of mexiletine to control trigeminal neuralgia. *Headache.* 1989;29(8):517–518.

67. Wallace MS, Magnuson S, Ridgeway B. Efficacy of oral mexiletine for neuropathic pain with allodynia: a double-blind, placebo-controlled, crossover study. *Reg Anesth Pain Med.* 2000;25(5):459–467.

68. Peraire M. Diagnosis and treatment of the patient with trigeminal neuralgia. *Neurologia.* 1997;12(1):12–22.

69. Jackson CE, Barohn RJ, Ptacek LJ. Paramyotonia congenita: abnormal short exercise test, and improvement after mexiletine therapy. *Muscle Nerve.* 1994;17(7):763–768.

70. Ghinea N, Lipworth W, Kerridge I. Evidence, regulation and 'rational' prescribing: the case of gabapentin for neuropathic pain. *J Eval Clin Pract.* 2015;21(1):28–33.

71. Kolotkin R, Gadde K, Crosby R, et al. Health-related quality of life in two randomized controlled trials of phentermine/topiramate for obesity: what mediates improvement? *Qual Life Res.* 2016;25(5):1237–1244. Available from: Academic Search Premier, Ipswich, MA. Accessed May 10, 2017.

72. Moore R, Wiffen PJ, Derry S, et al. Gabapentin for chronic neuropathic pain and fibromyalgia in adults. *Cochrane Database Syst Rev.* 2014;(4): CD007938. doi:10.1002/14651858.CD007938.pub3.

73. Hayashi T, Ichiyama T, Tanaka H, et al. Successful treatment of incontinence of feces in myotonic muscular dystrophy by mexiletine. *No To Hattatsu.* 1991;23(3):310–312.

74. Kwiecinski H, Ryniewicz B, Ostrzycki A. Treatment of myotonia with antiarrhythmic drugs. *Acta Neurol Scand.* 1992;86(4):371–375.

75. Taylor CP, Gee NS, Su TZ, et al. A summary of mechanistic hypotheses of gabapentin pharmacology. *Epilepsy Res.* 1998;29:233–249.

76. Eisenberg E, et al. Antiepileptic drugs in the treatment of neuropathic pain. *Drugs.* 2007;67:1265–1289.

77. Lal R, Sukbuntherng J, Luo W, et al. Clinical pharmacokinetic drug interaction studies of gabapentin enacarbil, a novel transported prodrug of gabapentin, with naproxen and cimetidine. *Br J Clin Pharmacol.* 2010;69(5):498–507. doi:10.1111/j.1365-2125.2010.03616.x.

78. Quintero GC. Review about gabapentin misuse, interactions, contraindications and side effects. *J Exp Pharmacol.* 2017;9:13–21. doi:10.2147/JEP.S124391.

79. Hansen C, Gilron I, Hong M. The effects of intrathecal gabapentin on spinal morphine tolerance in the rat tail-flick and paw pressure tests. *Anesth Analg.* 2004;99:1180–1184.

80. Hahn AF, Parkes AW, Bolton CF, et al. Neuromyotonia in hereditary motor neuropathy. *J Neurol Neurosurg Psychiatry.* 1991;54(3):230–235.

81. Guieu R, Mesdjian E, Rochat H, et al. Central analgesic effect of valproate in patients with epilepsy. *Seizure.* 1993;2(2):147–150.

82. Tremont-Lukats IW, Megeff C, Backonja MM. Anticonvulsants for neuropathic pain syndromes: mechanisms of action and place in therapy. *Drugs.* 2000;60(5):1029–1052.

83. Block F. Gabapentin zur Schmerztherapie. [Gabapentin for therapy of neuropathic pain.] *Schmerz.* 2001;15(4):280–288.

84. Backonja MM. Gabapentin monotherapy for the symptomatic treatment of painful neuropathy: a multicenter, double-blind, placebo-controlled trial in patients with diabetes mellitus. *Epilepsia.* 1999;40(suppl 6):S57–S59; discussion S73–S74.

85. Backonja M, Beydoun A, Edwards KR, et al. Gabapentin for the symptomatic treatment of painful neuropathy in patients with diabetes mellitus: a randomized controlled trial. *JAMA.* 1998;280(21):1831–1836.

86. Rowbotham M, Harden N, Stacey B, et al. Gabapentin for the treatment of postherpetic neuralgia: a randomized controlled trial. *JAMA.* 1998;280(21):1837–1842.

87. Rice AS, Maton S; the Postherpetic Neuralgia Study Group (UK). Gabapentin in postherpetic neuralgia: a randomized, double blind, placebo-controlled study. *Pain*. 2001;94:215–224. Comment in: *Pain*. 2002;96(3):411–412.

88. Priebe MM, Sherwood AM, Graves DE, et al. Effectiveness of gabapentin in controlling spasticity: a quantitative study. *Spinal Cord*. 1997;35(3):171–175

89. Jensen TS. Anticonvulsants in neuropathic pain: rationale and clinical evidence. *Eur J Pain*. 2002;6(suppl A):61–68.

90. di Vadi PP, Hamann W. The use of lamotrigine in neuropathic pain. *Anaesthesia*. 1998;53(8):808–809.

91. Zakrzewska JM. Trigeminal neuralgia. *Prim Dent Care*. 1997;4(1):17–19.

92. Simpson DM, Olney R, McArthur JC, et al. A placebo-controlled trial of lamotrigine for painful HIV-associated neuropathy. *Neurology*. 2000;54(11):2115–2119.

93. Vestergaard K, Andersen G, Gottrup H, et al. Lamotrigine for central poststroke pain: a randomized controlled trial. *Neurology*. 2001;56(2):184–190.

94. Backonja MM. Anticonvulsants (antineuropathics) for neuropathic pain syndromes. *Clin J Pain*. 2000;16(2 suppl):S67–S72.

95. McCleane G. 200 mg daily of lamotrigine has no analgesic effect in neuropathic pain: a randomised, double-blind, placebo controlled trial. *Pain*. 1999;83(1):105–107.

96. McCleane G. 200 mg daily of lamotrigine has no analgesic effect in neuropathic pain: a randomised, double-blind, placebo controlled trial. *Pain*. 1999;83(1): 105–107. Comment in: *Pain*. 2000;86(1–2):211–212.

97. Sindrup SH, Jensen TS. Pharmacotherapy of trigeminal neuralgia. *Clin J Pain*. 2002;18(1):22–27.

98. Rabinovich A, Fang J, Scrivani S. Diagnosis and management of trigeminal neuralgia. *Columbia Dental Rev*. 2000:5:4–7.

99. Beydoun A, Kutluay E. Oxcarbazepine. *Expert Opin Pharmacother*. 2002;3(1): 59–71.

100. Gonzalez-Darder JM, Ortega-Alvaro A, Ruz-Franzi I, et al. Antinociceptive effects of phenobarbital in "tail-flick" test and deafferentation pain. *Anesth Analg*. 1992;75(1):81–86.

101. Ipponi A, Lamberti C, Medica A, et al. Tiagabine antinociception in rodents depends on GABA(B) receptor activation: parallel antinociception testing and medial thalamus GABA microdialysis. *Eur J Pharmacol*. 1999;368(2–3):205–211.

102. Novak V, Kanard R, Kissel JT, et al. Treatment of painful sensory neuropathy with tiagabine: a pilot study. *Clin Auton Res*. 2001;11(6):357–361.

103. Meldrum BS, Chapman AG. Basic mechanisms of gabitril (tiagabine) and future potential developments. *Epilepsia*. 1999;40(suppl 9):S2–S6.

104. Martinez-Salio A, Porta-Etessam J, Berbel-Garcia A, et al. Antiepileptic drugs and neuropathic pain. *Rev Neurol*. 2001;32(4):345–350.

105. Bajwa ZH, Sami N, Warfield CA, et al. Topiramate relieves refractory intercostal neuralgia. *Neurology*. 1999;52(9):1917.

106. Canavero S, Bonicalzi V, Paolotti R. Lack of effect of topiramate for central pain. *Neurology*. 2002;58(5):831–832.

107. Rozen TD. Antiepileptic drugs in the management of cluster headache and trigeminal neuralgia. *Headache*. 2001;41(suppl 1):25–33.

108. Davies AN. Sodium valproate in cancer-related neuropathic pain. *J Pain Symptom Manage*. 2002;23(1):1.

109. Ekbom K, Hardebo JE. Cluster headache: aetiology, diagnosis and management. *Drugs*. 2002;62(1):61–69.

110. Hardy JR, Rees EA, Gwilliam B, et al. A phase II study to establish the efficacy and toxicity of sodium valproate in patients with cancer-related neuropathic pain. *J Pain Symptom Manage*. 2001;21(3):204–209.

111. Drewes AM, Andreasen A, Poulsen LH. Valproate for treatment of chronic central pain after spinal cord injury. A double-blind cross-over study. *Paraplegia*. 1994;32(8):565-569.

112. Grafova VN, Danilova EI, Reshetniak VK. The action of sodium valproate in central pain syndromes. *Eksp Klin Farmakol*. 1994;57(2):8–11.

113. Martin C, Martin A, Rud C, et al. Comparative study of sodium valproate and ketoprofen in the treatment of postoperative pain. *Ann Fr Anesth Reanim*. 1988;7(5):387–392.

114. Campostrini R, Paganini M, Boncinelli L, et al. Alterations of the state of consciousness induced by valproic acid: 6 case reports. *Riv Patol Nerv Ment*. 1983;104(1):23–34.

115. Kito M, Maehara M, Watanabe K. Mechanisms of T-type calcium channel blockade by zonisamide. *Seizure*. 1996;5(2):115–119.

116. Okada M, Kaneko S, Hirano T, et al. Effects of zonisamide on dopaminergic system. *Epilepsy Res*. 1995;22(3):193–205.

117. Devers A, Galer BS. Topical lidocaine patch relieves a variety of neuropathic pain conditions: an open-label study. *Clin J Pain*. 2000;16(3):205–208.

118. Argoff CE. New analgesics for neuropathic pain: the lidocaine patch. *Clin J Pain*. 2000;16(2 suppl):S62–S66.

119. Relieving the pain of postherpetic neuralgia with lidocaine patch 5%. *Drugs Ther Perspect*. 2000;16(9):1–3.

120. Christopher R, Buchanan L, Begalia K. Pain reduction in local anesthetic administration through pH buffering. *Ann Emerg Med*. 1988;17:117–120.

121. Moore R, Wiffen PJ, Derry S, et al. Zonisamide for neuropathic pain in adults. *Cochrane Database Syst Rev*. 2015;(1):CD011241. doi:10.1002/14651858. CD011241.pub2

122. Eggleston ST, Lush LW. Understanding allergic reactions to local anesthetics. *Ann Pharmacother*. 1996;30:851–857.

123. Covino BG. Pharmacology of local anaesthetic agents. *Br J Anaesth*. 1986;58(7):701–716.

124. Chahar P, Cummings KC. Liposomal bupivacaine: a review of a new bupivacaine formulation. *J Pain Res*. 2012;5:257–264.

125. Mather LE, Copeland SE, et al. Acute toxicity of local anesthetics: underlying pharmacokinetic and pharmacodynamic concepts. *Reg Anesth Pain Med*. 2005;30(6):553–566.

126. Weller WJ, Azzam MG, Smith RA, et al. Liposomal bupivacaine mixture has similar pain relief and significantly fewer complications at less cost compared to indwelling interscalene catheter in total shoulder arthroplasty. *J Arthroplasty*. 2017;32(11):3557–3562. pii: S0883-5403(17)30219-X.

127. Gazzotti F, Bertellini E, et al. Best indications for local anaesthetics: bupivacaine. *Minerva Anestesiol*. 2001;67(9 suppl 1):9–14.

128. Gulihar A, Robati S, Twaij H, et al. Articular cartilage and local anaesthetic: a systematic review of the current literature. *J Orthop*. 2015;12:200–210.

129. Anderson SL, Buchko JZ, Taillon MR, et al. Chondrolysis of the glenohumeral joint after infusion of bupivacaine through an intra-articular pain pump catheter: a report of 18 cases. *Arthroscopy*. 2010;26(4):451–461.

130. Breu A, Rosenmeier K, Kujat R, et al. The cytotoxicity of bupivacaine, ropivacaine, and mepivacaine on human chondrocytes and cartilage. *Anesth Analg*. 2013;117(2):514-522.

131. Dogan N, Erdem AF, Erman Z, et al. The effects of bupivacaine and neostigmine on articular cartilage and synovium in the rabbit knee joint. *J Int Med Res*. 2004;32:513–519.

132. Gommoll AH, Kang RW, Williams JM, et al. Chondrolysis after continuous intra-articular bupivacaine infusion: an experimental model investigating chondrotoxicity in the rabbit shoulder. *Arthroscopy*. 2006;22:813–819.

133. Piper SL, Kramer JD, Kim HT, et al. Effects of local anesthetics on articular cartilage. *Am J Sports Med*. 2011;39(10):2245–2253.

134. Dragoo JL, Braun HJ, Kim HJ, et al. The in vitro chondrotoxicity of single-dose local anesthetics. *Am J Sports Med*. 2012;40(4):794–799.

135. Syed HM, Green L, Bianski B, et al. Bupivacaine and triamcinolone may be toxic to human chondrocytes: a pilot study. *Clin Orthop Relat Res*. 2011;469 (10):2941–2947.

136. Gorfine SR, Onel E, Patou G, et al. Bupivacaine extended-release liposome injection for prolonged postsurgical analgesia in patients undergoing hemorrhoidectomy: a multicenter, randomized, double-blind, placebo-controlled trial. *Dis Colon Rectum*. 2011;54(12):1552–1559.

137. Onel E, Warnott K, Lambert W, et al. Pharmacokinetics of depobupivacaine (EXPARELTM), a novel bupivacaine extended release liposomal injection, in volunteers with moderate hepatic impairment. Poster presented at: 112th Annual Meeting of the American Society of Clinical Pharmacology and Therapeutics; March 3–6, 2011; Dallas, TX.

138. Davidson EM, Barenholz Y, Cohen R, et al. High-dose bupivacaine remotely loaded into multivesicular liposomes demonstrates slow drug release without systemic toxic plasma concentrations after subcutaneous administration in humans. *Anesth Analg*. 2010;110(4):1018–1023.

139. Heavner JE. Local anesthetics. *Curr Opin Anaesthesiol*. 2007;20(4):336–342.

140. Oda A, Ohashi H, et al. Characteristics of ropivacaine block of Na+ channels in rat dorsal root ganglion neurons. *Anesth Analg*. 2000;91(5):1213–1220.

141. Daykin H. The efficacy and safety of intravenous lidocaine for analgesia in the older adult: a literature review. *Br J Pain*. 2017;11(1):23–31.

142. Daubländer M, Kämmerer PW, Willershausen B, et al. Clinical use of an epinephrine-reduced (1/400,000) articaine solution in short-time dental routine treatments-a multicenter study. *Clin Oral Investig*. 2011;16(4):1289–1295.

143. Davenport RE, Porcelli RJ, Iacono VJ, et al. Effects of anesthetics containing epinephrine on catecholamine levels during periodontal surgery. *J Periodontol*. 1990;61(9):553–558.

144. Said Yekta-Michael S, Stein JM, Marioth-Wirtz E. Evaluation of the anesthetic effect of epinephrine-free articaine and mepivacaine through quantitative sensory testing. *Head Face Med*. 2015;11:2.

145. Gall H, Kaufmann R, et al. Adverse reactions to local anesthetics: analysis of 197 cases. *J Allergy Clin Immunol*. 1996;97(4):933–937.

146. McKay W, Morris R, et al. Sodium bicarbonate attenuates pain on skin infiltration with lidocaine, with or without epinephrine. *Anesth Analg*. 1987;66:572–574.

147. RD Miller, MC Pardo. *Basics of Anesthesia*. 6th ed. Philadelphia, PA: Elsevier Saunders; 2007:135.

148. Leone S, Di Cianni S, Casati A, et al. Pharmacology, toxicology, and clinical use of new long acting local anesthetics, ropivacaine and levobupivacaine. *Acta Biomed*. 2008;79:92–105.

149. Selbst SM, Fein JA. Sedation and analgesia. In: Fleisher GR, Ludwig S, Henretig FM, eds. *Textbook of Pediatric Emergency Medicine*. 5th ed. Philadelphia, PA: Lippincott Williams and Wilkins; 2006:69.

150. Watkins TW, Dupre S, Coucher JR. Ropivacaine and dexamethasone: a potentially dangerous combination for therapeutic pain injections. *J Med Imaging Radiat Oncol*. 2015;59:571–577.

151. MacMahon PJ, Eustace SJ, Kavanagh EC. Injectable corticosteroid and local anesthetic preparations: a review for radiologists. *Radiology*. 2009;252(3):647–661.

152. Becker DE, Reed KL. Essentials of local anesthetic pharmacology. *Anesth Prog*. 2006;53(3):98–109.

153. Chen Y, Jin Z, Xia Y, et al. The protective effect of lipid emulsion in preventing bupivacaine-induced mitochondrial injury and apoptosis of H9C2 cardiomyocytes. *Drug Deliv*. 2017;24:1, 430–436.

154. Rosenblatt MA, Abel M, et al. Successful use of a 20% lipid emulsion to resuscitate a patient after a presumed bupivacaine-related cardiac arrest. *Anesthesiology*. 2006;105(1):217–218.

155. Zygmunt M, Sapa J. Muscle relaxants—the current position in the treatment of spasticity in orthopedics. *Ortop Traumatol Rehabil*. 2015;17(4):423–430.

156. Khaliq W, Alam S, et al. Topical lidocaine for the treatment of postherpetic neuralgia. *Cochrane Database Syst Rev.* 2007;18(2):CD004846.

157. Dworkin RH, O'Connor AB, et al. Pharmacologic management of neuropathic pain: evidence-based recommendations. *Pain.* 2007;132(3):237–251.

158. Steward DJ. Eutectic mixture of local anesthetics (EMLA): what is it? What does it do? *J Pediatr.* 1993;122:S21.

159. Kumar M, Chawla R, Goyal M. Topical anesthesia. *J Anaesthesiol Clin Pharmacol.* 2015;31(4):450-456.

160. Miller KA, Balakrishnan G, et al. 1% lidocaine injection, EMLA cream, or "numby stuff" for topical analgesia associated with peripheral intravenous cannulation. *AANA J.* 2001;69(3):185-187.

161. Galinkin JL, Rose JB, et al. Lidocaine iontophoresis versus eutectic mixture of local anesthetics (EMUA®) for IV placement in children. *Anesth Analg.* 2002;94(6):1484–1488.

162. Eichenfield LF, Funk A, et al. A clinical study to evaluate the efficacy of ELA-Max (4% liposomal lidocaine) as compared with eutectic mixture of local anesthetics cream for pain reduction of venipuncture in children. *Pediatrics.* 2002;109:1093.

163. Meier T, et al. Efficacy of lidocaine patch 5% in the treatment of focal peripheral neuropathic pain syndromes: a randomized, double-blind, placebo-controlled study. *Pain.* 2003;106:151–158.

164. Neafsey PJ. Patching pain with lidocaine: new uses for the lidocaine 5% patch. *Home Healthc Nurse.* 2004;22(8):562–564.

165. Galer BS. Topical lidocaine patch relieves a variety of neuropathic pain conditions: an open-label pilot study. Paper presented at: American Academy of Neurology; May 6–13, 1995; Seattle.

166. Baron R, et al. 5% lidocaine medicated plaster versus pregabalin in post-herpetic neuralgia and diabetic polyneuropathy: an open-label, non-inferiority two-stage RCT study. *Curr Med Res Opin.* 2009;25(7):1663–1676.

167. Barbano EL, et al. Effectiveness, tolerability, and impact on quality of life of the 5% lidocaine patch in diabetic polyneuropathy. *Arch Neurol.* 2004;61(6):914–918.

168. Schilling CG, Bank DE, et al. Tetracaine, epinephrine (adrenalin), and cocaine (TAC) versus lidocaine, epinephrine, and tetracaine (LET) for anesthesia of lacerations in children. *Ann Emerg Med.* 1995;25(2):203–208.

169. Harman S, Zemek R, Duncan MJ, et al. Efficacy of pain control with topical lidocaine–epinephrine–tetracaine during laceration repair with tissue adhesive in children: a randomized controlled trial. *CMAJ.* 2013;185(13):E629–E634.

170. Sawyer J, Febbraro S, Masud S, et al. Heated lidocaine/tetracaine patch (Synera, Rapydan) compared with lidocaine/prilocaine cream (EMLA) for topical anaesthesia before vascular access. *Br J Anaesth.* 2009;102(2):210–215.

171. Radnovich R. Heated Lidocaine-Tetracaine Patch for management of shoulder impingement syndrome. *J Am Osteopath Assoc.* 2013;113(1):58–64.

172. Rauck R, Busch M, Marriott T. Effectiveness of a heated lidocaine/tetracaine topical patch for pain associated with myofascial trigger points: results of an open-label pilot study. *Pain Pract.* 2013;13(7):533–538.

173. Dalpiaz AS, Lordon SP, Lipman AG. Topical lidocaine patch therapy for myofascial pain. *J Pain Palliat Care Pharmacother.* 2004;18(3):15–34.

174. Kim WO, Song BM, Kil HK. Efficacy and safety of a lidocaine/tetracaine medicated patch or peel for dermatologic procedures: a meta-analysis. *Korean J Anesthesiol.* 2012;62(5):435–440.

175. Galer BS, Rowbotham MC, et al. Topical lidocaine patch relieves postherpetic neuralgia more effectively than a vehicle topical patch: results of an enriched enrollment study. *Pain.* 1999;80:533–538.

176. Wang Y, Mi J, Lu K, et al. Comparison of gating properties and use-dependent block of Nav1.5 and Nav1.7 channels by anti-arrhythmics mexiletine and lidocaine. *PLoS One.* 2015;10(6):e0128653.

177. See S, Ginzburg R. Choosing a skeletal muscle relaxant. *Am Fam Physician.* 2008;78(3):365–370.

178. Witenko C, Moorman-Li R, Motycka C, et al. Considerations for the appropriate use of skeletal muscle relaxants for the management of acute low back pain. *P T.* 2014;39(6):427–435.

179. Van Tulder MW, Touray T, Furlan A, et al. Muscle relaxants for nonspecific low back pain: a systematic review within the frame-work of the Cochrane Collaboration. *Spine.* 2003;28(17):1978–1992.

180. Chou R, Huffman LH. Medications for acute and chronic low back pain: a review of the evidence for an American Pain Society/American College of Physicians Clinical Practice Guideline. *Ann Intern Med.* 2007;147:505–514.

181. De Falla K. *Muscle Relaxants.* 2016. Available from: https://www.spine-health.com/treatment/pain-medication/muscle-relaxants. Accessed May 19, 2017.

182. Mann-Metzer P, Yarom Y. Pre- and postsynaptic inhibition mediated by GABA(B) receptors in cerebellar inhibitory interneurons. *J Neurophysiol.* 2002;87(1):183–190.

183. Chou R, et al. Comparative efficacy and safety of skeletal muscle relaxants for spasticity and musculoskeletal conditions: a systematic review. *J Pain Symptom Manag.* 2004;28(2):140–175.

184. Ertzgaard P, Campo C, Calabrese A. Efficacy and safety of oral baclofen in the management of spasticity: a rationale for intrathecal baclofen. *J Rehabil Med.* 2017;49:193–203.

185. Meythaler JM, Kowalski S. Pharmacologic management of spasticity: oral medications. In: Brashear A, Elovic EP, eds. *Spasticity: Diagnosis and Management.* 1st ed. New York: Demos Medical Publishing; 2011:199–227.

186. Katz RT. Management of spasticity. *Am J Phys Med Rehabil.* 1988;67:108–116.

187. Willerslev-Olsen M, Lundbye-Jensen J, Petersen TH, et al. The effect of baclofen and diazepam on motor skill acquisition in healthy subjects. *Exp Brain Res.* 2011;213(4):465–474.

188. Perez-Arrendondo A, Casares-Ramirez E, Carrillo-Mora P, et al. Baclofen in the therapeutic of sequelae of traumatic brain injury: spasticity. *Clin Neuropharmacol.* 2016;39(6):311–319.

189. Francisco GE, Yablon SA, Schiess MC, et al. Consensus panel guidelines for the use of intrathecal baclofen therapy in poststroke spastic hypertonia. *Top Stroke Rehabil.* 2006;13:74–85.

190. Boviatsis EJ, Kouyialis AT, Korfias S, et al. Functional outcome of intrathecal baclofen administration for severe spasticity. *Clin Neurol Neurosurg.* 2005;107:289–295.

191. Chow JW, Yablon SA, Stokic DS. Effect of intrathecal baclofen bolus injection on ankle muscle activation during gait in patients with acquired brain injury. *Neurorehabil Neural Repair.* 2015;29:163–173.

192. Heetla HW, Staal MJ, Proost JH, et al. Clinical relevance of pharmacological and physiological data in intrathecal baclofen therapy. *Arch Phys Med Rehabil.* 2014;95(11):2199–2206.

193. Ward A, Chaffman MO, Sorkin EM. Dantrolene. A review of its pharmacodynamic and pharmacokinetic properties and therapeutic use in malignant hyperthermia, the neuroleptic malignant syndrome and an update of its use in muscle spasticity. *Drugs.* 1986;32:130–168.

194. Krause T, Gerbershagen MU, Fiege M, et al. Dantrolene—a review of its pharmacology, therapeutic use and new developments. *Anaesthesia.* 2004;59(4):364–373.

195. Ketel WB, Kolb ME. Long-term treatment with dantrolene sodium of stroke patients with spasticity limiting the return of function. *Curr Med Res Opin.* 1984;9:161–169.

196. Rabchevsky AG, Kitzman PH. Latest approaches for the treatment of spasticity and autonomic dysreflexia in chronic spinal cord injury. *Neurotherapeutics.* 2011;8(2):274–282.

197. Kim JY, Chun S, Bang MS. Safety of low-dose oral dantrolene sodium on hepatic function. *Arch Phys Med Rehabil.* 2011;92(9):1359–1363.

198. Gatch M, Nguyen JD, Carbonaro T, et al. Carisoprodol tolerance and precipitated withdrawal. *Drug Alcohol Depend.* 2012;123(1–3):29–34.

199. "SOMA® COMPOUND" (PDF). Available from: accessdata.fda.gov. Meda Pharmaceuticals Inc. October 2009:5–17. Accessed April 16, 2017.

200. Hoiseth G, Karinen R, Sorlid HK, et al. The effect of scheduling and withdrawal of carisoprodol on prevalence of intoxications with the drug. *Basic Clin Pharmacol Toxicol.* 2009;105:345–349.

201. Bailey DN, Briggs JR. Carisoprodol: an unrecognized drug of abuse. *Am J Clin Pathol.* 2002;117:396–400.

202. Reeves RR, Burke RS. Carisoprodol: abuse potential and withdrawal syndrome. *Curr Drug Abuse Rev.* 2010;3:33–38.

203. Littrell RA, Sage T, Miller W. Meprobamate dependence secondary to carisoprodol (Soma) use. *Am J Drug Alcohol Abuse.* 1993;19:133–134.

204. Horsfall JT, Sprague JE. The Pharmacology and Toxicology of the 'Holy Trinity'. *Basic Clin Pharmacol Toxicol.* 2017;120(2):115–119.

205. Dean L. Carisoprodol therapy and CYP2C19 genotype. 2017 Apr 4. In: Pratt V, McLeod H, Dean L, et al., eds. *Medical Genetics Summaries [Internet].* Bethesda, MD: National Center for Biotechnology Information (US); 2012. Available from: https://www.ncbi.nlm.nih.gov/books/NBK425390/

206. Zacny JP, Paice JA, Coalson DW. Characterizing the subjective and psychomotor effects of carisoprodol in healthy volunteers. *Pharmacol Biochem Behav.* 2011;100(1):138–143.

207. Zacny JP, Paice JA, Coalson DW. Subjective and psychomotor effects of carisoprodol in combination with oxycodone in healthy volunteers. *Drug Alcohol Depend.* 2012;120(1–3):229–232.

208. Reeves RR, Liberto V. Abuse of combinations of carisoprodol and tramadol. *South Med J.* 2001;94:512–514.

209. Kobayashi H, Hasegawa Y, Ono H. Cyclobenzaprine, a centrally acting muscle relaxant, acts on descending serotonergic systems. *Eur J Pharmacol.* 1996;311(1):29–35.

210. Borenstein DG, Korn S. Efficacy of a low-dose regimen of cyclobenzaprine hydrochloride in acute skeletal muscle spasm: results of two placebo-controlled trials. *Clin Ther.* 2003;25(4):1056–1073.

211. Thomson Micromedex. 1974–2005. Available from: http://www.micromedex.com. Accessed May 17, 2017.

212. Meleger AL. Muscle relaxants and antispasticity agents. *Phys Med Rehabil Clin N Am.* 2006;17:401–413.

213. Helmy SA, El-Bedaiwy, H. Simultaneous determination of paracetamol and methocarbamol in human plasma by HPLC using UV detection with time programming: application to pharmacokinetic study. *Drug Res (Stuttg).* 2014;64(7):363–367.

214. Emrich OM, Milachowski KA, Strohmeier M. Methocarbamol in acute low back pain. A randomized double-blind controlled study. *MMW Fortschr Med.* 2015;157(suppl 5):9–16.

215. Aljuhani O, Kopp BJ, Patanwala AE. Effect of methocarbamol on acute pain after traumatic injury. *Am J Ther.* 2017;24(2):e202–e206.

216. Gonzalez-Perez LM, Infante-Cossio P, Granados-Nunez M, et al. Deep dry needling of trigger points located in the lateral pterygoid muscle: efficacy and safety of treatment for management of myofascial pain and temporomandibular dysfunction. *Med Oral Patol Oral Cir Bucal.* 2015;20(3):e326–e333.

217. Calcaterra NE, Barrow JC. Classics in chemical neuroscience: diazepam (Valium). *ACS Chem Nerosci.* 2014;5(4):253–260.

218. Valium (Diazepam), Physician's Desk Reference Online. Available from: http://www.pdr.net/drug-summary/valium?druglabelid=2100. Updated 2017. Accessed May 20, 2017.

219. Baenninger A, Costa e Silva JA, Hindmarch I, et al. *Good Chemistry: The Life and Legacy of Valium Inventor Leo Sternbach.* New York: McGraw Hill; 2004.

220. Valium (diazepam) Package Insert. Nutley, NJ: Roche Laboratories, Inc.; 2008.
221. Bosak AR, Skolnik AB. Serotonin syndrome associated with metaxalone overdose. *J Med Toxicol.* 2014;10(4):402–405.
222. Martini DI, Nacca N, Haswell D, et al. Serotonin syndrome following metaxalone overdose and therapeutic use of a selective serotonin reuptake inhibitor. *Clin Toxicol (Phila).* 2015;53(3):185–187.
223. Abeles M. Long-term effectiveness of orphenadrine citrate in the treatment of fibromyalgia. In: American College of Rheumatology Scientific Abstracts. 113–A270.
224. Hopf FW, Simms JA, Chang S-J, et al. Chlorzoxazone, an SK channel activator used in humans, reduces excessive alcohol intake in rats. *Biol Psychiatry.* 2011;69(7):618–624.
225. Bragstad A, Blikra G. Evaluation of a new skeletal muscle relaxant in the treatment of lower back pain (a comparison of DS 103-282 with chlorzoxazone). *Curr Ther Res Clin Exp.* 1979;26(1):39–43.
226. Zhou HY, Chen SR, Pan HL. Targeting *N*-methyl-D-aspartate receptors for treatment of neuropathic pain. *Expert Rev Clin Pharmacol.* 2011;4:379–388.
227. Pickering G, Morel V, Joly D, et al. Prevention of post-mastectomy neuropathic pain with memantine: study protocol for a randomized controlled trial. *Trials.* 2014;15:331.
228. Sang CN, Booher S, Gilron I, et al. Dextromethorphan and memantine in painful diabetic neuropathy and postherpetic neuralgia: efficacy and dose–response trials. *Anesthesiology.* 2002;96:1053–1061.
229. Jorum E, Warncke T, Stubhaug A. Cold allodynia and hyperalgesia in neuropathic pain: the effect of *N*-methyl-D-aspartate (NMDA) receptor antagonist ketamine-a double-blind, cross-over comparison with alfentanil and placebo. *Pain.* 2003;101:229–235.
230. Khan N, Smith MT. Multiple sclerosis-induced neuropathic pain: pharmacological management and pathophysiological insights from rodent EAE models. *Inflammopharmacology.* 2014;22(1):1–22.
231. Okon T. Ketamine: an introduction for the pain and palliative medicine physician. *Pain Physician.* 2007;10(3):493–500.
232. Gottschalk A, Schroeder F, et al. Amantadine, an *N*-methyl-D-aspartate receptor antagonist, does not enhance postoperative analgesia in women undergoing abdominal hysterectomy. *Anesth Analg.* 2001;93(1):192–196.
233. Helmy SA, Bali A. The effect of the preemptive use of the NMDA receptor antagonist dextromethorphan on postoperative analgesic requirements. *Anesth Analg.* 2001;92(3):739–744.
234. Yeh CC, Ho ST, et al. Absence of the preemptive analgesic effect of dextromethorphan in total knee replacement under epidural anesthesia. *Acta Anaesthesiol Sin.* 2000;38(4):187–193.
235. Himmelseher S, Ziegler-Pithamitsis D, et al. Small-dose S(+)-ketamine reduces postoperative pain when applied with ropivacaine in epidural anesthesia for total knee arthroplasty. *Anesth Analg.* 2001;92(5):1290–1295.
236. Weber C. NMDA-receptor antagonist in pain therapy. *Anasthesiol Intensivmed Notfallmed Schmerzther.* 1998;33(8):475–483.
237. Le DA, Lipton SA. Potential and current use of *N*-methyl-D-aspartate (NMDA) receptor antagonists in diseases of aging. *Drugs Aging.* 2001;18(10):717–724.
238. Parsons CG. NMDA receptors as targets for drug action in neuropathic pain. *Eur J Pharmacol.* 2001;429(1–3):71–78.
239. Fukui S, Komoda Y, Nosaka S. Clinical application of amantadine, an NMDA antagonist, for neuropathic pain. *J Anesth.* 2001;15(3):179–181.
240. White PF, Elig MR. Intravenous anaesthetics. In: Barash PG, ed. *Clinical Anaesthesia.* 6th ed. China: Lippincott Williams and Wilkins; 2013:478–500.
241. Persson J. Wherefore ketamine? *Curr Opin Anaesthesiol.* 2010;23:455–460.
242. Advisory Council on the Misuse of Drugs. Ketamine: a review of use and harm. 2013. Report. Available from: http://www.gov.uk/government/./ACMD_ketamine_report_dec13.pdf. Accessed July 8, 2014.
243. Hocking G, Cousins MJ. Ketamine in chronic pain management: an evidence-based review. *Anesth Analg.* 2003;97:1730–1739.
244. Ducharme J. No pain, no gain, big gain: effective pain management program and abstracts of the American College of Emergency Physicians 2011 Scientific Assembly; October 15–18, 2011; San Francisco, CA. Available from: http://www.webapps.acep.org/sa/syllabi/su-78.pdf. Accessed May 22, 2017.
245. Reves JG, Glass PS, Lubarsky DA, et al. Intravenous anaesthetics. In: Miller RD, ed. *Miller's Anaesthesia.* 7th ed. USA: Churchill Livingstone; 2010:719–771.
246. Domino EF. Taming the ketamine tiger. *Anesthesiology.* 2010;113:876–886.
247. Kiefer RT, Rohr P, Ploppa A, et al. Efficacy of ketamine in anesthetic dosage for the treatment of refractory complex regional pain syndrome: an open-label phase II study. *Pain Med.* 2008;9(8):1173–1201.
248. Kiefer RT, Rohr P, Ploppa A, et al. Complete recovery from intractable complex regional pain syndrome, CRPS-type I, following anesthetic ketamine and midazolam. *Pain Pract.* 2007;7(2):147–150.
249. Koffler SP, Hampstead BM, Irani F, et al. The neurocognitive effects of 5 day anesthetic ketamine for the treatment of refractory complex regional pain syndrome. *Arch Clin Neuropsychol.* 2007;22(6):719–729.
250. Kishimoto N, Kato J, et al. A case of RSD with complete disappearance of symptoms following intravenous ketamine infusion combined with stellate ganglion block and continuous epidural block. *Masui.* 1995;44(12):1680–1684.
251. Goldberg ME, Domsky R, Scaringe D, et al. Multi-day low dose ketamine infusion for the treatment of CRPS. *Pain Physician.* 2005;8:175–179.
252. Correll GE, Maleki J, Gracely EJ, et al. Subanesthetic ketamine infusion therapy: a retrospective analysis of a novel therapeutic approach to CRPS. *Pain Med.* 2004;5:263–275.
253. Zarate CA Jr, Singh JB, Carlson PJ, et al. A randomized trial of an *N*-methyl-D-aspartate antagonist in treatment-resistant major depression. *Arch Gen Psychiatry.* 2006;63:856–864.
254. Heresco-Levy U, Javitt DC, Gelfin Y, et al. Controlled trial of D-cycloserine adjuvant therapy for treatment-resistant major depressive disorder. *J Affect Disord.* 2006;93(1–3):239–243.
255. Schwartzman RJ, Alexander GM, Grothusen JR, et al. Outpatient intravenous ketamine for the treatment of complex regional pain syndrome: a double-blind placebo controlled study. *Pain.* 2009;147(1–3):107–115.
256. Collins S, Sigtermans MJ, Dahan A. NMDA receptor antagonists for the treatment of neuropathic pain. *Pain Med.* 2010;11(11):1726–1742.
257. Connolly SB, Prager JP, Harden RN. A systematic review of ketamine for complex regional pain syndrome. *Pain Med.* 2015;16(5):943–969.
258. Rabben T, Skjelbred P, et al. Prolonged analgesic effect of ketamine, an *N*-methyl-D-aspartate receptor inhibitor, in patients with chronic pain. *J Pharmacol Exp Ther.* 1999;289(2):1060–1066.
259. D'Arcy Y. Patching together transdermal pain control option (controlling pain). *Nursing.* 2005;35(9):17.
260. Weinbroum AA, Rudick V, et al. The role of dextromethorphan in pain control. *Can J Anaesth.* 2000;47(6):585–596.
261. Shin EJ, et al. Neuropsychotoxicity of abused drugs: potential of dextromethorphan and novel neuroprotective analogs of dextromethorphan with improved safety profiles in terms of abuse and neuroprotective effects. *J Pharmacol Sci.* 2008;106:22–27.
262. Werling LL, Lauterbach EC, et al. Dextromethorphan as a potential neuroprotective agent with unique mechanisms of action. *Neurologist.* 2007;13(5):272–293.
263. Linn KA, Long MT, Pagel PS. "Robo-Tripping": dextromethorphan abuse and its anesthetic implications. *Anesth Pain Med.* 2014;4(5):e20990.
264. Mack, A. Examination of the evidence for off-label use of gabapentin. *J Manag Care Pharm.* 2003;9(6):559–568.
265. Pud D, Eisenberg E, Spitzer A, et al. The NMDA receptor antagonist amantadine reduces surgical neuropathic pain in cancer patients: a double blind, randomized, placebo controlled trial. *Pain.* 1998;75(2-3):349–354.
266. Eisenberg E, Kleiser A, Dortort A, et al. The NMDA (*N*-methyl-D-aspartate) receptor antagonist memantine in the treatment of postherpetic neuralgia: a double-blind, placebo-controlled study. *Eur J Pain.* 1998;2:321–327.
267. Nikolajsen L, Gottrup H, Anders GD, et al. Memantine (a *N*-methyl-D-aspartate receptor antagonist) in the treatment of neuropathic pain after amputation or surgery: a randomized, double-blind, cross-over study. *Anesth Analg.* 2000;91:960–966.
268. Maier C, Dertwinkel R, Mansourian N, et al. Efficacy of the NMDA- receptor antagonist memantine in patients with chronic phantom limb pain-results of a randomized double-blinded, placebo-controlled trial. *Pain.* 2003;103:277–283.
269. Hackworth RJ, Tokarz KA, Fowler IM, et al. Profound pain reduction after induction of memantine treatment in two patients with severe phantom limb pain. *Anesth Analg.* 2008;107:1377–1379.
270. Sinis N, Birbaumer N, et al. Memantine treatment of complex regional pain syndrome: a preliminary report of six cases. *Clin J Pain.* 2007;23(3):237–243.
271. Schley M, Topfner S, Wiech K, et al. Continuous brachial plexus blockade in combination with the NMDA receptor antagonist memantine prevents phantom pain in acute traumatic upper limb amputees. *Eur J Pain.* 2007;11(3):299–308.
272. Hsu E, Cohen SP. Postamputation pain: epidemiology, mechanisms, and treatment. *J Pain Res.* 2013;6:121–136.
273. Morel V, Joly D, Villatte C, et al. Memantine before mastectomy prevents post-surgery pain: a randomized, blinded clinical trial in surgical patients. *PLoS One.* 2016;11(4):e0152741.
274. Tolbert D. Predicted versus actual steady-state plasma levels for oxaprozin, a new nonsteroidal anti-inflammatory drug. *Drug Ther.* 1993;(suppl):47–51.
275. Birmingham R. *Practical management of pain.* 2014. Available from: https://www-clinicalkey-com.proxy.libraries.rutgers.edu/#!/content/book/3-s2.0 B97803230834 09000402?scrollTo=%23hl0000470).
276. Targownik LE, Thompson PA. Gastroprotective strategies among NSAID users; guidelines for appropriate use in chronic illness. *Can Fam Physician.* 2006;52(9):100–1105.
277. Onk CK, Lirk P, et al. An evidence-based update on nonsteroidal anti-inflammatory drugs. *Clin Med Res.* 2007;5(1):19–34.
278. Arbuck DM. No perfect medicine—what you need to know about NSAID's and opioids. *Pract Pain Manag.* 2016;16(7).
279. Moore RA, Derry S, Wiffen PJ, et al. Effects of food on pharmacokinetics of immediate release oral formulations of aspirin, dipyrone, paracetamol and NSAIDs—a systematic review. 2015;80(3):381–388.
280. Taha AS, Hudson N, et al. Famotidine for the prevention of gastric and duodenal ulcers caused by nonsteroidal anti-inflammatory drugs. *N Engl J Med.* 1996;334:1435–1439.
281. Graham DY. Helicobacter pylori and nonsteroidal anti-inflammatory drugs: interaction with proton pump inhibitor therapy for prevention of nonsteroidal anti-inflammatory drug ulcers and ulcer complications-future research needs. *Am J Med.* 2001;110(1A):58S–61S.
282. Andrade RJ, Lucena MI, et al. Drug induced liver injury: an analysis of 461 incidences submitted to the Spanish registry over a 10 year period. *Gastroenterology.* 2005;129:512–521.
283. Product Information. In: Sifton DW, ed. *Physician's Desk Reference.* New Jersy: Moonvale; 2002.

284. Cohen DB, Kawamura S, Ehteshami JR, et al. Indomethacin and celecoxib impair rotator cuff tendon-to-bone healing. *Am J Sports Med*. 2006;34(3):362-369.

285. Coruzzi G, Venturi N, et al. Gastrointestinal safety of novel nonsteroidal anti-inflammatory drugs: selective COX-2 inhibitors and beyond. *Acta Biomed*. 2007;78(2):96-110.

286. Leese P, Hubbard R, Karim A, et al. Effects of celecoxib, a novel cyclooxygenase-2 inhibitor, on platelet function in healthy adults; a randomized, controlled trial. *J Clin Pharmacol*. 2000;40:124.

287. Harris RC, Breyer MD. Update on cyclooxygenase-2 inhibitors. *Clin J Am Soc Nephrol*. 2006;1(2):236-245.

288. Bombardier C, Laine L, Reicin A, et al. Comparison of upper intestinal toxicity of rofecoxib and naproxen in patients with rheumatoid arthritis. *N Engl J Med*. 2000;343:1520-1528.

289. Silverstein F, Faich G, Goldstein J, et al. Gastrointestinal toxicity with celecoxib vs. nonsteroidal anti-inflammatory drugs for osteoarthritis and rheumatoid arthritis. The CLASS Study: a randomized controlled trial. *JAMA*. 2000;284:1247-1255.

290. Schnitzer TJ, Mysler E, et al. Comparison of lumiracoxib with naproxen and ibuprofen in the Therapeutic Arthritis Research and Gastrointestinal Event Trial (TARGET), reduction in ulcer complications: randomised controlled trial. *Lancet*. 2004;363:665.

291. Wallace JL, McKnight W, et al. NSAID-induced gastric damage in rats: requirement for inhibition of both cyclooxygenase 1 and 2. *Gastroenterology*. 2000:119:706-714.

292. Yokota A, Taniguchi M, et al. Development of intestinal, but not gastric damage caused by a low dose of indomethacin in the presence of rofecoxib. *Inflammopharmacology*. 2005:13:209-216.

293. Fornai M, Blandizzi C, et al. Role of cyclooxygenases 1 and 2 in the modulation of neuromuscular functions in the distal colon of humans and mice. *Gut*. 1997;54:609-616.

294. Martinez-Gonzales J, Badimon L. Mechanisms underlying the cardiovascular effects of COX inhibition: benefits and names. *Curr Pharm Des*. 2007;13(22):2215-2227.

295. Caldwell B, Aldington S, et al. Risk of cardiovascular events and celecoxib: a systematic review and meta-analysis. *J R Soc Med*. 2006;99:132-140.

296. Bresalier RS, Sandler RS, et al. Cardiovascular events associated with rofecoxib in a colorectal adenoma chemoprevention trial. *N Engl J Med*. 2005;352(11):1092-1102.

297. Bertagnolli MM, Eagle CJ, et al. Celecoxib for the prevention of sporadic colorectal adenomas. *N Engl J Med*. 2006;355(9):873-884.

298. Salzberg DJ, Weir MR. COX-2 inhibitors and cardiovascular risk. *Subcell Biochem*. 2007;42:159-174.

299. Sopena F, Lanas A. How to advise aspirin use in patients who need NSAID's. *Curr Pharm Des*. 2007;13(22):2248-2260.

300. DuBois RN, Abramson SB, Crofford L, et al. Cyclooxygenase in biology and disease. *FASEB*. 1998;12:1063-1073.

301. Perazella M, Tray K. Selective cyclooxygenase-2 inhibitors: a pattern of nephrotoxicity similar to traditional NSAID's. *Am J Med*. 2001;111:64.

302. Swan SK, Rudy DW, et al. Effect of cyclooxygenase-2 inhibition on renal function in elderly persons receiving a low salt diet: a randomized, controlled trial. *Ann Intern Med*. 2000;133(1):1-9.

303. Dentali F, Douketis JD, et al. Does celecoxib potential the anticoagulation effect of warfarin? A randomized, double blind, controlled trial. *Ann Pharmacother*. 2006;40(7-8):1241-1247.

304. Layton D, Marshall V, et al. Serious skin reactions and selective COX-2 inhibitors: a case series from prescription event monitoring in England. *Drug Saf*. 2006;29(8):687-696.

305. Talhari C, Lauceviciute I, et al. COX-2 selective inhibitor valdecoxib induced severe allergic skin reactions. *J Allergy Clin Immunol*. 2005;115(5):1089-1090.

306. Radi ZA Khan NK. Effects of cyclooxygenase inhibition on bone, tendon and ligament healing. *Inflamm Res*. 2005;54(9):358-366.

307. Karachalios T, Boursinos L, et al. The effects of the short-term administration of low therapeutic doses of anti- COX-2 agents on the healing of fractures: an experimental study in rabbits. *J Bone Joint Surg Br*. 2007;89(9):1253-1269.

308. Górska J. Effects of back pain treatment with tizanidine. *Ortop Traumatol Rehabil*. 2005;7(3):306-309.

309. Delzell JE Jr, Grelle AR. Trigeminal neuralgia. New treatment options for a well-known cause of facial pain. *Arch Fam Med*. 1999;8(3):264-268.

310. Vorobeǐchik IaM, Kukushkin ML, et al. [The treatment of the phantom pain syndrome with tizanidine]. *Zh Nevropatol Psikhiatr Im S S Korsakova*. 1997; 97(3):36-39.

311. Hord AH, Chalfoun AG, et al. Systemic tizanidine hydrochloride (Zanaflex) relieves thermal hyperalgesia in rats with an experimental mononeuropathy. *Anesth Analg*. 2001;93(5):1310-1315.

312. Semenchuk MR, Sherman S. Effectiveness of tizanidine in neuropathic pain: an open-label study. *J Pain*. 2000;1(4):285-292.

313. Naeem M, Al Alem H, Al Shehri A, et al. Effect of *N*-methyl-D-aspartate receptor antagonist dextromethorphan on opioid analgesia in pediatric intensive care unit. *Pain Res Manag*. 2016;2016:1658172.

314. Thurlow W. Acetaminophen, aspirin, and renal failure. *N Engl J Med*. 2002;346:1588-1589.

315. Murros K, Kataja M, et al. Modified-release formulation of tizanidine in chronic tension-type headache. *Headache*. 2000;40(8):633-637.

316. Saper JR, Winner PK, et al. An open-label dose-titration study of the efficacy and tolerability of tizanidine hydrochloride tablets in the prophylaxis of chronic daily headache. *Headache*. 2001;41(4):357-368.

317. Smith TR. Low-dose tizanidine with nonsteroidal anti-inflammatory drugs for detoxification from analgesic rebound headache. *Headache*. 2002;42(3):175-177.

318. Talakoub R, Abbasi S, Maghami E, et al. The effect of oral tizanidine on postoperative pain relief after elective laparoscopic cholecystectomy. *Adv Biomed Res*. 2016;5:19.

319. Yang PP, Yeh G-C, Huang EY-K, et al. Effects of dextromethorphan and oxycodone on treatment of neuropathic pain in mice. *J Biomed Sci*. 2015;22(1):81.

320. Shah J, Wesnes KA, et al. Effects of food on the single-dose pharmacokinetics/pharmacodynamics of tizanidine capsules and tablets in healthy volunteers. *Clin Ther*. 2006;28(9):1308-1317.

321. ZANAFLEX® (tizanidine hydrochloride) capsules, tablets, for oral use Drug Information. Acorda Therapeutics Inc. Ardsley, NY 10502. Accessed September 1, 2016.

322. Smith HS, Barton AE. Tizanidine in the management of spasticity and musculoskeletal complaints in the palliative care population. *Am J Hosp Palliat Care*. 2000;17(1):50-58.

323. Granfors MT, Backman JT, Laitila J, et al. Tizanidine is mainly metabolized by cytochrome P450 1A2 in vitro. *Br J Clin Pharmacol*. 2004;57(3):349-353.

324. Momo K, Homma M, et al. Drug interaction of tizanidine and ciprofloxacin: case report. *Clin Pharmacol Ther*. 2006;80(6):717-719.

325. Momo K, Doki K, et al. Drug interaction of tizanidine and fluvoxamine. *Clin Pharmacol Ther*. 2004;76(5):509-510.

326. Granfors MT, Backman JT, et al. Oral contraceptives containing ethinyl estradiol and gestodene markedly increase plasma concentrations and effects of tizanidine by inhibiting cytochrome P450 1A2. *Clin Pharmacol Ther*. 2005;78(4):400-411.

327. Kao CD, Chang JB, et al. Hypotension due to interaction between lisinopril and tizanidine. *Ann Pharmacother*. 2004;38(11):1840-1843.

328. Raja SN, Haythornthwaite JA, et al. Opioids versus antidepressants in postherpetic neuralgia: a randomized, placebo-controlled trial. *Neurology*. 2002;59:1015-1021.

329. Huse E, Larbig W, et al. The effect of opioids on phantom limb pain and cortical reorganization. *Pain*. 2001;90:47-55.

330. Gimbel JS, Richards P, et al. Controlled-release oxycodone for pain in diabetic neuropathy: a randomized controlled trial. *Neurology*. 2003;60:927-934.

331. World Health Organization. *Cancer Pain Relief*. Geneva, Switzerland: WHO Office of Publications; 1986.

332. Dowell D, Haegerich TM, Chou R. CDC guideline for prescribing opioids for chronic pain—United States. *JAMA*. 2016;315(15):1624-1645.

333. Hojsted J, Sjogren P. An update on the role opioids in the management of chronic pain of nonmalignant origin. *Curr Opin Anaesthesiol*. 2007;20(5):451-455.

334. Martell BA, O'Connor PG, et al. Systemic review: opioid treatment for chronic back pain: prevalence, efficacy, and association with addiction. *Ann Intern Med*. 2007;146:116.

335. Eisenberg E, McNicol ED, et al. Efficacy and safety of opioid agonists in the treatment of neuropathic pain of nonmalignant origin: systematic review and meta-analysis of randomized controlled trials. *JAMA*. 2005;293(24):3043-3052.

336. Binder W, Mousa SA, et al. Sympathetic activation triggers endogenous opioid release and analgesia within peripheral inflamed tissue. *Eur J Neurosci*. 2004;20(1):92-100.

337. Schaible HG, Schmelz M, et al. Pathophysiology and treatment of pain in joint disease. *Adv Drug Deliv Rev*. 2006;58(2):323-342.

338. Ng HP, Nordstrom U, et al. Efficacy of intra-articular bupivacaine, ropivacaine, or a combination of ropivacaine, morphine, and ketorolac on postoperative pain relief after ambulatory arthroscopic knee surgery: a randomized double-blind study. *Reg Anesth Pain Med*. 2006;31(1):26-33.

339. Raj N, Sehgal A, et al. Comparison of the analgesic efficacy and plasma concentrations of high-dose intra-articular and intramuscular morphine for knee arthroscopy. *Eur J Anaesthesiol*. 2004;21(12):932-937.

340. Koulousakis A, Kutcha J, et al. Intrathecal opioids for intractable pain syndromes. *Acta Neurochir Suppl*. 2007;97(patient 1):43-48.

341. Iwaszkiewicz KS, Schneider JJ, Hua S. Targeting peripheral opioid receptors to promote analgesic and anti-inflammatory actions. *Front Pharmacol*. 2013;4:132. doi:10.3389/fphar.2013.00132.

342. Sharp BM. Multiple opioid receptors on immune cells modulate intracellular signaling. *Brain Behav Immun*. 2006;20(1):9-14.

343. Stein C, Schafer M, et al. Peripheral opioid receptors. *Ann Med*. 1995;27(2):219-221.

344. Stanos S. Appropriate use of opioid analgesics in chronic pain. *J Fam Pract*. 2007;56(2 suppl Pain):23-32.

345. Rowbotham MC, Twilling L, et al. Oral opioid therapy for chronic peripheral and central neuropathic pain. *N Engl J Med*. 2003;348(13):1223-1232.

346. Kalso E, Edwards JE, et al. Opioids in chronic non-cancer pain: systematic review of efficacy and safety. *Pain*. 2004;112:372-380.

347. Mercadante S. Opioid rotation for cancer pain: rationale and clinical aspects. *Cancer*. 1999;86(9):1856-1866.

348. De Leon-Casasola OA. Cellular mechanisms of opioid tolerance and the clinical approach to the opioid tolerant patient in the post-operative period. *Best Pract Res Clin Anaesthesiol*. 2005;16(4):521-525.

349. Rubinstein AL, Carpenter DM. Association between commonly prescribed opioids and androgen deficiency in men: a retrospective cohort analysis. *Pain Med*. 2017;18(4):637-644. doi:10.1093/pm/pnw182.

350. Seiferi S. Opioid medications. In: Dart RC, ed. *Medical Toxicology*. Philadelphia, PA: Lippincott Williams & Wilkins; 2003:753-788.

351. Peloso PM, Bellamy N, et al. Double blind randomized placebo control trial of controlled release codeine in the treatment of osteoarthritis of the hip or knee. *J Rheumatol.* 2000;27(3):764–771.

352. Food Drug Administration. FDA recommends against the continued use of propoxyphene website. Available from: https://www.fda.gov/Drugs/DrugSafety/ucm234338.htm. Nov 19, 2010. Accessed May 22, 2017.

353. Kornick CA, Santiago-Palma J, et al. Benefit-risk assessment of transdermal fentanyl for treatment of chronic pain. *Drug Saf.* 2003;26(13):951–973.

354. Herndon CM. Iontophoretic drug delivery system: focus on fentanyl. *Pharmacotherapy.* 2007;27(5):745–754.

355. Mayes S, Ferrone M. Fentanyl HCl patient-controlled iontophoretic transdermal system for the management of acute postoperative pain. *Ann Pharmacother.* 2006;40(12):2178–2186.

356. Hartrick CT, Pestano CR, Ding L, et al. Patient considerations in the use of transdermal iontophoretic fentanyl for acute postoperative pain. *J Pain Res.* 2016;9: 215–222. doi:10.2147/JPR.S89278.

357. Marquardt KA, Tharratt RS, et al. Fentanyl transdermal (Durogesic, Janssen). *Intensive Crit Care Nurs.* 1995;11(6):360–361.

358. Paice JA, Fine PG. Pain at the end of life. In: Ferrell B, Coyle N, eds. *Textbook of Palliative Nursing (Ferrell, Palliative Nursing).* New York: Oxford University Press; 2005.

359. Kotwal RS, O'Connor KC, et al. A novel pain management strategy for combat casualty care. *Ann Emerg Med.* 2004;44(2):121–127.

360. Ashburn MA, Ling GH, et al. Oral transmucosal fentanyl citrate (OTFC) for the treatment of postoperative pain. *Anesth Analg.* 1993;76(2):377–381.

361. Mahar PJ, Rana JA, et al. A randomized clinical trial of oral transmucosal fentanyl citrate versus intravenous morphine sulfate for initial control of pain in children with extremity injuries. *Pediatr Emerg Care.* 2007;23(8):544–548.

362. Blick SK, Wagstaff AJ. Fentanyl buccal tablet: in breakthrough pain in opioid-tolerant patients with cancer. *Drugs.* 2006;66(18):2387–2393; discussion 2394–2395.

363. Aronoff GM, Brennan MJ. Evidence-based oral transmucosal fentanyl citrate (OTFC) dosing guidelines. *Pain Med.* 2005;6(4):305–314.

364. Portenoy RK, Taylor D. A randomized, placebo-controlled study of fentanyl buccal tablet for breakthrough pain in opioid-treated patients with cancer. *Clin J Pain.* 2006;22(9):805–811.

365. Wirz S, Wartenberg HC, Nadstawek J. Less nausea, emesis, and constipation comparing hydromorphone and morphine? A prospective open-labeled investigation on cancer pain. *Support Care Cancer.* 2008;16(9):999–1009.

366. Quigley C. Hydromorphone for acute and chronic pain. *Cochrane Database Syst Rev.* 2002;(1):CD003447.

367. Guedes AG, Papich MG, et al. Comparison of plasma histamine levels after intravenous administration of hydromorphone and morphine in dogs. *J Vet Pharmacol Ther.* 2007;30(6):516–522.

368. Razaq M, Balicas M, et al. Use of hydromorphone (Dilaudid) and morphine for patients with hepatic and renal impairment. *Am J Ther.* 2007;14(4):414–416.

369. Shirk MB, Donahue KR, et al. Unlabeled uses of nebulized medications. *Am J Health Syst Pharm.* 2006;63(18):1704–1716.

370. Mitka M. FDA bans sale of unapproved cough suppressants containing hydrocodone. *JAMA.* 2007;298(19):2251–2252.

371. Isbell H, Fraser HF. Addiction to analgesics and barbiturates. *Pharm Rev.* 1950;2:355–397.

372. Mannino R, Coyne P, et al. Methadone for cancer-related neuropathic pain: a review of the literature. *J Opioid Manag.* 2006;2(5):269–276.

373. Moulin DE, Clark AJ, et al. Pharmacological management of chronic neuropathic pain-consensus statement and guidelines from the Canadian Pain Society. *Pain Res Manag.* 2007;12(1):13–21.

374. Moulin DE, Palma D, et al. Methadone in the management of intractable neuropathic noncancer pain. *Can J Neurol Sci.* 2005;32(3):340–343.

375. Inturrisi CE. Clinical pharmacology of opioids for pain. *Clin J Pain.* 2002;18 (4 suppl):S3–S13.

376. Ayonrinde OT, Bridge DR. The rediscovery of methadone for cancer pain management. *Med J Aust.* 2000;173(10):536–540.

377. Gupta A, Lawrence AT, et al. Current concepts in the mechanisms and management of drug-induced QT prolongation and torsade de pointes. *Am Heart J.* 2007;153(6):891–899.

378. Riley J, Eisenberg E. Oxycodone: a review of its use in the management of pain. *Curr Med Res Opin.* 2008;24(1):175–192.

379. Cicero TJ, Inciardi JA, et al. Trends in abuse of Oxycontin and other opioid analgesics in the United States: 2002-2004. *J Pain.* 2005;6(10):662–672.

380. Stambaugh JE, Reder RF, et al. Double-blind, randomized comparison of the analgesic and pharmacokinetic profiles of controlled- and immediate-release oral oxycodone in cancer pain patients. *J Clin Pharmacol.* 2001;41(5):500–506.

381. Hale ME, Fleischmann R, et al. Efficacy and safety of controlled-release versus immediate-release oxycodone: randomized, double-blind evaluation in patients with chronic back pain. *Clin J Pain.* 1999;15(3):179–183.

382. Ackerman SJ, Knight T, et al. Risk of constipation in patients prescribed fentanyl transdermal system or oxycodone hydrochloride controlled-release in a California Medicaid population. *Consult Pharm.* 2004;19(2):118–132.

383. Reisfield GM, Wilson GR. Rational use of sublingual opioids in palliative medicine. *J Palliat Med.* 2007;10(2):465–475.

384. Hans G. Buprenorphine—a review of its role in neuropathic pain. *J Opioid Manag.* 2007;3(4):195–206.

385. Koppert W, Ihmsen H, et al. Different profiles of buprenorphine-induced analgesia and antihyperalgesia in a human pain model. *Pain.* 2005;118(1–2):15–22.

386. Sarton E, Teppema L, et al. Naloxone reversal of opioid-induced respiratory depression with special emphasis on the partial agonist/antagonist buprenorphine. *Adv Exp Med Biol.* 2008;605:486–491.

387. Megarbane B, Hreiche R, et al. Does high-dose buprenorphine cause respiratory depression?: possible mechanisms and therapeutic consequences. *Toxicol Rev.* 2006;25(2):79–85.

388. Wolford R, Kahler J, et al. A prospective comparison of transnasal butorphanol and acetaminophen with codeine for the relief of acute musculoskeletal pain. *Am J Emerg Med.* 1997;15(1):101–103.

389. Gillis JC, Benfield P, et al. Transnasal butorphanol. A review of its pharmacodynamic and pharmacokinetic properties, and therapeutic potential in acute pain management. *Drugs.* 1995;50(1):157–175.

390. Zacny J, Bigelow G, et al. College on Problems of Drug Dependence taskforce on prescription opioid non-medical use and abuse: position statement. *Drug Alcohol Depend.* 2003;69(3):215–232.

391. Brown RL, Patterson JJ, et al. Substance abuse among patients with chronic back pain. *J Fam Pract.* 1996;43(2):152–160.

392. Breckenridge J, Clark JD. Patient characteristics associated with opioid versus nonsteroidal anti-inflammatory drug management of chronic low back pain. *J Pain.* 2003;4(6):344–350.

393. Martell BA, O'Connor PG. Systematic review: opioid treatment for chronic back pain: prevalence, efficacy, and association with addiction. *Ann Intern Med.* 2007;146(2):116–127.

394. Coluzzi F, Pappagallo M, et al. Opioid therapy for chronic noncancer pain: practice guidelines for initiation and maintenance of therapy. *Minerva Anestesiol.* 2005;71(7–8):425–433.

395. Agency Medical Directors Group. *Interagency Guidelines on Opioid Dosing for Chronic Non-cancer Pain: An Educational Pilot to improve Career and Safety with Opioid Treatment.* Washington, DC; 2007. Available from: http://www.agency-medicaldirectors.wa.gov/

396. Trescot AM, Boswell MV, et al. Opioid guidelines in the management of chronic non-cancer pain. *Pain Physician.* 2006;9(1):1–39.

397. DuPen A, Shen D, et al. Mechanisms of opioid-induced tolerance and hyperalgesia. *Pain Manag Nurs.* 2007;8(3):113–121.

398. Bhansali A, Velayutham P, et al. Effect of opiates on growth hormone secretion in acromegaly. *Horm Metab Res.* 2005;37(7):425–427.

399. Roberts LJ, Finch PM, et al. Sex hormone suppression by intrathecal opioids: a prospective study. *Clin J Pain.* 2002;18(3):144–148.

400. Page GG. Immunological effects of opioids in the presence or absence of pain. *J Pain Symptom Manag.* 2005;29(suppl):S25–S31.

401. Angst MS, Koppert W, et al. Short-term infusion of the mu-opioid agonist remifentanil in humans causes hyperalgesia during withdrawal. *Pain.* 2003;106(1–2): 49–57.

402. Mao J, Sung B, et al. Chronic morphine induces downregulation of spinal glutamate transporters: implications in morphine tolerance and abnormal pain sensitivity. *J Neurosci.* 2002;22(18):8312–8323.

403. Ebell M. Tramadol relieves neuropathic pain. *Am Fam Physician.* 2007;75(9): 1335–1336.

404. Boureau F, Legallicier P, et al. Tramadol in post-herpetic neuralgia: a randomized, double-blind, placebo-controlled trial. *Pain.* 2003;104(1–2):323–331.

405. Sindrup SH, Andersen G, et al. Tramadol relieves pain and allodynia in polyneuropathy: a randomised, double-blind, controlled trial. *Pain.* 1999;83(1): 85–90.

406. Harati Y, Gooch C, et al. Double-blind randomized trial of tramadol for the treatment of the pain of diabetic neuropathy. *Neurology.* 1998;50(6):1842–1846.

407. Wilder-Smith CH, Hill LT, et al. Postamputation pain and sensory changes in treatment-naive patients: characteristics and responses to treatment with tramadol, amitriptyline, and placebo. *Anesthesiology.* 2005;103(3):619–628.

408. Altman R, Hochberg M, et al. American College of Rheumatology 2012 recommendations for the use of nonpharmacologic and pharmacologic therapies in osteoarthritis of the hand, hip, and knee. *Arthritis Care Res (Hoboken).* 2012;64(4):465–474.

409. Roth SH. Efficacy and safety of tramadol HCl in breakthrough musculoskeletal pain attributed to osteoarthritis. *J Rheumatol.* 1998;25(7):1358–1363.

410. Alemdar M, Pekdemir M, et al. Single-dose intravenous tramadol for acute migraine pain in adults: a single-blind, prospective, randomized, placebo-controlled clinical trial. *Clin Ther.* 2007;29(7):1441–1447.

411. Tagarro I, Herrera J, et al. Effect of a simple dose-escalation schedule on tramadol tolerability: assessment in the clinical setting. *Clin Drug Investig.* 2005;25(1): 23–31.

412. Peloso PM, Fortin L, et al. Analgesic efficacy and safety of tramadol/acetaminophen combination tablets (Ultracet) in treatment of chronic low back pain: a multicenter, outpatient, randomized, double blind, placebo controlled trial. *J Rheumatol.* 2004;31(12):2454–2463.

413. Emkey R, Rosenthal N, et al. Efficacy and safety of tramadol/acetaminophen tablets (Ultracet) as add-on therapy for osteoarthritis pain in subjects receiving a COX-2 nonsteroidal antiinflammatory drug: a multicenter, randomized, double-blind, placebo-controlled trial. *J Rheumatol.* 2004;31(1):150–156.

414. Bennett RM, Kamin M, et al. Tramadol and acetaminophen combination tablets in the treatment of fibromyalgia pain: a double-blind, placebo-controlled study. *Am J Med.* 2003;114(7):537–545.

415. Lee EY, Lee EB, et al. Tramadol 37.5-mg/acetaminophen 325-mg combination tablets added to regular therapy for rheumatoid arthritis pain: a 1-week,

randomized, double-blind, placebo-controlled trial. *Clin Ther.* 2006;28(12): 2052–2060.

416. Hair PI, Curran MP, et al. Tramadol ER tablets. *Drugs.* 2006;66(15):2017–2027.

417. Lazebnik LB, Kotsiubinskaia OB, et al. Non-steroidal anti-inflammatory drugs and tramadol in the treatment of osteoarthrosis deformans in patients with arterial hypertension. *Klin Med (Mosk).* 2004;82(10):56–61.

418. Malonne H, Coffiner M, et al. Long-term tolerability of tramadol LP, a new once-daily formulation, in patients with osteoarthritis or low back pain. *J Clin Pharm Ther.* 2005;30(2):113–120.

419. Malonne H, Coffiner M, et al. Efficacy and tolerability of sustained-release tramadol in the treatment of symptomatic osteoarthritis of the hip or knee: a multicenter, randomized, double-blind, placebo-controlled study. *Clin Ther.* 2004;26(11):1774–1782.

420. Wallace MS, Staats P, et al. *Pain Medicine and Management: Just the Facts.* New York, NY: McGraw-Hill Professional; 2004.

421. Pascual ML, Fleming RR, et al. Open-label study of the safety and effectiveness of long-term therapy with extended-release tramadol in the management of chronic nonmalignant pain. *Curr Med Res Opin.* 2007;23(10):2531–2542.

422. Mongin G. Tramadol extended-release formulations in the management of pain due to osteoarthritis. *Expert Rev Neurother.* 2007;7(12):1775–1784.

423. Close BR. Tramadol: does it have a role in emergency medicine. *Emerg Med Australas.* 2005;17(1):73–83.

424. Moore RA, McQuay HJ, et al. Single-patient data meta-analysis of 3453 postoperative patients: oral tramadol versus placebo, codeine and combination analgesics. *Pain.* 1997;69(3):287–294.

425. FDA Drug Safety Communication: FDA restricts use of prescription codeine pain and cough medicines and tramadol pain medicines in children; recommends against use in breastfeeding women website. Published April 20, 2017. Available from: https://www.fda.gov/downloads/Drugs/DrugSafety/UCM553814.pdf. Accessed May 22, 2017.

426. Senay EC, Adams EH, et al. Physical dependence on Ultram (tramadol hydrochloride): both opioid-like and atypical withdrawal symptoms occur. *Drug Alcohol Depend.* 2003;69(3):233–241.

427. Substance Abuse and Mental Health Services Administration (SAMHSA). *Key Substance Use and Mental Health Indicators in the United States: Results from the 2015 National Survey on Drug Use and Health.* Rockville, MD: US Department of Health and Human Services; 2016. HHS Publication No. (SMA) 16-4984.

428. Centers for Disease Control and Prevention. Wide-ranging online data for epidemiologic research (WONDER), multiple cause of death data. Available from: http://www.cdc.gov/nchs/data/health_policy/AADR_drug_poisoning_involving_OA_Heroin_US_2000-2014.pdf. Accessed April 25, 2016.

429. O'Neill R, Lor K, et al. Abuse-Deterrent Opioid Formulations #329. *J Palliat Med.* 2017;20(6):676–678. doi:10.1089/jpm.2017.0088. Available from: http://online.liebertpub.com/doi/abs/10.1089/jpm.2017.0088

430. FDA Hysingla ER Factsheet. Published August 2015. Available from: https://www.accessdata.fda.gov/drugsatfda_docs/label/2015/022272s027lbl.pdf. Accessed May 22, 2017.

431. FDA Ventrela ER Factsheet. Published January 2017. Available from: https://www.accessdata.fda.gov/drugsatfda_docs/label/2017/207975s000lbl.pdf. Accessed May 22, 2017.

432. FDA Arymo ER Factsheet. Available from: https://www.accessdata.fda.gov/drugsatfda_docs/label/2017/208603s000lbl.pdf

433. FDA Embeda ER Factsheet. Published October 2014. Available from: https://www.accessdata.fda.gov/drugsatfda_docs/label/2014/022321s016lbl.pdf. Accessed May 22, 2017.

434. FDA MorphaBond ER Factsheet. Published October 2015. Available from: https://www.accessdata.fda.gov/drugsatfda_docs/label/2015/206544lbl.pdf. Accessed May 22, 2017.

435. Mercadante S. Oxycodone extended release capsules for the treatment of chronic pain. *Expert Rev Neurother.* 2017;17(5):427–431. doi:10.1080/14737175.2017.1 302331.

436. FDA OxyContin ER Factsheet. Published August 2015. Available from: https://www.accessdata.fda.gov/drugsatfda_docs/label/2015/022272s027lbl.pdf. Accessed May 22, 2017.

437. FDA Targiniq ER Factsheet. Published July 2014. Available from: https://www.accessdata.fda.gov/drugsatfda_docs/label/2014/205777lbl.pdf. Accessed May 22, 2017.

438. FDA Troxyca ER Factsheet. Published August 2016. Available from: https://www.accessdata.fda.gov/drugsatfda_docs/label/2016/207621s000lbl.pdf. Accessed May 22, 2017.

439. FDA RoxyBond ER Factsheet. Published April 2017. Available from: https://www.accessdata.fda.gov/drugsatfda_docs/label/2017/209777lbl.pdf. Accessed May 22, 2017.

440. FDA Xtampza ER Factsheet. Published April 2016. Available from: https://www.accessdata.fda.gov/drugsatfda_docs/label/2016/208090s000lbl.pdf. Accessed May 22, 2017.

441. Trevana Inc. OLINVO™ (oliceridine injection): The first μ receptor G protein Pathway Selective modulator (μGPS). Available from: http://www.trevena.com/OLINVO.php

442. Higo N. Recent trend of transdermal drug delivery system development. *Yakugaku Zasshi.* 2007;127(4):655–662.

443. Vandervoort J, Ludwig A. Microneedles for transdermal drug delivery: a minireview. *Front Biosci.* 2008;1(13)1711–1715.

444. Bikowski K, Shroot B. Multivesicular emulsion: a novel, controlled-release delivery system for topical dermatological agents. *J Drugs Dermatol.* 2006;5(10): 942–946.

445. Bruhlmann P, Michel BA. Topical diclofenac patch in patients with knee OA: a randomized, double blind, controlled clinical trial. *Clin Exp Rheumatol.* 2003;21(12):193–198.

446. Solignac M. Assessment of a topical NSAIDs in the treatment of pain and inflammation. The example of Flector Plaster: a local bioadhesive plaster containing diclofenac epolamine. *Presse Med.* 2004;33(14 Pt 2):3S10–23S13.

447. Stanos S. Osteoarthritis guidelines: a progressive role for topical NSAIDs. *J Am Osteopath Assoc.* 2013 Feb;113(2);123–127.

448. Belcaro G, Cesarone MR, et al. A plaster combining diclofenac and heparin: microcirculatory evaluation in 2 models of high perfusion microangiopathy. *Angiology.* 2005;56(6):707–713.

449. Mahler P, Mahler F, et al. Double blind, randomized, controlled study on the efficacy and safety of a novel diclofenac epolamine gel formulated with lecithin for the treatment of sprains, strains, and contusions. *Drug Exp Clin Res.* 2003;29(1):45–52.

450. FDA CDER Databases. Flector Patch. 2007. Available from: www.fda.gov/cder/foi/label/2007/021234lbl.pdf

451. Chong MS, Hester J. Diabetic painful neuropathy: current and future treatment options. *Drugs.* 2007;67(4):569–585.

452. Pospisilova E, Palecek J. Post-operative pain behavior in rats is reduced after single high-concentration capsaicin application. *Pain.* 2006;125(3):233–243.

453. Schnitzer TJ, Morton C, et al. Topical capsaicin therapy for OA pain: achieving a maintenance regime. *Semin Arthritis Rheum.* 1994;23(suppl):34–40.

454. Rapoport AM, Bigal ME. Intranasal medications for the treatment of migraine and cluster headache. *CNS Drugs.* 2004;18(10)671–685.

455. Rains C, Bryson HM. Topical capsaicin: a review of its pharmacological properties and therapeutic potential in post-herpetic neuralgia, diabetic neuropathy and OA. *Drugs Aging.* 1995;7(4):317–328.

456. Hautkappe M, Roizen MF, et al. Review of the effectiveness of capsaicin for painful cutaneous disorders and neural dysfunction. *Clin J Pain.* 1998;14(2):97–106.

457. Ribbers GM, Stam HJ. Complex regional pain syndrome type I treated with topical capsaicin: a case report. *Arch Phys Med Rehabil.* 2001;82(6):851–852.

458. Cannon DT, Wu Y. Topical capsaicin as an adjuvant analgesic for the treatment of traumatic amputee neurogenic residual limb pain. *Arch Phys Med Rehabil.* 1998;79(5):591–593.

459. Mason L, Moore RA, et al. Systematic review of topical capsaicin for the treatment of chronic pain. *BMJ.* 2004;328(7446):991.

460. Jann MW, Slade JH. Antidepressant agents for the treatment of chronic pain and depression. *Pharmacotherapy.* 2007;27(11):1571–1587.

461. Watson CPN, Vernich L, et al. Nortriptyline versus amitriptyline in postherpetic neuralgia: a randomized trial. *Neurology.* 1998;51:1166–1171.

462. Harding LM, Murphy A, Kinnman E, et al. Characterization of secondary hyperalgesia produced by topical capsaicin jelly—a new experimental tool for pain research. *Eur J Pain.* 2001;5(4):363–371.

463. Malisza KL, Docherty JC. Capsaicin as a source for painful stimulation in functional MRI. *J Magn Reson Imaging.* 2001;14(4):341–347.

464. Gazerani P, Anderson OK, et al. A human experimental capsaicin model for trigeminal sensitization: gender specific differences. *Pain.* 2005;118(1–2):155–161.

465. Kwak JY, Jung JY, Hwang SW, et al. A capsaicin-receptor antagonist, capsazepine, reduces inflammation-induced hyperalgesic responses in the rat: evidence for an endogenous capsaicin-like substance. *Neuroscience.* 1998;86(2):619–626.

466. Tominaga M, Julius D. Capsaicin receptor in the pain pathway. *Jpn J Pharmacol.* 2000;83(1):20–24.

467. Pascual DW, Bost KL, et al. The cytokine-like action of substance P upon B-cell differentiation. *Reg Immunol.* 1992;4(2):100–104.

468. Scardina GA, Augello L, et al. The role of neuromodulators (substance P and calcitonin gene-related peptide) in the development of neurogenic inflammation in the oral mucosa. *Minerva Stomatol.* 2004;53(1–2);21–32.

469. Minami T, Bakoshi S, Nakano H, et al. The effects of capsaicin cream on prostaglandin-induced allodynia. *Anesth Analg.* 2001;93(2):419–423.

470. Yang K, Kumamoto E, Furue H, et al. Capsaicin induces a slow inward current which is not mediated by substance P in substantia gelatinosa neurons of the rat spinal cord. *Neuropharmacology.* 2000;39(11):2185–2194.

471. Sullivan WJ, Panagos A, et al. Industrial medicine and acute MSK rehabilitation. 2. Medications for the treatment of acute MSK pain. *Arch Phys Med Rehabil.* 2007;88(3 suppl):S10–S13.

472. Forst T, Pohlmann T, et al. The influence of local capsaicin treatment on small nerve fibre function and neurovascular control in symptomatic diabetic neuropathy. *Acta Diabetol.* 2002;39(1):1–6.

473. Argoff CE. Topical analgesics in the management of acute and chronic pain. *Mayo Clin Proc.* 2013;88(2):195–205.

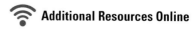 **Additional Resources Online**

CHAPTER 53

Lisa Huynh
Zachary L. McCormick
David J. Kennedy

Joint and Spinal Injection Procedures

Peripheral musculoskeletal and spine pain are two of the most common reasons for physician visits in the United States. Studies have shown that over 50% of adults have musculoskeletal pain (1), and the lifetime prevalence of spine pain in the United States approaches 80% to 90% (2). Combined, they are the leading cause of disability in the United States and represent a significant burden on the health care system (3,4). Although many treatment options exist for these conditions, targeted injections have consistently gained popularity in modern medicine since Hollander et al. demonstrated the effects of corticosteroid injections in the 1950s (5).

In clinical practice, the goal of an injection is to deliver an aliquot of medication directly to a specific target tissue. Given the focused nature of injections, they can be used for both diagnostic and therapeutic purposes. In order to maximize the likelihood of a safe and successful outcome from an injection, practitioners must have a wide range of knowledge. This knowledge includes but is not limited to superficial and deep anatomy, appropriate patient selection, indications/contraindications, pharmacology, risks, benefits, numerous procedure-specific technical details, as well as a general understanding of the limitations and role of diagnostic and therapeutic nature of these procedures. This chapter will serve as a guide to understanding the basic concepts of musculoskeletal and spine injections while also offering a broad overview of the evidence surrounding various aspects of injections. It will start with general considerations regarding the role of diagnostic and therapeutic injections, before delving into contraindications, medications, adverse reactions, the role of image guidance, and target-specific considerations.

THE ROLE OF INJECTIONS

Key Considerations for Ideal Interpretation of Diagnostic Injections

Diagnostic injections are generally done via gauging the degree of pain relief immediately following an injection of a local anesthetic (6). This immediate pain response can offer significant insights, although several key factors must be recognized in order to appropriately interpret the results.

Once a decision has been made to perform a diagnostic procedure, the practitioner must recognize the potential for a false negative. Historically, the main reason for a false negative was procedural inaccuracy. Anatomic landmark–guided,

otherwise known as "blind," injections have been repeatedly shown to be inaccurate in the spine, peripheral joints, and even soft tissues (7–12). While the miss rate has varied significantly between 10% and 80%, a unifying theme in the literature has emerged. Specifically, the data have shown that even in experienced hands, practitioners cannot be guaranteed that an anatomic landmark–guided procedure is 100% accurate. This inaccuracy is further potentially compounded by other factors such as unrecognized vascular uptake that can result in the anesthetic not reaching the target tissue (13,14). Therefore, if a patient fails to obtain pain relief following a procedure, the inaccuracy of the procedure must be considered as a possible reason for the lack of response. This ambiguity may be overcome through the use of image guidance during procedures. Ultrasound (US), fluoroscopy, computed tomography (CT), and magnetic resonance imaging (MRI) have all been used to guide and/or assure accuracy of these procedures. While each of these imaging modalities has its respective pros/cons and limitations, there is a robust volume of literature showing that appropriately selected imaging modalities can confirm accurate medication placement with a high degree of certainty (8,10,15). Therefore, the use of appropriate imaging to confirm the anesthetic actually reaches the target tissue could help significantly diminish the concerns regarding inaccuracy causing a false-negative response.

Another key feature in the interpretation of anesthetic blocks is the potential of false-positive responses. These also can occur from several sources. The first is through the potential for a lack of specificity with an injectate. Studies have shown that even with appropriate needle placement, the subsequent injectate frequently reaches additional tissues that were not intended (16–18). Simple examples include capsular defects in joint injections that allow the anesthetic to reach extra-articular structures or flow of anesthetic to adjacent structures in spine and soft tissue injections. In certain instances, this can be mitigated through the use of appropriate imaging modalities or the use of low-volume injections (19). These techniques, however, do not prevent the more common cause of false-positive responses, the placebo or nonspecific response. Placebo responses have been shown to occur in 20% to 40% of patients receiving injections (20,21). There are multiple techniques that can reduce the false-positive rate such as having an independent assessor determine the efficacy of the block, performing repeated blocks, or even performing dual comparative blocks utilizing anesthetics of varying duration of effects at each injection (22,23). While these techniques do decrease the likelihood of a false positive, they do not result in 100% specificity and sensitivity. Therefore, practitioners must acknowledge the possibility of a false positive from a diagnostic injection.

Inappropriate procedural follow-up can also result in misinterpretation of the diagnostic block. It is imperative to assess the response to the injection at a time when the anesthetic actually has a physiologic effect (24). While they do vary, local anesthetics generally have an onset within seconds to minutes and durations in the nature of several hours. Unfortunately, there are many studies in the literature that assess the diagnostic response at time intervals beyond the expected physiologic effects, often at days to weeks after the injection, thus adding errors through nonphysiologic effects (6). Therefore, to minimize recall errors and reduce the potential for nonphysiologic effects, the assessment of pain relief should be done immediately after an injection or through the appropriate use of postprocedure pain logs.

The combination of the clear potential for a false positive, along with the ability to significantly mitigate the potential for a false negative through appropriate imaging guidance and follow-up time frames, leads to the real utility of diagnostic injections: the negative response. If a specific target tissue is anesthetized and confirmed with the appropriate imaging modality, the patient should not have nociceptive responses from that tissue. Therefore, if a patient does not obtain relief of pain after such an injection, then one can assume that the targeted tissue is not the sole source of pain (6). In this case, other pain generators may be partially or fully contributing to the patient's symptoms. This is in contrast to a positive response, where even complete relief of pain may be due to placebo or nonspecific responses.

While the negative response to an appropriately done image-guided diagnostic injection does offer the highest degree of diagnostic confidence, the positive response also has value, but it must be placed in appropriate context. In addition to the sensitivity and specificity of a given procedure, the diagnostic confidence of a positive response is also contingent on the prevalence of the medical condition. In highly prevalent diseases, practitioners may have high confidence from a positive response following a single injection or even no injection. Conversely in diseases with low prevalence, where the placebo rate may be higher than the actual prevalence, practitioners may have low confidence in the results of a single block, thus necessitating more rigorous diagnostic standards.

A simple example of this concept would be the relative high degree of diagnostic confidence of the knee being the source of pain in a 70-year-old patient with unilateral knee pain during ambulation and Kellgren-Lawrence grade 4 knee osteoarthritis on radiographs. In this patient population, osteoarthritis has a high prevalence, such that practitioners may have high diagnostic confidence. In fact in this example, the confidence is high enough that diagnostic injections are likely not even needed. This would be in contrast to a 50-year-old with chronic buttock pain without radiation that has multiple positive physical exam maneuvers of the pelvis, hips, and spine and diffuse radiographic abnormalities in the hip and spine. In this patient population, there is not a single disease process that has a high prevalence. The patient could have pain arising from the hip, the posterior pelvis, or even the spine. Thus, a

positive single block to any given target would likely result in the practitioner having lower diagnostic confidence. However, an appropriately done injection, with negative results, could be believed for the reasons outlined above.

These examples raise the last major issue with diagnostic injections. Specifically, diagnostic injections should only be performed when the results of such injection would change the treatment course. In a 50-year-old with chronic buttock pain and a diverse differential diagnosis, the first treatment may be conservative exercise-based care. This type of care would not be predicated on the injection outcome. This may be in contrast to a patient who has failed conservative care and is being worked up for a potential invasive treatment such as radiofrequency neurotomy (RFN) of the lumbar zygapophyseal joints (Z-joints). Additionally, risks of the diagnostic injection must always be weighed against any potential benefits gained.

Therapeutic Injections

The second and more common major indication for interventional procedures is to offer a therapeutic effect to a specific target tissue. These are frequently done in combination with diagnostic injections, although therapeutic injections do have different goals, risks, indications, and appropriate follow-up times. Additionally, while therapeutic injections can be successful in isolation, they are generally considered adjuvant therapy to be implemented as part of a multifaceted treatment regimen. They also are typically done either after failing appropriate exercise-based conservative therapy or to help selected patients that are unable to tolerate such treatments.

Before being considered a viable treatment options, many factors must be considered. These include the relative risks of the procedure, the efficacy of the procedure, the natural history of the underlying disease process, and the risks and benefits of other available treatment options. It is only through consideration of all of these multiple facets that an appropriate treatment regimen can be given to an individual patient.

The risks/benefit of a given procedure clearly varies by the anatomic location and the medication being injected. For example, due to the proximity of the spinal cord, injections targeting the cervical epidural space would have a higher innate risk than injections targeting the knee. Additionally, corticosteroids have additional risks beyond local anesthetics. A detailed knowledge of these risks is essential and will thus be covered in more detail later in the chapter.

While essential, knowledge of procedural risks alone is insufficient for a full risk/benefit discussion. Practitioners must also be aware of the natural history of the disease process to determine if the patient is receiving an appropriate therapeutic effect. While anesthetic blocks offer diagnostic insights immediately, mere hours of relief would be considered insufficient for a therapeutic effect. A short-term effect of days/weeks/months may, however, be very appropriate for disease processes with a favorable natural history. In this example, the short-term relief may be sufficient to offer pain relief while the body is going through a natural healing process. In contrast, longer-term results are necessary in those with a chronic condition. Examples of disease processes with favorable natural histories in which a short-term effect would be reasonable are abundant in medicine. A simple example in the musculoskeletal world would be postoperative pain, where pain medications would be effective and beneficial immediately. However, longer-term follow-up of months to years in this patient population would show no differences in outcomes. Conversely, while short-term results may be appropriate in disease pathology with favorable natural histories, they would be insufficient for chronic conditions. Adding further confusion is that many disease processes, in the spine and musculoskeletal system, have a strong potential to reoccur.

An example will help elucidate this point. Urinary tract infections (UTIs) can be effectively treated with antibiotics within days. In this example, the appropriate time to determine effectiveness of the antibiotic is in the short term (days to weeks), as longer-term follow-up would likely fail to show any effect. Given UTIs can reoccur, it is possible to acquire another UTI 12 months later, regardless of the success of the initial treatment. Therefore, if a patient were to reacquire a UTI at 12 months, it would be erroneous to conclude that the current infection represents a failure of the original antibiotics. Similarly, while it is correct to state that the antibiotics only offered a "short-term" benefit, it would be incorrect to conclude that repeat antibiotics are not indicated for the 12-month infection recurrence since their benefits are only short term. In fact, short-term benefits are all that is expected and needed for this condition. Another erroneous perspective is to conclude that the original antibiotics were beneficial for 1 year or that these patients should now receive antibiotics annually. All of these are incorrect assumptions when considered in the context of the pharmacokinetics of the medications and the natural history of the disease. Unfortunately, this lack of understanding of the natural history of musculoskeletal and spine conditions has led many to erroneously conclude that the effects were only "short term" and thus imply that these procedures offer no benefit to the procedures (25).

In addition to the risks/benefits of a given therapeutic procedure and the natural history of the disease process, practitioners must also be aware of the risk/benefits and efficacy of available treatment alternatives. As discussed above, corticosteroid injections into the knee for osteoarthritis are generally thought to be low risk, although recurrent long-term corticosteroid dosing is clearly not ideal. For healthy patients with isolated advanced knee arthritis who have failed other conservative treatments, a total knee arthroplasty may be a viable option that has a generally favorable outcome. This, however, may not be a reasonable consideration for the same disease process in the unhealthy or very elderly. Thus, an otherwise healthy 70-year-old with unilateral knee osteoarthritis who obtains only short-term relief from an injection may be better suited for a more invasive knee replacement than years of recurrent injections. This may be in contrast to an unhealthy 99-year-old, who is not a surgical candidate but who gets some relief and increased mobility from injections. In the latter case, repeated interventions may be reasonable assuming the patient is truly obtaining benefits. Thus, even with the same underlying disease process, the same treatment response, and even the same theoretical treatment options, vastly different recommendations as to the usefulness of therapeutic injections would be made based on patient-specific factors.

It therefore requires a thorough understanding of the appropriate limitations and usefulness of diagnostic blocks, goals and alternative options for therapeutic procedures, risks and benefits of any given procedures, appropriate follow-up time frames based on expected natural history of a given disease, and pharmacology of the injected medications to appropriately implement intervention-based therapies into a treatment algorithm. The rest of the chapter will focus on more specific details surrounding these injections.

ADVERSE EVENTS ASSOCIATED WITH INJECTIONS

For any intervention, the risk versus benefit of the procedure should be considered in the context of each individual patient's complaint, comorbidities, and preferences. Injection procedures can target a wide variety of structures in the musculoskeletal system including but not limited to joints, tendons, ligaments, muscles, motor points, the epidural space, the intervertebral disks, and nerves. Clearly, these targets have varying levels of associated risks ranging from minor adverse events to serious complications. Minor adverse events are characterized as occurrences that require minimal if any medical intervention and result in no permanent sequelae (26). Such events are unavoidable to some extent in patients who undergo injections, regardless of the target tissue or medication injected. Examples would include injection site soreness, pain exacerbation, and vasovagal reaction. Serious complications are characterized as occurrences that require medical intervention and may result in permanent sequelae. These serious complications are generally rare, especially in peripheral injections. However, while techniques exist to mitigate these risks, they cannot be completely eliminated. Thus, it is vital for practitioners to properly counsel patients and to employ appropriate risk mitigation strategies. The following section addresses both minor adverse events and serious complications that can occur due to peripheral and spinal injections. The sections are divided into subsections based on causation, with adverse events due to needle insertion separated from those due to the subsequent procedure-specific injectate. Although a wide variety of medications have been utilized in musculoskeletal medicine, this chapter will focus on those commonly used including local anesthetics, corticosteroids, and viscosupplements.

Adverse Events Related to Needle Intervention
Minor Adverse Events Related to Needle Insertion

Vasovagal Reaction
The most common minor adverse event that may change or interrupt the procedure resulting from a needle intervention is a vasovagal reaction (27). Vasovagal reaction is a frequent response to injection procedures that is attributable to physiologic and psychological factors. This response may start with dizziness, faintness, sweating, and pallor and proceed to bradycardia, hypotension, and even loss of consciousness.

Vasovagal reaction occurs at a higher rate in patients who undergo spinal injection compared to peripheral joint injections. Systematic, prospectively collected adverse event data demonstrate vasovagal reaction incidence rates of 5% for transforaminal epidural steroid injection (TFESI) (28), 5% for lumbar medial branch blocks (MBBs) (29), 4% for intra-articular lumbar zygapophyseal joint injections (30), 3% for trigger point injection (29), 2% for sacroiliac joint injection (31), and 0.5% for intra-articular hip injections (29). Vasovagal reactions have also been shown to be more common in young males (29). Vasovagal reaction can be treated with ice packs to the head/neck, physical counterpressure maneuvers, Trendelenburg position, and IV fluids if the reaction is severe and sustained (32).

Other

Other minor adverse events include nonspinal hematoma, injection site soreness, and pain exacerbation. Nonspinal hematoma occurs at an approximate rate of 1% in association with intra-articular zygapophyseal joint injections (cervical > thoracic > lumbar) (33) and 0.1% in association with epidural steroid injections (ESIs) (interlaminar > transforaminal; thoracic > cervical > lumbar) (34). Incidence rates have not been defined for peripheral joint, tendon, and bursa injections. Bleeding can be minimized through proper technique, ideally with one pass of the needle through tissues, and assessment for any bleeding diathesis.

Serious Complications Related to Needle Insertion

Infection

While infections can be minimized through the use of a sterile technique, cellulitis, soft tissue infection, and abscesses are possible consequences any time a needle penetrates the skin. Joint infections have been estimated to occur at a frequency of 1 in 3,000 to 1 in 50,000 injections (35). Osteodiscitis, epidural abscess, or meningitis may result from needle trespass during spinal injection procedures. Osteodiscitis occurs most frequently as a result of discography, at a rate of approximately 0.1% per disk exposed to needle entry (36). Treatment with antibiotics and serial assessment during recovery are required in such cases. Osteodiscitis, epidural abscess, and meningitis are otherwise extremely rare adverse events. While case reports exist, several large published cohort studies of spinal injections, with over 10,000 consecutive injections, failed to demonstrate any infections (26,33,34).

The workup of a suspected infection depends on the injection site. For spine procedures, infections are generally evaluated by MRI scanning specifically looking for signs of infection or abscess. This is in contrast to peripheral joints, where an aspiration with subsequent fluid culture and analysis may be done to rule out an infection (37). Systemic blood markers of infection, such as an elevated white blood cell count, may be late findings, and thus a negative result does not rule out an active infectious process. Additionally, white blood cell counts may be elevated after administration of corticosteroids and may result in confusion regarding the presence of an infection. Lastly, an active infection must be differentiated from an aseptic flare that can occur following an injection of a corticosteroid or viscosupplement. Both an aseptic flare and a true infection can present with pain, swelling, and erythema. One noninvasive method to help differentiate these two entities is the time frame in which the symptoms start. Generally, aseptic reactions occur within the first 24 hours following an injection, while infections generally present later. However, this timing is not definitive for causation; thus, the provider must always consider the possibility of an infection in patients presenting with symptoms that could be due to an infection (38).

Bleeding

Bleeding as a result of needle trespass is rarely of clinical significance, but hemarthrosis is possible in association with joint injection, and epidural or subdural hematoma is possible as a result of some spinal injection. Patients receiving warfarin have a very small increased bleeding risk in association with joint injection if the international normalized ratio (INR) is at an appropriate therapeutic level. For this reason, many practitioners do not discontinue warfarin before a peripheral joint injection (39), so as to avoid an ischemic complication related to discontinuing anticoagulation, a potentially far more devastating consequence.

While most hematomas do not result in long-term complications, intraspinal hematomas can have devastating long-term consequences. The prognosis of neurologic recovery from epidural hematoma is improved if decompression is performed within 12 hours of symptom onset (40). However, approximately 50% of patients will still have permanent neurologic deficits even if decompressed within 8 hours. Thus, vigilance for neurologic changes by both the practitioner and patient/family/caregiver is vital. Formation of a hematoma that causes compromise of a peripheral nerve or nerve plexus is fortunately extremely rare, and they are estimated to occur with a frequency of 1/250,000 from interlaminar epidural injections (41).

Given this low frequency of a severe complication, anticoagulation in the periprocedure period is a more controversial issue with regard to spinal injections. The American Society of Regional Anesthesia (ASRA) guidelines recommend that anticoagulants be stopped prior to many spine injection procedures (42). However, the risk of stopping anticoagulation may be greater than the risk of bleeding complications due to continuation of such an agent. Specifically, discontinuation of therapeutic anticoagulation increases the risk of stroke and other major vascular thromboembolic events two- to sixfold during this period (43,44). Interlaminar epidural access is clearly associated with the potential for an epidural hematoma, but there are no case reports of epidural hematoma in association with cervical or lumbar TFESIs, lumbar intra-articular zygapophysial injections, and cervical or lumbar MBBs when appropriate technique is used. Thus, practitioners may consider continuing anticoagulant and antiplatelet medications before spine injections that do not involve interlaminar access, as the risk shifts to ischemic complications in this scenario.

Nerve Injury due to Needle Trauma

Nerve injuries may result from direct needle trauma. Direct trauma to a peripheral nerve may occur in the case of intentional nerve block procedures as well as soft tissue injections in the region of peripheral nerves. Intraneural or intrafascicular injection is likely more devastating to the nerve structure than needle trespass alone. The risk of both can be reduced with the use of ultrasound guidance more so than the use of a nerve stimulator (45). As such, it is now considered the standard of care to perform peripheral nerve blocks with ultrasound guidance. Ultrasound guidance should be used for joint or soft tissue injection in close proximity to neurovasculature, such as at the medial epicondyle of the elbow (ulnar nerve) and the scalene muscles (brachial plexus). Spine injections should all be done with imaging guidance that would allow the proceduralist to know the needle depth prior to injecting any medication. This is typically done with a depth view on fluoroscopy but may also be done with CT guidance.

Also, to further reduce this risk, the appropriate use of procedural sedation must be considered in discussion of neural trauma associated with injections. An alert patient can more readily detect needle proximity to neural structures; therefore, pain may serve as a warning to the proceduralist. While sedation may be used to improve a patient's experience of pain and anxiety during injection procedures, and decrease the possibility of vasovagal reaction (46), the sedation has also been associated with catastrophic complications cataloged in the American Society of Anesthesiologists' Closed Claims database (47,48). Thus, the minimal necessary amount of sedation should be given in order to prevent neurovascular injury and other serious adverse events.

Pneumothorax

Pneumothorax is possible with any procedures done in the proximity of the lung, including trigger point injections in the thoracic region, costovertebral joint injections, and intercostal nerve blocks. Pneumothorax is of greater concern in patients with low body mass index or minimal soft tissue in the target region. In such cases, ultrasound guidance may be considered to visualize the safe depth of needle advancement. Similar to many other serious adverse events associated with spinal and peripheral injections, the true incidence of pneumothorax is not well defined, as only case reports exist.

Most of these patients can be easily treated with administration of 100% oxygen, close monitoring (e.g., oxygen saturation, vital signs) of the patient, and, when necessary, needle aspiration of air. Only those pneumothoraces that result in significant dyspnea or those under tension require chest tube thoracostomy and vacuum drainage. Bilateral thoracic procedures should be undertaken with caution due to potential risk of bilateral pneumothorax.

Post-dural Puncture Headache

Inadvertent dural puncture may result from spine injection procedures, most commonly with the interlaminar approach. This event may result in post–dural puncture headache when cerebrospinal fluid (CSF) leak occurs. Dural punctures generally present with a position-dependent headache, where patients are worse when upright. They are generally self-limited and can be treated by conservatively with lying down and drinking caffeinated beverages. While generally not dangerous, the symptoms may be severe enough to lead some patients to seek medical care or present to the emergency room. In severe cases or those that do not resolve, an epidural blood patch may be needed.

Adverse Events Related to Medications Administered

Adverse events to medications also range from minor to serious. Allergic reactions epitomize this spectrum of severity, with some reactions being mild and self-limited while others can result in severe anaphylaxis or even death. The most common sources of allergic reactions are contrast medications, although other medications have been reported. Ester anesthetic agents (e.g., procaine, tetracaine) are more frequently associated with allergic reactions than amide anesthetic agents (e.g., lidocaine, ropivacaine), because esters are derivatives of para-aminobenzoic acid (PABA) (49). Preservatives such as methylparaben have also been shown to cause allergic reactions. Therefore, any medication that contains preservatives, including many corticosteroids and all multidose vials, has the potential to cause an allergic reaction.

TABLE 53-1	**Treatment of Anaphylactic Shock**
Airway	Establish clear airway; suction, if required
Breathing	• Oxygen with face mask or nasal cannula
	• Encourage adequate ventilation
	• Artificial ventilation, if required
Circulation	• Lie flat and elevate legs
	• IV fluids if ↓ blood pressure
	• CVS support drug if ↓ blood pressure persists (see below) or ↓ heart rate
	• Cardioversion if ventricular arrhythmias occur
Drugs	Intramuscular adrenaline, using 0.5 mg of 1:1,000 injected into mid–anterolateral thigh

Reprinted from Soar J, Pumphrey R, Cant A, et al. Emergency treatment of anaphylactic reactions-guidelines for healthcare providers. *Resuscitation.* 2008;77(2): 157–169. Copyright © 2008 Elsevier. With permission.

Although allergic reactions are rare, if there is a question of patient hypersensitivity to anesthetic agents, intradermal skin tests can be used successfully to diagnose the adverse responses. This can be helpful in instances when repeat injections are needed in a patient who previously had an allergic response after the injection of several types of medications at once.

Treatment depends on severity of symptoms. Allergic reactions are generally treated with general supportive measures, although at times may require the administration of fluids, antihistamine, steroids, and/or epinephrine. Anaphylactic shock is treated as a systemic toxic reaction with attention to maintaining cardiovascular and ventilatory function (**Table 53-1**).

Minor Adverse Events Related to Medications

Local Anesthetic

Nearly all patients experience a sensation of "burning" during deposition of local anesthetic into tissue structures; this is expected and is not considered a complication. Temporary motor block frequently occurs as an expected effect following the injection of a local anesthetic near a neural structure. Temporary partial motor block of the ipsilateral lumbosacral plexus may occur following sacroiliac joint injection as the anterior joint capsule often contains capsular defects that allow for escape of intra-articular injectate. While temporary motor block is not intrinsically hazardous, appropriate patient counseling, postprocedure monitoring, escort, transportation, and other precautions specific to the particular injection should be taken in order to prevent falls or other injury. Further workup for other more serious causes of neurologic dysfunction such as a hematoma may be warranted if the block lasts longer than the expected duration of the anesthetic. One caveat is that concurrent injection of dexamethasone may enhance the duration of the motor block, resulting in a longer than expected recovery time.

Corticosteroids

The use of corticosteroid may cause both local and systemic effects acutely or subacutely. Local effects include hypopigmentation of the skin (2 days to 2 months), skin atrophy (1 to 4 months), and lipoatrophy (50). While these changes may be permanent, they are largely cosmetic and have minimal health consequences. Systemic side effects of corticosteroids are shown in **Table 53-2**. Common self-limited systemic effects include headache, flushing, insomnia, and hyperglycemia.

TABLE 53-2	Systemic Effects of Corticosteroid Use	
	Acute/Subacute	**Chronic**
Neurologic/ psychiatric	Dizziness/vertigo Insomnia Irritability/agitation Headache	
Cardiovascular	Edema/fluid retention Hypertension Exacerbation of arrhythmias (rare)	
Endocrine/ metabolic	Adrenal suppression Vasomotor flushing Hyperglycemia Menstrual irregularities	Epidural lipomatosis (rare) Cushing's syndrome Insulin insensitivity Weight gain
Immunologic	Immunosuppression	Immunosuppression
Gastrointestinal	Nausea/vomiting Appetite loss	
Skin	Delayed wound healing	
Eye	Increased intraocular pressure	Cataracts
Skeletal/ musculoskeletal		Osteopenia/ osteoporosis Avascular necrosis Myopathy

Viscosupplements

Viscosupplement is generally not associated with systemic adverse events, as the hyaluronic acid molecule does not cross the joint capsule from the intra-articular space. A large cohort study of over 12,000 injections reported infrequent and minor adverse events, most commonly effusion (2.4%), arthralgia (1.2), joint warmth (0.6%), and erythema (0.3%) with one case of an acute aseptic arthritis (51). Another smaller cohort study (*n* = 734 injections) reported only minor adverse events in patients who underwent intra-articular hyaluronic injection of the hip (52). Aseptic arthritis is further addressed as a result of hyaluronic acid injection in the Serious Adverse Events Related to Medications section.

Serious Adverse Events Related to Medications

Local Anesthetic

Toxic Reactions. Various toxic reactions have been reported after use of local anesthetics, but with very low incidence (49). Local anesthetic agents are relatively lipid-soluble, low molecular weight compounds that readily cross the blood-brain barrier. As toxic levels are reached, disturbances of central nervous system (CNS) function are observed initially, producing signs of CNS excitation. Early symptoms of overdose include headache, ringing in the ears, numbness in the tongue and mouth, twitching of facial muscles, and restlessness (49). As blood levels increase, generalized tonic-clonic seizures may occur. If sufficiently high blood levels are reached, the initial excitation is followed by generalized CNS depression. Respiratory depression and ultimately respiratory arrest may occur secondary to the toxic effect of the local anesthetic agent on the respiratory center in the medulla. Occasionally, the excitatory phase may not occur and toxicity presents as CNS depression.

Cardiovascular system (CVS) effects either result indirectly from inhibition of autonomic pathways during regional anesthesia (as in high spinal or epidural block) or are directly due to depressant actions on the CVS. The CVS is generally more resistant to toxicity than the CNS. The CVS-to-CNS toxicity ratio is lower for bupivacaine than for lidocaine (49). Convulsive activity may initially be associated with an increase in heart rate, blood pressure, and cardiac output. As the blood concentration of a local anesthetic agent increases further, CVS depression occurs, resulting in a decrease in blood pressure secondary to myocardial depression, impaired cardiac conduction, and eventual peripheral vasodilation. Ultimately, circulatory collapse and cardiac arrest may result. In addition, certain agents such as bupivacaine may cause ventricular arrhythmias and fatal ventricular fibrillation. The onset of CVS depression with bupivacaine may occur relatively early and be resistant to usual therapeutic modalities. The pregnant patient is more sensitive to the cardiotoxic effects of bupivacaine (49).

Systemic toxicity may be due to unintentional intravascular injection or drug overdose. Intravascular injection produces signs of toxicity (usually seizures) during the injection itself, especially if injected directly into blood vessels supplying to the brain (e.g., vertebral artery during cervical TFESI or stellate ganglion block). A relative overdose results in toxic reactions when peak blood levels are reached, about 20 to 30 minutes after the injection. Factors that affect the blood concentration (site of injection, drug, dosage, addition of vasoconstrictor, speed of injection) influence the potential for systemic toxic reactions to develop.

Systemic toxicity is treated with general supportive measures (50). If early signs of toxicity occur, constant verbal contact should be maintained, oxygen administered, breathing encouraged, and CVS function monitored. If seizure activity occurs, a clear airway should be maintained and oxygen administered by assisted or controlled ventilation. If seizures continue, benzodiazepines should be administered. Alternative medications including small doses of succinylcholine, small doses of propofol, or thiopental are acceptable. Muscular convulsive activity is terminated with succinylcholine, but seizure activity in the brain is not affected. If CVS depression occurs, hypotension should be treated by increasing intravenous fluids, positioning the patient properly (elevate the legs), and using vasopressors such as ephedrine or epinephrine. A differential diagnosis of toxic reactions and mimicking events is shown in **Table 53-3**.

Spinal Block

Inadvertent subarachnoid or epidural blockade can occur with any injection that is performed close to the spine. These injections include intercostal nerve blocks, sympathetic blocks, and nerve root injections. High motor block is of particular concern when a cervical epidural injection is performed (**Table 53-4**) as respiratory compromise may result. As such, many providers avoid use of local anesthetics during cervical interlaminar ESIs. If anesthetic is included in the epidural injectate, it is vital that a subdural or intrathecal contrast pattern is recognized prior to injection of medication. Proper equipment and staff should always be available. This includes the ability to administer fluids and vasopressors if the patient develops hypotension from sympathetic blockade and to maintain ventilation with oxygen if the patient has impaired

TABLE 53-3	Differential Diagnosis of Local Anesthetic Reactions	
Etiology	**Major Clinical Feature**	**Comments**
Systemic toxic reaction		
Intravascular injection	Immediate convulsion and/or cardiac toxicity	Injection into vertebral or a carotid artery may cause convulsion even with administration of small dose
Relative overdose	Onset in 5–15 minutes with irritability, progressing to convulsions	
Epinephrine reaction	Tachycardia, hypertension, headache, apprehension	May vary with vasopressor used
Vasovagal reaction	Rapid onset	Rapidly reversible with Trendelenburg positioning and discontinuing the noxious stimulus
	Bradycardia Hypotension Pallor, faintness	
Allergy		
Immediate	Anaphylaxis (↓ blood pressure, bronchospasm, edema)	Allergy to amides extremely rare
Delayed	Urticaria	Cross-allergy, for example, with preservatives in local anesthetics and food
High spinal or epidural	Gradual onset Bradycardia[a] Hypotension Possible respiratory arrest	May lose consciousness with total spinal block; onset of cardiorespiratory effects more rapid than with high epidural or with subdural block
Concurrent medical episode (e.g., asthma attack, myocardial infarct)	May mimic local anesthetic reaction	Medical history important

[a]Sympathetic block above T4 adds cardioaccelerator nerve blockade to the vasodilation seen with blockade below T4; total spinal block may have rapid onset.
Reprinted with permission from Covino BG. Clinical pharmacology of local anesthetic agents. In: Cousins MJ, Bridenbaugh PO, eds. *Neural Blockade in Clinical Anesthesia and Management of Pain*. 2nd ed. Philadelphia, PA: Lippincott Williams & Wilkins; 1988:134.

respiratory function. For certain high-risk procedures, the proceduralist may consider utilizing a shorter-acting anesthetic in case such a reaction occurs.

Viscosupplements

Acute aseptic arthritis both related and unrelated to crystal formation after hyaluronic acid injection into the knee has been described in case reports or small case series (53–58). This reaction begins within hours of injection. Chronic synovitis related to granuloma formation after hyaluronic acid injection into the knee joint has also been reported (59). Hyaluronic acid had been postulated to cause calcium pyrophosphate dehydrate (CPPD) crystal precipitation, not all cases of aseptic arthritis show the presence of intra-articular crystals. The hyaluronic acid molecule has been shown to interact with a leukocyte adhesion molecule, CD44, that may account for

recruitment of an inflammatory response (60). Treatment is supportive as the reaction is generally self-limited.

Contrast Agent

Use of a contrast agent is the standard of care during the majority of spinal injection procedures in order to confirm appropriate needle tip placement in the target structure and to ensure lack of entry into an undesired structure (24). Iodinated contrast may cause an anaphylactic reaction, though this has rarely been described. If a patient has a known allergic reaction from contrast agents, several options exist if a repeat injection is needed. Premedication with oral steroids and diphenhydramine is generally effective, but has been shown to fail approximately 1% of the time (61). This has led some practitioners to use gadolinium-based contrast medium as a substitute in cases of known severe iodinated contrast allergy. However,

TABLE 53-4	Serious Immediate Adverse Events Associated with Epidural Steroid Injection	
	Presumed Mechanism	**Incidence**
Spinal Cord Injury	Particulate steroid obstruction of medullary arteriole, epidural hematoma, intramedullary injection	Extremely rare—case reports only
Stroke	Particulate steroid injection into, plaque disruption and embolization, or vasospasm of the vertebral artery; vertebral artery dissection	Extremely rare—case reports only
High Spinal Block	Inadvertent subarachnoid or intrathecal injection of local anesthetic in the cervical spine causing respiratory compromise	Extremely rare—case reports only
Seizure	Toxicity due to intravascular local anesthetic	Extremely rare—case reports only
Arrhythmia	Response to intravascular local anesthetic or possibly sympathetic blockade (T1-4) in a low cervical injection	Extremely rare—case reports only
Anaphylactic Reaction	Allergy	Extremely rare—case reports only

gadolinium contrast is contraindicated for intrathecal use, as it has been shown to be neurotoxic (62). Therefore, if a procedure has the risk of inadvertent intrathecal injection (e.g., interlaminar epidural injections), the practitioner must weigh these relative risks or allergic reaction versus neural toxicity. In some specific cases, the injection may even be done without the use of contrast.

Corticosteroids

A variety of serious systemic side effects have been described in association with corticosteroid use (**Table 53-2**). Hypothalamic-pituitary axis (HPA) suppression has been described following even a single corticosteroid injection (63). Additionally, a study has shown that the number of peripheral joints injected independently increases cortisol suppression more than the total steroid dose (64). Specifically, 80 mg of methylprednisolone injected into a single knee joint resulted in less HPA suppression than injecting 40 mg methylprednisolone into both knees. However, the clinical significance of this is unclear, as the majority of reported systemic complications are felt to require repeated high-dose injections, beyond the generally accepted maximum of three to four injections annually.

Conflicting evidence exists regarding an increased risk of osteoporotic vertebral compression fractures (65–67). Studies that have shown this correlation have been in patients receiving large numbers (e.g., >8) of corticosteroid injections annually. Other studies on less frequent injections have shown no increased risk of osteoporotic wrist or hip fracture following epidural or large joint steroid injections (66). Hyperglycemia is common following an injection of a corticosteroid. This is likely only potentially hazardous to a diabetic patient with baseline poor blood glucose control, as studies of both peripheral and spinal corticosteroid injections have failed to demonstrate clinically significant effects of transient hyperglycemia (68–70). Tendon rupture is a described complication of local corticosteroid injections, although the exact incidence is unclear (71).

Possibly, the most serious adverse event that may occur secondary to injection of corticosteroid is specific to the use of particulate steroid in transforaminal epidurals (**Table 53-4**). All cases of stroke and spinal cord injury associated with cervical TFESI have involved particulate corticosteroid, and all but one case associated with lumbar TFESI has involved particulate steroid (72–75). Animal studies demonstrate that intra-arterial injection of particulate steroid causes red blood cell aggregation and occlusion of downstream arterioles; this effect does not occur when dexamethasone (nonparticulate steroid) is injected (76). As such, the presumed mechanism of neurologic infarction is embolism of distal arterioles supplied by branches off of the vertebral artery (stroke) or embolism of arterioles originating from the radiculomedullary arteries that nourish the anterior spinal cord (spinal cord injury), due to inadvertent upstream arterial injection during transforaminal epidural access. As a result of these findings, the Multidisciplinary Pain Workgroup has recommended that dexamethasone be used exclusively for cervical TFESI and that particulate steroid be used in only rare cases during lumbar TFESI (77). Although beyond the scope of this chapter, there are fortunately multiple other safeguards that exist, which may help further decrease this risk. These include the use of real-time imaging with digital subtraction technology, an anesthetic test dose, extension tubing, various needle types, and nonparticulate corticosteroids.

TABLE 53-5	**Contraindications to Injections**	
Absolute	**Relative**
Patient refusal or inability to consent	Uncontrolled diabetes mellitus[b]
Pregnancy (fluoroscopic- or CT-guided)	Minor coagulopathy
Infection—local or systemic[a]	Anticoagulation therapy
Tumor at site	Severe osteoporosis[b]
Fracture/unstable joint	
Untreated major coagulopathy	
Acute medical Instability	
Septicemia	

[a]Aspiration excluded.
[b]For corticosteroid injections.

Of note, the addition of ropivacaine to dexamethasone may make this medication act as a particulate, thus resulting in permanent neurologic injury if injected into an artery that perfuses the spinal cord or brain.

CONTRAINDICATIONS FOR INTERVENTION

Clearly, the potential of developing a complication varies depending on the anatomic target and the medication utilized, thus resulting in differing specific contraindications. For example, a cervical interlaminar epidural injection clearly has a risk profile that includes bleeding and formation of an epidural hematoma resulting in permanent neurologic injury. Thus, while there are specific anatomic considerations and medication-based contraindications, there are also several generalizable contraindications that cross most procedures (see **Table 53-5**).

Physicians should have an established process to identify patients that are precluded from having an injection. Practitioners should be aware of current guidelines regarding anticoagulation and procedures and have developed a standard practice ahead of time in regard to anticoagulation and injections. If the procedure may cause weakness or sedation, then the patient should have transportation and a responsible adult who can care for the patient after the procedure. Although generally not required for most procedures, if sedation is utilized for anxiety, then the patient should fast appropriately to reduce the risk of aspiration. Any allergies to the injection medications or to material such as latex should be documented, and when appropriate alternatives should be used for the procedure.

INFORMED CONSENT

Although state laws vary in terms of the documentation required, informed consent involves providing enough information about the injection procedure and its associated risks so that the patient can intelligently decide whether or not to proceed (without external coercion or manipulation). This involves a thorough discussion of the procedure with the patient, including the common side effects, and risks of complications. Ideally, the possible benefits, alternative treatments, and risks of not proceeding with the injection should also be discussed. The patient should be given the opportunity to ask questions about details of the injection. The patient should not receive medications that could significantly impair responses or judgment before the consent is given.

UNIVERSAL PROTOCOL

In order to prevent wrong site, wrong procedure, or wrong person procedures from occurring, the Universal Protocol has been established and became a mandatory quality standard by the Joint Commission in 2004. A preprocedure verification process is conducted to verify the correct procedure, the correct patient, and the correct site. This entails marking the general area on the patient where the procedure will occur. Immediately before starting an invasive procedure, a time-out is conducted. All members in the room should stop, listen, and verify that the information is correct. A team member will then identify the patient, the correct site, the exact procedure to be done, the correct patient positioning, the need for periprocedural antibiotics/prophylaxis, and the presence of allergies.

COMMUNICATION

Communication with the patient is essential at all steps involved in patient care, including injection. Providing the patient with a complete explanation of the procedure will result in the individual having increased confidence and reduced anxiety. During the procedure, the physician should continually inform and reassure the patient as to the progress of the procedure.

UNIVERSAL PRECAUTIONS

Universal precautions are required for all injection techniques to reduce the incidence of transmission of infectious agents (24). These include the use of gloves and when needed protective eyewear and masks. Possible transmission of blood-borne pathogens during medical procedures is a common concern among patients and health care workers, owing to its potentially devastating consequences. Although this concern has largely focused on the human immunodeficiency virus (HIV), other agents, particularly

hepatitis B, C, and G viruses, are of significantly greater risk. The data show that the risk to health care workers from patients is far greater than the risk to patients from health care workers (78). It is important that proper sharps disposal containers are maintained in all areas where needles are used. Hollow needlesticks pose the greatest risk for occupational transmission, with studies following health care workers after such exposures finding the following seroconversion rates: hepatitis B, 5% to 37%; hepatitis C, 3% to 10%; and HIV, 0.2% to 0.8% (78). Research shows that recapping a needle increases the risk for needlestick; hence, needles should either be laid down in the sterile field or disposed uncapped in an appropriate container (78).

MEDICATION PHARMAKOKINETICS AND OTHER CONSIDERATIONS

Although a wide variety of medications have been utilized in musculoskeletal medicine, this chapter will focus on those commonly used including local anesthetics, corticosteroids, viscosupplements, and neurolytics.

Local Anesthetics

Local anesthetics exert their effect through a reversible blockade of sodium channels along the axonal membrane, which prevents neural signal transmission. Local anesthetics reduce or eliminate peripheral neurotransmission of pain stimuli, normalize the hyperalgesic state of the nervous system, and may prevent or reduce neuronal plasticity in the CNS that is partially driven by ongoing peripheral nociceptive input. This, in part, may explain the well-recognized clinical phenomenon of pain relief following injection of local anesthetic that outlasts the physiologic action of the anesthetic. The degree of neural blockade depends on the properties, absorption, amount, location, and other characteristics of the medication injected (79,80) (**Table 53-6**).

TABLE 53-6	**Anesthetic Agents**							
Characteristics	**Procaine (Novocain)**	**Lidocaine (Xylocaine)**	**Prilocaine (Citanest)**	**Mepivacaine (Carbocaine)**	**Bupivacaine (Marcaine)**	**Tetracaine (Pontocaine)**	**Etidocaine (Duranest)**	**Ropivacaine (Naropin)**
Physicochemical								
Relative potency[a]	1	3	3	3	15	15	15	15
Relative toxicity[a]	1	1.5	1.5	2.0	10	12	10	10
pH of solution	5–6.5	6.5	4.5	4.5	4.5–6	4.5–6.5	4.5	7.4
Clinical								
Onset	Moderate	Fast	Fast	Fast	Moderate	Very slow	Fast	Slow
Dispersion	Moderate	Marked	Marked	Marked	Moderate	Poor	Moderate	Moderate
Duration of action	Short	Intermediate	Intermediate	Intermediate	Long	Long	Long	Long
Relative duration[a]	1	1.5–2	1.75–2	2–2.5	6–8	6–8	5–8	6–8
Concentration of solution (%)	1–2	1–2	1–2	1–2	0.25–0.5	0.1–0.25	0.5–1	0.25–0.5
Maximum recommended dose (mg/kg, adult)	10–14	6–10	6	6–10	2–3	2	4–5	3–4
Total dose (mg, adult)	500	300	—	400	150	—	300	200
Toxic blood levels (μg/mL)								
CNS	—	18–21	20	22	4.5–5.5	—	4.3	4.3
CVS	—	35–50	—	—	6–10	—	—	—

[a]Procaine = 1.
CNS, central nervous system; CVS, cerebrovascular system.

Local anesthetics should be chosen appropriately based on their side effects, their half-life, and the site of injection. For example, some anesthetics such as high concentrations of Marcaine and lidocaine have been shown to be chondrotoxic (81). Thus, medications such as ropivacaine can be considered for intra-articular injections, especially if the viability of the chondrocytes is a consideration. Additionally, some commercial preparations may contain preservatives that have been associated with potential neurotoxicity (82). This would make these medications less than ideal to inject near vulnerable neural structures. This has led to most using preservative-free preparations for neural axial injections (see Adverse Events section for further discussion of local anesthetic toxicity).

Some local anesthetics have the propensity to precipitate crystals at physiologic pH (83). *In vitro* study shows that ropivacaine mixed with dexamethasone or betamethasone causes crystal precipitation at physiologic pH (7.0 to 7.5). Bupivacaine demonstrated much smaller crystal precipitates when mixed with betamethasone, and none with dexamethasone. No crystal precipitates were seen when lidocaine was mixed with triamcinolone, dexamethasone, or betamethasone. None of the three local anesthetics precipitated when mixed with triamcinolone. While *in vivo* confirmation is needed, based on these findings as noted above, it is advisable to avoid combination of ropivacaine with dexamethasone or betamethasone, as well as bupivacaine and betamethasone when injecting in close proximity to neurovascular structures; this is particularly relevant during TFESI when embolization of a radiculomedullary artery with crystal precipitate is theoretically possible.

The medication's half-life is also a consideration. Due to its rapid onset, agents such as lidocaine are generally considered useful for skin infiltration prior to larger needle insertion or for rapid confirmation/rule out of a suspected pain generator. Longer-duration anesthetics should be used with caution near adjacent neural structures, given the potential for a prolonged block.

Neurolytic Agents

While use of radio-frequency energy and cryoablation techniques have become the favored methods of therapeutic nerve destruction, neurolysis with injectable agents remains in clinical use. Alcohol (50% to 100%) and phenol (5% to 10%) are the most widely used neurolytic injectable agents in the United States. These agents indiscriminately destroy motor and sensory nerves via protein denaturation with subsequent Wallerian degeneration distal to the lesion.

Phenol can be used in the intrathecal and epidural spaces (typically for intractable cancer pain and short life expectancy), as well as for peripheral nerve and motor point nerve destruction. It is poorly soluble in water and is often added to glycerin to achieve concentrations higher than 7%. Radiopaque contrast can be added to phenol to allow fluoroscopic visualization of spread during injection. Phenol has a local anesthetic effect, resulting in less pain after the neurolytic injection. Because of this, long-term effects of denervation cannot be evaluated for 24 to 48 hours after the effects of the local anesthetic dissipate. Doses greater than 100 mg can result in serious toxicity (84). Careful patient positioning must be used with intrathecal use as phenol is hyperbaric compared to CSF.

Alcohol is used primarily in the intrathecal space, for nerve roots, and locally for sympathetic neurolysis. It is readily soluble in body tissues and produces an intense burning sensation upon injection. Patient positioning must also be carefully considered with use of alcohol, but opposite to phenol, it is hypobaric compared to CSF. Alcohol requires 12 to 24 hours before the denervation effects can be determined. Lastly, it should be noted that denervation of any neural tissue that has sensory input from the skin has an associated risk of painful dyskinesia at a rate of 20% to 30% (85).

Corticosteroids

Corticosteroids are among the most commonly injected medication in MSK medicine. They typically target the inflammatory process. These agents remain a mainstay of treatment despite known side effects (discussed in the Adverse Events section of this chapter) due to their ability to decrease inflammation through reduction of the capillary permeability and inhibit inflammatory mediators phospholipase A_2, TNF-a, and IL-1 (86,87). Furthermore, corticosteroids have been shown to inhibit neural transmission in nociceptive C fibers (88), thus also suggesting an additional mechanism of analgesia distinct from known anti-inflammatory properties. Commonly used commercially available corticosteroid preparations for injection therapy are shown in **Table 53-7**.

TABLE 53-7	**Properties of Commonly Used Corticosteroids**					
Characteristics	Hydrocortisone (Cortisol)	Prednisolone (Hydeltra)	Dexamethasone (Decadron)	Methylprednisolone (Depo-Medrol)	Triamcinolone (Aristospan, Kenalog)	Betamethasone (Celestone)
Physiochemical						
Relative anti-inflammatory potency[a]	1	4	25	5	5	25
Relative mineralocorticoid potency[a]	1	0.6	0	0.25	0	0
pH of solution	5.0–7.0	6.0–8.0	7.0–7.7	7.0–8.0	4.5–6.5	6.8–7.2
Clinical						
Onset	Rapid	Rapid	Rapid	Slow	Moderate	Rapid
Dispersion	Moderate	Low	High	Low	Moderate	Moderate
Salt retention	2+	1+	0	0	0	0
Plasma half-life (hrs)	1.5	2–3	36–54	18–26	1.5	6.5
Concentration (mg/mL)	50	20	4–10	40–80	10–40	6
Range of usual dose (mg)	25–100	10–40	4–15	10–40	5–20	1.5–8

[a]Relative to hydrocortisone.

Corticosteroids vary in concentration, duration, and side effects. Properties of commonly used corticosteroids are shown in **Table 53-7**. As discussed in the introduction, while these medications vary in duration, their effect on the disease process usually has no relationship to the half-life. Exact medications are chosen based on efficacy, side effect profile, costs, and site-specific details. All commercially available corticosteroids, except dexamethasone, have particles or aggregate into clusters that are larger than red blood cells. Therefore, if injected into an artery that perfuses neural structures such as the brain of spinal cord, they can result in infarct of this tissue with subsequent profound neurologic deficits (73). Thus, for procedures such as a transforaminal epidural injection, dexamethasone is usually considered the safer first-line treatment options (77,89). However, in peripheral joint injections where this is not considered a significant risk, triamcinolone hexacetonide and methylprednisolone acetate are often used because of their low costs and robust volume of literature showing efficacy (90). However, it must be acknowledged that there is minimal direct comparative literature of particulate versus nonparticulate steroid during intra-articulate injections to support the widely held belief that particulate steroids are associated with superior clinical outcomes.

Dose and Volume of Corticosteroid Injections

Dose of steroid and total injectate volume vary by target tissue and patient-specific factors such as age and presence of diabetes. Of these variables, relative dose effectiveness has been studied more commonly. For glenohumeral joint adhesive capsulitis, the available literature suggests that 20 mg compared to 40 mg of triamcinolone is no less effective, but 10 mg compared to 40 mg of triamcinolone is associated with inferior clinical outcomes (91,92). One study has demonstrated no difference between 80 and 40 mg of methylprednisolone for the treatment of symptomatic hip osteoarthritis at short-term follow-up, but a persistence of this effect was observed at 1-year follow-up with the 80-mg dose but not the 40-mg dose (93). For the treatment of symptomatic knee osteoarthritis, evidence suggests no clinical benefit of 80 mg compared to 40 mg of triamcinolone at 6-month follow-up (94). Minimal literature is available to guide corticosteroid dose selection for ESIs, but a reasonable approach is outlined in **Table 53-5**. One study in the spine showed no differences in varying doses of dexamethasone from 4, 8, or 12 mg (95) for a lumbar transforaminal epidural injection, and another study showed no outcome benefit of using doses greater than 10 mg of triamcinolone (96). For lumbar interlaminar epidural injections, one study showed no benefit of 80 mg compared to 40 mg of methylprednisolone (97). This variability in the literature regarding dosing has not effectively resulted in a universally agreed

upon dosing strategy. Therefore, practitioners must consider additional factors such as previous steroid dosages and overall patient health when considering the dose for a given patient.

Even less literature exists on injection volume. For peripheral joints only, one study to date has compared injectate volumes. This study showed no clinical outcome differences at 3-month follow-up associated with a total injectate volume of 3 versus 9 mL that included 40 mg of triamcinolone for the treatment of symptomatic hip osteoarthritis (98). For epidural injections, studies have shown that larger-volume injections are associated with better outcomes (99,100). Given these limited data, a reasonable approach to volume for epidural injections is outlined in **Table 53-8**. For other injection targets, practitioners should be mindful of the anatomic considerations such as joint volume. For example, the sacroiliac joint typically only holds 2 mL of fluid; thus, larger-volume injections would clearly result in the medication spreading to adjacent tissues. This may be a desired result for therapeutic purposes, but it would add additional difficulty in determining the value of a positive diagnostic block. Similarly, MBBs are commonly done with 0.2 mL to avoid anesthetizing adjacent structures (101). This would be in contrast to caudal epidural or even soft tissue injections where larger volumes of 10 to 20 mL are common to reach the desired target tissue.

To achieve a given volume, corticosteroid can be injected in a preservative-free diluent such as lidocaine (1% to 2%) or normal saline, though addition of a local anesthetic does carry the risk of spinal block if unintentional subdural or subarachnoid injection is unrecognized prior to administration of the injectate. This is particularly relevant during cervical interlaminar ESIs where the epidural space is narrow and the risk of unintended subdural or subarachnoid deposition of injectate is highest.

Viscosupplements

Hyaluronic acid (HA) is an endogenous glycosaminoglycan that is located in various tissues throughout the body. HA is a large molecule and, thus, does not readily cross cell membranes. Among other location-specific properties in the human body, HA serves to attenuate loading and sheering forces on joints as a component of synovial fluid. Thus, exogenous HA has historically been used via intra-articular injection to "supplement" the native synovial fluid in patients with symptomatic knee osteoarthritis in order to decrease forces on a painful joint. In addition to immediately increasing the amount of intra-articular HA, introduction of exogenous HA may stimulate endogenous production of more HA by the synovium (102). Evidence also suggests that HA may have anti-inflammatory properties and may stimulate production of articular cartilage matrix molecules (103–105). There is evidence that while high

TABLE 53-8	**Dosage of Corticosteroids for Epidural Injections**				
		Interlaminar ESI (mg)	Transforaminal ESI (mg)	Caudal ESI (mg)
Lumbar	Methylprednisolone	40–80	10–80	40–80
	Triamcinolone	40–80	10–80	40–80
	Betamethasone	6–12	6–12	6–12
	Dexamethasone	4–15	4–15[a]	4–15

[a]Recommended as first-line medication choice to help decrease the risk of permanent neurologic compromise as further discussed in the "Adverse Events" section.
ESI, epidural steroid injection.

TABLE 53-9	High Molecular Weight Versus Low Molecular Weight Viscosupplements	
High Molecular Weight Viscosupplements (6 kD)	**Low Molecular Weight Viscosupplements**
Synvisc	**0.5–1.0 kD**
	Suplasyn
Synvisc-One	Polireumin/Hyalgan
	Fermathron
	Suprahyal/Adant
	>1.0–1.8 kD
	Durolane
	Orthovisc
	Osteonil/Ostenil
	Viscoseal

molecular weight HA has anti-inflammatory properties, low molecular weight HA may be proinflammatory (106,107). This discrepancy has become a source of interest to clinicians as both high molecular weight (6 kD) and low molecular weight (0.5 to 1.8 kD) HA preparations are commercially available as joint viscosupplements (**Table 53-9**).

In the most recent clinical practice guidelines, the American Academy of Orthopaedic Surgeons (AAOS) did not recommend the use of intra-articular hyaluronic acid injection for symptomatic knee osteoarthritis based on a meta-analysis of 14 studies that indicated statistically but not clinically significant improvement in knee pain and function (108). These findings were based mostly upon non–image-guided injections of the knee. Of note, subanalysis showed that most of the studies that demonstrated favorable outcomes used high molecular weight cross-linked hyaluronic acid agents, yet comparative differences between agents did not reach statistical significance. Shortcomings of the methods used in the AAOS meta-analysis have been highlighted (109); thus, this recommendation remains controversial. Also given the known miss rate of knee injections (110), combined with the fact the supplement does not readily cross the joint capsule, these recommendations may only apply to a non–image-guided injection.

IMAGE GUIDANCE

The following section addresses image guidance modalities that are commonly used for peripheral and spinal injections, as well as their relative advantages and disadvantages. The benefits of image guidance for injections in relation to safety and efficacy are also discussed (see Chapter 5 for a discussion of imaging techniques).

Ultrasound

The use of ultrasound guidance for both diagnostic and therapeutic injections has increased substantially in recent years as quality of this technology has improved (see Chapter 6). Adoption of this guidance modality for injections may also be related to certain advantages including lack of radiation exposure, ease of bedside use, and ability to directly visualize neurovascular structures during simultaneous needle movement in real time. A 2015 report by the American Medical Society for Sports Medicine (AMSSM) states that ultrasound-guided injections are more accurate than landmark-guided injections of "large, intermediate, and small joints, tendon sheaths, peritendinous regions, deep gluteal muscles, pes anserinus bursa, sinus tarsi, and inflamed joints." Mounting evidence suggests equivalent accuracy of ultrasound guidance and fluoroscopic guidance for some injections that have historically been performed under fluoroscopic-guidance, such as for intra-articular hip joint (**Fig. 53-1A**) and glenohumeral joint injections (**Fig. 53-1B**) (111,112).

Beyond injection accuracy, the AMSSM report also addresses relative clinical effectiveness. The report states that ultrasound-guided injections are associated with superior clinical effectiveness compared to landmark-guided injections of large joints, inflamed joints, the subacromial-subdeltoid bursa, the carpal tunnel, and the first dorsal wrist compartment tendon sheath (113). There has been inadequate comparison of ultrasound guidance to landmark guidance with regard to relative clinical effectiveness in small joints.

While ultrasound guidance is generally considered advantageous for peripheral injections, this modality may be less useful when an injection target is shrouded by bone. Ultrasound

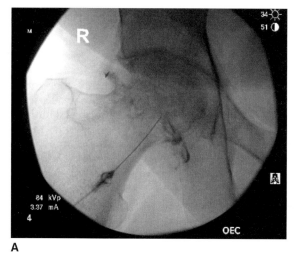

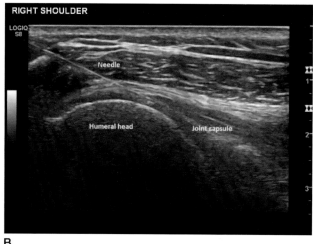

A   **B**

FIGURE 53-1.   **A:** Intra-articular hip injection using fluoroscopic guidance. **B:** Intra-articular glenohumeral joint injection using ultrasound guidance.

waves only reflect off of bone, and thus, the operator is unable to visualize tissue deep to osseous structures. For this reason, it is currently not standard of care to use ultrasound guidance for most spine injections when visualization of the needle position deep to axial bone structures is necessary to perform a safe and effective injection. For example, it is critical to visualize the needle tip immediately prior to injection of medication during a cervical TFESI in order to confidently avoid injection into a cervical radiculomedullary artery traversing through the neuroforamen or, furthermore, to avoid excessive needle advancement with possible direct cervical spinal cord trauma. Under ultrasound guidance, the needle tip cannot be adequately visualized through the bony confines of the axial cervical spine in relation to the cervical epidural space, and thus, a safe injection cannot be assured. With regard to certain diagnostic injections, ultrasound guidance alone may result in higher false-negative rates. Vascular trespass occurs in approximately 20% of medial branch nerve blocks when needle position is checked with the live injection of contrast dye viewed by digital subtraction angiography (114). In such cases, the needle can be repositioned until vascular flow is no longer visualized. If ultrasound guidance is used, without injection of contrast under live fluoroscopic guidance, nonvascular injection during medial branch nerve block for zygapophyseal joint anesthesia cannot be confirmed, and thus, a false-negative block may result. The utility of ultrasound may be further inhibited in obese patients where this modality may not offer sufficient visualization of the target tissues.

Fluoroscopy

Currently, fluoroscopic guidance is the standard of care for performing safe and effective spinal injections (24). Landmark guidance is associated with an unacceptably high rate of inaccurate injections and safety concerns (115,116), particularly with regard to ESIs. During a fluoroscopic-guided injection, the needle is advanced in a stepwise manner under serial imaging. Once the target of interest is reached, contrast agent is injected with the use of live fluoroscopy to confirm appropriate needle position at/in the structure. In the case of epidural injections, it is important to confirm epidural needle tip placement and lack of extradural, subdural, or subarachnoid placement prior to injection. In cases where vascular trespass is possible, contrast is injected and viewed in real time by live fluoroscopy to confirm a nonvascular flow pattern. Aspiration for "flashback" of blood is an inadequate safeguard for intravascular injection (13), as it has been shown to only be positive in approximately 40% of the cases that were shown to be vascular by live fluoroscopy.

Concerns exist regarding radiation exposure required during fluoroscopic-guided injections. However, studies have shown that the magnitude of radiation exposure during fluoroscopic-guided spine and appendicular injections is not clinically significant for a patient and represents a fraction of typical environmental exposure (117–120). Regardless, given that proceduralists are recurrently exposed, they should prevent any unnecessary radiation exposure to the patient, staff, and themselves by making specific adjustments to reduce radiation exposure (**Table 53-10**). Use of strategies to decrease radiation emission by the fluoroscopy unit as well as to decrease

TABLE 53-10	Strategies to Decrease Radiation Exposure to the Patient, Proceduralist, and Staff During Fluoroscopic-Guided Injections
Fluoroscopy unit adjustments to decrease emitted radiation	• Beam collimation • Automatic exposure control • Pulsed fluoroscopy • Use of "last image hold" function during needle advancement (decreases total images)
Barriers and distance to decrease exposure to emitted radiation	• Increase distance of patient from x-ray emitter side of C-arm (decrease distance of patient to the image intensifier) • Increase proceduralist and staff distance from the x-ray beam[a] • Lead barriers and table skirts • Personal shielding: lead aprons, thyroid shields, eyewear for the proceduralist and staff

[a]Dose of radiation exposure is inversely proportional to the distance squared; if the proceduralist moves from 1 to 3 ft away from the beam, his/her radiation exposure is decreased to one ninth of the original amount.

exposure to the emitted radiation has been demonstrated to decrease total radiation dose to the fluoroscopy suite staff by 97% (121).

Digital Subtraction Technology

Digital subtraction technology may be used in conjunction with live fluoroscopy. This technique involves first obtaining a static image (also known as a "mask" image) followed by injection of contrast agent. The original static image is "subtracted" from the imaging during contrast injection, such that the intensity/contrast of all static structures is minimized and the live contrast spread is highlighted (**Fig. 53-2**). This technique allows for improved detection of intravascular contrast flow by approximately 150% to 200% compared to live fluoroscopy alone during spine injections (114,122); this is particularly important for TFESIs, as discussed in the Adverse Events section of this chapter. While digital subtraction technology improves the sensitivity for detection of vascular injection, this assumes appropriate technique including visualization with lack of patient movement (breathing, swallowing, shifting, etc.) and adequate volume of contrast injection, as well as recognition by the proceduralist when vascular flow is present. As such, use of this technology does not inherently prevent vascular injection and subsequent consequences (123). Further, use of digital subtraction technology during TFESI procedures results in 200% to 400% greater radiation exposure to the patient compared to conventional live fluoroscopy (124). Therefore, judicious and not routine use of digital subtraction technology is currently recommended (77).

Computed Tomography

CT guidance may be used for injection guidance. CT guidance allows for direct visualization of deep neurovascular structures without the use of contrast media unlike other image guidance modalities. This technology has most

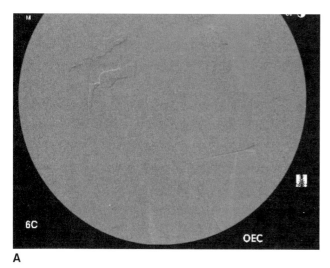

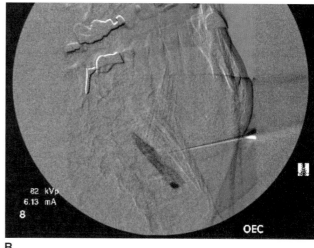

FIGURE 53-2. Precontrast digital subtraction technology "mask" image **(A)** is "subtracted" from live imaging during injection of contrast media **(B)**, which highlights the contrast spread and attenuates the visible background, during a left C5 selective nerve root block.

frequently been utilized during cervical TFESIs, where the vertebral artery can be directly visualized and avoided during needle advancement (**Fig. 53-3**). However, even with the use of a pulsed setting, it is associated with greater radiation exposure than conventional fluoroscopy by 800% to 1,900% during TFESI procedures (124). Use of CT guidance also results in longer procedure time compared with fluoroscopic-guided injection procedures (125,126). This technology is typically available to interventional radiologists, but rarely to other interventional specialists.

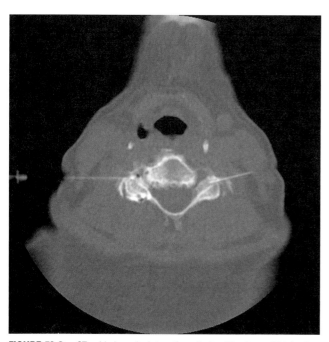

FIGURE 53-3. CT-guided cervical transforaminal epidural steroid injection. (Image courtesy of Vinil Shah, MD, University of California, San Francisco, Department of Radiology.)

SPECIAL CONSIDERATIONS

Below are common injections that warrant additional attention.

Epidural Steroid Injection

Background

Epidural steroid injections (ESIs) for the management of radicular pain provide the advantage of delivering potent anti-inflammatory agents in a localized fashion to the area of affected nerve roots, thereby decreasing the systemic side effects often seen with orally administered steroids. The primary indication for an ESI is radicular pain associated with a herniated nucleus pulposus or possibly spinal stenosis. A large variety of other indications have also been reported including radicular pain associated with lumbar spine compression fracture, facet or nerve root cysts, postlaminectomy back pain, cervical strain syndromes with associated myofascial pain, and postherpetic neuralgia. The outcomes in these disease conditions have been variable, and the overall evidence is poor for these conditions (127).

Optimal timing of ESIs is unknown, although there is evidence of better benefit if ESIs are performed within 3 months of radicular pain onset (127,128). The general consensus is that most patients with radicular symptoms should undergo a few weeks of treatment including oral medications and exercise-based therapy before undergoing ESIs (128). If a patient does not have success with such a program, or if the therapy cannot progress because the patient's pain is too severe, an ESI is indicated for pain control. ESIs may also be considered earlier in patients with severe radicular pain not responding to medication or with pain that is significantly interfering with a patient's sleep and/or function. Early ESIs also carry the theoretical benefit of controlling inflammation at an early stage and possibly preventing permanent neural damage such as nerve fibrosis from prolonged inflammation (129). The benefits of an early injection at disease prevention remain theoretical. However, as discussed in the General Considerations section, a full understanding of the natural history and available options is imperative. Although disk herniations tend to recur, they do have a favorable natural history. Therefore, short-term relief may be an acceptable outcome.

In general, it is felt that up to three to four ESIs within a year may be performed if clinically indicated. It is, however, unacceptable to proceed with a series of three ESIs, regardless of the clinical response to the first preceding injection(s). Evidence does show that the failure to obtain any relief with the first injection makes subsequent injections not likely to work also (72). Therefore, the standard is to assess the outcome from a given injection before proceeding with another injection. As detailed in the "Therapeutic Injections" section, the decision to proceed with any injection is based upon the response in context of the disease natural history, available treatment options, and risk/benefits of the procedure.

Fluoroscopic Guidance and Contrast

Fluoroscopic guidance with contrast dye is essential for accuracy and safety when performing ESIs (24). Published data show that even in experienced hands, epidural injections without fluoroscopic- and contrast-enhanced guidance (i.e., "blind injections") often result in inaccurate placement (8,10). These misplacements include the needle being inadvertently positioned into the subarachnoid, intravascular, or subcutaneous regions (caudal approach) or fascial plane superficial to the ligamentum flavum for interlaminar ESI. Misplacement into the subarachnoid or intravascular regions has major potential safety implications, particularly for those injections that include local anesthetics as part of the injectate. Use of detection of flash back of blood in the needle hub to gauge the intravascular placement of needle is not a reliable substitute for looking for a vascular pattern after contrast injection (130,131). Studies have also shown that accuracy increases efficacy. One such study demonstrated that fluoroscopic-guided transforaminal ESIs provided better pain relief than blind interlaminar ESIs (132). ESIs using fluoroscopic guidance have also been shown to reduce procedure-related complications compared to non–image-guided injections (127). As a result of these factors, it is recommended that ESIs be performed under fluoroscopic guidance and with radiographic contrast, documenting appropriate needle placement in order to improve their accuracy and, by extension, their safety and efficacy (24,77).

Evidence

Multiple high-quality studies, mostly involving the lumbar spine, have demonstrated efficacy of ESIs when performed on appropriate patients using image guidance and radiographic contrast (89,133,134). A recently published systematic review reveals up to 70% of patients achieve at least 50% relief of pain at 1 or 2 months after treatment, and about 30% achieve complete relief (127). By 12 months, the proportion of patients with continued relief decreases to 35% to 40%. Lumbar epidurals have also been shown to reduce the burden of disease by improving function (134–136) and reducing the need for surgery (137,138). In contrast to the lumbar spine, there are limited high-quality studies on efficacy of cervical epidurals. A recent systematic review suggests approximately 50% of patients experience 50% relief of radicular pain for at least 1 month following a cervical transforaminal epidural, though the available studies were of low quality (72).

Despite this robust literature, there are conflicting conclusions on the efficacy of ESIs. Some of these are due to methodologic flaws in the literature. Recurring flaws include failure to stratify by type of injection, failure to separate various underlying pathologies, failure to account for the use of image guidance, and even inappropriate follow-up time frames. Current data reveal that not all epidural approaches have equal efficacy (127,139–141) and should be evaluated as separate entities. Image guidance and radiographic contrast have been shown to result in improved efficacy and safety of epidurals (13,142). And injection at the level of pathology results in greater improvement compared to nonselective counterparts (129). Aside from technical considerations, response to ESIs has been shown to be related to several other factors such as the type and quantity of steroid preparation used, volume of injectate, underlying pathophysiology, and the duration of symptoms (127,129). Low-grade neural compression from intervertebral disk herniation appears to respond better than high-grade neural compression (133,143). There is greater evidence to suggest radicular pain induced by herniated nucleus pulposus appears to respond better to corticosteroid injection than that induced by spinal stenosis. A recently published randomized trial revealed no difference between epidural injection of glucocorticoids compared to anesthetic alone at 6 weeks, although at 3 weeks, the steroid group showed improved disability and intensity of leg pain compared to anesthetic alone (144). In lumbar spinal stenosis, the efficacy of ESI correlated with the degrees and the levels of stenosis categorized by MRI (129). ESIs provide better efficacy in reducing pain for patients with mild to moderate rather than severe stenosis. Patients with single-level lumbar spinal stenosis generally respond better than those with multilevel lumbar spinal stenosis.

Approaches

Cervical, thoracic, and lumbar epidural injections may be performed through interlaminar or transforaminal approaches. Lumbosacral epidurals may also be performed through a caudal approach. There is controversy over which technique provides the most effective delivery of medications with most evidence surrounding lumbar epidurals. Multiple studies and systematic reviews have attempted to show superiority of one technique over the other; however, there continues to be conflicting conclusions. Based on existing data, including a recently published systematic review comparing transforaminal versus interlaminar epidural injections, there are more studies that suggest superiority of transforaminal epidurals (127,139,140) over those only showing equivocal efficacy (132,145,146) with limited studies supporting interlaminar epidurals (147). Several studies suggest that the transforaminal approach is more effective compared to caudal or interlaminar approaches as they target the suspected spinal nerve in the neuroforaminal space (139). By placing medication in this area, there is increased likelihood of achieving ventral spread where radicular pain generators typically lie. Interlaminar injections, on the other hand, achieve ventral spread less frequently when performed at midline (115,148,149). Some recent studies suggest improved ventral flow with a parasagittal interlaminar approach (145).

Transforaminal Epidurals

Transforaminal epidurals are a more selective injection that theoretically targets a specific spinal nerve in the neuroforaminal space (**Fig. 53-4**). Careful attention should be undertaken

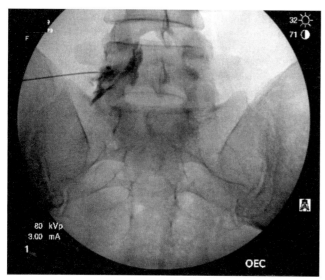

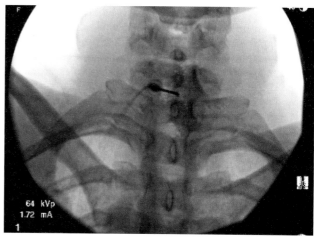

FIGURE 53-5. Epidural contrast pattern with "cobblestone" appearance during right paramedian C7-T1 interlaminar epidural steroid injection.

FIGURE 53-4. L5 neurogram with superomedial epidural contrast spread during left L5-S1 transforaminal epidural steroid injection.

to avoid vascular structures, particularly arterial vessels, which are more commonly encountered in transforaminal injections than with interlaminar injections. In the cervical spine, the vertebral artery enters deep to the transverse process at the sixth vertebrae or, occasionally, at the seventh vertebrae. The vertebral artery then runs through the transverse foramen of each vertebra, typically lying anterior to the ventral ramus (150). MRIs should be reviewed prior to injection to observe the vertebral artery course to avoid puncture. Radicular arteries are also of concern and may accompany nerve roots at all spinal levels. In the thoracolumbar spine, the artery of Adamkiewicz, the largest anterior segmental medullary artery, typically originates on the left side of the aorta between T8 and L1 vertebral levels, although may be present from T2 to L3 (151). If arterial injection is confirmed on contrast administration, the procedure should be terminated and resumed at a future encounter to allow the site of arterial puncture to heal.

Interlaminar Epidurals

Interlaminar epidurals target the posterior epidural space between the spinous processes in the midline (or paramedian) of two vertebrae through the ligamentum flavum through loss of resistance as the standard technique. While it is recommended that all epidurals be done under image guidance, some clinicians continue to perform interlaminar injections blindly using only loss of resistance as guidance of entry into the epidural space. Studies show, however, that false loss of resistance occurs frequently with one study quoting up to 53% (115). Loss of resistance is particularly difficult in degenerative conditions in which the dorsal epidural space is narrow or when a dense ligamentum flavum is absent. Given the potential to not actually place the medication in the epidural space (thus being ineffective), combined with the real possibility of a dural puncture or even direct spinal cord injection, cervical epidurals should be done with appropriate imaging guidance and utilization of a depth view. In general, cervical interlaminar injection should be performed at the C7-T1 level (**Fig. 53-5**)

or T1-2 level where the epidural space is typically more capacious (77). The anteroposterior depth of the epidural space cephalad to C7-T1 progressively diminishes, making dural puncture or even spinal cord puncture more likely (152). It is recommended to review the patient's MRI to evaluate the depth of epidural space prior to performing interlaminar injections. Lumbar spine injections can be done at any level after the safety of the proposed route is confirmed with CT or MRI scanning (24).

Caudal Epidurals

Caudal epidural is placed through the sacral hiatus (developmental absence of lamina resulting in a fissure at S5 and sometimes S4). Once through the sacral hiatus, the needle should be advanced approximately 1 to 2 cm into the caudal canal, and avoid advancing above the S3 level to prevent dural puncture. The caudal approach may be useful in patients who have previously undergone lumbar surgeries in which hardware or extensive scar tissue makes the lumbar approach difficult. A disadvantage to performing caudal injections is lack of control of where medications will flow. According to one study, epidural flow patterns in caudal injections include 68% bilaterally, 31% dorsally, 35% ventrally, and 34% dorsally and ventrally (153). Irrespective of the volume injected (10 vs. 50 cc), medication typically does not above the L3 vertebral level (154). To date, there is limited evidence to support superiority of caudal epidurals in comparison to transforaminal or interlaminar approaches.

Peripheral Joint Injection

Background

Injections into joints are common in outpatient musculoskeletal clinics. Specific techniques vary by joint, but similar planning and technical principles apply. As with all procedures, informed consent must be obtained with discussion of risks, benefits, and alternative treatments. When relevant, a discussion regarding continuation versus discontinuation of anticoagulation is necessary. Risk-versus-benefit analysis related to continuation of anticoagulation is described in the Adverse Events section; in nearly all cases of joint injection, continuation of anticoagulation is advised in the absence of a supratherapeutic INR or other comorbid bleeding diathesis.

The joint is usually injected from the extensor surface at a point where the synovium is closest to the skin. This site minimizes the interference from major neurovascular structures. When the ideal needle entry point has been determined, the tip of a retracted ballpoint pen or a needle hub may be used to create a temporary indentation. The skin is then prepared in a standard aseptic fashion over an area large enough to allow palpation of landmarks, and sterile technique is used throughout the procedure. While infection as a result of joint injection is rare (as discussed in the Adverse Events section), sterile technique is still recommended to minimize this possibility. The skin and subcutaneous tissue at the injection site may be anesthetized by injecting 1% lidocaine, using a 25- to 27- gauge needle. Alternatively, 5% lidocaine-prilocaine cream may be applied to the skin surface for 15 to 30 minutes prior to skin preparation, or a vapocoolant spray may be applied to the skin surface after preparation to provide adequate superficial anesthesia. A 1.5- to 3.5-in. 22- to 25-gauge needle is then advanced into the joint. Ultrasound or fluoroscopic guidance may be used depending on the regional anatomy of the specific joint. This consideration is discussed in the "Image Guidance" section. Local tissue and neurovascular trauma, as well as procedure-related pain, may be minimized by carefully directing the needle along a preplanned route, such that only one pass is necessary in ideal circumstances. This may represent another advantage of image guidance. Before injecting medication, aspiration should be performed to minimize the possibility of intravascular injection. After ensuring that the needle tip is located in the joint space, the medication is injected slowly, using constant pressure. The needle is then withdrawn, pressure is applied to minimize bleeding, and the puncture site is dressed. Specific technical considerations for intra-articular injections of the glenohumeral joint, hip joint, and knee joint are discussed below. Additionally, corticosteroid injections are discussed below, but other agents may be injected as detailed in the Medications section.

Indications for Intra-Articular Injection

Intra-articular injections may be used to diagnose the source of pain as articular or extra-articular. Aspiration of joint fluid with laboratory analysis may be helpful in determining the etiology of an intra-articular fluid collection; synovial fluid characteristics in various conditions are shown in **Table 53-11**. Intra-articular injections may also be used to provide an anti-inflammatory effect within the joint of interest when oral nonsteroidal anti-inflammatory drugs (NSAIDs) have failed to do so or are contraindicated. These injections are indicated to decrease morbidity in self-limited, sterile, inflammatory conditions. Joint injections may provide rapid relief of inflammatory pain and facilitate subsequent functional restoration; evidence suggests that joint pain results in inhibition of local muscle force output, particularly with regard to knee pain (155). Poorly controlled inflammation in more than three joints necessitates consideration of systemic anti-inflammatory agents.

Evidence

The evidence for clinical effectiveness of intra-articular injection depends on the underlying condition, the specific joint targeted, and the injectate. The majority of prospective studies of intra-articular steroid injections for the treatment of inflammatory conditions in major joints indicate effectiveness for moderate improvement in pain and function at short-term to intermediate follow-up duration (156–159). The evidence for clinical effectiveness in the treatment of joint pain is either limited or mixed when intra-articular hyaluronic acid is used. Intra-articular hyaluronic acid injection has been best studied for the indication of knee osteoarthritis; various systematic reviews have arrived at conflicting conclusions when recommending support versus avoidance of such injections (108,160). A detailed summary of this broad body of evidence is beyond the scope of the present chapter. However, further details related to the relative effectiveness of various injectable agents, as well as the influence of steroid type, dose, and total injectate volume, are discussed

TABLE 53-11	**Characteristics of Synovial Fluid in Various Conditions**				
			Inflammatory		
Characteristics	**Normal**	**Noninflammatory (e.g., osteoarthrosis, traumatic arthritis, osteochondritis dissecans, aseptic necrosis)**	**Group I rheumatoid arthritis (e.g., seropositive and seronegative spondyloarthritides)**	**Group II septic arthritis (e.g., bacterial infection tuberculosis)**	**Group III crystal synovitis (gout and pseudogout)**
Clarity	Transparent	Transparent	Transparent to opaque	Opaque, cloudy	Clear with flakes of fibrin
Color	Pale yellow	Yellow or straw	Yellow	Brown/green/yellow/gray	Yellow
Viscosity	High	High	Low	Very low (may be high with coagulase-positive *Staphylococcus*)	Low
WBC/mm³	<150	<3,000	3–50,000	50–300,000	3–50,000
Predominant cell	Mononuclear (<25% PMN)	Mononuclear (<25% PMN)	Neutrophil (>70% PMN)	Neutrophil (70%–100% PMN)	Neutrophil (>70% PMN)
Crystal	No	No	No	No	Yes
Culture	Negative	Negative	Negative	Often positive	Negative

in the Medications section. Evidence describing the utility versus lack of added value for image guidance is discussed in the "Image Guidance" section.

Technical Considerations of Common Major Joint Injections

Glenohumeral Joint

Technique

Multiple approaches to glenohumeral joint access are possible. When image guidance is not used, the posterior approach is used most commonly, although this technique has a demonstrated poor level of accuracy. After informed consent is obtained, the patient is placed in a seated position, with the humerus internally rotated. A needle trajectory into the glenohumeral joint capsule is defined by marking the skin two fingerbreadths inferior to the posterior angle of the acromion with a needle angled in an anteromedial direction toward the coracoid process (also identified by palpation). The patient is prepared in a standard aseptic fashion over an area large enough to allow palpation of landmarks, and sterile technique is used throughout the procedure. Needle gauge and length selection depends on the body habitus of the patient, but generally ranges from a 22- to 25-gauge, 1.5- to 2.5-in. needle. After optional use of vapocoolant spray or skin/superficial soft tissue local anesthetic administration, the needle is advanced along the planned trajectory, so as to avoid the neurovascular structures of the axilla that are located inferomedial to the ideal plane of needle advancement. The needle is gently advanced through the joint capsule, which can typically be appreciated by passage through a tough layer of tissue followed by a firm osseous endpoint (periosteum of the humeral head). Upon touch onto the humeral head, the needle tip is withdrawn 1 to 2 mm in order to avoid intraosseous injection and unnecessary pain. Aspiration is performed. If there is an effusion of the joint, aspiration should be completed and the fluid sent for laboratory analysis if clinically warranted. After negative aspiration, or if the aspirate is noninflammatory (clear and viscous), medication is administered. Considerations of medication type, dose, and volume selection are discussed in the Medications section. Typically, a 4- to 5-mL total injectate volume is used, with consideration of maximizing volume in the case of adhesive capsulitis in order to provide stretch/expansion to the joint capsule.

Comments

Fluoroscopic or ultrasound guidance is associated with superior injection accuracy compared to a blind approach, though superiority of clinical outcomes is unclear. Nonetheless, if diagnosis is in question, there is a clear advantage to the use of image guidance to confirm an intra-articular injectate. Further, image guidance allows avoidance of trauma to the articular cartilage by performing a more lateral injection on the humeral head, whereas trauma to the articular cartilage may be unavoidable in some cases using the blind-posterior technique as described above. If ultrasound guidance is used, a 3.5-in. spinal needle is typically used, as a more lateral entry point is generally necessary (greater tissue distance) to pass and visualize the needle deep to the ultrasound probe and into the joint capsule. Fluoroscopic guidance remains another alternative for confirmation of intra-articular injection given the ability to inject contrast agent until a positive arthrogram is visualized prior to injection of diagnostic/therapeutic agent(s).

If the indication for glenohumeral joint injection is adhesive capsulitis, it is generally helpful to plan for more aggressive range-of-motion and other physical therapy interventions during the window of greater treatment effect associated with the steroid injection (approximately 2 to 8 weeks). Intravascular injection and subsequent hematoma are possible, owing to the close proximity of the axillary vessels. If an arterial puncture occurs, prolonged direct pressure is usually adequate to prevent the development of a hematoma.

Hip Joint

Techniques

Image guidance is necessary to perform a safe and effective intra-articular hip joint injection as the rates of extracapsular injection and neurovascular trauma associated with a blind approach are unacceptably high (161,162). Considerations of ultrasound versus fluoroscopy for needle guidance are addressed in the "Image Guidance" section. After informed consent is obtained, the patient is placed in the supine position with the hip and knee joints extended and externally rotated. The femoral pulse in the inguinal crease is palpated and marked. The position of needle entry is selected after visualization with ultrasound or fluoroscopy to plan the appropriate trajectory from lateral to medial with a goal of needle tip position near the femoral head-neck junction; this position allows needle tip placement within the joint capsule without trauma to the articular cartilage or passage through the femoral neurovascular bundle located more medially. While individual anatomy is variable, the landmark of needle entry is typical located 2 cm inferior to the anterosuperior iliac spine (ASIS) and 3 cm lateral to the palpated femoral pulse at the level of the superior aspect of the greater trochanter. The patient is prepared in a standard aseptic fashion over an area large enough to allow palpation of landmarks, and sterile technique is used throughout the procedure. After injection of local anesthetic (typically 1% lidocaine) into the skin and soft tissue along the planned path of primary needle introduction, a 3.5-in. 22- to 25-gauge spinal needle is advanced in a posteromedial direction toward the femoral head-neck junction under ultrasound or fluoroscopic guidance. If ultrasound guidance is used, serial small-volume injections of local anesthetic or saline may be necessary to confirm needle tip position, as the spinal needle may appear less hyperechogenic during hip injection compared to injection of more superficial joints. This is a result of the steep needle angle that may be necessary to reach the deep hip joint; the needle appears most hyperechogenic under ultrasound visualization when advanced in parallel to the face of the probe, as ultrasound waves reflect perpendicular to the metal surface of the needle and are only detected if they return to the face of the probe. With steeper needle angles, fewer ultrasound waves are reflected back to the probe, and thus, the needle structure is more challenging to visualize. The needle is gently advanced through the joint capsule, which can typically be appreciated by passage through a tough layer of tissue followed by a firm osseous endpoint (periosteum of the femoral head/neck). Aspiration is then performed. If there is an effusion of the joint, the aspiration should be completed and the fluid sent for laboratory analysis if clinically warranted. If the aspirate is noninflammatory (clear and viscous), medication may be administered with observable flow into the joint evidenced by hyperechogenic signal below the capsule. Considerations of medication type, dose, and volume selection are discussed in the Medications section.

Comments

For intra-articular hip joint injections, there is no definitive advantage of one guidance technique compared to the other. However, as with other intra-articular joint injections, fluoroscopic guidance remains the gold standard for accuracy of placement within the joint capsule due to the ability to obtain an arthrogram using contrast agent prior to injection of diagnostic/therapeutic agent(s). Nevertheless, ultrasound guidance has the advantage of no radiation exposure and ability to perform procedure in a clinic setting as opposed to a surgical/fluoroscopy suite. Fluoroscopy has an advantage for visualization of target tissues in obese patients. Avascular necrosis of the hip has been reported as a result of repeated intra-articular injection of corticosteroids. Hematoma and intravascular injection are possible, owing to the close proximity of the femoral vessels. If an arterial puncture occurs, prolonged direct pressure is usually adequate to prevent the development of a hematoma.

Knee Joint

Techniques

A variety of approaches for intra-articular knee injection are possible, including approaches via the superolateral, superomedial, inferomedial, and inferolateral patellar recesses, as well as the lateral midpatellar approach; other less commonly performed techniques have also been described. The superolateral patellar recess approach is described here because this approach also facilitates in-plane ultrasound visualization of the needle during advancement and injection. After informed consent is obtained, the patient is placed in a supine position with the knee flexed to approximately 15 degrees. The patella is palpated in order to locate the superolateral angle. A site approximately 1 cm superior and 1 cm lateral to the ankle of the patella is marked for needle entry. The patient is prepared in a standard aseptic fashion over an area large enough to allow palpation of landmarks, and sterile technique is used throughout the procedure. As with all injections, needle gauge and length selection depends on the body habitus of the patient, but for intra-articular knee injection, needle gauge generally ranges between 22 and 25 gauge and length ranges between 1.5 and 2.0 in. After optional use of vapocoolant spray or skin/superficial soft tissue local anesthetic administration, the needle is advanced along a trajectory deep to the patella toward the intercondylar notch as shown (**Fig. 53-6**). Retracting the patella toward the needle in a lateral or superolateral direction may be helpful to allow the needle to pass under the patellar and into the knee joint without first encountering painful periosteum. If ultrasound guidance is used, similar technique may be applied, but with the needle insertion site planning based on visualization of the suprapatellar bursa using a short-axis view in relation to the quadriceps tendon. The needle is then advanced in parallel to the face of the ultrasound probe (in-plane) for direct visualization. If fluoroscopic guidance is used, the same principles apply, but site selection may be influenced by the bony anatomic variations of each individual patient. Regardless of a blind or image-guided approach, once the needle tip is believed to be located inside the joint capsule,

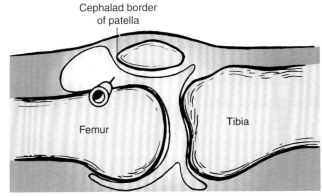

FIGURE 53-6. Knee joint injection. Medial approach to suprapatellar pouch for knee joint aspiration and injection. Note the connection between the suprapatellar pouch and main synovial cavity. (Reprinted with permission from Gatter RA. Arthrocentesis technique and intrasynovial therapy. In: Koopman WJ, ed. *Arthritis and Allied Conditions: A Textbook of Rheumatology.* 13th ed. Baltimore, MD: Lippincott Williams & Wilkins; 1997:752.)

aspiration is performed. If there is an effusion of the joint, the aspiration should be completed and the fluid sent for laboratory analysis if clinically warranted. After negative aspiration, or if the aspirate is noninflammatory (clear and viscous), medication is administered in the case of blind or ultrasound-guided injection. In the case of fluoroscopic guidance, contrast medium is first injected to confirm a positive arthrogram. Considerations of medication type, dose, and volume selection are discussed in the Medications section. Typically, a 5-mL total injectate volume is used.

Comments

As with glenohumeral joint injections, studies have shown mixed results with regard to superior clinical effectiveness when image guidance is used during intra-articular knee injections. However, if confirmation of intra-articular injection is desired, particularly when the purpose of the injection is at least in part diagnostic, image guidance is highly recommended (12). As with the joint injections discussed above, fluoroscopy remains the gold standard for confirmation of true intra-articular needle tip position given the ability to visualize an arthrogram immediately prior to injection of diagnostic/therapeutic agent(s). Image guidance may also allow avoidance of injection into Hoffa's fat pad during inferomedial, inferolateral, or lateral midpatellar approaches, which is possible if the needle remains superficial to the joint capsule and may cause steroid-related atrophy of this fat pad. Corticosteroid injection into the knee joint may impair epiphyseal growth in children, resulting in a significant leg length discrepancy.

Zygapophyseal Joint Injection/Radiofrequency Neurotomy

Background

The prevalence of lumbar zygapophyseal joint (Z-joint) pain has been reported to range from 6% in a primary care setting up to 40% in older populations in pain clinics (163,164). In individuals with chronic neck pain after a whiplash injury, Z-joint pain occurred in approximately 50% of patients (165). More recent literature examining 500 patients has reported a prevalence of 55% cervical facet joint pain, 42% thoracic facet joint pain, and 31% lumbar Z-joint pain in patients with *chronic* spine pain as identified with a double-block model (166). Lumbar facet joint pain has been reported in 16% of patients with *chronic postsurgical* lumbar spine pain (163). Studies of a larger population using a dual anesthetic block paradigm may be helpful in further identifying the prevalence in the general population for both acute and chronic low back pain.

Anatomy

Z-joints are pairs of small synovial joints in the posterior aspect of the spine, formed when the inferior articular process of one vertebra articulates with the superior articular process of the subjacent vertebra. The Z-joint at C2-3 is innervated by the third occipital nerve. For C3-7, each Z-joint is innervated by the medial branches of the corresponding joint (e.g., C3-4 zygapophyseal is innervated by C3 and C4 medial branches). The joints between C0-1 (atlanto-occipital) and C1-2 (atlantoaxial) joints are technically not Z-joints. They are innervated by the ventral rami of C1 and C2, respectively (150). In the thoracic and lumbar spine, the Z-joints are innervated by the medial branch from the level above and from the corresponding level (e.g., T3-4 Z-joint is innervated by the T2 and T3 medial branches; L4-5 Z-joint is innervated by the L3 and L4 medial branches). The exception is L5-S1, which is innervated by the L4 medial branch and the L5 dorsal primary ramus (150). Significant variability in the location of medial branches has been reported, particularly in the thoracic spine (167,168), which poses a challenge when performing and evaluating efficacy of diagnostic MBBs in the thoracic spine.

Pathophysiology of Z-Joint Pain

Zygapophyseal joint pain often derives from pathologic mechanical stress, inflammation, microtrauma, or osteoarthritis. There are no pathognomonic history or physical exam findings that reliably predict Z-joint pain (23,169). Imaging studies are also unable to confirm or refute the diagnosis of Z-joint pain (170). Given the lack of a clinical diagnostic gold standard, clinicians have used regional anesthesia to identify Z-joint pain. Abolishment of pain after anesthetic Z-joint injection or MBB confirms the Z-joint as the pain generator Z-joint injection is indicated in patients with acute or chronic back and neck pain of suspected Z-joint origin, with no evidence of neurologic deficits. However, since the majority of acute back and neck pain, including Z-joint pain, will resolve in several weeks, the injection is often reserved for individuals with severe pain that has failed to respond to 4 to 6 weeks of conservative therapy including oral analgesics, directed exercise-based therapy, and relative rest. Injection can be performed earlier if pain is inhibiting therapy progress.

Evidence

Intra-Articular Zygapophyseal Injection

The evidence for the therapeutic benefit of corticosteroids into the zygapophyseal joint injection remains controversial. While some uncontrolled studies have shown therapeutic efficacy (171), controlled studies have failed to demonstrate such efficacy (172–174). However, all of these studies had flaws in patient selection, thus limiting the ability to interpret the results. Therefore, there may still be a role for corticosteroid injections into the Z-joints, although likely only in a subset of patients with confirmed radiologic findings of active Z-joint inflammation (175,176).

Medial Branch Blocks

Medial branch blocks (MBBs) are considered the primary means of diagnosing zygapophyseal joint mediated pain. Since the degree of pain relief is a patient's subjective response, Z-joint injection or medial branch blockade is susceptible to false positives. Research has shown false-positive rates of 27% to 38% for lumbar blocks, 27% to 63% for cervical blocks, 55% for thoracic blocks, and a 32% placebo effect (20,165,169). To minimize false-positive rates, a double-block paradigm was proposed using two local anesthetics with different durations of action, one on each of two separate occasions (24). If each of the two injections relieves pain for the duration expected for the anesthetic used, Z-joint pain can be more reliably diagnosed. Published studies have validated this dual blockade paradigm, using comparative local anesthetics for MBBs to anesthetize Z-joints (177,178). Diagnostic blocks are therefore used as a precursor to help predict which patients will respond or not respond to a RFN.

Radiofrequency Neurotomy

Radiofrequency neurotomy (RFN) interrupts the nociceptive afferent from the Z-joint by thermally coagulating the two medial branches that innervate a given Z-joint. RFN can provide relative long-term benefit symptoms from persistent or recurrent Z-joint pain despite conservative care in a carefully selected subset of patients. One prospective study has demonstrated good efficacy from the procedures when patients with presumed Z-joint pain are selected using the double-block paradigm with comparative local anesthetic (179). The patients were diagnosed with lumbar Z-joint pain if they obtained at least 80% pain reduction after MBBs with 0.5 mL of 2% lidocaine on one occasion and 0.5% bupivacaine on another. At 12 months following the radiofrequency medial branch neurotomy, 60% of patients achieved at least 90% pain reduction and 87% of patients had 60% pain relief. Nerve regeneration may result in recurrence of pain though repeat RFN has been shown to be effective (180). Efficacy of RFN for cervical Z-joint pain (other than from the C2-3 joint that was excluded from this study) has also been demonstrated in a randomized, double-blinded, and placebo-controlled trial (22). A recently published systematic review on the effectiveness of fluoroscopically guided cervical medial branch RFN using a rigorous primary outcome of 100% pain relief showed 63% were pain free at 6 months and 38% were pain free at 1 year (181).

Sacroiliac Joint Injection

Background

The sacroiliac (SI) joint can be a significant source of low back pain (182–185). The SI joint is a true diarthrodial joint and with reported innervation by nerves from the L4 through S4 levels (150). Etiologies of SI pain include spondyloarthropathy, crystal arthropathy, septic arthritis, trauma, pregnancy, and abdominal diathesis. In addition, SI joint dysfunction (pain from a biomechanical disorder without a demonstrable lesion) has been proposed as a possible etiology of SI pain. The value of clinical data from history and physical examination in the diagnosis of SI joint pain remains controversial (186–188). Although SI joint pain frequently manifests as pain in the sacral sulcus areas, SI joint pain can refer to the buttock, lower lumbar region, groin, and lower limb (187). However, none of these symptoms, signs, or various provocative tests are pathognomonic for SI joint pain. Other sources of low back pain, such as lower lumbar Z-joint arthropathy or degenerative disk disease, can present similarly. This vague symptomology, combined with inaccuracy of blind and even ultrasound-guided injections for SI joint specifically (189,190), has made fluoroscopically guided SI joint blocks the most reliable available to diagnose those with suspected SI pain (24).

Among patients with chronic low back pain, a study using a single-block technique of the SI joint with a local anesthetic estimated the prevalence of SI joint pain as between 13% and 30% (191). A study on 54 patients with unilateral low back pain suspected from the SI joint, using a dual local anesthetic block technique, demonstrated an 18.5% prevalence of SI joint-based pain (192). Prevalence may be higher in the elderly (164) or lumbar fusion patients (192–194). Other studies show, however, that reproduced pain in at least three provocation exam maneuvers increases sensitivity and specificity of response to diagnostic injections (184,195,196). Diagnostic imaging, in the absence of sacroiliitis or trauma, has also been shown to have limited correlation with SI joint pain (17).

Evidence

The efficacy of SI joint corticosteroid injections has been reported in prospective and retrospective studies of patients with spondyloarthropathy (184,197). In a retrospective study, Slipman et al. reported a significant benefit from SI joint steroid injection in patients with SI joint syndrome (191). Thirty-one patients with chronic SI joint syndrome received an average of 2.1 fluoroscopic-guided SI joint corticosteroid injections. The average follow-up was 94.4 weeks. Of the 29 patients who completed the study, there was a significant improvement in the Oswestry Disability Score, VAS, and work status. This study was based off of a single anesthetic block. No studies to date have selected patients based on complete relief after dual comparative blocks using anesthetic only (184). Overall, there is only moderate evidence in support of therapeutic sacroiliac joint injections due to limited randomized controlled studies (184).

RFN has recently been proposed as a potential long-lasting treatment for SI joint pain and has been gaining more popularity along with other nonsurgical spinal procedures. RFN involves deinnervation of the SI joint nerves believed to be responsible for generating pain (198). It may be indicated as a treatment option for those patients who have failed more conservative measures, yet only received transient benefit from diagnostic and/or therapeutic injections of the SI joint (185). The true effectiveness of RFN of the SI joint is unclear, as of yet (185). In contrast to RFN in treating lumbar spine facet-mediated pain, which directly targets the medial branches of the dorsal rami, which innervate the facet joints (199), the SI joint has complex innervations (200). Therefore, no consistent procedural technique has been described in the literature. Multiple studies have, in fact, been done using various techniques for RFN of the SI joint all with variable outcomes (185). This underscores the fact that there is no standard pattern of ablation, and not enough available prospective data to determine which rami or branches should be

ablated, or if a specific technique is more efficacious. The studies do not show uniformity and additional studies to determine if RFN is useful for treating chronic SI joint pain are warranted.

Trigger Point Injection

Background

Trigger points may occur in any muscle or muscle group of the body. They are common in all muscles and have been found in 80% to 90% of the lower limbs in asymptomatic college students. This is further confounded by very poor inter- and intrarater reliability in detecting trigger points (201). This has led to some even questioning their existence and the utility of treatments targeting them (202). Additionally, the pathophysiology of a trigger point has not been well defined, but some investigators have proposed that trigger points are caused by abnormal endplate potentials that lead to greater or more frequent release of acetylcholine into the neuromuscular junction (203). Active trigger points are associated with higher concentrations of neurotransmitters and neuropeptides that are known to mediate pain signaling (204).

Trigger points are characterized by pain originating from small, circumscribed areas of local hyperirritability involving myofascial structures, resulting in local and referred pain. The most common definition is described by Simons and Travell as "a hyperirritable spot in skeletal muscle that is associated with a hypersensitive palpable nodule in a taut band" (205). Active trigger points are distinguished from "latent" trigger points by the presence of referred pain in addition to local pain without palpation; latent trigger points do not produce spontaneous pain and often do not cause referral of pain beyond a local tender spot (206). Characteristic pain referral patterns for many specific muscles/muscle complexes have been described (205). Trigger points may be associated with altered regional biomechanics (207), though it is unclear if the trigger point itself causes this or if the trigger point develops as a result of such changes.

Trigger points are best localized by deep palpation of the affected muscle, which reproduces the patient's typical local and referred pain. Passive or active stretching of the affected muscle may also provoke symptoms. Trigger point regions are often associated with "taut bands" of muscle tissue. The muscle in the immediate vicinity of the trigger point is often described as "ropey" or "tense." Since the interrater agreement of defining trigger points has been demonstrated as poor (208), it does cast further doubt into the exact definition and prevalence of the condition.

Evidence

The evidence for clinical effectiveness of trigger point injections is limited by heterogeneity of the definition of a trigger point (as alluded to above), heterogeneity of trigger point injection techniques, and lack of multiple high-quality studies for each specific treatment indication. However, systematic reviews do indicate that trigger point injections are associated with improved pain and disability for certain headache disorders, whiplash injury, as well as chronic neck, shoulder, and back pain (209,210). Collectively, the data typically fail to demonstrate evidence of a clinically detectable change when trigger point injections are compared to any other treatment. Further work is needed to better define optimal patient selection, needle technique and treatment protocol, as well as frequency of use, type, and volume of medications in the injectate. These injections also represent the largest source of lawsuits among interventional procedures, although this is more likely due to the large number of these procedures that are done annually rather than the safety profile of the procedure.

Technical Considerations

There is no evidence-based ideal technique for performing trigger point injections. Many providers follow the guidance provided by Simons and Travell (205), but various alternative techniques have not been compared in a head-to-head manner to determine relative safety and clinical effectiveness. The below description represents a common general technique that may be used based on the experience of the authors.

When treating an area of interest, palpation is used to identify trigger points according to the description above, and these sites are marked. This may be best achieved with the tip of a retracted ballpoint pen or needle hub in order to create a temporary indentation to mark the point of planned needle entry. The patient is prepared in a standard aseptic fashion over an area large enough to allow palpation of landmarks, and sterile technique is used throughout the procedure. Use of sterile gloves is required so that muscle in the sterile field may be palpated throughout the procedure. The skin and subcutaneous tissue at the injection site are usually not anesthetized.

Before the injection, the trigger point is repalpated and stabilized between the thumb and index finger for injection (**Fig. 53-7**). A 1.5- to 2.5-in., 22- to 27-gauge needle (depending on muscle depth) is advanced into the muscle at the point of maximum tenderness. Before injecting medication, aspiration should be performed to minimize the possibility of intravascular injection. If blood is aspirated, the needle should be repositioned. Presence of the "jump sign" (i.e., muscle twitch) or reproduction of typical pain may suggest that the needle has been successfully placed within the trigger point, though these signs are nonspecific. In cases where trigger points are located in close proximity to structures that must be avoided (e.g., rhomboid muscle overlaying the lung), ultrasound guidance may be useful to improve the safety of the procedure. Medication may be injected in a fanwise manner throughout the area of the trigger point (**Fig. 53-8**). Commonly, 1% lidocaine or 0.25% bupivacaine is injected without steroid, as there is insufficient evidence to suggest that steroid

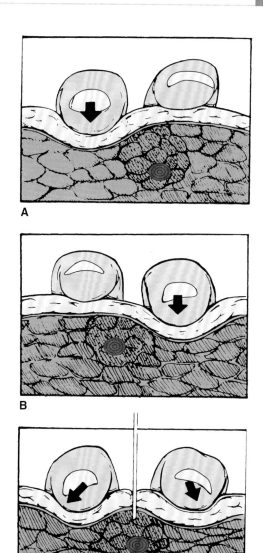

A

B

C

FIGURE 53-7. Trigger point palpation. **A and B:** Palpation and localization of trigger point by rolling beneath two fingers (*arrows*). **C:** Stabilization of trigger point for injection by spanning with two fingers (*arrows*). (Reprinted from Raj PP. Chronic pain. In: Raj PP, ed. *Clinical Practice of Regional Anesthesia.* 2nd ed. New York, NY; 1991:491. Copyright © 1991 Elsevier. With permission.)

FIGURE 53-8. Fanwise injection technique for trigger point. (Reprinted from Raj PP. Chronic pain. In: Raj PP, ed. *Clinical Practice of Regional Anesthesia.* 2nd ed. New York, NY; 1991:491. Copyright © 1991 Elsevier. With permission.)

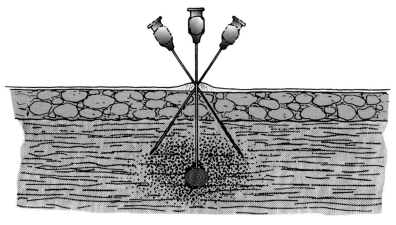

provides additional therapeutic benefit and can cause muscle atrophy. The needle is then withdrawn, pressure is applied to minimize bleeding, and the puncture site is dressed.

Comments

Adverse events associated with trigger point injections may occur depending on the specific treatment region. When performed in muscles overlaying the thorax, such as the rhomboids, serratus anterior, or lower trapezius, pneumothorax is possible. Intraneural injection is possible if injections are performed in regions where large nerves course in close proximity to muscles that may commonly be treated with trigger point injections, such as the anterior scalene or sternocleidomastoid muscles; ultrasound guidance is highly recommended when performing trigger point injections in such areas.

SUMMARY

Overall, injections can be a powerful tool in the diagnosis and treatment for a variety of musculoskeletal and spine conditions. However, they clearly do not work for every condition, and a thorough risk-versus-benefit discussion must be had before performing an injection. In order to maximize the likelihood of a safe and successful outcome from an injection, practitioners must have a full understanding of appropriate patient selection, indications/contraindications, pharmacology, risks, benefits, and numerous procedure-specific technical details, as well as a general understanding of the limitations and role of diagnostic and therapeutic nature of these procedures. It is only with this comprehensive understanding that these injections should be implemented.

REFERENCES

1. MacKay C, Canizares M, Davis AM, et al. Health care utilization for musculoskeletal disorders. *Arthritis Care Res.* 2010;62:161–169.
2. Freburger JK, et al. The rising prevalence of chronic low back pain. *Arch Intern Med.* 2009;169:251.
3. Weinstein SL. 2000-2010: the bone and joint decade. *J Bone Joint Surg Am.* 2000;82(1):1–3. Available from: https://www.ncbi.nlm.nih.gov/pubmed/10653078. Accessed July 13, 2017.
4. Kennedy DJ, Fredericson M. It is the most common form of arthritis and the leading cause of disability in older persons, affecting an estimated 27 million adults in the United States alone. Introduction. *PM R.* 2012;4:S1–S2.
5. Hollander JL. Hydrocortisone and cortisone injected into arthritic joints: comparative effects of and use of hydrocortisone as a local antiarthritic agent. *J Am Med Assoc.* 1951;147:1629.
6. Engel AJ, Bogduk N. Mathematical validation and credibility of diagnostic blocks for spinal pain. *Pain Med.* 2016;17(10):1821–1828. Available from: https://www.ncbi.nlm.nih.gov/pubmed/26995797. Accessed July 8, 2017.
7. Bisbinas I, Belthur M, Said HG, et al. Accuracy of needle placement in ACJ injections. *Knee Surg Sports Traumatol Arthrosc.* 2006;14:762–765.
8. Bartynski WS, Grahovac SZ, Rothfus WE. Incorrect needle position during lumbar epidural steroid administration: inaccuracy of loss of air pressure resistance and requirement of fluoroscopy and epidurography during needle insertion. *Am J Neuroradiol.* 2005;26:502–505.
9. Daley EL, Bajaj S, Bisson LJ, et al. Improving injection accuracy of the elbow, knee, and shoulder: does injection site and imaging make a difference? A systematic review. *Am J Sports Med.* 2011;39:656–662. doi:10.1177/0363546510390610.
10. Stitz MY, Sommer HM. Accuracy of blind versus fluoroscopically guided caudal epidural injection. *Spine.* 1999;24:1371–1376.
11. Yamakado K. The targeting accuracy of subacromial injection to the shoulder: an arthrographic evaluation. *Arthroscopy.* 2002;18:887–891.
12. Mattie R, Kennedy DJ. Importance of image guidance in glenohumeral joint injections: comparing rates of needle accuracy based on approach and physician level of training. *Am J Phys Med Rehabil.* 2016;95:57–61.
13. Sullivan WJ, et al. Incidence of intravascular uptake in lumbar spinal injection procedures. *Spine.* 2000;25:481–486.
14. Kaplan M, Dreyfuss P, Halbrook B, et al. The ability of lumbar medial branch blocks to anesthetize the zygapophysial joint. A physiologic challenge. *Spine.* 1998;23:1847–1852.
15. Finnoff JT, Hurdle MF, Smith J. Accuracy of ultrasound-guided versus fluoroscopically guided contrast-controlled piriformis injections: a cadaveric study. *J Ultrasound Med.* 2008;27:1157–1163.
16. Schwarzer AC, Aprill CN, Bogduk N. The sacroiliac joint in chronic low back pain. *Spine.* 1995;20:31–37.
17. Kennedy DJ, Shokat M, Visco CJ. Sacroiliac joint and lumbar zygapophysial joint corticosteroid injections. *Phys Med Rehabil Clin N Am.* 2010;21:835–842.
18. Bergman AG, Fredericson M. Shoulder MRI after impingement test injection. *Skeletal Radiol.* 1998;27:365–368.
19. Dreyfuss P, Schwarzer AC, Lau P, et al. Specificity of lumbar medial branch and L5 dorsal ramus blocks. A computed tomography study. *Spine.* 1997;22:895–902.
20. Fritzler A, Serafini M. Placebo response to interventional pain procedures and effect on patient outcome. *Tech Reg Anesth Pain Manag.* 2011;15:20–27.
21. Schwarzer AC, et al. The false-positive rate of uncontrolled diagnostic blocks of the lumbar zygapophysial joints. *Pain.* 1994;58:195–200.
22. Lord SM, Barnsley L, Wallis BJ, et al. Percutaneous radio-frequency neurotomy for chronic cervical zygapophyseal-joint pain. *N Engl J Med.* 1996;335:1721–1726.
23. Bogduk N, Dreyfuss P, Govind J. A narrative review of lumbar medial branch neurotomy for the treatment of back pain. *Pain Med.* 2009;10:1035–1045.
24. International Spine Intervention Society—2014. 22nd Annual scientific meeting research abstracts. *Pain Med.* 2014;15:1436–1446.
25. Chou R, et al. Interventional therapies, surgery, and interdisciplinary rehabilitation for low back pain: an evidence-based clinical practice guideline from the American Pain Society. *Spine.* 2009;34:1066–1077.
26. Kennedy DJ, Plastaras CT, Pingree MJ, et al. Delayed complications in interventional pain procedures: a multi-institutional study. *Pain Med.* 2014;15:1436–1446.
27. Kennedy DJ, et al. Vasovagal rates in fluoroscopically guided interventional procedures: a study of over 8,000 injections. *Spine J.* 2013;13:S23–S24.
28. Plastaras C, et al. Adverse events associated with fluoroscopically guided lumbosacral transforaminal epidural steroid injections. *Spine J.* 2015;15:2157–2165.
29. Kennedy DJ, et al. Vasovagal rates in fluoroscopically guided interventional procedures: a study of over 8,000 injections. *Pain Med.* 2013;14:1854–1859.
30. Plastaras C, McCormick Z, Macron D, et al. Adverse events associated with fluoroscopically guided zygapophyseal joint injections. *Pain Physician.* 2014;17(4):297–304. Available from: https://www-ncbi-nlm-nih-gov.laneproxy.stanford.edu/pubmed/25054389. Accessed July 18, 2017.
31. Plastaras CT, et al. Adverse events associated with fluoroscopically guided sacroiliac joint injections. *PM R.* 2012;4:473–478.
32. Sheldon RS, et al. 2015 heart rhythm society expert consensus statement on the diagnosis and treatment of postural tachycardia syndrome, inappropriate sinus tachycardia, and vasovagal syncope. *Heart Rhythm.* 2015;12:e41–e63.
33. Manchikanti L, Malla Y, Wargo BW. Complications of fluoroscopically directed facet joint nerve blocks: a prospective evaluation of 7,500 episodes with 43,000 nerve blocks. *Pain Physician.* 2012;15(2):E143–E150. Available from: https://www-ncbi-nlm-nih-gov.laneproxy.stanford.edu/pubmed/?term=Complications+of+fluoroscopically+directed+facet+joint+nerve+blocks%3A+a+prospective+evaluation+of+7%2C500+episodes+with+43%2C000+nerve+blocks. Accessed July 18, 2017.
34. Manchikanti L, et al. A prospective evaluation of complications of 10,000 fluoroscopically directed epidural injections. *Pain Physician.* 2012;15:131–140.
35. Charalambous CP, Tryfonidis M, Sadiq S, et al. Septic arthritis following intra-articular steroid injection of the knee? A survey of current practice regarding antiseptic technique used during intra-articular steroid injection of the knee. *Clin Rheumatol.* 2003;22:386–390.
36. Saboeiro GR, et al. Lumbar discography. *Radiol Clin North Am.* 2009;47(3):421–433. Available from: https://www-ncbi-nlm-nih-gov.laneproxy.stanford.edu/pubmed/?term=Guyer+RD%2C+Ohnmeiss+DD%3B+NASS.+Lumbar+discography.+Spine+J.+2003+May-Jun%3B3(3+Suppl)%3A11S-27S. Accessed July 18, 2017.
37. Schulz-Stübner S, Pottinger JM, Coffin SA, et al. Nosocomial infections and infection control in regional anesthesia. *Acta Anaesthesiol Scand.* 2008;52:1144–1157.
38. Schumacher HR, Chen LX. Injectable corticosteroids in treatment of arthritis of the knee. *Am J Med.* 2005;118:1208–1214.
39. Thumboo J, O'Duffy JD. A prospective study of the safety of joint and soft tissue aspirations and injections in patients taking warfarin sodium. *Arthritis Rheum.* 1998;41:736–739.
40. Mukerji N, Todd N. Spinal epidural haematoma; factors influencing outcome. *Br J Neurosurg.* 2013;27:712–717.
41. Faccenda KA, Finucane BT. Complications of regional anaesthesia Incidence and prevention. *Drug Saf.* 2001;24(6):413–442. Available from: https://www-ncbi-nlm-nih-gov.laneproxy.stanford.edu/pubmed/11368250. Accessed July 18, 2017.
42. Narouze S, et al. Interventional spine and pain procedures in patients on antiplatelet and anticoagulant medications: guidelines from the American Society of Regional Anesthesia and Pain Medicine, the European Society of Regional Anaesthesia and Pain Therapy, the American Academy of Pain Medicine, the International Neuromodulation Society, the North American Neuromodulation Society, and the World Institute of Pain. *Reg Anesth Pain Med.* 2015;40:182–212.
43. Authors/Task Force members; Windecker S, Kolh P, et al. 2014 ESC/EACTS Guidelines on myocardial revascularization: the Task Force on Myocardial Revascularization of the European Society of Cardiology (ESC) and the European Association for Cardio-Thoracic Surgery (EACTS) developed with the special contribution of the European Association of Percutaneous Cardiovascular Interventions (EAPCI). *Eur Heart J.* 2014;35:2541–2619.
44. Collet JP, Himbet F, Steg PG, et al. Myocardial infarction after aspirin cessation in stable coronary artery disease patients. *Int J Cardiol.* 2000;76(2-3):257–258.

Available from: https://www-ncbi-nlm-nih-gov.laneproxy.stanford.edu/pubmed/?term=Collet+Myocardial+infarction+after+aspirin+cessation+in+stable+coronary+artery+disease+patients. Accessed July 18, 2017.

45. Jeng CL, Rosenblatt MA. Intraneural injections and regional anesthesia: the known and the unknown. *Minerva Anestesiol.* 2011;77(1):54–58. Available from: https://www-ncbi-nlm-nih-gov.laneproxy.stanford.edu/pubmed/?term=Intraneural+injections+and+regional+anesthesia%3A+the+known+and+the+unknown. Accessed July 18, 2017.

46. Kennedy DJ, Schneider B, Smuck M, et al. The use of moderate sedation for the secondary prevention of adverse vasovagal reactions. *Pain Med.* 2015;16:673–679.

47. Fitzgibbon DR, Posner KL, Domino KB. Chronic pain management: American Society of Anesthesiologists Closed Claims Project. *Anesthesiology.* 2004;100(1):98–105. Available from: https://www-ncbi-nlm-nih-gov.laneproxy.stanford.edu/pubmed/?term=Chronic+pain+management%3A+American+Society+of+Anesthesiologists+Closed+Claims+Project. Accessed July 18, 2017.

48. Rathmell JP, et al. Injury and liability associated with cervical procedures for chronic pain. *Anesthesiology.* 2011;114:918–926.

49. Volcheck GW, Mertes PM. Local and general anesthetics immediate hypersensitivity reactions. *Immunol Allergy Clin North Am.* 2014;34:525–546.

50. Weinberg GL. Treatment of local anesthetic systemic toxicity (LAST). *Reg Anesth Pain Med.* 2010;35:188–193.

51. Kemper F, Gebhardt U, Meng T, et al. Tolerability and short-term effectiveness of hylan G-F 20 in 4253 patients with osteoarthritis of the knee in clinical practice. *Curr Med Res Opin.* 2005;21:1261–1269.

52. Migliore A, et al. Intra-articular administration of hylan G-F 20 in patients with symptomatic hip osteoarthritis: tolerability and effectiveness in a large cohort study in clinical practice. *Curr Med Res Opin.* 2008;24:1309–1316.

53. Bernardeau C, et al. Acute arthritis after intra-articular hyaluronate injection: onset of effusions without crystal. *Ann Rheum Dis.* 2001;60(5):518–520. Available from: https://www-ncbi-nlm-nih-gov.laneproxy.stanford.edu/pubmed/?term=Acute+arthritis+after+intra-articular+hyaluronate+injection%3A+onset+of+effusions+without+crystal. Accessed July 18, 2017.

54. Luzar MJ, Altawil B. Pseudogout following intraarticular injection of sodium hyaluronate. *Arthritis Rheum.* 1998;41:939–940.

55. Pullman-Mooar S, et al. Are there distinctive inflammatory flares after hylan g-f 20 intraarticular injections? *J Rheumatol.* 2002;29(12):2611–2614. Available from: https://www-ncbi-nlm-nih-gov.laneproxy.stanford.edu/pubmed/?term=Are+there+distinctive+inflammatory+flares+after+Hylan+GF+intra+articular+injections+%5Babstract%5D%3F. Accessed July 18, 2017.

56. Yacyshyn EA, Matteson EL. Gout after intraarticular injection of hylan GF-20 (Synvisc). *J Rheumatol.* 1999;26(12):2717. Available from: https://www-ncbi-nlm-nih-gov.laneproxy.stanford.edu/pubmed/?term=Gout+after+intra+articular+injection+of+Hylan+GF-20+(Synvisc). Accessed July 18, 2017.

57. Puttick MP, et al. Acute local reactions after intraarticular hylan for osteoarthritis of the knee. *J Rheumatol.* 1995;22(7):1311–1314. Available from: https://www-ncbi-nlm-nih-gov.laneproxy.stanford.edu/pubmed/7562764. Accessed July 18, 2017.

58. Maillefert JF, et al. Acute attack of chondrocalcinosis after an intraarticular injection of hyaluronan. *Rev Rhum Engl Ed.* 1997;64(10):593–594. Available from: https://www-ncbi-nlm-nih-gov.laneproxy.stanford.edu/pubmed/9385702. Accessed July 18, 2017.

59. Chen AL, et al. Granulomatous inflammation after Hylan G-F 20 viscosupplementation of the knee : a report of six cases. *J Bone Joint Surg Am.* 2002;84-A(7):1142–1147. Available from: https://www-ncbi-nlm-nih-gov.laneproxy.stanford.edu/pubmed/?term=Granulomatous+inflammation+after+Hylan+G-F+20+viscosupplementation+of+the+knee%3A+a+report+of+six+cases. Accessed July 18, 2017.

60. Kurosaka N, et al. Effects of hyaluronate on CD44 expression of infiltrating cells in exudate of rat air pouch, induced by sensitization with lipopolysaccharide. *J Rheumatol.* 1999;26(10):2186–2190. Available from: https://www-ncbi-nlm-nih-gov.laneproxy.stanford.edu/pubmed/?term=of+hyaluronate+on+CD44+expression+of+infiltrating+cells+in+exudate+of+rat+air+pouch+induced+by+sensitization+with+lipopolysaccharide.+Rheumatology. Accessed July 18, 2017.

61. Davenport MS, Cohan RH, Caoili EM, et al. Repeat contrast medium reactions in premedicated patients: frequency and severity. *Radiology.* 2009;253:372–379.

62. Kapoor R, Liu J, Devasenapathy A, et al. Gadolinium encephalopathy after intrathecal gadolinium injection. *Pain Physician.* 2010;13:E321–E326.

63. Duclos M, et al. High risk of adrenal insufficiency after a single articular steroid injection in athletes. *Med Sci Sports Exerc.* 2007;39:1036–1043.

64. Armstrong RD, et al. Serum methylprednisolone levels following intra-articular injection of methylprednisolone acetate. *Ann Rheum Dis.* 1981;40(6):571–574. Available from: https://www-ncbi-nlm-nih-gov.laneproxy.stanford.edu/pubmed/7332377. Accessed July 18, 2017.

65. Mandel S, Schilling J, Peterson E, et al. A retrospective analysis of vertebral body fractures following epidural steroid injections. *J Bone Joint Surg Am.* 2013;95:961–964.

66. Carreon L, Ong K, Lau E, et al. Risk of osteoporotic fracture after steroid injections in Medicare patients. *Scoliosis.* 2014;9:O46.

67. Friedly J, Chan L, Deyo R. Increases in lumbosacral injections in the medicare population: 1994 to 2001. *Spine.* 2007;32:1754–1760.

68. Gonzalez P, Laker SR, Sullivan W, et al. The effects of epidural betamethasone on blood glucose in patients with diabetes mellitus. *PM R.* 2009;1:340–345.

69. Even JL, Crosby CG, Song Y, et al. Effects of epidural steroid injections on blood glucose levels in patients with diabetes mellitus. *Spine.* 2012;37:E46–E50.

70. Younes M, et al. Systemic effects of epidural and intra-articular glucocorticoid injections in diabetic and non-diabetic patients. *Joint Bone Spine.* 2007;74:472–476.

71. Nichols AW. Complications associated with the use of corticosteroids in the treatment of athletic injuries. *Clin J Sport Med.* 2005;15(5):370–375. Available from: https://www-ncbi-nlm-nih-gov.laneproxy.stanford.edu/pubmed/16162982. Accessed July 18, 2017.

72. Engel A, King W, MacVicar J, et al. The effectiveness and risks of fluoroscopically guided cervical transforaminal injections of steroids: a systematic review with comprehensive analysis of the published data. *Pain Med.* 2014;15:386–402.

73. Kennedy DJ, Dreyfuss P, Aprill CN, et al. Paraplegia following image-guided transforaminal lumbar spine epidural steroid injection: two case reports. *Pain Med.* 2009;10:1389–1394.

74. Mehta P, Syrop I, Singh JR, et al. Systematic review of the efficacy of particulate versus nonparticulate corticosteroids in epidural injections. *PM R.* 2017;9:502–512.

75. Gharibo CG, et al. Conus medullaris infarction after a right l4 transforaminal epidural steroid injection using dexamethasone. *Pain Physician.* 2016;19(8):E1211–E1214. Available from: https://www-ncbi-nlm-nih-gov.laneproxy.stanford.edu/pubmed/?term=Conus+Medullaris+Infarction+After+a+Right+L4+Transforaminal+Epidural+Steroid+Injection+Using+Dexamethasone. Accessed July 18, 2017.

76. Laemmel E, et al. Deleterious effects of intra-arterial administration of particulate steroids on microvascular perfusion in a mouse model. *Radiology.* 2016;279:731–740.

77. Rathmell JP, et al. Safeguards to prevent neurologic complications after epidural steroid injections: consensus opinions from a multidisciplinary working group and national organizations. *Anesthesiology.* 2015;122:974–984.

78. Elseviers MM, Arias-Guillén M, Gorke A, et al. Sharps injuries amongst healthcare workers: review of incidence, transmissions and costs: sharps injuries amongst healthcare workers. *J Renal Care.* 2014;40:150–156.

79. Becker DE, Reed KL. Essentials of local anesthetic pharmacology. *Anesth Prog.* 2006;53:98–109.

80. Vadhanan P, Tripaty D, Adinarayanan S. Physiological and pharmacologic aspects of peripheral nerve blocks. *J Anaesthesiol Clin Pharmacol.* 2015;31:384.

81. Dragoo JL, Braun HJ, Kim HJ, et al. The in vitro chondrotoxicity of single-dose local anesthetics. *Am J Sports Med.* 2012;40:794–799.

82. Hodgson PS, et al. The neurotoxicity of drugs given intrathecally (spinal). *Anesth Analg.* 1999;88(4):797–809. Available from: https://www-ncbi-nlm-nih-gov.laneproxy.stanford.edu/pubmed/10195528. Accessed July 18, 2017.

83. Hwang H, et al. Crystallization of local anesthetics when mixed with corticosteroid solutions. *Ann Rehabil Med.* 2016;40:21.

84. Swerdlow M. Medico-legal aspects of complications following pain relieving blocks. *Pain.* 1982;13(4):321–331. Available from: https://www.ncbi.nlm.nih.gov/pubmed/?term=Swerdlow+M.+Medico-legal+aspects+of+complications+following+pain+relieving+block.+Pain.+1982%3B13%3A321%E2%80%93331. Accessed July 9, 2017.

85. Li R, et al. Peripheral nerve injuries treatment: a systematic review. *Cell Biochem Biophys.* 2014;68:449–454.

86. Takahashi H, et al. Inflammatory cytokines in the herniated disc of the lumbar spine. *Spine (Phila Pa 1976).* 1996;21(2):218–224. Available from: https://www-ncbi-nlm-nih-gov.laneproxy.stanford.edu/pubmed/8720407. Accessed July 18, 2017.

87. Mulleman D, Mammou S, Griffoul I, et al. Pathophysiology of disk-related sciatica. I.—Evidence supporting a chemical component. *Joint Bone Spine.* 2006;73:151–158.

88. Johansson A, Hao J, Sjölund B. Local corticosteroid application blocks transmission in normal nociceptive C-fibres. *Acta Anaesthesiol Scand.* 1990;34:335–338.

89. Kennedy DJ, et al. Comparative effectiveness of lumbar transforaminal epidural steroid injections with particulate versus nonparticulate corticosteroids for lumbar radicular pain due to intervertebral disc herniation: a prospective, randomized, double-blind trial. *Pain Med.* 2014;15:548–555.

90. Braddom R. *Physical Medicine and Rehabilitation.* Philadelphia, PA: Saunders; 2011.

91. Yoon S-H, Lee HY, Lee HJ, et al. Optimal dose of intra-articular corticosteroids for adhesive capsulitis: a randomized, triple-blind, placebo-controlled trial. *Am J Sports Med.* 2013;41:1133–1139.

92. de Jong BA, Dahmen R, Hogeweg JA, et al. Intra-articular triamcinolone acetonide injection in patients with capsulitis of the shoulder: a comparative study of two dose regimens. *Clin Rehabil.* 1998;12:211–215.

93. Robinson P, Keenan A-M, Conaghan PG. Clinical effectiveness and dose response of image-guided intra-articular corticosteroid injection for hip osteoarthritis. *Rheumatology.* 2006;46:285–291.

94. Popma JW, et al. Comparison of 2 dosages of intraarticular triamcinolone for the treatment of knee arthritis: results of a 12-week randomized controlled clinical trial. *J Rheumatol.* 2015;42(10):1865–18658. Available from: https://www-ncbi-nlm-nih-gov.laneproxy.stanford.edu/pubmed/?term=Popma+JW%2C+Snel+FW%2C+Haagsma+CJ%2C+et+al.+Comparison+of+2+Dosages+of+Intraarticular+Triamcinolone+for+the+Treatment+of+Knee+Arthritis%3A+Results+of+a+12-week+Randomized+Controlled+Clinical+Trial.+J+Rheumatol.+2015%3B42(10)%3A1865-1868. Accessed July 18, 2017.

95. Ahadian FM, McGreevy K, Schulteis G. Lumbar transforaminal epidural dexamethasone: a prospective, randomized, double-blind, dose-response trial. *Reg Anesth Pain Med.* 2011;36:572–578.

96. Kang SS, et al. The dosages of corticosteroid in transforaminal epidural steroid injections for lumbar radicular pain due to a herniated disc. *Pain Physician.* 2011;14:361–370.

97. Owlia MB, et al. Comparison of two doses of corticosteroid in epidural steroid injection for lumbar radicular pain. *Singapore Med J.* 2007;48(3):241–245. Available from: https://www-ncbi-nlm-nih-gov.laneproxy.stanford.edu/pubmed/?term=Comparison+of+two+doses+of+corticosteroid+in+epidural+steroid+injection+for+lumbar+radicular+pain. Accessed July 18, 2017.

98. Young R, Harding J, Kingsly A, et al. Therapeutic hip injections: is the injection volume important? *Clin Radiol.* 2012;67:55–60.

99. Chun EH, Park HS. Effect of high-volume injectate in lumbar transforaminal epidural steroid injections: a randomized, active control trial. *Pain Physician.* 2015;18(6):519–525. Available from: https://www.ncbi.nlm.nih.gov/pubmed/26606003. Accessed July 9, 2017.
100. Rabinovitch DL, Peliowski A, Furlan AD. Influence of lumbar epidural injection volume on pain relief for radicular leg pain and/or low back pain. *Spine J.* 2009;9:509–517.
101. Bogduk N. International Spinal Injection Society guidelines for the performance of spinal injection procedures. Part 1: Zygapophysial joint blocks. *Clin J Pain.* 1997;13:285–302.
102. Smith MM, Ghosh P. The synthesis of hyaluronic acid by human synovial fibroblasts is influenced by the nature of the hyaluronate in the extracellular environment. *Rheumatol Int.* 1987;7(3):113–122. Available from: https://www.ncbi.nlm.nih.gov/pubmed/?term=The+synthesis+of+hyaluronic+acid+by+human+synovial+fibroblasts+is+influenced+by+the+nature+of+the+hyaluronate+in+the+extracellular+environment. Accessed July 9, 2017.
103. Jiang D, Liang J, Noble PW. Hyaluronan as an immune regulator in human diseases. *Physiol Rev.* 2011;91:221–264.
104. Campo GM, et al. The inhibition of hyaluronan degradation reduced pro-inflammatory cytokines in mouse synovial fibroblasts subjected to collagen-induced arthritis. *J Cell Biochem.* 2012;113:1852–1867.
105. Guidolin DD, Ronchetti IP, Lini E, et al. Morphological analysis of articular cartilage biopsies from a randomized, clinical study comparing the effects of 500–730 kDa sodium hyaluronate (Hyalgan®) and methylprednisolone acetate on primary osteoarthritis of the knee. *Osteoarthritis Cartilage.* 2001;9:371–381.
106. Rayahin JE, Buhrman JS, Zhang Y, et al. High and low molecular weight hyaluronic acid differentially influence macrophage activation. *ACS Biomater Sci Eng.* 2015;1:481–493.
107. Campo GM, et al. Molecular size hyaluronan differently modulates toll-like receptor-4 in LPS-induced inflammation in mouse chondrocytes. *Biochimie.* 2010;92:204–215.
108. Jevsevar D, Donnelly P, Brown GA, et al. Viscosupplementation for osteoarthritis of the knee: a systematic review of the evidence. *J Bone Joint Surg Am.* 2015;97:2047–2060.
109. Miller LE, Altman R, McIntyre L. Unraveling the confusion behind hyaluronic acid efficacy in the treatment of symptomatic knee osteoarthritis. *J Pain Res.* 2016;9:421–423. doi:10.2147/JPR.S110675.
110. Telikicherla M. Accuracy of needle placement into the intra-articular space of the knee in osteoarthritis patients for viscosupplementation. *J Clin Diagn Res.* 2016;10(2):RC15–RC17. doi:10.7860/JCDR/2016/17127.7275.
111. Amber KT, Landy DC, Amber I, et al. Comparing the accuracy of ultrasound versus fluoroscopy in glenohumeral injections: a systematic review and meta-analysis: US versus Fluoro in Glenohumeral Injections. *J Clin Ultrasound.* 2014;42:411–416.
112. Martínez-Martínez A, et al. Comparison of ultrasound and fluoroscopic guidance for injection in CT arthrography and MR arthrography of the hip. *Radiologia.* 2016;58(6):454–459. Available from: https://www-ncbi-nlm-nih-gov.laneproxy.stanford.edu/pubmed/?term=Comparison+of+ultrasound+and+fluoroscopic+guidance+for+injection+in+CT+arthrography+and+MR+arthrography+of+the+hip. Accessed July 18, 2017.
113. Finnoff JT, et al. American Medical Society for Sports Medicine (AMSSM) position statement: interventional musculoskeletal ultrasound in sports medicine. *Br J Sports Med.* 2015;49:145–150.
114. Kennedy DJ, Mattie R, Scott Hamilton A, et al. Detection of intravascular injection during lumbar medial branch blocks: a comparison of aspiration, live fluoroscopy, and digital subtraction technology. *Pain Med.* 2016;17:1031–1036. doi:10.1093/pm/pnv073.
115. Stojanovic MP, et al. The role of fluoroscopy in cervical epidural steroid injections: an analysis of contrast dispersal patterns. *Spine (Phila Pa 1976).* 2002;27(5):509–514. Available from: https://www.ncbi.nlm.nih.gov/pubmed/?term=Stojanovic+M%2C+Vu+TN%2C+Caneris+O%2C+et+al+2002. Accessed July 18, 2017.
116. Renfrew DL, et al. Correct placement of epidural steroid injections: fluoroscopic guidance and contrast administration. *Am J Neuroradiol.* 1991;12:1003–1007.
117. Cushman DM, Mattie R, Clements ND, et al. The effect of body mass index on fluoroscopic time and radiation dose during intra-articular hip injections. *PM R.* 2016;8:876–882.
118. Cushman D, Mattie R, Curtis B, et al. The effect of body mass index on fluoroscopic time and radiation dose during lumbar transforaminal epidural steroid injections. *Spine J.* 2016;16:876–883.
119. McCormick ZL, et al. Is there a relationship between body mass index and fluoroscopy time during cervical interlaminar epidural steroid injections? *Pain Med.* 2017;18:1326–1333. doi:10.1093/pm/pnw264.
120. Mattie R, McCormick ZL, Fogg B, et al. The effect of body mass index on fluoroscopy time and radiation dose in intra-articular glenohumeral joint injections. *Clin Imaging.* 2017;42:19–24.
121. Plastaras C, et al. Fluoroscopy procedure and equipment changes to reduce staff radiation exposure in the interventional spine suite. *Pain Physician.* 2013;16(6):E731–E738. Available from: https://www.ncbi.nlm.nih.gov/pubmed/?term=fluoroscopy+procedure+and+equipment+changes+to+reduce+staff+radiation+exposure+in+the+interventional+spine+suite. Accessed July 18, 2017.
122. McLean JP, Sigler JD, Plastaras CT, et al. The rate of detection of intravascular injection in cervical transforaminal epidural steroid injections with and without digital subtraction angiography. *PM R.* 2009;1:636–642.
123. Chang Chien GC, Candido KD, et al. Digital subtraction angiography does not reliably prevent paraplegia associated with lumbar transforaminal epidural steroid injection. *Pain Physician.* 2012;15:515–523.
124. Maus T, et al. Radiation dose incurred in the exclusion of vascular filling in transforaminal epidural steroid injections: fluoroscopy, digital subtraction angiography, and CT/fluoroscopy. *Pain Med.* 2014;15:1328–1333.
125. Hoang JK, et al. Radiation dose exposure for lumbar spine epidural steroid injections: a comparison of conventional fluoroscopy data and CT fluoroscopy techniques. *Am J Roentgenol.* 2011;197:778–782.
126. Ng PP, Wilder MJ, Jenkins PA. CT fluoroscopy-guided cervical interlaminar steroid injections: is it overkill? *Am J Neuroradiol.* 2012;33:E138.
127. MacVicar J, King W, Landers MH, et al. The effectiveness of lumbar transforaminal injection of steroids: a comprehensive review with systematic analysis of the published data. *Pain Med.* 2013;14:14–28.
128. Kreiner DS, et al. An evidence-based clinical guideline for the diagnosis and treatment of lumbar disc herniation with radiculopathy. *Spine J.* 2014;14:180–191.
129. DePalma MJ, Slipman CW. Evidence-informed management of chronic low back pain with epidural steroid injections. *Spine J.* 2008;8:45–55.
130. Furman MB, O'Brien EM, Zgleszewski TM. Incidence of intravascular penetration in transforaminal lumbosacral epidural steroid injections. *Spine.* 2000;25:2628–2632.
131. Furman MB, Giovanniello MT, O'Brien EM. Incidence of intravascular penetration in transforaminal cervical epidural steroid injections. *Spine.* 2003;28:21–25.
132. Kolsi I, et al. Efficacy of nerve root versus interspinous injections of glucocorticoids in the treatment of disk-related sciatica. A pilot, prospective, randomized, double-blind study. *Joint Bone Spine.* 2000;67:113–118.
133. Ghahreman A, Bogduk N. Predictors of a favorable response to transforaminal injection of steroids in patients with lumbar radicular pain due to disc herniation. *Pain Med.* 2011;12:871–879.
134. Ghahreman A, Ferch R, Bogduk N. The efficacy of transforaminal injection of steroids for the treatment of lumbar radicular pain. *Pain Med.* 2010;11:1149–1168.
135. Lutz GE, Vad VB, Wisneski RJ. Fluoroscopic transforaminal lumbar epidural steroids: an outcome study. *Arch Phys Med Rehabil.* 1998;79:1362–1366.
136. Cyteval C, et al. Predictive factors of efficacy of periradicular corticosteroid injections for lumbar radiculopathy. *AJNR Am J Neuroradiol.* 2006;27:978–982.
137. Riew KD, et al. Nerve root blocks in the treatment of lumbar radicular pain. A minimum five-year follow-up. *J Bone Joint Surg Am.* 2006;88:1722–1725.
138. Riew KD, et al. The effect of nerve-root injections on the need for operative treatment of lumbar radicular pain. A prospective, randomized, controlled, double-blind study. *J Bone Joint Surg Am.* 2000;82–A:1589–1593.
139. Ackerman WE, Ahmad M. The efficacy of lumbar epidural steroid injections in patients with lumbar disc herniations. *Anesth Analg.* 2007;104:1217–1222.
140. Gharibo CG, et al. Interlaminar versus transforaminal epidural steroids for the treatment of subacute lumbar radicular pain: a randomized, blinded, prospective outcome study. *Pain Physician.* 2011;14:499–511.
141. Engel AJ, Kennedy DJ, Macvicar J, et al. Not all injections are the same. *Anesthesiology.* 2014;120:1282–1283.
142. Thomas E, et al. Efficacy of transforaminal versus interspinous corticosteroid injection in discal radiculalgia—a prospective, randomised, double-blind study. *Clin Rheumatol.* 2003;22(4–5):299–304. Available from: https://www-ncbi-nlm-nih-gov.laneproxy.stanford.edu/pubmed/?term=Thomas+E%2C+Cyteval+C%2C+Abiad+L%2C+et+al.+Efficacy+of+transforaminal+versus+interspinous+corticosteroid+injectionin+discal+radiculalgia+-+a+prospective%2C+randomised%2C+double-blind+study. Accessed July 18, 2017.
143. Choi SJ, et al. The use of magnetic resonance imaging to predict the clinical outcome of non-surgical treatment for lumbar intervertebral disc herniation. *Korean J Radiol.* 2007;8(2):156–163. Available from: https://www-ncbi-nlm-nih-gov.laneproxy.stanford.edu/pubmed/?term=(Choi+SJ%2C+Song+JS%2C+Kim+C+2007. Accessed July 18, 2017.
144. Friedly JL, et al. A randomized trial of epidural glucocorticoid injections for spinal stenosis. *N Engl J Med.* 2014;371:11–21.
145. Candido KD, Raghavendra MS, Chinthagada M, et al. A prospective evaluation of iodinated contrast flow patterns with fluoroscopically guided lumbar epidural steroid injections: the lateral parasagittal interlaminar epidural approach versus the transforaminal epidural approach. *Anesth Analg.* 2008;106:638–644.
146. Rados I, Sakic K, Fingler M, et al. Efficacy of interlaminar vs transforaminal epidural steroid injection for the treatment of chronic unilateral radicular pain: prospective, randomized study. *Pain Med.* 2011;12:1316–1321.
147. Chang-Chien GC, et al. Transforaminal versus interlaminar approaches to epidural steroid injections: a systematic review of comparative studies for lumbosacral radicular pain. *Pain Physician.* 2014;17:E509–E524.
148. Botwin KP, et al. Fluoroscopic guided lumbar interlaminar epidural injections: a prospective evaluation of epidurography contrast patterns and anatomical review of the epidural space. *Pain Physician.* 2004;7(1):77–80. Available from: https://www-ncbi-nlm-nih-gov.laneproxy.stanford.edu/pubmed/?term=Botwin+KP%2C+Natalicchio+J%2C+Hanna+A.+Fluoroscopic+guided+lumbar+interlaminar+epidural+injections%3A+a+prospective+evaluation+of+epidurography+contrast+patterns+and+anatomical+review+of+the+epidural+space. Accessed July 18, 2017.
149. Tomczak R, et al. Die epidurographie: vergleich mit CT-, spiral-CT- und MR-epidurographie. *RöFo.* 1996;165:123–129.
150. Bogduk N. *Clinical Anatomy of the Lumbar Spine and Sacrum.* Melbourne: Churchill Livingstone; 1997.
151. Murthy NS, Maus TP, Behrns CL. Intraforaminal location of the great anterior radiculomedullary artery (artery of Adamkiewicz): a retrospective review. *Pain Med.* 2010;11:1756–1764.
152. Hogan QH. Epidural anatomy examined by cryomicrotome section. Influence of age, vertebral level, and disease. *Reg Anesth.* 1996;21(5):395–406. Available from: https://www.ncbi.nlm.nih.gov/pubmed/?term=Hogan+QH.+Epidural+anatomy+

examined+by+cryomicrotome+section.++Anesthesiology+1996%3B21%3A395-406. Accessed July 18, 2017.

153. Barre L, Lutz GE, Southern D, et al. Fluoroscopically guided caudal epidural steroid injections for lumbar spinal stenosis: a retrospective evaluation of long term efficacy. *Pain Physician.* 2004;7:187–193.

154. Kim KM, et al. Cephalic spreading levels after volumetric caudal epidural injections in chronic low back pain. *J Korean Med Sci.* 2001;16(2):193–197. Available from: https://www-ncbi-nlm-nih-gov.laneproxy.stanford.edu/pubmed/?term=Kim+KM%2C+Kim+HS%2C+Choi+KH%2C+et+al.+Cephalic+spreading+levels+after+volumetric+caudal+epidural+injections+in+chronic+low+back+pain. Accessed July 18, 2017.

155. Henriksen M, Rosager S, Aaboe J, et al. Experimental knee pain reduces muscle strength. *J Pain.* 2011;12:460–467.

156. McCabe PS, Maricar N, Parkes MJ, et al. The efficacy of intra-articular steroids in hip osteoarthritis: a systematic review. *Osteoarthritis Cartilage.* 2016;24:1509–1517.

157. Zhang W, et al. OARSI recommendations for the management of hip and knee osteoarthritis, Part II: OARSI evidence-based, expert consensus guidelines. *Osteoarthritis Cartilage.* 2008;16:137–162.

158. Jüni P, et al. Intra-articular corticosteroid for knee osteoarthritis. *Cochrane Database Syst Rev.* 2015;(10):CD005328. doi:10.1002/14651858.CD005328.pub3.

159. Buchbinder R, Green S, Youd JM. Corticosteroid injections for shoulder pain. *Cochrane Database Syst Rev.* 2003;(1):CD004016. doi:10.1002/14651858.CD004016.

160. Bellamy N, et al. Viscosupplementation for the treatment of osteoarthritis of the knee. *Cochrane Database Syst Rev.* 2006;(2):CD005321. doi:10.1002/14651858.CD005321.pub2.

161. Dobson MM. A further anatomical check on the accuracy of intra-articular hip injections in relation to the therapy of coxarthritis. *Ann Rheum Dis.* 1950;9(3):237–240. Available from: https://www.ncbi.nlm.nih.gov/pubmed/?term=Dobson+M.+A+further+anatomical+check+on+the+accuracy+of+intra-+articular+hip+injections+in+relation+to+the+therapy+of+coxarthritis%2C+Ann+Rheum+Dis+1950%3B+9(3)%3A+237-240. Accessed July 18, 2017.

162. Leopold SS, et al. Safety and efficacy of intraarticular hip injection using anatomic landmarks. *Clin Orthop Relat Res.* 2001;(391):192–197. Available from: https://www.ncbi.nlm.nih.gov/pubmed/?term=Leopold+S%2C+Battista+V%2C+Oliverio+J.+Safety+and+efficacy+of+intraarticular+hip+injection+using+anatomic+landmarks.+Clin+Orthop+Relat+Res+2001%3B+391%3A+192-197. Accessed July 18, 2017.

163. Manchikanti L, Pampati V, Fellows B, et al. Prevalence of lumbar facet joint pain in chronic low back pain. *Pain Physician.* 1999;2:59–64.

164. DePalma MJ, Ketchum JM, Saullo TR. Multivariable analyses of the relationships between age, gender, and body mass index and the source of chronic low back pain. *Pain Med.* 2012;13:498–506.

165. Barnsley L, Lord SM, Wallis BJ, et al. The prevalence of chronic cervical zygapophysial joint pain after whiplash. *Spine.* 1995;20:20–25; discussion 26.

166. DePalma MJ, Ketchum JM, Saullo T. What is the source of chronic low back pain and does age play a role? *Pain Med.* 2011;12:224–233.

167. Chua WH, Bogduk N. The surgical anatomy of thoracic facet denervation. *Acta Neurochir (Wien).* 1995;136(3–4):140–144. Available from: https://www.ncbi-nlm-nih-gov.laneproxy.stanford.edu/pubmed/?term=Chua+WH%2C+Bogduk+N.+The+surgical+anatomy+of+thoracic+facet+denervation.+Acta+Neurochir+1995%3B136(3%E2%80%934)%3A140%E2%80%93144. Accessed July 18, 2017.

168. Furman M. *Atlas of Image-Guided Spinal Procedures.* Philadelphia, PA: Elsevier Saunders; 2013.

169. Bogduk N. On the rational use of diagnostic blocks for spinal pain. *Neurosurg Quart.* 2009;19:88–100.

170. Carrera GF, Williams AL. Current concepts in evaluation of the lumbar facet joints. *Crit Rev Diagn Imaging.* 1984;21:85–104.

171. Amoretti N, et al. Symptomatic lumbar facet joint cysts treated by CT-guided intracystic and intra-articular steroid injections. *Eur Radiol.* 2012;22:2836–2840.

172. Lilius G, Laasonen EM, Myllynen P, et al. Lumbar facet joint syndrome. A randomised clinical trial. *J Bone Joint Surg Br.* 1989;71:681–684.

173. Carette S, et al. A controlled trial of corticosteroid injections into facet joints for chronic low back pain. *N Engl J Med.* 1991;325:1002–1007.

174. Barnsley L, Lord SM, Wallis BJ, et al. Lack of effect of intraarticular corticosteroids for chronic pain in the cervical zygapophyseal joints. *N Engl J Med.* 1994;330:1047–1050.

175. Pneumaticos SG, Chatziioannou SN, Hipp JA, et al. Low back pain: prediction of short-term outcome of facet joint injection with bone scintigraphy. *Radiology.* 2006;238:693–698.

176. Dolan AL, et al. The value of SPECT scans in identifying back pain likely to benefit from facet joint injection. *Br J Rheumatol.* 1996;35:1269–1273.

177. Macvicar J, Borowczyk JM, Macvicar AM, et al. Lumbar medial branch radiofrequency neurotomy in New Zealand. *Pain Med.* 2013;14:639–645. doi:10.1111/pme.12000.

178. MacVicar J, Borowczyk JM, MacVicar AM, et al. Cervical medial branch radiofrequency neurotomy in New Zealand. *Pain Med.* 2012;13:647–654.

179. Dreyfuss P, et al. Radiofrequency facet joint denervation in the treatment of low back pain: a placebo-controlled clinical trial to assess efficacy. *Spine.* 2002;27:556–557.

180. Schofferman J, Kine G. Effectiveness of repeated radiofrequency neurotomy for lumbar facet pain. *Spine (Phila Pa 1976).* 2004;29(21):2471–2473. Available

181. Engel A, Rappard G, King W, et al. The effectiveness and risks of fluoroscopically-guided cervical medial branch thermal radiofrequency neurotomy: a systematic review with comprehensive analysis of the published data. *Pain Med.* 2016;17:658–669. doi:10.1111/pme.12928.

182. Fortin JD. Sacroiliac joint dysfunction A new perspective. *J Back Musculoskelet Rehabil.* 1993;3:31–43.

183. Dreyfuss P, Dreyer SJ, Cole A, et al. Sacroiliac joint pain. *J Am Acad Orthop Surg.* 2004;12:255.

184. Kennedy DJ, et al. Fluoroscopically guided diagnostic and therapeutic intra-articular sacroiliac joint injections: a systematic review. *Pain Med.* 2015;16:1500–1518.

185. King W, et al. Diagnosis and treatment of posterior sacroiliac complex pain: a systematic review with comprehensive analysis of the published data. *Pain Med.* 2015;16:257–265.

186. Dreyfuss P, Dryer S, Griffin J, et al. Positive sacroiliac screening tests in asymptomatic adults. *Spine.* 1994;19:1138–1143.

187. Dreyfuss P, Michaelsen M, Pauza K, et al. The value of medical history and physical examination in diagnosing sacroiliac joint pain. *Spine.* 1996;21:2594–2602.

188. Laslett M. The value of the physical examination in diagnosis of painful sacroiliac joint pathologies. *Spine.* 1998;23:962–964.

189. Jee H, Lee J-H, Park KD, et al. Ultrasound-guided versus fluoroscopy-guided sacroiliac joint intra-articular injections in the noninflammatory sacroiliac joint dysfunction: a prospective, randomized, single-blinded study. *Arch Phys Med Rehabil.* 2014;95:330–337.

190. Simopoulos TT, et al. A systematic evaluation of prevalence and diagnostic accuracy of sacroiliac joint interventions. *Pain Physician.* 2012;15:E305–E344.

191. Slipman CW, et al. Fluoroscopically guided therapeutic sacroiliac joint injections for sacroiliac joint syndrome. *Am J Phys Med Rehabil.* 2001;80:425–432.

192. Maigne JY, Planchon CA. Sacroiliac joint pain after lumbar fusion. A study with anesthetic blocks. *Eur Spine J.* 2005;14:654–658.

193. DePalma MJ, Ketchum JM, Saullo TR. Etiology of chronic low back pain in patients having undergone lumbar fusion. *Pain Med.* 2011;12:732–739.

194. Liliang PC, et al. Sacroiliac joint pain after lumbar and lumbosacral fusion: findings using dual diagnostic sacroiliac joint blocks. *Pain Med.* 2011;12:565–570.

195. Young S, Aprill C, Laslett M. Correlation of clinical examination characteristics with three sources of chronic low back pain. *Spine J.* 2003;3:460–465.

196. Slipman CW, Sterenfeld EB, Chou LH, et al. The predictive value of provocative sacroiliac joint stress maneuvers in the diagnosis of sacroiliac joint syndrome. *Arch Phys Med Rehabil.* 1998;79:288–292.

197. Hanly JG, Mitchell M, MacMillan L, et al. Efficacy of sacroiliac corticosteroid injections in patients with inflammatory spondyloarthropathy: results of a 6 month controlled study. *J Rheumatol.* 2000;27:719–722.

198. Cohen S, Abdi S. Lateral branch blocks as a treatment for sacroiliac joint pain: a pilot study. *Reg Anesth Pain Med.* 2003;28:113–119.

199. Burnham R, Yasui Y. An alternate method of radiofrequency neurotomy of the sacroiliac joint: a pilot study of the effect on pain, function, and satisfaction. *Reg Anesth Pain Med.* 2007;32:12–19.

200. Dreyfuss P, Henning T, Malladi N, et al. The ability of multi-site, multi-depth sacral lateral branch blocks to anesthetize the sacroiliac joint complex. *Pain Med.* 2009;10:679–688.

201. Myburgh C, Larsen AH, Hartvigsen J. A systematic, critical review of manual palpation for identifying myofascial trigger points: evidence and clinical significance. *Arch Phys Med Rehabil.* 2008;89:1169–1176.

202. Miles D. Re: "dry needling alters trigger points in the upper trapezius muscle and reduces pain in subjects with chronic myofascial pain". *PM R.* 2016;8:1225–1226.

203. Ge H-Y, Fernández-de-las-Peñas C, Yue S-W. Myofascial trigger points: spontaneous electrical activity and its consequences for pain induction and propagation. *Chin Med.* 2011;6:13.

204. Shah JP. An in vivo microanalytical technique for measuring the local biochemical milieu of human skeletal muscle. *J Appl Physiol.* 2005;99:1977–1984.

205. Simons DG, Travell JG, Simons LS. *Travell & Simons' Myofascial Pain and Dysfunction: Upper half of body.* Baltimore, MD: Lippincott Williams & Wilkins; 1999.

206. Celik D, Mutlu EK. Clinical implication of latent myofascial trigger point. *Curr Pain Headache Rep.* 2013;17:353.

207. Lucas KR, Polus BI, Rich PA. Latent myofascial trigger points: their effects on muscle activation and movement efficiency. *J Bodyw Mov Ther.* 2004;8:160–166.

208. Gerwin RD, et al. Interrater reliability in myofascial trigger point examination. *Pain.* 1997;69:65–73. Available from: https://www.ncbi.nlm.nih.gov/pubmed/9060014. Accessed July 18, 2017.

209. Scott NA, et al. Trigger point injections for chronic non-malignant musculoskeletal pain: a systematic review. *Pain Med.* 2009;10(1):54–69. Available from: https://www-ncbi-nlm-nih-gov.laneproxy.stanford.edu/pubmed/?term=Scott+NA%2C+Guo+B%2C+Barton+PM%2C+et+al.+Trigger+point+injections+for+chronic+non-malignant+musculoskeletal+pain%3A+a+systematic+review.+Pain+Med+2009%3B+10(1)%3A+54-69. Accessed July 18, 2017.

210. Robbins MS, et al. Trigger Point Injections for Headache Disorders: Expert Consensus Methodology and Narrative Review. *Headache.* 2014;54:1441–1459.

CHAPTER 54

Jayme S. Knutson
Steven W. Brose
Ela B. Plow

Richard D. Wilson
John Chae

Electrical Stimulation (Therapeutic and Functional)

Clinical applications of electrical stimulation (ES) to treat neurologic disease may be broadly classified as therapeutic or functional (1). Therapeutic ES is used to improve health or physical function by inducing physiologic changes that remain after the stimulation is used for a period of time and then discontinued. Therapeutic ES applications are temporary and may decrease impairment or prevent further impairment associated with immobility or disuse of a limb or organ system. By contrast, functional ES (FES) is used to replace impaired or lost neurologic function on a long-term basis. In FES applications, stimulation must be "on" to achieve a desired function; therefore, FES systems are usually designed to be worn by the user and are called neuroprostheses because they substitute for lost function (2). Some FES applications may have both neuroprosthetic and therapeutic benefits (3).

This chapter will review both therapeutic and functional applications of ES to treat neurologically based disorders encountered in the clinical practice of Physical Medicine and Rehabilitation. These applications include electrical stimulation for upper and lower extremity function, respiratory function, bladder and bowel function, and relief of neuropathic pain, as well as various applications involving stimulation of cortical and subcortical brain areas.

STIMULATION FOR LIMB MOVEMENT

Neuromuscular electrical stimulation (NMES) refers to the use of low-level electrical current to produce useful muscle contractions (4). In the field of Physical Medicine and Rehabilitation, NMES is used in cases of neurologic injury that result in muscle paralysis or paresis. NMES systems produce muscle contractions by activating motor neurons rather than muscle fibers directly (5). It follows then that for NMES to be effective, the peripheral nerves to the target muscles must be intact and the muscle physiology must be healthy. This typically excludes individuals who have muscle weakness or paralysis due to peripheral nerve injuries or muscular dystrophies. The patients for whom NMES can be used as a therapeutic and/or assistive device are those whose muscle paresis or paralysis is caused by injury or disease to upper motor neurons (i.e., central nervous system injuries). Therefore, most clinical NMES applications are designed for stroke or spinal cord injury (SCI) patients, and they may also be applicable to some individuals with cerebral palsy, traumatic brain injury, or multiple sclerosis. This section reviews therapeutic and functional NMES applications for restoration of upper and lower extremity function.

Upper Extremity

Stroke

Loss of arm and hand movement on one side of the body is common after stroke (6) (see also Chapter 18). Paretic upper limb extensors, hypertonic flexors, and loss of coordination often manifest as difficulty reaching forward and/or opening the hand in a functional manner (7). Therefore, NMES for upper limb stroke rehabilitation is usually applied to the elbow, wrist, and/or finger and thumb extensors. The purpose of most upper limb stroke NMES applications is to produce a persistent therapeutic effect, that is, improve recovery of volitional upper limb function. Therefore, these applications are temporary and noninvasive, with surface electrodes typically placed over the finger and wrist extensors. Elbow extensors or shoulder muscles may also be targeted in some applications. Three therapeutic NMES paradigms, distinguished by the method in which the stimulation is controlled, have been used for upper limb therapy: cyclic NMES, triggered NMES, and proportionally controlled NMES.

Cyclic NMES activates the paretic muscles according to an on-off cycle, with the timing, number of repetitions, and maximum intensity of stimulation preset by a therapist (8). When the device is turned on, stimulation elicits repeated muscle contractions and therefore repeated arm or hand movement lasting several seconds at a time. Cyclic NMES requires no input from the patient, who may simply relax and let the stimulator activate the muscles. Several two- or four-channel cyclic NMES stimulators are commercially available (e.g., Intelect Portable Electrotherapy NMES, DJO Global, Inc.) and are relatively inexpensive.

Triggered NMES also elicits repetitive muscle contractions but requires input from the patient (or therapist) in order for the stimulation to be delivered. EMG-triggered stimulators (e.g., NeuroMove, Zynex Medical, Inc.) prompt the patient to produce a suprathreshold electromyographic (EMG) signal by attempting to contract the paretic muscle, at least partially (9). If and when the amplitude of the EMG signal exceeds a preset threshold, the stimulator turns on and delivers a preset intensity of stimulation to the target muscle(s) for a preset duration, after which the stimulation turns off and the cycle repeats. Because stimulation and the corresponding cutaneous and proprioceptive feedback to the brain coincides with the patient's own effort to produce the stimulated movement, it is thought that this method may be more effective in promoting neurologic changes leading to better recovery. Switch-triggered stimulators (e.g., H200, Bioness, Inc.) have push buttons to trigger stimulation, which give the therapist (10) or the patient (11) control of the initiation and duration of stimulation, and thereby make it more feasible to incorporate NMES into task practice. Using NMES to assist task practice may lead to better outcomes than would be achieved with modalities like cyclic NMES or EMG-triggered NMES, which cannot be easily used to assist task practice because the duration of stimulation is preprogrammed (12).

Proportionally controlled NMES is an investigational modality in which the intensity and duration of stimulation are not preset but regulated *in real time by the patient* via a control strategy that translates the patient's desired movement into stimulation intensities. Contralaterally controlled functional electrical stimulation (CCFES) is an emerging approach in which the intensity of stimulation to the paretic finger and thumb extensors is proportionally controlled by an instrumented glove worn on the opposite (contralateral) hand (**Fig. 54-1A**). With the glove, the patient is able to control the degree of opening of their affected hand and practice using it in task-oriented therapy (13). A recent study showed CCFES to improve hand dexterity more than cyclic NMES (**Fig. 54-1B**). Another proportionally controlled NMES approach uses EMG signals from the impaired upper limb to deliver proportionally controlled stimulation (14). Proportionally controlled NMES may be more efficacious than other NMES methods because the approach capitalizes on the principle of intention-driven movement, linking the patient's motor commands to the stimulated movement and the resulting proprioceptive feedback to the brain. Proportionally controlled stimulators are not yet commercially available.

A recent review of 31 randomized controlled trials (RCTs) concluded that there is strong evidence that NMES applied in the context of task practice improves volitional upper extremity function in subacute and chronic stroke (15). This is corroborated by a recent meta-analysis of 18 RCTs (9 were upper limb studies) that concluded that NMES-assisted task training has a large therapeutic effect on upper limb activity compared with training alone (12). The most recent guidelines published by the American Heart Association recommend NMES in combination with task-specific training for stroke rehabilitation (16). The type of motor improvements that have been reported with NMES includes reductions in motor impairment (e.g., improvements in grip and extension strength, volitional EMG activity, Fugl-Meyer scores, active range of motion of wrist and fingers, spasticity) and improvements in motor function (e.g., Box and Blocks Test scores, Action Research Arm Test scores, Arm Motor Abilities Test scores, timed tasks). The persistence and magnitude of therapeutic effects are greatest in patients who have moderate to mild impairment and are less than 2 years poststroke when receiving treatment (13,17).

Only a few studies have directly compared NMES modalities. One such study of 122 subacute (≤6 months) stroke survivors found no significant differences between cyclic NMES, EMG-triggered NMES, and submotor threshold sensory stimulation, on upper limb function (18), a finding that confirmed

FIGURE 54-1. A: Contralaterally controlled functional electrical stimulation (CCFES) system in hemiparesis. Stimulation of the impaired right upper extremity is controlled via sensor glove worn on the left upper extremity. (Courtesy of Jayme S. Knutson, PhD, Cleveland FES Center.) **B:** Outcomes of CCFES and cyclic NMES (cNMES) groups for participants less than 2 years poststroke (and >6 months poststroke). Change in (*1*) Box and Block Test (BBT), (*2*) upper extremity Fugl-Meyer (UEFM), and (*3*) Arm Motor Abilities Test (AMAT). m, moderate hand impairment at baseline; s, severe hand impairment at baseline. (Data from Knutson JS, Gunzler DD, Wilson RD, et al. Contralaterally controlled functional electrical stimulation improves hand dexterity in chronic hemiparesis: a randomized trial. *Stroke*. 2016;47:2596–2602.)

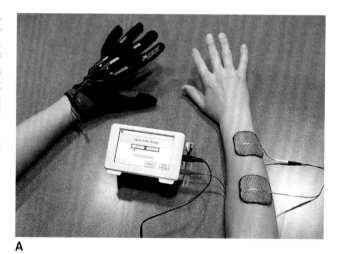

A

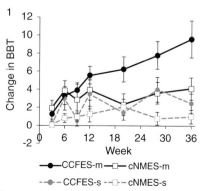
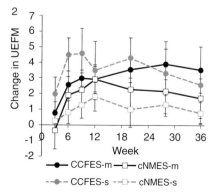
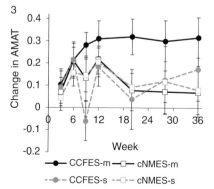

B

previous smaller studies (19,20). However, a recent study of 80 chronic (>6 months) patients found that CCFES improved hand dexterity more than cyclic NMES (13), which agrees with earlier CCFES studies in subacute patients (21,22). This finding suggests that effectiveness may depend on NMES modality.

While cyclic NMES and EMG- or switch-triggered NMES are commercially available, a clinically viable upper extremity neuroprosthesis for daily long-term use as an assistive device is not commercially available at the present time. Implantable microstimulator (23) or multichannel implantable pulse generator (24) approaches may be suitable long term, for stroke patients who have been carefully screened for prohibitive flexor hypertonia. Emerging technology, such as high-frequency stimulation to suppress hypertonia (25), and control strategies that provide seamless and intuitive methods by which patients control stimulation to their affected arm and hand are needed to successfully implement upper limb neuroprostheses in stroke.

Spinal Cord Injury

For individuals with tetraplegia after mid–cervical level SCI, restoration of hand function is their top priority (26) (see also Chapter 22). Patients with complete SCIs will typically not recover adequate volitional function even with NMES therapies; therefore, FES assistive devices are needed that can be used long term and produce significant neuroprosthetic effects. These systems may also be applicable to patients who do not adequately recover upper limb function after incomplete SCI or stroke. The existing alternatives for providing hand function for these individuals are limited, including braces, orthotics, and adapted equipment. Surgical interventions, such as tendon transfers, can be used to provide increased hand and arm function (27,28). However, neuroprostheses provide the most promising method for significant gain in hand and arm function for cervical level SCI (29). With FES, muscle contractions can be orchestrated to produce coordinated grasp opening and closing; thumb opening, closing, and positioning; wrist extension/flexion; forearm pronation; and elbow extension for individuals with fifth cervical (C5) and sixth cervical (C6) level SCI. The individual controls the coordinated muscle stimulation through movement of their voluntary musculature.

Neuroprostheses can be coupled with tendon transfers in order to maximize function (30). The objectives of these neuroprostheses are to reduce the need of individuals to rely on assistance from others, reduce the need for adaptive equipment, reduce the need to wear braces or other orthotic devices, and reduce the time it takes to perform tasks.

The first upper extremity neuroprostheses were developed in the 1960s using surface electrodes, in combination with a flexor hinge splint to open and close the hands of individuals with cervical SCI (31). This pioneering work led to the development and clinical testing of several surface NMES upper extremity neuroprostheses in SCI patients (32–34), but these systems have not been utilized for long-term function. Therefore, implanted neuroprostheses have been developed for permanent use.

The implanted stimulator-telemeter 12-channel (IST12) system is an implanted upper extremity FES system that has been evaluated in clinical trials conducted by researchers at Case Western Reserve University (CWRU) in Cleveland (35). This group has been developing implanted upper extremity neuroprostheses for SCI patients since 1986, when they implemented the first implanted hand grasp neuroprosthesis in a human volunteer (36,37). The IST12 system is an advanced version of the Freehand system, which underwent extensive assessment of clinical outcomes, received FDA approval for use in C5 and C6 tetraplegia, and was commercially available from 1997 to 2002. The IST12 system consists of a receiver/stimulator that is surgically implanted in the upper pectoral region and 12 epimysial and/or intramuscular electrodes implanted on or in the paralyzed muscles of the forearm and hand (**Fig. 54-2A**). An external radio-frequency (RF) coil transmits commands and power to the stimulator from an external control unit.

This implanted system approach was shown, in the multicenter clinical trial of the 8-channel Freehand system, to improve pinch force in every recipient (n = 50), grasp-release abilities in 98% of the participants, and independence in at least one task in 100% of the participants (38). More than 90% of the participants were satisfied with the neuroprosthesis and most used it regularly (39). Complication rates have been similar to the rates for pacemakers and include infection (<2%) and electrode lead failure (<1%) (40,41).

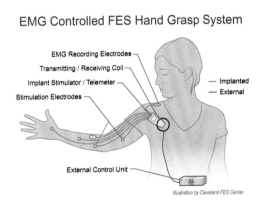

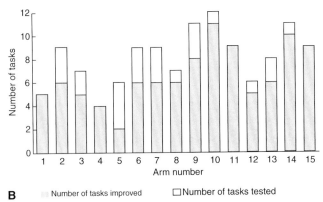

FIGURE 54-2. **A:** IST12 system for upper extremity function. (Courtesy of the Cleveland FES Center, Cleveland, OH.) **B:** Activities of daily living ability test performance across all arms in all subjects in the IST12 study. (Data from Kilgore KL. Hand grasp and reach in spinal cord injury. In: Kilgore K, ed. *Implantable Neuroprostheses for Restoring Function.* Cambridge: Elsevier; 2015:210–235.)

The IST12 system builds on the clinical success of the Freehand system by providing additional stimulus channels and incorporating implanted EMG control methods (35,42). The additional channels are used to activate hand intrinsic muscles, triceps, or pronator quadratus. Adding these muscles produces better hand opening, improved grasp-release function, increased reachable workspace, and better ability to orient the hand for tasks. The implanted EMG-recording electrodes eliminate the external shoulder-mounted transducer that was used to control hand opening and closing in the original Freehand system. Two EMG electrodes are implanted on muscles that the patient is able to contract and relax, for example, extensor carpi radialis longus or brachioradialis. A control algorithm then uses the EMG signals to enable the user to have proportional control of hand opening and closing. Because the EMG control strategy makes use of muscle signals derived from the ipsilateral side, it allows the neuroprosthesis to be implemented bilaterally (43).

The IST12 system has undergone clinical testing in 15 arms, in 12 individuals with C5 or C6 tetraplegia. Three of these participants had two systems implanted, one for each upper limb, in order to enable bimanual task performance. The longest follow-up has been 15 years. The functional results show that the neuroprosthesis provides significantly increased pinch force and grasp function for each research participant (43). All 12 participants (15 arms) demonstrated increased independence in at least 2 activities of daily living (**Fig. 54-2B**); 93% improved in 4 or more activities (44) with 1 demonstrating improvements in 11 out of 12 activities tested and 2 others demonstrating improvement in 9 out of 9 activities tested. Research participants with bilateral systems were able to perform activities such as using a fork and knife to cut food, using two hands to screw and unscrew a lid on a jar, and brushing the hair while blow-drying (43).

Current research topics in upper extremity neuroprostheses include incorporating proximal muscles for patients with higher cervical SCI to enable both arm and hand function (45) and evaluating alternative control inputs such as head orientation and movement (46), eye movements, and cortical signals (47), which may allow users to control stimulated limbs more naturally. Advances are also being made to eliminate all external components by implanting the control technology and powering the stimulator with a rechargeable implantable battery. Now in clinical trials at CWRU is a modular, totally implanted neuroprosthesis that can provide multiple functions, for example, upper and lower limb function, trunk support, and bladder, bowel, and diaphragm function (29). This "networked neuroprosthesis" is scalable to provide additional and advanced functions by adding different components, for example, stimulator and sensor modules. The advantage of the system is that multiple applications can be implemented in a single patient without the need for multiple devices that are specially designed for single applications and are difficult to integrate or upgrade (48). Also, two separate research groups recently conducted case studies of participants with tetraplegia from cervical SCI who had microelectrode arrays implanted in the hand area of the motor cortex and FES systems that produced arm and hand (49) or just hand movement (50). The participant in each study was able to control, via brain-computer interface (BCI) technology, the FES system and was able to perform functional tasks that require reaching, grasping,

and releasing objects, such as drinking from a mug and feeding oneself. These advances are expected to enhance and provide additional function, broaden the clinical indications, and facilitate clinical implementation.

Lower Extremity

There have been three main objectives in the application of NMES systems to the lower extremity: (a) eliminate foot drop and improve gait in poststroke hemiplegia, (b) enable standing and transfer after SCI, and (c) enable walking after SCI. Some of these approaches are being expanded to additional conditions, including multiple sclerosis (MS) and cerebral palsy.

Stroke

In the lower limb, hemiparesis, along with the inability to grade muscle contractions, poor motor coordination, poor endurance, spasticity, and impaired balance, has significant consequences on poststroke ambulation. At 6 months poststroke, approximately 30% of stroke survivors are unable to walk unassisted (51). Diminished ankle dorsiflexion, knee flexion, or hip flexion on one side can result in the inability to clear the floor with the affected limb during the swing phase of gait, resulting in difficult and unsafe ambulation or nonambulation.

Foot drop systems produce ankle dorsiflexion and eversion during the swing phase of gait by stimulating the peroneal nerve. There are three FDA-cleared NMES foot drop systems commercially available: Odstock dropped foot stimulator (ODFS, Odstock Medical, Ltd), WalkAide (Innovative Neurotronics, Inc.), and NESS L300 (Bioness, Inc.). All three systems use surface electrodes, with the active electrode placed over the common peroneal nerve just below the head of the fibula and the return (i.e., reference) electrode placed over the tibialis anterior. To synchronize the timing of stimulation to the swing phase of gait, these devices utilize either a wireless heel switch worn in the shoe of the paretic limb or a tilt sensor below the knee (52,53). Two foot drop systems with implanted electrodes and stimulator are commercially available in Europe. One is a dual-channel device (STIMuSTEP, Finetech Medical, Ltd) that stimulates the deep and superficial branches of the common peroneal nerve for better control of ankle dorsiflexion, eversion, and inversion (54,55). The other is a four-channel device (ActiGait, OttoBock) that uses a nerve cuff electrode surgically placed around the common peroneal nerve (56).

Peroneal nerve stimulation during gait has positive neuroprosthetic and therapeutic effects on ambulation. Neuroprosthetic effects have been shown in a number of case series studies and several RCTs, with improvements made on measures ranging from gait kinematic and spatiotemporal parameters to metabolic cost indices (52,53,57). A recent multicenter clinical trial of 99 chronic patients showed that after 42 weeks of peroneal nerve stimulation during gait, 67% of participants had a gain of ≥ 0.1 m/s (the minimal clinically important difference) in comfortable gait speed when walking with peroneal nerve stimulation (58). Therapeutic effects associated with peroneal nerve stimulation during gait have also been observed since the earliest studies. Such effects include improvements in ambulation function, normalization of EMG muscle activation patterns, emergence of EMG signals in previously silent muscles, and decreased cocontraction of antagonist muscles (52,53,59–61).

After 30 weeks of peroneal nerve stimulation during gait, 29% of 99 chronic stroke patients had a therapeutic effect on comfortable walking speed of ≥0.1 m/s (58).

Recently, four large RCTs compared the effects of a surface foot drop stimulator to an ankle-foot orthosis (AFO), which is usual care. Three of these studies evaluated participants after the subacute phase and demonstrated that peroneal nerve stimulation produced both therapeutic and neuroprosthetic improvements in gait that were comparable to an AFO (3,62,63). The fourth study focused on patients less than a year poststroke to capitalize on greater potential for early improvement (64). Again, the foot drop stimulator produced results similar to an AFO. Although the foot drop stimulator was not better than an AFO, these studies demonstrated noninferiority. When participants were asked about device preference, the majority preferred the foot drop stimulator to an AFO because they felt more confident, safer, and more comfortable and found the foot drop stimulator is easier to don and doff and use long term (65).

Multichannel NMES systems have been developed to address gait deficits that are not limited to ankle dysfunction but also involve impaired motor control at the hip and knee. Early work used surface electrodes and demonstrated improvements in qualitative and quantitative measures of gait after training with a 6-channel system that activated ankle, knee, and hip muscles (66). Recently, the NESS L300 Plus (Bioness, Inc.) has become available commercially, having two channels of stimulation—one for ankle dorsiflexion and another for knee flexion or extension. This may be useful if a patient cannot generate sufficient knee flexion for toe clearance during swing or knee extension for loading and stance (67). Multichannel percutaneous intramuscular electrode systems in combination with body weight–supported treadmill training have also shown positive therapeutic effects on gait kinematics (68).

An implanted multijoint lower extremity neuroprosthesis may provide long-term ambulation assistance on a daily basis in patients who need assistance at the hip, knee, and ankle. Recently, a case study of an 8-channel implanted stimulator with intramuscular electrodes implanted in hip, knee, and ankle muscles and with heel switch–triggered stimulation sequences for swing and stance demonstrated significant neuroprosthetic effect on walking speed (>0.2 m/s) and associated improvements in gait kinematics (69).

Spinal Cord Injury

For persons with paraplegia due to thoracic or lower cervical level SCI, standing from a seated position and transferring to another surface independently are primary objectives of some FES systems. The functional goals associated with standing include reaching for high objects, having face-to-face interactions with other people, performing tasks that require standing, and transferring between surfaces (e.g., bed to wheelchair and back) independently or with only minimal assistance.

An implanted neuroprosthesis for standing and transferring (70) being developed and evaluated in clinical trials at CWRU and the Cleveland VA Medical Center (CWRU/VA) uses an 8-channel implantable stimulator (37). Epimysial or intramuscular electrodes are implanted bilaterally on the vastus lateralis (knee extension), gluteus maximus (hip extension), semimembranosus (hip extension), and erector spinae (trunk extension).

The stimulator is implanted in the anterior lower abdomen. The user triggers stimulation by pressing a button mounted on a walker, which is used to assist with balance. An external control unit worn around the waist communicates with the stimulator through an RF-transmitting coil. When the button is pressed, a short delay allows the participant to comfortably position their hands on the walker before stimulation to the trunk, hip, and knee extensors increases to a level sufficient to raise the body from the seated position and maintain continuous standing. Another press of the button reverses the process and lowers the participant to a seated position in a controlled fashion.

In a case series study of 15 research participants with C6-T9 SCI, the CWRU/VA standing system achieved standing in all participants (71). On average, the subjects supported more than 85% of their body weight on their legs and could stand for 10 minutes. While standing, some participants were able to release one hand from the walker and reach objects overhead. Some were even able to use the system for limited swing-through gait with a walker. The neuroprosthesis also reduced the effort and assistance required to transfer, especially from a lower surface to a higher one. Use of the device had secondary benefits on general health and quality of life as well (72,73). Stimulation thresholds were stable, and internal components proved to be reliable with survival rates of epimysial electrodes in the extremities approaching 95% (74). At 1 year follow-up, during a 28-day monitoring period, data from 12 participants showed the device continued to be used by 11 of the 12 participants. Of the 11 who continued to use the device, the number of days used out of 28 ranged from 3 to 26 (average, 13.8 days). This is equivalent to an average of approximately 3.5 days a week. The total number of hours the device was used during the 28 days ranged from 0.1 to 48.6 (average, 12.4 hours). The average hours used per day ranged from 0 to 1.9 (average, 0.7 hours/day); 20% of the usage time was spent standing and 80% was spent exercising (71).

To increase maximum standing duration and reduce variability across patients, researchers at CWRU/VA are using stimulators with more channels to activate more muscles and/or more fully activate muscles using multicontact cuff electrodes on the femoral nerve (75). Also, advanced closed-loop controllers are being developed to enable patients to maintain balance longer by automatically adjusting the stimulation intensities when the patient is bumped or desires to maintain a leaning posture (76,77).

Stepping has been achieved with surface and implanted FES systems. These systems work by delivering preprogrammed patterns of stimulation that produce stepping movements in response to pressing buttons mounted to a walker. A single button press may initiate a repetitive cycle of stimulation, producing continuous stepping; or each successive step can be triggered by sequential button presses. The Parastep system (Sigmedics, Inc.) is an FDA-approved surface FES system that uses six channels of bilateral surface stimulation of the quadriceps, peroneal nerves, and glutei (78). A stride is produced by stimulating the quadriceps of one leg while initiating a flexion withdrawal reflex in the opposite leg by stimulating the peroneal nerve. To complete the stride, the knee extensors on the swinging leg are activated while the reflex is still flexing the hip. When stimulation that produces the flexion withdrawal reflex is turned off, the user is one step forward in double-limb support with bilateral quadriceps stimulation on. Parastep has been fitted to more than 1,000 people with SCI, with the majority achieving standing and at least 30 ft of ambulation (79). In spite of its ease of operation, the Parastep approach has limited applications for mobility in daily life because of its modest immediate benefit, lack of or habituation of adequate flexion withdrawal reflex, and high metabolic cost of walking (78).

Implanted FES systems may be a more effective way of providing functional ambulation. Rather than eliciting a reflex to produce stepping, an 8- or 16-channel neuroprosthesis stimulates multiple hip, knee, and ankle muscles. A case study of an individual with complete paraplegia, who was unable to stand prior to implant, received a 16-channel implanted FES system that enabled him to stand and walk short distances (80). But such a neuroprosthesis may have its greatest impact in people with motor incomplete injuries. Two individuals with incomplete SCI received an implanted 8-channel stimulator and after training experienced therapeutic effects that enabled them to walk with a walker without stimulation (81,82). In addition, when walking with stimulation, substantial neuroprosthetic benefits were realized, including increased walking speed (**Fig. 54-3**), distance, endurance, and joint kinematics. Another participant with incomplete SCI received a 12-channel stimulator with EMG-recording electrodes on the right gastrocnemius and quadriceps, which were used to trigger successive steps and resulted in greater walking speed and distance than a preprogrammed cyclic stimulation pattern (83). Two more research participants with incomplete SCI have implanted neuroprostheses with stepping that are triggered by accelerometers that detect walker placement or bilateral forearm crutch strike (84).

Some practical difficulties using NMES in general, but particularly for walking, include insufficient (depending on body mass) force production, fatigue of stimulated muscle, and limited ability to smoothly grade the force of contraction. These limitations are related in part to the fact that with NMES, large fast-fatiguing muscle fibers are recruited before low-force fatigue-resistant fibers (85), which is opposite of the natural order (i.e., physiologic size principle (86)). Techniques to mitigate these potential difficulties depend on the specific application, but most applications that involve chronically implanted NMES systems define a muscle conditioning protocol that is

designed to convert fast-twitch fast-fatiguing fibers to more fatigue-resistant fibers (87). Since fatigue occurs more rapidly with increasing stimulus pulse frequencies, the pulse frequency should be reduced to that just required to produce a fused muscle contraction (1). To increase force production from large muscles (i.e., quadriceps), recruitment of more motor units is possible with nerve cuff electrodes placed more proximally than intramuscular electrodes (75). Fatigue can also be delayed with multicontact nerve cuff electrodes that selectively activate independent motor unit pools of the same muscle in a sequence, allowing some motor units to rest while other motor units are active (88).

Hybrid neuroprosthetic systems combine FES with passive or powered bracing to reduce the energy required for walking and improve endurance, stability, and torque generation (89). For example, combining multijoint implanted FES with a variable impedance knee mechanism to provide stiffness in stance and freedom to move during swing reduced the intensity of stimulation needed for knee extension during stance (90). Likewise, a variable hip restraint reduced both forward lean and load on the upper limbs (91). Similarly, combining a hip and knee state-controlled brace with multijoint FES improved the stand-to-sit transition in SCI participants over FES alone (92). Other hybrid approaches combine motorized exoskeletons with surface FES. Surface FES applied to knee flexors and extensors reduces the necessary torque output from motors at the hip and knee relative to the motorized exoskeleton alone (93).

STIMULATION FOR RESPIRATORY FUNCTION

Respiratory complications remain among the most significant medical challenges faced by persons with neurologic sources of disability such as SCI, amyotrophic lateral sclerosis (ALS), and multiple sclerosis (see also Chapter 34). In SCI, pneumonia and septicemia continue to be the greatest contributors to decreased life expectancy (94). Persons with high cervical SCI may suffer from lost diaphragm function, which is innervated by phrenic nerve fibers stemming primarily from the C4 nerve root, as well as C3, C5, and potentially C6 roots (95). Therefore, high tetraplegia may result in respiratory failure requiring ventilatory assistance. Chronic mechanical ventilation is associated with several challenges, including substantial morbidity and mortality, encumbered mobility and physical discomfort, fear of social disconnection, difficulty with speech, and impaired sense of smell (96). Both tetraplegia and paraplegia may also result in loss of cough function.

Phrenic Nerve Stimulation for Inspiratory Function

Phrenic nerve pacing allows for decreased or even discontinued use of mechanical ventilation, and multiple reports have been published of positive user feedback (97–100). The Avery Mark IV Breathing Pacemaker system (Avery Biomedical Devices) and the Atrostim Phrenic Nerve Stimulator (97,101) (Atrotech Ltd) are two RF receiver/stimulator systems in clinical implementation (**Fig. 54-4**). In one long-term follow-up study of the Avery system in 12 persons with tetraplegia, 6 continued to use it full time (mean 13.7 years), 1 used it part time, and 3 stopped using it (102). An international study of 64 patients using the Atrostim system showed 94% of the 35 pediatric patients and 86% of the 29 adult patients eventually achieved complication-free successful pacing (103).

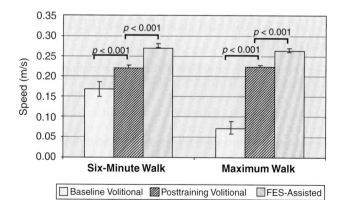

FIGURE 54-3. Walking speed during 6-minute walk test and maximum walk test improved posttraining compared with baseline volitional; speed additionally improved with functional electrical stimulation (FES). (Data from Bailey SN, Hardin EC, Kobetic R, et al. Neurotherapeutic and neuroprosthetic effects of implanted functional electrical stimulation for ambulation after incomplete spinal cord injury. *J Rehabil Res Dev.* 2010;47(1):7–16, with permission.)

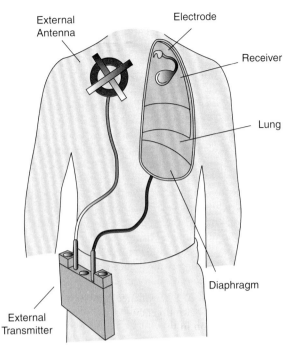

External Antenna

Electrode

Receiver

Lung

Diaphragm

External Transmitter

FIGURE 54-4. Avery Breathing Pacemaker system. (Courtesy of Avery Biomedical Devices, Commack, NY.)

Both systems involve bilateral synchronous stimulation of the phrenic nerves, causing contraction and descent of each hemidiaphragm, which subsequently drops intrathoracic pressure and induces inspiration. Cessation of stimulation results in relaxation of the diaphragm, an increase in intrathoracic pressure, and exhalation. Before implantation, a fluoroscopic examination of the chest is performed to verify adequate diaphragmatic excursion in response to stimulation (104). Surgical placement of the electrodes behind or over the phrenic nerves is achieved by accessing the nerves through a thoracic or cervical approach. The stimulator is positioned in a subcutaneous pocket on the anterior chest wall. Approximately 2 weeks after implantation, diaphragmatic reconditioning is achieved with low-frequency stimulation (105), followed by gradually increasing pacing times (96).

For patients with only a single intact phrenic nerve, it may be possible to achieve respiration by activating the inspiratory intercostal muscles in addition to the functioning phrenic nerve (106). In cases of significant injury to both phrenic nerves, an intercostal to phrenic nerve transfer may restore phrenic nerve viability and return possibility for diaphragm pacing (107).

Minimally invasive laparoscopic approaches may be used to position intramuscular electrodes bilaterally near the motor points of each hemidiaphragm for direct stimulation of the diaphragm (108). The NeuRx DPS system (Synapse Biomedical, Inc.), a percutaneous diaphragm pacing system (DPS), has been prospectively studied in at least 50 persons with SCI. Over 90% of the SCI subjects studied achieved significant independence from mechanical ventilation, and over 50% eliminated mechanical ventilation. This percutaneous system is also being studied as a means of prolonging survival in patients with ALS who already have chronic hypoventilation but have intact lower motor neurons innervating the diaphragm bilaterally.

Magnetic stimulation via magnetic coil placed over the C7-T1 or T9-T10 spinous processes is an alternative

noninvasive technique for inspiratory and expiratory muscle conditioning, respectively (109). Preliminary findings of this work are promising, with improvements in a variety of respiratory parameters, including peak inspiratory flow and peak expiratory flow. It remains to be demonstrated, however, whether this work can decrease caregiver burden—or do so sufficiently to offset the cost and complexity of investigating this work.

Restoration of Cough Function

The ability to clear secretions through effective cough is a crucial function for persons with neurologic disability and is frequently impaired in conditions such as SCI. Restoration of cough function has been achieved with electrical stimulation through 4-mm disk electrodes placed at the T9, T11, and L1 levels (midline) via hemilaminectomy incisions and routed to an RF stimulator/receiver implanted in the anterior chest wall (110,111). Recent long-term follow-up of a series of 10 persons with SCI by DiMarco et al. (112) using lower thoracic spinal cord stimulation (SCS) indicated continued maintenance of mean maximum airway pressures after 1 year and a mean of 4.6 years after implantation. This study indicated a significantly lower incidence of acute respiratory tract infections compared to preimplant levels, decreased caregiver training burden, and improved secretion clearance and respiratory care–related life quality.

Other Applications

Several other electrical stimulation approaches have been applied for pulmonary function. Work by Walter et al. (113) in animal models recently combined multiple sources of extradiaphragmatic muscle group stimulation; large respiratory responses were achieved, indicating potential for clinical implementation. Animal models indicate the potential for using high-frequency SCS to restore cough (114) or inspiratory function, potentially presenting an alternative to phrenic and diaphragmatic pacing techniques (115). Sleep apnea is treatable with electrical stimulation: the INSPIRE device (116) (Inspire Medical Systems, Inc.) is a clinically available sleep apnea electrical stimulation system; further investigation is needed to understand its range of applications in persons with neurologic disability.

STIMULATION FOR BLADDER AND BOWEL FUNCTION

Neurogenic bladder and bowel functions are among the most significant medical issues for persons with neurologic disability, particularly in SCI (26,117) (see also Chapter 22). Neurogenic bladder dysfunction can result in urinary tract infection (UTI), renal deterioration, bladder or kidney stones, urinary incontinence with skin injury and social isolation, and autonomic dysreflexia. Neurogenic bowel dysfunction can similarly result in skin injury, social isolation, autonomic dysreflexia, and structural injury to the bowel.

Sacral Anterior Root Stimulation: Finetech-Brindley Approach

The Finetech-Brindley Bladder Control system (118) (Finetech Medical, Ltd, Hertfordshire, UK) (**Fig. 54-5**) is an implanted system that enables micturition by producing a bladder

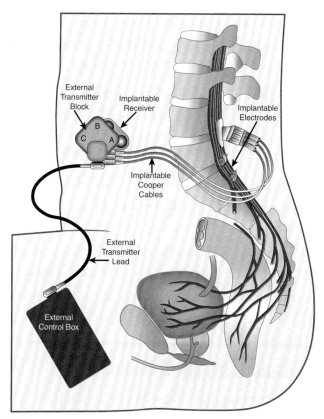

FIGURE 54-5. Finetech-Brindley Bladder Control system. (Courtesy of Finetech Medical, Ltd, Hertfordshire, UK.)

contraction with stimulation of the sacral anterior spinal nerve roots. Although not currently being implanted in the United States, the system has been implanted in more than 2,500 patients in at least 20 countries (119,120).

The electrodes are implanted bilaterally on the sacral spinal nerve roots either intradurally on the anterior (motor) roots in the cauda equina via a lower lumbar laminectomy (121) or extradurally on the mixed sacral nerves in the sacral canal via a laminectomy of S1-S3 (122). Bilateral posterior rhizotomies of the S2-S4 spinal nerves are usually performed to eliminate involuntary detrusor contractions (associated with neurogenic detrusor overactivity) and improve continence. While these interventions allow implantation of the system and reduction in side effects, they also add to the invasiveness and irreversibility of the approach.

The system is generally well-tolerated and effective, with a multicenter study reporting greater than 85% of implant recipients choosing to use the system as the primary means of bladder emptying and a similar percentage of continence achieved (119,120). Residual volume in the bladder was low, with decreases in UTI frequency (119,123). Satisfaction with the system has been reported to be high (124), an infection rate of about 1% in the first 500 implants, and the hardware was reported to be reliable with an average of one failure per 20 implant years (125). Cost savings are described due to less medication, supply use, and complications (126).

Bowel evacuation and penile erection are secondary uses of the Finetech-Brindley Bladder system. Some users are able to defecate by using longer intervals between bursts of stimulation to allow passage of stool, and decreased laxative use has been reported (127). Penile erection has been reported with intradural (120) and extradural root stimulation (128), with reports indicating higher percentages of erectile function from intradural stimulation.

Nonselective Sacral Root Stimulation

Bladder inhibition and continence can be improved in some patients by nonselectively stimulating sacral nerves, in contrast with the selective anterior root stimulation associated with rhizotomy of the Brindley approach. Kirkham et al. (129) investigated sacral nerve root stimulation with a Finetech-Brindley stimulator to increase bladder capacity without rhizotomy, although there was some concern of detrusor-sphincter dyssynergia, with inhibition likely achieved through afferent-mediated pathways. Concurrent activation of motor nerves to the sphincter may also assist in maintaining continence; however, the external sphincter fatigues rapidly with chronic stimulation.

There is evidence that continence can be improved in some *able-bodied* subjects with urgency, frequency, and urge incontinence by stimulation in the S3 foramen (Medtronic InterStim device) (130). Recent evaluation of the InterStim in multiple sclerosis suggests potential use of sacral neuromodulation strategies in other populations with neurogenic bladder such as SCI (131). Further investigation is needed, however, as the powerful bladder spasticity encountered in SCI may require stronger and more direct inhibition. Sacral neuromodulation has also been used to effect bowel function in certain populations such as idiopathic fecal incontinence (132). As with bladder function, however, further investigation is needed to evaluate its potential for persons with neurogenic bowel.

Tibial Nerve Stimulation

Percutaneous electrical stimulation of the tibial nerve, proximal and posterior to the medial malleolus, may be clinically conducted in the office setting for management of overactive bladder. Studies are being conducted to elucidate the mechanisms by which the technique achieves afferent-mediated neuromodulation, resulting in reflex inhibition of the detrusor; of interest are the overlapping spinal levels of the detrusor (receiving S2-S4 parasympathetic innervation) and the tibial nerve (L4-S3 spinal levels). Work in multiple sclerosis (133) highlights its potential for bladder management in neurologically injured populations. Further studies are required to evaluate whether episodic tibial stimulation can have a lasting impact on the powerful bladder spasticity seen in SCI and other conditions resulting in neurogenic bladder dysfunction.

Research Approaches to Neurogenic Bladder Management

A number of electrical stimulation laboratories are investigating alternative methods to obtain less invasive means of applying electrical stimulation to obtain neural control and thereby enhance the potential for near-term clinical translation.

Genital Nerve Stimulation

A promising approach to inhibiting bladder contractions and improving continence involves surface stimulation of the genital nerve (**Fig. 54-6**), a terminal branch of the pudendal nerve.

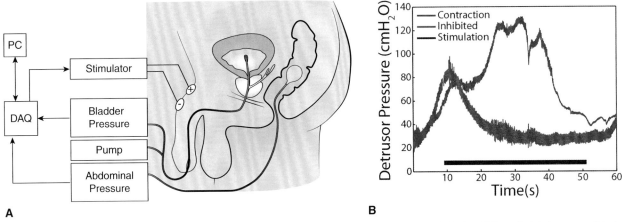

FIGURE 54-6. Genital nerve stimulation (GNS) acutely inhibits bladder contractions. **A:** Typical testing of GNS. Surface GNS applied during acute clinical urodynamics testing. Urethral and anal catheters measure bladder and abdominal pressures, respectively. A host computer (PC) controls data acquisition (DAQ) and stimulation. Two surface electrodes placed on the dorsum of the penis in males (clitoris in females) target the genital nerves. (From: Brose SW, Bourbeau DJ, Gustafson KJ. Genital nerve stimulation is tolerable and effective for bladder inhibition in sensate individuals with incomplete SCI. *J Spinal Cord Med.* 2018;41:1–8. Reprinted by permission of Taylor & Francis Ltd. http://www.tandfonline.com) **B:** An example of bladder inhibition in a patient with SCI. The bladder reflexively contracts during filling (*blue* (*top*) = control). When GNS is applied (*black bar bottom*), the hyperreflexic bladder contraction is inhibited (*red lower*). (From: Bourbeau DJ, Gustafson KJ, Brose SW. At-home genital nerve stimulation for individuals with SCI and neurogenic detrusor overactivity: a feasibility plot study. *J Spinal Cord Med.* 2018:1–11. Reprinted by permission of Taylor & Francis Ltd. http://www.tandfonline.com)

This surface sensory nerve stimulation technique, achieved through surface electrodes placed on the base of the penis or clitoris, is thought to induce bladder inhibition by activating sensory afferents that travel through the pudendal nerves and enter the spinal cord through the sacral dorsal root ganglia (134,135). Multiple studies during acute urodynamic procedures have demonstrated its effectiveness in inhibiting bladder contractions in persons with SCI-related neurogenic detrusor overactivity (136,137). It has been shown to be well-tolerated, even in persons with incomplete SCI who have sensation present in the area of electrical stimulation (138). Early longer-term/take-home studies in SCI are promising, providing a nonpharmacologic and noninvasive alternative to medical and surgical management for neurogenic bladder (139,140). Genital nerve stimulation has been demonstrated to reduce episodes of idiopathic fecal incontinence (141), but additional studies are needed for applications in neurogenic bowel dysfunction.

Other Techniques

A variety of other techniques have been investigated to manage different aspects of neurogenic bladder dysfunction. *Epidural spinal cord stimulation* is among the most promising approaches. The approach is capable of inducing urinary voiding in animal models (142). Work in human subjects has also indicated possible improvements in bladder, bowel, and sexual function (143). *Intraurethral stimulation* is a novel approach that has been demonstrated in animal (144) and human (145) models to induce bladder contractions without need for spinal surgery through stimulation of pudendal afferent fibers. *High-frequency pudendal nerve block* has potential to achieve inhibition of the external urethral sphincter; in combination with sacral root stimulation, it may remove the need for rhizotomy (146). *Dermatomal afferent stimulation* to decrease outlet resistance and allow voiding in chronic SCI in conjunction with sacral root stimulation has been demonstrated in animal models for the chronic management of neurogenic bladder (147). Early human SCI work indicates need for further investigation of the stimulus parameter space to achieve clinical viability (148).

ELECTRICAL STIMULATION FOR PAIN

Transcutaneous Electrical Nerve Stimulation

Transcutaneous electrical nerve stimulation (TENS) is a nonpharmacologic pain intervention in which an electrical current is delivered through the intact skin surface to peripheral sensory nerves to reduce pain (see also Chapter 39). TENS is commonly delivered by a portable, battery-powered electronic pulse generator that provides low-voltage electrical current through transcutaneous electrodes. The mechanism of pain relief associated with TENS is controversial, but it is believed that different analgesic effects can be produced by selectively activating different populations of afferents via different electrical stimulation parameters. The afferent stimulation is thought to alter the function of the peripheral and central nervous system to produce analgesia (149). Optimal settings for a TENS device are determined based on the symptomatic response of the individual patient. The parameters for TENS include stimulation intensity (0 to 50 mA), pulse frequency (range 1 to 250 Hz), and pulse duration (10 to 1,000 µs). While many different TENS or TENS-like techniques have been described in the literature, the most commonly prescribed include conventional, acupuncture-like, and intense TENS.

Conventional TENS is characterized by relatively high stimulation frequency (50 to 200 Hz) and low-intensity (submotor threshold) pulsed currents, with pulse duration between 100 and 200 µs and pulse amplitude adjusted to produce a strong comfortable paresthesia. The targeted nerves for conventional TENS are large diameter, low-threshold nonnoxious afferent (Aβ) nerve fibers in the painful dermatome (150). Stimulation of Aβ nerve fibers is believed to inhibit noxious pain information at the level of the dorsal horns of the spinal cord, preventing it from reaching the brain, thereby reducing the sensation of pain within the stimulated dermatome. Stimulation can be delivered whenever pain is experienced.

Acupuncture-like TENS is characterized by low-frequency (2 to 4 Hz), higher-intensity stimulation with longer pulse durations (100 to 400 µs) delivered through surface electrodes over motor points within the myotome that is associated with pain. Stimulation amplitude is adjusted to a level that produces a muscle contraction. The targeted nerve fibers are Aα efferent fibers, which induce a muscle twitch. If the low stimulation frequency is uncomfortable, bursts of pulses may be used to generate phasic contractions. The muscle contractions activate small diameter afferent fibers (Aδ or group III) within the muscle, which induce activation of descending pain inhibitory pathways (150).

Intense TENS is characterized by high-frequency (approximately 200 Hz), high-intensity (just tolerable) stimulation, with long pulse durations (1,000 μs) delivered via surface electrodes over peripheral nerves arising from the painful area. The targeted nerve fibers are small diameter cutaneous afferent (Aδ) fibers that produce peripheral block of nociceptive afferent activity (150). Stimulation is delivered for a few minutes at a time to act as a counterirritant, primarily during wound dressing changes or minor procedures that can be painful.

Interferential current therapy is a technique that is sometimes classified as TENS because it is typically delivered through surface electrodes. However, rather than a single pulsed current, two high-frequency (2,000 to 4,000 Hz) out-of-phase currents (carrier waves) are applied through two pairs of surface electrodes so that they interfere with each other to produce a low-amplitude–modulated wave with a frequency that is equal to the difference between the two carrier waves (151). The high-frequency carrier waves do not activate the cutaneous sensory nerves, making continuous stimulation more comfortable, while the resultant current penetrates deeper than conventional TENS, allowing activation of deeper nerves. The targeted nerves depend on the frequency of the resultant current. At 100 Hz, large diameter, low-threshold, nonnoxious afferent (Aβ) nerve fibers in the painful dermatome are stimulated, similar to conventional TENS, to reduce pain within that dermatome. At 15 Hz, afferent fibers (Aδ and C) are stimulated, which induce activation of descending pain inhibitory pathways (similar to acupuncture-like TENS) (151).

Indications for the use of TENS include both neurogenic pain (e.g., deafferentation pain, phantom pain, sympathetically mediated pain, postherpetic neuralgia, trigeminal neuralgia, atypical facial pain, brachial plexus avulsion) and musculoskeletal pain (e.g., joint pain, myofascial pain, acute posttraumatic pain). Placement of TENS electrodes is contraindicated on or near the eyes, in the mouth, transcerebrally, over the carotid sinuses (vasovagal reflex), on the anterior neck (laryngospasm), or on areas of decreased or absent sensation. TENS should not be used in epilepsy or pregnancy, on insensate skin, or in patients with an implanted electrical device, due to risk of interference or failure. Skin irritation and electrical burn are the most commonly reported complications, but in general, TENS is well-tolerated.

Despite widespread usage and a 50-year history as an adjunctive treatment to pharmacologic pain management, the therapeutic efficacy of TENS remains controversial. A systematic review (152) analyzed 25 RCTs (1,281 subjects) to determine the efficacy of TENS for chronic pain. In 13 of 22 controlled studies, there was a positive analgesic outcome in favor of TENS. Two systematic reviews (153,154) and a meta-analysis (155) were inconsistent on the effects of TENS on low back pain, with conclusions that ranged from not recommended (154) to effective (155). Similarly, one systematic review of 27 trials of electrical stimulation for pain relief in

knee osteoarthritis that included multiple TENS modalities did not find evidence to support pain relief with TENS (156), where another meta-analysis showed a significant reduction in knee pain due to osteoarthritis (157). A meta-analysis of three trials of TENS in treatment of painful diabetic polyneuropathy found pain reduction greater than that of placebo, along with improvement in secondary outcomes (158). In summary, TENS is a noninvasive, widely used modality for pain that is easy to apply with relatively few contraindications. There is mixed evidence due to methodologic quality and heterogeneity of studies within the literature that prevents clear guidance on how best to incorporate TENS into treatment of pain (159). High-quality RCTs remain necessary to definitively assess the therapeutic role of TENS in the management of pain.

Sensory Peripheral Nerve Stimulation

Implanted sensory peripheral nerve stimulation (sPNS) is utilized to stimulate sensory nerves for pain conditions in which there is a focal, chronic pain condition affecting one or two dermatomes. Electrode leads are placed beneath the skin near the target nerve to elicit paresthesias in the innervated territory. The electrodes can be placed with a needle introducer or by surgical dissection. Conditions treated by sPNS include headaches, complex regional pain syndrome (CRPS) type 2, and traumatic injury. In sensory peripheral nerve field stimulation (sPNfS), multiple electrodes can be placed within the region of maximal pain, where small distal branches of nerves are targeted within the subcutaneous space to elicit paresthesias in the painful region (160). sPNfS can stimulate a larger area and therefore is more commonly used to treat pain on the trunk, neck, or axial back. The mechanism of both techniques is thought to be the gate theory proposed by Melzack and Wall (161), though mechanisms similar to those of TENS may also be present. Initially, percutaneous electrodes are placed for a trial period of a few days or up to 2 weeks to evaluate pain reduction. If successful pain reduction is attained, often 50% pain relief, permanent leads are placed in the same region and connected to a permanent implantable pulse generator.

Limited research has been done to guide clinicians in the use of sPNS or sPNfS. The greatest amount of evidence is in the use of sPNS to treat chronic, refractory headache. The Congress of Neurological Surgeons performed a systematic review of the evidence and found nine nonrandomized trials in which sPNS was used to treat chronic occipital neuralgia (162). The conclusion of the review was that occipital nerve stimulation is recommended for chronic, refractory headache due to this condition. There is evidence for the use of occipital nerve stimulation for chronic, refractory migraine. A systematic review of 12 trials, in which 5 were RCTs, found efficacy when used in this population, though with a high rate of complications (66%). A RCT of severe, intractable pain of peripheral nerve origin from posttraumatic or postsurgical neuralgia found implanted sPNS to be effective in pain reduction (163).

Motor Peripheral Nerve Stimulation for Hemiplegic Shoulder Subluxation and Pain

Peripheral motor nerve stimulation has been used for the treatment of shoulder subluxation and pain following stroke. Poststroke shoulder dysfunction is characterized by early spasticity and weakness, which may progress over time to result in mechanical instability and diminished mobility at the glenohumeral joint. Even though it is not clear that poststroke shoulder subluxation is the cause of hemiplegic shoulder pain (HSP), treatment of subluxation continues to be the standard of care for treating HSP. In some patients, the subluxation is painful and reduction of subluxation improves pain. Shoulder subluxation may also interfere with recovery by limiting range of motion and therefore should be treated.

Surface NMES has been used to treat shoulder subluxation, often delivered through electrodes placed over the posterior deltoid and supraspinatus muscles for 6 hours daily for several weeks. Surface NMES is performed at frequencies between 35 and 50 Hz at an intensity that is comfortable and causes phasic muscle contractions (164). NMES applied to the shoulder has the ability to reduce poststroke shoulder subluxation during stimulation and may also provide long-term reduction of subluxation if it is combined with conventional therapy and begins within 6 months of the stroke (165). A meta-analysis determined that surface NMES applied to the shoulder and combined with conventional therapy prevented on an average 6.5 mm of shoulder subluxation as compared to 1.9 mm with conventional therapy alone (166). NMES may be beneficial for subluxation when used early after stroke (165). Although data suggest that surface NMES reduces shoulder subluxation, clinical implementation has been difficult due to the need for skilled personnel to ensure proper electrode placement and tolerable and reliable stimulation. This has limited the use of surface NMES for shoulder subluxation.

HSP, distinct from shoulder subluxation, is a frequent poststroke complication that is associated with a reduced quality of life for stroke survivors (167). The incidence of HSP may be 40% within the first 6 months poststroke (168). Surface NMES has long been utilized for HSP though there is little evidence for efficacy. A systematic review of all forms of electrical stimulation for shoulder pain, including surface NMES and TENS, did not find evidence that the addition of electrical stimulation to conventional therapy improved pain more than conventional therapy alone (169). A review and meta-analysis of 10 RCTs included nine studies evaluating the effect of NMES for HSP (165). Pooled analyses demonstrated no significant difference in pain compared to conventional therapy.

Percutaneous motor peripheral nerve stimulation (mPNS) to stimulate motor nerves with intramuscular electrodes is a treatment that has shown success in pain reduction for HSP. In a RCT, Yu et al. studied 61 chronic stroke survivors with shoulder pain and subluxation (170). The treatment group received percutaneous mPNS to stimulate the motor nerves of the supraspinatus, posterior deltoid, middle deltoid, and trapezius for 6 hours a day for 6 weeks. The treatment group exhibited a significant reduction in shoulder pain, which persisted for 6 months posttreatment, as compared to controls. A follow-up study found that pain reduction was maintained for $\geq$12 months posttreatment (171). Post hoc analysis revealed that treatment within 18 months of stroke was a predictor of treatment success (172). The percutaneous mPNS treatment has been simplified to 6 hours/day of stimulation via a single electrode for 3 weeks, with the target of stimulation being the axillary nerve that innervates the middle and posterior deltoid muscles (SPRINT system, SPR Therapeutics Corp., **Fig. 54-7A**). An RCT of single-electrode mPNS to treat HSP, with or without subluxation, showed greater pain relief than

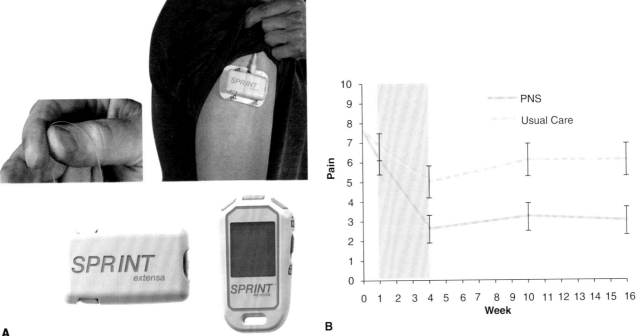

A   **B**

FIGURE 54-7. A: SPRINT peripheral nerve stimulation system for hemiplegic shoulder pain uses a percutaneous electrode placed intramuscularly near the axillary nerve. The electrode lead exits the skin and is connected to the stimulator control unit, which is adhered to the skin of the upper arm. (Courtesy of SPR Therapeutics Corp.) **B:** Worst pain in the last week on a 0 to 10 scale reported by 25 participants with chronic hemiplegic shoulder pain (12 to usual care, 13 to peripheral nerve stimulation). After 3 weeks of treatment for 6 hours/day (*shaded region*), the PNS group had significantly greater pain reductions at weeks 4, 10, and 16 than usual care. (Data from Wilson RD, Gunzler DD, Bennett ME, et al. Peripheral nerve stimulation compared with usual care for pain relief of hemiplegic shoulder pain: a randomized controlled trial. *Am J Phys Med Rehabil.* 2014;93(1):17–28.)

treatment with physical therapy (**Fig. 54-7B**) (173), and both percutaneous mPNS and physical therapy improved strength, range of motion, and function (174).

In summary, the use of surface NMES can reduce shoulder subluxation when provided in the first 6 months from stroke. Clinical usage of surface NMES systems may be limited by issues of stimulation-induced pain, difficult access of deeper muscles, and inconsistent surface electrode placement. Percutaneous intramuscular mPNS has been shown to reduce shoulder pain for up to 1 year posttreatment and has shown superiority over physical therapy.

Spinal Cord Stimulation

Spinal cord stimulation (SCS), also called dorsal column stimulation, has been used to treat a variety of pain syndromes. Human studies have demonstrated the clinical efficacy of dorsal column stimulation in relieving multiple chronic pain disorders. The proposed mechanism of action of SCS for reduction of neuropathic pain remains poorly understood. A review of mechanisms of SCS concluded that multiple mechanisms likely operate sequentially or simultaneously to relieve pain (175), though the effects of SCS appear to be mediated through the peripheral, spinal, and supraspinal systems. Stimulation is delivered through electrode leads that are placed percutaneously into the epidural space or, less commonly, through a paddle lead that is placed surgically through a laminotomy (**Fig. 54-8**). The spinal level of the electrodes is chosen based on the area of pathology, such as cervical spine for arm pain or low thoracic spine for leg pain. The first 6 to 10 days are a trial phase with an external stimulator. If an adequate response is achieved (often 50% pain reduction), a permanent implantable pulse generator will be connected to the electrode leads.

Multiple SCS stimulation patterns have been developed for the treatment of pain. Traditional SCS is delivered at frequencies

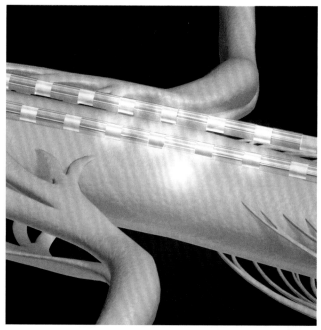

FIGURE 54-8. Stimulation of the dorsal horn of the spinal cord with two cylindrical leads with multiple evenly spaced electrode contacts. (Reprinted with permission from Hoppenfeld JD. *Fundamentals of Pain Medicine: How to Diagnose and Treat Your Patients.* 1st ed. Philadelphia, PA: Wolters Kluwer; 2014.)

lower than 1 kHz with the goal to replace the experience of pain with paresthesia in the same location (176). Some patients describe the paresthesia as unpleasant or intermittently unpleasant and associated with changes in position. Higher-frequency (10 kHz) stimulation does not induce paresthesia or cause discomfort with changes in position (176). Burst stimulation delivers traditional SCS in bursts of five pulses delivered at a frequency of 40 Hz and the pulse frequency of 500 Hz. A lower amplitude is utilized to provide pain relief with minimal or no paresthesia (177). Dorsal root ganglion stimulation is a technique in which the SCS electrode is placed adjacent to the spinal ganglion. A single electrode is able to provide paresthesia in a single dermatome; thus, this technique is most useful for a focal area of pain and for those areas in which traditional SCS is difficult to achieve paresthesia (178).

It is recommended that SCS be used in those who have failed adequate relief from conservative, medical management (176). Successful reduction of pain, secondary to SCS, is associated with appropriate patient selection. Psychological factors may contribute to dorsal column stimulation failure, which underscores the need for specific criteria for patient selection. Preoperative psychiatric evaluation is recommended before proceeding with SCS (176).

The use of SCS for chronic pain is common, though few high-quality trials have been conducted to demonstrate efficacy. Much of the available evidence is for traditional SCS, as alternative delivery methods are newer and therefore less studied. A review of six RCTs of SCS for chronic lumbar pain, in which three assessed efficacy, found evidence of the efficacy in pain reduction with traditional SCS, with moderate evidence for kilohertz frequency stimulation (179). Multiple reviews with lower levels of evidence have summarized the efficacy of SCS for treatment of chronic pain associated with angina (180), CRPS (181), and chronic pain from lower limb ischemia (182). In the clinical care of chronic pain patients, SCS is a viable treatment option for refractory low back pain. It may be effective in reducing pain in select patients with other chronic pain syndromes, but additional research needs to be completed to determine recommendations in those cases.

BRAIN STIMULATION

The last decade has seen a growing interest in the use of brain stimulation in the rehabilitation of patients with neurologic conditions. The technique involves application of electrical currents to the brain. Targeted structures may include superficial cortices (cortical stimulation) (183) or deeper nuclei (deep brain stimulation or DBS) (184). Brain stimulation is delivered based on the premise that electrical current applied to targeted regions may enhance their contribution toward recovery or help modify neural activity to alleviate symptoms (i.e., neuromodulation). As such, application of brain stimulation may serve to enhance the effects achieved with rehabilitative therapies (185). Here, we discuss the most common approaches.

Deep Brain Stimulation

Parkinson's Disease

The most common brain stimulation technique involves surgically implanted DBS, which is FDA approved for management of symptoms associated with Parkinson's disease (PD), such as bradykinesia and tremor. A neurostimulator or a pacemaker-like device is used to send electrical currents through an electrode implanted in the globus pallidus pars interna or the subthalamic nucleus (185,186). Because PD is a progressive neurodegenerative disorder, for which pharmacologic management carries significant side effects, DBS has emerged as a promising alternative. The technique is reversible and lacks side effects typically associated with ablative surgeries (185,186). Evidence accumulated over several randomized clinical trials has suggested that DBS may be superior to the best medical management in PD patients. Controversies still exist however regarding what is the most suitable target. While some trials report greater reduction of levodopa use and improvement in dyskinesia with pallidal targeting, others report reduction of use of dopaminergic agents with subthalamic stimulation. The technique overall is well-tolerated with few, infrequent complications such as intracranial hemorrhage and seizures (185,186).

Chronic Pain

Chronic pain is another neurologic condition addressed using DBS. For management of neuropathic syndromes, traditionally, sensory nuclei of the thalamus are targeted, while for nociceptive syndromes (such as low back pain), periventricular gray (PVG) and periaqueductal gray (PAG) are targeted. Despite evidence of efficacy, use of DBS for management of chronic pain is considered investigational. Long-term outcomes vary considerably (187). Levy et al. (188) originally reported that out of 141 patients, approximately 60% respond favorably. But at 6-year follow-up, less than a third of responders retained significant pain relief. Prospective multicenter clinical trials, similarly, report retention of greater than 50% relief in only 14% of the sample (187). Inclusion of a mix of etiologies introduces high variability among studies. Higher retention rates are noted in studies using homogenous samples (189). Overall, management of chronic neuropathic pain with DBS

is off-label given that findings have been mixed. Response and retention rates could be improved if ideal targets are identified for different etiologic conditions and heterogeneity of study samples is minimized.

Cortical Stimulation

Cortical stimulation is a "less invasive" or a "noninvasive" alternative to DBS. As the name suggests, currents are delivered to superficial cortical regions (190,191). Primary motor cortices are the most widely investigated targets. One method of delivering cortical stimulation involves surgical implantation of an epidural grid of stimulating electrodes and is known as epidural cortical stimulation (ECS). Other approaches involve noninvasive or "transcranial" delivery. Without requiring surgery, transcranial techniques can deliver currents through the scalp and skull (192,193). Transcranial techniques thus offer safer and inexpensive alternatives to surgical techniques.

Transcranial magnetic stimulation (TMS) uses an insulated coil of wire (magnetic coil) held in place over the scalp to produce a focused magnetic field that induces strong brief pulses of electrical current that depolarize and produce action potentials in motor cortical neurons lying immediately underneath the skull (**Fig. 54-9A**). Repetitive TMS pulses (rTMS) can modulate the excitability of cortical networks. Low-frequency (approximately 1 Hz) rTMS is believed to decrease excitability, while high-frequency rTMS (approximately 5 Hz) is believed to increase excitability of targeted cortices (194).

Transcranial direct current stimulation (tDCS) is a noninvasive brain stimulation technique that is administered with a simple portable DC stimulator (e.g., iontophoresis unit). The stimulator applies a low constant direct current through a pair of sponge electrodes (typically 5 × 5 cm) soaked in saline and placed over the scalp (**Fig. 54-9B**). Rather than triggering action potentials, tDCS modulates neuronal excitability by

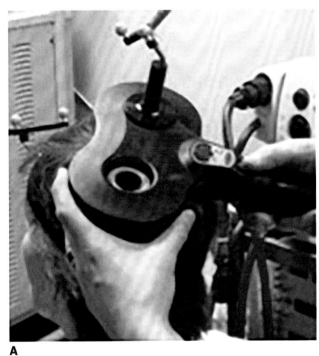
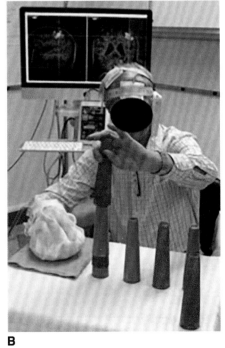

A   B

FIGURE 54-9. **A:** Repetitive transcranial magnetic stimulation (rTMS). **B:** Transcranial direct current stimulation (tDCS). Direct current is applied while the subject performs therapy with the left hand. (Courtesy of Ela B. Plow, PhD, Reprinted with permission from Cleveland Clinic Center for Medical Art & Photography © 2019. All Rights Reserved.)

hyperpolarizing or depolarizing the resting membrane potentials of underlying neurons (195). Changing the polarity of the current is widely reported to produce either inhibitory or excitatory effects. Cathodal tDCS, where the cathode is placed over the target area and the anode is placed remotely, is believed to decrease excitability, while anodal tDCS, where the anode is placed over the target area and the cathode is placed remotely, is thought to increase excitability of targeted cortices. Direct current is ramped on over several seconds to a maximum of 1 to 2 mA and then maintained at that level for approximately 20 minutes. Below, we discuss applications and evidence concerning cortical stimulation techniques.

Chronic Pain

One of the earliest applications of ECS was for management of pain due to central and peripheral deafferentation (196). Initial results in both types of pain were encouraging. In a subsequent series, however, improvements were only achieved in patients with peripheral syndromes. Several groups around the world similarly reported mixed results with trends favoring patients having pain of peripheral etiology (183). Use of ECS thus is considered off-label (183) because reliable outcomes across etiologies are lacking. Also, the procedure to implant the epidural electrode array is costly, is invasive, requires at least a burr hole or craniotomy even for placement of trial leads, and carries risks associated with surgical implantation, such as intracranial hemorrhages and infections (197).

The predominant use of rTMS in chronic neuropathic pain involves stimulation of the motor cortex (197). In a pioneering placebo-controlled trial, patients with chronic neuropathic pain immediately benefitted from a single session of 10 Hz rTMS delivered at an intensity below that needed to produce muscle twitches (197). The effect, however, was small (i.e., average reduction of two points on a visual analogue scale) and was achieved in only 7 of 18 patients (approximately 39% of sample). In subsequent studies, the long-term benefit of rTMS (198) has not been clinically meaningful (197). High variance in responsiveness to rTMS may be related to similar clinicopathologic factors as with ECS (199,200). Patients with peripheral trigeminal neuropathic pain experience good-to-excellent (201) pain relief (58% reduction in rating of pain severity) (202), benefits that are greater than those found in patients with central thalamic stroke pain (202,203). Site of pain also exaggerates differential responsiveness; facial pain appears to benefit the most with 64.3% of patients showing significant pain relief, while brainstem stroke with limb pain is associated with the worst prognosis, likely due to thalamocortical deafferentation (202). Influence of the etiology of pain and the site of pain thus should be considered when determining suitability of patients for rTMS therapies.

Anodal tDCS has also been explored for treating chronic pain (204,205). Although the reduction in pain following tDCS (approximately 63% improvement in pain rating) (204) is slightly lower than that following 20 Hz rTMS (approximately 71% improvement in pain rating), retention is comparable, lasting several weeks with only a 5-day treatment (204,205). Importantly, the mean reduction in pain (i.e., decrease in pain ratings) appears to be greater following 5 days of tDCS (58% and 63% in two different studies (204,205)) versus 5 days of rTMS (20% and 45% in the two different studies). In fact, longer treatment protocols generate even greater cumulative effects, with retention of benefit for almost

up to 60 days. These seemingly advantageous applications of tDCS, versus rTMS, should, however, be interpreted with some caution because effects of tDCS have only been demonstrated in studies of single etiology, such as SCI and multiple sclerosis (204,205).

Stroke Motor Rehabilitation

Perhaps, one of the most popular applications of ECS has been in the rehabilitation of the upper extremity following stroke. The goal is to affect residual cortical maps located in the vicinity of the lesion, with the idea that residual maps located in the territory of the motor cortex would have the potential to exhibit plastic changes that facilitate recovery. Submotor threshold, high-frequency (50 to 250 Hz) electrical stimulation is delivered during training of the impaired limb. Despite invariably encouraging results in animal studies (206), translation of ECS to human studies has had mixed success. Preliminary studies and phase I/II prospective clinical trials were able to replicate findings from animal studies. But a pivotal phase III trial failed to demonstrate any advantage of ECS in rehabilitation (190,191,207). This was likely due to inclusion of patients who had experienced extreme levels of damage to subcortical pathways to the paretic upper limb (190). Future studies must take into account these patient factors and tailor the stimulation accordingly.

rTMS and tDCS have been more widely investigated than ECS in the context of stroke rehabilitation. While ECS has been intended to tap into restorative processes within the vicinity of the lesion, rTMS and tDCS have, in addition, been intended to correct interhemispheric imbalances of neural activity that follow stroke. After stroke, the contralesional motor cortex exerts strong, persistent inhibition upon the ipsilesional motor cortex via transcallosal pathways. This further limits ipsilesional motor output and thereby contributes to upper limb paresis (208). This concept of interhemispheric rivalry has formed the basis for present-day transcranial electrical stimulation applications in stroke. Studies have focused on either reducing the inhibitory influence of the contralesional motor cortex with low-frequency rTMS (209) or cathodal tDCS or on increasing the excitatory activity of the ipsilesional motor cortex with high-frequency rTMS or anodal tDCS. These approaches have shown promise for recovery of function in many studies (193). However, significant improvements are evident mainly in less severely impaired patients (190,191,207,210,211). Patients with extensive damage to ipsilesional corticospinal pathways, in whom single-pulse TMS cannot produce a motor-evoked potential in paretic muscles, fail to show improvement in response to ECS or rTMS intended to increase excitatory activity of the ipsilesional motor cortex. By contrast, patients with sufficiently spared pathways, who demonstrate motor-evoked potentials in paretic muscles in response to single-pulse TMS, show significant improvement with these approaches (190,191,207,210,211). Therefore, degree of baseline impairment and damage may influence improvements that can be achieved with cortical stimulation.

SUMMARY

Decades of research and development have led to clinically effective therapeutic and functional applications of ES to treat neurologically based disorders encountered in the clinical practice of PM&R. ES systems that activate paralyzed arm and hand muscles can improve recovery of upper limb movement and function after stroke and can replace lost hand function after SCI. ES foot drop systems have both a therapeutic and neuroprosthetic effect on walking speed in stroke patients. ES systems that activate multiple leg muscles can enable SCI patients with paraplegia to stand and transfer and enable incomplete SCI patients to walk using a walker. ES systems that stimulate the phrenic nerves to activate the diaphragm may be an option for patients with high cervical SCI who require ventilatory assistance. Restoration of cough in patients with high SCI is being developed using SCS. ES systems that stimulate the sacral spinal nerve roots can enable micturition or improve continence and bowel function. ES systems that activate sensory nerves to elicit paresthesias, or motor nerves to produce muscle contractions, or the dorsal columns of the spinal cord may provide short- or long-term pain relief, depending on the pain syndrome. Cortical and DBS techniques are available or being developed to treat a growing list of movement disorders and other neurologic problems.

ES technology that is used to treat these medical problems ranges from simple handheld battery-operated units with surface electrodes to complex multichannel implanted stimulators and electrodes interfaced with implanted and external sensors and sophisticated programming stations and control algorithms that make the neuroprosthesis operate seamlessly in response to signals sensed from the patient. Many ES devices are now commercially available and are becoming routinely prescribed and utilized in PM&R clinics and therapy facilities. For more complex implanted ES systems, the pathway to commercialization and clinical availability is a greater challenge, but more and more are emerging out of research laboratories and into clinical environments. The establishment of efficacy of a broad spectrum of transcutaneous ES devices as well as implanted neuroprostheses and neuromodulators clearly expands the armamentarium of the physiatrist in the clinical care of patients. Future research will undoubtedly focus on further defining the patient populations, applications, and mechanisms by which ES may impart therapeutic and functional benefit. Ongoing basic and clinical research offers promise for an even broader spectrum of ES solutions to neurologically based disorders.

ACKNOWLEDGMENTS

The preparation of this chapter was supported in part by grants from the National Institutes of Health (NIH); National Institute of Child Health and Human Development (NICHD) grants R01HD068588, R01HD075542, R01HD084564, and K01HD069504; the Department of Veterans Affairs Rehabilitation Research and Development grants IK2RX001962 and I01RX000822; and the Society of Urodynamics, Female Pelvic Medicine, and Urogenital Reconstruction.

REFERENCES

1. Peckham PH. Principles of electrical stimulation. *Top Spinal Cord Inj Rehabil*. 1999;5(1):1–5.
2. Chae J, Kilgore K, Triolo R, et al. Neuromuscular stimulation for motor neuroprosthesis in hemiplegia. *Crit Rev Phys Rehabil Med*. 2000;12:1–23.
3. Kluding PM, Dunning K, O'Dell MW, et al. Foot drop stimulation versus ankle foot orthosis after stroke: 30-week outcomes. *Stroke*. 2013;44(6):1660–1669.
4. Sheffler LR, Chae J. Neuromuscular electrical stimulation in neurorehabilitation. *Muscle Nerve*. 2007;35(5):562–590.
5. Mortimer JT. Motor prostheses. In: Brookshart JM, Mountcastle VB, eds. *Handbook of Physiology—The Nervous System II*. Bethesda, MD: American Physiological Society; 1981:155–187.
6. Dobkin BH. Rehabilitation after stroke. *N Engl J Med*. 2005;352(16):1677–1684.
7. Lang CE, DeJong SL, Beebe JA. Recovery of thumb and finger extension and its relation to grasp performance after stroke. *J Neurophysiol*. 2009;102(1):451–459.
8. Rosewilliam S, Malhotra S, Roffe C, et al. Can surface neuromuscular electrical stimulation of the wrist and hand combined with routine therapy facilitate recovery of arm function in patients with stroke? *Arch Phys Med Rehabil*. 2012;93(10):1715.e1–1721.e1.
9. Meilink A, Hemmen B, Seelen HA, et al. Impact of EMG-triggered neuromuscular stimulation of the wrist and finger extensors of the paretic hand after stroke: a systematic review of the literature. *Clin Rehabil*. 2008;22(4):291–305.
10. Thrasher TA, Zivanovic V, McIlroy W, et al. Rehabilitation of reaching and grasping function in severe hemiplegic patients using functional electrical stimulation therapy. *Neurorehabil Neural Repair*. 2008;22(6):706–714.
11. Alon G, Levitt AF, McCarthy PA. Functional electrical stimulation enhancement of upper extremity functional recovery during stroke rehabilitation: a pilot study. *Neurorehabil Neural Repair*. 2007;21(3):207–215.
12. Howlett OA, Lannin NA, Ada L, et al. Functional electrical stimulation improves activity after stroke: a systematic review with meta-analysis. *Arch Phys Med Rehabil*. 2015;96(5):934–943.
13. Knutson JS, Gunzler DD, Wilson RD, et al. Contralaterally controlled functional electrical stimulation improves hand dexterity in chronic hemiparesis: a randomized trial. *Stroke*. 2016;47:2696–02.
14. Thorsen R, Cortesi M, Jonsdottir J, et al. Myoelectrically driven functional electrical stimulation may increase motor recovery of upper limb in poststroke subjects: a randomized controlled pilot study. *J Rehabil Res Dev*. 2013;50(6):785–794.
15. Foley N, Mehta S, Jutai J, et al. Upper extremity interventions. In: Teasell R, ed. *Evidence-Based Review of Stroke Rehabilitation*. 16th ed. London: Heart & Stroke Foundation Canadian Partnership for Stroke Recovery; 2014.
16. Winstein CJ, Stein J, Arena R, et al. Guidelines for adult stroke rehabilitation and recovery: a guideline for healthcare professionals from the American Heart Association/American Stroke Association. *Stroke*. 2016;47(6):e98–e169.
17. Hsu SS, Hu MH, Luh JJ, et al. Dosage of neuromuscular electrical stimulation: is it a determinant of upper limb functional improvement in stroke patients? *J Rehabil Med*. 2012;44(2):125–130.
18. Wilson RD, Page SJ, Delahanty M, et al. Upper-limb recovery after stroke: a randomized controlled trial comparing EMG-triggered, cyclic, and sensory electrical stimulation. *Neurorehabil Neural Repair*. 2016;30:978–987.
19. de Kroon JR, Ijzerman MJ. Electrical stimulation of the upper extremity in stroke: cyclic versus EMG-triggered stimulation. *Clin Rehabil*. 2008;22(8):690–697.
20. Boyaci A, Topuz O, Alkan H, et al. Comparison of the effectiveness of active and passive neuromuscular electrical stimulation of hemiplegic upper extremities: a randomized, controlled trial. *Int J Rehabil Res*. 2013;36(4):315–322.
21. Knutson JS, Harley MY, Hisel TZ, et al. Contralaterally controlled functional electrical stimulation for upper extremity hemiplegia: an early-phase randomized clinical trial in subacute stroke patients. *Neurorehabil Neural Repair*. 2012;26(3):239–246.
22. Shen Y, Yin Z, Fan Y, et al. Comparison of the effects of contralaterally controlled functional electrical stimulation and neuromuscular electrical stimulation on upper extremity functions in patients with stroke. *CNS Neurol Disord Drug Targets*. 2015;14(10):1260–1266.
23. Burridge JH, Turk R, Merrill D, et al. A personalized sensor-controlled microstimulator system for arm rehabilitation poststroke. Part 2: objective outcomes and patients' perspectives. *Neuromodulation*. 2011;14(1):80–88; discussion 8.
24. Knutson JS, Chae J, Hart RL, et al. Implanted neuroprosthesis for assisting arm and hand function after stroke: a case study. *J Rehabil Res Dev*. 2012;49(10):1505–1516.
25. Kilgore KL, Bhadra N. Reversible nerve conduction block using kilohertz frequency alternating current. *Neuromodulation*. 2014;17:242–254.
26. Anderson KD. Targeting recovery: priorities of the spinal cord-injured population. *J Neurotrauma*. 2004;21(10):1371–1383.
27. Ejeskar A, Hentz VR, Holst-Nielsen F, et al. Reconstructive hand surgery. *Spinal Cord*. 1999;37(7):475–479.
28. Keith MW, Peljovich AE. Rehabilitation of the hand and upper extremity in tetraplegia. In: Hunter JM, MacKin EJ, Callahan AD, et al., eds. *Rehabilitation of the Hand and Upper Extremity*. St. Louis, MO: Mosby, Inc.; 2002.
29. Peckham PH, Kilgore KL. Challenges and opportunities in restoring function after paralysis. *IEEE Trans Biomed Eng*. 2013;60(3):602–609.
30. Keith MW, Kilgore KL, Peckham PH, et al. Tendon transfers and functional electrical stimulation for restoration of hand function in spinal cord injury. *J Hand Surg [Am]*. 1996;21(1):89–99.
31. Long C II, Masciarelli VD. An electrophysiologic splint for the hand. *Arch Phys Med Rehabil*. 1963;44:499–503.
32. Alon G, McBride K. Persons with C5 or C6 tetraplegia achieve selected functional gains using a neuroprosthesis. *Arch Phys Med Rehabil*. 2003;84(1):119–124.
33. Snoek GJ, IJzerman MJ, in 't Groen FA, et al. Use of the NESS handmaster to restore handfunction in tetraplegia: clinical experiences in ten patients. *Spinal Cord*. 2000;38(4):244–249.
34. Prochazka A, Gauthier M, Wieler M, et al. The bionic glove: an electrical stimulator garment that provides controlled grasp and hand opening in quadriplegia. *Arch Phys Med Rehabil*. 1997;78(6):608–614.
35. Kilgore KL, Hoyen HA, Bryden AM, et al. An implanted upper-extremity neuroprosthesis using myoelectric control. *J Hand Surg [Am]*. 2008;33(4):539–550.
36. Keith MW, Peckham PH, Thrope GB, et al. Implantable functional neuromuscular stimulation in the tetraplegic hand. *J Hand Surg [Am]*. 1989;14(3):524–530.

37. Smith B, Peckham PH, Keith MW, et al. An externally powered, multichannel, implantable stimulator for versatile control of paralyzed muscle. *IEEE Trans Biomed Eng.* 1987;34(7):499–508.

38. Peckham PH, Keith MW, Kilgore KL, et al. Efficacy of an implanted neuroprosthesis for restoring hand grasp in tetraplegia: a multicenter study. *Arch Phys Med Rehabil.* 2001;82(10):1380–1388.

39. Stroh Wuolle K, Van Doren CL, Bryden AM, et al. Satisfaction with and usage of a hand neuroprosthesis. *Arch Phys Med Rehabil.* 1999;80(2):206–213.

40. Kilgore KL, Peckham PH, Keith MW, et al. Durability of implanted electrodes and leads in an upper-limb neuroprosthesis. *J Rehabil Res Dev.* 2003;40(6):457–468.

41. Kilgore KL, Peckham P, Keith MW. Twenty year experience with implanted neuroprostheses. *Conf Proc IEEE Eng Med Biol Soc.* 2009;2009:7212–7215.

42. Hart RL, Bhadra N, Montague FW, et al. Design and testing of an advanced implantable neuroprosthesis with myoelectric control. *IEEE Trans Neural Syst Rehabil Eng.* 2011;19(1):45–53.

43. Kilgore KL. Hand grasp and reach in spinal cord injury. In: Kilgore K, ed. *Implantable Neuroprostheses for Restoring Function.* Cambridge: Elsevier; 2015:210–235.

44. Bryden AM, Kilgore K, Keith MW, et al. Assessing activity of daily living performance after implantation of an upper extremity neuroprosthesis. *Top Spinal Cord Inj Rehabil.* 2008;13(4):37–53.

45. Bryden AM, Kilgore KL, Kirsch RF, et al. An implanted neuroprosthesis for high tetraplegia. *Top Spinal Cord Inj Rehabil.* 2005;10(3):38–52.

46. Williams MR, Kirsch RF. Case study: head orientation and neck electromyography for cursor control in persons with high cervical tetraplegia. *J Rehabil Res Dev.* 2016;53(4):519–530.

47. Collinger JL, Kryger MA, Barbara R, et al. Collaborative approach in the development of high-performance brain-computer interfaces for a neuroprosthetic arm: translation from animal models to human control. *Clin Transl Sci.* 2014;7(1):52–59.

48. Smith B, Campean A, Buckett JR, et al. Development of an implantable networked neuroprosthesis. *12th Annual Conference of the International Functional Electrical Stimulation Society.* Philadelphia, PA; 2007.

49. Ajiboye AB, Willett FR, Young DR, et al. Restoration of reaching and grasping movements through brain-controlled muscle stimulation in a person with tetraplegia: a proof-of-concept demonstration. *Lancet.* 2017;389(10081):1821–1830.

50. Bouton CE, Shaikhouni A, Annetta NV, et al. Restoring cortical control of functional movement in a human with quadriplegia. *Nature.* 2016;533(7602):247–250.

51. Kelly-Hayes M, Beiser A, Kase CS, et al. The influence of gender and age on disability following ischemic stroke: the Framingham study. *J Stroke Cerebrovasc Dis.* 2003;12(3):119–126.

52. Burridge JH, Taylor PN, Hagan SA, et al. The effects of common peroneal stimulation on the effort and speed of walking: a randomized controlled trial with chronic hemiplegic patients. *Clin Rehabil.* 1997;11(3):201–210.

53. Stein RB, Chong S, Everaert DG, et al. A multicenter trial of a footdrop stimulator controlled by a tilt sensor. *Neurorehabil Neural Repair.* 2006;20(3):371–379.

54. Kottink AI, Hermens HJ, Nene AV, et al. A randomized controlled trial of an implantable 2-channel peroneal nerve stimulator on walking speed and activity in poststroke hemiplegia. *Arch Phys Med Rehabil.* 2007;88(8):971–978.

55. Martin KD, Polanski WH, Schulz AK, et al. Restoration of ankle movements with the ActiGait implantable drop foot stimulator: a safe and reliable treatment option for permanent central leg palsy. *J Neurosurg.* 2016;124(1):70–76.

56. Burridge JH, Haugland M, Larsen B, et al. Phase II trial to evaluate the ActiGait implanted drop-foot stimulator in established hemiplegia. *J Rehabil Med.* 2007;39(3):212–218.

57. Kottink AI, Oostendorp LJ, Buurke JH, et al. The orthotic effect of functional electrical stimulation on the improvement of walking in stroke patients with a dropped foot: a systematic review. *Artif Organs.* 2004;28(6):577–586.

58. O'Dell MW, Dunning K, Kluding P, et al. Response and prediction of improvement in gait speed from functional electrical stimulation in persons with poststroke drop foot. *PM R.* 2014;6(7):587–601; quiz.

59. Taylor PN, Burridge JH, Dunkerley AL, et al. Clinical use of the Odstock dropped foot stimulator: its effect on the speed and effort of walking. *Arch Phys Med Rehabil.* 1999;80(12):1577–1583.

60. Robbins SM, Houghton PE, Woodbury MG, et al. The therapeutic effect of functional and transcutaneous electric stimulation on improving gait speed in stroke patients: a meta-analysis. *Arch Phys Med Rehabil.* 2006;87(6):853–859.

61. Stein RB, Everaert DG, Thompson AK, et al. Long-term therapeutic and orthotic effects of a foot drop stimulator on walking performance in progressive and nonprogressive neurological disorders. *Neurorehabil Neural Repair.* 2010;24(2):152–167.

62. Sheffler LR, Taylor PN, Gunzler DD, et al. Randomized controlled trial of surface peroneal nerve stimulation for motor relearning in lower limb hemiparesis. *Arch Phys Med Rehabil.* 2013;94(6):1007–1014.

63. Bethoux F, Rogers HL, Nolan KJ, et al. The effects of peroneal nerve functional electrical stimulation versus ankle-foot orthosis in patients with chronic stroke: a randomized controlled trial. *Neurorehabil Neural Repair.* 2014;28(7):688–697.

64. Everaert DG, Stein RB, Abrams GM, et al. Effect of a foot-drop stimulator and ankle-foot orthosis on walking performance after stroke: a multicenter randomized controlled trial. *Neurorehabil Neural Repair.* 2013;27(7):579–591.

65. Prenton S, Hollands KL, Kenney LP. Functional electrical stimulation versus ankle foot orthoses for foot-drop: a meta-analysis of orthotic effects. *J Rehabil Med.* 2016;48(8):646–656.

66. Bogataj U, Gros N, Kljajic M, et al. The rehabilitation of gait in patients with hemiplegia: a comparison between conventional therapy and multichannel functional electrical stimulation therapy. *Phys Ther.* 1995;75:490–502.

67. Springer S, Vatine JJ, Lipson R, et al. Effects of dual-channel functional electrical stimulation on gait performance in patients with hemiparesis. *Scientific World J.* 2012;2012:530906.

68. Daly JJ, Zimbelman J, Roenigk KL, et al. Recovery of coordinated gait: randomized controlled stroke trial of functional electrical stimulation (FES) versus no FES, with weight-supported treadmill and over-ground training. *Neurorehabil Neural Repair.* 2011;25(7):588–596.

69. Makowski NS, Kobetic R, Lombardo LM, et al. Improving walking with an implanted neuroprosthesis for hip, knee, and ankle control after stroke. *Am J Phys Med Rehabil.* 2016;95:880–888.

70. Davis JA Jr, Triolo RJ, Uhlir J, et al. Preliminary performance of a surgically implanted neuroprosthesis for standing and transfers—where do we stand? *J Rehabil Res Dev.* 2001;38(6):609–617.

71. Triolo RJ, Bailey SN, Miller ME, et al. Longitudinal performance of a surgically implanted neuroprosthesis for lower-extremity exercise, standing, and transfers after spinal cord injury. *Arch Phys Med Rehabil.* 2012;93(5):896–904.

72. Rohde LM, Bonder BR, Triolo RJ. Exploratory study of perceived quality of life with implanted standing neuroprostheses. *J Rehabil Res Dev.* 2012;49(2):265–278.

73. Agarwal S, Triolo RJ, Kobetic R, et al. Long-term user perceptions of an implanted neuroprosthesis for exercise, standing, and transfers after spinal cord injury. *J Rehabil Res Dev.* 2003;40(3):241–252.

74. Uhlir JP, Triolo RJ, Davis JA Jr, et al. Performance of epimysial stimulating electrodes in the lower extremities of individuals with spinal cord injury. *IEEE Trans Neural Syst Rehabil Eng.* 2004;12(2):279–287.

75. Fisher LE, Miller ME, Bailey SN, et al. Standing after spinal cord injury with four-contact nerve-cuff electrodes for quadriceps stimulation. *IEEE Trans Neural Syst Rehabil Eng.* 2008;16(5):473–478.

76. Nataraj R, Audu ML, Triolo RJ. Center of mass acceleration feedback control of functional neuromuscular stimulation for standing in presence of internal postural perturbations. *J Rehabil Res Dev.* 2012;49(6):889–911.

77. Nataraj R, Audu ML, Triolo RJ. Simulating the restoration of standing balance at leaning postures with functional neuromuscular stimulation following spinal cord injury. *Med Biol Eng Comput.* 2016;54(1):163–176.

78. Brissot R, Gallien P, Le Bot MP, et al. Clinical experience with functional electrical stimulation-assisted gait with Parastep in spinal cord-injured patients. *Spine.* 2000;25(4):501–508.

79. Graupe D, Kohn KH. Functional neuromuscular stimulator for short-distance ambulation by certain thoracic-level spinal-cord-injured paraplegics. *Surg Neurol.* 1998;50(3):202–207.

80. Kobetic R, Triolo RJ, Uhlir JP, et al. Implanted functional electrical stimulation system for mobility in paraplegia: a follow-up case report. *IEEE Trans Rehabil Eng.* 1999;7(4):390–398.

81. Hardin E, Kobetic R, Murray L, et al. Walking after incomplete spinal cord injury using an implanted FES system: a case report. *J Rehabil Res Dev.* 2007;44(3):333–346.

82. Bailey SN, Hardin EC, Kobetic R, et al. Neurotherapeutic and neuroprosthetic effects of implanted functional electrical stimulation for ambulation after incomplete spinal cord injury. *J Rehabil Res Dev.* 2010;47(1):7–16.

83. Lombardo LM, Bailey SN, Foglyano KM, et al. A preliminary comparison of myoelectric and cyclic control of an implanted neuroprosthesis to modulate gait speed in incomplete SCI. *J Spinal Cord Med.* 2015;38(1):115–122.

84. Foglyano KM, Schnellenberger JR, Kobetic R, et al. Accelerometer-based step initiation control for gait-assist neuroprostheses. *J Rehabil Res Dev.* 2016;53(6):919–932.

85. McNeal DR. Analysis of a model for excitation of myelinated nerve. *IEEE Trans Biomed Eng.* 1976;23(4):329–337.

86. Henneman E, Somjen G, Carpenter DO. Functional significance of cell size in spinal motoneurons. *J Neurophysiol.* 1965;28:560–580.

87. Peckham PH, Mortimer JT, Marsolais EB. Alteration in the force and fatigability of skeletal muscle in quadriplegic humans following exercise induced by chronic electrical stimulation. *Clin Orthop Relat Res.* 1976;(114):326–333.

88. Fisher LE, Tyler DJ, Triolo RJ. Optimization of selective stimulation parameters for multi-contact electrodes. *J Neuroeng Rehabil.* 2013;10:25.

89. Kobetic R, To CS, Schnellenberger JR, et al. Development of hybrid orthosis for standing, walking, and stair climbing after spinal cord injury. *J Rehabil Res Dev.* 2009;46(3):447–462.

90. Bulea TC, Kobetic R, Audu ML, et al. Stance controlled knee flexion improves stimulation driven walking after spinal cord injury. *J Neuroeng Rehabil.* 2013;10:68.

91. To CS, Kobetic R, Bulea TC, et al. Sensor-based hip control with hybrid neuroprosthesis for walking in paraplegia. *J Rehabil Res Dev.* 2014;51(2):229–244.

92. Chang SR, Nandor MJ, Kobetic R, et al. Improving stand-to-sit maneuver for individuals with spinal cord injury. *J Neuroeng Rehabil.* 2016;13:27.

93. Ha KH, Murray SA, Goldfarb M. An approach for the cooperative control of FES with a powered exoskeleton during level walking for persons with paraplegia. *IEEE Trans Neural Syst Rehabil Eng.* 2016;24(4):455–466.

94. Spinal Cord Injury (SCI) 2016 facts and figures at a glance. *J Spinal Cord Med.* 2016;39(4):493–494.

95. Ragnarsson KT. Functional electrical stimulation after spinal cord injury: current use, therapeutic effects and future directions. *Spinal Cord.* 2008;46:255–274.

96. DiMarco AF. Diaphragm pacing in patients with spinal cord injury. *Top Spinal Cord Inj Rehabil.* 1999;5(1):6–20.

97. Glenn WW, Hageman JH, Mauro A, et al. Electrical stimulation of excitable tissue by radio-frequency transmission. *Ann Surg.* 1964;160:338–350.

98. Glenn WW, Phelps ML, Elefteriades JA, et al. Twenty years of experience in phrenic nerve stimulation to pace the diaphragm. *Pacing Clin Electrophysiol.* 1986;9 (6 Pt 1):780–784.

99. Dobelle WH, D'Angelo MS, Goetz BF, et al. 200 cases with a new breathing pacemaker dispel myths about diaphragm pacing. *ASAIO J.* 1994;40(3):M244–M252.

100. Whiteneck GG, Charlifue SW, Frankel HL, et al. Mortality, morbidity, and psychosocial outcomes of persons spinal cord injured more than 20 years ago. *Paraplegia.* 1992;30(9):617–630.

101. Baer GA, Talonen PP, Shneerson JM, et al. Phrenic nerve stimulation for central ventilatory failure with bipolar and four-pole electrode systems. *Pacing Clin Electrophysiol.* 1990;13(8):1061–1072.

102. Elefteriades JA, Quin JA, Hogan JF, et al. Long-term follow-up of pacing of the conditioned diaphragm in quadriplegia. *Pacing Clin Electrophysiol.* 2002;25(6):897–906.

103. Weese-Mayer DE, Silvestri JM, Kenny AS, et al. Diaphragm pacing with a quadripolar phrenic nerve electrode: an international study. *Pacing Clin Electrophysiol.* 1996;19(9):1311–1319.

104. Carter RE, Menter R, Wood M, et al. Available respiratory options. In: Whiteneck G, Adler C, Carter RE, eds. *The Management of High Quadriplegia.* New York: Demos Publications; 1989:166–169.

105. Nochomovitz ML, Hopkins M, Brodkey J, et al. Conditioning of the diaphragm with phrenic nerve stimulation after prolonged disuse. *Am Rev Respir Dis.* 1984;130(4):685–688.

106. DiMarco AF, Takaoka Y, Kowalski KE. Combined intercostal and diaphragm pacing to provide artificial ventilation in patients with tetraplegia. *Arch Phys Med Rehabil.* 2005;86(6):1200–1207.

107. Krieger LM, Krieger AJ. The intercostal to phrenic nerve transfer: an effective means of reanimating the diaphragm in patients with high cervical spine injury. *Plast Reconstr Surg.* 2000;105(4):1255–1261.

108. DiMarco AF, Onders RP, Ignagni A, et al. Phrenic nerve pacing via intramuscular diaphragm electrodes in tetraplegic subjects. *Chest.* 2005;127(2):671–678.

109. Zhang X, Plow E, Ranganthan V, et al. Functional magnetic stimulation of inspiratory and expiratory muscles in subjects with tetraplegia. *PM R.* 2016;8(7):651–659.

110. Linder SH. Functional electrical stimulation to enhance cough in quadriplegia. *Chest.* 1993;103(1):166–169.

111. Jaeger RJ, Turba RM, Yarkony GM, et al. Cough in spinal cord injured patients: comparison of three methods to produce cough. *Arch Phys Med Rehabil.* 1993;74(12):1358–1361.

112. DiMarco AF, Kowalski KE, Hromyak DR, et al. Long-term follow-up of spinal cord stimulation to restore cough in subjects with spinal cord injury. *J Spinal Cord Med.* 2014;37(4):380–388.

113. Walter JS, Thomas D, Sayers S, et al. Respiratory responses to stimulation of abdominal and upper-thorax intercostal muscles using multiple Permaloc electrodes. *J Rehabil Res Dev.* 2015;52(1):85–96.

114. Kowalski KE, Romaniuk JR, Brose S, et al. High frequency spinal cord stimulation-New method to restore cough. *Respir Physiol Neurobiol.* 2016;232:54–56.

115. DiMarco AF, Kowalski KE. Activation of inspiratory muscles via spinal cord stimulation. *Respir Physiol Neurobiol.* 2013;189(2):438–449.

116. Green KK, Woodson BT. Upper airway stimulation therapy. *Otolaryngol Clin North Am.* 2016;49(6):1425–1431.

117. Lee JS, Kim SW, Jee SH, et al. Factors affecting quality of life among spinal cord injury patients in Korea. *Int Neurourol J.* 2016;20(4):316–320.

118. Brindley GS. History of the sacral anterior root stimulator, 1969-1982. *Neurourol Urodyn.* 1993;12(5):481–483.

119. Van Kerrebroeck PE, Koldewijn EL, Debruyne FM. Worldwide experience with the Finetech-Brindley sacral anterior root stimulator. *Neurourol Urodyn.* 1993;12(5):497–503.

120. Brindley GS. The first 500 patients with sacral anterior root stimulator implants: general description. *Paraplegia.* 1994;32(12):795–805.

121. Brindley GS, Polkey CE, Rushton DN. Sacral anterior root stimulators for bladder control in paraplegia. *Paraplegia.* 1982;20(6):365–381.

122. Sauerwein D, Ingunza W, Fischer J, et al. Extradural implantation of sacral anterior root stimulators. *J Neurol Neurosurg Psychiatry.* 1990;53(8):681–684.

123. Egon G, Barat M, Colombel P, et al. Implantation of anterior sacral root stimulators combined with posterior sacral rhizotomy in spinal injury patients. *World J Urol.* 1998;16(5):342–349.

124. Creasey GH, Grill JH, Korsten M, et al. An implantable neuroprosthesis for restoring bladder and bowel control to patients with spinal cord injuries: a multicenter trial. *Arch Phys Med Rehabil.* 2001;82(11):1512–1519.

125. Brindley GS. The first 500 sacral anterior root stimulators: implant failures and their repair. *Paraplegia.* 1995;33(1):5–9.

126. Creasey GH, Kilgore KL, Brown-Triolo DL, et al. Reduction of costs of disability using neuroprostheses. *Assist Technol.* 2000;12(1):67–75.

127. MacDonagh RP, Sun WM, Smallwood R, et al. Control of defecation in patients with spinal injuries by stimulation of sacral anterior nerve roots. *BMJ.* 1990;300(6738):1494–1497.

128. Creasey GH. Restoration of bladder, bowel, and sexual function. *Top Spinal Cord Inj Rehabil.* 1999;5:21–32.

129. Kirkham AP, Knight SL, Craggs MD, et al. Neuromodulation through sacral nerve roots 2 to 4 with a Finetech-Brindley sacral posterior and anterior root stimulator. *Spinal Cord.* 2002;40(6):272–281.

130. Kohli N, Patterson D. InterStim therapy: a contemporary approach to overactive bladder. *Rev Obstet Gynecol.* 2009;2(1):18–27.

131. Minardi D, Muzzonigro G. Sacral neuromodulation in patients with multiple sclerosis. *World J Urol.* 2012;30(1):123–128.

132. Devane LA, Evers J, Jones JF, et al. A review of sacral nerve stimulation parameters used in the treatment of faecal incontinence. *Surgeon.* 2015;13(3):156–162.

133. de Seze M, Raibaut P, Gallien P, et al. Transcutaneous posterior tibial nerve stimulation for treatment of the overactive bladder syndrome in multiple sclerosis: results of a multicenter prospective study. *Neurourol Urodyn.* 2011;30(3):306–311.

134. de Groat WC, Ryall RW. Reflexes to sacral parasympathetic neurones concerned with micturition in the cat. *J Physiol.* 1969;200(1):87–108.

135. Walter JS, Wheeler JS, Robinson CJ, et al. Inhibiting the hyperreflexic bladder with electrical stimulation in a spinal animal model. *Neurourol Urodyn.* 1993;12(3):241–252; discussion 53.

136. Farag FF, Martens FM, Rijkhoff NJ, et al. Dorsal genital nerve stimulation in patients with detrusor overactivity: a systematic review. *Curr Urol Rep.* 2012;13(5):385–388.

137. Bourbeau DJ, Creasey GH, Sidik S, et al. Genital nerve stimulation increases bladder capacity after SCI: meta-analysis. *J Spinal Cord Med.* 2018;41:426–434.

138. Brose SW, Bourbeau DJ, Gustafson KJ. Genital nerve stimulation is tolerable and effective for bladder inhibition in sensate individuals with incomplete SCI. *J Spinal Cord Med.* 2018;41:174–181.

139. Lee YH, Creasey GH. Self-controlled dorsal penile nerve stimulation to inhibit bladder hyperreflexia in incomplete spinal cord injury: a case report. *Arch Phys Med Rehabil.* 2002;83(2):273–277.

140. Opisso E, Borau A, Rijkhoff NJ. Subject-controlled stimulation of dorsal genital nerve to treat neurogenic detrusor overactivity at home. *Neurourol Urodyn.* 2013;32(7):1004–1009.

141. Worsoe J, Fynne L, Laurberg S, et al. Electrical stimulation of the dorsal clitoral nerve reduces incontinence episodes in idiopathic faecal incontinent patients: a pilot study. *Colorectal Dis.* 2012;14(3):349–355.

142. Gad PN, Roy RR, Zhong H, et al. Initiation of bladder voiding with epidural stimulation in paralyzed, step trained rats. *PLoS One.* 2014;9(9):e108184.

143. Harkema S, Gerasimenko Y, Hodes J, et al. Effect of epidural stimulation of the lumbosacral spinal cord on voluntary movement, standing, and assisted stepping after motor complete paraplegia: a case study. *Lancet.* 2011;377(9781):1938–1947.

144. Bruns TM, Bhadra N, Gustafson KJ. Intraurethral stimulation for reflex bladder activation depends on stimulation pattern and location. *Neurourol Urodyn.* 2009;28(6):561–566.

145. Kennelly MJ, Bennett ME, Grill WM, et al. Electrical stimulation of the urethra evokes bladder contractions and emptying in spinal cord injury men: case studies. *J Spinal Cord Med.* 2011;34(3):315–321.

146. Boger A, Bhadra N, Gustafson KJ. Bladder voiding by combined high frequency electrical pudendal nerve block and sacral root stimulation. *Neurourol Urodyn.* 2008;27(5):435–439.

147. McCoin JL, Bhadra N, Gustafson KJ. Electrical stimulation of sacral dermatomes can suppress aberrant urethral reflexes in felines with chronic spinal cord injury. *Neurourol Urodyn.* 2013;32(1):92–97.

148. McCoin JL, Bhadra N, Brose SW, et al. Does patterned afferent stimulation of sacral dermatomes suppress urethral sphincter reflexes in individuals with spinal cord injury? *Neurourol Urodyn.* 2015;34(3):219–223.

149. Vance CG, Dailey DL, Rakel BA, et al. Using TENS for pain control: the state of the evidence. *Pain Manag.* 2014;4(3):197–209.

150. Johnson M. Transcutaneous electrical nerve stimulation: mechanisms, clinical application and evidence. *Rev Pain.* 2007;1(1):7–11.

151. Goats GC. Interferential current therapy. *Br J Sports Med.* 1990;24(2):87–92.

152. Nnoaham KE, Kumbang J. Transcutaneous electrical nerve stimulation (TENS) for chronic pain. *Cochrane Database Syst Rev.* 2008;(3):CD003222.

153. Khadilkar A, Odebiyi DO, Brosseau L, et al. Transcutaneous electrical nerve stimulation (TENS) versus placebo for chronic low-back pain. *Cochrane Database Syst Rev.* 2008;(4):CD003008.

154. Dubinsky RM, Miyasaki J. Assessment: efficacy of transcutaneous electric nerve stimulation in the treatment of pain in neurologic disorders (an evidence-based review): report of the Therapeutics and Technology Assessment Subcommittee of the American Academy of Neurology. *Neurology.* 2010;74(2):173–176.

155. Machado LA, Kamper SJ, Herbert RD, et al. Analgesic effects of treatments for non-specific low back pain: a meta-analysis of placebo-controlled randomized trials. *Rheumatology (Oxford).* 2009;48(5):520–527.

156. Zeng C, Li H, Yang T, et al. Electrical stimulation for pain relief in knee osteoarthritis: systematic review and network meta-analysis. *Osteoarthritis Cartilage.* 2015;23(2):189–202.

157. Bjordal JM, Johnson MI, Lopes-Martins RA, et al. Short-term efficacy of physical interventions in osteoarthritic knee pain. A systematic review and meta-analysis of randomised placebo-controlled trials. *BMC Musculoskelet Disord.* 2007;8:51.

158. Jin DM, Xu Y, Geng DF, et al. Effect of transcutaneous electrical nerve stimulation on symptomatic diabetic peripheral neuropathy: a meta-analysis of randomized controlled trials. *Diabetes Res Clin Pract.* 2010;89(1):10–15.

159. Bennett MI, Hughes N, Johnson MI. Methodological quality in randomised controlled trials of transcutaneous electric nerve stimulation for pain: low fidelity may explain negative findings. *Pain.* 2011;152(6):1226–1232.

160. Petersen EA, Slavin KV. Peripheral nerve/field stimulation for chronic pain. *Neurosurg Clin N Am.* 2014;25(4):789–797.

161. Melzack R, Wall PD. Pain mechanisms: a new theory. *Science.* 1965;150(3699):971–979.

162. Sweet JA, Mitchell LS, Narouze S, et al. Occipital nerve stimulation for the treatment of patients with medically refractory occipital neuralgia: congress of neurological surgeons systematic review and evidence-based guideline. *Neurosurgery.* 2015;77(3):332–341.

163. Deer T, Pope J, Benyamin R, et al. Prospective, multicenter, randomized, double-blinded, partial crossover study to assess the safety and efficacy of the novel neuromodulation system in the treatment of patients with chronic pain of peripheral nerve origin. *Neuromodulation*. 2016;19(1):91–100.

164. Paci M, Nannetti L, Rinaldi LA. Glenohumeral subluxation in hemiplegia: an overview. *J Rehabil Res Dev*. 2005;42(4):557–568.

165. Vafadar AK, Cote JN, Archambault PS. Effectiveness of functional electrical stimulation in improving clinical outcomes in the upper arm following stroke: a systematic review and meta-analysis. *Biomed Res Int*. 2015;2015:729768.

166. Ada L, Foonghchomcheay A. Efficacy of electrical stimulation in preventing or reducing subluxation of the shoulder after stroke: a meta-analysis. *Aust J Physiother*. 2002;48:257–267.

167. Chae J, Mascarenhas D, Yu DT, et al. Poststroke shoulder pain: its relationship to motor impairment, activity limitation, and quality of life. *Arch Phys Med Rehabil*. 2007;88(3):298–301.

168. Gamble GE, Barberan E, Laasch HU, et al. Poststroke shoulder pain: a prospective study of the association and risk factors in 152 patients from a consecutive cohort of 205 patients presenting with stroke. *Eur J Pain*. 2002;6(6):467–474.

169. Price CI, Pandyan AD. Electrical stimulation for preventing and treating poststroke shoulder pain: a systematic Cochrane review. *Clin Rehabil*. 2001;15(1):5–19.

170. Yu DT, Chae J, Walker ME, et al. Intramuscular neuromuscular electric stimulation for poststroke shoulder pain: a multicenter randomized clinical trial. *Arch Phys Med Rehabil*. 2004;85(5):695–704.

171. Chae J, Yu DT, Walker ME, et al. Intramuscular electrical stimulation for hemiplegic shoulder pain: a 12-month follow-up of a multiple-center, randomized clinical trial. *Am J Phys Med Rehabil*. 2005;84(11):832–842.

172. Chae J, Ng A, Yu DT, et al. Intramuscular electrical stimulation for shoulder pain in hemiplegia: does time from stroke onset predict treatment success? *Neurorehabil Neural Repair*. 2007;21(6):561–567.

173. Wilson RD, Gunzler DD, Bennett ME, et al. Peripheral nerve stimulation compared with usual care for pain relief of hemiplegic shoulder pain: a randomized controlled trial. *Am J Phys Med Rehabil*. 2014;93(1):17–28.

174. Wilson RD, Knutson JS, Bennett ME, et al. The effect of peripheral nerve stimulation on shoulder biomechanics: a randomized controlled trial in comparison to physical therapy. *Am J Phys Med Rehabil*. 2017;96:191–198.

175. Oakley JC, Prager JP. Spinal cord stimulation: mechanisms of action. *Spine (Phila Pa 1976)*. 2002;27(22):2574–2583.

176. Deer TR, Mekhail N, Provenzano D, et al. The appropriate use of neurostimulation of the spinal cord and peripheral nervous system for the treatment of chronic pain and ischemic diseases: the Neuromodulation Appropriateness Consensus Committee. *Neuromodulation*. 2014;17(6):515–550; discussion 50.

177. Verrills P, Sinclair C, Barnard A. A review of spinal cord stimulation systems for chronic pain. *J Pain Res*. 2016;9:481–492.

178. Wolter T. Spinal cord stimulation for neuropathic pain: current perspectives. *J Pain Res*. 2014;7:651–663.

179. Grider JS, Manchikanti L, Carayannopoulos A, et al. Effectiveness of spinal cord stimulation in chronic spinal pain: a systematic review. *Pain Physician*. 2016;19(1):E33–E54.

180. Tsigaridas N, Naka K, Tsapogas P, et al. Spinal cord stimulation in refractory angina. A systematic review of randomized controlled trials. *Acta Cardiol*. 2015;70(2):233–243.

181. Visnjevac O, Costandi S, Patel BA, et al. A comprehensive outcome-specific review of the use of spinal cord stimulation for complex regional pain syndrome. *Pain Pract*. 2017;17:533–545.

182. Ubbink DT, Vermeulen H. Spinal cord stimulation for non-reconstructable chronic critical leg ischaemia. *Cochrane Database Syst Rev*. 2013;(2):CD004001.

183. Machado AG, Mogilner AY, Rezai A. Motor cortex stimulation for persistent non-cancer pain. In: Lozano AM, Gildenberg PL, Tasker RR, eds. *Textbook of Functional and Stereotactic Neurosurgery*. Berlin, Heidelberg: Springer-Verlag; 2009:2239–2249.

184. Benabid AL, Pollak P, Seigneuret E, et al. Chronic VIM thalamic stimulation in Parkinson's disease, essential tremor and extra-pyramidal dyskinesias. *Acta Neurochir Suppl (Wien)*. 1993;58:39–44.

185. Martinez-Ramirez D, Hu W, Bona AR, et al. Update on deep brain stimulation in Parkinson's disease. *Transl Neurodegener*. 2015;4:12.

186. Machado A, Rezai AR, Kopell BH, et al. Deep brain stimulation for Parkinson's disease: surgical technique and perioperative management. *Mov Disord*. 2006;21(suppl 14):S247–S258.

187. Coffey RJ. Deep brain stimulation for chronic pain: results of two multicenter trials and a structured review. *Pain Med*. 2001;2(3):183–192.

188. Levy RM, Lamb S, Adams JE. Treatment of chronic pain by deep brain stimulation: long term follow-up and review of the literature. *Neurosurgery*. 1987;21(6):885–893.

189. Kumar K, Toth C, Nath RK. Deep brain stimulation for intractable pain: a 15-year experience. *Neurosurgery*. 1997;40(4):736–746; discussion 46–47.

190. Plow EB, Carey JR, Nudo RJ, et al. Invasive cortical stimulation to promote recovery of function after stroke. *Stroke*. 2009;40(5):1926–1931.

191. Plow EB, Machado A. Invasive neurostimulation in stroke rehabilitation. *Neurotherapeutics*. 2014;11:572–582.

192. Fregni F, Pascual-Leone A. Technology insight: noninvasive brain stimulation in neurology-perspectives on the therapeutic potential of rTMS and tDCS. *Nat Clin Pract Neurol*. 2007;3(7):383–393.

193. Hummel FC, Cohen LG. Non-invasive brain stimulation. *Lancet Neurol*. 2006;5(8):708–712.

194. Rossi S, Hallett M, Rossini PM, et al. Safety, ethical considerations, and application guidelines for the use of transcranial magnetic stimulation in clinical practice and research. *Clin Neurophysiol*. 2009;120(12):2008–2039.

195. Nitsche MA, Fricke K, Henschke U, et al. Pharmacological modulation of cortical excitability shifts induced by transcranial direct current stimulation in humans. *J Physiol*. 2003;553(Pt 1):293–301.

196. Tsubokawa T, Katayama Y, Yamamoto T, et al. Chronic motor cortex stimulation in patients with thalamic pain. *J Neurosurg*. 1993;78(3):393–401.

197. Lefaucheur JP, Drouot X, Keravel Y, et al. Pain relief induced by repetitive transcranial magnetic stimulation of precentral cortex. *Neuroreport*. 2001;12(13):2963–2965.

198. Leung A, Donohue M, Xu R, et al. rTMS for suppressing neuropathic pain: a meta-analysis. *J Pain*. 2009;10(12):1205–1216.

199. Rasche D, Ruppolt M, Stippich C, et al. Motor cortex stimulation for long-term relief of chronic neuropathic pain: a 10 year experience. *Pain*. 2006;121(1–2):43–52.

200. Saitoh Y, Shibata M, Hirano S, et al. Motor cortex stimulation for central and peripheral deafferentation pain. Report of eight cases. *J Neurosurg*. 2000;92(1):150–155.

201. Nguyen JP, Lefaucheur JP, Decq P, et al. Chronic motor cortex stimulation in the treatment of central and neuropathic pain. Correlations between clinical, electrophysiological and anatomical data. *Pain*. 1999;82(3):245–251.

202. Lefaucheur JP, Drouot X, Menard-Lefaucheur I, et al. Neurogenic pain relief by repetitive transcranial magnetic cortical stimulation depends on the origin and the site of pain. *J Neurol Neurosurg Psychiatry*. 2004;75(4):612–616.

203. Lefaucheur JP, Drouot X, Nguyen JP. Interventional neurophysiology for pain control: duration of pain relief following repetitive transcranial magnetic stimulation of the motor cortex. *Neurophysiol Clin*. 2001;31(4):247–252.

204. Fregni F, Boggio PS, Lima MC, et al. A sham-controlled, phase II trial of transcranial direct current stimulation for the treatment of central pain in traumatic spinal cord injury. *Pain*. 2006;122(1–2):197–209.

205. Mori F, Codeca C, Kusayanagi H, et al. Effects of anodal transcranial direct current stimulation on chronic neuropathic pain in patients with multiple sclerosis. *J Pain*. 2010;11(5):436–442.

206. Kleim JA, Bruneau R, VandenBerg P, et al. Motor cortex stimulation enhances motor recovery and reduces peri-infarct dysfunction following ischemic insult. *Neurol Res*. 2003;25(8):789–793.

207. Levy RM, Harvey RL, Kissela BM, et al. Epidural electrical stimulation for stroke rehabilitation: results of the prospective, multicenter, randomized, single-blinded everest trial. *Neurorehabil Neural Repair*. 2016;30:107–119.

208. Murase N, Duque J, Mazzocchio R, et al. Influence of interhemispheric interactions on motor function in chronic stroke. *Ann Neurol*. 2004;55(3):400–409.

209. Fregni F, Boggio PS, Valle AC, et al. A sham-controlled trial of a 5-day course of repetitive transcranial magnetic stimulation of the unaffected hemisphere in stroke patients. *Stroke*. 2006;37(8):2115–2122.

210. Plow EB, Cunningham DA, Varnerin N, et al. Rethinking stimulation of the brain in stroke rehabilitation: why higher motor areas might be better alternatives for patients with greater impairments. *Neuroscientist*. 2015;21(3):225–240.

211. Sankarasubramanian V, Machado AG, Conforto AB, et al. Inhibition versus facilitation of contralesional motor cortices in stroke: deriving a model to tailor brain stimulation. *Clin Neurophysiol*. 2017;128(6):892–902.

CHAPTER 55

Cathy Bodine

Assistive Technology

HISTORICAL BACKGROUND AND PERSPECTIVE ON ASSISTIVE TECHNOLOGY

Humans have used tools to accomplish everyday tasks throughout history (and prehistory), but the perception remains that the use of technology as a tool for persons with disabilities and the elderly is a fairly recent phenomenon. In fact, James and Thorpe described any number of assistive devices used as early as the 6th or 7th century B.C. (1). Their descriptions include partial dentures, artificial legs and hands and drinking tubes, or straws. The earliest documented account of optical and lens technologies, or eyeglasses, came from Venice around A.D. 1300 (2). The term *assistive technology* (AT) to describe devices used to facilitate the accomplishment of everyday tasks by persons with disabilities is actually a more recent development (3).

In 1988, Public Law 100-407 defined AT as "Any item, piece of equipment or product system whether acquired commercially off the shelf, modified, or customized that is used to increase or improve functional capabilities of individuals with disabilities." This definition also included a second component defining AT services as any service that directly assists an individual with a disability in the selection, acquisition, or use of an AT device. This includes the following:

1. The evaluation of the needs of individuals with a disability, including a functional evaluation of the individual in his or her customary environment
2. Purchasing, leasing, or otherwise providing for the acquisition of AT by persons with disabilities
3. Selecting, designing, fitting, customizing, adapting, applying, retaining, repairing, or replacing AT devices
4. Coordinating and using other therapies, interventions, or services with AT devices, such as those associated with existing education and rehabilitation plans and programs
5. Training or technical assistance for the person with a disability, or, if appropriate, his or her family
6. Training or technical assistance for professionals (including individuals providing education or rehabilitation services), employers, or other individuals who provide services to, employ or otherwise are substantially involved in the major life functions of persons with disabilities (3)

This definition has also been included in other U.S. federal legislation authorizing services or supports for persons with disabilities, including the Rehabilitation Act (4) and the Individuals with Disabilities Act (5).

So what is AT? In short, AT is *a tool* used by someone with a disability to perform everyday tasks such as getting dressed,

moving around, controlling his or her environment, learning, working, or engaging in recreational activities. As a tool, AT is no different than using a hammer to drive a nail. Less than 40 years ago, there were fewer than 100 devices commercially available. Today, more than 42,000 assistive devices are listed on the AbleData Web site (www.abledata.com). AT use often begins shortly after birth, or after an illness or accident necessitates its use, and continues throughout the life span of someone with a disability.

Included within this textbook are chapters on wheelchairs and other mobility devices, recreational therapies and tools, orthotics and prosthetics, and many other rehabilitation devices or tools. The devices described by the authors of these chapters also fall within the definition of AT and are considered as such. This chapter covers basic information on other categories of AT products, evaluation, prescription and funding for AT, use of a team approach, and outcomes measurement in the field of AT devices and services. Readers are referred to the appropriate chapter for more in-depth information on those devices covered elsewhere in this textbook.

ASSISTIVE TECHNOLOGY MYTHS

AT tends to be divided into two major categories: low technology and high technology. Low technology or "low-tech" devices tend to be simple, non-electronic devices. Items such as dressing aids, pencil grips, picture-based communication boards for persons who are non-speaking, and magnifiers for persons with visual impairments fall within the category of low-tech devices. High technology or "high-tech" devices are typically described as sophisticated, electronic devices such as power wheelchairs, computers, or augmentative and alternative communication (AAC) devices that provide voice output for persons who are non-speaking. These devices are usually rather expensive and often require extensive training to ensure they are used to their full potential (6).

There are a number of myths surrounding the provision of AT that tend to reflect common misperceptions about both the technology and individuals with disabilities. These myths include:

1. AT is the "be all and end all."
2. AT is complicated and expensive.
3. Persons with the same disability benefit from the same devices.
4. Professionals are the best source of information for AT.
5. AT descriptions are always accurate and helpful.
6. A user's AT requirements need to be assessed just once.
7. AT devices will always be used.

8. Individuals with disabilities want the latest, most expensive device available.
9. AT is a luxury.
10. Only people with certain types of disabilities find AT useful.

Although AT does hold a great deal of promise for persons with disabilities and the elderly who would like to pursue everyday tasks that most of us take for granted, myths such as these have a tendency to cause practitioners and those they serve to disregard the potential utility of assistive devices. Tasks such as navigating freely throughout the community, talking with a loved one, texting or writing an e-mail or often out of reach for persons with disabilities. Proper prescription of AT can enable persons with disabilities to learn, work, and play, just like everyone else. Dispelling these myths can do much to ensure that those who can benefit from assistive devices and services receive appropriate supports (7–11).

AT AND ABANDONMENT

It is important to recognize that not everyone with a disability enjoys using technology, however, useful it might appear. Depending on the type of technology, nonuse or abandonment can be as low as 8% (life support technology) and as high as 78% (hearing aids). On average, one third of more optional ATs are abandoned, most within the first 3 months of acquiring the device. To date, research has not been done to ascertain the number of individuals who must continue to use devices they are not pleased with simply because they cannot abandon the technology without severe consequences (12–14). For example, an individual who has just received a new wheelchair that does not meet expectations simply cannot stop using the chair to navigate independently within his or her community. Rather, he or she must wait until third-party funding becomes available again (often as long as 3 to 6 years) or engage in potentially difficult and unproductive discussions with the vendor who has more than likely provided the chair as it was prescribed by the assessment team.

Research does tell us the number one reason individuals with disabilities choose not to use assistive devices is because practitioners failed to consider their opinions and preferences during the device selection process. In other words, the person with a disability was not included as an active member of the team during the evaluation process (12,15).

HUMAN FACTORS AND AT

A growing body of research in the field of human factors is being applied to the design and development of AT devices for persons with disabilities. Analysis of human factors in a global sense is concerned with how humans interact with various technologies. When you sit in a new car and notice how comfortable it is—how well the seat contours with your body and how accessible the controls are for the stereo system—you have experienced the growing information derived from human factors research.

Dr. King (16), a professor at the University of Wisconsin, Eau Claire, has expanded key points found in the literature on human factors and applied them to research and development in AT. He tells us that human factors in AT must be concerned with how human beings who have special needs, limitations or disabilities interact with devices and tools that may support, supplement, or replace some process or ability that has been lost or impaired by illness, injury, or aging. We must be concerned not only with how the user interacts with the devices but also with how the family or other close care providers react to the use of tools and devices in their settings. The interactions of the AT user alone with the technology does not tell us the whole story because persons who use assistive technologies must interact closely and frequently with, or depend upon others, for daily care and other aspects of their lives. The larger impact on those around the user must also be considered because they are key players in the implementation of any AT in the user's life. Across all component areas of AT, human factors must be concerned with how the potential user—as well as his or her family, personal care providers, education and therapy aides, teachers, and clinicians—interact with the assistive devices and technologic systems.

Analysis of human factors in AT is concerned with identifying special needs, capabilities, and limitations of users and then matching devices and controls to each individual user. Heterogeneity and individualization are primary considerations when dealing with persons who have specialized needs. However, mass-produced technologies, such as computers, must be designed for mass-market use, rather than for each unique individual. Flexibility and adaptability of technology to a wide range of user characteristics are critically important.

Human factor considerations in AT are especially focused on reducing user exertion, as well as stress and anxiety about relying on technology. We all have a bit of "technophobia" when it comes to use of new tools and devices—especially complex, high-tech devices. The fear and stress, particularly when they relate to devices that may be difficult to set up or require a great deal of exertion to use, can be deleterious to the AT user. Persons relying on AT have some type of limitation or disability. Expecting an individual with a disability to become skilled in additional tools, devices, or technology can be highly stressful to users as well as caregivers, because it adds more complexity to their life.

Human factors also focus on reducing danger caused by a device to the user and persons around them. AT professionals should also strive to reduce the possibility of failure during use, which can lead to rejection or abandonment of the device for future use, even when the system has considerable merit for the person with a disability (16).

AT AND THE INTERNATIONAL CLASSIFICATION OF FUNCTIONING, DISABILITY AND HEALTH

Disability itself is not precise and quantifiable. The concept of disability is not always agreed on by persons who self-identify as having a disability, persons who study disability, or the general public (17). This lack of agreement creates obstacles for studies focused on disability and to the equitable and effective administration of programs and policies intended for persons with disabilities. To facilitate agreement about the concept of disability, the World Health Organization (WHO) developed a global common language—one that is understood to include physical, mental, and social well-being. The WHO first published the International Classification of Impairment,

Disabilities, and Handicaps (ICIDH) in 1980 as a tool for classification of the "consequences of disease."

The newest version, International Classification of Functioning, Disability and Health, known as ICF (19), moves away from a "consequences of diseases" classification to a "component of health" classification (see Chapter 9). This latest model is designed to provide a common framework and language for the description of health domains and health-related domains. Using the common language of the ICF can help health care professionals to communicate the need for health care and related services, such as the provision of AT for persons with disabilities (18,19).

In the context of health, the following language is used:

- *Body functions* are the physiologic and psychological functions of body systems.
- *Body structures* are anatomic parts of the body, such as organs, limbs, and their components.
- *Impairments* are problems in body function or structure, such as significant deviation or loss.
- *Activity* is the execution of a task or action by an individual.
- *Participation* is involvement in a life situation.
- *Activity limitations* are difficulties an individual may have in executing activities.
- *Participation restrictions* are problems an individual may experience in involvement in life situations.
- *Environmental factors* make up the physical, social, and attitudinal environments in which people live and conduct their lives (19).

Application of the WHO global common health language makes possible the definition of the need for health care and related services; defines health outcomes in terms of body, person, and social functioning; provides a common framework for research, clinical work, and social policy; ensures the cost-effective provision and management of health care and related services; and characterizes physical, mental, social, economic, or environmental interventions that will improve lives and levels of functioning. Provision of AT for persons with disabilities is an intervention that has the potential to diminish activity limitations and participation restrictions, and in turn, improve the quality of life of individuals with disabilities. Throughout this chapter, the use of the WHO common health language is used to discuss the potential impact of AT.

AT FOR MOBILITY IMPAIRMENTS

Individuals with mobility impairments often present with unique needs and abilities. Some may demonstrate only lower body impairment, such as a spinal cord injury or spina bifida, with no other complications. AT solutions might include crutches, a scooter, or a wheelchair (see Chapter 58). Simple modifications or adaptations to the environment, such as removing physical barriers to access (wide doorway or a ramp instead of stairs) may be all that is needed. For others, automobile hand controls, adapted saddles for horseback riding, sit skis for downhill skiing, or even placing bricks under a desk or table to allow the wheelchair user to work comfortably at a workstation may be necessary accommodations.

Other adaptive equipment for persons with mobility impairments might include a van with an attached lift. Many individuals who use wheelchairs drive a wide range of motor vehicles as well as bicycles using specially customized hand controls for

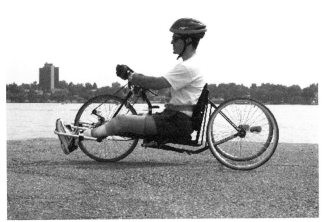

FIGURE 55-1.   AT for mobility impairments. (Courtesy of Marlin Cohrs, Assistive Technology Partners, Department of Rehabilitation Medicine, University of Colorado Health Sciences Center.)

turning and braking (**Fig. 55-1**). Chapters 57 and 58 provide in-depth discussions of a wide range of assistive technologies for persons with mobility impairments that interfere with ambulation and other activities of daily living (ADLs).

For someone with upper-body mobility impairment, such as poor hand control or paralysis, assistive devices might include alternative keyboards or other input methods to access a computer. Alternate keyboards come in many shapes and sizes. There are expanded keyboards, such as the Clevy Keyboard (**Fig. 55-2**), which provides larger, color-coded keys than a standard keyboard; the EZ See large print keyboard with large, high-contrast letters, and options such as a delayed response of the activated key for individuals who have difficulty either initiating touch or removing their finger after they have activated a key. For individuals who have never used a standard QWERTY keyboard layout, letters on the keyboard can be arranged alphabetically on some keyboards. This key arrangement is often helpful for young children who are developing literacy skills, as well as for adults who have cognitive or visual impairments that necessitate additional supports for reading and writing.

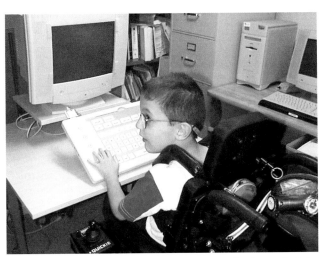

FIGURE 55-2.   Intellikeys keyboard. (Courtesy of Jim Sandstrum, Assistive Technology Partners, Department of Rehabilitation Medicine, University of Colorado Health Sciences Center.)

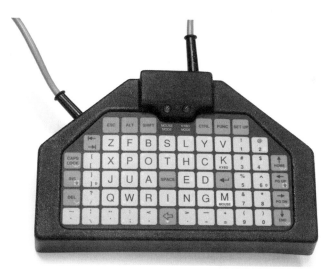

FIGURE 55-3. Tash Mini keyboard. (Courtesy of Marlin Cohrs, Department of Bioengineering, University of Colorado.)

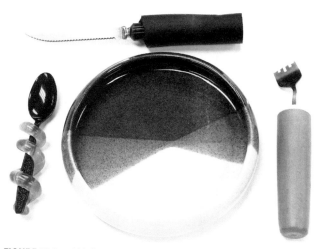

FIGURE 55-5. Aids for daily living. (Courtesy of Marlin Cohrs, Department of Bioengineering, University of Colorado.)

There are also small hands-free keyboards, such as the TouchFree Keyboard (**Fig. 55-3**). This keyboard was originally designed for individuals with repetitive stress injuries. It uses an infrared light beam detection technology. When an opaque object (i.e., a finger or pencil head) is placed inside a cell (key), a key-down signal is triggered and the character or function is activated. Individuals who are one-handed typists, or who use a head stick or mouth stick to type, frequently prefer a smaller-sized keyboard such as this one.

For individuals who are unable to use any type of keyboard or other device that requires hand mobility or finger pointing, there are a wide range of switches available that provide access not only to the computer but also to battery-operated electric toys and home-based or work appliances. The switches may be as simple as a "rocking lever" switch (**Fig. 55-4**) designed to be activated through a gross motor movement that involves touching or hitting the switch with the head, hand, arm, leg, or knee. Other switches can be activated by tongue touch, sipping and puffing on a straw, or through very fine movements, such as an eye blink or a single muscle twitch.

Fairly recent developments include eye gaze switches that calibrate intentional eye movement patterns and select targets such as individual keys on an on-screen keyboard and also brain wave technology (eye and muscle operated switch or EMOS) that responds to the excitation of alpha waves to trigger the selection. Other input methods for the computer include devices such as the HeadMouse Nano. This device translates natural head movements into directly proportional mouse pointer movement. Once the mouse arrives at the selected destination selections, mouse operations can be readily controlled by a variety of adaptive switches or mouse button software, such as Dragger. When combined with an onscreen keyboard, persons who are severely physically impaired can readily type on a computer or use this with an AAC device for speech output. He or she can also control an almost unlimited array of smart home, gaming, and other educational devices.

There are literally thousands of low-tech assistive devices available for persons with motor impairments. Commonly referred to as aids for daily living (ADLs), these include such things as weighted spoons, scoop plates, and other devices used to facilitate eating (**Fig. 55-5**); aids for personal hygiene, such as bath chairs and long-handled hairbrushes; adapted toys for play; built-up pencil grips for writing and drawing tasks; items for dressing, such as sock aids and one-handed buttoners; and many others. Prices and availability cover a wide range for items such as these. Many low-tech mobility aids can be handmade for just a few dollars, whereas others, such as an adult bath chair, may cost several hundred dollars. All share the common goal or utility of reducing activity limitations and increasing participation in daily life activities.

AT FOR COMMUNICATION DISORDERS

For individuals with severe expressive communication impairments, there is a wide range of AT devices available (see also Chapter 13). For persons who have reduced phonation or breath support, and speak very quietly, there are a number of portable amplification systems available that work much like a sound system in a large lecture hall. Called Voice Enhancers, these devices work as personal voice amplifiers. Individuals with medical conditions such as Parkinson disease, multiple

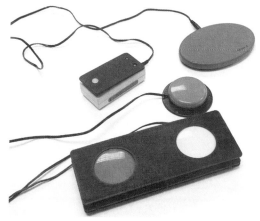

FIGURE 55-4. Switches. (Courtesy of Marlin Cohrs, Assistive Technology Partners, Department of Rehabilitation Medicine, University of Colorado Health Sciences Center.)

sclerosis (MS), Guillain-Barré syndrome, amyotrophic lateral sclerosis (ALS), and stroke may benefit. The VM Inline Voice Magnifier works with a telephone to add as much as 25 decibels of volume to the user's voice. There are lightweight headset models, such as the ADDvox FeatherLite Pro Headset, that works well for persons who prefer a hands-free device.

For those who are unable to talk at all or who have such severe expressive communication difficulties that only their most intimate associates understand them, there are a wide range of AAC devices on the market. These devices can range from very simple picture books to high-end sophisticated electronic communication devices with digitally recorded or synthetic speech output. Children and adults with complex communication needs (CCN) can benefit academically, vocationally, emotionally, and socially from the provision of a device that allows them to communicate their thoughts, learn, and share information and ideas, and otherwise participate in life activities.

It is important to note these AAC devices, although extremely useful and important to the lifestyles of many individuals who are nonspeaking, do not replace natural speech. Instead they *augment* or provide an *alternate* form of communication. Other communicative modalities, including vocalizations, gestures, sign language systems, eye gaze, etc., remain valid and acceptable forms of communication, and should be encouraged to develop along with the facility to communicate out loud using an AAC device.

Congenital conditions such as autism, cerebral palsy, reduced intellectual functioning, developmental verbal apraxia, and developmental language disorders can result in severe expressive communication impairments, necessitating the need for AAC interventions (20,21). Acquired disorders for which AAC is often used include traumatic brain injury (see Chapter 19), stroke (see Chapter 18), ALS (see Chapter 23), MS (see Chapter 20), and laryngectomy following surgical removal or alteration of the larynx (22–25). Augmentative communication systems have also been used successfully for individuals who are temporarily nonspeaking as a result of ventilator dependency (26).

There are two common myths surrounding the use of AAC. The first is that individuals who are nonspeaking must demonstrate certain developmental prerequisites before the prescription of an AAC device. On the contrary, there are no strict sets of cognitive or physical prerequisites to the use of AAC devices. Specific AAC techniques that match the individual's needs and abilities are chosen on the basis of a comprehensive evaluation by a qualified team of clinicians, family members, teachers, and others. The second myth is that the use of an AAC device will stifle or preclude the development or return of natural speech. However, research tells us that use of an AAC device can actually support improved speech production, and it in no way creates barriers to the development or return of natural speech (27,28).

Low-tech picture and alphabet boards are often used either as a preliminary step before purchasing an electronic voice output system or as a backup system, should an electronic device break or its use not be convenient (e.g., during swim lessons). These low-tech systems (**Fig. 55-6**) can be made from picture library software available through commercial vendors (Boardmaker Pro from Tobbdynavox or LessonPix) or can be handmade using digital photographs, pictures from print or online materials, or by simply using a marker to write or draw

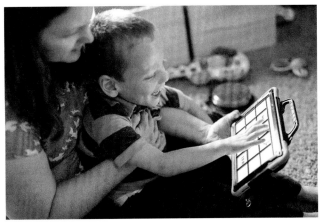

FIGURE 55-6.   AAC device. (Courtesy of Prentke Romich Company.)

letters, words, phrases, or pictures. Adults with progressive diseases such as ALS or MS frequently use low-tech picture or alphabet boards to clarify their meaning as communication abilities decrease or as they fatigue during the day. In any case, it is critical that the individual who is struggling to communicate serve as an integral decision-maker in the process of acquiring alternate strategies to vocal communication.

There are a number of electronic, low-tech voice output AAC devices available that are simple to program and use. The Talking Symbol Notepad, GoTalk, and TechTalk8 communication devices all use digital speech output (**Fig. 55-7**). Digital

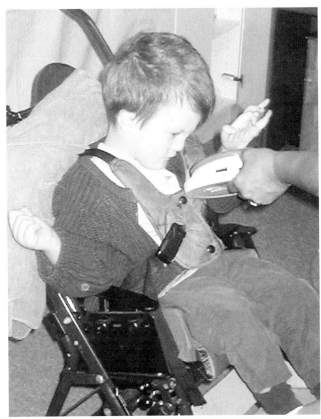

FIGURE 55-7.   Using the Big Mac. (Courtesy of Diane Brians, Assistive Technology Partners, Department of Rehabilitation Medicine, University of Colorado Health Sciences Center.)

speech devices work much like an old-school tape recorder. The person setting up the device simply holds down a button and records live voice into the microphone. The speech is digitized, or recorded, within the device. When the end user chooses to speak, he or she simply presses a button to activate the device. The good news is these devices are simple and fairly inexpensive to purchase. It is important to bear in mind, however, that they are intentionally designed to communicate quick, simple messages, such as "Hi," "let's play," or "leave me alone." These devices are not appropriate for individuals who have more than a few things to say or who have the ability to generate complex thoughts and feelings.

There are a number of more sophisticated AAC devices available as well. While stand-alone AAC devices are still common, many are now available as downloadable applications (apps) and can be used on either an android or IOS tablet device. They incorporate a synthetic voice system, with some also including digital recording capability to enable live voice recording. A synthetic voice system is essentially a "text-to-speech" device that speaks text that is typed or stored within the system. They are capable of encoding several thousand words, phrases, and sentences. AAC devices such as these are frequently designed to provide an alternate access to the computer and control appliances such as TV's, door openers, and other electrical items found in many environments.

Some of the more popular synthetic AAC devices include the NOVA chat 5, Tobii Dynavox I-12+, Accent 1400 with NuPoint and NuEye, and the Lightwriter SL40 Connect. The NOVA chat 5 is a good example of a system that is available on the Android platform. It incorporates a range of preloaded vocabulary configurations and includes a child's voice, a teen's voice, as well as a number of American, British English, and Australian adult options. The device also provides a bilingual Spanish/English option and speaks German, Dutch, and Canadian French.

In just the past 3 to 5 years, eye gaze technology has improved dramatically. For individuals who have no other option, such as those with end-stage ALS or locked in syndrome, eye gaze has reached a level that now makes it a useful tool. Systems with this feature typically have a built-in eye tracker that recognizes where on the screen eye gaze is focused. Using "dwell-time" (i.e., looking at an icon or character for a set length of time) or a secondary switch, users can select an icon or, with an onscreen keyboard, the character or function they desire and activate that option. Both the Tobii Dynavox I-12+ and the Accent 1400 with NuPoint and NuEye offer an eye gaze system for individuals who need to use their eyes to type or speak.

All AAC devices on the market can be activated through direct selection using either a finger or other pointing device, such as a head or mouth stick. A large number of the digital and text-to-speech devices can be activated using either direct selection or an alternate input mode. Alternate input includes all of the switches described above, as well as other additional infrared or wireless switches currently on the market. When an individual with a severe motor impairment and severe expressive communication impairment chooses to use a switch to activate an AAC device, the device can be preset to scan.

The most commonly used switch access method is called row column scanning. In this method, the end users start by activating a switch to begin the scan. When the correct row is

highlighted, he or she hits the switch again to start the lights scanning across the row (hence column). When the correct button is highlighted, the user hits the switch again to activate the chosen button. As can be surmised, using a scanning system to activate an AAC device can be a slow and tedious process. For many individuals however, this method provides the only available access to spoken and written communication, and for those select persons, it is highly prized as a window to the world.

One of the more vigorous debates within the field of AAC centers around the encoding or mapping strategies used to represent language on a communication device. Currently available systems vary greatly in vocabulary storage and retrieval methods, but all systems are based on communication symbols, whether orthographic or pictographic. Symbols vary in their transparency (guessability) and translucency (learnability). In order to select a set of symbols for an individual's communication system, it is important to match these factors with the individual's cognitive and perceptual abilities. It is important to ensure a speech language pathologist with training and experience in AAC is highly involved in working with the end user and their family to ensure an appropriate language, and language representation system is selected during the evaluation process.

AAC devices currently on the market have changed significantly in the past 5 years and are designed using today's technologies. They feature bluetooth with wireless control of home appliances, texting, phones, and numerous other features. There has also been a tremendous increase in the development of communication applications (apps) available for tablet devices such as the iPad as well as IOS and Android phones. These apps range from ready-made vocabulary sets with color-coded core words and symbols or pictures (most frequently used words) arranged in levels to encourage language development (Clicker Communicator App); to text-based communication apps that can work well for children and adults who are literate (Proloquo4Text). While there is much to be said for these mainstream devices and apps serving as communication systems, great care must be taken to ensure the selected app and hardware meet the communication and access needs of the end user.

AT FOR VISUAL IMPAIRMENTS, INCLUDING BLINDNESS

The term *visual impairment* technically encompasses all degrees of permanent vision loss, including total blindness, which affects a person's ability to perform the usual tasks of daily life. *Low vision* refers to a vision loss that is severe enough to impede performance of everyday tasks but still allows some useful visual discrimination. Low vision cannot be correct to normal by regular eyeglasses or contact lens.

For individuals with visual impairments, there are a variety of AT devices and strategies available to assist them to perform daily activities such as reading (**Fig. 55-8**), writing, daily care, mobility, and recreational activities. Among the low-tech solutions are simple handheld magnifiers, the use of large print, or mobility devices (e.g., long cane) for safe and efficient travel. High-contrast tape or markers can be used to indicate what an item is or where it is located within a physical plant.

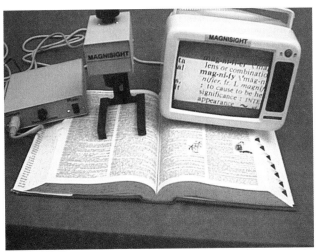

FIGURE 55-8. Low-tech magnification. (Courtesy of Marlin Cohrs, Department of Bioengineering, University of Colorado.)

Other low-tech devices, include items such as wind chimes to facilitate direction finding, using easily legible type fonts such as Verdana (16 pt or larger), and using vanilla- or beige-colored paper rather than white to improve visibility of text for individuals with severe visual impairments. Libraries that provide print materials in alternate formats for persons who have visual and learning impairments can arrange to have textbooks and other materials translated into various formats. For more information, contact the American Federation for the Blind (📶 **eTable 55-1**).

High-tech solutions for persons with visual impairments can include a computer, tablet or laptop outfitted with voice output software that allows text, software menus, and other tagged labels, graphics, figures, and/or pictures on the screen to be heard aloud by the person unable to see well enough to read the computer screen (Jaws, Outspoken). Brailled text, although somewhat less popular than in recent years, is still the first choice of many individuals to facilitate reading of print materials.

For individuals with some degree of visual ability, screen magnification software is available. ZoomText (**Fig. 55-9**) is one of the more popular versions of screen magnification programs. This software enables the end user to choose the amount and type of magnification he or she prefers for optimal computer access. As with mainstream commercial technology companies, AT companies have been engaging in buyouts and acquisitions of various companies and products. A good example of a merger is the inclusion of ZoomText and Jaws.

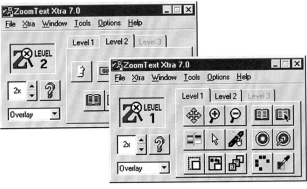

FIGURE 55-9. ZoomText Xtra. (Courtesy of Marlin Cohrs, Department of Bioengineering, University of Colorado.)

This package combines screen reading typically used by someone who cannot visualize text on a screen with ZoomText for magnification. Called "Fusion," this product is designed for individuals with advanced and/or progressive vision loss.

Technology for persons with visual impairment is an area to watch for rapid changes in the coming years. With the advent of built-in accessibility features in platforms such as Microsoft, Voice output, screen enlargement, and contrasting color features are all available at no cost to the end user. Additionally, accessibility to the Internet is improving daily. For Web sites to meet accessibility requirements, graphics must be tagged with relevant descriptions, web pages designed with less clutter, and the page must be set up in a tabbing order that is relevant for page navigation.

A number of organizations, most notably, Braille Institute (www.brailleinstitute.org), is developing free mobile phone apps to provide accessible smart phone user experiences. They have designed a product called Big Browser that supports low vision users as they navigate the web on the iPad. Most interestingly, they have developed an app call VIA (Visually Impaired Apps) for iPhone and iPad that helps blind and low-vision users sort through the more than 500,000 apps in the iTunes App Store to locate apps designed specifically for visually impaired users, or apps that might provide some functionality for this population. Finally, they have developed a simulation app called VisionSim that allows persons with vision within normal limits to experience one of nine degenerative eye diseases including macular degeneration, diabetic retinopathy, glaucoma, and cataracts.

There is also a great deal of exciting work going on in the navigation space for individuals with visual impairments. Traditional approaches to navigation include the long cane or a guide dog. With the advent of GPS, voice output, and improving indoor navigation technologies, apps are beginning to be developed to facilitate navigation (https://play.google.com/store/apps/details?id=com.lazarillo and http://www.popflock.com/learn?s=GPS_for_the_visually_impaired).

ALVU (Array of Lidars and Vibrotactile Units) is a contactless, intuitive, hands-free, and discreet wearable device that allows visually impaired users to detect low- and high-hanging obstacles as well as physical boundaries in their immediate environment. The solution allows for safe local navigation in both confined and open spaces by enabling the user to distinguish free space from obstacles. Using a sensor belt and a haptic strap, the device provides fairly reliable and accurate measurements of the distances between the user and surrounding obstacles or surfaces. The second iteration of this device includes a camera that can be worn and that is beginning to provide visual recognition of obstacles to provide additional feedback to the user. Other federally funded projects are investigating the use of haptic devices that can provide sensory positional and directional information to end users. In short, this technology space is rapidly evolving, and there will be many new options available for persons with visual impairments in the coming years.

AT FOR LEARNING AND COGNITION

Children and adults often present with a variety of learning and cognitive impairments resulting from either acquired or developmental disabilities. Not only can AT provide important accommodations for those with disabilities of all types, it can also become a critical tool to be used during recovery or acquisition of functional skill sets. For those with learning disabilities, there are a wide range of abilities that may benefit from an AT solution.

For example, many children with learning and cognitive impairments struggle with developing literacy skills. Fortunately, there are a number of both low- and high-technology solutions available to assist them. For those struggling to learn to read, there are products such as "Snap&Read Universal" (Don Johnston, Inc.); a tool that works with Google Chrome and the iPad that reads text aloud; including Web sites, PDFs, and Google Drive documents. It provides text highlighting, word definitions, a simplified summary of available text, and annotation features. Other software programs provide highlighted text and voice output, so the user can hear the words they are generating on the computer (Kurzweil 3000). Individuals who are unable to read print materials often use some of the software solutions mentioned in the previous section, such as Jaws for voice output or books available on devices such as the Kindle. While software alone cannot teach a child to read; software combined with appropriate instructional support can and often does lead to literacy.

There are hardware products such as the WhisperPhone Solo Headset (WhisperPhone) designed for children from kindergarten through fourth grade that provides voice amplification of the teacher who wears a microphone and filtering of external classroom sounds that may create disruptions for the child. There are also simple devices such as a bill and coin machine to teach money skills, simplified cookbooks, and switch operated toys for children who also have motor impairments (Attainment, Inc., AbleNet Technologies).

Voice recognition is a popular request both for persons with mobility impairments who are unable to type using their hands and for individuals whose learning disabilities are so significant they are unable to develop literacy skills. Voice recognition software such as Dragon Naturally Speaking (Nuance) enables an individual to speak into a microphone in order to input words, phrases, and sentences into standard computer word processing programs such as Microsoft Word. Although a bit trickier, voice recognition can be used for input and control functions for other software, such as database programs (Excel) and Windows.

Although voice recognition software is extremely popular, it is important to remember that it takes a fifth- to sixth-grade reading ability to train the standard software, simply because the individual's voice file cannot be developed unless he or she uses the standard training package that comes with the software. Nuance has developed a version for children, but its success rate for children with learning, and other cognitive disabilities, has not been provided. In addition, ambient noise such as in a typical classroom, as well as fluctuating vocal abilities (e.g., fatigue) found in many individuals with disabilities will have an impact on the accuracy of the voice recognition. In general, it takes more than 20 hours to train the software to an acceptable level of accuracy (>90%). This still means that for every 100 words, 10 will have to be identified as an error and corrected. Correcting errors within a voice recognition program requires facility with word processing programs. Although caution is in order when prescribing this type of software, the rapid pace of development bodes well for future use of this solution for persons with disabilities.

A very interesting development is the use of voice recognition to manage text messaging, e-mails, navigation, and web browsing through mainstream products such as Google's voice recognition system. Home automation tools, described later in this chapter, are also becoming extremely popular with consumers. For individuals who struggle with literacy or motor impairments, these tools are becoming ubiquitous as a viable strategy for managing much of the world around us. As voice recognition continues to improve for these products, ease-of-use and learnability will continue to improve leading to even more options for persons with cognitive and learning disabilities.

Low-tech adaptations for persons with learning and/or cognitive impairments can include simple solutions such as colored highlighter tape, pencil grips, enlarged text, and other easy modifications, such using a copy holder to hold print materials for easier viewing. Reminder lists with important times, places, and activities highlighted with a marker are often useful for individuals who need subtle memory prompts to be in the right place at the right time.

There are also a number of software packages available for these populations that focus on a range of topics, including academics, money management, personal skills development, behavior training, development of cognitive skills, memory improvement, problem solving, time concepts, safety awareness, speech and language therapy, telephone usage, recreational activities, and games. For individuals with cognitive and learning impairments, a number of simple techniques can be kept in mind when evaluating or designing activities and materials for use by persons with cognitive and learning impairments. **Table 55-1** includes some components of accessible interfaces to keep in mind.

Over the past decade, handheld smartphones and other digital assistants have also become ubiquitous. Utilizing avatars as well as video-prompting, these technologies have the capability of identifying precise steps in a task and providing auditory and visual prompts to facilitate task completion. For many of these technologies, a "most-to-least" prompting strategy is utilized. This means the individual requiring assistance is first given a simple prompt such as, "look again." If that doesn't work, the system will provide a more comprehensive prompt such as "look at the picture and make yours the same" (29,30). Nonlinear Context Aware Prompting (NCAP) is the latest entry in this arena. Using available features of smartphone and tablet devices such as calendars, along with newly developed capabilities such as indoor navigation, and knowledge of tasks to be completed, end users are prompted only when they need to be prompted and in a manner that works best for their cognitive capabilities (31).

These smart applications can be set up to remind someone to stay on task, return to work or studying after a break, and help them to locate where they need to be at any time. With sharing features, such as location and wayfinding, parents or other care providers can be alerted if their loved one is struggling. The technology and application space for cognitive impairments continues to evolve. At the national and international level, standards bodies, care providers, and technology companies are all recognizing the need to begin to address issues of cognitive impairment. This may be the fastest growing area of technology and support during the coming decade.

TABLE 55-1	Components of Accessible Interfaces

Simplicity of layout, operation, and appearance
- Is the interface crowded, complex, or otherwise overwhelming?
- Does the interface require complex mouse actions or keystroke combinations?
- Is the language level of the interface too complex for the user?

Consistency of critical elements in the interface
- Are interface elements and controls located consistently throughout the application?
- Are interface elements and controls activated in the same manner throughout the application?

Saliency of active elements
- Is the user directed visually or otherwise toward the central content of the interface?
- Is key information highlighted?
- Is there a minimum of competing information?
- Is it clear to the user when actions or changes occur in the interface?

Intuitive operation
- Is the operation of the software obvious to the user?
- Is the selection of user interface components simple and direct?
- Is it clear to the user that the interface is responding to his or her input?
- Is there clear feedback when the application is busy completing a task?

Organization
- Are similar functions grouped logically together?
- Does the organization of the interface make sense visually?

Adaptability
- Does the interface offer a choice of modalities for the user (e.g., can on-screen text be read aloud)?
- Can interface elements be added or removed easily to adjust to a user's abilities?
- Does the interface offer context-sensitive help, such as tool tips?
- Are on-screen instructions provided?
- Are cues provided automatically to the user if he or she waits for assistance?
- Is there a timed response?

Recoverability
- Can the user easily recover from an error?
- Is clear warning provided if an action cannot be undone?
- Can the user explore the interface safely without causing instability?

AT FOR HEARING

For an individual who is deaf or hard of hearing, there are two major effects of hearing loss, lack of auditory input and compromised ability to monitor speech output (see also Chapter 13). AT devices such as hearing aids and FM systems can often be used to facilitate both auditory input and speech output. Other types of AT devices provide a visual representation of the auditory signal. These include flashing lights to indicate an emergency alarm (fire, tornado), the phone ringing, or someone at the door.

Low-technology solutions or technology-free solutions might include use of sign language or other visual representations of the spoken word or providing information in a print format. Another recent adaptation is computer-assisted translation. Referred to by the acronym CART (Computer-Assisted Real-time Translation or Communication Access Real-time Technology), this solution involves a specially trained typist who captures or types the discourse of the speaker(s) on a computer that is then projected onto a monitor or other display. A variation of CART is computer-assisted note taking, when the primary purpose is to provide a written record for a student or employee.

Recent advances in the use of Avatars or Agents, as computer-based sign language interpreters, are being tested in real-world environments. A company named SignAll (www.signall.us) is pioneering one of the first fully automated sign language translation solutions using computer vision and natural language processing (NLP) to translate American Sign Language (ASL). Other researchers are working to develop sign language tutoring systems using a low-cost data glove and a software application. The system processes movement signals in real-time and uses Pattern Matching strategies to determine whether or not the trainee is processing the hand signal correctly (32). During the next few years, technology-based sign language interpreters are projected to be readily available in public locations and for private use.

Environmental adaptations can frequently support individuals who are deaf or hard-of-hearing. For example, when speaking to someone who has difficulty hearing, it is better not to stand in front of a light sources (windows, lamps, etc.) and to not over exaggerate lip movements. However, gestures can add richness to the dialogues. For individuals who wear hearing aids, there are a number of additional technologies that can facilitate hearing in large rooms or in crowded environments, such as in a restaurant or at a party. The Conference Mate and Whisper Voice are two products especially designed for this issue. The person with the hearing loss wears a neck loop (it looks much like a Bolo tie). In the case of the Conference Mate, a small octagonal device is placed on a convenient table. This device picks up voices within the room that are transmitted to the neck loop and then to the hearing aid for better reception. Although it may sound cumbersome, it can be an excellent solution for office- and school-based environments. The Whisper Voice works much the same way, except the device contains a small microphone and is portable. It can be passed from one speaker to another, with sound transmitted to the neck loop and then to the hearing aid for amplification. Chapter 13 contains additional information on hearing loss and auditory rehabilitation.

AT FOR ERGONOMICS AND PREVENTION OF SECONDARY INJURIES

A rapidly growing area of concern for AT practitioners is the development of repetitive motion disorders. For many persons with disabilities, the use of computer keyboards and other technologies presents an opportunity for secondary injuries to occur. Computer desks, tables, and chairs used in computer labs, classrooms, and at the office do not always match the physical needs of the end user. When those with disabilities (and those without) are not positioned properly and then spend hours repetitively performing the same motor movement, they can and do incur injuries.

An entire industry within AT has developed over the past few years dealing with repetitive motion disorders. Potential solutions for someone demonstrating this type of impairment include raising or lowering a chair or desk for the appropriate fit, implementing routine breaks within activities for the individual to move about or do something different, lumbar and other supports, specially designed ergonomic keyboards, and other ATs.

Many of the ATs described in earlier sections, such as voice recognition software, alternate and specially designed ergonomic keyboards, and strategies designed to minimize keystrokes and other repetitive movements, can also provide useful solutions for individuals with repetitive stress injuries. There are a number of Internet-based resources available that target ergonomic issues, such as those found in 🛜 **eTable 55-2**.

ENVIRONMENTAL AIDS TO DAILY LIVING AND SMART HOME TECHNOLOGIES

Electronic aids to daily living (EADLs), also described as environmental control units, provide alternative control of electrical and battery-operated devices within the environment. These devices may include the TV, DVD, music, lights, appliances, landlines, doors, electric hospital beds, and more. EADLs are designed to improve independence of ADLs. They are primarily used in the home but can also be used at work, school, and in hospitals.

EADLs provide alternative control to electronic devices and are designed for persons who are unable to use standard controls such as light switches or other electronic or battery-operated appliances and fixtures. EADLs can be helpful for persons with physical and/or cognitive disabilities. For example, a person with aphasia and motor impairments due to stroke may not be able to easily select a new TV channel. This person may benefit from a solution as simple as a standard TV remote operated through the EADL system.

A person with cerebral palsy on the other hand might have difficulty activating small buttons found on a remote control. This person may benefit from an EADL that is accessed by a switch to scan choices visible on a tablet device. Persons of all ages can benefit from this technology as well. For example, entry-level EADLs provide alternative control of toys for very young children.

EADLs are controlled by three different access methods: direct, switch, and voice. Direct access is generally finger-to-button, as on a standard remote control. Some EADLs have enlarged buttons or keyguards to assist direct access. Enlarged buttons can also make the buttons easier to see. Typically, individuals who use direct selection have fair to good fine motor control and vision.

In switch access, any type of switch can be placed at the best location for activation by the person. The first switch activation begins a scan of choices, usually of general categories (e.g., TV, lights, phone). The second switch activation chooses one of these categories. Choices within that category are now scanned (e.g., channel up, channel down, mute). A third switch activation selects the desired function, and the signal is sent to the TV. Most of these systems have visual displays with small text in English (although some are available in other languages) and no speech feedback. The person generally must have good sequencing skills and vision and be able to read.

Voice-operated EADLs respond to verbal commands. For example, if a user says "TV on," a signal is immediately sent to the TV to turn it on. The individual using the device needs to have a consistent, understandable voice to operate this option. They must also remember the available commands or be able to read a list to remind themselves. A person with a high-level spinal cord injury is a typical patient who could benefit from this device.

Many AAC devices are capable of sending signals to control devices within the home environment. This can be advantageous for several reasons. First, because EADL capability is built in, no additional technology or funding is needed. Second, these AAC devices allow the use of larger text, graphics, and auditory scanning. Auditory scanning verbally announces each choice as it is scanned. Depending on the AAC device, these auditory prompts can even be recorded in another language. This can be very helpful for individuals with low or no vision; who need prompts to assist with memory or sequencing challenges or who do not read (or do not read English). If they are already using a communication device, these features can be easily programmed to increase independence in the home. Some individuals who do not require an AAC device still use one solely for the EADL features because of the visual and cognitive advantages. AAC devices can be accessed directly by switch scanning, mouse control, or joystick.

Software and hardware are also available for computer users to provide control of devices within their personal environment. Typically, this technology is designed for computer users who are interested in automating their home and who do not wish to, or require use of an AAC device. It is imperative for people with disabilities to make their homes accessible in order to foster self-reliance and have the opportunity to live life as they choose.

One of the latest developments to enter the market has been labeled Smart Home Technologies. Driven by the mainstream market, these devices are designed to make life easier for persons with and without disabilities. Smart Home Technologies do not rely on disability-specific devices to carry out simple tasks. Based on the "Internet of Things," smartphones, and/or integrated systems such as Amazon Alexa, people with disabilities can now expand their smart home capabilities bit by bit, starting with what they need most. These technologies are evolving so rapidly, it is difficult to keep up. The paragraphs below describe options that are available now.

The Amazon Echo and its smaller iteration dubbed Echo Dot lets persons with good voice control manage devices in their home. Another option is the Amazon Alexa app for smartphones. It can be used to set alarms, reminders, and timers; produce a shopping list; and also carry out Internet searches while minimizing the need for hand use.

A smart lock is a relatively safer alternative to a keypad, especially if an individual needs to provide access to their home for housekeeping, care providers, or therapists. The August Smart Lock uses the individuals smartphone as a key, allowing them to give others temporary, guest or administrative access, and even restricts the number of times and days someone can have access to their home. The app monitors who entered the home and when, by keeping a log. Should access preferences change, individuals access privileges can be removed enhancing safety and security.

Smart doorbells and thermostats are also becoming popular. The Ring smart doorbell comes with a motion-sensor camera, providing a video feed to show who is at the door, allowing persons with disabilities to decide whether or not to answer. A Smart Thermostat keeps home environments at the exact temperature specified. For individuals with body temperature regulation issues, smart thermostats can facilitate constant environmental temperatures and can be adjusted easily through a tablet or smartphone app.

Poor home lighting can be an extreme risk factor for persons with low vision, cognitive or motor impairments. The Philips Hue light bulbs provide several options aside from just "on" and "off." These bulbs can change hues and can even be dimmed to decrease sensory overload. The Philips Hue starter kit is a smart strategy for testing the efficacy of these light bulbs in a variety of environments. Using either a smart light bulb or a plug that converts for a smart light bulb enables the use of a tablet device to activate the lighting system, creating a much more accessible environment for end users.

Operating curtains and shades can be difficult for individuals with restricted mobility. Smart window coverings incorporate either battery or electrically operated blinds and curtains that can be adjusted from a tablet device and even through voice commands using the Alexa or Echo systems. Some options include My Smart Blinds, Soma smart shades, and Slides for curtains.

Smart garage door openers allow individuals to open their garage from any location. Numerous brands including Nexx Garage, LiftMaster, and Chamberlain are compatible with most of the systems that do not come with their own branded smart add-on.

Smart home technologies can allow individuals with disabilities to live much more independently. When integrated with a smart home hub, these various devices can be integrated into a single app. This enables persons with and without disabilities to control any or all smart home technologies in a single place. Currently, available hub systems can be somewhat tricky to set up. However, this technology is changing very quickly to enable a hub to "recognize" all smart home technologies in a single environment and then organize and connect to them. As this capability improves, smart home technologies, either combined with existing EADL technologies or used on their own, will enable tremendous improvements in independence.

Considerations in EADL and Smart Home Selection

Features that are essential to consider in EADL and/or Smart Home technologies selection are (a) portability, (b) whether the client needs to use the technology from their bed, and (c) safety. A portable device is very important for an individual who is mobile within the home (i.e., driving a power wheelchair) and for people who need to use the device from more than one position, such as from a wheelchair and also from bed.

Accessing these options from bed is very important for many persons with disabilities. Alerting a caregiver of a need in the night, controlling an electric bed, turning on a light, and turning on some quiet music to help someone go to sleep are just a few examples. Motor control can change dramatically from sitting to lying down, which may require a different access method in general, or two different access methods (i.e., hand switch in the wheelchair and head switch in bed).

There are a number of important questions to be discussed during the EADL selection process. These include:
1. What environments will the person be in, and how much time is spent in each setting?
2. What appliances or devices need to be accessed?
3. Will needs and abilities change throughout the day or in different environments?
4. What are the individual's cognitive and sensory abilities? (17)

AT specialists should assess for the most appropriate EADL based on what devices the person would like to control, as well as motor, cognitive, and sensory skills. The AT specialist or the AT supplier or vendor can also assist with procuring funding, installing equipment in the home, and training the end user and caregivers in its use.

Appropriately prescribed EADLs/Smart Home technologies result in a more productive and satisfying lifestyle. In the hospital setting, EADLs allow patients to experience greater independence and can decrease the level of required nursing supervision and support. In the home, an EADL allows an individual more independence and flexibility while demonstrating the cost-benefit of decreased home health care and assistance. Traditional EADL's do not communicate activity information—so privacy concerns are not an issue. Medically designed EADLs are governed by HIPPA regulations.

SOCIALLY ASSISTIVE ROBOTICS

Socially assistive robotics (SARs) are at the forefront of new technologies designed to generate therapeutic benefit for children and adults with complex disabilities because they can be designed to be socially engaging and interactive. SARs facilitate social interaction, while at the same time, create opportunities for children to play and for adults to decrease feelings of social isolation.

SARs have been primarily used to mediate social interactions for children with autism spectrum disorders (ASD) (33–40). They have also been used therapeutically for adults with dementia (41–45) and individuals undergoing poststroke rehabilitation (46–49). In 2015, Rabbitt and collaborators provided a review of SAR use in mental health interventions, including ASD, and gave recommendations for clinical interventions employing SARs (50). They emphasized the importance of thinking about SARs as supplements to, not replacement of, human care providers. In other words, SARs are designed to serve as an extension of the therapist or educator. They utilize affective feedback to initiate and encourage interactions while using the adult or child's affective cues to maintain interactions.

The PARO (http://www.parorobots.com/) was designed specifically for adults with significant dementia. Based on a Harp seal, this attractive SAR has five kinds of sensors: tactile, light, audition, temperature, and posture. This enables the PARO to perceive both persons and the environment. For example, when held and stroked, he moves toward the individual and emits sounds of enjoyment. PARO remembers previous interactions. For example, if an individual typically pets PARO, he will nudge the user to pet again and blink his eyes. Results suggest that this SAR is capable of reducing patient and caregiver stress; stimulating interactions between patients and care providers; and facilitates improved socialization of individuals with advanced dementia (45,51,52).

Use of SARs as a therapeutic tool for children with ASD is one of the most widely recognized applications. This is due in large part because SARs are at the nexus between inanimate objects/toys and humans, whose attempts at social engagement are often stressful for a child with ASD (53). However, developing a SAR that is appropriately initiatory and responsive to a child with ASD is challenging because these children do not present a homogenous group.

Cabibihan et al. (54) reviewed the design features of available SARs and how these robots were used during therapeutic sessions with children with ASD. From the design perspective, they categorized requirements based on appearance, functionality, safety requirements, autonomy, modularity, and adaptability ((54), p. 618). They also looked at the types of behaviors targeted in therapy by various clinicians. These behaviors included imitation, eye contact, joint attention, turn-taking, emotion recognition and expression, self-initiated interactions, and triadic interactions. They concluded that SARs were used to achieve a variety of therapeutic intentions, among them, assisting in the diagnosis of ASD; as a friendly playmate; as a behavior eliciting agent; as a social mediator; as a social actor; and as a personal therapist (54). **Table 55-2** provides a summary overview of SARs and their components used for investigational research as well as those that are commercially available today. Each of these devices has been used to address therapeutic intervention goals for children with complex disabilities. At the University of Colorado, work is underway to design a SAR to be used as an augmentation of clinical interventions for children with complex cerebral palsy (55).

SARs are an exciting development in the field of assistive technology. Sensors, actuators, and processing capability are improving rapidly. These advances enable everyday clinicians to incorporate therapeutic objectives within the repertoire of the SAR; allowing them to provide much needed repetitions of therapeutic objectives at home, school, or in facilities serving the needs of adults with dementia.

TEAMING AND AT

"Teaming means you work together, no matter what. You do it because you'll come up with better ideas. And, if (or when) you disagree, you just figure it out—without fighting" (18).

Equal participation in the collaborative teamwork process by the person with a disability, family members, and service providers is critical for individuals to achieve their goals. As it is in so many areas of physical medicine and rehabilitation, AT services are delivered in a wide variety of settings, including comprehensive medical rehabilitation centers, university-affiliated clinics, state agency–based AT programs, private rehabilitation engineering and technology firms, and nonprofit disability organizations (56,57). Because AT is a relatively new field and preservice and in-service preparation is just beginning to register an impact, persons with disabilities may encounter difficulty locating experienced and credentialed professionals to deliver AT services.

A transdisciplinary model of service delivery is preferred as it provides a larger pool of resources and expertise. The team may include occupational and physical therapists, rehabilitation engineers, speech language pathologists, physiatrists, case managers, and other professionals identified as important to meeting the individualized goals of the person with a disability. It is critical that the team includes, as recognized members, the person with the disability(s), and his or her family and significant others when appropriate. It is also critical that at least one member of the team has some background knowledge and training in the field of AT. There are a number of university and online courses available for professionals to build expertise as well as resources in the field of AT.

The field of AT, like many other growing professions, is working to develop standards of practice and credentialing opportunities. The Rehabilitation Engineering and Assistive Technology Society of North America (RESNA), an interdisciplinary association for the advancement of rehabilitation and AT, has developed guidelines and credentialing examinations for three categories of specialists in AT (🛜 **eTable 55-3**).

For more information about the credentialing process and criteria for credentialing, contact RESNA at http://www.resna.org. A number of universities throughout the United States and Canada offer training in AT for a wide range of audiences. 🛜 **eTable 55-4** lists only a few of the available options. For more information, visit the Web and type assistive technology training into the search engine.

ASSESSMENT USING A TEAM APPROACH

The goal of any AT evaluation is to determine whether the individual receiving this service has the potential, and the desire, to benefit from AT devices and services at home, school, work, or play. Other outcomes of an AT evaluation include providing a safe and supportive environment for the person with a disability and his or her family to learn about and review available assistive devices; identifying necessary AT services such as training, modification, etc. that may be necessary for the equipment to be effective; and developing a potential list of recommended devices for trial usage before a final determination is made. Also, the individual and family, as well as the involved professionals, should specify exactly what they hope to achieve as a result of the evaluation (i.e., equipment ideas, potential success with vocational, or educational objectives).

When selecting team members to conduct an AT evaluation, appropriate disciplines should be chosen based on the identified needs of the person with the disability. For example, if the individual presents with both severe motor and

TABLE 55-2	Summary Table for Investigational and Commercial SARs				
Robot		**Vision System**	**Auditory System**	**Mobility System**	**Technology Readiness Level (TRL)**	**Development Status**
1	Bobus	Infrared	None	Wheeled base	7	Investigational (Université de Sherbrooke)
2	CHARLIE (Child-centered Adaptive Robot for Learning in an Interactive Environment)	Mono	1 Speaker	2 DOF head and arms	7	Investigational (University of South Carolina)
3	C-Pac	Infrared	Speaker	Wheeled base	7	Investigational (Université de Sherbrooke)
4	DiskCat	None	Speaker	Wheeled base	7	Investigational (Université de Sherbrooke)
5	FACE (Facial Automation for Conveying Emotions)	Mono	None	32 DOF facial movement	7	Investigational (University of Pisa)
6	HOAP-2	Stereo	None	25 DOF w/ humanoid legs	9	Commercial (Fujitsu Laboratories)
7	Infanoid	Foveated stereo	None	24 DOF torso	7	Investigational (Japan)
8	IROMEC (Interactive Robotic Social Mediators as Companions)	RGB-D	Microphones and speaker	Wheeled base	8	Investigational (European Union)
9	Jumbo	Infrared	Speaker	Wheeled base w/ moving trunk	7	Investigational (Université de Sherbrooke)
10	KASPAR	None	Speaker	8 DOF head, 3 DOF arms (2)	7	Investigational (University of Hertfordshire's)
11	Keepon	Stereo	Microphone	4 DOF (turn, nod, rock, bob)	7	Investigational (Carnegie Mellon University)
12	Kismet	Foveated stereo	Microphone and speaker	15 DOF expressive face	7	Investigational (MIT)
13	Labo-1	Infrared	Speaker	4 wheeled base	7	Investigational (University of Hertfordshire)
14	Lego Mindstorm NTX	None	Microphone	Wheeled base	6	Investigational
15	Maestro	Infrared	Speaker	Wheeled base	7	Investigational (Université de Sherbrooke)
16	Milo	RGB-D	8 microphones and speaker	18 DOF w/ legs	9	Commercial (Robokind)
17	Nao	Stereo	4 directional microphones and loudspeakers	25 DOFs w/ humanoid legs	9	Commercial (Aldebaran Robotics)
18	Pekee	Infrared	None	3 wheeled base	9	Commercial (Wany Robotics)
19	QueBall (formerly Roball)	None	Speaker	2 DOF sphere	9	Commercial (Que Innovations)
20	Robota	Infrared	2 Speakers	5 DOF (2 legs, 2 arms, 1 head)	9	Commercial (Didel SA)
21	Tito	Mono	Microphone and speaker	Wheeled base	7	Investigational (Université de Sherbrooke)
22	TREVOR (Triadic Relationship EVOking Robot)	None	None	3 DOF arms	7	Investigational (Brigham Young University)
23	Troy	None	Speaker	4 DOF arms, 2 DOF head	7	Investigational (Brigham Young University)

communication impairments, then an occupational or physical therapist with expertise in AT, as well as a speech-language pathologist with a background in working with persons with severe communication impairments and alternative forms of communication, should be included as members of the team. If a cognitive impairment has been identified during the intake process, someone versed in learning processes such as a psychologist, neurolinguist, teacher, or special educator might be appropriate members of the team. If there is an ergonomic issue (i.e., carpal tunnel syndrome), an evaluator with training in ergonomic assessment or a background in physical or occupational therapy is a necessary component for a successful experience.

It is *not* appropriate for an AT vendor to be called in to perform the AT evaluation. Although vendors can and should be considered as identified members of the team, it must be recognized that they have an inherent conflict of interest. They are there to sell products. When requested by the team, vendors should demonstrate their products, discuss pertinent features, and assist in setting up the equipment for evaluation and trial usage. However, other team members, including the end user and their family, should carry out the actual evaluation and make the final recommendation(s).

Phase I of the Assessment Process

Knowledge within the field of AT continues to grow and change, sometimes on a daily basis. As this evolution continues, a number of important variables are being identified that directly impact whether the AT recommended by the assessment team will be used or abandoned by the consumer (58,59). As a result of this information, the evaluation process continues to be refined. Many researchers are working to develop standardized AT measurement tools (60–62), but the fact remains that there are few available resources to guide practitioners who have not received formalized training in AT.

As mentioned earlier in this chapter, the number one reason AT is abandoned is because the needs and preferences of the consumer were not taken into account during the evaluation process. Other reasons cited for abandonment of devices include the following:

- Changes in consumer functional abilities or activities
- Lack of consumer motivation to use the device or do the task
- Lack of meaningful training on how to use the device
- Ineffective device performance or frequent breakdown
- Environmental obstacles to use, such as narrow doorways
- Lack of access to and information about repair and maintenance
- Lack of sufficient need for the device functions
- Device aesthetics, weight size, and appearance (62)

Careful review of these factors suggests that many of these issues can be considered during the evaluation process. At the University of Colorado Denver, School of Medicine, the assessment protocol has evolved from a group of practitioners trying any number of devices with the individual, to a team process that starts by leaving the technology out of sight. The process about to be described may sound laborious and cumbersome. With practice, we have reduced the time necessary for the evaluation process and have increased the likelihood that the individual who will be using it selects the appropriate technology. In addition, this process has decreased both

installation and follow-up training time and has resulted in improved outcomes for end users.

Phase I of the assessment process is initiated once a referral is received. Standard intake information is collected, usually over the phone that provides the name, primary diagnosis, age, reason for referral, etc. In the majority of cases, cognitive, motor, vision, and other standard clinical assessments have already been performed, and a release of information is requested from the individual or his or her caregivers for this information to be forwarded to the team. If it has not previously occurred, these evaluations are scheduled as a component of Phase II of the assessment process.

Based on the preliminary information, an appropriate team of professionals is assembled and a date chosen for the evaluation. The team leader takes responsibility for ensuring that the individual with the disability, his or her family, and any other significant individuals are invited to the evaluation. It is not unusual to vary the schedule to meet the needs of the family rather than the professionals.

When the time arrives for the evaluation, the team members are invited to gather and spend some time getting to know the individual. Using methods described by Cook and Polger (63) and Galvin and Scherer (64), the team first identifies the life roles of the consumer (e.g., student, brother, musician, etc.). Then, the specific activities engaged in by the individual to fulfill that life role are identified. For example, if he is a brother, then that means he may play hide and seek with a sibling, squabble over toys, or otherwise engage in brotherly activities. If he is a musician, then he may want or need to have access to musical instruments, sheet music, or simply a radio.

Next, the team identifies any problems that may occur during these activities. For example, the musician may not have enough hand control to play the piano or may experience visual or cognitive difficulties with sheet music. Specific questions are asked regarding where and when these difficulties occur (activity limitations). Perhaps problems occur when the individual is tired, or not properly positioned, or when he or she tries to communicate with others. The individual is also asked to describe instances of success with these activities and to discuss what made them successful (prior history with and without technology). Interestingly enough, the team by now is usually able to recognize patterns of success and failure from the individual's perspective, as common themes across environments emerge.

Finally, we ask the team to prioritize the order in which we can address identified barriers to participation, and a specific plan of action is developed. Within the specific plan of action, "must statements" are also developed. For example, the device must have a visible display in sunlight, or the technology chosen must weigh less than 2 lb. In one instance, the must statement read, "It must be purple."

It is at this point that the team may be reconfigured. For example, if the individual is not properly seated and positioned, they are referred first to the occupational or physical therapist for a seating and positioning evaluation before any other technology issues being addressed. At all times, the configuration of the team includes the individual being assessed and the caregivers, as the primary members to be consulted.

In many instances, various members of the team in collaboration with others determine that further assessment from their perspective is not warranted for the technology component to proceed. In other situations, it is determined that additional team members who were not previously considered should be invited to participate (e.g., vision specialist).

Phase II of the AT Assessment

Once the team has agreed on the specific plan of action and those things that must occur, phase II of the assessment process begins. The person with a disability and his/her caregivers are asked to preview any number of assistive devices that may serve to reduce activity limitations and increase participation in their chosen environments. These ATs are tried with the individual, and various adaptations, modifications, and setups are explored to ensure an appropriate match of the technology to the individual is made.

It is at this point that the AT skill sets of the clinician become critical. If trial devices are not properly configured or if the wrong information is given to the consumer, then they will be unable to make an appropriate selection. Because so many devices require extensive training and follow-up, it is also critical that realistic information regarding training issues (including learning time) is provided and appropriate resources within the local community be identified. In a number of instances, the technology that appears to be optimal for an individual does not carry with it the appropriate community supports. In those cases, it is often advantageous to work first to identify local resources or local AT professionals willing to receive additional training before sending the device home with the end user. At all times, the end user and his or her families should be informed and updated so that they can make the final decision regarding when and where they wish the equipment to be delivered.

With very few exceptions, the wise course of action involves borrowing or renting the equipment before a final purchase decision. For many individuals with disabilities, the actual use of various technologies on a day-to-day basis elicits new problems that must be resolved. Unexpected benefits, including changes in role and status, also occur as a result of improved functioning. In some cases, these unexpected benefits create an entirely new set of problems that must be addressed. For most, these disruptions can be resolved with time and energy. Others decide that they either prefer the old way of doing things or they are interested in adding or changing the technology once they have had a chance to experiment with it in different settings.

Writing the Evaluation Report

When writing the evaluation report for an AT assessment, it is important to ensure that a number of items are included. First and foremost, case managers, educators, and others unfamiliar with assistive technologies appreciate layman's terms when discussing the need for AT and what it will accomplish.

In cases in which medical insurance is being used to purchase the technology, it is critical to document the actual medical necessity for the device(s). For example, "Mrs. Smith will use this device to communicate her health care needs and to meet the functional goals outlined in the attached report." In instances when the evaluation was requested to determine educational or vocational benefit with assistive devices, it is important to document how these specific needs will be met with the prescribed equipment.

It is extremely important that all components of the assistive devices be included (e.g., cables, ancillary peripherals, or consumable supplies) in the list of recommended equipment. In many instances, devices are recommended for purchase as a "system." When this occurs, acquisition and implementation can be delayed for months because an item was not included in the initial list. It is also important to include contact information for the various vendors who sell the equipment. Many purchasers are unfamiliar with these companies, and acquisition can be delayed for months if this information is not included in the report.

FUNDING AT

The funding sources for AT fall into several basic categories (📶 eTable 55-5). One source to be investigated is private or government medical insurance. Medical insurance defines AT as medical equipment necessary for treatment of a specific illness or injury. A physician's prescription is usually required. When writing a prescription for an AT device, it is important that the physician is aware of the costs and benefits of the devices he or she is prescribing and is prepared to justify his or her prescriptions to third-party payers. Funding includes not only the initial cost of the device but also the expense involved in equipment maintenance and patient education, as well as the potential economic benefits it provides to the patient (e.g., return to work).

According to a publication sponsored by the American Medical Association (65), the following items (reprinted with permission) should be taken into account when prescribing AT and certifying medical necessity:

1. The physician must provide evidence of individual medical necessity.
2. An "appropriate" prescription is one that takes into consideration the comprehensive assessment process, including motivation and availability of training, the potential patient functional outcome, and the cost/benefit of available products.
3. Physicians should be prepared to provide sufficient information to insurance companies to ensure approval. Dialogue is often necessary to show medical necessity of complex assistive technologies (power wheelchairs, computer-based environmental control systems).
4. Basic knowledge of AT reimbursement for patient and physician includes familiarity with established medical necessity forms and prior authorization procedures.
5. Avoid making static decisions on a dynamic problem; anticipate future need.
6. Base decision on both expected performance and durability of the device.

Documentation in the Medical Record

In addition to prescribing and certifying medical necessity on various forms, physicians must be sure to maintain complete patient records that include the following information: Patient diagnosis or diagnoses; duration of the patient's condition; expected clinical course; prognosis; nature and extent of functional limitations; therapeutic interventions and results; past experience with related items; consultations and reports from other physicians, interdisciplinary team, home health agencies, etc.; complete listing of all assistive devices the patient is using, including copies of prescriptions and certification forms or letters; and tracking system for device performance, including follow-up assessment schedules and lists of professional and vendor names to contact if problems occur.

Letters of Medical Necessity

These letters should include the following areas: Diagnoses ICD-10-CM codes and functional limitation(s). In addition, it is critical to include the functional limitations he/she is unable to perform such as: ADLs, instrumental ADLs; ADLs and functional mobility; and work activities. For communication, indicate whether or not the patient can communicate verbally, in writing or independently over the phone. Finally, what access to the "use of the equipment will/allow the patient to: Function independently with the device/equipment; perform independent wheelchair mobility in the home; perform independent wheelchair mobility in the home and community; return home; be required as a lifetime medical need (if shorter duration, explain need); and/or improve the patient's functional ability."

The AT specialist involved in the assessment will be able to provide a description of equipment needed. This must include every single component necessary for a functioning device such as a complex wheelchair and seating system. If anything is left out of the letter of medical necessity, it will not be funded. Additionally, funding agencies require a "rationale" for all components. These rationales may include: Safety or safe positioning for an activity; cost-effectiveness in prevention of secondary complications (e.g., pressure sores); mobility restrictions preventing independent activity; access to areas in home, such as bathroom and kitchen; access to workplace or school; duration of expected use; past experience, interventions, and results (failure of less expensive solutions); duration of expected use; and the goals and benefits to patient.

AT is usually covered under policy provisions for durable medical equipment, orthotics and prosthetics, or daily living and mobility aids. With private insurance, AT providers request funding under the specific provisions of the individual policy, appealing any denials (an inevitable), and offering medical justification for coverage. With government insurance policies, such as Medicaid and Medicare, coverage is based on existing law and regulations. In 2002, regulations were promulgated by Medicare to include coverage of AAC devices (66,67).

Information on covered services and how to request funding is available from the Medicaid programs in individual states and from the regional offices for Medicare. AT professionals and other health care providers should continually advocate for adequate coverage of AT in all health care plans.

Funding of AT is also available from other federal and state government entities, such as the Veterans Administration, State Vocational Rehabilitation, Rehabilitation Services Administration, State Independent Living Rehabilitation Centers, and State Education Services. Local school districts may fund education-related AT for children. Each agency or program sets criteria for the funding of AT based on the mission of the agency and the purpose of the technology. For example, vocational rehabilitation agencies generally pay for devices to facilitate gainful employment, and education program funding is directed toward enhancing the client's performance in school.

Private funding is often available through subsidized loan programs, churches, charitable organizations, and disability-related nonprofit groups. The AT provider must keep abreast of the requirements of various funding sources in order to direct the client to appropriate organizations. Often a combination of funding from several sources is needed to reduce personal out-of-pocket costs. Because funding for replacement of AT devices is also difficult to obtain, careful selection of the initial device is required. Providers can also assist clients by considering funding when making equipment recommendations by including both low- and high-cost alternatives with their relative advantages. Funding is generally available for AT, but persistence and advocacy by the AT provider are required for success (68,69).

MEASURING OUTCOMES IN AT

The study of the impact of AT devices for individuals with disabilities poses a challenge in outcomes research. The field itself is a multidisciplinary area of study encompassing medicine, rehabilitation, psychology, education, engineering, and biotechnology specialties, and involves physical, cognitive, psychosocial, sensory, and physiologic effects. Consequently, there is a lack of consistency in what has been studied, how the outcomes have been measured, and where the results have been recorded. In the field of AT, there is also a paucity of outcomes measurement research in general (70).

Persons with functional limitations and the AT devices provided by professionals do not operate in a vacuum. They exist on a broad continuum and are impacted by such things as environmental and psychosocial issues, family finances, cultural differences, and other contextual factors. Services are often fragmented, with many consumers receiving interventions from any number of teams and facilities. General agreement within the field suggests that outcome measurement is a critical, unmet need. But a conceptual framework for developing measurement tools and measurement research has remained elusive (70–72). Studies of the treatment efficacy of AT devices and services have typically been relegated to single case study reports and occasional multiple case reports showing changes from baseline (73–77).

In recent years, the concept of AT has been broadened to encompass any technology that can improve a person's function (51,78–80). This is an important distinction, because it places nonoperative rehabilitation interventions, such as orthotics, prosthetics, robotics, smart home technologies, electrical stimulation, and functional neuromuscular stimulation, in the realm of AT.

The application of technology to improve human function has long been the goal of the AT professional. The AT specialist has the hands-on clinical experience to see what works and understands those factors leading to technology abandonment. Typical clinical practice, however, does not lend itself to the development of experimental methodologies to objectively evaluate patient performance with AT devices and services. Moreover, most AT clinicians do not have the resources to actively participate in a sustained program of research nor are these behaviors emphasized as a component of clinical intervention in most training programs.

Despite this limitation, AT professionals and the AT service delivery model have been effective in getting technology into the hands of the people who need it, creating a foundation for rehabilitation intervention service delivery in general. Because the AT specialist functions across disciplines, he or she is often the first to notice the impact of other treatment modalities. For example, it is typical for a child with an acquired disability to enter rehabilitation services with a variety of needs and assignments to various disciplines for treatment. It is often the AT specialist who notices incompatibilities between systems, such as a seating system with a lap tray that interferes with a child in the development of an alternate access method to a computer used to complete educational tasks.

In recent years, the National Institute on Independent Living Disability and Rehabilitation Research (NIDILRR) and the National Institutes of Health's National Center for Medical Rehabilitation Research (NIH NCMRR) have begun to fund various research activities devoted to developing standardized outcomes measurement systems in order to determine the efficacy of various AT devices and services. The plan for these activities calls for the dissemination of information to individuals with disabilities, their families, caregivers, funding sources, and manufacturers. Results from studies such as these are a welcome and necessary component for the continued development of this discipline.

THE FUTURE OF ASSISTIVE TECHNOLOGIES

The future of assistive technologies and universal design is exciting to contemplate. Intensive research and development activities are focusing on human-robot interaction (HRI), GPS, and a wide range of other context aware sensor technologies. Advances in the commercial manufacturing industry is leading the way by designing cheaper, less intrusive support systems for persons without disabilities.

Researchers and engineers focused on these technologies are quickly taking advantage of new discoveries as well as adding to the body of knowledge and the array of products available for persons with disabilities.

With over 600,000 people each year surviving a stroke, it has become the leading cause of serious long-term disability in the United States. In addition, the aging demographic worldwide is promoting an intense sense of urgency among government, public, and private entities. The need to create effective and safe strategies for aging in place is paramount and both public and private entities are rushing to invent new technologies and strategies to care for this very vulnerable population.

As technology advances, new therapy robots are developing that are increasingly compliant and captivating to use (77).

Context aware sensors and GPS systems are emerging technologies that can be useful in identifying where someone is; the status of his or her environment (temperature, location); and, changes in positioning, weight, etc. These same technologies are also proving to be an effective tool for persons with intellectual/developmental disabilities, MS, and other debilitating injuries or illnesses (79,81,82).

The field of AT is one of rapid change and growth. New technologies, new research possibilities, and a growing universal acceptance of AT devices and services support the recognition that persons with disabilities are persons with abilities who have much to contribute.

ACKNOWLEDGMENTS

Funding for this chapter is due in large part to NIILDRR grant no. H224A940014-01: Colorado Assistive Technology Project, State Grants for Technology Related Assistance.

Special thanks are also due to staff of Assistive Technology Partners, Department of Bioengineering, University of Colorado Anschutz Medical Campus, including Jim Sandstrum. The author also wishes to thank Dr. Thomas W. King, Department of Communication Disorders, University of Wisconsin-Eau Claire; Department of Geriatric Health, American Medical Association; Michelle Lange for her work on the EADL section; and previous AT chapter authors.

REFERENCES

1. James P, Thorpe I. *Centuries of Darkness: A Challenge to the Conventional Chronology of Old World Archaeology.* New Brunswick, NJ: Rutgers University Press; 1993.
2. Trease G. *Timechanges: The Evolution of Everyday Life.* New York: Warmick Press; 1985.
3. Public Law 100-407 and 103-218. Technology-related assistance for individuals with disabilities; 1988.
4. Weber MC. Towards access, accountability, procedural regularity and participation: the Rehabilitation Act Amendments of 1992 and 1993. *J Rehab.* 1994;60(3):21.
5. Ladenson R. *Individuals with Disabilities Education Act.* Greencastle, IN: Association for Practical and Professional Ethics; 2000.
6. Beukelman D, Mirenda P. *Augmentative and Alternative Communication: Supporting Children and Adults with Complex Communication Needs.* 4th ed. Baltimore, MD: Brookes Publishing; 2013.
7. Scherer MJ. *Living in the State of Stuck: How Technology Impacts the Lives of Persons with Disabilities.* Northampton, MA: Brookline Books; 1996.
8. Oishi MMK, Mitchell IM, Van der Loos HM. *Design and Use of Assistive Technology: Social, Technical, Ethical, and Economic Challenges.* New York, NY: Springer Science & Business Media; 2010.
9. Wilcox MJ, et al. Provider perspectives on the use of assistive technology for infants and toddlers with disabilities. *Top Early Child Spec Educ.* 2006;26(1):33–49.
10. Häggblom-Kronlöf G, Sonn U. Use of assistive devices—a reality full of contradictions in elderly persons' everyday life. *Disabil Rehab Assist Technol.* 2007;2(6):335–345.
11. Foley A, Ferri BA. Technology for people, not disabilities: ensuring access and inclusion. *J Res Spec Educ Needs.* 2012;12(4):192–200.
12. Scherer MJ. *Living in the State of Stuck: How Assistive Technology Impacts the Lives of People with Disabilities.* Northampton, MA: Brookline Books; 2005.
13. Koumpouros Y, et al. Translation and validation of the assistive technology device predisposition assessment in Greek in order to assess satisfaction with use of the selected assistive device. *Disabil Rehab Assist Technol.* 2017;12(5):535–542.
14. Brady E, Bigham JP. Crowdsourcing accessibility: human-powered access technologies. *Foundations Trends Hum–Comput Interact.* 2015;8(4):273–372.
15. Cruz D, et al. Assistive technology accessibility and abandonment: challenges for occupational therapists. *Open J Occup Ther.* 2016;4(1):10.
16. King T. *Assistive Technology—Essential Human Factors.* Boston, MA: Allyn & Bacon; 1999.
17. LaPlante MP. The demographics of disability. *Milbank Q.* 1991;69:55–77.
18. Rosenbaum P, Stewart D. The World Health Organization International Classification of Functioning, Disability, and Health: a model to guide clinical thinking, practice and research in the field of cerebral palsy. *Semin Pediatr Neurol.* 2004;11(1):5–10.
19. World Health Organization. *International Classification of Functioning, Disability and Health: ICF.* Geneva, Switzerland: WHO; 2001.
20. Light J, McNaughton D. *Communicative Competence for Individuals who Require Augmentative and Alternative Communication: A New Definition for a New Era of Communication?* Milton, England: Taylor & Francis; 2014.
21. Sigafoos J, et al. Augmentative and alternative communication (AAC) in intellectual and developmental disabilities. In: Luiselli JK, Fischer AJ, eds. *Computer-Assisted and Web-Based Innovations in Psychology, Special Education, and Health.* London, England: Elsevier; 2016:255–285.
22. Makkonen T, et al. Speech deterioration in amyotrophic lateral sclerosis (ALS) after manifestation of bulbar symptoms. *Int J Lang Commun Disord.* 2018;53(2):385–392.
23. Creer S, et al. Prevalence of people who could benefit from augmentative and alternative communication (AAC) in the UK: determining the need. *Int J Lang Commun Disord.* 2016;51(6):639–653.
24. Amundsen S. *Augmentative-Alternative Communication Access for Individuals with Communication Disorders in Medical Settings.* Orlando, FL: University of Central Florida, Electronic Theses and Dissertations; 2014.
25. Bahia MM, Chun RYS. Quality of life in aphasia: differences between fluent and non-fluent aphasic augmentative and alternative communication users. *Audiol Commun Res.* 2014;19(4):352–359.
26. Carruthers H, Astin F, Munro W. Which alternative communication methods are effective for voiceless patients in Intensive Care Units? A systematic review. *Intensive Critical Care Nurs.* 2017;42:88–96.

27. Light J, McNaughton D. Communicative competence for individuals who require augmentative and alternative communication: a new definition for a new era of communication? *Augment Altern Commun.* 2014;30(1):1–18.

28. Kangas K, Lloyd L. Early cognitive skills as prerequisites to augmentative and alternative communication use: what are we waiting for? *Augment Altern Commun.* 1988;4(4):211–221.

29. Lancioni GE. *Assistive Technology for People with Developmental Disabilities.* Milton, England: Taylor & Francis; 2017.

30. Wu P-F, Wheaton JE, Cannella-Malone HI. Effects of video prompting and activity schedules on the acquisition of independent living skills of students who are deaf and have developmental disabilities. *Educ Train Autism Dev Disabil.* 2016;51(4):366.

31. Heyn PC, Cassidy JL, Bodine C. The rehabilitation engineering research center for the advancement of cognitive technologies. *Am J Alzheimers Dis Other Demen.* 2015;30(1):6–12.

32. Ritchings T, Khadragi A, Saeb M. An intelligent computer-based system for sign language tutoring. *Assist Technol.* 2012;24(4):299–308.

33. FeilSeifer D, Mataric MJ. Towards the integration of socially assistive robots into the lives of children with ASD. In: *Human-Robot Interaction'09.* San Diego, CA; 2009.

34. Feil-Seifer DJ, Mataric MJ. Robot-assisted therapy for children with autism spectrum disorders. In: *Refereed Workshop Conference on Interaction Design for Children: Children with Special Needs.* Chicago, IL; 2008.

35. Feil-Seifer DJ, Mataric MJ. B3IA: an architecture for autonomous robot-assisted behavior intervention for children with autism spectrum disorders. In: *IEEE Proceedings of the International Workshop on Robot and Human Interactive Communication, August 2008.* Munich, Germany; 2008.

36. Robins B, et al. Scenarios of robot-assisted play for children with cognitive and physical disabilities. *Interact Stud.* 2012;13(2):189–234.

37. Robins B, et al. Robotic assistants in therapy and education of children with autism: can a small humanoid robot help encourage social interaction skills? *Univ Access Inform Soc.* 2005;4:105–120.

38. Costa S, et al. "Where is your nose?": developing body awareness skills among children with autism using a humanoid robot In: *ACHI 2013: The Sixth International Conference on Advances in Computer-Human Interactions.* Wilmington, DE: IARIA; 2013.

39. Dickerson P, Robins B, Dautenhahn K. Where the action is: a conversation analytic perspective on interaction between a humanoid robot, a co-present adult and a child with an ASD. *Interact Stud.* 2013;14(2):297–316.

40. Ferrari E, Robins B, Dautenhahn K. Therapeutic and educational objectives in robot assisted play for children with autism. In: *18th IEEE International Symposium on Robot and Human Interactive Communication.* Toyama, Japan. New York, NY: IEEE; 2009.

41. Marti P, et al. Socially assistive robotics in the treatment of behavioural and psychological symptoms of dementia. In: *BioRob 2006. The First IEEE/RAS-EMBS International Conference on Biomedical Robotics and Biomechatronics.* IEEE; 2006.

42. Tapus A, Tapus C, Mataric MJ. The use of socially assistive robots in the design of intelligent cognitive therapies for people with dementia. In: *2009 IEEE International Conference on Rehabilitation Robotics.* Kyoto, Japan. New York, NY: IEEE; 2009.

43. Wada K, et al. Robot therapy for elders affected by dementia. *IEEE Eng Med Biol.* 2008;27(4):53–60.

44. Felzmann H, et al. Robot-assisted care for elderly with dementia: is there a potential for genuine end-user empowerment? In: *Proceedings of ACM/IEEE International Conference on Human-Robot Interaction Workshops.* New York, NY: IEEE; 2015.

45. Sabanovic S, et al. PARO robot affects diverse interaction modalities in group sensory therapy for older adults with dementia. In: *2013 IEEE International Conference on Rehabilitation Robotics (ICORR).* New York, NY: IEEE; 2013.

46. Mataric M, et al. Socially assistive robotics for post-stroke rehabilitation. *J Neuroeng Rehabil.* 2007;4:5.

47. Mataric M, et al. Socially assistive robotics for stroke and mild TBI rehabilitation. *Stud Health Technol Inform.* 2009;145:249–262.

48. Tapus A, Tapus C, Mataric MJ. Hands-off therapist robot behavior adaptation to user personality for post-stroke rehabilitation therapy. In: *Proceedings 2007 IEEE International Conference on Robotics and Automation (ICRA).* Rome, Italy. New York, NY: IEEE; 2007.

49. Swift-Spong K, et al. Effects of comparative feedback from a Socially Assistive Robot on self-efficacy in post-stroke rehabilitation. In: *2015 IEEE International Conference on Rehabilitation Robotics (ICORR).* New York, NY: IEEE; 2015.

50. Rabbitt SM, Kazdin AE, Scassellati B. Integrating socially assistive robotics into mental healthcare interventions: applications and recommendations for expanded use. *Clin Psychol Rev.* 2015;35:35–46.

51. Collins S, et al. Sensing companions: potential clinical uses of robot sensor data for home care of older adults with depression. In: *Companion of the 2018 ACM/IEEE International Conference on Human-Robot Interaction.* New York, NY: ACM; 2018.

52. Moyle W, et al. Care staff perceptions of a social robot called Paro and a look-alike Plush Toy: a descriptive qualitative approach. *Aging Ment Health.* 2018;22(3):330–335.

53. Scassellati B, Admoni H, Mataric M. Robots for use in autism research. *Annu Rev Biomed Eng.* 2012;14:275–294.

54. Cabibihan J-J, et al. Why robots? A survey on the roles and benefits of social robots in the therapy of children with autism. *Int J Soc Robot.* 2013;5(4):593–618.

55. Encarnação P, Cook A. *Robotic Assistive Technologies: Principles and Practice.* Boca Raton, FL: CRC Press; 2017.

56. Kanada Y, et al. Reliability of clinical competency evaluation list for novice physical and occupational therapists requiring assistance. *J Phys Ther Sci.* 2015;27(10):3177.

57. Campbell PH, Milbourne S, Wilcox MJ. Adaptation interventions to promote participation in natural settings. *Infants & Young Children.* 2008;21(2):94–106.

58. Scherer MJ. *Living in the State of Stuck: How Technology Impacts the Lives of People with Disabilities.* 3rd ed. Cambridge, MA: Brookline Books; 2000.

59. Phillips B, Zhao H. Predictors of assistive technology abandonment. *Assist Technol.* 1993;5(1):36–45.

60. Sablier J, et al. Ecological assessments of activities of daily living and personal experiences with Mobus, an assistive technology for cognition: a pilot study in schizophrenia. *Assist Technol.* 2012;24(2):67–77.

61. Watts EH, O'Brian M, Wojcik BW. Four models of assistive technology consideration: how do they compare to recommended educational assessment practices? *J Spec Educ.* 2004;19(1):43–56.

62. Westby CE. Considerations in working successfully with culturally/linguistically diverse families in assessment and intervention of communicative disorders. *Semin Speech Lang.* 2009;30:279–289.

63. Galvin JC, Scherer M. *Evaluating, Selecting, and Using Appropriate Assistive Technology.* Gaithersburg, MD: Aspen Publishers, Inc.; 1996:394.

64. Cook AM, Polgar JM. *Assistive Technologies-E-Book: Principles and Practice.* St. Louis, MO: Elsevier Health Sciences; 2014.

65. Schwartzberg J, Kakavas K, Malking S. *Guidelines for the Use of Assistive Technology: Evaluation, Referral, Prescription.* Chicago, IL: American Medical Association; 1996:37–41.

66. Golinker L. Medicare eliminates computer-based device exclusion: a new class of AAC devices emerges. SIG 12. *Perspect Augment Altern Commun.* 2001;10(2):29–32.

67. Golinker L. *Key Questions for Medicare Coverage & Funding for AAC Devices.* National Coverage Determination 50.1: MCD Speech Generating Devices. Ithaca, NY; 2001.

68. Berry BE, Ignash S. Assistive technology: providing independence for individuals with disabilities. *Rehabil Nurs.* 2003;28(1):6–14.

69. Center on Technology and Disability. Republished with permission from Tots-n-Tech. (2009, April). *Resource Brief 3: Funding Assistive Technology.* Retrieved from https://www.ctdinstitute.org/sites/default/files/file_attachments/Brief_3_Funding_AT.pdf.

70. Jutai JW, et al. Toward a taxonomy of assistive technology device outcomes. *Am J Phys Med Rehabil.* 2005;84(4):294–302.

71. Lenker JA, et al. Psychometric and administrative properties of measures used in assistive technology device outcomes research. *Assist Technol.* 2005;17(1):7–22.

72. Jutai JW, et al. Article 11: predicting assistive technology device outcomes. *Arch Phys Med Rehabil.* 2006;87(10):e3.

73. Jutai J, et al. Outcomes measurement of assistive technologies: an institutional case study. *Assist Technol.* 1996;8(2):110–120.

74. Edyburn DL. Measuring assistive technology outcomes: key concepts. *J Spec Educ Technol.* 2003;18(2):53–55.

75. Fuhrer MJ, et al. A framework for the conceptual modelling of assistive technology device outcomes. *Disabil Rehabil.* 2003;25(22):1243–1251.

76. Light J, McNaughton D. From basic to applied research to improve outcomes for individuals who require augmentative alternative communication: potential contributions of eye tracking research methods. *Augment Altern Commun.* 2014;30(2):99–105.

77. Light J, McNaughton D. Designing AAC research and intervention to improve outcomes for individuals with complex communication needs. *Augment Altern Commun.* 2015;31(2):85–96.

78. Gray DB, Quatrano LA, Lieberman M. *Designing and Using Assistive Technology: The Human Perspective.* Baltimore, MD: Paul H. Brooks; 1998.

79. Gunther EJ, Sliker LJ, Bodine C. A UHF RFID positioning system for use in warehouse navigation by employees with cognitive disability. *Disabil Rehabil Assist Technol.* 2017;12(8):832–842.

80. Bodine C, et al. Social assistive robots for children with complex disabilities. In: Encarnacao P, Cook AM, eds. *Robotic Assistive Technologies: Principles and Practice.* Boca Raton, FL: CRC Press; 2017:261–308.

81. Jovanov E, et al. A wireless body area network of intelligent motion sensors for computer assisted physical rehabilitation. *J Neuroeng Rehabil.* 2005;2(1):6.

82. Fuentes JA, et al. Towards usability evaluation of multimodal assistive technologies using RGB-D sensors. In: Fuentes JA, ed. *Natural and Artificial Computation in Engineering and Medical Applications.* Berlin, Heidelberg: Springer; 2013:210–219.

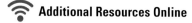 **Additional Resources Online**

Upper and Lower Limb Prosthetics

PROSTHETIC FITTING AND TRAINING

An understanding of the functional needs of the individual with an amputation, his/her interest and motivation in pursuing prosthetic fitting, and an assessment of his/her ambulatory potential are required to set realistic goals for prosthetic fitting and training. Not all the individuals with an amputation are candidates for prostheses. Although the factors that predict success in prosthetic use are partially understood, a number of factors have been associated with a poor outcome in returning the individual with an amputation to functional ambulation at household or community levels. Negative prognostic factors include a delay in wound healing, the presence of joint contractures, dementia or cognitive disorders, medical comorbidities, and higher levels of limb amputation (transfemoral) (1–3). Age has inconsistently been identified as a predictor of prosthetic success, implying that except in advanced age (>80 to 85 years) other factors play a more important role in determining the rehabilitation potential of the individual with an amputation.

As a result of the uncertainty in identifying prosthetic candidates, considerable clinical judgment is required. Some general guidelines can be followed. An individual with an amputation should have reasonable cardiovascular reserve, adequate wound healing, and good soft tissue coverage, range of motion, muscle strength, motor control, and learning ability to achieve useful prosthetic function. Individuals with a lower extremity (LE) amputation who can walk with a walker or crutches without a prosthesis usually possess the necessary balance, strength, and cardiovascular reserve to walk with a prosthesis. Examples of poor candidates for functional prosthetic fitting would be an individual with a dysvascular LE amputation with an open or poorly healed incision, an individual with a transfemoral amputation with a 30-degree flexion contracture at the hip, or an individual with a transradial amputation with a flail elbow and shoulder. Generally, individuals with a bilateral, short, transfemoral amputation over the age of 45 years are considered unlikely candidates for full-length prosthetic fitting. Additional medical problems such as severe coronary artery disease, pulmonary disease, severe polyneuropathy, or multiple joint arthritis may result in an individual with an amputation who could be fitted with a prosthesis but who may not be a functional prosthetic user. Patients in whom prognosis is poor, life expectancy is short, or with a disease that results in significant fluctuations in body weight are not good candidates. In borderline cases, it may be necessary to proceed with actual prosthetic fitting to determine the eventual prosthetic function. The use of a less costly rigid removable dressing (RRD) with pylon and foot or a preparatory prosthesis is appropriate

before a decision is made about fitting such a person with a more costly definitive prosthesis. The overall success rate in restoring functional ambulation in the individual with a lower limb amputation varies approximately from 36% to 70%. Amputation resulting from vascular disease is a manifestation of a severe systemic vasculopathy. The early mortality following major LE amputation is 15% to 20%, largely related to myocardial infarction. Overall, the individuals with dysvascular amputation have a 3- to 5-year 50% mortality, which underlies the importance of successful early rehabilitation to allow for an improved quality of life in their remaining years. Of the survivors, 50% develop vascular complications in the remaining limb within 5 years.

The timing of prosthetic fitting for the individual with an LE amputation remains controversial, reflecting the clinical uncertainty over early versus delayed weight bearing. Because the majority of LE amputations occur as a result of peripheral vascular disease (PVD), primary wound healing at the amputation site is of paramount importance. When the rigid dressing was introduced on a wide scale in the 1970s, it was used to implement immediate postoperative prosthesis (IPOP) (a rigid dressing with a pylon and foot) as a means to speed rehabilitation for individuals with LE amputation (4). Problems with wound healing and residual limb trauma from poorly fabricated devices and a lack of experienced teams to manage this approach to early postoperative care led to abandoning their use in the individual with a dysvascular amputation. Despite these problems, in selected centers with adequate experience and a process to monitor closely the residual limb, an immediate or early postoperative prosthesis fabricated several weeks after surgery has been used safely in individuals with a dysvascular amputation (5). Immediate fitting in the younger patient with traumatic amputation has been more successful and is a reasonable method of treatment. Immediate and early postoperative prostheses are, in effect, an RRD with a pylon and foot attached. This device is used to achieve limited partial to full weight bearing, reduce edema, and accomplish initial gait training. Because the fit of these devices is always suboptimal compared to a custom-molded socket, they are not recommended for extended use.

When concern over wound healing dominates clinical care in the postoperative period, prosthetic fitting is delayed until the residual limb has healed adequately to allow unrestricted weight bearing. Providing a prosthesis is typically performed in two stages: a preparatory prosthetic limb phase is followed by the provision of a definitive prosthesis. The preparatory prosthesis is often of simple design, lower performance, and more adjustable to changes in residual limb volume than is the definitive limb. It allows the individual with an amputation to gain skill and confidence in walking with prosthesis, facilitates residual limb maturation, and affords the rehabilitation team the opportunity to better define the ultimate functional level of the individual. The definitive prosthesis is provided when the residual limb shape has stabilized and the patient has reached a functional plateau with the preliminary prosthesis.

Stump maturation is an imprecisely defined concept that occurs when the volume of the residual limb has stabilized, soft tissue atrophy has occurred, and the residual limb has been molded into a cylindrical shape that optimizes prosthetic fitting. This can usually be determined when the individual with an amputation reports a plateau in the number of sock plies worn from day to day and by clinical exam that shows edema resolution. Residual limb maturation, typically, takes about 4 months (6) but may extend substantially longer depending on the activity level, amount of prosthetic limb use, and coexisting medical disease. After stump maturation occurs, a definitive prosthesis is prescribed to specifically meet the activities of daily living (ADLs) and vocational and avocational needs of the individual with an amputation. In the case of young children, the prosthesis prescription must also meet any needs related to the development of age-appropriate motor milestones. Although a two-stage approach (preparatory followed by definite limb) is commonly used, financial considerations are becoming increasingly important with many health insurance programs allowing for only a single limb. Under these situations, the prosthetic team may recommend as the initial prosthesis a limb that is projected to meet all the long-term needs of the individual with an amputation. Patients who are not candidates for functional prosthetic use may choose to have a cosmetic prosthesis that has an appearance similar to that of the opposite limb.

GAIT TRAINING

After completing the final prosthetic evaluation, the individual with a new amputation will require a period of gait training under the supervision of a physical therapist. The individual with an amputation is instructed on how to put on and take off the prosthesis, how to determine the appropriate number of limb socks to be worn, when and how to check the skin for evidence of irritation, and how to clean and care for the prosthesis. For the individual with a new amputation, it is best if the initial gait training occurs while the prosthesis is still capable of being adjusted to permit alignment or length changes that may become apparent during gait training. Gait training often occurs on an outpatient basis and may last from weeks to months. The more proximal levels of amputation require lengthier gait training.

Gait training begins with weight shifting and balance activities while still in the parallel bars. Once weight shifting and balance activities have been mastered, a program of progressive ambulation begins in the parallel bars and progresses to the most independent level of ambulation possible with or without gait aids. Specific training should focus on transfers, knee stability, equal step lengths, and avoiding lateral trunk bending. Following mastery of ambulation on flat, level surfaces, techniques for managing uneven terrain, stairs, ramps, curbs, and falling and getting up off the ground are learned. Moving from a walker to less cumbersome gait aids can be achieved for most individuals with an LE amputation. For higher functioning individuals with an amputation, prosthetic training should include instruction and practice in driving, recreation, and vocational pursuits. Developing the optimal benefit from a prosthesis must take into account the specific mechanical attributes of the components used. For example, using a dynamic response (i.e., energy-storing) prosthetic foot requires loading the prosthetic toe during mid-stance and late stance to capture energy for push-off assistance or to activate a prosthetic knee to initiate the swing phase.

Wearing tolerance for the prosthesis must be gradually increased. Initially, the individual with an amputation will wear the prosthesis only for 15 to 20 minutes, removing it to check the condition of the skin. As tolerance to weight bearing increases, the length of wearing time is gradually increased. Several weeks may be required before the individual with an amputation is able to wear the prosthesis full time. The individual with an amputation may take the prosthesis home when safe and independent ambulation has been demonstrated and residual limb skin checks are assured. Common gait deviations and their causes are highlighted in **Table 56-1**.

LE PROSTHETIC FOLLOW-UP

During the initial 6 to 18 months, most individuals with an amputation will experience continued loss of residual limb volume, resulting in a prosthetic socket that will be too large. During this period, return visits should occur frequently enough to ensure that this loss of residual limb volume is being compensated for by the use of additional limb socks or by appropriate modifications of the prosthetic socket. It is usual for an individual with a new amputation to require replacement of the prosthetic socket during this time because of the significant loss of soft tissue volume. During follow-up visits, the condition of the residual limb, the prosthesis, the individual's gait, and the level of function are reviewed (7). Appropriate medical treatment, prosthetic modifications, or additional therapies are prescribed as needed. When the residual limb volume has stabilized sufficiently and the patient is doing well with the prosthesis, yearly visits to the amputee clinic are appropriate. Once the residual limb has stabilized, the average life expectancy for an LE prosthesis before replacement should be 3 to 5 years.

LE Prostheses

The LE prosthetic prescription must balance the individual's need for stability, mobility, durability, and cosmesis with available resources and cost. Understanding the role and importance of prosthetic ambulation in achieving the mobility goals of the individual with an amputation is essential for correctly prescribing a prosthetic device. Prosthetic ambulation is usually the primary mode of mobility for the younger individual with an amputation as well as for other patients across a wider age range when the amputation is at the transtibial and more distal levels. For the elderly, with dysvascular amputation above the knee and a more proximal level of amputation, prosthetic ambulation is often limited to transfers, indoors, or short community distances. The prescription of the LE prosthesis is based on several principles: maximizing comfort, matching specific components to the mobility needs of the individual with an amputation, and providing acceptable cosmesis.

TABLE 56-1	Abnormalities of Amputee's Gait		
Gait Cycle	**Observed Gait Abnormality**	**Possible Cause**	**Suggested Modifications**
Transtibial Amputee Gait			
Initial contact to loading response	Abrupt heel contact, rapid knee flexion	Excessive heel lever[a]	Realign prosthetic foot, change heel stiffness
	Prolonged heel contact, knee remains fully extended	Inadequate heel lever[b] or heel worn out	Increase heel stiffness
		Improper socket flexion	Realign prosthesis
		Learned gait pattern, quadriceps weakness	Gait training and strengthening
	Jerky knee motion	Socket loose, poor alignment, inadequate suspension	
Mid-stance	Medial or lateral socket thrust, lateral trunk shift over prosthesis	Foot too far outset or inset, socket loose	Realign prosthesis, replace socket or adjust socks
	Pelvis drops or elevates	Prosthesis too short/too long	Adjust prosthetic length
Mid-stance to terminal stance	Early knee flexion or "drop off"	Inadequate toe lever[c]	Realign prosthesis, replace foot
Terminal stance	Heel off too early	Excessive toe lever,[d] too much socket extension	Realign prosthesis
	Heel off excessively delayed	Inadequate toe lever,[c] too much socket flexion	Realign prosthesis
Swing phase	Prosthetic foot drags	Prosthesis too long, inadequate suspension	Shorten limb, modify suspension
Successive double support	Uneven step length	Hip flexion contracture, gait insecurity	Physical therapy
		Uncomfortable socket	Adjust socket fit
Transfemoral Amputee Gait			
Initial contact to loading response	Foot rotation at heel strike	Poor socket fit/rotation	Adjust socket fit, add belt for rotation control
		Heel too firm	Reduce heel stiffness
	Knee buckling	Excessive heel lever[a]	Realign limb, reduce heel stiffness
		Incorrect prosthetic knee alignment	Realign TKA relationship
		Weak hip extensors	Gait training and strengthening
Mid-stance	Lateral trunk bend or shift over prosthesis	Prosthetic limb abducted	
		Too much socket abduction, foot too far outset	Realign prosthesis
		Prosthesis too long	Shorten prosthesis
		Medial groin pain	Adjust socket fit
		Poor medial-lateral prosthetic control	
		Poor socket fit	Adjust socket fit
		Weak hip abductors	Gait training and strengthening
		Short residual limb	Accept, possibly add hip joint
		Prosthesis too short	Adjust prosthetic length
Initial swing	Uneven heel rise	Knee friction too tight or loose	Adjust knee friction or damping
		Knee extension	
Swing phase	Circumduction or prosthetic limb	Inadequate knee flexion, knee too stiff	Adjust knee friction or damping
		Prosthesis too long, inadequate suspension	Adjust prosthesis length
		Poor gait pattern	Physical therapy
		Improper knee rotational alignment	Realign prosthesis
	Whips	Excessive socket rotation	Adjust socket fit
Successive double support	Uneven step length	Hip flexion contracture	Physical therapy
		Insufficient socket flexion	Realign prosthesis

[a]Causes of excessive heel lever—foot dorsiflexed too much, foot too far posterior, heel cushion too hard, shoe heel too hard.

[b]Causes of inadequate heel lever—foot plantarflexed too much, foot too far anterior, heel cushion too soft.

[c]Causes of inadequate toe lever—foot dorsiflexed too much, foot too far posterior, foot keel too soft/flexible.

[d]Causes of excessive toe lever—foot plantar flexed too much, foot too far anterior, foot keel too stiff.

Comfort is the most critical aspect and depends on achieving an appropriate distribution of forces between the residual limb and the socket. A poorly fitting or uncomfortable socket will limit the mobility and often lead to rejection of the prosthesis. Once comfort has been established, the appropriate choice of components facilitates achieving maximal independence and function during sitting, standing, transferring, walking, and running. Lastly, cosmetic concerns are considered. Cosmesis is influenced by personal preferences and psychosocial dynamics but is usually satisfactorily achieved using contoured foam

TABLE 56-2	Medicare Guidelines for Functional Classification of Patients with Prosthesis	
K Code Level	**Functional Level**	**Activity Level**
K0	Not a potential user for ambulation or transfer	Does not have the ability or potential to ambulate or transfer safely with or without assistance, and a prosthesis does not enhance their quality of life or mobility.
K1	A potential household ambulator including transfers	Has the ability or potential to use a prosthesis for transfer or ambulation on level surfaces at fixed cadence. Typical of the limited and unlimited household ambulator.
K2	A potential limited community ambulatory	Has the ability or potential for ambulation with the ability to traverse low level environmental barriers such as curbs, stairs, or uneven surfaces. Typical of the limited community ambulator.
K3	Community ambulator using variable cadence, including therapeutic exercise or vocation	Has the ability or potential for ambulation with variable cadence. Typical of the community ambulator that has the ability to traverse most environmental barriers and may have vocation, therapeutic, or exercise activity that demands prosthetic utilization beyond simple locomotion.
K4	High activity user that exceeds normal ambulation skills	Has the ability or potential for ambulation that exceeds basic ambulation skills, exhibiting high impact, stress, or energy levels. Typical of the prosthetic demands of the child, active adult, or athlete.

Data from MERC Medicare Advisory Bulletin, Columbia SC, 1994;12:95–145.

and a nylon or rubber skin tone cover. Some individuals with an amputation prefer not to have their prosthesis covered because of the possible interference with prosthetic component function.

Medicare, a major funding source for prosthetic limbs in the United States, requires that the functional level of the individual with an amputation be taken into account when prescribing a prosthesis. The functional index is referred to as the Medicare "K" code and limits the components that can be used when fabricating the prosthesis. Although only required for Medicare, the "K" code classification is a simple but useful hierarchical framework for classifying the mobility potential of all individuals with an LE amputation (**Table 56-2**).

LE Prosthetic Components

The continual introduction of new component designs and the overlap of functional features of components from various manufacturers make it difficult to stay abreast of available prosthetic options. Collaboration between health care providers (physician, prosthetist, and therapist) is essential in developing an appropriate, individualized limb prescription. Seldom is there a single correct choice of components for a prosthesis, rather most individuals with an amputation can be successfully fit using components that span a reasonable range of mechanical and functional characteristics. Because objective data, linking prosthetic component characteristics to the demographics of individuals with an amputation, are limited, empiric approaches and experience play a major role in limb prescription. The prescription for an LE prosthesis should include the Medicare "K" code, diagnosis including level of amputation and underlying medical conditions, type of prosthesis (with modifiers), socket type, liner, suspension method, foot, knee and hip systems (as required by amputation level), diagnostic or check socket, and supplies. The patient, ordering physician, and prosthetic provider should be clearly documented on the prescription.

Prosthetic Feet

Prostheses for amputations at or proximal to the ankle require the use of a prosthetic foot. The selection of an appropriate prosthetic foot is complicated by the wide range of foot designs, marketing-driven claims of performance, and the limited availability of objective data comparing the relative biomechanical and functional advantages of different feet. In the clinical setting, the selection of a prosthetic foot is largely empirically based on the conceptual goal of matching the functional characteristics of the foot to the expected activity needs of the individual (8–13). Within this approach, it is useful to group feet by their major functional feature(s) as belonging to rigid keel, flexible keel, single/multiaxial, or dynamic response (or energy-storing) categories. It is acceptable for the prescribing physician to define the functional features desired in the foot and to rely on the prosthetist who typically has a better working understanding of the commercially available feet to select the specific manufacturer and foot within the desired functional class. This multidisciplinary approach is increasingly important as foot designs become more sophisticated, more costly, and combine different functional characteristics into a single foot. Occasionally, another characteristic of a foot such as an adjustable heel height, cosmesis, or being waterproof is the primary determinate in its selection.

The solid ankle cushion heel (SACH) foot (**Fig. 56-1**) is the least expensive and most commonly prescribed prosthetic foot. It is durable and lightweight, which accounts in part for its usefulness. The SACH foot has no moving parts and consists of a wooden or composite keel with a compressible foam heel and toes that flex under load, allowing limited simulation of the effects of the heel and forefoot rocker mechanisms of the normal foot. A SACH foot is appropriate for individuals with an amputation who have a lower activity level (K1 to K2), with ambulation primarily limited to level surfaces. It can be used in a wide range of individuals with an amputation for the preparatory prosthesis and upgraded as the individual with an amputation progresses to a higher activity level. For a juvenile with an amputation, the SACH foot is often the most cost-effective foot due to the need for frequent foot changes because of rapid growth.

The flexible keel foot (see **Fig. 56-1**) is designed to mimic the motion of the forefoot rocker mechanism by replacing the rigid keel of the SACH foot with a flexible keel. The keel bends with controlled stiffness as the foot moves from

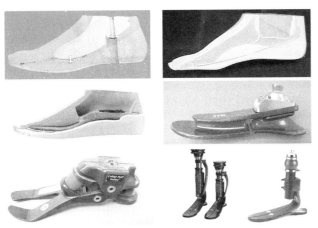

FIGURE 56-1. Prosthetic feet from the solid ankle cushion heel (SACH) and stationary attachment flexible endoskeletal (safe II flexible keel) foot (*top*). The impulse foot (dynamic response) and Luxon Max (dynamic response with multiaxis) (*middle*). The College Park TruStep (dynamic response, with some inversion, eversion, and transverse motion), the FlexFoot VSP (vertical shock pylon, dynamic response, multiaxis), and the Ceterus (VSP, dynamic response, multiaxis, and transverse motion) (*bottom*). The prosthetic manufactures have numerous feet available from the homebound to the paralympic patient. (Courtesy of Kingsley, Ohio Willow Wood, Otto Bock, CPI, OSSUR and Freedom Innovations. See prosthetic manufacture WEB Site Listings.)

mid-stance through preswing. Several versions of flexible keel feet are commercially available, each with different construction but sharing similar function. The stationary-ankle-flexible endoskeletal (SAFE) II foot is a commonly used flexible keel foot. The flexible keel foot allows some inversion and eversion and gives a smoother rollover than a SACH foot, making it appropriate for general mobility needs in the individual with an amputation with a low to moderate activity level. However, the more active individual with an amputation may perceive the flexible keel foot as being too soft, especially for fast walking or running activities.

Articulating prosthetic feet include both single axis and multiaxis designs. The single axis foot allows controlled movement in the sagittal plane (plantar flexion and dorsiflexion), adjusted by using different durometer bumpers. The primary advantage of the single axis foot is its ability to reduce knee-bending movements during limb loading, thus improving knee stability. Disadvantages include a greater weight than many other feet and more maintenance to ensure correct function. This foot is primarily used in the individual with a proximal amputation that requires better knee stabilization, such as the elderly individual with a transfemoral amputation or the individual with a transfemoral amputation and a short residual limb. Prosthetic feet with integral hydraulic ankles can provide similar sagittal plane motion but with the advantages of easier and faster adjustments for plantar flexion and dorsiflexion resistance.

Multiaxial foot designs allow for varying degrees of controlled movement in the sagittal, coronal, and transverse planes (plantar/dorsiflexion, inversion/eversion, some degree of transverse rotation). Multiaxis feet can use mechanical joints to supply motion such as the Greissinger foot or the College Park TruStep foot (see **Fig. 56-1**) but increasingly rely on the inherent flexibility of rubber and polymer materials to provide multiaxial motion. Using material flexibility improves durability

and reduces both weight and maintenance compared to mechanical jointed feet. Multiaxis "ankle" motion can be integrated into the foot or added to other feet through the use of separate multiaxial ankle components. Multiaxis capabilities are appropriate for the individual with an amputation who needs improved ankle motion to accommodate to uneven terrain and for the active individual with an amputation who requires greater ankle movement to adjust to different speeds or for cutting and pivoting quickly.

Dynamic response feet represent the largest category of prosthetic feet commercially available. Dynamic response (i.e., energy-storing) prosthetic feet incorporate elastic (spring-like) elements that store energy in the foot during limb loading and mid-stance as the elastic material compresses or flexes. Energy is returned at the time of push-off as the spring components of the foot return to its normal shape or configuration. Materials used to achieve dynamic response include carbon fiber, fiberglass, and composite materials (see **Fig. 56-1**). The dynamic energy characteristics of these feet make them particularly suitable for individuals with an amputation involved in activities requiring fast walking, running, and jumping. Many individuals with an amputation believe that they are more functional with a dynamic response foot. Dynamic elastic response (DER) feet were expected to make ambulation more efficient by reducing the oxygen consumption of individuals with an amputation, but the results of objective studies have been mixed (12,14). The metabolic benefits of DER designs are limited and primarily seen at faster walking speeds. Hybrid feet with some combination of controlled motion and dynamic response are becoming more popular. Vertical shock pylons (VSPs) and torque absorbers can be incorporated into prosthetic feet or added to existing feet to minimize vertical and rotational forces on the residual limb.

Prostheses by Level of Amputation

Partial Foot Amputation

Toe amputations, ray resections, and transmetatarsal amputations require minimal prosthetic/orthotic intervention. At the more distal foot amputation levels and for the less active individual with a transmetatarsal amputation, accommodative shoes with custom insoles, arch supports, and toe fillers are usually adequate. More active individuals with a transmetatarsal amputation may benefit from orthotic modifications that better substitute for the lost anterior foot lever arm. Options include the addition of carbon fiber or spring steel sole shanks, rocker soles, or short ankle foot orthosis. Partial foot amputations at the tarsal-metatarsal and transtarsal levels (e.g., Lisfranc, Chopart) are relatively uncommon and have historically been associated with equinovarus contracture of the hind foot, increasing the likelihood of skin breakdown over the plantar surface of the foot. However, improved surgical techniques that include Achilles tendon lengthening/resection and anterior tibialis and peroneus tendon transfers have reduced equinovarus deformities and result in a functional and useful amputation level (15,16). Prosthetic/orthotic devices for the individual with a proximal partial foot amputation need to supply medial-lateral stabilization of the hind foot and substitute for the lost forefoot lever. Options include (a) an extra depth shoe with toe filler, steel shank, and rocker bottom modifications; (b) custom posterior leaf-spring ankle-foot orthosis with toe filler; or (c) a custom prosthetic foot with a self-suspending rear-opening split socket (15,16). A major advantage of all partial foot amputations is the ability to be fully end bearing, allowing ambulation without any devices.

Syme Amputation

Similar to the hind foot amputation, the modified Syme (tibiotarsal disarticulation) amputation is capable of full weight end bearing. The heel flap is anchored to the distal end of the tibia and fibula, and following healing, allows short distance ambulation without a prosthesis. The substantial leg length discrepancy makes long distance ambulation without a prosthesis impractical. Over time, posterior migration of the distal heel pad occurs in some individuals with a Syme amputation leading to problems with skin breakdown and difficulty in prosthetic fitting (17–19). The relatively bulbous distal end of the residual limb has the advantage of enabling the use of self-suspending prosthetic designs; however, it also contributes to the major disadvantage of the Syme amputation—poor cosmesis due to the bulkiness of the prosthesis around the ankle joint. There are several different types of prostheses available for individuals with a Syme amputation.

The most common prosthetic style uses a total contact socket with a removable medial window (**Fig. 56-2**). The distal removable medial window allows the distal bulbous portion of the residual to slip easily into the socket, which is then held in place by closing and securing the window with Velcro straps. The major disadvantages to this prosthesis style are the poor cosmesis and the reduced strength of the socket due to the window. A second option uses a fixed posterior opening socket. This type of prosthesis is used for a very bulbous residual limb. This prosthesis is prone to breakage at the ankle joint and is not recommended for heavy duty users.

Alternative designs to window sockets use a flexible socket wall or liner to allow donning the prosthesis around the distal bulbous end of the residual limb. In the "stovepipe" design, a pelite or similar liner is used that is built up proximal to the ankle area, creating a cylindrical stovepipe-shaped inner liner. To don the prosthesis, the patient slips the distal bulbous residual past the narrow center of the liner that can then be easily inserted into the socket. This style of prosthesis is somewhat bulky but can be easily modified and is durable, making it suitable for use as a preparatory prosthesis or in active or obese patients.

The expandable wall prosthesis uses a double-wall socket that has a flexible, expandable inside liner and a rigid outer frame. The inner wall is made of silicone or other elastomers that are flexible enough to allow the bulbous residual limb to slide into the prosthesis. This prosthesis is typically difficult to modify but has the advantage of being very strong and useful for active users or obese patients, and is generally easy to don and doff, making it suitable for individuals with upper limb impairment or cognitive impairment.

Low-profile feet are needed for Syme prosthesis due to the limited space available beneath the socket. Acceptable foot options range from the rigid keel SACH feet through multiaxial and dynamic response feet.

Transtibial Amputation

Transtibial amputations are the most common amputation level seen in general practice. Considerable effort over the past several decades has gone into designing components to address the needs of individuals with transtibial amputations. The large number of options available increases the uncertainty when choosing components, but if approached systematically, straightforward reasoned decisions can be used to generate a prosthetic prescription. The following discussion of transtibial prosthetic components parallels the recommended approach for prescribing prostheses. Initially, the socket and liner system that will optimize comfort and skin protection is determined. Next, the suspension system is chosen and finally pylon and foot/ankle components are selected. All of these decisions are based on the physician's history and examination of the patient and the functional goals established by the rehabilitation team.

The patella tendon-bearing (PTB) total contact socket has been the internationally accepted standard transtibial socket since the 1960s (20). The PTB total contact socket is fabricated from a cast or scan of the residual limb, which is modified to specific weight-bearing (SWB) regions that are pressure tolerant and correspondingly modified to decrease pressure over bony prominences such as the tibia crest, fibula, and distal portion of the tibia (**Fig. 56-3**).

The standard PTB design has several variations (21,22). The PTB-supracondylar (PTBSC) socket has high medial and lateral sidewalls that extend above and over the femoral condyles, providing enhanced mediolateral stability and self-suspension of the prosthesis. The PTB-supracondylar/suprapatellar (PTBSCSP) socket further extends the PTBSC

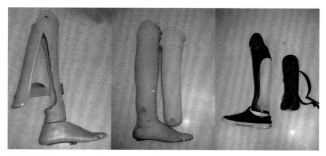

FIGURE 56-2. *From left to right*: The posterior opening Symes for bulbous distal end; PTB Symes with pelite liner; Canadian-type Syme prosthesis as modified by the Veterans Administration Prosthetic Center.

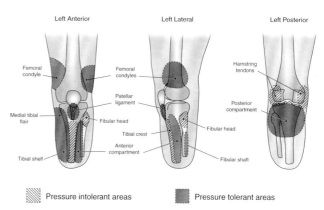

FIGURE 56-3. Areas that are pressure intolerant and tolerant for modification and fabrication of a specific weight-bearing (SWB) or PTB socket.

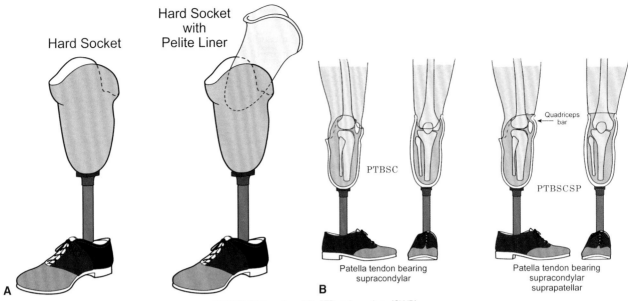

FIGURE 56-4.   A and B: PTB style sockets (SWB).

socket concept by also extending the anterior aspect of the socket so that the patellar is encompassed within the socket. The PTBSCSP gives additional stiffness to the mediolateral walls and applies force proximal to the patella during stance to provide sensory feedback to limit genu recurvatum. Both the PTBSC and PTBSCSP are primarily used in individuals with short residual limbs to improve varus/valgus control and to provide greater surface area for weight distribution (**Fig. 56-4**).

An alternative socket design for individuals with a transtibial amputation is the total surface-bearing (TSB) socket made practical by the development of gel and elastomeric liner systems (discussed below). The TSB socket is made from a cast or scan of the residual limb with minimal modifications. When used with gel liners, the TSB socket is believed to distribute pressure more uniformly within the socket. The relative advantages and disadvantages of TSB versus PTB total contact sockets remain poorly understood. When a comfortable fit cannot be achieved with one type of socket, empirically switching to the other can be successful.

Socket fit coupled with the choice of a liner are key considerations in assuring comfort and acceptance of the prosthetic limb. The liner functions as the primary interface between the residual limb and the remainder of the prosthesis. In this role, it must complement socket fit to ensure optimal pressure distribution while also eliminating harmful shear forces and providing a favorable moisture, heat, and chemical environment that prevents skin breakdown. PTB total contact sockets can be fit as hard sockets that do not use a liner or more commonly use a liner made from closed cell foam such as Pe-Lite for improved comfort. Using PTB total contact sockets and pelite liners are often an advantage in the preparatory prosthesis because of the relative ease with which the liner can be modified to accommodate changes in residual limb volume (20,21,23). Roll-on silicone or elastomeric gel liners are another option that can be used with a PTB total contact socket but are generally recommended for use with TSB socket designs. Gel liners are thought to enhance comfort and reduce shear, making them the initial choice for residual limbs with scarring or skin grafts

that compromise skin integrity (20,23). Gel liners result in more sweating and are generally less tolerated in warm climates than other liners. Contraindications to the use of gel liners are residual limbs with open wounds, poor hygiene, or a history of contact dermatitis.

The suspension system for the transtibial prosthesis must securely attach the limb during activities, minimize pistoning, and be comfortable when sitting. When working with individuals with an amputation who run, play sports, or are involved in climbing activities, ensuring effective suspension is especially important. Suspension systems can be grouped into categories that include straps, sleeves, gel liners with locking mechanisms, and suction (**Fig. 56-5**). A previously commonly used suspension system is the supracondylar cuff strap. Several variants exist, all of which consist of a multipart strap that attaches to the sidewalls of the socket and encircles the distal thigh using the normal anatomic flare of the supracondylar portion of the femur to maintain suspension. Thigh corset and side joints attached to the socket are a more rigid suspension option. The weight and bulk of the resulting limb makes it a poor initial choice for a contemporary prosthetic limb; however, individuals with an amputation who may benefit from this type of limb are those with a short transtibial amputation who require maximal medial-lateral stability for outdoor or work activities. This type of limb may also be preferred when coexisting ligamentous instability of the knee is present or to partially off-load a painful or weight-intolerant residual limb.

Sleeve suspension systems consist of rubber, neoprene, or elastic sleeves that are pulled up onto the distal thigh after donning the prosthesis (23). Sleeves are a general purpose suspension system that is inexpensive and effective for individuals with an amputation across a wide spectrum of activity levels. The primary disadvantages are related to excessive heat or sweating, the need for good grip strength to pull the sleeve up, and the occasional occurrence of contact dermatitis, especially with the use of neoprene-based sleeves. Silicone and elastomeric gel liners are prosthetic sock-shaped sleeves made from a variety of silicone and urethane elastomeric

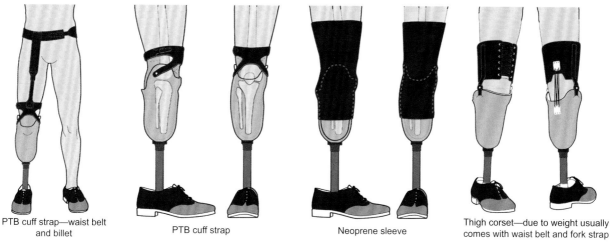

PTB cuff strap—waist belt
and billet

PTB cuff strap

Neoprene sleeve

Thigh corset—due to weight usually
comes with waist belt and fork strap

FIGURE 56-5. Suspension systems used for the transtibial prosthesis.

compounds that are rolled onto the residual limb. They function as both an interface and suspension method. The suspension function requires either a metal pin attached to the distal end of the liner that inserts into a locking mechanism in the bottom of the socket or by a Velcro lanyard strap that passes through a slot in the socket and connects with its counterpart attached to the outside of the socket. The suspension pin or lanyard securely anchors the liner to the socket, and the subsequent friction and suction that develops between the liner and the residual limb supplies the force required for suspension (**Fig. 56-6**). This approach provides excellent suspension for a wide range of activities and is increasingly being used as a general purpose suspension system. Gel liners are available in a wide range of sizes and thicknesses but can also be custom designed. The main disadvantages of gel liners are their high cost compared to straps or sleeves and their limited durability, which necessitates replacement of the liners every 6 to 12 months. In the presence of loose or excessive soft tissue in the residual limb, elongation and stretching of the distal tissues during swing phase can occur that may lead to pain.

The last option for suspension of the transtibial prosthesis uses suction. By combining a one-way air valve ported to the bottom of the socket with an airtight sleeve, a partial vacuum is created within the socket effectively suspending the prosthesis during the swing phase (24). The vacuum needed to hold the residual limb can be generated through a pistoning action of the residual limb within the socket or by a vacuum pump built into the prosthetic shank or foot that is activated at heel strike or by an electric-operated vacuum pump attached to the socket. These later options are known as vacuum-assisted socket suspension (VASS) (**Fig. 56-7**).

Most contemporary prostheses are endoskeletal in design. Using an endoskeletal pylon allows alignment changes after prosthetic fabrication and enables the use of additional components that can absorb forces or allow motion between the socket and the remainder of residual limb. Commonly used components include transverse rotators that reduce axial torques and vertical shock absorbers that cushion impact loading and may reduce oxygen consumption (14,25). The selection of a prosthetic foot completes the transtibial prosthesis prescription.

Knee Disarticulation

Knee disarticulation (KD) amputations share some of the same advantages and disadvantages as the Syme amputation (ankle disarticulation) (26). Similar to the Syme amputation, full weight bearing on the distal end of the KD residual limb is usually possible and the anatomic flare of the femoral

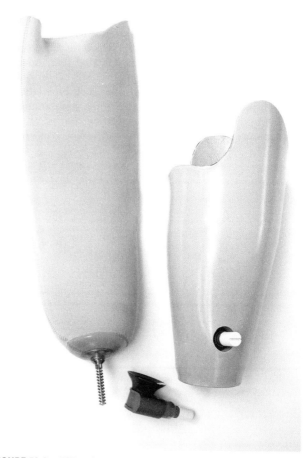

FIGURE 56-6. TSB socket with gel liner and pin system, and custom-fabricated liners to accommodate any irregularities of the residual limb. If pin or lanyard system is not being used, then the socket will be held by a suspension sleeve. (Courtesy of Otto Bock and Evolution Liners, see Web site listing.)

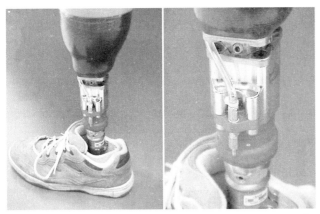

FIGURE 56-7. VASS works by use of a vertical shock pylon that acts like a vacuum pump and continually withdraws air from the sealed socket while ambulating. (Courtesy of Otto Bock, see Web site listing.)

condyles can be used for self-suspension of the prosthesis. Because of the improved distal weight bearing, the KD amputation does not require an ischial weight-bearing socket leading to enhanced comfort and sitting tolerance compared to a transfemoral socket. The KD has a bulbous distal end, which compromises prosthetic cosmesis. Compared to the individual with a transfemoral amputation, the long length of the KD residual improves the prosthetic control and allows a greater degree of dynamic muscular stability. However, the long residual limb limits the choice of prosthetic knee units that can be used to maintain symmetric knee centers between the amputated and nonamputated side. Advances in the design and development of the four-bar linkage or polycentric knee units (**Fig. 56-8**) offer good biomechanical function and acceptable limb cosmesis. KD, while an uncommon amputation level, is reemerging as an alternative to the transfemoral amputation when wound healing concerns are

acceptable because of the improved sitting balance, reduced energy cost of walking, and better acceptance rate than that for a transfemoral amputation (27).

Transfemoral Amputation

The development of new technology, materials, and prosthetic components over the past decade has arguably had the greatest impact on the care of the individual with an amputation at the transfemoral level. The following discussion of transfemoral prosthetic components is organized to parallel a reasonable approach to prescribing a prosthesis. Initially, the socket style is specified. Next, the residual limb interface/liner and suspension system are determined. Because liner and suspension options are closely linked at the transfemoral level, they are discussed together. Following selection of socket and suspension, the knee unit is selected and finally pylon and foot/ankle components are chosen.

The quadrilateral socket introduced following World War II had been the standard socket design for transfemoral prostheses until the emergence of a new socket design, the ischial containment socket (ICS) during the past 15 years. The quadrilateral socket, named for its quadrilateral shape as viewed in the transverse plane, is designed for ischial weight bearing on the posterior brim. Quadrilateral sockets are still used for long-term wearers who have become accustomed to its weight-bearing and control characteristics (28) (**Fig. 56-9**). Unfortunately, the quad socket design allowed femoral abduction and lateral shift during ambulation. The majority of individuals with new transfemoral amputations, the ICS, are believed to provide a more normal anatomic alignment of the femur inside

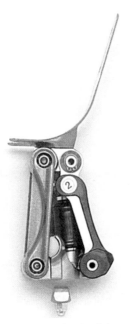

FIGURE 56-8. The 3R46 modular four-bar linkage or polycentric knee joint for KD. (Courtesy of Otto Bock, see Web site listing.)

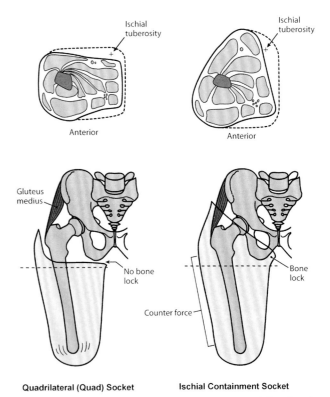

Quadrilateral (Quad) Socket   **Ischial Containment Socket**

FIGURE 56-9. Note the shapes between the quadrilateral (Quad) socket and the ICS. Also note the ischium sites inside the ICS socket rather than the socket brim (as does the quad socket).

the prosthesis. This is accomplished by extending the socket trimlines proximally and contouring the medial aspect of the socket to capture the ischial tuberosity inside the socket rather than allowing the tuberosity to sit on the posterior brim as in the quadrilateral socket. The ICS allows more effective hip and pelvic stabilizing forces to be developed during stance phase (28–30), which improves the medial-lateral control of the trunk. While the ICS is useful for all individuals with transfemoral amputations, the improved stability is especially beneficial for those with a short residual limb.

Several variants of the ICS have been introduced that include the normal shape-normal alignment, contoured adducted trochanter-controlled alignment method, the Sabolich ICS, and the Northwestern ICS and the M.A.S. (Marlo Anatomical Socket) ICS (28–32). These options vary somewhat in contour details, but all retain the basic functional characteristics of ICS. No clear consensus has emerged favoring one-design variant over the others, but all require considerable skill to fabricate correctly. Both the ISC and quadrilateral sockets can be fabricated as a rigid socket or by using a flexible thermoplastic inner socket supported by graphite-reinforced, laminated open framework (33,34). The advantages of the rigid frame-flexible liner type of socket designs are flexible walls that increase comfort, especially at the proximal brim, improved proprioception, accommodation of minor volume changes, less heat build-up, and enhanced suspension as the inner socket warms during use increasing its flexibility and improving the intimacy of the fit (30). The newest transfemoral socket designs use a strut frame with a flexible inner socket and adjustable straps, allowing the patient some control of the socket fit.

A number of interface liner systems and suspension options exist for the transfemoral prosthesis (**Fig. 56-10**) (23). The simplest liner system uses a hard socket with wool or cotton socks adjusted in plies to achieve a comfortable fit. Suspension for this type of prosthesis most commonly uses a Silesian belt or total elastic suspension (TES) belt. The Silesian belt attaches to the anterior and lateral portions of the proximal prosthetic socket and passes over the opposite iliac crest. The TES belt is made of the same neoprene material used for transtibial suspension sleeves. It slips over the outside of the prosthetic socket and surrounds the waist above the iliac crests to provide suspension. Both Silesian and TES suspension systems are simple to don, can be adapted for use by individuals with impaired hand function, and usually provide acceptable prosthetic limb suspension for low activity level patients. Disadvantages

include some inevitable pistoning of the prosthesis, reduced comfort due to bandage pressure, and heat or occasional dermatitis, especially with the TES belt. The TES and Silesian suspension systems can be used as a primary suspension system or coupled with other suspension options (discussed below) as an axillary suspension system when additional suspension security or rotation control is needed. Other suspension belt options include the pelvic band and hip joint. This option uses a single axis hip joint integrated into the lateral socket wall, which is attached to a pelvic band and belt closely contoured about the iliac crest. The side joint and band discourage rotation of the prosthesis and extend the lateral lever arm stabilizing the prosthesis, making it especially useful for the short residual transfemoral prosthesis.

Suction socket suspension is the second major type of suspension for the individual with a transfemoral amputation and, whenever feasible, is generally the preferred option (23). Suction sockets are total contact sockets worn directly against the skin of the residual limb that incorporate a one-way air valve in the distal socket. To don the prosthesis, the individual with an amputation has to pull the residual limb into the socket. This "dry fit" suction can be accomplished using an elastic stockinette, an Ace bandage, or an "EZ pull" sock made from a thin slippery nylon fabric. An alternative method is the "wet fit" process in which a liquid powder is applied to the residual limb, temporarily lubricating the skin, which can then be slipped into the socket. As the socket is being donned, the suction valve is functional and the remaining air is expelled through the valve, creating a small vacuum that holds the socket on the limb. For most users, suction suspension provides a very secure and comfortable suspension effect free from external belts or straps. Suction suspension requires a stable residual limb volume, and as a result is not a good option for preparatory prostheses when rapid limb shrinkage is expected. The presence of scar tissue can compromise the ability to maintain suction and may be poorly tolerated by the inherent high skin friction present in the socket. Prostheses that use suction sockets must be donned while standing and require both good balance and adequate hand strength and coordination to manipulate the pull sock and to install the valve. Difficulty with consistently pulling all of the proximal soft tissues of the thigh into the socket can lead to an adductor roll (a compression of the soft tissues of the medial groin between the proximal socket and the pelvis) that is painful and can lead to skin breakdown. Correcting this problem may require

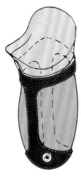 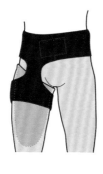 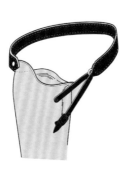 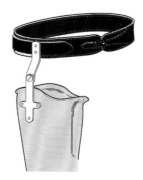 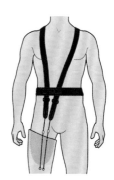

| Suction Suspension | TES Belt (Total Elastic Suspension) | Silesian Belt | Pelvic Belt and Band and Hip Joint | Suspenders |

FIGURE 56-10.   Possible suspensions that could be used for the transfemoral amputee.

socket modifications, changes to the donning technique, or the use of external vacuum pumps to help elongate the tissue of the residual limb to promote a better fit (35).

A variant of the hard socket uses hypobaric gel liners with an impregnated silicone band near the proximal end of the sock. The silicone band provides a seal to prevent air leak, allowing for a suction suspension effect that can accommodate changing residual limb volume secondary to limb shrinkage or weight change.

Similar to a transtibial prosthesis, silicone and elastomeric gel suspension liners with a lanyard strap or pin attachment can be used to provide a positive mechanical type of suspension. This suspension system provides good suspension, minimal pistoning, effective control of adductor rolls, and good comfort across a wide range of activity levels. Socks can be added over the suspension liner to accommodate for volume change of the residual limb. Effective use of gel liners can be problematic in the residual limb with excess or loose soft tissue because of difficulties in consistently donning the liner, excessive traction on soft tissue during swing, and poor rotational control of the prosthesis. The use of auxiliary TES or Silesian suspension may be needed in this situation.

During the last decade, a wide variety of prosthetic knee joints have been designed, fabricated, and made commercially available. A recent survey cataloged over 200 knee units, ranging from the simple single axis knee joints to the completely computerized knee units (**Fig. 56-11**). The primary purposes of the prosthetic knee are to provide stability during stance (to prevent knee buckling), either through alignment or mechanical means, knee motion during swing to permit clearance of the toe, and adequate flexion to allow the knee to bend when sitting. The knee unit should control the heel rise of the shank, assisting or resisting the acceleration and deceleration of the shank during the swing phase. The selection of an appropriate knee unit is primarily based on matching the stance phase stability features and the swing control aspects of the knee to the anticipated activity level and usage of the prosthesis (36–38). Hydraulic or pneumatic knee units are used for the K3 and K4 individual with an amputation and provide either swing phase control or swing and stance phase control for individuals who change their cadence frequently. Hydraulic knees can provide variable cadence and controlled stance flexion. Pneumatic knees have variable cadence in swing phase but limited stance phase control. For the K1 or K2 individual with an amputation who has difficulty maintaining knee stability during stance, locking knees and weight-activated stance control knees are available.

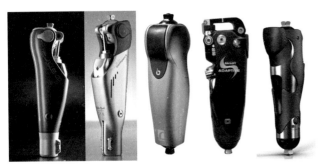

FIGURE 56-11. Some of the computerized knees available. *Left to right* is the C-leg, Compact knee, Rheo Knee, Smart Adaptive knee, and the Plie knee. (Courtesy of Otto Bock, Ossur, Endolite and Freedom Innovations. See prosthetic manufacture Web site listing.)

The four-bar, five-bar, and six-bar knee units are becoming increasingly popular due to the moveable centroid, which gives better stability of the knee. **Table 56-3** outlines the major types of knee joints and their advantages and disadvantages.

The same pylon components (VSPs and rotators) that are available for the individual with an amputation at the transtibial level are also available at the transfemoral level. In addition, a thigh rotator can be added for the individual with a transfemoral amputation who has a need to cross the prosthetic leg for ADLs (i.e., riding in a car, donning and doffing clothing or shoes, etc.) (**Fig. 56-12**).

Hip Disarticulation/Hemipelvectomy

Individuals with a transfemoral amputation, with less than 5 cm of residual femur, usually are fitted at hip disarticulation level. The standard prosthesis for a hip disarticulation is the Canadian hip disarticulation prosthesis (**Fig. 56-13**). The socket of this prosthesis encloses the hemipelvis on the side of the amputation and extends around the hemipelvis of the nonamputated side, leaving an opening for the nonamputated LE. There is a flexible anterior wall with an opening that allows the prosthesis to be donned. Weight is borne on the ischial tuberosity of the amputated side. Endoskeletal prosthetic components are preferred for this level of amputation to reduce the overall weight. The endoskeletal hip joint has an extension assist, as does the knee unit, which usually is a constant friction knee. Endoskeletal components may be made from aluminum, titanium, or carbon graphite composite materials. Traditionally, a single axis or SACH foot with a soft heel has been the most common choice for the prosthetic foot. A cosmetic cover completes the prosthetic prescription. If necessary, locking hip or knee joints can be used. For high functional level hip disarticulation patients, microprocessor knees may be a good choice to enhance stability.

The prosthesis for a hemipelvectomy resembles that for the hip disarticulation except in the interior configuration of the socket. In the hemipelvectomy, most of the weight is borne by the soft tissues on the amputated side, with some of the weight being borne by the sacrum, the rib cage, and the opposite ischial tuberosity.

Hemicorporectomy

Although rare, the hemicorporectomy (HCP), or translumbar amputation, has the most significant physiologic and psychological implications. During this procedure, the bony pelvis, pelvic contents, lower extremities, and external genitalia are removed following disarticulation of the lumbar spine and transection of the spinal cord. HCP is usually a last resort for patients with life-threatening conditions such as advanced pelvic tumors, pelvic osteomyelitis, crushing pelvic trauma, or intractable decubiti in the pelvic region. Once the amputation site is adequately healed, then a prosthetist should begin fabrication of the prosthesis.

The prosthesis is bucket shaped with two cut apertures to accommodate the patient's colostomy and ileostomy sites. This type of prosthesis is similar to those used in other cases of HCP (39). When using the prosthesis for the first time, the patient must limit the use and allow frequent checks for skin breakdown for the next several weeks. At first, the base of the prosthesis is attached to a flat board to provide a level seating surface and possibly later replaced with a rocker type board for greater mobility when transferring to and from a wheelchair and promoting easier wheelchair use.

TABLE 56-3	General Information on Prosthetic Knees and Usage		
Type of Knee	**Advantage**	**Disadvantage**	**Possible Usage**
Single axis constant friction	Simple Durable	Only constant swing phase control No stance control	Excellent for pediatrics Having good voluntary control of swing and stance phase but single cadence
Polycentric (not fluid control)	Low maintenance Varying stability through stance Shortens shank during swing for better toe clearance While sitting, some give natural and better cosmetic appearance	Single cadence Increased weight and bulk Complex mechanism Single cadence	Knee disartics Long transfemoral for appearance and short transfemoral for knee stability Weak hip extensors
Weight-activated stance control	Do not have adequate control to manage a bending knee or good enough hip control to stabilize braking mechanism if weight applied with knee flexed 0–20 degrees	Requires regular maintenance	Geriatrics
	Helpful for slower clients	Not very responsive for active walker Gait modified to unload knee Single cadence	Short residual limb General debility Uneven surfaces
Manual lock	Total stability in stance phase	No swing phase flexion, resulting in stiff knee gait Awkward in sitting	Patient requires mechanical stability in stance Last resort
Fluid control			
Single axis pneumatic control	Responds to changing gait speeds	Higher cost May need more maintenance Heavier	From pediatrics to adults, with good control
Single axis hydraulic control	Swing respond to changing gait speeds If stance phase has hydraulic resistance to knee flexion during weight bearing	Higher cost May need more maintenance Heavier	From pediatrics to adults, with go control Excellent reliability
Polycentric and multiaxis fluid control	Varying stability through stance Shortens shank during swing for better toe clearance While sitting some give natural and better cosmetic appearance Variable cadence	Higher cost May need more maintenance Heavier	For the more active amputee Knee disartics Long transfemoral for appearance and short transfemoral for knee stability Range from homebound to highly active amputee
Microprocessor control			
Single axis or multiaxis fluid control	On board computer adjusting knee for variable gait cycles Energy saving	Highest cost Heavy Unproven track record for dependability	For the more active patients Some computerized knees use a computer-regulated valve to adjust the swing phase resistance of a pneumatic cylinder Some use the computer to control swing phase function and stance phase stability Some systems using multiple sensors to send messages about changes walking back to the microchip 50 times a second

UPPER EXTREMITY AMPUTATION

General Principles of UE Amputation Management

The general approach to the care of the individual with a upper extremity (UE) amputation parallels that used in treating a lower limb amputation outlined in Chapter 37. The main differences will be highlighted and areas of unique management discussed.

Preprosthetic Patient Evaluation and Management

The preprosthetic evaluation, whether performed preoperatively or postoperatively, should focus on identifying factors that will affect rehabilitation and prosthetic fitting. Of particular importance is the presence of coexisting musculoskeletal or neurologic compromise such as significant shoulder range of motion loss or brachial plexus injury that would compromise or prevent the successful use of prosthesis. Initial education

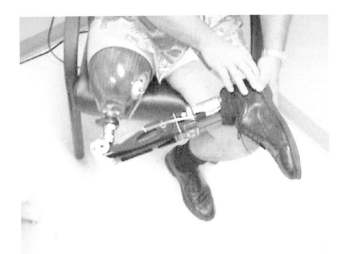

FIGURE 56-12. Rotator adaptor for rotation to allow better access for donning and doffing clothing or comfort while in a vehicle. (Courtesy of Otto Bock, see Web site listing.)

about the rehabilitation process, prosthetic options, and a discussion of realistic expectations should occur during this stage.

Postoperative Care

The options for postoperative care of the residual limb are similar to those used in the LE. Soft dressings along with stump shrinkers or elastic compressive stockinettes are the most com-

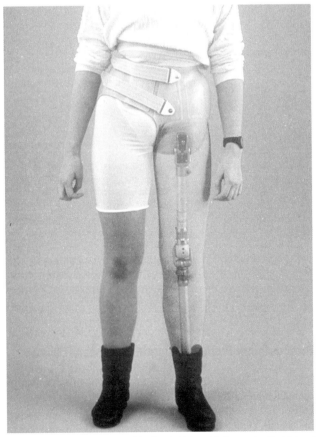

FIGURE 56-13. Canadian-type hip disarticulation with free motion hip joint and four-bar knee with outline of cover. (Courtesy of Otto Bock, see Web site listing.)

monly used wound care approach. In centers with experience in the application of RRDs, their use in the immediate and early postoperative period is advocated because of presumed benefits of better residual limb protection, edema control, and pain reduction. RRDs work best at the transradial amputation level because of the ease in suspending the cast. An additional advantage of RRDs is the ability to implement immediate or early postprosthetic fitting by attaching a hook, harness, and control system to the cast. Early prosthetic fitting is particularly important for the individual with a bilateral UE amputation to avoid the potentially profound psychology consequences resulting from the complete dependence that accompanies the loss of both UEs.

Prosthetic Fitting

Even more so than in the individual with an LE amputation, an understanding of the individual's vocational and avocational needs, motivation in pursuing prosthetic fitting, availability of a supportive social network, and cosmetic concerns are critical in goal setting and decision-making regarding prosthetic prescription. There are no fixed guidelines for deciding which individual with an upper limb amputation will benefit from a prosthetic limb. Factors that often prevent successful fitting and training include significant cognitive deficits, upper motor neuron syndromes that impair volitional coordination of the residual limb, plexopathies or peripheral nerve injuries, significant sensory loss, hyperpathia of the residual limb, or range of motion loss in the shoulder. The typical sequence of prosthetic rehabilitation involves initial fitting and training with a body-powered preparatory prostheses followed by a definite prosthesis when residual limb maturation has occurred 3 to 6 months postsurgery. Advantages of using a body-powered preparatory prosthesis include the greater ease of fitting, greater adaptability to changes in residual limb volume, early training in ADLs, and a lower cost compared to external-powered devices. Since it is difficult to predict either the likelihood of long-term acceptance of an upper limb prosthesis or an individual's preferred type of prosthetic system (body or external powered), the preparatory prosthetic phase should be used to explore various prosthetic options. Different types of terminal devices should be tried, and the individual with a UE amputation given enough time to explore the advantages and disadvantages of using the prosthesis in a variety of home, work, and social settings. This type of clinical trial allows more informed decision-making and participation of the patient at the time of definitive prosthetic prescription.

The overall acceptance and continued use of a prosthetic limb is influenced by a number of factors (40–43). Similar to the LE, as the amputation level moves more proximal, the prosthetic rejection rate increases. The majority of individuals with an amputation at the shoulder disarticulation or forequarter level ultimately reject prostheses. Approximately 40% of individuals with a transhumeral amputation (THA) become long-term users of a prosthetic limb. At the transradial amputation level, approximately 90% of individuals continue to use a prosthesis occasionally. More distal amputations in the hand have a lower rate of prosthetic limb acceptance, typically because of the greater preserved function of the residual limb. Individuals with bilateral amputations at all levels tend to have a higher acceptance rate for prosthetic limb use. Early work by Malone et al. (40) indicated that early fitting within

30 days postoperatively was associated with higher long-term acceptance. More recent studies (41,42) have not shown as strong a correlation, suggesting that even delayed fitting can be successful. Common reasons for rejecting a prosthetic limb include limited usefulness, excessive weight, residual limb pain, and poor durability (myoelectric prosthesis). It is also important to note that unilateral upper limb amputee can be totally independent in all self-care, and many other activities, without a prosthesis. Bilateral upper limb amputees are much more dependent on prosthetic devices for self-care tasks.

Final Prosthetic Evaluation and Control Training

Prosthetic training is an important component of the rehabilitation process and affects the successful use and acceptance of the prosthesis (44). General strengthening and range of motion exercises for the proximal residual limb started in the preprosthetic phase should continue. After the prosthesis has been fabricated, it should be checked by the members of the prosthetic team to ensure that the fit is comfortable and that the control system is properly adjusted for maximum functional operation. During initial use and training, the prosthesis should be removed every 15 to 30 minutes to check for signs of excessive pressure or irritation that may occur with poor socket fit or overuse. As the skin tolerance increases, wearing time is gradually increased during the first few days of wear and thereafter more quickly. With a well-fitting prosthesis, an individual with a UE amputation can wear the limb for an entire day within a week or 2 of receiving it.

Specific training involves instruction in how to put on and remove the prosthesis, adjusting the number of sock plies, and how to clean and care for the residual limb and prosthesis. Initial skills are acquired to control the terminal device and to activate position and lock the elbow in the individual with a THA. Grasping and releasing objects, transferring objects, and positioning of the terminal device for functional activities should be practiced under the guidance and feedback of an experienced therapist. ADLs, homemaking, and occupational and recreational activities should be undertaken and simulated in the training sessions. Successful prosthetic users rely on basic skills learned in therapy, which are supplemented and polished by practice at home during everyday tasks. The individual who is a long-term user of the upper limb often has very specific use patterns and preferences for components, harness type, and control cable adjustments. It is prudent to incorporate the desires of the individual into the decision-making and prescription process.

Control training for externally powered prostheses is more complex than for body-powered UE prostheses. The same goals as outlined for conventional prostheses are appropriate for myoelectric controlled prostheses. In addition, the individual must learn to separate, modulate, and sustain voluntary muscle contractions in the muscles selected to control the powered functions of the prosthesis. Training with an externally powered (electric) prosthesis often requires more time than with a body-powered prosthesis because more exacting individual muscle motions and quantity of muscle contraction are required for control of the prosthesis.

Adults and older children can be expected to practice specific tasks and routines, both in therapy and at home, as outlined by the therapist to achieve the necessary skills for independent function. The training time in a young child with a UE prosthesis will be significantly longer than that for an adult or older child.

UE Prosthetic Follow-Up

The routine follow-up visits for an individual with a new amputation should occur initially 4 to 6 weeks after delivery of the prosthesis, then every 2 to 6 months until a definite prosthesis is prescribed. Once clinically stable in a definitive prosthesis, yearly clinic visits, or whenever a problem arises, are usually adequate. At these follow-up visits, the individual's use and function with the prosthesis should be reviewed, difficulties or problems resolved, the fit and condition of the prosthesis evaluated, and the condition of the residual limb noted. If necessary, additional therapy may be suggested, repairs to the prosthesis made, medical problems with the residual limb addressed, and a new prosthesis prescribed if indicated. With average use, a UE prosthesis can be expected to be worn for 3 to 5 years before total replacement is necessary. The socket itself may need to be replaced more frequently than the other components.

Although our emphasis has been on prosthetic restoration, the focus of rehabilitation should remain on the individual with the UE amputation and his or her desired lifestyle following limb loss. Many individuals with a UE amputation do well without the aid of a prosthesis and should not be viewed as having failed if they choose not to wear a prosthesis.

Bilateral UE Amputations

The individual with a bilateral UE amputation is immediately faced with the loss of ability to perform almost every ADL. Early restoration of any ADL is important. Providing a utensil cuff, which can be attached to a residual arm, can assist the patient with feeding and tooth brushing. In the individual with a bilateral UE amputation, early prosthetic fitting should be accomplished, even with temporary or preparatory prostheses. In the individual with a bilateral amputation, the longer residual limb usually assumes dominance. Special component considerations apply in this case. Wrist flexion units, at least on the dominant side or perhaps bilaterally, will permit midline activities such as shirt buttoning, belt buckling, and toileting. Also wrist rotator units, which provide terminal device positioning, provide for easier bilateral prosthetic use. Special toileting techniques must be taught for patient independence. In addition, foot skills should be reviewed, and LE mobilizing exercises should be performed. Specialized bathroom equipment such as a bidet for toileting, a "shower tree" with multiple nozzles, and wall-mounted blow dryers may be needed.

UE Prostheses

A UE prosthesis attempts to replace very complex functions. The hand is able to perform a wide range of functional activities ranging from fine dexterity tasks requiring light prehensile forces to gross grasping movements with great prehensile forces, all under the guidance of sensory feedback. To accomplish these tasks in the dynamic world around us, the coordinated movements of the proximal muscles and joints of the UE must position the hand for functional activities. The prosthetic replacement for the UE is a limited substitute for the lost body part. With practice, it can replace several of the simple grasping and manipulating functions of the hand through a mildly to moderately restricted sphere of functional reach. A critical limitation of all UE prosthetic limbs is the severe restriction in sensory feedback from the terminal device relegating its use to that of simply assisting bimanual activities. The limited ability of the prosthetic limb to replace normal hand function typically results in a shift in hand dominance with amputation of the dominant hand.

UE prostheses can be divided into three groups: conventional or body powered, external powered or electric, and passive or cosmetic.

Body-Powered Prostheses

Since the majority of individuals with UE amputation first learn to use a body-powered limb, an initial discussion of the function of various components (45,46) used in this type of prosthetic limb follows. Understanding the role, use, and limitations of body-powered prosthetic limbs forms the framework for subsequent discussions of externally powered devices. All conventional body-powered UE prostheses have these component parts: socket, suspension, control cable system, terminal device, and interposing joints.

Socket

Traditionally, UE prostheses have used a dual-wall socket design fabricated from lightweight plastic or graphite composite materials. In dual wall designs, a rigid inner socket is fabricated from a custom mold of the residual limb and is the primary interface between the user and the prosthesis. Comfort and function are directly tied to the quality of the fit of the inner socket. The outer socket wall is fabricated to have the general shape, length, and contour of the normal arm or forearm and serves a cosmetic function and also supplies the foundation for the mounting of required components. This type of socket is durable and easily accommodates variation in residual limb volume using socks to adjust the fit.

An alternative approach to the design of the socket parallels the rigid frame, flexible liner approach used in lower limb prostheses. An inner socket is fabricated from flexible plastic materials to provide a total contact fit and is optimized for the use of suction suspension. Surrounding the inner socket is a rigid frame that provides the structural integrity of the socket. Windows in the outer socket allow for the movement of the muscles of residual limb to enhance comfort.

Suspension

The suspension system must hold the prosthesis securely to the residual limb and accommodate and distribute the forces associated with the weight of the prosthesis and any superimposed lifting loads. Suspension systems can be classified as harness-based, self-suspending sockets, or suction.

The most commonly used suspension for body-powered prostheses are variants of the harness-based system. The most commonly used harness is the figure-of-8 strap (**Fig. 56-14**). On the intact side, the harness loops around the axilla anchoring the limb and providing the counterforce for suspension and control cable forces. On the prosthetic side, the anterior strap carries the major suspending forces to the prosthesis by attaching directly to the socket (transhumeral) or indirectly through an intermediate Y-strap and triceps pad (transradial).

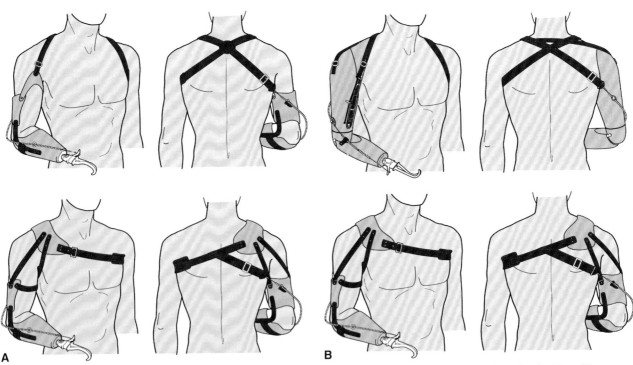

FIGURE 56-14. The transradial amputee has two types of harnessing. **A:** The figure-of-8 harness and the next shows the shoulder saddle and chest strap harness. The terminal device is activated by arm flexion or by biscapular abduction. **B:** For the transhumeral amputee, the same motion stated above will move the elbow and operate the terminal device once the elbow is in the locked position. To lock or unlock the elbow, the amputee must simultaneously use arm extension, shoulder depression, and arm abduction. Figure-of-8 and shoulder saddle for the transradial and transhumeral body powered harness. Shoulder saddle harnessing is used for the heavier lifting activities, or axillary pressure cannot be tolerated.

The posterior strap on the prosthetic side attaches to the control cable. For heavier lifting activities or when axillary pressure from a figure-of-8 harness is unacceptable, a shoulder saddle with chest strap system is a useful alternative suspension system. A leather or flexible plastic saddle is positioned over the prosthetic side shoulder and is secured using a chest strap that wraps around the intact chest wall in an infra-axillary location. The suspension of the prosthesis occurs through an inverted U-shaped cable or strap that is anchored to the top of the saddle and drapes downward to attach to the front and back of the prosthetic socket (transhumeral) or triceps pad (transradial). The control cable attaches to the posterior aspect of the chest strap.

Self-suspending socket designs are used when the bony configuration of the residual limb allows suspension, similar to the effect used in Syme amputations. Self-suspending sockets are largely limited to wrist and elbow disarticulations. In both harness and self-suspending systems, socks can be worn to optimize fit and improve comfort.

Suction suspension sockets are similar to those available to the individual with an LE amputation and use either a total contact socket with a one-way air valve or a roll-on gel liner with a locking pin. Suction sockets are appropriate primarily for the transhumeral residual limb with good soft tissue envelope, an absence of invaginated scarring, and a stable volume. Donning the suction socket with air valve involves the use of water-based lubricants or a pull sock to seat the residual limb into the socket. The one-way air valve creates suction inside of the socket, maintaining suspension. When using a gel liner with a distal attachment pin, the sleeve is rolled onto the residual limb and inserted into the socket where the pin mates with a locking mechanism. Suspension is accomplished through a combination of suction and skin friction.

Control Cable Mechanism

Body-powered prosthetic limbs use cables to link movements of the shoulder and humerus to activation of the terminal device and elbow. The movements that are captured for control include scapular abduction, shoulder depression and abduction, and humeral flexion. Control cables used to activate a single prosthetic component such as the terminal device are known as single control cables or Bowden cables. Dual control cable systems use the same cable to control two prosthetic functions, typically elbow flexion and terminal device opening in the transhumeral prosthesis. The control cable is attached to the figure-of-8 or chest strap harness used for suspension of the prosthesis. When a body-powered prosthesis incorporates a self-suspending socket design or suction suspension, a simple figure-of-8 or figure-of-9 harness strap system is still required to allow control functions to be performed.

Terminal Device

Terminal devices for body-powered prostheses can be hooks, functional or active hands, cosmetic or passive hands, or special terminal devices designed for specific activities (e.g., bowling ball terminal device, golf club holder). Hook-style terminal devices provide the equivalent of a lateral pinch grip, while active hand terminal devices provide a three-point chuck action (47). The most commonly used active terminal device is the voluntary-opening hook. While different

voluntary-opening hook designs are available for various applications, the most commonly prescribed design for general use is the Dorrance 5X, 5XA, and 7 (Hosmer Dorrance, Campbell, CA) (**Fig. 56-15**). With voluntary-opening devices, the individual with a UE amputation provides power through a cabling system to open the terminal device and relies on springs or rubber bands to provide the closing prehensile force. Typical closing forces range from 5 to 10 lb. Voluntary-opening active hands are available and in general are more cosmetic, but are heavier, interfere with visualizing the object being grasped, and provide lower prehensile forces. Voluntary-closing terminal devices allow the individual to provide a variable prehensile force transmitted through the control cable to the terminal device. Voluntary closing devices are capable of providing larger prehensile forces up to 20 to 25 lb (9 to 11 kg) and provide indirect sensory feedback through the force exerted on the control cable. A significant disadvantage of voluntary-closing devices is the need for a constant pull on the control cable during prolonged grasping, a skill that is difficult to accomplish during dynamic tasks. Passive

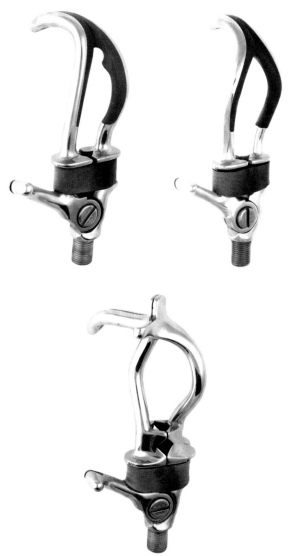

FIGURE 56-15. Most common terminal devices. (Images courtesy of Fillauer Companies.)

(cosmetic) hands are lighter than active hands and can be passively positioned. A passive hand does not provide grasp but can be useful for holding, lifting, pushing, or pulling. A cosmetic glove tinted to approximate the individual's skin color covers both functional and passive hands.

Wrist Unit

Wrist units provide a receptacle for connecting the terminal device to the prosthesis and permit prepositioning of the terminal device for functional activities (i.e., rotation for all units and flexion if the appropriate unit is used). Wrist rotation is performed using the intact hand or by pushing the terminal device against a firm surface and is held in place with either friction or a mechanical lock. Friction control wrist units are easily positioned but can slip when lifting heavier loads. A locking wrist unit enhances the use of the terminal device with heavier objects or where leverage with the terminal device is important for function. A wrist flexion unit allows the terminal device to be positioned in flexion, enhancing the ability to perform activities close to the body, a feature that is important for the individual with a bilateral UE amputation. A quick disconnect option permits the easy interchange of different terminal devices, such as a hook for a hand.

Additional details regarding components, sockets, suspension, and control systems are discussed where appropriate in the following sections relating to specific levels of amputation.

Prostheses by Level of Amputation

Partial Hand

For partial hand amputations (e.g., phalanges, ray resections, transmetacarpal), a prosthesis may not be necessary if the remaining hand has functional grasp. To be functionally useful, the residual hand needs to be able to provide a rudimentary grasp. This requires two opposing posts that can be moved into contact with each other to provide a prehensile force. When possible, surgical reconstruction of the remaining hand is often the preferred approach to preserving or enhancing function while maintaining sensation. When only one movable digit remains, as in a transmetacarpal amputation of digits 2 through 5, either an open or mitt-shaped prosthetic opposition post can be used to provide a stable surface for opposition with the thumb. In general, the substantial variability in the anatomy of the remaining partial hand requires creative custom solutions to optimize function (**Fig. 56-16**). At times, an individual with a UE amputation may require devices customized for specific activities. A cosmetic prosthesis is frequently provided for this level of amputation. Long-term usage varies, but the majority of individuals continue to wear them at least occasionally for social situations (47).

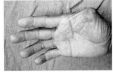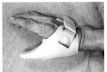

FIGURE 56-16. Thumb prosthesis set in position to allow for grasping and object manipulation.

Transradial Amputation/Wrist Disarticulation

The length of the bony forearm, measured from the medial epicondyle, classifies transradial amputations as very short (<35%), short (35% to 55%), and long (55% to 90%). Longer residual limb length enhances the forearm lever, making lifting easier, and allows capturing residual pronation-supination motion of the forearm. Long transradial residual limbs retain from 60 to 120 degrees of supination-pronation, which decreases to less than 60 degrees in short transradial residual limbs. For short and long transradial amputations, a dual-wall socket is attached to a triceps pad with flexible elbow hinges (straps) to allow pronation-supination. The triceps pad helps to distribute suspension forces and is needed to anchor the control cable. Most commonly, a figure-of-8 harness system is used for suspension and control. For very short transradial amputation levels, rigid hinges are generally used to provide greater stability of the socket on the residual limb. With transradial amputations, in which range of motion is limited at the elbow, polycentric elbow joints or a split socket with step-up hinges can be used to provide additional flexion. The additional flexion gained with the use of these elbow hinges is offset by a loss of elbow flexion power and lifting ability.

The wrist disarticulation (WD) prosthesis is a variant of the transradial prosthesis. Because WD spares the distal radial-ulnar joint, most forearm supination-pronation is preserved. Socket designs for the WD level are flattened distally to form an oval to capture supination-pronation, allowing active rotational positioning of the terminal device during activities. The distal flare of the residual limb can be taken advantage of to fabricate a self-suspending socket, but this usually leads to a bulbous, cosmetically compromised appearance similar to that occurring in the LE Syme amputation. The long residual limb necessitates the use of a special thin wrist unit to minimize the overall length of the prosthesis. If cosmesis is of primary importance to the patient, a long transradial amputation may be a more appropriate amputation level.

An example for the prescription of a transradial/WD limb could read as follows: *dual-wall total contact socket, flexible elbow hinges, triceps pad, figure-of-8 harness, single control cable, constant friction wrist unit with quick disconnect, 5XA hook, and cosmetic hand.*

Transhumeral Amputation/Elbow Disarticulation

The length of the residual humerus measured from the acromion classifies the THA as humeral neck (<30%), short transhumeral (30% to 50%), standard transhumeral (50% to 90%), and elbow disarticulation (90% to 100%). For short and standard transhumeral residual limb lengths, the traditional dual-wall socket extends to just below the acromion and attaches to either a figure-of-8 or a shoulder saddle and chest strap harness for suspension. With shorter residual limbs, securing the socket to the residual, especially under load, is more difficult. To accommodate this problem, the socket extends proximal and medial to the acromion, creating a partial shoulder cap. This socket design often can be suspended with only a chest strap, but other harness systems can be used for additional security or to improve control functions. However, with the shoulder cap socket, humeral abduction will be limited. Suction socket suspension systems are becoming the preferred system for individuals with a THA because of the improved suspension and greater ability to position the limb for activities. Even when suction suspension systems are used, an axillary harness is needed for control and can augment suspension, especially when lifting larger loads. Suction suspension, when used with externally powered myoelectric components, can result in a self-suspending prosthesis free of any harness.

The standard elbow component for the transhumeral prosthesis is the internal elbow joint. Internal elbow units allow for 135 degrees of flexion and can be manually locked into a number of preset flexed positions. The standard internal elbow unit incorporates a turntable that allows passive internal or external rotation of the forearm. Elbow spring-lift assist units are available and are generally recommended for internal elbow units to help counterbalance the weight of the forearm, making elbow flexion easier for the individual with an amputation. This unit requires approximately 5 cm of length. If the level of amputation is less than 2 in (5 cm) proximal to the epicondyles, then an internal elbow unit cannot be used unless an asymmetric elbow position compared to the intact limb is cosmetically acceptable. When the internal elbow unit cannot be used, locking external elbow joints are available but these are less cosmetic.

The control system for the transhumeral prosthesis uses two cables: a dual control cable that controls the elbow and terminal device and a secondary elbow locking cable. To control the prosthetic limb, the individual with an amputation uses scapular protraction and humeral flexion to flex the elbow into the desired position. The elbow is locked using the secondary control cable. Once locked, the same shoulder movements that powered the elbow are now available to activate the terminal device. Locking the elbow is typically accomplished by using a control cable that is routed along the anterior aspect of the socket and attaches to the front of the harness. Shoulder depression, humeral extension, or abduction movements are used to lock-unlock the elbow.

An elbow disarticulation prosthesis is a variant of the transhumeral prosthesis. The socket is flat and broad distally to conform to the anatomic configuration of the epicondyles of the distal humerus. This design provides some self-suspension and allows the individual with an amputation active rotation of the prosthesis (internal and external rotation of the humerus). The length of the residual limb requires the use of external elbow joints and a cable-operated locking mechanism. The harness is either a figure-of-8 or a shoulder saddle and chest strap. The control system for this level is the same as for the individual with a more proximal THA.

Example prescription for a short transhumeral prosthetic limb read as follows: *flexible wall/rigid frame suction socket, figure-of-8 axillary suspension and control harness, dual control cable, internal locking elbow with turntable and flexion assist, lightweight forearm shell, constant friction wrist unit with quick disconnect, 5XA hook, and cosmetic hand.*

Shoulder Disarticulation/Forequarter Amputation

For shoulder disarticulation and forequarter amputation, the socket extends onto the thorax to suspend and stabilize the prosthesis. The portion of the thorax covered by the socket is more extensive for the forequarter amputation. In some cases, an open frame socket rather than a plastic-laminated socket is chosen for these levels to reduce prosthetic weight and to minimize heat buildup by reducing the amount of skin coverage.

Prosthetic components are similar to those for the transhumeral prosthesis with the addition of a shoulder unit, which allows passive positioning of the shoulder joint in flexion-extension and abduction-adduction. Chest straps are attached to the anterior and posterior socket for suspension. The loss of ipsilateral shoulder motion for control purposes severely compromises the use of the prosthesis. A harness and control cable system that uses three individual cables can be used. Individual cables use intact side humeral flexion for prosthetic elbow control, chest expansion for terminal device control, and a manual nudge or pull cable for elbow locking. The body-powered prosthesis is cumbersome to don, has limited functionality, and is often used mainly for cosmesis. The difficulty in providing suitable body-powered prostheses at these proximal amputation levels argues against their routine use. For many individuals, a cosmetic limb is sufficient. For the highly motivated individual, externally powered prostheses may be more functional and hence can be considered.

Externally Powered Prostheses

Externally powered prosthetic limbs use small electric motors incorporated into the prosthetic component to control its function. Reliable external power units are available for terminal device operation, wrist rotation, and elbow flexion-extension. Myoelectric signals or switches control these electric motors. It is often difficult to predict the preferred type of power for the prosthetic limb for a particular individual until trial use of both has occurred. Compared to body-powered prostheses, external-powered prostheses are typically heavier, more costly, and less durable, especially if manual labor activities are frequently performed. Important advantages of external-powered prostheses compared to body-powered devices include improved comfort due to the reduced harness needs, better control, and lifting capacity for short transhumeral and shoulder disarticulation amputation levels, and the greater terminal device grip force of electric hooks and hands. In the case of the transradial level amputation, the prosthesis can use a self-suspending socket that eliminates the need for a harness (**Fig. 56-17**).

The preferred control system for external-powered prostheses is myoelectrical control. Myoelectrical control uses surface electrodes embedded in the prosthetic socket that make contact with the skin and detect muscle action potentials from voluntarily contracting muscles in the residual limb. The myoelectric signal controls an electric motor to provide a function (e.g., terminal device operation, wrist rotation, elbow flexion).

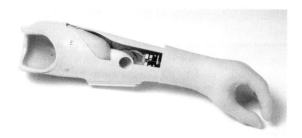

FIGURE 56-17. Otto Bock self-suspending transradial myo-prosthesis and the internal placement of the electronic components. (Courtesy of Otto Bock, see Web site listing.)

Prior to the prescription and fitting of a myoelectric prosthesis, the individual's ability to reliably contract and relax at least one muscle group in the residual limb should be ascertained. This can be accomplished using electromyographic biofeedback equipment or a myoelectric tester to identify the most appropriate electrode control location(s). Several different types of myoelectric controllers are available depending on the number of prosthetic functions that need to be controlled and the number of useful electrode sites identified. The dual-electrode system uses two sets of electrodes positioned over antagonist muscles allowing natural and intuitive myoelectric control to occur. For example, at the transradial level, activation of the forearm flexor muscles closes the terminal device while activation of the forearm extensors opens the terminal device. Most contemporary myoelectric control systems use proportional control so that the speed or strength of terminal device activation varies with the intensity of muscle contraction. When there are an inadequate number of usable electrode sites available to control all desired functions of the prosthesis, alternative control strategies can be used. Single site controllers use the strength of voluntary contraction from a single electrode (i.e., amplitude of the myoelectric signal) to control the motion (i.e., a weak contraction will close the terminal device and a strong contraction will open the terminal device) (48). Sequential or multistate controllers use the same electrode pair to control several functions (e.g., terminal device control and elbow activation). This type of controller uses a brief co-contraction to switch between control modes. Therefore, two myoelectric sites in the transhumeral amputee (biceps, triceps) can be used to control the terminal device open/close and elbow flex/extend. Any of the alternative control schemes take longer to learn and are not consistently mastered by all individuals with an amputation.

Proximal upper limb amputation (short transhumeral, shoulder disarticulation, and forequarter) may leave few choices for available muscle sites for myoelectric control. Targeted muscle reinnervation (TMR) is a surgical procedure to move peripheral nerves in the shoulder or residual limb that no longer have a target muscle, and implanting the nerve endings into a remaining muscle, such as the pectoralis. Once the nerve establishes a myoneural junction, then contraction of that muscle segment can become a new potential myoelectric site for prosthetic control. There can be multiple myoelectric sites in a large segmented muscle like the pectoralis. The surgical procedure is complex and the time to new muscle activation may be many months, thereby delaying prosthetic fitting. This surgical alternative currently remains best suited for the patient with bilateral proximal amputations when traditional prosthetic fitting provides little or no function.

When myoelectric control is not available or there are not enough electrode sites available, switches incorporated into the prosthetic socket or the harness can be used to implement or augment the control of various components. Simple on-off switches can be used to implement basic control of a powered component. More sophisticated servo control techniques based on position or force switches in the harness systems can be used to provide proportional control (49).

Myoelectric prosthetic components are available and sized to fit a wide range of people, from infants to adults. Most myoelectric terminal devices are hands, but electric hook and robotic designs are also available. Myoelectrically controlled prostheses can and have been fit immediately after surgery (50), but it is generally recommended that fitting be delayed until the residual limb is healed and the limb volume has stabilized. A stable limb volume is needed to ensure a consistent socket fit and reproducible electrode position and skin contact. Myoelectric components have been combined with body-powered components to result in a hybrid prosthesis, which may provide better function for some individuals with an amputation than either myoelectric or body-powered control used alone.

The newest generation of myoelectric hands provides multiple grasping modes, which are selected by the patient. Twenty or more options (such as gross grasp, tip pinch, three jaw chuck, lateral key pinch, point, peck) are available, but typically only three to four modes can be active at one time. The patient selects the mode by activating a special sequence of myoelectric signals in the residual limb or by scrolling through a menu on a smartphone. Individual finger control is not currently available but may be available in the next generation of "smart hands."

Cosmetic Prosthesis

A conventional body-powered or myoelectric prosthesis with a hand terminal device supplies adequate cosmesis for many individuals with a UE amputation. Using custom covers that are color and texture matched to the skin of the intact side can enhance cosmesis. These covers are expensive and have a limited life expectancy if used during functional activities. When an individual with an amputation is not a candidate for an active prosthetic limb, a cosmetic prosthetic can be fabricated using lightweight components that can be passively positioned to create a symmetric body image while wearing clothing.

Three-Dimensional Printing

The incorporation of 3-D printing in the fabrication of upper limb prosthetic sockets and components is gaining popularity but still has significant limitations. The 3-D printing process for a custom socket requires an electronic file from a digital scan of the residual limb, which is then modified by the prosthetist before it is sent to the 3-D printer. The 3-D printer uses these electronic instructions to fabricate the socket to a specified size and thickness, using a specified material (typically plastics). The primary advantage of 3-D printing is the ability to duplicate the same socket, or similar socket with minor modifications, quickly and easily. The cost of a 3-D printer depends on the size of the item being fabricated. The main disadvantage of 3-D printing of sockets is still the need for an experienced prosthetist or technician to capture the digital scan and modify the file. Each patient will need their unique electronic file to create their socket.

The use of 3-D printing for an entire cosmetic prosthesis may have some value, but now the electronic file must include digital information about the portion of the limb that is absent. Therefore, a digital scan of the remaining limb contralateral limb will be needed to define the shape of the prosthesis. Sometimes, a standard "model hand" file can be used for the hand based on measurements.

Three-dimensional printing is less useful for most lower limb prosthetic applications because it cannot fabricate functional knees or feet to the same standard as currently available commercially. Some simple joints or components, particularly in the pediatric population, can be fabricated quickly and easily using a standard open source file from the internet, but the durability and quality remains to be proven. Three-dimensional printing of upper limb prosthetics and orthotics in the pediatric population may have more application because the durability can be less, and the replacement rate is more frequent due to growth.

SPECIAL ISSUES IN THE CARE OF INDIVIDUALS WITH AN AMPUTATION

Pain

Pain is a common problem following amputation. Identifying the etiology of a pain complaint is often challenging because of the limited ability to examine the residual limb during prosthetic use and overlapping symptoms from different pain sources. The initial decision required in addressing pain complaints is to differentiate phantom limb pain from residual limb pain.

Phantom Limb Sensation/Pain

Phantom sensation, defined as the awareness of a nonpainful sensation in the amputated part of the limb, occurs in nearly all acquired amputations (51–53). Phantom sensation is most prominent immediately after amputation and generally diminishes over time, often in a telescoping fashion. The most vivid sensations are typically in the distal portion of the limb. Generally, phantom limb sensations that persist do not require treatment. An occasional problem with phantom sensation occurs when individuals are confused by the phantom sensation and attempt to walk without using a prosthesis.

Phantom pain is pain perceived in the amputated portion of the extremity. The incidence of phantom pain has been difficult to determine with reported frequency ranging from 4% to 80% (37,52,53). Like phantom sensation, phantom pain is most common immediately after amputation and usually becomes less frequent, less intense, and shorter in duration over time. Persistent phantom pain requiring treatment occurs in approximately 5% of individuals with an amputation. Phantom pain is often described as burning, cramping, stabbing, or squeezing but is sometimes reported as bizarre contortions of the limb. The pain may be generalized, but more commonly, it is experienced mainly in the distal parts of the missing limb. The cause and underlying physiology of phantom pain remain poorly understood, but the incidence of phantom pain has been associated with the presence of preamputation pain, phantom sensation, and residual limb pain. The correlation between preamputation pain and the subsequent development of phantom pain has led to attempts at preventing phantom pain by controlling periamputation limb pain with continuous epidural or peripheral nerve anesthesia. These attempts have shown mixed effectiveness (53). Once established, the successful treatment of phantom pain can be difficult and many therapeutic modalities have been tried (37,54–57). Although convincing evidence-based algorithms for the treatment of phantom pain do not exist, empiric clinical guidelines are frequently used. Medication is usually the first line of treatment employing tricyclic antidepressants

(amitriptyline) and anticonvulsants (e.g., carbamazepine, gabapentin, pregabalin), either alone or in combination. Other drugs that have been used with some success include mexiletine, calcitonin, N-methyl-D-aspartate (NMDA) receptor antagonists (ketamine, dextromethorphan, tramadol), and opioids. Evaluation and correction of any coexisting residual limb pain or prosthetic fit problems is also an important component of the initial management of phantom pain. Range of motion exercises, relaxation exercises, residual limb massage, transcutaneous electrical nerve stimulation (TENS), compressive stocking, and encouraging prosthesis use have little risk and may be useful adjuncts to medical management. Since problematic phantom pain often occurs only intermittently and is typically short lived, the patient's participation in decision-making is essential to weigh possible benefits of drug trials with the inconvenience and possible side effects of medications that need to be taken on a regular, continuous basis. Surgical treatments have not been shown to provide lasting pain relief and are rarely used.

Residual Limb Pain

In contrast to phantom limb pain, residual limb pain is the pain perceived as originating in and affecting the residual portion of the limb. Persistent residual limb pain occurs in up to 70% of individuals with lower limb amputation with about half reporting the pain as moderately to severely bothersome (52–55). Residual limb pain is commonly described as aching, sharp, throbbing, and burning in character. The underlying causes of residual limb pain can be classified as intrinsic or extrinsic.

Intrinsic residual limb pain is caused by changes or complications in the underlying neurovascular, bony, or soft tissues of the residual limb. Neuromas develop in all residual limbs after amputation but may only become problematic when entrapped in scar or positioned such that they are exposed to external mechanical loading. Diagnosing an underlying neuroma as the cause of pain can be difficult. When present, neuropathic symptoms including typical dysesthetic pain descriptors, radiation of pain in a specific nerve distribution, and the presence of pain when not using a prosthesis are helpful diagnostic aids, but at times, the pain location and description is nonspecific. Neuroma-related pain may be precipitated by tapping (Tinel's sign), direct compression from manual palpation or socket pressure, or traction on an adherent scarred nerve. Larger neuromas can be imaged with magnetic resonance imaging (58). When prosthetic use exacerbates neuroma pain, initial treatment interventions should include prosthetic modifications that attempt to reduce loading of pressure-sensitive areas. Useful approaches include the use of gel socks or liners to better distribute loads and to reduce shearing of adherent tissues, flexible sockets, or socket modification to relieve sensitive areas. Infiltration of the perineuromal region with local anesthetics combined with steroids can be a useful diagnostic and therapeutic procedure. If the injection relieves the pain, a series of similar injections over several months can be attempted to try to achieve lasting relief. When neuroma pain persists and limits function, surgery to resect and move the neuroma to a more protected location can often be helpful. However, following neuroma resection, the neuroma will reform and, on occasion, again become symptomatic.

Bony overgrowth from the distal end of the residual limb skeletal elements occasionally occurs in adults but is primarily a problem that occurs in children with an amputation. Heterotopic bone can form in the soft tissues of the residual limb and may follow trauma, hematoma, or fracture of the residual limb. Poorly contoured bone edges following surgery can lead to regions of high-pressure concentration. In any of these situations, the abnormal bone leads to localized tissue compression, pain, and tenderness that can progress to the development of adventitial bursa or soft tissue ulceration. Diagnosis is made with plain radiographs of the residual limb. Management is focused on prosthetic socket modifications to offload painful areas, but achieving a lasting comfortable fit can be difficult. Imaging the residual limb while weight bearing in the socket may provide greater insight to the limb/socket pressures. When prosthetic approaches fail, surgical revision is typically needed.

Osteomyelitis, tumor recurrence, stress fractures, and persistent limb ischemia also may occur in patients after amputation. These may cause more generalized residual limb pain and require medical and surgical management.

Extrinsic residual limb pain is caused by a mismatch between residual limb tissue tolerance and prosthetic loads imposed on the soft tissues. Poor socket fit and limb malalignment are the main causes. The coexistence of a compromised residual limb from intrinsic pathology reduces the safety margin between tissue tolerance and prosthetic socket loads, making it more difficult to achieve and maintain a comfortable fit. The ability to attain a comfortable socket fit is one of the most important aspects of prosthetic acceptance and function. Most contemporary prosthetic sockets are designed for total contact with modifications to the socket shape to preferentially load weight tolerance tissues. Socket fit is inevitably compromised with body weight changes or residual limb soft tissue atrophy over time. Clinical manifestations of poor fit or excessive local tissue loading include a gradual onset of pain while using a previously comfortable prosthesis, erythema persisting more than 15 to 20 minutes after wearing the limb, or the development of blisters, bursas, calluses, or skin ulceration. Changing the number of sock plies, adding pads to the socket, relieving high-pressure areas, or substituting a gel liner for socks can often restore a comfortable fit and prolong the useful life of a socket. When minor modifications fail, a replacement socket will need to be fabricated.

Malalignment of lower limb prostheses can create abnormally high or prolonged loading forces in the residual limb leading to pain even when the socket fit is acceptable. In the individual with a transtibial amputation, sagittal plane alignment problems most commonly affect the distal tibia region while frontal plane malalignment primarily affects loading forces along the fibula. In the individual with a transfemoral amputation, distal femur pain is often seen with alignment problems or with poor ischial capture allowing femoral abduction.

Choke Syndrome

A specific socket fit problem, almost exclusively seen in the individual with an LE amputation, is the choke syndrome. A choke syndrome develops when there is a simultaneous impairment of venous return from a prosthetic socket that is too tight proximally and a lack of total contact between the distal

residual limb and the socket. Edema develops in the residual limb where total contact is lost. Most commonly, this occurs in the distal aspect of the transtibial residual limb as atrophy takes place over time and additional socks are used to fill in for the loss of soft tissue volume. Because there is no corresponding volume change in the proximal bony aspect of the limb, the fit becomes too tight and constricts the venous return. Initially, a circumscribed indurated region develops while wearing the prosthesis. If significant edema develops acutely, there can be associated weeping or blistering of the skin. The area of choke is tender to palpation and is prone to developing cellulitis. As the choke syndrome becomes chronic, the tissues become increasingly thickened and indurated, verrucous hyperplasia develops, and skin becomes hyperpigmented because of hemosiderin deposition. Choke syndromes are treated by relieving the proximal constriction and restoring total contact between the residual limb and the socket (57,59). When the choke syndrome is mild, reducing the number of socks to decrease proximal residual limb constriction and adding or modifying the distal end pad may be adequate but typically a new total contact socket is needed.

Dermatologic Disorders

Dermatologic problems are common, particularly in the individual with an LE amputation, with surveys estimating that 30% to 50% of individuals with amputations experience one or more skin problems because of a prosthesis (58–61). Dermatologic complaints can be classified as related to hyperhidrosis, physical effects of prosthetic use, contact dermatitis, and infection.

Hyperhidrosis, while not indicative of underlying disease, is one of the most common skin-related complaints and has become more common with the introduction of silicone liners in the 1990s. An increase in sweating is reported by about half of the patients with the use of gel liners. Over several weeks, adaptation typically occurs and excessive sweating often resolves. Persistent hyperhidrosis makes it more difficult to maintain hygiene, increases the likelihood of skin maceration, and may contribute to the development of contact dermatitis (59–62). When using suction sockets, suspension effectiveness can be compromised. Problematic sweating can be controlled by using concentrated antiperspirants, such as Drysol (Person & Covey, Glendale, CA), on the residual limb or by changing to a liner system that allows the individual with an amputation to wear socks directly against the skin. A silver-impregnated sock under the gel liner may also control perspiration without abandoning the socket.

The skin of the residual limb is subjected to repeated shear, frictional, and loading forces. The physical effects of these repetitive loads can lead to keratin plugging of sebaceous glands and follicular hyperkeratosis, leading to the development of epidermoid cysts, folliculitis, and dermal granulomas. Cysts are frequently very tender and can spontaneously break open or become secondarily infected. Commonly affected areas are those that are subjected to high loading and shearing forces such as the groin region in the individual with a transfemoral amputation and the medial tibial flare and popliteal fossa in the individual with a transtibial amputation. Treatment is directed at local skin care as well as prosthetic modifications to reduce mechanical skin forces. Meticulous hygiene needs to be encouraged to keep skin, socks, and liner clean. Cosmetic or acne scrub pads can be used to help keep skin pores open. Warm compresses to promote drainage and oral antibiotics are useful in managing folliculitis and infected cysts. Larger and more persistent sebaceous cysts may require surgical drainage or excision. Concurrent with medical management, a review of prosthetic fit and alignment to ensure that loading of the affected region is optimized should be undertaken. Recurring problems can be helped with the use of prosthetic components that reduce residual limb shear and loading forces. These include gel liners, rotators, VSPs, and multiaxis ankle/foot devices.

Allergic or contact dermatitis accounts for approximately 20% of prosthetic-related dermatoses (60). Clinical symptoms range from mild lichenification or scaling to weeping eczema. A wide variety of offending agents has been identified. Detergents, scented emollients, creams, and talcs used for skin care should be considered as possible allergens and discontinued or changed. The use of gel sheaths and liners may result in contact dermatitis. The exact allergen is difficult to identify and is probably residual soap used in cleaning or chemical additives used in liner manufacturing rather than the hypoallergenic silicone material itself. If continued use of gel-type liners is needed, it is reasonable to switch to a different manufacturer or change to a different liner base material (e.g., silicone to urethane) to empirically attempt to resolve the rash. Neoprene, resins used in socket fabrication, and dyes and tanning agents used in leather are also potential allergens. If empiric trials of different materials cannot identify the allergen, patch testing for 24 to 48 hours with a small piece of the suspected material on the forearm may be helpful.

The use of gel sheaths, liners, and suspension sleeves can create a moist warm environment that may contribute to contact dermatitis, bacterial, and fungal skin infections. Attention to proper skin care and liner cleansing can minimize skin disorders. At times, wearing natural fiber socks or a nylon sheath between the liner and residual limb can absorb or wick away moisture and reduce skin problems. Removal of the prosthesis at midday to clean and dry the skin may also help.

Osseous Integration or Direct Skeletal Attachment

Many of the complications encountered with prosthetic fitting are related to fitting of the socket. In both upper and lower limb prosthetic fitting, the socket is attempting to capture the movement of the bony elements of the residual limb to control the prosthesis. However, the forces and movements of the bony elements are transmitted through the soft tissue elements of the residual limb (skin, subcutaneous tissue, muscle) to the socket. The pressure and sheer force on the soft tissue elements can result in pain and injury. The ideal connection of bony elements to the prosthesis would be direct skeletal attachment, essentially bypassing the soft tissue. Mechanical prosthetic implants into the bony elements of the residual limb have been proposed and attempted in animal and human subjects for three decades. There are four designs of mechanical implant that have been used at centers around the world with variable results. The common concern and complication is infection at the site where the mechanical implant exits the skin to attach to the prosthetic components. The frequency of

superficial infection is quite high (up to 50% of subjects), and deeper infection is frequent enough (up to 10%) to make this procedure unacceptable to most surgeons and patients. There is also a significant delay in prosthetic fitting (3 to 12 months), which also presents a new set of complications including deconditioning, joint contractures, and falls while the implant heals and matures. The surgical procedure has only been FDA approved on a limited basis in the United States since 2016, with several clinical trials underway at present. If the surgical procedure can be further refined, and the infection rate significantly reduced, then direct skeletal attachment of prosthetic devices will become the standard of care in the future.

Pediatric Limb Deficiency or Amputation

When amputations are performed in children for disease, tumor, trauma, or congenital skeletal deficiency for prosthetic fitting, a disarticulation level amputation is preferred rather than an amputation through a long bone when the resulting level of function with a prosthesis will be similar. Approximately 12% of children with acquired amputations experience a condition known as bony overgrowth. Bony overgrowth is the appositional deposition of bone at the end of the amputated long bone. This bone growth results in a spike-like formation at the end of the bone that has a thin cortex and no medullary canal. The bone frequently grows faster than the overlying skin and soft tissues; a bursa may develop over the sharp end, or the bone actually may protrude through the skin with subsequent development of cellulitis and osteomyelitis. Overgrowth is seen (in decreasing frequency) most frequently in the humerus, fibula, tibia, and femur. It has been reported in the congenital limb deficiencies but rarely. Several treatment approaches have been advocated for the management of this problem. Success is limited, but the technique proposed by Marquardt in which the distal end of the bone is capped with a cartilage epiphysis is the best of the surgical options available to manage this problem (63).

For the child with a congenital skeletal deficiency, the initial prosthesis for the UE usually is fitted when the child has attained independent sitting balance or at approximately 6 months of age (64–67) (**Table 56-4**). For the LE, the initial prosthesis is fitted when the child begins to pull to a stand, which generally is between 9 and 14 months. Young children and infants usually learn to use their prostheses by incorporating them as part of play activities rather than through specific exercises. Prosthetic training periods for children may last only for several minutes at a time because of limited attention span, and they may require much longer periods of free play interspersed between actual training sessions. It is important that parents be instructed in techniques to help their children attain the necessary prosthetic skills because much of the training in the use of the prosthesis will occur in the home rather than in the clinic. It is also important to understand when working with children who have a limb deficiency or amputation of the UE that the prosthesis becomes an aid rather than a replacement (**Table 56-5**). If the child cannot habilitate to the prosthesis, then it will be discarded.

The age at which to fit children with a myoelectric prosthesis is a controversial and complex issue beyond the scope of this chapter. This subject is reviewed in detail elsewhere (64,65,70,71).

TABLE 56-4	**Guidelines for Pediatric Prosthetic Fitting**		
Amputation Level	**Age for Prosthetic Fitting**	**Developmental Milestones**	**Prosthetic Prescription**
Transradial	6–7 mo	Sitting balance, reaches across mid-line for bimanual object manipulation	Body powered—passive mitt, self-suspending socket
	9–15 mo		Externally powered for greater grip strength, single control site (voluntary opening, auto close)
	24–36 mo		Change to two site control for voluntary opening and closing
Transhumeral	6–7 mo	Same as for transradial	Body powered—passive mitt and elbow, activate elbow at 18 mo
	24–48 mo		Externally powered terminal device, when terminal device control mastered, activate the elbow
Transtibial	9–12 mo	Child pulls to stand	PTB, supracondylar strap
Transfemoral	9–12 mo	Child pulls to stand	ICS, belt suspension, no knee unit until ages 3–4

TABLE 56-5	**Comparison of Children Versus Adults with an Amputation (63,67–69)**	
General		
Dynamic (growing)	vs.	Adynamic (decelerates—aging)
Dependent	vs.	Independent
Untrained (life disciplines)	vs.	Trained
Irresponsible	vs.	Responsible
Malleable	vs.	Less malleable
Physical		
Growing	vs.	Static
Immature	vs.	Mature
Longitudinal growth	vs.	Nonlongitudinal growth
Circumferential growth	vs.	Circumferential growth (dietary)
Circulation and tissue tolerance are ideal	vs.	Circulation and tolerance vary with age and health
	Influences surgical indications, site of amputation, and goals of training	
Social		
Member of family group	vs.	Independent person
Few independent social responsibilities	vs.	Variable responsibilities; depends on age, marriage, parenthood, etc.
Adjustment relatively easy	vs.	Adjustment less easy because of fixed social environment
Economic		
By family	vs.	By patient
Not self-supporting	vs.	Self-supporting or at least contributes to the economic welfare of the family
Amputation not of economic importance	vs.	Amputation may interfere with established economic status
Education		
Process of obtaining basic education	vs.	Usually completed
Advanced education can be planned to include handicap and its limitation and needs	vs.	Age often makes long reeducation and training difficult, if not impossible
Vocational		
Not selected or established	vs.	Established
Oriented around handicap	vs.	Must reorient vocationally because of handicap
Psychological		
Because of immaturity of development, may not have the profound changes sometimes seen in the adult. Usually reflects family (parental) reaction to the amputation or deformity. In general, is not a great problem in a stable family situation	vs.	Great variation. All the way from profound psychoneurosis to mature, reasonable acceptance of the disability. The impact of the amputation on the socioeconomic areas of the patient's existence are generally profound

PROSTHETIC PRESCRIPTION EXAMPLE CASES

The prosthetic prescriptions presented for these cases are as examples only. They do not represent the standard or typical prosthetic prescriptions for these levels of amputation. We want to be clear that a specific prosthetic prescription must be tailored to meet the specific needs of an individual with an amputation. The examples presented here serve to highlight the decision process that might be followed to arrive at an appropriate prosthetic prescription.

Case 74-1: Transradial Amputation

A 24-year-old, right-handed man sustains a work-related crush injury to his right hand, resulting in a long transradial level of amputation. He plans to return to work operating a drill press.
   Possible prosthetic prescriptions include the following:
- Body power prosthesis with double wall plastic laminate socket, quick-change locking wrist unit, no. 7 (heavy duty, "Farmer's hook") voluntary opening terminal device, flexible elbow hinges, triceps pad, figure-of-8 harness for suspension, and Bowden single control cable
- External power prosthesis with double-wall plastic laminate socket with self-suspending design and Otto Bock Greifer (myoelectric hook) terminal device

In this person, body power will be lightest in weight, most durable, and least expensive. If more than 6 to 7 lb (2.7 to 3.2 kg) of pinch force is necessary from the terminal device for functional activities, then a voluntary closing hook may be needed. The Greifer will provide up to 35 lb of pinch force.

Case 74-2: Transhumeral Amputation

A 35-year-old, right-handed female homemaker sustains a short transhumeral level of amputation following a motor vehicle accident. Possible prosthetic prescriptions include the following:
- Body power prosthesis with double-wall plastic laminate socket, constant friction wrist unit, no. 5XA (lightest weight) terminal device and a mechanical hand, internal, alternating locking elbow with turntable, figure-of-8 harness, and Bowden double control cable
- External power prosthesis with double-wall plastic laminate socket, myoelectric hand, myoelectric elbow, and figure-of-8 harness

In this woman, because of the short residual limb, external power may be more comfortable and functional but will be heavier and much more expensive than body power.

Case 74-3: Transtibial Amputation

A 72-year-old-retired man with type II diabetes and PVD has a transtibial amputation for an infected nonhealing ulcer and gangrenous foot. Use the Medicare functional level guidelines to help determine the foot selection. Possible prosthetic prescriptions include the following:
- Provisional prosthesis with total contact PTB thermoplastic socket, foam liner (soft insert), neoprene sleeve suspension, lightweight alignable shank, and SACH or single axis foot
- Definitive prosthesis with endoskeletal design, total contact laminated PTB socket, gel liner with pin suspension, and lightweight multiaxial foot

The provisional prosthesis is a lightweight design that provides a stable support base on which to learn to walk with a prosthesis. The soft liner will make modifications for changes in residual limb volume that are expected to be easier to accomplish. The definitive prosthesis has a gel liner with pin suspension to minimize the bulk around the knee and ease the donning process. Minimal changes in the residual limb volume and shape are expected, therefore major adjustments are not anticipated. The multi-axial foot will allow improved stability on uneven terrain in the yard and community.

Case 74-4: Transfemoral Amputation

A 28-year-old female day care teacher sustained an open comminuted distal femur fracture while mountain climbing and ultimately had a mid-thigh level transfemoral amputation after developing osteomyelitis. Possible prosthetic prescriptions include the following:
- Provisional prosthesis with total contact thermoplastic ICS, gel liner with strap suspension, hydraulic knee unit, lightweight dynamic response foot, and cosmetic foam cover
- Definitive prosthesis with total contact, carbon fiber reinforced, ischial containment, suction suspension, frame socket with thermoflex liner, thigh rotator, swing and stance phase control hydraulic knee unit hydraulic knee unit with microprocessor control, split-toe carbon fiber dynamic response foot, and cosmetic foam cover

The provisional prosthesis, an endoskeletal design with a gel liner, strap suspension, and hydraulic knee unit, was chosen to allow easy accommodation for anticipated major changes in residual limb volume that were expected to occur quickly with prosthetic use, while at the same time recognizing this individual's high level of physical activity. The cosmetic cover was added to the provisional prosthesis, not usually done, recognizing her work with small children and her desire not to scare them with the prosthesis. The changes in the definitive prosthesis include the true suction socket for more intimate fit and control, along with the microprocessor control knee to maximize stability and achieve a more secure suspension, and accommodate her recreational and competitive sports activities. The thigh rotator was added so that she could sit on the floor and work with the children in her class.

INTERNET RESOURCES

Company

Animated Prosthetics	www.animatedprosthetics.com
Becker Orthopedics	www.beckerorthopedic.com
CPI	www.college-park.com
Daw Industries	www.daw-usa.com
Endolite	www.endolite.com
Evolution Liners	www.evolutionliners.com
Fillauer	www.fillauer.com
Freedom Innovations	www.freedom-innovations.com
Hosmer	www.hosmer.com
Kingsley	www.kingsleymfg.com
Liberating Technologies	www.liberatingtechnologies.com
Living Skin	www.livingskin.com
Motion Control	www.utaharm.com
Ohio Willow Wood	www.owwco.com
Ossur	www.ossur.com
Otto Bock	www.ottobockus.com
T.R.S. Inc.	www.oandp.com/products/trs/

Amputee Athletes

Active Amp.org	www.activeamp.org
American Amputee Soccer Assoc.	www.ampsoccer.org
Challenged Athletes Foundation	www.challengedathletes.org/caf/
Disabled Sports USA	www.dsusa.org
International Paralympics Committee	www.paralympic.org

Other

American Academy of Orthotists and Prosthetists	www.oandp.org
Amputee Coalition of America	www.amputee-coalition.org
Amputee Resource Foundation of America, Inc.	www.amputeeresource.org
Barr Foundation	www.oandp.com/resources/organizations/barr
International Society for Prosthetics and Orthotics	www.i-s-p-o.org
National Limb Loss Information Center	www.amputee-coalition.org/nllic_about.html

ACKNOWLEDGMENTS

I would like to thank Nicolas E. Walsh, Gordon Bosker, and Daniel Santa Maria for their contributions to the earlier editions of this chapter.

REFERENCES

1. Cutson TM, Bongiorini DR. Rehabilitation of the older lower limb amputee: a brief review. *J Am Geriatr Soc.* 1996;44:1388–1393.
2. Fletcher DD, Andrews KL, Butters MA, et al. Rehabilitation of the geriatric vascular amputee patient: a population-based study. *Arch Phys Med Rehabil.* 2001;82:776–779.
3. Munin MC, Espejo-De Guzman MC, Boninger ML, et al. Predictive factors for successful early prosthetic ambulation among lower-limb amputees. *J Rehabil Res Dev.* 2001;38(4):379–384.
4. Burgess EM, Romano RL, Zetti JH. *The Management of Lower Extremity Amputations.* Washington, DC: US Government Printing Office; 1969.
5. Goldberg T. Postoperative management of lower extremity amputations. *Phys Med Rehabil Clin N Am.* 2006;17(1):173–180.
6. Carroll K, Edelstein JE. *Prosthetic and Patient Management: A Comprehensive Clinical Approach.* Thorofare, NJ: Slack Inc.; 2006.
7. Pasquina PF, Bryant PR, Huang ME, et al. Advances in amputee care. *Arch Phys Med Rehabil.* 2006;87(3 suppl 1):S34–S43.
8. Hafner BJ, Sanders JE, Czerniecki JM, et al. Transtibial energy storage and return prosthetic devices: a review of energy concepts and a proposed nomenclature. *J Rehabil Res Dev.* 2002;39:1–11.
9. Hofstad CH, Linde H, Limbeck J, et al. Prescription of prosthetic ankle-foot mechanisms after lower limb amputation. *Cochrane Database Syst Rev.* 2004;(1):CD003978.
10. Van der Linde H, Hofstad CJ, Guerts AC, et al. A systematic literature review of the effect of different prosthetic components on human functioning with a lower-limb prosthesis. *J Rehabil Res Dev.* 2004;41(4):555–570.
11. Nassan S. The latest designs in prosthetic feet. *Phys Med Rehabil Clin N Am.* 2000;11:609–625.
12. Czerniecki JM, Gitter A. Prosthetic feet: a scientific and clinical review of current components. *Phys Med Rehabil State Art Rev.* 1994;8:109–129.
13. Zmitrewicz RJ, Neptune RR, Walden JG, et al. The effect of foot and ankle prosthetic components on braking and propulsive impulses during transtibial amputee gait. *Arch Phys Med Rehabil.* 2006;87(10):1334–1339.
14. Hofstad C, Van der Linde H, Van Limbeek J, et al. Prescription of prosthetic ankle-foot mechanisms after lower limb amputation. *Cochrane Database Syst Rev.* 2004;(1):CD003978.
15. Tang SFT, Chen CPC, Chen MJL, et al. Transmetatarsal amputation prosthesis with carbon-fiber plate enhanced gait function. *Am J Phys Med Rehabil.* 2004;83(2):124–130.
16. Frykberg RG, Abraham S, Tierney E, et al. Syme amputation for limb salvage: early experience with 26 cases. *J Foot Ankle Surg.* 2007;46(2):93–100.
17. Stuck RM. Syme's ankle disarticulation. *Clin Podiatr Med Surg.* 1997;14:763–773.
18. Pinzur M. Restoration of walking ability with Syme's ankle disarticulation. *Clin Orthop.* 1999;361:71–75.
19. Hudson JR, Yu GV, Marzano R, et al. Syme's amputation. Surgical technique, prosthetic considerations, and case reports. *J Am Podiatr Med Assoc.* 2002;92(4):232–246.
20. Feragson J, Smith DG. Socket considerations for the patient with a transtibial amputation. *Clin Orthop.* 1999;361:76–84.
21. Kahle JT. Conventional and hydrostatic interface comparison. *J Prosthet Orthot.* 1999;11:85–90.
22. Selles RW, Janssens PJ, Jongnengel CD, et al. A randomized controlled trial comparing functional outcome and cost efficiency of a total surface-bearing socket versus a conventional patellar tendon-bearing socket in transtibial amputees. *Arch Phys Med Rehabil.* 2005;86:154–161.
23. Kapp S. Suspension systems for prostheses. *Clin Orthop.* 1999;361:55–62.
24. Board WJ, Street GM, Caspers C. A comparison of trans-tibial amputee suction and vacuum socket conditions. *Prosthet Orthot Int.* 2001;25(3):202–209.
25. Buckley JG, Jone SF, Birch KM. Oxygen consumption during ambulation: comparison of using a prosthesis fitted with and without a tele-torsion device. *Arch Phys Med Rehabil.* 2002;83(4):576–580.
26. Pinzur MS, Bowker JH. Knee disarticulation. *Clin Orthop.* 1999;361:23–28.
27. Hagberg E, Berlin OK, Renström P. Function after through knee compared with below knee and above knee amputation. *Prosthet Orthot Int.* 1992;16(3):168–173.
28. Schuch CM, Pritham CH. Current transfemoral sockets. *Clin Orthop.* 1999;361:48–54.
29. Gottschalk FA, Stills M. The biomechanics of transfemoral amputation. *Prosthet Orthot Int.* 1994;18:12–17.
30. Pritham CH. Biomechanics and shape of the above knee and above knee amputation. *Prosthet Orthot Int.* 1992;16(3):9–21.
31. Long IA. Normal shape-normal alignment (NSNA) above-knee prosthesis. *Clin Prosthet Orthot.* 1985;9:168–173.
32. Sabolich J. Contoured adducted trochanteric-controlled alignment method (CAT-CAM): introduction and basic principles. *Clin Prosthet Orthot.* 1985;9:15–26.
33. Kristinsson O. Flexible above-knee socket made from low-density polyethylene suspended by a weight-transmitting frame. *Prosthet Orthot.* 1983;37:25–27.
34. Pritham CH. Biomechanics and shape of the above-knee socket considered in light of the ischial containment concept. *Prosthet Orthot Int.* 1990;14:9–21.
35. Layton H. A vacuum donning procedure for transfemoral suction suspension prostheses. *J Prosthet Orthot.* 1998;10(1):21–24.
36. van de Veen PG. *Above Knee Prosthetic Technology.* The Netherlands: P.G. van de Veen Consultancy; 2001.
37. Esquenazi A, Meier RH. Rehabilitation in limb deficiency. 4. Limb amputation. *Arch Phys Med Rehabil.* 1996;77:S18–S28.
38. Michael JW. Modern prosthetic knee mechanisms. *Clin Orthop.* 1999;361:39–47.
39. Smith J, Tuel SM, Meythaler JM, et al. Prosthetic management of hemicorporectomy patients: new approaches. *Arch Phys Med Rehabil.* 1992;73(5):493–497.
40. Malone JM, Fleming LL, Robenson J, et al. Immediate, early, and late postsurgical management of upper-limb amputation. *J Rehabil Res Dev.* 1984;21:3–41.
41. Wright TW, Hagen AD, Wood MB. Prosthetic usage in major upper extremity amputations. *J Hand Surg Am.* 1995;20A:619–622.
42. Biddiss E, Chau T. Upper-limb prosthesis: critical factors in device abandonment. *Am J Phys Med Rehabil.* 2007;86(12):977–987.
43. Silcox DH, Rooks MD, Vogel RR, et al. Myoelectric prostheses: a long-term follow-up and a study of the use of alternate prostheses. *J Bone Joint Surg Am.* 1993;75A:1781–1789.
44. Lake C. Effects of prosthetic training on upper-extremity prosthesis use. *J Prosthet Orthot.* 1997;9:3–9.
45. Meier RH. Upper limb amputee rehabilitation. *Phys Med Rehabil Stars.* 1994;8(1):165–185.
46. Millsten S, Heger H, Hunter A. Prosthetic use in adult upper limb amputees: a comparison of the body powered and electrically powered prosthesis. *Prosthet Orthot Int.* 1986;10:27–34.
47. LeBlanc M. Use of prosthetic prehensors. *Prosthet Orthot Int.* 1988;12(3):152–154.
48. Leow ME, Pho RWH, Pereira BP. Esthetic prostheses in minor and major upper limb amputations. *Hand Clin.* 2001;17:489–497.
49. Michael JW. Upper limb powered components and controls: current concepts. *Clin Prosthet Orthot.* 1986;10:66–77.
50. Uellendahl JE. Upper extremity myoelectric prosthetics. *Phys Med Rehabil Clin N Am.* 2000;11:639–652.
51. Malone JM, Childers SJ, Underwood J, et al. Immediate postsurgical management of upper extremity amputation: conventional, electric, and myoelectric prostheses. *Orthot Prosthet.* 1981;35:1–9.
52. Nikolajsen L, Jenson TS. Phantom limb pain. *Br J Anaesth.* 2001;87:107–116.
53. Hill A. Phantom limb pain: a review of the literature on attributes and potential mechanisms. *J Pain Symptom Manage.* 1999;17:125–142.
54. Halbert J, Crotty M, Camerson ID. Evidence for the optimal management of acute and chronic phantom pain: a systematic review. *Clin J Pain.* 2002;18:84–92.
55. Sherman RA. Published treatments of phantom limb pain. *Am J Phys Med.* 1980;59:232–244.
56. Sherman RA, Sherman CJ, Gail NA. Survey of current phantom limb treatment in the United States. *Pain.* 1980;8:85–99.
57. Spire MC, Leonard JA. Prosthetic pearls: solutions to thorny problems. *Phys Med Rehabil Clin N Am.* 1996;7:509–516.
58. Boutin RD, Pathria MN, Resnick D. Disorders in the stumps of amputee patients: MR imaging. *AJR Am J Roentgenol.* 1998;171:497–501.
59. Levy SW. *Skin Problems of the Amputee.* St. Louis, MO: Warren H. Green; 1983.

60. Lyon CC, Kulkami J, Zimerson E, et al. Skin disorders in amputees. *J Am Acad Dermatol.* 2000;42:501–507.

61. Lake C, Supan TJ. The incidence of dermatologic problems in the silicone sleeve user. *J Prosthet Orthot.* 1997;9:97–106.

62. Dudek NL, Marks MB, Marshall SC, et al. Skin problems in an amputee clinic. *Am J Phys Med Rehabil.* 2006;85(5):424–429.

63. Smith DG, Michael JW, Bowker JH. *Atlas of Amputations and Limb Deficiencies: Surgical, Prosthetic, and Rehabilitation Principles.* 3rd ed. Rosemont, IL: American Academy of Orthopedic Surgeons; 2004.

64. Shaperman J, Landsberger SE, Setoguchi Y. Early upper limb prosthesis fitting: when and what do we fit. *J Prosthet Orthot.* 2003;15:11–17.

65. Scott RN. *Myoelectric Prostheses for Infants.* 4th ed. Fredrickton, NB: University of New Brunswick; 1992.

66. Jain S. Rehabilitation in limb deficiency. 2. The pediatric amputee. *Arch Phys Med Rehabil.* 1995;77:S9–S13.

67. Cummings DR. Pediatric prosthetics: an update. *Phys Med Rehabil Clin N Am.* 2006;17(1):15–21.

68. Nagarajan R, Neglia JP, Clohisy DR, et al. Education, employment, insurance, and marital status among 694 survivors of pediatric lower extremity bone tumors: a report from the childhood cancer survivor study. *Cancer.* 2003;97(10):2554–2564.

69. Lusardi MM, Nielsen CC. *Orthotics and Prosthetics in Rehabilitation.* Woburn, MA: Butterworth-Heinemann; 2007.

70. Day HJ. The ISO/ISPO classification of congenital limb deficiency. *Prosthet Orthot Int.* 1991;15(2):67–69.

71. Atkins DJ, Meier RH, eds. *Comprehensive Management of the Upper-Limb Amputee.* New York: Springer-Verlag; 1989.

Orthotics for the Lower and Upper Limb and Spine

Limb orthoses, with their many variations, are among the most commonly prescribed biomechanical rehabilitation devices intended to assist individuals with gait dysfunction, upper limb weakness, or spine pathology caused by musculoskeletal or neuromuscular diseases (1). They are intended to increase function and facilitate mobility for patients in the early or chronic stages of rehabilitation or as an intervention to improve comfort.

ROLE AND USE OF ORTHOTICS

Orthoses are devices applied to the external surface of the body to achieve one or more of the following: relieve pain, immobilize musculoskeletal segments, prevent or correct a deformity, and improve function. Orthoses provide a direct support component to the braced segment and limit the range of motion of one or more joints. This mechanism largely gives rise to reduction of axial loads and joint motion, thus aiding in pain relief. Orthosis also may be used to attempt to fully immobilize a joint and, in this manner, improve function and reduce pain. In conjunction with the above two mechanisms, a more difficult mechanism to visualize is the fact that orthoses modify the total static and dynamic force/moment distributions in the braced segment particularly evident in the lower limb more distal segments ("in" joints or about a joint center) or spine where counterforces are utilized to provide support or substitution for weak muscles while maintaining functional mobility. In some instances, these mechanisms when applied to the lower limb can make walking more efficient.

Overall, orthotics can be divided into two major categories, namely, corrective and accommodative devices; in the near future, orthotic technology will also provide artificial strength through externally powered effectors (direct or distant motors). Corrective devices are meant to improve the position of the limb segment, whether by stretching a contracture or improving the alignment of skeletal structures (1). Accommodative devices are meant to provide additional support to already deformed tissues, to prevent further deformity, and ultimately to improve function. Orthoses can be further classified as static (resting) or dynamic devices, the latter permitting movement of the involved joint(s) while controlling the direction, range, or alignment of the movement and, at times, providing a substitute power source for weak muscles, while a static device may also serve to protect. The spectrum of orthotic devices available in clinical practice is quite broad, ranging from a simple plastic device applied across one joint such as a proximal interphalangeal (PIP) joint immobilizer to a much more complex device made of a variety of materials and crossing multiple joints (hybrid knee-ankle-foot orthosis [KAFO]) (2); some also may include microprocessors for movement control or even power generators to move a joint. Knowledge of the disease or disorder being addressed with a particular orthosis, functional anatomy, biomechanics, orthotic components, and manufacturing materials and, finally, recognition of the expected outcome are essential for proper orthotic prescription (3,4).

TERMINOLOGY AND BIOMECHANICAL PRINCIPLES

In the past, the lexicon of terms used to describe orthoses was very confusing; often, clinicians used different terms to describe even the most basic similar device. Orthoses or parts of devices were given names that might describe their purpose, the body part to which they were applied, the inventor of the device, or the town or institution where they were developed. To facilitate communication and minimize the use of acronyms, a logical, easy-to-use system of standard universal terminology for orthotic devices was developed by the International Committee of Prosthetics and Orthotics toward the end of the 20th century (3). Orthotic devices are now named by the joints they encompass in correct sequence from proximal to distal followed by the word orthosis. For example, an orthosis that crosses the ankle and the foot is named an ankle-foot orthosis (AFO), while an orthosis that crosses the wrist and the fingers is named a wrist-finger orthosis (WFO). One that crosses the knee, ankle, and foot is called a KAFO. The intended biomechanical function and material may complement the terminology (i.e., dorsiflexion assist plastic AFO or extension assist WFO). More elaborate names or eponyms with regional variation are frequently given to such devices (3), but such language whenever possible should be avoided.

The three-point pressure biomechanical concept is integrated to most brace designs. Generally, a strong force is applied at a joint or rotational axis and a counterforce applied proximal and distal to that joint. The location of the force and counterforce may be clearly identified as a specific, pad, strap, or bar in the orthotic design (**Fig. 57-1**).

However, in many instances, the force and counterforces may be integrated into the design of the orthotic device and not as evident. The precise point of application and the magnitude

3 Points of Pressure Control Design

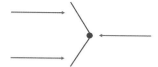

FIGURE 57-1. Three-point control concept. A strong force is applied at a joint and a counterforce is applied proximal and distal to the joint to control motion.

of the force and counterforce are critical to achieve the desired control. Ideally, the closer to the point of rotation one can apply the force, the more effective it will be, but occasionally, the required forces may be too large to be tolerated by the soft tissues. In that situation, one can simply move the point of pressure application farther from the joint to decrease the magnitude of the applied pressure. In other words, by increasing the lever distance, less pressure can generate the same force across the joint. The angle of pull of force is also very important to produce effective control of the identified joint and to prevent damage to ligamentous or structures and disruption of the joint integrity.

MATERIALS

The orthotic components chosen depend on which functions they fulfill, but most orthoses consist of three basic elements: interface components, structural components, and, if intended to be articulated, the type of joints. In orthoses of newer design, it may be impossible to differentiate the joints from the structural and interface components, for example, plastic AFO or thermoplastic wrist orthosis (2).

The choice of materials and techniques for the fabrication of orthotics continues to expand rapidly, and a full review of them is beyond the scope of this chapter. The reader is encouraged to read on the subject by reviewing other sections about this topic (5). The three primary material categories for the fabrication of orthosis are plastics, metals, and carbon graphite. Plastics have the benefits of lightweight, total contact, adjustable flexibility, the ability to adjust in shape, and a more cosmetic appearance. Metal orthoses often have the advantage of increased durability and, in the hands of a skilled orthotist, built-in adjustability but variable weight based on the selected metal (aluminum vs. stainless steel). For carbon graphite materials, the advantages of maximal tension strength, lightweight design are counterpoised to difficulty with adjustability and cost (6). Factors that dictate the type of material used in orthotic fabrication include the length of time the orthosis will be used, the amount of forces applied across the orthosis, user skin condition, sensation, and the amount of axial loading. Cost may be another factor to consider.

A complete orthotic prescription should include the anatomical joints it encompasses and side and indicate the desired biomechanical alignment and materials of fabrication and materials to use for closures (e.g., leather straps, Velcro, etc.) and where they should be used for correction as exemplified in **Figure 57-2.**

When the orthosis is ready for delivery to the user, it should be evaluated off and on the patient to ensure proper construction, fit, and function. When these characteristics

are achieved, appropriate training and review of the potential adverse effects, use, and care should be provided to patient and family. A wearing schedule that gradually increases use time and monitors the skin integrity should also be provided.

Modern orthotic management is best accomplished in the majority of patients with the use of plastic-molded orthoses. They provide more intimate contact with better distribution of the controlling/corrective forces over a larger surface area. These devices generally are more cosmetic in appearance because they can fit inside the user's shoe or underclothing and hence better accepted. Insurance coverage pressures in the United States have promoted the use of prefabricated non-molded devices, which may not be ideal for many patients (7).

For the lower limb, plastic braces allow the patient to interchange shoes, as long as constant heel height is maintained to avoid altering the intended dynamic alignment (position) of the device. Plastic materials are lighter in weight and easier to maintain. The availability of adjustable ankle joints that can be integrated to plastic orthoses developed in the last three decades has eliminated a major disadvantage of these devices when compared to those constructed out of metal/leather. Lack of skin integrity or sensation and fluctuating edema are relative contraindications to the prescription of intimately molded or fitted plastic devices. If the patient has adequate cognition, visual perception, and social support, he or she can receive the added benefits provided by plastic braces. Two major types of plastic materials are used in orthotics: thermosetting and thermoplastic materials. Thermosetting plastics include formaldehyde, epoxy, and polyester resins as well as carbon graphite that are typically used as laminates in a similar manner than that used for limb prosthetic socket fabrication. They require heat produced by a chemical reaction to set and harden a multilayer of weaved fibers of different products applied in a specific sequence and position.

Thermoplastics soften when they are heated, making the material moldable. Within limits, subsequent heating will soften the material for further modification, and lowering the temperature hardens the material once again.

High-temperature thermoplastics that generally are available in sheets, such as polyethylene, polypropylene, copolymers, ortholene, thermoplastic elastomers (TPEs), and vinyl polymers, require heating to temperatures greater than 300°F (150°C) to make it pliable to mold. Fabrication of an orthosis made of any of these materials requires an exact plaster mold of the desired body part since direct application to the body would risk burns. The heated plastic is applied to the positive mold for proper shaping under vacuum. These materials are durable, and they have "good elastic memory," returning to their original position after flexible deformation. Fabrication and adjustments to the biomechanical alignment and fit of an orthosis require the intervention of an orthotist. Based on the trim lines of the material (amount of plastic surrounding the joint), orthosis provided support and may simulate joint motion, and because of the elastic characteristics of the materials, they may produce a spring-action force (**Fig. 57-3**).

Because of their strength, durability, and ease of modification, orthoses manufactured out of metal/leather continue to have a definite place in the treatment of many patients such as those with soft tissue wounds, hyperhidrosis, fluctuating edema, or intolerance to plastics. The metals primarily used are steel and aluminum, mostly in alloy forms with various

EINSTEIN HEALTHCARE NETWORK

Lower Limb Orthotic Prescription

Name:_____   Age:_____   Date:_____

Diagnosis:_____   Patient ready: yes   no   Room#_____

Orthotist: _____   Third Party Coverage:_____

Circle and complete as necessary

Type: Foot   Ankle/Foot   PTB   Knee/Ankle/Foot   Knee   Hip/Knee/Ankle/Foot

Side: Right   Left   Bilateral   **Design:**   Articulated   Non Articulated   Anterior   Floor Reaction

Construction: Plastic:_____   Metal:_____   Graphyte:_____ Other:_____

Closures: Velcro   "D Ring"   Overlap   Laces   Buckles   Elastic   Right hand pull   Left Hand pull

Ankle joints: Gaffney   Gillet   Tamerak   Lawrence   Scottis   Double Adjustable   Other:_____

Ankle control: Plantarflexion:_____ °   Dorsiflexion:_____ °   Dacron strap   Inversion:_____ Eversion:_____

Resistance: PLS   Minimum   Moderate   Maximum   **Assistance:** Dorsiflexion   Extension

Foot plate: Long   Longitudinal arch   Padded   Metatarsal pad   UCBL   Tone reducing

Straps: Ankle   Mid foot   Forefoot   Inversion / eversion control   Valgus / varus control   Padded

Knee: Single axis   Non Protuding   Polycentric   Offset   Unloader   Stance Phase Control   Electronic

Knee lock: Drop locks   Bail locks   Retainers   Spring loaded   Stance phase locking   Other:_____

Knee control: Varus   Valgus   Flexion   Hyperextension   Infrapatelar strap   Suprapatelar   Knee Pad

Thigh section: Traditional   Quadrilateral   Narrow ML   Gluteal   Ischial WB   Anterior   Extended lateral wall

Hip control: Flexion   Abduction   Adduction   Silesian   External hip joint

Shoes: Orthopedic   Canvas   Soft extradepth   High top   Molded   Velcro   Other:_____

Special Instructions:_____

Please answer all questions:		Yes	No
	Patient can not be fitted with prefababricated brace	Yes	No
	Condition is longlasting lasting > 6 months	Yes	No
	Need to control joints in more than one plain	Yes	No
	Patient has neurological, vascular or orthopedic diagnosis	Yes	No

Signature _____ **M.D./D.O.**

®AE2017

FIGURE 57-2.   Example of a lower limb orthotic prescription form.

other metals to further increase their strength and to resist corrosion; straps and padding are made of leather. Although metal orthoses are heavier and are cosmetically less appealing to many patients, their durability and adjustability allow them to accommodate for longitudinal growth in children and the changing needs of the patient recovering from injury. The choice of orthotic material depends on the clinical purpose and the characteristics of the patient (**Fig. 57-4**).

Proper biomechanical alignment of lower limb orthoses is critical to maximize the ambulatory capability of a patient. Biomechanical malalignment can and does prevent a patient with borderline functional capacity from the value intended by the device; those patients with better recovery or less deficit may be able to compensate for inadequate orthotic alignment or designs. In those patients for whom orthotic joint motion is required, close correlation between the orthotic and the

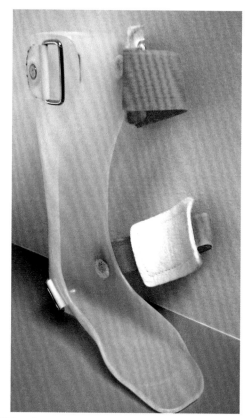

FIGURE 57-3. Example of a thermoplastic orthosis.

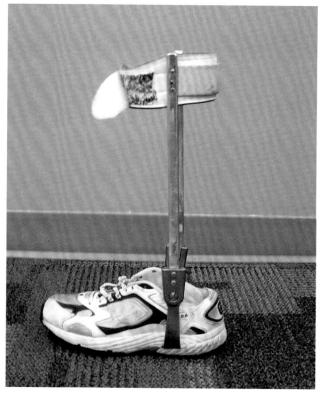

FIGURE 57-4. Metal ankle foot orthosis.

anatomic joint centers of rotation is of great importance to avoid a discrepancy in the axis of motion, which could produce pain, joint swelling, skin breakdown, and other preventable adverse effects.

Adjustability of brace alignment is a significant advantage to current practice patterns where patients are being transferred to inpatient rehabilitation programs much earlier than in the past and the length of stay in the rehabilitation programs has decreased significantly. Predicting the final rehabilitation outcome of these patients so early in their recovery may be very difficult. The ability to adjust the biomechanical alignment of the orthosis with simple tools or to convert a controlling force into an assistive one in order to respond to the patient's changing needs is an important advantage. This is also a potential problem as individuals or patients without the needed knowledge may alter the alignment of the brace, or in some cases, simple use over time may loosen the components changing the desired alignment features (2).

THE SHOE AS A COMPONENT

The shoe is an integral part of any lower limb orthosis that includes the foot, as it serves as the foundation for the device and directly impacts its function (8). The basic function of the shoe is to protect the foot from walking surfaces, the weather, and the environment as well as to provide support for the feet during standing and walking. The use of properly fitting shoes is essential to the success of any foot orthosis or AFO (9). Factors to consider when selecting a shoe are size, shape, fit, and function. Proper shoe size must take into consideration fit while standing, as the foot configuration changes with weight bearing and pathologic phenomenon such as spasticity (10). The foot may swell with prolonged sitting or activity and is often best fitted at the end of the day and after walking. If a plastic brace will be used, then the shoe may need to be slightly longer and or wider to accommodate for this additional space-occupying material. The parts of a shoe consist of the sole, the heel, the counter (heel and longitudinal arch), the upper, the linings, and reinforcements (11).

Each shoe component can be made of a wide variety of materials and designs, depending on the quality and specific use. The construction material of the shoe is very important when considering the function and the modifiability of a shoe.

Shoes are built around a positive model or replica of the weight-bearing foot, which is called a last (7). The shoe last, which is made of solid maple or plastic materials, determines the shape and fit, walking comfort, appearance, and style of the shoe when produced. During fabrication, the insole is nailed to the last, the lining is tucked to the inner sole rim, and the reinforcements (i.e., counter, toe box) are attached. The upper of the shoe is softened by humidity for easier molding and fitted snugly to the last to conform to its every detail and then nailed or glued to the inner sole. Finally, the outer sole and heel are added. The Goodyear welt construction of a shoe is a method used in production of high-quality shoes in which the upper is sewn to the sole.

The upper is that part of the shoe that is above the sole. It is most commonly made of leather, although any soft and durable material may be used. Deerskin is significantly softer than leather. It stretches more easily and is generally more accommodative but is not nearly as durable. Recently heat-moldable uppers have been introduced to the fabrication of shoes. The material is capable of easily stretching around anatomical deformities such as bunions or hammer toes; this material does not dissipate heat and moisture well.

The upper consists of the vamp, quarters, and lace stay. The vamp is the anterior portion of the upper, which covers the toes and the instep. The tongue, a strip of leather lying under the laces, and the throat, the opening at the base of the tongue, are parts of the vamp. Anteriorly, the vamp has a reinforced toe box or toe cap to maintain its appearance and to protect the toes against trauma. The lace stay or the portion containing the eyelets for laces is usually part of the vamp, but it may be part of the quarters. The two quarters make up the posterior part of the shoe, usually reinforced by the heel counter, which stabilizes the foot by supporting the calcaneus and giving structural stability to the shoe. The counter is made of firm leather or synthetic material. Sometimes, a band of leather, referred to as a collar, is stitched to the top of the quarters to reduce foot pistoning and to also stiffen the shoe. Laterally, the quarter is cut lower to avoid impinging on the malleolus.

The heel of the shoe is attached to the outer sole under the anatomic heel and is made of leather, wood, plastic, rubber, or metal. The most anterior edged of the heel is called the breast. The height and design of the heel vary greatly and measured at the breast. The flat heel has a broad base and measures 0.75 to 1.25 in. (2 to 4 cm) in height. A Thomas heel is a flat heel that has a medial anterior extension to support a weak longitudinal foot arch. Heels up to 3 in. (7 cm) high are available, but they are mainly used for fashionable appearance rather than for extended walking. Shoes with lower heels also exist. The clinician should be aware that the height of the heel has a direct impact on the foot and ankle positions as well as affecting the proximal joints and general posture of the trunk. When a brace is manufactured, and aligned, this is done with a particular shoe heel height as part of the design (4). High heels, especially those with a tapered, narrow striking point, make the ankle and foot more unstable to rotational forces and thereby contribute to foot stress, ankle injuries, and falls. Some studies have linked the use of such shoes to abnormal forces in the foot and more proximal joints (12).

Types and Styles

There are innumerable shoe types and styles (**Fig. 57-5**), although basic designs are relatively few and determined mainly by the shape of the upper, particularly the design of the toe and the height of the quarters. The low-quarter shoe, also known as Oxford shoe, is characterized by the quarters finishing approximately 1 in. below the malleoli with no restriction of ankle or subtalar movement. In high-quarter shoes, the quarters may extend up to barely cover the malleoli, as in the chukka shoe, or extend to the lower third of the tibia or higher, as in boots. The most common shoe style is the blucher type, in which the lace stay is not directly fastened to the vamp. This style gives a wide opening for the foot for easy foot insertion and greater adjustability over the midfoot. For ease of access to the shoe, the surgical opening shoe allows exposure of the entire foot by opening up to the toes. Shoe closure usually is accomplished by laces, which thread through two or more pairs of eyelets, although closure also can be achieved by buckles, zippers, Velcro flaps, or elastics.

Modifications to commercial footwear and in some instances, custom footwear are an important aspect of lower limb orthotic practice. Shoe modifications can successfully treat simple problems that affect walking as well as be an integral part of any lower limb orthotic prescription (7,13).

The shoe can be modified by adding a variety of alterations including changes to the heel, the addition of metatarsal pads and rockers, and other modifications.

Sole Materials

Materials used in the construction of shoe soles vary greatly and have significantly different properties with regard to weight, durability, shock absorption and attenuation, flexibility, and support. Leather soles are extremely durable, tend to be stiff and

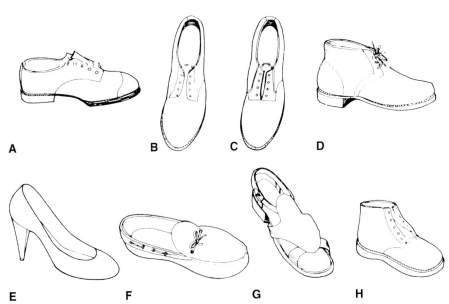

FIGURE 57-5. Shoe types and styles. **A:** Oxford or low quarter. **B:** Blucher-type Oxford. **C:** Bal-type Oxford. **D:** Chukka or high quarter. **E:** Pump. **F:** Moccasin. **G:** Sandal. **H:** Child's shoe.

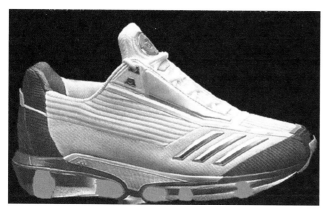

FIGURE 57-6. Athletic shoe.

heavy, and offer little or no shock absorption when compared to other materials and can be slippery in wet conditions.

Hard rubber is a great alternative to leather, especially when used to attach an AFO as it has some degree of impact absorption at heel strike and it is less slippery when used to walk on wet surfaces.

In recent years, athletic shoes (**Fig. 57-6**) have dramatically changed the design and materials used for their fabrication. The outer sole usually is made of highly durable rubber compounds that provide a good grip on the ground, whereas the inner sole is designed to closely fit the foot. Between the outer and inner soles, fluid, gel, or cavitated materials are placed for cushioning and shock dampening. The outer sole often is designed to flare out laterally at the heel and toward the mid foot to improve mediolateral stability at the ankle band, there is the option of using high-top design.

Due to their natural increase in coefficient of friction, rubber soles have more traction than leather shoes when walking on carpeted or dry surfaces. Sometimes, it is desirable to reduce friction, and the application of an external leather toe slider covering the front 1/3 of the sole can be of great benefit to facilitate limb advancement when limb clearance is impaired.

Shoe Fitting

The first requirement of a shoe is that it fits and does not cause pain, skin problems, or deformities. Ideally, both feet should be measured in length and width and the shoes tried on both feet in case of size discrepancy. If more than a one size difference exists, using split size shoes should be recommended (10,14). Footwear preferably should be purchased at the end of the day, when the feet are slightly swollen. When shoes are fitted, each shoe should be judged individually in a fully weight-bearing position. Shoes should be carefully tested for fit, both in length and width, not only by standing but by walking for several steps and stopping fast. The shoe length should extend at least a half-inch (1.2 cm) beyond the longest toe, usually the hallux or the second toe. The first metatarsal joint should be located at the inner curve of the shoe, and on toe dorsiflexion, the shoe should bend easily at the toe break that should run directly across the ball of the foot. The widest part of the shoe should coincide with the broadest part of the foot, leaving enough free space medial and lateral to the heads of the first and fifth metatarsal, respectively. The shoe widths measured at the ball are available in different sizes, ranging from A (narrow) to EEE (extra wide). Each size represents a

0.25-in. (0.6 cm) increase in width. If the material is soft and pliable, it should be possible to fold some material from the top of the toe box to confirm appropriate space for the toes. Extra-depth shoes and shoes with removable insoles are available to accommodate foot abnormalities and shoe inserts. The real proof of fit, however, is if the shoe is comfortable after hours of continuous wear or walking (15).

If there is a pathologic condition with loss of sensation in the feet, new shoes should be worn using a gradually increasing schedule starting at 2 hours/day only, after which shoes and socks should be removed and the feet carefully inspected.

Shoe Modifications

Stock shoes may require minor or major modifications by various methods to support the abnormal foot during weight bearing, to reduce pressure on painful areas, and to limit motion or accommodate deformed, weak, unstable, or painful joints. For these purposes, the clinician may select a special type of shoe, order certain alterations in the construction of the shoe, or apply corrections directly to the foot.

Although certain simple external modifications may be applied to many types of commercial shoes, welt shoes are more suitable to work with, especially for major internal modifications, because the process of removing and reattaching the sole to the upper usually does not alter the structure of the shoe.

Flares and Wedges

A flare is an extension attached, either medially or laterally, to the sole of the shoe intended to increase mediolateral ankle stability. The flare can be added to the heel only, or it can extend to the entire length of the shoe. A flare is not intended to correct a deformity but rather only to control motion. Widening the base of support with a flare (usually lateral sole flare) may provide a more stable platform for the foot (16). A wedge is used to help accommodate a rigid deformity or correct flexible deformities of the hindfoot. A shoe with a lateral wedge has more material under the lateral border of the foot than the medial border.

Flares and wedges may be combined in more severe cases, but in general, avoid medial flares that exceed ½ in. (1.2 cm) as the patient may trip with his other foot. For lateral flairs in excess of ½ in. (1.2 cm), a buttress should be included for better control (**Fig. 57-7**).

Lifts or Elevations

Elevations of the shoe can be used to address a variety of clinical problems. Most commonly, they are used to compensate for limb-length discrepancy. In a patient with a neurologic disorder who has impairment in limb clearance, a shoe lift added to the nonparetic limb can facilitate the swing phase of the affected limb. Elevations are applied either under the heel only or under the whole sole. They can be applied internally or added to the outer sole of the shoe. A heel-only elevation is appropriate for accommodating a fixed equinus position or reducing the strain on the Achilles tendon. A buildup less than ½ in. (1.2 cm) can be easily added inside the shoe. Greater corrections will need to be distributed between the inside and outside of the shoe.

Increasing the width of the sole of the shoe as the heel height increases should be considered in order to reduce the

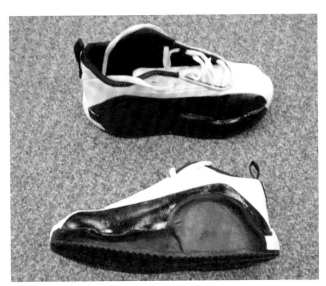

FIGURE 57-7. Shoe with medial flair and buttress.

possibility of mediolateral instability. A heel-only buildup greater than 1.5 in. (3.8 cm) is not recommended unless accompanied by a high-top shoe or an AFO to reduce the likelihood of ankle instability. A buildup that extends from heel to ball (shoe lift) is the more biomechanical appropriate intervention to compensate for a limb-length discrepancy or when attempting to decrease a swing phase foot drag (17). Creating a small rocker in the metatarsal area may be necessary if the lift stiffens the sole excessively.

Rigid Shanks

An extended rigid shank is traditionally a strip of spring steel or carbon graphite of varying rigidities that is placed between the layers of the outer sole or in some cases inside the shoe, extending from the heel to the toe brake of the shoe. An extended rigid shank, as its name indicates, extends to the tip of the shoe to make it rigid reducing bending stresses in the midfoot and forefoot, and it must be used in conjunction with a rocker sole. Some of the clinical indications for this shoe modification include metatarsalgia, hallux rigidus, and some arthropathies or Charcot-related joint deformities or pathologies.

Rocker Soles

The rocker sole is one of the most commonly prescribed shoe modifications (7,18). As implied by the name, the basic function of a rocker sole is to rock the foot from heel strike to toe-off without metatarsal bending. Rocker soles can reduce pressure under the metatarsal heads and can assist gait by easing and increasing forward propulsion in midstance to terminal stance. It can also be used to replace some of the motion lost due to the use of an extended steel shank. If the rocker sole is being implemented to offload an area of plantar pressure, then the apex of the rocker must be placed proximal to the pressure area.

The actual shape and height of the rocker sole depend on the specific problem to be treated and the expected biomechanical effect of the rocker sole (18,19). Care should be taken to assure that the rocker does not produce midstance anterior/posterior instability and to encourage the wearer to walk with shorter steps to enhance the efficacy of the modification.

Cushion Heel

Another useful shoe modification is the cushion heel, which consists of a wedge of shock-absorbing foam that is sandwiched between the heel and the sole of a shoe. The purpose of a cushion heel is to provide increased shock absorption and reduce the knee flexion forces occurring at heel strike. A cushion heel may be indicated for patients after ankle fusion or following a calcaneal fracture. It can also reduce knee flexion in early stance for those with quadriceps weakness.

FOOT ORTHOSES

In the hands of the experienced clinician, custom orthotics are an effective tool in the management of many of the abnormal biomechanics of the foot. As such, orthotics are designed in principle to be corrective or accommodative devices (20).

Corrective devices are meant to improve the position of the foot by changing the alignment of skeletal structures. Rigid materials such as thermoplastics, acrylic laminates, and carbon graphite composites are frequently used for this. Cork and polyethylene are example of materials used for semirigid orthotic devices that are corrective. Accommodative devices made of soft open or closed cell foams alone or in combination with semirigid materials provide cushioning and support to an already deformed foot structure while ultimately improving function.

Appropriate posting, longitudinal or transverse arch buildups, heel lifts, pressure relief areas, or other special modifications as well as the use of various materials in the same orthotic device can be integrated in the design and combined at the time of fabrication.

Custom foot orthoses (FOs) are superior to prefabricated ones because they can be designed to provide corrective forces to the affected joint(s) with more control. In addition, they can be configured to match precisely the patient's anatomy (of particular importance in the presence of impaired sensation) and activity requirements, and they can be manufactured from a variety of materials singly or in combination. Consideration should be given to the fact that external loads act as dynamic forces that may require different orthotic prescription and materials for different activities. One example of this careful application is the use of TPE for the longitudinal arch, Pelite as a molded substrate, and Poron for shock absorption in the same device (**Fig. 57-8**).

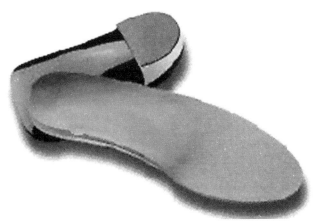

FIGURE 57-8. Hybrid material FO.

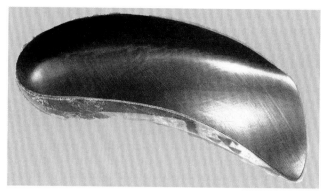

FIGURE 57-9. Carbon graphite–laminated foot orthotic.

Corrective FOs made of rigid materials can be extremely difficult to fit and require meticulous attention to detail during molding and fabrication (21). Progressive wearing periods of several weeks with close monitoring of the skin integrity is encouraged.

Figure 57-9 depicts a carbon graphite–laminated foot orthotic. FOs have not been investigated widely in controlled studies, and much of their design variance is founded on clinical experience.

ANKLE-FOOT ORTHOSES

Ankle-foot orthoses (AFOs) because of their mechanical lever arm are more effective in controlling the ankle complex and, when appropriately designed, can influence the knee joint as well.

The clinician must choose from metal/leather, plastic, carbon graphite, or a hybrid design assembly incorporating some or all the mentioned materials for an AFO. In general, plastic or hybrid systems predominate in North America and Europe because of the greater degree of client acceptance and control they offer (1). The choice of materials in the fabrication of orthotics is expanding rapidly, and a detail review of them is beyond the scope of this section. It is very unfortunate that insurance funding restrictions in general prevent open access to some of the recently introduce orthotic technology such as the use of composite or graphite and new advanced design devices. The older-style metal and leather orthoses usually are reserved for selected applications, such as when minimal soft tissue contact is desirable due to fluctuating edema, for wounds or for heat-sensitive individuals who cannot tolerate plastics, or when fitting large or heavy individuals (2). One of the most significant factors in material selection is cosmetic appearance, which heavily affects device acceptance.

A thermoplastic or laminated patellar tendon bearing ankle-foot orthosis (PTB-AFO) is indicated for patients who lack knee and ankle muscle power but have adequate hip extension strength, full knee extension range of motion, and no significant flexor spasticity or deformity (8). A molded footplate and a solid nonarticulated ankle design immobilize the foot and ankle in slight equinus, which produces a knee extension force during stance phase. Genu recurvatum is controlled by the ligamentous structures of the knee joint or adding a supracondylar anterior shell and a counteracting posteriorly placed popliteal shell. Limiting plantar flexion of the ankle can limit genu recurvatum as well.

Successful use of AFOs based upon electrical stimulation of weak or paralyzed muscles has been reported (17,22,23). In the United States and Europe, several commercial versions of such orthoses that incorporate neuromuscular electrical stimulation (NMES) for functional purposes have become available for clinical application (2). As with any other therapeutic intervention, to achieve their intended use, these devices require appropriate patient selection, no significant range of motion limitations or spasticity, and a clear understanding of the disease process and gait biomechanics as they relate to the system activation mechanism.

Equinovarus deformity is the most common pathologic lower limb posture seen in the population affected by central nervous system injuries (24). This abnormal posture results in an unstable base of support during stance phase. The contact with the ground occurs with the forefoot first, and weight is borne primarily on the lateral border of the foot; this position may be maintained during the stance phase. Heel contact may be limited or absent. Limitation in ankle dorsiflexion prevents forward progression of the tibia over the stationary foot in stance phase, causing compensatory knee hyperextension, hip flexion, and interference with terminal stance and preswing where lack of a propulsive phase is evident (8). During the swing phase, there is a sustained plantar flexed and inverted posture of the foot, possibly resulting in a limb clearance problem. The lack of adequate base of support results in instability of the whole body. For this reason, the correction of the abnormal ankle-foot posture is essential and usually can be achieved through the use of an orthotic device. The use of an AFO to control the abnormal posture of the ankle during stance and swing phase may require an ankle inversion strap or pad to assist in controlling the ankle inversion attitude. The orthosis should be attached preferentially to an orthopedic shoe, and the orthotic ankle should include a plantar flexion stop to control ankle plantar flexion during swing and stance phases (4). If ankle clonus is triggered during stance phase, a dorsiflexion stop will need to be considered as well to prevent the stretch response triggering this phenomenon. The stop angle should be set just before the clonus appears. A molded padded long plastic footplate in combination with a toe strap and an extra-depth shoe with high toe box can be used as an option to accommodate abnormal, painful, flexed toe posture (16).

KNEE-ANKLE-FOOT ORTHOSES

Below the knee, the components of the standard knee-ankle-foot orthoses (KAFOs) are the same as those of metal or plastic AFOs, except that the uprights extend to the knee joint, where they join the thigh uprights. A free flexing knee joint is indicated when mediolateral instability or genu recurvatum may be present but knee extension strength is adequate for stance phase weight-bearing stability.

If knee extensor muscles are weak, and knee flexion buckling occurs, a posterior offset knee joint may be indicated. In the absence of knee flexion contracture or spasticity, an offset knee joint provides a mechanical stable knee during stance while allowing knee flexion during the swing phase. This type of joint can provide stance phase knee stability if weight bearing is applied to the limb by placing the orthotic knee joint axis behind the anatomical knee joint. This results in anterior placement of the line of gravity in relationship to the knee.

Frequently, this will need to be combined with an ankle joint that limits dorsiflexion. This is not a fail proof system since knee instability may occur if the floor is uneven, the knee is not fully extended or loaded, or the ankle is allowed to dorsiflex more than 10 degrees (2). In such case, a knee lock may be a better choice. The drop-ring knee lock is most commonly used; it is placed on the proximal section of the upright bar and drops over the joint when it is fully extended. A spring-loaded pull rod may be added to the ring to facilitate locking and unlocking, especially when the patient is unable to flex at the hip to reach the knee or lacks hand or finger strength and dexterity. A knee with a spring-loaded cam that fits into a groove in full extension is easier to release but still gives good stability and may be used in patients with flexor spasticity. A bail lock (i.e., Swiss lock) is a lever bow that snaps into locked position on full extension and unlocks automatically when pressed upward. In the presence of a knee flexion contracture, an adjustable knee joint that makes use of either a fan or dial lock may be appropriate. Even when mechanically locked, the anatomical knee with weak extensors would bend some on weight bearing if not stabilized by straps above and below the patella or by a patellar pad or strap; a soft leather pad covering the kneecap and secured to the uprights works best. The thigh uprights are connected by a rigid, padded, upper thigh band with an anterior soft closure. This band should be 1.5 in. (3.7 cm) below the ischium, unless ischial weight bearing is prescribed. Usually, a second, rigid lower thigh band may also be used with soft anterior straps.

The Scott-Craig orthosis eliminates the lower thigh and calf bands and the hip joint typical of a HKAFO used in persons with spinal cord injuries, which facilitates donning and doffing and reduces its weight (**Fig. 57-10**) (25). It consists of two uprights with four rigid connections: posterior rigid upper thigh band, bail-type knee lock, rigid anterior upper tibial band with soft posterior strap, and, at the lower end, a stirrup with a rigid sole plate built into the shoe extending to the metatarsal heads. It is connected to the uprights by double-stop ankle joints that are adjusted to place the orthosis in 5 degrees of dorsiflexion for optimum balance (26). The shoe sole is perfectly flat from the heel to the metatarsal bar, where it becomes slightly rounded up to the toe. It is a stable orthosis that biomechanically functions as the standard KAFO but with fewer encumbrances from straps.

Because the anatomic knee joint has a changing axis of rotation, polycentric designed knee joints have the ability to maintain a better alignment during knee movement than single-axis knee joints and should be prescribed if the knee is to be allowed to flex in swing phase.

Plastic Knee-Ankle-Foot Orthoses

Plastic-molded or laminated KAFOs may incorporate standard ankle and knee components, but the uprights and bands are made of lightweight laminated or thermoplastics that closely fit the limb (**Fig. 57-11**). The thigh piece consists of a posterior quadrilateral shaped shell with or without an ischial weight-bearing or gluteal seat or have a narrow mediolateral shape thigh section if it is to be used bilaterally for improved comfort. The thigh section is closed anteriorly by a plastic band and a Velcro strap or a pair of padded straps. A suprapatellar or pretibial shell provides knee extension force, which eliminates the need for patellar strap and supplies mediolateral knee stability. At the lower end, the uprights are connected to a molded plastic footplate to be worn inside a shoe. Lightweight modular KAFOs have been designed for quick and easy assembly and provided for children with Duchenne muscular dystrophy in order to extend their walking ability (27).

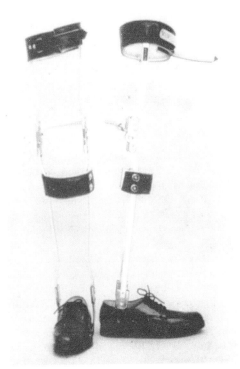

FIGURE 57-10.   The Scott-Craig knee-ankle-foot orthosis.

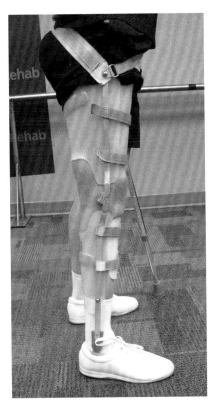

FIGURE 57-11.   Plastic-molded KAFO with hip belt.

KNEE ORTHOSES

Knee orthoses (KOs) are prescribed to control genu recurvatum and to provide mediolateral stability. With improvements in design and application, KOs have gained recognition by many as a treatment and prevention modality. The use of KOs for the prevention of knee injury in athletes is controversial. They may be used during sports and other physical activities to functionally support the unstable knee or during the rehabilitation phase following knee injury or surgery. However, there are many different categories of KOs leading to confusion for many prescribers (6,28).

The Swedish knee cage has no knee joint and prevents genu recurvatum but permits flexion. The three-way knee stabilizer orthosis looks similar and gives good control of structural knee instability in the lateral, medial, and posterior directions and is indicated for osteoarthritis, flexible genu valgum, and genu varum and for genu recurvatum of moderate severity. The standard KOs have short lever arms and may not be effective when strong forces are required for joint control. Most KOs tend to slip or migrate down the leg during movement resulting in discomfort from pressure or lack of joint alignment. Chew and colleges classified KOs as unloaders, prophylactic, and patellofemoral orthoses (28). No long-term study is available to support the benefit of the use of the unloader brace in osteoarthritis, but its effectiveness in short-term use has been documented by Pollo (6,29). Several KOs designed with longer lever arms and rotational control components have been commercially produced and prescribed for high-level athletics activities (**Fig. 57-12**).

HIP-KNEE-ANKLE-FOOT ORTHOSES

Hip-knee-ankle-foot orthoses (HKAFOs) consist of the same components as described for the standard AFOs and KAFOs, with the addition of an attached lockable hip joint and a pelvic band to control movements at the anatomic hip joint. The movement in the mediolateral plane is controlled with a single-axis design, while the sagittal motion may be controlled usually with a drop-ring lock. The pelvic band, which may be unilateral or bilateral, encompasses the pelvis between the iliac crest and greater trochanter laterally, curves down over the buttocks, and then passes up again over the sacrum. The indications for prescribing a pelvic band have been controversial because several studies indicate that it increases lumbar excursion and displacement of the center of gravity during ambulation, likely increasing energy cost. For persons with paraplegia, pelvic bands probably are not necessary if they are candidates for Scott-Craig–type orthosis, although they may improve standing balance, especially if flexor spasticity is severe.

The Louisiana State University reciprocating gait orthosis (**Fig. 57-13**) consists of bilateral KAFOs with knee locks, posterior plastic ankle-foot and thigh pieces, a custom-molded pelvic girdle, and special thrust-bearing hip joints, coupled together with a cam and a thoracic extension with Velcro straps (30,31). The cam mechanism provides hip stability by preventing simultaneous bilateral hip flexion yet allows free hip flexion coupled with reciprocal extension of the contralateral hip when weight shift during a step is attempted. Using two crutches, persons with paraplegia are able to ambulate with a four-point reciprocal gait pattern.

Newer orthotic systems that allow the knee joint to flex in the swing phase of walking and provide stability in the stance

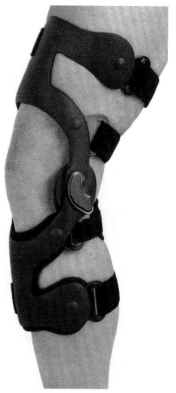

FIGURE 57-12. Knee orthosis to control instability.

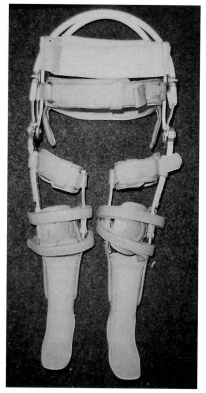

FIGURE 57-13. Louisiana State University reciprocating gait orthosis.

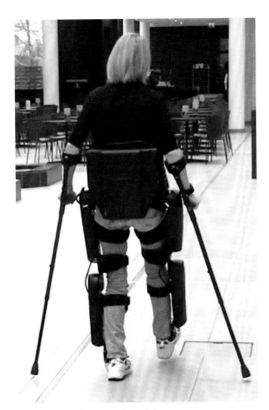

FIGURE 57-14. ReWalk-powered exoskeletons.

phase (stance stabilized orthosis) are becoming more common. The system may use mechanical or electronic systems to achieve knee locking in stance and unlocking in swing phase. Increase weight, cost, and maintenance are the main disadvantages, while normalization of gait pattern with likely reduction of energy consumption in the well-trained subject is the principal advantage (32).

Powered HKAFOs that supply independent hip and knee movement through computer-controlled motors in swing phase and joint stability in stance phase are now in clinical use; ReWalk and Indigo are approved by the Food and Drug Administration for home use and Ekso is approved for institutional training (24,33).

This device affords individuals with paraplegia independent sit to stand transfers, a reciprocal gait pattern on level surfaces, ramps, and curbs while using crutches. **Figure 57-14** here Subject walking with a ReWalk-powered HKAFO.

ORTHOTIC PRESCRIPTION

Orthoses should be prescribed based on the desired biomechanical function (2). A functional problem-oriented–based prescription, such as "orthosis to compensate for ankle dorsiflexion weakness," ensures that the communication with the orthotist is accurate producing the best solution for a particular patient (4). Further specifying the desired materials or specific joint type, function or motion limitations should be pursued when clear understanding of gait biomechanics and knowledge of available orthotic components exist. If this knowledge is not readily available, the prescription should be discussed with the orthotist. Physicians should aim at expanding their knowledge of such information to issue the most appropriate prescription.

A complete lower limb orthotic prescription should consider the diagnosis and type of footwear to be used, include the joints it encompasses, and suggest the desired biomechanical alignment and materials of fabrication for the orthosis (**Fig. 57-2**).

CLINICAL ORTHOTIC ALIGNMENT

Informal visual analysis of gait is routinely used by clinicians to improve the dynamic alignment of an orthosis. This type of analysis does not provide quantitative information and has many limitations due to the speed and complexity of human locomotion (2). Gait deviations and compensations present in the walking pattern of individuals who use orthotic devices further complicate the alignment methodology. Traditionally, a trial and error system is used to attain the best dynamic alignment of a brace (34).

Commonly, clinical observation and patient feedback are the primary sources of information on orthotic alignment. Usually, joint position and range of motion are continually adjusted until both the clinician and the patient are satisfied. Even under the ideal circumstances, orthotic alignment cannot be completely and accurately evaluated until patient stabilization of the compensatory muscle strategies to the device and symptoms has occurred over time.

Gait Analysis

Gait analysis affords the clinical team the opportunity to infuse objectivity into the process of orthotic alignment assessment. Experienced clinicians may assist their biomechanical orthotic prescription process with the use of special quantitative and semiquantitative assessment methods including slow-motion video recording and instrumented kinematic and kinetic gait analysis and dynamic electromyography and energetics (2,34,35).

In some laboratories, force platforms when combined with special hardware permit real-time visualization of a force vector (2,34). This technology provides an excellent visual estimate of the magnitude and polarity of a joint stance-phase moment. Based on its semiquantitative nature, simplicity, and no need for instrumentation of the subject, this information is of significant importance when attempting to optimize biomechanical orthotic alignment (**Fig. 57-15**).

UPPER LIMB

The upper limb is vastly different from the lower limb because of the unique and critical functioning of the hand. It is the role of the shoulder, elbow, and wrist to position the hand properly in space to provide the essential function of gross motor grasp and fine motor skills. The primary purpose of all upper limb orthoses, and the rehabilitation program related to their prescription, is to regain or to preserve prehension of the hand for use in activities of daily living (ADLs). A very common indication for upper limb orthoses is to substitute for weak or absent muscles at the wrist, elbow, or shoulder that fail to properly position the hand or substitute for weak musculature within the hand itself that fails to provide proper prehension and release. Common clinical examples would include brain injury, stroke, cervical spinal injury, brachial plexus injury, or peripheral nerve injury to the median, ulnar, or radial nerves.

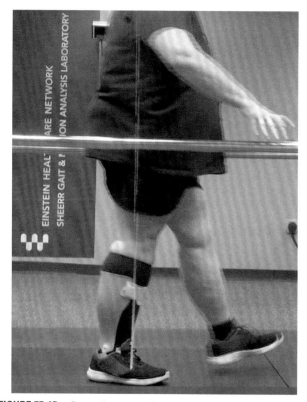

FIGURE 57-15. Brace alignment optimization using force line visualization.

The second goal is to protect damaged or impaired segments such as those commonly seen in cases of surgical repairs, trauma, rheumatoid arthritis, etc. With posttrauma or surgical repair, the orthosis is designed to control loading across injured bony segments or sprained/strained soft tissues, to promote proper healing. This goal is commonly achieved through a series of progressive static or dynamic orthoses, each allowing increasing forces or movement across a joint. In the case of rheumatoid arthritis and other progressive diseases, such as scleroderma, the goal may be slowing the progression of the disease. In these conditions, orthoses are also used as an adjuvant for pain control when inflamed joints must be temporarily immobilized and then over time slowly return to motion.

There are many clinical conditions of upper and lower motor neuron disease or injury affecting the upper limb where proper positioning is critical to prevent contracture or deformity. In these cases, there is no actual disease or injury to the segment included in the orthosis, but there has been proximal neurologic injury creating the risk of muscle force imbalance resulting in deformity or contracture. When contracture is present, efforts should be made to regain range of motion at the affected joints through progressive stretching orthoses.

Alternatively, a patient may be provided with a universal cuff, which wraps around the hand to provide an attachment for eating utensils or other grooming devices or devices to interact with a keyboard or writing.

The balanced forearm orthosis (BFO) is a wheelchair or table-mounted accessory, which attaches to a forearm trough that provides unweighing assistance to the patient arm addressing shoulder weakness to facilitate ADLs, such as feeding and grooming, and even access to household technologies.

ANATOMICAL PRINCIPLES FOR UPPER LIMB

Proper upper limb positioning requires understanding of anatomical plains, particularly when a joint is to be immobilized. The wrist should be immobilized in slight extension and neutral pronation/supination. This position facilitates hand prehension activities to reach the face and midline for ADLs.

The interphalangeal (IP) joints of the fingers should be immobilized in extension, but the metacarpophalangeal (MCP) joints should be immobilized in flexion to maintain the length of the collateral ligaments. The IP and MCP joints should be mobilized as soon as feasible to prevent contractures and adhesions of the tendons.

The thumb should be immobilized opposite the fingers in palmar abduction and extension. The web space should be maximized to maintain both gross grasp and fine motor pinch (**Fig. 57-16**). The hand itself has two transverse arches (proximal and distal metacarpals) with two different radii. These arches must be preserved to maintain proper finger positioning. As each finger is flexed individually, its fingertip points to the scaphoid bone. An orthosis that provides finger flexion must also follow the angle to the scaphoid. Forces across a finger or any other segment should be perpendicular to that segment and follow the anatomical angle of the joint involved to reduce abnormal torque.

COMMON UPPER LIMB ORTHOTIC DESIGNS

Finger and Thumb Orthoses

Simple static orthoses for the fingers or thumb are commonly used to treat sprains, fractures, and burns. They can be partial or circumferential providing both flexion-extension and mediolateral stability across the IP joints. Static finger orthoses with a flexion or extension block allow motion in one direction, but not the other. The best example of this is the finger ring orthoses, commonly used in rheumatoid arthritis (**Fig. 57-17**). The boutonniere's deformity creates flexion at the proximal IP (PIP) joint and hyperextension at the distal IP (DIP) joint. This can be controlled using a ring orthoses to block flexion at the PIP joint. The swan-neck deformity causes hyperextension at the PIP and flexion at the DIP joint. The same ring orthoses design can be reversed to address this problem. A variety of dynamic orthoses across the IP joints of the fingers are used for the purpose of stretching flexion contracture (**Fig. 57-18**). Traction is placed across the contracted joint using spring wire or rubber bands. A progressive

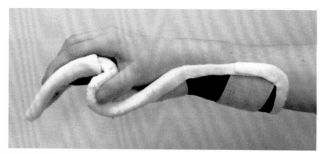

FIGURE 57-16. Proper positioning of the wrist, hand, and finger when immobilized.

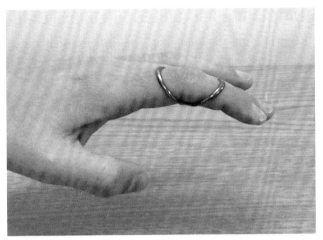

FIGURE 57-17. Static finger ring orthosis.

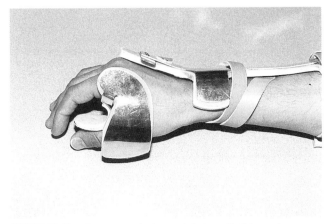

FIGURE 57-19. Opponens orthosis metal design with C-bar and opponens bar to stabilize thumb.

static orthotic program can accomplish the same result with periodic modifications of a static orthosis to stretch the contracture.

Hand-Finger Orthosis

The most common indication for a hand-finger orthosis is to gain control of the MCP joint of the fingers or thumb. Historically, the traditional static hand-finger orthosis consisted of a short opponens orthosis fabricate from metal, which wrapped around the medial or lateral side of the hand, preserving the arch of the hand. This would then act as a platform for outriggers or additional features, which would control the thumb, the MCP joints, or the fingers. A traditional short opponens orthosis would include a C-bar to maintain the web space between the thumb and fingers and an opponens bar to position the thumb opposite the fingers for gross grasp and fine motor pinch (**Fig. 57-19**). This is most commonly used for median nerve injuries where control of opposition is lost. An MCP extension block can also be incorporated into this orthosis to prevent MCP hyperextension (claw-hand deformity), which occurs in both median and ulnar nerve injuries. This modification allows the remaining intrinsic hand muscles to function more effectively. The design can be replicated using plastics with a circumferential design to maintain the transverse arches of the hand, place the thumb in opposition, and act as a platform for other attachments. The term "thumb spica" refers to a hand-finger orthosis, which is based on the hand and extends circumferentially around the thumb to fix the thumb in opposition (**Fig. 57-20**). This is commonly

prescribed for inflammatory conditions affecting the thumb and can also be used for fracture of the first metacarpal.

Dynamic hand-finger orthoses are most commonly used for flexion or extension contracture across the MCP joints using a three-point control principle with a force applied close to the MCP joint and opposing counterforces proximal and distal. The common "knuckle-bender orthosis" is used to stretch the extension contracture at the MCP joints when collateral ligaments have been allowed to shorten due to immobilization (**Fig. 57-21**). Dynamic hand-finger orthoses can also be used for more vigorous stretching of flexion contracture at the PIP joints.

As the flexion contracture improves, the positioning of the outrigger must be adjusted to maintain proper joint alignment. Failure to provide MCP extension block may simply create hyperextension across the MCP and failure to stretch the PIP contracture.

Wrist-Hand-Finger Orthosis

Static wrist-hand orthoses are used for the treatment of carpal tunnel syndrome, which commonly results from overuse of the wrist causing inflammation within the carpal tunnel. Immobilization of the wrist in neutral (i.e., 0 degrees of extension) while allowing freedom of thumb and finger movement can help reduce symptoms (**Fig. 57-22**). Static wrist-hand-finger orthoses are also commonly used as the first step following injury or repair to hand flexor or extensor tendons. A short period of protective immobilization is often

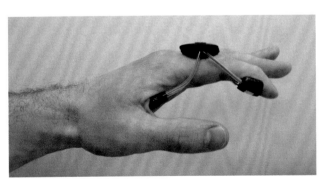

FIGURE 57-18. Dynamic finger orthoses.

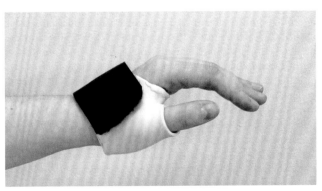

FIGURE 57-20. Thumb spica.

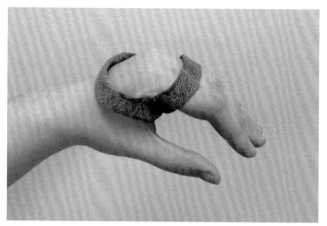

FIGURE 57-21. "Knuckle-bender" orthosis. Dynamic design to promote flexion at the MCP joint.

followed by limited motion to prevent tendon adhesions and joint contracture. With flexor tendon repair, the wrist is commonly positioned in neutral or slight flexion with the MCP joint motion blocked in flexion and the IP joints allowed to go to full extension. Often, flexion traction may be applied across the fingers to eliminate tension across the repair and promote a protective position (**Fig. 57-23**). As healing progresses, further motion of the MCP is allowed with full extension at the wrist until the healing is complete. The wrist-hand-finger orthosis for extensor tendon repair includes a reverse approach to the design where the wrist is positioned in neutral or extension position with a flexion block at the MCP and IP joints of the involved fingers. Flexion traction may be applied to reduce tension across the tendon repair site (**Fig. 57-24**). As healing progresses, further flexion is allowed at the MCP and IP joints and, once healing is complete, full motion allowed.

Radial nerve injury also requires a wrist-hand-finger orthosis to assist wrist and finger extension with rubber bands or spring wire providing extension at the wrist and outriggers with rubber bands providing extension at the fingers while maintaining the thumb in opposition.

The tenodesis prehension orthosis or flexor hinge orthosis is a dynamic wrist-hand-finger orthosis incorporating active wrist extension movement to promote gross grasp and fine motor pinch of the thumb and fingers. This is used for C6-level quadriplegia where wrist extension strength is maintained and can be used to supplement grasp (**Fig. 57-25**).

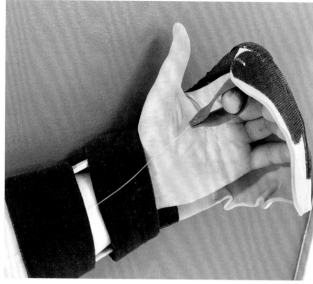

FIGURE 57-23. Dynamic wrist-hand-finger orthosis with extension block at MCP joint and fingers and dynamic traction at the index finger.

Static wrist-hand-finger orthoses can be used for positioning of the hand following stroke, brain injury, or brachial plexus injury. The MCP joints are positioned in flexion and the IP joints in full extension to prevent contracture of the collateral ligaments.

Elbow Orthoses

Dynamic elbow orthoses are commonly used for flexion or extension contracture across the elbow. If burn scars are involved, total contact across the burn scar area should be attempted for compression.

Various spring-loaded elbow orthoses are commercially available, which can be adjusted to steadily increase tension across the elbow as stretching progresses (**Fig. 57-26**). Spring-assisted elbow orthoses may be useful to augment elbow flexion when weakness or paralysis of the elbow flexor muscles exists. Static circumferential orthoses across the elbow are often used for fractures at or near the elbow. Fracture splinting of the radius and ulna should incorporate the elbow, wrist, and hand to control pronation and supination. An adjustable elbow lock

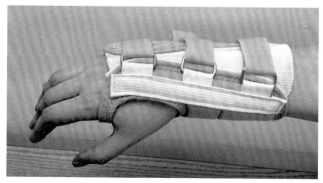

FIGURE 57-22. Static wrist-hand orthosis.

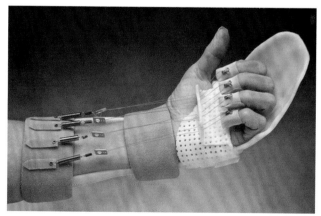

FIGURE 57-24. Dynamic wrist-hand-finger orthosis with flexion block at MCP joint and fingers and traction at fingers.

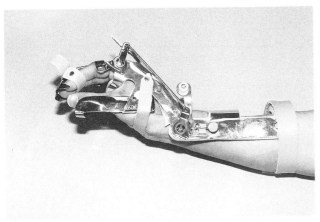

FIGURE 57-25. Dynamic wrist-hand-finger tenodesis orthosis with traditional metal flexor hinge design.

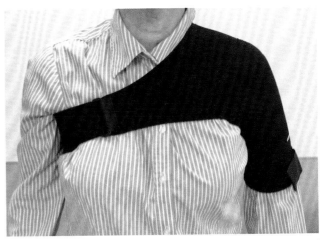

FIGURE 57-27. Flexible shoulder orthosis used to control humeral subluxation.

can be incorporated to steadily allow increase flexion or extension motion. Humeral fracture management may include a circumferential orthosis across the entire humeral segment and forearm. This would slowly progress allowing movement at the elbow as healing of the humeral fracture occurs.

Shoulder Orthoses

Flexible arm slings of various sorts have been used for a variety of shoulder problems including clavicular fracture, acromioclavicular joint injury, proximal humeral fracture, and glenohumeral subluxation due to hemiparesis.

These orthoses commonly consist of fabrics and straps that encompass the mid to proximal humerus and then extend across the shoulder anteriorly and posteriorly to the opposite axilla (**Fig. 57-27**). The primary goal is to maintain glenohumeral integrity and to limit motion across the AC and glenohumeral joints.

A true static shoulder-elbow-wrist-hand orthosis, such as the airplane splint or arm abduction orthosis, can prevent movement across the glenohumeral joint (**Fig. 57-28**). Care must be taken to mobilize the glenohumeral joint as soon as possible to prevent adhesive capsulitis.

Other specialized orthoses in this category include the BFO for patients with C5-level spinal injury. This device includes a forearm trough, which is suspended on a series of brackets and swivels mounted on the wheelchair. This significantly reduces the weight of the arm and allows the patient to use elbow flexion and shoulder adduction/abduction for limited ADLs. A universal cuff or hand orthosis can attach a swivel spoon or other device, which would allow independent feeding (**Fig. 57-29**). Finally, a combination of prosthetic and orthotic components can be used for the patient with brachial plexus injury to create a shoulder-elbow-wrist-hand orthosis to regain some limited prehension at the hand once the elbow is locked and stabilized. A dual control cable actuated by a

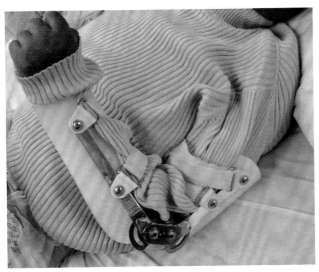

FIGURE 57-26. Dynamic elbow orthosis.

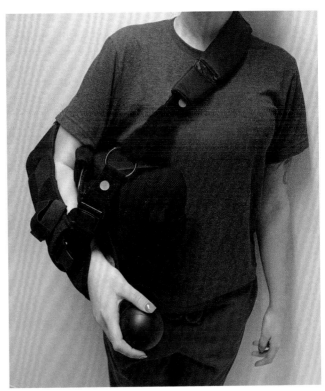

FIGURE 57-28. "Airplane splint" for static humeral abduction positioning.

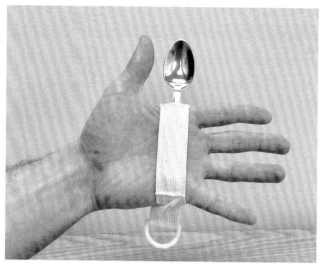

FIGURE 57-29. Universal cuff with spoon inserted.

figure-of-8 harness can use biscapular abduction to position the elbow and activate a prehension terminal device at the hand when there is complete paralysis at the elbow and hand (**Fig. 57-30**). The paralyzed limb can then be used as a gross assist or stabilizer.

Not different than the lower limb, the concept of neural activation has recently been incorporated into upper limb orthoses. Commercially available devices are now being used to create prehension or gross grasp in the paralyzed limb. These devices detect a myoelectric signal from an intact proximal muscle and then send a stimulating signal to distal paralyzed

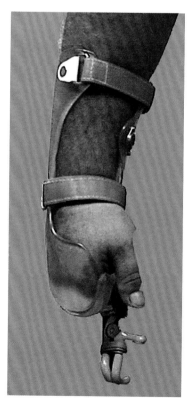

FIGURE 57-30. Wrist-hand orthosis with prosthetic hook for prehension.

muscles to contract via surface-based or implanted electrical stimulation. Stimulating electrodes for the finger flexor and extensor muscle groups create grasp and release maneuvers. For some devices, the wrist-hand orthotic component supports the wrist. The usefulness of these devices is variable and is dependent upon multiple factors such as muscle tone, target muscle excitability, and the presence of contractures as well as tolerance to the stimulation. Good strength and control at the shoulder and elbow greatly enhance the functionality of these devices.

A team approach with communication between the prescribing physician, patient, and therapist/orthotist will ensure fabrication and fit of a proper upper limb orthosis. Adequate instruction to the patient and appropriate therapy and follow-up will help reduce possible complications and achieve a favorable outcome.

SPINAL ORTHOSIS

Trunk support can be achieved by an increase in the intra-abdominal pressure reducing the demand on the spinal extensor musculature and the vertical loading and intradiscal pressure on the thoracolumbar spine (see also Chapters 27 and 28).

Spinal alignment and stability are achieved by the application of the previously discussed three-point force biomechanical principle inherent in all bracing. The corrective component ideally is located midway between the opposing forces above and below it. At each spinal level, orthoses require different designs to achieve their expected function. The desired physiologic effect must be considered when prescribing an orthosis so that the least restrictive device capable of achieving the desire goal is prescribed. For example, if trunk support by thoracoabdominal containment is sufficient to reduce compressive forces on the spine and stress on the musculature, then joint motion stabilization may not be necessary (14). Before orthotic prescription, determining the indication and goals for it is imperative. Once the treatment goal has been achieved and the device is no longer needed, it should be discontinued. There is no consensus, and much controversy surrounding the orthosis choice and the time length needed for immobilization.

Spinal orthoses are grouped by the anatomical joints they encompass. They may further be differentiated by the motion they restrict or allow. Within each group, there are multiple designs (**Table 57-1**).

Effective spinal bracing is complicated and needs to take into account multiple factors. It is influenced by achieving correct fit, body habitus, ability to restrict gross and segmental vertebral motion, and having patient compliance and willingness to tolerate a snug-fitting appliance. The effectiveness of the brace may be compromised if they loosen the straps. Individuals

TABLE 57-1	**Categories of Orthoses**

Cervical (CO)—soft or rigid head cervical (Philadelphia, Aspen, Miami, Newport)
Cervicothoracic (CTO)—Halo, SOMI, Minerva, any rigid collar with an anterior or posterior extension
Thoracolumbosacral (TLSO)—custom-molded body jacket, CASH, Jewitt
Lumbosacral (LSO)—chairback, Knight, corsets/binders
Sacroiliac (SO)—trochanteric belt, sacral belt, sacral corset

TABLE 57-2	**Effects of Cervical Collars on Percent Mean Motion Permitted**			
	Flexion/Extension	**Lateral Flexion**	**Rotation**	**Source**
Soft collar	74.2	92	83	Johnson
	91	91	89	Sandler
	92	92	91	Carter
Philadelphia	29	67	44	Johnson
	58/53	78	52	Lunsford
	60	89	73	Sandler
Miami J	41	—	20	Richter[a]
	52/62	65	52	Lunsford
	40/46			Gavin
Malibu	47/43	59	39	Lunsford
Newport	63/62	73	51	Lunsford
Aspen	31/48	—	—	Gavin
Aspen 2 post CTO	16/39	—	—	Gavin
Aspen 4 post CTO	12/20	—	—	Gavin
Minerva	46		14	Richter[a]
SOMI	28	66	34	Johnson
	39	82	82	Sandler
Halo	4	4	1	Johnson

[a]Richter only studied the upper cervical spine.

with a short stout neck and no defined chin are harder to fit with certain devices such as a cervical collar.

Pendulous breasts, short trunk, thoracic kyphosis, or an obese abdomen make it difficult to fit cervicothoracic or thoracolumbosacral orthoses. Two braces may need to be given to the patient so that one can be washed on a regular basis in order to maintain hygiene. Skin under the brace needs to be checked and washed daily. While using the brace, an exercise program should be implemented, if no contraindication exists to prevent disuse. In addition, the patient or caregiver must be instructed in donning and doffing techniques and its wearing schedule.

Cervical Orthoses

Cervical bracing can be categorized in two broad categories: cervical and cervicothoracic. Cervical devices encircle the cervical spine, whereas cervicothoracic braces extend into the thoracic spine. When adding a thoracic extension piece, the cervical orthosis (CO) provides greater motion control of the lower cervical spine. To limit extension and hyperextension of the cervical spine, an intimate fit under the occiput must be achieved. With cervical appliances, motion control varies based on the type of device. Soft collar provides minimal restriction, while a halo offers significant movement control. Several studies have examined the effects of various orthoses on cervical range of motion. These studies used different methods to quantify the amount of motion (e.g., radiographic analysis, goniometric assessment, and computerized spinal motion analysis). In addition, the sample size and population characteristics varied widely (i.e., cadaver models, healthy spines vs. injured spines). **Table 57-2** outlines motion allowed (3,13,16,18,19,28). For the orthosis to provide motion control, it must fit properly and be worn by the user.

It is essential to be aware of the potential adverse effects of bracing. Weakness, atrophy, and joint contracture may follow restriction of motion and inactivity. Skin irritation from poor fit, hygiene, perspiration, and shear and pressure can result in pressure sores, pain, and infection. Impaired ambulation and balance can result from the limitation in motion and weight of the device such as with a halo device, which in turn may make an individual more dependent in their activities of daily living. There can be a decrease in pulmonary capacity due to the restricted chest wall motion and potential increase in energy consumption. Eating and swallowing may be compromised due to the position of the head and neck. Psychological dependence on the brace can also develop, particularly for those using the device for pain control. Patients with certain medical conditions (e.g., neuromuscular disease), body types, and personalities may not be able to tolerate them.

SUMMARY

We have reviewed the basic principles of orthotic interventions for the upper and lower limb and spine, as they apply to the rehabilitation of patients with central and peripheral neurologic pathology and musculoskeletal disorders. The majority of patients may use orthoses to attempt to optimize their functional capabilities and improved quality of life. Orthoses are devices that are applied to the external surface of the body to achieve one or more of the following: relieve pain, immobilize musculoskeletal segments, reduce axial load, prevent or correct deformity, and improve function. Orthotics for the lower limbs are an integral part of the rehabilitative medical management of the patient population we serve.

REFERENCES

1. Kumar R, Roe MC, Scremin OU. Methods to estimate the proper length of a cane. *Arch Phys Med Rehabil.* 1995;76:1173–1175.
2. Esquenazi, A. Assessment and orthotic management of gait dysfunction in individuals with traumatic brain injury. In: Hsu J, Michael JW, Fisk J, eds. *AAOS Atlas of Orthoses and Assistive Devices.* 4th ed. Philadelphia, PA: Mosby, Elsevier Inc.; 2008:441–447. Chapter 34.
3. Condie ND. International Organization for Standardization (ISO) of terminology. In: Hsu J, Michael JW, Fisk J, eds. *AAOS Atlas of Orthoses and Assistive Devices.* 4th ed. Philadelphia, PA: Mosby, Elsevier Inc.; 2008:3–7. Chapter 1.

4. Esquenazi A, Hirai B. Gait analysis in stroke and head injury. In: Craik RL, Oatis CA, eds. *Gait Analysis, Theory and Application*. St. Louis, MO: Mosby; 1995:412–419.

5. Lunsford TR, Contoyannis B. Materials science. In: Hsu J, Michael JW, Fisk J, eds. *AAOS Atlas of Orthoses and Assistive Devices*. 4th ed. Philadelphia, PA: Mosby, Elsevier Inc.; 2008:15–51. Chapter 3.

6. Micheo W, Esquenazi A. Orthoses in the Prevention and Rehabilitation of Injuries. In: Frontera WR, ed. *Rehabilitation of Sports Injuries: Scientific Basis*. International Olympic Committee; 2003:301–315. Chapter 15.

7. Fisk JR, DeMuth S, Campbell J, et al. Suggested guidelines for the prescription of orthotic services, device delivery, education, and follow-up care: a multidisciplinary white paper. *Mil Med*. 2016;181(2):11–17.

8. Esquenazi A, Wikoff E, Hirai B, et al. Effects of a plantar flexed plastic molded ankle foot orthosis on gait pattern and lower limb muscle strength. Proceedings of the VI World Congress of the International Society for Prosthetics and Orthotics; 1989:208.

9. Lehmann JF. Biomechanics of ankle foot orthoses: prescription and design. *Arch Phys Med Rehabil*. 1979;160:200–207.

10. Staheli LT. Shoes for children: a review. *Pediatrics*. 1991;88:371–375.

11. Janisse DJ. Picking the shoe to fit the occasion. In: Hantula R, ed. *The Best of Diabetes Self Management*. New York: DSM Books; 2002:1130.

12. Kerrigan DC, Johansson JL, Bryant MG, et al. Moderate-heeled shoes and knee joint torques relevant to the development and progression of knee osteoarthritis. *Arch Phys Med Rehabil*. 2005;86(5):871–875.

13. Chen RCC, Lord M. A comparison of trial shoe and shell shoe fitting techniques. *Prosthet Orthot Int*. 1995;19:181–187.

14. Boulton AJM, Betts RP, Franks CI, et al. The natural history of foot pressure abnormalities in neuropathic diabetic subjects. *Diabetes Res*. 1987;5:73–77.

15. Esquenazi A, Talaty M, Jayaraman A. Powered exoskeletons for walking assistance in persons with central nervous system injuries. A narrative review. *PM R*. 2017;9: 46–62. doi:10.1016/j.pmr.2016.07.534.

16. Decker W, Albert S. *Contemporary Pedorthics*. Seattle, WA: Elton-Wolf; 2002:1070.

17. Robbins S, Waked E, McClaran J. Proprioception and stability: foot position awareness as a function of age and footwear. *Age Ageing*. 1995;24:67–72.

18. David S. Sims, Jr, Peter R. Cavanagh, Jan S. Ulbrecht. Risk factors in the diabetic foot: recognition and management. Physical Therapy. 1 December 1988;68(12): 1887–1902. Available at: https://doi.org/10.1093/ptj/68.12.1887

19. Brown M, Rudicel S, Esquenazi A. Measurement of dynamic pressures at the shoe-foot interface during normal walking with various foot orthosis using a new version of the FSCAN system. *Foot Ankle Int*. 1991:152–156.

20. Zamosky I, Licht S, Redford JB. Shoes and their modifications. In: Redford JB, ed. *Orthotics Etcetera*. Baltimore, MD: Williams & Wilkins; 1980:368–431.

21. Zhu H, Wertsch JJ, Harris GF, et al. Sensate and insensate in-shoe plantar pressures. *Arch Phys Med Rehabil*. 1993;74:1362–1368.

22. Janisse DJ, Wertsch J, Del Toro D. Foot orthoses and prescription footwear. In: Redford J, Basmajian J, Trautman P, eds. *Orthotics: Clinical Practice and Rehabilitation Technology*. Kansas City, MO: Churchill Livingstone; 1995:1120.

23. Sheffler LR, Hennessey MT, Naples GG, et al. Peroneal nerve stimulation versus an ankle foot orthosis for correction of footdrop in stroke: impact on functional ambulation. *Neurorehabil Neural Repair*. 2006;20(3):355–360.

24. Esquenazi A, Mayer N, Lee S, et al.; PROS Study Group. Patient registry of outcomes in spasticity care. *Am J Phys Med Rehabil*. 2012;91:729–746.

25. O'Daniel WE, Hahn HR. Follow-up usage of the Scott-Craig orthosis in paraplegia. *Paraplegia*. 1981;19:373–378.

26. Lehneis HR. New developments in lower limb orthotics through bioengineering. *Arch Phys Med Rehabil*. 1972;53:303–310.

27. Taktak DM, Bowker P. Lightweight modular knee-ankle-foot orthosis for Duchenne muscular dystrophy: design, development and evaluation. *Arch Phys Med Rehabil*. 1995;76:1156–1162.

28. Chew KTL, Lew HL, Date E, et al. Current evidence and clinical applications of therapeutic knee braces. *Am J Phys Med Rehabil*. 2007;86(8):678–686.

29. Pollo FE, Otis JC, Backus SI, et al. Reduction of medial compartment loads with valgus bracing of the osteoarthritic knee. *Am J Sports Med*. 2002;30:414–421.

30. Douglas R, Larson PF, D'Ambrosia R, et al. The LSU reciprocation-gait orthosis. *Orthopedics*. 1983;6:834–839.

31. Durr-Fillauer Medical, Inc. *LSU Reciprocating Gait Orthoses: A Pictorial Description and Application Manual*. Chattanooga, TN: Durr-Fillauer Medical, Inc.; 1983.

32. Michael JW. Lower limb orthoses. In: Hsu J, Michael JW, Fisk J, eds. *AAOS Atlas of Orthoses and Assistive Devices*. 4th ed. Philadelphia, PA: Mosby, Elsevier Inc.; 2008:343–355. Chapter 26.

33. Zeilig G, Levy A, Goffer A. A study for testing safety and tolerance of the ReWalk™, a walking device for people with complete long standing spinal cord injury. Proceedings of the International Spinal Cord Society; 2008; Durban, South Africa.

34. Esquenazi A, Talaty M, Seliktar R, et al. Dynamic electromyography during walking as an objective measurement of lower limb orthotic alignment. *Basic Appl Myol*. 1997;7(2):103–110.

35. Bampton S. *A Guide to the Visual Examination of Pathological Gait*. Temple University-Moss Rehabilitation Hospital, Rehabilitation Research and Training Center #8. Philadelphia, PA: 1979.

Lynn A. Worobey
Stephanie K. Rigot
Michael L. Boninger

CHAPTER 58

Wheelchairs

Freedom of movement is an essential component of human independence. In the National Academy of Medicine model on the enablement/disablement process (1), a wheelchair and its components are fundamental for altering the interaction a person with a mobility limitation has with the environment. Not surprisingly, studies in various populations and cultures have repeatedly shown that mobility is closely tied to quality of life (2–6). It is therefore critical that the physiatrist takes an active role in the wheelchair prescription process. Fundamental to this role is knowledge related to the understanding of the complex components that make up seating and wheelchairs. In this chapter, the readers will find information to help them gain an understanding of different manual, power, and hybrid wheelchairs. The importance of the wheelchair-user interface, ride comfort, durability, selection of accessories, and powered wheelchair control devices is also stressed. The readers are introduced to wheelchair and seating measurements and a variety of cushions and postural supports.

PRESCRIPTION PROCESS

The World Health Organization has been working to increase the access to wheelchairs for people with disabilities around the globe. The WHO Wheelchair Service Training package outlines eight necessary steps for wheelchair delivery: referral, assessment, prescription, funding, wheelchair preparation, fitting, user training, and maintenance repairs and follow-up (7). Each of these steps is presented in this chapter.

Team Approach

The complexity of wheelchair and seating components combined with the nuances of individuals and various disease processes make it virtually impossible for a single clinician to act independently when prescribing assistive technology for mobility. For this reason, it is important to involve an interdisciplinary team in the decision-making process (8). The most important team member is the patient. The opinions and desires of the patient are critical to a successful fitting but must be assessed in terms of their level of knowledge and insight. Some patients have been using a wheelchair for years and know exactly what they are looking for. For these individuals, team members act to provide unbiased information. Alternatively, a novice patient may have little knowledge of what is available and the trade-offs of each decision. For this individual, the team will need to be more directive. The family and caregiver should also provide input, as they will be the next most affected by the choice of wheelchair. Client involvement may lead to less equipment abandonment and increased satisfaction and perceived benefit from the equipment (9,10).

The assessment team can consist of a variety of rehabilitation professionals (eBox 58-1). Currently, Medicare and the majority of private insurance companies in the United States require a face-to-face physician assessment before providing a wheelchair. This face-to-face visit is a physician appointment that specifically addresses the need for the wheelchair as presented in the steps below. Given the training on function and mobility, a physiatrist can be the most appropriate physician to complete this assessment. Often an occupational or physical therapist working with the physician will conduct an evaluation. Ideally, the therapist will be certified by The Rehabilitation Engineering and Assistive Technology Society of North America (RESNA) as an assistive technology practitioner (ATP). An additional certification by RESNA as a Seating and Mobility Specialist (SMS) is also now available focused specifically on seating, mobility, and positioning. Other professionals who can be certified and may be part of the team include a rehabilitation engineer, an Assistive Technology Supplier (ATS), or Certified Rehabilitation Technology Supplier (CRTS, National Association of Rehabilitation Technology Suppliers). Those involved in the wheelchair selection process should have knowledge about the technology available in the market.

Patient History

The interview process must obtain standard information such as age, past medical history, and current medical diagnosis. It is essential to determine if the individual's physical impairment is changing rapidly or is stable. It is also important to establish the diagnosis that requires the wheelchair and to assure that there are no ongoing medical problems or complications that can affect the wheelchair prescription and the patient's health. However, unless the medical picture does not make sense or a condition has not been fully evaluated, this is not a diagnostic evaluation.

The most important aspect of the history is evaluating and documenting the user's functional goals and how their current assistive technology or lack thereof, meets these needs. The process involves obtaining critical information from the user about his or her environment, family support, and past use of assistive technology. It is important to understand both the intentions and the abilities of the user (11) to ensure that the wheelchair will be accepted and used. Also, if the patient has been using wheeled mobility, historical information about his or her current device should be addressed, including problems he or she may be having.

Additional necessary information includes type of insurance, physical capabilities, if the individual is able to transport a wheelchair and the environment in which the chair will be used. For example, access to a range of heights might be important to reach objects in the home and other environments. To support vocational needs, specific requirements may exist for mobility within a laboratory, operating room, courtroom, or machine shop. Leisure activities, pursued in such places as community centers, restaurants, movie theaters, and recreational environments, often place the most demands on the wheelchair. The surface conditions may impose restrictions on the type of wheelchair that is most appropriate. The regularity of the surface and its firmness and stability are important in determining the tire size, drive wheel location, and wheel diameter. The wheelchair model chosen should also be compatible with the user's public and private transportation needs (such as a bus, train, car, van, or airplane) and home/activities of daily living (ADL) environment.

Physical Examination

With an understanding of the individual's need or desire to perform different activities, the next step is examining the user. The history likely provided significant insight related to his or her physical abilities. To verify this, a physical examination should focus on aspects of the patient that will help (a) justify the wheelchair and seating system, (b) determine the most appropriate wheelchair and seating system, and (c) assure that medical issues are appropriately addressed. Based on the interview of the patient, it may be possible to omit some portions of the examination listed below.

Often individuals require a wheelchair because of cardiopulmonary disease. For these individuals, it is important to document a heart and lung examination. Attention should be paid to dyspnea on exertion and changes in vital signs with activity. These findings can be used to justify a power wheelchair, as the energy cost of wheelchair propulsion is not less than that of walking (12). Other common reasons for requiring a wheelchair are musculoskeletal and neurologic deficits. The clinician should document the neurologic and musculoskeletal deficits in a methodical fashion. In a patient with a stroke, for example, an examination to check for neglect or visual field deficit is important because it can impact the ability to independently drive a chair.

Obvious examination items include strength and range of motion. For individuals with chronic arthritis problems, the examination should document the painful, swollen, or malaligned joints. When no strength deficit is seen, it is important to document issues with coordination, tone, and proprioception. For example, a study by Fay et al. found that many individuals with multiple sclerosis were unable to effectively propel manual wheelchairs due to increased tone and decreased coordination (13). Participants also showed an inability to maintain a speed comparable to community walking speed (1 m/s). This type of finding can provide justification for the device selected.

While completing the examination, the rehabilitation team should be thinking about how the individual will control the wheelchair. If there is poor hand coordination, head or switch control may be needed. In certain cases, a foot joystick may be possible. Stability should be assessed by observing the individual in a current wheelchair or by asking him or her to sit unsupported on a mat table. Ask the patient to perform simple reaching tasks to determine the lateral and forward stability of the trunk, hand and arm strength, and hand fine motor skills.

Poor stability usually indicates the need for special attention to seating and positioning. Appropriate seating can enhance reach and stability, thus improving the performance of manual activities from the wheelchair. A critical point to evaluate is hip, knee, and ankle range of motion because contractures may need to be accommodated. The presence of kyphosis, scoliosis, or other fixed deformities should also be determined. It is well known that various groups of wheelchair users, such as individuals with tetraplegia and cerebral palsy, will develop kyphosis or scoliosis over time (14). What is less well known is whether spinal deformities can be prevented with appropriate seating. Even if prevention is not a goal, accommodation is needed for comfortable seating.

Finally, a thorough check of the individual's skin is important. This may not be needed for individuals with cardiopulmonary disease, but it is essential for individuals with neurologic deficits or those with previous history of pressure sores. The examination should include not only the buttocks but also the feet and calves, which can be affected by pressure against a leg rest. Attention should be paid to bony prominences and previous scars. This examination will help with cushion selection and wheelchair setup. Large, previously untreated ulcers are sometimes discovered, ultimately leading to treatment before seating plans can be implemented. Pressure mapping can also be completed with the user seated in their chair or on other demo cushions to determine if there are high-pressure areas.

For many people, a few simple measurements can be used to determine the proper dimensions for a wheelchair (15). Body measurements are typically made with the patient in the seated position. Probably the most obvious body measurements are the patient's height and weight. Weight is critical to obtaining a wheelchair that is sufficiently strong as many wheelchairs are only rated to hold up to 113 kg (250 lb). The height of the wheelchair user provides information about the person's size and can be used to check the final wheelchair measurements. For example, the sum of the sitting height, sitting depth, and lower-leg length should be close to the person's supine height. Additional measurements and definitions are used when specialized seating and postural support systems are required.

Other Considerations

For some individuals, the examination and history will not necessarily establish a clear need for a wheelchair. In these cases, it is important to consider alternative options that meet the individual's functional needs. It is important to establish how long the individual will be using the chair. If from the history and examination it is determined that the deficit will be transient, then a rental chair may be appropriate. Medicare will rent chairs for its beneficiaries. If during the history and physical examination medical issues that require intervention are identified, it may be appropriate to delay wheelchair prescription so that changes in the patient status do not necessitate changes in the prescription. In such case, a rental may provide short-term mobility.

The evaluation process should include a home assessment to make sure the device selected will work in the home environment. A home assessment conducted by the supplier is required by Medicare to ensure that the individual can navigate his or her home environment including doorways, thresholds, and different floor surfaces (16). This requirement highlights the importance of working with qualified suppliers such as those with the ATS credentials. If a home visit is conducted, a report of the visit should be included in the documentation.

Outcome measures should be used whenever possible to assess the users' baseline as well as the success of the wheelchair provision process. Some examples of outcome measures available at no cost include Goal Attainment Scale (GAS), Community Integration Measure (CIM), Impact on Participation and Autonomy (IPA), WHO Quality of Life—BREF (WHOQOL-BREF), Individually Prioritized Problem Assessment (IPPA), Wheelchair Users Shoulder Pain Index (WUSPI), Craig Handicap Assessment and Reporting Technique (CHART), IPA Questionnaire, Wheelchair Outcome Measure (WhOM), Wheelchair Skills Test (WST), and Functional Mobility Assessment (FMA) (9,17).

Documentation

Providing appropriate and quality wheelchairs requires well-organized and often extensive documentation. At the very least, a prescription and various insurance forms must be provided as well as a note that documents a face-to-face evaluation with the physician. For more expensive and complex interventions, a letter of medical necessity (LMN), which more specifically documents the team's findings and justifies the details of the wheelchair prescription, is required. eBox 58-2 in the electronic appendix lists Medicare-recommended assessment findings for power wheelchair provision. This letter usually consists of two components: a cover letter and the "client/patient evaluation and intake form." The cover letter summarizes the person's disability, problems with existing equipment or method of mobility, evaluation procedures, conclusions, explanation of why lower-cost alternatives will not suffice, risks of not providing the equipment, and a line-item justification for each of the various components being recommended. The "client/patient evaluation and intake form" guides the evaluation process and captures in-depth information of the evaluation findings required to support recommendations of the appropriate seating and mobility interventions. Often, a part of this examination will be completed by an occupational or physical therapist. The therapist will perform clinical trials and simulations, which allow the patient to try many different devices. Information from the patient's medical record including laboratory tests, imaging, and other diagnostic tests may be relevant to include (18).

In order for any health insurance provider to approve coverage for a wheelchair and seating system, the practitioner must establish and document medical necessity. Each funding source may have its own definition of "medically necessary," however; in general when it comes to wheelchairs, it is necessary to accommodate or replace a malfunctioning body part (i.e., paralysis or weakness of the lower extremities) or to reduce or manage disability. Many funding sources also require the recommended intervention to be the least costly, reasonable alternative. Therefore, as part of an evaluation, it is helpful to document that lower-cost alternatives have been tried and were unsuccessful and to cite specific reasons for the higher-cost choice. It is also helpful to document the potential outcomes if the person is not provided with the equipment. Examples of these risks include falls and fractures, development of pressure sores, joint contractures and musculoskeletal deformities, increased pain and discomfort, loss of function,

and ultimately being more restricted to a bed or chair. The final letter is reviewed and cosigned by both the therapist and physician.

Follow-Up

It is important that the delivery and the final fitting of the device is documented and verified by a follow-up visit with the team or one of the team members. With the support of the team, this visit ensures the client is comfortable providing final acceptance and approval of the device and provides the supplier with appropriate clinical delivery documentation. Finally, this visit can be used to refine the patient's wheelchair driving skills to enable safe operation. These skills can include driving, operation, maintenance, basic skills like proper propulsion technique and turning, as well as community level skills such as wheelies or threshold and curb negotiation. The Wheelchair Skills Training Program (WSTP, Dalhousie University) offers freely available evidence-based training materials grounded in motor learning principles (http://www.wheelchairskillsprogram.ca). These materials are accompanied by validated outcome measures for capacity and performance as evaluated by a rater, the WST, and the self-reported, Wheelchair Skills Test Questionnaire (WST-Q). The effectiveness of WSTP interventions has been demonstrated in 1:1 training, pairs, and group training to improve capacity among wheelchair users and clinicians (19–24).

MANUAL WHEELCHAIRS

Manual wheelchairs offer many advantages over powered mobility. Manual wheelchairs are much easier to transport because of their lighter weight. No special equipment is needed to place a manual wheelchair in a backseat, and individuals with paraplegia and tetraplegia are often capable of transporting their wheelchairs independently without additional technology. In addition, manual wheelchairs generally require less maintenance than do power devices, as there are no concerns related to batteries or controllers. Finally, manual wheelchairs offer a degree of physical exercise that can benefit the wheelchair user.

Depot Wheelchairs

The depot or institutional wheelchair is essentially the same wheelchair that was produced in the 1940s. This type of chair corresponds to the Medicare category of K0001 and, despite its numerous shortcomings, is the default chair for many insurance companies and Medicare. Today's depot wheelchairs may be a bit lighter than the 1940s models, but the basic frame design is unchanged, and they continue to weigh greater than 16 kg (36 lb). The weight of these devices is an important factor to consider with prescription as older adults report weight of the chair being a primary factor in abandonment (25). Depot wheelchairs are intended for institutional use, where many people may use the same wheelchair. These wheelchairs are typically used in airports, hospitals, and nursing care facilities. They are inappropriate for active people who use wheelchairs for personal mobility, including older persons in nursing homes. Depot wheelchairs are designed to be inexpensive, low maintenance, and attendant propelled and accommodate large variations in body size. Unlike the attendant-propelled chairs described below, depot chairs are designed neither for the comfort of the person being transported nor for that of

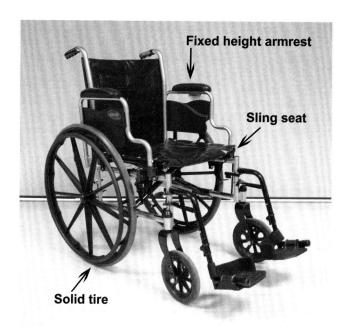

FIGURE 58-1. K0001 depot-style wheelchair.

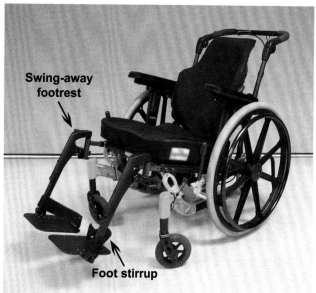

FIGURE 58-2. Attendant-propelled wheelchair with tilt-in-space.

the person pushing the chair. A typical depot wheelchair will have swing-away footrests, often removable armrests, a single cross-brace frame, and solid tires (**Fig. 58-1**). Depot wheelchairs have sling seats and back supports, which are uncomfortable and provide little support. Swing-away footrests add weight to the wheelchair; however, they make transferring into and out of the wheelchair easier. Armrests provide some comfort and stability to the depot wheelchair user and can aid in keeping clothing off the wheels. Depot chairs typically fold to reduce the area for storage and transportation. Solid tires are commonly used to reduce maintenance. Solid tires typically dramatically reduce ride comfort, increase rolling resistance, and add weight. There is very little, if anything, that can be adjusted to fit the user on a depot chair. Typically, only the legrest length is adjustable. Depot chairs are available in various seat widths, seat depths, and backrest heights.

Attendant-Propelled Chairs

Not all wheelchairs are propelled by the person sitting in the wheelchair. In many hospitals and long-term care facilities, wheelchairs are expected to be propelled by attendants. In addition, some individuals with severe disabilities are unable to propel a wheelchair or control a power wheelchair. For children who use attendant-propelled chairs, it is necessary to continually reassess if they may be able to use independent mobility. The primary consideration in the attendant-propelled chair is that the wheelchair has two users: the rider and the attendant. If the wheelchair is propelled solely by attendants with no assistance from the rider, then there may be no need for the larger drive wheels (**Fig. 58-2**). To keep the attendant comfortable, the weight of the chair should be kept as light as possible and the push handles adjusted to the height of the attendant. If the occupant will be sitting in the chair for prolonged periods of time, then attention must be paid to comfort. For this reason, attendant-propelled chairs often have tilt-in-space as an option. Tilt-in-space wheelchairs can help prevent pressure sores when they are tilted greater than 25 degrees (26).

When deciding between manual tilt-in-space chairs and power seating features, it is worthwhile to note that powered seating options will provide increased independence for the users if they are able to operate them.

A variant of the attendant-propelled wheelchair is sometimes called a "geri" chair in reference to geriatric users. This type of attendant-propelled wheelchair is typically designed to make transferring out of the chair difficult. The rider is seated in a large recliner-type wheelchair. The soft padding, reclined position, small wheels, and large size make it impossible for the rider to move the wheelchair and difficult for most riders to exit the wheelchair. This helps long-term care facility to exercise control over their clients with cognitive dysfunction. There has been considerable discussion about the appropriate use of attendant-propelled chairs that significantly restrain the rider's independence (26).

Lightweight and Ultralightweight Wheelchairs

The terms *lightweight* and *ultralightweight (referred to as ultralight) wheelchairs* are derived from the Medicare categories K0004 and K0005, respectively. K0004 wheelchairs must weigh less than 15.5 kg (34 lb) without footrests or armrests, and K0005 must weigh less than 13.6 kg (30 lb) without foot or arm supports. K0004 wheelchairs have very limited adjustability (**Fig. 58-3**). Like depot chairs, they can be sized to the user, but many of these chairs do not offer features such as adjustable axle plates, quick-release wheels, or a method to change the seat to back angle of the wheelchair. Because of the way Medicare reimbursement works, manufacturers attempt to build the best wheelchair possible under a certain Medicare reimbursable cost. Unfortunately, this practice of cost engineering does not necessarily lead to improvements in design. In addition, this Medicare policy may cause dealers to push wheelchair users toward K0001 and K0004 chairs, which have higher profit margins.

The ultralight wheelchair, K0005, is the highest-quality chair that is designed specifically as an active mobility device (**Fig. 58-4**). These chairs, which can easily cost more than $2,000, are usually highly adjustable and incorporate

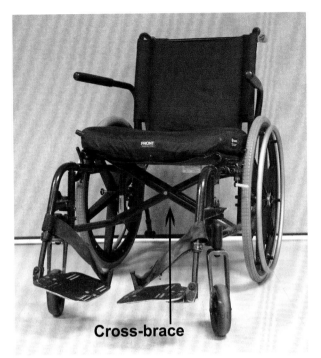

FIGURE 58-3. K0004 lightweight wheelchair with folding cross-brace design.

numerous design features made to enhance the ease of propulsion and increase the comfort of the wheelchair user. Despite high costs, when ultralight chairs undergo ANSI/RESNA testing, they have the longest fatigue life, indicating better

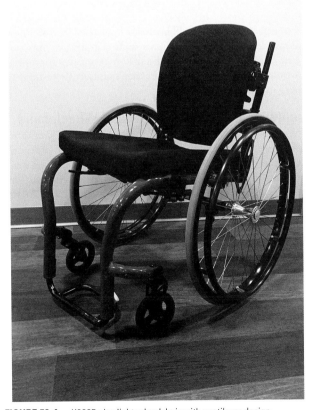

FIGURE 58-4. K0005 ultralight wheelchair with cantilever design.

cost-effectiveness (27–29). Frequent repairs and replacement needs secondary to poor wheelchair quality add to costs associated with the wheelchair; as such, while a user may pay more initially for a better quality chair, he or she may pay less to maintain the chair because of improved durability (30). When made of titanium or high-strength aluminum, this chair can easily weigh less than 9 kg (20 lb). At present, it is necessary to justify the need for a K0004 or K0005 wheelchair instead of a standard K0001. Unfortunately, it may not be possible to get prior authorization—resulting in the vendor potentially not being guaranteed ahead of time to be reimbursed for the wheelchair. As a result, vendors are often unwilling to take the risk that a $2,000 item will be reimbursed. Currently, Medicare allows vendors to ask for preauthorization of these chairs; however, few vendors take advantage of this opportunity.

Ultralight wheelchairs usually have a number of options and adjustments that can be made to appropriately fit the user. Following is a list of many of the components of chairs and options that are available. It is important to remember that every component adds weight to the chair. A balance must be reached between providing the optimal equipment to maximize the individual's function, while keeping the chair as light as possible. Some of these options are also available on lightweight and depot-type chairs; however, the components used on ultralight chairs are generally lighter and better in quality.

Frames

There are two basic frame types: folding and rigid. Within these two frame types, there are a number of different varieties. The most common type of manual wheelchair frame is the folding cross-brace frame (see **Fig. 58-3**). When viewed from the back of the frame, the cross members form an X with a hinge located in the middle. The chair is folded by pulling upward on the seat upholstery. Cross-member folding mechanisms are simple and easy to use. However, the wheelchair may collapse when tilted sideways, and the frame becomes taller when folded. Some chairs incorporate snaps or over-center locking mechanisms to reduce the problem of frame folding while on a side slope.

The most common rigid chair is the box frame. The box frame is named for its rectangular shape and the frame tubes that form a "box" (13). Box frames can be very strong and durable. These frames can also be collapsed to relatively small dimensions. The backrest usually folds forward, and when used with quick-release wheels, the chair becomes a rather compact shape. An alternative to the box frame is a cantilever frame that can act a suspension element (i.e., there is some flexibility purposely built into the frame). These cantilever frames may also have fewer tubes and parts and thus be more aesthetically pleasing (see **Fig. 58-4**).

Wheelchair users are exposed to vibration as they traverse uneven terrain such as a brick sidewalk. This vibration exposure can exceed an established health caution zone and can increase their risk for injury (31). In response, some manufacturers offer suspension elements on the frame. The frame material also affects vibrations, with carbon fiber shown to have the lowest transmission (32). In addition to decreasing vibration exposure, suspension can decrease head acceleration and seat forces during curb descent (33). The flexible element for the suspension can use either metal springs or polymer dampeners. Elastic elements on manual wheelchairs have not necessarily resulted in lower levels of vibration being transmitted to the user (34) and add to the overall weight of the wheelchair. In addition, the shock absorption can result in lost energy during propulsion. This can occur because the force generated by the wheelchair user during propulsion goes toward compressing the elastic elements rather than forward motion. Therefore, the decision to purchase a suspension wheelchair should depend on patient's preferences for the drive, feel, and comfort of the wheelchair.

COMPONENTS

A number of components can be attached to both manual and power wheelchairs. The following list is focused on manual wheelchairs, but many of the components are found on power wheelchairs as well.

Footrests

Most wheelchair users require support for their feet and lower legs. This support is provided by footrests. Footrests may be fixed, folding, swing-away (see **Fig. 58-2**), or elevating. The footrests must provide sufficient support for the lower legs and feet and must hold the feet in proper position to prevent foot drop or other deformities. It is essential to assess limitations in knee and foot range of motion. Some users have very tight hamstrings, requiring that the feet be positioned closer to or under the front edge of the seat. This is difficult to accomplish in most configurations. Extending the knees to accommodate the standard design of the footrest position in front of the seat results in a sitting posture with a posterior pelvic tilt and a tendency to slide forward in the seat. This is commonly seen in older adults in nursing homes using depot-type wheelchairs.

The feet must remain on the footrests at all times during propulsion, and therefore some type of cradle is recommended. Some wheelchairs (primarily those with swing-away footrests) use foot stirrups behind the heels of each foot (see **Fig. 58-2**). However, for other wheelchairs, it is best to use a continuous strap behind both feet because the rider's feet sometimes come over the stirrups during active use. The frame should be selected and configured so that the feet sit firmly upon the footrests, with shoes on, without lifting the upper legs from the seat cushion. Footrests are commonly placed between 25 and 50 mm (1 to 2 in.) from the ground to ensure that sufficient ground clearance is maintained. Footrest position has been correlated to sitting pressures on the ischial tuberosities (35). To prevent increased sitting pressure, it is critical to assure that the footrest height allows for weight bearing along the undersurface of the thigh. Often, the footrests are the first part of the chair to come in contact with an obstacle (such as a door, wall, or another chair), so they must be durable.

Rigid wheelchairs often use simple tubes across the front of the wheelchair. By using a tubular rigid footrest, the wheelchair becomes stiffer and stronger (see **Fig. 58-4**). Rigid footrests are used during sports activities and work well for people who are very active in their wheelchair. Folding wheelchairs often use footrests that fold up and leg rests that swing out of the way to ease in transfers. Swing-away leg rests are not as durable as rigid ones. In some cases, manufacturers design swing-away leg rests that will flexibly bend on impact. This helps to absorb the energy of the impact and possibly prevent serious injury to the wheelchair rider. Elevating leg rests can be used for people who

cannot maintain a 90-degree knee angle or who need their legs elevated for venous return. However, elevating leg rests make the wheelchair longer and heavier. This also has the effect of making the wheelchair less maneuverable by increasing the turning radius. Therefore, if elevating leg rests are needed, a power wheelchair should be strongly considered.

Armrests and Clothing Guards

Armrests provide a form of support and are convenient handles to hold onto when the rider leans to one side or the other to perform ADL like reaching. Armrests are also helpful when attempting to reach higher places. For example, some people use their removable armrests as a tool to nudge items off high shelves. Armrests are commonly used to perform a "push-up" to assist with seat pressure relief. However, this is not the preferred method of pressure relief because of the significant stress it puts on the upper extremity (36).

There are three basic styles of armrests: wraparound, full-length, and desk-length. Wraparound armrests mount at the back of the wheelchair onto the frame below the backrest in most cases (**Fig. 58-3**). The armrest comes up along the back of the backrest supports and wraps around to the front of the wheelchair. The major advantage of this design is that the armrest does not increase the width of the wheelchair like the other types of armrests. They are also lighter weight than other armrest options. Wraparound armrests are popular among active wheelchair users. The most significant drawback of this design is that the armrest does not serve as a side guard to keep the rider's clothing away from the wheels, although a removable piece of plastic called a clothing guard can be attached to the wheelchair frame to prevent clothes from getting caught in the wheels. Additionally, these armrests are often designed to swing away, and it is important to ensure that they are appropriately locked in before transferring if they are used as a position for hand placement.

Full-length and desk-length armrests are similar in design, the main difference being the length of the armrest (**Fig. 58-1**). Full-length armrests provide support for nearly the entire upper arm. They are popular on electric-powered wheelchairs because they provide a convenient and functional location for a joystick or other input device. Full-length armrests make it difficult to get close to some tables and desks. This is why manufacturers produce shorter desk-length armrests. Both of these types of armrests include clothing guards to protect clothing from the wheels. These types of armrests are mounted to the side of the wheelchair and may add as much as 5 cm to the width of the wheelchair.

Armrests can be fixed or height-adjustable. Height-adjustable armrests may move up and down to accommodate the length of the rider's trunk and arms. Most armrests can be moved in order to provide clearance for transferring in and out of the wheelchair and to allow a person to lean over the sides of the wheelchair. Armrests are either removed or flipped back. Both styles commonly use a latch, which is operated by the user. It is important to have secure latches on the armrests because armrests form convenient places for the user to hold onto during transfers. It should be noted that armrests could alter the way in which a person propels a wheelchair. The hands and arms must clear the armrest in order to reach the push rim. This can force the user into excessive abduction at the shoulder, which could be a risk factor for injury.

Wheel Locks

Wheel locks act as parking brakes to stabilize the wheelchair when the rider transfers to other seats and when the rider wishes to remain in a particular spot. When locked, they keep the wheelchair stable to allow the rider to push things from the chair. There are a variety of wheel locks used to restrain wheelchairs when transferring or parking. High-lock brakes, which are located near the front corner of the seat, on the upper tube of the wheelchair's side frame, are most common; however, location can vary. High-lock brakes require the least dexterity to operate. Extension levers can be added for people with limited reach or minimal strength. Wheel locks are standard equipment on wheelchairs, and they are simple to mount if the wheelchair does not come equipped with locks from the manufacturer.

Wheel locks may be push-to-lock or pull-to-lock. Most people prefer push-to-lock because wheel locks are more difficult to engage than to disengage. Riders often find it easier to push with the palm than pull with the fingers. Low wheel locks are usually mounted to the lower tube of the wheelchair's side frame. Low wheel locks require more mobility to operate. They also alleviate the common problem that is seen with high wheel locks of the user hitting his or her thumb against the lock when propelling the chair. This problem can be addressed for high wheel lock users by selecting retractable (i.e., scissors or butterfly) wheel locks. The retractable type of wheel lock helps to prevent jamming the thumbs and can also accommodate a wide variety of camber angles. The major drawback of retractable wheel locks is that they are more difficult to use than other types of wheel locks. The wheel lock must be positioned properly with respect to the wheel in order to operate effectively. If the wheels are repositioned, then the wheel locks must be repositioned. Tire pressure also affects the locking grip of these wheel locks. Although these devices can be convenient, any equipment added will increase the overall weight of the chair, making propulsion more difficult. Thus, many active manual wheelchair users will choose not to use armrests or wheel locks.

Tires

A variety of options exist with respect to tires. The most common and recommended type of tire is pneumatic. These tires are lightweight and provide cushioning against impact and vibration from rolling over surfaces. This cushioning may increase rider comfort and improve wheelchair durability. The main downside of pneumatic tires is that they require maintenance and they can puncture. Tire pressure needs to be kept at a predetermined level because it is critical to rolling resistance, which can be related to risk of secondary injury associated with manual wheelchair use; this pressure varies between brands and types and is printed on the tire for reference. A study has shown that when propelling on tires that were deflated by 50%, energy expenditure increases by 25% and deceleration increases by 16% with straight propulsion and 28% with turns (37,38). Similar effects are noted with tires on power-assist wheels (39). Clinicians involved with wheelchair users should squeeze their patients' tires to assure that they are keeping up with this important regular maintenance issue.

An alternative to pneumatic tires is solid inserts. These foam inserts fit into the pneumatic tire and replace the air-filled inner tube that would normally be there. They add some weight to the chair and may slightly worsen rolling resistance but are a good alternative for individuals who do not want to be responsible for maintenance of air pressure (40). A less viable alternative is solid tires. These tires require no maintenance and are low in cost. Unfortunately, rolling resistance is higher, and they make for an uncomfortable ride as all ground shocks are transmitted to the wheelchair user.

Additional Features

Anti-tippers

Anti-tippers are often placed on wheelchairs to assure they do not tip over backward. These can inhibit the ability to climb curbs, but they offer a measure of safety. It is suggested that these be ordered for all new wheelchairs and then have the user take them off when they are comfortable with the stability of the chair. Anti-tippers are available with pin settings that can adjust their height and allow them to be removed. Additionally, a flip-up option is available that allows the anti-tippers to be easily moved out of the way when the user is working on mobility skills such as curbs or wheelies.

Push Rims

A number of different push rims are currently available, and new styles are likely to be introduced into the market. Anodized aluminum rims are the current standard on most K0004 and K0005 chairs. Less expensive chairs may come with plastic push rims. For individuals with difficulty gripping the rim, alternative rims should be considered. These can include vinyl-coated rims, rims with projections (eFig. 58-1), and rims wrapped with surgical tubing. All of these rims have the advantage of increased friction, making it easier to push the chair forward. Unfortunately, this increased friction can lead to burns when the wheelchair user attempts to slow down the chair. There is ongoing research into advanced ergonomic push-rim designs that allow for easier and more comfortable propulsion as well as braking (41,42). For individuals who have good hand function, a push rim called the "Natural-Fit" (Out-Front, Mesa, AZ) is an ergonomically designed hand rim that has been shown to decrease fatigue, pain, and stresses placed on the upper extremity during wheelchair propulsion, (41,43). The "FlexRim" (Spinergy, Lyons, CO) is a durable rubber surface that bridges the gap between the wheel and push rim, conforming when gripped and has been shown to increase power and decrease impact loading, energy use, and grip forces (44,45).

Wheels

The standard wheels on lightweight and ultralightweight wheelchairs have spokes. Plastic wheels may be found on low-end chairs; however, they increase weight and decrease performance. High-end wheels are available with flexible spokes or with graphite and composite materials. A study performed by Hughes et al. (46) found that high-end wheels did not improve efficiency but did significantly improve comfort of the rider. These wheels can be easier to maintain than standard spokes and also offer improved aesthetics.

Caster Wheels

Caster wheels are available in a variety of shapes and sizes. Pneumatic wheels are larger than solid casters and may interfere with the footrests when turning. Pneumatics offers the advantage of easier propulsion over rough terrain and increased shock absorption. Many wheelchair users are using narrow rollerblade-type wheels, which allow quicker turns and reduce rolling resistance. Unfortunately, they can get caught in sewer grates or other small obstacles. Adding an elastomer shock absorber "frog-legs" in series with the caster can provide a means of shock absorption and vibration reduction (34).

Push Handles

Push handles, also known as canes, are attached to the back of the chair with the primary purpose of making it easier for an assistant to propel the wheelchair. Canes can also be used by the wheelchair occupant to help with pressure relief. The wheelchair user can hook an arm around the cane and pull to raise the contralateral hip, even in the absence of strong triceps muscles. Canes can also be used to hang a book bag or backpack onto the back of the chair.

Grade-Aids

Grade-aids are devices that attach to the wheel and allow it to roll forward but not back. In this manner, they can make it easier to roll up a hill. These should be considered for individuals who have upper-limb weakness and who must negotiate hills.

MANUAL WHEELCHAIR SELECTION AND SETUP

As stated previously, a number of the features described above and the adjustments described below are available only for ultralight wheelchairs. Best practice dictates that any individual who will propel a wheelchair as a primary means of mobility should receive this type of chair. The optimal setup for a manual wheelchair is described in the Clinical Practice Guideline (CPG) for preservation of upper limb function (36) (**Fig. 58-5**). The chair should be as narrow as possible without causing undue pressure on the thighs. Rear axle position should be adjustable to fit the user, as it can affect caster flutter, rolling resistance, stability, control, and maneuverability. With a longer wheel base or more rearward axle position, the chair has more stability; however, rolling resistance (47), caster flutter, and downward turning on side slopes are increased. These changes are primarily related to the proportion of the weight that is placed onto the back, or larger, wheels. As the rear wheels are moved backward, more weight is placed on the front casters, which have a smaller diameter and higher rolling resistance. Axle position is an important factor with

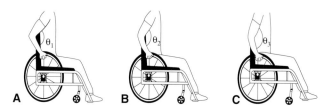

FIGURE 58-5. Optimal manual wheelchair setup. Illustrations **A–C** show differences in the elbow flexion angle (θ) from adjusting the height of the axle. Illustration **B** depicts the recommended elbow angle (θ2 = 100 to 120 degrees). Angle θ1 (illustration **A**) is smaller because the seat is too low (axle too high). Angle θ3 (illustration **C**) is larger because the seat is too high (axle too low).

community level skills of wheelies and curb negotiation, as a more posterior axle will require more effort on the part of the user to get the casters off the ground. A forward axle position has been found to be associated with improved propulsion biomechanics such as increased contact angle (access to more of the hand rim) (48). The cadence of the propulsive stroke is also higher with a more rearward axle position. This has been implicated relating to the risk of repetitive strain injury. Given these issues, the axle should be as far forward as possible, providing that the wheelchair user still feels stable. Most wheelchairs come in a factory-set position, with the axle most rearward. This should be gradually adjusted forward to maximize performance of the chair.

Axle height, or the distance between the shoulder and the axle, is an important parameter that is also described in the CPG (36). If the seat is too high, the wheelchair user will not be able to reach much of the push rim and so will push with shorter strokes and a faster cadence. If the seat is too low, the user will be forced to abduct at the shoulder during the propulsive stroke, which may cause rotator cuff impingement. In general, while sitting upright with the hands resting on the top of the wheels, the elbow angle should be between 100 and 120 degrees for optimal mobility (49,50). Alternatively, if the arms are left to hang freely at the side while sitting on the chair, the fingertips should be just past the axle of the wheel to maximize contact angle (48).

Camber describes the angle of the wheel with respect to the chair. Increasing camber has several advantages: the footprint of the chair is widened, creating greater side-to-side stability; it allows quicker turning; and positions the push rims more ergonomically for propulsion (it is more natural to push down and out). In addition, by having a wider base, the area where the hands are in contact with the push rims is less likely to come into contact with the wall (51). Finally, adding camber to the rear wheels reduces effective stiffness between the rolling surface and frame, thus reducing the vibration exposure of the user. A disadvantage to increasing camber is that it adds width to the chair. Generally, for daily use, the chair should be as narrow as possible without substantially diminishing the handling characteristics. The wheels should be offset enough from the seat to avoid rubbing against the clothing or body. Between 2 and 4 degrees of camber is appropriate for everyday use.

There are many other aspects of a wheelchair that can be adjusted to improve fit and performance. Some of these adjustments are discussed in the seating section that follows.

Alternative Manual Wheelchairs

Two alternatives worth mentioning are chairs for amputees and chairs for individuals with hemiparesis. Wheelchairs for individuals with amputations are typically designed with the rear axle set farther behind the user. This is needed because the absence of a leg causes the body's center of gravity to be shifted posteriorly, thus reducing rearward stability. Unfortunately, all of the negative aspects of a rearward axle are present. An alternative can be to add weight to the front of the wheelchair. Unfortunately, increased weight means increased rolling resistance. There is no simple answer as to what is best, and individual patients should make this decision for themselves.

For individuals with hemiparesis or other disabilities that propel better with one or both legs compared to propulsion with the arms, a "hemiheight" chair is an alternative. In this chair, there is typically one footrest or none at all, and the seat is low enough to the ground so that the feet can reach the floor. For an individual with hemiparesis, the use of the uninvolved arm and leg can provide limited, but functional, propulsion.

Another alternative for an individual with hemiparesis is a one-arm drive chair. This chair has two push rims on one side that control separate wheels. One-arm drives are heavier than standard chairs and can be difficult to control (52). These limitations make them less than ideal for an elderly stroke patient. Although not popular in the United States, lever drive wheelchairs are seen in Europe. These chairs offer a mechanical advantage by using a lever to make propulsion more efficient (50). Unfortunately, they do not offer the direct proprioceptive feedback of hand rim contact and can be difficult to maneuver in tight spaces and when traveling backward. Lever drive chairs are heavier and often wider than standard chairs. The Neater Uni-Wheelchair (NUW) is a unique system that allows the individual to steer with the footplate and propel with just one hand. Both lever drive and NUW chairs have improved mechanical efficiency than a standard chair among individuals with hemiparesis (53).

Propulsion Assistance

Propulsion assistance for manual wheelchairs can be achieved by adding power mechanisms or gearing to the wheels or through power add-ons to the front or rear of the chair. Propulsion assistance allows the user to push the wheelchair as one would normally while providing assistance. These devices allow individuals to perform tasks faster and easier. In addition, people who normally would need to use a power wheelchair may be able to self-propel a wheelchair with propulsion assistance despite obstacles such as steep ramps (54–56). When using propulsion assistance, oxygen consumption, heart rate, and push frequency are significantly lower (57,58). For individuals with upper-limb pain or tetraplegia, propulsion assistance may prove to be a good compromise between a manual wheelchair and a power wheelchair (59). Patients may encounter difficulty transferring from a chair equipped with certain propulsion assistance and in disassembling the power-equipped chair for transport.

The most studied devices sense torque in the push rim and provides addition propulsive force as the torque is applied (see **Fig. 58-6**). Performing wheelchair skills that require great control, such as a wheelie, may be more difficult with a power-assisted push rim (60). Another study of individuals using power assist in their real-life environment did not show a significant difference in the amount of time individuals used the device and the distance they traveled (61). Another power-assist option is the SmartDrive (Permobil, Inc., Lebanon, TN). It is a removable single wheel add-on system that latches on to the axle bar of a manual wheelchair. It works in combination with a wristband that communicates starting, stopping, and coasting. A wheelie can be performed with the SmartDrive. The Firefly (Rio Mobility, San Francisco, CA) is a fully powered handcycle that latches on to the front of a manual wheelchair. It has both forward and reverse throttles and folds up for

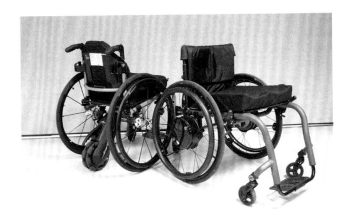

FIGURE 58-6.   Power-assist options: *Left:* SmartDrive, *Right:* power-assisted push rims.

storage. It increases the length of the chair, so it may not be as appropriate for indoor mobility and tight turning. It is important to remember that under current Medicare guidelines, a power-assisted device will not be funded unless the patient has used a manual wheelchair for 1 year. This should not prevent recommending the device but must be kept in mind when producing the LMN.

Add-on lever drive options also exist such as the Pivot Lever Drive (RIO Mobility, CA) that use bilateral levers to propel forward/backward, brake, and turn. ROWHEELS REV (Rowheels, Inc., Middleton, WI) are an alternative wheel option that utilizes pulling on the push rim for forward propulsion, rather than pushing. Based on this alternative design, groups of larger back and shoulder muscles are utilized for propulsion. The lack of batteries and motors make these a lighter option.

Manual Wheelchair Propulsion Technique

The most appropriate way to propel a wheelchair has been informed by studies that have found an association between upper-limb injuries and wheelchair propulsion biomechanics (47). Manual wheelchair users should propel with long smooth strokes that minimize the cadence with which they push and maximize the length of the stroke or contact angle (36,47). A greater contact angle should be achieved by reaching back further for initial hand contact. The wheelchair user should attempt to impact the rim smoothly and match the speed of the hand to the rotating speed of the push rim. During the recovery stage of the propulsive stroke, the user should let the hand drop below the push rim and stay below the push rim until he or she is ready to begin propulsion again (62) (**Fig. 58-7**). This approach can improve mechanics regardless of propulsion surface type or speed (63,64).

Wheelchair propulsion techniques can be evaluated by the wheelchair propulsion test consisting of 10 items that evaluate propulsion (65). The only requirements for this test are a 10-m runway and a stopwatch. While this test has good psychometric properties (reliability, validity, and inter-/intra-rater reliability), it only addresses some aspects of correct propulsion technique. Movement-based apps also exist that allow clinicians to record propulsion and analyze it in stop frames on either a smartphone or tablet.

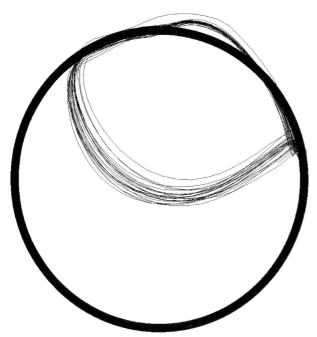

FIGURE 58-7. Recovery pattern. This represents data from a wheelchair user. The *dark circle* is the push rim. The *thinner lines* are from a marker placed on the wrist. This recovery pattern was found to provide the best efficiency. Direction of travel is left.

POWER WHEELCHAIRS

There is strong evidence in the literature to indicate that the use of powered mobility facilitates independence, improves occupational performance, and is correlated with a higher sense of quality of life for people who cannot ambulate or propel a manual wheelchair effectively (2,4,6). However, there are some disadvantages to powered mobility devices that need to be factored into the decision of powered versus manual wheelchair mobility (**Table 58-1**). Power wheelchairs come in a number of configurations. Two types are those with a power base and those with integrated seating systems. In general, wheelchairs with integrated seating systems are less expensive and offer less with respect to seating options.

TABLE 58-1	Powered Versus Manual Wheelchair Mobility
Advantages of Manual Wheelchairs	**Advantages of Power Wheelchairs**
Transportation: Easy to transport; can travel with friends without special vehicles	Distance: Can travel long distances without fatigue
Maintenance: Can be worked on independently	Speed: Can travel at higher speed without fatigue
Exercise: Theoretical benefit to the user from using own force to propel	Terrain: May be able to traverse rougher terrain
Aesthetics: Less appearance of disability	Protect the arm: Avoid repetitive strain injuries that are due to manual wheelchair propulsion

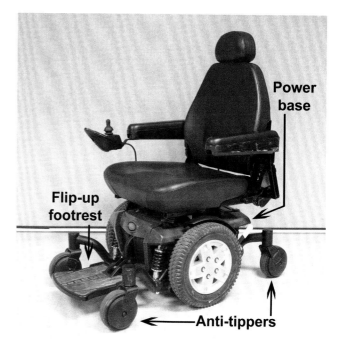

FIGURE 58-8. Mid-wheel-drive power wheelchair with power base. The seating system can be removed and replaced with a different seating configuration.

Power Bases

The power base is the lower portion of a power wheelchair that houses the motors, batteries, drive wheels, casters, and electronics to which a seating system is attached (**Fig. 58-8**). The base allows for the mounting of any variety or combination of different seating systems and seat functions, including tilt-in-space, reclining back, elevating leg rests, and seat elevator.

Drive Classification

Power wheelchair bases can be classified as rear wheel drive (RWD), mid-wheel drive (MWD), and front wheel drive (FWD). The classification of these three drive systems is based on the drive wheel location relative to the system's center of gravity. The drive wheel position defines the basic handling characteristic of any power wheelchair. Each system has unique driving and handling characteristics. In RWD power bases (**Fig. 58-9**), the drive wheels are behind the user's center of gravity, and the casters are in the front. RWD systems are the traditional design, and therefore many long-term power wheelchair users are familiar with their performance and prefer them to other designs. A major advantage of an RWD system is its predictable drive characteristic and stability. A potential drawback to an RWD system is its maneuverability in tight areas because of a larger turning radius (66).

In MWD power bases (see **Fig. 58-8**), the drive wheels are directly below the user's center of gravity and generally have a set of casters or anti-tippers in the front and rear of the drive wheels. The advantage of the MWD system is a smaller turning radius to maneuver in tight spaces. The turning radius required for a MWD is similar to that of an ultralight manual wheelchair (66). A disadvantage is a tendency to rock or pitch forward, especially with sudden stops or fast turns. When transitioning from a steep slope to a level surface (like coming off a curb cut), the front and rear casters

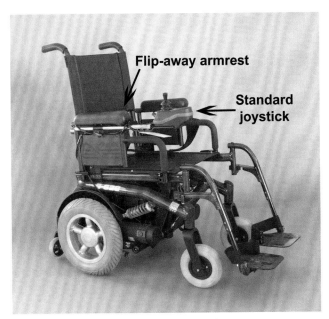

FIGURE 58-9. Rear-wheel-drive power wheelchair.

can hang up, leaving less traction on the drive wheels in the middle. However, manufactures have addressed these shortcomings and have updated designs of MWD that now are available with a wheelbase consisting of six wheels touching the ground; with two small wheels in the front and back. These wheels are equipped with suspension and shock absorbance systems that enhance forward stability and small obstacle climbing capability.

A FWD power base (**Fig. 58-10**) has the drive wheels in front of the user's center of gravity, and the rear wheels are casters. The advantage of an FWD system is that it tends to be quite stable and provides a tight turning radius. FWD systems

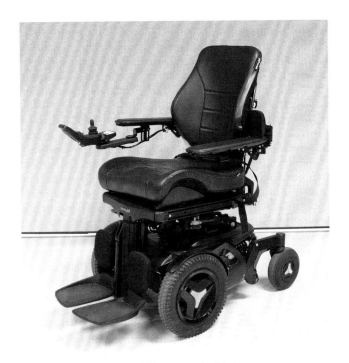

FIGURE 58-10. Front-wheel-drive power wheelchair.

may climb obstacles or curbs more easily as the large front wheels hit the obstacle first. A disadvantage is that an FWD system has more rearward center of gravity; therefore, the system may tend to fishtail and be difficult to drive in a straight line, especially on uneven surfaces.

Controls

The device that is used to control a powered mobility system is called an access device. The primary function of the access device is to drive the chair. The majority of input controls are programmable, allowing changes in speed and the amount of movement to determine the direction of the wheelchair. Many power wheelchair users brace some portion of their hand against the control box and use their hand and arm coordination to operate the joystick. Gross arm function, in many cases, can be used to operate a joystick. If the user does not have the hand function or coordination to operate a joystick input device, other options are available. Other parts of the body, such as the chin or foot, can operate a modified joystick.

The cognitive abilities required to operate an alternative control typically increase as the physical and functional abilities of the user decrease. Programmable wheelchair controllers allow reduction of the maximum velocity and modification of the acceleration and deceleration rates of the wheelchair. To assist persons with more severe cognitive or visual limitations, technologies are being developed that enable the wheelchair to follow walls, navigate through doorways, and stop when other objects are contacted (67). For persons with spasticity or tremor impacting the hand, modern controllers have filters that can be adjusted to give smoother wheelchair control. Positioning technology enables the joystick to be placed in a variety of locations to optimize the user's ability to operate it (68).

Joysticks

Joysticks are the most common access devices for powered wheelchair systems. Most joysticks are proportional; meaning the control's speed output to the wheelchair from the joystick is in proportion to how far the joystick is pushed from the center position. Joysticks can be fitted with a template that only allows motion in certain directions, which is useful for people with poor motor control. The end of the joystick can also be modified for easier grip. One common modification is a goalpost-shaped attachment (T-bar) with the upright section of the joystick on either side of the hand. Alternatively, a tennis ball cut to fit over a traditional joystick can make gripping easier.

Mini Joystick

The Mini Joystick, a type of microproportional joystick, may be a good alternative for a user who has lost gross arm function and is unable to use a conventional joystick but still possesses small distal motor function within the fingers. The Mini Joystick has the same proportional and directional features of a conventional joystick; however, the tuning and the physical displacement of the joystick is scaled down and requires significantly less effort to achieve small joystick displacement (i.e., wiggle of the tip of a finger). Its smaller size also permits more freedom in its placement to meet the functional/comfort needs of the user (i.e., custom fitted on a stable arm support for independent single finger control or custom fitted through the "horn" of a palmer support for thumb control). Its tuning and custom programmability capabilities allow head control drive option when faced with complete loss of upper extremity and lower extremity functions. Used as a chin interface, it requires minimal effort of facial and cervical musculature to operate the control.

Sip-and-Puff

Sip-and-puff switches are used primarily by people with tetraplegia. A sip-and-puff access device consists of a replaceable straw located near the mouth. Pulling and pushing air through the straw with the mouth controls the wheelchair. These systems can be set up in a variety of configurations. Generally, the user will sip a specific number of times to indicate a direction and puff to confirm the choice and activate the movement of the wheelchair. It is common for an auxiliary visual display to be used with sip-and-puff to provide feedback on which command was selected. Sip-and-puff is becoming somewhat antiquated now that microproportional joysticks, head array sensors, and gyroscopic-based joysticks are available.

Switches and Buttons

An array of switches or a single switch can be used to control a chair. The more switches, the greater the motor control needed to operate the equipment. Using scanning, a single switch can control a wheelchair. In scanning, choices are presented to the user on the wheelchair controller. When the desired choice is presented, the user activates the switch to select that command. Two switches can fully control a wheelchair in a fashion similar to the one described above for sip-and-puff systems. An array of switches can be used for quicker control. There is no proportional control of the wheelchair's speed with switched control. Thus, users are forced to travel at the same, rather slow velocity at all times.

Additional Control Options

Other technologies that are under current development include an eye gaze system with a live image of the environment and superimposed arrows on the screen that allow the user to steer (69). Intraoral systems like a tongue drive system that utilizes a magnetic barbell or chip in a dental retainer are in the prototype phase; however, further refinement is required before these are commercially available options (70–72).

Many of the input devices described in this section can be used for more than the control of the wheelchairs. Two common additional uses are environmental control and computer or smart phone access. In some cases, the computer is mounted to the wheelchair, but often it is at a fixed site. A critical consideration when selecting or designing a user interface is that the ability of the user to accurately control the interface is heavily dependent on the stability of the user within the wheelchair. Often custom seating and postural support systems are required for a user interface to be effective. The position and stability of the user interface are also critical to its efficacy as a functional access device. Bluetooth add-ons are commonly used to transmit commands from the wheelchair controller to other devices.

Cueing Systems

The Virtual Seating Coach (Permobil, TN) is a cueing system that prompts users to adjust their positioning for pressure relief through a smartphone app. The system also features a Web-facing clinician portal through which compliance and usage of power seating features (tilt, recline and leg elevation) can be tracked (73).

Considerations in Selection of Electric-Powered Mobility

There are many considerations in defining the correct power wheelchair for a given individual. Important factors include the means of transportation of the wheelchair, surface conditions the chair must negotiate, need to negotiate thresholds and curbs, and clearance widths in the environment. In addition, subject preference is important, as well as maximum speed and range. Transitions from manual to power wheelchairs can be for reasons such as upper extremity pain, injury or weakness as well as poor cardiopulmonary function or inability to maintain proper positioning (59). Users have indicated desires for future driving systems that allow for path following, obstacle avoidance, and target following (74,75). Some of the features exist currently such as the Drive Safe System (DSS) which is an obstacle avoidance system (76).

SEATING AND POSITIONING

Seating systems can be organized into three general categories: off-the-shelf systems, modular systems, and custom-molded systems. Overlap exists between the categories, and a given seating system should be prescribed and designed specific to the user's medical, functional, and personal preference needs. Medically, a system should address issues of soft tissue management, comfort, reducing the potential for or accommodating orthopedic deformities, and maintaining vital organ capacity. Functionally, the system should address the movements and supports the user needs to reach or access objects, transfer, get under tables, and perform ADL. The chair must become an extension of the user's body, much like an orthosis. This requires careful matching of critical chair dimensions to body dimensions, user abilities, and intended uses. The user's preference as to one system over another should be paramount in the prescription process. For example, a user may choose to forgo pressure relief and comfort for a firmer seating system that provides greater stability and allows him or her to have a firm surface to slide on the seat for ease with repositioning when transferring in/out of the device. The simplest form of seating system is a linear seating system that involves a planar seat and back with fixed angles and orientations.

Soft Tissue Management

Soft tissue management is a concern for all people who sit for prolonged periods of time and who have compromised sensation or the inability to perform weight shifts. External causes of skin breakdown or pressure sores include excessive prolonged pressure over bony prominences, friction and shear, as well as heat and moisture. Intrinsic factors include the inability to move, poor nutrition, vascular problems, and the loss of soft tissue elasticity (77). Loss of sensation is a key factor because discomfort is the usual trigger for shifting and moving. Because the causes of pressure ulcer vary, the choice of seat cushion will vary based on the client's risk factors and the characteristics of the cushion.

The fit of the wheelchair also contributes to pressure distribution. Footrests mounted too high increase the pressure over the ischial tuberosities. Properly adjusted armrest height allows weight to be distributed through the upper extremities. The angle of the back, relative to the seat, affects the stability and orientation of the pelvis and is reflected in how much a person will slouch, thus affecting pressure over the sacrococcygeal regions.

Material Properties of Seating Systems

Cushions are chosen based on their characteristics, which are related to the properties of the materials used in their construction. Materials specific to those used in the design and manufacturing of seating systems have certain characteristics, as shown in **Table 58-2**. Manufacturers make cushions that possess these qualities using flat and contoured foams, air-filled bladders, combinations of air and foam, flotation, viscous fluids, contoured plastic honeycombs, custom-contoured foam, and alternating pressure systems. These cushions vary in efficacy of pressure distribution, provision of postural stability, ability to insulate or conduct heat, and the reliability of their performance over time. Finding a cushion with good airflow and pressure distribution would be important for an immobile client who perspires heavily or is incontinent. Alternately, for a client prone to pressure ulcers, a practitioner would identify cushions with optimal redistribution of peak pressures. Active manual wheelchair users may not like an air-filled cushion because it does not provide a stable base for propulsion-related activities. Cushion design can also impact how easy or difficult it is for users to transfer to and from their chair. If all the needed features cannot be found in one cushion, trade-offs are necessary. Research evidence supports that a properly fitted pressure-reducing cushion, in contrast to a low-cost foam cushion, reduces the probability of a pressure sore (78).

TABLE 58-2	Characteristics of Materials Used in the Design and Manufacture of Seating Systems
Property	**Application**
Density: The ratio of mass or quantity of material to the volume of the cushion	A cushion filled with air will be much lighter than one composed of gel. Weight may be a problem for someone who has to lift it or propel a manual wheelchair.
Stiffness: The strength of the resistance to compression	Foam has low stiffness and does not resist body weight compared with a solid seat base. A solid surface provides greater pelvic stabilization; foam may allow better pressure distribution.
Thermal characteristics: The ability of the material to insulate or conduct heat	Dense foam cushions retain body heat. Honeycomb-designed cushions hold less heat. Gel and fluids tend to pull heat away from the body.
Friction: The ability to maintain position and to reposition if needed	Cushions with solid bases and slick covers make sliding in lateral transfers easier but may promote sacral sitting.

Pressure Mapping

Pressure-mapping technology estimates interface pressure. A thin mat with pressure sensors is placed between the client and the seating surface. The mat connects to a computer and presents data in both graphic and numeric forms. As part of a skilled clinical assessment, it can be predictive of potential risk for pressure sores (79). This technology can help a clinician decide which cushion provides the best pressure distribution for a particular client. It can also be used to educate clients on proper pressure relief techniques such as how far they need to lean or how far they need to tilt back and recline in a power wheelchair for adequate relief. It is important to remember that pressure-mapping devices do not measure shear forces, heat, moisture, postural stability, or maintenance of the cushion. These factors must also be considered.

Custom-Contoured Seating

Custom-contoured seating systems are necessary when all available off-the-shelf or modular seating systems cannot address the needs of the individual. This may occur in individuals with moderate to severe fixed and semiflexible structural deformities of the spine and extremities. In addition, individuals who require significant off-loading of soft tissue because of pressure sore issues may need a custom-contoured seat. Custom-molded systems are not capable of correcting deformities. Custom-contoured seating involves a process of capturing a specific mold of a person's body. The mold can be obtained through several methods, including liquid foam in place, plaster molds, or through computer-aided design/computer-aided manufacturing (CAD/CAM) with greater control and accuracy. CAD/CAM usually involves the use of a seating simulator composed of bead bags for the seat and backrest supports. The bead bags are manually and gravitationally contoured around the shape of the person's deformities or pressure points, followed by vacuum evacuation of the air from the bags to produce a rigid mold. This mold is then scanned, using sensors that send data to a robotic milling machine for the production of a positive mold.

Careful skin inspections should be performed, and pressure-mapping systems should be used as appropriate to verify that the custom-molded seat contours are applied properly. Inappropriately applied contours can lead to pressure sores. Careful consideration of transfer technique is needed with these seating systems because proper positioning in the seat is essential to performance, and the custom contours usually make transfers more difficult.

Back Support

A back support should conform to the normal spinal curvature while allowing movement as required by the user. The typical back support in a folding-frame wheelchair is sling upholstery, not because it is good back support, but because it bends to allow the chair to fold. Sling seats provide little in the way of support. In individuals with tetraplegia, the stretching of the sling back can mean that the wheelchair user adopts a more posterior tilt of the pelvis, and this may contribute to a kyphotic spine (14). Like cushions, wheelchair backs are chosen based on the client's seating goals. For clients with truncal weakness, the stability from a contoured backrest with or without modular lateral supports is needed to maintain head and neck position. Some clients may only need the soft contouring of an adjustable tension sling backrest, whereas others with significant kyphoscoliosis may need a custom-molded backrest to enable sitting in a more upright posture. Clients with this level of weakness or deformity will most likely use this seating in a powered mobility base or an attendant-operated base.

Back support is also important for manual wheelchair users. In addition to concerns about posterior pelvic sitting with a sling-back support, this back support stretches before a propulsive force is effectively applied to the rim, resulting in inefficiencies during wheelchair mobility. Unlike power wheelchairs, weight and range of motion are important factors to balance with the need for increased support in manual wheelchairs. Increased weight will increase the rolling resistance of the wheelchair; lighter-weight materials such as carbon fiber can be selected and are good choices for active manual wheelchair users. Impaired shoulder range of motion will affect the user's access to the push rim and can compromise propulsion biomechanics (80). Shape, fit, and adjustment of rigid backrests are important to address user comfort (81).

Recline and Tilt-in-Space

Recline and tilt-in-space technologies relieve pressure, manage posture, provide comfort, and help with personal care activities. Recline helps stretch hip flexors and also assists with attending to catheters, toileting, and dependent transfers. Because reclining the seat back creates shear, the user often shifts in the wheelchair into a sacral-seated position. For a patient who is unable to reposition without help, adding tilt may help the user reposition independently. Tilt-in-space keeps the hip and knee angles constant when tilting the client back. Unlike reclining systems, the position of the user is maintained in the tilt seating system.

It is essential that individuals who are unable to independently shift weight, unable to transfer independently, or have pain as a result of prolonged sitting, have a tilt-in-space and recline system on their chair (82). Tilt-in-space is also necessary for individuals with progressive disorders (82). An individual with amyotrophic lateral sclerosis may find it easy to perform weight shift and repositioning at an initial evaluation, but this can change quickly, leading to the need for modifications. Tilt and recline are also available in manual wheelchairs. For the most part, these chairs are only used for patients who require attendant control. As in recline, tilt-in-space greatly reduces pressure on the ischial tuberosities by shifting the pressure to the back. Several recent research studies support the combination of tilt-in-space and recline together. Using a combination of tilt-in-space and recline will maximize the function of both devices, enhance the ability of the individual to use the system for positioning, perform personal care tasks, reduce pressure and increase comfort (82). Tilting at least 20 to 35 degrees of tilt in combination with 100 to 120 degrees of recline is recommended for ischial pressure relief (83,84). It is worthwhile to note that these seating functions will increase the turning radius of the chair if the user drives with the chair in any amount of tilt and/or recline for comfort (66).

Other Positioning Systems

Stand-up wheelchairs are an alternative manual and power wheelchair that deserves mention. The benefits of standing for individuals normally unable to do so may include decreased bladder infections, reduced osteoporosis, and decreased spasticity (85). In addition, there are likely psychological benefits that result from the feeling of upright posture and the ability to interact at eye level (86). Certain people cannot use a stand-up wheelchair because they do not have adequate joint range of motion. Some of the benefits of a stand-up wheelchair can be obtained by using a variable-seat-height wheelchair. The most common function of variable-seat-height wheelchairs is to provide seat elevation. A seat elevator has many useful functions that will improve the quality of life of the user. The device can help individuals avoid positioning their hand above the shoulder, which can help to reduce shoulder pain (87). The individuals will be able to reach heights that would have been impossible in the past, thus increasing independence. By allowing the individual to change his or her seat height, an easier, downhill transfer can be performed. A downhill transfer may be beneficial because it can decrease the forces placed on the upper extremity (88). Finally, a seat elevator will allow the individual to interact with peers at eye level, thus improving the individual's ability to interact in a social situation. Seat elevators are strongly recommended by the CPG on preservation of upper limb function (36) and have been advocated by RESNA (86). Finally, some chairs offer lateral tilt-in-space. This feature allows the user to be leaned to either side and offers an alternative for people with difficult pressure sore or pain issues or the need for postural drainage.

Seating Setup

Setting up the wheelchair is critical to optimizing performance. A therapist or rehabilitation supplier working with the clinic commonly performs this. Seat height can be adjusted on most chairs. The seat height is dependent on the total body length of the user. Users with longer leg lengths will require higher seat heights to achieve sufficient clearance for the footrests. There is some flexibility when selecting seat height, even for taller individuals, because most active users prefer some seat angle or dump. Dump is achieved by tilting the seat down toward the backrest, thus the end closest to the backrest is lower than the front of the cushion. Dump allows the user to fit more securely in the chair, increasing the user's trunk stability and making the chair more responsive to the user's body movements. Increasing dump can make transfers more difficult. Seat depth is determined from the length of the upper legs. Generally, no more than a 75-mm (3 in.) gap should be between the front of the seat and the back of the knees when the person is in the wheelchair. This will help ensure broad distribution of the trunk weight over the buttocks and upper legs, without placing undue pressure behind the knee. Some gap is required to allow the user some freedom to adjust his or her position. Seat width is determined from the width of the person's hips, the intended use, and whether the person prefers to use side guards. Generally, the wheelchair should be as narrow as possible; thus, a chair about 1 in. wider than the user's hips is desirable.

Scooters

Scooters (**Fig. 58-11**) are another option for certain individuals. These devices typically have a single front wheel for steering and two drive wheels in the back. Possibly because scooters are available to help shoppers in many large department stores, they seem to have a greater degree of social acceptability than do wheelchairs. This leads many clients to request these devices. Steering is accomplished via hand bars that are intuitive to users who have previously used a bicycle. Seating is provided in a chair having foam padding typical of a car seat.

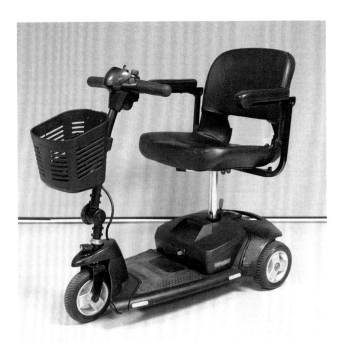

FIGURE 58-11. Scooter.

The backrest height ends at the level of the shoulder blades, which allows for unencumbered rotation of the trunk.

Scooters have a number of advantages and disadvantages that must be critically considered when prescribing this device (**Table 58-3**). In general, scooters are a reasonable option for individuals who retain some ability to ambulate, such as those with cardiopulmonary disease limiting the ability to walk. Scooters are a poor option for individuals with progressive neuromuscular disorders because they have few options to accommodate progressive disability. They are also a poor choice if one needs to stay in the chair all day because seating options are limited. If a scooter is found to be the appropriate device, it is important that the scooter is trialed in the patient's home environment. Scooters require a large turning radius and often do not fit well into a person's home.

Power Wheelchair Training

New wheelchair users should go through a wheelchair training program. Wheelchair users can first practice basic maneuvers in controlled environments and then transition to uneven surfaces and slope transitions (i.e., level to sloped surfaces) in both the uphill and downhill directions and maneuvering through tight environments. Once these skills are mastered, they should gradually tackle more challenging environments, such as steep grades

TABLE 58-3	**Scooters**
Advantages	**Disadvantages**
Lower cost	Less stability
Easier to assemble and disassemble for transportation	Require greater arm strength and control to drive
Better than some chairs at rough terrain	Fewer seating options
Less perceived stigma of disability	Poor turning radius. Must transfer out of chair for many activities

and step transitions that exceed Americans with Disabilities Act (ADA) Accessibility Guidelines. The rider should always practice with an appropriate lap belt (89) and chest support in place and a spotter (therapist) to assist if needed.

PEDIATRICS

In many ways, the seating and mobility needs of children with disabilities are similar to those of adults. Comfort, stability, and function are paramount, and there is no one perfect position for every activity or situation. There is a tendency to be aggressive with children and force them to sit upright with many postural supports in the hope of preventing or delaying deformities. This tendency in the design of the seating system may force postures that are not tolerated or desired over time. It is important to seek input from both the child and the caregivers who will be dealing with the seating system on an hourly basis. Several variables in system design need to be considered with children, including developmental status, mobility, growth, age-appropriate activities, school, therapies, the environment, and family issues. Children not only change in size, but their disability also often changes as they grow, even in nonprogressive disorders such as cerebral palsy.

Pediatric Seating Systems

Pediatric seating systems can be classified in the same manner as outlined for adults in the previous section, with off-the-shelf, modular, and custom-molded systems available. The issue of growth should not be overvalued over function or other points of concern. There are some systems that can accommodate growth to a certain degree; however, these modular systems tend to be heavier and bulkier than the lighter, more compact, off-the-shelf systems or custom system that cannot change with growth. Clinicians need to consider the impact on current function of a heavier system and make their recommendations accordingly. It is possible to justify a new chair in a shorter period of time based on growth.

In certain cases, such as when a child lacks muscle control, modular systems can offer advantages. Trunk lateral supports may need to be removed while the child is engaged in a dynamic reaching activity or in therapy working on trunk control but replaced to sit more passively when he or she fatigues. A child should also be allowed to passively sit when focused on other activities, such as schoolwork, or relaxing while riding in a vehicle or watching television. If the child has to focus all his or her energy on balance and stability, then he or she will have no energy to devote to the task at hand. If a seating system is too confining or restrictive with multiple supports, the child may fight the system to be able to move and be dynamic. Thus, the pediatric seating specialist must find a balance between appropriate amounts of support without overly restricting movement. An anterior chest harness or support may be needed for stabilization during transportation but removed to engage in schoolwork. It is important to educate all parties as to when a certain support is appropriate and when it is inappropriate. Inappropriate use of chest harnesses has resulted in strangulation when the child slid down in the seat because he or she was becoming uncomfortable and trying to fight the restrictions of the seating system (90). It is often difficult to find a balance between providing enough support and still allowing for some freedom of movement. Having systems that are modular and flexible, as well as educating caregivers, can help find this balance. Dynamic seating is another option that allows the chair to move in response to user-generated force, such as with fluctuating high tone or spasticity, and then returns them to a functional position. Examples of dynamic seating components include footrests, backrests, and headrests.

Custom-molded systems are indicated when a child's postural deformities are so severe that they cannot be supported by a modular or off-the-shelf seating system. Custom-molded systems are not as common with children as they are with adults, as children's deformities tend not to be as severe. As with off-the-shelf systems, custom-molded systems have no growth capabilities.

Mobility

Mobility is the precursor to all childhood development. Children need to explore their environment to know where things are and how to get them. The need for specific types of mobility bases, such as strollers, self-propelled systems, and powered systems, will depend on the age and the physical, developmental, and functional capabilities of the child, as well as the environmental and transportation resources of the family. Very young children may need a seating system that can be transferred and attached to a variety of bases for different activities. For play, children want to be close to the floor near their toys and peers. For eating, they need to be up where a caregiver can have access. Some manufacturers make seating systems that can be transferred to various mobile and stationary bases that are height adjustable. For example, one seating system can be transferred between a folding-style stroller-type base, a higher eating base, and a power-wheelchair base and can also serve as crash-tested car seat.

There has been a historical tendency to push children with disabilities to ambulate with braces and other aids. The practitioner, however, needs to consider the mobility needs of the child, including the expected surfaces and distances. A manual or power wheelchair may be more efficient and actually provide greater independence. Children often abandon cumbersome upright ambulation in favor of a wheelchair when they are able to make their own choice. Consider a child with cerebral palsy trying to ambulate with braces and crutches as well as carry a bag full of books through a crowded hallway. Manual wheelchairs are sometimes a useful option for children; however, the weight of the chair may be an issue. Even an ultralight manual wheelchair weighing 20 lb is going to be heavy for a 30- to 40-lb child. Proper chair selection and training are essential to the long-term health of the child.

Powered mobility is important for children who cannot effectively self-propel a manual system; however, families often do not have the resources or psychological readiness either to make the necessary home modifications or to purchase an accessible vehicle that can transport a powered system. Research and clinical intuition indicate that children without cognitive disability should be offered mobility devices such as power wheelchairs or adapted ride-on power toys as early as 12 to 18 months—about the time able-bodied children begin ambulating on their own (91–93). A study of children of age 14 to 30 months showed that those with powered mobility had improved scores compared to baseline for the Battelle Developmental Inventory and several scales of the Pediatric Evaluation of Disability Inventory (94). Even with a power wheelchair, there is often the need for a transportable folding supportive stroller-type base, as described previously, for use in family outings.

Psychosocial and Family Issues

There are many psychosocial and family-related issues practitioners need to be cognizant of and respect. Having a child with a birth or acquired disability can devastate a family. Initially, there tends to be focus on the search for a cure to the problem, and the family may be a reluctant to accept use of a wheelchair, place a ramp in front of the home, or purchase a van with a ramp. The practitioner needs to counsel the family regarding the realistically expected short- and long-term outcomes of the child's situation. There is also a tendency to "care for" a child with a disability, especially in certain cultures and religions. It is common for children with disabilities to develop learned helplessness and for parents to develop a codependency in the relationship with their child (95). Later in life, this can result in lack of ability to make decisions or function in society. Children with disabilities need to experience the same stages of development—including successes as well as failures—as their able-bodied peers within the norms and values of that culture. Practitioners again need to counsel families so that they can effectively use this equipment to facilitate development and promote active participation by the child as appropriate based on their current and potential capabilities.

STANDARDS AND DURABILITY

International standards are applied to mobility devices. The standards are formulated by ISO, the International Standards Organization; the American National Standards Institute; and by RESNA (96). The standards concern many aspects of wheelchairs, including electrical systems, durability, dimensions, flammability, strength of armrests, ability to withstand an impact, and stability, to name a few. These standards can be requested from the manufacturer and can serve as a method of comparing classes of wheelchair as well as individual wheelchairs to each other. Wheelchair users should be confident of the structural integrity of their wheelchair. Failure of any component is more than an inconvenience for the wheelchair users—it is the limitation of their mobility and can be life-threatening.

A study by Fitzgerald et al. (97) compares the results of standards testing on three classifications of manual wheelchairs. The classes followed Medicare definitions of K0001, depot or hospital-type (27); K0004, lightweight (98); and K0005, ultralight (28). Using ISO equivalent number of testing cycles, curb-drop and double-drum tests were expressed as a single variable, and Kaplan-Meier survival curves were determined. The fatigue life of ultralight wheelchairs was significantly greater than both the lightweight or hospital-type wheelchairs. Of a cohort of lightweight chairs, greater than 75% did not meet ANSI/RENSA standards in spite of improvements in design and manufacturing (30). Because ISO testing is based on a 5-year life cycle, it was concluded that lightweight and hospital-type wheelchairs might not last for the typical 3- to 5-year period expected by health insurers. A better investment for an individual patient was shown to be the ultralight, despite its initial high cost. This analysis did not take into account the other advantages of ultralight wheelchairs described in this chapter. Similar testing is being done on power wheelchairs. In general, similar to manual wheelchairs, results indicate that higher-quality power wheelchairs will be less costly over the life span of the chairs (57).

Survey-based studies have revealed increases in the percentage of users that report experiencing wheelchair failures. In the most recent report, 62% of wheelchair users reported experiencing breakdown in a 6-month period (99). These failures result in unwanted adverse consequences including injuries, missed school, work, and medical appointments (99–102).

WHEELCHAIR MAINTENANCE

Typically, a wheelchair will be used on a daily basis and, as such, has a life expectancy of 3 to 5 years. Just like maintaining a car, preventative maintenance is an essential activity for wheelchair users. However, Medicare policies, which are followed by many other insurers, do not cover preventative maintenance. As such, users may experience adverse consequences secondary to breakdown such as missing work or school, being stranded, or sustaining an injury. Educating users on how and when to complete preventative maintenance should be part of the provision process. A resource for clinicians on how and what to teach wheelchair users regarding basic maintenance can be found here: http://www.upmc-sci.org/wmtp (103).

SECONDARY INJURY/ACCIDENTS

Unfortunately, wheelchair users are at risk for other injuries as a direct result of their wheelchair use (104). In 2003, over 100,000 wheelchair-related injuries were treated in the emergency department. Of individuals treated, 68.9% were more than 65 years old, and 65.0% were female. The highest percentage of injures reported were fractures, contusions, and lacerations, and the leading cause of injury was from tips and falls (65% of injuries). A 2015 systematic review found that falls were most often caused by wheelchair design characteristic, transfer performance, poor balance, and negotiating uneven terrain or a cross-slope (105). Another important area of concern is that most wheelchairs are not crashworthy for use as seats in motor vehicles, as their seat belts and other seating components are not designed to withstand the forces occurring in motor vehicle accidents. Additional seat belts and tie downs must be used to individually hold both the patient and the wheelchair secure (106). Clinicians should be aware of this and discuss transportation directly with the patient.

Possibly the most important area of concern for manual wheelchair users are repetitive strain injuries of the upper extremities. These injuries are so significant that some researchers have gone so far as to say that damage to the upper limbs may be functionally and economically equivalent to a spinal cord injury of a higher neurologic level (107). The two most common areas of injury are the shoulder, with rotator cuff disease (108) and degenerative arthritis (109), and the wrist, in the form of carpal tunnel syndrome (110,111). These studies have found injury rates as high as 70%. Studies have found a direct link between manual wheelchair propulsion and injury to both the shoulder and wrist (47). Clinicians must be aware that an appropriately prescribed and setup wheelchair, which is propelled in an appropriate manner, can reduce the risk of injury. In addition, for some individuals, it may be appropriate to discuss power-assisted or power wheelchairs as a means for preserving the upper limb for activities such as transfers. As mentioned earlier, the CPG for preservation of upper limb function specifically details the proper manual wheelchair setup and propulsion techniques to prevent repetitive strain injuries (36).

FUNDING/INSURANCE

For many individuals, funding can present a major limitation to the type and quality of the wheelchair they can receive through their health insurance. It is tempting as a practitioner to determine the wheelchair that insurance will cover and then work from this limitation. This path can be poor for the patient and in the long term will not lead to changes in policy. Therefore, it is important that the clinician working with the patient determines the optimal mobility device. After making this determination, the team can then assess what is the best way to convince insurance that the device is medically necessary and should be covered.

Having stated this, it is helpful to know current policies and their impact on patients. The section below is focused on the United States, but policies differ markedly from one country to another. In the United States, wheelchairs and seating systems are covered in whole or part by health insurance plans, including Medicare Part B, state Medicaid programs, commercial insurance, and managed care plans, unless the policy stipulates no durable medical equipment coverage. Other funding sources also exist. If the device is needed for work-related activities, state vocational rehabilitation programs can be utilized. In addition, the Veteran's Administration for veterans with both service- and non–service-related disabilities can be a very valuable funding source.

Medicare funding policy for mobility-assistive equipment (MAE, the term they use to include canes, crutches, walkers, manual wheelchairs, scooters, and power wheelchairs) is important to understand and follow, as equipment can be denied if the practitioner's documentation does not reflect what is being requested in the policy. Medicare policy is also generally adopted by most other funding sources including State Medicaid programs and private health insurance. Medicare policy approaches the need for MAE from a functional perspective and uses mobility-related activities of daily living (MRADLs, meaning how mobility impacts a person's ability to participate in ADLs). In order to qualify for any MAE, a person has to have an impairment in "one or more" MRADL in the "home." The "in the home" language does, however, continue to be a restriction meaning that a manual wheelchair, scooter, or power wheelchair will not be covered if it is "only" to perform MRADLs outside the home. Medicare defines a mobility limitation as one that

- Prevents the patient from accomplishing an MRADL entirely (i.e., independence).
- The patient is at reasonably determined heightened risk of morbidity or mortality secondary to the attempts to perform an MRADL (i.e., safety).
- The patient is unable to complete the MRADL within a reasonable time frame (i.e., quality).

Requirements for documentation in the medical record are very specific and must be furnished to the company that supplies the equipment as they need to keep records on file in the event of an audit. Failure to provide the necessary documentation to the supplier will result in the supplier refusing to dispense the equipment. Physicians are also not permitted to complete forms provided by suppliers or manufacturers as a substitute for what is documented in the medical record. Medicare policy states that the medical record can include (but is not limited to) the items listed in 🛜 **eBox 58-2**. The policy also recognizes and encourages physicians to refer patients with mobility limitations to an occupational or physical therapist for assessment in identifying the appropriate MAE intervention and to provide necessary documentation.

The qualifying criteria for the various types of wheeled mobility devices are as follows:

The patient has limited ability to ambulate even with the use of a cane, crutch, or walker. For this, it is usually sufficient to explain that an individual can only ambulate short distances or is unsafe ambulating. Placing these limitations in the context of his or her current living situation and usual activities can help persuade payers of the need.

Lightweight and ultralightweight wheelchairs. To qualify for either of these wheelchairs, it is necessary to document that the person is unable to propel a lower-cost alternative standard wheelchair or use a cane or walker in an effective manner. It also helps document the person's lifestyle situation and how the wheelchair will facilitate his or her ability to engage in activities.

Power wheelchairs and power-operated vehicles. Powered mobility devices include power wheelchairs and power-operated vehicles (POVs) or scooters. To qualify for a power wheelchair or POV, one must document that the person cannot effectively propel any type of manual wheelchair. For individuals with upper-extremity paralysis, it is obvious that they cannot propel a manual chair. However, many other individuals can require a power wheelchair. People with upper-extremity pain that limits propulsion meet this criterion because pain and risk of aggravating injury may make them incapable of propelling a manual chair. This is also true for individuals with cardiopulmonary disease or obesity. Both of these conditions make functional manual wheelchair propulsion difficult and, in some cases, impossible. These deficits and risks should be documented and explained in the LMN.

Power wheelchairs are categorized into five groups. Group 1 power wheelchairs can only accommodate people up to a weight of 136 kg (300 lb) and cannot accommodate any seat functions such as tilt-in-space or a seat elevator. They can accommodate nonpowered options such as recline-only backs or manually elevating leg rests. They are also not well suited to negotiate uneven surfaces or thresholds more than 20 mm in height. Group 2 power wheelchairs can accommodate multiple weight capacities up to 272 kg (600 lb); however, they are only designed to accommodate a single power seat function such as a seat elevator or tilt-in-space. Group 2 chairs can also accommodate seating and positioning supports such as trunk or thigh supports, except for captain's chair seats. Group 3 power wheelchairs can handle multiple weight capacities up to 272 kg (600 lb) and multiple seat functions including a vent tray and alternative controls. Group 3 power wheelchairs require a person to have a neuromuscular, myopathy, or congenital orthopedic anomaly. Group 4 power wheelchairs are similar to Groups 2 and 3 power wheelchairs; however, they have features that are inherent to outdoor mobility such as larger motors and a suspension and therefore are not covered by Medicare and many other payer sources. Group 5 power wheelchairs are classified as pediatric products.

Scooters are only covered when a patient resides in a home where there is sufficient maneuvering space to operate a scooter, the patient can safely transfer in and out of a scooter, a scooter seating system will address the patient's postural needs, and the patient has sufficient upper extremity function to operate the scooter steering mechanism. Scooters are broken down into two groups. Group 1 POVs can handle multiple weight capacities and are generally designed to negotiate most level indoor and outdoor surfaces. Group 2 POVs have designed features such as larger motors and suspensions that are inherent to outdoor mobility only and therefore not covered by Medicare and many other health insurance plans.

Medicare requires that any Group 2 power wheelchair with a single power seat function, any Groups 3 or 4 power wheelchairs, or a pushrim-activated, power-assisted wheelchair be provided by a company that employs a RESNA-certified ATS. The beneficiary receiving the equipment must also be evaluated by a qualified medical practitioner (such as an occupational or physical therapists) with experience and knowledge in complex wheelchair seating and mobility equipment. As stated early, Medicare also requires that the supplier of wheeled MAE ensures that the patient's home and environment are suitable for the MAE and that there is sufficient maneuvering space to operate the device.

There are documented disparities in the quality and equity of wheelchairs provided to end users based on income level, age, race, and funding source. Minorities are less likely to have a working backup chair, less likely to have seating functions on power wheelchairs, and more likely to suffer adverse consequences secondary to breakdown (101). Individuals from lower socioeconomic statuses as well as older adults are less likely to have customized wheelchairs (112). There remain groups of individuals with disabilities who are not adequately supported by programs with financing for assistive technology, emphasizing the importance of advocating for one's patients (112–114).

SUMMARY

Prescription of wheelchairs is a complex and time-consuming task. Many parties need to be involved, and technology is constantly changing. In an ideal world, all wheelchairs would be prescribed using all the members of the team described earlier in this chapter, and clinicians would be reimbursed at a level that allowed for appropriate evaluation and training. Unfortunately, wheelchair clinics are costly to run; therefore, the team approach described may not be possible in many settings. It is essential that the physician signing the prescription understands the equipment well enough to explain the choices made as well as the trade-offs involved, limitations, and safety issues. Most importantly, the patient should be able to make informed choices.

A clinician practicing without a clinic can still provide good care. The best approach is to find a therapist in the rehabilitation team who has an interest in wheelchairs. If possible, the therapist should attend meetings such as RESNA (www.resna.org), the International Seating Symposium (www.iss.pitt.edu), or Medtrade (www.medtrade.com) to learn about new technology. In addition, the therapist should consider taking the ATP examination for certification. This can be sold to the hospital as a value-added service that their institution has and others do not. The other key team member then becomes the dealer. The doctor and therapist team should request (or require) that the dealer become a CRTS. The team can also ask the dealer to have equipment available for trials and to visit the patient's house. This team can be very effective at wheelchair delivery and can improve the function and quality of life of their patients.

FUTURE

New and exciting products are placed on the market each day. As mobility products improve, the line between needing the device because of a disability and wanting the device because it enhances mobility can become blurred. Mainstream use of assistive devices is a great thing for wheelchair users as it expands the market and lowers costs. In addition, it blurs the line between disability and normal function. In the future, it would not be uncommon for everyone to have a personal mobility device, such as the Segway (115), and the only difference between individuals with disabilities and individuals without impairments is that individuals with disabilities always use their vehicle. With these advances, it will be important for health care professionals to continue to lobby on behalf of their patients to increase funding for wheelchairs so that function dictates the prescription.

Note: Michael Boninger is an inventor of the Natural-Fit hand rim and receives a royalty from the University of Pittsburgh.

REFERENCES

1. Institute of Medicine (US) Committee on Assessing Rehabilitation Science and Engineering. Models of Disability and Rehabilitation. In: Brandt EN, Pope AM, eds. *Enabling America: Assessing the Role of Rehabilitation Science and Engineering.* Washington, DC: National Academies Press (US); 1997.
2. Evans R. The effect of electrically powered indoor/outdoor wheelchairs on occupation: a study of users' views. *Br J Occup Ther.* 2000;63(11):547–553.
3. Aronson KJ. Quality of life among persons with multiple sclerosis and their caregivers. *Neurology.* 1997;48(1):74–80.
4. Bottos M, Bolcati C, Sciuto L, et al. Powered wheelchairs and independence in young children with tetraplegia. *Dev Med Child Neurol.* 2001;43(11):769–777.
5. Buning ME, Angelo JA, Schmeler MR. Occupational performance and the transition to powered mobility: a pilot study. *Am J Occup Ther.* 2001;55(3):339–344.
6. Miles-Tapping C. Power wheelchairs and independent life styles. *Can J Rehabil.* 1996;10:137–146.
7. World Health Organization. *Guidelines on the Provision of Manual Wheelchairs in Less Resourced Settings.* Geneva, Switzerland: World Health Organization; 2008.
8. Cooper RA, Ohnabe H, Hobson DA. *An Introduction to Rehabilitation Engineering.* Boca Raton, FL: CRC Press; 2006.
9. Lukersmith S, Radbron L, Hopman K. Development of clinical guidelines for the prescription of a seated wheelchair or mobility scooter for people with traumatic brain injury or spinal cord injury. *Aust Occup Ther J.* 2013;60(6):378–386.
10. Wielandt T, Strong J. Compliance with prescribed adaptive equipment: a literature review. *Br J Occup Ther.* 2000;63(2):65–75.
11. Cooper RA. *Rehabilitation Engineering Applied to Mobility and Manipulation.* New York, NY: CRC Press; 1995.
12. Glaser RM, Simsen-Harold CA, Petrofsky JS, et al. Metabolic and cardiopulmonary responses of older wheelchair-dependent and ambulatory patients during locomotion. *Ergonomics.* 1983;26(7):687–697.
13. Fay BT, Boninger ML, Fitzgerald SG, et al. Manual wheelchair pushrim dynamics in people with multiple sclerosis. *Arch Phys Med Rehabil.* 2004;85(6):935–942.
14. Boninger ML, Saur T, Trefler E, et al. Postural changes with aging in tetraplegia: effects on life satisfaction and pain. *Arch Phys Med Rehabil.* 1998;79(12):1577–1581.
15. Grieco A. Sitting posture: an old problem and a new one. *Ergonomics.* 1986;29(3):345–362.
16. Greer N, Brasure M, Wilt TJ. Wheeled mobility (wheelchair) service delivery: scope of the evidence. *Ann Intern Med.* 2012;156(2):141–146.
17. Kumar A, Schmeler MR, Karmarkar AM, et al. Test-retest reliability of the functional mobility assessment (FMA): a pilot study. *Disabil Rehabil Assist Technol.* 2013;8(3):213–219.
18. Centers for Medicare & Medicaid Services, Medicare Learning Network. *Power Mobility Devices.* US Department of Health and Human Services; 2017. Available from: https://www.cms.gov/Outreach-and-Education/Medicare-Learning-Network-MLN/MLNProducts/Downloads/PMD_DocCvg_FactSheet_ICN905063.pdf
19. Best KL, Kirby RL, Smith C, et al. Wheelchair skills training for community-based manual wheelchair users: a randomized controlled trial. *Arch Phys Med Rehabil.* 2005;86(12):2316–2323.
20. Coolen AL, Kirby RL, Landry J, et al. Wheelchair skills training program for clinicians: a randomized controlled trial with occupational therapy students. *Arch Phys Med Rehabil.* 2004;85(7):1160–1167.
21. Kirby RL, Crawford KA, Smith C, et al. A wheelchair workshop for medical students improves knowledge and skills: a randomized controlled trial. *Am J Phys Med Rehabil.* 2011;90(3):197–206.
22. Kirby RL, Miller WC, Routhier F, et al. Effectiveness of a wheelchair skills training program for powered wheelchair users: a randomized controlled trial. *Arch Phys Med Rehabil.* 2015;96(11):2017.e2013–2026.e2013.
23. MacPhee AH, Kirby RL, Coolen AL, et al. Wheelchair skills training program: a randomized clinical trial of wheelchair users undergoing initial rehabilitation. *Arch Phys Med Rehabil.* 2004;85(1):41–50.
24. Worobey LA, Kirby RL, Heinemann AW, et al. Effectiveness of group wheelchair skills training for people with spinal cord injury: a randomized controlled trial. *Arch Phys Med Rehabil.* 2016;97(10):1777.e1773–1784.e1773.
25. Mann WC, Goodall S, Justiss MD, et al. Dissatisfaction and nonuse of assistive devices among frail elders. *Assist Technol.* 2002;14(2):130–139.
26. Shankar S, Mortenson WB, Wallace J. Taking control: an exploratory study of the use of tilt-in-space wheelchairs in residential care. *Am J Occup Ther.* 2015;69(2):6902290040.
27. Cooper RA, Robertson RN, Lawrence B, et al. Life-cycle analysis of depot versus rehabilitation manual wheelchairs. *J Rehabil Res Dev.* 1996;33(1):45.
28. Cooper RA, Boninger ML, Rentschler A. Evaluation of selected ultralight manual wheelchairs using ANSI/RESNA standards. *Arch Phys Med Rehabil.* 1999;80(4):462–467.
29. Liu H-Y, Hong E-K, Wang H, et al. Evaluation of aluminum ultralight rigid wheelchairs versus other ultralight wheelchairs using ANSI/RESNA standards. *J Rehabil Res Dev.* 2010;47(5):441.
30. Gebrosky B, Pearlman J, Cooper RA, et al. Evaluation of lightweight wheelchairs using ANSI/RESNA testing standards. *J Rehabil Res Dev.* 2013;50(10):1373–1389.
31. Garcia-Mendez Y, Pearlman JL, Boninger ML, et al. Health risks of vibration exposure to wheelchair users in the community. *J Spinal Cord Med.* 2013;36(4):365–375.
32. Chénier F, Aissaoui R. Effect of wheelchair frame material on users' mechanical work and transmitted vibration. *Biomed Res Int.* 2014;2014:609369.
33. Requejo PS, Maneekobkunwong S, McNitt-Gray J, et al. Influence of hand-rim wheelchairs with rear suspension on seat forces and head acceleration during curb descent landings. *J Rehabil Med.* 2009;41(6):459–466.
34. Cooper RA, Wolf E, Fitzgerald SG, et al. Seat and footrest shocks and vibrations in manual wheelchairs with and without suspension. *Arch Phys Med Rehabil.* 2003;84(1):96–102.
35. Tederko P, Besowski T, Jakubiak K, et al. Influence of wheelchair footrest height on ischial tuberosity pressure in individuals with paraplegia. *Spinal Cord.* 2015;53(6):471–475.
36. Paralyzed Veterans of America Consortium for Spinal Cord Medicine. Preservation of upper limb function following spinal cord injury: a clinical practice guideline for health-care professionals. *J Spinal Cord Med.* 2005;28(5):434–470.
37. Sawatzky B, Miller W, Denison I. Measuring energy expenditure using heart rate to assess the effects of wheelchair tyre pressure. *Clin Rehabil.* 2005;19(2):182–187.
38. Lin JT, Huang M, Sprigle S. Evaluation of wheelchair resistive forces during straight and turning trajectories across different wheelchair configurations using free-wheeling coast-down test. *J Rehabil Res Dev.* 2015;52(7):763.
39. Pavlidou E, Kloosterman MG, Buurke JH, et al. Rolling resistance and propulsion efficiency of manual and power-assisted wheelchairs. *Med Eng Phys.* 2015;37(11):1105–1110.
40. de Groot S, Vegter RJ, van der Woude LH. Effect of wheelchair mass, tire type and tire pressure on physical strain and wheelchair propulsion technique. *Med Eng Phys.* 2013;35(10):1476–1482.
41. Koontz AM, Yang Y, Boninger DS, et al. Investigation of the performance of an ergonomic handrim as a pain-relieving intervention for manual wheelchair users. *Assist Technol.* 2006;18(2):123–145.
42. Medola FO, Fortulan CA, Purquerio BDM, et al. A new design for an old concept of wheelchair pushrim. *Disabil Rehabil Assist Technol.* 2012;7(3):234–241.
43. Dieruf K, Ewer L, Boninger D. The natural-fit handrim: factors related to improvement in symptoms and function in wheelchair users. *J Spinal Cord Med.* 2008;31(5):578–585.
44. Richter M, Karpinski A, Rodriguez R, et al. Impact attenuation and efficiency characteristics of a flexible wheelchair handrim. *Top Spinal Cord Inj Rehabil.* 2009;15(2):71–78.
45. Richter WM, Rodriguez R, Woods KR, et al. Reduced finger and wrist flexor activity during propulsion with a new flexible handrim. *Arch Phys Med Rehabil.* 2006;87(12):1643–1647.
46. Hughes B, Sawatzky BJ, Hol AT. A comparison of spinergy versus standard steel-spoke wheelchair wheels. *Arch Phys Med Rehabil.* 2005;86(3):596–601.
47. Boninger ML, Koontz AM, Sisto SA, et al. Pushrim biomechanics and injury prevention in spinal cord injury: recommendations based on CULP-SCI investigations. *J Rehabil Res Dev.* 2005;42(3):9.
48. Gorce P, Louis N. Wheelchair propulsion kinematics in beginners and expert users: influence of wheelchair settings. *Clin Biomech.* 2012;27(1):7–15.
49. Boninger ML, Baldwin M, Cooper RA, et al. Manual wheelchair pushrim biomechanics and axle position. *Arch Phys Med Rehabil.* 2000;81(5):608–613.
50. Van der Woude L, Hendrich K, Veeger H, et al. Manual wheelchair propulsion: effects of power output on physiology and technique. *Med Sci Sports Exerc.* 1988;20(1):70–78.
51. Veeger D, Van der Woude L, Rozendal RH. The effect of rear wheel camber in manual wheelchair propulsion. *J Rehabil Res Dev.* 1989;26(2):37–46.
52. BKin JL, Sadeghi M. Mechanical efficiency of two commercial lever-propulsion mechanisms for manual wheelchair locomotion. *J Rehabil Res Dev.* 2013;50(10):1363.
53. Mandy A, Redhead L, McCudden C, et al. A comparison of vertical reaction forces during propulsion of three different one-arm drive wheelchairs by hemiplegic users. *Disabil Rehabil Assist Technol.* 2014;9(3):242–247.

54. Best KL, Kirby RL, Smith C, et al. Comparison between performance with a push-rim-activated power-assisted wheelchair and a manual wheelchair on the Wheelchair Skills Test. *Disabil Rehabil.* 2006;28(4):213–220.

55. Fitzgerald SG, Arva J, Cooper RA, et al. A pilot study on community usage of a pushrim-activated, power-assisted wheelchair. *Assist Technol.* 2003;15(2):113–119.

56. Cooper RA, Fitzgerald SG, Boninger ML, et al. Evaluation of a pushrim-activated, power-assisted wheelchair. *Arch Phys Med Rehabil.* 2001;82(5):702–708.

57. Algood SD, Cooper RA, Fitzgerald SG, et al. Impact of a pushrim-activated power-assisted wheelchair on the metabolic demands, stroke frequency, and range of motion among subjects with tetraplegia. *Arch Phys Med Rehabil.* 2004;85(11):1865–1871.

58. Guillon B, Van-Hecke G, Iddir J, et al. Evaluation of 3 pushrim-activated power-assisted wheelchairs in patients with spinal cord injury. *Arch Phys Med Rehabil.* 2015;96(5):894–904.

59. Kloosterman MG, Snoek GJ, van der Woude LH, et al. A systematic review on the pros and cons of using a pushrim-activated power-assisted wheelchair. *Clin Rehabil.* 2013;27(4):299–313.

60. Algood SD, Cooper RA, Fitzgerald SG, et al. Effect of a pushrim-activated power-assist wheelchair on the functional capabilities of persons with tetraplegia. *Arch Phys Med Rehabil.* 2005;86(3):380–386.

61. Levy CE, Chow JW, Tillman MD, et al. Variable-ratio pushrim-activated power-assist wheelchair eases wheeling over a variety of terrains for elders. *Arch Phys Med Rehabil.* 2004;85(1):104–112.

62. Boninger ML, Souza AL, Cooper RA, et al. Propulsion patterns and pushrim biomechanics in manual wheelchair propulsion. *Arch Phys Med Rehabil.* 2002;83(5):718–723.

63. Rice I, Gagnon D, Gallagher J, et al. Hand rim wheelchair propulsion training using biomechanical real-time visual feedback based on motor learning theory principles. *J Spinal Cord Med.* 2010;33(1):33–42.

64. Rice IM, Pohlig RT, Gallagher JD, et al. Handrim wheelchair propulsion training effect on overground propulsion using biomechanical real-time visual feedback. *Arch Phys Med Rehabil.* 2013;94(2):256–263.

65. Askari S, Kirby RL, Parker K, et al. Wheelchair propulsion test: development and measurement properties of a new test for manual wheelchair users. *Arch Phys Med Rehabil.* 2013;94(9):1690–1698.

66. Koontz AM, Brindle ED, Kankipati P, et al. Design features that affect the maneuverability of wheelchairs and scooters. *Arch Phys Med Rehabil.* 2010;91(5):759–764.

67. Simpson R, LoPresti E, Hayashi S, et al. A prototype power assist wheelchair that provides for obstacle detection and avoidance for those with visual impairments. *J Neuroeng Rehabil.* 2005;2(1):30.

68. Ding D, Cooper RA, Kaminski BA, et al. Integrated control and related technology of assistive devices. *Assist Technol.* 2003;15(2):89–97.

69. Wästlund E, Sponseller K, Pettersson O, et al. Evaluating gaze-driven power wheelchair with navigation support for persons with disabilities. *J Rehabil Res Dev.* 2015;52(7):815–826.

70. Kim J, Park H, Bruce J, et al. Qualitative assessment of tongue drive system by people with high-level spinal cord injury. *J Rehabil Res Dev.* 2014;51(3):451.

71. Kim J, Park H, Bruce J, et al. The tongue enables computer and wheelchair control for people with spinal cord injury. *Sci Transl Med.* 2013;5(213):213ra166.

72. Park H, Kiani M, Lee H-M, et al. A wireless magnetoresistive sensing system for an intraoral tongue-computer interface. *IEEE Trans Biomed Circuits Syst.* 2012;6(6):571–585.

73. Liu H-Y, Cooper R, Cooper R, et al. Seating virtual coach: a smart reminder for power seat function usage. *Technol Disabil.* 2010;22(1,2):53–60.

74. Boucher P, Atrash A, Kelouwani S, et al. Design and validation of an intelligent wheelchair towards a clinically-functional outcome. *J Neuroeng Rehabil.* 2013;10(1):58.

75. Rushton PW, Kairy D, Archambault P, et al. The potential impact of intelligent power wheelchair use on social participation: perspectives of users, caregivers and clinicians. *Disabil Rehabil Assist Technol.* 2015;10(3):191–197.

76. Mostowy LC. Performance testing of collision-avoidance system for power wheelchairs. *J Rehabil Res Dev.* 2011;48(5):529.

77. Byrne D, Salzberg C. Major risk factors for pressure ulcers in the spinal cord disabled. *Spinal Cord.* 1996;34:255–263.

78. Geyer MJ, Brienza DM, Karg P, et al. A randomized control trial to evaluate pressure-reducing seat cushions for elderly wheelchair users. *Adv Skin Wound Care.* 2001;14(3):120–129.

79. Brienza DM, Karg PE, Geyer MJ, et al. The relationship between pressure ulcer incidence and buttock-seat cushion interface pressure in at-risk elderly wheelchair users. *Arch Phys Med Rehabil.* 2001;82(4):529–533.

80. Medola FO, Elui VM, Santana Cda S, et al. Aspects of manual wheelchair configuration affecting mobility: a review. *J Phys Ther Sci.* 2014;26(2):313–318.

81. Hong E-K, Dicianno BE, Pearlman J, et al. Comfort and stability of wheelchair backrests according to the TAWC (tool for assessing wheelchair discomfort). *Disabil Rehabil Assist Technol.* 2016;11(3):223–227.

82. Dicianno BE, Lieberman J, Schmeler M, et al. *RESNA Position on the Application of Tilt, Recline, and Elevating Leg Rests for Wheelchairs: 2015 Current State of the Literature.* Arlington, VA: RESNA; 2015.

83. Jan Y-K, Crane BA, Liao F, et al. Comparison of muscle and skin perfusion over the ischial tuberosities in response to wheelchair tilt-in-space and recline angles in people with spinal cord injury. *Arch Phys Med Rehabil.* 2013;94(10):1990–1996.

84. Chen Y, Wang J, Lung C-W, et al. Effect of tilt and recline on ischial and coccygeal interface pressures in people with spinal cord injury. *Am J Phys Med Rehabil.* 2014;93(12):1019–1030.

85. Eng JJ, Levins SM, Townson AF, et al. Use of prolonged standing for individuals with spinal cord injuries. *Phys Ther.* 2001;81(8):1392.

86. Arva J, Schmeler MR, Lange ML, et al. RESNA position on the application of seat-elevating devices for wheelchair users. *Assist Technol.* 2009;21(2):69–72.

87. Sigholm G, Herberts P, Almström C, et al. Electromyographic analysis of shoulder muscle load. *J Orthop Res.* 1983;1(4):379–386.

88. Weiner DK, Long R, Hughes MA, et al. When older adults face the chair-rise challenge: a study of chair height availability and height-modified chair-rise performance in the elderly. *J Am Geriatr Soc.* 1993;41(1):6–10.

89. Cooper RA, Dvorznak MJ, O'Connor TJ, et al. Braking electric-powered wheelchairs: effect of braking method, seatbelt, and legrests. *Arch Phys Med Rehabil.* 1998;79(10):1244–1249.

90. Chaves ES, Cooper RA, Collins DM, et al. Review of the use of physical restraints and lap belts with wheelchair users. *Assist Technol.* 2007;19(2):94–107.

91. Butler C. Effects of powered mobility on self-initiated behaviors of very young children with locomotor disability. *Dev Med Child Neurol.* 1986;28(3):325–332.

92. Tefft D, Guerette P, Furumasu J. Cognitive predictors of young children's readiness for powered mobility. *Dev Med Child Neurol.* 1999;41(10):665–670.

93. Frank A, Ward J, Orwell N, et al. *Introduction of a New NHS Electric-Powered Indoor/Outdoor Chair (EPIOC) Service: Benefits, Risks and Implications for Prescribers.* Thousand Oaks, CA: SAGE Publications; 2000.

94. Jones MA, McEwen IR, Neas BR. Effects of power wheelchairs on the development and function of young children with severe motor impairments. *Pediatr Phys Ther.* 2012;24(2):131–140.

95. Holmbeck GN, Johnson SZ, Wills KE, et al. Observed and perceived parental overprotection in relation to psychosocial adjustment in preadolescents with a physical disability: the mediational role of behavioral autonomy. *J Consult Clin Psychol.* 2002;70(1):96.

96. Axelson P, Minkel J, Chesney D, et al. *A Guide to Wheelchair Selection: How to Use the ANSI/RESNA Wheelchair Standards to Buy a Wheelchair.* Washington, DC: Paralyzed Veterans of America; 1994.

97. Fitzgerald SG, Cooper RA, Boninger ML, et al. Comparison of fatigue life for 3 types of manual wheelchairs. *Arch Phys Med Rehabil.* 2001;82(10):1484–1488.

98. Cooper RA, Gonzalez J, Lawrence B, et al. Performance of selected lightweight wheelchairs on ANSI/RESNA tests. *Arch Phys Med Rehabil.* 1997;78(10):1138–1144.

99. Toro ML, Worobey L, Boninger ML, et al. Type and frequency of reported wheelchair repairs and related adverse consequences among people with spinal cord injury. *Arch Phys Med Rehabil.* 2016;97(10):1753–1760.

100. McClure LA, Boninger ML, Oyster ML, et al. Wheelchair repairs, breakdown, and adverse consequences for people with traumatic spinal cord injury. *Arch Phys Med Rehabil.* 2009;90(12):2034–2038.

101. Worobey L, Oyster M, Nemunaitis G, et al. Increases in wheelchair breakdowns, repairs, and adverse consequences for people with traumatic spinal cord injury. *Am J Phys Med Rehabil.* 2012;91(6):463.

102. Worobey L, Oyster M, Pearlman J, et al. Differences between manufacturers in reported power wheelchair repairs and adverse consequences among people with spinal cord injury. *Arch Phys Med Rehabil.* 2014;95(4):597–603.

103. Toro ML, Bird E, Oyster M, et al. Development of a wheelchair maintenance training programme and questionnaire for clinicians and wheelchair users. *Disabil Rehabil Assist Technol.* 2017;12(8):843–851.

104. Xiang H, Chany A, Smith GA. Wheelchair related injuries treated in US emergency departments. *Inj Prev.* 2006;12(1):8–11.

105. Rice LA, Ousley C, Sosnoff JJ. A systematic review of risk factors associated with accidental falls, outcome measures and interventions to manage fall risk in non-ambulatory adults. *Disabil Rehabil.* 2015;37(19):1697–1705.

106. VanRoosmalen L, Bertocci GE, Ha D, et al. Wheelchair integrated occupant restraints: feasibility in frontal impact. *Med Eng Phys.* 2001;23(10):687–698.

107. Sie IH, Waters RL, Adkins RH, et al. Upper extremity pain in the postrehabilitation spinal cord injured patient. *Arch Phys Med Rehabil.* 1992;73(1):44–48.

108. Escobedo EM, Hunter JC, Hollister MC, et al. MR imaging of rotator cuff tears in individuals with paraplegia. *Am J Roentgenol.* 1997;168(4):919–923.

109. Boninger ML, Towers JD, Cooper RA, et al. Shoulder imaging abnormalities in individuals with paraplegia. *J Rehabil Res Dev.* 2001;38(4):401.

110. Davidoff G, Werner R, Waring W. Compressive mononeuropathies of the upper extremity in chronic paraplegia. *Paraplegia.* 1991;29(1):17–24.

111. Aljure J, Eltorai I, Bradley WE, et al. Carpal tunnel syndrome in paraplegic patients. *Spinal Cord.* 1985;23(3):182–186.

112. Hunt PC, Boninger ML, Cooper RA, et al. Demographic and socioeconomic factors associated with disparity in wheelchair customizability among people with traumatic spinal cord injury. *Arch Phys Med Rehabil.* 2004;85(11):1859–1864.

113. Hubbard SL, Fitzgerald SG, Reker DM, et al. Demographic characteristics of veterans who received wheelchairs and scooters from Veterans Health Administration. *J Rehabil Res Dev.* 2006;43(7):831.

114. National Council on Disability. *Study on the Financing of Assistive Technology Devices and Services for Individuals with Disabilities: A Report to the President and the Congress of the United States of America;* 2012. Available from: http://www.ncd.gov/newsroom/publications/1993/assistive.htm

115. Sawatzky B, Denison I, Langrish S, et al. The Segway personal transporter as an alternative mobility device for people with disabilities: a pilot study. *Arch Phys Med Rehabil.* 2007;88(11):1423–1428.

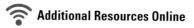 **Additional Resources Online**

Integrative Medicine in PM&R

Caring for the patient from a whole person perspective is one of the cornerstones of the practice of physical medicine and rehabilitation (PM&R); this means assessing not only the physical aspects of health but also acknowledging how social, emotional, and psychospiritual factors will play a significant role in health and healing. PM&R, as a field, is a leader in integrating these concepts of holism and a diverse spectrum of therapeutic modalities into the conventional medical paradigm. Similarly, the field of integrative health, which the Academic Consortium for Integrative Medicine and Health defines as "Integrative medicine and health reaffirms the importance of the relationship between practitioner and patient, focuses on the whole person, is informed by evidence, and makes use of all appropriate therapeutic and lifestyle approaches, healthcare professionals, and disciplines to achieve optimal health and healing" (1), expresses some parallel ideologies. Shared concepts between these fields include the focus on relationship-centered care, interprofessional team–based models, engaging the whole person to promote healing, the importance of self-efficacy, and a focus on quality of life (QOL) including functional goals. Because of the similarities between the theoretical underpinnings and models of PM&R and Integrative Health, these two fields dovetail well.

According to the National Health Information Survey (NHIS) conducted in 2012, 33.2% of U.S. adults and 11.6% of children utilized complementary health approaches (2). Natural products were the most commonly employed modality, with fish oil supplementation being the most popular among both adults and children. Mind-body approaches most commonly utilized were yoga, chiropractic care, osteopathic manual manipulation, massage therapy, and meditation. About 25 million adults reported daily pain, which is one of the most common reasons to seek integrative care (2–4).

After World War II, the distinctive field of PM&R evolved in response to the fact that mainstream medicine was not providing adequate care and treatment for patients who had sustained injuries to the musculoskeletal and central nervous systems. In his pioneering book, *The Knife Is Not Enough*, Dr. Henry H. Kessler clearly espoused the need for what are today being called "complementary and alternative" therapies (5). He not only included physical and dietary interventions in his multidisciplinary approach but also recognized the important role that spirituality played in healing. This approach has marked PM&R with more openness to integrative health than other specialties.

The NIH National Center for Integrative Health and Medicine (NCCIH) defines complementary medicine as an approach to medical care that is used together with conventional medicine. Integrative medicine combines treatments from conventional medicine and complementary practices for which there is evidence of safety and effectiveness. Typically, an integrative health intake involves a comprehensive discussion of all relevant topics in the patient's life, using a holistic model such as the Wheel of Health (**Fig. 59-1**). Alternative medicine is an older term denoting the substitution of unconventional therapies for conventional modalities and is no longer current.

This chapter is written as a descriptive and practical guide for the physiatrist with literature cited for further reading. **Table 59-1** presents a classification system of integrative therapies.

Because of the broad range of therapies within the realm of integrative medicine, this chapter focuses primarily on those therapies that are currently applied in common rehabilitation conditions and settings. The goals of this chapter are to provide (a) a brief introduction to the major integrative therapies that may be employed by physiatrists and used by patients and (b) a theoretical and research basis and where appropriate, clinical strategies for use of integrative therapies in the PM&R setting.

WHOLE MEDICAL SYSTEMS

The NIH NCCIH describes whole medical systems as approaches to care that are built upon complete systems of theory and practice that have evolved independently of the conventional medical approach used in North America and Europe.

Examples of whole medical systems include Traditional Chinese Medicine (TCM), which includes acupuncture, Ayurvedic medicine, and naturopathic medicine. Each of these approaches may have relevance to the practice of physiatry. Of these approaches, acupuncture is the most widely studied as an adjunctive therapy for the management of musculoskeletal pain, and therefore, this modality will be highlighted below.

Traditional Chinese Medicine

Traditional Chinese Medicine is over 3,000 years old and is based on the theory that there is a vital life force (qi) that supports physiologic functioning. qi is concentrated in multiple pathways or channels called meridians that run longitudinally throughout the body. Health is the state in which qi is flowing abundantly and harmoniously, and illness is believed to result from an improper amount distribution or imbalance of this energy, which then precipitates physiologic change (6). TCM encompasses multiple components including acupuncture, herbal medicines, and mind-body practices such as T'ai Chi and qigong. Acupuncture is the insertion of thin, noncutting needles into specific acupuncture points along the meridians in order to correct aberrant energy flow. T'ai Chi, a movement

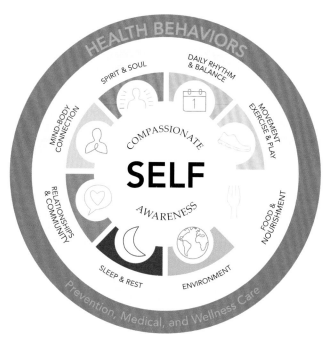

FIGURE 59-1. Wheel of Health. (© 2015 Osher Center for Integrative Medicine. Vanderbilt University Medical Center. Used with permission.)

therapy, and qigong, an energy therapy, are all based on this concept and are discussed in separate sections.

Acupuncture

Acupuncture has numerous applications in PM&R. It is utilized for both acute and chronic musculoskeletal and neurologic problems. Needles are placed both locally, near the anatomic location of the problem, as well as in other areas of the body. A typical acupuncture session lasts 30 to 60 minutes including examination and needle insertion. The number of sessions required depends on the intensity and chronicity of a condition as well as the age and general health of the patient.

For example, for a young otherwise healthy patient experiencing an acute muscular back spasm, one to two sessions may be sufficient. In comparison, for long-standing pain, such as radicular pain secondary to lumbar spinal stenosis, a greater number of sessions followed by less frequent maintenance sessions may be required to achieve optimum results.

Mechanistic research has begun to highlight promising avenues of exploration regarding the physiologic nature of the acupuncture channels and the points themselves (7). Histologic studies have suggested that some 80% of acupuncture points consist of a characteristic subcutaneous column of loose connective tissue, with a looped core bundle of neurovascular and lymphatic vessels that may help propagate the influence of superficial needle inputs to deeper structures (6). Decreased electrical resistance and increased capacitance have been reported between acupuncture points sharing energy channels (8). Additionally, nuclear medicine studies have shown that subcutaneous injection of technetium-99m into the low-resistance acupoints of humans and dogs results in a rapid migration of the radioactive tracer along the associated meridians; this movement is distinct from the trajectory of blood vessels, lymphatics, and peripheral nerves and is not observed with nonacupuncture points (9,10). Similar results using gadolinium injections and MRI have been reported in humans (11). There is substantial overlap in the locations and properties of myofascial trigger points, which react to needling with a local twitch response and predictable pain radiation patterns, and acupuncture points, which react to needling with a local ache (called "*de qi*") and radiation of this sensation along the associated acupuncture channels (12). However, as acupoints are not always tender to palpation and are often used for other indications aside from local pain, debate exists about whether trigger points may merely represent a smaller subset of acupuncture points called "*a shi*" points (13–15).

Anatomic studies *in vivo* and postmortem section in the upper arm have revealed that more than 80% of acupuncture points and 50% of meridians correspond to intermuscular and intramuscular connective tissue cleavage planes (16). Microscopic images show that the tissue resistance "needle grasp" effect (a sensation of resistance felt by the practitioner when the acupuncture needle has been advanced to its desired depth in some acupoints) that is clinically recognized upon twisting an inserted needle actually corresponds to the winding of collagen fibers and fibroblasts in the connective tissue around the surface of that rotated needle (16–19). Needle grasp of acupoints may thus propagate a mechanical stretch to the deeper fascial matrix, which ultimately invests structures such as the peritoneum of the viscera, the pleura, the perineurium, and the meninges (16,20). Mechanotransduction of this stretch converts into a potentially gene transcription–altering intracellular signal by deforming the cytoskeletons of fibroblasts and directly influencing actin and microtubule remodeling, as shown in a murine model (21,22). Related studies have demonstrated that cyclical stretching of fibroblasts in this fashion decreases TGF-β1 production and type 1 procollagen deposition (both factors normally promote fibrosis), which begins to suggest a common hypothesis explaining the therapeutic benefits of fascial stretching modalities such as physical therapy, massage, osteopathy, Rolfing, yoga, and acupuncture (23,24).

TABLE 59-1	Integrative Health and Medicine Techniques	
Categories of Integrative Health and Medicine	**Examples**
Whole medical systems	
Traditional systems	Ayurvedic medicine, traditional Chinese medicine (TCM includes acupuncture)
Other	Homeopathy, naturopathy
Mind-body therapies	Meditation, hypnosis, biofeedback, guided imagery, music therapy, art therapy, yoga, T'ai Chi
Natural products	
Vitamins and supplements	CoQ10, glucosamine/chondroitin, fish oil
Herbal medicines	Ginger, turmeric, lemon balm
Manual medicine	Osteopathic manual manipulation, massage therapy, chiropractic, craniosacral
Biofield therapies	Reiki, healing touch, qigong, Jin Shin Jyutsu

It has long been known that acupuncture stimulation acts on the autonomic nervous system and causes the release of endogenous endorphins, enkephalins, monoamines, and other neurotransmitters that play central roles in acupuncture analgesia (6,25). Neuroimaging has revealed a glimpse into the CNS networks that are manipulated via acupuncture stimulation (26,27). Studies using functional MR have demonstrated that needling certain acupuncture points activates areas of the somatosensory cortex that do not correspond anatomically but do correspond functionally under classical East Asian medical theory, although these data are still under debate (28–34). Major acupuncture points traditionally needled for pain management have been shown on fMRI to modulate activity in areas such as the hypothalamus, prefrontal cortex, insula, limbic system, and periaqueductal gray matter (35–38), which may help attenuate both the sensory and the emotional perception of pain and coordinate an autonomic response (26). Even after acupuncture stimulation is terminated, changes persist in the central connections among the limbic areas for pain, affect, and memory (35). These results may have implications for the rehabilitation of other disorders involving cerebral cortical remodeling, such as stroke, phantom limb pain, and neurodegenerative syndromes.

Controlled clinical trials have shown acupuncture to be effective for osteoarthritis (39,40) neurogenic pain following spinal cord injury (SCI) (41), neurogenic bladder (42), lateral epicondylitis, addiction, headache, tennis elbow, fibromyalgia, myofascial pain, low back pain, and carpal tunnel syndrome (43). Further randomized controlled trials looking at specific diagnosis may help elucidate length of response to treatment. Meta-analyses have reported that acupuncture has shown efficacy in the treatment of tension headache (44) in migraine prophylaxis (45), and as an adjunct to low back pain rehabilitation (46,47), but that further study is required to make conclusive statements regarding benefit or lack thereof in stroke rehabilitation (48–51) and rheumatoid arthritis (52,53). In practice, acupuncture is used to treat multiple conditions including osteoarthritis, lumbar spinal stenosis, tension headaches, muscle and ligament sprains, carpal tunnel syndrome, lateral epicondylitis, motor recovery after stroke, neurogenic pain, bowel and bladder dysfunction following SCI, early peripheral neuropathy, and migraine headaches among other conditions. Acupressure is a technique based on the concept of meridians and acupoints, but instead of needle insertion, pressure is applied to the acupoint. In practice, acupressure may be thought of as a weaker form of acupuncture. Patients may be given acupressure points as a part of their home exercise program to enhance the rehabilitation process.

Acupuncture in general is well accepted, well tolerated, and without significant adverse events (46). One study did indicate that blood pressure should be monitored in SCI patient (54). Acupuncture can be combined with traditional rehabilitation, for example, it can be utilized in low back pain patients to enhance improvements in function (46). In general, acupuncture is the most utilized approach for patients with chronic pain seeking care at integrative medicine clinics (55). Based on the current available evidence, acupuncture is typically well tolerated, is safe, and can be a useful tool in the physiatry practitioner's armamentarium.

Ayurvedic Medicine

The indigenous healing system native to India, Ayurvedic medicine (also called Ayurveda) translates as the "science of life," and is one of the oldest systems of medicine in the world. As the NCCIH website outlines, "Key concepts of Ayurvedic medicine include universal interconnectedness (among people, their health, and the universe), the body's constitution (*prakriti*), and life forces (*dosha*), which are often compared to the biologic humors of the ancient Greek system. Using these concepts, Ayurvedic physicians prescribe individualized treatments, including compounds of herbs or proprietary ingredients, and diet, exercise, and lifestyle recommendations (56). Like the field of PM&R, Ayurveda teaches that disease and healing occur on all levels: physical, emotional, mental, and spiritual. According to Ayurveda, five elements—earth, air, water, fire, and space—also occur in people in varying proportions that are grouped into types functionally classified as *doshas*. These proportions make up the individual's *prakriti*, or individual constitution, and determine the mental and physical makeup of each individual. Illness is thought to occur when there is an imbalance in the *doshas*. Each dosha has corresponding symptoms and illnesses that occur during imbalance. Treatments are individualized by constitutional type and include herbs, yoga postures, diet, pranayama or breathing techniques, purification techniques, meditation, and mantras (30). Ayurveda is not well integrated into the PM&R setting at this time. However, one tool used by Ayurvedic practitioners, yoga, is discussed in separate sections below.

Naturopathy

Naturopathy is a system that stresses health maintenance and disease prevention through patient education and acceptance of responsibility for one's own health. Underlying the various treatments in naturopathic medicine is the belief in the healing power of nature and the innate intelligence of the body. Naturopathic physicians are trained in the medical sciences as well as combinations of disciplines such as herbology, nutrition, homeopathy, or acupuncture. A naturopathic doctor holds the degree ND and has 4 years of training followed by an internship. Naturopathic physicians are licensed in some states and Canadian provinces, and scope of practice for some includes limited drug prescription (57).

MIND-BODY INTERVENTIONS

The basic premise of mind-body interventions is that the mind and body are not dualistically distinct entities but exist on a continuum. Thus, thoughts and emotions influence the body, and physical processes have an impact on the mental, emotional, and spiritual state. Mind-body interventions may be separated into either a mental or physical process that influences this mind-body continuum. "Mind"-based techniques including visual imagery, art and music therapy, biofeedback, hypnosis, meditation, and prayer are designed to act through the mind to alter its state and thus physical conditions including muscle tension, endorphin levels, and pain. Body-based techniques use the body as a vehicle and act to increase strength, flexibility, and body awareness, and in so doing, impact upon mental/psychological/spiritual states such as level of mental focus, anxiety, or compassion for self and others. These interventions are most efficacious when practiced in tandem, serving to reinforce each other, and for body-based interventions to allow experiential practice and integration of "mind"-based techniques. An example of this is mindful movement practiced in Mindfulness-Based Stress Reduction (MBSR) courses. Modern day usage and supporting evidence are listed for mind-body techniques separately below.

Mindfulness-Based Interventions

Mindfulness practice has a deep history across cultures and religions encompassing two millennia. Mindfulness involves qualities of attention and awareness that can be cultivated and developed through meditation and breath work, having deep roots in Buddhism. Jon Kabat-Zinn, a medical scientist and mindfulness practitioner partially responsible for the evolution of this treatment in Western culture and medicine over the past 30 years, operationalizes mindfulness as "the awareness that emerges through paying attention on purpose, in the present moment, and nonjudgmentally to the unfolding experience moment to moment" (58). There are two common meditative practices in mindfulness meditation, one as focused-attention meditation (samanthi) and the second being open-monitoring meditation (vipassana) (59). Regarding pain, both practices are taught and considered tools for self-regulation through enhancing attention and regulating distraction and to decrease reactivity to pain and/or difficult emotional experiences.

Over time, mindfulness training has been adapted into various clinical intervention programs and incorporated into psychosocial treatments for pain control, which are now considered a part of the "third-wave" cognitive-behavioral therapy (CBT) movement (60). These include MBSR (61), Mindfulness-Based Cognitive Therapy (MBCT) (62), and Acceptance and Commitment Therapy (ACT) (63). Importantly, with appropriate training, MBSR can be learned and practiced by nonpsychologist providers. Mindfulness interventions are helpful for patients with musculoskeletal and chronic pain disorders, and newer investigations show trends toward improvements for patients with neurocognitive and neuromotor disorders (64). The literature evaluating mindfulness-based interventions for chronic pain is promising, showing improvements in both chronic pain and depressive symptoms—however, due to limitations in historical research lacking randomization and small sample sizes, further studies are needed to provide sufficient evidence of these reports (65,66). Preliminary investigations incorporating MBSR and mindfulness-based techniques into rehabilitation programs are a new line of investigation, with researchers encouraging incorporating mindfulness and self-compassion practices into both physical and occupational therapy (64,67).

Hypnosis

Clinical hypnosis can be an extremely useful adjunctive intervention in the treatment of acute pain, chronic pain, and procedural distress. In hypnosis, one person (the practitioner) guides another (the subject) through an initial induction followed by a series of suggestions for experiences involving alterations in perception, memory, and voluntary action (68). During hypnosis, subjects obtain a state of consciousness involving focused attention and reduced peripheral awareness, having increased ability to respond to suggestion in this state (69). Hypnosis incorporates a number of components including relaxation, focused attention, imagery, interpersonal processing, and suggestion (70). It has been most widely studied

in the treatment of pain through the use of hypnotic analgesia. Regarding neurophysiology, hypnosis has been found to both (a) alter cortical activity in the brain and (b) impact specific areas of the brain consistent with pain relief—such as the ACC, somatosensory cortices, and insula (70,71).

In the treatment of acute pain, hypnosis is brief and addresses intense fleeting pain often induced by a medical procedure. Hypnosis has been applied in these settings and utilized in a range of procedures across ages extending from minor to major surgical procedures (72), lumbar punctures (73), and for burn wound care (74) as examples. Its application is found to result in reduced procedural time, less use of anesthesia, a reduction of postsurgical side effects, and shorter hospital stays—resulting in substantial cost savings (72).

In hypnosis for chronic pain, treatment is longer in duration. Treatment includes the use of recordings outside of sessions and the patient being instructed in self-hypnosis to provide additional tools for self-management of pain. Treatment also addresses other biopsychosocial aspects of the pain experience, such as motivation, fear of movement, social engagement, and sleep improvement. In the rehabilitation population, hypnosis has been applied to the treatment of chronic back pain (75), multiple sclerosis (76), SCI (77), and headaches (78). Meta-analyses conclude that hypnosis is an effective intervention for chronic pain, with benefits extending beyond pain relief (70,79). For example, with the use of hypnosis, over time, chronic pain patients report an increased sense of control over pain, improved sleep, stress reduction, and an improvement in overall well-being—even when their pain remained unchanged after the intervention (80).

Cognitive-Behavioral Therapy

Cognitive-behavioral therapy for chronic pain is considered the "gold standard" psychological treatment for individuals with a wide range of pain problems and a "first-line" treatment for chronic pain conditions. It has shown substantial evidence in improving pain and pain-related problems across a wide spectrum of pain conditions from a plethora of randomized controlled trials (81). In its biopsychosocial model, physical disorders are conceptualized a result of a complex and dynamic interaction among interdependent physiologic, psychological, social, and environmental factors influencing the development, course, and/or resolution of illnesses (82). Treatment is short term in nature, multimodal, and has overarching goals of improving mood, increasing physical functioning, and decreasing the subjective experience of pain (83). Patients are provided with a repertoire of techniques to help gain a sense of control over the effects of pain on their lives as well as modifying the affective, behavioral, cognitive, and sensory facets of the pain experience (84). Treatment generally follows three phases: (a) education, (b) skills training, and (c) application/maintenance (83). In CBT for chronic pain, historically treatment has been delivered in individual and/or group formats. In recent innovations, CBT has been successfully integrated into rehabilitation treatments including physical therapy, via telephone (85), and modified for use in online formats (81). For example, interventionists have successfully implemented a randomized trial of modified CBT/physical therapy program after lumbar surgical procedures, with significant and clinically meaningful improvement in postoperative outcomes (86). In the rehabilitation context, when used as a part of a multidisciplinary treatment, this intervention has been shown particularly helpful in reducing kinesiophobia, fear-avoidance behaviors, and increasing engagement in exercise programs in patients with spinal problems (87).

Biofeedback

Biofeedback is an established intervention often utilized in the context of CBT as a trained self-management skill. It is a procedure in which patients' bodily responses including heart rate, skin temperature, or muscle tension are monitored, reported, and visible during the procedure through a visual or auditory mechanism (88). This immediate feedback is theorized to improve patients' mind-body connections through improved self-monitoring and ultimately improves an individual's sense of efficacy as patients learn to harness their ability to self-regulate (89). It has two primary forms of delivery: electromyographic (EMG) feedback and electroencephalographic (EEG) feedback. Through EMG, patients learn to control and alleviate muscle tension. In EEG feedback, sometimes referred to as "neurofeedback," patients learn to regulate cognitive systems through observing their EEG brainwaves. Biofeedback has been heavily studied for use with chronic headache/migraine (90) and has been utilized and determined as efficacious in the treatment of low back pain (91) and chronic pain syndromes such as fibromyalgia (88).

MIND-BODY MOVEMENT THERAPIES

Described below are six of the more popular therapeutic movement modalities in use today: yoga, T'ai Chi, the Alexander technique, the Feldenkrais method, Pilates, and body-mind

centering (BMC). These techniques are similar in that they aim to improve a patient's kinesthetic ability, coordination of motion and breathing, and ease, control, and joy in everyday movement. All may be useful for a wide spectrum of patients from severely physically challenged to high-performance athletes.

Yoga and T'ai Chi are frequently referred to as "mind-body" techniques, because they actively seek to balance both the physical and nonphysical aspects of the person. Both are meditative in nature and are part of a larger philosophy or way of life. Each is derived from a broader system of health with an underlying model differing from those of the West. The other techniques discussed were developed in the 20th century. All of the techniques take a less focal and more global approach to rehabilitation of specific conditions based on the rationale that the whole body is involved in all movement. A summary of movement therapies and indications is listed in **Table 59-2**.

Yoga

Yoga is an ancient Indian art first brought to the United States in the mid-1800s. In Sanskrit, the word "*yoga*" means "union" (with the divine) and is a way of life involving a number of different spiritual practices and encompasses ethical conduct, social responsibility, nutrition, and physical health practices. The branch of yoga that is best known in the West is *hatha yoga* and is often simply referred to as "yoga." Originally intended to prepare the body for divine experience, it is practiced in the United States for the achievement of physical strength, flexibility, and relaxation through postures known as *asanas* (a-sa-nas). *Pranayama* (pra-na-ya-ma), or breathing techniques, and meditation are also often practiced along with hatha yoga. The many forms of yoga practiced in the United States are diverse

TABLE 59-2	Movement Therapies	
Technique	**Focus**	**Indications, Precautions, Considerations**
Anusara yoga (Sanskrit for "flowing with grace")	Alignment, smooth flow of poses, use of yoga to maintain health	General health, balanced combination of alignment, posture flow, and heart-centered approach; rigorous certification process
Kripalu yoga (Sanskrit for "compassion")	Gentle movement, strength and flexibility, awareness and care of the body, release of emotions	Deconditioning, neck and back pain, ROM deficits, fibromyalgia, initial rehabilitation phase of recovery from illness esp. postcardiac, postsurgical, increasing general strength and flexibility; broad-based certification process
Iyengar yoga	Alignment, correct execution of poses, use of yoga to correct physical health problems	Back and neck pain, scoliosis, sports rehabilitation; significant use of props and modifications for physical limitations; rigorous certification process
Viniyoga	Tailoring practice to the individual, therapeutic linking of breath with movement	Severe deconditioning, general conditioning, neck and back pain
Ashtanga yoga, Bikram yoga	Strength building	Athletic and mental conditioning; not to be used in serious injury, deconditioning, or rehabilitation
T'ai Chi	Balance, flexibility, stress reduction, body awareness	Fall-prone patients, peripheral neuropathy neck and back pain, general deconditioning. Requires ability to stand; may be modified to patient needs
Feldenkrais	Exploration and choice of useful movement; application to functional tasks	Neurologic disorders, orthopedic rehab, neck and back pain; rehabilitation of dance and musician injuries
Alexander technique	Posture and alignment, release of maladaptive movement habits, low back and neck pain	Neck injuries, scoliosis, low back pain, neck pain, rehabilitation of dancer and musician injuries, and any activity in which proper posture is important
Pilates	Core strengthening, balanced strengthening, ease of movement	Athletic rehabilitation, general strengthening, neck and back pain, postural awareness; avoid with moderate to severe injury unless practitioner has rehab experience

in terms of focus, strenuousness, and applications. A few of the forms most relevant to PM&R are described in **Table 59-2**.

Yoga has been extensively studied both in India and the West, with thousands of studies reporting positive health effects, including lowering of blood pressure (92), and decreased cholesterol levels (93). Yoga has been applied to programs for rheumatoid arthritis (94), osteoarthritis (95), chronic back pain (96–98), neck pain (98,99), cardiac rehabilitation (100), carpal tunnel syndrome (95), and improved athletic performance (101). Yoga is increasingly being integrated into the office and inpatient settings by instructors who are experienced in teaching rehabilitation patients (102). Individual sessions and classes are a convenient way to transition from physical therapy supervision to a home-based program (103).

T'ai Chi

T'ai Chi is a form of postures and movements that dates back to 17th century China. It consists of a series of flowing contrasting movements, with constant weight shifting from one leg to another, changing of direction, and moving the limbs in space. In these flowing movements, subjects transition from one posture to another with the goal of seamless, flowing motions focusing on achieving balanced and graceful movement. Since it is a slow, rhythmic and weight-bearing exercise, participants are able to improve balance, coordination, concentration, and relieve stress in a safe manner. Randomized trials report that benefits of T'ai Chi include improved cardiorespiratory function, improved strength and balance, decreased falls in the elderly (104–107), and improved psychological parameters (107). It has been well studied in patients with fibromyalgia (108–110) and has shown promise in the treatment of low back pain (111). Additionally, T'ai Chi has been modified for the elderly (T'ai Chi Chih), and the arthritis population and instructors are now certified by the Arthritis Foundation.

Movement Awareness Techniques

Movement awareness techniques focus less on strengthening isolated muscles and more on ease and comfort in functional movement. Each technique promotes body awareness and balance and may be taught in one-on-one or in a group format. The Alexander technique was developed by FM Alexander, a Shakespearean actor, in his attempts to heal his own recurrent loss of voice. Alexander found that his voice improved when he decreased his cervical tension. His technique attempts to improve posture and movement by focusing on developing a balance between the head and neck in static and dynamic situations, as well as proper breathing (112). Most sessions are one-on-one, with the practitioner directing the student verbally and with light touch into postures that will help him or her to experience the state of being in proper alignment. Alexander practitioners are consulted for any patient with postural difficulties or chronic and occupational back and neck pain (113,114). Clinical reports include effectiveness in increasing respiratory capacity (115) in Parkinson's (116) or for improved performance in athletics and the performing arts.

The Feldenkrais Method

The Feldenkrais method is a movement therapy that capitalizes on the ability of the human nervous system to develop new engrams or movement patterns. It was developed by Moshe Feldenkrais, PhD, a physicist and judo black belt who studied Alexander technique, yoga, psychology, and other disciplines and applied them to injury rehabilitation. This method teaches the patient to break down and examine functional movement habits and to choose new patterns based on their usefulness and efficiency. The technique helps patients to learn to use efficient and pain-free movement. Feldenkrais sessions are conducted in two formats. Awareness through movement is a verbally directed group lesson in which movements are gentle and slow, within comfort range. Lessons are based on a function (getting up from a chair, rolling from supine to prone). The second variation, functional integration, is a one on-one, hands-on technique in which the practitioner gently guides the student through various movement sequences. Feldenkrais has been used with various conditions, including cerebral palsy, hemiplegia, and multiple sclerosis. There are reports of the successful use of the Feldenkrais method in multiple sclerosis (117), orthopedic injuries (117), Parkinson's disease (118), and neck and low back pain (119–122) and evidence that it is cost effective in the management of chronic pain (123). A review of the numerous studies on Feldenkrais in rehabilitation concluded that with a great number of positive case reports, further research with rigorous methodology is warranted (124).

The Pilates Method

The Pilates method was developed by Joseph Pilates during and after World War I and combines the experiences he gained as a result of his contact with dancers, athletes, and disabled soldiers. The technique is now used by many high level athletes and dancers as well as those undergoing rehabilitation, especially for musculoskeletal conditions. This popular technique is characterized by use of proper body mechanics, stabilization of the shoulder and pelvic girdles, and coordinated breathing to promote strengthening with minimal increase in bulk. A typical rehabilitation program using a Pilates-based approach may begin not by focusing on the area that is injured but by teaching exercises to enhance awareness that the body works as a whole and that the injured part is weak link in the entire kinetic chain (125). Clinical reports of the use of Pilates-based protocols are in the area of sports training and rehabilitation (126,127).

The BMC Method

Bonnie Bainbridge-Cohen developed BMC, a unique approach to movement analysis and reeducation (128). Cohen drew on her training in occupational therapy, and Bobath's neurodevelopmental therapy, dance therapy, bodywork, martial arts, voice, and yoga. The primary goal of BMC is the integration of body and mind and the development of an ability to sense this connectedness. BMC teaches students to tune into the body and feel at the tissue and cellular levels. BMC holds that the body's tissues have the ability to respond to messages given to them (128). Thus, body tissues can be affected by the practitioner's hands as well as the patient's actions, thoughts, and intentions. The result is the modulation of pain and restrictions preventing optimal movement. BMC is used for patients affected by any neurologic or musculoskeletal condition including developmental issues, stroke, SCI, TBI, and orthopedic conditions.

SUPPLEMENTS AND NUTRITION

Dietary supplements (DS) are appealing to the public because of their accessibility and perceived efficacy and safety. According to the most recent National Health Interview Survey (NHIS) report in 2012, 17.7% of adults and 4.9% of children age 4 to 17 used natural products (129). Fish oil use increased significantly compared to the previous survey in 2007, while glucosamine chondroitin use was slightly lower though still ranked among the top 10 (130). Because of patient request for natural therapies, wide usage, increasing literature support, and their unique side effect profiles and interactions, physicians should be familiar with the most commonly used supplements for musculoskeletal disorders, as well as basic guidelines in choosing high-quality products and researching options.

Unlike conventional pharmacologic treatments, which undergo rigorous testing for safety and efficacy and must be approved by the FDA before they are marketed, DS are regulated under a Congressional Act, which places them in their own category—falling along the spectrum between drugs and food. The 1994 Dietary Supplement Health and Education Act defines a "dietary supplement" as a product taken by mouth, which contains one or a combination of vitamins, minerals, herbs or other botanicals, amino acids, concentrates, metabolites, constituents, or extracts (131). The Act makes manufacturers responsible for ensuring the safety and efficacy of their products by listing all ingredients and including a disclaimer stating that the product has not been evaluated by the FDA and "is not intended to diagnose, treat, cure, or prevent any disease." A 2007 addendum requires DS manufacturers to comply with current Good Manufacturing Practices (132).

The agents discussed here were chosen from a long list of supplements as those that have the most literature support and which are relevant specifically to PM&R musculoskeletal and pain conditions. A plethora of other DS is available for other conditions commonly treated by physiatrists such as post-stroke and traumatic brain injury, and cancer and cardiovascular rehabilitation but will not be reviewed here. Collaboration with physicians fellowship trained in integrative medicine and naturopathic doctors can help ensure patients use of DS supports their individual goals and preferences, without interfering with pharmaceuticals.

Herbal Medicines

Many botanicals have anti-inflammatory and analgesic properties *in vitro* and are promoted for musculoskeletal conditions. Clinical data are often lacking, though some supplements that show promise and have a reasonable safety profile are highlighted here.

Turmeric (*Curcuma longa*)

Turmeric extracts have been shown *in vitro* to act as a strong inhibitor of inflammatory and catabolic mediators, nitric oxide stimulated by IL-1β, IL-6, IL-8, TNF-α, PGE$_2$, and matrix metalloproteinases (133). Some evidence shows that it might be helpful for symptoms of osteoarthritis. Two clinical research studies shows that taking specific turmeric extracts 500 mg twice daily may significantly reduce pain and reliance on nonsteroidal anti-inflammatory drugs (NSAIDs) and improves functionality after 8 weeks compared to baseline in patients with knee osteoarthritis (134,135). In comparisons to

pharmaceuticals, a turmeric extract 500 mg four times daily was comparable to ibuprofen 400 mg twice daily after 6 weeks for reducing knee pain in osteoarthritis patients (136).

Ginger (*Zingiber officinale*)

Compounds in ginger can inhibit COX and LOX pathways. A 2015 systematic review of RCTs of ginger versus placebo concluded that ginger was modestly efficacious and reasonably safe for treatment of OA (137). Outcomes included significant reductions in pain upon standing, pain after walking, and stiffness. Several studies have also compared ginger to NSAIDs such as ibuprofen with mixed results (138,139). Doses of ginger extracts typically range from 250 mg 2 to 4 times daily to 500 mg twice daily; consistent use for 3 weeks may be needed to achieve the benefits. Topical gels and massage oil contained ginger extract also may provide short-term benefits for joint pain (140).

Capsicum

Capsicum peppers contain the constituent "capsaicin." It's this compound that makes the peppers fiery hot. Capsaicin is approved by the FDA and Health Canada as an OTC and prescription drug. Topical capsaicin in strengths of 0.25% to 0.75% is effective for temporary relief of pain related to osteoarthritis. Capsaicin works by depleting and inhibiting the reaccumulation of substance P, which is involved in pain transmission, in sensory nerves when it is repeatedly applied (141). At least 3 days of multiple daily capsaicin applications are typically required to achieve significant pain relief, and up to 2 weeks for maximum effect. Topical capsaicin can cause sensations of burning and irritation where applied, which may lead to discontinuation.

Additional Herbal Supplements

Many other herbal medicines have *in vitro* analgesic and anti-inflammatory properties, though good quality interventional studies in humans are limited, and have potential utility in osteoarthritis, lumbago, and other pain conditions. Examples include the following:

- Cat's claw (*Uncaria guianensis*)
- Devil's claw (*Harpagophytum procumbens*)
- Indian frankincense (*Boswellia serrata*)
- Phellodendron (*Phellodendron amurense*)
- Stinging nettle (*Urtica dioica*)
- Willow bark (*Salix* species)

Nonbotanical Dietary Supplements

Glucosamine Sulfate

Glucosamine, widely used for joint pain, is speculated to potentially modify joint structure and reverse or slow disease progression, as well as have analgesic effects. Endogenous glucosamine is found in hyaluronic acid, the major mucopolysaccharide (MPS) of synovial fluid in joints. It is required for production of glycosaminoglycan, which has a highly charged and acidic nature that attracts water and produces the gel-like matrix that gives connective tissue and joints resilience after compression and also reduces friction between bones, tendon, and cartilage. Conceptually, using glucosamine supplements could increase the availability of precursors leading to increased production of MPS and synovial fluid to repair eroded tissue or stimulate new cartilage synthesis.

Over 20 clinical studies lasting up to 3 years and enrolling over 2,500 patients have been conducted, evaluating glucosamine for osteoarthritis (142). Some of the important variables in such trials, which may contribute to varied findings, include glucosamine preparation (glucosamine sulfate vs. glucosamine hydrochloride), dosing schedule, and outcome measures (pain, function, radiographic change). A 2015 systematic review suggests that the long-term use of both glucosamine and chondroitin sulfate may have a small but significant effect on slowing disease progression in patients with knee OA based on changes in joint space assessed on plain radiographs and changes in tibiofemoral cartilage volume assessed by MRI. Other meta-analyses conclude that glucosamine sulfate decreases pain scores by 28% to 41%, improves functionality scores by 21% to 46%, and reduces risk or disease progression by 54% (143). In contrast, the American Academy of Orthopaedic Surgeons (AAOS) published clinical practice guidelines in 2013 for the treatment of symptomatic OA, which stated that use of glucosamine and chondroitin cannot be recommended based on current evidence (144). The AAOS included 21 prospective studies; 12 on glucosamine alone, 8 on chondroitin sulfate alone, and one assessed both. Eleven of 52 outcomes were reported as statistically significant in favor of glucosamine when compared to placebo. However, when meta-analyses were run for WOMAC pain, function, stiffness, and total subscale scores, all meta-analyses showed that the overall effect of glucosamine compared to placebo was not statistically significant.

Despite conflicting studies, glucosamine sulfate remains a reasonable option given its potential for both pain relief and disease modification. The suggested dose is 1,500 mg once daily or in divided doses +/– chondroitin sulfate. Initial concerns that glucosamine supplements could impact glucose control or HgbA1C have since been refuted. Additionally, while glucosamine is derived from the exoskeletons of shrimp, lobster, and crabs, patients with shellfish allergy should not have any issues, since those reactions are caused by IgE antibodies to antigens in the shellfish meat, not the shell.

S-adenosylmethionine

S-adenosylmethionine (SAMe) is an endogenous compound produced in the liver from the amino acid methionine. It has been used in Europe for over 25 years for the treatment of a broad range of conditions including osteoarthritis, depression, and fibromyalgia. The mechanism of action appears to be its involvement in several metabolic processes including those that synthesize proteins and detoxify substances in the liver, stimulate chondrocyte growth and repair, increase cartilage thickness, enhance proteoglycan synthesis, and reduce TNF-α (145,146). SAMe has been found in clinical trials to be significantly more effective than placebo for osteoarthritis symptom relief, and as effective as NSAIDs, including celecoxib, naproxen, indomethacin, piroxicam, and ibuprofen (145). Doses range from 400 to 1,600 mg, preferably in the butanedisulfonate salt form, which has the highest bioavailability at 5% and is more stable than other forms. It can take several days to several weeks for significant improvement. It is generally very well tolerated with few significant side effects—typically only mild gastrointestinal distress and insomnia is taken too late in day. It also should be avoided in patients with manic disorders and attention paid to potential serotonergic interactions.

Avocado/Soybean Unsaponifiables

A preparation of the unsaponifiable fractions of avocado and soybean is reported to repress the catabolic activities of chondrocytes and to increase proteoglycan accumulation by OA chondrocytes. Avocado/soybean unsaponifiables (ASU) have been shown to inhibit basal MMP-3 production and inflammatory cytokine production and to have a chondroprotective effect via IL-1-repression (147). ASU is available as a drug in some countries; in the United States, it is available as a dietary supplement. Early multicenter RCTs showed that patients with hip and knee OA taking ASU had slightly lower NSAID use and improvement in functional disability, but the more recent ERADIAS study showed no significant difference in mean joint space width loss or clinical outcomes after 3 years, though there was less progression of OA in the treatment group (148,149). The typical ASU dosage is 300 mg/d, standardized to 30% phytosterols; precautions include cross-reactivity in patients with latex allergies.

Fish Oil

One of the most discussed supplements in medicine today is the use of fish oil. Fish oil contains eicosapentaenoic acid (EPA) and docosapentaenoic (DHA), both precursors in the manufacture of anti-inflammatory compounds. EPA and DHA are necessary to the development and maintenance of healthy membranes and deficits associated with aberrant receptor binding capacity, cell signaling, and neural development. The use of fish oil has been well studied in the rheumatoid arthritis population, and patients tolerate high doses (5.5 g/d) with no negative incidents in 3 years of follow-up (150). Patients should be started at approximately 2 g/d and titrated upward as tolerated. Clinical evidence suggests that taking fish oil in combination with a glucosamine sulfate supplement does not significantly decrease osteoarthritis symptoms such as morning stiffness or pain in the hips and knees compared to glucosamine alone (151).

In summary, the physiatrist should advise patients that "natural" does not mean "safe" and that research on supplements is in its infancy. Just as with some pharmaceutical treatments, "nutraceutical" agents designed for therapeutic benefit may later prove to be unsafe under certain circumstances or of no benefit. It is important to make the decision to use both pharmaceuticals and supplements after balancing the patient's specific needs with data on efficacy, safety, and drug-drug and drug-supplement interactions (152). Electronic evidence-based resources are available for reference in patient care such as Natural Medicines and Consumerlab.com. When available, consultation with health professions with expertise in integrative medicine, naturopathic medicine, and pharmacy is an important step to ensuring patient safety and maximizing positive outcomes.

Nutrition

Nutrition is one of the core lifestyle factors that should be a part of any holistic treatment plan. Patients should be counseled on the profound influence of diet in healing the neuromusculoskeletal system. Because the Standard American Diet (SAD) contains significant amounts of precursors to proinflammatory fatty acids (saturated fat, vegetable oils, most nuts), with lesser proportions of foods that give rise to the manufacture of anti-inflammatory compounds (fruits and vegetables, omega-3–containing nuts, cold water fish), many patients ingest a diet that contributes to a high inflammatory load (153). Since many pain syndromes are associated with inflammation, an anti-inflammatory diet is a prudent choice for patients in pain or with healing neuromusculoskeletal systems (154). The basic principles of an anti-inflammatory diet include reduction of sources of arachidonic acid (mainly saturated fat from animal sources), elimination of trans fats, which interfere with essential fatty acid (EFA) metabolism, optimization of omega-6 to omega-3 ratios, consumption of abundant and variety of phytochemicals from fruits and vegetables, and use of anti-inflammatory herbs and spices. Many popular guides to an anti-inflammatory diet exist (155).

Evidence supports that anti-inflammatory Mediterranean and plant-based diets have a favorable impact on serum markers of systemic inflammation, with a few studies supported clinical impact. A 2016 publication in the *American Journal of Clinical Nutrition* followed 4,470 participants (mean age: 61.3) from the Osteoarthritis Initiative showed that those reporting a higher adherence to a Mediterranean diet had significantly more favorable scores on all outcomes investigated including better QOL and decreased pain, disability, and depression (156). There is evidence that anti-inflammatory vegetarian diets support the actions of anti-inflammatory supplements and decrease symptomatology in patients with systemic inflammatory conditions such as rheumatoid arthritis (157,158).

Intermittent fasting and fasting mimicking diets are gaining increased visibility as research findings show benefits including decreases in inflammatory markers, improved oxidative stress, and clinical benefits including rheumatoid arthritis (159,160).

The physiatrist who becomes educated about current nutrition knowledge and encourages patients to incorporate healthy, whole-food anti-inflammatory strategies may help patients not only address acute physiologic disturbances but also improve their QOL and prevent chronic disease.

MANIPULATIVE AND BODY-BASED THERAPIES

Manipulative and body-based therapies are employed to improve the structure and functioning of the body by manipulation of the musculoskeletal structure. Although often considered to be "unconventional" in mainstream medicine, many forms of physical manipulation and massage have been utilized for years in PM&R and osteopathic manual medicine. Typically, massage done in the context of PM&R is based on neuromuscular massage. Less conventional bodywork concepts and techniques are briefly reviewed below. An excellent introduction to a number of bodywork, mind-body, and energy techniques applied to the rehabilitation process can be found elsewhere (161–163).

Eastern massage styles, such as acupressure, shiatsu, cupping, and tuina, are derived from the original Chinese massage/manipulation technique known as anmo ("press and stroke"). Multiple studies have documented that myofascial trigger points are significantly correlated with acupressure with one study finding over 92% of trigger points correlated to acupressure points (97,164,165).

These techniques involve hand movements familiar to Western practitioners such as pressing, stroking, kneading, and grasping, as well as others such as joint manipulation and knuckle rolling, which are outside the scope of Western massage therapy. As with acupuncture, smooth and adequate flow of energy (chi) is considered the basis for good health. The most widespread use of Eastern massage techniques in the United States is by massage therapists trained in Western massage technique, integrating these additional skills into their practice. Licensed acupuncturists also routinely use Eastern manual techniques. Acupressure usually takes place on a treatment table, and lubricants are not ordinarily used. Case studies report it to be effective for the treatment of headache and temporomandibular joint pain, postoperative pain, and as an adjunct to pulmonary rehabilitation (166). *Shiatsu* means "finger pressure" in Japanese. Although the term is used synonymously with acupressure, the two are distinctly different therapies. In shiatsu massage, the session is often performed on the floor on a blanket or futon rather than on a table. This allows the practitioner to use various parts of his or her own body (feet, legs, or full body weight) for efficient application of pressure over points and along meridians. Passive stretching and range of motion are also a part of the session. *Tuina* ("push and pull" or "push and squeeze") is a massage/manipulation technique encompassing a variety of hand strokes, ranging from gentle and superficial movements to techniques with vigorous articulatory maneuvers. It may be roughly equated with Western manipulative techniques. Tuina is taught in the North America as a part of Chinese bodywork training in schools of oriental medicine.

Craniosacral Therapy

Craniosacral therapy is an osteopathic technique developed by William Sutherland DO in the early 1900s (163). It is a gentle, noninvasive manipulative technique applied to the spinal cord and cranium to correct disruptions in the craniosacral rhythmic activity. This activity is believed to be disrupted in orthopedic trauma, spinal cord, and traumatic brain injury; so one of the major focuses of this technique has been this type of injury (166,167). Upledger reports success in treating chronic pain, chronic brain dysfunction, spasticity, and other conditions associated with SCI. Craniosacral therapy has shown some benefit for chronic neck pain not caused by traumatic injury (168).

Rolfing

Rolfing was developed in the 1950s by Ida Rolf, a chemist who approached the body as a group of units (head, shoulders, trunk, pelvis, and limbs) connected to each other by the fascial network and with gravity (162). She used this concept in her approach to help clients achieve proper vertical alignment and efficient movement. The method is characterized by the release of restrictions in the deep fascial planes in the body, allowing shortened and tense muscles to relax and lengthen. The goal is to balance and align the body in the gravitational field. The practitioner uses a series of ten 60- to 90-minute sessions, working from superficial to progressively deeper structures, each session building upon the previous one. These may be followed by additional sessions after the client has had time to incorporate the changes into daily habit. Movement education may also be used in conjunction with hands-on work. Traditionally, the Rolfing treatment consists of a series of sessions, each concentrating on specific body regions. The intensity of pressure on muscle and connective tissue that characterizes the original style used by Rolf has been refined by many subsequent practitioners of Rolfing. In the rehabilitation setting, Rolfing has been used by therapists integrating the techniques into musculoskeletal and neurologic rehabilitation. A case series of patients with cerebral palsy and varying levels of motor impairment suggested that Rolfing was of benefit in improving locomotor capacity in patients with mild CP involvement (169). *Structural integration*, developed by a student of Rolf, uses a similar approach and philosophy. Increasing recognition of the importance of the fascia in structural and metabolic health (22) gives a new appreciation for the work of Ida Rolf and her colleagues.

Active Release Technique

Active Release Technique was developed by Michael Leahy D.C. and includes over 500 different protocols targeted at specific myofascial junctures in the body. This approach is frequently used in treatment for elite athletes. Training involves a thorough understanding of anatomy and highly specific palpation skills. Pressure is applied by the hands of the provider and is often accompanied by specific active movement by the patient as instructed by the provider. Antidotal reports suggest that this approach promotes faster recovery time, restores normal tissue function, and may prevent injury. More research is needed to determine safety and efficacy of this technique (170).

Trager Psychophysical Integration

Trager therapy involves a combination of gentle, hands-on tissue technique movement, reeducation, and relaxation exercises (171). It is similar to Feldenkrais and the Alexander technique. Developed by Milton Trager, MD, in the 1940s, it attempts to teach patients to move with ease and efficiency. The work consists of gentle rocking, stretching, and rolling movements intended to relax and enliven tense areas of the body. The Trager therapist attains a calm and focused state of mind in order to be in contact with the client's needs and responses. The practitioner manually communicates this light and energetic state to the client's body so that the body may relearn a feeling of ease in movement. Trager work may be used for the rehabilitation of sports and musculoskeletal conditions. In a controlled trial, Trager was equal to acupuncture for relief of chronic shoulder pain in spinal cord injured patients (172). Case studies suggest its usefulness as a useful adjunct in rehabilitation of chronic obstructive pulmonary disease (173) and cerebral palsy (173).

Biofield Therapies

Biofield therapies are a broad term encompassing modalities grounded in the concept that subtle energy may influence the mind and body. Some of the most commonly utilized therapies include Reiki, therapeutic touch (TT), and healing touch.

Biofield therapies are based on the postulate that there exists a subtle energy field within and around the body. Though this concept is largely limited in Western medical models, the existence of this subtle energy is an integral part of almost every traditional ethnic medical system, and the concept dates back thousands of years. The energy field is known as the vital life force in Western metaphysical traditions, and as *qi* or *chi* (Chinese), *ki* (Japanese), and *prana* (Sanskrit) in Eastern traditions. All of the techniques have as a basic underlying concept—the idea that illness is a result of, or at least associated with, imbalances and blockages in this energy field (174).

The various techniques included in this group of therapies involve a practitioner placing his/her hands on or near the physical body and either actively or passively altering the energy in the recipient's field. Although light physical touch may be involved, its purpose is to modulate the energy field not to manipulate the skin, muscle, or other organ, and the mechanism of action is quite different from that usually proposed in manual manipulation techniques (174,175). It should be noted, however, that a number of techniques (e.g., Jin Shin Jyutsu [JSJ] and Polarity Therapy, described below) have been developed during the past few decades that combine physical manipulation with subtle energy healing (176,177). In traditional systems of medicine, such as Chinese Medicine and Ayurveda, massage and energy healing, while seen as separate techniques, are often used together. Although generally used to promote the overall health of the individual, these techniques have also been used to treat specific diseases and medical conditions (175).

As written in *Primary Care: Clinics in Office Practice on Integrative Medicine,* "Varying conclusions have been drawn regarding the efficacy of these healing modalities in the treatment of pain." One systematic review examined the evidence for biofield therapies in various patient populations (178), including 13 studies related to different pain syndromes. The authors summarized that biofield studies examining impact for pain populations demonstrated level 1 evidence (strong) for these therapies to decrease measures of pain intensity. In contrast, they found only level 4 evidence (equivocal) for these therapies impacting more comprehensive assessments of pain (affective measures). While there have been variations in length of treatment across studies, there is evidence for decreased use of pain medications when employing these strategies (179). Interestingly, a Cochrane review performed in 2008 demonstrated that more advanced practitioners yielded greater improvements in pain that could not be attributed to placebo effect alone (180,181).

Therapeutic Touch

Therapeutic touch is a technique first described in 1979 and developed by a nurse academician, Dolores Krieger, PhD, Professor of Nursing at New York University, and Dora Kunz, a natural healer. The practitioner uses the hands to sense and locate problems and then serves as a conduit for universal energy, consciously transferring energy into the client's energy field in rhythmical, sweeping motions (182). TT is a credentialed nursing skill, and it is taught in over 80 universities in over 30 countries (183). As written in *Primary Care: Clinics in Office Practice on Integrative Medicine,* "There is ongoing interest in further research investigating the use of these modalities for musculoskeletal concerns." A pilot study examining the impact of healing touch on pain and mobility in those with osteoarthritis demonstrated significant improvements in both pain intensity and life interference (184), while another study showed improvements in shoulder range of motion (185). While there hasn't been significant research investigating TT, no significant side effects have been identified making it safe for those suffering with pain (186).

Qigong

Qigong (pronounced chee-*gong*) is an ancient Chinese philosophical system of harmonious integration of the human body with the universe (187,188). When qigong is practiced, the goal is to balance the qi or vital energy within the body, thus preventing or reducing energy imbalance, which can give rise to illness. In self-administered qigong (internal qigong), the individual uses a variety of means, including breathing, visualization, and physical movements, to bring the qi into balance. Qi can also be directed toward a recipient by a qigong practitioner, who consciously emits and directs the qi to another person (external qigong). The general healing nature of the qi is such as to suggest that it can be applied with some success to almost any medical or health problem. Rigorous research is sparse, but McGee and Chow relate a number of case studies for many different conditions, including stroke, paralysis, and cerebral palsy (189). Work evaluating the potential genomic modulatory effects if qigong and other mind-body practices are in early phases (190).

Other Energy Therapies

Reiki (pronounced *ray*-key) is a form of energy healing that usually involves a practitioner laying his or her hands slightly off of 12 specific locations on the body of the person being treated, allowing the "ki" or vital life force to flow through the Reiki practitioner into the body of the patient being treated (191). Having originated in Japan in the 1800s, Reiki has become an increasingly popular and accessible healing technique throughout the Western world. It can also be administered from a distance or self-administered. JSJ or "acupuncture without needles" is an energy healing technique that uses pulse diagnosis and meridian theory to correct imbalances along energy channels. It is practiced one-on-one and is recommended for patients who may not tolerate acupuncture needles. Practitioners place their hands on specific combinations of acupuncture points to release energy blockages. Self-administration can also be taught (176). In comparison to acupressure, there is significantly less emphasis on using physical pressure and more on adjusting the energy along the meridians. There have been no significant side effects identified, making it safe for application on both mild and severely ill patients. A meta-analysis involving 24 randomized controlled or controlled clinical trials involving 1,153 participants examining energy therapies such as TT and Reiki for pain showed a modest effect on pain (180).

SPECIAL TOPICS: SPORTS MEDICINE, FUNCTIONAL MEDICINE, INTEGRATIVE MEDICINE IN THE INPATIENT SETTING

Sports Medicine

The role of the sports medicine physician is to return the athlete to play as quickly and safely as possible after injury and to prevent injury and illness. Integrative therapies provide the sports physician with valuable tools to achieve these goals while avoiding the overuse of medications. The use of integrative strategies is readily accepted by elite athletes: in a study of Division I NCAA Intercollegiate athletes, 56% of subjects reported using integrative modalities over a 12-month time period, higher than the prevalence of these strategies being utilized by all adults in the United States (36%) (192).

Some of the more commonly used modalities are acupuncture, manual therapies (massage, osteopathic manual therapies, and chiropractic), nutritional supplements, meditation and visualization techniques, and movement therapies (114) for the treatment or prevention of injuries (193). In this brief review, only acupuncture, use of nutritional supplements for muscle recovery, and movement therapies, all discussed more fully above, are addressed.

Acupuncture is widely available and used by athletes at all levels for acute and chronic musculoskeletal conditions. In the office setting or on the sidelines, it is used in acute injuries for the rapid reduction of pain and swelling (193). This treatment of injuries within the first 48 hours is referred to as a tendinomuscular treatment (6). Used on a regular basis for nonacute conditions, acupuncture is helpful for restoration of flexibility, joint pain, and ligament sprains (194). Investigations are ongoing examining the exact mechanisms for pain modulation via acupuncture. The endogenous opioid system may be involved (48,195). A properly trained and licensed physician/acupuncturist should perform all treatments.

Proper nutrition and adequate caloric intake are extremely important in ensuring optimal performance. Athletes are strongly encouraged to follow the guidelines and basic principles of the anti-inflammatory diet (above). A sports medicine dietician/nutritionist with background in the nutrition and physical requirements of a particular sport is an integral part of the elite athlete's sports medicine team and should design a basic team program with modifications for each athlete based on caloric intake, gender, metabolism, and sport-specific needs. The same parameters are used in considering supplements. Athletes should, of course, be replete in basic vitamins and minerals. Examining supplements for their quality and safety is also imperative (196,197); additionally, the world doping agency has established an exhaustive list of banned substance supplements for the use in sports (198). There has been much interest in supplementation to enhance athletic performance. Of those examined, creatine, when used at safe doses, has demonstrated promise in the use of high-intensity exercise (199). While there are many multi-ingredient supplements on the market, investigation is ongoing in terms of both safety and efficacy (199).

There are various minerals advocated for use in athletes, especially those who experience greater loss due to excessive sweat. The majority of athletes can obtain adequate amounts with a well-balanced diet (200). Low levels of magnesium and sodium have been implicated in exercise-induced muscle cramps and poor exercise performance (200). It should be noted that serum magnesium levels are not a good measure of magnesium status; erythrocyte magnesium or urine levels after a magnesium challenge have been recommended as a better measure of actual magnesium levels (201,202). Various anti-inflammatory and antioxidant supplements described previously may be incorporated in the athlete's regimen.

Alexander and Feldenkrais techniques as well as other movement practices such as yoga and T'ai Chi, described above, are movement therapies that increasingly have a place in the treatment of sports injuries. These are especially helpful in restoring or implementing efficient movement patterns, which help the athlete heal and prevent injuries (203). The authors incorporate multiple modalities such as yoga, nutrition, physical therapy, and acupuncture to improve strength, flexibility, and balance and as part of the recovery and treatment of sport-related injuries.

Functional Medicine

Functional medicine is an emerging approach to complex and chronic disease. The term was first coined in 1993 by Jeffrey Bland, PhD, nutritional biochemist and previous Director of Nutritional Research at the Linus Pauling Institute of Science and Medicine. Functional medicine is an emerging paradigm that, instead of focusing on the primacy of pathology and differential diagnosis, focuses on the antecedent physiologic processes that ultimately find their expression in health and disease. This concept of "upstream medicine" was first elaborated by Leo Galland, MD, in his unpublished but widely disseminated paper, Patient Centered Diagnosis: *A Guide to the Treatment of Patients as Individuals* and published in 1997 as *The Four Pillars of Healing* (204). The tenets of functional medicine as outlined by the Institute of Functional Medicine are as follows:

- An understanding of the biochemical individuality of each human being based on the concepts of genetic and environmental uniqueness
- Awareness of the evidence that supports a patient-centered rather than a disease-centered approach to treatment
- Search for a dynamic balance among the internal and external body, mind, and spirit
- Interconnections of internal physiologic factors
- Identification of health as a positive vitality, not merely the absence of disease, and emphasizing those factors that encourage the enhancement of a vigorous physiology
- Promotion of organ reserve as the means to enhance the health span, not just the life span, of each patient (205,206)

Functional medicine reflects a system's biology approach to health care; a comprehensive analysis of the manner in which all components of the human biologic system interact functionally with the environment over time (207,208). Just as the physiatrist recognizes multiple interdependent macro aspects of function such as impairment, disability, and handicap, the functional medicine practitioner considers human function on a more fundamental level. These include processes such as communication inside and outside the cell, bioenergetics and energy transformation, issues of replication, repair and maintenance, structural integrity, elimination of waste, protection and defense, issues of transport and circulation, and the influence of environmental inputs such as nutrients and pollutants, as well as psychosocial stressors and the influence of both past physical and psychological trauma. All of these factors determine where the individual sits with respect to the continuum between vitality and disease. Nutritional medicine or "food as medicine" is a central hub of the functional medicine approach.

An example of how a physiatrist may practice functional medicine is the approach to a patient with osteoarthritis who wants to avoid surgery. In addition to recommending weight loss and physical therapy, the physiatrist would request detailed information on concurrent medical conditions, family history of inflammatory and other disease, lifestyle, environment,

and nutrition habits. Laboratory values for basic chemistry, metabolic indicators, nutrients, and toxic substances would be evaluated. If suspected, gluten and other food sensitivities, which can result in an overall increase in inflammatory load, would be ruled out. Nutritional, pharmaceutical, and lifestyle interventions would be implemented to return the patient to optimal functioning on structural, biochemical, and mental-spiritual levels. This is but one example of where a comprehensive approach and dietary modification may have a profound effect on health.

Because both physiatry and functional medicine see the patient with chronic disease at the center of a complex web of interactions, physiatrists and their patients may find this approach intellectually and clinically rewarding.

Use of Integrative Health Techniques in the Inpatient Setting

Integrative modalities are increasingly integrated into standard medical care, and there are examples of hospital systems, which have employed integrative strategies in an inpatient setting. Advantages of using integrative modalities within an inpatient rehabilitation hospital include increased variety of modalities, ability to treat across the continuum of care, and increased patient interest and confidence (209,210). Barriers to integration of conventional and integrative therapies include lack of established standards for practitioner licensing for some modalities, absence of protocols for management of specific conditions, and inconsistent third-party reimbursement. Suggestions for minimizing such barriers include hiring practitioners with experience in both conventional and integrative management of chronic musculoskeletal conditions, informed oversight and education of practitioners, ongoing education of therapists, physicians, and third-party payers. While integration of these therapies into the rehabilitation setting remains in its infancy, it likely holds great promise for expanded management options and patient satisfaction.

An example of utilizing integrative therapies in the inpatient setting is the University of California, San Diego. Inpatients are offered fee-based acupuncture and massage therapy by professionals in conjunction with standard medical care. They are also offered healing touch for free by trained nursing staff. Spaulding Rehabilitation Hospital is another example—they have a number of cross-trained practitioners, for example, physical therapists who also have training in Reiki and psychologists with training in hypnotherapy (210).

SUMMARY

The techniques discussed in this chapter represent only some of the more common integrative therapies available, which can be utilized in the rehabilitation setting. Integrative health modalities can be safely employed and may provide patients with hope and empowerment. Managing expectations and collaborative goal setting around improvements in function and QOL at each visit are important in promoting self-efficacy. Engaging patients in active self-care is linked to improvements in outcomes including increased self-efficacy, decreased health care costs, and higher patient satisfaction (211,212). Additionally, we recommend focusing on no more than 2 to 3 modalities at a given time, as each modality can take time and sometimes a financial commitment on the part of the patient.

Team-based, interprofessional models of care have long been a hallmark of the physiatric approach. As we continue to innovate as a field, we are well poised to employ integrative health strategies and partner with integrative health experts in order to provide optimal, efficient, and cost-effective care to our patients.

REFERENCES

1. Kligler B, Chesney M. Academic health centers and the growth of integrative medicine. *J Natl Cancer Inst Monogr*. 2014;2014(50):292–293. doi:10.1093/jncimonographs/lgu039.
2. Clarke TC, Black LI, Stussman BJ, et al. Trends in the use of complementary health approaches among adults: United States, 2002–2012. *Natl Health Stat Report*. 2015;10(79):1–16.
3. Chou R, Huffman LH; American Pain Society; American College of Physicians. Nonpharmacologic therapies for acute and chronic low back pain: a review of the evidence for an American Pain Society/American College of Physicians clinical practice guideline. *Ann Intern Med*. 2007;147(7):492–504. doi: org/10.7326/0003-4819-147-7-200710020-00007.
4. Nahin RL, Barnes PM, Stussman BJ, et al. Costs of complementary and alternative medicine (CAM) and frequency of visits to CAM practitioners: United States, 2007. *Natl Health Stat Report*. 2009;18(18):1–14.
5. Kessler HH. *The Knife Is Not Enough*. New York: WW Norton; 1968.
6. Helms JM. *Acupuncture Energetics: A Clinical Approach for Physicians*. Berkeley, CA: Medical Acupuncture Publishers; 1995.
7. Napadow V, Ahn A, Longhurst J. The status and future of acupuncture mechanism research. *J Altern Complement Med*. 2008;14(7):861–869.
8. Ahn AC, Colbert AP, Anderson BJ, et al. Electrical properties of acupuncture points and meridians: a systematic review. *Bioelectromagnetics*. 2008;29(4):245–256.
9. de Vernejoul P, Albarède P, Darras JC. Nuclear medicine and acupuncture message transmission. *J Nucl Med*. 1992;33(3):409–412.
10. Kovacs FM, Gotzens V, García A, et al. Experimental study on radioactive pathways of hypodermically injected technetium-99m. *J Nucl Med*. 1992;33(3):403–407.
11. Li HY, Yang JF, Chen M, et al. Visualized regional hypodermic migration channels of interstitial fluid in human beings: are these ancient meridians? *J Altern Complement Med*. 2008;14(6):621–628. doi:10.1089/acm.2007.0606.
12. Melzack R, Stillwell DM, Fox EJ. Trigger points and acupuncture points for pain: correlations and implications. *Pain*. 1977;3(1):3–23.
13. Birch S. Trigger point—acupuncture point correlations revisited. *J Altern Complement Med*. 2003;9(1):91–103.
14. Dorsher PT. Can classical acupuncture points and trigger points be compared in the treatment of pain disorders? Birch's analysis revisited. *J Altern Complement Med*. 2008;14(4):353–359. doi:10.1089/acm.2007.0810.
15. Birch S. On the impossibility of trigger point-acupoint equivalence: a commentary on Peter Dorsher's analysis. *J Altern Complement Med*. 2008;14(4):343–345.
16. Langevin HM, Yandow JA. Relationship of acupuncture points and meridians to connective tissue planes. *Anat Rec*. 2002;269(6):257–265.
17. Langevin HM, Churchill DL, Cipolla MJ. Mechanical signaling through connective tissue: a mechanism for the therapeutic effect of acupuncture. *FASEB J*. 2001;15:2275–2282.
18. Langevin HM, Churchill DL, Fox JR, et al. Biomechanical response to acupuncture needling in humans. *J Appl Physiol*. 2001;91:2471–2478.
19. Langevin HM, Churchill DL, Wu J, et al. Evidence of connective tissue involvement in acupuncture. *FASEB J*. 2002;16:872–874.
20. Kwon S, Lee Y, Park HJ, et al. Coarse needle surface potentiates analgesic effect elicited by acupuncture with twirling manipulation in rats with nociceptive pain. *BMC Complement Altern Med*. 2017;17(1):1. doi:10.1186/s12906-016-1505-2.
21. Langevin HM, Bouffard NA, Badger GJ, et al. Dynamic fibroblast cytoskeletal response to subcutaneous tissue stretch ex vivo and in vivo. *Am J Physiol Cell Physiol*. 2005;288:C747–C756.
22. Langevin HM, Bouffard NA, Badger GJ, et al. Subcutaneous tissue fibroblast cytoskeletal remodeling induced by acupuncture: evidence for a mechanotransduction-based mechanism. *J Cell Physiol*. 2006;207:767–774.
23. Bouffard NA, Cutroneo KR, Badger GJ, et al. Tissue stretch decreases soluble TGF-b1 and type-1 procollagen in mouse subcutaneous connective tissue: evidence from ex vivo and in vivo models. *J Cell Physiol*. 2008;214:389–395.
24. Langevin HM, Sherman KJ. Pathophysiological model for chronic low back pain integrating connective tissue and nervous system mechanisms. *Med Hypotheses*. 2007;68:74–80.
25. Soligo M, Nori SL, Protto V, et al. Acupuncture and neurotrophin modulation. *Int Rev Neurobiol*. 2013;111(1):91–124. doi:10.1016/B978-0-12-411545-3.00005-5.
26. Dhond RP, Kettner N, Napadow V. Neuroimaging acupuncture effects in the human brain. *J Altern Complement Med*. 2007;13:603–616.
27. Scheffold BE, Hsieh CL, Litscher G. Neuroimaging and neuromonitoring effects of electro and manual acupuncture on the central nervous system: a literature review and analysis. *Evid Based Complement Alternat Med*. 2015;2015:641742. doi:10.1155/2015/641742.
28. Cho ZH, Chung SC, Jones JP, et al. New findings of the correlation between acupoints and corresponding brain cortices using functional MRI. *Proc Natl Acad Sci U S A*. 1998;95(5):2670–2673.
29. Siedentopf CM, Golaszewski SM, Mottaghy FM, et al. Functional magnetic resonance imaging detects activation of the visual association cortex during laser acupuncture of the foot in humans. *Neurosci Lett*. 2002;327(1):53–56.
30. Gareus IK, Lacour M, Schulte AC, et al. Is there a BOLD response of the visual cortex on stimulation of the vision-related acupoint GB 37? *J Magn Reson Imaging*. 2002;15(3):227–232.
31. Li G, Cheung RT, Ma QY, et al. Visual cortical activations on fMRI upon stimulation of the vision-implicated acupoints. *Neuroreport*. 2003;14(5):669–673.
32. Yan B, Li K, Xu J, et al. Acupoint-specific fMRI patterns in human brain. *Neurosci Lett*. 2005;383(3):236–240.
33. Nakagoshi A, Fukunaga M, Umeda M, et al. Somatotopic representation of acupoints in human primary somatosensory cortex: an FMRI study. *Magn Reson Med Sci*. 2005;4(4):187–189.
34. Li L, Liu H, Li YZ, et al. The human brain response to acupuncture on same-meridian acupoints: evidence from an fMRI study. *J Altern Complement Med*. 2008;14(6):673–678.
35. Dhond RP, Yeh C, Park K, et al. Acupuncture modulates resting state connectivity in default and sensorimotor brain networks. *Pain*. 2008;136(3):407–418.
36. Hui KK, Liu J, Marina O, et al. The integrated response of the human cerebro-cerebellar and limbic systems to acupuncture stimulation at ST 36 as evidenced by fMRI. *Neuroimage*. 2005;27(3):479–496.
37. Liu WC, Feldman SC, Cook DB, et al. fMRI study of acupuncture-induced periaqueductal gray activity in humans. *Neuroreport*. 2004;15(12):1937–1940.
38. Chae Y, Lee H, Kim H, et al. The neural substrates of verum acupuncture compared to non-penetrating placebo needle: an fMRI study. *Neurosci Lett*. 2009;450(2):80–84.
39. Manyanga T, Froese M, Zarychanski R, et al. Pain management with acupuncture in osteoarthritis: a systematic review and meta-analysis. *BMC Complement Altern Med*. 2014;14(1):312. doi:10.1186/1472-6882-14-312.
40. Berman BM, Swyers JP, Ezzo J. The evidence for acupuncture as a treatment for rheumatologic conditions. *Rheum Dis Clin North Am*. 2000;26(1):103–115.
41. Nayak S, Shiflett SC, Schoenberger NE, et al. Is acupuncture effective in treating chronic pain after spinal cord injury? *Arch Phys Med Rehabil*. 2001;82(11):1578–1586.
42. Cheng PT, Wong MK, Chang PL. A therapeutic trial of acupuncture in neurogenic bladder of spinal cord injured patients—a preliminary report. *Spinal Cord*. 1998;36(7):476.
43. Anonymous. NIH Consensus development panel on acupuncture. Acupuncture. *JAMA*. 1998;280:1518–1524.
44. Nielsen A. Acupuncture for the prevention of tension-type headache (2016). *Explore (NY)*. 2017;13(3):228–231. doi:10.1016/j.explore.2017.03.007.
45. Lee MS, Ernst E. Acupuncture for pain: an overview of Cochrane reviews. *Chin J Integr Med*. 2011;17(3):187–189.
46. Weiss J, Quante S, Xue F, et al. Effectiveness and acceptance of acupuncture in patients with chronic low back pain: results of a prospective, randomized, controlled trial. *J Altern Complement Med*. 2013;19(12):935–941. doi:10.1089/acm.2012.0338.
47. Furlan AD, van Tulder MW, Cherkin DC, et al. Acupuncture and dry-needling for low back pain. *Cochrane Database Syst Rev*. 2005;(1):CD001351.
48. Hsieh Y-L, Hong C-Z, Liu S-Y, et al. Acupuncture at distant myofascial trigger spots enhances endogenous opioids in rabbits: a possible mechanism for managing myofascial pain. *Acupunct Med*. 2016;34(4):302–309. doi:10.1136/acupmed-2015-011026.
49. Xie Y, Wang L, He J, et al. Acupuncture for dysphagia in acute stroke. *Cochrane Database Syst Rev*. 2008;(3):CD006076.
50. Thomas LH, Cross S, Barrett J, et al. Treatment of urinary incontinence after stroke in adults. *Cochrane Database Syst Rev*. 2008;(1):CD004462. doi:10.1002/14651858.CD004462.pub3.
51. Yang A, Wu HM, Tang JL, et al. Acupuncture for stroke rehabilitation. *Cochrane Database Syst Rev*. 2016;(8):CD004131. doi:10.1002/14651858.CD004131.pub3.
52. Seca S, Miranda D, Cardoso D, et al. The effectiveness of acupuncture on pain, physical function and health-related quality of life in patients with rheumatoid arthritis. *JBI Database System Rev Implement Rep*. 2016;14(5):18–26. doi:10.11124/JBISRIR-2016-002543.
53. Casimiro L, Barnsley L, Brosseau L, et al. Acupuncture and electroacupuncture for the treatment of rheumatoid arthritis. *Cochrane Database Syst Rev*. 2005;(4):CD003788.
54. Averill A, Cotter AC, Nayak S, et al. Blood pressure response to acupuncture in a population at risk for autonomic dysreflexia. *Arch Phys Med Rehabil*. 2000;81(11):1494–1497.
55. Abrams DI, Dolor R, Roberts R, et al. The BraveNet prospective observational study on integrative medicine treatment approaches for pain. *BMC Complement Altern Med*. 2013;13(1):146. doi:10.1186/1472-6882-13-146.
56. Pole S. *Ayurvedic Medicine: The Principles of Traditional Practice*. Philadelphia, PA/London: Elsevier Health Sciences; 2006.
57. NCCAM Website. Questions and Answers about Homeopathy. April 2003. Available from: http://nccam.nih.gov/health/homeopathy/
58. Kabat-Zinn J. Mindfulness-based interventions in context: past, present, and future. *Clin Psychol Sci Pr*. 2003;10(2):144–156.
59. Lutz A, Slagter HA, Dunne JD, et al. Attention regulation and monitoring in meditation. *Trends Cogn Sci*. 2008;12(4):163–169.
60. Ost LG. Efficacy of the third wave of behavioral therapies: a systematic review and meta-analysis. *Behav Res Ther*. 2008;46(3):296–321.
61. Kabat-Zinn J, Lipworth L, Burney R. The clinical use of mindfulness meditation for the self-regulation of chronic pain. *J Behav Med*. 1985;8(2):163–190.

62. Teasdale JD, Segal ZV, Williams JM, et al. Prevention of relapse/recurrence in major depression by mindfulness-based cognitive therapy. *J Consult Clin Psychol.* 2000;68(4):615–623.

63. Hayes SC, Strosahl K, Wilson KG. *Acceptance and Commitment Therapy: An Experiential Approach to Behavior Change.* New York: Guilford Press; 1999: xvi, 304 p.

64. Hardison ME, Roll SC. Mindfulness interventions in physical rehabilitation: a scoping review. *Am J Occup Ther.* 2016;70(3):7003290030p1–7003290030p9.

65. Chiesa A, Serretti A. Mindfulness-based interventions for chronic pain: a systematic review of the evidence. *J Altern Complement Med.* 2011;17(1):83–93.

66. Rosenzweig S, Greeson JM, Reibel DK, et al. Mindfulness-based stress reduction for chronic pain conditions: variation in treatment outcomes and role of home meditation practice. *J Psychosom Res.* 2010;68(1):29–36.

67. Hill RJ, McKernan LC, Wang L, et al. Changes in psychosocial well-being after mindfulness-based stress reduction: a prospective cohort study. *J Man Manip Ther.* 2017;25:128–136.

68. Kihlstrom JF. Hypnosis. *Ann Rev Psychol.* 1985;36:385–418.

69. Elkins GR, Barabasz AF, Council JR, et al. Advancing research and practice: the revised APA Division 30 definition of hypnosis. *Int J Clin Exp Hypn.* 2015;63(1):1–9.

70. Jensen MP, Patterson DR. Hypnotic approaches for chronic pain management: clinical implications of recent research findings. *Am Psychol.* 2014;69(2):167–177.

71. Jensen MP, Adachi T, Tomé-Pires C, et al. Mechanisms of hypnosis: toward the development of a biopsychosocial model. *Int J Clin Exp Hypn.* 2015;63(1):34–75.

72. Montgomery GH, David D, Winkel G, et al. The effectiveness of adjunctive hypnosis with surgical patients: a meta-analysis. *Anesth Analg.* 2002;94(6):1639–1645.

73. Liossi C, Hatira P. Clinical hypnosis in the alleviation of procedure-related pain in pediatric oncology patients. *Int J Clin Exp Hypn.* 2003;51(1):4–28.

74. Patterson DR, Everett JJ, Burns GL, et al. Hypnosis for the treatment of burn pain. *J Consult Clin Psychol.* 1992;60(5):713–717.

75. Spinhoven P, Linssen AC. Education and self-hypnosis in the management of low back pain: a component analysis. *Br J Clin Psychol.* 1989;28(Pt 2):145–153.

76. Jensen MP, Barber J, Romano JM, et al. A comparison of self-hypnosis versus progressive muscle relaxation in patients with multiple sclerosis and chronic pain. *Int J Clin Exp Hypn.* 2009;57(2):198–221.

77. Jensen MP, Barber J, Romano JM, et al. Effects of self-hypnosis training and EMG biofeedback relaxation training on chronic pain in persons with spinal-cord injury. *Int J Clin Exp Hypn.* 2009;57(3):239–268.

78. Hammond DC. Review of the efficacy of clinical hypnosis with headaches and migraines. *Int J Clin Exp Hypn.* 2007;55(2):207–219.

79. Adachi T, Fujino H, Nakae A, et al. A meta-analysis of hypnosis for chronic pain problems: a comparison between hypnosis, standard care, and other psychological interventions. *Int J Clin Exp Hypn.* 2014;62(1):1–28.

80. Jensen MP, McArthur KD, Barber J, et al. Satisfaction with, and the beneficial side effects of, hypnotic analgesia. *Int J Clin Exp Hypn.* 2006;54(4):432–447.

81. Ehde DM, Dillworth TM, Turner JA. Cognitive-behavioral therapy for individuals with chronic pain: efficacy, innovations, and directions for research. *Am Psychol.* 2014;69(2):153–166.

82. Turk DC. A cognitive-behavioral perspective on treatment of chronic pain patients. In: Turk DC, Gatchel RJ, eds. *Psychological Approaches to Pain Management: A Practitioners Guide.* London: Guilford Press; 2002:138–158.

83. Williams DA. Cognitive and behavioral approaches to chronic pain. In: Wallace DJ, Clauw DJ, eds. *Fibromyalgia and Other Central Pain Syndromes.* Philadelphia, PA: Lippincott Williams & Wilkins; 2005:343–352.

84. Turk DC, Monarch ES. Biopsychosocial perspective on chronic pain. In: Turk DC, Gatchel RJ, eds. *Psychological Approaches to Pain Management.* 2nd ed. New York: Guilford Press; 2002:3–30.

85. Archer KR, Motzny N, Abraham CM, et al. Cognitive-behavioral-based physical therapy to improve surgical spine outcomes: a case series. *Phys Ther.* 2013;93(8):1130.

86. Archer KR, Devin CJ, Vanston SW, et al. Cognitive-behavioral-based physical therapy for patients with chronic pain undergoing lumbar spine surgery: a randomized controlled trial. *J Pain.* 2016;17(1):76–89.

87. Monticone M, Ferrante S, Rocca B, et al. Effect of a long-lasting multidisciplinary program on disability and fear-avoidance behaviors in patients with chronic low back pain: results of a randomized controlled trial. *Clin J Pain.* 2013;29(11):929–938.

88. Glombiewski JA, Bernardy K, Häuser W. Efficacy of EMG- and EEG-biofeedback in fibromyalgia syndrome: a meta-analysis and a systematic review of randomized controlled trials. *Evid Based Complement Alternat Med.* 2013;2013:962741.

89. Rains JC. Change mechanisms in EMG biofeedback training: cognitive changes underlying improvements in tension headache. *Headache.* 2008;48(5):735–736; discussion 6–7.

90. Morley S, Eccleston C, Williams A. Systematic review and meta-analysis of randomized controlled trails of cognitive behavior therapy and behavior therapy for chronic pain in adults, excluding headache. *Pain.* 1999;80(1):1–13.

91. Hoffman BM, Papas RK, Chatkoff DK, et al. Meta-analysis of psychological interventions for chronic low back pain. *Health Psychol.* 2007;26:1–9.

92. Sundar S, Agrawal SK, Singh VP, et al. Role of yoga in management of essential hypertension. *Acta Cardiol.* 1984;39(3):203–208.

93. Ornish D, Brown SE, Billings JH, et al. Can lifestyle changes reverse coronary heart disease?: the lifestyle heart trial. *Lancet.* 1990;336(8708):129–133.

94. Haslock I, Monro R, Nagarathna R, et al. Measuring the effects of yoga in rheumatoid arthritis. *Rheumatology.* 1994;33(8):787–788.

95. Garfinkel MS, Schumacher JH, Husain AB, et al. Evaluation of a yoga based regimen for treatment of osteoarthritis of the hands. *J Rheumatol.* 1994;21(12):2341–2343.

96. Schatz MP. *Back Care Basics: A Doctor's Gentle Yoga Program for Back and Neck Pain Relief.* Boulder: Shambhala Publications; 2016.

97. Groessl EJ, Schmalzl L, Maiya M, et al. Yoga for veterans with chronic low back pain: design and methods of a randomized clinical trial. *Contemp Clin Trials.* 2016;48(1):110–118. doi:10.1016/j.cct.2016.04.006.

98. Cramer H, Lauche R, Hohmann C, et al. Randomized-controlled trial comparing yoga and home-based exercise for chronic neck pain. *Clin J Pain.* 2013;29(3):216–223. doi:10.1097/AJP.0b013e318251026c.

99. Kim S-D. Effects of yoga on chronic neck pain: a systematic review of randomized controlled trials. *J Phys Ther Sci.* 2016;28(7):2171–2174. doi:10.1589/jpts.28.2171.

100. Levy JK. Standard and alternative adjunctive treatments in cardiac rehabilitation. *Tex Heart Inst J.* 1993;20(3):198.

101. Raju PS, Madhavi S, Prasad KV, et al. Comparison of effects of yoga & physical exercise in athletes. *Indian J Med Res.* 1994;100:81.

102. Taylor MJ, Majundmar M. Incorporating yoga therapeutics into orthopaedic physical therapy. *Orthop Phys Ther Clin North Am.* 2000;9(3):341–360.

103. Cotter AC. Western movement therapies. *Phys Med Rehabil Clin N Am.* 1999;10(3):603–616.

104. Voukelatos A, Cumming RG, Lord SR, et al. A randomized, controlled trial of tai chi for the prevention of falls: the Central Sydney tai chi trial. *J Am Geriatr Soc.* 2007;55(8):1185–1191.

105. Province MA, Hadley EC, Hornbrook MC, et al. The effects of exercise on falls in elderly patients: a preplanned meta-analysis of the FICSIT trials. *JAMA.* 1995;273(17):1341–1347.

106. Wolfson L, Whipple R, Derby C, et al. Balance and strength training in older adults: intervention gains and Tai Chi maintenance. *J Am Geriatr Soc.* 1996;44(5):498–506.

107. Plummer JP. Acupuncture and homeostasis: physiological, physical (postural) and psychological. *Am J Chin Med.* 1981;9(1):1–14.

108. Jones KD, Sherman CA, Mist SD, et al. A randomized controlled trial of 8-form Tai chi improves symptoms and functional mobility in fibromyalgia patients. *Clin Rheumatol.* 2012;31(8):1205–1214. doi:10.1007/s10067-012-1996-2.

109. Langhorst J, Klose P, Dobos GJ, et al. Efficacy and safety of meditative movement therapies in fibromyalgia syndrome: a systematic review and meta-analysis of randomized controlled trials. *Rheumatol Int.* 2013;33(1):193–207. doi:10.1007/s00296-012-2360-1.

110. Wang C, Schmid CH, Rones R, et al. A randomized trial of tai chi for fibromyalgia. *N Engl J Med.* 2010;363(8):743–754. doi:10.1056/NEJMoa0912611.

111. Hall AM, Maher CG, Lam P, et al. Tai chi exercise for treatment of pain and disability in people with persistent low back pain: a randomized controlled trial. *Arthritis Care Res (Hoboken).* 2011;63(11):1576–1583. doi:10.1002/acr.20594.

112. Harer JB, Munden S. *The Alexander Technique Resource Book: A Reference Guide.* Lanham, MD: Scarecrow Press; 2008.

113. MacPherson H, Tilbrook H, Richmond S, et al. Alexander technique lessons or acupuncture sessions for persons with chronic neck pain: a randomized trial. *Ann Intern Med.* 2015;163(9):653–662. doi:10.7326/M15-0667.

114. Kamalikhah T, Morowatisharifabad MA, Rezaei-Moghaddam F, et al. Alexander technique training coupled with an integrative model of behavioral prediction in teachers with low back pain. *Iran Red Crescent Med J.* 2016;18(9):e31218. doi:10.5812/ircmj.31218.

115. Austin JH, Ausubel P. Enhanced respiratory muscular function in normal adults after lessons in proprioceptive musculoskeletal education without exercises. *Chest.* 1992;102(2):486–490.

116. Stallibrass C. An evaluation of the Alexander Technique for the management of disability in Parkinson's disease—a preliminary study. *Clin Rehabil.* 1997;11(1):8–12.

117. Stephens J, Call S, Evans K, et al. Responses to ten Feldenkrais awareness through movement lessons by four women with multiple sclerosis: improved quality of life. *Phys Ther Case Rep.* 1999;2(1):58–69.

118. Schenkman M, Donovan J, Tsubota J, et al. Management of individuals with Parkinson's disease: rationale and case studies. *Phys Ther.* 1989;69(11):944–955.

119. Smith AL, Kolt GS, McConville JC. The effect of the Feldenkrais method on pain and anxiety in people experiencing chronic low back pain. *New Zeal J Phys Ther.* 2001;1:6–14.

120. Paolucci T, Zangrando F, Iosa M, et al. Improved interoceptive awareness in chronic low back pain: a comparison of Back school versus Feldenkrais method. *Disabil Rehabil.* 2017;39(10):994–1001. doi:10.1080/09638288.2016.1175035.

121. Hillier S, Worley A. The effectiveness of the Feldenkrais method: a systematic review of the evidence. *Evid Based Complement Alternat Med.* 2015;2015:752160. doi:10.1155/2015/752160.

122. Lundblad I, Elert J, Gerdle B. Randomized controlled trial of physiotherapy and Feldenkrais interventions in female workers with neck-shoulder complaints. *J Occup Rehabil.* 1999;9(3):179–194.

123. Bearman D, Shafarman S. The Feldenkrais Method in the treatment of chronic pain: a study of efficacy and cost effectiveness. *Am J Pain Manage.* 1999;9:22–27.

124. Ives JC, Shelley GA. The Feldenkrais Method® in rehabilitation: a review. *Work.* 1998;11(1):75–90.

125. Loosli AR, Herold D. Knee rehabilitation for dancers using a Pilates-based technique. *Kinesiol Med Dance.* 1992;14(2):1–2.

126. Hutchinson MR, Tremain L, Christiansen J, et al. Improving leaping ability in elite rhythmic gymnasts. *Med Sci Sports Exerc.* 1998;30(1):1543–1547.

127. Brown SE, Clippinger K. Rehabilitation of anterior cruciate ligament insufficiency in a dancer using the clinical reformer and a balanced body exercise method. *Work.* 1996;7(2):109–114.

128. Hartley L. *Wisdom of the Body Moving*. Berkeley, CA: North Atlantic Books; 1995.

129. Clarke TC, Black LI, Stussman BJ, et al. Trends in the use of complementary health approaches among adults: United States, 2002–2012. *Natl Health Stat Report*. 2015;(79):1–16.

130. National Institutes of Health. Nationwide study reports shifts in Americans' use of natural products. Updated February 10, 2015. Available from: www.nih.gov/news/health/feb2015/nccih-10.htm. Accessed January 1, 2019.

131. *Dietary Supplement Health and Education Act of 1994*. Available from: https://ods.od.nih.gov/About/DSHEA_Wording.aspx

132. U.S. Food and Drug Administration (FDA). Dietary supplement current good manufacturing practices (CGMPs) and interim final rule (IFR) facts. Updated September 19, 2014. Available from: www.fda.gov/Food/GuidanceRegulation/CGMP/ucm110858.htm. Accessed January 1, 2019.

133. Lantz RC, Chen GJ, Solyom AM, et al. The effect of turmeric extracts on inflammatory mediator production. *Phytomedicine*. 2005;12(6-7):445–452.

134. Belcaro G, Cesarone MR, Dugall M, et al. Efficacy and safety of Meriva®, a curcumin-phosphatidylcholine complex, during extended administration in osteoarthritis patients. *Altern Med Rev*. 2010;15(4):337–344.

135. Madhu K, Chanda K, Saji MJ. Safety and efficacy of *Curcuma longa* extract in the treatment of painful knee osteoarthritis: a randomized placebo-controlled trial. *Inflammopharmacology*. 2013;21(2):129–136. doi:10.1007/s10787-012-0163-3.

136. Kuptniratsaikul V, Dajpratham P, Taechaarpornkul W, et al. Efficacy and safety of *Curcuma domestica* extracts compared with ibuprofen in patients with knee osteoarthritis: a multicenter study. *Clin Interv Aging*. 2014;20(9):451–458. doi:10.2147/CIA.S58535.

137. Bartels EM, Folmer VN, Bliddal H, et al. Efficacy and safety of ginger in osteoarthritis patients: a meta-analysis of randomized placebo-controlled trials. *Osteoarthr Cartil*. 2015;23(1):13–21.

138. Haghighi M, Khalva A, Toliat T, et al. Comparing the effects of ginger (*Zingiber officinale*) extract and ibuprofen on patients with osteoarthritis. *Arch Iran Med*. 2005;8(1):267–271.

139. Bliddal H, Rosetzsky A, Schlichting P, et al. A randomized, placebo-controlled, cross-over study of ginger extracts and ibuprofen in osteoarthritis. *Osteoarthr Cartil*. 2000;8(1):9–12. doi:10.1053/joca.1999.0264.

140. Yip YB, Tam AC. An experimental study on the effectiveness of massage with aromatic ginger and orange essential oil for moderate-to-severe knee pain among the elderly in Hong Kong. *Complement Ther Med*. 2008;16(3):131–138. doi:10.1016/j.ctim.2007.12.003.

141. Schwarz NA, Spillane M, La Bounty P, et al. Capsaicin and evodiamine ingestion does not augment energy expenditure and fat oxidation at rest or after moderately-intense exercise. *Nutr Res*. 2013;33(12):1034–1042. doi:10.1016/j.nutres.2013.08.007.

142. Towheed TE, Maxwell L, Anastassiades TP, et al. Glucosamine therapy for treating osteoarthritis. *Cochrane Database Syst Rev*. 2005;(2):CD002946.

143. Poolsup N, Suthisisang C, Channark P, et al. Glucosamine long-term treatment and the progression of knee osteoarthritis: systematic review of randomized controlled trials. *Ann Pharmacother*. 2005;39(6):1080–1087.

144. Weber KL, Jevsevar DS, McGrory BJ. AAOS clinical practice guideline: surgical management of osteoarthritis of the knee: evidence-based guideline. *J Am Acad Orthop Surg*. 2016;24(8):e94–e96. doi:10.5435/JAAOS-D-16-00160.

145. Harmand MF, Vilamitjana J, Maloche E, et al. Effects of *S*-adenosylmethionine on human articular chondrocyte differentiation. An in vitro study. *Am J Med*. 1987;83(5A):48–54.

146. Chavez M. SAMe: *S*-adenosylmethionine. *Am J Health Syst Pharm*. 2000;57(2):119–123.

147. Khayyal MT, El-Ghazaly MA. The possible "chondroprotective" effect of the unsaponifiable constituents of avocado and soya in vivo. *Drugs Exp Clin Res*. 1998;24(1):41–50.

148. Maheu E, Cadet C, Marty M, et al. Randomised, controlled trial of avocado-soybean unsaponifiable (Piascledine) effect on structure modification in hip osteoarthritis: the ERADIAS study. *Ann Rheum Dis*. 2014;73(2):376–384. doi:10.1136/annrheumdis-2012-202485.

149. Christiansen BA, Bhatti S, Goudarzi R, et al. Erratum: response to the letter to the editor for "Management of Osteoarthritis with Avocado/Soybean Unsaponifiables". *Cartilage*. 2016;7(1):114–115. doi:10.1177/1947603515623157.

150. Kremer JM, Lawrence DA, Jubiz W, et al. Dietary fish oil and olive oil supplementation in patients with rheumatoid arthritis. Clinical and immunologic effects. *Arthritis Rheum*. 1990;33(6):810–820.

151. Gruenwald J, Petzold E, Busch R, et al. Effect of glucosamine sulfate with or without omega-3 fatty acids in patients with osteoarthritis. *Adv Ther*. 2009;26(9):858–871. doi:10.1007/s12325-009-0060-3.

152. Rotblatt M. Herbal medicine: expanded commission E monographs. *Ann Intern Med*. 2000;133(6):487.

153. Omoigui S. The biochemical origin of pain: the origin of all pain is inflammation and the inflammatory response. Part 2 of 3—inflammatory profile of pain syndromes. *Med Hypotheses*. 2007;69(6):1169–1178.

154. O'Keefe JH, Gheewala NM, O'Keefe JO. Dietary strategies for improving postprandial glucose, lipids, inflammation, and cardiovascular health. *J Am Coll Cardiol*. 2008;51(3):249–255. doi:10.1016/j.jacc.2007.10.016.

155. Weil A. *Eating Well for Optimum Health*. New York: Knopf; 2001.

156. Veronese N. Adherence to the Mediterranean diet is associated with better quality of life: data from the Osteoarthritis Initiative. *Am J Clin Nutr*. 2016;104(5):1403–1409.

157. Kjeldsen-Kragh J. Rheumatoid arthritis treated with vegetarian diets. *Am J Clin Nutr*. 1999;70(3 suppl):594S–600S. doi:10.1093/ajcn/70.3.594s.

158. Adam O. Nutrition as adjuvant therapy in chronic polyarthritis. *Rheumatol Int*. 1993;52(5):275–280.

159. Longo VD. Fasting: molecular mechanisms and clinical applications. *Cell Metab*. 2014;19(2):181–192.

160. Müller H, de Toledo FW, Resch KL. Fasting followed by vegetarian diet in patients with rheumatoid arthritis: a systematic review. *Scand J Rheumatol*. 2001;30(1):1–10.

161. Huang HY, Caballero B, Chang S, et al. The efficacy and safety of multivitamin and mineral supplement use to prevent cancer and chronic disease in adults: a systematic review for a NIH state-of-the-science conference. *Ann Intern Med*. 2006;145(5):372–385.

162. Cotter AC, Bartoli L, Schulman R. An overview of massage and touch therapies. *Phys Med Rehabil*. 2000;14(1):43–64.

163. McPartland J, Miller B. Bodywork therapy systems. *Phys Med Rehabil Clin N Am*. 1999;10(3):583–602.

164. Peng ZF. Comparison between western trigger point of acupuncture and traditional acupoints. *Zhongguo Zhen Jiu*. 2008;28(5):349–352.

165. Liu L, Skinner M, McDonough S, et al. Acupuncture for low back pain: an overview of systematic reviews. *Evid Based Complement Alternat Med*. 2015;2015:328196.

166. Upledger J, Vredevoogd J. *Craniosacral Therapy*. Seattle, WA: Eastland Press; 1983.

167. Upledger JE. Craniosacral therapy. *Phys Ther*. 1995;75:328–330.

168. King HH. Craniosacral therapy shown beneficial in management of chronic neck pain. *J Am Osteopath Assoc*. 2016;116(7):486–487. doi:10.7556/jaoa.2016.095.

169. Perry J, Jones M, Thomas L. Functional evaluation of Rolfing in cerebral palsy. *Dev Med Child Neurol*. 1981;23:717–729.

170. Kim JH, Lee HS, Park SW. Effects of the active release technique on pain and range of motion of patients with chronic neck pain. *J Phys Ther Sci*. 2015;27(8):2461–2464. doi:10.1589/jpts.27.2461.

171. Pavelka K, Gatterova J. Glucosamine sulfate use and delay of progression of knee osteoarthritis: a 3-year, randomized, placebo-controlled, double blind study. *Arch Intern Med*. 2002;(162):2113–2123.

172. Dyson-Hudson TA, Shiflett SC, Kirshblum SC. Acupuncture and Trager psychophysical integration in the treatment of wheelchair user's shoulder pain in individuals with spinal cord injury. *Arch Phys Med Rehabil*. 2001;82:1038–1046.

173. Witt P, MacKinnon J. Trager psychophysical integration: a method to improve chest mobility of patients with chronic lung disease. *Phys Ther*. 1986;66(2):214–217.

174. Rosch PJ. Bioelectromagnetic and subtle energy medicine: the interface between mind and matter. *Ann N Y Acad Sci*. 2009;1172(1):297–311. doi:10.1111/j.1749-6632.2009.04535.x.

175. Hammerschlag R, Marx BL, Aickin M. Nontouch biofield therapy: a systematic review of human randomized controlled trials reporting use of only nonphysical contact treatment. *J Altern Complement Med*. 2014;20(12):881–892. doi:http://doi.org/10.1089/acm.2014.0017.

176. Burmeister A. *The Touch of Healing: Energizing Body, Mind, and Spirit with the Art of Jin Shin Jyutsu*. New York: Bantam Books; 1997.

177. Sood A, Barton DL, Bauer BA, et al. A critical review of complementary therapies for cancer-related fatigue. *Integr Cancer Ther*. 2007;6(1):8–13.

178. Jain S, Mills PJ. Biofield therapies: helpful or full of hype? A best evidence synthesis. *Int J Behav Med*. 2010;17(1):1–16. doi:10.1007/s12529-009-9062-4.

179. Fazzino DL, Griffin MT, McNulty RS, et al. Energy healing and pain: a review of the literature. *Holist Nurs Pract*. 2010;24(2):79–88. doi:10.1097/HNP.0b013e3181d39718.

180. So PS, Jiang Y, Qin Y. Touch therapies for pain relief in adults. *Cochrane Database Syst Rev*. 2008;(4):CD006535. doi:http://doi.org/10.1002/14651858.CD006535.pub2.

181. Hillinger MG, Wolever RQ, McKernan LC, et al. Integrative medicine for the treatment of persistent pain. *Prim Care*. 2017;44(2):247–264.

182. Krieger D. *The Therapeutic Touch: How to Use Your Hands to Help or to Heal*. Englewood Cliffs, NJ: Prentice-Hall; 1979.

183. Therapeutic Touch International Association. The process of therapeutic touch Therapeutic Touch International Organization [Internet]. 2017. Available from: http://therapeutictouch.org/what-is-tt/history-of-tt

184. Lu D-F, Hart LK, Lutgendorf SK, et al. The effect of healing touch on the pain and mobility of persons with osteoarthritis: a feasibility study. *Geriatr Nurs*. 2013;34(4):314–322. doi:10.1016/j.gerinurse.2013.05.003.

185. Baldwin AL, Fullmer K, Schwartz GE. Comparison of physical therapy with energy healing for improving range of motion in subjects with restricted shoulder mobility. *Evid Based Complement Alternat Med*. 2013;2013:329731. doi:http://doi.org/10.1155/2013/329731.

186. Monroe CM. The effects of therapeutic touch on pain. *J Holist Nurs*. 2009;27(2):85–92. doi:10.1177/0898010108327213.

187. Eisenberg D, Wright TL. *Encounters with Qi*. New York: Viking Penguin; 1987.

188. Posadzki P. The sociology of Qi Gong: a qualitative study. *Complement Ther Med*. 2010;18(2):87–94. doi:http://doi.org/10.1016/j.ctim.2009.12.002.

189. McGee CT, Chow EPY. *Miracle Healing from China: Qigong*. Coeur d'Alene, ID: MediPress; 1994.

190. Saatcioglu F. Regulation of gene expression by yoga, meditation and related practices: a review of recent studies. *Asian J Psychiatr*. 2013;6(1):74–77. doi:10.1016/j.ajp.2012.10.002.

191. Rand W. *Reiki: The Healing Touch*. Southfield, MI: Vision Publications; 1991.

192. Nichols AW, Harrigan R. Complementary and alternative medicine usage by intercollegiate athletes. *Clin J Sport Med*. 2006;16(3):232–237.

193. Malone MA, Gloyer K. Complementary and alternative treatments in sports medicine. *Prim Care*. 2013;40(4):945–968, ix. doi:10.1016/j.pop.2013.08.010.
194. Wadsworth LT. Acupuncture in sports medicine. *Curr Sports Med Rep*. 2006;5(1):1–3.
195. Leung A, Khadivi B, Duann J-R, et al. The effect of ting point (tendinomuscular meridians) electroacupuncture on thermal pain: a model for studying the neuronal mechanism of acupuncture analgesia. *J Altern Complement Med*. 2005;11(4):653–661. doi:10.1089/acm.2005.11.653.
196. Deldicque L, Francaux M. Potential harmful effects of dietary supplements in sports medicine. *Curr Opin Clin Nutr Metab Care*. 2016;19(6):439–445. doi:10.1097/MCO.0000000000000321.
197. Kavukcu E, Burgazlı KM. Preventive health perspective in sports medicine: the trend at the use of medications and nutritional supplements during 5 years period between 2003 and 2008 in football. *Balkan Med J*. 2013;30(1):74–79. doi:10.5152/balkanmedj.2012.090.
198. Mazzoni I, Barroso O, Rabin O. The list of prohibited substances and methods in sport: structure and review process by the world anti-doping agency. *J Anal Toxicol*. 2011;35(9):608–612.
199. Naderi A, Earnest CP, Lowery RP, et al. Co-ingestion of nutritional ergogenic aids and high-intensity exercise performance. *Sports Med*. 2016;46(10):1407–1418. doi:http://doi.org/10.1007/s40279-016-0525-x.
200. Volpe S. Minerals as ergogenic aids. *Curr Sports Med Rep*. 2008;7(4):224–229.
201. Fillmore C, Bartoli L, Bach R, et al. Nutrition and dietary supplements. *Phys Med Rehabil Clin N Am*. 1999;10(2):673–703.
202. Bergeron MF. Muscle cramps during exercise—is it fatigue or electrolyte deficit? *Curr Sports Med Rep*. 2008;7(4):S50–S55.
203. Polsgrove MJ, Eggleston B, Lockyer R. Impact of 10-weeks of yoga practice on flexibility and balance of college athletes. *Int J Yoga*. 2016;9(1):27. doi:10.4103/0973-6131.171710.
204. Galland L. *The Four Pillars of Healing: How the New integrative—The Best of Conventional Medicine and Alternative Approaches—Can Cure You*. New York: Random House; 1997.
205. Jones D, ed. *Textbook of Functional Medicine*. Gig Harbor, WA: Institute for Functional Medicine; 2005:5.
206. Institute for Functional Medicine. Principles of Functional Medicine. Available from: https://www.functionalmedicine.org/What_is_Functional_Medicine/AboutFM/Principles/. Accessed February 16, 2017.
207. Bork P, Serrano L. Towards cellular systems in 4D. *Cell*. 2005;121:511–513.
208. Liu ET. Systems biology, integrative biology, predictive biology. *Cell*. 2005;121:505–506.
209. Fang J, Chen L, Ma R, et al. Comprehensive rehabilitation with integrative medicine for subacute stroke: a multicenter randomized controlled trial. *Sci Rep*. 2016;6:25850. doi:10.1038/srep25850.
210. Sierpina VS, Kreitzer MJ, Leskowitz E. Innovations in integrative healthcare education: Spaulding Rehabilitation Hospital—the integrative medicine project. *Explore (NY)*. 2007;3(1):70–71. doi:10.1016/j.explore.2006.10.012.
211. Charmel PA, Frampton SB. Building the business case for patient-centered care. *Healthc Financ Manage*. 2008;62(3):80–85.
212. Marks R, Allegrante JP, Lorig K. A review and synthesis of research evidence for self-efficacy-enhancing interventions for reducing chronic disability: implications for health education practice (part I). *Health Promot Pract*. 2005;6(1):37–43. doi:10.1177/1524839904266790.

CHAPTER 60

Mary D. Slavin
Alan M. Jette

Evidence-Based Practice in Rehabilitation (Including Clinical Trials)

Knowing is not enough; we must apply. Willing is not enough; we must do.

Goethe, 1829

HISTORY AND BACKGROUND

Since the 1990s, evidence-based medicine (EBM) has been promoted as an approach to bridge the gap between scientific research and clinical practice. David Sackett and leaders of the EBM movement sought to ground medical decision-making in rigorous scientific evidence. Based on principles and methods derived from clinical epidemiology, EBM systematically selects and applies research evidence as part of the clinical decision-making process. EBM uses an explicit framework to guide clinicians in the selection of diagnostic tests, clinical interventions, and methods for determining prognosis that represent the best available evidence. Since its introduction, EBM has been widely acknowledged as an important component of clinical practice. The 1990 Institute of Medicine report, *Crossing the Quality Chasm*, noted that an evidence-based approach to clinical practice provides a sound method for making clinical decisions, reduces idiosyncratic variations in practice, and bridges the gap between knowledge and practice (1). In 2011, the Institute of Medicine's (IOM) Roundtable on Value & Science-Driven Health Care set an ambitious goal: By 2020, 90% of clinical decisions will be supported by accurate, timely, and up-to-date clinical information and will reflect the best available evidence (2).

EBM should play an important role in promoting the translation of research into practice (3); however, the gap between the availability of research evidence and use of evidence in practice is widely acknowledged (4,5). While numerous rehabilitation scientific meetings and professional associations have focused on advancing EBM, the promise of EBM has not been fully realized. Indeed, decades after EBM was introduced, there are concerns about the degree to which current research

evidence is used in clinical practice (6). While considerable effort has been devoted to increasing EBM knowledge and skills of individual clinicians, implementation strategies to promote use of research in clinical settings have not been adequately addressed. The last several decades have witnessed an explosion of medical research, but the ability to identify, synthesize, and integrate these research findings into clinical practice has lagged behind.

The current state of scientific research and clinical practice is well articulated in Atul Gawande's 2014 Reith Lectures on *The Future of Medicine* (7). Gawande maintains that progress in medical research, a major achievement of the 20th century, has created the conditions that allow for a significant number of treatment failures due to lack of awareness. He further argues the major cause of treatment failure in 21st century will result from the poor or absent application of relevant research knowledge. We are at a critical juncture. An emphasis on understanding and implementing effective processes to adopt research evidence into clinical practice is needed to advance the EBM movement. This chapter focuses on the following: applying and adapting EBM principles to rehabilitation; gaining the knowledge needed understand how to incorporate research evidence into the clinical decision-making process; and understanding implementation issues that impact adoption and use of research evidence.

ADAPTING EVIDENCE-BASED MEDICINE FOR USE IN REHABILITATION

EBM was developed for use in general medicine, which has a primary focus on binary outcomes such as the presence/absence of disease. In contrast, increasing function and reducing disability are the primary goals of rehabilitation. Rehabilitation is a unique area of medicine focused on function, both as an outcome and as an area for clinical assessment (8). Rehabilitation

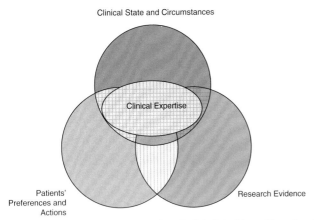

Clinical State and Circumstances

Clinical Expertise

Patients' Preferences and Actions

Research Evidence

FIGURE 60-1. Model for evidence-based clinical decisions. (Reproduced with permission from Haynes RB, Devereaux PJ, Guyatt GH. Clinical expertise in the era of evidence-based medicine and patient choice. *Evid Based Med.* 2002;7(2):36–38, with permission from BMJ Publishing Group Ltd.)

or capacity, and the environment" (9). The ICF provides a unifying model and defines rehabilitation as a health strategy that aims to help people "achieve and maintain optimal functioning in interaction with their environment" (10). Due to differences between the goals of general medicine and rehabilitation, one needs to translate EBM concepts for use in rehabilitation. EBM is grounded in clinical epidemiology (11), a field of study that uses epidemiologic methods to solve clinical problems (12). Rehabilitation professionals need to understand clinical epidemiology to acquire EBM skills to fully realize what EBM can offer the rehabilitation field. The remainder of this chapter uses the term evidence-based practice (EBP) to describe the adaptation of EBM principles to the rehabilitation field.

EBP DECISIONS

Evidence-based decisions are defined as the integration of best research evidence with clinical expertise and patient values (13). A model for evidence-based clinical decisions emphasizes three elements—*clinical state and circumstances*, *patient preferences and actions*, and *research evidence*—along with the fourth element, *clinical expertise*, that overlies the other three (**Fig. 60-1**) (14). This model recognizes the important role that clinical expertise plays in the clinical decision-making process. Clinical expertise is required to size up the patient's clinical state, communicate with patients to determine their preferences, and determine how to best apply research findings to the individual patient (14).

is based on a biopsychosocial model where treatment interventions interact with complex personal factors to produce multifaceted outcomes. The rehabilitation field has adopted the International Classification of Functioning Disability and Health (ICF) as a conceptual framework (see Chapter 9 on ICF). The ICF describes disability as the "interaction between a health condition, a person's decrease in body function, structure,

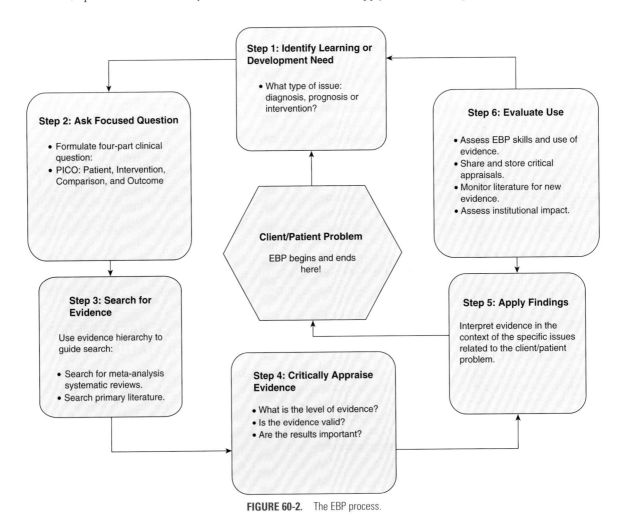

Step 1: Identify Learning or Development Need

• What type of issue: diagnosis, prognosis or intervention?

Step 2: Ask Focused Question

• Formulate four-part clinical question:
• PICO: Patient, Intervention, Comparison, and Outcome

Step 6: Evaluate Use

• Assess EBP skills and use of evidence.
• Share and store critical appraisals.
• Monitor literature for new evidence.
• Assess institutional impact.

Client/Patient Problem

EBP begins and ends here!

Step 3: Search for Evidence

Use evidence hierarchy to guide search:

• Search for meta-analysis systematic reviews.
• Search primary literature.

Step 4: Critically Appraise Evidence

• What is the level of evidence?
• Is the evidence valid?
• Are the results important?

Step 5: Apply Findings

Interpret evidence in the context of the specific issues related to the client/patient problem.

FIGURE 60-2. The EBP process.

EBP PROCESS

Figure 60-2 presents a schematic diagram of the steps involved in the EBP process. As the figure illustrates, EBP is patient focused. The first five steps in the EBP process—identifying the learning or development need, asking a focused question, searching for evidence, applying research evidence, and critically appraising evidence—begin and end with the patient. A sixth step, evaluating the use of evidence, adds a quality improvement component to the process. Clinicians interested in adopting an evidence-based approach will find a variety of resources on the Internet. 📶 **eTable 60-1** summarizes general EPB information. 📶 **eTable 60-2** summarizes Internet resources that serve as a guide to each step of the EPB process.

Step 1: Identify Learning or Development Need

The first step in the EBP process is to identify the learning issue and select the category of research evidence appropriate for the issue. For example, the learning issue may be uncertainty about which tests or clinical examination findings to consider in determining the presence or absence of a disease, impairment, or disorder—*evidence related to diagnosis*. A learning issue may arise when the patient inquires about the ability to return to work or the family inquires about the likelihood of a patient being able to return to home or to her/his previous level of functioning—*evidence related to prognosis*. Questions about other rehabilitation interventions that may yield a better outcome present another type of learning issue—*evidence related to intervention*. For each category of evidence—diagnosis, prognosis, or intervention—it is important to understand specific EBP concepts and terms.

Step 2: Ask a Focused Question

Once the learning issue and the appropriate category of research—diagnosis, prognosis, or intervention—are identified, a focused clinical question is formulated. A clinical question consists of four parts: patient, intervention, comparison, outcome (PICO). **Table 60-1** provides an example of the four-part clinical question. Clinical questions are constructed for each category of evidence. For example, a question related to diagnosis is framed as: For patients with shoulder pain, can clinical tests, compared to arthroscopy, identify patients with rotator cuff tears? A question related to prognosis is posed: For patients with a quadriceps contusion injury, can clinical tests predict the time to return to sports? And a question related to intervention is structured as follows: For elderly individuals with chronic disease, can a strength training exercise program reduce disability? Thus, a well-constructed clinical question establishes a link between patient problems, research evidence, and the clinical decision.

Step 3: Search for Research Evidence

Medicine has witnessed tremendous growth in research over the last century and this growth is particularly evident in the volume of available information. Each year, Medline indexes over 560,000 new articles and the Cochrane Center adds 20,000

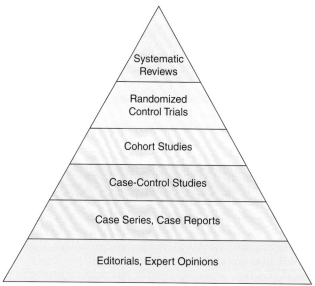

FIGURE 60-3. EBP research hierarchy.

new clinical trials. The volume of information presents a challenge because published research includes many preliminary or exploratory studies. Knowledge that has been rigorously tested and is of sufficient importance to influence practice represents only a small fraction of the published research (15). Thus, we do not suffer from a lack of information but from an inability to efficiently process and organize the plethora of available information. EBP provides useful strategies for the daunting task of keeping up-to-date on research literature. There are three strategies for conducting an effective and efficient search: (a) organize the search based on the hierarchy of research evidence quality; (b) use EBP search engines; and (c) search for evidence that has been summarized and rated for quality.

Research Evidence Hierarchy

Since the goal of EBP is to apply the best available evidence, the literature search begins by looking for the highest quality evidence. A key concept in EBP is that research evidence is not equal in value. EBP ranks research evidence based on a hierarchy that considers the degree to which the study design reduces bias and threats to validity. Professional organizations and EBP work groups have devised specific guidelines for rating evidence (16) that reflect the following values: controlled studies are ranked higher than uncontrolled studies; prospective studies are considered stronger than retrospective studies; and randomized studies are better than nonrandomized studies (17). Based on quality considerations, research evidence is categorized on a scale from Level I to VI: high-quality research with strong methodology is rated at the highest level (Level I) and expert opinion is ranked at the lowest level of evidence (Level V). Studies with weaknesses in research design and implementation or large confidence intervals (CIs) are ranked as Level II to IV (**Fig. 60-3**).

TABLE 60-1	**Four-Part Clinical Question**		
	P	**I**	**C**	**O**
Elements	Patient problem/ learning need	Intervention, diagnosis or Prognosis	Comparison (if indicated)	Outcome

Systematic reviews play an important role in EBP. In contrast to traditional opinion-based literature reviews, systematic reviews use a specific protocol to identify, critique, and summarize relevant studies that address a similar clinical question. Bias is minimized in systematic reviews because a comprehensive and reproducible process for searching the literature is outlined. Systematic reviews also assess the methodologic quality of studies (18), which is defined as "all aspects of a study's design and conduct can be shown to protect against systematic bias, nonsystematic bias, and inferential error" (19).

It is important to consider the type of research—diagnosis, prognosis, or intervention—when evaluating the strength of research evidence. For all types of evidence, a valid systematic review of quality research is the highest level of evidence while expert opinion is the lowest. However, for the other levels of evidence, the criteria for research quality are somewhat different for diagnosis, prognosis, or intervention studies. Evidence related to diagnosis compares the diagnostic test results to a "*gold*" standard, which is generally an accepted proof of the presence or absence of the disease or disorder. Therefore, an important consideration for ranking evidence from diagnostic studies is to determine how the gold, or reference, standard is applied (17). Studies in which the gold standard is consistently applied blindly or objectively to all subjects are ranked higher than studies in which the reference standard is not applied in such a manner. Furthermore, studies that validate diagnostic test results from a previous study are ranked higher than exploratory studies (16). Prognosis studies are concerned with examining the effect of patient characteristics on outcomes (17). Inception or prospective studies are rated higher than retrospective studies or studies using untreated subjects from randomized controlled trials (RCTs) (16). Intervention studies evaluate the effect of treatments on outcomes. RCTs help to eliminate potential bias and studies using RCTs are rated higher than cohort and case-controlled studies.

Role of Pragmatic Clinical Trials in EBP

The established EBP research evidence hierarchy, as presented in the previous section, is not without controversy. Some argue that the EBP preference for explanatory RCTs prioritizes experimental designs requiring homogenous samples in controlled research environments over more clinically relevant designs. Furthermore, the fact that significant EBP knowledge gaps exist suggests the presence of systematic flaws in the production of scientific evidence (20). While early-phase RCTs are rigorously designed to limit bias and promote internal validity, they are not designed to produce knowledge that can be directly generalized to the clinical settings. Consequently, it can be difficult to apply results from RCTs to clinical practice. RCTs are also expensive to conduct and may not be appropriate for late-phase trials. Pragmatic or practical clinical trials (PCTs) have received attention, in part, because these studies have the potential to fill a significant EBP knowledge gap. PCTs are conducted in realistic clinical environments, which may mitigate some implementation barriers associated with RCTs. PCTs are based on clinically relevant hypotheses and employ study designs that aim to answer specific clinical questions. While most RCTs focus on examining the *efficacy* of interventions, PCTs focus on examining the *effectiveness* of interventions in clinical practice. Study design features of PCTs differ from those of RCTs as follows: clinically relevant interventions are selected for comparison; study participants are diverse and can be recruited from heterogeneous

practice settings; and data are collected on a broad range of health outcomes. **Figure 60-4** delineates differences between PCTs and RCTs, highlighting the fact that RCTs emphasize internal validity, while PCTs emphasize external validity. In 1967, Schwartz and Lellouch described considerations when selecting the optimal clinical trial design and observed that "Most real problems contain both explanatory and pragmatic elements, for ethical reasons. Most trials hitherto have adopted the explanatory approach without question; the pragmatic approach would often have been more justifiable" (p. 505) (21). It is important to note that there is not always a clear distinction between explanatory and pragmatic trials; instead there is a continuum. The PRagmatic Explanatory Continuum Indicator Summary (PRECIS-2) is a tool that can be used to inform selection of a clinical trial design element. The PRECIS-2 framework is used to assess the following nine domains: (a) Eligibility, (b) Recruitment, (c) Setting, (d) Organization, (e) Flexibility (delivery), (f) Flexibility (adherence), (g) Follow-up, (h) Primary outcome, and (i) Primary analysis (22). Each domain is scored based on a 5-point Likert scale where 1 = very explanatory and 5 = very pragmatic. The PRECIS-2 toolkit is available for download from www.precis-2.org. This resource can be used during the design selection process to make sure that the trial design is appropriate for the research question and purpose.

Search Engines

The EBP hierarchy of research evidence is used to provide an efficient literature search strategy. The search begins by looking for systematic reviews that summarize the results of many different studies and provide an overview of the body of research evidence that addresses a clinical question. If no appropriate systematic reviews are located, the search continues by focusing on specific well-designed individual studies until the best studies are located. The EBP movement spawned the development of search engines designed to streamline the literature search process. Some search engines incorporate an EBP framework. The search is organized by the type of research evidence, and

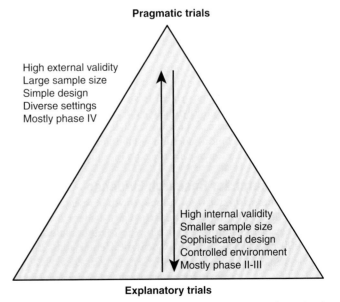

FIGURE 60-4. Comparison of pragmatic and explanatory trials. (Reproduced with the permission of the publisher, Les Laboratoires Servier, from: Patsopoulos NA. A pragmatic view on pragmatic trials. *Dialogues Clin Neurosci.* 2011;13(2):217–224. © 2011 Les Laboratoires Servier.)

the results are presented in order, based on the hierarchy of research evidence. One useful resource is SUMsearch, which is described as a "meta" search engine because it searches multiple databases. SUMsearch results are then organized according to the hierarchy of evidence. SUMsearch is a good starting point for conducting a literature search because it is an efficient strategy for viewing a summary of the available evidence in a specific area and it is especially effective for locating information on systematic reviews and guidelines (23).

Databases of systematic reviews can also be searched directly. The Cochrane Collaboration, an international group dedicated to combining similar randomized trials to produce a more statistically sound evidence through systematic reviews, is one of the best resources for systematic reviews. Complete systematic reviews require a subscription, but abstracts of the reviews are available via a searchable database at the Cochrane Web site. The Cochrane Library includes reviews for the top ten causes of disability in developed and developing nations, and, therefore, it is an important resource for evidence-based rehabilitation (24). Moreover, the Cochrane Collaboration includes study groups dedicated to examining topics relevant to rehabilitation such as bone joint and muscle trauma, movement disorders, multiple sclerosis, musculoskeletal and neuromuscular disorders, and stroke (25). Additional resources are available through Cochrane Rehabilitation whose aim is to ensure that all rehabilitation professionals can apply evidence-based clinical practice, combining the best available evidence as gathered by high-quality Cochrane systematic reviews, with their own clinical expertise and the values of patients (http://rehabilitation.cochrane.org/).

If the search fails to yield a relevant and valid systematic review or evidence summary, the next step is to search the primary literature. PubMed, a service of the U.S. National Library of Medicine and the National Institutes of Health, provides an extensive database of research abstracts (26). PubMed is widely recognized as the best resource for information from original studies (23). PubMed recently added an EBM search filter termed "clinical queries." This feature allows the user to conduct a search based on the category of evidence (diagnosis, prognosis, or therapy) and to request results that are "focused" to include a few of the most relevant studies (specific) or "expanded" to include a wider range of studies (sensitive).

Evidence Summaries

Searching for evidence that has already been summarized and critiqued is an effective strategy for busy clinicians. The EBP movement fostered the development of secondary resources or "predigested" evidence summaries (see 🛜 eTable 60-2). Evidence summaries help to address concerns that EBP demands too much time and requires research assessment skills beyond the ability of most clinicians. One example, the Database of Abstracts of Reviews of Effects (DARE), is a free, searchable database that includes evidence summaries relevant to rehabilitation (27). Each summary must meet specific quality criteria to be included in the DARE database. The evidence summary displays key elements of the study and concludes with a critical commentary. Discipline-specific evidence summaries are also available. The Physiotherapy Evidence Database (28) comprises abstracts of evidence-based clinical practice guidelines, systematic reviews, and clinical trials. The methods for the clinical trials are reviewed and rated on a ten-point scale (28). OTseeker is another database with abstracts of systematic reviews and clinical trials relevant to occupational therapy.

The clinical trials are rated on an eight-point internal validity score and a two-point statistical reporting score (29). Online journals, such as APC Journal Club and Evidence-Based Medicine, also summarize results of clinical trials. Secondary sources present clinically relevant research that has been critically appraised and provide an important resource for busy clinicians. However, it is still important to examine the source and consider the validity and accuracy of the research summary and appraisal. Evidence summaries streamline the EBP process by simplifying the critical appraisal of evidence, which is described in the next step. As databases of evidence summaries continue to grow, one can imagine a future where clinicians routinely use wireless, handheld devices for point-of-care access to relevant information that has been critiqued and summarized (30,31).

Step 4: Critically Appraise the Evidence

Once the highest level of evidence for a specific clinical question is located, the evidence is critically appraised. The first item of the critical appraisal process is to assess the validity of the research evidence. Unfortunately, specific standards for determining the validity of a study have not been established and a proliferation of critical appraisal tools has led to considerable confusion. One systematic review identified 121 published critical appraisal tools. While the tools vary somewhat, the most frequently cited areas evaluated to establish the validity of research evidence for efficacy studies were: eligibility criteria, statistical analysis, allocation of subjects, consideration of outcome measures used, sample size justification/power calculations, study design, and blinding (32). The critical appraisal process, which varies for different types of research evidence, is described in the following sections.

Systematic Reviews and Meta-Analyses

Similar to systematic reviews, meta-analyses use a specific protocol to locate and assess research articles addressing a specific question. However, meta-analyses go one step further by combining data to yield a summary statistic. The focus of the meta-analysis or systematic review should be clear with detailed information on the population, intervention, and outcomes. Systematic reviews should meet criteria for establishing homogeneity. Specifically, the studies should be similar in terms of patient characteristics (e.g., age, type of disease/disorders), interventions used, outcomes measured, and the study methods (e.g., randomized trials, cohort studies) (33). The search strategy used to identify research articles should include multiple search engines to ensure that all relevant studies are considered (34). The process used to include studies should be outlined and the criteria used to evaluate studies clearly stated (35). Each study should be evaluated in terms of the methodologic quality, precision or the width of the CI around the result and the external validity, or the extent to which the results can be generalized (34).

As the number of systematic reviews continues to grow, it is important to ensure that the information is up-to-date. Unfortunately, there is little research to support how and when to update systematic reviews, so it is important to consider if the information presented is still relevant (36).

Evidence Related to Diagnosis

Evidence related to diagnosis is concerned with determining the extent to which tests for specific conditions distinguish individuals with and without a specific disease, impairment, or disorder. Results from the diagnostic test and the "gold" standard are organized in a 2 × 2 contingency table and analyzed to

TABLE 60-2	Contingency Table: Summarizing Results from a Diagnostic Test			
	Gold standard identifies that disease/disorder is present	Gold standard identifies that disease/disorder is absent		Total
Test positive	A: Correct (identifies condition)	B: Incorrect (over identifies condition)		A + B
Test negative	C: Incorrect (misses condition)	D: Correct (identifies absence of condition)		C + D
Totals	A + C	B + D		

Sensitivity = A/A + C. Does a test correctly identify when the condition is present?
Specificity = D/B + D. Does a test correctly identify absence of the condition?

determine how well the diagnostic test sorts patients into the appropriate "bins," based on findings from the gold standard test. Often clinical tests are compared to an invasive surgical, radiologic, or electrodiagnostic gold standard test. Therefore, substituting a less invasive or less expensive clinical test is preferable. There are four possible outcomes when a diagnostic test is evaluated (**Table 60-2**): A, the test is positive and correctly identifies persons with the condition; B, the test is positive but the person does not have the condition; C, the test is negative but the person has the condition; D, the test is negative and the person does not have the condition.

The ability of a diagnostic test to correctly identify patients *with* a disease, impairment, or disorder is termed the test's *sensitivity*, which is calculated as the proportion of patients with the disorder who have a positive test result. The test's ability to identify patients without a disease, impairment, or disorder is termed as the test's *specificity*, which is calculated as the proportion of patients without the disorder who have a negative test result. Ideally, tests are sufficiently sensitive and specific so that individuals with the disease, impairment, or disorder are identified and receive the appropriate interventions and individuals without the disorder are identified and not subjected to unnecessary treatments or restrictions.

Likelihood ratios combine sensitivity and specificity and provide another way to summarize the value of a diagnostic test. A positive likelihood ratio is the odds that a patient with a condition will have a positive test result compared to a patient without the condition. A negative likelihood ratio is the odds that a patient without a condition will have a negative clinical test result compared to a patient with the condition.

The *positive predictive value* is the proportion of patients with positive test results who have the condition, and *negative predictive value* is the proportion of patients with negative test results who do not have the condition. Positive and negative predictive values provide a simple and clear way to represent diagnostic findings; however, because these values are affected by prevalence they must be interpreted with caution. A high prevalence will inflate the positive predictive values and lower the negative predictive values. Conversely, a low prevalence will lower the positive predictive value and inflate the negative predictive value. *Prevalence*, or pretest probability, estimates how common a disease or disorder is in the population. Prevalence estimates are derived from the study sample, the literature, or data from a specific clinical setting.

Several criteria must be met to establish the validity of research on a diagnostic test. First, the study should include an independent, blind comparison of the diagnostic test with a gold standard. It is important to critique the gold standard to ensure that it is, in fact, an accurate measure of the presence or absence of a disease or condition and that it was consistently applied to all test subjects. Next, consider the study design and

characteristics of the subjects. Ideally, a prospective cohort design is used and the sample includes subjects who represent the continuum of severity for the disease or disorder. If a study includes subjects without symptoms or is composed mainly of subjects with severe symptoms, the study may misrepresent the ability of the diagnostic test to identify persons with and without the disease or disorder. Before applying the results of a diagnostic study, examine the characteristics of the subjects to be sure that they are similar to the patient group for whom you intend to use the diagnostic test. Also, examine the methods section to determine if the diagnostic test was conducted in a manner consistent with its intended use. Finally, determine if the test was validated in a second, independent group of patients. If all of these criteria were met, the validity of the diagnostic study is established (37).

The next question is to determine the clinical importance of the diagnostic test by examining the ability of the test to correctly categorize patients with the condition of interest. Individual research studies may report results in terms of sensitivity, specificity, likelihood ratios, or predictive values (38). If results of the diagnostic study are not reported using the desired statistics, it may be possible to extract relevant data and calculate the variables of interest. With the use of calculators, which are available online, it is relatively easy to calculate different diagnostic variables.

Results from tests with continuous numeric scores can also be used to categorize patients for diagnostic purposes. A specific score is used as a cut-off point, and patients with scores above or at and below the cut-off point are categorized based on the presence or absence of a trait, condition, or functional ability. For example, a prospective study followed elderly individuals for 1 year and used their scores on the Tinetti balance scale to identify elderly individuals who fell within the year (39). A *receiver-operator characteristic curve*, which plots sensitivity and specificity of the different test scores, was examined to select a cut-off score that maximized the sensitivity and specificity of the test. As noted in 📶 **eFigure 60-1**, a cut-off point score of 33 on the Tinetti scale yields a sensitivity of 51% and a specificity of 74%. This means that only 51% of elderly subjects with Tinetti scores at or below 33 were correctly identified as fallers, while 74% of nonfallers were correctly categorized. Increasing the cut-off point to a score at or below 36 increased the sensitivity to 70%. With a more stringent cut-off point, more fallers were correctly identified. As noted in the previous example, sensitivity increases when the test is effective in ruling out the disorder. However, the increase in sensitivity was accompanied by a loss of specificity; now only 52% of nonfallers were correctly identified. This example illustrates the importance of considering the goal of the diagnostic test when selecting a cut-off point.

An example of a critical appraisal of a diagnostic study is presented in **Table 60-3**. In this study, clinical tests are compared to the gold standard that used joint arthroscopy to

TABLE 60-3 **Critical Appraisal: Diagnostic Study**

1. Is this diagnostic study valid? (7)

Was there an independent, blind comparison with a reference (gold) standard of diagnosis?

Prospective study using arthroscopic results as the gold standard. The authors completed clinical tests prior to grouping by arthroscopic results.

Was the diagnostic test evaluated in an appropriate spectrum of clients (like those in whom it would be used in practice)?

Yes

Was the reference standard applied regardless of the diagnostic test result?

Yes

Was the test (or cluster of tests) validated in a second, independent group of clients?

Yes

Interpretation: This diagnostic study is valid.

2. Are the results of this valid diagnostic study important?

Diagnosis of rotator cuff tear by three positive clinical tests: supraspinatus weakness, weakness in external rotation, positive impingement

	Gold standard diagnosis of rotator cuff tear by arthroscopy				Total
	Present		Absent		
Positive	48	a	b	1	49
Negative	152	c	d	199	351
Total	200		200		400

	Definition	Formula	Example
Sensitivity	Ability to correctly identify someone with the disorder	$\dfrac{a}{a+c}$	$\dfrac{48}{48+152} = 0.24 = 24\%$
Specificity	Ability to correctly identify someone without the disorder	$\dfrac{d}{b+d}$	$\dfrac{199}{1+199} = 0.995 = 99.5\%$
Likelihood ratio (positive test result)	The likelihood that a positive test result was observed for someone with a rotator cuff tear compared to someone without a rotator cuff tear.	$\dfrac{sens}{1-spec}$	$\dfrac{0.24}{1-0.995} = 48$
Likelihood ratio (negative test result)	The likelihood that a negative test result was observed for someone without a rotator cuff tear compared to someone with a rotator cuff tear.	$\dfrac{1-sens}{spec}$	$\dfrac{1-0.24}{0.995} = 0.76$
Positive predictive value	The proportion of subjects with positive results who have confirmed rotator cuff tears.	$\dfrac{a}{a+b}$	$\dfrac{48}{48+1} = 0.98 = 98\%$
Negative predictive value	The proportion of subjects with negative test results who do not have confirmed rotator cuff tears.	$\dfrac{d}{c+d}$	$\dfrac{199}{152+199} = 0.57 = 57\%$
Pretest probability (prevalence)	How common is the diagnosis of rotator cuff tear within the population (of this study)?	$\dfrac{a+c}{a+b+c+d}$	Estimate patient's pretest probability based on age (e.g., prevalence for ages 30–39 = 0.20)
Pretest odds	The odds of a rotator cuff tear before the tests are done.	$\dfrac{prev}{1-prev}$	$\dfrac{0.20}{1-0.2} = 0.25$
Posttest odds	The odds of a rotator cuff tear after the test has been carried out.	Pretest odds × +LR	$0.25 \times 48 = 12$
Posttest probability	The probability of a rotator cuff tear after the results are obtained	$\dfrac{posttest\ odds}{posttest\ odds + 1}$	$\dfrac{12}{12+1} = 0.92 = 92\%$ (or use nomogram)
Diagnostic accuracy	Percentage of people correctly diagnosed	$100 \times \dfrac{a+d}{a+b+c+d}$	$100 \times \dfrac{48+199}{400} = 61.7\%$

Continued

TABLE 60-3	**Critical Appraisal: Diagnostic Study** *(Continued)*	

CIs (95%)	Formula	Example
Positive predictive value	$SE = \sqrt{\dfrac{p \times (1-p)}{n}}$	$SE = \sqrt{\dfrac{0.98 \times (1-0.98)}{400}} = 0.01$
Note: This formula is also used for sensitivity and specificity	95% CI = $p \pm (1.96 \times SE)$	95% CI = $0.98 \pm 0.01 = 0.97$–99

Value of a Test—Based on Likelihood Ratio

+Likelihood Ratio	−Likelihood Ratio	Test Value
1.0	1.0	Useless (pretest probability = posttest disease probability)
1.0–2.0	0.5–1.0	Usually none to small
2.0–5.0	0.2–0.5	Small to moderate
5.0–10.0	0.1–0.2	Moderate to large
>10.0	0.0–0.1	Large

Adapted from Critical Appraisal Worksheets provided by the Centre for Evidence-Based Medicine, http://www.cebm.utoronto.ca/practise/ca/diagnosis. Murrell GAC, Walton JR. Diagnosis of rotator cuff tears. *Lancet*. 2001;357:769–770.

identify which patients had rotator cuff tears. This example shows that the clinical tests have low sensitivity (24%). Of the 200 patients with confirmed rotator cuff tears, only 48 were correctly identified with the clinical tests. The clinical tests were negative in 152 cases where arthroscopic findings showed a confirmed rotator cuff tear. Thus, a negative result on this clinical test was not effective in ruling out this condition. The sensitivity of a test increases when a *negative result* is able to *rule out* a disease or disorder. In this example with low sensitivity, more than 75% of the cases with negative results actually had a rotator cuff tear. In contrast, the specificity for the clinical tests is high (99%). There was only one case where the clinical tests indicated a rotator cuff tear that was not confirmed by arthroscopic findings. So it is likely that a patient with a positive test *does* have a rotator cuff tear. When a test has high specificity, a *positive result* is able to effectively *rule in* the target condition. This example demonstrates the importance of considering both sensitivity and specificity when selecting a diagnostic test. Because this test has high specificity, a positive result on the clinical tests is a good indication that the patient has a rotator cuff tear; however, due to the low sensitivity a large percentage of cases with negative test results will actually have a rotator cuff tear that is missed.

In this example, the positive likelihood ratio was large (40) and the negative likelihood ratio was useless (0.76). The positive predictive value showed that 98% of study subjects with positive clinical test results had rotator cuff tears and the negative predictive value showed that 57% of study subjects with negative tests did not have rotator cuff tears. However, the predictive values are affected by the prevalence of the condition. The pretest probability (prevalence) for rotator cuff tears for subjects between the ages of 30 and 39 was approximately 20%. After the three clinical tests were conducted and results obtained, the probability of having a rotator cuff tear increased to 92% and the overall diagnostic accuracy was 61.7%. The diagnostic information presented in this study can help clinicians understand the benefits and limitations of using clinical tests in patients with a suspected rotator cuff tear. This information can also be communicated to patients when explaining the clinical findings.

Evidence Related to Prognosis

Clinicians directly consider questions about a patient's prognosis all the time. At times prognostic questions are posed by patients such as "Will I regain my pre-fracture level of function?" or "How long will it take for me to recover from this injury and return to work?" At other times clinicians will consider prognosis less directly, such as when deciding where to discharge a patient at the end of an acute hospital stay. A question such as "Is this patient a good fit for inpatient rehabilitation?" is often based on a clinician's judgment of prognosis. Prognosis reflects a clinician's estimation of a patient's likely clinical course over time taking into account the likely complications of his or her disease, injury, or impairment. There are several different aspects to prognosis: a *qualitative aspect* (i.e., What outcomes could happen to this patient?); a *quantitative aspect* (i.e., How likely are the outcomes to occur to this patient?); a *temporal aspect* (i.e., Over what time period are the anticipated outcomes likely to occur?); and an *evaluative aspect* (i.e., What is likely to influence the outcomes?).

In rehabilitation, clinicians frequently base their prognostic judgments and advice on their clinical experience and less often on the basis of scientific evidence. Later in this section, we will consider a framework for appraising the validity, importance, and applicability of evidence using similar guidelines applied to evidence regarding diagnosis and treatment.

To evaluate prognostic evidence, the clinician needs to appraise three distinct and important elements: the validity of the evidence, the importance, and the applicability of evidence to the patient(s).

In determining whether prognostic evidence is valid, several different factors must be considered. First, the clinician must appraise if the evidence is based on a defined, representative sample of patients assembled at a common point in the course of their disease or episode of care (usually at the start). A second validity issue is the degree to which patient follow-up was complete and sufficiently long enough in duration. This judgment must be made in relation to the outcome being considered. A short follow-up with just a select few subjects would not be sufficient evidence to use for advising patients.

If the follow-up is long enough, the clinician still needs to assess which subjects entered the study but were lost to follow-up since a substantial loss to follow-up can significantly affect conclusions drawn about patient prognosis. For example, if patients who perform poorly are lost to follow-up, this would introduce significant bias into any prognostic determination.

The next issue is whether objective outcome criteria were defined and tracked with adequate validity. To minimize the potential effects of bias in outcome measurement, objective criteria should have been established and implemented in the collection of outcome data. In the best case, those making outcome measurements are kept in the dark (i.e., blind) to a patient's clinical characteristics and prognostic factors to minimize the likelihood of bias creeping into the assessment.

Once the validity of a prognostic investigation has been established, the next issue is to determine its importance and appropriateness by examining the characteristics of the study subjects and evaluating the degree to which the prognostic information is relevant to an individual patient's situation and/or condition. Finally, the CI around the prognostic estimate should be examined. A prognostic estimate with a relatively small CI provides greater assurance that the information will be important and useful to patients.

An example of a critical appraisal of a prognosis study is presented in **Table 60-4**. The study examined the ability of the Orpington prognostic scale (OPS) to predict functional recovery for patients at 3 and 6 months after a stroke. The study met most validity criteria, but it was noted that patients with severe and mild symptoms were not well represented. Therefore, when this evidence is applied to an individual patient, it is important to remember that the findings may differ for patients with severe or mild symptoms. At 6 months post stroke, patients with initial OPS scores of 3.6 achieved the following levels of functional ability (note: range includes 95% CIs): 56% to 71% were independent in personal care; 52% to 68% were independent in meal preparation; 48% to 63% were independent in medication administration; and 30% to 46% were independent in community mobility. This information can be useful when discussing expectations for functional outcomes with individual patients and their families.

Evidence Related to Intervention

Clinicians have many options in determining a course of care for their patients, but too often treatment decisions are based on a clinician's experience or preference. Many studies demonstrate disparities in clinical care and point to the need for

---

TABLE 60-4 **Critical Appraisal: Prognosis Study**

1. Are the results of this prognosis study valid?

Were the study subjects representative?	Yes—the sample consisted of patients with a broad age range with good representation of minorities. Subjects were drawn from 12 area hospitals. Rehabilitation occurred in a variety of settings.
Did the research study a broad spectrum of patients with the disorder?	No—patients with severe and mild stroke were underrepresented.
Were patients at a similar point in the course of their disease?	Yes—all subjects had baseline OPS measures completed between 3 and 14 days poststroke. Follow-up functional assessments were at 3- and 6-month intervals.
Were researchers recording the outcomes blinded to the prognostic factors?	Not clear
Were outcomes well defined and relevant? Were criteria for measuring outcomes preestablished?	Outcome measures were functional activities identified as important to individuals of both genders.
Were outcome measures established prior to the start of the study?	Yes
Was follow-up sufficiently long enough and complete?	Yes
What was the dropout rate? Were reasons for dropout documented?	Dropout rate was <20%. Reasons were documented. Characteristics of patients who did not complete the 6-month follow-up indicate that they were more severely involved.
Did the authors adjust for differences between groups?	No

2. Are the results of this prognostic study important?

Prevalence of independence in functional activities based on OPS baseline score of 3.6

Function	3 months	6 months
Personal care	51%	64%
	95% CI = 47%–54%	95% CI = 56%–71%
Meal preparation	53%	60%
	95% CI = 45%–61%	95% CI = 52%–68%
Medication administration	54%	56%
	95% CI = 46%–61%	95% CI = 48%–63%
Community mobility	29%	38%
	95% CI = 22%–36%	95% CI = 30%–46%

Adapted from Critical Appraisal Worksheets provided by the Centre for Evidence-Based Medicine, http://www.cebm.utoronto.ca/practise/ca/prognosis. Studenski SA, Wallace D, Duncan PW, et al. Predicting stroke recovery: three- and six-month rates of patient-centered functional outcomes based on the Orpington prognostic scale. *J Am Geriatr Soc.* 2001;49(3):308–312.

more equitable and evidence-based care (1). The goal of EBP is to help clinicians work with their patients to select interventions that are likely to produce the desired outcomes, are worth the costs and the efforts of using them, and fit with patient preferences. EBP provides an objective framework and a systematic approach to guide the clinical decision-making process. EBP focuses on determining the importance and clinical significance of research related to interventions so that their relative benefits can be better understood, communicated to the patient, and used to make decisions.

Critical appraisal of intervention studies begins by examining the outcome measure used in the study to determine if it is appropriate for answering the clinical question. Specifically, the dimension of outcome measure (e.g., impairment, functional limitation, disability) should match the outcome identified in the clinical question. It is also important to establish that the outcome measure used is valid and reliable.

The critical appraisal process continues by examining the methods section. Were subjects randomly assigned to groups? Were researchers (single) and, if possible, subjects (double) blind to group? Next, review the baseline characteristics and demographic information for the control and experimental groups to see if they are similar. If differences exist, could they affect the study results? Were subjects who withdrew or did not complete the study accounted for? And were subjects analyzed in the groups to which they were randomized (intention to treat analysis)?

Review the methods section to determine if both groups were treated equally, except for the experimental intervention. Determine if the follow-up was sufficiently long and complete. If the results were not statistically significant, the study should include a power analysis to determine if the number of subjects in the study was sufficient to find a difference if, in fact, one existed (41).

Once the validity of a study is established, the next step is to determine if the results are of sufficient magnitude to warrant a change in practice. Research studies comparing outcomes for different interventions, typically, report results in terms of *statistical significance* or *p-values*. The statistical significance is determined before the study begins and, most often, the significance level is set at $p < 0.05$. The *p*-value is the actual probability of obtaining the observed result if the null hypothesis (that there is no difference) is true. If the *p*-value is less than the identified significance level, the null hypothesis is rejected. Statistical significance is regularly reported in research studies and is the primary factor used to evaluate research findings. However, there is a difference between statistical significance and the magnitude of the treatment effect or *clinical significance*. Statistical significance assesses the probability of the difference between groups based on chance. However, since sample size affects statistical significance, a rather small treatment effect can yield statistically significant results if the sample size is large enough. EBP focuses on the magnitude of the effect or clinical significance of research findings so that they can guide in clinical decision-making.

Results from an intervention study in which data are reported as proportions can be summarized as the proportion of patients with good or bad outcomes. The *experimental event rate* (EER) and the *control event rate* (CER) represent the proportion of subjects who achieve the desired outcome in the respective groups. Using these values, one can determine the *relative benefit increase* (RBI), or increase in good outcomes in the experimental group. This useful statistic helps quantify the magnitude or clinical

significance of the intervention. The EER and CER are also used to calculate the absolute benefit increase (ABI), which is the absolute difference between rates of good outcomes in experimental and control groups. Finally, ABI can be used to calculate the *number needed to treat* (NNT) to achieve one additional good outcome. The NNT calculation is a useful statistic that captures the effort required to see the effect of an intervention (42). Moreover, the NNT statistic, in conjunction with financial data, can be used to determine cost/benefit ratios.

In EBP examples, treatment effects are often described in terms of dichotomous variables, such as the proportion or percentage of subjects that lived/died or were cured/not cured. Rehabilitation outcomes are not usually defined in terms of life and death or cures but the following are examples of dichotomous variables that are relevant to the rehabilitation field: returning to work or not, being discharged to home or skilled nursing facility, or achieving a target level on a functional test or not. When dichotomous variables are reported as percentages or proportions, these data can be used to quantify the magnitude or clinical significance of the treatment effect by calculating the ABI and the NNT.

The NNT calculation is not often reported in rehabilitation literature; however, it is a useful calculation. For example, if the effectiveness of an intervention is examined based on the proportion of patients discharged to home versus skilled nursing facility, the NNT calculation can estimate the number of patients that would have to be treated with this intervention to yield one additional discharge to home. The NNT calculation helps answer questions about the efficacy and clinical importance of an intervention. It is reported with CIs to indicate the precision of the estimate. Because NNT summarizes the effort required to produce positive outcomes, it can be used to calculate the costs and benefits of an intervention (43).

If data in a study are summarized as means and standard deviations, clinical importance is assessed by calculating the *effect size*, which considers the size of the difference between two groups relative to the variability of the outcome in the patient group without the confounding influence of sample size. The effect size, which is the standardized mean difference between two groups, is not often mentioned in research reports but is relatively easy to calculate (44).

$$\text{Effect size} = \frac{\left[\begin{array}{c}\text{Mean of experimental}\\ \text{group}\end{array}\right] - \left[\begin{array}{c}\text{Mean of control}\\ \text{group}\end{array}\right]}{\text{Standard deviation (pooled)}}.$$

Effect sizes are reported with CIs and they are used to categorize the magnitude of the treatment effect as follows: *large* (anything >0.5), *moderate* (0.5 to 0.3), *small* 0.3 to 0.1, and *trivial* (anything <0.1). Knowledge of the effect size is helpful when determining if the evidence is strong enough to change practice. It is also important to consider other aspects of the research design when evaluating the strength of evidence. A small or moderate effect size may be more meaningful in rehabilitation research because the variability among subjects (standard deviation) reduces the effect size.

EBP calculators can ease the burden of determining the clinical significance of research evidence. Free, online calculators are available for diagnostic tests, and for calculating the NNT and effect size (see **eTable 60-2**).

An example of a critical appraisal of an intervention study is presented in **Table 60-5**. The study examines the effect of

TABLE 60-5   Critical Appraisal: Intervention Study

1. Are the results of this therapy study valid?

Was randomization maintained?	Yes
Were all patients who entered into the trial accounted for?	Yes
Were all patients analyzed in the groups to which they were randomized (intention to treat analysis)?	Yes
Were researchers (single) and patients (double) blind to treatment group?	Not specified, but data collectors were not involved in the intervention.
Were baseline characteristics of the two groups similar?	No, more intervention subjects were women, not married, living along, had diabetes, were more restricted in activity days at baseline. Baseline status on outcome, gender, and age were adjusted in analyses.
Except for the experimental intervention, were both groups treated equally?	Yes, but difficult to control in this community-based study.
Was follow-up sufficiently long and complete?	Only 1 year. Previous study showed effects were not sustained after 1 year.
Was a power analysis performed?	Yes.
Level of evidence?	Individual randomized control trial
Dimension of outcome measure? Are the measures appropriate for answering the clinical question?	Study includes administrative, impairment, activity, and participation measures; all are appropriate for answering the clinical question.
Were the measures valid and reliable and used in other studies?	Yes.

Interpretation: This intervention study is valid.

2. Are the results of this valid intervention study important? How large and precise is the treatment effect?

Number of bed disability days for patients with ≥1 bed disability day at baseline

	Improved		Same or Worse		Total
Experimental	7	a	b	17	24
Control	0	c	d	15	15
Total	7		32		39

Experimental event rate (EER)	Proportion of patients in the experimental group who showed a positive effect	$EER = \dfrac{a}{a+b}$	$EER = \dfrac{7}{7+17} = 0.29 = 29\%$	
Control event rate (CER)	Proportion of patients in the control group who showed a positive effect	$CER = \dfrac{c}{c+d}$	$CER = \dfrac{0}{0+15} = 0 = 0\%$	
Relative benefit increase (RBI)	Proportional increase in rates of good outcomes between experimental and control patients	RBI = EER – CER/CER	RBI = 29 – 0/0 = cannot calculate	
Absolute benefit increase (ABI)	The absolute difference in rates of good outcomes between experimental and control patients	ABI = EER – CER	ABI = 29 – 0 = 29 = 29% 95% CI = 11%–47%	
Number needed to treat (NNT)	The number of patients needed to be treated to achieve one additional good outcome	NNT = 1/ABI	NNT = 100/29 = 4 95% CI = 2–9	

95% CI for ABI. 95% CI for NNT (calculated from ABI). 100/CI of lower limits of ABI = 100/11 = 9. 100/CI of upper limits of ABI 100/47 = 2.
Adapted from Critical Appraisal Worksheets provided by the Centre for Evidence-Based Medicine, http://www.cebm.utoronto.ca/practise/ca/therapyst. Leveille SG, Wagner EH, Davis C, et al. Preventing disability and managing chronic illness in frail older adults: a randomized trial of a community-based partnership with primary care. *J Am Geriatr Soc.* 1998;46:1191–1198.

an individual counseling and self-management program on bed disability days in elderly individuals. The EER shows that subjects with one or more bed disability day at baseline had a 29% increase in the rate of improving the number of bed disability days compared to the control group. According to the ABI calculation, we can be 95% confident that the increase in the rate of good outcomes is between 11% and 47%. For every three elderly individuals who participated in the program, one additional person improved in bed disability days. The NNT calculation indicates that we can be 95% confident that we will see one additional good outcome for every two to nine elderly individuals who participate in the program. These calculations can help determine the importance and economic impact of interventions. This information can also be part of patient communication.

Step 5: Apply Research Evidence

Applying research evidence to individual patients is one of the most challenging aspects of EBP. While specific rules and procedures serve as a guide in the preceding EBP steps, applying research evidence to individual patient cases requires sound clinical judgment. Indeed, applying evidence to patients assumes that results from research studies can be generalized when, in fact, patients present with a wide range of differences (45). One of the greatest challenges of EBP is to determine how an individual patient's age, disease characteristics, or comorbidities, which may differ from subjects in the study sample, affect the applicability of the evidence. For this reason, clinical expertise is a critical component of EBP.

The eligibility criteria for subjects in clinical trials must be considered when applying research findings to individual patients. For example, effectiveness studies (PCTs) have wide eligibility criteria and participation is extended to a heterogenous group of subjects. And, because the results were seen in a heterogenous group of subjects, it is easier to make a case that similar results will be seen in a wide range of patients. In contrast, efficacy studies (RCTs) have narrow eligibility criteria and participation limited to a homogenous group of highly responsive patients (46). Consequently, one must be cautious about applying the results of an efficacy study to the general population that includes a range of individuals who are not likely to be as responsive (47).

Communication with patients to explain options and determine their preferences is an important part of the decision-making process. The recent increase in consumerism and emphasis on patient-centered care reinforces the need to consider patient preferences when deciding on treatment choices. Patient involvement is a significant component of EBP, and there are many related benefits. Active patient involvement in care is associated with improved outcomes and enhanced quality of life (40,48). Informed patients are more likely to participate in their care and make better decisions (49). Since patients and their families often have access to a wealth of information through the Internet, they frequently bring along the results of their searches and provide the impetus to begin a discussion of diagnostic, prognostic, and treatment options.

Clinicians can effectively communicate with patients by clearly summarizing research evidence, outlining treatment options, and discussing estimates of potential benefits and risks. The discussion should explore the patient's values about the therapy and potential options (47). It is important to build a partnership and understand the patient's experience and expectations. The discussion of evidence should include a balanced presentation of options and, after consideration of the clinical evidence and patient's values, the clinician can recommend an option and explain how the choice is consistent with the patient's values. Finally, it is important to make sure that the patient understands and agrees with the recommendation (49).

Step 6: Evaluate the Use of Evidence

The final step in the EBP process involves an evaluation of the process and the use of evidence. The evaluation includes a reflection on how well the process worked. This step presents an opportunity to identify areas for improvement and to implement strategies for continued growth in becoming an evidence-based practitioner. The evaluation step also presents an opportunity to investigate the impact of evidence-based decisions to determine if changes in practice had an effect on outcomes.

BECOMING AN EVIDENCE-BASED PRACTITIONER

A recent systematic review identified multiple barriers to EBP, organized by specialty area. The top five barriers for rehabilitative care are (a) lack of research (conflicting study results, poor generalizability); (b) lack of resources (lack of institutional support); (c) lack of time; (d) inadequate access (too difficult to find information); and (e) lack of training (4).

Assessing Knowledge and Skill

The first step in becoming an evidence-based practitioner is to identify individual learning needs. Specific EBP competencies, such as conducting literature searches (50) and critically appraising literature (51–53) are often assessed. 📶 **eTable 60-3** presents a list of EBP competencies that can be used as a guide to gaining knowledge and skill. Validated tests of EBP, such as the Berlin Test (54) or the Fresno Test (55), are available, but they emphasize general medical cases and examples.

The prospect of developing expertise in all of the skills needed to be a competent evidence-based practitioner can seem overwhelming. It may also be helpful to consider stages of developing EBP abilities, as described below.

- **Stage 1:** I use EBP guidelines or protocols developed by colleagues but do not search the literature or critically appraise research.
- **Stage 2:** I seek and apply evidence-based summaries that give a clinical "bottom line," but I am not comfortable appraising and applying findings from primary literature.
- **Stage 3:** I have expertise in all EBP knowledge and skills. I am able to locate, appraise, and apply findings from primary literature and systematic reviews.

Considering EBP skills as stages makes it possible for every clinician to begin the process of becoming an evidence-based practitioner, even though some of areas of knowledge and skill have not been mastered yet.

Strategies to promote adoption of research evidence into clinical practice can be developed at three different levels: individual, professional, and organizational. On an individual level, clinicians can identify knowledge gaps and learning issues. These issues can be addressed by collaborative learning among colleagues, by attending workshops and courses, or by developing a self-study program using the online resources. Forming a group where members contribute different areas of expertise is an effective strategy to promote teamwork and individual learning. For example, organizing an EBP journal club allows members to gain knowledge and skill while working to create an EBP culture. An RCT to examine the effects of journal club participation on medical residents' EBP knowledge and skills showed the following significant changes: improved ability to critique the methods sections of articles; increased ability to read and incorporate medical literature in practice; and greater skepticism of results and conclusions (56). There are several options for creating effective journal clubs, but it is important to have identified roles, particularly with respect to the facilitator and specific presenter. Group members can begin by assessing their EBP strengths and weaknesses. Then, the group can work together and capitalize on the strengths of group members by sharing different areas of expertise (57). EBP work groups can develop systematic approaches to incorporate an evidence-based approach into scheduled activities. The group can identify a common place for recording clinical questions and select one question for critical appraisal and present the results during an in-service. Discussion of research evidence and patient preferences can also be incorporated into patient education activities.

EVIDENCE-BASED PRACTICE IMPLEMENTATION

The previous sections of this chapter describe the processes involved in EBP and outline the skills required to become an EBP practitioner. While this content is important to ensure that individual clinicians have the capacity to apply research findings to the clinical decision-making process, it cannot be assumed that important clinical knowledge will be adopted and used in clinical practice. EBP implementation is an area of critical importance that has not received adequate attention. Studies demonstrate that EBP professional education programs yield significant improvements in EBP knowledge but do not the impact evidence-seeking behavior in clinical practice. Clearly, a focus on EBP implementation is needed (58,59).

From Dissemination to Implementation

Strategies to promote use of evidence in clinical practice differ in terms of the level of sophistication and focus. At the most basic level, *dissemination* spreads new knowledge using planned strategies for specific target audiences. For example, research findings are widely disseminated via professional journals, but it is the responsibility of the EBP practitioner to review, digest and interpret the research literature, and appropriately apply this knowledge as part of the clinical decision-making process. At the next level, *knowledge translation* involves a "dynamic and iterative process that includes the synthesis, dissemination, exchange and ethically sound application of knowledge to improve health, provide more effective health services and products and strengthen the healthcare system" (60). Knowledge translation efforts may involve dissemination of "predigested" evidence summaries with clinical recommendations along with efforts to promote use of this knowledge in patient care. However, a primary focus on identifying implementation strategies to promote adoption of research evidence in clinical practice has been a missing ingredient. A relatively new area of study, *implementation science*, has emerged out of the need to better understand and mitigate challenges to adopting research evidence in clinical practice. Implementation science is defined as the "study of methods to promote the integration of research findings and evidence into healthcare policy and practice. Implementation science seeks to understand the behavior of healthcare professionals and other stakeholders as a key variable in the sustainable uptake, adoption, and implementation of evidence-based interventions" (61). As a new field, implementation science research was initially empirically driven, lacking sound theoretical frameworks for proposed interventions (62). As the field of implementation science has become more established (63), there has been a proliferation of theories and frameworks (64). The fact that implementation science covers a wide range of disciplines—from public health to surgery—likely contributes to this proliferation. In fact, since 2004, at least 10 peer-reviewed journals representing various scientific disciplines have devoted special issues or sections focused on EBP dissemination or implementation (65).

Implementation Science: Conceptual Frameworks

Various theories and frameworks have been used to develop interventions to promote the use of evidence in clinical practice and health systems and policies. In general, different implementation science approaches focus on the following: (a) *Process models* describe the steps involved (e.g., Graham's knowledge to action cycle) (66); (b) *determinant frameworks* focus on the influence of barriers and facilitators on desired outcomes; (c) *classic theories* are based on principles from other disciplines (e.g., psychology and sociology) such as Rogers Diffusion of Innovation theory (67); (d) *implementation theories* examine organizational readiness; and (e) *evaluation* frameworks emphasize the aspect of implementation to be evaluated. Acknowledging that the proliferation of different frameworks and inconsistent use of terminology hinders development of theory-based interventions, the Terminology Working Group was convened in September 2012 in Ottawa, Canada. The group developed a simple "meta-framework" to link with existing, more detailed and specific intervention frameworks. They identified four essential components that can be used to describe implementation interventions: Aims, Ingredients, Mechanism and Delivery (AIMD), as described in 🛜 **eTable 60-4**.

Numerous reviews of implementation research demonstrate moderate effects showing improvements in care with considerable variation, both within and across interventions. Few studies identify the rationale for the choice of intervention, and only limited contextual data is provided. Thus, there may be important differences between studies in terms of the context and barriers assessed in studies that purport use of homogenous interventions. For example, studies may address behaviors that are simple or complex and may focus on desirable or undesirable behaviors (63). Furthermore, implementation interventions can target the behavior of individuals, or operate at the organizational level.

EBP and Behavioral Change

Everett Rogers's seminal work on diffusion of innovation emphasized that evidence of an effective intervention is not sufficient to change behavior. The process of implementing change in clinical practice service is difficult, even when benefits have been clearly demonstrated (67,68). The process of implementing EBP in clinical practice often requires clinicians to change behavior (69). Behavioral change is a complicated process often overlooked as an important component of EBP. Grol and Grimshaw identify categories of theories used to explain why clinicians fail to adopt changes in practice (70). The first category of theories addresses cognitive issues with a focus on lack of knowledge about available research evidence. Knowledge issues can be addressed by strategies discussed in previous sections of this chapter. Other theories involve EBP implementation issues. As the Implementation Clinical Example 1 illustrates (**Box 60-1**), knowledge of evidence alone is not sufficient to guarantee that evidence will be adopted. In fact, there is often resistance to change. Another group of theories maintain that behavioral factors, such as feedback, incentives, modeling, and reinforcement influence the use of evidence in clinical practice. Social influence theories focus on the impact of group educational sessions and key opinion leaders on EBP implementation. Research studies examine the impact of interventions focused on promoting behavioral change as a strategy to improve the adoption of research evidence in practice. Unfortunately, systematic reviews reveal that interventions to promote behavioral change are often poorly designed and inadequately described (71,72). Consequently, it is difficult to examine the efficacy of these interventions (73,74). A systematic review of methods describing behavioral change interventions identified the following common elements among the interventions examined: barrier identification, linking barriers to intervention component selection, use of theory, and user engagement (i.e., seeking input on feasibility or acceptability of the intervention from the potential targets) (75). A final group of theories address organizational theories. These theories attribute problems integrating research evidence into clinical practice to broad systemic issues such as the organization of care and the culture of the organization.

EBP and Organizational Change

There is great potential for organizational interventions to promote adoption of research evidence in clinical practice. At the organizational level, the success of interventions may depend on contextual factors and characteristics of the organization or health system (76). One important factor is organizational readiness for change (77). Holt and Helfrich define readiness as "the degree to which those involved are individually and collectively primed, motivated and technically capable of executing the change" (p. S50) (78). According to Weiner, organizational readiness for change is a construct that is both multilevel (individual, group, unit, department) and multifaceted (psychological and behavioral readiness) (77). Organizational readiness for change considers the nature of the change, the change process, the context of the organization, and characteristics of individuals (79). An EBP implementation intervention that is based on organizational change theory would employ following the following elements: (a) highlight the discrepancy between current and desired performance levels; (b) support others expressing dissatisfaction with the status quo, and (c) increase the degree to which organizational members perceive the change is needed, important, or worthwhile (77).

As the Implementation Clinical Example 2 illustrates (**Box 60-1**), it may be difficult for an individual clinician to introduce a change in clinical practice. It is often easier to accept the status quo. Addressing EBP implementation at the organizational level has the potential to be a powerful tool for change. The culture of the organization is an important factor to consider. The following steps are recommended to create an EBP culture at an organizational level: (a) target a problem deemed to be important (e.g., high prevalence, high cost); (b) synthesize information about best practice; (c) summarize current practice information; (d) identify discrepancies between best practice and current practice; (e) develop a

practice improvement plan; (f) assess the potential impact of the improvement plan in terms of efficacy and cost; and (g) decide to implement or not and continue improvement efforts (80). While implementation interventions are often directed at the organizational level, evidence to support these interventions is limited. Systematic reviews of implementation interventions reveal few studies focused on organization and system level issues. One systematic review of organizational strategies to improve patient care found that the implementation strategies used resulted in inconsistent effects; however, the general findings were as follows: revision of professional roles and computer systems for knowledge management improved professional performance; patient outcomes were improved by multidisciplinary teams, integrated care services, and computer systems; and cost savings were reported from integrated care services. As these findings demonstrate, at the organizational level, computer systems and information technology solutions can provide evidence-based recommendations at the point of care and can be integrated with patient electronic health records (EHRs).

One strategy to increase adoption of evidence in clinical practice is to tailor implementation interventions to the clinical practice setting. This approach has been shown to increase use of research evidence (81). Tailoring implementation interventions involves three key steps: (a) identify determinants of practice, (b) design implementation interventions appropriate for the determinants identified, and (c) apply and assess of implementation interventions matched to the identified determinants (82). A systematic review of determinants to consider for tailored implementation interventions to improve use of clinical practice guidelines included guideline factors; individual health professional factors; patient factors; professional interactions; incentives and resources; capacity for organizational change; and social, political, and legal factors (83).

EBP and Health Systems

EBP is often viewed as an individualistic endeavor; however, EBP implementation approaches focused on increasing use of evidence within an organization or health system can have a wide-reaching impact and ultimately may be more effective. One promising area for future development is the use of knowledge gained from collecting and analyzing data within health systems. Health systems skills involve collecting data, devising solutions based on data, and disseminating results (84). Don Berwick, former director of the Centers of the US Medicare and Medicaid Services (CMS), acknowledges the powerful benefit to the health care system of deepening systems knowledge and taking action based on that knowledge. Berwick argues that one of the major challenges to adopting this approach is recognizing the value of dynamic learning and local adaptation as scientific learning progresses. Dynamic learning refers to learning achieved through the application "Plan-Do-Study-Act" cycles, a form of inquiry that capitalizes on processes and knowledge growth in a nonlinear fashion (85). It is an approach to continuous quality improvement in medicine that Berwick popularized through his Institute for Healthcare Improvement (86).

Berwick noted that dynamic systems learning requires a reexamination of the traditional hierarchy of scientific evidence as the basis for evaluating clinical practices. He contended that placing RCTs at the top of the scientific hierarchy—as typically done when considering against other forms of traditional inquiry—does not acknowledge the fact that most learning in complex systems occurs in local and individual settings. Berwick argues that the chasm between formal clinical trials and local improvement strategies is enormous, and scientific journals need to open their review process and pages to systems science and the knowledge it produces. There are some promising developments in systems science and significant steps toward deepening systems knowledge. For example, the High Value Healthcare Collaborative (HVHC), a consortium of 17 health care delivery systems and The Dartmouth Institute for Health Policy and Clinical Practice, is focused on improving health care quality and outcomes. The HVHC follows a systems science approach advocated by Gawande (among others), which includes (87) the following:

- *Measure*: Define, test, and disseminate advanced measures and tools to support clinicians, health care systems, and payers in their efforts to deliver high-value care.

- *Innovate*: Identify, test, and rapidly disseminate best-practice care models and payment models that are safe, improve care, have better outcomes, and reduce costs.

- *Replicate*: By establishing a collaborative "learning network," encourage membership by other organizations, help implement best practices in new member organizations (and learn from them), and distribute findings publicly so that they can be more broadly considered for implementation.

SUMMARY

EBM, a term coined in the 1990s by a group of clinicians and epidemiologists at McMaster University in Ontario, Canada, has evolved into an international movement that has been adopted across all heath care disciplines, including the disciplines that constitute the rehabilitation field. Continued growth of EBP in rehabilitation is needed to achieve the IOM goal that 90% of clinical decisions will be supported by research evidence by 2020. Primary barriers to EBP in rehabilitation include lack of research evidence and difficulty interpreting published research (4). Knowledge translation of rehabilitation research will be facilitated by use of EBP methods and terminology (e.g., NNT, effect size, likelihood ratios) in published manuscripts. Efforts to advance EBP in rehabilitation field would benefit from agreement on criteria for critiquing, evaluating, and grading the quality of rehabilitation research. Developing relevant patient cases and tools to assess EBP knowledge and skills with examples from rehabilitation will advance EBP training. Finally, there is a great need to develop and disseminate effective strategies to promote EBP implementation within organizations and health systems. The quote by Goethe at the beginning of this chapter is an apt reflection of the challenge facing rehabilitation professionals. We have witnessed tremendous advances in rehabilitation research and greatly expanded our knowledge base and scientific foundation. But knowing is not sufficient, and greater effort is needed to ensure that knowledge gained through research is applied. Reducing the gap between knowledge and practice will improve the care provided to patients receiving rehabilitation services.

ACKNOWLEDGMENTS

This chapter includes many insights gained during the Faculty Summer Institute: Integrating an Evidence-Based Approach into Rehabilitation Professional Education. The Institute, sponsored by the Center for Measuring Rehabilitation Outcomes at Boston University and supported by the National Institute of Disability and Rehabilitation Research, was held for three consecutive years (2001–2003). The following individuals participated in the Faculty Institute, and we acknowledge their contributions: Wendy J. Coster, PhD, OTR; Nancy Baker, ScD, OTR; Stephen M. Haley, PhD, PT; Julie Keysor, PhD, PT; Mary Law, PhD, OT(C); Robert Meenan, MD, MPH; Ken Ottenbacher, PhD, OTR; Hilary Siebens, MD; Patti Solomon PhD, PT; and Linda Tickle-Degnen, PhD, OTR.

REFERENCES

1. Institute of Medicine. *Crossing the Quality Chasm.* Washington, DC: The National Academies Press; 1990:2
2. Grossman C, Goolsby A, Olsen L, et al. *Engineering a Learning Healthcare System: A Look at the Future. Workshop Summary.* Washington, DC: The National Academies Press; 2011.
3. Schulkin J. Decision sciences and evidence-based medicine—two intellectual movements to support clinical decision making. *Acad Med.* 2000;75(8):816–818.
4. Sadeghi-Bazargani H, Tabrizi JS, Azami-Aghdash S. Barriers to evidence-based medicine: a systematic review. *J Eval Clin Pract.* 2014;20(6):793–802.
5. Bodenheimer T. The American health care system—the movement for improved quality in health care. *N Engl J Med.* 1999;340(6):488–492.
6. Jette AM. Moving research from the bedside into practice. *Phys Ther.* 2016; 96(5):594–596.
7. Gawande A. *The Future of Medicine. 2014 Reith Lecture.* Lecture presented at John F. Kennedy Presidential Library, Boston, MA, October 16, 2014.
8. Cieza A, Stucki G. Understanding functioning, disability and health in rheumatoid arthritis: the basis for rehabilitative care. *Curr Opin Rheumatol.* 2005;17:183–189.
9. World Health Organization. *International Classification of Functioning, Disability and Health.* Geneva, Switzerland: World Health Organization; 2001.
10. Stucki G, Cieza A, Melvin J. The International Classification of Functioning, Disability and Health (ICF): a unifying model for the conceptual description of the rehabilitation strategy. *J Rehabil Med.* 2007;39(4):279–285.
11. Maher CG, Sherrington C, Elkins M, et al. Challenges for evidence-based physical therapy: accessing and interpreting high-quality evidence on therapy. *Phys Ther.* 2004;84(7):644–654.
12. Jockel KH, Stang A. Perspectives of clinical epidemiology in Germany. *J Clin Epidemiol.* 1999;52(4):375–378.
13. Sackett DL, Richardson WS, Rosenberg W, et al. *Evidence Based Medicine. How to Practice and Teach EBM.* 2nd ed. London, UK: Churchill Livingstone; 2000.
14. Haynes RB, Devereaux PJ, Guyatt GH. Clinical expertise in the era of evidence-based medicine and patient choice. *Evid Based Med.* 2002;7(2):36–38.
15. Haynes RB. What kind of evidence is it that evidence-based medicine advocates want health care providers and consumers to pay attention to? *BMC Health Serv Res.* 2002;2(1):3.
16. Phillips B, Ball C, Sackett DL, et al. *Oxford Centre for Evidence-Based Medicine Levels of Evidence; Updated by Jeremy Howick*; 2009. Available from: http://www.cebm.net/index.aspx?o=1025. Accessed August 4, 2010.
17. Wright JG. A practical guide to assigning levels of evidence. *J Bone Joint Surg Am.* 2007;89(5):1128–1130.
18. West S, King V, Carey TS, et al. Systems to rate the strength of scientific evidence. *Evid Rep Technol Assess (Summ).* 2002;(47):1–11.
19. Lohr KN, Carey TS. Assessing "best evidence": issues in grading the quality of studies for systematic reviews. *Jt Comm J Qual Improv.* 1999;25(9):470–479.
20. Patsopoulos NA. A pragmatic view on pragmatic trials. *Dialogues Clin Neurosci.* 2011;13(2):217–224.
21. Schwartz D, Lellouch J. Explanatory and pragmatic attitudes in therapeutical trials. *J Clin Epidemiol.* 2009;62:499–505 (reprint from 1967).
22. Loudon K, Treweek S, Sullivan F, et al. The PRECIS-2 tool: designing trials that are fit for purpose. *BMJ.* 2015;350:h2147.
23. Booth A, O'Rourke A. SUMSearch and PubMed. *Evid Based Med.* 2000;5(3):71. doi:10.1136/ebm.5.3.71.
24. Grimshaw J. So what has the Cochrane Collaboration ever done for us? A report card on the first 10 years. *Can Med Assoc J.* 2004;171(7):747–749.
25. Cochrane Collaboration. Available from: http://www.cochrane.org/reviews/. Accessed December 1, 2008.
26. PubMed. Available from: http://www.ncbi.nlm.nih.gov/pubmed. Accessed December 1, 2008.

27. DARE. Available from: http://www.crd.york.ac.uk/crdweb/. Accessed December 1, 2008.
28. PEDro. Available from: http://www.pedro.fhs.usyd.edu.au/index.html. Accessed December 1, 2008.
29. OTseeker. Available from: http://www.otseeker.com/resources/default.asp. Accessed December 1, 2008.
30. White B. Making evidence-based medicine doable in everyday practice. *Fam Pract Manag.* 2004;11(2):51–58.
31. Geyman JP, Deyo R, Ramsey SD. *Evidence-Based Clinical Practice: Concepts and Approaches.* Boston, MA: Butterworth-Heinemann; 2000.
32. Katrak P, Bialocerkowski AE, Massy-Westropp N, et al. A systematic review of the content of critical appraisal tools. *BMC Med Res Methodol.* 2004;4(1):22.
33. Hatala R, Keitz S, Wyer P, et al. Tips for learners of evidence-based medicine: 4. Assessing heterogeneity of primary studies in systematic reviews and whether to combine their results. *Can Med Assoc J.* 2005;172(5):661–665.
34. Greenhalgh T. How to read a paper: papers that summarise other papers (systematic reviews and meta-analyses). *BMJ.* 1997;315(7109):672–675.
35. Helmer D, Savoie I, Green C, et al. Evidence-based practice: extending the search to find material for the systematic review. *Bull Med Libr Assoc.* 2001;89(4):346–352.
36. Moher D, Tsertsvadze A, Tricco AC, et al. A systematic review identified few methods and strategies describing when and how to update systematic reviews. *J Clin Epidemiol.* 2007;60(11):1095–1104.
37. Jaeschke R, Guyatt G, Sackett DL. Users' guides to the medical literature. III. How to use an article about a diagnostic test. A. Are the results of the study valid? Evidence-Based Medicine Working Group. *JAMA.* 1994;271(5):389–391.
38. Jaeschke R, Guyatt GH, Sackett DL. Users' guides to the medical literature. III. How to use an article about a diagnostic test. B. What are the results and will they help me in caring for my patients? The Evidence-Based Medicine Working Group. *JAMA.* 1994;271(9):703–707.
39. Raiche M, Hébert R, Prince F, et al. Screening older adults at risk of falling with the Tinetti balance scale. *Lancet.* 2000;356(9234):1001–1002.
40. Kaplan SH, Greenfield S, Ware JE Jr. Assessing the effects of physician-patient interactions on the outcomes of chronic disease. *Med Care.* 1989;27(3 suppl):S110–S127.
41. Guyatt GH, Sackett DL, Cook DJ. Users' guides to the medical literature. II. How to use an article about therapy or prevention. A. Are the results of the study valid? Evidence-Based Medicine Working Group. *JAMA.* 1993;270:2598–2601.
42. Guyatt GH, Sackett DL, Cook DJ. Users' guides to the medical literature. II. How to use an article about therapy or prevention. B. What were the results and will they help me in caring for my patients? Evidence-Based Medicine Working Group. *JAMA.* 1994;271(1):59–63.
43. Sackett D, Haynes RB, Guyatt GH, et al. *Clinical Epidemiology: A Basic Science for Clinical Medicine.* Boston, MA: Little, Brown and Company; 1991.
44. Cohen J. *Statistical Power Analysis for the Behavioral Sciences.* New Jersey: Laurence Earlham; 1988.
45. Sarasin FP. Decision analysis and the implementation of evidence-based medicine. *QJM.* 1999;92(11):669–671.
46. Yusuf S, Held P, Teo KK, et al. Selection of patients for randomized controlled trials: implications of wide or narrow eligibility criteria. *Stat Med.* 1990;9(1–2):73–83; discussion 83–86.
47. McAlister FA, Straus SE, Guyatt GH, et al. Helping patients integrate research evidence. *JAMA.* 2000;284(20):2594–2595.
48. Stewart MA. Effective physician-patient communication and health outcomes: a review. *Can Med Assoc J.* 1995;152(9):1423–1433.
49. Epstein RM, Alper BS, Quill TE. Communicating evidence for participatory decision making. *JAMA.* 2004;291(19):2359–2366.
50. Burrows SC, Tylman V. Evaluating medical student searches of MEDLINE for evidence-based information: process and application of results. *Bull Med Libr Assoc.* 1999;87(4):471–476.
51. Stern DT, Linzer M, O'Sullivan PS, et al. Evaluating medical residents' literature-appraisal skills. *Acad Med.* 1995;70(2):152–154.
52. Bennett KJ, Sackett D, Haynes RB, et al. A controlled trial of teaching critical appraisal of the clinical literature to medical students. *JAMA.* 1987;257(18):2451–2454.
53. Norman GR, Shannon SI. Effectiveness of instruction in critical appraisal (evidence-based medicine) skills: a critical appraisal. *Can Med Assoc J.* 1998;158:177–181.
54. Fritsche L, Greenhalgh T, Falck-Ytter Y, et al. Do short courses in evidence based medicine improve knowledge and skills? Validation of Berlin questionnaire and before and after study of courses in evidence based medicine. *BMJ.* 2002;325(7376):1338–1341.
55. Ramos KD, Schafer S, Tracz SM. Validation of the Fresno test of competence in evidence based medicine. *BMJ.* 2003;326(7384):319–321.
56. Linzer M, Brown JT, Frazier LM, et al. Impact of a medical journal club on house-staff reading habits, knowledge, and critical appraisal skills. A randomized control trial. *JAMA.* 1988;260(17):2537–2541.
57. Phillips RS, Glasziou P. What makes evidence-based journal clubs succeed? *Evid Based Med.* 2004;9(2):36–37.
58. McCluskey A, Lovarini M. Providing education on evidence-based practice improved knowledge but did not change behaviour: a before and after study. *BMC Med Educ.* 2005;5:40.
59. Taylor R, Reeves B, Ewings P, et al. Critical appraisal skills training for health care professionals: a randomized controlled trial. *BMC Med Educ.* 2004;4(30):1–10.
60. About knowledge translation; 2008. Canadian Institutes of Health Research website. Available from: http://www.cihr-irsc.gc.ca/e/29418.html#2
61. NIH Fogarty International Center, Frequently Asked Questions about Implementation Sciences (cited February 10, 2012).
62. Nilsen P. Making sense of implementation theories, models and frameworks. *Implement Sci.* 2015;10:53.
63. Eccles M, Grimshaw J, Walker A, et al. Changing the behavior of healthcare professionals: the use of theory in promoting the uptake of research findings. *J Clin Epidemiol.* 2005;58(2):107–112.
64. Bragge P, Grimshaw JM, Lokker C, et al. AIMD—a validated, simplified framework of interventions to promote and integrate evidence into health practices, systems, and policies. *BMC Med Res Methodol.* 2017;17(1):38.
65. Tabak RG, Khoong EC, Chambers DA, et al. Bridging research and practice: models for dissemination and implementation research. *Am J Prev Med.* 2012;43(3):337–350.
66. Graham ID, Logan J, Harrison MB, et al. Lost in knowledge translation: time for a map? *J Contin Educ Health Prof.* 2006;26(1):13–24.
67. Rogers EM. *Diffusion of Innovations.* The Free Press: New York; 2003.
68. Doran D, Sidani S. Outcomes-focused knowledge translation: a framework for knowledge translation and patient outcomes improvement. *Worldviews Evid Based Nurs.* 2007;4:3–13.
69. Grimshaw J, Eccles M, Lavis J, et al. Knowledge translation of research findings. *Implement Sci.* 2012;7(1):50.
70. Grol R, Grimshaw J. From best evidence to best practice: effective implementation of change in patients' care. *Lancet.* 2003;362(9391):1225–1230.
71. Eccles M, Flodgren G, Parmelli E, et al. Local opinion leaders: effects on professional practice and health care outcomes. *Cochrane Database Syst Rev.* 2011(8):CD000125.
72. Michie S, Johnston M. Theories and techniques of behaviour change: developing a cumulative science of behaviour change. *Health Psychol Rev.* 2012;6(1):1–6.
73. Gardner B, Whittington C, McAteer J, et al. Using theory to synthesise evidence from behaviour change interventions: the example of audit and feedback. *Soc Sci Med.* 2010;70(10):1618–1625.
74. Hoof TV, Miller N, Meehan T. Do published studies of educational outreach provide documentation of potentially important characteristics? *Am J Med Qual.* 2013;28(6):480–484.
75. Colquhoun HL, Squires JE, Kolehmainen N, et al. Methods for designing interventions to change healthcare professionals' behaviour: a systematic review. *Implement Sci.* 2017;12(1):30.
76. Spall HGCV, Shanbhag D, Gabizon I, et al. Effectiveness of implementation strategies in improving physician adherence to guideline recommendations in heart failure: a systematic review protocol. *BMJ Open.* 2016;6.
77. Weiner BJ. A theory of organizational readiness for change. *Implement Sci.* 2009;4(1):67.
78. Holt DT, Helfrich CD, Hall CG, et al. Are you ready? How health professionals can comprehensively conceptualize readiness for change. *J Gen Intern Med.* 2010;25(suppl 1):50–55.
79. Holt DT, Armenakis AA, Harris SG, et al. Toward a comprehensive definition of readiness for change: a review of research and instrumentation. *Res Organ Change Dev.* 2007;16:289–336.
80. Matchar DB, Samsa GP. The role of evidence reports in evidence-based medicine: a mechanism for linking scientific evidence and practice improvement. *Jt Comm J Qual Improv.* 1999;25(10):522–528.
81. Baker R, Camosso-Stefinovic J, Gillies C, et al. Tailored interventions to overcome identified barriers to change: effects on professional practice and health care outcomes. *Cochrane Database Syst Rev.* 2010;(3):CD005470.
82. Wensing M, Oxman A, Baker R, et al. Tailored implementation for chronic diseases (TICD): a project protocol. *Implement Sci.* 2011;(6):103.
83. Flottorp SA, Oxman AD, Krause J, et al. A checklist for identifying determinants of practice: a systematic review and synthesis of frameworks and taxonomies of factors that prevent or enable improvements in healthcare professional practice. *Implement Sci.* 2013;(8):35.
84. Gawande A. Cowboys and pit crews. *The New Yorker.* May 26, 2011. Available from: http://www.newyorker.com/online/blogs/newsdesk/2011/05/atul-gawande-harvard-medical-school-commencementaddress.html. Accessed January 29, 2016.
85. Grossman C, Goolsby A, Olsen L, et al. *Engineering: A Learning Healthcare System: A Look at the Future.* Institute of Medicine and National Academy of Engineering of the National Academies. Washington, DC; 2011.
86. Institute for Healthcare Improvement website. Available from: http://www.ihi.org/. Accessed January 29, 2016.
87. High Value Healthcare Collaborative website. Available from: http://highvalue-healthcare.org/. Accessed January 29, 2016.

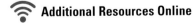 **Additional Resources Online**

Neural Repair and Plasticity

Increasing evidence suggests that behavioral recovery in neurological disease and injury is associated with neural plasticity. This premise has led to the development of numerous interventions that purportedly maximize recovery via neural repair processes. This chapter reviews these concepts, with an emphasis on stroke and on motor deficits. Stroke remains a leading cause of adult disability and illustrates many of the key principles that likely generalize to other conditions, such as multiple sclerosis (MS), spinal cord injury (SCI), and traumatic brain injury (TBI). Some degree of natural behavioral recovery (sometimes called spontaneous recovery) is usually seen in the weeks following stroke onset. Animal studies have provided insight into underlying molecular and neurophysiological events. Brain mapping studies in human patients have provided observations at the systems level that often parallel the findings in animals. The best outcomes are associated with the greatest return toward the normal state of brain functional organization. As our understanding of neural repair and plasticity processes becomes more sophisticated, it is anticipated that these underlying mechanisms will shape optimal methods to prescribe therapies.

STROKE

Natural Behavioral Recovery After Stroke in Humans

In the weeks following a stroke, survivors generally display some degree of natural behavioral recovery. Considerable variability exists, however (1). Key principles identified to date are that most recovery tends to occur within the first 3 months after stroke onset, cognitive deficits are more likely than motor deficits to show spontaneous gains beyond these 3 months (2,3), stroke survivors with more mild deficits achieve recovery quicker than those with more severe deficits (4–6), and different patterns of recovery can exist across different neurological domains within the same patient (7,8). Because of the differences in the rate and extent of recovery across neurological domains, restorative stroke trials might need to use behavioral outcome measures that focus on a single neurological domain rather than the global behavioral scales employed in acute stroke studies (7).

Despite individual differences in recovery rate and extent, a proportional recovery rule has been proposed (9). This rule maintains that in the first 3 months after stroke, survivors should regain approximately 70% of their maximum potential recovery. This rule was first established for motor recovery on the upper extremity subset of the Fugl-Meyer (FM) Scale, whose maximum score is 66. Thus, a stroke survivor with an initial FM upper extremity score of 50 is expected to regain 70% of the difference between the initial score and the maximum score, or 0.7 × 16 = 11 points. Hence, the FM upper extremity score at 3 months is expected to be 50 + 11 = 61 points. This rule appears to generalize to recovery of lower limb impairment, aphasia recovery, and visuospatial neglect (10–12). However, a subset of stroke survivors, specifically those with the most severe initial impairments, fall short of the proportionality trajectory, at least for upper extremity recovery. Stroke anatomy may play an important role in the ability of the CNS to undergo repair processes. Thus, in addition to the initial severity of impairment, extent of injury to the corticospinal tract may be an independent predictor of natural recovery (13).

Insights from Animal Studies

Studies in animal models have particular value because they are able to provide insight at the molecular and cellular levels. Also, unlike in clinical populations, within-subject study designs allow functional endpoints to be studied before and after injury.

Based on evidence from animal models, it is now well known that stroke triggers structural and functional plasticity that is remarkably widespread. Molecular cascades related to plasticity and repair mechanisms occur locally, in the peri-infarct cortex, in distant cortical areas, as well as in subcortical structures. These molecular cascades lead to altered axonal connections, dendritic branching, and synaptogenesis (14–22). In many cases, similar events occur in the opposite, intact hemisphere (📶 eTable 61-1).

Evidence is emerging for the role of exosomes after stroke (23). Exosomes are nanometer-sized lipid microvesicles derived from endosomes and released into extracellular fluids, such as blood and cerebrospinal fluid. Both rodent and human brain cells release exosomes into the extracellular space. Their ability to transfer DNAs, mRNAs, microRNAs, noncoding RNAs, proteins, and lipids among cells is thought to represent a novel intercellular communication mechanism (24). In particular, miRNAs and mRNAs play an important role in brain repair processes, including cerebral angiogenesis, neurogenesis, and potentially axonal growth and myelination (25). Future therapeutic approaches have been envisioned that take advantage of this unique communication system between neurons and astrocytes.

Insights have also come from studies of cortical representational maps. Nudo et al. (26) described changes in the hand motor map after stroke in nonhuman primates. Hand motor training after stroke was associated with expansion of the motor cortex hand representation (**Fig. 61-1**). This reorganization was later found to be related to local synaptogenesis (27).

Preinfarct

Postinfarct and rehabilitative therapy

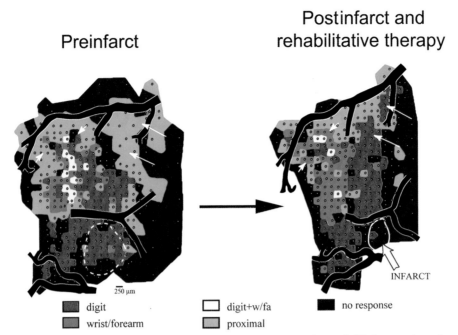

INFARCT

■ digit   □ digit+w/fa   ■ no response
■ wrist/forearm   ▦ proximal

250 μm

FIGURE 61-1. Serial findings using intracortical microstimulation mapping in nonhuman primates (*left*) before experimental stroke and (*right*) after stroke plus a program of rehabilitative training focused on hand training. The rehabilitative training prevented loss of hand territory adjacent to the infarct, when compared to animals not receiving this training. In some instances, the hand representations expanded into regions formerly occupied by representations of the elbow and shoulder (*white arrows*). This study demonstrated that rehabilitative training can shape subsequent reorganization in the adjacent intact cortex and suggested that the undamaged motor cortex may play an important role in motor recovery (26). The *long thin arrows* point to regions of undamaged cortex in which digit representations have invaded regions formerly occupied by representations of the elbow and shoulder. (Redrawn from Fig. 2 in Nudo RJ, Wise BM, SiFuentes F, et al. Neural substrates for the effects of rehabilitative training on motor recovery after ischemic infarct. *Science*. 1996;272(5269):1791–1794. Reprinted with permission from AAAS.)

When injuries occur in the primary motor cortex, cortical representational maps expand in cortical areas connected to the injured zone, such as premotor areas (28,29). The expansion is directly related to the size of the injury in the primary motor cortex, suggesting a possible vicarious role for the premotor cortex after injury. More recent studies have demonstrated that cortical representational map plasticity after injury is differentially modified by enriched environments, specific rehabilitative training regimens, medications, electrical stimulation, lesion size, and age (30–41).

Magnetic resonance imaging (MRI) studies have documented changes in representational maps noninvasively, and thus, the outcomes can be compared more directly with analogous results reported in human studies. These approaches may prove to be of great value in effective translation of therapeutic interventions (42–44). These findings are closely aligned with findings from serial fMRI exams in human subjects with stroke (45,46). New imaging methodologies in animal models have also demonstrated that normally stable dendritic spine morphology becomes remarkably dynamic after focal ischemia and that spine turnover plays an important role in shaping synaptic signaling. (47,48). While human imaging cannot yet achieve this subcellular resolution *in vivo*, these new methodologies have provided important insight into the structural elements that are remodeled during the recovery phase after stroke and provide a platform for testing hypotheses regarding therapeutic interventions.

Recovery Versus Compensation

A key issue that sparks significant controversy is whether functional gains after stroke or other brain injuries are the result of recovery or compensation. Whether in a research or clinical setting, recovery is gauged by improvements on various outcome measures that typically reflect impairments, limitations, or degree of participation, paralleling the International Classification of Functioning, Disability and Health (ICF) (49). However, as one moves from specific measures of impairment in body functions and structures, the influence of compensatory mechanisms becomes greater. The important clinical question to be addressed is whether patients should undergo rehabilitative training protocols that require that movements be performed in a near-normal manner or whether compensatory behavioral strategies should be encouraged. The answer to this question is not simple, as compensatory motor patterns contribute to improved function as well as persistent impairment after brain injury (50).

Recovery refers to the restitution of function back to a near-normal state (50). True recovery requires that the normal repertoire of behaviors that was available before the injury is restored (51). Thus, complete recovery after any substantial neural damage is rarely achieved. Short of future regenerative medicine approaches that might literally replace damaged brain tissue, virtually all clinical improvement in motor function contains some element of compensatory strategies. However, in the clinical literature, recovery is often used both to describe restitution of function and to clinically improve a particular outcome measure, regardless of how the improvement occurred (52).

To understand the distinction between recovery and compensation at different ICF levels, consider a stroke patient with a hemiparetic arm seated in a chair and reaching out to grab a drinking cup. Recovery at the impairment (body function/structure) level would refer to return to a premorbid condition in which the patient can reach and grab the cup with the same movement patterns as before the injury—that is, the same range of motion of all upper extremity joints, the same interjoint coordination, the same muscle force, etc. It should be obvious that not only does such recovery at the body function/activity level rarely occur, but it is difficult to assess the specific impairments outside of specialized laboratories. Compensation at the impairment level would refer to performance of the task using alternative movement patterns, with altered agonist/antagonist coactivation, delays in timing, and different muscle force profiles. The patient might reach for the cup by first propelling their trunk forward to compensate for reduced range of motion in the arm (53). Such compensatory strategies can be quite functional and often are not easily distinguished from true recovery by casual observation. At the functional limitation (activity) level, one might consider recovery as the successful accomplishment of the reach task by using end effectors that healthy individuals would use. Compensation might be represented by the successful completion of the task but by using the less-impaired limb. Such compensation at this level would be obvious even to the casual observer.

Focal infarcts induce widespread changes in connected networks that reorganize in ways that are not entirely predictable. These changes in distant areas and their interconnected fibers are considered compensatory. Alternative brain areas might reorganize to adopt at least some of the original function of the damaged tissue, a so-called vicarious process. Whether improved functional performance results from recovery or compensation, it is highly likely that neural plasticity is part of the process. Learning to use compensatory motor strategies requires the development of new skills and is accompanied by neural reorganization. Thus, after any finite damage to the nervous system, compensation must occur at least at the neural level.

Compensation begins as soon as the first movement is attempted after injury (50,54). The particular compensatory movement patterns that eventually develop and become part of the new motor repertoire are dependent upon the extent of the injury and initial severity and well-known motor learning and reward mechanisms that are engaged during the early relearning period. Motor patterns that are ineffective, effortful, or painful are negatively rewarded and tend to be used less frequently (learned nonuse). Motor patterns that are rewarded early in the relearning process tend to be used more frequently.

Animal studies have shed light on the neural remodeling that occurs when compensatory motor patterns are used. For example, after lesions in the forelimb motor cortex, unless specifically retrained to use the impaired limb, rats will rely on the nonparetic limb for reaching and grasping. In this case, the motor cortex in the intact hemisphere undergoes structural plasticity both due to the release of inhibition from the injured hemisphere as well as dendritic and synaptic growth induced by the overreliance on the nonparetic limb. In contrast, training strategies that encourage the use of the paretic limb result in structural changes in the peri-infarct region in the injured hemisphere. Behavioral function on the paretic side is improved by such postinjury early use of the paretic limb.

While typically motor rehabilitation emphasizes better motor performance as an endpoint, compensatory movement patterns can, to some extent, be encouraged or discouraged by specific interventions (55). But depending on the specificity of the functional endpoint, task-oriented practice protocols such as constraint-induced movement therapy may in some instances increase compensatory movements (56). Thus, while possibly the only option for severe impairments, improved performance accomplished through compensation can come at a cost (57,58). The clinical implications of these studies suggest that when an individual's capacity allows it, compensatory use of the nonparetic limb should be weighed against the negative effects on long-term function of the paretic limb.

System Insights from Brain Mapping Studies in Human Subjects

The molecular and subcellular measurements from animal studies are difficult to obtain in humans, though occasionally specific questions can be probed with molecular imaging methods such as positron emission tomography (PET). But *in vivo*, noninvasive brain mapping techniques in humans have provided important correlative information regarding remodeling of system-wide brain networks underlying stroke recovery in clinical populations. A number of functional neuroimaging methods have been used to this extent.

Overall, after stroke in humans, tissue function is reduced within the injured (or for deep strokes, overlying/corresponding) neocortex (59,60). Behaviors that rely on the dysfunctional cortex suffer. The best natural return of behavioral performance is associated with resolution of such reductions of cortical function. A number of compensatory brain responses also contribute to natural behavioral recovery. These include increased activation in secondary areas that are normally connected to the injured zones through a distributed network, a shift in interhemispheric lateralization toward the contralesional hemisphere, and shifts in representational maps surrounding the infarcted zone. In many cases, the larger the injury or greater the deficits, the more these compensatory events are seen. While many have argued that these compensatory responses do not represent true recovery of neuronal function, in patients with injury-related deficits, they can support greater daily life activities, and, in that sense, are adaptive. However, the best behavioral outcomes after stroke are associated with the greatest return of brain function toward the normal state of organization (61–63). These findings take on particular importance when it is realized that the same events that support natural recovery are likely those to be measured to assist studies aiming to therapeutically improve recovery.

Stroke Injury Reduces Cortical Activity Locally

When a stroke injures primary sensorimotor cortex and/or its underlying white matter, cortical function is reduced initially, increasing over time (45,63). Thus, several lines of evidence suggest that final behavioral outcome at the end of the stroke recovery period is related to the degree of neural activity in primary sensorimotor cortex. Similar findings have also been described in language (62,64,65) and right hemisphere attentional networks (63). Consistent with this, transcranial magnetic stimulation (TMS) studies of motor cortex after stroke have generally found that cortical motor maps are smaller and corticospinal tract physiological integrity is reduced in proportion to the severity of clinical deficits (66).

Viable cortical regions that surround an infarct might have special importance to repair and recovery. In animals, this peri-infarct zone often shows the greatest levels of growth-related molecular changes after stroke (15,26,67–69). Furthermore, therapeutic amplification of peri-infarct repair-related events has been associated with improved behavioral outcome (70–76). In humans, the volume of threatened but surviving peri-infarct tissue is directly related to the final clinical outcome (77,78).

Stroke Injury Incites Increased Cortical Activity at Distant Sites

Three main forms of reorganization at sites distant from stroke have been described: (a) increased activity in brain regions distant from, but connected to, the stroke zone; (b) increased activity in the contralesional hemisphere, which reduces the extent to which interhemispheric balance is lateralized; and (c) somatotopic shifts within intact cortical regions. Each has been associated with behavioral improvement after stroke.

The first form of reorganization involves increased activation within cortical areas that, prior to stroke, are part of an interconnected distributed network (54,79–84). This has been described in many studies, indeed since the first poststroke functional imaging study by Brion et al. (85). Reaction across a distributed network has been reported across many neurological domains including motor, language, attention, and visual functions.

A second form of reaction to stroke is reduced laterality of brain activity (64,79,80,82,85). Reduced laterality is a cardinal pattern of brain response to injury, having also been described in other neurological contexts such as epilepsy (86), TBI (87), primary progressive aphasia (88), and MS (89). The degree of brain insult needed to incite reduced laterality might be much lower than previously appreciated.

The exact function served by increased contralesional activity after stroke remains to be clarified. To some extent, this can be seen as simply a contralesional example of increased brain activation at sites distant from the stroke (**Fig. 61-2**) (90,91). Another interpretation is that this is a passive event, reflecting a reduced interhemispheric inhibition resulting from the stroke (92–96). Changes in interhemispheric inhibition are the focus of much discussion (95), and possibly of therapeutic value (96–98), though the significance of such findings might differ across patient subgroups (96). Another hypothesis is that

Movements of the stroke-affected (right) hand

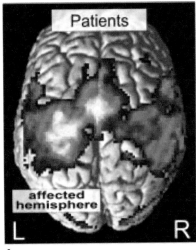
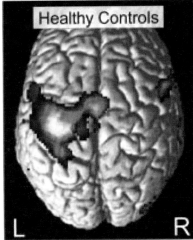

A

FIGURE 61-2. Pathophysiological disturbances in interhemispheric balance after stroke (90). In normal subjects, movements of the right hand result in neural activity predominantly in the left (i.e., contralateral) motor cortex (**A**, *right*). In stroke patients, movements of the stroke-affected (*right*) hand result in activation of both hemispheres. This imbalance is due, in part, to the reduction of normal inhibition conveyed by the corpus callosum from the affected hemisphere to the nonaffected hemisphere (i.e., contralesional hemisphere; **A**, *left*). Movements of the unaffected hand result in the normal contralateral activation of the motor cortex in both patients and healthy controls (**B**). (From Grefkes C, Nowak DA, Eickhoff SB, et al. Cortical connectivity after subcortical stroke assessed with functional magnetic resonance imaging. *Ann Neurol.* 2008;63:236–246. Copyright © 2007 American Neurological Association. Reprinted by permission of John Wiley & Sons, Inc.)

Movements of the unaffected (left) hand

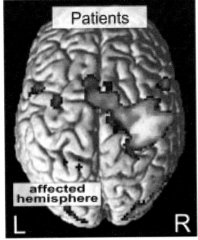
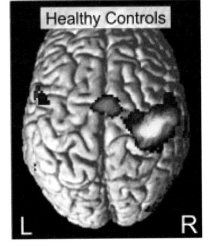

B

the contralesional hemisphere assumes functions that were previously based in the ipsilesional hemisphere. However, the data do not support this, at least not directly and completely. For example, stimulating contralesional motor cortex with TMS does not result in movement of the affected hand (99) and indeed might indicate greater pathology if such a response is seen (100). Contralesional hemisphere functions might be more substantial when stroke is prenatal (101).

A third compensatory response to focal injury is reorganization of somatotopic maps. Such maps are normally present in multiple cortical areas including motor, sensory, auditory, and visual cortex, and such somatotopic organization also exists in white matter, basal ganglia, secondary neocortex, and the hemisphere ipsilateral to movement (102–104). Nonhuman primate studies have provided rich characterization of cortical map changes after ischemic injury, providing insight into the effects of rehabilitation as well as infarct size and also describing novel axonal projections that can arise in this context, (14,26,29,34,105,106). While it is thought that the process of reorganization is initiated very early after focal injury, animal studies have demonstrated that early improvements in motor function are not reflected in spared motor maps until substantially later (39). Such delayed changes in motor maps may reflect either full maturation of synaptic connections in distant areas, more subtle changes in movement quality not captured in typical functional assessments of motor performance, or both. This process has been less studied in humans after a stroke, where most, but not all (54,107,108), investigations have focused on the motor system. The large scale features of motor cortex somatotopy that are normally present are preserved though occasional exceptions have been described (109). A shift of the motor cortex hand representation after stroke in the dorsal (110), ventral (83,111), or posterior (112,113) direction has been reported. Sites assuming such a shift in brain activation can demonstrate increased cortical thickness (108).

The motor cortex map relationships between face and hand may be among the most plastic in the brain, a suggestion that is supported by reports of invasion of hand motor representation into face motor area (83,109,111,114) and face into hand (115,116), in a variety of settings, first described after stroke by Weiller et al. (82). This process might reflect survival of distinct subsets of corticospinal tract fibers (117) that have key axonal connections between hand and face areas (118) and so could theoretically represent an approach to identify a biologically distinct subgroup of stroke patients in whom a particular therapy (one that encourages a ventral hand map shift) might be most likely to succeed.

These forms of poststroke increased activation have certain principles in common. These changes are not epiphenomena, as suggested by virtual lesion and other approaches (119–125), but rather directly contribute to natural behavioral recovery. Increased activity in distant areas (83,126) and reduced laterality (61,109,127,128) are time-dependent, increasing in the early weeks after stroke and generally declining thereafter. This decline is greater among subjects with better behavioral outcome, as the degree of persistently increased activity in both instances is generally highest in those with the poorest behavioral outcome (61,109,129). However, persistent, increased reorganization is not always helpful, as persistence of poststroke plasticity can be associated with induction of epilepsy (130) or chronic pain (131).

Diaschisis

The changes arising in areas distant from injury might in part be related to diaschisis or its resolution. Diaschisis refers to reduced activity, typically measured in terms of blood flow and/or metabolism, in uninjured brain areas that have rich connections with injured brain areas (132,133). Some data suggest that natural behavioral recovery is facilitated by the resolution of diaschisis, that is, restitution of brain activity in these uninjured areas that are distant from, but connected to, the site of infarct (46,134,135). The optimal method for defining, and thus for measuring, diaschisis remains unclear.

Time Window Influences Application of Restorative Therapies After Stroke

The time window that defines a restorative therapy likely varies according to the therapy and biological target. The biological targets for restorative agents vary over time, with brain levels spontaneously rising then falling dramatically in the weeks following a stroke. Some conceptual models have broken down poststroke brain changes into three epochs that overlap at least in part: (a) acute injury, taking place in the initial hours after a stroke; (b) repair, starting in the first days after stroke onset and lasting several weeks (This is a golden period for initiating exogenous restorative therapies, as the greatest degree of natural behavioral recovery is seen, and endogenous repair-related events [see Table 62-1] reach peak levels [📶 **eFig. 61-1**] (136,137). Note that exogenous therapies, from pharmacotherapies to behavioral interventions, must be examined in a two-tailed manner, as each can be deleterious as well as potentially helpful, as discussed below.), and (c) a plateau, starting weeks-months after stroke and representing a stable but still modifiable chronic phase. This third phase might have two temporal components (83): one representing the beginning of the chronic phase, with associated loss of treatment windows from phase 2, and the other arising many months-years after stroke onset, associated with late changes and complications. Late changes and complications of a "late plateau" epoch include new dystonias, cognitive/affective changes, and spasticity/contracture.

Other Factors Influencing Recovery

A number of general factors can influence outcome after stroke (45,117,138–148). The quality and intensity of behavioral experience during the weeks-months following a stroke, and the environment in which this experience takes place, are well established as having a major influence on behavioral outcome after stroke (35,149–154). The nature of the physical and social environment also influences the brain, in health (155) and after stroke (156). Genetic factors might also be important (157,158). Note that a number of factors can also *reduce* behavioral recovery after stroke. One example is drugs such as neuroleptics or antiepileptics (159–162). Other drugs, such as benzodiazepines, can induce an anamnestic state: a patient can have poststroke deficits, recover spontaneously, and then have the deficits reemerge years later.

Small Molecules

Many chemical events in the poststroke brain are relevant to repair. After injury, molecular programs set into motion. Genes are differentially regulated especially in sprouting neurons, leading to the concept of "the sprouting transcriptome"

(163). Genes are up-regulated that are related to axonal guidance, calcium signaling, extracellular matrix function, growth factors, transcription factors, and cytoskeletal modifying genes (163,164). Not surprisingly, a number of small molecules have been examined as potential therapies in this context (165–167). The mechanism for some of these small molecules revolves around direct manipulation of a specific neurotransmitter axis, such as increasing tone at serotoninergic (168,169) or monoaminergic (170–172) receptors. Results with the latter example, such as with amphetamine and related drugs (173–175), have been mixed. Other small molecule approaches have examined the administration of certain drugs (165,166). The brain events that support behavioral recovery appear to have a vulnerability (167) that lasts a lifetime.

Restorative Therapies

Restorative therapies aim to promote behavioral recovery after stroke. Numerous therapies, devices, and interventions for modifying function after stroke have been evaluated and are considered below (176–180).

Growth Factors

Growth factors, both growth-promoting and growth-inhibiting factors, play an important role in the development and spontaneous brain remodeling and, thus, might have great promise as therapies to improve function after stroke. A wide range of potential mechanisms exist, including promoting activity-dependent synaptic competition, long-term potentiation, facilitating key protein synthesis and synaptic transmission, and more. Several positive preclinical studies have been published (181), including those employing a hematopoietic growth factor (182–184). Kolb et al. (184) found that sequential administration of epidermal growth factor and erythropoietin to rats with experimental infarct reduced deficits, in some cases when treatment was initiated 7 days after stroke onset. A number of other guidance cues are provided by ligands that have dual roles in growth cone guidance and thus can either attract or repel growth cones. These include semaphorins, netrins, ephrins, and reactive glial and scare-derived axon growth inhibitors (185).

A great deal of interest has focused on myelin-associated proteins, such as NogoA and myelin-associated glycoprotein (MAG). While myelin-associated proteins normally inhibit axonal growth, their effects are modulated by experience. It has been suggested that activity or experience triggers a transient insensitivity to the inhibitory effects of myelin-associated proteins, resulting in synaptic reorganization. A novel monoclonal antibody against MAG has shown moderately positive effects in rodents with experimental stroke, but a nonhuman primate preclinical trial resulted in no effect (38,186). A clinical trial of this antibody was stopped at the predetermined interim analysis, as no change was found in gait velocity (187).

In most cases, these growth factors have been initiated 24 hours or longer after stroke onset in a rodent model of experimental stroke and were found to improve long-term behavioral outcome. This long therapeutic time window, the large number of examples of successful preclinical studies, the use of compounds that are endogenous to humans, and reliance on compounds that in many cases have a long history of safe application in humans are all factors that predict future successful application of growth factors to restoring function after stroke in humans.

For large molecules such as growth factors, access to the brain might prove to be a significant challenge. One potential solution to this involves the use of a "Trojan horse" approach. This approach enables larger molecules to be reformulated to allow them to be transported across the blood-brain barrier (BBB) via receptor-mediated transport. For example, brain-derived neurotrophic factor (BDNF) results in reduced lesion volume and improved functional outcome in rodent models of stroke. However, BDNF alone cannot easily cross the BBB. But a monoclonal antibody to the transferrin receptor can undergo receptor-mediated transport across the BBB. By conjugating BDNF to the antibody, BDNF can effectively be transported into the brain despite its size (188).

Cell-Based Therapies

A number of forms of exogenous cells, including induced pluripotent (189) and embryonic stem cells (190), have been examined in preclinical stroke models (191). Mobilization of endothelial progenitor cells (192) might also help repair after stroke (193). Limited data are available on treatment of human subjects with stroke using exogenous cells (191). The safety and feasibility of intracerebral transplantation of cultured neuronal cells in humans were established in two trials of Layton BioScience-neurons (194,195), with at best modest results. A small trial in human patients with subacute stroke found intravenous mesenchymal stromal cell (MSC, also referred to as marrow stromal cell) infusion to be safe and possibly effective for reducing disability (196). Microglia/macrophages are specifically modulated by cell-based therapies (197). MSC can be prepared autologously, eliminating the need for immunosuppression, and might have a therapeutic time window of up to 1 month poststroke (197). MSC might also prove useful as a conduit for therapies targeting specific genes (198–201). A number of issues require addressing whatever the cell used, such as establishing biological identity, activity, purity, and stability over time. There still remain significant challenges in conducting clinical trials with cell-based therapies, including the need to use immunosuppressive agents that pose risk for adverse events (202).

Electrical and Electromagnetic Brain Stimulation

Electrical and electromagnetic stimulation has been used to modulate a number of brain functions; indeed a brain-wide form of electrical stimulation, electroconvulsive therapy, remains the gold standard for the treatment of major depression (203). Several forms of brain stimulation intervention are under evaluation to improve function after stroke, though in most cases studies are at an early phase. One such form of noninvasive brain stimulation is repetitive TMS, which, depending on the frequency of stimulation, can have inhibitory or excitatory effects on cortical activity (204). As such, goals can include increased activity in ipsilesional cortical regions that are underactive (205–207) or decreased activity in contralesional cortical regions that are overactive and a source of potentially harmful inhibition (98). Repetitive TMS has been applied alone or in combination with rehabilitative training. Most studies have been conducted in the chronic phase after stroke. Transcranial electrical stimulation, including transcranial direct current stimulation (tDCS) and transcranial alternating current stimulation, has also shown promise in initial studies and might be less focal in its brain effects (206,207). Epidural motor cortex stimulation might also improve motor function after stroke (208), though a phase III study in 164 patients with chronic stroke found that the effects on motor status of epidural motor cortex stimulation plus rehabilitation therapy did not significantly differ from rehabilitation therapy alone at 4 weeks posttreatment. However, secondary analyses demonstrated that a greater proportion of stroke participants treated with epidural stimulation maintained or achieved the primary efficacy endpoint at 24 weeks posttreatment (209).

There is currently considerable interest in the use of another noninvasive brain stimulation approach, called tDCS. tDCS has gained popularity primarily because the system is relatively inexpensive and easy to implement. tDCS utilizes low-intensity direct current delivered through saline-soaked sponges over the skull. Currents under the anodal pole are thought to increase neuronal excitability, and currents under the cathodal pole are thought to decrease excitability (210). Excitability changes are typically assessed by using TMS to measure motor-evoked potentials elicited by TMS over the area of interest. However, it should be emphasized that the current flow through the brain is not straightforward, and much of the current is shunted through the skin. tDCS probably does not produce direct depolarization of neurons or axons, in contrast to TMS. However, a recent animal study suggests that tDCS may result in astrocytic calcium surges specifically in astrocytes and not neurons (211). Astrocytic signaling can have a significant effect on synaptic excitability.

Many relatively small tDCS trials have been conducted to evaluate its benefit in activities of daily living and arm function (212), in improving aphasia (213), and in improving hemispatial neglect (214) after stroke. At the current levels typically used (1 to 2 mA), tDCS appears to be safe. While the efficacy results to date are mixed, especially with regard to duration of effect, tDCS is currently considered a safe, potential treatment to modulate brain activity noninvasively after stroke. As standards for rigor and reproducibility are developed in the research community, and a better understanding of its mechanisms of action is achieved, it is hoped that recommendations regarding its clinical utility can be rendered with confidence in the future.

Device-Based Therapies

Numerous devices are under study to improve function after stroke, some employed external to the body and others surgically internalized. Some devices aim to substitute for the injured CNS, such as via a brain-computer interface (215,216). For others, such as via a laser-based device (217), functional electrical stimulation (218), neuroprosthetics, and robotic devices (219), the goal is to improve function in surviving CNS elements. Electrical stimulation and neuroprostheses are further discussed in Chapters 55 and 57, respectively. A number of different robotic devices have been examined (220–223). These devices have been largely focused on motor function, where mild-moderate gains have been documented. Robotic therapy offers potential advantages in that robotic devices can be active without fatigue for very long time periods, perform in a consistent and precise manner, can be programmed, have the capacity to measure a range of behaviors, and are enabled for telerehabilitation. Robotic therapy is further discussed in Chapter 63. Combination approaches employing a robotic therapy alongside a second restorative therapy such as a drug or neuromuscular stimulation have been less studied but might prove fruitful.

Task-Oriented and Repetitive Training-Based Interventions

Interventions based on task repetition are important to the repair process for at least two reasons: first, behavioral experience influences effectiveness of other interventions such as pharmacological therapy and noninvasive brain stimulation. Second, task-oriented and repetitive training-based interventions might have significant value as the main therapy of interest (224–226). A number of forms of therapy have been studied, with uncertain results at this time as to which is best. Cognitive-based strategies, such as those based on motor imagery or action observation, have shown promise (153,227–232). Interventions in the motor system have included bilateral training (233), use of a gravity-reduced environment (234), EMG trigger coupling (235), incorporating passive movement (236), or manipulating movement speed (237). The structure (238) and intensity (151,152) of the training program can influence extent of gains, but linear dose-response relationships are often elusive (239).

One such therapy of note is constraint-induced movement therapy, which is based on overcoming learned nonuse of the affected hand after stroke (240). Constraint-induced movement therapy has the nonaffected hand restrained while the affected hand undergoes an intense course of therapy. A multi-site phase III trial (241) found that 2 weeks of this therapy produced gains that remained significant 2 years after the end of the intervention (242) (🛜 eFig. 61-2). Modified forms of this therapy might increase the fraction of chronic stroke patients who are eligible (235). In addition, studies are examining this approach in other neurological domains such as language (243). An important question is the percentage of patients who can derive gain from this and other task-oriented and repetitive training-based interventions.

Key questions remain. When is the goal to simply provide a return of function via any means versus when is the goal to precisely restore CNS operations to a prestroke state? Indeed, disentangling behavioral compensation from true recovery of the specific behavior measured as an endpoint (57,244,245) might be important to some studies. What is the optimal time for safe and effective initiation? Application of intensive therapy very early after stroke might be deleterious (137,246). How extensive will concomitant experience and behavioral shaping need to be? What is the optimal dose of rehabilitation and how do we define dose? How will the target population be defined? Some of these questions might be best answered by incorporating studies of brain injury and function into therapeutic decision-making.

Utility of Brain Mapping Data for Restorative Therapy Clinical Trials After Stroke

Clinical stroke trials often enroll patients based on behavioral entry criteria. However, behavioral performance can arise on the basis of many different neurobiological states, only some of which are likely to respond to restorative therapy. Several studies suggest that human brain mapping can provide additional insights useful for optimal implementation of restorative therapies. By providing measures of injury and brain functional state, data from fMRI, PET, TMS, magnetoencephalography, electroencephalography, and other methods might be of value to clinical trials.

There are several functions that functional neuroimaging measures might play. One might be to guide particular details of a restorative intervention. If a therapy achieves its effect by targeting a specific functional brain region, such as the hand motor area, anatomical localization might be insufficient because localization of a specific function in the brain often has an inconsistent relationship with brain anatomy (247–250). Serial measurement of brain function might also guide therapy dose or duration (251,252). This approach has been demonstrated in clinical (253) and research (254) settings. A second role for functional neuroimaging measures might be to guide dose of therapy, for example, via measurement of fMRI laterality measurements (251) or motor-evoked potential by TMS (252).

An additional potential value of functional neuroimaging methods is to serve as entry criteria. Having a measure of CNS functional status and injury might assist usual behavioral and demographic measures (149,152) to identify patients most likely to respond to a given intervention. Functional measures of brain state have been incorporated into early-phase restorative stroke trials and found to predict response to therapy (7,251,252,255). A study by Stinear et al. (256) achieved good success at predicting arm motor gains from therapy using measures of demographics, CNS function, and injury. This model, and so many others, requires validation and further investigation, for example, of clinometrics. However, likely some measures beyond those obtainable at the bedside will likely prove useful for optimal prescription of restorative therapies after stroke.

Functional neuroimaging measures might also 1 day serve as surrogate endpoints in the evaluation of restorative therapies. Surrogate markers can be of considerable value to early-phase trials. A proof-of-principle functional neuroimaging study in a small target population could be very useful when considering proceeding to a late-phase trial (257). However, important concerns exist in the use of functional neuroimaging measures as a surrogate endpoint for restorative stroke therapeutics. Many more studies are needed to examine the performance of such measures in this context. A number of issues, such as the extent and specificity with which a surrogate marker captures treatment effect, require examination (258,259).

SUMMARY

Studies in animals and humans are providing new insights into the biological basis of natural recovery after stroke. On the backbone of this knowledge, a number of restorative therapies are entering human trials to promote improved outcomes. Measures of CNS injury and function might be useful toward these efforts. Further study is needed on a number of questions to optimally prescribe restorative therapies and reduce disability after stroke.

MULTIPLE SCLEROSIS

Multiple sclerosis (MS) is also a common source of disability, frequently affecting motor function (Chapter 20). Deficits are acquired over a much longer time in MS as compared to stroke. For example, in one study of a broad range of subjects with MS, the median time to reach irreversible limited walking ability for more than 500 m without aid or rest was 8 years, to

walk with unilateral support for not more than 100 m without rest was 20 years, and to walk for not more than 10 m without rest while leaning against a wall or support was 30 years (260). Upper extremity motor deficits, such as those related to ataxia and paresis, are also a common source of disability in MS (261).

Brain plasticity is an important functional determinant in MS over two time scales. First, steady destruction of myelin and axons over the years results in disability. During this period, reorganization of brain function can reduce the impact that such injury has on behavioral decline. Second, over the ensuing weeks to months, approximately 85% of patients with MS have a relapsing, remitting course (262) in which a relapse peaks at an interval of about 1 to 2 months and then improves over a similar time period. The resolution of these MS flares has been attributed to a number of brain events, such as neurological reserve and resolution of inflammatory insult, and a number of studies suggest that brain plasticity is also important. Note too that there are numerous asymptomatic brain lesions for each symptomatic one in most patients with MS, a fact that might further support the importance of brain plasticity in the maintenance of behavioral status in this condition.

Thus, it is possible that brain plasticity minimizes the debilitating effects of MS injury accrual over the long-term period by promoting recovery from silent or symptomatic MS flares over the short-term period. A number of studies have provided insights into the brain events important in this regard, with substantial overlap as compared to findings in patients with stroke. This information gains importance in the current discussion because events important to maximizing behavioral status in the natural course of the disease are likely to be many of the same measures whose measurement can guide optimization of therapy-derived recovery.

fMRI studies of brain plasticity in MS have found that early in the course of the disease, brain activation is larger and more widespread as compared to healthy controls. Later in the disease, laterality of activation is reduced (i.e., activation is more bilateral) (263–265), akin to stroke patients who have larger infarcts or greater deficits. Bilateral sensorimotor cortical regions are activated to a greater extent in the setting of MS-related white matter injury (266,267). This increased degree of bilateral organization persists to the greatest extent in subjects with persistent deficits after an acute MS relapse and returns to a normal, lateralized (i.e., contralateral-predominant) form of organization in subjects with the least degree of persistent disability (268,269). The pattern of brain activation during performance of a simple motor task in subjects recovered from stroke has been considered similar to the pattern seen in healthy subjects during performance of a complex task (79); a similar analogy has been made in subjects with MS (270).

A number of repair-based therapeutic strategies are also being explored in MS, though considerably less knowledge exists on this approach in MS as compared to in stroke. Many of these overlap with approaches described for stroke, above, such as stem cells and growth factors. Manipulation of myelin growth inhibitory molecules such as Nogo, as well as other myelin components, might also be an important avenue to promote repair in this demyelinating disease. A range of immune-based approaches, which constitute the centerpiece of acute MS therapies, might also have a role in promoting repair (271–274).

An increasing number of studies have examined the utility of brain mapping data for restorative therapies in patients with MS. Parry et al. (275) tested the effects of increased cholinergic tone on the pattern of fMRI activation during performance of the Stroop test, a cognitive task. At baseline, patients with MS and moderate disability had similar behavioral performance as compared to controls but on fMRI showed increased left medial prefrontal, and decreased right frontal, activation. Treatment with the cholinesterase inhibitor rivastigmine normalized both of these fMRI abnormalities in patients but had little effect on a small cohort of healthy control subjects. Mainero et al. (276) found that administration of 3,4-diaminopyridine to patients with MS was associated with reduced intracortical inhibition and increased intracortical facilitation. Though no behavioral correlates were noted in relation to these physiological changes, a favorable effect on behavior would be expected by analogy (206,277).

More recent cross-sectional fMRI studies have shown the brain changes at different stages of the disease, allowing speculation about the role of neuroplasticity in functional status. Abnormalities in fMRI images appear early in the course of MS but are variable at different stages (278). Increased recruitment of brain areas normally involved with a motor task occurs at the beginning of the disease and is typically related to the extent and severity of CNS damage (279). Later, activation decreased. It has been observed that a relapse temporarily alters functional organization of motor networks (280). Finally, rehabilitation interventions have been shown to alter resting state functional connectivity in people with MS (281). Inroads are also being made in understanding the interaction between the immune system and neural plasticity based on common molecular mechanisms.

SPINAL CORD INJURY

Though spinal cord injury (SCI) can be associated with a variety of functional impairments, motor deficits are generally a prominent feature (Chapter 22) (282). The most frequent neurologic category is incomplete tetraplegia (47.2%), followed by incomplete paraplegia (20.4%), complete paraplegia (20.2%), and complete tetraplegia (11.5%). Less than 1% of persons experience complete neurologic recovery by hospital discharge (283).

Persons with SCI generally show modest spontaneous sensory and motor improvement in the first 3 to 6 months following injury (284), although significant spontaneous improvement beyond the 1st year post SCI is uncommon (285). Motor deficits are thus common and persistent after SCI and impact a number of health, quality of life, and other issues in subjects with SCI (286–288). For example, by 10 years after SCI, 68% of persons with paraplegia, and 76% of those with tetraplegia, remain unemployed (283). Concerns over sexual and bowel/bladder function are also prevalent (289,290).

There has been limited study of the changes in the function of the human CNS after SCI. Some studies have found a broad decrease in brain activation (291–293), particularly in primary sensorimotor cortex, whereas others have found supranormal brain activation (294). The basis for these discrepancies remains unclear but could be due to differences in age or injury pattern of the population studied, years post SCI at time of study, or the nature of the task used to probe motor

system function, some uncovering deficient processing and others emphasizing supranormal efforts to compensate (292). A commonly described feature is a change in somatotopic organization within primary sensorimotor cortex, with representation of supralesional body regions expanding at the expense of infralesional body regions (84,295–298). Spontaneous changes in laterality, so prominent in studies of stroke or MS, as above, are generally not prominent after SCI, perhaps due in part to the fact that injury typically affects the CNS bilaterally or perhaps due in part to the fact that SCI spares brain commissural fibers whose integrity helps maintain normal hemispheric balance. As such, a laterality index is unlikely to be a useful variable in brain mapping studies of subjects with SCI. Widespread abnormalities in the limbic system have also been described (299,300), the full impact of which has yet to be appreciated. The temporal sequence of brain changes after CNS is just beginning to be understood (292). Also, the direct study of spinal cord function and plasticity at the level of the spinal cord is an emerging approach that might provide novel insights after SCI and after other forms of SCI (177,300).

A small number of studies have examined changes in CNS function in relation to therapy after SCI. Wolfe et al. (301) found that 4-diaminopyridine can improve central conduction time in subjects with SCI. Winchester et al. (302) studied body weight–supported treadmill training in four patients with motor incomplete SCI. These authors compared fMRI during attempted unilateral foot and toe movement before versus after training. This therapy was associated with increased activation within several bilateral areas, including primary sensorimotor cortex and cerebellum, though to a variable extent. The authors observed that, although all participants demonstrated a change in the blood-oxygen level–dependent signal following training, only those patients who demonstrated a substantial increase in activation of the cerebellum demonstrated an improvement in their ability to walk overground, suggesting that this measure in this brain region, at least when examined using this task during fMRI, might be useful as a biological marker of successful treatment effect. A small study suggests that gains from treadmill training correlate with improvements in motor system physiology (303). Similarly, a case reports motor cortex hand map expansion in relation to gains from hand sensorimotor physiotherapy (304), though this result was not found in a larger study (305). These initial findings anticipate that many of the principles under discussion for use of brain mapping to improve physiotherapy effects in trials of recovery after stroke, such as use of physiology or brain map measures as entry criteria or as treatment biomarkers, might also pertain to SCI.

Another form of intervention that has been evaluated after SCI is motor imagery. Motor imagery normally activates many of the same brain regions as motor execution and has been associated with improvements in motor performance (227,306). The effects of 1 week of motor imagery training to the tongue and to the foot were evaluated in 10 subjects with chronic, complete tetraplegia/paraplegia plus 10 healthy controls (307). The behavioral outcome measure was speed of performance of a complex sequence. Motor imagery training was associated with a significant improvement in this behavior in a nonparalyzed muscle group, the tongue, for both groups. In both the healthy controls and the subjects with SCI, serial fMRI scanning (before vs. after training) during attempted right foot movement was associated with increased fMRI activation in left putamen, an area associated with motor learning, despite foot movements being present in controls and absent in subjects with SCI. Training effects on brain plasticity can thus be measured independent of behavior effects, a finding that might be important for designing biological markers in trials targeting severely disabled patient populations. Note that this fMRI change was absent in a second healthy control group serially imaged without training. The main conclusion from this study is that motor imagery training improves brain function whether or not sensorimotor function is present in the trained limb. An additional conclusion is that motor imagery, by virtue of its favorable effects on brain motor system organization, might have value as an adjunct motor restorative therapy. Another key point from this study is that brain plasticity related to plegic limbs can be studied in subjects with chronic SCI. The above study examined, as a first step, the effects of a pure motor imagery intervention, but, as with subjects with stroke, motor imagery might have its greatest effect when directly combined with physiotherapy interventions.

Finally, neurotechnology-based approaches have advanced over the past several years. Robot-mediated therapy may aid walking in some patients following SCI, but results have been mixed (308). However, plasticity in spinal cord physiology resulting from lower limb robotic training has been demonstrated both in rodent and human populations (309–311). Neuroprosthetic technologies employing novel epidural stimulation paradigms have also shown promise as adjuncts to traditional rehabilitation (312).

TRAUMATIC BRAIN INJURY (SEE CHAPTER 19)

Traumatic brain injury (TBI) is a common, heterogeneous condition that is the source of much human suffering. Patients can present with wide-ranging impairments, including cognitive, visual, and motor. Despite a number of advances in neurorehabilitation, substantial morbidity and mortality remain (313–316). TBI shares some clinical features of other forms of CNS injury. For example, predictors of outcome after TBI, such as severity of initial deficits, are similar to those described in other forms of CNS injury, though social aspects may play a larger role in TBI (313).

Treatment of TBI has been reviewed elsewhere (315). In the more chronic phase, physiotherapy regimens targeting TBI may not be as developed as with other conditions (316). More intensive rehabilitation programs are associated with earlier function gains (317,318). There have been limited advances in therapies that promote brain repair after TBI, with relatively few studies examining restorative medications in the setting of human TBI (319). Small studies suggest that some of the treatments potentially useful for promoting brain repair after stroke might have utility after TBI (320–323), and similarly, brain stimulation (324), cognitive rehabilitation (325), and progesterone (326) may also have some efficacy. Spontaneous increases in growth factor levels that have been observed after TBI might indicate a therapeutic role for this family of restorative therapies (327). Cellular therapies might also have promise in reducing disability after TBI (328,329).

Brain imaging is providing new insights into the pathophysiology of TBI as well as of the brain repair that arises secondarily (330). Diffusion tensor imaging (DTI) measures injury, particularly in the white matter. DTI sometimes discloses injury that was completely inapparent with standard anatomical MRI scanning (331,332) or discloses evidence of repair (333). fMRI provides information about function that, as with stroke (334), sometimes vastly exceeds what can be determined with behavioral exam (335) or anatomical imaging (336). Insights with fMRI (337–340) and other functional neuroimaging methods (341–344) extend across brain functional systems as well as injury severities (343,345). Functional imaging studies of TBI have been criticized for lack of protocol standardization (346), a concern common to the study of many neurological conditions (347).

An improved understanding of the pathophysiology of TBI will be useful to better define and target repair-related processes (346,347). In parallel, a need exists for advances in functional neuroimaging. Such advances should permit continued growth (348) in the ability to use measures of brain plasticity in humans to improve application of restorative therapies to reduce disability after TBI.

SUMMARY

The CNS possesses innate responses to injury; some are adaptive, while others are maladaptive. Increased attention is being paid to these responses. The result is a better understanding of CNS repair in humans. A wide range of therapies are under investigation with the aim of promoting CNS repair. Together, these advances anticipate regular use of restorative therapies to promote CNS repair and reduce disability in patients with stroke, MS, SCI, TBI, and other neurological conditions.

ACKNOWLEDGMENTS

Dr. Nudo is supported by grants from NIH (NS30853 and HD057850), the Department of Defense (W81XWH-15-JWMRP), Paralyzed Veterans of America, and the Ronald D. Deffenbaugh Family Foundation.

REFERENCES

1. Twitchell TE. The restoration of motor function following hemiplegia in man. *Brain*. 1951;74:443–480.
2. Kertesz A. What do we learn from recovery from aphasia? *Adv Neurol*. 1988;47:277–292.
3. Desmond DW, Moroney JT, Sano M, et al. Recovery of cognitive function after stroke. *Stroke*. 1996;27:1798–1803.
4. Duncan PW, Goldstein LB, Matchar D, et al. Measurement of motor recovery after stroke. Outcome assessment and sample size requirements. *Stroke*. 1992;23:1084–1089.
5. Wade DT, Langton-Hewer R, Wood VA, et al. The hemiplegic arm after stroke: measurement and recovery. *J Neurol Neurosurg Psychiatry*. 1983;46:521–524.
6. Pedersen PM, Jørgensen HS, Nakayama H, et al. Aphasia in acute stroke: incidence, determinants, and recovery. *Ann Neurol*. 1995;38:659–666.
7. Cramer SC, Koroshetz WJ, Finklestein SP. The case for modality-specific outcome measures in clinical trials of stroke recovery-promoting agents. *Stroke*. 2007;38:1393–1395.
8. Hier DB, Mondlock J, Caplan LR. Recovery of behavioral abnormalities after right hemisphere stroke. *Neurology*. 1983;33:345–350.
9. Prabhakaran S, Zarahn E, Riley C. Inter-individual variability in the capacity for motor recovery after ischemic stroke. *Neurorehabil Neural Repair*. 2008;22:64–71.
10. Lazar RM, Minzer B, Antoniello D, et al. Improvement in aphasia scores after stroke is well predicted by initial severity. *Stroke*. 2010;41(7):1485–1488.
11. Winters C, van Wegen EE, Daffertshofer A, et al. Generalizability of the proportional recovery model for the upper extremity after an ischemic stroke. *Neurorehabil Neural Repair*. 2017;29(7):614–622.
12. Smith MC, Byblow WD, Barber PA, et al. Proportional recovery from lower limb motor impairment after stroke. *Stroke*. 2017;48:1400–1403.
13. Rondina JM, Park C, Ward NS. Brain regions important for recovery after severe post-stroke upper limb paresis. *J Neurol Neurosurg Psychiatry*. 2017;88:737–743.
14. Nudo RJ. Postinfarct cortical plasticity and behavioral recovery. *Stroke*. 2007;38:840–845.

15. Carmichael ST. Cellular and molecular mechanisms of neural repair after stroke: making waves. *Ann Neurol.* 2006;59:735–742.

16. Komitova M, Johansson BB, Eriksson PS. On neural plasticity, new neurons and the postischemic milieu: an integrated view on experimental rehabilitation. *Exp Neurol.* 2006;199:42–55.

17. Chopp M, Zhang ZG, Jiang Q. Neurogenesis, angiogenesis, and MRI indices of functional recovery from stroke. *Stroke.* 2007;38:827–831.

18. Wieloch T, Nikolich K. Mechanisms of neural plasticity following brain injury. *Curr Opin Neurobiol.* 2006;16:258–264.

19. Nudo RJ. Recovery after brain injury: mechanisms and principles. *Front Hum Neurosci.* 2013;7:887.

20. Redecker C, Wang W, Fritschy J, et al. Widespread and long-lasting alterations in GABA(A)-receptor subtypes after focal cortical infarcts in rats: mediation by NMDA-dependent processes. *J Cereb Blood Flow Metab.* 2002;22:1463–1475.

21. Carmichael ST. Gene expression changes after focal stroke, traumatic brain and spinal cord injuries. *Curr Opin Neurol.* 2003;16:699–704.

22. Carmichael ST, Kathirvelu B, Schweppe CA. Molecular, cellular and functional events in axonal sprouting after stroke. *Exp Neurol.* 2017;287:384–394.

23. Zhang ZG, Chopp M. Exosomes in stroke pathogenesis and therapy. *J Clin Investig.* 2016;126:1190–1197.

24. Lai PK, Breakefield XO. Role of exosomes/microvesicles in the nervous system and use in emerging therapies. *Front Physiol.* 2012;3:1–14.

25. He X, Yu Y, Awatramani R, et al. Unwrapping myelination by microRNAs. *Neuroscientist.* 2012;18:45–55.

26. Nudo RJ, Wise BM, SiFuentes F, et al. Neural substrates for the effects of rehabilitative training on motor recovery after ischemic infarct. *Science.* 1996;272:1791–1794.

27. Kleim J, Barbay S, Cooper N. Motor learning-dependent synaptogenesis is localized to functionally reorganized motor cortex. *Neurobiol Learn Mem.* 2002;77:63–77.

28. Frost SB, Barbay S, Friel KM, et al. Reorganization of remote cortical regions after ischemic brain injury: a potential substrate for stroke recovery. *J Neurophysiol.* 2003;89:3205–3214.

29. Dancause N, Barbay S, Frost SB, et al. Effects of small ischemic lesions in the primary motor cortex on neurophysiological organization in ventral premotor cortex. *J Neurophysiol.* 2006;96:3506–3511.

30. Zhang L, Zhang RL, Wang Y. Functional recovery in aged and young rats after embolic stroke: treatment with a phosphodiesterase type 5 inhibitor. *Stroke.* 2005;36:847–852.

31. Popa-Wagner A, Carmichael ST, Kokaia Z, et al. The response of the aged brain to stroke: too much, too soon? *Curr Neurovasc Res.* 2007;4:216–227.

32. Napieralski JA, Butler AK, Chesselet MF, et al. Anatomical and functional evidence for lesion-specific sprouting of corticostriatal input in the adult rat. *J Comp Neurol.* 1996;373:484–497.

33. Voorhies AC, Jones TA. The behavioral and dendritic growth effects of focal sensorimotor cortical damage depend on the method of lesion induction. *Behav Brain Res.* 2002;133:237–246.

34. Nudo RJ, Milliken GW. Reorganization of movement representations in primary motor cortex following focal ischemic infarcts in adult squirrel monkeys. *J Neurophysiol.* 1996;75:2144–2149.

35. Johansson BB. Brain plasticity and stroke rehabilitation. The Willis lecture. *Stroke.* 2000;31:223–230.

36. Hicks AU, Hewlett K, Windle V, et al. Enriched environment enhances transplanted subventricular zone stem cell migration and functional recovery after stroke. *Neuroscience.* 2007;146:31–40.

37. Plautz EJ, Barbay S, Frost SB. Effects of subdural monopolar cortical stimulation paired with rehabilitative training on behavioral and neurophysiological recovery after cortical ischemic stroke in adult squirrel monkeys. *Neurorehabil Neural Repair.* 2016;30:159–172.

38. Barbay S, Plautz EJ, Zoubina E, et al. Effects of postinfarct myelin-associated glycoprotein antibody treatment on motor recovery and motor map plasticity in squirrel monkeys. *Stroke.* 2015;46:1620–1625.

39. Nishibe M, Rd UE, Barbay S, et al. Rehabilitative training promotes rapid motor recovery but delayed motor map reorganization in a rat cortical ischemic infarct model. *Neurorehabil Neural Repair.* 2015;29:472–482.

40. Touvykine B, Mansoori BK, Jean-Charles L, et al. The effect of lesion size on the organization of the ipsilesional and contralesional motor cortex. *Neurorehabil Neural Repair.* 2016;30:280–292.

41. Tennant KA, Kerr AL, Adkins DL, et al. Age-dependent reorganization of peri-infarct "premotor" cortex with task-specific rehabilitative training in mice. *Neurorehabil Neural Repair.* 2015;29:193–202.

42. van der Zijden JP, Wu O, van der Toorn A, et al. Changes in neuronal connectivity after stroke in rats as studied by serial manganese-enhanced MRI. *Neuroimage.* 2007;34:1650–1657.

43. Dijkhuizen R, Ren J, Mandeville J, et al. Functional magnetic resonance imaging of reorganization in rat brain after stroke. *Proc Natl Acad Sci U S A.* 2001;98:12766–12771.

44. Dijkhuizen RM, Singhal AB, Mandeville JB, et al. Correlation between brain reorganization, ischemic damage, and neurologic status after transient focal cerebral ischemia in rats: a functional magnetic resonance imaging study. *J Neurosci.* 2003;23:510–517.

45. Feydy A, Carlier R, Roby-Brami A, et al. Longitudinal study of motor recovery after stroke: recruitment and focusing of brain activation. *Stroke.* 2002;33:1610–1617.

46. Nhan H, Barquist K, Bell K, et al. Brain function early after stroke in relation to subsequent recovery. *J Cereb Blood Flow Metab.* 2004;24:756–763.

47. Enright LE, Zhang S, Murphy TH, et al. Fine mapping of the spatial relationship between acute ischemia and dendritic structure indicates selective vulnerability of layer V neuron dendritic tufts within single neurons in vivo. *J Cereb Blood Flow Metab.* 2007;27:1185–1200.

48. Brown CE, Li P, Boyd JD, et al. Extensive turnover of dendritic spines and vascular remodeling in cortical tissues recovering from stroke. *J Neurosci.* 2007;27:4101–4109.

49. Salter K, Jutai JW, Teasell R, et al. Issues for selection of outcome measures in stroke rehabilitation: ICF Body Functions. *Disabil Rehabil.* 2005;27:191–207.

50. Jones TA. Motor compensation and its effects on neural reorganization after stroke. *Nat Rev Neurosci.* 2017;18:267–280.

51. Bernhardt J, Hayward KS, Kwakkel G, et al. Agreed definitions and a shared vision for new standards in stroke recovery research: the stroke recovery and rehabilitation roundtable taskforce. *Neurorehabil Neural Repair.* 2017;31:793–799.

52. Levin MF, Kleim JA, Wolf SL. What do motor "recovery" and "compensation" mean in patients following stroke? *Neurorehabil Neural Repair.* 2009;23:313–319.

53. Levin MF, Cirstea MC. Improvement of arm movement patterns and endpoint control depends on type of feedback during practice in stroke survivors. *Neurorehabil Neural Repair.* 2007;21(5):398–411.

54. Rosen HJ, Petersen SE, Linenweber MR, et al. Neural correlates of recovery from aphasia after damage to left inferior frontal cortex. *Neurology.* 2000;55:1883–1894.

55. Valdes BA, Schneider AN, Van der Loos HFM. Reducing trunk compensation in stroke survivors: a randomized crossover trial comparing visual and force feedback modalities. *Arch Phys Med Rehabil.* 2017;98:1932–1940.

56. Massie C, Malcolm MP, Greene D, et al. The effects of constraint-induced therapy on kinematic outcomes and compensatory movement patterns: an exploratory study. *Arch Phys Med Rehabil.* 2009;90:571–579.

57. Friel KM, Nudo RJ. Recovery of motor function after focal cortical injury in primates: compensatory movement patterns used during rehabilitative training. *Somatosens Mot Res.* 1998;15:173–189.

58. Allred RP, Maldonado MA, Hsu And JE, et al. Training the "less-affected" forelimb after unilateral cortical infarcts interferes with functional recovery of the impaired forelimb in rats. *Restor Neurol Neurosci.* 2005;23:297–302.

59. Chu W-J, Mason GF, Pan JW, et al. Regional cerebral blood flow and magnetic resonance spectroscopic imaging findings in diaschisis from stroke. *Stroke.* 2002;33:1243–1248.

60. Thickbroom GW, Byrnes ML, Archer SA. Motor outcome after subcortical stroke correlates with the degree of cortical reorganization. *Clin Neurophysiol.* 2004;115:2144–2150.

61. Ward NS, Brown MM, Thompson AJ, et al. Neural correlates of outcome after stroke: a cross-sectional fMRI study. *Brain.* 2003;126:1430–1448.

62. Warburton E, Price CJ, Swinburn K, et al. Mechanisms of recovery from aphasia: evidence from positron emission tomography studies. *J Neurol Neurosurg Psychiatry.* 1999;66:155–161.

63. Corbetta M, Kincade MJ, Lewis C, et al. Neural basis and recovery of spatial attention deficits in spatial neglect. *Nat Neurosci.* 2005;8:1603–1610.

64. Blank SC, Bird H, Turkheimer F, et al. Speech production after stroke: the role of the right pars opercularis. *Ann Neurol.* 2003;54(3):310–320.

65. Hillis AE, Wityk RJ, Tuffiash E, et al. Hypoperfusion of Wernicke's area predicts severity of semantic deficit in acute stroke. *Ann Neurol.* 2001;50:561–566.

66. Talelli P, Greenwood RJ, Rothwell JC. Arm function after stroke: neurophysiological correlates and recovery mechanisms assessed by transcranial magnetic stimulation. *Clin Neurophysiol.* 2006;117:1641–1659.

67. Carmichael ST. Plasticity of cortical projections after stroke. *Neuroscientist.* 2003;9:64–75.

68. Carmichael ST, Archibeque I, Luke L. Growth-associated gene expression after stroke: evidence for a growth-promoting region in peri-infarct cortex. *Exp Neurol.* 2005;193:291–311.

69. Kleim J, Bruneau R, VandenBerg P. Motor cortex stimulation enhances motor recovery and reduces peri-infarct dysfunction following ischemic insult. *Neurol Res.* 2003;25:789–793.

70. Kleim JA, Jones TA, Schallert T. Motor enrichment and the induction of plasticity before or after brain injury. *Neurochem Res.* 2003;28:1757–1769.

71. Stroemer RP, Kent TA, Hulsebosch CE. Enhanced neocortical neural sprouting, synaptogenesis, and behavioral recovery with D-amphetamine therapy after neocortical infarction in rats. *Stroke.* 1998;29:2381–2393.

72. Li Y, Chen J, Zhang CL. Gliosis and brain remodeling after treatment of stroke in rats with marrow stromal cells. *Glia.* 2005;49:407–417.

73. Speliotes EK, Caday CG, Do T, et al. Increased expression of basic fibroblast growth factor (bFGF) following focal cerebral infarction in the rat. Brain research. *Mol Brain Res.* 1996;39:31–42.

74. Witte OW, Bidmon H, Schiene K, et al. Functional differentiation of multiple perilesional zones after focal cerebral ischemia. *J Cereb Blood Flow Metab.* 2000;20:1149–1165.

75. Eysel UT. Perilesional cortical dysfunction and reorganization. *Adv Neurol.* 1997;73:195–206.

76. Plautz E, Barbay S, Frost S. Post-infarct cortical plasticity and behavioral recovery using concurrent cortical stimulation and rehabilitative training: a feasibility study in primates. *Neurol Res.* 2003;25:801–810.

77. Furlan M, Marchal G, Viader F. Spontaneous neurological recovery after stroke and the fate of the ischemic penumbra. *Ann Neurol.* 1996;40:216–226.

78. Heiss WD, Grond M, Thiel A, et al. Tissue at risk of infarction rescued by early reperfusion: a positron emission tomography study in systemic recombinant tissue plasminogen activator thrombolysis of acute stroke. *J Cereb Blood Flow Metab.* 1998;18:1298–1307.

79. Cramer SC, Nelles G, Benson RR, et al. A functional MRI study of subjects recovered from hemiparetic stroke. *Stroke.* 1997;28:2518–2527.

80. Chollet F, DiPiero V, Wise RJ, et al. The functional anatomy of motor recovery after stroke in humans: a study with positron emission tomography. *Ann Neurol.* 1991;29:63–71.

81. Kleiser R, Wittsack HJ, Butefisch CM, et al. Functional activation within the PI-DWI mismatch region in recovery from ischemic stroke: preliminary observations. *Neuroimage.* 2005;24:515–523.

82. Weiller C, Ramsay SC, Wise RJ, et al. Individual patterns of functional reorganization in the human cerebral cortex after capsular infarction. *Ann Neurol.* 1993;33:181–189.

83. Tombari D, Loubinoux I, Pariente J, et al. A longitudinal fMRI study: in recovering and then in clinically stable sub-cortical stroke patients. *Neuroimage.* 2004;23:827–839.

84. Corbetta M, Burton H, Sinclair RJ, et al. Functional reorganization and stability of somatosensory-motor cortical topography in a tetraplegic subject with late recovery. *Proc Natl Acad Sci U S A.* 2002;99:17066–17071.

85. Brion JP, Demuerisse G, Capon A. Evidence of cortical reorganization in hemiparetic patients. *Stroke.* 1989;20:1079–1084.

86. Detre JA. fMRI: applications in epilepsy. *Epilepsia.* 2004;45(suppl 4):26–31.

87. Christodoulou C, DeLuca J, Ricker JH, et al. Functional magnetic resonance imaging of working memory impairment after traumatic brain injury. *J Neurol Neurosurg Psychiatry.* 2001;71:161–168.

88. Vandenbulcke M, Peeters R, Van Hecke P, et al. Anterior temporal laterality in primary progressive aphasia shifts to the right. *Ann Neurol.* 2005;58:362–370.

89. Lee M, Reddy H, Johansen-Berg H, et al. The motor cortex shows adaptive functional changes to brain injury from multiple sclerosis. *Ann Neurol.* 2000;47:606–613.

90. Grefkes C, Nowak DA, Eickhoff SB, et al. Cortical connectivity after subcortical stroke assessed with functional magnetic resonance imaging. *Ann Neurol.* 2008;63:236–246.

91. Shimizu T, Hosaki A, Hino T, et al. Motor cortical disinhibition in the unaffected hemisphere after unilateral cortical stroke. *Brain.* 2002;125:1896–1907.

92. Manganotti P, Patuzzo S, Cortese F, et al. Motor disinhibition in affected and unaffected hemisphere in the early period of recovery after stroke. *Clin Neurophysiol.* 2002;113:936–943.

93. Liepert J, Hamzei F, Weiller C. Motor cortex disinhibition of the unaffected hemisphere after acute stroke. *Muscle Nerve.* 2000;23:1761–1763.

94. Butefisch CM, Netz J, Wessling M, et al. Remote changes in cortical excitability after stroke. *Brain.* 2003;126:470–481.

95. Murase N, Duque J, Mazzocchio R, et al. Influence of interhemispheric interactions on motor function in chronic stroke. *Ann Neurol.* 2004;55:400–409.

96. Butefisch CM, Wessling M, Netz J, et al. Relationship between interhemispheric inhibition and motor cortex excitability in subacute stroke patients. *Neurorehabil Neural Repair.* 2008;22:4–21.

97. Mansur CG, Fregni F, Boggio PS, et al. A sham stimulation-controlled trial of rTMS of the unaffected hemisphere in stroke patients. *Neurology.* 2005;64:1802–1804.

98. Fregni F, Boggio PS, Valle AC, et al. A sham-controlled trial of a 5-day course of repetitive transcranial magnetic stimulation of the unaffected hemisphere in stroke patients. *Stroke.* 2006;37:2115–2122.

99. Palmer E, Ashby P, Hajek VE. Ipsilateral fast corticospinal pathways do not account for recovery in stroke. *Ann Neurol.* 1992;32:519–525.

100. Turton A, Wroe S, Trepte N, et al. Contralateral and ipsilateral EMG responses to transcranial magnetic stimulation during recovery of arm and hand function after stroke. *Electroencephalogr Clin Neurophysiol.* 1996;101:316–328.

101. Staudt M, Grodd W, Gerloff C, et al. Two types of ipsilateral reorganization in congenital hemiparesis: a TMS and fMRI study. *Brain.* 2002;125:2222–2237.

102. Alkadhi H, Crelier GR, Boendermaker SH, et al. Somatotopy in the ipsilateral primary motor cortex. *Neuroreport.* 2002;13:2065–2070.

103. Fontaine D, Capelle L, Duffau H. Somatotopy of the supplementary motor area: evidence from correlation of the extent of surgical resection with the clinical patterns of deficit. *Neurosurgery.* 2002;50:297–303.

104. Godschalk M, Mitz AR, van Duin B, et al. Somatotopy of monkey premotor cortex examined with microstimulation. *Neurosci Res.* 1995;23:269–279.

105. Frost SB, Chen D, Barbay S, et al. Effects of forced use on the ventral premotor cortex distal forelimb representation after ischemic infarct in primary motor cortex. *PM R.* 2016;8:S158.

106. Dancause N, Barbay S, Frost SB, et al. Extensive cortical rewiring after brain injury. *J Neurosci.* 2005;25:10167–10179.

107. Nelles G, de Greiff A, Pscherer A, et al. Cortical activation in hemianopia after stroke. *Neurosci Lett.* 2007;426:34–38.

108. Schaechter JD, Moore CI, Connell BD, et al. Structural and functional plasticity in the somatosensory cortex of chronic stroke patients. *Brain.* 2006;129:2722–2733.

109. Cramer SC, Crafton KR. Somatotopy and movement representation sites following cortical stroke. *Exp Brain Res.* 2006;168:25–32.

110. Jaillard A, Martin CD, Garambois K, et al. Vicarious function within the human primary motor cortex? A longitudinal fMRI stroke study. *Brain.* 2005;128:1122–1138.

111. Schaechter JD, Perdue KL, Wang R. Structural damage to the corticospinal tract correlates with bilateral sensorimotor cortex reorganization in stroke patients. *Neuroimage.* 2008;39:1370–1382.

112. Pineiro R, Pendlebury S, Johansen-Berg H, et al. Functional MRI detects posterior shifts in primary sensorimotor cortex activation after stroke: evidence of local adaptive reorganization? *Stroke.* 2001;32:1134–1139.

113. Calautti C, Leroy F, Guincestre JY, et al. Displacement of primary sensorimotor cortex activation after subcortical stroke: a longitudinal PET study with clinical correlation. *Neuroimage.* 2003;19:1650–1654.

114. Rijntjes M, Tegenthoff M, Liepert J, et al. Cortical reorganization in patients with facial palsy. *Ann Neurol.* 1997;41:621–630.

115. Lotze M, Flor H, Grodd W, et al. Phantom movements and pain. An fMRI study in upper limb amputees. *Brain.* 2001;124:2268–2277.

116. Elbert T, Flor H, Birbaumer N, et al. Extensive reorganization of the somatosensory cortex in adult humans after nervous system injury. *Neuroreport.* 1994;5:2593–2597.

117. Newton JM, Ward NS, Parker GJ, et al. Non-invasive mapping of corticofugal fibres from multiple motor areas—relevance to stroke recovery. *Brain.* 2006;129:1844–1858.

118. Manger PR, Woods TM, Munoz A, et al. Hand/face border as a limiting boundary in the body representation in monkey somatosensory cortex. *J Neurosci.* 1997;17:6338–6351.

119. Lotze M, Markert J, Sauseng P, et al. The role of multiple contralesional motor areas for complex hand movements after internal capsular lesion. *J Neurosci.* 2006;26:6096–6102.

120. Winhuisen L, Thiel A, Schumacher B, et al. Role of the contralateral inferior frontal gyrus in recovery of language function in poststroke aphasia: a combined repetitive transcranial magnetic stimulation and positron emission tomography study. *Stroke.* 2005;36:1759–1763.

121. Johansen-Berg H, Rushworth MF, Bogdanovic MD, et al. The role of ipsilateral premotor cortex in hand movement after stroke. *Proc Natl Acad Sci U S A.* 2002;99:14518–14523.

122. Werhahn KJ, Conforto AB, Kadom N, et al. Contribution of the ipsilateral motor cortex to recovery after chronic stroke. *Ann Neurol.* 2003;54:464–472.

123. Butefisch CM, Kleiser R, Korber B, et al. Recruitment of contralesional motor cortex in stroke patients with recovery of hand function. *Neurology.* 2005;64:1067–1069.

124. Serrien DJ, Strens LH, Cassidy MJ, et al. Functional significance of the ipsilateral hemisphere during movement of the affected hand after stroke. *Exp Neurol.* 2004;190:425–432.

125. Gerloff C, Bushara K, Sailer A, et al. Multimodal imaging of brain reorganization in motor areas of the contralesional hemisphere of well recovered patients after capsular stroke. *Brain.* 2006;129:791–808.

126. Ward NS, Brown MM, Thompson AJ, et al. The influence of time after stroke on brain activations during a motor task. *Ann Neurol.* 2004;55:829–834.

127. Small SL, Hlustik P, Noll DC, et al. Cerebellar hemispheric activation ipsilateral to the paretic hand correlates with functional recovery after stroke. *Brain.* 2002;125:1544–1557.

128. Saur D, Lange R, Baumgaertner A, et al. Dynamics of language reorganization after stroke. *Brain.* 2006;129:1371–1384.

129. Ward NS, Brown MM, Thompson AJ, et al. Neural correlates of motor recovery after stroke: a longitudinal fMRI study. *Brain.* 2003;126:2476–2496.

130. Witte OW, Stoll G. Delayed and remote effects of focal cortical infarctions: secondary damage and reactive plasticity. *Adv Neurol.* 1997;73:207–227.

131. Chen R, Cohen LG, Hallett M. Nervous system reorganization following injury. *Neuroscience.* 2002;111:761–773.

132. von Monakow C. Diaschisis, 1914. In: Pribram K, ed. *Brain and Behavior I. Mood, States and Mind.* Baltimore, MD: Penguin Books; 1969:26–34.

133. Feeney DM, Baron JC. Diaschisis. *Stroke.* 1986;17:817–830.

134. Carmichael ST, Tatsukawa K, Katsman D, et al. Evolution of diaschisis in a focal stroke model. *Stroke.* 2004;35:758–763.

135. Seitz RJ, Azari NP, Knorr U, et al. The role of diaschisis in stroke recovery. *Stroke.* 1999;30:1844–1850.

136. Biernaskie J, Chernenko G, Corbett D. Efficacy of rehabilitative experience declines with time after focal ischemic brain injury. *J Neurosci.* 2004;24:1245–1254.

137. Dromerick A, Lang C, Powers W. Very early constraint-induced movement therapy (VECTORS): A single-center RCT. *Neurology.* 2009;73:195–201.

138. Hinkle JL. Variables explaining functional recovery following motor stroke. *J Neurosci Nurs.* 2006;38:6–12.

139. Kwakkel G, Kollen BJ, van der Grond J, et al. Probability of regaining dexterity in the flaccid upper limb: impact of severity of paresis and time since onset in acute stroke. *Stroke.* 2003;34:2181–2186.

140. Feys H, Van Hees J, Bruyninckx F, et al. Value of somatosensory and motor evoked potentials in predicting arm recovery after a stroke. *J Neurol Neurosurg Psychiatry.* 2000;68:323–331.

141. Escudero JV, Sancho J, Bautista D, et al. Prognostic value of motor evoked potential obtained by transcranial magnetic brain stimulation in motor function recovery in patients with acute ischemic stroke. *Stroke.* 1998;29:1854–1859.

142. Watanabe T, Honda Y, Fujii Y, et al. Three-dimensional anisotropy contrast magnetic resonance axonography to predict the prognosis for motor function in patients suffering from stroke. *J Neurosurg.* 2001;94:955–960.

143. Heald A, Bates D, Cartlidge NE, et al. Longitudinal study of central motor conduction time following stroke. 2. Central motor conduction measured within 72 h after stroke as a predictor of functional outcome at 12 months. *Brain.* 1993;116(Pt 6):1371–1385.

144. Crafton K, Mark A, Cramer S. Improved understanding of cortical injury by incorporating measures of functional anatomy. *Brain.* 2003;126:1650–1659.

145. Tilling K, Sterne JA, Rudd AG, et al. A new method for predicting recovery after stroke. *Stroke.* 2001;32:2867–2873.

146. Uchino K, Billheimer D, Cramer SC. Entry criteria and baseline characteristics predict outcome in acute stroke trials. *Stroke.* 2001;32:909–916.

147. Gainotti G, Antonucci G, Marra C, et al. Relation between depression after stroke, antidepressant therapy, and functional recovery. *J Neurol Neurosurg Psychiatry.* 2001;71:258–261.

148. Kotila M, Waltimo O, Niemi ML, et al. The profile of recovery from stroke and factors influencing outcome. *Stroke.* 1984;15:1039–1044.

149. Kwakkel G. Impact of intensity of practice after stroke: issues for consideration. *Disabil Rehabil.* 2006;28:823–830.

150. Dobkin BH. The clinical science of neurologic rehabilitation. *Oxford Univ Press.* 2003;74:466–467.

151. Kwakkel G, Wagenaar R, Twisk J. Intensity of leg and arm training after primary middle-cerebral-artery stroke: a randomised trial. *Lancet.* 1999;354:191–196.

152. Van Peppen RP, Kwakkel G, Wood-Dauphinee S, et al. The impact of physical therapy on functional outcomes after stroke: what's the evidence? *Clin Rehabil.* 2004;18:833–862.

153. Cicerone KD, Dahlberg C, Malec JF, et al. Evidence-based cognitive rehabilitation: updated review of the literature from 1998 through 2002. *Arch Phys Med Rehabil.* 2005;86:1681–1692.

154. Bhogal S, Teasell R, Speechley M. Intensity of aphasia therapy, impact on recovery. *Stroke.* 2003;34:987–993.

155. Globus A, Rosenzweig MR, Bennett EL, et al. Effects of differential experience on dendritic spine counts in rat cerebral cortex. *J Comp Physiol Psychol.* 1973;82:175–181.

156. Will BE, Rosenzweig MR, Bennett EL, et al. Relatively brief environmental enrichment aids recovery of learning capacity and alters brain measures after postweaning brain lesions in rats. *J Comp Physiol Psychol.* 1977;91:33–50.

157. Kleim JA, Chan S, Pringle E, et al. BDNF val66met polymorphism is associated with modified experience-dependent plasticity in human motor cortex. *Nat Neurosci.* 2006;9:735–737.

158. Siironen J, Juvela S, Kanarek K, et al. The Met allele of the BDNF Val66Met polymorphism predicts poor outcome among survivors of aneurysmal subarachnoid hemorrhage. *Stroke.* 2007;38(10):2858–2860.

159. Goldstein LB. Common drugs may influence motor recovery after stroke. The Sygen In Acute Stroke Study Investigators. *Neurology.* 1995;45:865–871.

160. Troisi E, Paolucci S, Silvestrini M, et al. Prognostic factors in stroke rehabilitation: the possible role of pharmacological treatment. *Acta Neurol Scand.* 2002;105:100–106.

161. Conroy B, Zorowitz R, Horn SD, et al. An exploration of central nervous system medication use and outcomes in stroke rehabilitation. *Arch Phys Med Rehabil.* 2005;86:73–81.

162. Zhao CS, Hartikainen S, Schallert T, et al. CNS-active drugs in aging population at high risk of cerebrovascular events: Evidence from preclinical and clinical studies. *Neurosci Biobehav Rev.* 2008;32:56–71.

163. Overman JJ, Carmichael ST. Plasticity in the injured brain: more than molecules matter. *Neuroscientist.* 2014;20:15–28.

164. Urban ETRI, Bury SD, Guggenmos DJ. Gene expression changes of interconnected spared cortical neurons 7 days after ischemic infarct of the primary motor cortex in the rat. *Mol Cell Biochem.* 2012;369:267–286.

165. Lazar RM, Fitzsimmons B-F, Marshall RS, et al. Reemergence of stroke deficits with midazolam challenge. *Stroke.* 2002;33:283–285.

166. Thal GD, Szabo MD, Lopez-Bresnahan M, et al. Exacerbation or unmasking of focal neurologic deficits by sedatives. *Anesthesiology.* 1996;85:21–25.

167. Kleim JA, Bruneau R, Calder K, et al. Functional organization of adult motor cortex is dependent upon continued protein synthesis. *Neuron.* 2003;40:167–176.

168. Miyai I, Reding MJ. Effects of antidepressants on functional recovery following stroke. *Neurorehabil Neural Repair.* 1998;12:5–13.

169. Dam M, Tonin P, De Boni A, et al. Effects of fluoxetine and maprotiline on functional recovery in poststroke hemiplegic patients undergoing rehabilitation therapy. *Stroke.* 1996;27:1211–1214.

170. Sivenius J, Sarasoja T, Aaltonen H. Selegiline treatment facilitates recovery after stroke. *Neurorehabil Neural Repair.* 2001;15:183–190.

171. Grade C, Redford B, Chrostowski J, et al. Methylphenidate in early poststroke recovery: a double-blind, placebo-controlled study. *Arch Phys Med Rehabil.* 1998;79:1047–1050.

172. Scheidtmann K, Fries W, Müller F, et al. Effect of levodopa in combination with physiotherapy on functional motor recovery after stroke: a prospective, randomised, double-blind study. *Lancet.* 2001;358:787–790.

173. Crisostomo EA, Duncan PW, Propst M, et al. Evidence that amphetamine with physical therapy promotes recovery of motor function in stroke patients. *Ann Neurol.* 1988;23:94–97.

174. Walker-Batson D, Smith P, Curtis S, et al. Amphetamine paired with physical therapy accelerates motor recovery after stroke. Further evidence. *Stroke.* 1995;26:2254–2259.

175. Gladstone DJ, Danells CJ, Armesto A, et al. Physiotherapy coupled with dextroamphetamine for rehabilitation after hemiparetic stroke: a randomized, double-blind, placebo-controlled trial. *Stroke.* 2006;37:179–185.

176. Chen P, Goldberg DE, Kolb B, et al. Inosine induces axonal rewiring and improves behavioral outcome after stroke. *Proc Natl Acad Sci U S A.* 2002;99(13):9031–9036.

177. Chen MDJ, Xu C, Zacharek MSA, et al. Niaspan increases angiogenesis and improves functional recovery after stroke. *Ann Neurol.* 2007;62:49–58.

178. Wahlgren NG, Martinsson L. New concepts for drug therapy after stroke. Can we enhance recovery? *Cerebrovasc Dis.* 1998;8:33–38.

179. Phillips JP, Devier DJ, Feeney DM. Rehabilitation pharmacology: bridging laboratory work to clinical application. *J Head Trauma Rehabil.* 2003;18:342–356.

180. Gu Q. Neuromodulatory transmitter systems in the cortex and their role in cortical plasticity. *Neuroscience.* 2002;111:815–835.

181. Schabitz WR, Berger C, Kollmar R. Effect of brain-derived neurotrophic factor treatment and forced arm use on functional motor recovery after small cortical ischemia. *Stroke.* 2004;35:992–997.

182. Wang L, Zhang Z, Wang Y, et al. Treatment of stroke with erythropoietin enhances neurogenesis and angiogenesis and improves neurological function in rats. *Stroke.* 2004;35:1732–1737.

183. Schneider UC, Schilling L, Schroeck H, et al. Granulocyte-macrophage colony-stimulating factor-induced vessel growth restores cerebral blood supply after bilateral carotid artery occlusion. *Stroke.* 2007;38:1320–1328.

184. Kolb B, Morshead C, Gonzalez C, et al. Growth factor-stimulated generation of new cortical tissue and functional recovery after stroke damage to the motor cortex of rats. *J Cereb Blood Flow Metab.* 2007;27:983–997.

185. Hou ST, Jiang SX, Smith RA. Permissive and repulsive cues and signalling pathways of axonal outgrowth and regeneration. *Int Rev Cell Mol Biol.* 2008;267:125–181.

186. Cash D, Easton AC, Mesquita M, et al. GSK249320, a monoclonal antibody against the axon outgrowth inhibition molecule myelin-associated glycoprotein, improves outcome of rodents with experimental stroke. *J Neurol Exp Neurosci.* 2016;2:28–33.

187. Cramer SC, Enney LA, Russell CK. Proof-of-concept randomization trial of the monoclonal antibody GSK249320 versus placebo in stroke patients. *Stroke.* 2017;48:692–698.

188. Zhang Y, Pardridge WM. Blood-brain barrier targeting of BDNF improves motor function in rats with middle cerebral artery occlusion. *Brain Res.* 2006;1111:227–229.

189. Yu J, Vodyanik MA, Smuga-Otto K. Induced pluripotent stem cell lines derived from human somatic cells. *Science.* 2007;318:1917–1920.

190. Chen CP, Lee YJ, Chiu ST. The application of stem cells in the treatment of ischemic diseases. *Histol Histopathol.* 2006;21:1209–1216.

191. Savitz SI, Dinsmore JH, Wechsler LR. Cell therapy for stroke. *NeuroRx.* 2004;1:406–414.

192. Yip HK, Chang LT, Chang WN. Level and value of circulating endothelial progenitor cells in patients after acute ischemic stroke. *Stroke.* 2008;39:69–74.

193. Lapergue B, Mohammad A, Shuaib A. Endothelial progenitor cells and cerebrovascular diseases. *Prog Neurobiol.* 2007;83:349–362.

194. Kondziolka D, Steinberg GK, Wechsler L, et al. Neurotransplantation for patients with subcortical motor stroke: a phase 2 randomized trial. *J Neurosurg.* 2005;103(1):38–45.

195. Kondziolka D, Wechsler L, Goldstein S, et al. Transplantation of cultured human neuronal cells for patients with stroke. *Neurology.* 2000;55:565–569.

196. Bang OY, Lee JS, Lee PH, et al. Autologous mesenchymal stem cell transplantation in stroke patients. *Ann Neurol.* 2005;58:653–654.

197. Shen LH, Li Y, Chen J, et al. Therapeutic benefit of bone marrow stromal cells administered 1 month after stroke. *J Cereb Blood Flow Metab.* 2007;27:6–13.

198. Kurozumi K, Nakamura K, Tamiya T. BDNF gene-modified mesenchymal stem cells promote functional recovery and reduce infarct size in the rat middle cerebral artery occlusion model. *Mol Ther.* 2004;9:189–197.

199. Liu H, Honmou O, Harada K. Neuroprotection by PlGF gene-modified human mesenchymal stem cells after cerebral ischaemia. *Brain.* 2006;129:2734–2745.

200. Zhao MZ, Nonoguchi N, Ikeda N, et al. Novel therapeutic strategy for stroke in rats by bone marrow stromal cells and ex vivo HGF gene transfer with HSV-1 vector. *J Cereb Blood Flow Metab.* 2006;26:1176–1188.

201. Horita Y, Honmou O, Harada K, et al. Intravenous administration of glial cell line-derived neurotrophic factor gene-modified human mesenchymal stem cells protects against injury in a cerebral ischemia model in the adult rat. *J Neurosci Res.* 2006;84:1495–1504.

202. Savitz SI. Developing cellular therapies for stroke. *Stroke.* 2015;46:2026–2031.

203. Christopher EJ. Electroconvulsive therapy in the medically ill. *Curr Psychiatry Rep.* 2003;5:225–230.

204. Valero-Cabre A, Payne BR, Pascual-Leone A. Opposite impact on (14)C-2-deoxyglucose brain metabolism following patterns of high and low frequency repetitive transcranial magnetic stimulation in the posterior parietal cortex. *Exp Brain Res.* 2007;176:603–615.

205. Khedr EM, Ahmed MA, Fathy N, et al. Therapeutic trial of repetitive transcranial magnetic stimulation after acute ischemic stroke. *Neurology.* 2005;65:466–468.

206. Hummel F, Celnik P, Giraux P. Effects of non-invasive cortical stimulation on skilled motor function in chronic stroke. *Brain.* 2005;128:490–499.

207. Graef P, Dadalt ML, Rodrigues DA, et al. Transcranial magnetic stimulation combined with upper-limb training for improving function after stroke: a systematic review and meta-analysis. *J Neurol Sci.* 2016;369:149–158.

208. Brown JA, Lutsep HL, Weinand M, et al. Motor cortex stimulation for the enhancement of recovery from stroke: a prospective, multicenter safety study. *Neurosurgery.* 2006;58:464–473.

209. Levy RM, Harvey RL, Kissela BM, et al. Epidural electrical stimulation for stroke rehabilitation: results of the prospective, multicenter, randomized, single-blinded Everest trial. *Neurorehabil Neural Repair.* 2016;30:107–119.

210. Nitsche MA, Paulus W. Excitability changes induced in the human motor cortex by weak transcranial direct current stimulation. *J Physiol.* 2000;527(Pt 3):633–639.

211. Monai H, Ohkura M, Tanaka M, et al. Calcium imaging reveals glial involvement in transcranial direct current stimulation-induced plasticity in mouse brain. *Nat Commun.* 2016;7:11100.

212. Elsner B, Kwakkel G, Kugler J, et al. Transcranial direct current stimulation (tDCS) for improving capacity in activities and arm function after stroke: a network meta-analysis of randomised controlled trials. *J Neuroeng Rehabil.* 2017;14:95.

213. Elsner B, Kugler J, Pohl M, et al. Transcranial direct current stimulation (tDCS) for improving aphasia in patients after stroke. *Cochrane Database Syst Rev.* 2013;(6):CD009760.

214. Salazar APS, Vaz PG, Marchese RR, et al. Noninvasive brain stimulation improves hemispatial neglect after stroke: a systematic review and meta-analysis. *Arch Phys Med Rehabil.* 2018;99:355.e1–366.e1.

215. Hochberg LR, Serruya MD, Friehs GM, et al. Neuronal ensemble control of prosthetic devices by a human with tetraplegia. *Nature*. 2006;442:164–171.
216. Schiff ND, Giacino JT, Kalmar K, et al. Behavioural improvements with thalamic stimulation after severe traumatic brain injury. *Nature*. 2007;448:600–603.
217. Lampl Y, Zivin JA, Fisher M. Infrared laser therapy for ischemic stroke: a new treatment strategy: results of the NeuroThera Effectiveness and Safety Trial-1 (NEST-1). *Stroke*. 2007;38:1843–1849.
218. Ring H, Rosenthal N. Controlled study of neuroprosthetic functional electrical stimulation in sub-acute post-stroke. *J Rehabilitation Med*. 2005;37:32–36.
219. Sheffler LR, Chae MDJ. Neuromuscular electrical stimulation in neurorehabilitation. *Muscle Nerve*. 2007;35:562–590.
220. Kwakkel G, Kollen BJ, Krebs HI. Effects of robot-assisted therapy on upper limb recovery after stroke: a systematic review. *Neurorehabil Neural Repair*. 2008;22:111–121.
221. Volpe BT, Ferraro M, Lynch D, et al. Robotics and other devices in the treatment of patients recovering from stroke. *Curr Neurol Neurosci Rep*. 2005;5:465–470.
222. Reinkensmeyer D, Emken J, Cramer S. Robotics, motor learning, and neurologic recovery. *Annu Rev Biomed Eng*. 2004;6:497–525.
223. Deutsch JE, Lewis JA, Burdea G, et al. Technical and patient performance using a virtual reality-integrated telerehabilitation system: preliminary finding. *IEEE Trans Neural Syst Rehabil Eng*. 2007;15:30–35.
224. Duncan P, Studenski S, Richards L. Randomized clinical trial of therapeutic exercise in subacute stroke. *Stroke*. 2003;34:2173–2180.
225. Woldag H, Hummelsheim H. Evidence-based physiotherapeutic concepts for improving arm and hand function in stroke patients: a review. *J Neurol*. 2002;249:518–528.
226. French B, Forster A, Langhorne P, et al. Repetitive task training for improving functional ability after stroke. *Cochrane Database Syst Rev*. 2007;(4):CD006073.
227. Sharma N, Pomeroy VM, Baron JC. Motor imagery: a backdoor to the motor system after stroke? *Stroke*. 2006;37:1941–1952.
228. Rode G, Pisella L, Rossetti Y, et al. Bottom-up transfer of sensory-motor plasticity to recovery of spatial cognition: visuomotor adaptation and spatial neglect. *Prog Brain Res*. 2003;142:273–287.
229. Butefisch C, Khurana V, Kopylev L, et al. Enhancing encoding of a motor memory in the primary motor cortex by cortical stimulation. *J Neurophysiol*. 2004;91:2110–2116.
230. Page SJ, Levine P, Leonard A. Mental practice in chronic stroke: results of a randomized, placebo-controlled trial. *Stroke*. 2007;38:1293–1297.
231. Johnson-Frey SH. Stimulation through simulation? Motor imagery and functional reorganization in hemiplegic stroke patients. *Brain Cogn*. 2004;55:328–331.
232. Mulder T. Motor imagery and action observation: cognitive tools for rehabilitation. *J Neural Transm (Vienna)*. 2007;114:1265–1278.
233. Luft A, McCombe-Waller S, Whitall J. Repetitive bilateral arm training and motor cortex activation in chronic stroke: a randomized controlled trial. *JAMA*. 2004;292:1853–1861.
234. Sanchez RJ, Liu J, Rao S, et al. Automating arm movement training following severe stroke: functional exercises with quantitative feedback in a gravity-reduced environment. *IEEE Trans Neural Syst Rehabil Eng*. 2006;14:378–389.
235. Page SJ, Levine P. Back from the brink: electromyography-triggered stimulation combined with modified constraint-induced movement therapy in chronic stroke. *Arch Phys Med Rehabil*. 2006;87(1):27–31.
236. Lindberg P, Schmitz C, Forssberg H, et al. Effects of passive-active movement training on upper limb motor function and cortical activation in chronic patients with stroke: a pilot study. *J Rehabil Med*. 2004;36:117–123.
237. Pohl M, Mehrholz J, Ritschel C, et al. Speed-dependent treadmill training in ambulatory hemiparetic stroke patients: a randomized controlled trial. *Stroke*. 2002;33:553–558.
238. Sullivan KJ, Knowlton BJ, Dobkin BH. Step training with body weight support: effect of treadmill speed and practice paradigms on poststroke locomotor recovery. *Arch Phys Med Rehabil*. 2002;83:683–691.
239. Lang CE, Strube MJ, Bland MD. Does response of task-specific upper limb training in people at least 6 months poststroke: a phase II, single-blind, randomized, controlled trial. *Ann Neurol*. 2016;80(3):342–354.
240. Taub E, Uswatte G, Mark VW, et al. The learned nonuse phenomenon: implications for rehabilitation. *Eura Medicophys*. 2006;42:241–256.
241. Wolf SL, Winstein CJ, Miller JP. Effect of constraint-induced movement therapy on upper extremity function 3 to 9 months after stroke: the EXCITE randomized clinical trial. *JAMA*. 2006;296:2095–2104.
242. Wolf SL, Winstein CJ, Miller JP, et al. Retention of upper limb function in stroke survivors who have received constraint-induced movement therapy: the EXCITE randomised trial. *Lancet Neurol*. 2008;7:33–40.
243. Meinzer M, Elbert T, Djundja D, et al. Extending the constraint-induced movement therapy (CIMT) approach to cognitive functions: constraint-induced aphasia therapy (CIAT) of chronic aphasia. *NeuroRehabilitation*. 2007;22:311–318.
244. McKenna JE, Whishaw IQ. Complete compensation in skilled reaching success with associated impairments in limb synergies, after dorsal column lesion in the rat. *J Neurosci*. 1999;19:1885–1894.
245. Cirstea MC, Levin MF. Improvement of arm movement patterns and endpoint control depends on type of feedback during practice in stroke survivors. *Neurorehabil Neural Repair*. 2007;21(5):398–411.
246. Kozlowski DA, James DC, Schallert T. Use-dependent exaggeration of neuronal injury after unilateral sensorimotor cortex lesions. *J Neurosci*. 1996;16:4776–4786.
247. Penfield W, Boldrey E. Somatic motor and sensory representation in the cerebral cortex of man as studied by electrical stimulation. *Brain*. 1937;60:389–443.
248. Whitaker HA, Selnes OA. Anatomic variations in the cortex: individual differences and the problem of the localization of language functions. *Ann N Y Acad Sci*. 1976;280:844–854.
249. Van Essen DC, Drury HA, Joshi S, et al. Functional and structural mapping of human cerebral cortex: solutions are in the surfaces. *Proc Natl Acad Sci U S A*. 1998;95:788–795.
250. Cramer S, Benson R, Burra V. Mapping individual brains to guide restorative therapy after stroke: rationale and pilot studies. *Neurol Res*. 2003;25:811–814.
251. Dong Y, Dobkin BH, Cen SY. Motor cortex activation during treatment may predict therapeutic gains in paretic hand function after stroke. *Stroke*. 2006;37:1552–1555.
252. Koski L, Mernar TJ, Dobkin BH. Immediate and long-term changes in corticomotor output in response to rehabilitation: correlation with functional improvements in chronic stroke. *Neurorehabil Neural Repair*. 2004;18:230–249.
253. Kombos T, Suess O, Funk T, et al. Intra-operative mapping of the motor cortex during surgery in and around the motor cortex. *Acta Neurochir*. 2000;142:263–268.
254. Cramer SC, Benson RR, Himes DM, et al. Use of functional MRI to guide decisions in a clinical stroke trial. *Stroke*. 2005;36:50–52.
255. Platz T, Kim IH, Engel U, et al. Brain activation pattern as assessed with multi-modal EEG analysis predict motor recovery among stroke patients with mild arm paresis who receive the Arm Ability Training. *Restor Neurol Neurosci*. 2002;20:21–35.
256. Stinear CM, Barber PA, Smale PR, et al. Functional potential in chronic stroke patients depends on corticospinal tract integrity. *Brain*. 2007;130:170–180.
257. Stephen RM, Gillies RJ. Promise and progress for functional and molecular imaging of response to targeted therapies. *Pharm Res*. 2007;24:1172–1185.
258. Fleming TR, DeMets DL. Surrogate end points in clinical trials: are we being misled? *Ann Intern Med*. 1996;125:605–613.
259. Bucher HC, Guyatt GH, Cook DJ, et al. Users' guides to the medical literature: XIX. Applying clinical trial results. A How to use an article measuring the effect of an intervention on surrogate end points Evidence-Based Medicine Working Group. *JAMA*. 1999;282:771–778.
260. Vukusic S, Confavreux C. Natural history of multiple sclerosis: risk factors and prognostic indicators. *Curr Opin Neurol*. 2007;20:269–274.
261. Quintern J, Immisch I, Albrecht H, et al. Influence of visual and proprioceptive afferences on upper limb ataxia in patients with multiple sclerosis. *J Neurol Sci*. 1999;163:61–69.
262. Vollmer T. The natural history of relapses in multiple sclerosis. *J Neurol Sci*. 2007;256(suppl 1):S5–S13.
263. Rocca MA, Colombo B, Falini A. Cortical adaptation in patients with MS: a cross-sectional functional MRI study of disease phenotypes. *Lancet Neurol*. 2005;4:618–626.
264. Wang J, Hier DB. Motor reorganization in multiple sclerosis. *Neurol Res*. 2007;29:3–8.
265. Pantano P, Mainero C, Caramia F, et al. Functional brain reorganization in multiple sclerosis: evidence from fMRI studies. *J Neuroimaging*. 2006;16(2):104–114.
266. Lenzi D, Conte A, Mainero C, et al. Effect of corpus callosum damage on ipsilateral motor activation in patients with multiple sclerosis: a functional and anatomical study. *Hum Brain Mapp*. 2007;28(7):636–644.
267. Rocca MA, Gallo A, Colombo B, et al. Pyramidal tract lesions and movement-associated cortical recruitment in patients with MS. *Neuroimage*. 2004;23:141–147.
268. Reddy H, Narayanan S, Matthews PM, et al. Relating axonal injury to functional recovery in MS. *Neurology*. 2000;54:236–239.
269. Mezzapesa DM, Rocca MA, Rodegher M, et al. Functional cortical changes of the sensorimotor network are associated with clinical recovery in multiple sclerosis. *Hum Brain Mapp*. 2008;29(5):562–573.
270. Filippi M, Rocca MA, Mezzapesa DM, et al. A functional MRI study of cortical activations associated with object manipulation in patients with MS. *Neuroimage*. 2004;21(3):1147–1154.
271. Gallo V, Armstrong RC. Myelin repair strategies: a cellular view. *Curr Opin Neurol*. 2008;21:278–283.
272. Popovich PG, Longbrake EE. Can the immune system be harnessed to repair the CNS? *Nat Rev Neurosci*. 2008;9:481–493.
273. Payne N, Siatskas C, Bernard CC. The promise of stem cell and regenerative therapies for multiple sclerosis. *J Autoimmun*. 2008;31:288–294.
274. Hohlfeld R, Neurotrophic cross-talk between the nervous and immune systems: relevance for repair strategies in multiple sclerosis? *J Neurol Sci*. 2008;265(1–2):93–96.
275. Parry AM, Scott RB, Palace J. Potentially adaptive functional changes in cognitive processing for patients with multiple sclerosis and their acute modulation by rivastigmine. *Brain*. 2003;126:2750–2760.
276. Mainero C, Inghilleri M, Pantano P, et al. Enhanced brain motor activity in patients with MS after a single dose of 3,4-diaminopyridine. *Neurology*. 2004;62:2044–2050.
277. Celnik P, Hummel F, Harris-Love M, et al. Somatosensory stimulation enhances the effects of training functional hand tasks in patients with chronic stroke. *Arch Phys Med Rehabil*. 2007;88:1369–1376.
278. Rocca MA, Absinta M, Moiola L, et al. Functional and structural connectivity of the motor network in pediatric and adult-onset relapsing-remitting multiple sclerosis. *Radiology*. 2010;254:541–550.
279. Enzinger C, Pinter D, Rocca MA. Longitudinal fMRI studies: exploring brain plasticity and repair in MS. *Mult Scler*. 2016;22(3):269–278.
280. Pantano P, Bernardi S, Tinelli E. Impaired cortical deactivation during hand movement in the relapsing phase of multiple sclerosis: a cross-sectional and longitudinal fMRI study. *Mult Scler*. 2011;17:1177–1184.
281. Parisi L, Rocca MA, Mattioli F. Changes of brain resting state functional connectivity predict the persistence of cognitive rehabilitation effects in patients with multiple sclerosis. *Mult Scler*. 2014;20:686–694.
282. Ma VY, Chan L, Carruthers KJ. Incidence, prevalence, costs, and impact on disability of common conditions requiring rehabilitation in the United States: stroke, spinal cord injury, traumatic brain injury, multiple sclerosis, osteoarthritis, rheumatoid arthritis, limb loss, and back pain. *Arch Phys Med Rehabil*. 2014;95:986–995.

283. Ditunno JF, Stover SL, Freed MM, et al. Motor recovery of the upper extremities in traumatic quadriplegia: a multicenter study. *Arch Phys Med Rehabil.* 1992;73:431–436.

284. *Facts and Figures at a Glance-June 2006*; 2007. Available from: www.spinalcord.uab.edu

285. Kirshblum S, Millis S, McKinley W, et al. Late neurologic recovery after traumatic spinal cord injury. *Arch Phys Med Rehabil.* 2004;85:1811–1817.

286. Jayaraman A, Gregory CM, Bowden M, et al. Lower extremity skeletal muscle function in persons with incomplete spinal cord injury. *Spinal Cord.* 2006;44(11):680–687.

287. DeVivo MJ, Richards JS. Community reintegration and quality of life following spinal cord injury. *Paraplegia.* 1992;30:108–112.

288. Frankel HL, Coll JR, Charlifue SW, et al. Long-term survival in spinal cord injury: a fifty year investigation. *Spinal Cord.* 1998;36:266–274.

289. Anderson KD. Targeting recovery: priorities of the spinal cord-injured population. *J Neurotrauma.* 2004;21(10):1371–1383.

290. Cramer SC, Lastra L, Lacourse MG, et al. Brain motor system function after chronic, complete spinal cord injury. *Brain.* 2005;128:2941–2950.

291. Jurkiewicz MT, Mikulis DJ, McIlroy WE, et al. Sensorimotor cortical plasticity during recovery following spinal cord injury: a longitudinal fMRI study. *Neurorehabil Neural Repair.* 2007;21:527–538.

292. Sabbah P, de Schonen S, Leveque C, et al. Sensorimotor cortical activity in patients with complete spinal cord injury: a functional magnetic resonance imaging study. *J Neurotrauma.* 2002;19:53–60.

293. Alkadhi H, Brugger P, Boendermaker SH, et al. What disconnection tells about motor imagery: evidence from paraplegic patients. *Cereb Cortex.* 2005;15(2):131–140.

294. Topka H, Cohen LG, Cole RA, et al. Reorganization of corticospinal pathways following spinal cord injury. *Neurology.* 1991;41:1276–1283.

295. Bruehlmeier M, Dietz V, Leenders KL, et al. How does the human brain deal with a spinal cord injury? *Eur J Neurosci.* 1998;10:3918–3922.

296. Mikulis DJ, Jurkiewicz MT, McIlroy WE, et al. Adaptation in the motor cortex following cervical spinal cord injury. *Neurology.* 2002;58:794–801.

297. Turner J, Lee J, Martinez O, et al. Somatotopy of the motor cortex after long-term spinal cord injury or amputation. *IEEE Trans Neural Syst Rehabil Eng.* 2001;9(2):154–160.

298. Wrigley PJ, Gustin SM, Macey PM, et al. Anatomical changes in human motor cortex and motor pathways following complete thoracic spinal cord injury. *Cereb Cortex.* 2009;19(1):224–232.

299. Nicotra A, Critchley HD, Mathias CJ, et al. Emotional and autonomic consequences of spinal cord injury explored using functional brain imaging. *Brain.* 2006;129(Pt 3):718–728.

300. Harkema SJ. Neural plasticity after human spinal cord injury: application of locomotor training to the rehabilitation of walking. *Neuroscientist.* 2001;7:455–468.

301. Wolfe DL, Hayes KC, Hsieh JT, et al. Effects of 4-aminopyridine on motor evoked potentials in patients with spinal cord injury: a double-blinded, placebo-controlled crossover trial. *J Neurotrauma.* 2001;18:757–771.

302. Winchester P, McColl R, Querry R, et al. Changes in supraspinal activation patterns following robotic locomotor therapy in motor-incomplete spinal cord injury. *Neurorehabil Neural Repair.* 2005;19:313–324.

303. Thomas SL, Gorassini MA. Increases in corticospinal tract function by treadmill training after incomplete spinal cord injury. *J Neurophysiol.* 2005;94:2844–2855.

304. Hoffman LR, Field-Fote EC. Cortical reorganization following bimanual training and somatosensory stimulation in cervical spinal cord injury: a case report. *Phys Ther.* 2007;87:208–223.

305. Beekhuizen KS, Field-Fote EC. Massed practice versus massed practice with stimulation: effects on upper extremity function and cortical plasticity in individuals with incomplete cervical spinal cord injury. *Neurorehabil Neural Repair.* 2005;19:33–45.

306. Lacourse MG, Turner JA, Randolph-Orr E, et al. Cerebral and cerebellar sensorimotor plasticity following motor imagery-based mental practice of a sequential movement. *J Rehabil Res Dev.* 2004;41:505–524.

307. Cramer SC, Orr EL, Cohen MJ, et al. Effects of motor imagery training after chronic, complete spinal cord injury. *Exp Brain Res.* 2007;177:233–242.

308. Stevenson AJ, Mrachaczkersting N, van Asseldonk E, et al. Spinal plasticity in robot-mediated therapy for the lower limbs. *J Neuroeng Rehabil.* 2015;12:81.

309. Edgerton VR, Roy RR. Robotic training and spinal cord plasticity. *Brain Res Bull.* 2009;78:4–12.

310. Knikou M, Brand R, Mignardot JB, et al. Functional reorganization of soleus H-reflex modulation during stepping after robotic-assisted step training in people with complete and incomplete spinal cord injury. *Exp Brain Res.* 2013;228(3):279–296.

311. van den Brand R, Mignardot JB, von Zitzewitz J, et al. Neuroprosthetic technologies to augment the impact of neurorehabilitation after spinal cord injury. *Ann Phys Rehabil Med.* 2015;58(4):232–237.

312. Angeli CA, Boakye M, Morton RA, et al. Recovery of over-ground walking after chronic motor complete spinal cord injury. *N Engl J Med.* 2018;379:1244–1250.

313. Willemse-van Son AH, Ribbers GM, Verhagen AP, et al. Prognostic factors of long-term functioning and productivity after traumatic brain injury: a systematic review of prospective cohort studies. *Clin Rehabil.* 2007;21:1024–1037.

314. Nortje J, Menon DK. Traumatic brain injury: physiology, mechanisms, and outcome. *Curr Opin Neurol.* 2004;17:711–718.

315. Crooks CY, Zumsteg JM, Bell KR. Traumatic brain injury: a review of practice management and recent advances. *Phys Med Rehabil Clin N Am.* 2007;18(4):681–710, vi.

316. Hellweg S, Johannes S. Physiotherapy after traumatic brain injury: a systematic review of the literature. *Brain Inj.* 2008;22(5):365–373.

317. Goldstein LB. Neuropharmacology of TBI-induced plasticity. *Brain Inj.* 2003;17(8):685–694.

318. Turner-Stokes L, Pick A, Nair A, et al. Multi-disciplinary rehabilitation for acquired brain injury in adults of working age. *Cochrane Database Syst Rev.* 2005;(12):CD004170.

319. Raghupathi R, McIntosh TK. Pharmacotherapy for traumatic brain injury: a review. *Proc West Pharmacol Soc.* 1998;41:241–246.

320. Chandler MC, Barnhill JL, Gualtieri CT. Amantadine for the agitated head-injury patient. *Brain Inj.* 1988;2:309–311.

321. Gualtieri CT, Evans RW. Stimulant treatment for the neurobehavioural sequelae of traumatic brain injury. *Brain Inj.* 1988;2:273–290.

322. Smith JM, Lunga P, Story D, et al. Inosine promotes recovery of skilled motor function in a model of focal brain injury. *Brain.* 2007;130(Pt 4):915–925.

323. Mostert JP, Koch MW, Heerings M, et al. Therapeutic potential of fluoxetine in neurological disorders. *CNS Neurosci Ther.* 2008;14:153–164.

324. Pape TL-B, Rosenow J, Lewis G. Transcranial magnetic stimulation: a possible treatment for TBI. *J Head Trauma Rehabil.* 2006;21:437–451.

325. Cicerone K, Levin H, Malec J, et al. Cognitive rehabilitation interventions for executive function: moving from bench to bedside in patients with traumatic brain injury. *J Cogn Neurosci.* 2006;18:1212–1222.

326. Stein DG. Progesterone exerts neuroprotective effects after brain injury. *Brain Res Rev.* 2008;57:386–397.

327. Chiaretti A, Antonelli A, Genovese O, et al. Nerve growth factor and doublecortin expression correlates with improved outcome in children with severe traumatic brain injury. *J Trauma.* 2008;65:80–85.

328. Maegele M, Schaefer U. Stem cell-based cellular replacement strategies following traumatic brain injury (TBI). *Minim Invasive Ther Allied Technol.* 2008;17(2):119–131.

329. Mahmood A, Lu D, Chopp M. Intravenous administration of marrow stromal cells (MSCs) increases the expression of growth factors in rat brain after traumatic brain injury. *J Neurotrauma.* 2004;21:33–39.

330. Levin HS. Neuroplasticity following non-penetrating traumatic brain injury. *Brain Inj.* 2003;17:665–674.

331. Sidaros A, Engberg AW, Sidaros K, et al. Diffusion tensor imaging during recovery from severe traumatic brain injury and relation to clinical outcome: a longitudinal study. *Brain.* 2008;131:559–572.

332. Levin HS, Wilde EA, Chu Z, et al. Diffusion tensor imaging in relation to cognitive and functional outcome of traumatic brain injury in children. *J Head Trauma Rehabil.* 2008;23(4):197–208.

333. Voss HU, Ulug AM, Dyke JP, et al. Possible axonal regrowth in late recovery from the minimally conscious state. *J Clin Invest.* 2006;116:2005–2011.

334. Cramer S, Mark A, Barquist K. Motor cortex activation is preserved in patients with chronic hemiplegic stroke. *Ann Neurol.* 2002;52:607–616.

335. Enzinger C, Ropele S, Fazekas F. Brain motor system function in a patient with complete spinal cord injury following extensive brain-computer interface training. *Exp Brain Res.* 2008;190:215–223.

336. Fontaine A, Azouvi P, Remy P, et al. Functional anatomy of neuropsychological deficits after severe traumatic brain injury. *Neurology.* 1999;53:1963–1968.

337. Lotze M, Grodd W, Rodden FA, et al. Neuroimaging patterns associated with motor control in traumatic brain injury. *Neurorehabil Neural Repair.* 2006;20:14–23.

338. Newsome MR, Scheibel RS, Steinberg JL, et al. Working memory brain activation following severe traumatic brain injury. *Cortex.* 2007;43:95–111.

339. Mani TM, Miller LS, Yanasak N, et al. Evaluation of changes in motor and visual functional activation over time following moderate-to-severe brain injury. *Brain Inj.* 2007;21:1155–1163.

340. Sanchez-Carrion R, Gomez PV, Junque C, et al. Frontal hypoactivation on functional magnetic resonance imaging in working memory after severe diffuse traumatic brain injury. *J Neurotrauma.* 2008;25:479–494.

341. Cihangiroglu M, Ramsey RG, Dohrmann GJ. Brain injury: analysis of imaging modalities. *Neurol Res.* 2002;24:7–18.

342. Hunter JV, Thornton RJ, Wang ZJ, et al. Late proton MR spectroscopy in children after traumatic brain injury: correlation with cognitive outcomes. AJNR. *Am J Neuroradiol.* 2005;26:482–488.

343. Belanger HG, Vanderploeg RD, Curtiss G, et al. Recent neuroimaging techniques in mild traumatic brain injury. *J Neuropsychiatry Clin Neurosci.* 2007;19:5–20.

344. Gallagher CN, Hutchinson PJ, Pickard JD. Neuroimaging in trauma. *Curr Opin Neurol.* 2007;20:403–409.

345. Forbes ML. Rare window: functional magnetic resonance imaging and mild traumatic brain injury. *Crit Care Med.* 2007;35:2659–2661.

346. Saatman KE, Duhaime AC, Bullock R, et al. Classification of traumatic brain injury for targeted therapies. *J Neurotrauma.* 2008;25(7):719–738.

347. Cramer SC. Repairing the human brain after stroke. II Restorative therapies. *Ann Neurol.* 2008;63:549–560.

348. Kraus MF, Smith GS, Butters M, et al. Effects of the dopaminergic agent and NMDA receptor antagonist amantadine on cognitive function, cerebral glucose metabolism and D2 receptor availability in chronic traumatic brain injury: a study using positron emission tomography (PET). *Brain Inj.* 2005;19:471–479.

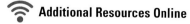 **Additional Resources Online**

62

Shuo-Hsiu (James) Chang
Jennifer L. Sullivan   Marcia K. O'Malley
Zahra Kadivar   Gerard E. Francisco

Rehabilitation Robotics

Following a neurologic injury or disease, the resultant impairments and subsequent decrease in community participation negatively impact quality of life and can account for staggering financial burden. Thus, while the aspirational goals of neurologic therapeutics to reverse a disease or repair injured neural tissue are still not achieved, interventions should focus on restoration of functional capabilities through either provision of assistance or induction of neuroplasticity in the meantime. Rehabilitation plays a major role in reversing the consequences of functional loss through various means, including the teaching of compensatory strategies, motor relearning, and functional retraining. In the last few decades, following discovery that the central nervous system remains plastic after an insult or disease, much emphasis has been placed on targeting neuroplasticity during rehabilitation process (1) (see also Chapter 61). Investigations in animals and humans have demonstrated that task-specific activities of sufficient dosage, intensity, and repetition have the potential to induce or facilitate neuroplastic processes (2). Over time, it has also been recognized that, in general, the effective rehabilitation strategies are ones that involve early intervention and multisensory and multimodality approach (3). The latter may involve human-machine interaction through the use of prostheses, orthoses, or robots.

Robotics has garnered significant attention in rehabilitation, largely due to its demonstrated ability and potential to augment rehabilitation and recovery (4). Already widely employed in other industries, robots have been reliable tools in substituting for lost function, augmenting power and physical capabilities, and minimizing efforts (e.g., robots as orthoses). Initially, the reputed role of robots in rehabilitation was their ability to present a specific task whose intensity (through either variable resistance or high repetition) could be modulated. Robots can relieve therapists of some of the work, thus decreasing personnel costs, minimizing work-related injuries, and promoting consistency of training (5). They can also provide long-term, frequent therapy that may not be affordable given the constraints of the current reimbursement structure for rehabilitation.

To state that the only salient features of robots in augmenting rehabilitation and recovery are their capability to modify intensity and repetition is an oversimplification of their potential as effective rehabilitative tools. Already robots are being seen as agents to heighten sensorimotor/robot-patient interaction through sensory (visual, auditory, proprioceptive, and haptic) feedback and cognitive engagement, which may be critical elements in a multimodality approach to influence neuroplasticity (5). In addition, robots offer a novel method of progressive motor training based on the ability to modify the program to provide increasing levels of resistance while performing a task. These features make robots potent tools that can influence experience-induced neuroplasticity.

Other useful features of robots, that make them attractive in rehabilitation, include their ability to provide objective measurements to document progress and treatment outcomes. Many robots have measurement features that can assess a user's functional capabilities. Most robots have tracking sensors that monitor performance of the robot and, therefore, the user's movements as well. **Figure 62-1** summarizes the features that make robots attractive rehabilitation tools. The objective of this chapter is to introduce the field of rehabilitation robotics. In this chapter, we will provide an overview of robotics terminology, key features, and functions, and a summary of robotic rehabilitation innovations, including clinical applications and future directions, challenges, and opportunities.

A PRIMER ON ROBOTICS

Overview: Robots in the Rehabilitation Domain

In its most generic form, a robot is a machine that can sense, think, and then act: it senses certain aspects of its behavior and/or environment, evaluates those sensory inputs, and then uses that information to choose and perform an action. Rehabilitation robots, more specifically, tend to be controllable electromechanical devices designed for human interaction during rehabilitation exercises. They typically utilize active assistance, guidance, or resistance to train movement and increase strength, although some are designed for assessment purposes only. The vast majority are specific to either the upper limb (UL) or lower limb (LL). UL devices typically utilize some form of target-hitting task to train shoulder, elbow, forearm, wrist, or hand movement. LL devices are often designed to facilitate walking. This section provides an overview of robotic systems, highlighting key fundamental concepts (see Siciliano and Khatib (6) for more details).

Robot Components

Most robots are a collection of link segments that are connected with movable *joints*. Like the majority of human joints, robot joints are often rotational, allowing a link segment to pivot around a joint; however, robots can also have linear joints, which allow for extension and retraction. Joints can also be actuated or nonactuated. Actuated joints are connected to an *actuator*, for example, a motor, which allows them to be controlled programmatically. Actuators are analogous to muscles: they produce a force in response to a command signal, which

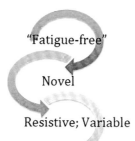

FIGURE 62-1. Features of robots useful in rehabilitation.

causes movement about one or more joints. When joints are not connected to an actuation mechanism, they are called nonactuated joints and must be moved manually. Hinges and sliders are examples of nonactuated joints. In rehabilitation robots, nonactuated joints are often used for adjustability, for example, to accommodate users of various sizes and limb lengths.

The most distal part of the robot is usually what interacts with the environment; for this reason, it is referred to as the *end-effector*. In manufacturing robots, the end effector is often a tool or gripper, depending on the intended function. In rehabilitation robots, especially those designed for ULs, the end effector is usually a handle for the user to grasp. The spatial area that the end effector can reach is called the robot's *workspace*. The size and dimensionality of the workspace depend on a number of design characteristics, but the two main factors are the *range of motion (ROM)* of each joint and how many *degrees of freedom (DOFs)* the robot has. Broadly speaking, a DOF is a direction along which something can move (**Fig. 62-2**). For example, the human knee has only one DOF, flexion/extension, whereas the hip has three DOF (flexion/extension, abduction/adduction, and internal/external rotation). Motions that only utilize one DOF are called

single-DOF movements, whereas motions that combine two or more DOFs are called *multi-DOF* movements. Typically, robots with more DOFs have larger workspaces because they have the flexibility to assume more poses than do robots with fewer DOFs.

Drive System

Actuated joints often utilize some sort of *transmission* between the joint and the actuator. One of the most common purposes of a transmission is to adjust the speed and torque outputs of the motor. Since rehabilitation robots typically need to drive heavy loads at low speeds, the transmission is usually designed to increase the torque and decrease the movement speed at the joint. In other cases, transmissions are used so that the motors, which are heavy, can be mounted on some sort of stationary base instead of on the robot itself. The alternative to a transmission is a *direct drive* implementation, where the actuator is directly connected to its respective joint. The benefit of direct drive is that it is easier to ensure that the movement of the joint will match the (commanded) movement of the actuator, whereas a transmission can introduce undesirable effects such as backlash and additional friction. However, in most direct drive configurations, the actuator needs to be mounted on the robot itself, which will increase the weight of the device compared to a design in which the motors are mounted on a stationary base.

Form Factor

There are three broad classifications that categorize different types of rehabilitation robots: end-effector devices, exoskeletons, and soft robots.

In *end-effector devices*, the contact between the user and the robot is only at the end-effector. A joystick is an example of a very simple, end-effector device. For UL devices, the end-effector is typically a handle for the user to grasp. The main limitation of end-effector devices is that while the robot does track the motion of the end effector (i.e., the user's hand), there is usually no way to measure or track the movement of the user's other joints. Thus, there is no way to prevent compensatory movements without therapist supervision or physical restraints.

Exoskeletons are devices with anatomically-inspired form factors that mimic the structure and movement of human limbs. They are called exoskeletons because they are usually mounted on or around the limb like a brace. The majority of exoskeleton devices designed for rehabilitation purposes are made for either the upper or the lower limb. While LL exoskeletons are typically intended for gait training, there is more diversity among UL devices, which can include any subset of joints from the shoulder to the wrist. Hand exoskeletons are usually separate devices due to the complexity of finger manipulation. Although exoskeletons are usually much more cumbersome than end-effector devices, the advantage they offer is the ability to measure and control the movement at each joint.

Soft robots are not defined by their structure but by their materials. As the name suggests, soft robots are nonrigid devices that are made of compliant materials, often to make them more comfortable to wear. These devices often mount the actuators on a stationary base or in a backpack and utilize some sort of cable transmission system to control the joints.

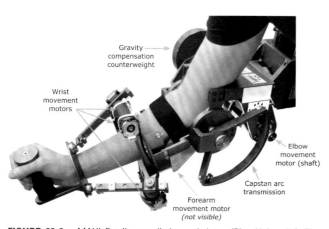

FIGURE 62-2. MAHI Exo-II upper-limb exoskeleton (Rice University). The MAHI Exo-II has four active DOFs: elbow flexion/extension, forearm pronation/supination, wrist flexion/extension, and wrist radial/ulnar deviation. The capstan arc serves as a transmission element between the rotation of the elbow motor and the flexion/extension movement of the user.

The challenge that comes with compliant materials is precise actuation and control; the lack of rigidity makes it difficult to secure the device in a way that ensures accurate tracking of all joint movements.

Dynamics and Control

Rehabilitation exercises that involve active guidance, assistance, or resistance require a means of controlling the robot to produce the desired behavior at the desired time. This means understanding how the force produced by each actuator will affect the movement of the associated joint and how this movement, in turn, will change the overall pose of the robot and the interaction between the robot and the environment. This framework for robot-aided exercise is analogous to human motor control, where the central nervous system determines what command signal should be sent to each muscle to produce a specific action, such as reaching out to grasp an object.

The mathematics required to model and control a robot can be broken into three portions: kinematics, dynamics, and control.

Kinematics broadly refers to the motion of a robot, neglecting the forces that cause it. More specifically, kinematic models describe the relationship between the position, orientation, and movement of each joint and the position, orientation, and movement of the end effector. These equations are based solely on the physical design and geometry of the robot. *Forward* kinematic equations use the position and orientation of the individual joints to compute the resulting pose of the end effector. *Inverse* kinematic equations start with a desired end-effector pose and back-calculate the required position and orientation of each joint.

Building on the kinematics, a robot's *dynamic* equations define the relationship between joint *torques* and *forces* and the ensuing *motion* of the end effector. Similar to forward and inverse kinematics, *forward* dynamic equations use known actuator torques to compute the behavior of the end effector, while *inverse* dynamics start with the desired behavior of the end effector and back-calculate the required joint torques.

The *controller* is the mathematical algorithm that determines what command signal should be sent to each joint actuator to drive the robot to the desired state. The command signal is computed based on the robot's dynamics as well as the difference between the actual and the target value of the parameter of interest. For example, a control law designed to manipulate the position of the end effector would use the position *error*—that is, the difference between the actual position and the desired position—to compute a value of joint torque to command to the actuator(s). The direction of the output torque would drive the end effector toward the desired position, and the magnitude of the output torque would decrease as the position error decreases.

User Interaction

Rehabilitation robots usually have multiple modes of operation in order to accommodate both training and assessment tasks, as well as a wide variety of user ability levels.

For assessment tasks, the robot is typically in *backdrive* mode, which allows the user to move the end effector without any assistance or resistance from the robot. Many rehabilitation robots also incorporate active or passive *gravity*

compensation, which counteracts the weight of the limb and robot so the user can execute movements without having to overcome gravity. Gravity compensation can be achieved passively through mechanical design, like a counterweight, or actively through motor programming and knowledge of the robot's dynamics.

The types of exercises vary significantly across platforms, but one of the most common training modes is *assist-as-needed* (7). As the name implies, an assist-as-needed controller only helps the users when they are struggling to complete the task on their own. As the user moves through the prescribed task, the controller compares his or her behavior (e.g., joint position at a certain time, movement velocity, muscle activation) to a previously recorded reference level. If the user is too far below that reference level, the robot will provide assistance. If the user's behavior catches up to the reference level, the robot will stop assisting. Specifics such as the choice of control parameter (position, velocity, etc.), the reference signal (is it a constant value or a function of time or space?), when the robot assistance kicks in, and how much assistance is provided will all depend on the design of the controller.

CURRENT ROLE OF ROBOTS IN PHYSICAL MEDICINE AND REHABILITATION

Recovery and the rehabilitation strategy for enhancing UL and LL function in patients with neurologic disorders depends on the type and location (cerebral or spinal cord injury [SCI]) and severity of the damage. Improvement of sensorimotor function is attributed largely to spontaneous recovery in the initial phases (i.e., first 3 months) (8,9) and can be achieved by therapies that influence neuroplasticity. The critical elements for facilitating neuroplasticity include the number of tasks/movements, repetition, and task specificity (10), and since robotic systems can offer repetitive, reproducible movements, they are considered as a tool to deliver the therapies efficiently and effectively. Compared to conventional therapies where patients with stroke or SCI perform less than 50 movement repetitions with the training limbs in a typical therapy session, robot-assisted intervention could achieve over 1,000 repetitions per 45- to 60-minute session (11). Moreover, robot-assisted intervention could also promote active physical and cognitive engagement and provide feedback of the movement/task that can enhance motivation and facilitate plasticity (12,13). The proposed functional recovery model of robot-assisted intervention is shown in **Figure 62-3**. Several robotic devices have been used to investigate their effectiveness in neurologic recovery. These robotic devices vary greatly in terms of design. The majority of research for the neurologic population has focused on stroke survivors (see Chapter 18) with more limited efforts devoted to other neurologic diagnoses such as SCI (see Chapter 22), traumatic brain injury (TBI; see Chapter 19), and cerebral palsy (CP; see Chapter 45). In addition to assisting in therapeutic intervention, robotic systems can also assist in (a) activities of daily living (ADLs) to restore independence and function, such as reaching and grasping and overground walking and (b) assessment of function and monitoring the recovery progress. More specific information can be found in the next section.

Robot-assisted rehabilitation can further be developed and analyzed in the context of the International Classification of Functioning, Disability, and Health (ICF) framework

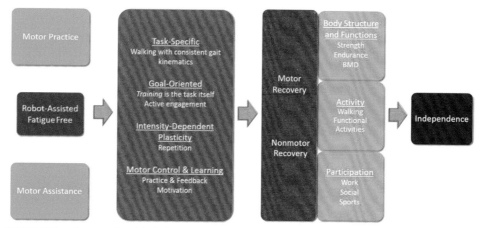

FIGURE 62-3. A proposed model of robot-assisted rehabilitation in promoting functional recovery and independence.

(see Chapter 9) with an emphasis on person-centered rehabilitation (14). For example, powered orthoses and wearable exoskeletons could promote mobility and community reintegration (activity and participation domain); using robotic technology could promote motivation (personal factor domain) and public policy and health care reimbursement that is conducive to the use of rehabilitation robots (environmental factor domain).

CURRENT EVIDENCE

Upper Limb Rehabilitation with Robots

Utilization of robotic devices for UL rehabilitation is considered a novel, reliable, and efficient approach in delivering therapy following impairments impacting UL movement and function. Regaining UL function is an important indicator of quality of life (15,16). Current literature on rehabilitation robotic devices for UL research indicates that task-specific (17) and task-intensive practice (18) could significantly improve motor recovery and neuroplasticity after neurologic injuries. The greater effectiveness of intensive, task-specific practice relative to standard therapy techniques suggests that repetitive motor practice is a crucial rehabilitation component and presents a key opportunity for the introduction of robotics in rehabilitation.

Upper Limb Robotic Devices

Numerous UL robotic devices have been made commercially available for clinical use. These devices offer different types of motion assistance and target specific UL joints. **Table 62-1** provides a summary of the commercially available robotic devices with details including joint movements they support. We identified the following joints for the purpose of this chapter: shoulder, elbow, forearm, wrist, and fingers. This table also includes details on the types of motions these devices support as well as the patient population they are intended for. The specified population as well as FDA status is based on what was listed for device marketing including publications.

Robot-Assisted Assessment

Evaluation and assessment of UL function are the key to understanding the effectiveness of rehabilitation as well as justifying reimbursement for insurance purposes. Although assessments vary depending on the impairment type, certain outcomes are commonly used for assessment of UL function in individuals

with neurologic injuries. Some of these assessments include range-of-motion testing, grip strength, box and blocks test (19), Fugl-Meyer Arm Motor Scale (20), Jebsen-Taylor hand function test (21), Action Research Arm test (22), and Wolf motor function test (23). The aforementioned tools can sometimes lack the sensitivity to quantify dysfunction and can also be time consuming. This could impact appropriate utilization of outcome tools, the ability to demonstrate effectiveness of treatments, and/or identifying improvement. Integration of robotic technology into the clinical setting could improve the quality of assessments and significantly reduce the amount of required time to complete assessments as well.

Assessment of movement quality has been widely researched in robotic and nonrobotic settings. While numerous metrics have been proposed to measure movement quality and motor planning, more research is needed to provide guidelines on clinical meaningfulness of these measures. Some of the "movement planning" metrics and measures include the angle at which one can reach a target, time to peak velocity, response latency, and initial direction error. Other measures that indicate movement quality include variability of movement, phase differences in velocity profile, time efficiency, movement accuracy, movement trajectory, mean velocity, trajectory length, acceleration profile, joint angle correlation, and movement smoothness. While describing all of the above metrics is beyond the scope of this chapter, it is important to note that many of the measures above are extracted from velocity and trajectory profiles easily collected by the robotic device. Generally speaking, the differences between healthy and impaired movement kinematics are evident in velocity signals. A point-to-point reaching movement should produce a bell-shaped velocity curve with respect to time, where velocity is 0 at the beginning of the movement, reaches its maximum value at the halfway point, and returns to 0 at the end of the movement. In contrast, impaired movements tend to have multiple peaks, indicating fragmented, jerky movement with numerous stops or pauses. These smaller bell curves are called ***sub-movement*** (**Fig. 62-4**). As recovery progresses, the submovements tend to become more blended and decrease in number, resulting in larger and larger sub-movement until the point-to-point movement is one motion (24). Intuitively, it is suggested that as submovements become increasingly more blended, the movement becomes "smoother." However, quantifying this smoothness is not

TABLE 62-1 **UL Rehabilitation Robotic Systems**

Device Name	Company (HQ)	FDA Approved?	Type	Shoulder	Elbow	Forearm	Wrist	Finger/Hand	Target Populations/ "Indications"
ArmeoSpring + ManovoSpring	Hocoma (Switzerland)	Yes	Arm exoskeleton + hand module	X	X	X	X	X	Stroke, MS, CP, SCI, TBI, muscle diseases, Parkinson's, UL ataxia, neuropathies, neurosurgical interventions
ArmeoPower + ManovoPower	Hocoma (Switzerland)		Arm exoskeleton + hand module	X	X	X	X	X	Stroke, MS, CP, SCI, TBI, muscle diseases, Parkinson's, UL ataxia, neuropathies, neurosurgical interventions
ReoGo	Motorika (United States)		End-effector device	X	X				Stroke, SCI, neurologic conditions
InMotion ARM	Bionik (Canada)		End-effector device	X	X				Stroke, CP, TBI
InMotion WRIST	Bionik (Canada)		Wrist exoskeleton			X	X		Stroke, CP, SCI, MS, Parkinson's
Bi-Manu-Track	Reha-Stim (Germany)		Wrist exoskeleton			X	X		Stroke
Hand Mentor Pro	Motus Nova (United States)	Yes	Wrist exoskeleton				X	X	Stroke
Amadeo	Tyromotion (Austria)		End-effector device					X	Stroke, SCI, TBI, CP, MS
Sinfonia	Gloreha (Italy)		Soft exoskeleton/ glove					X	CNS injuries, SCI, peripheral neuropathies, musculoskeletal dysfunctions
Hand of Hope	Rehab-Robotics (China)		Hand exoskeleton					X	Stroke, SCI

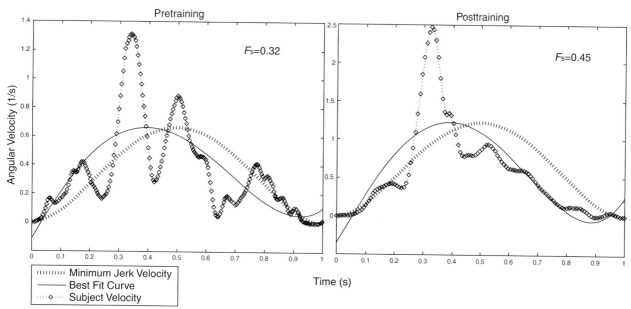

FIGURE 62-4. Angular velocity profiles of a single target hit task during wrist radial deviation before **(left panel)** and after **(right panel)** training with the RiceWrist robotic device. This figure also depicts the minimum jerk velocity. The minimum jerk velocity profile is a function of the actual distance traveled by the individual's hand between two target hits, as well as the total time of that motion, and represents the velocity profile of an ideally smooth movement over the specified distance in the specified amount of time. The best-fit curves of the velocity profiles are also presented. F_S describes the correlation between an individual's velocity profile and the corresponding minimum jerk velocity profile. (From Kadivar Z, Sullivan JL, Eng DP, et al. Robotic training and kinematic analysis of arm and hand after incomplete spinal cord injury: a case study. *IEEE Int Conf Rehabil Robot.* 2011;2011:5975429.)

straightforward, as it is difficult to pinpoint the many nuances that constitute a healthy, "normal" movement. Consequently, there is currently no single metric that serves as the preeminent, definitive indicator of movement quality.

Robotic assessment of motor planning has been reported from end-effector robotic studies including the ARM-Guide (25,26), KINARM (27,28), and HapticMaster (27) devices. Additional evidence supports the effectiveness of robotic devices in measuring other movement quality metrics. Robotic devices such as the RiceWrist (29,30) and ARM-Guide (31) have been shown effective in measuring movement smoothness. Temporal efficiency has been measured through devices such as KINARM (28). Other measures such as movement synergy, movement accuracy, and ROM have been also successfully measured through robotic devices such as MIME (32), MIT-MANUS (33), and REHAROB (34), respectively.

Robot-Assisted UL Function

Robotic devices can offer different levels of assistance to guide the patient during movement and ADLs. Depending on the state of the recovery, the level of required assistance may vary. While many UL robotic devices such as MIT-MANUS, MEMOS, InMotion 2 and 3, ARM-Guide, MIME, BFIAMT, ARMIN, and ARMEO can move the limb in a full user-passive mode, the assist-as-needed mode is only offered through some robotic devices including MAHI Exo-II, RiceWrist, InMotion 2 and 3, ARMEO, MEMOS, and MIME.

Robot-Assisted Therapy

Existing research includes two main approaches when utilizing robotic devices for rehabilitation purposes: robotic training alone and robotic training combined with other interventions.

Robotic Training Alone

Although UL function is impaired in individuals with a variety of neurologic injuries (e.g., stroke, TBI, SCI, multiple sclerosis (MS), CP, Parkinson's disease), the majority of research is focused on UL robotic rehabilitation after stroke (see Chapter 18). This could be due to the high prevalence of stroke and the resulting hemiparesis as well as the financial implication it has on patients, families, and the health care system.

According to American Heart Association (AHA), varied repetitive task practice with robotic devices for the UL has class I level evidence for outpatient stroke rehabilitation and class IIA evidence for inpatient stroke care for individuals who possess some voluntary figure extension (35). There are numerous publications on robotic rehabilitation of the UL after stroke. However the majority of these publications are case studies and feasibility studies. There are limited randomized controlled trials or large clinical trials to help us understand the overall effectiveness of robotic rehabilitation after stroke and other neurological conditions (36,37,31).

Robotic Training Combined with Electrical Stimulation

There is evidence that robotic training combined with electrical stimulation (ES) of distal and proximal segments of the UL could lead to significant improvements in motor function in individuals with stroke. In a randomized controlled trial, 20 sessions of Electromyography-driven wrist robotic training with ES led to more significant improvements in Fugl-Meyer score as well as improvements in Action Research Arm test that did not occur with robotic training alone (38). Another randomized control trial has shown the benefit of combining shoulder/elbow robotic training with MIT-MANUS/InMotion 2 and

ES in achieving greater active ROM compared to robotic training alone (39). A smaller study has also shown the benefits of adding ES to robotic training based on improvements observed combining ES with ArmeoSpring (40).

In summary, robotic training combined with ES is more effective than robotic training alone and can lead to improvements in Fugl-Meyer scores, reduced needs for functional ES, and increased joint ROM. These studies are limited, as they do not compare the above mentioned interventions to conventional therapy alone. However, systematic reviews suggest that robotic training alone is only as effective as conventional therapy in improving overall UL function (41–43). Furthermore, it is suggested that robotic training may only be of more benefit (when compared to conventional therapy) in improving UL motor control (43). Given that during conventional therapy, ES is usually combined with active, passive, or functional movements, one can assume that the advantage of combining ES with robotic devices is reducing labor costs and potentially allowing patients to receive more automated therapy in environments other than clinical settings.

Robotic Training Combined with Transcranial Direct Current Stimulation

A systematic review of the literature suggests that robotic training combined with transcranial direct current stimulation (tDCS) does not result in greater improvements than robotic training alone (44). A small study combining robotic-assisted wrist movements with tDCS in chronic stroke survivors showed improvements in movement smoothness and movement speed when combined with tDCS (45). However, a similar study using the same concept in chronic stroke survivors found no benefits in adding tDCS to robotic training (46). It appears that multiple factors contribute to the effectiveness of this combination including the timing of the application of tDCS (before or during robotic rehabilitation) as well as the phase of stroke. Given that tDCS is not commonly used in clinical settings, further research is required to better understand the effectiveness tDCS combined with robotic rehabilitation as well as conventional therapy.

Robotic Training Combined with Virtual Reality

There is some evidence regarding the effectiveness of virtual reality training in overall motor function as well as on ADL. The combination of virtual reality with robotic devices is promising but unsubstantiated. Exoskeleton robotic devices (e.g., PERCRO L-Exos) have been used to not only assist patients (assist as needed) during movement but to also provide kinematic feedback (47). It is believed that the combination of visual and kinematic feedback could result in improvements in simple (e.g., reaching) and complex (object manipulation) tasks (48).

Robotic Training Combined with Botulinum Toxin

The use of robotic devices after botulinum toxin (BoNT) injection is a new concept with minimal scientific support. Very few studies have been done in this area. Existing studies in this area suggest improvements in motor function and reduction in spasticity in children with CP (49) and stroke (50). Given that a usual rehabilitation protocol after BoNT injection primarily involves repeated ROM and stretching exercise of the limb, it is reasonable to assume that robotic devices would be beneficial if they can move the limb in the desired ROM.

Lower Limb Rehabilitation with Robots

The primary role and function of the LL is locomotion (see Chapter 4). Locomotion is very complicated, laboriously acquired, and becomes almost entirely automatic. Disturbances of gait are commonly observed in individuals with neuromuscular and musculoskeletal injuries, and loss of mobility is the activity of daily living in which patients place the greatest value. The impact on patients is enormous, with negative ramifications on their participation in social, vocational, and recreational activities. In this section, the most reported and commercially available LL rehabilitation robotic systems and clinical findings are summarized.

Lower Limb Robotic Devices

Robot-assisted gait rehabilitation is an emerging therapeutic practice. Several robotic orthoses have been proposed during the last two decades for gait training of neurologically impaired patients. It should be noted that this idea is not new; earlier robotic devices were developed in 1910 (51) and 1970 (52,53). Around 1994, development of LL rehabilitation robotic systems started with the Lokomat, a robotic gait orthosis combined with a body weight–supported treadmill (54). Currently, LL rehabilitation robotic systems include, powered protheses, static robots, wearable robotic orthhoses, and exoskeletons (**Fig. 62-5**).

Powered prostheses have also been developed for patients with LL amputations (see Chapters 37 and 56). Two commonly seen active prostheses are knee-ankle and ankle-foot prosthesis. Active prostheses that replace missing LLs have the potential to greatly improve the quality of life of persons with LL impairments (55). Design of actuator and control strategies are two of the most important aspects to reach maximal power output and voluntary control over the prosthesis, and more clinical evaluation is needed (55).

There are two types of static robots: end-effector (see **Fig. 62-5**) and treadmill-based exoskeleton (see **Fig. 62-5**). Static end-effector LL robotic devices are a type of device in which users stand on a footplate without wearing the device. The end-effector systems use footplates to generate a motion of a limb in space (56,57). The movement is generated from the most distal segment of the extremity, and no alignment between patient-robot joint is required.

Robotic orthoses can be divided into full LL, or multijoint robotic orthoses and single-joint robotic orthoses. Single-joint robotic orthoses have increasingly been developed to address gait problems, such as drop foot. A well-known robotic ankle orthosis is MIT's Anklebot (58) (see **Fig. 62-5**).

Multiple-joint wearable exoskeleton can be combined with a treadmill system (static robot) or overground robot. Wearable overground exoskeletons allow the patients to walk overground and explore the environment. The predefined gait trajectory exoskeletons are designed for mobility and the devices can be either assistive or rehabilitation devices. The characteristics of FDA-approved wearable exoskeletons, that are also commercially available, are summarized in **Table 62-2**.

Robot-Assisted Assessment

Besides using robotic devices for neurorehabilitation, robotic devices can be utilized to provide more objective, sensitive, reliable, and time-efficient clinical assessment. Similar to UL assessment, qualitative measures (i.e., ROM, muscle strength,

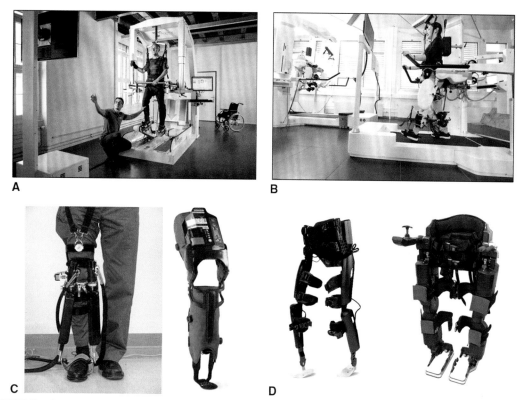

FIGURE 62-5. Examples of lower limb robotic devices. **A:** Static end-effector treadmill (G-EO System, Reha Technology AG, Switzerland). **B:** Static exoskeleton treadmill (Picture: Hocoma, Switzerland). **C:** Wearable powered orthosis: Anklebot (*left*) and AlterG Bionic Leg (*right*, AlterG, Inc.). **D.** Wearable overground exoskeleton. ReWalk Personal 6.0 (*left*, ReWalk Robotics) and REX (*right*, Rex Bionics Ltd.).

torque, proprioception) and functional measures (i.e., gait kinematics and balance) can be performed with LL robotic devices. Specifically for LL assessment, robotic assistance can improve assessment of severely affected patients (low functioning). Comprehensive reviews and more detailed descriptions of robot-assisted clinical assessment procedures can be found in Maggioni et al. (59), Shirota et al. (60), and Carpino et al. (61). In LL function, assessment of balance remains crude and has limited value in the treatment of patients with neurologic impairment. Due to the complexity of balance control and the body systems involved, it is critical to understand how neurologic impairments have affected its various components (static, dynamic, reactive balance) (60,62–65) (**Table 62-3**).

Robot-Assisted Overground Walking

Powered orthoses and overground exoskeletons may assist individuals with neurologic disorders, such as SCI (see Chapter 22) and stroke, to restore walking function. Powered orthoses for LL rehabilitation have been critically and extensively reviewed previously (66). In general, the physiologic cost can be reduced during ambulation with robotic assistance (67,68). Studies also have indicated that persons with SCI (69–77), stroke (75,76), and MS (77,78) could walk with a wearable overground exoskeleton safely in a real-world setting, after training, and possibly to use exoskeletons for independent ambulation at home and community environments depending on the injury level and severity. While it is generally thought that users need to have sufficient UL strength to use an assistive device (i.e., walker or cane) when ambulating with an overground exoskeleton, a self-supported robot, such as

REX, controlled by a joystick, requires minimal hand function (79), or devices combined with other types of robotic body weight–support device (80) could allow persons with severe impairment (i.e., tetraplegia) to ambulate for a short distance. Furthermore, self-supporting exoskeletons, such as REX, also raise the possibility of integrating brain-machine interfaces that may allow users to perform specific LL functional activities and therapeutic exercises without the use of manual control (81).

Robot-Assisted Locomotion Training

Clinical efficacy and effectiveness of robot-assisted training on LL function with various rehabilitation robotic devices have been investigated, and more studies, particularly during different recovery stages, are ongoing. Robot-assisted training is considered safe and feasible, and the intensity of the exercise is safe for (neurologic) patients at risk of cardiovascular diseases (82).

According to reviews and meta-analyses, treadmill-based robot-assisted gait training may improve gait function, including gait speed and walking distance in patients with SCI (69,83), stroke (84,85), TBI (86), MS (87), and CP (88). These effects could be either greater than or equivalent to conventional therapy. It has been suggested that neuromuscular adaptation responding to the training, such as LL muscular activation, may lead to gait improvement (89–91).

Lefeber et al. (82) analyzed the effects of robot assistance on energy consumption and cardiorespiratory load during walking. They evaluated studies on healthy subjects and stroke and SCI patients with end effectors, treadmill-based, and wearable

TABLE 62-2	Characteristics of Commercially Available Wearable Exoskeleton Devices[a]				
Device	**ReWalk**	**Ekso (Version 1.1) and Ekso GT (Version 1.2)**	**Indego**	**HAL for Medical Use (Lower Limb Type)**	**REX**
Classification name/ regulatory class Institutional use	Powered exoskeleton Device class II SCI T4-6	Powered exoskeleton Device class II SCI T4-L5, SCI C7-T3 (ASIA D), stroke (hemiplegia)	Powered exoskeleton Device class II SCI C7-L5; stroke (hemiplegia)	Powered exoskeleton Device class II SCI C4-L5 (ASIA C, ASIA D); T11-L5 (ASIA A with Zones of Partial Preservation, ASIA B)	Powered exerciser Device class I Lower limb weakness
Home/community use	SCI T7-L5	No	SCI T3-L5	No	No
CE marking	Yes	Yes	Yes	Yes	Yes
Stepping	Tilting motion at the trunk and weight shifting center of mass	Manual button pushes on controller; weight shifting center of mass; weight shifting and active forward progression of limb	Forward and backward lean or tilting of the upper leg over the feet; active forward progression of limb	Surface electromyography bioelectrical signals of the hip and knee extensor and flexor muscles; postural cues and sensor shoe measurements; joint motion	29 onboard computer processors control movement and balance through joystick control
Hip-knee	Motors at the hip and knee	Motors at the hip and knee	Motors at the hip and knee	Motors at the hip and knee	Motors at the hip, knee, and ankle
Ankle	Double-action orthotic joint with adjustable spring-assisted dorsiflexion	Adjustable resting ankle angle and adjustable dorsiflexion stiffness	Ankle-foot orthoses	Ankle-foot orthoses	Motors at the ankle for inversion, eversion, and dorsiflexion
Weight	30 kg	23 kg	11.8 kg	14 kg	45 kg
User limitation[b]	Height: 160–190 cm Weight: <100 kg	Height: 158–188 cm Weight: <100 kg	Height: 155–195 cm Weight: <113 kg	Height: 150–190 cm Weight: 40–100 kg	Height: 142–193 cm Weight: 40–100 kg
Prerequisites	The ability to use hands and shoulders (manipulate assistive device). Healthy cardiovascular system and bone density. Sufficient range of motion to attain normal, reciprocal gait pattern and sit to/from stand transitions	Sufficient upper body and lower body strength to assist with standing and weight shifting. If no lower extremity function, must have near normal upper extremity motor function at the shoulder and hands to manipulate assistive device. Healthy cardiovascular system and bone density. Sufficient range of motion to attain normal, reciprocal gait pattern and sit to/from stand transitions	Sufficient upper body and lower body strength to assist with standing and weight shifting. If no lower extremity function, must have near normal upper extremity motor function at the shoulder and hands to manipulate assistive device. Healthy cardiovascular system and bone density. Sufficient range of motion to attain normal, reciprocal gait pattern and sit to/from stand transition	The user must exhibit sufficient residual motor and movement-related functions of the hip and knee to trigger and control HAL. The user must be supported by a body weight–support (BWS) system before donning the device and during device use. The BWS must not be detached from the patient before doffing this device. HAL is not intended to provide sit-stand or stand-sit movements	The manual dexterity to control the joystick. Healthy cardiovascular system and bone density. Sufficient range of motion to attain normal, reciprocal gait pattern and sit to/from stand transitions
Mobility aid	Forearm crutches	Walker, forearm crutches, cane	Walker, forearm crutches, cane	No	No

[a]The information listed is based on the FDA database or/and device user manuals.
[b]In addition to body height and weight limitation, each device has its specification on upper and lower leg length and hip width.

TABLE 62-3 Example of LL Rehabilitation Robotic Systems That Are Suitable for Balance Assessment

Example Robotic Devices	Feasibility Balance Assessment			Type of Assessment Suitability			Type of Perturbation Suitability			Quantitative Measurements Suitability		
	Steady-state	Anticipatory	Reactive	Severely Affected Patients	Balance Assessment in Walking	Balance Assessment in Walking	Moving Ground	Horizontal Pushes	Joint	Embedded Sensors	Wearable Sensors	External Sensors
Treadmill-based end effector	S, W	S, W	S, W	Y	Y	Y	Y	N	N	CK CIF	(CIF) BK	BK
Treadmill-based exoskeletons	S, W	S, W	UK	Y	Y	Y	Y	Y	Y	GRF CK (CIF)	GRF BK	GRF
Wearable exoskeletons	S, W	S, W	S, W (depending on the model)	Y	Y	Y	N	N	Y	CK CIF	GRF BK	GRF

S, standing; W, walking; BK, body kinematics; UK, unknown; COM/sacrum, configuration of a segmental representation of the body (position, speed, acceleration); CK, connection point(s) kinematics: points where the robotic device is connected to the body (position, speed, acceleration); CIF, connection point(s) interaction forces: points where the robotic device is connected (6D-, 3D-, 1D-force or pressure distribution); GRF, ground reaction forces: contact between foot and standing surface (6D-, 3D-, 1D-force or pressure distribution).

Adapted from Shirota C, van Asseldonk E, Matjacic Z, et al. Robot-supported assessment of balance in standing and walking. *J Neuroeng Rehabil.* 2017;14(1):80.

exoskeletons. The results suggest that walking with robot assistance, especially when of short duration, is less energy consuming and cardiorespiratory stressful than walking without robot assistance, but results depend on factors such as robot type, walking speed, amount of body weight support, and level of effort (82).

As for wearable exoskeletons, most of the literature includes prospective case series, and there is minimal clinical evidence regarding the efficacy and effectiveness on locomotion, as compared to other forms of gait training in SCI (72) and stroke (92). In a recent study, Chang et al. (93) investigated the effects of exoskeleton-assisted gait training (15 sessions with Ekso 1.1) in persons with incomplete SCI as compared to conventional gait training (**Fig. 62-6**). The results showed that gait endurance (distance of a 6-minute walk test) and stride length were improved in the exoskeleton group, but not in the conventional group. In a randomized clinical trial by Watanabe et al., stroke survivors who received robot-assisted gait training with a wearable exoskeleton (HAL) improved functional ambulation category after 12 training sessions, and at 8 and 12 weeks after training, compared to conventional gait training (92). In addition to improvement in LL function, secondary physiologic improvements such as a reduction in spasticity, increase in bone mineral density, and increase in quality of life were reported (94–96).

User Feedback

The trials mentioned above have suggested that rehabilitation robotic systems have the potential to improve the functional capabilities of persons with neurologic impairment, particularly in relation to ambulatory outcomes. Most of the literature focuses on the design specification of the technology, and there is minimal involvement of users in the development of the design of rehabilitation robotic systems, especially exoskeleton technology. It has been acknowledged that the wide acceptance of robotic exoskeleton for both rehabilitation and function is dependent on the end users being central to the design and the development of the technology (97). However, the establishment of the feasibility and effectiveness of user-centered design, in relation to exoskeleton technology, is lacking. Studies have investigated the end users' (including persons with impairment and clinicians) feedback and experiences in robotic technology, and, in general, the feedback has been positive in terms of the device, robot-assisted locomotion training program, and perceived health benefits such as overall health status, UL strength, endurance, and their sleep and psychological well-being (98–101). In terms of the feedback with regard to the wearable exoskeleton design and functionality, in a small study using two wearable overground exoskeletons (Ekso 1.1 and REX), differences in user satisfaction between these two devices were reported. The users indicated that many changes should be made to both exoskeletons; some suggestions were made for the REX (i.e., changing the speed, ability to walk over uneven surfaces, and transportability) and others were more necessary for the Esko (i.e., ability to drive and manage toileting needs while wearing the device). Interestingly, participants reported that they would be somewhat likely to use both exoskeletons at home and in the community if they were available (102).

CHALLENGES, FUTURE DIRECTIONS, AND OPPORTUNITIES

The developments in robotic technology described above are impressive and demonstrate the ability to realize in-clinic and wearable systems that are capable of assessing, supporting, and

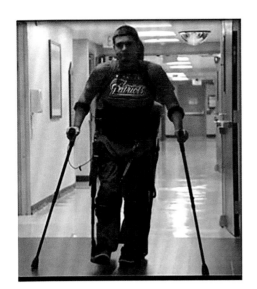
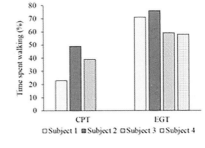
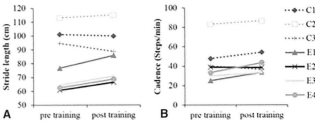

FIGURE 62-6. Changes in gait characteristics after gait training with a wearable overground exoskeleton in persons with incomplete SCI. **A:** A subject walked with the exoskeleton (Ekso 1.1) during a typical training session. During training, a physical therapist stood behind the subject. **B:** Subjects walking with the exoskeleton (EGT) spent substantially more time 66% ± 9% on walking compared to subjects in conventional physical therapy (CPT) group who spent 37% ± 13% of the time in weight-bearing activities (i.e., standing and walking). **C:** EGT group showed significant increased stride length at post-training assessment (pre-training 66 ± 7 cm, post-training 72 ± 9 cm) (*a*). EGT group also increased cadence from 32 ± 6 steps/min at pre-training assessment to 37 ± 5 steps/min at post-training assessment; however, the increase was not statistically significant (*b*). *Dotted lines* represent the CPT group. *Solid lines* represent the EGT group. (Adapted from Chang SH, Afzal T; Group TSCE, Berliner J, Francisco GE. Exoskeleton-assisted gait training to improve gait in individuals with spinal cord injury: a pilot randomized study. *Pilot Feasibility Stud.* 2018;4:62. http://creativecommons.org/licenses/by/4.0/)

restoring human movement following neurologic injury. Still, there are several challenges in rehabilitation robotic systems.

In terms of the use of robots for assessment, some of the key challenges are in framing assessment in ways that are clinically relevant. For example, how do metrics derived from the robot's sensors correlate to more widely understood and accepted clinical metrics? How does assessment conducted with a robotic device translate to functional improvements in ADL? To advance the applications of robotic systems for assessment of motor impairment, it is vital that the measurements and metrics taken with the robot demonstrate clinical relevance and that capabilities measured with a robot translate to improvements in functional independence.

Among therapeutic robotic systems, there is an underlying challenge of determining how best to use robots to promote plasticity and recovery. Many of the studies surveyed here focus solely on the effectiveness of a robot for delivery of therapy. Still, we don't yet have a good understanding of the dosage, intensity, and duration of therapy that are most effectively delivered with our robotic technology. Second, it would be beneficial to understand what is it about the interaction of the therapist with the patient that promotes recovery, what aspects of these interactions can be replicated in robotic rehabilitation, and what is the most effective means to realize these goals. During robotic rehabilitation, we are just starting to explore ways of ensuring the cognitive and physical engagement of the patient, detecting their intent to move, and making the robot responsive to the patient's intentions, all of which are known to be beneficial to therapy outcomes (103,104). Finally, combinatorial treatments, where robotic systems are used in conjunction with pharmacologic, electrophysiologic, or neuroimaging techniques, offer great promise and are just beginning to be studied.

In the space of assistive robotic systems, the primary challenges lie in the translation from the laboratory to clinical and real-life settings. For example, wearability and portability are a significant challenge, especially for assistive devices that are intended for use in everyday settings, in the home, and for mobility. Issues like battery life, weight, compliance, and fit to the body must all be considered. The potential for new frontiers such as soft robotic systems is particularly exciting. Beyond physical wearability and portability, robotic technology must be easy and intuitive for the user to control, such as the capability of the robot to detect a user's intent and respond with the appropriate amount of support to complete the desired movement. Providing sensory feedback, either auditory or haptic, to the user could improve the intuitiveness of a robot's control.

A good number of these future challenges are technological. Regardless of the intended use of the robot (assessment, assistance, or therapy), the technology remains cost-prohibitive for many clinical environments. Costs are directly associated with the capability and complexity of the robot. Simple, low-cost robotic devices may only support a single degree of freedom of movement or offer limited force or torque output, both of which impact the utility of the robot in rehabilitation applications.

Finally, there remain practical clinical issues. Robotic interventions are not necessarily reimbursed by insurance companies, limiting the proliferation of these technologies. As with any new technology, education and training of the clinical staff who will use these robotic tools are necessary to ensure their best use. Clinicians need to understand the underlying technology, systems, and applications to know which robotic solution is right for their particular patient needs.

SUMMARY

In this chapter, we have provided an overview of rehabilitation robotic systems and clinical evidence to date. Development of the robotic technology, including the wearability, portability, and intuitive user control of these robotic systems, could further advance the application of robot-assisted rehabilitation and provide more person-centered and cost-effective rehabilitation approaches. Current literature suggests that rehabilitation robotic system design should be an iterative process whereby user perspectives are sought early in the process, and incorporated and continually refined by experience with robotic devices to ensure that devices developed are acceptable and usable by the target populations. This requires close collaboration among stakeholders, clinicians, roboticists, patients, policy-makers, and insurance company representatives. The devices described in this chapter illustrate how the integration of rehabilitation robotic systems to assist UL and LL function can be implemented along the continuum of recovery and reintegration. Other opportunities for integration of robots in the rehabilitation continuum are best defined by user capabilities and functional objectives as milestones for application of various robotic rehabilitation systems. Although the cost-effectiveness of robot-assisted rehabilitation has not been determined and randomized control trials with larger sample sizes are needed, current studies show promise that rehabilitation robotic systems can be used to augment rehabilitation outcomes and support functional independence for range of neurologic impairments.

REFERENCES

1. Bayona NA, Bitensky J, Salter K, et al. The role of task-specific training in rehabilitation therapies. *Top Stroke Rehabil*. 2005;12(3):58–65.
2. Lang CE, Lohse KR, Birkenmeier RL. Dose and timing in neurorehabilitation: prescribing motor therapy after stroke. *Curr Opin Neurol*. 2015;28(6):549–555.
3. Purpura G, Cioni G, Tinelli F. Multisensory-based rehabilitation approach: translational insights from animal models to early intervention. *Front Neurosci*. 2017;11:430.
4. Gassert R, Dietz V. Rehabilitation robots for the treatment of sensorimotor deficits: a neurophysiological perspective. *J Neuroeng Rehabil*. 2018;15(1):46.
5. Ona ED, Cano-de la Cuerda R, et al. A review of robotics in neurorehabilitation: towards an automated process for upper limb. *J Healthc Eng*. 2018;2018:9758939.
6. Siciliano B, Khatib O, eds. *Springer Handbook of Robotics*. Springer; 2016 Jul 27.
7. Marchal-Crespo L, Reinkensmeyer DJ. Review of control strategies for robotic movement training after neurologic injury. *J Neuroeng Rehabil*. 2009 Dec;6(1):20.
8. Curt A, Van Hedel HJ, Klaus D, et al. Recovery from a spinal cord injury: significance of compensation, neural plasticity, and repair. *J Neurotrauma*. 2008;25(6):677–685.
9. Zarahn E, Alon L, Ryan SL, et al. Prediction of motor recovery using initial impairment and fMRI 48 h poststroke. *Cereb Cortex*. 2011;21(12):2712–2721.
10. Kleim JA, Jones TA. Principles of experience-dependent neural plasticity: implications for rehabilitation after brain damage. *J Speech Lang Hear Res*. 2008;51(1):S225–S239.
11. Lang CE, Macdonald JR, Reisman DS, et al. Observation of amounts of movement practice provided during stroke rehabilitation. *Arch Phys Med Rehabil*. 2009;90(10):1692–1698.
12. Danzl MM, Etter NM, Andreatta RD, et al. Facilitating neurorehabilitation through principles of engagement. *J Allied Health*. 2012;41(1):35–41.
13. Mawase F, Uehara S, Bastian AJ, et al. Motor learning enhances use-dependent plasticity. *J Neurosci*. 2017;37(10):2673–2685.
14. Sivan M, Gallagher J, Holt R, et al. Investigating the International Classification of Functioning, Disability, and Health (ICF) framework to capture user needs in the concept stage of rehabilitation technology development. *Assist Technol*. 2014;26(3):164–173.

15. Bailey R, Kaskutas V, Fox I, et al. Effect of upper extremity nerve damage on activity participation, pain, depression, and quality of life. *J Hand Surg Am.* 2009; 34(9):1682–1688.

16. Snoek GJ, IJzerman MJ, Hermens HJ, et al. Survey of the needs of patients with spinal cord injury: impact and priority for improvement in hand function in tetraplegics. *Spinal Cord.* 2004;42(9):526–532.

17. Hubbard IJ, Parsons MW, Neilson C, et al. Task-specific training: evidence for and translation to clinical practice. *Occup Ther Int.* 2009;16(3–4):175–189.

18. Shaw SE, Morris DM, Uswatte G, et al. Constraint-induced movement therapy for recovery of upper-limb function following traumatic brain injury. *J Rehabil Res Dev.* 2005;42(6):769–778.

19. Desrosiers J, Bravo G, Hebert R, et al. Validation of the Box and Block Test as a measure of dexterity of elderly people: reliability, validity, and norms studies. *Arch Phys Med Rehabil.* 1994;75(7):751–755.

20. Fugl-Meyer AR, Jaasko L, Leyman I, et al. The post-stroke hemiplegic patient. 1. a method for evaluation of physical performance. *Scand J Rehabil Med.* 1975;7(1):13–31.

21. Sears ED, Chung KC. Validity and responsiveness of the Jebsen-Taylor Hand Function Test. *J Hand Surg Am.* 2010;35(1):30–37.

22. Hsieh CL, Hsueh IP, Chiang FM, et al. Inter-rater reliability and validity of the action research arm test in stroke patients. *Age Ageing.* 1998;27(2):107–113.

23. Wolf SL, Catlin PA, Ellis M, et al. Assessing Wolf motor function test as outcome measure for research in patients after stroke. *Stroke.* 2001;32(7):1635–1639.

24. Rohrer B, Fasoli S, Krebs HI, et al. Submovements grow larger, fewer, and more blended during stroke recovery. *Motor control.* 2004 Oct;8(4):472–483.

25. Kahn LE, Lum PS, Rymer WZ, et al. Robot-assisted movement training for the stroke-impaired arm: Does it matter what the robot does? *J Rehabil Res Dev.* 2006; 43(5):619–630.

26. Reinkensmeyer DJ, Kahn LE, Averbuch M, et al. Understanding and treating arm movement impairment after chronic brain injury: progress with the ARM guide. *J Rehabil Res Dev.* 2000;37(6):653–662.

27. Dukelow SP, Herter TM, Bagg SD, et al. The independence of deficits in position sense and visually guided reaching following stroke. *J Neuroeng Rehabil.* 2012;9:72.

28. Semrau JA, Herter TM, Scott SH, et al. Robotic identification of kinesthetic deficits after stroke. *Stroke.* 2013;44(12):3414–3421.

29. Kadivar Z, Sullivan JL, Eng DP, et al. Robotic training and kinematic analysis of arm and hand after incomplete spinal cord injury: a case study. *IEEE Int Conf Rehabil Robot.* 2011;2011:5975429.

30. Pehlivan AU, Sergi F, Erwin A, et al. Design and validation of the RiceWrist-S exoskeleton for robotic rehabilitation after incomplete spinal cord injury. *Robotica.* 2014;32(8):1415–1431.

31. Kahn LE, Zygman ML, Rymer WZ, et al. Robot-assisted reaching exercise promotes arm movement recovery in chronic hemiparetic stroke: a randomized controlled pilot study. *J Neuroeng Rehabil.* 2006;3:12.

32. Lum PS, Burgar CG, Van der Loos M, et al. MIME robotic device for upper-limb neurorehabilitation in subacute stroke subjects: a follow-up study. *J Rehabil Res Dev.* 2006;43(5):631–642.

33. Dipietro L, Krebs HI, Fasoli SE, et al. Changing motor synergies in chronic stroke. *J Neurophysiol.* 2007;98(2):757–768.

34. Toth A, Fazekas G, Arz G, Jurak M, Horvath M. Passive robotic movement therapy of the spastic hemiparetic arm with REHAROB: report of the first clinical test and the follow-up system improvement. In 9th International Conference on Rehabilitation Robotics, 2005. ICORR 2005. 2005 Jun 28 (pp. 127–130). IEEE.

35. Miller EL, Murray L, Richards L, et al. Comprehensive overview of nursing and interdisciplinary rehabilitation care of the stroke patient: a scientific statement from the American Heart Association. *Stroke.* 2010;41(10):2402–2448.

36. Masiero S, Celia A, Rosati G, et al. Robotic-assisted rehabilitation of the upper limb after acute stroke. *Arch Phys Med Rehabil.* 2007;88:142–149.

37. Volpe BT, Lynch D, Rykman-Berland A, et al. Intensive sensorimotor arm training mediated by therapist or robot improves hemiparesis in patients with chronic stroke. *Neurorehabil Neural Repair.* 2008;22:305–310.

38. Hu XL, Tong RK, Ho NS, et al. Wrist rehabilitation assisted by an electromyography-driven neuromuscular electrical stimulation robot after stroke. *Neurorehabil Neural Repair.* 2015;29(8):767–776.

39. Miyasaka H, Orand A, Ohnishi H, et al. Ability of electrical stimulation therapy to improve the effectiveness of robotic training for paretic upper limbs in patients with stroke. *Med Eng Phys.* 2016;38(11):1172–1175.

40. Meadmore KL, Hughes AM, Freeman CT, et al. Functional electrical stimulation mediated by iterative learning control and 3D robotics reduces motor impairment in chronic stroke. *J Neuroeng Rehabil.* 2012;9:32.

41. Kwakkel G, Kollen BJ, Krebs HI. Effects of robot-assisted therapy on upper limb recovery after stroke: a systematic review. *Neurorehabil Neural Repair.* 2008;22(2):111–121.

42. Norouzi-Gheidari N, Archambault PS, Fung J. Effects of robot-assisted therapy on stroke rehabilitation in upper limbs: systematic review and meta-analysis of the literature. *J Rehabil Res Dev.* 2012;49(4):479–496.

43. Lo AC, Guarino PD, Richards LG, et al. Robot-assisted therapy for long-term upper-limb impairment after stroke. *N Engl J Med.* 2010;362(19):1772–1783.

44. Hesse S, Waldner A, Mehrholz J, et al. Combined transcranial direct current stimulation and robot-assisted arm training in subacute stroke patients: an exploratory, randomized multicenter trial. *Neurorehabil Neural Repair.* 2011;25(9):838–846.

45. Giacobbe V, Krebs HI, Volpe BT, et al. Transcranial direct current stimulation (tDCS) and robotic practice in chronic stroke: the dimension of timing. *NeuroRehabilitation.* 2013;33(1):49–56.

46. Geroin C, Picelli A, Munari D, et al. Combined transcranial direct current stimulation and robot-assisted gait training in patients with chronic stroke: a preliminary comparison. *Clin Rehabil.* 2011;25(6):537–548.

47. Frisoli A, Sotgiu E, Procopio C, et al. Design and implementation of a training strategy in chronic stroke with an arm robotic exoskeleton. *IEEE Int Conf Rehabil Robot.* 2011;2011:5975512.

48. Frisoli A, Borelli L, Montagner A, et al. Arm rehabilitation with a robotic exoskeleton in Virtual Reality. In 2007 IEEE 10th International Conference on Rehabilitation Robotics 2007 Jun 13 (pp. 631–642). IEEE.

49. Frascarelli F, Masia L, Di Rosa G, et al. Robot-mediated and clinical scales evaluation after upper limb botulinum toxin type A injection in children with hemiplegia. *J Rehabil Med.* 2009;41(12):988–994.

50. Takebayashi T, Amano S, Hanada K, et al. Therapeutic synergism in the treatment of post-stroke arm paresis utilizing botulinum toxin, robotic therapy, and constraint-induced movement therapy. *PM R.* 2014;6(11):1054–1058.

51. Khalili D, Zomlefer M. An intelligent robotic system for rehabilitation of joints and estimation of body segment parameters. *IEEE Trans Biomed Eng.* 1988;35(2): 138–146.

52. Seireg A, Grundmann J. Design of a multitask exoskeletal walking device for paraplegics. *Biomech Med Dev.* 1981:569–644.

53. Vukobratovic M, Hristic D, Stojiljkovic Z. Development of active anthropomorphic exoskeletons. *Med Biol Eng.* 1974;12(1):66–80.

54. Colombo G, Joerg M, Schreier R, et al. Treadmill training of paraplegic patients using a robotic orthosis. *J Rehabil Res Dev.* 2000;37(6):693–700.

55. Windrich M, Grimmer M, Christ O, et al. Active lower limb prosthetics: a systematic review of design issues and solutions. *Biomed Eng Online.* 2016;15 (suppl 3):140.

56. Freivogel S, Mehrholz J, Husak-Sotomayor T, et al. Gait training with the newly developed 'LokoHelp'-system is feasible for non-ambulatory patients after stroke, spinal cord and brain injury. A feasibility study. *Brain Inj.* 2008;22(7–8): 625–632.

57. Hesse S, Uhlenbrock D. A mechanized gait trainer for restoration of gait. *J Rehabil Res Dev.* 2000;37(6):701–708.

58. Khanna I, Roy A, Rodgers MM, et al. Effects of unilateral robotic limb loading on gait characteristics in subjects with chronic stroke. *J Neuroeng Rehabil.* 2010;7(1):23.

59. Maggioni S, Melendez-Calderon A, van Asseldonk E, et al. Robot-aided assessment of lower extremity functions: a review. *J Neuroeng Rehabil.* 2016;13(1):72.

60. Shirota C, van Asseldonk E, Matjacic Z, et al. Robot-supported assessment of balance in standing and walking. *J Neuroeng Rehabil.* 2017;14(1):80.

61. Carpino G, Pezzola A, Urbano M, et al. Assessing effectiveness and costs in robot-mediated lower limbs rehabilitation: a meta-analysis and state of the art. *J Healthc Eng.* 2018;2018:7492024.

62. Horak FB. Postural orientation and equilibrium: what do we need to know about neural control of balance to prevent falls? *Age Ageing.* 2006;35(suppl 2):ii7–ii11.

63. Horak FB, Shupert CL, Mirka A. Components of postural dyscontrol in the elderly: a review. *Neurobiol Aging.* 1989;10(6):727–738.

64. Horak FB, Wrisley DM, Frank J. The balance evaluation systems test (BESTest) to differentiate balance deficits. *Phys Ther.* 2009;89(5):484–498.

65. Mancini M, Horak FB. The relevance of clinical balance assessment tools to differentiate balance deficits. *Eur J Phys Rehabil Med.* 2010;46(2):239.

66. Krebs HI, Volpe BT, Hesse S, et al. Rehabilitation robotics. In: Frontera WR, ed. *Delisa's Physical Medicine Rehabilitation.* 5th ed. Riverwoods, IL: Lippincott Williams & Wilkins; 2010. 2187–2200.

67. Arazpour M, Bani MA, Hutchins SW, et al. The physiological cost index of walking with mechanical and powered gait orthosis in patients with spinal cord injury. *Spinal Cord.* 2013;51(5):356–359.

68. Lefeber N, De Keersmaecker E, Henderix S, et al. Physiological responses and perceived exertion during robot-assisted and body weight-supported gait after stroke. *Neurorehabil Neural Repair.* 2018;32(12):1043–1054.

69. Cheung EYY, Ng TKW, Yu KKK, et al. Robot-assisted training for people with spinal cord injury: a meta-analysis. *Arch Phys Med Rehabil.* 2017;98(11): 2320–2331.e12.

70. Geigle PR, Kallins M. Exoskeleton-assisted walking for people with spinal cord injury. *Arch Phys Med Rehabil.* 2017;98(7):1493–1495.

71. Louie DR, Eng JJ, Lam T; Spinal Cord Injury Research Evidence Research Team. Gait speed using powered robotic exoskeletons after spinal cord injury: a systematic review and correlational study. *J Neuroeng Rehabil.* 2015;12:82.

72. Miller LE, Zimmermann AK, Herbert WG. Clinical effectiveness and safety of powered exoskeleton-assisted walking in patients with spinal cord injury: systematic review with meta-analysis. *Med Devices (Auckl).* 2016;9:455–466.

73. Tefertiller C, Hays K, Jones J, et al. Initial outcomes from a multicenter study utilizing the indego powered exoskeleton in spinal cord injury. *Top Spinal Cord Inj Rehabil.* 2018;24(1):78–85.

74. Asselin PK, Avedissian M, Knezevic S, et al. Training persons with spinal cord injury to ambulate using a powered exoskeleton. *J Vis Exp.* 2016;112.

75. Morone G, Paolucci S, Cherubini A, et al. Robot-assisted gait training for stroke patients: current state of the art and perspectives of robotics. *Neuropsychiatr Dis Treat.* 2017;13:1303.

76. Louie DR, Eng JJ. Powered robotic exoskeletons in post-stroke rehabilitation of gait: a scoping review. *J Neuroeng Rehabil.* 2016;13(1):53.

77. Chang S-H, Kern M, Afzal T, et al. Wearable exoskeleton assisted rehabilitation in multiple sclerosis: feasibility and experience. In: González-Vargas J, Ibáñez J, Contreras-Vidal J, van der Kooij H, Pons J. eds. *Wearable Robotics: Challenges and Trends.* Biosystems & Biorobotics. Vol 16. Cham: Springer; 2017:15–19.

78. Kozlowski AJ, Fabian M, Lad D, et al. Feasibility and safety of a powered exoskeleton for assisted walking for persons with multiple sclerosis: a single-group preliminary study. *Arch Phys Med Rehabil.* 2017;98(7):1300–1307.

79. Birch N, Graham J, Priestley T, et al. Results of the first interim analysis of the RAPPER II trial in patients with spinal cord injury: ambulation and functional exercise programs in the REX powered walking aid. *J Neuroeng Rehabil.* 2017;14(1):60.

80. Chang SH, Zhu F, Patel N, et al. Combining robotic exoskeleton and body weight unweighing technology to promote walking activity in tetraplegia following SCI: a case study. *J Spinal Cord Med.* 2018:1–4.

81. He Y, Eguren D, Azorin JM, et al. Brain-machine interfaces for controlling lower-limb powered robotic systems. *J Neural Eng.* 2018;15(2):021004.

82. Lefeber N, Swinnen E, Kerckhofs E. The immediate effects of robot-assistance on energy consumption and cardiorespiratory load during walking compared to walking without robot-assistance: a systematic review. *Disabil Rehabil Assist Technol.* 2017;12(7):657–671.

83. Nam KY, Kim HJ, Kwon BS, et al. Robot-assisted gait training (Lokomat) improves walking function and activity in people with spinal cord injury: a systematic review. *J Neuroeng Rehabil.* 2017;14(1):24.

84. Mehrholz J, Thomas S, Werner C, et al. Electromechanical-assisted training for walking after stroke. *Cochrane Database Syst Rev.* 2017;5:CD006185.

85. Bruni MF, Melegari C, De Cola MC, et al. What does best evidence tell us about robotic gait rehabilitation in stroke patients: a systematic review and meta-analysis. *J Clin Neurosci.* 2018;48:11–17.

86. Esquenazi A, Lee S, Wikoff A, et al. A comparison of locomotor therapy interventions: partial-body weight-supported Treadmill, Lokomat, and G-EO training in people with traumatic brain injury. *PM R.* 2017;9(9):839–846.

87. Straudi S, Fanciullacci C, Martinuzzi C, et al. The effects of robot-assisted gait training in progressive multiple sclerosis: a randomized controlled trial. *Mult Scler.* 2016;22(3):373–384.

88. Bayon C, Martin-Lorenzo T, Moral-Saiz B, et al. A robot-based gait training therapy for pediatric population with cerebral palsy: goal setting, proposal and preliminary clinical implementation. *J Neuroeng Rehabil.* 2018;15(1):69.

89. Androwis GJ, Pilkar R, Ramanujam A, et al. Electromyography assessment during gait in a robotic exoskeleton for acute stroke. *Front Neurol.* 2018;9:630.

90. Chisari C, Bertolucci F, Monaco V, et al. Robot-assisted gait training improves motor performances and modifies Motor Unit firing in poststroke patients. *Eur J Phys Rehabil Med.* 2015;51(1):59–69.

91. Ramanujam A, Cirnigliaro CM, Garbarini E, et al. Neuromechanical adaptations during a robotic powered exoskeleton assisted walking session. *J Spinal Cord Med.* 2018;41(5):518–528.

92. Watanabe H, Goto R, Tanaka N, et al. Effects of gait training using the Hybrid Assistive Limb® in recovery-phase stroke patients: a 2-month follow-up, randomized, controlled study. *NeuroRehabilitation.* 2017;40(3):363–367.

93. Chang SH, Afzal T; Group TSCE, Berliner J, Francisco GE. Exoskeleton-assisted gait training to improve gait in individuals with spinal cord injury: a pilot randomized study. *Pilot Feasibility Stud.* 2018;4:62.

94. Karelis AD, Carvalho LP, Castillo MJ, et al. Effect on body composition and bone mineral density of walking with a robotic exoskeleton in adults with chronic spinal cord injury. *J Rehabil Med.* 2017;49(1):84–87.

95. Baunsgaard CB, Nissen UV, Brust AK, et al. Exoskeleton gait training after spinal cord injury: An exploratory study on secondary health conditions. *J Rehabil Med.* 2018;50(9):806–813.

96. Juszczak M, Gallo E, Bushnik T. Examining the effects of a powered exoskeleton on quality of life and secondary impairments in people living with spinal cord injury. *Top Spinal Cord Inj Rehabil.* 2018;24(4):336–342.

97. Pons JL. Rehabilitation exoskeletal robotics. The promise of an emerging field. *IEEE Eng Med Biol Mag.* 2010;29(3):57–63.

98. Cahill A, Ginley OM, Bertrand C, et al. Gym-based exoskeleton walking: a preliminary exploration of non-ambulatory end-user perspectives. *Disabil Health J.* 2018;11(3):478–485.

99. Hill D, Holloway CS, Morgado Ramirez DZ, et al. What are user perspectives of exoskeleton technology? A literature review. *Int J Technol Assess Health Care.* 2017;33(2):160–167.

100. Heinemann AW, Jayaraman A, Mummidisetty CK, et al. Experience of robotic exoskeleton use at four spinal cord injury model systems centers. *J Neurol Phys Ther.* 2018;42(4):256–267.

101. Gagnon DH, Vermette M, Duclos C, et al. Satisfaction and perceptions of long-term manual wheelchair users with a spinal cord injury upon completion of a locomotor training program with an overground robotic exoskeleton. *Disabil Rehabil Assist Technol.* 2017:1–8.

102. Poritz JM, Taylor HB, Francisco GE, et al. User satisfaction with lower limb wearable robotic exoskeletons. *Disabil Rehabil Assist Technol.* 2019 Feb 15:1–6.

103. Blank AA, French JA, Pehlivan AU, et al. Current trends in robot-assisted upper-limb stroke rehabilitation: promoting patient engagement in therapy. *Curr Phys Med Rehabil Rep.* 2014 Sep 1;2(3):184–195.

104. Losey DP, McDonald CG, Battaglia E, et al. A review of intent detection, arbitration, and communication aspects of shared control for physical human–robot interaction. *Appl Mech Rev.* 2018 Jan 1;70(1):010804.

Note: Page numbers followed by *f* indicate figure. Page numbers followed by *t* indicate table.